Transplantation of the Liver

Second Edition

Transplantation of the Liver

Ronald W. Busuttil, MD, PhD
Professor and Chief
Division of Liver and Pancreas Transplantation
Dumont Chair in Transplantation Surgery
David Geffen School of Medicine at UCLA
Los Angeles, California

Goran K. Klintmalm, MD, PhD
Chairman and Chief, Baylor Regional Transplant Institute
Director, Transplantation Services;
Director, Dallas Liver Transplant Program
Baylor University Medical Center
Dallas, Texas

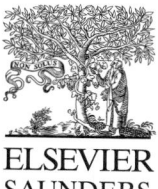

ELSEVIER
SAUNDERS

ELSEVIER
SAUNDERS

1600 John F. Kennedy Blvd.
Ste. 1800
Philadelphia, PA 19103-2899

Library of Congress Cataloging-in-Publication Data
Transplantation of the liver/[edited by] Ronald W. Busuttil, Goran B. Klintmalm.—2nd ed.
    p. ; cm.
Includes bibliographical references and index.
ISBN 0-7216-0118-9
    1. Liver—Transplantation. I. Busuttil, Ronald W. II. Klintmalm, Goran B.
    [DNLM: 1. Liver Transplantation. WI 770 T7725 2005]
RD546.T643 2005
617.5'5620592—dc22

2004053661

Acquisitions Editor: Judith Fletcher
Developmental Editor: Agnes Byrne
Publishing Services Manager: Tina Rebane
Project Manager: Jodi Kaye
Design Coordinator: Ellen Zanolle

Printed in the United States of America
Last digit is the print number: 9 8 7 6 5 4 3 2 1

Contributors

Anantharaju Abhinandana, MD
Gastroenterologist, Shoals Hospital,
  Muscle Shoals, Alabama
*Unusual Indications for Liver
  Transplantation*

Kareem Abu-Elmagd, MD, PhD
Professor of Surgery, University of
  Pittsburgh School of Medicine;
  Director of Intestinal Transplant Services,
  Thomas E. Starzl Transplantation
  Institute, University of Pittsburgh
  Medical Center, Pittsburgh, Pennsylvania
*Cell Migration, Chimerism, and Graft
  Acceptance, With Particular Reference to
  the Liver*

Estella M. Alonso, MD
Associate Professor of Pediatrics,
  Northwestern University Feinberg School
  of Medicine; Director of Liver
  Transplantation, Department of
  Pediatrics, Division of Gastroenterology,
  Hepatology and Nutrition, Children's
  Memorial Hospital, Chicago, Illinois
*General Criteria for Pediatric
  Transplantation*

Maria H. Alonso, MD
Assistant Professor of Surgery, University
  of Cincinnati College of Medicine;
  Pediatric Surgeon, Cincinnati Children's
  Hospital Medical Center, Cincinnati, Ohio
*Transplantation for Hepatic Malignancy in
  Children*

Edwin C. Amos III, MD
Associate Clinical Professor of Neurology,
  David Geffen School of Medicine at
  UCLA, Los Angeles; Attending
  Neurologist, St. John's Hospital and
  Health Center, and Santa Monica UCLA
  Medical Center, Santa Monica,
  California
*Postoperative Neurological Disorders and
  Prognosis*

Paula Andreani, MD
Surgeon, Hôpital Paul Brousse, Villejuif,
  France
Split-Liver Transplantation for Two Adults

Nancy L. Ascher, MD, PhD
Professor and Chair of Surgery,
  Department of Surgery, University of
  California, San Francisco School of
  Medicine, San Francisco, California
Rejection After Transplantation

Daniel Azoulay, MD
Professor of Surgery, Université Paris-Sud;
  Hôpital Paul Brousse, Villejuif, France
*Split-Liver Transplantation for
  Two Adults*

Lars Bäckman, MD, PhD
Associate Professor, Karolinska Institute,
  Stockholm; Director of Liver
  Transplantation, Department of
  Transplantation and Liver Surgery,
  Sahlgrenska University Hospital,
  Gothenburg, Sweden
*Liver Organ Allocation: The European
  Models*

William F. Balistreri, MD
Dorothy M. M. Kersten Professor of
  Pediatrics, University of Cincinnati
  College of Medicine; Director, Division
  of Gastroenterology, Hepatology, and
  Nutrition; and Medical Director,
  Pediatric Liver Care Center,
  Cincinnati Children's Hospital Medical
  Center, Cincinnati, Ohio
*Transplantation for Cholestatic Liver
  Disease in the Pediatric Patient*

Mehdi Baluch, MD
Fellow in Gastroenterology, Loyola
  University Medical Center, Maywood,
  Illinois
*Unusual Indications for Liver
  Transplantation*

Thomas M. Beebe, BSN, RN
Database Manager, Israel Penn
   International Transplant Tumor Registry;
   Department of Surgery, Division of
   Transplantation, University of Cincinnati
   College of Medicine, Cincinnati, Ohio
Transplant-Related Malignancies

Steven H. Belle, PhD, MScHyg
Associate Professor, Departments of
   Epidemiology and Biostatistics,
   University of Pittsburgh Graduate School
   of Public Health, Pittsburgh,
   Pennsylvania
*U.S. Trends in Liver Transplantation,
   1988 to 2001*

Marina Berenguer, MD
Staff, Hospital Universitario La Fe,
   Valencia, Spain
Hepatitis C and Liver Transplantation

Andres Besedovsky, MD
Clinical Research Scholar, Siragusa
   Transplantation Center, Children's
   Memorial Hospital, Chicago, Illinois
*General Criteria for Pediatric
   Transplantation*

Jorge A. Bezerra, MD
Associate Professor of Pediatrics, University
   of Cincinnati College of Medicine;
   Director, Biliary Atresia Center, and
   Associate Director, NIH-Digestive
   Research Development Center, Cincinnati
   Children's Hospital Medical Center,
   Cincinnati, Ohio
*Transplantation for Cholestatic Liver
   Disease in the Pediatric Patient*

Henri Bismuth, MD
Professor, Université Paris-Sud; Hôpital
   Paul Brousse, Villejuif, France
Split-Liver Transplantation for Two Adults

Kevin E. Bove, MD
Professor of Pathology and Pediatrics,
   University of Cincinnati College of
   Medicine; Staff Pathologist, Cincinnati
   Children's Hospital Medical Center,
   Cincinnati, Ohio
*Transplantation for Hepatic Malignancy in
   Children*

Lynda Brady, MD
Assistant Professor of Pediatrics,
   The University of Chicago Stritch School
   of Medicine, Chicago, Illinois
Transplantation for Biliary Atresia

John Brems, MD
Associate Professor of Surgery, Loyola
   University Medical School; Surgical
   Director, Abdominal Transplantation,
   Loyola University Medical Center,
   Maywood, Illinois
*Unusual Indications for Liver
   Transplantation*

Robert S. Brown, Jr., MD, MPH
Associate Professor of Clinical Medicine
   and Pediatrics, Columbia University
   College of Physicians and Surgeons;
   Chief, Center for Liver Disease and
   Transplantation, New York-Presbyterian
   Hospital, New York, New York
*Current Indications, Contraindications,
   Delisting Criteria, and Timing for Liver
   Transplantation*

Joseph F. Buell, MD, FACS
Director, Israel Penn International
   Transplant Tumor Registry, Division of
   Transplantation; Assistant Professor of
   Surgery, Department of Surgery, Division
   of Transplantation, University of
   Cincinnati College of Medicine,
   Cincinnati, Ohio
Transplant-Related Malignancies

Ronald W. Busuttil, MD, PhD
Professor and Chief, Division of Liver
   and Pancreas Transplantation and
   Dumont Chair in Transplantation Surgery,
   David Geffen School of Medicine at
   UCLA, Los Angeles, California
*Management of Portal Hypertensive
   Hemorrhage in the Era of Liver
   Transplantation; The Recipient
   Hepatectomy and Grafting; Liver
   Transplantation and Situs Inversus;
   Retransplantation; Ischemia-Reperfusion
   Injury of the Liver*

José Cañón, MD
Medical Staff, Organizacion Nacional de
   Transplantes, Madrid, Spain
*Liver Organ Allocation: The European
   Models*

Ian C. Carmody, MD, FRCS(C)
Clinical Instructor, Department of Liver
   and Pancreas Transplantation,
   David Geffen School of Medicine at
   UCLA, Los Angeles, California
*Treatment of Acute and Chronic Rejection;
   Arterial Complications After Liver
   Transplantation*

J. Michael Cecka, PhD
Professor and Director of Clinical Research, Department of Pathology and Laboratory Medicine, David Geffen School of Medicine at UCLA, Los Angeles, California
ABO, Tissue Typing, and Cross-match Incompatibility in Liver Transplantation

Ravi S. Chari, MD
Surgical Oncologist, Vanderbilt University Medical Center, Nashville, Tennessee
Extracorporeal Xenogeneic Liver Support

Michael R. Charlton, MD
Associate Professor of Medicine, William J. Von Liebig Transplant Center, Mayo Clinic College of Medicine, Rochester, Minnesota
Late Complications of Liver Transplantation and Recurrence of Disease

Pauline W. Chen, MD
Assistant Professor, Division of Liver and Pancreas Transplantation, David Geffen School of Medicine at UCLA; Surgeon, Dumont-UCLA Liver Cancer Center and Dumont-UCLA Transplant Center, Los Angeles, California
Treatment of Acute and Chronic Rejection

Wing S. Cheung, MD, MBA
Staff, Harvard Medical School; Research Fellow and Resident in General Surgery, Massachusetts General Hospital, Boston, Massachusetts
Development of Bioartificial Liver

Srinath Chinnakotla, MBBS, MCh
Attending Transplant Surgeon, Baylor University Medical Center, Dallas, Texas
Induction and Maintenance of Immunosuppression

Byung-Ho Choe, MD, PhD
Associate Professor, Section of Gastroenterology, Department of Pediatrics, Kyungpook National University School of Medicine, Daegu, Republic of Korea
Transplantation for Cholestatic Liver Disease in the Pediatric Patient

Pierre-Alain Clavien, MD, PhD
Chairman, Department of Visceral and Transplantation Surgery, University of Zurich Faculty of Medicine; Chairman, Department of Visceral and Transplantation Surgery, Cantonal Hospital of Zurich, Zurich, Switzerland
Principles of Liver Preservation

Steven D. Colquhoun, MD
Associate Professor, Department of Surgery, David Geffen School of Medicine at UCLA; Director of Liver Transplantation, Cedars-Sinai Medical Center, Los Angeles, California
Graft Failure: Etiology, Recognition, and Treatment

A. Benedict Cosimi, MD
Claude E. Welch Professor of Surgery, Harvard Medical School; Chief, Transplantation Unit, Massachusetts General Hospital, Boston, Massachusetts
New Approaches in Immunosuppression

Terianne Cowling, BA
Research Associate, Baylor University Medical Center, Dallas, Texas
Long-Term Functional Recovery and Quality of Life: Childhood, Adulthood, Employment, Pregnancy, and Family Planning

Jeffrey S. Crippin, MD
Professor of Medicine and Medical Director of Liver Transplantation, Washington University in St. Louis School of Medicine, St. Louis, Missouri
Transplantation for Sclerosing Cholangitis

David C. Cronin II, MD, PhD, FACS
Associate Professor and Director, Liver Transplantation, Department of Surgery, Yale University School of Medicine, New Haven, Connecticut
Ethics of Living Donor Liver Transplantation

Natividad Cuende, MD, PhD
Medical Staff, Organizacion Nacional de Transplantes, Madrid, Spain
Liver Organ Allocation: The European Models

Timothy J. Davern II, MD
Associate Professor of Medicine, University of California, San Francisco, School of Medicine; Attending Hepatologist, UCSF Medical Center, San Francisco, California
Molecular and Cellular Basis of Hepatic Failure

Gary L. Davis, MD
Director, Division of Hepatology, Baylor University Medical Center; Medical Director, Liver Transplantation, Baylor Regional Transplant Institute, Dallas, Texas
Natural History of Hepatitis C

Jean de Ville de Goyet, MD, PhD, FRCS
Professor of Surgery, Université Catholique de Louvain; Director of Abdominal Transplant and Pediatric Surgery Department, St. Luc University Hospital, Brussels, Belgium
Split-Liver Transplantation for the Pediatric and Adult Recipient

Massimo Del Gaudio, MD
Professor, Université Paris-Sud; Hôpital Paul Brousse, Villejuif, France
Split-Liver Transplantation for Two Adults

Anthony J. Demetris, MD
Professor of Pathology, University of Pittsburgh School of Medicine; Director, Division of Transplantation Pathology, Thomas E. Starzl Transplantation Institute, University of Pittsburgh Medical Center, Pittsburgh, Pennsylvania
Histological Patterns of Rejection and Other Causes of Liver Dysfunction; Cell Migration, Chimerism, and Graft Acceptance, With Particular Reference to the Liver

Niraj M. Desai, MD
Assistant Professor of Surgery, Washington University in St. Louis School of Medicine; Staff Surgeon, Barnes-Jewish Hospital and St. Louis Children's Hospital, St. Louis, Missouri
Portal Vein Thrombosis and Other Venous Anomalies in Liver Transplantation

Sonu Dhillon, MD
Fellow in Gastroenterology, Loyola University Medical Center, Maywood, Illinois
Unusual Indications for Liver Transplantation

E. Roland Dickson, MD
Mary Lowell Leary Professor of Medicine, Mayo Clinic College of Medicine; Consultant, Mayo Clinic and Foundation, Rochester, Minnesota
Liver Transplantation for Primary Biliary Cirrhosis

Vivek Dixit, PhD
Professor of Medicine, Department of Medicine, Division of Digestive Diseases, David Geffen School of Medicine at UCLA, Los Angeles, California
Hepatocyte Transplantation in Liver Disease

Bijan Eghtesad, MD
Associate Professor of Surgery, University of Pittsburgh School of Medicine, Pittsburgh, Pennsylvania
Cell Migration, Chimerism, and Graft Acceptance, With Particular Reference to the Liver

Karan Emerick, MD
Assistant Professor of Pediatrics, Northwestern University Feinberg School of Medicine; Attending Physician, Division of Gastroenterology, Hepatology, and Nutrition, Department of Pediatrics, Children's Memorial Hospital, Chicago, Illinois
General Criteria for Pediatric Transplantation

Jean C. Emond, MD
Thomas S. Zimmer Professor of Surgery, Columbia University College of Physicians and Surgeons; Vice Chairman of Transplantation and Chief of Transplantation, Center for Liver Disease and Transplantation, New York-Presbyterian Hospital, New York, New York
Surgical Anatomy of the Liver; Outcomes of Living Donor Liver Transplantation; Postoperative Care of Pediatric Liver Transplant Recipients

Carlos O. Esquivel, MD, PhD
Arnold and Barbara Silverman Professor of Pediatric Transplantation, Professor of Surgery, and Associate Director, Institute on Immunity, Transplantation, and Infection, Stanford University School of Medicine; Chief, Division of Transplantation, and Director of Liver and Intestinal Transplantation, Stanford Hospital & Clinics, and Lucile Salter Packard Children's Hospital, Stanford University Medical Center, Palo Alto, California
Results: Survival and Quality of Life After Orthotopic Liver Transplantation in Children

Idris V. R. Evans, MSc
Professor, Department of Epidemiology, University of Pittsburgh Graduate School of Public Health, Pittsburgh, Pennsylvania
U.S. Trends in Liver Transplantation, 1988 to 2001

Douglas G. Farmer, MD
Associate Professor of Surgery, David
  Geffen School of Medicine at UCLA;
  Director, Intestinal Transplantation Center,
  UCLA Medical Center, Los Angeles,
  California
Liver Transplantation and Situs Inversus

Scott A. Fink, MD, MPH
Clinical Fellow, Harvard Medical School;
  Clinical Fellow, Division of
  Gastroenterology, Brigham and Women's
  Hospital, Boston, Massachusetts
*Current Indications, Contraindications,
  Delisting Criteria, and Timing for Liver
  Transplantation*

Sander S. Florman, MD
Assistant Professor of Surgery and
  Pediatrics and Associate Residency
  Program Director, Tulane University
  School of Medicine; Director of Liver
  Transplantation, Tulane University
  Hospital and Clinic, New Orleans,
  Louisiana
*Adult Living Donor Hepatectomy and
  Recipient Operation*

Constantino Fondevila, MD, PhD
Assistant Researcher, Division of Liver and
  Pancreas Transplantation, David Geffen
  School of Medicine at UCLA, Los Angeles,
  California; Transplant Surgeon,
  Liver Unit, Digestive Disease Institute
  University of Barcelona Hospital Clinic,
  Barcelona, Spain
*Donor Selection and Management;
  Ischemia-Reperfusion Injury of the Liver*

Paulo Fontes, MD
Assistant Professor of Surgery, University
  of Pittsburgh School of Medicine;
  Co-Director, Liver Transplantation,
  Thomas E. Starzl Transplantation
  Institute, University of Pittsburgh
  Medical Center, Pittsburgh, Pennsylvania
*Cell Migration, Chimerism, and Graft
  Acceptance, With Particular Reference to
  the Liver*

**John L. R. Forsythe, MBBS, MD,
FRCS(Ed), FRCS(Eng)**
Senior Lecturer, University of Edinburgh
  Faculty of Medicine, Edinburgh;
  Consultant Transplant Surgeon and
  Clinical Director, Royal Infirmary of
  Edinburgh, Edinburgh, Scotland
Liver Organ Allocation: The European Models

Ira J. Fox, MD
Charles W. McLaughlin Professor of
  Surgery, University of Nebraska College
  of Medicine, Omaha, Nebraska
Xenotransplantation and the Liver

Richard B. Freeman, Jr., MD
Professor of Surgery, Tufts University
  School of Medicine; Surgeon, Division of
  Transplant Surgery, Tufts-New England
  Medical Center, Boston, Massachusetts
Liver Allocation: The U.S. Model

J. Mark Fulmer, MD
Staff Radiologist, Baylor University Medical
  Center; President, American Radiology
  Associates, P.A., Dallas, Texas
*Transplantation for Primary Hepatic
  Malignancy; Transplantation for
  Budd-Chiari Syndrome*

John J. Fung, MD, PhD
Professor of Surgery, Department of
  General Surgery, Cleveland Clinic
  Foundation, Cleveland, Ohio
*History of Liver and Multivisceral
  Transplantation; Cell Migration,
  Chimerism, and Graft Acceptance,
  With Particular Reference to the Liver*

Sunil K. Geevarghese, MD
Division of Surgical Oncology, Division of
  Hepatobiliary Surgery and Liver
  Transplantation, Vanderbilt Transplant
  Center and Vanderbilt-Ingram Cancer
  Center, Vanderbilt University School of
  Medicine, Nashville, Tennessee
*Management of Portal Hypertensive
  Hemorrhage in the Era of Liver
  Transplantation*

Magdalene M. George, PhD
Research Associate, St. Luke's Medical
  Center, Milwaukee, Wisconsin
*Unusual Indications for Liver
  Transplantation*

Till Gerling, MD, PhD
Medical Staff, Eurotransplant International
  Foundation, Leiden, The Netherlands
Liver Organ Allocation: The European Models

Rafik M. Ghobrial, MD, PhD
Professor of Surgery, Division of Liver and
  Pancreas Transplantation, David Geffen
  School of Medicine at UCLA,
  Los Angeles, California
*Donor Selection and Management; Outcome
  Predictors in Liver Transplantation*

Antoinette S. Gomes, MD
Professor, Radiological Sciences and
  Medicine, David Geffen School of Medicine
  at UCLA; Physician, Cardiovascular and
  Interventional Radiology, UCLA Medical
  Center, Los Angeles, California
*Radiologic Evaluation in the Liver
  Transplant Patient*

Thomas A. Gonwa, MD, FACP
Professor of Medicine, Mayo Clinic College
  of Medicine, Rochester, Minnesota;
  Medical Director, Kidney/Pancreas
  Transplantation, and Director, Division of
  Transplant Medicine, Department of
  Transplantation Mayo Clinic Jacksonville
  and St. Luke's Hospital, Jacksonville,
  Florida
*Pretransplantation Evaluation: Pulmonary,
  Cardiac, and Renal*

Sherilyn A. Gordon, MD
Assistant Professor of Surgery, Division of
  Liver and Pancreas Transplantation,
  David Geffen School of Medicine at
  UCLA; Dumont-UCLA Transplant Center,
  Los Angeles, California
*Surgical Anatomy of the Liver; Arterial
  Complications After Liver Transplantation*

Michael D. Green, MD, MPH
Professor of Pediatrics and Surgery,
  University of Pittsburgh School of
  Medicine; Staff, Children's Hospital of
  Pittsburgh, Pittsburgh, Pennsylvania
*Pretransplantation Infectious Disease
  Screening for Liver Transplantation:
  Candidates and Donors*

Raza Hamdani, MD
Staff Hepatologist, St. Luke's Medical
  Center, Milwaukee, Wisconsin
*Unusual Indications for Liver
  Transplantation*

Michael J. Hanaway, MD
Director of Pancreas Transplantation,
  Department of Surgery, University of
  Cincinnati College of Medicine, Cincinnati,
  Ohio
Transplant-Related Malignancies

Rick Harrison, MD
Professor of Clinical Pediatrics, David
  Geffen School of Medicine at UCLA;
  Co-Director, Pediatric Intensive Care Unit,
  Mattel Children's Hospital, Los Angeles,
  California
*Postoperative Intensive Care Management
  in Children*

Jeanette Hasse, PhD, RD, FADA, CNSD
Transplant Nutrition Specialist, Transplant
  Services, Baylor University Medical
  Center, Dallas, Texas
*Nutritional Aspects of Adult Liver
  Transplantation*

Paul H. Hayashi, MD
Transplant Hepatology Fellow, University of
  Colorado Health Sciences Center, Denver,
  Colorado
*Donor and Recipient Evaluation and
  Selection for Adult-to-Adult Right Hepatic
  Lobe Liver Transplantation*

Martin Hertl, MD
Assistant Professor of Surgery, Harvard
  Medical School; Surgical Director,
  Liver Transplantation, Massachusetts
  General Hospital, Boston,
  Massachusetts
New Approaches in Immunosuppression

Jonathan R. Hiatt, MD
Professor of Surgery and Director of
  Surgical Education, Division of Liver and
  Pancreas Transplantation, David Geffen
  School of Medicine at UCLA,
  Los Angeles, California
*Influence of Liver Transplantation on Liver
  Surgery; Management of Portal
  Hypertensive Hemorrhage in the Era of
  Liver Transplantation*

Ryutaro Hirose, MD, FACS
Assistant Professor in Residence, Division
  of Transplantation, Department of
  Surgery, University of California,
  San Francisco, School of Medicine,
  San Francisco, California
Novel Immunosuppressive Agents

Garrett M. Hisatake, MD
Surgeon, Department of Transplantation,
  California Pacific Medical Center,
  San Francisco, California
*Influence of Liver Transplantation on Liver
  Surgery*

Curtis D. Holt, PharmD
Associate Clinical Professor, Department of
  Surgery, David Geffen School of
  Medicine at UCLA, Los Angeles;
  Associate Clinical Professor,
  University of California, San Francisco,
  School of Pharmacy, San Francisco,
  California
Infections After Liver Transplantation

Yukihiro Inomata, MD
Professor and Director, Kumamoto University Faculty of Medicine and Pharmaceutical Sciences, Department of Pediatric Surgery, Kumamoto, Japan
Living Related Liver Transplantation in Pediatric Recipients

Sheila Jowsey, MD
Assistant Professor, Mayo Clinic College of Medicine; Consultant, Saint Mary's Hospital and Rochester Methodist Hospital, Rochester, Minnesota
Psychosocial Assessment of Adult Liver Transplant Recipients

Oded Jurim, MD
Staff, Hadassah University Medical Center, Hebrew University of Jerusalem, Jerusalem, Israel
Retransplantation

Igal Kam, MD
Professor, Division of Transplant Surgery, University of Colorado School of Medicine; Chief, Liver Transplantation, University of Colorado Health Sciences Center, Denver, Colorado
Donor and Recipient Evaluation and Selection for Adult-to-Adult Right Hepatic Lobe Liver Transplantation

Tomoaki Kato, MD
Associate Professor of Surgery, University of Miami College of Medicine, Miami, Florida
Transplantation of the Liver with Digestive Organs

Cesar A. Keller, MD, FCCP
Professor of Medicine, Mayo Clinic College of Medicine, Rochester, Minnesota; Medical Director, Heart-Lung and Lung Transplant Program, Transplant Center, Mayo Clinic, Jacksonville, Florida
Pretransplantation Evaluation: Pulmonary, Cardiac, and Renal

W. Ray Kim, MD, MBA
Associate Professor of Medicine, Mayo Clinic College of Medicine; Consultant, Mayo Clinic, Rochester, Minnesota
Liver Transplantation for Primary Biliary Cirrhosis

Cindy J. Kin, BA
Medical Student, Columbia University College of Physicians and Surgeons, New York, New York
Outcomes of Living Donor Liver Transplantation

Goran B. Klintmalm, MD, PhD
Chairman and Chief, Baylor Regional Transplant Institute; Director, Transplantation Services; Director, Dallas Liver Transplant Program, Baylor University Medical Center, Dallas, Texas
Transplantation for Primary Hepatic Malignancy; Transplantation for Budd-Chiari Syndrome; The Recipient Hepatectomy and Grafting; Combined Liver-Kidney Transplantation; Postoperative Intensive Care Unit Management: Adult Liver Transplant Recipients; Postoperative Management Beyond the Intensive Care Unit: Adults; Induction and Maintenance of Immunosuppression; Outcome Predictors in Liver Transplantation; Long-Term Functional Recovery and Quality of Life: Childhood, Adulthood, Employment, Pregnancy, and Family Planning

Gregg Kunder, BS, BSN, CCTC
Transplant Coordinator, The Pfleger Liver Institute and Dumont–UCLA Transplant Center, UCLA Medical Center, Los Angeles, California
Role of the Posttransplant Coordinator

Jerzy W. Kupiec-Weglinski, MD, PhD
Professor of Surgery and Pathology, David Geffen School of Medicine at UCLA; Director, Dumont-UCLA Transplantation Research Laboratories, Los Angeles, California
Ischemia-Reperfusion Injury of the Liver

Chi Lai, MD
Transplant Pathology Fellow, University of Pittsburgh Medical Center, Pittsburgh, Pennsylvania
Histological Patterns of Rejection and Other Causes of Liver Dysfunction

John Lake, MD
Professor of Medicine and Surgery, University of Minnesota Medical School–Minneapolis; Director, Division of Gastroenterology, Hepatology and Nutrition; Director, Liver Transplantation Program, Fairview-University Medical Center, Minneapolis, Minnesota
Hepatitis C and Liver Transplantation

Charles R. Lassman, MD, PhD
Associate Professor of Pathology and
  Laboratory Medicine, David Geffen
  School of Medicine at UCLA; Chief,
  Hepatobiliary Pathology, Chief, Renal
  Pathology, and Associate Chief,
  Autopsy Pathology, UCLA Medical
  Center, Los Angeles, California
*Pathology of Recurrence of Non-Neoplastic
  Disease After Liver Transplantation*

Susan M. Lerner, MD
Assistant Professor of Surgery and Director,
  Surgery Clerkship, Penn State University
  College of Medicine; Surgical Director,
  Liver Transplantation, Penn State Milton S.
  Hershey Medical Center, Hershey,
  Pennsylvania
Retransplantation

Marlon F. Levy, MD
Assistant Director and Transplant Surgeon,
  Baylor University Medical Center, Dallas,
  Texas; Surgical Director of Transplantation,
  Baylor All Saints Medical Center,
  Fort Worth, Texas
*Long-Term Functional Recovery and Quality
  of Life: Childhood, Adulthood,
  Employment, Pregnancy, and Family
  Planning; Extracorporeal Xenogeneic
  Liver Support*

S. David Li, MD
Staff, Immanuel St. Joseph's-Mayo Health
  System, Mankato, Minnesota
Unusual Indications for Liver Transplantation

Piyaporn Limanond, MD
Instructor, Department of Radiology,
  Mahidol University Faculty of Medicine;
  Radiologist, Siriraj Hospital, Bangkok,
  Thailand
*Imaging Techniques in Living Donor
  Transplantation*

Gerald S. Lipshutz, MD, MS
Assistant Professor of Surgery, Division of
  Liver and Pancreas Transplantation,
  David Geffen School of Medicine at
  UCLA, Los Angeles, California
Rejection After Transplantation

Steven J. Lobritto, MD
Associate Professor of Medicine and
  Pediatrics, Columbia University College
  of Physicians and Surgeons; Pediatric
  Medical Director, New York-Presbyterian
  Hospital, New York, New York
*Postoperative Care of Pediatric Liver
  Transplant Recipients*

David S. K. Lu, MD
Professor of Radiology, David Geffen
  School of Medicine at UCLA; Director,
  Computed Tomography, and Chief,
  Cross Sectional Interventional Service,
  UCLA Medical Center, Los Angeles,
  California
*Imaging Techniques in Living Donor
  Transplantation*

Zhengbin Lu, MD, PhD
Hepatic and Gastric Pathologist,
  Ameripath, Inc., Indianapolis,
  Indiana
*Histological Patterns of Rejection and Other
  Causes of Liver Dysfunction*

Michael R. Lucey, MD, FRCPI
Professor of Medicine, Department of
  Medicine, University of Wisconsin
  Medical School; Chief, Section of
  Gastroenterology and Hepatology,
  University Hospital and Clinic,
  Madison, Wisconsin
*Liver Transplantation for Alcoholic
  Liver Disease*

Martin L. Mai, MD
Assistant Professor of Medicine, Mayo
  Clinic College of Medicine, Rochester,
  Minnesota; Consultant, Department of
  Transplantation, Mayo Clinic, Jacksonville,
  Florida
*Pretransplantation Evaluation: Pulmonary,
  Cardiac, and Renal*

Cosme Y. Manzarbeitia, MD, FACS
Chairman, Division of Transplantation,
  and Director, Liver Transplantation and
  Hepatobiliary Surgery Program,
  Department of Surgery, Albert Einstein
  Medical Center, Philadelphia,
  Pennsylvania
*Non–Heart-Beating Donor Liver
  Transplantation*

Amadeo Marcos, MD
Professor of Surgery, University of
  Pittsburgh School of Medicine; Clinical
  Director of Transplantation, Thomas E.
  Starzl Transplantation Institute,
  University of Pittsburgh Medical Center,
  Pittsburgh, Pennsylvania
*History of Liver and Multivisceral
  Transplantation; Cell Migration,
  Chimerism, and Graft Acceptance,
  with Particular Reference to the Liver*

Victor J. Marder, MD
Professor of Clinical Medicine, David Geffen School of Medicine at UCLA; Director, Vascular Medicine Program, Orthopaedic Hospital, Los Angeles, California
Liver Transplantation for Hematological Disorders

Carlos Margarit, MD, PhD
Professor of Surgery, Universidad Autonoma de Barcelona; Director, Liver Transplantation Unit, Hospital Vall Hebron, Barcelona, Spain
Liver Organ Allocation: The European Models; Auxiliary Liver Transplantation

James Markmann, MD, PhD
Associate Professor of Surgery, University of Pennsylvania School of Medicine; Surgeon, University of Pennsylvania Hospital, Philadelphia, Pennsylvania
Retransplantation

Suzanne V. McDiarmid, MD
Professor of Pediatrics and Surgery, David Geffen School of Medicine at UCLA; Director, Pediatric Liver Transplantation, ULCA Medical Center, Los Angeles, California
Liver Transplantation for Metabolic Disease; Special Considerations for Pediatric Immunosuppression After Liver Transplantation

K. V. Narayanan Menon, MD
Assistant Professor of Medicine, William J. Von Liebig Transplant Center, Mayo Medical School, Rochester, Minnesota
Late Complications of Liver Transplantation and Recurrence of Disease

William C. Meyers, MD
Professor of Surgery, Duke University School of Medicine; Associate Director, Endosurgical Center, Duke University Medical Center, Durham, North Carolina
Extracorporeal Xenogeneic Liver Support

Marian G. Michaels, MD, MPH
Associate Professor of Pediatrics and Surgery, University of Pittsburgh School of Medicine; Staff, Children's Hospital of Pittsburgh, Pittsburgh, Pennsylvania
Pretransplantation Infectious Disease Screening for Liver Transplantation: Candidates and Donors

Charles M. Miller, MD
Associate Professor of Surgery, Cleveland Clinic Lerner College of Medicine, Case Western Reserve University; Director, Liver Transplantation, Department of General Surgery, Cleveland Clinic Foundation, Cleveland, Ohio
Adult Living Donor Hepatectomy and Recipient Operation

J. Michael Millis, MD
Professor of Surgery, The University of Chicago Pritzker School of Medicine; Chief, Section of Transplantation, The University of Chicago Hospitals, Chicago, Illinois
Transplantation for Biliary Atresia

Ayse L. Mindikoglu, MD
AASLD Research Fellow, University of Miami School of Medicine, Center for Liver Disease; Research Fellow, Miami VA Medical Center, Miami, Florida
Unusual Indications for Liver Transplantation

Marida Minervini
Staff, University of Pittsburgh Medical Center; Pittsburgh, Pennsylvania
Histological Patterns of Rejection and Other Causes of Liver Dysfunction

Bianca Miranda, MD, PhD
Medical Director, Organizacion Nacional de Trasplantes, Madrid, Spain
Liver Organ Allocation: The European Models

Ernesto P. Molmenti, MD, PhD
Associate Professor of Surgery, Transplantation and General Surgery, Johns Hopkins University School of Medicine; Consultant, Johns Hopkins Hospital, Baltimore, Maryland
Clinical Management of the Necrotic Liver During Transplantation

Ferdinand Mühlbacher, MD
Professor of Surgery, Medical University of Vienna; Staff, Vienna General Hospital, Vienna, Austria
Liver Transplantation for Metastases of the Liver

Noriko Murase, MD
Associate Professor of Surgery, University of Pittsburgh School of Medicine; Surgeon, Thomas E. Starzl Transplantation Institute, University of Pittsburgh Medical Center, Pittsburgh, Pennsylvania
History of Liver and Multivisceral Transplantation; Cell Migration, Chimerism, and Graft Acceptance, with Particular Reference to the Liver

Mike Nalesnik, MD
Professor of Pathology, University of Pittsburgh School of Medicine, Pittsburgh, Pennsylvania
Histological Patterns of Rejection and Other Causes of Liver Dysfunction

Peter Neuhaus, MD
Professor of Surgery, Charité-Universitaetsmedizin Berlin, Humboldt Universitaet zu Berlin; Professor of Surgery and Chief, Department of General, Visceral, and Transplantation Surgery, Campus Virchow Clinic, Berlin, Germany
Technical Problems: Biliary

Jose M. Nieto, DO
Hepatology Fellow, David Geffen School of Medicine at UCLA; Staff, West Los Angeles Veterans Affairs Medical Center, Los Angeles, California
Liver Transplantation for Autoimmune Hepatitis

Nicholas N. Nissen, MD
Assistant Clinical Professor of Surgery, David Geffen School of Medicine at UCLA; Assistant Surgical Director, Multi-Organ Transplant Program, Cedars-Sinai Medical Center, Los Angeles, California
Graft Failure: Etiology, Recognition, and Treatment

Kim M. Olthoff, MD
Associate Professor of Surgery, University of Pennsylvania School of Medicine; Director, Liver Transplantation, Hospital of the University of Pennsylvania and The Children's Hospital of Philadelphia, Philadelphia, Pennsylvania
Portal Vein Thrombosis and Other Venous Anomalies in Liver Transplantation

Jean-Bernard Otte, MD
Professor Emeritus of Surgery, Université Catholique de Couvain; Former Head, Department of Pediatric Surgery, Cliniques Saint-Luc, Brussels, Belgium
Split-Liver Transplantation for the Pediatric and Adult Recipient

Andreas Pascher, MD
Professor of Surgery, Charité-Universitaetsmedizin Berlin, Humboldt Universitaet zu Berlin; Professor of Surgery, Department of General, Visceral, and Transplantation Surgery, Campus Virchow Clinic, Berlin, Germany
Technical Problems: Biliary

Guido G. Persijn, MD, PhD
Medical Director, Eurotransplant International Foundation, Leiden, The Netherlands
Liver Organ Allocation: The European Models

Phuong-Chi T. Pham, MD
Associate Professor of Medicine, David Geffen School of Medicine at UCLA, Los Angeles; Staff, Olive View–UCLA Medical Center, Sylmar, California
Renal Failure in Adult Liver Transplant Recipients

Phuong-Thu T. Pham, MD
Assistant Professor of Medicine, David Geffen School of Medicine at UCLA, Los Angeles, California
Renal Failure in Adult Liver Transplant Recipients

Jeffrey L. Platt, MD
Professor of Surgery, Immunology, and Pediatrics, Mayo Clinic College of Medicine; Director, Transplantation Biology Program, Mayo Clinic, Rochester, Minnesota
Xenotransplantation and the Liver

Jorge Rakela, MD
Professor of Medicine, Mayo Clinic College of Medicine; Chair, Department of Internal Medicine, Mayo Clinic, Scottsdale, Arizona
Monitoring and Care of the Patient Before Liver Transplantation

Steven S. Raman, MD
Radiologist, The Pfleger Liver Institute and Gastrointestinal and Genitourinary Radiology Program, David Geffen School of Medicine at UCLA, Los Angeles, California
Imaging Techniques for Living Donor Transplantation

Michael A. E. Ramsay, MD, FRCA
Clinical Professor, University of Texas
 Southwestern Medical School; Chairman,
 Department of Anesthesiology, Baylor
 University Medical Center at Dallas,
 Dallas, Texas
*Anesthesia for Liver
 Transplantation*

Henry B. Randall, MD
Attending Transplant Surgeon, Baylor
 Regional Transplant Institute, Baylor
 University Medical Center; Pediatric
 Transplant Surgeon, Children's Medical
 Center and University of Texas
 Southwestern Medical Center, Dallas,
 Texas
*Postoperative Intensive Care Unit
 Management: Adult Liver Transplant
 Recipients*

Parmjeet Randhawa, MD
Professor of Pathology, University of
 Pittsburgh School of Medicine,
 Pittsburgh, Pennsylvania
*Histological Patterns of Rejection
 and Other Causes of Liver
 Dysfunction*

Elaine F. Reed, MS, PhD
Professor of Pathology and Director,
 UCLA Immunogenetics Center,
 Department of Pathology and Laboratory
 Medicine, David Geffen School of
 Medicine at UCLA, Los Angeles,
 California
*ABO, Tissue Typing, and Cross-match
 Incompatibility in Liver
 Transplantation*

David J. Reich, MD, FACS
Associate Director, Liver Transplantation
 and Hepatobiliary Surgery Program,
 Albert Einstein Medical Center;
 Associate Professor of Surgery,
 Jefferson Medical College,
 Thomas Jefferson University,
 Philadelphia, Pennsylvania
*Non–Heart-Beating Donor Liver
 Transplantation*

Paulo R. Reichert, MD
Professor of Surgery, Department of
 Anatomy, Universidade de Passo Fundo,
 Passo Fundo, Brazil
Surgical Anatomy of the Liver

John F. Renz, MD, PhD
Assistant Professor of Surgery, Columbia
 University College of Physicians and
 Surgeons; Center for Liver Disease
 and Transplantation, New York,
 New York
*Surgical Anatomy of the Liver; The Donor
 Operation; Outcomes of Living Donor
 Liver Transplantation*

Stephen M. Riordan, MD, FRACP, FRCP
Associate Professor, Department of
 Medicine, The University of New South
 Wales Faculty of Medicine;
 Director, Gastrointestinal and
 Liver Unit, The Prince of Wales Hospital,
 Sydney, New South Wales,
 Australia
*Transplantation for Fulminant Hepatic
 Failure*

John P. Roberts, MD
Professor of Surgery, University of
 California, San Francisco, School of
 Medicine; Chief, Division of
 Transplantation UCSF Comprehensive
 Cancer Center, San Francisco,
 California
Rejection After Transplantation

Bruno Roche, MD
Universite Paris-Sud; Hospital Staff, Hôpital
 Paul Brousse, Centre Hepato-Biliaire,
 Villejuif, France
*Transplantation for Viral Hepatitis
 A and B*

Susanne Rasoul Rockenschaub, MD
Staff, Vienna General Hospital, Vienna,
 Austria
*Liver Transplantation for Metastases of the
 Liver*

Xavier Rogiers, MD
Professor of Surgery, University of
 Hamburg Medical School; Director of
 Klinik und Poliklinik, Universitäts
 Klinikum Hamburg-Eppendorf, Hamburg,
 Germany
*Spilt-Liver Transplantation for the Pediatric
 and Adult Recipient*

L. S. Rothenberg, JD
Associate Professor of Clinical Medicine,
 David Geffen School of Medicine at
 UCLA; Ethicist, UCLA Healthcare,
 Los Angeles, California
*Ethical Decisions in Liver
 Transplantation*

Steven M. Rudich, MD
Associate Professor of Surgery, University
  of Cincinnati College of Medicine;
  Director of Liver Transplant Services,
  Division of Transplantation,
  University of Cincinnati University
  Hospital, Cincinnati, Ohio
Transplant-Related Malignancies

Frederick C. Ryckman, MD
Professor of Surgery, University of
  Cincinnati College of Medicine;
  Surgical Director, Liver Transplantation,
  Cincinnati Children's Hospital Medical
  Center, Cincinnati, Ohio
*Transplantation for Hepatic Malignancy in
  Children*

Sammy Saab, MD, MPH
Assistant Professor of Medicine and
  Surgery, David Geffen School of
  Medicine at UCLA, Los Angeles,
  California
*Liver Transplantation for Autoimmune
  Hepatitis*

Bob H. Saggi, MD
Assistant Professor of Surgery, University
  of Texas Medical School at Houston,
  Houston, Texas
*Outcomes of Living Donor Liver
  Transplantation*

Didier Samuel, MD, PhD
Professor of Hepatology, Université
  Paris-Sud; Hospital Staff, Hôpital Paul
  Brousse, Centre Hepato-Biliaire, Villejuif,
  France
*Transplantation for Viral Hepatitis
  A and B*

Edmund Q. Sanchez, MD, FACS
Attending Transplant Surgeon and
  Fellowship Director, Baylor Regional
  Transplant Institute, Baylor University
  Medical Center, Dallas, Texas
*Combined Liver-Kidney Transplantation;
  Postoperative Management Beyond the
  Intensive Care Unit: Adults*

Randolph Schaffer III, MD
Surgical Director, Living Donor Organ
  Transplant Program, Scripps Clinic/
  Green Hospital, La Jolla,
  California
Transplantation for Biliary Atresia

Paul J. Scheel, Jr., MD
Associate Professor of Medicine and
  Vice Chairman, Department of Medicine,
  Johns Hopkins University School of
  Medicine; Director, Division of
  Nephrology, Johns Hopkins Hospital,
  Baltimore, Maryland
*Clinical Management of the Necrotic Liver
  During Transplantation*

Terry Schneekloth, MD
Assistant Professor, Mayo Clinic College
  of Medicine; Director of Addiction
  Services, Mayo Clinic, Rochester,
  Minnesota
*Psychosocial Assessment of Adult Liver
  Transplant Recipients*

Dawn Sears, MD
Assistant Professor, Texas A&M University
  Health Science Center College of
  Medicine, College Station, Texas; Staff
  Physician, Scott & White Memorial
  Hospital, Temple, Texas
Natural History of Hepatitis C

Nazia Selzner, MD, PhD
Research Fellow, Department of Visceral
  Surgery and Transplantation, University
  Hospital of Zurich, Zurich, Switzerland
Principles of Liver Preservation

Abraham Shaked, MD, PhD
Professor of Surgery, University of
  Pennsylvania School of Medicine;
  Chief, Division of Transplantation
  Surgery, Director, PENN Transplant
  Center, Philadelphia,
  Pennsylvania
*Genetic Modulation in
  Transplantation*

Pratima Sharma, MD
Medical Director, Emory Transplant Center,
  Atlanta, Georgia
*Monitoring and Care of the Patient Before
  Liver Transplantation*

Mark Siegler, MD
Professor of Medicine and Director,
  MacLean Center for Clinical Medical
  Ethics, The University of Chicago
  Pritzker School of Medicine, Chicago,
  Illinois
*Ethics of Living Donor Liver
  Transplantation*

Thomas E. Starzl, MD, PhD
Professor of Surgery, University of
Pittsburgh School of Medicine;
Staff, University of Pittsburgh
Medical Center, Pittsburgh,
Pennsylvania
*History of Liver and Multivisceral
Transplantation; Cell Migration,
Chimerism, and Graft Acceptance,
with Particular Reference to the
Liver*

Marvin J. Stone, MD, MACP
Chief of Oncology and Director,
Baylor Charles A. Sammons Cancer
Center, Baylor University Medical Center,
Dallas, Texas
*Transplantation for Primary Hepatic
Malignancy; Transplantation for
Budd–Chiari Syndrome*

**Steven M. Strasberg, MD,
FRCS(C), FACS**
Professor of Surgery, Washington
University in St. Louis; Head, Section of
Hepatobiliary-Pancreatic Surgery,
Barnes-Jewish Hospital, St. Louis,
Missouri
Principles of Liver Preservation

Thomas B. Strouse, MD
Assistant Clinical Professor of Psychiatry,
David Geffen School of Medicine at
UCLA; Director, Psychosocial Services
and Cancer Pain Management Service,
Cedars-Sinai Medical Center,
Los Angeles, California
*Neuropsychiatric Outcomes in Liver
Transplant Recipients*

Jayant A. Talwalkar, MD, MPH
Assistant Professor of Medicine,
Mayo Clinic College of Medicine;
Consultant, Mayo Clinic, Rochester,
Minnesota
*Liver Transplantation for Primary Biliary
Cirrhosis*

Koichi Tanaka, MD
Professor and Director, Transplantation
and Immunology, Kyoto University
Faculty of Medicine, Kyoto,
Japan
*Living Related Liver Transplantation in
Pediatric Recipients*

William D. Tap, MD
Hematology-Oncology Fellow, David Geffen
School of Medicine at UCLA,
Los Angeles, California
*Liver Transplantation for Hematological
Disorders*

Mark J. Thomas, MD
Assistant Professor of Surgery, Division of
Transplantation, University of Cincinnati
College of Medicine, Cincinnati,
Ohio
Transplant-Related Malignancies

Gregory M. Tiao, MD
Assistant Professor of Surgery, University
of Cincinnati College of Medicine;
Attending Surgeon, Pediatric and
Transplant Surgery, Cincinnati Children's
Hospital Medical Center, Cincinnati, Ohio
*Transplantation for Hepatic Malignancy in
Children*

James F. Trotter, MD
Associate Professor, Division of
Gastroenterology/Hepatology, University
of Colorado School of Medicine, Denver,
Colorado
*Donor and Recipient Evaluation and
Selection for Adult-to-Adult Right Hepatic
Lobe Liver Transplantation*

Massimo Trucco, MD
Professor of Pediatric Immunology,
University of Pittsburgh School of
Medicine; Staff, Children's Hospital of
Pittsburgh, Pittsburgh, Pennsylvania
*Cell Migration, Chimerism, and Graft
Acceptance, with Particular Reference to
the Liver*

Andreas G. Tzakis, MD
Professor of Surgery, University of
Miami School of Medicine, Miami,
Florida
*Transplantation of the Liver with Digestive
Organs*

Joseph P. Vacanti, MD
Johns Homans Professor of Surgery,
Harvard Medical School; Surgeon in
Chief, Massachusetts General Hospital
for Children; Chief of Pediatric
Transplantation, Massachusetts
General Hospital, Boston,
Massachusetts
Development of Bioartificial Liver

David H. van Thiel, MD
Medical Director of Liver Transplantation and Director of Hepatology, St. Luke's Medical Center; Gastroenterologist, Abdominal Transplant and Liver Disease Clinic, Milwaukee, Wisconsin
Unusual Indications for Liver Transplantation

Hugo E. Vargas, MD
Associate Professor of Medicine, Mayo Clinic College of Medicine; Consultant, Mayo Clinic, Scottsdale, and Mayo Clinic Hospital, Phoenix, Arizona
Monitoring and Care of the Patient Before Liver Transplantation

Flavio Vincenti, MD
Professor of Clinical Medicine, Department of Surgery, University of California, San Francisco, School of Medicine, San Francisco, California
Novel Immunosuppressive Agents

Robert M. Weinrieb, MD
Associate Professor of Psychiatry, University of Pennsylvania School of Medicine, Philadelphia, Pennsylvania
Liver Transplantation for Alcoholic Liver Disease

Peter F. Whitington, MD
Professor of Pediatrics and Transplantation, Northwestern University Feinberg School of Medicine; Division Chief, Pediatric Gastroenterology, Hepatology and Nutrition, and Director, Siragusa Transplantation Center, Children's Memorial Hospital, Chicago, Illinois
General Criteria for Pediatric Transplantation

Kelly Wicker, RN, BSN
Program Manager, Liver/Kidney/Pancreas Transplantation, Baylor University Medical Center, Dallas, Texas
Clinical Nurse Coordinator: Nursing Focus on Care of Patients with End-Stage Liver Disease

Alan H. Wilkinson, MD
Professor of Medicine, David Geffen School of Medicine at UCLA; Medical Director, Kidney and Pancreas Transplantation, UCLA Medical Center, Los Angeles, California
Renal Failure in Adult Liver Transplant Recipients

Roger Williams, MD, CBE, FRCP, FRCS, FRCPE, FRACP, FMedSci, FRCPI(Hon), FACP(Hon)
Professor, University College London; Director, The Institute of Hepatology, London, England
Transplantation for Fulminant Hepatic Failure

Drew J. Winston, MD
Associate Clinical Professor of Medicine, David Geffen School of Medicine at UCLA; Physician, UCLA Medical Center, Los Angeles, California
Infections after Liver Transplantation

E. Steve Woodle, MD
Professor of Surgery and Director, Division of Transplantation, University of Cincinnati College of Medicine; Chairman, Board of Directors, Israel Penn International Transplant Tumor Registry, Cincinnati, Ohio
Transplant-Related Malignancies

Tong Wu, MD, PhD
Assistant Professor of Pathology, University of Pittsburgh School of Medicine, Pittsburgh, Pennsylvania
Histological Patterns of Rejection and Other Causes of Liver Dysfunction

Hal F. Yee, Jr., MD, PhD,
Professor of Medicine, University of California, San Francisco, School of Medicine; Chief, Gastroenterology and Hepatology, San Francisco General Hospital, San Francisco, California
Molecular and Cellular Basis of Hepatic Failure

Heidi Yeh, MD
Instructor of Surgery, University of Pennsylvania School of Medicine, Philadelphia, Pennsylvania
Genetic Modulation in Transplantation

Hasan Yersiz, MD
Assistant Professor of Surgery, David Geffen School of Medicine at UCLA, Los Angeles, California
The Donor Operation

Daniel S. Yip, MD
Assistant Professor of Medicine, Mayo Clinic College of Medicine, Rochester, Minnesota; Medical Director, Heart Failure and Transplantation, Mayo Clinic Jacksonville/St. Luke's Hospital, Jacksonville, Florida
Pretransplantation Evaluation: Pulmonary, Cardiac, and Renal

Foreword

No sense of accomplishment can exceed that of seeing a robust liver transplant recipient who, a few weeks earlier, was seemingly near death from end-stage hepatic failure. Witnessing such miraculous transitions was what sustained efforts to replace the liver in the 1960s and 1970s when therapeutic triumph was not the usual outcome. Although the longest surviving liver recipient is currently in her 36th posttransplant year, the high mortality and morbidity in the early experience suggested that liver transplantation was a feasible, but not practical, form of treatment. Sea changes occurred with the advent in 1980 of cyclosporine, and again a decade later with the arrival of tacrolimus.

With the better immunosuppression, a rapid proliferation of new centers began in the mid-1980s. Two of the largest and most successful programs were founded by Ronald Busuttil in 1983 and Goran Klintmalm in 1985. In 1995, the two men published a state-of-the-art book on liver transplantation. The various chapters were contributed by surgeons, internists, and pediatricians with extensive experience and expertise in various aspects of patient selection, the operation itself, and pre- and postoperative care. Immunologists and others who provided essential components of the substructure also were represented. The book was a great success at every level of the healthcare hierarchy, from students to professors.

By the time of the book's launch in 1995, the combination of acceptable results and the number of centers with well-trained surgeons, had made liver replacement the universally accepted "last court of appeal" for virtually all patients dying of non-neoplastic liver disease, and for a selected subgroup of those with malignant hepatic tumors that could not be removed with conventional subtotal hepatic resection. It also was apparent, even from a casual reading of the first edition of *Liver Transplantation,* that organ supply already had become the principal deterrent to further expansion of these services. Liver xenotransplantation was discussed as a potential way to deal with the impending crisis; however, with the opposition by the public, as well as within the profession, to using closely related species (e.g., the baboon) as donors, this possibility was and remains remote.

In their second edition, therefore, Busuttil, Klintmalm, and their contributing authors have emphasized practical ways of expanding, or more efficiently utilizing, the human organ pool. These include the acceptance of cadaveric livers that were once discarded, the division of one organ for transplantation into two recipients, and the scrupulously careful use of live volunteer donors. Another way of stretching the supply is to reduce the need for retransplantation. In the past, such hopes have depended almost exclusively on the development of more potent immunosuppressive drugs. This new edition of *Liver Transplantation* contains a full account of agents that have been developed since 1995. Almost all were designed to attack specific targets in the immunologic cascade of rejection. However, some of the most promising possibilities are instead based on strategies that exploit leukocyte chimerism-dependent mechanisms of alloengraftment and acquired tolerance.

Other topics also are more completely covered than in the first edition. Intestinal, cluster, and multivisceral transplant operations were direct outgrowths of liver transplantation and are now part of the standard armamentarium in advanced centers. The management of patients with failure of one or all of these visceral organs has been expanded, with particular emphasis on events in the intensive care environment and in patients under anesthesia. No matter what the focus, the *Pearls and Pitfalls* section at the end of each chapter alerts the reader to specific points that might otherwise be missed. Some of these sections are so helpful that it may be beneficial to peruse the *Pearls and Pitfalls* before tackling the main text.

In 1995, I concluded my Foreword to the inaugural edition of *Liver Transplantation* as follows: *"The creation of a genuine classic is a cause for wonder, which inevitably increases with time. Years from now, Drs. Busuttil and Klintmalm are apt to look back at their work product and to ask themselves how they had been able in their earlier life to construct something this good".* They have, in fact, now made the work product even better.

THOMAS E. STARZL

Preface

It has been 9 years since *Transplantation of the Liver* was first published. The goal of the text was to provide a "comprehensive and up-to-date treatise covering all aspects of liver transplantation" that would have a broad application to all transplant professionals, as well as physicians, scientists, students and patients who have an interest in the discipline. Moreover, we hoped that this book would serve as a platform for new advances in the field.

Since the first edition, an explosion of new discoveries has significantly changed transplantation and the ways in which it is applied. Many of these were barely considered in the previous edition, as their influence on treatment and outcome was untested or unknown. In the new edition, we have attempted to address the latest discoveries and knowledge by providing expanded and in-depth coverage of hepatitis C, hepatocellular malignancy, adult living donor transplantation, new immunosuppression strategies, and ischemic reperfusion injury.

Deceased organ allocation policy has undergone significant change since the final rule for operation of the Organ Procurement and Transplantation Network was enacted in 2000. Currently, the Model for End-Stage Liver Disease (MELD) and the Pediatric Model for End-Stage Liver Disease (PELD) are used to allocate livers in the United States. In this edition, the impact of these allocation models on waiting list mortality, survival after transplantation, and prioritization by disease is discussed in great detail and is also compared to and contrasted with different allocation schemes used in other countries.

The basic format of the new edition is the same as that of the first, in that we have recruited a wide authorship from world experts. We attempted to select authors with a strong track record in their particular area of endeavor, as well as a sense of opposing views, thus enabling them to articulate a consensus of opinion.

Most of the chapters have been thoroughly modified, and many new ones have been added. A new section, "Pearls and Pitfalls," is found at the end of most chapters and serves as a bullet point summary of the salient topics. Examples of areas that are totally new to this edition include a chapter on the molecular and cellular basis of hepatic failure (Section I) and a treatise on allocation, timing, and delisting criteria for liver transplantation. In Section II, we have included two chapters on hepatitis C, covering natural history, new indications for transplantation, risk factors for recurrence, and the controversial issue of retransplantation. Chapters on transplantation for hepatocellular carcinoma have been extensively enhanced to fully discuss the new selection criteria and their effect on long-term outcomes; extended criteria also are considered in detail. Sections III and IV deal with evaluation of the pediatric recipient and special considerations in patient evaluation. The chapter on liver transplantation for metabolic disease has been thoroughly updated to ensure the most current information on diagnosis, molecular markers, timing, monitoring, and outcomes in these difficult cases. Evaluation of patients with preexisting cardiac and pulmonary disease, with an emphasis on primary pulmonary hypertension and portopulmonary syndrome, is also extensively covered.

Section V, "The Operation," has been extensively reworked, with an emphasis on the various flexible techniques in organ procurement and a new chapter on donor selection criteria and management, particularly as they relate to the successful use of marginal donors. Additionally, a new chapter on non–heart-beating donors has been included. An entire section has been added for comprehensive coverage of split and living donor transplantation. Authorship in this section is truly international and emphasizes the tremendous new strides that have been made with these procedures over the past 5 to 6 years.

In Section IX, "Pathology," a chapter on the important topic of disease recurrence exclusive of malignancy has been added. This topic reflects recognition of the importance of viral recurrence on long-term graft function. In Section XI, new strategies in liver transplant immunosuppression are covered, with special emphasis on multi-drug regimens, calcineurin inhibitors, withdrawal, and antibody induction. The impact of immunosuppression on disease recurrence and the induction of tolerance are also addressed.

Section XII is concerned with survival, results, and preoperative predictors, as well as models for outcome prediction. These topics are particularly cogent in times when only the patients with highest severity scores are chosen to receive organs. Further developments in liver transplantation, including xenotransplantation and hepatocyte transplantation, have been completely updated, and a new chapter on ischemia-reperfusion injury as it affects marginal organ utilization has been added.

As you can see, we have attempted to include all aspects of the liver transplant process from anatomy to xenotransplantation. We set the same standard for the second edition as for the first: We believe the text will serve as the state-of-the-art reference and a platform for new advances and innovations that will continue to improve therapy for end-stage liver disease.

RONALD W. BUSUTTIL

GORAN B. KLINTMALM

Acknowledgment

To Colleen Devaney and Karen Hanie for their tireless efforts and dedication to this book. Without their work, this publication would not have been possible.

RONALD W. BUSUTTIL
GORAN B. KLINTMALM

Contents

I ▪ General Considerations 1

1 History of Liver and Multivisceral Transplantation 3
THOMAS E. STARZL • NORIKO MURASE • AMADEO MARCOS • JOHN J. FUNG

2 Surgical Anatomy of the Liver 23
JOHN F. RENZ • PAULO R. REICHERT • SHERYLIN A. GORDON • JEAN C. EMOND

3 Molecular and Cellular Basis of Hepatic Failure 43
HAL F. YEE, JR. • TIMOTHY J. DAVERN II

4 Influence of Liver Transplantation on Liver Surgery 57
GARRETT M. HISATAKE • JONATHAN R. HIATT

5 Liver Allocation: The U.S. Model 63
RICHARD B. FREEMAN, JR.

6 Liver Organ Allocation: The European Models 79
LARS BÄCKMAN • JOHN L. R. FORSYTHE • BIANCA MIRANDA • NATIVIDAD CUENDE
JOSE CAÑÓN • CARLOS MARGARIT • TILL GERLING • GUIDO G. PERSIJN

II ▪ Patient Evaluation: Adult 93

7 Current Indications, Contraindications, Delisting Criteria, and Timing for Liver
Transplantaion 95
SCOTT A. FINK • ROBERT S. BROWN, JR.

8 Transplantation for Viral Hepatitis A and B 115
BRUNO ROCHE • DIDIER SAMUEL

9 Natural History of Hepatitis C 129
DAWN SEARS • GARY L. DAVIS

10 Hepatitis C and Liver Transplantation 143
MARINA BERENGUER • JOHN LAKE

11 Transplantation for Fulminant Hepatic Failure 161
STEPHEN M. RIORDAN • ROGER WILLIAMS

12 Liver Transplantation for Primary Biliary Cirrhosis 177
JAYANT A. TALWALKAR • W. RAY KIM • E. ROLAND DICKSON

13 Transplantation for Sclerosing Cholangitis 187
JEFFREY S. CRIPPIN

14 Liver Transplantation for Autoimmune Hepatitis 195
JOSE M. NIETO • SAMMY SAAB

15 Transplantation for Primary Hepatic Malignancy 211
MARVIN J. STONE • J. MARK FULMER • GORAN B. KLINTMALM

16 Liver Transplantation for Metastases of the Liver 233
FERDINAND MÜHLBACHER • SUSANNE RASOUL ROCKENSCHAUB

17 Liver Transplantation for Hematological Disorders 239
WILLIAM D. TAP • VICTOR J. MARDER

18 Transplantation for Budd-Chiari Syndrome 249
MARVIN J. STONE • J. MARK FULMER • GORAN B. KLINTMALM

19 Liver Transplantation for Alcoholic Liver Disease 265
ROBERT M. WEINRIEB • MICHAEL R. LUCEY

20 Unusual Indications for Liver Transplantation 275
DAVID H. van THIEL • AYSE L. MINDIKOGLU
ANANTHARAJU ABHINANDANA • MEHDI BALUCH • SONU DHILLON
MAGDALENE M. GEORGE • JOHN BREMS • S. DAVID LI • RAZA HAMDANI

III ▪ Patient Evaluation: Pediatric 285

21 General Criteria for Pediatric Transplantation 287
ESTELLA M. ALONSO • ANDRES BESEDOVSKY • KARAN EMERICK • PETER F. WHITINGTON

22 Transplantation for Cholestatic Liver Disease in the Pediatric Patient 303
BYUNG-HO CHOE • JORGE A. BEZERRA • WILLIAM F. BALISTRERI

23 Transplantation for Biliary Atresia 323
RANDOLPH SCHAFFER III • LYNDA BRADY • J. MICHAEL MILLIS

24 Liver Transplantation for Metabolic Disease 337
SUZANNE V. McDIARMID

25 Transplantation for Hepatic Malignancy in Children 367
FREDERICK C. RYCKMAN • MARIA H. ALONSO • GREGORY M. TIAO • KEVIN E. BOVE

IV ▪ Special Considerations in Patient Evaluation 379

26 Ethical Decisions in Liver Transplantation 381
L. S. ROTHENBERG

27 Psychosocial Assessment of Adult Liver Transplant Recipients 395
SHEILA JOWSEY • TERRY SCHNEEKLOTH

28 Pretransplantation Evaluation: Pulmonary, Cardiac, and Renal 405
MARTIN L. MAI • DANIEL S. YIP • CESAR A. KELLER • THOMAS A. GONWA

29 Pretransplantation Infectious Disease Screening for Liver Transplantation:
Candidates and Donors 429
MARIAN G. MICHAELS • MICHAEL D. GREEN

30 Clinical Nurse Coordinator: Nursing Focus on Care of Patients with
End-Stage Liver Disease 439
KELLY WICKER

31 Radiologic Evaluation in the Liver Transplant Patient 447
ANTOINETTE S. GOMES

32 Monitoring and Care of the Patient Before Liver Transplantation 473
PRATIMA SHARMA • HUGO E. VARGAS • JORGE RAKELA

33 Nutritional Aspects of Adult Liver Transplantation 491
JEANETTE HASSE

34 Management of Portal Hypertensive Hemorrhage in the Era of Liver
Transplantation 507
SUNIL K. GEEVARGHESE • JONATHAN R. HIATT • RONALD W. BUSUTTIL

V ■ Operation 513

35 Donor Selection and Management 515
CONSTANTINO FONDEVILA • RAFIK M. GHOBRIAL

36 Non–Heart-Beating Donor Liver Transplantation 529
DAVID J. REICH • COSME Y. MANZARBEITIA

37 The Donor Operation 545
JOHN F. RENZ • HASAN YERSIZ

38 Principles of Liver Preservation 561
STEVEN M. STRASBERG • NAZIA SELZNER • PIERRE-ALAIN CLAVIEN

39 The Recipient Hepatectomy and Grafting 575
GORAN B. KLINTMALM • RONALD W. BUSUTTIL

40 Anesthesia for Liver Transplantation 589
MICHAEL A. E. RAMSAY

VI ■ Split and Living Donor Transplantation 607

41 Split-Liver Transplantation for the Pediatric and Adult Recipient 609
JEAN DE VILLE DE GOYET • XAVIER ROGIERS • JEAN-BERNARD OTTE

42 Living Related Liver Transplantation in Pediatric Recipients 629
KOICHI TANAKA • YUKIHIRO INOMATA

43 Split-Liver Transplantation for Two Adults 647
DANIEL AZOULAY • MASSIMO DEL GAUDIO • PAULA ANDREANI • HENRI BISMUTH

44 Donor and Recipient Evaluation and Selection for Adult-to-Adult Right
Hepatic Lobe Liver Transplantation 655
JAMES F. TROTTER • PAUL H. HAYASHI • IGAL KAM

45 Adult Living Donor Hepatectomy and Recipient Operation 675
SANDER S. FLORMAN • CHARLES M. MILLER

46 Imaging Techniques for Living Donor Transplantation 703
PIYAPORN LIMANOND • STEVEN S. RAMAN • DAVID S. K. LU

47 Outcomes of Living Donor Liver Transplantation 713
JOHN F. RENZ • CINDY J. KIN • BOB H. SAGGI • JEAN C. EMOND

48 Ethics of Living Donor Liver Transplantation 725
DAVID C. CRONIN II • MARK SIEGLER

VII ▪ Unusual Operative Problems 741

49 Portal Vein Thrombosis and Other Venous Anomalies in
Liver Transplantation 743
NIRAJ M. DESAI • KIM M. OLTHOFF

50 Liver Transplantation and Situs Inversus 755
DOUGLAS G. FARMER • RONALD W. BUSUTTIL

51 Retransplantation 767
SUSAN M. LERNER • JAMES MARKMANN • ODED JURIM • RONALD W. BUSUTTIL

52 Clinical Management of the Necrotic Liver During Transplantation 777
ERNESTO P. MOLMENTI • PAUL J. SCHEEL, JR.

53 Transplantation of the Liver with Digestive Organs 787
TOMOAKI KATO • ANDREAS G. TZAKIS

54 Combined Liver-Kidney Transplantation 803
EDMUND Q. SANCHEZ • GORAN B. KLINTMALM

55 Auxiliary Liver Transplantation 815
CARLOS MARGARIT

VIII ▪ Postoperative Care 831

56 Postoperative Intensive Care Unit Management: Adult Liver Transplant
Recipients 833
HENRY B. RANDALL • GORAN B. KLINTMALM

57 Postoperative Intensive Care Management in Children 853
RICK HARRISON

58 Postoperative Management Beyond the Intensive Care Unit: Adults 865
EDMUND Q. SANCHEZ • GORAN B. KLINTMALM

59 Postoperative Care of Pediatric Liver Transplant Recipients 881
STEVEN J. LOBRITTO • JEAN C. EMOND

60 Renal Failure in Adult Liver Transplant Recipients 891
PHUONG-THU T. PHAM • PHUONG-CHI T. PHAM • ALAN H. WILKINSON

61 Graft Failure: Etiology, Recognition, and Treatment 915
NICHOLAS N. NISSEN • STEVEN D. COLQUHOUN

62 Technical Problems: Biliary 929
PETER NEUHAUS • ANDREAS PASCHER

63 Arterial Complications After Liver Transplantation 953
SHERILYN A. GORDON • IAN C. CARMODY

64 Infections After Liver Transplantation 963
CURTIS D. HOLT • DREW J. WINSTON

65 Late Complications of Liver Transplantation and Recurrence of Disease 995
MICHAEL R. CHARLTON • K. V. NARAYANAN MENON

66 Neuropsychiatric Outcomes in Liver Transplant Recipients 1019
THOMAS B. STROUSE

67 Postoperative Neurological Disorders and Prognosis 1029
EDWIN C. AMOS III

68 Role of the Posttransplant Coordinator 1037
GREGG KUNDER

IX ▪ Liver Transplant Pathology 1055

69 Histological Patterns of Rejection and Other Causes of Liver Dysfunction 1057
ANTHONY J. DEMETRIS • MIKE NALESNIK • PARMJEET RANDHAWA • TONG WU
MARIDA MINERVINI • CHI LAI • ZHENGBIN LU

70 Pathology of Recurrence of Non-Neoplastic Disease After Liver
Transplantation 1129
CHARLES R. LASSMAN

71 Transplant-Related Malignancies 1149
JOSEPH F. BUELL • THOMAS M. BEEBE • MICHAEL J. HANAWAY • MARK J. THOMAS
STEVEN M. RUDICH • E. STEVE WOODLE

X ▪ Immunology of Liver Transplantation 1165

72 Rejection After Transplantation 1167
GERALD S. LIPSHUTZ • NANCY L. ASCHER • JOHN P. ROBERTS

73 Cell Migration, Chimerism, and Graft Acceptance, with Particular
Reference to the Liver 1183
THOMAS E. STARZL • NORIKO MURASE • ANTHONY J. DEMETRIS • MASSIMO TRUCCO
BIJAN EGHTESAD • PAULO FONTES • KAREEM ABU-ELMAGD • AMADEO MARCOS
JOHN J. FUNG

74 ABO, Tissue Typing, and Cross-match Incompatibility in
Liver Transplantation 1199
J. MICHAEL CECKA • ELAINE F. REED

XI ▪ Immunosuppression 1211

75 Induction and Maintenance of Immunosuppression 1213
SRINATH CHINNAKOTLA • GORAN B. KLINTMALM

76 Special Considerations for Pediatric Immunosuppression After
Liver Transplantation 1235
SUZANNE V. McDIARMID

77 Treatment of Acute and Chronic Rejection 1263
IAN C. CARMODY • PAULINE W. CHEN

78 Novel Immunosuppressive Agents 1275
RYUTARO HIROSE • FLAVIO VINCENTI

XII ■ Survival and Results 1283

79 Outcome Predictors in Liver Transplantation 1285
RAFIK M. GHOBRIAL • GORAN B. KLINTMALM

80 U.S. Trends in Liver Transplantation, 1988 to 2001 1299
IDRIS V. R. EVANS • STEVEN H. BELLE

81 Long-Term Functional Recovery and Quality of Life: Childhood, Adulthood,
Employment, Pregnancy, and Family Planning 1323
MARLON F. LEVY • TERIANNE COWLING • GORAN B. KLINTMALM

82 Results: Survival and Quality of Life After Orthotopic Liver
Transplantation in Children 1335
CARLOS O. ESQUIVEL

XIII ■ Future Developments in Liver Transplantation 1355

83 Genetic Modulation in Transplantation 1357
HEIDI YEH • ABRAHAM SHAKED

84 Xenotransplantation and the Liver 1365
JEFFREY L. PLATT • IRA J. FOX

85 Hepatocyte Transplantation in Liver Disease 1379
VIVEK DIXIT

86 New Approaches in Immunosuppression 1387
MARTIN HERTL • A. BENEDICT COSIMI

87 Ischemia-Reperfusion Injury of the Liver 1403
CONSTANTINO FONDEVILA • RONALD W. BUSUTTIL • JERZY W. KUPIEC-WEGLINSKI

88 Extracorporeal Xenogeneic Liver Support 1415
RAVI S. CHARI • WILLIAM C. MEYERS • MARLON F. LEVY

89 Development of Bioartificial Liver 1425
WING S. CHEUNG • JOSEPH P. VACANTI

Index 1437

General Considerations

History of Liver and Multivisceral Transplantation*

THOMAS E. STARZL
NORIKO MURASE
AMADEO MARCOS
JOHN J. FUNG

Genesis of liver transplantation   5

Prerequisites for canine liver replacement   7

Pathology of liver rejection   7

Variant liver transplant procedures   7

Immunosuppression by host cytoablation   8

Drug immunosuppression for clinical
   kidney transplantation   9

Human liver trials of 1963   10

Liver transplant moratorium   12
   Role of human leukocyte antigen
      (HLA) matching   12
   Development of antilymphocyte
      globulin (ALG)   12
   Demonstration of hepatic tolerogenicity   12
   Reassessment of the auxiliary liver graft   13
   Improved organ preservation   13

Resumption of human liver replacement   13

Advent of better drugs   14

Technical innovations   15
   Donor procedures   15
   Recipient operation   16

Indications for liver transplantation   17

Benign disease   17
Neoplastic diseases   17
Organ shortage   17
   Use of marginal donors   17
   Living donor transplantation   18
   Split-liver procedures   19
Xenotransplantation   19

Between 1955 and the end of 1967, the framework of clinical organ transplantation that exists today was established in a small number of centers in continental Europe, Great Britain, and North America. The kidney was, at first, the forerunner organ, but liver transplantation soon became the driving force in discoveries and advances that were applicable for other kinds

*The work was supported by National Institutes of Health (NIH) grants DK 29961 and DK 6420. The development of liver transplantation was supported continuously over a 40-year period by grants from the National Institutes of Health and from the Denver Veterans Administration. The chapter was prepared with the indispensable assistance of Ms. Terry L. Mangan (*mangantl@msx.upmc.edu*), Executive Secretary, of the liver transplant program from 1982 to the present.

of organs. These accomplishments included the development of better methods of organ preservation, the evolution of present-day immunosuppression, and the elucidation of the seminal mechanisms of alloengraftment and acquired tolerance. In addition, research in liver transplantation is responsible for insight into the metabolic interrelations of the intra-abdominal viscera in disease and health, progress in the understanding and treatment of liver-based inborn errors of metabolism, and identification of growth factors that influence hepatic growth control and regeneration. Table 1–1 summarizes and annotates most of the major milestones and events in this complex chain of events.[1-58]

Table 1–1. MILESTONES OF LIVER TRANSPLANTATION

Year	Description	Reference
1955	First article in the literature on auxiliary liver transplantation	1
1956	First mention of concept of liver replacement	2
1958–1960	Formal research programs of total hepatectomy and liver replacement in dogs	3,4
1960	Abdominal multivisceral transplantation described in dogs	5
1963	Azathioprine-prednisone cocktail introduced (kidneys first, then livers) and recognition of organ-induced tolerance	6
1963	Description of in situ preservation-procurement method	7
1963	First human liver transplantations (University of Colorado)	8
1964–1965	Evidence of hepatropic (liver-supporting) factor(s) in portal venous blood	9,10
1965	First clear evidence of hepatic tolerogenicity	11
1966	First liver xenotransplantation on July 15, 1966 (chimpanzee donor)	12
1966	Clinical introduction of antilymphocyte globulin (ALG) (kidneys, then livers)	13
1966–1970	Proof that human leukocyte antigen (HLA) matching would not be a major factor in organ transplantation	14,15
1967	First successful human liver replacements: under azathioprine, prednisone, and ALG	16
1967–1968	Acceptance of brain death concept	17
1969	First use of liver transplantation to cure inborn error of metabolism	18
1973	Recognition that the liver resists antibody-mediated rejection	19
1973–1975	Principal portal venous hepatotrophic factor identified as insulin	20,21
1976	Improved slush liver preservation permits long-distance procurement	22,23
1979	Systematic use of arterial and venous grafts for cadaver organ revascularization	24
1979	Cyclosporine introduced for organ transplantation including two liver recipients	25
1980	Cyclosporine-steroid cocktail introduced clinically	26
1981	80% 1-year liver recipient survival reported using cyclosporine-prednisone	27
1983	Introduction of pump-driven venovenous bypass without anticoagulation	28–30
1983–1984	US consensus development conference conclusion that liver transplantation is a service (1983) is followed by rapid proliferation of transplant centers worldwide	31
1984	Standardization of in situ preservation-procurement-preservation techniques for multiple cadaver organs	32,33
1984	Reversibility demonstrated of B-cell malignancies—post-transplant lymphoproliferative disease (PTLD)—in liver and other organ recipients	34
1984	First reports of reduced-size liver grafts	35,36
1987–1989	First successful transplantation of liver-containing multivisceral grafts	37,38
1987	University of Wisconsin (UW) solution improves liver and other organ preservation	39–41
1987	Report of successful extensive use of livers from marginal donors	42
1988	Compliance with Organ Transplant Act of 1984 by national adoption of Pittsburgh point system for cadaver kidney and liver distribution	43,44

Continued

Table 1-1. MILESTONES OF LIVER TRANSPLANTATION—cont'd

Year	Description	Reference
1989	Popularization of the piggyback variation of liver transplantation	45
1989	Clinical introduction of FK506 (tacrolimus)-based immunosuppression	46,47
1989	First report of splitting cadaver livers for 2 recipients	48
1990	First successful use of live liver donors (left-side fragments)	49,50
1992-1998	Discovery of donor leukocyte microchimerism in liver (and other organ) recipients with recognition of clonal exhaustion-deletion as the seminal mechanism of organ engraftment	51-53
1994-1999	Live-donor transplantation of right-side liver fragments	54-56
2001	Development of mechanism-based tolerogenic immunosuppression	57
2003	Double knockout of porcine α1,3-galactosyltransferase (GT) gene, revitalizing hopes of clinical xenotransplantation	58

Genesis of Liver Transplantation

Transplantation of all the major organs except the liver can be traced back to the early 1900s.[59,60] In contrast, the first report of liver transplantation did not appear until 1955 in a journal called *Transplantation Bulletin*, the forerunner of the present day *Transplantation*.

The Auxiliary Liver Concept. In a one-page article, C. Stuart Welch of Albany Medical College described the insertion of a hepatic allograft in the right paravertebral gutter of dogs, without disturbing the native liver.[1] More complete information was published in *Surgery* the following year.[61] The auxiliary livers were revascularized by anastomosing the graft hepatic artery to the recipient aortoiliac system and by end-to-end anastomosis of the graft portal vein to the host inferior vena cava (Fig. 1–1). Welch obviated the need to anastomose multiple hepatic veins by including the short length of donor retrohepatic vena cava into which all of these hepatic veins empty as part of his auxiliary allografts. The upper end of the caval segment of the graft was anastomosed to the recipient vena cava, and the lower end was ligated or sutured (see Fig. 1–1).

Unlike other kinds of transplanted organs, the auxiliary allografts underwent dramatic shrinkage. The atrophy, which began within 3 or 4 days, was attributed at the time to liver rejection. The view was consistent with the current dogma of the time, that liver size and regeneration are governed by the volume of portal venous inflow (the "flow hypothesis" of hepatic homeostasis). Because the portal vein of the transplanted extra livers had been provided with an ample amount of systemic (i.e., vena caval) blood (see Fig. 1–1), the acute allograft atrophy was ascribed to immunological factors. A decade passed before it was demonstrated that the liver shrinkage actually was due to the dearth in vena caval and other systemic blood of molecules (especially

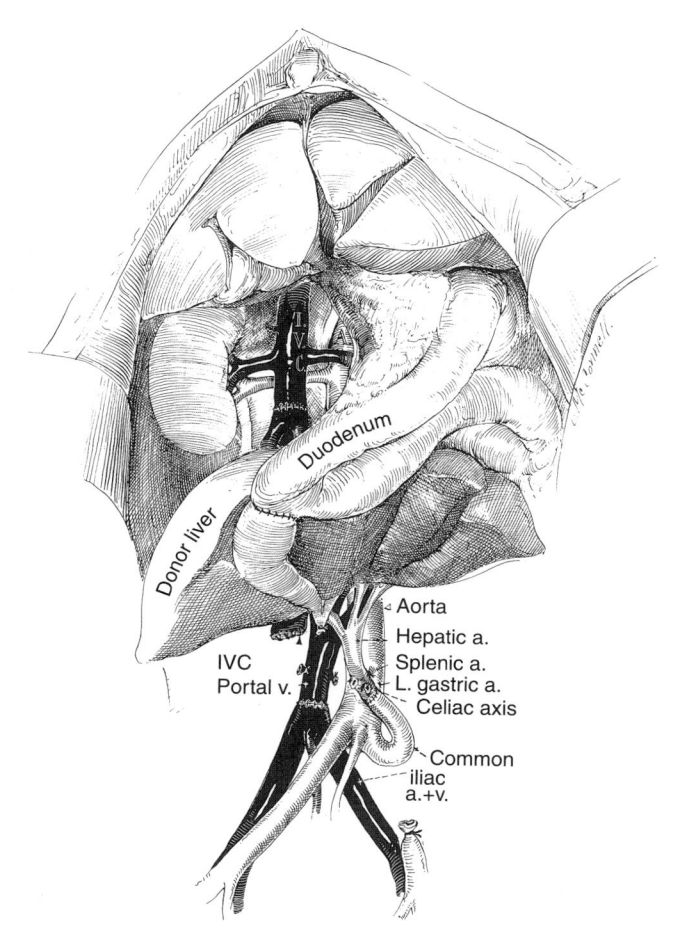

FIGURE 1–1

Auxiliary liver homotransplantation in dogs (the Welch procedure). Note that the reconstituted portal venous inflow is from the inferior vena caval bed rather than from the splanchnic organs. Biliary drainage was with cholecystoduodenostomy. (From Starzl TE, Marchioro TL, Rowlands DT Jr, et al: Immunosuppression after experimental and clinical homotransplantation of the liver. Ann Surg 160:411-439, 1964.)

insulin) that are normally presented to liver in high concentrations in splanchnic venous blood (see Reassessment of the Auxiliary Liver Graft).[9,10,20,21]

Orthotopic Liver Transplantation. The concept of liver replacement (orthotopic transplantation) was first mentioned by Jack Cannon in a one-page account of the transplant activities in the surgery department of the recently founded University of California, Los Angeles (UCLA) School of Medicine.[2] The species studied was not mentioned (presumably dog), and there was no specific information about the procedure. It is noteworthy that Cannon's article (entitled "Brief Report") and the two articles on auxiliary hepatic transplantation by Welch and colleagues[1,61] were the sole references to the liver in M.F.A. Woodruff's compendium of work in the transplantation field up to 1959.[62]

By the time Woodruff's book was published in 1960, extensive investigations of liver replacement in dogs had been completed in independent studies started in the summer of 1958 at both Northwestern University in Chicago[3] and the Peter Bent Brigham Hospital in Boston.[4] The Boston studies,[4,63,64] under the direction of Francis D. Moore, were a natural extension of an immunologically oriented institutional commitment to organ transplantation that initially was preoccupied with the kidney. In contrast, the Northwestern initiative[3,65] stemmed from an earlier investigation at the

University of Miami of the metabolic interrelationships of the liver with the pancreas and intestine.[66,67] To facilitate these studies, a new method of total hepatectomy was developed in which the unique feature was preservation of the host retrohepatic inferior vena cava.[68]

The canine host hepatectomy developed in Miami was essentially the same as that in today's *piggyback* variation of liver transplantation.[45,69,70] For liver transplantation in the dog, however, it was simpler to excise the host retrohepatic vena cava along with the native liver and to replace it with the comparable caval segment of the donor liver into which the hepatic veins empty. After completing the vena caval anastomoses above and below the liver, hepatic arterial and biliary tract anastomoses were performed with conventional methods (Fig. 1–2).[3,4] When different means of portal revascularization were systematically tested in the Northwestern laboratory (Fig. 1–3), any deviation from normal of the portal supply resulted in reduced survival.

The research teams at Northwestern and Brigham Hospital were unaware of each other's activities until late 1959, and direct contact was not established until the 1960 meeting of the American Surgical Association. By then, the cumulative total of liver replacements in unmodified (nonimmunosuppressed) dogs had increased to 80 in Chicago[3] and 31 in Boston.[4] The results were published separately in 1960 in different journals.

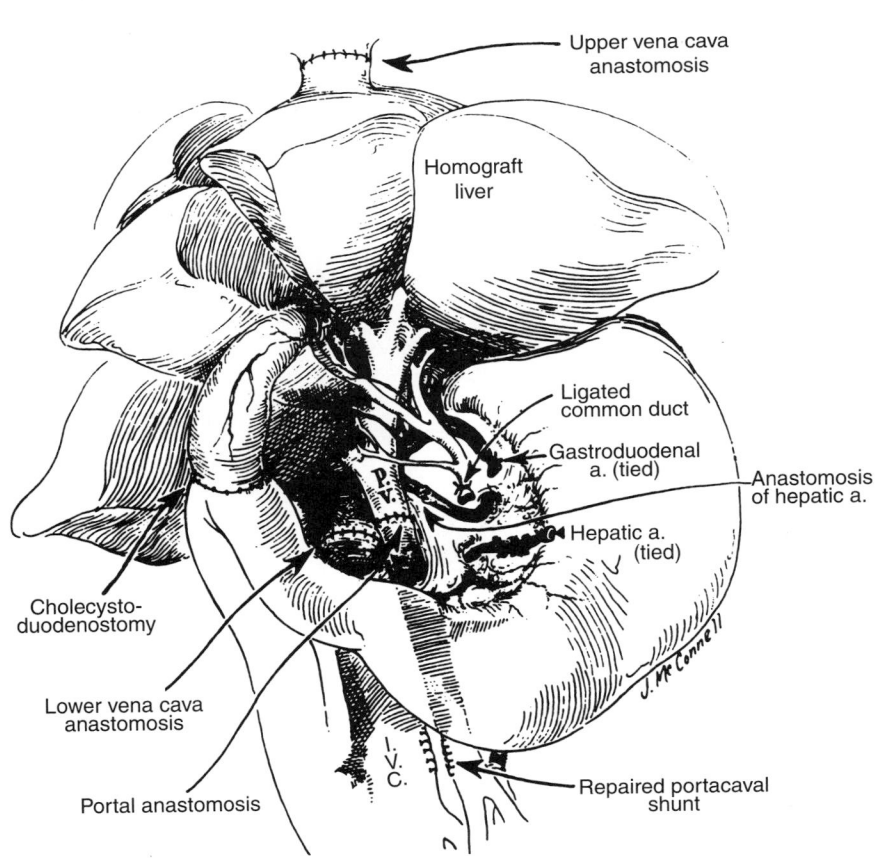

FIGURE 1–2

Completed liver replacement in the dog. The fact that the recipient was a dog rather than a human is identifiable only by the multilobar appearance of the liver. (From Brettschneider L, Daloze PM, Huguet C, et al: The use of combined preservation techniques for extended storage of orthotopic liver homografts. Surg Gynecol Obstet 126:263-274, 1968.)

Upper vena cava anastomosis

Homograft liver

Ligated common duct

Gastroduodenal a. (tied)

Anastomosis of hepatic a.

Hepatic a. (tied)

Cholecysto-duodenostomy

Lower vena cava anastomosis

Portal anastomosis

Repaired portacaval shunt

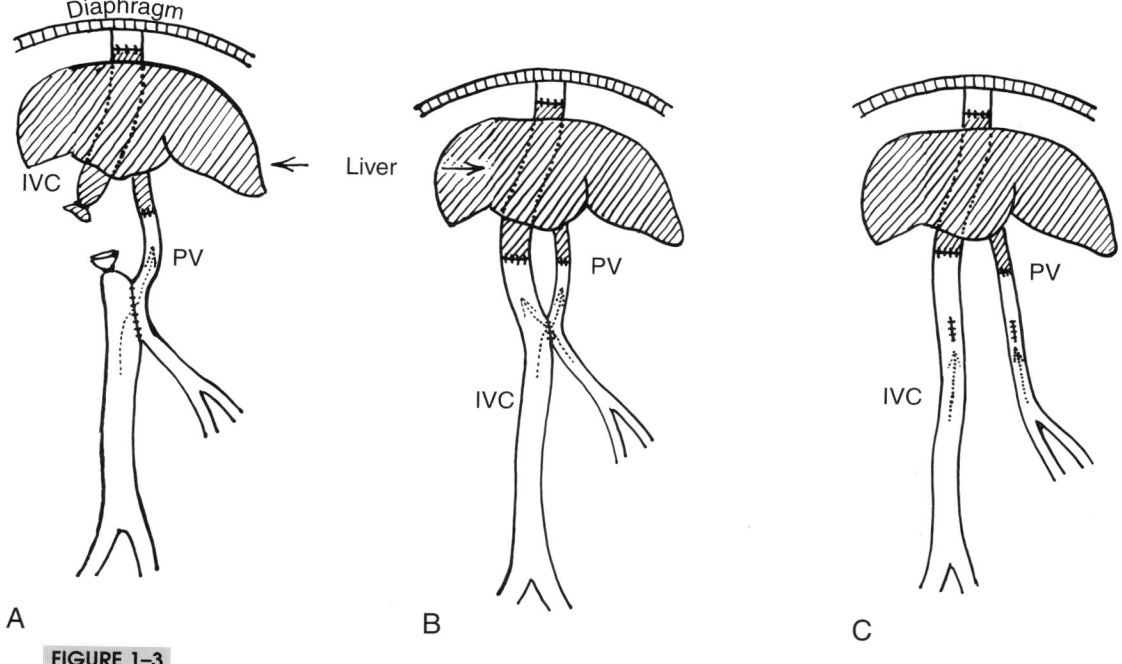

FIGURE 1–3

Alternative methods of portal vein revascularization: *A*, reverse Eck fistula; *B*, with small side-to-side porta-caval shunt; *C*, anatomically normal. Survival was best with C. (From Starzl TE, Kaupp HA Jr, Brock DR, et al: Reconstructive problems in canine liver homotransplantation with special reference to the postoperative role of hepatic venous flow. Surg Gynecol Obstet 111:733-743, 1960.) IVC, inferior vena cava; PV, portal vein.

Prerequisites for Canine Liver Replacement

The two prerequisites for perioperative survival of the canine recipients had been identified in both laboratories. The first requirement was prevention of ischemic injury to the allograft. This was accomplished in Boston by immersing the liver in iced saline. At Northwestern, the livers were cooled by the intravascular infusion of chilled lactated Ringer's solution (Fig. 1–4). This now universal first step in preservation of all organs had never been used before, apparently because of fear of damaging the microcirculation. Better liver preservation was later obtained with infusates of differing osmotic, oncotic, and electrolyte composition (e.g., the Collins,[22] Schalm,[23] and University of Wisconsin [UW] solutions).[39-41]

The second prerequisite for successful canine liver transplantation was avoidance of damage to the recipient splanchnic and systemic venous beds, the drainage of which was obstructed during host hepatectomy and graft implantation. This was accomplished in both laboratories by decompressing external venovenous bypasses, which differed in detail.

Pathology of Liver Rejection

Until 1960, the kidney had been the only organ allograft whose unmodified rejection had been systematically studied. Most of the transplanted canine livers were destroyed in 5 to 10 days. Typically, a heavy concentration of mononuclear cells was seen in the portal triads and within and around the central veins. Hepatocyte necrosis was extensive.[64,65] A curious exception was noted, however, in the 63rd liver replacement experiment.

In the exceptional recipient, the serum bilirubin reached a peak at 11 days, but then progressively declined (Fig. 1–5, dashed line).[65] The predominant histopathological findings in the allograft by day 21 were more those of repair and regeneration than of rejection. *This was the first recorded exception to the existing dogma (based on skin graft research) that rejection, once begun, was inexorable.* Five years later, similar observations were made in allografts of long-surviving canine liver recipients in Denver, whose rejections had developed and then spontaneously reversed under stable daily doses of azathioprine.[11]

Variant Liver Transplant Procedures

The studies completed by the end of 1959 in Boston and Chicago defined almost to the last detail the liver replacement operation soon to be performed in humans. The operation of multivisceral transplantation, in which the allograft consisted of the liver and all of the other intraperitoneal organs, also was perfected (Fig. 1–6, center).[5] It was noted that rejection of the different splanchnic organs transplanted with the liver was

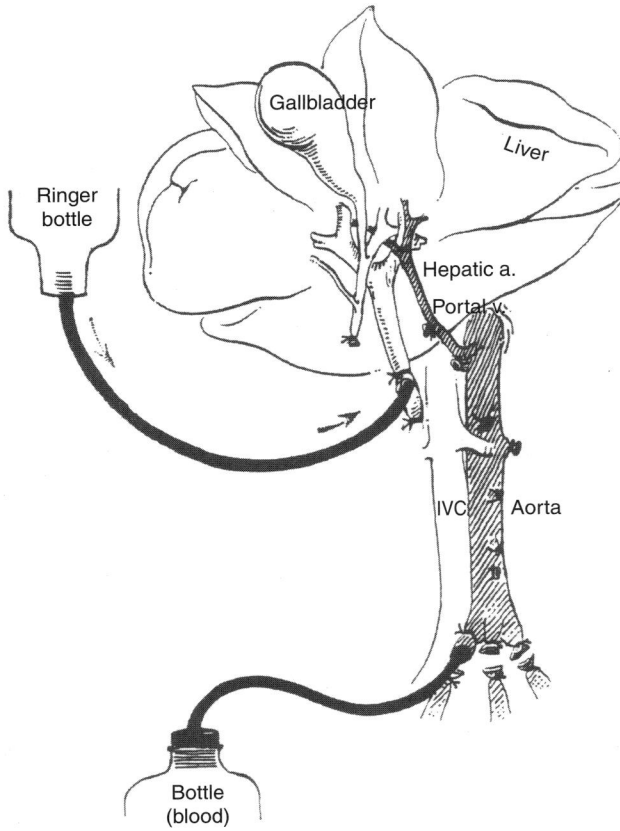

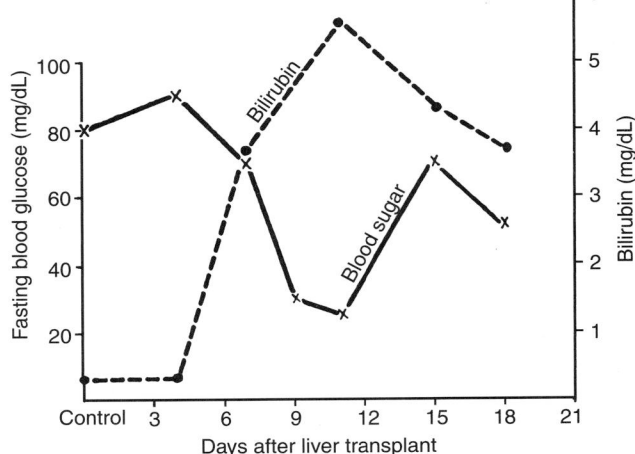

FIGURE 1–5

Serial blood glucose and serum bilirubin levels in a nonimmuno-suppressed canine liver recipient who survived for 3 weeks. Note the decline of bilirubin after the eleventh day. This evidence of the spontaneous reversal of rejection was consistent with the histopathology of the autopsy liver at 21 days. (From Starzl TE, Kaupp HA Jr, Brock DR, Linman JW: Studies on the rejection of the transplanted homologous dog liver. Surg Gynecol Obstet 112: 135-144, 1961.)

FIGURE 1–4

Cooling of the canine hepatic allograft by infusion of chilled lactated Ringer's solution into the donor portal vein. The animals were simultaneously exsanguinated. (From Starzl TE, Kaupp HA Jr, Brock DR, et al: Reconstructive problems in canine liver homotransplantation with special reference to the postoperative role of hepatic venous flow. Surg Gynecol Obstet 111:733-743, 1960.)

much less severe than the rejection of the individual organs transplanted alone,[71] an observation that was validated much later in rodent studies[72,73] and in humans.[74] In addition, the recipients had histopathological evidence of a widespread graft-versus-host reaction in their tissues, but without overt graft-versus-host disease (GVHD). This was the first clue that GVHD might not blight intestinal or liver transplantation, or both, if such procedures were ever to become feasible.

Multivisceral transplantation and its modifications (see Fig. 1–6) were applied in humans 30 years later[37,38,75,76] and are now part of the conventional armamentarium of advanced organ transplant centers. However, when the canine operation was first presented at the Surgical Forum of the American College of Surgeons in October 1960,[5] it was ridiculed. In fact, all research in whole-organ transplantation (including of the kidney) during 1958 to 1960 was considered naïve or wasteful by many critics and especially by basic

immunologists, most of whom viewed the immune barrier to transplantation as impenetrable.

Immunosuppression by Host Cytoablation

Just as this kind of surgical research in unmodified dogs was losing momentum, it was dramatically revitalized by six successful human kidney transplantations performed between January 1959 and February 1962, first by Joseph Murray in Boston[77] and then five more times by the independent teams of Jean Hamburger[78] and Rene Kuss[79] in Paris. The first cases were compiled under circumstances that would not be acceptable in today's climate of institutional review board (IRB) regulation (i.e., before long-term survival had been accomplished in animals). All six patients were preconditioned with sublethal doses of 4.5 Gy total-body irradiation (Table 1–2, above the dashed line). Although *success* was defined as survival for at least 1 year, the first two recipients (both of fraternal twin kidneys) had continuous graft function for more than 2 decades without the need for posttransplant immunosuppression. These were the first examples of acquired immunological tolerance in humans. However, the drug-free state was not considered to be *real tolerance* for reasons described in Chapter 73, "Cell Migration, Chimerism, and Graft Acceptance, with Particular Reference to the Liver."

In an effort to replace irradiation for conditioning, the UCLA urologist Willard Goodwin pretreated six

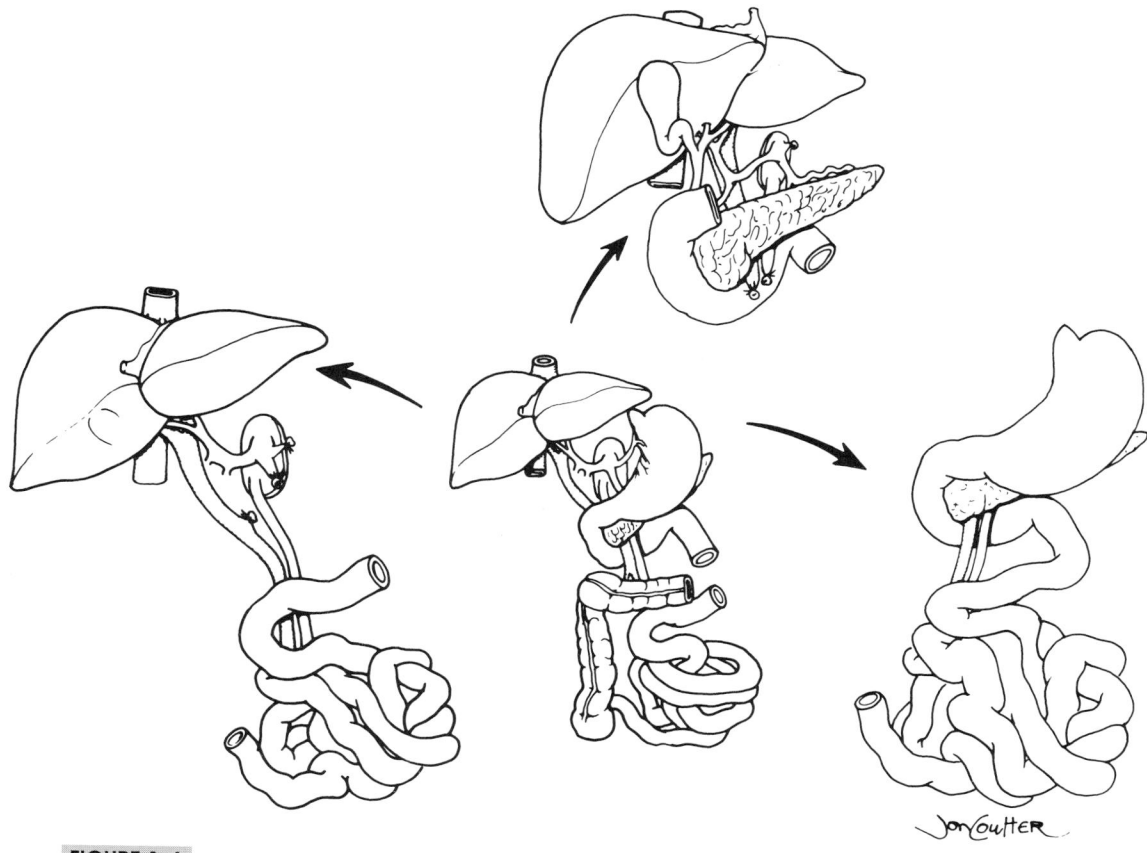

FIGURE 1-6

The original canine multivisceral allograft (*bottom center*) and its variations (*arrows*). All are used clinically today. (From Starzl TE: The saga of liver replacement, with particular reference to the reciprocal influence of liver and kidney transplantation (1955-1967). J Am Coll Surg 195:587-610, 2002.)

human kidney recipients in 1960 to 1961 with myelotoxic doses of cyclophosphamide and methotrexate.[80] One patient had prolonged survival (143 days), during which rejection was successfully reversed several times with prednisone. This important observation was not reported until 1963. In any event, it quickly became apparent that cytoablation would not be the means by which liver transplantation could be accomplished.

In our hands, total-body irradiation precluded even perioperative, much less extended, survival of canine liver recipients.[81]

Drug Immunosuppression for Clinical Kidney Transplantation

Since the early 1950s, skin graft survival in rabbits was slightly prolonged by treatment with adrenal cortical steroids.[82,83] However, the era of drug immunosuppression usually is designated to begin on the arrival of the drug 6-mercaptopurine (6-MP). After establishing that 6-MP was immunosuppressive without a need for overt bone marrow depression,[84] Schwartz and Dameshek at Tufts Medical School in Boston[85] and Meeker and Good and colleagues at the University of Minnesota[86] demonstrated modest prolongation of skin allograft survival in rabbits. Survival of canine kidney allografts for up to 40 days under 6-MP was then reported by Calne in London[87] and independently for similar times by Zukoski in Richmond.[88] By the end of 1960, Calne

Table 1-2. KIDNEY TRANSPLANTATION: 6 MONTHS OR GREATER SURVIVAL AS OF MARCH 1963

	City (Ref)*	Date	Donor	Survival (mo)
1	Boston (77)	1/24/59	Fraternal twin	>50
2	Paris (78)	6/29/59	Fraternal twin	>45
3	Paris (79)	6/22/60	Unrelated	18 (Died)
4	Paris (78)	12/19/60	Mother	>12 (Died)
5	Paris (79)	3/12/61	Unrelated	18 (Died)
6	Paris (78)	2/12/62	Cousin	>13
7	Boston (93)	4/5/62	Unrelated	11

*Boston: Joseph E Murray (patients 1 and 7); Paris: Jean Hamburger (patients 2, 4, and 6), R Küss (patients 3 and 5).

(by now in Boston with Murray)[89,90] and Zukoski (with David Hume in Richmond)[91] obtained even longer survival of canine kidney recipients. In Calne's report, the best results were obtained with the imidazole derivative of 6-MP, azathioprine (Imuran).[89] However, survival for as long as 100 days was unusual (i.e., < 5% of the experiments).

When clinical kidney transplant trials with the new drugs were begun in Boston in 1960 to 1961 with initially high expectations,[92] the possibility of transplanting the human liver no longer seemed so remote. In 1961, William R. Waddell left Massachusetts General Hospital to become Chair of Surgery at the University of Colorado, where one of us (T.E.S) joined him from Northwestern. Armed with more than 3 years of experience in Chicago with canine hepatic replacement, we settled on liver transplantation as our highest priority for clinical development. The plan was tabled when we learned that the Boston clinical trial of kidney transplantation had yielded disappointing results. A ray of hope could be found, however, in a report by the future Nobel laureate, Joseph Murray, in the September 1962 issue of *Annals of Surgery*.[92]

The article included a description of a kidney allograft that was still functioning under azathioprine immunosuppression 120 days after its transplantation from an unrelated donor on April 6, 1962. The kidney was still functioning at 10 months when next reported in June 1963.[93] Although the patient's blood urea nitrogen (BUN) was now elevated (110 mg/dL), the graft was destined to support dialysis-free life for another 7 months (total of 17 months). It was the first example of 1-year survival of a human organ allograft without host conditioning with total-body irradiation (see Table 1–2, number 7). However, this was the only kidney recipient of the first 13 treated solely with chemical immunosuppression who survived for as long as 6 months.[92-94]

In the meantime, we had obtained our own supply of azathioprine in the spring of 1962 and began systematically evaluating it at the Denver VA Hospital laboratory with the simpler canine kidney model instead of liver transplantation. As in other laboratories, our yield of survivals of as long as 100 days was small. However, two crucial findings were clinically relevant. The first was that the kidney rejections that developed with azathioprine invariably could be reversed by the delayed addition of large doses of prednisone.[95]

The second key observation was that a mean survival of 36 days in dogs treated with azathioprine was almost doubled when the animals also were pretreated with the drug for 7 to 30 days.[96] We now committed to clinical trials of kidney and liver transplantation, in that order. Daily doses of azathioprine were given to the kidney recipients for 1 to 2 weeks before, as well as after, kidney transplantation from living donors, adding

prednisone only to treat rejection. The human renal transplantation program was opened in the autumn of 1962.

The two features of the adaptive immune response to allografts that would make transplantation of all kinds of organs feasible were described in the title of the report of the first 10 kidney cases: "The Reversal of Rejection in Human Renal Homografts with Subsequent Development of Homograft Tolerance."[6] The term *tolerance* referred to the time-related decline of need for maintenance immunosuppression. Largely because of this observation, we already had concluded that renal transplantation had reached the level of a bona fide, albeit still flawed, clinical service. At the time, there were only three clinically active kidney transplant centers in the United States: the long-standing Brigham program and the two centers opened in 1962—ours at the University of Colorado and David Hume's in Richmond, Virginia.

One year later, nearly 50 kidney teams had started or were gearing up, including the program at UCLA that had opened in 1960 and closed in 1961. A similar proliferation of kidney centers also was under way throughout Europe. Moreover, the benefits of kidney transplantation proved to be truly long-lasting in some cases. Eight of the Colorado kidney recipients of the 1962 to 1963 era still bear their original transplants 40 years later and are the longest surviving organ allograft recipients in the world.[97]

Human Liver Trials of 1963

Although the follow-ups were still short, our encouraging kidney experience triggered the decision to go forward with the infinitely more difficult initiative of liver transplantation. The first attempt on March 1, 1963 was in an unconscious and ventilator-bound child with biliary atresia who bled to death during operation. The next two recipients, both adults, died 22 and 7.5 days after their transplantations on May 5 and June 3, 1963 for the indication of primary liver malignancies (Table 1–3). These two patients were found at autopsy to have extrahepatic micrometastases.[8]

As in the kidney recipients, azathioprine was administered before as well as after transplantation, adding a high-dose course of prednisone with the onset of rejections. The rejections were easily reversed (Fig. 1–7), and the transplanted livers retrieved at autopsy after 7.5 and 22 days were remarkably free of rejection. Good allograft preservation was accomplished by transfemoral infusion of a chilled perfusate into the aorta of the non–heart-beating donors after cross-clamping the aorta at the diaphragm (Fig. 1–8), in much the same way as in the first stage of the *flexible* multiple organ procurement operation used today.[32,33] There was little ischemic damage to the allografts during the cold ischemia of

Table 1-3. THE FIRST SEVEN HUMAN LIVER RECIPIENTS

Age	Date	City (Ref)	Liver Disease	Survival (Days)	Main Cause of Death
3	3/1/63	Denver (8)	Biliary atresia	0	Intraoperative bleeding
48	5/5/63	Denver (8)	Hepatoma, cirrhosis	22	Pulmonary emboli, sepsis
68	6/3/63	Denver (8)	Duct cell carcinoma	75	Pulmonary emboli
52	7/10/63	Denver (9)	Hepatoma, cirrhosis	65	Gastrointestinal bleeding, pulmonary emboli/edema, liver failure
58	9/16/63	Boston (98)	Colon metastases	11	Pneumonitis, hepatic abscesses, failure
29	10/4/63	Denver (9)	Hepatoma	23	Sepsis, bile peritonitis, pulmonary emboli
75	1/?/64	Paris (99)	Colon metastases	0	Intraoperative hemorrhage

2.5 and 8 hours, as judged by modest increases in the liver injury tests.

The various anastomoses were performed in the same way as in the dog experiments except for the biliary tract reconstruction. The complete operation was drawn in 1963 (Fig. 1–9). The picture could be used today, and often is, to depict a perfectly executed human liver transplantation. The flaw in the trial was the use of passive venovenous bypasses. Blood clots formed in the bypass tubing, migrated to the lungs, and caused or contributed to the deaths of all four of the 1963 Denver recipients who survived the operation (see Table 1–3). Overzealous correction of clotting abnormalities probably contributed to the formation of the emboli. Coagulation had been monitored with serial thromboelastograms and corrected with blood components and with ε-aminocaproic acid (an analogue of the currently used aprotinine).

Ironically, the venous decompression that had been critical for survival in the dog experiments is not mandatory in most human liver recipients. The motor-driven venovenous bypass system, which was introduced in Pittsburgh in the 1980s,[28-30] made the procedure easier; but in many centers, it now is used only selectively and

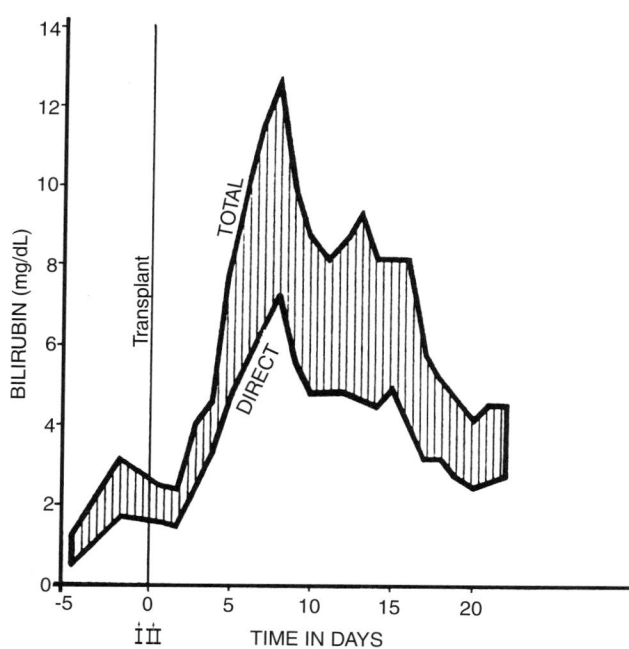

FIGURE 1-7

Rise in serum bilirubin to 12.8 mg/dL in the first patient who survived liver replacement. The bilirubin declined after institution of high-dose prednisone therapy. The patient died of pulmonary emboli after 22 days. (From Starzl TE, Marchioro TL, Von Kaulla KN, et al: Homotransplantation of the liver in humans. Surg Gynecol Obstet 117:659–676, 1963.)

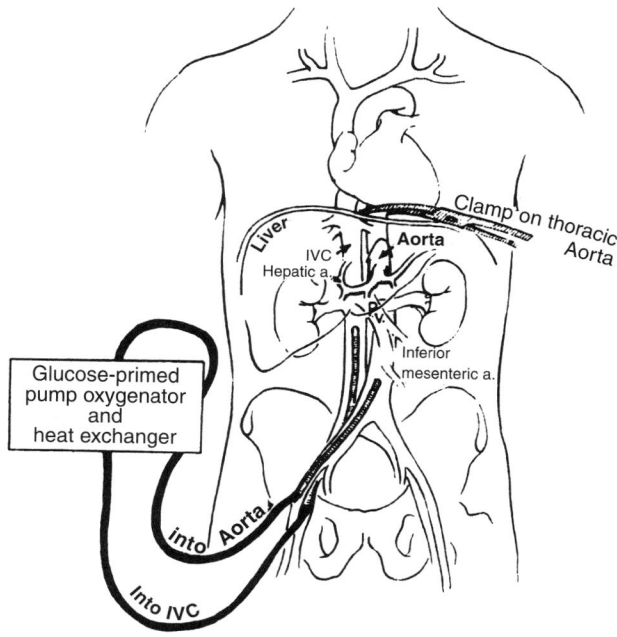

FIGURE 1-8

Extracorporeal perfusion of the deceased donors reported in 1963. "The venous drainage was from the inferior vena cava and the arterial inflow was through the aorta after insertion of the catheters through the femoral vessels. Note clamp on thoracic aorta to perfuse the lower half of the corpse selectively. A glucose-primed pump oxygenator was used with a heat exchanger."[8]

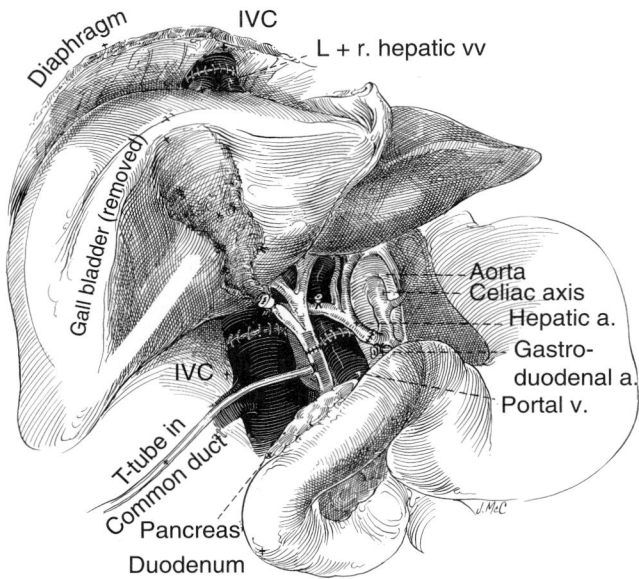

FIGURE 1–9

The operation carried out in the first two patients who survived liver replacement on May 5 and June 3, 1963. The patients lived for 22 and 7.5 days. (From Starzl TE: Experience in Hepatic Transplantation. Philadelphia, Saunders, 1969, p 138.)

almost never in infants or small children. In fact, venous decompression was later shown to be expendable in dogs that were submitted to common bile duct ligation several weeks in advance of transplantation. With the development of venous collaterals in these animals, it was possible at a second stage to carry out liver replacement without venovenous bypass.[100]

Liver Transplant Moratorium

During the last half of 1963, two more liver transplantations were performed in Denver,[9] and one each in Boston[98] and Paris[99] (see Table 1–3). After the deaths of these patients, clinical activity ceased for 3.5 years, between January 1964 and the summer of 1967. The worldwide moratorium was voluntary, but the decision to stop was reinforced by widespread criticism of attempting to replace an unpaired vital organ with an operation that had come to be perceived as too formidable to be practical. During the moratorium, advances were made, most of which were applicable to all organs.

Role of Human Leukocyte Antigen (HLA) Matching

In a clinical collaboration with Paul Terasaki of UCLA, it was shown that the quality of human leukocyte antigen (HLA) matching, short of perfect compatibility, had little association with kidney transplant outcome.[14,15,101] By inference, desperately ill liver, heart, and other transplant candidates who could not wait for a well-matched organ would not suffer a significant penalty by receiving a mismatched one.

Development of Antilymphocyte Globulin (ALG)

A second objective was to improve immunosuppression. Between 1963 and 1966, antilymphocyte globulin (ALG) was prepared from antilymphocyte serum (ALS) obtained from horses immunized against dog or human lymphoid cells.[102] After extensive preclinical studies, human-specific ALG was introduced clinically in 1966 in combination with azathioprine and prednisone (the *triple drug cocktail*).[13,16] In the preclinical canine studies, the efficacy of dog-specific ALG had been demonstrated when it was given before, at the time of, or after kidney and liver transplantation. Because pretreatment appeared to be valuable, it was incorporated for the patients whenever possible.

Demonstration of Hepatic Tolerogenicity

The feasibility of liver transplantation reflected during this period was increasingly evidenced by a growing kennel population of long-surviving canine recipients (Fig. 1–10), none of which was treated with more than a 4-month course of azathioprine[11] or a few doses of ALG.[13] In presenting the results of 143 canine liver replacements to the Society of University Surgeons in February 1965, it was emphasized that "Although the early recovery after liver homotransplantations has many hazards … the frequency and rapidity with which dogs could be withdrawn from immunosuppression without an ensuing fatal rejection is remarkable …. The consistency of this state of host-graft nonreactivity and the rapidity with which it seemed to develop exceeds that reported after canine renal homotransplantations."[11]

A year later, the French surgeon, Henri Garnier, reported (with Cordier) that a significant percentage of *untreated* outbred pig liver recipients did not reject their allografts.[103] This observation promptly was confirmed and extended in England by Calne at Cambridge,[104] Peacock and Terblanche in Bristol,[105] and us.[106] Calne and colleagues subsequently demonstrated that the tolerance self-induced by the liver extended to other tissues and organs from the liver donor, but not from third-party pigs.[107]

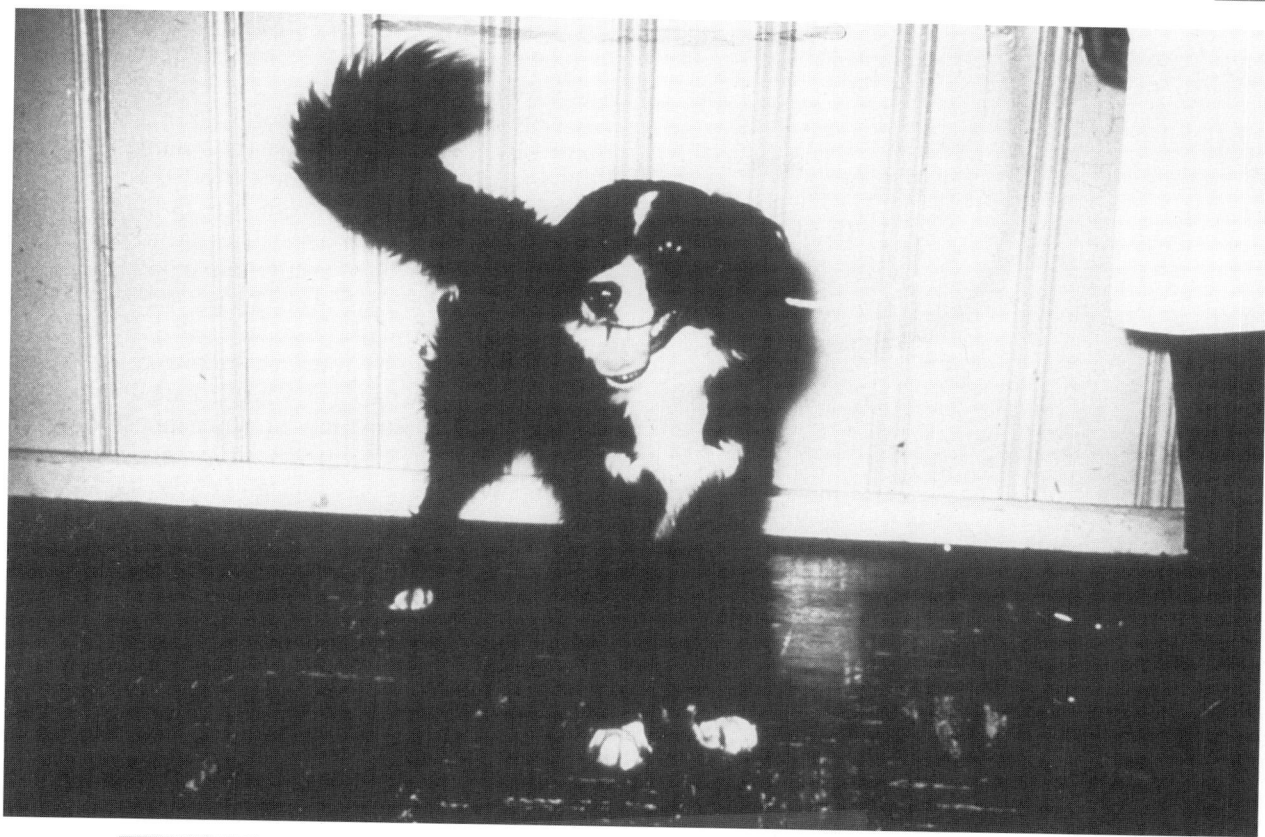

FIGURE 1–10

Canine recipient of an orthotopic liver homograft, 5 years later. The operation was on March 23, 1964. The dog was treated for only 120 days with azathioprine and died of old age 13 years after transplantation.

Reassessment of the Auxiliary Liver Graft

Although the primary focus during the moratorium was on liver replacement, the ostensibly less radical auxiliary liver transplantation (Welch's operation) was reevaluated. After showing that rejection could be completely prevented in some dogs with high doses of azathioprine, it was proved that the acute atrophy of Welch's auxiliary livers was caused by depriving the allografts of liver-supporting constituents of splanchnic venous blood (see Fig. 1–1).[9,10] The technical difficulties of obtaining optimal portal vein revascularization finalized the decision to proceed clinically with liver replacement.

However, the *hepatotropic* qualities of splanchnic venous blood were not fully explained until the mid-1970s. Eventually, it was established that endogenous insulin was the most important factor.[20,21] This was a decisive step in understanding the pathophysiology of Eck's fistula (portacaval shunt).[108] Only then could it be readily understood why total splanchnic venous diversion (i.e., portacaval shunting) was such a severe insult to the already damaged liver of patients with hepatic disease, particularly if there had been significant portal

flow prior to the shunt. In addition, the demonstration that insulin is a liver growth factor was the beginning of the field of hepatotropic physiology (i.e., studies of the effect of growth factors on liver structure, size, function, and the capacity for regeneration).[109]

Improved Organ Preservation

The potential pitfall of organ preservation remained. It would still be necessary to obtain livers from non–heart-beating donors. To help surmount this difficulty, we developed an ex vivo perfusion system in 1966 and 1967 that permitted reliable preservation of canine livers for as long as a day.[110] Now, it was time to try again.

Resumption of Human Liver Replacement

The liver program was reopened in July 1967 and was reinforced by a powerful new member, Carl Gustav Groth, a 2-year National Institutes of Health (NIH) fellow

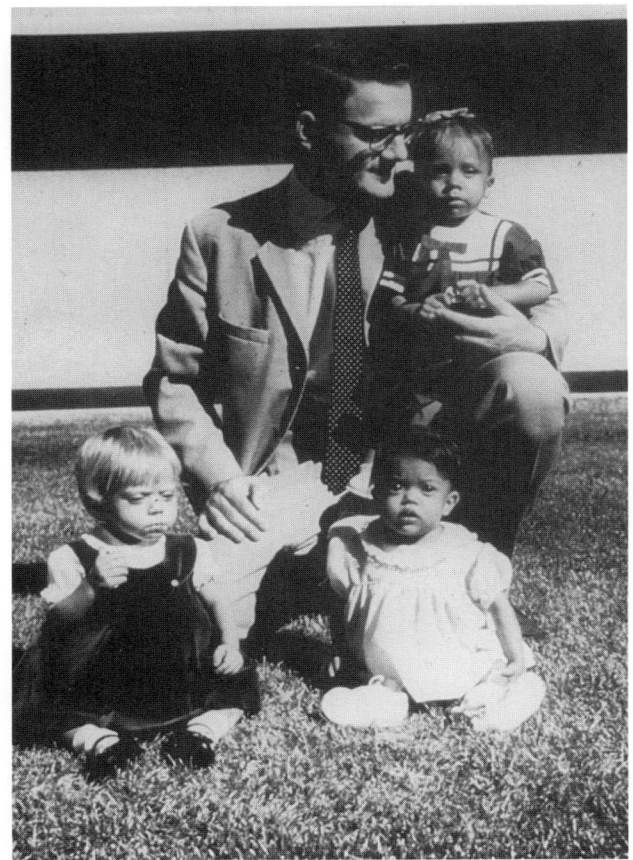

FIGURE 1–11

The first three human recipients to have prolonged survival after liver replacements in July and August, 1967. The adult, Carl Groth, was then an NIH-supported fellow.

from Stockholm. Multiple examples of prolonged human liver recipient survival promptly were produced under triple-drug immunosuppression with azathioprine, prednisone, and ALG (Fig. 1–11).[16]

The liver transplant beachhead was reinforced by the opening of Roy Calne's clinical program in Cambridge, England in February 1968.[69] By the time

the first textbook on liver transplantation was written in 1969,[111] there had been 33 human liver replacements in the world: 25 in Denver and 8 elsewhere (4 by Calne). The German and French teams of Rudolf Pichlmayr and Henri Bismuth began to make important contributions to liver transplantation in the early 1970s, followed by the Dutch group of Rudi Krom later in the decade.

Transplantation of other extrarenal organs followed close behind the liver, using similar immunosuppression (Table 1–4). Hearts were successfully transplanted in 1968 in Capetown by Barnard[112] and in Palo Alto by Shumway.[113] In 1969, the first prolonged survival after human lung[114] and pancreas transplantation[115] was accomplished in Ghent, Belgium and Minneapolis, respectively. Despite these achievements, transplantation of the extrarenal organs, and especially of the liver, remained controversial for another decade, because of the high mortality rate. Only 34 (20%) of the 170 liver recipients treated at the University of Colorado through 1979 survived for 5 years or longer.[52]

The unusual tolerogenicity of the hepatic allograft previously demonstrated in dogs and pigs was evident in human liver recipients of the 1970s. In 1995, 12 (28%) of the 42 Colorado patients still surviving from this era already had been off all immunosuppression for 1 to 17 years.[116] Since then, the majority of the remaining 30, some of whom are now beyond the third of a century posttransplant milestone, also have stopped drugs without rejection.[117,118] Such drug-free tolerance was almost unheard of with the other kinds of deceased-donor organs.

Advent of Better Drugs

Although the feasibility of transplanting the liver and other extrarenal organs had been established, the widespread use of these procedures was precluded until cyclosporine was introduced clinically in England in 1978 by Calne[25] and combined with prednisone in Denver 1 year later.[26] Results further improved with all

Table 1-4. FIRST SUCCESSFUL TRANSPLANTATION OF HUMAN ALLOGRAFTS (SURVIVAL >6 MONTHS)				
Organ	City	Date	Physician/Surgeon	Ref
Kidney	Boston	1/24/59	Murray	77
Liver	Denver	7/23/67	Starzl	16
Heart	Cape Town	1/2/68	Barnard/Shumway	112,113
Lung*	Ghent	11/14/68	Derom	114
Pancreas†	Minneapolis	6/3/69	Lillehei	115

*Patient died after 10 months; all others in table lived more than 1 year with functioning graft. The first more than 1-year survival of isolated lung recipients was not reported until 1987.
†Kidney and pancreas allografts in uremic patient.

organs when tacrolimus was substituted for cyclosporine in the 1990s.[46,47] The stepwise increases in liver recipient survival, first with cyclosporine-based[27,119] and then with tacrolimus-based immunosuppression,[46,47] were particularly striking (Fig. 1–12). Thus, by the end of the 20th century, transplantation of the liver and all of the other vital organs had become an integral part of sophisticated medical practice in every developed country in the world. The dramatic spread of liver transplantation that began in the mid-1980s was made possible by a supremely talented new generation of surgeons who in turn began to instruct their own competent trainees.

There was, however, one disappointment. With the better immunosuppressants, drug-free liver recipients such as those treated with azathioprine (or cyclophosphamide), prednisone, and ALG in the mortality-plagued 1970s were expected to become common. Yet, this was seen less frequently than before. It was clear that the goal of deliberate production of drug-free liver recipients would remain out of reach until the mechanisms leading to organ-induced tolerance were understood. Insight into these mechanisms of tolerance began to emerge in 1992 when low-level donor leukocyte chimerism (microchimerism) was demonstrated in all 30 kidney and liver recipients studied from 3 to

30 years after successful transplantation. Chapter 73 describes how this new information permitted the development of more tolerogenic strategies of immunosuppression applicable to transplantation of all organ allografts.

Technical Innovations

Although the ascension of liver transplantation was dominated by improvements in immunosuppression, there were other significant developments, including modifications in the details of both the donor and recipient operations.

Donor Procedures

Cooling of deceased-donor organs is done today by variations of the in situ technique originally developed before the acceptance of brain death conditions (see Fig. 1–8), but with simple infusion without a bypass.[7] These methods[32,33] allow removal of all thoracic and abdominal organs, including the liver, without jeopardizing any of the individual organs—even with unstable donors, including those whose hearts have ceased

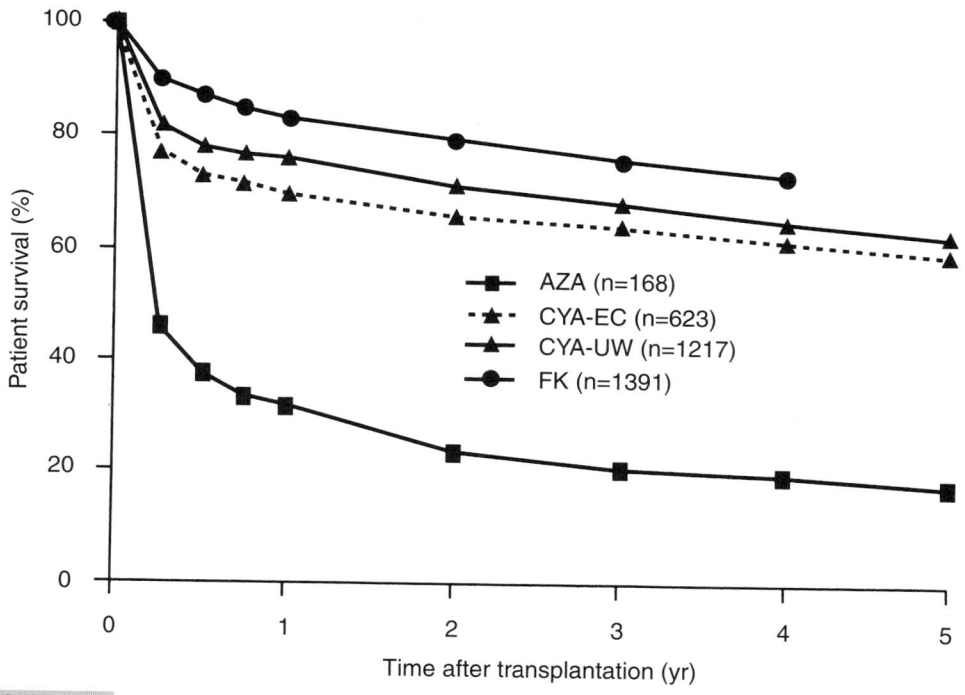

FIGURE 1-12

Stepwise improvements in patient survival after liver replacement. These were associated with the advent of increasingly potent immunosuppressive drugs. AZA, azathioprine; CYA, cyclosporine before [*dashed line*] and after [*continuous line*] the availability of UW solution; FK, tacrolimus. Most of the difference between the dashed and continuous lines was because of the availability of FK for the rescue of cyclosporine failures. The data shown here were presented to the American Surgical Association in April 1994.

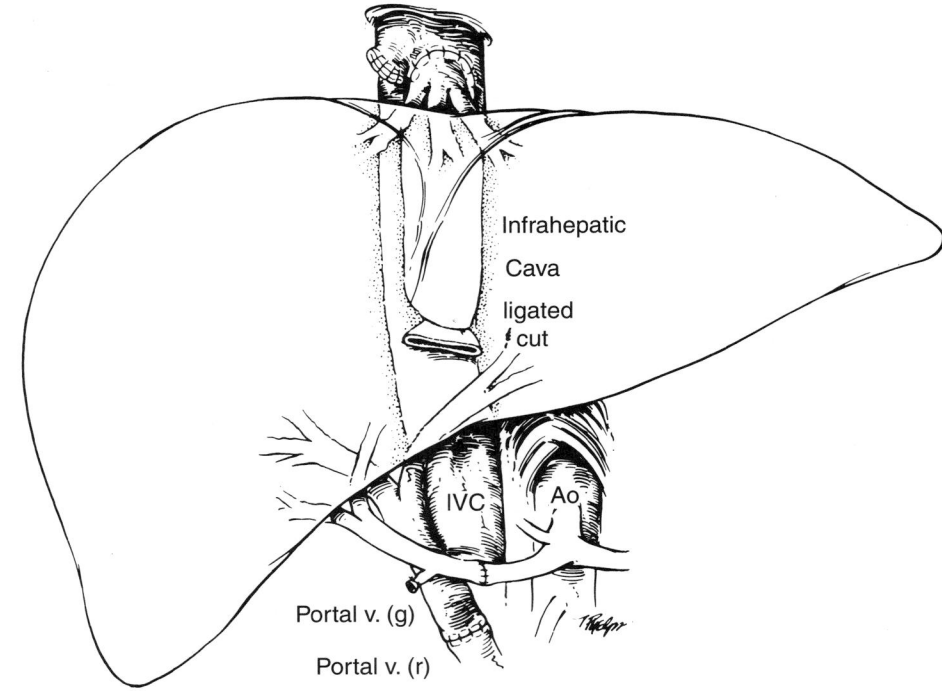

FIGURE 1-13

Transplantation of a liver piggybacked onto an inferior vena cava, which is preserved through its length. Note that the suprahepatic vena cava of the homograft is anastomosed to the anterior wall of the recipient vena cava. The retrohepatic vena cava of the homograft is sutured or ligated, leaving a blind sac into which empty numerous hepatic veins. (From Tzakis A, Todo S, Starzl TE: Orthotopic liver transplantation with preservation of the inferior vena cava. Ann Surg 210:649-652, 1989.) Ao, aorta; IVC, inferior vena cava.

to beat. By 1987, multiple organ procurement techniques had become so standardized that they were interchangeable not only from city to city but also from country to country. After the chilled organs are removed, subsequent preservation usually is performed by simple refrigeration rather than by sophisticated methods of continuous perfusion that were developed in the 1960s.

Recipient Operation

The incidence of biliary duct complications (obstruction, fistula, and cholangitis), which had been more than 30%, was reduced by the use of choledochocholedochostomy with a T-tube stent or, if this was not feasible, by choledochojejunostomy to a Roux limb.[119] The systematic use of venovenous bypasses without anticoagulation in adult recipients greatly diminished the occurrence of hemorrhages of nightmare proportions that were common at one time. Management of coagulopathies continued to be facilitated by the use of the thromboelastogram to follow the minute-to-minute clotting changes in the operating room.[120] With better control of bleeding, scarring from multiple upper abdominal operations, as well as prior portosystemic shunts, were

eliminated as serious adverse factors in major centers. The systematic use of arterial and venous grafts that was introduced in the 1970s[24] eliminated extensive thrombosis of the portal and superior mesenteric veins as a contraindication to liver transplantation[121] and has facilitated arterialization in complex cases.

The shortage of appropriate-sized donors for very small pediatric recipients was greatly ameliorated by the use of partial livers. The introduction of such operations followed the development of sophisticated techniques of hepatic resection for neoplasms.[122,123] The first known reduced liver transplant graft operation was performed in Denver in 1975.[124] This case was not reported, however, until long after the description of the technique by Bismuth and Houssin in Paris[35] and by Broelsch and Pichlmayr and colleagues in Hanover.[36] Implantation of liver fragments has been facilitated by use of the piggyback principle,[49] by which the recipient retrohepatic vena cava is kept intact and the venous outflow of the graft is anastomosed to cuffs of the host hepatic veins (Fig. 1-13). The piggyback modification was first used as early as 1968 in Cambridge, England[69] and in Denver[70] for the transplantation of pediatric livers, but the operation was rarely used for full-sized adult livers until its popularization by Tzakis and colleagues.[45]

Indications for Liver Transplantation

By the early 1990s, liver transplantation had become the accepted court of last appeal for essentially all non-neoplastic end-stage liver diseases and for selected patients with otherwise nonresectable hepatic malignancies.

Benign Disease

Parenchymal and Cholestatic Disorder

By the end of the 1980s, diagnoses that had precluded liver transplantation, such as the diagnosis of alcoholic cirrhosis, were no longer absolute contraindications. The list of benign diseases treatable by transplantation had become so long (nearly 100) that it was being divided into broad categories (Table 1–5) (e.g., cholestatic and parenchymal diseases).[125,126]

Inborn Errors of Metabolism

Products of hepatic synthesis permanently retain the original metabolic specificity of the donor after transplantation. Consequently, the correction of inborn errors by liver transplantation can be expected to endure for the life of the graft. By 1989, 16 liver-based or liver-influenced inborn errors of metabolism had been compiled (Table 1–6). Many others have been added since.

Neoplastic Diseases

The early use of conventional liver transplantation to treat otherwise nonresectable primary or metastatic hepatic cancers resulted in a high rate of recurrence.[8,119,127] Nevertheless, the use of liver transplantation to treat less-advanced cancers has continued, almost invariably in combination with adjuvant chemotherapy or other protocols. Certain kinds of neoplasms have a better prognosis than others. In an attempt to increase the perimeter of resectability, upper abdominal exenteration (i.e., en bloc removal of the liver, pancreas, spleen, stomach, duodenum, proximal jejunum, and ascending colon) has been used to treat extensive sarcomas, carcinoid tumors, and other malignancies that are still regionally confined.[76,128] The excised organs are replaced with hepatopancreaticoduodenal grafts (see Fig. 1–6, top) or, in some cases, by the liver alone.

Organ Shortage

By the late 1980s, there were enough liver transplant teams to use the available supply of deceased-donor organs. Efforts to equitably allocate livers to competing teams began officially in November 1987, when the United Network of Organ Sharing (UNOS) attempted to apply at a national level a *point system* based on urgency of need, size match, and logistic considerations that had been in effect in western Pennsylvania for most of the 1980s.[44] Neither the system nor its many modifications has satisfied all of the caregivers, patient advocacy groups, and other stakeholders. However, all interested groups, including surgeons, have tried to increase the pool of available organs.

Use of Marginal Donors

As early as 1986, Makowka and colleagues[42] identified the impending organ shortage and reported the feasibility of systematically using livers from older donors, donors with biochemical or histopathological evidence of liver injury, and those whose terminal course was characterized by management errors, physiological abnormalities, or the administration of potentially damaging pharmacological agents. At first criticized, this means of expanding the donor pool became widely

Table 1-5. GENERIC LISTING OF LIVER DISEASE TREATABLE BY LIVER TRANSPLANTATION
Disease Category
PARENCHYMAL
Postnecrotic cirrhosis
Alcoholic cirrhosis
Acute liver failure
Budd-Chiari syndrome
Congenital hepatic fibrosis
Cystic fibrosis
Neonatal hepatitis
Hepatic trauma
Others
CHOLESTATIC
Biliary atresia
Primary biliary cirrhosis
Sclerosing cholangitis
Secondary biliary cirrhosis
Familial cholestasis
Others
Inborn Errors of Metabolism
TUMORS
Benign
Primary malignant
Metastatic

Table 1–6. INBORN ERRORS OF METABOLISM TREATED WITH LIVER TRANSPLANTATION*

Disease	Explanation of Disease	Survival	Disease
α_1-Antitrypsin deficiency	Structural abnormality of the protease inhibitor synthesized in the liver	13 yr	Cirrhosis
Wilson's disease	Abnormal biliary copper excretion, decreased copper binding to ceruloplasmin, and copper accumulation in tissues; autosomal recessive gene mapped to chromosome 13	16.5 yr	Cirrhosis
Tyrosinemia	Fumaroylacetoacetate hydrolase deficiency	7.5 yr	Cirrhosis, hepatoma
Type I glycogen storage disease	Glucose-6-phosphatase deficiency	7 yr	Glycogen storage, fibrosis, tumors
Type IV glycogen storage disease	Amylo-1:4,1:6-transglucosidase (branching enzyme) defect	4.5 yr	Cirrhosis
Cystic fibrosis	Unknown; pancellular disease, liver often affected	4.5 yr	Cirrhosis
Niemann-Pick disease	Sphingomyelinase deficiency, sphingomyelin storage	2 yr (died)	None
Sea-blue histiocyte syndrome	Unknown, neurovisceral lipochrome	7 yr	Cirrhosis
Erythropoietic protoporphyria	Hepatic ferrochelatase deficiency, ?overproduction of protoporphyrin by erythropoietic tissues	1.5 yr	Cirrhosis
Crigler-Najjer syndrome	Glucuronyl transferase deficiency	4 yr	None
Type I hyperoxaluria	Peroxisomal alanine: glyoxylate aminotransferase deficiency	8 mo	None
Urea cycle enzyme deficiency (three types)	Ornithine carbamoyltransferase	8 mo	None
C protein deficiency	Defective C protein synthesis	2.5 yr	None
Familial hypercholesterolemia	Low-density lipoprotein receptor deficiency, low-density lipoprotein overproduction	6 yr	None
Hemophilia A	Factor VIII deficiency	4 yr	Cirrhosis, a complication of blood component therapy
Hemophilia B	Factor IX deficiency	6 mo	Cirrhosis, a complication of blood component therapy

*Most of the patients were in the University of Colorado–University of Pittsburgh series. This is a follow-up to January 1989. More inborn errors have been added since 1989.
From Starzl TE, Demetris AJ, Van Thiel DH: Liver transplantation (1). N Engl J Med 321:1014-1022, 1989. Reprinted by permission of The New England Journal of Medicine, 1989. Copyright 1989. Massachusetts Medical Society.

accepted once the magnitude of the supply problem was appreciated. Serious and frequently contentious efforts are still being made to define what constitutes a *marginal* donor and how to decide who gets the liver.[129]

Living Donor Transplantation

In an extension of the reduced liver graft procedures developed in deceased donors,[35,36] portions of liver ranging from the left lateral segment to the extended right lobe have been removed from volunteer adult donors for transplantation to pediatric recipients. Living donor liver transplantation from an adult liver to a child was first done successfully by Strong and Lynch in Adelaide, Australia.[49] The operation for pediatric recipients was subsequently popularized by Christoph Broelsch and associates at the University of Chicago,[50] who reported their results at the American Surgical Association conference in 1990 along with their experience with reduced-size deceased-donor organs and deceased-donor split livers.

To obtain an adequate liver mass for recipient body weight in adult-to-adult living donor transplantation, the size of the transected liver fragment was first increased from the left lateral segment to a full left lobe. The more common operation today is transplantation of a right lobe. This was first carried out in Japan when unexpected anatomical findings were encountered in the donor.[54] The first cases and series of right lobe transplantation in the United States were not published until 1998-1999.[55,56] Since then, more than 1500 right lobe transplantations have been performed in more than 40 American centers with patient and graft survival equivalent to that with whole-organ, deceased-donor transplantation or with various kinds of partial liver transplantation, including the predecessor adult-to-child procedure.

Despite its utility, liver donation from a living donor has been used with caution by many liver transplant surgeons because it has had a mortality of approximately 0.5%.

Split-Liver Procedures

More efficient use of deceased-donor organs has been made possible by sharing one liver between two recipients. The split-liver procedure was first reported from Europe by Rudolf Pichlmayr in 1989 and soon thereafter by Bismuth (Paris) and Broelsch (Chicago). The results were inferior at first to those obtained with whole livers.[50] But after a learning curve and incorporation of the lessons learned from living donors, the results with livers split between adult and pediatric recipients have been comparable to standard deceased-donor transplantation of whole organs. This practice may make the use of living donors for pediatric recipients unnecessary.

Moreover, splitting of the adult liver into full left and right lobes for transplantation into two adults (or even the sharing of a pediatric liver by two infants or children) could further relieve the organ shortage. This has been done successfully in a small number of adult cases.[130,131] Full implementation of this technique will require restriction of its use to optimal donors, careful assessment of the donor's physiological status before hepatectomy, careful consideration of the logistics involved, and the intelligent application of allocation rules for recipient selection.[132]

Xenotransplantation

Clinical transplantation of chimpanzee livers[12] was attempted three times between 1966 and 1973, with deaths after 0, 9, and 14 days.[133] The clinical course and pathological findings in the two patients who survived the operation were indistinguishable from those after allotransplantation. Two additional hepatic xenotransplantations were attempted, in June 1992 and January 1993, with more phylogenetically distant baboon donors. Survival was 70 and 26 days.[134,135] Neither humoral nor cell-mediated rejection could be

indicted as the cause of failure in these cases. However, there was evidence of continuous complement activation in both. The xenografts did not function optimally, and both developed findings of intrahepatic cholestasis within the first postoperative week. It also was suspected that synthetic products of the baboon liver may have been incompatible with the human metabolic environment.

The anthropomorphic qualities of chimpanzees and baboons and the perception that these animals pose a high risk from zoonotic infections have all but precluded further trials with primate donors. Hopes of using lower mammalian donors have been raised recently by the knockout in cloned pigs of both copies of the α1,3-galactosyltransferase gene.[58] The enzyme product of this gene is required for the synthesis of the sugar chain epitope α-gal, against which humans and other higher primates have preformed antibodies.

Elimination (double knockout) of the α-gal epitope avoids the immediate innate immune response to pig organs (i.e., hyperacute rejection does not occur), but it is almost certain that other genetic modifications will be needed before pig organs will be suitable for clinical use. Even if the immune barrier to livers is controlled, the multiple synthetic products of the porcine liver could make pig-to-human liver xenotransplantation tantamount to endowment of an inborn error (or errors) of metabolism.

References

1. Welch CS: A note on transplantation of the whole liver in dogs. Transplant Bull 2:54-55, 1955.
2. Cannon JA: Brief report. Transplant Bull 3:7, 1956.
3. Starzl TE, Kaupp HA Jr, Brock DR, et al: Reconstructive problems in canine liver homotransplantation with special reference to the postoperative role of hepatic venous flow. Surg Gynecol Obstet 111:733-743, 1960.
4. Moore FD, Wheeler HB, Demissianos HV, et al: Experimental whole organ transplantation of the liver and of the spleen. Ann Surg 152:374-387, 1960.
5. Starzl TE, Kaupp HA Jr: Mass homotransplantation of abdominal organs in dogs. Surg Forum 11:28-30, 1960.
6. Starzl TE, Marchioro TL, Waddell WR: The reversal of rejection in human renal homografts with subsequent development of homograft tolerance. Surg Gynecol Obstet 117:385-395, 1963.
7. Marchioro TL, Huntley RT, Waddell WR, Starzl TE: Extracorporeal perfusion for obtaining postmortem homografts. Surgery 54:900-911, 1963.
8. Starzl TE, Marchioro TL, Von Kaulla KN, et al: Homotransplantation of the liver in humans. Surg Gynecol Obstet 117:659-676, 1963.
9. Starzl TE, Marchioro TL, Rowlands DT Jr, et al: Immunosuppression after experimental and clinical homotransplantation of the liver. Ann Surg 160:411-439, 1964.
10. Marchioro TL, Porter KA, Dickinson TC, et al: Physiologic requirements for auxiliary liver homotransplantation. Surg Gynecol Obstet 121:17-31, 1965.
11. Starzl TE, Marchioro TL, Porter KA, et al: Factors determining short- and long-term survival after orthotopic liver homotransplantation in the dog. Surgery 58:131-155, 1965.
12. Starzl TE: Orthotopic heterotransplantation. In Starzl TE, (ed): Experience in Hepatic Transplantation. Philadelphia, WB Saunders, 1969, pp 408-421.

13. Starzl TE, Marchioro TL, Porter KA, et al: The use of heterologous antilymphoid agents in canine renal and liver homotransplantation and in human renal homotransplantation. Surg Gynecol Obstet 124:301-318, 1967.
14. Terasaki PI, Vredevoe DL, Mickey MR, et al: Serotyping for homotransplantation. VI. Selection of kidney donors for thirty-two recipients. Ann N Y Acad Sci 129:500-520, 1966.
15. Starzl TE, Porter KA, Andres G, et al: Long-term survival after renal transplantation in humans: With special reference to histocompatibility matching, thymectomy, homograft glomerulonephritis, heterologous ALG, and recipient malignancy. Ann Surg 172:437-472, 1970.
16. Starzl TE, Groth CG, Brettschneider L, et al: Orthotopic homotransplantation of the human liver. Ann Surg 168:392-415, 1968.
17. Definition of irreversible coma: Report of the ad hoc committee of the Harvard Medical School to examine the definition of brain death. JAMA 205:337, 1968.
18. DuBois RS, Giles G, Rodgerson DO, et al: Orthotopic liver transplantation for Wilson's disease. Lancet 1:505-508, 1971.
19. Starzl TE, Ishikawa M, Putnam CW, et al: Progress in and deterrents to orthotopic liver transplantation, with special reference to survival, resistance to hyperacute rejection, and biliary duct reconstruction. Transplant Proc 6:129-139, 1974.
20. Starzl TE, Francavilla A, Halgrimson CG, et al: The origin, hormonal nature, and action of hepatotrophic substances in portal venous blood. Surg Gynecol Obstet 137:179-199, 1973.
21. Starzl TE, Porter KA, Putnam CW: Intraportal insulin protects from the liver injury of portacaval shunt in dogs. Lancet 2:1241-1246, 1975.
22. Benichou J, Halgrimson CG, Weil R III, et al: Canine and human liver preservation for 6 to 18 hours by cold infusion. Transplantation 24:407-411, 1977.
23. Wall WJ, Calne RY, Herbertson BM, et al: Simple hypothermic preservation for transporting human livers long distance for homotransplantation. Transplantation 23:210-216, 1977.
24. Starzl TE, Halgrimson CG, Koep LJ, et al: Vascular homografts from cadaveric organ donors. Surg Gynecol Obstet 149:737, 1979.
25. Calne RY, Rolles K, White DJ, et al: Cyclosporin A initially as the only immunosuppressant in 34 recipients of cadaveric organs: 32 kidneys, 2 pancreases, and 2 livers. Lancet 2:1033-1036, 1979.
26. Starzl TE, Weil R III, Iwatsuki S, et al: The use of cyclosporin A and prednisone in cadaver kidney transplantation. Surg Gynecol Obstet 151:17-26, 1980.
27. Starzl TE, Klintmalm GBG, Porter KA, et al: Liver transplantation with use of cyclosporin A and prednisone. N Engl J Med 305:266-269, 1981.
28. Denmark SW, Shaw BW Jr, Starzl TE, Griffith BP: Veno-venous bypass without systemic anticoagulation in canine and human liver transplantation. Surg Forum 34:380-382, 1983.
29. Shaw BW Jr, Martin DJ, Marquez JM, et al: Venous bypass in clinical liver transplantation. Ann Surg 200:524-534, 1984.
30. Griffith BP, Shaw BW Jr, Hardesty RL, et al: Veno-venous bypass without systemic anticoagulation for transplantation of the human liver. Surg Gynecol Obstet 160:270-272, 1985.
31. National Institutes of Health Consensus Development Conference on Liver Transplantation. Sponsored by the National Institute of Arthritis, Diabetes, and Digestive and Kidney Diseases and the National Institutes of Health Office of Medical Applications of Research. Hepatology (1 Suppl) 1S-110S, 1984.
32. Starzl TE, Hakala TR, Shaw BW Jr, et al: A flexible procedure for multiple cadaveric organ procurement. Surg Gynecol Obstet 158:223-230, 1984.
33. Starzl TE, Miller C, Broznick B, Makowka L: An improved technique for multiple organ harvesting. Surg Gynecol Obstet 165:343-348, 1987.

34. Starzl TE, Nalesnik MA, Porter KA, et al: Reversibility of lymphomas and lymphoproliferative lesions developing under cyclosporin-steroid therapy. Lancet 1:583-587, 1984.
35. Bismuth H, Houssin D: Reduced-sized orthotopic liver graft in hepatic transplantation in children. Surgery. 95:367-370, 1984.
36. Broelsch CE, Neuhaus P, Burdelski M, et al: Orthotope transplantation von Lebegmenten bei mit Gallengangsatresien. (Orthotopic transplantation of hepatic segments in infants with biliary atresia). In Kolsowski L (ed): Chirurgisches Forum 1984, F Experim U Klimische Forschung Hrsga. Berline, Springer-Verlag, 1984, pp 105-109.
37. Starzl TE, Rowe MI, Todo S, et al: Transplantation of multiple abdominal viscera. JAMA 261:1449-1457, 1989.
38. Grant D, Wall W, Mimeault R, et al: Successful small-bowel/liver transplantation. Lancet 335:181-184, 1990.
39. Jamieson NV, Sundberg R, Lindell S, et al: Successful 24- to 30-hour preservation of the canine liver: a preliminary report. Transplant Proc 20 (Suppl 1):945-947, 1988.
40. Kalayoglu M, Sollinger HW, Stratta RJ, et al: Extended preservation of the liver for clinical transplantation. Lancet 1:617-619, 1988.
41. Todo S, Nery J, Yanaga K, et al: Extended preservation of human liver grafts with UW solution. JAMA 261:711-714, 1989.
42. Makowka L, Gordon RD, Todo S, et al: Analysis of donor criteria for the prediction of outcome in clinical liver transplantation. Transplant Proc 19:2378-2382, 1987.
43. Starzl TE, Hakala T, Tzakis A, et al: A multifactorial system for equitable selection of cadaveric kidney recipients. JAMA 257:3073-3075, 1987.
44. Starzl TE, Gordon RD, Tzakis A, et al: Equitable allocation of extrarenal organs: With special reference to the liver. Transplant Proc 20:131-138, 1988.
45. Tzakis A, Todo S, Starzl TE: Orthotopic liver transplantation with preservation of the inferior vena cava. Ann Surg 210:649-652, 1989.
46. Starzl TE, Todo S, Fung J, et al: FK 506 for human liver, kidney and pancreas transplantation. Lancet 2:1000-1004, 1989.
47. Todo S, Fung JJ, Starzl TE, et al: Liver, kidney, and thoracic organ transplantation under FK 506. Ann Surg 212:295-305, 1990.
48. Pichlmayr R, Ringe B, Gubernatis G, et al: Transplantation einer spenderleber auf Zwis Empfanger (Split liver transplantation) Eine neue Methode in der Weitzentwicklung der Lebesegment transplantation. Langenbecks Arch Surg 373:127-130, 1989.
49. Strong RW, Lynch SV, Ong TH, et al: Successful liver transplantation from a living donor to her son. N Engl J Med 322:1505-1507, 1990.
50. Broelsch CE, Emond JC, Whitington PF, et al: Application of reduced-size liver transplants as split grafts, auxiliary orthotopic grafts, and living related segmental transplants. Ann Surg 212:368-375, 1990.
51. Starzl TE, Demetris AJ, Murase N, et al: Cell migration, chimerism, and graft acceptance. Lancet 339:1579-1582, 1992.
52. Starzl TE, Demetris AJ, Trucco M, et al: Cell migration and chimerism after whole-organ transplantation: The basis of graft acceptance. Hepatology 17(6):1127-1152, 1993.
53. Starzl TE, Zinkernagel R: Antigen localization and migration in immunity and tolerance. New Engl J Med 339:1905-1913, 1998.
54. Yamaoka Y, Washida M, Honda K, et al: Liver transplantation using a right lobe graft from a living related donor. Transplantation 57:1127-1130, 1994.
55. Wachs M, Bak T, Karrer F, et al: Adult Living donor liver transplantation using a right hepatic lobe. Transplantation 66:1313-1316, 1998.
56. Marcos A, Fisher RA, Ham JM, et al: Right lobe living donor liver transplantation. Transplantation 68:798-803, 1999.
57. Starzl TE, Murase N, Abu-Elmagd K, et al: Tolerogenic immunosuppression for organ transplantation. Lancet 361:1502-1510, 2003.

58. Phelps CJ, Koike C, Vaught TD, et al: Production of α1,3-galac-tosyltransferase-deficient pigs. Science 299:411-414, 2003.
59. Brent L: A History of Transplantation Immunology. London, Academic Press, 1997, pp 1-482.
60. Hamilton D: Towards the Impossible. Philadelphia, Lippincott Williams & Wilkins.
61. Goodrich EO Jr, Welch HF, Nelson JA, et al: Homotransplantation of the canine liver. Surgery 39:244-251, 1956.
62. Woodruff MFA: The Transplantation of Tissues and Organs. Springfield, Illinois, Charles C Thomas, 1960, pp 1-777.
63. Moore FD, Smith LL, Burnap TK, et al: One-stage homotransplantation of the liver following total hepatectomy in dogs. Transplant Bull 6:103-110, 1959.
64. McBride RA, Wheeler HB, Smith LL, et al: Homotransplantation of the canine liver as an orthotopic vascularized graft. Histologic and functional correlations during residence in the new host. Am J Pathol 41:501-515, 1962.
65. Starzl TE, Kaupp HA Jr, Brock DR, Linman JW: Studies on the rejection of the transplanted homologous dog liver. Surg Gynecol Obstet 112:135-144, 1961.
66. Meyer WH Jr, Starzl TE: The effect of Eck and reverse Eck fistula in dogs with experimental diabetes mellitus. Surgery 45:760-764, 1959.
67. Meyer WH Jr, Starzl TE: The reverse portacaval shunt. Surgery 45:531-534, 1959.
68. Starzl TE, Bernhard VM, Benvenuto R, Cortes N: A new method for one-stage hepatectomy in dogs. Surgery 46:880-886, 1959.
69. Calne RY, Williams R: Liver transplantation in man. I. Observations on technique and organization in five cases. Br Med J 4:535-540, 1968.
70. Starzl TE: Experience in Hepatic Transplantation. Philadelphia, WB Saunders, 1969, pp 131-135.
71. Starzl TE, Kaupp HA Jr, Brock DR, et al: Homotransplantation of multiple visceral organs. Am J Surg 103:219-229, 1962.
72. Murase N, Demetris AJ, Kim DG, et al: Rejection of the multivisceral allografts in rats: A sequential analysis with comparison to isolated orthotopic small bowel and liver grafts. Surgery 108:880-889, 1990.
73. Murase N, Demetris AJ, Matsuzaki T, et al: Long survival in rats after multivisceral versus isolated small bowel allotransplantation under FK 506. Surgery 110:87-98, 1991.
74. Todo S, Reyes J, Furukawa H, et al: Outcome analysis of 71 clinical intestinal transplantations. Ann Surg 222:270-282, 1995.
75. Starzl TE, Todo S, Tzakis A, et al: The many faces of multivisceral transplantation. Surg Gynecol Obstet 172:335-344, 1991.
76. Starzl TE, Todo S, Tzakis A, et al: Abdominal organ cluster transplantation for the treatment of upper abdominal malignancies. Ann Surg 210:374-386, 1989.
77. Murray JE, Merrill JP, Dammin GJ, et al: Study of transplantation immunity after total body irradiation: Clinical and experimental investigation. Surgery 48:272-284, 1960.
78. Hamburger J, Vaysse J, Crosnier J, et al: Renal homotransplantation in man after radiation of the recipient. Am J Med 32:854-871, 1962.
79. Küss R, Legrain M, Mathé G, et al: Homologous human kidney transplantation: Experience with six patients. Postgrad Med J 38:528-531, 1962.
80. Goodwin WE, Kaufman JJ, Mims MM, et al: Human renal transplantation. I. Clinical experience with six cases of renal homotransplantation. J Urology 89:13-24, 1963.
81. Starzl TE, Butz GW Jr, Brock DR, et al: Canine liver homotransplants: The effect of host and graft irradiation. Arch Surg 85:460-464, 1962.
82. Billingham RE, Krohn PL, Medawar PB: Effect of cortisone on survival of skin homografts in rabbits. Br Med J 1:1157-1163, 1951.
83. Morgan JA: The influence of cortisone on the survival of homografts of skin in the rabbit. Surgery 30:506-515, 1951.
84. Schwartz R, Dameshek W: Drug-induced immunological tolerance. Nature 183:1682-1683, 1959.
85. Schwartz R, Dameshek W: The effects of 6-mercaptopurine on homograft reactions. J Clin Invest 39:952-958, 1960.
86. Meeker W, Condie R, Weiner D, et al: Prolongation of skin homograft survival in rabbits by 6-mercaptopurine. Proc Soc Exp Biol Med 102:459-461, 1959.
87. Calne RY: The rejection of renal homografts: Inhibition in dogs by 6-mercaptopurine. Lancet 1:417-418, 1960.
88. Zukoski CF, Lee HM, Hume DM: The prolongation of functional survival of canine renal homografts by 6-mercaptopurine. Surg Forum 11:470-472, 1960.
89. Calne RY: Inhibition of the rejection of renal homografts in dogs by purine analogues. Transplant Bull 28:445-461, 1961.
90. Calne RY, Alexandre GPJ, Murray JE: A study of the effects of drugs in prolonging survival of homologous renal transplants in dogs. Ann NY Acad Sci 99:743-761, 1962.
91. Zukoski CF, Callaway JM: Tolerance to a canine renal homograft induced by 6-methyl mercaptopurine. Surg Forum 13:62-64, 1962.
92. Murray JE, Merrill JP, Dammin GJ, et al: Kidney transplantation in modified recipients. Ann Surg 156:337-355, 1962.
93. Murray JE, Merrill JP, Harrison JH, et al: Prolonged survival of human-kidney homografts by immunosuppressive drug therapy. New Engl J Med 268:1315-1323, 1963.
94. Hopewell J, Calne RY, Beswick I: Three clinical cases of renal transplantation. Br Med J I:411-413, 1964.
95. Marchioro TL, Axtell HK, LaVia MF, et al: The role of adrenocortical steroids in reversing established homograft rejection. Surgery 55:412-417, 1964.
96. Starzl TE: Experience in Renal Transplantation. Philadelphia, WB Saunders, 1964, pp 131-133.
97. Starzl TE: The saga of liver replacement, with particular reference to the reciprocal influence of liver and kidney transplantation (1955-1967). J Am Coll Surg 195:587-610, 2002.
98. Moore FD, Birtch AG, Dagher F, et al: Immunosuppression and vascular insufficiency in liver transplantation. NY Ann Acad Sci 120:729-738, 1964.
99. Demirleau, Noureddine, Vignes, et al: Tentative d'homogreffe hepatique [Attempted hepatic homograft]. Mem Acad Chir (Paris) 90:177, 1964.
100. Picache RS, Kapur BML, Starzl TE: The effect of liver disease on the need for venous decompression during the anhepatic phase of canine orthotopic liver transplantation. Surgery 67:319-321, 1970.
101. Terasaki PI, Marchioro TL, Starzl TE: Sero-typing of human lymphocyte antigens: Preliminary trials on long-term kidney homograft survivors. In: Histocompatibility Testing. Washington, DC, National Academy Science–National Research Council, 1965, pp 83-96.
102. Iwasaki Y, Porter KA, Amend JR, et al: The preparation and testing of horse antidog and antihuman antilymphoid plasma or serum and its protein fractions. Surg Gynecol Obstet 124:1-24, 1967.
103. Cordier G, Garnier H, Clot JP, et al: La greffe de foie orthotopique chez le porc. Mem Acad Chir (Paris) 92:799-807, 1966.
104. Calne RY, White HJO, Yoffa DE, et al: Observations of orthotopic liver transplantation in the pig. Br Med J 2:478-480, 1967.
105. Peacock JH, Terblanche J: Orthotopic homotransplantation of the liver in the pig. In Read AE (ed): The Liver. London, Butterworth. 1967, p 333.
106. Starzl TE: Experience in Hepatic Transplantation. Philadelphia, WB Saunders, 1969, pp 184-190.
107. Calne RY, Sells RA, Pena Jr, et al: Induction of immunological tolerance by porcine liver allografts. Nature 223:472-474, 1969.

108. Starzl TE, Porter KA, Francavilla A: The Eck fistula in animals and humans. Curr Probl Surg 20:687-752, 1983.

109. Francavilla A, Hagiya M, Porter KA, et al: Augmenter of liver regeneration (ALR): Its place in the universe of hepatic growth factors. Hepatology 20:747-757, 1994.

110. Brettschneider L, Daloze PM, Huguet C, et al: The use of combined preservation techniques for extended storage of orthotopic liver homografts. Surg Gynecol Obstet 126:263-274, 1968.

111. Starzl TE: Experience in Hepatic Transplantation. Philadelphia, WB Saunders, 1969, pp 1-553.

112. Barnard CN: What we have learned about heart transplants. J Thorac Cardiovasc Surg 56:457-468, 1968.

113. Stinson EB, Griepp RB, Clark DA, et al: Cardiac transplantation in man. VIII. Survival and function. J Thorac Cardiovasc Surg 60:303-321, 1970.

114. Derom F, Barbier F, Ringoir S, et al: Ten-month survival after lung homotransplantation in man. J Thorac Cardiovasc Surg 61:835-846, 1971.

115. Lillehei RC, Simmons RL, Najarian JS, et al: Pancreaticoduodenal allotransplantation: Experimental and clinical observations. Ann Surg 172:405-436, 1970.

116. Starzl TE, Demetris AJ, Murase N, et al: The lost chord: Microchimerism. Immunol Today 17: 577-584;588, 1996.

117. Ramos HC, Reyes J, Abu-Elmagd K, et al: Weaning of immuno-suppression in long-term liver transplant recipients. Transplantation 59:212-217, 1995.

118. Mazariegos GV, Reyes J, Marino I, et al: Weaning of immuno-suppression in liver transplant recipients. Transplantation 63:243-249, 1997.

119. Starzl TE, Iwatsuki S, Van Thiel DH, et al: Evolution of liver transplantation. Hepatology 2:614-636, 1982.

120. Kang YG, Martin DJ, Marquez J, et al: Intraoperative changes in blood coagulation and thrombelastographic monitoring in liver transplantation. Anesth Analg 64:888-896, 1985.

121. Stieber AC, Zetti G, Todo S, et al: The spectrum of portal vein thrombosis in liver transplantation. Ann Surg 213:199-206, 1991.

122. Starzl TE, Bell RH, Beart RW, Putnam CW: Hepatic trisegmen-tectomy and other liver resections. Surg Gynecol Obstet 141:429-437, 1975.

123. Starzl TE, Iwatsuki S, Shaw BW Jr, et al: Left hepatic triseg-mentectomy. Surg Gynecol Obstet 155:21-27, 1982.

124. Starzl TE, Demetris AJ: Liver transplantation: A 31 year per-spective. Chicago, Year Book, 1990, pp 38-41.

125. Starzl TE, Demetris AJ, Van Thiel DH: Liver transplantation (1). N Engl J Med 321:1014-1022, 1989.

126. Starzl TE, Demetris AJ, Van Thiel DH: Liver transplantation (2). N Engl J Med 321:1092-1099, 1989.

127. Iwatsuki S, Gordon RD, Shaw BW Jr, Starzl TE: Role of liver transplantation in cancer therapy. Ann Surg 202:401-407, 1985.

128. Alessiani M, Tzakis A, Todo S, et al: Assessment of 5-year experience with abdominal organ cluster transplantation. J Am Coll Surg 180:1-9, 1995.

129. Busuttil RW, Tanaka K: The utility of marginal donors in liver transplantation. Liver Transpl 9:651-663, 2003.

130. Rogiers X, Malago M, Gawad K, et al: In situ splitting of cadaveric livers. The ultimate expansion of a limited donor pool. Ann Surg 224:331-339, 1996.

131. Gundlach M, Broering D, Topp S, Sterneck M, Rogiers X: Split-cava technique: Liver splitting for two adult recipients. Liver Transpl 6:703-706, 2000.

132. Marcos A: Split-liver transplantation for adult recipients. Liver Transpl 6:707-709, 2000.

133. Starzl TE: Baboon renal and chimpanzee liver heterotransplan-tation. In Hardy MA (ed): Xenograft 25. Amsterdam & New York, Excerpta-Medical, Elsevier Science (Biomedical Division), 1989, pp 17-28.

134. Starzl TE, Fung J, Tzakis A, et al: Baboon-to-human liver trans-plantation. Lancet 341:65-71, 1993.

135. Starzl TE, Valdivia LA, Murase N, et al: The biologic basis of and strategies for clinical xenotransplantation. Immunol Rev 141:213-244, 1994.

Surgical Anatomy of the Liver

JOHN F. RENZ
PAULO R. REICHERT
SHERYLIN GORDON
JEAN C. EMOND

Embryology 24

Topographic anatomy 25

Lobar anatomy 25

Segmental anatomy 26

Applied surgical anatomy 27
  Anatomy of the hepatic hilum 27
  Couinaud segment II/III allograft 28
  Hemiliver allografts 31

Although an early chapter on anatomy is a prerequisite for a surgical text, the brief period since the previous edition of *Transplantation of the Liver* has seen such a dramatic change in the practice of clinical liver transplantation that the relevance of such a review is significantly increased. The integration of hepatobiliary surgery and liver transplantation, coupled with advances in critical care of the patient afflicted with liver disease, has expanded the role of major hepatic resection[1] and permitted the routine application of partial-liver allografts derived from living or deceased donors to adults and children.[2,3] In less than a decade, partial-liver allografts have become the most common allograft for pediatric patients,[4] whereas the application of partial-liver allografts to adults from living or deceased donors has dominated recent surgical interest in the transplantation community.[5-8] Fundamental to the successful outcome of major hepatic resection or partial-liver transplantation is the avoidance of technical complications. Recognition of this tenet has stimulated intense interest in the intrahepatic architecture of the liver so as to perform procedures that maximize viable hepatic mass and minimize blood loss while averting a biliary or vascular complication. The increased application of major hepatic resection and partial-liver allografts has also created confusion with respect to nomenclature, as several systems are currently applied within the literature.[9,10] In this setting, a concise anatomic review with direct application to clinical transplant surgery is particularly relevant.

Embryology

Review of the embryologic development of the liver is prerequisite to understanding intrahepatic anatomy and present nomenclature systems. The hepatobiliary system originates from the hepatic diverticulum, a ventral outpouching of the distal foregut early in the fourth week of gestation (3-mm embryo). The outgrowth of proliferating endodermal cells infiltrates the embryonal ventral mesentery and extends into the septum transversum to form the early liver primordium.[11,12] The rapidly proliferating primordium continues to expand, ultimately invading the left and right vitelline veins (omphalomesenteric veins). The intrahepatic left and right vitelline veins undergo extensive remodeling to create *separate* liver chords and portal sinusoids from the primordium mass,[9,11,13] a distinction that will persist as separate right and left intrahepatic portal circulations.[9] Through this process, the vitelline veins are divided into an intrahepatic component containing hepatic chords and portal sinusoids, a cranial component delivering blood from the embryonic liver to the heart, and a caudal component carrying blood from the yolk sac to the liver. Further endodermal cell proliferation stems from hepatic cords and biliary epithelia that coalesce to create sinusoids, whereas hemopoietic tissue, Kupffer cells, and interstitial connective tissue originate from the splanchnic mesenchyme of the septum transversum.[12]

The hepatic veins originate from the vitelline venous system. The cranial component of the left vitelline vein initially involutes, shunting all returning blood to the heart through the cranial component of the right vitelline vein, known as the *embryonic common hepatic vein.* The common hepatic vein functions as an early single outflow source from the liver to the heart and persists as the later right hepatic vein. The vitelline venous system of the left side of the liver later reconstitutes channels that mature into left and middle hepatic veins to augment venous return from the liver to the heart and define the permanent anatomic arrangement. Vitelline venous system development is manifested by the surgical findings of a distinct right hepatic vein emptying directly into the vena cava as compared with the middle and left hepatic veins that typically empty via a common channel.[13,14]

The embryological development of the extrahepatic main portal vein is a complex process involving fusion of left and right vitelline venous elements returning blood from the gut-yolk sac complex. Details of this process are beyond the scope of this review, but have been expertly detailed.[9,13,14] The principal objectives are to create a single inflow source to the liver from the bilateral vitelline veins and to preserve the anatomic relationship of the main portal vein to the developing duodenum. As the yolk sac regresses, the omphalic portions of the vitelline veins disappear, whereas the mesenteric branches proliferate with increasing length and complexity of the intestinal tract.[15] Between the fourth and sixth weeks (4.5- to 9-mm embryo), caudal elements of both vitelline veins unite through intravenous channels and undergo segmental involution to form a composite, S-shaped vessel, located posterior to the first portion of the duodenum, that drains both vitelline venous beds as a single inflow to the liver.[9,13,14]

The intrahepatic, left portal vein is also a composite vessel originating from a communication between the vitelline veins and a segment of the left umbilical vein.[14] The umbilical veins, which carry blood from the placenta to the fetus, are originally paired; however, the left umbilical vein is invaded by hepatic tissue and hypertrophies, whereas the right atrophies prior to contact with the liver. Umbilical blood initially flows through a meshwork of intrahepatic sinusoids; however, as volume increases, these sinusoids coalesce to receive the proximal portion of the developing left portal vein and form a single channel shunt through the liver, termed the *ductus venosus*.[14,15] The ductus venosus receives branches from the liver before joining the hepatic veins to empty into the inferior vena cava.[13] After birth, the ductus venosus closes to form the ligamentum venosum.

The biliary and arterial systems develop later, along the latticework provided by the established portal venous system. The right biliary and arterial branches follow the portal system exactly, whereas the left biliary and arterial systems divide into equal-size branches on either side of the intrahepatic portion of the umbilical vein.[9]

The embryonal liver develops rapidly to occupy most of the abdominal cavity. By 9 weeks' gestation, the liver accounts for approximately 10% of the embryo's total weight with relatively equal hepatic mass on each side of the falciform ligament. The initial equality in volume between topographic lobes is lost by 12 weeks as the topographic right lobe hypertrophies to spawn the caudate lobe (initially recognizable at 6 weeks) and represent the majority of hepatic mass.[11,12]

The ventral mesentery persists as the gastrohepatic ligament[16] and the fibrous visceral peritoneum of the liver, first described by Glisson in 1659,[17] that envelopes the organ, except for a "bare area" on the superoposterior surface of the right lobe where the organ is in direct contact with the inferior vena cava, diaphragm, and superior aspect of the right adrenal gland. Glisson's capsule extends into the parenchyma as intrahepatic septa or trabeculae that support vascular structures and serve as surgical landmarks.[18,19]

Functional milestones in embryonic development include intrahepatic hematopoiesis during the 6th week, hepatocyte bile formation at the 12th week, and excretion of bile into the duodenum by the 16th week.[11] The third trimester marks the cessation of hematopoiesis with a concomitant decrease in liver growth to account for approximately 5% of the newborn's body weight.[12,18]

Topographic Anatomy

Topographic anatomy, initially described in early Babylon (3000-2000 BC), divides the liver according to external landmarks. This anatomic system dominated through the late 19th century but is only of historical interest today. The principal landmarks defining topographic anatomy include the falciform ligament, umbilical fissure, gallbladder fossa, and transverse hilar fissure.[18,20] These landmarks delineate four lobes (Fig. 2-1): left (medial to falciform), right (lateral to falciform), quadrate, and caudate (spigelian).[21]

The liver is supported in position through peritoneal reflections continuous with Glisson's capsule that attach to the duodenum, stomach, diaphragm, and anterior abdominal wall. These peritoneal reflections include the falciform ligament, right and left triangular ligaments, and right and left coronary ligaments, as well as the lesser omentum. The falciform ligament extends from the ligamentum teres superiorly along the anterior liver surface in continuity with both the diaphragm and anterior abdominal wall above the umbilicus.[18] The ligamentum teres, a remnant of the vestigial umbilical vein, frequently undergoes recanalization in cirrhotic patients to decompress the portal system through collaterals of the periumbilical superficial venous plexus, producing the characteristic "caput medusa." As the falciform ligament continues toward the diaphragm, the peritoneal sheets composing the ligament separate to adopt a triangular shape that broadly covers the entry of the hepatic veins into the inferior vena cava.[19]

Over the inferior vena cava, the peritoneal reflections progress laterally to become the anterior layers of the left and right coronary ligaments. The coronary ligaments anchor the superior surface of the liver through anterior and posterior reflections to the diaphragm. As the right and left coronary ligaments extend laterally, each unites with the posterior reflections to form the respective right and left triangular ligaments. The right coronary ligament may continue and fuse to the superior pole of the right kidney to form the hepatorenal ligament.[18]

The lesser omentum is a continuous fold of peritoneum arising from the posterior reflection of the left triangular ligament. The lesser omentum extends from the liver onto the lesser curvature of the stomach and first 2 cm of the duodenum to form the gastrohepatic and hepatoduodenal ligaments, respectively. The hepatoduodenal ligament forms the anterior border of the epiploic foramen of Winslow and contains the porta hepatis.

Lobar Anatomy

Galen (130-201 AD) initially postulated the hepatic arterial and portal venous systems terminated as minute connections that gradually reconstituted into hepatic veins draining to the inferior vena cava.[21] The concept of *separate* hepatic arterial and portal venous systems reconstituting through the hepatic veins resurfaced in 1888, when Hugo Rex studied hepatic corrosion casts from mammals.[22] Rex concluded that the right and left branches of the portal vein functioned as unique vascular systems, dividing the liver into separate halves. James Cantlie, in 1898, extended these findings to humans, proposing a functional division of the liver into two lobes (Cantlie's term) of relatively equal size based on the branching of the portal vein and hepatic ducts.[23] The proposed plane of demarcation was a connective tissue layer, indistinguishable from surface topography, that bisects the gallbladder fossa and inferior vena cava, incorrectly termed *Cantlie's line.* Cantlie's description shifted the entire quadrate lobe (topographic term), as well as a large component of the caudate lobe (topographic term), into the anatomic boundaries of Cantlie's left lobe. This classification system, founded on intrahepatic functional anatomy, resulted in a surgical revolution through the performance of successful anatomic resections.[24] Tiffany reported the first liver resection performed in the United States in 1890[25] (although the accuracy of this

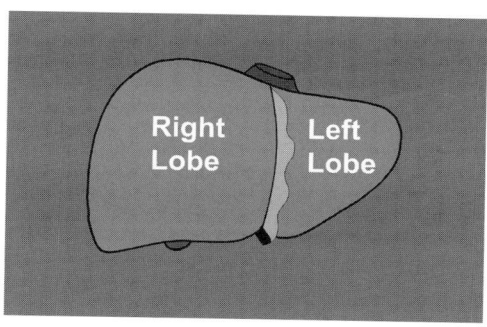

A

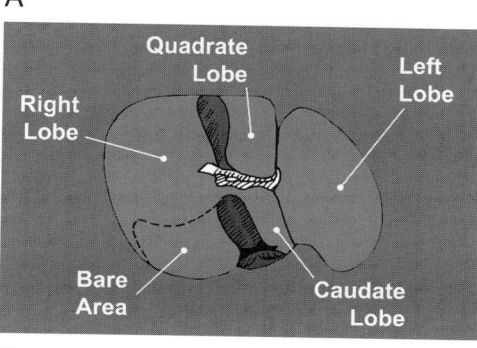

B

FIGURE 2–1

Topographic anatomy of the liver. The landmarks defining topographic anatomy include the falciform ligament, umbilical fissure, gallbladder fossa, and transverse hilar fissure. These delineate four hepatic lobes: left, right, quadrate, and caudate (spigelian). **A,** Anterior view; **B,** posterior view.

publication is widely disputed) and Professor William Keen of Jefferson Medical College confidently proclaimed to members of the Pennsylvania State Medical Society on May 17, 1899 "after my experience with these three cases [liver resections], I should hardly hesitate to attack almost any hepatic tumor without regard to its size."[21]

Cantlie's reference to hepatic lobes created two definitions for the same term and has been the source of continuing confusion.[9] Europeans continue to describe hepatic lobes based on topographic anatomy, whereas North American surgeons adopted "lobectomy" as the hemiliver defined by Cantlie. One must be certain as to the reference system in use (topographic anatomy or Cantlie's anatomic classification) when applying the term *lobe* or *lobectomy*. A more appropriate scheme is to refer to Cantlie's anatomic lobes as hemilivers, thus describing a right or left hepatectomy. The anatomic system of Cantlie was later expanded by the North American anatomists Healey and Schroy, who based their nomenclature on biliary anatomy, rather than on Cantlie's description of portal venous anatomy, while retaining the term lobe.[26] Each lobe is independent with respect to portal supply, arterial vascularization, and biliary drainage; however, a lobar fissure, rather than Cantlie's line, separates the right and left hepatic lobes that were each subdivided into two segments according to second-order biliary anatomy. The right lobe was divided into anterior and posterior segments by a right segmental fissure, whereas the left lobe was divided into medial and lateral segments by a left segmental fissure.[9] The left segmental fissure corresponds to the travel of the falciform ligament, whereas the right segmental fissure is not discernible by topography. Within this system, the medial segment of the left lobe contains the entire quadrate lobe as well as the major portion of the caudate lobe. Healey and Schroy's classification scheme became the foundation for anatomic liver surgery and led to the descriptive but anatomically imprecise term *hepatic trisegmentectomy* for extended right or left hepatectomy, as well as the term *left lateral segment* for the topographic left lobe.[27]

Segmental Anatomy

The most sophisticated classification of intrahepatic anatomy is by Couinaud, who in 1954 founded his anatomic description on the portal venous system.[28] Portal vein distribution within the liver was subdivided into eight "segments." Individual segments each receive a "portal pedicle" consisting of a portal venous branch, hepatic arterial branch, and a bile duct radicle with segmental drainage through a dedicated hepatic venous branch. The eight functional units embrace the hepatic veins that provide outflow to the inferior vena cava (Fig. 2–2).

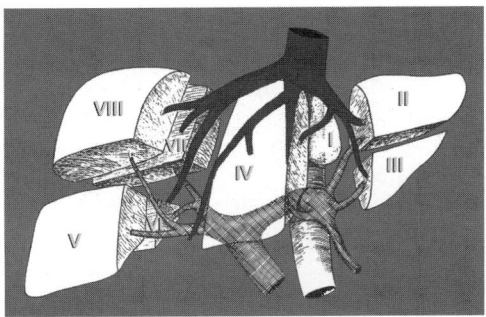

FIGURE 2–2

Segmental liver anatomy. The segmental anatomy of the liver as described by Couinaud. Each anatomic segment (*Roman numeral*) receives a unique portal pedicle (*light gray*) consisting of a portal venous branch, hepatic arterial inflow, and bile duct. Venous drainage occurs via a major hepatic venous outflow branch (*dark gray*).

The hepatic veins travel in connective tissue planes, termed *fissures* or *scissurae*, dividing the liver into four sectors (see Fig. 2–2). The left portal fissure contains the left hepatic vein, the main portal fissure corresponds to Cantlie's line and contains the middle hepatic vein, and the lateral-most (right) portal fissure contains the right hepatic vein. Three of the four sectors contain smaller fissures that subdivide each into two segments to form a total of seven segments. Of the accessory lobes, only the caudate (segment I) is a functionally autonomous segment. Segment I is supplied by both the left and right branches of the portal vein and hepatic artery and empties directly into the vena cava.[28] This relationship is well demonstrated in patients with Budd-Chiari disease who augment hepatic outflow through hypertrophic veins that drain directly from segment I into the vena cava. Biliary drainage of segment I occurs via small anterior radicles draining directly into the posterior surface of the biliary confluence. Segments II and III correspond to the posterior and anterior segments of the topographic left lobe, respectively. Segment IV, the largest segment and the only one derived from an undivided hepatic sector, extends from the left portal fissure to the main portal fissure (Cantlie's line) and includes the entire volume of the quadrate lobe. The right portal fissure divides the right lobe into an anteromedial sector and a posterolateral sector, each of which is subdivided into anterior and posterior segments. Of the anteromedial sector, the anterior segment is designated segment V, with segment VIII located posteriorly. The posterolateral sector is composed of segment VI anteriorly and segment VII posteriorly (see Fig. 2–2).[28]

The recognition of the segmental anatomy of the liver was a significant advancement for hepatic surgery. In 1982, Bismuth integrated Couinaud's classification scheme into a formal anatomic approach to hepatectomy[24] that has been widely adopted by liver surgeons in Europe, Asia, and North America. Rather than perform atypical resections based on the size or location of a lesion, hepatic resections could be performed along functional planes that would minimize intraoperative blood loss and postoperative necrosis of devitalized tissue. This classification revolutionized hepatic surgery by providing a foundation for the development of highly selective anatomic resections as well as innovations in transplantation using surgically created partial-liver grafts.

Applied Surgical Anatomy

Couinaud's anatomic classification permits the creation of partial-liver allografts from either deceased or living donors (Fig. 2–3). The successful application of partial-liver allografts mandates detailed anatomic considerations because these procedures predispose to unique complications. Fundamental to the application of these techniques is an understanding of intrahepatic vascular and biliary anatomy. Although the incidence of vascular complications has declined with the widespread application of microsurgical techniques,[29-34] the relatively high incidence of biliary complications that has persisted with the application of partial-liver allografts[3,7,35] often does not reflect inherent technical failures but originates from an incomplete understanding of variation within the biliary system, as well as inaccuracies of noninvasive techniques to assess intrahepatic biliary territories preoperatively.

Four distinct allografts have been used routinely in partial-liver transplantation (see Fig. 2–3). These include the right hemiliver (Couinaud segments V to VIII), the left hemiliver (Couinaud segments II to IV), the topographic left lobe (Couinaud segments II to III), and the topographic right lobe (Couinaud segments IV to VIII). This chapter describes the surgical anatomy applicable to each of these allografts based on the available English literature as well as the authors' examination of 75 hepatic corrosion casts, 60 anatomic dissections, 25 split-liver procedures, 150 living donor procedures, and hundreds of deceased donor procurements.

Anatomy of the Hepatic Hilum

All partial-liver allograft preparation includes a hilar dissection. The objective is to specifically isolate vascular and biliary supply with minimal disruption to surrounding structures. Figure 2–4 depicts the anatomic relation of the proper hepatic artery, common hepatic duct, and portal vein. The conventional anatomic relationship of the hilum is the portal vein located posterior with the proper hepatic artery anteromedial and the common hepatic duct anterolateral. Following bifurcation of the proper hepatic artery, the right hepatic artery progresses laterally and courses posterior to the common hepatic duct (see Fig. 2–4). Arterial variations within the hilum are common,[36,37] particularly in the setting of superior mesenteric artery–derived arterial supply. In classic descriptions, the proper hepatic originates distal to the takeoff of the gastroduodenal artery and receives aortic inflow via the celiac trunk. When arterial inflow

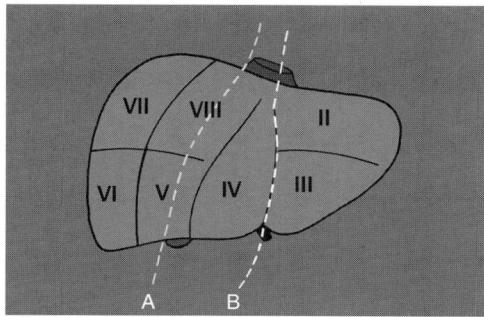

FIGURE 2–3

Surgical division of the liver along Cantlie's line (*dashed line labeled "A"*) yields a left hemiliver (segments I to IV or II to IV) and right hemiliver (segments V to VIII) allograft that can be used in adult-to-adult living donor and split-liver transplantation between two adults. Division along the falciform ligament (*dashed line labeled "B"*) yields a segment II/III allograft, also termed a *left lateral segment allograft* or *topographic left lobe*, and remnant segments I, IV to VIII allograft, also termed a *right trisegment allograft* or *topographic right lobe*.

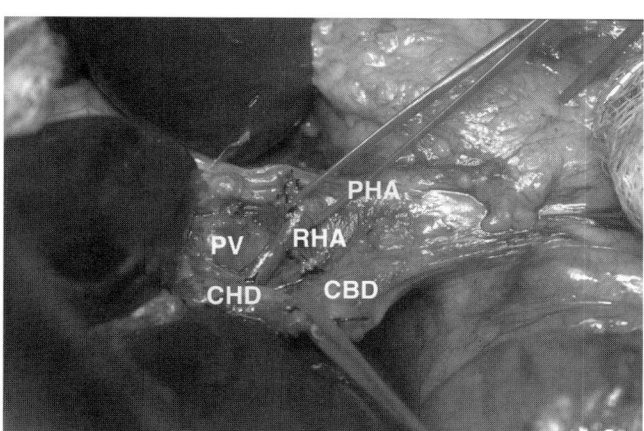

FIGURE 2–4

Intraoperative hilar dissection. The three principal elements of the porta hepatis—the common hepatic duct (CHD), the portal vein (PV), and the proper hepatic artery (PHA)—are demonstrated in this intraoperative photograph. The anterolateral CHD is retracted (lower vessel loop) just prior to the origin of the cystic duct signaling the beginning of the common bile duct (CBD). The bifurcation of the anteromedial PHA to form the right hepatic artery (RHA) is retracted medial (upper vessel loop). The RHA (center) is immediately anterior to the PV and courses posterior to the CHD in celiac-derived hepatic arterial supply.

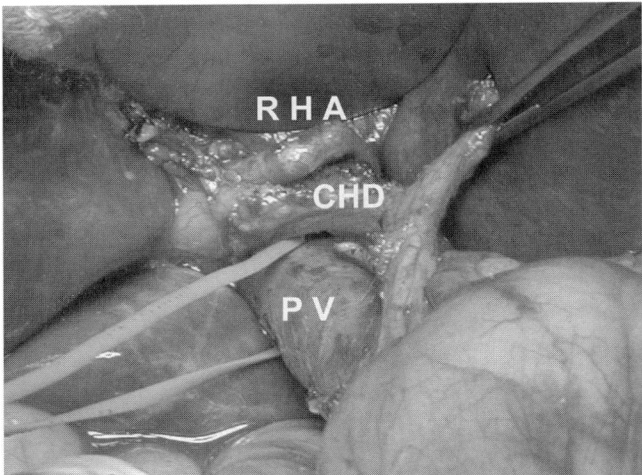

FIGURE 2-5

Anatomy of the hilum. The main portal vein (PV) is dissected and encircled with a vessel loop. The cystic duct is retracted with the forceps and the right hepatic artery (RHA) lies above the common hepatic duct (CHD). Note that the course of the right hepatic artery anterior to the common hepatic duct is rare except in the setting of replaced arterial anatomy.

originates from the superior mesenteric artery, anatomy is termed *replaced*. Thus, the entire proper hepatic artery may be replaced, or the right hepatic artery may independently originate from the superior mesenteric, rather than the proper hepatic, to be replaced. Replaced anatomy is readily identifiable preoperatively by computed tomography, magnetic resonance arteriography, or angiography, and is clinically relevant as hilar arterial variations, with respect to the common hepatic duct, are common in the setting of replaced anatomy (Fig. 2-5).

Couinaud Segment II/III Allograft

Division of the hepatic parenchyma at the falciform ligament yields a segment II/III allograft, commonly referred to as a *left lateral segment* or *topographic left lobe*, of approximately 250 cc volume for pediatric recipients.[38-40] The segment II/III allograft can be further reduced to a "monosegment" allograft (segment III) for very small infants and neonates.[41]

Dissection of the portal triad originates at the base of the round ligament with isolation of the left hepatic artery, left portal vein, and left hepatic duct. The left hepatic vein is isolated and encircled with a vessel loop. With vascular control achieved, parenchymal transection typically occurs within 1 cm to the right of the falciform ligament and progresses to within 1 cm of the left hepatic duct in the umbilical fissure.[7,42] The following anatomic description is based on the procedure described.

At its origin, the left hepatic artery courses outside the liver along the inferior aspect of segment IV with the left hepatic duct and left portal vein for approximately 3 cm prior to entering the liver at the level of the umbilical fissure. The left hepatic artery originates anteromedial and inferior to the origin of the left portal vein but ascends to be anterosuperior to the left portal vein by the point of parenchyma entrance. Although extrahepatic, the left hepatic artery sends a major and several minor branches to segment IV. Accompanying the left hepatic artery is the left portal vein that sends branches to segments I and IV along its extrahepatic course.

Principal segment IV arterial branches may originate proximal, near the origin of the left hepatic artery, or distal at the level of the umbilical fissure (Fig. 2-6). Furthermore, principal segment IV arterial branches may originate independently, distal to the origin of the left hepatic artery, to create parallel arteries across segment IV with superior branches servicing segment II (Fig. 2-7).[42,43] Segment IV penetrating arteries provide significant inflow, and particular attention should be devoted to their preservation. In split-liver transplantation, principal segment IV arteries that originate near the umbilical fissure may be anastomosed to the segment I, IV to VIII allograft's gastroduodenal remnant to preserve arterial inflow.

Arterial supply to the segment II/III allograft may originate from the left gastric artery. A single artery courses transversely across the gastrohepatic ligament from the left gastric artery on the lesser curvature of the stomach to enter the inferior surface of segment III just anterior to segment I (caudate lobe) in approximately 15% to 23% of deceased donors.[36,37,44,45] This anatomic variant can be the principal arterial supply to

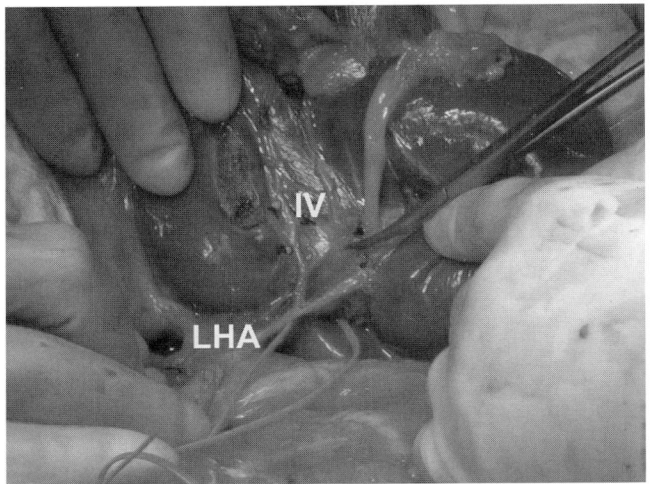

FIGURE 2-6

Segment IV arterial branches originating from the left hepatic artery (LHA).

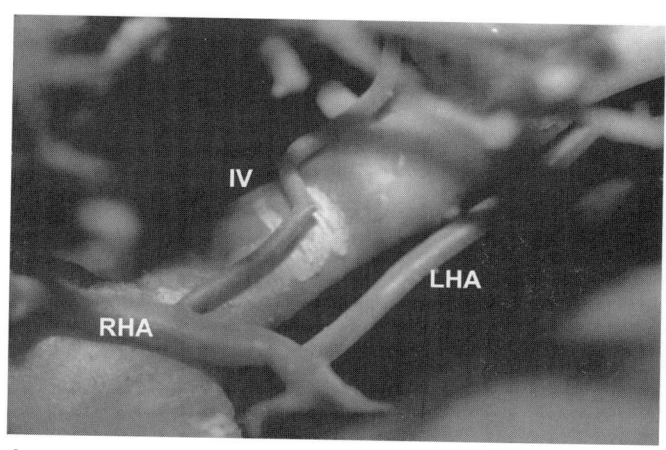
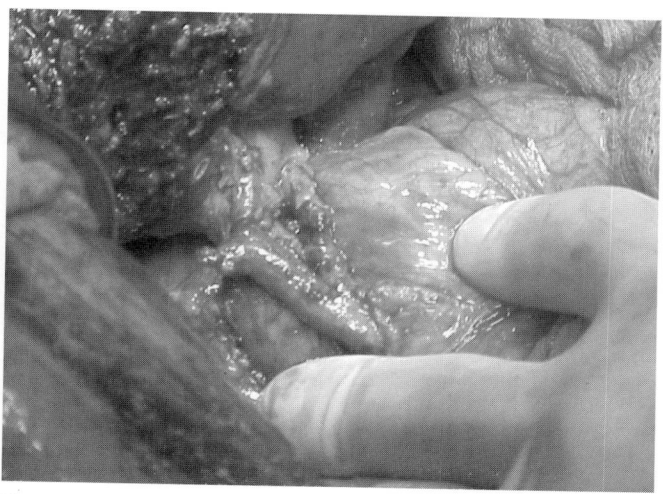

A

B

FIGURE 2–7

Independent segment IV hepatic artery. A large segment IV artery, diameter greater than 1 mm, originates distal to the origin of the left hepatic artery (LHA) and courses anterosuperior to the left portal vein to supply segments IV and II. **A**, Corrosion cast; **B**, intraoperative photograph. RHA, right hepatic artery.

the segment II/III allograft, as a replaced vessel, or augment arterial supply to the allograft as an accessory vessel.

Arterial and biliary structures are superior to the extrahepatic portion of the left portal vein with the orientation of the portal pedicle at the umbilical fissure preserved as the structures penetrate the hepatic parenchyma. The left hepatic artery is anterosuperior to the left portal vein, whereas the orientation of the left hepatic duct system, with respect to the left portal vein, is variable. The anatomic relationship of the left hepatic duct to the left portal vein at the umbilical fissure is anterosuperior (35%), superoposterior (35%), and midline on the left portal vein (20%). Separate ducts from segments II and III that unite greater than 1 cm lateral to the umbilical fissure to form the left hepatic duct occur in approximately 10% of study specimens.[42,46] In this anatomic variant, the segment II duct remains posterosuperior while the segment III and IV ducts course anterosuperior to join just prior to the hilum (Fig. 2-8C).

The union of biliary ducts from segments II and III forms the segment II/III duct. The segment II/III duct receives biliary drainage from segment IV to become the left hepatic duct. The anatomy of the segment II/III duct, as well as segment IV ducts that cross the plane of the umbilical fissure, has been documented.[42,46] The most commonly observed biliary pattern (55%) is the union of segment II and segment III ducts within 1 cm of the umbilical fissure (see Fig. 2–8A). For this variant, the segment II/III duct receives a single segment IV

duct between the umbilical fissure and the hilum to form the left hepatic duct. The union of segment II and segment III ducts was at the umbilical fissure in 5% of specimens, lateral to the umbilical fissure within segment IV in 50% of specimens, and medial to the umbilical fissure in 45% of specimens. Healey and Schroy have described the union of segment II and segment III bile ducts within the umbilical fissure in 50%, lateral to the umbilical fissure in 42%, and medial to the fissure in 8% of autopsy specimens.[47]

The second most frequent anatomic pattern (30%) is creation of the segment II/III duct close to the umbilical fissure followed by the union of two parallel ducts from segment IV to form the left hepatic duct (see Fig. 2–8B). Typically, one segment IV duct is on the umbilical portion of the left portal vein and one is close to the union of the right hepatic duct. Thus, biliary radicles originating in segment IV cross the umbilical fissure to drain the anteroinferior component of segment III in approximately 30% of specimens. Healey and Schroy reported a 20% incidence of segment IV ducts crossing the umbilical fissure in a study of 100 autopsy specimens.[47] Segment IV biliary radicles crossing the umbilical fissure are a potential source of parenchymal leaks. Segment IV biliary radicles that cross the umbilical fissure are consistently located anterior to the left portal vein and the segment II/III duct (see Fig. 2–8B). They are terminal in nature without a distinct connection to the principal segment III duct; however, their significance in biliary drainage is trivial and they are readily amenable to suture ligation.

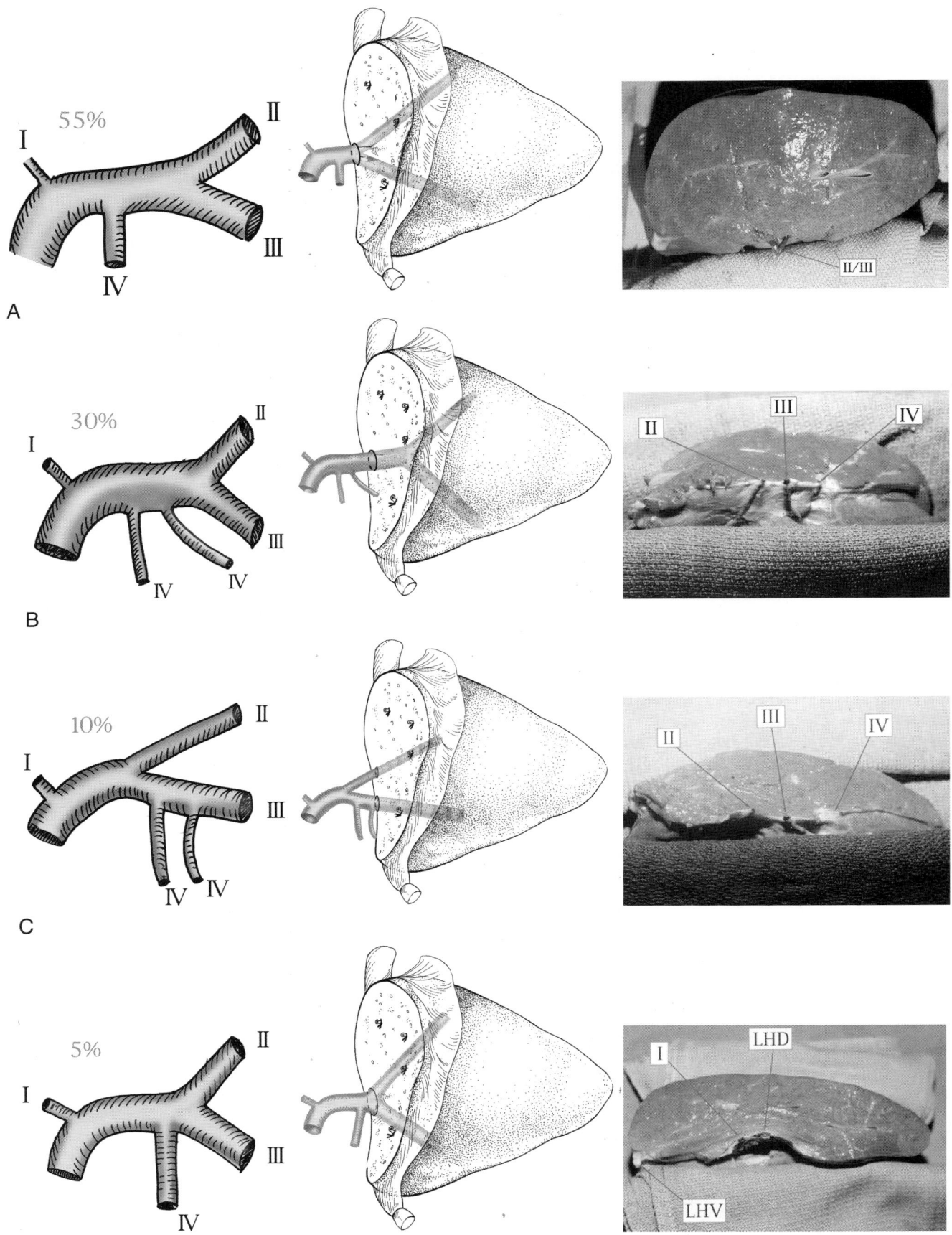

The third biliary pattern is a single segment III duct, which receives a duct from segment IV and joins segment II close to the hepatic hilum (see Fig. 2–8C). This pattern was identified in 10% of specimens. In this anatomic variant, there is absence of a distinct segment II/III duct.

The least observed biliary pattern (5%) is defined by segment II and segment III ducts joining immediately lateral to the umbilical fissure to form a very short segment II/III duct that receives the segment IV duct just after crossing the umbilical fissure, becoming the left hepatic duct (see Fig. 2–8D). In our analysis, a single segment II/III duct had formed within 1 cm lateral to the umbilical fissure in 90% of specimens. Russell, in a review of 838 cholangiograms and 15 liver autopsy specimens, likewise described the union of segment II and segment III bile ducts immediately lateral to the plane of the falciform ligament in most specimens.[48]

The union of segment II and segment III ducts occurs within a connective tissue sheath to form a bile duct plate that can be identified clinically (see Fig. 2–8A to D). The connective tissue plate at the origin of the segment II/III duct is analogous to the hilar plate at the main biliary confluence. An essential element to identification of biliary anatomy is recognition of the bile duct plate as a connective tissue interface that envelops the ducts and guides dissection.

The anatomy of the left hepatic vein can be broadly described by three distinct anatomic patterns (Fig. 2–9). The most common pattern, observed in 73% of specimens, was union of segment II and segment III veins to form a principal left hepatic vein at the umbilical fissure (see Fig. 2–9A). Notably, this pattern receives significant tributaries draining the posterior aspect of segment IV as it approaches the inferior vena cava. The second most frequently observed pattern, observed in 14% of anatomic specimens, involved separate large veins, each draining an individual segment, that unite to form the left hepatic vein at the level of the inferior vena cava (see Fig. 2–9B). In this pattern, each venous channel receives tributaries from the posterior aspects of segment IV before uniting just prior to the inferior vena cava. The third anatomic pattern, identified in 13% of specimens, is a union of segment II and segment III draining veins within the parenchyma of the segment II/III allograft to form the left hepatic vein medial to the umbilical fissure. In this pattern, the left hepatic vein is a large single vessel that empties directly into the inferior vena cava without receiving significant tributaries from segment IV (see Fig. 2–9C). The middle and left hepatic veins fuse to form a common channel prior to the vena cava; however, dissection at or slightly within the parenchyma will delineate a plane of separation between the venous structures. Rarely, segments II and III will independently drain into the inferior vena cava. Recognition of separate segment II and segment III hepatic veins is critical to maintain adequate venous outflow from the allograft and requires both orifices to be incorporated on a common caval patch.[42]

The anatomy of the remnant segment I, IV to VIII allograft is straightforward because division of the portal pedicle occurs distal to the hilar bifurcation at the umbilical fissure.

Hemiliver Allografts

For transplantation of two adults from one adult deceased donor or a living donor liver transplantation between two adults, the liver is divided along Cantlie's line to create two nearly equal-size hemilivers (see Fig. 2–3). Left hemiliver allografts of approximately 400-cc volume can be created with (segments I to IV) or without the caudate lobe (segments II to IV) for recipients who are children, teenagers, and adults who typically weigh less than 60 kg. Right hemiliver allografts (segments I, V/VIII, or V/VIII) have a typical volume of approximately 800 to 1000 cc and are generally suitable for candidates who weigh less than 80 kg.[49-52] The applied surgical anatomy for these procedures focuses on hilar anatomy at the bifurcation, as well as the relationship of the middle and right hepatic veins.

Bifurcation of the proper hepatic artery into the right and left hepatic arteries occurs outside the hepatic parenchyma, permitting direct isolation of each vessel. Classic descriptions emphasize distinction; however, the region of the hilar plate and the junction of segments IV and V is best understood as a network of vascular supply involving both left and right hepatic arteries. Following bifurcation of the proper hepatic artery, the right hepatic artery courses posterior and lateral to the common hepatic duct to enter the right

FIGURE 2–8

Biliary variation within segments II and III. The four biliary variants of segments II and III are depicted in panels **A** through **D**. Each variant is depicted as an illustration (*left*), in relation to the segment II/III allograft (*center*), and by actual photograph (*right*) within the panel. **B** depicts segment IV biliary radicles crossing the umbilical fissure to drain the anterior aspect of segment III. Segment IV radicles are located anterior to the principal duct of segment III outside of the biliary connective tissue sheath and may be the source of posttransplantation biliary leaks if not identified.

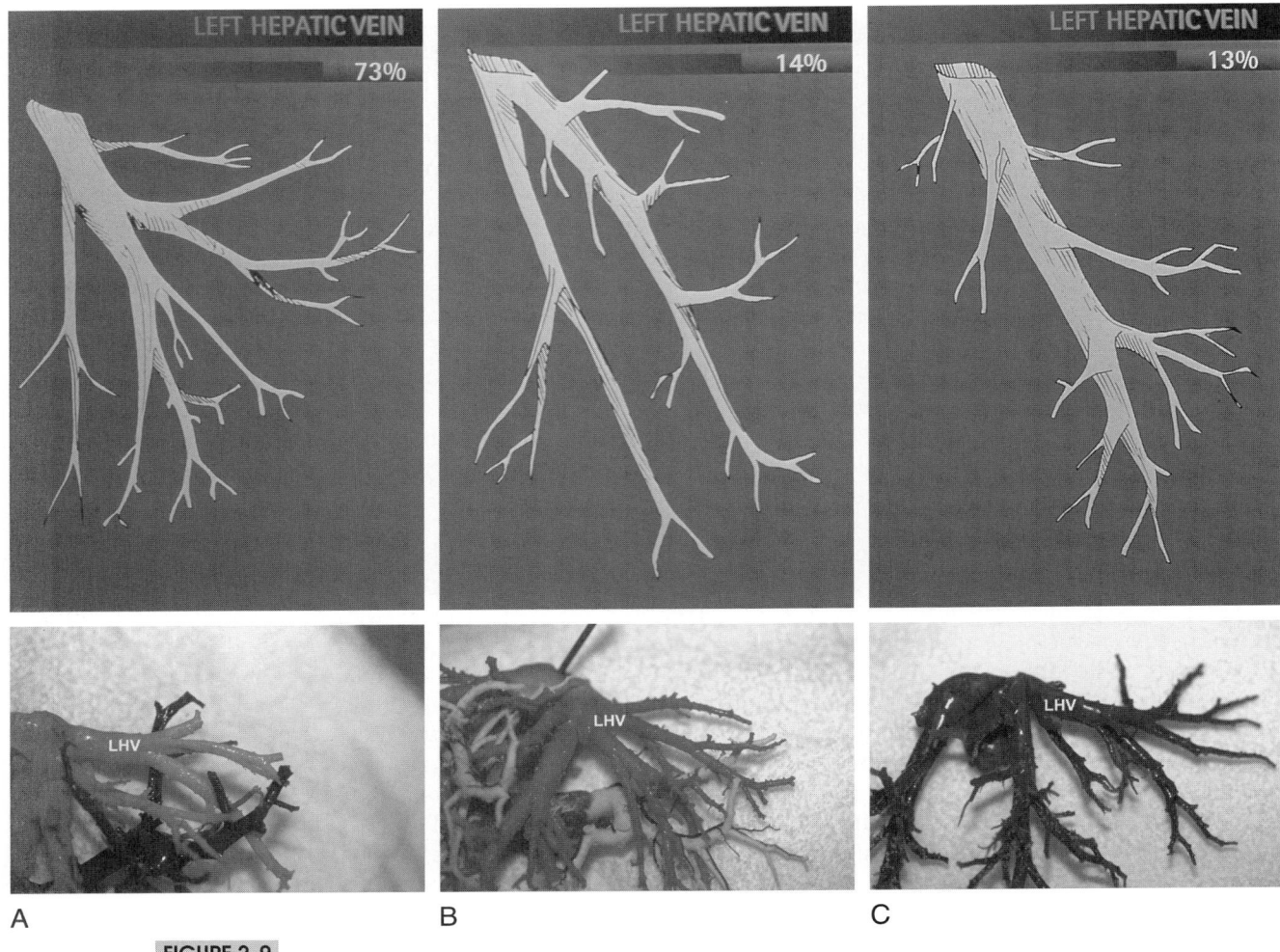

FIGURE 2–9

Anatomic variation of the left hepatic vein is depicted in schematic form with an accompanying corrosion cast.

hemiliver directly. As described earlier, the left hepatic artery courses extrahepatic along the inferior aspect of segment IV with the left hepatic duct before entering the parenchyma at the umbilical fissure. The occurrence of a significant (>1 mm) arterial branch or branches derived from the right hepatic artery that cross Cantlie's line to supply segment IV was identified in 15% of specimens (Fig. 2–10). These branches may be extraparenchymal or intraparenchymal and pass anterior or posterior to the left portal vein coursing along the inferior aspect of segment IV. Segment IV receives the principal supply of these branches; however, the authors have identified small branches to segments II and III (see Figs. 2–7A and 2–10). Marcos has described the clinical occurrence of this anatomic variant in living donor liver transplantation and has advocated a modified arterial dissection to preserve the vascular supply to segment IV.[53]

The right hepatic artery sends numerous small branches of less than 1 mm diameter across Cantlie's

line to supply segment IV (see Fig. 2–10). The authors assert these are surgically significant as aggressive dissection in the tissue plane defined by the bifurcation of the right and left hepatic arteries will disrupt these small vessels servicing segment IV and may contribute to the occurrence of segment IV bile leaks.[53] To minimize segment IV ischemia, identification and exposure of the right hepatic artery *lateral* to the common hepatic duct is advocated. Lateral exposure avoids devascularization of the bifurcation and preserves arterial supply to segment IV. In split-liver transplantation, the authors maintain this practice by preserving the celiac axis with the left graft. An accessory right hepatic artery, originating extraparenchymal from the proper hepatic artery and traveling lateral for approximately 2 cm before penetrating the right hemiliver to supply the inferior portions of segments V and VI, is observed in approximately 5% of specimens (Fig. 2–11).

In 1963, Parke provided a detailed description of the vascular supply of the common bile duct that has

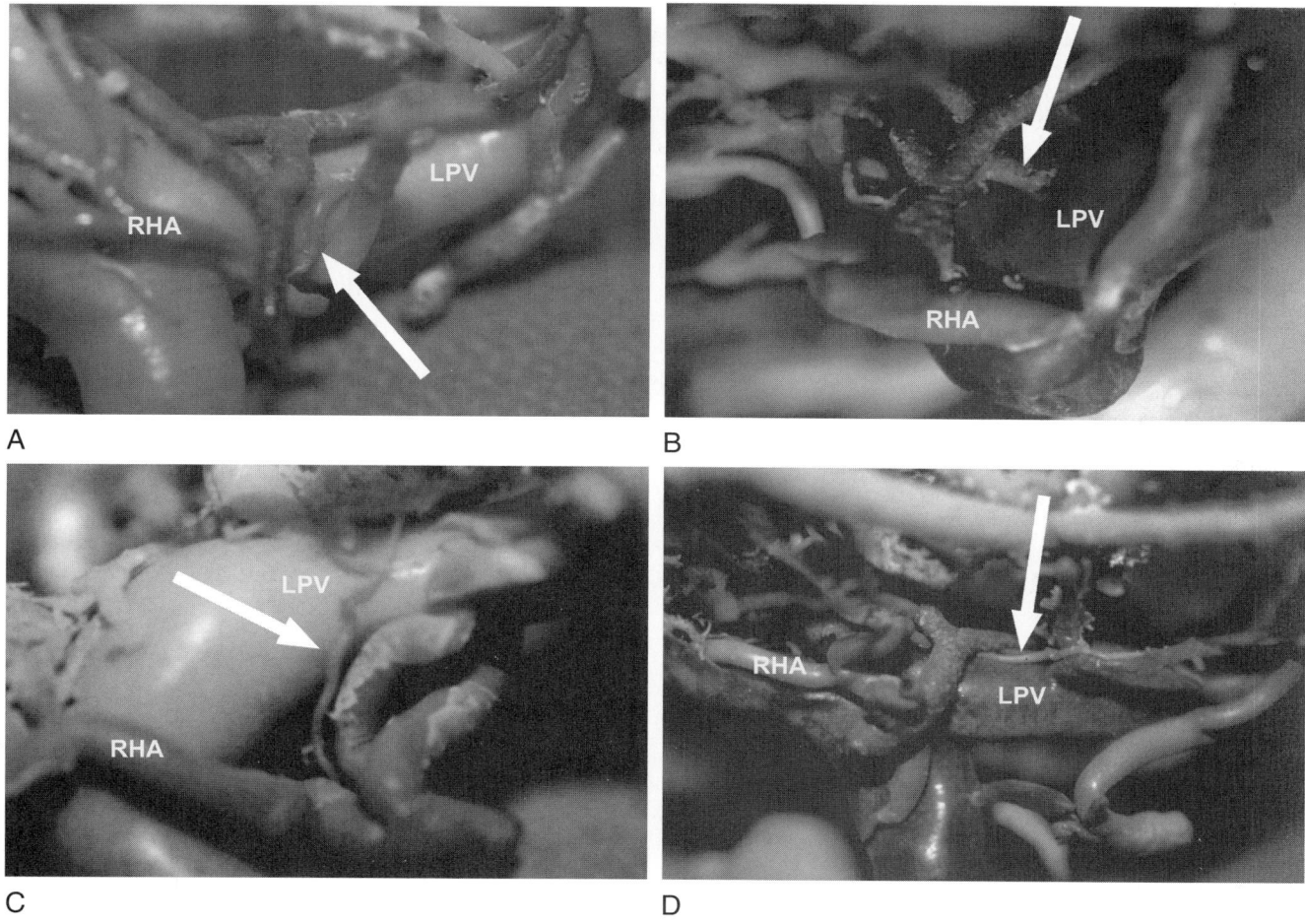

FIGURE 2–10

Right hepatic arterial supply to the left hemiliver. The anatomic relationship of the hilum is confirmed in each cast with the common hepatic duct anterior to the right hepatic artery (RHA) and portal vein bifurcation. **A,** A 1-mm branch of the right hepatic artery (*arrow*) extends anterior to the portal vein to supply segment IV. *Note the trifurcated portal vein and posterior right hepatic duct to be discussed.* **B,** A 2-mm branch of the right hepatic artery (*arrow*) crosses Cantlie's line posterior to the left portal vein (LPV) to supply segments II, III, and IV. **C** and **D,** The right hepatic artery sends small branches of less than 1 mm diameter (*arrow*) across Cantlie's line to supply segment IV both anterior (**C**) and posterior (**D**) to the left portal vein.

become a landmark manuscript.[54] The common hepatic and common bile ducts share an epicholedochal plexus that is multiply supplied by the pancreaticoduodenal, gastroduodenal, cystic, and hepatic arteries.[54] The left and right hepatic arteries contribute equally to the common hepatic duct bifurcation, underscoring the recommendation for the dissection strategy discussed earlier. In addition, the cystic artery typically originates from the right hepatic artery posterior to the common hepatic duct and bifurcates to supply the anterior and posterior aspects of the gallbladder. This artery is of minimal clinical significance in split-liver or living donor liver transplantation.

The bifurcation of the main portal vein is superior and posterior to the bifurcation of the proper hepatic artery and immediately inferior to the hilar connective tissue plate. As it ascends, the main portal vein gives several minor branches to the hilum above the origin of the left gastric vein. As described earlier, the left portal vein remains extrahepatic, whereas the right portal vein immediately enters the parenchyma of the right hemiliver. The right portal vein branches within 3 cm of the origin into an anterior and posterior segmental branch in addition to sending a large branch directly posterior into segment VIII. This may manifest as an intraparenchymal main portal vein trifurcation (see Fig. 2–10A). The anterior

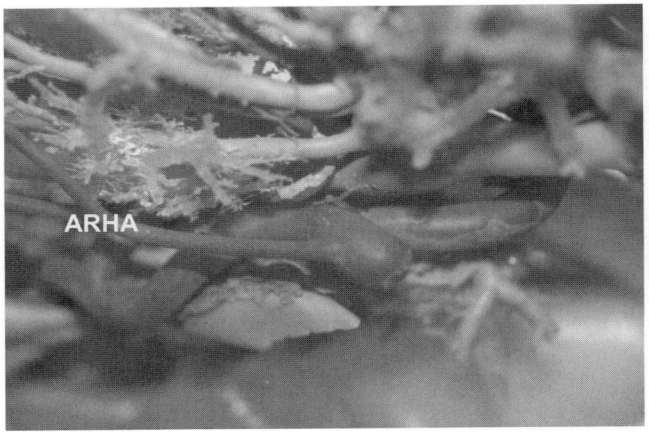

FIGURE 2–11

An accessory right hepatic artery (ARHA) originates from the proper hepatic artery proximal to its bifurcation and courses laterally to supply segments V and VI.

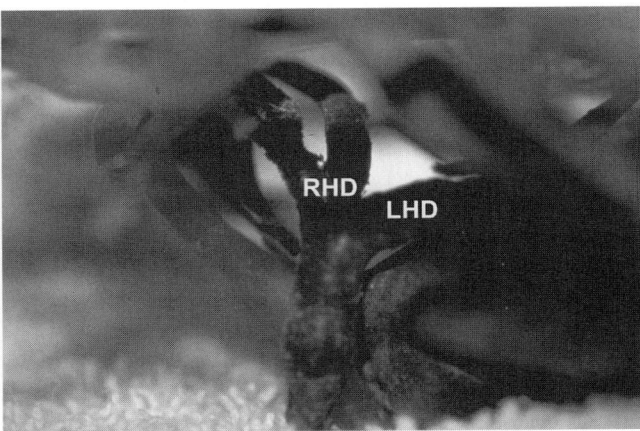

FIGURE 2–12

Anatomy of the common hepatic duct bifurcation. The common hepatic duct bifurcates at the hilar plate to form the left (LHD) and right hepatic ducts (RHD). The left hepatic duct remains extrahepatic with the left portal pedicle whereas the right hepatic duct directly enters the hepatic parenchyma, dividing early into its secondary branches. Union of anterior and posterior branches of the right hepatic duct occurs within 5 mm of the common hepatic duct bifurcation in 33% of specimens.

branch services segments V and VI, whereas the posterior branch services segments VII and VIII. The bifurcation of the anterior and posterior segmental branches occurs within the parenchyma; however, the origin of the posterior portal vein branch to segment VIII can be isolated high in the hilum and divided to enhance exposure in particularly difficult dissections.

Faithful to Couinaud's anatomic description,[28] the biliary tree parallels hepatic venous anatomy within the right lobe and segment IV. At the bifurcation, the common hepatic duct is sheathed in connective tissue to create a surgically identifiable hilar plate within the transverse fissure. In reconstructive biliary surgery, it is possible to expose the confluence of the right and left hepatic ducts by dissecting anteriorly in the portal plate at the base of segment IV.[19] Thus, it is possible to access high bile duct cancers or biliary strictures above the confluence.

The common hepatic duct bifurcation is the most superior landmark of the hilum. The left hepatic duct, like other components of the left portal pedicle, courses approximately 3 cm along the inferior border of segment IV superior to the left portal vein and is available for high anastomosis in the treatment of hilar obstruction. The right hepatic duct directly enters the hepatic parenchyma and, similar to the portal vein, divides early into its secondary branches. Union of anterior and posterior branches of the right hepatic duct occurs within 5 mm of the common hepatic duct bifurcation in 33% of specimens and within 1.5 cm of the common hepatic duct bifurcation in 90% of specimens (Fig. 2–12). A very significant surgical variant found in approximately 15% of specimens is the separate origination of the posterior branch of the right hepatic duct directly from the left hepatic duct (Fig. 2–13). In this variant, the posterior branch of the right hepatic duct

originates approximately 1 cm beyond the hilar plate from the left hepatic duct and crosses Cantlie's line to drain segments VII and VIII.[46] This branch cannot be ignored in right hemiliver grafts and requires a separate biliary anastomosis. In left hemiliver grafts, the duct should be gently probed to verify it does not lead to segment II (as detailed by Fig. 2–8C) with connection to the left hepatic duct verified by gentle flushing of saline prior to ligation.

Paramount to the successful application of partial-liver allografts is an appreciation of hepatic venous anatomy and the interplay between the left, middle, and right hepatic veins in providing sufficient outflow to each vascular territory. The "transition zones" are principally segment IV for the left hemiliver allograft and segments V and VIII for the right hemiliver allograft. The middle hepatic vein is essential to preservation of adequate liver mass to meet the metabolic demands of the transplant recipient. For the left hemiliver allograft, segment IV has a relative excess of venous capacity with preservation of the left and middle hepatic veins. Segment IV venous outflow was principally derived from the left hepatic vein in 9%, middle hepatic vein in 55%, and equally between left and middle in 36% of cast specimens.[46]

Figure 2-14 details the anatomy of the middle hepatic vein. The most frequently observed anatomic pattern (70%) is approximately equal venous drainage from segments IV, V, and VIII via large secondary branches that unite deep within the hepatic parenchyma (see Fig. 2–14A). In 20% of specimens, the middle hepatic

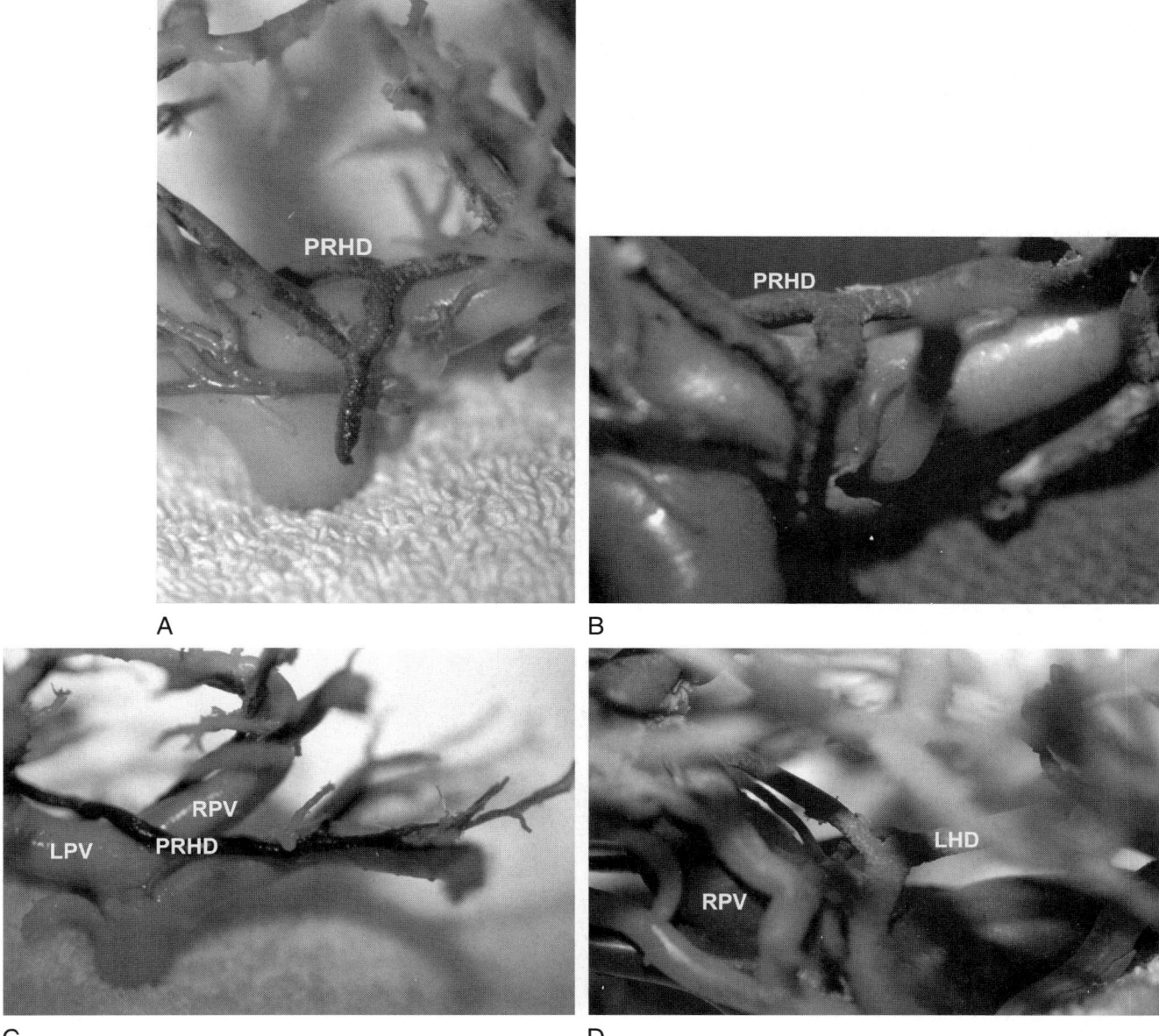

FIGURE 2-13

A posterior right hepatic duct (PRHD) originates from the left hepatic duct (LHD) and crosses Cantlie's line to enter the right lobe (**A** and **B**) (see also Fig. 2–10A). **C,** Dorsal view of posterior right hepatic duct branch as it courses to drain segments VII and VIII. Note the trifurcated portal vein (PV). **D,** Anatomic variant with two anterior right hepatic branches uniting at the bifurcation and a posterior hepatic duct branch originating from the left hepatic duct.

vein is a single large vessel receiving secondary branches from segments IV, V, and VIII throughout its course (see Fig. 2–14B). A very significant variant observed in 10% of specimens consists of a broad, dominant middle hepatic vein that sweeps laterally to service the entire anterolateral surface of the right hemiliver. This variant provides the principal venous outflow to segments V

and VI in addition to drainage of segments VIII and IV (see Fig. 2–14C).

Right hemiliver allografts may not have sufficient venous outflow without the middle hepatic vein. Consequently, it is essential to understand the relationship between the right and middle hepatic veins in providing sufficient venous outflow. Figure 2–15 illustrates

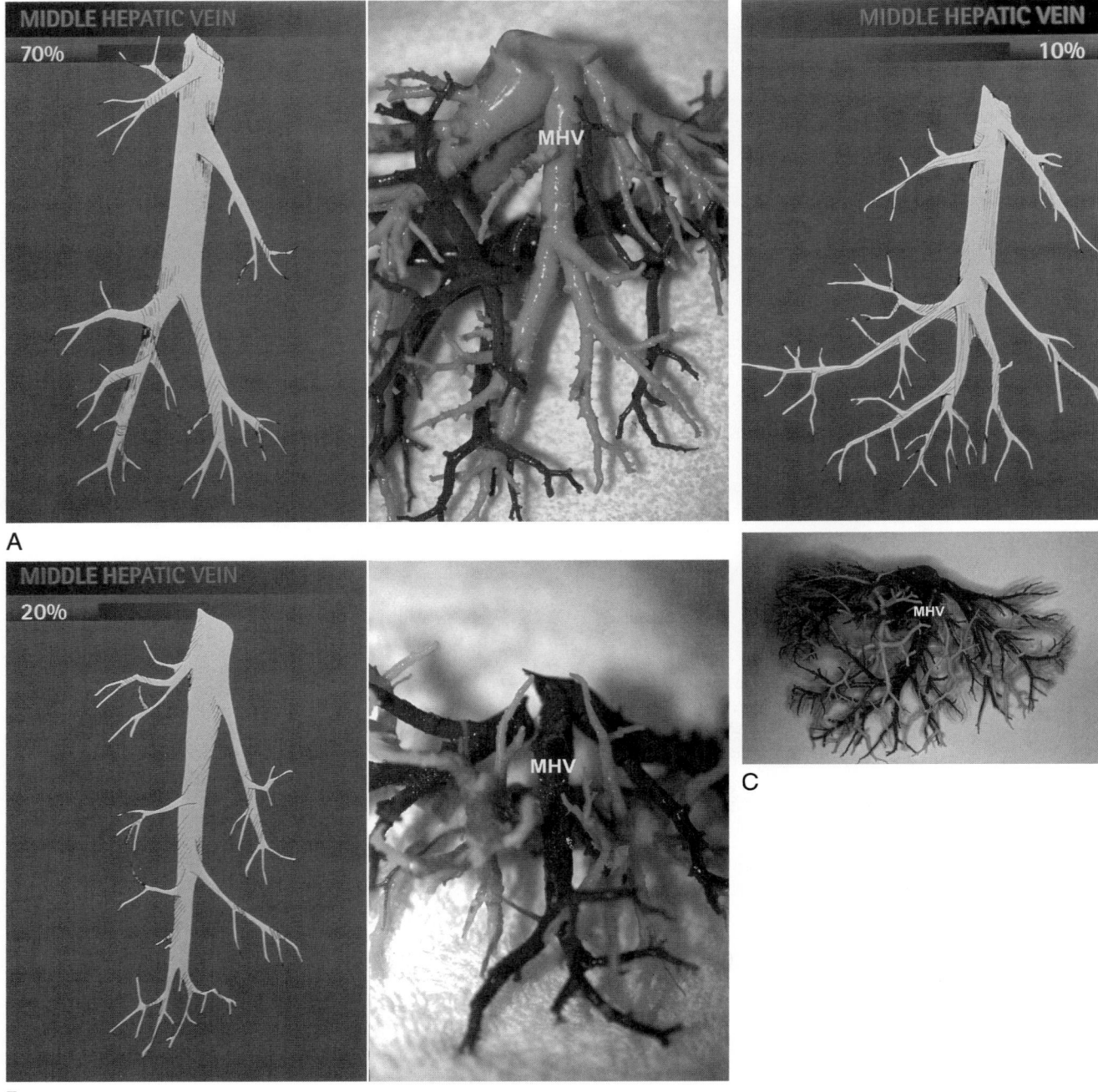

MIDDLE HEPATIC VEIN
70%

A

B

C

FIGURE 2–14

The anatomy of the middle hepatic vein (MHV) is depicted as a diagram with a corresponding corrosion cast.

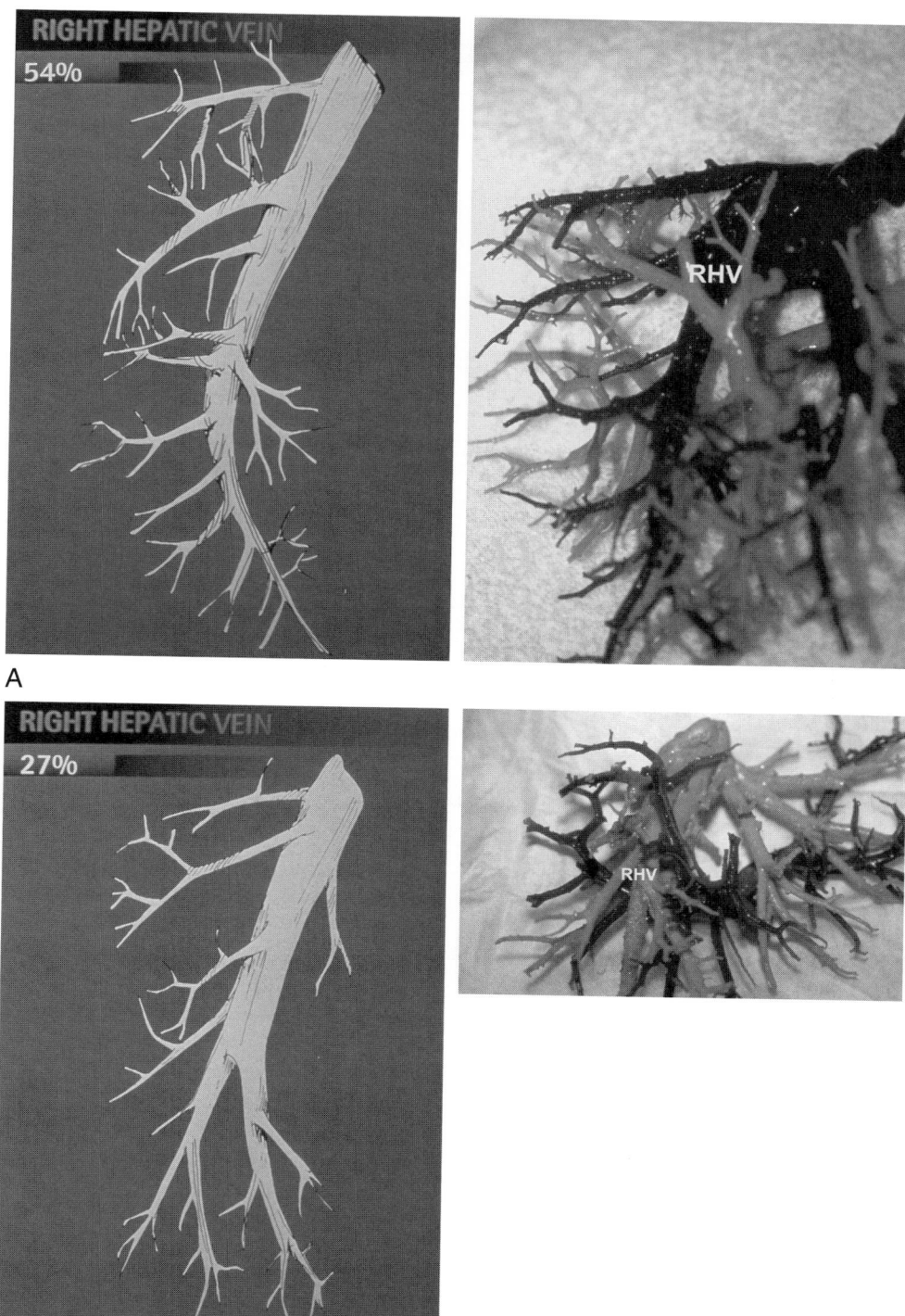

Continued

FIGURE 2–15

The anatomy of the right hepatic vein (RHV) is depicted as a diagram with a corresponding corrosion cast.

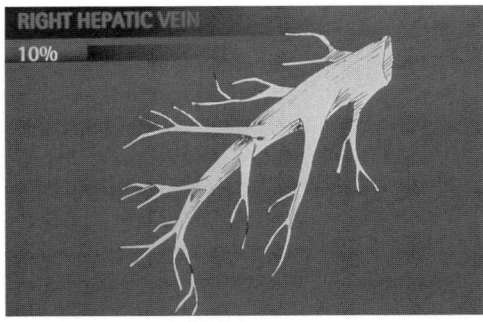
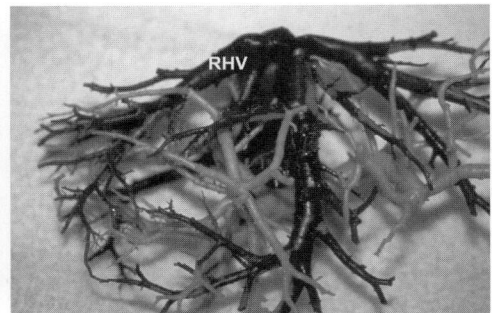

C

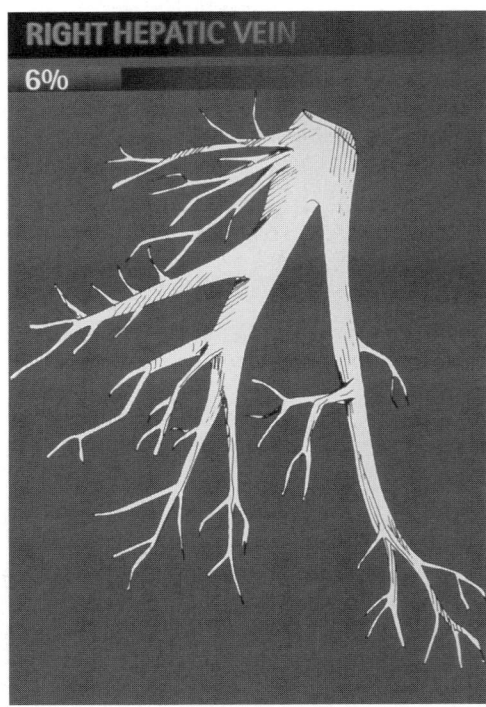
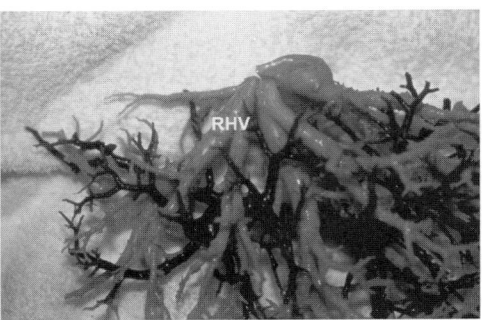

D

FIGURE 2–15, cont'd

the right hepatic venous anatomy. In 90% of specimens (see Fig. 2–15A, B, and D), the right hepatic vein courses throughout the right hemiliver to provide venous drainage; however, as demonstrated in Fig. 2–15C, there is a variant where the right hepatic vein is very short and posterior, providing limited venous drainage to segments VII and VIII with no involvement of the anterolateral surface of the right hemiliver (segments V and VI). This anatomic variation occurs in conjunction with a broad anterior middle hepatic vein that sweeps lateral as depicted in Figure 2–14C. The drainage provided by these two variants (Fig. 2–16) neglects the posterior aspect of segments V and VI that are serviced by large accessory hepatic veins that drain

directly into the inferior vena cava (Fig. 2–17). Accessory hepatic veins with a diameter larger than 5 mm occur with an incidence of approximately 10% to 15%, particularly in the setting of a single, short, posterior right hepatic vein that principally drains segments VII and VIII (see Fig. 2–15C). Identification of large, accessory hepatic veins from segments V and VI during hepatectomy is a predictor of this anatomic venous pattern. Middle hepatic venous branches draining segments V and VIII[55-57] as well as accessory hepatic veins larger than 5 mm in diameter are clinically significant and should be preserved through a caval patch or individually for implantation into the recipient vena cava.

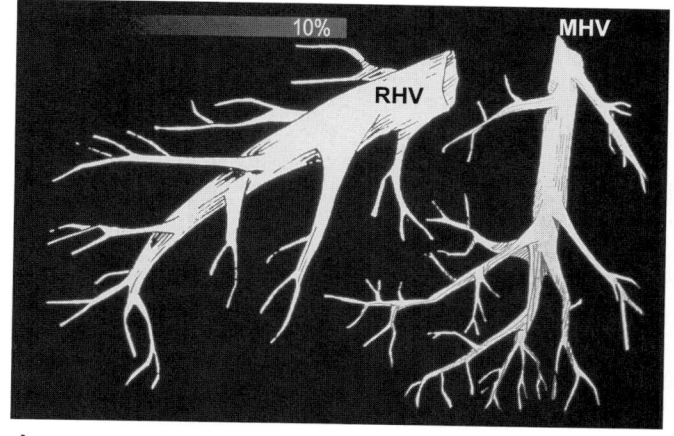

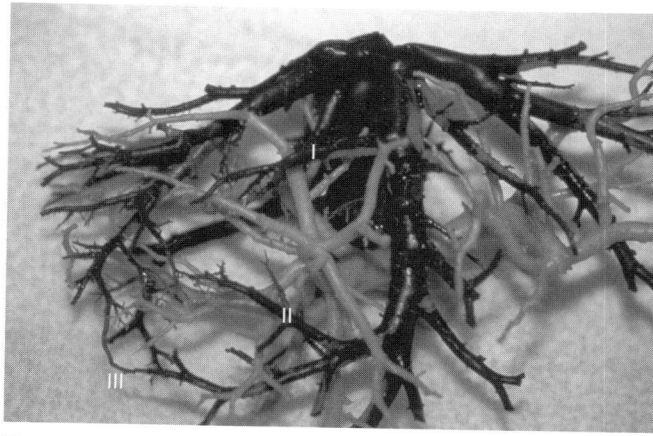

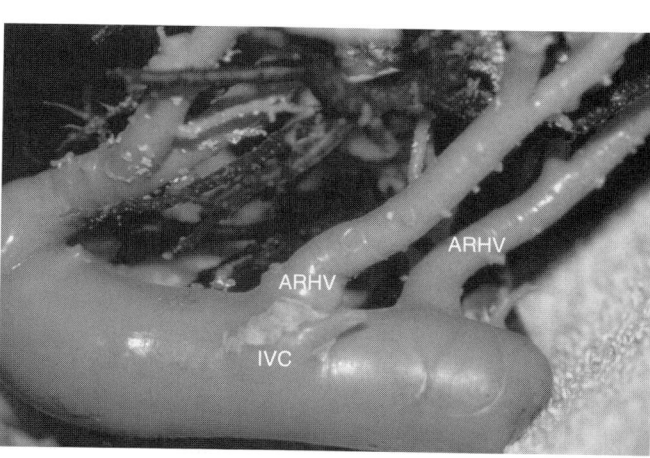

FIGURE 2–16

Interaction of the right and left hepatic veins. A broad, anterior middle hepatic vein (MHV) sweeps lateral to provide the principal drainage to the anterolateral aspect of the right hemiliver. This occurs in conjunction with a short, posterior right hepatic vein (RHV) that principally drains segments VII and VIII. Notice the multiple venous arcades (**B**, numbered *I*, *II*, and *III*) that interconnect the two venous systems. **C**, Intraoperative ultrasound demonstrates the venous drainage of segment VIII by the middle hepatic vein.

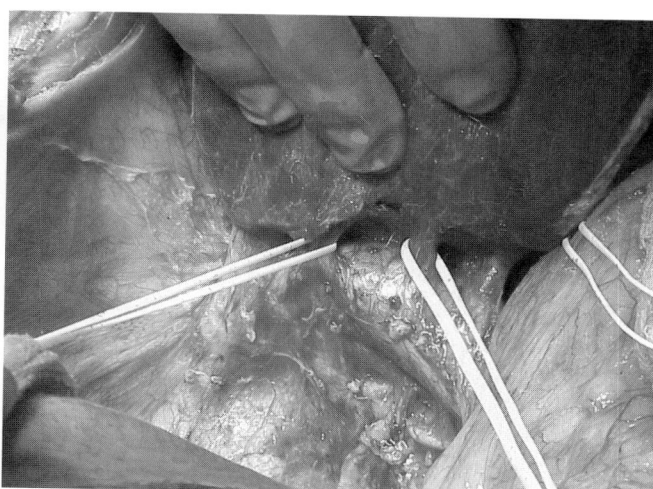

FIGURE 2–17

Accessory right hepatic veins (ARHV) originating from the posterior surface of the liver and draining directly into the inferior vena cava (IVC) are demonstrated by a corrosion cast (**A**) and intraoperative photograph (**B**).

Pearls and Pitfalls

- Successful application of partial-liver allografts mandates detailed understanding of intrahepatic anatomy.
- Review of the embryology and nomenclature systems described in this chapter provides a foundation for appreciating the origin of anatomic variants and their affect on surgical procedures.

Hilar Anatomy

- Arterial variations with respect to orientation and destination are frequent in the presence of *replaced* anatomy.
- Trifurcation of the portal vein is often approachable with a high hilar dissection.

Couinaud Segment II/III Allograft

- Dissection of the portal pedicle at the base of the round ligament isolates the left hepatic artery, left portal vein, and left hepatic duct. Branches of the left portal vein servicing the caudate lobe should be divided during the dissection.
- Parenchyma transection 1 cm lateral of the falciform ligament yields a single segment II/III duct in approximately 90% of surgical specimens.
- Biliary radicles from segment IV may cross the umbilical fissure anterior to the segment II/III bile duct outside of the biliary connective tissue sheath. These are terminal ducts that are amenable to suture ligation.
- Segment IV penetrating arteries provide significant inflow and particular attention should be devoted to their preservation.

Hemiliver Allografts

- The hilar plate and junction of segments IV and V compose a vascular network involving both left and right hepatic arteries. To minimize segment IV ischemia, identification and exposure of the right hepatic artery *lateral* to the common hepatic duct during living donor liver transplantation of segment IV to VIII allografts is advocated. Lateral exposure avoids devascularization of the bifurcation and preserves arterial supply to segment IV. In split-liver transplantation, this practice preserves the celiac axis with the left graft.
- At the bifurcation, the common hepatic duct is sheathed in connective tissue to create an

Pearls and Pitfalls—cont'd

identifiable hilar plate within the transverse fissure. It is possible to expose the confluence of the right and left hepatic ducts by dissecting anteriorly in the portal plate at the base of segment IV. This provides access to high bile duct cancers or biliary strictures above the confluence.

- A very significant surgical variant is the separate origination of the posterior branch of the right hepatic duct directly from the left hepatic duct. The posterior branch of the right hepatic duct originates approximately 1 cm beyond the hilar plate from the left hepatic duct and crosses Cantlie's line to drain segments VII and VIII. This branch cannot be ignored in right hemiliver grafts and requires a separate biliary anastomosis.
- Hepatic venous anatomy can be broadly categorized and is easily recognizable with preoperative imaging. The presence of an anterior, broadly sweeping lateral middle hepatic vein that services segments V and VI occurs with a short, posteriorly located right hepatic vein. With this anatomy, clinically significant accessory hepatic veins drain the posterior surface of the liver directly to the inferior vena cava.

References

1. Fortner J, Blumgart L: A historic perspective of liver surgery for tumors at the end of the millennium. J Am Coll Surg 193:210-222, 2001.
2. Marcos A, Ham JM, Fisher RA, et al: Single-center analysis of the first 40 adult-to-adult living donor liver transplants using the right lobe. Liver Transpl 6:296-301, 2000.
3. Yersiz H, Renz J, Farmer D, et al: One-hundred in situ split-liver transplantations: A single center experience. Ann Surg 238:496-505, 2003.
4. UNOS: United Network for Organ Sharing. Available at http://www.UNOS.org, 2004.
5. Humar A, Kandaswamy R, Sielaff T, et al: Split-liver transplants for 2 adult recipients: An initial experience. American Transplant Congress, Transplant 2001, May 12-16, 2001, Chicago, Illinois.
6. Brown R, Russo M, Lai M, et al: A survey of liver transplantation from living adult donors in the United States. N Engl J Med 348:818-825, 2003.
7. Renz J, Yersiz H, Farmer D, et al: Changing faces of liver transplantation: Partial-liver grafts for adults. J Hepatobiliary Pancreat Surg 10:31-44, 2003.
8. Renz JF, Emond JC, Yersiz H, et al: Split-liver transplantation in the United States: Outcomes of a national survey. Ann Surg 239:172-181, 2004.
9. Strasberg S: Terminology of liver anatomy and liver resections: Coming to grips with hepatic Babel. J Am Coll Surg 184:413-434, 1997.

10. Botero A, Strasberg S: Division of the left hemiliver in man-segments, sectors, or sections. Liver Transpl Surg 4:226-231, 1998.
11. Jordan H, Kindred J: The liver. In Jordan H, Kindred J (eds): Textbook of Embryology. New York, Appleton-Century, 1942, pp 156-160.
12. Moore K: The digestive system. In Moore K (ed): The Developing Human. Philadelphia, WB Saunders, 1982, pp 227-252.
13. Arey L: Development of the veins. In Rea R (ed): Developmental Anatomy. Philadelphia, WB Saunders, 1965, pp 360-368.
14. Jordan H, Kindred J: Development of the hepatic portal system. In: Jordan H, Kindred J (eds): Textbook of Embryology. New York, Appleton-Century, 1942, pp 214-217.
15. Patten B, Carlson B: The portal vein. In Patten B, Carlson B (eds): Foundations of Embryology. New York, McGraw-Hill, 1974, pp 564-565.
16. Jordan H, Kindred J: The intestines. In Jordan H, Kindred J (eds): Textbook of Embryology. New York, Appleton-Century, 1942, pp 145-148.
17. Glisson F: Anatomia Hepatis. Amsterdam, Ravesteyn, 1659.
18. Meyers W: Anatomy and physiology. In Sabiston DJ (ed): Textbook of Surgery. Philadelphia, WB Saunders, 1991, pp 976-992.
19. Emond JC, Renz JF: Surgical anatomy of the liver and its application to hepatobiliary surgery and transplantation. Semin Liver Dis 14:158-168, 1994.
20. Jastrow M: The liver in antiquity and the beginnings of anatomy. Philadelphia, Transactions of the College of Physicians, 1907.
21. McClusky D III, Skandalakis L, Colborn G, Skandalakis J: Hepatic surgery and hepatic surgical anatomy: Historical partners in progress. World J Surg 21:330-342, 1997.
22. Rex H: Beitrage zur Morphologie der Saugerleber. Morphol Jahrb 14:517-615, 1888.
23. Cantlie J: On a new arrangement of the right and left lobes of the liver. Proc Anat Soc Great Britain Ireland 32:4-9, 1897.
24. Bismuth H: Surgical anatomy and anatomical surgery of the liver. World J Surg 6:3-9, 1982.
25. Tiffany L: Surgery of the liver. Boston Med Surg J 23:557, 1890.
26. Healey J Jr, Schroy P: Anatomy of the biliary ducts within the human liver; analysis of the prevailing pattern of branchings and the major variations of the biliary ducts. Arch Surg 66:599-616, 1953.
27. Starzl TE, Bell R, Beart R, Putnam C: Hepatic trisegmentectomy and other liver resections. Surg Gynecol Obstet 141:429-437, 1975.
28. Couinaud C: Les enveloppes vasculobiliares de foie ou capsule de Glisson. Leur interet dans la chirurgie vesiculaire, les resections hepatiques et l'abord du hile du foie. Lyon Chir 49:589-615, 1954.
29. Tanaka K, Uemoto S, Tokunaga Y, et al: Surgical techniques and innovations in living related liver transplantation. Ann Surg 217:82-91, 1993.
30. Emond JC, Heffron TG, Whitington PF, Broelsch CE: Reconstruction of the hepatic vein in reduced size hepatic transplantation. Surg Gynecol Obstet 176:11-17, 1993.
31. Ozaki C, Katz S, Monsour H, Wood R: Vascular reconstruction in living-related liver transplantation. Transplant Proc 26:167-168, 1994.
32. Kuang AA, Rosenthal P, Roberts JP, et al: Decreased mortality from technical failure improves results in pediatric liver transplantation. Arch Surg 131:887-892; discussion 892-893, 1996.
33. Inomoto T, Nishizawa F, Sasaki H, et al: Experiences of 120 microsurgical reconstructions of hepatic artery in living related liver transplantation. Surgery 119:20-26, 1996.
34. Furuta S, Ikegami T, Nakazawa Y, et al: Hepatic artery reconstruction in living donor liver transplantation from the microsurgeon's point of view. Liver Transpl Surg 3:388-393, 1997.
35. Reichert PR, Renz JF, Rosenthal P, et al: Biliary complications of reduced-organ liver transplantation. Liver Transpl Surg 4:343-349, 1998.
36. Todo S, Makowka L, Tzakis A, et al: Hepatic artery in liver transplantation. Transplant Proc 19:2406-2411, 1987.
37. Hiatt J, Gabbay J, Busuttil RW: Surgical anatomy of the hepatic artery in 1000 cases. Ann Surg 220:50-52, 1994.
38. Raia S, Nery J, Mies S: Liver transplantation from live donors. Lancet 2:497, 1989.
39. Strong RW, Lynch SV, Ong TH, et al: Successful liver transplantation from a living donor to her son. N Engl J Med 322:1505-1507, 1990.
40. Emond JC, Renz JF, Ferrell LD, et al: Functional analysis of grafts from living donors. Implications for the treatment of older recipients. Ann Surg 224:544-552; discussion 552-554, 1996.
41. Oike F, Sakamoto S, Kasahara M, et al: Monosegment graft in living donor liver transplantation. American Transplant Congress, Transplant 2001, May 12-16, 2001, Chicago, Illinois.
42. Reichert PR, Renz JF, D'Albuquerque LA, et al: Surgical anatomy of the left lateral segment as applied to living-donor and split-liver transplantation: A clinicopathologic study. Ann Surg 232:658-664, 2000.
43. Renz JF, Reichert PR, Emond JC: Hepatic arterial anatomy as applied to living-donor and split-liver transplantation. Liver Transpl 6:367-369, 2000.
44. Healey J, Hodge J: Surgical anatomy. Philadelphia, BC Decker, 1990.
45. Emre S, Schwartz M, Miller C: The donor operation. In Busuttil R, Klintmalm G (eds): Transplantation of the Liver. Philadelphia, WB Saunders, 1996, pp 392-404.
46. Renz JF, Reichert PR, Emond JC: Biliary anatomy as applied to pediatric living donor and split-liver transplantation. Liver Transpl 6:801-804, 2000.
47. Healey J Jr, Schroy P: Anatomy of the biliary ducts within the human liver. Arch Surg 66:599-616, 1953.
48. Russell E, Yrizzary J, Montalvo B, et al: Left hepatic duct anatomy: Implications. Radiology 174:353-356, 1990.
49. Sommacale D, Farges O, Ettorre GM, et al: In situ split liver transplantation for two adult recipients. Transplantation 69:1005-1007, 2000.
50. Yersiz H, Renz JF, Hisatake G, et al: Technical and logistical considerations of in situ split-liver transplantation for two adults: Part I. Creation of left segment II, III, IV and right segment I, V-VIII grafts. Liver Transpl 7:1077-1080, 2001.
51. Yersiz H, Renz JF, Hisatake G, et al: Technical and logistical considerations of in situ split-liver transplantation for two adults: Part II. Creation of left segment I-IV and right segment V-VIII grafts. Liver Transpl 8:78-81, 2002.
52. Humar A, Khwaja K, Sielaff TD, et al: Technique of split-liver transplant for two adult recipients. Liver Transpl 8:725-729, 2002.
53. Marcos A: Right lobe living donor liver transplantation: A review. Liver Transpl 6:3-20, 2000.
54. Parke WW, Michels MA, Ghosh GM: Blood supply of the common bile duct. Surg Gynecol Obstet 117:47-55, 1963.
55. Renz J: Normal and variant anatomy of the liver. National Institutes of Health Workshop on Living-Donor Liver Transplantation, December, 2000, Washington, DC.
56. Ghobrial RM, Hsieh CB, Lerner S, et al: Technical challenges of hepatic venous outflow reconstruction in right lobe adult living donor liver transplantation. Liver Transpl 7:551-555, 2001.
57. Marcos A, Orloff M, Mieles L, et al: Functional venous anatomy for right-lobe grafting and techniques to optimize outflow. Liver Transpl 7:845-852, 2001.

3

Molecular and Cellular Basis of Hepatic Failure

HAL F. YEE, JR
TIMOTHY J. DAVERN II

Definitions   44

Acute liver failure   44
   Clinical manifestations   44
   Etiology   45
   Pathogenesis   45

Cirrhosis   48
   Clinical manifestations   48
   Etiology   50
   Pathogenesis   50

Perspectives and Future Directions   55

Hepatic failure is the principal indication for liver transplantation. It arises from the loss of functional hepatic parenchyma that can result from either acute liver failure or cirrhosis. In the United States, acute liver failure affects approximately 2000 to 4000 individuals per year and is the indication for approximately 5% of liver transplants. Cirrhosis, which kills approximately 25,000 Americans per year, is responsible for the vast majority of liver transplants performed. Although impaired hepatic function characterizes both acute liver failure and cirrhosis, the mechanisms underlying the pathogenesis of these two disorders are, in general, distinct. In this chapter, we briefly review the molecular and cellular basis of acute liver failure and cirrhosis, recognizing that the separation of liver failure into acute and chronic is somewhat artificial. Many patients with chronic liver disease succumb to *acute on chronic* liver failure when an acute insult (e.g., hepatitis A) is superimposed on hitherto compensated cirrhosis (e.g., hepatitis C). In addition, many of the clinical manifestations (Table 3–1) and causes (Table 3–2) of acute and chronic liver failure are shared. Nonetheless, we separate these two ends of a spectrum in this chapter for clarity. Space limitations dictate that many important areas of research in this field are not addressed. Similarly, worthy contributions from many laboratories are not cited. Accordingly, references to several recent reviews are provided for readers interested in a more detailed treatment.

Table 3-1. CLINICAL MANIFESTATIONS OF ACUTE LIVER FAILURE AND DECOMPENSATED CIRRHOSIS

	Acute Liver Failure	Decompensated Cirrhosis
Fluid retention	+	+++
Portal hypertensive bleeding	–	+++
Coagulopathy	+++	++
Jaundice	++	+++
Hepatic encephalopathy	+++	++
Cerebral edema	+++	–
Infection	+++	++
Renal failure	+++	++
Hepatocellular carcinoma	–	++

–, unusual; +, infrequent; ++, common; +++, characteristic of the syndrome.

Definitions

Acute liver failure (ALF) is a clinical syndrome characterized by severe liver injury complicated by encephalopathy. Essential for the diagnosis of ALF are the absence of clinically overt chronic liver disease and the presence of encephalopathy not caused by sedation or some other nonhepatic cause. Most studies of ALF include patients that develop encephalopathy within 8 weeks of the onset of symptoms, which are often nonspecific and flu-like, or within 2 weeks of the onset of jaundice. A variant of ALF with a more insidious onset, called subfulminant hepatic failure, is usually defined by liver failure with hepatic encephalopathy that develops between 2 weeks and 3 months from the onset of jaundice.

Cirrhosis is a pathological diagnosis that is defined by the presence of extensive hepatic fibrosis associated with derangement of the liver's normal lobular and vascular architecture. It is characterized by the presence of nodules of regenerating hepatocytes surrounded by exuberant extracellular matrix (ECM) in the form of fibrotic bands. Hepatic function can be impaired to a clinically significant degree when the structural abnormalities that distinguish cirrhosis are sufficiently advanced. This potentially life-threatening condition is the final common pathway through which nearly all forms of chronic liver disease cause morbidity and mortality.

Acute Liver Failure

Clinical Manifestations

Hepatic encephalopathy is, by definition, present to some degree in all patients with ALF. Other common clinical manifestations of ALF include cerebral edema, infection, renal failure, hypotension, hypoglycemia, jaundice, and electrolyte abnormalities, whereas portal

Table 3-2. ETIOLOGIES THAT LEAD TO LIVER FAILURE

	Acute Liver Failure	Decompensated Cirrhosis
Drugs/toxins	Acetaminophen Isoniazid	Ethanol Methotrexate Excess vitamin A
Infections	Hepatitis A Hepatitis B (±Hepatitis Δ) Hepatitis E	Hepatitis B Hepatitis C Schistosomiasis
Vascular	Shock (i.e., acute ischemia) Hepatic vein occlusion (Budd-Chiari syndrome)	Congestive heart failure Hepatic vein occlusion (Budd-Chiari syndrome)
Metabolic and genetic disorders	Wilson's disease Reye's syndrome Tyrosinemia Pregnancy-associated (Acute fatty liver/HELLP syndrome)	Nonalcoholic steatohepatitis Hereditary hemochromatosis α_1-antitrypsin deficiency Wilson's disease Tyrosinemia
Autoimmune	Autoimmune hepatitis	Autoimmune hepatitis Primary biliary cirrhosis Primary sclerosing cholangitis
Biliary disorders		Chronic obstruction of the biliary tract Byler disease
Unknown	Indeterminate acute liver failure	Cryptogenic cirrhosis

HELLP, hemolysis, elevated liver enzymes, and low platelet (count).

hypertensive bleeding and severe fluid retention are distinctly unusual (see Table 3–1). The syndrome of ALF is associated with high mortality, with most patients dying from cerebral edema and sepsis. However, some causes of ALF are associated with a better prognosis than are other causes. In general, the more rapid onset forms of ALF, such as that associated with acetaminophen hepatotoxicity, have a higher incidence of cerebral edema but an overall better prognosis, probably reflecting the lack of liver architectural derangement and, thus, more favorable conditions for hepatic regeneration. In contrast, ALF caused by idiosyncratic drug reactions, Wilson's disease, and indeterminate cause, which tend to follow a subfulminant course, carries a particularly poor prognosis.[1]

Etiology

ALF results from the abrupt loss of liver function secondary to severe injury from a variety of causes that may be grouped into several general categories (see Table 3–2). The most common causes of ALF in the United States currently are drugs and toxins, in particular, acetaminophen, and ALF of indeterminate cause, presumably a heterogeneous group of occult viral infections, autoimmune disorders, toxic exposures, and metabolic insults. The incidence of ALF from viral hepatitis A and B in the United States appears to be decreasing, perhaps in part the result of an active vaccination program, and together they now account for less than 10% of ALF cases per year.[2]

Pathogenesis

The lack of suitable animal models has hampered research on the mechanisms of ALF and, as a result, the pathophysiological basis for the syndrome of ALF is incompletely understood. Nevertheless, based on the available data, it appears that ALF usually reflects the effects of inflammatory cytokines and cells initiating a cascade of events culminating in massive liver cell death while inhibiting cell replication. Although the hepatocyte is often the focus of attention in ALF, all of the various liver cell types (Table 3–3) undoubtedly play important roles. Liver injury usually results from a complex interaction between the injurious agent (e.g., virus, chemical, self-reactive immune cells) and the response of host cells to the insult, including activation of both liver parenchymal and nonparenchymal cells with cytokine release.

Acute infection with hepatitis B (HBV) illustrates the importance of the host cell response in the pathogenesis of ALF. Under most circumstances, HBV is a noncytopathic virus, although overexpression of certain viral proteins in cultured cells may cause toxicity. In vivo liver damage from HBV appears to result largely from the host immune responses to virally infected cells rather than from a direct result of viral injury per se. For example, in a transgenic mouse model expressing HBV proteins, severe acute liver damage occurs only after HBV-specific cytotoxic T-lymphocytes (CTLs) are infused that target and destroy HBV surface antigen (HBsAg)-positive hepatocytes. Prior to such a challenge, the mice have little or no demonstrable liver pathology.

Table 3–3. THE ROLES OF THE MAJOR CELL POPULATIONS IN THE HEALTHY LIVER

Cell Type	Approximate Fraction in the Healthy Liver	Roles in the Healthy Liver
Hepatocytes	60%	Uptake, storage, metabolism, and release of carbohyrates, proteins, lipids, and vitamins Synthesis of plasma proteins, lipoproteins, fatty acids, cholesterol, phospholipids, and glucose Bile synthesis and secretion Degradation and detoxification of exogenous and endogenous compounds
Stellate cells	5%	Storage of vitamin A Synthesis of extracellular matrix Support of homeostasis of hepatocytes and endothelial cells
Cholangiocytes	3%	Fluid and electroyte secretion/resorption Protein translocation
Kupffer cells	15%	Phagocytosis and clearance of microrganisms, endotoxins, tumor cells, particulate matter Immune defense Tumor cell surveillance
Endothelial cells	15%	Endocytic uptake of glycoproteins Scavenging of denatured circulating proteins
Immune cells	2%	Cytotoxicity toward virus-infected and tumor cells

Full recovery from ALF is possible, and this suggests that outcomes may be improved if cell death can be curtailed and hepatic repair enhanced. Ultimately, prognosis in ALF depends on the balance of liver cell death with liver repair and regeneration. Indeed, survival critically depends upon rapid and robust recovery of liver cell function before the life-threatening complications, such as cerebral edema and sepsis, of ALF supervene.

Liver Regeneration and Repair

The adequacy of liver repair and regeneration following acute liver injury appears to be as important as the extent of the injury in determining outcome. The molecular mechanisms underlying hepatic regeneration have been elucidated primarily in the partial hepatectomy rodent model, in which two thirds of the liver, including the left lateral and medial lobes, are removed intact.[3] However, relatively little is known about liver regeneration in the setting of ALF, particularly in humans, and it is likely that this process differs in many important ways from regeneration associated with partial hepatectomy because, for example, with partial hepatectomy the remaining liver is intact and normal, whereas in ALF the entire liver is involved. Illustrating this point, the roles of hepatocyte growth factor (HGF) and transforming growth factor-β (TGF-β), which are relatively well-characterized positive and negative regulators of hepatocyte proliferation following partial hepatectomy, are unclear in the setting of ALF. Indeed, paradoxically, serum HGF levels, which rise within an hour of partial hepatectomy, appear to correlate inversely with prognosis in the setting of ALF.

Hepatic regeneration represents the culmination of a complex interaction among liver cells, matrix, cytokines, and hormones.[4,5] Under normal conditions, only a small fraction of hepatocytes ($\sim$1/20,000) are in mitosis. When hepatocytes are injured and die, they are usually replaced by mature hepatocytes. Experiments in several different murine models suggest that mature hepatocytes have the ability to undergo multiple rounds of replication.[6] Whether this is also true of fully differentiated human hepatocytes, which (unlike mice) lack active telomerase—the enzyme responsible for maintaining chromosome end length with DNA replication—is currently unclear. Under certain situations, including when protein synthesis is inhibited, perisinusoidal oval cells, which have some stem cell properties, also participate in hepatic regeneration. Furthermore, recent experiments both in murine models of liver injury and histological studies of liver transplant explants suggest that extrahepatic cells derived from the bone marrow also appear to have the ability to contribute to hepatic regeneration, but the molecular mechanisms of this process are currently controversial.[7]

After partial hepatectomy, the onset of liver cell replication is rapid, with the peak of hepatocyte DNA synthesis occurring within approximately 24 hours, and the peak of nonparenchymal cell DNA synthesis occurring approximately 24 hours later.[4] Amazingly, normal liver mass is restored after only 7 to 10 days following 50% partial hepatectomy in rats, although the regenerative capacity of hepatocytes is in part related to the age of the animal.[8] Liver regeneration, encompassing both hypertrophy and hyperplasia, is characterized by the activation of more than 100 genes encoding cytokines, growth factors, transcription factors, and cellular constituents.[8] HGF, epidermal growth factor (EGF), TGF-β, tumor necrosis factor-α (TNF-α), and interleukin (IL)-6 appear to have particularly important roles in hepatic regeneration. The plasma concentration of HGF, produced primarily by stellate cells, increases dramatically within 1 hour of a partial hepatectomy, and it acts through its receptor, c-met, which is highly expressed on hepatocytes.[3] The role of TGF-β, a potent growth inhibitor factor produced by sinusoidal endothelial cells and hepatocytes, in possibly terminating hepatic regeneration once complete is still unclear.

During the so-called priming phase of replication, normally quiescent hepatocytes enter the cell cycle—moving from the G_0 to the G_1 phase—and become replication competent. This early phase, which lasts 4 to 6 hours following partial hepatectomy, is marked by increased circulating levels of TNF-α and IL-6, as well as other cytokines, matrix remodeling in the remaining liver, and the activation of a series of immediate early genes including the proto-oncogenes *c-fos*, *c-jun*, and *c-myc*.[8] Activation of these and other genes ultimately leads to progression through the early to mid-G_1 phase of the cell cycle.[3] Progression through the cell cycle (G_1 through S phases) is regulated by growth factors and activation of early (D and E) and late (A and B) cyclins and their associated cyclin-dependent kinases (CDKs). Inactivation of cell cycle inhibitory proteins, retinoblastoma (Rb) protein and p130, is also required to release the transcription factor E2F that stimulates cell cycle progression and DNA replication (S phase).

TNF-α, released primarily from Kupffer cells, appears to play a critical role in the initiation of the transcriptional cascade contributing to hepatocyte replication. Transcription factors activated as part of this cascade include, among others[8]:

- Nuclear factor-κ B (NF-κB)
- Signal transducer and activator of transcription 3 (STAT3)

- Activating protein-1 (AP-1)
- CAAT enhancer binding protein β (C/EBP-β)
- Extracellular signal-regulated kinase (ERK)
- c-Jun N-terminal kinase (JNK) kinases

The early activation of NF-κB by a rapid posttranscriptional mechanism activates expression of IL-6, which in turn activates STAT3 and other genes. When NF-κB activity is blocked after partial hepatectomy, the residual liver undergoes massive apoptosis.[4] Genetically modified mice that lack IL-6 or the receptor for TNF-α have deficient liver regeneration and develop liver failure following partial hepatectomy that is ameliorated by recombinant IL-6 administration, strongly suggesting that IL-6 is acting downstream of TNF-α in the regeneration cascade. In the setting of severe ALF, hepatic regeneration is impaired despite high serum levels of IL-6, TNF-α, and HGF.

Liver Cell Death

Like other cells, liver cells die from apoptosis and necrosis, two pathways of cell death that are morphologically distinct but interrelated and that probably should be viewed as two ends of a cell death continuum. The cell death pathway taken, either apoptosis or necrosis, appears to be related to the nature and severity of the inciting insult, the cell type, its metabolic status, and the integrity of the cell death machinery. Both types of cell death probably occur simultaneously in most forms of ALF.[9] Necrosis involves severe depletion of cellular adenosine triphosphate (ATP) and results in cell swelling, loss of cell membrane integrity, and lysis, which invariably elicits a secondary immune response. In contrast, apoptosis, or programmed cell death, is characterized by a more orderly process of nuclear and cytoplasmic shrinkage, condensation, and blebbing without loss of cell membrane integrity or release of intracellular contents; thus it allows cellular debris to be removed without intense secondary inflammation and marked perturbation of neighboring cells. Again, both processes (apoptosis and necrosis) may, and probably often do, occur simultaneously, and the same stimuli in varying intensities can trigger both processes. In general, liver cell necrosis rather than apoptosis tends to predominate, with extensive oxidative damage to mitochondria because this depletes cellular ATP stores and also may inhibit caspase activity, both of which are necessary for the successful execution of the apoptosis pathway.

Apoptosis is a highly conserved process essential to organogenesis and immune cell homeostasis that was first recognized pathologically in liver 3 decades ago as acidophilic (Councilman) bodies. However, fundamental insights into the molecular details of the apoptosis pathway are more recent, initially gleaned from experiments in the worm *Caenorhabditis elegans* and only later in mammalian cells. The apoptosis cascade involves the sequential activation of a series of cysteine proteases called caspases. This cascade can be triggered by a variety of insults that may be extrinsic or intrinsic to the cell undergoing apoptosis. Extrinsic triggers involve activation of cell surface *death* receptors, whereas intrinsic triggers signal apoptosis via oxidative stress of mitochondria and possibly other cellular organelles.[10]

Diverse factors trigger liver cell death, such as hypoxia (e.g., with ischemia–reperfusion), reactive oxygen species (e.g., generated during drug metabolism), viral infection, and autoimmune injury; however, they generally induce cell death via cell surface death receptors or by injuring mitochondria, although both processes often occur simultaneously. Indeed, participation of mitochondria appears to be essential to death receptor–mediated apoptosis in hepatocytes.[11] Oxidative injury to mitochondria secondary to TNF-α, for example, results in opening of mitochondrial permeability transition (MPT) pores at the junction of the inner and outer mitochondrial membranes. Opening of the MPT pores, in turn, leads to release of intramitochondrial cytochrome *c* and apoptosis-inducing factor (AIF) and to initiation of the apoptosis cascade via caspase-9. Loss of the mitochondrial membrane potential also results in disruption of oxidative phosphorylation and ATP depletion, and this may also contribute to liver cell death.[12]

Focus on Fas. Perhaps the best-studied extrinsic trigger of hepatocyte apoptosis is engagement of the cell surface receptor, Fas (CD95/APO-1), a member of the tumor necrosis/nerve growth factor receptor family that is highly expressed on activated lymphocytes, and also constitutively expressed on a variety of nonlymphoid cells, including hepatocytes. The ligand for Fas, Fas ligand (FasL/CD95L), is a cell surface protein that is expressed by activated T cells in which it mediates lymphocyte homeostasis and, together with the perforin/granzyme system, T-cell cytotoxicity. In addition to lymphocytes, hepatocytes also appear to be capable of expressing FasL in certain situations. Binding of FasL or agonist antibodies (e.g., Jo2) to Fas causes the latter to trimerize, resulting in the recruitment of a series of intracellular molecules in a signaling cascade that activates caspases responsible for degrading cellular components and ultimately results in the morphological features of apoptosis.

A physiological role for Fas in liver homeostasis is suggested by the observation that mice deficient in Fas develop, among other abnormalities, significant liver hyperplasia.[13] Based on immunohistological studies,

Fas is expressed at low levels in a normal human liver, but expression appears to be upregulated in the setting of both acute and chronic liver disease.[14] In particular, Fas-mediated apoptosis plays a major role in development of liver failure from Wilson's disease and viral hepatitis B.[10,15] Hepatocytes constitutively express a lower level of certain antiapoptotic proteins (e.g., Bcl-2 and Bcl-xL) than most other cells, which may partly explain their special sensitivity to Fas-mediated apoptosis. In addition, FasL expression on hepatocytes has also given rise to the idea that under certain circumstances hepatocytes may actively induce apoptosis in neighboring cells, a process termed *fratricide.*

The expression of death receptors, including Fas, on hepatocytes is relatively well established, but expression of these receptors on nonparenchymal cells is less well defined. Fas expression has been demonstrated on murine endothelial cells, stellate cells, and cholangiocytes.[16] When it was reported more than a decade ago that intravenous administration of an activating anti-Fas antibody to mice results in ALF secondary to massive hepatocyte apoptosis and death, it was initially assumed that direct engagement and activation of hepatocyte Fas was responsible. However, injury to sinusoidal endothelial cells appears to play a predominant role in the development of FasL-induced ALF in this model, highlighting that injury and death of nonparenchymal cells, as opposed to hepatocytes, may be critical to the development of some forms of ALF.[17]

Recent studies in murine models suggest that inhibiting Fas expression in the liver may prevent or ameliorate ALF (Fig. 3–1). For example, a recent report showed that liver Fas expression could be reduced by RNA interference (RNAi), now a popular method of experimentally knocking down gene expression in cultured cells and in mouse models.[18] Knocking down expression of Fas in this fashion largely protected mice against an otherwise lethal challenge with either an apoptosis-inducing anti-Fas antibody, or concavalin A, which causes immune-mediated liver damage.[19] This work not only directly implicates Fas-mediated apoptosis in liver injury but also suggests that selectively inhibiting this process, in this case by RNAi, may be therapeutic. A similar study using RNAi to decrease expression of caspase-8, a key enzyme in death receptor–mediated apoptosis, also demonstrates a significant therapeutic effect even if the RNAi was initiated after liver injury, in this case by a viral (adenovirus) infection.[20] Likewise, prior studies show that expression of antiapoptotic proteins (e.g., Bcl-2) in hepatocytes may also prevent liver cell apoptosis secondary to a variety of noxious agents. Caution must be exercised with any of these potential therapeutic approaches, however, as inhibition of the apoptosis pathway may redirect cells to the necrosis pathway and also may predispose to neoplasia.

Summary of the Pathogenesis of Acute Liver Failure

The preceding discussion is by necessity incomplete and largely ignores several important areas of research relevant to the pathogenesis of ALF. For example, both pro- and anti-inflammatory cytokines play critical roles in the pathogenesis of ALF. Interferon-γ, a proinflammatory cytokine involved in macrophage and T-lymphocyte activation, mediates liver cell injury in a mouse model of hepatitis B. Similarly, by acting through interferon-γ, IL-12 appears to play a role in liver injury in some murine models of ALF.[10]

A variety of cytokines, including IL-10, IL-11, IL-13, and IL-4, protect against liver injury when administered to mice, presumably by downregulating proinflammatory cytokines, nitric oxide, and reactive oxygen species. Preliminary immunocytochemical analysis of livers from patients with ALF suggests that an imbalance of proinflammatory (interferon-γ) and anti-inflammatory (IL-12 and IL-10) cytokines may, in fact, contribute to the pathogenesis of liver failure.[21] Nitric oxide—a gas that is generated during enzymatic conversion of L-arginine to L-citrulline by hepatocytes, Kupffer cells, and endothelial cells—is both constitutively expressed and induced by proinflammatory cytokines (e.g., TNF-α) in the liver and may contribute to oxidative stress in certain situations (e.g., acetaminophen toxicity).[10] However, nitric oxide may also have protective effects, and its role in liver injury is still incompletely defined.

The relative rarity of ALF speaks to the resiliency of the liver, which is normally capable of withstanding tremendous insults caused by an impressive array or protective, repair, and regenerative mechanisms. It is only in the rare situations, when these mechanisms are critically impaired or have been overwhelmed, that clinically overt liver failure becomes manifest. Despite its relative rarity, ALF represents an important medical problem because it typically affects young, otherwise healthy individuals and is associated with high mortality. A more complete understanding of the fundamental molecular mechanisms underlying development of ALF, particularly those responsible for liver cell death and regeneration, is clearly needed before rational therapeutics can be developed. Until that time liver transplantation must continue to be considered for any patient developing ALF.

Cirrhosis

Clinical Manifestations

The majority of individuals whose liver biopsies demonstrate cirrhosis exhibit no symptoms or signs of

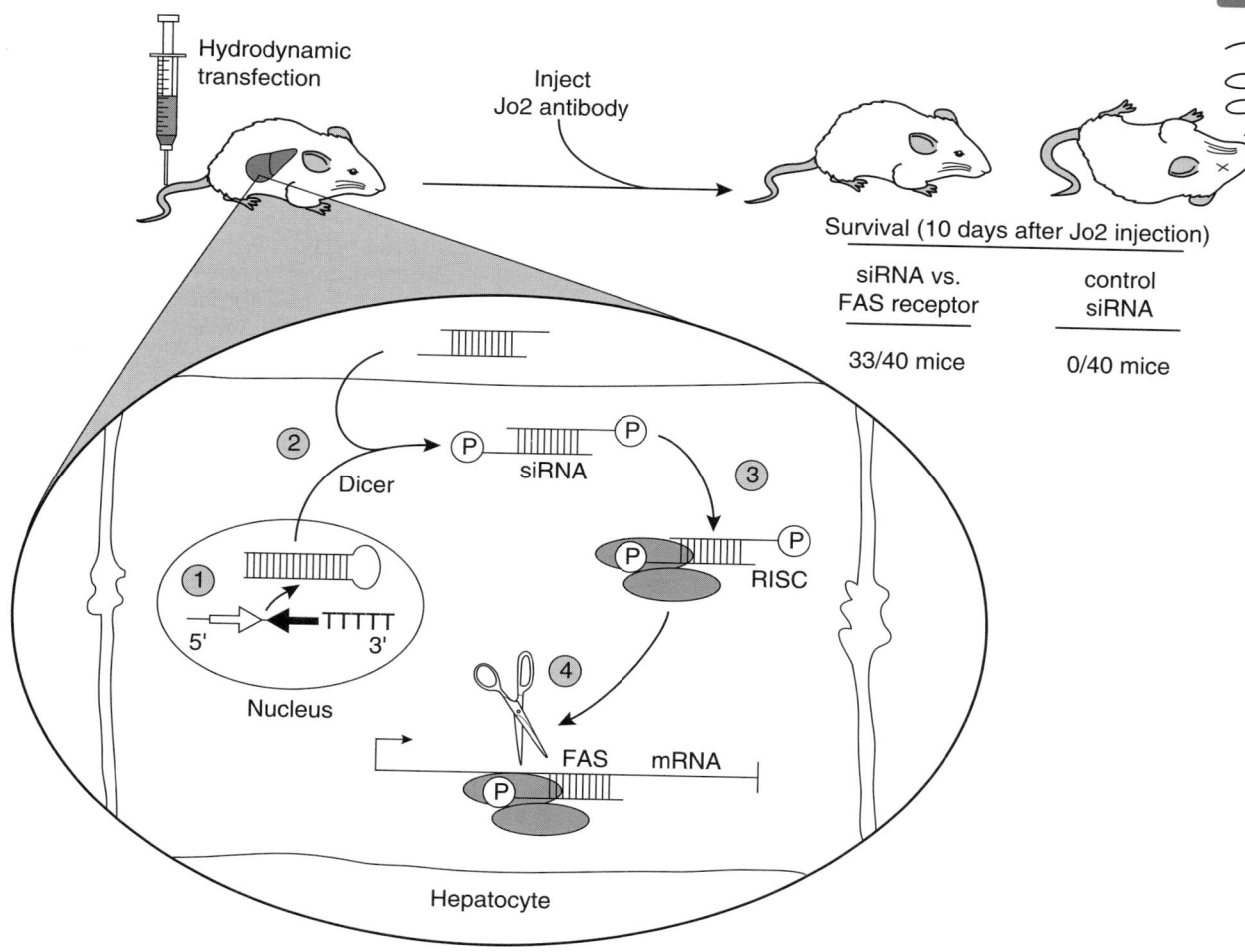

FIGURE 3–1

Knocking down Fas expression improves outcome of mice with acute liver failure (ALF). RNA interference (RNAi) is an evolutionarily conserved, posttranscriptional, homology-dependent gene-silencing mechanism used by eukaryotic cells to target destruction of mRNA. RNAi has been exploited as a powerful and popular experimental method to knock down gene expression with great precision both in cultured cells and in mice.[18] Within cells, RNAi is initiated by small interfering RNA (siRNA), a double-stranded form of RNA that is 21 to 23 bases in length, usually generated by cleavage of larger double-stranded transcripts by an endonuclease complex (*Dicer*). Experimentally, RNAi can also be accomplished by expressing siRNA precursors (small, hairpin RNAs) from DNA templates *(1)* or by introducing synthetic siRNA directly into cells *(2)* by transfection. siRNAs introduced into cells by either route assemble with a multiprotein complex, termed *RNA-inducing silencing complex* (RISC), *(3)* that uses the siRNA as a guide to identify and degrade homologous mRNA target sequence, thus acting as a sequence-specific nuclease *(4)*. In the study by Song and colleagues,[19] investigators used a technique called hydrodynamic transfection to deliver and express anti-Fas siRNAs in a mouse liver to specifically decrease Fas expression. Mice treated in this fashion were largely resistant to the subsequent administration of an activating anti-Fas antibody (Jo2), which otherwise results in uniformly lethal ALF by inducing massive hepatocyte apoptosis.

liver disease, and their tests for liver synthetic function are intact. Clinically silent cirrhosis, however, can progress, eventually compromising hepatocyte function and hepatic circulation. If cirrhosis becomes sufficiently severe, liver failure and portal hypertension can occur. The first signs of advanced cirrhosis are commonly laboratory abnormalities, which can include thrombocytopenia, prolonged prothrombin time, hyperbilirubinemia, or hypoalbuminemia. When cirrhosis causes hepatic

decompensation, any or all of the following clinical manifestations can occur (see Table 3–1):

- Encephalopathy
- Variceal bleeding
- Peripheral edema, ascites, and spontaneous bacterial peritonitis
- Hepatorenal and hepatopulmonary syndromes
- Muscle atrophy

- Coagulopathy
- Jaundice

Although some of these complications (e.g., variceal bleeding, spontaneous bacterial peritonitis, hepatorenal syndrome) are in themselves life-threatening, the prognosis for any patient with decompensated cirrhosis is poor and warrants consideration for liver transplantation.

Etiology

Nearly all causes of chronic liver injury can produce fibrosis and lead to the development of cirrhosis (see Table 3–2). Hepatitis B is the most common cause of cirrhosis worldwide. Cirrhosis will develop in 25% to 33% of the estimated 400 million individuals chronically infected with hepatitis B throughout the world. In the United States, the most common causes of cirrhosis are nonalcoholic fatty liver (NAFL), alcoholism, and hepatitis C. NAFL was recently recognized as a major cause of cirrhosis in industrialized nations, in which up to 5% of the population has NAFL. The proportion of those with NAFL that progresses to cirrhosis is not known, but emerging data indicate that NAFL may be the principal cause of cryptogenic cirrhosis among those undergoing evaluation for liver transplantation. Alcoholism is reported to contribute to 40% to 90% of cases of cirrhosis in North America and Europe. Alcohol-associated cirrhosis is a leading indication for this surgery. Hepatitis C is the primary indication for liver transplantation. One hundred million persons around the world are chronically infected with hepatitis C, with approximately 4 million cases in the United States. Of those with hepatitis C, 15% to 20% of livers are believed to progress to cirrhosis. Currently, approximately 60% of those receiving liver transplants are chronically infected with hepatitis C. Table 3–2 lists other less common causes of cirrhosis.

Pathogenesis

Over the past 2 decades, substantial effort has been made to elucidate the molecular and cellular mechanisms underlying the development of cirrhosis. Because space constraints only permit us to provide an overview, the reader is directed to a number of excellent reviews for a deeper examination of the pathogenesis of cirrhosis.[22-32] In the discussion to follow, primary references are provided for data that are not already found in these comprehensive review articles. Cirrhosis is distinguished by increased deposition and altered composition of ECM components in the portal tracts, around the central veins, or in the perisinusoidal spaces of the liver. This pathological surplus of ECM, termed *fibrosis*, can progress to distort the liver's lobular and microvascular

architecture (i.e., cirrhosis). If sufficiently severe, fibrosis can result in compromised hepatocyte function. The alterations in hepatic structure and function associated with cirrhosis are similar regardless of the cause of chronic liver injury, which indicates that the general mechanisms underlying fibrosis of the liver are shared. Two populations of fibrogenic cell types, hepatic stellate cells and hepatic myofibroblasts, mediate hepatic fibrosis.

Hepatic Stellate Cells and Myofibroblasts Mediate the Liver's Response to Injury

Hepatic stellate cells, also called Ito cells or hepatic lipocytes, occupy the space of Disse (i.e., perisinusoidal space). In a normal liver, these cells have a star-like appearance radially extending numerous cytoplasmic protrusions that contact the basal face of the hepatocytes and run along and encircle the endothelial cells that line the sinusoids (Fig. 3–2). It is partly the anatomic location of stellate cells, along with circumstantial experimental evidence, that suggests these cells modulate sinusoidal blood flow and enhance solute exchange within the perisinusoidal space. Stellate cells also synthesize small amounts of extracellular matrix proteins, including laminin and type IV collagen, which make up the basement membrane. A notable attribute of this cell type is that it displays prominent cytosolic vesicles in which retinoids, including vitamin A, are stored. In addition, stellate cells release soluble growth factors, cytokines, and peptides that contribute to liver

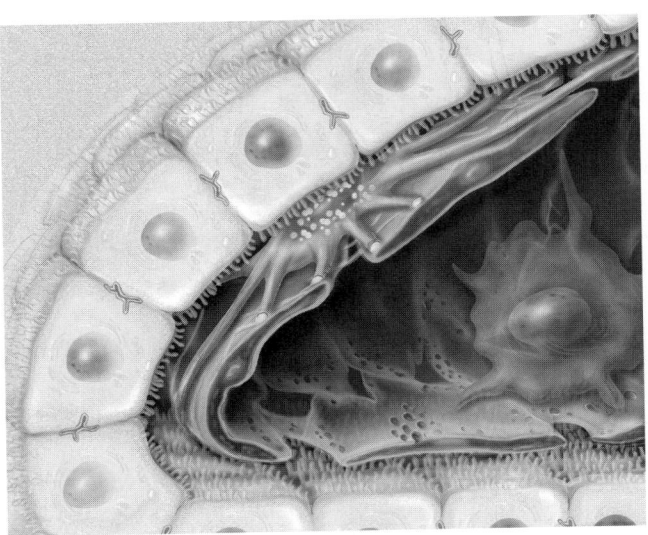

FIGURE 3–2

The three-dimensional microanatomy of the liver. The stellate cell occupies the perisinusoidal space between the hepatocytes and sinusoidal endothelial cells. Note the defining star-like shape with protrusions extending around the sinusoid. (From Friedman SL, Arthur MJP: Targeting hepatic fibrosis. Sci Med 8:194-205, 2002.)

cell development, differentiation, and survival. Thus, under normal conditions, stellate cells store vitamin A, support the homeostasis of hepatocytes and the endothelium, and may contribute to regulation of the microcirculation.

Hepatic injury provokes the release of diverse soluble and insoluble mediators generated by hepatocytes, sinusoidal endothelia, biliary epithelia, Kupffer cells and other leukocytes, stellate cells and hepatic myofibroblasts, and platelets. These injury-induced factors stimulate a wound-healing response in which stellate cells migrate to the site of insult, proliferate at that site, produce ECM (fibrogenesis), and place tension across the ECM. These stellate cell responses facilitate parenchymal restitution after an acute hepatic insult. If liver injury resolves, stellate cell chemotaxis and proliferation end, excess stellate cells undergo apoptosis, and surplus ECM is broken down (fibrolysis) by extracellular matrix metalloproteinases (MMPs). In this way, the wound-repair response is terminated once injury has resolved and tissue healing has been accomplished.

However, if liver injury persists, hepatic myofibroblasts (mesenchymally derived cells located primarily adjacent to the portal triads and central veins) are also recruited to affected sites. Chronic hepatic injury stimulates both hepatic myofibroblasts and stellate cells to proliferate, lay down ECM, and mediate contraction-dependent remodeling of ECM. Clearly, synthesis of extracellular matrix components (e.g., collagens and fibronectins) is essential for the development of fibrosis, but other properties of these fibrogenic cells are also necessary. For example, chemotaxis and proliferation augment the number of stellate cells and hepatic myofibroblasts located within areas of liver injury, which intensifies the synthesis and remodeling of ECM. Remodeling of ECM also requires regulation of extracellular MMP activity and the contractile tension generated by the fibrogenic cells. Accumulation of excess ECM in the form of contracted fibrotic bands can result from chronic liver injury. Thus, fibrosis occurs when injury-induced stimuli persist and keep the homeostatic balance tipped toward migration, proliferation, fibrogenesis, and contraction and away from apoptosis, fibrolysis, and relaxation. From a molecular perspective, fibrosis is the combined result of the sustained effects of a series of diverse extracellular stimuli on many interconnected signaling pathways that differentially modulate critical dynamic and well-coordinated behaviors of the fibrogenic cells of the liver (Fig. 3–3).

Fibrosis is a Consequence of the Liver's Response to Chronic Injury

During injury, the behavior of stellate cells and hepatic myofibroblasts is regulated by paracrine interactions with damaged hepatocytes and endothelial cells; activated

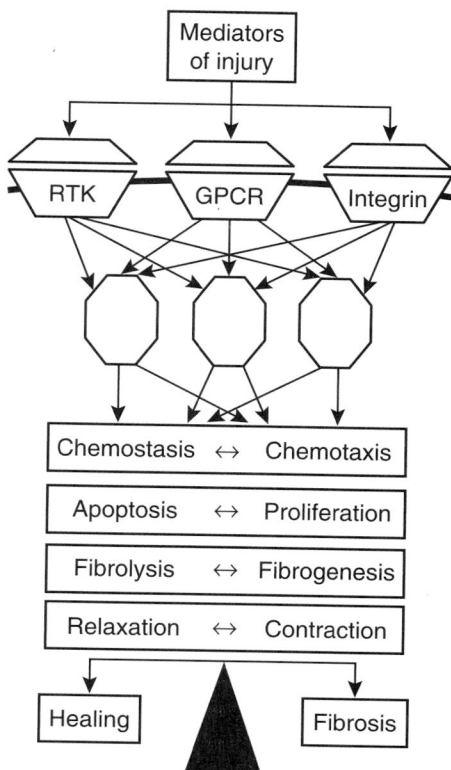

FIGURE 3–3

In this proposed model for the liver's injury response, fibrosis is the combined result of the effects of a series of diverse extracellular mediators of injury on many interconnected signaling pathways that differentially modulate dynamic and well-coordinated behaviors of the fibrogenic cells of the liver. Whether normal healing or fibrosis occurs depends on the location, duration, and intensity of the injury response.

platelets, Kupffer cells, and infiltrating leukocytes; and other stellate cells and hepatic myofibroblasts. These interactions are mediated by growth factors, regulatory peptides and lipids, cytokines, extracellular matrix components, and toxic metabolites (Table 3–4). Injured hepatocytes can release highly toxic compounds, such as reactive oxygen intermediates (ROI) and lipid peroxides, that can induce activation of Kupffer cells and leukocytes. Hepatocytes can also produce inflammatory mediators including insulin-like growth factor-1 and vascular endothelial growth factor. Activated Kupffer cells and other leukocytes can also generate ROI and lipid peroxides, as well as soluble agents such as TGF-β, platelet-derived growth factor (PDGF), TNF-α, interferon-γ, and IL-1, IL-2, IL-6, IL-10, and IL-13. Sinusoidal endothelial cells can influence the injury response by producing laminin and a splice variant of fibronectin (EIIIA isoform), converting latent TGF-β to the active form through the activation of plasmin, and secreting ET-1 and nitric oxide. Platelets also produce TGF-β and PDGF and are the principal source of regulatory lipids,

Table 3–4. EFFECTS OF SELECTED MEDIATORS OF HEPATIC FIBROSIS

Molecule	Source	Effects on Fibrogenic Cell Functions
RECEPTOR TYROSINE KINASE LIGANDS		
Transforming GF-β	K, F, E, P	(+) fibrogenesis, migration; (−) proliferation, fibrolysis
Platelet-derived GF	B, K, F, P	(+) proliferation; (±) migration; (−) contraction
Insulin-like GF-1	H, E, P	(+) proliferation
Epidermal GF	P	(+) proliferation, migration
Vascular endothelial GF	H, F, E, P	(+) proliferation; (−) contraction
G-PROTEIN–COUPLED RECEPTOR LIGANDS		
Endothelin-1	E, F	(+) migration, contraction; (±) proliferation
Lysophosphatidic acid	P	(+) migration, contraction
Angiotensin II	F	(+) proliferation, fibrogenesis, contraction
Thrombin	F	(+) proliferation, contraction
Leptin	F	(+) fibrogenesis; (−) fibrolysis
Tumor necrosis factor-α (TNF-α)	K	(+) apoptosis
Interleukin-1	K, E	(+) fibrogenesis
Interleukin-4	K	(+) fibrogenesis
Interleukin-6	K	(+) fibrogenesis
Interleukin-10	K	(−) fibrogenesis
Interleukin-13	K	(+) fibrogenesis
Interferon-γ	K	(−) fibrogenesis, migration
Monocyte chemotactic protein-1	F	(+) migration
INTEGRIN RECEPTOR LIGANDS		
Collagen I	F	(+) proliferation, migration, fibrolysis
Collagen III	F	(+) proliferation
Collagen IV	F	(+) proliferation, fibrolysis; (−) fibrogenesis
Fibronectin	E, F	(+) fibrogenesis
MISCELLANEOUS FACTORS		
Reactive oxygen intermediates	H, K, E	(+) fibrogenesis
Lipid peroxides	H, K	(+) fibrogenesis
Nitric oxide	E, H, K	(−) proliferation, contraction

B, biliary epithelium; E, sinusoidal endothelium; F, stellate cells and myofibroblasts; GF, growth factor; H, hepatocytes; K, Kuppfer and other inflammatory cells; P, platelets; (+), stimulate; (−), inhibit.

including lysophosphatidic acid and sphingosine-1-phosphate. Stellate cells and hepatic myofibroblasts themselves can secrete soluble and insoluble factors that can act in paracrine or autocrine fashion, including:

- TGF-β
- PDGF
- Vascular endothelial growth factor (VEGF)
- Endothelin-1
- Leptin
- IL-8
- Monocyte chemotactic protein

- Cytokine-induced neutrophil chemoattractant
- Fibronectin
- Laminin
- Collagens I, III, IV, VI, XIV, and XVIII

In addition, significant amounts of certain factors, including PDGF, HGF, VEGF, and TNF-α, can bind to the ECM and be released, particularly during fibrolysis.

The effects of these injury-associated extracellular mediators are primarily transduced by plasma membrane receptors (i.e., receptor tyrosine kinases, G-protein–coupled receptors, and integrins) or intracellular receptors (i.e., nuclear receptors). These receptors in turn act through intracellular signaling pathways that control protein expression or directly regulate the physical behavior of stellate cells and hepatic myofibroblasts. It has become clear that no single mediator or signaling pathway is sufficient to trigger hepatic fibrosis. Moreover, the functional consequence of any given mediator or signaling pathway is not stereotypical, but depends on the timing and subcellular localization of the signal, as well as cross-talk from other pathways. The emerging model for wound healing in the liver is one in which diverse stimuli orchestrate the activation and inhibition of multiple interconnected signal transduction pathways that regulate distinct cellular responses (e.g., chemotaxis-chemostasis, proliferation-apoptosis, fibrogenesis-fibrolysis, contraction-relaxation). In this dynamic model, acute hepatic damage leads to injury-induced signaling that regulates a wound-healing response that requires accumulation of the liver's fibrogenic cells and ECM at the site of injury. If this damage is transient, the injury response ceases once healing has occurred, and normal homeostatic mechanisms result in the removal of surplus fibrogenic cells and ECM. Conversely, during chronic liver disease injury-induced signaling persists, causing a continuing wound-healing response that results in the pathological accumulation of fibrogenic cells and ECM at sites of injury. With time, this sustained wound-healing response can result in the development of fibrosis and, subsequently, cirrhosis. In other words, fibrosis occurs when the net balance of injury-induced signaling is tipped toward the wound-healing response for too long.

Fibrosis Results From a Complex Cascade in Interconnected Signaling Events

Current knowledge is insufficient to provide a complete picture of the pathogenesis of fibrosis. However, a plethora of studies over the past 15 years provides a glimpse into the intricate signaling pathways that govern the wound-healing response. Much of this research has depended on well-characterized stellate cell and hepatic myofibroblast culture models. The relevance of this work is not entirely certain, but key elements have been validated by animal and human studies of liver injury. It is impossible in a short chapter to detail even a modest portion of the myriad molecular and cellular signals that have already been shown to participate in the development of fibrosis. However, it is instructive to discuss the elaborately regulated pleiotropic effects of three injury-associated mediators that play important roles in the liver's wound-healing response.

Effects of Platelet-Derived Growth Factor. PDGF, particularly PDGF-BB, is the strongest chemotactic and mitogenic agent for the fibrogenic cells of the liver. During liver injury, expression of this growth factor and its cognate receptor are highest in areas of greatest damage.

PDGF is secreted in response to injury by platelets, Kupffer cells, stellate cells, and hepatic myofibroblasts. Moreover, it is sequestered by the ECM and can be released during fibrolysis. An early response to injury is the upregulation of PDGF receptors, which enhances the sensitivity of stellate cells to this growth factor. PDGF receptors are members of the receptor tyrosine kinase superfamily that acts via protein phosphorylation cascades. It has been reported that PDGF has an unusual bell-shaped effect on the migration of hepatic myofibroblasts.[33] At lower concentrations of PDGF, migration is stimulated, but at higher concentrations migration is inhibited. PDGF induces migration through signaling pathways that involve phosphatidylinositol-3 (PI3) kinase, p38 mitogen-activated protein (MAP) kinase, and focal adhesion proteins, including focal adhesion kinase (FAK) and paxillin. Specifically, the effects of p38 MAP kinase on migration are transduced by actin-dependent membrane ruffling and cell spreading.[34] At higher concentrations, PDGF inhibits migration by provoking depolymerization of the actin cytoskeleton and reducing the activity of focal adhesion proteins. Hence, we suggest that early in the injury response, or distant from the injured region, PDGF concentrations are relatively low and stimulate chemotaxis toward the site of damage. Later, during the injury response after fibrogenic cells have migrated into the affected area, PDGF concentrations would be relatively high and the migratory response should be attenuated. Thus, the bell-shaped PDGF dose-response relationship for migration suggests a novel mechanism for accumulating fibrogenic cells within injured areas.

PDGF is also a potent stimulus for the proliferation of fibrogenic cells in the liver. However, PDGF-induced proliferation is mediated primarily by pathways that signal through Ras/MEK (mitogen-activating protein ERK kinase)/ERK, rather than p38 MAP kinase.[34] Additionally, Ca^{2+} and H^+ signaling pathways appear to be required for the mitogenic response to PDGF. Involvement by phosphoinositol-3 kinase has also been suggested, possibly by enhancing the activity of ERK. It is notable that PDGF does not have a bell-shaped effect on proliferation. One might predict that fibrogenic cells would continue to proliferate within injured areas where the PDGF concentration is relatively high, even though chemotaxis would have been shut down at those concentrations. To make matters even more complex, PDGF increases the synthesis of prostaglandin E2, which inhibits proliferation through a cyclic 3′,5′-adenosine monophosphate (cAMP)-dependent mechanism. This implies the possibility of a PDGF-triggered negative feedback loop that would self-limit the growth of these cells. Taken together, these data suggest that PDGF facilitates accumulation of fibrogenic cells within injured areas of the liver through distinct effects on chemotaxis and proliferation that are mediated by discrete signal transduction pathways.

Effects of Transforming Growth Factor-β. TGF-β is the principal stimulus for ECM accumulation. In the cirrhotic livers of humans, the expression of TGF-β is greatest in areas where ECM is most abundant. This cytokine, which is produced by Kupffer cells, platelets, and sinusoidal endothelial cells in response to injury, has paracrine actions on the endothelial cells and fibrogenic cells of the liver. Moreover, TGF-β induces sinusoidal endothelial cells to express a fibronectin splice variant that stimulates stellate cell fibrogenesis. In fibrogenic cells, TGF-β stimulates its own expression, which permits the development of a powerful autocrine-positive feedback loop. TGF-β signaling can also be modulated by the conversion of TGF-β from its latent to its active form by sinusoidal endothelial cells and by augmenting the expression and ligand affinity of TGF-β receptors in the fibrogenic cells of the liver. TGF-β induces the accumulation of ECM by enhancing ECM synthesis and reducing ECM degradation. First, TGF-β enhances the transcription of collagen I, the predominant ECM component observed in cirrhosis, probably by reducing the expression of negative regulators of transcription and through putative TGF-β responsive elements in the gene encoding for collagen I. TGF-β also upregulates synthesis of other ECM components, including fibronectin and proteoglycan. Second, TGF-β inhibits ECM degradation by reducing synthesis of important matrix metalloproteinases (e.g., MMP-1, MMP-2, MMP-3) and by upregulating plasminogen activator inhibitor (PAI) and tissue inhibitors of metalloproteinases (TIMPs), which are proteins that inhibit the breakdown of ECM.

In addition to regulating the accumulation of ECM, TGF-β also modulates other processes important for the development of fibrosis. TGF-β stimulates the migration of stellate cells and inhibits apoptosis. Surprisingly, in different studies, TGF-β stimulated, inhibited, or had no effect on proliferation. It is uncertain whether this phenomenon has physiological importance or is simply a technical artifact. It is significant, however, that TGF-β upregulates the expression of PDGF receptors, which play a fundamental role in fibrosis, as described previously. Although the molecular mechanisms linking TGF-β to its observed effects on fibrogenic cells are incompletely understood, evidence suggests that they involve the regulation of transcription by pathways that signal through Sma and Mad (SMAD)-related proteins, MEK and ERK, and hydrogen peroxide and C/EBP-β.

Effects of Endothelin-1. Endothelin-1 (ET-1) is a vasoactive peptide that strongly stimulates generation of contractile tension by the fibrogenic cells of the liver. Sinusoidal endothelial cells and fibrogenic cells secrete this peptide in response to hepatic injury. ET-1 binds to ET_A and ET_B receptors, which are G-protein–coupled seven-transmembrane receptors. Binding of ET-1 to its cognate receptors causes an augmentation of myosin light-chain phosphorylation through G-protein–coupled activation of Ca^{2+}-dependent myosin light-chain kinase and rho-dependent inhibition of myosin phosphatase.[35] Phosphorylation of the myosin light chain activates myosin, which interacts with bundles of polymerized actin, resulting in the generation of tension. The tension generated by these fibrogenic cells permits orientation and remodeling of the ECM. Evidence also suggests that alterations in the tension generated by stellate cells, which encircle the sinusoids, modulates hepatic blood flow.[30,36]

In addition to its role in the regulation of contractile tension, ET-1 modulates the migration and proliferation of fibrogenic cells in the liver. The effect of ET-1 on migration is predicted by the essential role that retrograde contraction plays in cellular locomotion. As expected, ET-1 stimulates migration through a rho-associated, kinase-dependent pathway. The role that this peptide plays in the regulation of proliferation is more complex. ET_A stimulates proliferation through Ras/MEK/ERK-signaling pathways, whereas ET_B inhibits proliferation through a prostaglandin/cAMP-signaling pathway. Since the relative ratio of ET_B:ET_A increases with time after injury, the effects of ET-1 on cell growth change with the duration of injury.

As discussed, PDGF, TGF-β, and ET-1 each act via multiple signal transduction pathways to regulate patterns of cellular behavior that are essential for the development of cirrhosis:

- PDGF is a powerful regulator of chemotaxis and proliferation.
- TGF-β strongly induces the accumulation of ECM, but also facilitates migration and inhibits apoptosis.
- ET-1 is a strong agonist for contraction, but also affects chemotaxis and proliferation.

Yet, PDGF, TGF-β, and ET-1 represent only three of the numerous soluble and insoluble molecules that are produced in response to hepatic injury (see Table 3–4). All of these other injury mediators also have pleiotropic effects that are mediated by signal transduction pathways that work in a coordinated manner. Thus, the molecular and cellular mechanisms underlying the development of cirrhosis are incredibly complex. Despite this complexity, there have been advances to develop preventive and therapeutic strategies for the management of cirrhosis. Indeed, pharmacological antagonists of each of the three injury mediators discussed here prevent or reduce fibrosis in animal models of chronic liver injury.[23,26,32]

Summary of the Pathogenesis of Cirrhosis

It is increasingly clear that fibrosis of the liver is mediated by the same molecular signals and cellular processes that govern the normal wound-healing response. It is the location, duration, and intensity of liver injury that dictate clinical outcome. For example, in most forms of chronic liver injury, including hepatitis C and autoimmune hepatitis, fibrosis is initially most prominent in the portal region, the location most affected by these diseases. In contrast, alcoholic and nonalcoholic steatohepatitis, both of which are characterized by early lobular injury, initially display lobular fibrosis, especially around the sinusoids. If hepatic injury is transient, such as occurs with hepatitis A, complete healing occurs without any evidence of excess accumulation of ECM. Conversely, liver fibrosis occurs only months to decades after onset of chronic hepatic injury. The clinical observation that only a portion of patients suffering from chronic liver diseases—such as hepatitis B and C, alcoholic and nonalcoholic steatohepatitis, and hereditary hemochromatosis—develop cirrhosis suggests that there may be an intensity threshold for a given individual that must be crossed in order for fibrosis to ensue. Finally, it has become generally recognized that if the source of chronic liver injury is removed, fibrosis can be reversed.[27,32,37] This has been demonstrated in a number of liver diseases, including biliary obstruction, hepatitis C, and autoimmune hepatitis. Whether cirrhosis itself can be significantly reversed remains controversial. The pathogenesis of cirrhosis is complex and is mediated by the dynamic and multifaceted response of the fibrogenic cells of the liver to chronic injury.

Perspectives and Future Directions

Why some patients develop ALF rather than self-limited hepatitis remains an important, but as yet unanswered, question. The same questions can be applied to cirrhosis; a large majority of patients with chronic liver disease never develop cirrhosis. There are undoubtedly genetic polymorphisms that predispose to ALF or cirrhosis. Indeed, the host response to injury is as likely as or even more important than the inciting agent or disease. If these genetic differences can be elucidated, it is likely that novel and therapeutic strategies for ALF and cirrhosis will be developed. At a minimum, an improved ability to assess prognosis would enhance the management of patients with acute and chronic liver disease.

A better understanding of the molecular pathogenesis of ALF and cirrhosis will undoubtedly translate into improved therapies in the future. In the case of ALF, such therapy will be directed toward limiting cell death by blocking harmful responses while preserving or even enhancing the liver's innate ability to repair and regenerate. For example, new forms of therapy might focus on modifying the early inflammatory events, interrupting apoptotic- and growth-inhibitory pathways, and providing temporary liver support to allow time for hepatic regeneration and repair. However, as noted earlier, specifically inhibiting apoptosis may be problematic in that this may redirect cells toward the generally more destructive necrotic cell death pathway and also potentially promote cancer. Likewise, cytokines may have both detrimental and protective roles in ALF, and anti-cytokine therapy may thus have unanticipated consequences. For example, in a clinical trial of sepsis, a TNF-α antagonist increased mortality, and it is conceivable that such therapy used for ALF might also inhibit hepatic regeneration and worsen outcomes. Because some of the same molecular pathways critical in liver regeneration are also involved in cell death, therapeutic targets will need to be chosen with great care.

In the case of cirrhosis, efforts will be directed toward the prevention or reversal of fibrosis. This will not be a simple task for two major reasons. First, fibrosis results from the liver's response to injury, albeit a sustained and exuberant response. Thus, safe and effective therapies for cirrhosis must blunt the injury response that causes fibrosis without compromising the normal wound-healing response. Second, the large majority of patients with chronic liver disease do not develop cirrhosis, and even those who do, often live many years before developing clinical disease. Therefore, improved strategies for determining which patients have the greatest disposition to progressing to decompensated cirrhosis are critical. Otherwise, any successful therapy for prevention must be very safe, because a large number of patients need to be treated for one to benefit. It is likely that a greatly increased understanding of the molecular and cellular mechanisms underlying fibrosis will be required to overcome the hurdles necessary to create effective and safe therapies for cirrhosis.

References

1. Ostapowicz G, Fontana RJ, Schiodt FV, et al: Results of a prospective study of acute liver failure at 17 tertiary care centers in the United States. Ann Intern Med 137:947-954, 2002.
2. Schiodt FV, Davern TJ, Shakil AO, et al: Viral hepatitis-related acute liver failure. Am J Gastroenterol 98:448-453, 2003.
3. Rozga J: Hepatocyte proliferation in health and in liver failure. Med Sci Monit 8:RA32-38, 2002.
4. Thomson RK, Arthur MJ: Mechanisms of liver cell damage and repair. Eur J Gastroenterol Hepatol 11:949-955, 1999.
5. Tangkijvanich P, Melton AC, Santiskulvong C, et al: Rho and p38 MAP kinase signaling pathways mediate LPA-stimulated hepatic myofibroblast migration. J Biomed Sci 10:352-358, 2003.
6. Grompe M, Laconi E, Shafritz DA: Principles of therapeutic liver repopulation. Semin Liver Dis 19:7-14, 1999.
7. Lagasse EH, Connors M, Al-Dhalimy, et al: Purified hematopoietic stem cells can differentiate into hepatocytes in vivo. Nat Med 6:1229-1234, 2000.
8. Fausto N: Liver regeneration: From laboratory to clinic. Liver Transpl 7:835-844, 2001.
9. Kaplowitz N: Biochemical and cellular mechanisms of toxic liver injury. Semin Liver Dis 22:137-144, 2002.
10. Riordan SM, Williams R: Mechanisms of hepatocyte injury, multiorgan failure, and prognostic criteria in acute liver failure. Semin Liver Dis 23:203-215, 2003.

11. Ockner RK: Apoptosis and liver diseases: Recent concepts of mechanism and significance. J Gastroenterol Hepatol 16:248-260, 2001.
12. Losser MR, Payen D: Mechanisms of liver damage. Semin Liver Dis 16:357-367, 1996.
13. Galle PR, Krammer PH: CD95-induced apoptosis in human liver disease. Semin Liver Dis 18:141-151, 1998.
14. Ryo K, Kamogawa Y, Ikeda I, et al: Significance of Fas antigen-mediated apoptosis in human fulminant hepatic failure. Am J Gastroenterol 95:2047-2055, 2000.
15. Galle PR, Hofmann WK, Walczak H, et al: Involvement of the CD95 (APO-1/Fas) receptor and ligand in liver damage. J Exp Med 182:1223-1230, 1995.
16. Yoon JH, Gores GJ: Death receptor-mediated apoptosis and the liver. J Hepatol 37:400-410, 2002.
17. Kaplowitz N: Mechanisms of liver cell injury. J Hepatol 32(1 Suppl):39-47, 2000.
18. Davern TJ: Increasing the RISC for HCV. Gastroenterology 125:1546-1548, 2003.
19. Song E, Lee SK, Wang J, et al: RNA interference targeting Fas protects mice from fulminant hepatitis. Nat Med 9:347-351, 2003.
20. Zender L, Hutker S, Liedtke C, et al: Caspase 8 small interfering RNA prevents acute liver failure in mice. Proc Natl Acad Sci U S A 100(13):7797-7802, 2003.
21. Leifeld L, Cheng S, Ramakers J, et al: Imbalanced intrahepatic expression of interleukin 12, interferon gamma, and interleukin 10 in fulminant hepatitis B. Hepatology 36(4 Pt 1):1001-1008, 2002.
22. Benyon RC, Arthur MJ: Extracellular matrix degradation and the role of hepatic stellate cells. Semin Liver Dis 21(3):373-384, 2001.
23. Bissell DM, Maher JJ: Hepatic fibrosis and cirrhosis. In Zakim D, Boyer TD (eds): Hepatology: A Textbook of Liver Disease. Philadelphia, WB Saunders, 2003, pp 395-416.
24. Brenner DA, Rippe RA: Pathogenesis of hepatic fibrosis. In Yamada T (ed): Textbook of Gastroenterology. Philadelphia, Lippincott Williams & Wilkins, 2003, pp 605-620.
25. Friedman SL: Molecular regulation of hepatic fibrosis, an integrated cellular response to tissue injury. J Biol Chem 275:2247-2250, 2000.
26. Friedman SL: Hepatic Fibrosis. In Schiff ER, Sorrell MF, Maddrey WC (eds): Schiff's Diseases of the Liver. Philadelphia, Lippincott Williams & Wilkins, 2003, pp 409-427.
27. Iredale JP: Cirrhosis: New research provides a basis for rational and targeted treatments. BMJ 327:143-147, 2003.
28. Pinzani M, Marra F: Cytokine receptors and signaling in hepatic stellate cells. Semin Liver Dis 21:397-416, 2001.
29. Ramadori G, Armbrust T: Cytokines in the liver. Eur J Gastroenterol Hepatol 13:777-784, 2001.
30. Rockey DC: Hepatic blood flow regulation by stellate cells in normal and injured liver. Semin Liver Dis 21(3):337-349, 2001.
31. Schuppan D, Ruehl M, Somasundaram R, et al: Matrix as a modulator of hepatic fibrogenesis. Semin Liver Dis 21:351-372, 2001.
32. Tangkijvanich P, Yee HF Jr: Cirrhosis—Can we reverse hepatic fibrosis? Eur J Surg (Suppl) 587:100-112, 2002.
33. Tangkijvanich P, Melton AC, Chitapanarux T, et al: Platelet-derived growth factor-Bβ and lysophosphatidic acid distinctly regulate hepatic myofibroblast migration through focal adhesion kinase. Exp Cell Res 281:140-147, 2002.
34. Tangkijvanich P, Santiskulvong C, Melton AC, et al: p38 MAP kinase mediates platelet-derived growth factor–stimulated migration of hepatic myofibroblasts. J Cell Physiol 191:351-561, 2002.
35. Saab S, Tam SP, Tran BN, et al: Myosin mediates contractile force generation by hepatic stellate cells in response to endothelin-1. J Biomed Sci 9(6 Pt 2):607-612, 2002.
36. Thimgan MS, Yee HF Jr: Quantitation of rat hepatic stellate cell contraction: Stellate cells' contribution to sinusoidal resistance. Am J Physiol 277(1 Pt 1):G137-143, 1999.
37. Friedman SL, Arthur MJP: Targeting hepatic fibrosis. Sci Med 8:194-205, 2002.

4

Influence of Liver Transplantation on Liver Surgery

GARRETT M. HISATAKE
JONATHAN R. HIATT

Physiology and anatomy of the liver and biliary system 57
  Liver growth and regeneration 57
  Hepatic vascular and biliary anatomy 58

Operative techniques 58
  Exposure and mobilization of the liver 58
  Liver trauma 59
  Liver resection 60
  Biliary reconstruction 61

Surgical education 61

Summary 61

Liver transplantation is now accepted as the gold standard treatment for patients with end-stage liver disease. The tremendous success of liver transplantation has produced a ripple effect on many other medical and scientific disciplines and, in particular, on conventional liver surgery. The anatomic principles, technical refinements, and basic scientific underpinnings of liver transplantation have immediate relevance to the work of surgeons with interests in nontransplant hepatobiliary surgery, trauma surgery, surgical critical care, and surgical education. The addition of transplantation as a therapeutic option for patients who were previously considered at high risk for standard surgical therapy (such as those with potentially resectable hepatic malignancies complicated by cirrhosis) has changed management algorithms and timing of interventions that alter portal and biliary anatomy prior to definitive therapy. This chapter examines the effects of the liver transplantation experience on modern hepatobiliary surgery.

Physiology and Anatomy of the Liver and Biliary System

Liver Growth and Regeneration

It is commonly accepted that the liver occupies a central role in the complex metabolic interactions among organ systems occurring during stress and illness. This delicate homeostasis is further balanced by the remarkable capacity of the liver to expand hepatocyte mass rapidly in response to changing metabolic demands or significant hepatic injury. Simultaneous advances in critical care, anesthetic management, pharmacology, and oncology have paralleled the advances in liver transplantation over the last 4 decades, stimulating a rapid growth of research in hepatic regeneration, ischemia-reperfusion (I-R) injury, and fulminant hepatic failure.[1,2]

Gene expression in the regenerating hepatocytes has been studied, and hepatocyte growth factors, which accumulate in the serum after partial resections, have been identified and characterized.[3] These hepatotropic factors may be synthesized in the liver or other tissues and include epidermal growth factor, insulin, glucagon, norepinephrine, vasopressin, transforming growth factors, and others. Of particular importance is the recent discovery that early activation of the cytokines interleukin (IL)-6 and tumor necrosis factor-alpha (TNF-α) serves to trigger the regenerative response.[4] These factors are produced in large quantities immediately following liver injury; preliminary evidence supports the bone marrow–derived Kupffer cells as their primary source.[5] Finally, growing evidence suggests that the same cytokine-dependent activation processes that drive hepatic regeneration are also responsible for the physiological and histological changes typically seen in post-transplant I-R injury.[6]

This research is potentially applicable to treatment of patients with loss of liver substance from a variety of causes, including inflammation, infection, trauma, and surgical resection. It also may offer a better understanding of the phenomenon of *small-for-size* syndrome, characterized by prolonged cholestasis and graft dysfunction after partial and living donor liver grafts.[7]

Hepatic Vascular and Biliary Anatomy

The donor and recipient hepatectomy procedures offer a broad experience in upper abdominal surgery and provide supreme lessons in surgical anatomy, including exposure, surgical approach, mobilization techniques, and hepatic vascular isolation, as well as an appreciation for the variations of hepatic vascular and biliary anatomy.

Although deviations from standard hepatic arterial anatomy have been long recognized,[8] the UCLA series of donor hepatectomies shows that these variations are particularly common (Fig. 4–1). In this series,[9] updated to include more than 1500 cases, 26% of donor livers had anomalous hepatic arterial supply, most often a replaced right hepatic artery arising from the superior mesenteric artery (14%), followed by an accessory left hepatic artery arising from the left gastric artery (13%). Arterial patterns, in order of frequency, included:

- Type 1 anatomy, which is normal (n=1,135), with the common hepatic artery arising from the celiac axis to form the gastroduodenal and proper hepatic arteries, and the proper hepatic dividing distally into right and left branches
- Type 3 (n=168), with a replaced or accessory right hepatic artery originating from the superior mesenteric artery
- Type 2 (n=153), with a replaced or accessory left hepatic artery arising from the left gastric artery
- Type 4 (n=43), with both right and left hepatic arteries arising from the superior mesenteric and left gastric arteries, respectively
- Type 5 (n=27), with the entire common hepatic artery arising as a branch of the superior mesenteric artery
- Type 6 (n=3), with the common hepatic artery originating directly from the aorta

Although less common, portal venous and biliary anomalies are also recognized with growing frequency. Nakamura[10] reviewed right lobe hepatectomies for living donor liver transplantation and reported aberrant portal venous anatomy in 7.5% of donors; portal vein trifurcation or an aberrant branch from the left portal vein supplying the right anterior lobe was the most frequent anomaly. Common variants of biliary anatomy include trifurcation of the common hepatic duct into left, right anterior, and right posterior ducts, with no significant length of right hepatic duct (20%), and aberrant drainage of the right posterior duct into the left hepatic duct (5%).[11]

An increasing experience with split-liver and living donor liver transplantation and wider application of surgical treatment for hepatic malignancies obligates familiarity with these anatomic variations, which will provide challenges in complex reconstructions.

Operative Techniques

Exposure and Mobilization of the Liver

Both the donor and recipient operations depend on precise mobilization of the liver by division of the major ligamentous attachments. The approach in which total exposure of the upper abdomen is gained via a transverse upper abdominal incision, with selective use of a sternal extension, has largely eliminated the highly morbid right thoracotomy as a component of elective liver surgery.[12] The principles of liver mobilization and hepatic vascular isolation are particularly applicable to liver trauma and liver resection.

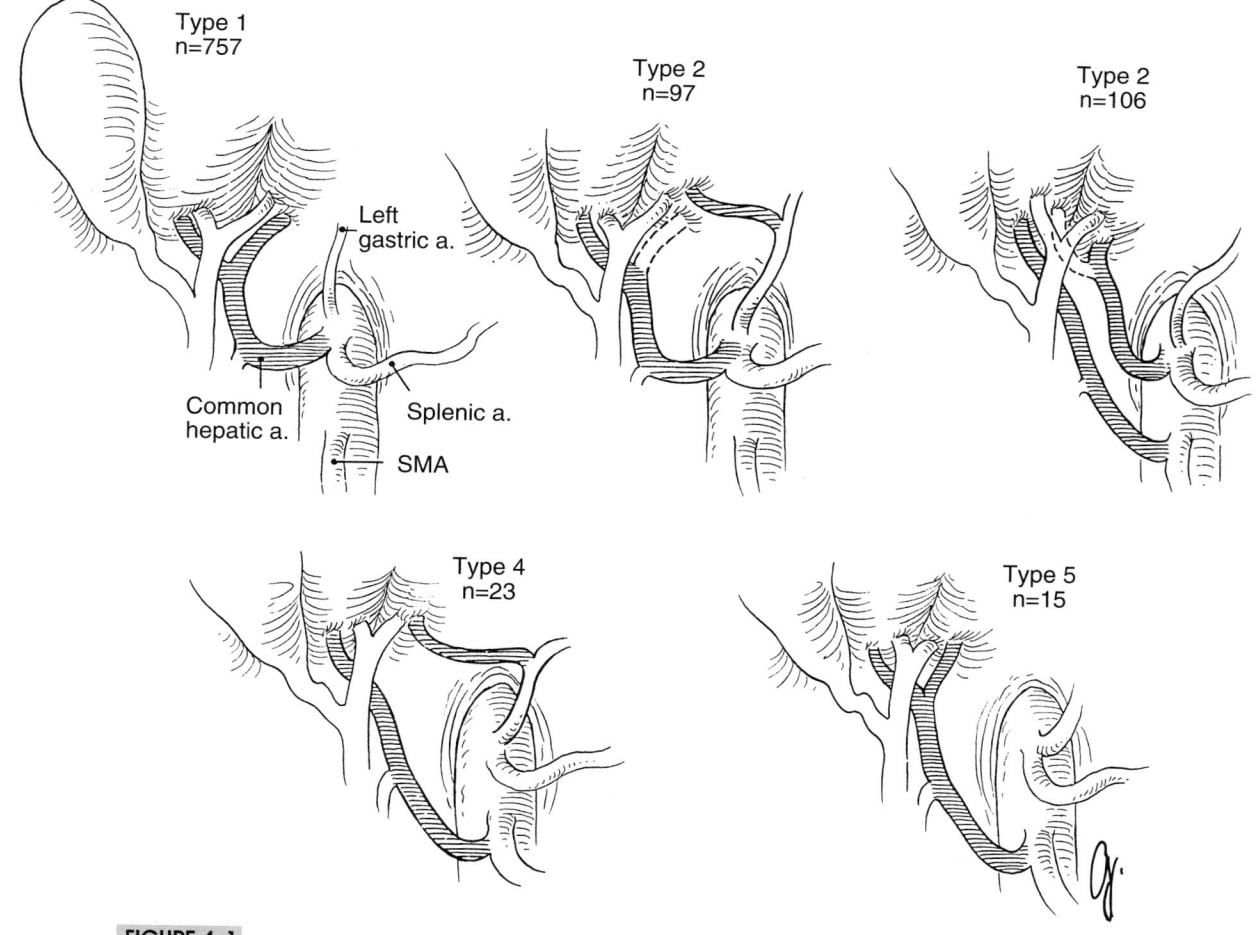

FIGURE 4–1

Hepatic arterial anatomy in 998 cases.[9] Dotted lines indicate that the variant artery may be accessory (if branch shown by dotted line is present) or replaced (if absent). Type 1—normal; Type 2—replaced (accessory) left hepatic artery from left gastric; Type 3—replaced (accessory) right hepatic artery from superior mesenteric artery (SMA); Type 4—double replaced system; Type 5—common hepatic artery (CHA) from SMA. In two patients (not shown), the CHA arose directly from the aorta. (From Hiatt JR, Gabbay J, Busuttil RW: Surgical anatomy of the hepatic arteries in 1000 cases. Ann Surg 220:50-52, Fig. 1, 1994.)

Liver Trauma

The liver and spleen are the solid viscera most commonly injured in major abdominal trauma. Although infrequent, retrohepatic vena caval and hepatic venous injuries are particularly devastating, in part because of difficulty in gaining access to the privileged portion of the right subphrenic space containing the segment of the inferior vena cava (IVC) between the renal veins and the right atrium (Fig. 4–2). In hypovolemic trauma patients, elimination of venous return via the suprahepatic IVC produces cardiac arrest. In contrast, experience from dedicated liver transplant centers demonstrates that in resuscitated euvolemic patients, temporary total occlusion of the portal structures and the vena cavae (Fig. 4–3) is well tolerated[13] and can be combined with a portosystemic shunt procedure to permit treatment of

other injuries or delay of definitive repair until resuscitation is completed. With the addition of aortic occlusion for the hypovolemic patient, vascular isolation continues to play a critical role in management of injuries to the retrohepatic IVC.[14,15] Several reports[16] document the efficacy of total hepatic vascular isolation with selective addition of a portal decompressive procedure for major hepatic trauma.[17,18] In addition, recent evidence suggests that in situ cold perfusion may significantly extend the duration of total vascular isolation tolerated in these patients. For major liver injuries with massive parenchymal destruction, liver avulsion, or unreconstructable damage to the porta hepatis, total hepatectomy with orthotopic transplantation is a potential treatment that has been used occasionally (Fig. 4–4).[19] Taken together, these methods derived from liver transplantation have given surgeons greater

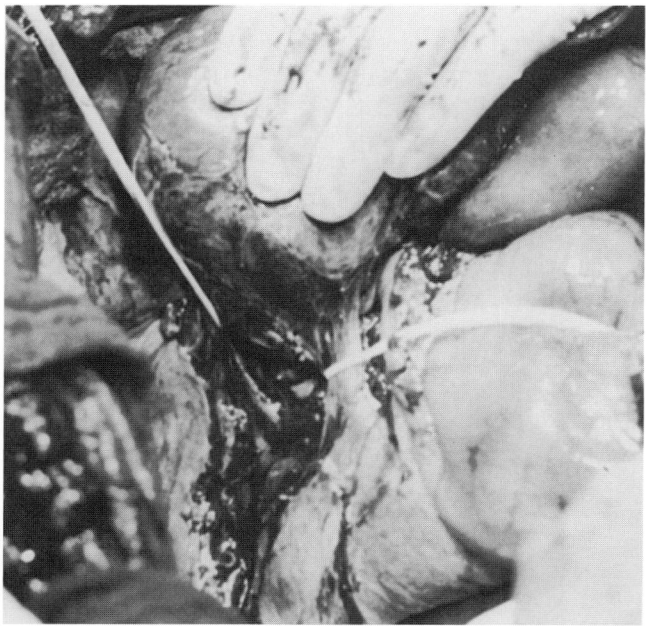

FIGURE 4–2

Dissection of the right retrohepatic space during recipient hepatectomy demonstrates complete access to the retrohepatic vena cava. The right triangular ligament has been divided, the liver is elevated upward and to the left, and the supra- and infrahepatic venae cavae are surrounded with tapes.

ability to treat patients with severe traumatic liver injuries and improved the outlook for patients who previously had few treatment options.

Liver Resection

During the past 25 years, developments in liver resection and liver transplantation have been intertwined.[20] The transplant surgeon's intimate familiarity with subsegmental liver anatomy, further strengthened by experience using reduced-size grafts for transplantation, has immediate application to techniques of liver resection for benign and malignant processes. As an example, the surgical treatment of isolated caudate lobe lesions, once considered extremely hazardous, is now easily accomplished using methods of caval preservation (the *piggyback* technique) and generous exposure gained by dividing the gastrohepatic ligament.[21,22] An emerging concept is one of liver resection and transplantation as a continuum within an *obligatory* armamentarium.[20]

New resectional techniques have improved the surgical approach to challenging liver tumors,[23,24] whereas the use of portal clamping, with or without caval occlusion, diminishes blood loss and allows for safe management of the hepatic veins involved or abutted by the tumor mass.[25] More recent experience using

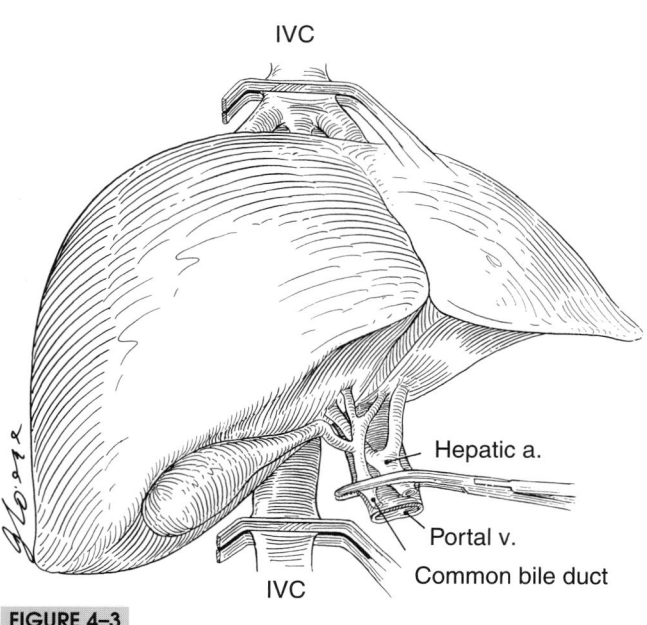

FIGURE 4–3

Technique of hepatic vascular isolation with occlusion of porta hepatis and vena cavae above and below the liver. These methods are used for hepatic resection in euvolemic patients. In the hypovolemic trauma patient, aortic occlusion is added to facilitate repair of injured hepatic veins or retrohepatic vena cava (see Fig. 4–2). IVC, inferior vena cava.

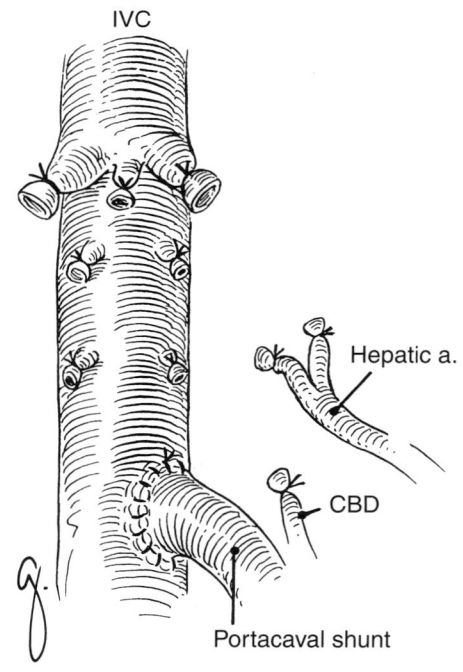

FIGURE 4–4

Total hepatectomy with temporary end-to-side portacaval shunt allows maintenance of portal venous return during an extended anhepatic phase. CBD, common bile duct; IVC, inferior vena cava.

intermittent portal occlusion for major resection procedures shows that hepatic parenchymal ischemia is well tolerated and significantly extends the safe period of ischemia while simultaneously reducing the subsequent reperfusion injury.[26] Experience with in situ hypothermic perfusion for hepatic resection[27] has stimulated the development of the more radical ex situ, or extracorporeal, bench procedures for resection of tumors otherwise deemed untreatable by conventional means.[28]

Biliary Reconstruction

Construction of the biliary anastomosis is a crucial component of the transplant operation. Although early experience relied almost exclusively on drainage through a Roux-en-Y choledochojejunostomy,[29] later studies indicate that preservation of the delicate blood supply to the bile duct would allow reconstruction using a direct biliary anastomosis.

To investigate healing of the biliary anastomosis, Northover and Terblanche performed polyester resin cast studies of the vascular supply to the supraduodenal common bile duct.[30] These data are of interest to all biliary surgeons. The blood supply was found to arise from the right hepatic and cystic arteries above and the retroduodenal branch of the gastroduodenal artery below. A previously undescribed retroportal artery also was identified.

Currently the preferred reconstruction is by choledochocholedochostomy when the recipient common bile duct is available, reserving the more difficult and time-consuming Roux-en-Y choledochojejunostomy for a donor-recipient size mismatch or an inadequate recipient bile duct situation. Considerable experience in bile duct reconstruction has grown from the living donor liver transplantation, in which multiple small-caliber ducts are frequently encountered.[31] Important advances include the use of magnification to facilitate the precise placement of fine sutures, the use of stents in small choledochojejunal anastomoses, and an algorithmic approach to the evaluation and treatment of biliary complications.

Biliary complications include leaks, strictures, and problems with the Roux-en-Y limb.[32] Various radiological procedures are important for diagnosis and management. These include nuclide cholescintigraphy to demonstrate routes of bile flow and invasive procedures such as percutaneous transhepatic cholangiography, endoscopic retrograde cholangiography, stricture dilatation, and stent placement for definitive therapy of specific complications.[33,34]

Surgical Education

As a consequence of the recent explosion in application of laparoendoscopic techniques to general surgical procedures, most common biliary operations are now performed laparoscopically, and training of open biliary surgery is in jeopardy. The concept of a hepatobiliary service that performs advanced procedures—including liver resection, complex biliary reconstruction, and liver transplantation—is important to surgical training, affords the trainees a concentrated exposure to open biliary surgery, and provides a balance to the laparoscopic methods.

Summary

The discipline of liver transplantation has grown remarkably over the last three decades and now represents the most effective treatment for patients with advanced liver disease. Largely because of the innovations derived from the liver transplant experience, the face of liver surgery has evolved from infrequent, exceedingly risky operations fraught with high mortality to complex procedures regularly performed in most tertiary centers. Liver transplantation encompasses crucial anatomic and technical lessons for the general surgeon, represents an important component of surgical training in the era of minimally invasive surgery, and has provided a profound stimulus to technical and scientific innovation in the surgery of liver disease. This fertile interaction among related surgical disciplines should not be overlooked when the benefits of the procedure are tallied.

References

1. Fausto N: Liver regeneration. J Hepatol 32 (Suppl) 1:19-31, 2000.
2. Taub R, Greenbaum LE, Peng Y: Transcriptional regulatory signals define cytokine-dependent and -independent pathways in liver regeneration. Semin Liver Dis 19:117-127, 1999.
3. Starzl TE, Terblanche J: Heptatotrophic substances. Prog Liver Dis 6:135-152, 1979.
4. Galun E, Axelrod JH: The role of cytokines in liver failure and regeneration: Potential new molecular therapies. Biochim Biophys Acta 1592:345-358, 2002.
5. Aldeguer X, Debonera F, Shaked A, et al: Interleukin-6 from intrahepatic cells of bone marrow origin is required for normal murine liver regeneration. Hepatology 35:40-48, 2001.
6. Olthoff K: Molecular pathways of regeneration and repair after liver transplantation. World J Surg 26:831-837, 2002.
7. Kiuchi T, Kasahara M, Uryuhara K, et al: Impact of graft size mismatching on graft prognosis in liver transplantation from living donors. Transplantation 67:321-327,1999.
8. Brems JJ, Millis JM, Hiatt JR, et al: Hepatic artery reconstruction during liver transplantation. Transplantation 47:403-406, 1989.
9. Hiatt JR, Gabbay J, Busuttil RW: Surgical anatomy of the hepatic arteries in 1000 cases. Ann Surg 220:50-52, 1994.
10. Nakamura T, Tanaka K, Kiuchi T, et al: Anatomical variations and surgical strategies in right lobe living donor liver transplantation: Lessons from 120 cases. Transplantation 73:1896-1903, 2002.
11. Deshpande RR, Heaton ND, Rela M: Surgical anatomy of segmental liver transplantation. Br J Surg 89:1078-1088, 2002.

12. Stimson RE, Pellegrini CA, Way LW: Factors affecting the morbidity of elective liver resection. Am J Surg 153:189-196, 1987.

13. Shaw BW, Martin DJ, Marquez JM, et al: Venous bypass in clinical liver transplantation. Ann Surg 200:524-534, 1984.

14. Baumgartner F, Scudamore C, Nair C, et al: Venovenous bypass for major hepatic and caval trauma. J Trauma 39:671-673, 1995.

15. Broering DC, Al-Shurafa A, Mueller L, et al: Total vascular isolation and in situ cold perfusion for management of severe liver trauma. J Trauma 53: 564-567, 2002.

16. Ringe B, Pichlmayr R, Ziegler H, et al: Management of severe hepatic trauma by two-stage total hepatectomy and subsequent liver transplantation. Surgery 109:792-795, 1991.

17. Rogers FB, Reese J, Shackford SR, Osler TM: The use of venovenous bypass and total vascular isolation of the liver in the surgical management of juxtahepatic venous injuries in blunt hepatic trauma. J Trauma 43:530-533, 1997.

18. Biffl WL, Moore EE, Franciose RJ: Venovenous bypass and hepatic vascular isolation as adjuncts in the repair of destructive wounds to the retrohepatic inferior vena cava. J Trauma 45:400-403, 1998.

19. Angstadt J, Jarrell B, Moritz M, et al: Surgical management of severe liver trauma: A role for liver transplantation. J Trauma 29:606-608,1989.

20. Iwatsuki S, Starzl TE: Personal experience with 411 hepatic resections. Ann Surg 208:421-434, 1985.

21. Tzakis A, Todo S, Starzl TE: Orthotopic liver transplantation with preservation of the inferior vena cava. Ann Surg 210:649-652, 1989.

22. Colonna JO, Shaked A, Gelabert HA, Busuttil RW: Resection of the caudate lobe through "bloody gulch." Surg Gynecol Obstet 176:401-402, 1993.

23. Ryan JA, Faulkner J: Liver resection without blood transfusion. Am J Surg 157:472-475, 1989.

24. Emre S, Schwartz ME, Katz E, Miller CM: Liver resection under total vascular isolation: Variations on a theme. Ann Surg 217:15-19, 1993.

25. Delva E, Camus Y, Nordlinger B, et al: Vascular occlusions for liver resections. Operative management and tolerance to hepatic ischemia: 142 cases. Ann Surg 209:211-218, 1989.

26. Belghiti J, Noun R, Malafosse R, et al: Continuous versus intermittent portal triad clamping for liver resection: A controlled study. Ann Surg 229:369-375, 1999.

27. Delriviere L, Hannoun L: In situ and ex situ in vivo procedures for complex major liver resections requiring prolonged hepatic vascular exclusion in normal and diseased livers. J Am Coll Surg 181:272-276, 1995.

28. Sauvanet A, Dousset B, Belghiti J: A simplified technique of ex situ hepatic surgical treatment. J Am Coll Surg 178:79-82, 1994.

29. Hiatt JR, Quinones-Baldrich WJ, Ramming KP, et al: Operations upon the biliary tract during transplantation of the liver. Surg Gynecol Obstet 165:89-93, 1987.

30. Northover J, Terblanche J: Bile duct blood supply: Its importance in human liver transplantation. Transplantation 26:67-79, 1978.

31. Renz JF, Reichert PR, Emond JC: Biliary anatomy as applied to pediatric living donor and split-liver transplantation. Liver Transpl 6:801-804, 2000.

32. Moser MAJ, Wall WJ: Management of biliary problems after liver transplantation. Liver Transpl 7 (Suppl 1):S46-S52, 2001.

33. Shah SR, Dooley J, Agarwal R, et al: Routine endoscopic retrograde cholangiography in the detection of early biliary complications after liver transplantation. Liver Transpl 8:491-494, 2002.

34. Colonna JO, Shaked A, Gomes A, et al: Biliary strictures complicating liver transplantation: Incidence, pathogenesis, management, and outcome. Ann Surg 216:344-352, 1992.

5

Liver Allocation: The U.S. Model

RICHARD B. FREEMAN, JR

Historical perspective   63
   Early liver allocation   63
   Legislation   64

General principles of liver allocation   66
   Justice and utility, individual rights versus
      good of the whole   66
   Definitions of need and outcome   68

Models for liver allocation   69
   Center-based allocation   69
   Patient-based allocation   69

Methods of patient-based allocation   69
   Distribution units   70
   Allocation protocols   71

Current U.S. policy   72

Future U.S. policy   75

Historical Perspective

Early Liver Allocation

Dr. Starzl and the liver transplant pioneers performed the first liver transplants with organs procured from donors declared dead by cardiopulmonary criteria.[1] In those early days, before adoption of the acceptance of brain death criteria, the donor had to be in close proximity to the recipient because donor liver preservation was extremely limited. Most liver procurement and allocation processes were contained within transplant center hospitals. Moreover, at this stage, liver transplantation was an experimental procedure, and few candidates were available. Investigators made all allocation decisions within their institution, with no need to consider larger regional or national allocation issues. At the same time, renal transplantation began to grow, and in Richmond, Boston, and Los Angeles, hospitals began to band together to improve identification and acquisition of donor kidneys. In addition, as renal transplantation expanded, legislators crafted the Uniform Anatomical Gift Act[2] in 1968, which defined a legal means to enable those who wished to do so to donate their organs or allow their next of kin to carry out their wishes. At the same time, the Ad Hoc Committee of the Harvard Medical School to Examine the Definition of Brain Death published their findings and defined standards by which individuals could be declared dead by neurological criteria alone.[3] This development reduced the amount of ischemic damage to transplantable organs and allowed donor organs to be maintained for longer periods after declaration of death, thus opening the possibility of procuring organs from donors located in hospitals at greater distances from the transplant center. As the brain death definition became more widely accepted, legislation followed in the form of the Uniform Brain Death Act in 1978[4] and the Uniform Determination of Death Act in 1980.[5] Clinical use of cyclosporine was also introduced in 1978, which brought liver transplantation out of the realm of experimental to accepted standard of care. All these events helped advance liver transplantation, make its practice more widespread, and increase the demand for donor organs. As for kidneys, liver transplant centers broadened their efforts to increase donation and recognized the need to increase the number of hospitals capable of identifying donors. Regional sharing of donor kidneys evolved, and regional boundaries were established among geographically contiguous regions. The need for coordinated efforts for organ retrieval through better-structured organizations was also recognized, and organ procurement organizations (OPOs) were established in Richmond and Boston, and others soon followed. The organization based in Richmond, called the South East Organ Procurement Foundation (SEOPF), developed a computer registry, first for renal transplant patients and later for patients waiting for any organ type. Further improvements in surgical technique and candidate selection and refinements in immunosuppressive therapy increased the success rate of liver transplantation and thus intensified demand. Personal relationships among transplant professionals and interhospital relationships and agreements with hospitals sometimes far removed from local transplant centers served to increase organ availability during the late 1970s and early 1980s. In the late 1970s SEOPF expanded its computer registry to a more national scope, but there was still no formal method for matching donors to recipients, nor were there formal guidelines for determining priority on the waiting list. Liver transplantation allocation prioritization systems evolved along with renal transplantation and, for the most part, used a first-come, first-served, waiting time–based system. At the same time, media attention was focused on some candidates for whom donor livers could not be found, and several pleas for directed donation were promulgated through the media in an effort to draw from a nationwide potential donor pool.

Legislation

As the cases in the media at that time dramatically illustrated, there was no formal way to facilitate sharing of organs among OPOs or matching of donors to liver recipients, nor were there standardized rules for determining which patients were eligible for liver

transplantation and what type of priority any given patient should receive within an OPO or geographic region or nationally. Based on these intersecting developments, Congress recognized the need for a national system for organ transplantation and passed the National Organ Transplant Act (NOTA), which was signed into law by President Reagan in 1984.[6] Among other provisions, NOTA mandated that a national task force address the distribution of organs and standardization of national practice.[7] This important piece of legislation and the task force established that a national system for organ procurement and distribution must be formed, as well as a national registry of transplant recipients. NOTA also made it illegal to obtain human organs for transplantation through financial considerations. In addition, NOTA required the secretary of the Department of Health and Human Services (DHHS) to issue a final rule for regulations to oversee organ transplant allocation and policy development. Subsequent to passage of NOTA, the National Transplant Task Force determined that donor organs are a national resource to be used for the public good and outlined the framework for a national system called the Organ Procurement and Transplantation Network (OPTN). In 1987, the United Network for Organ Sharing (UNOS), a private not-for-profit corporation derived from the SEOPF OPO, was awarded the first federal contract to administer the OPTN and the national Scientific Registry of Transplant Recipients (SRTR). As administrator of the OPTN, UNOS is responsible for development and implementation of all allocation policy and assessment of compliance.

NOTA was amended in 1988 to require that all OPOs and transplant centers be members of the OPTN and that all members of the OPTN abide by OPTN policies to remain Medicare or Medicaid eligible.[8] Federal regulation of OPOs authorized by the NOTA amendment was promulgated in 1988; the regulations specified performance and quality measures that OPOs were required to meet to qualify for federal reimbursement by Medicare and Medicaid.[9] These regulations also required that OPOs document agreements with the hospitals from which they would be soliciting donors, as well as the transplant centers to which organs procured by that OPO would be offered. In addition, OPOs were required to designate areas that they were willing to serve and have these service areas certified by the Center for Medicare and Medicaid Service (CMS) (Fig. 5–1). Table 5–1 summarizes U.S. federal legislative and regulatory action relevant to liver transplantation allocation.

Subsequent legislation, the Omnibus Budget Reconciliation Act of 1988,[10] required all hospitals to have a written protocol for identification of potential donors and report all such cases to the OPO with which the hospital has a service agreement. UNOS, as the holder of the federal contract to administer the OPTN,

ORGAN PROCUREMENT ORGANIZATION SERVICE AREAS

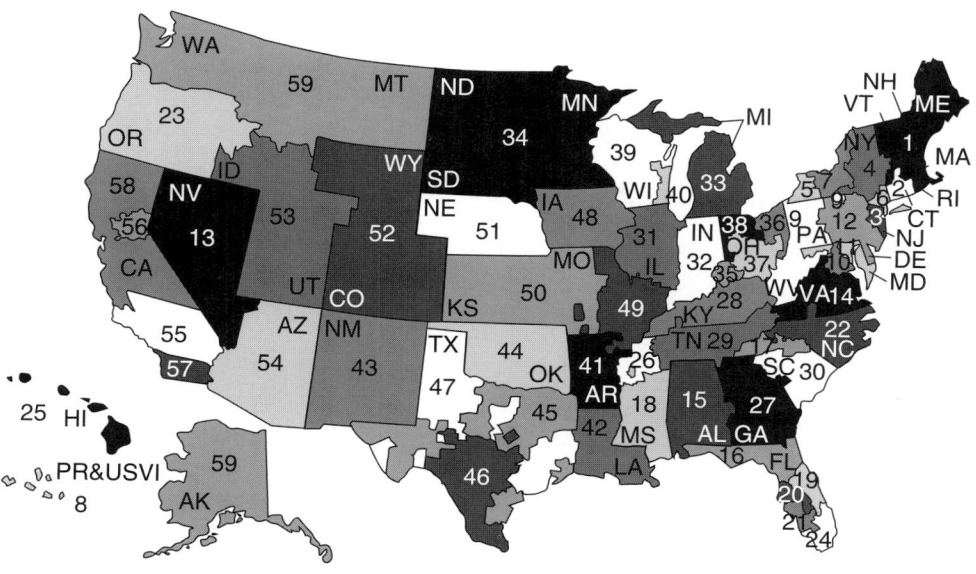

1. New England Organ Bank
2. Northeast OPO and Tissue Bank
3. NJ Organ and Tissue Sharing Network
4. Center for Donation and Transplant
5. Upstate New York Transplant Services
6. New York Organ Donor Network
7. Finger Lakes Donor Recovery Network
8. Lifelink of Puerto Rico
9. Center for Organ Recovery and Education
10. Washington Regional Transplant Consortium
11. Transplant Resource Center of Maryland
12. Gift of Life Donor Program
13. Nevada Donor Network
14. LifeNet
15. Alabama Organ Center
16. The OPO at the University of Florida
17. Life Share of the Carolinas
18. Mississippi Organ Recovery Agency
19. Translife/Florida Hospital
20. Lifelink of Florida

21. Lifelink of Southwest Florida
22. Carolina Donor Services
23. Pacific Northwest Transplant Bank
24. University of Miami OPO
25. Organ Donor Center of Hawaii
26. Mid-South Transplant Foundation
27. Lifelink of Georgia
28. Kentucky Organ Donor Affiliates
29. Tennessee Donor Services
30. SC Organ Procurement Agency
31. Regional Organ Bank of Illinois
32. Indiana OPO
33. Transplantation Society of Michigan
34. Lifesource Upper Midwest OPO
35. Ohio Valley Life Center
36. Lifebanc
37. Lifeline of Ohio Organ Procurement
38. Life Connection of Ohio
39. University of Wisconsin Hospital and Clinic
40. Wisconsin Donor Network

41. Arkansas Regional Organ Recovery Agency
42. Louisiana Organ Procurement Agency
43. New Mexico Donor Services
44. Oklahoma Organ Sharing Network
45. Southwest Transplant Alliance
46. Texas Organ Sharing Alliance
47. Life Gift Organ Donation Center
48. Iowa Donor Network
49. Mid-America Transplant Services
50. Midwest Transplant Network
51. Nebraska Organ Retrieval System
52. Donor Alliance
53. Intermountain Organ Recovery Systems
54. Donor Network of Arizona
55. Southern CA Organ Procurement Center
56. Golden State Transplant Services
57. Organ and Tissue Acquisition Center of Southern CA
58. California Transplant Donor Network
59. LifeCenter Northwest

FIGURE 5–1

Organ procurement organization service areas as of July 2001 as certified by the Center for Medicare and Medicaid Service.

developed national policies for organ allocation and program certification and examined candidate prioritization systems and distribution units. The initial UNOS liver allocation policy was founded on renal transplantation principles; however, it immediately became clear that waiting time alone would be insufficient to prioritize liver candidates and that some measure of disease severity would need to be used to better categorize these patients. Liver distribution units, or the area from which a potential recipient has the opportunity to receive a deceased donor liver, were defined similar to renal transplant areas and were based on the OPO service area as the smallest unit of distribution. UNOS, in an effort to organize liver distribution into larger areas for administrative and organ distribution purposes,

also created 10 regions by combining geographically contiguous OPO service areas along the lines of the nascent renal distribution regions (Fig. 5–2). These boundaries were loosely based on the federally funded end-stage renal disease geographic regions that were designed to define areas of similar population density. During this time, an informal system for allocation of donor livers to the most gravely ill candidates was developed in the form of the "UNOS Stat" designation. This system was ostensibly designed to allow potential candidates who met certain criteria to receive a liver from anywhere in the country. Unfortunately, these criteria were not well defined or objective, and there was a perception of abuse of this system that led to its abolishment in 1993. However, in 1997, the need to expand

Table 5–1. SIGNIFICANT LEGISLATION AND REGULATION FOR THE U.S. ORGAN ALLOCATION SYSTEM

Year	Legislation/Regulation	Result
1968	Uniform Anatomical Gift Act	Provided legal framework to allow donation of organs
1978	Uniform Declaration of Brain Death Act	Provided legal acceptance of declaration of death by neurological criteria
1980	Uniform Determination of Death Act	Provided that death could be legally declared by cardiopulmonary or neurological criteria
1984	National Organ Transplant Act (NOTA)	Required the Secretary of the Department of Health and Human Services to:
		Appoint a task force to study transplantation
		Develop a network for transplantation nationwide (OPTN)
		Establish a computer system for matching donors and recipients
		Create a national transplant registry
		Required that all OPOs have a policy for allocation of organs
		Made it unlawful to transfer human organs for financial considerations
1988	NOTA amended	Required the OPTN to develop:
		Membership criteria
		Medical criteria for listing candidates and allocating organs
		Standards to prevent transmission of diseases by donated organs
		Criteria to distribute organs on a regional or national basis
1988	OPO Regulations 42 CFR Chapter IV § 486.301	Performance standards and quality criteria for OPOs are set: OPOs must meet to maintain Medicare/Medicaid eligibility for reimbursement
2000	Organ Procurement Organization Certification Act	Revised OPO performance standards
2000	"Final Rule" 42 CFR Part 121	Codified regulations for the OPTN and scientific registry
		Set performance standards for organ allocation policies
		Revised data release regulations

OPO, organ procurement organization; OPTN, Organ Procurement and Transplantation Network.

the liver distribution units for acutely ill liver candidates and the recognition that there was wide disparity among the various regions of the country in waiting time for liver transplant organ offers led to considerable controversy and stimulated the DHHS to issue the regulations specified by NOTA that would provide organ transplant oversight.[11] The initial proposed form of this "Final Rule" raised even more controversy that resulted in congressional action in which the Institute of Medicine (IOM) was commissioned to study organ allocation and pay specific attention to liver allocation. The IOM published its findings in 1999.[12] Based on the recommendations of this IOM report, the proposed "Final Rule" was amended and became effective November 19, 1999. The main points of the amended "Final Rule" established

performance goals for bringing about: standardized criteria for placing patients on transplant lists, standardized criteria for defining a patient's medical status, and allocation policies that make most effective use of

organs, especially by making them available whenever feasible to the most medically urgent patients who are appropriate candidates for transplantation.

The "Final Rule" also sets standards for availability of organ transplantation data, and it addressed the governing structure of the OPTN.[13] Since implementation, much progress has been made in using objective criteria for defining the medical status of liver candidates.

General Principles of Liver Allocation

Justice and Utility, Individual Rights versus Good of the Whole

Equitable and effective allocation of scarce resources has been a problem for caregivers since the earliest forms of medical care. Determining who should receive

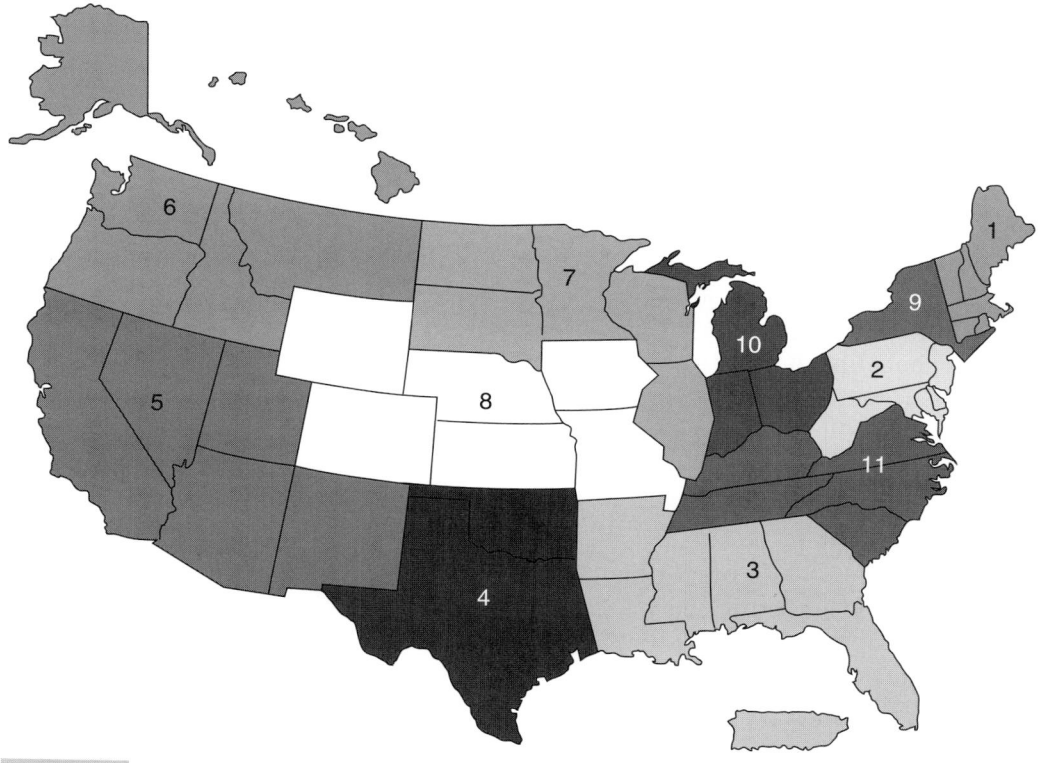

FIGURE 5–2

United Network for Organ Sharing regions.

medical attention and what goals for individual patients and for overall groups of patients should be achieved by the application of allocation policies requires knowledge of ethical and clinical principles. Justice, or what is fair for the individual,[14] is one measure that must be addressed by any system for disbursement of scarce medical resources. Allocation decisions based on medical justice place emphasis on using individual characteristics to assign priority for care. Individual characteristics that might be taken into consideration include individuals' societal worth, their status as a provider for others, their ability to compensate their caregivers, the urgency of the medical conditions requiring intervention, or various combinations of these characteristics.[15] Other measures of fairness might be based on timing—that is, a first-come, first-served type of justice. However, many of these characteristics are extremely subjective and arbitrary. The timing of an individual's entry into a medical system may be influenced by many factors unrelated to that person's medical condition. Furthermore, other individual characteristics, such as societal worth, for example, are often in the eye of the beholder.

To try to provide a just system for the delivery of scarce medical resources, the concept of triage was developed on the battlefield to use individual medical characteristics to select injured soldiers for care.[16]

Surgeons, overwhelmed by casualties, separated the injured into three groups: those who were injured beyond hope and thus could not benefit from medical care, those who had less serious injuries that did not require immediate attention and could wait for care, and those who could be saved, but only if medical resources were applied expeditiously. In this example, individual characteristics based on medical urgency or medical need were used to allocate the battlefield medical resources.

More recently, individual medical need has been a driving force for the application of medical justice in American health care policy. Medical justice was the foundation for establishment of the Medicare/Medicaid system and was the basis for the federal government ensuring that renal dialysis care would be provided for all individuals in need, largely without regard to optimizing outcome for the whole.[17] However, for transplantation, and most acutely for liver transplantation, donor resources are much more constrained than other health care resources, which are mostly limited by financial constraints. Because of these more confounding resource restrictions, use of a donor organ for a given individual based solely on medical justice criteria has direct potential to affect another individual's access to care. Furthermore, if only individual needs were used as the criterion for allocation, it is possible that resources would be wasted. If under the system of triage all the medical resources were directed to the most severely injured soldiers who carried a much higher mortality rate even when they received medical care, many salvageable injuries would be deprived of life-saving care with an overall increase in mortality rates.

Thus, the principle of triage has a utilitarian component.[18] A utilitarian approach to resource allocation stipulates that that scarce medical resources be allocated for the good of the whole group.[19] In this sense, the scarce resources should be directed to achieve the best overall outcome. There are many possible measures of the "best outcome" for a group. On the battlefield, the best application of scarce resources might be to treat the injured who are most likely to recover and fight another day. One might use cost of care as a measure of "best outcome" for a population and apply scarce resources only to those likely to cost the least. Alternatively, quality of life may be the outcome priority, and scarce resources might be given to those most likely to achieve a high level of quality of life even though others might die without the treatment. In the case of transplantation, a purely utilitarian approach might allocate scarce organs to recipients least likely to experience graft failure or most likely to survive long-term. These two partially competing forces for scarce medical resources, individual need and overall population results, or medical justice versus medical utility, must be resolved to some degree in any allocation policy, but they are of critical importance in liver transplantation policy.

Definitions of Need and Outcome

To design an efficient, objective, and reproducible system of resource allocation, precise definitions of need and outcome must be established. Conflicts between physicians' obligation to meet their patients' individual medical needs and physicians' need to use the scarce resource in the most equitable and efficient way for the betterment of all are unavoidable. Although some have argued that this basic dichotomy for physicians should disqualify them from making these decisions,[20] others have argued that only physicians are uniquely qualified to wrestle with these problems.[21] Providing objective measures of need and outcome helps make the system much more transparent, thereby enabling a much more enlightened assessment of physicians' obligations to their patients and their role as stewards of a scarce resource and whatever success is achieved in balancing these issues.

Measuring need for patients with chronic liver disease has evolved from the first-come, first-served approach derived from renal allocation systems to an

Table 5–2. CHILD-TURCOTTE-PUGH SCORE AS USED IN LIVER ALLOCATION POLICY BEFORE FEBRUARY 2001

Criterion	Points		
	1	2	3
Albumin (g/dL)	>3.5	2.8–3.5	<2.8
Total bilirubin (mg/dL)	<2	2–3	>3
International normalized ratio	<1.7	1.71–2.24	>2.25
Ascites	None	Controlled medically	Poorly controlled
Encephalopathy	None	Controlled medically	Poorly controlled

understanding that severity of liver disease is a better measure of medical justice for liver transplant candidates. Initially, the setting in which the liver transplant candidate was receiving care was used as a surrogate for severity of liver disease, with patients being treated in intensive care units receiving higher priority than those treated in routine inpatient settings, who in turn received higher priority than those being treated at home. Eventually, this arrangement was recognized to be more of a measure of physician practice behavior and not a direct measure of a patient's condition. Soon thereafter, the well-established Child-Turcotte-Pugh (CTP) score (Table 5–2) was adopted as a more direct measure of a patient's condition. Although the CTP score had been used in clinical practice for more than 20 years, several limitations were recognized as the care of waiting liver transplant candidates improved and evolved. The CTP score was never developed or validated as a good measure of severity for patients waiting for liver transplantation. Moreover, as care of patients with end-stage liver disease has improved, it has become apparent that the CTP score does not adequately segregate patients with progressively abnormal laboratory test values. For example, patients with serum bilirubin values of 3.5 mg/dL were assigned the same score as those with values of 10, 20, or 40 mg/dL. The CTP score also includes subjective clinical measures, encephalopathy and ascites, which are subject to clinical interpretation and less objective. These deficiencies led to adoption of a continuous measurement of liver disease severity based on the Model for End-Stage Liver Disease (MELD) score. The MELD score, by defining the severity of liver disease as the risk of dying within 3 months based on three routine laboratory tests, provides a continuous measurement of need based on objective criteria.[22] Use of continuous disease scores for liver allocation is discussed in later sections in this chapter.

Outcome results are also important measures of both justice and utility for any allocation system. For patients with life-threatening illness, the mortality rate is the most profound, easiest to define and measure parameter of outcome. For the liver allocation system, individual justice is served by measuring individual mortality with and without performance of transplantation. However, it is difficult to accurately estimate individual risks based on individual characteristics, which means that population statistics become necessary. By using population-based assessments it becomes possible to measure utilitarian outcomes and the effectiveness of the allocation system in its stewardship of scarce resources for the benefit of society. For these reasons, the efficacy of organ allocation has been measured by patient and graft survival rates. For liver transplantation, we can divide patient survival into survival while waiting for a transplant and survival after transplantation. Survival while on the waiting list can be seen as a utilitarian measure of the successful recognition of individual need. Survival after transplantation is a utilitarian measure of the application of distributive justice. Ultimately, the liver allocation system must strive to maximize both outcome measures.

Models for Liver Allocation

Center-Based Allocation

In the early period of liver transplantation, donors were usually identified by the transplant center and the donor organ then allocated by the center to whatever candidate the center believed most appropriate. This model of liver allocation can be termed center-based allocation. When there is little competition among centers for organs and physicians act responsibly, justice and utility can be well served by such a model. Today, many areas in the world allocate livers according to center-based allocation models. For example, in Britain, in cases in which no emergency candidate exists, each center rotates in turn to receive the next donor liver, and transplant clinicians within that center choose whatever recipient they deem appropriate. Individual patient justice is served by caregivers' obligation to care for their patients, and the overall efficacy of these systems has been quite good.[23] Liver allocation models outside the United States are discussed in detail elsewhere in this textbook.

In the case of the U.S. system, however, large distances, numerous centers, and extreme heterogeneity in the size of waiting lists at various centers and heterogeneity in organ availability around the country made center-based allocation less desirable. Furthermore, NOTA and the "Final Rule" mandated that donors be allocated to patients, not centers or physicians. For these reasons, patient-specific criteria were developed to prioritize patients, and the UNOS computer system was implemented to manage patients and their data.

Patient-Based Allocation

In previous U.S. liver allocation systems, candidates were categorized by individual characteristics and grouped into status categories. Within each category and stratified by blood type, candidates were further segregated by time waiting on the list. As discussed previously, early status definitions were based on the location at which the transplant candidate was receiving care. Use of these location-based criteria, however, was an indirect method of defining candidates' characteristics and was as much a reflection of physicians' behavior as it was a measure of candidates' severity of disease. More recent revisions to the system have incorporated progressively more objective measures of disease severity that are more directly specific to a given patient's condition. For each organ donor in the United States, the UNOS computer system categorizes potential recipients by these individual patient characteristics to determine which candidates should receive the organ offer within the local OPO, then within the region, and finally nationally. Thus, each so-called match run for a given donor potentially ranks every appropriate liver candidate with that donor according to the patient's characteristics. However, in areas where the local OPO serves only one transplant center, the donor is effectively allocated to the center, not an individual, because all waiting patients at that center will be ranked ahead of patients in other centers in outside OPOs. This situation remains controversial in the U.S. organ allocation policy and is discussed in more detail in the section on distribution units in this chapter.

Methods of Patient-Based Allocation

In considering the U.S. model for liver allocation, two important elements that are intertwined must be appreciated. The first element, the liver distribution unit, is defined as the group of patients to whom a donor organ is first allocated. These distribution units are progressively expanded if there is no recipient willing to accept a donor liver offer in the smallest distribution unit. Current UNOS/OPTN policy stipulates that the OPO service area is the smallest distribution unit (see Fig. 5–1). The second important element of liver allocation is the prioritization system. Prioritization rules are applied within distribution units to rank waiting candidates and determine to whom the donor liver will be allocated.

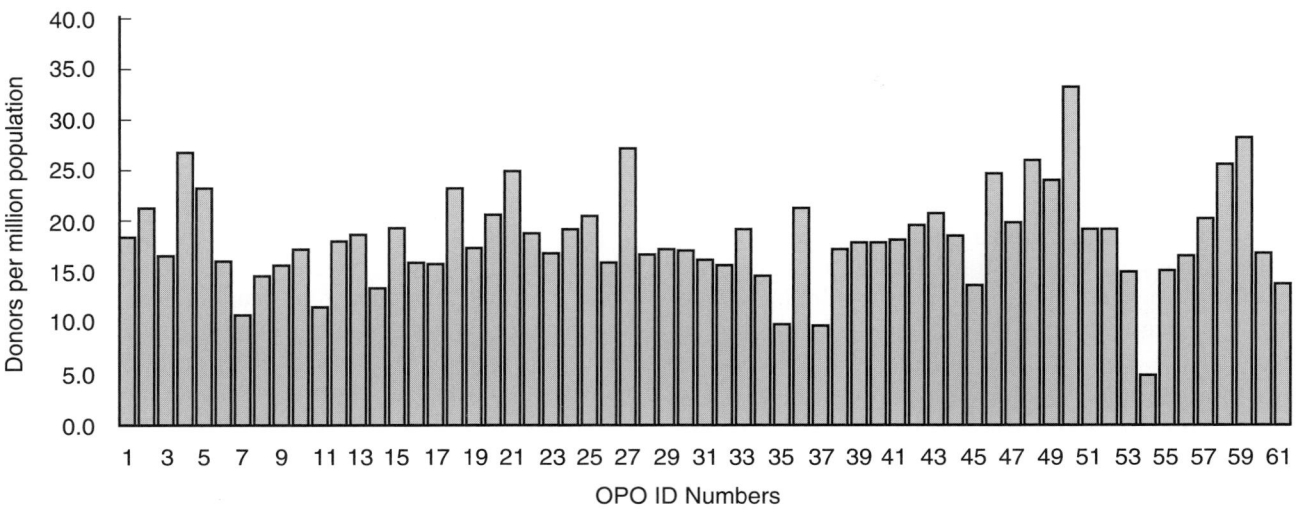

FIGURE 5-3

Donors per million population for organ procurement organizations in the United States as of 2000 (www.UNOS.org).

Distribution Units

Liver distribution units can be designed in many possible ways. As mentioned earlier, the current U.S. system specifies the OPO service areas (see Fig. 5-1) as the smallest liver distribution units. Hence, donor livers are first allocated to all candidates waiting at centers served by the OPO that is procuring the donor liver. If no centers accept this donor organ for their patients, the donor is offered to the next largest liver distribution unit, the UNOS region (see Figs. 5-1 and 5-2), and finally to the national liver distribution unit. Thus, U.S. distribution units are geographically based. This form of allocation is for the most part based on historical practice and the development of renal distribution units in the late 1970s and early 1980s. It has created one of the problems inherent in the U.S. system in that these geographically defined units are extremely heterogeneous in number of transplant centers served, number of donors identified and procured (Fig. 5-3), and number of patients waiting for a liver transplant.

Historical, political, and local loyalties notwithstanding, it is possible to envisage that other units of distribution might be defined. Donor organs could be distributed over a portion of the total national waiting list. For example, when a donor is identified, the computer could generate a list of all waiting candidates in centers in the general region of the donor hospital until a certain percentage of the total waiting list has been listed. This group of patients could then be ranked according to prevailing prioritization rules. Another alternative would be to distribute livers over a certain proportion of the total population in a given area.

Such a system is in place for renal transplant allocation in New England, where population distance points are calculated according to the population between the donor hospital and the candidates' transplant centers.[24] Candidates waiting at centers with less population between the center and the donor hospital get increasing priority.

Tremendous historical precedents and existing geopolitical boundaries make proposals to alter existing distribution units controversial and politically charged. In 1997 to 1999, discrepancies in waiting times for liver transplant candidates among various distribution units raised enormous media attention and political rancor. Much of this debate and controversy centered on the potential that existing boundaries might be redrawn to reduce waiting time discrepancies. The IOM report was commissioned to address some of these concerns and recommended that distribution unit lines be redrawn.[25] However, subsequent studies using computer model simulations pointed out that redrawing distribution unit boundaries according to new geographic configurations would not result in substantial differences in overall results for the transplant system.[26] Furthermore, these computer simulations suggested that such reconfiguration would result in a shift of donor organs out of some OPOs and into others and would not necessarily overcome the regional differences in organ availability, OPO efficiency, and size of liver candidate waiting lists. These highly charged issues have led policymakers to focus more recent efforts on allocation protocols that more objectively define patient need for transplantation.

Allocation Protocols

Early in the history of liver transplantation, candidates were prioritized by a first-come, first-served system in which time on the list was the only criterion for ranking these patients. Waiting time is a reasonable form of egalitarian medical justice to rank candidates if all candidates enter the system with similar needs.[27] In the case of renal transplantation, this system remains a just method because most patients enter the renal transplant waiting list with renal failure of similar severity. In addition, complete loss of renal organ function can be treated effectively with dialysis and does not result in death, thus making renal transplantation much less urgent than liver transplantation. Patients with end-stage liver disease enter the system with widely varying severity of liver disease, with widely varying rates of progression of their disease, and with no artificial means to sustain them. Use of waiting time as a major criterion for allocation of livers serves to select patients who enter the system early in the course of their disease or patients who have very slowly progressive disease. Patients with more severe liver failure or rapidly progressive disease cannot wait for long periods. Waiting time then, to use the battlefield triage analogy, directs medical resources to liver transplant candidates with disease that can wait for treatment by giving significant priority for time on the list. This method of allocation results in more patients dying than necessary and, in some cases, directs livers to candidates whose mortality risk is greater with the transplant than without it. Preliminary results from a system in which waiting time was significantly de-emphasized as an allocation criterion substantiated the reduction in waiting list mortality.[28] Early results of the new MELD/Pediatric (model) for End-Stage Liver Disease (PELD) system for liver allocation suggest reduced waiting list death rates as well.[28a]

In part, waiting time was used as a surrogate because it is difficult to define measures of liver disease severity in patients with diverse diagnoses and rates of progression who enter the system at widely variable points in their disease history. Ordering patients into categorical groups or status definitions, as was the previous practice, failed to take these wide variations into account, and within the status definitions, waiting time became the most important discriminator. For these reasons, many clinicians and the IOM recognized that de-emphasizing waiting time and using a continuous disease severity scale without categorical status definitions would be a better system for liver candidate prioritization.[25] Such a continuous scale using the CTP score in a continuous fashion was successful in better ranking patients.[28]

Although the CTP score has been an accepted measure of liver disease severity, it had never been independently validated as a predictive measure of liver transplant waiting list mortality. As discussed earlier, a liver transplant candidate's risk of death while waiting is one measure of disease severity that can be easily quantified. Previous studies that developed statistical models to select patients for the transjugular portosystemic stent procedure based on the risk of dying within 3 months afterward showed that the MELD score was highly predictive of mortality.[29] Subsequent studies validated the MELD score as predictive of 3-month mortality in a variety of cohorts of adult patients with chronic liver disease.[22,30] Similarly, a risk score for pediatric patients with chronic liver disease that defined the risk of death within 3 months was developed and called the Pediatric End-Stage Liver Disease score.[31] Policymakers selected the risk of dying within 3 months (as predicted by the MELD/PELD score) as a measure of chronic liver disease severity that is appropriate for candidates waiting for liver transplantation for several reasons. The MELD/PELD scores (Table 5–3) are measures of individual patient risk based on objective laboratory values. Use of the MELD/PELD scores for defining individual mortality risk to prioritize liver transplant candidates is a much more precise way to define individual need. By doing so, arbitrary categorization is removed, variables subject to physician interpretation such as the degree of encephalopathy or ascites are eliminated, and de-emphasizing waiting time removes an arbitrary measure of entry time on the waiting list. Thus, the MELD and PELD scores are more objective measures of individual need as defined by the risk of death, and they reflect a further refinement of application of individual justice in liver allocation.

The MELD/PELD scores have limitations in liver allocation, however. Several studies have shown that the concordance[32] (a measure of the predictive value of a test) of the MELD score to predict mortality is approximately 0.80, which suggests that, for as many as 20% of patients, the MELD score will not be highly accurate in predicting mortality.[22] In addition, mortality risk is not the only measure of disease severity that should be

---

Table 5–3. MELD AND PELD EQUATIONS

MELD = 6.3 + (0.957 × ln (creatinine) + 0.378 × ln (bilirubin) + 1.12 × ln (INR) + 0.643) × 10

PELD = (0.436 × Age*) − (0.687 × ln (albumin)) + (0.480 × ln (bilirubin)) + (1.857 × ln (INR)) + (0.667 × Growth failure†) × 10

*PELD: Age younger than 1 year is assigned a value of 1; age older than 1 year is assigned 0.

†PELD: Growth failure is assigned a value of 1; no growth failure is assigned 0.

INR, international normalized ratio; ln, natural logarithm; MELD, Model for End-Stage Liver Disease; PELD, Pediatric (model) for End-Stage Liver Disease.

considered when ranking candidates for liver transplantation. Recent studies have shown that for patients with cirrhosis and early-stage hepatocellular cancer (HCC), liver transplantation provides better long-term cure rates.[33] However, patients with favorable HCC tumor stages may not have severe intrinsic liver disease and thus do not have an increased risk of death that is greater than their risk of tumor progression. Therefore, an appropriate outcome measure for these patients is the risk of progression beyond a favorable stage for transplantation. Unfortunately, this endpoint is more imprecise and requires statistical study of natural history data to develop equations similar to the MELD/PELD scores. Such data are not available, although computer simulations of HCC progression have been developed and published.[34] The risk of progression beyond a favorable stage for transplantation has been termed the liver waiting list "dropout rate" by several investigators.[35] They have conclusively shown that the longer candidates with HCC wait, the more likely they are to progress beyond a favorable stage for transplantation. Other similarly difficult-to-define endpoints for risk assessment can be imagined for other diagnoses that are treatable by liver transplantation but for which the MELD/PELD scores might not apply. Metabolic diseases with a risk of HCC development or familial amyloid syndromes with a risk of severe myocardial or neurological impairment might have risk scores developed to predict these endpoints. Unfortunately, good natural history data essential for developing these risk models are sorely lacking for these other conditions. Ultimately, risk scores might be developed for all diagnoses based on the risk of development of conditions that carry an unacceptably high risk of posttransplant failure. Consensus on what constitutes an unacceptable risk of failure remains to be achieved.

Alternatively, a utilitarian approach could be taken by designing allocation algorithms to maximize outcome after transplantation. There may be some benefit to such an approach inasmuch as many of the pretransplant variables associated with a high risk of death while waiting are also associated with a high risk of death after transplantation. Taken to extreme, however, a purely utilitarian system would potentially allocate organs to patients with a relatively low risk of dying of liver failure without a transplant to maximize the success rate after transplantation. In this extreme case, many patients who would probably survive the transplant procedure would die while waiting because their chance of success was not as high as that of a less ill candidate. This also becomes important when quality of life is considered in liver allocation. It is possible to conceive of allocation plans designed to maximize the quality of life either while waiting or after transplantation, or both. However, it is difficult to imagine a system where the risk of deterioration in quality of life would receive higher priority for liver allocation than the risk of dying of liver disease.

Current U.S. Policy

A complete description of current U.S. liver allocation policy has been published recently,[36] and the policy language is available online.[37] Because of the deficiencies of waiting time and categorical stratification of candidates outlined earlier, the U.S. OPTN/UNOS instituted the so-called MELD/PELD system for liver allocation in February 2002. This system is based on the MELD score for adults and the PELD score for pediatric patients (candidates 18 years or younger). The current policy retains an emergency status category (status 1) for patients with acute liver failure or for those with primary graft failure within a week of transplantation. The distribution unit for candidates meeting the status 1 definition is the OPO followed by the UNOS/OPTN region (Table 5–4). Thus, donor organs procured by an OPO are first offered to candidates meeting the status 1 criteria listed at centers served by that OPO. Then, any candidate meeting the status 1 definitions listed at a center within the UNOS/OPTN region containing the procuring OPO is next offered the liver. Pediatric candidates who progress to require intensive care can also be designated status 1 and receive the benefit of the regional distribution unit. If no regional candidate accepts the donor organ, it is offered to candidates at centers served by the procuring OPO according to their MELD/PELD score. All other candidates are prioritized by their MELD or PELD scores. The primary distribution unit for these candidates is the local OPO (see Fig. 5–1).* All candidates at centers served by the OPO are offered donor livers by descending MELD/PELD scores, and livers are distributed first in the OPO distribution unit by descending MELD/PELD scores. If no candidate accepts the organ offer, it is offered to all candidates waiting at centers within that region in descending MELD/PELD order and then nationally to all candidates, first to those meeting status 1 and then by descending MELD/PELD score (see Table 5–4).

The original MELD score as developed by Malinchoc and colleagues[29] was altered in several minor ways for implementation as part of liver allocation policy. The disease etiology variable that controlled for cholestatic and noncholestatic liver disease was removed from the original version. Removal of this variable did not change the predictive power of the MELD equation,[22] and by doing so, any causative discrimination was

---

*In some cases, agreements among OPOs or with larger OPOs establish alternative local distribution units.

Table 5-4. DONOR LIVER ALLOCATION SEQUENCE

Adult Donor Older than 18 Years

Local

1. Status 1 patients in descending point order

Regional

2. Status 1 patients in descending point order

Local

3. All other patients in descending order of mortality risk scores (MELD/PELD)

Regional

4. All other patients in descending order of mortality risk scores (MELD/PELD)

National

5. Status 1 patients in descending point order

6. All other patients in descending order of mortality risk scores (MELD/PELD)

Pediatric Donor 18 Years or Younger

Local

1. Status 1 pediatric patients in descending point order

2. Status 1 adult patients in descending point order

Regional

3. Status 1 pediatric patients in descending point order

4. Status 1 adult patients in descending point order

Local

5. Pediatric patients with ≥ 50% mortality

6. Adult patients with ≥ 50% mortality

7. Pediatric patients with < 50% mortality

8. Adult patients with < 50% mortality

Regional

9. Pediatric patients with ≥ 50% mortality

10. Adult patients with ≥ 50% mortality

11. Pediatric patients with < 50% mortality

12. Adult patients with < 50% mortality

National

13. Status 1 pediatric patients in descending point order

14. Status 1 adult patients in descending point order

15. Pediatric patients with ≥ 50% mortality

16. Adult patients with ≥ 50% mortality

17. Pediatric patients with < 50% mortality

18. Adult patients with < 50% mortality

MELD, Model for End-Stage Liver Disease; PELD, Pediatric (model) for End-Stage Liver Disease.

The serum creatinine value in the MELD score is capped at a maximum of 4.0 mg/dL because policy designers believed that since serum creatinine is a good independent predictor of poor outcome after transplantation,[38] candidates with significantly elevated serum creatinine values should not receive extra priority to avoid futile transplants. Candidates with higher creatinine levels have their serum creatinine values set to 4.0 mg/dL for calculation of the MELD score. The overall MELD score is also capped at a maximum of 40 points to limit the priority given candidates whose MELD scores total greater than 40 and who are thus subject to extremely high pretransplant and posttransplant mortality. Adult patients with MELD scores higher than 40 have their scores set to 40 but may still be listed if a center believes that such a candidate is an appropriate risk. In addition, approximately 3% of candidates on the liver transplant waiting list require renal dialysis. Because serum creatinine values in these patients may be artificially low, the policy assigns all patients maintained on dialysis a serum creatinine value of 4 mg/dL for calculation of MELD scores. Pediatric patients do not have laboratory values less than 1 rounded up, nor are limits placed on their laboratory values or overall PELD score. Centers can update a patient's MELD/ PELD score whenever a change in laboratory data occurs. Furthermore, existing MELD/PELD scores must be recertified by new laboratory data with increasing frequency for higher scores (Table 5–5). Pediatric and adult candidates are ranked on one list according to their MELD/PELD scores even though for any given PELD score, a pediatric candidate has a lower risk of mortality than an adult does with the identical MELD score (Fig. 5–4). As a result, pediatric patients with lower mortality are ranked equal to adults with higher mortality in an effort to allow children a slight advantage overall. In addition, pediatric donor livers are

Table 5-5. RECERTIFICATION SCHEDULE FOR LIVER TRANSPLANT CANDIDATES ON THE WAITING LIST ACCORDING TO THEIR MELD OR PELD SCORES

Score	Frequency
MELD/PELD ≥ 25	Every 7 days
MELD/PELD ≤ 24 but > 18	Every 30 days
MELD/PELD ≤ 18 but ≥ 11	Every 90 days
MELD/PELD ≤ 10	Every year

If recertification is not performed by the center, the patient reverts to last available MELD/PELD score.

If no previous MELD/PELD score, the patient is assigned 6 MELD/PELD points.

Recertification requires re-entry of new laboratory tests within 48 hours of the due date.

MELD, Model for End-Stage Liver Disease; PELD, Pediatric (model) for End-Stage Liver Disease.

eliminated from the allocation policy. Laboratory values less than 1 are rounded up to 1 to avoid a calculation of negative MELD scores because of the natural logarithm expressions in the MELD equation. The actual score derived by either the MELD or PELD equation is multiplied by 10 to obtain a whole integer.

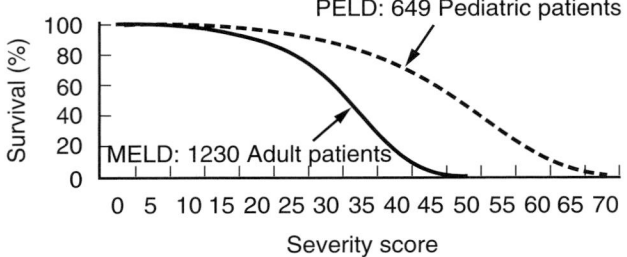

FIGURE 5–4

MELD and PELD scores plotted as a function of mortality risk.

preferentially allocated to pediatric recipients (see Table 5–4).

Waiting time is used only to rank candidates with identical MELD/PELD scores. Waiting time is carried "backward," but not "forward." Thus, when a candidate has been waiting for 2 weeks at a MELD score of 10 and then moves to a MELD score of 15 because of a change in laboratory values, the 2 weeks of waiting time is not carried forward and a new waiting time clock starts for that patient at the MELD score of 15. If after 2 additional weeks at a score of 15 the patient's laboratory values improve such that the MELD score is now 12, the 2 weeks of time waiting at 15 are carried "backward" and added to the time accrued at the MELD score of 12. This time affects priority ranking only if there are other patients with MELD/PELD scores equal to 12 when an organ is offered. The patient with the longest waiting time at that score, including any time accrued at a score higher than that score, is offered the organ first. Time waiting at inactive status does not accumulate.

As discussed earlier, MELD and PELD scores are good measures of need if need is defined as risk of dying of liver disease. Also, as mentioned previously, there are many conditions for which liver transplantation is appropriate and effective therapy but for which mortality risk is not a good measure of need. For these reasons, the current policy allows centers to request increased MELD or PELD scores for liver transplant candidates whom the center believes warrant increased priority. The largest group of such patients consists of candidates with HCC. Regional review boards (RRBs) assess each request for increased priority prospectively and grant approval or deny the application. The current policy recognizes that excellent outcomes can be achieved in candidates with HCC who meet the so-called Milan criteria with a single tumor nodule less than 5 cm in size or three or fewer tumors with the largest no greater than 3 cm in size.[39] The policy allows RRBs to assign 24 MELD points to candidates with more extensive tumors within the Milan criteria. Selection of these initial priority levels was based on best estimates of risk of tumor progression beyond the

Milan criteria with the understanding that they will probably need to be adjusted as more data become available.

For other conditions that may be appropriately treated by liver transplantation, centers may apply to their RRBs with specific requests for increased MELD/PELD points if they can justify the increased priority. This mechanism allows for peer review of all cases that might not be well served by the MELD/PELD scores and allows patients with unusual circumstances access to liver transplantation.

Early results of this plan have yielded a reduction in the number of patients dying and being removed from the waiting list for being too sick when compared with the corresponding 6 months in the preceding year under the previous allocation system.[40] In addition, more transplants were performed, and there were fewer registrations on the liver waiting list (Fig. 5–5). These results may not all be attributable to the new system; however, removal of waiting time as a major determinant of rank on the list eliminates significant

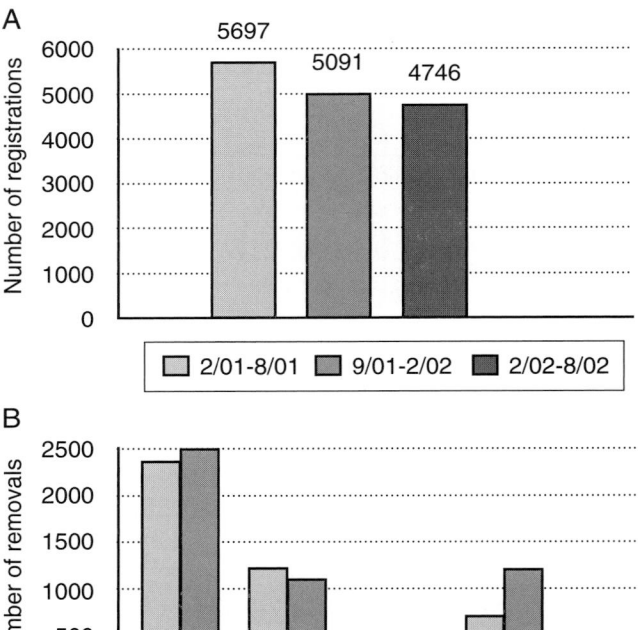

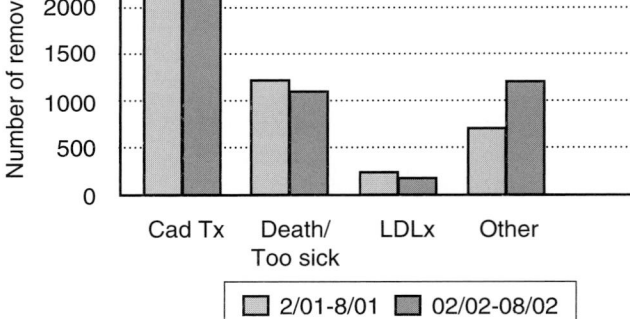

FIGURE 5–5

Comparison of the early results of the new MELD allocation system in the first 6 months (February 2002 to August 2002) with the corresponding 6 months (February 2001 to August 2001) of the previous year. **A,** New registrations on the liver transplant waiting list. **B,** Removals from the waiting list.

Cad Tx, cadaveric transplant; LDLx, living donor liver transplant.

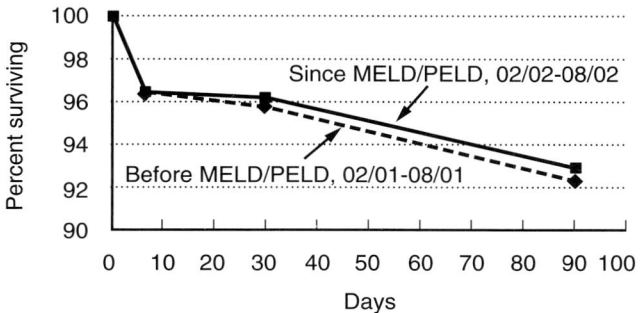

FIGURE 5–6

Early posttransplant results since implementation of the MELD/PELD system compared with the period February 2001 to August 2001.

incentive to "list patients early" and probably reduces the number of new registrations. Moreover, because the MELD score more accurately estimates the risk of dying, the new system can identify patients for whom the risk of death without a transplant is small relative to their risk of death with a transplant, hence leading centers to remove them from the active waiting list.

When waiting candidates are stratified by race, gender, or age, the new allocation system has not resulted in disproportionate increases or decreases in the numbers of transplants performed or the number of patients removed from the list. However, the new system has increased the proportion of patients who receive transplants for a diagnosis of HCC, as was intended. Early posttransplant survival results suggest that there has not been a significant change in 30- and 90-day survival rates under the MELD/PELD system relative to the previous year (Fig. 5–6).[28a]

Future U.S. Policy

One of the most important developments in the evolution of liver transplant policy has been an increasing effort to use evidence-based decision-making to develop policy. Whole sessions at national meetings are now devoted to scientific study of organ allocation, whereas in the past, policy development was much more empirical. Explicit in implementing new allocation policy is the commitment to constantly evaluate the results of changes, make the system as transparent and understandable to all users as possible, and try to continuously improve the system. To this end, it is essential to have the regulatory framework under which the OPTN operates specify enough authority to oversee the policy and collect the data, but not to impede evaluation, development, and promulgation of new policy efforts as they are deemed necessary or warranted.

Areas where future U.S. liver allocation policy will need attention are many. With as many as 16,000 new

cases of HCC diagnosed in the United States each year,[41] candidates with HCC will continue to potentially overwhelm the donor pool. Determining what proportion of the donor pool should be directed to these patients will remain a critical issue. In addition, as more data are published that better define the natural history of HCC and better selection criteria are developed for liver transplantation in candidates with HCC, new risk models, listing criteria, and priority systems for HCC will need to be developed and implemented. Moreover, as ablative treatments improve and more short- and long-term results are available, timing and selection of liver transplantation as treatment of HCC within the sequence of all these treatments will become critical, and the allocation system will need to be adjusted to reflect these developments.

As more data accumulate for all conditions treatable by liver transplantation, other objective variables may be defined to improve the risk models. Recent reports indicating that the rate of change in the MELD score may be more predictive than any one static score[42] suggest that incorporation of this dynamic variable into the allocation algorithm may be helpful. Other dichotomous variables such as mechanical ventilation or dialysis may likewise be included after prospectively validating their predictive value in the MELD/PELD equations. Re-examination of the coefficients within the MELD and PELD equations may also be necessary to improve the accuracy of the models. Revision of minimum listing criteria may become necessary to avoid placement of patients with an extremely low risk of death on the waiting list. Because risk models can define which patients are not likely to experience the endpoint defined as need for a liver transplant (i.e., death from chronic liver disease, progression beyond favorable tumor stage for HCC, etc.), minimum listing criteria may need to be established to limit the waiting list to candidates most likely to benefit. This modification should reduce the number of transplants performed in patients with low levels of need and enable more organs to be directed to those with higher risk. Implementation of these minimum criteria will help reduce regional and local disparities caused by relative differences in organ availability and waiting list size.

Differences in rates of transplantation and waiting list deaths across regional and OPO boundaries will remain difficult problems. Current distribution unit boundaries are arbitrarily based on OPO service areas, many of which are rooted in long-standing relationships between hospitals and OPOs. Differences across boundaries are related to differences in rates of brain death, identification of potential organ donors, procurement and OPO efficiency, and vastly different waiting list dynamics based on liver candidate referral patterns, insurer contracts, and the number of transplant programs competing for scarce resources within the local liver distribution unit. In many cases, simply redrawing the distribution unit boundaries does not alter some or all of these factors[26] and involves many far-reaching concerns surrounding local versus state versus federal regulation, local loyalties, and disruption of current organ procurement efforts. Use of more objective measures of need for prioritization of liver candidates may, however, allow for identification of potential candidates with a high risk of death but good chance of a successful outcome for whom neighboring OPOs would be willing to share organs.

Ultimately, as discussed throughout this chapter, allocation must balance reduction in waiting list mortality through identification and quantification of individual medical justice and maximization of post-transplant outcome through selection of candidates with the best chance of success. Thus, liver allocation should not only select candidates for transplantation with the highest risk of dying (or the highest risk of progression beyond a favorable stage of disease) but also select candidates with the best chance of long-term survival. Development of risk models that use objective, patient-specific pretransplant variables to predict who is at highest risk of dying without the transplant has progressed significantly and will continue to do so. Unfortunately, no models that use only objective, patient-specific pretransplant variables that are highly predictive of posttransplant mortality have been developed to date. Future liver allocation depends on these posttransplant predictive models. Combining pretransplant risk scores with posttransplant risk scores to direct the organs to those most in need but who are most likely to survive represents a combination of individual justice with resource utilitarianism to achieve the best possible balance. As with medical care in general, U.S. organ allocation policy should not be viewed as a static, rigid, or codified doctrine, but it is better understood as a constantly evolving and improving process as more information becomes available and advances in the field require refinements. Continuously striving to improve these policies is the only just way to improve liver transplantation in the future.

References

1. Starzl TE, Marchioro TL, Faris TD: Liver transplantation. Ann Intern Med 64:473-477, 1966.
2. Sadler AM Jr, Sadler BL, Stason EB: The uniform anatomical gift act. A model for reform. JAMA 206:2505-2506, 1968.
3. A definition of irreversible coma. Report of the Ad Hoc Committee of the Harvard Medical School to Examine the Definition of Brain Death. JAMA 205:85-88, 1968.
4. Uniform Brain Death Act. Uniform Laws Annotated, vol 12. St. Paul, MN, West Publishing, 1996, p 65.
5. Uniform Declaration of Death Act. Uniform Laws Annotated, vol 12A. St. Paul, MN, West Publishing, 1996, p 593.
6. National Organ Transplant Act (NOTA) sections 371-376 of the Public Health Service Act, 1984.
7. National Task Force on Organ Transplantation: Organ Transplantation: Issues and Recommendations. Rockville, MD, Office of Organ Transplantation, Health Resources and Services Administration, Department of health and Human Services, 1986.
8. PL 100-607, 42 USC 273.
9. 42 CFR Part 486, Subpart G, see 53 FR 6549, March 1, 1988.
10. PL 99-509 § 9318.
11. Section 121.8, Federal Register [FR Doc. 98-8191], 42 CFR Part 121 April 2, 1998, p 16296.
12. Organ Procurement and Transplantation: Assessing Current Policies and the Potential Impact of the DHHS Final Rule. Washington, DC, National Academy Press, 1999.
13. 64 FR 56658, October 20, 1999.
14. Outka G: Social justice and equal access to health care. J Religious Ethics 2:11-32, 1974.
15. Daniels NJ: Just Health Care. New York, Cambridge University Press, 1985.
16. Crumplin MK: [Surgery in the English army at Waterloo.] Ann Chir 51:68-75, 1997.
17. Daniels N: Why saying no to patients in the United States is so hard. Cost containment, justice, and provider autonomy. N Engl J Med 314:1380-1383, 1986.
18. Baker R, Strosberg M: Triage and equality: An historical reassessment of utilitarian analyses of triage. Kennedy Inst Ethics J 2:103-123, 1992.
19. Mill JS: Utilitarianism. London, Collins, 1863.
20. Daniels NJ: The ideal advocate and limited resources. Theor Med 8:69-80, 1987.
21. Purtilo RB: What kind of good is a donor liver anyway, and should we care? Liver Transpl Surg 1:75-80, 1995.
22. Weisner RH, McDiarmid SV, Kamath PS, et al: MELD and PELD: Application of survival models to liver allocation. Liver Transpl 7:567-580, 2001.
23. Neuberger J, James O: Guidelines for selection of patients for liver transplantation in the era of donor-organ shortage. Lancet 354:1636-1639, 1999.
24. Delmonico FL, Harmon WE, Lorber MI, et al: A new allocation plan for renal transplantation. Transplant Proc 31:358-359, 1999.
25. Organ Procurement and Transplantation: Assessing Current Policies and the Potential Impact of the DHHS Final Rule. Washington, DC, National Academy Press, 1999, p 6.
26. Freeman RB, Harper AM, Edwards EB: Redrawing organ distribution boundaries: Results of a computer simulated analysis for liver transplantation. Liver Transpl 8:659-666, 2002.
27. Calabresi G, Bobbit P: Tragic Choices: The Conflicts Society Confronts in the Allocation of Tragically Scarce Resources. New York, WW Norton, 1978.
28. Freeman RB, Rohrer RJ, Katz E, et al: Preliminary results of a liver allocation plan using a continuous medical severity score that de-emphasizes waiting time. Liver Transpl 7:173-178, 2001.
28a. Freeman RB, Wiesner RH, Harper A, et al: Results of the first year of the new liver allocation plan. Liver Transpl 10:7-15, 2004.
29. Malinchoc M, Kamath PS, Gordon FD, et al: A model to predict poor survival in patients undergoing transjugular intrahepatic portosystemic shunts. Hepatology 31:864-871, 2000.
30. Wiesner RH, Edwards EB, Freeman RB, et al: Model for end stage liver disease (MELD) and allocation of donor livers. Gastroenterology 124:91-96, 2003.
31. McDiarmid SV, Anand R, Lindblad AS: The Principal Investigators and Institutions of the Studies of Pediatric Liver Transplantation (SPLIT) Research Group. Development of a pediatric end-stage liver disease score to predict poor outcome in children awaiting liver transplantation. Transplantation 74:173-181, 2002.

32. Hanley JA, McNeil BJ: The meaning and use of the area under a receiver operating characteristic (ROC) curve. Radiology 143:29-36, 1982.

33. Wong LL: Current status of liver transplantation for hepatocellular cancer. Am J Surg 183:309-316, 2002.

34. Cheng SJ, Freeman RB, Wong JB: Predicting the probability of progression free survival in patients with small hepatocellular carcinoma. Liver Transpl 8:323-328, 2002.

35. Lovelet JM, Foster J, Briux J: Intention to treat analysis of surgical treatment of early hepatocellular carcinoma: Resection versus transplantation. Hepatology 30:1434-1440, 1999.

36. Freeman RB, Wiesner RH, Harper A, et al: The new liver allocation system: Moving towards evidence based transplantation policy. Liver Transpl 8:851-858, 2002.

37. www.UNOS.org.

38. Bennett-Guerrero E, Feierman DE, Barclay GR, et al: Preoperative and intraoperative predictors of postoperative morbidity, poor graft function, and early rejection in 190 patients undergoing liver transplantation. Arch Surg 136:1177-1183, 2001.

39. Mazzaferro V, Regalia E, Doci R, et al: Liver transplantation for the treatment of small hepatocellular carcinomas in patients with cirrhosis. N Engl J Med 334:693-699, 1996.

40. http://www.unos.org/news/newsDetail.asp?id=227, accessed March 10, 2003.

41. Cancer Facts & Figures 2001, www.cancer.org, accessed January 18, 2003.

42. Merion RM, Wolfe RA, Dykstra DM, et al: Longitudinal assessment of mortality risk among candidates for liver transplantation. Liver Transpl 9:12-18, 2003.

6

Liver Organ Allocation: The European Models

LARS BÄCKMAN
JOHN L. R. FORSYTHE
BIANCA MIRANDA
NATIVIDAD CUENDE
JOSE CAÑÓN
CARLOS MARGARIT
TILL GERLING
GUIDO G. PERSIJN

Liver transplantation in Europe   79

Organ allocation   80

Spain   81

United Kingdom Transplant   83
  Fast track   86

Scandiatransplant   86

The Eurotransplant liver allocation system   87

Discussion   90

Liver Transplantation in Europe

The number of liver transplants performed in Europe has increased, reaching a plateau of close to 4000 liver transplants performed annually (Fig. 6–1).[1] The number of listed patients waiting for a liver transplant continues to increase, and the gap is widening between them and the number of available liver grafts. Table 6–1 lists the liver transplant activity and organ donation rates in different European countries and regions.[2] It is obvious from Table 6–1 that the liver transplantation activity and organ donation rates vary in the different countries and regions in Europe. Table 6–2 lists the main indications for end-stage liver disease and liver transplantation. As in the United States, liver cirrhosis resulting from chronic hepatitis C and alcoholic cirrhosis are the main and increasing indications for liver transplantation.

This chapter gives an overview and description of some different European organ allocation systems

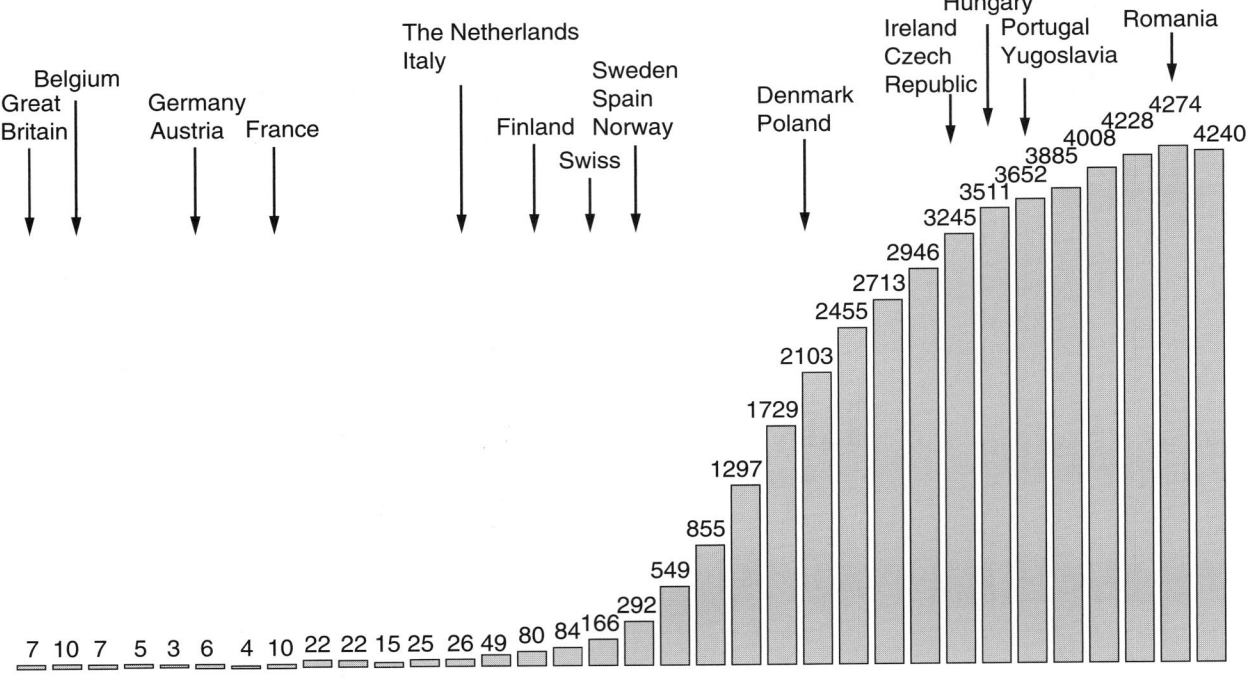

FIGURE 6–1

Development of liver transplantation in Europe between 1968 and 2001. Evolution of 46,530 liver transplantations in Europe.

and organizations. The differences presented reflect differences in legislation, organ donation rates, indications for liver transplantation, and traditions in the practice of medicine in different countries and regions of Europe.

Organ Allocation

There are no uniform rules or systems for organ allocation in Europe or within the European Union.

Table 6–1. LIVER TRANSPLANTATION ACTIVITY AND NUMBER OF PATIENTS ON WAITING LISTS IN DIFFERENT COUNTRIES AND REGIONS IN EUROPE IN 2001

	Population (Millions)	Liver Transplantation Per Million Inhabitants	Liver Transplants/Waiting List (Absolute Number)	Overall Mortality From Chronic Liver Disease (Expressed Per 100,000 Inhabitants in 1996)
France	60	13.4	803/457	16.5
Eurotransplant*	117	10.2	1193/1089	20.2
Scandiatransplant†	24	8.7	209/45	8.9
UKT‡	63	11.1	700/180	7.5
Organizacion Nacional de Transplantes§	43	23.3	972/522	17.3

*Germany, Austria, Belgium, the Netherlands, Luxembourg, and Slovenia
†Sweden, Norway, Finland, Denmark, and Iceland
‡United Kingdom Transplant—Great Britain and Ireland
§Spain

Table 6–2. INDICATIONS FOR ADULT LIVER TRANSPLANTATION IN EUROPE OCTOBER 1991 TO DECEMBER 2002*

Diagnosis	LD	DD	P-Value
Acute hepatic failure	4%	7%	ns
Cirrhosis	55%	53%	ns
Cancers	25%	13%	P<0.0001
Retransplantation	1%	10%	P<0.0001
Others	17%	15%	ns

*Data from the European Liver Transplant Registry. D, deceased donor; LD, living donor; ns, not significant.

There are different organ exchange organizations for different countries and geographical areas, including:

- Organizacion Nacional de Transplantes (ONT) in Spain
- United Kingdom Transplant (UKT) for the United Kingdom and Ireland
- Eurotransplant (Germany, the Netherlands, Belgium, Luxembourg, Austria, and Slovenia)
- Scandiatransplant (Sweden, Norway, Finland, Denmark, and Iceland)
- North Italian Transplant (NIT)
- Etablissement francais des Greffes (EfG) in France

The majority of livers are allocated and transplanted within each procurement and exchange organization, but there is collaboration in case of surplus organs among these organizations.

Most organizations have similar rules with an urgent priority group that includes acute hepatic failure and early retransplantation following vascular thrombosis as well as primary nonfunction. There are, however, important differences as well.

Although no universally accepted liver allocation rules exist, two methods are primarily followed. Organ allocation can be patient-directed, as is the case in the United States and some European countries (Eurotransplant), or center-directed, which is the case in other European countries (Spain, Scandiatransplant, and United Kingdom Transplant). An organ allocation system is a matter of consensus among transplant teams, organizational structures, health authorities, and customer and patient organizations. Regardless of the model chosen, all systems work with two factor categories. The first category includes medical criteria such as blood group, human leukocyte antigen (HLA) compatibility (kidney transplantation), primary disease, donor and recipient matching, donor virology status, severity of recipient status, and others. The second category is nonmedical criteria, which include geographical distance and resources consumed. Waiting time or cold ischemia time may appear in either category.

The Committee of Ministers of the Council of Europe, considering that organ transplantation is severely restricted by availability of organs for transplantation, recognizes the need to set up a public system with an officially recognized network of transplant centers and an official register of patients on waiting lists.[2] The committee also recommends that such a system provide complete information for health care professionals and the general public. This information should include criteria for registration and allocation, figures and flows of registered patients, and average waiting times for different groups of patients. The system must ensure, as far as possible, that no group of patients waits longer than another group.

Currently, few livers are exchanged between the different organizations. There is, however, an increasing collaboration with some former eastern European countries with recognized allocation systems and organizations. The goal is to use donor organs fully and, more importantly, to develop the field of organ transplantation in these countries to the level of the rest of Europe.

Spain

Spain has 17 autonomous regions, with a public health service in each, providing health care for 99% of the population. There are currently 22 active liver transplant centers in Spain. There is a requirement for official hospital authorization to perform a liver transplant with an obligation to officially record all patients registered on the waiting list. The ONT provides the services necessary for organ procurement, allocation support, and waiting list management.[3] Spain has the highest organ donation rate in the world—partly because of outstanding donor detection and organ procurement organizations—which is often referred to as "the Spanish model for organ donation." Deceased-donor organ donation rates achieved the level of 33 donors per million population without large differences among regions (average range in the different years is between 30 and 40 donors per million population). In addition, non–heart-beating donor (NHBD) programs are available and account for 2% to 3% of all donors.

Organ allocation in Spain is center-oriented. All available organs are referred to the coordinating offices, which are in Barcelona for the Catalonia region and in Madrid for the rest of Spain. The rules for allocation are decided by consensus among transplant centers and representatives from regional health authorities. Currently, national priority is given to lung, heart, and liver emergencies, and it is publicly and clearly stated what is considered an emergency and the circumstances under which a patient can be listed as an urgent patient.[4] In the absence of urgent patients, the organ is allocated to the hospital, city, region, or area. If no recipient is available in Spain, the liver is offered internationally. In any event, medical matching rules are obeyed. Finally, once an organ is offered to the transplant center, the final decision about the recipient is made internally by the transplant team. Rates of indications and transplantation, as well as waiting times and probabilities of being transplanted for the different groups of patients, are analyzed annually.

An urgent liver transplant recipient is defined as having fulminant liver failure in the absence of any previous liver disease or retransplantation within the first 7 postoperative days. In pediatric recipients, 30 days are accepted. The urgent recipient gets national priority with the possibility of blood group and body weight selection within the first 48 hours. The patient can be listed as urgent for only 3 days. In case of coincidental urgencies, livers are allocated first to pediatric recipients (younger than 15 years of age) and next to patients according to the time they have been on the waiting list.

The Spanish organ procurement system achieves similar donation rates among the different regions, leading to a point at which liver transplantation does not correlate with organ donation rates but with the number of listed patients (Fig. 6–2). The larger the candidate pool, the higher the absolute number of liver transplants performed.

A review of the outcomes of all patients admitted to the liver transplant waiting lists in Spain from 1999 through 2002 (Figs. 6–3 and 6–4) shows that a total of 4950 patients were registered during that period. Of these, 322 were urgent patients. Between 1.5 and 2 liver urgencies per million population were registered every year. Among them, most were fulminant liver failures. Primary graft failure within the first 7 days after surgery accounted for only 2% to 3% of all transplants. Urgent cases were excluded from the analysis of clearance from the waiting list, given their priority. Of the remaining patients, 546 were still on waiting lists at the end of the period, 558 had died, and 3524 had received transplants. The median waiting time for the grafted patients was 95 days; the median waiting time for the deceased patients was 93 days, which was less than the median time of 159 days for those still waiting. These data indicate that patients are undergoing transplantation following medical criteria, with the sickest patients undergoing transplantation first.[5] No significant differences were observed in clearance rates from the waiting lists in relation to blood, age, or weight groups; region where the patient lives; primary liver disease; and other studied variables. Use of living donor livers and split-liver procedures performed during the review period accounted for 5% to 6% of the activity. During 2003, of the 1037 registered liver transplants, 31 were living donor livers, 16 were split livers, 11 were domino livers, and only 3 were from NHBDs.

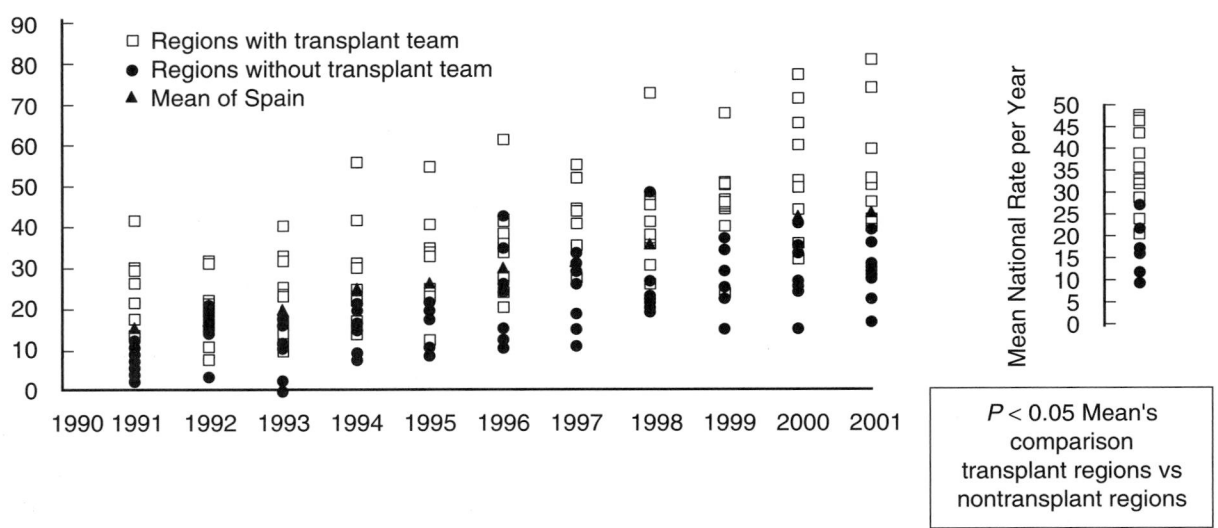

FIGURE 6–2

The rate of listing patients for liver transplantation in Spain between 1990 and 2001. Data from regions with and without liver transplant centers are presented.

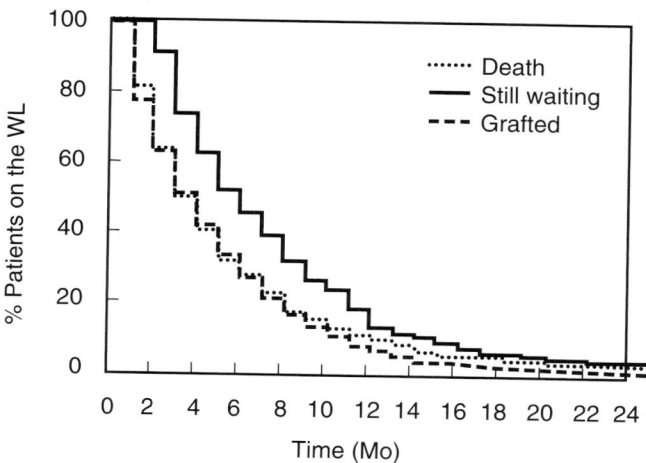

FIGURE 6-3

Clearance of patients from the liver transplant waiting list in Spain, 1999-2002: Overall analysis (urgent patients are excluded).

	N	Mean	Median
Grafted	3524	137,5925	95,0000
Still waiting	546	228,4908	159,0000
Death	558	155,4624	92,5000
Total	4628	150,4710	102,0000

Global Wilcoxon test *P* < 0.01
Still vs the rest *P* < 0.01

United Kingdom Transplant

In the United Kingdom liver transplantation is provided by the National Health Service (NHS) through top-sliced funding from the health budget. There are seven designated transplant centers in the United Kingdom, and the unit in the Republic of Ireland (Dublin) works closely on organizational issues. United Kingdom Transplant is a special health authority with a dual responsibility to:

• Organize and monitor organ allocation systems

• Increase the number of individuals whose lives are saved or transformed through organ transplantation

The Liver Advisory Group of UKT consists of a chairperson who is a clinician from a liver transplant center, two representatives from each liver transplant unit, individuals who give statistical advice, personnel from UKT, and patient representatives. This advisory group is the main forum for discussion regarding patient assessment and liver retrieval and allocation. Episodes of noncompliance with rules are rare and are dealt with by the advisory group and the UKT Medical Director.

The numbers of donors and liver transplants have remained largely static over the last few years, although the total number in 2002 to 2003 reached a new high at 705 (Fig. 6–5).[6] The rate of liver transplantation in the United Kingdom is 11.1 per million population, which is lower than in other parts of Europe such as France (19.3 per million population) and Spain (24.3 per million population). The different figures in these countries may be because of a different disease burden but may also reflect the donor rates in these countries. These figures also should be seen against a background of increased incidence of liver disease in the United Kingdom. For instance, in Scotland (population 5 million) the mortality from liver disease almost doubled between 1991 and 1999, from 556 to 994, respectively.

The donor rate in the United Kingdom in 2002 to 2003 was 13.1 donors per million inhabitants. This varied between 11.4 donors per million inhabitants in Wales to 18.9 donors per million inhabitants in Northern Ireland. This compares poorly with some other European countries, most notably Spain where the rate is 33 donors per million inhabitants. The United Kingdom Department of Health acknowledged this fact in 2000 when UKT was reorganized and various initiatives to improve the organ donation rate were undertaken. These included review of transplant coordination services and the appointment of donor liaison nursing staffs in major intensive care units across the United Kingdom. In addition, a potential donor audit was carried out, and the initial results from this audit show an alarming increase in the rate of refusal when relatives are approached to consider organ donation from a family member who has been confirmed dead by brain stem death testing.[7] Forty-eight percent of relatives have refused to allow organ donation in these circumstances. The cause for this increase in relatives' refusals is unclear but may be linked to high profile cases of general medical malpractice, which have eroded the trust that existed between those who deliver care and those who receive it in the NHS.

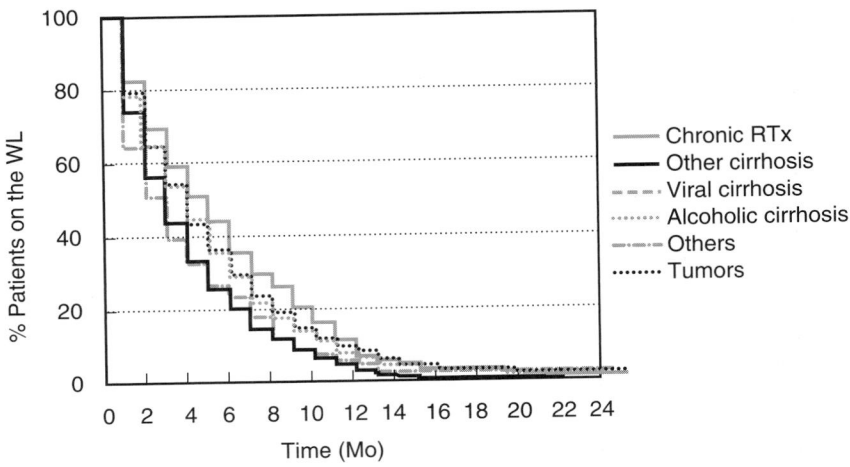

	N	Mean	Median
Tumors	633	109,1912	77,0000
Others	225	166,0756	125,0000
Alcoholic cirrhosis	1235	143,9449	105,0000
Other cirrhosis	1130	149,7726	105,0000
Chronic RTx	149	108,6577	61,0000
Total	3372	139,2912	97,0000

Global Wilcoxon test $P < 0.01$
Tumors vs Other and cirrhosis $P < 0.01$
RTx vs Others and cirrhosis $P < 0.01$

FIGURE 6–4

Clearance of patients from the liver transplant waiting list in Spain, 1999-2002: grouped by primary diagnosis (urgent patients are excluded).

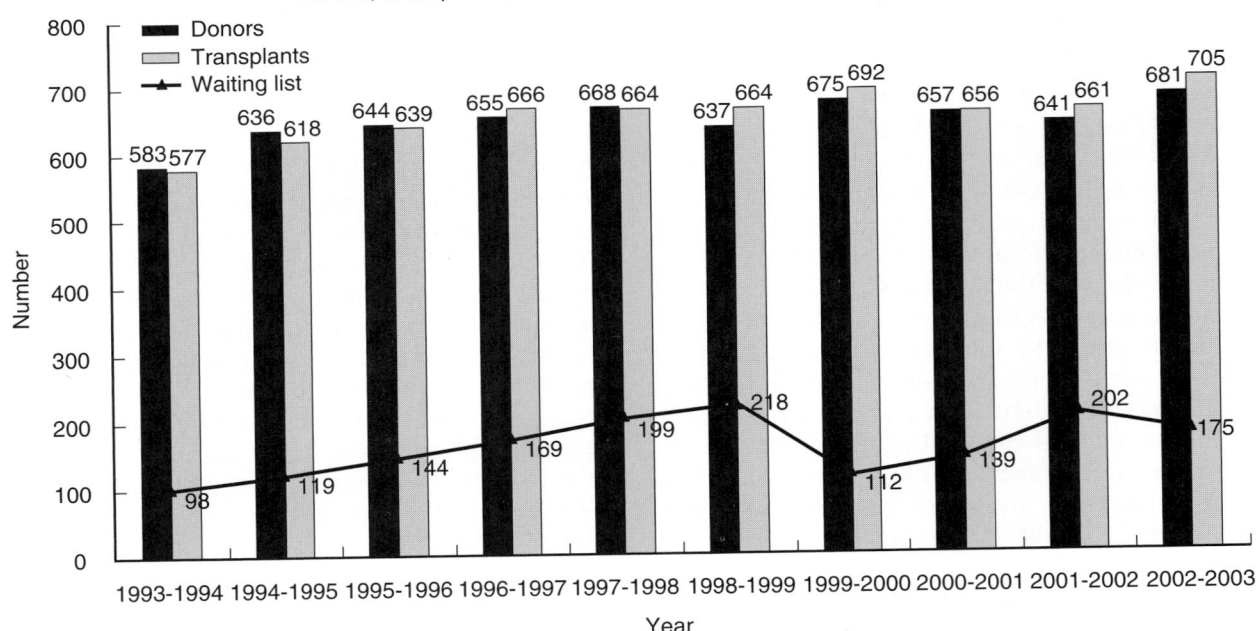

Cadaveric Liver Program in the UK, April 1, 1993 - March 31, 2003: Number of Donors, Transplants, and Patients on the Active Waiting List on March 31, 2003

FIGURE 6–5

Evolution of liver transplantation in the United Kingdom between 1993 and 2003.

In 1993, zonal retrieval was introduced across the UK, operated by the designated liver transplant centers. At that time only 62% of livers donated were retrieved by their future designated zonal teams. Now more than 90% of livers are retrieved by the local zonal team. This is considered a successful development by both the transplant units carrying out retrieval and donor hospitals, which can establish a relationship with their local team. The size of the zone is reviewed annually by the Liver Advisory Group of UKT. Originally these zones were delineated on the basis of population size, but since 2001 they have been designed based on recent donor numbers. It is of note that in 2002 to 2003, 23 livers were retrieved from NHBDs.

To be admitted to the liver transplant waiting list, a patient must be referred for consideration of transplantation to the local transplant unit. Unfortunately, not all patients who would benefit from transplantation are referred for assessment.[8] However, once patients are admitted to any transplant unit in the UK, the evaluation period is very similar in all centers. The diagnosis of liver disease is confirmed and staged. If any contraindications to transplantation are discovered, an alternative treatment is sought. The patient is seen by numerous members of the multidisciplinary team, and the patient's own view regarding transplantation is sought. Next, a team assessment meeting is held, a decision is made, and the decision is communicated to the patient and his or her relatives. After discussion at the Liver Advisory Group of UKT, it has been agreed by all centers that a patient must have a greater than 50% survival probability of 5 years after transplantation, with a quality of life acceptable to the patient, before placement on the active transplant list.[9]

For certain primary liver diseases, special conditions apply. In alcoholic liver disease, it is important that the patient accept responsibility for the liver disease and demonstrate the ability to abstain from alcohol. Most units also carry out an assessment of the risk of recidivism. Those felt to be a high risk of returning to harmful drinking are either given further counseling and help, if they will accept this, or are excluded from the active waiting list. For those with hepatocellular carcinoma, either as the primary disease or secondary to hepatitis or chronic liver disease, there is general acceptance of the Milan criteria,[10] which is that a patient who has a single tumor greater than 5 cm or two tumors that are each greater than 2 cm should not be placed on the active waiting list. There is no stipulation as to which modality should be used to measure the tumor, although most units use magnetic resonance imaging (MRI) for this purpose.

There is no audit of the chronic waiting list; however, there apparently is significant similarity of patient profiles from center to center. In a 1-year period ending March 2003, 69% of patients who had been listed for transplant had received at least one liver, 19% were still on the waiting list either in active or suspended form, 6% of the patients had died, and another 6% had been removed from the waiting list. It is likely that most patients removed from the list were too sick for liver transplantation.

The allocation rules, which are defined by the Liver Advisory Group in UKT, evolve and change over the years as innovative techniques in liver transplantation are introduced. For example, in 2002 to 2003, 705 liver transplants were performed, 66 of which were split-liver transplants. The current agreed-upon splitting criteria are:

- Age 40 years and younger
- Weight 50 kg (110 pounds) or more
- Short intensive care unit (ICU) stay (less than 5 days)
- No deranged liver function tests
- Hemodynamically stable—no prolonged hypertension, no high-dose inotropes, no systemic sepsis

These are only guidelines, but on each occasion that these criteria have been fulfilled and splitting has not occurred, the Liver Advisory Group is informed and may review the circumstances of the case.

In the UK, the offering sequence for receiving a liver transplant is:

- Super urgent liver patients in the order of registration
- Local zonal center regardless of their position in the offering rotation
- All other designated centers by order of the rotation
- Other European exchange organizations
- Super urgent—for patients who received a liver transplant that failed in the early postoperative period (because of primary nonfunction or vascular thrombosis), or who have fulminant hepatic failure

The last category, super urgent, entitles the patient to the next available blood-group–compatible liver wherever that liver is retrieved in the United Kingdom. It is obvious that such a system is open to abuse and, therefore, the criteria are carefully defined and closely monitored. In essence the patient should be expected to live not more than 3 days without a liver transplant. For patients with fulminant hepatic failure, the King's criteria (Table 6–3) are used.[11]

The logistics of a super urgent listing are straightforward: A form is completed, signed by the consultant in charge of the patient, and sent to UKT, from which the information is forwarded to each center in the United Kingdom. If there are any unusual circumstances, other centers may challenge the urgent listing. Otherwise the patient is placed on the super urgent list and will be offered the next blood-group–compatible liver. If two

Table 6–3. KING'S COLLEGE CRITERIA FOR ACUTE HEPATIC FAILURE

Acetaminophen Patients

pH < 7.30 (irrespective of encephalopathy grade)

or

Prothrombin time >100 seconds and serum creatinine >300 μmol/L in patients with grade III or IV encephalopathy

Nonacetominophen Patients

Prothrombin time >100 seconds (irrespective of encephalopathy grade)

or

Any 3 of the following variables (irrespective of encephalopathy grade)

Age < 10 or > 40 years

Etiology: non-A, non-B hepatitis, halothane hepatitis, idiosyncratic drug reactions

Duration of jaundice before onset of encephalopathy >7 days

Prothrombin time > 50 seconds

Serum bilirubin > 300 μmol/L

super urgent patients are listed in the United Kingdom concurrently, the time of listing governs allocation.

When a deceased-donor liver is retrieved, the local zonal team has first refusal for any blood group that is identical to patients on their list. If that center does not have a suitable recipient (for instance because there is no individual with an identical blood group or the clinician feels that the donor liver is too marginal for any recipients on their list), the liver is then offered to other centers within the United Kingdom. The order of offering is decided on by a strict rotation system that is based on point allocation; the center gains points by exporting livers and loses points by importing.

The Duty Office in UKT is encouraged to offer all livers to centers, even when there are relative contraindications, such as virological problems. Clinical urgency can overrule practice guidelines in many circumstances, even when there are relative contraindications.[12]

For any one center, the allocation of a liver within a list of blood-group–compatible individuals is decided on by local policy. However, most units in the United Kingdom choose the recipient based on the size and match between donor and recipient and the patient's time on the waiting list, in addition to the clinical urgency. Most liver transplant surgeons acknowledge that a sick recipient will need a good liver, whereas a stable recipient can likely withstand an expanded criteria liver following transplantation.[13]

Fast Track

On certain occasions it is advantageous for a liver to be offered quickly to all centers to allow transport to the accepting center as quickly as possible; this reduces cold ischemic time to a minimum. For this reason, a fast track liver offer scheme exists in the UK. This can be brought into operation when 4 hours of cold ischemic time has already elapsed and a whole liver or lobe is on offer, or in circumstances when there are domino donors or NHBDs. Common examples of when the fast track system is used include:

- A right lobe donated following splitting of a whole liver
- A liver that has become available when initial laparotomy has revealed that the intended recipient is not fit for surgery

Relevant information is entered on a form especially designed for this situation, and the form is then sent simultaneously to all centers in the United Kingdom. Centers are given 30 minutes to respond, and those who have indicated acceptance are ranked in the rotation used for the chronic liver waiting list.

Living donor liver transplantation was first successfully performed in a child in 1990.[13] An adult-to-adult living donor procedure followed this success in 1993.[14] There continue to be developments of this surgical technique, but there are also many ethical considerations because of the donor morbidity and mortality associated with it. Therefore, this technique is not currently available to patients within the United Kingdom via the National Health Service (although nearly one third of liver transplants in other parts of Europe are living donor procedures), but its use and development are being debated.[1,15] A few of these procedures have been performed in the United Kingdom, but these were carried out on foreign nationals.

Many UK clinicians feel that living donor transplantation is very likely to be introduced in large part because of patient pressure. Opinion is divided on whether the procedure should be only for patients who are already eligible for liver transplantation or whether living donor livers should also be used for patients who do not meet the current criteria. Whichever course is decided, it is imperative that the donor advocate team be well established in any program. This was one of the main recommendations that came out of a donor disaster, in which a donor died after giving a portion of his liver to his brother. This was the subject of a December 2002 report to the New York State Transplant Council and New York State Department of Health.

Scandiatransplant

Scandiatransplant was founded in 1969 and has its headquarters in Århus, Denmark. As with other organ exchange organizations, its initial purpose was to allocate kidneys. Scandiatransplant is a collaboration of all organ transplant centers in the Nordic countries—Sweden,

Table 6–5. URGENCY CODES IN THE EUROTRANSPLANT LIVER ALLOCATION SYSTEM (ELAS)

Medical Urgency		Priority	Mandatory Exchange
HU	High urgency	Internationally first	Yes
CO	Approved combined organ	Internationally second	Yes
T2	Chronic disease, acute deterioration	Nationally over T3/T4	No
T3	Chronic disease, complications	Based on point score	No
T4	Chronic disease, no complications	Based on point score	No
NT	Temporarily not transplantable	Not matched	—

without transplantation, and has a CTP score of 11 or higher, and one or more of the following complications:

- Unresponsive variceal bleeding
- Hepatorenal syndrome
- Refractory ascites/hepatohydrothorax
- Encephalopathy grade III/IV that is unresponsive to medical therapy
- Repeated spontaneous bacterial peritonitis

T2 patients also are audited prospectively. The ET medical staff evaluates the request according to the current criteria. After approval, status T2 is granted and the urgency code is changed. A patient is granted the T2 status for the duration of 28 days.

Patients are listed as T3 if they have a CTP score of 10 or more, or a CTP of 7 and one or more of the following complications:

- Known hepatocellular carcinoma (HCC), assessment according to state-of-the-art rules
- Tumor diameter 5 cm or less
- Three or fewer nodes involved
- Tumor less than 3 cm in diameter and no macrovascular invasion or extrahepatic spread

T4 patients include all other patients with a CTP score of at least 7 (T4 criteria). Patients temporarily not transplantable (NT) should be placed in urgency NT. Patients can accumulate waiting time points in NT up to a maximum of 30 days. The maximum number of waiting time points remains 400 points (i.e., 360 days). All previously accumulated waiting time is retained in NT. Patients appearing on the national waiting list without urgency points are not selected in matching procedures.

Elective pediatric patients (<16 years of age) are stratified into only two categories. Patients in T2 are hospitalized in the transplant center or are eligible for transplantation with a left lateral segment (i.e., a left split-liver procedure), or both. Patients in T3 comprise all other pediatric patients. A pediatric donor (<46 kg [101.4 lb]) is preferentially allocated to pediatric patients.

ET countries can be divided into regions comprising one or more transplant centers. Transplant candidates in urgencies T3 and T4 receive 200 extra points if they are from the same donor center or region. ET countries with regions are Austria (three regions) and Germany (seven regions). ABO-incompatible liver transplants

Table 6–6. THE EUROTRANSPLANT POINT SCORING SYSTEM FOR LIVER ALLOCATION, STRATIFIED BY ACTIVE URGENCY*

	High Urgency (HU)	Combined Organ (CO)	T2	T3	T4
Match selection	First international	Second international	First national	According to individual point score	According to individual point score
Match ranking	Time spent in HU, longest waiting first	Time spent in CO, longest waiting first	Time spent in T2, longest waiting first	According to individual point score	According to individual point score
Waiting time				1.11 points per active waiting day (counter stops after 365 days)	1.11 points per active waiting day (counter stops after 365 days)
Urgency				200 points	100 points
Region†				200 points	200 points

*Patients temporarily not transplantable (NT) are not selected in the matching; patients in HU, CO, and T2 are selected and ranked based on the higher urgency and not on point score.

†Germany is the only ET country with seven regions. Only recipients registered in a center in the same region as the donor receive regional points.

are not allowed. Full ABO compatibility applies to pediatric HU, pediatric and adult combined organ (CO), pediatric T2 and T3, and split-liver transplantations. ET-compatible is defined as a restricted compatibility (i.e., ABO-O to ABO-O and ABO-B recipients). This rule applies to adult HU, adult T2, and domino liver transplantations.

Split-liver transplantation (SLT) is encouraged. Each liver donor who meets the conditions (weight ≥50 kg [110 lb] and ≤50 years of age) is considered a potential split-liver donor. If a transplant center does not consider a split procedure, a reason must be given. The splitting center is allowed to keep the second split and allocate it to a suitable recipient from its own waiting list. If the second split cannot be allocated or transplanted in the splitting center, the second split is reported to the ET duty desk for allocation through ELAS.

Livers from NHBDs are allocated according to the same allocation algorithm as postmortem heart-beating donors. However, according to the German law on transplantation (Transplantationsgesetz), organs from NHBDs must not be harvested or allocated in Germany.

As a consequence of a gradually increasing waiting list mortality under the current ELAS, and following the positive experience with the implementation of the MELD/PELD scores in UNOS in 2002,[21] the Board of ET issued a recommendation in 2003 to adapt and implement both scores in ET in the near future.

Discussion

The increasing number of patients waiting and listed for liver transplantation and the gap between demand and supply will increase unless there are dramatic changes in the donation rates in Europe. In addition, as in the United States, liver cirrhosis from chronic hepatitis C is an increasing indication for liver transplantation. In the future, splitting of liver grafts may play an important role in increasing the number of transplants by optimizing the utilization of donor livers. Splitting will definitely also increase the exchange of organs between the different exchange and allocation organizations in Europe. An increase in the number of living donors (adult to adult) would also certainly result in reduced morbidity and mortality on the waiting lists. As pointed out, there are no uniform rules or systems for liver allocation in Europe. Different systems are used, ranging from center-oriented to patient-oriented. Some systems are constructed using rigorous rules based on points and scores, whereas others are based on the clinical judgment of the responsible transplant surgeon. The current diversity makes it impossible to adopt a uniform organ allocation system in Europe in the foreseeable future.

Pearls and Pitfalls

- There is no uniform liver or organ allocation system within Europe or the European Union.
- There are different large organ allocation organizations covering several countries.
- There are varying donation and transplantation rates in the allocation organizations.
- Liver allocation is center-directed in Spain, in the Scandiatransplant system, and in the United Kingdom Transplant system.
- Liver allocation is patient-directed in the Eurotransplant system.
- There is potential to increase the number of grafts by developing split-liver and living related donor transplantation.

References

1. European Liver Transplant Registry online: Available at http://www.eltr.org/publi/index_rv.php3
2. International figures for organ donation and transplantation activities. Newsletter Transplant, Council of Europe 7(12), 2002.
3. Miranda B, Vilardell J, Grinyó JM: Optimizing cadaveric organ procurement: The Catalan and Spanish experience. Am J Transplant 3:1-8, 2003.
4. www.ont.es/esp/informacion/J_informacion.htm (updated Sept, 2004).
5. Cuende MN, Miranda SB, Cañón CJF, et al: Criterios de priorización para el acceso al trasplante. El caso del trasplante hepático en España. Med Clin (Barc) 120:380-386, 2003.
6. UK Transplant Activity Report 2002-2003: Available at http://www.uktransplant.org.uk/ukt/statistics/transplant_activity/transplant_activity_uk.jsp
7. Gore GM, Cable DJ, Holland AJB: Organ donation from intensive care units. Br Med J 304:349-355, 1992.
8. Davies M, Langman M, Elias E, Neuberger J: Liver disease in a district hospital remote from a transplant centre: A study of admissions and deaths. Gut 33:1397-1399, 1992.
9. Neuberger J, James O: Guidelines for selection of patients for liver transplantation in the era of donor organ shortage. Lancet 354:1636-1639, 1999.
10. Mazzaferro V, et al: Liver transplantation for the treatment of small hepatocellular carcinomas in patients with cirrhosis. N Eng J Med 334:693-699, 1996.
11. O'Grady JG, Alexander GJM, Hallyar KM, Williams R: Early indicators of prognosis in fulminant hepatic failure. Gastroenterology 97:439-445, 1988.
12. Department of Health [UK] Advisory Committee on the Microbiological Safety of Blood and Tissues for Transplantation: Guidance on the Microbiological Safety of Human Organs, Tissues and Cells used in Transplantation. Her Majesty's Stationery Office, London, August 2000.
13. Strong RW, Lynch SV, Ong TH, et al: Successful liver transplantation from a liver donor to her son. N Engl J Med 322:1505-1507, 1993.
14. Achida T, Matsunami H, Kawasaki S, et al: Living related donor liver transplantation from adult to adult for primary biliary cirrhosis. Ann Intern Med 122:275-176, 1995.
15. Neuberger J, Price D: Role of living liver donation in the United Kingdom. BMJ 327:676-679, 2003.

16. Scandiatransplant online: Available at
http://www.scandiatransplant.org/

17. Björö K, Friman S, Höckerstedt K, et al: Liver transplantation in
the Nordic countries 1982-1998: Changes of indications and
improving results. Scand J Gastroenterol 34:714-722, 1999.

18. Björö K, Ericzon BG, Kirkegaard P, et al: Liver transplantation for
fulminant hepatic failure: Impact of donor-recipient ABO-matching
on the outcome. Transplantation 75:347-353, 2003.

19. De Meester J, Persijn GG, Wujciak T, et al. for the Eurotransplant
International Foundation: The new Eurotransplant kidney allocation
system. Report one year after implementation. Transplantation
66:1154-1159, 1998.

20. Neuberger J, Ubel PA: Finding a place for public preferences
in liver allocation decisions. Transplantation 70:1411-1413, 2000.

21. Freeman RB, Wiesner RH, Edwards E, et al: Results of the first year
of the new liver allocation plan. Liver Transpl 10:7-15, 2004.

II

Patient Evaluation: Adult

Current Indications, Contraindications, Delisting Criteria, and Timing for Liver Transplantation

SCOTT A. FINK
ROBERT S. BROWN, JR

Philosophy   96

The evaluation process   96

Listing for transplantation   96
  Scoring systems and prioritization on the waiting list   97
  Impact of MELD on outcomes and transplant benefit   98

Indications for transplantation   98
  Alcoholic liver disease   98
  Viral hepatitis   100
  Cholestatic liver disease   101
  Malignant diseases of the liver   101
  Metabolic liver diseases   103
  Vascular diseases of the liver   103
  Fulminant hepatic failure   104

Indications for liver transplantation in children   104
  Pediatric cholestatic diseases   104
  Pediatric metabolic liver diseases   105
  Viral and nonviral hepatitis in children   105
  Hepatic malignancy in children   105
  Retransplantation in children   105

Listing and evaluation   105

Contraindications   107
  Age   107
  Psychosocial contraindications   107
  Cardiopulmonary contraindications   107
  Infectious contraindications   108

Management on the waiting list   108
  Timing of transplantation   109
  Delisting criteria   110
  Timing of living donor liver transplantation   110

Summary   111

On a November afternoon in 2004, 17,489 patients were awaiting liver transplantation. To this point in the year, only 4132 liver transplants had been performed.[1] The fact that more than four times as many patients awaited a new liver as had received a transplant over the previous 11 months illustrates the cold calculus of transplantation: Far fewer organs are available than there are patients who need them.

This deficit places the transplant team in a unique position in the medical field. Unlike other diseases, where resources are relatively plentiful, the transplant physician must make choices regarding the best candidates for transplantation. Often these choices are difficult and require rigorous evaluation of the patient, the patient's support structure, the progress of disease, and prospects for recovery. Recently, mathematical models that assess risk by combining medical facts with disease epidemiology have assisted these decisions. However, in the end, the transplant enterprise involves rationing organs and care to those who are perceived to benefit most. This chapter focuses on the broad aspects of this process, particularly patient selection and timing for listing and transplantation. The philosophical principles behind transplantation are introduced, and the process behind listing a patient for transplantation is discussed. Finally, aspects of the decision to remove a patient from the transplant list are discussed, in particular, for transplant "futility."

Philosophy

By necessity, transplantation decisions are guided by a utilitarian philosophy. In the best of all possible worlds, a treatment modality would be without risk and available to all who would benefit from it. Vaccination and prenatal vitamins for pregnant mothers are examples of this type of therapy, with virtually no risk and a probable benefit that is high.

At the other end of the spectrum are therapies that are so severe in nature, so dangerous in their implications, that they are reserved for only the most hopeless of cases. Emergency portocaval shunting for many years was the only therapy for severe variceal bleeding that failed balloon tamponade. Fortunately, the higher effectiveness combined with the minimal associated morbidity of interventional endoscopic therapy and, when needed, transjugular intrahepatic portosystemic shunting has obviated the need for major surgery as a therapy for almost all gastrointestinal bleeding. The risks associated with emergency surgery in cirrhotic patients are such that it is rarely performed today.

A liver transplant is a far more complicated decision for both the physician and patient. A terminal illness is being replaced by a new and different chronic condition by way of a major surgical procedure. The transplant team needs to ensure that the patient is neither too ill nor too healthy to merit a transplant. The patient must have sufficient medical reserve to survive through and thrive after liver transplant surgery. The risks are not only to the patient undergoing the procedure, but also to the remainder of the waiting list who do not receive the graft and are still at risk for adverse pretransplant outcomes.

Utilitarian philosophy dictates that the resources be focused on applications for which they would do the most good. Maximal good at minimal cost is a common mantra of utilitarian thinkers. When rationing a limited supply of organs to a large pool of eligible recipients, utilitarian philosophy becomes quite important. These principles guide the transplant team in making decisions.

The Evaluation Process

The first step toward liver transplantation is recognition by the patient's primary medical care team that the patient would potentially benefit from liver transplantation. Oftentimes, patients are referred to a liver transplant center by a gastroenterologist or hepatologist, although primary care physicians or other specialists may pursue the referral. Physicians who are not specialists in transplantation need to be educated in recognizing when a patient with liver disease is a candidate for evaluation.

Once a referral is made, the patient is evaluated by the liver transplant center. Questions need to be answered regarding the patient's fitness for surgery, psychosocial preparedness, and potential for recovery. Does the patient have preexisting medical conditions unrelated to the liver disease that would make transplantation unnecessarily risky? Does the patient have the social support structure in place to adequately ensure compliance with the rigorous medical regimen required of a liver transplant recipient? Is the patient's liver disease at a sufficiently early stage that no survival benefit would be derived and thus the patient should not be listed for transplantation? Conversely, has the patient's liver disease progressed to such an advanced state or are coexistent medical conditions so severe that transplantation would prove too risky?

Once the transplant workup along with the psychosocial and medical evaluations, which are the focus of other chapters in this text, have been completed, the transplant center must process this information and make a decision regarding whether the patient should be placed on the transplant list. Frequently, this decision involves an objective evaluation by a committee of transplant surgeons, hepatologists, psychiatrists, social workers, transplant coordinators, nurses, and others who will decide whether the patient would benefit from and merits listing.

Listing for Transplantation

On being accepted onto a transplant center's waiting list, the patient is registered with the United Network for Organ Sharing (UNOS) Organ Center. UNOS runs a centralized computer network that includes all transplant hospitals' waiting lists and links all organ procurement organizations (OPOs).[1] Once entered onto a transplant center's waiting list, the patient is made part of the national organ allocation infrastructure from which decisions about organ allocation are made. However, organs

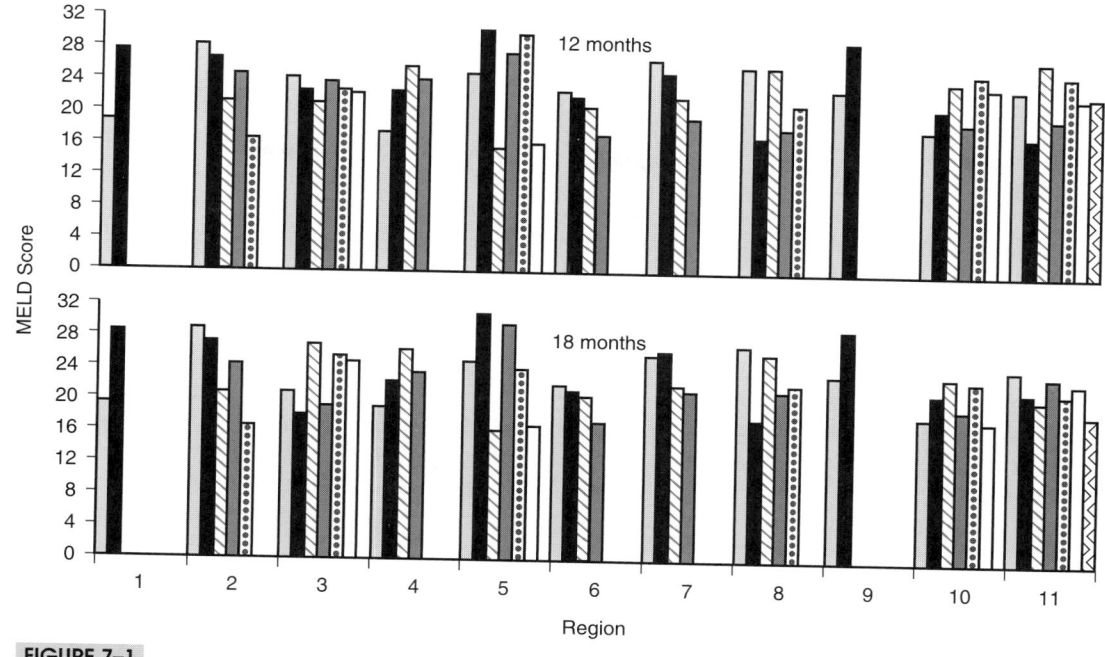

FIGURE 7–1

Mean MELD score at deceased donor transplantation by region, by organ procurement organization, all cases.

are allocated locally within the OPO first, followed by regionally within the 11 UNOS regions, and then nationally for all patients with chronic liver disease. Currently, there are wide variations in the Model for End-Stage Liver Disease (MELD) score at transplantation across OPOs (Fig. 7–1). In an attempt to achieve equity among candidates for orthotopic liver transplantation (OLT), broader regional sharing arrangements are available for UNOS status 1 patients with acute liver failure in most regions, and sharing for patients with MELD scores higher than 15 is awaiting approval and implementation by the UNOS board.

Scoring Systems and Prioritization on the Waiting List

To optimize the allocation and distribution of organs, an organ allocation system should be built on evidence-based outcome measures and principles of justice and equity, maximal utility, and transparency.[2] Whereas in previous years organ allocation was predicated principally on location (at home, hospitalized, or intensive care unit bound) and on waiting time, it has recently shifted to a risk-based system using the MELD score.

For more than 30 years, the Child-Pugh classification system has been used to predict mortality and morbidity in patients with liver disease.[3] Although variations of the Child-Pugh classification have been integral in stratifying patients for liver transplantation, it poorly prioritizes patients on the liver transplant list.[4] The Child-Pugh score and waiting time were previously used in a complex mechanism to allocate organs. However, the system did

not differentiate medical urgency well and thus was largely a waiting time–based system. As a result, as discussed in other chapters, organ allocation is now based on the MELD and the Pediatric End-Stage Liver Disease (PELD) model, mathematical regression models that more accurately predict short-term mortality on the waiting list and benefit from transplantation. MELD is based on logarithmic transformation of the recipient's international normalized ratio (INR), bilirubin, and creatinine into a validated mathematical model. PELD includes albumin, bilirubin, INR, age (< 1 year, > 1 year), and the presence of growth failure to risk-stratify children with chronic liver disease on the waiting list.

MELD and PELD objectively assess the patient's need for transplantation, the temporal likelihood of transplantation, and most importantly, the short-term prognosis while waiting for a transplant. By imparting a simple mechanism by which to assess these factors, these models have provided physicians involved in the care of pretransplant patients with a tool to link patients' prognosis with their probability of transplantation. These tools are invaluable when selecting patients for transplantation.

MELD is based on a patient's parameters at a single point in time. As a result, the risk of death while on the transplant list is more accurately predicted by serial than by single scores. The change in MELD, or delta MELD, does add to the MELD score in accurately predicting outcome. It provides valuable information regarding the progression of disease while at the same time prognosticating on the patient's course.[5] Delta MELD has been proposed to enhance prioritization for transplantation, but difficulties in defining standard intervals for delta MELD have hampered proposals for its implementation.

Impact of MELD on Outcomes and Transplant Benefit

Donor organs should be allocated to patients with the highest likelihood of a transplant benefit.[6] After the implementation of MELD, the survival benefit of liver transplantation within 1 year of the procedure has been concentrated among patients at the highest risk for pre-transplant death. Consequently, patients who are at the lowest risk of pretransplant death and would have little or no demonstrable benefit from transplantation continue to remain on the waiting list.[7]

In the first 18 months after introduction of the MELD-based allocation system, there was a direct relationship between the risk of death while awaiting a transplant and the MELD score and a decrease in the overall pretransplant mortality rate. Patient and graft survival rates were also slightly better after the implementation of MELD.[7] MELD and PELD scores provide physicians with a snapshot of the patient at a given time, so they need to be updated by periodic data capture. In this way, they provide the physician with a continuous picture of the patient's status.

Because MELD is based on objective biochemical tests and results in a large, continuous scale of severity, it better estimates the short-term prognosis of patients with end-stage liver disease.[8,9] Transplantation of patients with low MELD scores (< 15) has been associated with higher mortality after transplantation than would be expected on the waiting list, thus suggesting that transplantation of patients with low MELD scores is not the best use of the donor pool.[7]

Although MELD scores have had tremendous value for physicians involved in patient selection as a tool for predicting survival of patients with end-stage liver disease, it is poor at predicting posttransplant outcomes.[5] Its purpose is to aid transplant specialists in selecting those who would benefit most from transplantation by taking into account their risk of mortality from living with their end-stage liver disease. It does not provide a highly accurate measure of the patient's chance for survival after liver transplantation, although posttransplant survival is modestly worse at very high (> 30) MELD scores.

Indications for Transplantation

Patients should be considered for transplantation only if they are thought to be capable of surviving the perioperative period and complying with the intense chronic medical regimen and follow-up required of transplant recipients. They must refrain from addictive behavior such as recidivism to alcohol or drug abuse. Furthermore, they should have no other major medical illnesses significantly curtailing life expectancy.

The list of indications for liver transplantation is as wide as the spectrum of liver disease itself. Generally, any form of end-stage liver disease that is irreversible and curable with liver transplantation is an indication for transplantation. If the disease is a systemic disease involving the liver, systemic cure must be achieved with liver transplantation or the systemic effects must be minor in implication.[1]

Because of concern in the late 1990s over regional disparities in the character of patients waiting for a transplant and concern about wide variance in criteria for placing a patient on the waiting list for transplantation, the American Society of Transplant Physicians and the American Association for the Study of Liver Diseases formulated recommendations that outlined minimal criteria for placement of adults on the liver transplant waiting list in 1997.[10] The guidelines recommended that when a patient is placed on the waiting list, it indicates that both the center and the patient are ready to proceed with transplantation immediately should an organ become available. To qualify for listing, the patient's expected survival rate should be 90% or less within 1 year without transplantation. Exceptions were recommended for patients who do not meet these survival criteria but have other indications for immediate transplantation such as impaired quality of life.

Based on the panel's review of published data, they recommended that a Child-Pugh score of 7 or higher be correlated with a survival rate of 90% or less at 1 year as a result of the morbidity associated with decompensation, including intractable ascites, jaundice, hepatic encephalopathy, and bleeding. Patients with a Child-Pugh score of 7 or higher or with bleeding associated with portal hypertension should be listed for transplantation. The authors thought that these criteria were sufficient for patients with chronic hepatitis B and C and went on to make disease-specific recommendations.

In 2003, the most common diagnoses in patients waiting for liver transplantation were cirrhosis (42%), alcoholic liver disease (20%), hepatitis (20%), hepatocellular carcinoma (5%), and primary sclerosing cholangitis (5%). As indicated in Figure 7–2, the diagnoses in patients on the waiting list and at time of transplantation are quite similar. What follows is a discussion regarding the issues surrounding the more common indications for liver transplantation.

Alcoholic Liver Disease

A history of alcohol use is very common in patients evaluated for liver transplantation. Moreover, alcohol

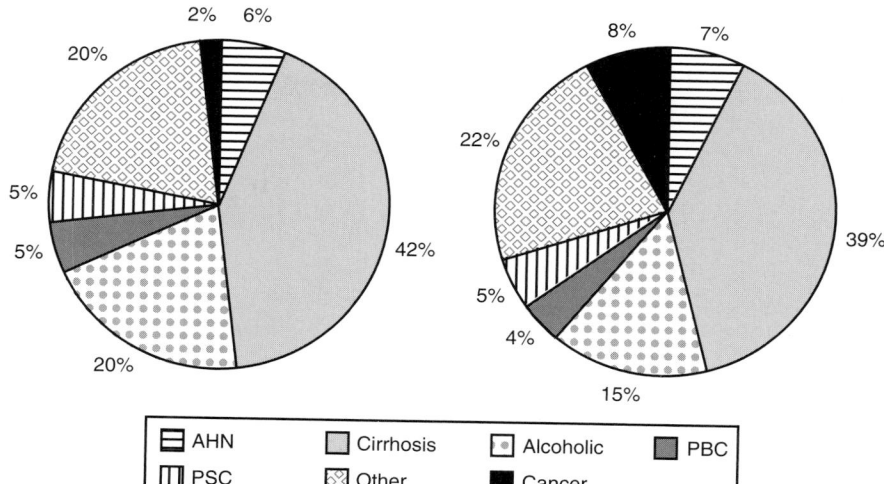

Liver Diagnosis Waiting vs. Transplanted 2003

FIGURE 7–2

In 2003, the most common diagnoses in patients waiting for liver transplantation were cirrhosis and alcoholic liver disease. AHN, acute hepatic necrosis; PBC, primary biliary cirrhosis; PSC, primary sclerosing cholangitis. (Redrawn from United Network for Organ Sharing web data, 2003.)

use is frequently an issue in patients who receive transplants for other reasons (e.g., hepatitis C). In these cases, alcohol frequently acts a cofactor in the development of end-stage liver disease.

It is only recently that health care professionals outside psychiatry and addiction medicine have clearly accepted alcohol abuse as a disease. Yet many unanswered questions remain. Does a personal tendency toward alcohol addiction predispose patients to resume alcohol use even after a period of abstinence before transplantation? Will any amount of alcohol use after transplantation affect the new organ and, if so, how much and to what degree? For the transplant physician, these questions make the issue complex, especially since data on the adverse effects of recurrent alcoholic liver disease are much more limited than for recurrence of hepatitis C or other liver diseases. As a result, alcohol use, abuse, and dependence all touch on the ethical issues at the center of candidate selection for liver transplantation. Given the stigma associated with alcoholism and addiction in general, this issue is highly charged, particularly in the public eye.

Risk factors for the development of alcoholic liver disease include drinking outside meal times, drinking on a daily basis, and consuming multiple drinks at a single sitting. Obesity, advancing age, and genetic factors also play a role in the advance toward end-stage liver disease.[11]

The survival benefit from transplantation for alcoholic liver disease is greatest in the sickest patients. Patients with Child-Pugh class B and C cirrhosis and those with intractable encephalopathy, a history of variceal bleeding, poor quality of life, and a life expectancy of less than a year seem to benefit most from transplantation.[11]

Current recommendations for minimal listing criteria for patients with alcoholic liver disease include a Child-Pugh score of 7 or higher, portal hypertensive bleeding, or an episode of spontaneous bacterial peritonitis. Candidates must undergo assessment by an addiction specialist that the risk of recidivism is low, as well as 6 concurrent months of abstinence, or they could be referred to a regional review board if the program believes that they are candidates for transplantation, regardless of whether 6 months of abstinence was achieved.[10] These same criteria should also be applied to patients in whom dual liver diseases, including alcoholic liver disease, have been diagnosed.

A key concern when considering patients with alcoholic liver disease remains whether they will relapse into their previous alcohol use patterns. A secondary question becomes whether reversion to previous deleterious behavior will prove detrimental to the transplanted liver.

It is generally accepted that a period of abstinence during the liver transplantation evaluation period is necessary for listing. Because many patients with alcoholic liver disease do not stop drinking or die soon after the diagnosis is made and because others who become abstinent at the time of diagnosis may improve their liver function to such an extent that transplantation is not required, most patients with alcoholic liver disease do not undergo OLT.[12] Abstinence for 6 months in effect excludes from transplantation patients with reversible liver failure as a result of alcoholic hepatitis.

The generally accepted period of abstinence required by many centers is 6 months, with 85% of U.S. and European liver transplant programs requiring some period of abstinence before listing patients for transplantation.[13] The rationale for requiring a period of abstinence by patients before transplantation is based on (1) ensuring that the patient's liver will not recover function as a result of abstaining from alcohol, thus negating the need for transplantation, (2) identifying patients who are at high risk for relapse to drinking, and (3) allowing time for alcohol addiction and relapse prevention therapy before transplantation.[11]

The 6-month period is not based on established epidemiological evidence, nor has abstinence before transplantation been shown to adequately predict abstinence after liver transplantation, although longer periods of abstinence do correlate with lower rates of recidivism. Most surprisingly, little evidence exists to support the fact that abstinence has an impact on patient or graft survival.[11] Although it is sensible to generally follow the 6-month rule, strict enforcement clearly hurts patients who die during the abstinence period or experience complications of their liver disease before the 6-month period is completed. Decisions regarding alcohol use should therefore be made on a case-by-case basis.[14]

Finally, the evaluating team needs to keep in mind that alcohol use is a powerful cofactor in the progression of other liver disease. Use of alcohol after transplantation could have a negative impact on survival of the graft in patients who underwent transplantation for cirrhosis primarily related to hepatitis C, for example.[11]

Viral Hepatitis

Hepatitis C

Viral hepatitis remains a leading cause of end-stage liver disease. In addition to considering readiness for transplantation, the transplant team needs to take into account the state of disease and treat accordingly to promote graft survival after transplantation. It has been shown, for example, that a higher hepatitis C virus (HCV) load before transplantation correlates with lower survival rates after transplantation. One study showed that patients with an HCV RNA titer of 1×10^6 copies/mL or higher before transplantation had a cumulative 5-year survival rate of 57% versus 84% for those with HCV RNA titers of less than 1×10^6 copies/mL ($P = .0001$).[15]

HCV is a particularly vexing problem for the transplant physician because the nearly universal recurrence of viremia after transplantation has an adverse outcome on overall graft survival rates. Evaluation requires not only detecting patients who would benefit most from transplantation but also developing antiviral strategies to reduce or eliminate the viral burden before transplantation and thus decrease posttransplant recurrence. Pretransplant viral load, advanced recipient age, hyperbilirubinemia, elevated INR, pretransplant cytomegalovirus status, and advanced donor age have an adverse impact on patient survival after transplantation.[16]

Because recurrence of HCV disease is nearly universal and often follows an accelerated posttransplant course, the issue of whether to retransplant patients with graft failure as a result of recurrent hepatitis C is highly controversial. Should those who need a second transplant receive less of a priority than those having their first? The criteria that establish the standards for retransplantation for recurrent hepatitis C vary from center to center, including some centers that no longer perform the procedure because of poor patient and graft survival. Patients undergoing retransplantation for HCV disease do have worse outcomes than recipients of primary transplants do. However, the outcomes are not clearly worse than retransplantation for other causes. Thus, it does not seem reasonable to systematically exclude patients with recurrent hepatitis C from retransplantation. However, patients with early aggressive recurrence and graft failure within the first year have very poor outcomes after retransplantation, as do patients with very high MELD scores. These patients should not undergo repeat transplantation except under highly selected conditions.

Hepatitis B

Transplantation for hepatitis B had been plagued by universal recurrence and had been abandoned in the late 1980s, before prophylaxis, because of poor outcomes with severe hepatitis B virus (HBV) recurrence. Recurrence of hepatitis B surface antigen (HBsAg) in serum was associated with fibrosing cholestatic hepatitis and aggressive graft loss with 1-year mortality higher than 50%. Recurrence was related to the degree of viremia; patients who were hepatitis B early antigen (HBeAg) positive and those with detectable HBV DNA by solution hybridization ($> 10^6$ copies/mL) had high rates of recurrence, whereas patients with fulminant HBV, those with delta coinfection, and HBeAg-negative patients all had lower pretransplant viral loads and lower rates of recurrence. Fortunately, hepatitis B immune globulin (HBIG) prophylaxis with oral nucleoside or nucleotide therapy can prevent reinfection of the graft, and significant hepatitis B recurrence after transplantation is rare. Thus, currently, recurrence of significant hepatitis B disease after transplantation is not nearly as common as it is with hepatitis C. This therapy has revitalized transplantation for this indication. Questions remain regarding the duration of HBIG prophylaxis and the optimal antiviral therapy to use. The use of nucleoside monotherapy with lamivudine after transplantation was associated with a recurrence rate of greater than 20%. Most programs are using HBIG for at least 1 year, and many programs administer HBIG indefinitely with nucleoside/nucleotide therapy. Levels of HBsAb higher than 500 IU/mL are associated with very low rates of recurrence when used with or without oral antiviral agents. We use combination therapy indefinitely at the current time in the absence of long-term data on emergence of resistant HBV when antiviral therapy is used without HBIG.

Cholestatic Liver Disease

To assess severity in primary biliary cirrhosis (PBC) and primary sclerosing cholangitis (PSC), the cholestatic liver diseases, the Mayo models for PSC and PBC are frequently used. Patients with a Child-Pugh score of 7 or higher or the advent of portal hypertensive bleeding are eligible by current criteria for listing for transplantation. In addition, patients with a Mayo model risk score predicting greater than 10% mortality at 1 year should be listed for transplantation.[10] Patients with recurrent cholangitis may have MELD scores that inadequately predict their risk for the development of resistant bacterial or fungal infections and thus their mortality. They also suffer from greatly impaired quality of life because of the need for frequent endoscopic or percutaneous procedures and often require external drainage. Added priority for OLT may be obtained in these cases by petitioning the regional review board. A similar approach can be taken for impairment in quality of life as a result of xanthomatous neuropathy, intractable pruritus, or severe metabolic bone disease in patients with PBC. Alternatively, these complications can be viewed as indications for proceeding to living donor liver transplantation (LDLT) if an acceptable volunteer donor exists.

Malignant Diseases of the Liver

Another group of diseases for which the issues regarding listing criteria for transplantation are complicated are the malignant diseases. Theoretically, primary malignant diseases of the hepatobiliary tract, namely, hepatocellular carcinoma (HCC) and cholangiocarcinoma, could be cured by surgical resection. Since a transplanted organ would often be required to replace the resected organ because of liver insufficiency in the remnant as a result of bilobar or severe liver disease, transplantation has evolved as a crucial therapy for these diseases.

Because extrahepatic disease would render transplantation futile and because of difficulty in predicting whether the malignancy has spread, criteria have been developed to stratify the risk of recurrence of tumor based on size and other characteristics. The transplant team uses these criteria to decide whether to list patients with a malignancy for transplantation.

Cholangiocarcinoma

Cholangiocarcinoma is a highly malignant neoplasm that arises from the bile duct epithelia. Sixty percent occur in the perihilar region at the confluence of the right and left hepatic ducts (Klatskin tumor). PSC is the most common risk factor for the development of cholangiocarcinoma. Currently, no medical therapies are effective for cholangiocarcinoma. Median survival is 9 to 12 months, with long-term survival being infrequent. Even with resection, local recurrence is common. Patients with PSC and cholangiocarcinoma are poor candidates for resection because their disease is more frequently multifocal and they often have fibrotic/cirrhotic liver disease, which makes the risk of liver failure and death after resection prohibitive.[17]

Cholangiocarcinoma has been viewed in the past as a contraindication to transplantation because of reported long-term survival rates after transplantation ranging from 20% to 30%, significantly lower than rates in patients transplanted for cirrhosis.[18] Treatment of cholangiocarcinoma, however, has changed somewhat over the past decade.

Although previous studies showed poor outcomes and high recurrence rates in patients with cholangiocarcinoma who received transplants, these older data originated from patients with various stages of disease, selection criteria were poorly defined, and no adjuvant and neoadjuvant chemotherapy was given. In 1994, a new management protocol involving preoperative chemoradiotherapy followed by liver transplantation for patients with localized perihilar cholangiocarcinoma and regional lymph node–negative disease was begun. With this new protocol, 88% of patients were alive 1 year after transplantation and 82% were alive at 5 years.[17] These data suggested that the use of neoadjuvant therapy selects a group of patients with cholangiocarcinoma who will probably achieve a clear survival benefit from transplantation. However, this indication remains controversial, and OLT in such patients should probably be performed in the context of clinical studies at experienced centers at the current time.

Hepatocellular Carcinoma

HCC, which frequently coexists with cirrhosis or viral hepatitis, presents similar difficulties. Unlike cholangiocarcinoma, it is accepted, based on a large body of data, that patients with limited HCC can undergo transplantation with a low recurrence rate. Controversy in this area pertains to the stage of tumor beyond which OLT should not be performed. Current recommendations are that liver transplantation is indicated in patients with limited HCC (stage I to II, i.e., T1 or T2, N0, M0 disease) and no evidence of invasion of large vascular structures or extrahepatic disease.[19] The prognostic value of high α-fetoprotein (AFP) levels is controversial, although recurrence is more frequent with higher AFP values, especially values greater than 1000 to 2000, probably because of either more extensive disease in the liver than noted on preoperative imaging or occult extrahepatic disease. Although no cutoff value of AFP is recommended for excluding patients from OLT, caution and planned exploration with an identified back-up candidate before OLT are prudent for patients with AFP values greater than 1000, especially if the levels are rising despite locoregional therapy. If patients clearly have no evidence of extrahepatic spread and the tumor appears small enough that such metastasis would seem unlikely, transplantation has offered high long-term cure rates with low recurrence rates after OLT.

Controversy exists, however, regarding the optimal diagnostic criteria for HCC and the role of pretransplant therapy. Although it is thought that lesions above a certain size can clearly be defined as HCC based on imaging only, smaller lesions present diagnostic dilemmas. Some experts have called for biopsy with histological confirmation of all lesions in patients being evaluated for transplantation, whereas others advocate biopsy only for nodules smaller than 2 cm, the protocol supported by the guidelines put forth by the European Association for the Study of Liver Disease.[20] There are concerns on the other side about false-negative results with biopsy, especially given rates of "incidental" HCC of up to 20% on explants in HCV-infected patients.

We recommend biopsy of all lesions in patients who have no other independent indication for OLT, for example, a patient with Child's class A cirrhosis, a small lesion (<2 cm), and a low AFP value. Serial imaging and close follow-up are required in such patients because some will turn out to have HCC even with a negative biopsy. However, in patients with decompensated disease and a new hypervascular lesion larger than 2 cm that is characteristic of HCC, the risk associated with core biopsy as well as the risk of needle track spreading and false-negative results makes a presumptive diagnosis of HCC an appropriate choice. It is important to note that fine-needle aspiration does not provide the architectural detail required for the diagnosis of well-differentiated HCC; core needle biopsy is required.

Tumor size, AFP level, the presence of vascular or capsular invasion, bilobular location, and the number of nodules are poor prognostic factors and independently predict mortality and recurrence of HCC. AFP is also a predictor of recurrence—an AFP level greater than 300 ng/dL indicates a high chance of recurrence.[19]

The TNM system of staging cannot be used with 100% accuracy to evaluate candidates for transplantation because it is based on a postoperative scoring system rather than pre-OLT imaging. In one of the largest studies to date involving an international registry of hepatic tumors in liver transplantation, Klintmalm and colleagues showed that tumor size greater than 5 cm, the presence of vascular invasion, and a poorly differentiated histological grade of the tumor were strong negative predictors of patient survival after transplantation for HCC.[21]

If selection of candidates is limited to patients with solitary tumors smaller than 5 cm or to subjects with up to three nodules, each under 3 cm in size, the 5-year survival rate may exceed 70% and the recurrence rate is usually less than 15% after transplantation.[20,22-25]

Priority on the Waiting List for Orthotopic Liver Transplantation in Patients with Hepatocellular Carcinoma. The current MELD-based scoring used by UNOS allows an exception to be made for additional MELD priority in patients with HCC. The rationale behind this rule is that patients with HCC may not have cirrhosis or intrinsic liver disease and thus would have lower MELD scores based on laboratory values that do not accurately predict their mortality risk. They would consequently have less chance of transplantation and more progression of their tumors on the waiting list. The low priority for HCC in the previous allocation scheme had led to a high dropout rate because of tumor progression. Because patients with HCC benefit from early transplantation before metastasis or growth of the lesion, the allocation system was altered to take this factor into account. T1 lesions were given a MELD score of 24 and T2 lesions a score of 29. The priority was increased every 3 months. No priority was given to tumors that exceeded these guidelines. This modification resulted in a marked increase in the number of HCC patients receiving transplants with very short waiting times and a decrease in the dropout rate to close to zero.

Surprisingly, up to 25% of patients with HCC who underwent transplantation in the United States in the first MELD era did not have evidence of HCC in the explanted liver, thus suggesting incorrect interpretation of the findings or imaging results that led to the diagnosis of HCC and leading some to postulate that encouragement for early transplantation in the MELD era might provide incentive for limited workups in these patients.[20,26] Most of these tumors were T1 lesions smaller than 2 cm. Additional modification has led to a reduced MELD priority than previously for T2 lesions (24 points) and no additional priority for T1 lesions. This adjustment should reduce the proportion of HCC patients among transplant recipients and the rate of HCC cases without histological confirmation.

LDLT is increasingly being sought for patients with HCC. With LDLT, transplantation can be performed earlier, before HCC has metastasized. Patients with tumors smaller than 5 cm, fewer than three nodules, and no evidence of concurrent malignant disease can be considered for LDLT, which may be the best option for the growing number of patients with cirrhosis and small tumors.[27] LDLT results in a better outcome for patients with HCC and a lower risk of death (relative risk, 0.35). LDLT patients are younger and tend to have lower MELD scores.[28] Furthermore, by limiting use of the donor pool, LDLT allows more patients to undergo transplantation.[28]

Therapy for Hepatocellular Carcinoma Before Orthotopic Liver Transplantation. The role of pretransplant locoregional or systemic therapy is unclear.

The goal of pretransplant therapy is to reduce the tumor burden to prevent recurrence and progression while on the waiting list. Theoretically, necrotic tumor would also be less likely to be spread during mobilization and removal of the liver at the transplant procedure.

In the past, chemotherapy directed at lesions via an intra-arterial pump and embolization of the arterial supply of a lesion have been used with varying degrees of success. Transarterial chemoembolization (TACE), whereby a chemotherapeutic agent is injected along with a compound that limits circulation to just the tumor, has shown some effectiveness with survival benefits outside the transplant setting for HCC. In 1995, Venook and coworkers showed that selected patients with limited HCC (less than three lesions with the largest < 3 cm or one lesion < 5 cm) who receive preoperative chemoembolization followed by OLT achieved excellent long-term survival. Ten of the 11 patients with unresectable HCC who received preoperative chemoembolization and later underwent OLT remained tumor free at a median time of 40 months.[29] Because this and most other studies have used routine chemoembolization to prevent progression during the waiting period, it is widely accepted at the current time.

Randomized data on the efficacy of TACE are limited. However, lower posttransplant recurrence rates in patients who underwent chemoembolization for known tumors than in those with incidental tumors, despite larger tumor size in the chemoembolization group,[29] may represent an effect of TACE on lowering recurrence rates, although it may also reflect differences in tumor biology in the two groups. TACE also treats tumors that might be too small to be seen on imaging because it treats entire lobes of the liver.

Percutaneous ethanol, acetic acid, and radiofrequency ablation (RFA) are also being used increasing for a wide variety of malignant diseases of the liver. Ethanol injection can be performed with a very small-bore needle but is effective only for small lesions (generally less than 2 to 3 cm). RFA and acetic acid can be used for lesions up to 5 cm; RFA can also be performed in the operating room with laparoscopy or laparotomy, usually under ultrasound guidance. For larger lesions, directed ablation usually achieves a higher degree of necrosis than TACE does, although needle track spread can occur. The risk of recurrence after percutaneous catheter ablative therapy is less well studied and cannot be predicted.[19,30] Frequently, a combination of approaches is used, particularly if the lesion is larger (e.g., beyond the UNOS criteria for additional priority) or the waiting time is predicted to be long.

Recent data indicate that neoadjuvant therapy for HCC improves posttransplant survival. A study looking at pretransplant ablative therapy (ethanol injection, embolization, TACE, or RFA) in patients listed in the International Registry of Hepatic Tumors in Liver Transplantation showed a dramatic increase in recurrence-free survival after OLT in patients with HCC who had undergone ablation therapy: 69% of patients were alive free of tumor in the ablation group as compared with 31% in the group that did not receive ablation therapy ($P < .0001$).[31] Interestingly, the positive impact increased with worsening tumor characteristics, and the survival benefit increased as the number of nodules in the tumor grew.

Metabolic Liver Diseases

The metabolic liver diseases, including Wilson's disease, hereditary hemochromatosis, and α_1-antitrypsin disease, are all indications for transplantation once the liver has irreversible damage. Because all these diseases have systemic effects, the pretransplant workup must include a coordinated systemic workup to allow for identification of systemic disease that would preclude transplantation. Hemochromatosis can lead to iron deposition in the myocardium and thereby result in irreversible cardiomyopathy or conduction system damage with arrhythmia. Cardiac dysfunction is a primary reason why mortality after transplantation is higher for hemochromatosis than for other indications. α_1-Antitrypsin deficiency can lead to pulmonary emphysema, which requires careful cardiopulmonary evaluation to exclude pulmonary insufficiency or pulmonary hypertension. Occasionally, combined liver-lung transplantation is required, but end-stage liver and lung disease rarely coexist.

Vascular Diseases of the Liver

Vascular abnormalities such as Budd-Chiari syndrome or veno-occlusive disease frequently result in acute hepatic failure because of the abrupt nature of development of the disease. Portal vein thrombosis is much better tolerated and rarely causes liver failure; it is usually the result of chronic liver disease and is characterized by sudden worsening of portal hypertension. Because of its frequent association with HCC, careful screening for HCC should be undertaken in all new cases of portal vein thrombosis. The workup for all patients with vascular thrombosis without a clear underlying cause must include evaluation for a hypercoagulable state or underlying malignancy that could have led to the disease. Many of these patients have underlying hematological disorders such as polycythemia vera and, in addition to blood testing, bone marrow biopsy is frequently needed.

Addressing and treating any discovered hypercoagulable state are crucial to the success of transplantation. Patients who undergo transplantation for Budd-Chiari syndrome should be treated for life after OLT because of the high rate of recurrent clotting in this cohort. As discussed in a later chapter, 65% to 80% of patients do well with hydroxyurea and aspirin and may not require long-term anticoagulation.

Fulminant Hepatic Failure

Fulminant hepatic failure, or the rapid development of encephalopathy, coagulopathy, and jaundice in those without a history of chronic liver disease, is an indication for liver transplantation after the onset of stage 2 encephalopathy.[10] Criteria for the definition of fulminant hepatic failure include the development of hepatic encephalopathy within 8 weeks of the onset of symptoms in a patient without a history of liver disease, whereas subacute hepatic failure is defined as the development of hepatic encephalopathy within 6 months but after 8 weeks of the onset of symptoms in a patient not previously known to have liver disease. Patients with subacute failure have virtually universal mortality without organ replacement, and all should be considered for transplantation.[10] Acetaminophen toxicity is the most common cause of fulminant liver failure, followed by viral causes; drug toxicity is the most common form of subfulminant liver failure with a known cause.

Patients with fulminant hepatic failure need to be observed closely because a portion who meet criteria for the diagnosis will recover full liver function without therapy.[32] It is critical to understand the chances of recovery in patients with fulminant hepatic failure before transplantation. If the patient has a clear opportunity for full recovery, transplantation may become unnecessary. However, waiting too long may lead to irreversible cerebral edema and death. Use of the King's College criteria and other prognostic scoring systems, as well as transjugular liver biopsy to look for massive or submassive necrosis, may assist clinicians in differentiating patients with a low chance of spontaneous recovery who should undergo expedited transplantation.

A more difficult dilemma is that of acute alcoholic hepatitis. If a patient has a known drinking history and the liver failure is clearly secondary to alcoholic hepatitis after a binge drinking episode, the transplant team is faced with a dilemma regarding whether to transplant a liver into an individual with a known predilection for alcohol abuse without knowing the patient's chances for recovery from addiction. Most centers have viewed alcoholic hepatitis as a contraindication to OLT, although exceptions are occasionally made on a case-by-case basis in acute settings, particularly in young patients or those with an unclear cause (e.g., alcohol plus acetaminophen toxicity).

Indications for Liver Transplantation in Children

Indications for pediatric liver transplantation include cholestatic diseases (predominantly biliary atresia), metabolic diseases, fulminant hepatic failure, chronic active hepatitis, malignancy, Budd-Chiari syndrome, parenteral nutrition–induced cirrhosis, trauma, and Caroli's disease.[33] Children should be listed for transplantation if decompensation has either already occurred or is considered inevitable. Decompensation is characterized by intractable cholestasis; portal hypertension with or without variceal bleeding; multiple episodes of ascending cholangitis; failure of synthetic function, including coagulopathy or low serum albumin or low cholesterol; failure to thrive; growth failure or malnutrition; intractable ascites; encephalopathy; unacceptable quality of life, including school failure or intractable pruritus; metabolic defects for which liver transplantation will reverse life-threatening complications or prevent irreversible central nervous system damage; or life-threatening complications of stable liver disease, such as hepatopulmonary syndrome. Failure of growth or normal development is an indication for transplantation because it will reverse growth failure and result in significant catch-up growth if OLT is performed early in the course of disease.

Pediatric Cholestatic Diseases

Cholestatic syndromes are the most common indications for liver transplantation in children. Obstructive cholestasis includes biliary atresia and sclerosing cholangitis. Biliary atresia is the indication in 60% to 70% of pediatric liver transplant candidates. Although lifesaving when performed in the first 45 days of life, the Kasai procedure to treat congenital biliary atresia does not completely obviate the need for transplantation in the vast majority of cases. Even with timely performance of the procedure, around 75% of patients will require a transplant, and children who have undergone the Kasai procedure should be listed for transplantation when any general indication for transplantation occurs or the surgeon deems the operation to have a high probability of failure.[33] Without the Kasai procedure, death is inevitable before 2 years of age, and children who do not undergo the procedure or who have significant portal hypertension that precludes the procedure should be listed as soon as the diagnosis is made.[33]

Intrahepatic cholestasis may be mild or severe. Even with mild forms, however, pruritus may be so severe that transplantation is required. Severe forms of intrahepatic cholestasis, such as Byler's disease and Alagille syndrome, can lead to cirrhosis and require transplantation. With Alagille syndrome, the frequent cardiomyopathy associated with the disease may make transplantation impossible, and thus careful cardiac evaluation is essential.[33]

Pediatric Metabolic Liver Diseases

Metabolic diseases of childhood that are indications for transplantation include urea cycle defects, Crigler-Najjar syndrome, tyrosinemia, Wilson's disease, and cystic fibrosis.[1] The presence of any metabolic defect in children with liver disease needs to be investigated before transplantation because some metabolic defects have extrahepatic manifestations or involve defects in extrahepatic tissue that may not be reversible with liver transplantation. Therefore, liver transplantation should be considered only if the defect is localized to the liver or, if it occurs in extrahepatic tissue, the defect does not include the central nervous system and will be overridden by a normally functioning liver. Finally, the extrahepatic manifestations of the metabolic defect should not be so severe that liver transplantation is precluded. Tyrosinemia is associated with a high rate of HCC, and thus this possibility needs to be investigated carefully.[33]

Viral and Nonviral Hepatitis in Children

Hepatitis is a relatively infrequent indication for transplantation in children. Nevertheless, children should be listed for transplantation if one or more of the general indications for liver transplantation are met. Autoimmune hepatitis, which often overlaps with sclerosing cholangitis (overlap syndrome, autoimmune cholangiopathy), can lead to a need for transplantation, especially in adolescence, if immunosuppressive therapy fails.

Hepatic Malignancy in Children

With regard to malignancy, hepatoblastoma is the most frequent primary liver malignancy in children. Because hepatoblastoma is locally invasive with late distant metastases and a better long-term prognosis than seen with HCC, children should be immediately listed if the disease is confined to the liver but unresectable or if recurrent tumor is found after resection.[33] Neoadjuvant chemotherapy is frequently used before transplantation in patients with extensive disease. HCC is a rare indication, except as a complication of metabolic liver disease (e.g., tyrosinemia).

Retransplantation in Children

The most common indication for retransplantation in children is hepatic artery thrombosis, which occurs at a higher frequency than after adult OLT and may be manifested very acutely and require urgent retransplantation.[1,34] Other indications for retransplantation include acute rejection (rare), delayed graft function or primary nonfunction, chronic rejection, and recurrent disease.[33] Chronic rejection is frequently due to medication noncompliance during adolescence.

Listing and Evaluation

Once the decision to evaluate a patient for transplantation is made and the patient has been referred to a transplant center for assessment, the pretransplant workup is undertaken (Table 7–1). Although the protocol and requirements vary from hospital to hospital, most programs require a basic battery of laboratory tests to examine the patient's general chemistry and hematological counts. In addition, laboratory examinations frequently include elements of the liver disease workup that have not been previously performed.

The workup also includes a search for occult infection that could be reactivated with immunosuppression. Chest radiographs and tests for purified protein derivative are performed to ensure that the patient does not have latent tuberculosis. Rapid plasma reagin testing is performed to look for evidence of syphilis. Testing for human immunodeficiency virus (HIV) is performed. Any infections should be treated or under control before transplantation.

A thorough workup includes an evaluation of the patient's general medical condition and fitness for major surgery. An electrocardiogram, chest radiograph, echocardiogram (frequently a saline contrast or "bubble" echocardiogram to exclude intrapulmonary shunting), cardiac stress testing, and pulmonary function testing (including D_{LCO} and arterial blood gases), are common elements of the workup. Close coordination with referring physicians and specialists is frequently required to best understand the patient's preoperative risk.

Imaging of the abdomen and hepatic parenchyma and vasculature is routinely performed on all pretransplant patients. Ultrasound is used to assess the patency of the portal and hepatic vasculature and to determine liver size. Computed tomography and magnetic resonance imaging are frequently performed to exclude HCC or for clarification of abnormalities on ultrasound. Additional tests, such as right heart catheterization to exclude pulmonary hypertension, may be required for follow-up of the results of the aforementioned workup (see Table 7–1 for pretransplant evaluation).

Mortality and morbidity after transplantation may be related to compliance with medication.[35] Addictive behavior that could adversely affect survival of the graft may continue after transplantation if not treated beforehand. Because the patient's psychosocial status and social support may have an impact on compliance

Table 7-1. EVALUATION FOR TRANSPLANTATION

	Required	Optional	Test/Procedure
PHASE I			
A. Triage	X		Review records and medical history
B. Pathology	X		Review biopsy if available
C. Evaluations	X		Transplant coordinator/nurse practitioner
	X		Hepatologist
	X		Surgeon
	X		Social services
	X		Financial counselor
		X	Psychiatry
D. Laboratory	X		Chemistry, hematology, serology, tumor markers, ABO, HIV, virology
PHASE II			
A. Radiology	X		Doppler ultrasound to assess portal vein patency
	X		Triple-phase spiral abdominal CT scan/MRI (? only elevated AFP)
	X		ECG
	X		Bone density
	X		Chest x-ray: PA and lateral
		X	Chest CT (patients with HCC) to r/o metastasis
		X	Bone scan (patients with HCC) to r/o metastasis
B. Cardiology		X	Bubble Echo (if age > 50 yr or previous IVDA) to r/o pulmonary HTN, hepatopulmonary syndrome
		X	Adenosine stress test (age > 50 yr or positive risk factors) to r/o ischemia
		X	Coronary angiography (if positive stress test or significant history)
		X	Cardiology consultation (recipients > 50 yr or positive workup)
C. Pulmonary	X		ABG on room air
		X	PFT with D_{LCO} (smokers or positive bubble Echo)
		X	ABG on 100% O_2 (if bubble Echo positive)
D. Neurology: > 60 yr with encephalopathy, history of seizures, CVA, neurological disorders, or CAD	X		MRI/MRA of brain
	X		Carotid Doppler
	X		Neurology consultation
E. Gastrointestinal		X	Colonoscopy (> 50 yr or elevated CEA)
		X	Upper endoscopy
		X	ERCP
F. Gynecological	X		PAP smears on all females
		X	Mammography (women > 40 yr)
G. Consultations		X	Dental
		X	Nutritional
PHASE III: WAITING FOR A TRANSPLANT			
A. HCC screening	X		AFP every 3 mo
	X		Abdominal imaging every 6 mo (more frequent if suspicious region requires closer follow-up)
B. Treatment of HCV		X	Pegylated interferon and ribavirin (on case-by-case basis)
C. Update MELD according to severity of illness (UNOS guidelines)	X		MELD score $\geq$ 25: check laboratory values every 7 days 24–19: every 30 days 18–11: every 90 days $\leq$ 10: every year

ABG, arterial blood gases; ABO, blood type; AFP, α-fetoprotein; CAD, coronary artery disease; CEA, carcinoembryonic antigen; CT, computed tomography; CVA, cerebrovascular accident; ECG, electrocardiogram; Echo, echocardiogram; ERCP, endoscopic retrograde cholangiopancreatography; HCC, hepatocellular carcinoma; HIV, human immunodeficiency virus; HTN, hypertension; IVDA, intravenous drug abuse; MELD, Model for End-Stage Liver Disease; MRA, magnetic resonance angiography; MRI, magnetic resonance imaging; PA, posteroanterior; PFT, pulmonary function tests; r/o, rule out; UNOS, United Network for Organ Sharing.

and outcome, a thorough evaluation of the patient's psychiatric and socioeconomic challenges is important.

A thorough psychosocial assessment is part of every transplant workup. Forty-three percent of candidates for liver transplantation have at least one psychiatric disorder. Because the severity of psychiatric disorders often correlates with the severity of liver disease, an understanding of the patient's psychiatric state is crucial to assessing suitability for transplantation.[36] Dedicated social workers and psychiatrists are integral members of the transplant team, and their evaluation is critical in transplant selection and management.

Socioeconomic status has been hypothesized to correlate with graft survival. If immunosuppressive medications cannot be obtained because of economic barriers, failure of the graft is likely. Socioeconomic barriers can make follow-up difficult and lead to recidivism to addictive behavior. In one study, however, socioeconomic status did not affect patient or graft survival.[35] Needless to say, a thorough evaluation can detect future challenges that could be avoided. Financial coordinators assess the adequacy of transplant coverage and, with the social workers, assist patients in obtaining additional financial support for transplantation and appropriate follow-up. The goal should be to provide care to all who require it and to identify adequate resources for patients to undergo and be successful with organ replacement therapy.

Contraindications

When dealing with a scarce resource such as a donated organ, the team should perform liver transplantation only on candidates in whom a reasonable chance of graft and patient survival is predicted. For this reason, there are individuals in whom, for one reason or another, transplantation is contraindicated. Some contraindications are relative; if ameliorated before transplantation, the transplant operation can proceed. Others are absolute. In such cases, either there is no reasonable expectation that either the patient or the graft will survive the transplant procedure, or justice prevents allocation to an individual who is unlikely to ever meet the criteria for OLT.

It is important to note that relative contraindications, particularly for LDLT, vary from center to center. Most contraindications to liver transplantation relate to comorbid conditions.[37] Relative contraindications to transplantation include alcohol use within 6 months in a patient with a history of alcohol abuse, illicit drug use within 6 months in a patient with a history of illicit drug abuse, extrahepatic malignancy in the past (not including nonmelanoma skin cancer or those who meet the oncological definition of cure), and systemic sepsis.[10]

Age

Advancing age is an important relative contraindication to liver transplantation. Data suggest that patients older than 70 years need to undergo liver transplantation at a less severe level of disease to have a good outcome. If these patients are allowed to wait, their chances of debility or development of comorbid medical conditions that would preclude transplantation rise.[37]

Psychosocial Contraindications

As discussed, alcohol abuse can be a relative contraindication to liver transplantation. Although some patients are able to preserve the graft if they continue to drink after transplantation, recurrence of disease with resumption of alcohol use remains a concern in the vast majority of patients transplanted for alcohol-induced liver disease. Unfortunately, there are few reliable predictors of relapse in alcoholic patients, which makes it difficult to identify before transplantation those patients at greatest risk for relapse after transplantation.[14,38]

Cardiopulmonary Contraindications

The presence of pulmonary disease, particularly pulmonary hypertension, can be an absolute contraindication to liver transplantation because severe pulmonary hypertension or severe hypoxemia from hepatopulmonary syndrome makes the patient an unacceptable operable risk. During the transplant procedure, various hemodynamic challenges occur, particularly during the time of vena caval clamping and reperfusion of the newly implanted graft after restoration of caval flow. These changes challenge patients whose right ventricular function is impaired.[39] A mean pulmonary artery pressure greater than 35 mm Hg is a contraindication if it is impossible to lower with medications before transplantation.

The presence of hepatopulmonary syndrome does predict morbidity and mortality in patients with end-stage liver disease. Patients with hepatopulmonary syndrome have nearly twice the death rate of all other transplant recipients 1 year after surgery. However, early hepatopulmonary syndrome is reversed with OLT and can be viewed as an indication to proceed with organ replacement. Because of markedly different estimates of prevalence of the disease, it has been suggested that there is inadequate diagnostic accuracy in identifying the syndrome. No strict definitions of the diagnostic criteria have been established.[40] Criteria currently accepted by most centers include the presence of liver disease combined with a Po_2 of 70 mm Hg or less while breathing room air and evidence of intrapulmonary vascular dilatation.

Response to breathing 100% oxygen and calculation of shunt ratios do not adequately predict outcomes in patients with hepatopulmonary syndrome.[41] Because Doppler echocardiography has a poor predictive value in estimating pulmonary artery pressure, right heart catheterization is recommended to assess for the presence of portopulmonary hypertension in patients at risk.[40]

Infectious Contraindications

HIV Infection

It was previously thought that HIV infection was an absolute contraindication to liver transplantation. Although still controversial, with many centers regarding transplantation of HIV-infected individuals as experimental, it is now a relative contraindication to OLT. Concerns have included the cumulative impact of virological and pharmacological immunosuppression, inability to control HIV viremia, and decreased life expectancy after transplantation. In the era of highly active antiretroviral therapy (HAART), however, these ideas have been reassessed. Transplantation of selected HIV-positive patients with suppressed HIV viral load is now being performed and is the subject of a National Institutes of Health (NIH)-sponsored multicenter study.

Thus, HIV disease is no longer considered to be an absolute contraindication to liver transplantation as long as attention is paid to comorbid conditions. It has been shown, for example, that HIV-positive patients with HBV who receive prophylaxis against recurrence of hepatitis B after transplantation have excellent short- and long-term survival rates.[42] Various centers have published results showing that 1-year survival rates are no different for HIV-positive and HIV-negative patients.[43]

Because of their chronic disease, however, caution has to be exercised during transplant evaluations to ensure the absence of occult infection or other HIV-associated comorbid conditions that could contraindicate transplantation. The current absolute contraindications to liver transplantation in HIV-infected patients include uncontrollable HIV disease as a result of multidrug resistance, renal failure, leukoencephalopathy, advanced malnutrition, requirement for life support, and the presence of opportunistic infections.

Requirements for life support and advanced malnutrition, in particular, are risk factors for decreased survival after transplantation. Opportunistic infection exclusions include an opportunistic infection within 6 to 12 months, previous Kaposi's sarcoma, and JC polyomavirus infection. Of note, a history of *Pneumocystis carinii* pneumonia is not a contraindication to transplantation.[44]

It is also important to recall that because liver patients have hypersplenism, their CD4 counts may appear to be artificially low. Lower CD4 counts can be accepted if based on a relative comparison with the absolute neutrophil count.[44]

Another relative contraindication for patients with HIV disease includes a history of noncompliance with medications. Patients who are ineligible for HAART because of intolerance of the medication as a result of severe liver dysfunction should be considered for transplantation if they have previously shown responsiveness to HAART.[44] In addition, it is unclear what the contraindications would be for patients with HIV disease who are characterized as long-term nonprogressors and have low, stable viral counts despite the absence of HAART.

HIV-infected patients should therefore be considered for transplantation if they meet standard criteria. Centers that transplant patients with HIV disease should have particular expertise in HIV management and be working with a transplant pharmacologist who has particular expertise in drug interactions given the complex drug combinations inherent in HAART. A transplant infectious disease specialist who has worked with issues involving HIV and transplantation is recommended.[44]

Other Infectious Contraindications

Patients with an active, uncontrolled infection cannot undergo transplantation. Infection presents a higher risk when one considers the high-dose immunosuppression required of patients acutely after transplantation. Patients who have spontaneous bacterial peritonitis need to be treated before transplantation. Infection with drug-resistant bacteria or fungi may require delisting or deactivation until these pathogens are eradicated because the outcome of transplantation can be poor in this setting (see "Delisting Criteria"). Recommendations for treatment of resistant bacteria (methicillin-resistant *Staphylococcus aureus* and vancomycin-resistant enterococci being the most common) or fungi are 4 to 6 weeks of appropriate antibiotics/antifungals with surveillance cultures and documentation of eradication.

Management on the Waiting List

It is crucial that the transplant team assist in the medical care of the patient's end-stage liver disease while the patient is being evaluated for liver transplantation or after the patient has been listed for transplantation and is awaiting an organ. One study investigating the care of potential transplant candidates showed deficiencies in attending to the pretransplant medical needs of patients. Screening rates for HCC were found to be poor. Standard preventive procedures for patients with end-stage liver disease, including endoscopic screening for esophageal varices and primary or secondary prophylaxis against variceal bleeding, were not followed.[45] MELD scores need to be updated regularly, every 3 months on average, or when any clinical deterioration occurs. Thus, the appropriate timing of transplantation, including consideration of LDLT, is more likely to be achieved in appropriate candidates.

Timing of Transplantation

Timing of transplantation involves determining the period when the patient will derive the maximum benefit from receiving a new liver. Because the goal is to avoid futile transplantation, it is a subject of active investigation with considerable attention from the transplant community.

If the transplant is performed too early, before liver failure develops, for example, the risks of transplantation in terms of morbidity and mortality will outweigh the benefits. In contrast, if the transplant team waits too long to list a patient for transplantation, the risks of the procedure can overshadow its benefits.

MELD scoring, although helpful in assessing patient survival while waiting for a transplant, does not appear to correlate with posttransplant survival in all subsets of patients. Recent data suggest that patients with MELD scores less than 15 do not derive a survival benefit in the first year, particularly those with scores less than 12. The survival benefit increases with each increase in MELD score above 15 (Fig. 7–3).[7] In a separate study by Desai and colleagues, the MELD score was found to be a relatively poor predictor of posttransplant outcomes in all but patients with the highest 20% of MELD scores.[46]

If a patient is moribund as a result of end-stage liver disease, comatose, in renal failure, or on a ventilator (or any combination of these factors), the risk of dying regardless of the procedure outweighs the now-diminished benefit of transplantation. In a study by Abt and associates, analysis of UNOS data showed that location in the intensive care unit before transplantation, retransplantation, female donor to male recipient, age older than 44 years, and recipient race increased the rate of allograft failure, specifically, the need for retransplantation, in patients receiving adult-to-adult LDLT.[47] However, there is no absolute MELD cutoff for transplant futility. Although the posttransplant risk of dying increases by 50% at high MELD scores (>30) and there is a higher rate of waiting list removal for the reason of "death/too sick," outcomes in a select group of the sickest patients are still reasonable, especially given the more than 300-fold increase in mortality before transplantation in candidates with high MELD scores (Table 7–2).

The optimal time for liver transplantation is once patients begin to show evidence of decompensation or achieve a MELD score of 15 or greater. Synthetic dysfunction, malnutrition, or onset of the first complication

FIGURE 7–3

MELD has been shown to predict survival of patients while awaiting transplantation. Patients with MELD scores higher than 15 derive a survival benefit with each subsequent point increase in their score.

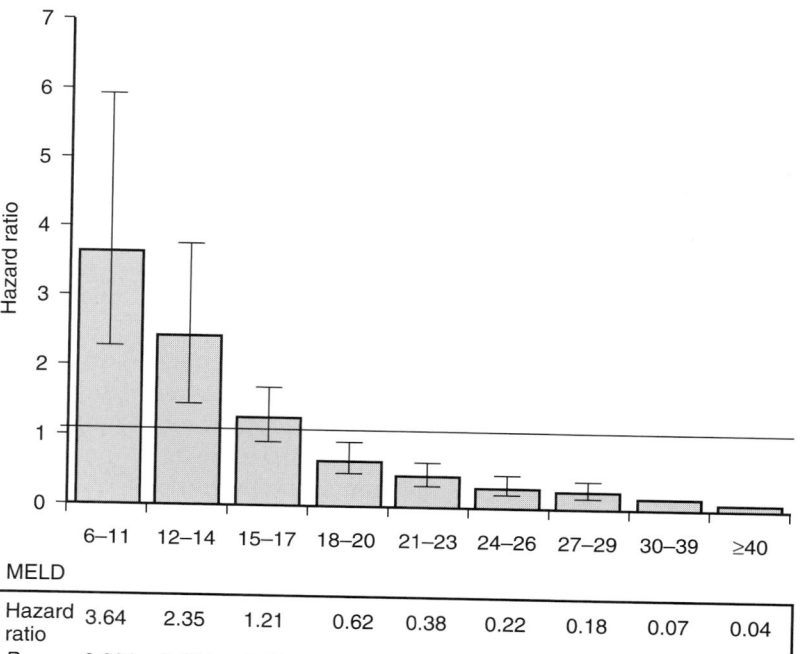

MELD	6–11	12–14	15–17	18–20	21–23	24–26	27–29	30–39	≥40
Hazard ratio	3.64	2.35	1.21	0.62	0.38	0.22	0.18	0.07	0.04
P-values	<0.001	<0.001	0.41	<0.01	<0.001	<0.001	<0.001	<0.001	<0.001

Table 7-2. UNADJUSTED WAITING LIST AND TRANSPLANT MORTALITY RATES BY MELD CATEGORY

MELD	Waiting List			Transplantation (1-Year Follow-up)		
	DEATHS	PY	RATE PER 1000 PY	DEATHS	PY	RATE PER 1000 PY
6–11	130	2901	44.8	19	116	163.3
12–14	96	1830	52.5	23	180	127.4
15–17	181	1237	146.4	38	231	164.7
18–20	150	552	271.9	33	190	174.1
21–23	142	276	514.9	31	174	178.4
24–26	105	125	840.7	21	119	176.9
27–29	99	60	1663.8	18	92	195.9
30–39	348	75	4634.1	54	220	245.5
40*	287	22	13,152.7	18	68	264.6
Total	1538	7078	217.3	255	1390	183.5

*Includes patients whose MELD score was capped at 40.
MELD, Model for End-Stage Liver Disease; PY, patient-years.
From Merion M, Schaubel DE, Dykstra DM, et al: The survival benefit of liver transplantation. Am J Transplant 5:307-313, 2005.

of cirrhosis indicates the commencement of decompensation. Patients should be expected to survive the waiting time required to procure an organ based on their MELD score. Patients with HCC should be referred for transplant evaluation as soon as the tumor is discovered because transplantation should be performed as early as possible in all appropriate HCC candidates. Children should be referred for transplant evaluation at the point that they fall off their growth curve.[48] Therefore, although there is no longer an advantage to early referral in terms of waiting time, early referral allows pretransplant problems to be addressed and management and the timing of transplantation to be optimized.

Delisting Criteria

Delisting or temporarily deactivating patients from the transplant list involves a calculation that the patient would not derive a survival benefit from the transplant, either because the patient's condition has worsened to the point that the procedure's risks would now outweigh its benefits or, rarely, because the patient's condition has improved. Recent guidelines have called for the development of absolute minimum cutoff survival rates for acceptable predicted posttransplant survival. These rates would probably range from 40% to 60%.[6] Guidelines have also called for the development of an intermediate category such as a temporary deactivation status or a modification of the patient's MELD score with a decrease in points for critical complications.[6] Mechanical ventilation, requirement for hemodialysis, fungal or resistant bacterial infections, and a previous

transplant all have an adverse impact on the likelihood of posttransplant survival. When several of these factors are present, the posttransplant risk becomes prohibitive and transplantation should be deferred. Current research is directed at developing evidence-based recommendations for delisting.

Additionally, patients should be removed from the transplant list if their condition deteriorates to the extent that it is unlikely that they would survive the procedure. All absolute contraindications to listing are adequate reasons for delisting if they occur while a patient is awaiting transplantation, including resumption of alcohol use while awaiting transplantation.[10]

Timing of Living Donor Liver Transplantation

First performed by Yamaoka and colleagues in Japan in 1994, centers in the United States have performed more than 1500 LDLT procedures since 1989 in children and 1998 in adults.[1] Because living donation permits the timing of transplantation independent of waiting time and the severity of liver disease, criteria for transplantation in these patients are somewhat different than in patients waiting for deceased donor organs.

Timing of LDLT is a great deal more flexible and allows the transplant team to tailor the transplant time for a particular patient. Because a living donor organ has significantly less cold ischemia time than a deceased donor organ does as a consequence of moving immediately from the donor to the recipient and being from a healthy, extensively screened individual, living donor livers are potentially of better quality than deceased donor livers. However, a living donor allograft has significantly less hepatic mass than a full-sized deceased donor organ does. To date, outcomes of living donation and deceased donor liver transplantation (DDLT) have been similar. Furthermore, every transplantation with a liver obtained from a living donor potentially frees up a deceased donor organ for transplantation into another recipient because living donor recipients are not part of the deceased donor recipient pool.[27]

A reduced waiting period for a living donor organ, the principal benefit of living donor transplants, may decrease the risk for decompensation or death before transplantation and thus improve the chance for success. Data have shown shorter waiting times and improved survival on the waiting list for patients with potential donors for LDLT, with mortality being half that of those listed for DDLT (Fig 7–4).[49,50] Because the transplant is performed on an elective basis, the operation can proceed immediately after the workup is performed. As a result of the flexibility of the waiting period before transplantation in living donor recipients, the team has time to stabilize the patient's comorbid conditions, which also improves the chance for success.[27]

LDLT has tremendous growth potential; the graft doubles in size within 4 weeks of transplantation, with more than 150,000 hepatocytes generated every second for the first week after transplantation.[51,52] Questions have risen regarding whether there are any negative implications of the accelerated growth rate found in the liver segment transplanted in LDLT. It has been thought, for example, that this growth potential may predispose to more aggressive recurrence of hepatitis C in patients transplanted for HCV-related cirrhosis. Several recent large studies have shown that the incidence and severity of hepatitis C recurrence were not different between DDLT and LDLT recipients.[53-55] However, in one study, the incidence of cholestatic hepatitis, a particularly virulent and rapidly destructive form of recurrent hepatitis C, was found to be significantly greater in LDLT patients.[54]

Schiffman and coworkers examined liver biopsy specimens from 23 LDLT and 53 DDLT patients and found no significant differences in the degree of hepatic inflammation between the two groups over a period of 3 years. The mean fibrosis score increased in a stepwise manner in the DDLT patients but reached a plateau after 12 months in the LDLT patients, thus indicating that more severe progression of fibrosis secondary to recurrent hepatitis C did not occur in LDLT patients.[55]

Patients with decompensated cirrhosis and Child-Pugh scores of 10 or higher are the most appropriate patients for LDLT. Acute hepatic failure is also an acceptable indication, but concern regarding coercion and adequacy of the donor workup given the time constraints has made this indication somewhat controversial. Recipients should meet standard indications for OLT and not have any contraindications. Using the current donor and recipient criteria, it has been estimated that approximately 5% of patients listed for DDLT would be able to undergo LDLT, mainly because of lack of appropriate donors.[27]

As with DDLT, the ideal candidate for LDLT is one who is sick enough to derive a benefit from transplantation but not so sick that a potentially high posttransplant mortality risk is incurred. A simple rule of thumb is that an appropriate LDLT candidate is a patient in whom transplantation would be performed today if organs were unlimited. MELD can help identify candidates for LDLT who are not likely to benefit because they are either too sick or too well to undergo transplantation.[56] In a study by Trotter and colleagues, between 1997 and 1999, 51% of 100 potential LDLT recipients evaluated at one center were rejected. The most frequent reasons for rejection included medical comorbidity, high-risk psychosocial issues, obesity, financial issues, and procurement of a deceased donor organ during the evaluation.[57] Overall, in experienced centers, it appears that about a third of adult patients on the waiting list may have a potential donor and half will undergo the procedure, thus indicating that LDLT may be applicable in up to 15% of patients on the waiting list.[58] The reluctance to perform LDLT may relate to highly publicized donor death; between 2001 and 2003 the number of centers performing the procedure and the number of cases dropped drastically (Fig. 7–5).[59,60] With increased experience and the NIH-funded living donor cohort study A2ALL, it is hoped that living donation will expand to better meet organ demand in the future.

Summary

Transplant physicians continue to struggle with a scarcity of organs relative to the number of patients

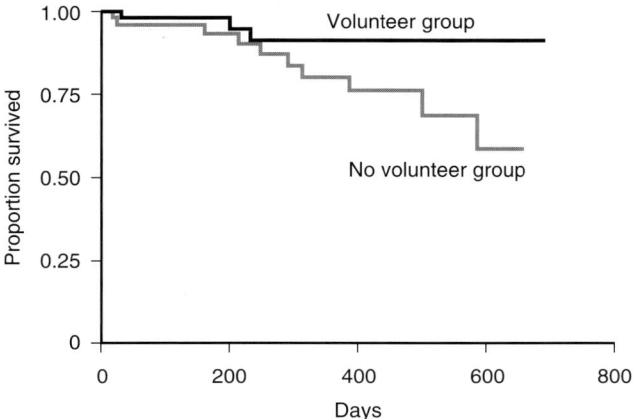

FIGURE 7–4

Intent-to-treat analysis of overall survival from the time of listing in individuals with and without volunteers for potential living donation. A clear survival benefit is indicated for the potential living donor group.

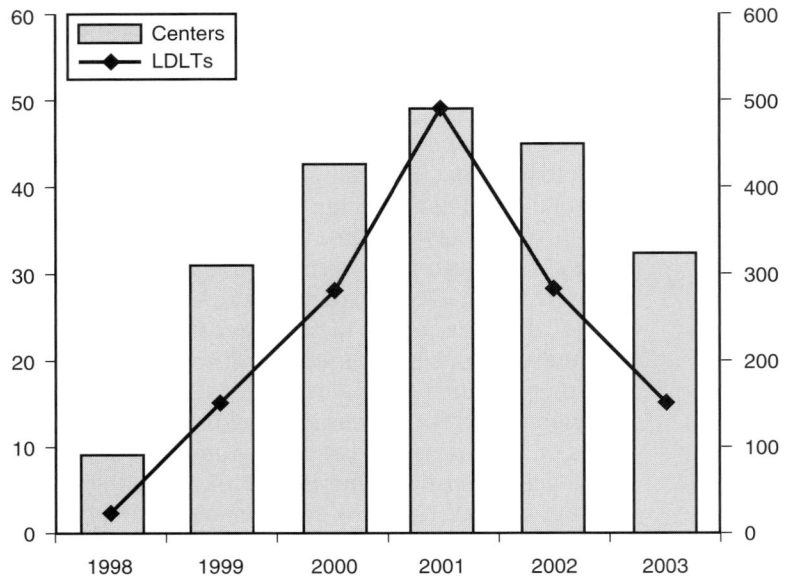

FIGURE 7–5

Number of centers and number of adult living donor liver transplants performed from 1998 to 2003 in the United States. Between 2000 and 2003, the number of centers performing living donor liver transplantation dropped drastically.

awaiting transplantation. This problem has created the impetus to select patients for transplantation who are most likely to benefit and least likely to be harmed by the process. Mathematical models such as MELD and PELD have assisted physicians in prognosticating and choosing the most appropriate candidates for transplantation. If conditions that would have contraindicated initial placement on the transplant list develop in patients on the waiting list or if patients revisit self-destructive addictive or noncompliant behavior, they should be removed from the transplant list. LDLT necessitates a workup distinct from that of DDLT and requires unique consideration of timing of the transplant procedure.

Pearls and Pitfalls

- Decisions regarding suitability for transplantation should be guided by a desire to achieve maximal cure with minimal morbidity and mortality.
- Prompt referral to a transplant center and communication with the transplant team are essential for timely patient evaluation.
- Implementation of the MELD scoring system has decreased pretransplant mortality without diminishing posttransplant survival rates.
- Contraindications to transplantation are shrinking, but the development of relative contraindications to OLT while on the list is rising as patients become more ill during the waiting period.

Pearls and Pitfalls—cont'd

- The transplant evaluation should include an extensive medical and psychosocial evaluation to look for social and medical impediments to transplantation.
- Living and deceased donor transplantation should optimally be performed between a MELD score of 15 and 30 whenever possible to achieve maximal transplant benefit.
- Living donor liver transplantation offers more timely transplantation with reduced waiting time mortality, but less than 15% of recipients will have donors and undergo such transplantation.
- Criteria for removing a patient from the transplant list are similar to those that would preclude the patient's initial listing, as well as the development of medical contraindications, including coma with a need for ventilation and resistant bacterial or fungal infections.

References

1. United Network for Organ Sharing [UNOS] web data.
2. Brown RS, Lake JR: The survival impact of liver transplantation in the MELD era, and the future for organ allocation and distribution. Am J Transplant 5:203-205, 2005.
3. Pugh RNH, Murray-Lion IM, Dawson JC, et al: Transection of the oesophagus for bleeding oesophageal varices. Br J Surg 60: 640-646, 1979.
4. Wiesner RM, McDiarmid SV, Karath PS, et al: Application of survival models to liver allocation. Liver Transpl 7:567-580, 2001.
5. Merion RM, Wolfe RA, Dykstra DM, et al: Longitudinal assessment of mortality risk among candidates for liver transplantation. Liver Transpl 9:12-18, 2003.

6. Olthoff KM, Brown RS, Delmonico FL, et al: Summary report of a national conference: Evolving concepts in liver allocation in the MELD and PELD era. Liver Transpl 10:A6-A22, 2004.
7. Merion M, Schaubel DE, Dykstra DM, et al: The survival benefit of liver transplantation. Am J Transplant 5:307-313, 2005.
8. Kamath PS, Wiesner RH, Malinchoc M, et al: A model to predict survival in patients with end-stage liver disease. Hepatology 33:464-470, 2001.
9. Longheval G, Vereerstraeten P, Thiry P: Predictive models of short- and long-term survival in patients with nonbiliary cirrhosis. Liver Transpl 9:260-267, 2003.
10. Lucey MR, Brown KA, Everson GT, et al: Minimal criteria for placement of adults on the liver transplant waiting list. Liver Transpl Surg 3:628-637, 1997.
11. Neuberger J, Schulz KH, Day C, et al: Treatment for alcoholic liver disease. J Hepatol 36:130-137, 2002.
12. Veldt BJ, Laine F, Guillygoamarc'h A, et al: Indications of liver transplantation in severe alcoholic liver cirrhosis. J Hepatol 36:93-98, 2002.
13. Everhart JE, Beresford TP: Liver transplantation in the United States. Liver Transpl Surg 3:220-226, 1997.
14. Lim JK, Keefe EB: Liver transplantation for alcoholic liver disease. Liver Transpl 10:S31-S38, 2004.
15. Charlton M, Seaberg E, Wiesner R, et al: Predictors of patient and graft survival following liver transplantation for hepatitis C. Hepatology 28:823-830, 1998.
16. Charlton M, Ruppert K, Belle SH, et al: Long-term results and modeling to predict outcomes in recipients with HCV infection. Liver Transpl 10:1120-1130, 2004.
17. Heimbach JK, Haddock MG, Alberts SR, et al: Transplantation for hilar cholangiocarcinoma. Liver Transpl 10:565-568, 2004.
18. Shimoda M, Farmer DG, Colquhoun SD, et al: Liver transplantation for cholangiocarcinoma. Liver Transpl 7:1023-1033, 2001.
19. Figueras J, Ibanez L, Ramos E, et al: Selection criteria for liver transplantation in early-stage hepatocellular carcinoma with cirrhosis. Liver Transpl 7:877-883, 2001.
20. Sala M, Varela M, Bruix J: Selection of candidates with hepatocellular carcinoma in the MELD era. Liver Transpl 10:54-59, 2004.
21. Klintmalm GB: Liver transplantation for hepatocellular carcinoma. Ann Surg 228:479-490, 1998.
22. Bismuth H, Majno PE, Adam R: Liver transplantation for hepatocellular carcinoma. Semin Liver Dis 19:311-322, 1999.
23. Mazzafero V, Regalia E, Doci R, et al: Liver transplantation for hepatocellular carcinoma in patients with cirrhosis. N Engl J Med 334:693-699, 1996.
24. Llovet JM, Fuster J, Bruix J, et al: Intention-to-treat analysis of surgical treatment for early hepatocellular carcinoma. Hepatology 30:1434-1440, 1999.
25. Jonas S, Bechstein WO, Steinmuller T, et al: Vascular invasion and histopathologic grading to determine outcome after liver transplantation for hepatocellular carcinoma in cirrhosis. Hepatology 33:1080-1086, 2001.
26. Freeman RB, Wiesner RH, Edwards E, et al: Results of the first year of the new liver allocation plan. Liver Transpl 10:7-15, 2004.
27. Trotter JF: Selection of donors and recipients for living donor liver transplantation. Liver Transpl 6:S52-S58, 2000.
28. Lo CM, Fan S, Liu C, et al: The role and limitation of living donor liver transplantation for hepatocellular carcinoma. Liver Transpl 10:440-447, 2004.
29. Venook AP, Ferrell LD, Roberts JP: Liver transplantation for hepatocellular carcinoma. Liver Transpl Surg 4:242-248, 1995.
30. Sala M, Fuster J, Llovet J, et al: Pathological risk of recurrence after surgical resection for HCC. Liver Transpl 10:1296-1302, 2004.
31. Klintmalm GB: The outcome of neoadjuvant therapy for hepatocellular carcinoma in liver transplantation (personal communication).
32. O'Grady J, Alexander GJ, Hayllar KM, et al: Early indicators of prognosis in fulminant hepatic failure. Gastroenterology 97:439-445, 1989.
33. UNOS Policy 3 Appendix 3B, accessed 1/13/05 http://www.unos.org/PoliciesandBylaws/policies/docs/policy_15.doc.
34. D'Alessandro AM, Ploeg RJ, Knechtle SJ, et al: Retransplantation of the liver—a seven-year experience. Transplantation 55:1083-1087, 1993.
35. Yoo HY, Galabova V, Edwin D, et al: Socioeconomic status does not affect the outcome of liver transplantation. Liver Transpl 8:1133-1137, 2002.
36. Rocca P, Cocuzza E, Rasetti R, et al: Predictors of psychiatric disorders in liver transplantation candidates. Liver Transpl 9:721-726, 2003.
37. Safdar K, Neff GW, Montalano M, et al: Liver transplant for the septuagenarians. Transplant Proc 36:1445-1448, 2004.
38. Bellamy CO, DiMartini AM, Ruppert K, et al: Liver transplantation for alcoholic cirrhosis. Transplantation 72:619-626, 2001.
39. Colle IO, Moreau R, Godinho E, et al: Diagnosis of portopulmonary hypertension in candidates for liver transplantation. Hepatology 37:401-409, 2003.
40. Arguedas MR, Abrams GA, Krowka MJ, et al: Prospective evaluation of outcomes and predictors of mortality in patients with hepatopulmonary syndrome undergoing liver transplantation. Hepatology 37:192-197, 2003.
41. Mandell MS: Hepatopulmonary syndrome and portopulmonary hypertension in the model for end-stage liver disease era. Liver Transpl 10(10 Suppl 2):S54-S58, 2004.
42. Yoshida EM, Erb SR, Partovi N, et al: Liver transplantation for chronic hepatitis B infection with the use of combination lamivudine and low-dose hepatitis B immune globulin. Liver Transpl Surg 5:520-525, 1999.
43. Ragni M, Belle SH, Im KA, et al: Survival of human immunodeficiency virus–infected liver transplant recipients. J Infect Dis 188:1412-1420, 2003.
44. Fung J, Eghtesad B, Patel-Tom K, et al: Liver transplantation in patients with HIV infection. Liver Transpl 10:S39-S53, 2004.
45. Macedo G, Lopes S, Barroso S, et al: Implementation of screening and preventive strategies in liver transplant candidates [abstract]. Transplant Proc 35:115, 2003.
46. Desai NJ, Mange KC, Crawford MD, et al: Predicting outcome after liver transplantation. Transplantation 2004:99-106, 2004.
47. Abt PL, Mange KC, Olthoff KM, et al: Allograft survival following adult-to-adult living donor liver transplantation. Am J Transplant 4: 1302-1307, 2004.
48. Carithers RC: Liver transplantation. Liver Transpl 6:122-135, 2000.
49. Liu CL, Lam B, Lo CM: Impact of right-lobe live donor liver transplantation on patients waiting for liver transplantation. Liver Transpl 9:863-869, 2003.
50. Russo MW, LaPointe-Rudow D, Kinkhabwala M, et al: Impact of adult living donor liver transplantation on waiting time survival in candidates listed for liver transplantation. Am J Transplant 4:427-431, 2004.
51. Baltz AC, Trotter JF: Living donor liver transplantation and hepatitis C. Clin Liver Dis 7:651-665, 2003.
52. Marcos A, Fisher RA, Han JM, et al: Liver regeneration and function in donor and recipient right lobe adult living donor liver transplantation. Transplantation 69:1375-1379, 2000.
53. Russo MW, Galanko J, Beavers K, et al: Patient and graft survival in hepatitis C recipients after adult living donor liver transplantation in the United States. Liver Transpl 10:340-346, 2004.
54. Gaglio PJ, Malireddy S, Levitt BS, et al: Increased risk of cholestatic hepatitis C in recipients of grafts from living versus cadaveric liver donors. Liver Transpl 9:1028-1035, 2003.
55. Shiffman ML, Stravitz RT, Contos MJ, et al: Histologic recurrence of chronic hepatitis C virus in patients after living donor and

deceased donor liver transplantation. Liver Transpl 10: 1248-1255, 2004.

56. Freeman RB: The impact of the model for end-stage liver disease on recipient selection for adult living donor liver donation. Liver Transpl 9(10 Suppl 2):S54-S59, 2003.

57. Trotter JF, Wachs M, Trouillot T, et al: Evaluation of 100 patients for living donor liver transplantation. Liver Transpl 6:290-295, 2000.

58. Rudow DL, Russo MW, Hafliger S, et al: Clinical and ethnic differences in candidates listed for liver transplantation with and without potential living donors. Liver Transpl 9:254-259, 2003.

59. Russo MW, Brown RS Jr: Adult living donor liver transplantation. Am J Transplant 4:458-465, 2004.

60. Brown RS Jr, Russo MW, Lai M, et al: A survey of adult living donor living transplantation in the United States. N Engl J Med 348:818-825, 2003.

Transplantation for Viral Hepatitis A and B

BRUNO ROCHE
DIDIER SAMUEL

Transplantation for hepatitis B   116
    Indications for liver transplantation   116
    Mechanisms of hepatitis B virus recurrence
        after liver transplantation   116
    Prevention of hepatitis B virus recurrence   116
    Hepatitis B virus recurrence   122
    Survival of patients who undergo transplantation
        for hepatitis B virus cirrhosis   123
    Liver transplantation in patients with
        hepatitis D virus liver cirrhosis   124
    Liver transplantation for fulminant
        hepatitis B   124

Transplantation for hepatitis A   124

Conclusion   125

In the United States and Europe, 5% to 10% of patients undergoing orthotopic liver transplantation (OLT) have hepatitis B virus (HBV)-associated chronic or fulminant liver disease.[1,2] Results of OLT have been hampered by recurrent infection. Acute or chronic liver disease on the graft secondary to viral reinfection may lead to graft failure, retransplantation, or death.[3,4]

Historically, the spontaneous risk for HBV reinfection was about 80% when related to the initial liver disease (i.e., acute versus chronic) and to the presence of HBV replication at the time of transplantation.[3,4] Over the last decade, there have been major advances in the management of HBV transplant candidates. Using a combination of prophylaxis with hepatitis B immune globulin (HBIg) and lamivudine, which is administered before and after transplantation, OLT in patients with hepatitis B produces excellent survival and recurrence rates even in patients with preoperative viral replication.[5,6] Several effective drugs have been developed for the management of HBV disease on the graft so that outcome is currently good.

Indications for transplantation in hepatitis A are limited to fulminant hepatitis.

In this chapter, we review indications, prevention of recurrence, and results of OLT for HBV-related liver disease and indications and results of OLT for hepatitis A.

Transplantation for Hepatitis B

Indications for Liver Transplantation

Liver transplantation should be considered when the expected median term survival is less than 2 years. Transplantation is indicated in patients with a history of spontaneous bacterial peritonitis, chronic encephalopathy, refractory ascites, or recurrent variceal bleeding despite endoscopic treatments. Hepatocellular carcinoma is also a common indication for liver transplantation in patients infected with HBV.

Mechanisms of Hepatitis B Virus Recurrence After Liver Transplantation

HBV reinfection is the consequence of an immediate reinfection of the graft caused by circulating HBV particles, reinfection of the graft from HBV particles coming from extrahepatic sites, or both. In patients receiving HBIg, HBV reinfection may be the consequence of:

- HBV overproduction coming from extrahepatic sites
- An insufficient protective titer of anti-hepatitis B surface (HBs) antibodies
- The emergence of escape mutants

This latter mechanism is probably important because mutations in the pre-S/S genome of HBV and in the "a" determinant have been described secondary to administration of HBIg.[7,8]

Peripheral mononuclear cells may be implicated in this immune pressure selection mechanism; for example, we have shown that the HBV strain predominant in a patient after reinfection was the strain predominating in the mononuclear cells of this patient before liver transplantation.[9] This mechanism of escape mutation is not exclusive—HBV reinfection with a nonmutated form of HBV occurs in patients receiving HBIg.[8]

In patients receiving lamivudine monoprophylaxis, HBV surface antigen (HBsAg) remained positive, progressively declining over a period of a few months after transplantation to become undetectable. Lo and colleagues[10] described active anti-HBs production in some patients after transplantation. The increase of antibody level occurred in these patients when the donor was anti-HBs positive, which supports the hypothesis of anti-HBs production arising from the lymphocytes of the donor.

Prevention of Hepatitis B Virus Recurrence

Hepatitis B Immune Globulins Monoprophylaxis

The mechanism or mechanisms by which HBIg protects the transplanted liver against HBV reinfection are poorly understood. One hypothesis suggests that HBIg protects naïve hepatocytes against HBV that is released from extrahepatic sites through the blocking of a putative HBV receptor. Regardless of the mechanism involved, there is evidence for a dose-dependent response to HBIg treatment that protects patients against HBV reinfection of the graft.[6,11,12] In some studies, the administration of HBIg during the anhepatic phase and short-term posttransplantation period gave disappointing results; most patients developed HBV recurrence.[3,4,11] The Hanover group subsequently adjusted HBIg dosages to maintain the anti-HBs titer at greater than 100 IU/L for a minimum of 6 months after OLT.[13]

We and other European transplant centers adopted indefinite immunoprophylaxis.[12] Patients received 10,000 IU/L during the anhepatic phase and 10,000 IU/L daily during the 6 postoperative days. After that, the level of anti-HBs was assessed weekly, and 10,000 IU of HBIg was readministered when the anti-HBs level was less than 100 IU/L. In a European multicenter study reporting 372 HBsAg-positive patients, the effect of long-term administration of HBIg was clearly evidenced—there was a dramatic decrease in the rate of HBV recurrence, from 75% in patients receiving no or short-term administration of HBIg to 33% in those receiving long-term administration of HBIg ($P < 0.001$).[11] Recurrence of HBV occurred in[11]:

- 67% of patients who underwent transplantation for HBV cirrhosis
- 40% of patients who underwent transplantation for fulminant hepatitis B-delta
- 32% of patients who underwent transplantation for hepatitis D virus (HDV) cirrhosis
- 17% of patients who underwent transplantation for fulminant hepatitis B

The HBV recurrence rate related to the presence of HBV replication, which was assessed by both hepatitis B e antigen (HBeAg) and HBV-DNA detection in serum using conventional hybridization techniques at the time of transplantation. The recurrence rates measured were ($P = 0.05$)[11]:

- 83% in HBV DNA and HBeAg-positive HBV-cirrhosis patients
- 58% in HBV DNA and HBeAg-negative HBV-cirrhosis patients

These results were confirmed by other clinical trials in the United States and Europe and by long-term follow-up studies (Table 8–1).[14-16] In our series, reporting on 284 HBsAg-positive patients, the 10-year rate of HBV recurrence was 56.5% of patients who underwent transplantation for HBV cirrhosis, 37.5% of those who underwent transplantation for fulminant hepatitis B-delta, 15.5% of those who underwent transplantation for HDV cirrhosis, and nil for those who underwent transplantation for fulminant hepatitis B.[14]

Table 8-1. RATE OF HBV RECURRENCE AFTER LIVER TRANSPLANTATION FOR NONREPLICATIVE OR REPLICATIVE HBV CIRRHOSIS USING HEPATITIS B IMMUNE GLOBULIN

Authors	Patients	Prevention of HBV Recurrence*	Rate of HBV Recurrence	Follow-Up (Months)
NONREPLICATIVE HBV CIRRHOSIS				
O'Grady[4]	9	Short-term HBIg	78%	40
Samuel[11]	15	None	67%	36
	13	Short-term HBIg	92%	36
Muller[16]	14	HBIg >100 IU/L (6-12 months)	28%	24
Samuel[12]	24	Long-term HBIg >100 IU/L	29%	24
Samuel[11]	37	Long-term HBIg >100 IU/L	38%	36
Samuel[14]	52	Long-term HBIg >100 IU/L	36.9%	120
Gugenheim[18]	30	Long-term HBIg >500 IU/L	15.2%	60
McGory[17]	9	Long-term HBIg >500 IU/L	0	24
REPLICATIVE HBV CIRRHOSIS				
O'Grady[4]	11	Short-term HBIg	100%	15
Samuel[11]	16	None	75%	36
	14	Short-term HBIg	71%	36
Muller[16]	9	HBIg >100 IU/L (6-12 months)	89%	24
Samuel[12]	16	Long-term HBIg >100 IU/L	96%	24
Samuel[11]	47	Long-term HBIg >100 IU/L	70%	36
Samuel[14]	30	Long-term HBIg >100 IU/L	79%	60
McGory[17]	19	Long-term HBIg >500 IU/L	16%	18
Sawyer[19]	26	Long-term HBIg >500 IU/L	35%	36
Samuel[14]	10	Long-term HBIg >500 IU/L and antiviral drugs	20%	60

*Prevention of HBV recurrence with short- or long-term hepatitis B immune globulin (HBIg) to maintain anti-HBs levels of at least 100 or >500 IU/L.
HBIg, hepatitis B immune globulin; HBV, hepatitis B virus.

For patients who were HBV-DNA–positive preoperatively, the rate of HBV reinfection was significantly reduced by using higher HBIg doses and maintaining a serum anti-HBs level greater than 500 IU/L, or by using pre- or post-OLT supplemental antiviral therapy, or both. Several reports using very high doses of HBIg and maintenance titers of more than 500 IU/L showed promising results, even in patients who were HBV-DNA–positive before transplantation.[15,17] HBV recurrence occurred in 0 to 15.2% and 16% to 35% of patients transplanted for nonreplicative and replicative HBV cirrhosis, respectively (see Table 8–1).[14,17-19]

Taking into consideration the inter- and intrapatient variations in pharmacokinetics of HBIg, monitoring serum anti-HBs levels is required. An alternative approach, proposed by Terrault and colleagues, gives a fixed monthly dose of 10,000 IU HBIg intravenously, irrespective of preoperative viral replication status.[15] HBV recurrence at 2 years was observed in 19% and 76% of patients who received and did not receive this dosage of HBIg, respectively.

Most data support long-term intravenous administration of HBIg. Efforts to use intramuscular HBIg have been motivated by a substantial cost benefit and unavailability of intravenous HBIg, but experience with the intramuscular route of HBIg is limited to a small number of patients.

HBIg administration has a very satisfactory record of safety, and adverse events observed are usually minor and rare. Mercury poisoning occurs anecdotally in patients receiving an intramuscular form of HBIg via perfusion by the intravenous route.[20] Some cases of immune reactions occur but are easily prevented by infusion of steroids, antihistaminic drugs, and a longer duration of perfusion. Long-term HBIg administration has several drawbacks, however, including the following:

- HBIg administration on a long-term basis is expensive, but the cost is highly variable depending on the country and the manufacturer.[6]
- HBIg administration is constraining because of the need for close monitoring of the level of anti-HBs antibodies and the frequent reinjection requirement (every 1 or 2 months, depending on these levels).

- The HBV reinfection rate remains high in high-risk groups (i.e., patients with HBV replication at time of transplantation).
- Emergence of escape mutants has been described.[7,8]

Pretransplantation Antiviral Therapies

Until the end of the 1990s, the presence of HBV replication was considered a contraindication to OLT by most centers. Thus an antiviral treatment to clear HBV DNA from serum before performing OLT is logical and can reduce the rate of posttransplant infection. However, patients who are candidates for OLT are difficult to treat because of the severity of the liver disease. An ideal treatment in this setting should have a rapid, potent antiviral action without provoking deterioration of liver function. A major limitation of using interferon before OLT has been its poor tolerability in cirrhotic patients and its modest antiviral effect. Interferon has actually been supplanted by new antiviral analogues.

Famciclovir. Famciclovir has good bioavailability after oral administration, but its activity against HBV is modest, so use of famciclovir in prevention of HBV recurrence is limited.[21]

Lamivudine. Lamivudine (LAM) is well tolerated even in decompensated cirrhosis, and it achieves a negative HBV DNA result (by molecular hybridization) in 90% of patients.[22-26] However, viremia occurs in more than 80% of patients following cessation of therapy, and mutations in the YMDD motif of the HBV-DNA polymerase gene increases with treatment duration.

Villeneuve and colleagues[22] reported 35 patients with severely decompensated HBV cirrhosis and replicative HBV infection, who were treated with LAM at a dose of 100 or 150 mg daily. Within 6 months of treatment initiation, 7 patients underwent liver transplantation and 5 patients died. In 23 patients who were treated for at least 6 months (mean = 19 months), there was a slow but marked improvement in liver function in 22 patients, and 2 patients were taken off the transplant list. The rate of development of resistance to LAM was 10% at 1 year and 25% after 2 years of treatment with stable liver function. These results are confirmed in other studies, which show that LAM slowly improves hepatic function of patients with decompensated cirrhosis and replicating HBV,[23,24] and it may confer a significant survival advantage compared with a matched, untreated cohort.[25]

Fontana and colleagues,[26] in a multicenter study of 309 patients, found that LAM did not improve overall pre-OLT or OLT-free survival. However, a subset of patients, with less advanced liver failure, may have derived clinical benefit from LAM treatment. The baseline Child-Pugh score was the only variable significantly associated with death before OLT and was also a significant predictor of OLT-free survival.[26] In a prospective multicenter study reported by Fontana and colleagues, 154 patients listed for OLT received LAM for a median of 16 months.[27] The majority of deaths, 78%, occurred within the first 6 months of therapy. The estimated 3-year survival of patients who survived at least 6 months was 88% on continued treatment. Elevated serum bilirubin, creatinine levels, and the presence of detectable serum HBV DNA were strong and independent predictors of 6-month mortality. Virologic response to LAM was similar in both survivors and nonsurvivors. The severity of liver disease at the time of starting therapy is a better predictor of early mortality than the virologic response to LAM. Thus, patients with advanced liver failure should be prioritized for OLT, irrespective of the antiviral response.

A question that emerges is when to initiate therapy in patients listed for OLT. Prolonged administration of LAM usually is necessary to obtain significant clinical benefits, but the risk for developing drug-resistant mutations increases with the duration of treatment and may exacerbate liver failure. The advent of new antiviral agents such as adefovir dipivoxil, which has antiviral activity against YMDD-mutant HBV, may resolve the question and serve as *rescue* therapy for patients with LAM resistance.[28] Schiff and colleagues used adefovir dipivoxil, 10 mg per day for a median of 18 weeks, in 128 patients with decompensated cirrhosis who failed LAM therapy before OLT.[29] A median reduction of serum HBV-DNA levels of 2.2 log after 4 weeks and 4.1 log after 24 weeks and an associated Child-Pugh score improvement were observed. Cases of liver transplantation in patients with YMDD mutants were reported with controversial results. In two cases, recurrence of HBV was successfully prevented by administering a prophylaxis combining HBIg and LAM.[30,31] Conversely, Rosenau and colleagues reported on HBV recurrence after transplantation for two patients with YMDD mutants despite the same combination prophylaxis.[32] This suggests that transplantation should either be contraindicated in case of emergence of HBV escape mutations before transplantation or performed only after use of new antiviral treatment.

Posttransplantation Antiviral Therapies

Lamivudine Monotherapy. The administration of LAM alone before and after OLT gave promising results at 1 year, with only 1 case of HBV recurrence in 10 patients.[33] A longer follow-up, however, showed a rate of recurrence of 5 of 10 patients because of the emergence of escape mutations in the YMDD part of the polymerase gene and sometimes a severe clinical course.[34] Similar results were reported in other studies,

Table 8–2. PREVENTION OF HBV RECURRENCE WITH LAMIVUDINE MONOTHERAPY BEFORE AND AFTER LIVER TRANSPLANTATION

Authors	No. of Patients	Pretreatment Virologic Status of Transplanted Patients		Duration of Treatment Before OLT (Months)*	No. Pts HBV-DNA Positive at Time of OLT	No. of Trnsp	No. of HBV Recurrences (%)	Follow-Up after OLT (Months)*	Deaths Related to HBV Recurrence
		No. Pts HBV-DNA Positive	No. Pts HBeAg Positive						
Grellier[33,†]	17	8	4	2 (1.2-5.6)	0	12	5 (50%)	32 (16-51)	2
Mutimer[34,†]	23	9	11	NA	3	17	5 (29.4%)	37 (22-50)	2
Malkan[36]	13	3	2	8 (1-31)	0	13	4 (30.7%)	22 (4-37)	2
Lo[35]	31	11	18	1.6 (0.03-20.4)	6	31	7‡ (22.6%)	16 (6-47)	0
Perillo[24]	77	26	24	2.1 (0.03-20.9)	6	47	17 (36.1%)	38 (2.7-48.5)	1

*Mean (range).
†These two studies report common patients.
‡6 of these patients were HBsAg positive, HBV DNA negative by PCR.
HBeAg, hepatitis B e antigen; HBV, hepatitis B virus; NA, not available; OLT, orthotopic liver transplantation; Pts, patients; trnsp, transplants.

with HBV recurrence in 22.6% to 50% of patients (Table 8–2).[24,35,36] Thus, the administration of LAM alone as a prophylaxis after liver transplantation is probably insufficient, particularly in replicative patients.

Combination of Lamivudine and Hepatitis B Immune Globulin. Several groups developed a more rational approach by giving LAM before transplantation and a combination of LAM and HBIg after OLT. The initial results were very encouraging, demonstrating disappearance of HBV DNA prior to OLT and absence of HBV recurrence.[37] In these studies, the HBV recurrence rates at 1 to 2 years were less than 10% (Table 8–3).[32,37-46] In addition, HBV DNA was found to be negative by polymerase chain reaction (PCR) in most cases at 1 year after OLT. Lamivudine coadministration permits the reduction of the overall amount of HBIg given after transplantation compared with giving HBIg alone.[32,38] The good results of combination treatment may be the consequence of a synergistic effect with reduction of the production of HBsAg by LAM and with a decreased rate of escape mutations in the pre-S/S and YMDD regions.

Passive immunoprophylaxis protocols used in different centers are heterogeneous in regard to both dosing and routes of administration of HBIg (see Table 8–3). The major limitation of intravenous (IV) HBIg protocols is its cost. Therefore, a reduction in high doses of HBIg, which appear unnecessary for the majority of patients receiving combination therapy, reduces treatment costs. Han and colleagues[47] showed that conversion from IV to intramuscular (IM) HBIg in combination with LAM resulted in an absence of HBV recurrence in 58 of 59 (98%) treated patients. Taking efficacy and cost-effectiveness into consideration, IM HBIg plus LAM seems to be superior to IV HBIg plus LAM. The optimal HBIg protocol in the LAM era is yet to be defined.

Guidelines and Future Prospects

Patients who are considered OLT candidates should be subdivided into patients who have active viral replication and those who do not. For patients without viral replication (i.e., hepatitis B-delta cirrhosis, fulminant hepatitis B), there is no evidence that preoperative antiviral therapy is useful. These patients should receive HBIg, 10,000 IU given daily for 7 days, including the anhepatic period, and then every 6 to 8 weeks indefinitely to maintain anti-HBs titers that are more than 100 IU/L. For patients with viral replication (i.e., viral B cirrhosis), LAM therapy should be started at least 4 weeks before OLT. Patients with advanced liver failure should be prioritized for OLT, irrespective of the antiviral response. Patients who develop resistance to LAM may respond to adefovir dipivoxil. Transplantation may be performed for negative HBV-DNA (by molecular hybridization) patients. After transplantation, these high-risk patients should receive a combination of HBIg (10,000 IU daily for 7 days, and then indefinitely every 4 weeks to maintain anti-HBs titers of more than 500 IU/L, especially during the first 2 years after surgery) and antiviral therapy (lamivudine ± adefovir dipivoxil) (Fig. 8–1).

Discontinuation of Hepatitis B Immune Globulin

Future prospects, especially in patients without replication before transplantation, will be the possibility of stopping HBIg therapy and replacing it with LAM or vaccination.

Table 8-3. PREVENTION OF HBV RECURRENCE AFTER LIVER TRANSPLANTATION WITH LAMIVUDINE AND ANTI-HBsAg

Authors	Pretreatment Virologic Status of Transplant Patients					Prevention of HBV Recurrence Pre-OLT Duration (Months)	Post-OLT	No. of HBV Recurrences (%)*	Follow-Up (Months)*
	No. of Patients	No. Pts HBV-DNA Positive	No. Pts HBeAg Positive	No. Pts HBV-DNA Positive at OLT	No. of Trnsp				
Markowitz[37]	14	5	1	1	14	Lamivudine 3 (0.7-7.8)	LAM[a]+HBIg IV	0	13
Yao[40]	10	9[b]	6	2	10	Lamivudine 8.6 (1-22)	LAM+HBIg IM[c]	1 (10%)	15 (10-21)
Yoshida[41]	7	4	NA	0	7	Lamivudine NA	LAM+HBIg IM[d]	0	17 (13-21)
Angus[39]	37	36	19	NA	37	Lamivudine 3.2	LAM+HBIg IM	1 (2.7%)	18 (5-45)
Marzano[38]	33	26	7	0	26[e]	Lamivudine 4.6 (0.6-14.1)	LAM+HBIg IV[f]	1 (4%)	30 ± 8
McCaughan[42]	9	9	0	NA	9	0	LAM+HBIg IM[g]	0	17 (9-24)
Rosenau[32]	21	11	3	5[h]	21	Lamivudine 4.6 (0.06-14.1)	LAM+HBIg IV[i]	2 (9.5%)	21 (2.4-49.1)
Roche[46]	15	15	5	4	15	Lamivudine 4.6 (0.3-13)	LAM+HBIg IV[j]	1 (6.6%)	15 (3-36)
Han[43]	59	NA	NA	NA	59	Lamivudine NA	LAM+HBIg IV[k]	0	15 (1-61.8)
Seehofer[44]	17	17	9	5	17	Lamivudine 10.6 (1-28)	LAM+HBIg IV[l]	3 (18%)	25 (9-49)
Gane[45]	107	79	39	35	107	Lamivudine 2 (0.5-3.5)	LAM+HBIg IM[m]	4 (3.7%)	26 (0.5-76)

*Mean (range)

[a] Lamivudine initiated at OLT in four patients, HBIg 80,000 IU first month, then 10,000 IU/month.

[b] One patient developed lamivudine resistance.

[c] For patients who are HBV-DNA positive, 80,000 IU IV + 3,300 IU IM first month, then 1480 IU IM/month. For patients who are HBV-DNA negative, 10,000 IU IV + 4400 IU IM first month, then 1480 IU IM/month.

[d] Use 43,400 IU IM first month, then 4300 to 6800 IU IM/month.

[e] Seven patients were not transplanted—four died from liver failure, three had improved liver function.

[f] Use 46,500 IU IV first month then 5000 IU IV/month.

[g] Use 3200 IU IM first month then 400 IU IM/month.

[h] Two patients with YMDD mutation before OLT.

[i] Use 45,000 IU IV first week then reinjection to maintain anti-HBsAg >500 IU/L until day 14, then >200 IU/L.

[j] Use 80,000 IU IV first month then 10,000 IU IV/month.

[k] Use 80,000 IU IV first week then 10,000 IU IV/month.

[l] Use 80,000 IU IV first week then 1,500-2,000 IU IV to maintain anti-HBsAg>100 IU/L.

[m] Use 400-800 IU IM first week then monthly thereafter.

HBIg = hepatitis B immune globulin; HBeAg = hepatitis B e antigen; HBsAg = hepatitis B surface antigen; HBV = hepatitis B virus; IM = intramuscular; IV = intravenous; LAM = lamivudine; NA = not available; OLT = orthotopic liver transplantation; Pts = patients; trnsp = transplants.

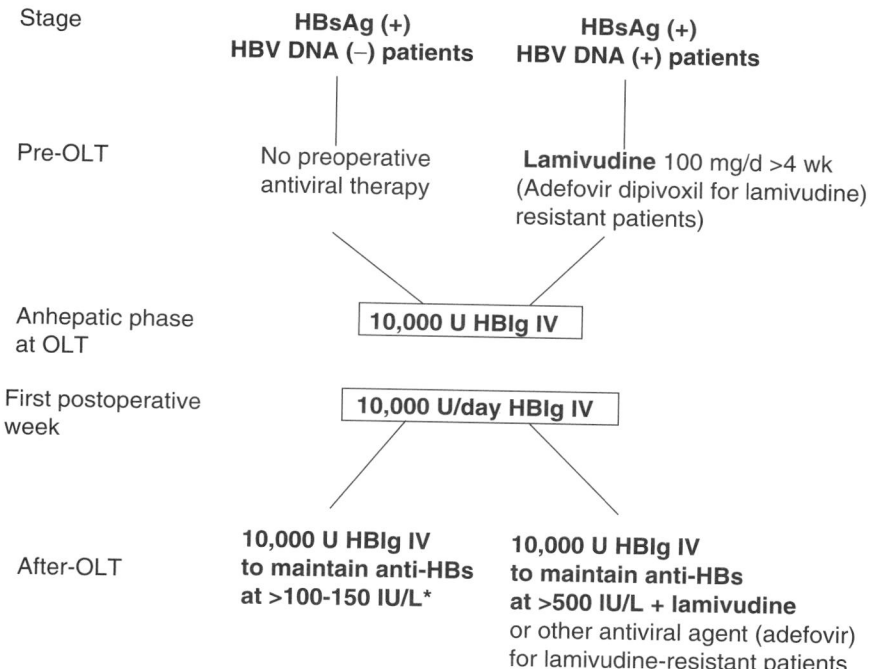

Stage	HBsAg (+) HBV DNA (−) patients	HBsAg (+) HBV DNA (+) patients
Pre-OLT	No preoperative antiviral therapy	**Lamivudine** 100 mg/d >4 wk (Adefovir dipivoxil for lamivudine) resistant patients)
Anhepatic phase at OLT	**10,000 U HBIg IV**	
First postoperative week	**10,000 U/day HBIg IV**	
After-OLT	**10,000 U HBIg IV to maintain anti-HBs at >100-150 IU/L***	**10,000 U HBIg IV to maintain anti-HBs at >500 IU/L + lamivudine** or other antiviral agent (adefovir) for lamivudine-resistant patients

*It may be possible to stop HBIg after 2-3 years in selected patients and replace it by lamivudine or HBV vaccination

FIGURE 8–1

Hepatitis B immune globulin prophylaxis for prevention of HBV graft recurrence following orthotopic liver transplantation (OLT).

The aims are to reduce the long-term costs and the constraint of HBIg administration. In a recent study, HBIg administration was discontinued in a select group of 17 patients and replaced by anti-HBV vaccination.[48] The authors claim good results with anti-HBs production and absence of HBV reinfection. However, the antibody level is low and declining with time in most of the patients. These results are confirmed with a longer follow-up[49] and in another study.[50] Conflicting results are reported by Angelico using a triple course of hepatitis B vaccination, also in 17 patients who underwent transplantation for HBV cirrhosis after cessation of HBIg.[51] An anti-HBs titer greater than 100 IU/L was observed in only two patients (12%). Patient populations, methodologies, and definitions are different in these studies.

Two studies compared the HBV reinfection rate in a group of patients who had undergone transplantation and were randomized to receive HBIg or LAM after a period of administration of HBIg.[52,53] In the study by Naoumov,[53] 24 patients were selected who were considered a low risk for HBV reinfection (i.e., absence of detectable HBV DNA at time of transplantation and no HBV reinfection after a minimal follow-up of 6 months after transplantation). At 1 year, the HBV reinfection rate was not significantly different: 2 of 12 patients and 1 of 12 patients in the LAM and HBIg groups, respectively. However, HBV DNA was detected by PCR in the serum of patients without HBV recurrence in 2 of 11 patients in the HBIg group and in 5 of 10 patients in the LAM group. This should keep us alert. Indeed, the follow-up of these studies is limited, only 1 to 2 years, and it has been clearly shown that the risk of escape mutations with LAM increases with time.

HBIg withdrawal has also been explored in patients receiving combination prophylaxis. Buti and colleagues studied 29 patients who were HBV-DNA–negative at time of OLT, 12 spontaneously and 17 LAM-induced.[54] HBIg doses given were 10,000 IU IV during the anhepatic phase and on the first postoperative day, followed by 5000 IU per day until day 7 and then 4000 IU IM weekly until the end of the first month. Patients were then randomized to receive either LAM monotherapy (14 patients) or LAM plus HBIg at 2000 IU IM monthly (15 patients) until month 18. None of the patients developed HBV recurrence during the study period. Indeed, HBV DNA was positive by PCR at month 18 in 3 patients who received HBIg plus LAM and in 1 who received LAM monotherapy. Polymerase mutants were detected in 3 of these 4 patients.

It is important to determine which patients should be chosen for cessation of HBIg therapy—patients without replication at the time of transplantation, patients with a minimal delay of 2 to 3 years after transplantation, or patients with no detection of HBV DNA by PCR. The arguments against the withdrawal of HBIg are:

- The possibility that irreversible HBV infection might recur after cessation of HBIg
- The persistence of HBV DNA in serum, liver, or peripheral blood mononuclear cells in 50% of HBV-transplanted patients who are HBsAg-negative and on HBIg long-term therapy 10 years after transplantation,[14] or who are receiving combination prophylaxis with HBIg and LAM[38,53]
- The inability to identify patients who have cleared HBV after transplantation

Hepatitis B Virus Recurrence

Spontaneous Outcome of Hepatitis B Virus Recurrence

Most cases of HBV reinfection occur during the first 3 years after transplantation and rarely thereafter. HBV reinfection is characterized by the appearance of HBsAg in serum. The HBV replication level is usually high, and large amounts of HBV particles are present in the graft.[55] Historically, HBV reinfection had a major impact on graft and patient survival[11] because almost all patients with HBV reinfection developed graft disease.[3,4,12] In most cases, acute lobular hepatitis occurred with an evolution to chronic active hepatitis. In some cases, acute liver failure was observed. This severe evolution was probably related to the high amount of HBsAg, HBeAg, and hepatitis B core antigen (HBcAg) present in the nuclei and the cytoplasm of the hepatocytes, suggesting that liver injury is caused by a direct cytopathic effect of the virus.

A particular form of virus is called fibrosing cholestatic hepatitis.[56] It is characterized clinically by a severe outcome and histologically by:

- A cholestatic pattern
- Limited necrosis
- Rapid development of fibrosis
- An enormous amount of HBsAg and HBcAg in the liver

Also, fibrosing cholestatic hepatitis is found mainly in patients not receiving anti-HBs immunoprophylaxis.[56] This high amount of virion particles within the graft is probably the consequence of immunosuppressive therapy, which enhances HBV replication.[57] Rapid reduction in the dose of corticosteroids in liver transplant recipients with HBV infection is a common practice in many transplant programs.[58]

Antiviral treatments have dramatically improved the prognosis of HBV graft reinfection.

Treatment of Hepatitis B Virus Graft Infection

Treatment of HBV graft infection is indicated:

- In patients with recurrent HBV infection without prophylaxis
- In patients with recurrent HBV infection despite prevention with HBIg or LAM, or both
- In patients with de novo HBV infection

In general the treatment of HBV infection is mandatory because of the severity of the liver graft disease in relation to a high viral load. Selection of therapy for HBV infection depends on treatments previously received by patients (i.e., no therapy, HBIg alone, LAM alone, or HBIg and LAM in combination). In the context of protocols that include LAM as prophylaxis, posttransplantation HBV breakthrough involves resistant HBV species.

Interferon is not very efficient in this setting and there is a risk of graft rejection.[59] Nucleoside analogues such as ganciclovir,[60,61] famciclovir,[62] and LAM[62-66] do not augment the risk of rejection, have an antiviral effect, and are well tolerated. The advent of all these agents considerably changed the outcome of liver transplant patients infected with HBV. The main disadvantage of these treatments is that they should be used for long periods, which is a limiting factor especially for ganciclovir because it is administered intravenously. There is a risk of a viral replication rebound when these agents are stopped. Lamivudine is the most widely used nucleoside analogue because it has a much more potent antiviral effect than ganciclovir and famciclovir. Lamivudine, 100 mg daily, is well tolerated and achieves a rapid loss of HBV DNA in serum. In a multicenter study of 52 HBV-DNA–positive transplanted patients, LAM for 1 year resulted in a 60% loss of HBV DNA in serum, 11% HBe seroconversion, 4% HBs seroconversion, and a histological improvement.[63] These results are confirmed in other studies showing negative HBV DNA in 68% to 100% of patients and HBe seroconversion in 3% to 30% of patients treated for periods of 12 to 36 months (Table 8–4). Prolonged therapy (i.e., more than 6 months) is associated with the development of breakthrough (i.e., a rise in serum HBV DNA and alanine aminotransferase [ALT]) levels caused by the emergence of HBV escape mutants in 14% to 62% of patients (see Table 8–4) and clinical deterioration in some cases.[65] Thus with longer follow-up, it seems likely that the majority of treated patients would develop HBV-DNA breakthrough.

Molecular analysis of mutations observed during LAM or famciclovir monotherapy shows changes in the gene for the viral DNA polymerase (B or C domains,

Table 8–4. LAMIVUDINE TREATMENT OF HEPATITIS B AFTER TRANSPLANTATION

| Authors | No. of Patients | Pretreatment | | Treatment Duration (Months)* | No. Pts HBV-DNA Negative | Seroconversion | | No. Pts With Breakthrough | Average Time to Breakthrough (Months)* |
		No. Pts HBV-DNA Positive	No. Pts HBeAg Positive			No. Pts HBeAg	No. Pts HBsAg		
Perillo[63]	52	47	45	12	32 (68%)	5 (11%)	2 (4%)	14 (27%)	8 (NA)
Roche[64]	16	16	10	15.5 (1-30)	13 (81%)	3 (30%)	3 (18.7%)	6 (50%)	8 (6-12)
Rayes[62]	41	41	NA	12 to 36	31 (75.6%)	NA	NA	14 (45%)	NA/(3.7-13)
Malkan[36]	15	14	6	21.2 (4-39)	14 (100%)	0	1 (6.6%)	2 (14.2%)	11.5 (7-16)
Fontana[65]	33	29	24	21 (4-36)	22 (72%)	1 (3%)	0	13 (45%)	15 (6-29)

*Mean (range).
HBeAg = hepatitis B e antigen; HBsAg = hepatitis B surface antigen; HBV = hepatitis B virus; NA = not available; Pts = patients.

or both). Thus famciclovir-resistant virus may not be sensitive to LAM. When antiviral drugs are stopped, the wild-type HBV becomes the dominant viral population, but retreatment is associated with the development of resistant mutants at an accelerated rate.[66] Bock and colleagues[67] reported severe posttransplantation HBV disease in patients receiving combination prophylaxis with LAM and HBIg related to a drug-dependent, enhanced replication of LAM-resistant HBV mutants. HBV sequence analysis of these patients shows both mutations in the "a" determinant of the envelope and the YMDD motif (domain C) of the polymerase protein. In vitro experiments indicate that combinations of mutations enhance replication in vitro in the presence of LAM. This suggests that continuation of LAM could be deleterious in these patients. The prevalence of patients with LAM-resistant HBV infection will continue to increase because of the increasing number of patients treated with LAM before or after transplantation.

Fortunately, new HBV antivirals such as adefovir dipivoxil are effective in viral suppression of LAM-resistant variants.[29,68,69] Use of adefovir dipivoxil at a dose of 10 mg per day may be limited by toxicity, possibly associated with impaired renal function. Schiff and colleagues reported 121 patients treated with adefovir dipivoxil, 10 mg per day, for a median of 33 weeks (range, 1-88 weeks).[29] Treatment for 48 weeks resulted in a significant decline in HBV-DNA levels by 4 log copies/mL. Dose reductions are required if creatinine clearance is less than 50 mL/minute, whereas no dose adjustment is needed for hepatic dysfunction. Successful treatment by adefovir dipivoxil for liver failure, such as cholestatic fibrosing hepatitis resulting from LAM-resistant HBV, was reported in the transplant setting.[69-72] For these patients, sustained inhibition of replication was not achieved with high-dose LAM, ganciclovir, or famciclovir treatment. It is not known if patients who are treated for LAM resistance with adefovir dipivoxil need to continue on LAM, but it seems better to continue

both drugs for some period after the initiation of adefovir dipivoxil. Until now, resistance to adefovir dipivoxil has not been reported,[73] but it could be expected with prolonged exposure. The indication for treatment with adefovir dipivoxil after emergence of HBV mutants resistant to LAM should be further explored. After emergence of mutation, there are several possibilities:

- Continue LAM treatment alone in case of normal liver enzymes and no disease progression.
- Start adefovir dipivoxil in addition to LAM.
- Start adefovir dipivoxil in place of LAM.

The discontinuation of LAM without replacement by adefovir dipivoxil may put the patient at risk for hepatitis exacerbation. Experience with entecavir[74] or tenofovir[75] is limited, but these antivirals may be effective in treatment of LAM variants in transplanted patients.

Retransplantation for Hepatitis B Virus Recurrence

Historically, liver retransplantation for HBV recurrence was highly controversial and considered a contraindication for surgery because of the high risk of recurrence on the second graft and because of overall poor results.[76] The advent of combining HBIg with new antiviral agents has completely changed this outcome, so good results are now achievable.[77]

Survival of Patients Who Undergo Transplantation for Hepatitis B Virus Cirrhosis

In the absence of prophylaxis of HBV reinfection, the 5-year survival rate is low (between 40% and 60%) and HBV-related deaths are frequent 6 months after transplant surgery. In 206 patients receiving adequate immunoprophylaxis, results of OLT for HBV infection in Berlin were similar to those results achieved with other indications. In the Berlin series, the 2-year patient survival increased from 85% in 1988-1993 to 94% after 1997 ($P < 0.05$) using prevention of HBV recurrence with HBIg and LAM. The 2-year recurrence rates in the two periods were 42% and 8% ($P < 0.05$).[5] In the multivariate analysis for patient survival, only the covariates hepatocarcinoma and HBV recurrence were statistically significant. In our own series, the 10-year survival rate of patients who underwent transplantation for HBV cirrhosis and HDV cirrhosis was 70.9% and 89%, respectively.[14]

Liver Transplantation in Patients with Hepatitis D Virus Liver Cirrhosis

Patients chronically infected with HBV and HDV are less at risk of HBsAg reappearance than patients infected with HBV alone. The rate of HBsAg reappearance in patients with viral B-delta cirrhosis is approximately 50% in patients who do not receive long-term HBIg.[4,78] In the European multicenter study, HBV recurrence in HDV cirrhotic patients was 17% and 60% in those receiving and those not receiving long-term HBIg, respectively.[11] The overall lower HBV recurrence rate in these patients is probably because almost all patients were HBV-DNA–negative at the time of liver transplantation and because HDV has an inhibitory effect on HBV replication.

However, delta patients are at risk of reinfection by HBV or HDV, or both. HDV reinfection, assessed by the presence of HDV RNA and hepatitis D antigen (HDAg) in serum or liver, is frequent and was observed in 80% of cases after transplantation in the first posttransplant months.[79] The course of HDV reinfection varies depending on whether or not HBsAg is present. In the few cases where HBsAg reappeared, it was associated with a combined HBV-HDV replication; HBV DNA and HDV RNA were present in serum or HDAg was present in the liver, or both.[79] Acute hepatitis, followed by chronic hepatitis, developed.[79] HBV-HDV recurrence is, in general, less severe than HBV recurrence alone.[11] In the patients who remained HBsAg-negative after transplantation, the amount of HDAg in the liver graft was low, and the liver graft remained histologically normal. At long-term follow-up, HDV markers progressively disappeared from liver and serum when HBsAg did not recur.[79] The hypotheses for explaining the presence of HDV replication in HBsAg-negative patients are:

- HBV markers could be present but not detectable.
- HDV is present in the hepatocytes in the absence of HBsAg but either cannot replicate or has a low replication level.
- The level of HDV RNA in the liver is much lower in patients without HBsAg than those with HBsAg,

and this low level of delta virus may explain the absence of liver graft lesions.

In conclusion, the risk of HBsAg reappearance after liver transplantation in viral B-delta cirrhotic patients who received long-term HBIg is low, and the 10-year survival rate is good.

Liver Transplantation for Fulminant Hepatitis B

Hepatitis B virus is a common cause of fulminant hepatic failure (FHF), which occurs in 1% to 4% of patients with acute hepatitis B. Acute HBV infection is diagnosed by detection of immunoglobulin (Ig) M antibodies against hepatitis B core antigen because a substantial number of patients have negative HBsAg and serum HBV DNA. Coinfection with HBV and HDV, or superinfection by HDV in patients with chronic hepatitis B, can also cause FHF. The incidence of such coinfection is higher in intravenous drug users. FHF following reactivation of chronic hepatitis B has been described mainly in patients with diverse immunosuppressant conditions. Emergency liver transplantation is the treatment of choice for the most severe forms of fulminant hepatitis B. Indeed, transplantation was shown to be associated with survival rates of 60% to 70%, whereas only 5% to 10% of the patients were expected to survive spontaneously.[80] In Europe, 17% of patients undergoing liver transplantation for fulminant hepatitis have fulminant hepatitis B.[2] In patients with fulminant hepatitis B, the risk of HBV reinfection is controlled by immunoprophylaxis. The European multicenter study showed that whatever the treatment administered, HBV infection recurred in 17% of patients undergoing transplantation for fulminant hepatitis B.[11] In our patients who underwent transplantation for fulminant hepatitis B and were receiving long-term HBIg, the rate of HBV reinfection was 0.[14] The lower recurrence rate of HBV infection in fulminant hepatitis B patients may be because most of these patients were HBV-DNA–negative at the time of OLT.

Transplantation for Hepatitis A

Hepatitis A virus (HAV), a nonenveloped RNA virus, is particularly resistant and contagious. The infection is spread chiefly by fecal-oral transmission and is a public health problem throughout the world. The main complication of HAV infection is fulminant hepatitis (acute liver failure with encephalopathy), which occurs in less than 1% of cases. It appears to be more frequent in adults than in children.[81] In the United States, approximately one third of adults have anti-HAV antibodies, and 100 deaths per year are attributed to fulminant hepatitis A. In Europe, 0.2% of patients undergoing liver transplantation have fulminant hepatitis A (this represents 2% of transplantation for fulminant hepatitis).[2] Fulminant hepatitis A is also a frequent cause of death due to FHF among children in developing countries. The mechanisms of fulminant outcome are unknown. Low HAV viremia was associated with a severe course in our series.[82] This suggests that a strong immune response may be associated with a severe or a fulminant course. Other factors such as age, gender, and acetaminophen toxicity may also play a role in the course of hepatitis A.[82] However, fulminant hepatitis A resolves spontaneously more frequently than fulminant hepatitis of other origins, and the decision to perform transplantation or not is thus particularly difficult.[83] OLT has markedly changed the prognosis of fulminant hepatitis A in industrialized countries and is currently indicated for patients with deep coma and low factor V levels.[80] Because of the high possibility of liver regeneration in fulminant hepatitis A, however, the possibility of auxiliary orthotopic liver transplantation should be raised, particularly in young patients.[84,85] However, as described by our group, auxiliary partial orthotopic liver transplant (APOLT) is associated with higher morbidity and should be reserved for patients with a low-grade coma.[86]

Conclusion

During the past decade, major advances have been made in the management of HBV transplant candidates. The advent of long-term HBIg administration as a prophylaxis of HBV recurrence was a major breakthrough in the management of patients, especially those without replication at the time of transplantation. By using LAM before transplantation and a combination of LAM and HBIg after transplantation it is possible to reduce the rate of HBV reinfection in HBV replicative cirrhotic patients. Future research should:

- Test new protocols using lower HBIg doses given intravenously or intramuscularly alone or in combination with additional antiviral agents.
- Identify patients in whom HBIg prophylaxis can be stopped safely.
- Develop new antiviral agents with activity for patients with LAM resistance.

Currently, treatment of posttransplantation hepatitis B is a less important clinical problem than it was historically. However, in the context of protocols that include LAM as prophylaxis, posttransplantation HBV breakthrough involves LAM-resistant variants. LAM is the most widely used nucleoside analogue in *naïve* patients, but prolonged therapy is limited by the development of breakthrough because of the emergence of HBV escape mutants. Fortunately, new HBV antivirals such as adefovir dipivoxil, entecavir, and tenofovir are effective in viral suppression of LAM-resistant variants. Future prospects should compare combinations of antivirals to monotherapy, define duration of therapy, and develop criteria for safe discontinuation of drug therapy.

Pearls and Pitfalls

- Patients undergoing OLT for hepatitis B without prophylaxis are at high risk for HBV recurrence and severe graft lesions.
- Long-term monoprophylaxis with HBIg significantly reduces the risk for HBV recurrences and increases survival. However, HBV reinfection rates remain high in patients with HBV replication before OLT (presence of HBeAg or HBV DNA, or both).
- Lamivudine (LAM) therapy for decompensated HBV cirrhosis before OLT results in inhibition of viral replication and clinical improvement. Efficacy of LAM is limited by the emergence of LAM-resistant YMDD mutants.
- Prophylaxis of HBV recurrence with LAM monotherapy is associated with a risk for drug resistance and an overall 3-year rate of reinfection of 50%.
- Combination prophylaxis with HBIg and LAM can reduce the overall rate of recurrent hepatitis B to 0 to 10%.
- Dose, duration, and route of administration of HBIg needed when used in combination with LAM remains to be determined. Future prospects, mainly in patients without replication before OLT, will include the possibility of stopping HBIg therapy and replacing it with LAM or HBV vaccination.
- LAM is highly effective in the treatment of recurrent HBV infection, but its efficacy is limited by the emergence of LAM-resistant YMDD mutants.
- Adefovir dipivoxil appears safe and effective in the treatment of liver recipients with LAM-resistant HBV disease.

References

1. Seaberg EC, Belle SH, Beringer KC, et al: Liver transplantation in the United States from 1987-1998: Updated results from the Pitt-UNOS liver transplant registry. In Cecka JM, Terasaki PI (eds.): Clinical Transplants 1998, Los Angeles, UCLA Tissue Typing Laboratory, 1999, pp 17-37.

2. European Liver Transplant Registry (ELTR)—Registry for the European liver transplant association, data analysis, 05/1968-6/2002, online: Available at http://www.eltr.org

3. Todo S, Demetris AJ, Van Thiel D, et al: Orthotopic liver transplantation for patients with hepatitis B virus related liver disease. Hepatology 13:619-626, 1991.

4. O'Grady JG, Smith HM, Davies SE, et al: Hepatitis B virus re-infection after orthotopic liver transplantation: Serological and clinical implications. J Hepatol 14:104-111, 1992.

5. Steinmuller T, Seehofer D, Rayes N, et al: Increasing applicability of liver transplantation for patients with hepatitis B–related liver disease. Hepatology 35:1528-1535, 2002.

6. Shouval D, Samuel D: Hepatitis B immune globulin to prevent HBV graft reinfection following liver transplantation: A concise review. Hepatology 32:1189-1195, 2000.

7. Ghany MG, Ayola B, Villamil FG, et al: Hepatitis B virus S mutants in liver transplant recipients who were reinfected despite hepatitis B immune globulin prophylaxis. Hepatology 27:213-222, 1998.

8. Terrault NA, Zhiou S, McCory RW, et al: Incidence and clinical consequences of surface and polymerase gene mutations in liver transplant recipients on hepatitis B immunoglobulin. Hepatology 28:555-561, 1998.

9. Brind A, Jiang JJ, Samuel D, et al: Evidence for selection of hepatitis B mutants after liver transplantation through peripheral blood mononuclear cell infection. J Hepatol 26:228-235, 1997.

10. Lo CM, Fung JTK, Lau GKK, et al: Development of antibody to hepatitis B surface antigen after liver transplantation for chronic hepatitis B. Hepatology 37:36-43, 2003.

11. Samuel D, Muller R, Alexander G, et al: Liver transplantation in European patients with the hepatitis B surface antigen. N Engl J Med 329:1842-1847, 1993.

12. Samuel D, Bismuth A, Mathieu D, et al: Passive immunoprophylaxis after liver transplantation in HBsAg-positive patients. Lancet 337:813-815, 1991.

13. Lauchart W, Muller R, Pichlmayr R: Long-term immunoprophylaxis of hepatitis B virus (HBV) re-infection in recipients of human liver allografts. Transplant Proc 19:4051-4053, 1987.

14. Roche B, Feray C, Gigou M, et al: HBV DNA persistence 10 years after liver transplantation despite successful anti-HBs immunoprophylaxis. Hepatology 38:86-95, 2003.

15. Terrault NA, Zhou S, Combs C, et al: Prophylaxis in liver transplant recipients using a fixed dosing schedule of hepatitis B immunoglobulins. Hepatology 24:1327-1333, 1996.

16. Muller R, Gubernatis G, Farle M, et al: Liver transplantation in HBs antigen (HBsAg) carriers. Prevention of hepatitis B virus (HBV) recurrence by passive immunisation. J Hepatol 13:90-96, 1991.

17. McGory RW, Ishitani MB, Oliveira WM, et al: Improved outcome of orthotopic liver transplantation for chronic hepatitis B cirrhosis with aggressive passive immunization. Transplantation 61:1358-1364, 1996.

18. Gugenheim J, Crafa F, Fabiani P, et al: Récidive du virus de l'hépatite B après transplantation hépatique. Gastroenterol Clin Biol 16:430-433, 1992.

19. Sawyer RG, McGory RW, Gaffey MJ, et al: Improved clinical outcome with liver transplantation for hepatitis B related cirrhosis. Ann Surg 227:841-850, 1998.

20. Lowell JA, Burgess S, Shenoy S, et al: Mercury poisoning associated with high dose hepatitis B immune globulin administration after liver transplantation. Liver Transpl Surg 2:475-478, 1996.

21. DeMan RA, Marcellin P, Habal F, et al: A randomized placebo-controlled study to evaluate the efficacy of 12-month famciclovir treatment in patients with chronic hepatitis B e antigen–positive hepatitis B. Hepatology 32:413-417, 2000.

22. Villeneuve JP, Condreay LD, Willems B, et al: Lamivudine treatment for decompensated cirrhosis resulting from chronic hepatitis B. Hepatology 31:207-210, 2000.

23. Kapoor D, Guptan RC, Wakil SM, et al: Beneficial effects of lamivudine in hepatitis B virus–related decompensated cirrhosis. J Hepatol 33:308-312, 2000.

24. Perrillo RP, Wright T, Rakela J, et al: A multicenter United States–Canadian trial to assess lamivudine monotherapy before and after transplantation for chronic hepatitis B. Hepatology 33:424-432, 2001.

25. Yao FY, Terrault NA, Freise C, et al: Lamivudine treatment is beneficial in patients with severely decompensated cirrhosis and actively replicating hepatitis B infection awaiting liver transplantation: A comparative study using a matched, untreated cohort. Hepatology 34:411-416, 2001.

26. Fontana R, Keeffe E, Carey W, et al: Effect of lamivudine treatment on survival of 309 North American patients awaiting liver transplantation for chronic hepatitis B. Liver Transpl 8:433-439, 2002.

27. Fontana R, Hann H, Perrillo R, et al: Determinants of early mortality in patients with decompensated chronic hepatitis B treated with antiviral therapy. Gastroenterology 123:719-727, 2002.

28. Perrillo R, Schiff E, Yoshida E, et al: Adefovir dipivoxil for the treatment of lamivudine-resistant hepatitis B mutants. Hepatology 32:129-134, 2000.

29. Schiff E, Lai CL, Neuhaus P, et al: Adefovir dipivoxil for the treatment of chronic hepatitis B in patients pre- and post-liver transplantation with lamivudine-resistant hepatitis B virus. Hepatology 36:371A, 2002.

30. Stärkel P, Horsmans Y, Geubel A, et al: Favorable outcome of orthotopic liver transplantation in a patient with subacute liver failure due to emergence of a hepatitis B YMDD escape mutant virus. J Hepatol 35:679-681, 2001.

31. Saab S, Kim M, Wright T, et al: Successful orthotopic liver transplantation for lamivudine associated YMDD mutant hepatitis B virus. Gastroenterology 119:1382-1384, 2000.

32. Rosenau J, Bahr M, Tillmann HL, et al: Lamivudine and low-dose hepatitis B immune globulin for prophylaxis of hepatitis B reinfection after liver transplantation: Possible role of mutations in the YMDD motif prior to transplantation as a risk factor for reinfection. J Hepatol 34:895-902, 2001.

33. Grellier L, Mutimer D, Ahmed M, et al: Lamivudine prophylaxis against reinfection in liver transplantation for hepatitis B cirrhosis. Lancet 348:1212-1215, 1996.

34. Mutimer D, Dusheiko G, Barrett C, et al: Lamivudine without HBIg for prevention of graft reinfection by hepatitis B: Long-term follow-up. Transplantation 70:809-815, 2000.

35. Lo CM, Cheung ST, Lai CL, et al: Liver transplantation in Asian patients with chronic hepatitis B using Lamivudine prophylaxis. Ann Surg 233:276-281, 2001.

36. Malkan G, Cattral M, Humar A, et al: Lamivudine for hepatitis B in liver transplantation. Transplantation 69:1403-1407, 2000.

37. Markowitz JS, Martin P, Conrad AJ, et al: Prophylaxis against hepatitis B recurrence following liver transplantation using combination lamivudine and hepatitis B immune globulin. Hepatology 28:585-589, 1998.

38. Marzano A, Salizzoni M, Debernardi-Venon W, et al: Prevention of hepatitis B virus recurrence after liver transplantation in cirrhotic patients treated with lamivudine and passive immunoprophylaxis. J Hepatol 34:903-910, 2001.

39. Angus PW, McCaughan GW, Gane EJ, et al: Combination low-dose hepatitis B immune globulin and lamivudine therapy provides effective prophylaxis against posttransplantation hepatitis B. Liver Transpl 6:429-433, 2000.

40. Yao FY, Osorio RW, Roberts JP, et al: Intramuscular hepatitis B immune globulin combined with lamivudine for prophylaxis against hepatitis B recurrence after liver transplantation. Liver Transpl Surg 5:491-496, 1999.

41. Yoshida EM, Erb SR, Partovi N, et al: Liver transplantation for chronic hepatitis B infection with the use of combination

lamivudine and low-dose hepatitis B immune globulin. Liver Transpl Surg 5:520-525, 1999.

42. McCaughan GW, Spencer J, Koorey D, et al: Lamivudine therapy in patients undergoing liver transplantation for hepatitis B virus precore mutant-associated infection: High resistance rates in treatment of recurrence but universal prevention if used as prophylaxis with very low dose hepatitis B immune globulin. Liver Transpl Surg 6:512-519, 1999.

43. Han SH, Ofman J, Holt C, et al: An efficacy and cost-effectiveness analysis of combination hepatitis B immune globulin and lamivudine to prevent recurrent hepatitis B after orthotopic liver transplantation compared with hepatitis B immune globulin monotherapy. Liver Transpl 6:741-748, 2001.

44. Seehofer D, Rayes N, Naumann U, et al: Preoperative antiviral treatment and postoperative prophylaxis in HBV-DNA positive patients undergoing liver transplantation. Transplantation 72:1381-1385, 2001.

45. Gane EJ, McCaughan G, Crawford D, et al: Combination lamivudine plus low dose intramuscular hepatitis B immunoglobulin prevents recurrent hepatitis B and may eradicate residual graft infection. Hepatology 36:221A, 2002.

46. Roche B, Samuel D, Roque AM, et al: Intravenous anti-HBs Ig combined with oral lamivudine for prophylaxis against HBV recurrence after liver transplantation (abstract). J Hepatol 30: A80, 1999.

47. Han SH, Martin P, Edelstein M, et al: Conversion from intravenous to intramuscular hepatitis B immune globulin in combination with lamivudine is safe and cost-effective in patients receiving long-term prophylaxis to prevent hepatitis B recurrence after liver transplantation. Liver Transpl 9:182-187, 2003.

48. Sanchez-Fueyo A, Rimola A, Grande L, et al: Hepatitis B immunoglobulin discontinuation followed by hepatitis B virus vaccination: A new strategy in the prophylaxis of hepatitis B virus recurrence after liver transplantation. Hepatology 31:496-501, 2000.

49. Sanchez-Fueyo A, Martinez-Bauer E, Rimola A: Hepatitis B vaccination after liver transplantation. Hepatology 36:257-258, 2002.

50. Bienzle U, Gunther M, Neuhaus R, et al: Successful hepatitis B vaccination in patients who underwent transplantation for hepatitis B virus-related cirrhosis: Preliminary results. Liver Transpl 8:562-564, 2002.

51. Angelico M, Di Paolo D, Trinito M, et al: Failure of a reinforced triple course of hepatitis B vaccination in patients transplanted for HBV-related cirrhosis. Hepatology 35:176-181, 2002.

52. Dodson SF, De Vera ME, Bonham CA, et al: Lamivudine after hepatitis B immune globulin is effective in preventing hepatitis B recurrence after liver transplantation. Liver Transpl 6:434-439, 2000.

53. Naoumov NV, Lopes AR, Burra P, et al: Randomized trial of lamivudine versus hepatitis B immunoglobulin for long-term prophylaxis of hepatitis B recurrence after liver transplantation. J Hepatol 34:888-894, 2001.

54. Buti M, Mas A, Prieto M, et al: A randomized study comparing lamivudine monotherapy after a short course of hepatitis B immune globulin (HBIg) and lamivudine with long-term lamivudine plus HBIg in the prevention of hepatitis B virus recurrence after liver transplantation. J Hepatol 38:811-817, 2003.

55. Phillips MJ, Cameron R, Flowers MA, et al: Post-transplant recurrent hepatitis B viral liver disease. Viral-burden, steato-viral, and fibroviral hepatitis. Am J Pathol 140:1295-1308, 1992.

56. Davies SE, Portmann BC, O'Grady JG, et al: Hepatic histologic findings after transplantation for chronic hepatitis B virus infection, including a unique pattern of fibrosing cholestatic hepatitis. Hepatology 13:150-157, 1991.

57. Tur-Kaspa R, Laub O: Corticosteroids stimulate hepatitis B virus DNA, mRNA and protein production in a stable expression system. J Hepatol 11:34-36, 1990.

58. Gish RG, Keefe EB, Lim J, et al: Survival after liver transplantation for chronic hepatitis B using reduced immunosuppression. J Hepatol 22:257-262, 1995.

59. Terrault NA, Combs Holland C, Ferrel L, et al: Interferon alpha for recurrent hepatitis B infection after liver transplantation. Liver Transpl Surg 2:132-138, 1996.

60. Gish RG, Lau JYN, Brooks L, et al: Ganciclovir treatment of hepatitis B virus (HBV) infection in liver transplant patients. Hepatology 23:1-7, 1996.

61. Roche B, Samuel D, Gigou M, et al: Long-term ganciclovir therapy for hepatitis B virus infection after liver transplantation. J Hepatol 31:584-592, 1999.

62. Rayes N, Seehofer D, Hopf U, et al: Comparison of famciclovir and lamivudine in the long-term treatment of hepatitis B infection after liver transplantation. Transplantation 71:96-101, 2001.

63. Perrillo R, Rakela J, Dienstag J, et al: Multicenter study of lamivudine therapy for hepatitis B after liver transplantation. Hepatology 29:1581-1586, 1999.

64. Roche B, Samuel D, Roque AM, et al: Lamivudine therapy for HBV infection after liver transplantation (abstract). J Hepatol 30:78, 1999.

65. Fontana RJ, Hann HW, Wright T, et al: A multicenter study of lamivudine treatment in 33 patients with hepatitis B after liver transplantation. Liver Transpl 6:504-510, 2001.

66. Chayama K, Suzuki Y, Kobayashi M, et al: Emergence and takeover of YMDD motif mutant hepatitis B virus during long-term lamivudine therapy and re-takeover by wild type after cessation of therapy. Hepatology 27:1711-1716, 1998.

67. Bock CT, Tillmann HL, Torresi J, et al: Selection of hepatitis B virus polymerase mutants with enhanced replication by lamivudine treatment after liver transplantation. Gastroenterology 22:264-273, 2002.

68. Perrillo R, Schiff E, Yoshida E, et al: Adefovir dipivoxil for the treatment of lamivudine-resistant hepatitis B mutants. Hepatology 32:129-134 2000.

69. Benhamou Y, Bochet M, Thibault V, et al: Safety and efficacy of adefovir dipivoxil in patients co-infected with HIV-1 and lamivudine-resistant hepatitis B virus: An open-label pilot study. Lancet 358:718-723, 2001.

70. Peters MG, Singer G, Howard T, et al: Fulminant hepatic failure resulting from lamivudine-resistant hepatitis B virus in a renal transplant recipient: Durable response after orthotopic liver transplantation on adefovir dipivoxil and hepatitis B immune globulin. Transplantation 68:1912-1914, 1999.

71. Mutimer D, Feraz-Neto BH, Harrison R, et al: Acute liver graft failure due to emergence of lamivudine resistant hepatitis B virus: Rapid resolution during treatment with adefovir. Gut 49: 860-863, 2001.

72. Walsh KM, Woodall T, Lamy P, et al: Successful treatment with adefovir dipivoxil in a patient with fibrosing cholestatic hepatitis and lamivudine resistant hepatitis B virus. Gut 49:436-440, 2001.

73. Yang H, Westland CE, Delaney WE, et al: Resistance surveillance in chronic hepatitis B patients treated with adefovir dipivoxil for up to 60 weeks. Hepatology 36:464-473, 2002.

74. Shakil AO, Lilly L, Angus P, et al: Entecavir reduces viral load in liver transplant patients who have failed prophylaxis or treatment for hepatitis B (abstract). Hepatology 34(suppl):619, 2001.

75. Van Bommel F, Wunsche T, Schurmann D, et al: Tenofovir treatment in patients with lamivudine-resistant hepatitis B mutants strongly affects viral replication. Hepatology 36:507-508, 2002.

76. Crippin J, Foster B, Carlen S, et al: Retransplantation in hepatitis B—a multicenter experience. Transplantation 57:823-826, 1994.

77. Roche B, Samuel D, Feray C, et al: Retransplantation of the liver for recurrent hepatitis B virus infection: The Paul Brousse experience. Liver Transpl Surg 5:166-174, 1999.

78. Ottobrelli A, Marzano A, Smedile A, et al: Patterns of hepatitis delta virus reinfection and disease in liver transplantation. Gastroenterology 101:1649-1655, 1991.

79. Samuel D, Zignego AL, Reynes M, et al: Long-term clinical and virologic outcome after liver transplantation for cirrhosis due to chronic delta hepatitis. Hepatology 21:333-339, 1995.

80. Bismuth H, Samuel D, Gugenheim J, et al: Emergency Liver transplantation for fulminant hepatitis. Ann Intern Med 107:337-341, 1987.

81. Lemon SM , Shapiro CN: The value of immunization against hepatitis A. Infect Agents Dis 3:38-49, 1994.

82. Rezende G, Roque-Afonso AM, Samuel D, et al: Viral and clinical factors associated with the fulminant course of hepatitis A infection. Hepatology 38:613-618, 2003.

83. Ostapowicz G, Fontana RJ, Schiodt FV, et al: Results of a prospective study of acute liver failure at 17 tertiary care centers in the United States. Ann Intern Med 137:947-954, 2002.

84. Chenard-Neu MP, Boudjema K, Bernuau J, et al: Auxiliary liver transplantation: Regeneration of the native liver and outcome in 30 patients with fulminant hepatic failure: A multicenter European Study. Hepatology 23:1119-1127, 1996.

85. Bismuth H, Azoulay D, Samuel D, et al: Auxiliary partial orthotopic liver transplantation for fulminant hepatitis. The Paul Brousse experience. Ann Surg 224:712-724, 1996.

86. Azoulay D, Samuel D, Ichai P, et al: Auxiliary partial orthotopic versus standard orthotopic whole liver transplantation for acute liver failure. Ann Surg 234:723-731, 2001.

9

Natural History of Hepatitis C

DAWN SEARS
GARY L. DAVIS

Hepatitis C virus   129
　Pathogenesis   130
　Incidence and prevalence of hepatitis C virus
　　infection   130

Progression to cirrhosis   131

Hepatic decompensation   132

Hepatocellular carcinoma   134

Antiviral treatment   134

Liver transplantation   136

**Assessment of disease severity and need for
　transplantation   137**

Summary   138

Chronic hepatitis C is perhaps the most common cause of chronic liver disease, at least in the United States and Europe. It is a major, if not *the* major, cause of hepatocellular carcinoma (HCC) and the leading indication for liver transplantation.[1,2] This chapter provides an overview of the hepatitis C virus (HCV) and an understanding of the natural history of the infection. The natural history of HCV infection has changed in recent years, and this has significant implications for liver transplantations.

Hepatitis C Virus

Although a virus was long suspected as the cause of a hepatitis that was not caused by either hepatitis A or hepatitis B, its identity was elusive and it was not identified until 1989.[3] Nonetheless, the agent responsible for non-A, non-B hepatitis was well characterized before this time by careful observation of infectious isolates in humans and chimpanzees. The agent was known to be lipid-encapsidated and approximately 50 nm.[4] These characteristics were suggestive of an RNA virus, most likely of the *Flaviviridae* family. Eventually, blind cloning methods were able to identify a portion of the virus and eventually assemble the complete 9.6 kb genome.[3] Indeed, the agent responsible for non-A, non-B hepatitis turned out to be an RNA virus resembling *Flaviviridae*, and it was named hepatitis C.[3,5]

Several characteristics of HCV deserve mention because they affect the natural history of the virus and our ability to treat it. The virus is a single-stranded RNA virus and as such lacks the ability to proofread and correct errors during replication.[6] It replicates at an extremely high rate, producing up to 10^{12} virions per day.[7] As a result, considerable genomic heterogeneity occurs, which probably contributes to escape from immune surveillance and viral survival in the host. Over time, this heterogeneity has resulted in distinct populations of HCV, called genotypes, around the world.[8] These genotypes influence the response to antiviral treatment. Currently, there are six genotypes and more than 100 subtypes.[8] Genotype 1 is the most common worldwide, particularly in the United States and Europe, and is the most resistant to antiviral therapy.[9]

Pathogenesis

HCV is not felt to be directly cytopathic under ordinary circumstances.[10] In immunocompetent individuals, early activation and mobilization of the cellular immune response plays a large, pivotal role in early handling of the virus and, in most cases, progression of the disease once chronic infection has occurred.[11] The CD4+ cells appear to be activated early in the infection, and a vigorous CD4+ response may result in higher rates of viral eradication during acute hepatitis.[11] Although CD8+ cells (cytotoxic T-cell lymphocytes) may also contribute to acute viral clearance, their role is more significant after chronicity is established, at which time they appear to be responsible for hepatocyte injury.[11] However, patients with higher levels of virus-specific cellular immune response may also be more sensitive to the antiviral effects of interferon-based therapies.[12] In contrast to the situation in immune competent individuals, HCV may become directly cytopathic to infected hepatocytes in a small number of immune compromised patients, including those receiving antirejection medications.[13] In these immunosuppressed patients, virus levels are typically extremely high and immunochemical stains show that hepatocytes are stuffed with the virus, which results in a clinical picture of fibrosing cholestatic hepatitis similar to that sometimes seen in recurrent hepatitis B following transplantation.[14]

The majority of acutely infected persons mount an antibody response to HCV within weeks of exposure. However, the presence of antibody does not appear to influence the outcome of infection and, in fact, persists in chronic infection.[15] It has been suggested that the viral heterogeneity allows the virus to escape from the humoral immune response.[16]

Incidence and Prevalence of Hepatitis C Virus Infection

Acute infection is uncommon and, because it is usually asymptomatic, typically goes unrecognized.[17] Table 9–1 lists the characteristics of HCV and the infection resulting from it. The incubation period ranges from 5 to 12 weeks.[18] When symptomatic, the presentation is nonspecific and cannot be clinically distinguished from other forms of hepatitis without serological testing. Because antibody to HCV may be undetectable in a sizable proportion of patients with acute hepatitis,[19] either repeat antibody testing or sensitive molecular tests—such as polymerase chain reaction (PCR) or transcription-mediated amplification (TMA)—should be used to confirm the diagnosis if the anti-HCV result is initially negative. Fulminant hepatitis from hepatitis C is extremely rare and is not even listed in most series of fulminant hepatic failure.[20] All patients with acute hepatitis C require serial monitoring of liver enzymes and virus levels to seek evidence of spontaneous resolution of infection. Spontaneous recovery occurs in 10% to 50% of cases and appears to be age and gender dependent.[21,22] Spontaneous recovery should be assumed only if serum aminotransferase levels and HCV RNA remain normal and undetectable, respectively, for at least 6 months after infection. It is important to recognize that serum ALT may return to the normal range and HCV RNA may transiently become undetectable in some patients whononetheless go on to develop chronic infection.[23]

Chronic hepatitis C is a common liver disease because chronic infection eventuates in 50% to 90% of acutely infected individuals.[21,22] The worldwide prevalence of the infection is estimated to be approximately

Table 9–1. CHARACTERISTICS OF HEPATITIS C VIRUS AND INFECTION

Acute Hepatitis	
Incidence (U.S.)	<30,000/yr
Incubation period	5-12 wk
Diagnosis	Serial anti-HCV determinations HCV RNA by amplification
Spontaneous resolution	10%-50%
Chronic Hepatitis	
Prevalence estimates	U.S.: 3-4 million Global: 170 million
Risk factors	Intravenous drug use: 60% High-risk sexual behavior: 20% Other (occupational, perinatal): 10% Unknown: 10%
Diagnosis	Anti-HCV
Risk of cirrhosis	10%-30% by 20 yr

170 million persons (approximately 3%), but there is considerable geographic variation.[24] For example, up to 7% of the populations of some West African nations are infected.[25] This is thought to result from iatrogenic spread caused by cultural and medical practices because risk factors common in the United States and European populations are absent. In the United States, 4 million (approximately 1.8%) individuals have chronic hepatitis C virus (HCV) infection.[26]

The high prevalence of infection results from two factors. First, the incidence of acute infection before the mid-1980s was extremely high, largely because of transfusion transmission.[27] For example, in the 1960s, the incidence of acute posttransfusion hepatitis among patients undergoing open-heart surgery was 30% because paid blood donors were common, biochemical tests for screening donors were insensitive, and patients received multiple units of blood (average 17 units).[28] It has been estimated that 200,000 to 300,000 cases of acute hepatitis C occurred per year during the 1960s.

This trend continued at least until the early 1970s when a volunteer blood donor system was introduced in the United States and serological testing for the recently identified hepatitis A and B viruses became available. However, transfusion-associated hepatitis, although inconsistently reported, continued to account for approximately 50% of reported cases of acute non-A, non-B hepatitis until blood use declined and more intensive screening of donor risk factors was introduced because of a concern about the risk of HIV transmission.[29] Finally, the identification of HCV allowed introduction of specific antibody screening for the virus in potential blood donors in 1990.[3] Since that time, transfusion-associated hepatitis C has been uncommon. Now that third-generation antibody tests are required in blood donation centers, the risk of transfusion-associated HCV infection is less than 1 per 270,000 (0.00037%) units transfused in the United States.[30] Nucleic acid testing in some blood banks has reduced the risk of hepatitis C to nearly zero. Furthermore, the overall annual incidence of acute hepatitis C has fallen to about 30,000 cases.[31] More than 50% of the acute infections involve easily identifiable risk factors, the most common being intravenous (IV) drug use (>30%).[30,31] Other causes of acquiring infection include other percutaneous or sexual exposures, although these are probably uncommon. The second factor responsible for the high prevalence of HCV infection is the tendency for acute infection to persist. Chronic HCV infection results in 50% to 90% of acutely infected individuals.[21,22] Lower chronicity rates occur in the young, particularly in young women, whereas the average risk of chronicity in older adults is probably 80% to 85%. Thus, most of the many cases of acute hepatitis acquired over the last 4 decades

resulted in chronic hepatitis C. Given the incidence of acute infection since 1960 and the observed chronicity rates, mathematical models estimate the current prevalence of chronic infection to be approximately 3.1 million in the United States, a figure that is remarkably close to the prevalence estimated by the recent NHANES III (National Health and Nutrition Examination Survey) serological survey of the population.[32]

Progression to Cirrhosis

Chronic hepatitis C is usually a slowly progressive disease (Fig. 9–1). Only 20% to 30% of infected patients develop cirrhosis after 10 to 20 years of infection.[33-35] Many patients demonstrate little fibrosis even after decades of infection. Several factors increase the risk of developing hepatic fibrosis or cirrhosis (Table 9–2). The duration of infection is perhaps the most important of these.[36] Most patients who develop cirrhosis have had infection for more than 20 years.[37] In the year 2000, approximately 30% of patients with chronic hepatitis C had a history of infection for at least this long.[38] That proportion will increase in the future as the cohort of chronically infected patients ages. It is estimated that by the year 2010, more than 60% of patients will have had infection for more than 2 decades.[32,38] This has obvious and significant implications for the prevalence

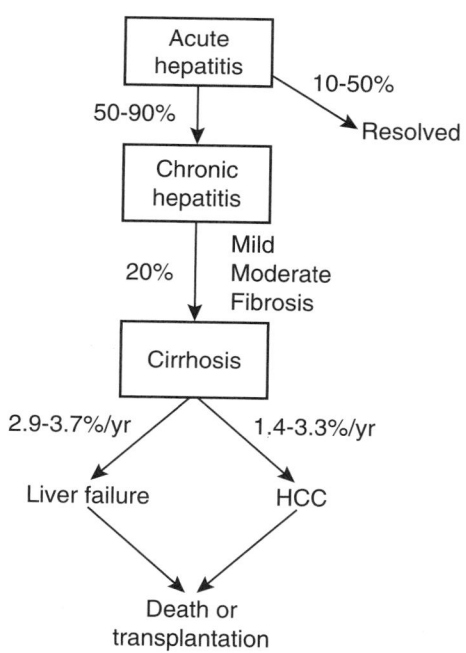

FIGURE 9–1

Natural history of hepatitis C virus (HCV) infection. HCC, hepatocellular carcinoma.

Table 9-2. FACTORS INFLUENCING THE PROGRESSION OF FIBROSIS IN CHRONIC HEPATITIS C
Duration of infection
Degree of hepatic inflammation
Presence of hepatic fibrosis
Alcohol intake
Age greater than 40-50 yr
Male gender
Obesity
Hepatic steatosis
Coinfection with HIV
Coinfection with the hepatitis B virus (HBV)

Table 9-3. ANNUAL RISK OF HEPATIC DECOMPENSATION IN CIRRHOTIC PATIENTS WITH CHRONIC HEPATITIS C	
Clinical decompensation (all causes)	2.9%-3.7%
Ascites	2.7%
Jaundice	1.4%
Gastrointestinal bleeding	1.0%
Hepatocellular carcinoma	1.4%-3.3%
Death (overall)	3.0%
Compensated cirrhosis	1.3%-2.1%
Decompensated cirrhosis	3.0%-10.0%

of cirrhosis in the infected population. Mathematical models estimate that the proportion of infected patients with cirrhosis will increase by more than 50% (from 22% of infected cases to 35%) and that complications of cirrhosis such as liver failure and hepatocellular carcinoma (HCC) will nearly double.[32]

Alcohol is another important factor associated with more rapid progression to fibrosis and cirrhosis. The relative risk of cirrhosis increases at least threefold among regular alcohol consumers.[39,40] This is the single most important factor in disease progression that is entirely preventable. Other factors that may influence progression to a lesser degree are age older than 40 to 50 years, male gender, obesity, coinfection with hepatitis B or HIV, and hepatic steatosis.[41-43] Fibrosis itself may also independently predict further progression.[35] Patients found to have periportal or bridging fibrosis on liver biopsy progress to cirrhosis at a much faster rate than those with no or only portal fibrosis. Virological factors themselves do not appear to contribute to progression of the disease process but do affect response rates to therapy.[44]

Hepatic Decompensation

Most patients who develop cirrhosis will remain well compensated for the remainder of their lives. Decompensation, manifested by development of ascites, encephalopathy, jaundice, variceal bleeding, or significant synthetic dysfunction, occurs in 2.9% to 3.7% of patients per year (Table 9–3).[45,46] Decompensation is of great prognostic importance, even if the decompensation event is transient or easily managed. Only half of patients with chronic hepatitis C and cirrhosis survive 5 years after the initial episode of decompensation (Fig. 9–2).[45] Although the complications of decompensated cirrhosis can usually be adequately managed over the short term, they signal a change in patient prognosis and, thus, usually warrant consideration of liver

transplantation when the first episode of decompensation occurs.

Decompensation most commonly presents as ascites or variceal hemorrhage, both manifestations of portal hypertension.[45] At least one third of deaths in patients with cirrhosis occur as a consequence of these two complications. When ascites first presents, it can usually be managed easily with diuretics and salt restriction. One should not be lulled into complacency with patients who are easily managed medically, however, because the excess mortality is still 10% to 33% after 3 years.[47] Thus, such patients should usually be considered for transplantation at the time that ascites first appears. In addition, careful monitoring for spontaneous bacterial peritonitis (SBP), intravascular volume depletion, metabolic derangements, and renal failure are absolutely necessary because infection or over-diuresis,

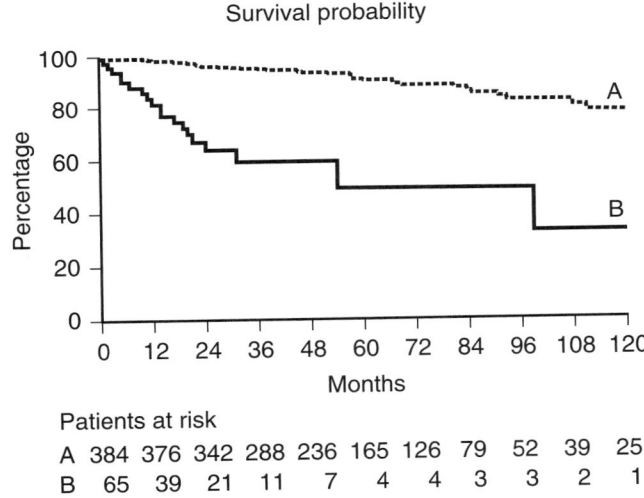

Survival probability

Patients at risk

| A | 384 | 376 | 342 | 288 | 236 | 165 | 126 | 79 | 52 | 39 | 25 |
| B | 65 | 39 | 21 | 11 | 7 | 4 | 4 | 3 | 3 | 2 | 1 |

FIGURE 9–2

Survival in patients with cirrhosis caused by chronic hepatitis C. Compensated cirrhosis is shown as line A and decompensated cirrhosis as line B. (From Fattovich G, Giustina G, Degos F, et al: Effectiveness of interferon alfa on incidence of hepatocellular carcinoma and decompensation in cirrhosis type C. J Hepatol 27:201-205, 1997.)

or both, are associated with further decompensation and risk of death. Interventions such as large-volume paracentesis and transvenous intrahepatic portosystemic shunting (TIPS) are reserved for patients who are either refractory to maximal doses of diuretics or are unable to tolerate diuretics, usually because of renal insufficiency or recurrent electrolyte abnormalities. If ascites is truly refractory to medical management, mean survival is only 12 months in patients who cannot undergo transplantation.[48] Spontaneous bacterial peritonitis is the most common infection in patients, with cirrhosis occurring in approximately 10% of those with ascites.[49] It is an extremely serious complication that has an average mortality rate of approximately 25% per episode.[50] Furthermore, the median survival is only 9 months after an episode of SBP.[51] Short-term mortality is greatly influenced by the severity of the underlying liver disease, concurrent gastrointestinal (GI) bleeding, and, especially, renal failure. Mortality is 100% if SBP is associated with worsening renal failure, 31% with stable renal insufficiency, and 5% in those without renal impairment.[50] The use of prophylactic antibiotics to prevent SBP is controversial.[52] The risk of SBP is extremely low if the ascitic protein is more than 1.0 g/dL, but is approximately 20% in those with lower protein content.[50,52] Nonetheless, in the latter group the only controlled trial of prophylactic antibiotics failed to show a significant benefit in reducing the risk of SBP, and the risk of bacterial resistance is a concern.[53] Conversely, the risk of recurrent SBP is 68% in those who have already had an episode, and prophylactic daily use of a quinolone antibiotic such as norfloxacin reduces the 1-year risk of another episode to approximately 20%.[54]

Bleeding from esophageal or gastric varices is a major complication of portal hypertension. Varices develop in 4% to 8% of patients with cirrhosis per year and enlarge in nearly 50% of cases over a 10-year period.[55,56] The overall incidence of variceal bleeding in patients with cirrhosis caused by chronic hepatitis C is approximately 1% per year, but this risk appears to be higher in patients with large or enlarging varices.[46] Nonselective β-blockers reduce the chance of the first episode of variceal hemorrhage in such patients by approximately half.[57] The first episode of bleeding is higher in those with large varices, advanced hepatic decompensation, ascites, and infection.[58] Mortality from the first variceal bleed is high and is dependent on the severity of liver disease.[58] Furthermore, approximately 45% of cirrhotic patients with GI hemorrhage develop bacterial infections, and this event is associated with very high in-hospital mortality.[59] Sepsis is a major cause of mortality in cirrhotic patients with GI bleeding.[60] Infection also increases the chance of recurrent hemorrhage.[61] Thus, all patients with cirrhosis who are hospitalized for GI bleeding should receive antibiotic prophylaxis.[52] Generally, a 7-day course of an oral quinolone is preferable,

although alternate therapy should be considered in patients who have been on chronic quinolone prophylaxis for SBP. Antibiotics reduce the chance of bacterial infection from 45% to 14% and improve short-term survival.[52]

Before the widespread availability of endoscopic interventions such as variceal sclerosis or banding, the mortality was 50% or more within 6 weeks of a variceal bleed. Currently 60% of patients presenting with variceal hemorrhage survive 1 year.[62] Once the first episode of bleeding has occurred, recurrent hemorrhage occurs in approximately 70% of patients.[63] Therefore, patients who bleed from varices and survive the initial hospitalization should be managed by endoscopic intervention with obliteration of visible varices. TIPS should be considered in patients with concurrent ascites or rebleeding despite aggressive endoscopic therapy. Both options significantly reduce the risk of rebleeding. As a result, the chance of surviving each subsequent year following intervention with medical, endoscopic, or radiologic therapy is 87%.[62,64] Thus, the decision to proceed to transplantation evaluation in patients who have had a variceal hemorrhage should be driven by the degree of hepatic decompensation and not simply by the history of GI bleeding. Finally, it is particularly important to recognize that 26% to 56% of patients with portal hypertension and GI bleeding will have a nonvariceal source,[65] particularly from peptic ulcers and portal hypertensive gastropathy. Thus, early endoscopy is necessary to make a precise diagnosis to guide immediate and long-term therapy.

Symptoms of hepatic encephalopathy may range from minor sleep disturbances or personality change to overt cognitive dysfunction and coma. Encephalopathy is an uncommon initial manifestation of decompensation in patients with chronic hepatitis C,[45,46] but it is typically present to some degree in most patients as their disease progresses. Generally, hepatic encephalopathy occurs in patients with advanced hepatic synthetic dysfunction and other manifestations of decompensation. It is associated with an extremely poor prognosis. Among patients with cirrhosis of any cause, encephalopathy is associated with 68% excess mortality in the first year after onset.[65] As such, it is a symptom that requires consideration for transplantation.

Most symptoms of chronic encephalopathy are controllable, and the standard treatment consists of administration of a poorly absorbable disaccharide, such as lactulose (β-galactosidofructose). Lactulose has several potential mechanisms of action that may contribute to its effectiveness.[66] Metabolism of lactulose to lactate and acetate in the colon reduces colonic pH and thereby reduces intestinal absorption and portal concentrations of nitrogen. This is associated with decreased plasma ammonia levels. Lactulose also acts as a cathartic, which is important in removing nitrogenous substrate from the bowel. Oral neomycin may be helpful in patients who either do not tolerate or fail to respond to lactulose. Its mechanism of action is not known. Generally, it should not be used for long periods because it has a small but real risk of renal and ototoxicity. Careful monitoring is necessary in patients receiving the drug. Acute exacerbations of encephalopathy may be precipitated by infection, GI bleeding, renal insufficiency, alkalosis, hypokalemia, constipation, or portal vein thrombosis. Such episodes are best managed by correcting the precipitating cause, if possible. Short-term protein restriction may be necessary, but long-term protein restriction in patients with cirrhosis may be detrimental and should be avoided.

Hepatocellular Carcinoma

HCC is the fifth most common cancer worldwide. Chronic HCV infection is the most common risk factor for HCC in the United States.[67] HCC in patients with chronic hepatitis C almost always occurs in the setting of cirrhosis and after a duration of infection of 20 to 30 years.[37,67,68] Additional risk factors for HCC in these patients include male gender, alcohol use, immunocompromised state, longer duration of infection, and decompensated liver disease.[68,69] The risk of HCC in patients with HCV-related cirrhosis is 1.4% to 3.3% per year and appears to be increasing.[2,45,46] It is estimated that the number of cases of HCC in the United States will continue to increase for at least another 2 decades.[32]

Imaging studies of the liver and α-fetoprotein (AFP) levels can be useful in detecting early HCC.[70,71] However, AFP alone is a poor predictor of the presence of tumor. It is both insensitive by not being elevated in many patients with HCC and nonspecific in that elevation of the AFP level is common in patients with chronic hepatitis without tumor.[72,73] The most predictive AFP level in patients with chronic hepatitis C and cirrhosis is approximately 50 ng/mL.[72,73] Cost-effectiveness studies have previously argued against surveillance for HCC; however, the current availability of effective interventions such as transarterial chemoembolization, radiofrequency ablation, or liver transplantation justifies screening.[74-76] In the absence of intervention, case fatality for HCC is 97%, second only to pancreatic malignancy.[77] Survival following liver transplantation for patients with HCC and cirrhosis is 64% at 3 years compared with 76% in patients with chronic hepatitis C and cirrhosis without tumor.[78]

Antiviral Treatment

Antiviral treatment of chronic hepatitis C became available in 1990, and the efficacy of the regimens has improved steadily since then.[79] Currently, treatment with pegylated interferon and oral ribavirin results in eradication of HCV in more than half of treated patients.[80,81] Pegylated interferons consist of standard recombinant interferon attached to polyethylene glycol (PEG) chains. Two preparations of pegylated interferon are currently available. They differ by:

- The type of standard interferon (recombinant interferon alfa-2a or -2b)
- Polyethylene glycol (PEG) chain size (40 kd or 12 kd) and configuration (branched or linear)
- Pharmacokinetic properties ($t_{1/2}$ of 80 and 40 hours, respectively)
- Dose (fixed and weight-based, respectively)

Both are administered subcutaneously once per week (as compared to three times per week for unmodified interferon), and both appear to have similar efficacy when combined with oral ribavirin, a synthetic guanosine analogue.[82] The mechanisms by which this combination of drugs inhibits HCV is not clearly understood, but interferons have several antiviral properties including[83]:

- Direct antiviral mechanisms (inhibition of virus attachment and uncoating; induction of intracellular proteins and ribonucleases)
- Indirect antiviral mechanisms that work via amplification of specific (cytotoxic T-lymphocyte [CTL]) and nonspecific (natural killer cell) immune responses

The results of recent clinical trials with the combination of pegylated interferon and ribavirin are encouraging. Manns and colleagues reported a trial in which some patients were given peginterferon alfa-2b (1.5 μg/kg administered once weekly) plus ribavirin (800 mg per day) for 1 year and other patients were given standard interferon plus ribavirin.[80] The overall sustained virologic response rate in the peginterferon plus ribavirin arm was 54%. Sustained virologic response (SVR) was achieved in 42% of patients infected with HCV genotype 1 and 82% of those with genotype 2 or 3.[80] In the second study, Fried and colleagues evaluated a fixed dose of peginterferon alfa-2a (180 μg given once weekly) plus ribavirin (1000-1200 mg/daily) for 1 year compared with standard interferon plus ribavirin.[81] The overall SVR rate in the pegylated interferon plus ribavirin arm was 56%. SVR was attained in 46% of patients infected with genotype 1 and 76% of those with genotype 2 or 3.[81] Although there were significant differences in the drug characteristics, study design, and patient characteristics in these two trials, the outcomes are remarkably similar.

The optimal dosing of these drugs has not yet been defined. In retrospect, the dose of ribavirin used in the Manns study was suboptimal.[80] Hadziyannis and colleagues demonstrated that the optimal dose of ribavirin for genotype 1 patients was 1000-1200 mg per day (for those weighing less than or more than 75 kg [165 lb], respectively), and the optimal duration of treatment was 1 year.[84] By contrast, patients with genotype 2 or 3 responded as well with doses of 800 mg per day and just 6 months of treatment (78% SVR) as they did with higher doses for a longer duration (77% SVR).[84] Thus, it is important to determine viral genotype before treatment to enable the optimal treatment regimen to be administered. Finally, failure to respond to treatment can be confirmed by measurement of HCV RNA after the first 12 weeks of treatment.[85] If the virus level does not drop by at least 2 logs (99%) from baseline, sustained response is unlikely with further therapy and discontinuation of treatment can be considered.

Post hoc analyses of these studies show that certain baseline patient characteristics may affect treatment outcomes.[86] Patients with low HCV RNA levels (<2 million copies/mL) had higher SVR rates than those with higher viral levels (56% to 75% versus 41% to 49%), particularly those infected with viral genotype 1. The presence of bridging fibrosis or cirrhosis reduces the response to antiviral therapy (41% to 44% versus 54% to 55%), but this effect is small compared with that previously observed with interferon monotherapy.[86] Advancing age also appears to reduce response. Sustained responses in those younger than 35 years exceeded 60% but declined to less than 50% after age 45 years. Weight negatively influences response, regardless of whether fixed-dose or weight-based dosing is used, with the greatest inhibition of response being in those weighing more than 98 kg (216 lb). Given the upward trend in the prevalence of obesity in the United States, this is an obvious limitation of this form of therapy.[87] Finally, the SVR rate is lower in blacks than in whites (26% versus 39%).[88]

Successful treatment requires a motivated and compliant patient. Patients must be informed of potential side effects and the need for close monitoring of therapy.[89] Alcohol must be avoided because it impairs treatment response and accelerates disease progression. Depression can limit treatment adherence and, if present, should be treated before interferon is started. Ribavirin is potentially teratogenic and embryotoxic; therefore, patients and sexual partners must practice effective contraception during and for 6 months after treatment. Renal failure is a contraindication because ribavirin is renally excreted.

Most treated patients experience at least temporary side effects. Cytopenia is common in treated patients and requires close monitoring of blood counts during the first 8 weeks of treatment. Neutropenia (absolute neutrophil count [ANC] <750) occurs in 18% to 20% of treated patients, usually during the first 2 weeks of therapy, but is not associated with infections and typically responds to a 25% to 50% reduction in the interferon dose.[80,81] Thus, less than 1% of patients require discontinuation of treatment for profound neutropenia not prevented by dose reduction (ANC <500). Platelet counts decrease little during combination therapy.[80,81] Up to 3% of cases require interferon dose reductions for platelet counts less than 50,000, but it is rare (<1%) that therapy needs to be stopped (i.e., when platelet count reaches <30,000).

Anemia occurs in response to ribavirin accumulation in red cells.[80,81] The mean hemoglobin drop is about 2.5 g/dL, and it is observed during the first 8 weeks of treatment. Hemoglobin levels less than 10 g/dL usually require ribavirin dose reductions; this occurs in 1% to 9% of cases. Discontinuation for anemia is unusual. The benefit of using growth factors such as erythropoietin or granulocyte colony stimulating factor (G-CSF) to maintain full doses of the two drugs (i.e., peginterferon plus ribavirin) remains unproved and controversial. No trials comparing early dose reduction to full dosing using growth factors have been carried out. However, dose reductions during the first 3 months of treatment can significantly impair treatment response in contrast to late dose reductions, so there may be at least theoretical justification for using growth factors.[85]

Almost all patients experience some degree of flu-like symptoms such as fever, myalgias, body aches, and nausea.[89] Treatment is stopped for adverse symptoms twice as often as for laboratory abnormalities. These symptoms may lead to dose reductions as well. The most common reasons are depression, insomnia, irritability, and fatigue. Many of these adverse effects are more tolerable if patients are educated about them, remain well hydrated, and exercise during the treatment course. Depression symptoms are improved by antidepressants, and taking them often avoids the need for dose changes. Every effort should be made to maintain full dosing during the first 3 months of treatment because dose reductions during this early period can significantly reduce the chance of a treatment response. Dose reductions after 12 weeks appear to have less effect on treatment outcome.

Although the immediate goal of antiviral therapy in patients with chronic hepatitis C is to eradicate infection, the long-term goal is prevention of cirrhosis or its complications.[90] Treatment should be considered for all patients with chronic hepatitis C (Table 9–4). However, treatment of patients who have already developed fibrosis has the greatest impact on reducing the complications of cirrhosis and, therefore, the need for liver transplantation in coming years.[32] Thus, finding cirrhosis or bridging fibrosis on liver biopsy should not deter a decision to treat, but rather provide a stronger rationale for it.[90] Although, as discussed earlier, rates of response to treatment are on average approximately 10% less in patients with advanced fibrosis, eradication of virus in these patients slows or stops the progression of fibrosis.[86] Indeed, fibrosis regresses in many patients followed over time after successful treatment.[91-93] Furthermore, studies such as Hepatitis C Antiviral Long-Term Treatment Against Cirrhosis (HALT-C) and COlchicine versus Peg-Intron LOngterm Trial (COPILOT) are under way to assess whether maintenance interferon treatment may

Table 9-4. APPROACHES TO AND ISSUES IN ANTIVIRAL TREATMENT OF CHRONIC HEPATITIS C WITH CIRRHOSIS

Chronic Hepatitis Without Fibrosis

Pegylated interferon plus ribavirin.

Duration determined by genotype.

Lack of EVR identifies nonresponders.

SVR achieved in approximately 55%.

Short-term effect on decompensation rate is low.

Chronic Hepatitis With Bridging Fibrosis or Cirrhosis

Treat like patients without fibrosis (see above).

Increased risk of cytopenia.

SVR achieved in 41%-44%.

SVR more likely to affect natural history.

Chronic Hepatitis With Decompensated Cirrhosis

Preexisting cytopenia or tenuous clinical status may preclude treatment in 30%-50%.

Treatment is difficult and labor intensive.

Cytopenia limits treatment:
    Thrombocytopenia most common (36%-53%).
    40% do not achieve full dose.
    Dose reductions in >20%.
    Growth factors may be required.

Treatment discontinuations in >20%.

HCV RNA becomes negative in 27%-40%.

SVR in approximately 20%.

HCV loss may prevent recurrence after transplant.

EVR, early viral response; SVR, sustained viral response.

prevent progression of fibrosis and complications of cirrhosis in patients who do not clear the virus.[94]

Although treatment is encouraged in those with compensated cirrhosis, it is challenging and potentially dangerous in patients with more advanced disease, particularly those with decompensated cirrhosis (see Table 9-4).[95,96] Treatment in such cases is best overseen by experienced hepatologists. Everson and colleagues used an increasing dose regimen of combination therapy with interferon and ribavirin in patients with both compensated and decompensated cirrhosis caused by HCV who were listed for liver transplantation.[95] It was hoped that this low, accelerated-dose regimen would result in less cytopenia. However, thrombocytopenia occurred in 36% of cases, growth factors were required to maintain blood counts in approximately 30% of patients, and 40% of patients still failed to reach the full dose. Nonetheless, a preliminary report of the results suggests that on-treatment virological responses could be achieved in nearly 40% of patients and SVR in more than 20% of patients.[95] None of the eight patients who became HCV RNA negative on treatment and went on to transplantation experienced viral recurrence after transplantation.

Less favorable outcomes have been reported by Crippen and colleagues, although the study group of patients listed for transplantation had more advanced decompensation than the Everson study group (Child-Turcotte-Pugh [CTP] score 11.9 versus 7.1).[96] Only 15 of 32 patients screened for this study met entry criteria. Thrombocytopenia developed in 53% of patients in the Crippen study, leukopenia in 27% of patients, encephalopathy in 20% of patients, infections in 13% of patients, and death in 7% of patients. Treatment was stopped prematurely in almost all subjects, and the study was terminated early. Nonetheless, HCV RNA became undetectable in 4 of 15 (27%) of patients, and 55% had a decrease in viral levels during therapy. Only two patients in the study underwent liver transplantation (neither was HCV RNA negative) and both developed viral recurrence. Clearly, patients with advanced decompensation such as in the Crippen study tolerate interferon-based therapy extremely poorly and would probably benefit more from consideration of treatment when HCV disease recurs after transplantation. Decompensated patients who are more stable, such as those in the Everson study, can be considered for treatment. There are currently no data on the tolerability and efficacy of pegylated interferons in patients with decompensated cirrhosis. The addition of pegylated interferons and the potential advantage of growth factors on maintaining adequate antiviral dosing regimens may improve responses in this difficult-to-treat population and needs to be studied prospectively.

In summary, sustained clearance of HCV is now possible in more than 50% of patients with chronic hepatitis C.[80,81] This is a remarkable achievement for a pharmacological treatment of a chronic viral infection. Virological response is associated with a reduction of hepatic inflammation on liver biopsy, often to normal.[91-93] Because progression to fibrosis and cirrhosis is at least partly dependent on the severity of periportal inflammation, one would expect that virological response would slow the rate of fibrosis. Indeed, treatment response causes a striking reduction in the rate of hepatic fibrosis and regression of septal fibrosis in more than 50% of cases.[97] It is reasonable to assume that these short-term benefits would translate into a reduction in morbidity and mortality. Several studies also suggest that the risk of HCC is reduced by treatment of the infection, although this remains controversial.[98] The likely impact of combination treatment on disease mortality and the future need for liver transplantation has been demonstrated by mathematical modeling and cost-benefit analyses.[32]

Liver Transplantation

Chronic hepatitis C is a slowly progressive disease that often results in cirrhosis and its complications. Hepatitis C

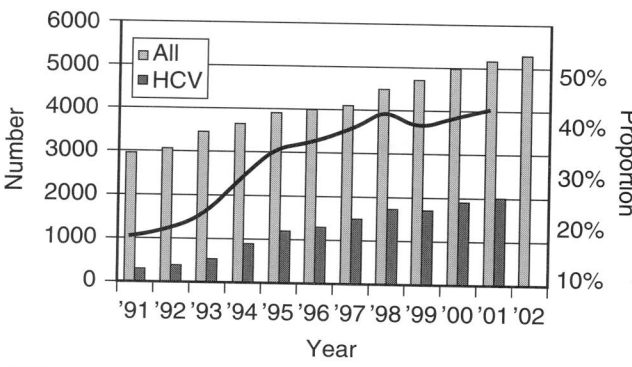

FIGURE 9–3

Number of liver transplants performed yearly in the United States since 1991. Total number of transplants shown as shaded bar. The number performed because of HCV-related cirrhosis, with or without hepatocellular carcinoma (HCC), is shown as a solid bar. The proportion performed because of HCV-related cirrhosis, with or without HCC, is shown as a solid line.

is the leading indication for liver transplantation in the United States today.[1] Patients with chronic hepatitis C have made up an ever-increasing proportion of cases on the transplant waiting list since 1991 (Fig. 9–3).[1] Mathematical models predict that this trend will continue for at least the next 20 years (Table 9–5).[32,99] It is estimated that the number of cases of decompensated cirrhosis, HCC, and liver-related death will increase by more than 60% over that period.[32] More than 17,000 individuals were on the waiting list for a liver transplant in the United States in 2003, and slightly more than 5000 liver transplants took place that year. At least 40% of these transplants were related to chronic hepatitis C (decompensated cirrhosis or HCC).[1] Current donor supply meets less than one third of the demand. This gap will inevitably continue to widen if new treatment modalities for hepatitis C are not found and if novel transplant options are not found.[32]

Table 9–5. PROJECTED IMPACT OF CHRONIC HEPATITIS C ON LIVER TRANSPLANTATION NEED

	Year 2000	Year 2020
HCV prevalence (U.S.)	2,904,678	2,681,556
Cirrhosis, total	472,103	858,788
Decompensated cirrhosis	65,294	134,743
Hepatocellular carcinoma	7,271	13,183
Liver-related deaths	13,000	36,483
Transplant listings	10,893	—
Transplants performed	4,893	—
Transplants performed for HCV	1,900 (~40%)	—

Assessment of Disease Severity and Need for Transplantation

Survival is excellent in patients with well-compensated cirrhosis caused by chronic hepatitis C.[45] The decision about when to refer a patient for liver transplant evaluation can, therefore, be confusing. The time of onset of hepatic decompensation signals a striking change in short-term prognosis.[45] Five-year survival after onset of decompensation is only 50%.[45] Decompensation may present as either significant hepatic synthetic dysfunction (coagulopathy, hypoalbuminemia, or jaundice) or complications of portal hypertension such as ascites, hepatic encephalopathy, or variceal hemorrhage. As described earlier, all of these demand consideration of transplantation.

Several scoring systems have been developed to estimate short-term survival, and these have proved helpful in assessing the need for transplantation and priority for receipt of a donor organ. The CTP classification is a measurement of severity of liver disease that was originally developed to estimate survival after portosystemic shunting.[100,101] It was the scoring system originally used as the basis for donor organ allocation.[102] The five factors used in this calculation are:

1. Presence of ascites
2. Degree of encephalopathy
3. Bilirubin levels
4. Albumin levels
5. Prothrombin time

A CTP score of at least 7 is generally required for listing for liver transplantation, although there are exceptions, such as for patients with HCC.

The Model for Endstage Liver Disease (MELD) score is also useful.[103] This is a mathematical score derived from the serum bilirubin, prothrombin time, and creatinine:

$$\text{MELD score} = (0.957 \times \log_e [\text{creatinine mg/dL}] + 3.78 \\ \times \log_e [\text{bilirubin mg/dL}] + 11.20 \\ \times \log_e [\text{INR}] + 6.43) \times 10$$

where INR is the international normalized ratio.

The MELD score is more predictive of short-term survival than the CTP score. The area under the receiver operating characteristic (ROC) curve for the MELD score is 0.83 (95% confidence interval: 0.81-0.84) versus 0.76 (95% confidence interval: 0.74-0.79) for the CTP score, and increasing scores predict a higher 3-month mortality in a stepwise manner.[103] The MELD score is the measure currently used to determine priority on the liver transplant waiting list with deceased-donor organs being offered to those patients with the highest score in their blood group.

Patients presenting with HCC often have good liver function as determined by both the CTP and MELD scores. Thus, an organ allocation system based wholly on synthetic function would significantly reduce the chance that these patients would receive a transplant.[104,105] The solution would be to offer a MELD score to these patients that would equate their chance of surviving an additional 3 months with dying or becoming inoperable. Currently transplantation is not offered when a single tumor is larger than 5 cm or when more than three lesions are present. Unfortunately, there are no studies that estimate the likelihood of a patient dying or exceeding this definition of inoperability over 3 months, although there are mathematical models based on mean tumor doubling times in order to provide such an estimate.[105] Initially, the MELD system gave high organ priority to patients with T2 lesions and a lower priority to those with T1 lesions. As data have become available on waiting list mortality, the MELD advantage offered to patients has been decreased, and further refinements are likely to occur in coming years.[106,107] Finally, the effect of pretransplant interventions (e.g., transarterial chemoembolization and radiofrequency ablation of tumor growth rate) and survival before transplant need to be considered, especially for smaller tumors.[107]

Summary

Chronic hepatitis C is a common and usually slowly progressive liver disease. Most patients with this infection will live long and healthy lives without clinical evidence of significant liver disease. However, left untreated, cirrhosis eventuates in 20% to 30% of cases after decades of chronic infection. Most patients who develop significant fibrosis or cirrhosis continue to do well for many years. However, complications of cirrhosis such as decompensation (ascites, encephalopathy, variceal hemorrhage, or hepatic synthetic dysfunction) or HCC appear in 2% to 5% of patients with cirrhosis per year and significantly affect survival. Liver transplantation is often the only option for these patients.

Antiviral therapy consisting of long-acting pegylated interferon and ribavirin is highly effective against HCV and is capable of permanently eradicating infection in approximately 50% of cases. Successful treatment appears to halt the progression of liver disease and often results in regression of established fibrosis. Thus, successful treatment probably prevents the complications of liver disease that would ultimately require consideration of transplantation, although this remains unproved in prospective studies.

Pearls and Pitfalls

- The incidence of chronic hepatitis C is 4 million in the United States and 170 million worldwide. It is the most common form of chronic liver disease in the United States and Europe.
- Cirrhosis develops in more than 20% of patients with chronic hepatitis C, but it may take decades to evolve.
- Manifestations of decompensated cirrhosis (ascites, encephalopathy, variceal hemorrhage, or synthetic dysfunction) occur in 2.9% to 3.7% of cirrhotic patients per year. The onset of any of these manifestations of hepatic decompensation is associated with a marked reduction in 5-year survival and warrants consideration of liver transplantation.
- Chronic hepatitis C is the most common cause of HCC in the United States and Europe. Liver transplantation is usually curative in such cases.
- The number of cases of chronic hepatitis C with decompensated cirrhosis or HCC is projected to increase up to twofold over the next 20 years.
- Patients with fibrosis or cirrhosis on liver biopsy should be educated about potential complications of cirrhosis and followed expectantly. Complications should be managed aggressively as follows, but should also prompt referral for transplant evaluation.
  - Endoscopy should be performed in patients with cirrhosis, and those with large varices should be prophylactically treated with β-blockade.
  - Acute variceal hemorrhage requires resuscitation and control of hemorrhage, but long-term management should include repeated band ligation, β-blockade, and/or transvenous intrahepatic portosystemic shunting (TIPS).
  - Ascites should be managed with diuretics, salt restriction, and careful monitoring of renal function and electrolytes. Prophylactic antibiotics should be reserved for patients who have already had an episode of spontaneous bacterial peritonitis. Ascites that is refractory to diuretic management (does not respond or is complicated by electrolyte abnormalities or renal insufficiency) can be managed by large-volume paracentesis or TIPS.

Pearls and Pitfalls—cont'd

- Encephalopathy should be managed by lactulose. Protein restriction should be avoided except for management of acute episodes of encephalopathy.

- Surveillance for HCC should include imaging of the liver and α-fetoprotein levels at least annually.

- Antiviral treatment with pegylated interferon and ribavirin can permanently eradicate virus in approximately half of treated cases and should be considered in all cases of chronic hepatitis C. Sustained viral response to therapy stops the progression of liver disease and can result in regression of established fibrosis or cirrhosis. Viral response may also reduce the risk of HCC.

- Whenever possible, treatment should be considered before patients develop advanced liver disease. Once decompensation develops, antiviral treatment is difficult, labor intensive, and less well tolerated. Low doses that are gradually increased may be better tolerated, and growth factors, such as erythropoietin, may reduce cytopenia that could otherwise limit treatment. These patients should be monitored by an experienced hepatologist.

References

1. Organ Procurement and Transplantation Network (OPTN) database online: Available at http://www.optn.org/
2. El Serag H: Hepatocellular carcinoma and hepatitis C in the United States. Hepatology 36(Suppl 1):S74-S83, 2002.
3. Choo QL, Kuo G, Weiner AJ, et al: Isolation of a CDNA clone derived from a blood-borne non-A, non-B viral hepatitis genome. Science 244:359, 1989.
4. Bradley DW, Maynard JE, Popper H, et al: Post transfusion NANBH: Physicochemical properties of two distinct agents. J Infect Dis 148:254-265, 1983.
5. Miller RH, Purcell RH: Hepatitis C virus shares amino acid sequence similarity with pestiviruses and flaviviruses as well as members of two plant virus supergroups. Proc Natl Acad Sci U S A 87:2057-2061, 1990.
6. Ogata N, Alter HJ, Miller RH, et al: Nucleotide sequence and mutation rate of the H strain of hepatitis C virus. Proc Natl Acad Sci U S A 88:3391-3396, 1991.
7. Neumann AU, Lam NP, Dahari H, et al: Hepatitis C viral dynamics in vivo and the antiviral efficacy of interferon alfa therapy. Science 282:103-107, 1998.
8. Simmonds P, Alberti A, Alter HJ, et al: A proposed system for the nomenclature of hepatitis C viral genotypes (Letter). Hepatology 19:1321-1324, 1994.
9. Lau JYN, Davis GL, Prescott LE, et al: Distribution of hepatitis C virus genotypes determined by line probe assay in patients with chronic hepatitis C seen in tertiary referral centers in the United States. Ann Intern Med 124:868-876, 1996.
10. Lau GGK, Davis GL, Wu PC, et al: Hepatic expression of hepatitis C virus RNA in chronic hepatitis C: Study by in-situ reverse-transcription polymerase chain reaction. Hepatology 23:1318, 1996.
11. Nelson DR: The immunopathogenesis of hepatitis C virus infection. Clin Liver Dis 5:931-953, 2001.
12. Nelson DR, Marousis CG, Ohno, et al: Intrahepatic hepatitis C virus–specific cytotoxic T lymphocyte activity and response to interferon alfa therapy in chronic hepatitis C. Hepatology 28:225-230, 1998.
13. Lim HL, Lau GKK, Davis GL, et al: Cholestatic hepatitis leading to hepatic failure in a patient with organ-transmitted hepatitis C virus infection. Gastroenterology 106:248, 1994.
14. Cooksley WG, McIvor CA: Fibrosing cholestatic hepatitis and HBV after bone marrow transplantation. Biomed Pharmacother 49:117-124, 1995.
15. Baumert TF, Wellnitz S, Aono S, et al: Antibodies against hepatitis C virus–like particles and viral clearance in acute and chronic hepatitis C. Hepatology 32:610-617, 2000.
16. Farci P, Alter HJ, Wong DC, et al: Prevention of hepatitis C virus infection in chimpanzees after antibody-mediated in vitro neutralization. Proc Natl Acad Sci U S A 91:7792-7796, 1994.
17. Alter MJ, Margolis HS, Krawczynski K, et al: The natural history of community-acquired hepatitis C in the United States. N Engl J Med 327:1899-1905, 1992.
18. Dienstag JL: Non-A, non-B hepatitis. I. Recognition, epidemiology, and clinical features. Gastroenterology 85:439-462, 1983.
19. Vrielink H, Reesink HW, van den Burg PJ, et al: Performance of three generations of anti-hepatitis C virus enzyme linked immunosorbent assays in donors and patients. Transfusion 37:845-849, 1997.
20. Mutimer D, Shaw J, Neuberger J, et al: Failure to incriminate hepatitis B, hepatitis C, and hepatitis E viruses in the aetiology of fulminant non-A, non-B hepatitis. Gut 36:433-436, 1995.
21. Bradley DW, Maynard JE: Etiology and natural history of posttransfusion non A, non B hepatitis. Semin Liver Dis 6:56-66, 1986.
22. Kenny-Walsh E, for the Irish Hepatology Research Group: Clinical outcomes after hepatitis infection from contaminated anti-globulin. N Engl J Med 340:1228-1233, 1999.
23. Alter MJ: The detection, transmission, and outcome of hepatitis C virus infection. Infect Agents Dis 2:155-166, 1993.
24. World Health Organization (WHO) Global Surveillance and Control of Hepatitis C: Report of a WHO consultation organized in collaboration with the Viral Hepatitis Prevention Board, Antwerp, Belgium. J Viral Hepat 6:35-47, 1999.
25. Wasley A, Alter MJ: Epidemiology of hepatitis C: Geographic differences and temporal trends. Semin Liver Dis 20:1-16, 2000.
26. National Center for Health Statistics: Third National Health and Nutrition Examination Survey (NHANES III) (CD-ROM Catalog No. PB97-502959). Hyattsville, Md, Public Health Service. 1996.
27. Alter HJ, Purcell RH, Shih JW, et al: Detection of antibody to hepatitis C virus in prospectively followed transfusion recipients with acute and chronic non-A, non-B hepatitis. N Engl J Med 321:1494-1500, 1989.
28. Alter HJ, Houghton M: Hepatitis C virus and eliminating posttransfusion hepatitis. Nat Med 6:1082-1086, 2000.
29. Donahue JG, Munoz A, Ness PM, et al: The declining risk of post-transfusion hepatitis C virus infection. N Engl J Med 327:369-373, 1992.
30. Schreiber GB, Busch MP, Kleinman SH, et al: The risk of transfusion-transmitted viral infections. N Engl J Med 334:1685-1690, 1996.
31. Alter MJ: Hepatitis C virus infection in the United States. J Hepatol 31(Suppl 1):88-91, 1999.
32. Davis GL, Albright JE, Cook SF, Rosenberg DM: Projecting the future healthcare burden from hepatitis C in the United States. Liver Transpl 9:331-338, 2003.

33. Di Bisceglie AM, Goodman ZD, Ishak KG, et al: Long-term clinical and histopathological follow-up of chronic post-transfusion hepatitis. Hepatology 14:969-974, 1991.

34. Hopf U, Moller B, Kuther D, et al: Long-term follow-up of post-transfusion and sporadic chronic hepatitis non-A, non-B and frequency of circulating antibodies to hepatitis C virus (HCV). J Hepatol 10:69-76, 1990.

35. Yano M, Kumada H, Kage M, et al: The long-term pathological evolution of chronic hepatitis C. Hepatology 23:1334-1340, 1996.

36. Poynard R, Ratziu V, Charlotte R, Goodman Z, et al: Rates and risk factors of liver fibrosis progression in patients with chronic hepatitis C. J Hepatol 34:730-739, 2001.

37. Tong MJ, EL-Farra NS, Reikes AR, Co RI: Clinical outcomes after transfusion-associated hepatitis C. N Engl J Med 332:1463-1466, 1995.

38. Armstrong GL, Alter MJ, McQuillan GM, Margolis HS: The past incidence of hepatitis C virus infection: Implications for the future burden of chronic liver disease in the United States. Hepatology 2000; 31:777-782.

39. Wiley TE, McCarthy M, Breidi L, et al: Impact of alcohol on the histological and clinical progression of hepatitis C infection. Hepatology 28:805-809, 1998.

40. Corrao G, Arico S: Independent and combined action of hepatitis C virus infection and alcohol consumption on the risk of symptomatic liver cirrhosis. Hepatology 27:914-919, 1998.

41. Poynard T, Bedossa P, Opolon P: Natural history of liver fibrosis progression in patients with chronic hepatitis C. Lancet 349: 825-832, 1997.

42. Benhamou Y, Bochet M, Di Martino V, et al: Liver fibrosis progression in human immunodeficiency virus and hepatitis C virus coinfected patients. The Multivirc Group. Hepatology 30: 1054-1058, 1999.

43. Castera L, Pawlotsky JM, Dhumeaux D: Worsening of steatosis and fibrosis progression in hepatitis C. Gut 52:1531, 2003.

44. Vargas HE, Wang LF, Laskus T, et al: Distribution of infecting hepatitis C virus genotypes in end-stage liver disease patients at a large American transplantation center. J Infect Dis 175:448-450, 1997.

45. Fattovich G, Giustina G, Degos F, et al: Effectiveness of interferon alfa on incidence of hepatocellular carcinoma and decompensation in cirrhosis type C. J Hepatol 27:201-205, 1997.

46. Sangiovanni A, Fasani P, Ronchi G, et al: The long-term course of hepatitis C related cirrhosis (abstract). J Hepatol 36(Suppl 1): S177-S178, 2002.

47. Salerno F, Borroni G, Moser P, et al: Survival and prognostic factors of cirrhotic patients with ascites. Am J Gastroenterol 88: 514-519, 1993.

48. Sanyal AJ, Genning C, Reddy KR, et al: The North American study for the treatment of refractory ascites. Gastroenterology 124:634-641, 2003.

49. Llach J, Rimola A, Navasa M, et al: Incidence and predictive factors of first episode of spontaneous bacterial peritonitis in cirrhosis with ascites: Relevance of ascitic fluid protein concentration. Hepatology 16:724-727, 1992.

50. Follo A, Llovet JM, Navasa M, et al: Renal impairment following spontaneous bacterial peritonitis in cirrhosis: Incidence, clinical course, predictive factors and prognosis. Hepatology 20:1495-1501, 1994.

51. Tito L, Rimola A, Gines P, et al: Recurrence of spontaneous bacterial peritonitis in cirrhosis: Frequency and predictive factors. Hepatology 8:27-31, 1988.

52. Garcia-Tsao G: Bacterial infections and antibiotics in cirrhosis. In Arroyo V, Forns X, Garcia-Pagan JC, Rodes J (eds): Progress in the Treatment of Liver Diseases. Barcelona, Spain, Arts Medica, 2003, pp 43-50.

53. Grange JD, Roulot D, Pelletier F, et al: Norfloxacin primary prophylaxis of bacterial infections in cirrhotic patients with ascites—a double blind randomized trial. J Hepatol 29:430-436, 1998.

54. Gines P, Rimola A, Planas R, et al: Norfloxacin prevents bacterial peritonitis recurrence in cirrhosis: Results of a double blind, placebo-controlled trial. Hepatology 12:716-724, 1990.

55. Cales P, Desmorat H, Vinel JP: Incidence of large oesophageal varices in patients with cirrhosis; application to prophylaxis of first bleeding. Gut 31:1298-1302, 1990.

56. Pagliaro L, D'Amico G, Pasta L, et al: Portal hypertension in cirrhosis: Natural history. In Bosch J, Groszmann R (eds): Portal Hypertension: Pathophysiology and Treatment. Cambridge, MA, Blackwell Scientific, 1994, pp 72-92.

57. Poynard T, Cales P, Pasta L, et al: Beta-adrenergic antagonist drugs in the prevention of gastrointestinal bleeding in patients with cirrhosis and oesophageal varices. N Engl J Med 324:1532-1538, 1991.

58. Grace ND, Groszman RJ, Garcia-Tsao G, et al: Portal hypertension and variceal bleeding: An AASLD single topic symposium. Hepatology 28:868-880, 1998.

59. Deschenes M, Villeneuve JP: Risk factors for the development of bacterial infections in hospitalized patients with cirrhosis. Am J Gastroenterol 94:2193-2197, 1999.

60. Bleicher G, Boulanger R, Squara P, et al: Frequency of infections in cirrhotic patients presenting with acute gastrointestinal hemorrhage. Br J Surg 73:724-726, 1986.

61. Bernard B, Cadranel JF, Valla D, et al: Prognostic significance of bacterial infection in bleeding cirrhotic patients: A prospective study. Gastroenterology 108:1828-1834, 1995.

62. Veterans Affairs Cooperative Variceal Sclerotherapy Group: Sclerotherapy for male alcoholic cirrhotic patients who have bled from esophageal varices: Results of a randomized, multicenter clinical trial. Hepatology 20:618-625, 1994.

63. D'Amico G, Pagliaro L, Bosch J: The treatment of portal hypertension: A meta-analytic review. Hepatology 22:332-354, 1995.

64. Christensen E, Krintel JJ, Hansen S, et al: Prognosis after the first episode of gastrointestinal bleeding or coma in cirrhosis: Survival and prognostic factors. Scand J Gastroenterol 24:999-1006, 1989.

65. Mitchell K, Theodossi A, Williams R: Endoscopy in patients with portal hypertension and upper gastrointestinal bleeding. In Westaby D, MacDougall BR, Williams R (eds): Variceal Bleeding. London, Pitman, 1982, pp 62-67.

66. Weber FL Jr: Effects of lactulose on nitrogen metabolism. Scand J Gastroenterol 222(Suppl):83-87, 1997.

67. Liang TJ, Jeffers LJ, Reddy KR, et al: Viral pathogenesis of hepatocellular carcinoma in the United States. Hepatology 18: 1326-1333, 1993.

68. Degos F, Christidis C, Ganne-Carrie N, et al: Hepatitis C virus related cirrhosis: Time to occurrence of hepatocellular carcinoma and death. Gut 47:131-136, 2000.

69. Dutta U, Byth K, Kench J, et al: Risk factors for development of hepatocellular carcinoma among Australians with hepatitis C: A case-control study. Aust N Z J Med 29:300-307, 1999.

70. Arguedas MR, Chen VK, Eloubeidi MA, Fallon MB: Screening for hepatocellular carcinoma in patients with hepatitis C cirrhosis: A cost-utility analysis. Am J Gastroenterol 98:679-690, 2003.

71. Gebo KA, Chander G, Jenckes MW, et al: Screening tests for hepatocellular carcinoma in patients with chronic hepatitis C: A systematic review. Hepatology 36(Suppl):S84-S92, 2002.

72. Trevisani F, D'Intino PE, Morselli-Labate AM, et al: Serum alpha-fetoprotein for diagnosis of hepatocellular carcinoma in patients with chronic liver disease: Influence of HBsAg and anti-HCV status. J Hepatol 34:570-575, 2001.

73. Gupta S, Bent S, Kohlwes J: Test characteristics of alpha-fetoprotein for detecting hepatocellular carcinoma in patients with hepatitis C. A systematic review and critical analysis. Ann Intern Med 139:46-50, 2003.

74. Qian J, Feng GS, Vogl T: Combined interventional therapies of hepatocellular carcinoma. World J Gastroenterol 9:1885-1891, 2003.

75. Donckier V, Van Laethem JL, Van Gansbeke D, et al: New considerations for an overall approach to treat hepatocellular carcinoma in cirrhotic patients. J Surg Oncol 84:36-44, 2003.

76. Saab S, Ly D, Nieto J, et al: Hepatocellular carcinoma screening in patients waiting for liver transplantation: A decision analytic model. Liver Transpl 9:672-681, 2003.

77. Ferlay J, Bray F, Pisani P, et al: GLOBOCAN 2000. Cancer incidence, mortality and prevalence worldwide. Version 1.0. International Agency for Research on Cancer (IARC) Cancer Base No. 5. Lyon, IARC, 2001.

78. United Network of Organ Sharing (UNOS): 2003 Annual Report of the U.S. Organ Procurement and Transplantation Network and the Scientific Registry of Transplant Recipients: Table 9.9a: Unadjusted graft survival, deceased donor liver transplant survival at 3 months, 1 year, 3 years, and 5 years. 2003 (online) Rockville, MD. Available at: http://www.optn.org/AR2003/909a_rec_dgn_li.htm.

79. McHutchison JG, Fried MW: Current therapy for hepatitis C: Pegylated interferon and ribavirin. Clin Liver Dis 7:149-161, 2003.

80. Manns MP, McHutchison JG, Gordon S, et al: Peginterferon alfa-2b plus ribavirin compared to interferon alfa-2b plus ribavirin for the treatment of chronic hepatitis C: A randomized trial. Lancet 358:958-965, 2001.

81. Fried MW, Shiffman ML, Reddy R, et al: Peginterferon alfa-2a plus ribavirin for chronic hepatitis C virus infection. N Engl J Med 347:975-982, 2002.

82. Baker DE: Pegylated interferons. Rev Gastroenterol Disord 1:87-99, 2001.

83. Peters M, Davis GL, Dooley JS, et al: The interferon system in acute and chronic viral hepatitis. In Popper H, Schaffner F (eds): Progress in Liver Diseases, vol. 8. New York, Grune and Stratton, 1986, pp 453-467.

84. Hadziyannis SJ, Cheinquer H, Morgan T, et al: Peg-interferon alfa-2a (40KD) (Pegasys) in combination with ribavirin: Efficacy and safety results from a phase III, randomized, double-blind, multicentre study examining the effect of duration of treatment and ribavirin dose (abstract). J Hepatol 37:536A, 2002.

85. Davis GL, Wong JB, McHutchison JG, et al: Early virologic response to treatment with pegylated interferon alfa-2b plus ribavirin in patients with chronic hepatitis C. Hepatology 38:645-652, 2003.

86. Davis GL: Treatment of hepatitis C: State of the art. In Phair JP, King E, Goldhagen H (eds): Hepatitis Annual Update 2003. Milford, MA, iMedOptions, 2003, pp 41-56,

87. McCullough AJ: Obesity and its nurturing effect on hepatitis C. Hepatology 38:557-559, 2003.

88. Jeffers LJ, Cassidy W, Howell C, et al: Peginterferon alfa-2A (40KD) (PEGASYS®) in combination with ribavirin in African American and Caucasian patients with chronic hepatitis C virus genotype 1: Results of a multicenter study (abstract). Hepatology 38(Suppl 1):54A, 2003.

89. Russo MW, Fried MW: Side effects of therapy for chronic hepatitis C. Gastroenterology 124:1711-1719, 2003.

90. Davis GL: Interferon treatment of cirrhotic patients with chronic hepatitis C: A logical intervention (editorial). Am J Gastroenterol 89:658-660, 1994.

91. Shiratori Y, Imazeki F, Moriyama M, et al: Histologic improvement of fibrosis in patients with hepatitis C who have sustained response to interferon therapy. Ann Intern Med 132:517-524, 2000.

92. Marcellin P, Boyer N, Gervais A, et al: Long-term histologic improvement and loss of detectable intrahepatic HCV RNA in patients with chronic hepatitis C and sustained response to interferon-alpha therapy. Ann Intern Med 127:875-881, 1997.

93. Shindo M, Di Bisceglie AM, Hoofnagle JH: Long-term follow-up of patients with chronic hepatitis C treated with alpha-interferon. Hepatology 15:1013-1016, 1992.

94. Anonymous: This month from the NIH: HALT-C study. Hepatology 36:792-793, 2002.

95. Everson GT, Troillet T, Trotter T, et al: Treatment of decompensated cirrhotics with a low-accelerating dose regimen of interferon alfa-2b plus ribavirin: Safety and efficacy (abstract). Hepatology 32:308A, 2000.

96. Crippin JS, Sheiner P, Terrault N, et al: A pilot study of the tolerability and efficacy of antiviral therapy in patients awaiting liver transplantation for hepatitis C (abstract). Hepatology 32:308A, 2000.

97. Poynard T, McHutchison J, Davis GL, et al: Impact of interferon alfa-2b and ribavirin on progression of liver fibrosis in patients with chronic hepatitis C. Hepatology 32:1131-1137, 2000.

98. Everson GT: Maintenance interferon for chronic hepatitis C: More issues than answers? Hepatology 32:436-438, 2000.

99. Rakela J, Vargas HE: Hepatitis C: Magnitude of the problem. Liver Transpl 8(Suppl 1):S3-S6, 2002.

100. Child CG II, Turcotte JG: Surgery and portal hypertension. In Child CG III (ed): The Liver and Portal Hypertension. Philadelphia, Saunders, 1964, pp 50-58.

101. Angermayr B, Cejna M, Karnel F, et al: Child-Pugh versus MELD score in predicting survival in patients undergoing transjugular intrahepatic portosystemic shunt. Gut 52:879-885, 2003.

102. Freeman RB, Rohrer RJ, Katz E, et al: Preliminary results of a liver allocation plan using a continuous medical severity score that de-emphasizes waiting time. Liver Transpl 7:173-178, 2001.

103. Wiesner R, Edwards E, Freeman R, et al: Model for end-stage liver disease (MELD) and allocation of donor livers. Gastroenterology 124:91-96, 2003.

104. Roberts JP: Prioritization of patients with liver cancer within the MELD system. Liver Transpl 8:329-330, 2002.

105. Cheng SJ, Freeman RB Jr, Wong JB: Predicting the probability of progression-free survival in patients with small hepatocellular carcinoma. Liver Transpl 8:323-328, 2002.

106. United Network for Organ Sharing online. Policy 3.6.4.4, Allocation of livers. Liver transplant candidates with hepatocellular carcinoma (HCC): Available at http://www.unos.org/PoliciesandBylaws/policies/docs/policy_8.doc. Accessed: September 15, 2004.

107. Yao FY, Bass NM, Nikolai B, et al: A follow-up analysis of the pattern and predictors of dropout from the waiting list for liver transplantation in patients with hepatocellular carcinoma: Implications for the current organ allocation policy. Liver Transpl 9:684-692, 2003.

Hepatitis C and Liver Transplantation

MARINA BERENGUER
JOHN LAKE

Pretransplant hepatitis C virus infection   144
   Natural history of hepatitis C virus
     infection   144
   Indications for liver transplantation   144

Posttransplant hepatitis C virus infection   145
   Source of infection   145
   Definition of viral recurrence as opposed to
     histological recurrence   145
   Natural history of hepatitis C virus infection
     after liver transplantation   146
   Factors influencing disease severity and
     progression or survival   147

Patient management   152
   Pretransplantation antiviral therapy   152
   Preemptive therapy in the early
     posttransplant period   153
   Treatment of hepatitis C virus–related
     graft disease   153

Retransplantation   155

Conclusion   155

Cirrhosis secondary to chronic hepatitis C virus (HCV) infection is the most common disease indication for liver transplantation among adults in most European and North American centers. In 2002, HCV infection was present in 44% of all adults who underwent liver transplantation in the United States.[1] Recurrence of HCV infection in the allograft is universal in these patients and leads to the development of chronic histological liver damage in the majority of recipients. However, the natural history of hepatitis C recurrence is variable. Whereas some patients have an accelerated course leading to early allograft failure, in others significant fibrosis may take years to develop. Overall, however, the natural history of hepatitis C is significantly more aggressive in liver transplant recipients than in patients whose immunity is intact, with progression to cirrhosis reported in 8% to 44% after the fifth postoperative year. The enhanced disease progression is probably multifactorial in etiology and depends on the interaction between several host, donor, viral, and external factors. Short-term graft survival is not affected by hepatitis C recurrence. However, by 5 years, survival is decreased in comparison to other nonviral disease indications. In addition, based on one preliminary report, concern has been raised that the outcome after living related liver transplantation for HCV-related cirrhosis may be worse than when deceased donors are used. This observation, however, requires additional study.

The current therapeutic options available to either prevent or treat reinfection or recurrent disease (or both) are relatively ineffective. Given this lack of effective antiviral therapy and the progressive nature of recurrent hepatitis C in a significant subset, it is expected that the number of recipients in need of retransplantation because of HCV-related graft cirrhosis will continue to rise in the coming years. This prospect is problematic inasmuch as the results of retransplantation are inferior to those of primary transplantation. For this reason, concern is beginning to be raised regarding whether retransplantation should be an option for all recipients in whom recurrent HCV-related allograft failure develops.

Pretransplant Hepatitis C Virus Infection

Natural History of Hepatitis C Virus Infection

HCV infection is a prevalent infection in most developed countries; it affects 1.5% to 2% of the general population, with at least 2.7 million carriers in the United States and an estimated 170 million carriers worldwide. The natural history of this infection has been extensively evaluated.[2] One of the most striking features is the high risk of persistence after viral acquisition and progression to chronic hepatitis, a condition that develops in 65% to 85% of those exposed to the virus. Eventually, cirrhosis develops in 15% to 25% of chronically infected patients. The time frame between infection and the development of cirrhosis is calculated in decades and appears to be influenced by alcohol abuse, age at infection, gender, and genetic background. However, not all cases of chronic hepatitis C are progressive or lead to severe complications. Indeed, a significant proportion of patients, typically those with minimal or no elevations in alanine aminotransferase (ALT) levels and a milder degree of necro-inflammation, remain asymptomatic and without significant liver disease for many decades, if not for life.[3] The prognosis of those who progress to HCV-related cirrhosis depends primarily on the development of two events, clinical decompensation (e.g., development of ascites) and hepatocellular carcinoma (HCC). Although the 10-year patient survival rate reaches 80% in the absence of these events, it drops to less than 50% once complications develop.[4] The risk of decompensation unrelated to HCC has been estimated to be on the order of 15% to 20% after 4 years of follow-up.[4-6] The annual incidence of HCC in HCV-infected cirrhotic patients ranges between 1.5% and 3.3%.[4-6]

Indications for Liver Transplantation

Liver transplantation should be considered when the course of the disease is sufficiently advanced that medium-term (2 to 5 years) survival is unlikely without this intervention. Since the outcome of compensated HCV-related cirrhosis is sufficiently good, cirrhosis per se should not be considered an indication for liver transplantation. In fact, recent data have shown that patients with compensated cirrhosis or transition to cirrhosis can be successfully treated by antiviral therapy, with manageable, but significant, side effects. In such cases, treatment often leads to disease stabilization, and in a few cases, it has been suggested to reverse established cirrhosis.[7] A sustained response can be achieved with the use of pegylated interferon-alfa in combination with ribavirin in approximately 40% of these patients, with unfortunately lower response rates in those infected with HCV genotype 1, the most prevalent genotype in patients with cirrhosis, than in those infected with genotypes 2 and 3 ($\approx$45% versus 80%, respectively). Interestingly, histological analysis in these studies has shown that half the patients with advanced fibrosis who attain a sustained virological response have an improvement in their fibrosis score on follow-up biopsy.[8] It remains to be shown whether improvement in fibrosis can be reliably achieved in patients without a virological response who are treated with long-term, maintenance interferon therapy. There are at least two ongoing large multicenter trials that should provide answers to these questions. Since the trends in hepatitis C predict that the proportion of HCV-infected patients with cirrhosis, decompensated cirrhosis, and HCC will double in the next 20 years,[9] it would seem prudent to be aggressive with antiviral therapy in this population.

Once decompensation occurs, liver transplantation is the treatment of choice. This is the case for patients with hepatic insufficiency who have attained a Child-Turcotte-Pugh score greater than 7, or have a history of spontaneous bacterial peritonitis, refractory ascites, encephalopathy, or recurrent variceal bleeding unresponsive to traditional endoscopic or radiological treatment. The growing discrepancy between available donor organs and the need for transplantation has led to recent reevaluation of selection and listing criteria for liver transplantation, as well as priorities for organ allocation. For this purpose, a new system or disease severity index called the Model for End-Stage Liver Disease (MELD) was recently created (see Chapter 5).[10] It is still unclear whether MELD will better predict which HCV-infected candidates are at high risk for pretransplant or posttransplant mortality.[11]

The coexistence of HCC is an increasingly frequent complication of HCV-related cirrhosis. The criteria applied to select patients for transplantation in these circumstances have been fully evaluated and generally include absence of vascular invasion, diameter less than 5 cm, and fewer than three nodules. With these selection criteria, survival rates do not differ from those achieved in HCV-infected patients without HCC (see Chapter 15). In many centers, these patients are listed for liver transplantation in the absence of hepatic decompensation. For example, in the MELD system, patients with stage 1 or stage 2 tumors are assigned MELD scores of 20 and 24, respectively. However, immediate listing for transplantation might not be the optimal approach to those with resectable HCC and compensated cirrhosis. Given the long waiting times for liver transplantation in many parts of the world, patients with small tumors, who are initially good candidates, may be susceptible to the development of progressive disease before a donor organ is found. To address this problem, a variety of methods have been used in an attempt to gain control of the tumor or tumors while on the waiting list, including liver resection, alcohol injection, chemoembolization, percutaneous radiofrequency ablation, and systemic chemotherapy. The efficacy of these approaches is still unknown given the lack of prospective randomized trials. A recent publication suggests that in centers with long waiting list times (>6 months), resection should be considered as initial treatment in patients with compensated cirrhosis and liver transplantation reserved as "adjuvant" therapy.[12] In these circumstances, antiviral therapy could also be attempted. Transplantation could then potentially be obviated in patients with successful tumor ablation who achieve a complete response.

Posttransplant Hepatitis C Virus Infection

Source of Infection

The most common source of posttransplant HCV infection is pretransplantation infection. Indeed, recurrent infection, defined as the reappearance of HCV RNA in serum, is nearly universal. A rapid decrease in HCV RNA occurs immediately after removal of the infected liver, followed by an even sharper decline after implantation of the allograft, presumably representing virus uptake by the new liver.[13] This decline is followed by a progressive increase in serum HCV RNA levels such that pretransplantation levels are reached as soon as day 4 and increase up to 10- to 20-fold higher 1 month after transplantation.[14] The virus may also be acquired by those without evidence of previous HCV infection from contaminated blood or donor organs. However, de novo acquisition of HCV infection has become extremely uncommon (<1% of HCV-negative recipients) as a result of routine and efficient screening for HCV in blood and organ donors.[15]

In the current era of organ shortage and given the progressive increase in the number of HCV-infected patients in need of transplantation, some authors have advocated the use of organs from anti-HCV–positive donors. In these cases, viral transmission to the recipient depends primarily on the donor's HCV RNA status. HCV RNA–positive donors invariably transmit HCV to recipients, whereas organs from anti-HCV–positive, HCV RNA–negative donors transmit infection at a much lower rate. The appropriateness of using these organs largely depends on the prognosis of recipients receiving HCV-infected grafts (see later).

Definition of Viral Recurrence as Opposed to Histological Recurrence

Antibody assays for HCV are of little value after transplantation. The diagnosis of HCV reinfection should be established by a virological assay, typically a qualitative polymerase chain reaction assay. With quantitative assays becoming more sensitive, these generally suffice. Levels of viremia after transplantation are higher than pretransplant levels.[14] Viral load, although not generally associated with the severity of liver disease in the nontransplant setting, may be useful to predict outcome (i.e., the development of cholestatic hepatitis) and monitor therapy. Standardized quantitative assays with results given in international units should be used to allow comparison between studies and longitudinal evaluation in individual patients.

Both pretransplant and early posttransplant viral loads[16,17] are predictors of severe posttransplant liver disease. They are also predictors of response to therapy. Thus, it may be useful to monitor HCV RNA levels.

The diagnosis of recurrent HCV disease, in contrast to reinfection, is based on histological findings. Indeed, standard liver tests lack specificity and sensitivity in this setting and may underestimate the presence of liver damage. In particular, there is generally a poor correlation between the severity of histological disease and serum transaminase levels.[18-21]

Histologically, acute hepatitis typically develops between the second and fourth month after transplantation, whereas changes consistent with chronic hepatitis are usually seen after the third posttransplant month.[22] The histopathological features of recurrent acute and chronic HCV disease include many of the features seen in nonimmunocompromised patients. Early liver changes seen in the acute phase include minimal lobular inflammation with scattered apoptotic bodies, minimal cell swelling, and steatosis. This lesion progresses within 2 to 4 weeks to a more fully developed hepatitis, with portal and lobular inflammation of varying degrees in association with hepatocyte necrosis and midzonal macrovesicular steatosis. The portal infiltrates are typically mononuclear cells, which may form lymphoid aggregates. Fatty change, bile duct damage, and patchy parenchymal lymphocytic infiltrates are also common. Fatty change alone may be an early marker of recurrence. Atypical histological findings, including marked bile duct epithelial injury, venulitis, profound cholestasis, bile duct proliferation, and perivenular ballooning of hepatocytes, may also be seen in patients with recurrent HCV infection and can mimic other entities such as acute cellular rejection, obstruction, and ischemia.[23] Exclusion of other causative factors such as CMV hepatitis, obstruction, ischemia, and drug toxicity may require serological, immunohistochemical, radiological, and endoscopic studies; drug discontinuation; or serial biopsy. Immunohistochemical and in situ methods to detect HCV antigens or HCV RNA, or both, in liver tissue have been evaluated as a means of differentiating recurrent hepatitis C from other conditions and as a predictor of disease severity. In general, the results are conflicting, with relatively poor correlation with histological findings.

A major issue in clinical practice is to distinguish recurrent hepatitis from rejection with hepatitis.[24] Rejection does not occur more frequently in patients with hepatitis C, but it can certainly be difficult to differentiate recurrence of hepatitis C from acute cellular rejection at time points beyond 2 months after transplantation. However, one could argue that this dilemma has not been framed appropriately. The challenge should not be to differentiate recurrence of hepatitis C from rejection, but rather to determine whether alloimmunity is also playing a role in posttransplant hepatitis C and how it should best be treated. This issue is important because although the occurrence of acute cellular rejection does not have an important impact on long-term outcomes in HCV-negative liver recipients, such is not the case in patients who undergo liver transplantation for HCV disease. HCV-negative recipients who experience an episode of rejection have only half the mortality rate of HCV-negative recipients who do not experience an episode of rejection. By contrast, HCV-positive recipients have a threefold increased risk of death if they are treated with steroids for a single episode of rejection and more than a fivefold increased risk of death if they experience steroid-refractory acute cellular rejection.[25] For this reason, many centers have now decided to not treat mild acute rejection, defined as Banff grade 1 rejection in HCV-positive recipients, particularly when it occurs more than 2 months after transplantation. A recent study involving the use of gene microarray technology suggests that in the future, evaluation of overexpression of specific proinflammatory proteins may help differentiate whether rejection or hepatitis is predominant.[26]

Table 10–1. RECURRENT HEPATITIS C: HISTOLOGICAL EVOLUTION*

Author	N	Follow-up (mo)	Chronic Hepatitis (%)	Cirrhosis (%)
Feray, 1994	60	42 (mean)	68	7.5
Gane, 1996	149	36 (median)	88	8
Johnson, 1996	67	—	46	16
Prieto, 1999	81	32 (mean)	97	15
Feray, 1999	652	42 (mean)	80	10
Testa, 2000	300	23 (median)	40	6
Sanchez-Fueyos, 2002	122	43 (median)	95	23
Berenguer, 2002	283	6 (median)	97	23

*Studies based on protocol biopsy.

In the meantime, such differentiation should be based on timing and clinical and histological grounds (Table 10–1).

Natural History of Hepatitis C Virus Infection after Liver Transplantation

Histological Outcome

HCV replication, as measured by negative-strand HCV RNA, generally begins in the first week after transplantation (Fig. 10–1). It is typically followed by the development of histological liver damage or recurrent hepatitis, which occurs in the majority of patients (see Table 10–1). Indeed, by month 6, acute hepatitis develops in more than 50% of patients, and by month 12, more than 80% have progressed to chronic hepatitis. The rate of progression to cirrhosis, however, is quite variable. Although some patients maintain minimal to moderate histological changes, others progress rapidly to end-stage liver disease and allograft failure. Based on published studies, cirrhosis develops within the first 5 to 7 years after transplantation in 8% to 44% of recipients.[18,19,22,27-30] This wide range of results probably relates to the use of different case definitions, as mentioned previously. Indeed, protocol liver biopsies are generally needed to identify progression to severe forms of chronic hepatitis. In one study based on yearly liver biopsies, the probability of HCV-related graft cirrhosis developing was 28% at 5 years.[19] In addition, an accelerated course of liver injury leading to early allograft failure develops in a small proportion of patients (<10%).[31] These cases are marked by striking elevations in serum alkaline phosphatase activity and very high HCV RNA levels (generally >2,000,000 IU/mL).[32] The histological findings are those of cholestatic hepatitis manifested by cholestasis, marked lobular disarray, centrizonal hepatocyte ballooning,

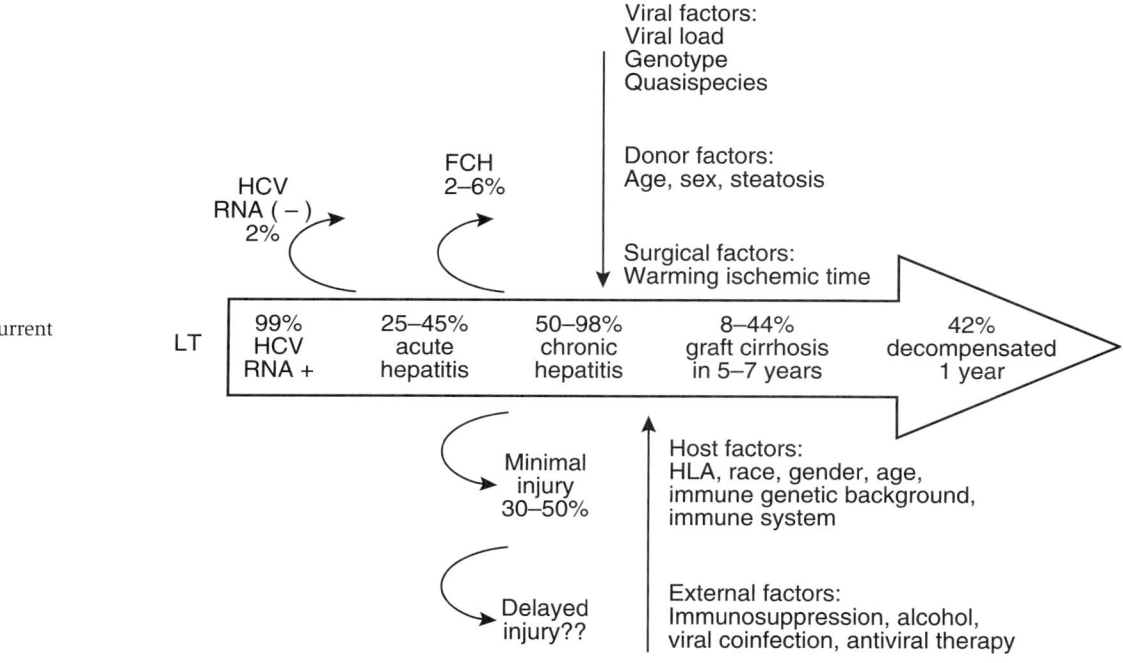

FIGURE 10–1

Natural history of recurrent hepatitis C.

and relative lack of inflammation. Immunologically, there appears to be a relatively inept cellular immune response against HCV that may allow the virus to become cytopathic.[33] Once cholestatic hepatitis develops, survival is relatively short and treatment is generally ineffective.

The course of hepatitis C is generally more aggressive in immunocompromised than in immunocompetent patients, with the rate of progression of fibrosis significantly higher (0.3 fibrosis units/yr [0.004 to 2.19] versus 0.2 fibrosis units/yr [0.09 to 0.8], P <.0001) and, as a consequence, the interval until the development of cirrhosis shorter (9 to 12 years versus 20 to 30 years).[34] This accelerated disease course continues even after cirrhosis is established such that the risk for clinical decompensation is higher in these patients (42% versus 5% to 10% in 1 year).[35]

Finally, recent data have shown that the frequency of disease progression and the risk for severe HCV-related hepatitis after transplantation are increasing in recent years.[30,34,36]

Clinical Outcome

The negative impact of HCV infection on posttransplant outcomes has been documented in several recent studies in which it has been shown that HCV infection significantly impairs patient and graft survival (60% to 70% versus 76% to 77% in non-HCV controls at 5 years) (Fig. 10–2).[30,37] In addition, the more aggressive histological disease seen in recent years is beginning to translate in some centers to a further reduction in graft

survival, with recurrence of HCV-related cirrhosis being the main cause of death.[30]

Factors Influencing Disease Severity and Progression or Survival

At present, although short- and medium-term graft survival rates have been reasonable, it is important that we define factors associated with a poor outcome to improve long-term results. With this knowledge, conditions contributing to worse outcomes that are present before or develop after transplantation could optimally be addressed or avoided. In addition, patients in whom poor outcomes are inevitable would not be subjected to the trauma of undergoing transplantation.

Factors that have been tested for an association with disease severity/progression or survival (or both) include those related to the host (demographics, genetic background, immune status, comorbidity, hepatic function at transplantation), the virus (genotype, HCV RNA levels, viral quasispecies), and environment (immunosuppression, alcohol, viral coinfection) (Table 10–2). In addition, certain variables are unique to the transplant setting, including those related to the donor (age, degree of hepatic steatosis, liver volume, living versus deceased) and surgery.[22] In most studies performed to date, the focus has been on viral and iatrogenic parameters, but relatively little is published on host factors. Interestingly, in the immunocompetent population, the most powerful predictors of disease severity are those related to the host, whereas

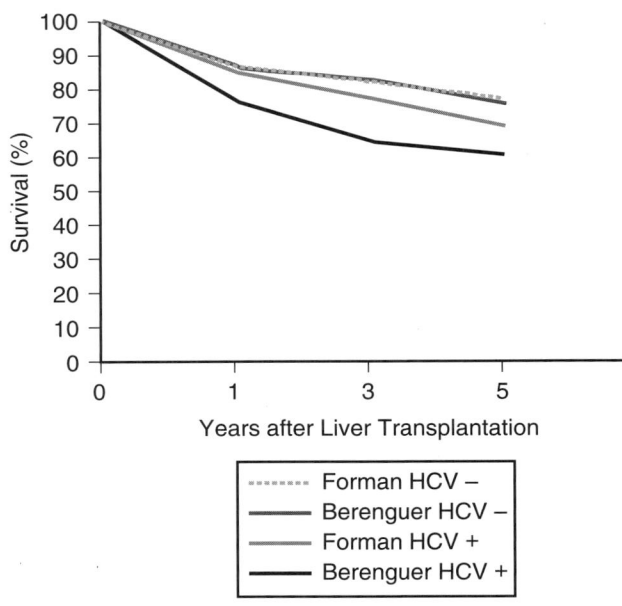

FIGURE 10–2

Patient survival in hepatitis C virus (HCV)-infected and non–HCV-infected liver transplant recipients. (Adapted from Berenguer M, Prieto M, San Juan F, et al: Contribution of donor age to the recent decrease in patient survival among HCV-infected liver transplant recipients. Hepatology 36:202-210, 2002; and Forman LM, Lewis JD, Berlin JA, et al: The association between hepatitis C infection and survival after orthotopic liver transplantation. Gastroenterology 122:889-896, 2002.)

virus-related factors (e.g., genotype and HCV RNA) do not appear to play a major role in determining outcome. However, age at the time of infection, gender, the existence of any type of immunodeficiency (Table 10–3), and most importantly, alcohol use strongly

Table 10–3. IMMUNOSUPPRESSION: EFFECTS ON VIRAL LOAD AND DISEASE SEVERITY/PROGRESSION

	Effect on Viral Load	Effect on Disease Progression
Corticosteroids	Increase	Negative
Cyclosporine	Unknown	Controversial
Tacrolimus	Unknown	Controversial
OKT3	Unknown	Negative
Anti–IL-2 receptor antibody	Unknown	Unknown
MMF	Controversial	Controversial
MMF + Anti–IL-2 receptor	Increase	Negative

IL-2, interleukin-2; MMF, mycophenolate mofetil.

affect disease progression.[2] In the liver transplant setting, similar variables have been found to influence the outcome, although the type and strength of these associations are not strictly the same.

Host-Related Variables

Immune Status. Several indirect findings highlight the deleterious effect of the immunosuppressed state, a variable intrinsically related to the transplant setting. Indeed, the course of HCV infection is clearly accelerated in liver transplant recipients in comparison to immunocompetent patients, with a higher rate of fibrogenesis and a greater risk of early clinical decompensation and allograft failure after transplantation.[34,35] Moreover, the posttransplant outcome in HCV-positive recipients,

Table 10–2. FACTORS INFLUENCING DISEASE SEVERITY/PROGRESSION OR SURVIVIAL

Factors	Association	Type of Association
Pretransplant Factors		
Donor age	Established	45–50 yr
Living donor	Unknown insufficient data	Negative
HLA-DR matching	Controversial	
Donor genetic factors	Unknown insufficient data	
Recipient-Related Factors		
Gender	Established	Female: worse survival
Age	Established	Survival
Nonwhite	Insufficient	Survival, FP?
Severity of illness	Established	Survival
Virological-Related Factors		
Genotype	Controversial	1b: worse
Pre–liver transplant viral load	Established	Survival, FP
Early post–liver transplant viral load	Established	Survival, Hx

FP, fibrosis progression; Hx, history.

including both histological progression and graft survival, has worsened in recent years at a time when more potent immunosuppressive agents are being used for both induction and maintenance of immunosuppression.[30,34,36] Furthermore, HCV-related disease progression appears to be of particular concern in those coinfected with human immunodeficiency virus (HIV) both before and after transplantation,[38,39] again emphasizing the negative impact of the immunosuppressed state. Finally, several studies have highlighted the negative impact of the development of infection with cytomegalovirus, a virus with immunosuppressive properties, on both histological outcome and survival.[40,41]

Treatment of Rejection and Hepatitis C. In terms of the impact of immunosuppression on long-term outcomes in patients transplanted for hepatitis C, there is little doubt that the use of corticosteroid boluses to treat acute cellular rejection is harmful to HCV-infected recipients.[18,19,25,34,42,43] Corticosteroid boluses are associated with an increase in serum HCV RNA concentrations of 4- to 100-fold.[44] One study showed that corticosteroid boluses are also associated with an increased frequency of acute hepatitis and an earlier time to recurrence.[28] The higher HCV RNA levels are additionally associated with increased histological severity of recurrent hepatitis. As mentioned earlier, HCV-positive recipients who are administered steroids for the treatment of rejection have a threefold greater risk of early posttransplant mortality.[25]

Similarly, the use of OKT3 to treat rejection is associated with a greater chance of recurrence of hepatitis C and also a greater risk of posttransplant graft loss.[19,30,36,43,45]

Maintenance Immunosuppression and Hepatitis C Virus Infection. Although the impact of additional immunosuppression for the treatment of rejection on hepatitis C is clear, when one looks at the agents used for induction or maintenance of immunosuppression, the conclusions are not so clear. For example, some data suggest that complete avoidance of corticosteroids may be beneficial in patients with HCV infection undergoing liver transplantation.[46] However, there is also evidence that complete withdrawal of corticosteroids may be harmful to HCV-infected patients undergoing liver transplantation.[36,47]

Similarly, the data with mycophenolate mofetil (MMF) are confusing. Several studies have found a correlation between the use of MMF and worse outcomes in HCV-positive recipients.[36,41,48] A study from Berlin showed that if MMF is added to the posttransplant regimen, there is no change in HCV RNA levels or severity of disease.[49] This finding is significant in that inosine-5′-monophosphate dehydrogenase inhibitors have been tested as antiviral agents in hepatitis C. Two large randomized trials compared MMF with azathioprine in a maintenance immunosuppressive regimen. Neither of these studies showed significant differences in either rates of recurrence of hepatitis C or outcomes in the study patients versus controls.[50,51]

One interesting study suggests that patients who receive a relatively high exposure to MMF have improved outcomes over patients who receive a lower exposure to MMF. Patients never exposed to MMF have an intermediate response in terms of severity of recurrent disease.[52]

Finally, the data on antibody induction are also mixed. One uncontrolled trial has suggested that the use of anti-CD25 induction therapy has a negative impact on long-term outcomes in patients transplanted for hepatitis C.[48] By contrast, two controlled and randomized trials have suggested no impact.[53,54]

Given these confusing and occasionally conflicting results regarding the impact of immunosuppression on the outcome of patients who undergo liver transplantation for HCV disease, how can one generate a unifying hypothesis that will help guide our use of immunosuppressive agents in this difficult population? The "classic" paradigm is that greater immunosuppression leads to more severe posttransplant hepatitis C. One could argue that it may not be simply the degree of immunosuppression that has an impact on long-term outcomes in patients transplanted for hepatitis C but, rather, dramatic *changes in immunosuppression* may be the factor that has a negative impact on outcomes in patients transplanted for hepatitis C. This could explain why the use of corticosteroid boluses and OKT3 for the treatment of rejection is particularly harmful to HCV-infected patients, whereas either steroid avoidance or maintenance of low levels of corticosteroids, but not late steroid withdrawal, may be beneficial.[55] It may also help explain why greater exposure to MMF appears to be better than less MMF exposure. It is likely that in that study the principal difference was not in the dose of MMF used, but rather whether MMF was discontinued after a relatively short period (e.g., 3 months), which has generally been the standard in liver transplant recipients in the United States.

Immunogenetic Background. There is now strong evidence for the important role of heredity in the host immune response to infectious pathogens and for susceptibility and outcome after exposure to microbial agents. Both the major histocompatibility complex (MHC) genes and non-MHC genes are increasingly being identified as candidate genes with significant importance in the outcome of infectious diseases. In HCV, specific HLA class II alleles such as HLA-B14 and HLA-DRB1*04 have emerged as possible modulators of disease severity. Regulatory mechanisms that control cytokine production, including tumor necrosis factor-α (TNF-α), are in part genetically influenced.

For example, it has been shown that cytokine genes are polymorphic at specific sites. These polymorphisms may have an effect on cytokine production. In one study, Rosen and colleagues evaluated the impact of polymorphisms at positions -238 and -308 of the TNF-α gene promoter (mutations associated with susceptibility to active hepatitis after HCV exposure in immunocompetent patients) in liver donors on the severity and outcome of recurrent hepatitis C.[56] They found that time to recurrence was shorter and the hepatic activity index greater in those who received an organ from donors with the TNF-α -308 allele, suggesting that a specific donor TNF-α genotype known to be associated with high TNF-α production may contribute to accelerated graft injury in liver transplant recipients with HCV infection.

Furthermore, some but not all authors have suggested that donor/recipient matching at the HLA-B locus reduces the incidence of acute cellular rejection but also promotes the recurrence of viral hepatitis.[57,58] Discrepancies may be explained by differences between studies in HLA typing methods, selection and ethnic backgrounds of patients, and the immunosuppressive regimen used.

Finally, race has also been found to influence outcome in patients with recurrent HCV infection, with nonwhites doing worse than whites.[16,34]

Viral-Related Variables

Hepatitis C Virus Genotypes. Studies evaluating the relationship between severity of liver disease after transplantation and HCV genotype are conflicting.[22] Some but not all studies have implicated genotype 1, and in particular subtype 1b, in more aggressive post-transplant disease than seen with non–genotype 1 viruses.[27,59-61] A recent study has also shown that genotype 1b may induce more severe apoptosis than occurs with other genotypes.[62] Factors that could account for these discrepant results include differences in genotype distribution in the study population, the presence of unmeasured confounding variables such as the type and amount of immunosuppressive agents administered, the length of histological follow-up, and differences in case definitions. Strains with differing virulence but within the genotype 1b subset may also be implicated.[63]

HCV RNA Levels. Levels of viremia before and early after transplantation appear to correlate with the development and severity of hepatitis C in the graft. In the National Institute for Diabetes and Digestive and Kidney Diseases Liver Transplantation Database, the relative risk of graft loss was 3.6-fold higher in patients with a pretransplant viral load greater than 1 million viral Eq/mL than in those with a lower viral load, with

5-year cumulative patient survival rates of 57% and 84%, respectively ($P = .001$).[16]

One study has longitudinally assessed hepatic HCV RNA levels. Paralleling a decrease in the amount of immunosuppression, intrahepatic HCV RNA levels declined with time despite progression to severe liver disease, thus suggesting an immune-mediated injury in this situation.[59] High levels of viremia and intrahepatic HCV RNA, however, have been described in the setting of cholestatic hepatitis and during the acute phase of recurrent hepatitis C.[32,59] This finding suggests that during the early phase of recurrent hepatitis C or in cholestatic hepatitis C, the liver damage may be due to a direct cytopathic effect of HCV.[33]

Hepatitis C Virus Heterogeneity. HCV heterogeneity may play a role in the pathogenesis of progressive HCV disease.[64-67] A high viral load before transplantation may influence the distribution of HCV quasispecies and yield a greater chance for new and "more fit" variants to expand and dominate the viral population once cellular immunity is impaired by immunosuppression.[67] Genetic divergence of emerging variants has been found to be higher in immunosuppressed patients than in immunocompetent controls, with higher divergence occurring in those with the most severe forms of post-transplant cholestatic hepatitis.[66] Interestingly, one study has shown an increased number of pretransplantation major variants in recipients with recurrent hepatitis versus those without recurrent hepatitis.[67] Altogether, these data suggest that immunosuppression plays a role in the evolution of new, potentially more pathogenic variants. This situation may have an increased likelihood of occurring in the setting of a higher replication rate before transplantation.[68]

Donor-Related Variables

Several studies have found an association between the *age of the donor* and the severity of recurrent hepatitis C, the rate of disease progression, and posttransplant survival.[30,36,41,69] In a recent series, only 14% of the recipients who received an organ from a donor younger than 30 years contracted cirrhosis. By contrast, 45% and 52% of those receiving an organ from donors aged 31 to 59 or older than 59, respectively ($P < .0001$), contracted cirrhosis.[30] The recent trend toward increasing age of deceased donors may explain the worsening outcome in HCV-positive recipients seen in recent years.[30,36,69] This observation may have important implications for donor liver allocation. In addition, it correlates with data from the immunocompetent population, where age at the time of infection is an important and powerful determinant of the natural history of the disease. Age-related changes in the liver's response to infection may be a key factor that determines the increased susceptibility of an older liver to HCV-related fibrosis. Alternatively, it could be explained by the existence of a higher degree of steatosis found in older donors.

Similar to what has recently been suggested in the immunocompetent population, steatosis also appears to be detrimental in liver transplant recipients. In one study, for instance, 60% of the patients with worse outcomes were characterized by a high degree of macrovesicular steatosis in early posttransplant biopsies performed during the first 28 days after transplantation.[17] In contrast, none of the control patients with benign recurrence was found to have steatosis in early biopsy specimens. More data are awaited on this important issue. In fact, one potential factor that could explain different outcomes in different centers could be the difference in practice policies regarding the use of fatty livers.[70]

The *anti-HCV status of the donor* may also influence the posttransplant outcome. Superinfection has been described in this setting, with ultimate prevalence of genotype 1 viruses in all recipient-donor pairs in which superinfection occurred.[71] It appears, however, that both histological outcome and survival rates in HCV-positive recipients are not affected by receiving an organ from an anti-HCV–positive donor.[72-74] Interestingly, patients retaining their own strain had more severe liver disease than did those who became infected by the donor strain, thus suggesting either different pathogenic capabilities of different HCV strains or that learned pretransplant immune responses may also contribute to more severe posttransplant disease. Until more data become available, the use of these organs provides a life-saving option in some cases and does not appear to place the recipient at higher risk for graft damage or loss, at least in the short and medium term.

Surgical-Related Variables

Prolonged rewarming time during allograft implantation has been associated with severe recurrent hepatitis C.[75] If these data are confirmed, special emphasis should be placed on minimizing rewarming time, for instance, by using surgical techniques associated with a decreased period of graft rewarming, such as vena cava preservation.

Histology-Related Variables

The histological findings observed in the initial liver biopsy specimen have been shown in some studies to be reliable predictors of subsequent outcome. In two studies, for instance, the grade of necro-inflammatory activity observed in the first-year liver transplant biopsy was associated with the risk for development of cirrhosis. Only 3% to 10% of those with mild hepatitis contracted cirrhosis, whereas this percentage increased to 30% to 60% in those who showed moderate to severe activity in the first year.[18,19] Furthermore, not only is the severity of inflammation predictive but also other specific histological features such as steatosis, ballooning degeneration, cholestasis, and confluent necrosis[76,77] may be helpful in predicting progression to severe hepatitis or cirrhosis, or to both. In addition, timing of recurrence appears to be important in predicting outcome, with recurrence within the first 6 months being associated with a worse prognosis.[28]

External Factors

Patients coinfected with hepatitis B virus (HBV) appear to have milder disease and better survival than those infected with HCV alone do.[27] Although interactions between both viruses may explain this improved outcome, a second explanation may be the benefits of passive transmission of antibodies against HCV in coinfected patients receiving hepatitis B immune globulin in the era before specific HCV screening of blood products.[78] In contrast, coinfection with hepatitis G virus does not seem to influence the posttransplant course of HCV disease.[79]

Alcohol Intake. A substantial proportion of patients have end-stage liver disease caused by both alcohol and chronic HCV infection. The histological findings are typically indistinguishable from those found in patients with HCV alone. However, the liver disease is clearly more severe and accelerated in patients with concomitant alcohol abuse and chronic HCV infection than in those with HCV who have never abused alcohol. The same may hold true after liver transplantation, but data on this issue are surprisingly limited, and of course most recipients are counseled against posttransplant alcohol use.[28,80]

Year of Transplantation. Recently, the year of transplantation was found to be predictive of progression of fibrosis, time to cirrhosis, and even survival, with patients undergoing transplantation more recently progressing at a faster rate to allograft failure than those transplanted earlier.[30,34,36] Reasons that explain the worse outcome seen in HCV-infected patients in recent years are not fully understood. Possible factors contributing to this observation have been discussed earlier.

Knowing the pretransplant variables associated with a poor outcome is important so that specific measures might be taken before the surgery. For instance, and given the association between the age of the donor, HIV coinfection, and more aggressive histological disease, organs from younger donors should be used for these patients. Alternatively, minimizing warm ischemia time may also have a positive effect on the natural history of HCV-related disease after transplantation. Prophylaxis of HCV-infected patients with ganciclovir or valganciclovir reduces the risk of cytomegalovirus disease and, in doing so, may also reduce the severity of recurrent hepatitis C. Finally, therapeutic interventions such as antiviral therapy with interferon in patients with high levels of viremia awaiting transplantation may be tried. Although all these interventions are of potential benefit for HCV candidates, no study has as yet documented their positive impact on posttransplant hepatitis C.

Patient Management

There is little consensus on the optimal approach to antiviral therapy for HCV-positive patients undergoing liver transplantation for two reasons: (1) limited efficacy of the available therapies and (2) inability to interpret current studies because of a lack of appropriate control patients.

Although preventing HCV reinfection should be the major goal, there is currently no available intervention to effectively prevent reinfection. A retrospective review of the use of hepatitis B immune globulin, obtained in the era before routine HCV screening of blood and plasma donors, in patients coinfected with HCV and HBV suggested that passive immunoprophylaxis might be effective in reducing recurrent infection.[78] However, in a recent Canadian study, hepatitis C immune globulin had no demonstrable effect on HCV reinfection.[81]

Four potential approaches to antiviral therapy can be used in HCV-positive recipients: (1) treatment of the patient before transplantation, with the goal of suppressing viral replication so that viral recurrence is prevented or at least the risk of aggressive recurrent HCV disease is reduced; (2) preemptive early posttransplant antiviral therapy before histological damage has occurred in an attempt to avoid the development of histological hepatitis or prevent its progression; (3) treatment of disease when and if it does occur; and (4) no treatment, with retransplantation in those progressing to allograft failure.

Pretransplantation Antiviral Therapy

Antiviral therapy may be attempted before transplantation to clear the virus and prevent recurrence. Alternatively, it may be used to alter the posttransplant course, since HCV RNA levels before transplantation have been shown to correlate with posttransplant outcomes. This approach is likely to be successful only if effective pretransplant doses of antivirals can be administered and if lowering HCV RNA levels before transplantation does indeed improve posttransplant outcomes. However, the currently available antiviral agents (interferon and ribavirin) are difficult to use in decompensated patients because of the risk of further decompensation of disease or development of bacterial sepsis or the occurrence of dangerous leukopenia or thrombocytopenia. Moreover, despite some reports of success with this approach,[82] the patients treated to date represent a highly selected group such that most HCV-positive patients on the waiting list would not meet the criteria for initiation of treatment. Two studies have tested this approach to treatment.[82,83] Both used a protocol that started with low doses of interferon with or without ribavirin and slowly increased the drug dosages as tolerated. These studies emphasize the advantages and disadvantages of this approach. In a multicenter study by Crippin and colleagues,[82] HCV-infected patients at or near the top of their respective waiting lists were randomly assigned to one of three treatment arms, two involving therapy with interferon as monotherapy and one involving interferon in combination with ribavirin. Less than half the patients screened met the entry criteria, with thrombocytopenia and leukopenia being the most common reasons for exclusion. Eventually, only 15 patients from five large transplant centers received antiviral therapy. Nine patients were treated with interferon monotherapy, whereas six received combination therapy with ribavirin (400 mg twice daily). During treatment, loss of detectable HCV RNA was seen in 33%. Unfortunately, recurrence of infection was not prevented in the only patient undergoing transplantation with undetectable viremia (by bDNA) at the time of transplantation. In addition, a significant number of adverse effects occurred (n = 23), many of which were considered severe. Although thrombocytopenia was the most frequent adverse event, infection was the most severe. These side effects, particularly life-threatening infection, ultimately led to early termination of the study.[82] Two conclusions can be drawn from this study: (1) a large proportion of patients awaiting transplantation will not benefit from this approach because of the presence of contraindications, particularly thrombocytopenia and neutropenia, and (2) awareness of the potential complications is important when treating the small proportion who meet the initiation criteria.

In the second study, conducted by Everson and associates,[83] patients with cirrhosis (mean Child-Pugh score of 7) were initially given low doses of interferon (1.5 mU three times weekly) and ribavirin (600 mg daily) with a slow increase in the dose of both drugs every 2 weeks as tolerated. Growth factors, including granulocyte colony-stimulating factor and erythropoietin, were administered if needed to support peripheral blood cell counts. Results in the first 91 patients, the majority infected with genotype 1 viruses, were recently reported. During treatment, virological responses occurred in 38% and sustained virological responses occurred in 22% of patients, with responses being significantly more common in patients with a non–genotype 1 virus and in those treated for more than 6 months. Posttransplant reinfection was prevented in eight recipients who were HCV RNA negative at the time of transplantation. Twenty-eight percent of the patients had treatment discontinued because of the development of severe side effects.

The main difference between the two studies lies in the severity of liver disease at initiation of therapy and the regimen used. In the study by Crippin and colleagues, the mean Child-Pugh score was 12.[82] Patients in the study of Everson and colleagues had significantly less advanced disease. In addition, lower doses were used at initiation in the latter study. These studies suggest that (1) pretransplant treatment with combination therapy is feasible in selected patients, those with Child-Pugh scores less than 9 or 10, and a group of patients who may benefit from this approach are those with coexistent HCC, since typically these candidates have less advanced liver disease; (2) use of growth factors is commonly required to complete the course of therapy; (3) reinfection can be prevented if HCV RNA is absent at the time of transplantation; although no data are yet available, it is possible that a reduction in HCV RNA levels will reduce the severity of posttransplant liver disease; and (4) responses were generally achievable in those infected with HCV genotypes 2 and 3, who unfortunately represent the minority of liver transplant candidates.

Preemptive Therapy in the Early Posttransplant Period

Preemptive therapy with interferon either alone or in combination with ribavirin in the early posttransplant period has also been used in an attempt to reduce the incidence or severity (or both) of recurrent hepatitis C. The rationale for this approach comes from our knowledge of predictors of response in the immunocompetent population, in whom low viral load and absence of bridging fibrosis or cirrhosis are predictive of response. In that sense, the early posttransplant period is characterized by a lower viral load within the first month and absence of fibrosis. In two early studies, recipients were randomized within 2 weeks of transplantation to receive either interferon alone or placebo for 1 year.[84,85] Although patient and graft survival did not differ between groups and the rate of reinfection was not affected by treatment, histological disease recurrence was observed less frequently in interferon-treated patients in one study (8 of 30 evaluable at 1 year) than in those who were not treated (22 of 41; $P = .01$).[84] In the second study, histological recurrence and its severity did not differ between groups, and the only difference between groups was a delay in the

development of HCV-related hepatitis in treated patients (408 versus 193 days, $P = .05$).[85] Although side effects were common in these studies, with leukopenia being the most frequently observed, the incidence of rejection was not increased by interferon therapy.

In another case series, 36 recipients were treated with interferon alfa-2b and ribavirin starting at the third posttransplant week and continuing for 1 year. After a median follow-up of 52 months, actuarial 5-year survival was excellent (87.5%). At 36 months after discontinuation of therapy, a sustained virological and biochemical response was achieved in 12 patients (33%), 20% in those infected with HCV genotype 1 and 100% in those with genotype 2. Liver biopsy findings were normal in patients with a sustained response. By contrast, progression to severe hepatitis C was observed in four of the nonresponders (11% of the overall series). Common side effects included hemolytic anemia and asthenia, which were treated by dose reduction.[86]

Although these results are promising, they need to be confirmed in larger series. Recent data suggest that the applicability of this approach is limited given the frequent development of side effects that lead to discontinuation of therapy and the relatively low proportion of patients meeting the entry criteria, particularly with regard to anemia, neutropenia, and thrombocytopenia.[87] In addition, efficacy is limited in those infected with HCV genotype 1, who constitute the majority of patients undergoing transplantation for HCV-related cirrhosis.

Treatment of Hepatitis C Virus–Related Graft Disease

Treatment of recurrent HCV disease with interferon or ribavirin as single agents has thus far been disappointing, but initial results from combination therapy with interferon/pegylated interferon and ribavirin are slightly encouraging.

Interferon alone, at doses of 3 mU three times weekly for 6 months, has failed to clear serum HCV RNA despite transient normalization of ALT values in a subset of treated patients (0% to 28%) with minor or no histological improvement. Moreover, since interferon can upregulate expression of HLA class I and II antigens and thus increase the risk of allograft rejection, there has been concern about using it in solid-organ transplant recipients. In contrast to the renal transplant experience, interferon-induced rejection occurs uncommonly liver transplant recipients.[88-90]

To improve the response rate, several approaches have been tried. Ribavirin monotherapy has been evaluated in liver transplant recipients, with biochemical improvement observed in many, but virological clearance seen in none. Relapse after withdrawal was universal, and no improvement in rates of fibrosis was demonstrated. The main side effect was hemolysis, which resolved after cessation of therapy.[90]

Combination therapy is the most recent approach, and results have been better, although far from good. In the first pilot study, 21 patients with early documented recurrent HCV disease were treated with interferon alfa-2b (3 mU three times weekly) and ribavirin (1000 mg/day) for 6 months and then maintained on ribavirin monotherapy for 6 additional months.[91] The median time between transplantation and initiation of therapy was 9 months (range, 3 to 24). All patients normalized their ALT values, and 50% cleared HCV RNA from serum at the end of the combination treatment period. The remaining patients, although viremic, experienced a 50% reduction in viral load. Only one patient had a biochemical relapse during the 6-month period of ribavirin alone despite reappearance of serum HCV RNA in 50% who had initially cleared HCV RNA. Most importantly, all but one patient who tolerated the drug showed an improvement in liver histology. Safety and tolerability were satisfactory, with reversible hemolytic anemia being the most common side effect. This side effect is probably related to rapid accumulation of the drug inside red cells, and one factor that appears to predict its occurrence is renal dysfunction, a condition extremely common in liver recipients. Three patients needed interruption of therapy and administration of erythropoietin because of anemia. No patient experienced allograft rejection. Early intervention

combined with therapy at a stage when patients had not progressed to more advanced degrees of liver injury may explain why they obtained good results.

Additional recently published studies evaluating the effect of combination therapy in liver transplant recipients with recurrent hepatitis C have yielded similar results: a sustained virological response rate ranging from 9% to 33%; dose adjustments in 35% of the patients; drug discontinuation, mainly ribavirin, in 30% to 40%; and severe adverse effects, particularly decompensation, in 5% of treated recipients (Table 10–4).[92-98] Data on posttreatment histology are generally lacking.

In a recent randomized study, there were no major differences in fibrosis activity and stage before treatment and at the end of follow-up.[98] It is possible, however, that an effect on histology will be seen with longer follow-up. In a recent study, 6 versus 12 months of combination therapy was compared in 57 transplant patients. A sustained virological response was achieved in 6 of 27 patients treated for 6 months (22%) and in 5 of 30 treated for 12 months (17%) ($P = .4$).[97] In addition, greater response rates were found in those infected with non–genotype 1 HCV versus genotype 1 after both 6 and 12 months of therapy (43% versus 15% and 43% versus 9%, respectively). Moreover, the identical response rates at 6 and 12 months in the non–genotype 1 group suggest that 6 months of therapy is sufficient for recurrent hepatitis C.

These preliminary findings imply that response rates to standard interferon and ribavirin are generally lower

Table 10–4. COMBINATION THERAPY WITH INTERFERON-α AND RIBAVIRIN IN PATIENTS WITH RECURRENT HEPATITIS C

Author	Treatment Regimen	Biochemical Response/Virological Response (%)	Sustained Biochemical Response/Sustained Virological Response* (%)	Histological Improvement	D/C (%)
Bizollon,[91] 1997	6 mo IFN + Rbv + 6 mo Rbv	100/48	86/24	Yes	14
Alberti,[92] 2001	12 mo IFN + Rbv + long-term Rbv	83/44	78/3	Yes	22
Gopal,[93] 2001	IFN + Rbv indefinitely	NA/50	NA/8	NA	0
Ahmad,[94] 2001	6 mo IFN (n = 40) vs 12 mo combination (n = 20)	20 vs 25/15 vs 40	NA vs NA/2.5 vs 20	No	25
De Vera,[95] 2001	IFN + Rbv ≥ 12 mo	77/9	71/9	No	40
Narayanan,[96] 2002	12 mo IFN + Rbv	42/35	NA	Yes	50
Lavezzo,[97] 2002	12 mo IFN-Rbv (n = 30) vs 6 mo IFN-Rbv (n = 27)	66 vs 53/23 vs 33	37 vs 30/17 vs 22	Yes	5
Samuel,[98] 2003	IFN + Rbv (n = 28) vs placebo (n = 24)	NA/32	18/21	No	43

*The sustained virological response was significantly higher in patients infected with HCV genotypes 2, 3, and 4 than in those infected with HCV genotype 1.
D/C, discontinuation; IFN, interferon; NA, not available; Rbv, ribavirin.

after liver transplantation than in immunocompetent patients. Reasons for this lower rate include high levels of viremia, high frequency of HCV genotype 1 in these patients, and low tolerability of interferon and ribavirin leading to frequent dose reductions. Many patients have renal insufficiency secondary to immunosuppressive agents, and because of impaired renal clearance of ribavirin, drug-associated hemolysis can be profound. Thus, if ribavirin is initiated as part of combination therapy, the dose should be 600 to 800 mg, depending on renal function and the presence of anemia. There are no clear data to support one specific immunosuppressive agent over another in patients receiving HCV antiviral therapy.

In summary, although the results with combination therapy are better than those with monotherapy, they are clearly insufficient for a patient population characterized by a more aggressive course of hepatitis. Although the side effects are comparable to those seen in nontransplant patients, the rate of drug discontinuation is significantly higher, mainly because of anemia. The use of erythropoietin and dosage adjustment of ribavirin may help reduce this rate of discontinuation. Many aspects still need to be addressed, such as the optimal dose and duration, whether ribavirin maintenance is needed after discontinuation of interferon, or the potential benefit of using stimulating factors.

In conclusion, each of the strategies has advantages and disadvantages. Prophylactic therapy while the patient is awaiting transplantation is the best theoretical approach. It is, however, limited by the low tolerability of antiviral agents. It is unlikely that this approach will have a major impact on posttransplant recurrence of HCV, since only a relatively small proportion of patients qualify for therapy. In addition, treatment with interferon may result in the selection of more virulent or resistant viral strains and ultimately lead to a more aggressive course of the disease or to a posttransplant situation in which no antivirals are available if needed.

Preemptive posttransplant therapy is also attractive. However, it is unknown whether this approach reduces the risk of recurrent hepatitis C or whether it only delays its recurrence. In addition, HCV RNA levels increase rapidly after transplantation, so the window for initiation of treatment with a low viral load is narrow. Finally, a significant proportion of patients are not candidates for therapy in the early posttransplant period, and tolerance of full doses of both drugs is unlikely. With the currently available treatments, treating established disease is probably the most cost-effective option. Although limited by relatively low efficacy, tolerance appears to be better, and treatment is offered only to patients in whom progressive disease develops.[99] In that sense, protocol liver biopsies may identify early histological changes that herald an aggressive course, and in these cases, therapeutic interventions may be implemented at earlier stages when a response appears to occur more frequently.

We anxiously await the development of true antiviral agents targeted specifically against HCV. With such therapies, one could anticipate a revolution in the outcome of patients transplanted for hepatitis C similar to that seen with the introduction of lamivudine for the management of patients undergoing transplantation for hepatitis B.

Retransplantation

With the continuing increase in the number of HCV-infected recipients potentially in need of retransplantation, it has become imperative to determine whether some or all patients with graft failure as a result of recurrent HCV disease are candidates for retransplantation. To date, there is reluctance to accept these patients for retransplantation, particularly those in whom recurrent disease leading to graft failure develops over a short period. Concern regarding retransplantation in this population relates to four issues: (1) early reports suggesting a worse outcome after retransplantation in these patients than in those undergoing retransplantation for other indications[100,101]; (2) uncertainty regarding the natural history of recurrent hepatitis C in the second graft; (3) advanced age of the recipient, since most had their first transplant in their late forties to early fifties; and (4) the ever-present organ shortage. However, some recent reports have indicated improved outcomes, particularly when retransplantation is performed before the development of infectious and renal complications[102,103] or the occurrence of advanced liver dysfunction as indicated by their MELD score. Still, the results of retransplantation are inferior to those of primary transplantation regardless of cause.[1,103] In addition, preliminary data suggest that the severity of recurrent hepatitis C in the second graft is related to that observed in the first graft.[104] Some consensus regarding this issue is urgently needed, since retransplantation on a large scale for recurrent hepatitis C would have a significant impact on outcomes, resource utilization, and perhaps even donation.[105]

Conclusion

There are a certain number of proven concepts regarding HCV infection in the setting of liver transplantation, including (1) a progressive increase in the number of patients infected with HCV who are in need of a first or second transplant; (2) universal viral reinfection; (3) extremely low risk of de novo HCV infection; (4) recurrent hepatitis C in the majority with progression to cirrhosis in a substantial proportion of patients over time; (5) a variable natural history of disease measured histologically that ranges from minimal damage to cholestatic hepatitis; (7) acceptable graft and patient survival with short- and medium-term follow-up, but inferior to that of uninfected controls; (8) lack of effective prophylactic therapies to prevent recurrence; and (9) limited efficacy of current antivirals in the treatment of posttransplant HCV disease.

A number of important issues remain to be investigated, including (1) optimal management of HCV-infected patients awaiting liver transplantation, in particular, decreasing waiting list mortality with the use of HCV-infected organ donors or antiviral drugs (or both) before transplantation; (2) expansion of the donor pool; (3) improved understanding of the long-term outcome of HCV-positive liver transplant recipients and the variables associated with outcome; (4) improving the management of recurrent hepatitis C, particularly with regard to immunosuppression; (5) evaluation of new approaches to the prevention or treatment (or both) of HCV reinfection; (6) defining the outcome of HCV-positive patients undergoing living related liver transplantation; and (7) development of a consensus regarding retransplantation in patients with allograft failure secondary to recurrent HCV disease.

Pearls and Pitfalls

- Chronic HCV infection leading to cirrhosis and hepatocellular carcinoma is the most common indication for liver transplantation in Western countries.

- Long-term posttransplant survival is reduced in comparison to that in patients with nonmalignant indications.

- Viral recurrence is universal and leads to chronic graft hepatitis in the majority of recipients.

- Progression of hepatitis C to cirrhosis is accelerated in liver transplant recipients when compared with immunocompetent patients.

- The interaction between host, viral, and external factors, particularly the rate of viral replication before and early after transplantation, the age of the donor, and the degree of immunosuppression, determines the natural history of recurrent hepatitis C.

- Treatment of established recurrent hepatitis C with (pegylated) interferon in combination with ribavirin yields lower rates of sustained virological response (ranging from 8% to 33%) than in the nontransplant population.

References

1. United Network for Organ Sharing. Available at http://www.unet.org. Accessed May 2002.
2. Seeff LB: Natural history of chronic hepatitis C. Hepatology 36 (5 Suppl 1):S35-S46, 2002.
3. Ghany MG, Kleiner DE, Alter H, et al: Progression of fibrosis in chronic hepatitis C. Gastroenterology 124:97-104, 2003.
4. Fattovitch G, Giustina G, Degos F, et al: Morbidity and mortality in compensated cirrhosis type C: A retrospective follow-up study of 384 patients. Gastroenterology 112:463-472, 1997.
5. Serfaty L, Aumaître H, Chazouillères O, et al: Determinants of outcome of compensated hepatitis C virus–related cirrhosis. Hepatology 27:1435-1440, 1998.
6. Hu KQ, Tong MJ: The long-term outcomes of patients with compensated hepatitis C virus–related cirrhosis and history of parenteral exposure in the United States. Hepatology 29:1311-1316, 1999.
7. Poynard T, McHutchison J, Manns M, et al: Impact of pegylated interferon alfa-2b and ribavirin on liver fibrosis in patients with chronic hepatitis C. Gastroenterology 122:1303-1313, 2002.
8. Wright TL: Treatment of patients with hepatitis C and cirrhosis. Hepatology 36(5 Suppl 1):S185-S194, 2002.
9. Davis GL, Albright JE, Cook SF, Rosenberg DM: Projecting future complications of chronic hepatitis C in the United States. Liver Transpl 9:331-338, 2003.
10. Wiesner RH, McDiarmid SV, Kamath PS: MELD and PELD: Application of survival models to liver allocation. Liver Transpl 7:567-580, 2001.
11. Onaca NN, Levy MF, Netto GJ, et al: Pretransplant MELD score as a predictor of outcome after liver transplantation for chronic hepatitis C. Am J Transplant 3:626-630, 2003.
12. Suarez Y, Franca ACV, Llovet JM, et al: The current status of liver transplantation for primary hepatic malignancy. Clin Liver Dis 4:591-605, 2000.
13. Garcia-Retortillo M, Forns X, Feliu A, et al: Hepatitis C virus kinetics during and immediately after liver transplantation. Hepatology 35:680-687, 2002.
14. Chazouilleres O, Kim M, Combs C, et al: Quantitation of hepatitis C virus RNA in liver transplant recipients. Gastroenterology 106:994-999, 1994.
15. Everhart JE, Wei Y, Eng H, et al: Recurrent and new hepatitis C virus infection after liver transplantation. Hepatology 29:1220-1226, 1999.
16. Charlton M, Seaberg E, Wiesner R, et al: Predictors of patient and graft survival following liver transplantation for hepatitis C. Hepatology 28:823-830, 1998.
17. Sreekumar R, Gonzalez-Koch A, Maor-Kendler Y, et al: Early identification of recipients with progressive histologic recurrence of hepatitis C after liver transplantation. Hepatology 32:1125-1130, 2000.
18. Gane E, Portmann B, Naoumov N, et al: Long-term outcome of hepatitis C infection after liver transplantation. N Engl J Med 334:815-820, 1996.
19. Prieto M, Berenguer M, Rayón M, et al: High incidence of allograft cirrhosis in hepatitis C virus genotype 1b infection following transplantation: Relationship with rejection episodes. Hepatology 29:250-256, 1999.
20. Berenguer M, Rayón M, Prieto M, et al: Are post-transplantation protocol liver biopsies useful in the long-term? Liver Transpl 7:790-796, 2001.
21. Sebagh M, Rifai K, Feray C, et al: All liver recipients benefit from the protocol 10-year liver biopsies. Hepatology 37:1293-1301, 2003.
22. Berenguer M, Lopez-Labrador FX, Wright TL: Hepatitis C and liver transplantation. J Hepatol 35:666-678, 2001.

23. Petrovic LM, Villamil FG, Vierling JM, et al: Comparison of histopathology in acute allograft rejection and recurrent hepatitis C infection after liver transplantation. Liver Transpl Surg 3:398-406, 1997.

24. Guido M, Thung SN: Distinguishing rejection from recurrent viral hepatitis on liver biopsy. Viral Hepatitis 4:127-136, 1998.

25. Charlton M, Seaberg E: Impact of immunosuppression and acute rejection on recurrence of hepatitis C: Results of the National Institute of Diabetes and Digestive and Kidney Diseases Liver Transplantation Database. Liver Transpl Surg 5(Suppl):S107-S114, 1999.

26. Sreekumar R, Rasmussen DL, Wiesner RH, Charlton MR: Differential allograft gene expression in acute cellular rejection and recurrence of hepatitis C after liver transplantation. Liver Transpl 8:814-821, 2002.

27. Feray C, Caccamo L, Alexander GJM, et al: European Collaborative Study on factors influencing the outcome after liver transplantation for hepatitis C. Gastroenterology 117:619-625, 1999.

28. Testa G, Crippin JS, Netto GJ, et al: Liver transplantation for hepatitis C: Recurrence and disease progression in 300 patients. Liver Transpl 6:553-561, 2000.

29. Sanchez-Fueyos A, Restrepo J-C, Quintó L, et al: Impact of the recurrence of hepatitis C infection after liver transplantation on the long term viability of the graft. Transplantation 73:56-63, 2002.

30. Berenguer M, Prieto M, San Juan F, et al: Contribution of donor age to the recent decrease in patient survival among HCV-infected liver transplant recipients. Hepatology 36:202-210, 2002.

31. Schluger L, Sheiner P, Thung S, et al: Severe recurrent cholestatic hepatitis C following orthotopic liver transplantation. Hepatology 23:971-976, 1996.

32. Doughty AL, Spencer JD, Cossart YE, McCaughan GW: Cholestatic hepatitis after liver transplantation is associated with persistently high serum hepatitis C virus RNA levels. Liver Transpl Surg 4:15-21, 1998.

33. McCaughan GW, Zekry A: Pathogenesis of hepatitis C virus recurrence in the liver allograft. Liver Transpl 8(Suppl 1):S7-S13, 2002.

34. Berenguer M, Ferrell L, Watson J, et al: HCV-related fibrosis progression following liver transplantation: Increase in recent years. J Hepatol 32:673-684, 2000.

35. Berenguer M, Prieto M, Rayon JM, et al: Natural history of clinically compensated HCV-related graft cirrhosis following liver transplantation. Hepatology 32:852-858, 2000.

36. Berenguer M, Crippin J, Gish R, et al: A model to predict severe HCV-related disease following liver transplantation. Hepatology 38:34-41, 2003.

37. Forman LM, Lewis JD, Berlin JA, et al: The association between hepatitis C infection and survival after orthotopic liver transplantation. Gastroenterology 122:889-896, 2002.

38. Prachalias AA, Pozniak A, Taylor C, et al: Liver transplantation in adults coinfected with HIV. Transplantation 72:1684-1688, 2001.

39. Neff GW, Bonham A, Tzakis AG, et al: Orthotopic liver transplantation in patients with human immunodeficiency virus and end-stage liver disease. Liver Transpl 9:239-247, 2003.

40. Rosen H, Chou S, Corless C, et al: Cytomegalovirus viremia. Risk factor for allograft cirrhosis after liver transplantation for hepatitis C. Transplantation 64:721-726, 1997.

41. Burak KW, Kremers WK, Batts KP, et al: Impact of cytomegalovirus infection, year of transplantation, and donor age on outcomes after liver transplantation for hepatitis C. Liver Transpl 8:362-369, 2002.

42. Sheiner PA, Schwartz ME, Mor E, et al: Severe or multiple rejection episodes are associated with early recurrence of hepatitis C after orthotopic liver transplantation. Hepatology 21:30-34, 1995.

43. Berenguer M, Prieto M, Córdoba J, et al: Early development of chronic active hepatitis in recurrent hepatitis C virus infection after liver transplantation: Association with treatment of rejection. J Hepatol 28:756-763, 1998.

44. Gane E, Naoumov N, Qian K, et al: A longitudinal analysis of hepatitis C virus replication following liver transplantation. Gastroenterology 110:167-177, 1996.

45. Rosen HR, Shackleton CR, Higa L, et al: Use of OKT3 is associated with early and severe recurrence of hepatitis C after liver transplantation. Am J Gastroenterol 92:1453-1457, 1997.

46. Eason JD, Nair S, Cohen AJ, et al: Steroid-free liver transplantation using rabbit antithymocyte globulin and early tacrolimus monotherapy. Transplantation 75:1396-1399, 2003.

47. Brillanti S, Vivarelli M, De Ruvo N, et al: Slowly tapering off steroids protects the graft against hepatitis C recurrence after liver transplantation. Liver Transpl 8:884-888, 2002.

48. Nelson DR, Soldevila-Pico C, Reed A, et al: The effect of anti–interleukin-2 receptor therapy on the course of hepatitis C recurrence after liver transplantation. Liver Transpl 7:1064-1070, 2001.

49. Bahra M, Neumann UP, Harren M, et al: Significance of mycophenolate mofetil treatment in patients with HCV reinfection after liver transplantation: Impact on clinical course and histologic damage. Transplant Proc 34:2934-2935, 2002.

50. Fischer L, Sterneck M, Gahlemann CG, et al: Prospective study comparing safety and efficacy of mycophenolate mofetil versus azathioprine in primary liver transplant recipients. Transplant Proc 32:2125-2127, 2000.

51. Jain A, Kashyap R, Demetris AJ, et al: A prospective randomized trial of mycophenolate mofetil in liver transplant recipients with hepatitis C. Liver Transpl 8:40-46, 2002.

52. Fasola CG, Netto GJ, Jennings LW, et al: Recurrence of hepatitis C in liver transplant recipients treated with mycophenolate mofetil. Transplant Proc 34:1563-1564, 2002.

53. Calmus Y, Scheele JR, Gonzalez-Pinto I, et al: Immuno-prophylaxis with basiliximab, a chimeric anti–interleukin-2 receptor monoclonal antibody, in combination with azathioprine-containing triple therapy in liver transplant recipients. Liver Transpl 8:123-131, 2002.

54. Neuhaus P, Clavien PA, Kittur D, et al: Improved treatment response with basiliximab immunoprophylaxis after liver transplantation: Results from a double-blind randomized placebo-controlled trial. Liver Transpl 8:132-142, 2002.

55. Berenguer M: Outcome of post-transplantation HCV-disease—is it the host, the virus or how we modify the host and/or the virus? Liver Transpl 8:889-891, 2002.

56. Rosen HR, Lentz JJ, Rose SL, et al: Donor polymorphism of tumor necrosis factor gene. Relationship with variable severity of hepatitis C recurrence after liver transplantation. Transplantation 68:1898-1902, 1999.

57. Manez R, Mateo R, Tabasco J, et al: The influence of HLA donor-recipient compatibility on the recurrence of HBV and HCV hepatitis after transplantation. Transplantation 59:640-642, 1994.

58. Cotler SJ, Gaur LK, Gretch DR, et al: Donor-recipient sharing of HLA class II alleles predicts earlier recurrence and accelerated progression of hepatitis C following liver transplantation. Tissue Antigens 52:435-443, 1998.

59. Di Martino V, Saurini F, Samuel D, et al: Long-term longitudinal study of intrahepatic hepatitis C virus replication after liver transplantation. Hepatology 26:1343-1350, 1997.

60. Zhou S, Terrault N, Ferrell L, et al: Severity of liver disease in liver transplantation recipients with hepatitis C virus infection: Relationship to genotype and level of viremia. Hepatology 24:1041-1046, 1996.

61. Vargas HE, Laskus T, Wang LF, et al: The influence of hepatitis C virus genotypes on the outcome of liver transplantation. Liver Transpl Surg 4:22-27, 1998.

62. Di Martino V, Brenot C, Samuel D, et al: Influence of liver hepatitis C virus RNA and hepatitis C virus genotype on Fas-mediated apoptosis after liver transplantation for hepatitis C. Transplantation 70:1390-1396, 2000.

63. Gigou M, Roque-Alfonso AM, Falissard B, et al: Genetic clustering of hepatitis C virus strains and severity of recurrent hepatitis after liver transplantation. J Virol 75:11,292-11,297, 2001.

64. Sullivan DG, Wilson JJ, Carithers RL Jr, et al: Multigene tracking of hepatitis C virus quasispecies after liver transplantation: Correlation of genetic diversification in the envelope region with asymptomatic or mild disease patterns. J Virol 72:10,036-10,043, 1998.

65. Doughty AL, Painter DM, McCaughan GW: Post-transplant quasispecies pattern remains stable over time in patients with recurrent cholestatic hepatitis due to hepatitis C virus. J Hepatol 32:10-20, 2000.

66. Pessoa MG, Bzowej NH, Berenguer M, et al: Evolution of hepatitis C (HCV) quasispecies in patients with severe cholestatic hepatitis following liver transplantation. Hepatology 30:1513-1520, 1999.

67. Pelletier SJ, Raymond DP, Crabtree TD, et al: Pretransplantation hepatitis C virus quasispecies may be predictive of outcome after liver transplantation. Hepatology 32:375-381, 2000.

68. Pelletier SJ, Raymond DP, Crabtree TD, et al: Hepatitis C–induced hepatic allograft injury is associated with a pre-transplantation elevated viral replication rate. Hepatology 32:418-426, 2000.

69. Wali M, Harrison RF, Gow PJ, Mutimer D: Advancing donor liver age and rapid fibrosis progression following transplantation for hepatitis C. Gut 51:248-252, 2002.

70. Imber CJ, St Peter SD, Lopez I, et al: Current practice regarding the use of fatty livers: A trans-Atlantic survey. Liver Transpl 8:545-549, 2002.

71. Laskus T, Wang LF, Rakela J, et al: Dynamic behavior of hepatitis C virus in chronically infected patients receiving liver graft from infected donors. Virology 220:171-176, 1996.

72. Testa G, Goldstein RM, Netto G, et al: Long-term outcome of patients transplanted with livers from hepatitis C–positive donors. Transplantation 65:925-929, 1998.

73. Vargas HE, Laskus T, Wang LF, et al: Outcome of liver transplantation in hepatitis C virus–infected patients who received hepatitis C virus–infected grafts. Gastroenterology 117:149-153, 1999.

74. Velidedeoglu E, Desai NM, Campos L, et al: The outcome of liver grafts procured from hepatitis C–positive donors. Transplantation 73:582-587, 2002.

75. Baron PW, Sindram D, Higdon D, et al: Prolonged rewarming time during allograft implantation predisposes to recurrent hepatitis C infection after liver transplantation. Liver Transpl 6:407-412, 2000.

76. Rosen HR, Gretch DR, Oehlke M, et al: Timing and severity of initial hepatitis C recurrence as predictors of long-term liver allograft injury. Transplantation 65:1178-1182, 1998.

77. Guido M, Fagiuoli S, Tessari G, et al: Histology predicts cirrhotic evolution of post transplant hepatitis C. Gut 50:697-700, 2002.

78. Feray C, Gigou M, Samuel D, et al: Incidence of hepatitis C in patients receiving different preparations of hepatitis B immunoglobulins after liver transplantation. Ann Intern Med 128:810-816, 1998.

79. Berenguer M, Terrault NA, Piatak M, et al: Hepatitis G virus infection in patients with hepatitis C virus infection undergoing liver transplantation. Gastroenterology 111:1569-1575, 1996.

80. Neuberger J, Schulz KH, Day C, et al: Transplantation for alcoholic liver disease. J Hepatol 36:130-137, 2002.

81. Willems B, Ede M, Marotta P, et al: Anti-HCV human immunoglobulins for the prevention of graft infection in HCV-related liver transplantation, a pilot study [abstract]. J Hepatol 36(Suppl 1):96, 2002.

82. Crippin JS, Sheiner P, Terrault NA, et al: A pilot study of the tolerability and efficacy of antiviral therapy in patients awaiting liver transplantation for hepatitis C. Liver Transpl 8:350-355, 2002.

83. Everson GT, Trouillot T, Trotter J, et al: Treatment of decompensated cirrhotics with a slow-accelerating dose regimen (LADR) of interferon-alfa-2b plus ribavirin: Safety and efficacy [abstract]. Hepatology 32:308A, 2000.

84. Sheiner P, Boros P, Klion FM, et al: The efficacy of prophylactic interferon alfa-2b in preventing recurrent hepatitis C after liver transplantation. Hepatology 28:831-838, 1998.

85. Singh N, Gayowski T, Wannstedt C, et al: Interferon-α for prophylaxis of recurrent viral hepatitis C in liver transplant recipients. Transplantation 65:82-86, 1998.

86. Mazzaferro V, Tagger A, Schiavo M, et al: Prevention of recurrent hepatitis C after liver transplantation with early interferon and ribavirin treatment. Transplant Proc 33:1355-1357, 2001.

87. Terrault N, Khalili M, Bollinger K, et al: Limitations in the use of a prophylactic antiviral strategy in hepatitis C infected patients undergoing liver transplantation [abstract]. Hepatology 36:177A, 2002.

88. Wright TL, Combs C, Kim M, et al: Interferon alpha therapy for hepatitis C virus infection following liver transplantation. Hepatology 20:773-779, 1994.

89. Feray C, Samuel D, Gigou M, et al: An open trial of interferon alfa recombinant for hepatitis C after liver transplantation: Antiviral effects and risk of rejection. Hepatology 22:1084-1089, 1995.

90. Gane EJ, Lo SK, Riordan SM, et al: A randomized study comparing ribavirin and interferon alfa monotherapy for hepatitis C recurrence after liver transplantation. Hepatology 27:1403-1407, 1998.

91. Bizollon T, Palazzo U, Ducerf C, et al: Pilot study of the combination of interferon alfa and ribavirin as therapy of recurrent hepatitis C after liver transplantation. Hepatology 26:500-504, 1997.

92. Alberti AB, Belli LS, Airoldi A, et al: Combined therapy with interferon and low-dose ribavirin in posttransplantation recurrent hepatitis C: A pragmatic study. Liver Transpl 7:870-876, 2001.

93. Gopal DV, Rabkin JM, Berk BS, et al: Treatment of progressive hepatitis C recurrence after liver transplantation with combination interferon plus ribavirin. Liver Transpl 7:181-190, 2001.

94. Ahmad J, Dodson SF, Demetris AJ, et al: Recurrent hepatitis C after liver transplantation: A nonrandomized trial of interferon alfa alone versus interferon alfa and ribavirin. Liver Transpl 7:863-869, 2001.

95. De Vera ME, Smallwood GA, Rosado K, et al: Interferon-alpha and ribavirin for the treatment of recurrent hepatitis C after liver transplantation. Transplantation 71:678-686, 2001.

96. Narayanan M, Poterucha JJ, El-Amin OM, et al: Treatment of posttransplantation recurrence of hepatitis C with interferon and ribavirin: Lessons on tolerability and efficacy. Liver Transpl 8:623-629, 2002.

97. Lavezzo B, Franchello A, Smedile A, et al: Treatment of recurrent hepatitis C in liver transplants: Efficacy of a six versus twelve month course of interferon alfa 2b with ribavirin. J Hepatol 37:247-252, 2002.

98. Samuel D, Bizollon T, Feray C, et al: Interferon-alfa 2b plus ribavirin in patients with chronic hepatitis C after liver transplantation: A randomized study. Gastroenterology 124:642-650, 2003.

99. Saab S, Ly D, Han SB, et al: Is it cost-effective to treat recurrent hepatitis C infection in orthotopic liver transplantation patients? Liver Transpl 8:449-457, 2002.

100. Sheiner PA, Schluger LK, Emre S, et al: Retransplantation for recurrent hepatitis C. Liver Transpl Surg 3:130-136, 1997.
101. Rosen H, O'Reilly P, Shackleton C, et al: Graft loss following liver transplantation in patients with chronic hepatitis C. Transplantation 62:1773-1776, 1997.
102. Rosen HR, Madden JP, Martin P: A model to predict survival following liver retransplantation. Hepatology 29:365-370, 1999.
103. Busuttil RW, Shaked A, Millis JM, et al: One thousand liver transplants. The lessons learned. Ann Surg 219:490-499, 1994.
104. Berenguer M, Prieto M, Palau A, et al: Severe recurrent hepatitis C following liver retransplantation for HCV-related graft failure. Liver Transpl 9:228-235, 2002.
105. Biggins SW, Beldecos A, Rabkin JM, Rosen HR: Retransplantation for hepatic allograft failure: Prognostic modeling and ethical considerations. Liver Transpl 8:313-322, 2002.

Transplantation for Fulminant Hepatic Failure

STEPHEN M. RIORDAN
ROGER WILLIAMS

Etiological considerations   162
  Acetaminophen   163
  Hepatitis viruses   163
  Other causes   165

Selection criteria for transplantation   165
  King's College criteria   165
  Other prognostic criteria   167

Trends in transplantation activity   169

Outcome of transplantation   169
  Auxiliary partial transplantation   170
  Living related transplantation   170

Supportive treatment in the pretransplant
  period   171

Role of extracorporeal and cell-based liver
  support   173

Fulminant hepatic failure (FHF) is defined by the presence of hepatic encephalopathy occurring as the consequence of severe liver damage in patients without previous, clinically overt liver disease. Components of the clinical syndrome may include cerebral edema, hemodynamic instability, renal failure, coagulopathy, metabolic disturbances, and susceptibility to bacterial and fungal infection. The causes of FHF vary according to geographical location, although hepatotoxicity caused by acetaminophen is now the most common cause in many Western countries, followed by drug reactions. In a small proportion of FHF patients the cause cannot be determined, and there is speculation that the source may be an as yet unknown hepatitis virus. Despite considerable investigation, however, a new non–A-to-non–E hepatitis virus has not been identified.

In its most severe form, FHF carries a high mortality unless urgent liver transplantation is performed. When a patient does not satisfy the selection criteria that are currently used to qualify for orthotopic liver transplantation (OLT), it is not a reliable predictor that the patient will experience spontaneous survival. There is an urgent need to refine prognostic criteria to improve the identification of patients who can confidently be managed by medical means alone. The most recent analysis from the European Liver Transplant Registry (ELTR) documents 1-, 5-, and 10-year survival rates following deceased-donor OLT for FHF of 63%, 59%, and 54%, respectively. The plateau in mortality rate 3 months after transplantation reflects the fact that patients who undergo transplantation are critically ill before the procedure and often undergo a complicated early postoperative period. Patients who survive beyond the first 3 months after transplantation follow a survival curve comparable to that seen following elective transplantation performed for cirrhosis. Despite much enthusiasm for temporary liver support strategies based on extracorporeal perfusion or transplantation of hepatocytes, none of those techniques (which have been used clinically to date) are of proven overall benefit either in enhancing spontaneous survival or as a bridge to liver transplantation.

FHF was originally described as occurring within 8 weeks of the onset of symptoms in patients without preexisting liver disease.[1] It is a potentially devastating syndrome that may include cerebral edema, hemodynamic instability, renal failure, coagulopathy, profound metabolic disturbances, and a particular susceptibility to bacterial and fungal infection. Other definitions have alternatively been proposed that recognize the jaundice-to-encephalopathy time as an important prognostic index.[2] In contrast to the original description, these other classifications allow for the inclusion of cases with previously asymptomatic chronic liver conditions, such as fulminant presentations of Wilson's disease with underlying cirrhosis and fulminant reactivation of hepatitis B in chronic carriers.

Increasing evidence suggests that liver damage in FHF results both as a direct consequence of the initiating drug, toxin, virus, or other cause and from the subsequent activation of various nonparenchymal cells with release of cytokines. Accumulation of toxins such as ammonia and lactate, along with deleterious effects of vasoactive cytokines produced in response to the initiating cause of liver injury or complicating sepsis, or both, contribute to the development of multiorgan dysfunction in FHF. Adrenal insufficiency may contribute to the propensity for systemic hypotension,[3] as occurs in severe sepsis. The recent finding of a normal hepatic venous pyruvate-to-lactate ratio suggests that accelerated glycolysis, rather than tissue hypoxia, accounts for accumulation of lactate,[4] which has been implicated in the pathogenesis of cerebral edema in FHF.[5] Increased glycolysis is a known consequence of the systemic inflammatory response syndrome (SIRS), and may be the mechanism underlying the observation of a significant association between the severity of the SIRS and the grade of hepatic encephalopathy in FHF.[6] Sepsis is a major cause of SIRS in FHF, and sepsis-related oxidative stress both promotes hepatocellular necrosis and inhibits liver cell regeneration, upon which spontaneous recovery ultimately depends. Complicating sepsis also exacerbates the already increased energy requirements of FHF.

Although advances in supportive medical care have improved survival, FHF in its most severe form continues to carry a high mortality rate unless emergency OLT is performed. FHF currently accounts for approximately 10% of all primary indications for OLT in Europe, the United States, and Australia. Nonetheless, the rapidity with which the clinical syndrome often progresses, along with a worldwide shortage of deceased-donor organs, so that many patients die or develop contraindications to transplantation (such as sepsis) before a donor liver becomes available, even with priority listing, limits the applicability of OLT in the FHF setting. To help overcome this problem, using living related donors for OLT has been introduced as a therapeutic option for FHF both in pediatric and, more recently, adult patients.

Irrespective of the source of the donor liver, the risk of serious side effects from long-term pharmacological immunosuppression means that conventional OLT cannot be considered a panacea for FHF. Consequently, recent interest has centered on the possibility of providing temporary liver support in the form of auxiliary partial organ transplantation, use of extracorporeal artificial or bioartificial devices, or hepatocyte transplantation. The goal is not only that these solutions become a *bridge* to OLT but also that they allow time for, or even actively promote, native liver regeneration, thereby rendering OLT unnecessary.

Etiological Considerations

The prevalence of the various causes of FHF varies according to geographical location. This has relevance in that the likelihood of survival with supportive medical care, without need for transplantation, varies according to the cause. In particular, the rate of progression of the clinical syndrome varies according to its cause and, somewhat paradoxically, spontaneous survival with medical management alone is inversely related to the rapidity of onset of encephalopathy.[7] In a nontransplant series, survival was 36% when encephalopathy was hyperacute in onset, occurring within 1 week of the development of jaundice, but no more than 14% with longer jaundice-to-encephalopathy times. FHF caused by acetaminophen hepatotoxicity is nearly always hyperacute in onset, although the majority of cases related to infection with hepatitis A virus (HAV) and hepatitis B virus (HBV) (but a lower proportion of patients with the other etiologies discussed further on) also conform to this pattern.[2] Because of the rapidity of progression of encephalopathy in these hyperacute groups, patients may become comatose before deep jaundice has developed. Within the acetaminophen hepatotoxicity group, survival with medical management is inversely correlated with the grade of encephalopathy at admission, at least in nonacidotic patients.[8]

Acetaminophen

Hepatotoxicity caused by acetaminophen is by far the most frequent cause of FHF, and hence indication for emergency OLT for FHF, in the United Kingdom, accounting for 60% to 70% of cases in recent series.[9] Recent series from Denmark and the United States reported that acetaminophen is the most prevalent cause of FHF, in keeping with a trend toward greater numbers of cases in many Western countries and reflecting that acetaminophen remains the most commonly used substance in self-poisoning in these countries. An estimated 100,000 cases of intentional acetaminophen overdose are reported annually in the United States. Increasing numbers of overdose cases are also being recorded in Australia and many other parts of the world.

There is no evidence that increasing general awareness of the serious toxicity that acetaminophen can cause leads to a reduced frequency of overdose. Indeed, experience reported until the late 1990s in the United Kingdom is that rates of acetaminophen overdose with deliberate intent increased in both men and women in comparison to the late 1980s, with rates in males showing a relatively larger increase and approaching those in females. Nonetheless, a recent change in packaging and the introduction of measures designed to limit the quantity of acetaminophen that can be purchased without a prescription have had substantial impact, presumably by reducing the number of cases of FHF caused by overdose taken on impulse.[10] The direct result is that more donor organs are available for transplantation in patients with FHF from other causes.

Most instances of acetaminophen-induced FHF in the United Kingdom and Australia are the consequence of an overdose of the drug taken at a single time with suicidal or parasuicidal intent. Serious psychiatric disturbance contraindicates transplantation in only a minority of such patients. Cases of severe hepatotoxicity after ingestion of recommended (or near-recommended) doses of acetaminophen, mostly over several days to weeks, have also been reported, including in patients with chronic exposure to alcohol or to enzyme-inducing drugs, such as antituberculous chemotherapy (rifampicin and isoniazid) and anticonvulsants (phenytoin, carbamazepine, and phenobarbital). Clinicians in the United States place considerable emphasis on this, because the combination of alcohol and acetaminophen accounted for up to two thirds of all cases of acute liver failure (ALF) admitted to one center.[11]

The possibility that FHF may occur in chronic alcoholics who take acetaminophen for therapeutic reasons at recommended (or near-recommended) daily doses is addressed in a number of reports, mainly from the United States. In the studies, acetaminophen has generally been taken over periods of several days or longer. There are delays in presentation and recognition of the causative connection between acetaminophen use and hepatotoxicity in many of the reports of unintentional acetaminophen-induced hepatotoxicity at relatively low doses in association with chronic alcohol exposure. Such patients have often presented only after liver damage has been established, contributing to a poor prognosis without transplantation. Severe hepatotoxicity at recommended or near-recommended daily doses of acetaminophen has also been reported in the absence of chronic alcohol use or enzyme induction because of other causes, particularly in the context of prior starvation or malnutrition.[12]

Hepatitis Viruses

Any virus that can cause acute hepatitis may potentially give rise to FHF. Such viruses can be broadly categorized as those that primarily affect the liver, such as the hepatitis viruses (A to E), and those in which liver involvement may occur as part of disseminated infection. These include Epstein-Barr virus, cytomegalovirus (CMV), varicella-zoster virus, enteroviruses, parvovirus B19, adenovirus, and herpes simplex virus (HSV). The latter occurs mainly, although not exclusively, in immunosuppressed individuals and in children. FHF also occurs with infection with togavirus-like particles, papillomavirus, paramyxoviruses, and hemorrhagic fever viruses. Although viral hepatitis is decreasing as a cause of FHF in the West, where hepatotoxicity caused by acetaminophen predominates, it remains the major causative factor in a large part of the world, including Asia, the Western Pacific region, the Middle East, Africa, South America, and European centers.

In general, the frequency with which the different hepatitis viruses are responsible for FHF in a particular geographical location is a reflection of their underlying prevalence. HAV infection is common in countries where there is overcrowding and poor standards of sanitation. Nonetheless, HAV infection accounts for fewer than 10% of cases of FHF in most series. The risk of FHF caused by HAV infection increases markedly in those older than 40 years of age and in the setting of preexisting chronic liver disease. An increased prevalence of FHF following HAV superinfection in patients with chronic hepatitis C virus (HCV) infection in one series was attributed to an effect of HAV, in view of a reduced rate of HCV replication observed during acute HAV infection.[13]

A more prevalent cause of FHF on a worldwide basis is HBV. More than one third of the world's population has been infected with HBV, with an estimated 400 million chronic carriers of HBV throughout the world. HBV infection is highly endemic in Southeast Asia and the Western Pacific region, along with parts of the Mediterranean littoral, the Middle East, and sub-Saharan Africa. Accordingly, HBV infection is a particularly common cause of FHF in such areas. Infection with HBV is the most prevalent cause of FHF, and hence transplantation for FHF, in the Far East, France, and many other southern European countries. Nonetheless, universal childhood immunization programs undertaken in some countries over the past 10 to 15 years have had a substantial impact in reducing HBV surface antigen (HBsAg) carriage rates in preschool and early school-aged children, and it is hoped that FHF caused by this agent will, accordingly, become less common in the future. Reactivation of HBV, such as after withdrawal of immunosuppressive or cytotoxic chemotherapy for various hematological and other malignancies, is a well-recognized cause of FHF. Reactivation occurring in the context of chronic HBV carriage, unrelated to immunosuppression withdrawal, is more common than de novo HBV infection as a cause of FHF in Taiwan and other Far East countries. Use of antiviral agents, such as lamivudine or adefovir dipivoxil, may have a role in patients with detectable circulating HBV DNA levels, although viral replication is characteristically low or absent by the time of clinical presentation with FHF, and reports are conflicting as to their value. These agents should certainly be used prophylactically in HBV carriers undergoing chemotherapy or immunosuppressive treatment to reduce the likelihood of the development of FHF following immune reconstitution.[14]

Fulminant HBV infection results from an exaggerated host immune response in an attempt to clear the virus. Indeed, 50% to 66.6% of cases have lost HBsAg by or within a few days of clinical presentation. The diagnosis of acute HBV infection in such cases rests on the presence of anti-hepatitis B core (HBc) immunoglobulin (Ig) M in serum. However, a Japanese study of patients with FHF found that anti-HBc IgM was not measurable in serum in nearly 50% of patients in whom HBV was detected by a sensitive polymerase chain reaction (PCR) technique.[15] Evidence of HBV infection in seronegative individuals with FHF apparently caused by non-A, non-B hepatitis was first reported in San Francisco, where HBV DNA was detected in serum or liver tissue of 6 of 17 (35%) such patients.[16] HBV DNA was found in liver, but not in serum, in 50% of those for whom both serum and liver were available for analysis. HBV viral sequences may even be evident in liver tissue when immunohistochemical staining for HBsAg and hepatitis B core antigen (HBcAg) is negative. The potential clinical relevance of this latter situation is suggested by experience in the posttransplantation setting, in which serum markers may become positive in association with the use of immunosuppressive regimens. Nonetheless, evidence of *occult* HBV infection was not found in any patient with FHF of otherwise indeterminant cause in a more recent multicenter series of 22 such patients from the United States.[17]

There is an association between FHF and the precore mutant HBV strain, which has a point mutation at nucleotide 1896 in the precore region that results in a translational stop codon (preventing secretion of HBeAg). This mutant is highly prevalent in Asia, Africa, and the Middle East, especially in relation to HBV genotype D. Nonetheless, studies from the United States, France, and India, where the prevalence of the precore mutant is low, demonstrate that this mutation is not necessary for the development of fulminant hepatitis B. Additional HBV mutations involving nucleotides 1762 and 1764 within the precore promoter region can also result in increased viral replication and similarly impaired HBeAg synthesis. An association between such mutations and FHF has been reported in Japanese patients. Aritomi and colleagues[18] have demonstrated a correlation between mutations in the core promoter and precore regions of the HBV genome and the severity of HBV infection in Japan, with at least one such mutation present in all 7 patients with HBV-related FHF compared with 4 of 41 (9.8%) patients with self-limited, acute hepatitis B.

Both coinfection with HBV and hepatitis D virus (HDV) and superinfection of chronic HBV carriers with HDV are associated with development of FHF. Cases of FHF caused by dual HBV and HDV infection are becoming less common in southern Europe because the prevalence of HDV has decreased substantially in recent years. Evidence from India suggests a worse outcome in dual HBV- and HDV-infected FHF patients compared with those infected with HBV alone. Coinfection with HAV and HBV and superinfection of chronic HBV carriers with HAV leading to FHF have also been reported.

Hepatitis E virus (HEV) is an enterally transmitted RNA virus of the Calicivirus group for which no specific antiviral treatment is available. It is the most common cause of epidemic hepatitis and FHF in tropical countries such as India and other developing countries of Southeast Asia, accounting for 50% of cases of FHF in a recent series.[19] A particularly high prevalence of infection with HEV, along with a high mortality rate, occurs in pregnant women, especially during the second and third trimesters. HEV infection has also occasionally been implicated in a relatively small number of sporadic cases of FHF in the West. A vaccine for HEV is currently under development.

There is also a striking geographical difference in the prevalence of FHF related to HCV infection. In Japan and Taiwan, HCV positivity occurs in up to 59% of patients with FHF of presumed viral origin, but in whom markers for HAV and HBV are not present. Conversely, infection with HCV alone is an uncommon cause of FHF in the West and in India. Instances of FHF related to HCV have also been reported in Italian patients with chronic HCV infection following the withdrawal of chemotherapy, a situation analogous to that seen with chronic HBV infection. As in the latter circumstance, levels of HCV viremia were typically low at the time of the fulminant illness.

Although an as yet unidentified hepatitis virus has been presumed to be the cause of at least some of the cases in which no definite cause can be established, there is no evidence that it exists, and the prevalence of these indeterminate cases has fallen in many countries in recent years. The "no definite cause" group accounts for less than 10% of cases in a series from King's College Hospital, London.[20] The sporadic nature of such cases raises the possibility that exposure to an undisclosed drug or other toxin may be responsible. Figures are higher elsewhere, including 19% in the United States,[21] 14% to 18% in India,[22] and 16% in Taiwan.[23] Initial enthusiasm that three described viruses—namely GB virus-C (GBV-C)/hepatitis G virus (HGV), transfusion-transmitted virus (TTV), and the SEN virus—may account for some such cases has, to date, not been proved.

Other Causes

Documentation of cases of FHF caused by ingestion of food contaminated with the *Bacillus cereus* emetic toxin, which inhibits hepatic mitochondrial fatty-acid oxidation, raises the possibility that other hitherto poorly categorized mitochondrial toxins may be responsible for many cases currently considered of indeterminate cause. Nonacetaminophen drug reactions, mostly idiosyncratic, account for approximately 10% to 15% of cases of FHF in Western countries. Ecstasy (3,4-methylenedioxymethamphetamine) and other illicit drugs are increasingly recognized causes in our experience. Instances of severe liver damage with use of antiretroviral agents in patients with human immunodeficiency virus (HIV) infection are also recognized, either as a direct drug effect or in relation to immune reconstitution in the setting of associated chronic HBV or HCV infections.

Other uncommon causes of FHF include autoimmune hepatitis, pregnancy-related disorders such as acute fatty liver of pregnancy (AFLP) and the HELLP (hemolysis, elevated liver enzymes and low platelet count) syndrome, *Amanita phalloides* poisoning, veno-occlusive disease, acute Budd-Chiari syndrome, hepatic ischemia related to heart failure or septic shock, heatstroke, and Wilson's disease.

Selection Criteria for Transplantation

Selection criteria for OLT are based on indices that identify the most severely affected patients—those who have a poor prognosis with medical management alone. Reliable, clinically applicable, early markers of prognosis are required to accurately stratify risk in individual patients and ensure that those who are highly likely to die without OLT are listed as early as possible. The goals of the selection criteria are to maximize the time for a donor organ to be procured and, at the same time, to spare the patients in whom spontaneous recovery will otherwise occur from unnecessary transplantation.

King's College Criteria

Selection criteria for OLT in the setting of FHF are not currently standardized. Nonetheless, those formulated at King's College Hospital in London, following retrospective, multivariate analysis of possible prognostic factors in 588 patients treated medically between 1973 and 1985,[24] are the most widely applied (Table 11–1). The original assessment of accuracy of these indicators was based on consideration of outcome, again retrospective, in a further consecutive series of patients managed during 1986 and 1987, including 121 with FHF caused by acetaminophen and 54 with other causes. Positive predictive values for death (the proportions of those patients

Table 11–1. KING'S COLLEGE SELECTION CRITERIA FOR ORTHOTOPIC LIVER TRANSPLANTATION (OLT) ACCORDING TO CAUSE OF FULMINANT HEPATIC FAILURE

Cause	Selection Criteria for Orthotopic Liver Transplantation (OLT)
Acetaminophen	Arterial pH <7.30 despite normal intravascular filling pressures (irrespective of grade of encephalopathy) OR Prothrombin time >100 seconds + serum creatinine >300 μmol/L in patients with grade III or IV encephalopathy

Nonacetaminophen	Prothrombin time >100 seconds (irrespective of grade of encephalopathy) OR
	Any three of the following (irrespective of grade of encephalopathy):
	  Non-A, non-B hepatitis (cryptogenic), halothane hepatitis, or other drug toxicity
	  Age <10 years or >40 years
	  Jaundice-to-encephalopathy interval >7 days
	  Prothrombin time >50 seconds
	  Serum bilirubin >300 μmol/L

From O'Grady JG, Alexander GJM, Hayllar KM, et al: Early indicators of prognosis in fulminant hepatic failure. Gastroenterology 97:439-445, 1989.

fulfilling criteria who died) in the acetaminophen and nonacetaminophen groups were 84% and 98%, respectively, whereas negative predictive values (the proportions of those patients not fulfilling criteria who survived) were 86% and 82%, respectively. Predictive accuracies (the proportions of all patients in whom outcome was correctly predicted) were 85% and 94%, respectively.

Several subsequent reports from other centers using the King's College criteria indicated that although fulfillment of criteria carries a poor prognosis for spontaneous survival, lack of fulfillment carries a less favorable outlook than originally suggested,[7,9] leading to much uncertainty as to which patients can be managed without listing for urgent transplantation[25] (Table 11–2).

Table 11–2. VALIDATION OF THE KING'S COLLEGE PROGNOSTIC CRITERIA IN PATIENTS WITH FULMINANT HEPATIC FAILURE

	PPV (%)	NPV (%)	PA (%)
FHF Caused by Acetaminophen			
O'Grady et al: 1989 (London)[24]			
Arterial pH <7.3	95	78	81
PT >100 sec, serum creatinine >300 μmol/L, and grade III or IV encephalopathy	67	86	83
Overall	84	86	85
Anand et al: 1997 (Birmingham)[9]			
Arterial pH <7.3	77	64	70
PT >100 sec, serum creatinine >300 μmol/L, and grade III or IV encephalopathy	79	72	73
Overall	73	71	72
Shakil et al: 2000 (Pittsburgh)[7]			
Arterial pH <7.3	69	80	72
INR >6.5, serum creatinine >300 μmol/L, and grade III or IV encephalopathy	100	79	86
Bernal et al: 2002 (London)[27]			
Overall	80	94	—
Schmidt and Dalhoff, 2002 (Denmark)[29]			
Overall	80	93	92
FHF Caused by Nonacetaminophen Sources			
O'Grady et al: 1989 (London)[24]			
PT >100 sec	100	26	46
Any 3 of 5 variables*	96	82	92
Overall	98	82	94
Pauwels et al: 1993 (Paris)[26]			
Overall At admission	96	50	80
48 hours before death	89	47	79
Anand et al: 1997 (Birmingham)[9]			
PT >100 sec	100	37	52
Any 3 of 5 variables*	65	17	52
Overall	68	25	61
Shakil et al: 2000 (Pittsburgh)[7]			
PT >100 sec	98	50	79
Any 3 of 5 variables*	91	42	74

*PT >50 seconds; jaundice-to-encephalopathy time >7 days; non-A, non-B hepatitis, or drug-induced cause; age <10 years or >40 years; serum bilirubin >300 μmol/L.
PPV, positive predictive value; NPV, negative predictive value; PA, predictive accuracy; PT, prothrombin time; INR, international normalized ratio.
From Riordan SM, Williams R: Mechanisms of hepatocyte injury, multiorgan failure and prognostic criteria in acute liver failure. Semin Liver Dis 23:203-215, 2003.

Shakil and colleagues[7] reported retrospectively on the Pittsburgh experience with these criteria in 177 patients over a 13-year period to 1995, the first such assessment to be performed in the United States (adding to two previously published validation studies from the United Kingdom and Europe).[26] Nearly 50% of the patients in the Pittsburgh series underwent OLT a median of 3 days after admission. The spontaneous survival rate was 14%, whereas almost 40% of the patients who did not undergo OLT died a median of 6 days after admission. Patients who died without OLT were significantly more likely than those who survived spontaneously to have grade III or grade IV encephalopathy at the time of admission, in keeping with previous reports from the United Kingdom and the United States.[7,9,24] The large majority of patients who died without OLT had been considered transplant candidates, at least early in their clinical course. This is compatible with experience in the United Kingdom where approximately 35% of those initially suitable for OLT rapidly develop contraindications—such as uncontrolled cerebral edema, sepsis, severe hemodynamic disturbance, and multiorgan failure—and thus become unsuited for transplantation.[27]

The Pittsburgh analysis found that the King's College prognostic criteria carry acceptably high positive predictive values for death in patients with FHF caused by both acetaminophen and other sources. Negative predictive values in the acetaminophen group were also acceptably high in the Pittsburgh series, comparable to those documented in the original report. However, the negative predictive value in the nonacetaminophen group was found to be seriously lacking.

This observation—that the ability of the King's College criteria to predict which patients will survive without the need for urgent OLT was substantially lower than in the original report, especially in cases with nonacetaminophen causes—is in accord with previously reported studies. Two such studies were[9,26]:

- 81 patients managed at Hospital Saint-Antoine, Paris, between 1978 and 1988
- 145 patients treated at Queen Elizabeth Hospital, Birmingham, between 1990 and 1994

Overall predictive accuracies were somewhat reduced in each of these series in comparison to the original assessment (see Table 11–2).

These findings raised the possibility that other factors not currently included in the King's College criteria must also have prognostic importance. Indeed, Anand and colleagues[9] identified peak white cell count and hyperkalemia as additional, independent indicators of poor prognosis in patients with acetaminophen-related FHF. Although it is possible that the accuracy of prognostic criteria in this group may be improved by the inclusion of these parameters, any practical significance in terms of identifying patients whose prognosis would be improved by emergency OLT would likely be limited. This is because such abnormalities often occur relatively late in the clinical course and in the setting of contraindications such as sepsis and hemodynamic disturbance. In the nonacetaminophen group, negative predictive value was marginally improved without compromising positive predictive value by reducing the cut-off for prothrombin time from 100 seconds to 75 seconds.

The King's College criteria were recently reevaluated in another cohort of patients with FHF caused by acetaminophen managed at that center.[28] The positive predictive value was 80% compared with 84% in the original series, whereas the negative predictive value was 94%, even higher than the 86% found in the original series and in keeping with the figure of 93% in a recent series from Denmark.[29] With additional consideration of a postresuscitation arterial blood lactate level greater than 3.0 mmol/L, or either a postresuscitation or an *early* value greater than 3.5 mmol/L, negative predictive values were 97% and 99%, respectively. Positive predictive values fell to 79% and 74%, respectively. Additional consideration of blood lactate levels modestly improved the negative predictive value, but the positive predictive value remained higher with the initial King's College criteria alone (see Table 11–2). Nonetheless, patients with a poor outcome were identified earlier when blood lactate levels were taken into consideration.[28]

Other Prognostic Criteria

Alternate prognostic indices have been proposed. In a series of 58 nontransplanted patients (managed between 1986 and 1990) with acute viral hepatitis, mostly related to HBV infection, Bernuau and colleagues[29] in Clichy found that criteria based on the presence of coma or confusion in association with reduced factor V levels carried positive and negative predictive values for death of 82% and 98%, respectively. Clinically apparent encephalopathy was present on admission or subsequently in most, but not all, patients. However, a subsequently reported French study of 81 encephalopathic patients with nonacetaminophen-related FHF, mostly caused by acute viral hepatitis B as in the Clichy series, found a substantially lower ability of the Clichy criteria to identify correctly patients who will survive without OLT.[26] Furthermore, the Clichy criteria performed less well in this regard than the King's College criteria when both sets of indicators were applied to the same nonacetaminophen study population. The negative predictive values were 28% and 50%, respectively, on admission, and 36% and 47%, respectively, when reevaluated 48 hours before death,[26] a time chosen to approximate the mean waiting time for a donor liver in some European transplant series. By contrast, positive predictive values of the two sets of criteria were comparably high,[26] in keeping with a subsequent report on 17 patients from London.[30]

Nevens and colleagues,[31] in a Belgian series of 28 patients with nonacetaminophen-related FHF, found that overall predictive accuracy was modestly increased when both sets of criteria were considered in combination, although the ability to identify patients who will recover spontaneously remained low even in this circumstance. In the only reported comparative assessment of the two sets of criteria in acetaminophen-related FHF, Izumi and colleagues,[30] in a series of 81 patients, found that the Clichy criteria performed less well, with lower positive predictive value (49% versus 92%) and predictive accuracy (56% versus 83%). The negative predictive value was, however, acceptably high.

Taken together, these findings suggest that patients with either acetaminophen- or nonacetaminophen-related FHF who fulfill the King's College criteria and those with nonacetaminophen-related causes meeting the Clichy criteria should be listed for urgent OLT; an exception is nonacidotic patients with acetaminophen-related disease, when the encephalopathy grade is not advanced. Lack of fulfillment of prognostic criteria in current use may not reliably predict spontaneous survival, especially in cases unrelated to acetaminophen, and OLT should still be considered for this group. There is an urgent need to refine prognostic criteria in this group to improve the identification of patients who can confidently be managed by medical means alone. This already difficult issue will likely become even more complex as the use of temporary liver support based on extracorporeal perfusion or transplantation of hepatocytes or stem cells (as discussed further on) are proved to be of benefit.

Proposed alternate prognostic indices for FHF are:

- Factor VIII–to–factor V ratios
- Serial prothrombin times
- Assessment of liver size on computed tomography (CT) scanning
- Liver histology
- Acute Physiology and Chronic Health Evaluation (APACHE) score
- Sensory evoked potentials
- Serum levels of Gc-globulin (vitamin D–binding protein), which is an important liver-derived component of the extracellular actin-scavenging system
- Severity of the SIRS

There are varying degrees of applicability and reports of efficacy with all of these methods.[32]

In tropical areas of India, in which viral hepatitis is the most common cause of FHF, older age, cerebral edema, and degree of prolongation of prothrombin time are factors indicative of poor prognosis. As already referred to, fulminant presentations (with encephalopathy) of

Wilson's disease and Budd-Chiari syndrome in association with extensive hepatocellular necrosis are generally considered to represent indications for urgent OLT. Primary myeloproliferative disorders responsible for the Budd-Chiari syndrome should not be considered a contraindication to OLT.[32]

The possible prognostic value of circulating and intrahepatic cytokine levels is the subject of several recent reports. Circulating levels of both interleukin (IL)-6 and IL-8, but not tumor necrosis factor-α (TNF-α), were significantly higher in patients who subsequently died than in those who survived in a report from the United Kingdom.[33] The lack of correlation to degree of liver failure, as reflected by prothrombin time, serum bilirubin level, or degree of hepatic encephalopathy, suggests that these parameters do not reflect the severity of acute liver failure per se, but rather its complications (such as circulatory disturbance and resultant extrahepatic multiorgan failure). The value of incorporating such indices in prognostic modeling with the aim of selecting patients for transplantation is limited because the hemodynamic instability of which they are reflective otherwise precludes such intervention. A Japanese study found that circulating levels at hospital admission of TNF-α and IL-10, but not IL-6, were significantly higher in patients who died than in those who survived. In keeping with the United Kingdom experience, levels did not correlate significantly with degree of liver injury as reflected by serum transaminase values.[34] A German series found no significant correlations between intrahepatic levels of IL-12, interferon (IFN)-γ, or IL-10, at either protein or mRNA levels, and jaundice-to-encephalopathy time, encephalopathy grade, requirement for inotrope support, serum bilirubin level, prothrombin time, or APACHE II score.[35]

Hyperphosphatemia—possibly as a consequence of renal impairment and lack of substrate utilization because of blunted hepatic regenerative activity—has been reported to be an early predictor of poor outcome in severe acetaminophen-related liver injury.[29] In a series of 125 patients, including 30 with hepatic encephalopathy, a threshold phosphate concentration of 1.2 mmol/L or more at 48 to 96 hours after overdose had higher sensitivity (89% versus 67%), predictive accuracy (98% versus 92%), and positive (100% versus 80%) and negative (98% versus 93%) predictive values for death than the King's College criteria. Specificity was 100%. Consideration of the King's College criteria in combination with the phosphate level led to improvement in sensitivity to 94%. As with consideration of blood lactate levels,[28] patients with a poor outcome were identified substantially earlier using the phosphate criteria (median 1 hour after referral) than with the King's College guidelines (median of 12 hours).

The association between adrenal insufficiency and outcome has been assessed. Patients who did not survive to discharge from the intensive care unit or who underwent liver transplantation had significantly lower increment and peak cortisol levels after stimulation with synanthem than patients who survived. Higher incidences of subnormal increment and peak cortisol levels were found in nonsurvivors (55%) than in survivors (21%).[3] Nonetheless, the relative lack of both sensitivity and specificity limits the usefulness of these parameters for prognostic modeling in individual patients, at least when considered in isolation.

Trends in Transplantation Activity

Data from the National Transplant Database of the United Kingdom and Ireland indicate that the number of patients with acetaminophen-induced FHF who were listed for super-urgent OLT increased by more than 75% during the period from 1995 to 1998, accounting for 40% of all super-urgent listings and 38% of all super-urgent transplants in the 12 months preceding and including August 1998. Numbers have fallen progressively in recent years, with the proportion of patients listed and undergoing transplantation in 2001-2002 falling to 53% and 56% of their 1997-1998 values, respectively. As a corollary, the number of patients listed and undergoing transplantation for FHF of other causes has increased, including a more than 50% increase during 2001 to 2002 compared with 1997 to 1998 in the number of patients listed for acute graft dysfunction following transplantation.[20] This presumably reflects a greater use of expanded criteria liver grafts in elective circumstances. The number of patients undergoing transplantation for FHF caused by non–A-to-non–E hepatitis has also increased over this time.[20] This is a result of greater organ availability for super-urgent transplantation because of the reduction in acetaminophen-related procedures, rather than an increase in prevalence of FHF caused by seronegative hepatitis, as discussed earlier. Priority listing within the super-urgent category in the United Kingdom and Ireland offers the possibility of ABO-matched grafts being available within 24 to 72 hours.

Recent experience from the United States is that 66% of FHF patients listed for transplantation received a graft after a median waiting time of 3 days. Eighteen percent of those listed for urgent transplantation died on the waiting list after a median of 5 days. These findings indicate that lack of early donor organ availability remains a crucial factor that limits survival.[36] As in the United Kingdom, a relatively low percentage of acetaminophen-related cases compared with those with FHF caused by other causes come to transplantation because of the relatively high spontaneous survival rate.[36]

Outcome of Transplantation

The most recent analysis from the European Liver Transplant Registry (ELTR) (Hospital Paul Brousse, Villejuif, France) documents 1-, 5-, and 10-year survival rates following deceased-donor OLT for FHF of 63%, 59%, and 54%, respectively. The plateau in mortality rate 3 months after transplant surgery reflects the fact that patients who undergo transplantation are critically ill before the procedure and often undergo a complicated early postoperative period. Survival is substantially reduced in patients with sepsis and multiorgan failure prior to OLT.[37] Nonetheless, ELTR data indicate that patients who survive beyond the first 3 months follow a survival curve comparable to that seen following elective OLT performed for cirrhosis. A center workload of fewer than 25 transplants per year and fewer than 20 split-liver grafts per year was among risk factors for poor outcome following liver transplantation.[38] In the best centers, outcome with split-liver grafts is comparable to outcome following the use of full-sized organs.[39]

An important issue is the potential for virus-related cases of FHF to recur after transplantation, especially under the influence of immunosuppression. Patients who undergo transplantation for fulminant HBV infection have a significantly reduced rate of hepatitis B recurrence than those who undergo transplantation for HBV-related cirrhosis.[40] This presumably relates to the high prevalence of viral clearance prior to the procedure in the former setting. Recurrent HBV-related FHF is distinctly uncommon. Reports are conflicting as to whether coinfection with HDV favors a reduced incidence of hepatitis B recurrence following OLT, because of an inhibitory effect on HBV replication.[41,42] In patients in whom viral eradication is not attained before OLT, infection with the precore mutant HBV strain may be associated with more severe disease following OLT, with a substantially increased risk of HBV-related graft loss compared with that associated with wild-type infection reported in one study, although experience in patients who underwent transplantation specifically for fulminant hepatitis B is limited. Hepatitis B immunoglobulin, along with antiviral agents such as lamivudine, has an important role in prophylaxis against recurrent HBV infection in the posttransplant period.

Graft damage caused by recurrent HAV and other viral infections, including those described with togavirus-like particles, is occasionally seen following OLT for fulminant disease.[43] Although some degree of hepatitis C recurrence is almost universal following OLT for cirrhosis, there are few data in the FHF setting. Recurrence of hepatitis E has not been observed, although only a small number of patients have undergone transplantation for fulminant HEV infection to date.

To minimize the risk of clinically relevant viral recurrence, every effort is made to taper corticosteroid dosage rapidly in patients who undergo transplantation for virus-related FHF, with the aim of complete withdrawal within 3 months provided that graft function remains stable.

A retrospective comparison of costs and cost-effectiveness of OLT performed for FHF and cirrhosis has been reported.[44] Costs for up to 1 year after OLT were estimated to be Euro 107,675 for the cirrhosis group and Euro 90,792 for those who underwent transplantation for FHF. Nonetheless, OLT was considered less cost-effective when performed for FHF than when performed for cirrhosis because of the lower 1-year survival following OLT in the FHF group.

Auxiliary Partial Transplantation

An auxiliary partial OLT is performed when there is undoubted potential for spontaneous liver regeneration in FHF and may be considered a form of temporary liver support in most recipients. This technique involves the removal of the left or right lobe segment of the diseased liver and replacing it with the equivalent segment of the donor organ. Right lobe transplantation is generally used in adults, whereas a left lobe harvested from an adult may suffice for a child. Results published from a European Auxiliary Liver Transplant (EURALT) Registry cooperative study[45] show that:

- Survival rate with auxiliary partial OLT is comparable to that for conventional OLT in qualified patients.
- Immunosuppressive therapy can be withdrawn, leading to graft atrophy. This occurred in 65% of patients surviving at 1 year, in whom adequate regeneration of the native liver had occurred.

Similarly, full regeneration of the native liver was documented in 8 of 11 (74%) surviving patients in a series of 17 auxiliary partial OLT recipients from two French centers.[46] Immunosuppressive treatment was subsequently withdrawn or the dosage tapered in seven of these eight patients.

A different experience is reported by Azoulay and colleagues,[47] who compared auxiliary partial OLT with standard whole-liver transplantation in a consecutive series of 49 patients who underwent transplantation for fulminant or subfulminant hepatitis at another French center. OLT was performed in 37 patients and auxiliary partial OLT in 12. Each patient treated with auxiliary partial OLT was matched to 2 patients undergoing OLT according to age, coma grade, cause of liver failure, and clinical course. Although 1-year patient survival was identical (66%) in the two groups, the complication rate was higher in the auxiliary partial

OLT recipients. In particular, patients undergoing the auxiliary procedure experienced significantly more technical complications (1 ± 1.3 versus 0.3 ± 0.5), episodes of bacteriemia, requirement of retransplantation (3 of 12 patients versus 0 of 24 patients), and neurological sequelae or brain death (4 of 12 patients versus 2 of 24 patients). In only 2 of 12 auxiliary partial OLT recipients (17%) was the procedure a complete success, which was reflected by the ability to withdraw immunosuppression and patient survival. Experience with auxiliary partial OLT in the United States is limited.

Living Related Transplantation

In parts of the world where deceased-donor organ donation is not widely accepted, recourse has been made to the living related donor procedure, especially in children. The 1-year survival rates following living related OLT for FHF in a total of 35 pediatric cases in three reported series,[48-50] using left lobe and left lateral segments, ranged from 59% to 90%. Living related, left lobe, right lobe, and extended right lobe OLT also have been used successfully in adults with FHF. The 1-year survival rate in the largest reported series of 53 adult patients in Japan was 75%.[51] Pioneering work in Hong Kong demonstrates that a graft in excess of 40% of standard liver volume is often required to reverse the severe metabolic derangements that occur in FHF.[52,53] This can translate to the requirement for an extended right lobe graft for adult recipients, although few centers go as far as this. At least some degree of live donor graft injury is common in small-for-size adult recipients. In particular, patients receiving a right lobe graft less than 40% of standard liver weight often develop transient portal hypertension after reperfusion, accompanied by intragraft upregulation of endothelin-1 and ultrastructural evidence of sinusoidal damage.[54] A relatively high rate of biliary complications ranging from 15% to 64% has also been reported.[55] Nonetheless, availability of right lobe living related transplantation substantially improves the survival rate of adults with FHF, with 50% of patients enrolled in such a program surviving compared with only 6% of patients managed medically while awaiting a deceased-donor graft in a series from Hong Kong.[56]

Rigorous donor selection criteria, both physical and psychological, and expert postoperative care are required if the safety of the donor is not to be compromised. The reported incidence of donor death in the United States is approximately 0.2%.[57] This is substantially higher than that for kidney donation, which carries a risk of death of approximately 0.03%. No donor deaths have yet been reported from Asian centers.[58] There is concern about the ability to assess potential donors properly on an emergency basis, as is necessary when dealing with FHF. Although in the pediatric setting parents approach the possibility of living related liver transplantation with enthusiasm, a recent analysis found that almost two thirds of potential donors were ultimately considered unsuitable for organ donation, with both parents deemed unsuitable in more than 20% of cases.[59]

Living related adult-to-adult transplantation is increasingly performed in the United States, although concentrated in a few large-volume centers,[57] but the procedure still accounts for only a small proportion of transplants performed in the United States and the United Kingdom.

Supportive Treatment in the Pretransplant Period

Supportive medical interventions are aimed at maintaining hemodynamic, cerebral, and renal function; reversing metabolic derangements; preventing or

treating infection; preventing stress ulceration of gastric mucosa; and, when appropriate, treating coagulopathy. The overall aims are to allow time for liver regeneration to occur and to prevent contraindications to OLT, as discussed further on[60] (Table 11-3).

Controversy continues about the role of extradural pressure monitoring. In our experience, this procedure is of value in guiding therapy in ventilated patients with grade III or grade IV encephalopathy, particularly during OLT. This is because the increase in cerebral blood flow (CBF) that occurs with reperfusion may be deleterious, especially in those with defective autoregulation. The monitoring transducer must be inserted with sufficient clotting factor support to achieve an international normalized ratio (INR) of 2 or less, and platelet transfusions are needed to achieve a count of 50×10^9/L or more.[61] Nonetheless, such monitoring does carry some risk of hemorrhage at the time of insertion of the transducer or later, and the transducer should be removed no longer than 5 days after insertion because of the risk of infection.

Table 11-3. SUPPORTIVE MEDICAL MANAGEMENT IN THE PRETRANSPLANT PERIOD IN FULMINANT HEPATIC FAILURE

System	Aim	Intervention and Comments
Cardiovascular	Maintain hemodynamic stability	Exclude sepsis and ensure adequate intravascular filling; substantial volumes of colloid may be required given the often profound vasodilation; epinephrine or norepinephrine infusions are indicated if mean arterial pressure (MAP) is <60 mmHg despite adequate intravascular volumes. In FHF related to acetaminophen, N-acetylcysteine infusion was associated with improved systemic hemodynamic stability, a reduced incidence of multiorgan failure, and improved survival, even with late administration. Others have found a more variable systemic hemodynamic response to N-acetylcysteine, with clear responders and nonresponders. Improvement in indocyanine green clearance following N-acetylcysteine infusion in patients with a range of etiologies of FHF (in many instances out of proportion to changes in systemic hemodynamics) suggests a beneficial regional effect on the hepatosplanchnic circulation.
	Optimize oxygen delivery and consumption parameters	Based on the data claculated by the Fick method, N-acetylcysteine infusion was shown to significantly improve oxygen delivery and facilitate mean 46% and 29% increases in global tissue oxygen consumption after 30 min in patients with acetaminophen and other etiologies, respectively. Prostacyclin infusion also improved oxygen delivery and consumption, while combined infusions led to a significant increase in oxygen delivery but not consumption compared to infusion of N-acetylcysteine alone. Prostacyclin infusion prevented a fall in global tissue oxygen consumption related to use of inotropes. A recent study using indirect calorimetry rather than the Fick method found a smaller (6%) early improvement in global tissue oxygen consumption with N-acetylcysteine, which was not sustained throughout a 5-hour period of monitoring.
Neurological	Optimize cerebral blood flow (CBF), cerebral perfusion pressure (CPP), and oxygen consumption; prevent cerebral edema	Treatment with N-acetylcysteine has been reported to increase CBF and cerebral oxygen consumption, with a fall in anaerobic metabolism. Infusion of prostacyclin also improves CBF. A fall in CPP to <50 mmHg because of arterial hypotension should be managed with inotropes, provided that intravascular volume status is adequate. A reverse jugular venous oxygen saturation of 55%-75% and an arteriojugular venous lactate difference ≤35 mmol/L suggest an adequate CPP. Cooling of core body temperature to 32°-33° C is of value.

Continued

Table 11-3. SUPPORTIVE MEDICAL MANAGEMENT IN THE PRETRANSPLANT PERIOD IN FULMINANT HEPATIC FAILURE—cont'd

System	Aim	Intervention and Comments
	Treat established cerebral edema	Manage with the head raised by 20 to 30 degrees. Elective sedation and paralysis prevent surges in intracranial pressure (ICP). Bolus injection of mannitol is first-line treatment, leading to improved CBF and oxygen consumption with a fall in anaerobic metabolism. Prophylactic phenytoin reduces the incidence of exacerbating subclinical epilepsy. Thiopentone is used for intractable cerebral hypertension. Indomethacin may be effective. Consider hepatectomy during the period between organ retrieval and transplantation in cases for whom a donor liver has become available. Hyperventilation is appropriate in the subgroup with increased jugular venous oxygen saturation and elevated ICP suggestive of cerebral hyperemia. Extradural pressure monitoring is of particular value in transplant candidates, as a sudden increase in CBF occurs with reperfusion and may be deleterious, especially in those with defective autoregulation.
Renal	Maintain renal function or provide renal replacement therapy	Ensure adequate intravascular volume status and treat complicating infection. Therapeutic trials of low-dose dopamine and furosemide are often instituted, although efficacy is not proved. In patients with FHF related to acetaminophen, the incidence of renal failure requiring dialysis is reduced with N-acetylcysteine infusion, even after severe liver damage has occurred. When dialysis is required in FHF patients, continuous venovenous hemodialysis (CVVHD) is preferable to intermittent hemodialysis, as complicating hypotension with the latter results in a fall in CPP and exacerbates or precipitates cerebral edema. Indications for CVVHD include uncontrolled acidosis, hyperkalemia, fluid overload, and oliguria associated with a serum creatinine >300 μmol/L or cerebral edema requiring treatment with mannitol.
Metabolic	Meet caloric and nutritional demands	Caloric requirements of 35-50 kcal/kg are required to meet resting metabolic demand. Protein intakes in excess of 1g/kg/day are necessary to maintain nitrogen balance. Up to 50% of nonprotein calories should be delivered as lipid, using medium chain triglyceride supplements only in proven cases of steatorrhea. Hypoglycemia, hypophosphatemia, hypokalemia, and hypomagnesemia require aggressive replacement. Enteral nutrition is preferable to parenteral in view of maintained integrity of gut mucosa and reduced bacterial translocation and incidence of sepsis.
Immune	Prevent or treat infection	Prophylactic parenteral broad-spectrum antibiotic regimens combined with enteral amphotericin B and clotrimazole pessaries reduce the incidence of infection 20%. The latter approach is as effective as more intensive enteral decontamination regimens. Proven bacterial infection should be treated according to in vitro sensitivities, while invasive fungal infection requires parenteral treatment with an appropriate antifungal agent. In the absence of a positive isolate, consider fungal infection if fever is unresponsive to broad-spectrum antibiotics or if there is leukocytosis or deterioration in neurological status after initial improvement, especially in the presence of renal failure. Granulocyte colony stimulating factor improves neutrophil function in FHF and may have a role in preventing and treating infection in this group.
Gastrointestinal	Prevent stress ulceration	Prophylactic use of sucralfate is preferable to antisecretory drugs, which predispose to gastric bacterial overgrowth and nosocomial pneumonia.
Hematological	Reverse coagulopathy (in selected circumstances)	Because the prothrombin time is an important prognostic variable, infusion of fresh-frozen plasma is indicated only for bleeding or at the time of invasive procedures, such as insertion of intracranial pressure monitors. Platelet transfusions are required in the latter circumstances if the count is $<50 \times 10^9/L$ and prophylactically if the count is $<20 \times 10^9/L$.

From Riordan SM, Williams R: Fulminant hepatic failure. Clin Liver Dis 4:25-45, 2000.

Specific therapies and interventions to be considered include:

- A therapeutic trial of immunosuppression in autoimmune hepatitis and HELLP syndrome
- Urgent delivery of the fetus in AFLP
- Use of penicillin and silibinin as antidotes in *Amanita* poisoning
- Decompressive vascular shunting (surgically or radiologically achieved) in selected patients with veno-occlusive disease and acute Budd-Chiari syndrome

Investigation for an underlying procoagulant disorder is mandatory in patients with Budd-Chiari syndrome. Interventional radiology, including not only placement of a transjugular intrahepatic portosystemic shunt (TIPS) but also hepatic venous angioplasty and stenting of the inferior vena cava, may have a role in patients with hepatic venous outflow block, depending on the exact clinical context. Recognition of the rare fulminant presentation of Wilson's disease, suggested clinically by the presence of hemolysis, splenomegaly, and Kayser-Fleischer rings, is crucial as mortality in those with severe encephalopathy is virtually 100% without urgent OLT. By contrast, survival without transplantation can be achieved with early D-penicillamine treatment in most nonencephalopathic Wilson's disease patients who present acutely with other manifestations of severe hepatic insufficiency, which highlights the importance of early recognition of this disorder.[62] Lymphomatous infiltration of the liver is another rare but potentially treatable cause of FHF. Making a specific diagnosis is also important in view of the potential for recurrence after OLT if not recognized before such intervention. Treatment of precipitating cardiac dysfunction is necessary in ischemic FHF due to left ventricular failure, along with appropriate antibiotics and vasopressor agents in septic shock. Transplantation is invariably contraindicated in these latter groups unless heart failure can be reversed.

Role of Extracorporeal and Cell-Based Liver Support

As discussed elsewhere, an ever-increasing number of extracorporeal devices of varying complexity and strategies for transplantation of hepatocytes and stem cells are being developed as potential alternatives to auxiliary partial OLT for providing temporary liver support in FHF.

Successful experiences have been reported, including instances of spontaneous survival without OLT. However, definite answers as to the efficacy of these devices will be obtained only with controlled, multicenter clinical trials using well-defined patient groups and standardized outcome measures.

Pearls and Pitfalls

- Fulminant hepatic failure (FHF) is defined by the presence of hepatic encephalopathy occurring as the consequence of severe liver damage in patients without previous, clinically overt liver disease.
- Components of the clinical syndrome may include cerebral edema, hemodynamic instability, renal failure, coagulopathy, metabolic disturbance, and susceptibility to bacterial and fungal infection.
- The relative prevalence of causes of FHF vary according to geographical location, although hepatotoxicity caused by acetaminophen is now the most common cause in many Western countries, followed by drug reactions. The cause is not established in a small proportion of patients, and, despite considerable investigation, a new non–A-to-non–E hepatitis virus has not been identified.
- In its most severe form, FHF carries a high mortality, unless urgent liver transplantation is performed.
- Lack of fulfillment of selection criteria in current use does not reliably predict spontaneous survival, and there is an urgent need to refine prognostic criteria to improve the identification of patients who can confidently be managed by medical means alone.
- The most recent analysis from the European Liver Transplant Registry documents 1-, 5-, and 10-year survival rates following deceased-donor orthotopic liver transplantation for FHF of 63%, 59%, and 54%, respectively.
- The plateau in mortality rate 3 months after transplantation reflects the fact that patients who undergo transplantation are critically ill before the procedure and often undergo a complicated early postoperative period. Those patients who survive beyond the first 3 months follow a survival curve comparable to that seen after elective transplantation performed for cirrhosis.
- Despite much enthusiasm for temporary liver support strategies based on extracorporeal perfusion or transplantation of hepatocytes, none of the techniques that have been used clinically to date is of proven overall benefit, either in enhancing spontaneous survival or as a bridge to liver transplantation.

References

1. Trey C, Davidson CS: The management of fulminant hepatic failure. In Popper H, Schaffner F (eds): Progress in Liver Failure. New York, Grune and Stratton, 1970, pp 282-298.
2. O'Grady JG, Schalm S, Williams R: Acute liver failure: Redefining the syndromes. Lancet 342:373-375, 1993.
3. Harry R, Auzinger G, Wendon J: The clinical importance of adrenal insufficiency in acute hepatic dysfunction. Hepatology 36:395-402, 2002.

4. Clemmesen O: Splanchnic circulation and metabolism in patients with acute liver failure. Dan Med Bull 49:177-193, 2002.

5. Tofteng F, Jorgensen L, Hamsen BA, et al: Cerebral microdialysis in patients with fulminant hepatic failure. Hepatology 36:1333-1340, 2002.

6. Rolando N, Wade J, Davalos M, et al: The systemic inflammatory response syndrome in acute liver failure. Hepatology 32:734-739, 2000.

7. Shakil AO, Kramer D, Mazariegos GV, et al: Acute liver failure: Clinical features, outcome analysis, and applicability of prognostic criteria. Liver Transpl Surg 6:163-169, 2000.

8. Schiodt FV, Atillasoy E, Shakil AO, et al: Etiology and outcome for 295 patients with acute liver failure in the United States. Liver Transpl Surg 5:29-34, 1999.

9. Anand AC, Nightingale P, Neuberger JM: Early indicators of prognosis in fulminant hepatic failure: An assessment of the King's criteria. J Hepatol 26:62-68, 1997.

10. Hawton K, Townsend E, Deeks J, et al: Effects of legislation restricting pack sizes of paracetamol and salicylate on self-poisoning in the United Kingdom: Before and after study. BMJ 322:1203-1207, 2001.

11. Lee WM: Acute liver failure. N Engl J Med 329:1862-1872, 1993.

12. Kurtovic J, Riordan SM: Paracetamol-induced hepatotoxicity at recommended dosage. J Int Med 253:240-243, 2003.

13. Vento S, Garofano T, Renzini C, et al: Fulminant hepatitis associated with hepatitis A virus superinfection in patients with chronic hepatitis C. N Engl J Med 338:286-290, 1998.

14. Lau GK, He M-L, Fong DY, et al: Preemptive use of lamivudine reduces hepatitis B exacerbation after allogeneic hematopoietic cell transplantation. Hepatology 36:702-709, 2002.

15. Inokuchi K, Nakata K, Hamasaki K, et al: Prevalence of hepatitis B or C virus infection in patients with fulminant viral hepatitis. J Hepatol 24:258-264, 1996.

16. Wright TL, Mamish D, Combs C, et al: Hepatitis B virus and apparent fulminant non-A, non-B hepatitis. Lancet 339:952-955, 1992.

17. Teo EK, Ostapowicz G, Hussain M, et al: Hepatitis B infection in patients with acute liver failure in the United States. Hepatology 33:972-976, 2001.

18. Aritomi T, Yatsuhashi H, Fujino T, et al: Association of mutations in the core promoter and precore region of hepatitis virus with fulminant and severe acute hepatitis in Japan. J Gastroenterol Hepatol 13:1125-1132, 1998.

19. Madan K, Gopalkrishna V, Kar P, et al: Detection of hepatitis C and E virus genomes in sera of patients with acute viral hepatitis and fulminant hepatitis by their simultaneous amplification in PCR. J Gastroenterol Hepatol 13:125-130, 1998.

20. Bernal W: Changing patterns of causation and the use of transplantation in the United Kingdom (USA). Semin Liver Dis 23(3):227-237, 2003.

21. Ostapowicz G, Fontana RJ, Larson AM, et al: Etiology and outcome of acute liver failure in the USA: Preliminary results of a prospective multi-center study. Hepatology 30:221A, 1999.

22. Jain A, Kar P, Madan K, et al: Hepatitis C virus infection in sporadic fulminant viral hepatitis in North India: Cause or co-factor? Eur J Gastroenterol Hepatol 11:1231-1237, 1999.

23. Liu C-J, Kao J-H, Lai M-Y, et al: Minimal role of GB virus-C/hepatitis G virus in fulminant and subfulminant hepatitis in Taiwan. J Gastroenterol Hepatol 14:352-357, 1999.

24. O'Grady JG, Alexander GJM, Hayllar KM, et al: Early indicators of prognosis in fulminant hepatic failure. Gastroenterology 97:439-445, 1989.

25. Riordan SM, Williams R: Mechanisms of hepatocyte injury, multiorgan failure and prognostic criteria in acute liver failure. Semin Liver Dis 23:203-215, 2003.

26. Pauwels A, Mostefa-Kara N, Florent C, Levy VG: Emergency liver transplantation for acute liver failure. J Hepatol 17:124-127, 1993.

27. Bernal W, Wendon J, Rela M, et al: Use and outcome of liver transplantation in acetaminophen-induced acute liver failure. Hepatology 27:1050-1055, 1998.

28. Bernal W, Donaldson N, Wyncoll D, Wendon J: Blood lactate as an early predictor of outcome in paracetamol-induced acute liver failure: A cohort study. Lancet 359:558-563, 2002.

29. Schmidt LE, Dalhoff K: Serum phosphate is an early predictor of outcome in severe acetaminophen-induced hepatotoxicity. Hepatology 36:659-665, 2002.

30. Izumi S, Langley PG, Wendon J, et al: Coagulation factor V levels as a prognostic indicator in fulminant hepatic failure. Hepatology 23:1507-1511, 1996.

31. Nevens F, Schepens D, Wilmer A, et al: Evaluation of the King's and the Clichy criteria for the selection of OLTX in patients with non-paracetamol induced acute liver failure. Hepatology 28:223A, 1998.

32. Williams R, Riordan SM: Fulminant hepatic failure. In Schiff E, Sorrell M, Madrey W (eds): Schiff's Diseases of the Liver (9th ed). New Jersey, Lippincott, Williams & Wilkins, 2003. In press.

33. Sheron N, Keane H, Goka J, et al: Circulating acute phase cytokines and cytokine inhibitors in fulminant hepatic failure: Associations with mortality and haemodynamics. Clin Intensive Care 12:127-131, 2001.

34. Nagaki M, Iwai H, Naiki T, et al: High levels of serum interleukin-10 and tumour necrosis factor-α are associated with fatality in fulminant hepatitis. J Infect Dis 182:1103-1108, 2000.

35. Leifeld L, Cheng S, Ramakers J, et al: Imbalanced intrahepatic expression of interleukin 12, interferon gamma, and interleukin 10 in fulminant hepatitis B. Hepatology 36:1001-1008, 2002.

36. Shakil AO, Hay JE, Hynan L, et al: Results of a prospective study of acute liver failure at 17 tertiary care centers in the United States. Ann Intern Med 137:947-954, 2002.

37. Pitre J, Soubrane O, Dousset B, et al: How valid is emergency liver transplantation for acute liver necrosis in patients with multiple-organ failure? Liver Transpl Surg 2:1-7, 1996.

38. Adam R, Cailliez V, Majno P, et al: Normalised intrinsic mortality risk in liver transplantation: European Liver Transplant Registry study. Lancet 356:621-627, 2000.

39. Deshpande RR, Bowles MJ, Vilca-Melendez H, et al: Results of split liver transplantation in children. Ann Surg 236:248-253, 2002.

40. Samuel D, Muller G, Alexander G, et al: Liver transplantation in European patients with hepatitis B surface antigen. N Engl J Med 329:1842-1847, 1993.

41. O'Grady JG, Smith HM, Davies SE, et al: Hepatitis B virus reinfection after orthotopic liver transplantation. J Hepatol 14:104-111, 1992.

42. Marsman WA, Wiesner RW, Batts KP, et al: Fulminant hepatitis B virus: Recurrence after liver transplantation in two patients also infected with hepatitis delta virus. Hepatology 25:434-438, 1997.

43. Fagan EA, Ellis D, Toovey D, et al: Toga virus-like particles in fulminant sporadic non-A, non-B hepatitis and after transplantation. J Med Virol 38:71-77, 1992.

44. Van Agthoven M, Metselaar HJ, Tilanus HW, et al: A comparison of the costs and effects of liver transplantation for acute and for chronic liver failure. Transpl Int 14:87-94, 2001.

45. van Hoek B, de Boer J, Boudjema K, et al: Auxiliary versus orthotopic liver transplantation for acute liver failure. J Hepatol 30:699-705, 1999.

46. Boudjema K, Bachellier P, Wolf P, et al: Auxiliary liver transplantation and bioartificial bridging procedures in treatment of acute liver failure. World J Surg 26:264-274, 2002.

47. Azoulay D, Samuel D, Ichai P, et al: Auxiliary partial orthotopic versus standard orthotopic whole liver transplantation for acute liver failure: A reappraisal from a single center by a case-control study. Ann Surg 234:723-731, 2001.

48. Emre S, Schwartz ME, Shneider B, et al: Living related liver transplantation for acute liver failure in children. Liver Transpl Surg 5:161-165, 1999.

49. Miwa S, Hasikura Y, Mita A, et al: Living-related liver transplantation for patients with fulminant and subfulminant hepatic failure. Hepatology 30:1521-1526, 1999.

50. Uemoto S, Inomata Y, Sakurai T, et al: Living donor liver transplantation for fulminant hepatic failure. Transplantation 70:152-157, 2000.

51. Ichida T, Todo S, Fujiwara K, et al: Living related donor liver transplantation for adult fulminant hepatic failure. Hepatology 32:340A, 2000.

52. Lo C-M, Fan S-T, Liu C-L, et al: Adult-to-adult living donor transplantation using extended right lobe grafts. Ann Surg 226:261-270, 1997.

53. Lo C-M, Fan S-T, Liu C-L, et al: Increased risk for living liver donors after extended right hepatectomy. Transplant Proc 31:533-534, 1999.

54. Man K, Fan ST, Lo CM, et al: Graft injury in relation to graft size in right lobe live donor liver transplantation: A study of hepatic sinusoidal injury in correlation with portal hemodynamics and intragraft gene expression. Ann Surg 237:256-264, 2003.

55. Fan ST, Lo CM, Liu CL, et al: Biliary reconstruction and complications of right lobe live donor liver transplantation. Ann Surg 236:676-683, 2002.

56. Liu CL, Fan ST, Lo CM, et al: Right-lobe live donor liver transplantation improves survival of patients with acute liver failure. Br J Surg 89:317-322, 2002.

57. Brown RS Jr, Russo MW, Lai M, et al: A survey of liver transplantation from living adult donors in the United States. N Engl J Med 348:818-825, 2003.

58. Liu CL, Fan ST, Lo CM, Wong J: Living-donor liver transplantation for high-urgency situations. Transplantation 75:S33-S36, 2003.

59. Baker A, Dhawan A, Devlin J, et al: Assessment of potential donors for living related liver transplantation. Br J Surg 86:200-205, 1999.

60. Riordan SM, Williams R: Fulminant hepatic failure. Clin Liver Dis 4:25-45, 2000.

61. Philips B, Armstrong IR, Pollock A, et al: Cerebral blood flow and metabolism in patients with chronic liver disease under-going orthotopic liver transplantation. Hepatology 27:369-376, 1998.

62. Durand F, Bernuau J, Giostra E, et al: Wilson's disease with severe hepatic insufficiency: Beneficial effects of early administration of D-penicillamine. Gut 41:849-852, 2001.

Liver Transplantation for Primary Biliary Cirrhosis

JAYANT A. TALWALKAR
W. RAY KIM
E. ROLAND DICKSON

Epidemiology and etiology   177

Clinical features   178
  Presymptomatic disease   178
  Symptomatic disease   178
  Disease complications   179

Diagnosis   179

Natural history and prognosis   179

Medical treatment of primary biliary
  cirrhosis   180

Liver transplantation for primary biliary
  cirrhosis   180
  Outcome of orthotopic liver transplantation
    for primary biliary cirrhosis   180
  Quality of life after orthotopic liver
    transplantation   182
  MELD scores in patients with primary biliary
    cirrhosis   182

Posttransplant issues in primary biliary
  cirrhosis   183
  Recurrent primary biliary cirrhosis   183
  Bone disease in recipients of orthotopic
    liver transplantation for primary biliary
    cirrhosis   183

Conclusion   184

Primary biliary cirrhosis (PBC) is a chronic cholestatic liver disease characterized by the destruction of interlobular and septal bile ducts. The natural history is usually one of gradual progression to cirrhosis and death. Although ursodeoxycholic acid (UDCA) has been shown to prolong survival free of liver transplantation, not all patients benefit from this therapy, and PBC remains an important indication for orthotopic liver transplantation (OLT). As therapy for end-stage PBC, OLT has been shown to prolong survival and improve quality of life. Recurrence of PBC after liver transplantation is not uncommon, yet there is little evidence to date that recurrent PBC is of major clinical importance.

Epidemiology and Etiology

PBC has been reported from virtually all parts of the world and affects all races. In the United States, population-based data on the epidemiology of PBC have been sparse. We have recently conducted a study in which the incidence and prevalence of PBC were determined in Olmsted County, Minnesota.[1] Among patients in whom PBC was diagnosed between 1975 and 1995 in this predominantly white community, 89% were women with a median age at diagnosis of 52 years. The overall age- and gender-adjusted incidence was 2.7 cases per 100,000 person-years. The incidence in women was 4.5 per 100,000 person-years, versus only 0.7 per 100,000 for men. The age- and gender-adjusted prevalence in Olmsted County as of December 1995 was 40.2 cases per 100,000 persons. These data compare with European studies, which have estimated incidence rates ranging from 0.4 to 5.8 per 100,000 person-years and a prevalence 0.5 to 39 per 100,000 population.[2-11] If our results are projected nationally, about 3500 new cases are expected to be diagnosed each year, with some 47,000 prevalent cases of PBC among the white population in the United States.

Evidence to date strongly suggests that PBC is an immune-mediated process. The hallmark of humoral immunity in patients with PBC is the presence of anti-mitochondrial antibody (AMA).[12-14] In greater than 95% of PBC patients AMA is directed against the E2 subunit of the pyruvate dehydrogenase complex (PDC-E2).[15] However, the mechanisms by which AMA or other immunological abnormalities result in bile duct inflammation and fibrosis remain incompletely understood.

Epidemiological studies have demonstrated an association between PBC and a variety of factors,[16] such as a family history of PBC, urinary tract infection, cigarette smoking, and previous tonsillectomy. By using serum AMA as a screening test in family members of PBC patients, a 2% to 4% prevalence rate of seropositivity has been observed in asymptomatic related individuals.[17,18] The risk is highest in daughters of women with PBC, in whom the development of PBC is as high as 60 times that of controls.[19]

With regard to environmental factors, the concept of "molecular mimicry" by microbial antigens has been proposed as a pathogenetic mechanism for PBC.[20,21] This theory hypothesizes that cross-reactivity between self and microbial antigens causes the immune system to recognize and attack the biliary epithelium as though it were a foreign antigen. For example, T-cell clones from PBC patients could be activated by peptides from *Escherichia coli* analogous to sequences within the PDC-E2 subunit.[22] Molecular mimicry offers a potential explanation for the association between urinary tract infection and PBC. In addition to *E. coli*, other organisms such as *Helicobacter pylori* and *Chlamydia* species have also been implicated.[23] Although attractive in concept, this theory remains to be proved with empirical data.

Clinical Features

Presymptomatic Disease

The increased use of multichannel automated chemical analyzers in laboratories has led to an increase in the number of asymptomatic patients who have an isolated elevation in serum alkaline phosphatase at initial evaluation. Other patients are identified by an elevation in cholesterol or during evaluation of another disease,

such as Hashimoto's thyroiditis or keratoconjunctivitis sicca.

Whether patients with asymptomatic PBC are biologically distinct from those with symptomatic disease has been debated.[24] Early reports suggested that not all people with asymptomatic PBC manifest symptoms and that their long-term survival is no different from that of the general population.[3] However, more recent data based on longer-term follow-up indicate that the previous findings probably represented lead-time bias. Namely, the favorable prognosis and prolonged survival observed in patients with asymptomatic PBC were due to the fact that the diagnosis was made early in the course of the disease. Nonetheless, when symptomatic disease develops later in patients with asymptomatic PBC, their course parallels that of patients who initially have symptoms.[10] Most presymptomatic patients seen at tertiary referral centers appear to manifest symptoms after 2 to 4 years of follow-up.

Symptomatic Disease

The classic manifestation of PBC is that of a middle-aged woman in whom fatigue and pruritus gradually develop. The relative order of frequency of initial symptoms and signs is given in Table 12–1.

The neurophysiological mechanism for fatigue in patients with PBC is not well understood, although alterations in central neurotransmission[25] and impaired corticotropin-releasing hormone release have been hypothesized.[26] The severity of fatigue appears to be independent of the degree of hepatic reserve and may spontaneously remit and reappear. Patients with PBC may also have conditions that affect their energy level, such as depression or sleep disturbance.[27,28]

Pruritus in PBC is presumed to be related to accumulation of bile acids in serum.[29] Endogenous opioids may also play a role.[30] The severity of pruritus in PBC is independent of histological stage and may be persistent or recurring. Most patients report more severe symptoms at nighttime than in daylight hours. Curiously, pruritus

Table 12–1. SYMPTOMS AND SIGNS OF PRIMARY BILIARY CIRRHOSIS AT INITIAL EVALUATION

Feature	Prevalence (%)
Asymptomatic	40
Fatigue	65
Pruritus	35
Hepatomegaly	25
Hyperpigmentation	25
Splenomegaly	15
Jaundice	10
Xanthelasma	10

tends to gradually resolve with progression of hepatic disease.[31]

Jaundice is usually a late symptom that heralds the onset of advanced histological disease, but it was seen in 20% of patients at initial evaluation in earlier series. Other symptoms are more nonspecific and may include right upper quadrant abdominal pain, nausea, and anorexia. Complications from cirrhosis and portal hypertension, such as ascites, variceal bleeding, and hepatic encephalopathy, occur late in the course of disease.

As many as 70% of individuals with PBC have coexistent extrahepatic autoimmune disease states.[32] Keratoconjunctivitis sicca resulting in dry eyes and xerostomia (Sjögren's syndrome) is the most prevalent autoimmune disease and occurs in about 75% of cases.[33,34] Arthritis, including inflammatory joint disorders, has been observed in 10% to 40% of instances.[35,36] Scleroderma or any component of the CREST syndrome (calcinosis, Raynaud's phenomenon, esophageal dysmotility, sclerodactyly, and telangiectasia) may be found in up to 10% of patients.[37] Thyroid disease affects 15% to 20% of individuals and consists primarily of lymphocytic (Hashimoto's) thyroiditis.[38]

Disease Complications

Hypercholesterolemia and hyperlipidemia are present in up to 85% of patients with PBC.[39] In early-stage disease, lipoprotein abnormalities are commonly found,[40] including elevated high-density lipoprotein rather than low-density lipoprotein. This ratio may reverse with disease progression. However, despite markedly altered serum lipid values, there is no evidence for an increased prevalence of atherosclerotic disease.[39,41]

Metabolic bone disease is also common in patients with PBC and for the most part results from decreased bone mass (osteopenia and osteoporosis) rather than osteomalacia (defective bone mineralization).[42] Approximately one third of patients with PBC have osteopenia (defined as greater than 1.5 SD lower than controls), and 11% have osteoporosis (lower than 2.5 SD) by lumbar spine bone mineral densitometry.[43] Hence, many patients are at an increased risk for bone fractures, which adds to the morbidity and decreased quality of life. In addition to chronically impaired liver function, which in general has been associated with osteopenia, the subsequent cholestasis and predilection for females are thought to underlie the high prevalence of bone disease in patients with PBC.[44]

Steatorrhea is a common finding in patients with advanced hepatic disease from PBC.[45] Impairment in bile acid delivery and insufficient critical micellar concentrations in the small intestine represent the most common cause, although the coexistence of celiac disease, exocrine pancreatic insufficiency, and bacterial overgrowth syndrome (in patients with scleroderma)

may also contribute. In patients with advanced disease, steatorrhea may lead to malabsorption of fat-soluble vitamins.[46]

The increased occurrence of hepatocellular carcinoma (HCC) in PBC is increasingly being recognized in the late stages of disease.[47-49] The clinical effectiveness of HCC surveillance by abdominal ultrasound and determination of serum α-fetoprotein levels every 6 to 12 months in end-stage PBC patients, however, remains unknown. An increased risk for extrahepatic malignancy such as breast cancer remains controversial.[47,50,51]

Diagnosis

The diagnosis of PBC is usually based on a clinical syndrome consisting of chronic cholestasis, including increased alkaline phosphatase, the presence of AMA, and characteristic histological features of nonsuppurative inflammation of the bile ducts on liver biopsy. In addition to elevated serum alkaline phosphatase, modestly increased values of alanine aminotransferase and aspartate aminotransferase are common. Serum total bilirubin levels often rise during disease progression but are commonly within normal limits at diagnosis.

Serum AMA is found in 95% of patients with PBC. However, AMAs in low titer may be seen in patients with other liver diseases, including patients with autoimmune hepatitis and, less frequently, primary sclerosing cholangitis or drug-induced hepatotoxicity. Other autoantibodies that may be found in patients with PBC include anticentromere antibodies, rheumatoid factor and antithyroid antibodies, antinuclear antibody (ANA), and anti–smooth muscle antibody. The presence of serum ANA and clinical features suggestive of PBC in the absence of AMA has been termed AMA-negative PBC.[52-54]

Histologically, PBC is defined as a chronic nonsuppurative destructive cholangitis.[55,56] The characteristic florid duct lesion consists of granulomatous destruction of the interlobular and septal bile ducts. Although histological confirmation of the diagnosis may not be necessary for a typical patient with positive AMA, liver biopsy is needed for determining the histological stage of the disease. Histological classification schemes have been developed for staging PBC; such schemes describe the characteristic progression of liver injury in PBC, including both focal and segmental destruction of intralobular bile ducts resulting in cholestasis and eventually biliary cirrhosis.[55,56]

Natural History and Prognosis

In the majority of patients with PBC, a progressive clinical course resulting in fibrosis and eventually cirrhosis is often observed. Estimates of overall median survival range between 10 and 15 years from the time of diagnosis, whereas advanced histological disease (stage 3 or 4) imparts a median survival approaching 8 years.[57] Elevations in total bilirubin above 8 to 10 mg/dL have been associated with a median life expectancy of 2 years.[58] To account for these clinical variables as determinants of survival, a number of mathematical models simulating the natural history of PBC have been developed and refined for clinical use.[59,60]

Most of these models are based on proportional hazards regression analysis and typically incorporate clinical and biochemical variables to compute a summary index of disease severity, which in turn may be applied to an equation to arrive at a prediction of survival. Of these models, the prognostic models developed by investigators at the Mayo Clinic have been extensively validated and widely used.

The Mayo model for PBC was based on the results of 312 patients in whom PBC had been carefully diagnosed and who were enrolled in clinical trials of D-penicillamine.[61] Because this medication was found to not provide therapeutic benefit and the study protocol stipulated that patients not take any other medications that might potentially influence the clinical course of disease, the progression of disease in this group of patients was deemed appropriate to represent the natural history of PBC. Of the 312 patients, 125 died after a median follow-up of 66 months. Nineteen underwent liver transplantation, and 160 were alive and being monitored. From an array of demographic, clinical, biochemical, and histological variables in these patients, five were identified as statistically and clinically significant predictors of survival. Based on these variables, a summary score, or risk score, was obtained and patient survival estimated. This model subsequently underwent a number of validation studies.[62-64] The strength of the Mayo model includes the advantage of not requiring liver histology and the rigorous validation to which the model was subjected.

Medical Treatment of Primary Biliary Cirrhosis

Five randomized controlled trials of adequate size and duration have provided extensive information regarding the effectiveness of UDCA for PBC.[65-69] Improvements in symptom and hepatic biochemical parameters were demonstrated in all five studies. A combined analysis of three studies using UDCA at doses of 13 to 15 mg/kg/day revealed improvement in survival free of liver transplantation in patients receiving active drug.[70] Long-term (10-year) survival with UDCA has also been observed to exceed Mayo PBC model predictions in selected populations.[71] In addition, UDCA has been shown to reduce the risk for development of esophageal varices and cirrhosis[72] while being a cost-effective therapy.

The mechanism of action of UDCA therapy for PBC is not completely understood. UDCA essentially replaces endogenous hydrophobic bile acids and probably inhibits apoptosis and mitochondrial dysfunction.[73] Moreover, there is evidence to suggest that UDCA is associated with membrane stabilization,[74] reduced aberrant HLA class I expression on hepatocytes,[75] and decreased cytokine production.[76]

Although some degree of response is seen almost universally in PBC patients receiving UDCA therapy, up to two thirds of patients may be classified as incomplete responders, defined as the failure to normalize serum hepatic biochemistry or histological progression, or both, despite treatment with UDCA. Higher levels of serum alkaline phosphatase and advanced fibrosis at baseline have been associated with incomplete responses.

A number of agents have been evaluated for further treatment of PBC, particularly in patients who fail to achieve a complete response. These agents include immunosuppressants such as corticosteroids, azathioprine, cyclosporine, and methotrexate; antifibrotic agents such as D-penicillamine; and colchicine alone or in combination with UDCA. Other novel agents currently being evaluated include malotilate, chlorambucil, thalidomide, silymarin, and bezafibrate, none of which, however, have been shown to be effective to date.

Liver Transplantation for Primary Biliary Cirrhosis

As of today, PBC remains among the most common indications for liver transplantation in the United States. Clearly, the most effective therapeutic alternative for patients with end-stage PBC is liver transplantation. Indications for OLT in PBC include complications of portal hypertension, such as hepatic encephalopathy, refractory ascites, spontaneous bacterial peritonitis, and hepatorenal syndrome. In addition, intractable pruritus and disabling fatigue have been considered a justifiable indication for patients with PBC, although the increasing donor organ shortage has made it difficult to perform OLT for quality-of-life issues alone.

Outcome of Orthotopic Liver Transplantation for Primary Biliary Cirrhosis

In 1989, Markus and colleagues examined the efficacy of liver transplantation by comparing actual patient survival after liver transplantation with expected survival according to the Mayo natural history model

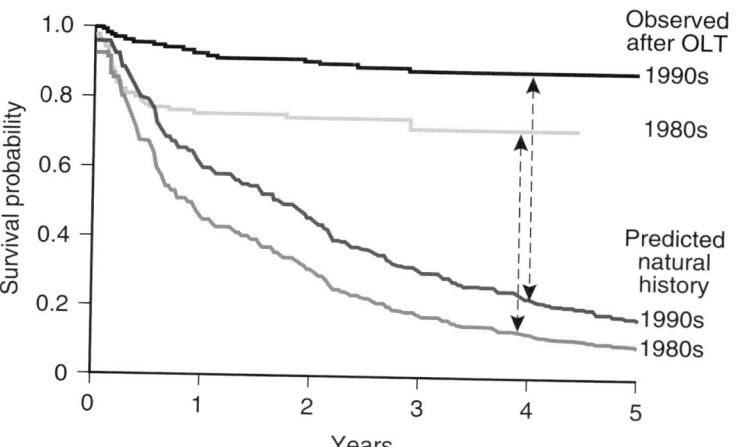

FIGURE 12–1

Patient survival after liver transplantation in the 1980s and 1990s.

for PBC.[77] The patient population in which posttransplant survival was assessed consisted of 161 subjects who underwent liver transplantation at the University of Pittsburgh and Baylor University Medical Center between 1980 and 1987. These patients were monitored for a median duration of 25 months. In the comparison between actual posttransplant survival and survival without transplantation as predicted by the Mayo natural history model, a highly significant difference was found (2-year survival rate of 74% with transplantation versus 31% without transplantation, $P < .01$).

In 1998, a follow-up report was published on 143 patients with PBC who underwent liver transplantation at Baylor University Medical Center and the Mayo Clinic between 1987 and 1994.[78] Patients were monitored for a minimum of 18 months (median, 35.8 months). Figure 12–1 compares the survival of patients from the 1980s[77] and 1990s.[78] Several important points may be made. First, there was a significant improvement in posttransplant survival between the two series. For example, survival rates at 1 year increased from 75% to 93% and at 3 years from 72% to 88%. Second, this gain in survival was in part due to better timing of liver transplantation, as shown by the predicted natural history curves demonstrating that patients from the 1990s had a better predicted survival without OLT, thus indicating that they received transplants earlier in their natural history than did patients from the previous era. However, the estimated gain in survival after OLT (dashed lines in Fig. 12–1) seems to be larger in the latter era.

In both studies, pretransplant disease severity had a significant impact on posttransplant survival. When data from the two studies were analyzed together, there was a threshold in the risk score above which the risk of death increased significantly (Fig. 12–2). A risk score threshold of 7.8 was common to both the first and the current series, thus indicating that patients with a higher risk score had a worse outcome than those with a lower risk score regardless of the era of transplantation.

A similar study that analyzed the outcome of liver transplantation in 70 PBC patients was conducted by Neuberger and coworkers.[78a] Patients were divided into three groups according to their bilirubin level and the European prognostic index. The 1-year posttransplant survival rate in patients from the low-risk group (median bilirubin concentration of 4.9 mg/dL and expected survival without a transplant of longer than 9 months) was 78%, whereas that of the high-risk group (median bilirubin concentration of 27.3 mg/dL and expected survival of less than 4 months) was only 50%.

In summary, the Mayo natural history model and other measures to reflect the degree of liver damage are informative in estimating outcomes after liver transplantation in patients with PBC. To the extent that modern transplant techniques can consistently replace the diseased organ, the outcome of liver transplantation today is determined not only by the severity of liver

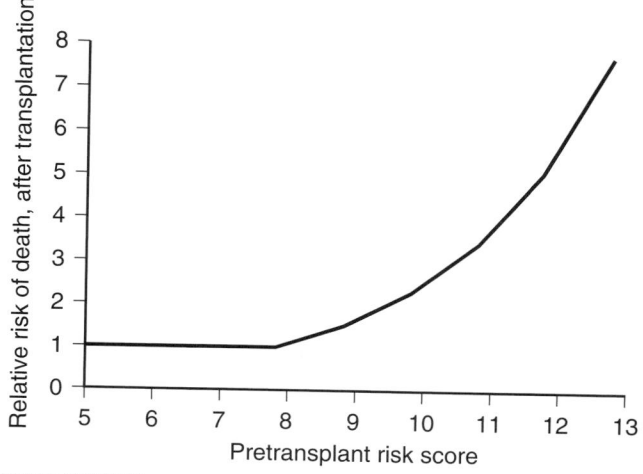

FIGURE 12–2

Effect of pretransplantation disease on posttransplantation survival.

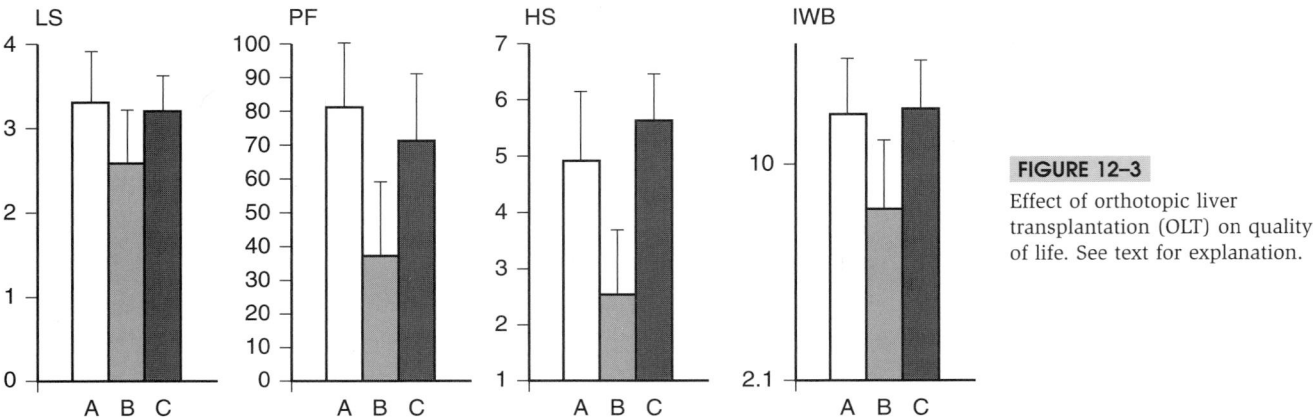

FIGURE 12–3

Effect of orthotopic liver transplantation (OLT) on quality of life. See text for explanation.

disease but also by the integrity of extrahepatic organ systems. Pretransplant disease severity has the greatest impact on short-term outcome because patients with higher risk scores are likely to have multisystem dysfunction and be at higher risk for perioperative mortality and morbidity.[79-82] Once patients survive the initial insult from the transplant operation, their longevity may not be greatly affected by the extent of injury to the replaced liver.

Quality of Life after Orthotopic Liver Transplantation

A number of investigators have demonstrated that OLT significantly improves quality of life.[83,84] Figure 12–3 illustrates the evolution of quality of life in patients with PBC or primary sclerosing cholangitis from the early ambulatory phase (column A), to end-stage disease (before OLT) (column B), to post-OLT status (column C). The instrument with which quality of life was measured is known as the NIDDK-QA form, an instrument that has been demonstrated to be reliable and valid. This instrument entails four domains (LS, liver symptoms; PF, physical functioning; HS, health satisfaction; and IWB, overall well-being). In Figure 12–3, the increase in disease severity between A and B resulted in a significant decrement in quality of life, which recovered almost fully 1 year after OLT (C).[83] An interesting observation was that when compared with ambulatory patients, OLT recipients were worse off from the standpoint of physical function, but they were equally happy (IWB) and more satisfied with their health (HS).

MELD Scores in Patients with Primary Biliary Cirrhosis

In February 2002, the United Network for Organ Sharing (UNOS) adopted the Model for End-Stage Liver Disease (MELD) as the disease severity index by which organ allocation priorities for liver transplantation should be determined.[85,86] MELD had originally been derived from a predictive model for survival of patients undergoing the transjugular intrahepatic portosystemic shunt (TIPS) procedure.[87] Although these patients constitute a very select subgroup among those with end-stage liver disease, it was subsequently shown that the index was an accurate measure of disease severity in patients with a wide spectrum of severity. MELD is based on three laboratory-based variables: serum total bilirubin, creatinine, and the international normalized ratio. The measure with which the validity of the model was determined was the c (concordance)-statistic, a widely used tool to assess prognostic models for their ability to rank individuals according to their mortality risk.[88] This statistic may range from 0 to 1, with 1 corresponding to perfect discrimination and 0.5 to what is expected by chance alone.

The validity of MELD was examined in a number of groups of patients with liver disease. One of these consisted of PBC patients, based on whose data the Mayo PBC natural history model was created. These patients were accrued at Mayo Clinic between 1973 and 1984. Of these 418 patients, 92 lacked variables necessary for the MELD score, which left 326 for analysis. Subsequent to initial enrollment in the study, patients were monitored prospectively. Of the 326 patients, 127, or 39%, died without liver transplantation, whereas 25 received liver transplants.

The c-statistic for the MELD score's prediction of 3-month mortality was 0.87 (95% confidence interval [CI], 0.71 to 1.00), and that for 1-year mortality remained at 0.87 (95% CI, 0.80 to 0.93). These concordances are respectable in comparison to the Mayo PBC model, which had a c-statistic of 0.91 (0.83 to 0.99) in this group.

In the original TIPS study, liver disease diagnosis (cholestatic or alcoholic versus other categories) was part of the model in that for a given score, patients with cholestatic liver disease had better survival than those with other types of liver disease. However, when MELD was implemented, liver disease diagnosis was eliminated from the model for a number of mostly practical reasons. One of the justifications was that patients with cholestatic disease may experience types of complications different from those in patients with parenchymal liver disease, such as pruritus, osteoporosis, fat malabsorption, and fatigue. In addition, patients with primary sclerosing cholangitis may have further complications such as ascending cholangitis, cholangiocarcinoma, or problems related to inflammatory bowel disease.[89,90] When this issue was formally tested, there was a minimal decrease in the c-statistic with the elimination of liver disease diagnosis.

Posttransplant Issues in Primary Biliary Cirrhosis

Recurrent Primary Biliary Cirrhosis

Whether PBC recurs after OLT has been a matter of debate, in part because of difficulties in making a firm diagnosis. More recently, however, it is generally accepted that PBC recurs in some patients.[91-94] To appreciate the incidence of recurrent PBC, one needs long-term follow-up in a sufficiently large number of patients. Reports to date estimate that evidence of recurrence is found in 8% to 25% of patients at 5 years and 22% to 30% at 10 years.[95,96]

Initial reports of allograft histological features consistent with stage I PBC were limited by the absence of explicit criteria for recurrent disease, including the exclusion of acute cellular rejection.[91] Diagnostic criteria for recurrent PBC have been proposed but have not been validated.[93] Difficulties in the diagnosis of recurrence include a high prevalence of pathological lesions involving the bile ducts of liver transplant recipients, including acute and chronic rejection, changes secondary to large bile duct strictures, and infectious processes. Serum AMA status appears to have no role in assessing recurrence risk. This antibody may disappear soon after transplantation, only to return later with or without recurrent disease.[97] Finally, the size of the liver biopsy specimen may affect the sensitivity of the diagnosis of recurrence.

Published reports to date suggest that recurrent PBC is not a significant clinical problem. Garcia and coauthors reported that of 400 OLT recipients with PBC, significant liver disease as a result of recurrence developed in only 2 patients after a mean follow-up of 56 months.[95] Other studies with shorter follow-up rarely report serious consequences of recurrent disease.[92,94,98,99] However, as increasingly large numbers of recipients survive long-term after OLT, recurrent disease may prove to be a significant issue in the future.

Tapering of corticosteroids from immunosuppression regimens after liver transplantation has been suggested to be a potential risk factor for recurrent PBC.[100] In addition, one report found that tacrolimus was associated with a shorter time to recurrence than was cyclosporine, although this observation may simply reflect the fact that more recent patients tend to be treated with lower levels of immunosuppression.[95] The role of UDCA in patients with recurrent PBC remains controversial. No published information is available regarding the efficacy of UDCA therapy in halting disease progression from early-stage recurrent disease. Anecdotal experience suggests that UDCA improves liver biochemistry. However, the significance of such improvement in terms of overall survival and natural history remains uncertain.

Bone Disease in Recipients of Orthotopic Liver Transplantation for Primary Biliary Cirrhosis

In patients undergoing liver transplantation, a 20% decline in bone mineral density may occur up to 6 months after surgery and can significantly increase the risk for osseous fractures (particularly those involving vertebral bodies).[101] Because of the high prevalence of metabolic bone disease in PBC before OLT, these patients tend to experience more problems with osteopenia/osteoporosis after OLT.[102]

In patients with osteopenia (defined by T scores between −1.5 and −2.5) and osteoporosis (defined by T scores less than −2.5), several therapeutic modalities are available, although clinical evidence based on randomized trials is scarce. Ensuring adequate intake of calcium (1000 to 1200 mg daily) along with weight-bearing activity is recommended as initial treatment of all patients.[103] Measurement of serum vitamin D levels may be helpful in patients with fat-soluble vitamin malabsorption. Oral replacement therapy must be instituted if measured serum levels are reduced. Hormone replacement therapy has also been used for the prevention of osteoporosis in patients with PBC.[104] However, in individual patients, the risks and benefits of such therapy need to be considered before it is initiated. Raloxifene, an estrogen analogue that is devoid of the systemic side effects of the more commonly used estrogen preparations, may be beneficial. The use of calcitonin in this setting remains controversial, whereas oral bisphosphonates (including alendronate, risedronate, and etidronate) have been commonly used to halt or reverse bone loss in OLT recipients.[105,106] A randomized study comparing calcitonin (40 IU intramuscularly daily) and cyclical etidronate showed a significant increase in vertebral bone mass in both groups (6.4% and 8.2% per year, respectively). Unfortunately, there was no control (no treatment) group in that study, which makes it difficult to interpret these results. However, based on data from renal and cardiac transplantation, bisphosphonates are a reasonable choice for patients with documented osteoporosis after OLT.[107]

Conclusion

OLT represents a major advance in the care of patients with PBC. Although there will undoubtedly be more clinical trials to assess the efficacy of medical therapies, no studies to date have demonstrated that these therapies ultimately preclude death or the need for OLT. Mathematical models provide a reliable estimate of a patient's survival with and without transplantation. As the trend continues toward progressively more favorable survival with OLT, the tendency will be to offer transplantation earlier in the course of the disease. Studies are currently under way to better assess quality-of-life and cost-effectiveness issues in liver transplantation. Most patients appear to enjoy extended periods of good health and productive work after transplantation.

Pearls and Pitfalls

- The diagnosis of PBC should be considered when the following clinical features are present:
  - Cholestatic serum liver profile
  - Serum AMA positivity
  - Liver histology compatible with PBC
- Initial therapy with UDCA at 13 to 15 mg/kg/day for a minimum treatment period of 6 months is recommended. The treatment goal is to achieve a reduction in the serum alkaline phosphatase level that is less than or equal to 1.5 times the upper limit of normal (complete response).
- Survival after liver transplantation in PBC exceeds 90% at 1 year and 80% at 3 years.
- Recurrent PBC may occur in up to 25% of patients after liver transplantation.

References

1. Kim WR, Lindor K, Locke G, et al: Epidemiology and natural history of primary biliary cirrhosis in a U.S. community. Gastroenterology 119:1631-1636, 2000.
2. Myszor M, James OF: The epidemiology of primary biliary cirrhosis in north-east England: An increasingly common disease? QJM 75:377-385, 1990.
3. Lofgren J, Jarnerot G, Danielsson D, Hemdal I: Incidence and prevalence of primary biliary cirrhosis in a defined population in Sweden. Scand J Gastroenterol 20:647-650, 1985.
4. Danielsson A, Boqvist L, Uddenfeldt P: Epidemiology of primary biliary cirrhosis in a defined rural population in the northern part of Sweden. Hepatology 11:458-464, 1990.
5. Hamlyn AN, Sherlock S: The epidemiology of primary biliary cirrhosis: A survey of mortality in England and Wales. Gut 15:473-479, 1974.
6. Witt-Sullivan H, Heathcote J, Cauch K, et al: The demography of primary biliary cirrhosis in Ontario, Canada. Hepatology 12:98-105, 1990.
7. Triger DR, Berg PA, Rodes J: Epidemiology of primary biliary cirrhosis. Liver 4:195-200, 1984.
8. Boberg KM, Aadland E, Jahnsen J, et al: Incidence and prevalence of primary biliary cirrhosis, primary sclerosing cholangitis, and autoimmune hepatitis in a Norwegian population. Scand J Gastroenterol 33:99-103, 1998.
9. Eriksson S, Lindgren S: The prevalence and clinical spectrum of primary biliary cirrhosis in a defined population. Scand J Gastroenterol 19:971-976, 1984.
10. Metcalf JV, Bhopal RS, Gray J, et al: Incidence and prevalence of primary biliary cirrhosis in the city of Newcastle upon Tyne, England. Int J Epidemiol 26:830-836, 1997.
11. James OF, Bhopal R, Howel D, et al: Primary biliary cirrhosis once rare, now common in the United Kingdom? Hepatology 30:390-394, 1999.
12. Van de Water J, Ansari AA, Surh CD, et al: Evidence for the targeting by 2-oxo-dehydrogenase enzymes in the T cell response of primary biliary cirrhosis. J Immunol 146:89-94, 1991.
13. Leung PS, Chuang DT, Wynn RM, et al: Autoantibodies to BCOADC-E2 in patients with primary biliary cirrhosis recognize a conformational epitope. Hepatology 22:505-513, 1995.
14. Maeda T, Loveland BE, Rowley MJ, Mackay IR: Autoantibody against dihydrolipoamide dehydrogenase, the E3 subunit of the 2-oxoacid dehydrogenase complexes: Significance for primary biliary cirrhosis. Hepatology 14:994-999, 1991.
15. Gershwin ME, Rowley M, Davis PA, et al: Molecular biology of the 2-oxo-acid dehydrogenase complexes and anti-mitochondrial antibodies. Prog Liver Dis 10:47-61, 1992.
16. Parikh-Patel A, Gold EB, Worman H, et al: Risk factors for primary biliary cirrhosis in a cohort of patients from the United States. Hepatology 33:16-21, 2001.
17. Feizi T, Naccarato R, Sherlock S, Doniach D: Mitochondrial and other tissue antibodies in relatives of patients with primary biliary cirrhosis. Clin Exp Immunol 10:609-622, 1972.
18. Caldwell SH, Leung PS, Spivey JR, et al: Antimitochondrial antibodies in kindreds of patients with primary biliary cirrhosis: Antimitochondrial antibodies are unique to clinical disease and are absent in asymptomatic family members. Hepatology 16:899-905, 1992.
19. Jones DE, Watt FE, Metcalf JV, et al: Familial primary biliary cirrhosis reassessed: A geographically-based population study. J Hepatol 30:402-407, 1999.
20. Shimoda S, Nakamura M, Ishibashi H, et al: HLA DRB4 0101–restricted immunodominant T cell autoepitope of pyruvate dehydrogenase complex in primary biliary cirrhosis: Evidence of molecular mimicry in human autoimmune diseases. J Exp Med 181:1835-1845, 1995.
21. Burroughs AK, Butler P, Sternberg MJ, Baum H: Molecular mimicry in liver disease. Nature 358:377-378, 1992.
22. Shigematsu H, Shimoda S, Nakamura M, et al: Fine specificity of T cells reactive to human PDC-E2 163-176 peptide, the immunodominant autoantigen in primary biliary cirrhosis: Implications for molecular mimicry and cross-recognition among mitochondrial autoantigens. Hepatology 32:901-909, 2000.
23. Trauner M, Boyer JL: Cholestatic syndromes. Curr Opin Gastroenterol 17:242, 2001.

24. Springer J, Cauch-Dudek K, O'Rourke K, et al: Asymptomatic primary biliary cirrhosis: A study of its natural history and prognosis. Am J Gastroenterol 94:47-53, 1999.

25. Jones EA, Yurdaydin C: Is fatigue associated with cholestasis mediated by altered central neurotransmission? Hepatology 25:492-494, 1997.

26. Swain MG, Maric M: Defective corticotropin-releasing hormone mediated neuroendocrine and behavioral responses in cholestatic rats: Implications for cholestatic liver disease–related sickness behaviors. Hepatology 22:1560-1564, 1995.

27. Cauch-Dudek K, Abbey S, Stewart DE, Heathcote EJ: Fatigue in primary biliary cirrhosis. Gut 43:705-710, 1998.

28. Huet PM, Deslauriers J, Tran A, et al: Impact of fatigue on the quality of life of patients with primary biliary cirrhosis. Am J Gastroenterol 95:760-767, 2000.

29. Kirby J, Heaton KW, Burton JL: Pruritic effect of bile salts. BMJ 4:693-695, 1974.

30. Jones EA, Bergasa NV: The pruritus of cholestasis: From bile acids to opiate agonists. Hepatology 11:884-887, 1990.

31. Lloyd-Thomas H, Sherlock S: Testosterone therapy for the pruritus of obstructive jaundice. BMJ 2:1289, 1952.

32. Golding PL, Smith M, Williams R: Multisystem involvement in chronic liver disease. Studies on the incidence and pathogenesis. Am J Med 55:772-782, 1973.

33. Alarcon-Segovia D, Diaz-Jouanen E, Fishbein E: Features of Sjögren's syndrome in primary biliary cirrhosis. Ann Intern Med 79:31-36, 1973.

34. Tsianos EV, Hoofnagle JH, Fox PC, et al: Sjögren's syndrome in patients with primary biliary cirrhosis. Hepatology 11:730-734, 1990.

35. Child DL, Mathews JA, Thompson RP: Arthritis and primary biliary cirrhosis. BMJ 2:557, 1977.

36. Uddenfeldt P, Danielsson A: Evaluation of rheumatic disorders in patients with primary biliary cirrhosis. Ann Clin Res 18:148-153, 1986.

37. Murray-Lyon IM, Thompson RP, Ansell ID, Williams R: Scleroderma and primary biliary cirrhosis. BMJ 1:258-259, 1970.

38. Crowe JP, Christensen E, Butler J: Primary biliary cirrhosis and the prevalence of hypothyroidism and its relationship to thyroid autoantibodies and sicca syndrome. Gastroenterology 78:1437, 1980.

39. Crippin JS, Lindor KD, Jorgensen R, et al: Hypercholesterolemia and atherosclerosis in primary biliary cirrhosis: What is the risk? Hepatology 15:858-862, 1992.

40. Jahn CE, Schaefer EJ, Taam LA, et al: Lipoprotein abnormalities in primary biliary cirrhosis. Association with hepatic lipase inhibition as well as altered cholesterol esterification. Gastroenterology 89:1266-1278, 1985.

41. Longo M, Crosignani A, Battezzati M: Hyperlipidemic state and cardiovascular risk in primary biliary cirrhosis [abstract]. Gastroenterology 118:A1008, 2000.

42. Hodgson SF, Dickson ER, Wahner HW, et al: Bone loss and reduced osteoblast function in primary biliary cirrhosis. Ann Intern Med 103:855-860, 1985.

43. Hay JE: Bone disease in cholestatic liver disease. Gastroenterology 108:276-283, 1995.

44. Angulo P, Lindor KD: Primary biliary cirrhosis and primary sclerosing cholangitis. Clin Liver Dis 3:529-570, 1999.

45. Lanspa SJ, Chan AT, Bell JS 3rd, et al: Pathogenesis of steatorrhea in primary biliary cirrhosis. Hepatology 5:837-842, 1985.

46. Kaplan MM, Elta GH, Furie B, et al: Fat-soluble vitamin nutriture in primary biliary cirrhosis. Gastroenterology 95:787-792, 1988.

47. Nijhawan PK, Therneau TM, Dickson ER, et al: Incidence of cancer in primary biliary cirrhosis: The Mayo experience. Hepatology 29:1396-1398, 1999.

48. Loof L, Adami HO, Sparen P, et al: Cancer risk in primary biliary cirrhosis: A population-based study from Sweden. Hepatology 20:101-104, 1994.

49. Farinati F, Floreani A, De Maria N, et al: Hepatocellular carcinoma in primary biliary cirrhosis. J Hepatol 21:315-316, 1994.

50. Goudie BM, Burt AD, Boyle P, et al: Breast cancer in women with primary biliary cirrhosis. Br Med J (Clin Res Ed) 291:1597-1598, 1985.

51. Wolke AM, Schaffner F, Kapelman B, Sacks HS: Malignancy in primary biliary cirrhosis. High incidence of breast cancer in affected women. Am J Med 76:1075-1078, 1984.

52. Goodman ZD, McNally PR, Davis DR, Ishak KG: Autoimmune cholangitis: A variant of primary biliary cirrhosis. Clinicopathologic and serologic correlations in 200 cases. Dig Dis Sci 40:1232-1242, 1995.

53. Ben-Ari Z, Dhillon AP, Sherlock S: Autoimmune cholangiopathy: Part of the spectrum of autoimmune chronic active hepatitis. Hepatology 18:10-15, 1993.

54. Michieletti P, Wanless IR, Katz A, et al: Antimitochondrial antibody–negative primary biliary cirrhosis: A distinct syndrome of autoimmune cholangitis. Gut 35:260-265, 1994.

55. Ludwig J, Dickson ER, McDonald GS: Staging of chronic nonsuppurative destructive cholangitis (syndrome of primary biliary cirrhosis). Virchows Arch A Pathol Anat Histol 379:103-112, 1978.

56. Scheuer PJ: Primary biliary cirrhosis: Chronic non-suppurative destructive cholangitis. Am J Pathol 46:387, 1965.

57. Christensen E, Crowe J, Doniach D: Clinical pattern and course of disease in primary biliary cirrhosis based on an analysis of 236 patients. Gastroenterology 78:236, 1980.

58. Shapiro J, Smith H, Schaffner R: Serum bilirubin: A prognostic factor in primary biliary cirrhosis. Gut 20:137, 1979.

59. Kim W, Dickson ER: Predictive model of natural history of cholestatic liver disease. Clin Liver Dis North Am 2:313-332, 1998.

60. Kim W, Dickson ER: Natural history models of primary biliary cirrhosis. In Lindor KD, Poupon RE, Heathcote EJ (eds): Primary Biliary Cirrhosis. Dordrecht, The Netherlands, Kluwer, 1999.

61. Dickson ER, Grambsch PM, Fleming TR, et al: Prognosis in primary biliary cirrhosis: Model for decision making. Hepatology 10:1-7, 1989.

62. Grambsch PM, Dickson ER, Kaplan M, et al: Extramural cross-validation of the Mayo primary biliary cirrhosis survival model establishes its generalizability. Hepatology 10:846-850, 1989.

63. Murtaugh P, Dickson ER, Van Dam GM, et al: Primary biliary cirrhosis: Prediction of short-term survival based on repeated patient visits. Hepatology 20:126-134, 1994.

64. Grambsch PM, Dickson ER, Wiesner RH, Langworthy A: Application of the Mayo primary biliary cirrhosis survival model to Mayo liver transplant patients. Mayo Clin Proc 64:699-704, 1989.

65. Lindor KD, Dickson ER, Baldus WP, et al: Ursodeoxycholic acid in the treatment of primary biliary cirrhosis. Gastroenterology 106:1284-1290, 1994.

66. Poupon RE, Balkau B, Eschwege E, Poupon R: A multicenter, controlled trial of ursodiol for the treatment of primary biliary cirrhosis. UDCA-PBC Study Group. N Engl J Med 324:1548-1554, 1991.

67. Heathcote EJ, Cauch-Dudek K, Walker V, et al: The Canadian Multicenter Double-Blind Randomized Controlled Trial of ursodeoxycholic acid in primary biliary cirrhosis. Hepatology 19:1149-1156, 1994.

68. Pares A, Caballeria L, Rodes J, et al: Long-term effects of ursodeoxycholic acid in primary biliary cirrhosis: Results of a double-blind controlled multicentric trial. UDCA-Cooperative Group from the Spanish Association for the Study of the Liver. J Hepatol 32:561-566, 2000.

69. Combes B, Carithers RL Jr, Maddrey WC, et al: A randomized, double-blind, placebo-controlled trial of ursodeoxycholic acid in primary biliary cirrhosis. Hepatology 22:759-766, 1995.

70. Poupon RE, Lindor KD, Cauch-Dudek K, et al: Combined analysis of randomized controlled trials of ursodeoxycholic acid in primary biliary cirrhosis. Gastroenterology 113:884-890, 1997.

71. Poupon RE, Bonnand AM, Chretien Y, Poupon R: Ten-year survival in ursodeoxycholic acid–treated patients with primary biliary cirrhosis. The UDCA-PBC Study Group. Hepatology 29:1668-1671, 1999.

72. Lindor KD, Jorgensen RA, Therneau TM, et al: Ursodeoxycholic acid delays the onset of esophageal varices in primary biliary cirrhosis. Mayo Clin Proc 72:1137-1140, 1997.

73. Rodrigues CM, Steer CJ: Mitochondrial membrane perturbations in cholestasis. J Hepatol 32:135-141, 2000.

74. Heuman DM, Bajaj R: Ursodeoxycholate conjugates protect against disruption of cholesterol-rich membranes by bile salts. Gastroenterology 106:1333-1341, 1994.

75. Hillaire S, Boucher E, Calmus Y, et al: Effects of bile acids and cholestasis on major histocompatibility complex class I in human and rat hepatocytes. Gastroenterology 107:781-788, 1994.

76. Yoshikawa M, Tsujii T, Matsumura K, et al: Immunomodulatory effects of ursodeoxycholic acid on immune responses. Hepatology 16:358-364, 1992.

77. Markus BH, Dickson ER, Grambsch PM, et al: Efficiency of liver transplantation in patients with primary biliary cirrhosis. N Engl J Med 320:1709-1713, 1989.

78. Kim WR, Wiesner RH, Therneau TM, et al: Optimal timing of liver transplantation for primary biliary cirrhosis. Hepatology 28:33-38, 1998.

78a. Neuberger JM, Gunson BK, Buckels JA, et al: Referral of patients with primary biliary cirrhosis for liver transplantation. Gut 31:1069-1072, 1990.

79. Ricci P, Therneau TM, Malinchoc M, et al: A prognostic model for the outcome of liver transplantation in patients with cholestatic liver disease. Hepatology 25:672-677, 1997.

80. Spanier TB, Klein RD, Nasraway SA, et al: Multiple organ failure after liver transplantation. Crit Care Med 23:466-473, 1995.

81. Cuervas-Mons V, Millan I, Gavaler JS, et al: Prognostic value of preoperatively obtained clinical and laboratory data in predicting survival following orthotopic liver transplantation. Hepatology 6:922-927, 1986.

82. Doyle HR, Marino IR, Jabbour N, et al: Early death or retransplantation in adults after orthotopic liver transplantation. Can outcome be predicted? Transplantation 57:1028-1036, 1994.

83. Gross CR, Malinchoc M, Kim WR, et al: Quality of life before and after liver transplantation for cholestatic liver disease. Hepatology 29:356-364, 1999.

84. Kim WR, Lindor KD, Malinchoc M, et al: Reliability and validity of the NIDDK-QA Instrument in the assessment of quality of life in ambulatory patients with cholestatic liver disease. Hepatology 32:924-929, 2000.

85. Kamath P, Wiesner R, Malinchoc M, et al: Model to predict survival in patients with end-stage liver disease. Hepatology 33:464-470, 2001.

86. Wiesner RH, Kamath PS, Malinchoc M, et al: MELD and PELD: Application of survival models to liver allocation. Liver Transpl 7:567-580, 2001.

87. Malinchoc M, Kamath PS, Gordon FD, et al: A model to predict poor survival in patients undergoing transjugular intrahepatic portosystemic shunts. Hepatology 31:864-871, 2000.

88. Hanley JA, McNeil BJ: The meaning and use of the area under a receiver operating characteristic (ROC) curve. Radiology 143:29-36, 1982.

89. Angulo-Hernandez P, Lindor K: Primary sclerosing cholangitis. Hepatology 30:325-332, 1999.

90. deGroen P, Gores G, LaRusso N, et al: Medical progress—biliary tract cancers. N Engl J Med 28:1368-1378, 1999.

91. Neuberger J, Portmann B, Macdougall BR, et al: Recurrence of primary biliary cirrhosis after liver transplantation. N Engl J Med 306:1-4, 1982.

92. Polson RJ, Portmann B, Neuberger J, et al: Evidence for disease recurrence after liver transplantation for primary biliary cirrhosis. Clinical and histologic follow-up studies. Gastroenterology 97:715-725, 1989.

93. Hubscher SG, Elias E, Buckels JA, et al: Primary biliary cirrhosis. Histological evidence of disease recurrence after liver transplantation. J Hepatol 18:173-184, 1993.

94. Balan V, Batts KP, Porayko MK, et al: Histological evidence for recurrence of primary biliary cirrhosis after liver transplantation. Hepatology 18:1392-1398, 1993.

95. Liermann RF, Evangelista C, Garcia C, et al: Transplantation for primary biliary cirrhosis: Retrospective analysis of 400 patients in a single centre. Hepatology 33:22-27, 2001.

96. Abu-Elmagd KDJ, Rakela J, Balan V, et al: Transplantation for primary biliary cirrhosis: Recurrence and outcome in 421 patients [abstract]. Hepatology 26:176A, 1997.

97. Dubel L, Farges O, Bismuth H, et al: Kinetics of anti-M2 antibodies after liver transplantation for primary biliary cirrhosis. J Hepatol 23:674-680, 1995.

98. Knoop M, Bechstein WO, Schrem H, et al: Clinical significance of recurrent primary biliary cirrhosis after liver transplantation. Transpl Int 9(Suppl 1):S115-S119, 1996.

99. Khettry U, Anand N, Faul PN, et al: Liver transplantation for primary biliary cirrhosis: A long-term pathologic study. Liver Transpl 9:87-96, 2003.

100. Neuberger J: Recurrent primary biliary cirrhosis. Best Pract Res Clin Gastroenterol 14:669, 2000.

101. Eastell R, Dickson ER, Hodgson SF: Rates of vertebral bone loss before and after liver transplantation in women with primary biliary cirrhosis. Hepatology 14:296, 1991.

102. Newton J, Francis R, Prince M, et al: Osteoporosis in primary biliary cirrhosis revisited. Gut 49:282-287, 2001.

103. Neuhaus R, Kubo A, Lohmann R, et al: Calcitriol in prevention and therapy of osteoporosis after liver transplantation. Transplant Proc 31:472-473, 1999.

104. Crippin J, Jorgensen RA, Dickson ER: Hepatic osteodystrophy in primary biliary cirrhosis: Effects on medical treatment. Am J Gastroenterol 89:47, 1994.

105. Riemens SC, Oostdijk A, van Doormaal JJ, et al: Bone loss after liver transplantation is not prevented by cyclical etidronate, calcium and alphacalcidol. The Liver Transplant Group, Groningen. Osteopor Int 6:213-218, 1996.

106. Valero MA, Loinaz C, Larrodera L, et al: Calcitonin and bisphosphonates treatment in bone loss after liver transplantation. Calcif Tissue Int 57:15-19, 1995.

107. Shane E, Thys-Jacobs S, Papadopoulos A: Antiresorptive therapy prevents bone loss after cardiac transplantation. J Bone Miner Res 11:635, 1996.

Transplantation for Sclerosing Cholangitis

JEFFREY S. CRIPPIN

Issues prior to transplantation   188
   Bacterial cholangitis   188
   Pruritus   188
   Hepatic osteodystrophy   188
   Inflammatory bowel disease   188
   Cholangiocarcinoma   189
   Prognostic models for survival   189

Transplant surgery   189

Posttransplant survival   189

Posttransplant complications   190
   Acute cellular and chronic/ductopenic
      rejection   190
   Inflammatory bowel disease following
      transplantation   190
   Recurrent disease and biliary strictures   190

Summary   192

Sclerosing cholangitis is characterized by chronic biliary duct inflammation, subsequently resulting in fibrotic stricturing and duct obliteration. Biliary cirrhosis follows, with progression to complications of end-stage liver disease, liver failure, and the need for liver transplantation. Although there are many possible explanations for this process—biliary obstruction from previous biliary duct surgery or injury, choledocholithiasis, congenital biliary tract anomalies, hepatic arterial infusion of chemotherapeutic agents, and ischemic injury from hepatic arterial stenosis and thrombosis—the vast majority of patients presenting to transplant centers have primary sclerosing cholangitis (PSC).

In addition to biliary duct injury and the typical cholangiographic findings, PSC has a number of other characteristics. Approximately 70% of patients with PSC have inflammatory bowel disease, predominantly in the form of ulcerative colitis, although the disease can appear following liver transplantation. The disease more often affects men and is progressive in nature.[1-3] Presentation is usually at the time of symptoms and fibrotic bile ductule changes, with little in the way of hope for medical management. Multiple medical therapies have been studied; however, trials of bile acid therapy and immunosuppressive agents have not led to prolonged survival or any improvement in quality of life. Surgical therapies or endoscopically placed stents may relieve obstruction associated with a dominant stricture, but there is no long-term effect on survival or disease progression. Thus, liver transplantation ultimately remains the only option for patients with PSC with complications of end-stage liver disease or recurrent episodes of bacterial cholangitis caused by chronic biliary obstruction, or both.

Issues Prior to Transplantation

The general criteria for liver transplantation are no different for PSC than for other chronic liver diseases. Furthermore, the Model for End-stage Liver Disease (MELD) score calculation is identical to that used for patients on the waiting list with other diseases. However, disease-specific complications may arise and may lead to a request for additional MELD points from the regional review board.

Bacterial Cholangitis

The presence of fibrotic stricturing resulting in impaired bile flow may lead to recurrent episodes of bacterial cholangitis. Cholangiographic evaluation may identify a dominant stricture amenable to balloon dilation. However, diffuse involvement of the intrahepatic biliary tree can lead to recurrent episodes of cholangitis and biliary sepsis. Broad-spectrum antibiotic coverage for gram-negative bacteria and *Enterococcus* usually leads to improvement, but hepatic abscesses may occur in the face of obliterated bile ducts. Recurrent episodes should prompt referral to a transplant center, even in the absence of complications of end-stage liver disease.

Pruritus

Pruritus is a common complication of cholestatic liver diseases. Although dilation of a dominant stricture may lead to improvement or resolution, some patients may complain of pruritus in the absence of jaundice or a dominant stricture. This is likely related to an increase in central opioid receptors.[4] Treatment may range from the simple to the bizarre:

- Antihistamines and topical lotions are rarely helpful.
- Cholestyramine has historically been the treatment of choice.
- Ursodeoxycholic acid is helpful in a small percentage of patients.
- Rifampin, in a dose of 150 to 300 mg twice a day, can decrease the pruritus.[5] If decompensation occurs in a patient using rifampin therapy who has otherwise stable PSC, the patient may have rifampin hepatotoxicity.

- Opiate antagonists, such as naltrexone in a dose of 25 to 50 mg daily to twice a day, can lead to immediate resolution of pruritus.[6]
- Serotonin uptake inhibitors decreased symptoms in one small study.[7]
- Plasmapheresis can lead to transient resolution of symptoms if medical therapy does not lead to improvement.[8] However, plasmapheresis should be used only for patients with severe symptoms, such as soft tissue abscesses related to skin excoriations or suicidal ideation.
- Liver transplantation is another option; however, the current MELD prioritization system does not give "extra" points for pruritus, unless approved by a regional review board.

Hepatic Osteodystrophy

Hepatic osteodystrophy, which is a common complication of cholestatic liver disease, can lead to vertebral body compression fractures resulting in severe, immobilizing back pain and atraumatic fractures of the axial skeleton.[9] Thus, bone densitometry should be measured in all patients with PSC being evaluated for a liver transplant. Calcium and vitamin D supplementation, particularly in deficient patients, should be instituted, although evidence that this actually improves bone density in patients with PSC is lacking. The use of antiresorptive agents (such as bisphosphonates or calcitonin) or hormone replacement therapy in postmenopausal or oophorectomized women is also not of proven benefit, although these therapies are frequently used. Debilitating bone disease was once considered an indication for transplantation; however, the worsening of bone density over the course of the first 3 postoperative months, with as many as one third of patients with PSC suffering pathological fractures,[10] has actually led many transplant centers to consider this a contraindication to transplantation.

Inflammatory Bowel Disease

The common association of inflammatory bowel disease with PSC often raises management issues before transplantation. The potential for colonic malignancy in patients with ulcerative colitis should result in a screening colonoscopy during the initial evaluation. If colonic dysplasia is present, a practical issue regarding management may be problematic. Although colonic resection in the face of end-stage liver disease may be associated with increased morbidity and even mortality, the issue of delaying resection until a suitable time after the transplant is plagued by concern that malignancy may be present and, if so, its behavior in the presence of immunosuppression. Each case must be considered individually, with careful assessment of the potential risks and benefits. Medical management of the patient with active colitis should be no different from that for any other patient with ulcerative colitis; however, severe cases should be controlled before the patient assumes a position at the top of the list. Attempts to minimize immunosuppressive therapy in a patient at the top of the list to reduce the chance of an opportunistic infection should be carefully weighed against the potential for a disease flare.

Cholangiocarcinoma

The risk of cholangiocarcinoma is increased in patients with PSC, occurring in 10% to 20% of cases.[11,12] Unfortunately, predictive factors are lacking, with conflicting studies regarding the risk of more advanced disease as measured by survival models,[13,14] a history of significant alcohol intake or tobacco use,[15,16] and the presence of colorectal neoplasia.[15,17] Ideally, a serum tumor marker would allow early detection of cholangiocarcinoma, but results have been less than perfect. A cancer antigen (CA) 19-9 level greater than 100 U/mL has a sensitivity ranging from 75% to 89% and a specificity ranging from 80% to 86%.[15,18] Another measure using the CA 19-9 level and the carcinoembryonic antigen (CEA) (CA 19-9 + [CEA × 40]) found that a level greater than 400 had a specificity of more than 90% for cholangiocarcinoma in patients with PSC.[19] Another study, using the area under the curve for this score, found it no better than the CA 19-9 alone.[15] Endoscopic screening with brushings of the biliary tree may detect otherwise undetectable cases; however, access is limited and no study has shown an increased detection or survival rate using this technique.[20]

Magnetic resonance cholangiopancreatography (MRCP) is a less invasive method of evaluating the biliary tree, but to date no evidence exists of any effect on early detection. If the diagnosis is made, surgical resection is often impossible in the face of PSC, particularly in advanced stages. Chemotherapeutic options are ineffective, and transplantation appears life-saving in highly selected patients.[21] Patients on the list should be screened regularly, despite the inability to deal with this tumor, if only to prevent a transplant from being performed if the potential risk of recurrence and spread is deemed unacceptably high.

Prognostic Models for Survival

The MELD scoring system is the standard for prioritization on the waiting list in the United States. Before MELD, several other disease-specific mathematical models for survival in patients with PSC existed, although their practical use in clinical practice was unclear. The Mayo Clinic devised a model using serum bilirubin, age, histological stage, and splenomegaly.[22] King's College used hepatomegaly, splenomegaly, histological stage, age, and alkaline phosphatase in their model.[23] Although these models may have a place in the management of patients with PSC, their exact role in the management and timing of transplantation requires further study.

Transplant Surgery

The principles of liver transplant surgery for sclerosing cholangitis differ little from those for other liver diseases. Any remaining recipient biliary duct tissue could subsequently develop fibrotic changes, if not already present, so it is standard practice to avoid the use of native duct tissue. A Roux-en-Y choledochojejunostomy is the procedure of choice. Although the optimal length of the jejunal limb has not been established, 40 cm of defunctionalized jejunum is routinely used. The importance of a Roux limb of adequate length is illustrated by a single case report of a patient with PSC and intrahepatic strictures after liver transplantation. Although recurrent PSC in the liver allograft was considered, the presence of partially digested vegetable matter embedded in a severely inflamed duct was thought to be responsible, presumably the result of food refluxing up the 20-cm jejunal limb and across the biliary enteric anastomosis.[25] The transplant surgery may be complicated by previous biliary surgery, although this is much less common currently because of an apparent decrease in attempts at surgical management.

Posttransplant Survival

Survival following transplantation for PSC is excellent. Although an initial series had an actuarial 1-year survival of 71%, these results were compromised by patients with cholangiocarcinoma.[26] Recent studies show 1-year survival rates ranging from 90% to 94%, with 5-year survival rates ranging from 84% to 86%.[27-29] One center reported a 10-year survival of 70%.[29] The most common cause of death is infection, with 26% of deaths caused by this complication in one series.[29]

Cholangiocarcinoma clearly affects survival rates, particularly in patients with tumors found incidentally. A study of 169 patients undergoing transplantation over a 9-year period found a 10.6% incidence of cholangiocarcinoma.[30] Although the 1-year survival rate was not different for patients with cholangiocarcinoma versus patients without, the 5-year survival of patients with PSC alone was 75.8%, whereas 26.7% of those with malignant changes survived the same period.

More of those with cholangiocarcinoma known before the transplant died than those with incidental tumors at 2 years (26.7% survival versus 54.6% survival), although the small numbers prevented this from reaching statistical significance. Overall, incidental cholangiocarcinomas are found in 1.5% to 8% of cases.[27,29,30]

Posttransplant Complications

Other sections of this book address general complications seen in liver transplant recipients. Patients undergoing transplantation for PSC have disease-specific complications that may lead to increased morbidity and mortality.

Acute Cellular and Chronic/Ductopenic Rejection

Acute rejection of the transplanted liver is a risk for all transplant recipients. Several centers have identified an increased incidence of acute rejection in patients undergoing transplantation for PSC. In one series, an increased incidence of acute rejection was seen when compared with patients undergoing transplantation for other diseases (68.7% versus 59.3% [$P=0.04$]).[29] Coexistent inflammatory bowel disease may also increase the risk of rejection. One group showed more episodes of acute cellular rejection per patient,[29] whereas another group saw a trend toward more severe episodes of acute rejection, based on the use of monoclonal T-cell antibody, the need to switch from cyclosporine to tacrolimus, or the need for another transplant.[27]

Chronic/ductopenic rejection can also occur in patients undergoing transplantation for PSC. The largest series showed an incidence of 8%, with a significant decrease in patient and allograft survival.[29] A similar decrease in patient and allograft survival was seen in another series in which 13% of patients developed chronic/ductopenic rejection.[31] The timing of the transplant likely influences the risk, as patients undergoing transplantation earlier in one series had a higher rate of chronic/ductopenic rejection, likely caused by the development of additional immunosuppressive agents.[29]

Inflammatory Bowel Disease Following Transplantation

The course of inflammatory bowel disease following a liver transplant is variable. Many patients have improvement in symptoms or may be maintained on lower doses of anti-inflammatory agents, which are thought to be related to the immunosuppressive agents required to prevent rejection. However, some patients actually have worsening of their disease or the new onset of inflammatory bowel disease after transplantation. No specific events related to the transplant have been identified as precipitating factors.

Follow-up of ulcerative colitis should include an annual screening colonoscopy to monitor for malignant disease. One series of 31 PSC transplant recipients with a history of ulcerative colitis, with a mean follow-up of 45 months, revealed a 6.5% incidence of colorectal carcinoma. Whether the presence of immunosuppressive medication increases the risk of colorectal carcinoma is unclear.

Recurrent Disease and Biliary Strictures

The presence of biliary strictures following liver transplantation may be secondary to any number of problems. In the patient who undergoes transplantation for PSC, the question of disease recurrence in the transplanted liver must be considered. Isolated strictures at the biliary enteric anastomosis are sometimes a technical complication, occurring in approximately 5% of patients. These can be treated effectively via a percutaneous approach by an interventional radiologist with balloon dilation and indwelling stent placement. If unsuccessful, reconstructive biliary surgery may be necessary.

Recurrence of PSC in the transplanted liver has been a topic of debate for a number of reasons. The absence of other contributing factors must be ruled out before PCS recurrence is considered. For example, the biliary system of the transplanted liver receives its blood supply from the hepatic artery. Thus, any compromise in hepatic arterial blood flow, such as profound hypotension, hepatic artery thrombosis, or hepatic artery stenosis, may lead to ischemic bile duct injury. Cholangiographically, the appearance of ischemic bile duct injury is no different from the classic appearance of PSC, although one series found an increased incidence of biliary sludge in patients with ischemic biliary injury.[31] Severe preservation injury and an ABO-incompatible donor liver can also lead to biliary strictures. Chronic/ductopenic rejection, with its characteristic arteriopathy, could also lead to bile duct ischemia, although one study did not demonstrate bile duct stricturing in patients with PSC with ductopenic rejection.[31] Chronic/ductopenic rejection occurred earlier than what was defined as recurrent PSC (mean of 5 months versus 25 months), and was associated with a significant decrease in both patient and allograft survival. Thus, although fibro-obliterative bile duct changes may be seen in both chronic/ductopenic rejection and recurrent PSC, an early appearance of these changes may be more consistent with ductopenic rejection.

The Mayo Clinic group looked at their experience with patients undergoing transplantation for PSC and attempted to define disease recurrence in the absence of compromised hepatic arterial blood flow, established chronic/ductopenic rejection, ABO incompatibility between the donor and the recipient, and an anastomotic stricture without other biliary strictures.[29] Their proposal included patients with an established diagnosis of PSC at least 90 days following the transplant with either of the following:

1. A cholangiogram marked by nonanastomotic biliary strictures of the intrahepatic and/or extrahepatic biliary tree

2. A liver biopsy with fibrous cholangitis and/or fibro-obliterative lesions with or without ductopenia, biliary fibrosis, or biliary cirrhosis.

Cholangiographic evidence was seen at a mean of 421 days (range 92 to 1275 days) following a transplant in 18.3% of patients. Histological evidence was seen at a mean of 1380 days following the transplant (range 420 to 3240 days) in 9.2% of the patients. Cholangiographic *and* histological changes were seen in 7.5% of the study group. No obvious precipitating factors could be identified (i.e., patients with recurrent disease had no evidence of more frequent episodes of prolonged cold ischemia time, different preservation solutions, cytomegalovirus [CMV] infections, or positive lymphocytotoxic crossmatches). However, inflammatory bowel disease was seen more frequently in the patients with recurrent disease. No difference in patient or allograft survival was seen at 5 years in those with recurrent disease versus those without based on this definition.

The findings in the Mayo Clinic study raise a number of questions regarding the natural history of recurrent PSC. One could theorize that bile ductule injury must be present, albeit at the microscopic level, for some time prior to the fibrotic changes characteristic of disease recurrence. A recent series of nontransplant patients with autoimmune hepatitis evolving to cholangiographically proven PSC suggests that microscopic ductule injury precedes the macroscopic changes seen radiographically.[32] However, the timing of the cholangiographic changes in the Mayo Clinic series was actually much earlier than the mean time to the histological changes. This raises several possibilities. Some cases of recurrent disease may occur in an accelerated fashion, without evidence of earlier histological change. However, the possibility that histological changes were indeed present before the radiographic changes must be considered as well. In Figure 13–1A, note the biliary stricturing in a patient 2 years after undergoing transplantation for PSC, with no evidence of abnormal hepatic arterial flow or ductopenia. However, the histological changes are rather bland and without evidence of the characteristic onion skin fibrosis (Fig. 13–1B). In Figure 13–2, another patient with recurrent PSC has histological changes (from the liver allograft explant for a retransplant) that were seen in association with biliary stricturing. This leaves the question of histological changes preceding cholangiographic changes unanswered. Furthermore, the possibility of a sampling error may also be a factor.

Ideally, the identification of recurrent disease in its earliest stages could lead to medical therapy that, theoretically, could slow disease progression or stop it all together.

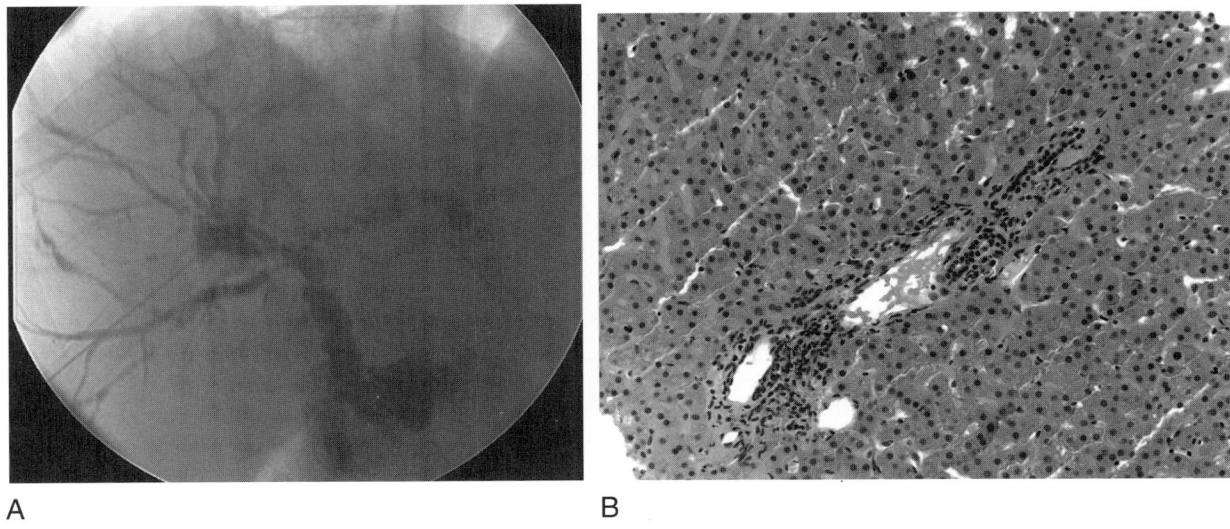

A   B

FIGURE 13–1

A, Percutaneous cholangiogram from a patient who underwent transplantation for primary sclerosing cholangitis (PSC) with characteristic biliary stricturing. This patient had no evidence of compromised hepatic arterial flow. **B,** Liver biopsy from the same patient showing a mild portal lymphocytic infiltrate and an absence of significant biliary duct damage and fibrosis.

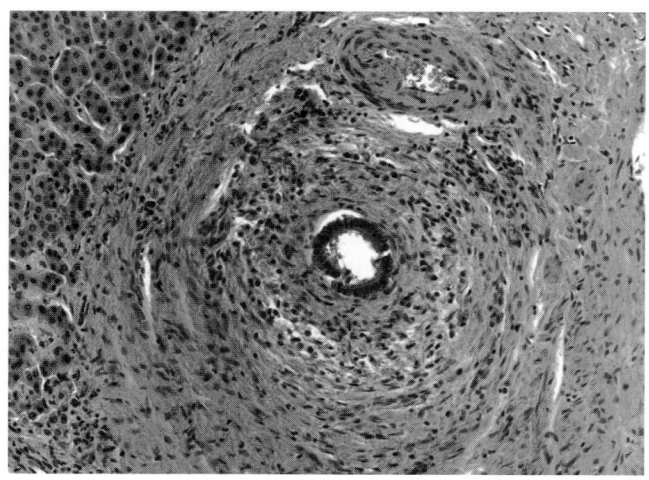

FIGURE 13–2

Liver biopsy from the allograft explant of a patient transplanted for recurrent primary sclerosing cholangitis (PSC). Note the periductal fibrosis and lymphocytic infiltrate.

Unfortunately, the lack of an identifiable medical therapy for this disease, at any stage, makes it impossible to make definitive recommendations. Potential medical interventions include additional immunosuppressive agents or bile acid therapy, or both. Controlled trials will have to be performed before definitive recommendations can be made regarding preemptive medical therapy immediately following the transplant or at the time histological changes are identified.

Summary

Since the first edition of this book was published in 1996, we have gained a better understanding of the potential problems associated with liver transplantation for PSC. One-year survival rates of 90% or more are now seen, with 10-year survival rates of 70%. Despite this success, we continue to struggle with the issues of disease recurrence, the risk of cholangiocarcinoma prior to transplantation, and the optimal management of coexistent inflammatory bowel disease. Hopefully, by the time the third edition of this book is released, we will have defined the natural history of disease recurrence, have early medical therapies that will affect and slow disease progression, and be able to identify the factors that lead to exacerbation of inflammatory bowel disease. If the next 5 to 10 years are anything like the last, these goals will be achieved.

Acknowledgments

Thank you to Hanlin Wang, MD, for his assistance with the histological images and to Dan Brown, MD, for his assistance with the radiographic image.

> ## Pearls and Pitfalls
>
> - Cholangiocarcinoma occurs in 10% to 20% of patients with PSC.
> - Although screening for cholangiocarcinoma is frequently practiced, the optimal screening tool remains to be defined.
> - Other causes of biliary strictures must be ruled out before PSC can *recur* in the liver allograft.
> - Patients undergoing transplantation for PSC should be screened for colorectal carcinoma annually.

References

1. Porayko MK, Wiesner RH, LaRusso NF, et al: Patients with asymptomatic primary sclerosing cholangitis frequently have progressive disease. Gastroenterology 98:1594-1602, 1990.
2. Broome U, Olsson R, Loof L, Bodemar G, et al: Natural history and prognostic factors in 305 Swedish patients with primary sclerosing cholangitis. Gut 38: 610-615, 1996.
3. Angulo P, Larson DR, Therneau TM, et al: Time course of histological progression in primary sclerosing cholangitis. Am J Gastroenterol 94:3310-3313, 1999.
4. Jones EA, Bergasa NV: The pruritus of cholestasis: From bile acids to opiate agonists. Hepatology 11:884-887, 1990.
5. Ghent CN, Carruthers SG: Treatment of pruritus in primary biliary cirrhosis with rifampin. Gastroenterology 94:488-493, 1988.
6. Wolfhagen FHJ, Sternieris E, Hop WCJ, et al: Oral naltrexone treatment for cholestatic pruritus: A double blind, placebo-controlled study. Gastroenterology 113:1264-1269, 1997.
7. Schworer H, Hartman H, Ramadori G: Relief of cholestatic pruritus by a novel class of drugs: 5-Hydroxytryptamine type 3 (5-HT$_3$) receptor antagonists. Effectiveness of odansetron. Pain 61:33-37, 1995.
8. Cohen LB, Ambinder EP, Wolke AM, et al: Role of plasmapheresis in primary biliary cirrhosis. Gut 26:291-294, 1985.
9. Angulo P, Therneau TM, Jorgensen RA, et al: Bone disease in patients with primary sclerosing cholangitis: Prevalence, severity, and prediction of severity. J Hepatol 29:729-735, 1998.
10. Porayko MK, Wiesner RH, Hay JE, et al: Bone disease in liver transplant recipients: Incidence, timing, and risk factors. Transplant Proc 23:1462-1465, 1991.
11. Rosen CB, Nagorney DM, Wiesner RH, et al: Cholangiocarcinoma complicating primary sclerosing cholangitis. Ann Surg 213: 21-25, 1991.
12. Ahrendt SA, Pitt HA, Nakeeb A, et al: Diagnosis and management of cholangiocarcinoma in primary sclerosing cholangitis. J Gastrointest Surg 3:357-368, 1999.
13. Nashan B, Schlitt HJ, Tusch G, et al: Biliary malignancies in primary sclerosing cholangitis: Timing for liver transplantation. Hepatology 23:1105-1111, 1996.
14. Olivera MA, McCashland TM, Ruby L, et al: Mayo risk score is not predictive of cholangiocarcinoma associated with primary sclerosing cholangitis [Abstract]. Gastroenterology 114:A1316, 1998.
15. Chalasani N, Baluyut A, Ismail A, et al: Cholangiocarcinoma in patients with primary sclerosing cholangitis: A multicenter case-control study. Hepatology 31:7-11, 2000.
16. Bergquist A, Glaumann H, Persson B, et al: Risk factors and clinical presentation of hepatobiliary carcinoma in patients with

primary sclerosing cholangitis: A case-control study. Hepatology 27:311-316, 1998.

17. Broome U, Lofberg R, Veress B, et al: Primary sclerosing cholangitis and ulcerative colitis: Evidence for increased neoplastic potential. Hepatology 22:1404-1408, 1995.

18. Nichols JC, Gores GJ, LaRusso NF, et al: Predicting cholangiocarcinoma in patients with primary sclerosing cholangitis: An analysis of the serological marker CA 19-9. Mayo Clin Proc 68:874-879, 1993.

19. Ramage JK, Donaghy A, Farrant JM, et al: Serum tumor markers for the diagnosis of cholangiocarcinoma in primary sclerosing cholangitis. Gastroenterology 108:865-869, 1995.

20. Ponsioen CY, Vrouenraets SM, van Milligen de Wit AW, et al: Value of brush cytology for dominant strictures in primary sclerosing cholangitis. Endoscopy 31:305-309, 1999.

21. De Vreede I, Steers JL, Burch PA, et al: Prolonged disease-free survival after orthotopic liver transplantation plus adjuvant chemoirradiation for cholangiocarcinoma. Liver Transpl 6: 309-316, 2000.

22. Kim WR, Therneau TM, Wiesner RH, et al: A revised natural history model for primary sclerosing cholangitis obviates the need for liver histology. Mayo Clin Proc 75:688-694, 2000.

23. Farrant JM, Hayllar KM, Wilkinson ML, et al: Natural history and prognostic variables in primary sclerosing cholangitis. Gastroenterology 100:1710-1717, 1991.

24. Lerut J, Demetris AJ, Stieber AC, et al: Intrahepatic bile duct strictures after human orthotopic liver transplantation: Recurrence of primary sclerosing cholangitis or unusual presentation of allograft rejection. Transpl Int 1:127-130, 1988.

25. Hartmann GG, Gordon R, Lerut J, et al: Intrahepatic bile duct strictures in a liver allograft recipient mimicking recurrent PSC: Follow-up of a case report. Transpl Int 4:191-192, 1991.

26. Marsh JW, Iwatsuki S, Makowka L, et al: Orthotopic liver transplantation for primary sclerosing cholangitis. Ann Surg 207: 21-25, 1988.

27. Narumi S, Roberts JP, Emond JC, et al: Liver transplantation for sclerosing cholangitis. Hepatology 22:451-457, 1995.

28. Goss JS, Shackleton CR, Farmer DG, et al: Orthotopic liver transplantation for primary sclerosing cholangitis: A 12 year single center experience. Ann Surg 225:472-483, 1997.

29. Graziadei IW, Wiesner RH, Marotta PJ, et al: Long-term results of patients undergoing liver transplantation for primary sclerosing cholangitis. Hepatology 30:1121-1127, 1999.

30. Abu Elmagd KM, Selby R, Iwatsuki S, et al: Cholangiocarcinoma and sclerosing cholangitis: Clinical characteristics and effect on survival after liver transplantation. Transplant Proc 25:1124-1125, 1993.

31. Jeyarajah TR, Netto GJ, Lee SP, et al: Recurrent PSC after orthotopic liver transplantation. Transplantation 66:1300-1306, 1998.

32. Abdo AA, Bain VG, Kichian K, et al: Evolution of autoimmune hepatitis to primary sclerosing cholangitis: A sequential syndrome. Hepatology 36:1393-1399, 2002.

Liver Transplantation for Autoimmune Hepatitis

JOSE M. NIETO
SAMMY SAAB

Historical perspective   195

Epidemiology   196

Diagnostic criteria   196

Immunoserological subclassifications   197

Pathophysiology   199

Clinical manifestations   199
  Clinical symptoms   199
  Physical findings   200
  Associated autoimmune disorders   200
  Laboratory findings   200
  Histological features   201

Medical treatment   201
  First-line medical regimen   201
  Adjunctive medical treatment   203
  New pharmacotherapies   203

Role of liver transplantation   204

Immunosuppression after liver transplantation   204

Acute and chronic allograft rejection   204

Recurrent autoimmune hepatitis after
  transplantation   204
  Risk factors for recurrence   205
  Pathogenesis   206

De novo autoimmune hepatitis after liver
  transplantation (graft dysfunction mimicking
  autoimmune hepatitis)   206
  Pathogenesis   207

Autoimmune hepatitis (AIH) is a chronic, necroinflammatory liver disease of unknown etiology characterized by the presence of various circulating autoantibodies, hypergammaglobulinemia, and interface hepatitis of predominant lymphoplasmacytic necroinflammatory infiltration on histologic examination.[1,2] AIH reflects complex interactions among triggering factors, autoantigens, genetic predispositions, and immunoregulatory networks.[3] There is a higher prevalence among females,[4] an immunogenetic connection with the human leukocyte antigen (HLA) A1-B8-DR3 or DR4 haplotype,[5] and an association with extrahepatic conditions.[6] AIH tends to respond well to immunosuppressive therapy.[7] Patients who do not achieve remission are at risk of developing liver cirrhosis.[8] Liver transplantation is the treatment of choice in patients with decompensated AIH,[9] but acute allograft rejection and recurrence of primary disease is common.[10,11] De novo AIH after transplantation can occur in both pediatric and adult populations.[12,15]

Historical Perspective

Hyperproteinemia and idiopathic recurrent jaundice with unresolving hepatic inflammation were first described in the early 1940s,[13,14] but idiopathic AIH was not recognized until 1950 when Waldenström described the constellation of cirrhosis, plasma cell infiltration of the liver, and hypergammaglobulinemia in young women.[16] In 1955, the lupus erythematosus (LE) cell phenomenon[17] and the presence of antinuclear antibodies (ANAs) led Mackay and colleagues[18] to introduce the term *lupoid hepatitis*. In the 1960s, subgroups of patients were distinguished by specific immunoserological findings, and Page and colleagues[19] demonstrated that treatment with 6-mercaptopurine improved clinical symptoms and decreased the level of hypergammaglobulinemia. Whittingham and colleagues[20] distinguished among chronic active hepatitis and systemic lupus erythematosus and introduced the term *autoimmune hepatitis*. In 1973, Rizzetto and colleagues described an autoantibody reacting with the microsomal fraction of hepatocytes and renal tubular epithelium in patients with chronic active hepatitis.[21] In 1987, the first formal proposal to subclassify AIH was introduced. The same year, Manns and colleagues described anti–soluble liver antigen (SLA)/anti–liver-pancreas antigen (LP), which occurred in approximately 30% of patients who presented with seronegative conventional autoantibodies, and type 3 classifications for AIH were suggested.[22]

Epidemiology

In early reports on the prevalence of AIH, the condition was included within the spectrum of chronic active hepatitis. Early epidemiological studies from 1970 to 1995 in Western European populations showed a mean annual incidence of AIH ranging from 1.9 to 16.9 cases per 100,000 persons.[23-27] AIH accounts for 2.6% of liver transplantations in Europe[28] and 5.9% in the United States.[29] The incidence and characteristics of AIH differ in various geographical regions. Based on recent, limited epidemiological studies, the incidence of type 1 AIH in the white populations of Europe and North America ranges from 0.1 to 1.9 cases per 100,000 persons per year; it is less frequent in Japan.[29] Type 2 AIH is most prevalent in Southern Europe, and type 3, which is characterized by the occurrence of anti–SLA/LP, is also higher in Europe. The frequency of HLA markers varies among ethnic groups. HLA DR3 and DR4 are the major risk factors for type 1 AIH in white European and North American populations. HLA DR4 is a principal risk factor in Japanese patients. Females are affected more than males (3.6:1), and all ages and ethnic groups are susceptible.

The mortality of untreated AIH is high. Up to 40% of untreated patients with decompensated liver disease expire within 6 months.[30] Cirrhosis develops in approximately 40% of diagnosed, untreated patients.[31] Of patients with cirrhosis, 54% develop esophageal varices within 2 years, and 20% expire from variceal hemorrhage.[32] In patients with sustained serum aminotransferase levels more than 10-fold normal or more than 5-fold normal in conjunction with serum γ-globulin concentrations that are elevated at least 2-fold, mortality without treatment is 90% at 10 years.[30] The risk of developing cirrhosis is associated with histological findings. In patients with periportal hepatitis, cirrhosis develops in 17% within 5 years, bridging necrosis or multiacinar necrosis progresses to cirrhosis in 82% within 5 years, and mortality is 45%.[33] Patients with moderate laboratory findings—serum aminotransferase levels less than 10-fold normal or less than 5-fold normal in conjunction with serum γ-globulin concentrations that are elevated less than 2-fold—develop cirrhosis in 49% of cases within 15 years, and death from fulminant hepatic failure occurs in 10%.[34] Hepatocellular carcinoma occurs in 11% of patients with cirrhosis after 18 years and increases to 29% after 13 years in these patients. With immunosuppression treatment, 65% of patients achieve clinical, biochemical, and histological remission within 18 months, and 80% do so within 3 years. The 20-year survival rate of treated patients is 80%, in contrast to a 10-year survival rate of 10% in untreated patients.[35] Although immunosuppression remains the mainstay of therapy for AIH, 9% of patients deteriorate on traditional regimens, 13% develop treatment-related side effects that warrant premature discontinuation of medication, and 13% have an incomplete response. Of patients who experience remission and discontinue therapy, 74% to 85% relapse within 3 years.[36,37]

Diagnostic Criteria

The trigger or cause of AIH is unknown and no pathognomonic features have been identified. Therefore, diagnosis requires the presence of a combination of clinical, histological, and laboratory abnormalities together with the exclusion of other possible causes of liver disease (Table 14–1). All patients suspected of having AIH must be evaluated for hereditary (Wilson's disease, genetic hemochromatosis, and α_1-antitrypsin deficiency), infectious, and drug-induced liver injury because of overlapping features with AIH.[38]

An international panel has proposed a diagnostic criteria, and its validity has been confirmed by six major studies evaluating a total of 983 patients.[39] A scoring system also has been proposed to assess the certainty of the diagnosis (Table 14–2).[38] The diagnostic criteria include gender, serum γ-globulin levels, autoantibodies, alcohol use, medications, viral markers, histology, HLA, and immunosuppression treatment response. These variables help rule out other possible causes of chronic active hepatitis. The score is based on pretreatment features; therefore, it can be adjusted by the response to treatment. By taking into account each component of the syndrome, discrepant features and

Table 14-1. DIAGNOSTIC CRITERIA FOR AUTOIMMUNE HEPATITIS

Requisites	Diagnostic Criteria	
	Definite	**Probable**
No genetic liver disease	Normal α_1-antitrypsin phenotype	Partial α_1-antitrypsin deficiency
	Normal serum ceruloplasmin, iron, and ferritin levels	Nonspecific serum copper, ceruloplasmin, iron, and/or ferritin abnormalities
No active viral infection	No markers of current infection with hepatitis A, B, and C viruses	No markers of current infection with hepatitis A, B, and C viruses
No toxic or alcohol injury	Daily alcohol <25 g/day and no recent use of hepatotoxic drugs	Daily alcohol <50 g/day and no recent use of hepatotoxic drugs
Laboratory features	Predominant serum aminotransferase abnormality	Predominant serum aminotransferase abnormality
	Globulin, γ-globulin or immunoglobulin G level ≥1.5 times normal	Hypergammaglobulinemia of any degree
Autoantibodies	ANAs, SMAs, or anti–LKM-1 ≥1:80 in adults and ≥1:20 in children; no AMAs	ANAs, SMAs, or anti–LKM-1 ≥1:40 in adults or other autoantibodies*
Histological findings	Interface hepatitis	Interface hepatitis
	No biliary lesions, granulomas, or prominent changes suggestive of another disease	No biliary lesions, granulomas, or prominent changes suggestive of another disease

*Includes perinuclear antineutrophil cytoplasmic antibodies and the not generally available antibodies to soluble liver antigen/liver pancreas, actin, liver cytosol type 1, and asialoglycoprotein receptor. AMAs, antimitochondrial antibodies; ANAs, antinuclear antibodies; LKM, liver-kidney microsome; SMAs, smooth muscle antibodies.
Based on recommendations from Alvarez F, Berg PA, Bianchi FB, et al: International Autoimmune Hepatitis Group Report: Review of criteria for diagnosis of autoimmune hepatitis. J Hepatol 31:929-938, 1999.

biases associated with isolated inconsistencies can be avoided.[39] The sensitivity of the scoring system for AIH ranges from 97% to 100%,[40-42] and its specificity for excluding AIH in patients with chronic hepatitis C ranges from 66% to 92%.[43,44]

In most cases, the scoring system is not needed for diagnosis of AIH when the clinical, laboratory, and histological features of the syndrome are well defined. The importance of the scoring system is in its assessment of variant or atypical syndromes that resemble the classic diagnosis.[45] A limitation of the scoring system is its ability to exclude cholestatic syndromes, such as cholestatic overlap syndromes (primary sclerosing cholangitis [PSC] and primary biliary cirrhosis [PBC]), that present with autoimmune features. Excluding biliary disease has shown a better performance in the scoring system, and cholangiography is recommended for all patients with definite or probable AIH scores that do not respond to standard steroid therapy.[46]

Immunoserological Subclassifications

Three types of AIH subclassificaions have been proposed based on immunoserological markers. The subclasses do not have different causes or responses to corticosteroid therapy. Transplantation outcomes are similar among the different subclassifications (Table 14–3).

Type 1 is the most common subclass of AIH worldwide, representing 80% of cases. It is associated with non–organ-specific ANAs or anti–smooth muscle antibodies (SMAs), or both. It affects all age groups with a bimodal age distribution of 10 to 20 years and 45 to 75 years and a female prevalence of 78%. It is associated with HLA DR3 (*DRB1*0301*) and DR4 (*DRB1*0401*) in white Northern European and North American patients. White patients with type 1 AIH and DR3 are younger, have a higher treatment failure rate, relapse after corticosteroid withdrawal, and require liver transplantation. Patients with DR4 are older, frequently have concurrent autoimmune diseases (48%), and have a better corticosteroid response.[47] The clinical course is often unremarkable, and acute onset is very rare. Approximately 25% have cirrhosis at the time of diagnosis.

Type 2 AIH is a rare disorder that affects 20% of AIH patients in Europe, but only 4% in the United States, and it is characterized by anti–liver-kidney microsome (LKM)-1. Serum immunoglobulin (Ig) levels are moderately elevated with a reduction in IgA, and susceptibility may relate to *DRB *0701*. Perinuclear antineutrophil cytoplasmic antibody (pANCA) is common in type 1 but is not detected in type 2 AIH. The anti–LKM-1 autoantibodies inhibit cytochrome P450 (CYP) 2D6 activity and may occur with chronic hepatitis C virus (HCV) infection. Female predominance is 89%. Extrahepatic autoimmune syndromes are less common than AIH type 1.

Table 14–2. DIAGNOSTIC SCORING SYSTEM FOR ATYPICAL AUTOIMMUNE HEPATITIS IN ADULTS

Category	Factor	Score	Category	Factor	Score
Gender	Female	+2	Concurrent immune disease	Any nonhepatic disease of an immune nature	+2
Alk phos: AST (or ALT) ratio	>3 <1.5	−2 +2	Other autoantibodies*	Anti–SLA/LP, actin, LC1, pANCA	+2
γ-globulin or IgG (times above upper limit of normal)	>2.0 1.5-2.0 1.0-1.5 <1.0	+3 +2 +1 0	Histological features	Interface hepatitis Plasma cells Rosettes None of above Biliary changes† Atypical features‡	+3 +1 +1 −5 −3 −3
ANAs, SMAs, or anti–LKM-1 titers	>1:80 1:80 1:40 <1:40	+3 +2 +1 0	HLA	DR3 or DR4	+1
AMAs	Positive	−4	Treatment response	Remission alone Remission with relapse	+2 +3
Viral markers of active infection	Positive Negative	−3 +3			
Hepatotoxic drugs	Yes No	−4 +1	Pretreatment score Definite diagnosis Probable diagnosis		>15 10-15
Alcohol	<25 g/d >60 g/d	+2 −2	Posttreatment score Definite diagnosis Probable diagnosis		>17 12-17

*Unconventional or generally unavailable antibodies associated with liver disease include perinuclear antineutrophil cytoplasmic antibodies (pANCAs) and antibodies to actin, anti–soluble liver antigen/liver pancreas (anti–SLA/LP), asialoglycoprotein receptor (ASGPR), and liver cytosol type 1 (LC-1).
†Includes destructive cholangitis, nondestructive cholangitis, or ductopenia.
‡Includes steatosis, iron overload consistent with genetic hemochromatosis, alcohol-induced hepatitis, viral features (ground-glass hepatocytes), or inclusions (cytomegalovirus, herpes simplex).
Alk phos, (serum) alkaline phosphatase (level); ALT, (serum) alanine aminotransferase (level); AMAs, antimitochondrial antibodies; ANAs, antinuclear antibodies; AST, (serum) aspartate aminotransferase (level); HLA, human leukocyte antigen; IgG, (serum) immunoglobulin G (level); LKM, liver-kidney microsome; SMAs, smooth muscle antibodies.
Based on recommendations from Alvarez F, Berg PA, Bianchi FB, et al: International Autoimmune Hepatitis Group Report: Review of criteria for diagnosis of autoimmune hepatitis. J Hepatol 31(5):929-938, 1999.

Table 14–3. IMMUNOSEROLOGICAL CLASSIFICATIONS

Clinical Features	Type 1	Type 2a	Type 2b	Type 3
Diagnostic autoantibodies	ANA SMA pANCA	Anti–LKM	Anti–LKM (low titers) HCV Ab	Anti–SLA/LP
Age	Bimodal (10-20 y and 45-75 y)	Pediatric (2-14 y) Rare in adults	Adults	Adults (30-50 y)
Women (%)	78	89	<50	90
Concurrent immune disease (%)	48	34	Unknown	58
γ-globulin elevation	+++	+	+	++
Low IgA	No	Occasional	No	No
HLA association	B8, DR3, DR4	B14, DR3, C4AQO	B8, DR3, DR4	Uncertain
Steroid response	+++	++	±	+++
Progression to cirrhosis (%)	45	82	Unknown	75

ANA, antinuclear antibody; HLA, human leukocyte antigen; IgA, immunoglobulin A; LKM, liver-kidney microsome; pANCA, perinuclear antineutrophil cytoplasmic antibody; SLA/LP, soluble liver antigen/liver pancreas; SMA, smooth muscle antibody.

The age range is from 2 to 14 years, but type 2 is also reported in adults in Europe. Type 2 carries a higher risk of progression to cirrhosis and fulminant hepatitis at presentation. It has been proposed that type 2 be subdivided into 2a (HCV-negative young women with severe liver disease and high titers of anti–LKM-1) and 2b (HCV-positive, predominantly older males, with low anti–LKM-1 titers).

A distinct form of LKM-positive AIH has been recognized in association with autoimmune polyglandular syndrome (APS)-1, which is characterized by autoimmune polyendocrinopathy, candidiasis, ectodermal dystrophy (APECED). APECED is characterized by ectodermal disorders, chronic mucocutaneous candidiasis, immune-mediated destruction of endocrine tissues (parathyroid gland, adrenal gland, ovaries), autoantibody production to CYP1A2, and AIH (10% to 18%). It is caused by a mutation in the autoimmune regulator (AIRE) gene.[48] Patients with AIH and APECED have no gender predominance and have particularly aggressive liver disease that does not respond well to immunosuppressive therapy.

A second type of LKM autoantibodies, anti–LKM-2, is directed against CYP2C9 and is induced in ticrynafen-associated hepatitis. A third group, anti–LKM-3, occurs in 6% to 10% of patients with chronic hepatitis D virus (HDV).

Type 3 AIH is characterized by the presence of anti–SLA/LP, a urogenital atrophy (UGA)-suppressor, tRNA-associated protein. This subclass is clinically and biochemically indistinguishable from AIH type 1. The age range of patients is between 30 and 50 years, and 90% of cases are females. Patients respond well to corticosteroid treatment.[49]

Pathophysiology

The most accepted hypothesis for the cause of AIH suggests that an environmental agent triggers an autoimmune process against the liver in a genetically predisposed individual. Multiple triggering factors have been implicated such as viruses, drugs, and toxins. Proposed viral triggers include measles virus; hepatitis A, B, and C; and the Epstein-Barr virus.[50-55] Drugs associated with AIH include diclofenac, methyldopa, oxyphenisatin, nitrofurantoin, and minocycline.[56] The actual mechanisms by which these environmental agents can initiate autoimmunity and trigger AIH are unknown. Molecular mimicry is currently the most popular theory.

During immunological development, individuals are protected against self-reactive T and B cells by negative clonal selection and apoptosis of these cells. Many studies support the idea of epitope mimicry, in which a susceptible individual is presented with an environmental agent, which exhibits antigens that share homologies with host antigens. These shared homologies result in a cross-reaction and loss of self-tolerance leading to an immune response generated against the host tissue. There can potentially be a long lag time between exposure to the trigger and onset of disease, and the environmental agent may or may not be present when the autoimmune disease becomes clinically apparent.[57]

Genetic predisposition is determined by genes that encode HLAs on the major histocompatibility complex, immunoglobulins, and T-cell receptor molecules. Type 1 AIH is associated with the HLA-DR3 and HLA-DR4 serotypes. The HLA-class II susceptibility alleles of AIH are located on the *DRB1* gene, and in whites they are *DRB1*0301* and *DRB1*0401*.[58-60] Different ethnic groups have different susceptibility alleles. For example, the predominant DR4 allele in Japanese patients is *DRB1*0405*.[61] How these alleles confer susceptibility to AIH is not well understood, but the risk of disease seems to relate to the amino acid sequences in the HLA-class II antigen-binding groove carried by the *DRB1*0301* and *DRB1*0401* alleles in whites.

Both cellular and humoral immunity are involved in the autoimmune destruction of hepatocytes. It is mediated by CD4$^+$ helper T cells that recognize self-antigen.[62] Cytokines such as interferon (INF)-γ, tumor necrosis factor-α (TNF-α), and interleukin (IL) 2 in the environment will lead to the differentiation of different effector cells. CD8$^+$ cytotoxic T cells are involved in both cell-mediated and humoral autoimmunity in AIH. Antibody-dependent cytotoxic activity mainly involves antibodies against the asialoglycoprotein receptor (ASGPR), a hepatocyte membrane protein.[63,64] Natural killer cells are present in the normal liver and may be involved with liver destruction possibly through the expression of the Fas ligand and the binding of its Fc receptor with an antigen-antibody complex on the hepatocyte.

Clinical Manifestations

Clinical Symptoms

Autoimmune hepatitis is typically an insidious disease of young females, who constitute approximately 70% of all cases, and as many as 50% of patients are younger than 30 years of age. Onset usually occurs in the third and fifth decades of life, but patient ages range from 9 months to 77 years. An acute presentation that mimics acute viral hepatitis clinically and biochemically occurs in approximately 30% of patients.[65] A rare fulminant presentation with severe encephalopathy has been described, particularly among the anti–LKM-1 group.[66] Postmenopausal women constitute a subgroup that derives less net benefit from corticosteroid therapy and has a greater frequency of associated complications.[67]

Many patients with AIH may be asymptomatic for a long period. In most cases, the clinical presentation does not differ from that of other forms of chronic hepatitis.[68] Fatigability is the most common symptom at presentation (85%), and 77% of patients also describe features of jaundice (scleral icterus, change in color of urine and stool). Mild right upper quadrant pain (48%), pruritus (36%), anorexia (30%), polymyalgias (30%), diarrhea (28%), and constant pyrexia (18%) are frequent complaints.[69] Menstrual abnormalities (89%) include delayed menarche, irregular menstrual cycles, and amenorrhea. In later stages, the consequences of portal hypertension dominate, including ascites, bleeding esophageal varices, and encephalopathy.[69]

Physical Findings

Physical findings depend on the duration and severity of the disease. Hepatomegaly (78%) and jaundice (69%) are the most common physical findings at the time of diagnosis. Splenomegaly can be present in patients with and without portal hypertension (56% and 32%, respectively). Ascites (20%) and hepatic encephalopathy (14%) are recognized less frequently, but when they occur they are highly suggestive of cirrhosis.[70] Esophageal varices (8%) are not common initial findings.[71] Rare cutaneous manifestations include acne, facial rounding, hirsutism, hyperpigmented striae, xanthelasmas, and spider nevi. Gynecomastia occasionally is present in men.

Associated Autoimmune Disorders

A specific feature of AIH is the association of extrahepatic, autoimmune-mediated syndromes (40% to 50%), including autoimmune thyroiditis, rheumatoid arthritis, and diabetes mellitus.[68] Other disorders include Sjögren's syndrome, polymyositis, IgA deficiency, idiopathic thrombocytopenia, urticaria, vitiligo, CREST syndrome (calcinosis cutis, Raynaud's phenomenon, esophageal motility disorder, sclerodactyly, and telangiectasia), Addison's disease, lichen planus, and nail dystrophy. Inflammatory bowel disease is also common, and screening for antiendomysial antibodies is advisable to exclude celiac sprue.[72] Associated ulcerative colitis raises suspicions about the diagnosis of AIH; therefore, a cholangiography is indicated to exclude PSC. The presence of concurrent extrahepatic immunological disorders in the patient or family member supports the diagnosis.

Laboratory Findings

The major biochemical abnormalities include elevated serum aminotransferase activity and bilirubin concentrations with normal or only moderately elevated serum alkaline phosphatase with hypergammaglobulinemia. Serum aminotransferase elevations greater than 1000 IU/L are more typical of viral, drug-induced, or ischemic hepatitis. It is now recognized that aminotransferase and bilirubin levels vary widely among individuals and fluctuate or normalize at times; therefore, a threefold elevation is no longer considered diagnostic of AIH.[38] Hypergammaglobulinemia is characteristically caused by a disproportionate increase in the IgG fraction, which may be elevated even if total globulin concentrations are normal.

Autoantibodies are the serological hallmark of AIH, therefore ANAs, SMAs, and anti–LKM should be determined in all patients with clinical, laboratory, and/or histological suspicion of AIH. When these autoantibodies are undetectable and AIH is still considered, the SLA/LP antigens may be helpful. ANAs are present alone (13%) or with SMAs (54%) in 67% of patients with AIH.[73] They represent the most common autoantibody in AIH and occur in high titers, usually exceeding 1:160. ANA is nonspecific and can be found in PBC, PSC, chronic viral hepatitis, drug-induced hepatitis, and alcohol liver disease. SMAs are directed against actin and nonactin components and are present in 87% of patients with AIH, either alone (33%) or in conjunction with ANAs (54%).[73] SMA autoantibodies are also nonspecific and occur in titers lower than 1:80 in other liver diseases, rheumatological disorders, and infectious diseases. SMA is associated with HLA DR3 in actin-positive patients and with HLA DR4 with non–actin-positive patients.[74]

Anti–LKM typically occurs in the absence of SMAs and ANAs.[75,76] LKM-1 autoantibodies inhibit CYP2D6 activity in vitro.[77] Anti–LKM-1 can be found in hepatitis C infection.[77] Antibodies to LKM-1 occur in only 4% of adults with AIH in the United States.[75] They are usually described in pediatric patients in Europe; 20% of patients with anti–LKM-1 in France and Germany are adults.[76] Anti–LKM-2 is directed against CYP2C9. Anti–LKM-3 has been identified in 6% to 10% of patients with chronic hepatitis D virus infection.[78]

Anti–SLA/LPs are highly specific markers of AIH and are present as the only marker in 10% to 30% of patients.[79] In approximately 75% of cases, SLAs/LPs are present simultaneously with other autoantibodies and appear in 12% of cases with SMA- and/or ANA-positive patients. Asialoglycoprotein receptor (ASGPR) is observed in 88% of all patients with AIH[80]; however, it can also be found in chronic hepatitis B, hepatitis C, PBC, and alcoholic hepatitis. Its presence correlates with histological activity, its disappearance connotes response to treatment, and its persistence signifies relapse after corticosteroid treatment. Anti–liver-cytosol type 1 autoantibodies (anti–LC-1) are present in 32% of type 2 AIH, and their presence may correlate with disease activity. Perinuclear antineutrophil cytoplasm occurs in 92% of type 1 AIH, but its role is not clear and routine determination is not recommended.

Histological Features

There are no pathognomonic histological features of AIH. Interface (periportal or paraseptal) hepatitis, with a predominantly lymphoplasmacytic necroinflammatory infiltrate, is the most common histological finding in AIH. *Piecemeal*, or periportal, hepatitis is characterized by disruption of the limiting hepatocyte plate, where the interface among the parenchyma and portal tracts is the site of active inflammation and hepatocellular necrosis.

Plasma cell infiltration is abundant at the interface and through the acinus, but 34% of patients with AIH have few or no plasma cells. *Rosettes* are small clusters of hepatocytes surrounded by inflammatory cells that are prominent in the periportal regions. Pyknotic (apoptotic) cell necrosis and ballooning degeneration of hepatocytes are present in 39% of patients, and scattered multinucleated hepatocytes are nonspecific findings of AIH. Other nonspecific findings of AIH include steatosis, lymphoid aggregates, copper deposits, siderosis, and bile ductile proliferation.

Cirrhosis in patients with AIH is described as active or inactive depending on whether periportal (piecemeal) necrosis is present or not. These various patterns of necrosis represent fluctuations in the degree and extent of disease activity.

Medical Treatment

First-Line Medical Regimen

The fundamental goals of medical treatment (Fig. 14–1) are induction and maintenance of remission. Multiple randomized, controlled trials demonstrate clinical, biochemical, and histological improvement of severe AIH, as well as survival with corticosteroids or in conjunction with azathioprine treatment.[30,32,47] Although corticosteroid therapy improves histological parameters and survival, there is no evidence that it hinders disease progression to cirrhosis.[36] All immunoserological subtypes of AIH respond to standard medical treatment, but currently there are no randomized, controlled trials for subtypes 2 and 3. Treatment success depends on the appropriate selection of patients, treatment to complete endpoints (histological remission), and effective management of suboptimal treatment outcomes, such

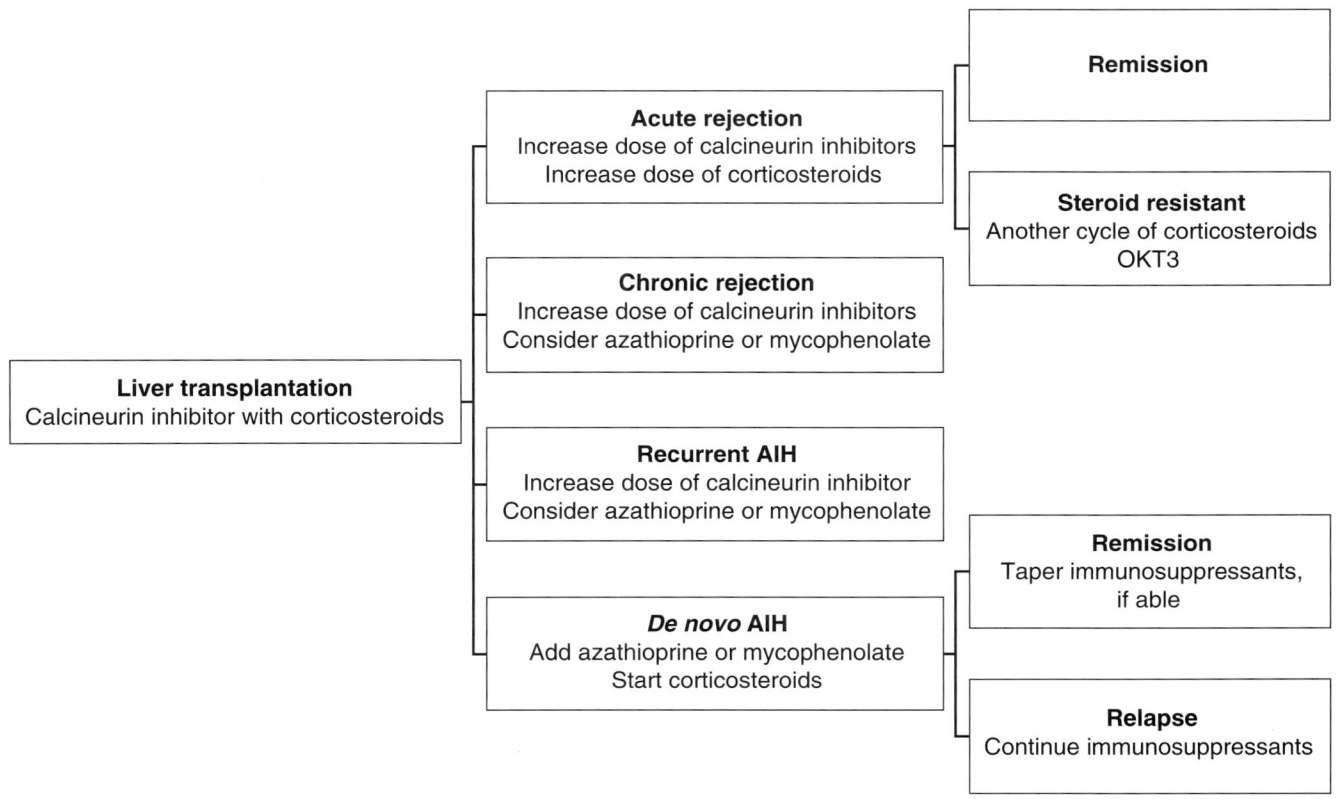

FIGURE 14–1

Decision Tree: Management of autoimmune hepatitis after liver transplantation. AIH, autoimmune hepatitis.

as incomplete response, drug toxicity, and treatment failures.

The absolute indications for therapy include acute onset or fulminant AIH, aminotransferase levels that are 10-fold greater than normal or aminotransferase levels 5-fold greater than normal and γ-globulin levels 2-fold greater than normal, and histological evidence of bridging necrosis or multilobular necrosis.[81] In patients with asymptomatic or mild AIH, the indication for corticosteroid therapy is currently uncertain.[82] Therefore, indications for corticosteroid treatment in patients with mild AIH must be individualized according to the clinical symptoms; disease progression and potential drug-related risks and benefits must be weighed against each other. Patients with inactive cirrhosis, complications of portal hypertension without hepatocellular inflammation, or mild interface hepatitis in the absence of symptoms are not candidates for drug therapy.

The standard initial treatment of AIH is prednisone monotherapy or combination therapy with lower dose prednisone and azathioprine (Table 14–4). Both treatment strategies are equally effective. Prednisolone or prednisone can be used and both are effective. Combination treatment is generally preferred because it decreases the adverse effect profile (10% versus 44% in monotherapy). The approach on which strategy to use involves the consideration of the individual patient:

- Combination therapy is more appropriate for the elderly, patients with osteoporosis, patients with a metabolic syndrome (postmenopausal, diabetes, hypertension, obesity, acne), and/or psychiatric instability.
- Monotherapy with corticosteroids is preferred in patients with hematological abnormalities (cytopenia), thiopurine methyltransferase deficiency, malignancy, pregnancy, and in young, fertile patients.

A brief treatment trial can be used as a diagnostic tool. Patients receiving corticosteroids should undergo routine eye examinations for cataracts and glaucoma, and those receiving azathioprine should be monitored for leukopenia and thrombocytopenia (see Table 14–3).

The goal of treatment is aminotransferase normalization, histological resolution, and clinical remission of symptoms. Liver biopsy assessment before termination of treatment is suggested but not essential if clinical and laboratory criteria for remission are satisfied. Liver biopsy can accurately identify histological remission and avoids premature drug withdrawal, which produces a higher incidence of relapse. After remission, a normal liver biopsy result has a relapse rate of 20%, compared with portal hepatitis, which has a 50% frequency of relapse at 6 months. A sustained response without relapse occurs in only 17% of the treated patients.

Relapse is the recrudescence of disease activity after remission and drug withdrawal. It is characterized by both clinical symptoms (fatigue, arthralgias), a biochemical increase in the serum aminotransferase to threefold greater than normal, and/or an increase in serum γ-globulin to more than 2 g/dL. These biochemical

Table 14–4. TREATMENT REGIMENS FOR ADULTS

	Monotherapy	Combination	
	Prednisone Only (mg/d)	Prednisone (mg/d)	Azathioprine (mg/d)
Week 1	60	30	50
Week 2	40	20	50
Week 3	30	15	50
Week 4	30	15	50
Maintenance until endpoint	20	10	50
Reasons for preference	Cytopenia	Postmenopausal State	
	Thiopurine methyltransferase deficiency	Osteoporosis	
	Pregnancy	Brittle diabetes	
	Malignancy	Obesity	
	Short course (≤6 mo)	Acne	
		Emotional lability	
		Hypertension	

From Czaja AJ, Freese DK: American Association for the Study of Liver Disease. Diagnosis and treatment of autoimmune hepatitis. Hepatology 36(2):479-497, 2002.
d, day.

changes are associated with interface hepatitis and re-treatment when standard medical therapy is indicated. Patients who relapse have a higher rate of esophageal varices (25% versus 15%), progression to cirrhosis (40% versus 18%), and death from hepatic failure (15% versus 4%) than patients with sustained remission.[83]

Two treatment strategies for patients who have relapsed more than two times have been established. One strategy is the indefinite use of the lowest dose of prednisone that prevents symptoms and maintains biochemical remission. Another strategy is indefinite azathioprine administration after remission has been achieved. The long-term use of these two strategies has not been compared head to head, but both strategies have shown inactive or minimal histological disease in 94% of follow-up liver biopsies. Twelve percent of patients treated with these schedules were able to be permanently withdrawn from medications after 70 months of follow-up.[83]

Treatment failure is characterized by sustained disease activity, which can lead to the development of or progression to cirrhosis with portal hypertension. The complications of this lead to liver transplantation or death. Treatment failures are treated with high-dose prednisone (60 mg) or combination treatment with prednisone (30 mg) and azathioprine (150 mg). Doses are reduced after each month of clinical and biochemical improvement until conventional maintenance levels of the medications are reached. Seventy-five percent of patients treated with high doses attain clinical and laboratory remission, but only 20% achieve histological resolution.[39] Treatment is, therefore, indefinite and patients who fail this regimen are at risk of liver failure and drug toxicity; they commonly become candidates for liver transplantation and investigational protocols. Alternative treatment strategies include cyclosporine, 6-mercaptopurine, methotrexate, tacrolimus, and mycophenolate mofetil.[39]

Incomplete responders achieve moderate clinical, laboratory, and histological improvement that is insufficient to satisfy remission criteria within 3 years. Treatment extended beyond 3 years is associated with a 7% per year probability of remission and an increasing risk of drug-related toxicity.[39] Benefit-risk analysis calculations suggest that standard therapy should be terminated in these patients after 3 years, and long-term low-dose prednisone or an every-other-day regimen and/or azathioprine should be started and maintained indefinitely.

Drug toxicity is the development of severe, drug-related complications, which may require premature drug withdrawal or dose reduction. Corticosteroid-related intolerances are the most common causes of drug discontinuation. Cytopenia, nausea, emotional lability, hypertension, cosmetic changes, and diabetes are dose-related complications. The corticosteroids should be reduced to the lowest dose possible to attenuate symptoms, and azathioprine may be co-administered. Appropriate therapy of the complication must be included, which may consist of antihypertensive medication, diabetic regimens, bone maintenance schedules, gastric acid suppression, and antidepressants. If severe reactions occur, the offending drug must be discontinued.

Adjunctive Medical Treatment

Adjunctive medical treatment should be implemented in patients who are receiving chronic corticosteroid treatment or are at high risk for developing steroid-induced complications, or both. Adjunctive therapies may prevent or minimize the side effects associated with AIH and its treatments. Regular exercise (e.g., walking, biking, swimming) and weight control should be emphasized because of the high incidence of osteoporosis. Vitamin supplementation, including vitamin K for hypoprothrombinemia (10 mg per day), calcium supplementation (1-1.5 g per day), and vitamin D (50,000 IU once per week) should be included with chronic steroid treatment. Postmenopausal women should consider hormonal replacement therapy. Symptomatic osteoporosis or progressive osteopenia should be treated with bisphosphonates, such as alendronate (70 mg per week).[84] Antihypertensive medications, diabetes treatments, gastric acid suppression, and/or antidepressants should be administered if corticosteroid complications arise. Patients should also be monitored for bone disease with an annual bone mineral densitometry, and standard yearly health maintenance checkups should also be emphasized.

New Pharmacotherapies

Immunosuppression with corticosteroids and azathioprine are effective in the majority of patients with AIH, but 10% to 20% of treated patients do not respond or cannot tolerate doses required for optimal inhibition of hepatocellular inflammation and fibrogenesis. New immunosuppressive agents have been developed, but currently there is limited experience with their use. Cyclosporine is used successfully and is well tolerated as a primary treatment in pediatric and adult patients. Cyclosporine inhibits clonal expansion of activated CD4 helper T cells, blocks the release on IL-2, impairs activation and expansion of cytotoxic T cells, and decreases antibody production. Currently there are 13 reported trials and cases with a total of 96 patients using cyclosporine, which report a biochemical response ranging from 67% to 100%.[85]

Tacrolimus (FK506) inhibits expression of the IL-2 receptor and prevents expansion of cytotoxic T cells. Currently two trials, with a total of 28 patients, report biochemical improvement in the majority of patients.[85] Mycophenolate mofetil inhibits inosine monophosphate dehydrogenase, which results in the depletion of guanine nucleotides and inhibition of DNA synthesis. Its use has been reported in a case series of 7 patients, in which 5 of 7 patients had biochemical normalization at 3 months, and 6 patients discontinued prednisone by 16 months.[86]

Role of Liver Transplantation

Liver transplantation should be considered in all patients who develop decompensated liver disease from AIH. Liver transplantation is associated with a 5-year patient and graft survival, ranging from 83% to 92%, and a 10-year survival of approximately 75%.[37] Recurrent disease after transplantation occurs in approximately 12% to 36%, but it is usually mild and manageable.[87] HLA DR3 or DR4 is found in 100% of patients with recurrent disease compared with 40% in those without recurrence; however, recurrent disease is unrelated to the HLA status of the donor.[87] De novo AIH occurs in 0.7% and 1.4% of adults and in 2.3% and 5.2% of children after transplantation.[88]

A multivariate analysis to look for prognostic factors associated with a more rapid progression of AIH before transplantation demonstrated that age greater than 60 years, male gender, type 2 AIH, HLA A1-B8 DR3, and concurrent extrahepatic autoimmune diseases are more likely to progress to liver failure. These patients, when undergoing transplantation, are not at a greater risk for decompensation.[83] The histological and biochemical indicators associated with a higher mortality from liver failure are multilobular necrosis and progressive hyperbilirubinemia.

Immunosuppression After Liver Transplantation

Patients with AIH require more aggressive immunosuppression because of the higher incidence of acute, chronic rejection and disease recurrence in the allograft. The optimal regimen is not established, but most centers use a calcineurin inhibitor together with azathioprine or mycophenolate and corticosteroids. It seems sensible to maintain minimal effective immunosuppression, but these patients must be carefully monitored with both serological (serum autoantibodies and immunoglobulins) and histological examination. Withdrawal of immunosuppression is rarely possible in these patients, and the majority of recipients require long-term steroid treatment.[89,90]

Immunosuppressive treatment must be titrated not only to allograft function but also to its adverse effects.

Acute and Chronic Allograft Rejection

Patients who undergo grafting for AIH are at greater risk for both acute and chronic rejection.[29,91] There is no evidence that acute rejection is associated with an ominous impact on graft survival, and there is some evidence suggesting that it may actually promote tolerance. Acute rejection occurs in approximately 56% to 83% of patients and is steroid-resistant in 23% to 59%, which requires ornithine-ketoacid transaminase (OKT3) treatment. Patients are also at higher risk for multiple acute rejections. Molmenti and colleagues reported an incidence of acute allograft rejection of 75% in the first 3 months and 80% in the first year in patients with a pre-OLT diagnosis of AIH compared with 57% and 60% in patients without AIH, respectively.[92] Multiple episodes of acute cellular rejection are associated with AIH recurrence after transplantation.[92] Sasaki and colleagues reported on a patient with AIH who developed accelerated rejection during antirejection therapy with OKT3.[93] The recipient had matched its donor at one HLA-DR locus. The authors speculated that this, in combination with an autoimmune diathesis, may have provided a milieu for severe rejection that led to graft loss in the recipient. The immunosuppressive regimen should address this concern for acute allograft rejection, and any reduction in immunosuppression should be performed cautiously, particularly in the first several months after liver transplantation.

Chronic rejection after liver transplantation is a cause of allograft dysfunction leading to graft failure and retransplantation. Milkiewicz and colleagues reported that patients with AIH have an incidence of 15.6% chronic rejection compared with 2% in alcoholic liver disease patients.[91] The authors identified that the risk factors of young age at time of transplantation and moderate to severe acute rejection on liver biopsy results predispose to a higher rate of progression to chronic rejection.[91] Patients who undergo transplantation for AIH are more prone to develop chronic rejection and therefore may require more intensive immunosuppression after liver transplantation.

Recurrent Autoimmune Hepatitis After Transplantation

Recurrent AIH after liver transplantation is characterized by the combination of clinical symptoms, biochemical changes, circulating autoantibodies, histological features (portal and/or lobular hepatitis with lymphoplasmacytic infiltration, plasma cells, piecemeal necrosis, and bridging fibrosis), steroid dependence, and exclusion of other causes of allograft dysfunction.[94] Recurrence of AIH after liver transplantation was initially reported by Neuberger and colleagues in 1984. They reported a case of a 26-year-old HLA-B8-DR3–positive woman with AIH who received an HLA-B8-DR3–negative graft.[95] Recurrent AIH has been reported in several studies with an incidence ranging from 0 to 80%, but in the majority of large studies the range is from 12% to 36% (Table 14–5).[107,116]

In many cases, recurrent AIH is related to suboptimal immunosuppression, and both biochemical and histological features rapidly resolve once adequate immunosuppression is restored. In other cases, however, recurrent AIH is more aggressive with progression to cirrhosis and graft failure leading to retransplantation. Recurrence in the pediatric populations is reported to be more aggressive leading to retransplantation more often. Recurrence tends to occur more aggressively in patients who have undergone retransplantation.

Currently there are no established diagnostic criteria for recurrent AIH. Its diagnosis is based on the constellation of symptoms, autoantibodies, steroid dependence, increased serum transaminase levels, and hypergammaglobulinemia. The histological diagnosis of recurrent AIH is based on evidence of portal or lobular hepatitis, or both, in the presence of lymphatic, plasmacytic, or lymphoplasmacytic infiltrates; acidophilic bodies in the liver and the absence of other histological changes including those of viral hepatitis, drug toxicity, alcoholic hepatitis, and acute or chronic rejection.[38,94]

It is important to differentiate acute cellular rejection from AIH recurrence. Most acute rejection episodes occur during the first month after transplantation, whereas most cases of recurrent AIH are diagnosed more than 12 months after transplantation. Recurrent AIH can be distinguished from acute cellular rejection by the presence of periportal and lobular hepatocellular necrosis, lack of portal or centrilobular venulitis, lack of immunoblasts in the inflammatory infiltrate, and cholestasis. Both recurrent AIH and acute rejection can be treated with either increasing doses of immunosuppressants or corticosteroids, depending on the disease severity. The difference is in the duration of treatment. Recurrent AIH requires a slower taper and potentially continual use of additional immunosuppressants.

Risk Factors for Recurrence

Recurrence of AIH is found to be more commonly associated with HLA-DR3– or HLA-DR4–positive recipients

Table 14–5. RECURRENT AUTOIMMUNE HEPATITIS AFTER LIVER TRANSPLANTATION

Reference	Patients	Recurrent AIH	Onset After LT (Months)	Response to Treatment	Risk Factors Identified
Gonzalez-Koch et al.[87]	41	7 (17%)	52	Yes	Recipient HLA DR 3/DR 4
Prados et al.[107]	27	9 (33%)	30	Yes 5 of 9	LKM-1 negative pre-LT
Ratziu et al.[12]	25	3 (12%)			
Milkiewicz et al.[28]	47	13 (27%)		3 regraph	
Bahar et al.[108]	40	13 (32%)			
Reich et al.[109]	32	6 (19%)		3 regraph	
Ayata et al.[96]	14	5 (36%)			
Neuberger et al.[109]	1		18	Yes	
Birnbaum et al.[110]	6	5 (83%)	11.4	3 regraph	
Sempoux et al.[111]	1		4	Yes	
Narumi et al.[11]	40	5 (13%)	17.5	Yes 4/5	Recipient HLA DR3
Sanchez-Urdazpal et al.[37]	24	0 (0%)			
Ahmed et al.[9]	33	20 (60%)	24	Yes	
Wright et al.[10]	43	11 (26%)	18		Recipient HLA DR 3
Gotz et al.[112]	24	12 (50%)		Yes	
Yusoff et al.[113]	12	2 (17%)			
Molmenti et al.[92]	55	11 (20%)	Adults	Yes	ACR episodes

ACR, acute cellular rejection; AIH, autoimmune hepatitis; HLA, human leukocyte antigen; LT, liver transplantation; LKM, liver-kidney-microsome.

regardless of donor status, but these findings have not been universally confirmed. There was no increased risk associated with the immunosuppression used. A number of studies suggest that recurrent AIH is associated with a reduction in immunosuppressive medication dosage. However, corticosteroids have been successfully withdrawn in some patients after transplantation. In a review of 89 cases, only 5% with AIH type 2 developed recurrent disease compared with 34% of AIH type 1.[94] The presence of severe necroinflammatory activity in the native hepatectomy specimen at the time of transplantation was found to be a strong predictor of recurrent AIH.[96] There is no evidence to support that liver allograft rejection is a risk factor for the development of recurrent AIH.

Acute cellular rejection is also associated with AIH recurrence. Ayata and colleagues first described a high incidence of acute cellular rejection (10 of 12 patients) in patients with recurrent AIH.[96] Recently, Molmenti and colleagues demonstrated a greater incidence of acute cellular rejection during the first year after OLT in patients with recurrent AIH; however, graft failure was not increased.[92]

Pathogenesis

One hypothesis of recurrent AIH involves the existence of memory T cells in the recipient that can be reactivated by antigens expressed by the donor liver that are processed and presented by the antigen-presenting cells (APCs) of the recipient.[64] The speed of replacement of APCs of the donor allograft with APCs of the recipient or the number of recipient APCs outside the liver in lymph nodes and spleen, or both, may in part determine the onset and/or severity of AIH recurrence.

Another hypothesis is direct activation of the recipient T-cell receptors by the major histocompatibility complex (MHC) molecules expressed by the APCs of the allograft.[64] Consequently, the existence of other autoimmune promoters must be postulated, for example,

polymorphisms of the genes producing the cytokines may facilitate direct cytotoxicity and/or regulate immunocyte activation.[97]

Another hypothesis is that molecular mimicry among unidentified hepatotropic viruses infecting the allograft and self-antigens is a basis for recurrence. There is also a possibility of undiscovered viruses that could trigger immunoreactivity.[98]

In summary, patients who are immunosuppressed respond well to increased immunosuppression treatment by restarting corticosteroids plus or minus azathioprine. In patients who have progressive disease, tacrolimus may offer an advantage over cyclosporine-based immunosuppression.[99]

De Novo Autoimmune Hepatitis After Liver Transplantation (Graft Dysfunction Mimicking Autoimmune Hepatitis)

De novo AIH is a posttransplantation clinical syndrome that rarely occurs unpredictably in patients who undergo transplantation for nonautoimmune liver disease (Table 14–6).[100] This syndrome was originally reported in 7 of 180 pediatric liver allografts that developed graft dysfunction at a median posttransplant period of 24 months.[88] None of the patients originally underwent grafting for AIH, but their features were reminiscent of classic AIH, including:

- High IgG
- Serum autoantibodies (one patient with ANA, two patients with ANA/SMA, three patients with atypical LKM, one patient with gastric parietal cell antibody)
- Histological findings of interface hepatitis, perivenular cell necrosis, bridging fibrosis, and collapse

Table 14–6. DE NOVO AUTOIMMUNE HEPATITIS AFTER LIVER TRANSPLANTATION

Reference	Patients	De Novo AIH	Group	Response to Treatment
Heneghan et al.[101]	1000	7 (0.7%)	Adults	2 lost grafts
Andries et al.[114]	471	11 (2.3%)	Children	Yes, 7 of 11
Gupta et al.[115]	115	6 (5.2%)	Children	2 lost grafts
Kerkar et al.[88]	180	7 (3.8%)	Children	Yes
Hernandez et al.[116]	155	5 (3.2%)	Children	Yes, 3 of 5
Spada et al.[15]	116	5 (4.3%)	Children	Yes
Salcedo et al.[100]	350	12 (3.4%)	Children	Yes
Jones et al.[102]	2		Adults	Yes
Tan et al.[103]	1		Adult	Yes

AIH, autoimmune hepatitis.

The presence of autoantibodies is associated with an unfavorable posttransplant clinical course that includes chronic hepatitis, graft dysfunction, chronic rejection, and death.[100] Interestingly, the reported cases did not respond to high-dose steroids and an increased dose of calcineurin inhibitors, but only to standard treatment for AIH, which led to excellent graft and patient survival.[88] Relapse tends to occur after decreasing or withdrawing steroid maintenance therapy.[100] De novo AIH was also identified in seven adult patients after transplantation, and two patterns of disease were identified. One was characterized by low transaminase levels and ANA or SMA positivity at low titers, and the other had high transaminase levels and high titer LKM-1.[101] All patients were treated for immunosuppression but, unlike the pediatric group, two patients developed graft failure. There are also two reported cases out of three patients who underwent transplantation for primary biliary cirrhosis and developed concurrent de novo AIH and recurrent PBC; they responded well to corticosteroids.[102,103]

Salcedo and colleagues propose that the following be used in the evaluation of de novo AIH[100]:

- Allograft dysfunction not associated with other known causes of graft dysfunction, such as vascular or biliary disease, rejection, or viral hepatitis
- Presence of autoantibodies
- Histological evidence of portal and periportal hepatitis with or without centrilobular necrosis, and lymphoplasmacytic portal tract infiltrate with a variable degree of plasma cells
- Response to standard therapy

Pathogenesis

The pathogenesis and development of posttransplant de novo autoimmunity in patients transplanted for nonautoimmune conditions remains unclear. In addition to release of autoantigens from damaged tissues, a possible mechanism is molecular mimicry, in which exposure to viruses with autoantigens leads to cross-reactive immunity.[57] Viral infections may also lead to autoimmunity through other mechanisms, including polyclonal stimulation, enhancement and induction of membrane expression of MHC class I and II antigens, and interference with immunoregulatory cells or idiotype anti-idiotype networks, or both.[58] Another possible mechanism suggested by animal experiments is that calcineurin inhibitors predispose to autoimmunity and autoimmune disease, possibly by interfering with the maturation of T lymphocytes or the function of regulatory T cells, with consequent emergence and activation of autoaggressive T-cell clones.[104] Tacrolimus affects the thymic microenvironment in a fashion like cyclosporine,

and it also can induce a graft-versus-host–like reaction after syngeneic bone marrow transplantation in rats.[105]

Aguilera and colleagues described an association among the occurrence of de novo immune-mediated hepatitis with the presence of antibodies to glutathione-S-transferase T1 (GSTT1) in recipients of liver transplants bearing a GSTT1-null genotype, suggesting that these newly developed antibodies could be the consequence of an antibody-mediated immune response against a foreign protein present in the graft and not the result of an autoimmune reaction.[106]

In summary, de novo AIH can develop in both children and adults at any stage after transplantation. Currently no risk factors have been identified, and the type of immunosuppression and indication do not appear to be implicated. Patients tend to respond to conventional therapy for AIH, and should be maintained on long-term treatment because relapse may develop after steroid withdrawal.

Pearls and Pitfalls

- De novo AIH after liver transplantation is uncommon and is identified in less than 5% of recipients.
- Recipients undergoing transplantation for AIH generally require at least two immunosuppressive agents to maintain graft function.
- Recurrent AIH is usually related to suboptimal immunosuppression.
- Autoimmune hepatitis may be a risk factor for acute cellular rejection in the first year after transplantation.
- Acute cellular rejection and severe recurrent AIH are treated similarly with high-dose corticosteroids.

References

1. Czaja AJ: Autoimmune hepatitis: Evolving concepts and treatment strategies. Dig Dis Sci 40:435-456, 1995.
2. Czaja AJ, Carpenter HA: Sensitivity, specificity and predictability of biopsy interpretations in chronic hepatitis. Gastroenterology 105:1824-1832, 1993.
3. Czaja AJ, Donaldson PT: Genetic susceptibilities for immune expression and liver cell injury in autoimmune hepatitis. Immunol Rev 174:250-259, 2000.
4. Johnson PJ, McFarle IG, Eddleson AL: The natural course and heterogeneity of autoimmune-type chronic active hepatitis. Semin Liver Dis 11:187-196, 1991.
5. Manns MP, Krüger M: Genetics in liver diseases. Gastroenterology 106:1676-1697, 1994.
6. Gregorio GV, Portman B, Reid F, et al: Autoimmune hepatitis in childhood: A 20-year experience. Hepatology 25:541-547, 1997.

7. Roberts SK, Therneau TM, Czaja AJ: Prognosis of histological cirrhosis in type 1 autoimmune hepatitis. Gastroenterology 110:848-857, 1996.

8. Czaja AJ, Rakela J, Ludwig J: Features reflective of early prognosis in corticosteroid-treated severe autoimmune chronic active hepatitis. Gastroenterology 95:448-453, 1998.

9. Ahmed M, Mutimer D, Hathaway M, et al: Liver transplantation for autoimmune hepatitis: A 12 year experience. Transplant Proc 29:496, 1997.

10. Wright HL, Bou-Abboud CF, Hassanein T, et al: Disease recurrence and rejection following liver transplantation for autoimmune chronic active liver disease. Transplantation 53:136-139, 1992.

11. Narumi S, Hakamada K, Sasaki M, et al: Liver transplantation for autoimmune hepatitis: Rejection and recurrence. Transplant Proc 31:1955-1956, 1999.

12. Ratziu V, Samuel D, Sebagh M, et al: Long-term follow-up after liver transplantation for autoimmune hepatitis: Evidence of recurrence of primary disease. Hepatology 30:131-141, 1999.

13. Cullinan ER: Idiopathic jaundice associated with subacute necrosis of the liver. St Barth Hosp Rep 69:55-142, 1936.

14. Amberg S: Hyperproteinemia associated with severe liver damage. Proc Staff Meet Mayo Clin 17:360-362, 1942.

15. Spada M, Bertani A, Sonzogni A, et al: A cause of late graft dysfunction after liver transplantation in children: De novo autoimmune hepatitis. Transplant Proc 33:1747-1748, 2001.

16. Waldenstrom J: Leber, Blutproteine und Nahrungseiweiss. Dutch Gesellsch Verdau Stoffwechselkr 15:113-121, 1950.

17. Joske RA, King WE: The "LE cell" phenomenon in active chronic viral hepatitis. Lancet 2:477-480, 1955.

18. Mackay IR, Taft LI, Cowling DC: Lupoid hepatitis and the hepatic lesions of systemic lupus erythematosus. Lancet 2:1323-1326, 1956.

19. Page AR, Condie RM, Good RA: Suppression of plasma cell hepatitis with 6-mercaptopurine. Am J Med 36:200-213, 1964.

20. Whittingham SF, Irwin J, Mackay IR: Smooth muscle autoantibody in "auto-immune" hepatitis. Gastroenterology 51:499-505, 1966.

21. Rizzetto M, Swana G, Doniach D, et al: Microsomal antibodies in active chronic hepatitis and other disorders. Clin Exp Immunol 15:331-334, 1973.

22. Manns M, Gerken G, Kyriasoulis A, et al: Characterization of a new subgroup of autoimmune chronic active hepatitis by autoantibodies against a soluble liver antigen. Lancet 1:1333-1339, 1987.

23. Hodges JR, Millward-Sadler GH, Wright R: Chronic active hepatitis: The spectrum of disease. Lancet 1:550-552, 1982.

24. Bjarnason I, Magnusson B, Bjornsson S: Idiopathic chronic active hepatitis in Iceland. Acta Med Scand 211:305-307, 1982.

25. Ritland S: The incidence of chronic active hepatitis in Norway: A retrospective study. Scand J Gastroenterol 20 (Suppl 107):58-60, 1985.

26. Olsson R, Lindberg J, Weiland O, et al: Chronic active hepatitis in Sweden. The etiologic spectrum, clinical presentation, and laboratory profile. Scand J Gastroenterol 23:463-470, 1988.

27. Boberg KM, Asdland E, Hahnsen J, et al: Incidence and prevalence of primary biliary cirrhosis, primary sclerosing cholangitis, and autoimmune hepatitis in a Norwegian population. Scand J Gastroenterol 33:99-103, 1998.

28. Milkiewicz P, Hubscher SG, Skiba G, et al: Recurrence of autoimmune hepatitis after liver transplantation. Transplantation 68:253-256, 1999.

29. Wiesner RH, Demetris AJ, Belle SH, et al: Acute allograft rejection: Incidence, risk factors, and impact on outcome. Hepatology 28:638-645, 1998.

30. Soloway RD, Summerskill WHJ, Baggenstoss AH, et al: Clinical, biochemical, and histological remission of severe chronic active liver disease: A controlled study of treatments and early prognosis. Gastroenterology 63:820-833, 1972.

31. Mistilis SP, Skyring AP, Blackburn CRB: Natural history of active chronic hepatitis. I. Clinical features, course, diagnostic criteria, morbidity, mortality, and survival. Australas Ann Med 17:214-223, 1968.

32. Murray-Lyon IM, Stern RB, Williams R: Controlled trial of prednisone and azathioprine in active chronic hepatitis. Lancet 1:735-737, 1973.

33. Schalm SW, Korman MG, Summerskill WHJ, et al: Severe chronic active liver disease. Prognostic significance of initial morphologic patterns. Am J Dig Dis 22:973-980, 1977.

34. DeGroote J, Fevery J, Lepoutre L: Long-term follow-up of chronic active hepatitis of moderate severity. Gut 19:510-513, 1978.

35. Czaja AJ: Therapy of autoimmune hepatitis-state of the art. In Manns MP, Paumgartner G, Leuschner U (eds): Immunology and Liver, Falk Symposium 114. Dordrecht, Kluwer Academic Publishers, BV; 2000, pp 311-324.

36. Davis GL, Czaja AJ: Immediate and long-term results of corticosteroid therapy for severe idiopathic chronic active hepatitis. In Czaja AJ, Dickson ER (eds): Chronic Active Hepatitis. The Mayo Clinic Experience. New York, Marcel Dekker, 1986, pp 269-283.

37. Sanchez-Urdazpal L, Czaja AJ, van Hoek B, et al: Prognostic features and role of liver transplantation in severe corticosteroid-treated autoimmune chronic active hepatitis. Hepatology 15:215-221, 1992.

38. Alvarez F, Berg PA, Bianchi FB, et al: International Autoimmune Hepatitis Group Report: Review of criteria for diagnosis of autoimmune hepatitis. J Hepatol 31:929-938, 1999.

39. Czaja AJ, Freese DK, American Association for the Study of Liver Disease (AASLD): Diagnosis and treatment of autoimmune hepatitis. Hepatology 35:890-897, 2002.

40. Czaja AJ, Carpenter HA: Validation of a scoring system for the diagnosis of autoimmune hepatitis. Dig Dis Sci 41:305-314, 1996.

41. Bianchi FB, Cassani F, Lenzi M, et al: Impact of International Autoimmune Hepatitis Group scoring system in definition of autoimmune hepatitis. An Italian experience. Dig Dis Sci 41:166-171, 1996.

42. Toda G, Zeniya M, Watanabe F, Imawari M, et al: Present status of autoimmune hepatitis in Japan correlating the characteristics with intenational criteria in an area with a high rate of HCV infection. J Hepatol 26:1207-1212, 1997.

43. Miyakawa H, Kitazawa E, Abe K, et al: Chronic hepatitis C associated with anti-liver/kidney microsome-1 antibody is not a subgroup of autoimmune hepatitis. J Gastroenterol 32:769-776, 1997.

44. Dickson RC, Gaffey MJ, Ishitani MB, et al: The international autoimmune hepatitis score in chronic hepatitis C. J Viral Hepat 4:121-128, 1997.

45. Boberg KM, Fausa O, Haaland T, et al: Features of autoimmune hepatitis in primary sclerosing cholangitis: An evaluation of 114 primary sclerosing cholangitis patients according to a scoring system for the diagnosis of autoimmune hepatitis. Hepatology 23:1369-1376, 1996.

46. Omagari K, Masuda J, Kato Y, et al: Re-analysis of clinical features of 89 patients with autoimmune hepatitis using the revised scoring system proposed by the International Autoimmune Hepatitis Group. Intern Med 39:1008-1012, 2000.

47. Cook GC, Mulligan R, Sherlock S: Controlled prospective trial of corticosteroid therapy in active chronic hepatitis. QJM 40:159-185, 1971.

48. Nagamine K, Peterson P, Scott HS, et al: Positional cloning of the APECED gene. Nat Genet 17:393-398, 1997.

49. Kanzler S, Weidemann C, Gerken G, et al: Clinical significance of autoantibodies to soluble liver antigen in autoimmune hepatitis. J Hepatol 31:635-640, 1999.

50. Robertson DA, Zhang SL, Guy EC, et al: Persistent measles virus genome in autoimmune chronic active hepatitis. Lancet 2:9-11, 1997.

51. Rahaman SM, Chira P, Koff RS: Idiopathic autoimmune chronic hepatitis triggered by hepatitis A. Am J Gastroenterol 89:106-108, 1994.

52. Vento S, Garafano T, Di Perri G, et al: Identification of hepatitis A virus as a trigger for autoimmune chronic hepatitis type 1 in susceptible individuals. Lancet 337:1183-1187, 1997.

53. Cianciara J, Laskus T: Development of transient autoimmune hepatitis during interferon treatment of chronic hepatitis B. Dig Dis Sci 40:1852-1854, 1995.

54. Vento S, Cainelli F, Renzini C, et al: Autoimmune hepatitis type 2 induced by HCV and persisting after viral clearance. Lancet 350:1298-1299, 1997.

55. Vento S, Guella L, Mirandola F, et al: Epstein-Barr virus as a trigger for autoimmune hepatitis in susceptible individuals. Lancet 346:608-609, 1995.

56. Gough A, Chapman S, Wagstaff K, et al: Minocycline induced autoimmune hepatitis and systemic lupus erythematosus-like syndrome. BMJ 312:169-172, 1996.

57. Vogel A, Manns MP, Strassburg C: Autoimmunity and viruses. Clin Liver Dis 6:451-465, 2002.

58. Strettell MD, Donaldson PT, Thomson LJ, et al: Allelic basis for HLA-encoded susceptibility to type 1 autoimmune hepatitis. Gastroenterology 112:2028-2035, 1997.

59. Czaja AJ, Carpenter HA, Santrach PJ, et al: Significance of HLA DR4 in type 1 autoimmune hepatitis. Gastroenterology 105:1502-1507, 1993.

60. Czaja AJ, Strettell MD, Thomson LJ, et al: Associations among alleles of the major histocompatibility complex and type 1 autoimmune hepatitis. Hepatology 25:317-323, 1997.

61. Seki T, Ota M, Furuta S, et al: HLA class II molecules and autoimmune hepatitis susceptibility in Japanese patients. Gastroenterology 103:1041-1047, 1992.

62. Wen L, Peakman M, Lobo-Yeo A, et al: T-cell–directed hepatocyte damage in autoimmune chronic active hepatitis. Lancet 336:1527-1530, 1999.

63. Lohr HF, Schlaak JF, Lohse AW, et al: Autoreactive CD4+ LKM-specific and anticlonotypic T-cell responses in LKM-1 antibody-positive autoimmune hepatitis. Hepatology 24:1416-1421, 1996.

64. Vierling JM: Immunology of acute and chronic hepatic allograft rejection. Liver Transpl Surg 5:S1-S20, 1999.

65. Nikias GA, Batta KP, Czaja AJ: The nature and prognostic implications of autoimmune hepatitis with an acute presentation. J Hepatol 20:1374-1380, 1994.

66. Hay JE, Czaja AJ, Rakela J: The nature of unexplained chronic aminotransferase elevations of a mild to moderate degree in asymptomatic patients. Hepatology 2:193-197, 1989.

67. Lebovics E, Schaffner F, Klion FM, et al. Autoimmune chronic active hepatitis in postmenopausal women. Dig Dis Sci 30:824-882, 1985.

68. Desmet VJ, Gerber M, Hoofnaagle JH, et al: Classification of chronic hepatitis: Diagnosis, grading, and staging. Hepatology 19:1513-1520, 1994.

69. Thaler H: The natural history of chronic hepatitis. In Schaffner F, Sherlock S, Leevy CM (eds): The Liver and Its Disease. New York, Stratton Intercontinental Medical Books, 1974, pp 207-215.

70. Czaja AL, Wolf AM, Baggenstoss AH: Clinical assessment of cirrhosis in severe chronic active liver disease. Mayo Clin Proc 55:360-364, 1980.

71. Czaja AJ, Wolf AM, Summerskill WHJ: Development and early prognosis of esophageal varices in severe chronic active liver disease (CALD) treated with prednisone. Gastroenterology 77:629-633, 1979.

72. Volta U, De Franceschi L, Molinaro N, et al: Frequency and significance of anti-gliadin and anti-endomysial antibodies in autoimmune hepatitis. J Hepatol 14:325-331, 1992.

73. Czaja AJ: Behavior significance of autoantibodies in type 1 autoimmune hepatitis. J Hepatol 30:394-401, 1999.

74. Czaja AJ, Cassani F, Cataleta M, et al: Frequency and significance of antibodies to actin in type 1 autoimmune hepatitis. Hepatology 24:1068-1073, 1996.

75. Czaja AJ, Manns MP, Homburger HA: Frequency and significance of antibodies to liver/kidney microsome type 1 in adults with chronic active hepatitis. Gastroenterology 103:1290-1295, 1992.

76. Homberg JC, Abuaf N, Bernard O, et al: Chronic active hepatitis associated with anti liver/kidney microsome antibody type 1: A second type of "autoimmune" hepatitis. Hepatology 7:1333-1339, 1987.

77. Manns MP, Griffin KJ, Sullivan KF, et al: LKM-1 autoantibodies recognize a short linear sequence in P450IID6, a cytochrome P-450 monooxygenase. J Clin Invest 88:1370-1378, 1991.

78. Crivelli O, Lavarini C, Chiaberge E, et al: Microsomal autoantibodies in chronic infection with HBsAg associated delta agent. Clin Exp Immunol 54:232-238, 1983.

79. Czaja AJ, Carpenter HA, Manns MP: Antibodies to soluble liver antigen, P450IID6 and mitochondrial complexes in chronic hepatitis. Gastroenterology 105:1522-1528, 1993.

80. Portalla T, Treichel U, Löhr H, et al: The asialoglycoprotein receptor as target structure in autoimmune liver disease. Semin Liver Dis 11:215-222, 1991.

81. Manns MP, Strassburg CP: Autoimmune hepatitis. In O'Grady JG, Lake JR, Howdle DP (eds): Comprehensive Clinical Hepatology, vol. 16. London, Mosby, 2000, pp 1-14.

82. Koretz RL, Lewin KJ, Higgins J, et al: Chronic active hepatitis. Who meets treatment criteria? Dig Dis Sci 25:695-699, 1980.

83. Czaja AJ, Menon KVN, Carpenter HA: Sustained remission after corticosteroid therapy of type 1 autoimmune hepatitis: A retrospective analysis. Hepatology 35:215-219, 2000.

84. Liberman UA, Weiss SR, Broll J, et al: Effect of oral alendronate on bone mineral density and the incidence of fractures in postmenopausal osteoporosis. N Engl J Med 333:1437-1443, 1995.

85. Vierling JM, Flores PA: Evolving new therapies of autoimmune hepatitis. Clin Liver Dis 6:1-15, 2002.

86. Richardson PD, James PD, Ryder SD: Mycophenolate mofetil for maintenance of remission in autoimmune hepatitis in patients resistant to or intolerant to azathioprine. J Hepatol 33:371-375, 2000.

87. González-Koch A, Czaja AJ, Carpenter HA, et al: Recurrent autoimmune hepatitis after orthotopic liver transplantation. Liver Transpl 4:302-310, 2001.

88. Kerkar N, Hadzic N, Davies ET, Portmann B, et al: De-novo autoimmune hepatitis after liver transplantation. Lancet 353:409-413, 1998.

89. Trouillot TE, Shrestha R, Kam I, et al: Successful withdrawal of prednisolone after adult liver transplantation for autoimmune hepatitis. Liver Transpl Surg 5:375-380, 1999.

90. Devlin J, Doherty D, Thomson L, et al: Defining the outcome of immunosuppression withdrawal after liver transplantation. Hepatology 27:926-933, 1998.

91. Milkiewicz P, Gunson B, Saksena S, et al: Increased incidence of chronic rejection in patients transplanted for autoimmune hepatitis: Assessment of risk factors. Transplantation 70:477-480, 2000.

92. Molmenti EP, Netto FS, Murray NG, et al: Incidence and recurrence of autoimmune/alloimmune hepatitis in liver transplant recipients. Liver Transpl 8:519-526, 2002.

93. Sasaki AW, Lee RG, Porayko MK, et al: Accelerated liver allograft rejection during prophylactic immunosuppression with OKT3. Transplantation 55:216-219, 1993.

94. Mann MP, Bahr MJ: Recurrent autoimmune hepatitis after liver transplantation: When self becomes non-self. Hepatology 32:868-870, 2000.

95. Neuberger J, Portmann B, Calne RY, Williams R: Recurrence of autoimmune chronic active hepatitis following orthotopic liver grafting. Transplantation 37:363-365, 1984.

96. Ayata G, Gordon FD, Lewis WD, et al: Liver transplantation for autoimmune hepatitis: A long-term pathologic study. Hepatology 32:185-192, 2000.

97. Agarwal K, Czaja AJ, Jones DEJ, et al: CTLA-4 gene polymorphisms and susceptibility to type 1 autoimmune hepatitis. Hepatology 31:49-53, 2000.

98. Albert LJ, Inman RD: Molecular mimicry and autoimmunity. N Engl J Med 341:2068-2074, 1999.

99. Hurtova M, Duclos-Vallee JC, Johanet C, et al: Successful tacrolimus therapy for a severe recurrence of type 1 autoimmune hepatitis in a liver allograft recipient. Liver Transpl 7:556-558, 2001.

100. Salcedo M, Vaquero J, Banares R, et al: Response to steroids in *de novo* autoimmune hepatitis after transplantation. Hepatology 35:349-356, 2002.

101. Heneghan MA, Portmann BC, Norris SM, et al: Graft dysfunction mimicking autoimmune hepatitis following liver transplantation in adults. Hepatology 34:464-470, 2001.

102. Jones DE, James OF, Portmann B, et al: Development of autoimmune hepatitis following liver transplantation for primary biliary cirrhosis. Hepatology 30:53-57, 2000.

103. Tan CK, Sian Ho M: Concurrent *de novo* autoimmune hepatitis and recurrence of primary biliary cirrhosis post liver transplantation. Liver Transpl 7:461-465, 2001.

104. Bucy PB, Yan Xu X, Li J, et al: Cyclosporin A induced autoimmune disease in mice. J Immunol 151:1039-1050, 2000.

105. Cooper MH, Hartman GG, Starzl TE, et al: The induction of pseudo-graft-versus-host disease following syngeneic bone marrow transplantation using FK 506. Transplant Proc 23:3234-3235, 1991.

106. Aguilera I, Wichman I, Sousa JM, et al: Antibodies against glutathione-S-transferase TI (GSTTI) in patients with *de novo* immune hepatitis following liver transplantation. Clin Exp Immunol 126:535-539, 2001.

107. Prados E, Cuervas-Mons V, de la Matat M, et al: Outcome of autoimmune hepatitis after liver transplantation. Transplantation 66:1645-1650, 1998.

108. Bahar RJ, Yanni GS, Martin MG, et al: Orthotopic liver transplantation for autoimmune hepatitis and cryptogenic chronic hepatitis in children. Transplantation 72:829-833, 2001.

109. Reich DJ, Fiel I, Guarrera JV, et al: Liver transplantation for autoimmune hepatitis. Hepatology 32:693-700, 2000.

110. Birbaum AH, Benkov KJ, Pittman NS, et al: Recurrence of autoimmune hepatitis in children after liver transplantation. J Pediatr Gastroenterol Nutr 25:20-25, 1997.

111. Sempoux C, Horsmans Y, Lerut J, et al: Acute lobular hepatitis as the first manifestation of recurrent autoimmune hepatitis after orthotopic liver transplantation. Liver 17:311-315, 1997.

112. Gotz G, Neuhaus R, Bechstein WO, et al: Recurrence of autoimmune hepatitis after liver transplantation. Transplant Proc 31:430-431, 1994.

113. Yusoff IF, House AK, De Boer WB, et al: Disease recurrence after liver transplantation in Western Australia. J Gastroenterol Hepatol 17:203-207, 2002.

114. Andries S, Casamayou L, Sempoux C, et al: Posttransplant immune hepatitis in pediatric liver transplant recipients: Incidence and maintenance therapy with azathioprine. Transplantation 72:267-272, 2001.

115. Gupta P, Hart J, Millis JM, et al: De novo hepatitis with autoimmune antibodies and atypical histology: A rare cause of late graft dysfunction after pediatric liver transplantation. Transplantation 71:664-668, 2001.

116. Hernandez HM, Kovarik P, Whitington PF, et al: Autoimmune hepatitis as a late complication of liver transplantation. J Pediatr Gastroenterol Nutr 32:131-136, 2001.

Transplantation for Primary Hepatic Malignancy

MARVIN J. STONE
J. MARK FULMER
GORAN B. KLINTMALM

Diagnostic medical imaging evaluation of solid hepatic masses   212

Hepatocellular carcinoma   214
   Epidemiology   214
   Clinical presentation and diagnosis   215
   Staging   216
   Prognostic factors and organ allocation   217
   Orthotopic liver transplantation   218
   International Liver Transplant Tumor
     Registry   219

Cholangiocarcinoma   222

Epithelioid hemangioendothelioma   223

Other hepatic tumors   224

Discussion   224

Summary   225

In July 1967, a liver transplant was performed on a 19-month-old girl with hepatocellular carcinoma (HCC). She was the 10th hepatic transplant recipient in the world and the first to achieve extended survival. This patient developed tumor recurrence 3 months after surgery, but survived 400 days before dying of disseminated metastatic disease.[1,2] During the past 4 decades, enthusiasm for total hepatectomy for primary hepatic malignancy has waxed and waned. Although most transplant centers had some patients who survived for long periods and were probably cured, this was the exception rather than the rule.[3-9] The initial enthusiasm for transplantation in patients with hepatobiliary cancer soon faded as early recurrences appeared in the majority of cases.[4] These recurrences usually appeared within 2 years after transplant, the most common site being the liver allograft. Such recurrences were probably caused by the presence of micrometastases not apparent at surgery. This experience led to a pessimistic attitude about using precious donor livers for treatment of malignant disease.[10,11] Such poor early outcomes for patients with HCC treated by orthotopic liver transplantation (OLT) led to the decision in 1989 by the U.S. Department of Health and Human Services that HCC was a contraindication for liver transplantation. The use of a multimodality approach with neoadjuvant systemic chemotherapy during the late 1980s and early 1990s appeared promising, although its efficacy has not been confirmed in controlled clinical trials.[12-15] These early neoadjuvant studies included patients with very large or multifocal tumors, or both. About the same time, the waiting time for donor livers in many centers increased to more than 1 year, making liver transplantation for primary hepatic malignancy impractical because such prolonged waits were more than twice the median survival for hepatocellular carcinoma. Various locoregional holding maneuvers were developed, including transarterial chemoembolization (TACE),[16-22] ethanol injection,[23-25] cryosurgery,[24,25] and radiofrequency thermal ablation (RFA).[24-27]

Since the late 1990s, enthusiasm for liver transplantation for primary hepatic malignancy, principally hepatocellular carcinoma, has increased again as it was demonstrated that better results might be achieved if patients were selected more rigorously. The priorities for such patients have improved, and so the consequent waiting time for donor livers has decreased to 90 days or less for many patients.

The role of various neoadjuvant approaches, whether locoregional techniques or systemic chemotherapy, needs further evaluation and integration into the overall objective of tumor removal and hepatic replacement.[28-33] The purpose of this chapter is to review the status of OLT for primary hepatic malignancy.

Diagnostic Medical Imaging Evaluation of Solid Hepatic Masses

Evaluation of solid hepatic masses has evolved to include the entire armamentarium of medical imaging.[34-38] Although the study of space-occupying lesions of the liver is most often performed with a multimodality approach, the focus of that imaging evaluation is to answer several fundamental questions. Those questions include the precise location of the lesion within the hepatic parenchyma, characteristics of the lesion's internal structure, exact number of lesions visible, margins of the lesions, and any associated findings that might give clues regarding the spread of neoplasm beyond the liver.

Definition of the location of a lesion in the liver is performed by defining surgical planes related to hepatic vascular and biliary landmarks. Elucidating the precise location of the lesion allows for preoperative planning for segmental or nonanatomic resection. Lesion localization is particularly critical before thermal ablation or cryotherapy. Exact delineation of the lesion's location is best provided with magnetic resonance imaging (MRI) or contrast-enhanced computed tomography (CT) (Figs. 15–1 to 15–5). Newer three-dimensional modeling techniques with bolus infusion CT allows for surface rendering and precise therapeutic planning.

Defining the imaging characteristics of the lesion in question helps clarify its benign or malignant nature. Although neoplastic hepatic lesions vary in appearance, there are features that, if present, lead to a strong suspicion of a malignant process (see Fig. 15–1). These features include a lesion that is round and solid, and an enhancement pattern with hepatic arterial supply (see Fig. 15–2 A and B). The margins of malignant lesions are usually associated with an area of adjacent hepatic compression and may often demonstrate edema in the normal hepatic parenchyma, resulting in a somewhat *feathered* or indistinct appearance. Primary malignant lesions, which are adjacent to the hepatic capsule, often result in capsular retraction, resulting in deformity of the liver margin. Similarly, hepatocellular carcinoma may demonstrate intravascular extension with resultant occlusion of portal venous branches. This is often caused by direct invasion of the vein rather than compressive, bland thrombosis. Positron emission tomography (PET) scanning is particularly helpful in evaluation of extrahepatic metastases. This whole-body technique allows for staging of known disseminated malignancy.

Primary biliary malignancy centrally located within the liver is notoriously difficult to image. The classic Klatskin tumor of the biliary confluence is often isoechoic at sonographic imaging, isodense when visualized with computed tomographic scanning, and isointense to the surrounding hepatic parenchyma with MRI. Clues to this lesion are usually manifested by a distal biliary obstructive pattern and the common finding of porta hepatis lymphadenopathy. Some centrally located lesions can be visualized on MRI (see Figs. 15–3 and 15–4). Peripheral primary cholangiocarcinoma is

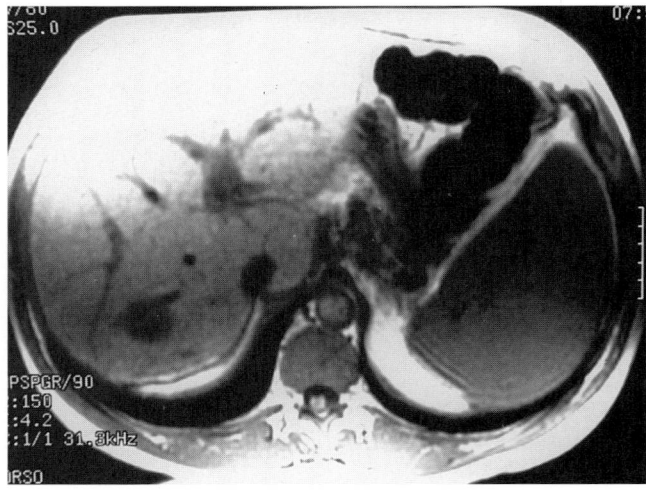

FIGURE 15–1

Solitary hepatoma. Magnetic resonance imaging (MRI) evaluation demonstrates focal solid mass in the posterior segment of the right hepatic lobe in a patient with long-standing cirrhosis.

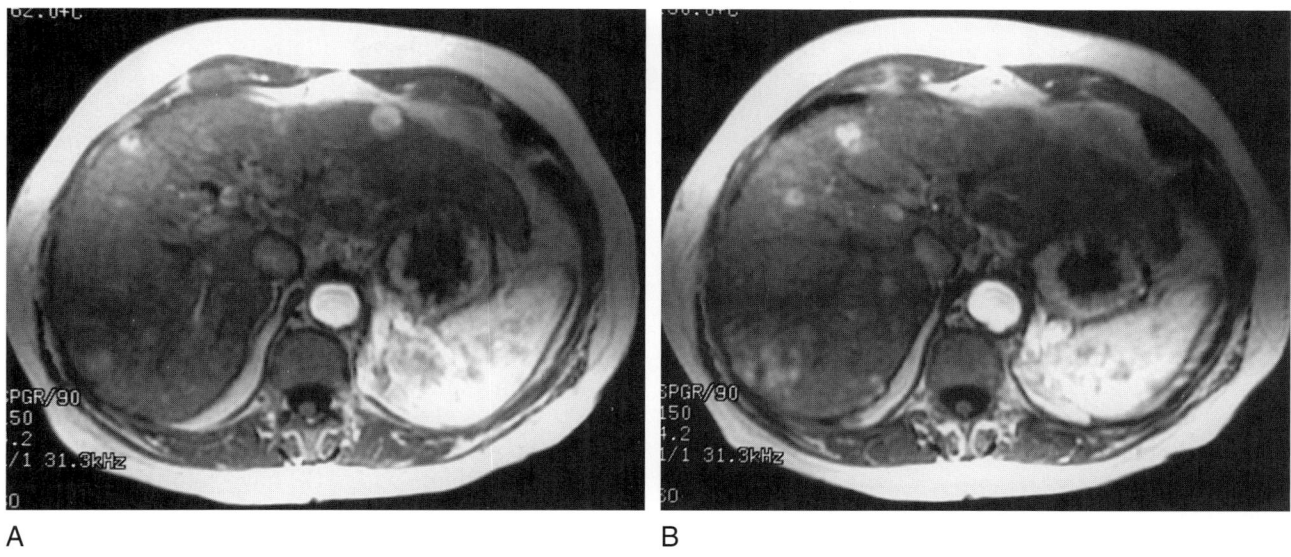

FIGURE 15-2

A and **B**, Multifocal hepatoma. Contrast-enhanced magnetic resonance imaging (MRI) evaluation demonstrates multiple arterially enhancing masses in a patient with long-standing cirrhosis.

more typical in its appearance. These are often large lesions with brisk contrast enhancement during arterial imaging, with associated high signal intensity on T_2-weighted MRI sequences.

During the initial evaluation of any space-occupying mass in the liver, it is helpful to ensure that the imaging features of the identified lesion do not meet the criteria for well-known, benign processes. Cavernous hemangioma, hepatic cyst, focal nodular hyperplasia, and focal infiltration of fat are often identified in the liver parenchyma. These may mimic solid space-occupying masses with malignant features, and care must be taken to evaluate any lesion thoroughly to identify typical features of common benign processes.

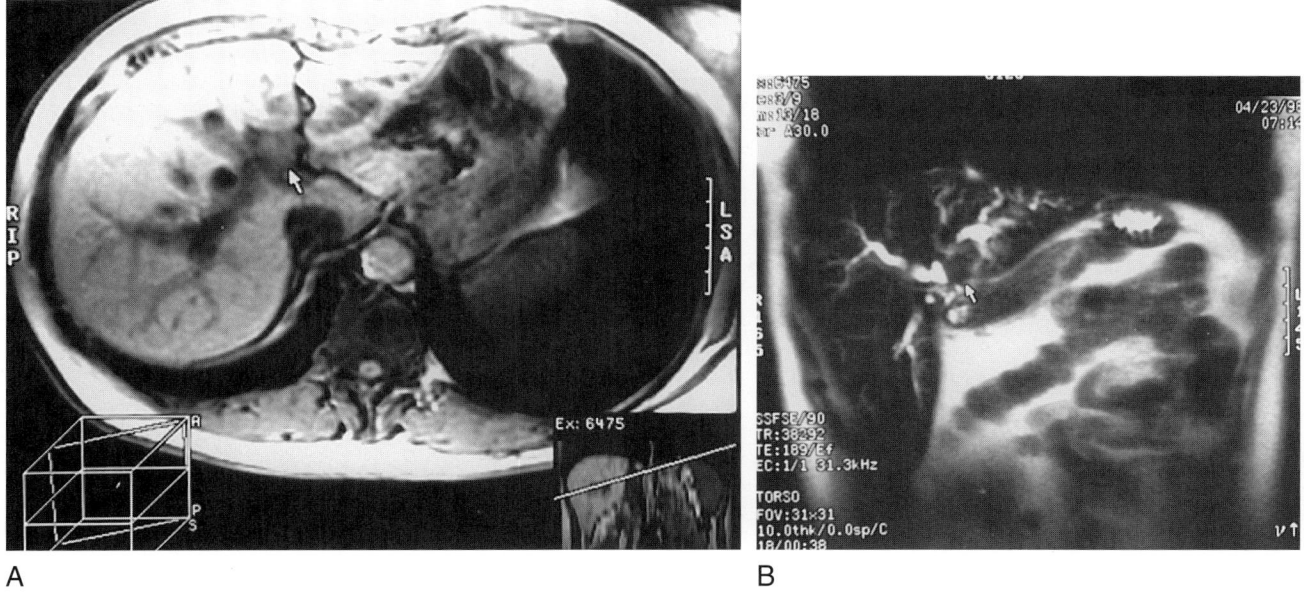

FIGURE 15-3

A, Central primary cholangiocarcinoma. Axial MRI demonstrates a central soft tissue mass *(white arrow)* with associated biliary obstruction. **B**, MRI cholangiopancreatography in the same patient demonstrates the central mass *(white arrow)* with intrahepatic bile duct obstruction.

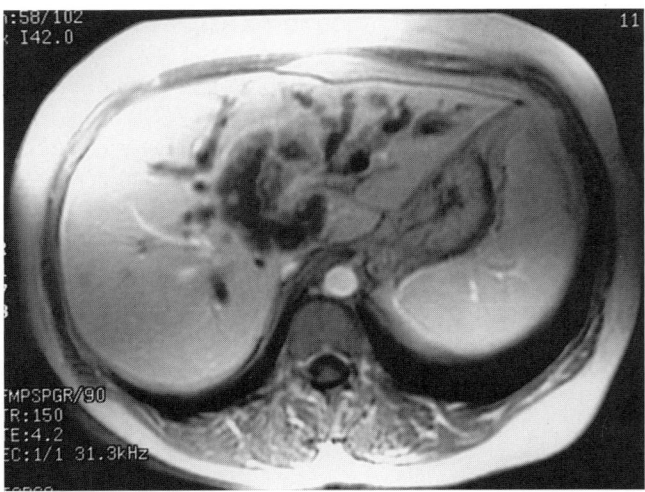

FIGURE 15–4

Large central cholangiocarcinoma. Contrast-enhanced MRI evaluation demonstrates a large, central cholangiocarcinoma with associated intrahepatic bile duct obstruction.

A complete evaluation of a solid mass in the liver will result in thorough delineation of the lesion's location, imaging characteristics, background hepatic parenchyma, and evidence of additional foci of suspected malignancy within the abdominal lymph nodes, pulmonary parenchyma, and skeleton. If the lesion in the liver exhibits nonbenign features, histological confirmation of the nature of the lesion may be necessary (see Fig. 15–5).

Evaluation of hepatic masses requires a multidisciplinary, multimodality paradigm. Thorough characterization

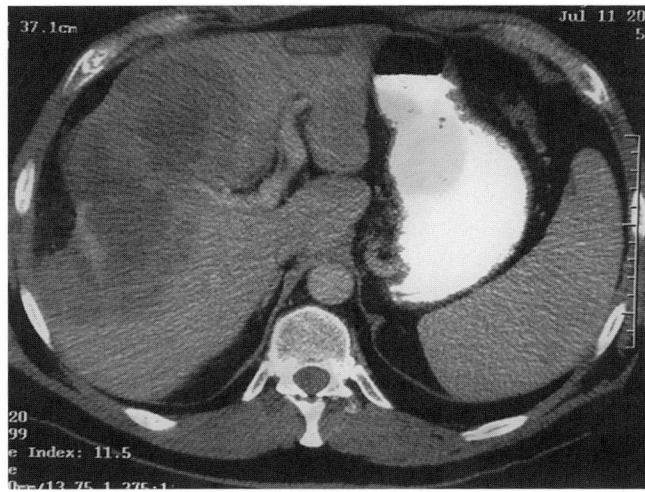

FIGURE 15–5

Epithelioid hemangioendothelioma. Contrast-enhanced computed tomographic evaluation demonstrates a large hepatic mass within homogeneous enhancement and capsular retraction. Biopsy demonstrated the nature of the lesion.

of hepatic masses will help direct planning for hepatic replacement, primary lesion resection, ablative procedures, percutaneous biopsy, or imaging follow-up.

Hepatocellular Carcinoma

Epidemiology

In the United States, metastatic carcinoma is much more common than primary hepatic malignancy. HCC accounts for 80% to 90% of primary hepatic cancers, with intrahepatic cholangiocarcinoma making up most of the others.[39-42] Mixed hepatocholangiocarcinomas also occur along with other rare tumors. Eighty percent to 90% of patients with HCC have some type of cirrhosis, most commonly related to viral hepatitis or alcohol. HCC is one of the most common tumors in the world, especially in West Africa and Asia, and is responsible for more than 1 million new cases per year worldwide (Table 15–1).[40-44] It is three times more frequent in men than in women. Untreated HCC has a median survival of 6 months from diagnosis. Most patients are in the advanced stages of their disease by the time the tumor is recognized. Patients with established cirrhosis have an annual HCC incidence of 3% to 10% per year. Chronic inflammatory disease with necrosis results in increased cell division and mutation. Ongoing hepatocellular turnover also leads to reduced time for DNA repair. The cycles of inflammation, necrosis, and fibrosis distort the normal hepatic architecture. It is thought that HCC originates from adenomatous hyperplasia that becomes atypical hyperplasia and then undergoes transformation to overt malignancy. These changes are associated with marked alterations in the apoptosis-to-mitosis ratio that ultimately contribute to loss of cell growth control.[45] As is true of other types of cancer, hepatic

Table 15–1. INCIDENCE OF HEPATOCELLULAR CARCINOMA BY GEOGRAPHICAL REGION

Region	Incidence
Western Africa	30-48 per 100,000
China	27-36 per 100,000
Mediterranean	5-20 per 100,000
Northern Europe	5 per 100,000
United States	4 per 100,000
South America	0.2-5.0 per 100,000

Modified from Russo MW, Jacobson IM: Hepatocellular cancer: Screening, surveillance, and prevention. In Kelsen DP, Daly JM, Levin B, et al (eds): Gastrointestinal Oncology: Principles & Practice. Philadelphia, Lippincott Williams & Wilkins, 2002, p. 560.

carcinogenesis is a multistep and multifocal process. Vascular invasion is the strongest predictor of tumor recurrence and correlates with tumor number and size. In Asia the distribution of HCC is closely related to hepatitis B virus (HBV) incidence, whereas in the United States approximately 50% of all HCC cases are associated with hepatitis C virus (HCV) (see Table 15–1).[40-44] The incidence of HCC in the United States doubled between 1975 and 1998 and continues to rise, especially in white, middle-aged men.[46] The risk of HCC appears maximal 30 years after infection with HCV.[47-49] Projections indicate that the number of HCC cases caused by HCV in the United States will increase from approximately 7000 in the year 2000 to more than 13,000 in 2020 and then remain essentially unchanged until 2040.[49] Unlike HBV, HCV does not integrate into host DNA. HCC develops in as many as 45% of individuals with cirrhosis resulting from genetic hemochromatosis.[50] Multiple chromosome abnormalities and specific genetic mutations have been described in HCC, but a unifying molecular pathogenesis has thus far not emerged.[39,51-53] A variety of other risk factors for HCC include aflatoxins, azo dyes, aromatic amines, N-nitroso compounds, chlorinated hydrocarbons, hydrosol compounds, pesticides, radiation, Thorotrast, smoking, porphyria, Budd-Chiari syndrome, oral contraceptives, anabolic androgenic steroids, and α_1-antitrypsin deficiency.[40-44] Transgenic and knockout mouse models appear valuable in the study of mechanisms of interaction of the various risk factors in human HCC.[45,54]

HCC is one of the most common fatal tumors worldwide, with an estimated annual incidence of 1 million cases; it may be the most frequent malignancy in males.[40-44] In the United States, approximately 17,000 new cases were predicted in 2004; the case-fatality ratio is 0.8, and the median survival generally is less than 6 months. α-Fetoprotein (AFP) serum levels are helpful in the diagnosis if they are very high or if values rise with time.[55] Elevated AFP levels also occur in pregnancy, hepatitis, and germ cell tumors. The prognosis for patients with AFP-negative HCC is somewhat better, but median survival in this subgroup is still less than 1 year.[55,56] Des-γ-carboxy prothrombin (DCP) has been reported to be a useful tumor marker for HCC and also may have prognostic significance.[57] Chronic hepatitis B virus infection appears to be the major cause of HCC, although tumor incidence in those individuals with asymptomatic infection with this virus is low.[58] Hepatitis C virus appears to be an independent risk factor in Japan and the Western hemisphere.[47-49] Other causative factors include aflatoxins and multiple types of cirrhosis, especially those associated with genetic hemochromatosis and alcohol.[39-42] HCC is uncommon in patients with cirrhosis because of autoimmune chronic active hepatitis, Wilson's disease, and primary biliary cirrhosis.

Clinical Presentation and Diagnosis

Patients with HCC may present with a palpable liver mass, abdominal pain, or deterioration in a patient with chronic liver disease, or the tumor may be found incidentally. Rarely, an arterial bruit may be audible over the mass. Signs of chronic liver disease (ascites, jaundice, splenomegaly) may be present. Serum α-fetoprotein is elevated in approximately 70% of patients with HCC, and values in excess of 400 ng/mL are virtually diagnostic if the patient does not have a germ cell tumor.[55] Various paraneoplastic syndromes occur including secondary polycythemia, polymyositis, hypoglycemia, and diarrhea.[39,59] Imaging procedures are valuable in the diagnosis of HCC. Twenty percent to 60% of small HCCs are multifocal. Ultrasonography, CT, and MRI are helpful (see Figs. 15–1 and 15–2).[34-38] However, imaging studies do not always distinguish focal nodular hyperplasia (FNH) from HCC. Iron colloid injection may be useful in making this distinction. The indications for liver biopsy in patients with suspected HCC are controversial because there appears to be a 2% to 3% incidence of needle-tract seeding following such invasive procedures.[60,61] The decision about biopsy is complicated by the evidence that the histological grade may be an important prognostic factor in HCC. If so, it may be necessary to obtain a biopsy to determine which tumor patients are *not* candidates for transplantation.

Many patients are referred for transplant evaluation after a liver biopsy has revealed the presence of malignancy. The difficulty in histologically determining primary versus metastatic tumor, particularly with small specimens, should not be underestimated.[62] Moreover, it is sometimes difficult to distinguish HCC from cholangiocarcinoma. Even when multiple immunohistochemical stains using monoclonal antibodies are used, the differential diagnosis of HCC versus cholangiocarcinoma versus metastatic carcinoma may be equivocal.[62,63] The hepatocyte paraffin (Hep Par 1) monoclonal antibody is sensitive but not specific for HCC.[64,65] Using a battery of immunohistochemical stains (e.g., AFP, CD10, epithelial membrane antigen, monoclonal carcinoembryonic antigen [CEA], polyclonal CEA, and CD15) allows a more precise diagnosis. With rare exceptions, patients with metastatic disease of the liver or those with primary liver malignancy and extrahepatic tumor spread are not candidates for OLT. Thus it is crucial to interpret histology in the context of clinical and other laboratory data. For the patient with a large hepatic mass and marked elevation (>400 ng/mL) of AFP, the diagnosis of HCC is relatively simple, even without histological confirmation. Because of possible extrahepatic seeding, a biopsy may even be contraindicated. By contrast, the patient having one or more hepatic mass lesions and no or only mild AFP elevation may require liver biopsy for diagnosis. However, it should be realized that it may be easier to determine that a malignancy is present than it is to specify the cell of origin accurately or whether the tumor is primary or metastatic.

Staging

Multiple staging systems have been developed for HCC and other primary hepatic malignancies.[25] The TNM system, which is recommended by the International Joint Staging Agency of the American College of Surgery, is based on tumor (T), node (N), and metastatic (M) involvement (Table 15–2).[66] Multiple revisions were made in the 2002 version of the TNM staging system (Table 15–3). Recipients with stage I and stage II involvement benefit most from OLT. However, this classification relies on imaging procedures that may understage as many as 33.3% of patients. Moreover, it does not take into account the presence of underlying liver disease. Some studies have found a lack of correlation between TNM stage and tumor-free survival following OLT. Because of such discordance, alternative staging systems have been proposed. The Okuda staging system classifies patients according to tumor size, serum albumin and bilirubin levels, and the presence of ascites to determine stage I, II, or III disease.[25,67] Another system developed by the Cancer of the Liver Italian Program (CLIP) is simple to use and based on Child-Pugh class, tumor morphology and extension, AFP level, and the presence of portal vein thrombosis (Table 15–4).[68-70] The computed CLIP score (range: 0 to 6) correlates with median and 1-year survival. None of the staging systems uses molecular markers (e.g., p53, gene expression profiling), which may prove to have important prognostic significance.

Table 15–2. DEFINITION OF TUMOR, NODE, METASTASIS (TNM) STAGING SYSTEM

Extent of Disease	Definition		
TX	Primary tumor cannot be assessed.		
T0	No evidence of primary tumor.		
T1	Solitary tumor without vascular invasion.		
T2	Solitary tumor with vascular invasion or multiple tumors, none more than 5 cm.		
T3	Multiple tumors more than 5 cm or tumor involving a major branch of the portal or hepatic vein(s).		
T4	Tumor(s) with direct invasion of adjacent organs other than the gallbladder or with perforation of visceral peritoneum.		
NX	Regional lymph nodes cannot be assessed.		
N0	No regional lymph node metastasis.		
N1	Regional lymph node metastasis.		
MX	Distant metastasis cannot be assessed.		
M0	No distant metastasis.		
M1	Distant metastasis.		
STAGE GROUPING			
Stage I	T1	N0	M0
Stage II	T2	N0	M0
Stage IIIA	T3	N0	M0
Stage IIIB	T4	N0	M0
Stage IIIC	Any T	N1	M0
Stage IV	Any T	Any N	M1

From Greene FL, Balch CM, Page DL, et al (eds): Liver (Including Intrahepatic Bile Ducts). American Joint Committee on Cancer. New York, Springer-Verlag, 6th ed, 2002, pp. 131-138.

Table 15–3. TUMOR, NODE, METASTASIS (TNM) SUMMARY OF CHANGES

The T categories in the 6th edition (2002) have been redefined and simplified.

All solitary tumors without vascular invasion, regardless of size, are classified as T1 because of similar prognosis.

All solitary tumors with vascular invasion (again regardless of size) are combined with multiple tumors ≤5 cm and classified as T2 because of similar prognosis.

Multiple tumors >5 cm and tumors with evidence of major vascular invasion are combined and classified as T3 because of similarly poor prognosis.

Tumor(s) with direct invasion of adjacent organs other than the gallbladder or with perforation of visceral peritoneum are classified separately as T4.

The separate subcategory for multiple bilobar tumors has been eliminated because of a lack of distinct prognostic value.

T3 N0 tumors and tumors with lymph node involvement are combined into stage III because of similar prognosis.

Stage IV defines metastatic disease only. The subcategories IVA and IVB have been eliminated.

From Greene FL, Balch CM, Page DL, et al (eds): Liver (Including Intrahepatic Bile Ducts). American Joint Committee on Cancer. New York, Springer-Verlag, 6th ed, 2002, pp. 131-138.

Table 15–4. CANCER OF THE LIVER ITALIAN PROGRAM (CLIP) SCORING SYSTEM

Variable	Score
Child-Pugh stage	
A	0
B	1
C	2
Tumor morphology	
Uninodular and extension ≤50%	0
Multinodular and extension ≤50%	1
Massive or extension >50%	2
α-Fetoprotein (AFP)	
<400 ng/mL	0
≥400 ng/mL	1
Portal vein thrombosis	
No	0
Yes	1

CLIP Score	Median Survival (Mo)	One-Year Survival (%)
0	35.7	84
1	22.1	66
2	8.5	45
3	6.9	36
4-6	3.2	9

This scoring information previously appeared in Nguyen MH, Keeffe EB: Treatment of Hepatocellular Cancer. In Rustgi AK, Crawford JM (eds): Gastrointestinal Cancers. Edinburgh: WB Saunders, 2003, p. 607. It is adapted from the following articles:

The Cancer of the Liver Italian Program (CLIP) Investigators. A new prognostic system for hepatocellular carcinoma: A retrospective study of 435 patients. Hepatology 28:751, 1998.

The Cancer of the Liver Italian Program (CLIP) Investigators. Prospective validation of the CLIP score: A new prognostic system for patients with cirrhosis and hepatocellular carcinoma. Hepatology 31:840, 2000.

Levy I, Sherman M: Staging of hepatocellular carcinoma: Assessment of the CLIP, Okuda, and Child-Pugh staging systems in a cohort of 257 patients in Toronto. Gut 50:881-885, 2002.

Prognostic Factors and Organ Allocation

Findings that appear to be important in prognosis include clinical status, liver function, tumor size and grade, and serum levels of AFP, DCP, and vascular endothelial growth factor. In general, patients with tumors greater than 5 cm in diameter, node involvement, vascular invasion, and high histological grade have a poor prognosis.[71-74] A number of molecular markers have been described but remain to be validated prospectively.

In 1996, Mazzaferro and colleagues reported improved survival and reduced recurrence after OLT using what became known as the *Milan criteria*, which included cirrhotic patients having a single tumor 5 cm or less in diameter or patients with no more than three tumors, each 3 cm or less in diameter.[71] Patients with evidence of vascular invasion or nodal involvement preoperatively were excluded. Nevertheless, 27% of patients had tumors that were understaged before surgery. Twenty-eight of the 48 patients who underwent transplantation had preoperative chemoembolization. The recurrence rate was 8% and recurrence-free survival was 83% at 4 years. Actuarial 4-year overall survival was 75%. These results argued strongly that careful selection of patients with smaller HCCs yield survival rates nearly similar to those observed in patients who underwent transplantation for nonmalignant conditions. Further studies using the Milan and similar selection criteria have confirmed these impressive results. In 2001, the Department of Health and Human Services approved HCC as an indication for OLT.[75]

As noted, the TNM staging system does not consider the severity of underlying liver disease, and several studies indicate this method of staging correlates poorly with survival of patients with HCC. The other staging systems were proposed in order to improve this prognostication. In February 2002, the model for end-stage liver disease (MELD) was implemented in view of its excellent ability to predict patient life span during a 3-month period.[76-80] This model uses total serum bilirubin, serum creatinine, and prothrombin time international normalized ratio (INR) to calculate a risk score for mortality on the waiting list. Patients with the highest scores (range: 6 to 40) are given the highest priority. An adjustment to the MELD score was accepted by United Network of Organ Sharing (UNOS) for patients with HCC awaiting OLT according to tumor size less than 2 cm or 2 to 5 cm, or two to three nodules, all 3 cm or less. These new organ allocation criteria have significantly reduced the waiting time for HCC patients. With shorter waiting times, modification of tumor size criteria has been proposed so that patients with larger tumors might be considered for OLT.[74,81,82] MELD scores continue to be adjusted and refined as experience with this new system of donor organ allocation is acquired.[83-90]

Efforts to shorten waiting times by expanding the donor pool have also been explored.[77] These include use of marginal donors, which include those older than 50 years of age, those with fatty infiltration of the liver, and viral hepatitis (B and C)–positive donors. Split-liver transplants, *domino* transplants in patients with hereditary transthyretin amyloidosis, and living donors are other possible modes of enlarging the donor pool.[91] Xenotransplantation potentially offers the best solution for the donor problem but is not yet feasible.[59,77,92]

The use of living donors has been reported from several centers in Asia and the United States.[91,93-97] Such donors usually are relatives of the recipient. Major ethical issues exist in these situations. Moreover, significant morbidity and some deaths have occurred in donors. Because of these complications, and the reduced waiting time for deceased-donor livers through the use of MELD score, it remains to be seen how widely living donors will be used for transplantation in patients with hepatic malignancy in the United States. Because of societal factors, it is likely that living donors will continue to be used in Asia.

Orthotopic Liver Transplantation

The resurgence of interest in OLT for HCC has led to a plethora of reviews during the past few years.[97-109] Treatment options for most patients with HCC are palliative because of the advanced stage of their disease at diagnosis (Table 15–5). Only surgical removal by hepatic resection and total hepatectomy with liver replacement are potentially curable maneuvers. Transplantation has several advantages over resection. First, it is the only option for patients with poor hepatic function—an important consideration because approximately 80% to 90% of HCC patients have cirrhosis. Second, both the tumor and the underlying liver disease are removed simultaneously. Third, HCC is frequently multifocal, especially with hepatitis C, and total hepatectomy removes the source of potentially later-developing tumors, whereas partial hepatic resection does not.

As noted, early on it was hoped that primary hepatic tumors might become one of the prime indications for OLT. However, poor results with most patients in centers worldwide led to a decline in enthusiasm. Multiple studies have shown that hepatic resection is associated with a 5-year survival of only approximately 30%. Moreover, most patients with HCC are not candidates for resection because of underlying liver disease or multifocal tumors, or both. Enthusiasm for liver transplantation has increased because of significantly better outcomes observed in more recent years as compared with earlier experience. More stringent selection of patients is likely to be one factor responsible for this improvement. Other components, including adjunctive treatment, also may have a role. Early results with neoadjuvant (pre- and intraoperative) or postoperative adjuvant systemic chemotherapy, or both, appeared promising, but controlled studies have not been performed, in part because of the prolonged waiting time for donor livers that developed in the mid-1990s.[12-15] Additional reports have suggested that adjuvant chemotherapy or chemoembolization improves patient survival in conjunction with OLT for HCC.[110,111] Unfortunately, currently available cytotoxic chemotherapy

Table 15–5. TREATMENT OPTIONS FOR HEPATOCELLULAR CARCINOMA
Potentially curative options
Total hepatectomy with orthotopic liver transplantation
Partial hepatectomy
(Each with combined modality neo/postoperative adjuvant therapy)
Palliative treatments
Systemic therapies
Chemotherapy
Hormonal therapy
Immunotherapy
Other biological therapy
Locoregional therapies
Hepatic artery transcatheter treatments
Transarterial chemotherapy
Transarterial embolization
Transarterial chemoembolization
Transarterial radioembolization
Ablative/cytoreductive therapies
Ethanol injection
Cryosurgery
Radiofrequency ablation
Palliative resection
External beam radiation
Brachytherapy
Supportive care
Future approaches
Gene therapy
Hepatocyte transplantation
Xenotransplantation

Revised from Fong Y, Venook AP, Lawrence T: Hepatocellular cancer: Clinical management. In Kelsen DP, Daly JM, Levin B, et al (eds): Gastrointestinal Oncology: Principles & Practice. Philadelphia, Lippincott Williams & Wilkins, 2002, p 582.

for advanced HCC is of little value. Neoadjuvant radiation therapy just prior to OLT has been reported from France.[110] Radioisotopes are sometimes used with embolization. More recently, a variety of locoregional techniques have been used in HCC patients. These include embolization with lipiodol or chemotherapy drugs, ethanol injection, cryosurgery, and RFA.[16-27,110,111] The superiority of any one of these procedures over the others is unclear, as no prospective controlled, randomized trials have addressed this point. In addition, it is not clear whether any of them improve overall survival in HCC patients, although two studies suggest that TACE does.[17-19] The optimal multimodality therapeutic regimen for HCC is unknown, but appropriate selection of patients combined with neoadjuvant chemotherapy or a locoregional pretransplant procedure, or both, may prove to be the most effective approach.[28-33,110-114] As noted, long-term survivors after OLT alone were seen in most centers, but were few in number before the mid-1990s. The general experience was that there was a high incidence of recurrence, usually 60% to 70%, within the first 2 years after transplantation. The most likely site of recurrence was in the liver allograft, followed by lungs and bone. At least 25 different series have been reported during the last 15 years with 3- or 5-year, or both, actuarial survival results after OLT for HCC (Table 15–6).[6,8,9,13,14,71,73,81,95,98,106,115-128] Notable improvement has been evident from many centers since the mid-1990s. In general, higher survival figures are reported in the more recent studies. A number of suggested prognostic factors have emerged from these studies, namely tumor size, multifocality, bilobar distribution, lymphovascular invasion, presence of a capsule, stage, lymph node status, metastatic disease, and histological grade.

Analysis of UNOS data—comprising 985 patients undergoing transplantation for HCC in the United States between 1987 and 2001—has confirmed the steady improvement in overall and graft survival during the eras 1987 to 1991, 1992 to 1995, and 1996 to 2001 (Fig. 15–6).[129,130] Five-year survival was 25% for 1987 to 1991, 47% for 1992 to 1995, and 61% during the period from 1996 to 2001. The control group consisted of 33,339 patients who underwent transplantation for benign disease; these patients had a 5-year survival rate of 75%, a figure that did not change significantly during the 15-year study period. Figure 15–6 shows the improvement in patient and graft survival for each succeeding 5-year interval. The reasons for this improvement are unclear. Better patient selection and delineation of prognostic factors likely account for some of the upswing.[129-140] The influence of various types of adjunctive therapy may be an important factor as well, and this possibility merits rigorous examination.

International Liver Transplant Tumor Registry

In 1992 the International Liver Transplant Tumor Registry was established at Baylor University Medical Center in Dallas; it now lists more than 1000 patients with HCC.[72,141] Analysis of the data from the first 790 patients with HCC indicated that recurrence-free 5-year survival was 49% and overall 5-year survival was 62% (Fig. 15–7). Patient survival was influenced by tumor size greater than 5 cm, vascular invasion, node involvement, and histological grade. Figure 15–8 shows the effect of vascular invasion on reduced patient survival. No difference in survival was observed with

Table 15–6. RESULTS OF LIVER TRANSPLANTATION FOR HEPATOCELLULAR CARCINOMA*

Study	No. of Patients	Actuarial Survival (%)		
		1 yr	3 yr	5 yr
O'Grady et al. 1988[6]	50	40	—	—
Ringe et al. 1989[8]	52	—	37	—
Yokoyama et al. 1990[115]	80	64	45	45
Penn et al. 1991[9]	365	30	—	18
Iwatsuki et al. 1991[116]	71	—	43	—
Pichlmayr et al. 1992[117]	87	—	—	20
Bismuth et al. 1993[118]	60	75	49	—
Stone et al. 1993[13]	20	70	55	45
Dalgic et al. 1994[119]	39	56	32	26
Farmer et al. 1994[120]	44	71	42	—
Selby et al. 1995[121]	105	66	39	36
Schwartz et al. 1995[122]	57	72	57	—
Olthoff et al. 1995[14]	25	78	46	—
Mazzaferro et al. 1996[71]	48	90	75 at 4 yr	—
Pichlmayr et al. 1998[98]	126	54	32	27
Bechstein et al. 1998[123]	52	88	—	71
Llovet et al. 1999[124]	58	84	74	74
Iwatsuki et al. 2000[73]	344	73	59	49
Figueras et al. 2000[125]	85	84	74	60
Yao et al. 2001[81]	70	91	—	72
Hemming et al. 2001[126]	112	78	63	57
Tamura et al. 2001[127]	53	79	65	61
Jones et al. 2001[128]	120	90	—	71
Margarit et al. 2002[106]	103	81	66	58
Kaihara et al. 2003[95]	56 (living donors)	73	55	—

*Many patients with tumors >5 cm were included in studies prior to 1996. Variable numbers of patients received combined modality therapy given as pretransplant (locoregional procedures or systemic chemotherapy) and/or postoperative adjuvant systemic chemotherapy. Waiting times for donor livers are generally not listed in these reports.

fibrolamellar variant versus nonfibrolamellar HCC beyond 2 years (Fig. 15–9). Histological grade appeared to have a negative impact on overall survival in patients with known tumors. Incidental tumors accounted for 45% of the entire group and tended to be smaller, more likely to be of lower histological grade, less likely to be multifocal or bilobar, and less likely to have vascular invasion. Bilobar spread and age greater than 60 years were negative prognostic factors for survival in patients with incidental tumors.

When all HCC tumors (known and incidental) were analyzed, tumor size greater than 5 cm, histological

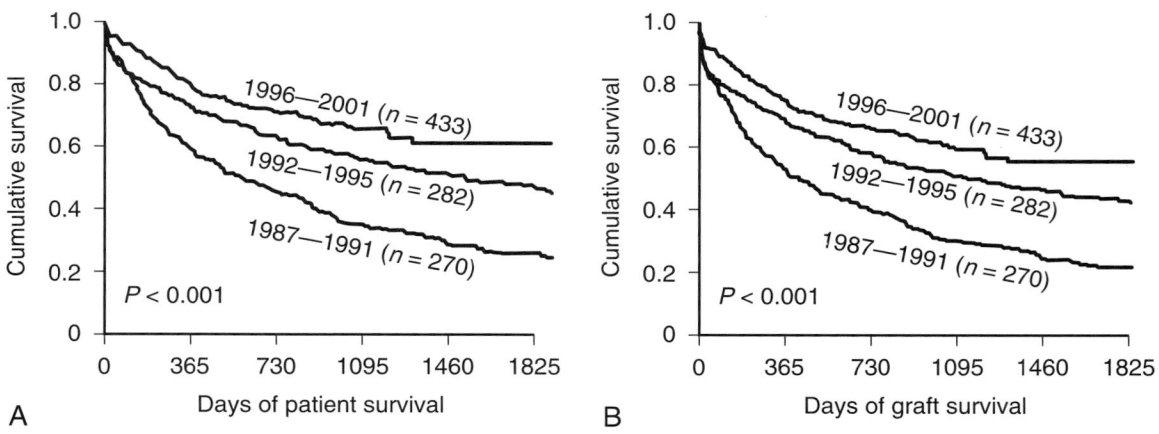

FIGURE 15–6

Patient (**A**) and graft (**B**) survival by Kaplan-Meier analysis for patients who underwent transplantation for HCC at different time periods. (United Network of Organ Sharing [UNOS] data from Yoo HY, Patt CH, Geschwind JF, et al: The outcome of liver transplantation in patients with hepatocellular carcinoma in the United States between 1987 and 2001: 5-year survival has improved significantly with time. J Clin Oncol 21:4329-4335, 2003.)

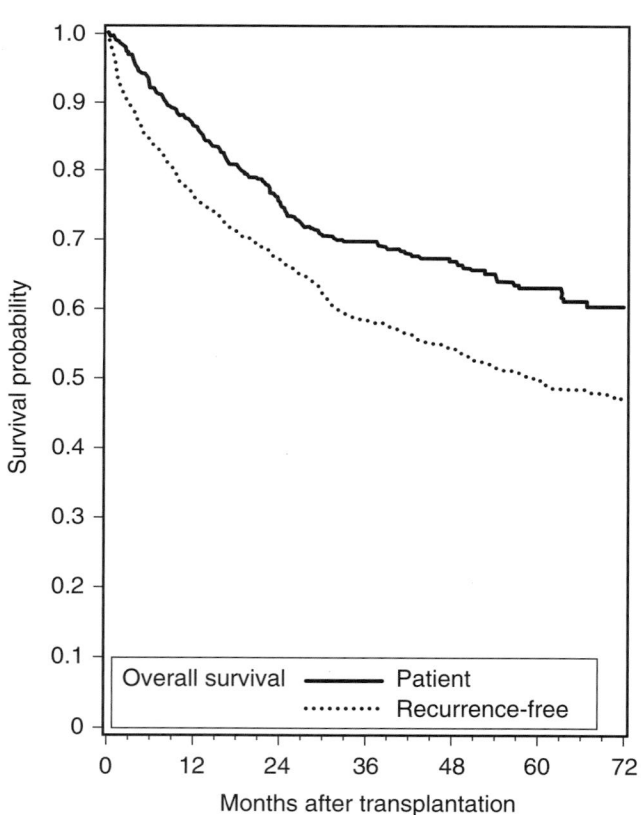

FIGURE 15–7

Patient and recurrence-free survival probability after liver transplantation. (Data from Molmenti EP, Klintmalm GB: Liver transplantation in association with hepatocellular carcinoma: An update of the International Tumor Registry. Liver Transpl 8:736-748, 2002.)

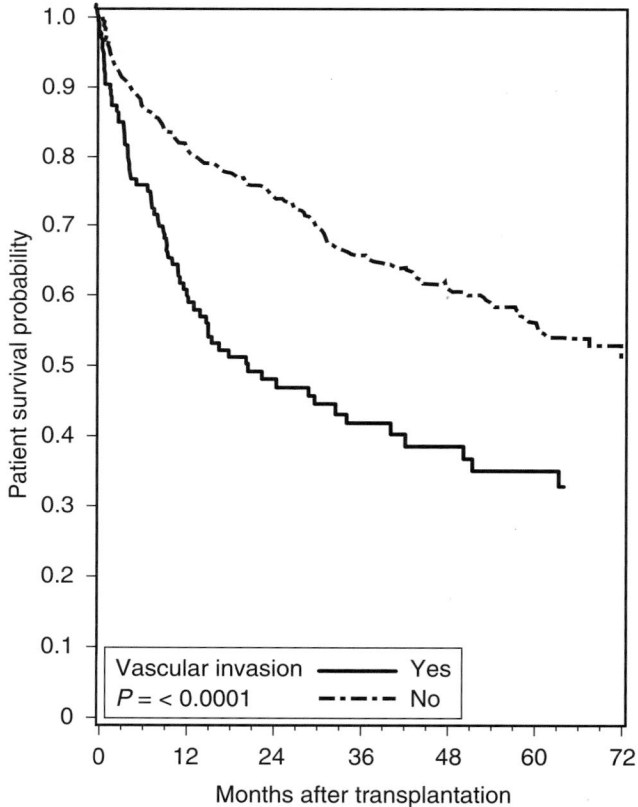

FIGURE 15–8

Patient survival probability after liver transplantation according to vascular invasion of the tumor. (Data from Molmenti EP, Klintmalm GB: Liver transplantation in association with hepatocellular carcinoma: An update of the International Tumor Registry. Liver Transpl 8:736-748, 2002.)

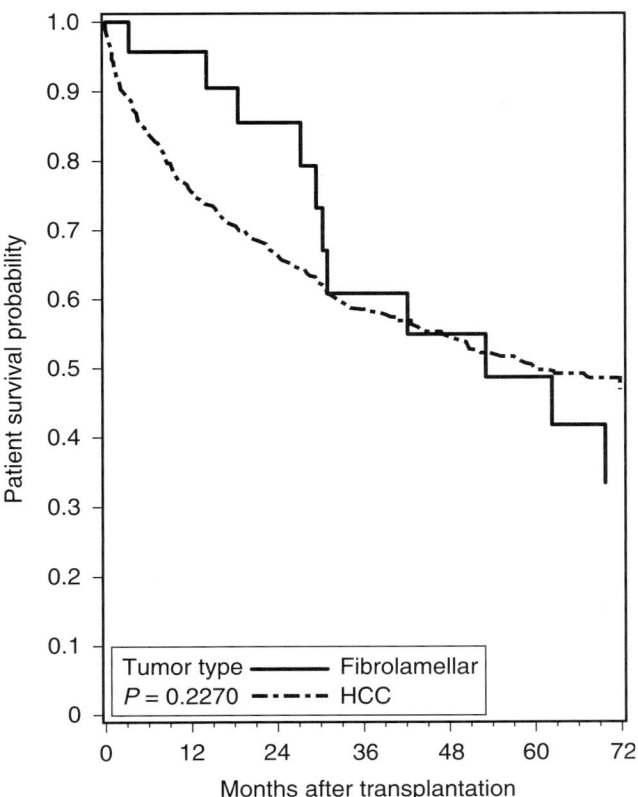

FIGURE 15–9

Patient survival probability after liver transplantation for fibrolamellar and nonfibrolamellar HCC. (Data from Molmenti EP, Klintmalm GB: Liver transplantation in association with hepatocellular carcinoma: An update of the International Tumor Registry. Liver Transpl 8:736-748, 2002.)

Table 15–7. LIVER TRANSPLANTATION FOR HEPATOCELLULAR CARCINOMA: SOME PROGNOSTIC FACTORS

Tumor size

Lymph node involvement

Vascular invasion

   Imaging

   Microscopic

Histologic grade

Multifocality

Age >60 years

Des-γ-carboxy prothrombin serum level

Molecular assays including reverse transcriptase polymerase chain reaction and gene expression profiling (under active investigation)

biopsy, is limited. Table 15–7 lists important prognostic factors in HCC.

Early experience in Dallas suggests that RFA combined with OLT may improve the overall outlook. However, needle-tract seeding has been reported in 12% of patients undergoing percutaneous RFA by the Barcelona group.[142] Risk of seeding is probably reduced by laparoscopic RFA. Intraoperative low-dose doxorubicin is given to patients with known HCC at OLT.[13,15] The role of preoperative, intraoperative, and/or postoperative chemotherapy requires further study to establish whether this approach should be integrated into the overall transplant schema. It will require prospective, controlled trials at multiple institutions to address these important questions and define the optimal multimodality regimen. Because of the projected significant increase in prevalence of hepatocellular carcinoma in the United States caused by HCV during the next 20 years,[49] such trials assume even more importance. Vaccination programs for hepatitis B ultimately can be expected to have a positive impact on the worldwide incidence of HCC, but it will be some time before this is achieved.

As of June 2003, the International Liver Transplant Tumor Registry listed 1141 patients, of whom 1019 (85.6%) had HCC; 22 (1.9%) of the cases were fibrolamellar. The registry data suggest that incidental HCC discovered in the native liver after transplantation has essentially the same long-term prognosis as a tumor removed, which was the reason for the transplant. If so, an incidental HCC in a transplant patient should be treated as aggressively as if the transplant had been undertaken for HCC. Further data should help clarify the type, indications, prognostic factors, and timing of total hepatectomy for HCC. It should be emphasized that the registry data obtained thus far do not specify

grade, and positive nodes were significantly predictive of patient survival. Recurrence-free survival for all tumors was significantly influenced by tumor size greater than 5 cm, positive nodes, bilobar spread, and vascular invasion. The latter was significantly more likely in low-grade tumors greater than 5 cm in diameter when compared with higher grade tumors. Approximately 50% of deaths after liver transplantation for HCC were tumor-related. Notably, 40% of deaths in the incidental subgroup were also tumor related.

If histological grade is confirmed as an important prognostic factor, the importance of pretransplant biopsy may necessitate obtaining a histological specimen, despite the risk of needle-tract implantation, because identification of a high-grade tumor would place that patient in a poor prognostic group.[60,61,136] By contrast, more differentiated tumors less than 5 cm without lymphovascular invasion suggest that the patient would be a good candidate for liver replacement. It should be kept in mind that accurate determination of the presence of vascular invasion by preoperative studies, even what adjunctive therapy patients received, although approximately 50% received some. It will be important to determine whether some particular type and schedule of therapy (e.g., locoregional or systemic adjuvant) yield superior results. Tumor-free survival in the 564 patients with HCC entered since 1996 is approximately 60% at 5 years. The reasons for these improved results compared with early historical controls are unclear, but they are in accord with the UNOS data.[129,130] They likely relate to better selection of patients as well as possible benefit from adjunctive therapy. It will be important to delineate prognostic factors further, refine selection criteria, and define optimal adjuvant combined modality therapy in the future. The historical evolution of OLT for HCC has been marked by high hopes and dismal disappointments in various eras (Table 15–8). However, significant progress has been made, and it seems likely that liver transplantation will be used increasingly because it offers the best chance for cure in selected patients with HCC.

Cholangiocarcinoma

Cholangiocarcinomas (CCs) arise from bile duct epithelium and are generally divided into two types[143,144]:

1. Peripheral (arising from intrahepatic bile ducts)

2. Extrahepatic (arising near the confluence of the major hepatic ducts in the liver hilum or more distally in the common bile duct)

The central or hilar cholangiocarcinoma is also known as the Klatskin tumor. Cholangiocarcinomas can be centrally located intrahepatic lesions as well (see Figs. 15–3 and 15–4). These tumors usually are mucin-secreting adenocarcinomas; they are difficult to distinguish from metastatic adenocarcinomas even with a panel of immunohistochemical stains using monoclonal antibodies to keratin and other antigens.[63-65] Cholangiocarcinoma may be mixed with elements of HCC.[43,145] Most cholangiocarcinomas are multicentric, indolent, and locally invasive. Extrahepatic metastases occur more frequently with peripheral cholangiocarcinomas (80%) than with the hilar type (40%). Causative factors include clonorchiasis, ulcerative colitis, primary sclerosing cholangitis (PSC), fibrocystic diseases, and exposure to the radiocontrast agent Thorotrast. Presenting symptoms often consist of jaundice, pruritus, and weight loss. Patients with PSC who develop cholangiocarcinoma frequently have abrupt deterioration of hepatic function, principally with a cholestatic picture.[144] Surgical resection for hilar or peripheral cholangiocarcinoma has yielded an average survival of 18 to 24 months. In many patients these tumors are unresectable. Intrahepatic cholangiocarcinoma is much less common than HCC but even more

Table 15–8. THE EVOLUTION OF LIVER TRANSPLANTATION FOR HEPATOCELLULAR CARCINOMA	
1967-1989	Liver replacement only in patients with advanced disease resulted in early recurrence within 2 years in majority of recipients, most often in the allograft.
	Long-term survival in occasional patients.
	OLT not indicated for HCC.
1989-1995	Early attempts at combined modality therapy—adjuvant systemic chemotherapy, radiation therapy, locoregional maneuvers (chemoembolization, alcohol injection).
	Promising results in some uncontrolled studies.
1996-2001	Donor waiting times for tumor patients greatly prolonged (>1 year).
	Improved definition of selection and staging criteria.
	OLT for HCC approved in 2001.
	Use of marginal and living donors to expand donor pool.
	Additional locoregional techniques (cryosurgery, radiofrequency ablation).
2002-present	UNOS implements MELD system for organ allocation with adjustments for patients with HCC: shorter donor waiting times for tumor patients.
	Better definition and refinement of prognostic factors/selection criteria.
	Delineation of timing and sequence of adjuvant combined modality therapy ongoing; optimal regimen unknown.
	Identification of molecular markers/gene expression profiling.
	Future development of artificial liver cells and xenotransplantation.

HCC, hepatocellular carcinoma; MELD, Model for End-stage Liver Disease; OLT, orthotopic liver transplantation; UNOS, United Network of Organ Sharing.

difficult to treat; chemotherapy has not proved beneficial, and radiation is of marginal value. Intrahepatic cholangiocarcinoma is staged by the same TNM system used for HCC (see Tables 15–2 and 15–3). As prognostic factors for cholangiocarcinoma become better delineated, it is likely that distinct staging criteria for this unusual tumor will be developed. Imaging studies as previously delineated are important aspects of staging cholangiocarcinoma (see Figs. 15–3 and 15–4). PET scanning may also be useful.[145] An elevated serum cancer antigen (CA) 19-9 value may be helpful, although nonspecific.

Results of liver transplantation alone for cholangiocarcinoma have been poor, with median survival generally less than 1 year.[4-9,143-162] As with HCC, however, occasional patients have had prolonged survival (>5 years) at multiple centers. Jenkins and colleagues[147] summarized the experience with 45 patients from six institutions. These patients included those with both intrahepatic and extrahepatic (Klatskin) cholangiocarcinomas. Median survival for the group was 8 months, and 1-year survival was 36%; these results were not substantially different from those for untreated patients with cholangiocarcinoma. Penn's series included 109 patients from liver transplant centers throughout the world and reported to the Cincinnati Transplant Tumor Registry.[9] Overall survival was 30% 2 years after transplantation.

The Hannover experience included 10 patients with peripheral cancer and 20 with central bile duct cancer.[8] Four of the former had evidence of extrahepatic metastases at the time of surgery. Eight of the 10 patients with peripheral tumors survived more than 30 days, but metastatic disease in the liver, lung, or bone developed in all. Metastatic involvement of regional lymph nodes was present in 7 of the 20 patients with central cholangiocarcinoma. Median survival in this group was 7 months. By contrast, median survival in 13 patients without regional node disease was 35 months, with an actuarial 2-year survival of 64%. Initial sites of recurrence included lymph nodes (6 patients), peritoneum (2 patients), and liver (1 patient).

Our group in Dallas investigated a combined modality approach for patients with cholangiocarcinoma using 5-fluorouracil radiosensitization.[148,149] Within 5 to 9 weeks after OLT, radiation therapy was initiated to the porta hepatis and regional lymph nodes. Using 24-MeV x-rays via multiple-field techniques, 55.8 Gy was delivered over a 6-week interval. Concurrent 5-fluorouracil was administered by 96-hour intravenous infusion at a dose of 450 mg/m^2 during weeks 1 and 4 of radiation. Patients received the standard immunosuppressive drug regimen. Analysis of the results in 17 patients treated with this protocol indicated only questionable benefit.[149] Eleven of 14 evaluable patients experienced recurrence; 3 others were alive without evidence of tumor 44 months,

31 months, and 28 months, respectively, after OLT. One-year survival for the group was 53%.

The UCLA group reported results of 25 patients (9 with extrahepatic disease and 16 intrahepatic disease) who had OLT for unresectable cholangiocarcinoma. Nine patients received adjuvant postoperative chemotherapy. Overall and disease-free survival rates were 71% and 67% at 1 year and 35% and 32% at 3 years, respectively. Favorable prognostic factors were absence of contiguous organ invasion at OLT, small tumor size, and single-tumor foci. No significant difference in disease-free or overall survival was observed between patients with extrahepatic and those with intrahepatic cholangiocarcinoma.

Investigators at the Mayo Clinic have used neoadjuvant radiochemotherapy followed by OLT in selected patients with unresectable early stage cholangiocarcinoma. They reported 20 patients with favorable outcome (mean follow-up 47 months), with only 1 patient having recurrence at the time of the report.[77,150] Results from Omaha and Pittsburgh also support the use of combined modality treatment for cholangiocarcinoma.[153,161]

Controlled clinical trials using new multimodality protocols are indicated before patients with cholangiocarcinoma can be considered to benefit from OLT. In the absence of such trials, OLT cannot be recommended for this patient group.[146,156]

Epithelioid Hemangioendothelioma

Epithelioid hemangioendothelioma (EH) is a rare malignant tumor of endothelial origin that may arise in the liver.[163-172] An association with oral contraceptive use has been reported. Imaging evaluation, as previously described, is useful and may suggest the diagnosis (see Fig. 15–5). The microscopic appearance may suggest other primary liver or metastatic tumors, but the endothelial nature of the tumor cells revealed by the presence of positive immunohistochemical staining for factor VIII–related antigen, CD34, and/or CD31 confirms the diagnosis.[167-169] The prognosis is unpredictable, and the morphological appearance does not correlate well with biological behavior. The tumor grows slowly but aggressively. Eighty-eight patients with EH treated with OLT have been reported, with 1- and 5-year survival rates of 61% and 44%, respectively.[4,169,171] Unlike the circumstance with other primary liver neoplasms, the presence of extrahepatic EH does not correlate with survival, so this finding is not necessarily a contraindication to liver replacement. Five patients with metastatic involvement at the time of transplantation were alive a mean of 41 months after surgery in the report by Marino and colleagues.[166] Extrahepatic sites included hilar lymph nodes, rib, lungs, pleura, and diaphragm. One patient was alive 11 years after OLT. Because long-term survival is possible despite the presence of extra-hepatic metastasis, selected patients with hepatic EH should be considered candidates for liver transplantation. The role of adjuvant chemotherapy, radiation, or biological therapy is unclear. Interferon has been reported to cause tumor regression, but it may increase the likelihood of graft rejection.[171]

Other Hepatic Tumors

As expected, results of OLT in patients with metastatic tumors to the liver have been dismal. Transplantation for these patients, therefore, cannot be recommended.[98,103,106] A possible exception is the group of patients with metastatic carcinoid and other neuroendocrine tumors (NETs). Favorable results have been obtained in some patients.[3,4,8,10,173-178] In a review of 103 patients with malignant NETs who underwent OLT, the 2- and 5-year survival rates were 60% and 47%, respectively. Recurrence-free survival was less than 24%, however.[173,174] Favorable prognostic factors included age younger than 50 years, primary tumor in lung or bowel, and pretreatment with somatostatin analogues (univariate). Age older than 50 years and OLT combined with upper abdominal exenteration or a Whipple procedure were adverse prognostic factors (multivariate). The role of OLT remains unclear for malignant NETs but may be considered for younger patients with disease confined to the liver. Carcinoids are frequently slow-growing tumors, and dramatic benefit from disabling symptoms has been achieved by OLT in some patients. Carcinoid tumors of the common bile duct are rarely reported.[177]

In contrast to the surprisingly good results with OLT in patients with EH, transplantation for hepatic angiosarcoma has not proved successful.[98,103] However, only a few patients with angiosarcoma have undergone transplantation, and firm conclusions cannot be drawn. Because angiosarcoma of the liver is a rare tumor,[179] it is unlikely that the role of transplantation in treatment of this aggressive neoplasm will be clarified in the near future.

Discussion

Liver resection and transplantation are currently the only curative treatments for patients with primary hepatic malignancies. Because 90% of hepatic cancers are HCC and 80% of those patients have cirrhosis, resection is an option for only a small number of patients and is associated with a high recurrence rate. Thus the only realistic chance for cure for the vast majority of patients is transplantation. Since the first edition of this book in 1996, a rebirth of interest in OLT for liver malignancies,

especially HCC, has occurred. The previous pessimistic attitude was based on experience from many centers throughout the world that early recurrence after OLT alone, usually in the allograft within the first 2 years, was the rule. During the past decade, there has been a clear improvement in outcome, although the reasons for this are not clearly defined (see Table 15–6).[71,73,81,95,98,106,120-130,141] Better patient selection based on identification of key prognostic factors appears to be partially responsible. The emergence of multimodality neoadjuvant therapy, both systemic chemotherapy and various locoregional maneuvers, also may play a significant role; however, the optimal technique and schedule for such approaches remain undefined. The importance of reduction in waiting time for donor livers made possible by adoption of the MELD organ allocation system cannot be overemphasized.[75-90] Use of living donors obviously shortens waiting time as well, but it introduces significant ethical dilemmas and potential significant medical risks for the donor. Other attempts to increase the donor pool have met with some success, but their overall impact appears limited. Liver-assist devices may prove useful as a bridge to transplantation in certain acutely ill patients. Hepatocyte transplantation and xenotransplantation are potential solutions for the donor problem and eventually may become feasible.[77,91,92]

Pichlmayr has pointed out that patients and their families ride an emotional roller coaster as their hopes wax and wane, with the patient enduring major surgery and its related complications and then experiencing early recurrence before finally succumbing to the original neoplasm.[10] Nevertheless, transplantation offers the only chance for cure in the majority of patients with unresectable tumors, and long-term survival, which occurred only rarely prior to 1990, is now being observed at major transplant centers throughout the world.[4-10] The recurrences after OLT appear, in part, to be caused by small numbers of tumor cells undetectable at surgery that are present outside the liver or are related to manipulation of the tumor during total hepatectomy. The high initial recurrence rate in the allograft suggests that tumor cells having metastatic potential circulate before taking up residence in the new liver, where they proliferate and develop into ultimately fatal gross metastases.[13,14,180-183] If true, such a circumstance may be prevented or delayed significantly by the use of effective adjunctive systemic chemotherapy. Efforts in this regard are limited by the lack of available chemotherapy drugs having significant antitumor activity in patients with advanced HCC or cholangiocarcinoma. Despite these limitations, it is known that drugs with only modest activity in advanced disease may be more effective when the tumor burden is low.[184] The value of systemic chemotherapy as an adjunct to surgery has been proved in other types of malignancy, notably breast and colon cancer.[185] Such experience provides the rationale for attempts at combined modality therapy using systemic chemotherapy in conjunction with OLT for patients with unresectable primary hepatic malignancies. The necessity of using postoperative immunosuppression in the transplant recipient poses an additional potential risk for recurrence and makes the use of cytotoxic chemotherapy drugs (which are also immunosuppressive) difficult but not insurmountable.[71,186] The "more is better" approach may not be wise in tumor patients who are allograft recipients. Immunosuppressive agents may also lead to enhancement of growth of micrometastatic foci, as it has been reported that tumor doubling times are more rapid in transplant recipients than in patients not receiving immunosuppressive therapy who undergo resection for HCC.[187] Too much immunosuppression also predisposes to posttransplant lymphoproliferative disorders and other malignancies.[9,188,189] A predictable definition of tolerance in the transplant patient could allow withdrawal of immunosuppressive therapy, a highly desirable goal. Early attempts appear promising.[190]

During the past decade a variety of locoregional techniques have been developed in an effort to treat primary liver neoplasms and limit their spread (see Table 15–5).[16-27,98-106] These include various hepatic artery transcatheter approaches, with or without chemotherapy or radioisotopes, in order to embolize the vessels providing blood to the tumor. A number of ablative or cytoreductive methods are also in use and include ethanol injection, cryosurgery, and radiofrequency (thermal) ablation. Each approach has its own advantages and limitations, and it is not clear which is superior because no controlled prospective trials comparing them have been conducted. Such procedures have been used as palliative maneuvers or as a *bridge* to transplantation. Hepatic resection followed by *salvage* OLT also has been proposed. Definition of the optimal role and timing of these various procedures is needed so that a combined modality program, with neoadjuvant and postoperative components, can be developed to maximize the chance for cure (see Pearls and Pitfalls). With the recent change in organ allocation for tumor patients, waiting times have been shortened. Despite this important development, it would be a mistake to assume that no adjunctive therapy is necessary. Optimal combinations and sequence of locoregional and systemic chemotherapeutic regimens need to be investigated and delineated.[12-15,28-33,105,110-114] The use of biological therapeutic approaches also should be explored. Improvement in results of OLT for HCC appears to be clearly evident and likely is related to better selection criteria and definition of important prognostic factors.

Another possible component requiring close examination is the type and timing of neoadjuvant and postoperative adjuvant treatment that has been given to many patients. Future data derived from the International Liver Transplant Tumor Registry may yield important information regarding direction and design of prospective trials.

Clearly, the prevention of tumor recurrence in a liver transplant recipient involves a delicate balance among susceptibility of residual tumor cells to administered cytotoxic drugs, maintenance of the functioning allograft, and the unwanted effects of immunosuppression on host resistance. New biological approaches, including gene therapy, have the ability to modulate cell physiology and enhance specificity.[97] Initial attempts to induce a graft-versus-tumor effect by means of a nonmyeloablative hematopoietic stem cell transplant following OLT also have been reported.[191]

Liver transplantation remains the only option for cure in the majority of patients with HCC. Delineation of prognostic factors and refinement of selection criteria will improve outcomes for this otherwise fatal disease, which will increase in incidence during the next 2 decades in Western countries. Identification and validation of molecular genetic markers in pathogenesis and prognosis are under active investigation.[192-198] In all probability, such markers will contribute significantly to our understanding and management of HCC. It seems likely that combined systemic adjuvant, perhaps neoadjuvant, chemotherapy and locoregional techniques will be beneficial as more is learned about their timing and scheduling.

Although the revised system of organ allocation for tumor patients has made transplantation/liver replacement much more feasible, donor availability remains a serious problem. The number of potential deceased organ donors in the United States is less than 14,000 per year and, in July 2003, more than 82,000 patients were waiting for a solid-organ transplant.[199] Various strategies to enlarge the donor pool have helped somewhat. One such strategy, the use of living donors, carries with it both medical risk and ethical dilemmas. Hepatocyte transplants and xenotransplants remain experimental and their ultimate clinical role undefined.

Indefinite immunosuppression poses a risk to all transplant recipients, especially tumor patients. Recurrence of the original neoplasm as well as posttransplant lymphoproliferative disorders and other de novo tumors are serious problems that are more likely to occur with long-term immunosuppression.[200] Thus attempts to identify immune tolerance accurately and wean patients from immunosuppressive therapy would have major impact and hopefully will become successful in the future.[190]

Summary

The early results of hepatic transplantation for patients with primary hepatic malignancies were disappointing.

Although occasional patients achieved long-term disease-free survival and were probably cured, most experienced early tumor recurrence and died from the original neoplasm. Recurrences usually appeared during the first 2 years, often in the allograft. Better definition of prognostic factors and more rigorous patient selection have resulted in significant improvement in 5-year survival for patients receiving transplants for HCC during the past decade. This enhanced survival rate for tumor patients is approaching the survival rate that is seen in patients transplanted for benign disease. Liver transplantation has emerged as the therapy of choice for most HCC patients and offers their only chance for cure. Adequate staging is essential to identify suitable candidates for transplantation as well as to compare results obtained at different institutions. Additional prognostic factors obtained through the application of molecular biological techniques such as microarray analysis are likely to be valuable in the future and are eagerly awaited. For patients with small HCC confined to the liver, recent data indicate that transplantation, perhaps combined with multimodal therapy using locoregional procedures and neoadjuvant systemic chemotherapy, results in improved disease-free survival. Such a combined modality approach, when optimized, could have a further significant favorable impact on outcome for patients with this neoplasm. The management of patients with HCC remains complex and challenging. However, there is progress in this enormous problem, and it is becoming increasingly clear that liver transplantation is the therapy of choice for some patients with limited-stage disease. Further advances in our ability to define clinical immune tolerance and thus permit reduction of immunosuppression are highly sought. Effective treatment for patients with advanced HCC and prevention remain future goals.

New adjunctive approaches are needed for patients with cholangiocarcinoma. Indications for hepatic

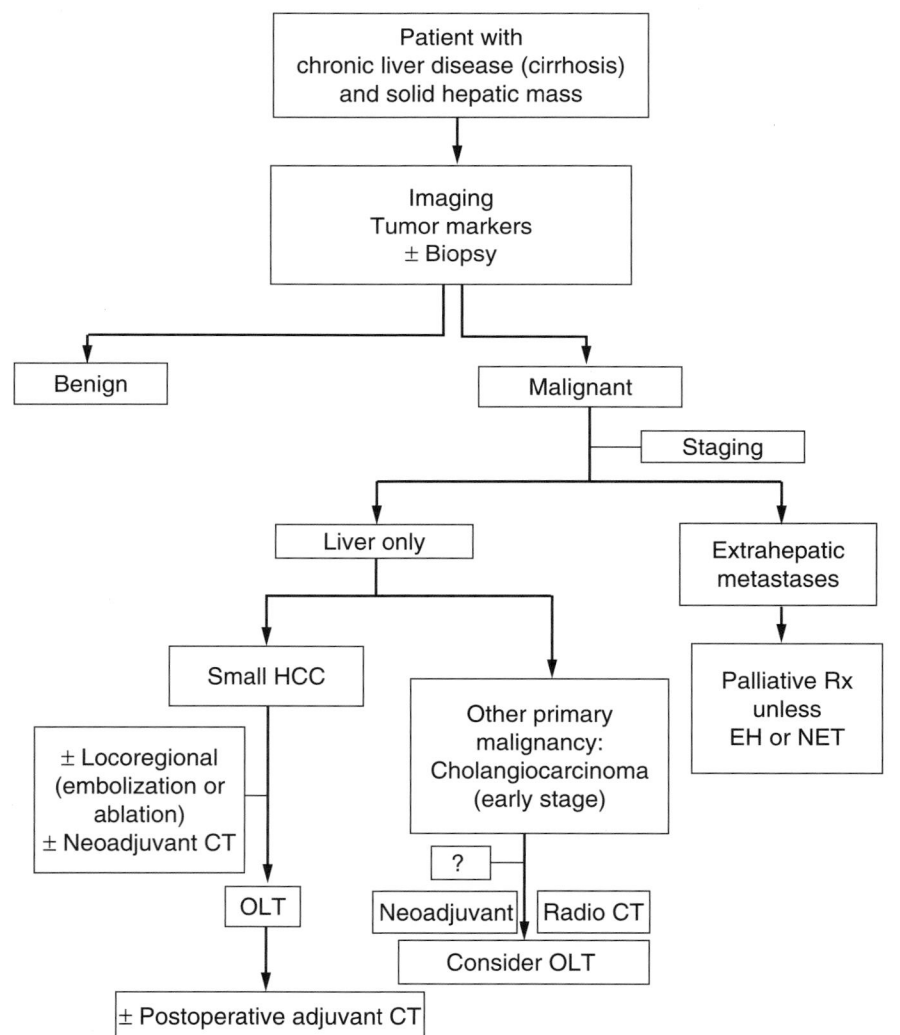

FIGURE 15–10

Decision tree: primary hepatic malignancy. Patients with advanced HCC or cholangiocarcinoma should be considered for experimental clinical trials or palliative care. CT, chemotherapy; EH, epithelioid hemangioendothelioma; NET, neuroendocrine tumor; OLT, orthotopic liver transplant.

transplantation in patients with other primary hepatic malignancies are marginal, with the exception of EH and certain NETs.

Improvement in the results of treatment for primary hepatic malignancies constitutes one of the major challenges facing the transplant community during the next decade (Fig. 15–10). Delineation of the most advantageous adjunctive therapy to use in combination with transplantation may have a major positive impact on survival for patients. Future progress in the treatment of primary liver cancer depends on close interaction and cooperation between transplant surgeons, oncologists, and other specialists in the setting of prospective, controlled clinical trials.

Acknowledgments

Supported in part by the Robert Schanbaum Memorial Fund, the James E. Nauss Cancer Research Fund, and the Edward and Ruth Wilkof Foundation. Linda Miller provided expert help with manuscript preparation.

Pearls and Pitfalls

- Subcentimeter lesion is not HCC until proved by histology, continued growth, or AFP levels greater than 400 ng/mL.
- FNH can easily be confused with HCC.
- Liver biopsy yields morphology and tumor grade at the risk (low) of tumor seeding.
- A negative brush biopsy result from the bile duct does not rule out cholangiocarcinoma.
- After transplant, one half of the deaths are from recurrent HCC, also for incidental tumors. Consider chemotherapy for all patients with HCC after transplantation.
- Underimmunosuppression is unusual in tumor patients; rejection is not a problem in these patients.
- Consider aggressive therapy if HCC recurs.
- Adjunct pretransplant therapy is intended to stop growth and spread pretransplant *and* prevent posttransplant recurrence.

References

1. Starzl TE: Experience in Hepatic Transplantation. Philadelphia, WB Saunders, 1969, pp 350-355.
2. Starzl TE: The Puzzle People. Pittsburgh, University of Pittsburgh, 1992, pp 166-167.
3. Starzl TE, Demetris AJ, Van Thiel D: Liver transplantation. N Engl J Med 321:1014-1022, 1092-1099, 1989.
4. Klintmalm GB, Stone MJ: Liver transplantation for malignancy. Transplant Rev 4:52-58, 1990.
5. Iwatsuki S, Gordon RD, Shaw BW Jr, Starzl TE: Role of liver transplantation in cancer therapy. Ann Surg 202:401-407, 1985.
6. O'Grady JG, Polson RJ, Rolles K, et al: Liver transplantation for malignant disease. Ann Surg 207:373-379, 1988.
7. Pichlmayr R, Ringe B, Bechstein WO, et al: Approach to primary liver cancer. Recent Results Cancer Res 110:65-73, 1988.
8. Ringe B, Wittekind C, Bechstein WO, et al: The role of liver transplantation in hepatobiliary malignancy. Ann Surg 209:88-98, 1989.
9. Penn I: Hepatic transplantation for primary and metastatic cancers of the liver. Surgery 110:726-735, 1991.
10. Pichlmayr R: Is there a place for liver grafting for malignancy? Transplant Proc 20(Suppl 1):478-482, 1988.
11. Olthoff KM, Millis JM, Rosove MH, et al: Is liver transplantation justified for the treatment of hepatic malignancies? Arch Surg 125:1261-1268, 1990.
12. Stone MJ, Klintmalm G, Polter D, et al: Neoadjuvant chemotherapy and orthotopic liver transplantation for hepatocellular carcinoma. Transplantation 48:344-347, 1989.
13. Stone MJ, Klintmalm GBG, Polter D, et al: Neoadjuvant chemotherapy and liver transplantation for hepatocellular carcinoma: A pilot study in 20 patients. Gastroenterology 104:196-202, 1993.
14. Olthoff KM, Rosove MH, Shackleton CR, et al: Adjuvant chemotherapy improves survival after liver transplantation for hepatocellular carcinoma. Ann Surg 221:734-743, 1995.
15. Stone MJ: Transplantation for Primary Hepatic Malignancy. In Busuttil RW, Klintmalm GB (eds): Ttransplantation of the Liver. Philadelphia, WB Saunders, 1996, pp 125-129.
16. Bismuth H, Morino M, Sherlock D, et al: Primary treatment of hepatocellular carcinoma by arterial chemoembolization. Am J Surg 163:387-394, 1992.
17. Llovet J, Real MI, Montana X, et al: Arterial embolization or chemoembolization versus symptomatic treatment in patients with unresectable hepatocellular carcinoma: A randomized controlled trial. Lancet 359:1734-1739, 2002.
18. Lo CM, Ngan H, Tso WK, et al: Randomized controlled trial of transarterial lipoidal chemoembolization for unresectable hepatocellular carcinoma. Hepatology 35:1164-1171, 2002.
19. Geschwind JFH: Chemoembolization for hepatocellular carcinoma: Where does the truth lie? J Vasc Interv Radiol 13:991-994, 2002.
20. Ramsey DE, Kernagis LY, Soulen MC, et al: Chemoembolization of hepatocellular carcinoma. J Vasc Interv Radiol 13:S211-S221, 2002.
21. Ebied OM, Federle MP, Carr BI, et al: Evaluation of responses to chemoembolization in patients with unresectable hepatocellular carcinoma. Cancer 97:1042-1050, 2003.
22. Stuart K: Chemoembolization in the management of liver tumors. The Oncologist 8:425-437, 2003.
23. Shiina S, Tagawa K, Niwa Y, et al: Percutaneous ethanol injection therapy for hepatocellular carcinoma: Results in 146 patients. Am J Roentgenol 160:1023-1028, 1993.
24. Fong Y, Venook AP, Lawrence T: Hepatocellular cancer: Clinical management. In Kelsen DP, Daly JM, Levin B, et al. (eds): Gastrointestinal Oncology Principles & Practice. Philadelphia, Lippincott Williams & Wilkins, 2002, pp 579-600.
25. Nguyen MH, Keeffe EB: Treatment of hepatocellular cancer. In Rustgi AK, Crawford JM (eds): Gastrointestinal Cancers. Edinburgh, Saunders, 2003, pp 605-622.
26. Fontana RJ, Hamidullah H, Nghiem H, et al: Percutaneous radiofrequency thermal ablation of hepatocellular carcinoma: A safe and effective bridge to liver transplantation. Liver Transpl 8:1165-1174, 2002.
27. Komorizono Y, Oketani M, Sako K, et al: Risk factors for local recurrence of small hepatocellular carcinoma tumors after a single session, single application of percutaneous radiofrequency ablation. Cancer 97:1253-1262, 2003.

28. Christians KK, Pitt HA, Rilling WS, et al: Hepatocellular carcinoma: Multimodality management. Surgery 130:554-560, 2001.
29. Medina-Franco H, Sellers MT, Eckhoff DE, et al: Multimodality treatment for patients with hepatocellular carcinoma: analysis of prognostic factors in a single western institution series. J Gastrointest Surg 5:638-645, 2001.
30. Patt CH, Thuluvath PJ: Role of liver transplantation in the management of hepatocellular carcinoma. J Vasc Interv Radiol 13:S205-S210, 2002.
31. Rilling WS, Drooz A: Multidisciplinary management of hepatocellular carcinoma. J Vasc Interv Radiol 13:S259-S263, 2002.
32. Maluf D, Fisher RA, Maroney T, et al: Non-resective ablation and liver transplantation in patients with cirrhosis and hepatocellular carcinoma (HCC): Safety and efficacy. Am J Transplant 3:312-317, 2003.
33. Chui AKK, Rao ARN, Island RE, et al: Multi-modality tumor control prior to liver transplantation in patients with hepatocellular carcinoma (HCC). J Gastrointest Surg 7:269, 2003.
34. Mortelé KJ, De Keukeleire K, Praet M, et al: Malignant focal hepatic lesions complicating underlying liver disease: Dual-phase contrast-enhanced spiral CT sensitivity and specificity in orthotopic liver transplant patients. Eur Radiol 11:1631-1638, 2001.
35. Bhartia B, Ward J, Guthrie JA, et al: Hepatocellular carcinoma in cirrhotic livers: Double-contrast thin-section MR imaging with pathologic correlation of explanted tissue. Am J Roentgenol 180:577-584, 2003.
36. Teefey SA, Hildeboldt CC, Dehadashti F, et al: Detection of primary hepatic malignancy in liver transplant candidates: Prospective comparison of CT, MR Imaging, US, and PET. Radiology 226:533-542, 2003.
37. Krinsky GA, Israel G: Nondysplastic nodules that are hyperintense on T_1-weighted gradient-echo MR imaging: Frequency in cirrhotic patients undergoing transplantation. Am J Roentgenol 180:1023-1027, 2003.
38. Freeman RB: Diagnosing hepatocellular carcinoma: A virtual reality. Liver Transpl 8:762-764, 2002.
39. Engstrom PF, Sigurdson ER, Evans AA, et al: Primary neoplasms of the liver. In Holland-Frei (ed): Cancer Medicine 6. Hamilton, Ontario, BC Decker, 2003.
40. Befeler AS, Di Bisceglie AM: Hepatocellular carcinoma: Diagnosis and treatment. Gastroenterology 122:1609-1619, 2002.
41. Zhu AX: Hepatocellular carcinoma: Are we making progress? Cancer Invest 21:418-428, 2003.
42. Llovet JM, Burroughs A, Bruix J, et al: Hepatocellular carcinoma. Lancet 362:1907-1917, 2003.
43. Russo MW, Jacobson IM: Hepatocellular cancer: Screening, surveillance, and prevention. In Kelsen DP, Daly JM, Levin B, et al. (eds): Gastrointestinal Oncology Principles & Practice. Philadelphia, Lippincott Williams & Wilkins, 2002, pp 559-568.
44. Kew MC: Hepatocellular cancer: Epidemiology and risk factors. In Kelsen DP, Daly JM, Levin B, et al. (eds): Gastrointestinal Oncology Principles & Practice. Philadelphia, Lippincott Williams & Wilkins, 2002, pp 529-538.
45. Kirimlioglu H, Dvorchick I, Ruppert K, et al: Hepatocellular carcinomas in native livers from patients treated with orthotopic liver transplantation: Biologic and therapeutic implications. Hepatology 34:502-510, 2001.
46. El-Serag HB, Davila JA, Petersen NJ, et al: The continuing increase in the incidence of hepatocellular carcinoma in the United States: An update. Ann Intern Med 139:817-823, 2003.
47. Simonetti RG, Cammà C, Fiorello F, et al: Hepatitis C virus infection as a risk factor for hepatocellular carcinoma in patients with cirrhosis. Ann Intern Med 116:97-103, 1992.
48. Flamm SL: Chronic hepatitis C virus infection. JAMA 18:2413-2417, 2003.
49. Davis GL, Albright JE, Cook SF, et al: Projecting future complications of chronic hepatitis C in the United States. Liver Transpl 9:331-338, 2003.
50. Deugnier YM, Guyader D, Cranstock L, et al: Primary liver cancer in genetic hemochromatosis: a clinical pathological, and pathogenetic study of 54 cases. Gastroenterology 104:228-234, 1993.
51. Hofseth LJ, Perwez H, Wang XW, et al: Hepatocellular cancer: Molecular biology and genetics. In Kelsen DP, Daly JM, Levin B, et al. (eds): Gastrointestinal Oncology Principles & Practice. Philadelphia, Lippincott Williams & Wilkins, 2002, pp 539-558.
52. Ozturk M, Cetin-Atalay R: Biology of hepatocellular cancer. In Rustgi AK, Crawford JM (eds): Gastrointestinal Cancers. Edinburgh, Saunders, 2003, pp 575-592.
53. Moon WS, Tarnawski AS: Nuclear translocation of survivin in hepatocellular carcinoma: A key to cancer cell growth? Hum Pathol 34:1119-1126, 2003.
54. Sell S: Mouse models to study the interaction of risk factors for human liver cancer. Cancer Res 63:7553-7562, 2003.
55. Taketa K: α-Fetoprotein: Reevaluation in hepatology. Hepatology 12:1420-1432, 1990.
56. Epstein B, Ettinger D, Leichner PK, Order SE: Multimodality cisplatin treatment in nonresectable alpha-fetoprotein-positive hepatoma. Cancer 67:896-900, 1991.
57. Nagaoka S, Yatsuhashi H, Hamada H, et al: The des-γ-carboxy prothrombin index is a new prognostic indicator for hepatocellular carcinoma. Cancer 98:2671-2677, 2003.
58. de Franchis R, Meucci G, Vecchi M, et al: The natural history of asymptomatic hepatitis B surface antigen carriers. Ann Intern Med 118:191-194, 1993.
59. Kew MC: Clinical aspects of hepatocellular cancer. In Rustgi AK, Crawford JM (eds): Gastrointestinal Cancers. Edinburgh, Saunders, 2003, pp 563-574.
60. Molmenti EP, Klintmalm GB: Hepatocellular cancer in liver transplantation. J Hepatobiliary Pancreat Surg 8:427-434, 2001.
61. Dumortier J, Lombard-Bohas C, Valette PJ, et al: Needle tract recurrence of hepatocellular carcinoma after liver transplantation. Gut 47:301, 2000.
62. Kung ITM, Chan S-K, Fung K-H: Fine-needle aspiration in hepatocellular carcinoma. Cancer 67:673-680, 1991.
63. Lau SK, Prakash S, Geller SA, et al: Comparative immunohistochemical profile of hepatocellular carcinoma, cholangiocarcinoma, and metastatic adenocarcinoma. Hum Pathol 33:1175-1181, 2002.
64. Kakar S, Muir T, Murphy LM, et al: Immunoreactivity of Hep Par 1 in hepatic and extrahepatic tumors and its correlation with albumin in situ hybridization in hepatocellular carcinoma. Am J Clin Pathol 119:361-366, 2003.
65. Fan Z, van de Rijn M, Montgomery K, et al: Hep Par 1 antibody stain for the differential diagnosis of hepatocellular carcinoma: 676 tumors tested using tissue microassays and conventional tissue selections. Mod Pathol 16:137-144, 2003.
66. Greene FL, Balch CM, Page DL, et al (eds): Liver (Including Intrahepatic Bile Ducts), American Joint Committee on Cancer, 6th ed. New York, Springer-Verlag, 2002, pp131-138.
67. Okuda K, Ohtukic T, Obata H, et al: National history of hepatocellular carcinoma and prognosis in relation to treatment: Study of 850 patients. Cancer 56:918, 1985.
68. The Cancer of the Liver Italian Program (CLIP) Investigators. A new prognostic system for hepatocellular carcinoma: A retrospective study of 435 patients. Hepatology 28:751, 1998.
69. The Cancer of the Liver Italian Program (CLIP) Investigators. Prospective validation of the CLIP score: A new prognostic system for patients with cirrhosis and hepatocellular carcinoma. Hepatology 31:840, 2000.
70. Levy I, Sherman M: Staging of hepatocellular carcinoma: Assessment of the CLIP, Okuda, and Child-Pugh staging systems in a cohort of 257 patients in Toronto. Gut 50:881-885, 2002.

71. Mazzaferro V, Regalia E, Doci R, et al: Liver transplantation for the treatment of small hepatocellular carcinomas in patients with cirrhosis. N Engl J Med 334:693-699, 1996.

72. Klintmalm GB: Liver transplantation for hepatocellular carcinoma. A registry report of the impact of tumor characteristics on outcome. Ann Surg 228:479-490, 1998.

73. Iwatsuki S, Dvorchik I, Marsh JW, et al: Liver transplantation for hepatocellular carcinoma: A proposal of a prognostic scoring system. J Am Coll Surg 191:389-394, 2000.

74. Bruix J, Llovet JM: Prognostic prediction and treatment strategy in hepatocellular carcinoma. Hepatology 35:519-524, 2002.

75. Fung J, Marsh W: The quandary over liver transplantation for hepatocellular carcinoma: The greater sin? Liver Transpl 8:775-777, 2002.

76. Wiesner RH, McDiarmid SV, Kamath PS, et al: MELD and PELD: Application of survival models to liver allocation. Liver Transpl 7:567-580, 2001.

77. Weisner RH, Rakela J, Ishitani MB, et al: Recent advances in liver transplantation. Mayo Clin Proc 78:197-210, 2003.

78. Cheng SJ, Freeman RB, Wong JB: Predicting the probability of progression-free survival in patients with small hepatocellular carcinoma. Liver Transpl 8:323-328, 2002.

79. Roberts JP: Prioritization of patients with liver cancer within the MELD system. Liver Transpl 8:329-330, 2002.

80. Yao FY, Bass NM, Nikolai B, et al: Liver transplantation for hepatocellular carcinoma: Analysis of survival according to the intention-to-treat principle and dropout from the waiting list. Liver Transpl 8:873-883, 2002.

81. Yao FY, Ferrell L, Bass NM, et al: Liver transplantation for hepatocellular carcinoma: expansion of the tumor size limits does not adversely impact survival. Hepatology 33:1394-1403, 2001.

82. Yao FY, Ferrell L, Bass NM, et al: Liver transplantation for hepatocellular carcinoma: comparison of the proposed UCSF criteria with the Milan criteria and the Pittsburgh modified TNM criteria. Liver Transpl 8:765-774, 2002.

83. Llado L, Figueras J, Memba R, et al: Is MELD really the definitive score for liver allocation? Liver Transpl 8:795-798, 2002.

84. Freeman RB: In pursuit of the ideal liver allocation model. Liver Transpl 8:799-801, 2002.

85. Yao FY, Bass NM, Nikolai B, et al: A follow-up analysis of the pattern and predictors of dropout from the waiting list for liver transplantation in patients with hepatocellular carcinoma: implications for the current organ allocation policy. Liver Transpl 9:684-692, 2003.

86. Marsh JW, Dvorchik I: Liver organ allocation for hepatocellular carcinoma: Are we sure? Liver Transpl 9:693-696, 2003.

87. Durand F, Belghiti J: Liver transplantation for hepatocellular carcinoma: Should we push the limits? Liver Transpl 9:697-699, 2003.

88. Bruix J, Fuster J, Llovet JM: Liver transplantation for hepatocellular carcinoma: Foucault pendulum versus evidence-based decision. Liver Transpl 9:700-702, 2003.

89. Freeman RB: MELD/PELD: One year later. Transplant Proc 35:2425-2427, 2003.

90. Wiesner R, Edwards E, Freeman R, et al: Model for end-stage liver disease (MELD) and allocation of donor livers. Gastroenterology 124:91-96, 2003.

91. Grewal HP: Impact of surgical innovation on liver transplantation. Lancet 359:368-370, 2002.

92. Cooper DK: Clinical xenotransplantation—how close are we? Lancet 362:557-559, 2003.

93. Tan KC: Surgery for hepatocellular carcinoma. J Gastroenterol Hepatol 17:S421-S423, 2002.

94. Gondolesi G, Muñoz L, Matsumoto C, et al: Hepatocellular carcinoma: A prime indication for living donor transplantation. J Gastrointest Surg 6:102-107, 2002.

95. Kaihara S, Kiuchi T, Ueda M, et al: Living-donor liver transplantation for hepatocellular carcinoma. Transplantation 75:S37-S40, 2003.

96. Hess D, Humar A, Sielaff TD: Living related liver transplantation for recurrent hepatocellular carcinoma in a normal liver. Clin Transplant 16:240-242, 2002.

97. Suehiro T, Terashi T, Shiotani S, et al: Liver transplantation for hepatocellular carcinoma. Surgery 131:S190-S194, 2002.

98. Pichlmayr R, Weimann A, Oldhafer KJ, et al: Appraisal of transplantation for malignant tumours of the liver with special reference to early stage hepatocellular carcinoma. Eur J Surg Oncol 24:60-67, 1998.

99. Molmenti EP, March JW, Dvorchik I, et al: Liver transplantation: Current management. Surg Clin North Am 79:43-57, 1999.

100. Strong RW: Transplantation for liver and biliary cancer. Semin Surg Oncol 19:189-199, 2000.

101. Kashef E, Roberts JP: Transplantation for hepatocellular carcinoma. Semin Oncol 28:497-502, 2001.

102. Little SA, Fong Y: Hepatocellular carcinoma: Current surgical management. Semin Oncol 28:474-486, 2001.

103. Koffran A, Fryer JP, Abecassis M: Indications and results of liver transplantation for primary and metastatic liver cancer. Cancer Treat Res 109:77-99, 2001.

104. Durand F, Belghiti J: Liver transplantation for hepatocellular carcinoma. Hepatogastroenterology 49:47-52, 2002.

105. Wong LL: Current status of liver transplantation for hepatocellular cancer. Am J Surg 183:309-316, 2002.

106. Margarit C, Charco R, Hidalgo E, et al: Liver transplantation for malignant diseases: Selection and pattern of recurrence. World J Surg 26:257-263, 2002.

107. Figueras J, Ibañez L, Ramos E, et al: Selection criteria for liver transplantation in early-stage hepatocellular carcinoma with cirrhosis: Results of a multicenter study. Liver Transpl 7:877-883, 2001.

108. De Carlis L, Giocomoni A, Lauterio A, et al: Liver transplantation for hepatocellular cancer: Should the current indication criteria be changed? Transpl Int 16:115-122, 2003.

109. Steinmüller T, Jonas S, Neuhaus P: Review article: Liver transplantation for hepatocellular carcinoma. Aliment Pharmacol Ther 17:138-144, 2003.

110. Cherqui D: Role of adjuvant treatment in liver transplantation for advanced hepatocellular carcinoma. J Hepatobiliary Pancreat Surg 5:35-40, 1998.

111. Troisi R, Defreyne L, Hesse UJ, et al: Multimodal treatment for hepatocellular carcinoma on cirrhosis: The role of chemoembolization and alcoholization before liver transplantation. Clin Transplant 12:313-319, 1998.

112. Llovet JM, Aponte JJ, Fuster J, et al: Cost effectiveness of adjuvant therapy for hepatocellular carcinoma during the waiting list for liver transplantation. Gut 50:123-128, 2002.

113. Fisher RA, Maroney TP, Fulcher AS, et al: Hepatocellular carcinoma: Strategy for optimizing surgical resection, transplantation and palliation. Clin Transplant 16:52-58, 2002.

114. Roayaie S, Frischer SJ, Emre SH, et al: Long-term results with multimodal adjuvant therapy and liver transplantation for the treatment of hepatocellular carcinomas larger than 5 centimeters. Ann Surg 235:533-539, 2002.

115. Yokoyama I, Todo S, Iwatsuki S, Starzl TE: Liver transplantation in the treatment of primary liver cancer. Hepatogastroenterology 37:188-193, 1990.

116. Iwatsuki S, Starzl TE, Sheahan DG, et al: Hepatic resection versus transplantation for hepatocellular carcinoma. Ann Surg 214:221-229, 1991.

117. Pichlmayr R, Weimann A, Steinhoff G, et al: Liver transplantation for hepatocellular carcinoma: Clinical results and future aspects. Cancer Chemother Pharmacol 21(Suppl 1):S157-S161, 1992.

118. Bismuth H, Chiche L, Adam R, et al: Liver resection versus transplantation for hepatocellular carcinoma in cirrhotic patients. Ann Surg 218:145-151, 1993.

119. Dalgic A, Mirza DF, Gunson BK, et al: Role of total hepatectomy and transplantation in hepatocellular carcinoma. Transplant Proc 26:3564-3565, 1994.

120. Farmer DG, Rosove MH, Shaked A, et al: Treatment of hepatocellular carcinoma. Ann Surg 219:236-247, 1994.

121. Selby R, Kadry Z, Carr B, et al: Liver transplantation for hepatocellular carcinoma. World J Surg 19:53-58, 1995.

122. Schwartz ME, Sung M, Mor E, et al: A multidisciplinary approach to hepatocellular carcinoma in patients with cirrhosis. J Am Coll Surg 180:596-603, 1995.

123. Bechstein WO, Guckelberger O, Kling N, et al: Recurrence-free survival after liver transplantation for small hepatocellular carcinoma. Transpl Int 11:S189-S192, 1998.

124. Llovet JM, Fuster J, Bruix J: Intention-to-treat analysis of surgical treatment for early hepatocellular carcinoma: Resection versus transplantation. Hepatology 30:1434-1440, 1999.

125. Figueras J, Jaurrieta E, Valls C, et al: Resection or transplantation for hepatocellular carcinoma in cirrhotic patients: Outcomes based on indicated treatment strategy. J Am Coll Surg 190:580-587, 2000.

126. Hemming AW, Cattral MS, Reed AI, et al: Liver transplantation for hepatocellular carcinoma: A proposal of a prognostic scoring system. Ann Surg 233:652-659, 2001.

127. Tamura S, Kato T, Berho M, et al: Impact of histological grade of hepatocellular carcinoma on the outcome of liver transplantation. Arch Surg 136:25-30, 2001.

128. Jones S, Bechstein WO, Steinmuller T, et al: Vascular invasion and histopathologic grading determine outcome after liver transplantation for hepatocellular carcinoma. Hepatology 33:1080-1086, 2001.

129. Yoo HY, Patt CH, Geschwind JF, et al: The outcome of liver transplantation in patients with hepatocellular carcinoma in the United States between 1987 and 2001: 5-year survival has improved significantly with time. J Clin Oncol 21:4329-4335, 2003.

130. Vauthey J-N, Ajani JA: Liver transplantation and hepatocellular carcinoma biology: Beginning of the end of the era of educated guesses. J Clin Oncol 21:4265-4267, 2003.

131. Vauthey JN, Lauwers GY, Esnaola NF, et al: Simplified staging for hepatocellular carcinoma. J Clin Oncol 20:1527-1536, 2002.

132. Esnaola NF, Lauwers GY, Mirza NQ, et al: Predictors of microvascular invasion in patients with hepatocellular carcinoma who are candidates for orthotopic liver transplantation. J Gastrointest Surg 6:224-232, 2002.

133. Poon RT, Fan ST, Lo CM, et al: Long-term survival and pattern of recurrence after resection of small hepatocellular carcinoma in patients with preserved liver function: Implications for a strategy of salvage transplantation. Ann Surg 235:373-382, 2002.

134. Fong Y, Sun RL, Jarnagin W, et al: An analysis of 412 cases of hepatocellular carcinoma at a Western center. Ann Surg 229:790-799, 1999.

135. Wayne JD, Lauwers GY, Ikai I, et al: Preoperative predictors of survival after resection of small hepatocellular carcinomas. Ann Surg 235:722-731, 2002.

136. Durand F, Regimbeau JM, Belghiti J, et al: Assessment of the benefits and risks of percutaneous biopsy before surgical resection of hepatocellular carcinoma. J Hepatol 35:254-258, 2001.

137. Iizuka N, Oka M, Yamada-Okabe H, et al: Oligonucleotide microarray for prediction of early intrahepatic recurrence of hepatocellular carcinoma after curative resection. Lancet 361:923-929, 2003.

138. Poon RT, Ng IO, Lau C, et al: Serum vascular endothelial growth factor predicts venous invasion in hepatocellular carcinoma: A prospective study. Ann Surg 233:227-235, 2001.

139. Chao Y, Li CP, Chau GY, et al: Prognostic significance of vascular endothelial growth factor, basic fibroblast growth factor, and angiogenin in patients with resectable hepatocellular carcinoma after surgery. Ann Surg Oncol 10:355-362, 2003.

140. Miyamoto A, Fujiwara Y, Sakon M, et al: Development of a multiple-marker RT-PCR assay for detection of micrometastases of hepatocellular carcinoma. Dig Dis Sci 45:1376-1382, 2000.

141. Molmenti EP, Klintmalm GB: Liver transplantation in association with hepatocellular carcinoma: An update of the International Tumor Registry. Liver Transpl 8:736-748, 2002.

142. Llovet JM, Vilana R, Bru C, et al: Increased Risk of tumor seeding after percutaneous radiofrequency ablation for single hepatocellular carcinoma. Hepatology 33:1124-1129, 2001.

143. Jarnagin WR, Koea JB, Klimstra DS: Cancers of the biliary tree: Staging, technique, and pathology. In Kelsen DP, Daly JM, Kern SE, et al. (eds): Gastrointestinal Oncology: Principles and Practice. Philadelphia, Lippincott Williams & Wilkins, 2002, pp 615-643.

144. Lillemoe KD, Schulick RD, Kennedy AS, et al: Cancers of the biliary tree: Clinical management. In Kelsen DP, Daly JM, Kern SE, et al. (eds): Gastrointestinal Oncology: Principles and Practice. Philadelphia, Lippincott Williams & Wilkins, 2002, pp 645-661.

145. Kwon Y, Lee SK, Kim J-S, et al: Synchronous hepatocellular carcinoma and cholangiocarcinoma arising in two different dysplastic nodules. Mod Pathol 15:1096-1101, 2002.

146. Yoon J-H, Gores GJ: Diagnosis, staging, and treatment of cholangiocarcinoma. Curr Treat Options Gastroenterol 6:105-112, 2003.

147. Jenkins RL, Pinson CW, Stone MD: Experience with transplantation in the treatment of liver cancer. Cancer Chemother Pharmacol 23(Suppl):S104-S109, 1989.

148. Senzer NN, Stone MJ, Klintmalm GB, Polter D: Adjuvant radiochemotherapy following orthotopic liver transplantation for bile duct cancer. Transplantation 50:1045-1047, 1990.

149. Goldstein RM, Stone MJ, Tillery GW, et al: Is liver transplantation indicated for cholangiocarcinoma? Am J Surg 166:768-772, 1993.

150. De Vreede I, Steers JL, Burch PA, et al: Prolonged disease-free survival after orthotopic liver transplantation plus adjuvant chemoirradiation for cholangiocarcinoma. Liver Transpl 6:309-316, 2000.

151. Shimoda M, Farmer DG, Colquhoun SD, et al: Liver transplantation for cholangiocellular carcinoma: Analysis of a single-center experience and review of the literature. Liver Transpl 7:1023-1033, 2001.

152. Shirabe K, Shimada M, Harimoto N, et al: Intrahepatic cholangiocarcinoma: Its mode of spreading and therapeutic modalities. Surgery 131:S159-S164, 2002.

153. Sudan D, DeRoover A, Chinnakotla S, et al: Radiochemotherapy and transplantation allow long-term survival for nonresectable hilar cholangiocarcinoma. Am J Transpl 2:774-779, 2002.

154. Hassoun Z, Gores GJ, Rosen CB: Preliminary experience with liver transplantation in selected patients with unresectable hilar cholangiocarcinoma. Surg Oncol Clin N Am 11:909-921, 2002.

155. Kokudo N, Makuuchi M: Extent of resection and outcome after curative resection for intrahepatic cholangiocarcinoma. Surg Oncol Clin N Am 11:969-983, 2002.

156. Neuberger J: Liver transplantation for cholestatic liver disease. Curr Treat Options Gastroenterol 6:113-121, 2003.

157. Lindnér P, Norrby J, Olausson M, et al: Survival after liver transplantation for cholangiocarcinoma has increased during the last decade. Transplant Proc 35:811-812, 2003.

158. Robles R, Figueras J, Turrión VS, et al: Liver transplantation for hilar cholangiocarcinoma: Spanish experience. Transplant Proc 35:1821-1822, 2003.

159. Robles R, Figueras J, Turrión VS, et al: Liver transplantation for peripheral cholangiocarcinoma: Spanish experience. Transplant Proc 35:1823-1824, 2003.

160. Kadry Z, Mullhaupt B, Renner EL, et al: Living donor liver transplantation and tolerance: A potential strategy in cholangiocarcinoma. Transplantation 76:1003-1006, 2003.

161. Urego M, Flickinger JC, Carr BI: Radiotherapy and multimodality management of cholangiocarcinoma. Int J Radiat Oncol Biol Phys 44:121-126, 1999.

162. Iwatsuki S, Todo S, Marsh JW, et al: Treatment of hilar cholangiocarcinoma (Klatskin tumors) with hepatic resection or transplantation. J Am Coll Surg 187:358-364, 1998.

163. Craig JR, Peters RL, Edmondson HA: Tumors of the Liver and Intrahepatic Bile Ducts. Washington, DC, Armed Forces Institute of Pathology, 1989.

164. Ishak KG, Sesterhenn IA, Goodman ZD, et al: Epithelioid hemangioendothelioma of the liver. A clinicopathologic and follow-up study of 32 cases. Hum Pathol 15:839-852, 1984.

165. Furui S, Itai Y, Ohtomo K, et al: Hepatic epithelioid hemangioendothelioma: Report of five cases. Radiology 171:63-68, 1989.

166. Marino IR, Todo S, Tzakis AG, et al: Treatment of hepatic epithelioid hemangioendothelioma with liver transplantation. Cancer 62:2079-2084, 1988.

167. Demetris AJ, Minervini M, Raikow RB, et al: Hepatic epithelioid hemangioendothelioma. Biological questions based on pattern of recurrence in an allograft and tumor immunophenotype. Am J Surg Pathol 21:263-270, 1997.

168. Walsh MM, Hytiroglou P, Thung SN, et al: Epithelioid hemangioendothelioma of the liver mimicking Budd-Chiari syndrome. Arch Pathol Lab Med 122:846-848, 1998.

169. Makhlouf HR, Ishak KG, Goodman ZD: Epithelioid hemangioendothelioma of the liver. A clinicopathologic study of 137 cases. Cancer 85:562-582, 1999.

170. Ben-Haim M, Roayaie S, Ye MQ, et al: Hepatic epithelioid hemangioendothelioma: Resection or transplantation, which and when? Liver Transpl Surg 5:526-531, 1999.

171. Kayler LK, Merion RM, Arenas JD, et al: Epithelioid hemangioendothelioma of the liver disseminated to the peritoneum treated with liver transplantation and Interferon alpha-2b. Transplantation 74:128-130, 2002.

172. Simpson ND, Ahmed AM, Simpson PW, et al: Living donor liver transplantation in a patient with hepatic epithelioid hemangioendothelioma. J Clin Gastroenterol 37:349-350, 2003.

173. Jensen RT: Carcinoid and pancreatic endocrine tumors: recent advances in molecular pathogenesis, localization, and treatment. Curr Opin Oncol 12:368-377, 2000.

174. Lehnert T: Liver transplantation for metastatic neuroendocrine carcinoma: An analysis of 103 patients. Transplantation 66:1307-1312, 1998.

175. de Vries H, Verschueren RCJ, Willemse PHB, et al: Diagnostic, surgical and medical aspect of the midgut carcinoids. Cancer Treat Rev 28:11-25, 2002.

176. El Rassi ZS, Ferdinand L, Mohsine RM, et al: Primary and secondary liver endocrine tumors: Clinical presentation, surgical approach and outcome. Hepatogastroenterology 49:1340-1346, 2002.

177. Podnos YD, Jimenez JC, Zainabadi K, et al: Carcinoid tumors of the common bile duct: Report of two cases. Surg Today 33:553-555, 2003.

178. Fernández JA, Robles R, Marín C, et al: Role of liver transplantation in the management of metastatic neuroendocrine tumors. Transplant Proc 35:1832-1833, 2003.

179. Neshiwat LF, Friedland ML, Schorr-Lesnick B, et al: Hepatic angiosarcoma. Am J Med 93:219-222, 1992.

180. Gores GJ, Steers JL: Progress in orthotopic liver transplantation for hepatocellular carcinoma. Gastroenterology 104:317-320, 1993.

181. Tong AW, Su D, Mues G, et al: Chemosensitization of human hepatocellular carcinoma cells with cyclosporin A in post-liver transplant patient plasma. Clin Cancer Res 2:531-539, 1996.

182. Klintmalm GB, Stone MJ: The results of liver transplantation with adjuvant chemotherapy for hepatobiliary surgery. J Hepatobiliary Pancreat Surg 2:141-144, 1994.

183. Yamanaka N, Okamoto E, Fujihara S, et al: Do the tumor cells of hepatocellular carcinomas dislodge into the portal venous stream during hepatic resection? Cancer 70:2263-2267, 1992.

184. Harris DT, Mastrangelo MJ: Theory and application of early systemic therapy. Semin Oncol 18:493-503, 1991.

185. Perry MC, Anderson CM, Donehower RC: Chemotherapy. In Abeloff MD, Armitage JO, Lichter AS, et al. (eds): Clinical Oncology, 2nd ed. New York, Churchill Livingstone, 2000, pp 378-422.

186. Horn M, Phebus C, Blatt J: Cancer chemotherapy after solid organ transplantation. Cancer 66:1468-1471, 1990.

187. Yokoyama I, Carr B, Saitsu H, et al: Accelerated growth rates of recurrent hepatocellular carcinoma after liver transplantation. Cancer 68:2095-2100, 1991.

188. Sanchez EQ, Marubashi S, Jung G, et al: De novo tumors after liver transplantation: A single-institution experience. Liver Transpl 8:285-291, 2002.

189. Menachem Y, Safadi R, Ashuir Y, et al: Malignancy after liver transplantation in patients with premalignant conditions. J Clin Gastroenterol 36:436-439, 2003.

190. Starzl TE, Murase N, Abu-Elmagd K, et al: Tolerogenic immunosuppression for organ transplantation. Lancet 361:1502-1510, 2003.

191. Söderdahl G, Barkholt L, Hentschke P, et al: Liver transplantation followed by adjuvant nonmyeloablative hemopoietic stem cell transplantation for advanced primary liver cancer in humans. Transplantation 75:1061-1066, 2003.

192. Delpuech O, Trabut JB, Carnot F, et al: Identification, using cDNA macroarray analysis, of distinct gene expression profiles associated with pathological and virological features of hepatocellular carcinoma. Oncogene 21:2926-2937, 2002.

193. Qiu W, David D, Zhou B, et al: Down-regulation of growth arrest DNA damage-inducible gene 45β expression is associated with human hepatocellular carcinoma. Am J Pathol 162:1961-1974, 2003.

194. Kaneko S, Kobayashi K: Clinical application of a DNA chip in the field of liver disease. J Gastroenterol 38(Suppl 15):85-88, 2003.

195. Kim JW, Wang XW: Gene expression profiling of preneoplastic liver disease and liver cancer: A new era for improved early detection and treatment of these deadly diseases? Carcinogenesis 24:363-369, 2003.

196. Iizuka N, Oka M, Yamada-Okabe H, et al: Differential gene expression in distinct virologic types of hepatocellular carcinoma: Association with liver cirrhosis. Oncogene 22:3007-3014, 2003.

197. Paradis V, Bièche I, Dargère D, et al: Molecular profiling of hepatocellular carcinomas (HCC) using a large-scale real-time RT-PCR approach. Am J Pathol 163:733-741, 2003.

198. Iizuka N, Oka M, Yamada-Okabe H, et al: Oligonucleotide microarray for prediction of early intrahepatic recurrence of hepatocellular carcinoma after curative resection. Lancet 361:923-929, 2003.

199. Sheehy E, Conrad SL, Brigham LE, et al: Estimating the number of potential organ donors in the United States. N Engl J Med 349:667-674, 2003.

200. Vivarelli M, Bellusci R, Cucchetti A, et al: Low recurrence rate of hepatocellular carcinoma after liver transplantation: Better patient selection or lower immunosuppression? Transplantation 74:1746-1751, 2002.

Liver Transplantation for Metastases of the Liver

FERDINAND MÜHLBACHER
SUSANNE RASOUL ROCKENSCHAUB

Transplant indications for secondary
   malignancies in the past   233
   Surgery-only approach   233

Lessons learned from the European Liver
   Transplant Registry   234

Does immunosuppression stimulate tumor
   growth?   235

Donor shortage and liver transplantation for
   malignant disease—use of living donor
   organs   235

Alternative methods of treating liver
   metastases   235

Are there tumors with metastases that warrant
   liver transplantation?   236

Summary   236

Transplant Indications for Secondary Malignancies in the Past

Liver transplantation has been considered a therapeutic option for metastatic liver disease if the primary tumor is successfully removed and no extrahepatic tumor is evident. Reports consist of anecdotal observations from personal series or preliminary findings from registries. Liver transplantation for metastases from cancer of the colon and tail of the pancreas, hypernephroma, meningioma, and duodenal leiomyosarcoma has been reported by Calne.[1] The Denver-Cincinnati registry reported procedures for liver metastases from colon cancer, small bowel or bronchial tree carcinoids, leiomyosarcoma of the small bowel, breast carcinoma, gastrinoma, glucagonoma, meningioma, neuroblastoma, renal cell carcinoma, cystosarcoma of the pancreas, hemangiopericytoma, seminoma, VIPoma, melanoma, acute myeloid leukemia, and unknown primaries.[2] The common denominator was an unfavorable outcome in that most of the patients died (59%) of tumor recurrence[2] or suffered surgical complications.

Surgery-Only Approach

Selection of transplant candidates was based on the presence of histologically tumor-free central aortic lymph

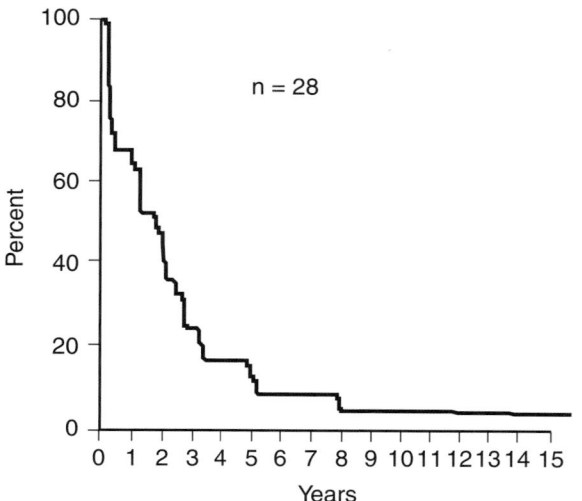

FIGURE 16-1

Patient survival after orthotopic liver transplantation for colorectal metastatic liver disease (N = 28).

nodes at primary surgery and radiologically confirmed limitation of tumor to the liver. No adjuvant chemotherapy was administered.[3] In a larger single-center series of patients with liver metastases from colon carcinoma reported by the group in Vienna, the actuarial 1-year tumor-free survival rate was 68%; however, with the larger experience of 19 patients, median survival did not exceed 13.1 months.[3] The group terminated this "surgery-only" program after 28 cases, with the longest survival being 21 years (alive in 2004) and the second longest being 7 years, the latter patient dying of recurrence of the tumor (Fig. 16-1).

A combined approach of debulking by liver transplantation combined with myelotoxic chemotherapy, total-body irradiation, and then autologous bone marrow transplantation was reported from Innsbruck.[4] Five patients who suffered from metastatic breast cancer were treated according to this protocol, the longest survival time being 5 years. All patients gained several years of quality life extension.[5]

Scattered experience with orthotopic liver transplantation (OLT) for liver metastases originating from neuroendocrine tumors[1,2,4,6,7] and the observation that neuroendocrine tumors of the pancreas seem to be a different biological entity because of their slow progression[8] stimulated several programs to attempt a more systematic approach. Pancreas resection combined with OLT was reported to relieve symptoms for up to 34 months[9,10] in three cases.

A more radical surgical approach in four patients consisting of multivisceral resection combined with OLT was reported from Frankfurt; two patients were free of tumor after 6 months, one patient died of tumor progression after 11 months, and one died of surgical complications. All four had far-advanced tumor disease before OLT.[11]

In a multimodal protocol developed at the Mount Sinai center, hepatic artery chemoembolization was used to control symptoms; OLT was performed in those with persistent symptoms or evidence of progression. Three patients underwent transplantation, with no recurrence at a follow-up of 12 to 30 months.[12]

Lessons Learned from the European Liver Transplant Registry

The European Liver Transplant Registry (ELTR) collected operative and follow-up data on 46,530 transplantations in 41,522 patients from 124 institutions in 21 European countries from May 1968 to December 2001.[13] Data are transmitted to the ELTR twice a year, including follow-up data, and centers are audited for accuracy of the data. Of these transplantations, 4417 (11% of the total) were performed for malignancy indications:

Hepatocellular carcinoma: 3364 (76%)

Cholangiocarcinoma: 196 (4%)

Bile duct carcinoma: 177 (4%)

Metastatic liver disease: 313 (7%)

Other types of carcinoma: 367 (8%)

Figure 16-2 shows Kaplan-Meier patient survival estimates after OLT for the main malignancy indications. Expected survival rates for hepatoma patients are 77%, 53%, and 43% after 1, 5, and 10 years, respectively.

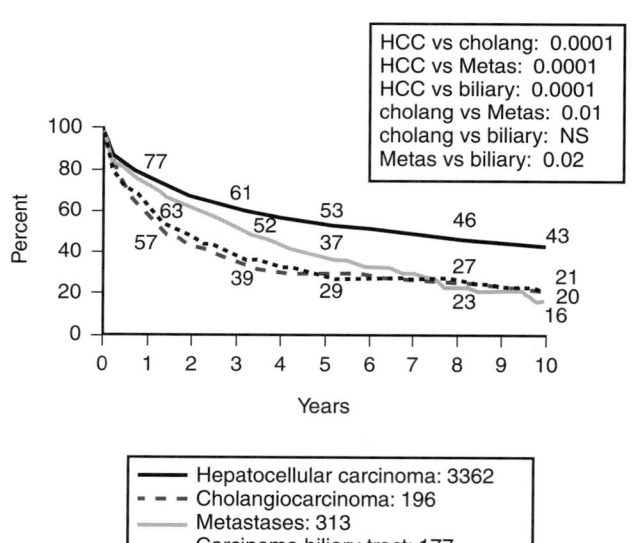

FIGURE 16-2

Patient survival after orthotopic liver transplantation for different hepatic malignancies. (Data from the European Liver Transplant Registry, January 1988 to December 2001.)

Their chance of survival has markedly improved, probably because of patient selection according to the Milan criteria.[14] Similarly, patients undergoing transplantation for metastatic disease have improved survival rates: 63%, 37%, and 21% after 1, 5, and 10 years, respectively. There is a statistically significant difference between all malignancies except for cholangiocarcinoma and biliary tract carcinoma. Patients with metastases do worse than hepatoma patients because their tumor stage is certainly inferior to that of hepatoma patients, but the results are determined mostly by the type of metastases in the majority of patients, with neuroendocrine metastases exhibiting biological behavior different from that of other metastases.

A comparison between metastases from neuroendocrine and colorectal carcinoma shows the biological difference between these tumors even more clearly. Survival rates with neuroendocrine metastases are 73%, 42%, and 25% after 1, 5, and 10 years, respectively, whereas patients with colorectal metastases have survival rates of 66% and 19% after 1 and 5 years, with virtually no one surviving for 10 years (Fig. 16–3).

Does Immunosuppression Stimulate Tumor Growth?

The risk of de novo tumor development, both posttransplant lymphoproliferative disorder[15] and solid tumors, is increased in transplant patients. Recipients of liver and kidney transplants have a 7% to 8% risk of de novo tumor development within 10 years after transplantation, and the risk is almost 15% in heart transplant recipients.[16] Of these lesions, 50% are skin tumors. There is no direct evidence that immunosuppression stimulates tumor growth after liver transplantation for malignant liver disease. In a nonrandomized comparison between liver transplantation and liver

resection for hepatocellular carcinoma (HCC), the survival rates after 1 and 5 years were identical, thus indicating no dramatic effect of immunosuppression on the development of residual tumor disease.[17] In addition, a nonrandomized retrospective analysis of survival data in patients with unresectable liver metastases from colorectal cancer treated by either liver transplantation or local transarterial chemotherapy revealed a marked survival benefit in favor of transplantation, with no signs of accelerated tumor growth.[4]

Donor Shortage and Liver Transplantation for Malignant Disease—Use of Living Donor Organs

Organ shortage currently limits liver transplantation. With malignant disease as an indication for OLT, there seems to be a consensus that patient survival after OLT for malignancies should match the short-term and midterm results of transplantation for other nonmalignant indications,[18] and even retransplantation has to meet this standard.[19] As seen in the Kaplan-Meier curves derived from ELTR data, OLT for liver metastases from colorectal carcinoma has by far not yet met these criteria and should, for the time being, no longer be considered an appropriate indication (see Fig. 16–2). However, a multimodal approach consisting of OLT combined with adjuvant or neoadjuvant chemotherapy has never been attempted in any case. Multimodal strategies combining OLT and adjuvant treatment have been partly successful in patients with cholangiocarcinoma,[20] but not in HCC patients[21] because of the lack of efficacious chemotherapy. A variety of powerful drugs are available for the treatment of colorectal tumors, and adjuvant drug treatment in conjunction with OLT and proper patient selection may be an alternative in the future.

Living donors as a source of liver transplant organs may also change the attitude toward transplantation because it obviates the argument of organ shortage. Liver transplantation for HCC surpassing the Milan criteria will not usually be considered an appropriate indication because of the organ shortage and outcomes inferior to those for nonmalignant indications. With living donors, the Milan criteria are sometimes exceeded by up to 48% in HCC patients.[22]

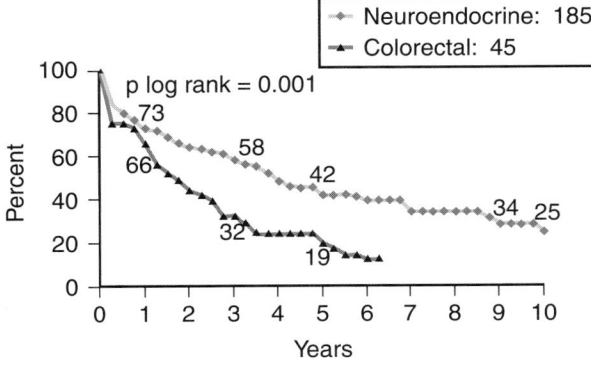

FIGURE 16–3

Patient survival after orthotopic liver transplantation for liver metastases from neuroendocrine and colorectal cancer. (Data from the European Liver Transplant Registry, January 1988 to December 2001.)

Alternative Methods of Treating Liver Metastases

Many alternative methods[23] are available for treating liver metastases after colorectal carcinoma. Liver resection can be combined with cryotherapy,[24] radiofrequency ablation,[25,26] or transarterial catheter embolization,[27] and some of these methods can also be applied percutaneously.[28] Alternative treatment is of course also available for metastases from neuroendocrine tumors.[29-32] These alternatives are associated with lower procedural mortality than OLT is and may be oncologically equally effective as far as colorectal metastases are concerned.

However, alternative methods have their limitations.[33,34] In general, large tumor size, numerous lesions, or unresponsiveness to treatment should suggest reconsideration of liver transplantation. There are a few long-term survivors after OLT for colorectal liver metastases: one patient is now free of recurrence after 21 years[35] and an additional patient for 11 years.[36] Common to these two patients is the sequential appearance of liver metastases after resection of the primary tumor without involvement of any lymphatic tissue. In both cases, the liver tumor was too large for alternative treatment.

Are There Tumors with Metastases That Warrant Liver Transplantation?

Neuroendocrine tumor metastases have been treated with locoregional methods[37-39] as well as OLT.[40-44] One has to consider the risk-benefit ratio of liver transplantation versus its alternatives. OLT attempts oncological cure. Because of the biological behavior of neuroendocrine liver metastases, tumor recurrence is not the predominant issue. Patients are free of symptoms without repeated intervention, and survival is certainly comparable to that of alternative treatment, provided that the 1-year patient survival rate is higher than 90%. In a series of 57 patients who received multimodal (not OLT) therapy for liver metastases after radical local surgery, patient survival rates after 5 and 10 years were 64% and 28%, respectively.[32] OLT series are rather small[38-40]; however, one series of 19 cases from Hannover showed survival rates of 80% and 50% after 5 and 10 years, respectively, but only 3 patients were free of tumor recurrence after 8 years.[45]

Summary

- OLT for the treatment of metastatic liver disease has been performed in substantial numbers for only two different tumor types: (1) liver metastases from neuroendocrine tumors with an origin in the gastrointestinal tract and the pancreas and (2) liver metastases from colorectal cancer.
- Short-term results and quality of life were satisfactory, but the 5- and 10-year survival rates were inferior to those for nonmalignant indications and, with regard to the dramatic organ shortage, were unacceptably low. Organ shortage may be irrelevant in case of organs from living donors.
- Because of the availability of alternative treatment methods for liver metastases, the actual need for OLT is very low.
- Liver metastases from neuroendocrine tumors may be an indication for OLT if the size and location of the lesions are unsuitable for alternative treatment and the symptoms cannot be controlled pharmacologically.
- Liver metastases from colorectal cancer should be considered an indication for OLT only if all alternative procedures fail; with cancer-free lymph nodes, adjuvant chemotherapy should be considered if ongoing trials of adjuvant chemotherapy combined with liver resection show a beneficial survival effect of adjuvant chemotherapy.

References

1. Calne RY: Liver transplantation: The recent Cambridge–King's College Hospital experience. Clin Transpl 51, 1987.
2. Penn I: Hepatic transplantation for primary and metastatic cancers of the liver. Surgery 110:726, 1991.
3. Mühlbacher F, Huk I, Steininger R, et al: Is orthotopic liver transplantation a feasible treatment for secondary cancer of the liver? Transplant Proc 23:1567, 1991.
4. Huber C, Niederwieser D, Schonitzer D, et al: Liver transplantation followed by high-dose cyclophosphamide, total-body irradiation, and autologous bone marrow transplantation for treatment of metastatic breast cancer. A case report. Transplantation 37:311, 1984.
5. Margreiter R, Niederwieser D, Frommhold H, et al: Tumor recurrence after liver transplantation followed by high-dose cyclophosphamide, total body irradiation, and autologous bone marrow transplantation for treatment of metastatic liver disease. Transplant Proc 19:2403, 1987.
6. Makowka L, Tzakis AG, Mazzaferro V, et al: Transplantation of the liver for metastatic endocrine tumors of the intestine and pancreas. Surg Gynecol Obstet 168:107, 1989.
7. Pichlmayr R: Is there a place for liver grafting for malignancy? Transplant Proc 20(Suppl 1):478, 1988.
8. Eckhauser FE, Cheung PS, Vinik AI, et al: Nonfunctioning malignant neuroendocrine tumors of the pancreas. Surgery 100:978, 1986.
9. Alsina AE, Bartus S, Hull D, et al: Liver transplant for metastatic neuroendocrine tumor. J Clin Gastroenterol 12:533, 1990.
10. Schweizer RT, Alsina AE, Rosson R, Bartus SA: Liver transplantation for metastatic neuroendocrine tumors. Transplant Proc 25:1973, 1993.
11. Wenisch HJ, Markus BH, Herrmann GH, et al: [Multi-visceral upper abdominal resection and orthotopic liver transplantation—a surgical treatment concept for regionally metastatic tumors of the endocrine pancreas.] Zentralbl Chir 117:334, 1992.
12. Curtiss SI, Mor E, Schwartz ME, et al: A rational approach to the use of hepatic transplantation in the treatment of metastatic neuroendocrine tumors. J Am Coll Surg 180:184, 1995.

13. Adam R, for the European Liver Transplant Registry: European Liver Transplant Registry Data Analysis Booklet 05/68-12/01. Available at http://www.eltr.org 2002.

14. Mazzaferro V, Regalia E, Doci R, et al: Liver transplantation for the treatment of small hepatocellular carcinomas in patients with cirrhosis. N Engl J Med 334:693, 1996.

15. Opelz G, Dohler B: Lymphomas after solid organ transplantation: A collaborative transplant study report. Am J Transplant 4: 222, 2004.

16. Opelz G: Tumor risk. Transpl Int(Suppl), 2000.

17. Steininger R, Herbst F, Fugger R, et al: Immunosuppression does not enhance tumor growth after orthotopic liver transplantation for hepatoma. Transplant Proc 24:2690, 1992.

18. Margarit C, Charco R, Hidalgo E, et al: Liver transplantation for malignant diseases: Selection and pattern of recurrence. World J Surg 26:257, 2002.

19. Azoulay D, Linhares MM, Huguet E, et al: Decision for retransplantation of the liver: An experience- and cost-based analysis. Ann Surg 236:713, 2002.

20. De Vreede I, Steers JL, Burch PA, et al: Prolonged disease-free survival after orthotopic liver transplantation plus adjuvant chemoirradiation for cholangiocarcinoma. Liver Transpl 6: 309, 2000.

21. Pokorny H, Gnant M, Langer F, et al: Failure of doxorubicin adjuvant chemotherapy in OLT for HCCA to prolong patient survival. Am J Transplant 2005 (in press).

22. Kaihara S, Kiuchi T, Ueda M, et al: Living-donor liver transplantation for hepatocellular carcinoma. Transplantation 75(Suppl 3):S37, 2003.

23. Fusai G, Davidson BR: Management of colorectal liver metastases. Colorectal Dis 5:2, 2003.

24. Yan DB, Clingan P, Morris DL: Hepatic cryotherapy and regional chemotherapy with or without resection for liver metastases from colorectal carcinoma: How many are too many? Cancer 98:320, 2003.

25. Moffat FL, Falk RE, Calhoun K, et al: Effect of radiofrequency hyperthermia and chemotherapy on primary and secondary hepatic malignancies when used with metronidazole. Surgery 94: 536, 1983.

26. Hansler J, Neureiter D, Wasserburger M, et al: Percutaneous US-guided radiofrequency ablation with perfused needle applicators: Improved survival with the VX2 tumor model in rabbits. Radiology 230:169, 2004.

27. Bloomston M, Binitie O, Fraiji E, et al: Transcatheter arterial chemoembolization with or without radiofrequency ablation in the management of patients with advanced hepatic malignancy. Am Surg 68:827, 2002.

28. Livraghi T: Guidelines for treatment of liver cancer. Eur J Ultrasound 13:167, 2001.

29. Ahlman H, Wangberg B, Jansson S, et al: Interventional treatment of gastrointestinal neuroendocrine tumours. Digestion 62(Suppl 1):59, 2000.

30. Siperstein AE, Berber E: Cryoablation, percutaneous alcohol injection, and radiofrequency ablation for treatment of neuroendocrine liver metastases. World J Surg 25:693, 2001.

31. Schindl M, Kaczirek K, Passler C, et al: Treatment of small intestinal neuroendocrine tumors: Is an extended multimodal approach justified? World J Surg 26:976, 2002.

32. Sutcliffe R, Maguire D, Ramage J, et al: Management of neuroendocrine liver metastases. Am J Surg 187:39, 2004.

33. Scaife CL, Curley SA: Complication, local recurrence, and survival rates after radiofrequency ablation for hepatic malignancies. Surg Oncol Clin N Am 12:243, 2003.

34. Steinke K, Glenn D, King J, Morris DL: Percutaneous pulmonary radiofrequency ablation: Difficulty achieving complete ablations in big lung lesions. Br J Radiol 76:742, 2003.

35. Mühlbacher F Sr, Berlakovich G: Unpublished observation, 2004.

36. Honore C, Detry O, De Roover A, et al: Liver transplantation for metastatic colon adenocarcinoma: Report of a case with 10 years of follow-up without recurrence. Transpl Int 16:692, 2003.

37. Sutcliffe R, Maguire D, Ramage J, et al: Management of neuroendocrine liver metastases. Am J Surg 187:39, 2004.

38. Loewe C, Schindl M, Cejna M, et al: Permanent transarterial embolization of neuroendocrine metastases of the liver using cyanoacrylate and Lipiodol: Assessment of mid- and long-term results. AJR Am J Roentgenol 180:1379, 2003.

39. Henn AR, Levine EA, McNulty W, Zagoria RJ: Percutaneous radiofrequency ablation of hepatic metastases for symptomatic relief of neuroendocrine syndromes. AJR Am J Roentgenol 181:1005, 2003.

40. Alsina AE, Bartus S, Hull D, et al: Liver transplant for metastatic neuroendocrine tumor. J Clin Gastroenterol 12:533, 1990.

41. Bechstein WO, Neuhaus P: Liver transplantation for hepatic metastases of neuroendocrine tumors. Ann N Y Acad Sci 733: 507, 1994.

42. Frilling A, Rogiers X, Knofel WT, Broelsch CE: Liver transplantation for metastatic carcinoid tumors. Digestion 55(Suppl 3):104, 1994.

43. Lang H, Oldhafer KJ, Weimann A, et al: Liver transplantation for metastatic neuroendocrine tumors. Ann Surg 225:347, 1997.

44. Olausson M, Friman S, Cahlin C, et al: Indications and results of liver transplantation in patients with neuroendocrine tumors. World J Surg 26:998, 2002.

45. Rosenau J, Bahr MJ, von Wasielewski R, et al: Ki67, E-cadherin, and p53 as prognostic indicators of long-term outcome after liver transplantation for metastatic neuroendocrine tumors. Transplantation 73:386, 2002.

Liver Transplantation for Hematological Disorders

WILLIAM D. TAP
VICTOR J. MARDER

Hereditary amyloidosis   239

Hemochromatosis   240

Blood coagulation disorders   241
   Hemophilia   241
   Thrombophilia   243

Erythropoietic protoporphyria   243

Disorders transmitted by orthotopic liver
   transplantation   245

Summary   245

Orthotopic liver transplantation (OLT) often affords a last-ditch treatment option for a disparate group of disorders that may be managed by the hematologist. In some cases, OLT cures the patient by correcting the root cause of the problem, whereas in other cases, patients may benefit only transiently because the induced organ damage is irreversible. Atypically, OLT may subject the patient to a new illness, as when an affected liver is replaced by one carrying a new genetic defect. This chapter reviews the need for and results of OLT in patients with hereditary amyloidosis, hemochromatosis, coagulation disorders, and protoporphyria; most cases have a genetic foundation, with the illnesses following distinct paths that may lead to hepatic decompensation.

Hereditary Amyloidosis

The most common genetic defect that causes systemic amyloid deposition derives from the transthyretin (*TTR*) gene, mutation of which results in an autosomal dominant disease pattern. TTR, also called prealbumin, is a tetrameric plasma protein that is mostly synthesized by hepatocytes and transports thyroxin, triiodothyronine, and retinol binding protein. More than 80 *TTR* gene mutations have been identified as amyloidogenic (ATTR), or inducing the deposition of insoluble amyloid fibers.[1] The most common mutation is seen in patients with familial amyloid polyneuropathy

(FAP); such patients have a point mutation in the *TTR* gene at amino acid 30 (V30M).[1-3] FAP affects the peripheral and autonomic nervous systems in adults and is often fatal within 10 years of development. Patients suffer renal failure, cardiomyopathy with arrhythmias, vitreal opacity, and severe gastrointestinal complications.

OLT was first used as a curative modality for FAP in 1990.[4] After OLT, only normal TTR is synthesized, and improvement in gastrointestinal pathology and clinical findings follows.[5] In 54 centers worldwide, 579 OLTs have been performed on 539 patients with FAP, with 128 reported deaths and an overall 5-year survival rate of 77%.[1] One-year survival rates have increased from 77% in those transplanted between 1990 and 1994 to 90% in those transplanted between 1995 and 2000. The improvement is attributed to better intraoperative and postoperative care and a change in the selection process such that transplantation is performed in patients with a more favorable nutritional status earlier in their disease course.[1] A significant proportion of transplanted patients had regression of symptoms relative to the gastrointestinal tract (52%), sensory neuropathy (41%), motor and muscular function (37%), and nutritional status (40%), but only 21% showed improvement in cardiovascular symptoms (Fig. 17–1).[1]

Data suggest that removal of the mutated *TTR* gene can reverse tissue injury secondary to amyloid deposition and that neuronal regeneration may occur.[5,6] However, reversal of myocardial injury is problematic, thus explaining the high rate of cardiac death in patients with FAP (39%) versus that after OLT for other indications (9%).[1] The refractory nature of amyloid-induced cardiovascular disease warrants more vigorous screening and selection criteria before OLT, especially since the modified body mass index and duration of disease may not be sufficient to predict transplant outcome.[1] Two other transplant-related complications deserve attention, namely, refractory intraoperative orthostatic hypotension and sudden cardiac death as a result of amyloid-induced conduction abnormalities.

OLT has been applied successfully to treat other hereditary forms of amyloidosis, such as the autosomal dominant form caused by mutation of the fibrinogen A alpha chain. Since plasma fibrinogen derives overwhelmingly from hepatic synthesis, OLT should be curative, and successful correction by OLT has been documented in a single case report.[7] OLT has not been a viable therapeutic approach to date for the most common form of acquired systemic amyloidosis, that caused by deposition of monoclonal immunoglobulin light-chain fragments produced by a malignant clone of plasma cells in bone marrow.

Hemochromatosis

Hereditary hemochromatosis (HHC), an autosomal recessive disorder linked to chromosome 6,[8] has a carrier rate of 10% and prevalence of 0.5%.[9] A disruption in iron homeostasis leads to widespread tissue deposition and the clinical effects of cirrhosis, increased risk of hepatocellular carcinoma, cardiomyopathy, arrhythmias, diabetes mellitus, skin hyperpigmentation, endocrine failure, and arthropathy. Clinical manifestations are highly variable, evolve slowly, are rarely present before the second decade, and are less evident in women who are protected by menstrual blood loss.

In 1996, Feder and colleagues cloned the gene responsible for HHC[10] and described two missense mutations (C282Y and H63D) in the *HFE* gene, whose function is to facilitate iron homeostasis via its interaction with transferrin receptor 1 (TfR1)[11] or by modulation of hepcidin synthesis.[12] The *HFE* gene is expressed in the liver, as well as in the intestine, pancreas, ovary, kidney, and placenta.[10,11] The loss of cysteine in the C282Y mutation, which affects 80% to 90% of patients with clinical HHC,[10] prevents disulfide bond formation and induces aberrant folding of the molecule. This altered tertiary structure prevents binding of the major histocompatibility class I–like HFE complex to β_2-microglobulin, a step necessary for transport to and eventual expression on the cell surface.[11,12] Mutation of the *HFE* gene may indirectly cause reticuloendothelial cells and villous enterocytes to release excess iron into an already overloaded system, thus leading to pathological organ

HEREDITARY (FAMILIAL) AMYLOIDOSIS

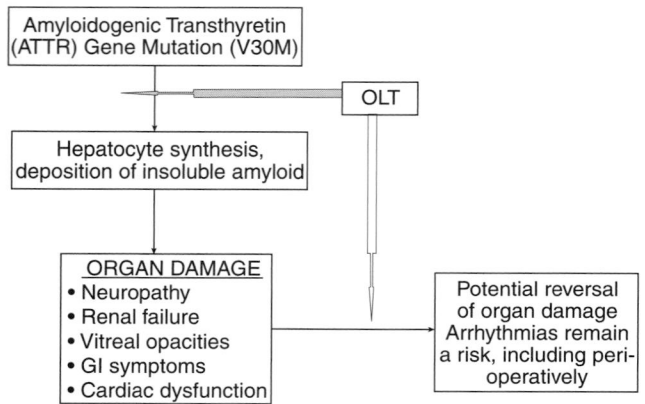

FIGURE 17–1

Hereditary (familial) amyloidosis. Amyloidogenic mutations in the transthyretin gene induce hepatic synthesis of insoluble amyloid, which accumulates in various organs, notably the heart, peripheral nerves, and kidneys. Othotopic liver transplantation (OLT) substitutes wild-type (normal) transthyretin synthesis for the amyloidogenic form, thereby halting further amyloid deposition. Over time, amyloid may be recycled and the tissue damage corrected, but the risk of cardiac arrhythmia remains, especially in the perioperative period. GI, gastrointestinal.

iron accumulation.[12] The H63D mutation does convey some propensity for iron accumulation, but it does not have the same clinical impact as the C282Y mutation.[13]

OLT has provided interesting biological outcomes that provide insight into the pathogenesis of iron accumulation. After inadvertent transplantation of a homozygous C282Y liver and intestine into a wild-type host, the recipient showed a tendency for iron overload,[14] thus providing strong evidence for a genetic influence of HHC. In a case report, transplantation of a C282Y heterozygous liver into a patient who was negative for the C282Y and the H63D mutations led to hemochromatosis. Sequencing of the recipient's *HFE* genotype characterized a novel mutation in the *HFE* gene (R6S); the C282Y/R6S compound heterozygote expressed disease, perhaps showing the additive effect of different mutations.[15] Even with transplantation of an affected liver, most (five of seven) patients do not show iron accumulation that is not explainable by concurrent medical illness.[9,14]

About 50% to 75% of homozygous C282Y patients have clinical evidence of disease,[16,17] which has been classified into four stages[17]:

- Genetic predisposition but no other abnormality
- Iron overload without symptoms
- Iron overload with early symptoms (lethargy, arthralgia)
- Iron overload with organ damage, especially cirrhosis

Before discovery of the *HFE* gene, the diagnosis of primary hemochromatosis was often based on the hepatic iron index (hepatic iron concentration divided by age), and a value greater than 1.9 was thought to define HHC. However, a review of more than 450 OLT patients showed that only 10% of patients with a hepatic iron index greater than 1.9 were homozygous for the C282Y mutation.[18] Other inherited disorders of iron metabolism have been associated with severe iron loading, including juvenile hemochromatosis[19] and mutations in the ferroportin[20] and TfR2 genes.[21] Acquired (secondary) iron overload also leads to substantial hepatic iron deposition, perhaps as a byproduct of inflammation or viral invasion.[22] Of 197 homozygous C282Y patients, none with a serum ferritin level less than 1000 μg/L, normal aspartate transaminase, and no evidence of hepatomegaly had severe fibrosis,[23] thus justifying conservative management without liver biopsy. Determination of *HFE* status is a priority because phlebotomy and chelator therapy before significant systemic iron deposition occurs can prevent clinical sequelae.[24] In a patient with clinical, radiographic, or biochemical markers consistent with substantial iron overload who is not C282Y$^+$/C282Y$^+$, diagnostic liver biopsy is mandated.[17]

Hereditary hemochromatosis and secondary hemochromatosis are uncommon indications for OLT,

representing only 0.5% to 1% of cases.[25] The 5-year survival rate may or may not be inferior in patients with hepatic iron overload,[9,25] although younger subjects may have some degree of protection against subsequent iron deposition.[26] Patients are susceptible to bacterial and fungal infection,[27] which is postulated to result from a deleterious effect of iron on cellular immunity.[28] Cardiac iron deposition can be manifested as dilated or restrictive cardiomyopathy with an increased risk for arrhythmias, heart failure, or myocardial infarction, often with only minimal pretransplant electrocardiographic warning signs.[29] Some data suggest that the *HFE* gene mutation itself is a risk factor for acute myocardial infarction or idiopathic dilated cardiomyopathy,[30,31] although this view is not universal.[32] Furthermore, patients with iron-loading anemia are at increased risk for myocardial dysfunction and death, and an increased systemic iron load, regardless of cause, may contribute to the atherosclerotic burden.[33]

Regarding long-term outcomes after OLT, the underlying disorder is the principal determinant of success. Patients with secondary hemochromatosis will have temporary relief of liver disease, but ultimately, recurrent iron accumulation may follow if the primary disorder is not corrected. The post-OLT course for patients with HHC depends on whether the hereditary defect affects HFE protein synthesis in the liver or in other organs (Fig. 17–2). Absent irreversible cardiac disease, a patient with a mutation affecting hepatic synthesis should have an excellent response to OLT. The hepatocytes of the allograft would produce a wild-type HFE protein that should correctly regulate iron homeostasis, thereby preventing further abnormal iron accumulation. However, if the primary defect stems from aberrant HFE proteins made in the duodenal mucosa, OLT would be only a palliative measure because pathological iron accumulation would not be controlled and recurrence of hepatic iron deposition and hepatic failure would follow.

By biochemical measures, the results of OLT have been gratifying. A review of 22 patients who underwent OLT for hemochromatosis showed that serum markers remained normal for 2.8 years.[34] Early hepatic biopsy in 41 patients with pretransplant hemochromatosis showed no statistical difference in iron deposition in the new liver from that of a control population, and 2 of 3 C282Y homozygous patients had no iron accumulation.[35]

Blood Coagulation Disorders

Hemophilia

Cirrhosis in Patients with Hemophilia. Hemophiliacs who received clotting factor concentrates derived from pooled human plasma before the mid-1980s were

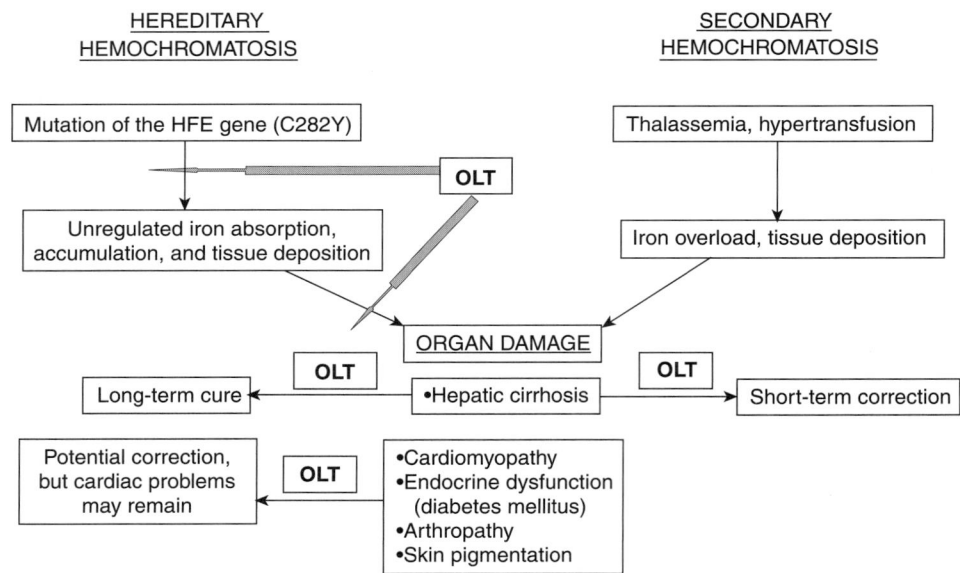

FIGURE 17–2

Hereditary and secondary hemochromatosis. In hereditary hemochromatosis (*left*), mutations in the *HFE* gene disrupt iron homeostasis and cause tissue iron accumulation and damage. Hepatic iron deposits can cause panlobular necrosis, cirrhosis, and overt liver failure, for which orthotopic liver transplantation (OLT) may be a life-saving and even curative modality. In secondary hemochromatosis (*right*), systemic iron overload and organ damage can result from various acquired processes, for example, hypertransfusion for severe and lifelong anemia. OLT can restore hepatic function temporarily, but continued iron accumulation usually follows unless the underlying cause is corrected.

almost invariably exposed to hepatitis C virus (HCV) and human immunodeficiency virus (HIV). The cumulative risk of hepatic decompensation in hemophiliacs with hepatitis C after initial exposure to the virus is 1.7% in 10 years and 10.8% in 20 years,[36] and cirrhosis develops in 30% of patients with persistent chronic hepatitis.[37] Hemophiliac patients with HCV are often coinfected with HIV, a combination that increases the risk and rate of incurring substantial hepatic injury.[38]

Liver transplantation has two uses in hemophiliac patients (Fig. 17–3). It can be a life-saving technique for cirrhosis, and since synthesis of factor VIII and

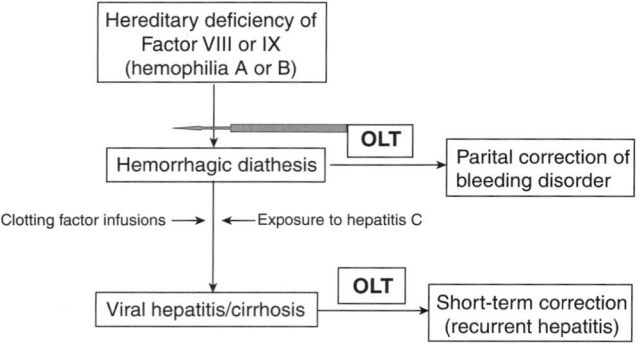

FIGURE 17–3

Hemophilia. Exposure of hemophiliac patients to blood product concentrates can result in viral hepatitis, cirrhosis, and liver failure. Orthotopic liver transplantation (OLT) can be a life-saving modality, but self-recurrence of viral hepatitis is common. Since coagulation factors are produced by hepatocytes, endothelial cells, or both, OLT will partially correct the bleeding disorder, at least to the degree that spontaneous hemorrhages do not occur.

factor IX occurs in hepatocytes, it is a potentially curative modality for hemophiliac bleeding. The first liver transplant in a patient with hemophilia A and end-stage liver disease was performed in 1985,[39] with allograft function maintaining plasma factor VIII levels in the normal range by 18 hours after surgery; these findings were reproduced in a patient with hemophilia B in 1987.[40]

Of 26 patients with hemophilia who underwent OLT for liver failure between 1982 and 1996, all had their underlying factor deficiency corrected, and replacement infusions were discontinued 24 hours after surgery,[41] coincident with the onset of de novo factor production. One- and 3-year survival rates were 83% and 68%, respectively, consistent with data for non-hemophiliac patients who undergo OLT for hepatitis.[42,43] One- and 3-year survival rates for patients with HIV were significantly lower than those for patients without HIV, 67% versus 90% and 23% versus 83%, respectively.[41] Although OLT cures the coagulation disorder, hemophiliac patients are at risk for recurrent hepatitis, which was noted after a mean of 9 months in 6 of 20 patients transplanted for hepatitis C.[41]

Bleeding should not be a major risk for hemophiliac patients undergoing OLT, provided that appropriate factor replacement is administered. Tissue damage from chronic previous bleeding may present a nidus for postoperative complications despite adequate factor replacement, as reported in a patient who died of a subdural hemorrhage at the site of a small chronic hematoma.[41] Supportive clotting factor administration generally consists of a preoperative bolus, followed by bolus injections or a continuous infusion; the latter regimen produces a constant plasma factor level that can be maintained at 100% until healing, which usually requires at least 2 weeks. Adjustments in dosage should be made according to blood clotting factor levels, to which some contribution is probably made by the transplanted liver. Antifibrinolytic agents such as ε-aminocaproic acid or aprotinin are useful adjuncts since fibrinolysis may be a significant factor in operative and postoperative bleeding.

Hemorrhagic Diatheses Other than Hemophilia. OLT has been used to correct severe bleeding diatheses caused by factor deficiencies in individuals with normal hepatic function. Since virtually all the clotting factors are synthesized in hepatocytes, transplantation should be able to cure hereditary deficiencies,[41] as documented in twin sisters with severe bleeding symptoms who underwent OLT to correct factor VII deficiency.[44] Allograft function restored factor VII levels within 48 hours of transplantation. OLT for correction of bleeding in patients with von Willebrand's disease is slightly more controversial. Transplantation in these patients, who are only poorly controlled with factor replacement therapy, has shown an increase in production of von Willebrand factor, but without an improvement in ristocetin cofactor activity or bleeding time.[45,46]

Thrombophilia

Homozygous protein C deficiency causes a hypercoagulable state that is manifested in the neonatal period as disseminated intravascular coagulation, purpura fulminans, and thromboembolism. Treatment involves the administration of anticoagulant drugs plus intermittent transfusion of blood products containing protein C (plasma or protein C concentrate). These approaches are not curative, and OLT has been attempted in two cases, both of which showed dramatic and lasting benefit (Fig. 17–4). A 20-month-old child received a liver transplant because of perinatal thrombotic problems that were inadequately controlled with fresh-frozen plasma.[47] Postoperatively, the child suffered hepatic artery and portal vein thrombosis, but gradually improved with anticoagulation as the allograft restored protein C levels to normal. Another case concerned an 8-year-old child who was a compound heterozygote for protein C deficiency and protein C dysfunction.[48] Renal failure had developed as a result of bilateral renal vein thrombosis, and intracranial hemorrhages and gastrointestinal bleeding complicated chronic anticoagulant therapy. Protein C concentrate was effective, but end-stage renal failure and refractory malignant hypertension developed. After a combined renal-liver transplant, the patient did well and was weaned off protein C concentrate by 2 weeks after transplantation.

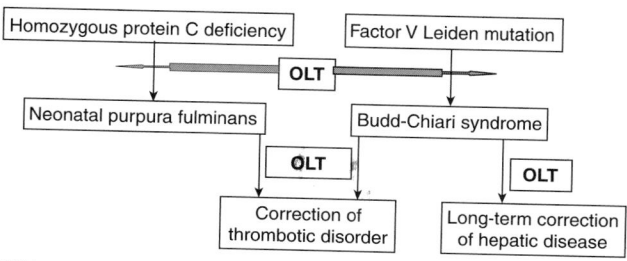

THROMBOPHILIA

FIGURE 17–4

Thrombophilia. Homozygous protein C deficiency (*left*) is manifested in the peripartum period as life-threatening purpura fulminans. Because protein C is synthesized entirely in the liver, orthotopic liver transplantation (OLT) cures the thrombophilia. Other thrombophilias, such as factor V (Leiden) (*right*), are not usually apparent until adulthood, Budd-Chiari syndrome being a particularly aggressive thrombotic manifestation. OLT can partially modulate this thrombophilia by synthesis of normal factor V, but OLT is used primarily to reverse the hepatic failure caused by Budd-Chiari syndrome.

Patients who are heterozygous for the *factor V Leiden (FVL) mutation* have a 7-fold increased risk for venous thrombosis, and patients homozygous for this condition have an 80-fold higher risk.[49] This mutation affects coagulation factor V so that it cannot be degraded by activated protein C (hence the term "activated protein C resistance"). The result of factor V resistance is a hypercoagulable state caused by unregulated coagulant activity. Transplantation for FVL is not usually warranted because the thrombophilia can be managed with long-term coumarin anticoagulation. However, FVL is a significant risk factor for Budd-Chiari syndrome, and six such patients have undergone OLT, all with curative results.[50]

Erythropoietic Protoporphyria

Erythropoietic protoporphyria (EPP) is a rare genetic disorder of heme metabolism that causes the accumulation and increased excretion of protoporphyrin IX, the lipid-soluble photosensitive precursor of hemoglobin. The porphyrias are divided into hepatic and erythropoietic, depending on whether the liver or bone marrow is responsible for producing the excess porphyrins, EPP being one of the erythropoietic class. Heme synthesis occurs in almost every cell, the vast majority (85%) devoted to hemoglobin production in erythropoietic tissue. Initially, glycine and succinyl coenzyme A are combined into δ-aminolevulinic acid (ALA) by the mitochondrial-based enzyme ALA synthase, which is the rate-limiting enzyme and under negative feedback control by the heme end product.

After ALA formation, three reactions occur in the cytoplasm, and synthesis is completed in the mitochondria, where ferrochelatase catalyzes the complexing of protoporphyrin IX with iron to form the heme molecule.[51] Seven enzymes are required in the heme pathway, and deficiencies of each relate to a specific porphyrial disease.

EPP is caused by the absence of ferrochelatase and subsequent disruption of the last step in the heme pathway.[52] The lack of ferrochelatase results in a vicious cycle of excessive protoporphyrin IX production, the end product of an unregulated cascade of constitutive reactions caused by the absence of heme feedback inhibition. The ferrochelatase gene has been mapped to chromosome 18, region q21.3,[53,54] and has significant genetic heterogeneity that allows phenotypic expression of more than 65 different mutations in EPP patients.[55] Ferrochelatase levels in affected individuals are lower than would be expected by a simple autosomal dominant inheritance pattern, symptomatic individuals usually having less than 50% activity,[56] perhaps explained by inheritance of defects from each parent that cause absent expression or expression of an abnormal variant, or both.[56,57] Some cases of EPP are transmitted in an autosomal recessive pattern, but they may still be associated with severe hepatic dysfunction.[58]

EPP is a devastating disease that results in an increase in erythrocyte, hepatic, plasma, and fecal protoporphyrin concentrations.[59] The disease is usually manifested as childhood photosensitivity, with erythema, edema, pruritus, and chronic deforming skin damage developing in affected individuals as a result of ultraviolet light–initiated photoreaction of the protoporphyrin that has accumulated in dermal blood vessels and skin.[60] Accumulation of lipid-soluble protoporphyrin molecules also causes axonal neuropathy, abdominal pain, anemia, and hepatic dysfunction.[61-63]

Excess protoporphyrin is excreted in feces via the biliary system and may precipitate in bile and crystallize in the hepatic parenchyma.[64] Such precipitation can lead to micronodular and panlobular necrosis, with detectable birefringent red-brown porphyrin pigment accompanied by the clinical sequelae of end-stage liver disease. Worsening hepatic injury may further decrease ferrochelatase activity and create a vicious cycle that leads to progressive hepatic failure.[65] Mild abnormalities in liver function are present in 10% of patients; hepatic failure occurs in only 5%,

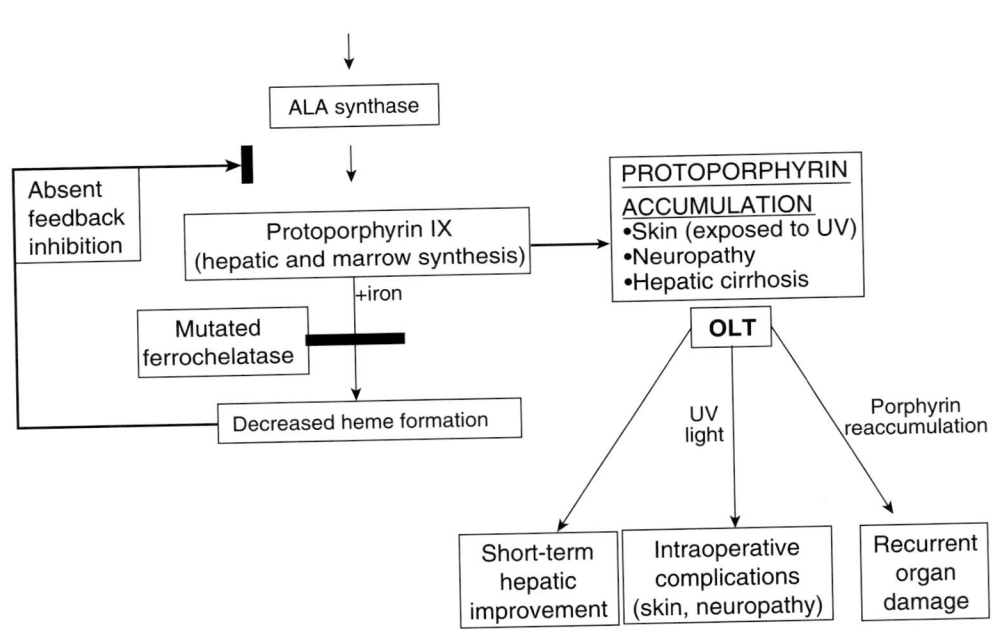

FIGURE 17–5

Erythropoietic protoporphyria. A mutated ferrochelatase prevents heme synthesis and causes accumulation of protoporphyrin IX. Without heme, there is insufficient feedback inhibition of δ-aminolevulinic acid (ALA) synthase to modulate the multiple-step pathway of heme synthesis. The toxic product, protoporphyrin IX, accumulates and causes skin reactions secondary to ultraviolet (UV) exposure, neuropathy, and cirrhosis. Orthotopic liver transplantation (OLT) can be life-saving, but since protoporphyrin IX production occurs in bone marrow as well as the liver, reaccumulation occurs. Intraoperative precautions are required to prevent patient exposure to UV light, which can induce acute skin and neurological complications.

but when failure does occur, it is life-threatening and may warrant OLT.

Once hepatic failure develops, OLT can be life-saving,[65-67] but not without significant intraoperative and postoperative problems (Fig. 17–5).[68] Bloomer and coauthors reported a cohort of nine such patients: two died within the first 2 months as a result of operative complications, two suffered skin burns from operating room lights, three were left with axonal neuropathies, and two had recurrent protoporphyric liver damage.[69] Phototoxic burns on the abdomen and viscera from intense light exposure during surgery are the result of intraoperative exposure of protoporphyrin to ultraviolet light, which causes free radical formation and tissue damage, biliary fistulas, intestinal perforation, and even death.[63,68,69] Polyneuropathy may be exacerbated post-operatively,[68] as in the case of a 54-year-old man in whom profound postoperative axonal neuropathy developed despite a reduction in operating room light and halogen head lamp intensity with filters.[70] Three days postoperatively, the patient required reintubation for progressive muscle weakness, and the hospital course was complicated by a severe polyneuropathy that required a year to resolve. Plasmapheresis and exchange transfusion have been used preoperatively to reduce protoporphyrin levels, but even an 80% reduction in circulating protoporphyrins may not guarantee a safe outcome.[68,70]

EPP patients undergoing OLT fall into an intermediate-risk group when compared with the general liver transplant population. OLT is not curative because protoporphyrins are still produced by bone marrow post-operatively and systemic levels usually remain elevated. It is not uncommon for porphyrins to accumulate in the allograft, sometimes leading to fulminant allograft failure. The liver allograft may outperform the native organ in protoporphyrin clearance, so in some patients serum protoporphyrin levels fall after OLT, even while the erythrocyte protoporphyrin concentration remains high.[67]

Hematin has been administered preoperatively to decrease protoporphyrin levels.[71,72] This iron-containing metalloporphyrin decreases hepatic and marrow heme synthesis by inhibiting δ-ALA synthase, the rate-limiting enzyme in heme production. The effect that hematin has on hepatic disease is still unclear, but a decrease in postadministration plasma protoporphyrin levels has been correlated with increased excretion in feces and urine.[73] Hematin has been used in the postoperative setting for cholestasis and allograft salvage,[74] as illustrated in a 59-year-old man with hepatic allograft dysfunction after OLT.[75] Hematin was initiated after unsuccessful use of plasmapheresis and hypertransfusion, and the graft was kept free of measurable disease by a chronic maintenance schedule of intravenous hematin.

Murine bone marrow transplant models are being evaluated as therapy for EPP,[76] which may be a target for gene therapy.[77] OLT remains a potential life-saving option, but it is not curative, and currently only reactive measures such as hematin infusion and plasma exchange are available for managing the devastating clinical outcomes of the disease.

Disorders Transmitted by Orthotopic Liver Transplantation

Because the prevalence of FVL in the white population is 4% to 6%, occasional transplantation of a liver that synthesizes this mutant is not unexpected. In a retrospective survey of 276 donor livers, 19 were heterozygous and none were homozygous for the FVL mutation. There were 41 episodes of thrombosis, 6 in patients who were heterozygous for the FVL mutation, and the FVL mutation was present in 4 of 31 cases of hepatic vessel thrombosis.[78] The presence of FVL confers an increased risk of postoperative thrombosis, but the relative risk for hepatic vessel thrombosis is low.

Bleeding Disorders. OLT-related transmission of a hemorrhagic diathesis has been described in a young female who had a prolonged prothrombin time after transplantation of a liver that was deficient in factor VII synthesis[79]; a factor XI deficiency via this mechanism has also been described.[80] An unusual case of acquired hemophilia A resulting from a factor VIII inhibitor was caused by transport of antibody-producing "passenger" lymphocytes in the transplanted liver.[81]

Summary

OLT it is the only current curative modality for patients with hereditary forms of amyloidosis. This treatment is appropriate for hereditary hemochromatosis with advanced liver disease, but it may not alleviate iron-related damage in other organs or the underlying genetic defect. OLT may be performed in patients with severe hemophilia A and B for liver failure caused by viral infection after transfusion of contaminated blood products; in these cases, OLT relieves the sequelae of hepatic injury and may also cure the hemorrhagic disorder. OLT has cured the life-threatening thrombophilia caused by homozygous protein C deficiency. It is appropriate for erythropoietic protoporphyria with liver failure, although the metabolic defect is not cured and attention must be paid to avoiding phototoxic injury during surgery (Table 17–1).

Table 17-1. ANTICIPATED RESULTS OF LIVER TRANSPLANTATION IN HEMATOLOGICAL DISORDERS

Disorder	Underlying Defect	Clinical Result	Potential Problems
Hereditary amyloidosis	Completely corrected	Improved organ function if further amyloid deposition prevented	Cardiac function may not improve because of irreversible amyloid deposits
Hereditary hemochromatosis	Probably not corrected	Immediate correction of hepatic failure	Reaccumulation of tissue iron
Hemophilia A and B	Correction of factor deficiency to a variable degree	Hepatic failure corrected. Prevention of spontaneous bleeding	May still require factor for surgical procedures. Recurrent viral hepatitis
Protein C deficiency	Completely corrected	Thrombophilia cured, no need for anticoagulation	Induced deficiency if affected liver is transplanted
Erythropoietic protoporphyria	Partial correction (liver but not other tissues)	Resolution of hepatic failure	Possible phototoxic injury (neuropathy) during surgery. Recurrent disease

Pearls and Pitfalls

Pearls

- In patients with hereditary amyloidosis, along with the modified body mass index and the duration of disease, the refractory nature of amyloid-induced cardiovascular disease warrants consideration in the selection criteria for OLT.

- Determination of HFE status in patients with hemochromatosis is a priority because phlebotomy and chelator therapy before significant systemic iron deposition occurs can prevent clinical sequelae of the disease.

- Bleeding should not be a major risk for hemophiliac patients undergoing OLT, provided that appropriate factor replacement is administered: preoperative bolus followed by a continuous infusion.

- In patients with erythropoietic protoporphyria, hematin has been used in the postoperative setting for cholestasis and allograft salvage. Postoperative maintenance hematin may be a way to keep the allograft free of measurable disease.

Pitfalls

- In patients with hereditary amyloidosis, refractory intraoperative orthostatic hypotension and sudden cardiac death as a result of amyloid-induced conduction abnormalities are two transplant-related complications that deserve attention.

Pearls and Pitfalls—cont'd

- Liver transplantation is appropriate for hereditary hemochromatosis with advanced liver disease, but it may not alleviate iron-related damage in other organs or the underlying genetic defect.

- In hemophiliacs, tissue damage from chronic previous bleeding may present a nidus for postoperative complications despite adequate factor replacement.

- In patients with erythropoietic protoporphyria, intraoperative exposure of the protoporphyrin moieties to ultraviolet light causes free radical formation and tissue damage, biliary fistulas, intestinal perforation, and even death. Polyneuropathy may be exacerbated postoperatively.

References

1. Herlenius G, Wilczek HE, Larsson M, et al: Ten years of international experience with liver transplantation for familial amyloidotic polyneuropathy: Results from the Familial Amyloidotic Polyneuropathy World Transplant Registry. Transplantation 77:64-71, 2004.
2. Tawara S, Nakazato M, Kangawa K, et al: Identification of amyloid prealbumin variant in familial amyloidotic polyneuropathy (Japanese type). Biochem Biophys Res Commun 116:880-888, 1983.
3. Saraiva MJ, Costa PP, Birken S, et al: Presence of an abnormal transthyretin (prealbumin) in Portuguese patients with familial amyloidotic polyneuropathy. Trans Assoc Am Physicians 96:261-270, 1983.
4. Holmgren G, Steen L, Ekstedt J, et al: Biochemical effect of liver transplantation in two Swedish patients with familial amyloidotic polyneuropathy (FAP-met30). Clin Genet 40:242-246, 1991.

5. Holmgren G, Ericzon BG, Groth CG, et al: Clinical improvement and amyloid regression after liver transplantation in hereditary transthyretin amyloidosis. Lancet 341:1113-1116, 1993.

6. Ikeda S, Takei Y, Yanagisawa N, et al: Peripheral nerves regenerated in familial amyloid polyneuropathy after liver transplantation. Ann Intern Med 127:618-620, 1997.

7. Zeldenrust S, Gertz M, Uemichi T, et al: Orthotopic liver transplantation for hereditary fibrinogen amyloidosis. Transplantation 75:560-561, 2003.

8. Simon M, Bourel M, Genetet B, et al: Idiopathic hemochromatosis. Demonstration of recessive transmission and early detection by family HLA typing. N Engl J Med 297:1017-1021, 1977.

9. Brandhagen DJ: Liver transplantation for hereditary hemochromatosis. Liver Transpl 7:663-672, 2001.

10. Feder JN, Gnirke A, Thomas W, et al: A novel MHC class I–like gene is mutated in patients with hereditary haemochromatosis. Nat Genet 13:399-409, 1996.

11. Enns CA: Pumping iron: The strange partnership of the hemochromatosis protein, a class I MHC homolog, with the transferrin receptor. Traffic 2:167-174, 2001.

12. Pietrangelo A: Hereditary haemochromatosis—a new look at an old disease. N Engl J Med 350:2383-2397, 2004.

13. Gochee PA, Powell LW, Cullen DJ, et al: A population-based study of the biochemical and clinical expression of the H63D hemochromatosis mutation. Gastroenterology 122:646-651, 2002.

14. Adams PC, Jeffrey G, Alanen K, et al: Transplantation of haemochromatosis liver and intestine into a normal recipient. Gut 45:783, 1999.

15. Wigg AJ, Harley H, Casey G: Heterozygous recipient and donor HFE mutations associated with hereditary hemochromatosis phenotype after liver transplantation. Gut 52:433-435, 2003.

16. Olynyk JK, Cullen DJ, Aquilia S, et al: A population-based study of the clinical expression of the hemochromatosis gene. N Engl J Med 341:718-724, 1999.

17. Adams P, Brissot P, Powell LW: EASL International Consensus Conference on Haemochromatosis. J Hepatol 33:485-504, 2000.

18. Brandhagen DJ, Alvarez W, Therneau TM, et al: Iron overload in cirrhosis—*HFE* genotypes and outcome after liver transplantation. Hepatology 31:456-460, 2000.

19. Roetto A, Totaro A, Cazzola M, et al: Juvenile hemochromatosis locus maps to chromosome 1q. Am J Hum Genet 64:1388-1393, 1999.

20. Montosi G, Donovan A, Totaro A, et al: Autosomal-dominant hemochromatosis is associated with a mutation in the ferroportin (*SLC11A3*) gene. J Clin Invest 108:619-623, 2001.

21. Roetto A, Totaro A, Piperno A, et al: New mutations inactivating transferrin receptor 2 in hemochromatosis type 3. Blood 97:2555-2560, 2001.

22. Bottomley SS: Secondary iron overload disorders. Semin Hematol 35:77-86, 1998.

23. Guyader D, Jacquelinet C, Moirand R, et al: Noninvasive prediction of fibrosis in C282Y homozygous haemochromatosis. Gastroenterology 115:929-936, 1998.

24. Niederau C, Fischer R, Sonnenberg A, et al: Survival and causes of death in cirrhotic and in noncirrhotic patients with primary hemochromatosis. N Engl J Med 313:1256-1262, 1985.

25. Kilpe VE, Krakauer H, Wren RE: An analysis of liver transplant experience from 37 transplant centers as reported to Medicare. Transplantation 56:554-561, 1993.

26. Keefe EB: Liver transplantation in patients with hepatic iron overload: Favorable or unfavorable outcome? Hepatology 32:1396-1398, 2000.

27. Weinberg ED: Iron, infection, and neoplasia. Clin Physiol Biochem 4:50-60, 1986.

28. Weiss G, Wachter H, Fuchs D: Linkage of cell-mediated immunity to iron metabolism. Immunol Today 16:495-500, 1995.

29. Farrell FJ, Nguyen M, Woodley S, et al: Outcome of liver transplantation in patients with hemochromatosis. Hepatology 20:404-410, 1994.

30. Tuomainen TP, Kontula K, Nyyssonen K, et al: increased risk of acute myocardial infarction in carriers of the hemochromatosis gene Cys282Tyr mutation: A prospective cohort study in men in eastern Finland. Circulation 100:1274-1279, 1999.

31. Mahon NG, Coonar AS, Jeffery S, et al: Haemochromatosis gene mutations in idiopathic dilated cardiomyopathy. Heart 84:541-547, 2000.

32. Gunn IR, Maxwell FK, Gaffney D, et al: Haemochromatosis gene mutations and risk of coronary heart disease: A West of Scotland Coronary Prevention Study (WOSCOPS) substudy. Heart 90:304-306, 2004.

33. de Valk B, Marx JJ: Iron, atherosclerosis, and ischemic heart disease. Arch Intern Med 159:1542-1548, 1999.

34. Powell LW: Does transplantation of the liver cure genetic hemochromatosis? J Hepatol 16:259-261, 1992.

35. Parolin MB, Batts KP, Wiesner RH, et al: Liver allograft iron accumulation in patients with and without pretransplantation hepatic hemosiderosis. Liver Transpl 8:331-339, 2002.

36. Telfer P, Sabin C, Devereux H, et al: The progression of HCV-associated liver disease in a cohort of haemophiliac patients. Br J Haematol 87:555-561, 1994.

37. Makris M, Preston, FE, Rosendaal FR, et al: The natural history of chronic hepatitis C in haemophiliacs. Br J Haematol 94:746-752, 1996.

38. Eyster ME, Fried MW, Di Bisceglie AM, et al: Increasing hepatitis C virus RNA levels in hemophiliacs: Relationship to human immunodeficiency virus infection and liver disease. Multicenter Hemophilia Cohort Study. Blood 84:1020-1023, 1994.

39. Lewis JH, Bontempo FA, Spero JA, et al: Liver transplantation in a haemophiliac [letter]. N Engl J Med 312:1189-1190, 1985.

40. Merion RM, Delius RE, Campebell DA, et al: Orthotopic liver transplantation totally corrects factor IX deficiency in haemophilia B. Surgery 104:929-931, 1988.

41. Gordon FH, Mistry PK, Sabin CA, et al: Outcome of orthotopic liver transplantation in patients with haemophilia. Gut 42:744-749, 1998.

42. Gane EJ, Portmann BC, Naoumov NV, et al: Long-term outcome of hepatitis C infection after liver transplantation. N Engl J Med 334:815-820, 1996.

43. Samuel D, Muller R, Alexander G, et al: Liver transplantation in European patients with the hepatitis B surface antigen. N Engl J Med 329:1842-1847, 1993.

44. Levi D, Pefkarou A, Fort JA, et al: Liver transplantation for factor VII deficiency. Transplantation 72:1836-1837, 2001.

45. Mannuccio MP, Federici A, Cattaneo M, et al: Liver transplantation in severe von Willebrand's disease. Lancet 337:1105, 1991.

46. Hunt BJ: Liver transplantation for severe von Willebrand's disease. Lancet 337:1553, 1991.

47. Casella JF, Lewis JH, Bontempo FA, et al: Successful treatment of homozygous protein C deficiency by hepatic transplantation. Lancet 1:435-438, 1988.

48. Angelis M, Pegelow CH, Khan FA, et al: En bloc heterotopic auxiliary liver and bilateral renal transplant in a patient with homozygous protein C deficiency. J Pediatr 138:120-122, 2001.

49. Rosendaal FR, Koster T, Vandenbroucke JP, et al: High risk of thrombosis in patients homozygous for FVL (activated protein C resistance). Blood 85:1504-1508, 1995.

50. Nezakatgoo N, Shokouh-Amiri MH, Gaber AO, et al: Liver transplantation for acute Budd-Chiari syndrome in identical twin sisters with factor V Leiden mutation. Transplantation 76:195-198, 2003.

51. Harbin BM, Dailey HA: Orientation of ferrochelatase in bovine liver mitochondria. Biochemistry 24:366-370, 1985.

52. Bottomley SS, Tanaka M, Everett MA: Diminished erythroid ferrochelatase activity in protoporphyria. J Lab Clin Med 86: 126-131, 1975.

53. Taketani S, Inazawa J, Nakahashi Y, et al: Structure of the human ferrochelatase gene. Exon/intron gene organization and location of the gene to chromosome 18. Eur J Biochem 205:217-222, 1992.

54. Brenner DA, Didier JM, Frasier F, et al: A molecular defect in human protoporphyria. Am J Hum Genet 50:1203-1210, 1992.

55. Schneider-Yin X, Gouya L, Meier-Weinand A, et al: New insights into the pathogenesis of erythropoietic protoporphyria and their impact on patient care. Eur J Pediatr 159:719-725, 2000.

56. Gouya L, Puy H, Lamoril J, et al: Inheritance in erythropoietic protoporphyria: A common wild-type ferrochelatase allelic variant with low expression accounts for clinical manifestation. Blood 93:2105-2110, 1999.

57. Went LN, Klasen EC: Genetic aspects of erythropoietic protoporphyria. Ann Hum Genet 48:105-117, 1984.

58. Sarkany RP, Cox TM: Autosomal recessive erythropoietic protoporphyria: A syndrome of severe photosensitivity and liver failure. QJM 88:541-549, 1995.

59. Scholnick P, Marver HS, Schmid R: Erythropoietic protoporphyria: Evidence for multiple sites of excess protoporphyrin formation. J Clin Invest 50:203-207, 1971.

60. Gigli I, Schotharst AA, Soter NA, et al: Erythropoietic protoporphyria. Photoactivation of the complement system. J Clin Invest 66:517-520, 1980.

61. Bloomer JR, Phillips MJ, Davidson DL, et al: Hepatic disease in erythropoietic protoporphyria. Am J Med 58:869-882, 1975.

62. Rank JM, Carithers R, Bloomer JR: Evidence for neurological dysfunction in end-stage protoporphyric liver disease. Hepatology 18:1404-1409, 1993.

63. Key NS, Rank JM, Freese D, et al: Hemolytic anemia in protoporphyria: Possible precipitating role of liver failure and photic stress. Am J Hematol 39:220-227, 1992.

64. Bloomer JR, Enriquez R: Evidence that hepatic crystalline deposits in a patient with protoporphyria are composed of protoporphyrin. Gastroenterology 82:569-573, 1982.

65. Bloomer J, Bruzzone C, Zhu L, et al: Molecular defects in ferrochelatase in patients with protoporphyria requiring liver transplantation. J Clin Invest 102:107-114, 1998.

66. Mion FB, Faure JL, Berger F, et al: Liver transplantation for protoporphyria. Report of a new case with subsequent medium-term follow-up. J Hepatol 16:203-207, 1992.

67. Polson RJ, Lim CK, Rolles K, et al: The effect of liver transplantation in a 13-year old boy with erythropoietic protoporphyria. Transplantation 46:386-389, 1988.

68. Herbert A, Corbin D, Williams A, et al: Erythropoietic protoporphyria: Unusual skin and neurological problems after liver transplantation. Gastroenterology 100:1753-1757, 1991.

69. Bloomer JR, Rank JM, Payne WD, et al: Follow-up after liver transplantation for protoporphyric liver disease. Liver Transpl Surg 2:269-275, 1996.

70. Nguyen L, Blust M, Bailin M, et al: Photosensitivity and perioperative polyneuropathy complicating orthotopic liver transplantation in a patient with erythropoietic protoporphyria. Anesthesiology 91:1173-1175, 1999.

71. Bloomer JR, Pierach CA: Effect of hematin administration to patients with protoporphyria and liver disease. Hepatology 2: 817-821, 1982.

72. Reichheld JH, Katz E, Banner BF, et al: The value of intravenous heme-albumin and plasmapheresis in reducing postoperative complications of orthotopic liver transplantation for erythropoietic protoporphyria. Transplantation 67:922-928, 1999.

73. Watson CJ, Bossenmaier I, Cardinal R, et al: Repression by hematin of porphyrin biosynthesis in erythrocyte precursors in congenital erythropoietic porphyria. Proc Natl Acad Sci U S A 71:278-282, 1974.

74. Do KD, Banner BF, Katz E, et al: Benefits of chronic plasmapheresis and intravenous heme-albumin in erythropoietic protoporphyria after orthotopic liver transplantation. Transplantation 73:469-472, 2002.

75. Dellon ES, Szczepiorkowski ZM, Dzik WH, et al: Treatment of recurrent allograft dysfunction with intravenous hematin after liver transplantation for erythropoietic protoporphyria. Transplantation 73:911-915, 2002.

76. Pawliuk R, Bachelot T, Wise RJ, et al: Long-term cure of the photosensitivity of murine erythropoietic protoporphyria by preselective gene therapy. Nat Med 5:768-773, 1999.

77. Richard E, Mendez M, Mazurier F, et al: Gene therapy of a mouse model of protoporphyria with a self-inactivating erythroid-specific lentiviral vector without preselection. Mol Ther 4:331-338, 2001.

78. Hirshfield G, Collier JD, Brown K, et al: Donor factor V Leiden mutation and vascular thrombosis following liver transplantation. Liver Transpl Surg 4:58-61, 1998.

79. Guy SR, Magliocca JF, Fruchtman S, et al: Transmission of factor VII deficiency through liver transplantation. Transpl Int 12: 278-280, 1999.

80. Clarkson K, Rosenfeld B, Fair J, et al: Factor XI deficiency acquired by liver transplantation. Ann Intern Med 115:877-879, 1991.

81. Hisatake GM, Chen TW, Renz JF, et al: Acquired hemophilia A after liver transplantation: A case report. Liver Transpl 9:523-526, 2003.

Transplantation for Budd-Chiari Syndrome*

MARVIN J. STONE
J. MARK FULMER
GORAN B. KLINTMALM

Etiology   250

Pathology and pathophysiology   250

Clinical presentation and diagnostic
    evaluation   251
    Diagnostic imaging   251

Etiological diagnosis: myeloproliferative
    disorders and other conditions   254

Liver transplantation   254
    Consideration for transplantation: indications
        and contraindications   254
    Surgical considerations   256
    Long-term results   257

Antithrombotic therapy   257

Case Histories   259
    Case 10—undiagnosed myeloproliferative
        disorder   259
    Case 6—polycythemia vera in a
        16-year-old girl   260
    Case 16—unclassified myeloproliferative
        disorder and factor V Leiden   260
    Case 17—prothrombin gene mutation   260
    Case 15—sarcoidosis   261

Summary   261

In 1845 George Budd, a British internist, described a patient with hepatic venous thrombosis who developed abdominal pain, hepatomegaly, and ascites.[1] William Osler reported the first case of a membranous web causing vena caval and hepatic vein obstruction in 1879.[2] The Austrian pathologist, Hans Chiari, specified the clinicopathological features of the syndrome emphasizing occlusion of the intrahepatic veins in 1899.[3]

Budd-Chiari syndrome (BCS) results from obstruction of hepatic venous drainage because of various causes and leads to progressive liver damage and portal hypertension. The venous occlusion is usually thrombotic and occurs at the level of the major hepatic veins or the inferior vena cava at any point proximal to the right atrium.[4,5] Histologically, there is centrolobular congestion, sinusoidal dilatation, hepatocyte necrosis, and varying degrees of fibrosis.[5-7] Portal vein areas remain intact. The clinical presentation depends on the tempo and extent of hepatic vein occlusion. As recently as 1996, it was stated that "as many as 70% of patients with occlusion of the hepatic veins may not have a primary

*Supported in part by the Edward and Ruth Wilkof Foundation, the Robert A. Schanbaum Fund, and the James E. Nauss Cancer Research Fund.

detectable cause."[7] This is no longer true. A variety of causative mechanisms have been identified in BCS. Because these mechanisms have important bearing on long-term patient management and outcome, it is important to identify the specific cause responsible for hepatic vein occlusion in individual patients. With thorough evaluation, the proportion of idiopathic BCS should be no greater than 10% of all cases.

Etiology

BCS results from diverse causative factors (Table 18–1).[4-22] Their incidence varies significantly in different parts of the world. In India and other parts of Asia, many cases are idiopathic or caused by vena caval webs. Thus in a study of 71 BCS patients in India seen between 1992

Table 18–1. ETIOLOGICAL CONSIDERATIONS IN THE BUDD-CHIARI SYNDROME

Myeloproliferative disorders
  Polycythemia vera
  Essential thrombocythemia
  Paroxysmal nocturnal hemoglobinuria
  Others rare

Factor V Leiden mutation

Prothrombin gene mutation G20210A

Protein C deficiency

Protein S deficiency

Antithrombin III deficiency

Antiphospholipid syndrome
  Lupus-like anticoagulant
  Anticardiolipin antibodies

Pregnancy and postpartum

Oral contraceptives

Dysfibrinogenemia

Hyperhomocysteinemia

Membranous webs

Behçet's disease

Polycystic liver disease

Myeloma/amyloidosis

Sarcoidosis

Benign and malignant tumors

Infections

Trauma

Veno-occlusive disease

Herbal teas (pyrrolizidine alkaloids)

  After gemtuzumab and high-dose chemotherapy with hematopoietic stem cell transplantation

Combinations of above

and 1997, 42 were idiopathic and 18 had vena caval membranes.[18] Membranous webs may be congenital or caused by fibrosis from chronic thrombosis. Hepatic vein obstruction because of hepatocellular carcinoma is common in South Africa. Myeloproliferative disorders (MPDs) and other definable hypercoagulable states account for the majority of BCS cases in Europe and Western countries.[4,5,8-17,22-40] The specific cause should be sought in every patient because the pre- and postsurgical management and outcome are, to a large extent, dependent on prevention of further hepatic vein occlusion.

Pathology and Pathophysiology

The multiple underlying conditions listed in Table 18–1 do not define the morphology of the obstruction or the site involved. In Asian countries, the common finding is a membranous web in the inferior vena cava, specifically at the suprahepatic region, resulting in progressive thrombosis of the inferior vena cava and the liver ostia.[2,3,6,7,13,18] In the United States and Europe, hematological disorders leading to thrombosis are the most frequent underlying mechanisms responsible for occlusion of the main hepatic veins.[8-14,22-38] This thrombotic form of the syndrome accounts for up to 80% of the patients presenting for surgical treatment of BCS.[8,22] Compression or invasion of the hepatic veins by tumors or granulomas occasionally results in acute or chronic occlusion or thrombosis of the hepatic vein, leading to clinical expression of BCS.[17,18,39,40] The reason for the predominant localization of thrombosis at the level of the liver portion of the vena cava is not known, although for many years the underlying mechanism was believed to be an endophlebitis of the hepatic vein. The weight of the clinical evidence now indicates that the primary process is thrombotic rather than inflammatory. This conclusion is supported by autopsy studies demonstrating fibrous obstruction as the final product of thrombus organization.[41]

Histopathological findings characteristic of rapidly progressive hepatic vein occlusion include intense congestion and cellular atrophy (Fig. 18–1). Areas of necrosis and cell dropout are often superimposed. Centrilobular extravasation of red cells and necrosis can extend to the periphery of the lobules; however, the portal areas are preserved.[7] In patients with chronic hepatic vein thromboses, cardiac-type cirrhosis develops. The typical finding in this group of patients is fibrosis in the parenchyma-free center of the liver lobules.[10]

Hepatic veno-occlusive disease is a distinct form of BCS characterized by central venous dilatation, centrilobular necrosis, and intimal thickening throughout

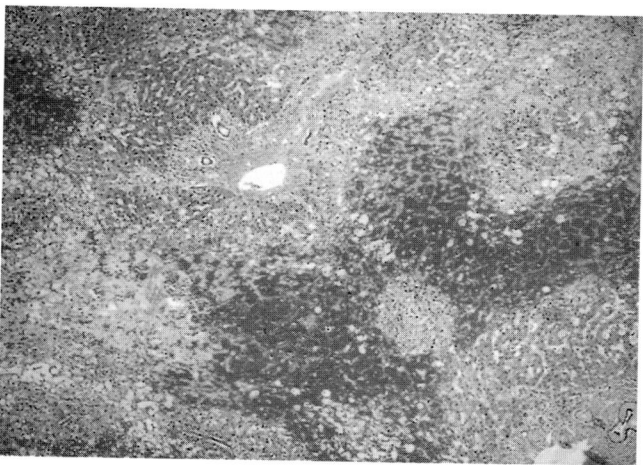

FIGURE 18-1

Native liver from patient 11 showing extensive hepatocellular necrosis, hemorrhage, and architectural collapse characteristic of Budd-Chiari syndrome (BCS). (H&E ×100)

the smaller liver venules at the microscopic level. The principal cause of this disease is continuous exposure to hepatotoxic pyrrolizidine alkaloids.[11] Hepatic veno-occlusive disease has also been reported to develop after high-dose chemotherapy and in the setting of hematopoietic stem cell transplantation.[42]

The wide range of topographical and pathological causes encompassed under the BCS label merits a better classification to facilitate patient evaluation, prognostic prediction, and rational treatment. Ludwig and colleagues[43] suggested a more accurate and simplified classification of BCS on the basis of morphological features (thrombotic versus nonthrombotic), site of the lesion (inferior vena cava, major or small hepatic veins), and cause. Such a classification would help clarify the pathophysiology, histopathology, and spectrum of diseases that lead to the hepatic venous outflow obstruction and would aid in the selection of the appropriate medical management of patients with BCS.

Clinical Presentation and Diagnostic Evaluation

The clinical picture depends on the tempo and extent of hepatic vein occlusion and is directly related to liver congestion with subsequent hepatocyte necrosis and, ultimately, fibrosis.

Although the presentation of patients suffering from BCS is variable, the clinical history correlates with the acuity of disease onset. Most patients with BCS present with gradual onset of right upper quadrant abdominal pain, tender hepatomegaly, and ascites. The right upper quadrant pain is often preceded by weeks to months of vague abdominal distress. Splenomegaly and an enlarged caudate lobe (palpable epigastric mass) are frequent additional findings. Patients with occlusion of the inferior vena cava have lower extremity edema, distended abdominal flank and back veins, and albuminuria. Sudden-onset upper abdominal pain with vomiting and rapid accumulation of ascites with an enlarged, tender liver are less common and are associated with acute onset of disease. Only rarely will these patients experience fulminant liver failure, which is characterized by massive liver necrosis and consequent liver coma, severe coagulopathy, and hypoglycemia.[44] In the chronic type of BCS, the development of end-stage liver disease may not be associated with the typical stigmata of chronic liver disease seen in cirrhotic patients. Fatigue and poor nutritional status are common; however, spider angiomas and palmar erythema are unusual, and jaundice is usually mild. A common physical finding is lower extremity edema resulting from partial or complete occlusion of the retrohepatic vena cava by the hypertrophied caudate lobe. Caval obstruction may decrease kidney perfusion pressure, thereby contributing to the development of kidney failure. Despite severe portal hypertension in this patient population, variceal bleeding is uncommon.

Routine laboratory tests indicate variable degrees of liver dysfunction. Serum transaminase, bilirubin, and alkaline phosphatase levels are normal or mildly elevated. Serum albumin may be decreased, and albumin levels correlate well with the severity of liver injury and the magnitude of protein loss into ascitic fluid. Prothrombin time may be mildly prolonged.

Liver biopsy typically demonstrates intense centrilobular congestion and pressure necrosis of the liver parenchyma. Cardiac-type cirrhosis is seen in the advanced stage of the disease. Liver biopsy may not be necessary in every patient; however, chronic BCS patients with biopsy findings of cirrhosis and marginal liver reserve should be considered for liver transplantation rather than a decompressive procedure.

Diagnostic Imaging

Noninvasive hepatic imaging has assumed a progressively important role in the diagnostic evaluation of BCS. Duplex ultrasonography and color Doppler ultrasound imaging accurately define the flow parameters of the hepatic veins, the portal vein, and the inferior vena cava in most patients (Fig. 18–2). Often, ultrasound is the initial imaging modality in patients being evaluated for hepatic veno-occlusive disease. Ultrasound is less sensitive for the detection of hepatic masses than computed tomography (CT) or magnetic resonance imaging (MRI).

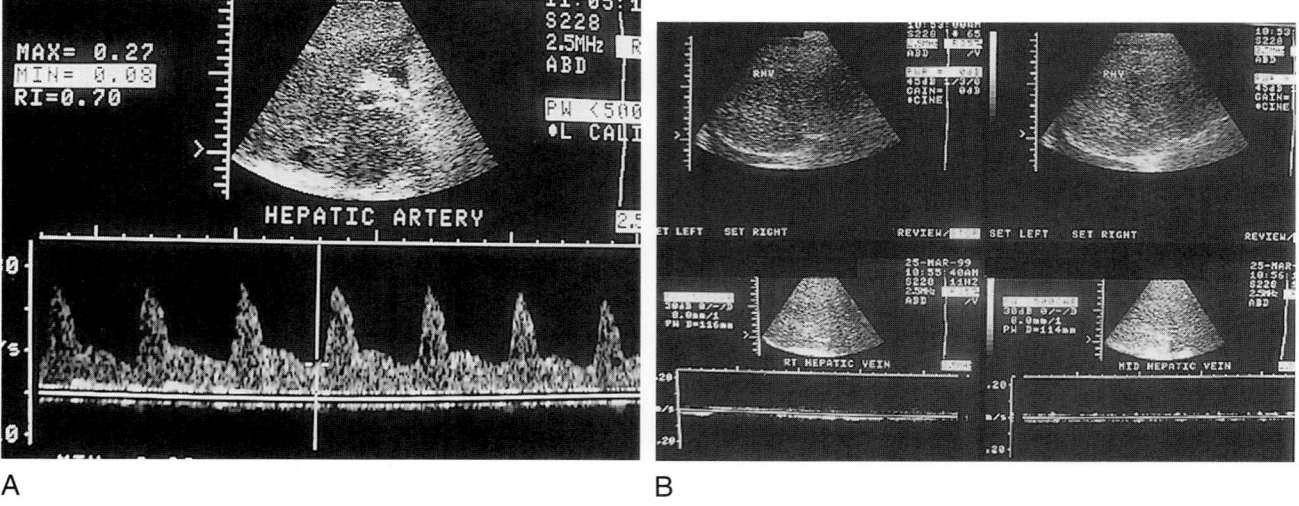

A   B

FIGURE 18–2

A, Doppler evaluation of hepatic artery demonstrates normal visibility and normal Doppler wave-form.
B, The same patient demonstrates nonvisualization of hepatic veins, and no Doppler signal from hepatic venous structures. These are the sonographic findings of BCS.

Multiphase infusion CT evaluation accurately images the hepatic parenchyma and gives valuable information regarding hepatic venous and portal venous flow (Fig. 18–3). An enlarged caudate lobe is characteristically observed. CT arteriography and venography accurately assess the anatomic features of hepatic vasculature. CT also defines hepatic morphology and helps distinguish BCS from other processes that may mimic veno-occlusive disease.[45]

MRI is very sensitive in the detection of hepatic mass disease, as well as in evaluating flow characteristics in the hepatic vasculature (Fig. 18–4). MRI also provides insight into diffuse hepatic disease.[46] Both gadolinium-based contrast agents and iron-based contrast agents are commercially available. These agents are particularly valuable in assessing hepatic heterogeneity demonstrated on ultrasound or CT studies.

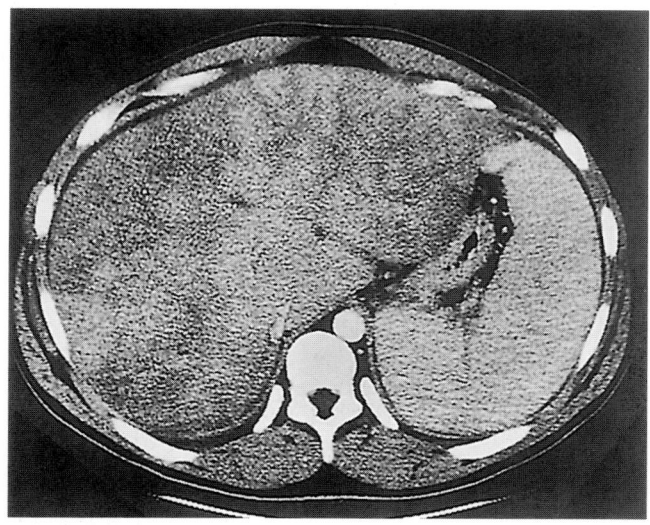

FIGURE 18–3

Computed tomographic scan demonstrating enlarged caudate lobe and compressed inferior vena cava. (From Shaked A, Goldstein R: Transplantation for Budd-Chiari syndrome. In Busuttil RW, Klintmalm GB (eds): Transplantation of the Liver. Philadelphia, WB Saunders, 1996, p 140.)

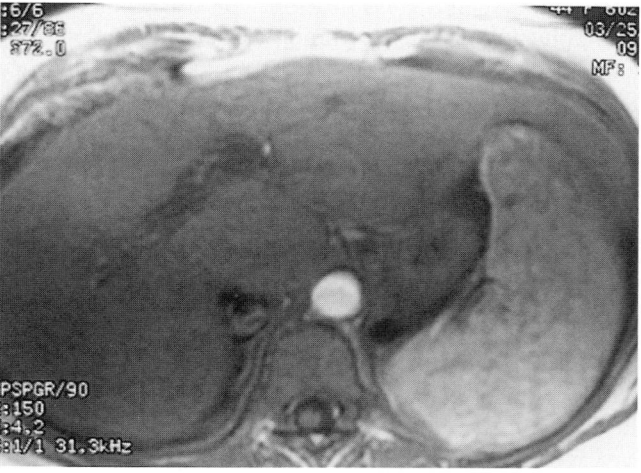

FIGURE 18–4

Contrast-enhanced MRI evaluation demonstrates no visible enhancement of normal hepatic veins. Notice inhomogeneous enhancement of hepatic parenchyma and caudate lobe enlargement.

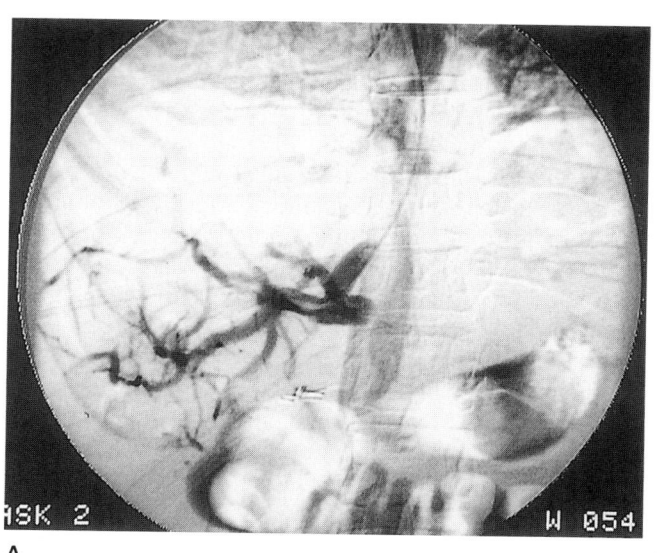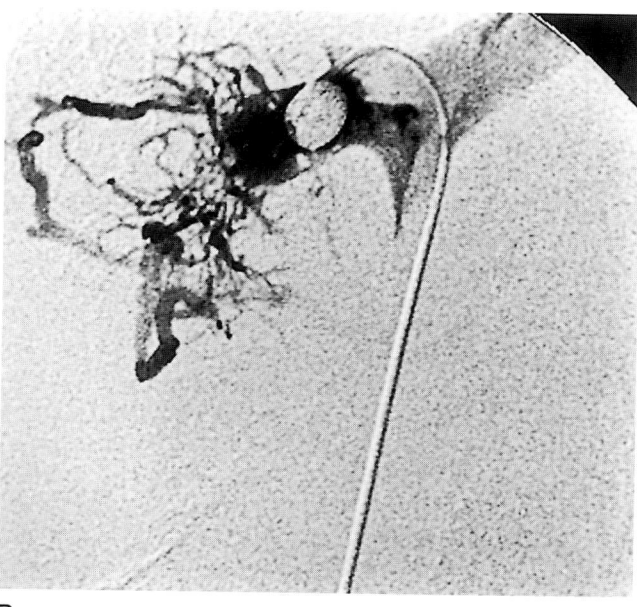

A   B

FIGURE 18–5

A, Hepatic venogram demonstrates cannulation of right hepatic vein. Middle and left hepatic veins are completely occluded. **B,** Hepatic venogram on another patient demonstrates irregular "spiderweb" appearance of BCS. (**B** from Shaked A, Goldstein R: Transplantation for Budd-Chiari syndrome. In Busuttil RW, Klintmalm GB (eds): Transplantation of the Liver, Philadelphia, WB Saunders, 1996, p 139.)

In patients with known or suspected BCS, the noninvasive imaging evaluation is used to confirm the diagnosis and uncover unsuspected malignancies. This is particularly important because hepatic malignancy is more common in patients with BCS than in the general population.

Hepatic venography remains the gold standard for the imaging diagnosis of BCS. The hepatic veins may be cannulated from a femoral or jugular approach. A spiderweb appearance of the intrahepatic veins is confirmatory (Fig. 18–5). Hepatic venography also allows measurement of the hepatic wedge pressure, and inferior venacavography can be performed during the same catheterization. These more invasive procedures are usually reserved for patients in whom shunt therapy rather than transplantation is contemplated.

Thorough radiological evaluation of BCS is best accomplished with a multimodality approach. Cross-sectional imaging (CT or MRI) is used to examine the entire abdominal contents as well as to confirm and characterize hepatic blood flow. The measurement of flow parameters is usually accomplished with sonography. In patients who are not transplant candidates, venography confirms the diagnosis of BCS and provides preoperative assessment prior to shunt therapy.

Once hepatic vein obstruction is demonstrated, its cause should be established. Table 18–2 lists suggested diagnostic studies.

Table 18–2. DIAGNOSTIC TESTS FOR EVALUATION OF CAUSE OF BUDD-CHIARI SYNDROME

Complete blood count (CBC) and peripheral blood smear
Liver function blood tests
Liver imaging studies
Liver biopsy
Bone marrow aspiration and biopsy
Factor V Leiden mutation
Prothrombin gene mutation
Antithrombin III
Protein C (total + functional)
Protein S (total + functional)
Lupus-like anticoagulant
Anticardiolipin antibodies
Homocysteine level
Serum protein electrophoresis
Sucrose hemolysis test
Ham test
Flow cytometry for CD55, CD59 expression

Etiological Diagnosis: Myeloproliferative Disorders and Other Conditions

In Western countries, the recognition of overt or occult MPDs—especially polycythemia vera, essential thrombocythemia, and paroxysmal nocturnal hemoglobinuria—as causes of BCS has been documented for more than 20 years. Other MPDs (agnogenic myeloid metaplasia, chronic granulocytic leukemia, and erythroleukemia) are rarely associated with BCS. MPDs are the cause of 40% to 70% of BCS cases in the United States and Europe.[8,22] Coagulation abnormalities, both hereditary and acquired, are also causes of BCS. Some of these disorders were recognized during the 1990s. If prevention of further thrombosis is to be achieved, complete hematological evaluation of each patient with BCS for evidence of MPDs and other hypercoagulable states becomes imperative. Consideration of one series of patients studied serially illustrates several pertinent points in this regard.

Between January 1987 and March 2000, 17 patients with BCS underwent orthotopic liver transplantation (OLT) at Baylor University Medical Center in Dallas, Texas (Table 18–3).[8,26] Data for this study were collected through a prospectively maintained longitudinal database and chart review. The diagnosis of BCS was confirmed by imaging studies, including MRI, CT, Doppler ultrasonography, and angiography. Pathological examination of the native liver after transplantation was performed in all cases.

Bone marrow examination was performed in all patients except the first. The diagnosis of MPDs was based on bone marrow morphological abnormalities in conjunction with peripheral blood counts.[47,48] Spontaneous erythroid colony-forming assays were not performed.[22,23] Hypercoagulability evaluation was conducted in all patients. An expanded battery of studies was used as new causes for thrombophilia were established (see Table 18–2). The first 13 patients underwent transplantation before 1996, prior to widespread recognition of factor V Leiden (the prothrombin gene mutation) and hyperhomocysteinemia as causes of the hypercoagulable state. Laboratory studies performed on the earlier patients included functional and total protein C and protein S, antithrombin III, anticardiolipin immunoglobulin G and M antibodies, lupus-like anticoagulant, sucrose hemolysis, and serum protein electrophoresis. This protocol was not in place when the first patient with BCS was seen, but it was used subsequently. Causative diagnoses were established in 15 of the 16 remaining patients (94%).

The purpose of this study was to identify the origin of BCS and to determine whether antiplatelet treatment rather than anticoagulation would be effective in patients with underlying MPDs.

Table 18–3 lists demographics and bone marrow findings of the 17 patients in this study. Twelve patients were women, and 5 were men. Age at time of orthotopic liver transplantation (OLT) ranged from 17 to 53 years. Time from onset of BCS to OLT ranged from approximately 4 months to 4 years. Twelve patients (71%) had evidence of an MPD as the cause of their BCS. Six of these patients had a clinical picture that was consistent with polycythemia vera, 2 patients had essential thrombocythemia, and 4 patients had unclassifiable MPDs. Cytogenetic analysis was performed in 5 patients (patients 2, 7, 8, 11, and 16), and all were normal. Two patients (patients 1 and 7) were classified as having idiopathic BCS. The 3 remaining patients had protein C deficiency (patient 13), sarcoidosis (patient 15), and the prothrombin gene (G20210A) mutation (patient 17). One patient (patient 16) was found to be heterozygous for factor V Leiden in addition to having an MPD.

Thus it was possible to arrive at a causative diagnosis in nearly all patients with BCS. Seventy-one percent had evidence of an MPD.[8]

Liver Transplantation

Consideration for Transplantation: Indications and Contraindications

The first liver transplant for BCS was performed in 1974.[49] The selection of patients to undergo OLT for BCS must be made on an individual basis. Long-term results of OLT versus portosystemic shunting are similar in terms of patient outcome.[4,12,17,19-21,50-52] Patients selected for shunt surgery should have relatively well preserved synthetic function, with OLT being indicated when synthetic function is poor. Development of encephalopathy is an indicator of poor residual liver function; thus, a portosystemic shunt is usually contraindicated. Therefore, appropriate surgical therapy for BCS should be performed after consideration of the reversibility of the liver disease and the fitness of the candidate to withstand surgery.

Once surgical therapy is accepted as the preferred treatment, two issues must be addressed. First, assessment of the severity of the liver disease at the time of presentation is essential, after which the predicted course of the disease after a shunt procedure versus liver replacement must be considered. In recent years, these issues have gained increasing relevance because total hepatectomy and OLT can reverse the liver failure and restore normal blood flow through the inferior vena cava.

Several liver transplantation centers have reported good results in BCS patients undergoing OLT.[7,8,12-21,51-54] The 3-year survival rate after transplantation was greater than 75%, with surviving patients returning to

Table 18-3. CHARACTERISTICS OF PATIENTS TREATED WITH OLT FOR BCS

Patient	Age (yr)/Gender	Bone Marrow, Megakaryocyte Findings	Cause of BCS	Date of OLT	Follow-Up After OLT (Months)
No. 1	41/F	Not done	Idiopathic	1/31/87	120
No. 2	23/F	Increased, clustered, dysplastic	Polycythemia vera	2/23/87 3/27/87	158
No. 3	34/M	Increased, clustered	MPD unclassified	9/14//87	119
No. 4	24/M	Increased, dysplastic	Polycythemia vera	11/01/87	7
No. 5*	20/F	Increased	Polycythemia vera	9/03/88	120
No. 6	16/F	Increased, clustered	Polycythemia vera	12/16/88 5/9/95	124
No. 7	34/M	Normal	Idiopathic‡	5/12/90	123
No. 8	23/F	Increased, clustered, dysplastic	MPD unclassified	11/22/91	84
No. 9	28/F	Dysplastic	MPD unclassified	12/06/91	3
No. 10	34/F	Clustered, dysplastic	Essential thrombocythemia	4/20/92	84
No. 11	26/F	Increased, clustered	Polycythemia vera	6/30/94	41
No. 12†	18/F	Increased (marked)	Polycythemia vera	10/08/94	45
No. 13	53/F	Normal	Protein C deficiency	8/27/95	40
No. 14	31/F	Increased, dysplastic	Essential thrombocythemia	8/18/96	45
No. 15	44/M	Normal	Sarcoidosis	1/16/97	39
No. 16	36/F	Increased, clustered	MPD unclassified and factor V Leiden	10/04/98	11
No. 17	25/M	Normal	Prothrombin gene mutation	3/22/00	1

*Patient 5 had a white blood cell count of $16.1 \times 10^3/\mu L$, a hematocrit of 48%, and a platelet count of $1040 \times 10^3/\mu L$ at the time of bone marrow examination.
†Patient 12 had a white blood cell count of $12.5 \times 10^3/\mu L$, hematocrit 60%, and platelet count of $563 \times 10^3/\mu L$ at the time of bone marrow examination.
‡An elevated homocysteine level was found in this patient after transplantation.
BCS, Budd-Chiari syndrome; MPD, myeloproliferative disorder; OLT, orthotopic liver transplantation.
Modified from Melear JM, Goldstein RM, Levy MF, et al: Hematologic aspects of liver transplantation for Budd-Chiari syndrome with special reference to myeloproliferative disorders. Transplantation 74:1090-1095, 2002.

a functional lifestyle. Although these reports may be interpreted as an unequivocal recommendation for OLT as therapy for patients with BCS, excellent long-term results have also been reported after portosystemic shunts.[13,50-53] Furthermore, liver function tests may return to normal after shunting, with stabilization or even improvement of the parenchymal injury, as indicated by postoperative liver biopsies. These reports demonstrate a central dilemma in the management of patients with BCS and indicate the need to establish

standards for determining which patients should undergo decompressive shunting versus liver transplantation. Such criteria should include reversibility of liver injury, primary disease leading to the hepatic venous obstruction, and fitness of the patient to withstand either surgical procedure.

The severity of liver failure and the functional liver reserve should be determined by clinical and laboratory data, aided by liver biopsy. Hepatocyte synthetic failure is reflected by serum levels of albumin less than

3 g/dL, prolonged coagulation times (prothrombin time greater than 3 seconds more than control), and the inability to conjugate bilirubin and secrete bile (conjugated bilirubin greater than 3 mg/dL). Patients selected for shunt surgery should have relatively well preserved synthetic function. In contrast, OLT is indicated when liver synthetic function is poor.[50-53] Assessment of liver reserve is critical; patients with no reserve (i.e., irreversible parenchymal injury) may rapidly decompensate after portosystemic shunt, resulting in high mortality.[51,55,56] Acute or chronic liver failure after portosystemic shunt, therefore, indicates poor liver reserve and signals the need for urgent liver transplantation.

Development of encephalopathy in end-stage liver disease is generally regarded as an indicator of poor residual liver function. Portosystemic shunt is usually contraindicated in encephalopathic patients because further neurological deterioration may be a consequence of the procedure. For this reason, encephalopathy complicating acute or long-standing BCS should be considered an indicator for OLT.

The role of the liver biopsy in determining the extent of injury caused by long-standing hepatic venous occlusion is not clear. However, liver biopsy alone should not be the dominant focus of decision-making. The ambiguity of biopsy findings is illustrated by the favorable clinical course of some shunt patients whose biopsies showed fibrosis at initial presentation.[51,57] There are conflicting reports about the role of portosystemic shunting in arresting the progression of cirrhosis, but progressive fibrosis and cirrhosis dominate the course of at least a small group of shunt patients.[57-59]

The primary disease causing obstruction of the hepatic vein may also determine appropriate surgical intervention. A number of reports have identified BCS as a potential risk factor for the development of hepatoma.[60,61] The finding of a small incidental hepatoma should prompt consideration of OLT. In contrast, results of transplantation for stage IV hepatocellular carcinoma (tumor invading the portal or hepatic veins) are dismal, and shunt surgery is more appropriate therapy. Other similar exclusion criteria for transplantation are hepatic venous occlusion secondary to locally invasive tumors or metastatic extrahepatic malignancies.

Several studies outline clinical criteria to distinguish shunt versus transplantation candidates.[51,52] These studies suggest that patients with fulminant or chronic forms of BCS should undergo transplantation, and those with acute or subacute BCS should undergo portosystemic decompressive procedures. These clinical criteria, when considered with assessment of residual liver function, provide a therapeutic framework for successful management of this otherwise fatal syndrome. Screening for coexisting medical conditions in this group of patients is similar to that in other OLT candidates. In addition, thrombosis of the hepatic veins in the setting of a hypercoagulable state mandates careful evaluation of the portal system, and the absence of clots in the cava and iliac veins should be confirmed before surgery to anticipate the need for portal venous grafts and access sites for venovenous bypass.

In summary, appropriate surgical therapy for BCS should be performed only after consideration of the reversibility of the liver disease and the fitness of the candidate to withstand surgery. The operation must be individualized to the unique expression of the disease for each patient.

Surgical Considerations

The standard operative technique of liver transplantation is recommended for most cases of BCS.[4] Exposure of the suprahepatic vena cava is best achieved via bilateral subcostal incision with midline extension to the xiphoid. Institution of venovenous bypass before abdominal skin incision and placement on portal bypass early in the operation clearly decrease blood loss related to severe portal hypertension and obstruction of the caval blood flow by the hypertrophied caudate lobe. The dissection is characteristically difficult when approaching the suprahepatic vena cava because of dense adhesions between the liver and the diaphragm. In most cases, the suprahepatic vena cava can be encircled and a clamp applied. Occasionally, the diaphragm must be dissected off the inferior vena cava up to the right atrium. This approach avoids splitting of the diaphragm or thoracic extension.

The surgical approach can be modified in the presence of complete obstruction of the suprahepatic vena cava caused by an organized thrombus that is not amenable to thrombectomy. The suprahepatic clamp is removed, and a curvilinear incision through the tendinous portion of the diaphragm exposes the pericardium. An end-to-end anastomosis is performed to the intrapericardial portion of the inferior vena cava.[62] Similarly, a previous hepatoatrial anastomosis can be taken down via an inferior median sternotomy and median laparotomy.[63] To avoid venous air embolism during dissection, the patient can be placed on cardiopulmonary bypass with short periods of induced fibrillation. The diaphragm is split through the central fibrous body, and the cuff of the donor atrium is brought to the chest followed by standard anastomosis. (Despite removal of the liver with a long suprahepatic or atrial cuff, transplantation of the heart from the same donor is still possible.)

As noted previously, it is not uncommon to perform transplantation in patients with prior portosystemic shunting, most commonly end-to-end portacaval or mesoatrial shunts. Dissection of end-to-side portacaval shunts is performed as previously described.[64]

Recent modifications include the placement of a portal cannula through the inferior mesenteric vein followed by simple ligation of the mesoportacaval shunt immediately after reperfusion. Mesoatrial shunts should be ligated; however, the portal outflow can still be used in case of portal vein occlusion. A word of caution, BCS patients can be the most technically challenging patients for liver transplant surgery, especially if they have had previous surgeries that have caused adhesions to the surface of the liver, producing huge and friable varices. Such patients need to be approached with utmost caution and care.

The incidence of portal vein thrombosis or occlusion of the infrahepatic inferior vena cava is reported to be higher in patients with BCS than in other transplant recipients.[65] Restoration of portal blood flow is usually successful after thrombectomy; rarely is a portal vein graft required.[64] The infrahepatic inferior vena cava can either be thrombectomized or allowed to remain occluded if the organized thrombus extends below the renal veins.

Long-Term Results

Reported 3-year survival of patients who underwent transplantation for BCS range from 45% to 88%. The European Liver Transplant Registry recorded 82 patients who underwent transplantation for BCS, with a 3-year survival of 57%.[66] These long-term results are comparable to survival after portosystemic shunt procedures, but these data should be interpreted with the knowledge that different patient populations undergo shunt versus OLT and that selection criteria for OLT may vary among centers. Furthermore, OLT may not be an option in some centers performing shunt procedures.

In our study, with both options available, proper preoperative assessment of liver reserve resulted in similar survival in both groups. Furthermore, patients who deteriorated after shunting could be rescued by urgent OLT. The pattern of liver function tests after shunt surgery was variable. In some patients liver function tests stabilized, but others showed further deterioration in synthetic function; in a few patients extensive fibrosis developed. In contrast, successful OLT resulted in completely normal liver function. Patients undergoing OLT for curable parasitic disease had no evidence of recurrence within 2 years after surgery, whereas disseminated disease recurred and progressed slowly over 3 to 19 months after transplantation.[67] Despite these advantages of transplantation, significant drawbacks are well known and include complications related to lifelong immunosuppression and the development of acute or chronic rejection.

A randomized study comparing OLT and shunt procedures is unlikely to be performed for patients suffering from various types of BCS in a single center,

in part because of the rarity of the syndrome. The message emerging from the surgical literature is that patients with BCS must not be inserted into any preconceived surgical approach. Various options for the treatment of the BCS should be individualized to the particular underlying causative diagnosis, disease, and clinical presentation.

Antithrombotic Therapy

The effectiveness of OLT in patients with BCS has been complicated by recurrent thrombosis and difficulties in establishing a cause for the thrombosis.[6,19-22,53,54,68-74] Anticoagulation with heparin followed by warfarin has been the therapy of choice to prevent posttransplant thrombosis.[6,12,19-22,54,69,70,72-74] Recent advances in understanding the origin of the BCS indicate that overt or occult MPDs are a frequent cause in the United States and Europe.[22-25] Despite the recognition that MPDs are major causative disorders of BCS in Western countries, therapeutic recommendations continue to focus on anticoagulation.[22,75] The pathophysiological abnormalities in MPDs include qualitative and quantitative platelet defects that are associated with both abnormal bleeding and clotting. Thus treatment directed toward altering platelet production and function may be more rational and effective than anticoagulation.

In the Dallas study, patients with MPDs (see Table 18–3) were given aspirin, 325 mg per day, and hydroxyurea, 500 to 1500 mg per day, 4 to 7 days after OLT.[8] Neither heparin nor any other anticoagulation was routinely given after OLT. The hydroxyurea dose was titrated to maintain platelet counts between $100 \times 10^3/\mu L$ and $250 \times 10^3/\mu L$. Patients were maintained on these medications. Patients who were recognized as having an MPD before transplantation received the same regimen. Thrombolytic therapy was attempted unsuccessfully in two patients thought to have acute BCS. However, such thrombolytic treatment has been reported to have efficacy in occasional patients.[20] After anagrelide became available, it was used in place of hydroxyurea in 2 patients who developed anemia or granulocytopenia on the latter agent. Patients without MPDs were treated on the basis of their underlying condition. Standard immunosuppressive therapy was used after OLT and consisted of cyclosporine and prednisolone for the first 12 patients and cyclosporine microemulsion and prednisolone for the last 5 patients.

Anticoagulation with warfarin and heparin has generally been the therapy used to prevent recurrent thrombosis in patients who have BCS and are undergoing OLT or portosystemic shunting.[6,12,19-22,52-54,69] In 1991, we reported the use of hydroxyurea and aspirin in 5 patients who underwent transplantation for BCS associated with MPDs.[26] This treatment approach was predicated on our experience and those of others, that MPDs were a common cause of BCS. Twelve of 17 patients (71%) in the Dallas study had evident MPDs, which are hematopoietic clonal stem cell disorders associated with a paradoxical propensity to bleed and clot abnormally.[8] Recently, a classification system has been proposed that relies heavily on megakaryocyte morphology in diagnosing MPDs.[48] In polycythemia vera patients with BCS, peripheral blood counts may not be elevated because of splenomegaly and hypersplenism. Therefore, bone marrow morphological findings are crucial. Several authors have reported finding a high percentage of occult MPDs by using spontaneous erythroid colony-forming assays in vitro.[23-25,76] All of our 12 patients with MPDs had morphological abnormalities of the megakaryocyte lineage (see Table 18–3). Thus, spontaneous erythroid colony-forming assays were not necessary for the diagnosis of MPDs in these patients. However, such studies may have been helpful in the two patients with idiopathic BCS.

Of the 17 patients, 3 were given warfarin after OLT for various reasons. Patient 1 was receiving warfarin before this study was initiated. Patient 2 had recurrent thrombus in a brachial artery that had been damaged at cardiac catheterization during pretransplant evaluation. She developed recurrent thrombosis in this artery while receiving aspirin and hydroxyurea therapy, so warfarin was added. Patient 10 had a pretransplant diagnosis of cryptogenic cirrhosis but was later determined to have BCS. The diagnosis of an MPD in patient 10 was subsequently made on histological review of the spleen (removed 1 month after OLT) and after she had two episodes of thrombosis after OLT with retained thrombus in the portal vein (see case 10 report further on). Therefore, warfarin was continued. These 3 patients were not given aspirin because of anticoagulation.

Follow-up of the 17 patients ranged from 1 to 158 months, with a mean of 68.4 months and median of 45 months. Two of the 17 patients died. Patient 4 died secondary to acute hepatitis B and multisystem organ failure 7 months after OLT while receiving hydroxyurea. Patient 6 died secondary to portal vein thrombosis while receiving hydroxyurea and aspirin 124 months after initial OLT (see case report further on). Two allografts were lost—one secondary to hepatitis C 78 months after OLT (patient 6) and the other as a result of vanishing bile duct syndrome 1 month after OLT (patient 2). Neither allograft showed evidence of recurrent thrombosis.

Mean follow-up of the 10 patients treated with only hydroxyurea and aspirin was 59.9 months.[8] Of these 10 patients, 1 patient (patient 6) had a recurrent thrombus manifested as portal vein thrombosis 124 months after the first OLT. No other instances of thromboembolic complications occurred in this group, and no major bleeding complications were identified. Moreover, the patients treated with antiplatelet therapy only underwent multiple liver biopsies to monitor allograft status with no bleeding complications. In 2 patients from the group of 17 (patients 14 and 16), anagrelide was administered after initial therapy with hydroxyurea; aspirin was continued in both patients. Observed side effects included transient cytopenias secondary, in part, to hydroxyurea. No clinical sequelae were noted, and these cytopenias were managed by temporarily discontinuing hydroxyurea or, in the later patients, by substituting anagrelide for hydroxyurea.

In patients presenting with BCS, a complete hematological workup, including bone marrow examination, is mandatory, because this procedure may yield important information for guiding therapy.[8] The underlying drive to thrombosis in patients with MPDs may not be adequately treated using heparin and warfarin. These agents also expose patients to risks associated with anticoagulation. Our approach consisted of managing patients diagnosed with BCS secondary to an MPD in a different manner. The use of hydroxyurea and aspirin directed treatment toward abnormal platelets and appears to be a more rational approach that is a safe and effective alternative to anticoagulation therapy. Anagrelide may be superior to hydroxyurea for the treatment of thrombocytosis because its action is primarily on megakaryocytes and platelets, with less effect on normal erythroid and granulocytic precursors. None of our MPD patients has developed leukemia, although this remains a future possibility.[22,77,78]

The recurrent thrombosis rate in Baylor Dallas patients treated with hydroxyurea and aspirin compares favorably with other series. Ninety percent (9 of 10) of our patients have not had evidence of recurrent thrombosis with a median follow-up of 59.9 months. One series in which 7 patients on warfarin were followed after OLT revealed that all 7 patients remained alive, but 2 patients required retransplantation because of recurrent BCS, and 1 patient had major gastrointestinal bleeding.[69] Another study[54] examined 16 patients with BCS who had undergone anticoagulation after OLT. Mean follow-up was 28.2 months. The authors found a 31% rate of thrombosis (three in the portal vein, one in the hepatic artery, and one in the axillary vein). A 44% rate of bleeding complications also was observed.

Antiplatelet therapy with hydroxyurea and aspirin appears to be an effective, safe, and preferable alternative to anticoagulation in preventing recurrent thrombosis in transplant recipients who have BCS and an MPD (Fig. 18–6). Patients treated with warfarin therapy to prevent recurrent thrombosis are at substantial risk when their prothrombin time falls to subtherapeutic levels.[10,53,69] Warfarin was discontinued in a patient who was seen in 1981 by one of this chapter's authors (G.B.K.) in preparation for liver biopsy and experienced recurrent thromboses. The patient was hospitalized and

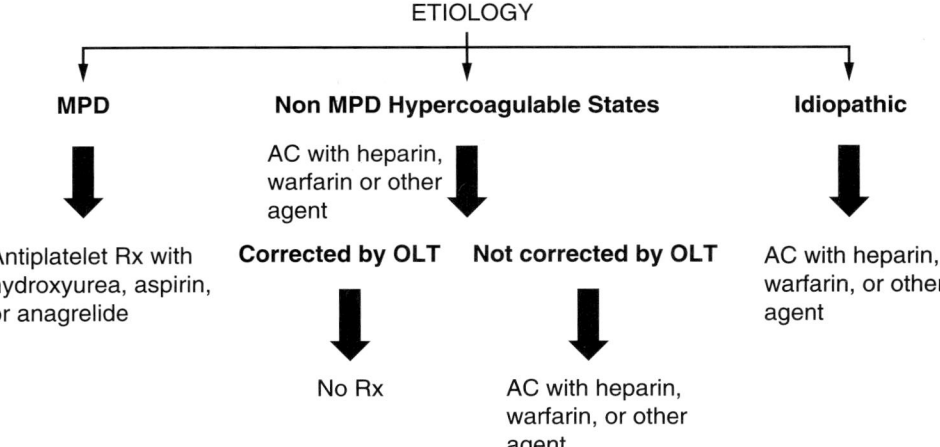

FIGURE 18–6

Decision tree for antithrombotic treatment in BCS. Note: Thrombolytic therapy is a consideration for patients presenting with acute BCS. Some patients with BCS, because of polycythemia vera, do not have elevated hematocrits. If the hematocrit is greater than 45%, phlebotomy should be performed with antiplatelet medications. MPD, myeloproliferative disorder; AC, anticoagulation.

died after a prolonged course. This experience was one of the initial motivating factors in our current therapeutic approach to patients who have BCS and are undergoing OLT.

In patients not having an MPD, posttransplant antithrombotic therapy may not be necessary if an underlying hereditary defect is corrected by liver transplantation, for example, protein C deficiency or the prothrombin gene mutation.[8,79] For patients with acquired thrombophilia, posttransplant therapy will vary (see Fig. 18–6). The patient with sarcoidosis was being followed without antiplatelet or anticoagulant treatment. By contrast, individuals with BCS caused by antiphospholipid antibodies should be maintained on anticoagulation. For BCS patients in whom a thorough hypercoagulable evaluation and bone marrow examination are negative and who, therefore, have idiopathic BCS, long-term anticoagulation seems prudent.

Case Histories

The following case reports illustrate the causative spectrum and clinical presentation of patients with BCS.[8] Table 18–3 lists the case numbers.

Case 10—Undiagnosed Myeloproliferative Disorder

This 34-year-old white woman began having symptoms of liver dysfunction in March 1990. Evaluation failed to reveal the cause of her liver failure, and she underwent transplantation in April 1992 with the diagnosis of cryptogenic cirrhosis. Pretreatment platelet count was normal. This patient developed a thrombus in the portal and splenic veins 1 month after OLT, and splenectomy

was performed. Recurrent thrombus of the portal vein graft and marked postsplenectomy thrombocytosis aroused suspicion of an MPD. Additional histological review of the spleen disclosed trilineage extramedullary hematopoiesis, a finding strongly suggestive of an MPD (Fig. 18–7). Subsequent bone marrow examination was consistent with essential thrombocythemia. Administration of warfarin began when the recurrent thrombus in the portal vein occurred. Hydroxyurea was added after the diagnosis of essential thrombocythemia was made.

This case illustrates the value of bone marrow examination to establish the diagnosis of MPDs in patients who present with BCS. Had the underlying MPD been

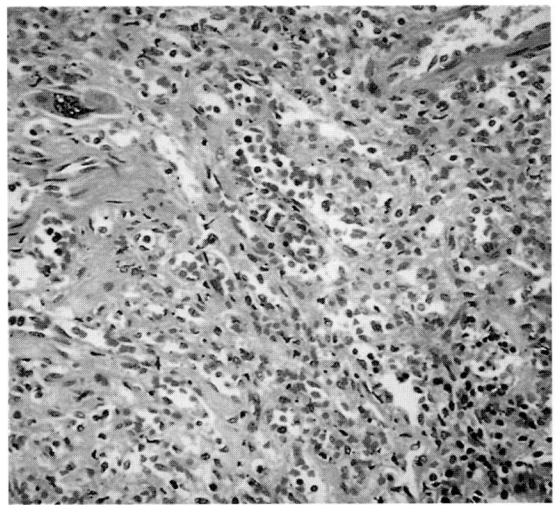

FIGURE 18–7

Spleen from patient 10 showing extramedullary hematopoiesis with red cell precursors (right lower corner) and a megakaryocyte (left upper corner). (H&E × 200)

recognized earlier, splenectomy would not have been performed. Despite multiple thromboses soon after OLT, this patient has not had a recurrent thrombus since starting hydroxyurea and warfarin more than 7 years ago. Her platelet count has been well controlled and has ranged from $130 \times 10^3/\mu L$ to $306 \times 10^3/\mu L$.

Case 6—Polycythemia Vera in a 16-Year-Old Girl

This young patient abruptly developed abdominal pain and nausea in April 1988. She was found to have ascites and elevation of liver enzyme levels. A CT, an MRI, and a Doppler sonogram revealed hepatic venous thrombosis. A complete blood count disclosed a white blood cell count of $14 \times 10^3/\mu L$, a hematocrit of 41%, and a platelet count of $600 \times 10^3/\mu L$. Leukocyte alkaline phosphatase was elevated at 200 (normal 16 to 77). Bone marrow examination showed a hypercellular marrow with erythroid hyperplasia and absent iron stores. Megakaryocytes were increased in number and clustered in multiple areas. The diagnosis of polycythemia vera was made. Treatment with hydroxyurea and aspirin was instituted.

The patient underwent liver transplantation in December 1988. Pathological examination of the native liver confirmed hepatic venous thrombosis. A second transplant 78 months after the first was necessitated by the development of hepatitis C. The excised allograft showed no evidence of recurrent thrombosis. Liver biopsy in March 1998 disclosed ductopenia and fibrosis consistent with chronic rejection. One year later, the patient developed abdominal pain as a result of portal vein thrombosis. She died while waiting for her third liver transplant. Hydroxyurea and aspirin therapy were well tolerated for 10 years until she became symptomatic from a portal vein thrombus and eventually died of this complication. This patient was the only one with an MPD in our study to experience documented recurrent thrombosis. It occurred more than 10 years after the institution of antiplatelet therapy and developed in the setting of liver dysfunction from recurrent hepatitis C and chronic rejection.

Case 16—Unclassified Myeloproliferative Disorder and Factor V Leiden

A 36-year-old white woman presented with a 1-year history of nausea and vomiting and intermittent right upper quadrant pain. Her only medication at the time of presentation in March 1997 was an oral contraceptive. Hepatic venogram showed thrombosed hepatic veins.

Bone marrow examination disclosed a 75% cellular specimen, megakaryocytic hyperplasia with clustering, and an increase in reticulin. She was believed to have an early MPD of unclassified type. A DNA assay for factor V Leiden mutation was reported as heterozygous positive.

The patient underwent OLT in October 1998. Native liver pathology confirmed hepatic vein thrombosis. Hydroxyurea and aspirin were continued after surgery. Anagrelide was substituted subsequently because of the development of anemia on hydroxyurea. She is currently doing well 11 months after OLT with no evidence of recurrent thrombosis.

This patient had evidence of an MPD and also factor V Leiden mutation. Combinations of MPDs and other hypercoagulable states have been reported.[25,27-29] The factor V Leiden mutation was recognized in patients with BCS in 1997.[27] Homozygous factor V Leiden has also been described as the cause of BCS.[30-32] Therefore, it is important to perform a thorough hypercoagulable workup in addition to a bone marrow evaluation in patients with BCS.

Oral contraceptives, pregnancy, and the postpartum state may be risk factors for BCS.[23,33,34] Valla and colleagues[34] examined 33 women with BCS who were 15 to 45 years of age and found that 21 had underlying MPDs or suspected early MPDs on the basis of the spontaneous proliferation of erythroid progenitor cells of colony-forming assays. Fifty-four percent of these women were oral contraceptive users, and their relative risk of developing BCS was 2.37 when compared to controls. In another report, Valla and colleagues[34] noted a female preponderance of BCS in patients younger than 50 years and suggested that this finding may be related to the thrombogenic effect of estrogen. Of the 11 women in our study younger than 45 years of age, 4 were taking oral contraceptives (36%) and 1 (patient 8) had delivered a child only 2 months before the onset of symptoms.

Case 17—Prothrombin Gene Mutation

This 25-year-old man from Israel was transferred to our institution for urgent OLT as a result of refractory ascites, renal insufficiency, and hepatic encephalopathy. The patient was first diagnosed with BCS 18 months previously when he presented with ascites. Hematological evaluation, including bone marrow examination, was negative for MPDs. Warfarin therapy was initiated. Multiple surgical procedures were unsuccessful in controlling the ascites. Evaluation at Baylor University Medical Center in Dallas disclosed normal bone marrow. However, a G20210A mutation of the prothrombin gene was detected. Other hypercoagulable studies were negative.

The patient underwent OLT in March 2000 and returned to Israel 1 month after OLT in good condition. He was not given hydroxyurea or warfarin after transplantation because it is probable that the hypercoagulable defect was corrected by the liver allograft. The prothrombin gene mutation has been reported in patients with BCS,[35,36] but its incidence is unknown. Interestingly, this condition can be detected even after OLT, because the test is performed on DNA from leukocytes.

Case 15—Sarcoidosis

This 44-year-old black man received a transplant because of BCS 3.5 years after elevated liver biochemistry values were detected. Six months before OLT, liver function worsened and a Doppler study disclosed thrombosis of the hepatic veins. Hypercoagulable workup and bone marrow examination were negative. OLT was performed in January 1997. Native liver pathology revealed noncaseating granulomas that compressed veins within the liver and thrombosis of the hepatic veins. Special stains for acid-fast bacilli and fungi were negative. The diagnosis of sarcoidosis was made, and the patient did well after OLT. To the best of our knowledge, this is only the third reported case of sarcoid involvement of the liver causing BCS.[39,40] In this circumstance, neither warfarin nor antiplatelet therapy was given to prevent recurrent thrombosis because the granulomas that compressed the hepatic veins were removed.

Summary

Thorough evaluation will establish the cause of hepatic vein thrombosis in nearly all patients who present with BCS. In Western countries, MPDs and other definable hypercoagulable states account for the majority of BCS. Treatment of patients with MPDs using hydroxyurea and aspirin appears to be a safe and effective regimen, without exposing them to the risks of anticoagulation with warfarin. Anagrelide may be preferable to hydroxyurea in certain patients. After transplantation, patients can continue antiplatelet therapy when undergoing liver biopsy to monitor allograft function, which is another major advantage of this approach. Some patients who present with BCS require warfarin therapy after OLT. The type of antithrombotic therapy used should be based on the cause of the BCS. Patients in whom there is correction of the hypercoagulable state by liver allografting probably do not require anticoagulation or other antithrombotic treatment.

Pearls and Pitfalls

- Clinical presentation depends on the extent and rapidity of hepatic venous outflow obstruction.
- Imaging studies show:
  - Hypertrophied caudate lobe
  - Spiderweb pattern of hepatic veins
- Complete hematological evaluation, including bone marrow examination, should be performed. Many, perhaps most, patients with BCS in Western countries have underlying MPDs.
- Optimal antithrombotic therapy depends on the cause.

References

1. Budd G: Diseases of the liver, 1st ed. London, John Churchill, 1845, pp 136-148.
2. Osler W: Case of obstruction of vena cava inferior, with great stenosis of orifices of hepatic veins. J Anat Physiol 13:291-304, 1879.
3. Chiari H: Ueber die selbstandige Phlebitis Obliterans der Haupstamme der venae hepaticae als Todesursache. Beitr Path Anat 26:1-18, 1899.
4. Shaked A, Goldstein R: Transplantation for Budd-Chiari syndrome. In Busuttil RW, Klintmalm GB (eds): Transplantation of the Liver. Philadelphia, Saunders, 1996, pp 138-144.
5. Sherlock S, Dooley J: Diseases of the Liver and Biliary System, 11th ed. Oxford, Blackwell Science Ltd., 2002, pp 192-198.
6. Tilanus HW: Budd-Chiari syndrome. Br J Surg 82:1023-1030, 1995.
7. Wang ZG, Jones RS: Budd-Chiari syndrome. Curr Probl Surg 33:83-211, 1996.
8. Melear JM, Goldstein RM, Levy MF, et al: Hematologic aspects of liver transplantation for Budd-Chiari syndrome with special reference to myeloproliferative disorders. Transplantation 74:1090-1095, 2002.
9. Powell-Jackson PR, Melia W, Canalese J, et al: Budd-Chiari syndrome: Clinical patterns and therapy. QJM 201:79-88, 1982.
10. Mitchell MA, Boitnott JK, Kaufman S, et al: Budd-Chiari syndrome: Etiology, diagnosis and management. Medicine 61:199-218, 1982.
11. McDermott WV, Ridker PM: The Budd-Chiari syndrome and hepatic venoocclusive disease: Recognition and treatment. Arch Surg 125:525-527, 1990.
12. Halff G, Todo S, Tzakis AG, et al: Liver transplantation for the Budd-Chiari syndrome. Ann Surg 211:43-49, 1990.
13. Klein AS, Cameron JL: Diagnosis and management of the Budd-Chiari syndrome. Am J Surg 160:128-133, 1990.
14. Langnas AN, Sorrell MF: The Budd-Chiari syndrome: A therapeutic Gordian knot? Semin Liver Dis 13:352-359, 1993.
15. Dilwari JB, Bambery P, Chawla Y, et al: Hepatic outflow obstruction (Budd-Chiari syndrome): Experience with 177 patients and a review of the literature. Medicine 73:21-36, 1994.
16. Mahmoud AE, Mendoza A, Meshikhes AN, et al: Clinical spectrum, investigations and treatment of Budd-Chiari syndrome. QJM 89:37-43, 1996.

17. Faust TW: Budd-Chiari syndrome. Curr Treat Options Gastroenterol 2:491-504, 1999.
18. Singh V, Sinha SK, Nain CK, et al: Budd-Chiari syndrome: Our experience of 71 patients. J Gastroenterol Hepatol 15:550-554, 2000.
19. Orloff MJ, Daily PO, Orloff SL, et al: A 27-year experience with surgical treatment of Budd-Chiari syndrome. Ann Surg 232: 340-352, 2000.
20. Slakey DP, Klein AS, Venbrux AC, et al: Budd-Chiari syndrome: Current management options. Ann Surg 233:522-527, 2001.
21. Srinivasan P, Rela M, Prachalias A, et al: Liver transplantation for Budd-Chiari syndrome. Transplantation 73:973-977, 2002.
22. Valla DC: Hepatic vein thrombosis (Budd-Chiari syndrome). Semin Liver Dis 22:5-14, 2002.
23. Valla D, Casadelvall N, Lacombe C, et al: Primary myeloproliferative disorder and hepatic vein thrombosis. Ann Intern Med 103:329-334, 1985.
24. De Stefano V, Teofili L, Leone G, et al: Spontaneous erythroid colony formation as the clue to an underlying myeloproliferative disorder in patients with Budd-Chiari syndrome or portal vein thrombosis. Semin Thromb Hemost 23:411-418, 1997.
25. Hirshberg B, Shouval D, Fibach E, et al: Flow cytometric analysis of autonomous growth of erythroid precursors in liquid culture detects occult polycythemia vera in the Budd-Chiari syndrome. J Hepatol 32:574-578, 2000.
26. Goldstein R, Clark P, Klintmalm G, et al: Prevention of recurrent thrombosis following liver transplantation for Budd-Chiari syndrome associated with myeloproliferative disorders: Treatment with hydroxyurea and aspirin. Transplant Proc 23:1559-1560, 1991.
27. Mahmoud AE, Elias E, Beauchamp N, et al: Prevalence of the factor V Leiden mutation in hepatic and portal vein thrombosis. Gut 40:798-800, 1997.
28. Hoffman R, Nimer A, Lanir N, et al: Budd-Chiari syndrome associated with factor V Leiden mutation: A report of 6 patients. Liver Transpl Surg 5:96-100, 1999.
29. Janssen HL, Meinardi JR, Vleggaar FP, et al: Factor V Leiden mutation, prothrombin gene mutation, and deficiencies in coagulation inhibitors associated with Budd-Chiari syndrome and portal vein thrombosis: Results of a case-control study. Blood 96:2364-2368, 2000.
30. Tan HP, Markowitz JS, Maley WR, et al: Successful liver transplantation in a patient with Budd-Chiari syndrome caused by homozygous factor V Leiden. Liver Transpl 6:654-656, 2000.
31. Garewal GG, Das R, Chawla Y, et al: Budd-Chiari syndrome associated with homozygous factor V Leiden mutation. Br J Haematol 105:842, 1999.
32. Leebek FW, Lameris JS, Van Buuren HR, et al: Budd-Chiari syndrome, portal vein and mesenteric vein thrombosis in a patient homozygous for factor V Leiden mutation treated by TIPS and thrombolysis. Br J Haematol 102:929-931, 1998.
33. Maddrey W: Hepatic vein thrombosis (Budd-Chiari syndrome): Possible association with the use of oral contraceptives. Semin Liver Dis 7:32-39, 1987.
34. Valla D, Le MG, Poynard T, et al: Risk of hepatic vein thrombosis in relation to recent use of oral contraceptives: A case control study. Gastroenterology 90:807-811, 1986.
35. Oner AF, Arslan S, Caksen H, et al: Budd-Chiari syndrome in a patient heterozygous for both factor V Leiden and the G20210A mutation on the prothrombin gene. Thromb Haemost 82:1366-1367, 1999.
36. Buccairelli P, Franchi F, Alatri A, et al: Budd-Chiari syndrome in a patient heterozygous for the G20210A mutation on the prothrombin gene. Thromb Haemost 79:445-446, 1998.
37. Junge U, Wienke J, Shuler A: Acute Budd-Chiari syndrome, portal and splenic vein thrombosis in a patient with ulcerative colitis associated with antiphospholipid antibodies and protein C deficiency. Z Gastroenterol 39:845-852, 2001.
38. Espinosa G, Font J, Garcia-Pagan JC, et al: Budd-Chiari syndrome secondary to antiphospholipid syndrome. Medicine 80:345-354, 2001.
39. Nataline MR, Goyette RE, Owensby LC, et al: The Budd-Chiari syndrome in sarcoidosis. JAMA 239:2657-2658, 1978.
40. Russi EW, Bansky G, Pfaltz M, et al: Budd-Chiari syndrome in sarcoidosis. Gastroenterology 81:71-75, 1986.
41. Kage M, Arakawa M, Kojiro M, et al: Histopathology of membranous obstruction of the inferior vena cava in the BCS. Gastroenterology 102:2081-2090, 1992.
42. Kumar S, DeLeve LD, Kamath PS, et al: Hepatic veno-occlusive disease (sinusoidal obstruction syndrome) after hematopoietic stem cell transplantation. Mayo Clin Proc 78:589-598, 2003.
43. Ludwig J, Hashimoto E, McGill DB, et al: Classification of hepatic venous outflow obstruction: Ambiguous terminology of the Budd-Chiari syndrome. Mayo Clin Proc 65:51-55, 1990.
44. Powell-Jackson PR, Ede RJ, Williams R: The BCS presenting as fulminant liver failure. Gut 27:1101-1105, 1986.
45. McKusick MS: Imaging findings in Budd-Chiari syndrome. Liver Transpl 7:743-744, 2001.
46. Noone TC, Semelka RC, Siegalman ES, et al: Budd-Chiari syndrome: Spectrum of appearances of acute, subacute, and chronic disease with magnetic resonance imaging. J Magn Reson Imaging 11:44-50, 2000.
47. Brunning RD, McKenna RW: Chronic myeloproliferative diseases. Atlas of tumor pathology: Tumors of the bone marrow. Washington, DC, Armed Forces Institute of Pathology, 1993, pp 193-254.
48. Michiels JJ, Juvonen E: Proposal for revised diagnostic criteria of essential thrombocythemia and polycythemia vera by the thrombocythemia vera study group. Semin Thromb Hemost 23:339-347, 1997.
49. Putnam CW, Porter KA, Weil R, et al: Liver transplantation for Budd-Chiari syndrome. JAMA 236:1142-1143, 1976.
50. Orloff MJ, Orloff MS, Daily PO: Long-term results of treatment of BCS with portal decompression. Arch Surg 127:1182-1188, 1992.
51. Shaked A, Goldstein RM, Klintmalm GB, et al: Portosystemic shunt versus liver transplantation for the BCS. Surg Gynecol Obstet 17:453-459, 1992.
52. Bismuth H, Sherlock DJ: Portasystemic shunting versus liver transplantation for the BCS. Ann Surg 214:581-589, 1991.
53. Zeitoun G, Escolando S, Hadengue A, et al: Outcome of the Budd-Chiari syndrome: A multivariate analysis of factors related to survival including surgical portosystemic shunting. Hepatology 30:84-89, 1999.
54. Campbell DA Jr, Rolles K, Jamieson N, et al: Hepatic transplantation with perioperative and long-term anticoagulation as treatment for Budd-Chiari syndrome. Surg Gynecol Obstet 166: 511-518, 1988.
55. Ahn SS, Yellin A, Sheng FC, et al: Selective surgical therapy of the BCS provides superior rates than conservative medical treatment. J Vasc Surg 5:28-37, 1987.
56. Oldhafer KJ, Ringe K, Wittekind C, et al: BCS: Portocaval shunt and subsequent liver transplantation. Surgery 107:471-474, 1990.
57. Henderson JM, Warren WD, Milikan JW Jr, et al: Surgical options, hematologic evaluation, and pathologic changes in BCS. Am J Surg 159:41-50, 1990.
58. Orloff M, Girard B: Long term results of treatment of BCS by side-to-side portocaval shunt. Surg Gynecol Obstet 168:33-41, 1989.
59. Vons C, Bourstyn E, Bonnet P, et al: Results of portal systemic shunts in BCS. Ann Surg 203:366-370, 1986.
60. Nakamura T, Nakamura S, Aikawa T, et al: Obstruction of the inferior vena cava in the hepatic portion and the hepatic veins. Angiology 19:479-498, 1968.
61. Van der Merve CF, Arts MS: Primary liver cancer in the Transvaal. Hepatogastroenterology 28:233-235, 1981.
62. Burtch GD, Merion RM: Transdiaphragmatic exposure for direct atrial-caval anastomosis in liver transplantation for BCS. Transplantation 48:161-163, 1989.

63. Carrel T, Decurtins M, Laske A, et al: Liver transplantation with atrioatrial anastomosis for the BCS. Ann Thorac Surg 50:658-660, 1990.
64. Shaked A, Busuttil RW: Liver transplantation in patients with portal vein thrombosis and central portocaval shunts. Ann Surg 214:696-702, 1991.
65. Nonami T, Yokoyama I, Iwatsuki S, et al: The incidence of portal vein thrombosis at liver transplantation. Hepatology 16:1195-1198, 1992.
66. Committee for the European Liver Transplant Registry. European Live Transplant Registry 1989. Paris, Hospital Paul Brousse, 1989.
67. Bresson-Hadni S, Franza A, Miguet JP, et al: Orthotopic liver transplantation for incurable alveolar echinococcosis of the liver. Report of 17 cases. Hepatology 13:1061-1070, 1990.
68. Seltman HJ, Dekker A, Van Thiel DH, et al: Budd-Chiari syndrome recurring in a transplanted liver. Gastroenterology 84:640-643, 1983.
69. Knoop M, Lemmens HP, Bechstein WO, et al: Treatment of the Budd-Chiari syndrome with orthotopic liver transplantation and long-term anticoagulation. Clin Transplant 8:67-72, 1994.
70. Schattenfroh N, Bechstein WO, Blumhardt G, et al: Liver transplantation for PNH with Budd-Chiari syndrome. Transpl Int 6:354-358, 1993.
71. Rückert JC, Rückert RI, Rudolph B, et al: Recurrence of the Budd-Chiari syndrome after orthotopic liver transplantation. Hepatogastroenterology 46:867-871, 1999.
72. Rao ARN, Chui AKK, Gurkhan A, et al: Orthotopic liver transplantation for treatment of patients with Budd-Chiari syndrome: A single-center experience. Transplant Proc 32:2206-2207, 2000.
73. Malkowski P, Michalowicz B, Pawlak J, et al: Liver transplantation in patients with Budd-Chiari syndrome. Transplant Proc 34:629-630, 2002.
74. Ulrich F, Steinmüller T, Lang M, et al: Liver transplantation in patients with advanced Budd-Chiari syndrome. Transplant Proc 34:2278, 2002.
75. Kitchens CS: Venous thromboses in unusual sites. In Kitchens CS, Alving BM, Kessler CM (eds): Consultative Hemostasis and Thrombosis. Philadelphia, Saunders, 2002, pp 232-234.
76. Pagliuca A, Mufti GJ, Janossa-Tahernia M, et al: In vitro colony culture and chromosomal studies in hepatic and portal vein thrombosis—possible evidence of an occult myeloproliferative state. QJM, New Series 76:981-989, 1990.
77. Saigal S, Norria S, Srinivasan P, et al: Successful outcome of orthotopic liver transplantation in patients with preexisting malignant states. Liver Transpl 7:11-15, 2001.
78. Bahr MJ, Rosenau J, Tietge UJF, et al: Immunosuppression and the prognosis of patients suffering from myeloproliferative disorders after liver transplantation. Transplant Proc 34:1493-1494, 2002.
79. Ganguli SC, Ramzan NN, McKusick MA, et al: Budd-Chiari Syndrome in patients with hematological disease: A therapeutic challenge. Hepatology 27:1157-1161, 1998.

Liver Transplantation for Alcoholic Liver Disease

ROBERT M. WEINRIEB
MICHAEL R. LUCEY

Historical perspective   266

Current status of liver transplantation for alcoholic liver disease   266

National Institutes of Health Workshop: Liver transplantation for alcoholic liver disease   266
Factors increasing or diminishing the risk of developing alcoholic liver disease   267
The use of diagnostic criteria   267
Referral biases for liver transplantation of patients with alcoholic liver disease   268
Quality of life in patients undergoing transplantation for alcoholic liver disease   268
Rate of posttransplant alcohol relapse   268
Studies of treatment for alcoholism in liver transplant patients   269

Treatment of alcoholism: An overview   270
Alcoholism treatment in the liver transplant setting   270
An approach to the alcoholic liver transplant recipient   271

Approximately 4% of women and 11% of men in the United States are either problem drinkers or are addicted to alcohol.[1] Unfortunately, less than 10% of alcoholics are receiving alcoholism treatment at any given time.[2] The aggregate financial cost of alcoholism to our society is estimated to exceed $200 billion per year because of treatment costs, lost wages, motor vehicle accidents, legal fees, and alcohol-related medical care.[3] End-stage liver disease is one of the most financially, physically, and psychologically debilitating effects of alcohol misuse. Nearly 20% of men who drink between 80 g and 100 g of alcohol (8 drinks) per day, or women who drink as little as 20 g (2 drinks) per day for more than 10 years have the greatest risk of developing cirrhosis.[4] Although alcoholism is currently the second most common cause of end-stage liver disease that necessitates liver transplantation in the United States, there is considerable overlap with the prevailing cause of end-stage liver disease, which is hepatitis C virus (HCV) infection.[5] Furthermore, alcoholics infected with HCV are thought to be at risk of accelerating the development of end-stage liver disease because of the synergistically damaging effects of alcohol and HCV to the liver.[6] Liver transplantation is often the only option for survival when individuals reach end-stage liver failure. Patient and graft survival after liver transplantation in patients with alcoholic liver disease are as good or better than for many other indications.

Historical Perspective

Liver transplantation was first recognized as an appropriate treatment for advanced liver disease at the National Institutes of Health (NIH) Consensus Development Conference in 1983.[7] Ostensibly, the NIH's acceptance of alcoholics for liver transplantation was predicated on the assumption that very few alcoholics would ever meet the medical and psychosocial criteria necessary for transplant candidacy.[7] In 1988, Starzl reported a 1- to 3-year survival rate of 68% in a cohort of 41 alcoholics who underwent transplantation and were treated during the cyclosporine era, which was similar to the survival rate of recipients who had undergone transplantation for diseases other than alcoholic liver disease (ALD) over the same period.[8] Furthermore, only 2 of the 35 surviving alcoholic liver transplant recipients were thought to have returned to drinking, thus prompting Dr. Starzl to remark that "liver transplantation was the ultimate sobering experience."[8]

That alcoholics could be eligible to receive as costly and limited a resource as a liver transplant instead of patients who required transplant "through no fault of their own," has provoked a continuing debate regarding the moral and ethical issues raised by Starzl's unconventional use of the liver transplant procedure. Much of the debate has focused on the significance of sobriety in the alcoholic patient in need of liver transplantation and what duration of abstinence constitutes a reasonable requirement as a prerequisite to transplantation. This is well shown by the landmark case of *Allen versus Mansour*. The presiding judge of the United States District Court ruled that the 2-year abstinence requirement mandated by Medicaid was "arbitrary and unreasonable," because such a proscription might reasonably exceed the life span of an alcoholic patient who would die without a liver transplant.[9] The judge challenged the transplant community to develop reasonable guidelines for the provision of liver transplantation to alcoholics that did not compromise the lives of the patients or the integrity of the medical community.

Current Status of Liver Transplantation for Alcoholic Liver Disease

ALD is the most common or second most common diagnosis in patients undergoing liver transplantation in North America and Europe. The outcome of these highly selected patients is excellent. One-year and 5-year survival rates are approximately 85% and 60%, respectively, and are similar among alcoholics and nonalcoholics.[10-17] Furthermore, there is a significant survival advantage in alcoholics with transplants compared with alcoholic patients who were refused transplants on psychiatric grounds in uncontrolled studies.[11]

The ideal time for transplantation of patients with ALD is based on a balance of outcome from medical management compared with the outcome of liver transplantation. In the absence of randomized, controlled clinical trials, Poynard estimated the efficacy of liver transplantation for alcoholic cirrhosis using matched and simulated controls.[18] There was a significant benefit among patients with advanced cirrhosis (class C, 11 to 15 points, on the Child-Pugh scoring system) only. In patients with medium risk (class B, 8 to 10 points, on the Child-Pugh scoring system) there was no significant survival difference in comparison to controls. Poynard's data would suggest that liver transplantation be confined to patients with advanced alcoholic liver failure.

The data cited in the previous paragraph refer to decompensated and compensated alcoholic cirrhosis. Acute alcoholic hepatitis presents particular difficulties in this summary because it is associated with features of decompensated liver failure and because some patients recover with abstinence. Severe acute alcoholic hepatitis has a poor outcome with standard supportive management. The mortality rate of the patients with severe alcoholic hepatitis was 35% and 46% in two studies.[19,20] The addition of acute renal failure further worsens the prognosis.[21] However, data do not exist on the chance of success with transplantation for patients affected by acute alcoholic hepatitis. Conversely, Veldt and colleagues suggested that failure to recover from acute alcoholic hepatitis after 3 months of abstinence indicates that spontaneous recovery is unlikely and that transplantation should become a consideration in persons who maintain 3 months of abstinence without resolution of decompensation.[22]

National Institutes of Health Workshop: Liver Transplantation for Alcoholic Liver Disease

In 1996, the NIH National Institute on Diabetes and Digestive and Kidney Diseases, together with the National Institute on Alcohol Abuse and Alcoholism, sponsored a 2-day workshop entitled "Liver Transplantation for Alcoholic Liver Disease" in which the major issues of liver transplantation for alcoholics were presented and discussed in a public forum.[23] The organizers concluded the meeting with an executive statement and recommendations for areas of further research related to ALD. Table 19-1 contains the six items suggested by the workshop. This chapter reviews the degree that the transplant community has addressed these six areas of study in subsequent years.

Table 19-1. AREAS OF STUDY PROPOSED BY NIDDK/NIAAA WORKSHOP IN 1996

1. Clinical or natural history studies on factors increasing or diminishing the risk of developing ALD

2. The use of strict and widely applicable diagnostic criteria for alcohol abuse and dependence to provide reliable information on the proportion of patients receiving transplants for ALD

3. Investigations into the reasons for referral or lack of referral for liver transplantation of patients with ALD

4. Evaluation of quality of life in patients undergoing transplantation for ALD

5. The accurate determination of posttransplant alcohol relapse, using definitions in practice in the addiction literature

6. Studies of treatment for alcoholism in liver transplant patients

ALD, alcoholic liver disease; NIAAA, National Institute on Alcohol Abuse and Alcoholism;
NIDDK, National Institute of Diabetes and Digestive and Kidney Diseases.
From Hoofnagle JH, Kresina T, Fuller RK, et al: Liver transplantation for alcoholic liver disease: Executive statement and recommendations. Summary of a National Institutes of Health workshop held December 6-7, 1996, Bethesda, Md, Liver Transpl Surg 3:347-350, 1997.

Factors Increasing or Diminishing the Risk of Developing Alcoholic Liver Disease

There have been major advances in our basic understanding of alcohol-mediated liver injury since 1996. Acetaldehyde is proposed as the primary ethanol metabolite agent that leads to alcohol-induced liver damage.[24] The immune response to acetaldehyde delivery, and the hypermetabolic state caused by increased oxygen consumption secondary to perturbance of the nicotinamide-adenine dinucleotide (reduced form)/nicotinamide-adenine dinucleotide (NADH/NAD) ratio may be crucial developing steps. Oxidative stress has also been implicated in alcohol-induced tissue damage, because administration of alcohol to healthy humans leads to the generation of reactive oxygen species (products of lipid peroxidation), and acute alcoholic hepatitis is a condition of marked oxidative stress.[25] Oxidative stress in ALD is caused by pro-oxidant formation, by inadequate intake of antioxidants, and by alcohol's inhibition of glutathione synthesis. The pro-oxidants involved in alcohol-induced liver disease are reactive oxygen species (ROS) and reactive nitrogen species (RNS). The sources for these antioxidants include mitochondria and cytochrome P450 (CYP) 2E1 in hepatocytes, NAD(p)H in oxidases, and induced nitric oxide synthase (iNOS) in inflammatory cells. Some studies show that iNOS knockout mice are

protected completely against oxidative stress caused by ethanol.[26] Activation of Kupffer cells is an important element in the sequence of events leading to alcoholic liver injury. Circulating endotoxin levels, which are increased after alcohol intake, may activate Kupffer cells.[27]

Fibrogenesis within the liver is a consequence of activation of collagen-producing stellate cells. The pathway leading to the activation of stellate cells is not certain and may include a number of simultaneous processes such as direct injury from reactive oxidative species or through intermediate steps, which include the expression of interleukins (ILs) such as tumor necrosis factor-α (TNF-α), IL1, IL6, IL8, and the transforming growth factors. The profile of cytokine released in response to alcohol, lipid peroxidation/oxidant stress, circulating endotoxin, and Kupffer cell activation is influenced by genetic polymorphisms.[28] These observations are of potential importance in the discovery of therapies for ALD, which include antioxidant agents and blocking the release of cytokines and growth factors that precipitate the collagen deposition.[29]

The Use of Diagnostic Criteria

The second recommendation made by the NIH executive committee was for clinicians to implement strict and widely applicable diagnostic criteria regarding alcohol addiction to provide reliable information on the proportion of patients receiving transplants for ALD. To the best of our knowledge, this has not been put into general practice. A survey of 69 U.S. liver transplant programs found that although 83% of centers rely on a psychiatrist or addiction specialist to see each patient with ALD during the evaluation phase, rarely are standardized psychiatric diagnoses reported in the literature.[30] One study found that 71% of patients undergoing liver transplantation for ALD met the Diagnostic and Statistical Manual of Mental Disorders-Fourth Edition (DSM-IV) criteria for *Alcohol Dependence* when standardized criteria were used.[31] This means that almost one third of the patients evaluated in that study either had *Alcohol Abuse*, a less severe form of an alcohol-use disorder than alcohol dependence, or perhaps no diagnosable alcohol use disorder whatsoever.

Alcohol dependence is distinguished from alcohol abuse in the DSM-IV in that dependence is thought of in terms of biological symptoms, such as tolerance and withdrawal, and psychosocial consequences, such as interference with important role obligations.[32] Alcohol abuse is a moderately severe problem compared with alcohol dependence, which has more serious psychosocial and physical consequences. The DSM-IV does not use the amount of alcohol consumed as a criterion for making either diagnosis. By contrast, the National Institute on Alcohol Abuse and Alcoholism (NIAAA) convened a panel of experts at a conference on "Measuring Outcome in Alcohol Treatment Trials" and defined heavy drinking for men as any day of consumption of six or more standard drinks, whereas for women the definition is four or more drinks.[33] For the purposes of the NIAAA definitions, one drink is equivalent to 14 g of alcohol or 12 oz of beer, 4 oz of wine, or 1 oz of distilled spirits. An individual who regularly consumes alcohol in excess of these heavy drinking thresholds is above the 90th percentile for adult alcohol consumption in the United States.

Making a standardized diagnosis of alcohol abuse or dependence in liver transplant patients is important because by the time most patients with ALD are seen for liver transplant evaluation, they have stopped drinking on their own without the benefit of formal alcoholism treatment.[34] For many patients with ALD, quitting drinking on their own often represents a source of great pride; however, it also seems to reinforce for them the misconception that they never really had an alcohol problem. Furthermore, for patients with ALD who are reluctant to be honest with the transplant team for fear of being rejected for transplantation, the failure by the transplant team to make an accurate diagnosis of an alcohol or drug use disorder at the initial transplant evaluation could cause such patients to balk at the opportunity to ask transplant team members for additional support for their substance abuse problem for fear of being rejected for transplantation. Finally, the use of standardized criteria may be the only way to determine whether carrying the diagnosis of abuse versus dependence has differential clinical or prognostic significance. Presumably, patients with alcohol abuse should be at less risk of recidivism than those with dependence, but at this point data are needed to support this contention.

The gold standard for diagnosing psychiatric disorders is the Structured Clinical Interview for the DSM-IV (SCID).[35] Training to properly administer the entire SCID is difficult, and the full instrument takes 45 minutes to 1 hour to administer by experienced diagnosticians. This might explain why so few reports of standardized psychiatric diagnoses are in the transplant literature. The Mini International Neuropsychiatric Interview (MINI)[36] is much easier to learn and can take less than 20 minutes for an experienced clinician to administer to an uncomplicated patient. Perhaps the best way for psychiatric clinicians to abide by the recommendations of the NIH committee would be for them to administer only the alcohol and drug diagnoses modules of the MINI, a process that could take less than 5 minutes.

Referral Biases for Liver Transplantation of Patients with Alcoholic Liver Disease

There are few data regarding referral biases for ALD liver transplantation. We suspect that patients with

ALD in liver transplant centers represent the tip of a very large iceberg. Davies and colleagues retrospectively reviewed referrals for liver transplantation in a community-based hospital in South Wales, United Kingdom and found a failure to refer that was most marked among patients with ALD.[37] This may have changed in the following years, although an opinion survey among the lay public and doctors conducted by the Birmingham, England group showed widespread bias against offering liver transplantation to alcoholics.[38] Although continued drinking or substance abuse is a reasonable and legitimate reason for deferral of transplant evaluation, the effects on transplant eligibility of social support or psychiatric illnesses have not been systematically identified and empirically tested.

Quality of Life in Patients Undergoing Transplantation for Alcoholic Liver Disease

Many studies have shown that carefully selected alcoholics fare as well as nonalcoholics on survival and quality of life indices 1 year to 5 years after transplantation.[39,40] The NIH conference drew on quality of life outcomes in a prospective study using the National Institute of Diabetes and Digestive and Kidney Diseases (NIDDK) Liver Transplant Database (LTD) in which 48 to 50 patients with ALD were compared with 158 to 164 adult liver transplant recipients without ALD.[41] In this study, statistically significant differences in mean scores were found for general health perception, general well being, and the effects and stresses of psychological symptoms in the ALD and non-ALD patients. The authors concluded that patients with ALD had somewhat worse outcomes than those without ALD during the initial 3 years after transplantation. We reviewed the subsequent literature, and, despite follow-ups of approximately 2 years, none of the studies we found replicated the increasing impairment in health-related quality of life indices reported by Wiesner and colleagues.[41] It is not clear why there should be such a discrepancy between the NIH-LTD study and all others. Prospective studies with follow-up of recipients for 5 years or more will be necessary to determine whether quality of life in liver transplant recipients with ALD is worse than in a comparable group of non-ALD liver transplant recipients.

Rate of Posttransplant Alcohol Relapse

The fifth proposal the NIH Executive Committee sought to define was the actual rate of posttransplantation alcohol relapse and to identify predictive factors and consequences of posttransplantation drinking. To evaluate the research that has addressed this question, it is important to understand that there are differences in the way alcoholism treatment and research professionals view a relapse compared with the way in which the majority of transplant treatment providers define it. Before 1990, most alcoholism treatment studies defined *relapse* as any drinking, whether it be a fifth of liquor taken daily for a month or a sip of wine on a person's birthday. In a landmark study using naltrexone to reduce craving for alcohol, relapse was operationally defined as a heavy drinking episode in which a study subject drank more than five drinks in one sitting, drank more than 5 days in a row, or came to a research visit with a positive blood alcohol level. In contrast, a *slip* was defined as one or more isolated incidents in which a study subject did not lose control of his or her drinking. Unlike a slip, research has shown that a relapse of 60 to 90 g of alcohol is a good predictor of acute alcohol-related problems that are associated with harmful consequences to an individual's health and well-being.[42,43] Alcoholism is viewed by substance abuse professionals as a multifactorial, chronic, relapsing disorder in which drinking is likely to occur in a majority of alcoholics, with or without treatment. Thus, when considering clinical management for a patient, making the distinction between a slip and a relapse makes clinical and scientific sense.

Determining the quantity and frequency of drinking in alcoholic liver transplant patients is not an easy task. Most of us in the transplant field have seen that a minor slip in the posttransplant phase does not usually cause harm to the graft, although it should alert the transplant team that the patient is at significant risk of transitioning into a pattern of heavier, more harmful drinking. By contrast, a slip in the pretransplant phase may be far more harmful to a patient. Whether a pretransplant slip predicts posttransplant drinking is not currently known. Indeed, the pretransplant patient who drinks must face the dilemma posed by the following "either/or" questions:

- Do I approach the transplant team for help knowing that telling them puts me at risk of being removed from the waiting list?

- Should I be dishonest by not telling the transplant team and take the chance that I can control my drinking?

We have argued previously that this kind of double-bind dilemma places patients in a potentially dire position in which they face the very real possibility of death as a consequence of their choice to seek care.[44]

Consequently, our review prompts the following question: Are reliable, valid predictors of posttransplant drinking available to guide the clinician in the selection of appropriate liver transplant candidates? The short answer is no. The most extensively studied predictor variable is the *6-month rule.* This is an arbitrary period during which 6 months of alcohol abstinence is required by most transplant programs for liver transplant candidates with ALD to become eligible for the waiting list. Based on clinical experience, participants of the 1996 NIH conference on alcoholism and liver transplantation concurred that 6 months of alcohol abstinence is an ideal time frame for a sufficient return of liver function to obviate the need for liver transplantation in a subset of patients with acute alcoholic hepatitis who were well enough for their livers to rebound. Subsequent to the 1996 conference, Veldt and colleagues showed that failure to recover from severe acute alcoholic hepatitis within 3 months of initiation of abstinence from alcohol carries a poor prognosis for spontaneous recovery.[22] However, consensus on whether the 6-month rule predicts posttransplant abstinence or rates of posttransplant morbidity and mortality was not reached either at or subsequent to the 1996 conference. A review by Tome and colleagues of 21 studies concluded that 20% to 50% of alcoholic patients selected to receive a liver transplant acknowledge some alcohol use in the first 5 years after liver transplantation.[45] More importantly, of those who drank, 10% to 15% resumed heavy drinking (relapsed) and died, injured their graft, or experienced other serious medical problems associated with alcoholism. There are many limitations to the studies included in this composite review. Most were retrospective, short-term, and compromised by a failure to contact representative samples of all patients who had undergone transplantation. Importantly, most studies measured *any* alcohol use—not severe or problematic alcohol use. All studies had problems getting accurate data about drinking. Few studies used breathalyzers or serum alcohol levels, and there is reason to believe that most of the self-reports underestimated actual drinking. In summary, we believe there is insufficient evidence to conclude whether 6 months stable pretransplant abstinence in alcoholic liver transplant patients is an adequate sole criterion to prevent alcohol relapse after transplantation.

Studies of Treatment for Alcoholism in Liver Transplant Patients

At the 1996 NIH workshop, there was a paucity of information on treating alcoholism in liver transplant candidates and recipients. Nevertheless, it was assumed that what was known about alcoholism treatment research outside the transplantation context would be directly applicable to liver transplant patients. By contrast, clinically important differences between non–liver transplant alcoholics and liver-transplant alcoholics were beginning to be recognized by some investigators. For example, Wagner and colleagues[46] pointed out that unlike the majority of alcoholics who do not undergo transplantation, most of the liver transplant alcoholics quit drinking on their own and do not need further intervention. These observations were subsequently validated by a study of alcoholic patients who underwent liver transplantation and who displayed significantly lower measures of motivation for alcoholism treatment, often receiving no alcoholism treatment and not even attending an Alcoholics Anonymous (AA) meeting.[47,48]

Nelson and colleagues recommend that alcoholic liver transplant candidates sign a contract assuring lifelong abstinence from substances of abuse in order to earn a place on the waiting list.[49] This practice was rated as "very important" by 45% of the participants in a survey of 69 U.S. liver transplant programs.[30] Although this form of contingency contracting may have therapeutic benefit, to date there is no research to support or refute such a practice. By comparison, it has been reasoned that making placement on the transplant waiting list contingent on a scientifically unsubstantiated belief is unethical, and given the fact that 20% to 50% of patients return to drinking after liver transplant,[45] it may also be unrealistic. Furthermore, an AA member who refuses to sign a lifelong abstinence contract in order to be eligible for a liver transplant may be expressing legitimate insight into their recovery and not telegraphing any intent to drink in the future.

Treatment of Alcoholism: An Overview

Berglund and colleagues summarized the proceedings of a symposium on the treatment of alcoholism held at the 2002 annual meeting of the Research Society on Alcoholism.[50] A brief description of the findings is given here, but interested readers are urged to read the complete report.[51] We present the findings from three main treatment topics: prevention of hazardous drinking, psychosocial treatment interventions, and pharmacological interventions.

1. *Preventive Interventions*—Twenty-seven randomized studies composed of more than 10,000 persons were assessed. Most of the interventions were based on secondary prevention and carried out in primary care settings by physicians or nurses. More extensive interventions did not consistently result in greater treatment benefits. Brief interventions were shown to be effective in reducing drinking for up to 2 years in most studies.

2. *Psychosocial Interventions*—Sixteen of 23 studies involving psychosocial intervention were evaluable by meta-analyses. The analyses determined that treatment was effective, especially specific treatment derived from theoretical models using standardized methods of treatment delivery (from manuals and systematic supervision). Examples included motivational enhancement therapy, cognitive behavioral therapy, and 12-step

facilitation. One caveat was that most studies evaluated effectiveness between 3 and 12 months only, with occasional contacts after 1 year. In addition to recommending that alcoholism intervention studies be aimed at gauging the stability of treatment success in the long-term, the reviewers suggested that interventions of different intensity and focus be tested according to the severity of an individual's alcohol problem.

Two additional studies found that patients with greater problem severity did better if they received inpatient treatment, whereas patients with less severe problems fared better with outpatient care. In addition these studies found that extensive treatment is more cost-effective than short-term treatment among patients with poor prognostic factors (psychiatric comorbidity or more severe alcohol dependence).[52]

3. *Pharmacological Interventions*—Randomized clinical trials, conducted up to June 2002, were surveyed. Each study was of at least 4 weeks' duration and included at least 15 subjects. A total of 122 published and 15 unpublished studies were reviewed. Four studies compared aversive treatment agents (e.g., disulfiram) with placebo. Only one study showed a positive benefit from this aversive agent, and only when the drug was distributed under supervision.

Acamprosate, whose mechanism of action is not completely understood, is thought to be an N-methyl-D-aspartate (NMDA)/glutamate (glu) antagonist that may reduce the craving for alcohol. Although acamprosate was rejected by the U.S. Food and Drug Administration (FDA) for approval in the United States because of insufficient efficacy, it is widely used in Europe, where it has been studied extensively. A meta-analysis of 15 studies in this review found that using abstinence or any continued drinking as an endpoint, produced an effect size (fixed model) of 0.2. (95% confidence interval [CI], .20 to .32), independent of treatment duration (3 to 12 months), with a negative test of heterogeneity.

Naltrexone and nalmefene are opiate antagonists; naltrexone is FDA approved for the treatment of alcoholism. Of 21 studies (n = 2253), 8 (n = 870) showed positive effects, 2 (n = 255) showed positive effects only in the completers' analyses, and 3 (n = 926) had negative results. In all, the meta-analysis showed an effect size (fixed model), of 0.28 (95% CI, .13 to .44) with a negative test of heterogeneity. Thus, in the short-term treatment of alcohol dependence, naltrexone and acamprosate have confirmed effects, as does disulfiram, if given under supervision.

Alcoholism Treatment in the Liver Transplant Setting

Based on the finding that motivation for alcoholism treatment in liver transplant patients was low,[48] Weinrieb and colleagues chose Motivational Enhancement Therapy (MET) as a nonpharmacological intervention. MET was adapted to the needs of liver transplant recipients and compared with naltrexone and placebo in a three-arm pilot study. Naltrexone was selected because of its ability to reduce craving and to reduce relapse rates in those who slip.[53] We found that only 5 of 60 patients screened for the study consented, and of those, none completed the 6-month posttransplant alcoholism treatment trial. Recruitment was hampered by severe illness, fear of naltrexone-induced hepatotoxicity, and the belief that alcoholism was no longer a problem for the patients. The lack of conviction that alcohol remains a problem mirrors our observations and those of others that craving for alcohol and motivation for treatment occur less among the alcoholics selected for liver transplantation than among their peers who enter conventional alcoholism treatment studies.

The Birmingham group has described a pilot investigation into the feasibility of providing a psychosocial intervention for alcoholism in liver transplant recipients. Georgiou and colleagues evaluated three 1-hour outpatient sessions of Social Behavior and Network Therapy (SBNT), which used techniques of Motivational Interviewing (MI) in 20 alcoholic liver transplant recipients.[54] The focus of the intervention was to foster a positive social network via a supportive person in the alcoholic's life. There were no negative consequences for patients who refused to be in the study. The mean duration of pretransplant abstinence was 29.7 months (range: 6 to 96 months). Measures of alcohol consumption were taken by random self-report and blood alcohol levels before transplant and repeated once 6 months after transplantation. Five patients refused participation, but results were available for 17 of 19 patients who completed the study. Eight patients (42%) reported drinking some alcohol after transplantation. Of those, 4 (21%) drank weekly and 1 (5%) drank more than 21 units per week (1 unit = 10 g ethyl alcohol [EtOH] per drink). Patients who drank were enrolled in an intensive treatment program. Patients also reported that the sessions were less judgmental and more constructive than what they had received in the community. Although the study was not a randomized clinical trial and did not have a control group, the results suggest that alcoholic liver transplant patients are amenable to therapy when it is provided in a nonjudgmental and supportive construct. It is premature to say what form of alcoholism therapy will be most effective in alcoholic liver transplant recipients. Nevertheless, the high rates of drinking while awaiting transplant (approximately 15%) or after transplantation (30% to 50%) and the potential for serious adverse health consequences make it clear that some form of an alcoholism treatment intervention is warranted either before or after transplantation in many alcoholic recipients.

An Approach to the Alcoholic Liver Transplant Recipient

When considering alcoholic liver transplant patients, we believe the focus should be on trying to identify patients at risk. Current knowledge suggests that most alcoholics do not return to drinking after transplantation, and among those that do, the majority will not develop devastating alcohol-related injuries, at least in the short term. The fact that 10% to 15% will suffer grave consequences presents an alarming risk and, therefore, we must continue to give our patients the message that they must strive for total abstinence. As we said previously, many patients make it a point of pride that they quit drinking on their own without the benefit of treatment intervention. Many are also resistant to attending AA meetings because of perceived bad experiences or the fear of expressing themselves in public. On further questioning, however, we have learned that it is not uncommon for patients to resist AA simply because talking about drinking makes them feel vulnerable to drink. In general, we believe that at the time of transplant evaluation, most patients with less than 2 years of sobriety should receive alcoholism treatment. Exceptions to this guideline are patients who have:

- Abstained from alcohol more than 6 months
- No psychiatric or drug use history
- Strong support networks
- No family history of addictions
- No prior alcoholism treatment

Conversely, there will also be people with more than 2 years of sobriety with poor social supports, limited insight into their alcoholism, and a plethora of psychiatric problems for whom a course of alcoholism treatment would be strongly indicated.

Inquiries into a patient's recent use of alcohol or drugs, or both, by transplant team members, blood alcohol level measurements, and urine drug screens for illicit substances at each visit are underused tools. Although transplant recipients may question the value of this approach—because of the misconception that "all alcoholics and drug addicts lie"—in fact, many recovering persons would welcome this approach as another method of support in their struggle to maintain sobriety. This should be as routine as a blood pressure check or blood glucose monitoring. For patients who admit to using alcohol who are on the waiting list or are being evaluated for transplant, the transplant team must take care not to shame the patient into addiction treatment. Patients are keenly aware of the risks of being removed from the transplant list for being honest about their problems; therefore, we must respect the courage it takes for them to tell us about their use and do everything we can to assist them in obtaining addiction treatment without the fear of losing every opportunity for a transplant. Although such patients require additional time and effort by the transplant team, this approach cultivates trust between the patient and the transplant team because it shows the patient that the transplant team is both fair and open-minded. We believe that to remove an addicted patient permanently from the waiting list for a slip or relapse without any opportunity for recovery is unethical and hypocritical. Addiction, after all, is a chronic, relapsing disorder; if we accept addicts onto our transplant list, we should treat them accordingly.

Finally, we and others have found that depression, anxiety, medication adherence, job counseling, family therapy, and financial counseling are also important areas of intervention in end-stage liver disease patients with alcohol use disorders. The importance of maintaining stability in these areas of a patient's life to their addiction recovery cannot be overstated. In summary, being a liver transplant treatment provider means taking on the care of alcoholics and drug addicts, a task requiring sensitivity and specialized knowledge and experience.

Pearls and Pitfalls

- Every evaluation for liver transplantation should include careful assessment by a specialist in addiction medicine, and alcohol dependence or abuse should be diagnosed by strict criteria whenever appropriate.

- The utility of the 6-month abstinence rule as a predictor of future drinking is not well established.

- Alcoholism treatment should be selected on a case-by-case basis, but many candidates with less than 2 years of sobriety should be referred for alcoholism treatment.

- Alcoholism relapse should be defined by severity and distinguished from slips. All slips should trigger reassessment and referral for therapy, when necessary.

- We do not know how many alcoholics with liver disease are screened out before they reach a liver transplant center.

- Alcoholics awaiting or following transplantation often do not acknowledge any ongoing craving for alcohol and show low motivation for alcohol use treatment.

- Up to 50% of alcoholic liver transplant recipients will use some alcohol in the first 5 years after transplantation; 10% to 15% relapse into addictive or harmful drinking.

References

1. Grant B: Epidemiologic Bulletin No. 35: Prevalence of DSM-IV alcohol abuse and dependence, United States 1992. Alcohol Health Res World 3:243-248, 1994.
2. Sparks R, Babor R, Blum R, et al: Broadening the base of treatment for alcohol problems: Report of a study by a committee of the Institute of Medicine, Division of Mental Health and Behavioral Medicine. Washington, DC, National Academy Press, 1990.
3. Harwood H, Kristiansen P, Rachel J, et al: Social and economic costs of alcohol abuse and alcoholism, Research Park Triangle, NC, Research Triangle Institute, 1985.
4. Bellentani S, Tiribelli C, Saccoccio G, et al: Prevalence of chronic liver disease in the general population of northern Italy: The Dionysus study. Hepatology 20:1442-1449, 1994.
5. Anonymous: The United Network of Organ Sharing, 2004. See http://www.UNOS.org
6. Wiley T, McCarthy M, Breidi L, et al: Impact of alcohol on the histological and clinical progression of hepatitis C infection. Hepatology 28:805-809, 1998.
7. Scharschmidt BF: Human liver transplantation: Analysis of data on 540 patients from four centers. Hepatology 4(Suppl):95S-101S, 1984.
8. Starzl TE, Van TD, Tzakis AG, et al: Orthotopic liver transplantation for alcoholic cirrhosis. JAMA 260:2542-2544, 1988.
9. *Allen v Mansour*, in Federal Suppl 681, District Court for the Eastern District of Michigan, Southern Division, 1986, pp 1232-1239.
10. Lucey MR, Carr K, Beresford TP, et al: Alcohol use after liver transplantation in alcoholics: A clinical cohort follow-up study. Hepatology 25:1223-1227, 1997.
11. Lucey MR, Merion RM, Henley KS, et al: Selection for and outcome of liver transplantation in alcoholic liver disease. Gastroenterology 10:1736-1741, 1992.
12. Kumar S, Stauber RE, Gavaler JS, et al: Orthotopic liver transplantation for alcoholic liver disease. Hepatology 11:159-164, 1990.
13. Knechtle SJ, Fleming MF, Barry KL, et al: Liver Transplantation in alcoholics: Assessment of psychological health and work activity. Transplant Proc 25:1916-1918, 1993.
14. Gish R, Lee A, Keefe E, et al: Liver transplantation for patients with alcoholism and end-stage liver disease. Am J Gastroenterol 88:1337-1342, 1993.
15. Neuberger J, Schulz K, Day C, et al: Transplantation for alcoholic liver disease. J Hepatol 36:130-137, 2002.
16. Pageaux G, Michel J, Coste V, et al: Alcoholic cirrhosis is a good indication for liver transplantation, even for cases of recidivism. Gut 45:421-426 1999.
17. Bellamy C, DiMartini A, Ruppert K, et al: Liver transplantation for alcoholic cirrhosis: Long term follow-up and impact of disease recurrence. Transplantation 27:619-626, 2001.
18. Poynard T, Naveau S, Doffoel M, et al: Evaluation of efficacy of liver transplantation in alcoholic cirrhosis using matched and simulated controls: 5-year survival. Multi-centre group. J Hepatol 30:1130-1137, 1999.
19. Akriviadis E, Botla R, Briggs W, et al: Pentoxifylline improves short-term survival in severe acute alcoholic hepatitis: A double-blind, placebo-controlled trial. Gastroenterology 119:1637-1648, 2000.
20. Carithers RJ, Herlong H, Diehl A, et al: Methylprednisolone therapy in patients with severe alcoholic hepatitis. A randomized multicenter trial. Ann Intern Med 110:685-690, 1989.
21. Mutimer D, Burra P, Neuberger J, et al: Managing severe alcoholic hepatitis complicated by renal failure. QJM 86:649-656, 1993.
22. Veldt B, Laine F, Guillygomarc'h A, et al: Indication of liver transplantation in severe alcoholic liver cirrhosis: Quantitative evaluation and optimal timing. J Hepatol 36:93-98, 2002.

23. Hoofnagle JH, Kresina T, Fuller RK, et al: Liver transplantation for alcoholic liver disease: Executive statement and recommendations. Summary of a National Institutes of Health workshop held December 6-7, 1996, Bethesda, Md. Liver Transpl Surg 3:347-350, 1997.

24. Lieber C: Biochemical factors in alcoholic liver disease. Semin Liver Dis 13:136-153, 1993.

25. Meagher E, Barry O, Burke A, et al: Alcohol-induced generation of lipid peroxidation products in humans. J Clin Invest 104:805-813, 1999.

26. McKim S, Gabele E, Isayama F, et al: Inducible nitric oxide synthase is required in alcohol-induced liver injury: Studies with knockout mice. Gastroenterology 125:1834-1844, 2003.

27. Uesugi T, Froh M, Arteel G, et al: Role of lipopolysaccharide-binding protein in early alcohol-induced liver injury in mice. J Immunol 168:2963-2969, 2002.

28. Grove J, Daly A, Bassendine M, et al: Interleukin 10 promoter region polymorphisms and susceptibility to advanced alcoholic liver disease. Gut 46:540-545, 2000.

29. Tome S, Lucey M: Current management of alcoholic liver disease. Aliment Pharmacol Ther 19:1-8, 2004.

30. Everhart JE, Beresford TP: Liver transplantation for alcoholic liver disease: A survey of transplantation programs in the United States. Liver Transpl Surg 3:220-226, 1997.

31. DiMartini A, Beresford T: Alcoholism and liver transplantation. Curr Opin Organ Transplant 4:117-181, 1999.

32. Staab J, Datto C, Weinrieb R, et al: Detection and diagnosis of psychiatric disorders in primary medical care settings. Med Clin North Am 85:579-596, 2001.

33. Sobell L, Sobell M, Connors G, Agrawal S: Assessing drinking outcomes in alcohol treatment efficacy studies: Selecting a yardstick of success. Alcohol Clin Exp Res 27:1661-1666, 2003.

34. Weinrieb RM, Van Horn DH, McLellan AT, et al: Alcoholism treatment after liver transplantation: Lessons learned from a clinical trial that failed. Psychosomatics 42:110-116, 2001.

35. First M, Spitzer R, Gibbon M, Williams J: Structured Clinical Interview for DSM-IV Axis I Disorders, Version 2.0, Patient Edition (SCID-I/P). New York, Biometrics Research, New York Psychiatric Institute, 1996.

36. Sheehan D, Lecrubier Y, Harnett K, et al: The validity of the Mini International Neuropsychiatric Interview (MINI) according to the SCID-P and its reliability. Eur Psychiatry 12:232-241, 1997.

37. Davies M, Langman M, Elias E, Neuberger J: Liver disease in a district hospital remote from a transplant centre: A study of admissions and deaths. Gut 33:1397-1399, 1992.

38. Neuberger J, Adams D, MacMaster P, et al: Assessing priorities for allocation of donor liver grafts: Survey of public and clinicians. BMJ 317:172-175, 1998.

39. Beresford TP, Schwartz J, Wilson D, et al: The short-term psychological health of alcoholic and non-alcoholic liver transplant recipients. Alcohol Clin Exp Res 16:996-999, 1992.

40. Howard L, Fahy T, Wong P, et al: Psychiatric outcome in alcoholic liver transplant patients. QJM 87:731-736, 1994.

41. Wiesner RH, Lombardero M, Lake J, et al: Liver transplantation for end-stage alcoholic liver disease: An assessment of outcomes. Liver Transpl Surg 3:231-240, 1997.

42. Smith DS, Collins M, Kreisberg JP, et al: Screening for problem drinking in college freshman. J Am Coll Health 36:89-94, 1987.

43. O'Brien C, McLellan A: Myths about the treatment of addiction. Lancet 347:237-240, 1996.

44. Weinrieb R, Van Horn D, Lucey M, McLellan A: Interpreting the significance of drinking by alcohol dependent liver transplant patients: Fostering candor is the key to recovery. Liver Transpl 6:769-776, 2000.

45. Tome S, Lucey M: Timing of liver transplantation in alcoholic cirrhosis. J Hepatol 39:302-307, 2003.

46. Wagner CC, Haller DL, Olbrisch ME: Relapse prevention treatment for liver transplant patients. J Clin Psychol 3:387-398, 1996.

47. DiMartini A, Day N, Dew M, et al: Alcohol use following liver transplantation: A comparison of follow-up methods. Psychosomatics 42:55-62, 2001.

48. Weinrieb RM, Van Horn DH, McLellan AT, et al: Drinking behavior and motivation for treatment among alcohol-dependent liver transplant candidates. J Addict Dis 20:105-119, 2001.

49. Nelson M, Presberg B, Olbrisch M, Levenson J: Behavioral contingency contracting to reduce substance abuse and other high-risk health behaviors in organ transplant patients. J Transpl Coord 5:35-40, 1995.

50. Berglund M, Thelander S, Salaspuro M, et al: Treatment of alcohol abuse: An evidence-based review. Alcohol Clin Exp Res 27:1645-1656, 2003.

51. Berglund M, Johnsson E, Thelander S (eds): Treatment of Alcohol and Drug Abuse: An Evidence-Based Review. Weinheim, UK, Wiley-VCH, 2003.

52. Holder H, Cisler R, Longabaugh R, et al: Alcohol treatment and medical care costs from Project MATCH. Addiction 95:999-1013, 2000.

53. Volpicelli JR, Alterman AI, Hayashida M, O'Brien CP: Naltrexone in the treatment of alcohol dependence. Arch Gen Psychiatry 49:876-880, 1992.

54. Georgiou G, Webb K, Griggs K, et al: First report of a psychosocial intervention for patients with alcohol-related liver disease undergoing liver transplantation. Liver Transpl 9:772-775, 2003.

Unusual Indications for Liver Transplantation

DAVID H. VAN THIEL
AYSE L. MINDIKOGLU
ANANTHARAJU ABHINANDANA
MEHDI BALUCH
SONU DHILLON
MAGDALENE M. GEORGE
JOHN BREMS
S. DAVID LI
RAZA HAMDANI

Inborn errors of metabolism and heritable diseases 276
  Oxalosis 276
  Familial homozygous hypercholesterolemia 276
  Familial amyloid polyneuropathy 277
  Protoporphyria 277
  Deficits in fatty acid metabolism 278
  Urea cycle defects 279
  Cystic fibrosis 279

Acute hepatic failure 279
  Drugs 279
  Infectious agents 279

Vascular disorders 280
  Budd-Chiari syndrome 280
  Giant hemangioma with Kasabach-Merritt syndrome 281
  Hereditary hemorrhagic telangiectasia 281
  Veno-occlusive disease 281

Miscellaneous disorders 281
  Polycystic liver disease 281
  Sarcoidosis 281

Neuroendocrine tumors 282
Diffuse bile duct stenosis/idiopathic adult bile ductopenia 282
Benign hepatic tumors 282
Hepatic lymphangiomatosis 282

Liver transplantation is a widely available and accepted procedure for the treatment of advanced-stage liver disease.[1] The leading indications for liver transplantation in adults are chronic hepatitis C, alcoholic liver disease, and the cholestatic liver diseases primary biliary cirrhosis (PBC) and primary sclerosing cholangitis (PSC).[2] In children, the leading disease indication for liver transplantation is biliary atresia.[3] Liver transplantation is also used as a life-saving procedure in adults and children with acute hepatic failure.[4,5]

In addition to these usual indications for liver transplantation, a great number of unusual indications exist.

These conditions are rarely seen at any given transplant center and, as a result, may not be recognized as an indication for liver transplantation. This chapter identifies specific reasons for liver transplantation in various unusual conditions for which liver transplantation has been shown to be effective therapy.

Inborn Errors of Metabolism and Heritable Diseases

Oxalosis

Type 1 oxalosis is a rare autosomal recessive disorder caused by a deficiency of the liver-specific enzyme alanine glyoxylate aminotransferase.[6-8] As a result of this deficiency, overproduction of oxalate from glycine occurs in the liver and leads to progressive calcium oxalate formation, nephrocalcinosis, and eventually, renal failure.

Isolated kidney transplantation in patients with oxalosis has failed universally because of rapid reaccumulation of calcium oxalate in the kidney graft. Although the liver is histologically and biochemically normal in oxalosis, the enzymatic defect within the liver results in systemic hyperoxalosis. To prevent recurrent renal failure in cases of oxalosis, combined simultaneous or sequential liver transplantation followed by kidney transplantation is performed. Typically, hyperdialysis is used to reduce serum oxalate levels either after liver transplantation and before kidney transplantation or after combined kidney and liver transplantation. Ideally, hyperdialysis should be initiated before kidney and liver transplantation.

Because of the mixed experience with simultaneous liver-kidney transplantation, the current most widely used approach is to perform the liver transplant first. This sequence eliminates the overproduction of oxalate. Once overproduction of oxalate is eliminated, 6 to 12 months of high-intensity hemodialysis is used to remove sequestered oxalate stores in the body and control the serum oxalate level. When the body's oxalate pool is reduced to normal levels, kidney transplantation is performed to free the individual from the need for continued renal dialysis.

A few cases of simultaneous liver-kidney transplantation after a period of intense hemodialysis to normalize oxalate levels have been reported. The approach in such cases has been to vigorously hydrate the individual, provide pharmacological doses of pyridoxine, and force a diuresis after combined liver-kidney transplantation to maximize urinary excretion of mobilizable stores of oxalate while preventing solubilized oxalate from accumulating in the kidney graft. This approach, although more attractive to patients because it involves a single transplant procedure, is associated with an increased risk of posttransplant renal failure as a consequence of the

massive quantities of oxalate that are mobilized after transplantation and deposited in the kidney graft. A domino liver transplant can be performed in which a liver from a patient with oxalosis is transplanted into another individual with hepatic disease. Transplantation of a liver with oxalosis results in the development of oxalosis in the recipient of the domino liver transplant. This risk may be acceptable in elderly recipients or those with hepatic cancer because they are unlikely to receive a deceased donor liver graft if existing protocols for graft allocation are followed. In the former case, patients may not survive long enough after hepatic transplantation for oxalate-induced renal failure to develop. In the latter case, such transplantation provides extended life potentially free of cancer but at the cost of renal failure secondary to oxalosis if long-term survival is achieved.

Familial Homozygous Hypercholesterolemia

Familial homozygous hypercholesterolemia is an autosomal recessive disease characterized by hypercholesterolemia and accelerated atherosclerosis leading to severe coronary artery disease.[9-11] In severe cases (less than 2% of normal low-density lipoprotein [LDL] receptor activity), cardiovascular death is likely to occur within the first decade of life. In patients with a less severe deficiency of the LDL receptor (2% to 30% of normal activity), the disease is likely to produce cardiovascular death within the second or third decade of life.

Aggressive use of statin drugs may delay the development of atherosclerosis and overt cardiac disease in patients with familial homozygous hypercholesterolemia. In the past, two surgical procedures have been used to treat this condition in an effort to delay liver transplantation: end-to-side portocaval shunting and ileal bypass. Both these procedures have been discarded and replaced with the use of statin drugs. The current approach to familial homozygous hypercholesterolemia with severe cardiovascular disease is to perform either simultaneous or sequential heart-liver transplantation. Simultaneous transplantation is preferred if the heart graft functions immediately. In cases in which such is not the case, sequential transplantation can be accomplished. In both situations, the heart relieves the cardiac disease (usually advanced coronary artery disease with ischemic cardiomyopathy), whereas the liver graft removes the underlying defect, a hepatic deficiency of LDL receptors. In most cases after liver transplantation, the serum cholesterol level declines markedly and, in some cases, can actually normalize. In patients who continue to have moderate degrees of hypercholesterolemia, statin drugs can be used to normalize the serum cholesterol level.

Familial Amyloid Polyneuropathy

Familial amyloid polyneuropathy is a dominantly inherited neuropathic form of amyloidosis caused by the hepatic production of a mutant transthyretin (TTR).[12-14] Because TTR is produced almost exclusively by the liver, liver transplantation eliminates the underlying cause of the disease: production of an insoluble β-pleated mutant TTR that accumulates in peripheral and autonomic nerves. The disease is fatal with an expected survival of 12 to 15 years after the onset of clinical disease. The initial symptom is usually a peripheral neuropathy, although autonomic neuropathy with gastrointestinal and cardiovascular symptoms is also common. The presence of clinical autonomic neuropathy has a negative impact on both morbidity and mortality before and after liver transplantation.

Initially, liver transplantation was performed in patients who were severely malnourished and those who had advanced peripheral or autonomic neuropathy. Because the disease resolves very slowly, if at all, as the deposited amyloid material is resolubilized and removed, these patients continue to experience their disease manifestations after transplantation. Thus, the results are poor, and some recipients actually die of posttransplant malnutrition, sepsis (usually urosepsis), or cardiac arrhythmias as a consequence of their persistent amyloid-induced disease processes.

The current approach to patients with familial amyloid polyneuropathy is to perform transplantation early after the initial onset of clinical manifestations of their disease.

Because the liver of these patients is normal except for its production of a mutant TTR protein, the liver explant in such cases is often used as part of a domino transplant despite the fact that the recipient of the explant domino liver will, with sufficient time, acquire the disease process (amyloid polyneuropathy). The period before the onset of clinical disease is long, between 10 and 50 years depending on variations in phenotypic expression of amyloid polyneuropathy in different endemic areas, so acceptance of a liver from a donor with familial amyloid polyneuropathy can be expected to provide the recipient of the domino liver with 10- to 50-year disease-free (polyneuropathy) posttransplant survival. For most transplant recipients in their mid-40s or 50s, this extra risk represents a minimal addition to the inherent risks of liver transplantation.

Protoporphyria

Protoporphyria is a metabolic disease wherein iron is not inserted into the protoporphyrin precursor of heme as a result of a mutant ferrochelatase protein.[15-17] Many different mutations of the ferrochelatase gene have been identified in cases of protoporphyria. In most, the mutation observed is limited to a single family. Classically, the disease is described as an autosomal dominant trait with incomplete penetrance. However, most patients have severely reduced ferrochelatase levels, thus suggesting the presence of two rather than one abnormal gene. Cases have been described in which both parents of an affected patient have a different gene defect with little or no clinical disease but the combination of both abnormal genes in their offspring results in the phenotypic expression of overt protoporphyria. Regardless of the specific method of inheritance, affected patients have a unique form of immediate hypersensitivity to sun exposure characterized by a burning or stinging sensation coupled with erythema and edema.

It has been estimated that 10% of patients with severe protoporphyria experience clinically evident hepatic injury that progresses to hepatic fibrosis and, ultimately, hepatic failure. Once hepatic decompensation occurs, the disease progresses rapidly to death unless hepatic transplantation is accomplished.

Hepatic accumulation of protoporphyrin can be reduced but not eliminated by the administration of oral charcoal, cholestyramine, or colestipol. Additional measures that have been used include frequent red blood cell transfusions to suppress erythropoiesis, administration of hematin to suppress porphyrin synthesis, and plasmapheresis to remove free protoporphyrin in plasma.

When liver transplantation is used as a life-saving procedure in individuals with protoporphyria, the patient needs to be prepared for surgery with aggressive plasmapheresis to remove protoporphyrin from the blood, and the operating room must be modified to reduce light exposure to exposed tissues during the transplant procedure by using red lights, which do not activate the protoporphyrin in light-exposed tissues.

The ideal theoretical therapy for protoporphyria with developing liver failure is a combined bone marrow and liver transplant procedure. Unfortunately, once the liver disease is sufficiently advanced to justify liver transplantation, there is insufficient time to perform a bone marrow transplant and allow the individual to recover normal hematological status before the liver transplant because of rapid progression of the liver disease.

Protoporphyrin-induced liver disease recurs in the transplanted liver despite the reduction in hepatic protoporphyrin production as a result of the liver transplant. Persistent production of excess protoporphyrin by bone marrow results in recurrent photosensitivity and hepatic disease. This fact strongly supports sequential transplantation of the liver followed by a bone marrow transplant in patients with protoporphyria once early clinical hepatic involvement becomes manifest.

Deficits in Fatty Acid Metabolism

Disorders of Fatty Acid Oxidation

Hepatic mitochondria are responsible for the metabolism of fatty acids and the production of ketone bodies (3-hydroxybutyrate and acetoacetate), which serve as alternative fuel for the central nervous system during fasting.[18-22] Inherited disorders of fatty acid oxidation are clinically heterogeneous but are typically manifested by hypoglycemia, intolerance of fasting, seizures, hepatic disease, skeletal and cardiac myopathy, and occasionally, sudden death.

The symptoms and signs of these various disorders can develop at any age. When they occur, they can lead to life-threatening metabolic decompensation as a result of accumulation of toxic intermediates in serum and energy deprivation at involved tissue sites.

Neonatal Liver Failure Caused by Deficiencies in the Respiratory Chain of Mitochondria. These diseases can occur in the first few months of life and are characterized by lactic acidosis, jaundice, conjugated hyperbilirubinemia, abnormal serum alanine aminotransferase levels, coagulopathy, ketotic hypoglycemia, and hyperammonemia. Early clinical symptoms are lethargy, hypotonia, and vomiting.

Liver biopsy specimens from affected patients show microvesicular steatosis, canalicular cholestasis, and bile duct proliferation. The periportal and centrilobular fibrosis in these cases can progress to overt micronodular cirrhosis. Glycogen depletion and iron deposition within the liver are common in these disease processes. The abnormal mitochondria in these diseases are evident on electron microscopy. Once initiated, the disease process is rapidly progressive and leads to death from liver failure or sepsis, or from both. These diseases are heterogeneous in terms of their extrahepatic manifestations. Most patients have severe neurological involvement with weakness, hypotonia, poor cry and suck responses, recurrent episodes of apnea, and myoclonic seizures. Patients with neurological signs and symptoms are not candidates for liver transplantation because these findings do not revert but can continue and lead to severe neurological disease and death. Some patients, however, do not have neurological findings, and these few can undergo successful liver transplantation.

Congenital Mitochondrial DNA Depletion Syndrome. This disorder is manifested within the first week of life as hypotonia, hepatic failure, renal dysfunction, and lactic acidosis. It is characterized by an increased number of mitochondria with reduced mitochondrial DNA content. The diagnosis is established by documenting a reduced mitochondrial DNA–to–nuclear DNA ratio in affected tissues. Reduced activity of the respiratory chain complexes I, III, and IV can be documented in patients, whereas the activity of complex II remains normal. In a few cases, the disease appears to be liver specific and spares the muscle, brain, kidneys, and heart. In such cases, liver transplantation is life-saving.

Reye's Syndrome. This acquired form of hepatic mitochondrial disease is due to an interaction between a viral illness (influenza, varicella, enteroviruses, other viruses) and salicylate therapy and results in defective ureagenesis, ketogenesis, hyperammonemia, hypoglycemia, elevated free fatty acids, lactic acidosis, and the production of various dicarboxylic acids. Most cases occur in the autumn and winter, when viral illnesses in children aged 5 to 15 years are most frequent.

The symptoms of hepatic disease in children with Reye's syndrome develop after the clinical onset of the viral illness, often after the child appears to be recovering from the prodromal viral illness. After several hours of vomiting, which can be severe and lead to dehydration, encephalopathy develops. Serum alanine and aspartate aminotransferase levels increase, as does the blood ammonia level. Mild to moderate prolongation of the prothrombin time and hypoglycemia also occur. It is important to note that despite the potentially lethal disease, the serum bilirubin level remains normal. Liver biopsy samples show microvesicular steatosis in the absence of hepatic inflammation or necrosis. Electron microscopy can demonstrate abnormal mitochondria. In patients with suggested Reye's syndrome and overt liver failure, it may be that Reye's syndrome is in actuality a consequence of a defect in fatty acid oxidation rather than true Reye's syndrome. In these latter cases, liver transplantation is indicated as a life-saving procedure.

Long-Chain 3-Hydroxyacyl-Coenzyme A Dehydrogenase Deficiency. Women who are heterozygotes for this enzyme deficiency are at risk for third-trimester life-threatening complications of pregnancy, including acute fatty liver of pregnancy and the HELLP syndrome (hemolysis, elevated liver enzymes, low platelets). In addition, they are at risk for preeclampsia/eclampsia. These disorders are associated with variable degrees of hepatic steatosis, hyperammonemia, an elevated lactate-pyruvate ratio, lactic acidosis, ketosis, and hepatic disease that occurs suddenly and progresses rapidly to coma and death in the absence of hyperbilirubinemia. In these more advanced cases, liver transplantation is life-saving and may need to be performed either before or after delivery.

Other defects in fatty acid oxidation that can occur rarely and cause liver failure in pregnant women include trifunctional protein deficiency, carnitine palmitoyltransferase deficiency, and short-chain acyl-CoA dehydrogenase deficiency.

Urea Cycle Defects

These disorders are inherited as autosomal recessive disorders except for ornithine transcarbamylase deficiency,[23-25] which is inherited as an X-linked recessive disorder. No single mutation in any of these disorders has been shown to define the disease. Rather, a large number of different mutations have been identified for each disorder. Thus, the diagnosis of a urea cycle defect relies on enzymatic assays of blood and urine for the metabolites that characterize each disorder.

Liver transplantation for a urea cycle deficiency is essentially curative. Episodes of hyperammonemia no longer occur, dietary restriction is no longer necessary, and alternative pathway medications can be discontinued. It is important to note that liver transplantation does not correct the low levels of plasma arginine and citrulline present in individuals with carbamyl phosphate synthetase deficiency or ornithine transcarbamylase deficiency because most of the citrulline in plasma is a product of intestinal rather than hepatic synthesis. Thus, individuals with either of these two disorders, even after successful liver transplantation, continue to require supplements of either citrulline or arginine.

Cystic Fibrosis

Cystic fibrosis is the most common fatal, autosomal recessively inherited disease in the white population, with a frequency of 1 in 2000 to 3000 live births.[26,27] It is usually initially manifested as recurrent/persistent pulmonary infections, pancreatic insufficiency, intestinal obstruction, or reproductive tract obstruction resulting in infertility. It is caused by one or another mutation in the cystic fibrosis transmembrane conductance regulator protein, a complex chloride channel present in exocrine tissues. Intrahepatic focal or diffuse biliary tract obstruction leads to focal or diffuse secondary biliary cirrhosis in patients with cystic fibrosis and hepatic involvement.

Specifically, focal biliary cirrhosis occurs in 2% to 5% of patients with cystic fibrosis. More diffuse hepatic involvement can lead to clinically evident secondary biliary cirrhosis and, when present, is an indication for liver transplantation either in the absence or, more often, in association with pulmonary transplantation.

Acute Hepatic Failure

Drugs

Valproic Acid

Valproic acid is metabolized to a mitochondrial toxin, 4-ene-valproic acid, that can cause fulminant hepatic failure necessitating liver transplantation.[28] As with most mitochondrial diseases, a severe microvesicular steatosis characterizes the hepatic histology in patients with valproic acid hepatotoxicity. Vomiting, hypoglycemia, coma, and lactic acidosis often without hyperbilirubinemia characterize this disease process.

Other toxins that can poison the respiratory chain may also result in fulminant hepatic failure, including cyanide, antimycin A, and rotenone. Intravenous tetracycline and overdoses of iron can rarely produce hepatic failure necessitating liver transplantation.

Nucleoside Analogues

A unique drug toxicity caused by the use of nucleoside analogues for the treatment of viral infections such as human immunodeficiency virus and hepatitis B virus (HBV) and characterized by the experience with fialuridine can produce mitochondrial toxicity.[29] The use of these drugs leads to depletion of mitochondrial DNA and hepatic steatosis, fatigue, nausea, abdominal pain, coagulopathy, hyperammonemia, lactic acidosis, and pancreatitis with minimal or no hyperbilirubinemia. Liver transplantation has been life-saving in some of these cases.

Infectious Agents

Bacterial Toxins and Fulminant Hepatic Failure

Cereulide, the emetic toxin of *Bacillus cereus*, has been shown to inhibit the respiratory chain and lead to hepatic steatosis and a picture of fulminant hepatic failure that can be treated by liver transplantation and antibiotics directed at the responsible bacterial infection.[30]

Fulminant Herpes or Cytomegalovirus Infection

Orthotopic liver transplantation has been used for the treatment of fulminant herpes simplex virus or cytomegalovirus infection in children and pregnant women who acquire disseminated infection.[31,32] In these cases, early diagnosis with the initiation of high-dose intravenous acyclovir therapy and occasionally liver transplantation is life-saving.

Hepatic Failure Caused by Emergence of the YMDD Escape Mutant of Hepatitis B Virus

Chronic HBV infection is often treated with lamivudine.[33,34] In up to 30% of cases, mutant forms of HBV can be detected after 1 year or more of continuous lamivudine therapy. These mutants are resistant to lamivudine and other drugs such as famciclovir. The originally identified mutant virus had a mutation in the YMDD locus of the HBV DNA polymerase gene.

One of the approaches to these mutant viruses is to stop the lamivudine therapy and allow the wild-type virus to replicate and eliminate the less replicative-sufficient mutant virus. Rarely, sudden discontinuation of therapy with a nucleoside analogue such as lamivudine results in the initiation of an episode of severe hepatitis and acute hepatic failure necessitating emergency liver transplantation. In cases in which lamivudine therapy is not discontinued and adefovir therapy is not initiated, the mutant viral infection can lead to progressive liver disease and recurrent cirrhosis. Liver transplantation is possible in cases resulting in advanced liver disease with the combined use of hepatitis B immune globulin and adefovir. Several agents in addition to adefovir are being developed that should reduce the problem associated with the development of mutant HBV infections in patients treated with lamivudine and other nucleoside analogues.

Fulminant Hepatic Failure Caused by Hepatitis A or Hepatitis E

These two forms of viral hepatitis rarely cause fulminant hepatic failure except in older individuals (>40 years of age) in the case of hepatitis A and pregnant malnourished women in the case of hepatitis E.[35,36] Both conditions can result in acute hepatic failure in individuals with underlying chronic hepatitis B or C or other forms of chronic parenchymal liver disease. Liver transplantation for such cases of acute liver failure occurring in an individual with preexisting chronic hepatitis B or C is the only available successful therapy.

Fulminant non-A, non-B, non-C Hepatitis

Fulminant hepatic failure in cases of non-A, non-B, non-C hepatitis can occur in young adults (mean age, 32 years), especially if the individual is either pregnant or malnourished.[37-41] Liver transplantation is life-saving in these cases. Unfortunately, in 15% of such cases, the fulminant hepatic failure recurs after transplantation and thus necessitates a second liver transplant procedure within days to weeks. Moreover, aplastic anemia is a late complication of the disease process.

Chronic Fungal Infections of the Biliary Tract

Rarely, chronic biliary candidiasis or cryptococcal infection can be mistaken for PSC.[42] When such a patient is correctly identified, antifungal therapy should be administered and liver transplantation may be avoided.

In rare cases, the diagnosis of fungal cholangiopathy is not made preoperatively, and an incorrect diagnosis of either PSC or idiopathic bile duct paucity (a form of the idiopathic vanishing bile duct syndrome seen in adults) is made and hepatic transplantation is performed. These patients require prolonged antifungal therapy after transplantation for a minimum of 4 to 6 weeks and possibly longer (3 months to a year), depending on the presence or absence of recurrent fungal disease in the allograft.

Echinococcus granulosus Hydatid Cyst Disease

This parasitic disease is common in parts of France, Germany, Poland, and extensive areas of the former Soviet Union.[43,44] The natural host for this infection is the fox. Once acquired by humans as a result of the ingestion of cysts, the disease can progress to liver failure as a result of vascular disease (Budd-Chiari syndrome), hepatobiliary disease (pseudosclerosing cholangitis), or secondary biliary cirrhosis. With any of these manifestations of the disease, liver transplantation may be an appropriate therapeutic option. Postoperative complications in patients who receive transplants for echinococcal infection are common and can be catastrophic if the hepatic tumor is violated and cysts contaminate the operative field.

Vascular Disorders

Budd-Chiari Syndrome

Budd-Chiari syndrome consists pathologically of focal or diffuse venous thrombosis of the hepatic veins.[45-47] This process can occur as a consequence of a congenital web in the inferior vena cava (IVC) between the right atrium and the entry site of the hepatic veins and has been observed most often in Asian Indians and Japanese women. The IVC web leads to stasis and hepatic venous vascular injury, which can progress to vascular thrombosis within the hepatic veins as well as the subdiaphragmatic IVC caudal to the web.

It can also develop as a consequence of a congenital defect in either coagulation or fibrinolysis, as occurs in patients with factor V Leiden mutation or a prothrombin mutation or in those homozygous for methylene tetrahydrofolate reductase (MTHFR), antithrombin III, protein C, or protein S deficiency. Often, the use of oral contraceptives, estrogen replacement therapy, or pregnancy is responsible for precipitating the venous thrombosis in such cases.

Yet another cause of Budd-Chiari syndrome is the presence of a myeloproliferative disorder such as polycythemia rubra vera, essential thrombocytosis, or paroxysmal nocturnal hemoglobinuria.

Finally, Behçet's syndrome and antiphospholipid or anticardiolipin autoantibodies (or both) have been reported as a cause of Budd-Chiari syndrome.

Liver transplantation for the treatment of Budd-Chiari syndrome is accomplished at two chronological ends of the natural history of the disease process. Specifically, in acute cases of Budd-Chiari syndrome associated with acute or subacute hepatic failure, liver transplantation can be life-saving. In patients with end-stage Budd-Chiari disease and cirrhosis secondary to chronic venous outlet obstruction, liver transplantation is also life-saving. In these latter cases, previous mesocaval portal shunts, side-to-side portal shunts, or portal-atrial vascular shunts may have been created earlier in the natural history of the disease and are complicating the recipient hepatectomy.

With resection of the initiating IVC web and thrombosis as part of the recipient hepatectomy or replacement of the diseased liver with a liver that does not have a mutant process such as factor V Leiden, a prothrombin mutation, MTHFR homozygosity, or antithrombin III, protein C, or protein S deficiency, the vasculopathy is resolved and no special posttransplant care is needed. In patients in whom the primary disease process exists outside the liver, as for example with polycythemia rubra vera and other myeloproliferative diseases, Behçet's disease, and other rare vasculopathies, lifelong anticoagulation is necessary after transplantation.

It needs to be pointed out that diagnosis of the forme fruste of polycythemia rubra vera requires bone marrow aspiration and culture of the marrow for detection of erythroid colony-forming units in the absence of erythropoietin, a factor that is normally required for the proliferation of erythropoietic colonies in culture.

Giant Hemangioma with Kasabach-Merritt Syndrome

Patients with giant hemangiomas and coagulopathy consisting of thrombocytopenia, prolongation of the prothrombin and activated partial thromboplastin time, and laboratory evidence of disseminated intravascular coagulopathy (Kasabach-Merritt syndrome) have occasionally been treated by transplantation.[48-51]

Hereditary Hemorrhagic Telangiectasia

Hereditary hemorrhagic telangiectasia, or Rendu-Osler-Weber syndrome, is an inherited autosomal dominant disease characterized by arteriovenous malformations that occur in multiple organs.[52,53] Hepatic involvement is uncommon but can be complicated by portal hypertension, hepatic encephalopathy, high-output congestive heart failure, and rarely, hemobilia. When these complications occur, liver transplantation is one of several therapeutic options that also include vascular embolization and partial hepatic resection, depending on the extent of disease within the liver.

Veno-occlusive Disease

Bone marrow transplantation and kidney transplantation are occasionally complicated by hepatic dysfunction leading to hepatic failure as a consequence of veno-occlusive disease. Graft-versus-host disease can also be an indication for liver transplantation in patients with a previous bone marrow transplant.[54-58]

Miscellaneous Disorders

Polycystic Liver Disease

Polycystic liver disease can progress to massive hepatomegaly resulting in severe physical and social disability.[59] Liver transplantation can reverse the malnutrition, cachexia, and quality-of-life dysfunction associated with this disease. Simultaneous renal transplantation is not required unless renal failure is present, and it can often be delayed for many years.

Sarcoidosis

Sarcoidosis is a multisystem disease characterized by the presence of noncaseating granuloma and fibrosis.[60-62] Most deaths attributable to sarcoidosis are a result of cardiac disease (50%), with pulmonary disease accounting for most of the remaining deaths (43%). Noncardiac, nonpulmonary disease is responsible for less than 7% of the total deaths from sarcoidosis. Thus, advanced liver disease as a result of sarcoidosis is an extremely unusual indication for liver transplantation.

Liver transplantation for sarcoidosis is generally performed when the sarcoidosis complicates cases of chronic hepatitis C or other disease processes involving the liver. Liver transplantation has also been performed for cases of hepatic sarcoidosis in which the sarcoidosis has severely affected the individual's quality of life in a negative manner such that movement, self-care, and eating are made difficult, as occurs in patients with polycystic liver disease.

Disease recurrence within the liver and exacerbations of extrahepatic sarcoidosis have been reported after liver transplantation. Recurrent sarcoidosis or an exacerbation of preexisting sarcoidosis in the lung can be difficult to differentiate from tuberculosis or lymphoma (or both) after liver transplantation in a patient who received a transplant for sarcoidosis.

Neuroendocrine Tumors

Patients with metastatic carcinoid/neuroendocrine tumors and severe symptoms unresponsive to octreotide therapy or those with massive hepatic tumor and no evidence of extrahepatic disease can be treated by liver transplantation.[63,64] In such cases, the primary lesion should have been either resected previously or removed at the time of the liver transplant procedure.

Diffuse Bile Duct Stenosis/Idiopathic Adult Bile Ductopenia

These two rare conditions are associated with a reduced size and number of bile ducts within or outside the liver.[65] The clinical picture in each is similar to that of other chronic cholestatic disorders such as PSC or PBC. The specific indications for transplantation in these disorders are also identical to those for PSC or PBC.

Benign Hepatic Tumors

Hepatic Adenoma

Hepatic adenoma can occur as an isolated lesion (most often) or as multiple adenomas (unusual).[66,67] The more typical case consists of a single adenoma and is seen in individuals with glycogen storage disease (type I), women who use oral contraceptive agents, or men and women who have used sex steroids for any of a number of legitimate clinical or illicit indications. These tumors, although benign, can undergo central necrosis or hemorrhage and cause pain, or they can be strategically located and cause biliary or vascular injury to the rest of the liver, thus necessitating their removal. In centrally located lesions or lesions that involve such a large fraction of the liver that hepatic resection is precluded, liver transplantation is indicated.

Multiple hepatic adenomatosis can occur as an isolated disease process or as part of a familial disorder. Repetitive segmental hepatic resection of these lesions is unlikely to remove all the lesions safely and may enhance the growth of residual tumors in the liver. In some of these patients, especially those with adenomas that are growing or causing symptoms, liver transplantation is an appropriate therapy.

Mesenchymal Hamartomas

These lesions can be of such size that they incapacitate the patient or cause recurrent abdominal pain and, rarely, hepatic failure.[68] If these lesions either cannot be resected with a standard surgical procedure or recur after such surgery, liver transplantation is an appropriate course of action.

Massive Hepatic Hemangiomas

Occasionally, hepatic hemangiomas are of sufficient size or centrally located in the hilar area of the liver that resection without liver transplantation is not possible.[69] In general, these lesions do not require surgical intervention unless they are causing pain, enlarging progressively, or consuming platelets and clotting factors and resulting in thrombocytopenia and disseminated intravascular coagulation (Kasabach-Merritt syndrome).

Hepatic Lymphangiomatosis

This extremely rare condition has caused hepatic dysfunction, as well as intractable dyspnea, fatigue, and malnutrition as a result of the inability of affected individuals to eat; it can also be associated with debilitating chronic abdominal pain.[70] As with other benign tumors, sequential hepatic resection is the treatment of choice unless the lesion has recurred after a previous attempt at resection, is centrally located with involvement of the hilar structures, or is of such size that resection without transplantation is not possible.

Inflammatory Pseudotumor of the Liver

This "tumor" can occur in many different tissues. In rare cases, it involves the liver.[71] When it is located in a hilar location, it can lead to secondary biliary cirrhosis as a result of recurrent episodes of cholangitis. The presence of this lesion along with hepatic failure, portal hypertension with bleeding, or a combination of these two problems can be a rare indication for liver transplantation.

Focal Nodular Hyperplasia

As with the other benign lesions, focal nodular hyperplasia can be treated by liver transplantation if the lesion is centrally located (which is often the case) and is causing hilar strictures with resultant portal hypertension, biliary obstruction with recurrent cholangitis, or hepatic failure as a result of hilar vascular involvement.[72,73] This disease is often associated with vascular abnormalities involving the liver or collagen vascular disease processes. Rarely, nodular hyperplasia is a diffuse phenomenon in the liver. This too can be an indication for transplantation and is often mistaken preoperatively for cryptogenic cirrhosis.

Biliary Papillomatosis

Biliary papillomatosis is a rare entity associated with recurrent episodes of cholangitis and the development of secondary biliary cirrhosis; it can be complicated by recurrent episodes of sepsis or portal hypertension, or both.[74] In very rare cases, cholangiolar carcinoma can arise from the chronically inflamed epithelium that exists in these cases. Liver transplantation with a Roux-en-Y choledochojejunostomy can be a treatment option and should be performed before malignant transformation of the adenomatous biliary epithelium.

References

1. Starzl TE, Demetris AJ, Van Thiel DH: Medical progress: Liver transplantation (Part I). N Engl J Med 321:1014-1022, 1989.
2. Starzl TE, Demetris AJ, Van Thiel DH: Medical progress: Liver transplantation (Part II). N Engl J Med 321:1092-1099, 1989.
3. Kelly DA: Current results and evolving indications for liver transplantation in children. J Pediatr Gastroenterol Nutr 27:214-221, 1998.
4. Van Thiel DH, Brems J, Nadir A, et al: Liver transplantation for fulminant hepatic failure. J Gastroenterol 37(Suppl 13):78-81, 2002.
5. Devictor D, Desplangues L, Debray D, et al: Emergency liver transplantation for fulminant liver failure in infants and children. Hepatology 16:1156-1162, 1992.
6. Monico CG, Milliner DS: Combined liver-kidney and kidney-alone transplantation in primary hyperoxaluria. Liver Transpl 7:954-963, 2001.
7. Donckier V, El Nakadi I, Closset J, et al: Domino hepatic transplantation using the liver from a patient with primary hyperoxaluria. Transplantation 71:1346-1348, 2001.
8. Shapiro R, Weismann I, Mandel H, et al: Primary hyperoxaluria type 1: Improved outcome with timely liver transplantation: A single-center report of 36 children. Transplantation 15:428-432, 2001.
9. Bilheimer DW, Goldstein JL, Grundy SM, et al: Liver transplantation to provide low-density-lipoprotein receptors and lower plasma cholesterol in a child with homozygous familial hypercholesterolemia. N Engl J Med 311:1658-1664, 1984.
10. Lopez-Santamaria M, Migliazza L, Gamez M, et al: Liver transplantation in patients with homozygotic familial hypercholesterolemia previously treated by end-to-side portocaval shunt and ileal bypass. J Pediatr Surg 35:630-633, 2000.
11. Castilla Cabezas JA, Lopez-Cillero P, Jiminez J, et al: Role of orthotopic liver transplant in the treatment of homozygous familial hypercholesterolemia. Rev Esp Enferm Dig 92:601-608, 2000.
12. Jonsen E, Suhr O, Tashima K, Athlin E: Early liver transplantation is essential for familial amyloidotic polyneuropathy patients' quality of life. Amyloid 8:52-57, 2001.
13. Suhr OB, Ericzon BG, Friman S: Long-term follow-up of survival of liver transplant recipients with familial myeloid polyneuropathy (Portuguese type). Liver Transpl 8:787-794, 2002.
14. Suhr OB, Ando Y, Holmgren G, et al: Liver transplantation in familial amyloidotic polyneuropathy (FAP). A comparative study of transplanted and non-transplanted patients' survival. Transpl Int 11(Suppl 1):S160-S163, 1998.
15. Meerman L: Erythropoietic protoporphyria. An overview with emphasis on the liver. Scand J Gastroenterol 79:79-85, 2000.
16. Bloomer JR, Rank JM, Payne WD, et al: Follow-up after liver transplantation for protoporphyric liver disease. Liver Transpl 2:269-275, 1996.
17. Bloomer JR, Weimer MK, Bossenmaier IC, et al: Liver transplantation in a patient with protoporphyria. Gastroenterology 97:188-194, 1989.
18. van't Hoff WG, Dixon M, Taylor J, et al: Combined liver-kidney transplantation in methylmalonic acidemia. J Pediatr 132:1043-1044, 1998.
19. Leonard JV, Walter JH, McKiernan PJ: The management of organic acidaemias: The role of transplantation. J Inherit Metab Dis 24:309-311, 2001.
20. Sokal EM, Sokol R, Cormier V, et al: Liver transplantation in mitochondrial respiratory chain disorders. Eur J Pediatr 158(Suppl 2):S81-S84, 1999.
21. Van Spronsen FJ, Bernard O, Saudubray JM: Liver transplantation in mitochondrial respiratory chain disorders. Eur J Pediatr 158(Suppl 2):S81-S84, 1999.
22. Thomson M, McKierman P, Buckels J, et al: Generalized mitochondrial cytopathy is an absolute contraindication to orthotopic liver transplantation. J Pediatr Gastroenterol Nutr 26:478-481, 1998.
23. Hasagawa T, Tzakis AG, Todo S, et al: Orthotopic liver transplantation for ornithine transcarbamylase deficiency with hyperammonemic encephalopathy. J Pediatr Surg 30:863-865, 1995.
24. Busuttil AA, Goss JA, Seu P, et al: The role of orthotopic liver transplantation in the treatment of ornithine transcarbamylase deficiency. Liver Transpl Surg 4:350-354, 1998.
25. Whitington PF, Alonso EM, Boyle JT, et al: Liver transplantation for the treatment of urea cycle disorders. J Inherit Metab Dis 1:112-118, 1998.
26. Cox KL, Ward RE, Rurgiuele TL, et al: Orthotopic liver transplantation in patients with cystic fibrosis. Pediatrics 80:570-574, 1987.
27. Noble-Jamieson G, Barnes N, Jamieson N, et al: Liver transplantation for hepatic cirrhosis in cystic fibrosis. J R Soc Med 89:31-37, 1996.
28. Bell EA, Shaefer MS, Markin RS: Treatment of valproic acid–associated hepatic failure with orthotopic liver transplantation. Ann Pharmacother 26:18, 1992.
29. McKenzie R, Fried MW, Sallie R, et al: Hepatic failure and lactic acidosis due to fialuridine (FIAU), an investigational nucleoside analogue for chronic hepatitis B. N Engl J Med 333:1099-1105, 1995.
30. Mahler H, Pasi A, Kramer JM, et al: Fulminant liver failure in association with the emetic toxin of *Bacillus cereus*. N Engl J Med 336:1142-1148, 1997.
31. Egawa H, Inomata Y, Nakayama S, et al: Fulminant hepatic failure secondary to herpes simplex virus infection in a neonate: A case report of successful treatment with liver transplantation and perioperative acyclovir. Liver Transpl Surg 4:513-516, 1998.
32. Chauveau E, Martin J, Saliba F, et al: Fatal fulminating hepatitis due to herpes simplex virus type 2 in a young immunocompetent female. Med Trop (Mars) 59:58-60, 1999.
33. Stärkel P, Horsmans Y, Geubel A, et al: Favorable outcome of orthotopic liver transplantation in a patient with subacute liver failure due to the emergence of a hepatitis B YMDD escape mutant virus. J Hepatol 35:679-681, 2001.
34. Saab S, Kim M, Wright TL, et al: Successful orthotopic liver transplantation for lamivudine-associated YMDD mutant hepatitis B virus. Gastroenterology 119:1382-1384, 2000.
35. Kyrlagkitsis I, Cramp ME, Smith H, et al: Acute hepatitis A virus infection: A review of prognostic factors from 25 years experience in a tertiary referral center. Hepatogastroenterology 49:524-528, 2002.
36. Nicoluzzi J, Mennecier D, Sogni P, et al: Hepatitis E–associated subacute liver failure: A rare indication for liver transplantation. Am J Gastroenterol 96:2278-2279, 2001.
37. Ferraz ML, Silva AE, Macdonald GA, et al: Fulminant hepatitis in patients undergoing liver transplantation: Evidence for a non-A, non-B, non-C, non-D, and non-E syndrome. Liver Transpl Surg 2:60-66, 1996.
38. Mutimer D, Shaw J, Neuberger J, et al: Failure to incriminate hepatitis B, hepatitis C, and hepatitis E viruses in the aetiology of fulminant non-A, non-B hepatitis. Gut 36:433-436, 1995.

39. Ellis AJ, Saleh M, Smith H, et al: Late-onset hepatic failure: Clinical features, serology and outcome following transplantation. J Hepatol 23:363-372, 1995.

40. Ben-Ari Z, Samuel D, Zemel R, et al: Fulminant non–A-G viral hepatitis leading to liver transplantation. Arch Intern Med 160:388-392, 2000.

41. Uemoto S, Inomata Y, Sakurai T, et al: Living donor liver transplantation for fulminant hepatic failure. Transplantation 70:152-157, 2000.

42. Noack KB, Osmon DR, Batts KP, et al: Successful orthotopic liver transplantation in a patient with refractory biliary candidiasis. Gastroenterology 101:1728-1730, 1991.

43. Moreno-Gonzalez E, Loinaz Segurola C, Garcia Urena MA, et al: Liver transplantation for *Echinococcus granulosus* hydatid disease. Transplantation 58:797-800, 1994.

44. Loinaz C, Moreno-Gonzalez E, Gomez R, et al: Liver transplantation in liver disease: *Echinococcus granulosus*. Transplant Proc 30:328-329, 1998.

45. Jamieson NV, Williams R, Calne RY: Liver transplantation for Budd-Chiari syndrome, 1976-1990. Ann Chir 45:362-365, 1991.

46. Tan HP, Markowitz JS, Maley WR, et al: Successful liver transplantation in a patient with Budd-Chiari syndrome caused by homozygous factor V Leiden. Liver Transpl 6:654-656, 2000.

47. Bucciarelli P, Franchi F, Alatri A, et al: Budd-Chiari syndrome in a patient heterozygous for the G20210A mutation of the pro-thrombin gene. Thromb Haemost 79:445-446, 1998.

48. Klompmaker IJ, Slooff MJH, van der Meer GM, et al: Orthotopic liver transplantation in a patient with a giant cavernous hemangioma of the liver and Kasabach-Merritt syndrome. Transplantation 48:149-151, 1989.

49. Moreno Egea A, Del Pozo Rodriguez M, Vicente Cantero M, Abellan Atenza J: Indications for surgery in the treatment of hepatic hemangioma. Hepatogastroenterology 43:422-426, 1996.

50. Kumashiro Y, Kasahara M, Nomoto K, et al: Living donor liver transplantation for giant hepatic hemangioma with Kasabach-Merritt syndrome with a posterior segment graft. Liver Transpl 8:721-724, 2002.

51. Hockwald SN, Blumgart LH: Giant hepatic hemangioma with Kasabach-Merritt syndrome: Is the appropriate treatment enucleation or liver transplantation? HPB Surg 11:413-419, 2000.

52. Hillert C, Broering DC, Gundlach M, et al: Hepatic involvement in hereditary hemorrhagic telangiectasia: An unusual indication for liver transplantation. Liver Transpl 7:266-268, 2001.

53. Odorico JS, Hakim MN, Becker YT, et al: Liver transplantation as definitive therapy for complications after arterial embolization for hepatic manifestations of hereditary hemorrhagic telangiectasia. Liver Transpl Surg 4:483-490, 1998.

54. Rosen HR, Martin P, Schiller GJ, et al: Orthotopic liver transplantation for bone-marrow transplant–associated veno-occlusive disease and graft-versus-host disease of the liver. Liver Transpl Surg 2:225-232, 1996.

55. Norris S, Crosbie O, McEntee G, et al: Orthotopic liver transplantation for veno-occlusive disease complicating autologous bone marrow transplantation. Transplantation 63:1521-1524, 1997.

56. Bunin N, Leahey A, Dunn S: Related donor liver transplant for veno-occlusive disease following T-depleted unrelated donor bone marrow transplantation. Transplantation 61:664-666, 1996.

57. Schlitt HJ, Tischler HJ, Ringe B, et al: Allogeneic liver transplantation for hepatic veno-occlusive disease after bone marrow transplantation—clinical and immunological considerations. Bone Marrow Transplant 16:473-478, 1995.

58. Hagglund H, Ringden O, Ericzon BG, et al: Treatment of hepatic venoocclusive disease with recombinant human tissue plasminogen activator or orthotopic liver transplantation after allogenic bone marrow transplantation. Transplantation 62:1076-1080, 1996.

59. Pirenne J, Aerts R, Yoong K, et al: Liver transplantation for polycystic liver disease. Liver Transpl 7:238-245, 2001.

60. Casavilla FA, Gordon R, Wright HI, et al: Clinical course after liver transplantation in patients with sarcoidosis. Ann Intern Med 118:865-866, 1993.

61. Barbers RG: Role of transplantation (lung, liver, and heart) in sarcoidosis. Clin Chest Med 18:865-873, 1997.

62. Pescovitz MD, Jones HM, Cummings OW, et al: Diffuse retroperitoneal lymphadenopathy following liver transplantation—a case of recurrent sarcoidosis. Transplantation 60:393-396, 1995.

63. Ramage JK, Catnach SM, Williams R: Overview: The management of metastatic carcinoid tumors. Liver Transpl Surg 1:107-110, 1995.

64. Routley D, Ramage JK, McPeake J, et al: Orthotopic liver transplantation in the treatment of metastatic neuroendocrine tumors of the liver. Liver Transpl Surg 1:118-121, 1995.

65. Camargo CA Jr, Washington MK, Fitz JG: Adult presentation of diffuse bile duct stenosis: Therapy with liver transplantation. Liver Transpl Surg 2:235-237, 1996.

66. Marino I, Scantlebury V, Bronsther O, et al: Total hepatectomy and liver transplantations for hepatocellular adenomatosis and focal nodular hyperplasia. Transpl Int 5(Suppl 1):201-205, 1992.

67. Yunta PJ, Moya A, San-Juan F, et al: A new case of hepatic adenomatosis treated with orthotopic liver transplantation. Ann Chir 126:672-674, 2001.

68. Kim HB, Maller E, Redd D, et al: Orthotopic liver transplantation for inflammatory myofibroblastic tumor of the liver hilum. J Pediatr Surg 31:840-842, 1996.

69. Belli L, DeCarlis L, Beati C, et al: Surgical treatment of symptomatic giant hemangiomas of the liver. Surg Gynecol Obstet 174:474-478, 1992.

70. Miller C, Mazzaferro V, Makowka L, et al: Orthotopic liver transplantation for massive hepatic lymphangiomatosis. Surgery 103:490-495, 1988.

71. Hemeghan MA, Kaplan CG, Priebe CJ Jr, Partin JS: Inflammatory pseudotumor of the liver: A rare cause of obstructive jaundice and portal hypertension in a child. Pediatr Radiol 14:433-435, 1984.

72. Radomski JS, Chojnacki KA, Mortiz MJ, et al: Results of liver transplantation for nodular regenerative hyperplasia. Am Surg 66:1067-1070, 2000.

73. Elariny HA Mizhai SS, Hayes DH, et al: Nodular regenerative hyperplasia: A controversial indication for orthotopic liver transplantation. Transpl Int 7:309-313, 1994.

74. Beavers KL, Fried MW, Johnson MW, et al: Orthotopic liver transplantation for biliary papillomatosis. Liver Transpl 7:264-266, 2001.

III

Patient Evaluation: Pediatric

General Criteria for Pediatric Transplantation

ESTELLA M. ALONSO
ANDRES BESEDOVSKY
KARAN EMERICK
PETER F. WHITINGTON

General indications for liver transplantation
   in children   288
   Primary liver disease expected to progress to
      hepatic failure   288
   Symptoms of nonprogressive primary liver
      disease   289
   Liver transplantation as primary therapy for
      inborn errors of metabolism   289
   Secondary liver disease   290
   Primary hepatic malignancy   290

General contraindications to liver
   transplantation   291

Management of specific diseases leading
   to liver transplantation in children   292

Referral to a transplant center   295

Evaluating the pediatric transplant
   candidate   295
   Issues unique to pediatric liver
      transplantation   297
   Liver transplantation in neonates   298

Liver transplantation is an effective and widely accepted treatment for children with liver disease. In just 2 decades pediatric liver transplantation has matured as a clinical therapy from one performed in only a few centers in the United States and Western Europe to one that is practiced worldwide in innumerable medical institutions. This transformation can be traced to a few critical developments. Improvements in immunosuppressive agents suitable for use in children have clearly been of key importance in improving survival after transplantation. The application of technical variant allografts overcame the shortage of suitable donors for children and permitted many more children to undergo transplantation. Finally, the understanding of where, when, and how to use transplant therapy in children has improved. The latter is an ongoing process that has been aided by the creation in 1995 of a nationwide database comprising the experiences of 38 centers in the United States.[1] As the data from "Studies of Pediatric Liver Transplantation" (SPLIT) are analyzed and disseminated, further improvements should be realized.

Several factors about liver transplantation must be kept in mind for the procedure to be used in a manner that is consistent with the best medical interests of a pediatric patient. First, it must be remembered that it is a high-risk procedure, carrying a significant risk for mortality under the best of circumstances. Second, there is potential for chronic disability and the requirement for long-term drug administration. A number of transplant critics believe that having a liver transplant represents trading one disease for another. The results in children, however, suggest that a long-term, high-quality life is the rule rather than the exception. Nonetheless, it cannot be denied that a population of potentially impaired children is being created by this therapy. Every effort should be made to follow the outcome of the recipients of hepatic allografts carefully over many years to determine the true value of the procedure. A third consideration is that liver transplantation is extremely expensive. In an age of managed care in the private sector and budget deficits in the public sector, every effort is being made to reduce the cost of transplant therapy and to seek alternative therapies.

Many of the ideas concerning specific indications for transplant discussed here are the result of intuition and empiricism. If certain factors have not yet been shown to have an impact on the outcome of transplantation, that should not be taken as proof that they have no impact. Better data are clearly needed. For example, analyses of outcome in relation to the condition of the patient at the time of the procedure have failed to demonstrate a negative effect. Notwithstanding the obvious scientific faults of this type of analysis, including the failure to randomize patients to receive early versus late transplantation, the results make no sense. It is obvious that performing this type of surgery in patients in relatively good health with good nutritional stores will have a better outcome than when performed in moribund patients. Many of the large number of remaining questions about how to use liver transplantation may never be answered with certainty, but it remains important to study them.

This chapter reviews liver transplantation as it is practiced now, with particular focus on the indications for liver transplantation in children. We provide a general overview, a discussion of some specific indications in children, and an overview of aspects of liver transplantation that are unique to the pediatric population.

General Indications for Liver Transplantation in Children

The indications for liver transplantation in children can be categorized within the following framework (Table 21–1):

- Primary liver disease that is expected to progress to hepatic failure
- Liver disease with symptoms of nonprogressive primary liver disease and morbidity that outweigh the risks of transplantation
- Primary therapy for liver-based metabolic diseases

Table 21–1. APPROXIMATE FREQUENCIES OF SPECIFIC INDICATIONS FOR 500 PEDIATRIC LIVER TRANSPLANT RECIPIENTS (IN THE AUTHORS' EXPERIENCE)

Indication	Frequency
HEPATIC FAILURE	**95%**
Biliary atresia	62%
α_1-Antitrypsin deficiency	8%
Progressive familial intrahepatic cholestasis	7%
Fulminant hepatic failure	5%
Primary sclerosing cholangitis	3%
Autoimmune hepatitis	2%
Neonatal hepatitis	2%
Postnecrotic cirrhosis	2%
Tyrosinemia	2%
Secondary biliary cirrhosis	1%
Wilson's disease	< 1%
Congenital hepatic fibrosis	< 1%
NONPROGRESSIVE LIVER DISEASE	**< 1%**
Arteriohepatic dysplasia (Alagille syndrome)	< 1%
PRIMARY THERAPY FOR INBORN ERRORS	**< 1%**
Glycogen storage disease	< 1%
Urea cycle defects	< 1%
Crigler-Najjar syndrome	< 1%
SECONDARY LIVER DISEASE	**2%**
Cystic fibrosis	1%
Langerhans cell histiocytosis	1%
PRIMARY HEPATIC MALIGNANCY	**1%**
Hepatoblastoma	1%

- Liver disease as part of a systemic illness (i.e., secondary liver disease)
- Primary hepatic malignancy

Primary Liver Disease Expected to Progress to Hepatic Failure

Hepatic failure, whether acute or the result of end-stage liver disease, is the major indication for liver transplantation in infants and children. Table 21–2 lists the pediatric liver diseases that fit into this indication. Progressive biliary cirrhosis caused by biliary atresia is the most frequent single disease indication in all series. Parenchymal liver diseases, including autoimmune and chronic viral hepatitis, certain metabolic diseases that lead to liver failure, and fulminant hepatic failure (FHF), are also common indications.

Cirrhosis is neither a specific disease entity nor a general indication. It is an anatomic diagnosis with functional implications, and its diagnosis has grave

Table 21–2. DISEASES FOR WHICH ORTHOTOPIC LIVER TRANSPLANTATION HAS BEEN PERFORMED IN INFANTS AND CHILDREN FOR THE INDICATION OF HEPATIC INSUFFICIENCY

Metabolic diseases

  α_1-Antitrypsin deficiency

  Tyrosinemia

  Glycogen storage diseases

    Type IV

    Type III

  Wilson's disease

  Neonatal hemochromatosis

Acute and chronic hepatitis

  Fulminant hepatic failure

    Viral

    Toxin/drug induced

    Autoimmune hepatitis

  Chronic hepatitis/cirrhosis

    Hepatitis B virus

    Hepatitis C virus

    Autoimmune hepatitis

    Idiopathic

Intrahepatic cholestasis

  Idiopathic neonatal hepatitis

  Alagille syndrome

  Progressive familial intrahepatic cholestasis

Obstructive biliary tract disease

  Extrahepatic biliary atresia

  Primary sclerosing cholangitis

  Traumatic/postsurgical biliary tract diseases

Miscellaneous

  Cryptogenic cirrhosis

  Congenital hepatic fibrosis

  Cystic fibrosis

  Cirrhosis secondary to prolonged total parenteral nutrition

prognostic implications. Transplantation may not improve the 5-year survival of some children with cirrhosis. For example, the development of portal hypertension and gastrointestinal bleeding in children with biliary atresia and successful portoenterostomy has been shown not to affect survival.[2] Directly addressing the complications of cirrhosis, such as performing distal splenorenal shunts for bleeding varices or hypersplenism, may be more appropriate treatment options than transplantation.[3] Cirrhosis should not be considered an indication for liver transplantation unless there is evidence of functional hepatic decompensation.

An important factor in determining when inevitable hepatic insufficiency will develop is the natural history of the patient's liver disease. Biliary atresia, for example, has a clearly defined natural history in patients who either did not receive a portoenterostomy or in whom surgery failed to produce effective biliary drainage. These patients typically reach end-stage at some point between 9 and 18 months of age and thus are clearly candidates for liver transplantation in infancy.[4,5] Unfortunately, few other chronic liver diseases in children have such a clearly defined natural history.

Liver transplantation holds the greatest potential for survival in children with FHF.[6] However, it is not possible to determine prospectively which children will recover without transplantation. The ongoing National Institutes of Health (NIH)-funded acute liver failure study should improve our ability to estimate the probabilities of recovery based on cause and other factors and should improve the decision-making process regarding transplantation. At present, every child with acute liver failure should be considered a candidate for emergency transplantation.

Symptoms of Nonprogressive Primary Liver Disease

Several chronic cholestatic disorders of childhood produce severe symptoms, but rarely result in the development of end-stage liver failure. Alagille syndrome represents the prototype of this indication. When estimating the value of liver transplantation in treating these diseases, the morbidity of the liver disease must be weighed carefully against the mortality associated with liver transplantation. Pruritus that results in cutaneous mutilation and poor school performance and is refractory to medical therapy can be a valid indication for liver transplantation. Other morbid effects of chronic cholestatic liver disease that may merit consideration for transplantation include severe growth failure and malnutrition, refractory bone disease, hypercholesterolemia, and xanthomatosis. All other avenues of therapy should be exhausted, however, before transplantation is considered in these cases. For example, partial cutaneous biliary diversion can alleviate severe pruritis as well as hypercholesterolemia and xanthomatosis in children with Alagille syndrome,[7] which is clearly preferable to transplantation.

Liver Transplantation as Primary Therapy for Inborn Errors of Metabolism

Many human diseases result from inborn errors of critical metabolic or synthetic processes that principally involve the liver. Some of these, including α_1-antitrypsin deficiency, hereditary tyrosinemia, glycogen storage disease (types III and IV), Wilson's disease, and hereditary hemochromatosis, cause structural liver injury (including cirrhosis) and constitute routine indications for orthotopic liver transplantation (OLT) in pediatric and adult patients. Transplantation is required for acute or chronic liver failure or to eliminate the potential for malignancy, a frequent complication of several metabolic disorders.[8] Replacement of the liver also results in correction of the metabolic defect.

Replacement of the liver can benefit children with inborn errors of metabolism that do not injure the liver, the principal goal of treatment being to correct the metabolic error. Examples of disorders that have been treated in this way include urea cycle defects, Crigler-Najjar syndrome, homozygous familial hypercholesterolemia, and primary hyperoxaluria. The decision whether to perform liver transplantation depends on knowing that it will correct the metabolic defect, that there is no effective alternative therapy, and that the patient has not experienced irreversible complications. Crigler-Najjar syndrome represents the prototype for this decision-making process.[9-12] The severe deficiency of bilirubin uridine diphosphate (UDP)-glucuronyl transferase results in the systemic accumulation of bilirubin, which, if untreated, leads to neurological injury. These patients can be effectively treated for a time with phototherapy and the enteric administration of bilirubin-binding agents.[11] However, medical therapy is very cumbersome and inevitably fails to maintain safe levels of bilirubin in teenagers. As a result, these patients are usually managed medically until they are 10 to 12 years of age, at which time liver transplantation is performed.

The decision-making process is different for urea cycle defects, which result in hyperammonemia and brain damage. Despite advances in medical management, severe defects such as ornithine transcarbamylase (OTC) deficiency in males still have a very poor outcome.[13] Boys with OTC deficiency should be considered for transplantation immediately on making the diagnosis. Even taking an aggressive approach, neurological outcome is poor if the child has experienced very high serum ammonia levels or has had significant brain injury.[14] Successful transplantation corrects the metabolic defect but cannot undo preexisting brain damage. OTC deficiency is an X-linked disease. Girls who are heterozygous for the condition have a spectrum of illnesses, from none to quite severe.[15,16] More severely affected girls should be considered for transplantation if medical therapy fails to prevent episodes of hyperammonemia. In contrast, obligate heterozygous mothers have provided living donor allografts for affected sons.[17] Diseases with variable expressions and responses to medical therapy, such as the glycogen storage disease type I and familial hypercholesterolemia, must be considered individually.

Complete replacement of the liver may not be necessary when considering the treatment of metabolic diseases in which there is deficient enzyme activity. The quantity of functioning liver mass needed to carry out critical metabolic functions may allow for the effective use of auxiliary transplants or hepatocyte transplants. Orthotopic replacement of the left lobe of the liver has been used to treat ornithine transcarbamylase deficiency and Crigler-Najjar syndrome with some success. Likewise, hepatocyte transplantation has shown some promise, although maintaining function over time is difficult.[10]

Primary hyperoxaluria is a metabolic liver disease that uniquely results from an abnormal metabolic pathway that produces excess metabolite. Overproduced oxalate is filtered by the kidney, crystallizes, and causes micro-obstructive renal failure.[18] Transplanted kidneys suffer the same fate if the liver is not replaced as well, whereas preemptive liver transplantation can prevent renal damage.[19-21]

Secondary Liver Disease

Many children and young adults with cystic fibrosis and biliary cirrhosis have undergone liver transplantation.[22,23] Initially, there was concern that the associated use of immunosuppressives might lead to more severe infectious complications in these patients. However, that has not been the case. Many patients have improved pulmonary function, probably as the result of improved strength and general health. Successful liver transplantation is performed in children with sclerosing cholangitis secondary to Langerhans cell histiocytosis.[24-26] It is imperative to gain control of the systemic disease before undertaking liver transplantation while understanding that the liver disease is irreversible. Thus, the appropriate use of chemotherapy should not be curtailed because of concerns about causing liver damage. This disease is notable for a significantly increased risk for posttransplant lymphoproliferative disease[26] and perhaps recurrence.[27] When dealing with secondary liver disease, each patient and set of circumstances must be weighed on an individual basis to determine whether this approach is justified.

Primary Hepatic Malignancy

The prognosis after liver transplantation for patients with hepatocellular carcinoma has improved dramatically. This is now a major indication in adults, whereas previously it was a near-absolute contraindication for transplantation (see Chapter 15, "Transplantation for Primary Hepatic Malignancy"). Hepatocellular carcinoma is extremely rare in children outside the context of metabolic liver disease. The experience in metabolic liver disease suggests that small lesions do not reduce survival after transplantation, whereas the prognosis for children with large or multifocal carcinomas is bleak. The incidence of hepatocellular carcinoma in tyrosinemia is so great that liver transplantation has been performed as preemptive therapy.[28-30] However, with improved metabolic control it now seems reasonable to use prolonged medical therapy while monitoring closely for the development of cancer, which is done by frequent measurement of α-fetoprotein.[31] Diseases associated with no significant increased risk for malignancy during the early stages of disease need not be monitored. For example, carcinoma can develop in patients with glycogen storage disease, but only after adenomas are present; thus, the development of adenomas marks the time when frequent monitoring of α-fetoprotein should be initiated and transplantation considered.

The experience with liver transplantation in hepatoblastoma is limited.[32-35] This malignancy often presents symptomatically with abdominal distention because of a large tumor. Treating similar cases of hepatocellular carcinoma would be futile. However, hepatoblastomas are often sensitive to chemotherapy, which should be used initially to shrink the tumor mass before resection is attempted.[36] Only if complete resection is not possible should transplantation be considered. There is some debate about transplantation in the presence of metastatic disease. With chemosensitive tumors, resection of lung lesions followed by transplantation and posttransplant chemotherapy has met with reasonable success.[34] Such cases should probably be managed in centers with substantial experience in dealing with this cancer.

General Contraindications to Liver Transplantation

Many patients referred for liver transplantation are found to be candidates for beneficial alternative therapies. The experienced personnel at referral centers are frequently better prepared to judge the relative risks and benefits of transplantation versus alternative therapies than are referring physicians in the community, so consultation in this regard should be a primary role of referral centers. Because liver transplantation carries a significant risk, any potentially effective alternate therapy should be pursued. However, there is also risk involved with pursuing another therapy that turns out to be ineffective. In some cases, it makes sense to place the patient on the active transplant waiting list while closely observing the effects of other therapeutic interventions.

If a poor quality of life is expected following transplantation, consideration should be given to withholding therapy. This particularly applies to diseases that injure the central nervous system. Many infants with advanced liver disease have poor psychomotor development, especially of gross motor skills, but these deficits seem to recover, although possibly not fully, after liver transplantation.[37-39] Most infants with severe motor delay prior to transplantation will fall within the normal range if tested a year after transplantation.[37] Social development is not impaired to as great a degree as physical development, and recovery is faster. Neither physical nor social disabilities are reasons to deny transplantation.

It may not be possible to make any predictions about neurological outcome in some cases, such as the previously healthy child who presents with FHF and deep hepatic coma. Liver transplantation almost always reverses encephalopathy, but the recovery of the patient with cerebral edema is often incomplete, and sometimes brain death follows successful transplantation.[40]

Impairment of other organ systems can preclude liver transplantation. Complex congenital heart disease often accompanies Alagille syndrome and is severalfold higher in patients with biliary atresia than in the general population.[41,42] Examples of involvement of other systems include severe congenital hepatic fibrosis and polycystic kidney disease presenting at a very early age, and nephropathy with α₁-antitrypsin deficiency and Alagille syndrome.[41,43] In these unusual situations, the strategy may include multiorgan transplantation or a decision not to offer the patient a liver transplant.

Chronic liver disease and hepatic insufficiency have profound effects on other organ system functions. Secondary organ failure can have a negative effect on outcome after liver transplantation, so some of the systemic effects of liver disease must be medically corrected before liver transplantation can be considered. For example, the patient with hepatic coma and secondary ventilatory insufficiency can be treated by liver transplantation. In contrast, the development of intrapulmonary shunts, with or without pulmonary hypertension, can result in respiratory failure that may not recover.[44] Patients presenting with chronic liver disease and chronic hemoglobin desaturation, as evidenced by cyanosis, digital clubbing, and other symptoms, should undergo a careful pulmonary function study and possible cardiac catheterization. Many children with advanced cirrhosis secondary to biliary atresia have cardiomegaly, which appears to be secondary to a mild dilated cardiomyopathy, probably the result of malnutrition and other factors. These patients occasionally exhibit heart failure and require therapy, but usually recover after transplantation. The patient with functional renal insufficiency (hepatorenal syndrome, urinary sodium <20 mEq/L, normal sediment) is managed by establishing an access for renal dialysis before or during the liver transplant procedure. Renal function recovers after liver replacement.[45] Major intra-abdominal vascular anomalies associated with biliary atresia were once considered absolute contraindications to liver transplantation, but surgical advances allow successful liver transplantation even in the child with congenital absence of the portal vein.[46] Thorough preoperative evaluation of the vascular anatomy of the abdomen is required to plan the operative approach.

Any major acute systemic infection is a relative contraindication to liver transplantation, but sometimes the transplant cannot be avoided. For example, one of the complications encountered in the patient with biliary atresia is ascending cholangitis, which can be refractory to all medical management. Continued antibiotic therapy is likely to be ineffective and liver function can deteriorate, rendering the patient a less favorable candidate. Although the risk for postoperative infectious complications is high in this group, it is appropriate to proceed with liver transplantation when a donor becomes available. Likewise, patients with end-stage liver disease frequently develop systemic infections, including spontaneous bacterial peritonitis and sepsis. If these infections result in rapid hepatic decompensation, a combined medical/surgical approach is usually justified. Liver transplantation should be deferred until any viral infection, no matter how trivial, is resolved. Possible exceptions to this involve infections with the herpesviruses, other than Epstein-Barr virus (EBV), which often can be controlled even in the face of immunosuppression (e.g., cytomegalovirus [CMV], varicella, herpes simplex virus [HSV]-1).

A final contraindication to liver transplantation is disease that is expected to recur after therapy. Metastatic carcinomas, to or from the liver, and some other cancers that involve the liver (such as sarcomas) also have a poor long-term outcome after transplantation. Chronic viral infections, including hepatitis B and C viruses (HBV and HCV) and HIV, persist or recur after liver transplantation. The management of these conditions in adult patients has improved and is discussed in Chapters 8 ("Transplantation for Viral Hepatitis A and B") and 10 ("Transplantation for Hepatitis C: Risk Factors and Treatment"). Data in children are limited, and treatment of children with these infections generally follows the paradigms established in adult populations. Despite a high recurrence rate after transplantation, children with autoimmune hepatitis are not denied transplant therapy if needed.[47-49]

Management of Specific Diseases Leading to Liver Transplantation in Children

The diseases that result in a need for liver transplantation in children can be classified under the general indications previously discussed. Table 21–1 presents an overall list of the indications for transplantation in 500 children in our experience. The frequency of indications is similar to most other series. The following discussion highlights some of the questions regarding application of this therapeutic modality in children with the more important specific diseases.

Biliary atresia is by far the most common specific indication for liver transplantation in children. Recent SPLIT data indicate that this single disease accounts for 42% of pediatric transplants performed and 65% of those performed in children younger than 1 year.[1] Given the incidence of this disease, 400 to 600 new cases will be seen in the United States yearly. Perhaps a third of these will have a successful Kasai portoenterostomy procedure that will delay the need for transplant until the child is older.[50] Patients with biliary atresia and failed portoenterostomy procedures will typically reach end-stage liver disease sometime between 9 and 18 months of age, which results in 250 to 400 infants with biliary atresia that need transplants yearly.

The general strategy in managing a patient with biliary atresia should be one that maximizes overall outcome. Successful portoenterostomy prolongs survival out of infancy, and performing this procedure does not seem to imperil the patient at the time of transplantation. The results in several series suggest that survival is significantly reduced when liver transplantation is performed in a patient younger than 1 year of age. Therefore, any patient who can benefit from a portoenterostomy, based on age at diagnosis and other clinical factors, should have that procedure as initial therapy.

It has been common practice by many pediatric surgeons to perform the Kasai procedure again when it has not worked previously. Some common sense must be applied in this regard, although there is no evidence on which to base recommendations. If the portoenterostomy results in only a brief period of bile drainage and the histology of the ductal remnants indicates little chance for effective drainage to begin with, there should be no attempt to repeat the procedure. If there has been long-term effective drainage that has abruptly stopped, suggesting local cicatrix formation, an experienced surgeon may attempt to remove the scar and reestablish bile flow. However, repeated attempts to redo portoenterostomies in hopeless situations should be avoided because the repeated surgery can make transplantation much more difficult.

In the evolution of the portoenterostomy, a number of variants have been introduced with the purported advantage of reducing the frequency of ascending cholangitis. Unfortunately, no data have emerged supporting their use, and ascending cholangitis remains an important factor in the long-term survival of patients who have undergone successful portoenterostomy procedures.[51,52] Intestinal complications after transplantation are more common in patients who have had complex bowel surgery. We have also found that both long loops and externalization of bile drainage interfere with nutrition before transplantation and that long loops are associated with posttransplant malabsorption.[53] Also, exteriorization of enterostomy loops is associated with bleeding from the stoma and infection at the time of transplantation. The portoenterostomy, therefore, should be done just as Kasai described it using a relatively short biliary limb entering the intestinal mainstream as close as possible to the Treitz ligament.

Hypoplastic portal veins, often only 1 to 2 mm in diameter, are seen in patients with failed portoenterostomies and can complicate transplantation. Patients with successful portoenterostomies who continue to grow and come to transplantation years later have normal portal veins, which argues for performing the procedure. Hypoplastic portal veins are also observed in small children undergoing liver transplantation without prior portoenterostomy. The hypoplasia appears to be a consequence of cirrhosis early in life. Portal hypertension does not distend the portal vein under these conditions because of its intrinsic small radius and the effect of Laplace's law on the wall tension. Also, collateral circulation might develop relatively more easily in early life, limiting the magnitude of the portal pressure. No matter what the reason for the portal vein hypoplasia, it should not be used as a reason for not performing portoenterostomy.

The infant with a failed portoenterostomy should be referred as early as possible for evaluation because there is a significant lag time for obtaining a donor, and there is little risk of performing liver transplantation in these children too early. In the patient with the successful portoenterostomy, the matter of timing is more difficult. Most will experience progressive cirrhosis, probably the result of the intrinsic biology of biliary atresia. It is not a failure of surgery that brings the patient to transplant after 5 to 10 years. Good medical management and prudent surgery can be used to overcome the complications of cirrhosis and extend life without transplantation in some cases. However, the development of end-stage liver disease should be considered an indication to proceed with transplantation.

α_1-Antitrypsin deficiency is the most common inborn error of metabolism that eventuates in the need for liver transplantation.[54] This genetic disease has a highly variable effect on the liver and other systems. There is no medical therapy that effectively prevents the progression of liver disease. Most individuals with the genetic defect have no liver disease. Approximately 10% have neonatal cholestasis, which usually resolves after a few months. A small proportion of these patients develop macronodular cirrhosis, characteristically before the age of 20 years.[55] Rarely, the disease causes rapidly progressive cirrhosis and liver failure in infancy and is associated with an increased incidence of hepatocellular carcinoma in children and adults. Other systems can be involved, such as the early onset of emphysema and membranoproliferative nephritis. Liver transplantation has a role only in the patient with hepatic insufficiency or early malignancy and cannot be justified for the treatment or prevention of lung or kidney disease.[56] Transplantation results in the recipient assuming the α_1-antitrypsin phenotype of the donor, but it cannot be justified simply to correct the metabolic error. It should be considered for the infant with progressive liver failure. Patients with neonatal cholestasis that resolves should simply be observed for the onset of cirrhosis with yearly physical and biochemical evaluations. If cirrhosis develops, the patient will probably develop hepatic insufficiency at some point, but usually after several years. All older patients with cirrhosis should have regular screening for hepatocellular carcinoma. Transplantation should be performed only when needed for liver failure or malignancy.

Tyrosinemia results from deficient fumarylacetoacetate hydrolase activity in several tissues. Sometimes the defect results in rapidly progressive liver disease or FHF in infancy, with subsequent need of emergency liver transplantation. Rapid diagnosis in patients suspected of having tyrosinemia by measurement of urinary succinylacetone is important because medical therapy can prevent progression of disease to liver failure. Administration of an inhibitor of tyrosine catabolism, 2-(2-nitro-4-trifluoromethylbenzoyl)-1,3-cyclohexanedione (NTBC), disrupts the metabolic pathway before toxic substances are produced.[31,57] It is usually used in conjunction with a low-tyrosine diet, which can reduce the very high plasma tyrosine levels that result from metabolic blockade. NTBC therapy is very effective if instituted before the onset of disease, such as with siblings of affected patients diagnosed prenatally or just after birth. It is also effective in patients presenting with acute or chronic tyrosinemia. However, many such patients have chronic liver disease, such as postnecrotic cirrhosis caused by toxic injury suffered before instituting therapy.[58] Untreated patients and patients treated with dietary restriction only have an extremely high risk for hepatocellular carcinoma.[28] It is unclear to what degree that risk is eliminated in NTBC-treated children. The current approach is to treat these patients with NTBC and diet. If the patient cannot be completely stabilized by medical means, transplantation must be performed. If the patient responds to therapy, transplantation can be delayed while the clinical course is monitored. Serum α-fetoprotein levels should be closely watched. Failure to maintain completely normal levels indicates incomplete metabolic control or irreversible genetic changes in the liver,[59] either of which predicts a high risk for the development of hepatocellular carcinoma. In these cases, liver transplantation should be performed by age 2 to 3 years because of the risk of malignancy. Liver transplantation reverses the clinical syndrome, but some patients continue to excrete succinylacetone into the urine, indicating that a renal tubular defect remains.

Liver transplantation holds the greatest life-saving potential for children with acute hepatic failure, but the decision to use it in this situation is complex.[6,60] Determining the cause of hepatic failure is an important factor in deciding whether transplantation is appropriate. The highest mortality is seen in children with non–A-E hepatitis (indeterminate), acute Wilson's disease, some hepatotoxicity such as mushroom poisoning, and some idiosyncratic, drug-induced hepatitis. Patients with these disorders who present with a rapid onset and progression to stage III or stage IV hepatic encephalopathy and coagulopathy should be considered for immediate transplantation. In contrast, children with hepatitis A, certain hepatotoxicity (particularly when caused by acetaminophen poisoning), and severe autoimmune hepatitis may make a complete recovery with medical therapy. Thus careful monitoring for poor prognostic factors is required before selection.

In contrast to adults, the duration of illness before the onset of encephalopathy or the degree of encephalopathy at the time of presentation carries little prognostic significance in children. Neither is there any significant difference in survival rate between patients who present with late-onset hepatic failure and those with acute fulminant hepatitis. Survival does correlate with degree of severity of encephalopathy; in one study survival was 18% for patients with stage IV hepatic coma, 48% for those with stage III coma, and 66% for stage II coma.[61] The development of cerebral edema and renal failure, particularly in association with collapsing liver mass, is associated with a grave prognosis.

Our work with children and adults who have FHF has led to an aggressive, empirical approach to management. It is appropriate to list for emergency liver transplantation all children who have reached stage III hepatic coma, and liver transplantation should be performed as soon as a donor is available.[60,61] A patient showing signs of stabilization (lack of progressive deterioration) or evidence of recovering function (improved coagulation parameters) while awaiting graft availability has an outlook for spontaneous recovery as good as with liver transplantation, so the decision to perform transplantation is reversed. However, most children with acute liver failure have a rapid downhill course and require maximal medical therapy until a donor becomes available.

Survival after liver transplantation performed for acute hepatic failure is somewhat reduced when compared with the general survival rates in children.[40,61-63] The causes for reduced survival are not entirely known. Because the development of irreversible brain damage is a major cause of reduced survival, it is essential to be certain that brain damage has not occurred before the operation. Current techniques are inadequate but

include monitoring intracranial pressure (ICP), the identification of cerebral infarction or intracranial hemorrhage by cerebral computed tomography (CT) or magnetic resonance imaging (MRI), and looking for evidence of midbrain coning, such as fixed, dilated pupils. Cerebral dysfunction or brain death following transplantation was the cause of death in all series, indicating the importance of not performing transplantation in patients with irreversible brain damage.

Another factor in poor posttransplant outcome is the development of aplastic anemia, a unique and common complication of acute hepatic failure secondary to non–A-E hepatitis. The mechanism is unknown, but presumably it represents involvement of the bone marrow with the same virus that caused the liver disease. Thrombocytopenia and leukopenia in association with non–A-E hepatitis portend a poor outcome if transplantation is performed.[64]

The shortage of donors affects survival. Not only do children die without transplantation, but less than ideal donor organs are often accepted because of the urgency of the situation. Improved survival in recent studies using living donor and split-liver transplants suggests that limited availability of deceased donor organs is a major factor in poor outcome.[65-67] The use of auxiliary liver transplants and hepatocyte transplantation shows promise and may be useful as a support measure, with some patients recovering without the need for full liver replacement.[68,69]

Chronic intrahepatic cholestasis syndromes represent a complex group of disorders in which liver transplantation has a variable role because symptoms are usually severe, but the diseases often are not life-threatening. Patients with Alagille syndrome may have debilitating pruritus and hypercholesterolemia with xanthomatosis, but infrequently develop end-stage liver disease.[41] The issue arises as to whether liver transplantation should be used to treat symptoms only, its risks weighed only against the degree of incapacitation from symptoms, which can in some cases result in social invalidism. Alternative forms of therapy, including administration of ursodeoxycholic acid and partial cutaneous biliary diversion,[7,70] may provide relief from pruritus in some patients, and many of the complications can be treated by specific administration of vitamins and other nutrients. However, in some instances, the cholestasis is refractory to all therapy, and liver transplantation should be considered. In the occasional patient with cirrhosis, transplantation should also be considered even before decompensation of function because these patients are usually refractory to other measures, and there seems little reason to delay therapy that can eliminate the severe symptoms. Patients with progressive familial intrahepatic cholestasis (PFIC) (e.g., gene defects in FIC-1 and BSEP [bile salt export pump]) develop cirrhosis early in life,[71,72] but there are effective alternative therapies available that have much lower risk than transplantation.[70,73] As a rule of thumb, if cirrhosis has developed in any patient with chronic intrahepatic cholestasis, there is little reason to avoid transplantation because these patients will progress to end-stage disease. It is better to perform transplantation early and improve the quality of life.

Liver transplantation may not be indicated in the management of liver structure. Congenital hepatic fibrosis is such a condition.[74,75] In this disease, there is dense fibrous scarring of the portal triads. Patients who have severe portal hypertension with hypersplenism and portosystemic collaterals may have little if any parenchymal dysfunction. In contrast to the patient with cirrhosis, other measures such as endoscopic sclerotherapy of varices and portosystemic shunts (e.g., a distal splenorenal shunt) should be used to treat these patients. Rarely, these patients can have hepatic insufficiency, in which case liver transplantation is indicated. Because they also have associated cystic disease of the kidney, combined liver-kidney transplant can be considered.

Referral to a Transplant Center

The best time for referral is as soon as the patient is identified as having a condition that will require transplantation. Examples of who should be referred are infants with biliary atresia who remain jaundiced after portoenterostomy, all children with acute hepatic failure, and patients with cirrhosis for any reason. An individual patient may not need transplantation right away, but it is in most patients' best interest not to wait until the complications of advanced liver disease have been encountered before referring them to a transplant center.

Early referral allows the transplant center to have maximal input into the management strategy. Transplant centers have extensive experience with children with advanced liver disease and can help the referring physician in the management of complications before transplantation, improving diagnosis and suggesting alternative therapies. In addition, a close working relationship between the transplant center and the family/referring physician can develop before the procedure takes place, which leads to improved ability to coordinate postoperative care.

Evaluating the Pediatric Transplant Candidate

The basic pretransplant evaluation involves the elements presented in Table 21–3. This evaluation can be performed in approximately half a day in an outpatient

Table 21–3. BASICS OF THE PRETRANSPLANT EVALUATION

Confirm the diagnosis and need for transplantation.

Determine the urgency for transplantation.

Look for possible contraindications to transplantation.

Look for processes that might present a problem after transplantation.

Establish a relationship with parents and primary care providers.

Arrange for finances.

Arrange a mechanism for contacting parents and providing transport.

Establish a plan for interim management.

setting, except in unusual or complex cases. A routine should be established and a checklist created for each patient evaluated. A multidisciplinary approach is preferred because it provides maximal input and balance to the evaluation.

Confirming the diagnosis and determining the urgency for transplantation are essential in the effort to avoid performing transplantation in a child with benign liver disease or who is in the early stages of progressive liver disease, when the prognosis without transplantation is excellent. Although patients with end-stage disease sometimes undergo transplantation without a specific diagnosis, there is need for the team to make every effort to confirm the diagnosis. Reasons for doing so include avoiding transplantation when it is not indicated, avoiding transplantation for disorders that will recur, and providing appropriate genetic counseling to the family. In addition, better alternative therapies can be found for many patients. Primary or secondary disease of other organ systems should result in consultation from other specialists.

The transplant surgeon should be involved in evaluating the patient for surgery as well as in participating in the general evaluation and becoming familiar to the child and family. The most important anatomic variables to be evaluated are the portal vein, the other intra-abdominal vasculature and, in the case of a patient with biliary atresia, the type of portoenterostomy performed. Thorough preoperative evaluation of the vascular anatomy of the abdomen is required to plan the operative approach. Some children with biliary atresia have associated congenital absence or thrombosis of the portal vein, hypoplastic portal veins, or other major vascular anomalies. Advanced knowledge of the anatomy is essential for proper planning. Variants of the Kasai portoenterostomy involve long biliary limbs of the Roux-en-Y or the creation of cutaneous stomas, or both. Advance knowledge of this anatomy is needed to plan the approach to choledochoenterostomy. Long limbs may need to be returned to the intestinal mainstream in order to avoid postoperative malabsorption. Cutaneous stomas should be taken down before transplantation to avoid postoperative infections, improve growth, and avoid hemorrhage from stomal varices.

Transplantation should be delayed until the point at which the likelihood of short-term survival is less than that expected with transplantation, but it should occur before the opportunity for maximal posttransplant survival and outcome has been lost. The level of illness at the time of transplantation directly influences posttransplant patient survival. For example, patients requiring intensive care, especially those requiring mechanical ventilation or dialysis, have a significantly diminished 1-year survival. Likewise, patients who develop multiple medical complications before transplantation may sustain injury to other organ systems, which is likely to have long-term health implications. Therefore, quantifying this illness at the time of transplant referral is a valuable step in planning the appropriate timing of transplantation. There is, at present, no reliable set of criteria for staging pediatric liver disease. The current method of liver allocation, however, does include a numerical system to calculate mortality risk that may be used to stage chronic liver disease in children. The Pediatric End-Stage Liver Disease (PELD) score was developed to prioritize patients for transplantation.[76] This system stages liver disease by waiting list mortality risk in patients that have already been accepted as transplant candidates. It is not known if this system will be a reliable indicator of posttransplant events.

The PELD score ability to predict the probability of waiting list mortality in children with chronic liver disease was validated.[76-78] Mathematical modeling was used to identify and weigh the impact of readily available clinical variables on 3-month survival. These variables were chosen from existing data submitted through the SPLIT project. The model was developed to predict two possible endpoints, namely, requirement for intensive care support and death. A cohort of 779 children was included in analyses of the impact of 17 disease-specific candidate variables, of which 5 were found to predict the selected endpoints. The receiver operating characteristics (ROCs) of the model at 3 and 6 months following listing for liver transplantation were 0.82 and 0.82, respectively, for death or transfer to an ICU; and 0.92 and 0.89, respectively, for death alone. As the PELD score increases, mortality risk increases, resulting in a 3-month mortality of 50% in patients with a PELD score equal to 46. The resulting model for liver allocation to children was adopted by the United Network of Organ Sharing (UNOS) in February 2002:

$$PELD\ Score = (0.436[age]) - 0.687\ \log_e [albumin\ g/dL]$$
$$+ 0.480\ \log_e [total\ bilirubin\ mg/dL]$$
$$+ 1.857\ \log_e [INR] + 0.667\ [growth\ failure]$$

where age < 1 year, score = 1; age > 1 year, score = 0; growth failure: 2 standard deviations below mean for age, score = 1; ≤2 standard deviations below the mean for age, score = 0. INR = international normalized ratio.

Many children develop complications that increase their mortality risk, but that are not captured by the scoring system. Examples include gastrointestinal bleeding that is refractory to medical intervention, hepatopulmonary syndrome, and advancing pulmonary disease in patients with cystic fibrosis. These complications were infrequent in the patient cohort used for model development and, therefore, their impact has not been fully tested. Patients who develop such complications may be given additional priority on the waiting list by determination of regional review boards. Such applications for review sidestep the philosophy of the new allocation system, which is to be objective and standardized, yet may be necessary to avoid waiting list mortality for individual patients. The current system is clearly an imperfect solution to a serious problem, and ongoing development is necessary to address these issues. When the patient may have access to a living donor or split-liver graft, all aspects must be considered and weighed before proceeding with transplantation.

Growth is an important feature of childhood that reflects the functional status of the liver. We have found that the demonstrated inability of the liver to support a child's growth and nutritional status is as good a measure as any for the need to proceed with transplantation. When it becomes evident that no further growth is possible despite maximal nutritional support, transplantation should be performed as soon as possible. A child with growth failure secondary to liver disease cannot improve as a transplant candidate.

The candidate must be evaluated with regard to the potential for the development of infections after transplantation. The serological CMV status determines the risk for serious infection after transplantation. EBV is also important because of its association with posttransplant lymphoproliferative disease. Naïve patients seem to be at much higher risk.[79,80] Varicella serological status should be known so that proper care can be provided in case of exposure. Potential recipients should be provided immunizations before transplantation if at all possible. This should include rubella, rubeola, mumps, HBV, hepatitis A virus (HAV), polio, varicella, DPT (diphtheria, pertussis, and tetanus), *Haemophilus influenzae* B, and *Streptococcus pneumoniae* vaccines. Limited experience with measles vaccine given after transplantation indicates that it is safe but has limited efficacy.

Dedicated social workers provide important insight into the family's resources and resourcefulness and can identify problems that deserve focused input. Travel arrangements and accommodations for the family at the time of transplantation should be established with the help of the center staff.

Issues Unique to Pediatric Liver Transplantation

Nutritional Consequences of Chronic Liver Disease and Their Impact on Transplantation

Children with chronic liver disease almost invariably develop evidence of malnutrition—which is obviously important to patient well-being—during the course of illness, and there is almost no understanding of the basis for liver-related nutritional disturbances. It is commonly believed that malabsorption is the major cause of malnutrition in these patients. It is indeed true that most infants with biliary atresia have malabsorption of fats and fat-soluble vitamins because of total disruption of bile flow into the intestine. However, patients with biliary atresia often demonstrate normal rates of growth for up to 6 months with support provided by elemental diets and supplemental fat-soluble vitamins. Clinical malnutrition becomes evident only when the liver disease has progressed to a more advanced stage, at which time patients do not gain weight or otherwise improve their general nutritional status, even if provided supranormal quantities of nutrients by intravenous infusion. This suggests that erosion of parenchymal function is the critical

phenomenon leading to disturbed nutrition. Similarly, wasting is characteristic in parenchymal liver disease, such as neonatal hepatitis (Fig. 21–1). The transplant center should:

- Routinely monitor the nutritional state of potential candidates by performing regular anthropometric examinations
- Provide advice and support to the primary physician with regard to nutritional support

Despite every effort, the majority of infants are severely malnourished at the time of transplantation. Thus, restoration of nutrition is a focus for medical postoperative care in most infants with biliary atresia.

Surgical Innovations Affecting Pediatric Liver Transplantation

Organ size is of utmost importance in pediatric transplantation. The majority of children with liver disease reach end-stage disease before 2 years of age, whereas relatively few do so between the ages of 2 and 10 years. There is a second mortality peak after age 10 that extends into adulthood.[81,82] The pattern of mortality from liver disease is in contrast to the epidemiology of accidents, which involve mainly preschool and school-aged children. Consequently, most pediatric liver donors are too large for the typical pediatric recipient, creating a donor-to-recipient mismatch that causes excessively long waiting times and high pretransplant

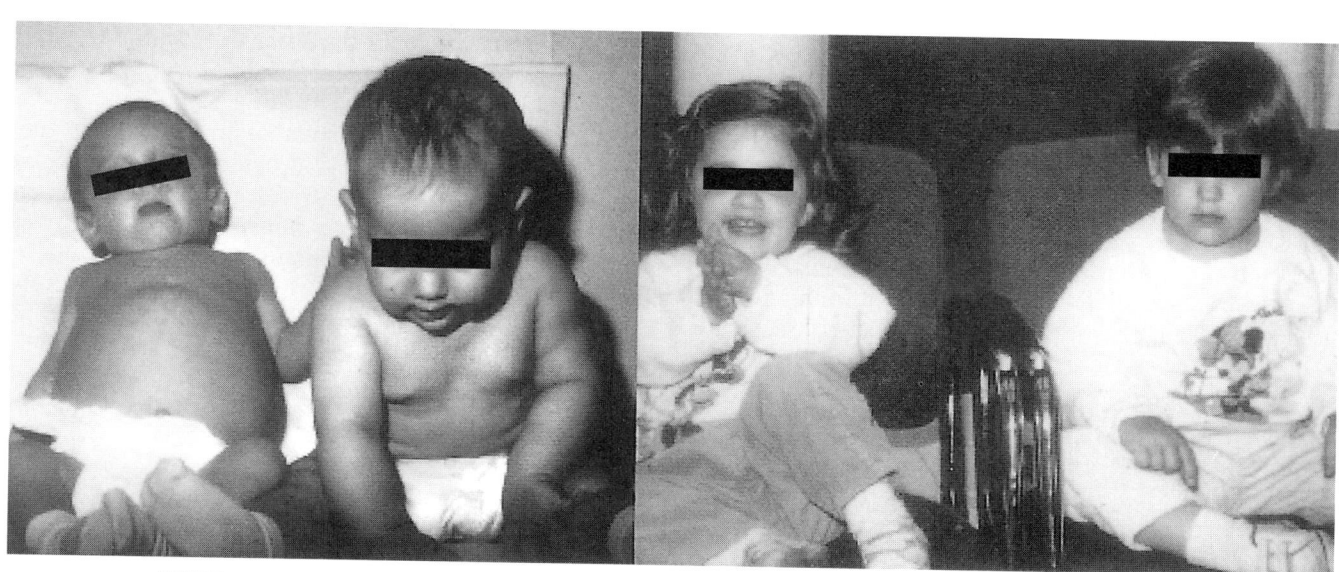

FIGURE 21–1

The effect of parenchymal liver disease on nutrition and the correcting effect of liver transplantation. The child on the left in each panel suffered malnutrition and failure to thrive as a result of severe progressive neonatal hepatitis (*left*) and received a liver transplant using the right lobe in a split-liver operation at 5 months of age. In follow-up at 2 years of age (*right*), she has achieved growth and general function equivalent to her twin (*shown on the right in each panel*).

mortality among small children. Furthermore, grafts from older children are used in adult transplant recipients. To overcome the inadequacy of donors for young children, the techniques for using larger donors were developed. Technical variant allograft surgery is discussed in detail in Chapters 41 and 42. Developed in the late 1980s and early 1990s, this surgery is now used in all major pediatric transplant centers.

Reduced-size liver transplantation is the technique by which the size of a donor liver is reduced to provide a hepatic allograft for a recipient who is usually somewhat smaller than the donor.[83] It was the most common approach to pediatric transplantation for several years until the shortage of deceased donors became critical. The techniques of technical variant allograft transplantation were further expanded to split-liver transplantation and transplantation using living related donors.[84,85] Split-liver transplantation is a technique in which a donor liver is divided to provide grafts for two recipients. Despite its complexity, its use in pediatric centers should be expanded because of the obvious advantage of being able to obtain a graft for an adult and child from a single deceased donor. At present, rules for organ sharing through split-liver procedures are being developed. Living donor transplantation, in which a healthy donor undergoes partial hepatectomy for the purpose of providing a graft for transplantation, was developed for application in young children. In more recent years, it has seen expanded application in adult-to-adult living donor transplantation.

In pediatric transplantation, it is necessary to compute the size of the graft needed and, therefore, select the resection required for the creation of an appropriate-sized graft. The crux of the issue is matching the graft to the size of the space in which it is to reside, and this must be done by visual inspection of the donor organ and the recipient's hepatic fossa. The anatomy of the liver is not uniform; some donors have relatively large or small livers, and some livers have relatively large or small lobes. Grafts can routinely be obtained from a donor up to 10 times the weight of the recipient and at times from donors larger than that. No formula can be used to determine the volume of the hepatic fossa from the recipient's size and weight. Left lateral lobe grafts are generally used when the donor-to-recipient weight ratio exceeds 4, and the left lobe graft is used when the ratio is between 2 and 4. Right lobe grafts have been used in teenagers as in adult-to-adult procedures.

There are several clear advantages to living donor liver transplantation for infants and young children.[86] First, the earlier and more elective transplantation of small infants provides a major advantage in that these children are not malnourished and have not encountered major complications of liver disease at the time of transplantation.[87,88] The quality of the graft is uniformly outstanding. Although the frequency of rejection has not been less than in recipients of deceased-donor allografts, the severity of rejection has been.[89] It has been accepted into practice in major centers in the United States, Japan, and Europe. Despite its apparent advantages, there remains considerable debate regarding whether the benefits of the procedure outweigh the potential risk to consenting donors.

Liver Transplantation in Neonates

Infants younger than 3 months of age, defined as neonates, present unique medical and technical challenges in transplantation.[90-94] Their small size coupled with their extremely critical condition at presentation results in high rates of operative and postoperative complications, leading to reduced survival of those who undergo transplantation. Liver transplantation of neonates is uncommon, with 8 to 14 cases performed nationally per year out of approximately 600 pediatric liver transplants. Patient and graft survival, 57% and 38% respectively, remain significantly lower than those of older children.[90,95]

All neonatal liver transplants are performed for acute liver failure. Table 21–4 provides epidemiological summary statistics from the literature and the experience at our center for neonatal liver transplantation. The most commonly reported indication is giant cell hepatitis. It accounts for more than half of liver transplants in this age group. Neonatal hemochromatosis (NH), or iron

Table 21–4. INDICATIONS FOR NEONATAL ORTHOTOPIC LIVER TRANSPLANTATION IN REPORTED SERIES AND AUTHORS' CENTER

Author	Total Patients	Giant Cell Hepatitis	Iron Storage Disease	Viral Hepatitis	Other
Woodle et al.[90]	23	12 (52%)	4 (17%)	0	7 (31%)
Bonatti et al.[91]	9	1 (12%)	3 (33%)	3 (33%)	2 (22%)
Noujaim et al.[92]	15	0	4 (27%)	4 (27%)	7 (4%)
Lund et al.[93]	3	0	3 (100%)	0	0
Srinivasan et al.[94]	6	0	4 (66%)	1 (17%)	1 (17%)
Children's Memorial Hospital	7	0	2 (29%)	1 (14%)	4 (57%)

storage disease, although underrepresented in the transplant literature, is the most frequently recognized cause of acute liver failure in newborns. Additional indications include HBV, echovirus or other enterovirus infection, total parenteral nutrition (TPN)-associated liver disease, and hepatic hemangioendotheliomatosis.[90,91]

The special considerations of neonatal OLT relate to the specific physiology of the neonates in liver failure and their small size. A neonate in acute liver failure is in a tenuous medical condition. Impaired respiratory function, severe coagulopathy, malnutrition, and ascites frequently complicate the picture in these patients. Depressed cardiac and renal function are also common, and patients frequently require hemodialysis or hemofiltration, both of which are difficult to perform in very small patients.

The small size of these patients makes graft selection difficult and uniquely important. The typical body weights of neonatal recipients range from 3.5 to 4.5 kg (7.7 to 9.9 lb). Full-sized grafts from donors weighing less than 6 kg (13.2 lb) are associated with high rates of graft failure. Therefore, all neonatal liver transplants are now performed with technical variant grafts, either from deceased or living donors. The use of oversized allografts should be avoided because it commonly results in delayed abdominal closure and increased intra-abdominal pressure with subsequent impairment of respiratory function and decreased graft perfusion. The impact of these complications should not be underestimated; an oversized graft often triggers a series of events that ultimately leads to graft failure and patient mortality.

Other challenges in neonatal liver transplantation are that technical variant grafts have a higher risk of both primary nonfunction and poor early function and are associated with increased risk for postoperative bleeding and bile leak. It also appears that the incidence of vascular thrombosis is very high in these patients, which may result from both technical difficulties and medical/physiological idiosyncrasies such as relatively low perfusion pressure.

Medically, these patients have a very high risk of infection. Bacterial and fungal infections affect up to 75% of patients and directly contribute to mortality in 50%.[95,96] Primary EBV and CMV infections are more likely to cause life-threatening multisystem disease in these naïve patients. Additionally, neonates are at increased risk for EBV-associated posttransplant lymphoproliferative disease.[79]

In most centers, neonates receive immunosuppressive regimens similar to those given older patients, with protocols based on either cyclosporine or tacrolimus. The long-term risks of rejection and the ongoing immunosuppressive needs of this population have not been systematically studied. At present, they are assumed to be similar to those of older children. Apart from relatively short-term survival, very little information is available regarding the outcome of neonatal patients who receive liver transplantation. The experience at our center suggests that intact long-term survival is unusual. There is a clear need for careful outcomes analysis to determine the value of neonatal liver transplantation and to identify areas in which improvements can be made.

Pearls and Pitfalls

- Progression to stage III encephalopathy in a patient with fulminant hepatic failure is an indication for emergent liver transplantation.

- In FHF in children, the duration of illness and degree of encephalopathy at the time of presentation carry little prognostic significance.

- Early referral to a transplant center allows a transplant hepatologist to assess and modify risk factors for morbidity and mortality in patients who will ultimately require OLT.

- One of the strongest predictors of outcomes in children with FHF is the cause of the liver injury.

- Growth failure in patients with biliary atresia can be an early and important indicator of liver synthetic insufficiency.

- One third of children with FHF of indeterminate cause (non–A-E hepatitis) will develop aplastic anemia, which is associated with a high rate of mortality.

- The most important contraindication to liver transplantation is effective alternative therapy.
  - Example 1: Biliary atresia with good synthetic function but portal hypertension may respond to distal splenorenal shunt.
  - Example 2: Progressive familial intrahepatic cholestasis or Alagille syndrome may respond to biliary diversion prior to requiring OLT.

- Systemic infections are usually contraindications for OLT, except in cases such as recalcitrant cholangitis and spontaneous bacterial peritonitis, which may require aggressive medical therapy and OLT for resolution.

- Systemic diseases such as Langerhans cell histiocytosis or malignant disease should be treated primarily (i.e., with chemotherapy) prior to OLT.

- Delaying transplantation in patients with metabolic diseases that cause elevated ammonia levels (e.g., OTC deficiency) risks irreversible neurological injury. Patients with intact neurological function should receive a transplant before significant crises occur.

References

1. Studies of Pediatric Liver Transplantation (SPLIT): Year 2000 outcomes. Transplantation 72:463-476, 2001.
2. Miga D, Sokol RJ, Mackenzie T, et al: Survival after first esophageal variceal hemorrhage in patients with biliary atresia. J Pediatr 139:291-296, 2001.
3. Shilyansky J, Roberts EA, Superina RA: Distal splenorenal shunts for the treatment of severe thrombocytopenia from portal hypertension in children. J Gastrointest Surg 3:167-172, 1999.
4. Grosfeld JL, Fitzgerald JF, Predaina R, et al: The efficacy of hepatoportoenterostomy in biliary atresia. Surgery 106:692-701, 1989.
5. Lilly JR, Karrer FM, Hall RJ, et al: The surgery of biliary atresia. Ann Surg 210:289-296, 1989.
6. Whitington PF, Soriano HE, Alonso EM: Fulminant hepatic failure in children. In Suchy FJ, Sokol RJ, Balistreri WF (eds): Liver Disease in Children. Philadelphia, Lippincott, Williams & Wilkins, 2001, pp 63-88.
7. Emerick KM, Whitington PF: Partial external biliary diversion for intractable pruritus and xanthomas in Alagille syndrome. Hepatology 35:1501-1506, 2002.
8. Ishak KG: Hepatocellular carcinoma associated with the inherited metabolic diseases. In Tabor E, DiBisceglie AM, Purcell RH (eds): Etiology, Pathology, and Treatment of Hepatocellular Carcinoma in North America. Houston, Gulf Publishing, 1991, pp 91-103.
9. Rela M, Muiesan P, Vilca-Melendez H, et al: Auxiliary partial orthotopic liver transplantation for Crigler-Najjar syndrome type I. Ann Surg 229:565-569, 1999.
10. Fox IJ, Chowdhury JR, Kaufman SS, et al: Treatment of the Crigler-Najjar syndrome type I with hepatocyte transplantation. N Engl J Med 338:1422-1426, 1998.
11. Van der Veere CN, Sinaasappel M, McDonagh AF, et al: Current therapy for Crigler-Najjar syndrome type 1: Report of a world registry. Hepatology 24:311-315, 1996.
12. Whitington PF, Emond JC, Heffron TG, Thistlethwaite JR: Orthotopic auxiliary liver transplantation for Crigler-Najjar syndrome type I. Lancet 342:779-780, 1993.
13. Maestri NE, Hauser ER, Bartholemew D, Brusilow SW: Prospective treatment of urea cycle disorders. J Pediatr 119:923-928, 1991.
14. Whitington PF, Alonso EM, Boyle JT, et al: Liver transplantation for the treatment of urea cycle disorders. J Inherit Metab Dis 21(Suppl 1):112-118, 1998.
15. Lee B, Yu H, Jahoor F, et al: In vivo urea cycle flux distinguishes and correlates with phenotypic severity in disorders of the urea cycle. Proc Natl Acad Sci U S A 97:8021-8026, 2000.
16. Heringlake S, Boker K, Manns M: Fatal clinical course of ornithine transcarbamylase deficiency in an adult heterozygous female patient. Digestion 58:83-86, 1997.
17. Nagasaka H, Yorifuji T, Egawa H, et al: Successful living-donor liver transplantation from an asymptomatic carrier mother in ornithine transcarbamylase deficiency. J Pediatr 138:432-434, 2001.
18. Watts RW: The clinical spectrum of the primary hyperoxalurias and their treatment. J Nephrol 11(Suppl 1):4-7, 1998.
19. Kemper MJ, Nolkemper D, Rogiers X, et al: Preemptive liver transplantation in primary hyperoxaluria type 1: Timing and preliminary results. J Nephrol 11(Suppl 1):46-48, 1998.
20. Ellis SR, Hulton SA, McKiernan PJ, et al: Combined liver-kidney transplantation for primary hyperoxaluria type 1 in young children. Nephrol Dial Transplant 16:348-354, 2001.
21. Astarcioglu I, Karademir S, Gulay H, et al: Primary hyperoxaluria: Simultaneous combined liver and kidney transplantation from a living related donor. Liver Transpl 9:433-436, 2003.
22. Noble-Jamieson G, Valente J, Barnes ND, et al: Liver transplantation for hepatic cirrhosis in cystic fibrosis. Arch Dis Child 71:349-352, 1994.
23. Mack DR, Traystman MD, Colombo JL, et al: Clinical denouement and mutation analysis of patients with cystic fibrosis undergoing liver transplantation for biliary cirrhosis. J Pediatr 127:881-887, 1995.
24. Rajwal SR, Stringer MD, Davison SM, et al: Use of basiliximab in pediatric liver transplantation for Langerhans cell histiocytosis. Pediatr Transplant 7:247-251, 2003.
25. Rand ER, Whitington PF: Successful orthotopic liver transplantation in two patients with liver failure due to sclerosing cholangitis in the setting of Langerhans cell histiocytosis. J Pediatr Gastroenterol Nutr 15:202-207, 1992.
26. Newell KA, Alonso EM, Kelly SM, et al: Association between liver transplantation for Langerhans cell histiocytosis, rejection, and development of posttransplant lymphoproliferative disease in children. J Pediatr 131:98-104, 1997.
27. Hadzic N, Pritchard J, Webb D, et al: Recurrence of Langerhans cell histiocytosis in the graft after pediatric liver transplantation. Transplantation 70:815-819, 2000.
28. Starzl TE, Zitelli BJ, Shaw BW Jr, et al: Changing concepts: Liver replacement for hereditary tyrosinemia and hepatoma. J Pediatr 106:604-606, 1985.
29. Esquivel CO, Mieles L, Marino IR, et al: Liver transplantation for hereditary tyrosinemia in the presence of hepatocellular carcinoma. Transplant Proc 21:2445-2446, 1989.
30. Freese DK, Tuchman M, Schwarzenberg SJ, et al: Early liver transplantation is indicated for tyrosinemia type I. J Pediatr Gastroenterol Nutr 13:10-15, 1991.
31. Grompe M: The pathophysiology and treatment of hereditary tyrosinemia type 1. Semin Liver Dis 21:563-571, 2001.
32. Tagge EP, Tagge DU, Reyes J, et al: Resection, including transplantation, for hepatoblastoma and hepatocellular carcinoma: Impact on survival. J Pediatr Surg 27:292-297, 1992.
33. Bilik R, Superina R: Transplantation for unresectable liver tumors in children. Transplant Proc 29:2834-2835, 1997.
34. Superina R, Bilik R: Results of liver transplantation in children with unresectable liver tumors. J Pediatr Surg 31:835-839, 1996.
35. Srinivasan P, McCall J, Pritchard J, et al: Orthotopic liver transplantation for unresectable hepatoblastoma. Transplantation 74:652-655, 2002.
36. Fuchs J, Rydzynski J, Von Schweinitz D, et al: Pretreatment prognostic factors and treatment results in children with hepatoblastoma: A report from the German Cooperative Pediatric Liver Tumor Study HB 94. Cancer 95:172-182, 2002.
37. Wayman KI, Cox KL, Esquivel CO: Neurodevelopmental outcome of young children with extrahepatic biliary atresia 1 year after liver transplantation. J Pediatr 131:894-898, 1997.
38. Stewart SM, Uauy R, Kennard BD, et al: Mental development and growth in children with chronic liver disease of early and late onset. Pediatrics 82:167-172, 1988.
39. Stewart SM, Uauy R, Waller DA, et al: Mental and motor development correlates in patients with end-stage biliary atresia awaiting liver transplantation. Pediatrics 79:882-888, 1987.
40. Durand P, Debray D, Mandel R, et al: Acute liver failure in infancy: A 14-year experience of a pediatric liver transplantation center. J Pediatr 139:871-876, 2001.
41. Emerick KM, Rand EB, Goldmuntz E, et al: Features of Alagille syndrome in 92 patients: Frequency and relation to prognosis. Hepatology 29:822-829, 1999.
42. Balistreri WF, Bove KE, Ryckman FC: Biliary atresia and other disorders of the extrahepatic bile ducts. In Suchy FJ, Sokol RJ, Balistreri WF (eds): Liver Disease in Children. Philadelphia, Lippincott, Williams & Wilkins, 2001, pp 253-274.
43. Lhotta K: Beyond hepatorenal syndrome: Glomerulonephritis in patients with liver disease. Semin Nephrol 22:302-308, 2002.
44. Uemoto S, Inomata Y, Egawa H, et al: Effects of hypoxemia on early postoperative course of liver transplantation in pediatric patients with intrapulmonary shunting. Transplantation 63:407-414, 1997.

45. Wood RP, Ellis D, Starzl TE: The reversal of the hepatorenal syndrome in four pediatric patients following successful orthotopic liver transplantation. Ann Surg 205:415-419, 1987.

46. Woodle ES, Thistlethwaite JR, Emond JC, et al: Successful orthotopic liver transplantation in congenital absence of the portal vein. Surgery 107:475-479, 1990.

47. Czaja AJ: Autoimmune hepatitis after liver transplantation and other lessons of self-intolerance. Liver Transpl 8:505-513, 2002.

48. Gonzalez-Koch A, Czaja AJ, Carpenter HA, et al: Recurrent autoimmune hepatitis after orthotopic liver transplantation. Liver Transpl 7:302-310, 2001.

49. Andries S, Casamayou L, Sempoux C, et al: Posttransplant immune hepatitis in pediatric liver transplant recipients: Incidence and maintenance therapy with azathioprine. Transplantation 72:267-272, 2001.

50. Chardot C, Carton M, Spire-Bendelac N, et al: Prognosis of biliary atresia in the era of liver transplantation: French national study from 1986 to 1996. Hepatology 30:606-611, 1999.

51. Lunzmann K, Schweizer P: The influence of cholangitis on the prognosis of extrahepatic biliary atresia. Eur J Pediatr Surg 9:19-23, 1999.

52. Rothenberg SS, Schroter GP, Karrer FM, Lilly JR: Cholangitis after the Kasai operation for biliary atresia. J Pediatr Surg 24:729-732, 1989.

53. Whitington PF, Emond JC, Whitington SH, et al: Small-bowel length and the dose of cyclosporine in children after liver transplantation. N Engl J Med 322:733-738, 1990.

54. Alagille D: α-1-Antitrypsin deficiency. Hepatology 4(1 Suppl): 11S-14S, 1984.

55. Perlmutter DH: Alpha(1)-antitrypsin deficiency. Curr Treat Options Gastroenterol 3:451-456, 2000.

56. Prachalias AA, Kalife M, Francavilla R, et al: Liver transplantation for alpha-1-antitrypsin deficiency in children. Transpl Int 13:207-210, 2000.

57. Holme E, Lindstedt S: Tyrosinaemia type I and NTBC (2-(2-nitro-4-trifluoromethylbenzoyl)-1,3-cyclohexanedione). J Inherit Metab Dis 21:507-517, 1998.

58. Crone J, Moslinger D, Bodamer OA, et al: Reversibility of cirrhotic regenerative liver nodules upon NTBC treatment in a child with tyrosinaemia type I. Acta Paediatr 92:625-628, 2003.

59. Luijerink MC, Jacobs SM, van Beurden EA, et al: Extensive changes in liver gene expression induced by Hereditary Tyrosinemia type I are not normalized by treatment with 2-(2-nitro-4-trifluoromethyl-benzoyl)-1,3-cyclohexanedione (NTBC). J Hepatol 39:901-909, 2003.

60. Whitington PF, Alonso EM: Fulminant hepatitis and acute liver failure. In Kelly DA (ed): Paediatric Liver Diseases. Oxford, Blackwell, 107-126, 2003.

61. Emond JC, Aran PP, Whitington PF, et al: Liver transplantation in the management of fulminant hepatic failure. Gastroenterology 96:1583-1588, 1989.

62. Superina RA, Pearl RH, Roberts EA, et al: Liver transplantation in children: The initial Toronto experience. J Pediatr Surg 24:1013-1019, 1989.

63. Brems JJ, Hiatt JR, Ramming KP, et al: Fulminant hepatic failure: The role of liver transplantation as primary therapy. Am J Surg 154:137-141, 1987.

64. Tzakis MG, Arditi M, Whitington PF, et al: Aplastic anemia complicating orthotopic liver transplantation for non-A, non-B hepatitis. N Engl J Med 319:393-396, 1988.

65. Mack CL, Ferrario M, Abecassis M, et al: Living donor liver transplantation for children with liver failure and concurrent multiple organ system failure. Liver Transpl 7:890-895, 2001.

66. Miwa S, Hashikura Y, Mita A, et al: Living-related liver transplantation for patients with fulminant and subfulminant hepatic failure. Hepatology 30:1521-1526, 1999.

67. Emre S, Schwartz ME, Shneider B, et al: Living related liver transplantation for acute liver failure in children. Liver Transpl Surg 5:161-165, 1999.

68. Azoulay D, Samuel D, Ichai P, et al: Auxiliary partial orthotopic versus standard orthotopic whole liver transplantation for acute liver failure: A reappraisal from a single center by a case-control study. Ann Surg 234:723-731, 2001.

69. Otte JB: Auxiliary partial orthotopic liver transplantation for acute liver failure in children. Pediatr Transplant 3:252-256, 1999.

70. Whitington PF, Whitington GL: Partial external diversion of bile for the treatment of intractable pruritus associated with intrahepatic cholestasis. Gastroenterology 95:130-136, 1988.

71. Whitington PF, Freese DK, Sharp HL, et al: Clinical and biochemical findings in progressive familial intrahepatic cholestasis. J Pediatr Gastroenterol Nutr 18:134-141, 1994.

72. Alonso EM, Snover DC, Montag A, et al: Histologic pathology of the liver in progressive familial intrahepatic cholestasis. J Pediatr Gastroenterol Nutr 18:128-133, 1994.

73. Emond JC, Whitington PF: Selective surgical management of progressive familial intrahepatic cholestasis (Byler's disease). J Pediatr Surg 30:1635-1641, 1995.

74. Rogers J, Bueno J, Shapiro R, et al: Results of simultaneous and sequential pediatric liver and kidney transplantation. Transplantation 72:1666-1670, 2001.

75. Khan K, Schwarzenberg SJ, Sharp HL, et al: Morbidity from congenital hepatic fibrosis after renal transplantation for autosomal recessive polycystic kidney disease. Am J Transplant 2:360-365, 2002.

76. McDiarmid SV, Anand R, Lindblad AS: Development of a pediatric end-stage liver disease score to predict poor outcome in children awaiting liver transplantation. Transplantation 74:173-181, 2002.

77. Freeman RB Jr, Wiesner RH, Harper A, et al: The new liver allocation system: Moving toward evidence-based transplantation policy. Liver Transpl 8:851-858, 2002.

78. Wiesner RH, McDiarmid SV, Kamath PS, et al: MELD and PELD: Application of survival models to liver allocation. Liver Transpl 7:567-580, 2001.

79. Newell KA, Alonso EM, Whitington PF, et al: Posttransplant lymphoproliferative disease in pediatric liver transplantation. Interplay between primary Epstein-Barr virus infection and immunosuppression. Transplantation 62:370-375, 1996.

80. McDiarmid SV, Jordan S, Lee GS, et al: Prevention and preemptive therapy of posttransplant lymphoproliferative disease in pediatric liver recipients. Transplantation 66:1604-1611, 1998.

81. United States Bureau of Vital Statistics: Vital statistics of the U.S. 1982. Mortality. Part A,B. Hyattsville, MD, 1986.

82. Lloyd-Still JD: Mortality from liver disease in children. Am J Dis Child 139:381-384, 1985.

83. Broelsch CE, Emond JC, Thistlethwaite JR, et al: Liver transplantation with reduced-sized donor organs. Transplantation 45:519-524, 1988.

84. Broelsch CE, Stevens LH, Whitington PF: The use of reduced-size liver transplants in children, including split livers and living related liver transplants. Eur J Pediatr Surg 1:166-171, 1991.

85. Broelsch CE, Whitington PF, Emond JC, et al: Liver transplantation in children from living related donors: Surgical techniques and results. Ann Surg 214:428-439, 1991.

86. Colombani PM, Lau H, Prabhakaran K, et al: Cumulative experience with pediatric living related liver transplantation. J Pediatr Surg 35:9-12, 2000.

87. Emond JC: Cinical application of living-related liver transplantation. Gastroenterol Clin North Am 22:301-315, 1993.

88. Emond JC, Heffron TG, Kortz EO, et al: Improved results of living-related liver transplantation with routine application in a pediatric program. Transplantation 55:835-840, 1993.

89. Alonso EM, Piper JB, Echols G, et al: Allograft rejection in pediatric recipients of living related liver transplants. Hepatology 23:40-43, 1996.

90. Woodle ES, Millis JM, So SKS, et al: Liver transplantation in the first three months of life. Transplantation 66:606-609, 1998.

91. Bonatti H, Muiesan P, Connelly S, et al: Hepatic transplantation in children under 3 months of age: A single centre's experience. J Pediatr Surg 32:486-488, 1997.

92. Noujaim HM, Mayer DA, Buckles JA, et al: Techniques for and outcome of liver transplantation in neonates and infants weighing up to 5 kilograms. J Pediatr Surg 37:159-164, 2002.

93. Lund DP, Lillehei CW, Kevy S, et al: Liver transplantation in newborn liver failure: Treatment for neonatal hemochromatosis. Transplant Proc 25:1068-1071, 1993.

94. Srinivasan P, Vilca-Melendez H, Muiesan P, et al: Liver transplantation with monosegments. Surgery 126:10-12, 1999.

95. Cacciarelli TV, Esquivel CO, Moore DH, et al: Factors affecting survival after orthotopic liver transplantation in infants. Transplantation 64:242-248, 1997.

96. Beath SV, Brook GD, Kelly DA, et al: Successful liver transplantation in babies under 1 year. BMJ 307:825-828, 1993.

Transplantation for Cholestatic Liver Disease in the Pediatric Patient

BYUNG-HO CHOE
JORGE A. BEZERRA
WILLIAM F. BALISTRERI

Differential diagnosis   303

Specific clinical conditions of intrahepatic cholestasis   305
   Neonatal hepatitis   306
   Alagille syndrome   308
   Progressive familial intrahepatic cholestasis   310
   Infectious hepatitis   314
   Total parenteral nutrition–associated cholestasis   315

Conclusions   316

Cholestasis, clinically defined as conjugated hyperbilirubinemia or elevated total serum bile acid levels, or both, is a common pediatric disorder, especially in the neonatal period. Cholestasis in the pediatric patient is multifactorial and frequently progresses to end-stage liver disease, often despite initial palliative treatment. The outcome has changed dramatically, however, with the advent of liver transplantation. Improvements in immunosuppressive regimens and the use of segmental liver transplantation not only have extended this treatment modality to a greater number of infants but also have improved the outcome.[1] Further improvement of the pre- and post-transplant outcomes are dependent on a better understanding of the underlying pathogenesis of the various forms of pediatric cholestasis and continued use of innovative surgical techniques, coupled with better control of organ rejection and infection. In this chapter we review the clinical aspects of different forms of diseases associated with prolonged cholestasis in the pediatric patient and the impact of liver transplantation.

Differential Diagnosis

Cholestasis in the pediatric patient is associated with infectious, toxic, metabolic, and anatomic conditions that directly or indirectly affect the liver and biliary tract; most commonly, however, no identifiable offending agent is detected. Tables 22–1 and 22–2 list the recognizable disease entities associated with cholestasis or elevated liver enzymes, or both, and the relative frequency of various causes of liver disease in pediatric patients. In view of the extensive differential diagnoses, the evaluation of the infant with cholestasis must be thorough, yet rapid, so that specific treatment can be initiated and temporizing procedures can be performed.

In the infant, cholestasis associated with severe hepatic synthetic dysfunction points to life-threatening metabolic disorders. Fortunately, cholestasis in infants presents more frequently with initially normal liver synthetic function. In those infants without evidence of infection, evaluation for patency of the biliary system is

Table 22–1. DISEASES CAUSING JAUNDICE/ELEVATED LIVER ENZYMES

Infants[181]

Infections

Bacterial: Sepsis (*Escherichia coli*)

Viral: Cytomegalovirus, rubella, coxsackievirus, echovirus, herpesvirus, adenovirus

Metabolic disorders

Inherited: α_1-antitrypsin deficiency, galactosemia, hereditary fructose intolerance, cystic fibrosis, Niemann-Pick disease, tyrosinemia

Acquired: Cholestasis and liver disease associated with total parenteral nutrition, hypothyroidism, panhypopituitarism

Idiopathic disorders: Neonatal hepatitis, progressive familial intrahepatic cholestasis (e.g., Byler's disease), cerebrohepatorenal (Zellweger) syndrome

Malformation of the bile ducts

Atresia/paucity: Biliary atresia, intrahepatic bile duct paucity nonsyndromic and syndromic (Alagille syndrome)

Cystic malformations: Choledochal cysts, cystic dilation of the intrahepatic bile ducts (Caroli's disease), congenital hepatic fibrosis, polycystic disease of the liver and kidneys

Children and Adolescents

Acute viral hepatitis (HAV)

Inherited disorders: Wilson's disease, cystic fibrosis, hepatic porphyrias, Dubin-Johnson syndrome, Rotor's syndrome

Malignancies: leukemia, lymphoma, liver tumors

Chemicals: hepatotoxic agents, toxins (insecticides, hydrocarbons, alcohol, organophosphates, hypervitaminosis A, mushrooms, acetaminophen)

Parasitic infections: schistosomiasis, leptospirosis, visceral larva migrans

Idiopathic or secondary lesions: chronic hepatitis, inflammatory bowel disease (ulcerative colitis), rheumatoid arthritis, obesity

Table 22–2. MOST FREQUENT CAUSES OF LIVER DISEASE IN PEDIATRIC PATIENTS ACCORDING TO AGE[181]

Neonates and Infants

Cholestatic disorders

Biliary atresia

Choledochal cyst

Paucity of intrahepatic bile ducts (e.g., Alagille syndrome)

Progressive familial intrahepatic cholestasis syndromes (Byler's disease and syndrome)

Benign recurrent intrahepatic cholestasis

Caroli's disease and syndrome

Inspissated bile (*Streptococcus pneumoniae*-related hemolytic disease)

Cholelithiasis

Idiopathic neonatal hepatitis and mimickers

Cystic fibrosis

α_1-antitrypsin deficiency

Hypopituitarism/hypothyroidism

Neonatal iron storage disease

Viral hepatitis or other infectious diseases in the neonate

Cytomegalovirus

Herpes simplex virus/herpes zoster virus/human herpesvirus 6

Epstein-Barr virus

Parvovirus B19

Rubella

Reovirus type 3

Adenovirus

Enterovirus

Bacterial sepsis/urinary tract infection

Syphilis

Tuberculosis

Toxoplasmosis

Metabolic disease

Disorders of peroxisomal function (Zellweger syndrome)

Disorders of bile acid metabolism

Disorders of urea cycle

Disorders of amino acid metabolism (tyrosinemia)

Disorders of lipid metabolism (Niemann-Pick type C/Gaucher/Wolman)

Disorders of carbohydrate metabolism (galactosemia, fructosemia, type IV glycogen storage disease)

Toxic/pharmacological injury (acetaminophen, total parenteral nutrition, hypervitaminosis A)

Tumors (intra- and extrahepatic)

Older Children and Adolescents

Hepatitis

Viral hepatitis (hepatitis B virus, hepatitis C virus)

Table 22-2. MOST FREQUENT CAUSES OF LIVER DISEASE IN PEDIATRIC PATIENTS ACCORDING TO AGE[181]—cont'd

Older Children and Adolescents—cont'd

Autoimmune hepatitis

Toxicity

Pharmacological (e.g., acetaminophen)

Liver disease associated with chronic inflammatory bowel disease, sclerosing cholangitis

Parasitic infections

Toxins and pharmacological remedies

Malignancies

Wilson's disease

Occlusion of the hepatic veins

Fatty liver of pregnancy

Fatty liver of obesity (nonalcoholic steatohepatitis)

Hypotension/ischemia/cardiac failure

---

a high priority because biliary atresia is seen in a significant portion of these patients.[2]

A specific treatment is available for less than 10% of the diseases associated with neonatal cholestasis (Table 22–3); however, in neonates whose treatable disorders are identified, potential adverse effects can be avoided. For example, neonates with bacteremia or galactosemia require either immediate antibiotic and supportive treatment or avoidance of lactose in the diet, respectively, to avoid septicemia or a metabolic catastrophe. Similarly, recognition of *nontreatable* disorders and the institution of palliative measures may be of short-term benefit. For example, portoenterostomy performed at an early stage improves the outcome of neonates with biliary atresia.[3,4]

Most neonatal cholestasis cases arise secondary to obstructive or inflammatory processes involving the hepatobiliary tree, or both; the underlying offending agent or agents often is unidentified.[5-7] A significant overlap among these entities and their separation into extra- and intrahepatic forms is probably too simplistic. For example, biliary atresia is a disease that mainly affects the extrahepatic bile ducts, yet it shares many characteristics with neonatal hepatitis, a primary parenchymal disease.[5,8-10] Likewise, progression of histological features of intrahepatic cholestasis and portal inflammation to paucity or absence of bile ducts occurs in patients with Alagille syndrome.[11-13]

Together, biliary atresia and idiopathic neonatal hepatitis account for the majority (60% to 70%) of cases of neonatal cholestasis, followed by α_1-antitrypsin deficiency and known causes of intrahepatic cholestasis.

This chapter focuses on descriptions of the clinical characteristics and potential treatment modalities, including the use of liver transplantation, for conditions associated with cholestasis. It does not contain discussions of biliary atresia or metabolic and genetic/chromosomal disorders, which are covered elsewhere in this book.

Specific Clinical Conditions of Intrahepatic Cholestasis

Intrahepatic cholestasis (IHC) represents a peculiar class of disorders characterized by marked cholestasis and specific phenotypic and epidemiological features.

Paucity syndromes may have a disparate genesis, representing congenital absence, partial failure to form, atrophy secondary to diminished bile flow, or progressive injury (immune, viral, ischemic) with disappearance. The histopathological changes may relate to presumed

Table 22-3. RELATIVE FREQUENCY OF THE VARIOUS CLINICAL FORMS OF NEONATAL CHOLESTASIS BASED ON SEVERAL PUBLISHED SERIES INCLUDING MORE THAN 500 CASES

Clinical Form	Cumulative (%)	Estimated Frequency (Per 10,000 Live Births)
Idiopathic neonatal hepatitis	35-40	1.25
Extrahepatic biliary atresia	25-30	0.70
α_1-Antitrypsin deficiency	7-10	0.25
Intrahepatic cholestasis (with or without paucity)	5-6	0.14
Bacterial sepsis	2	< 0.1
Cytomegalovirus hepatitis	3-5	< 0.1
Rubella, herpes simplex	1	< 0.1
Endocrine (hypothyroidism, panhypopituitarism)	1	< 0.1
Galactosemia	1	< 0.1

From Balistreri WF: Interrelationship between the infantile cholangiopathies and paucity of the intrahepatic bile ducts. In Balistreri WF, Stocker JT (eds): Pediatric Hepatology. New York, Hemisphere, 1990, pp 1-18.

physiological alterations; the ductular abnormalities associated with intrahepatic cholestasis may represent a primary functional or enzymatic defect or a change secondary to the toxic effects of retained compounds, such as bile acids. The pathogenesis of bile duct paucity is unknown. However, the progressive nature (segmental destructive changes or a progressive decrease in the number of bile ducts per portal tract seen in serial sectioning of biopsy specimens), from the early features of bile duct inflammation to the later observation of paucity, suggests immunological injury to existing ducts (similar to other syndromes of *disappearing* intrahepatic bile ducts) rather than failure of ducts to develop. Other postulated mechanisms include alterations in bile acid metabolism, chromosomal abnormalities, and intrauterine or postnatal infection.[4,14] Table 22–4 lists the many disorders in which bile duct paucity has been reported.

The heterogeneous subsets of cholestatic diseases, which are characterized by IHC with or without bile duct alterations (paucity), represent specific syndromes

Table 22–4. DISORDERS IN WHICH BILE DUCT PAUCITY HAS BEEN REPORTED

Infectious Diseases

Cytomegalovirus

Herpes simplex virus

Rubella

Syphilis

Metabolic or Endocrine Diseases

α_1-Antitrypsin deficiency

Cystic fibrosis

Inborn errors of bile acid metabolism

Peroxisomal disorders (Zellweger syndrome)

Panhypopituitarism

Chromosomal Disorders

Trisomy syndromes 17, 18, and 21

Turner's syndrome

Immunological Disorders

Graft-versus-host disease

Vanishing bile duct syndrome (after liver transplantation)

Idiopathic Disorders

Alagille syndrome

Nonsyndromic bile duct paucity

Byler's disease

Aagenaes syndrome

Sclerosing cholangitis (?)

Toxin Exposure

Data from Balistreri WF: Interrelationship between the infantile cholangiopathies and paucity of the intrahepatic bile ducts. In Balistreri WF, Stocker JT, (eds): Pediatric Hepatology. New York, Hemisphere, 1990, pp 1-18.

with different prognostic implications. The multiple forms of IHC have varying clinical features with a high degree of variability in presentation and prognosis. Certain progressive, familial forms, such as progressive familial intrahepatic cholestasia (PFIC), are often fatal; however, in patients with syndromic paucity of the ducts (Alagille syndrome), the prognosis is much more favorable.

Neonatal Hepatitis

Neonatal hepatitis is simply a descriptive term for patients with prolonged IHC of neonatal onset. There are at least three subgroups:

1. Viral hepatitis in the neonate
2. Metabolic liver disease mimicking viral hepatitis
3. Idiopathic neonatal hepatitis

All three forms share a characteristic liver histology[15]; however, hepatitis in the neonate and metabolic liver disease differ from idiopathic neonatal hepatitis by the presence of an identifiable offending agent.[16,17] Idiopathic neonatal hepatitis implies the existence of an unidentified pathophysiological process associated with inflammatory changes in the liver without evidence of mechanical obstruction. Although idiopathic neonatal hepatitis is a common cause of neonatal cholestasis, the fact that the etiopathogenesis is undefined should evoke a vigilant and insightful evaluation. These patients may have an undetected metabolic or infectious disease, because the clinical course and hepatic histopathology of metabolic and infectious diseases are sometimes indistinguishable from idiopathic neonatal hepatitis. For example, cholestasis associated with α_1-antitrypsin deficiency and cholestasis associated with inborn errors of bile acid biosynthesis were formerly included in this idiopathic category but are now clearly understood to be specific identifiable metabolic liver diseases.[14,18]

In the absence of a specific cause, idiopathic neonatal hepatitis is the only diagnosis that can be made in 35% to 40% of infants with prolonged neonatal cholestasis.

Familial idiopathic neonatal hepatitis must be differentiated from the IHC syndromes. The idiopathic category will continue to shrink with the discovery of new metabolic or viral origins of liver disease presenting in the neonatal period.[19]

Infants with idiopathic neonatal hepatitis present with jaundice, usually in the first week of life.[15,20] Affected infants may appear well and gain weight normally; however, approximately one third of them fail to thrive or present with a fulminant course.[20] Jaundice and hepatomegaly are the major physical findings; splenomegaly might also be present. Acholic stools may be present transiently; this is a clinical feature that patients with idiopathic neonatal hepatitis share with patients with biliary atresia. If associated features such as microcephaly, cataracts, chorioretinitis, hydrocephalus, and purpura are present, they should suggest an intrauterine infection. Two forms of idiopathic neonatal hepatitis have been identified based on their clinical course: *sporadic* and *familial*. In the more common sporadic (nonfamilial) form, the outcome is favorable; in the vast majority recovery is complete.[21-24] This pattern differs from familial cases, in which the mortality rate (or need for liver transplantation) is greater than 60%, spontaneous recovery is seen in less than 30%, and chronic liver disease develops in approximately 10% of patients.

Macroscopically (as often seen in core needle biopsies), the liver is green to black. Microscopic findings include a variable inflammatory infiltrate with lymphocytes, eosinophils and neutrophils, swelling of hepatocytes with marked variation in size and degenerative changes, individual cell necrosis, multinucleated giant cells, and extramedullary hematopoiesis.[25] Canalicular stasis is present, but ductular bile plugs are absent and bile duct proliferation is negligible.[15,26]

The clinical course of patients with idiopathic neonatal hepatitis is highly variable, and the treatment is primarily supportive. Emphasis is given to optimizing nutrition in order to maintain growth and prevent the consequences of vitamin deficiency by supplementation with fat-soluble vitamins. In both sporadic and familial forms of idiopathic neonatal hepatitis, the severe, progressive course of liver disease has been altered by liver transplantation.[27-34] Before liver transplantation, however, patients with idiopathic neonatal hepatitis must be thoroughly evaluated so that specific infectious and metabolic disorders (such as α_1-antitrypsin deficiency and inborn errors of bile acid metabolism) are ruled out. A close follow-up is needed, which is individualized to each patient, so that the pace of the disease can be established. Liver transplantation is indicated for patients with neonatal hepatitis with growth failure or end-stage liver disease. The frequency of neonatal hepatitis as an indication for liver transplantation varies among the published reports (Tables 22–5 and 22–6).[3]

In summary, patients with idiopathic neonatal hepatitis require a care plan that includes:

- Thorough evaluation to exclude specific infectious or metabolic disorders
- Nutritional support and vitamin supplementation
- Close follow-up to understand the pace of the disease
- Evaluation for liver transplantation when there is growth failure, portal hypertension, or end-stage liver disease

Table 22–5. INDICATIONS FOR PEDIATRIC LIVER TRANSPLANT AT CHILDREN'S HOSPITAL MEDICAL CENTER, CINCINNATI, OHIO (JULY 1986 TO FEBRUARY 1993)

Diagnosis	Evaluated (n = 188)	Listed for OLT (n = 102)	Died Waiting (n = 11)	Transplanted (n = 80)	
				Whole	Reduced
Extrahepatic biliary atresia	70	58	5	14	27
Intrahepatic cholestasis					
Idiopathic neonatal hepatitis	7	4	1	1	2
Alagille syndrome	1	0	0	—	—
Nonsyndromic bile duct paucity	1	1	0	—	1
Byler's disease	1	0	—	—	—
Metabolic disease					
α_1-Antitrypsin deficiency	15	13	1	9	1
Wilson's disease	3	2	0	2	—
Tyrosinemia	3	2	0	—	3
Crigler-Najjar type 1	1	1	0	—	—
Glycogen storage disease type IV	1	1	0	1	—
Hyperoxaluria	1	1	0	1	—
Inborn error of bile acid metabolism	2	0	0	—	—
Acute and chronic hepatitis					
Fulminant hepatic failure	13	13	4	3	6
Chronic active hepatitis	6	3	0	3	—
Acute autoimmune hepatitis	1	0	—	—	—
Miscellaneous/Other					

OLT, orthotopic liver transplantation.

Table 22-6. INDICATIONS FOR LIVER TRANSPLANTATION AT CHILDREN'S HOSPITAL MEDICAL CENTER, UNIVERSITY OF CINCINNATI, CINCINNATI, OHIO, 1986-1999

Diagnosis	No. of Patients	% Total
	180	100
Cholestatic conditions		54
Biliary atresia	89	
Alagille syndrome	1	
Biliary hypoplasia	1	
Cholestasis (idiopathic)	2	
Sclerosing cholangitis	1	
TPN-induced liver failure	3	
Fulminant hepatic failure	25	14
Metabolic disease		19
α_1-Antitrypsin deficiency	15	
Wilson's disease	2	
Tyrosinemia	4	
Neonatal iron storage disease	4	
Hyperoxaluria	3	
Cystic fibrosis	1	
Urea cycle defects	3	
Glycogen storage disease	2	
Niemann-Pick disease	1	
Other conditions		13
Hepatitis (neonatal)	2	
Hepatitis (autoimmune)	3	
Hepatoblastoma	3	
Cirrhosis (cryptogenic)	13	
Congenital hepatoid fibrosis	1	

TPN, total parenteral nutrition.
From Ryckman FC, Alonso MH, Bucuvalas JC, Balistreri WF: Liver transplantation in children. In Suchy FJ, Sokol RJ, Balistreri WF, (eds): Liver Disease in Children, 2nd ed. Philadelphia, Lippincott Williams & Wilkins, 2001, p 950.

Alagille Syndrome

Alagille and colleagues reported a unique constellation of clinical features of familial pulmonary stenosis and neonatal liver disease.[35] It became an easily recognizable entity following the extensive description of patients with cholestasis caused by paucity of interlobular bile ducts and commonly associated clinical manifestations of typical facial features (broad forehead; deeply set eyes; long, straight nose; and underdeveloped mandible) and various congenital malformations (e.g., cardiovascular malformations such as peripheral pulmonic stenosis, vertebral arch defects, renal disease, and posterior embryotoxon).[36,37] Serum levels of alkaline phosphatase (ALP), γ-glutamyl transpeptidase (GTP), and bile acids are increased, indicating a defect in biliary excretion. In a series of 111 patients with paucity of interlobular bile ducts, Alagille and colleagues identified 80 cases with syndromic features.[37] Twenty-six of these patients had all five features of the syndrome (complete syndrome), whereas 42 patients had four of the features, and 12 had three features (partial syndrome) (Table 22-7). With elucidation of the genetic basis for this syndrome, a broader spectrum of clinical manifestations can be compiled from subsequent reports by several authors; these features are seen less commonly and some of them may actually represent concomitant nutrient deficiencies secondary to chronic cholestasis (Table 22-8).[35-41]

The liver biopsy specimens obtained during early infancy may resemble any other form of neonatal hepatitis; the evolution to classic findings of paucity may occur over time.[11,40] Paucity is defined as an absence or marked reduction in the number of bile ducts in the portal triads (<0.5 interlobular bile ducts per triad) in the presence of normal-sized branches of the portal vein and hepatic artery. Early biopsies, obtained in the first few months of life, might show only IHC and portal inflammation; serial biopsies may demonstrate resolution of inflammation and fewer bile ducts.[42]

Further characterization of the responsible gene or genes was done and additional molecular tests performed to determine the pathophysiology of the disease and to diagnose the Alagille syndrome precisely. These studies

Table 22-7. THE ALAGILLE SYNDROME

Criteria and Features	Incidence (%)
MAJOR CRITERIA	
Decreased number of interlobular ducts/chronic cholestasis	91
Extrahepatic anomalies (variable expression)	
Unusual facies	95
Vertebral arch defects	87
Cardiovascular abnormalities	70
Posterior embryotoxon	89
ASSOCIATED FEATURES	
Growth retardation	50
Mental retardation	16
Renal abnormalities	68
Hypogonadism	<10
Bone disease	<10
High-pitched voice	<10

From Balistreri WF: Interrelationship between the infantile cholangiopathies and paucity of the intrahepatic bile ducts. In Balistreri WF, Stocker JT, (eds): Pediatric Hepatology. New York, Hemisphere, 1990, pp 1-18.

Table 22–8. CLINICAL, LABORATORY, AND RADIOGRAPHIC FINDINGS IN PATIENTS WITH ALAGILLE SYNDROME

ORGAN OR SYSTEM	FINDINGS
Hepatic	Neonatal cholestasis
	Hypercholesterolemia, often of extreme degree
	Paucity of intrahepatic bile ducts
	Attenuated extrahepatic bile ducts
Heart	Peripheral pulmonic stenosis
	Pulmonic valvular stenosis
	Ventricular septal defect
	Tetralogy of Fallot
Central nervous system	Absent reflexes (vitamin E deficiency)
	Poor school performance
Renal	Tubulointerstitial nephropathy
	Decreased creatinine clearance
	Increased uric acid, increased blood urea nitrogen
Eyes	Posterior embryotoxon
	Abnormal iris strands (Axenfeld's anomaly)
	Retinal pigmentary changes
	High myopia
	Posterior subcapsular cataracts
	Strabismus
Bones	Abnormal vertebrae (butterfly compression, pointed anterior process C1)
	Short distal phalanges
	Short ulnae
Lumbar spine	Decreased interpedicular distance
	Abnormal progression of interpedicular distance
Endocrine	Decreased thyroxine
	Increased testosterone
Skin	Porphyria cutanea tarda–like blistering
	Scarring of light-exposed skin

Modified from Balistreri WF: Interrelationship between the infantile cholangiopathies and paucity of the intrahepatic bile ducts. In Balistreri WF, Stocker JT, (eds): Pediatric Hepatology. New York, Hemisphere, 1990, pp 1-18.

have been of great clinical benefit in avoiding unnecessary surgery, in initiating proper therapy, and in instituting genetic counseling.

Alagille syndrome exhibits a complex phenotype and inheritance pattern. It has been reported in successive generations of single kindreds, strongly supporting an autosomal dominant mode of inheritance, with decreased penetrance and variable expressivity.[37]

Siblings and parents of probands often have mild expression of the disease gene, with only one or two abnormalities. A segregation analysis of 33 families collected through 43 probands corroborated the theory of autosomal dominant inheritance; penetrance was 94%, and 15% of the cases were sporadic.[43] Expressivity of the Alagille phenotype is variable; relatives who were considered affected if they exhibited any one of the major features were identified as presenting minor forms of the disease. The frequency of new mutations seems to be high (15% to 50%).[44] Therefore, in the absence of definitive clinical or genetic markers for carriers, counseling for recurrence risks is inaccurate.

The candidate region for the Alagille gene was narrowed to a 250-kb segment on chromosome 20p12; within this region the JAG1 gene (Jagged-1) was identified.[45,46] Mutations in human JAG1, which encodes a ligand for the Notch receptor, have thus been linked to Alagille syndrome.[45,46] Members of the Notch gene family that encode evolutionarily conserved transmembrane receptors are involved in cell fate specification during embryonic development. The Notch locus encodes a receptor that mediates cell-cell interactions. Diagnosis of Alagille syndrome, a condition that should be suspected in all patients with unexplained cholestasis, will thus be confirmed by genetic analysis for mutations of JAG1.[47]

The prognosis for prolonged survival is good, but patients with Alagille syndrome are at high risk for growth failure and morbidity because of pruritus, xanthomas, and complications of vitamin deficiency. Young patients usually do not develop cirrhosis; of the 80 patients in the Alagille series, 4 died of liver complications (2 each with liver failure and portal hypertension).[11,37] The outcome and survival of Alagille syndrome is influenced by multiple factors. Cardiac disease, hepatic disease, and intracranial bleeding account for the majority of the cases of mortality in Alagille syndrome.[37,48-50] Hoffenberg and colleagues reported that children with Alagille syndrome identified in infancy because of cholestasis have a 58% (15 of 26) probability of long-term survival without liver transplantation; this is a worse prognosis than other follow-up studies have reported.[50] Although early jaundice and higher bilirubin levels suggested a worse prognosis, the association between bilirubin and poor outcome was no longer significant when patients with complex congenital heart disease were excluded.[51] The 20-year predicted life expectancy is 75% for all patients, 80% for those not requiring liver transplantation, and 60% for those who required liver transplantation.[48] Lykavieris and colleagues have reviewed the outcome of 163 children with Alagille syndrome and liver involvement and reported that actuarial survival rates with native liver were 51% and 38% at 10 and 20 years, respectively.[55] Schwarzenberg and colleagues reported follow-up data of 6 adult patients with the Alagille syndrome.[52] In these patients, there was increased morbidity caused by cholelithiasis, pancreatic insufficiency, duodenal ulcer, and renal disease; liver-related mortality was also increased, with 2 of the 6 patients dying of liver failure and hepatocellular carcinoma. Hepatocellular carcinoma is a rare complication that has been reported in patients with the Alagille syndrome.[53,54] Severe liver complications are possible even after late onset of liver disease, demanding follow-up throughout life.[55]

Treatment of patients with the Alagille syndrome is aimed at improved nutrition, fat-soluble vitamin supplementation, and support of associated nonhepatic (cardiac, renal) complications. Therapy is often ineffective. In our experience, the use of ursodeoxycholic acid (UDCA; 15 to 30 mg/kg/day in divided doses) may help to decrease the severity of the pruritus, lower the cholesterol levels, reduce xanthomas, and improve biochemical parameters.[56] In cases of extreme, intractable pruritus, biliary diversion is a successful therapeutic option.[57]

The use of liver transplantation as a treatment modality for patients with the Alagille syndrome is rarely required. Although their symptoms might be severe, the disease usually is not life-threatening. It is important to establish a precise diagnosis and avoid unnecessary procedures; hepatoportoenterostomy in patients with Alagille syndrome is associated with a poor clinical course.[58,59] Liver transplantation has a clear indication when these therapeutic modalities fail to improve the debilitating pruritus and the quality of life or when the patient develops end-stage liver disease or portal hypertension. Marino and colleagues reported liver transplantation as the treatment in 13 patients with Alagille syndrome;[58] 3 of these patients had cirrhosis. The remaining indications were stated to be progressive portal fibrosis, severe and permanent cholestasis, growth retardation, failure of medical therapy to control the complications of the disease, and frequent and prolonged hospitalizations.[58] The overall mortality rate was 46%. Seven of the 13 patients had undergone portoenterostomy and represented the subgroup with the highest mortality rate (5 of 7). Ganschow and colleagues reported 23 children with Alagille syndrome, 14 of whom underwent liver transplantation. Patient and graft survival rate was 85.7%. Three of the 14 patients who underwent transplantation showed unexpected extrahepatic complications, such as severe bleeding (caused by intrathoracic arterial malformation) and hypoplastic aorta.[60] Despite the generally nonprogressive nature of the liver disease, liver transplantation has been performed in desperation to improve the quality of life. Liver transplantation is indicated in only a minority of patients (in approximately 15% of Alagille syndrome patients), and it may result in an increased risk of extrahepatic (vascular system) complications.[60] The timing of liver transplantation should be considered carefully because the risk of death associated with transplantation may not be justified to treat morbid cholestasis. Emerick and colleagues have reported that liver transplantation for hepatic decompensation was necessary in 21% (19 of 92) of patients.[48] The factors that contributed significantly to mortality were complex congenital heart disease (15%), intracranial bleeding (25%), and hepatic disease or hepatic transplantation (25%).

In summary, the primary goal in the management of patients with the Alagille syndrome is *do no harm*. The diagnosis must be established to avoid surgical procedures that will worsen the clinical course.[59] A well-delineated care plan should therefore include:

- Thorough evaluation
- Nutritional support and vitamin supplementation
- Treatment of associated pruritus with UDCA or partial external biliary diversion
- Close follow-up and treatment of nonhepatic complications
- Evaluation for liver transplantation when there is growth failure, portal hypertension, or end-stage liver disease

Progressive Familial Intrahepatic Cholestasis

Severe forms of intrahepatic cholestasis with progressive hepatocellular damage may occur sporadically or on an apparent familial basis. The clinical and pathological features and natural progression described in case reports vary, implying significant heterogeneity. Table 22–9 reflects a proposed classification scheme.[4] The term *progressive familial intrahepatic cholestasis* (PFIC) is used to refer to this group of disorders. The typical criteria include the presence of chronic, unremitting hepatocellular cholestasis; the exclusion of identifiable metabolic or anatomic disorders; an occurrence pattern consistent with autosomal recessive inheritance; and a characteristic combination of clinical, biochemical, and histological features.[4,6,61] PFIC typically presents in the first 6 months of life as cholestasis, hepatomegaly, severe pruritus, growth failure, pancreatic insufficiency, or fat-soluble vitamin deficiency.

In view of the progressive course of patients with PFIC, it is important to ascertain a precise diagnosis, provide nutritional support and vitamin supplementation, treat the associated pruritus, and evaluate for liver transplantation if end-stage liver disease supervenes.

Progressive Familial Intrahepatic Cholestasis, Type 1 (Byler's Disease)

Formally termed *Byler's disease*, PFIC type 1 (PFIC-1), is a severe form of familial intrahepatic cholestasis,

Table 22-9. PROPOSED CLASSIFICATION OF DISORDERS ASSOCIATED WITH CHRONIC INTRAHEPATIC CHOLESTASIS

Persistent

    Idiopathic neonatal hepatitis

    With intrahepatic bile duct paucity

        Alagille syndrome

        Nonsyndromic paucity

    Progressive familial intrahepatic cholestasis (PFIC)

        Disorders of canalicular transport

            Bile acid

            Byler's disease (PFIC-1) (*FIC1* deficiency)

          PFIC-2 (BSEP deficiency)

        Phospholipids (*MDR3* deficiency)

        Disorders of bile acid biosynthesis

Recurrent

    Benign recurrent intrahepatic cholestasis (BRIC)

    Hereditary cholestasis with lymphedema (Aagenaes syndrome)

BSEP, bile salt export pump.
From Balistreri WF: Intrahepatic cholestasis. J Pediatr Gastroenterol Nutr 35(Suppl 1):S17-S23, 2002.

most commonly manifested as neonatal cholestasis and characterized by progressive hepatocellular damage. The first detailed description of PFIC-1 involved members of Amish kindred, descended from Jacob Byler; therefore the eponym Byler's disease was used to describe this variant. Patients may have delayed clinical findings of cholestasis, with jaundice, pruritus, and hepatomegaly not noted until later in the first year of life. Patients with Byler's disease have progressive and persistent cholestasis with the development of end-stage liver disease. Neuromuscular manifestations and rickets may develop because of vitamin deficiencies secondary to chronic cholestasis; affected patients may also develop gallstones and hepatocellular carcinoma.[62-66] Death from cirrhosis and liver failure is likely in childhood or early adolescence.

Laboratory evaluation shows mild elevation of aminotransferase and alkaline phosphatase levels. Although there is a marked elevation of serum bile acids and bilirubin levels, serum cholesterol levels are normal or only mildly elevated. Serum γ-GTP levels may also be normal or low; this may be a relatively specific feature of PFIC-1.[67]

The gene for PFIC-1 was mapped to a 19-cM region of chromosome 18q21-q22. Haplotype analysis narrowed the candidate region for both diseases to the same interval of less than 1 cM, in which a gene mutated in patients with benign recurrent intrahepatic cholestasis (BRIC) and PFIC-1 was identified. Classically, PFIC-1

disease comprises two different disorders, PFIC-1 and BRIC. However, these two disorders may be considered as two ends of a continuum.[68] The *FIC1* gene is expressed in several epithelial tissues and, surprisingly, more strongly in the pancreas and the small intestine than in the liver.[69] ATP8B1 (initially named *FIC1*) is a canalicular P-type adenosine triphosphatase (ATPase) that participates in maintaining the distribution of aminophospholipids between the inner and outer leaflets of the plasma membrane.[70] In PFIC linked to *FIC1*, cholestasis and pruritus may initially wax and wane but may eventually persist.

The liver histology may show a variety of findings including early features of giant cell transformation and slight proliferation or paucity of bile ducts; later biopsies demonstrate periportal fibrosis or progression to biliary cirrhosis.[62,71,72] Hepatocanalicular cholestasis and disruption of the liver cell plate arrangement were early, uniform findings. Duct loss was a prominent finding. Proliferating ductules at the margins of portal tracts increased as fibrosis progressed and were especially prominent histologically in end-stage disease. The constellation of histological findings in PFIC forms a recognizable pattern, and the liver histology appears to have a predictable progression.[73] Light microscopy findings on liver biopsy specimens in infancy are indistinguishable in PFIC-1 and BRIC, but portal tract fibrosis and bridging are seen with advancing age in patients with PFIC-1. Electron microscopy in patients with PFIC-1 shows dilatation of the canalicular lumen, which is filled with coarse, particulate, amorphous, granular material; a decreased number of microvilli; and focal interruption of the canalicular membrane.[45] The coarsely granular bile found in canaliculi with transmission electron microscopy (TEM) in PFIC-1 has not been identified in BRIC or in other forms of PFIC. The phenotype is suggestive of a defect in bile acid transport at the canalicular membrane. The biliary bile acid concentrations are decreased, with a predominance of cholic acid. However, chenodeoxycholic acid (CDCA) predominates in the serum and in the urine.

The treatment is primarily supportive, with aggressive nutritional and vitamin supplementation. Symptomatic treatment of pruritus is important as it is a frequent, debilitating symptom. Partial external biliary diversion (PEBD) that diverts bile salts from the enterohepatic recirculation arrests the progression of disease and relieves pruritus in the majority of patients.[57] Hollands and colleagues applied ileal exclusion, which offers a stoma-free, completely reversible biliary diversion. Early results on a few patients are promising, but long-term evaluation of growth, development, and liver function and histology is needed before advocating this as the primary therapy for PFIC-1.[74] Liver transplantation is indicated in patients with decompensated cirrhosis or failed diversion with mutilating pruritus.[75-77] The surgical survival rate after transplantation is excellent.[78] External biliary diversion has been used successfully to control cholestasis[57]; when pruritus persists, the addition of UDCA may help resolve the symptom. Therapy with UDCA and PEBD may prevent evolution toward cirrhosis and therefore avoid, at least in the short term, the need for liver transplantation in some children.[77] Medical therapy was effective in the long term in 10% of the patients, resulting in clinical and biochemical normalization.[76] Both surgical therapeutic methods for PFIC, PEBD, and liver transplantation resulted in an 80% success rate, and therefore should be used as complementary therapies. In patients who have not progressed to liver cirrhosis, PEBD should be the first choice of treatment. Patients presenting with cirrhosis or after ineffective PEBD should qualify for liver transplantation.[76,79] Liver transplantation in patients with PFIC-1 has been performed by several centers.[28,31,80-84] Soubrane and colleagues reported improved growth and quality of life and low mortality (one death) in a group of 14 patients after a mean follow-up period of 17 months.[77]

Progressive Familial Intrahepatic Cholestasis, Type 2

A second distinct form of PFIC (PFIC-2) is caused by a defective function of the canalicular bile salt export pump (BSEP). Affected children present with cholestasis, high serum bile acids, and low γ-GTP activity. PFIC-2 patients seem to have a phenotype consistent with an isolated defect in ATP-dependent bile acid transport at the canalicular membrane level. In contrast to patients with PFIC-1 (who have a number of extrahepatic features that may continue to manifest after liver transplantation, including pancreatitis, diarrhea, and malabsorption), infants with PFIC-2 appear to have a defect restricted to the liver, which is readily corrected by liver transplantation.[85]

Jaundice appears during the first 3 weeks of life, and serum γ-GTP levels are normal. At presentation in infancy, liver biopsy findings uniformly show neonatal hepatitis with giant cell change rather than the bland intracanalicular cholestasis of PFIC-1. In hepatectomy and autopsy specimens, chronic hepatitis with lobular inflammation and portal-portal bridging fibrosis has been found. The phenotype suggests an isolated transport defect in bile acid excretion because CDCA concentrations in bile are decreased, as in patients with PFIC-1; the coarse granular bile seen by TEM in PFIC-1 is not present.

The gene responsible for this form of PFIC has been mapped to chromosome 2q24; provisionally this disorder has been termed PFIC-2. The ATP-dependent bile acid transporter, BSEP, formerly called the sister of P-glycoprotein, is responsible for active transport of bile acids across the hepatocyte canalicular membrane

into bile. It is now recognized that mutations in the gene encoding this protein, liver-specific, ATP-binding cassette transporter (ABCB11) are responsible for a subgroup of infants and children with PFIC-2.[86-88]

PFIC-2 is compatible with a loss of the ability to excrete bile acids efficiently into the bile canaliculus and a marked reduction in bile acid–dependent bile flow. Bile acids retained within hepatocytes cause progressive injury and, with efflux of bile salts back into the blood, a progressive increase in serum bile acid concentrations. The low biliary bile acid concentrations seen in patients with PFIC-2 may be insufficient to release γ-GTP from biliary epithelium, with the result that serum γ-GTP levels remain paradoxically normal in these severely cholestatic patients.[85]

Clinically, patients with PFIC-2 seem to lack the relapsing course seen in the early stages of PFIC-1 and, instead, have a more rapidly progressive course to fibrosis.[78] Therapy is ineffective, and relatively rapid progression to cirrhosis is the rule. The role of biliary diversion is unclear. Management is the same as that for PFIC-1.

Progressive Familial Intrahepatic Cholestasis, Type 3

Patients with PFIC type 3 (PFIC-3) can be distinguished from those with the other types by high serum γ-GTP activity and liver histology that shows portal fibrosis with ductular proliferation and inflammatory infiltrate in the early stages despite patency of intra- and extrahepatic bile ducts. PFIC-3 usually presents later in a patient's life, carries a higher risk of portal hypertension and gastrointestinal bleeding, and ends in liver failure at a later age. It is characterized by a mild and variable pruritus, moderately raised concentrations of serum primary bile acid, and normal concentrations of biliary primary bile acids.[89-91] It is postulated that a genetic defect in the MDR3 gene, which is located on chromosome 7q21, may be the cause of this type of PFIC, which shares biochemical, histological, and genetic features with Mdr2−/− mice.[89] As in the murine model, the liver pathology may be caused by a toxic effect of bile acids on bile canaliculi and the biliary epithelium in the absence of biliary phospholipids.[92,93] Indeed, biliary phospholipids normally protect ductular epithelial cells from the toxicity of bile acids by forming mixed micelles. As for PFIC-3, cholestasis would result from the toxicity of bile in which detergent bile salts are not inactivated by phospholipids.[79] The absence of phospholipid would be expected to destabilize micelles and promote lithogenic bile with crystallized cholesterol, which could produce small bile duct obstruction.[78] In children with cholestasis and high serum bile acid concentrations, a high serum γ-GTP value would indicate MDR3 deficiency, which should be excluded through biliary phospholipid determination and genetic analysis of *PGY3* gene.[47] De Vree and colleagues hypothesized that UDCA nonresponding patients have a complete defect in phospholipid secretion and that partial UDCA replacement is insufficient to reduce the increased bile salt toxicity in phospholipid-free bile of these patients. Patients who do respond to UDCA therapy may have a partial defect, and the residual phospholipid concentration in bile, combined with a partial UDCA replacement, may be sufficient to reduce the bile salt toxicity below a critical threshold.[89] Management is the same as for PFIC-1.

Inborn Errors of Bile Acid Biosynthesis

Defective bile acid biosynthesis occurs in the presence of a *primary* enzyme deficiency as well as a *secondary* consequence of specific organelle dysfunction. Defects in specific reactions have been identified via fast atom bombardment ionization–mass spectrometry (FAB-MS) and gas chromatography–mass spectrometry (GC-MS), which were used to screen for inborn errors of bile acid biosynthesis. Screening has been focused on patients considered to have idiopathic forms of intrahepatic cholestatic disease, such as PFIC and idiopathic neonatal hepatitis; recognition now allows for subsegmentation of those broader categories. At present, several distinct disorders related to defective transformation of the steroid *nucleus* or the cholesterol *side chain* have been delineated.[94]

Deficiency of 3β-hydroxy-Δ^5-C_{27}-steroid dehydrogenase (3β-HSDH), the enzyme that catalyzes the second reaction in the principal pathway for the synthesis of bile acids, is present with prolonged neonatal jaundice together with the biopsy features of neonatal hepatitis. It also presents between the ages of 4 and 46 months with jaundice, hepatosplenomegaly, and steatorrhea (a clinical picture resembling PFIC).[91] In children with cholestasis and low serum bile acid levels, an inborn error of bile acid synthesis should be excluded by urinary bile acid analysis by means of FAB-MS.[47]

Bile acid replacement resulted in considerable clinical and biochemical improvement in two children with 3β-HSDH deficiency who developed rickets during infancy and did not develop clinically evident liver disease until 3 years of age. The importance of thorough investigation of fat-soluble vitamin deficiencies in infancy is emphasized.[95]

North American Indian Cholestasis

North American Indian childhood cirrhosis (NAIC), closely resembling PFIC-1 , is a distinct, rapidly evolving form of familial cholestasis found in aboriginal children from northwestern Quebec. It typically presents with transient neonatal jaundice in a child who is otherwise healthy, and progresses to biliary cirrhosis and portal hypertension. Of 14 reported patients, 9 had an onset that resembled neonatal cholestasis; however, progressive deterioration was observed in all, with the development of portal fibrosis and neoductule proliferation. Genetic analysis suggests autosomal recessive inheritance and a carrier frequency of 10% in this population. Gene mapping studies showed that the NAIC gene is located on chromosome 16q22. The histological features of NAIC show early bile duct proliferation and rapid development of portal fibrosis and biliary cirrhosis, suggesting a cholangiopathic phenomenon. Ultrastructural analysis of liver specimens from children with NAIC suggests the existence of microfilament dysfunction.[96] Together with gene mapping studies showing that the NAIC gene is different from those of other familial cholestasis, these observations suggest that NAIC is a distinct entity that could be classified as progressive familial cholangiopathy.

Early onset of portal hypertension and variceal hemorrhage necessitated portosystemic shunts in 7 of the 14 children mentioned previously.[96] Currently, liver transplantation is the only effective therapy for patients with advanced disease. In transplanted livers, no recurrence of NAIC was observed after 1 to 10 years.[97,98]

Fatal Familial Cholestasis Syndrome in Greenland Eskimo Children

Cholestasis familiaris groenlandica (CFG), a Byler-like disease, is a common recessive disease and is a severe form of intrahepatic cholestasis described among indigenous Inuit families in Greenland. Patients present with jaundice, pruritus, bleeding episodes, malnutrition, growth retardation, steatorrhea, osteodystrophy, and dwarfism; they die in childhood because of end-stage liver disease. It is suggested to be a form of PFIC-1.[99] Different haplotypes follow the disease gene among Inuits in West Greenland and a possibility of locus heterogeneity of CFG between East and West Greenland exists, suggesting CFG is not a homogeneous disease.[100]

Despite marked cholestasis, the serum cholesterol levels are low to normal. Of the 16 patients described, 50% died by 3 years of age.[101] The reported early histological findings were variable, with canalicular cholestasis and rosette formation of the hepatocytes around dilatated canaliculi and centrilobular fibrosis. Ultrastructural examination revealed granular material in bile canaliculi with a band-like condensation of microfilaments.[101,102] There are no reports of liver transplantation for patients with fatal familial cholestasis syndrome in Greenland Eskimo children. A suggested care plan for these patients is the same as outlined for patients with PFIC-1.

Benign Recurrent Intrahepatic Cholestasis

BRIC is a syndrome characterized by multiple transient episodes of cholestasis of various duration followed by spontaneous remission.[103,104] Patients have several episodes of pronounced jaundice with intense pruritus and biochemical evidence of cholestasis, with increased serum bile acid levels and a mild increase in aminotransferase levels. Characteristically, serum γ-GTP activity is low and normal liver structure is preserved.

Approximately 20% of patients experience their first attack by 1 year of age; other patients have the onset during adolescence or in their late 20s. Multiple family members are affected. BRIC is an autosomal recessive liver disease. Additional clinical features overlap with those seen in patients with PFIC-1, but complete clinical and biochemical resolution followed by recurrent attacks establish the diagnosis. BRIC is also linked to specific mutations in the FIC1 gene.[47] Although PFIC and BRIC are clinically distinct diseases, they map to the same chromosomal region—they are allelic diseases caused by different mutations in the same gene.[105] Liver biopsy specimens may show bile plugs; intrahepatic and extrahepatic bile ducts are normal on cholangiography.[104]

The goal of the treatment is primarily nutritional support and relief of symptoms, specifically of pruritus, but this is generally unsatisfactory. Liver transplantation is not indicated in patients with benign recurrent intrahepatic cholestasis. A suggested care plan includes:

- Effort to ascertain a precise diagnosis
- Institution of nutritional support and vitamin supplementation
- Treatment of the associated pruritus
- Close follow-up

Hereditary Cholestasis With Lymphedema (Aagenaes Syndrome)

Hereditary cholestasis with lymphedema is a syndrome of intrahepatic cholestasis and lymphedema of the legs described by Aagenaes and associates in a group of patients of Norwegian extraction.[106] Jaundice is consistently present during the neonatal period, but occurs episodically in children. The cholestatic liver disease tends to improve with age, with most patients having a normal serum bilirubin concentration by 3 or 4 years of age. Lymphedema in the lower extremities begins in later childhood and has been attributed to lymphatic vessel hypoplasia. The relationship between the peripheral lymphatic obstruction and liver disease is uncertain; Aagenaes postulates a hepatic lymph hypoplasia or a functional defect in lymphatic flow leading to cholestasis.

Cholestasis of Aagenaes syndrome possibly is not caused by a primary defect of bile acids or other biliary constituents but might be a consequence of other factors, such as a primary defect in the lymphatic circulation.[107]

Diagnosis of a sporadic case of this syndrome has so far been impossible until lymphedema develops, which may be moderate and, therefore, overlooked in some cases. A possible lymphohypoplasia in the liver would probably not be observed in the histologic examination, not even through electron microscopy.[108] Study of reported cases supports an autosomal recessive mode of inheritance. Genetic linkage analysis points to abnormalities in chromosome 15q.[109] Liver histology shows giant cell transformation and cholestasis in infancy. Cirrhosis has been found in several adult patients.[110]

Treatment is limited to avoiding complications of malabsorption during episodes of cholestasis, particularly fat-soluble vitamin deficiency. Lymphedema tends to become the dominant symptom of disease later in life and can be disabling in some patients. It may improve later in life and can be controlled in some patients by symptomatic treatment such as physiotherapy and wrapping of the lower extremities.[78] Liver transplantation can potentially improve survival of patients with advanced cirrhosis and portal hypertension, but no data are available.[27-30,111]

Infectious Hepatitis

Various infectious agents are capable of causing cholestatic liver disease that mimics idiopathic neonatal hepatitis. Bacterial infections such as Weil's disease, cytomegalovirus (CMV), herpes simplex virus, and toxoplasmosis cause cholestasis, particularly in infants and immunocompromised individuals. Severe cholestatic jaundice caused by intrahepatic cholestasis (and not caused by hemolysis) has also been observed in patients suffering from acute *Plasmodium falciparum* infection.[112] Among the bacterial and parasitic agents, *Treponema pallidum* and *Toxoplasma gondii* are known to affect the liver as part of the multisystem disease that results from perinatal infection.[113-115] Likewise, the liver is also targeted by congenital viral infections that might have devastating long-lasting sequelae, such as cardiovascular malformations, hearing loss, and mental retardation. CMV and rubella are examples of such congenital infections; however, the liver injury resolves and progression to cirrhosis is extremely rare when the infant survives,[116,117] although death caused by acquired CMV infection has been reported.[118] Prolonged cholestasis associated with CMV infection has been observed.[119] Herpes simplex and coxsackievirus infections of the neonate potentially have a more aggressive pattern and may cause hepatic necrosis.[120-125] In these cases, the infections involve other organs and when the use of antiviral agents and supportive care achieve recovery, the liver disease subsides. Although there is a potential for large areas of necrosis and ensuing liver failure, there is no report of liver transplantation in this setting. Echovirus (types 11, 14, 19) causes hepatic necrosis (similar to that caused by herpes simplex virus) and progressive liver dysfunction, which occur in the first 5 days of life.[126-130] In one reported series, infection with echovirus 11 was associated with hepatic necrosis in 6 of 12 neonates.[131] Residual cirrhosis may be present after the infant recovers from the acute infection, and liver transplantation is a valuable therapeutic option. One patient with echovirus 11–associated liver failure underwent transplantation in our series with no recurrence of the infection to date (see Table 22–5). There are data to suggest that the hepatotropic viruses (hepatitis viruses A, B, C, delta, and E) are not responsible for a significant number of cases of neonatal cholestasis.[132,133]

Generalized or localized bacterial infections can lead to cholestasis without direct invasion of the liver by the infectious agent.[134] This type of cholestasis is caused by the systemic effects of inflammatory mediators released during the infectious process and is relatively frequent in neonates (33.3% of all cases of neonatal jaundice) and young children.[135] The most common cause of such infections reported in these age groups is urinary tract infections with *Escherichia coli*.[135] Jaundice may be the only clinical sign of infection in these patients.[134] In adults, sepsis-induced cholestasis occurs mostly in patients with gram-negative sepsis. In most cases, the primary site of infection is intra-abdominal (e.g. appendicitis, diverticulitis, peritonitis), but it has also been reported in association with other bacterial infections in the absence of sepsis (e.g., pneumonia).[134,136] Cholestasis usually develops within a few days of the onset of bacteremia, but can occur from 1 to 9 days before the initial positive blood culture in 33.3% of patients.[137] Disproportionate elevation of conjugated serum bilirubin is the predominant biochemical feature of jaundice of sepsis, with moderate elevations of serum ALP and γ-GTP levels and normal to slightly elevated serum transaminase levels. Serum bilirubin levels usually peak between 5 and 10 mg/dL (characteristically 75% to 80% conjugated bilirubin), but levels as high as 30 to 50 mg/dL have been reported.[134,138] Liver histology is nonspecific and shows intrahepatic cholestasis with little or no hepatocellular necrosis.[134] Liver biopsy usually is not indicated for the diagnosis.

Successful therapy of the underlying infection normally results in resolution of the liver function abnormalities in 2 to 30 days. If it persists, jaundice associated with sepsis carries a poor prognosis with mortality rates as high as 90%, but minor laboratory abnormalities without jaundice have a better prognosis with a much lower mortality rate of approximately 10%.[134,137,139] In the absence of sepsis, cholestasis accompanying extrahepatic bacterial infections is usually mild.[138]

Total Parenteral Nutrition–Associated Cholestasis

Total parenteral nutrition (TPN) has an important role in pediatric nutrition, especially for low-birth-weight premature neonates and for infants with short-gut syndrome secondary to extensive intestinal resection (because of congenital anomalies of the gut or necrotizing enterocolitis). In these patients, however, prolonged TPN has important hepatobiliary consequences that range from asymptomatic elevation of liver enzymes and reversible fatty liver to severe cholestasis and cirrhosis. Although the incidence and severity of TPN-associated hepatic dysfunction have decreased because of improvements in clinical management, hepatobiliary complications of TPN remain a major cause of morbidity and mortality in these patients. Hepatobiliary abnormalities not only may be caused by TPN but also may reflect underlying disease or effects of pharmacological agents. Despite these confounding factors, current evidence suggests that TPN contributes to intrahepatic cholestasis and biliary sludge in infants, and it may lead to steatosis, steatohepatitis, biliary sludge, cholelithiasis, and cholestasis in adults.[140]

Cholestasis is the most frequent, predictable complication, especially in premature, low-birth-weight infants.[141-143] In a series of 62 premature infants receiving TPN, cholestasis (defined as an elevated bilirubin level) was present in 23% of patients, with an incidence of 80% if exclusive TPN was used for more than 60 days, and 90% if used more than 90 days.[144] Abnormal liver test results are first evident within 2 weeks after TPN therapy is initiated and resolve in approximately 4 weeks following discontinuation of TPN therapy.[141,145] Continuance of TPN promotes persistence of cholestasis.[141,144,146] The onset of jaundice in infants receiving TPN is often associated with systemic illnesses and multisystem involvement, in which cholestasis is detected as part of routine laboratory tests. The increase in bilirubin, bile acids, and transaminases is insidious, and hepatomegaly may also be present[147-149]; sludge has been reported in 44% of neonates receiving TPN for a mean duration of 10 days[150] and in all adults receiving TPN for more than 6 weeks.[151]

The pathogenesis of TPN-associated cholestasis is poorly defined. Multiple factors have been considered, including direct toxicity of TPN to the liver, hepatic nutritional deficiencies resulting from the nutritional inadequacies of TPN, complications related to lack of enteral intake, and inadequate stimulation of the enterohepatic circulation and bowel function.[152] In premature infants, immaturity of the biliary secretory system probably plays a major role in the development of cholestasis.[153] The decreased size of the bile acid pool and the less well-developed hepatic mitochondrial function may make premature neonates more susceptible to the development of cholestasis.[142,154,155] Enteral starvation followed by a lack of cholecystokinin release contributes to production of biliary sludge, because a decreased emptying of the gallbladder promotes stasis of bile in the gallbladder.[156-158] The immature liver has lower basal and bile acid–stimulated bile flow rates and decreased response to choleretic hormones (secretin and glucagon).[159,160] Immature hepatocytes also produce abnormal, potentially toxic bile acid metabolites (monohydroxy bile acids, such as lithocholate).[143] There may be sequelae of hypoperfusion, by-products of intestinal injury such as bacterial toxins, or alterations in bile acid metabolism.[143] No consistent data clearly incriminate the absolute or relative concentration of glucose or fat, but free oxygen radicals generated from peroxidation of infused lipids may play a role.[161] There is indirect evidence for a deleterious effect of infused protein.[143,162] Liver biopsy specimens show fatty changes early in the course of TPN-associated cholestasis.[143,163-165] Other findings include accumulation of bile pigment in liver cells, canalicular bile plugs, and a mild, chronic inflammatory portal infiltrate. Portal expansion, ductular proliferation, and portal and lobular fibrosis similar to that seen in biliary atresia have been reported.[166] Overall, these clinical, biochemical, and histological criteria are not specific; and the diagnosis of TPN-associated cholestasis is made when these findings are present in the appropriate clinical setting (premature infant, short-gut syndrome, and so on) and a search for other causes of cholestasis is unrevealing. Approximately 10% of patients have an alternative, specific cause such as cystic fibrosis and galactosemia.[167]

In the neonatal setting, TPN can often be discontinued as the respiratory and multisystem diseases improve; clinical and histological changes are reversible if TPN has been used for less than 90 days.[164,165] The significant hepatobiliary consequences are seen in infants and children in whom TPN is the primary mode of nutrition (those with extensive intestinal resection or total aganglionosis). Every attempt should be made to initiate oral feeding; even continuous, slowly administered small volumes of any oral intake might aid in halting the progression to cholestasis or decrease the severity of hepatobiliary complications.[168,169] Interventions used to prevent TPN-related liver disease can be instituted even after liver abnormalities (discovered with liver testing) have developed. The caloric needs; constituents such as carbohydrates, proteins, and lipids; and the ratios of carbohydrates to lipids and calories to nitrogen need to be carefully assessed and readjusted. There should be an adequate calorie-to-nitrogen ratio in the infusate and no excessive parenteral infusion of nutrients. Cycling TPN to mimic physiological feeding and fasting stages resolves liver test abnormalities and reduces hepatomegaly.[140] Pharmacological stimulation

of bile flow with UDCA, L-glutamine, glucagon, or cholecystokinin may decrease hepatic steatosis[165,171] and prevent biliary sludge.[156] UDCA supplementation enriches the bile acid pool and reduces the potentially toxic lithocholic acid, favorably influencing cholestasis.[172] In TPN-related hepatic dysfunction, UDCA decreases liver enzymes, but its usefulness in reversing cholestasis is unproved.[140] Patients receiving TPN who lack enteral alimentation experience bacterial overgrowth. Altered mucosal defense mechanisms[173] and increased bacterial translocation[174,175] result in accumulation of hepatotoxic substances, such as endotoxin and bacterial by-products. Bowel decontamination with metronidazole or other possible antibiotics may decrease hepatic lipid accumulation.[176-178] With continued TPN in the face of progressive cholestasis, the cholestasis persists and may lead to severe portal fibrosis and micronodular cirrhosis.[165,179] Liver transplantation is a therapeutic option, but the outcome depends on the correction of the associated intestinal disease; improved outcome might be seen in combined liver plus small intestinal transplantation.

Conclusions

The development of jaundice secondary to conjugated hyperbilirubinemia in infancy and childhood requires immediate evaluation so that specific treatment may be initiated. For all patients other than those with biliary atresia, one needs to look for known causes of intrahepatic cholestasis, such as α_1-antitrypsin deficiency and cystic fibrosis. When the origin remains obscure, the differential diagnosis is aided by syndromic features, documentation of pruritus, serum levels of γ-GTP, and bile acids. Also, the liver biopsy specimen must be carefully examined, which will provide parameters for initial grouping into functional defects.[2]

The primary goal is to establish a precise diagnosis followed by aggressive medical therapy and follow-up by:

- Providing nutritional support and vitamin supplementation
- Using choleretic agents to alleviate pruritus
- Monitoring growth, clinical, and biochemical parameters
- Optimizing psychosocial development—assessing quality of life
- Gauging success, including searching for complications

Despite the success of transplantation, major challenges in childhood liver transplantation remain, including improved preoperative management to ensure adequate growth, more precise posttransplant management of immunosuppression to ensure graft viability and avoidance of lymphoproliferative disease, earlier recognition of CMV and Epstein-Barr virus infection, and provision of services in a more cost-effective manner.[180] Before liver transplantation is performed in a patient with a cholestatic disease, other surgical options should be considered, such as PEBD in patients with intractable pruritus and portocaval or intrahepatic shunts (transjugular intrahepatic portocaval shunt [TIPS]) in patients with portal hypertension. Indications for liver transplantation consist primarily of severe growth failure, poor quality of life, end-stage liver disease (bleeding, hypersplenism), or when the risks of complications outweigh the risks of liver transplantation.

Pearls and Pitfalls

- Cholestasis is a pathological state of reduced bile formation or flow. There is retention of substances normally excreted into bile (i.e., conjugated hyperbilirubinemia or elevated total serum bile acid levels, or both). Cholestasis in the pediatric patient is associated with infectious, toxic, metabolic, and anatomic conditions that directly or indirectly affect the liver and biliary tract.

- Hepatitis in the neonate and metabolic liver disease differ from idiopathic neonatal hepatitis by the presence of an identifiable offending agent. Patients with idiopathic neonatal hepatitis require a thorough evaluation to exclude specific infectious or metabolic disorders and evaluation for liver transplantation when there is growth failure, portal hypertension, or end-stage liver disease.

- Clinical features of the Alagille syndrome include cholestasis (caused by paucity of interlobular bile ducts) and various facial and congenital malformations (e.g., cardiovascular malformations, vertebral arch defects, and posterior embryotoxon).

- Patients with the Alagille syndrome are at high risk for growth failure and morbidity caused by pruritus, xanthomas, and complications of vitamin deficiency. The primary goal in the management is to do no harm—establish the diagnosis and avoid surgical procedures that will worsen the clinical course. The prognosis for prolonged survival is good.

- PFIC typically presents in the first 6 months of life as cholestasis, hepatomegaly, pruritus, and growth failure. Mutations in specific canalicular membrane transport proteins in a family of PFIC have been found. PFIC-1 and PFIC-2

Pearls and Pitfalls—cont'd

constitute a syndrome called low-γ-GTP PFIC. PFIC-3 can be distinguished by a high serum γ-GTP activity and liver histology that shows portal fibrosis with ductular proliferation and inflammatory infiltrate in the early stages despite patency of intra- and extrahepatic bile ducts.

- Therapy with UDCA and partial external biliary diversion could prevent evolution toward cirrhosis and therefore avoid, at least in the short term, the need for liver transplantation in some children with PFIC.

- In children with cholestasis and low serum bile acid levels, an inborn error of bile acid synthesis should be excluded by urinary bile acid analysis using FAB-MS. Bile acid replacement results in considerable clinical and biochemical improvement.

- In view of the neonatal immature processes of bile-acid uptake, transport, and excretion, sepsis or total parental nutrition could trigger cholestasis more easily.

- Even continuous, slowly administered, small volumes of any oral intake might aid in halting the progression to TPN-associated cholestasis or decrease the severity of hepatobiliary complications.

References

1. Ryckman FC, Flake AW, Fisher RA, et al: Segmental orthotopic hepatic transplantation as a means to improve patient survival and diminish waiting-list mortality. J Pediatr Surg 26:422-427; discussion 427-428, 1991.
2. Bezerra JA, Balistreri WF: Cholestatic syndromes of infancy and childhood. Semin Gastrointest Dis 12:54-65, 2001.
3. Ryckman FC, Alonso MH, Bucuvalas JC, Balistreri WF: Liver transplantation in children. In Suchy FJ, Sokol RJ, Balistreri WF (eds): Liver Disease in Children, 2nd ed. Philadelphia, Lippincott Williams & Wilkins, 2001, pp 949-973.
4. Balistreri WF: Intrahepatic cholestasis. J Pediatr Gastroenterol Nutr 35(Suppl 1):S17-S23, 2002.
5. Landing BH: Considerations of the pathogenesis of neonatal hepatitis, biliary atresia and choledochal cyst—the concept of infantile obstructive cholangiopathy. Prog Pediatr Surg 6:113-139, 1974.
6. Balistreri WF: Neonatal cholestasis. J Pediatr 106:171-184, 1985.
7. Balistreri WF: Neonatal cholestasis: Lessons from the past, issues for the future. Semin Liver Dis 7:61-66, 1987.
8. Eriksson S, Larsson C: Familial benign chronic intrahepatic cholestasis. Hepatology 3:391-398, 1983.
9. Desmet VJ: Intrahepatic bile ducts under the lens. J Hepatol 1:545-559, 1985.

10. Desmet VJ: Cholangiopathies: Past, present, and future. Semin Liver Dis 7:67-76, 1987.

11. Dahms BB, Petrelli M, Wyllie R, et al: Arteriohepatic dysplasia in infancy and childhood: A longitudinal study of six patients. Hepatology 2:350-358, 1982.

12. Berman MD, Ishak KG, Schaefer EJ, et al: Syndromatic hepatic ductular hypoplasia (arteriohepatic dysplasia): A clinical and hepatic histologic study of three patients. Dig Dis Sci 26:485-497, 1981.

13. Kahn E, Daum F, Markowitz J, et al: Nonsyndromatic paucity of interlobular bile ducts: Light and electron microscopic evaluation of sequential liver biopsies in early childhood. Hepatology 6:890-901, 1986.

14. Balistreri WF: Liver disease in infancy and childhood. In Schiff ER, Sorrell MF, Maddrey WC (eds): Schiff's Diseases of the Liver, 8th ed. Philadelphia, Lippincott Raven, 1999, pp 1357-1512.

15. Craig JM, Landing RH: Forms of hepatitis in neonatal period simulating biliary atresia. Arch Pathol 54:321, 1952.

16. Danks DM, Campbell PE, Jack I, et al: Studies of the aetiology of neonatal hepatitis and biliary atresia. Arch Dis Child 52:360-367, 1977.

17. Mowat AP, Psacharopoulos HT, Williams R: Extrahepatic biliary atresia versus neonatal hepatitis. Review of 137 prospectively investigated infants. Arch Dis Child 51:763-770, 1976.

18. Balistreri WF, Stocker JT (eds): Pediatric Hepatology. New York, Hemisphere, 1990.

19. Balistreri WF: Pediatric hepatology. A half-century of progress. Clin Liver Dis 4:191-210, 2000.

20. Alagille D: Cholestasis in the first three months of life. In Popper H, Schaffner F (eds): Progress in Liver Disease. New York, Grune & Stratton, 1979, p 471.

21. Danks DM, Campbell PE, Smith AL, Rogers J: Prognosis of babies with neonatal hepatitis. Arch Dis Child 52:368-372, 1977.

22. Deutsch J, Smith AL, Danks DM, Campbell PE: Long term prognosis for babies with neonatal liver disease. Arch Dis Child 60:447-451, 1985.

23. Odievre M, Hadchouel M, Landrieu P, et al: Long-term prognosis for infants with intrahepatic cholestasis and patent extrahepatic biliary tract. Arch Dis Child 56:373-376, 1981.

24. Dick MC, Mowat AP: Hepatitis syndrome in infancy—an epidemiological survey with 10 year follow up. Arch Dis Child 60:512-516, 1985.

25. Montgomery CK, Ruebner BH: Neonatal hepatocellular giant cell transformation: A review. Perspect Pediatr Pathol 3:85-101, 1976.

26. Brough AJ, Bernstein J: Conjugated hyperbilirubinemia in early infancy. A reassessment of liver biopsy. Hum Pathol 5:507-516, 1974.

27. Gartner JC Jr, Zitelli BJ, Malatack JJ, et al: Orthotopic liver transplantation in children: Two-year experience with 47 patients. Pediatrics 74:140-145, 1984.

28. Dominguez R, Young LW, Ledesma-Medina J, et al: Pediatric liver transplantation. Part II. Diagnostic imaging in postoperative management. Radiology 157:339-344, 1985.

29. Zitelli BJ, Malatack JJ, Gartner JC Jr, et al: Evaluation of the pediatric patient for liver transplantation. Pediatrics 78:559-565, 1986.

30. Malatack JJ, Schaid DJ, Urbach AH, et al: Choosing a pediatric recipient for orthotopic liver transplantation. J Pediatr 111:479-489, 1987.

31. Burdelski M, Schmidt K, Hoyer PF, et al: Liver transplantation in children: The Hannover experience. Transplant Proc 19:3277-3281, 1987.

32. Buckels JA: Paediatric liver transplantation: Review of current experience. J Inherit Metab Dis 14:596-603, 1991.

33. Langnas AN, Marujo WC, Inagaki M, et al: The results of reduced-size liver transplantation, including split livers, in patients with end-stage liver disease. Transplantation 53:387-391, 1992.

34. Tokunaga Y, Concepcion W, Berquist WE, et al: Graft involvement by *Legionella* in a liver transplant recipient. Arch Surg 127:475-477, 1992.

35. Watson GH, Miller V: Arteriohepatic dysplasia: Familial pulmonary arterial stenosis with neonatal liver disease. Arch Dis Child 48:459-466, 1973.

36. Alagille D, Odievre M, Gautier M, Dommergues JP: Hepatic ductular hypoplasia associated with characteristic facies, vertebral malformations, retarded physical, mental, and sexual development, and cardiac murmur. J Pediatr 86:63-71, 1975.

37. Alagille D, Estrada A, Hadchouel M, et al: Syndromic paucity of interlobular bile ducts (Alagille syndrome or arteriohepatic dysplasia): Review of 80 cases. J Pediatr 110:195-200, 1987.

38. Puklin JE, Riely CA, Simon RM, Cotlier E: Anterior segment and retinal pigmentary abnormalities in arteriohepatic dysplasia. Ophthalmology 88:337-347, 1981.

39. Hyams JS, Berman MM, Davis BH: Tubulointerstitial nephropathy associated with arteriohepatic dysplasia. Gastroenterology 85:430-434, 1983.

40. Deprettere A, Portmann B, Mowat AP: Syndromic paucity of the intrahepatic bile ducts: Diagnostic difficulty. Severe morbidity throughout early childhood. J Pediatr Gastroenterol Nutr 6:865-871, 1987.

41. Tolia V, Dubois RS, Watts FB Jr, Perrin E: Renal abnormalities in paucity of interlobular bile ducts. J Pediatr Gastroenterol Nutr 6:971-976, 1987.

42. Valencia-Mayoral P, Weber J, Cutz E, et al: Possible defect n the bile secretory apparatus in arteriohepatic dysplasia (Alagille's syndrome): A review with observations on the ultrastructure of liver. Hepatology 4:691-698, 1984.

43. Dhorne-Pollet S, Deleuze JF, Hadchouel M, Bonaiti-Pellie C: Segregation analysis of Alagille syndrome. J Med Genet 31:453-457, 1994.

44. Elmslie FV, Vivian AJ, Gardiner H, et al: Alagille syndrome: Family studies. J Med Genet 32:264-268, 1995.

45. Bull LN, Carlton VE, Stricker NL, et al: Genetic and morphological findings in progressive familial intrahepatic cholestasis (Byler disease [PFIC-1] and Byler syndrome): Evidence for heterogeneity. Hepatology 26:155-164, 1997.

46. Oda T, Elkahloun AG, Pike BL, et al: Mutations in the human Jagged1 gene are responsible for Alagille syndrome. Nat Genet 16:235-242, 1997.

47. Colombo C, Okolicsanyi L, Strazzabosco M: Advances in familial and congenital cholestatic diseases. Clinical and diagnostic implications. Dig Liver Dis 32:152-159, 2000.

48. Emerick KM, Rand EB, Goldmuntz E, et al: Features of Alagille syndrome in 92 patients: Frequency and relation to prognosis. Hepatology 29:822-829, 1999.

49. Quiros-Tejeira RE, Ament ME, Heyman MB, et al: Variable morbidity in Alagille syndrome: A review of 43 cases. J Pediatr Gastroenterol Nutr 29:431-437, 1999.

50. Hoffenberg EJ, Narkewicz MR, Sondheimer JM, et al: Outcome of syndromic paucity of interlobular bile ducts (Alagille syndrome) with onset of cholestasis in infancy. J Pediatr 127:220-224, 1995.

51. MacBride Emerick K: Outcome of liver disease in children with Alagille syndrome: A study of 163 patients. J Pediatr Gastroenterol Nutr 35:103-104, 2002.

52. Schwarzenberg SJ, Grothe RM, Sharp HL, et al: Long-term complications of arteriohepatic dysplasia. Am J Med 93:171-176, 1992.

53. Ong E, Williams SM, Anderson JC, Kaplan PA: MR imaging of a hepatoma associated with Alagille syndrome. J Comput Assist Tomogr 10:1047-1049, 1986.

54. Kaufman SS, Wood RP, Shaw BW Jr, et al: Hepatocarcinoma in a child with the Alagille syndrome. Am J Dis Child 141:698-700, 1987.

55. Lykavieris P, Hadchouel M, Chardot C, Bernard O: Outcome of liver disease in children with Alagille syndrome: A study of 163 patients. Gut 49:431-435, 2001.
56. Balistreri WF, A-Kader HH, Heubi JE: Ursodeoxycholic acid (UDCA) decreases serum cholesterol levels, ameliorates symptoms, and improves biochemical parameters in pediatric patients with chronic intrahepatic cholestasis. In Paumgartner G, Stiehl A, Gerok W (eds): Bile Acids as Therapeutic Agents. Falk Symposium # 58. Dordrecht, The Netherlands, Kluwer Academic Publishers, 1991, p 1.
57. Whitington PF, Whitington GL: Partial external diversion of bile for the treatment of intractable pruritus associated with intrahepatic cholestasis. Gastroenterology 95:130-136, 1988.
58. Marino IR, ChapChap P, Esquivel CO, et al: Liver transplantation for arteriohepatic dysplasia (Alagille's syndrome). Transpl Int 5:61-64, 1992.
59. Markowitz J, Daum F, Kahn EI, et al: Arteriohepatic dysplasia. I. Pitfalls in diagnosis and management. Hepatology 3:74-76, 1983.
60. Ganschow R, Grabhorn E, Helmke K, et al: Liver transplantation in children with Alagille syndrome. Transplant Proc 33:3608-3609, 2001.
61. Whitington PF, Freese DK, Alonso EM, et al: Clinical and biochemical findings in progressive familial intrahepatic cholestasis. J Pediatr Gastroenterol Nutr 18:134-141, 1994.
62. Odievre M, Gautier M, Hadchouel M, Alagille D: Severe familial intrahepatic cholestasis. Arch Dis Child 48:806-812, 1973.
63. Ugarte N, Gonzalez-Crussi F: Hepatoma in siblings with progressive familial cholestatic cirrhosis of childhood. Am J Clin Pathol 76:172-177, 1981.
64. Tazawa Y, Konno T: Familial cholestasis with gallstone, ataxia and visual disturbance. Tohoku J Exp Med 137:137-144, 1982.
65. Dahms BB: Hepatoma in familial cholestatic cirrhosis of childhood: Its occurrence in twin brothers. Arch Pathol Lab Med 103:30-33, 1979.
66. Schubert WK, Partin JS, Partin JC: Congenital cholestasis: Clinical and ultrastructural study. In Berenberg SR (ed): Liver Diseases in Infancy and Childhood. Baltimore, Williams & Wilkins, 1976, p 148.
67. Maggiore G, Bernard O, Riely CA, et al: Normal serum gamma-glutamyl-transpeptidase activity identifies groups of infants with idiopathic cholestasis with poor prognosis. J Pediatr 111:251-252, 1987.
68. Van Mil SW, Klomp LW, Bull LN, Houwen RH: FIC1 disease: A spectrum of intrahepatic cholestatic disorders. Semin Liver Dis 21:535-544, 2001.
69. Bull LN, van Eijk MJ, Pawlikowska L, et al: A gene encoding a P-type ATPase mutated in two forms of hereditary cholestasis. Nat Genet 18:219-224, 1998.
70. Ujhazy P, Ortiz D, Misra S, et al: Familial intrahepatic cholestasis 1: Studies of localization and function. Hepatology 34:768-775, 2001.
71. Clayton RJ, Iber FL, Ruebner BH, McKusick VA: Byler disease. Fatal familial intrahepatic cholestasis in an Amish kindred. Am J Dis Child 117:112-124, 1969.
72. Ballow M, Margolis CZ, Schachtel B, Hsia YE: Progressive familial intrahepatic cholestasis. Pediatrics 51:998-1007, 1973.
73. Alonso EM, Snover DC, Montag A, et al: Histologic pathology of the liver in progressive familial intrahepatic cholestasis. J Pediatr Gastroenterol Nutr 18:128-133, 1994.
74. Hollands CM, Rivera-Pedrogo FJ, Gonzalez-Vallina R, et al: Ileal exclusion for Byler's disease: An alternative surgical approach with promising early results for pruritus. J Pediatr Surg 33:220-224, 1998.
75. Emond JC, Whitington PF: Selective surgical management of progressive familial intrahepatic cholestasis (Byler's disease). J Pediatr Surg 30:1635-1641, 1995.
76. Ismail H, Kalicinski P, Markiewicz M, et al: Treatment of progressive familial intrahepatic cholestasis: Liver transplantation or partial external biliary diversion. Pediatr Transplant 3:219-224, 1999.
77. Soubrane O, Gauthier F, DeVictor D, et al: Orthotopic liver transplantation for Byler disease. Transplantation 50:804-806, 1990.
78. Whitington PF, Emerick KM, Suchy FJ: Familial hepatocellular cholestasis. In Suchy FJ, Sokol RJ, Balistreri WF (eds): Liver disease in children, 2nd ed. Philadelphia, Lippincott Williams & Wilkins, 2001, pp xii, 992.
79. Jacquemin E: Progressive familial intrahepatic cholestasis. Genetic basis and treatment. Clin Liver Dis 4:753-763, 2000.
80. Otte JB, de Ville de Goyet J, de Hemptinne B, et al: Liver transplantation in children: Report of 2 1/2 years' experience at the University of Louvain Medical School in Brussels. Transplant Proc 19:3289-3302, 1987.
81. Whitington PF, Balistreri WF: Liver transplantation in pediatrics: Indications, contraindications, and pretransplant management. J Pediatr 118:169-177, 1991.
82. Superina RA: Liver transplantation in children: An update. Surg Annu 24:195-226, 1992.
83. Bismuth H, Houssin D: Reduced-sized orthotopic liver graft in hepatic transplantation in children. Surgery 95:367-370, 1984.
84. Otte JB, Yandza T, de Ville de Goyet J, et al: Pediatric liver transplantation: Report on 52 patients with a 2-year survival of 86%. J Pediatr Surg 23:250-253, 1988.
85. Suchy FJ: Another form of familial intrahepatic cholestasis, another new gene. Hepatology 29:1911-1912, 1999.
86. Thompson R, Strautnieks S: BSEP: Function and role in progressive familial intrahepatic cholestasis. Semin Liver Dis 21:545-550, 2001.
87. Strautnieks SS, Bull LN, Knisely AS, et al: A gene encoding a liver-specific ABC transporter is mutated in progressive familial intrahepatic cholestasis. Nat Genet 20:233-238, 1998.
88. Strautnieks SS, Kagalwalla AF, Tanner MS, et al: Identification of a locus for progressive familial intrahepatic cholestasis PFIC2 on chromosome 2q24. Am J Hum Genet 61:630-633, 1997.
89. De Vree JM, Jacquemin E, Sturm E, et al: Mutations in the MDR3 gene cause progressive familial intrahepatic cholestasis. Proc Natl Acad Sci U S A 95:282-287, 1998.
90. Deleuze JF, Jacquemin E, Dubuisson C, et al: Defect of multidrug-resistance 3 gene expression in a subtype of progressive familial intrahepatic cholestasis. Hepatology 23:904-908, 1996.
91. Jacquemin E, Setchell KD, O'Connell NC, et al: A new cause of progressive intrahepatic cholestasis: 3 beta-hydroxy-C27-steroid dehydrogenase/isomerase deficiency. J Pediatr 125:379-384, 1994.
92. Smit JJ, Schinkel AH, Oude Elferink RP, et al: Homozygous disruption of the murine mdr2 P-glycoprotein gene leads to a complete absence of phospholipid from bile and to liver disease. Cell 75:451-462, 1993.
93. Smith AJ, de Vree JM, Ottenhoff R, et al: Hepatocyte-specific expression of the human MDR3 P-glycoprotein gene restores the biliary phosphatidylcholine excretion absent in Mdr2 (-/-) mice. Hepatology 28:530-536, 1998.
94. Balistreri WF: Inborn errors of bile acid biosynthesis and transport. Novel forms of metabolic liver disease. Gastroenterol Clin North Am 28:145-172, 1999.
95. Akobeng AK, Clayton PT, Miller V, et al: An inborn error of bile acid synthesis (3beta-hydroxy-delta5-C27-steroid dehydrogenase deficiency) presenting as malabsorption leading to rickets. Arch Dis Child 80:463-465, 1999.
96. Weber AM, Tuchweber B, Yousef I, et al: Severe familial cholestasis in North American Indian children: A clinical model of microfilament dysfunction? Gastroenterology 81:653-662, 1981.
97. Drouin E, Russo P, Tuchweber B, et al: North American Indian cirrhosis in children: A review of 30 cases. J Pediatr Gastroenterol Nutr 31:395-404, 2000.

98. Chagnon P, Michaud J, Mitchell G, et al: A missense mutation (R565W) in cirhin (FLJ14728) in North American Indian childhood cirrhosis. Am J Hum Genet 71:1443-1449, 2002.

99. Klomp LW, Bull LN, Knisely AS, et al: A missense mutation in FIC1 is associated with Greenland familial cholestasis. Hepatology 32:1337-1341, 2000.

100. Eiberg H, Nielsen IM: Linkage of Cholestasis familiaris groenlandica/Byler-like disease to chromosome 18. Int J Circumpolar Health 59:57-62, 2000.

101. Ornvold K, Nielsen IM, Poulsen H: Fatal familial cholestatic syndrome in Greenland Eskimo children. A histomorphological analysis of 16 cases. Virchows Arch A Pathol Anat Histopathol 415:275-281, 1989.

102. Nielsen IM, Ornvold K, Jacobsen BB, Ranek L: Fatal familial cholestatic syndrome in Greenland Eskimo children. Acta Paediatr Scand 75:1010-1016, 1986.

103. Summerskill WJH, Walshe JM: Benign recurrent intrahepatic "obstructive" jaundice. Lancet 2:686, 1959.

104. De Pagter AG, van Berge Henegouwen GP, ten Bokkel Huinink JA, Brandt KH: Familial benign recurrent intrahepatic cholestasis. Interrelation with intrahepatic cholestasis of pregnancy and from oral contraceptives? Gastroenterology 71:202-207, 1976.

105. Carlton VE, Knisely AS, Freimer NB: Mapping of a locus for progressive familial intrahepatic cholestasis (Byler disease) to 18q21-q22, the benign recurrent intrahepatic cholestasis region. Hum Mol Genet 4:1049-1053, 1995.

106. Aagenaes O: Hereditary recurrent cholestasis with lymphoedema—two new families. Acta Paediatr Scand 63:465-471, 1974.

107. Nemeth A, Aagenaes O, Strandvik B: Urinary bile acid excretion pattern in children with Aagenaes syndrome (abstract ESPGHAN-NASPGN 5th Joint Meeting). J Pediatr Gastroenterol Nutr 26:581, 1998.

108. Aagenaes O: Hereditary cholestasis with lymphoedema (Aagenaes syndrome, cholestasis-lymphoedema syndrome). New cases and follow-up from infancy to adult age. Scand J Gastroenterol 33:335-345, 1998.

109. Bull LN, Roche E, Song EJ, et al: Mapping of the locus for cholestasis-lymphedema syndrome (Aagenaes syndrome) to a 6.6-cM interval on chromosome 15q. Am J Hum Genet 67:994-999, 2000.

110. Aagenaes O, Henriksen T, Sorland S: Hereditary neonatal cholestasis combined with vascular malformations. In Berenberg SR (ed): Liver Diseases in Infancy and Childhood. Baltimore, Williams & Wilkins, 1976, pp 199-206.

111. Lloyd-Still JD: Mortality from liver disease in children. Implications for hepatic transplantation programs. Am J Dis Child 139:381-384, 1985.

112. Cook GC: Liver involvement in systemic infection. Eur J Gastroenterol Hepatol 9:1239-1247, 1997.

113. Callahan JWP, Russell WO, Smith MG: Human toxoplasmosis: A clinico-pathologic study with presentation of five cases and review of the literature. Medicine 25:343, 1946.

114. Desmonts G, Couvreur J: Congenital toxoplasmosis. A prospective study of 378 pregnancies. N Engl J Med 290:1110-1116, 1974.

115. Dorfman DH, Glaser JH: Congenital syphilis presenting in infants after the newborn period. N Engl J Med 323:1299-1302, 1990.

116. Binder ND, Buckmaster JW, Benda GI: Outcome for fetus with ascites and cytomegalovirus infection. Pediatrics 82:100-103, 1988.

117. Watson JRH: Hepatosplenomegaly as a complication of maternal rubella: Report of two cases. Med J Aust 1:516, 1952.

118. De Cates CR, Roberton NR, Walker JR: Fatal acquired cytomegalovirus infection in a neonate with maternal antibody. J Infect 17:235-239, 1988.

119. Takeuchi T, Yoshioka K, Hori A, et al: Cytomegalic inclusion disease presenting acute intrahepatic cholestasis. Intern Med 31:1376-1380, 1992.

120. Fechner RE, Smith MG, Middlekamp JN: Coxsackie B virus infection of the newborn. Am J Pathol 42:493, 1963.

121. Kilbrick S, Benirschke K: Severe generalized disease occurring in the newborn period and due to infection with coxsackie virus group B. Pediatrics 22:857, 1958.

122. Pugh RCB, Newns GH, Dudgeon JA: Hepatic necrosis in disseminated herpes simplex. Arch Dis Child 29:60, 1954.

123. Quilligan JJ, Wilson JL: Fatal herpes simplex infection in a newborn infant. J Lab Clin Med 38:742, 1951.

124. Zuelzer WW, Stulberg CS: Herpes simplex virus as the cause of fulminant visceral disease and hepatitis in infancy. Am J Dis Child 83:421, 1952.

125. Hass GM: Hepatoadrenal necrosis with intranuclear inclusions: Report of a case. Am J Pathol 11:127, 1935.

126. Berkovich S, Smithwick EM: Transplacental infection due to ECHO virus type 22. J Pediatr 72:94-96, 1968.

127. Hughes JR, Wilfert CM, Moore M, et al: Echovirus 14 infection associated with fatal neonatal hepatic necrosis. Am J Dis Child 123:61-67, 1972.

128. Philip AG, Larson EJ: Overwhelming neonatal infection with ECHO 19 virus. J Pediatr 82:391-397, 1973.

129. Modlin JF: Fatal echovirus 11 disease in premature neonates. Pediatrics 66:775-780, 1980.

130. Gitlin N, Visveshwara N, Kassel SH, et al: Fulminant neonatal hepatic necrosis associated with echovirus type 11 infection. West J Med 138:260-263, 1983.

131. Berry PJ, Nagington J: Fatal infection with echovirus 11. Arch Dis Child 57:22-29, 1982.

132. Balistreri WF, Tabor E, Gerety RJ: Negative serology for hepatitis A and B viruses in 18 cases of neonatal cholestasis. Pediatrics 66:269-271, 1980.

133. Andres JM: Neonatal hepatobiliary disorders. Clin Perinatol 23:321-352, 1996.

134. Zimmerman HJ, Fang M, Utili R, et al: Jaundice due to bacterial infection. Gastroenterology 77:362-374, 1979.

135. Escobedo MB, Barton LL, Marshall RE, Zarkowsky H: The frequency of jaundice in neonatal bacterial infections: Observation on 16 newborns without hemolytic disease. Clin Pediatr (Phila) 13:656-657, 1974.

136. Abrams GA, Trauner M, Nathanson MH: Nitric oxide and liver disease. Gastroenterologist 3:220-233, 1995.

137. Franson TR, LaBrecque DR, Buggy BP, et al: Serial bilirubin determinations as a prognostic marker in clinical infections. Am J Med Sci 297:149-152, 1989.

138. Miller DJ, Keeton DG, Webber BL, et al: Jaundice in severe bacterial infection. Gastroenterology 71:94-97, 1976.

139. Quale JM, Mandel LJ, Bergasa NV, Straus EW: Clinical significance and pathogenesis of hyperbilirubinemia associated with Staphylococcus aureus septicemia. Am J Med 85:615-618, 1988.

140. Sandhu IS, Jarvis C, Everson GT: Total parenteral nutrition and cholestasis. Clin Liver Dis 1999.3:489-508.

141. Postuma R, Trevenen CL: Liver disease in infants receiving total parenteral nutrition. Pediatrics 63:110-115, 1979.

142. Whitington PF: Cholestasis associated with total parenteral nutrition in infants. Hepatology 5:693-696, 1985.

143. Balistreri WF, Bove K: Hepatobiliary consequences of parenteral nutrition. In Popper H, Schaffner F (eds): Progress in liver disease, vol IX. Philadelphia, Saunders, 1989, p 567.

144. Beale EF, Nelson RM, Bucciarelli RL, et al: Intrahepatic cholestasis associated with parenteral nutrition in premature infants. Pediatrics 64:342-347, 1979.

145. Merritt RJ: Cholestasis associated with total parenteral nutrition. J Pediatr Gastroenterol Nutr 5:9-22, 1986.

146. Manginello FP, Javitt NB: Parenteral nutrition and neonatal cholestasis. J Pediatr 94:296-298, 1979.
147. Benjamin DR: Cholelithiasis in infants: The role of total parenteral nutrition and gastrointestinal dysfunction. J Pediatr Surg 17:386-389, 1982.
148. Roslyn JJ, Pitt HA, Mann LL, et al: Gallbladder disease in patients on long-term parenteral nutrition. Gastroenterology 84:148-154, 1983.
149. King DR, Ginn-Pease ME, Lloyd TV, et al: Parenteral nutrition with associated cholelithiasis: Another iatrogenic disease of infants and children. J Pediatr Surg 22:593-596, 1987.
150. Matos C, Avni EF, Van Gansbeke D, et al: Total parenteral nutrition (TPN) and gallbladder diseases in neonates. Sonographic assessment. J Ultrasound Med 6:243-248, 1987.
151. Messing B, Bories C, Kunstlinger F, Bernier JJ: Does total parenteral nutrition induce gallbladder sludge formation and lithiasis? Gastroenterology 84:1012-1019, 1983.
152. Quigley EM, Marsh MN, Shaffer JL, Markin RS: Hepatobiliary complications of total parenteral nutrition. Gastroenterology 104:286-301, 1993.
153. Fisher RL: Hepatobiliary abnormalities associated with total parenteral nutrition. Gastroenterol Clin North Am 18:645-666, 1989.
154. Brown MR, Thunberg BJ, Golub L, et al: Decreased cholestasis with enteral instead of intravenous protein in the very low-birth-weight infant. J Pediatr Gastroenterol Nutr 9:21-27, 1989.
155. Gleghorn EE, Merritt RJ, Henton DH, et al: A subacute rabbit model for hepatobiliary dysfunction during total parenteral nutrition. J Pediatr Gastroenterol Nutr 9:246-255, 1989.
156. Sitzmann JV, Pitt HA, Steinborn PA, et al: Cholecystokinin prevents parenteral nutrition induced biliary sludge in humans. Surg Gynecol Obstet 170:25-31, 1990.
157. Innis SM: Effect of cholecystokinin-octapeptide on total parenteral nutrition-induced changes in hepatic bile secretion and composition in the rat. J Pediatr Gastroenterol Nutr 5:793-798, 1986.
158. Carey MC, Cahalane MJ: Whither biliary sludge? Gastroenterology 95:508-523, 1988.
159. Shaffer EA, Zahavi I, Gall DG: Postnatal development of hepatic bile formation in the rabbit. Dig Dis Sci 30:558-563, 1985.
160. Tavoloni N: Bile secretion and its control in the newborn puppy. Pediatr Res 20:203-208, 1986.
161. Pitkanen O, Hallman M, Andersson S: Generation of free radicals in lipid emulsion used in parenteral nutrition. Pediatr Res 29:56-59, 1991.
162. Graham MF, Tavill AS, Halpin TC, Louis LN: Inhibition of bile flow in the isolated perfused rat liver by a synthetic parenteral amino acid mixture: associated net amino acid fluxes. Hepatology 4:69-73, 1984.
163. Benjamin DR: Hepatobiliary dysfunction in infants and children associated with long-term total parenteral nutrition. A clinicopathologic study. Am J Clin Pathol 76:276-283, 1981.
164. Bernstein J, Chang CH, Brough AJ, Heidelberger KP: Conjugated hyperbilirubinemia in infancy associated with parenteral alimentation. J Pediatr 90:361-367, 1977.
165. Cohen C, Olsen MM: Pediatric total parenteral nutrition. Liver histopathology. Arch Pathol Lab Med 105:152-156, 1981.
166. Body JJ, Bleiberg H, Bron D, et al: Total parenteral nutrition-induced cholestasis mimicking large bile duct obstruction. Histopathology 6:787-792, 1982.
167. Farrell MK, Balistreri WF: Parenteral nutrition and hepatobiliary dysfunction. Clin Perinatol 13:197-212, 1986.
168. Dunn L, Hulman S, Weiner J, Kliegman R: Beneficial effects of early hypocaloric enteral feeding on neonatal gastrointestinal function: Preliminary report of a randomized trial. J Pediatr 112:622-629, 1988.
169. Slagle TA, Gross SJ: Effect of early low-volume enteral substrate on subsequent feeding tolerance in very low birth weight infants. J Pediatr 113:526-531, 1988.
170. Li SJ, Nussbaum MS, McFadden DW, et al: Reversal of hepatic steatosis in rats by addition of glucagon to total parenteral nutrition (TPN). J Surg Res 46:557-566, 1989.
171. Li SJ, Nussbaum MS, McFadden DW, et al: Addition of L-glutamine to total parenteral nutrition and its effects on portal insulin and glucagon and the development of hepatic steatosis in rats. J Surg Res 48:421-426, 1990.
172. Heathcote EJ, Cauch-Dudek K, Walker V, et al: The Canadian multicenter double-blind randomized controlled trial of ursodeoxycholic acid in primary biliary cirrhosis. Hepatology 19:1149-1156, 1994.
173. Alverdy J, Chi HS, Sheldon GF: The effect of parenteral nutrition on gastrointestinal immunity. The importance of enteral stimulation. Ann Surg 202:681-684, 1985.
174. Spaeth G, Specian RD, Berg RD, Deitch EA: Bulk prevents bacterial translocation induced by the oral administration of total parenteral nutrition solution. JPEN J Parenter Enteral Nutr 14:442-447, 1990.
175. Spaeth G, Berg RD, Specian RD, Deitch EA: Food without fiber promotes bacterial translocation from the gut. Surgery 108:240-246; discussion 246-247, 1990.
176. Pappo I, Bercovier H, Berry EM, et al: Polymyxin B reduces total parenteral nutrition-associated hepatic steatosis by its antibacterial activity and by blocking deleterious effects of lipopolysaccharide. JPEN J Parenter Enteral Nutr 16:529-532, 1992.
177. Freund HR, Muggia-Sullam M, LaFrance R, et al: A possible beneficial effect of metronidazole in reducing TPN-associated liver function derangements. J Surg Res 38:356-363, 1985.
178. Capron JP, Gineston JL, Herve MA, Braillon A: Metronidazole in prevention of cholestasis associated with total parenteral nutrition. Lancet 1:446-447, 1983.
179. Dahms BB, Halpin TC Jr: Serial liver biopsies in parenteral nutrition-associated cholestasis of early infancy. Gastroenterology 81:136-144, 1981.
180. Balistreri WF: Transplantation for childhood liver disease: An overview. Liver Transpl Surg 4(Suppl 1):S18-S23, 1998.
181. D'Agata ID, Balistreri WF: Evaluation of liver disease in the pediatric patient. Pediatr Rev 20:376-390, 1999.

Transplantation for Biliary Atresia

RANDOLPH SCHAFFER III
LYNDA BRADY
J. MICHAEL MILLIS

History   323

Incidence   324

Etiology   324
  Viral infections   324
  Defect in morphogenesis   324
  Immune-mediated injury   324

Clinical forms   324
  Classification   325
  Histological features   325

Clinical findings and diagnostic evaluation   325

Medical management   327

Surgical management   328
  The Kasai operation and its modifications   328
  Liver transplantation   329

History

The first major review of biliary atresia (BA) was written by Thompson in 1891.[1] In his review of 50 reported cases from the literature, including 1 of his own, Thompson described the signs, symptoms, gross pathology, and natural history of this inflammatory lesion. Among the reported patients, 16% were thought to be theoretically amenable to surgical correction. Holmes[2] in 1916 added to this review and reinforced the concept of "correctable" and "noncorrectable" conditions. It was not until 1928, however, that the first successful reconstruction of the "correctable" type of BA was reported by Ladd.[3] In 1953, Gross[4] documented that BA was the most common cause of obstructive jaundice in infants, with most of Gross' patients having "noncorrectable" biliary ductal occlusion. Unfortunately, over the next 20 years, little progress was made in surgical management of the noncorrectable forms of BA.

Then, in 1968, Kasai[5] reported a 10-year experience in achieving operative relief of BA through hepatic portoenterostomy in infants previously thought to be noncorrectable. This report, along with results from others in Japan and elsewhere, ultimately led to the acceptance of hepatic portoenterostomy as the treatment of choice in patients with noncorrectable BA. With increased experience it became apparent that early diagnosis and timely operations were essential to successful restoration of bile flow, yet long-term success was still rare. Starzl and colleagues[6] introduced liver transplantation as a treatment option in 1963. However, it was not until the introduction of cyclosporine in the early 1980s that liver transplantation became a viable therapeutic option for patients with BA. Today, the strategy for surgical therapy in most patients involves an initial Kasai procedure and then subsequent liver transplantation, when necessary.

Incidence

BA is the most common cause of surgical jaundice in infants, and because of the high frequency of progression to end-stage liver disease, it is the most common indication for pediatric liver transplantation. The disease occurs worldwide and affects an estimated 1 in 8000 to 1 in 14,000 live births with a slight female preponderance.[7,8] At one time it was widely postulated that BA resulted from failed recanalization of embryonic bile ducts. This theory has since been abandoned. Although in some patients the lesion may be a true congenital malformation, in most it seems to be acquired in late gestation or postnatally.[7,9,10] The demonstration of significant seasonal clustering in several studies adds to the theory that BA may be caused by environmental exposure, such as to a virus, in the perinatal period.[8-10]

Etiology

BA is the end result of a destructive inflammatory process that affects the intrahepatic and extrahepatic bile ducts. Extensive research is being conducted to discover the etiology and pathophysiology of the disease. The genetics of BA is unclear. Although BA does not generally occur in siblings of children with BA and there are twins discordant for BA, several studies have suggested a genetic predisposition.[11,12] Genetic predisposition is not enough, however, to explain the obliterating process that characterizes BA. Three areas of research are ongoing: viral and environmental factors, defects in morphogenesis, and immune-mediated injury.

Viral Infections

Several viruses have been proposed to be the cause of BA; the two most extensively studied are reovirus type 3 and rotavirus type C. There are animal models in which these viruses can induce BA, but no consistent data support either virus as a cause of BA in humans.[13-15] The search for a viral cause or environmental toxin began after it was proposed that there was seasonal variation or time-space clustering of cases of BA.

At least two studies of the epidemiology of BA do not support the theory that there is time-space clustering of cases.[16,17]

Defect in Morphogenesis

The hypothesis of a defect in morphogenesis is particularly appealing for patients with BA polysplenia syndrome or fetal BA. These patients have multiple anomalies associated with BA.[18,19] Several investigators have described interruption in the normal remodeling of the biliary tree during fetal life.[20] These patients have ductal plate malformations on histological examination.[20] More recently, investigators have described abdominal situs inversus, severe jaundice, and death in transgenic mice with deletion of the inversin gene.[21] The pathology of the mice was similar in many respects to that of patients with BA. These results suggest a role of the inversin gene in development of the hepatobiliary system and raise the possibility that the human analogue of the inversin gene may play a role in BA, especially in patients with multiple anomalies.

Immune-Mediated Injury

It has been proposed that patients with BA may have an abnormality in their immune system,[21] and there is evidence of immune activation in BA patients in comparison to controls. Patients with BA have an increase in the number of CD68+ macrophages and a corresponding increase in serum interleukin-18.[22-24] Whether the immune system is reacting to a stimulus (viral or toxin) or whether BA is another example of an autoimmune disease is yet to be determined.

Clinical Forms

At least two different forms of biliary atresia are recognized: a *fetal* form and a *postnatal* form. The fetal form is the less common manifestation and occurs in 10% to 35% of all patients. These infants have no jaundice-free interval after birth and a high frequency of associated malformations (10% to 20%). The most commonly associated anomaly is the "polysplenia syndrome." In this syndrome, the combination of BA and splenic abnormalities is often accompanied by other malformations, including intestinal malrotation, abdominal situs inversus, cardiac defects, and vascular abnormalities (such as a preduodenal or absent portal vein, an interrupted retrohepatic vena cava, and anomalous hepatic arterial circulation).[20,25,26] Patients with this form of BA are assumed to have a true malformation syndrome resulting in defective organogenesis.

Patients with the fetal form also have poorer surgical outcomes.[19,25,27] In contrast, the postnatal form has no associated congenital anomalies. It is thought that this form may be a result of the insult occurring at a time different from that of the fetal form, or it may be due to a different cause altogether.

Classification

As stated earlier, BA has long been divided into correctable and noncorrectable types. The Japanese Society of Pediatric Surgeons replaced the traditional classification system (correctable and noncorrectable) with a more comprehensive system based on the macroscopic and cholangiographic appearance of the biliary ducts. Type 1 BA consists of atresia of the common bile duct with or without cystic dilatation of the distal patent duct. Type 2 is defined as atresia of the common hepatic duct, and type 3 has atresia of the right and left hepatic ducts up to the porta hepatis. Type 3 is the most common of the main types and occurs 70% to nearly 90% of the time. The three major types are then further divided into subtypes according to the pattern of the distal bile ducts and into subgroups based on the pattern of the hepatic hilar radicles. This further classification, however, appears to have no bearing on operative outcome.

Histological Features

Microscopically, three specific types of biliary structures appear at the transected hilar surface: bile ducts, collecting ductules, and biliary glands.[28] Only the microscopic bile ducts are believed to communicate with the intrahepatic biliary system. Bile flow may be anticipated after hepatic portoenterostomy when these ductal structures are present, even if they are severely deformed by inflammation. The number of these ducts, however, decreases progressively with age as they are replaced by fibrous tissue. It is thought that if flow can be maintained through these ducts for the first few months after surgery, they will ultimately act as internal biliary fistulas. Many studies have tried to correlate the number and size of these ductal structures with the success rate of hepatic portoenterostomy, unfortunately with conflicting results.[28,29] Although the presence of larger ducts usually portends success, the absence of such does not necessarily condemn one to failure.

Histopathological examination of the ductal remnant in BA demonstrates chronic inflammation and granulation resulting in complete obstruction. As with any obstructive process in this age group, there is initial hepatocellular and canalicular cholestasis and, eventually, an accompanying proliferation of the biliary ductules in the portal tracts. As the unrelieved obstruction progresses, focal hepatocyte necrosis occurs, multinucleated giant hepatocytes and an inflammatory infiltrate appear, portal tracts are widened by edema, and intralobular fibrosis develops. These findings, however, are also classic features of neonatal hepatitis, and the similarities between early BA and neonatal hepatitis result in decreased specificity of early percutaneous biopsy. Nonetheless, by 4 to 8 weeks of age, the three findings pathognomonic of BA can usually be seen: (1) bile plugs in the ductules, (2) portal fibrosis, and (3) biliary ductular proliferation.

Clinical Findings and Diagnostic Evaluation

Despite the various possible causes, BA has consistent clinical findings. The patient is a normal-sized, full-term baby who is gaining weight and is jaundiced past the age of 2 weeks. Hepatomegaly may be noted on physical examination. There may be dark urine, and initially stools will be intermittently acholic. If no intervention is performed, the liver disease will progress, and by 3 to 4 months, failure to thrive will be present. Later, as cirrhosis develops, the child will have muscle wasting, ascites, hepatosplenomegaly, and bleeding.

It is imperative to intervene early, before 8 weeks of age, for the Kasai operation to be successful.[30] All children with jaundice after 2 weeks of age need to undergo a laboratory evaluation to determine whether they have conjugated hyperbilirubinemia. Any child with conjugated hyperbilirubinemia should be referred to a pediatric gastroenterologist for further assessment.

Although the differential diagnosis of a neonate with cholestasis is extensive (Table 23–1), many of the diseases included do not have the same clinical features as BA. When presented with a relatively healthy newborn whose only symptom is cholestasis, the list of possible causes is much smaller. TORCH (toxoplasmosis, other agents, rubella, cytomegalovirus, herpes simplex) infections must be considered in a child with cholestasis, because most patients with TORCH infections have clinical features similar to those of BA (hepatosplenomegaly, jaundice, and petechial or purpuric rash in a premature or intrauterine growth–retarded infant). Children who acquire cytomegalovirus infection late in pregnancy may have cholestasis and mild hepatitis, which resolves.[31] Infants with enteral viral sepsis present in the first week of life with severe hepatitis and liver failure.[32,33] In addition to elevated transaminases, jaundice, and severe coagulopathy, these patients have thrombocytopenia. Like enteral viruses, herpesviruses and parvovirus B19 have been reported to cause significant liver disease and hepatic failure in the newborn period. The final viruses to affect the liver in the newborn period

Table 23-1. DIFFERENTIAL DIAGNOSIS OF CHOLESTATIC NEONATES

Biliary atresia

Neonatal hepatitis

Metabolic disease

   α_1-Antitrypsin deficiency

   Galactosemia

   Cystic fibrosis

   Disorders of bile acid synthesis

Choledochal cyst

Ductal paucity

   Alagille syndrome

   Nonsyndromic paucity of ducts

   Persistent familial intrahepatic cholestasis

Infection

   Escherichia coli

   TORCH

   Syphilis

   HHV-6

   HIV

   Enteric viral sepsis

Endocrine

   Hypopituitarism

HHV, human herpesvirus; HIV, human immunodeficiency virus; TORCH, toxoplasmosis, other agents, rubella, cytomegalovirus, herpes simplex.

are the hepatotropic viruses. Congenitally acquired hepatitis B and C are likely to cause chronic carrier states in these infants, but fulminant failure from hepatitis B has been reported, although is unlikely to occur in countries in which pregnant women are screened and children are treated with immune globulin and vaccine. The vast majority of cases of hepatitis A in pediatric patients are anicteric, but there have been three reported cases of cholestatic liver disease in patients with congenitally acquired hepatitis A infection.[34,35] In children with vomiting, encephalopathy, and hyperammonemia with or without severe coagulopathy, a workup for metabolic liver disease should be performed.

The vast majority of cholestatic neonates have BA or neonatal hepatitis, so the challenge in the diagnostic workup is to define the role of various laboratory and imaging studies and biopsy findings in differentiating the two. Figure 23–1 is an algorithm for the workup of a cholestatic neonate. The workup begins with laboratory evaluation. Alanine transaminase and aspartate transaminase are mildly elevated in patients with BA. Significantly elevated transaminases may indicate hepatocellular disease. Alkaline phosphatase levels are always elevated. In later manifestations of BA, alkaline

phosphatase may be very elevated secondary to bone disease. γ-Glutamyl transpeptidase (GGTP) is likewise always elevated in BA. Although elevated GGTP suggests BA, it is not enough to confirm the diagnosis. Persistent familial intrahepatic cholestasis types I and II and primary disorders of bile acid synthesis are associated with low or normal GGTP. The prothrombin time should be checked to ensure that there is no coagulopathy secondary to vitamin K deficiency. Patients with BA usually have normal serum, but it may be abnormal in those with hypopituitarism. Complete blood counts and platelets should be checked before any invasive procedure and may be abnormal in patients with neonatal hepatitis (hemolysis) or viral infection (thrombocytopenia). Serum α_1-antitrypsin levels should be determined. Urine should be sent for culture and testing for reducing substances. The presence of reducing substances is suggestive of galactosemia, in which case galactose 1-phosphate uridyltransferase levels should be determined. Ultrasound should be performed on every infant with cholestasis to rule out structural defects such as choledochal cysts. If no gallbladder is seen after a 4-hour fast, the findings are consistent with BA. Other findings on ultrasound, such as the triangular cord sign, the shape of the gallbladder, and the shape and thickness of the gallbladder wall, have been used to support the diagnosis of BA.[36,37]

After ultrasonography, the workup of BA depends on the expertise available at the institution. Technetium 99–labeled hepatoiminodiacetic acid (HIDA) scans can be performed. If they demonstrate excretion into the gut, the patient does not have BA. Several problems are associated with this test. The patient should be pretreated with phenobarbital (5 mg/kg/day for 5 days) before the test, and in patients with severe cholestasis and neonatal hepatitis, the liver may not excrete.[38] Recently, institutions have begun to perform magnetic resonance cholangiography (MRC) with various levels of sensitivity.[39,40] MRC has advantages over other modalities in that it is noninvasive and can be performed quickly. Endoscopic retrograde cholangiopancreatography (ERCP) can be used to demonstrate open biliary systems in children with cholestasis not caused by BA. In patients with BA the biliary tree is not visualized. This procedure is invasive, and few pediatric centers have the expertise to perform ERCP in children younger than 8 weeks. There have been reports of duodenal aspiration used to diagnose BA, but it is a cumbersome test for the patient and has less sensitivity and specificity than liver biopsy does.[41]

The most sensitive and specific test to delineate between BA and neonatal hepatitis is liver biopsy.[42] The procedure is safe and can yield results quickly. If the biopsy findings are consistent with BA, the child should undergo intraoperative cholangiography and a Kasai procedure. If the biopsy is consistent with neonatal

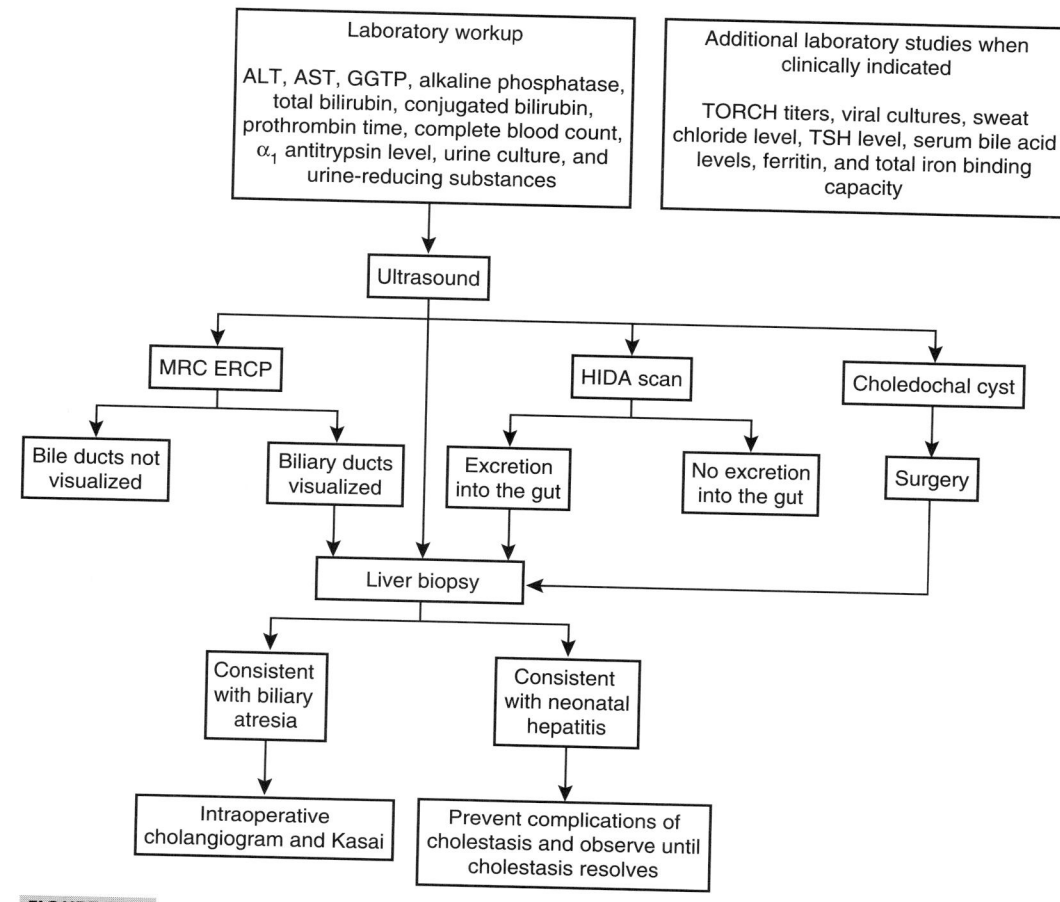

FIGURE 23-1

Algorithm for the workup of neonatal jaundice. ALT, alanine transaminase; AST, aspartate transaminase; ERCP, endoscopic retrograde cholangiopancreatography; GGTP, γ-glutamyl transpeptidase; HIDA, hepato-iminodiacetic acid; MRC, magnetic resonance cholangiography; TORCH, toxoplasmosis, other agents, rubella, cytomegalovirus, herpes simplex; TSH, thyroid-stimulating hormone.

(giant cell) hepatitis, the child should be treated and monitored until the problem resolves. If other biopsy findings are present, further workup should be pursued to elucidate the cause of the cholestasis.

Medical Management

Management of patients with BA should proceed in two phases. The first is to establish biliary drainage and manage the complications that result from drainage. The second is to treat those with cirrhosis and compromised liver function.

After Kasai portoenterostomy, adjunct steroid therapy has been used to help establish bile flow. Several studies have demonstrated improved survival in steroid-treated patients.[27,43,44] Meyers and associates compared 14 patients receiving steroids, ursodeoxycholic acid (UDCA), and a combination of intravenous and oral antibiotics with 14 patients receiving oral antibiotics and intermittent UDCA.[27] Survival without liver transplantation or cholestatic liver disease was significantly better in the first group. Although these studies suggest a beneficial effect of steroids, further controlled studies are needed to establish efficacy.

UDCA has been shown to improve biochemical and nutritional parameters without adverse effects in children with BA.[45,46] Improved survival without transplantation has not been demonstrated. In small studies, oral herbal and milk thistle supplements have shown comparable effects.[47,48] Although complementary medicines may have effects similar to those of UDCA, the production and content of these medicines are not controlled by the Food and Drug Administration, and inconsistencies in formulation can make these drugs potentially dangerous and difficult to study.

The most common complication after portoenterostomy is cholangitis, the diagnosis of which is suggested by fever and increasing bilirubin.[49] Cholangitis increases the risk for cirrhosis and decreases patient survival,[49,50] so it should be treated aggressively with parenteral antibiotics. Recent studies have demonstrated a benefit of prophylactic oral antibiotics in preventing cholangitis.[51] The study of Meyers and colleagues suggests that longer, more aggressive antibiotic therapy may increase the success of portoenterostomy.[27]

Cholestasis may be present for several weeks after successful portoenterostomy or may develop if bile flow stops. Cholestatic patients are unable to absorb fats or fat-soluble vitamins effectively, and complications of vitamin deficiency develop if vitamins A, D, E, and K are not supplemented. Cholestasis also causes a deficiency in essential phospholipids and fatty acids (linoleic acid and arachidonic acid), which improves with supplementation and treatment with UDCA.[52,53]

As liver disease progresses and energy expenditure increases, patients are not able to take in enough calories, so nutritional supplementation is needed. In infants, supplementation usually consists of a formula with medium-chain triglycerides. Some data, however, support the use of branched-chain amino acid–containing formulas in pediatric patients.[54]

Pruritus can also be a complication of cholestatic liver disease. UDCA relieves pruritus in a small percentage of patients.[45,46] In those who do not respond to UDCA, diphenhydramine, and local skin care, rifampin is the next treatment of choice and is effective in more then 50% of patients with pruritus.[55,56] Long-acting opiate antagonists can be used in patients who do not respond to rifampin.[57]

The final complication that arises in patients with BA is portal hypertension. It can be manifested as gastrointestinal bleeding, ascites, hypersplenism, and encephalopathy. Treatment of portal hypertension should be directed at preventing complications.

Ascites accumulates because of the poor synthetic function of the liver, with resultant hypoalbuminemia and the hyperaldosteronism of chronic liver disease. Treatment consists of nutritional supplementation, salt restriction, and diuretic therapy. Spontaneous bacterial peritonitis occurs in patients with ascites. Patients with abdominal pain and fever should be assessed and treated. The large spleen size may increase intra-abdominal pressure and exacerbate the ascites, respiratory distress, and poor oral intake. The thrombocytopenia secondary to the hypersplenism increases the risk of bleeding and should be monitored closely. Since the patient's hypersplenism will completely resolve after transplantation, splenectomy or partial splenectomy is unnecessary. Encephalopathy may be difficult to diagnose in small children but should be suspected in any child with insomnia, chronic irritability, or a change in personality. Treatment with lactulose or neomycin should be instituted in those with encephalopathy.

Gastrointestinal bleeding is the most significant manifestation of portal hypertension. Once gastrointestinal

hemorrhage occurs, initial management should focus on establishing hemodynamic stability. The bleeding can be controlled by the administration of octreotide and by endoscopic sclerotherapy or banding.[58,59] Endoscopic band ligation has been shown to be as effective as sclerotherapy and safer.[60] Bleeding that cannot be controlled by endoscopic or medical management may be controlled by a transjugular intrahepatic portosystemic shunt.[61]

Prophylaxis against variceal bleeding can be accomplished endoscopically.[59,60] Prophylaxis with pharmacological agents has been demonstrated to be effective in adults with cirrhosis. In two studies in pediatric patients, therapy with propranolol was safe, but further studies are needed to establish the efficacy of these treatments.[62]

Surgical Management

The Kasai Operation and Its Modifications

Before the development of adequate surgical therapy, the natural history of untreated BA was progressive cirrhosis and, in the overwhelming majority of patients, eventual death from variceal bleeding, infection, or hepatic decompensation by 3 years of age.[63] When Kasai and Suzuki first introduced hepatic portoenterostomy in 1959,[64] the procedure was regarded with skepticism. Since that time, the Kasai procedure has become the mainstay of initial surgical therapy by providing the dissected hepatic hilar plate with intestinal drainage.

Over the years, surgeons have attempted to modify the original Kasai procedure to overcome some of its technical shortcomings—specifically, problems with inadequate drainage and postoperative cholangitis. Drainage of the hilar plate depends on the presence of sufficient biliary structures in the transected surface of the hepatic hilum. To improve the probability of encountering such structures, the operation has evolved over time to incorporate a much wider dissection of the porta hepatis. Since the obliterated hepatic ducts usually form a cone-shaped fibrous remnant anterior and cranial to the bifurcation of the portal vein, many authors now advocate separating the bile duct remnants from the right and left portal vein branches and extending the dissection as posteriorly as possible between the right and left portal veins.[65-68] Extended medial and lateral dissection also appears to improve drainage.[69,70]

With regard to the role of reoperation, Ibrahim and coworkers[71] reviewed their early and late results and found that only patients with good bile drainage after their initial Kasai procedure went on to experience adequate bile drainage after reoperation. The general consensus now seems to be that reoperation is indicated only in patients who have good initial bile flow after the first operation and then experience sudden cessation of flow. Redo surgery may be appropriate in patients with mechanical obstruction as the cause of diminished bile drainage if they also have minimal hepatic impairment and no portal hypertension. Otherwise, such attempts at salvage are likely to cause unnecessary adhesions and may interfere with subsequent liver transplantation.

Cholangitis is the most common complication after hepatic portoenterostomy, and prevention of such bouts is crucial for maintaining long-term bile drainage. To reduce the incidence of this devastating complication, surgeons have used various forms of intestinal conduits for drainage. The original Kasai procedure used a 30-cm-long Roux-en-Y jejunal limb. Modifications of this reconstruction have included the use of a longer Roux-en-Y limb (40 to 70 cm in length), partial and total diversion of the biliary drainage limb with the use of various stomas, creation of intussuscepted intestinal valves, and the use of physiological intestinal valves (i.e., the ileocecal valve).[72] Although stomas can reduce the severity of cholangitis, they do not appear to lessen the incidence. Intussusception-type valves are associated with fewer bouts of cholangitis, but recently there has been a return to the original Kasai procedure and the use of a longer Roux-en-Y limb to avoid complicating subsequent liver transplantation if the portoenterostomy fails.

Timing and Outcome

Nearly every major series has confirmed the relationship between age at the time of hepatic portoenterostomy and subsequent clearance of jaundice. Although improved postoperative management, including the use of steroids and antibiotics after the Kasai procedure, has led to nearly comparable biliary drainage in patients undergoing surgery as late as 80 days of age at some centers,[73] clearly, survival rates are still dramatically affected by the timing of operative intervention. A recent review of the Tohoku University Hospital experience showed a steady decrease in 10-year survival rates with increased age at surgery (72% 10-year survival rate in patients operated on before the age of 60 days, 41% in patients 61 to 70 days old, 30% in patients 71 to 90 days old, and only 13% in those operated on after 3 months of age).[73] Other series show 5- and 10-year actuarial survival rates to vary widely (each ranging from around 25% to 60%) and to depend on such factors as age of the patient, extent of hepatic fibrosis, surgical decade, number of cholangitis episodes after surgery, and anatomy of the atretic bile ducts. In patients in whom hepatic portoenterostomy is

successful, long-term follow-up studies are now beginning to show no significant detrimental impact on their quality of life.[74,75] Barring the presence of severe fibrosis on liver biopsy, it is our recommendation that most patients with BA undergo hepatic portoenterostomy as the first surgical procedure.

Liver Transplantation

Indications

Although 5-year actuarial survival rates for all BA patients have been reported to be higher than 60% at some centers,[73] the 5-year survival rate without liver transplantation is around 20% in some studies[76,77] and at best approaches 40% in others.[78] Nonetheless, even in patients in whom progressive liver disease continues to develop as a result of an inadequate or failed Kasai procedure, the operation allows for continued growth and development, up to an average of 47 months in one study,[79] before undergoing liver transplantation. This additional time plus growth gives the patient access to more potential donors and enhances the chance for a less complicated postoperative course. However, signs and symptoms of a failing portoenterostomy, such as repeated episodes of cholangitis, jaundice, ascites, decreased synthetic function, variceal hemorrhage, and diminished growth and development, should result in prompt referral for transplantation.

Transplantation as Primary Therapy

With few exceptions, it appears that children older than 3 months gain little from hepatic portoenterostomy. With improvement in posttransplant outcomes and more accepted use of segmental grafts from both deceased and living donor sources, primary therapy with liver transplantation should be considered in children who manage to escape diagnosis before the onset of severe hepatic dysfunction.[80]

Technical Considerations

The fundamental principles of organ procurement, recipient hepatectomy, and liver grafting have been described extensively elsewhere. Several factors, however, are unique to children with BA, such as the frequent occurrence of previous portal dissection and anatomic anomalies. The majority of patients with BA have already had considerable dissection in the porta hepatis from their Kasai procedure. Such dissection can result in significant intra-abdominal adhesions, particularly if reoperative salvage has also been attempted. Dense, bloody portal hilar adhesions, especially in smaller patients, who do not tolerate significant blood loss, can make the operation challenging. As described by Goss and colleagues,[81] we recommend first approaching the hepatic hilum from the right posterolateral aspect by reflecting the transverse colon and second portion of the duodenum from the usually unscarred posterior right lobe. In doing so, the Roux-en-Y jejunal limb is then encountered crossing the transverse mesocolon and can be traced to the hilum. Here, the jejunal limb is transected with a linear stapler and reflected inferiorly to allow better exposure of the hilum and continued dissection of the hepatic arteries and portal vein. We typically ligate and divide the right and left hepatic arteries and both the right and left portal vein branches. If the portal vein is small and sclerotic from previous operations or bouts of cholangitis, the portal vein is dissected proximally to the confluence of the splenic and superior mesenteric veins. When transplanting a whole organ or a reduced-size graft with the donor cava, the recipient's retrohepatic cava is preferentially resected with the liver and replaced. When segmental grafts are used, the cava is left intact and the liver is dissected until only the hepatic vein branches remain intact. If the inferior vena cava is congenitally absent, control of the hepatic veins is achieved as they traverse the diaphragm and enter the right atrium.

When a whole organ is transplanted, we proceed with orthotopic transplantation in the standard fashion. With more pediatric patients receiving segmental grafts, however, certain adjustments in technique are made to accommodate the donor and recipient vessels. Venous outflow obstruction was a critical complication in many of the early recipients of segmental liver grafts. We use the technique first described by Emond and associates: triangulation of the recipient hepatic vein orifice along the anterior vena cava together with the corresponding wall of the donor hepatic vein and triangulation of the anastomosis.[82] By creating as short and as wide an anastomosis as possible, the incidence of hepatic vein stenosis can be minimized. This technique also allows the graft to be slightly rotated, which facilitates access to the hilar structures and better aligns the inflow vessels.

Portal inflow is accomplished with an end-to-end anastomosis of the donor and recipient portal veins whenever possible. If a size disparity exists, a branch patch of the recipient's right and left portal veins can be used. Often, however, the recipient portal vein is sclerotic or thrombosed as a result of previous hepatic portoenterostomy or cholangitis episodes. If the confluence of the splenic and superior mesenteric veins is patent and the donor portal vein will reach, this confluence is the next preferred site of anastomosis. If not technically feasible, an interposition vein graft can be performed by using standard deceased donor sources or a donor ovarian vein, inferior mesenteric vein, or saphenous vein if the graft was provided by a living donor.[83]

Successful hepatic arterial anastomosis is of the utmost importance. Like others, we have found that implementation of microvascular techniques and use of the operating microscope have dramatically improved results.[81,84,85] Smaller vessels, such as those encountered in infant recipients and with segmental grafts, are typically anastomosed in an end-to-end manner by using the operating microscope and interrupted 8–0 or 9–0 monofilament sutures. When the recipient is older and the vessels are larger (> 4 mm), we use the branch patch technique. In the case of aberrant arterial anatomy, the supraceliac aorta is the inflow vessel of choice. The use of arterial conduits and the infrarenal aorta is avoided if possible. We currently administer an intraoperative and postoperative heparin infusion along with aspirin therapy postoperatively. In all operations involving small vascular anastomoses, we now use implantable Doppler probes to monitor vessel patency in the postoperative period.[86] The probes are placed at the conclusion of the transplant, before closure of the abdomen, and are held in proximity to the vessel with fibrin glue (Fig. 23–2). The ability to continuously monitor hepatic arterial and portal venous flow has facilitated early recognition of impaired flow resulting from increased intra-abdominal pressure and other technical problems and has allowed early graft salvage in these instances. The technique has also minimized the postoperative use of operator-dependent ultrasonography, which was previously used to confirm vessel patency.

The biliary reconstruction is straightforward and uses the previous Roux-en-Y limb of the hepatic portoenterostomy if suitable; otherwise, a 40-cm Roux-en-Y jejunal limb is created. An internal stent and interrupted 6–0 absorbable monofilament sutures are used to create the choledochojejunostomy (or hepaticojejunostomy in the case of a segmental graft).

Technical Variants

Approximately 10% to 20% of BA patients have multiple other malformations, such as situs inversus, absent inferior vena cava, preduodenal portal vein, and other manifestations of the polysplenia syndrome (Fig. 23–3). Although such anatomic abnormalities make liver transplantation in these patients technically challenging, they do not appear to have a significant impact on outcome.[25,87-90]

Complications

The complications in patients transplanted for BA are the complications of any pediatric liver transplant patient. They include the usual vascular and biliary complications, infections, rejection episodes, and complications of long-term immunosuppression and are covered extensively in subsequent chapters.

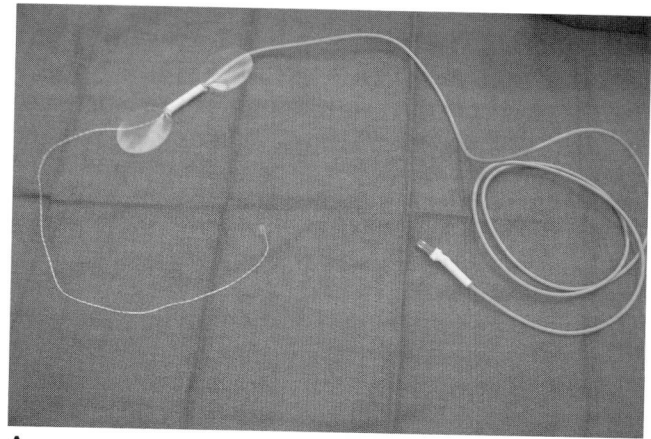

A

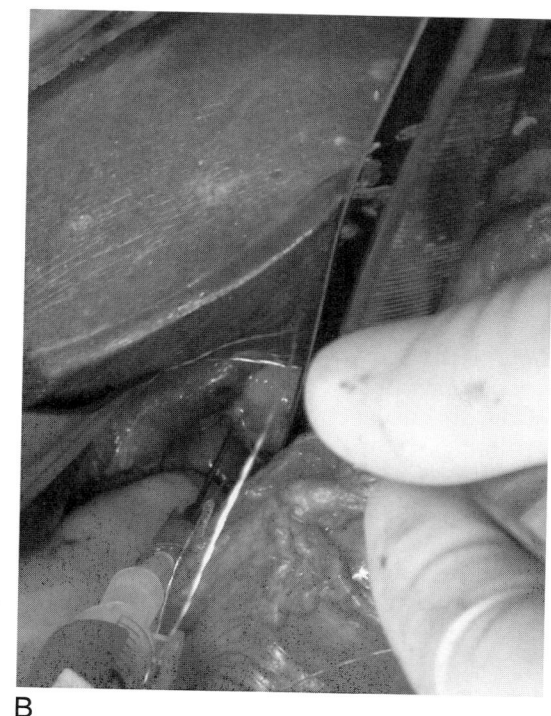

B

FIGURE 23–2

A, Implantable Doppler probe. **B,** Fibrin glue placed on probes located on the surface of the hepatic artery and portal vein to stabilize the probes.

Certainly, the most devastating early complication is hepatic artery thrombosis. The clinical findings can range from essentially no symptoms to episodes of relapsing bacteremia to fulminant graft necrosis and failure. Despite meticulous surgical technique and antiplatelet and anticoagulation therapy, arterial thrombosis is still reported in as many as 8% to 20% of pediatric liver transplants,[81,91,92] and it remains the leading cause of early graft failure and the primary indication for retransplantation. Most centers that have implemented microvascular techniques and use of the operating microscope, however, have noted a significant

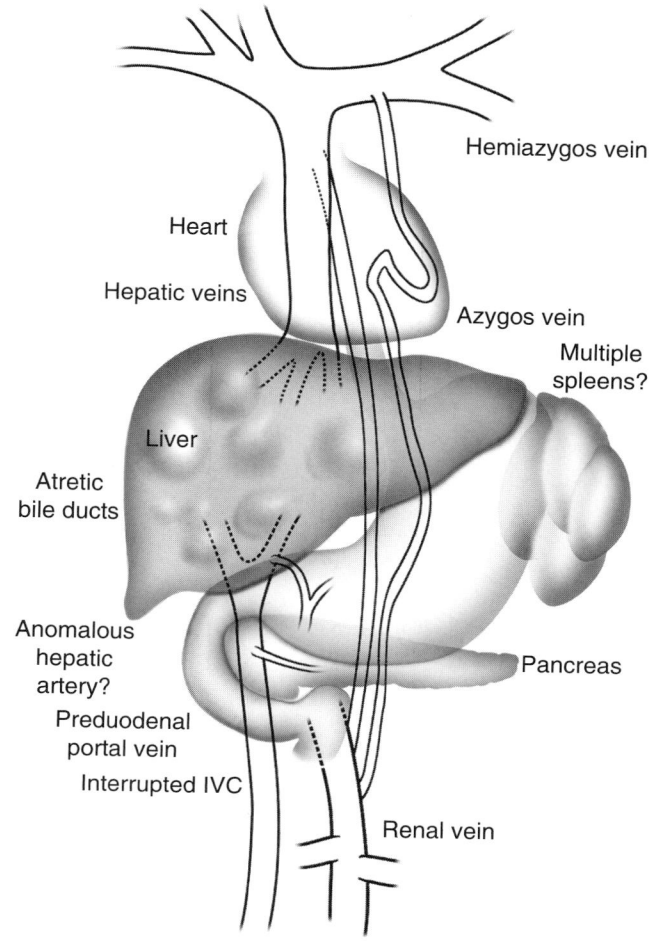

FIGURE 23–3

Anatomic variants associated with biliary atresia. IVC, inferior vena cava.

decline in the incidence of hepatic artery thrombosis.[84,93-95] Presumably, with use of the microscope, implantable Doppler probes, and avoidance of excessive intra-abdominal pressure in conjunction with continued attention to maximizing arterial inflow and adjunctive medical therapy, the rate of arterial thrombosis resulting in graft loss can continue to drop. At the same time, a better understanding of the hepatic microvasculature and its response to the damage caused by ischemia-reperfusion and acute rejection may permit the development of methods to further avoid this complication. More unusual arterial complications such as pseudoaneurysm and hepatic artery rupture are usually a result of infection (typically *Candida* or *Pseudomonas* species). Fortunately, these complications are rare, because they often result in fatal hemorrhage.

Vascular complications can involve both the portal inflow to the graft and the hepatic vein and vena cava outflow tracts. Venous outflow tract obstruction is a relatively rare event in the early postoperative period and occurs in approximately 4% to 7% of patients overall.[82,96] Attention to surgical technique and graft positioning can often prevent intraoperative and early outflow obstruction, whereas currently, little can be done to prevent late stenosis, which probably results from scarring. In the postoperative period, the onset of abdominal pain, ascites, hepatomegaly, splenomegaly, increased liver function test values, and coagulopathy may be clues to the diagnosis. Portal vein thrombosis and stenosis occur at a slightly higher rate than outflow problems do. Studies are conflicting regarding whether the incidence of vascular complications is higher in smaller pediatric recipients.[97-99] Early postoperative portal vein occlusion can be manifested in a variety of ways ranging from no overt symptoms to progressive liver failure. If diagnosed promptly, early reoperation and thrombectomy can potentially salvage the graft. In a single-center review of 600 pediatric liver transplants, long-term venous complications occurred in 50 of 524 grafts surviving more than 90 days.[85] Thirty-eight (7.2%) of these were portal vein complications, and 12 (2.3%) involved the hepatic vein or vena cava outflow. When patients requiring vein conduits for portal reconstruction were excluded, the incidence of late portal vein complications dropped to 1%. The majority of these patients were successfully managed with venous angioplasty and, occasionally, stenting. The remaining third required surgical shunting (eight patients) or retransplantation (five patients). The overall survival with retransplantation is lower, but there are reports of patients being retransplanted up to three times, and clearly, retransplantation plays a major role in the care of pediatric patients.

Biliary tract complications and intestinal perforation are fairly frequent, with each occurring in nearly 20% of patients after liver transplantation.[99] Leaks from the biliary enteric anastomosis are commonly associated with hepatic artery thrombosis, although they can also occur in the absence of a vascular complication. Late biliary strictures and cholestasis are often the result of chronic rejection or ischemia. Frequently, subtle elevations in serum alkaline phosphatase may be the only clue to the diagnosis. Noninvasive imaging may be unreliable, and percutaneous transhepatic cholangiography is often necessary, not only to confirm the diagnosis but also to provide drainage and allow for dilatation and stenting when necessary. Intrahepatic strictures pose a much greater problem and usually require retransplantation.

Leaks or breakdown of the jejunojejunostomy and the intestinal staple lines, or both, may also be seen in the early postoperative period. Spontaneous intestinal perforation occurs surprisingly often in the early postoperative period and appears to be independent of the number of previous surgical procedures or trauma at the time of liver transplantation.[100,101] A high index of suspicion, rapid diagnostic imaging, and early operative re-exploration may be the only means of effectively treating this often lethal complication.

Results

Since the first days of pediatric liver transplantation, surgeons and transplant centers have gained significant experience in the intraoperative and postoperative care of pediatric liver transplant recipients. Although complications after pediatric liver transplantation are frequent and often severe, the rewards are great and the results generally good. Improved surgical techniques, better intraoperative anesthetic management, and improvements in pediatric critical care, along with a greater understanding of the long-term sequelae of immunosuppression in children, have combined to yield ever-improving results after liver transplantation for BA. Table 23–2 summarizes some of the larger reported experience with liver transplantation for BA. The 5-year actuarial survival rates reported by these centers are comparable to those for pediatric patients undergoing liver transplantation for all reasons. Of note is the significant percentage of patients transplanted with segmental grafts at most centers, with some using segmental grafts exclusively in children younger than 2 years. The ability to expand the donor pool in this fashion has enabled many patients with BA to undergo liver transplantation before the development of

Table 23–2. RESULTS OF LIVER TRANSPLANTATION FOR BILIARY ATRESIA

Series	Number of Patients	Segmental Grafts (%)	Retransplantation (%)	5-Year Patient Survival Rate (%)	5-Year Graft Survival Rate (%)
Diem et al.,[102] 2003	328	62	16	83	72
Goss et al.,[81] 1996	190	18	16	78	76
Ishikawa et al.,[103] 1999	73	47	14	74	N/A
Nagral et al.,[79] 1997	64	63	23	84	69
Peeters et al.,[104] 2001	52	N/A	21	70	64

N/A, data not available.

decompensated hepatic failure. The use of segmental grafts from both living and deceased donors (usually of excellent quality) in conjunction with the ability to transplant these recipients in a generally healthier state has resulted in a significant survival benefit.

Pearls and Pitfalls

- Aggressive early diagnosis of biliary atresia is necessary in newborns.
- Hepatic portoenterostomy should be the first procedure; although 70% to 80% fail, it allows for growth and development of the child.
- On failure of the first Kasai procedure, patients should be referred for orthotopic liver transplantation; multiple attempts at salvage should be avoided.
- An operating microscope should be used for vessels smaller than 4 mm in diameter.
- Living donors and reduced-size liver transplants have helped overcome the shortage of pediatric donors and avoid end-stage liver disease and decompensation.

References

1. Thompson J: On congenital obliteration of the bile ducts. Edinb Med J 37:523, 1891.
2. Holmes J: Congenital obliteration of the bile ducts—diagnosis and suggestions for treatment. Am J Dis Child 11:405-431, 1916.
3. Ladd W: Congenital atresia and stenosis of the bile ducts. JAMA 91:1028-1031, 1928.
4. Gross R (ed): The Surgery of Infancy and Childhood. Philadelphia, WB Saunders, 1953.
5. Kasai M: [Surgery of anomalies of the bile ducts, with special reference to surgical techniques.] Geka Chiryo 19:942-950, 1968.
6. Starzl T, Marchioro TL, Vonkaulla KN, et al: Homotransplantation of the liver in humans. Surg Gynecol Obstet 117: 659-676, 1963.
7. Danks DM, Campbell PE, Jack I, et al: Studies of the aetiology of neonatal hepatitis and biliary atresia. Arch Dis Child 52:360-367, 1977.
8. Yoon PW, Bresee JS, Olney RS, et al: Epidemiology of biliary atresia: A population-based study. Pediatrics 99:376-382, 1997.
9. Balistreri WF: Neonatal cholestasis. J Pediatr 106:171-184, 1985.
10. Balistreri WF, Grand R, Hoofnagle JH, et al: Biliary atresia: Current concepts and research directions. Summary of a symposium. Hepatology 23:1682-1692, 1996.
11. Hyams JS, Glaser JH, Leichtner AM, Morecki R: Discordance for biliary atresia in two sets of monozygotic twins. J Pediatr 107:420-422, 1985.
12. Schweizer P, Kerremans J: Discordant findings in extrahepatic bile duct atresia in 6 sets of twins. Z Kinderchir 43:72-75, 1988.
13. Bobo L, Ojeh C, Chir D, et al: Lack of evidence for rotavirus by polymerase chain reaction/enzyme immunoassay of hepatobiliary samples from children with biliary atresia. Pediatr Res 41: 229-234, 1997.
14. Czech-Schmidt G, Verhagen W, Szavay P, et al: Immunological gap in the infectious animal model for biliary atresia. J Surg Res 101:62-67, 2001.
15. Szavay PO, Leonhardt J, Czech-Schmidt G, Petersen C: The role of reovirus type 3 infection in an established murine model for biliary atresia. Eur J Pediatr Surg 12:248-250, 2002.
16. Bezerra JA, Tiao G, Ryckman FC, et al: Genetic induction of proinflammatory immunity in children with biliary atresia. Lancet 360:1653-1659, 2002.
17. Davenport M, Dhawan A: Epidemiologic study of infants with biliary atresia. Pediatrics 101:729-730, 1998.
18. Desmet VJ: Congenital diseases of intrahepatic bile ducts: Variations on the theme "ductal plate malformation." Hepatology 16:1069-1083, 1992.
19. Davenport M, Savage M, Mowat AP, Howard ER: Biliary atresia splenic malformation syndrome: An etiologic and prognostic subgroup. Surgery 113:662-668, 1993.
20. Carmi R, Magee CA, Neill CA, Karrer FM: Extrahepatic biliary atresia and associated anomalies: Etiologic heterogeneity suggested by distinctive patterns of associations. Am J Med Genet 45:683-693, 1993.
21. Schreiber RA, Kleinman RE: Genetics, immunology, and biliary atresia: An opening or a diversion? J Pediatr Gastroenterol Nutr 16:111-113, 1993.
22. Tracy TF Jr, Dillon P, Fox ES, et al: The inflammatory response in pediatric biliary disease: Macrophage phenotype and distribution. J Pediatr Surg 31:121-125, discussion 125-126, 1996.
23. Kobayashi H, Puri P, O'Briain DS, et al: Hepatic overexpression of MHC class II antigens and macrophage-associated antigens (CD68) in patients with biliary atresia of poor prognosis. J Pediatr Surg 32:590-593, 1997.
24. Urushihara N, Iwagaki H, Yagi T, et al: Elevation of serum interleukin-18 levels and activation of Kupffer cells in biliary atresia. J Pediatr Surg 35:446-449, 2000.
25. Vazquez J, Lopez Gutierrez JC, Gomez M, et al: Biliary atresia and the polysplenia syndrome: Its impact on final outcome. J Pediatr Surg 30:485-487, 1995.
26. Lilly JR, Chandra RS: Surgical hazards of co-existing anomalies in biliary atresia. Surg Gynecol Obstet 139:49-54, 1974.
27. Meyers RL, Book LS, O'Gorman MA, et al: High-dose steroids, ursodeoxycholic acid, and chronic intravenous antibiotics improve bile flow after Kasai procedure in infants with biliary atresia. J Pediatr Surg 38:406-411, 2003.
28. Tan CE, Davenport M, Driver M, Howard ER: Does the morphology of the extrahepatic biliary remnants in biliary atresia influence survival? A review of 205 cases. J Pediatr Surg 29:1459-1464, 1994.
29. Gautier M, Jehan P, Odievre M: Histologic study of biliary fibrous remnants in 48 cases of extrahepatic biliary atresia: Correlation with postoperative bile flow restoration. J Pediatr 89:704-709, 1976.
30. Chardot C, Carton M, Spire-Bendelac N, et al: Epidemiology of biliary atresia in France: A national study 1986-96. J Hepatol 31:1006-1013, 1999.
31. McCracken GH Jr, Shinefield HM, Cobb K, et al: Congenital cytomegalic inclusion disease. A longitudinal study of 20 patients. Am J Dis Child 117:522-539, 1969.
32. Moldin J: Perinatal echovirus infection: Insights from a literature review of 61 cases and 16 outbreaks in nurseries. Rev Infect Dis 8:918-926, 1986.
33. Pruekprasert P, Stout C, Patamasucon P: Neonatal enterovirus infection. J Assoc Acad Minor Physicians 6(4):134-138, 1995.
34. Erkan T, Kutlu T, Cullu F, Tumay GT: A case of vertical transmission of hepatitis A virus infection. Acta Paediatr 87:1008-1009, 1998.

35. Renge RL, Dani VS, Chitambar SD, Arankalle VA: Vertical transmission of hepatitis A. Indian J Pediatr 69:535-536, 2002.

36. Park WH, Choi SO, Lee HJ: Technical innovation for noninvasive and early diagnosis of biliary atresia: The ultrasonographic "triangular cord" sign. J Hepatobiliary Pancreat Surg 8:337-341, 2001.

37. Farrant P, Meire HB, Mieli-Vergani G: Improved diagnosis of extraheptic biliary atresia by high frequency ultrasound of the gall bladder. Br J Radiol 74:952-954, 2001.

38. Gilmour SM, Hershkop M, Reifen R, et al: Outcome of hepatobiliary scanning in neonatal hepatitis syndrome. J Nucl Med 38:1279-1282, 1997.

39. Han SJ, Kim MJ, Han A, et al: Magnetic resonance cholangiography for the diagnosis of biliary atresia. J Pediatr Surg 37:599-604, 2002.

40. Norton KI, Glass RB, Kogan D, et al: MR cholangiography in the evaluation of neonatal cholestasis: Initial results. Radiology 222:687-691, 2002.

41. Larrosa-Haro A, Caro-Lopez AM, Coello-Ramirez P, et al: Duodenal tube test in the diagnosis of biliary atresia. J Pediatr Gastroenterol Nutr 32:311-315, 2001.

42. Ridaura Sanz C, Navarro Castilla E: [Role of liver biopsy in the diagnosis of prolonged cholestasis in infants.] Rev Invest Clin 44:193-202, 1992.

43. Muraji T, Higashimoto Y: The improved outlook for biliary atresia with corticosteroid therapy. J Pediatr Surg 32:1103-1106, discussion 1106-1107, 1997.

44. Dillon PW, Owings E, Cilley R, et al: Immunosuppression as adjuvant therapy for biliary atresia. J Pediatr Surg 36:80-85, 2001.

45. Balistreri WF: Bile acid therapy in pediatric hepatobiliary disease: The role of ursodeoxycholic acid. J Pediatr Gastroenterol Nutr 24:573-589, 1997.

46. Lebensztejn DM: Application of ursodeoxycholic acid (UDCA) in the therapy of liver and biliary duct diseases in children. Med Sci Monit 6:632-636, 2000.

47. Saller R, Meier R, Brignoli R: The use of silymarin in the treatment of liver diseases. Drugs 61:2035-2063, 2001.

48. Kobayashi H, Horikoshi K, Yamataka A, et al: Beneficial effect of a traditional herbal medicine (inchin-ko-to) in postoperative biliary atresia patients. Pediatr Surg Int 17:386-389, 2001.

49. Wu ET, Chen HL, Ni YH, et al: Bacterial cholangitis in patients with biliary atresia: Impact on short-term outcome. Pediatr Surg Int 17:390-395, 2001.

50. Lunzmann K, Schweizer P: The influence of cholangitis on the prognosis of extrahepatic biliary atresia. Eur J Pediatr Surg 9: 19-23, 1999.

51. Bu LN, Chen HL, Chang CJ, et al: Prophylactic oral antibiotics in prevention of recurrent cholangitis after the Kasai portoenterostomy. J Pediatr Surg 38:590-593, 2003.

52. Socha P, Koletzko B, Jankowska I, et al: Essential fatty acid metabolism in infants with cholestasis. Acta Paediatr 87:278-283, 1998.

53. Yamashiro Y, Ohtsuka Y, Shimizu T, et al: Effects of ursodeoxycholic acid treatment on essential fatty acid deficiency in patients with biliary atresia. J Pediatr Surg 29:425-428, 1994.

54. Pierro A, Koletzko B, Carnielli V, et al: Resting energy expenditure is increased in infants and children with extrahepatic biliary atresia. J Pediatr Surg 24:534-538, 1989.

55. Gregorio GV, Ball CS, Mowat AP, Mieli-Vergani G: Effect of rifampicin in the treatment of pruritus in hepatic cholestasis. Arch Dis Child 69:141-143, 1993.

56. Yerushalmi B, Sokol RJ, Narkewicz MR, et al: Use of rifampin for severe pruritus in children with chronic cholestasis. J Pediatr Gastroenterol Nutr 29:442-447, 1999.

57. Bergasa NV, Schmitt JM, Talbot TL, et al: Open-label trial of oral nalmefene therapy for the pruritus of cholestasis. Hepatology 27:679-684, 1998.

58. Corley DA, Cello JP, Adkisson W, et al: Octreotide for acute esophageal variceal bleeding: A meta-analysis. Gastroenterology 120:946-954, 2001.

59. Karrer FM, Narkewicz MR: Esophageal varices: Current management in children. Semin Pediatr Surg 8:193-201, 1999.

60. Zargar SA, Javid G, Khan BA, et al: Endoscopic ligation compared with sclerotherapy for bleeding esophageal varices in children with extrahepatic portal venous obstruction. Hepatology 36:666-672, 2002.

61. Hackworth CA, Leef JA, Rosenblum JD, et al: Transjugular intrahepatic portosystemic shunt creation in children: Initial clinical experience. Radiology 206:109-114, 1998.

62. Shashidhar H, Langhans N, Grand RJ: Propranolol in prevention of portal hypertensive hemorrhage in children: A pilot study. J Pediatr Gastroenterol Nutr 29:12-17, 1999.

63. Karrer FM, Lilly JR, Stewart BA, Hall RJ: Biliary atresia registry, 1976 to 1989. J Pediatr Surg 25:1076-1080, discussion 1081, 1990.

64. Kasai M, Suzuki S: A new operation for "non-correctable" biliary atresia: Hepatic portoenterostomy. Shujutsu 13:773-779, 1959.

65. Ohi R, Ibrahim M: Biliary atresia. Semin Pediatr Surg 1:115-124, 1992.

66. Endo M, Katsumata K, Yokoyama J, et al: Extended dissection of the porta hepatis and creation of an intussuscepted ileocolic conduit for biliary atresia. J Pediatr Surg 18:784-793, 1983.

67. Ito T, Nagaya M, Ando H, et al: Modified hepatic portal enterostomy for biliary atresia. Z Kinderchir 39:242-245, 1984.

68. Toyosaka A, Okamoto E, Okasora T, et al: Extensive dissection at the porta hepatis for biliary atresia. J Pediatr Surg 29:896-899, 1994.

69. Schweizer P, Kirschner HJ, Schittenhelm C: Anatomy of the porta hepatis (PH) as rational basis for the hepatoporto-enterostomy (HPE). Eur J Pediatr Surg 9:13-18, 1999.

70. Ando H, Seo T, Ito F, et al: A new hepatic portoenterostomy with division of the ligamentum venosum for treatment of biliary atresia: A preliminary report. J Pediatr Surg 32:1552-1554, 1997.

71. Ibrahim M, Ohi R, Chiba T: Indications and results of reoperation for biliary atresia. In Ohi R (ed): Biliary Atresia. Tokyo, Icom Associates, 1991, pp 96-100.

72. Ohi R: Biliary atresia. In Balistreri WF, Ohi R, Todani T, et al (eds): Hepatobiliary, Pancreatic, and Splenic Disease in Children: Medical and Surgical Management. New York, Elsevier, 1997, pp 249-251.

73. Ohi R: Surgery for biliary atresia. Liver 21:175-182, 2001.

74. Kuroda T, Saeki M, Nakano M, Morikawa N: Biliary atresia, the next generation: A review of liver function, social activity, and sexual development in the late postoperative period. J Pediatr Surg 37:1709-1712, 2002.

75. Howard ER, MacLean G, Nio M, et al: Survival patterns in biliary atresia and comparison of quality of life of long-term survivors in Japan and England. J Pediatr Surg 36:892-897, 2001.

76. Alagille D: Liver transplantation in children—indications in cholestatic states. Transplant Proc 19:3242-3248, 1987.

77. Miyano T, Fujimoto T, Ohya T, Shimomura H: Current concept of the treatment of biliary atresia. World J Surg 17:332-336, 1993.

78. Davenport M, Kerkar N, Mieli-Vergani G, et al: Biliary atresia: The King's College Hospital experience (1974-1995). J Pediatr Surg 32:479-485, 1997.

79. Nagral S, Muiesan P, Vilca-Melendez H, et al: Liver transplantation for extra hepatic biliary atresia. Tohoku J Exp Med 181: 117-127, 1997.

80. Wood RP, Langnas AN, Stratta RJ, et al: Optimal therapy for patients with biliary atresia: Portoenterostomy ("Kasai" procedures) versus primary transplantation. J Pediatr Surg 25:153-160, discussion 160-162, 1990.

81. Goss JA, Shackleton CR, Swenson K, et al: Orthotopic liver transplantation for congenital biliary atresia. An 11-year, single-center experience. Ann Surg 224:276-284, discussion 284-287, 1996.

82. Emond JC, Heffron TG, Whitington PF, Broelsch CE: Reconstruction of the hepatic vein in reduced size hepatic transplantation. Surg Gynecol Obstet 176:11-17, 1993.
83. Saad S, Tanaka K, Inomata Y, et al: Portal vein reconstruction in pediatric liver transplantation from living donors. Ann Surg 227:275-281, 1998.
84. Tanaka K, Uemoto S, Tokunaga Y, et al: Surgical techniques and innovations in living related liver transplantation. Ann Surg 217:82-91, 1993.
85. Buell JF, Funaki B, Cronin DC, et al: Long-term venous complications after full-size and segmental pediatric liver transplantation. Ann Surg 236:658-666, 2002.
86. Cronin DC 2nd, Schechter L, Lohman RF, et al: Advances in pediatric liver transplantation: Continuous monitoring of portal venous and hepatic artery flow with an implantable Doppler probe. Transplantation 74:887-890, 2002.
87. Farmer DG, Shaked A, Olthoff KM, et al: Evaluation, operative management, and outcome after liver transplantation in children with biliary atresia and situs inversus. Ann Surg 222:47-50, 1995.
88. Mattei P, Wise B, Schwarz K, et al: Orthotopic liver transplantation in patients with biliary atresia and situs inversus. Pediatr Surg Int 14:104-110, 1998.
89. Maggard MA, Goss JA, Swenson KL, et al: Liver transplantation in polysplenia syndrome: Use of a living-related donor. Transplantation 68:1206-1209, 1999.
90. Falchetti D, de Carvalho FB, Clapuyt P, et al: Liver transplantation in children with biliary atresia and polysplenia syndrome. J Pediatr Surg 26:528-531, 1991.
91. Stevens LH, Emond JC, Piper JB, et al: Hepatic artery thrombosis in infants. A comparison of whole livers, reduced-size grafts, and grafts from living-related donors. Transplantation 53:396-399, 1992.
92. Stringer MD, Marshall MM, Muiesan P, et al: Survival and outcome after hepatic artery thrombosis complicating pediatric liver transplantation. J Pediatr Surg 36:888-891, 2001.
93. Millis JM, Cronin DC, Brady LM, et al: Primary living-donor liver transplantation at the University of Chicago: Technical aspects of the first 104 recipients. Ann Surg 232:104-111, 2000.
94. Chan KL, Fan ST, Saing H, et al: Paediatric liver transplantation: Queen Mary Hospital experience. Chin Med J (Engl) 111: 610-614, 1998.
95. Shackleton CR, Goss JA, Swenson K, et al: The impact of microsurgical hepatic arterial reconstruction on the outcome of liver transplantation for congenital biliary atresia. Am J Surg 173: 431-435, 1997.
96. Egawa H, Inomata Y, Uemoto S, et al: Hepatic vein reconstruction in 152 living-related donor liver transplantation patients. Surgery 121:250-257, 1997.
97. Van der Werf WJ, D'Alessandro AM, Knechtle SJ, et al: Infant pediatric liver transplantation results equal those for older pediatric patients. J Pediatr Surg 33:20-23, 1998.
98. Inomata Y, Tanaka K, Okajima H, et al: Living related liver transplantation for children younger than one year old. Eur J Pediatr Surg 6:148-151, 1996.
99. Yamanaka J, Lynch SV, Ong TH, et al: Surgical complications and long-term outcome in pediatric liver transplantation. Hepatogastroenterology 47:1371-1374, 2000.
100. Shaked A, Vargas J, Csete ME, et al: Diagnosis and treatment of bowel perforation following pediatric orthotopic liver transplantation. Arch Surg 128:994-998, discussion 998-999, 1993.
101. Beierle EA, Nicolette LA, Billmire DF, et al: Gastrointestinal perforation after pediatric orthotopic liver transplantation. J Pediatr Surg 33:240-242, 1998.
102. Diem HV, Evrard V, Vinh HT, et al: Pediatric liver transplantation for biliary atresia: Results of primary grafts in 328 recipients. Transplantation 75:1692-1697, 2003.
103. Ishikawa M, Lynch SV, Balderson GA, et al: Liver transplantation in Japanese and Australian/New Zealand children with biliary atresia: A 10-year comparative study. Eur J Surg 165: 454-459, 1999.
104. Peeters PM, Sieders E, De Jong KP, et al: Comparison of outcome after pediatric liver transplantation for metabolic diseases and biliary atresia. Eur J Pediatr Surg 11:28-35, 2001.

Liver Transplantation for Metabolic Disease

SUZANNE V. McDIARMID

α_1-Antitrypsin deficiency   339
  Liver disease as a manifestation of
    α_1-antitrypsin deficiency   340
  Pathology   340
  Liver transplantation for α_1-antitrypsin
    deficiency   341

Wilson's disease   341
  Clinical features   342
  Liver transplantation for Wilson's
    disease   343

Disorders of amino acids   344
  Tyrosinemia   344
  Urea cycle defects   346
  Other disorders of amino acid
    metabolism   348

Disorders of carbohydrate metabolism   349
  Galactosemia and fructosemia   349
  Glycogen storage diseases   349

Disorders of lipid metabolism   351
  Familial hypercholesterolemia   351
  Lipoidoses   352

Disorders of bilirubin metabolism   353

Cystic fibrosis   354
  Clinical features   354
  Liver transplantation   355

Hyperoxaluria type 1   355
  Liver and kidney transplantation   355

Other metabolic diseases for which liver
transplantation has been performed   357
  Neonatal iron storage disease   357
  Defects of mitochondrial function   358
  Mucopolysaccharidoses   359

Liver transplantation has made possible the functional cure of several metabolic diseases characterized by inherited genetic defects.[1-8] In many pediatric transplantation centers, metabolic diseases, most notably α_1-antitrypsin deficiency, are the second most common indication for liver transplantation after biliary atresia.[9,10] The Studies of Pediatric Liver Transplantation (SPLIT) database shows that of 1187 children transplanted between 1995 and 2002, 11.9% received a transplant for a metabolic disease. The number of children who underwent liver transplantation for each metabolic disease diagnosis is shown in Table 24–1.[11] The long-term survival and quality of life of children who undergo liver transplantation for metabolic disease is similar to that of children with other liver diseases.[12,13] The manifestations of metabolic disease affecting the liver are diverse and range from acute liver failure to cirrhosis complicated by hepatoma. However, the indication for liver transplantation may go beyond the recognized complications of acute or chronic

Table 24-1. INDICATIONS FOR LIVER TRANSPLANTATION FOR CHILDREN WITH METABOLIC LIVER DISEASE

Total number of children transplanted	1187	
Transplantation for metabolic disease	141	11.9%*
α_1-Antitrypsin deficiency	39	27.7%†
Urea cycle defects	22	15.6%
Tyrosinemia	16	11.3%
Cystic fibrosis	12	8.5%
Wilson's disease	10	7.1%
Neonatal iron storage disease	9	6.4%
Primary hyperoxaluria	8	5.7%
Glycogen storage disease	7	5.0%
Crigler-Najjar syndrome	6	4.2%
Other	12	8.5%

*Percentage of total children transplanted who have metabolic liver disease.

†Percentage of children with a given diagnosis and transplanted for metabolic liver disease.

From McDiarmid S, Anand R, Lindblad AS, SPLIT Research Group: Studies of pediatric liver transplantation: 2002 update. An overview of demographics, indications, timing, and immunosuppressive practices in pediatric liver transplantation in the United States and Canada. Pediatr Transplant 8:284-294, 2004.

liver failure.[14] Life-threatening extrahepatic disease as a result of a deficient enzyme localized to hepatocytes, as occurs, for example, in central nervous system (CNS) manifestations of the urea cycle defects, can be cured by liver transplantation. Liver transplantation has also been advocated to improve the severely impaired quality of life in children who must endure rigidly enforced protein-restricted diets to control the potentially devastating neurological consequences of the organic acidurias.

To determine when liver transplantation is appropriate treatment of metabolic disorders, it is useful to consider two general categories of disease[3]: (1) metabolic disease with structural liver damage leading to end-stage liver disease (e.g., α_1-antitrypsin deficiency, familial tyrosinemia, and Wilson's disease) and (2) metabolic disease without structural liver damage (e.g., familial hypercholesterolemia, primary oxalosis, and urea cycle defects).

In the first group, the genetic defect may be localized to the liver itself, such as occurs in the familial cholestatic syndromes (see Chapter 22), but more commonly the liver is one of the end-organs damaged as a result of a more widespread defect (e.g., tyrosinemia and α_1-antitrypsin deficiency). When the liver is exclusively involved and also the only site of the metabolic defect, the decision to replace the liver is easily made, and liver transplantation can be expected to provide complete reversal of the metabolic defect. However, in diseases in which the liver is damaged as a consequence of a widespread enzymatic defect residing in a variety of cells other than hepatocytes, determination of whether liver transplantation is indicated is more complex. Essential to this decision is precise knowledge of the genetic defect itself, the somatic cells in which the cellular defect is expressed, the extent of organ involvement outside the liver, and whether liver replacement alone will be sufficient to either prevent further deterioration or improve dysfunction in extrahepatic organs. Tyrosinemia is illustrative of these principles.[15] The deficient enzyme, fumarylacetoacetate hydrolase (FAH), is not localized to hepatocytes, and the kidneys and CNS are two other major organs affected. However, tyrosinemia is associated with a spectrum of severe liver disease for which liver transplantation is indicated, ranging from fulminant hepatitis to cirrhosis with hepatoma formation. The Fanconi syndrome–like kidney disease associated with tyrosinemia often persists after liver transplantation, although some functional improvement usually occurs. The neurological crises do not appear to recur after transplantation. Thus, in tyrosinemia, liver replacement not only is life-saving but also ameliorates the extrahepatic manifestations of the disease.

In contrast, in the mucopolysaccharidoses, successful liver transplantation circumvents the consequences of unremitting liver fibrosis but is unable to overcome the widespread extrahepatic expression of the enzymatic defect and therefore allows continued accumulation, particularly in the CNS, of abnormal sphingomyelin. Ongoing neurological deterioration can be anticipated. In this instance, liver transplantation alone would not be indicated, but when combined with a bone marrow transplant, it may be a more successful approach if attempted early.[16]

Medical therapies that might preclude or delay transplantation should be optimized. In general, the success of these measures depends on early diagnosis. This is particularly relevant with the use of chelating agents in Wilson's disease; treatment with 2-nitro-4-trifluoromethylbenzoyl-1,3-cyclohexanedione (NTBC), a compound that blocks the formation of toxic metabolites in tyrosinemia; and phototherapy in Crigler-Najjar syndrome.[17]

In the future, total liver replacement may become obsolete for some categories of metabolic disease.[18] In metabolic diseases in which the liver is structurally normal, hepatocyte transplantation is an attractive option. Normal allogeneic hepatocytes have been able to provide temporary metabolic support in animal models,[19] as first shown in the Gunn rat model of Crigler-Najjar syndrome[20,21] and later in case studies of children with Crigler-Najjar syndrome[22] and those with ornithine transcarbamylase (OTC) deficiency.[23] However, a major disadvantage is that immunosuppression is still required. A more attractive option involves the use of gene therapy to modify the genetic program of the patient's own hepatocytes.[24] Harvested hepatocytes infected in vitro with a recombinant retrovirus or adenovirus carrying the normal human gene are then able to express the normal gene's protein products. Autologous transplantation of these genetically reconstituted hepatocytes is then performed. This approach has been used successfully in animal models for such diseases as familial hypercholesterolemia,[25] the urea cycle defects,[26] Crigler-Najjar syndrome,[27] and tyrosinemia.[28] Alternatively, in vivo modification of hepatocytes might be achieved by a vector containing the normal gene. Such approaches would avoid the significant morbidity and mortality associated with orthotopic liver transplantation and a lifetime of immunosuppression.

To reverse the metabolic defect, animal models have shown that only a small percentage of the total liver cell mass needs to be replaced with cells containing viable enzyme. However, in clinical reports of hepatocyte transplantation for Crigler-Najjar disease, urea cycle defects, and hypercholesterolemia, despite transplantation of what should have been an adequate cell mass, only partial correction of the defect has been reported. Not only is the long-term viability of transplanted cells a problem to be overcome, but a limitation of hepatocyte transplantation is that only about 1% of the liver mass can be replaced by transplanted cells.

Recently, attention has been focused on the concept of "liver repopulation" whereby the transplanted cells are given a growth advantage over the recipient's own cells.[29] To be successful in animal models, this technique has two specific requirements to provide "the space" for the transplanted cells to proliferate. First, the transplanted cells must have an advantage in either proliferation or survival in comparison to the endogenous hepatocyte population. Second, removal of endogenous hepatocytes, usually by partial hepatectomy, is required to provide the stimulus for liver regeneration, which selectively allows the transplanted hepatocytes to proliferate. In animal models, approaches used to decrease the regenerative capacity of endogenous hepatocytes include drugs blocking DNA syntheses and irradiation. By applying these two principles in animal studies, up to 90% of the host liver cells can be replaced by transplanted cells. If such techniques prove applicable to humans, hepatocyte transplantation, including the transplantation of genetically altered autologous hepatocytes, would become a clinical reality.

The rapidly advancing field of stem cell transplantation may also have important implications for the correction of some liver-localized metabolic diseases. Stem cells, whether of bone marrow or liver origin, may prove to be the best candidate cells for transplantation into the liver.[30,31]

The following sections systematically describe metabolic defects for which liver transplantation is indicated. For each disease entity, a description is provided of the metabolic defect and its genetics, inheritance and biochemical effects, pathology, clinical manifestations from infancy through the teenage years, indications for transplantation, and impact of transplantation on the course of the disease. Liver transplantation for familial cholestasis syndromes and hemopoietic metabolic disease is discussed in Chapters 22 and 24, respectively.

α_1-Antitrypsin Deficiency

α_1-Antitrypsin deficiency is one of the most common lethal inherited diseases that affect the white population. It is characterized by liver disease in children and emphysema in adults. There is a rare association of α_1-antitrypsin deficiency with glomerulonephritis in children and young adults.[32] The frequency of the disease is between 1 in 2000 and 1 in 7000[33] in populations of European descent. Liver disease associated with α_1-antitrypsin deficiency is the most common metabolic disease for which liver transplantation is performed in children.[34]

α_1-Antitrypsin is a major serine protease inhibitor that is produced primarily in the liver, but also to some extent in neutrophils and macrophages. Its most important function is inhibition of neutrophil elastase, a powerful proteolytic enzyme capable of degrading extracellular structural proteins, particularly elastin.[35] The effect of low circulating α_1-antitrypsin levels is most dramatically seen in the lung, where the unopposed action of neutrophil elastase leads to progressive destruction of the lung parenchyma, which becomes clinically manifested as emphysema. In contrast, liver disease is the result of retention of the abnormal α_1-antitrypsin molecule within hepatocytes.[36]

α_1-Antitrypsin is a small, 52-kD glycosylated protein. It is encoded for by a single gene located on chromosome 14 with codominant expression of the two inherited alleles. At least 75 allelic variants have been described.[37] Phenotyping, designated by the Pi (protease inhibitor) nomenclature, was originally described by the relative mobility of the α_1-antitrypsin molecule along an acid starch gel gradient.[38] Variants are described by letters of the alphabet. Approximately 70% to 80% of selected populations have the normal phenotype, PiMM. The α_1-antitrypsin deficiency state is most often characterized by PiZZ. Other variations have been described (e.g., PiMZ, PiMS) and are variably associated with low α_1-antitrypsin levels and clinical disease.[37-40]

Liver Disease as a Manifestation of α_1-Antitrypsin Deficiency

The first association of α_1-antitrypsin deficiency and liver disease was made by Freier and colleagues[41] in 1968 and expanded by Sharp and associates in 1969.[42] Soon thereafter, Sveger's large prospective screening of 200,000 newborns in Sweden provided the study that still stands as the best description of the natural history of the disease.[43,44] In this study, 120 PiZZ infants were identified, 12% of whom presented with cholestasis within the first 3 months and an additional 6% had clinical evidence of liver disease (hepatosplenomegaly). In a follow-up study, 73% of PiZZ infants had transaminitis by 6 months of age that persisted until age 8 in 59%.[45] Overall, about 3% of infants with the PiZZ phenotype progressed to cirrhosis, which represented about 20% of the PiZZ infants with neonatal cholestasis. Since these first observations, additional information has allowed an easily remembered generalization to be made. Of PiZZ infants with cholestasis, cirrhosis will develop in 25% in the first decade, 25% will show persistent transaminitis progressing to cirrhosis in the second decade, 25% will have mild transaminitis without cirrhosis, and the biochemical abnormality will resolve completely and show only mild fibrosis on liver biopsy in 25%.[38]

Typically, in an infant with α_1-antitrypsin deficiency and cholestasis, the jaundice resolves by about 6 months.[44] However, the transaminitis usually persists. In those who progress to cirrhosis, the clinical development of portal hypertension, with or without recrudescence of jaundice, is a common manifestation later in childhood.[39] In many children the progression to end-stage liver disease may be quite slow.[46] Rarely, however, the course progresses rapidly to end-stage liver disease. The early development of ascites with cirrhosis on liver biopsy is an ominous sign and has been reported as early as 2 weeks of age, thus suggesting that in some infants the liver insult begins in utero.[47]

The severity of the cholestatic liver disease in infancy correlates with the appearance of cirrhosis in later childhood.[48] However, α_1-antitrypsin deficiency must still be considered a cause of cirrhosis in childhood, even without an antecedent history of neonatal cholestasis.[49] Persistent abnormalities in urinary bile acids may also predict progression to cirrhosis.[50] Other risk factors are female sex and siblings in whom cirrhosis has also developed. Whether early breast-feeding is protective remains debatable.[48,51]

The PiZZ phenotype is most often correlated with liver disease. However, both PiMZ and PiSZ individuals have been reported with moderately depressed α_1-antitrypsin serum levels, as well as clinical and histological evidence of liver disease.[37,38,43,52-54] The association of hepatocellular carcinoma (HCC) in adults with "cryptogenic" cirrhosis has been linked to previously undiagnosed ZZ and MZ phenotypes.[55]

Pathology

The characteristic pathology of the liver in α_1-antitrypsin–deficient patients with liver disease provides insight into the mechanism of liver injury.[56] Abnormal globules of α_1-antitrypsin, characteristically periodic acid–Schiff positive and diastase resistant, accumulate in periportal lymphocytes, which are the site of α_1-antitrypsin production (Fig. 24–1).[38,52] On electron microscopy, the rough endoplasmic reticulum of such cells is distended with similar granules.[57,58] It has been postulated that abnormal folding of the mutant α_1-antitrypsin molecule leads to accumulation in the rough endoplasmic reticulum.[59] Retention of abnormally folded proteins in

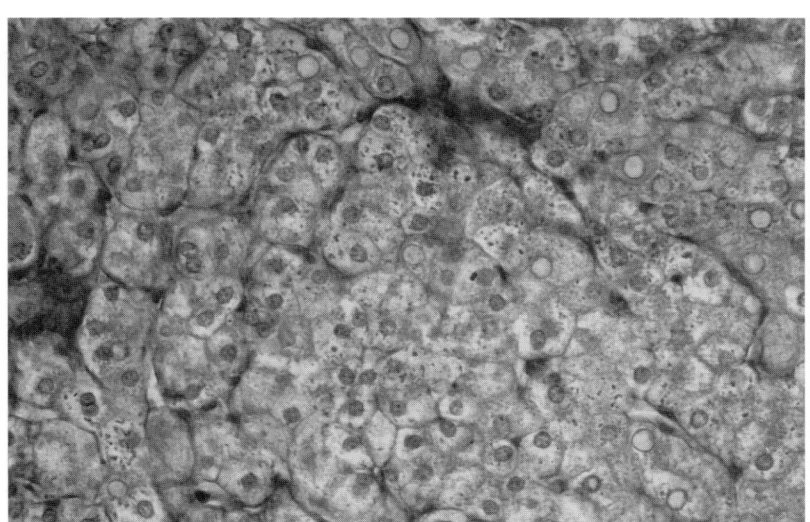

FIGURE 24–1

α_1-Antitrypsin deficiency. In a periodic acid–Schiff–stained section of the liver after diastase, pink, diastase-resistant globules of α_1-antitrypsin are apparent within hepatocytes, particularly in the periportal area. Fibrosis in the portal triad is also evident.

the endoplasmic reticulum is thought to be a protective mechanism that allows degradation of abnormal proteins to prevent further cellular damage. It is now proposed that patients with liver disease associated with α_1-antitrypsin deficiency have a defect in the degradative pathway that causes greater accumulation of the putatively hepatotoxic mutant α_1-antitrypsin molecule.[56] Because liver disease develops in only a small minority of patients with the ZZ genotype, the defect in degradation is thought to be controlled by either other unlinked genetic traits or environmental factors.

It is now clear that the mechanism of liver injury in α_1-antitrypsin deficiency is not analogous to the mechanism of injury in the lung, which is caused by low tissue levels of α_1-antitrypsin that allow destruction of the parenchyma by locally released proteases. This different mechanism is substantiated by studies of patients with the rare Pi-Null phenotype in which no detectable α_1-antitrypsin is present in serum or hepatocytes and no liver injury occurs.[37] Augmentation of α_1-antitrypsin serum levels by administering recombinant α_1-antitrypsin can be expected to improve lung function but has not been shown to either turn off or promote secretion of α_1-antitrypsin globules accumulated in the liver.[60,61]

Liver Transplantation for α_1-Antitrypsin Deficiency

Liver transplantation as an effective cure for α_1-antitrypsin deficiency was first performed in 1973.[62] The transplanted liver produced normal α_1-antitrypsin molecules, and the α_1-antitrypsin serum level normalized. The recipient's phenotype converted to that of the donor. As could be predicted by the restoration of circulating α_1-antitrypsin levels to normal, no patients to date have contracted emphysema. However, it should be remembered that the transplanted patient's original genotype is unchanged in the germ cell line, so when children transplanted for α_1-antitrypsin deficiency reach reproductive age, genetic counseling should be offered.[53]

The excellent outcomes now reported from many centers for children undergoing liver transplantation for α_1-antitrypsin deficiency associated with end-stage liver disease has changed the overall prognosis substantially for children with this disease.[63,64] In a large single-center experience in children with clinical liver disease secondary to α_1-antitrypsin deficiency, 27% underwent transplantation. The duration of jaundice and the severity of the histological features and biochemical abnormalities predicted outcome at an early stage of the disease.[65] As a group, children undergoing transplantation for α_1-antitrypsin deficiency have lower mortality and morbidity than other pediatric recipients do.[10,13] This better outcome can be attributed to their generally older age at initial evaluation, which often

shows portal hypertension and bleeding varices. Jaundice is usually mild and nutritional status better preserved than in younger children with biliary atresia. In addition, most have had no previous abdominal surgeries. However, like other conditions associated with cirrhosis and portal hypertension, children with α_1-antitrypsin deficiency have a propensity for the development of large arteriovenous pulmonary shunts and cyanosis before transplantation.[66] The degree of shunt and arterial oxygenation should be evaluated before transplantation. Although these problems may resolve over time, large shunts complicate the early postoperative period and compromise weaning from the ventilator.[67,68]

Rupture of a splenic artery aneurysm has also been described as a lethal complication after liver transplantation in a child with α_1-antitrypsin deficiency.[69] Such rupture is most likely a reflection of the commonly seen severe pretransplantation portal hypertension and not a function of the disease itself.

Other possibilities for the future treatment of liver disease associated with α_1-antitrypsin deficiency might include gene therapy to suppress the abnormal Z gene so that the mutant molecule is not produced. It will also be difficult to prospectively determine which patients to treat because clearly, liver disease does not develop in all these children. For such preventive strategies to be successful, a better understanding of the other genetic and environmental triggers that predispose patients with abnormal phenotypes to the development of liver disease will be needed.

Wilson's Disease

Copper accumulation in the liver, CNS, eyes, and kidneys is the cardinal clinical feature of Wilson's disease, an autosomal recessive disease of copper metabolism with a prevalence of about 1 in 30,000 in most populations. The liver plays an essential role in copper homeostasis inasmuch as about 95% of copper in the portal vein is taken up by the liver and biliary excretion of copper is the only physiologically important route of copper elimination. About 90% of serum copper is bound to ceruloplasmin. Newborn infants show concentrations of copper within the liver similar to those of patients with Wilson's disease.[70] Normally, the liver copper level falls toward adult levels by 6 months of age. In Wilson's disease, copper first accumulates in the liver and subsequently in the CNS and other extrahepatic tissues.[70-73]

In recent years, elucidation of the copper metabolic pathway in the liver and discovery of the genes that encode the proteins essential to normal copper metabolism have greatly enhanced our understanding of the molecular and genetic basis of Wilson's disease.[74,75] Mutations in the *ATP7B* gene give rise to Wilson's disease. The gene product for *ATP7B* is an adenosine triphosphate (ATP)-dependent copper transporter that is required for the intrahepatocyte delivery of copper to the secretory pathway that incorporates copper into apoceruloplasmin, with subsequent transport across the lipid bilayer of the hepatocyte into bile. The frequency of the abnormal gene, irrespective of race, is about 1 in 200 to 400.[70] Heterozygote carriers occur at a frequency of about 1 per 100 in the general population.[72]

Because more than 200 mutations have been described, it is currently difficult to screen populations for Wilson's disease. However, genetic analysis is useful in screening families of affected individuals. A single dominant mutation (H1069Q) is found primarily in Slavic populations but in only about a third of North American populations. In addition, there is often a poor correlation between patients homozygous for specific alleles and the clinical manifestations of disease, thus implying that additional genetic or environmental factors play a role.

Clinical Features

Evolution of the liver injury in Wilson's disease appears to be related to redistribution of copper within the liver, which may induce oxidant injury in hepatocyte mitochondria.[76] Clinical evidence of disease seldom occurs before 5 years of age, although one case of jaundice in a 2-year-old has been described.[71] In children, the liver manifestations of the disease are most frequently manifested in their teenage years,[71] whereas 40% of adults initially have neurological abnormalities.[70] The symptoms of neurological disease are usually subtle in children. Personality and behavior changes or poor school performance may be present. The predominantly motor abnormalities of tremor, dystonia, and dysarthria become more pronounced with age and are related to the effects of copper accumulation in the extrapyramidal system. In adult patients with primarily neurological manifestations of Wilson's disease, the condition may be misdiagnosed as mental retardation or psychiatric impairment, and the true origin of their neurological disease is never appreciated.[72]

The clinical manifestations of liver impairment in Wilson's disease are diverse and range from asymptomatic hepatosplenomegaly with an associated low-grade transaminitis to fulminant liver failure. The heterogenicity in findings frequently delays the diagnosis. Chronic active hepatitis progressing to cirrhosis[77] may remain clinically silent for years before becoming manifested as acute onset of jaundice, which is often misdiagnosed as acute hepatitis. In some adolescents, the acute hepatitis–like picture may progress over a period of weeks to severe liver failure, whereas in others, the first manifestation of the disease is fulminant liver failure.[70-72] Portal hypertension and bleeding varices are also frequent initial signs.

Physical examination may not be especially helpful in making the diagnosis of Wilson's disease. Hepatosplenomegaly is frequently present, but the liver may be shrunken in advanced cases. Kayser-Fleischer rings, seen as a rusty brown ring at the junction of the iris and cornea caused by deposition of copper in Descemet's membrane, are often said to be pathognomonic of Wilson's disease. The ring first appears as a crescent in the superior aspect of the eye but may be difficult to visualize in brown eyes.[78] Slit-lamp examination is often required. However, Kayser-Fleischer rings do not usually appear until midadolescence and are not unique to Wilson's disease.[79]

The diagnosis of Wilson's disease may also be confounded by an often-confusing constellation of test results.[70-73,79] Classically, serum ceruloplasmin is low (<20 mg/dL), serum copper is low (<80 mg/L), and 24-hour urine copper is high (>100 mg/24 hr). However, 15% of homozygotes with liver disease[79] have normal ceruloplasmin, and about 20% of carriers of the Wilson's disease gene[72] have low ceruloplasmin. Low ceruloplasmin levels are likewise seen in severe copper deficiency and fulminant liver failure. Because ceruloplasmin is also an acute phase reactant, it may be elevated with ongoing inflammatory liver injury and in pregnancy or with estrogen administration. Total serum copper is unreliable as well because free serum copper is often increased in untreated or fulminant Wilson's disease. The 24-hour urine copper level is also elevated in chronic liver disease with cholestasis, acute liver failure, and severe proteinuria. Careful collection in copper-free containers is required.

The copper content of the liver is the most reliable diagnostic test. In Wilson's disease, a copper content greater than 250 µg/g dry tissue (normal, <50 µg) is frequently seen. Values up to 3000 µg/g are not uncommon.[79] Although an increased copper concentration may also be seen with chronic active hepatitis and primary biliary cirrhosis, ceruloplasmin is either normal or increased in these diseases, and other distinctive features should allow differentiation.[77]

If ceruloplasmin is normal, a useful adjuvant test is to measure the incorporation of radioactive copper into ceruloplasmin. Wilson's disease is characterized by decreased accumulation of radioactive copper.[80] This test is of no value if the serum ceruloplasmin concentration is low.[72]

Abnormalities in liver function vary depending on the clinical manifestation. However, rapid diagnosis of Wilson's disease in patients with fulminant liver failure is of critical importance.[81] Acute hemolysis frequently accompanies fulminant Wilson's disease because massive amounts of copper are released into the circulation and lyse red blood cell membranes.[71] The association of acute hemolysis with liver failure in an adolescent should be diagnosed as Wilson's disease until proved otherwise. In addition, the characteristic pattern of mildly elevated transaminases with high serum bilirubin and an unexpectedly normal alkaline phosphatase concentration should prompt consideration of Wilson's disease over most other causes of acute fulminant liver failure.[82,83] In one study of emergency liver transplantation, 11.4% of children with fulminant liver failure had Wilson's disease.[84]

Deiss and coworkers describe four stages of Wilson's disease before treatment.[85] In stage 1, copper accumulates in the cytosol of the hepatocyte, and the patient remains asymptomatic. In stage 2, copper is redistributed into lysosomes, with some copper being released into the circulation. Liver fibrosis, cirrhosis, or liver failure may occur. In stage 3, copper accumulates asymptomatically in the CNS, which leads to neurological symptoms in stage 4.

In the liver, the histological appearance of early Wilson's disease includes fatty infiltration and glycogen-filled hepatocyte nuclei. Distinctive, but not unique, mitochondrial abnormalities are present on electron microscopy. As the disease progresses, there is continuing fibrosis, parenchymal collapse, inflammatory cell infiltrates, and nodular regeneration culminating in frank cirrhosis. In patients presenting with acute liver failure, liver necrosis is the predominant histological factor.[70]

Liver Transplantation for Wilson's Disease

Orthotopic liver transplantation provides a cure for Wilson's disease in patients in whom medical therapy has failed or in those found to have advanced decompensated liver disease at initial evaluation. Medical management in patients in whom Wilson's disease is diagnosed in the early stages of the disease—and continued lifelong—may abrogate the need for liver transplantation entirely. D-Penicillamine,[86] trientine dihydrochloride,[87] and tetrathiomolybdate[88] are chelating agents with proven success. More recently, the use of oral zinc has been advocated in asymptomatic patients after an initial cupruresis has been induced with chelating agents or in combination with a chelator in patients with symptoms related to either liver or neurological disease. In one report, combination therapy averted liver transplantation in several patients.[74] Oral zinc induces the formation of metallothionein, a copper-binding substrate, within the enterocyte. Ingested copper is then bound within the enterocyte to metallothionein and sloughed into the gastrointestinal tract, never reaching the systemic circulation.[89-91]

Various attempts have been made to ascertain which patients with Wilson's disease should be considered for transplantation.[92] Indications include failure of medical treatment to improve either liver or neurological function, fulminant liver failure, and decompensated cirrhosis at initial evaluation. On the basis of a scoring system, Nazer and colleagues accurately predicted which patients had a poor prognosis when treated medically. Elevations in bilirubin, serum glutamic-oxaloacetic transaminase, and prothrombin time predicted increased mortality. Jaundice and ascites also correlated with a poor outcome.[93]

Successful liver transplantation for Wilson's disease with complete reversal of the metabolic manifestations was first reported by Dubois and associates in 1971.[94] By the early 1980s, orthotopic liver transplantation had become the standard treatment of Wilson's disease manifested as fulminant liver failure or decompensated chronic disease. The results of transplantation, particularly in patients with fulminant Wilson's disease, have been impressive.[95,96] In reported series, fulminant liver failure, which occurs more frequently in females by a 2:1 ratio, is the indication for liver transplantation in the majority of patients.[97,98] In one of the largest single-center reports in which 45 patients underwent transplantation for Wilson's disease, 42.2% were younger than 18 years at transplantation, and two thirds of the patients received transplants for either fulminant or subfulminant liver failure; 73.3% of these patients survived more than 5 years after transplantation.[98] Aggressive temporizing strategies may be needed to maintain patients with acute fulminant liver failure secondary to Wilson's disease until a liver can be found. Treatments have included D-penicillamine in conjunction with hemofiltration in patients with kidney failure[99] and heterotopic transplantation.[100]

In successful liver recipients, an initial period of cupruresis is followed by normalization of serum copper, ceruloplasmin, and liver copper content.[101] The characteristic Kayser-Fleischer rings resolve slowly, in some cases more than 3 years.[102] Adult patients with neurological or psychological impairments have shown complete[103] or partial recovery,[104] although such recovery may take several months. In general, patients transplanted for Wilson's disease enjoy an excellent quality of life.[105] A still-contentious issue is whether liver transplantation is justified for neurological disease without severe liver disease. This debate is exemplified by a report of a 15-year-old without significant liver disease who was bedridden with severe incapacitating dysarthria despite maximal medical therapy. This patient reportedly returned almost to normal after liver transplantation.[106]

The use of a living related donor for Wilson's disease, usually a parent who is a heterozygote carrier, carries the risk that copper metabolism may remain abnormal after transplantation. In a recent report of two children who each received a graft from a parent, it was shown that the liver copper content was slightly elevated, not exceeding 250 μg/g dry weight. However, serum copper and ceruloplasmin levels were lower and urinary copper excretion higher than normal. The long-term outcome is as yet unknown.[107] It would seem prudent to avoid living related donors whenever possible for Wilson's disease or to perform gene analysis preoperatively if the procedure is to be attempted.[108]

The future holds the promise that gene therapy or isolated hepatocyte transplantation may offer definitive therapy for patients identified very early in the disease process. Transplantation of normal hepatocytes into Long-Evans cinnamon rats, an animal model of Wilson's disease, showed that a viable transplanted hepatocyte mass of 4% to 20% prevented the development of Wilson's disease.[109]

Identification of any child with Wilson's disease, regardless of whether liver transplantation is a therapeutic option, should always prompt a systematic investigation of all family members. Early detection and treatment of asymptomatic homozygotes may prevent the necessity for subsequent liver transplantation.

Disorders of Amino Acids

Tyrosinemia

Hereditary tyrosinemia type I is an autosomal recessive disease in which FAH, the terminal enzyme in tyrosine metabolism, is deficient. The more than 30 mutations of the gene located on chromosome 15[110] account for the wide clinical variability of the disease.[111] The distribution of the genetic abnormality varies considerably with population groups. In Quebec, where the disease was first described in 1967 by Larochelle and coworkers,[112] the incidence of the disease is 1 in 10,000 but rises to 1 in 800 births in one geographically isolated area. In comparison, the incidence in Scandinavia is 1 in 50,000.[15,113]

The diagnosis of tyrosinemia is made by demonstrating reduced activity of FAH, the enzyme responsible for cleaving fumarylacetoacetate into fumaric and acetoacetic acids.[114] In Quebec, neonatal screening programs on dried blood spots are important for early detection in this high-risk population.[115,116]

Clinical Features of Liver Disease in Tyrosinemia

Lethal liver disease, neurological crises, and a Fanconi syndrome with hypophosphatemic rickets characterize the disease. Although serum tyrosine, methionine, and phenylalanine are elevated in serum, these elevations are not thought to mediate the toxic injury. Accumulation of fumarylacetoacetate and maleylacetoacetate most likely mediates the cellular toxicity.[117-122]

Liver disease in tyrosinemia can be manifested as either acute or chronic disease. Tanguay and colleagues demonstrated no FAH activity in the acute form, whereas in the chronic form, FAH activity was about 20% of normal.[15]

Acute disease becomes apparent in infancy with the onset of fulminant liver failure. Frequently, infants present with a bleeding diathesis, and liver failure is diagnosed secondarily. Tyrosinemia should be considered in an infant with coagulopathy even without other clinical evidence of liver failure.[123] A few of these infants respond to a diet low in tyrosine, phenylalanine, and methionine, but most succumb if no other intervention is made. In these infants the liver may be pale and enlarged with already-apparent micronodular cirrhosis, bile duct proliferation, steatosis, and pseudoacinar arrangements of hepatocytes.[118]

The chronic form of tyrosinemia-induced liver disease has a more insidious onset. Although it often develops after the first year of life, it should be considered even in very young children—particularly those with unexplained rickets or Fanconi syndrome. The liver is enlarged and coarsely nodular with progression from micronodular to macronodular cirrhosis.[118,119] There may be clinical evidence of portal hypertension and decompensated cirrhosis with jaundice, ascites, and loss of synthetic function. Before the use of NTBC (see later), even with strict dietary management children with tyrosinemia showed a frightening propensity for the development of HCC after the age of 2 years. The malignancy is multifocal within the liver and may have metastasized at the time of diagnosis.[120]

Extrahepatic Manifestations

Neurological crises, which usually occur after 1 year of age, may also be a fatal consequence of tyrosinemia. The defining features of the syndrome are the acute onset of profound weakness or paralysis, painful dysesthesias, often with hypertonic posturing, and self-mutilation. Respiratory muscle paralysis may quickly lead to death. Seizures and sustained arterial hypertension are other common features. Mitchell and colleagues reported a 42% incidence of neurological crises with an associated mortality of 70% in 48 tyrosinemic children hospitalized in Quebec.[121]

The clinical features of the neurological crises closely resemble those of acute porphyria, and indeed, as in porphyria, elevated serum δ-aminolevulinic acid is common. These elevated levels are due to inhibition of aminolevulinic acid dehydrase by succinylacetone, a metabolite of tyrosine degradation. Treatment of neurological crises is largely supportive, although hematin, which decreases aminolevulinic acid production, may shorten the course.[122] Emergency liver transplantation may be required for severely affected children, particularly those in respiratory failure, and averts any further crises.[124]

The kidneys are the third major organ affected by hereditary tyrosinemia. Kidney biopsies have shown glomerulosclerosis and interstitial fibrosis.[118] Autotoxicity of the kidneys by the local production of succinylacetone has been proposed as the mechanism of tubular dysfunction.[125]

Medical Therapy

A major advance in the medical management of tyrosinemia has been made since 1991 when the first patient was treated with NTBC, a compound that inhibits tyrosine degradation and blocks the enzymes responsible for accumulation of the toxic metabolites (particularly succinylacetoacetate) that induce the liver injury (Fig. 24–2).[126]

By 2000, more than 300 patients had been enrolled in an international study,[127] and more than 100 of these patients had been treated for longer than 5 years. The starting dose is 1 mg/kg/day, but up to 2 mg/kg/day may be required in infants. The greatest benefit was seen in children in whom the disease was diagnosed and treated before 6 months of age. In this cohort, 90% responded—including some with an acute manifestation. Of the 10% with no clinical response, five children died and three others underwent liver transplantation. The least amount of benefit was seen in those beginning therapy after 2 years of age. This population was heterogeneous, with tyrosinemia newly diagnosed in some children and others managed for often long periods by diet restriction alone. In this group the main reason for withdrawal from NTBC therapy was suspicion of HCC. Maintenance of a tyrosine-restricted diet is still essential with NTBC treatment, as shown in both animal and human studies. Rigorous monitoring of tyrosine levels is required. It is important to avoid tyrosine levels greater than 500 µmol/L, which are associated with corneal lesions, hyperkeratotic lesions of the palms and soles, and perhaps nervous system abnormalities.

The critical question remains whether early NTBC treatment can eliminate the risk for HCC. In children treated early in life, HCC developed in 2 (1%) during the first year of treatment.[127] In a single-center report, 2 of 10 children failed NTBC treatment, with hepatic dysplasia developing in 1—the other was a nonresponder.[128] Until further information is available, it would seem prudent to be very vigilant in monitoring for the development of HCC in children treated with NTBC—particularly after 2 years of age. Serial imaging studies of the liver, immediate biopsy of any suspicious lesions, and frequent measurement of serum α-fetoprotein levels (in children with low levels during NTBC therapy) will be necessary.

Liver Transplantation for Tyrosinemia

Before the advent of NTBC therapy, liver transplantation was life-saving in children with hereditary tyrosinemia and remains so for children who are nonresponders to NTBC, those who already have cirrhosis at initial evaluation, and children with evidence of hepatic dysplasia or malignant change. In 1976, the first patient with tyrosinemia underwent transplantation.[129] The metabolic abnormalities were promptly reversed, although the patient did have HCC with a

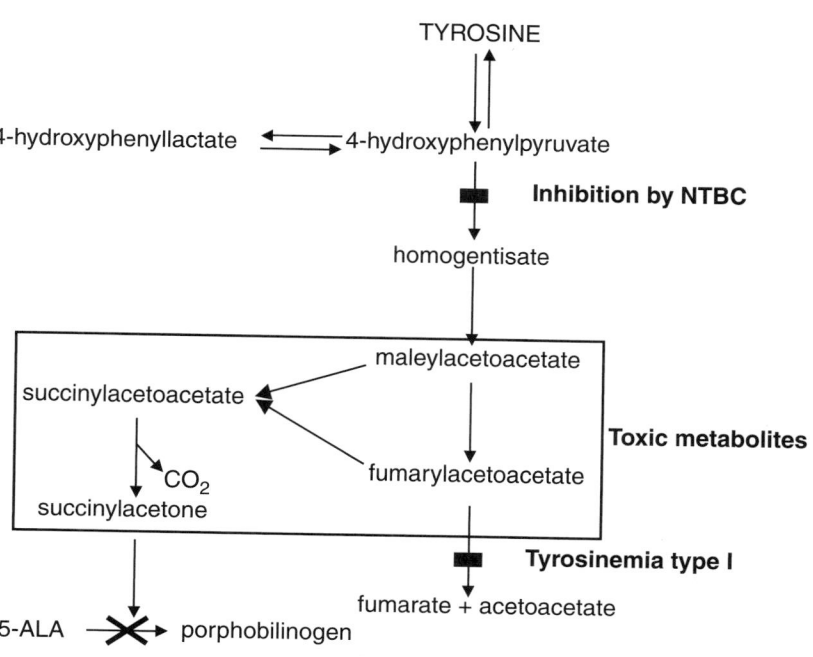

FIGURE 24–2

The metabolic pathway for tyrosine degradation. Note the proximal site of action of NTBC (2-nitro-4-trifluoromethylbenzoyl-1,3-cyclohexanedione), which blocks formation of the toxic metabolites. The site of the enzymatic defect is also shown. (Adapted from Holme E, Lindstedt S: Nontransplant treatment of tyrosinemia. Clin Liver Dis 4: 805-814, 2000.)

pulmonary metastasis at the time of transplantation. In 1985, Starzl and coauthors reported the successful outcome of four children with chronic tyrosinemia and made the important point that transplantation should be considered early, before hepatoma develops.[130] The concern for malignant transformation is further justified by reports of liver cell dysplasia and HCC in explanted livers from children undergoing transplantation.[131,132] Esquivel and associates reported tumor in 5 of 10 children who underwent transplantation for tyrosinemia. All five children were younger than 2 years at transplantation, and in three, both lobes were involved. Recurrent tumor has occurred in one child.[132] A further observation that 37% of children older than 2 years will have hepatoma[120] prompted most authors, before the use of NTBC therapy, to recommend elective transplantation at about 2 years of age, a concept supported by the excellent results reported from several centers.[133-136]

The dilemma still persists regarding when to offer transplantation to children with chronic tyrosinemia in whom decompensated end-stage liver disease has not yet occurred.[137] Evidence from NTBC studies suggests that children older than 2 years do not have a clear benefit from NTBC therapy, and because the risk for HCC is of increasing concern after 2 years of age, liver transplantation rather than NTBC therapy is the preferred choice. The diagnosis of hepatoma itself is fraught with difficulties because serum α-fetoprotein levels cannot generally be used as a marker. α-Fetoprotein levels, often in the thousands, are characteristic of children with tyrosinemia, even without tumor. Similarly, computed tomographic scans and ultrasonograms may show liver nodules, even very early in the course of the disease, that may not be malignant.

Unfortunately, maintenance of normal tyrosine levels by dietary means is no protection against the development of hepatoma or the progression of liver disease. In a review of 10 patients, 9 of whom had been on a strict diet, 3 had HCC before transplantation, 2 had incidental carcinoma diagnosed at transplantation, and 9 had hepatocyte dysplasia.[138]

The decision regarding transplantation is more easily made when the infant presents with fulminant liver failure.[136] In such infants the severity of their disease usually precludes a trial of NTBC. As experience has accrued with liver transplantation in small infants, the fear of a poor outcome in such young recipients has been allayed. Esquival and colleagues reported an 80% survival rate in infants younger than 1 year who underwent transplantation for tyrosinemia.[132] In very young infants, a trial of dietary management and NTBC is reasonable only if some stabilization in liver function can be achieved.

Although many of the clinical features of tyrosinemia resolve,[139,140] liver transplantation does not guarantee complete reversal of the kidney impairment seen in hereditary tyrosinemia. Not all patients reported[140] have shown complete normalization of tubular dysfunction or the glomerular filtration rate (GFR),[141] and many continue to have some, albeit reduced, amounts of succinylacetone in their urine. The ongoing endogenous production of succinylacetone is the most likely explanation, but heterogeneity in local expression of tyrosinemia in the kidney is evident by the variation in kidney function reported after liver transplantation.[142] However, because the GFR is frequently impaired before transplantation and ongoing posttransplant kidney impairment secondary to cyclosporine use is likely, careful posttransplant management of renal function is necessary. Paradis and coworkers monitored the GFR in tyrosinemic children after transplantation and fractionated their cyclosporine doses, which avoided further nephrotoxicity.[143]

A mouse model of FAH deficiency is now allowing experimental approaches to gene therapy for tyrosinemia.[144] This approach will be of particular benefit in high-risk populations in which routine screening of newborns, siblings of index cases, and infants with early manifestation of disease is performed.

Urea Cycle Defects

Biosynthesis of urea is dependent on six enzymes, all of which are localized in the liver.[145] Inherited defects of urea synthesis are frequently manifested soon after birth as severe and often fatal syndromes marked by hyperammonemia, coma, and devastating CNS impairment. The cornerstone of medical management is dietary protein restriction combined with attempts to increase the excretion of ammonia. Exchange transfusion, peritoneal dialysis, and hemodialysis can acutely lower ammonia concentrations but are impractical for long-term management. Sodium benzoate, either orally or intravenously, also lowers ammonia levels by allowing the excretion of nitrogen as hippurate. Phenylacetate, arginine, glucose, and insulin infusions have also been used.[146] However, medical interventions have high associated morbidity and mortality in the long-term amelioration of these disorders. Risks include protein deficiency, growth retardation, accidental overdose of drugs used to lower ammonia levels, and the unpredictable recurrence of coma leading to devastating neurological injury.[145,147]

Liver transplantation, either complete or auxiliary, could be predicted to cure urea cycle defects. Three of the six enzymopathies of urea synthesis have now been treated by liver transplantation.[148-150] The difficulty lies in successfully implementing the procedure in the neonatal period, when many of these infants are identified, before irreversible CNS damage occurs. The barrier to liver transplantation in the very young is being lowered as the technique of and expertise in transplantation have become perfected, as demonstrated by successful liver transplantation in a 14-day-old for a urea cycle defect.[148]

The liver in patients with urea cycle defects is structurally normal. Although either complete or auxiliary liver replacement can effect a metabolic cure because only about 3% to 5% of hepatocytes with normal OTC expression are required to reverse the clinical manifestations of the disease, isolated allogeneic hepatocyte transplantation or genetic modification of the patient's own hepatocytes could also achieve a functional cure. In a case report of an infant with OTC deficiency treated by infusion of batches of isolated hepatocytes over a 4-week period, hyperammonemia resolved temporarily but returned after 31 days. The viability of allogeneic hepatocytes, despite immunosuppression, remains the hurdle to overcome for this modality to be successful in the long term.[23] In a rodent model, virus-mediated transfer of human argininosuccinate synthetase has already been accomplished.[26] The helper-dependent adenoviral vectors may offer the best chance of long-term gene expression.[151] Once perfected in humans, this modality would allow correction of the metabolic defect in the first days of life, before neurological damage is evident and without the considerable risks of liver transplantation.

Ornithine Transcarbamylase Deficiency

The most common of the urea cycle defects, OTC deficiency is an X-linked dominant disease.[152] Affected males are usually seen in the first days of life with lethargy, irritability, and poor feeding rapidly progressing to convulsions, apnea, and coma. The diagnosis is suggested by markedly elevated serum ammonia levels, low or normal blood urea, low serum citrulline levels, and severe oroticaciduria. Liver biopsy is not necessary for diagnosis and, in fact, has been associated with precipitating hyperammonemic crises and subsequent death. Although liver dysfunction is not clinically significant in OTC deficiency, transaminitis with fibrosis and glycogenosis on liver biopsy has been described.[153]

With intensive early intervention, sometimes including hemodialysis, some boys with either the complete or incomplete form of OTC deficiency have survived beyond the neonatal period with protein restriction.[154] However, hyperammonemic crises frequently precipitated by catabolic stress such as acute illness may still occur with the attendant risk of further neurological damage.

Heterozygote girls may show a spectrum of clinical disease consistent with the Lyon hypothesis of random inactivation of the normal X chromosome.[155] Some are clinically normal, whereas others may be identified in either infancy or later childhood by episodes of lethargy,

irritability, and even coma precipitated by increased protein intake. A fatal clinical course of OTC deficiency was described in a heterozygous woman.[156] Diagnosis of OTC deficiency in female heterozygotes is often difficult and requires a high index of suspicion. Provocative testing with protein loads or allopurinol challenge is not always conclusive, and DNA analysis does not detect the mutation in some cases. Measures of in vivo urea cycle activity may be more sensitive.[157] Several reports of liver transplantation in girls have shown complete correction of the defect.[155]

The success of liver transplantation in reversing the metabolic defect in OTC deficiency is well described.[148,158] Early diagnosis and aggressive management to lower ammonia levels in the newborn period are essential to limit the degree of neurological injury sustained before transplantation.[149] Such injury can often be difficult to predict given that many of these children are evaluated for transplantation before 1 month of age. Generally, the younger the child at transplantation, the better the neurological prognosis. In our experience of three boys aged 40 to 223 days at the time of liver transplantation, all have survived, two with some mild neurological impairments that became more noticeable as they approached school age. In all, serum ammonia levels and serum arginine levels are normal, but before supplementation, citrulline levels were low because of the persistent deficiency of OTC in the intestinal mucosa.[159] Auxiliary liver transplantation has also been performed in both boys and heterozygous girls with OTC deficiency.[158,160] In the first report of this procedure,[158] an already neurologically impaired 14-month-old underwent transplantation to improve his quality of life. The recipient's left lobe was removed, and segments II and III of the liver graft were placed in an orthotopic position. Normalization of serum ammonia on a full diet without any medications was achieved. Both the native liver and the graft are functional. This case exemplifies the principle that only a portion of a normal liver is required to provide enough normal enzyme activity to reverse the metabolic deficit.

Liver transplantation using a related living donor, particularly a mother, raises the concern of using a heterozygous OTC-deficient graft. Death of a recipient who received a graft from a deceased donor with unsuspected OTC deficiency has already been reported.[161] Although success has been reported with the mother used as a donor, other living donor programs advocate allopurinol loading tests to exclude heterozygote donors.[162]

Carbamoyl-Phosphate Synthetase Deficiency

Inherited as an autosomal recessive trait, the neonatal form of carbamoyl-phosphate synthetase deficiency presents a clinical picture similar to OTC deficiency.

The diagnosis is differentiated from OTC deficiency by the absence of oroticaciduria.[145]

Partial carbamoyl-phosphate synthetase deficiency in which episodic hyperammonemia may be manifested in the first weeks or months of life has also been described. Developmental retardation is seen in both forms.

There are two reports of liver transplantation in children with carbamoyl-phosphate synthetase deficiency. A 14-day-old boy successfully underwent transplantation with a newborn deceased donor liver and has had complete normalization of serum ammonia on an unrestricted diet. He has some delay in developmental milestones, which the authors attribute to a brain abscess after transplantation.[148] The second child, who underwent transplantation at 20 months, already had developmental delay. Although his serum ammonia levels normalized, citrulline levels remained undetectable and dietary supplementation was needed.[163]

Argininosuccinate Synthetase Deficiency

High citrulline levels characterize the rare autosomal recessive condition of argininosuccinate synthetase deficiency. A severe neonatal form has been described, with some survivors beyond the neonatal period[145] who were successfully transplanted.[150,164] A variant, usually seen in adult patients of Japanese descent, has been treated by liver transplantation with reversal of the neurological defects associated with hyperammonemia.[23,148,165-167] Two Japanese children have received living donor grafts from heterozygous parents. In both, the hyperammonemic episodes resolved. In one, plasma citrulline levels remained high,[168] and in the other they normalized.[162]

Other Disorders of Amino Acid Metabolism

The more common organic acidurias methylmalonicacidemia, propionicacidemia, and maple syrup urine disease have in common a wide spectrum of clinical manifestations characterized by metabolic acidosis, lethargy, poor feeding, hepatomegaly, and various degrees of neurological impairment. Medical management primarily relies on very strict dietary protein restriction. However, despite good dietary compliance, these children may suffer life-threatening crises. Although the enzymatic defects are not confined to the liver, several children have undergone liver transplantation with variable success.

Methylmalonicacidemia and Propionicacidemia

Of the organic acidemias, liver transplantation for methylmalonicacidemia is the most commonly reported.

Children present with hepatomegaly, increased ammonia and transaminases, hypoglycemia, and variable degrees of neurological impairment. End-stage kidney disease develops in long-term survivors, thus prompting consideration for kidney transplantation. Despite medical management with dietary protein restriction and carnitine supplementation, disease exacerbations with vomiting, dehydration, acidosis, and hypoglycemia may occur and be manifested as acute emergencies.[169] Some children with methylmalonicacidemia appear to have minimal CNS involvement and have undergone liver or kidney transplantation (or both), but with mixed results.[170-172] Of particular concern is the late appearance of metabolic stroke reported in one patient and progressive neurological disability in another.[173,174] At this time, liver transplantation would appear to have a dubious role in providing long-term benefit to most of these patients.[172] However, others have considered the improvement in quality of life a justification for liver transplantation, even if some neurological impairment is present.[12]

The clinical manifestations of the propionic acidemias are very similar to those of the methylmalonic acidemias. A neonatal-onset form has been described. Several case reports in the literature, including a recipient of a living donor graft[175] and another of an auxiliary graft,[176] relate that liver transplantation reduced serum ammonia levels and allowed less restricted dietary protein intake.[177]

Maple Syrup Urine Disease

Maple syrup urine disease is an autosomal recessive disorder of branched-chain amino acid metabolism. Impaired activity of the branched-chain 2-oxoacid dehydrogenase complex results in the accumulation of branched chain L-amino acids (leucine, isoleucine, and valine) and 2-oxoacids. The increased leucine levels appear to exert most of the neurotoxic effects. Children often present in infancy with obtundation, coma, and seizures, with some succumbing to cerebral edema. Very high serum leucine levels are the diagnostic tip-off. Neurological sequelae can be averted by aggressive medical management during crises, including growth hormone and insulin infusions, hemofiltration or dialysis, and rigorous management of cerebral edema. With very strict control of dietary protein, which requires gastrostomy tube feeding in infants, further neurological crises can be avoided in some children. However, crises can occur even with full compliance with the protein-restricted diet and can be precipitated by any catabolic stress, such as an intercurrent illness, exercise, fasting, or dehydration. The risk of sustaining neurological damage from such episodes continues throughout life. Although modern management of maple syrup urine disease in dedicated centers has been associated with good neurological outcome,[178] the quality of life in these children as they grow older, combined with the ongoing risk of CNS injury, has led some specialists in this disease to recommend liver transplantation. Three case reports have been published worldwide—the first in a child with maple syrup urine disease in whom the indication for liver transplantation was hepatitis A–induced fulminant liver failure. After transplantation, although plasma concentrations of branched-chain amino acids and 2-oxoacids were two to three times normal, the child could resume a normal diet with no further neurologic sequelae.[179] Liver transplantation should be considered in children without significant neurological damage who have already proved difficult to control with dietary protein restriction alone.[180]

Disorders of Carbohydrate Metabolism

Galactosemia and Fructosemia

Galactosemia (galactose 1-phosphate uridyltransferase deficiency) and hereditary fructosemia (fructose 1-phosphate aldolase deficiency) can both be manifested in infancy as fulminant liver failure.[181] Galactosemia occurs in the first few days after milk feeding begins and produces a life-threatening illness with vomiting, jaundice, hepatomegaly, liver failure, and kidney-type Fanconi syndrome. Infants are acidotic, and galactose, a reducing substance, can be demonstrated in urine. Elimination of all milk products from the diet reverses the acute liver and kidney decompensation, and emergency liver transplantation is not necessary. The enzymatic defect also occurs in many other extrahepatic sites such as red blood cells, skin fibroblasts, and intestinal mucosal cells. Several clinically milder variants have been described. Although dietary management can control this disease, even small amounts of ingested galactose can apparently lead to progressive liver injury culminating in cirrhosis with the subsequent development of HCC. At least two young adults have now undergone liver transplantation for cirrhosis with HCC secondary to galactosemia.[182]

Hereditary fructosemia is recognized in the first few months of life after the introduction of fruit sugars and sucrose to the diet. The clinical features are quite similar to those of galactosemia and consist of failure to thrive, vomiting, fulminant liver failure, and Fanconi syndrome. The infants are characteristically hypoglycemic with hypophosphatemia and lactic acidosis. However, with the elimination of fructose, sucrose, and sorbitol from the diet, complete recovery occurs and liver transplantation is not necessary.[181]

Glycogen Storage Diseases

At least 12 glycogen storage diseases have been identified, most of which can be controlled by dietary means. Hepatomegaly and hypoglycemia are common to most of the variants. The enzymatic deficiency, however, is not localized to the liver, and glycogen storage is readily seen in biopsy samples of other tissues, particularly the heart, skeletal muscle, and CNS.[181] For this reason, caution should be practiced when recommending liver transplantation for the glycogen storage diseases.[182]

Type IV glycogen storage disease is a rare autosomal recessive condition caused by a brancher enzyme deficiency that results in the accumulation of an abnormal glycogen resembling amylopectin, a plant starch. The gene is located on chromosome 3p14, and several mutations have been described, thus accounting for the variability in clinical findings.[183] Usually, the disease develops early in life, with rapidly progressive liver injury leading to cirrhosis.[184] There is also evidence for amylopectin accumulation in the CNS, heart, and skeletal muscle. In such patients, dietary management is not successful, and death from cirrhotic liver disease occurs within the first few years of life unless liver transplantation is performed. However, because the enzymatic defect is not limited to hepatocytes, ongoing accumulation in extrahepatic tissue can occur. Selby and associates[185] reported seven children with type IV glycogenosis who underwent liver transplantation. No evidence was found of progressive amylopectin accumulation in extrahepatic sites, and a reduction in cardiac amylopectin was described in one child. However, Sokal and coauthors reported increasing amylopectin deposition in the heart after liver transplantation, which ultimately led to the patient's death.[186] In a more recent report of 13 children transplanted for type IV glycogen storage disease with up to 13 years of follow-up, only 1 had evidence of cardiac or neuromuscular complications.[187]

In 1993, Starzl and associates reported two children with type IV glycogen storage disease, both of whom had a decrease in cardiac amylopectin after liver transplantation. In both patients, donor-derived cells could be demonstrated in the heart and skin (Fig. 24–3). These authors postulated that microchimerism, in which enzymatically normal cells migrate from the graft to the periphery, may be the mechanism by which the diffuse cellular enzymatic defect can be ameliorated.[188]

Type IA glycogen storage disease, an autosomal recessive defect caused by glucose-6-phosphatase deficiency, was the first liver enzyme deficiency described. Normally, the enzyme is expressed in the liver, kidneys, and intestine. Hepatomegaly, hypoglycemia, lactic acidosis, and growth failure occur in infancy but can generally be well controlled by frequent glucose and starch

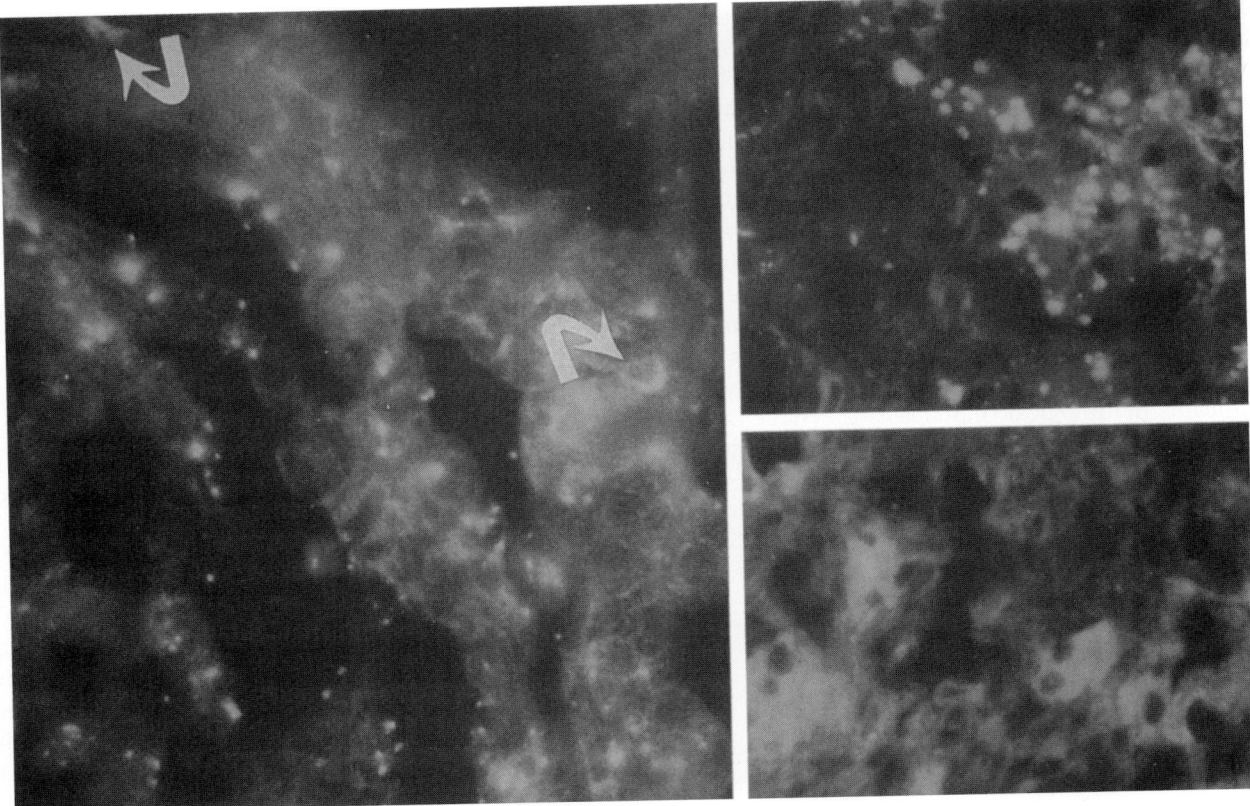

FIGURE 24–3

Type IV glycogen storage disease. Immunocytochemical analysis of the heart, transplanted liver, and native liver in a patient with type IV glycogen storage disease shows chimerism. In the left panel, green fluorescence (*arrows*) identifies cells with the donor's phenotype (HLA-DR1, HLA-DR4) in the interstitium of the heart. The upper right panel shows positive green-staining donor cells (HLA-DR1, HLA-DR4) in the transplanted liver. The lower right panel (negative control) shows absence of donor cells in the recipient's native liver. All sections were stained with a single monoclonal antibody specific for HLA-DR1 and HLA-DR4. The yellow globules are autofluorescent intracellular pigment. (Reprinted, by permission, from Starlz TE, Demetris AJ, Trucco M, et al: Chimerism after liver transplantation for type IV glycogen storage disease and type 1 Gaucher's disease. N Engl J Med 328:745-749, 1993.)

feeding and avoidance of lactose and sucrose. Hyperuricemia may lead to kidney stone formation and requires allopurinol treatment.[181]

Some patients with type IA glycogen storage disease have difficulty complying with restricted diets and almost continuous feedings as they enter childhood and are thus susceptible to episodes of severe hypoglycemia with seizures. For such life-threatening complications, liver transplantation has been successfully performed with complete resolution of the metabolic defect, good catch-up growth, and improved quality of life.[184,187,189] However, liver replacement cannot be expected to correct the intestinal and kidney deficiency of glucose-6-phosphatase. Focal segmental glomerulosclerosis, which has been associated with glycogen storage disease type IA, has occurred after liver transplantation.[189] In the type IB glycogen storage disease variant, the associated neutrophil dysfunction has also persisted after liver transplantation.[187]

The development of hepatic adenomas with malignant transformation has been described in type I glycogen storage diseases and is the other consideration for liver replacement. This complication generally occurs in postpubertal patients with an incidence varying between 22% and 75% and an estimated risk that 10% will undergo malignant transformation.[190] Whether assiduous control of hypoglycemia decreases the potential for malignancy is unknown.[191] This potentially fatal complication has already been averted by liver transplantation.[192] However, the difficulty lies in detecting when the malignant change occurs. Because the adenomas are usually multiple, surgical resection does not typically provide definitive treatment. As children with glucose-6-phosphatase deficiency survive longer, they should be regularly screened for the development of adenomas, with subsequent biopsy of discovered adenomas. If either dysplasia or malignant change is found, liver transplantation should be considered.

The clinical dilemma is how many lesions should undergo biopsy and how often.

A single experience of allogeneic hepatocyte transplantation was recently reported in a 47-year-old woman with glycogen storage disease type IA, who 9 months after hepatocyte transplantation could eat an unrestricted diet and fast for 71 hours without hypoglycemia. Two billion hepatocytes in two separate infusions were given through an indwelling portal vein catheter, and triple-drug immunosuppression was administered.[193] This report suggests that isolated hepatocyte transplantation may become a treatment option for patients before the development of adenomas.

Type III glycogen storage disease has clinical features similar to but less severe than those of type I disease. However, hepatic fibrosis leading to cirrhosis and adenomas is more common. Successful liver transplantation has been reported.[187,194]

Disorders of Lipid Metabolism

Familial Hypercholesterolemia

Type IIA familial hypercholesterolemia is an autosomal recessive disease characterized by markedly elevated serum low-density lipoprotein (LDL) cholesterol levels, early-onset atherosclerosis, multiple xanthomas, and left ventricular outflow obstruction.[195,196] As a consequence, premature death from myocardial infarction occurs in the second or third decade. The gene encoding for LDL receptors appears to be defective, so either LDL receptor expression is absent or the receptor itself is abnormal and unable to bind LDL.[197] As a consequence, LDL levels in plasma rise and total cholesterol may be as high as 700 to 1000 mg/dL in homozygotes. Disease in such patients is also refractory to treatment with drugs that lower plasma cholesterol because both bile-sequestrating agents and the 3-hydroxy-3-methylglutaryl coenzyme A reductase inhibitors (e.g., lovastatin) depend on induction of LDL receptors for their therapeutic effect.[198] In contrast, heterozygote carriers of the familial hypercholesterolemia gene are able to be successfully treated by medical means because their one normal gene allows adequate induction of LDL receptors.

The concept that liver replacement may be the therapy of choice was supported by evidence from animal studies in which it was shown that 50% to 70% of the body's total LDL receptors resided on hepatocytes.[199] Subsequently, in 1984 Starzl and coworkers reported successful simultaneous heart and liver transplantation in a 6-year-old girl with heart failure who had previously undergone two coronary bypass operations.[200] Within 10 weeks of transplantation, the girl's serum

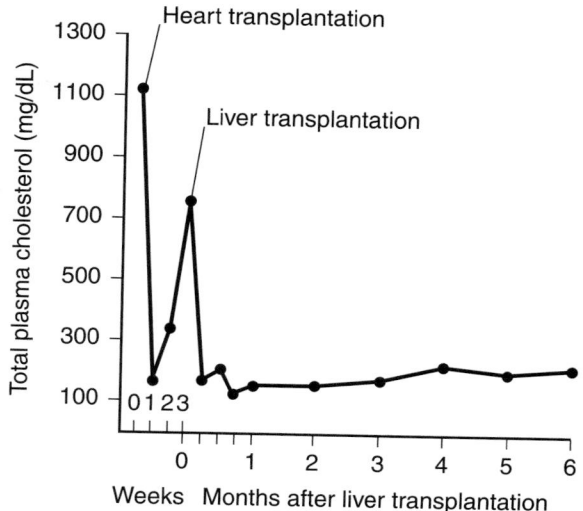

FIGURE 24–4

Familial hypercholesterolemia. Changes in total plasma cholesterol after liver transplantation for familial hypercholesterolemia type IIA are depicted. (Reproduced with permission from Valdivielso P, Escolar JL, Cuervas-Mons V, et al: Lipids and lipoprotein changes after heart and liver transplantation in a patient with homozygous familial hypercholesterolemia. Ann Intern Med 108:204-206, 1988.)

cholesterol levels had fallen from a pretransplant value of more than 1000 mg/dL to 270 mg/dL. One year after transplantations, the child's cholesterol levels were normalized with adjunctive lovastatin therapy.[201] The child remained asymptomatic with no evidence of recurrent coronary artery disease.

Other reports quickly followed of isolated liver transplantation with coronary bypass,[202] sequential heart and liver transplantation,[203] or combined heart-liver transplantation.[204,205] In all patients, LDL cholesterol, total cholesterol, and apolipoprotein B levels decreased. High-density lipoprotein (HDL) levels increased, and the LDL/HDL ratio was decreased.[204,206] The dramatic fall in serum cholesterol after sequential heart and liver transplantation is shown in Figure 24–4. Patients have had regression of their xanthomas and normal coronary angiograms. The majority have not required additional cholesterol-lowering medications or restrictive diets. Liver transplantation alone, before the onset of coronary artery disease, may be the optimal choice.[207,208] Some authors have advocated placement of a portocaval shunt early in life to at least partially reduce cholesterol levels, followed by liver transplantation.[209]

Although the liver in familial hypercholesterolemia is structurally normal, liver replacement provides normal numbers of LDL receptors so that serum cholesterol falls and the life-threatening complications of coronary artery disease are prevented. Two experimental models that might avoid the considerable risks of complete liver transplantation hold promise. The first is transplantation of allogeneic hepatocytes with normal expression of LDL. In the Watanabe rabbit model of heritable hyperlipidemia, intraperitoneal injection of normal hepatocytes lowered LDL cholesterol by 45% for 4 weeks.[210] Another approach is transfection of harvested hepatocytes with a recombinant retrovirus expressing a functional LDL receptor gene.[25] Again in the Watanabe rabbit model, this approach resulted in a temporary reduction in serum cholesterol. Unfortunately, in both these experimental models, cell death of the transplanted hepatocytes precluded a long-lasting effect, a problem that remains unsolved.

Lipoidoses

The lipoidoses are rare inherited defects in which abnormal lipid compounds are stored in multiple organs. In general, the enzymatic defects are widespread, and affected patients often suffer severe neurological impairment, with death occurring in infancy and childhood. Patients with milder clinical variants of two types of lipoidoses, Gaucher's disease, and Niemann-Pick disease, have undergone liver transplantation in an attempt to ameliorate the liver manifestations of the disease. In general, most reported patients have continued to show extrahepatic storage of the abnormal lipid.

Gaucher's Disease

Gaucher's disease is the most common lysosomal storage disease. This autosomally inherited deficiency of glucocerebrosidase results in the accumulation of glucosylceramide in the liposomes of reticuloendothelial cells distributed throughout the body.[211] The acute infantile forms are characterized by severe neurological impairment, as well as hepatosplenomegaly, osteolytic bone lesions, and pancytopenia. The adult variants of the disease (types 1 and 3) do not have significant neurological involvement, and the course of the disease is more insidious.[212]

The first patient who underwent liver transplantation for Gaucher's disease experienced portal hypertension secondary to hepatic fibrosis with subsequent life-threatening variceal hemorrhage. The patient was neurologically normal before transplantation, but died 2½ months afterward with intractable rejection.[213] At autopsy, the liver graft showed a threefold increase in glucosylceramide in comparison to controls, thus indicating only partial correction of the defect. A second patient also underwent transplantation for complications of cirrhosis, but 1 year later a liver biopsy showed a scattering of "wrinkled paper" Gaucher cells, although fibrosis had not yet been established.[214] A 61% increase in hepatic glucocerebrosidase activity 9 months after surgery was noted in a 42-year-old man.[215]

Recent evidence suggests that enzyme replacement therapy with alglucerase may be an effective, although very costly, treatment in some patients.[216]

However, 6 years of replacement therapy did not prevent severe hepatic fibrosis in a 15-year-old who underwent liver transplantation but subsequently died.[217]

Niemann-Pick Disease

This group of diseases has in common sphingomyelinase deficiency resulting in the deposition of sphingomyelin throughout the viscera and brain.[218] Inherited as an autosomal recessive trait, types IA and IIA are manifested in early childhood as severe progressive neurological damage, hepatosplenomegaly, and pulmonary infiltrates. Early death is inevitable. The subacute "adult" form has an onset in childhood and is characterized by hepatosplenomegaly progressing to cirrhosis.[219] Pulmonary involvement is also seen, but the CNS is spared.

Liver transplantation was reported in a woman with Niemann-Pick disease type B.[215] The sphingomyelin content in the liver graft was normal, but the peripheral blood leukocytes continued to show very low sphingomyelinase levels. Daloze and colleagues reported a boy with spasticity and myoclonus secondary to type A Niemann-Pick disease who received a liver transplant at 2 years of age.[220] For 2 years after transplantation the boy's neurological function improved, the lipid infiltrates in the retina regressed, and sphingomyelin did not reaccumulate in the graft. However, electron microscopic studies of the liver graft 540 days after transplantation continued to show the small lucent vacuoles described in Niemann-Pick disease (Fig. 24–5). He died of respiratory and infectious complications. At autopsy, several tissues, including the brain, showed accumulation of sphingomyelin.

Transplantation was also attempted for a variant of Niemann-Pick syndrome described as a neurovisceral storage disease characterized by sea-blue histiocytes in the bone marrow.[221] Liver cirrhosis and severe neurological impairment had occurred by 6 years of age, when the liver transplant was performed. An incidental HCC was found in the excised liver. After an initial period of stabilization, the patient continued to show progressive neurological deterioration, and Kupffer cells within the liver graft again reaccumulated the ceroid storage material.[222]

Wolman's Disease

Wolman's disease[223] is the severe infantile form of lysosomal acid lipase deficiency. Inherited absence of this enzyme results in the accumulation of lipids within lysosomes in the intestinal mucosa, vascular endothelium,

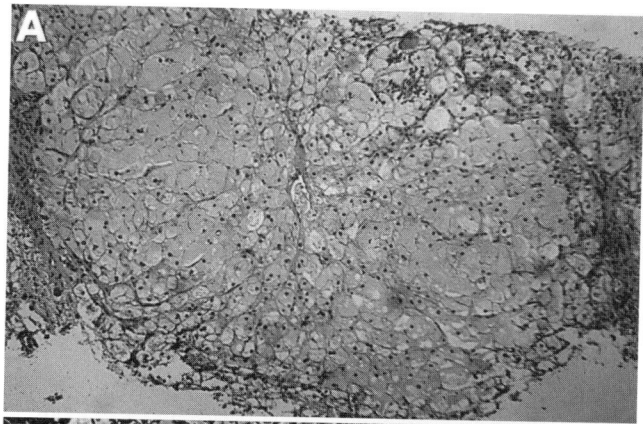

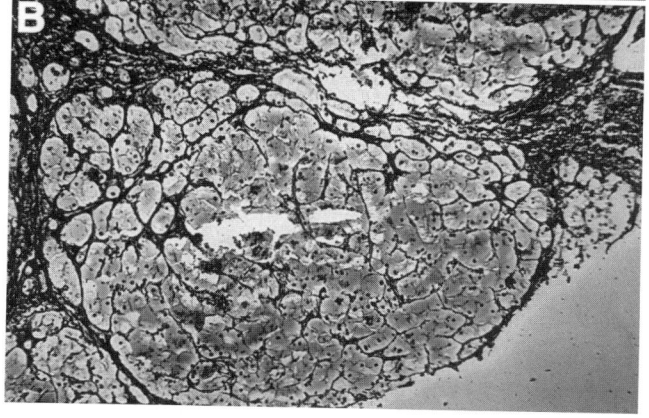

FIGURE 24–5

Niemann-Pick disease: electron micrographs of the liver before (**A**) and after (**B**) liver transplantation. The numerous large electron-lucent membrane-bound vacuoles seen before transplantation are no longer visible, but small storage vacuoles are seen in the graft 540 days after transplantation. (From Daloze P, Delvin EE, Florieux FA, et al: Replacement therapy for inherited enzyme deficiency: Liver orthotopic transplantation in Niemann-Pick disease type A. Am J Med Genet 1:229-239, 1977.)

lymph nodes, spleen, leukocytes, and bone marrow. Infants present with vomiting and diarrhea, abdominal distention, and marked hepatosplenomegaly. The diagnostic tip-off is bilateral adrenal calcification. Infants seldom survive beyond the first year. The condition may be amenable to future therapies with combined bone marrow and liver transplantation.[224] Research into these possibilities has been aided by the recent identification of an animal model resembling the human disease.

Cholesterol Ester Storage Disease

Cholesterol ester storage disease[223] is the mild form of acid lipase deficiency and typically occurs in adolescence or adulthood. In a few cases, accumulation of cholesteryl esters within hepatocytes has resulted in progressive fibrosis and portal hypertension. Liver transplantation has been successful in patients with life-threatening variceal bleeding but minimal extrahepatic involvement.[225,226]

Disorders of Bilirubin Metabolism

The hallmark of Crigler-Najjar syndrome, first described in 1952, is severe nonhemolytic unconjugated hyperbilirubinemia, usually beginning in the newborn period. The autosomal, recessively inherited enzyme defect lies within the group of uridine diphosphate glucuronyltransferases (UDPGTs), which conjugate bilirubin within the hepatocyte. Mutations in the *UGT1* gene complex encoding the defective enzyme have been identified and may facilitate prenatal diagnosis.[227] Two forms of the syndrome exist with quite different prognoses. In type I, UDPGT activity is undetectable, the profound hyperbilirubinemia is unresponsive to phenobarbital therapy, and without treatment kernicterus develops, which is inevitably fatal.[228] In type II Crigler-Najjar syndrome, some UDPGT activity is preserved and can be successfully induced by phenobarbital, thereby allowing successful medical management of these patients. Bilirubin levels fall to less than 4 mg/dL, and any long-term CNS sequelae are completely avoided.[229]

The mainstay of early therapy for type I Crigler-Najjar syndrome is phototherapy. With exposure to high-intensity irradiation, frequently for more than 12 hours per day, the total bilirubin level can initially be maintained at less than 20 mg/dL and the development of kernicterus averted.[230,231] However, intense long-term phototherapy, during which the infant's eyes are patched and activities are curtailed, is difficult to continue in an active toddler. A further problem is that as the child grows, subcutaneous tissue increases and surface area decreases, and as a result, phototherapy becomes less effective. Although it is not clearly established at what level of unconjugated bilirubin kernicterus develops, most experts recommend that total bilirubin not exceed 20 to 25 mg/dL in an older infant.[232] Of concern is that the devastating consequences of kernicterus have been noted to develop unpredictably.[233] Classically occurring in the neonatal period, a second incidence peak of kernicterus also occurs in puberty. Bilirubin-lowering medications such as tin protoporphyrin and oral calcium phosphate,[234] which bind unconjugated bilirubin, may have some benefit but are still under investigation.[235,236]

Although anatomic liver disease is mild and usually limited to elevated intracellular bilirubin with canalicular bile stasis, liver transplantation can be expected to cure type I Crigler-Najjar syndrome by replacing the UDPGT-deficient hepatocytes with normal cells. Kaufman and coauthors reported the first patient with type I Crigler-Najjar syndrome to undergo transplantation.[237] A permanent and rapid fall in total bilirubin occurred, and the patient thrived (Fig. 24–6). This experience was soon confirmed by others,[238,239] and at present, liver transplantation remains the only

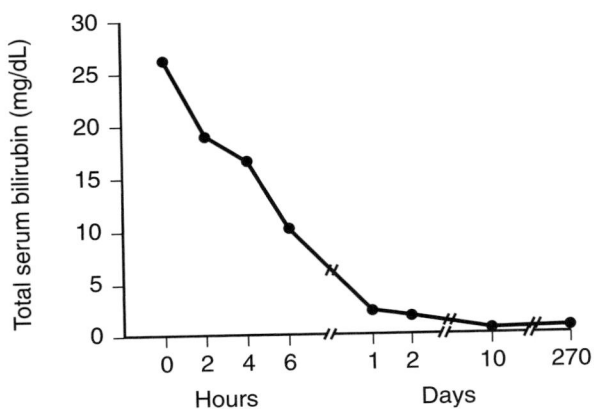

FIGURE 24–6

Crigler-Najjar syndrome: fall in serum bilirubin in a 3-year-old with Crigler-Najjar syndrome during and after liver transplantation. Hours 0 and 6 indicate the start and completion of surgery. Later lines represent postoperative days. (From Kaufman SS, Wood RP, Shaw BW, et al: Orthotopic liver transplantation for type I Crigler-Najjar syndrome. Hepatology 6:1259-1262, 1986.)

therapeutic option for these children once phototherapy becomes ineffective or impractical.[232] If liver transplantation is delayed beyond midchildhood, the risk of neurological damage increases.[232] In a report of 57 patients from the Crigler-Najjar world registry, brain damage had already occurred in 26%. Thirty-seven percent had received a liver transplant at an average age of 9.1 years, but of these patients a third already had neurological impairment. The children without neurological impairment were transplanted at a mean of 5.9 years as compared with a significantly higher mean age of 14.3 years in children transplanted with already-evident CNS damage.[234] In a single-center experience, six children underwent liver transplantation at a mean age of 52.5 months. All children survived with normal bilirubin levels, and all but one child transplanted at 8 years of age are developmentally normal.[240]

Particular attention should be paid to the anesthetic and perioperative care of children with Crigler-Najjar syndrome who are undergoing liver transplantation. Prager and colleagues outlined the drugs and metabolic conditions that may acutely elevate unconjugated bilirubin, displace bilirubin from albumin, or precipitate kernicterus. Phototherapy may be required until the transplanted liver is functioning sufficiently to conjugate the increased bilirubin load.[241]

Auxiliary partial orthotopic liver transplantation, although presenting technical challenges, is a procedure ideally suited to patients with Crigler-Najjar syndrome inasmuch as it has been shown in Gunn rats that only about 1% to 2% of the normal hepatocyte mass is needed for bilirubin conjugation.[20] In auxiliary transplantation, it was shown that a donor liver mass of 12% to 23% of the whole organ normalized serum bilirubin.[242] The advantage of the procedure is that the native liver remains in place should the graft fail. The King's College Hospital has reported a series of seven children who underwent this procedure. Median serum bilirubin levels were 50 and 23 μmol/L at 5 and 23 days, respectively, after auxiliary transplantation. Interestingly, rejection episodes were characterized by unconjugated hyperbilirubinemia as opposed to the usual conjugated hyperbilirubinemia typical of rejection.[243]

Type I Crigler-Najjar syndrome, in which the enzyme defect is localized in an architecturally nearly normal liver, would also be an ideal target disease for hepatocyte transplantation and gene therapy. The UDPGT-deficient Gunn rat, which is a model of the human syndrome, has allowed experimentation in these concepts.[244,245] Ex vivo gene therapy, in which genetically altered hepatocytes are transplanted into the liver, and in vivo gene transfer using recombinant adenovirus- or simian virus–based vectors have had reported success.[245] Both these modalities have been successful in lowering total bilirubin. These alternative therapies, if successful in humans, could avoid the significant risk associated with total-liver replacement.

Cystic Fibrosis

Cystic fibrosis, which has an estimated incidence of 1 in 2000 live births in the white population, is one of the most common inherited lethal diseases.[246] In 1989, the abnormal gene, the cystic fibrosis transmembrane conductance regulator (CFTR), was localized to the long arm of chromosome 7.[247] Now, more than 600 mutations have been described. The most common mutation in white populations is the ΔF508 mutation, which accounts for about 70% of CF alleles. About 2% to 15% of CF alleles account for 15 to 20 other mutations. CF mutation analysis, its relevance in different ethnic populations, and particularly its use in prenatal diagnosis are central topics in the unfolding understanding of this disease.[248,249]

Clinical Features

Cystic fibrosis is characterized by thick viscous secretions causing obstruction in the pancreas, lungs, liver, intestine and vas deferens.[250] In normal individuals, the chloride ion transporter gene allows chloride channels in cell membranes at the luminal surface to open, thereby facilitating passive transport of chloride and water. In patients with cystic fibrosis, the defective opening of chloride channels results in diminished chloride and water excretion.[251] Therefore, secretions become viscid and eventually obstructive.

In early childhood, chronic pulmonary infections and pancreatic insufficiency are the predominant manifestations. Previously, cystic fibrosis was usually fatal in childhood. Now, with improved antimicrobial drugs and nutritional support, the life expectancy of patients with cystic fibrosis is commonly extended into the third and even fourth decades of life. Therefore, the liver disease associated with cystic fibrosis, which typically becomes manifested in adolescence, is now more frequently encountered. Cirrhosis occurs in about 20% of older children, with portal hypertension developing in 2%.[252] The liver disease is often clinically silent, with nearly normal bilirubin and transaminase levels, and is diagnosed only with the onset of variceal bleeding. The characteristic histological appearance of the liver is nodular biliary cirrhosis with pathognomonic eosinophilic concretions in the small bile ducts.[246,253]

More unusual is the development of liver disease in infants with cystic fibrosis. In the largest reported experience, 12 infants, two thirds of whom were boys, were referred at a median age of 6.5 weeks. Conjugated hyperbilirubinemia was the initial finding in 11 infants and hypoalbuminemia in 1 other. Of these patients, all but one resolved the cholestasis without evidence of chronic liver disease at a median follow-up of 42 months. The long-term outcome is not yet evident.

Liver Transplantation

Shunt procedures have been the most often used surgical therapy for intractable variceal bleeding, but they are associated with life-threatening pulmonary and liver decompensation. Although they may delay the need for liver transplantation, the risk is that pulmonary disease will progress and prevent later transplantation.[254] The reluctance to perform liver transplantation in children with cystic fibrosis and established pulmonary disease is well founded and borne out by experience.[255] The first concern is the probable detrimental effect of immunosuppression on chronic pulmonary infection and the additional risk of systemic spread. Second, pancreatic insufficiency may cause impaired absorption of immunosuppressants and ongoing nutritional compromise. Third, although liver transplantation palliates the liver complications, it would not be expected to have an impact on other systems involved, particularly lung disease, which may eventually be life-threatening. However, in selected patients with mild to moderate pulmonary disease, some of these obstacles have been overcome, as demonstrated by the good survival rates and improved quality of life in children with cystic fibrosis who undergo liver transplantation.[256,257] Several authors[258,259] stress that the best results are obtained in younger children with relatively less severe manifestations of both their liver and lung disease. In one center's experience of 10 children, three of the four deaths were related to pulmonary infection, and all nonsurvivors were less than the 5th percentile for height and weight at transplantation.[259] Colonization

with *Aspergillus* was not associated with morbidity or mortality. It should be noted that the recipient bile duct still produces viscid bile, and cholestasis from inspissated bile in the recipient duct has been reported.[255] In a survey of transplant centers, 33 cystic fibrosis patients who underwent liver transplantation had an actuarial 5-year survival rate of 62%. Of concern is that *Pseudomonas* infection contributed to 5 of 11 deaths.[260]

Combined liver-lung transplantation (with or without the heart) either simultaneously or sequentially has been attempted with mixed results. A 70% actuarial 1-year survival rate was reported by one center,[250] another center reported one death in seven patients receiving combined transplants,[261] and in another experience, four of five patients died within 2 months.[258] Successful liver and intestinal transplantation was performed in a 7-month-old boy with extensive small bowel necrosis as a result of meconium ileus in the newborn period.[262] The greatest hope for better management of this disease lies not in transplantation but in the rapidly advancing area of gene therapy. Careful patient selection must be ensured when considering liver or combined liver-lung transplantation as a therapeutic option for this disease.

Hyperoxaluria Type 1

Primary hyperoxaluria type 1 is an autosomal recessive disease of oxalate overproduction that results in diffuse oxalate deposition, particularly prominent in the kidneys, bone, and heart.[263] Usually, kidney failure is the ultimate cause of death. However, kidney transplantation is not curative because the most commonly defective enzyme, alanine-glyoxylate aminotransferase, the gene for which is located on chromosome 2q37.5,[264] is specific to the peroxisomes of hepatocytes.[265] Medical therapy includes pyridoxine, high fluid intake in those not yet in renal failure, and crystallization inhibitors. Despite these treatments, end-stage renal failure occurs in 50% of children by 15 years of age, and the overall mortality has been estimated at 30%.[266]

Liver and Kidney Transplantation

Early in the consideration of transplant options for patients with primary hyperoxaluria, a considerable experience was reported for kidney transplantation alone. In some series, early renal allograft survival was superior to that in combined liver-kidney transplantation, but as would be expected from current knowledge of the enzyme defect site, kidney transplantation alone has repeatedly been proved to not prevent recurrent renal failure.[266,267] From registry data at 8 years after kidney-only transplantation, the kidney death–censored graft survival rate was 76% in patients receiving a liver-kidney transplant versus 48% for a kidney-alone transplant.[268] Kidney-alone transplantation can be considered only for pyridoxine-responsive type 1 disease or the less severe type 2 disease. In type 2 hyperoxaluria, the deficiency in glyoxylate reductase is not confined to the liver, and it is still uncertain whether liver replacement will correct the metabolic defect.[267]

Combined liver-kidney transplantation is the treatment of choice in hyperoxaluria when kidney failure has occurred or is imminent. This strategy was first attempted by Watts and colleagues in 1987.[269] Although the patient ultimately died of infectious complications, serum oxalate levels fell soon after transplantation. After this report, the successful outcome of combined liver-kidney transplantation, including that for the severe infantile form of hyperoxaluria,[270] has effected a cure for this disease.[270-274] A key principle is aggressive medical management before and after transplantation to decrease systemic oxalate concentrations.

In a large single-center experience of 36 children with primary hyperoxaluria type 1, combined liver-kidney transplantation was performed in 9 and preemptive liver-alone transplantation in 3. Renal function has improved to a mean GFR of 86 mL/min/1.73 m^2, but all three children with a liver-only transplant have oxalate deposits remaining in the kidney. This center's experience also emphasized the significant mortality associated with this disease without transplantation. Of 23 nontransplanted children, 9 have died of systemic complications of oxalosis, and 14 are alive, including 2 who are listed for transplantation.[275]

The debate continues regarding whether preemptive liver transplantation alone is justified before renal impairment becomes important. The clinical course of primary hyperoxaluria may be highly variable, with some children presenting in renal failure in infancy, whereas in its mildest forms, renal stones in adults may be the only manifestation. Even siblings with the same genotype may have widely varying clinical progression. In addition, projecting the rate of disease progression in some patients is speculative at best. Clearly, the risks of liver transplantation and long-term immunosuppression must be weighed carefully in a child with near-normal renal function whose evolution of disease may be quite slow.[276] In a series of four children undergoing preemptive liver transplantation, the GFR ranged from 27 to 98 mL/min/1.73 m^2.[277] No further deterioration in renal function was seen in 3 to 5 years of follow-up. One justification for liver-alone transplantation is to prevent further systemic accumulation of oxalate in a patient for whom renal transplantation is planned in the future, but organ availability is a problem.[278] However, using two different donors negates the reported protective immunological effect that the liver graft appears to confer on a renal graft from the same donor.[279,280]

After successful liver-kidney transplantation, the usual strategy to ensure ongoing depletion of the accumulated oxalate load is to induce high daily urine output with fluid loading. In young children, fluid loading via a gastrostomy tube is required. Posttransplant hemodialysis is now used only rarely. Hyperoxaluria may continue for months after transplantation, and very large amounts of urinary oxalate can be measured (up to 10,500 μmol/24 hr in one case). This increased urinary oxalate load is due to mobilization and excretion of the large body stores of oxalate and not to decreased activity of alanine-glyoxylate aminotransferase in the liver graft.[267,281] As the total-body oxalate load decreases, gradual radiological and histological improvement in serum oxalate osteoarthropathy is seen (Fig. 24–7).[274,282] Serial bone mineral density studies are useful to track the improvement in oxalate-associated bone disease after transplantation.[283] Also reported is reversal of oxalate-associated cardiomyopathy.[284]

In the severe infantile form of the disease, the extrarenal systemic complications of oxalate deposition may be particularly devastating. Deposition of oxalate in the bones results in multiple fractures, severe deformity, and debilitating chronic pain. Oxalate in the myocardium and pericardium can cause life-threatening heart failure. Compounded with the need for dialysis—not only for renal failure but also to continue to decrease the total-body oxalate load—these infants are often chronically ill and malnourished and have increased susceptibility to infection. The challenge of achieving early combined liver-kidney transplantation is to find appropriately sized organs for these often very small children. A kidney combined with a partial-liver graft from a larger child or teenager offers one of the best scenarios for success. Living donor transplantation—using one donor—has been reported[285] but carries with it increased risk for the donor and possible compromise in oxalate metabolism if the donor is a heterozygote (parent or sibling) for the disease. Success in four of six young children after combined liver-kidney, liver first followed by kidney, or isolated liver transplantation has been reported.[286]

Recommendations for liver or kidney transplantation or a combination have emerged from the European experience. Watts and colleagues[287] suggest that (1) when the GFR is less than 25 mL/min/1.73 m^2, combined liver-kidney transplantation is the treatment of choice; (2) isolated liver transplantation should be considered if the GFR is between 25 and 60 mL/min/1.73 m^2 and the disease is following an aggressive course; (3) avoidance of prolonged dialysis is important to prevent the necessity of excreting a large systemic oxalate load after transplantation, which might impair kidney graft function[288]; and (4) if liver transplantation is to be considered, the diagnosis must be confirmed by

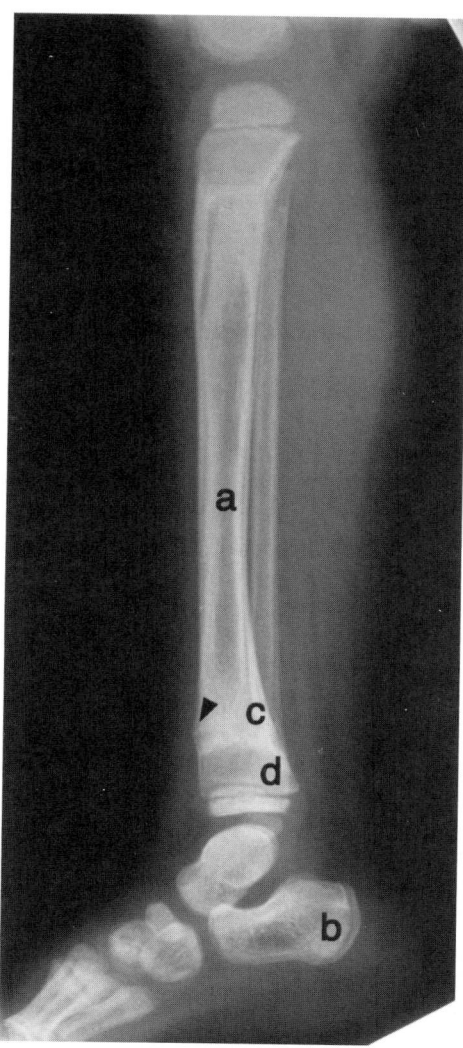

FIGURE 24–7

Primary hyperoxaluria. A radiograph of the lower extremity shows resolving bone disease after intensive dialysis followed by combined liver-kidney transplantation. Note the periosteal thickening with new bone (a), bone-within-a-bone appearance (b), and the previous hyperdense metaphysis (c) with new hypodense regions of bone growth (d). There is also an old fracture site at the metaphysis (*arrowhead*). (From McDiarmid SV: The liver and metabolic disease of childhood. Liver Transpl Surg 4:S34-S50, 1998.)

measuring alanine-glyoxylate aminotransferase activity in a liver biopsy specimen before transplantation.

Other Metabolic Diseases for Which Liver Transplantation Has Been Performed

Neonatal Iron Storage Disease

In neonatal iron storage disease (neonatal hemochromatosis),[289,290] severe liver insufficiency may be evident at birth or in the first weeks of life, thus suggesting that the process begins in utero.[291,292] Infants at risk are often severely affected with hydrops, coagulopathy, hypoalbuminemia, and kidney and liver failure. Progressive and severe cholestasis is usual with only a slight transaminitis. The histological findings in the liver are nonspecific and consist of diffuse fibrosis, loss of normal architecture, bile duct proliferation, and sometimes giant cell transformation. Death usually occurs within the first weeks or months of life.

Both sporadic and inherited cases have been described. The underlying defect remains unknown, although increased iron stores in other organs have been noted.[291] The diagnosis is made by excluding other causes of fulminant cholestatic liver failure in infants and by demonstrating elevated ferritin levels, increased transferrin saturation, and increased iron content, not only in the liver but in extrahepatic organs as well. In contrast to hereditary hemochromatosis (a disease of adults characterized by a specific genetic defect), the iron accumulation is predominantly within hepatocytes rather than reticuloendothelial cells. Magnetic resonance imaging with T2-weighted scans may be helpful to demonstrate the increased iron content in extrahepatic organs such as the pancreas, along with characteristic sparing of the spleen.[293]

Medical management with antioxidant and chelating agent "cocktails" has had variable success, with reports of amelioration of disease in some patients.[294] However, in a later experience of eight treated children, seven failed and died before liver transplantation could be attempted. Only one child stabilized sufficiently with therapy to allow later successful transplantation.[295]

Several authors have now described successful outcomes in infants who underwent liver replacement for neonatal iron storage disease.[8,296] Early recognition and aggressive management are necessary to support these severely ill infants through the first weeks of life until liver transplantation can be performed.[297] A single-center experience of eight children with neonatal iron storage disease reported that of five patients treated with antioxidant therapy, only two responded. Both responders started therapy by day 5 of life, had lower peak ferritin levels than nonresponders did, and did not require liver transplantation. Multisystem failure developed in two nonresponders, and liver transplantation could not be performed. A total of three children received transplants, with only one survivor. Of the remaining three children who were not treated with antioxidant therapy, two died before transplantation and one survived after transplantation.[298] This experience illustrates the high mortality associated with this disease and the variability in response to antioxidant therapy. Early diagnosis is essential to optimize the chance of response to therapy or to offer early transplantation before multisystem failure develops.

Careful follow-up of such children is needed because the metabolic basis of this disease is not yet known and it may represent the end stage of different disease processes beginning antenatally.[291]

Defects of Mitochondrial Function

In recent years there have been major advances in defining the key role that mitochondrial disorders play in the cause of pediatric liver disease of unknown cause. One of the first recognizable clinical entities was Reye's syndrome, which is characterized by previously well children presenting with hypoglycemia, vomiting, and lethargy progressing to coma, hyperammonemia, and liver failure.[299] Liver biopsy specimens showed microvesicular fat and structurally abnormal mitochondria. Soon after Reye's syndrome was described, several inherited diseases with similarities to Reye's syndrome were reported in which mitochondrial beta oxidation appeared to be the defect.[300-302] These diseases were the medium- and long-chain acyl coenzyme A dehydrogenase deficiencies. Frequently unmasked by fasting or infectious disease, these rare syndromes may be misdiagnosed as sudden infant death syndrome or Reye's syndrome. Infants may be comatose and in apparent noncholestatic liver failure.[303,304] Once the condition is diagnosed, these children can often be successfully managed by frequent high carbohydrate feedings and carnitine supplementation.

Mitochondrial function is essential to several metabolic pathways, including those requiring the key enzyme ATP synthase, which carries out oxidative phosphorylation and ATP synthesis. The mitochondrial matrix contains the enzymes of the tricarboxylic acid cycle, urea cycle, and fatty acid beta oxidation pathways. The inner mitochondrial membrane contains the electron transport chain, which is essential for mitochondrial respiration and provision of energy for adenosine phosphate synthesis. This diversity in mitochondrial function accounts for the many different metabolic diseases now attributed to mitochondrial disorders. The growing list can be divided into those in which the mitochondrial defect is the primary cause of the liver disorder and those in which there is an acquired mitochondrial injury mediated by toxins (e.g., cyanide), drugs (e.g., salicylic acid, valproic acid), or heavy metals (copper and iron overload). A complete list and discussion of the clinical manifestations and the site of the defect can be found in a comprehensive review by Sokal and Treem.[305]

It is now recognized that disorders of mitochondrial function may have a wide spectrum of manifestations—including both acute and chronic liver disease[306]—and should also be considered in the differential diagnosis of neonates with acute liver failure.[307]

However, mitochondrial disorders generally involve many other organs, particularly the nervous system and cardiac and skeletal muscle. Clinical involvement of the bone marrow, kidney, and colon has also been described. For this reason, few of the expanding list of diseases caused by mitochondrial defects will be amenable to a functional "cure" by liver transplantation.

The role of liver transplantation must be very carefully considered in children with suspected mitochondrial disease. Such evaluation is made even more difficult if the child presents in coma with evidence of fulminant liver failure without discernible cause. A good example is provided by the very similar features of Reye's syndrome, an acquired mitochondrial disorder (associated with varicella infection and salicylic acid ingestion), and the primary mitochondrial disorders of fatty acid oxidation (the medium- and long-chain acyl-CoA dehydrogenase deficiencies). In both conditions, the onset of coma is early, with severe hypoglycemia, hyperammonemia, and coagulopathy. On liver biopsy, the inflammation and necrosis are unimpressive, but diffuse microvesicular fat is characteristic. Cerebral edema is frequently severe and is most often the cause of death.[308] Liver transplantation is contraindicated because the mitochondrial dysfunction is diffuse, particularly that involving the CNS. With very aggressive medical therapy, many of these children—especially those with fatty acid oxidative defects—will survive without significant neurological impairment, although repeat episodes may occur with future catabolic stress.

In contrast, specific mitochondrial respiratory chain disorders (i.e., oxidative phosphorylation defects) have been successfully treated by liver transplantation, although selection of candidates remains problematic.[309] In a single-center study of five children with fulminant liver failure, a retrospective study of the explanted liver showed defects in the mitochondrial respiratory chain complexes I, III, and IV.[310] However, the clinical outcome after liver transplantation was variable, with two of the five children showing ongoing neurological impairment after transplantation that was fatal in one child. In a multicenter experience of 11 children with mitochondrial respiratory chain disorders, 6 died after liver transplantation, 3 of whom suffered further neurological injury after transplantation.[311] The key message from these experiences is that extrahepatic disease present before transplantation portends a poor outcome and should exclude children from consideration for liver transplantation—a point illustrated by the successful transplantation of a child with mitochondrial respiratory chain deficiency whose only manifestation of disease was end-stage liver disease.[312]

One of the problems in establishing the liver transplantation candidacy of a child in rapidly progressive acute liver failure is the difficulty in quickly establishing the diagnosis of a mitochondrial disorder. Readily available laboratory tests that are suggestive, but not diagnostic, are a persistent serum lactate level higher than 2.5 nM, an increased lactate-pyruvate ratio in plasma and cerebrospinal fluid (>20:1 mol/mol), a β-OH butyrate–acetoacetate ratio greater than 2:1 mol/mol, and diffuse microsteatosis on liver biopsy.[306] Children with chronic liver disease may have a history of vomiting, hypotonia, developmental delay, and hypoglycemia. Liver histology is more variable and includes steatosis, cholestasis, and cirrhosis. Electron microscopy studies often show the structural abnormalities of the mitochondria. Definitive diagnosis requires sophisticated biochemical studies of mitochondrial respiration on fresh liver or muscle tissue.

Mucopolysaccharidoses

Severe hepatomegaly progressing to fibrosis is a frequent finding in the spectrum of disease characterized by lysosomal storage of incompletely degraded mucopolysaccharides. The inherited enzyme deficiency is widespread in somatic cells. Affected children generally have varying degrees of progressive mental retardation, skeletal deformity, dwarfing, corneal clouding, and coarse facial features.[313] Liver transplantation was performed in one child with type IVB Sanfilippo syndrome (W. Berquist, M.D., personal communication, September 1986) in an attempt to treat the variceal bleeding associated with progressive liver fibrosis that is characteristic of many of the variants.[314] Although the procedure extended the child's life, gradual mental retardation continued, though at perhaps a slower rate than expected. The child subsequently died of chronic hepatitis C.

Bone marrow transplantation, performed before liver compromise occurs, appears to be a better treatment option, with resolution or improvement in some of the clinical features.[315-318] Resnick and coauthors reported that bone marrow engraftment was associated with a decrease in liver size and disappearance of lysosomal storage material in the donor-derived Kupffer cells that repopulate the liver, as well as in the hepatocytes themselves. Hepatocyte clearance was not achieved in two other cases.[16]

In conclusion, liver transplantation offers a unique opportunity to replace a metabolically defective organ and reverse the certain fatal outcome of several metabolic diseases, most notably α_1-antitrypsin deficiency, hereditary tyrosinemia, and Wilson's disease. Judgment must be exercised in the selection of patients and timing of liver replacement, particularly for metabolic diseases with significant extrahepatic manifestations. The future holds the promise that for at least some of these conditions, hepatocyte or stem cell transplantation or gene therapy will make liver transplantation obsolete.

Acknowledgment

The author wishes to thank Dinora Duarte for her invaluable expertise in preparation of this work.

References

1. Burdelski M, Rodeck B, Latta A, et al: Treatment of inherited metabolic disorders by liver transplantation. Inherit Metab Dis 14:604-618, 1991.
2. Mowat AP: Liver disorders in children: The indications for liver replacement in parenchymal and metabolic diseases. Transplant Proc 19:3236-3241, 1987.
3. Starzl TE, Demetris AJ, Van Thiel DH: Liver transplantation. (First of two parts). N Engl J Med 321:1014-1022, 1989.
4. Groth CG, Ringden O: Transplantation in relation to the treatment of inherited disease. Transplantation 38:319-327, 1984.
5. Shaw B, Wood RP, Kaufman SS, et al: Liver transplantation therapy for children: Part 1. J Pediatr Gastroenterol Nutr 7:157-166, 1988.
6. Starzl TE, Demetris AJ, Van Thiel DH: Liver transplantation. (Second of two parts). N Engl J Med 321:1092-1099, 1989.
7. Zitelli BJ, Malatack JJ, Gartner C Jr, et al: Orthotopic liver transplantation in children with hepatic-based metabolic disease. Transplant Proc 15:1284-1287, 1983.
8. Esquivel CO, Marino IR, Fioravanti V, Van Thiel DH: Liver transplantation for metabolic disease of the liver. Gastroenterology 17:167-175, 1988.
9. Esquivel CO, Iwatsuki S, Gordon R, et al: Indications for pediatric liver transplantation. J Pediatr 111:1039-1045, 1987.
10. Busuttil RW, Seu P, Millis JM, et al: Liver transplantation in children. Ann Surg 213:48-57, 1991.
11. Sho M, Sandner SE, Najafian N, et al: New insights into the interactions between T-cell costimulatory blockade and conventional immunosuppressive drugs. Ann Surg 236:667-675, 2002.
12. Kayler LK, Merion RM, Lee S, et al: Long-term survival after liver transplantation in children with metabolic disorders. Pediatr Transplant 6:295-300, 2002.
13. Peeters PM, Sieders E, de Jong KP, et al: Comparison of outcome after pediatric liver transplantation for metabolic diseases and biliary atresia. Eur J Pediatr Surg 11:28-35, 2001.
14. Burdelski M: Liver transplantation in metabolic diseases: Current status. Pediatr Transplant 6:361-363, 2002.
15. Tanguay RM, Valet JP, Lescault A, et al: Different molecular basis for fumarylacetoacetate hydrolase deficiency in the two clinical forms of hereditary tyrosinemia (type I). Am J Hum Genet 47:308-316, 1990.
16. Resnick JM, Krivit W, Snover DC, et al: Pathology of the liver in mucopolysaccharidosis: Light and electron microscopic assessment before and after bone marrow transplantation. Bone Marrow Transplant 10:273-280, 1992.
17. A-Kader HH, Balistreri WF: Nontransplant alternatives for the treatment of patients with metabolic disease. Semin Liver Dis 18:255-261, 1998.
18. Balistreri WF: Nontransplant options for the treatment of metabolic liver disease: Saving livers while saving lives. Hepatology 19:782-787, 1994.
19. Bumgardner GL, Fasola C, Sutherland DE: Prospects for hepatocyte transplantation. Hepatology 8:1158-1161, 1988.
20. Matas AJ, Sutherland DER, Steffes MW, et al: Hepatocellular transplantation for metabolic deficiencies: Decrease of plasma bilirubin in Gunn rats. Science 192:892-894, 1976.

21. Vroemen JP, Buurman WA, Heirwegh KP, et al: Hepatocyte transplantation for enzyme deficiency disease in congenic rats. Transplantation 42:130-135, 1986.

22. Fox IJ, Chowdhury JR, Kaufman SS, et al: Treatment of the Crigler-Najjar syndrome type I with hepatocyte transplantation. N Engl J Med 338:1422-1426, 1998.

23. Horslen SP, McCowan TC, Goertzen TC, et al: Isolated hepatocyte transplantation in an infant with a severe urea cycle disorder. Pediatrics 111:1262-1267, 2003.

24. Kay MA, Ponder KP, Woo SLC: Human gene therapy: Present and future. Breast Cancer Res Treat 21:83-93, 1992.

25. Wilson JM, Chowdhury NR, Grossman M, et al: Temporary amelioration of hyperlipidemia in low density lipoprotein receptor–deficient rabbits transplanted with genetically modified hepatocytes. Proc Natl Acad Sci U S A 87:8437-8441, 1990.

26. Wood PA, Herman GE, Chao CYJ, et al: Retrovirus-mediated gene transfer of argininosuccinate synthetase into cultured rodent cells and human citrullinemic fibroblasts. Cold Spring Harb Symp Quart Biol 51:1027-1034, 1986.

27. Tada K, Roy-Chowdhury N, Prasad V, et al: Long-term amelioration of bilirubin glucuronidation defect in Gunn rats by transplanting genetically modified immortalized autologous hepatocytes. Cell Transplant 7:607-616, 1998.

28. Overturf K, Al-Dhalimy M, Tanguay R, et al: Hepatocytes corrected by gene therapy are selected in vivo in a murine model of hereditary tyrosinaemia type 1. Nat Genet 12:266-273, 1996.

29. Grompe M: Liver repopulation for the treatment of metabolic disease. J Inherit Metab Dis 24:231-244, 2001.

30. Rosenthal N: Prometheus's vulture and the stem-cell promise. N Engl J Med 349:267-274, 2003.

31. Hochedlinger K, Jaenisch R: Nuclear transplantation, embryonic stem cells, and the potential for cell therapy. N Engl J Med 349:275-286, 2003.

32. Davis ID, Burke B, Freese D, et al: The pathologic spectrum of the nephropathy associated with alpha 1-antitrypsin deficiency. Hum Pathol 23:57-62, 1992.

33. Brantly M, Nukins T, Crystal RG: Molecular basis of alpha-1-antitrypsin deficiency. Am J Med 84:13-31, 1988.

34. Vennarecci G, Gunson BK, Ismail T, et al: Transplantation for end-stage liver disease related to alpha 1 antitrypsin. Transplantation 61:1488-1495, 1996.

35. Hussain M, Mieli-Vergani G, Mowat AP: Alpha-1-antitrypsin deficiency and liver disease: Clinical presentation, diagnosis and treatment. Inherit Metab Dis 14:497-511, 1991.

36. Eriksson S: Studies in alpha-1-antitrypsin deficiency. Acta Med Scand 432:1-85, 1965.

37. Birrer P, McElvaney NG, Chang-Stroman LM, Crystal RG: Alpha-1-antitrypsin deficiency and liver disease. Inherit Metab Dis 14:512-525, 1991.

38. Sharp HL: Alpha-1-antitrypsin: An ignored protein in understanding liver disease. Semin Liver Dis 2:314-328, 1982.

39. Buist AS: Alpha-1-antitrypsin deficiency in lung and liver disease. Hosp Pract 24:51-59, 1989.

40. Hodges JR, Millward-Sadler GH, Barbatis C, Wright R: Heterozygous MZ alpha-1-antitrypsin deficiency in adults with chronic active hepatitis and cryptogenic cirrhosis. N Engl J Med 304:557-560, 1982.

41. Freier E, Sharp HL, Bridges RA: Alpha-1-antitrypsin deficiency associated with familial infantile liver disease. Clin Chem 14:782, 1968.

42. Sharp HL, Bridges RA, Krivit W, Freier E: Cirrhosis associated with alpha-1-antitrypsin deficiency: A previously unrecognized disorder. J Lab Clin Med 73:934-939, 1969.

43. Sveger T: Alpha-1-antitrypsin deficiency in early childhood. Pediatrics 62:22-25, 1978.

44. Sveger T: The natural history of liver disease in alpha-1-antitrypsin deficiency in children. Acta Paediatr Scand 77:847-851, 1988.

45. Sveger T: Liver disease in alpha-1-antitrypsin deficiency detected by screening of 200,000 infants. N Engl J Med 294:1316-1321, 1976.

46. Volpert D, Molleston JP, Perlmutter DH: Alpha 1-antitrypsin deficiency–associated liver disease progresses slowly in some children. J Pediatr Gastroenterol Nutr 31:504-505, 2000.

47. Ghishan FK, Gray GF, Greene HL: Alpha-1-antitrypsin deficiency presenting with ascites and cirrhosis in the neonatal period. Gastroenterology 85:435-438, 1983.

48. Ghishan FK, Greene HL: Liver disease in children with PiZZ alpha-1-antitrypsin deficiency. Hepatology 8:307-310, 1988.

49. Nemeth A, Strandvik B: Liver disease in children with alpha-1-antitrypsin deficiency without neonatal cholestasis. Acta Paediatr Scand 71:1001-1005, 1982.

50. Nemeth A, Strandvik B: Natural history of children with alpha-1-antitrypsin deficiency and neonatal cholestasis. Acta Paediatr Scand 71:993-999, 1982.

51. Ibarguen E, Gross CR, Savik SK, Sharp HL: Liver disease in alpha-1-antitrypsin deficiency: Prognostic indicators. J Pediatr 117:864-870, 1990.

52. Bhan AK, Grand RJ, Colten HR, Alper CA: Liver in alpha-1-antitrypsin deficiency: Morphologic observations and in vitro synthesis of alpha-1-antitrypsin. Pediatr Res 10:40-45, 1976.

53. Hood JM, Koep LJ, Peters RL, et al: Liver transplantation for advanced liver disease with alpha-1-antitrypsin deficiency. N Engl J Med 302:272-275, 1980.

54. Odievre M, Martin JP, Hadchouel M, et al: Alpha-1-antitrypsin deficiency and liver disease in children: Phenotypes, manifestations, and prognosis. Pediatrics 57:226-231, 1976.

55. Eriksson S, Hagerstrand I: Cirrhosis and malignant hepatoma in alpha-1-antitrypsin deficiency. Acta Med Scand 195:451-458, 1974.

56. Perlmutter DH: Liver injury in alpha 1-antitrypsin deficiency. Clin Liver Dis 4:387-408, 2000.

57. Hultcrantz R, Mengarelli S: Ultrastructural liver pathology in patients with minimal liver disease and alpha-1-antitrypsin deficiency: A comparison between heterozygous and homozygous patients. Hepatology 4:937-945, 1984.

58. Nemeth A, Strandvik B, Glaumann H: Alpha-1-antitrypsin deficiency and juvenile liver disease. Ultrastructural observations compared to light microscopy and routine liver tests. Virchows Arch B Cell Pathol 44:15-33, 1983.

59. Kozutami Y, Segal M, Normington K, et al: The presence of malfolded proteins in the endoplasmic reticulum signals the induction of glucose-regulated proteins. Nature 332:462-464, 1988.

60. Gadek JE, Fells GA, Holland PV, Crystal RG: Replacement therapy of alpha-1-antitrypsin deficiency. Reversal of protease-antiprotease imbalance within the alveolar structures of PiZ subjects. J Clin Invest 68:1158-1165, 1982.

61. Cohen AB: Unraveling the mysteries of alpha-1-antitrypsin deficiency. N Engl J Med 314:778-779, 1986.

62. Putnam CW, Porter KA, Peters RL, et al: Liver replacement for alpha-1-antitrypsin deficiency. Surgery 81:258-261, 1977.

63. Filipponi F, Soubrane O, Labrousse F, et al: Liver transplantation for end-stage liver disease associated with alpha-1-antitrypsin deficiency in children: Pretransplant natural history, timing and results of transplantation. J Hepatol 20:72-78, 1994.

64. Prachalias AA, Kalife M, Francavilla R, et al: Liver transplantation for alpha-1-antitrypsin deficiency in children. Transpl Int 13:207-210, 2000.

65. Francavilla R, Castellaneta SP, Hadzic N, et al: Prognosis of alpha-1-antitrypsin deficiency–related liver disease in the era of paediatric liver transplantation. J Hepatol 32:986-992, 2000.

66. Krowka MJ, Cortese DA: Pulmonary aspects of chronic liver disease and liver transplantation. Mayo Clin Proc 60:407-418, 1985.

67. Sang OK, Bender TM, Bowen A, et al: Plain radiographic, nuclear medicine and angiographic observations of hepatogenic pulmonary angiodysplasia. Pediatr Radiol 13:111-115, 1983.

68. McCloskey JJ, Schleien C, Schwarz K, et al: Severe hypoxemia and intrapulmonary shunting resulting from cirrhosis reversed by liver transplantation in a pediatric patient. J Pediatr 118:902-904, 1991.

69. Brems JJ, Hiatt JR, Klein AS, et al: Splenic artery aneurysm rupture following orthotopic liver transplantation. Transplantation 45:1136-1137, 1988.

70. Sternlieb I, Scheinberg IH: Wilson's disease. In Schaffner F, Sherlock S, Leevy CM (eds): The Liver and Its Diseases. New York, Intercontinental Book Corp, 1974, pp 328-336.

71. Riely CA: Wilson's disease. Pediatr Rev 5:217-222, 1984.

72. Marsden CD: Wilson's disease. Q J Med 65:959-966, 1987.

73. Sternlieb I: Perspectives on Wilson's disease. Hepatology 12:1234-1239, 1980.

74. Schilsky ML: Diagnosis and treatment of Wilson's disease. Pediatr Transplant 6:15-19, 2002.

75. Ting Y, Gitlin JD: Hepatic copper metabolism: Insights from genetic disease. Hepatology 37:1241-1247, 2003.

76. Sokol RJ, Devereaux M, Mierau GW, et al: Oxidant injury to hepatic mitochondrial lipids in rats with dietary copper overload. Modification by vitamin E deficiency. Gastroenterology 99:1061-1071, 1990.

77. Scott JP, Gollan JL, Samourian S, Sherlock S: Wilson's disease, presenting as chronic active hepatitis. Gastroenterology 74:645-651, 1978.

78. Wiebers DO, Hollenhorst RW, Goldstein NP: The ophthalmologic manifestations of Wilson's disease. Mayo Clin Proc 50:409-416, 1977.

79. Sternlieb I: Diagnosis of Wilson's disease. Gastroenterology 74:787-793, 1978.

80. Sternlieb I, Scheinberg IH: The role of radiocopper in the diagnosis of Wilson's disease. Gastroenterology 77:138-142, 1979.

81. McCullough AJ, Fleming CR, Thistle JL, et al: Diagnosis of Wilson's disease presenting as fulminant hepatic failure. Gastroenterology 84:161-167, 1983.

82. Shaver WA, Bhatt H, Combes B: Low serum alkaline phosphatase activity in Wilson's disease. Hepatology 6:859-863, 1986.

83. Berman DH, Leventhal RI, Gavaler JS, et al: Rapid clinical identification of fulminant Wilson's disease from other causes of fulminant hepatic failure using readily available laboratory tests. Hepatology 10:574, 1989.

84. Devictor D, Desplanques L, Debray D, et al: Emergency liver transplantation for fulminant liver failure in infants and children. Hepatology 16:1156-1162, 1992.

85. Deiss A, Lynch RE, Lee GR: Long-term therapy of Wilson's disease. Ann Intern Med 75:57-65, 1971.

86. Walshe JM: Penicillamine, a new oral therapy for Wilson's disease. Am J Med 21:487-495, 1956.

87. Walshe JM: Treatment of Wilson's disease with trientine (triethylene tetramine) dihydrochloride. Lancet 1:643-647, 1982.

88. Brewer GJ, Hedera P, Kluin KJ, et al: Treatment of Wilson disease with ammonium tetrathiomolybdate: III. Initial therapy in total of 55 neurologically affected patients and follow-up with zinc therapy. Arch Neurol 60:379-385, 2003.

89. Lipsky MA, Gollan JL: Treatment of Wilson's disease: In D-penicillamine we trust. What about zinc? Hepatology 7:593-595, 1987.

90. Hill GM, Brewer GJ, Prasad AS, et al: Treatment of Wilson's disease with zinc. I. Oral zinc therapy regimens. Hepatology 7:522-528, 1987.

91. Brewer GJ, Hill GM, Prasad AS, et al: Oral zinc therapy for Wilson's disease. Ann Intern Med 994:314-320, 1983.

92. Sternlieb I: Wilson's disease: Indications for liver transplants. Hepatology 4:15S-17S, 1984.

93. Nazer H, Ede RJ, Mowat AP, Williams R: Wilson's disease: Clinical presentation and use of prognostic index. Gut 27:1377-1381, 1986.

94. Dubois RS, Giles G, Rodgerson DO, et al: Orthotopic liver transplantation for Wilson's disease. Lancet 1:505-508, 1971.

95. Sokal RJ, Francis PD, Gold SH, et al: Orthotopic liver transplantation for acute fulminant Wilson's disease. J Pediatr 107:549-552, 1985.

96. Ho TA, Hamilton JW, Kalayoglu M, Belzer FO: Liver transplantation and Wilson's disease. Wisc Med J 87:14-15, 1988.

97. Emre S, Atillasoy EO, Ozdemir S, et al: Orthotopic liver transplantation for Wilson's disease. A single-center experience. Transplantation 72:1232-1236, 2001.

98. Eghtesad B, Nezakatgoo N, Geraci LC, et al: Liver transplantation for Wilson's disease: A single-center experience. Liver Transpl 5:467-474, 1999.

99. Rakela J, Kurtz SB, McCarthy JT, et al: Fulminant Wilson's disease treated with postdilution hemofiltration and orthotopic liver transplantation. Gastroenterology 90:2004-2007, 1986.

100. Pett S, Pelham A, Tizard J, et al: Pediatric liver transplantation: Cambridge/King's series, December 1983 to August 1986. Transplant Proc 19:3256-3260, 1987.

101. Groth CG, Dubois RS, Corman JL, et al: Metabolic effects of hepatic replacement in Wilson's disease. Transplant Proc 5:829-833, 1973.

102. Song HC, Ku WC, Chen CL: Disappearance of Kayser-Fleischer rings following liver transplantation. Transplant Proc 24:1483-1485, 1992.

103. Polson RJ, Rolles K, Calne RY, et al: Reversal of severe neurological manifestations of Wilson's disease following orthotopic liver transplantation. Q J Med 64:685-691, 1987.

104. Schilsky ML, Scheinberg IH, Sternlieb I: Liver transplantation for Wilson's disease: Indications and outcomes. Hepatology 19:583-587, 1994.

105. Sutcliffe RP, Maguire DD, Muiesan P, et al: Liver transplantation for Wilson's disease: Long-term results and quality-of-life assessment. Transplantation 15:1003-1006, 2003.

106. Bax RT, Hassler A, Luck W, et al: Cerebral manifestation of Wilson's disease successfully treated with liver transplantation. Neurology 51:863-865, 1998.

107. Komatsu H, Fujisawa T, Inui A, et al: Hepatic copper concentration in children undergoing living related liver transplantation due to Wilsonian fulminant hepatic failure. Clin Transplant 16:227-232, 2002.

108. Kobayashi S, Ochiai T, Hori S, et al: Copper metabolism after living donor liver transplantation for hepatic failure of Wilson's disease from a gene mutated donor. Hepatogastroenterology 48:1259-1261, 2001.

109. Yoshida Y, Tokusashi Y, Ogawa K: Intrahepatic transplantation of normal hepatocytes prevents Wilson's disease in Long-Evans cinnamon rats. Gastroenterology 111:1654-1660, 1996.

110. Phaneuf D, Labelle Y, Berube D, et al: Cloning and expression of the cDNA encoding human fumarylacetoacetate hydrolase, the enzyme deficient in hereditary tyrosinemia: Assignment of the gene to chromosome 15. Am J Hum Genet 48:525-535, 1991.

111. Ploos van Amstel JK, Bergman AJ, van Beurden EA, et al: Hereditary tyrosinemia type 1: Novel missense, nonsense and splice consensus mutations in the human fumarylacetoacetate hydrolase gene; variability of the genotype-phenotype relationship. Hum Genet 97:51-59, 1996.

112. Larochelle J, Mortezai A, Belanger M, et al: Experience with 37 infants with tyrosinemia. Can Med Assoc J 97:1051-1054, 1967.

113. De Braekeleer M, Larochelle J: Genetic epidemiology of hereditary tyrosinemia in Quebec and in Sanguenay-Lac-St-Jean. Am J Hum Genet 47:302-307, 1990.

114. Lindblad B, Lindstedt S, Steen G: On the enzymic defects in hereditary tyrosinemia. Proc Natl Acad Sci U S A 74:4641-4645, 1977.

115. Grenier A, Laberge C: A modified automated fluorometric method for tyrosine determination in blood spotted on

paper: A mass screening procedure for tyrosinemia. Clin Chim Acta 57:71-75, 1974.

116. Laberge C, Grenier A, Valet JP, Morissette J: Fumarylacetoacetase measurement as a mass-screening procedure for hereditary tyrosinemia type I. Am J Hum Genet 47:325-328, 1990.

117. Kvittengen EA: Hereditary tyrosinemia type 1—an overview. Scand J Clin Invest 46:27-34, 1986.

118. Russo P, O'Regan S: Visceral pathology of hereditary tyrosinemia type I. Am J Hum Genet 47:317-324, 1990.

119. Dehner LP, Snover DC, Sharp HL, et al: Hereditary tyrosinemia type I (chronic form): Pathologic findings in the liver. Hum Pathol 20:149-158, 1989.

120. Weinberg AG, Mize CE, Worthen HG: The occurrence of hepatoma in the chronic form of hereditary tyrosinemia. J Pediatr 88:434-438, 1976.

121. Mitchell G, Larochelle J, Lambert M, et al: Neurologic crises in hereditary tyrosinemia. N Engl J Med 322:432-437, 1990.

122. Rank JM, Pascual-Leone A, Payne W, et al: Hematin therapy for the neurologic crisis of tyrosinemia. J Pediatr 118:136-139, 1991.

123. Croffie JM, Gupta SK, Chong SK, Fitzgerald JF: Tyrosinemia type 1 should be suspected in infants with severe coagulopathy even in the absence of other signs of liver failure. Pediatrics 103:675-678, 1999.

124. Noble-Jamieson G, Jamieson N, Clayton P, et al: Neurological crisis in hereditary tyrosinaemia and complete reversal after liver transplantation. Arch Dis Child 70:544-545, 1994.

125. Roth KS, Carter BE, Higgins ES: Succinylacetone effects on renal tubular phosphate metabolism: A model for experimental renal Fanconi syndrome. Proc Soc Exp Biol Med 196:428-431, 1991.

126. Lindstedt S, Holme E, Lock EA, et al: Treatment of hereditary tyrosinaemia type I by inhibition of 4-hydroxyphenylpyruvate dioxygenase. Lancet 340:813-817, 1992.

127. Holme E, Lindstedt S: Nontransplant treatment of tyrosinemia. Clin Liver Dis 4:805-814, 2000.

128. Mohan N, Mckiernan P, Preece MA, et al: Indications and outcome of liver transplantation in tyrosinaemia type 1. Eur J Pediatr 158:S49-S54, 1999.

129. Fisch RO, McCabe ERB, Doeden D, et al: Homotransplantation of the liver in a patient with hepatoma in hereditary tyrosinemia. J Pediatr 93:592-596, 1978.

130. Starzl TE, Zitelli BJ, Shaw BW, et al: Changing concepts: Liver replacement for hereditary tyrosinemia and hepatoma. J Pediatr 106:604-606, 1985.

131. Manowski Z, Silver MM, Roberts EA, et al: Liver cell dysplasia and early liver transplantation in hereditary tyrosinemia. Mod Pathol 3:694-701, 1990.

132. Esquivel CO, Mieles L, Marino IR, et al: Liver transplantation for hereditary tyrosinemia in the presence of hepatocellular carcinoma. Transplant Proc 21:2445-2446, 1989.

133. Paradis KJG, Weber A, Seidman EG, et al: Liver transplantation for hereditary tyrosinemia: The Quebec experience. Am J Hum Genet 47:338-342, 1991.

134. Freese D, Tuchman M, Schwarzenberg SJ, et al: Early liver transplantation is indicated for tyrosinemia type I. J Pediatr Gastroenterol Nutr 13:10-15, 1991.

135. Flye MW, Riely CA, Hainline BE, et al: The effects of early treatment of hereditary tryosinemia type I in infancy by orthotopic liver transplantation. Transplantation 49:916-921, 1990.

136. Sokal E, Bustos R, Van Hoof F, Otte JB: Liver transplantation for hereditary tyrosinemia—early transplantation following the patient's stabilization. Transplantation 54:937-939, 1992.

137. Salt A, Barnes ND, Rolles K, et al: Liver transplantation in tyrosinaemia type 1: The dilemma of timing the operation. Acta Paediatr 81:449-452, 1992.

138. Mieles L, Esquivel CO, Van Thiel DH, et al: Liver transplantation for tyrosinemia. A review of 10 cases from the University of Pittsburgh. Dig Dis Sci 35:153-157, 1990.

139. Van Thiel DH, Gartner C Jr, Thorp FK, et al: Resolution of the clinical features of tyrosinemia following orthotopic liver transplantation for hepatoma. J Hepatol 3:42-48, 1986.

140. Shoemaker LR, Strife CF, Balistreri WF, Ryckman FC: Rapid improvement in the renal tubular dysfunction associated with tyrosinemia following hepatic replacement. Pediatrics 89:251-255, 1992.

141. Laine J, Salo MK, Krogerus L, et al: Nephropathy of type I tyrosinemia after liver transplantation. Pediatr Res 37:640-645, 1995.

142. Tuchman M, Freese D, Sharp HL, et al: Contribution of extrahepatic tissues to biochemical abnormalities in hereditary tyrosinemia type I: Study of three patients after liver transplantation. J Pediatr 110:399-403, 1987.

143. Paradis KJG, O'Regan S, Seidman EG, et al: Improvement in true glomerular filtration rate after cyclosporine fractionation in pediatric liver transplant recipients. Transplantation 51:922-925, 1991.

144. Pitkanen ST, Salo MK, Heikenheimo M: Hereditary tyrosinaemia type I: From basics to progress in treatment. Ann Med 32:530-538, 2000.

145. Walser M: Urea cycle enzymopathies. Semin Liver Dis 2:329-339, 1982.

146. Brusilow SW, Danney M, Waber LJ, et al: Treatment of episodic hyperammonemia in children with inborn errors of urea synthesis. N Engl J Med 310:1630-1634, 1984.

147. Batshaw ML, MacArthur RB, Tuchman M: Alternative pathway therapy for urea cycle disorders: Twenty years later. J Pediatr 140:490, 2002.

148. Todo S, Starzl TE, Tzakis A, et al: Orthotopic liver transplantation for urea cycle enzyme deficiency. Hepatology 15:419-422, 1992.

149. Whitington PF, Alonso EM, Boyle JT, et al: Liver transplantation for the treatment of urea cycle disorders. J Inherit Metab Dis 21:112-118, 1998.

150. Saudubray JM, Touati G, Delonlay P, et al: Liver transplantation in urea cycle disorders. Eur J Pediatr 158:S55-S59, 1999.

151. Lee B, Goss J: Long-term correction of urea cycle disorders. J Pediatr 138:S62-S71, 2001.

152. Brusilow SW, Horwich A: Urea cycle enzymes. In Scriver CR, Baudet AL, Sly WS, Valle D (eds): The Metabolic Basis of Inherited Diseases. New York, McGraw-Hill, 1989, pp 629-663.

153. Badizadegan K, Perez-Atayde AR: Focal glycogenosis of the liver in disorders of ureagenesis: Its occurrence and diagnostic significance. Hepatology 26:365-373, 1997.

154. Largilliere C, Farriaux JP: Ornithine transcarbamylase deficiency in a boy with long survival [letter]. J Pediatr 113:952, 1988.

155. Largilliere C, Houssin D, Gottrand F, et al: Liver transplantation for ornithine transcarbamylase deficiency in a girl. J Pediatr 115:415-417, 1989.

156. Heringlake S, Boker K, Manns M: Fatal clinical course of ornithine transcarbamylase deficiency in adult heterozygous female patient. Digestion 58:83-86, 1997.

157. Scaglia F, Zheng Q, O'Brien WE, et al: An integrated approach to the diagnosis and prospective management of partial ornithine transcarbamylase deficiency. Pediatrics 109:150-152, 2002.

158. Broelsch CE, Emond JC, Whitington PF, et al: Application of reduced-size liver transplants as split grafts, auxiliary orthotopic grafts, and living related segmental transplants. Ann Surg 212:368-377, 1990.

159. Busuttil AA, Goss JA, Seu P, et al: The role of orthotopic liver transplantation in the treatment of ornithine transcarbamylase deficiency. Liver Transpl Surg 4:350-354, 1998.

160. Kasahara M, Kiuchi T, Uryuhara K, et al: Treatment of ornithine transcarbamylase deficiency in girls by auxiliary liver transplantation: Conceptual changes in a living-donor programs. J Pediatr Surg 33:1753-1756, 1998.

161. Plochl W, Spiss CK, Plochl E: Death after transplantation of a liver from a donor with unrecognized ornithine transcarbamylase deficiency. N Engl J Med 16:921-922, 1999.

162. Kasahara M, Ohwada S, Takeichi T, et al: Living-related liver transplantation for type II citrullinemia using a graft from heterozygote donor. Transplantation 71:157-159, 2001.

163. Tuchman M: Persistent acitrullinemia after liver transplantation for carbamylphosphate synthetase deficiency. N Engl J Med 320:1498-1499, 1989.

164. Fletcher JM, Couper R, Moore D, et al: Liver transplantation for citrullinaemia improves intellectual function. J Inherit Metab Dis 22:581-586, 1999.

165. Yazaki M, Ikeda S, Takei Y, et al: Complete neurological recovery of an adult patient with type II citrullinemia after living related partial liver transplantation. Transplantation 62:1679-1684, 1996.

166. Kawata A, Suda M, Tanabe H: Adult-onset type II citrullinemia: Clinical pictures before and after liver transplantation. Intern Med 36:408-412, 1997.

167. Ikeda S, Yazaki M, Takei Y, et al: Type II (adult onset) citrullinaemia: Clinical pictures and the therapeutic effect of liver transplantation. J Neurol Neurosurg Psychiatry 71:663-670, 2001.

168. Ban K, Sugiyama N, Sugiyama K, et al: A pediatric patient with classical citrullinemia who underwent living-related partial liver transplantation. Transplantation 71:1495-1497, 2001.

169. Henriquez H, el Din A, Ozand PT, et al: Emergency presentations of patients with methylmalonic acidemia, propionic acidemia and branched chain amino acidemia (MSUD). Brain Dev 16(Suppl):86-93, 1994.

170. van't Hoff WG, Dixon M, Taylor J, et al: Combined liver-kidney transplantation in methylmalonic acidemia. J Pediatr 132:1043-1044, 1998.

171. van't Hoff W, McKiernan PJ, Surtees RA, Leonard JV: Liver transplantation for methylmalonic acidemia. Eur J Pediatr 158:S70-S74, 1999.

172. Leonard JV, Walter JH, McKiernan PJ: The management of organic acidaemias: The role of transplantation. J Inherit Metab Dis 24:309-311, 2001.

173. Nyhan WL, Gargus JJ, Boyle K, et al: Progressive neurologic disability in methylmalonic acidemia despite transplantation of the liver. Eur J Pediatr 161:377-379, 2002.

174. Chakrapani A, Sivakumar P, McKiernan PJ, Leonard JV: Metabolic stroke in methylmalonic acidemia five years after liver transplantation. J Pediatr 140:261-263, 2002.

175. Yorifuji T, Muroi J, Uematsu A, et al: Living-related liver transplantation for neonatal-onset propionic acidemia. J Pediatr 137:572-574, 2000.

176. Rela M, Muiesan P, Andreani P, et al: Auxiliary liver transplantation for metabolic diseases. Transplant Proc 29:444-445, 1997.

177. Saudubray JM, Touati G, Delonlay P, et al: Liver transplantation in propionic acidaemia. Eur J Pediatr 158:S65-S69, 1999.

178. Morton DH, Strauss KA, Robinson DL, et al: Diagnosis and treatment of maple syrup disease: A study of 36 patients. Pediatrics 109:999-1008, 2002.

179. Bodner-Leidecker A, Wendel U, Saudubray JM, Schadewaldt P: Branched-chain L-amino acid metabolism in classical maple syrup urine disease after orthotopic liver transplantation. J Inherit Metab Dis 23:805-818, 2000.

180. Wendel U, Saudubray JM, Bodner A, Schadewaldt P: Liver transplantation in maple syrup urine disease. Eur J Pediatr 158:60-64, 1999.

181. Stanley CA: Disorders of carbohydrate metabolism. In Walker WA, Durie PR, Hamilton JR, et al (eds): Pediatric Gastrointestinal Disease. Philadelphia, BC Decker, 1991, pp 936-943.

182. Otto G, Herfarth C, Senninger N, et al: Hepatic transplantation in galactosemia. Transplantation 47:902-903, 1989.

183. Moses SW, Parvari R: The variable presentations of glycogen storage disease type IV: A review of clinical, enzymatic and molecular studies. Curr Mol Med 2:177-188, 2002.

184. Malatack JJ, Iwatsuki S, Gartner JC, et al: Liver transplantation for type I glycogen storage disease. Lancet 1:1073-1074, 1983.

185. Selby R, Starzl TE, Yunis B, et al: Liver transplantation for type IV glycogen storage disease. N Engl J Med 324:39-42, 1991.

186. Sokal E, Van Hoof F, Alberti D, et al: Progressive cardiac failure following orthotopic liver transplantation for type IV glycogenosis. Eur J Pediatr 151:200-203, 1992.

187. Matern D, Starzl TE, Arnaout W, et al: Liver transplantation for glycogen storage disease types I, III, and IV. Eur J Pediatr 158:S43-S48, 1999.

188. Starzl TE, Demetris AJ, Trucco M, et al: Chimerism after liver transplantation for type IV glycogen storage disease and type 1 Gaucher's disease. N Engl J Med 328:745-749, 1993.

189. Faivre L, Houssin D, Valayer J, et al: Long-term outcome of liver transplantation in patients with glycogen storage disease type IA. J Inherit Metab Dis 22:723-732, 1999.

190. Lee PJ: Glycogen storage disease type I: Pathophysiology of liver adenomas. Eur J Pediatr 161:S46-S49, 2002.

191. Howell RR: Glycogen storage disease research and clinical problems: A reappraisal. J Pediatr Gastroenterol Nutr 3:12-13, 1984.

192. Coire CI, Qizilbash AH, Castelli MF: Hepatic adenomata in type Ia glycogen storage disease. Arch Pathol Lab Med 111:166-169, 1987.

193. Muraca M, Gerunda G, Neri D, et al: Hepatocyte transplantation as a treatment for glycogen storage disease type IA. Lancet 359:317-318, 2002.

194. Labrune P, Trioche P, Duvaltier I, et al: Hepatocellular adenomas in glycogen storage disease type I and III: A series of 43 patients and review of the literature. J Pediatr Gastroenterol Nutr 24:276-279, 1997.

195. Allen JM, Thompson GR, Myant NB, et al: Cardiovascular complications of homozygous familial hypercholesterolaemia. Br Heart J 44:361-368, 1980.

196. Goldstein J, Brown MS: Familial hypercholesterolemia. In Stanbury JB, Wyngaarden JB, Fredrickson DS (eds): The Metabolic Basis of Inherited Disease. New York, McGraw-Hill, 1983, pp 1215-1250.

197. Brown MS, Goldstein J: Familial hypercholesterolemia: A genetic defect in the low-density lipoprotein receptor. N Engl J Med 294:1386-1390, 1976.

198. Bilheimer DW, Grundy SM, Brown MS, Goldstein J: Mevinolin and colestipol stimulate receptor-mediated clearance of low density lipoprotein from plasma in familial hypercholesterolemia heterozygotes. Proc Natl Acad Sci U S A 80:4124-4128, 1983.

199. Bilheimer DW: Portacaval shunt and liver transplantation in treatment of familial hypercholesterolemia. Arteriosclerosis Suppl 9:I158-I163, 1989.

200. Starzl TE, Bilheimer DW, Bahnson HT, et al: Heart-liver transplantation in a patient with familial hypercholesterolaemia. Lancet 1:1382-1383, 1984.

201. East C, Grundy SM, Bilheimer DW: Normal cholesterol levels with lovastatin (Mevinolin) therapy in a child with homozygous familial hypercholesterolemia following liver transplantation. JAMA 256:2843-2848, 1986.

202. Brush JE, Leon MB, Starzl TE, et al: Successful treatment of angina pectoris with liver transplantation and bilateral internal mammary bypass graft surgery in familial hypercholesterolemia. Am Heart J 116:1365-1367, 1988.

203. Figuera D, Ardaiz J, Martin-Judez V, et al: Combined transplantation of heart and liver from two different donors in a patient with familial type IIa hypercholesterolemia. J Heart Transplant 5:327-329, 1986.

204. Barbir M, Khaghani A, Kehely A, et al: Normal levels of lipoproteins including lipoprotein(a) after liver-heart transplantation in a patient with homozygous familial hypercholesterolaemia. Q J Med 85:307-308, 1992.

205. Shaw BW, Bahnson HT, Hardesty RL, et al: Combined transplantation of the heart and liver. Ann Surg 202:667-672, 1985.
206. Valdivielso P, Escolar JL, Cuervas-Mons V, et al: Lipids and lipoprotein changes after heart and liver transplantation in a patient with homozygous familial hypercholesterolemia. Ann Intern Med 108:204-206, 1988.
207. Sokal E, Ulla L, Harvengt C, Otte JB: Liver transplantation for familial hypercholesterolemia before the onset of cardiovascular complications. Transplantation 55:432-433, 1993.
208. Revell SP, Noble-Jamieson G, Johnston P, et al: Liver transplantation for homozygous familial hypercholesterolaemia. Arch Dis Child 73:456-458, 1995.
209. Lopez Santamaria M, Migliazza L, Gamez M, et al: Liver transplantation in patients with homozygotic familial hypercholesterolemia previously treated by end-to-side portocaval shunt and ileal bypass. J Pediatr Surg 35:630-633, 2000.
210. Wiederkehr JC, Kondos GT, Pollak R: Hepatocyte transplantation for the low-density lipoprotein receptor–deficient state. A study in the Watanabe rabbit. Transplantation 50:466-476, 1990.
211. Brady RO, Kanfer JN, Bradley RM, Shapiro D: Demonstration of a deficiency of glucocerebroside-cleaving enzyme in Gaucher's disease. J Clin Invest 45:1112-1115, 1966.
212. Barranger JA, Ginns EI: Glucosylceramide lipidosis: Gaucher's disease. In Scriver CR, Baudet AL, Sly WS, Valle D (eds): The Metabolic Basis of Inherited Disease. New York, McGraw-Hill, 1989, p 1677.
213. Carlson DE, Busuttil RW, Giudici TA, Barranger JA: Orthotopic liver transplantation in the treatment of complications of type 1 Gaucher disease. Transplantation 49:1192-1194, 1990.
214. DuCerf CK, Bancel B, Caillon P, et al: Orthotopic liver transplantation for type 1 Gaucher's Disease. Transplantation 53:1141-1143, 1992.
215. Smanik EJ, Tavill AS, Jacobs GH, et al: Orthotopic liver transplantation in two adults with Niemann-Pick and Gaucher's diseases: Implications for the treatment of inherited metabolic disease. Hepatology 17:42-49, 1993.
216. Figueroa ML, Rosenbloom BE, Kay AC, et al: A less costly regimen of alglucerase to treat Gaucher's disease. N Engl J Med 327:1632-1636, 1992.
217. Perel Y, Bioulac-Sage P, Chateil JF, et al: Gaucher's disease and fatal hepatic fibrosis despite prolonged enzyme replacement therapy. Pediatrics 109:1170-1173, 2002.
218. Spence MW, Callahan JW: Sphingomyelin-cholesterol lipidoses: The Niemann-Pick group of diseases. In Scriver CR, Baudet AL, Sly WS, Valle D (eds): The Metabolic Basis of Inherited Disease. New York, McGraw-Hill, 1989, pp 1655-1676.
219. Brady RO, Filling-Katz MR, Barton NW, Pentchev PG: Niemann-Pick disease types C and D. Neurol Clin 7:75-88, 1989.
220. Daloze P, Delvin EE, Glorieux FH, et al: Replacement therapy for inherited enzyme deficiency: Liver orthotopic transplantation in Niemann-Pick disease type A. Am J Med Genet 1:229-239, 1977.
221. Silverstein MN, Ellefson RD, Dhern EJ: The syndrome of the sea-blue histiocyte. N Engl J Med 282:1-4, 1970.
222. Gartner C Jr, Bergman I, Malatack JJ, et al: Progression of neurovisceral storage disease with supranuclear ophthalmoplegia following orthotopic liver transplantation. Pediatrics 77:104-106, 1986.
223. Schmitz G, Assmann G: Acid lipase deficiency: Wolman's disease. Cholesteryl ester storage disease. In Scriver CR, Baudet AL, Sly WS, Valle D (eds): The Metabolic Basis of Inherited Disease. New York, McGraw-Hill, 1989, pp 1623-1644.
224. Coates PM, Cortner JA: Lysosomal acid lipase deficiency: Cholesterol ester storage disease and Wolman's disease. In Walker WA, Durie PR, Hamilton JR, et al (eds): Pediatric Gastrointestinal Disease. Philadelphia, BC Decker, 1991, pp 957-965.
225. Ferry GD, Whisennand HH, Finegold MJ, et al: Liver transplantation for cholesteryl ester storage disease. J Pediatr Gastroenterol Nutr 12:376-378, 1991.
226. Martinez Ibanez V, Margarit C, Tormo R, et al: Liver transplantation in metabolic diseases. Report of five pediatric cases. Transplant Proc 19:3803-3804, 1987.
227. Ciotti M, Obaray R, Martin MG, Owens IS: Genetic defects at the UGT1 locus associated with Crigler-Najjar type I disease, including a prenatal diagnosis. Am J Med Genet 68:173-178, 1997.
228. Arias IM, Gartner LM, Cohen M, et al: Chronic non-hemolytic hyperbilirubinemia with glucuronyl transferase deficiency: Clinical, biochemical, pharmacodynamic and genetic evidence for heterogeneity. Am J Med 47:395-409, 1969.
229. Arias IM: Chronic unconjugated hyperbilirubinaemia without overt signs of haemolysis in adolescents and adults. J Clin Invest 41:2233-2245, 1962.
230. Yohannan MD, Terry HJ, Littlewood JM: Long-term phototherapy in Crigler-Najjar syndrome. Arch Dis Child 58:460-462, 1983.
231. Karoly S, Thomas D, Maria K, Margit T: Crigler-Najjar syndrome: Successful home care phototherapy with good results. Orv Hetil 5:2457, 1980.
232. Pett S, Mowat AP: Crigler-Najjar syndrome types I and II. Clinical experience—King's College Hospital 1972-1978. Phenobarbitone, phototherapy and liver transplantation. Mol Aspects Med 9:473-482, 1987.
233. Blaschke TF, Berk PD, Scharschmidt BF, et al: Crigler-Najjar syndrome: An unusual course with development of neurologic damage at age eighteen. Pediatr Res 8:573-590, 1974.
234. van der Veere CN, Sinaasappel M, McDonagh AF, et al: Current therapy for Crigler-Najjar syndrome type 1: Report of a world registry. Hepatology 24:311-315, 1996.
235. McDonagh AF: Tin-protoporphyrin in the management of children with Crigler-Najjar disease. Pediatrics 86:151-152, 1990.
236. Rubaltelli FF, Guerrini P, Reddi E, Jori G: Tin-protoporphyrin in the management of children with Crigler-Najjar disease. Pediatrics 84:728-731, 1989.
237. Kaufman SS, Wood RP, Shaw BW, et al: Orthotopic liver transplantation for type I Crigler-Najjar syndrome. Hepatology 6:1259-1262, 1986.
238. Shevell MI, Bernard B, Adelson JW, et al: Crigler-Najjar syndrome type I: Treatment by home phototherapy followed by orthotopic hepatic transplantation. J Pediatr 110:429-431, 1987.
239. Gartner JC, Zitelli BJ, Malatack JJ, et al: Orthotopic liver transplantation in children: Two-year experience with 47 patients. Pediatrics 74:140-145, 1984.
240. Sokal EM, Silva ES, Hermans D, et al: Orthotopic liver transplantation for Crigler-Najjar type I disease in six children. Transplantation 60:1095-1098, 1995.
241. Prager MC, Johnson KL, Ascher NL, Roberts JP: Anesthetic care of patients with Crigler-Najjar syndrome. Anesth Analg 74:162-164, 1992.
242. Asonuma K, Gilbert JC, Stein JE, et al: Quantitation of transplanted hepatic mass necessary to cure the Gunn rat model of hyperbilirubinemia. J Pediatr Surg 27:298-301, 1992.
243. Rela M, Muiesan P, Vilca-Melendez H, et al: Auxiliary partial orthotopic liver transplantation for Crigler-Najjar syndrome type I. Ann Surg 229:565-569, 1999.
244. Dixit V, Darvasi R, Arthur M, et al: Restoration of liver function in Gunn rats without immunosuppression using transplanted microencapsulated hepatocytes. Hepatology 12:1342-1349, 1990.
245. Askari FK, Hitomi Y, Mao M, Wilson JM: Complete correction of hyperbilirubinemia in the Gunn rat model of Crigler-Najjar syndrome type I following transient in vivo adenovirus-mediated expression of human bilirubin UDP-glucuronosyltransferase. Gene Ther 3:381-388, 1996.

246. Isenberg JN: Cystic fibrosis: Its influence on the liver, biliary tree, and bile salt metabolism. Semin Liver Dis 2:302-313, 1982.

247. Rommens JM, Iannuzzi MC, Kerem B, et al: Identification of the cystic fibrosis gene: Chromosome walking and jumping. Science 245:1059-1065, 1989.

248. Farrell PM, Fost N: Prenatal screening for cystic fibrosis: Where are we now? J Pediatr 141:758-763, 2002.

249. Genetic testing for cystic fibrosis. Arch Intern Med 159: 1529-1539, 1999.

250. Couetil JP, Houssin DP, Soubrane O, et al: Combined lung and liver transplantation in patients with cystic fibrosis. A 4½-year experience. J Thorac Cardiovasc Surg 110:1415-1422, 1995.

251. Quinton PM: Cystic fibrosis: A disease in electrolyte transport. FASEB J 4:2709-2717, 1990.

252. Schuster SR, Schwachman H, Toyama WM, et al: The management of portal hypertension in cystic fibrosis. J Pediatr Surg 12:201-206, 1977.

253. Psarcharopoulos HT, Portman B, Howard ER, et al: Hepatic complications of cystic fibrosis. Lancet 2:78-80, 1982.

254. Shapira R, Hadzic N, Francavilla R, et al: Retrospective review of cystic fibrosis presenting as infantile liver disease. Arch Dis Child 81:125-128, 1999.

255. Cox KL, Ward RE, Furguiele TL, et al: Orthotopic liver transplantation in patients with cystic fibrosis. Pediatrics 80:571-574, 1987.

256. Revell SP, Robertson NRC, Noble-Jamieson G, Barnes ND: Liver transplantation in cystic fibrosis. J R Soc Med 86:111-112, 1993.

257. Mieles L, Orenstein D, Teperman L, et al: Liver transplantation in cystic fibrosis. Lancet 1:1073, 1989.

258. Milkiewicz P, Skiba G, Kelly D, et al: Transplantation for cystic fibrosis: Outcome following early liver transplantation. J Gastroenterol Hepatol 17:208-213, 2002.

259. Molmenti EP, Squires RH, Nagata D, et al: Liver transplantation for cholestasis associated with cystic fibrosis in the pediatric population. Pediatr Transplant 7:93-97, 2003.

260. Cox KL: Liver transplantation in cystic fibrosis. Clin Res 39:6A, 1991.

261. Couetil JP, Soubrane O, Houssin DP, et al: Combined heart-lung-liver, double lung–liver, and isolated liver transplantation for cystic fibrosis in children. Transpl Int 10:33-39, 1997.

262. Fridell JA, Mazariegos GV, Orenstein D, et al: Liver and intestinal transplantation in a child with cystic fibrosis: A case report. Pediatr Transplant 7:240-242, 2003.

263. Williams HE, Smith LH: Primary hyperoxaluria. In Scriver CR, Baudet AL, Sly WS, Valle D (eds): The Metabolic Basis of Inherited Disease. New York, McGraw-Hill, 1989, pp 933-944.

264. Cochat P, Rolland MO, Bozon D, et al: [Molecular pathology of type 1 primary hyperoxaluria] Pathologie moleculaire de l'hyperoxalurie primitive de type 1. Nephrologie 15:375-380, 1994.

265. Danpure CJ, Jennings PR, Watts RWE: Enzymological diagnosis of primary hyperoxaluria type 1 by measurement of hepatic alanine:glyoxylate aminotransferase activity. Lancet 1:289-291, 1987.

266. Cochat P, Gaulier JM, Koch Nogueira PC, et al: Combined liver-kidney transplantation in primary hyperoxaluria type I. Eur J Pediatr 158:S75-S80, 1999.

267. Monico CG, Milliner DS: Combined liver-kidney and kidney-alone transplantation in primary hyperoxaluria. Liver Transpl 7:954-963, 2001.

268. Cibrik DM, Kaplan B, Arndorfer JA, Meier-Kriesche HU: Renal allograft survival in patients with oxalosis. Transplantation 15:707-710, 2002.

269. Watts RWE, Calne RY, Rolles K, et al: Successful treatment of primary hyperoxaluria type I by combined hepatic and renal transplantation. Lancet 2:474-475, 1987.

270. Schurmann G, Scharer K, Wingen AM, et al: Early liver transplantation for primary hyperoxaluria type I in an infant with chronic renal failure. Nephrol Dial Transplant 5:825-527, 1991.

271. Jamieson NV, Watts RWE, Evans DB, et al: Liver and kidney transplantation in the treatment of primary hyperoxaluria. Transplant Proc 23:1557-1558, 1991.

272. Polinsky MS, Dunn S, Kaiser BA, et al: Combined liver-kidney transplantation in a child with primary hyperoxaluria. Pediatr Nephrol 5:332-334, 1991.

273. Cochat P, Faure JL, Divry P, et al: Liver transplantation in primary hyperoxaluria type 1 [letter]. Lancet 1:1142-1143, 1989.

274. Gagnadoux MF, Lacaille F, Niaudet P, et al: Long term results of liver-kidney transplantation in children with primary hyperoxaluria. Pediatr Nephrol 16:946-950, 2001.

275. Shapiro R, Weismann I, Mandel H, et al: Primary hyperoxaluria type 1: Improved outcome with timely liver transplantation: A single-center report of 36 children. Transplantation 72: 428-432, 2001.

276. Leumann E, Hoppe B: Pre-emptive liver transplantation in primary hyperoxaluria type I: A controversial issue. Pediatr Transplant 4:161-164, 2000.

277. Nolkemper D, Kemper MJ, Burdelski M, et al: Long-term results of pre-emptive liver transplantation in primary hyperoxaluria type I. Pediatr Transplant 4:177-181, 2000.

278. Bastani B, Mistry BM, Nahass GT, et al: Oxalate kinetics and reversal of the complications after orthotopic liver transplantation in a patient with primary hyperoxalosis type I awaiting renal transplantation. Am J Nephrol 19:64-69, 1999.

279. Creput C, Durrbach A, Samuel D, et al: Incidence of renal and liver rejection and patient survival rate following combined liver and kidney transplantation. Am J Transplant 3:348-356, 2003.

280. Morrissey PE, Gordon F, Shaffer D, et al: Combined liver-kidney transplantation in patients with cirrhosis and renal failure: Effect of a positive cross-match and benefits of combined transplantation. Liver Transpl Surg 4:363-369, 1998.

281. Ruder H, Otto G, Schutgens RBH, et al: Excessive urinary oxalate excretion after combined renal and hepatic transplantation for correction of hyperoxaluria type 1. Eur J Pediatr 150:56-58, 1990.

282. Toussaint C, De Pauw L, Vienne A, et al: Radiological and histological improvement of oxalate osteopathy after combined liver-kidney transplantation in primary hyperoxaluria type 1. Am J Kidney Dis 21:54-63, 1993.

283. Behnke B, Kemper MJ, Kruse HP, Muller-Wiefel DE: Bone mineral density in children with primary hyperoxaluria type I. Nephrol Dial Transplant 16:2236-2239, 2001.

284. Detry O, Honore P, DeRoover A, et al: Reversal of oxalosis cardiomyopathy after combined liver and kidney transplantation. Transpl Int 15:50-52, 2002.

285. Astarcioglu I, Karademir S, Gulay H, et al: Primary hyperoxaluria: Simultaneous combined liver and kidney transplantation from living related donor. Liver Transpl 9:433-436, 2003.

286. Ellis SR, Hulton SA, McKiernan PJ, et al: Combined liver-kidney transplantation for primary hyperoxaluria type I in young children. Nephrol Dial Transplant 16:348-354, 2001.

287. Watts RWE, Danpure CJ, De Pauw L, et al: Combined liver-kidney and isolated liver transplantations for primary hyperoxaluria type 1: The European experience. Nephrol Dial Transplant 6:502-511, 1991.

288. Toussaint C, Vienne A, De Pauw L, et al: Combined liver-kidney transplantation in primary hyperoxaluria type I. Bone histopathology and oxalate body content. Transplantation 59:1700-1704, 1995.

289. Goldfischer S, Grotsky HW, Chang CH, et al: Idiopathic neonatal iron storage involving the liver, pancreas, heart, and endocrine and exocrine glands. Hepatology 1:58-64, 1982.

290. Murray KF, Kowdley KV: Neonatal hemochromatosis. Pediatrics 108:960-964, 2001.

291. Piccoli DA, Witzleben CA, Watkins JB: Neonatal iron storage disease. In Walker WA, Durie PR, Hamilton JR, et al (eds): Pediatric Gastrointestinal Disease. Philadelphia, BC Decker, 1991, pp 1063-1065.

292. Egawa H, Berquist W, Garcia-Kennedy R, et al: Rapid development of hepatocellular siderosis after liver transplantation for neonatal hemochromatosis. Transplantation 62:1511-1513, 1996.

293. Hayes AM, Jaramillo D, Levy HL, Knisely AS: Neonatal hemochromatosis: Diagnosis with MR imaging. AJR Am J Roentgenol 159:623-625, 1992.

294. Shamieh I, Kibort PK, Suchy FJ, Freese DK: Antioxidant therapy for neonatal iron storage disease [abstract]. Pediatr Res 33:109A, 1993.

295. Sigurdsson L, Reyes J, Kocoshis SA, et al: Neonatal hemochromatosis: Outcomes of pharmacologic and surgical therapies. J Pediatr Gastroenterol Nutr 26:85-89, 1998.

296. Muiesan P, Rela M, Kane P, et al: Liver transplantation for neonatal haemochromatosis. Arch Dis Child Fetal Neonatal Ed 73:F178-F180, 1995.

297. Vohra P, Haller C, Magid M, et al: Neonatal hemochromatosis: The importance of early recognition of liver failure. J Pediatr 136:537-541, 2000.

298. Flynn DM, Mohan N, McKiernan P, et al: Progress in treatment and outcome for children with neonatal haemochromatosis. Arch Dis Child Fetal Neonatal Ed 88:F124-F127, 2003.

299. Treem WR, Witzleben CA, Piccoli DA, et al: Medium-chain and long-chain acyl CoA dehydrogenase deficiency: Clinical, pathologic and ultrastructural differentiation from Reye's syndrome. Hepatology 6:1270-1278, 1986.

300. Taubman B, Hale DE, Kelley RI: Familial Reye-like syndrome: A presentation of medium-chain acyl coenzyme A dehydrogenase deficiency. Pediatrics 79:382-385, 1987.

301. Duran M, Mitchell G, de Klerk JBC, et al: Octanoic acidemia and octanoylcarnitine excretion with dicarboxylic aciduria due to defective oxidation of medium-chain fatty acids. J Pediatr 107:397-404, 1985.

302. Duran M, Hofkamp M, Rhead WJ, et al: Sudden child death and "healthy" affected family members with medium-chain acyl-coenzyme A dehydrogenase deficiency. Pediatrics 78:1052-1057, 1986.

303. Roe CR, Millington DS, Maltby DA, Kinnebrew P: Recognition of medium-chain acyl-CoA dehydrogenase deficiency in asymptomatic siblings of children dying of sudden infant death or Reye-like syndromes. J Pediatr 108:13-18, 1986.

304. Greene CL, Blitzer MG, Shapira E: Inborn errors of metabolism and Reye syndrome: Differential diagnosis. J Pediatr 113:156-159, 1988.

305. Sokal RJ, Treem WR: Mitochondria and childhood liver disease. J Pediatr Gastroenterol Nutr 28:4-16, 1999.

306. Munnich A, Rotig A, Chretien D, et al: Clinical presentation of mitochondrial disorders in childhood. J Inherit Metab Dis 19:521-527, 1996.

307. Cormier V, Rustin P, Bonnefont JP, et al: Hepatic failure in disorders of oxidative phosphorylation with neonatal onset. J Pediatr 119:951-954, 1991.

308. Heubi JE, Partin JC, Partin JS, Schubert WK: Reye's syndrome: Current concepts. Hepatology 7:155-164, 1987.

309. Goncalves I, Hermans D, Chretien D, et al: Mitochondrial respiratory chain defect: A new etiology for neonatal cholestasis and early liver insufficiency. J Hepatol 23:290-294, 1995.

310. Dubern B, Broue P, Dubuisson C, et al: Orthotopic liver transplantation for mitochondrial respiratory chain disorders: A study of 5 children. Transplantation 71:633-637, 2001.

311. Sokal EM, Sokol R, Cormier V, et al: Liver transplantation in mitochondrial respiratory chain disorders. Eur J Pediatr 158:S81-S84, 1999.

312. Rake JP, van Spronsen FJ, Visser G, et al: End-stage liver disease as the only consequence of a mitochondrial respiratory chain deficiency: No contra-indication for liver transplantation. Eur J Pediatr 159:523-526, 2000.

313. McKusick VA, Neufeld EF: The mucopolysaccharide storage diseases. In Stanbury JB, Wyngaarden JB, Fredrickson DS, et al (eds): The Metabolic Basis of Inherited Diseases. New York, McGraw-Hill, 1983, pp 751-777.

314. Parfrey MA, Hutchins GM: Hepatic fibrosis in the mucopolysaccharidoses. Am J Med 81:825-829, 1986.

315. Navarro C, Dominguez C, Costa M, Ortega JJ: Bone marrow transplant in a case of mucopolysaccharidosis I Scheie phenotype: Skin ultrastructure before and after transplantation. Acta Neuropathol 82:33-38, 1991.

316. Krivit W, Pierpont ME, Ayaz K, et al: Bone marrow transplantation in Maroteaux-Lamy disease (mucopolysaccharidosis VI): Correction of the enzymatic defect. N Engl J Med 31:1606-1611, 1984.

317. Whitley CB, Ramsay NKC, Kersey JH, Krivit W: Bone marrow transplantation for Hurler syndrome: Assessment of metabolic correction. Birth Defects 22:7-24, 1986.

318. McGovern MM, Ludman MD, Short MP, et al: Bone marrow transplantation in Maroteaux-Lamy syndrome (MPS type 6): Status 40 months after BMT. Birth Defects 22:41-53, 1986.

25

Transplantation for Hepatic Malignancy in Children

FREDERICK C. RYCKMAN
MARIA H. ALONSO
GREGORY M. TIAO
KEVIN E. BOVE

Transplantation for primary hepatocellular neoplasms 368
   Hepatoblastoma 368
   Hepatocellular carcinoma 371
   Hepatic malignancy related to preexisting metabolic disease 372

Transplantation for primary vascular neoplasms 373
   Benign vascular lesions 374
   Malignant vascular lesions 375

Summary 376

In the pediatric population, primary hepatic malignancy is an uncommon indication for liver transplantation; however, its use represents one of the benchmarks in the history of transplantation. A 3-year-old child with biliary atresia and incidentally discovered hepatocellular carcinoma (HCC) underwent transplantation on January 2, 1970, and that individual is the oldest surviving liver transplant recipient.[1]

Hepatoblastoma and HCC are the two most common primary hepatic malignancies found in children. Until recently, the outcome of children who underwent liver transplantation for these lesions was poor. However, new studies have documented the efficacy of liver transplantation in a subset of patients who have hepatoblastoma, and thus transplantation has been established as an integral part of the treatment strategy in these children.[2-6] The role of liver transplantation for HCC in the pediatric population remains unclear.

In this chapter we discuss the management of primary hepatic malignancy in children with a focus on recent developments in the use of liver transplantation. In addition, we discuss the role of transplantation for vascular neoplasms of the liver and the evolving role of transplantation in patients with preexisting metabolic disease who are at risk for the development of HCC.

Transplantation for Primary Hepatocellular Neoplasms

Hepatoblastoma

Hepatoblastoma is the most common primary malignancy found in the liver in childhood, with an annual incidence of one per million children. The median age at diagnosis is 1 year, and it is found more frequently in males. A child with hepatoblastoma can have a variety of manifestations ranging from an asymptomatic abdominal mass found by a primary caregiver to an acute abdomen secondary to tumor rupture. On occasion, the size of the tumor is so large that it causes respiratory distress or failure to thrive because of loss of abdominal domain. Rarely, a hepatoblastoma may produce the hormone β-human chorionic gonadotropin (β-HCG) and result in the paraneoplastic process of precocious puberty.[7]

Etiology

Hepatoblastomas arise from immature hepatic epithelium and are classified histologically into epithelial, anaplastic, and macrotrabecular cell types. The epithelial cell type can be further divided into fetal and embryonal variants. Children with the fetal cell type of hepatoblastoma have the best prognosis.

The cause of hepatoblastoma remains unknown. As with many malignancies, abnormalities in gene expression are thought to play a role; however, the specific mechanism by which the tumor develops remains unclear. Patients who are afflicted with the genetic conditions of Beckwith-Wiedemann syndrome, its variant hemihypertophy, and familial adenomatous polyposis are found to have an increased incidence of hepatoblastoma and need close surveillance in childhood.

Diagnosis

Blood tests in a child with hepatoblastoma often show anemia, thrombocytosis, and leukocytosis. Hepatocellular transaminases are usually within normal limits. Serum levels of α-fetoprotein (AFP) are elevated in more than 90% of patients with hepatoblastoma. On occasion, an elevated β-HCG level is found.

Radiographic analysis is essential in the diagnosis and treatment of a child in whom hepatoblastoma is suspected. Cross-sectional imaging of the abdomen with either computed tomography (CT) or magnetic resonance imaging (MRI) will identify the site from which a mass arises and will assist in determination of resectability of the lesion. The patency of the portal vein and hepatic artery and the proximity of the tumor

Table 25–1. STAGING SYSTEM ACCORDING TO THE EXTENT OF RESIDUAL DISEASE AFTER SURGERY AT THE TIME OF DIAGNOSIS

I	Complete resection
II	Microscopic residual tumor
III	Gross residual tumor
	Biopsy without resection
IV	Metastatic disease at diagnosis

to major hepatic veins can be determined by the same imaging modalities or by ultrasound. A computed tomographic scan of the chest should be used to rule out metastatic lung disease.

Tissue diagnosis by definitive resection or biopsy obtained via a percutaneous, open, or laparoscopic approach is necessary to establish the diagnosis.

Staging

Hepatoblastomas are staged according to two different systems. In North America, tumors are staged at the time of initial evaluation according to the extent of residual disease after surgical resection (Table 25–1). The prognosis varies with the stage of the tumor.

In Europe, tumors are staged according to the degree of intrahepatic tumor extension as demonstrated by radiographic analysis at the time of diagnosis.[8,9] In the *Pre Treatment Extent* of Disease (PRETEXT) staging system, the liver is divided into right anterior, right posterior, left medial, and left lateral sectors. Patients are classified into four stages: PRETEXT I, tumor in only one sector; PRETEXT II, tumor involving two adjoining sectors; PRETEXT III, tumor involving three contiguous sectors or two nonadjoining sectors; PRETEXT IV, tumor in all four sectors (Fig. 25–1). In addition to the intrahepatic extent of disease, involvement of a hepatic or portal vein, the presence of hilar lymphadenopathy, and the presence of metastatic disease are documented. Treatment algorithms are based on the stage of the lesion. The PRETEXT staging system has been shown to be a predictor of outcome in clinical trials in Europe.[8,9]

Treatment Strategy

Complete surgical resection of the primary liver lesion remains the most essential and crucial intervention for achieving long-term survival. In children with tumor confined to a single lobe of the liver, standard lobectomy followed by adjuvant chemotherapy is indicated. Historically, more than 50% of children presented with lesions unresectable by conventional surgery at the time of diagnosis, and the outcome was poor because

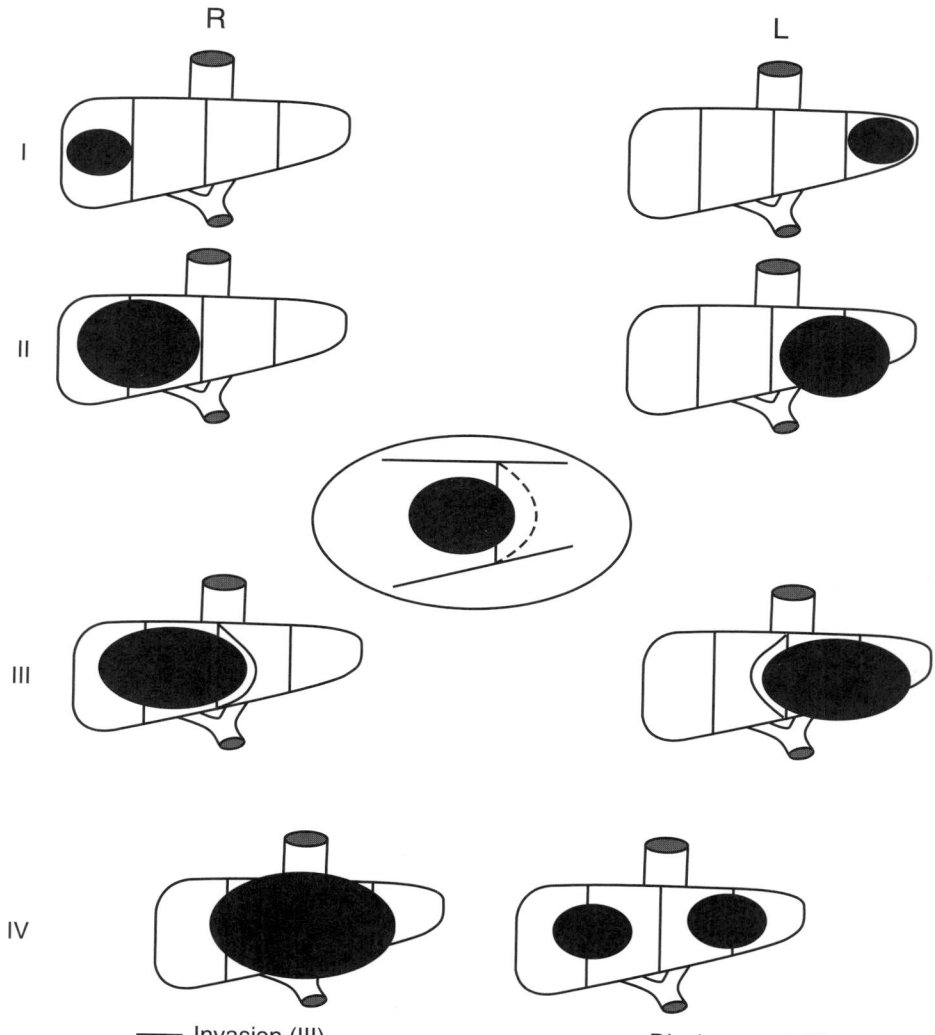

FIGURE 25–1

SIOPEL pretreatment extent of disease (PRETEXT).

of residual disease after attempted resection. In 1982, Evans and coauthors reported a significant improvement in the outcome of children treated with neoadjuvant chemotherapy followed by surgical resection.[10] This finding dramatically altered the treatment strategy in children with hepatoblastoma. More than 75% of lesions initially thought to be unresectable decrease sufficiently in size during neoadjuvant chemotherapy to allow subsequent conventional resection. The combination of neoadjuvant chemotherapy followed by conventional resection has improved the prognosis of children with hepatoblastoma such that 70% to 80% achieve long-term survival.[11-13]

Despite these improvements, some patients still have tumor that is too extensive for conventional resection after neoadjuvant chemotherapy. It is these patients who may benefit from total hepatectomy and orthotopic liver transplantation. Although initial studies on the outcome of orthotopic liver transplantation for

hepatoblastoma reported mixed results, multiple recent studies have documented the efficacy of this form of treatment (Table 25–2). Transplantation can be also be used for salvage after attempted conventional resection in which residual disease remains.

On occasion, the size of the tumor at initial evaluation is so large that it may compromise the respiratory status of the patient. The time required for adjuvant chemotherapy to induce tumor shrinkage may leave the patient ventilator dependent for a prolonged period. In these patients, early transplantation may be indicated.

Outcome

Initial accounts of liver transplantation for hepatoblastoma reported a 50% survival rate, with half the poor outcomes being due to tumor recurrence.[14,15] Most patients did not receive adjuvant chemotherapy.

Table 25-2. LIVER TRANSPLANTATION FOR HEPATOBLASTOMA

Study	No. of Patients	Preoperative Chemotherapy	Previous Resection (%)	Recurrence (%)	Mortality (%)	Overall Survival (%)
Penn,[14] 1991	18	No	N/A	50	N/A	50
Koneru,[15] 1991	12	No	33	25	25	50
Al-Qabandi,[16] 1999	8	Yes	25	25	12	63
Reyes,[2] 2000	12	Yes	8	17	0	83
Srinivasan,[4] 2002	13	Yes	8	8	7	93
Molmenti,[17] 2002	9	Yes	33	13	33	63
Pimpalwar,[3] 2002	12	Yes	0	17	8	83
Tiao,[6] 2003	8	Yes	38	0	12	88

More recent studies in which patients received chemotherapy both before and after transplantation have reported improved outcome after liver transplantation such that the 5-year survival rate after transplantation ranges from 63% to 93%.[2-6] Variables previously thought to be predictors of poor outcome, such as vascular invasion or metastatic disease at the time of diagnosis, have not been shown to have an impact on outcome after transplantation. Transplant-related complications have been the cause of mortality in less than 10% of patients since 1999. These studies demonstrate the efficacy of transplantation in patients who have what was once considered unresectable hepatoblastoma.

Tumor recurrence remains the most significant problem after transplantation, with recurrence rates of up to 25% in recent series. The outcome is usually poor if recurrence develops. Recurrence rates after transplantation, however, are similar to those after conventional resection. A recent study by Pimpalwar and colleagues addressed this observation.[3] They found that tumor susceptibility to chemotherapy as manifested by decreasing AFP levels or a reduction in tumor size on cross-sectional imaging better predicted outcome than did the manner in which the tumor was completely removed. Patients with a poor response to adjuvant chemotherapy had worse outcomes regardless of whether conventional resection or transplantation was performed than did those who had a good response to chemotherapy before surgery. The number of patients in this study was small, so a larger study will be necessary to confirm these findings.

Patients with extensive hepatic disease not amenable to conventional resection after chemotherapy who also had metastatic lung lesions at diagnosis may still be considered for transplantation. Although the overall prognosis is worse for this group of patients, a subset of patients respond well to adjuvant chemotherapy and, if complete clearance of their lung disease can be achieved, may do well after transplantation. Thoracoscopic or open resection may be necessary to remove all metastatic lesions. In the SIOPEL 1 study (International Society of Paediatric Oncology Liver Tumor Study Group) performed in Europe, three patients with metastatic lung disease and large lesions that responded well to chemotherapy subsequently underwent transplantation; they were disease free 3 years after transplantation.[17,18] In our own experience, we have performed transplants in two children who had lung lesions at the time of diagnosis, both of whom have done well since transplantation. The length of time that a patient needs to be free of metastatic disease before transplantation remains uncertain.

Our current algorithm for the management of a child with hepatoblastoma involves a combination of conventional resection, chemotherapy, and transplantation (Fig. 25-2). The treatment algorithm is tailored to the individual child. In children with unresectable lesions at the time of diagnosis, adjuvant cisplatin-based chemotherapy is administered, and after every two cycles of chemotherapy, the patient is restaged radiographically. If the lesion has decreased sufficiently in size to allow conventional resection, surgery is performed. At least two cycles of chemotherapy are administered after resection. If the lesion remains too large to resect after four cycles of chemotherapy, the patient is listed for transplantation. Chemotherapy is continued while the patient is waiting for transplantation. In some of our patients, we have used living related transplantation so that the use of chemotherapy is not prolonged while waiting for an appropriate organ. Ideally, two rounds of chemotherapy are administered after transplantation.

One area of controversy in the management of hepatoblastoma is the role of aggressive conventional resection (i.e., trisegmentectomy or central liver resection) in children who have bulky tumors despite adjuvant chemotherapy. Surgical radicality as defined by trisegmentectomy was shown to be a negative predictor of outcome in the German Cooperative Pediatric Liver Tumor Study HB 94.[19] In contrast, in the SIOPEL 1 study, aggressive conventional resection did not have a negative impact on outcome. Even in the 11 patients

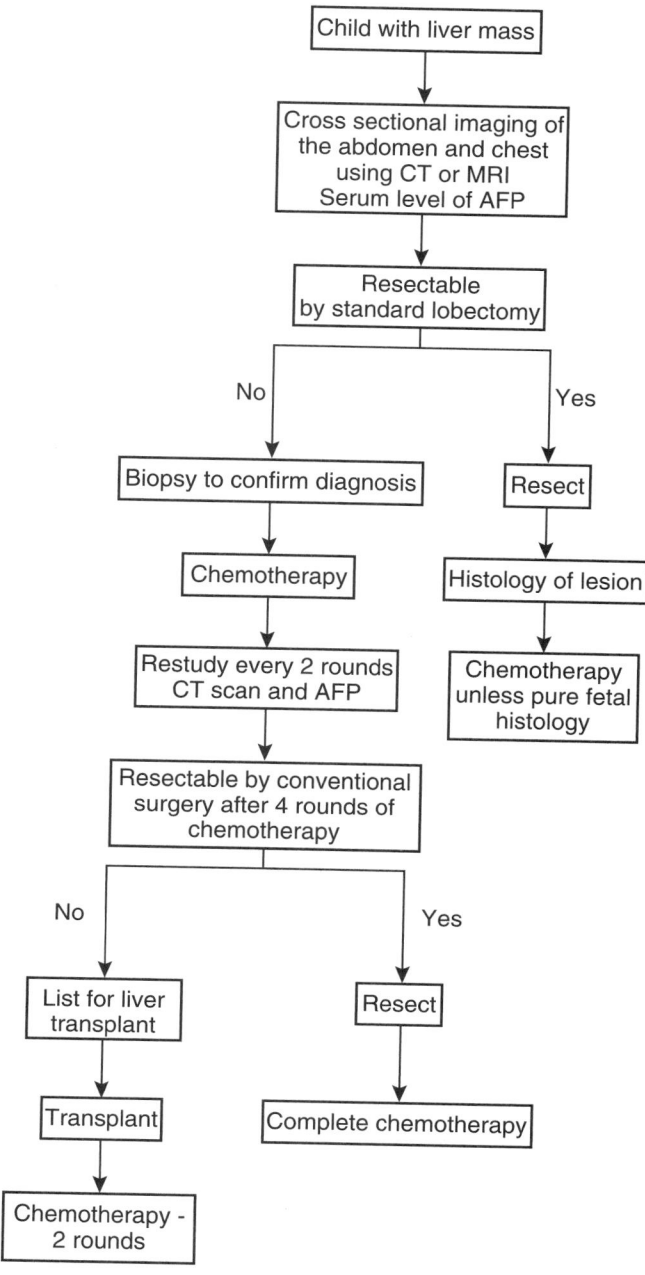

FIGURE 25–2

Algorithm for the management of a child with hepatoblastoma.

who had positive microscopic margins after resection, local tumor recurrence did not develop in any.[12] In our experience, three of six patients who underwent trisegmentectomy required liver transplantation, two for residual gross disease and one for hepatic insufficiency. We believe that primary transplantation is indicated if on radiographic analysis no margin can be visualized between the tumor and the left hepatic vein if right trisegmentectomy is being considered or between the tumor and the right hepatic vein if left trisegmentectomy is being considered. This issue requires further study.

Close follow-up is essential for all children who have undergone treatment of hepatoblastoma. Serial measurement of AFP levels and annual radiographic evaluation are important to facilitate early detection of recurrent disease (Table 25–3).

Hepatocellular Carcinoma

HCC is seen less frequently than hepatoblastoma in the pediatric population. Affected children present in two different fashions. De novo HCC is seen in older children with a median age at diagnosis of 10 years. These children have fatigue, weight loss, abdominal pain, and hepatomegaly. No underlying hepatic disease is present. Lesions tend to be large and are often accompanied by metastatic disease.

HCC that arises in the context of preexisting liver disease may occur at any age and is found in a third of children with HCC. Childhood disorders such as biliary atresia, tyrosinemia, Fanconi anemia, type I glycogen storage disorders, familial intrahepatic cholestasis syndromes, and viral hepatitis all result in chronic underlying hepatocellular damage that predisposes a child to the development of HCC. Multicentric lesions are often present. HCC that arises under these circumstances may be found incidentally at the time of transplantation or, preferably, may be detected by careful screening of at-risk children. Surveillance for a rise in AFP levels and imaging modalities such as ultrasound or MRI should be used when managing children with preexisting liver disease to enable early detection of malignancy.

Etiology

The cause of HCC is unknown. As in adults with cirrhosis, chronic hepatocellular injury from an underlying condition predisposes affected individuals to HCC, but the mechanism by which the malignancy arises is unknown.

The histological appearance of HCC in children is identical to that in adults and is divided into "classic" and fibrolamellar subtypes. The fibrolamellar variant is seen most often in adolescents and young adults. Its distinct histological appearance consists of polygonal cells with large oval vesicular nuclei. The fibrous stroma is characteristically arranged in a lamellar pattern between groups of tumor cells with a surrounding pseudocapsule. It has an indolent growth pattern, which affords the patient a better chance at primary resection and, hence, an improved prognosis.

Diagnosis

Laboratory studies in a child with HCC typically show anemia and mildly elevated hepatocellular transaminases. In 50% of children, serum levels of AFP

Table 25-3. LIVER TRANSPLANTATION FOR HEPATOCELLULAR CARCINOMA IN CHILDREN

Study	No. of Patients	Preoperative Chemotherapy	Preexisting Liver Disease (%)	Recurrence (%)	Transplant Mortality (%)	Overall 5-Year Survival (%)
Tagge,[20] 1992	9	Selected	N/A	45	11	44
Superina,[21] 1996	3	Yes	66	0	0	100
Achilleos,[22] 1996	2	Yes	100	50	50	0
Reyes,[2] 2000	19	Selected	79	32	10	68

are elevated, but not to the same degree as those found in a child with hepatoblastoma.

Cross-sectional imaging of the abdomen with either CT or MRI will identify the site from which a mass arises and will assist in determination of the resectability of the lesion. The patency of the portal vein and hepatic artery and the proximity of the tumor to major hepatic veins can also be determined. Metastatic disease is seen more frequently in patients with HCC, so CT of the chest is essential.

Tissue diagnosis by definitive resection or biopsy allows differentiation between HCC and hepatoblastoma, which is essential because the treatment strategies are markedly different. The TNM staging system used in the adult HCC population is also applied to children.

Treatment

Fewer treatment alternatives are available for a child with HCC than for one who has hepatoblastoma. Adjuvant chemotherapy is not effective treatment of this tumor. Chemoembolization may be used in an effort to reduce tumor size so that definitive resection can be attempted. Complete surgical resection offers the only opportunity for a good outcome; however, recurrence and extrahepatic spread are common even when total resection has been achieved. In contrast to children who have hepatoblastoma, the prognosis of a child with HCC is poor, with 5-year survival rates reaching only 20% to 30%.

Total hepatectomy and orthotopic liver transplantation have been used in the treatment of children and adolescents with HCC. Because of the relative infrequency of HCC in children, the experience of transplantation for HCC in the pediatric population is limited.[2,20-22]

Outcome

The outcome of liver transplantation for HCC in the pediatric population has been dependent on the initial findings. Children with incidental HCC identified at the time of transplantation for other liver diseases have an outcome consistent with their primary disease. Recurrence is uncommon. In patients with preexisting liver disease leading to HCC or in those with large lesions not amenable to conventional resection, the prognosis has been dependent on the features of the HCC. In a study from Pittsburgh of children with HCC who have undergone transplantation, variables that predicted outcome after liver transplantation, including extrahepatic spread, vascular invasion, and tumor size greater than 4 cm, mirrored the predictive variables reported in adults. Tumor recurrence was the most common cause of mortality.

Careful screening is essential when considering a child with HCC for liver transplantation. Extensive radiographic imaging, including a bone scan, should be used to rule out the presence of extrahepatic spread. If vascular invasion is suspected, arteriography may be necessary to better define vessel integrity. Diagnostic laparoscopy should be considered if hilar lymphadenopathy is present to rule out lymphatic spread. A "backup" recipient should be identified at the time of transplantation so that if extrahepatic spread is encountered during exploration, an alternate recipient is available.

Hepatic Malignancy Related to Preexisting Metabolic Disease

The association between preexisting metabolic disease affecting the liver and liver malignancy has been well recognized; however, adequate treatment options to prevent the evolution of neoplasia did not exist before liver transplantation. The use of liver transplantation for these syndromes now allows the option of planned replacement of the affected liver before the development of malignancy or, certainly, early in the course.

Hereditary Tyrosinemia

Hereditary tyrosinemia is a rare autosomal recessive disorder of amino acid metabolism characterized by a deficiency of fumarylacetoacetate hydrolase, which leads to the accumulation of abnormal metabolites of tyrosine toxic to both the liver and kidney.[23,24] This condition results in variable hepatocellular and renal dysfunction. Two differing manifestations of the disease occur, both of which can be seen within a single kindred. Acute tyrosinemia is manifested in infancy as fulminant hepatorenal failure associated with fatty degeneration of the liver and hepatic fibrosis. These infants have rapidly progressive hepatosplenomegaly, failure to thrive, and encephalopathy. The indolent form of the disease allows survival into childhood with slowly progressive cirrhosis. Dietary restriction of phenylalanine and tyrosine is partially effective in improving renal tubular function and may slow the development of liver disease. The use of 2-(2-nitro-4-trifluoromethyl-benzoyl)-1,3-cyclohexanedione (NTBC) inhibits 4-hydroxyphenylpyruvate dioxygenase and prevents formation of the toxic metabolites maleylacetoacetate and fumarylacetoacetate.[25] NTBC offers new hope for successful medical therapy. In the past, most infants with acute tyrosinemia required transplantation in the first year of life, before HCC developed. In those with the indolent form, cirrhosis inevitably developed, with an incidence of HCC ranging from 15% to 37% in children older than 2 years.[26] In a review of 220 children treated with NTBC, only 10% failed to respond clinically.[26] The role of this and future medications in preventing the formation of carcinogenic metabolites of tyrosine degradation remains to be completely defined.

With increasing age and liver damage, the development of HCC becomes a major concern. The high rate of malignant degeneration is thought to be related to inhibition of S-adenosylmethionase by accumulated fumarylacetoacetate, which presumably results in decreased methyl groups available for the methylation of DNA and RNA and thereby leads to mutagenesis and abnormal protein synthesis.[25] In addition, decreased activity of mixed-function oxidases has also been noted and may contribute to difficulty in the metabolism and excretion of hepatotoxins.[27] This presumed biochemical mechanism would make all children with tyrosinemia potentially susceptible to HCC secondary to these metabolic abnormalities. However, NTBC treatment improves hepatic injury and, thus far, seems to decrease and possibly eliminate the risk for development of HCC.[28] Although HCC has been reported in at least one infant who started NTBC therapy at 5 months of age and was treated for 1 year before transplantation, the data do show a diminished need for liver transplantation for liver disease and HCC.[29] In none of the 101 children, now between 2 and 8 years old, who started NTBC therapy before 2 years of age has hepatic malignancy developed.[26]

Although liver transplantation has been used as a treatment modality in children with known carcinoma, its more appropriate role is preventive; transplantation should be performed before the development of tumor. Several studies have detailed the natural history of tyrosinemia in an effort to identify an appropriate age for preemptive transplantation in the pre-NTBC era.[27] NTBC treatment has significantly diminished the need for liver transplantation for tyrosinemia. However, some children may present at such a late stage that treatment will be ineffective. In still others HCC may develop despite NTBC therapy. Therefore, children receiving NTBC should be monitored carefully for the development of progressive liver disease. Since routine screening for HCC is not reliable, liver transplantation should be considered when malignancy cannot be completely excluded.[28]

Glycogen Storage Disease

Glycogen storage disease type Ia is a deficiency of glucose-6-phosphatase that is transmitted by autosomal recessive inheritance; it leads to the accumulation of glycogen in the liver, kidneys, and intestine. Liver adenomas can develop within regenerative nodules at an age range at diagnosis of 3 to 40 years, especially when glucose metabolism is poorly balanced.[30,31] In several cases, serial liver biopsy has documented the development of HCC within a previously benign adenoma.[30,32-34] In a review by Coire and associates, malignant transformation to HCC occurred in 11% of reported cases[30]; in two additional patients aged 12 and 21 years, hepatoblastoma developed.[35] Liver transplantation would be appropriate when adenomas are progressively increasing in size despite dietary management and malignant change cannot be excluded or when patients have failed vigorous medical therapy.[30,36,37] In these patients, an additional advantage after liver transplantation is correction of the metabolic abnormalities characteristic of type Ia glycogen storage disease.

Glycogen storage disease type III is caused by a deficiency of glycogen debranching enzyme activity. With both liver and muscle involvement, it is designated type IIIa; approximately 15% of patients have isolated liver involvement, designated type IIIb.[38] Several case reports have documented HCC in both subtypes of type III glycogen storage disease in adult patients with cirrhosis and either an explant- or autopsy-proven malignancy.[39,40]

Transplantation for Primary Vascular Neoplasms

The spectrum of vascular lesions seen in children includes benign vascular malformations that possess no malignant potential but can be manifested as life-threatening progressive congestive heart failure or coagulopathy; benign capillary hemangioma; epithelioid hemangioendothelioma, a lesion of intermediate invasive potential; and rare aggressive malignant lesions such as angiosarcoma. The primary therapy for each is dictated by a proper initial histological diagnosis, which is often difficult because of the large size, variable radiological imaging, and complex histology of hepatic vascular lesions. Classification of vascular lesions at all sites in children is currently undergoing critical reassessment with the aid of imaging studies and immunophenotyping; the emerging consensus is that two major groups, malformations and neoplasms, embrace most, if not all lesions.[41]

Benign Vascular Lesions

Arteriovenous Malformations and Hemangiomas

Benign vascular lesions of the liver in infants and children include hemangiomas and vascular malformations, often with arteriovenous communications. Transplantation for either type of benign vascular lesion in pediatric patients is undertaken only when extensive multicentric involvement precludes partial hepatectomy and vascular complications endanger the life of the child.

Extensive solitary vascular lesions of the liver with arteriovenous shunting, in the past often termed "cavernous hemangiomas," have been responsible for congestive heart failure, platelet consumption, and diffuse intravascular coagulation.[42] This constellation of clinical symptoms in association with a large vascular lesion is known as Kasabach-Merritt syndrome. Initial attempts at medical management in these patients, usually infants, include diuretics and inotropic support for heart failure symptoms. Involution of the vascular anomalies has been reported to be hastened by the administration of steroids (methylprednisolone). Although the effectiveness of steroids has not been conclusively established, 2 to 5 mg/kg/day for 2 to 4 weeks followed by a 3- to 5-week taper is commonly used. Steroid-sensitive lesions should begin to respond within 1 week.[43-45] In refractory cases that do not reach the threshold for major hepatic resection or transplantation, interferon alfa and cyclophosphamide (Cytoxan) have been used.[46,47] Attempts at embolization and vaso-occlusion are frequently overcome by the recruitment of preexisting collateral circulation with recurrence of symptoms. In addition, hepatic necrosis after embolization can lead to poorly controlled or tolerated metabolic acidosis, thus further complicating subsequent surgical intervention. These procedures are occasionally beneficial in decreasing hyperperfusion before attempts at surgical resection. Individual experience with this lesion validates transplantation in these infants as the treatment of choice when the clinical manifestations of arteriovenous shunting are life-threatening and resection is not feasible. Recurrence or metastasis is not expected with this non-neoplastic lesion. Histological confirmation is necessary so that a vascular neoplasm, possibly of an aggressive type, can be excluded.

Infantile Hemangioendothelioma

Infantile hemangioendothelioma of the liver is most commonly recognized within the first 6 to 12 months of life, usually because of hepatomegaly. Cutaneous hemangiomas of similar histology may also be associated with the condition. Although the vast majority of hepatic hemangioendotheliomas are benign and smaller lesions may spontaneously regress, up to 40% are multicentric. Treatment options parallel those for "cavernous hemangiomas" with arteriovenous communication as described earlier, but Kasabach-Merritt syndrome and signs of arteriovenous shunting are much less common. Transplantation is rarely necessary.

Classically, infantile hemangioendotheliomas are divided into two histological types: type I lesions are composed of dilated vascular channels lined by plump endothelial cells that are benign, and type II lesions have more aggressive morphology with irregular branched vascular channels lined by plump, pleomorphic endothelial cells. Type II lesions may pursue a more aggressive course, as suggested by their morphology.[22,44,48] Several reports have identified malignant transformation of previously unremarkable type II lesions to angiosarcoma.[43,49-52] These patients have often enjoyed a favorable response to steroids or surgical resection and have had a previous benign biopsy before this evolution. Although such transformation is uncommon, it emphasizes the importance of continued follow-up of all infantile hemangioendotheliomas.

The endothelium of hepatic infantile hemangioendothelioma is strongly reactive with anti–Glut-1, which is also a reliable marker for postnatal infantile hemangiomas of the skin (classic "strawberry hemangioma"), but Glut-1 is absent in the endothelium of congenital hemangiomas, lymphatic endothelium, and vascular malformations, including those in the liver.[41] Thus, biopsy may be helpful in the classification of hepatic vascular lesions in cases in which the diagnosis is in doubt, before decisions about management are made.

Eight cases of transplantation for infantile hemangioendothelioma are detailed in Table 25–4. Indications for transplantation were progressive hepatomegaly and, frequently, congestive heart failure or vascular compression of the inferior vena cava. The overall survival rate was 63% in this small group. Two late deaths (25%) were due to non–tumor-related complications. One patient died 41 months after transplantation, with

Table 25–4. TRANSPLANTATION FOR INFANTILE HEMANGIOENDOTHELIOMA

Study	# Cases	Age at Surgery	Indication	Follow-up	Status
Ismail[53]	1	3 yr	Mass, growth	4 mo	No recurrence
Colonna[54]	1	1.5 yr	Mass, s/p embolization	15 mo	No recurrence
Hays[55]	1	2 yr	Mass, growth	6 mo	No recurrence
Egawa[56]	1	6 mo	Mass, CHF	12 mo	No recurrence
Achilleos[22] (also reported by Calder[48])	1	2.9 yr	Mass, IVC obstruction	41 mo	Vertebral body recurrence—36 mo, died at 41 mo
Daller[44]	1	14 days median	Mass, CHF	19 yr	No recurrence
	1	14 days median	Mass, CHF	6 yr	Died—IVH at 2203 days
	1	14 days median	Mass, CHF	2.6 yr	Died—PTLD at 940 days

CHF, congestive heart failure; IVC, inferior vena cava; IVH, intraventricular hemorrhage; PTLD, posttransplant lymphoproliferative disorder; s/p, status post.

tumor recurrence within a vertebral body first recognized 36 months after transplantation; this case represents the only instance of metastatic spread.

Malignant Vascular Lesions

Epithelial Hemangioendothelioma

Epithelial hemangioendothelioma is a tumor of vascular endothelial origin that is frequently multicentric in origin, thus precluding partial hepatectomy. It occurs in young adults without underlying cirrhosis, and its clinical course, characterized by slow growth and late metastatic potential, has made these patients candidates for total hepatectomy and transplantation.[57-61] Accurate definition and diagnosis of this tumor have been facilitated by the presence of several immunohistochemical markers, including staining for factor VIII–related antigen in the tumor and defined histological criteria. Accurate immunohistochemical identification of this tumor has shown that the conventional histopathological variables for grading malignancies, such as necrosis, cytological pleomorphism, and mitotic figures, are not reliable in this tumor.[58,61] Metastasis most often occurs in bones, pleura, and lymph nodes, with a natural disease span of 5 to 10 years.

Five children with epithelial hemangioendothelioma have successfully undergone transplantation (Table 25–5). The tumor was confined to the liver in four patients, with lymph node metastasis and vascular invasion in one. All five patients survived without recurrent disease. The true long-term survival cannot be assessed from this small series of case reports. The more extensive adult experience emphasizes important principles in management that can be applied to children and adolescents as well. Actuarial patient survival/disease-free survival rates at 1, 3, and 5 years were 100%/81%, 86%/69%, and 71%/60%; in 56%, hilar lymph node or vascular invasion was present. There was no difference in recurrence rates in patients with positive or negative nodes.[62] The development of new metastatic lesions should prompt local resection when feasible. The favorable prolonged natural history of this tumor makes it difficult to predict the ultimate outcome of such cases, although late recurrence is common. Inadequate information exists to define the role of adjuvant immunotherapy, radiotherapy, or chemotherapy in this disease.

Angiosarcoma

Angiosarcoma is a rapidly progressive, often multifocal, but rare malignant lesion seen in the liver in children. In all, less than 30 patients have been reported,

Table 25–5. TRANSPLANTATION FOR EPITHELIAL HEMANGIOENDOTHELIOMA IN CHILDHOOD

Study	No. Cases	Age at Surgery	Indication	Follow-up	Status
Olthoff[63]	2	"Child"	Multifocal mass	21, 39, 65 mo	No Recurrence
	1	"Child"	Multifocal mass, positive lymph nodes, vascular invasion		
Ismail[53]	1	3 yr	Mass, growth	Not recorded	Not recorded
	1	3 yr			

with 2 having undergone liver transplantation.[50] In both cases, the pretransplant diagnosis was benign epithelial hemangioendothelioma, thus emphasizing the difficulty in identifying this malignant component within a large hepatic lesion. One patient died of post-transplant cytomegalovirus infection 4 months after transplantation without residual or metastatic disease; the second patient had no recurrence or metastatic disease 4 months after transplantation. We have experience with a single patient who underwent emergency transplantation for a presumed ruptured hemangioendothelioma; on later pathological review the patient had angiosarcoma within the lesion. Metastasis developed 1 year after transplantation. This lesion does not respond to radiotherapy or chemotherapy, and it has been treated by transplantation only because of lack of preoperative identification.

Summary

Recent advances in chemotherapy have made liver transplantation in infants and children with hepatoblastoma an acceptable and successful mode of treatment in cases in which primary resection is not possible. The role of transplantation in central liver tumors and those requiring extensive resection remains controversial, although the initial results of total hepatectomy and transplantation may offer long-term survival advantages. HCC continues to present significant challenges in the occasional child in whom this lesion develops. Lessons learned in the more extensive adult experience will surely apply to children as well. Efforts to prevent the development of carcinoma in children with primary hepatic metabolic disease have been very successful; tyrosinemia represents the most significant example and serves as a template for future advances. Vascular abnormalities may require transplantation as a result of uncontrollable arteriovenous shunting or transformation of slowly progressive, initially benign lesions. Biopsy is key to developing treatment strategies because malignant lesions such as angiosarcoma do not benefit from transplantation at the present time.

Pearls and Pitfalls

Primary Hepatocellular Malignancies

- Hepatoblastoma is the most common primary hepatocellular malignancy in children. Because it is very sensitive to chemotherapy, originally unresectable lesions can undergo conventional resection after initial treatment.

Pearls and Pitfalls—cont'd

- Long-term survival after transplantation for hepatoblastoma is excellent, and it should be considered primary therapy in children with unresectable disease after two to three cycles of chemotherapy.
- Long-term survival in children after transplantation for hepatocellular carcinoma reflects the adult experience with this tumor.
- Initiation of NTBC treatment in the first weeks of infancy can prevent the early formation of hepatocellular carcinoma in patients with hereditary tyrosinemia.

Primary Vascular Lesions

- Benign vascular lesions with significant arteriovenous shunting and refractory congestive heart failure can be successfully treated by liver transplantation.
- Infantile hemangioendothelioma is often multifocal and rarely pursues an aggressive course.
- Epithelial hemangioendothelioma is characterized by slow growth and late malignant degeneration; resection or transplantation is indicated.
- Liver transplantation for angiosarcoma is not presently successful because of early recurrence and death.

References

1. Starzl TE, Demetris AJ: Liver Transplantation: A 31 year perspective. Chicago, Year Book, 1990, pp 119-130.
2. Reyes JD, Carr B, Dvorchik I, et al: Liver transplantation and chemotherapy for hepatoblastoma and hepatocellular cancer in childhood and adolescence. J Pediatr 136:795-804, 2000.
3. Pimpalwar AP, Sharif K, Ramani P, et al: Strategy for hepatoblastoma management: Transplant versus nontransplant surgery. J Pediatr Surg 37:240-245, 2002.
4. Srinivasan P, McCall J, Pritchard J, et al: Orthotopic liver transplantation for unresectable hepatoblastoma. Transplantation 74:652-655, 2002.
5. Molmenti EP, Nagata D, Roden J, et al: Liver transplantation for hepatoblastoma in the pediatric population. Transplant Proc 33:1749, 2001.
6. Tiao G, Allen S, Bobey N, et al: The current management of hepatoblastoma: A combination of chemotherapy, conventional resection and liver transplantation. J Pediatr, in press.
7. Heimann A, White PF, Riely CA, et al: Hepatoblastoma presenting as isosexual precocity. The clinical importance of histologic and serologic parameters. J Clin Gastroenterol 9:105-110, 1987.
8. Perilongo G, Shafford E, Plaschkes J: SIOPEL trials using preoperative chemotherapy in hepatoblastoma. Lancet Oncol 1:94-100, 2000.

9. Brown J, Perilongo G, Shafford E, et al: Pretreatment prognostic factors for children with hepatoblastoma—results from the International Society of Paediatric Oncology (SIOP) study SIOPEL 1. Eur J Cancer 36:1418-1425, 2000.

10. Evans AE, Land VJ, Newton WA, et al: Combination chemotherapy (vincristine, Adriamycin, cyclophosphamide, and 5-fluorouracil) in the treatment of children with malignant hepatoma. Cancer 50:821-826, 1982.

11. Reynolds M, Douglass EC, Finegold M, et al: Chemotherapy can convert unresectable hepatoblastoma. J Pediatr Surg 27:1080-1083, discussion 1083-1084, 1992.

12. Schnater JM, Aronson DC, Plaschkes J, et al: Surgical view of the treatment of patients with hepatoblastoma: Results from the first prospective trial of the International Society of Pediatric Oncology Liver Tumor Study Group. Cancer 94:1111-1120, 2002.

13. Fuchs J, Rydzynski J, Hecker H, et al: The influence of preoperative chemotherapy and surgical technique in the treatment of hepatoblastoma—a report from the German Cooperative Liver Tumour Studies HB 89 and HB 94. Eur J Pediatr Surg 12:255-261, 2002.

14. Penn I: Hepatic transplantation for primary and metastatic cancers of the liver. Surgery 110:726-734, discussion 734-735, 1991.

15. Koneru B, Flye MW, Busuttil RW, et al: Liver transplantation for hepatoblastoma. The American experience. Ann Surg 213:118-121, 1991.

16. Al-Qabandi W, Jenkinson HC, Buckels JA, et al: Orthotopic liver transplantation for unresectable hepatoblastoma: A single center's experience. J Pediatr Surg 34:1261-1264, 1999.

17. Molmenti EP, Wilkinson K, Molmenti H, et al: Treatment of unresectable hepatoblastoma with liver transplantation in the pediatric population. Am J Transplant 2:535-538, 2002.

18. Perilongo G, Brown J, Shafford E, et al: Hepatoblastoma presenting with lung metastases: Treatment results of the first cooperative, prospective study of the International Society of Paediatric Oncology on childhood liver tumors. Cancer 89:1845-1853, 2000.

19. Fuchs J, Rydzynski J, Von Schweinitz D, et al: Pretreatment prognostic factors and treatment results in children with hepatoblastoma: A report from the German Cooperative Pediatric Liver Tumor Study HB 94. Cancer 95:172-182, 2002.

20. Tagge EP, Tagge DU, Reyes J, et al: Resection, including transplantation, for hepatoblastoma and hepatocellular carcinoma: Impact on survival. J Pediatr Surg 27:292-296, discussion 297, 1992.

21. Superina R, Bilik R: Results of liver transplantation in children with unresectable liver tumors. J Pediatr Surg 31:835-839, 1996.

22. Achilleos OA, Buist LJ, Kelly DA, et al: Unresectable hepatic tumors in childhood and the role of liver transplantation. J Pediatr Surg 31:1563-1567, 1996.

23. Mieles LA, Esquivel CO, Van Thiel DH, et al: Liver transplantation for tyrosinemia. A review of 10 cases from the University of Pittsburgh. Dig Dis Sci 35:153-157, 1990.

24. Weinberg AG, Mize CE, Worthen HG: The occurrence of hepatoma in the chronic form of hereditary tyrosinemia. J Pediatr 88:434-438, 1976.

25. Lindstedt S, Holme E, Lock EA, et al: Treatment of hereditary tyrosinaemia type I by inhibition of 4-hydroxyphenylpyruvate dioxygenase. Lancet 340:813-817, 1992.

26. Russo PA, Mitchell GA, Tanguay RM: Tyrosinemia: A review. Pediatr Dev Pathol 4:212-221, 2001.

27. Freese DK, Tuchman M, Schwarzenberg SJ, et al: Early liver transplantation is indicated for tyrosinemia type I. J Pediatr Gastroenterol Nutr 13:10-15, 1991.

28. Shneider BL: Pediatric liver transplantation in metabolic disease: Clinical decision making. Pediatr Transplant 6:25-29, 2002.

29. Mohan N, McKiernan P, Preece MA, et al: Indications and outcome of liver transplantation in tyrosinaemia type 1. Eur J Pediatr 158(Suppl 2):S49-S54, 1999.

30. Coire CI, Qizilbash AH, Castelli MF: Hepatic adenomata in type Ia glycogen storage disease. Arch Pathol Lab Med 111:166-169, 1987.

31. Faivre L, Houssin D, Valayer J, et al: Long-term outcome of liver transplantation in patients with glycogen storage disease type Ia. J Inherit Metab Dis 22:723-732, 1999.

32. Conti JA, Kemeny N: Type Ia glycogenosis associated with hepatocellular carcinoma. Cancer 69:1320-1322, 1992.

33. Limmer J, Fleig WE, Leupold D, et al: Hepatocellular carcinoma in type I glycogen storage disease. Hepatology 8:531-537, 1988.

34. Fujiyama S, Sato K, Sakai M, et al: A case of type Ia glycogen storage disease complicated by hepatic adenoma. Hepatogastroenterology 37:432-435, 1990.

35. Ito E, Sato Y, Kawauchi K, et al: Type 1a glycogen storage disease with hepatoblastoma in siblings. Cancer 59:1776-1780, 1987.

36. Zitelli BJ, Gartner JC Jr, Malatack JJ, et al: Liver transplantation in children: A pediatrician's perspective. Pediatr Ann 20:691-698, 1991.

37. Malatack JJ, Finegold DN, Iwatsuki S, et al: Liver transplantation for type I glycogen storage disease. Lancet 1:1073-1075, 1983.

38. Matern D, Starzl TE, Arnaout W, et al: Liver transplantation for glycogen storage disease types I, III, and IV. Eur J Pediatr 158(Suppl 2):S43-S48, 1999.

39. Siciliano M, De Candia E, Ballarin S, et al: Hepatocellular carcinoma complicating liver cirrhosis in type IIIa glycogen storage disease. J Clin Gastroenterol 31:80-82, 2000.

40. Haagsma EB, Smit GP, Niezen-Koning KE, et al: Type IIIb glycogen storage disease associated with end-stage cirrhosis and hepatocellular carcinoma. The Liver Transplant Group. Hepatology 25:537-540, 1997.

41. Mo JQ, Dimashkieh HH, Bove KE: GLUT1 endothelial reactivity distinguishes hepatic infantile hemangioma from congenital hepatic vascular malformation with associated capillary proliferation. Hum Pathol 35:200-209, 2004.

42. Touloukian RJ: Nonmalignant liver tumors and hepatic infections. In Welch KJ, Randolph JG, Ravitch MM, et al (eds): Pediatric Surgery, 4th ed. Chicago, Year Book, 1986, pp 1067-1074.

43. Meyers RL, Scaife ER: Benign liver and biliary tract masses in infants and toddlers. Semin Pediatr Surg 9:146-155, 2000.

44. Daller JA, Bueno J, Gutierrez J, et al: Hepatic hemangioendothelioma: Clinical experience and management strategy. J Pediatr Surg 34:98-105, discussion 105-106, 1999.

45. Stanley P, Geer GD, Miller JH, et al: Infantile hepatic hemangiomas. Clinical features, radiologic investigations, and treatment of 20 patients. Cancer 64:936-949, 1989.

46. Woltering MC, Robben S, Egeler RM: Hepatic hemangioendothelioma of infancy: Treatment with interferon alpha. J Pediatr Gastroenterol Nutr 24:348-351, 1997.

47. Ezekowitz RA, Mulliken JB, Folkman J: Interferon alfa-2a therapy for life-threatening hemangiomas of infancy. N Engl J Med 326:1456-1463, 1992.

48. Calder CI, Raafat F, Buckels JA, Kelly DA: Orthotopic liver transplantation for type 2 hepatic infantile haemangioendothelioma. Histopathology 28:271-273, 1996.

49. Alt B, Hafez GR, Trigg M, et al: Angiosarcoma of the liver and spleen in an infant. Pediatr Pathol 4:331-339, 1985.

50. Awan S, Davenport M, Portmann B, Howard ER: Angiosarcoma of the liver in children. J Pediatr Surg 31:1729-1732, 1996.

51. Kirchner SG, Heller RM, Kasselberg AG, Greene HL: Infantile hepatic hemangioendothelioma with subsequent malignant degeneration. Pediatr Radiol 11:42-45, 1981.

52. Selby DM, Stocker JT, Ishak KG: Angiosarcoma of the liver in childhood: A clinicopathologic and follow-up study of 10 cases. Pediatr Pathol 12:485-498, 1992.

53. Ismail T, Angrisani L, Gunson BK, et al: Primary hepatic malignancy: The role of liver transplantation. Br J Surg 77:983-987, 1990.

54. Colonna JO 2nd, Ray RA, Goldstein LI, et al: Orthotopic liver transplantation for hepatobiliary malignancy. Report of three cases of special interest. Transplantation 42:561-562, 1986.
55. Hays D: Personal communication, 1995.
56. Egawa H, Berquist W, Garcia-Kennedy R, et al: Respiratory distress from benign liver tumors: A report of two unusual cases treated with hepatic transplantation. J Pediatr Gastroenterol Nutr 19:114-117, 1994.
57. Scoazec JY, Lamy P, Degott C, et al: Epithelioid hemangio-endothelioma of the liver. Diagnostic features and role of liver transplantation. Gastroenterology 94:1447-1453, 1988.
58. Marino IR, Todo S, Tzakis AG, et al: Treatment of hepatic epithelioid hemangioendothelioma with liver transplantation. Cancer 62:2079-2084, 1988.
59. Klompmaker IJ, Sloof MJ, van der Meer J, et al: Orthotopic liver transplantation in a patient with a giant cavernous hemangioma of the liver and Kasabach-Merritt syndrome. Transplantation 48:149-151, 1989.
60. van de Stadt J, Gelin M, Adler M, Lambilliotte JP: Epithelioid hemangioendothelioma and liver transplantation. Gastroenterology 96:275-276, 1989.
61. Dietze O, Davies SE, Williams R, Portmann B: Malignant epithelioid haemangioendothelioma of the liver: A clinicopathological and histochemical study of 12 cases. Histopathology 15:225-237, 1989.
62. Madariaga JR, Marino IR, Karavias DD, et al: Long-term results after liver transplantation for primary hepatic epithelioid hemangioendothelioma. Ann Surg Oncol 2:483-487, 1995.
63. Olthoff KM, Millis JM, Rosove MH, et al: Is liver transplantation justified for the treatment of hepatic malignancies? Arch Surg 125:1261-1266, discussion 1266-1268, 1990.

IV

Special Considerations in Patient Evaluation

Ethical Decisions in Liver Transplantation

L. S. ROTHENBERG

Donation and procurement of organs 381
Deceased-donor organs 381
Determination of death 382
Altruism versus duty or payment
 for organs 383
Anencephalic and xenograft organs 384
Allocation of organs among transplant
 centers 385
Family veto of organ donor cards 386
Required request laws 386

Selection of patients for transplantation 387
Equitable selection and access 387
Patients with end-stage alcoholic liver
 disease (cirrhosis) 388
Retransplantation 388
Role of perceived noncompliance in
 selection 389
Foreign nationals as potential recipients 390

Resource allocation issues 390
Future of federal funding for organ
 transplantation 390

Future of health care expenditures 391

As we start the 21st century, medicine and surgery are facing numerous ethical dilemmas, and the field of liver transplantation is no exception. These questions inevitably involve underlying ethical principles such as:

- Respecting the self-determination of patients with decision-making capacity (sometimes called *autonomy*)
- Acting to protect the patient's well-being (sometimes called *beneficence*)
- Acting in a manner that promotes fairness and equity to all involved (sometimes called *justice*).

The applications of these principles with regard to liver transplantation are explored in this chapter with reference to the donation and procurement of organs, the selection of patients for transplantation, and the place of liver transplantation in the allocation of health care resources and the development of national priorities.

Donation and Procurement of Organs

Deceased-Donor Organs

The United Network for Organ Sharing (UNOS), the organization that administers the U.S. Organ Procurement and Transplantation Network (OPTN), reported that as of August 15, 2004, more than 17,000 people on its national patient list were waiting for a liver, and that a total of 5671 liver transplants were performed at medical centers containing approximately 121 U.S. liver transplant programs during 2003. This latter figure was only slightly higher than the comparable figure for 2002 of 5330 liver transplants.[1]

Many end-stage liver disease patients die each year waiting for a transplant, and their numbers appear to be increasing each year. Based on the latest data available, of those liver patients registered on the UNOS/OPTN Transplant Waiting List, 1791 died in 2000 before a liver could be obtained, 2034 in 2001, and 1818 in 2002.[2] These deaths occurred despite the increasing number of deceased-donor livers obtained from 2000 to 2002: 4995 in 2000, 5107 in 2001, and 5292 in 2002.[3] Researchers estimate there is a potential supply of deceased-donor livers in the United States of 6900 to 9600 annually. Given "immunological considerations, size constraints, and other organ-specific donor selection criteria, subsets of individuals may always be at a disadvantage in efforts to identify suitable donors."[4] Moreover, in a recent study, researchers seeking to estimate the supply of potential organ donors generally in the United States have concluded that the number for all organs is 16,796, but the number of actual donors obtained by U.S. organ procurement agencies is about 35% of that.[4a]

The existing number of actual livers procured each year, therefore, is clearly inadequate to meet the current or future needs in the United States, given current procurement efficiency rates and the unique needs of certain liver transplant patients. Donor livers are a genuinely scarce resource, and questions of fairness in their procurement and distribution are inevitable. Although it is comforting to presume that increased educational programs, new legal approaches, or financial or other incentives can increase the supply of deceased-donor organs, there is no current evidence that such efforts will succeed.

Determination of Death

Acceptance of organ procurement and transplantation depends, in large part, on public confidence that deceased-donor organs, including livers, are being taken from people who are truly dead in the public's understanding of that term and not, as one pundit joked, "kind of dead." In other words, the often-quoted truism that the determination of death is a medical decision hides the reality that the concept of death, while given both a medical and legal rationale, is fundamentally a social and not a scientific concept, informed by cultural and religious beliefs.

The medical criteria for whole-brain death in the United States were authoritatively defined by a U.S. Presidential Commission in 1981 (see Chapter 38, "Principles of Liver Preservation"). The major principles are:

- Both cerebral and brain stem functions must be absent.
- The cause or causes of this total lack of brain functioning must have been identified and determined to be irreversible.
- The absence of all brain function must have persisted during a period of treatment and observation.[5,6]

The Uniform Determination of Death Act (1981) provided the legal framework by stating that "an individual is dead if there is irreversible cessation of circulatory and respiratory functions or if there is irreversible cessation of all brain functions of the entire brain, including the brain stem." This statutory definition has been adopted by an overwhelming majority of U.S. state legislatures; New York and North Carolina have adopted substantially similar versions. In other states, courts have upheld these "brain death" criteria in judicial rulings.

Yet difficulties persist. The very phrase *brain death* connotes to some the existence of two types of death, *regular death* and *brain death*. This distinction is aided by the perception that the death of patients who lose cardiac and respiratory functions and who are not on ventilator support is different from the death of patients on ventilators who are seen on bedside monitors with breathing and cardiac activity.

It might be helpful to stop using the phrase *brain death* and use only the single word *death* for persons on or off the ventilator, no matter how the determination of death is made. Yet, the phrase *brain death* is used precisely to explain how this breathing, heart-beating person could be said to be dead.

There have been efforts to broaden the category of what constitutes death in humans, including suggestions that babies with anencephaly and persons in persistent vegetative states be treated as though dead for purposes of organ donations. These efforts have met with significant public and professional resistance.[7] Indeed, there are two opposing streams of thought from those who are unhappy with the current definition of death for transplant procurement purposes:

- Some believe that the current whole-brain death criteria should be *narrowed* to require stricter criteria, prolonged observation, and more mandatory neurological testing.[8]
- Some believe that the criteria should be *widened* to include patients who have been declared dead by traditional cardiopulmonary criteria (i.e., the *regular dead* as contrasted with the *brain dead*, often referred to as the *non–heart-beating deceased*

donor)[9] or who are alive by current criteria but have been diagnosed with "permanent loss of consciousness" (i.e., the "higher brain" versus "whole brain" standard).[10]

- Arguments in favor of using organs from executed prisoners have been advanced, some in response to reports of the practice occurring in China.[11]

Altruism Versus Duty or Payment for Organs

Use of Living Donors

There are three categories of living donors:

1. Living related donors (such as parents, siblings, or children) who are genetically related to the recipient

2. Living emotionally related donors (such as spouses, significant others, and close friends) who are genetically unrelated

3. Living unrelated donors who are strangers to the recipient and who may or may not be compensated for their donated organ

The use of living donors began for kidney transplantations, and although living donors usually do well after donating a single kidney, there was initial resistance in some circles to using living kidney donors. The rare death of a living kidney donor, the potential morbidity risks for those who survive, and the uncertainty about the degree of improvement in recipient and graft survival compared with deceased-donor organs seemed to militate against their use. The continuing shortage of deceased-donor organs, however, pushed in the other direction. (See Chapter 52, "Clinical Management of Necrotic Liver During Transplantation," and Chapter 48, "Ethics of Living Donor Liver Transplantation.")

Segmental liver transplantation (also known as living donor liver transplants) was first reported in the early 1980s and first performed in the United States in 1985 by Broelsch. In 1988 to 1989 (before beginning an approved series of 20 experimental transplants at the University of Chicago Children's Hospital in 1990), Broelsch and colleagues conducted a year-long series of seminars at the university and published two articles exploring the ethics of liver transplantation with living donors.[12,13] Not only did such a dialogue reflect the best traditions of a scientific approach to conducting research but it also may have been a unique experience in publicly discussing the ethics of a procedure *prior* to a major clinical trial rather than in response to it. As a result, the issues of risks and benefits, informed consent procedures, and the selection of recipients and donors were carefully spelled out in a very public way and deliberately opened to comment and criticism before

the start of the experiment. These procedures were designed to give children needing elective rather emergent liver transplants a better chance of receiving a graft.

The ethical issues presented are similar to those involved in living related renal donation and appear to justify such a procedure when deceased donors are unavailable and when the careful model by Broelsch and colleagues is followed. Such procedures, however, are not without risk to the donors—the first live donor in the 1990 Chicago trials, a 29-year-old woman, lost her spleen and a liter of blood when a retractor slipped; she also suffered a bile duct injury, which was repaired.[14] The Chicago team has also reported outcomes for living donors that included two marital dissolutions and one serious psychiatric illness along with more minor problems.[15] The major ethical consideration concerning the use of living donors has been judged to be the estimate of the risk of performing a partial hepatectomy on the donor.[16] Questions also have been raised about the efficacy, necessity, and ethics of the approach.[17] Such transplants are also performed in other countries including Japan,[18,19] Brazil,[20] and Turkey.[21]

Organ donation by living donors brings into focus perplexing ethical problems because of the dangers of coercion and external as well as self-generated pressures on the donor. Liver transplant teams must evaluate the motives, capacities, and emotional feelings of prospective donors in a variety of factual contexts, while at the same time seeking to respect the freely made decisions of prospective donors with decision-making capacity and valuing the life-saving potential of this gift to the recipients and the satisfaction of donors. They have also struggled with the question as to what level of informed consent can be obtained in such situations and the role of altruism in such decisions.

For these reasons, various national guidelines have emphasized limiting living donation to those persons who are either genetically or emotionally related to the recipient, whose motives seem altruistic and not based on duty or coercion, and who can make informed decisions with a clear understanding of the risks and benefits involved. They typically require that potential donors not receive any economic reward other than payment of reasonable medical expenses and lost income. Such a guideline excludes almost all living unrelated donors (in contrast to living emotionally related donors). Finally, they seek to make clear to all parties that donors are not to be sacrificed for recipients.

The current number of liver transplants performed in the United States involving living donors remains small but has been growing steadily. The most recent statistics from UNOS/OPTN show an increase from 2 living donor transplants performed in 1989 to 252 in 1999, 385 in 2000, 506 in 2001, 353 in 2002, and 315 in 2003.[22]

Sale of Organs and Rewarded Gifting

The use of living unrelated organ donors may have begun, albeit unwittingly, in 1971 at the Christian Medical College in Vellore, India, when the kidney transplant surgeon, Dr. Mohan Rao, discovered that the donor, introduced to Dr. Rao as the recipient's *cousin*, was in fact a paid stranger.

There is a tradition in India of paying living related kidney donors. Media advertisements by both kidney donors and would-be recipients have been commonplace, as well as efforts to control the brokering of kidneys by carefully monitored programs in individual transplant centers. The argument is made that this practice is ethically acceptable in India because of the inability to provide dialysis for more than a small percentage of Indian patients with end-stage renal disease, and the social acceptance in India of paid donors as an alternative to the otherwise certain deaths of recipients.[23] Others have said that there is greater public sympathy in India for kidney donors in need of the money than for the hospitals and medical teams, who are viewed as exploitative.

There are also reports suggesting that wealthy recipients from the Middle East and western Asia who have gone to India or other countries in the developing world (such as the Philippines) for living unrelated kidney transplants have received inferior medical care, sustained higher than normal complication rates, and been financially exploited along with their donors. Such commercialized programs may inhibit the development of local transplant programs involving deceased donors because families of prospective donors see no reason to authorize the removal of organs if such organs are available elsewhere for purchase. This is particularly true if the society involved has cultural or religious objections to the concept of *brain death* and organ procurement.[24,25]

Western nations have been quick to condemn such practices. The National Organ Transplantation Act of 1984 in the United States makes the buying and selling of human organs illegal. The United Kingdom passed a similar law in 1989 after a scandal involving four paid Turkish donors hired by an organ broker was publicized. In 1990, three British physicians were disciplined for their role in those transplants.[26] Indeed, India in 1994 joined a list of more than 20 nations that have banned commercial payment for human organs used in transplantation.[27]

Yet, in the United States, donors of sperm and blood plasma are legally paid for their donations. It has been argued that given the chronic shortage of both deceased and even living related and emotionally related donors, there should be a program of *rewarded gifting* for organs just as there is for sperm and plasma.

Those arguing for such a program claim that even among related donors and recipients, money or some other reward is often secretly exchanged. Moreover, they suggest that persons should have the right to sell organs or tissues under controlled circumstances, and the benefit to recipients should be matched by a benefit to donors beyond abstract altruistic joy.

Those who argue most strenuously for a rewarded gifting program would exclude brokers and direct payment from recipients or transplant programs. They would change the nature of the reward from money to tax rebates or credits, burial grants, insurance policies, future medical coverage, or tuition subsidies for children. They would introduce a carefully regulated system in which both living related and living unrelated donors would be carefully evaluated by transplant centers under uniform medical and ethical guidelines with a third party, such as the government, independently handling the rewards after the transplant was completed.

Those opposed to rewarded gifting claim that such programs, even with the limits contemplated, would jeopardize public support for organ transplantation, particularly for deceased-donor organ donation. They claim that such programs would be costly and are unjustified without greater educational efforts to encourage donation. Some even argue that the use of living donors is increasingly unjustified in the face of improved techniques for deceased-donor organ transplantation and a failure to maximize the retrieval of deceased-donor organs.

The year 2003 saw possibly the high point in a flurry of reports of altruistic living unrelated donors when a donor in Philadelphia, having already given one kidney to a total stranger, publicly voiced his desire to give his remaining kidney to some other suitable recipient.[28]

Anencephalic and Xenograft Organs

Human organ transplants using anencephalic organ donors have been reported in the United States, Europe, and Japan. Xenograft organs have also been used, although largely in research on animals. Space does not permit a review of the ethical issues involving anencephalic and xenograft transplants, but there are concerns about the functional utility of the transplanted organs, the application of U.S. brain death standards in the case of anencephalic donors, the animal rights debate in the context of xenograft organs, and the currently unmet need each year for the many infants and children in the United States who require liver transplants.

The U.S. center with the greatest experience in seeking anencephalic organ donors (Loma Linda University Medical Center, California) concluded in 1989, after a research effort involving 12 infants and no successful transplants, that "it is usually not feasible, with the restrictions of current law [requiring total brain death], to procure solid organs for transplantation from anencephalic infants."[29]

Unfortunately, the experience with liver xenografts is no less problematic, although the issues are somewhat different. In the 20th century, more than 30 experiments were attempted with the goal of transplanting an animal organ into a human being, without long-term success. A team at the University of Pittsburgh in 1992 transplanted a liver from a 15-year-old male baboon into a 35-year-old white male with hepatitis B and human immunodeficiency virus who lived for 70 days after the procedure before suffering a fatal cerebral and subarachnoid hemorrhage that was caused by an *Aspergillus* infection.[30]

Xenografts have also been used as a bridge-to-transplantation device, and an experimental artificial liver system, called albumin dialysis, which uses an external filtering system incorporating living pig or human liver cells to remove toxic substances from the blood, has been used in early clinical trials in Germany (where the system was invented) and at the University of Michigan, among other sites.[31,32]

Questions remain as to the compatibility of nonhuman donors. Although chimpanzees are believed to be the most compatible to humans, they have been designated an endangered species and may not be imported into the United States. Dramatically increased breeding programs for donor animals would be necessary and would raise ethical concerns.[33] Those concerns include the objections to killing animals for this purpose and for the purpose of further research, as well as the pain and suffering the animals may endure during the research period. Arthur Caplan, an ethicist deeply involved in the transplantation field, argues that such xenograft research is ethically defensible "where no reasonable alternative therapy exists" and where appropriate ethical and scientific requirements have been met.[34]

Particularly relevant to the consideration of future xenograft experiments is the finding in blood samples from the 1992 Pittsburgh baboon-to-human liver recipient of infectious baboon cytomegalovirus.[35] Thus, careful preliminary research is necessary to justify inviting human participants in any such clinical xenograft trials.

Allocation of Organs Among Transplant Centers

In the United States, the OPTN is privately operated under government supervision. The National Organ Transplant Act (Public Law 98-507), passed by Congress in 1984, called for such a network to be established and administered by a nonprofit entity under contract to the U.S. Department of Health and Human Services (HHS).

UNOS was created as a legal entity in 1984 as an outgrowth of the South-Eastern Organ Procurement Foundation (SEOPF) of Richmond, Virginia. SEOPF was established in 1975 by several transplant centers as a means of sharing transplant information and protocols and of creating a shared computer registry system. Other U.S. transplant centers sought to join this computer registry, and in the late 1970s and early 1980s, a loosely formed national network was created with the SEOPF offices and computers as its center.

UNOS, beginning in September 1986, has administered the OPTN under contract with the Health Resources and Services Administration of the HHS. Following publication of an influential report by the National Academy of Science's Institute of Medicine,[36] HHS in March 2000 implemented a Final Rule (42 CFR Part 121) governing the operations of the OPTN and requiring OPTN policies to be submitted to the HHS Secretary for final approval.

The UNOS system for allocating the distribution of livers was originally developed during the late 1980s and early 1990s (see Chapter 38). Because of intense political as well as competitive pressures among national and regional liver transplant programs, which actually delayed the implementation of the Final Rule,[37] the liver allocation rules were changed in 2002 to promote a mandated sharing of donated livers (particularly for so-called status 1 patients) across large regions instead of sharing exclusively within local program priorities. The competition among liver transplant programs in itself raises important ethical questions worthy of consideration.[38]

In mid-2003, the OPTN/UNOS policy governing the allocation of livers (Policy 3.6) set out an allocation algorithm both for livers from adult donors (those 18 years of age and older) and for livers from pediatric donors. It also incorporates the Model for End-Stage Liver Disease (MELD) scoring system, first developed at the Mayo Clinic, as well as the Pediatric End-Stage Liver Disease (PELD) scoring system, both of which attempt to quantify through various factors the probability of the transplant candidate's death, that is, a mortality risk score. Points are also given to status 1 candidates for blood type similarity or compatibility and for time spent waiting on the OPTN/UNOS patient waiting list.

The current adult liver allocation algorithm gives first priority to status 1 patients—defined as "fulminant liver failure with a life expectancy, without a liver transplant, of less than 7 days"—as follows:

- First in descending point order at the local program
- Then to the same status 1 patients in descending point order at programs within the OPO region

- Then to local candidates in descending order of mortality risk (MELD) scores
- Then to regional candidates in the same order of MELD scores
- Finally to status 1 patients in descending point order nationally followed by all other national candidates in descending order of their MELD scores

The pediatric liver allocation algorithm is similar but permits pediatric donor livers to be given to adult candidates when feasible if there are no pediatric liver candidates: first to status 1 candidates at the local program level and then at the regional level.

The discussion in the early 1990s of the "feasibility, fairness, and enforceability" of a single national waiting list[39] has abated for the time being but may reemerge as competitive pressures among the programs ebb and flow.

Family Veto of Organ Donor Cards

The National Kidney Foundation and state motor vehicle departments in the United States have sought to portray the decision to donate organs as solely within the control of the would-be donor. Transplant programs or OPOs, however, have routinely permitted family members to veto such decisions. Even when properly signed organ donor cards were in the possession of transplant teams, the transplant teams or OPOs have routinely refused to honor such cards if family members objected, reportedly for public relations reasons. This occurs despite the Uniform Anatomical Gift Act (the model law written in 1968 to provide a legal basis for such gifts in advance of the death of the donor, and adopted in all of the states and the District of Columbia), which authorized such gifts by any person older than 18 years of age with decision-making capacity.

The mere fact that family members are even asked for their consent in the presence of a properly signed donor card suggests that the donor card process is misleadingly presented as a donor decision process. No warning is given to the donor card signer of the power of the family, in practice, to veto his or her decision to donate. It is in fact a family or next-of-kin decision process rather than a donor decision process. The ability of the family to veto raises ethical questions about campaigns to obtain signed donor cards.

As of mid-2004, 24 states* adopted a revised Uniform Anatomical Gift Act (1987), which specifically

provides that next of kin need not consent to organ donations if the document making the gift has not been revoked by the donor before death (section 2[h]). The new law also removes the previous legal requirement for a witness' signature on the donor card or other document (section 2[b]).

Required Request Laws

In the mid-1980s, many U.S. state legislatures began adopting laws requiring hospitals to develop policies that facilitated the possibility of organ donation. These policies required the identification as possible donors of all patients determined to be, or anticipated to soon become, "brain dead," and the offering to legal next of kin or other authorized person for such patients an opportunity to donate organs.

Almost all U.S. states have now adopted varying forms of such "routine inquiry/required request" laws, and federal law now mandates that all hospitals receiving Medicare or Medicaid funds have a process in place to make such donor inquiries. The theory behind this legal approach was that it would make more organs available, but that theory remains to be proved. Although organ donations have increased in some states and referrals to organ procurement agencies of potential donors have increased in all states, the actual number of all types of donor livers recovered has increased only slightly nationally (11.4%) from 2000 (5199) through 2003 (5997).

This result has prompted some commentators to suggest that the problem is not a legal one, but a psychological one on the part of attending physicians and nurses who do not wish either to be involved in or to see families *stressed* by organ donation requests at the time a loved one has died. Others, perhaps more pragmatic, have suggested that the better approach is to adopt *presumed consent* laws similar to those adopted in a number of U.S. states that permit the removal of pituitary glands and corneas from eligible cadavers unless the patient objected in writing prior to death or the family objected at the time of death. This approach assumes, of course, that public as well as judicial reaction will be equally tolerant to the removal of organs without explicit consent.

There appears to be a deeply felt preference among physicians for the organ procurement process to be a voluntary one. In France, which has presumed consent laws, physicians, for public relations reasons, continue to seek family consent despite the laws and refuse to take organs when families object. It also has been suggested that routine inquiry about organ donation preferences in the event of sudden death should become part of the standard medical history.

*Alabama, Arizona, Arkansas, California, Connecticut, Hawaii, Idaho, Indiana, Iowa, Minnesota, Montana, Nevada, New Hampshire, New Mexico, North Dakota, Oregon, Pennsylvania, Rhode Island, Tennessee, Utah, Vermont, Virginia, Washington, and Wisconsin

Selection of Patients for Transplantation

Equitable Selection and Access

The system of distribution of deceased-donor livers is theoretically blind to the possibility of discrimination based on age, race, gender, and socioeconomic status. In practice, this equity has not always proved to be the case, and unanticipated distortions in the allocation of donor organs may occur. There is evidence that women, African Americans, and low-income patients do not receive transplants at the same rate as white men with high incomes.

A patient must pass through several stages before actually receiving a transplant. First, he or she must be appropriately informed as to available treatment options (see Chapter 5, "Liver Allocation: The U.S. Model"). The patient is then referred for transplant evaluation (see Chapter 5). The transplant team, following a favorable consideration of relatively objective medical factors and subjective psychosocial factors, then offers the transplantation option to the patients they have helped educate. If the patient accepts, he or she is placed on the deceased-donor waiting list both locally and nationally. When a suitable liver becomes available, the patient receiving that organ must have priority over other patients based on the scoring system described previously (see Chapter 38).

Such a complex system is inevitably prone to distortion. Are all patients with liver failure equally educated as to their options? Do all primary physicians and hepatologists refer patients for evaluation expeditiously? Do all transplant programs distribute livers fairly? Similarly, we must assess the medical and biological factors (for example, the high levels of antibodies in multiparous women) that may affect organ distribution.

There are human factors that influence allocation decisions as well. Media stories in 1993 told of competition between large and small transplant programs that purportedly deprived the neediest end-stage liver disease patients of available organs,[40] the special relationships between certain hospitals and organ procurement agencies that lead to organs going to specific hospitals rather than patients with the greatest priority,[41] the accusation that being the governor of a state can help you jump to the head of the waiting list if you need a new liver and heart,[42] and the hefty markups by hospitals in the form of procurement charges for transplanted livers and other organs.[43] These controversial issues do not instill a public sense of fairness about the organ allocation process. Even professionals are unhappy. One surgeon-critic has written that "length of time on the waiting list is the least fair, most easily manipulated, and most mindless of all methods of organ allocation."[44] Others have complained of Medicare policies regarding accreditation of liver transplant programs that they claim amount to "rationing care on the basis of a program's statistics."[45] Some of the manipulation criticisms may have been alleviated by the adoption in 2002 of the OPTN/UNOS mandatory liver allocation algorithms mentioned earlier.

Age has also become a contentious issue, with some arguing that liver transplant patients older than 60 years do as well as younger patients and should not be excluded solely on grounds of age,[46] whereas others argue that in this "youth-oriented society," organs should go to the young on the basis of future productivity rather to older candidates on the basis of past productivity.[47] A survey in 1991 found that two thirds of the transplant centers polled had no specific age limit, whereas the remaining third excluded patients over a median age of 70 years.[48] OPTN/UNOS data as of 2002 showed that the number and percentage nationally of liver transplant recipients age 65 years and older has steadily increased from 1998 through 2002, with a slightly higher percentage of older recipients receiving living-donor organs—deceased-donor organs (1998, 316 recipients, 7.2%; 2002, 347 recipients, 7.0%), living donor organs (1998, 2 recipients, 2.1%; 2002, 15 recipients, 4.2%).[49,50]

Gender may also be a factor. In a study presented in 1993, researchers at the University of Pennsylvania Medical Center in Philadelphia found that there may be less obvious reasons to explain why of the 2700 cardiac transplants performed worldwide in 1992, 81% of the recipients were men. They found that 29% of all women accepted as cardiac transplant candidates at their own institution over a 4.5-year period refused the surgery, whereas only 9% of the men made that choice. In addition to their unwillingness to undergo transplantation, the age of these women was found to be more advanced when they developed cardiomyopathy, they had less favorable insurance status (less private insurance and more Medicaid coverage), and referring physicians were possibly more biased against transplants for women than for men.[51] Although the data for adults in the United States receiving liver transplants from all donor types between 1988 and 2003 show a smaller average percentage of women than men receiving transplants during this period (40.57% female recipients versus 59.43% male recipients), and 2003 data (the latest full year available) show one of the lowest percentages of female recipients in that 16-year period (34.1% female versus 65.9% male),[52] the possible relevance of extenuating factors remains unexplored. The data suggest that "there was a trend in 2002 toward a greater percentage of women receiving living donor liver transplants (43%) compared with deceased donors (34%), possibly because of size considerations."[52a]

Patients with End-Stage Alcoholic Liver Disease (Cirrhosis)

Although Starzl and colleagues argued that the policy of accepting patients with HIV for transplantation is more controversial than the practice of accepting carefully selected patients with a history of alcoholism,[53] some would challenge that assertion. Added to the stigma of alcoholism have been the medical arguments of:

- Typical multiorgan damage and severe malnutrition that could complicate the patient's ability to withstand the long surgical procedure and postoperative care
- The prospect of patient noncompliance with the lifelong immunosuppressive regimen in a manner (i.e., a return to alcohol) leading to rejection of the scarce organ[54]

A report from a transplant ethics committee at the University of Michigan suggested that the widespread unwillingness to consider such patients rests solely on the assumptions that alcoholics are "morally blameworthy" and that as a group, they will not "exhibit satisfactory rates of survival after transplantation"; such arguments were rejected by the university's observers.[55] Even so, a pair of ethicists have suggested that although not excluding them, transplant programs should *not* treat patients with alcohol-related end-stage liver disease as equal to other liver transplant candidates. Instead, they should be given a lower priority ranking on waiting lists than other patients and that only abstinent patients who have not previously been offered alcoholism treatment be accepted.[56] A counter argument is to *not* link the degree of responsibility for liver damage to medical priority for transplantation and to use more objective criteria for assessing responsibility for one's health[57] as well as to improve posttransplant techniques so as to reduce relapse to alcohol or substance abuse.[58]

A glance at the actual experience of liver programs around the world with such patients provides a generally positive picture. The University of Pittsburgh performed transplantations in 221 patients with alcoholic liver disease (cirrhosis and hepatitis) in a 6-year period between 1986 and 1992 and found that patients with alcoholic cirrhosis had a similar survival and posttransplant hospitalization rate as those with alcoholic hepatitis (with or without associated cirrhosis), but a much higher long-term (2-year) sobriety rate (80% to 90% versus 40% to 50%) than the hepatitis group.[59] A study at the University of California, San Francisco, of 43 patients with alcoholic liver disease over a 3-year period (composing 16.7% of all adult liver transplants performed at that institution during 1988 to 1991) showed a higher survival rate for this subgroup than for the entire group of orthotopic liver transplant patients (100% versus 81%), a lower retransplantation rate (0 versus 8%), and a pattern of similar outcomes in terms of compliance, return to employment, and a return to drinking alcohol after transplantation (approximately 19%).[60]

A University of Wisconsin study (41 patients with alcoholic cirrhosis who underwent transplantation from 1984 to 1990) also found no difference in alcohol use between posttransplant patients with alcoholic liver disease and nonalcoholic patients and a similar rate of survival, postoperative morbidity, depression, self-perceived health status, employment, and role functioning.[61] Similar positive reports have come from transplant programs in Germany,[62] France,[63] and Switzerland,[64] with the program in Geneva finding useful the involvement of an ethics committee in the selection of such patients. Finally, observations about the potentially greater risk of alcoholic liver disease for women[65] and the possibility that liver transplantation can improve cognitive functioning in patients with alcoholic cirrhosis, possibly reversing hepatic encephalopathy,[66] may be relevant to decisions about the ethics of accepting such patients for transplantation.

Retransplantation

As a generalization, one can observe a serious difference in perception of ethical duties toward specific patients on the part of transplant surgeons and other team members as compared with nontransplant team professionals. Transplant surgeons in particular almost invariably feel a greater duty toward patients on whom they have already operated in contrast to patients who have been accepted for transplantation and are awaiting their first organ, despite the fact that technically all are their patients at least in terms of the transplant programs in which they are involved or lead. This is particularly true with pediatric patients.

For this reason, the issue of retransplantation can become extremely controversial for some and totally routine for others, even if patients' lives hang in the balance. If donor livers are scarce and retransplantation of one patient is chosen over primary transplantation of another, the latter may die on the waiting list, and the issue of fairness or equity becomes relevant. Resource allocation and rationing decisions involved in such choices are difficult to sweep away by simple assertions of the principle of "first come, first served" because the avoidance of one patient's death may lead to the possible detriment, even death, of another.

Also, we are not simply talking about only *one* retransplanted liver. In a study of 151 retransplanted liver patients at the University of Pittsburgh between 1987 and 1990, 28 (19%) had a *second* retransplant, and 6 (4%) had a *third*.[67] Similarly, in a University of Wisconsin study of 58 retransplant patients from 1984 to 1992, 34 (77%) had *two* retransplants, 7 (16%) had *three*, 2 (5%) had *four*, and one (2%) had *five*.[68] Retransplantation can obviously be beneficial to patients if used selectively. Although the length of stay and cost of retransplantation is higher than that for primary transplants, the overall actuarial 1-year and 5-year survival in one program was found to be only slightly lower for retransplanted patients (86.6% versus 74.8% at 1 year, 71.4% versus 62.5% at 5 years).[68] Poorer outcomes have been associated with emergency retransplantation associated with primary nonfunction, early hepatic artery thrombosis, acute rejection, and other causes, including hepatitis B.[69,70] Even among these disease categories, those with primary nonfunction of the graft may have a longer survival rate after retransplantation than those with acute rejection or arterial thrombosis.[71] The timing of such retransplantation is also crucial to their success, particularly if emergent retransplantation is to be avoided.[72]

A 2003 study looking at data from 1988 through 2001 argues that retransplantation is associated with "a greater rate of complications and lower patient and graft survival" than primary liver transplantation, and that retransplantation for primary graft nonfunction and hepatitis C virus infection "was associated with lower patient and graft survival compared with retransplantation for other causes."[73]

All that said, however, the question remains whether any retransplantation is ever justified, (whether the initial liver disease was alcoholic in origin or of any other kind), much less retransplantation with an indefinite number of new livers to replace failing ones. Transplant surgeons have generally argued that as long as the patient and graft survival rates for retransplants were comparable to those of primary transplants (and survival rates for all have improved in recent years with new immunosuppressive regimens), such procedures were justified.[74] However, the most recent data, cited previously, suggest that the results are not, in fact, comparable. The UNOS Ethics Committee, although acknowledging "the issue of justice in considering repeat transplantation," has articulated the seemingly contradictory view that "Graft failure, particularly early or immediate failure, evokes significant concerns regarding repeat transplantation. However, the likelihood of long-term survival of a repeat transplant should receive strong consideration."[75]

Looking at the issue from a health economics vantage point, Roger Evans and colleagues published a study cosponsored by UNOS and the U.S. Health Care Financing Administration that reviewed the experience with all patients who underwent retransplantation in the United States during 1988. They found that the difference in the comparative median charges for primary liver grafts versus retransplanted grafts were significant ($132,282 versus $338,660) and that comparative 1-year survival figures for such grafts were also noteworthy (68.7% for primary grafts versus 50.1% for retransplanted grafts). They concluded that given the expense involved, the patients denied their chance for a primary graft, and the public's concern about scarce health care resources in general, "retransplantation constitutes a cost-ineffective use of scarce donor organs, the outcome of which is disconcerting."[76]

These issues can only become more inflammatory when patient noncompliance with immunosuppressive medication is seen as the cause of graft failure, but that only begs the question of whether any patient's death from graft failure related to an allocation decision can be more easily justified. Given the acknowledged scarcity in livers, this ethical question may be the most difficult one that liver transplant teams will be forced to face in the future, particularly because retransplantation now accounts for 10% of all liver transplants performed.[77]

Role of Perceived Noncompliance in Selection

One initial exclusionary factor that is not widely understood is the role of perceived or past noncompliance with medical regimens. This psychosocial issue affords great opportunity for discrimination because it can be used to deny access unfairly if used too loosely. Indeed, there is often no scientific study to establish that even relatively objective social factors correlate with outcome, thus affording a mask for utilitarian or prejudicial judgments.[78]

Noncompliance is best measured by looking to relatively objective criteria such as the patient's past record of keeping medical appointments, taking prescribed drugs in the proper regimen, stopping substance abuse (smoking, alcohol, and drugs) and maintaining abstinence with professional assistance, and obtaining psychological or psychiatric therapy for diagnosed mental health problems. Indeed, perhaps the most scientific assessment of this aspect of the selection process has been done by the specialist transplant psychiatrists, whose literature is insightful and candid.[79-81]

The presence of a social support system in the form of family or friends is obviously crucial and can overcome a patient's physical and learning disabilities. On the contrary, the absence of a support network and the inability of the patient to understand or comply with the demands of a lifelong treatment regimen and to make medical appointments can be a legitimate reason for denying a transplant to a patient based on the scarcity of the resource involved—the donor livers—and the other potential recipients waiting for such organs.

Foreign Nationals as Potential Recipients

Press reports during the 1980s of foreign nationals "buying their way to the front of the line" for kidney transplants raised the issue as to whether organs donated by U.S. citizens and residents ought to be restricted to U.S. recipients. In 1985, some 300 of the approximately 6000 deceased-donor kidneys transplanted in the United States went to nonresident patients who came to the United States for the procedures. There was a suggestion that in communities with extensive media publicity about foreign patients receiving transplanted kidneys, deceased-donor donations fell below previous levels.

Although some argued that humanitarian considerations precluded the use of national citizenship as a criterion for acceptance as a recipient, others suggested that the donated organs are a national resource and that U.S. citizens should at least have priority over foreign nationals. Others proposed a ceiling or cap on the number of nonresident aliens who could be put on any one program's waiting list, but then treating all on the list equally.

In response to this concern, the American Society of Transplant Surgeons adopted guidelines in 1986 limiting the transplantation of organs into foreign nationals "to an average of 5% per year of the organs transplanted at any single center" and mandating that the charges for such transplants be on the same basis as the charges to U.S. citizens. The UNOS board, in 1988, adopted a somewhat similar policy that provided for the potential review by a UNOS committee of any program's transplants involving foreign nationals, and the automatic review of any UNOS member center that has foreign nationals constituting more than 10% of its recipients. The UNOS policy also requires that patients accepted for organ transplants be treated equally under UNOS guidelines for the distribution of organs.

In 1993, the United States Congress was considering, as part of the reauthorization bill for the National Organ Transplant Act, a mandatory requirement that organ transplant centers place non-U.S. residents on a second, lower priority waiting list, which could only be reached after the main waiting list had been cleared of patients, a policy reportedly followed in other nations.[39] No such requirement was forthcoming, however, and the latest version of the pertinent OPTN/UNOS policy (Policy 6.0, *Transplantation of Non-Resident Aliens*, last revised in July 2004):

- Continues the policy of nondiscrimination in transplant allocation decisions regarding non-U.S. residents

- Allows for audits of transplant programs "where nonresident alien recipients constitute more than 5% of recipients of any particular type of deceased-donor organ"
- Reinforces the point that selection of patients "shall not be influenced by favoritism or discrimination based on political influence, national origin, race, sex, religion, or financial status" and that non-U.S. residents not be charged higher fees than domestic residents.[82]

Resource Allocation Issues

Future of Federal Funding for Organ Transplantation

Despite superficial similarities, there are differences in solid organ transplantation programs. Unlike any other solid organ transplantation effort, kidney transplantation usually has hemodialysis as a long-term fallback modality, whereas liver, heart, lung, and pancreas transplant recipients have no similar treatment mechanism at this time. Thus, although kidney transplantation led the way and remains the volume leader in the transplantation community (the UNOS figures for 2002 show 14,523 *kidneys* transplanted in the United States, 5060 *livers*, 2111 *hearts*, 31 *heart-lung combinations*, 1041 *lungs*, and 1778 *other organs or multiorgan procedures*),[83] there is a potential source of tension among the various transplant teams.

This competitiveness has been observed vividly when organ procurement teams jockeyed for position as to which organs were to be removed first. Collegial collaboration was mixed with a sense of a *pecking order* in which liver and heart teams were placed before kidney teams, partly because of their claim of a life-and-death time struggle and partly because of their greater recent media publicity. Fortunately, the technical aspects of multiorgan procurement have been resolved, and the capacity to store organs for longer periods has helped to defuse a potential source of tension. There may remain a sense of inequity over the full Medicare funding of kidney transplants in contrast to the more limited federal funding for liver, heart, and other organ or multiorgan transplants.

We stand on the verge of significant technological breakthroughs in clinical medicine that may radically alter the distribution of our resources. Human gene therapy has begun in closely monitored research trials at the National Institutes of Health and elsewhere. Those involved in the exploration and mapping of the human genome predict not only the identification of most of the genes but also the development of techniques to engineer proteins that can optimize gene functioning or even create new gene functions for particular kinds of organs. The combination of artificial devices and liver cell biology may replace surgical transplants of livers in the future.[84]

Thus, it may be possible to address end-stage liver disease as a disease process by totally different medical treatment approaches in the future without the use of whole or partial liver transplantation, at least for some patients. Will we then, as a society, be willing to invest the large sums of money required to produce and clinically apply such new treatment modalities? If the funding mechanism for health care is correctly perceived as a national combination of public and private funds, who will determine these priorities? Which diseases will get the greatest attention and funding? Will transplantation be as exciting as the new gene therapy and other aspects of molecular medicine that are developed in the next several decades?

Underlying these issues is a much more troublesome question, namely, should the sickest patients get the available organs? Are urgent or emergency transplants for acetaminophen overdose ever justified, particularly when the recipients cannot themselves consent to the procedure and agree to the lifelong drug and other regimens required to maintain the graft? Purely scientific studies of transplant efficacy might argue for giving grafts to those who are the least sick and the most likely to survive the longest and with the least complications with their new organ. This approach, however, conflicts with the symbolic idea of the "rescue at death's door," which currently controls the waiting list priorities. Also lurking in the background is the question of whether patients benefit from the presence of more than 120 liver transplant programs in the United States in addition to the 700 plus transplant programs at U.S. medical institutions. Also, do the financial and donor organ resources necessary to support them, while beneficial to the institutions and professionals involved and to their trainees, maximize the best possible outcome for individual patients and promote the most appropriate values for the society as a whole?

Two distinguished sociologists of science, who involved themselves in the transplantation field for decades, announced in 1992 that they were leaving the field, intentionally separating themselves from what they believed "has become an overly zealous medical and societal commitment to the endless perpetuation of life and to repairing and rebuilding people through organ replacement—and from the human suffering, and the social, cultural, and spiritual harm [they] believe such unexamined excess can, and already has, brought in its wake."[85]

There remains the possibility that those in a position to influence these decisions (which are as much political and business decisions as they are medical and scientific ones) may decide, as the Clinton administration hinted, that primary and preventive care should take precedence over acute care programs, such as organ transplantation, and thus receive funding priority and greater patient access. These resource allocation or rationing decisions, as they are sometimes labeled, are going to be particularly difficult when those competing for funding pit diseases with larger populations against those that are rarer, those with greater mortality against those with lesser morbidity, those that affect majority populations against those that only affect specific races or ethnic groups, and the like. Hospitals threatened with financial ruin or forced mergers may find in the future that transplant programs, currently a significant revenue enhancer, will be less attractive if funding patterns change or if patient populations shift. Changes to managed care systems have only exacerbated these problems despite the historical support by the public in the United States for *rescue* technology.

With health care spending spiraling ever higher and many patients and providers fighting for their share of that health care funding pie, these issues will have to be faced, and they have enormous ethical implications. They will also require the commitment by surgeons and others to justify existing and new approaches to liver transplantation by carefully designed clinical trials, such as those suggested for the treatment of severe liver disease.[86] This all assumes, however, that the health care portion of the societal budget maintains its present significant percentage and growth pattern.

Future of Health Care Expenditures

In the United States, the seeming primacy of health care costs over other government expenses is being increasingly questioned. The relevant statistics offer some insight. Recently published data show that overall health care costs in the United States have passed the trillion-dollar mark and are skyrocketing upward toward the 2 trillion dollar figure. In 2002 (the latest year for which statistics are available), the United States spent $1.6 trillion on health care, which translates to $5440 per capita or 14.9% of the gross national product.[87]

As talk of rationing and cost containment becomes more fashionable, particularly in a context of national economic budgetary constraints in the face of a massive federal deficit and debt, it will be interesting to see whether the U.S. public will continue to support such priorities for health care over potentially competing claims for law enforcement and prisons, education, and social welfare (to mention only three). Medicare and Medicaid budget cuts at the federal level and state government budget cuts may either reduce public funding for transplant programs or, at the very least, prevent their expansion to treat new patients.

Some commentators suggest that although Congress may have authorized Medicare funding for end-stage renal disease therapy in 1972 because it believed that saving life should take priority over other values, including cost and cost-effectiveness, the federal government's values may have shifted to place cost containment higher than the survival of individual citizens. If that is a correct assessment, future liver transplantation programs in the United States will have to cope with the same issues of funding equity and priority and patient access that similar programs in other parts of the world have been facing.

Acknowledgment

Portions of this chapter have been adapted, with permission of the publisher, from my chapter, "Ethical and Legal Issues in Kidney Transplantation." In Danovitch GM (ed): Handbook of Kidney Transplantation, 3rd ed. Philadelphia, Lippincott Williams & Wilkins, 2001, pp 380-393.

References

1. Organ Procurement and Transplantation Network online: Transplants by Donor, U.S. Transplants Performed: January 1, 1988 to June 30, 2004, For Organ = Liver, Format = Portrait. Availalbe at www.optn.org/data.
2. Organ Procurement and Transplantation Network online: 2003 Annual Report, Table 9.3, Reported deaths and annual death rates per 1,000 patient years at risk, 1993 to 2002, liver waiting list. Available at www.optn.org/AR2003/903_li.pdf.
3. Organ Procurement and Transplantation Network online: 2003 Annual Report, Table 2.4, Deceased donor characteristics, 1993 to 2002, liver donors. Available at www.optn.org/AR2003/204_age_dc.htm.
4. Orians CE, Evans RW, Ascher NL: Estimates of organ-specific donor availability for the United States. Transplant Proc 25:1541, 1993.
4a. Guadagnoli E, Christiansen CL, Beasley CL: Potential organ-donor supply and efficiency of organ procurement organizations. Health Care Financ Rev 24:101, 2003.
5. President's Commission for the Study of Ethical Problems in Medicine and Biomedical and Behavioral Research: Guidelines for determination of death. JAMA 246:2184, 1981.
6. President's Commission for the Study of Ethical Problems in Medicine and Biomedical and Behavioral Research: Defining Death: A Report on the Medical, Legal, and Ethical Issues in the Determination of Death. Washington D.C., U.S. Government Printing Office, 1981.
7. Rothenberg LS: The anencephalic neonate and brain death: An international review of medical, ethical, and legal issues. Transplant Proc 22:1037, 1990.
8. Byrne PA, Nilges RG: The brain stem in brain death: A critical view. Issues Law Med 9:3, 1993.
9. Arnold RM, Youngner SJ (eds): Ethical, psychosocial, and public policy implications of procuring organs from non-heart-beating cadavers. Kennedy Inst Ethics J 3:103, 1993.
10. Truog RF, Fackler JC: Rethinking brain death. Crit Care Med 20:1705, 1992.
11. Palmer LP Jr.: Organ Transplants from Executed Prisoners: An Argument for the Creation of Death Sentence Organ Removal Statutes. Jefferson, NC, McFarland, 1999.
12. Singer PA, Lantos JD, Whitington PF, et al: Equipoise and the ethics of segmental liver transplantation. Clin Res 36:539, 1988.
13. Singer PA, Siegler M, Whitington PF, et al: Ethics of liver transplantation with living donors. N Engl J Med 321:620, 1989.
14. Cotton P: Living-donor liver transplants cap surgical research for decade of 1980s: News. JAMA 263:13, 1990.
15. Goldman LS: Liver transplantation using living donors: Preliminary donor psychiatric outcomes. Psychosomatics 34:235, 1993.
16. Siegler M: Liver transplantation using living donors. Transplant Proc 24:2223, 1992.
17. McMaster P, Czerniak A: Living related liver transplantation: A note of caution. In Land W, Dossetor JB (eds): Organ Replacement Therapy: Ethics, Justice and Commerce. Berlin, Springer-Verlag, 1991, pp 130-135.
18. Shimahara Y, Awane M, Yamaoka Y, et al: Safety and operative stress for donors in living-related partial liver transplantation. Transplant Proc 25:1081, 1993.
19. Tanaka K, Uemoto S, Tokunaga Y, et al: Liver transplantation in children from living-related donors. Transplant Proc 25:1084, 1993.
20. Segre M: Partial liver transplantation from living donors. Camb Q Healthc Ethics 4:305, 1992.
21. Haberal M, Telatar H, Bilgin B, et al: Living related liver transplantation in an adult and child: Medical risk and benefit in non-renal donors. In Land W, Dossetor JB (eds): Organ Replacement Therapy: Ethics, Justice And Commerce. Berlin, Springer-Verlag, 1991, pp 83-92.
22. Organ Procurement and Transplantation Network online: Donors Recovered in the U.S. by donor type, donors recovered: January 1, 1988-June 30, 2004, for organ = liver. Available at www.optn.org/data.
23. Reddy KC, Thiagarajan CM, Shunmugasundaram D, et al: Unconventional renal transplantation in India. Transplant Proc 22:910, 1990.
24. Johny KV, Nesim J, Namboori N, Gupta RK: Values gained and lost in live unrelated renal transplantation. Transplant Proc 22:915, 1990.
25. Abouna GM, Kumar MSA, Samhan M, et al: Commercialization in human organs: A Middle Eastern perspective. Transplant Proc 21:918, 1990.
26. Gray M: 3 British physicians found guilty for roles in paid kidney donations. Am Med News 3:38, 1990.
27. Transplantation of Human Organs Act India Central (Act No. 42 of 1994), s.19.
28. Strom S: An organ donor's generosity raises the question of how much is too much. New York Times, August 17, 2003, sect. 1, p 13.
29. Peabody JL, Emery JR, Ashwal S: Experience with anencephalic infants as prospective organ donors. N Engl J Med 321:344, 1989.
30. Starzl TE, Fung J, Tzakis A, et al: Baboon-to-human liver transplantation. Lancet 341:65, 1993.
31. Awad SS, Swaniker F, Magee J, et al: Results of a phase I trial evaluating a liver support device utilizing albumin dialysis. Surgery 130:354, 2001.
32. Stange J, Hassanein TI, Mehta R, et al: The molecular adsorbents recycling system as a liver support system based on albumin dialysis: A summary of preclinical investigations, prospective, randomized, controlled clinical trial, and clinical experience from 19 centers. Artif Organs 26:103, 2002.
33. Reetsma K: Xenografts. Transplant Proc 24:2225, 1992.
34. Caplan AL: Ethical issues raised by research involving xenografts. In Caplan AL (ed): If I Were a Rich Man Could I Buy a Pancreas? and Other Essays on the Ethics of Health Care. Bloomington, IN, Indiana University Press, 1992, pp 178-191.

35. Michaels MG, Jenkins FJ, St George K, et al: Detection of infectious baboon cytomegalovirus after baboon-to-human liver xenotransplantation. J Virol 75:2825, 2001.

36. Institute of Medicine: Organ procurement and transplantation: Assessing current policies and the potential impact of the DHSS Final Rule. Washington, DC, National Academies Press, 1999.

37. Weimer DL: Values and interests in private regulation: The OPTN liver allocation rules [manuscript, 2002] online. Available at http://www.essex.ac.uk/ECPR/events/jointsessions/paper archive/ turin/ws18/Weimer.pdf.

38. Thomasma DC, Micetich KC, Brems J, Van Thiel D: The ethics of competition in liver transplantation. Camb Q Healthc Ethics 8:321, 1999.

39. McCartney S: Law may allow few transplants for foreigners. Wall St J B1, 1993 June 30.

40. McCartney S: People most needing transplantable livers now often miss out. Wall Street Journal, April 1, 1993:A1, A6.

41. McCartney S: Allocation of organs disregards needs of patient, may break law, GAO says. Wall Street Journal, April 23, 1993:B6.

42. Belkin L: Fairness debated in quick transplant. New York Times, June 16, 1993:A8.

43. Winslow R: Organ-transplant recipients often pay hospitals hefty markups, study asserts. Wall Street Journal, June 23, 1993:B4.

44. Jonasson O: Waiting in line: Should selected patients ever be moved up? Transplant Proc 21:3390, 1989.

45. Burck R, Sheldon M, Burton LA, et al: Limiting access and patient selection in liver transplantation: Letter. N Engl J Med 326:413, 1992.

46. Emre S, Mor E, Schwartz ME, et al: Liver transplantation in patients beyond age 60. Transplant Proc 25:1075, 1993.

47. Randall T: Successful liver transplantation in older patients raises new hopes, challenges, ethics questions: News. JAMA 264:428, 1990.

48. Randall T: Criteria for evaluating potential transplant recipients vary among centers, physicians: News. JAMA 269:3091, 1993.

49. Organ Procurement and Transplantation Network online: 2003 Annual Report, Table 9.4a, Transplant recipient characteristics, 1993 to 2002, recipients of deceased donor livers. Available at http://www.optn.org/AR2003/904a_age_li.htm.

50. Organ Procurement and Transplantation Network online: 2003 Annual Report, Table 9.4b, Transplant recipient characteristics, 1993 to 2002, recipients of living donor livers. Available at http://www.optn.org/AR2003/904b_age_li.htm.

51. Randall T: The gender gap in selection of cardiac transplantation candidates: Bogus or bias?: News. JAMA 269:2718, 1993.

52. Organ Procurement and Transplantation Network online: Transplants in the U.S. by recipient gender, U.S. transplants performed: January 1, 1998-June 30, 2004, for organ = liver, format = portrait. Available at www.optn.org/data.

52a. Organ Procurement and Transplantation Network online: 2003 Annual Report, Chap. VII ("Liver and Intestine Transplantation"). Available at http://www.optn.org/AR2003/Chapter_VII_AR_ CD.htm.

53. Starzl TE, Demetris AJ, Van Thiel D: Liver transplantation (pt. 1). N Engl J Med 321:1014, 1989.

54. Schwartzman K: In veno veritas?: Alcoholics and liver transplantation. Can Med Assoc J 141:1262, 1989.

55. Cohen C, Benjamin M, and the Ethics and Social Impact Committee of the Transplant and Health Policy Center, Ann Arbor, MI: Alcoholics and liver transplantation. JAMA 265:1299, 1991.

56. Moss AH, Siegler M: Should alcoholics compete equally for liver transplantation? JAMA 265:1295, 1991.

57. Martens W: Do alcoholic liver transplantation candidates merit lower medical priority than non-alcoholic candidates? Transpl Int 14:170, 2001.

58. DiMartini A, Weinrieb R, Fireman M: Liver transplantation in patients with alcohol and other substance abuse disorders. Psychiatr Clin North Am 25:195, 2002.

59. Bonet H, Manez R, Kramer D, et al: Survival of patients transplanted with alcoholic hepatitis plus cirrhosis as compared to those with cirrhosis alone. Transplant Proc 25:1126, 1993.

60. Osorio RW, Freise CE, Ascher NL, et al: Orthotopic liver transplantation for end-stage alcoholic liver disease. Transplant Proc 25:1133, 1993.

61. Knechtle SJ, Fleming MF, Barry KL, et al: Liver transplantation in alcoholics: Assessment of psychological health and work activity. Transplant Proc 25:1916, 1993.

62. Platz KP, Mueller AR, Spree E, et al: Liver transplantation for alcoholic cirrhosis. Transpl Int 13(Suppl 1):S127, 2000.

63. Pageaux GP, Souche B, Perney P, et al: Results and cost of orthotopic liver transplantation for alcoholic cirrhosis. Transplant Proc 25:1135, 1993.

64. Rohner A: La transplantation hepatique dans la cirrhose alcoolique est-elle legitime? [Is liver transplantation for alcoholic cirrhosis justified?]. Schweiz Med Wochenschr 122:628, 1992.

65. Killeen TK: Alcoholism and liver transplantation: Ethical and nursing implications. Perspect Psychiatr Care 29:7, 1993.

66. Arria AM, Tarter RE, Starzl TE, Van Thiel DH: Improvement in cognitive functioning of alcoholics following orthotopic liver transplantation. Alcohol Clin Exp Res 15:956, 1991.

67. Morel P, Rilo HLR, Tzakis AG, et al: Liver retransplantation in adults: Overall results and determinant factors affecting the outcome. Transplantation 23:3029, 1991.

68. D'Alessandro AM, Ploeg RJ, Knechtle SJ, et al: Retransplantation of the liver—a seven-year experience. Transplantation 55:1083, 1993.

69. Mora NP, Klintmalm GB, Cofer JB, et al: Results after liver transplantation (RETx): A comparative study between "elective" vs. "nonelective" RETx. Transplant Proc 22:1509, 1990.

70. Mora NP, Klintmalm GB, Cofer JB, et al: Results after liver retransplantation in a group of 50 regrafted patients: Two different concepts of elective versus emergency retransplantation. Transpl Int 4:231, 1991.

71. Fangmann J, Ringe B, Hauss J, Pichlmayr R: Hepatic retransplantation: The Hannover experience of two decades. Transplant Proc 25:1077, 1993.

72. Anthuber M, Pratschke E, Jauch KW, et al: Liver retransplantation—indications, frequency, results. Transplant Proc 24:1965, 1992.

73. Yoo HY, Maheshwari A, Thuluvath PJ: Retransplantation of liver: Primary graft nonfunction and hepatitis C virus are associated with worse outcome. Liver Transpl 9:897, 2003.

74. Almond PS, Matas AJ, Gillingham K, et al: Risk factors for second renal allografts immunosuppressed with cyclosporine. Transplantation 52:253, 1991.

75. Ethics Committee, United Network for Organ Sharing: General considerations in assessment for transplant candidacy (accesssed at www.optn.org/resources/bioethics.asp?index = 4).

76. Evans RW, Manninen DL, Dong FB, McLynne DA: Is retransplantation cost effective? Transplantation 25:1694, 1993.

77. Biggins SW, Beldecos A, Rabkin JM, Rosen HR: Retransplantation for hepatic allograft failure: Prognostic modeling and ethical considerations. Liver Transplant 8:313, 2002.

78. Robertson JA: Patient selection for organ transplantation: Age, incarceration, family support, and other social factors. Transplant Proc 21:3397, 1989.

79. Wolcott DE: Organ transplantation psychiatry. Psychosomatics 34:112, 1993.

80. Levenson JL, Olbrisch ME: Psychiatric aspects of heart transplantation. Psychosomatics 34:114, 1993.

81. Twillman RK, Manetto C, Wellisch DK, Wolcott DL: The transplant evaluation rating scale: A revision of the psychosocial levels system for evaluating organ transplant candidates. Psychosomatics 34:144, 1993.

82. Organ Procurement and Transplantation Network online: Policy 6.0, Transplantation of non-residents aliens. Available at http://www.unos.org/PoliciesandBylaws/policies/pdfs/policy_18.pdf.

83. Organ Procurement and Transplantation Network online: 2002 Annual Report, Table 1.8, Transplants by organ and donor type, 1993 to 2002. Available at http://www.optn.org/AR2003/108_dh.htm.

84. Di Campli C, Nestola M, Piscaglia AC, et al: Cell-based therapy for liver diseases. Eur Rev Med Pharmacol Sci 7:41, 2003.

85. Fox RC, Swazey JP: Leaving the field. Hastings Cent Rep 22:9, 1992.

86. Mullhaupt B, Kullak-Ublick GA, Ambuhl P, et al: First clinical experience with Molecular Adsorbent Recirculating System (MARS) in six patients with severe acute chronic liver failure. Liver 22(Suppl 2):59, 2002.

87. U.S. Centers for Medicare and Medicaid Services online: Highlights-National health expenditures, 2002. Available at cms.hhs.gov/statistics/nhe/historical/highlights.asp?

Psychosocial Assessment of Adult Liver Transplant Recipients

SHEILA JOWSEY
TERRY SCHNEEKLOTH

Psychiatrist's role   395
   Components of the psychiatric
      evaluation   396

Special issues in transplant patients   397
   Adapting to the waiting period   397
   Management of mood disorders   398
   Familial amyloidosis   399
   Cancer   399
   Hepatitis C   399
   Management of personality disorders   400
   Alcoholism and substance abuse   400
   Nicotine dependence   401
   Obesity   402
   Geriatric patients   402

Psychiatrist's Role

Individuals who undergo transplantation experience one of the most stressful and potentially rewarding interventions in modern medicine. Patients who are near death can be restored to health but will live with a demanding medical regimen of immunosuppressive medication and medical monitoring. It is understandable that patients need to be evaluated to determine how they are coping with their life-threatening illness and to evaluate if psychiatric comorbidities will diminish their ability to adapt to the transplant regimen. A consensus exists in the mental health community that pretransplant screening of transplant candidates is best provided by a multidisciplinary team that may include a psychiatrist, psychologist, social worker, chaplain, clinical nurse specialist, and chemical dependency counselors.[1,2] The goals of this multidisciplinary team are to understand the experience of the patient, assess the durability of the patient's support system, determine if psychiatric conditions preclude the patient's ability to comply with the transplant regimen, and support the mental health of the patient and the family during the waiting period.

Little has been written about how best to integrate the roles of mental health specialists striving to assess and intervene during the pretransplant period. There is no current standard for the psychosocial selection criteria for transplantation.[2] Ideally, both a psychiatrist or psychologist and a social worker will assess the patient. Psychiatrists can diagnose psychiatric conditions, recommend pharmacological interventions, detect neurocognitive impairments caused by encephalopathy that may otherwise be missed, and assess motivation and family support. Psychologists also perform diagnostic evaluations, recommend behavioral interventions, and provide counseling and psychometric testing. Social workers screen for past psychiatric problems, monitor for psychological distress on the part of the patient and family, and assist with the financial and insurance needs of the patients. Ill patients with complex medical conditions and distressed families benefit from a multidisciplinary team approach that brings the expertise of all these specialties to bear. A chaplain can provide crucial emotional support to transplant patients, and the use of religious coping can enhance adjustments for patients and their families. Chemical dependency counselors can provide diagnostic evaluations and ongoing monitoring of alcoholic cirrhotics, which is invaluable in detecting alcoholic relapse.

Because of the scarcity of organs, every transplant team struggles with the assessment of patients who appear to be at higher risk for noncompliance or poor adaptation to transplantation. The psychiatrist, psychologist, and social worker all assist in the evaluation of patients who have increased risk, including chemically dependent patients, patients with impulsive behavior or a history of poor compliance, and patients with a history of self-destructive behavior. Presenting the results of the multidisciplinary evaluation to the transplant team's selection conference provides an important opportunity for the discussion of factors suggestive of a poor outcome. Additionally, transplant nurse coordinators can contribute information about maladaptive behavior or evidence of limited coping skills noted as the patient interacts with the medical team. Figure 27–1 presents a possible decision-making process.

Components of the Psychiatric Evaluation

The psychiatrist's goal is to understand how the patient is adapting to his or her illness and to screen for psychiatric pathology. The psychiatrist conducts an extensive psychiatric interview (Table 27–1) and assesses how the patient's physical symptoms have affected his or her life. Typically, patients with end-stage liver disease complain of fatigue, insomnia, pruritus, discomfort from ascites, decreased concentration, or confusion because of encephalopathy. Often, their ability to work, drive, or perform household work diminishes. This may result in spouses, adult children, and other family

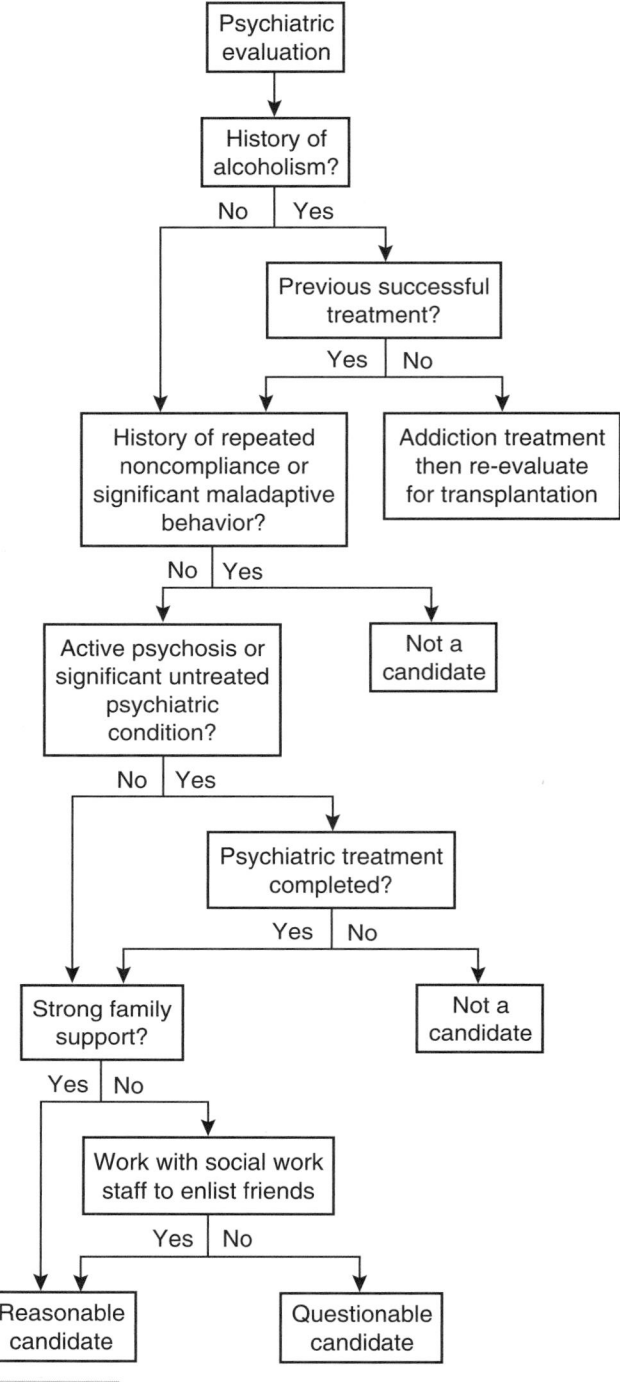

FIGURE 27–1

Decision Tree: Psychosocial Assessment of Adult Liver Transplant Candidates.

members assuming tasks for which the patient previously had been responsible. Potential loss of insurance, decreased wage earning capacity, and guilt over the inability to provide can all add to the patient's stress. Family relations can also be strained, as spouses assume more caretaking responsibilities and hold down jobs to maintain health care insurance.

Table 27–1. TRANSPLANT PSYCHIATRIC INTERVIEW
Patient's reaction to end-stage disease
Knowledge about transplantation
History of compliance
Acceptance of posttransplant medical regimen, including need for daily immunosuppressives, and medical follow-up
Family reaction to health
Psychiatric review of systems
Past psychiatric history
Family psychiatric history
Alcohol use history
Illicit substance history
Prescription drug use history
Nicotine use history
Developmental history
Mental status examination

Table 27–2. BEHAVIORAL CHECKLIST
Noncompliance with follow-up appointments
Limited support system
Family conflict
Expressed hostility to transplant team
Idealizing or devaluing members of the transplant team
Expectation of "special treatment" (i.e., rescheduling appointments repeatedly for insignificant reasons)
Excessive concern with physical appearance
Rigid expectations regarding patient education, medical information (i.e., repeated requests for detailed information despite reasonable efforts at education)
Indifference to medical teaching/instructions
Contradictory history provided to different members of the transplant team
Engaging in high-risk behavior (altercations with police, little concern about personal safety)
Switching transplant centers for unclear reasons
Marked ambivalence about transplantation

A thorough review of common psychiatric symptoms is performed to detect conditions that can affect the patient's ability to comply with posttransplant recommendations. Depression, adjustment disorders, anxiety, and insomnia are all common in transplant patients.[3] A past psychiatric history and family history can alert clinicians to patients at risk for developing psychiatric conditions while on the transplant list. Obtaining information from family members and local health care providers can be crucial in developing a full understanding of the patient's past psychiatric history and his or her current ability to cope with transplantation and to uncover behavior that the patient is reluctant to discuss, such as problematic alcohol or drug use.

The use of psychometric screening tools also identifies maladaptive personality traits, psychiatric symptoms, patterns of alcohol use, cognitive impairment, or increased levels of distress. Use of screening tools alone is not sufficient to determine the need for treatment intervention and should be accompanied by a thorough clinical evaluation before treatment is pursued. Common psychometric tools include depression screening tools, personality inventories, distress scales, and alcoholism screening tools.

Experienced transplant staff often report problematic behavior noted while the patient is on the transplant waiting list. This behavior (Table 27–2) can be informative about the patient's ability to interact with the team of individuals who provide services to transplant patients. Patients who are repeatedly noncompliant or who have little family support can be at increased risk of poor outcomes.[4]

Transplant-specific rating scales have been created to help assist transplant teams in understanding areas of concern. The Transplant Evaluation Rating Scale[5] and the Psychosocial Assessment of Candidates for Transplantation scale[6] rate the patients on family support and availability, past psychiatric history and coping, use of substances, history of compliance, and knowledge about transplantation. Very few studies have determined whether these scales predict poorer outcome after transplantation.[6]

There are few absolute psychiatric contraindications to transplantation. Most psychiatrists agree that patients with active or untreated mania, psychosis, or chemical dependency should not undergo transplantation. In one study, 60% of bipolar patients were compliant after transplant, but only 28.6% of schizophrenia patients were compliant.[7] Patients with progressive dementing conditions usually are not considered candidates.

Special Issues in Transplant Patients

Adapting to the Waiting Period

The Model for End-stage Liver Disease (MELD)[8] does not include encephalopathy and ascites as factors contributing to the probability of being transplanted. The MELD score has replaced the Child-Turcotte-Pugh score, which previously determined the United Network for Organ Sharing (UNOS) allocation policy and waiting time.[9] Patients with low MELD scores, which is determined by serum creatinine and total serum bilirubin levels, international normalized ratio of prothrombin time, and cause of liver disease, may have encephalopathy and ascites, which results in significant distress for the patients. Thus, detection of encephalopathy and symptomatic strategies to manage these symptoms is crucial. Assessing cognitive function in patients on the liver transplant waiting list can be easily performed using a standard battery of psychometric tests. The Trail Making Tests A and B and the Wechsler Adult Intelligence Scale–Revised (WAIS-R) block design and digit-symbol test[10] are reasonable psychometric tests to detect minimal encephalopathy. The West Haven criteria grade hepatic encephalopathy on a scale from I to IV based on changes in consciousness, intellectual function, and behavior,[11] but may not assist the clinician in perceiving the more subtle cognitive changes of patients with minimal encephalopathy. Muscle cramps and pruritus have been found to impair quality of life significantly for transplant candidates, as have subclinical encephalopathy, sleep disorders, and refractory ascites.[12] Sleep disorders of clinical significance occur in approximately 50% of cirrhotic patients.[13] The stress of the waiting period with the associated physical symptoms that impair quality of life can be demoralizing for the transplant recipient. Often patients will struggle to continue working despite increasing problems with concentration and increasing fatigue. Fear of losing insurance coverage can become a factor in the patient's distress. Spouses also will often need to carefully maintain insurance coverage if their insurance is the primary source of insurance for the patient. Thus, spouses may not be able to accompany the patient to appointments if the transplant center is far from where they live because of the need to be at work. The presence of a support system that involves more than a spouse or significant other can help the patient with transportation needs, assistance at medical appointments, and respite for the working spouse.

The spouse or other family members benefit from meeting with the transplant team members and participating in support groups. Some studies have found that spouses experience more distress before and after transplantation than patients do.[14] Other stressors for transplant candidates can include fear of death and worrying about family members and about the impending transplantation. Patients commonly cope by using psychological defenses such as humor, cognitive strategies to promote optimism, and behavioral strategies to maintain normal routines.[15]

During the waiting period, behavioral concerns that may not have been evident at the time of the initial assessment may become evident. Often patients have to return for ongoing medical reevaluation, and their resistance to follow-up care can be an important predictor of posttransplant noncompliance. Such noncompliance can occur in patients with personality disorders,[16] but also has been seen in medical populations with depression.[17] Treatment of depression, which is discussed in more detail in the next section, may result in improved compliance. Patients who repeatedly demonstrate noncompliance with medical care during the waiting period should be reviewed by the transplant team and their candidacy for transplantation reconsidered.

Patients are educated about transplantation by nurse coordinators, physicians, other transplant patients, and through patient literature. Many transplant centers use transplant support groups to foster the development of skills to cope with transplantation and provide information. Meetings can include topics such as medication, physical side effects, the healing process, and financial issues.[18] Patient education about transplantation may be impaired by language barriers, preexisting learning disabilities, and hepatic encephalopathy. Patients are more likely to remember if they understand the information presented and are more likely to adhere if their preferences are considered.[19] The relationship between the physician and the patient has been stressed as an important factor in the success of communicating information to patients,[20] and suggestions to improve communication include ascertaining if too much information is being provided, asking the patient to summarize the discussion, and understanding the patient's cognitive learning style (verbal or spatial and picture based).

Management of Mood Disorders

Many patients experience mood symptoms prior to transplantion. More than 50% of patients may experience depressive symptoms, and more than 30% experience anxiety symptoms, which are correlated with liver disease severity.[3] Patients with cirrhosis who also have depression perceive their quality of life as significantly poorer than nondepressed cirrhotic patients.[21] It is important to evaluate and monitor patients for mood symptoms, not only at the time of initial evaluation but also while the patient waits for transplantation. They may be reluctant to talk about these symptoms because of the stigma of mental illness or for fear of jeopardizing their chances of undergoing transplantation. Giving patients permission to speak about their mood symptoms and reassuring them that treatment is available is important. They should also be told that mood symptoms are common and will not preclude transplantation.

A common question about the management of mood disorders focuses on the dosing of psychoactive medications for transplant candidates with decreased liver function. Nontricyclic antidepressants appear to be relatively safe, but clearance of sertraline, paroxetine, fluvoxamine, fluoxetine, mirtazapine, and nefazodone is significantly prolonged in patients with liver disease.[22] Most psychiatrists would avoid nefazodone because of reported rare hepatotoxicity that resulted in a "black box" warning on the prescribing information. Nefazodone interacts with immunosuppressives and should be avoided for this reason as well.[23]

Anxiolytics have a limited role in the treatment of anxiety disorders for patients with end-stage liver disease. Benzodiazepines can potentially worsen encephalopathy and should be avoided if possible. Tricyclic antidepressants should also be avoided if possible. Increased serum levels of tricyclic antidepressants can occur because of decreased hepatic metabolism, and elevated levels of these medications can lead to cardiac conduction abnormalities. If used, careful monitoring of drug levels is necessary.

In recent years, the use of herbal agents for depressive and anxiety symptoms has become common. One in six adults taking prescription drugs reports taking an herbal product.[24] Kava, which is used as a sedative, causes hepatotoxicity. St. John's Wort, commonly used for depressive symptoms, is associated with reduced levels of cyclosporine and tacrolimus. Patients should be instructed about the possibility of drug interactions or toxicity with herbal medicines.

Nonpharmacological approaches can also be helpful to patients in managing anxiety and depressive symptoms pretransplant. Individual and group therapy can offer the patient the opportunity to talk about sadness, helplessness, hopelessness, ambivalence about transplantation, concern about families, and conflicted feelings about needing deceased donor organs.[25]

A syndrome has recently been described in the recipients of living donor organs. Depression, somatization, adjustment disorders, and conversion disorder may occur in recipients who were noted preoperatively to have elevated scores on psychometric testing, suggesting conflicted feelings about the living donor proceeding with the surgery.[26] Evaluating transplant candidates for their feelings about living donor transplantation prior to transplant surgery, especially in patients who have difficulty expressing their feelings, may help diminish the potential risk for this phenomenon, which has been called "the paradoxical psychiatric syndrome."

Familial Amyloidosis

Amyloidosis results from the deposition of insoluble, fibrous amyloid proteins in the extracellular spaces of organs. Heredofamilial amyloidosis involving the nervous system results in peripheral neuropathy, postural hypotension, inability to sweat, and sphincter incompetence. The average survival is 7 to 15 years.[27] Since the early 1990s, liver transplantation has been offered

to patients with familial amyloidosis in order to remove the site of synthesis of the mutant protein. Patients awaiting transplantation for amyloidosis may experience significant anxiety related to the debilitating effects of amyloidosis on their nervous system. Fear of becoming dependent on others because of neuropathy or anxiety from witnessing the devastating effects of amyloidosis on other family members contributes to increased levels of anxiety while awaiting transplantation. Supportive psychotherapy and monitoring for depressive symptoms is prudent in this population.

Cancer

Patients with hepatocellular carcinoma and cholangiocarcinoma may be candidates for transplantation. Patients with hepatocellular tumors smaller than 5 cm and up to three tumor nodules smaller than 3 cm have had a 3-year survival rate of 83%. The organ allocation policy for patients with tumors results in a MELD score of 29 for patients with tumors greater than 2 cm in diameter.[9] As a result, patients who otherwise are not experiencing end-stage liver disease may be diagnosed with a tumor and quickly be allocated an organ. Patients who have a short period to adapt to the knowledge that they need a transplant and those who have enjoyed a reasonable quality of life prior to transplant may find transplantation to be an aversive experience. They will have to adapt to ill health, medication regimens, and rehabilitation. These patients may benefit from reevaluation for anxiety and depression and adjustment disorders after transplantation.

Some patients with cholangiocarcinoma may successfully undergo transplantation after receiving radiation therapy and chemotherapy.[28] These patients often are experiencing a reasonable quality of life when they are suddenly confronted with the diagnosis of cancer and then the need for a transplant. They often experience anxiety as they await transplantation because of the fear that their disease will progress prior to transplantation. Family members can also appear distressed, and support from mental health providers, social workers, clinical nurse specialists, and chaplains can be especially valuable for these patients and their families. Patients describe "living with a time bomb" as the best metaphor for life with cancer prior to transplantation.

Hepatitis C

Hepatitis C is the most common cause of chronic liver disease and is found in 50% to 80% of intravenous (IV) drug users and occurs in as many as 46% of patients with alcoholic liver disease.[29] Depressive symptoms have been reported in up to 57% of hepatitis C–infected patients.[30] Patients complain of malaise and fatigue, and their quality of life is poor compared with unaffected patients.

Interferon (INF) alfa and ribavirin treatment is used for the treatment of hepatitis C but is associated with many side effects. Mood disorders can be serious, and completed suicides have been reported. Patients studied for 6 months on INF alfa-2b were noted to have a 58% incidence neuropsychiatric toxicity with significant depression, anxiety, and somatization scores.[31]

If psychiatric symptoms occur during IFN alfa therapy, dose reduction is recommended, and treatment should be discontinued if suicidal thinking occurs.[29] Antidepressants have been prescribed for the prevention of depression induced by IFN alfa and resulted in 11% of patients treated with antidepressants experiencing depression versus 45% in the placebo group.[32] Alternatively, close monitoring for depression and early treatment with antidepressants after starting INF has also been advocated.[33] Screening for depression prior to treatment with IFN alfa should be performed, and patients with depression should be treated before beginning IFN alfa treatment. Those without depression should be monitored for emergent mood symptoms.

Management of Personality Disorders

Patients with personality disorders have more compliance problems after transplantation[34]; however, in alcoholic transplant patients with personality disorders, survival was similar to patients with no personality disorders.[35] Few studies have established whether standardized personality tests can predict outcomes after transplant. Interviews with patients to determine the presence of personality disorders can be confounded by the significant distress the patients are experiencing at the time of evaluation, the coexistence of encephalopathy, and the patient's and family's desire to present the patient as an ideal candidate to the interviewer.

While the patient is waiting for a transplant, the transplant team can assess the patient's ability to cope with illness and comply with the expectations of the transplant team. Although mental health professionals often see patients at the time of the initial transplant evaluation, transplant coordinators, social workers, and nurses who continue caring for the patient may begin to detect problematic behavior that was not readily apparent initially. Transplant teams and psychiatrists need to develop a mechanism for communicating information about problematic behavior that becomes apparent while the patient awaits transplantation. Nurse coordinators who have extensive contact with the transplant candidate but no formal psychiatric training can be educated about maladaptive coping and

notify the psychiatrist to coordinate further evaluation of the patient. Patients whose behavior is incompatible with transplant (see Table 27–2) can be reassessed for psychiatric comorbidities that could exacerbate maladaptive coping, be offered psychiatric interventions, or can be reassessed for consideration of medical management instead of transplantation.

Psychiatrists, psychologists, and other mental health care workers evaluate patients in terms of psychopathology. Another paradigm is to determine whether the patient has fundamental problems in developing a relationship with the transplant team. Rating scales have been used to measure the quality of a patient's ability to develop trusting relationships. Patients who tend to rely on themselves and dismiss the input of others are at increased risk of noncompliance.[36,37] Detecting deficiencies in attachment to the transplant team early on may help identify patients who will resist the recommendations of the treatment team and thus be at greater risk of noncompliance. Interventions to help patients understand their resistance may yield improved compliance but as yet have not been studied in transplant populations.

Patients may have maladaptive coping because of the stress of living with chronic illness, which results in an adaptive triad of uncertainty, enduring change, and suffering.[38] Education, bibliotherapy, peer counseling, and a buddy system have all been found to be useful for decreasing uncertainty,[38] and supportive, expressive group therapy, including spiritual and existential approaches, often is helpful in addressing the psychological distress of chronic illness. For patients who live a significant distance from the transplant center, frequent communication between the transplant psychiatrist and the local mental health provider can help determine if the patient is responding to these interventions.

Alcoholism and Substance Abuse

Alcohol dependence is a major public health problem in the United States. However, problem drinkers underreport their alcohol consumption and rationalize or deny negative consequences of their alcohol use. A patient may go years, if not decades, without physician assessment and diagnosis of the alcoholism, even when the patient is hospitalized with alcohol-related medical problems.[39] Alcohol-related liver disease (ALD) may develop after a decade or more of high-dose drinking and is responsible for more than 50% of end-stage liver disease deaths in the United States.[40] Prior to 1983, ALD was a rare indication for liver transplantation; however, carefully selected abstinent patients with ALD increasingly underwent transplantation in the late 1980s.[23] Beginning in the 1990s, a series of American and European studies indicated that graft and patient survival in the ALD patient group mirrored that seen in patients who underwent transplantation for non-alcoholic liver disease.[41-48] The 7-year survival rate after liver transplantation for alcohol-induced liver disease has been reported at 60%, comparable to the rates for primary biliary cirrhosis (76%), chronic hepatitis C (57%), and chronic hepatitis B (47%).[49] Because of the high prevalence of the disease and favorable outcomes in graft recipients, ALD has become the second leading diagnosis among those receiving orthotopic liver transplantation (OLT) in the United States. Between 1988 and 1995, approximately 23% of liver transplants were carried out for ALD.[43,49]

There has been much debate about allocation of organs to persons with ALD.[41] The primary issue is the potential for posttransplant relapse to alcohol use, with consequent injury to the graft and increased morbidity and mortality. Depending on the definition of relapse and the methods used to follow patients, varying rates of relapse have been reported from several countries.[42,50,51] These figures have ranged from as low as 12% from data published by Kumar and associates to as high as 95% in a study from London.[42,52] Most single-center U.S. studies indicate relapse rates of approximately 10% to 15% per year for the first 3 years after transplantation. After 3 to 7 years of posttransplant abstinence, graft recipients have a much lower likelihood of subsequent relapse.[49] Given current shortages of donor organs, careful consideration of each candidate remains a pertinent issue for transplant selection committees.

Various criteria have been used by transplant centers to select patients with alcohol-related liver disease for OLT. These criteria have included duration of abstinence greater than 6 months, family or social support, absence of illicit substance or prescription medication abuse, and the absence of other psychiatric disorders, especially psychotic disorders or personality disorders, and compliance with treatment team recommendations (Table 27-3).[53]

Prior studies have examined the so-called 6-month abstinence rule and have found it unhelpful in predicting posttransplant relapse.[54-57] Other studies indicate that patients with personality disorders, prior failed attempts at addiction treatment, and limited social support are at greater risk of relapse.[58,59]

Table 27-3. RISKS FOR RELAPSE IN ALCOHOLIC LIVER TRANSPLANT PATIENTS

Polydrug dependence

Lack of stable social support

Lack of insight about diagnosis

Personality disorder

Past inability to maintain abstinence (previous failed treatment attempts)

Spouse/partner continues to use alcohol/substances

The roles of addiction treatment and Alcoholics Anonymous (AA) involvement, the primary means of establishing and maintaining abstinence in nontransplantation alcoholics, have received little attention in transplant research. Both interventions are targeted at improving a person's insight into the addictive behaviors and fostering an understanding of life-long abstinence. At this point, some U.S. transplantation programs do not require addiction treatment if patients have been abstinent for a predetermined number of months; other programs require successful completion of treatment prior to listing.

The diagnosis of alcoholism requires a careful psychiatric evaluation, including questioning the patient about past alcohol use, negative consequences of alcohol use, compulsive use, tolerance, attempts to cut down on use, withdrawal symptoms, and past treatment for alcoholism. History should also be obtained from family members. Laboratory tests such as γ-glutamyltransferase and mean corpuscular volume determinations are not sensitive enough to indicate clearly the current use of alcohol in patients with liver disease.[60] Carbohydrate-deficient transferrin (CDT) has been studied as a marker for high-dose alcohol consumption.[61] In a recent study, 50% of patients with end-stage liver disease who were abstaining from alcohol demonstrated false-positive elevations of CDT.[62]

Patients with untreated alcohol dependence need an intensive addiction treatment program. The goals of the treatment program include insight into the addictive pattern of use and its consequences, need for ongoing abstinence, and relapse prevention skills. Once treatment is completed, regular involvement in an ongoing addiction self-help group, such as AA, is a reasonable approach. An addictions professional should monitor patients for relapse while they await transplant. The treatment team should also perform periodic random urine screens to document ongoing abstinence.

Nicotine Dependence

Although alcohol dependence has received considerable attention in the liver transplant literature, concern about the impact of nicotine use is only beginning to be addressed as a risk for transplant complications. This is especially important in alcoholic cirrhotics because alcoholics have smoking rates of more than 85%.[63] In one study, vascular complications occurred in 17.8% of patients with a history of smoking versus 8% for non-smokers. The authors recommended that smoking cessation should be essential for liver transplant candidates.[64] Smoking cessation can prevent smoking-related morbidity and mortality from heart disease, lung disease, and cancer.[65] Patients should be asked about current nicotine use and encouraged to discontinue smoking using behavioral strategies, nicotine replacement products, and antidepressant agents. Bupropion has been noted to be effective for smoking cessation,[63] but in transplant recipients, the dose should be decreased because this medication is extensively metabolized by the liver.

Obesity

The prevalence of obesity in the United States is 19.8%.[66] Seven percent of patients undergoing orthotopic liver transplantation are severely or morbidly obese (BMI > 35 kg/m^2), resulting in adverse cardiovascular events and resulting in a significantly lower 5-year survival.[67] Complications of cardiovascular disease represent the third most common cause of late mortality after recurrent liver disease, and complications of immune suppression and efforts to correct reversible cardiovascular risk factors, such as obesity, are now being considered.[68] Also of note, 21.6% of patients who were nonobese before transplantation became obese within 2 years of transplantation.[69]

Obesity is frequently associated with nonalcoholic liver disease, including nonalcoholic steatohepatitis. It is estimated that about 30.1 million obese adults in the United States may have steatosis, and 8.6 million may have steatohepatitis. Improvement in liver function tests has been noted with weight loss in patients with nonalcoholic fatty liver disease.[70]

There are few studies addressing how to manage the obese pretransplant patient. Physical fatigue decreases the patient's ability to exercise, making weight loss more difficult. Generally, a 5% to 10% reduction in body weight for obese patients over 6 months may be reasonable with a combination of exercise and moderate caloric reduction. A referral to behavioral psychologists specializing in weight management can help patients acquire behavioral strategies that reinforce new approaches to food intake and exercise.

Geriatric Patients

Currently, 10.7% of patients waiting for liver transplantation are older than 65 years of age.[71] Older patients stay 3.9 days longer in the hospital, and, on average, use more services, resulting in an additional $32,795 in cost from both increased hospital stay and utilization of resources.[72] Older patients have poorer nutritional status, muscle wasting, encephalopathy, higher creatinine levels, longer intensive care unit stays, and total hospital days after transplantation,[73] but quality of life at 1 year is similar to nongeriatric patients. Older patients need more extensive support networks to assist them because of the increased complications and slower recovery after transplantation. Relying on an elderly spouse as the only support person may result in rehospitalizations for the patient when elderly caregivers fatigue during the rehabilitation process. Transplantation teams should anticipate the need to monitor these patients for encephalopathy and treat sleep deprivation, electrolyte imbalances, and toxicity from immunosuppressive agents early. Also, efforts to stimulate elderly patients' appetites using low doses of methylphenidate or mirtazapine may be helpful. We do not know whether elderly patients are at greater risk for depression after transplantation as a result of their longer hospital stays and debilitated state.

Pearls and Pitfalls

- Treat depression when it occurs before transplantation. Patients often can tolerate low-dose serotonin reuptake inhibitors.

- Alcoholic patients with no history of chemical dependency treatment should successfully complete a chemical dependency treatment program.

- Nicotine dependence can lead to increased morbidity after transplantation and should be screened for and treated.

- Obese patients increasingly are presenting for transplantation, and weight management should be addressed.

- Noncompliance or maladaptive behavior may best be detected while the patient is waiting for a transplant. Good communication between nurse coordinators and mental health staff is critical to identifying noncompliance and developing intervention strategies.

- A multidisciplinary approach that fosters good communication among psychiatry, psychology, social work and nursing disciplines, and chemical dependency counselors and chaplains is best suited to the complex needs of the transplant patient.

- Patients with months of abstinence may only be maintaining abstinence because they are too ill to drink. Chemical dependency treatment is still warranted.

- Some antidepressants can be toxic to the liver (nefazodone) or interact with immunosuppressants (nefazodone, fluvoxamine) and should be avoided in liver transplant patients.

- Noncompliance is difficult to assess initially because the patient is motivated to appear as an ideal candidate. Ongoing monitoring for noncompliance is needed.

Pearls and Pitfalls—cont'd

- Sleep disturbance is a common, untreated condition in transplant patients, which may respond well to low dosages of medications with sedating effects, such as trazodone.
- Irritability and depression often go undetected and can demoralize the patient and family. Ask the patient about these symptoms and consider treating if the patient reports persistent symptoms.

References

1. Skotzko C, Stowe J, Wright C, et al: Approaching a consensus: Psychosocial support services for solid organ transplantation programs. Prog Transplant 11:163-168, 2001.
2. Levenson J, Olbrisch M: Psychosocial evaluation of organ transplant candidates. A comparative survey of process, criteria, and outcomes in heart, liver, and kidney transplantation. Psychosomatics 34:314-323, 1993.
3. Streisand R, Rodrigue J, Sears S Jr, et al: A psychometric normative database for pre-liver transplantation evaluations. The Florida cohort 1991-1996. Psychosomatics 40:479-485, 1999.
4. Chacko R, Harper R, Gotto J, et al: Psychiatric interview and psychometric predictors of cardiac transplant survival. Am J Psychiatry 153:1607-1612, 1996.
5. Twillman R, Manetto C, Wellisch D, et al: The Transplant Evaluation Rating Scale. A revision of the psychosocial levels system for evaluating organ transplant candidates. Psychosomatics 34:144-153, 1993.
6. Olbrisch M, Levenson J, Hamer R: The PACT: A rating scale for the study of clinical decision-making in psychosocial screening of organ transplant candidates. Clin Transplant 3:164-169, 1989.
7. Coffman K, Crone C: Transplantation in patients with histories of psychotic disorder. Psychosomatics 40:139, 1999.
8. Malinchoc M, Kamath P, Gordon F, et al: A model to predict poor survival in patients undergoing transjugular intrahepatic portosystemic shunts. Hepatology 31:864-871, 2000.
9. Wiesner R, Rakela J, Ishitani M, et al: Recent advances in liver transplantation. Mayo Clin Proc 78:197-210, 2003.
10. Ferenci P, Lockwood A, Mullen K, et al: Hepatic encephalopathy—definition, nomenclature, diagnosis, and quantification: Final report of the working party at the 11th World Congresses of Gastroenterology, Vienna. Hepatology 35:716-721, 1998.
11. Atterbury C, Maddrey W, Conn H: Neomycin-sorbitol and lactulose in the treatment of acute portal-systemic encephalopathy. A controlled, double-blind clinical trial. Am J Dig Dis 23:398-406, 1978.
12. Marchesini G, Bianchi G, Amodio P, et al: The Italian Study Group for quality of life in cirrhosis. Factors associated with poor health-related quality of life of patients with cirrhosis. Gastroenterology 120:170-178, 2001.
13. Wiltfang J, Nolte W, Weissenborn K, et al: Psychiatric aspects of portal-systemic encephalopathy. Metab Brain Dis 13:379-389, 1998.
14. Bohachick P, Reeder S, Taylor M, et al: Psychosocial impact of heart transplantation on spouses. Clin Nurs Res 10:6-28, 2001.
15. Porter R, Krout L, Parks V, et al: Perceived stress and coping strategies among candidates for heart transplantation during the organ waiting period. J Heart Lung Transplant 13:102-107, 1994.
16. Dobbels F, De Geest S, Cleemput I, et al: Psychosocial and behavioral selection criteria for solid organ transplantation. Prog Transplant 11:121-130, 2001.
17. DiMatteo M, Lepper H, Croghan T: Depression is a risk factor for noncompliance with medical treatment: Meta-analysis of the effects of anxiety and depression on patient adherence. Arch Intern Med 160:2101-2107, 2000.
18. Kiedar R, Katz P, Nakache RJA: "Living again": Heterogeneous support group for transplant patients and their families. Transplant Proc 33:2930-2931, 2001.
19. Chisholm M: Enhancing transplant patients' adherence to medication therapy. Clin Transplant 16:30-38, 2002.
20. Pumilia C: Psychological impact of the physician-patient relationship on compliance: A case study and clinical strategies. Prog Transplant 12:10-16, 2002.
21. Singh N, Gayowski T, Wagener M, et al: Depression in patients with cirrhosis. Impact on outcome. Dig Dis Sci 42:1421-1427, 1997.
22. Robinson M, Levenson J: Psychopharmacology in Transplantation in Biopsychosocial Perspectives on Transplantation. New York, Kluwer Academic/Plenum Publishers, 2001.
23. Jowsey S, Taylor M, Schneekloth T, et al: Psychosocial challenges in transplantation. J Psychiatr Pract 7:404-414, 2001.
24. DeSmet P: Herbal remedies. N Engl J Med 347:2046-2056, 2002.
25. Abbey S, Farrow S: Group therapy and organ transplantation. Int J Group Psychother 48:163-185, 1998.
26. Fukunishi I, Sugawara Y, Takayama T, et al: Association between pretransplant psychological assessments and posttransplant psychiatric disorders in living-related transplantation. Psychosomatics 43:49-54, 2002.
27. Sipe J, Cohen A: Amyloidosis. In Fave A, Braunwald E, Isselbacher K, et al. (eds): Harrison's Textbook of Medicine. New York, McGraw-Hill, 1998.
28. De Vreede I, Steers J, Burch P, et al: Prolonged disease-free survival after orthotopic liver transplantation plus adjuvant chemoirradiation for cholangiocarcinoma. Liver Transpl 6:309-316, 2000.
29. Dieperink E, Willenbring M, Ho S: Neuropsychiatric symptoms associated with hepatitis C and interferon alpha: A review. Am J Psychiatry 157:867-876, 2000.
30. Zdilar D, Franco-Bronson K, Buchler N, et al: Hepatitis C, interferon alfa, and depression. Hepatology 31:1207-1211, 2000.
31. Fontana R, Schwartz S, Gebremariam A, et al: Emotional distress during interferon-alpha-2B and ribavirin treatment of chronic hepatitis C. Psychosomatics 43:378-385, 2002.
32. Musselman D, Lawson D, Gumnick J, et al: Paroxetine for the prevention of depression induced by high-dose interferon alfa. N Engl J Med 344:961-966, 2001.
33. Kraus M, Schafer A, Scheurlen M: Paroxetine for the prevention of depression induced by interferon alfa [letter]. N Engl J Med 345:375-376, 2001.
34. Levenson J, Olbrisch M: Psychosocial screening and selection of candidates for organ transplantation. In Trzepacz P, DiMartini A (eds): The Transplant Patient: Biological, Psychiatric and Ethical Issues in Organ Transplantation. Cambridge, MA, Cambridge University Press, 2000.
35. Fireman M, Rbkin J, Atkinson R: Personality traits and outcome of liver transplantation. Psychosomatics 40:143, 1999.
36. Griffin D, Bartholomew K: The metaphysics of measurement: The case of adult attachment. Adv Pers Relationships 5:17-52, 1994.
37. Ciechanowski P, Katon W, Russo J, et al: The patient-provider relationship: Attachment theory and adherence to treatment in diabetes. Am J Psychiatry 158:29-35, 2001.
38. Maunder R, Esplen M: Facilitating adjustment to inflammatory bowel disease: A model of psychosocial intervention in non-psychiatric patients. Psychother Psychosom 68:230-240, 1999.

39. Schneekloth T, Morse R, Herrick L, et al: Point prevalence of alcoholism in hospitalized patients: Continuing challenges of detection, assessment, and diagnosis. Mayo Clin Proc 76:460-466, 2001.

40. Grant B, Debakey S, Zobeck T: Liver cirrhosis mortality in the United States, 1973-1988. Washington, DC, U.S. Department of Health and Human Services, 1991.

41. Krom R: Liver transplantation and alcohol: Who should get transplants? Hepatology 20:28S-32S, 1994.

42. Kumar S, Stauber R, Gavaler J, et al: Orthotopic liver transplantation for alcoholic liver disease. Hepatology 11:159-164, 1990.

43. Belle S, Beringer K, Detre K: An update on liver transplantation in the United States: Recipient characteristics and outcome. In Cecka J, Terasaki P (eds): Clinical Transplants. Los Angeles, UCLA Tissue Typing Laboratory, 1995.

44. Lucey M, Merion R, Henley K, et al: Selection for and outcome of liver transplantation in alcoholic liver disease. Gastroenterology 102:1736-1741, 1992.

45. Berlakovich G, Steininger R, Herbst F, et al: Efficacy of liver transplantation for alcoholic cirrhosis with respect to recidivism and compliance. Transplantation 58:560-565, 1994.

46. Campbell D Jr, Magee J, Punch J, et al: One center's experience with liver transplantation: Alcohol use relapse over the long-term. Liver Transpl Surg 4:S58-S64, 1998.

47. Conjeevaram H, Hart J, Lissoos T, et al: Rapidly progressive liver injury and fatal alcoholic hepatitis occurring after liver transplantation in alcoholic patients. Transplantation 67:1562-1568, 1999.

48. Neuberger J, Tang H: Relapse after transplantation: European studies. Liver Transpl Surg 8:275-279, 1997.

49. Hoofnagle J, Kresina T, Fuller R, et al: Liver transplantation for alcoholic liver disease: Executive statement and recommendations. Summary of a National Institutes of Health workshop held December 6-7, 1996, Bethesda, Maryland. Liver Transpl Surg 3:347-350, 1997.

50. Pereira S, Williams R: Liver transplantation for alcoholic liver disease at King's College Hospital: Survival and quality of life. Liver Transpl 6:762-768, 2000.

51. Poynard T, Barthelemy P, Fratte S, et al: Evaluation of efficacy of liver transplantation in alcoholic cirrhosis by a case-control study and simulated controls. Lancet 344:502-507, 1994.

52. Howard L, Fahy T, Wong P, et al: Psychiatric outcome in alcoholic liver transplant patients. QJM 87:731-736, 1994.

53. Everhart J, Beresford T: Liver transplantation for alcoholic liver disease: A survey of transplantation programs in the United States. Liver Transpl Surg 3:220-226, 1997.

54. Platz K, Mueller A, Spree E, et al: Liver transplantation for alcoholic cirrhosis. Transpl Int 13:S127-S130, 2000.

55. Vaillant G: The natural history of alcoholism and its relationship to liver transplantation. Liver Transpl Surg 3:304-310, 1997.

56. Beresford T: Predictive factors for alcoholic relapse in the selection of alcohol-dependent persons for hepatic transplant. Liver Transpl Surg 3:280-291, 1997.

57. Yates W, Martin M, LaBrecque D, et al: A model to examine the validity of the 6-month abstinence criterion for liver transplantation. Alcohol Clin Exp Res 22:513-517, 1998.

58. Gish R, Lee A, Keeffe E, et al: Liver transplantation for patients with alcoholism and end-stage liver disease. Am J Gastroenterol 88:1337-1342, 1993.

59. Lucey M, Carr K, Beresford T, et al: Alcohol use after liver transplantation in alcoholics: A clinical cohort follow-up study. Hepatology 25:1223-1227, 1997.

60. DiMartini A, Trzepacz P: Alcoholism and organ transplantation. In DiMartini A, Trzepacz P (eds): The Transplant Patient. Cambridge, MA, Cambridge University Press, 2000, 214-238.

61. Stibler H, Borg S, Allgulander C: Clinical significance of abnormal heterogeneity of transferrin in relation to alcohol consumption. Acta Med Scand 206:275-281, 1979.

62. DiMartini A, Day N, Lane T, et al: Carbohydrate deficient transferrin in abstaining patients with end-stage liver disease. Alcohol Clin Exp Res 25:1729-1733, 2001.

63. Abrams D, King T, Clark M, et al: Behavioral management strategies: Management of nicotine dependence, obesity, and cardiopulmonary rehabilitation exercise. In Stoudemire A, Fogel B, Greenberg D (eds): Psychiatric Care of the Medical Patient. Oxford, Oxford University Press, 2000, 519-546.

64. Pungapong S, Manzarbeitia C, Ortiz J, et al: Cigarette smoking is associated with an increased incidence of vascular complications after liver transplantation. Liver Transpl 8:582-587, 2002.

65. Levy G, Marsden P: Cigarette smoking—Association with hepatic artery thrombosis. Liver Transpl 8:588-590, 2002.

66. Mokdad A, Bowman B, Ford E, et al: The continuing epidemics of obesity and diabetes in the United States. JAMA 286:1195-1200, 2001.

67. Nair S, Sumita V, Thuluvath P: Obesity and its effect on survival in patients undergoing orthotopic liver transplantation in the United States. Hepatology 35:105-109, 2002.

68. Reuben A: Long-term management of the liver transplant patient: Diabetes, hyperlipidemia, and obesity. Liver Transpl 7:513-521, 2001.

69. Everhart J, Lombardero M, Lake J, et al: Weight change and obesity after liver transplantation: Incidence and risk factors. Liver Transpl Surg 4:285-296, 1998.

70. Angulo P: Nonalcoholic fatty liver disease. N Engl J Med 346:1221-1231, 2002.

71. National data report for adults older than 65 on waiting list. Available at www.optn.org. Accessed December 1, 2004.

72. Showstack J, Katz P, Lake J, et al: Resource utilization in liver transplantation: Effects of patient characteristics and clinical practice. NIDDK Liver Transplantation Database Group. JAMA 281:1381-1386, 1999.

73. Zetterman R, Belle S, Hoofnagle J, et al: Age and liver transplantation: A report of the liver transplantation database. Transplantation 66:500-506, 1998.

Pretransplantation Evaluation: Pulmonary, Cardiac, and Renal

MARTIN L. MAI
DANIEL S. YIP
CESAR A. KELLER
THOMAS A. GONWA

Pulmonary 405
  Diagnosis of pleuropulmonary
    conditions 406
  Disease-related changes 410
  Evaluation 411
  Contraindications to liver
    transplantation 414

Cardiac 414
  Coronary artery disease 414
  Left ventricular dysfunction 415
  Arrhythmia 415
  Evaluation 415

Renal 417
  Diagnosis 417
  Disease-related changes 420
  Evaluation 420

Summary 422

Liver transplantation is now offered to a larger population of patients because of the growth and experience of transplant centers and the improvements in technology and technique. For example, renal insufficiency, severe hypoxemia, and pulmonary hypertension previously were considered absolute contraindications for liver transplantation.[1,2] It is now recognized that certain patients with these problems may be suitable recipients for liver transplant.[3] Preoperative evaluation thus becomes very important in selecting these individuals. In this chapter we review the pulmonary, cardiac, and renal preoperative evaluation of liver transplant candidates with special focus on particular illnesses associated with end-stage liver disease, necessary diagnostic and laboratory studies, and absolute and relative contraindications to transplantation.

Pulmonary

Pulmonary disease is prevalent in individuals with end-stage liver disease and takes many forms.[4,5] Identification of significant obstructive or restrictive pulmonary conditions that may alter the prognosis of liver transplantation is relevant to improve outcomes.

Clinical history of dyspnea on exertion, orthopnea, cough, and smoking history identifies patients at risk for complications. In guidelines published by the American College of Physicians in 1990, testing of pulmonary function by spirometry was recommended for patients with a history of tobacco use or dyspnea who were to undergo upper abdominal surgery.[6] Studies have defined that preoperative clinical factors that are independently associated with pulmonary complications following nonthoracic surgery include age of 65 years or more, smoking of 40 pack-years, history of chronic obstructive airways disease, and exercise capacity of two blocks or less or one flight of stairs.[7] In the same study, relevant preoperative physical examination findings predicting pulmonary risk included body mass index equal to or higher than 30, positive cough test, positive wheezing test, forced expiratory time of 9 seconds or longer, and maximal laryngeal height of 4 cm or less. These findings in clinical history and physical examination can help identify patients at higher potential surgical risk who may require more detailed evaluation. Seldom do pulmonary abnormalities alone contraindicate liver transplantation (unless the abnormalities are extreme). However, increased pulmonary surgical risk added to other risk factors may help the liver transplant team decide for or against listing a patient for liver transplantation, and identify those who will require intense pulmonary management following surgery.

Diagnosis of Pleuropulmonary Conditions

Hepatic Hydrothorax

Ascites and pleural effusions are common in liver disease and can affect oxygenation and ventilation. Hepatic hydrothorax is defined as the presence of pleural effusion in patients with liver cirrhosis in the absence of primary cardiopulmonary disease.[8] It is present in 5% to 10% of cirrhotic patients with ascites.[9] Ascites formation may result in an increase in intra-abdominal pressure causing a rise in the diaphragm and a concomitant decrease in lung volume and chest wall compliance.[10] Pleural effusions are seen in patients with end-stage liver disease and may be caused by hypoalbuminemia and azygos vein hypertension.[11] Formation of hepatic hydrothorax has been shown to be secondary to passage of ascitic fluid through defects in the diaphragm directly into the pleural space. This has been shown by injecting air and iodine-131–labeled albumin into the abdominal cavity, which they moves rapidly into the pleural space.[12] Diaphragmatic defects can be large or microscopic, and they may result from anatomic thinning and separation of the collagenous fibers of the diaphragmatic tendinous portion.

Factors such as congenital defects, cirrhotic cachexia, and emaciation contribute to diaphragmatic thinning, evaginations of the peritoneum, and formation of pleuroperitoneal blebs that may rupture following sudden increases in intra-abdominal pressure, occurring while coughing or straining.[13] The negative intrathoracic pressure of the pleural space compared with the positive pressure of the peritoneal cavity favors one-way transfer of fluid across the diaphragmatic defects with subsequent trapping of fluid in the pleural space. Hepatic hydrothorax will accumulate when the accumulation of peritoneal fluid in the pleural cavity exceeds the pleural space's absorptive capacity. For reasons poorly understood, the accumulation of fluid is much more common in the right hemithorax, with few cases accumulating fluid in the left space or bilaterally.[14] Although most patients with hepatic hydrothorax also have ascites, up to 20% of the cases may not have clinically detectable ascitic fluid accumulation.[15]

The clinical presentation of hepatic hydrothorax may range from an asymptomatic incidental finding in a patient being evaluated for chronic liver failure to a presentation of progressive shortness of breath, cough, and hypoxemia. These symptoms typically present gradually as the volume of pleural fluid increases. Rarely, the presentation may be one of acute respiratory failure following cough or exertion.[16] Rarely these effusions may also get infected, developing spontaneous bacterial empyema, which may occur as a result of infection of the peritoneal cavity or may result from transient bacteremia infecting the pleural space.[17]

Patients considered for liver transplantation who present with hepatic hydrothorax require the following workup[8]:

- Imaging, which includes chest radiograph and computerized scanning of the chest with contrast and computed tomography (CT) of the abdomen. This helps to rule out the presence of primary pulmonary pathology, which could explain the presence of pleural effusion. It also establishes the presence or absence of ascitic fluid. It is important to evaluate the absence of mediastinal or intra-abdominal lymphadenopathy that could be associated with a malignant effusion. The contrast computed tomographic scanning also screens out the possibility of pulmonary embolism as a cause of pleural effusion.

- Echocardiography, which helps rule out left ventricular failure, valvular disease, or pulmonary hypertension, all of which could be associated with accumulation of pleural fluid. Abdominal ultrasound with Doppler study are also part of the diagnostic process.

This preliminary workup is to be followed by a diagnostic thoracentesis. The typical fluid from hepatic hydrothorax is a sterile transudate with low cell counts, low protein levels (<2.5 g/dL) with a fluid protein-to-serum protein ratio less than 0.5, a lactate dehydrogenase (LDH) fluid-to-serum LDH ratio less than 0.6, and pleural fluid amylase lower than serum amylase.[18] The fluid should be processed using Gram stain, acid-fast bacilli stains, and fungal stains. Cultures should be obtained to rule out infectious processes. A pleural fluid cytologic examination should be included to rule out malignancy. Cases with pertinent clinical settings in which infection or malignancy is suspected may require thoracoscopic inspection and pleural biopsy. Patients with ascites should also be assessed by diagnostic paracentesis.

The management of hepatic hydrothorax includes daily sodium intake restriction to 90 mEq and diuretics (typically furosemide and spironolactone). Symptomatic patients in whom medical therapy fails transiently improve with therapeutic thoracentesis, but removal of more than 2 L should be avoided to minimize the risk of systemic hypotension and unilateral pulmonary edema.[8] Patients with large hepatic hydrothoraces who are being evaluated for possible liver transplant should have their pulmonary function tests and gas exchange evaluated following therapeutic thoracentesis, because at this time there is better opportunity to assess the true baseline function of the subject. Insertion of a chest tube should be avoided, because the associated protein and fluid loss carries a high morbidity and mortality.[19] When therapeutic thoracentesis is required more than once every 2 to 3 weeks in patients already on sodium restriction and optimal diuretic therapy, other alternatives need to be considered.

An alternative therapy is pleurodesis, which is performed by injecting sclerosing agents into the pleural space. This procedure is rarely successful, although reports indicate that chemical pleurodesis associated with continuous positive airway pressure (CPAP), to decrease the negative intrathoracic pressure, is associated with better outcomes.[20] Another approach is videothoracoscopy, which is used to identify diaphragmatic defects and use of sutures, placing biological glue and talc pleurodesis of the pleural cavity after the defects are closed.[20] Other therapeutic alternatives include placement of peritoneovenous shunts.[21] These shunts are frequently complicated by infection, thrombosis, and technical difficulties. Placing transjugular intrahepatic portosystemic shunts (TIPS) with expandable metal stents in the hepatic parenchyma between the hepatic and portal venous systems under fluoroscopic guidance can decrease the elevated hepatic sinusoidal pressure that is the main cause of fluid accumulation in cirrhosis. Some patients with hepatic hydrothorax improve with this approach.[22] A portion of patients undergoing the TIPS procedure progress into hepatic encephalopathy and worsening liver function. Therefore, this approach is best suited for centers where liver transplantation is

an option. For patients with severe hepatic hydrothorax who are otherwise good candidates for liver transplantation, this will be the best long-term solution. Hepatic hydrothorax is not a contraindication for liver transplantation per se, unless it is associated with an empyema.

Portal Pulmonary Shunts and Pleural Spider Angiomas

Portal pulmonary shunts and pleural spider angiomas are well documented in chronic liver disease and are associated with portal hypertension. Fortunately, they do not appear to have a significant effect on oxygenation, as their contribution to pulmonary shunting is small.[11,23] Hypoxemia in patients with chronic liver disease in the absence of parenchymal lung disease, obstructive lung disease, asthma, ascites, or pulmonary hypertension has been well described and is often referred to as *hepatopulmonary syndrome.*

Hepatopulmonary Syndrome

Hepatopulmonary syndrome (HPS) refers to a syndrome characterized by a triad composed of:

- Chronic liver disease
- Abnormal gas exchange resulting in an increased alveolar-arterial oxygen gradient and, in some cases, significant hypoxemia
- Evidence of intravascular pulmonary vasodilations[24-26]

The presence of intravascular pulmonary vasodilations can be assessed by detecting extrapulmonary (brain) uptake of ^{99m}Tc-labeled macroaggregated albumin (MAA) after lung scanning.[26] Contrast transthoracic echocardiography has been the preferred diagnostic tool. Agitated saline is used as a contrast by creating a stream of microbubbles after intravenous injection. These microbubbles are larger than the diameter of the capillary vascular structures. They opacify the right side of the heart in the normal subject and then are filtered into the pulmonary vascular bed; they should not appear in the left side of the heart. If microbubbles appear in the left side of the heart within three heart beats, an intracardiac right-to-left shunting is suspected. Appearance of microbubbles on the left side of the heart four to six beats after the appearance in the right side of the heart suggests the presence of pulmonary vascular dilatations or pulmonary vascular arteriovenous malformations, which allows right-to-left intrapulmonary shunting.[27] In patients in whom the surface echocardiogram may not be clear, a contrast transesophageal echocardiogram can be performed. This procedure is more sensitive and specific than a transthoracic echocardiogram in defining whether a right-to-left shunt is indeed present and will clearly define if the shunt is cardiac or intrapulmonary.[28] Some patients with hepatopulmonary syndrome additionally require the performance of such testing while in an upright position, because the shunting is more pronounced in an upright versus a recumbent position.

Hepatopulmonary syndrome occurs in 12% to 47% of patients,[29,30] depending on which criteria for hypoxemia is used. A study of 98 patients with biopsy-proven cirrhosis who were referred for transplantation reports the results of contrast echocardiography and gas exchange studies performed.[27] Thirty-three of them (34%) had a positive contrast echocardiography consistent with the presence of right-to-left intrapulmonary shunting. If an alveolar-arterial oxygen gradient greater than 20 mm Hg is used as criteria for abnormal gas exchange, the prevalence of HPS is 31%. If the threshold used is Pao_2 less than 70 mm Hg on room air while resting upright, the prevalence decreases to 15%. A Pao_2 less than 65 mm Hg in this population has a positive predictive value for the diagnosis of HPS of 100%. The clinical presentation of patients with significant HPS includes dyspnea. Also, in patients with predominant intrapulmonary shunting in the lower lobes, platypnea (increased dyspnea and hyperventilation in the upright position) and orthodeoxia (worsening hypoxemia in upright position compared with recumbency) occurs. In addition, spider nevi are more commonly present among patients with clinically significant HPS.[27] Many studies have attempted to define the pathophysiology of this process.[24,31-34] The hypoxemia may be caused by one of several entities including ventilation-perfusion mismatch, right-to-left intrapulmonary shunting, or diffusion defects. More recent reports describe a process of intrapulmonary vasodilation of pre- and postcapillary vessels creating arteriovenous channels. These channels result in impaired oxygenation via a true anatomic shunt or, more importantly, via physiological shunts created by a diffusion-perfusion impairment.[24,34,35,36] Diffusion-perfusion impairment is a term used to describe the inability of oxygen to reach all of the blood in the dilated arteriovenous channel. Demonstration of intrapulmonary vasodilation is discussed later in this section. It can be present in individuals who are normoxemic, or it can result in severe and life-threatening hypoxemia. The cause is not well understood, although attempts to improve oxygenation with almitrine bismesylate[37] and somatostatin[24,25] have met with minimal success.

The pulmonary vascular space is a direct recipient of venous blood flow and constituents arising from liver and portal systems. Various liver disorders are characterized by a hyperdynamic circulatory state manifested by elevated cardiac output and decreased systemic vascular resistance (SVR) and pulmonary vascular resistances (PVR),[38] in a fashion that closely resembles the hemodynamic picture of sepsis. It has been speculated that this phenomenon may be triggered by vasodilator substances released by the diseased liver, failure to clear normally produced vasodilating agents from circulation, or by failure of the diseased liver to release normal vasoconstrictive agents.[39] Animal studies have provided some insight into the possible cause. Ligation of the common bile duct in rats produces a model of cirrhosis with development of HPS, with intrapulmonary vascular dilatations, an increased alveolar-arterial oxygen difference, and a hyperdynamic state replicating the abnormalities seen in human hepatopulmonary syndrome.[40] The syndrome in these models occurs in large part from overproduction of nitric oxide (NO) in the lung. Induced nitric oxide synthase (iNOS) is expressed in pulmonary intravascular macrophages of cirrhotic rats, which may explain the increase in lung production of NO in this animal model.[41] In cirrhosis, intestinal bacterial overgrowth, impaired host defenses, and disruption of the mucosal barrier in the gut favors dissemination of gut lumen bacteria within the body. This process is called bacterial translocation. Bacterial translocation occurs in up to 75% of animals with experimental cirrhosis.[42] Normally the lung does not get exposed to large amounts of bacterial products because the liver, via Kupffer cells, clears nearly all bacteria and bacterial endotoxins from the bloodstream. In cirrhosis, however, portosystemic shunts and decreased phagocytic capacity develops, which allows circulating bacteria and bacterial endotoxins to enter the pulmonary circulation.[43] The lungs then become the site where clearance of gut bacteria and endotoxins is done through an increase in pulmonary phagocytic activity, which produces extensive accumulation of pulmonary intravascular macrophages adhering to the pulmonary endothelium.[41] During phagocytosis, activated macrophages release secretory products, including cytokines and NO, into the extracellular environment.[44] All these factors suggest that translocation of gut bacteria in cirrhotic rats is an important step in the pathogenesis of HPS.

A study investigated this issue further in a group of rats subjected to common bile duct ligation. Some rats received prophylactic norfloxacin therapy to prevent bacterial translocation and were compared with rats who did not receive antimicrobial therapy. Another group of rats receiving a sham operation was also included in the study.[45] The rats subjected to ligation of the bile duct developed cirrhosis as expected, and the lungs from these rats showed accumulation of mononuclear macrophage-like cells within the lumen of pulmonary vessels. The percent of vessels with large accumulations of adherent macrophages was significantly larger on untreated rats. Untreated rats also developed hemodynamic changes of vasodilation with lower SVR and PVR and higher cardiac index compared with rats receiving antibiotics and rats receiving a sham operation. Development of HPS with intravascular dilatations characterized by abnormal gas exchange and abnormal brain uptake (determined by [99mTc]-labeled macroaggregated albumin studies) revealed that HPS development was significantly higher among untreated rats compared with those receiving antibiotics. The activity and expression of the lung of iNOS were reduced to normal among treated rats. The study concluded that norfloxacin reduced HPS severity by inhibiting gram-negative bacterial translocation, thereby decreasing the NO production by intrapulmonary intravascular macrophages. It also concluded that bacterial translocation may be the key to the pathogenesis of HPS.

One case report describes a man with severe HPS complicated by the presence of a brain abscess. He was treated for 4 months with oral norfloxacin and the HPS was resolved with the 4-month treatment.[46] Further studies in this area may define more precisely the pathophysiology and potential medical therapy of HPS.

The reversibility of this abnormality via liver transplantation has been debated. Previously, severe hypoxemia secondary to hepatopulmonary syndrome was an absolute contraindication to liver transplantation.[1,2] However, liver transplantation in patients with severe hypoxemia secondary to HPS has been performed, and reversibility in some patients has been described.[34,46,47,47a] Reviews of the outcomes of liver transplantation among patients with HPS indicate increased posttransplantation mortality (16% to 29%)[48,49] compared with liver transplant recipients without HPS. The mortality is worse among patients with a pretransplantation PaO_2 less than 50 mm Hg (30%), compared with those with PaO_2 greater than 50 mm Hg (4%).[46] The resolution of HPS occurs in most patients surviving liver transplantation, and the shunt fraction may improve within a few days after transplantation or it may occur in a delayed fashion, with resolution requiring up to 15 months.[50] In a few patients, the HPS will not resolve following transplantation.

Evaluation and candidacy of patients with hepatopulmonary syndrome is discussed later.

Portopulmonary Hypertension

Pulmonary hypertension may occur in patients with chronic liver disease and portal hypertension.[51] Portopulmonary hypertension (POPH) is considered to be a pulmonary vascular constrictive/obliterative process believed to develop as a consequence of liver disease complicated by pulmonary hypertension.[39] Mild to moderate POPH may be entirely asymptomatic, yet the prognosis of the liver transplant candidate is compromised in the presence of pulmonary hypertension. Therefore, all candidates for liver transplantation are usually screened with Doppler echocardiography at the time of evaluation.[51-53] Continuous wave Doppler of the tricuspid regurgitant jet, when present, is used to calculate the right ventricular pressure with the formula:

$$\text{PA systolic} = (4 \times \text{maximum velocity of regurgitant jet}^2) + \text{mean right atrial pressure}$$

estimated as:

- 0 when the inferior vena cava is collapsed
- 5 when it is not collapsed
- 10 when it is clearly enlarged and fails to collapse during inspiration[54]

Patients with systolic pulmonary artery pressure greater than 30 mm Hg, calculated by echocardiogram, are considered to have pulmonary hypertension and should undergo cardiac catheterization to confirm the diagnosis.

Echo Doppler is considered to be highly sensitive for establishing the pulmonary hypertension diagnosis, but it is not specific. The diagnosis is established by catheterization of the right side of the heart when showing:

- Pulmonary artery mean (PAM) pressures greater than 25 mm Hg
- PVR greater than 120 dyne·sec·cm⁻⁵
- Pulmonary capillary wedge pressure less than 15 mm Hg[53]

In general terms, patients with POPH have higher cardiac output levels than patients with primary pulmonary hypertension with comparable elevations in pulmonary artery pressures.[54] The prevalence of POPH diagnosed by echocardiogram, performed on 165 patients who were referred for liver transplantation, has been reported at 10% (17 of 165 patients). Ten of the patients were confirmed to have POPH by right heart catheterization (6%).[51] Ramsay and colleagues reported on a review of 1205 consecutive liver transplant recipients, where the incidence of pulmonary hypertension, defined as PAM pressure greater than 25 mm Hg, was 8.5% (n = 102 cases).[55] In this report, the incidence of mild pulmonary hypertension (PA systolic >30 and <44 mm Hg) was 6.7%, moderate pulmonary hypertension (PA systolic 45 to 59 mm Hg) was 1.16%, and severe pulmonary hypertension (PA systolic >60 mm Hg) was 0.58%. Pathological findings in POPH are indistinguishable from those seen in primary pulmonary hypertension.[56] Although HPS and POPH were originally thought to be distinct and mutually exclusive entities, it has been increasingly recognized that these diseases coexist in some cases.[56,57] Some of these rare cases have been characterized by initial presentation with hypoxemia secondary to hepatopulmonary syndrome, which resolves or improves following liver transplantation, to become complicated by late development of severe pulmonary hypertension not present at the time of liver transplant.[58]

The medical management of portopulmonary hypertension involves the use of continuous intravenous infusion of epoprostenol (prostacyclin). Intravenous epoprostenol is a potent pulmonary vasodilator. Its short half-life (3 to 5 minutes) requires delivery through a permanent indwelling catheter with a continuous infusion pump. This agent is effective in the short- and long-term management of patients with severe primary pulmonary hypertension.[59] In addition to its vasodilating properties, it also has antiplatelet and antiproliferative properties that favor vascular remodeling.[60] Acute and long-term improvement in pulmonary hemodynamics in patients with moderate to severe POPH has been reported.[60a,61] The benefits of this approach have to be considered in the context of potentially serious adverse events, such as line-related sepsis and thrombosis. Experience with other vasodilator agents is limited. Patients with pulmonary hypertension and end-stage liver disease usually do not show vasodilator response to acute administration of nitric oxide.[62]

POPH presents a challenge in determining liver transplant candidacy. Plevak and colleagues[63] have reported 33 patients with mild to moderate pulmonary hypertension (PVR 120.5-270.7 dyne·sec·cm^{-5}) at the time of anesthetic induction for orthotopic liver transplant (OLT). Pulmonary hypertension was not exacerbated by surgery and had no appreciable influence on mortality. Some have reported severe pulmonary hypertension as a contraindication to liver transplantation, unless undertaken with a combined heart-lung transplant.[51,64] Krowka and coworkers have described the outcomes of 43 patients with POPH who underwent liver transplantation.[65] Overall mortality was 15 of 43 patients (35%), mostly because of cardiopulmonary dysfunction. PAM pressure greater than 50 mm Hg was associated with 100% cardiopulmonary mortality. In patients with PAM of 35 to 50 mm Hg and a PVR greater than 250 dyne·sec·cm^{-5}, the mortality rate was 50%. No mortality was reported in patients with mean PA pressure less than 35 mm Hg. Based on this evidence, a reasonable approach to follow with patients diagnosed with POPH is to proceed with liver transplantation in those with mild to moderate pulmonary hypertension. Those with severe POPH (PAM pressures higher than 40 to 50 mm Hg) should be initiated on chronic epoprostenol infusion with follow-up right side of the heart catheterization every 3 to 6 months, and proceed with transplantation on epoprostenol infusion only when the hemodynamic profile shows reduction of PAM below 35 mm Hg and PVR below 250 dyne·sec·cm^{-5}.[54] Use of intravenous epoprostenol in association with inhaled NO to reduce preoperative pulmonary hypertension to levels less than 35 mm Hg, followed by successful liver transplantation, has been described in a small group of 6 patients by Molmenti and coworkers.[66] Patients transplanted with infusion of epoprostenol should be continued on epoprostenol infusion after liver transplantation and progressively weaned from this medication under monitoring over at least 6 months after transplantation. This is because there is evidence of progressive right ventricular failure and persistent pulmonary hypertension among patients transplanted with significant pulmonary hypertension, suggesting persistent PVR, which will require time to undergo remodeling.[67,68]

Disease-Related Changes

Primary Biliary Cirrhosis

Several studies have described pulmonary dysfunction in patients with primary biliary cirrhosis.[4,11] The most common abnormality seen is a decreased diffusion capacity, and this may or may not be related to the presence of concurrent Sjögren's syndrome.[69,70] Obstructive and restrictive airway disease has been demonstrated in patients with primary biliary cirrhosis and Sjögren's syndrome. Evidence suggests that these pulmonary abnormalities may be related to the presence of Sjögren's syndrome and not to the liver disease.[4,70,71] Restrictive lung disease may be mimicked in the individual with severe osteopenia, which causes thorax deformity and reduced lung volumes.[11] Interstitial lung disease in the form of lymphocytic interstitial pneumonitis can occur and may be fatal.[4] Special consideration should be given to the possible overlap syndrome that exists between primary biliary cirrhosis and sarcoidosis when evaluating patients with interstitial lung disease.[4,72]

α_1-Antitrypsin Deficiency

α_1-Antitrypsin is a glycoprotein synthesized mainly by hepatocytes and alveolar macrophages. It is a protease inhibitor and protects tissues from proteolytic attack by leukocyte proteases such as elastase, cathepsin, and trypsin, which are present during inflammatory reactions.[73] Abnormal α_1 protein synthesis evolves from a single-point gene mutation located on chromosomes 14q31-32.2,[74] which is codominantly expressed in the hepatocyte. More than 90 alleles have been identified, but only a few are associated with low or undetectable serum level of the protein. α_1-Antitrypsin plays an important role in neutralizing neutrophil elastase in the lungs. Deficiency of α_1-antitrypsin allows neutrophil elastase to destroy the alveolar wall's connective tissue, resulting in emphysema.[75] The phenotype for the α_1-antitrypsin gene can be assessed.[76] Heterozygous phenotypes usually do not manifest clinical liver disease,[4] although hepatomegaly, spider nevi, and esophageal varices have been reported. Homozygotes of the PiZZ phenotype deposit abnormal α_1-antitrypsin protein within the hepatocyte, which is pathologically characterized by periodic acid–Schiff test–positive cytoplasmic globules. A significant portion of these individuals may have progression to cirrhosis and portal hypertension as children or adults.[4] The prominent pulmonary abnormality that occurs as an adult with the PiZZ phenotype is panacinar emphysema with severe expiratory airflow obstruction resulting in dyspnea. The emphysematous changes in these individuals occurs predominantly in the lower lobes, contrary to the usual upper lobe bullous emphysema that occurs in chronic smokers. Bullous emphysema is caused by the imbalance between protective α_1 protein and neutrophil elastase produced by leukocytes. This imbalance allows destruction of the supportive elastic tissues that tether open small airways.[39] Severe emphysema typically occurs in individuals younger than 50 years, and it will be accelerated in the α_1-antitrypsin-deficient patient who is also a smoker.[77]

The normal plasma level of α_1-antitrypsin is 150 to 350 mg/dL. Levels under 80 mg/dL are insufficient to protect the lung from developing emphysema. Most patients under this threshold will have the PiZZ phenotype. These patients can be managed with *augmentation* therapy, which involves weekly or monthly intravenous infusion of pooled human α_1-antiprotease for selected patients showing established airflow obstruction who are nonsmokers.[78] Patients selected for treatment receive purified pooled human antiprotease (Prolastin) 60 mg/kg for 1 hour per week or 250 mg/kg for 6 hours per month to maintain α_1-antitrypsin levels higher than 80 mg/dL. This therapy is costly (approximately $40,000 per year),[79] and may have adverse effects such as low-grade fever, anaphylaxis, and the consequences of using a blood product transfusion. Augmentation therapy does not improve liver function. Liver transplantation alone or in conjunction with a double-lung transplant has been reported in patients with α_1-antitrypsin deficiency who develop cirrhosis.[80,81] It is the most common metabolic disease leading to liver transplantation in children.[82] Most commonly, single- or double-lung transplantation has been a successful approach for patients with severe α_1-antitrypsin-related severe emphysema who do not have liver disease.[83]

Cystic Fibrosis

Cystic fibrosis (CF) is one of the most common homozygous genetic diseases among white individuals, with an approximate prevalence of 1 per 2000 births.[84] Although most CF patients eventually succumb to respiratory failure, cor pulmonale, and pulmonary hypertension, advances in their medical management has improved their survival into late adulthood. It is well recognized that significant deterioration in forced vital capacity, forced expiratory volume at 1 second (FEV$_1$), hypercapnia,

and hypoxemia are all markers of poor prognosis among patients with CF, which is part of the criteria for selecting candidates for bilateral lung transplantation. However, there is increasing recognition that associated chronic liver disease and hepatomegaly are also important negatives in correlation with survival.[85] Although only 8% of deaths among patients with both liver disease and CF are reported,[86] liver failure is nevertheless the second most common cause of death among these patients, following respiratory failure. Liver transplantation has been reported to be an effective therapy in patients with CF who develop portal hypertension and hepatic dysfunction. Liver transplant recipients with CF who do not have end-stage lung disease recover well from surgery and their lung function may even improve after undergoing the transplant.[87] For patients with advanced respiratory disease, combined transplantation—including heart, lung, and liver; sequential double-lung-liver; and bilateral lobar lung from a split left lung and a reduced liver—has been reported with variable success.[88]

Evaluation

Figure 28–1 summarizes the initial evaluation process of prospective liver transplant recipients. The evaluation should include:

- Posteroanterior and lateral chest radiographs
- Arterial blood gas measurements taken with the patient in an upright sitting position and breathing room air
- A baseline transthoracic echocardiogram

If obstructive or restrictive lung disease is suspected, the workup should proceed to establish the significance of pulmonary disease; the tests for this should include a computed tomographic scan of the chest, pulmonary function testing such as lung volumes, expiratory flows, maximal volume ventilation, and diffusion capacity. If arterial hypoxemia (room air Pao$_2$ <70 mm Hg), hypercapnia (Paco$_2$ >45 mm Hg), or a significant reduction in volumes and flows (FEV$_1$ <1 L) are found, the patient needs referral for further pulmonary evaluation prior to establishing candidacy for liver transplantation. If the chest radiograph finds significant pleural effusion present, the workup should include CT of chest to define underlying pleural or pulmonary disease and characteristics of the pleural effusion. A thoracentesis should be planned for diagnostic and therapeutic purposes. The fluid should be analyzed for cell counts, differential, protein, glucose, LDH and PH should be measured, and fluid should be submitted for bacteriological and cytological studies. If the fluid shows the characteristics of an exudate (elevated protein and LDH levels), then infection and neoplasia must be

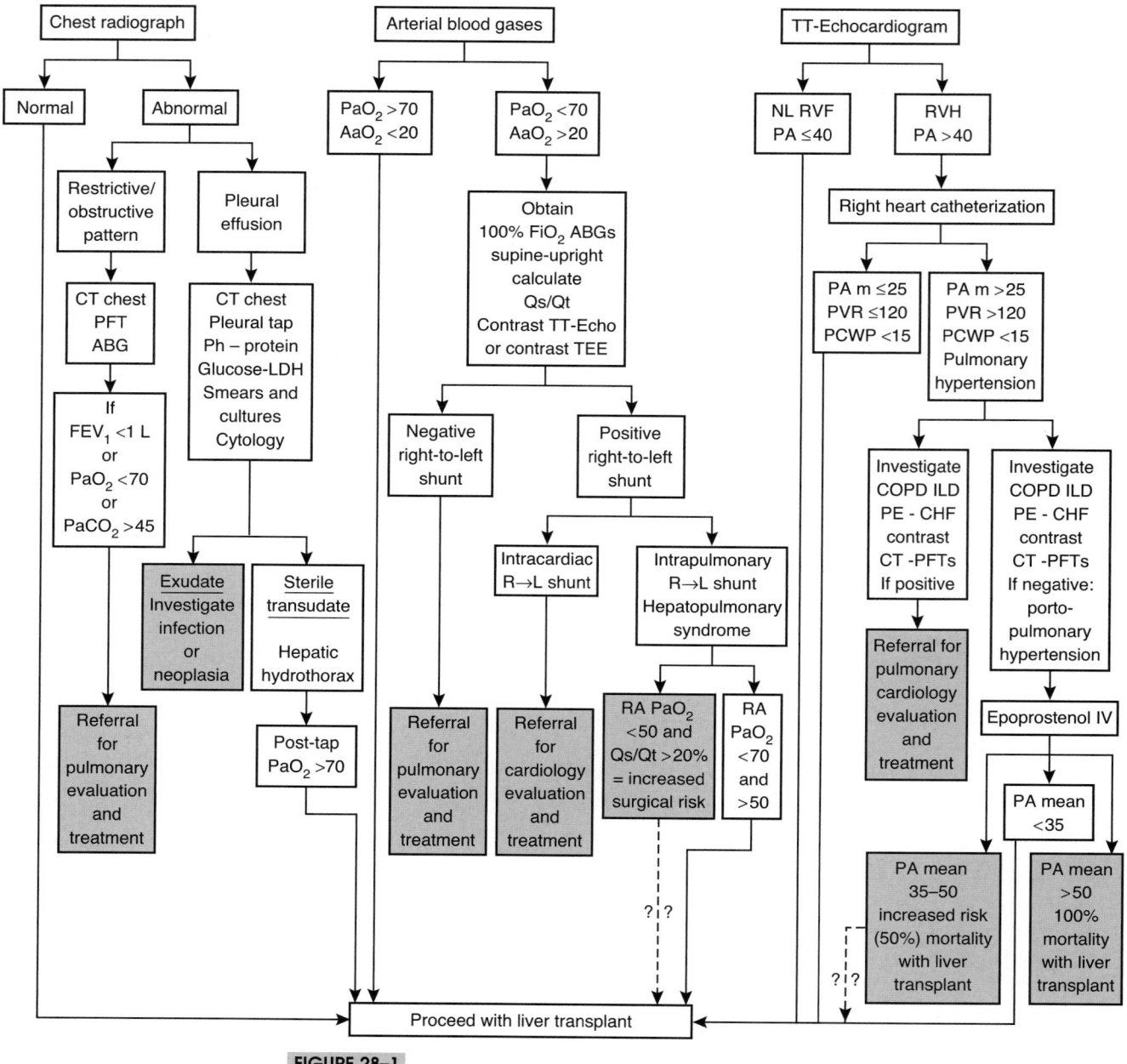

FIGURE 28–1

Liver transplant candidate: pulmonary diagnostic workup algorithm.

considered and further workup is indicated until these conditions are ruled out. If the fluid is found to be a sterile transudate, the diagnosis is hepatic hydrothorax. Patients with hepatic hydrothorax without significant gas exchange abnormalities (preferable if measured after the fluid is evacuated) should proceed with liver transplantation if otherwise indicated.

Patients showing hypoxemia in the baseline arterial blood gases, characterized by room air PaO_2 less than 70 mm Hg and or room air alveolar-arterial oxygen gradient greater than 20 mm Hg should have further studies including shunt studies with 100% inspired oxygen in the supine and standing positions to determine the presence of true anatomic shunt versus ventilation-perfusion mismatch versus diffusion-perfusion impairment.

Alveolar-arterial oxygen gradient (AaO_2) is calculated using the alveolar-air equation as

$$AaO_2 = P_{AO_2} - Pa_{O_2}$$

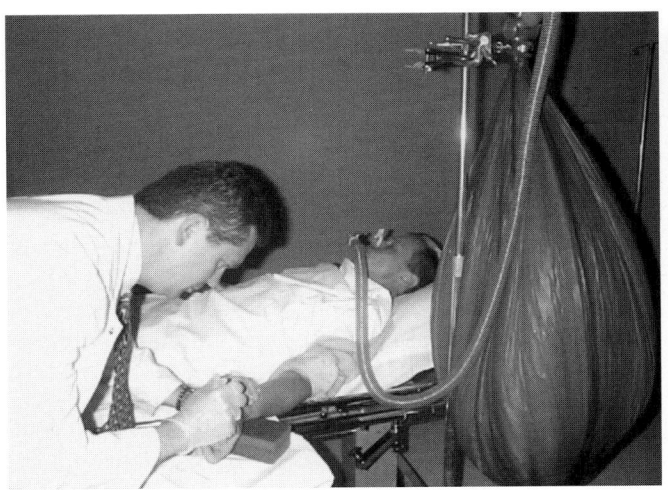
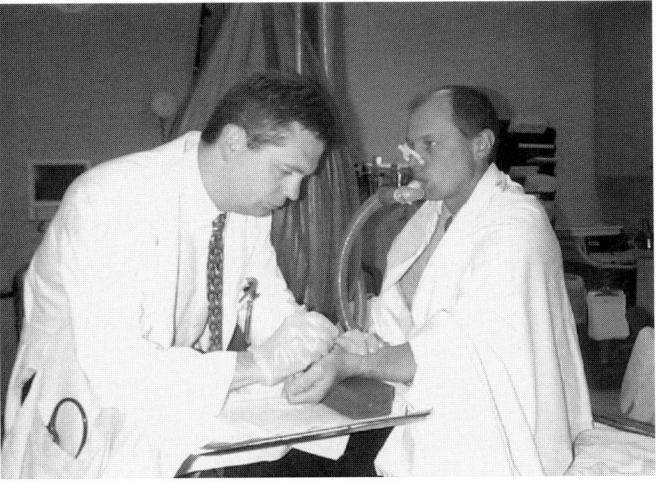

A   B

FIGURE 28–2

Shunt studies in the supine and upright positions. **A,** Patient breathes from a source of pure oxygen via a one-way valve mouthpiece with the nose clipped. After at least 15 minutes in the supine position, an arterial blood gas is drawn. **B,** The patient is then placed in the upright position where the process is repeated. Arterial blood gases are then used to calculate the shunt fraction (Qs/Qt). The patient with typical hepatopulmonary syndrome will show hypoxemia and increased Qs/Qt in the supine position that worsens in the upright position (orthodeoxia). In addition, compensatory hyperventilation (respiratory alkalosis) and dyspnea will occur in the upright position (platypnea).

where P_{AO_2} = (barometric pressure − 47) $\times F_{IO_2} - P_{aCO_2}/0.8.$

The normal gradient is calculated as A_{aO_2} = 2.5 + 0.21 × age. Most adults normally have an A_{aO_2} less than 20 mm Hg.

Calculation of the shunt fraction (Qs/Qt) requires administration of 100% F_{IO_2} via a one-way valve mouthpiece connected to a pure oxygen source (usually a large-volume balloon filled with 100% F_{IO_2}). The patient breathes from the oxygen source with the nose clipped in both the supine and upright positions (Fig. 28–2) and arterial blood gas measurements are obtained. The shunt fraction is calculated as:

$$\frac{Qs}{Qt} = \frac{((P_{AO_2} - P_{aO_2}) \times 0.0031) \times 100}{((P_{AO_2} - P_{aO_2}) \times 0.0031) + 5}$$

The normal Qs/Qt fraction is less than 5%. Values greater than 20% are consistent with severe hepatopulmonary syndrome. A preoperative P_{aO_2} in room air less than 50 mm Hg and a shunt fraction greater than 20% are the strongest predictors for postoperative mortality among these patients[50,51]; therefore, decisions about liver transplantation among these patients must be individualized by each transplant center.

Radioisotope scanning using ^{99m}Tc-labeled macro-aggregated albumin measures lung perfusion and extra-pulmonary uptake, or pulmonary angiography may also be helpful in demonstrating intrapulmonary vasodilation as a cause of hypoxemia.[28] True anatomic shunts show little or no improvement in P_{aO_2} on 100% oxygen. Ventilation-perfusion mismatch usually shows improvement on 100% oxygen, whereas individuals with diffusion-perfusion impairment may show a range of responses to 100% oxygen from little improvement to near normal increase in P_{aO_2}. Contrast-enhanced echocardiography using an injection of agitated saline to create microbubbles can further assist in the differentiation of these diagnoses as discussed in the section of hepatopulmonary syndrome. These tests help to confirm the physiological cause of hypoxemia.[24] If intrapulmonary shunting is suspected and a contrast transthoracic echocardiogram is not diagnostic, a contrast transesophageal echocardiogram is indicated.[27,28]

Screening patients for pulmonary hypertension can be performed with a chest radiograph and echocardiography. The chest radiograph may demonstrate an enlarged right atrium or plethoric pulmonary vessels suggestive of pulmonary hypertension. Two-dimensional echocardiography with Doppler showing enlarged chambers on the right side of the heart and estimated pulmonary pressures greater than 40 mm Hg indicate that a right heart catheterization should be performed, which is the gold standard in making the diagnosis of pulmonary hypertension. Pulmonary hypertension is defined as pulmonary artery mean pressure (PAM) greater than 25 mm Hg, with associated PVR greater than 120 dyne·sec·cm^{-5} with normal pulmonary capillary wedge pressures (PCWP) less than 15 mm Hg. If pulmonary hypertension is detected in these patients, a workup to rule out other causes of pulmonary hypertension (such as obstructive and restrictive lung disease, pulmonary thromboembolism, and cardiac disease) needs to be completed. Patients found to have associated causes need to be treated for those conditions; liver transplantation is deferred for these patients. Patients found to have either no explanation for or another explanation for pulmonary hypertension are diagnosed with HPS. Those found to have significant pulmonary hypertension may require medical therapy with intravenous epoprostenol (Flolan) in preparation for liver transplantation. Those with PAM pressures less than 35 mm Hg have a reasonable prognosis, those with PAM pressures in the range of 35 to 50 mm Hg are at risk for increased mortality, and those who remain with PAM pressures greater than 50 mm Hg face 100% mortality if subjected to liver transplantation without combined heart or heart lung transplant.

Contraindications to Liver Transplantation

The surgical risks for patients with significant asthma or obstructive lung disease are well described.[5] Assessing the candidacy of the patient with significant hypoxemia (PaO_2 <70 mm Hg) is much more difficult. As has been alluded to earlier, severe arterial hypoxemia (PaO_2 <50 mm Hg) is considered at least a relative, if not an absolute, contraindication to liver transplantation, and each center must make individualized decisions for these patients. Now there is a better pathophysiological understanding of what causes hypoxemia in chronic liver disease.[4,35] If the cause is felt to be secondary to intrapulmonary vascular dilatation and the response to 100% oxygen is fair to good, prognosis may be favorable. However, patients with poor response to 100% inspired oxygen, who maintain shunt fractions higher than 20% (either from true anatomical shunts or fixed intrapulmonary vasodilation) have a much higher surgical risk given the potential of postoperative complications, which may further exacerbate hypoxemia.

Patients with severe pulmonary hypertension (PVR > 250 dyne · sec · cm^{-5} and PAM pressures of 35 to 50 mm Hg) are at higher risk for cardiopulmonary-related mortality, and the indication for liver transplantation in these patients should be individualized by centers accustomed to treating them. Patients with PAM pressures greater than 50 mm Hg despite medical therapy face 100% mortality with liver transplantation.[37-41] They should not be transplanted, or consideration should be given to combined heart-lung-liver or lung-liver transplantation; but the outcome of patients using this approach is largely unknown because there are only anecdotal case reports available.

Cardiac

The heart of a patient undergoing liver transplantation must endure many stressors. Adequate myocardial reserve is vital to the success of liver transplantation. As liver transplantation has become more successful in the treatment of patients with end-stage liver disease, patients of advancing age and patients with extrahepatic organ dysfunction are being considered. The goal of the preoperative evaluation of cardiac function is to optimize myocardial function and minimize perioperative complications.

Preload reduction may occur from systemic hypotension related to blood loss, or from clamping of the inferior vena cava during resection of the native liver. Conversely, release of the inferior vena cava clamp at reperfusion in the absence of venovenous bypass will rapidly increase preload at the moment that contractility is most impaired. Furthermore, aortic cross-clamping may be required to place an arterial graft, and thus abruptly increase afterload. Ionized hypocalcemia from citrate complexing during blood transfusions may induce cardiac dysfunction or rhythm abnormalities.[89] Postreperfusion syndrome has been attributed to acute acidosis, hyperkalemia, and hypothermia following reperfusion of the transplanted liver. The resulting cardiovascular collapse, characterized by hypotension, myocardial depression, rhythm irregularities, or all of these, dramatically increases work placed on the heart.[90] Left and right ventricular dysfunction can occur during liver transplantation.[91-93] The resulting hypotension may be multifactorial, but can be poorly tolerated in patients with compromised coronary perfusion, valvular heart disease, cardiac arrhythmias, and myocardial infiltration with amyloid or iron. Anticipation of these changes during liver transplantation necessitates full cardiac evaluation preoperatively. Focus of the evaluation revolves around the presence of coronary artery disease, left ventricular dysfunction, valvular heart disease, and arrhythmias.

Coronary Artery Disease

Patients with end-stage liver disease frequently have risk factors associated with coronary artery disease (CAD) (Table 28–1). Indeed, Carey and colleagues found a 27% prevalence of angiographically moderate or severe CAD in liver transplant candidates older than the age of 50 years.[94] Moderate or severe CAD was defined as the presence of more than 30% stenosis. The presence of severe CAD (defined as stenosis >70%) was found to be 16.2%. After eliminating patients with a documented history of CAD, the authors found that 13.3% of the patients studied had significant asymptomatic CAD. Plotkin and colleagues studied a population of

Table 28-1. CORONARY ARTERY DISEASE RISK FACTORS
Diabetes mellitus
Hypertension
Hypercholesterolemia
Smoking
Obesity
Age
Family history of premature coronary artery disease

patients undergoing evaluation for liver transplantation who were suspected of being at risk for the presence of CAD with dobutamine stress echocardiography.[95] Coronary angiography was performed on those patients with abnormal studies (defined as electrocardiogram [ECG] changes with or without the development of chest pain, or the development of new wall motion abnormalities with dobutamine infusion). In this study, the prevalence of CAD was 5%. Both studies identified diabetes as a significant risk factor for the presence of CAD. When patients with CAD undergo liver transplantation, Plotkin and colleagues found the 3-year mortality to be 50%.[96]

Left Ventricular Dysfunction

The most common cause of left ventricular (LV) systolic dysfunction (poor LV ejection fraction) is preexisting CAD and previous myocardial infarction. Furthermore, uncompensated valvular heart disease, such as severe aortic stenosis, aortic insufficiency, or mitral insufficiency, can lead to LV systolic dysfunction. Severe tricuspid regurgitation, may lead to right ventricular systolic dysfunction. Long-standing, poorly controlled hypertension can lead to LV hypertrophy and diastolic dysfunction (abnormal LV relaxation). As this condition progresses, it is possible that the LV will begin to fail and result in decreased ejection fraction. Diastolic dysfunction is poorly tolerated if preload is significantly reduced. When combined with LV hypertrophy and decreased LV filling time caused by tachycardia, the cardiac output could be effectively reduced to the point that hypotension ensues.

Cardiomyopathy has been described in several different forms of liver disease. It is believed that alcohol's direct myocardial depressant effect is associated with dilated cardiomyopathy in Laënnec's cirrhosis.[97] Myofibroblastic proliferation of mitral valve chordae tendineae has also been described in patients with Laënnec's cirrhosis. Hemochromatosis can cause infiltration of the myocardium with iron, resulting in restrictive cardiomyopathy.[98] In addition, patients with hepatic tumors undergoing treatment with anthracycline

chemotherapeutic agents may develop toxicity leading to cardiomyopathy.

Arrhythmia

Preexisting dysrhythmias such as atrial fibrillation or supraventricular tachycardia may be aggravated by the increased adrenergic state found after surgery. This is further aggravated by volume, electrolyte (hypokalemia, hypomagnesemia, hypocalcemia), and acid-base imbalances that are found in the perioperative state. These circumstances could lead to hypotension, making postoperative management more difficult. Preexisting rhythm abnormalities have been described in patients with hemochromatosis and Wilson's disease. Patients with preexisting prolonged QT may be at particular risk with the use of tacrolimus (FK506, Prograf), a lincomycin.

Evaluation

Assessment of cardiac risk for liver transplantation begins with a detailed history with careful attention to the presence of cardiac risk factors (see Table 28–1) and symptoms suggestive of coronary ischemia or significant valvular heart disease. A history of tobacco use should be sought, particularly in patients with alcohol-related liver disease. Hyperlipidemia may occur in patients with primary biliary cirrhosis. Diabetes is a risk factor for nonalcoholic steatohepatitis (NASH) and may be secondarily present in patients with hemochromatosis. Patients with a history of hypertension may present with normal or decreased blood pressure caused by vasodilation from advanced liver disease, but are still at risk to develop preexisting coronary disease. Advanced liver disease is often associated with muscle wasting and weakness that result in profound fatigue with minimal exertion. This debilitated state may result in lack of stress placed on the coronary circulation to induce symptoms of angina. Thus, the lack of angina does not rule out the presence of CAD or preclude the need for ischemic evaluation.

Electrocardiogram

All patients undergoing evaluation for liver transplantation should receive an ECG. Rhythm abnormalities should be controlled prior to transplantation and warrant further investigation with stress testing. The presence of LV hypertrophy is associated with hypertension and warrants further investigation with stress testing. The presence of a right or left bundle-branch block may indicate the presence of underlying cardiac disease and should be further investigated with echocardiography and stress testing. A finding of Q-wave and ST-segment or T-wave abnormalities suggests the presence of underlying CAD and warrants echocardiography and stress testing. Electrocardiographic evidence of right atrial enlargement or right ventricular hypertension suggests the presence of pulmonary hypertension and should prompt a more precise measurement of pulmonary artery pressures.

Echocardiography

Echocardiography with Doppler should also be performed on all patients undergoing evaluation for liver transplantation. Two-dimensional echocardiography detects whether focal or diffuse LV wall motion abnormalities are present. Abnormal wall motion should be followed up with coronary angiography to determine if untreated CAD is the cause of abnormal LV function. Doppler evaluation of the cardiac valves detects whether significant valvular disease is present, which may have an adverse effect on the perioperative risk for cardiovascular complications. Doppler evaluation of the tricuspid valve could estimate right ventricular systolic pressure, thus correlating with an estimation of the systolic pulmonary artery pressure. Elevation of pulmonary artery pressure suggests the presence of POPH. This echocardiographic finding necessitates right heart catheterization with a balloon-tipped pulmonary artery catheter to confirm the presence of pulmonary hypertension. If such abnormalities are detected in the screening ECG or echocardiogram, evaluation by a cardiovascular specialist would be helpful both to further determine the risk for adverse cardiovascular events and to help identify treatment strategies that would assist in lowering the risk to an acceptable level.

Intravenous saline contrast should be given to detect the presence of right-to-left shunting while undergoing echocardiography. Bubbles from the intravenous saline contrast crossing the atrial septum seen within the first or second cardiac cycle suggest the presence of a patent foramen ovale (PFO), which would assist in fluid management preoperatively, perioperatively, and postoperatively. As preload increases, the right atrial pressure will increase and exacerbate right-to-left shunting across the PFO, possibly resulting in hypoxemia. Visualization of bubbles in the left ventricle late after administration of intravenous saline contrast (after the fourth or fifth cardiac cycle) suggests the presence of intrapulmonary shunting. Intrapulmonary shunting is common in liver disease, and when it is associated with hypoxemia (Pao_2 <60 in room air), the diagnosis of hepatopulmonary syndrome is suggested. The intravenous saline contrast should be given both with and without a Valsalva maneuver, as right-to-left shunting may be present only when the right atrial pressure is increased, as demonstrated by the Valsalva maneuver. Finally, administering the intravenous saline contrast from the left antecubital vein helps to detect the presence of a persistent left superior vena cava.

Stress Testing

Patients older than 45 years, patients with coronary risk factors (see Table 28–1), and patients with clinical predictors of increased perioperative risk for adverse cardiovascular events (Table 28–2) should undergo some form of noninvasive evaluation to assist in the determination of hemodynamically significant CAD. Patients with end-stage liver disease are frequently debilitated and may not develop angina, because they are unable to exert themselves to the extent that the myocardial oxygen demand exceeds the decreased supply caused by the presence of CAD. The debilitated state of these patients precludes them from performing a valid stress test using a treadmill or a bicycle, because they are unlikely to be able to exert themselves to the extent that they reach 85% of predicted maximal heart rate with physical exertion. Pharmacological stress testing has been used successfully in a strategy to detect the presence

Table 28–2. CLINICAL PREDICTORS OF ADVERSE PERIOPERATIVE CARDIAC COMPLICATIONS

Major Clinical Predictors

Recent myocardial infarction

Unstable angina

Decompensated congestive heart failure

Significant arrhythmias (high-grade atrioventricular block, symptomatic ventricular arrhythmias with coronary artery disease, supraventricular arrhythmias with uncontrolled ventricular rate)

Severe valvular disease

Intermediate Clinical Predictors

Mild angina

Prior myocardial infarction

Compensated or prior congestive heart failure

Diabetes mellitus

Minor Clinical Predictors

Advanced age

Abnormal electrocardiogram

Low functional capacity

History of stroke

Uncontrolled systemic hypertension

From Eagle KA, Berger PB, Calkins H, et al: ACC/AHA guideline update for perioperative cardiovascular evaluation for noncardiac surgery—executive summary: A report of the American College of Cardiology/American Heart Association Task Force on Practice Guidelines (Committee to Update the 1996 Guidelines on Perioperative Cardiovascular Evaluation for Noncardiac Surgery). Copyright © 2002 by American College of Cardiology and American Heart Association, Inc.

of CAD as part of a comprehensive cardiovascular evaluation for noncardiac surgery in those who cannot perform a maximal exercise stress test.[99] Dipyridamole, in combination with thallium-201 or ^{99m}Tc-labeled sestamibi, can assist in evaluating the risk of cardiac events in patients known or suspected of having CAD who are undergoing major noncardiovascular surgery.[100,101] Dobutamine stress echocardiography also is a useful aid for assessing the risk of adverse perioperative cardiac events in patients undergoing nonvascular surgery.[102] In patients who are unable to achieve an 85% predicted maximal heart rate, the addition of atropine to a dobutamine stress echocardiography improves the sensitivity for detecting CAD.[103] This is especially important because the use of β-blockers for portal hypertension may have a negative impact on the ability to achieve an 85% predicted maximal heart rate, and thus reduce the sensitivity of the dobutamine stress echocardiogram. Donovan and associates and Plotkin and colleagues have shown the utility of a dobutamine stress echo in detecting the presence of CAD and how the results may be used to assist with treatment strategies to manage these patients.[95,104] Both studies showed that patients with a dobutamine stress echo that did not reveal myocardial ischemia—defined as a new wall motion abnormality with dobutamine infusion—did not have excessive cardiovascular events. The negative predictive value was 100% in both studies.

In the event of an abnormal stress test, consultation with a cardiovascular specialist would be helpful to assist in determining the need for further evaluation, such as coronary angiography. The severity of coronary disease and LV function determines the risk for liver transplantation. Percutaneous coronary intervention (PCI) with balloon or stents, or both, typically requires the use of unfractionated heparin or antiplatelet agents, or both, such as aspirin, glycoprotein (GP) IIb/IIIa inhibitors, ticlopidine, or clopidogrel. The use of these agents prior to liver transplantation places the patient at increased risk for bleeding, as many patients with end-stage liver disease are coagulopathic or thrombocytopenic, or both. Furthermore, surgical intervention to repair severe CAD or valvular heart with coronary artery bypass grafting (CABG) or valve repair/replacement prior to liver transplantation is associated with high morbidity and mortality.[96,105] Simultaneous CABG and valve repair and replacement has been done, but it also carries high risk of morbidity and mortality.

Renal

Diagnosis

Renal disease is a common sequela of hepatic failure. Proper assessment of renal function is important in the patient undergoing evaluation for liver transplantation. Preoperative renal failure increases postoperative liver transplantation mortality.[106-108] In patients with severe or irreversible renal disease, or both, therapies such as preoperative or intraoperative dialysis, combined liver-kidney transplant, and altered postoperative renal-sparing immunosuppression may favorably affect postoperative mortality and morbidity.[109-111] Knowledge of the effects of liver disease on the kidney enables proper preoperative evaluation of liver transplant candidates.

Many metabolic abnormalities occur in the setting of hepatic failure, including disturbances in acid-base balance. Respiratory alkalosis is the most frequent acid-base abnormality, and the degree of alkalosis directly correlates with the severity of liver disease.[112,113] The cause is uncertain, with progesterone[114] and retained amines[112] implicated as possible causes. The degree of respiratory alkalosis does not appear to be associated with ammonia (NH_3) production or the development of hypoxemia.[114] Metabolic alkalosis may develop, most commonly as a consequence of diuretic therapy.[112] Metabolic alkalosis stimulates an increased formation of NH_3 from NH_4^+, which then more easily enters the blood-brain barrier and increases the risk of hepatic encephalopathy.[112] Metabolic acidosis can occur in the form of lactate and renal tubular acidosis. Lactic acidosis develops in acute and chronic forms of liver disease when insufficient hepatic tissue remains to metabolize lactate, or from overproduction of lactate caused by complications of infection, gastrointestinal bleeding, or hypotension.[115,116] Distal (type I) renal tubular acidosis has been reported in primary biliary cirrhosis, autoimmune hepatitis, alcoholic liver disease (ALD), and cryptogenic cirrhosis.[115,117] Proximal (type II) renal tubular acidosis is associated with Wilson's disease, often creating a true Fanconi syndrome.[118] Forms of hyperchloremic metabolic acidosis may develop with the use of spironolactone or cholestyramine.[119,120] Renal dysfunction may be a source of metabolic acidosis with advanced liver disease, and in both anion gap and nonanion gap forms.[115,121] The acid-base disturbances do not present a contraindication to hepatic transplantation, but recognition is important for providing adequate preoperative care.[115]

Other metabolic abnormalities that occur in the setting of hepatic failure are electrolyte changes. Hyponatremia develops secondary to hemodynamic changes occurring with hepatic failure and is most commonly found in the presence of ascites.[115,122] Splanchnic vasodilation leads to a decrease in effective arterial blood volume, stimulating baroreceptors, which in turn signal nonosmotic production of antidiuretic hormone.[123] Careful treatment of symptomatic hyponatremia and proper perioperative fluid management of hyponatremia are important in preventing demyelinating complications of the brain (central pontine myelinolysis) and are discussed in several reviews.[124,125] Treatment using an experimental vasopressin antagonist has been described.[126] Hypokalemia is most commonly caused by diuretic use, gastrointestinal losses associated with lactulose and, rarely, magnesium deficiency.[115] Hypokalemia is a confounding factor in the development and maintenance of metabolic alkalosis and, as mentioned earlier, may therefore increase the risk of hepatic encephalopathy. Potassium supplementation and the use of potassium-sparing diuretics are effective therapies. Renal dysfunction, β-blockers (used to prevent variceal bleeding), potassium-sparing diuretics, nonsteroidal anti-inflammatory drugs (NSAIDs), and the use of angiotensin-converting enzyme (ACE) inhibitor and angiotensin receptor blocker (ARB) medication may singly or in combination produce hyperkalemia.[127-129] Monitoring potassium, particularly in patients with renal dysfunction and concomitant use of these drugs, is important in preventing life-threatening hyperkalemia.

Clinical evaluation of renal dysfunction in patients with advanced hepatic disease is not always straightforward. Defining renal function remains important in establishing operative risk and candidacy for transplantation and may influence perioperative care, including postoperative immunosuppression. Creatinine is normally a useful marker of renal function. Yet, in this patient population, it has been found to be unreliable for several reasons. Creatine, a precursor of creatinine, is primarily synthesized by the liver and is produced at rates that are half that of healthy volunteers.[130] This decreases the substrate available for use by the muscles and other tissue to produce creatinine. Additionally, malnourishment and decreased muscle mass lead to decreased production of creatinine, with blood levels lower than one would expect for a particular given glomerular filtration rate (GFR).[131] Increased renal tubular secretion of creatinine may further reduce blood concentrations, particularly in a setting of renal dysfunction.[132,133] Some analytical methods of determining creatinine may underestimate true serum concentration in the presence of hyperbilirubinemia, although this appears to be laboratory dependent.[134] In cirrhotics with normal serum creatinine, 37% of patients are reported to have a GFR of less than 50 mL/min, and 31% have a GFR between 50 and 80 mL/min.[135] This is one of several studies confirming the poor relationship between creatinine and GFR.[134] Other serum markers such as cystatin C may prove valuable in assessing renal function in the future.[136,137]

Equations estimating GFR are used to assess renal function in other patient populations. These formulae use varying combinations of a patient's age, sex, weight, ethnicity, serum creatinine, serum urea nitrogen, and serum albumin to predict GFR. The popular Cockcroft-Gault equation is compared with inulin clearance (the gold standard for measuring GFR) in patients with advanced liver disease and is found to overestimate GFR, particularly in patients with inulin clearances less than 70 mL/min.[130,136] Other formulae, such as the Modification of Diet in Renal Disease (MDRD) and the Nankivell equation, have not been validated in cirrhotics and cannot be recommended for use at this time.[138,139]

Determining GFR by direct measurements is possible with several tools. As mentioned before, inulin clearance is recognized as the gold standard, but the scarcity of product, limited number of trained personnel, duration of the study, and the expense limit its use to research settings.[134] A 24-hour urine collection for measuring creatinine clearance is a common means of determining GFR. Unfortunately, measured creatinine clearance in cirrhotics overestimates GFR by 13% when inulin clearance is greater than 70 mL/min, and by 96% when inulin clearance is less than 70 mL/min.[130] Nonetheless, measured creatinine clearance, as an estimate of GFR, is superior to creatinine or calculated creatinine clearance.[130,134] Other options for determining GFR include use of isotope markers such as ^{125}I-iothalamate, ^{99m}Tc-DTPA, and ^{51}Cr-EDTA, and nonisotopes like cold iothalamate and iohexol.[138,140-142] These techniques are not widely available and none has been validated in cirrhotics to determine GFR, although they may be helpful.[110,134] Although flawed, 24-hour urine for creatinine is a community standard in measuring GFR. In the future, the validation of isotope and nonisotope markers for GFR listed previously will make the determination of renal function more precise and improve selection and care of liver transplant candidates.

Renal disease manifests in many ways, and one form is volume depletion. Diuretic therapy, paracentesis, diarrhea secondary to lactulose, and gastrointestinal bleeding may produce volume depletion and adversely affect renal function. Prevention of volume depletion in cirrhotics is important in maintaining renal health. Diuretic use for ascites should be limited to a maximal dose of 400 mg of spironolactone and/or 160 mg of furosemide daily in divided doses.[143] Blood urea nitrogen (BUN) and creatinine should be monitored on this therapy, particularly in ascitic patients without edema. The furosemide natriuresis test may help identify diuretic responders in advanced liver disease and avoid complications of diuretic use in nonresponders.[144] Hypovolemia after large-volume paracentesis may be prevented by albumin infusion after treatment. Wong and Blendis recommend determining plasma renin activity (PRA) levels to determine patients who are at high risk for renal dysfunction after large-volume paracentesis. In high-risk patients, intravenous administration of 6 to 8 g of albumin/L of ascites drained is recommended to preserve renal function, particularly for volume removal of more than 5 L of ascites.[143,145] Lactulose-induced diarrhea used to treat hepatic encephalopathy may produce volume depletion, particularly if the patient does not ingest adequate fluid because of confusion. Gastrointestinal bleeding that produces hypotension must be aggressively treated to limit detrimental effects on renal function. Additionally, patients with ascites and variceal bleeding should be administered prophylactic antibiotics to prevent subacute bacterial peritonitis and renal failure.[143]

Patients with advanced liver disease are exposed to nephrotoxins, which may alter renal function. Aminoglycosides are directly toxic to renal tubular cells.[146] Amphotericin and contrast agents are also toxic to these cells, but like NSAIDs (both nonselective and cyclooxygenase-2 [COX-2] inhibitors), they may produce renal dysfunction by vasoconstriction.[127,147-149] Another form of renal dysfunction induced by NSAIDs is acute interstitial nephritis, which may be accompanied by minimal-change glomerulopathy, producing nephrotic proteinuria.[150] Interestingly, cholestasis itself is nephrotoxic with links to renal vasoconstriction and direct tubular toxicity, perhaps from the effects of elevated blood concentrations of bile acids.[143] Prerenal physiology found in advanced liver disease may increase the toxicity of these agents, and they should be avoided if possible. When used, the patient should be properly hydrated and monitored to minimize adverse renal effects. A history of nephrotoxin exposure should be obtained in all cirrhotics with renal dysfunction.

Prerenal injury to the kidneys is common in cirrhosis and presents in its most severe form as hepatorenal syndrome (HRS). In 1996, the International Ascites Club provided a consensus definition of HRS (Table 28–3).[151] This consensus group further categorized HRS as type I and type II:[151]

- Type I HRS is defined by a doubling of serum creatinine to a level greater than 2.5 mg/dL or a halving of creatinine clearance to less than 20 mL/min in less than 2 weeks.

- Type II HRS is associated with a slowly progressive increase in serum creatinine to a level greater than 1.5 mg/dL or a creatinine clearance of less than 40 mL/min.

Type I HRS carries a worse prognosis, with a mortality of 80% at 2 weeks.[152] The pathophysiological hallmark of HRS is severe renovasoconstriction in a setting of high cardiac output and mild systemic hypotension. This functional disease of the kidneys usually causes no structural injury. Indeed, kidneys from patients with HRS have been successfully transplanted into patients with chronic kidney failure.[153] (The reader is referred to several excellent reviews of the pathophysiology of HRS.)[143,154-157] Briefly, splanchnic vasodilation occurs in a setting of presinusoidal hypertension caused by liver disease. Splanchnic vasodilation produces a fall in systemic vascular resistance and blood pressure, with

Table 28–3. DIAGNOSTIC CRITERIA FOR HEPATORENAL SYNDROME

Major

Chronic or acute liver disease with advanced hepatic failure and portal hypertension

Low glomerular filtration rate, as indicated by serum creatinine of > 1.5 mg/dL or 24-hour creatinine clearance < 40 mL/min

Absence of shock, ongoing bacterial infection, and current or recent treatment with nephrotoxic drugs

Absence of gastrointestinal fluid loss or renal fluid loss

No sustained improvement in renal function following diuretic withdrawal and expansion of plasma volume with 1.5 L of isotonic saline

Proteinuria < 500 mg/day and no sonogram evidence of obstruction or parenchymal renal disease

Additional Criteria (Not Required for Diagnosis)

Urine volume < 500 mL/day

Urine sodium < 10 mEq/L

Urine osmolality > plasma osmolality

Urine red blood cells < 50/HPF

Serum sodium concentration < 130 mEq/L

Based in part on information from reference 151.

increasing cardiac output. These hemodynamic changes decrease renal perfusion directly and also stimulate sympathetic nerve activity, the renin-aldosterone-angiotensin system, vasopressin, endothelin, and nitric oxide levels, and they may decrease renal vasodilators, producing renovasoconstriction. A better understanding of the pathophysiology of HRS has created opportunities for treatment. Therapy may stabilize or improve renal function, prolonging survival, and allow completion of liver transplant evaluation and transplantation itself in a patient who otherwise may not have survived.

Prerenal physiology (first hit) is present in advanced liver disease, and it is proposed that many cases of HRS develop as a consequence of the second hit of an additional factor precipitating more severe renovasoconstriction.[143] Prevention of the effects of the second hit may decrease the incidence of HRS. Recommendations include prophylactic antibiotics in the setting of variceal bleeding, prophylactic albumin infusion for large-volume paracentesis and as a part of the treatment for subacute bacterial peritonitis, judicious use of diuretics, and avoidance of nephrotoxic drugs and chemicals.[143] Once HRS develops, pharmacological treatment focuses on increasing systemic mean arterial pressure (MAP) and renal blood flow. Reports of vasopressin analogues acting preferentially to reverse splanchnic vasodilation and improve renal blood flow and function have been complicated by cutaneous necrosis, ischemic colitis, and extremity ischemia, which may limit their use.[158-161]

A pilot study of 12 patients reports success in reversing type I HRS, with noradrenaline, albumin, and furosemide complicated by one episode of reversible myocardial hypokinesis.[162] Long-term use of midodrine in combination with octreotide to produce a stable elevation of MAP of at least 15 mm Hg has reversed type I HRS in all of five patients studied without significant side effects.[163] A letter to the Lancet describes *N*-acetylcysteine administered intravenously in 12 patients with early HRS that improved renal function.[164] Endothelin antagonist BQ123 infusion increased inulin and PAH clearance in three patients with HRS.[165] Therapy with misoprostol, a synthetic analogue of prostaglandin E$_1$ or dopamine, has not produced improvement in patients with HRS.[166]

Nonpharmacological treatments to reverse HRS have been described. In one uncontrolled trial, most patients with HRS who were treated with an inserted transjugular intrahepatic portosystemic shunt (TIPS) had a dramatic improvement in renal function.[167] This study excluded patients with a bilirubin greater than or equal to 15 mg/dL, Child-Pugh score greater than 12, or severe encephalopathy. However, no randomized controlled trial has been performed using TIPS in HRS; therefore, its use is recommended for clinical trials only.[143] Molecular adsorbent recirculating system (MARS) is a nonpharmacological intervention studied for the treatment of HRS. Mitzner and colleagues performed a randomized control study in 13 patients with type I HRS using MARS with hemodiafiltration (HDF) versus HDF alone.[168] Each group received standard medical therapy. Creatinine was significantly lower, and MAP and survival were significantly higher in the MARS group. This may prove to be therapy providing an effective bridge to transplant, but more study is required.[143] Future controlled trials will establish standard treatment for hepatorenal syndrome, but until then many of the previously listed treatment options must be considered experimental.

Dialysis may provide support for patients with acute renal failure secondary to hepatorenal syndrome. Dialysis support is indicated with the expectation of reversible liver disease or liver transplantation;[169] otherwise, it should not be offered as it does not favorably affect long-term survival and may prolong suffering.[157,169] Patients with acute renal failure awaiting liver transplantation often require continuous forms of renal replacement therapy because of hemodynamic instability.[157,169] There is no consistent evidence of improved outcomes with continuous forms of dialysis when compared with conventional dialysis support, except in the setting of increased intracranial pressure.[157,170]

Renal dysfunction in the setting of cirrhosis not meeting criteria for HRS requires further evaluation. Acute tubular necrosis (ATN) must be considered if renal dysfunction does not respond favorably to fluid. ATN may result from ischemic or toxic injury from diuretics, paracentesis, infection, gastrointestinal losses, contrast, or nephrotoxic drugs.[169] Proteinuria is usually absent in ATN. Differences from HRS include elevated urine sodium, fractional excretion of sodium greater than 1%, and isosthenuric urine often accompanied by muddy brown granular casts.[171,172] Reports have described a low fractional excretion of sodium with an ATN injury because of underlying severe prerenal physiology of advanced liver disease.[172] This is a functional form of renal disease and is usually reversible, with 5% to 11% of the patients requiring long-term dialysis.[171]

In the presence of proteinuria, pyuria, or microscopic hematuria, fixed or intrinsic renal parenchymal disease has to be considered. Proteinuria or hematuria, or both, may represent renal injury from underlying hypertension or diabetes—the two most common causes of kidney disease.[173,174] De novo forms of glomerulonephritis and medication-induced allergic interstitial nephritis are included in the differential diagnoses, and often can be diagnosed only with kidney biopsy. Polycystic kidney disease, nephrolithiasis, obstructive nephropathy, and urinary tract cancer usually can be excluded with sonography or computerized tomography. Documentation of intrinsic renal disease is important because of the potential for progression of underlying renal disease after transplantation and the worry of calcineurin inhibitor toxicity[175] when used for immunosuppression. Knowledge of the degree of intrinsic disease and its potential to progress may be used to determine the patient's candidacy for combined liver/kidney transplant and posttransplant immunosuppression.

Disease-Related Changes

There are intrinsic renal diseases specifically associated with forms of advanced liver failure.[175,176] These diseases are listed in Table 28–4,[175-180] and the diagnosis requires renal biopsy.

There are little data describing the natural course of these kidney diseases in the setting of cirrhosis and subsequent liver transplantation.[175] Studies of the benefit of treatment for kidney disease and advanced liver failure have been limited to hepatitis B and hepatitis C patients, usually with antiviral agents.[175,176] There are no guidelines for the treatment of renal disease and advanced liver failure, and even standard nephrology treatment such as dietary protein restriction and the use of ACE inhibitors or ARBs may be contraindicated for some patients,[175] requiring highly individualized therapy.

Evaluation

Renal evaluation of liver transplant candidates requires integrated work of the transplant team to best serve

Table 28-4. RENAL DISEASES ASSOCIATED WITH ADVANCED LIVER FAILURE

Liver Disease	Renal Disease
Hepatitis B	Membranous nephropathy
	Membranoproliferative glomerulonephritis
	Polyarteritis nodosa
	IgA nephropathy
Hepatitis C	Membranoproliferative glomerulonephritis
	Membranous nephropathy
	Focal segmental glomerulonephritis
	Diabetic nephropathy
	Fibrillary glomerulonephritis
Primary biliary cirrhosis	Membranous nephropathy
	Antiglomerular basement membrane disease
	ANCA disease
	Interstitial nephritis
α_1-Antitrypsin deficiency	IgA nephropathy
	Membranoproliferative glomerulonephritis
	Antiglomerular basement membrane disease
Autoimmune hepatitis	Immune complex glomerulonephritis
Sarcoidosis	Interstitial nephritis
Laënnec's or cryptogenic cirrhosis	IgA nephropathy
	Hepatic glomerulosclerosis

ANCA, antineutrophil cytoplasmic antibody; Ig, immunoglobulin. Based in part on information from references 175–180.

Table 28-5. RENAL EVALUATION IN LIVER TRANSPLANT CANDIDATES

Electrolytes
Blood sugar
BUN
Creatinine
ABG, if necessary
Urinalysis
Urinary spot sodium and creatinine
24-hour urine for protein
GFR
Sonogram of kidneys
Kidney biopsy, if necessary

ABG, arterial blood gas; BUN, blood urea nitrogen; GFR, glomerular filtration rate.

the patient. Input from attending nephrologists, hepatologists, liver transplant surgeons, and transplant anesthetists is needed to determine not only the patient's candidacy for liver or liver-kidney transplantation but also the perioperative need for renal replacement therapy (pre- and intraoperative dialysis), or renal-sparing immunosuppression. Planning provides the best opportunity for renal success. Table 28–5 summarizes the renal evaluation in patients with advanced liver disease.

The history should include queries concerning diabetic or hypertensive history, exposure to contrast, need for paracentesis, complications of bacterial peritonitis and gastrointestinal hemorrhage, use of diuretics, lactulose, NSAIDs, and nephrotoxic antibiotics. On physical examination, careful assessment of volume is necessary with attention to blood pressure, weight, urine volume, skin turgor, mucous membranes, lung fields, heart sounds, and the presence of edema or ascites. Laboratory tests should include measurement of electrolytes, blood glucose, BUN and creatinine and, in the setting of suspected acid-base disturbances, an arterial blood gas determination. Urine should be inspected for protein, cells of inflammation, and casts. Spot urine for sodium and creatinine gives information for the calculation of fractional excretion of sodium, which may prove helpful in determining effective arterial blood volume, particularly in a setting of low urine output. GFR should be measured. A 24-hour urine for protein excretion should be collected with the creatinine clearance. Isotope and nonradioactive clearance studies have not been validated in advanced liver failure but may prove helpful in evaluating GFR. Ultrasonography of the kidney screens for structural abnormalities and, if found, additional tests, including CT, magnetic resonance imaging (MRI), cystoscopy with retrograde studies, and urology consultation should be considered. A renal biopsy should be performed in the presence of proteinuria greater than 500 mg per day, unexplained hematuria greater than six cells per high-powered field, red blood cell casts, sterile pyuria, or unexplained kidney dysfunction.[110] The coagulation status of the patient may influence whether a percutaneous, transjugular intravenous, or open biopsy technique is used.

In patients being evaluated for liver transplantation, concomitant kidney transplantation should be used for irreversible kidney failure or biopsy-proven intrinsic renal disease with a strong likelihood of progressing to chronic kidney failure.[110,175] Proposed guidelines recommend offering combined liver-kidney transplantation to patients with primary renal disease, biopsy-proven markers of disease progression, and true GFR less than 35 to 40 mL/min, with no functional renal impairment such as HRS.[110] The proposed histological markers of progression include interstitial volume with more than 30% composed of fibrosis, moderate arteriosclerosis, and 40% or more of glomeruli affected by glomerulosclerosis. These preliminary guidelines also suggest searching for atubular glomeruli, as this has been a risk factor for progressive disease in noncirrhotics.[110] In patients with concomitant primary and functional renal disease, such as HRS or ATN, it is recommended that reversibility with treatment or dialysis support be explored, and no kidney should be offered if GFR improves to greater than 40 mL/min.[110] In patients without primary renal disease who develop dialysis-requiring acute renal failure secondary to HRS or ATN, kidney transplantation should be considered if dialysis support continues for 12 weeks or more. In that setting, the proposed guidelines suggest that patients undergo assessment of renal cortical flow by duplex ultrasonography or renal scan.[110] If flow is present and kidney size is normal with low urine sodium, reversible functional disease is likely and no kidney transplant should be offered. If flow is absent or decreased, kidney size is decreased, and urine sodium levels are high, irreversible renal injury may be indicated. Biopsy should be performed (intraoperatively if necessary), and a kidney transplant should be performed in those with histological markers of progressive disease (as previously discussed).[110]

Patients with significant renal dysfunction or acute renal failure need to be carefully assessed for dialysis support immediately before liver transplantation. Liver transplant surgery is accompanied by intraoperative bleeding and acid-base changes managed by large volumes of blood products and crystalloid. Electrolyte shifts are common, particularly hyperkalemia with liver reperfusion. Volume changes and vasopressor administration may exacerbate underlying renal dysfunction during the operation, making medical management a challenge. Intraoperative dialysis with continuous renal replacement therapy managed by experienced staff should be considered in the high-risk patient. Setup of dialysis access, equipment, and personnel prior to the first incision may minimize complications.

Patients with recognized moderate to severe renal dysfunction preoperatively who undergo liver transplantation should be considered for renal-sparing immunosuppression. Reports have described prevention of liver rejection using delayed calcineurin immunosuppression with antibody induction.[181,182] Immunosuppression options for patients with significant renal dysfunction should be discussed preoperatively to reduce potential renal toxicity after surgery.

Summary

Preoperative evaluation of pulmonary, cardiac, and renal functions is a team effort. A thorough workup not only identifies those who are candidates for transplantation (including those for combined transplantation) but also helps direct perioperative and postoperative management.

Pearls and Pitfalls

- Pulmonary
  - Pretransplant evaluation should always include contrast-enhanced echocardiography to screen for hepatopulmonary syndrome and portopulmonary hypertension.
  - Patients with hypoxemia in baseline resting upright arterial blood gases, or with Aao_2 greater than 20 mm Hg, should have arterial blood gas measurements on 100% Fio_2 in supine and upright positions to calculate shunt fractions and differentiate between intrapulmonary hepatopulmonary syndrome and ventilation-perfusion mismatch.
  - If estimated right ventricular pressure is greater than 40 mm Hg by echocardiography, a right heart catheterization with full hemodynamic study should be performed to determine if portopulmonary hypertension is present.
  - Chronic liver disease patients with PAM pressure greater than 35 mm Hg and PVR greater than 250 dyne·sec·cm^{-5} despite medical therapy face a 50% or higher mortality rate if subjected to liver transplantation.
  - Patients with portopulmonary hypertension who achieve a PAM pressure of less than 35 mm Hg and a PVR of less than 250 dyne·sec·cm^{-5} on continuous intravenous epoprostenol therapy and undergo liver transplantation should have a slow weaning (6 months) from epoprostenol following surgery to avoid rebound pulmonary hypertension and severe right heart failure following transplantation.
- Cardiac
  - The highest sensitivity and specificity of dobutamine echo stress test is achieved when more than 85% of predicted maximal heart rate is achieved during dobutamine infusion.
  - If 85% of predicted heart rate is not achieved, an adenosine or dipyridamole stress test with nuclear imaging (i.e., sestamibi) should be performed.

Pearls and Pitfalls—cont'd

- If the echocardiographic images are suboptimal and the walls of the left ventricle are not adequately imaged, nuclear stress testing should be used as a screening tool for coronary ischemia.

- Abnormal electrocardiographic changes in the absence of wall motion abnormality at peak dobutamine infusion are nondiagnostic for detecting the presence of coronary ischemia.

- Renal
  - The patient's GFR should be measured.
  - Combined liver-kidney transplantation should be considered for patients with intrinsic renal disease, biopsy-proven markers of disease progression, and measured GFR less than 40 mL/min.
  - Intraoperative dialysis support should be considered for patients with significant renal dysfunction to minimize problems with volume excess and hyperkalemia.
  - Use of serum creatinine as a marker for GFR should be avoided.
  - Use of prediction or estimation equations to determine GFR should be avoided.
  - Offering combined liver-kidney transplantation to patients with a reversible kidney injury such as HRS or ATN should be avoided.

References

1. VanThiel DH, Schade RR, Gavaler JS, et al: Medical aspects of liver transplantation. Hepatology 4:S79-S83, 1984.
2. Busuttil RW, Goldstein LI, Danovitch GM, et al: Liver transplantation today. Ann Intern Med 104:377-389, 1986.
3. Donovan JP, Zetterman RK, Burnett DA, Sorrell MF: Preoperative evaluation, preparation, and timing of orthotopic liver transplantation in the adult. Semin Liver Dis 9:168-175, 1989.
4. Krowka MJ, Cortese DA: Pulmonary aspects of liver disease and liver transplantation. Clin Chest Med 10:593-616, 1989.
5. Siefka AD, Lillington GA: Pulmonary complications of surgery. In: Bolt RJ (ed): Medical Evaluation of the Surgical Patient. Mount Kisco, NY, Futura Publishing, 1987, pp 307-326.
6. Powell CA, Caplan C: Pulmonary function tests in preoperative pulmonary evaluation. Clin Chest Med 22:703-714, 2001.
7. McAlister FA, Khan NA, Straus SE, et al: Accuracy of the preoperative assessment in predicting pulmonary risk after nonthoracic surgery. Am J Respir Crit Care Med 167:741-744, 2003.
8. Lazaridis KN, Frank JW, Krowka MJ, et al: Hepatic hydrothorax: Pathogenesis, diagnosis and management. Am J Med 107:262-267, 1999.
9. Strauss RM, Boyer TD: Hepatic hydrothorax. Semin Liver Dis 17:227-232, 1997.
10. Abelman WH, Frank NR, Gaensler EA, Cugell DN: Effects of abdominal distention by ascites on lung volumes and ventilation. Arch Intern Med 93:528-540, 1954.
11. Krowka MT, Cortese DA: Pulmonary aspects of chronic liver disease and liver transplantation. Mayo Clin Proc 60:407-418, 1985.
12. Lieberman FL, Hidemura R, Peters RL, et al: Pathogenesis and treatment of hydrothorax complicating cirrhosis with ascites. Ann Int Med 64:341-351, 1966.
13. Albers WM, Salem AJ, Salomon DA, et al: Hepatic hydrothorax. Cause and management. Arch Intern Med 151:2383-2388, 1991.
14. Strauss RM, Boyer TD: Hepatic hydrothorax. Semin Liver Dis 17:227-232, 1997.
15. Rubinstein D, McInnes IE, Dudley FJ: Hepatic hydrothorax in the absence of clinical ascites: Diagnosis and management. Gastroenterology 88:188-191, 1985.
16. Castellote J, Gornals J, Lopez C, Xiol X: Acute tension hydrothorax: A life-threatening complication of cirrhosis. J Clin Gastroenterol 34:588-589, 2002.
17. Xiol X, Castellvi JM, Guardiola J, et al: Spontaneous bacterial empyema in cirrhotic patients: A prospective study. Hepatology 23:719-723, 1996.
18. Sahn SA: State of the art: The pleura. Am Rev Respir Dis 138:184-234, 1988.
19. Runyon BA, Greenblatt M, Mingh RH: Hepatic hydrothorax is a relative contraindication to chest tube insertion. Am J Gastroenterol 81:566-567, 1986.
20. Moroux J, Perrin C, Venissac N, et al: Management of pleural effusion of cirrhotic origin. Chest 109:1093-1096, 1996.
21. Ghandour E, Carter J, Feola M, et al: Management of hepatic hydrothorax with peritoneovenous shunt. South Med J 83:718-719, 1990.
22. Strauss RM, Martin LG, Kaufman SL, Boyer TD: Transjugular intrahepatic portosystemic shunt for the management of symptomatic cirrhotic hydrothorax. Am J Gastroenterol 89:1520-1522, 1994.
23. Berthelot P, Walker JG, Sherlock S, Reid L: Arterial changes in the lungs in cirrhosis of the liver—lung spider nevi. N Engl J Med 274:291-298, 1966.
24. Krowka MJ, Cortese DA: Hepatopulmonary syndrome: An evolving perspective in the era of liver transplantation. Hepatology 11:138-142, 1990.
25. Krowka MJ, Dickson ER, Cortese DA: Hepatopulmonary syndrome: Clinical observations and lack of therapeutic response to somatostatin analogue. Chest 104:515-521, 1993.
26. Krowka MJ, Wiseman GA, Burnet OL, et al: Hepatopulmonary syndrome: A prospective study of relationships between severity of liver disease, PaO_2, response to 100% oxygen and brain uptake after 99TC MAA lung scanning. Chest 118:615-624, 2000.
27. Schenk P, Fuhrman V, Madl C, et al: Hepatopulmonary syndrome: Prevalence and predictive value of various cut offs for arterial oxygenation and their clinical consequences. Gut 51:853-859, 2002.
28. Aller R, Moya JL, Moreira V, et al: Diagnosis of hepatopulmonary syndrome with contrast transesophageal echocardiography: Advantages over contrast transthoracic echocardiography. Dig Dis Sci 44:1243-1248, 1999.
29. Krowka MJ, Tajik J, Dickson ER, et al: Intrapulmonary vascular dilatations (IVPD) in liver transplant candidates: Screening by two-dimensional contrast-enhanced echocardiography. Chest 97:465-470, 1990.
30. Hopkins WE, Waggoner AD, Barzilai B: Frequency and significance of intrapulmonary right-to-left shunting in end-stage hepatic disease. Am J Cardiol 70:516-519, 1992.
31. Edell ES, Cortese DA, Krowka MT, Rehder K: Severe hypoxemia and liver disease. Am Rev Respir Dis 140:1631-1635, 1989.
32. Davis HH, Schwartz DJ, Lefrak SS, et al: Alveolar-capillary oxygen disequilibrium in hepatic cirrhosis. Chest 73:507-511, 1978.
33. Bank ER, Thrall JH, Dantzker DR: Radionuclide demonstration of intrapulmonary shunting in cirrhosis. Am J Roentgenol 140:967-969, 1983.

34. Stoller JK, Moodie D, Schiavone WA, et al: Reduction of intrapulmonary shunt and resolution of digital clubbing associated with primary biliary cirrhosis after liver transplantation. Hepatology 11:54-58, 1990.

35. Stoller JK: As the liver goes, so goes the lung. Chest 97:1028-1029, 1990.

36. Krowka MJ: Caveats concerning hepatopulmonary syndrome (editorial). J Hepatol 34:756-758, 2001.

37. Krowka MT, Cortese DA: Severe hypoxemia associated with liver disease: Mayo Clinic experience and the experimental use of almitrine bismesylate. Mayo Clin Proc 62:164-173, 1987.

38. Lange PA, Stoller JK: Hepatopulmonary syndrome. UpToDate online: Available at www.uptodate.com, keywords: "hepatopulmonary syndrome."

39. Krowka MJ: Hepatopulmonary syndromes. Gut 46:1-4, 2000.

40. Fallon MB, Abrams GA, McGrath JW, et al: Common bile duct ligation in the rat: A model of intrapulmonary vasodilatation and hepatopulmonary syndrome. Am J Physiol 272:G779-G784, 1997.

41. Nunes H, Lebrec D, Mazmaninan M, et al: Role of nitric oxide in hepatopulmonary syndrome in cirrhotic rats. Am J Respir Crit Care Med 164:879-885, 2001.

42. Wiest R, Das S, Garcia-Tsao G, et al: Bacterial translocation in cirrhotic rats stimulates eNOS-derived NO production and impairs mesenteric contractility. J Clin Invest 104:1223-1233, 1999.

43. Reynolds JV, Murchan P, Leonard N, et al: Gut barrier failure in experimental jaundice. J Surg Res 62:11-16, 1996.

44. Panos RJ, Backer SK: Mediators, cytokines and growth factors in liver-lung interactions. Clin Chest Med 17:151-169, 1996.

45. Rabiller A, Nunes H, Lebrec D, et al: Prevention of gram-negative translocation reduces the severity of hepatopulmonary syndrome. Am J Respir Crit Care Med 166:514-517, 2002.

46. Starzl TE, Groth CG, Brattschneider L, et al: Extended survival in three cases of orthotopic homo transplantation of the human liver. Surgery 63:549, 1968.

47. Eriksson LS, Söderman C, Ericzon B, et al: Normalization of ventilation/perfusion relationship after liver transplantation in patients with decompensated cirrhosis: Evidence for a hepatopulmonary syndrome. Hepatology 12:1350, 1990.

47a. Anel RM, Sheagren JN: Novel presentation and approach to management of hepatopulmonary syndrome with use of antimicrobial agents. Clin Infect Dis 32:E131-E136, 2001.

48. Krowka MJ, Porayko MK, Plevak DJ: Hepatopulmonary syndrome with progressive hypoxemia as an indication for liver transplantation. Case reports and literature review. Mayo Clin Proc 72:44-53, 1997.

49. Arguedas MR, Abrams GA, Krowka MJ, Fallon MB: Prospective evaluation of outcomes and predictors of mortality in patients with hepatopulmonary syndrome undergoing liver transplantation. Hepatology 37:192-197, 2003.

50. Battaglia SE, Pretto JJ, Irving LB, et al: Resolution of gas exchange abnormalities and intrapulmonary shunting following liver transplantation. Hepatology 25:1228, 1997.

51. Colle IO, Moreau R, Godinho E, et al: Diagnosis of portopulmonary hypertension in candidates for liver transplantation: A prospective study. Hepatology 37:401-409, 2003.

52. Jiang L, Wiegers SE, Weyman AE: Right ventricle. In Weymen AE (ed): Principles and practice of echocardiography, 2nd ed. Philadelphia, Lea & Febiger, 1994, pp 901-902.

53. Swanson K, Krowka M: Arterial oxygenation associated with portopulmonary hypertension. Chest 121:1869-1875, 2002.

54. Kuo P, Plotkin J, Sean G, et al: Portopulmonary hypertension and the liver transplant candidate. Transplantation 67:1087-1093, 1999.

55. Ramsay MAE, Simpson BR, Nguyen AT, et al: Severe pulmonary hypertension in liver transplant candidates. Liver Transpl Surg 3:494-500, 1997.

56. Edwards BS, Weir EK, Edwards WD, et al: Coexistent pulmonary and portal hypertension: Morphological and clinical features. J Am Coll Cardiol 10:1233-1238, 1987.

57. Jones F, Kuo PC, Johnson LB, et al: The coexistence of portopulmonary hypertension and hepatopulmonary syndrome. Anesthesiology 90:626-629, 1999.

58. Kaspar MD, Ramsay MAE, Shuey CB, et al: Severe pulmonary hypertension and amelioration of hepatopulmonary syndrome after liver transplantation. Liver Transpl Surg 4:177-179, 1998.

59. Barst RJ, Rubin LJ, Long WA, et al: A comparison of continuous intravenous epoprostenol with conventional therapy for primary pulmonary hypertension. N Engl J Med 334:296, 1998.

60. McLaughlin V, Genthner D, Panella M, et al: Reduction in pulmonary vascular resistance with long-term epoprostenol therapy in primary pulmonary hypertension. N Engl J Med 338:273, 1998.

60a. Martinez-Palli G, Barbera JA, Taura P, et al: Severe portopulmonary hypertension after liver transplantation in a patient with preexistent hepatopulmonary syndrome. J Hepatol 31:1075-1079, 1999.

61. Krowka MJ, Frantz RP, McGoon MD, et al: Improvement in pulmonary hemodynamics during intravenous epoprostenol (prostacyclin): A study of 15 patients with moderate to severe portopulmonary hypertension. Hepatology 30:641-648, 1999.

62. Ramsay MAE, Schmidt A, Hien HAT, et al: Nitric oxide does not reverse pulmonary hypertension associated with end-stage liver disease: A preliminary report. Hepatology 25:524-527, 1997.

63. Plevak D, Krowka M, Rettke S, et al: Successful liver transplantation in patients with mild to moderate pulmonary hypertension. Transplant Proc 25:1840, 1993.

64. DeWolf AM, Gasior T, Kang Y: Pulmonary hypertension in a patient undergoing liver transplant. Transplant Proc 23:2000-2001, 1991.

65. Krowka MJ, Plevak DJ, Findlay JY, et al: Pulmonary hemodynamics and perioperative cardiopulmonary related mortality in patients with portopulmonary hypertension undergoing liver transplantation. Liver Transpl 6:443-450, 2000.

66. Molmenti EP, Ramsay M, Lynch K, et al: Epoprostenol and nitric oxide therapy for severe pulmonary hypertension in liver transplantation. Transplant Proc 33:1332, 2001.

67. Ramsay MAE, Simpson BR, Nguyen KJ, et al: Nitric oxide does not reverse pulmonary hypertension associated with end stage liver disease: A preliminary report. Hepatology 25:254, 1997.

68. Ramsay MAE, Spikes C, East CA, et al: The perioperative management of portopulmonary hypertension with nitric oxide and epoprostenol. Anesthesiology 90:299-301, 1999.

69. Fishman AP (ed): Pulmonary Hypertension and Cor Pulmonale. Pulmonary Diseases and Disorders. New York, McGraw-Hill, 1988.

70. Rodriguez-Roisin R, Pares A, Bruguera M, et al: Pulmonary involvement in primary biliary cirrhosis. Thorax 36:208-212, 1981.

71. Uddenfeldt P, Bjerle P, Danielsson A, et al: Lung function abnormalities in patients with primary biliary cirrhosis. Acta Med Scand 223:549-555, 1988.

72. James DG, Williams WJ: Sarcoidosis and other granulomatous disorders. Philadelphia, WB Saunders, pp 144-148, 1985.

73. Francavilla R, Castellaneta S, Hadzic N, et al: Prognosis of alpha-1 antitrypsin deficiency-related liver disease in the era of paediatric liver transplantation. J Hepatol 32:986-992, 2000.

74. Lai EC, Kao FT, Law ML, et al: Assignment of the alpha 1 antitrypsin gene and sequence-related gene to human chromosome 14 by molecular hybridization. Am J Hum Genet 35:385-392, 1983.

75. Brantley ML, Paul LD, Miller BN, et al: Clinical features and alpha 1 antitrypsin deficiency of adults with symptoms. Am Rev Respir Dis 138:327-336, 1988.

76. Crystal RG, Brantly ML, Hubbard RC, et al: The alpha 1-antitrypsin gene and its mutations. Chest 95:196-208, 1989.
77. Alpha-1-Antitrypsin Deficiency Registry Study Group. Survival and FEV1 decline in individuals with severe deficiency of alpha-1-antitrypsin. Am J Respir Crit Care Med 158:49-59, 1998.
78. American Thoracic Society. Guidelines for the approach to the patient with severe hereditary alpha-1-antitrypsin deficiency. Am Rev Respir Dis 140:1494-1497, 1989.
79. Mullins CD, Huang X, Merchant S, et al: The direct medical costs of alpha(1) antitrypsin deficiency. Chest 119:745-752, 2001.
80. Hood JM, Koep LJ, Peters RL, et al: Liver transplantation for advanced liver disease with alpha-1-antitrypsin deficiency. N Engl J Med 302:272-275, 1980.
81. Cooper JD, Patterson GA, Grossman R, Maurer J: Double-lung transplant for advanced chronic obstructive lung disease. Am Rev Respir Dis 139:303-307, 1989.
82. Francavilla R, Castellaneta SP, Hadzic N, et al: Prognosis of alpha-1-antitrypsin deficiency-related liver disease in the era of paediatric liver transplantation. J Hepatol 32:986-992, 2000.
83. Patterson GA, Maurer JR, Williams TJ, et al: Comparison of outcomes of double and single lung transplantation for obstructive lung disease. J Thorac Cardiovasc Surg 101:623-631, 1991.
84. Wood RE, Boat TF, Doershuk CF: Cystic fibrosis. Am Rev Respir Dis 113:833-878, 1976.
85. Hayllar KM, Williams SG, Wise AE, et al: A prognostic model for the prediction of survival in cystic fibrosis. Thorax 52:313-317, 1997.
86. Scott-Jupp R, Lama M, Taenner MS: Prevalence of liver disease in cystic fibrosis. Arch Dis Child 66:690-701, 1991.
87. Milkiewicz P, Skiba G, Kelly D, et al: Transplantation for cystic fibrosis: Outcome following early liver transplantation. J Gastroenterol Hepatol 17:208-213, 2002.
88. Couetil JP, Soubrane O, Houssin DP, et al: Combined heart-lung-liver, double-lung-liver and isolated liver transplantation for cystic fibrosis in children. Transpl Int 10:33-39, 1997.
89. Marquez J, Martin D, Virji MA, et al: Cardiovascular depression secondary to ionic hypocalcemia during hepatic transplantation in humans. Anesthesiology 65:457-461, 1986.
90. Aggarwal S, Kang Y, Freeman JA, et al: Postreperfusion syndrome: Cardiovascular collapse following hepatic reperfusion during liver transplantation. Transplant Proc 19(suppl 3):54-55, 1987.
91. DeWolf AM: Does ventricular dysfunction occur during liver transplantation? Transplant Proc 23:1922-1923, 1991.
92. Lichtor JL: Ventricular dysfunction does occur during liver transplantation. Transplant Proc 23:1924-1926, 1991.
93. DeWolf A, Gasior T, Begliomini B, et al: Right ventricular function during orthotopic liver transplantation. Anesthesiology 73:A97, 1990.
94. Carey WD, Dumot JA, Pimentel RR, et al: The prevalence of coronary artery disease in liver transplant candidates over age 50. Transplantation 59:859-864, 1995.
95. Plotkin JS, Benitez RM, Kuo PC, et al: Dobutamine stress echocardiography for preoperative cardiac risk stratification in patients undergoing orthotopic liver transplantation. Liver Transplant Surg 4:253-257, 1998.
96. Plotkin JS, Scott VL, Pinna A, et al: Morbidity and mortality in patients with coronary artery disease undergoing orthotopic liver transplantation. Liver Transpl Surg 2:426-430, 1996.
97. Urbano-Marquez A, Estruch R, Navarro-Lopez F, et al: The effects of alcoholism on skeletal and cardiac muscle. N Engl J Med 320:409-419, 1989.
98. Dabestani A, Child JS, Henze E, et al: Primary hemachromatosis: Anatomic and physiological characteristics of the cardiac ventricles and their response to phlebotomy. Am J Cardiol 54:153, 1984.
99. Eagle KM, Berger PB, Calkins H, et al: ACC/AHA guideline update for perioperative cardiovascular evaluation for noncardiac surgery—Executive summary. J Am Coll Cardiol 39:542-553, 2002.
100. Younis L, Stratmann H, Takase B, et al: Preoperative clinical assessment and dipyridamole thallium-201 scintigraphy for prediction and prevention of cardiac events in patients having major noncardiovascular surgery and known or suspected coronary artery disease. Am J Cardiol 74:311-317, 1994.
101. Miller DD, Younis LT, Chaitman BR, et al: Diagnostic accuracy of dipyridamole technetium 99m-labeled sestamibi myocardial tomography for detection of coronary artery disease. J Nucl Cardiol 4:18-24, 1997.
102. Das MK, Pellikka PA, Mahoney DW, et al: Assessment of cardiac risk before nonvascular surgery. J Am Coll Cardiol 35:1647-1653, 2000.
103. McNeill AJ, Fioretti PM, El-Said EM: Enhanced sensitivity for detection of coronary artery disease by addition of atropine to dobutamine stress echocardiography. Am J Cardiol 70:41-46, 1992.
104. Donovan CL, Marcovitz PA, Punch JD, et al: Two-dimensional and dobutamine stress echocardiography in the preoperative assessment of patients with end-stage liver disease prior to orthotopic liver transplantation. Transplantation 61:1180-1188, 1996.
105. Schwartz AJ, Hensley FA: Three patients requiring both coronary artery bypass surgery and orthotopic liver transplantation. J Cardiothorac Vas Anesth 9:322-332, 1995.
106. Markmann JF, Markmann JW, Markmann DA, et al: Preoperative factors associated with outcome and their impact on resource use in 1148 consecutive primary liver transplants. Transplantation 72:1113-1122, 2001.
107. Nair S, Verma S, Thuluvath PJ: Pretransplant renal function predicts survival in patients undergoing orthotopic liver transplantation. Hepatology 35:1179-1185, 2002.
108. Gonwa TA, Mai ML, Melton LB, et al: End-stage renal disease (ESRD) after orthotopic liver transplantation (OLTX) using calcineurin-based immunotherapy. Transplantation 72:1934-1939, 2001.
109. Gonwa TA, Mai ML, Melton LB, et al: Renal replacement therapy and orthotopic liver transplantation: The role of continuous veno-venous hemodialysis. Transplantation 71:1424-1428, 2001.
110. Davis CL, Gonwa TA, Wilkinson AH: Identification of patients best suited for combined liver-kidney transplantation: Part II. Liver Transpl 8:193-211, 2002.
111. Moser MAJ: Options for induction immunosuppression in liver transplant recipients. Drugs 62:995-1011, 2002.
112. Milionis HJ, Elisaf MS: Acid-base abnormalities in a patient with hepatic cirrhosis. Nephrol Dial Transplant 14:1599-1601, 1999.
113. Prytz H, Thomsen AC: Acid-base status in liver cirrhosis. Disturbances in stable, terminal and portal-caval shunted patients. Scand J Gastroenterol 11:249-256, 1976.
114. Lustik SJ, Chhibber AK, Kolano JW, et al: The hyperventilation of cirrhosis: Progesterone and estradiol effects. Hepatology 25:55-58, 1997.
115. Merritt WT: Metabolism and liver transplantation: Review of perioperative issues. Liver Transpl 6(supp 1):S76-S84, 2000.
116. Oster JR, Perez GO: Acid-base disturbances in liver disease. J Hepatol 2:299-306, 1986.
117. Toblli JR, Findor J, Sorda J, et al: Latent distal renal tubular acidosis (dRTA) in primary biliary cirrhosis (PBC) and chronic autoimmune hepatitis (CAH). Acta Gastroenterol Latinoam 23:235-238, 1993.
118. Wilson DM, Goldstein NP: Bicarbonate excretion in Wilson's disease (hepatolenticular degeneration). Mayo Clin Proc 49:394-400, 1974.
119. Gabow PA, Moore S, Schrier RW: Spironolactone-induced hyperchloremic acidosis in cirrhosis. Ann Intern Med 90:338-340, 1979.

120. Eaves ER, Korman MG: Cholestyramine-induced hyperchloremic metabolic acidosis. Aust N Z J Med 14:670-672, 1984.

121. Post TW, Rose BD: Approach to the adult with metabolic acidosis. UpToDate Online, version 11.1, www.uptodate.com, 2001.

122. Borroni G, Maggi A, Sangiovanni A, et al: Clinical relevance of hyponatremia for the hospital outcome of cirrhotic patients. Dig Liver Dis 32:605-610, 2000.

123. Gross P, Wehrle R, Bussemaker E: Hyponatremia: Pathophysiology, differential diagnosis and new aspects of treatment. Clin Nephrol 46:273-276, 1996.

124. Sterns RH: Severe symptomatic hyponatremia: Treatment and outcome. A study of 64 cases. Ann Intern Med 107:656-664, 1987.

125. Sterns RH, Cappuccio JD, Silver SM, et al: Neurological sequelae after treatment of severe hyponatremia: A multicenter perspective. J Am Soc Nephrol 4:1522-1530, 1994.

126. Gines P, Jimenez W: Aquaretic agents: A new potential treatment of dilutional hyponatremia in cirrhosis. J Hepatol 24:506-512, 1996.

127. Rose BD, Post TW: Clinical Physiology of Acid-Base and Electrolyte Disorders, 5th ed. New York, McGraw-Hill, 2001, pp 192-196, 383-396, 898-910.

128. Castellino P, Bia MJ, DeFronzo RA: Adrenergic modulation of potassium metabolism in uremia. Kidney Int 37:793-798, 1990.

129. Schepkens H, Vanholder R, Billiouw J, et al: Life-threatening hyperkalemia using combined therapy with angiotensin-converting enzyme inhibitors and spironolactone: An analysis of 25 cases. Am J Med 15:438-441, 2001.

130. Papadakis MA, Arieff AL: Unpredictability of clinical evaluation of renal function in cirrhosis. Am J Med 82:945-952, 1987.

131. Gecelter GR, Comer CM: Nutritional support during liver failure. Crit Care Clin 11:675-683, 1995.

132. Levey AS: Measurement of renal function in chronic renal disease. Kidney Int 38:167-184, 1990.

133. Roy L, Legault L, Pomier-Layrargues G: Glomerular filtration rate measurement in cirrhotic patients with renal failure. Clin Nephrol 50:342-346, 1998.

134. Sherman DS, Fish DN, Teitelbaum I: Assessing renal function in cirrhotic patients: Problems and pitfalls. Am J Kidney Dis 41:269-278, 2003.

135. Amarapurkar DN, Dhawan P, Kalro RH: Role of routine estimation of creatinine clearance in patients with liver cirrhosis. Indian J Gastroenterol 13:79-82, 1994.

136. Orlando R, Mussap M, Plebani M, et al: Diagnostic value of plasma cystatin C as a glomerular filtration marker in decompensated liver cirrhosis. Clin Chem 48:850-858, 2002.

137. Demirtas S, Bozbas A, Akbay A, et al: Diagnostic value of serum cystatin C for evaluation of hepatorenal syndrome. Clin Chim Acta 311:81-89, 2001.

138. Levey AS, Bosch JP, Lewis JB, et al: A more accurate method to estimate glomerular filtration rate from serum creatinine. A new prediction equation. Ann Intern Med 130:461-470, 1999.

139. Nankivell BJ, Gruenewald SM, Allen RDM, et al: Predicting glomerular filtration rate after kidney transplantation. Transplantation 59:1683-1689, 1995.

140. Perrone RD, Steinman TI, Beck GJ, et al: Utilization of radioisotopic filtration markers in chronic renal insufficiency: Simultaneous comparison of ^{125}I-iothalamate, ^{169}Yb-DTPA, ^{99m}Tc -DTPA and inulin. Am J Kidney Dis 16:224-235, 1990.

141. Wilson DM, Bergert JH, Larson TS, et al: GFR determined by nonradiolabeled iothalamate using capillary electrophoresis. Am J Kidney Dis 30:646-652, 1997.

142. Gaspari F, Perico N, Remuzzi G: Application of newer clearance techniques for the determination of glomerular filtration rate. Curr Opin Nephrol Hypertension 7:675-680, 1998.

143. Wong F, Blendis L: New challenge of hepatorenal syndrome: Prevention and treatment. Hepatology 34:1242-1251, 2001.

144. Spahr L, Villeneuve JP, Tran HK, et al: Furosemide-induced natriuresis as a test to identify cirrhotic patients with refractory ascites. Hepatology 33:28-31, 2001.

145. Suzuki H, Stanley AJ: Current management and novel therapeutic strategies for refractory ascites and hepatorenal syndrome. QJM 94:293-300, 2001.

146. Humes HD: Aminoglycoside nephrotoxicity. Kidney Int 33:900-911, 1988

147. Branch RA: Prevention of amphotericin B-induced renal impairment. A review on the use of sodium supplementation. Arch Intern Med 148:2389-2394, 1988.

148. Russo D, Minutolo R, Cianciaruso B, et al: Early effects of contrast media on renal hemodynamics and tubular function in chronic renal failure. J Am Soc Nephrol 6:1451-1458, 1995.

149. Dunn MJ: Are COX-2 selective inhibitors nephrotoxic? Am J Kid Dis 35:976-977, 2000.

150. Warren GV, Korbet SM, Schwartz MM, et al: Minimal change glomerulopathy associated with nonsteroidal anti-inflammatory drugs. Am J Kidney Dis 13:127-130, 1989.

151. Arroyo V, Gines P, Gerbes A, et al: Definition and diagnostic criteria of refractory ascites and hepatorenal syndrome in cirrhosis. Hepatology 23:164-176, 1996.

152. Gines A, Escorsell A, Gines P, et al: Incidence, predictive factors, and prognosis of the hepatorenal syndrome in cirrhosis with ascites. Gastroenterology 105:229-236, 1993.

153. Koppel MH, Coburn JM, Mims MM, et al: Transplantation of cadaveric kidneys from patients with hepatorenal syndrome. New Engl J Med 280:1367-1371, 1969.

154. Dagher L, Moore K: The hepatorenal syndrome. Gut 49:729-737, 2001.

155. Cardenas A, Uriz J, Gines P, et al: Hepatorenal syndrome. Liver Transpl 6(supp 1):S63-S71, 2000.

156. Bataller R, Gines P, Arroyo V, et al: Hepatorenal syndrome. Clin Liv Dis 4:487-507, 2000.

157. Briglia AE, Anania FA: Hepatorenal syndrome: Definition, pathophysiology, and intervention. Crit Care Clin 18:345-373, 2002.

158. Guevara M, Gines P, Fernandez-Esparrach G, et al: Reversibility of hepatorenal syndrome by prolonged administration of ornipressin and plasma volume expansion. Hepatology 27:35-41, 1998.

159. Ganne-Carrie N, Hadengue A, Mathurin P, et al: Hepatorenal syndrome: Long-term treatment with terlipressin as a bridge to liver transplantation. Dig Dis Sci 41:1054-1056, 1996.

160. Moreau R, Durand F, Poynard T, et al: Terlipressin in patients with cirrhosis and type 1 hepatorenal syndrome: A retrospective multicenter study. Gastroenterology 122:923-930, 2002.

161. Halimi C, Bonnard P, Bernard B, et al: Effect of terlipressin (Glypressin) on hepatorenal syndrome in cirrhotic patients: Results of a multicentre pilot study. Eur J Gastroenterol Hepatol 14:153-158, 2002.

162. Duvoux C, Zanditenas D, Hezode C, et al: Effects of noradrenalin and albumin in patients with type I hepatorenal syndrome: A pilot study. Hepatology 36:374-380, 2002.

163. Angeli P, Volpin R, Gerunda G, et al: Reversal of type 1 hepatorenal syndrome with administration of midodrine and octreotide. Hepatology 29:1690-1697, 1999.

164. Holt S, Goodier D, Marley R, et al: Improvement in renal function in hepatorenal syndrome with N-acetylcysteine. Lancet 353:294-295, 1999.

165. Soper CP, Latif AB, Bending MR: Amelioration of hepatorenal syndrome with selective endothelin-A antagonist. Lancet 347:1842-1843, 1996.

166. Dagher L, Patch D, Marley R, et al: Review article: Pharmacological treatment of the hepatorenal syndrome in cirrhotic patients. Aliment Pharmacol Ther 14:515-521, 2000.

167. Brensing KA, Textor J, Perz J, et al: Long-term outcome after transjugular intrahepatic portosystemic stent-shunt in

non-transplant cirrhotics with hepatorenal syndrome: A phase II study. Gut 47:288-295, 2000.

168. Mitzner SR, Stange J, Klammt S, et al: Improvement of hepatorenal syndrome with extracorporeal albumin dialysis MARS: Results of a prospective, randomized, controlled clinical trial. Liver Transpl 6:277-286, 2000.

169. Eckhardt KU: Renal failure in liver disease. Intensive Care Med 25:5-14, 1999.

170. Vanholder R, Van Biesen W, Lameire N: What is the renal replacement method of first choice for intensive care patients? J Am Soc Nephrol 12(Suppl 17):S40-S43, 2001.

171. Esson ML, Schrier RW: Diagnosis and treatment of acute tubular necrosis. Ann Intern Med 137:744-752, 2002.

172. Zarich S, Fang LS, Diamond JR: Fractional excretion of sodium. Exceptions to its diagnostic value. Arch Intern Med 145:108-112, 1985.

173. Schlessinger SD, Tankersley MR, Curtis JJ: Clinical documentation of end-stage renal disease due to hypertension. Am J Kidney Dis 23:655-660, 1994.

174. United States Renal Data System. Excerpts from the USRDS 2000 annual data report: Atlas of end-stage renal disease in the United States. Am J Kidney Dis 36(Supp 2):S1, 2000.

175. Davis CL, Gonwa TA, Wilkinson AH: Pathophysiology of renal disease associated with liver disorders: Implications for liver transplantation. Part I. Liver Transpl 8:91-109, 2002.

176. Wong F: Liver and kidney diseases. Clin Liver Dis 6:981-1011, 2002.

177. DiBelgiojoso GB, Ferrario F, Landriani N: Virus related glomerular diseases: Histological and clinical aspects. J Nephrol 15:469-479, 2002.

178. Altraif IH, Abdulla AS, al Sebayel MI, et al: Hepatitis C associated glomerulonephritis. Am J Nephrol 15:407-410, 1995.

179. Os I, Skjorten F, Svalander C, et al: Alpha-1-antitrypsin deficiency associated with hepatic cirrhosis and IgA nephritis. Nephron 77:235-237, 1997.

180. Komatsu T, Utsunomiya K, Oyaizu T: Goodpasture's syndrome associated with primary biliary cirrhosis. Intern Med 37:611-613, 1998.

181. Emre S, Gondolesi G, Polat K, et al: Use of daclizumab as initial immunosuppression in liver transplant recipients with impaired renal function. Liver Transpl 7:220-225, 2001.

182. Nelson DR, Soldevila-Pico C, Reed A, et al: Anti-interleukin-2 receptor therapy in combination with mycophenolate mofetil is associated with more severe hepatitis C recurrence after liver transplantation. Liver Transpl 7:1064-1070, 2001.

Pretransplantation Infectious Disease Screening for Liver Transplantation: Candidates and Donors

MARIAN G. MICHAELS
MICHAEL D. GREEN

Pretransplant evaluation   430
    Prior infections   430
    Candidate immunizations   436
    Evaluating fever at time of transplant   436
Conclusion   437

Infections are a major cause of morbidity and mortality following liver transplantation, in part because of the immunosuppressive drugs required to prevent rejection of the new organ. Although not every infection can be anticipated, many types of infections can be predicted, and some can even be prevented. Accordingly, it is important to screen potential candidates and donors for the presence of risk factors for infections that may develop following transplantation. Experience has identified the major sources of pathogenic organisms, including the recipient's endogenous flora, the environment, and the donor organ. Pretransplant serological evaluation of the donor helps to predict risks of acquiring an infection from the donor organ. Similarly, performing a careful history, examination, and serological screening on the recipient further clarifies the risk of acquiring certain pathogens following the transplant procedure. The role of an infectious disease pretransplantation evaluation is therefore to identify host and donor risk factors that might predispose the patient to future infectious problems and to plan strategies to prevent the development of these complications. The decision to perform screening on a candidate or donor must consider the impact of potential disease, the availability of reliable testing methods, the cost of testing, and the amount of specimen that would be required. This chapter discusses the infectious disease approach to the pretransplantation evaluation of both candidates and donors.

Pretransplant Evaluation

The infectious disease evaluation of the liver transplantation candidate should help physicians (1) recognize potential pathogens with which the patient has previously been infected or colonized; (2) review antimicrobial sensitivities of potential bacterial pathogens to help guide prophylactic and treatment strategies; and (3) document the candidate's immunological experience that influences the risk of developing infection. Perhaps as important, the pretransplantation evaluation also provides an opportunity for the candidate and family to be educated about infections associated with transplantation. Patients can be made aware of the implications of immunosuppression, including its impact not only on infectious agents contracted following the transplantation procedure but also on the potential for reactivation of viruses and other latent pathogens. Patients can be further educated about the availability of preventive strategies and treatment regimens for many of the potential infectious complications that are associated with liver transplantation. Finally, the infectious disease evaluation provides the opportunity to document the patient's immunization history and to develop a plan for the delivery of appropriate vaccines prior to the institution of immune suppression (Tables 29–1 and 29–2).

Prior Infections

After transplantation, microbiological species that are harbored innocently in the candidate may reactivate under immunosuppression. Typically, these are organisms that exist in a latent state and can include viruses, bacteria, fungi, and parasites. Likewise, the donor organ can harbor transmissible agents within either hepatocytes or "passenger leukocytes" that can be passed to the transplant recipient. Many of these organisms are the same latent pathogens that can cause potential problems if reactivation occurs in the recipient.

Viruses

Herpesviruses

The most important of the viral pathogens are members of the herpesvirus family, including cytomegalovirus (CMV), Epstein-Barr virus (EBV), herpes simplex virus (HSV), and varicella-zoster virus (VZV).

Table 29–1. PRETRANSPLANT INFECTIOUS DISEASE EVALUATION OF CANDIDATES FOR LIVER TRANSPLANTATION

History
SPECIAL EMPHASIS ON:
Immunization history
Previous episodes of spontaneous bacterial peritonitis
Previous episodes of bacterial cholangitis
Travel history
Residence in areas endemic for specific organisms
Physical Examination
TUBERCULIN SKIN TEST
SEROLOGIC STUDIES
HIV 1 and 2
HTLV 1 and 2
Hepatitis A
Hepatitis B: sAg, sAb, cAb, eAg
Hepatitis C
Hepatitis D
CMV: IgG, IgM
EBV: VCA IgG, VCA IgM, EBNA, early antigen
VZV: IgG
Measles
RPR

Other herpesviruses, such as human herpesvirus 6 (HHV6), 7 (HHV7), and 8 (HHV8), are also increasingly recognized after transplantation. A healthy person usually acquires these viruses during childhood or young adulthood. These DNA viruses remain latent in target cells for the life of the host, long after symptoms of the primary infection have abated. Reactivation can occur at any time, with immunosuppression being recognized as a potent stimulator. Both the donor organ and the host cells can harbor viruses that can reactivate after transplantation. Obtaining pretransplant serological

Table 29–2. PRETRANSPLANT INFECTIOUS DISEASE EVALUATION OF LIVER TRANSPLANT ORGAN DONOR

Serologic Studies
HIV 1 and 2
HTLV 1 and 2
Hepatitis A
Hepatitis B: sAg, sAb, cAb, eAg
Hepatitis C (EIA, ± RIBA or PCR)
Hepatitis D
CMV: IgG, IgM
EBV: VCA IgG
RPR

Table 29-3. PROPHYLACTIC MANAGEMENT STRATEGY FOR PREEXISTING INFECTIONS IN LIVER TRANSPLANT CANDIDATES AFTER TRANSPLANTATION

Organism	Management Strategy
Cytomegalovirus	Ganciclovir alone or in combination with CMV-hyperimmune globulin or preemptive monitoring
Epstein-Barr virus	No prophylaxis currently proven to be effective; viral load monitoring advocated for at-risk patients
Herpes simplex virus	Oral acyclovir × 3 months after transplant, individualized treatment thereafter
Varicella-zoster virus	No prophylaxis
	Varicella-zoster immune globulin (VZIG) immediately after exposure, if nonimmune and exposed to varicella after transplant
Human immunodeficiency virus (HIV)	Relative contraindication to transplantation at many centers outside of investigational study
Hepatitis B virus: Eag (+)	Relative contraindication to transplantation at many centers
Hepatitis B virus: Eag (−)	Consider HBIG and antivirals (e.g., lamivudine)
Hepatitis C virus	Consider interferon and ribavirin
Previous peritonitis or cholangitis	Obtain antibiotic susceptibilities of microorganisms recovered from last episode of infection; devise perioperative antibiotic prophylaxis accordingly
Mycobacterium tuberculosis	Isoniazid with close follow-up of liver enzymes
Histoplasmosis	Long-term maintenance with azole therapy with or without induction with amphotericin B products
Coccidioidomycosis	Long-term maintenance with azole therapy with or without induction with amphotericin B products

measurements demonstrating seropositivity for these herpesviruses is important for predicting risk of developing, as well as preventing, disease caused by these pathogens (Table 29-3).

CMV is one of the most common causes of infection after liver transplantation.[1,2] Reactivation of CMV has been noted to cause symptomatic disease in 8% to 40% of previously immune liver transplant recipients.[3-5] Because prior seropositivity is common, especially in adult populations (approximately 60% to 70%), reactivation disease constitutes a significant component of clinical infection.[6,7] However, the major risk factor for severe CMV disease is primary infection, that is, transplantation of a seronegative recipient with an organ from a seropositive donor.[3] The source of the CMV has been documented as donor-derived both epidemiologically[3] and by restriction enzyme digests of donor and recipient CMV isolates.[8]

Serological screening for CMV should be performed in all candidates and donors. Various prophylactic treatment strategies for CMV disease using antiviral agents, such as ganciclovir or valganciclovir as well as CMV hyperimmune globulin, have been studied in solid-organ transplantation. Additional preventive strategies that monitor patients for the presence of specific risk factors for CMV disease (e.g., treatment of rejection) or the presence of subclinical infection (as demonstrated by pp65 antigenemia or quantitative CMV DNA monitoring) as an indicator for initiation of preemptive antiviral therapy have also been proposed.[9] In general, decisions regarding which approach to use, as well as the duration of prophylaxis, are frequently tied to results of serological screening on the donor and the recipient. Detailed descriptions of these preventive strategies, as well as treatment algorithms for those patients who develop disease following liver transplantation, are discussed in more detail in Chapter 64.

EBV, another cause of posttransplantation infection, often produces asymptomatic infection in young children or a self-limited mononucleosis syndrome in adolescents and adults. After the initial disease, the virus is maintained within B lymphocytes in a latent state. However, pharyngeal shedding of replicative virus can be found periodically in up to 23% of normal individuals.[10] In immunosuppressed populations, such as those with acquired immunodeficiency syndrome (AIDS) or those that have undergone organ transplantation, viral shedding may occur in 65% to 94% of seropositive patients.[10,11] More worrisome is the ability of EBV to cause B-cell proliferation or lymphoma in the context of impaired T-cell function. The highest risk for developing EBV-driven posttransplantation lymphoproliferative disorders (PTLD) is primary infection.[12-14] However, PTLD does occur in up to 2% of previously immune orthotopic liver transplantation (OLT) recipients. Most transplant centers perform EBV serologic tests on candidates. Increasingly available data suggest that the EBV-mismatched patients (EBV seropositive donor/seronegative recipient) are at the highest risk of developing EBV-associated disease. Accordingly, we also recommend screening donors for evidence of EBV to identify the mismatched donor-recipient pairs. As is the case with CMV, the availability of this information may guide the implementation of evolving strategies aimed at the prevention of EBV disease. These are discussed in greater detail in Chapter 64.

Reactivation of viral infection can also occur with HSV after transplantation. In one large series highlighting the potential of HSV disease after immunosuppression, 75% of adult liver transplantation recipients were noted to be seropositive for HSV.[1] Most often HSV causes persistent, localized lesions within the first month after transplantation or after treatment for rejection episodes. Disseminated HSV disease is rare but can occur. HSV hepatitis occurred in 8 of 1664 (0.5%) patients who underwent liver transplantation in the 1980s at the University of Pittsburgh.[15] Seven of the eight instances of HSV hepatitis were believed to be caused by reactivation of disease rather than primary acquisition. Prophylactic strategies using oral acyclovir or related compounds (e.g., valacyclovir, famciclovir) for patients found to have serological evidence of HSV prior to transplantation can safely decrease the incidence of reactivation. Although possible, donor-associated transmission of HSV is rare because this virus does not establish latent infection in the liver. Donor screening is therefore not recommended for HSV.

VZV can cause disease both from primary infection and from reactivation after transplantation. In one study of 121 adult liver transplant recipients, 8 patients developed VZV 19 to 575 days after transplantation.[1] One of these patients died of disseminated zoster despite acyclovir treatment. Patients without preexisting immunity are at risk for severe disease after transplantation if they are exposed to chickenpox. Pediatric transplantation recipients who are often still susceptible to VZV are at the highest risk, whereas most adults have previous immunity. In one study, 51 of 90 children undergoing liver transplantation were susceptible to chickenpox.[16] Twenty-five of the susceptible children were exposed to varicella and received varicella-zoster immune globulin (VZIG). Seven of these children and 7 others who did not receive VZIG developed chickenpox. Two of the 14 children died; both received acyclovir late in the course of their infection. Administration of VZIG within 72 hours of varicella exposure decreases the incidence of disease as well as the severity of infection in those who develop disease despite prophylaxis. Knowledge of the potential recipient's serological status against VZV is necessary to determine who should receive VZIG after such an exposure following transplantation. Furthermore, identification of transplant candidates as being susceptible to varicella provides the opportunity to immunize them with the varicella vaccine prior to transplantation. Although the efficacy of this vaccine has not been established in patients with end-stage liver disease, provision of the vaccine at this time would seem preferable to allowing such patients to be exposed to wild-type varicella virus while they are immunosuppressed following the transplant procedure. Because the VZV remains latent in ganglionic nerve endings, it could only be transmitted by a donor who was actively undergoing primary viremia. Only a single case of donor-associated transmission of VZV has been reported. Accordingly, donor screening is not recommended for VZV.

Infection with HHV6 and HHV7 universally occurs during the early years of life, and neither donors nor recipients have been routinely screened for these diseases before liver transplantation. Increasing data suggest that coincidental reactivation of one or both of these viruses with CMV can amplify the severity of disease typically seen with CMV alone.[17] In addition, case reports suggest that HHV6 in the absence of other pathogens can cause a febrile illness with or without a rash. Donor transmission of HHV6 was also found to cause febrile illnesses in young infants receiving living related liver transplants from their mothers. In all but one case, the illness attributed to HHV6 was self-limited.[18] At this time, routine screening for HHV6 and HHV7 is not recommended.

The most recently recognized human herpesvirus, HHV8, is a gamma herpesvirus that is endemic in Africa and has relatively high rates of prevalence in Mediterranean countries. The virus has been associated with development of Kaposi sarcoma. Currently, donor transmission and reactivation disease have been postulated to lead to disease for individuals (or their donors) who are from geographical areas with high prevalence rates of HHV8. Limitations in serological testing are a current problem for screening. Although it is reasonable to consider screening for recipients and donors that come from moderate to highly endemic areas, routine screening of transplant candidates and donors from North America, Asia, and much of Europe where rates of the virus are quite small cannot be endorsed at this time.[19]

Hepatitis Viruses

Hepatitis B is a pathogen that causes serious disease after transplantation. Screening of the candidate for hepatitis B should include the full panel of hepatitis B serology (see Table 29–1). Transplant candidates who have not had previous hepatitis B infection and are seronegative for hepatitis B surface antibody should receive the hepatitis B vaccination series prior to transplantation. Transplantation of patients found to have chronic hepatitis B infection has been associated with an increase in morbidity compared with transplant recipients without evidence of hepatitis B infection. This is true not only for patients undergoing liver transplantation but also for those undergoing a renal transplant. The use of prophylactic strategies using hepatitis B immunoglobulin (HBIG) and interferon alfa improved but did not prevent a high relapse rate in patients transplanted for chronic hepatitis B.[20] However, the availability of effective antiviral therapy (e.g., lamivudine) and more aggressive strategies with HBIG affect both the rate and the prevention of relapsed disease.[21] Relapses of HBV that occur after transplantation have more rapid progression of disease than natural disease. Furthermore, subsequent retransplantations result in increasingly rapid hepatic deterioration.[20] The availability of preventive and treatment strategies has led to the acceptance of hepatitis B–positive patients as appropriate recipients of liver transplantation.

In general, potential donors found to be positive for active hepatitis B infection should be disqualified. Organs from donors with antibody against hepatitis B surface antigen and negative for antihepatitis B core antigen are immune on the basis of previous vaccination and are safe to use for transplantation. Individuals with both antibody against hepatitis B surface and core antigens have been considered to be immune and low risk candidates for transplantation. However, even individuals who have developed antibodies against surface antigens can still maintain hepatitis B DNA in the liver and thus represent some risk for transmission after liver transplantation.[22] This is particularly true for donors with the presence of antihepatitis B core immunoglobulin (Ig) M antibody. Because there is a definite increased risk of transmitting hepatitis B to recipients of their livers,[23] avoidance of donors that are core antibody positive is recommended by many. Some centers, however, have been able to successfully use these livers as a result of an aggressive prophylaxis strategy.[24]

Hepatitis C is a major indication for liver transplantation. Although the presence of hepatitis C infection in the candidate prior to transplantation is associated with a nearly 100% reinfection rate of the allograft, and despite the fact that 50% to 80% of these patients will develop hepatitis of the allograft, the patient and graft survival of these recipients is not adversely affected for the first 5 to 10 years.[20,25,26] Although the impact of reinfection with hepatitis C appears to be limited for most patients, data exist that suggest the development of rapid progression to fibrosing cholestatic hepatitis in a subset of patients with very high viral loads.[26] Research regarding treatment to reduce the viral load prior to transplantation and increasing information on specific genetics of hepatitis C should assist with screening procedures to allow for more selective timing of transplantation in this group of patients. In the meantime, the overall reasonable survival rates for 5 and 10 years allow centers to perform liver transplantation for individuals with hepatitis C cirrhosis.

The potential for donor transmission of HCV is well established. In general, patients who are known to be HCV positive are not considered to be acceptable donors for liver transplantation. An exception to this appears to be the use of a hepatic allograft from a donor who is HCV positive for a recipient who is also known to have HCV. Although reinfection can occur, data from numerous studies suggest that the use of such organs is safe in the HCV-positive recipient.[22]

Hepatitis A virus can cause more severe liver disease in a patient whose liver function is already compromised.[20] In addition, a highly effective vaccine against hepatitis A virus is available. For these reasons, candidates for liver transplantation should be tested for previous immunity to hepatitis A. If they are negative for hepatitis A, they should be vaccinated. Routine testing and preventive strategies are not available for hepatitis E and G at this time.

Retroviruses

The human immunodeficiency virus (HIV) is a potential pathogen in transplant candidates and donors that may not be clinically apparent.[25,27-29] Since 1985, candidate screening for HIV infection has been part of the routine pretransplantation evaluation at most institutions. A retrospective study of 3023 solid-organ transplant recipients during the 1980s at the University of Pittsburgh identified 11 patients as seropositive for HIV prior to transplantation.[27] An additional 14 patients, who had not been previously screened, were seropositive for HIV shortly after transplantation. The AIDS-free time was shorter in these 25 patients compared with nontransplant and hemophiliac patients or transfusion-acquired HIV infection. Erice and colleagues from Minnesota identified 88 patients in the literature and at their own institution who had or developed HIV infection after transplantation.[28] Ten liver transplantation recipients were HIV-positive prior to transplantation. Mean follow-up was 19 months; all but one patient died after an average period of 14 months. However, both of these studies were performed prior to the availability of highly active antiretroviral therapies (HAART). In the current era of HAART, individuals with end-stage liver disease may benefit from liver transplantation despite infection with HIV.[30] Close monitoring is critical, and currently it is best done as part of an ongoing multicentered trial.

HIV may be transmitted to a transplant recipient via the organ or blood transfusions. Simonds and colleagues at the Centers for Disease Control reported the transmission of HIV from a single donor to all four recipients of solid organ grafts and three of four recipients of bone grafts.[29] The donor was seronegative during screening, indicating a very early stage of infection when HIV antibody was not yet detectable, highlighting limitations of screening methods that rely on antibody tests. Molecular assays are more sensitive but are not always available in a timely fashion and are costly. Screening by risk factors and using molecular assays when doubt is present have assisted in decreasing the inadvertent use of HIV-infected donors.

Human T-lymphotropic viruses (HTLV) are relatively rare infections that can lead to adult T-cell leukemia or neurological disorders. Most often, infection is asymptomatic; however, there is theoretical concern about increased pathogenicity under the immunosuppressive environment of transplantation. Although it is not a contraindication to being a candidate, it is worth knowing about the serological status so as to watch for disease afterward.[31,32] Although definite concern exists about transmitting HTLV 1 or 2 with an organ, this has not been proved to occur. In general, donors who are seropositive for either of these retroviruses are not used by any groups. However, in some cases, where time is of the essence and no other appropriate donor is available, some centers use HTLV-positive donors with proper consent.[22]

Other Viruses

A number of viruses can theoretically be transmitted if a donor is undergoing acute viremia at the time of harvest, but the ability to screen for these viruses is limited. However, it is conceivable that in the future nucleic assay–based assays may be designed for such a purpose. For this reason, the process of screening must remain flexible and responsive to emerging pathogens. This is noted by the recent transmission of West Nile virus to all four recipients of a single organ donor followed by several other case reports of donor transmission.[33] Although testing all donors for West Nile virus is not necessary, it does make sense to avoid or to test potential donors that have had an unexplained encephalitis process during months when mosquitoes are prevalent.

Bacteria

Frequently, patients awaiting liver transplantation have experienced one or more episodes of spontaneous bacterial peritonitis (SBP). The major risk factor for developing SBP is the presence of ascites. A careful history of previous episodes of SBP should be obtained. The clinician must anticipate the possible development of this complication in transplant candidates, as SBP results in substantial morbidity and mortality.[34] Infection is typically signaled by the presence of fever, abdominal pain, and hypoactive or absent bowel sounds. Bacteremia may be present in up to 50% of episodes. Diagnosis is confirmed by paracentesis (see Table 29–3).

Developing an episode of SBP before transplantation carries prognostic implications for patients after transplantation. In one series, SBP was identified in 25 of 277 adult liver transplant candidates who subsequently received a liver transplant.[34] A significant increase in the rate of postoperative complications (both technical and infectious) was noted in these patients compared with the 252 patients who did not experience an episode of SBP. The mortality rate in the SBP group was 76%, compared with 8% in the non-SBP group. Of interest, 5 of 14 patients experiencing postoperative peritonitis were infected with the same bacterial species identified during their pretransplant episode of SBP. However, a second series identified a rate of posttransplant sepsis in only 8.8% of liver transplant recipients with a history of SBP, compared with a 10% rate in controls. The authors of this second study concluded that the history of SBP did not lead to an increased rate of posttransplant sepsis if the patient had received 4 days or more of appropriate treatment prior to undergoing transplantation.[35]

Bacterial cholangitis is another infection observed in the candidate awaiting liver transplantation. This is particularly common in children who have undergone a Kasai procedure for biliary atresia.[36] Similarly, episodes of bacterial cholangitis are noted among adult transplant candidates with underlying liver diseases such as sclerosing cholangitis or secondary biliary cirrhosis. To date, there is no documentation of an increase in postoperative morbidity or mortality in patients with a pretransplant history of bacterial cholangitis. However, knowledge of the bacterial species causing infections prior to transplantation and their antimicrobial susceptibility might guide perioperative prophylaxis and subsequent empirical therapy.

Tuberculosis (TB) is a particular concern in immunosuppressed hosts. This is especially true with the recent increase in the prevalence of multidrug-resistant TB. Little published information is available describing the incidence and outcome of TB in liver transplant recipients.[37,38] All candidates should have a tuberculin skin test. Because of the high risk of TB after transplantation, induration greater than 5 mm at 48 to 72 hours should be interpreted as a positive skin test. Patients known to have a positive tuberculin skin test or who come from an endemic area are at increased risk for symptomatic reactivation of TB after transplantation.[37,38] Other risk factors for reactivation of latent TB after transplantation include severe hepatic failure at the time of transplant, aggressive antirejection therapy, and/or concurrent HIV infection.[37,38] Review of the larger experience of TB in renal transplant recipients offers additional insight. TB after renal transplantation has been reported as occurring as much as 15 times more commonly than the rate seen in the general population[39] and is also more likely in patients coming from areas endemic for TB. Although many of these cases represent reactivation of disease in patients with inadequate or no prior therapy,[40] active TB has also occurred in patients who received appropriate anti-TB therapy before transplantation.[40,41] Accordingly, there is a need for anti-TB therapy after transplantation independent of prior treatment, paralleling recommendations for patients undergoing prolonged corticosteroid or other immunosuppressive regimens even with a history of appropriately treated TB.[42] Concern exists with prophylaxis because of hepatic toxicity from isoniazid, especially in patients older than 35 years. Although it has generally been found to be safe after renal transplantation, extrapolation from the kidney transplant population is limited by differences in immunosuppressive regimens and the underlying health of liver transplant candidates. Thus, prophylaxis of liver transplant recipients for TB remains controversial. We believe that prophylaxis should be initiated and close monitoring of liver enzymes performed to assess potential toxicity.

Living related donors should be screened by history for infection or exposure to TB as well as by tuberculin skin testing. Donor transmission did occur when a mother with an unrecognized TB infection donated a lobe of her liver to her child. The recipient developed a hepatic abscess from *Mycobacterium tuberculosis* and the mother concomitantly was diagnosed with pulmonary TB.[43] Donation from someone with a positive history for TB or a positive skin test should not be considered without documentation of adequate anti-TB treatment. Time constraints do not permit skin testing of deceased donors, but information regarding a history of active TB and treatment should be elicited. In addition, the chest radiographs of potential donors should be reviewed for findings that suggest TB infection.

Current practice at the University of Pittsburgh includes obtaining a careful history of prior exposure and treatment of TB. A tuberculin skin test is performed on all candidates. Given the relative insensitivity of the skin testing in chronically ill patients, review of a chest radiograph for lesions consistent with healed TB is suggested for candidates from endemic areas. Patients with a positive TB history and/or a positive skin test receive isoniazid (or alternative therapy if from a geographical area with a high rate of resistance) for 9 to 12 months after transplantation, although some experts recommend continuing therapy indefinitely. Attempts at a more definitive diagnosis are indicated in patients from endemic areas with a negative skin test result but suspicious chest radiographs. Careful evaluation for evidence of side effects, particularly hepatotoxicity, is maintained, and isoniazid is discontinued when unacceptable toxicity is identified.

Transmission of bacterial pathogens from the donor to the recipient has long been a concern after transplantation. Cultures of blood, urine, and peritoneal fluid or perfusate are routinely obtained at most institutions. Two large studies retrospectively evaluated the finding of bacteremia in donors of solid organs, including livers.[44] Despite finding bacteremia in approximately 5% of donors in both series, no transmission occurred in the recipients. However, recipients in all cases were receiving antibiotic coverage, and caretakers were informed of the bacteremia so that appropriate changes in antibiotic regimens to cover these pathogens could be made. These studies suggest that prophylactic antibiotics can allow for the successful use of organs even from bacteremic donors. Blood cultures from the donor at the time of harvest are recommended. Another study evaluating the use of organs from donors with bacterial meningitis (*Escherichia coli, Streptococcus pneumoniae,* and *Neisseria meningitidis*) also found an absence of adverse events in recipients; donors had been treated prior to organ harvest, and recipients received 5 to 10 days of antibiotic treatment.[45]

Serological assays are typically obtained on both donors and candidates for syphilis using a nontreponemal test (e.g., rapid plasma regain [RPR]) and Venereal Disease Research Laboratory ([VDRL] slide test) as the screen and a specific treponemal test if the screen is positive. In the past, a confirmed positive test for syphilis was considered a contraindication to use of the organ. However, successful transplantation has been carried out by giving penicillin to the deceased donor prior to harvest and by then treating the recipients.[46]

Parasites and Fungi

Parasitic or fungal pathogens harbored with few or no symptoms in the normal host can cause disease (both primary and reactivation) after transplantation. Examples of these infections include toxoplasmosis, cryptococcosis, coccidioidomycosis and histoplasmosis. More exotic diseases (e.g., malaria, Chagas' disease, strongyloidiasis) have been reported after organ transplantation in patients from countries with endemic disease.[47] Because patients often travel to transplant centers distant from their homes, it is imperative that transplant physicians be aware of the local environmental risks of each patient (see Table 29–3).

Screening of candidates should include a careful history of prior illness with fungal or parasitic infections. Stool should be screened for ova and parasites in patients coming from areas where parasitic diseases are frequently encountered. Routine serological screening for *Toxoplasma gondii* is not universally recommended for those undergoing liver transplantation but is advocated by some. Likewise, liver donors are not routinely screened, as *T. gondii* does not have a propensity to remain latent in this organ; this contrasts with cardiac donors, from whom the risk of transmission is considerably higher. However, on rare occasions, donor transmission of *T. gondii* has occurred in noncardiac transplant recipients, leading some experts to recommend screening for all organ donors.[48] Trimethoprim sulfamethoxazole used at most centers as prophylaxis against *Pneumocystis jiroveci* also has activity against toxoplasmosis and can protect against reactivation of donor-transmitted disease.

Antifungal prophylaxis should be considered in candidates with a positive history of prior fungal infection with pathogens known to recur after resolution of the primary infection. Experience with coccidioidomycosis in transplant recipients suggests that antifungal therapy, such as an azole agent, should be given in transplant recipients with this history to prevent reactivation.[49] Similarly, reactivation of histoplasmosis after organ transplantation can occur; therefore, prophylaxis with an azole agent should also be given indefinitely. Donor transmission of histoplasmosis has also been documented in a recipient of a kidney transplant whose donor was from an endemic area.[50] Blastomycosis has been noted on rare occasion after transplantation. Amphotericin B is the most reliable therapy in the immunocompromised host, although azoles (itraconazole, fluconazole, and voriconazole) that have good in vitro activity against *Blastomyces dermatitidis* may be effective.[51] *Aspergillus* can reactivate or infect patients after liver transplantation, causing substantial morbidity and mortality. Accordingly, individuals known to have active disease with *Aspergillus* should receive aggressive therapy aimed at eradication prior to the time of transplantation. In addition, patients with cystic fibrosis undergoing liver transplantation can be colonized with *Aspergillus*. Data are limited for disease after liver transplantation, but the diseases have been shown to occur after lung transplantation. For this reason, prophylaxis with agents active against *Aspergillus* should be used. Colonization with *Candida* species can occasionally be found prior to liver transplantation, particularly in patients who have been on broad spectrum antibiotic treatment. If yeast is found, low-dose amphotericin or azoles should be used to treat disease or eradicate colonization. The use of azoles in patients awaiting liver transplantation can be dangerous because of hepatotoxicity, and accordingly, most would prefer the use of low-dose amphotericin or liposomal formulations over fluconazole. Screening for past fungal disease for liver transplantation recipients has not been routine, but it should be considered in patients from endemic areas or those who have high-risk factors.

Candidate Immunizations

It is critical to document the immunization history of the transplant candidate. This is often overlooked in the adult patient population. For children, the history should identify the status of immunizations against diphtheria, pertussis, tetanus, polio, measles, mumps, rubella, *S. pneumoniae,* and *Haemophilus influenzae* type B. Likewise, for both pediatric and adult candidates for liver transplantation, vaccination history for hepatitis A and hepatitis B should be obtained. Attempts to update the patient's immunization status should be made prior to transplantation when vaccination is more likely to be effective. Seasonal influenza vaccination is also recommended for candidates and household contacts. Measles vaccination prior to transplantation is controversial, as this is a live virus and the time until an organ becomes available is difficult to predict. If patients do not have measles antibody present and 1 to 2 months are anticipated between the time of evaluation and transplantation, we generally recommend administration of measles-mumps-rubella (MMR) vaccine. Patients expected to undergo transplantation within several weeks of the evaluation should not receive live virus vaccine. Inactivated vaccines (e.g., hepatitis A, hepatitis B, diphtheria, tetanus toxoid, and acellular pertussis [DTP], or tetanus-diphtheria [Td] for adults) may be given in the hospital during the evaluation. Ensuring adequate immunization against tetanus and diphtheria should be routine for adults as well as children. Acellular pertussis vaccines may be useful when licensed for adult use. Likewise it is prudent to update hepatitis A and B immunizations.

Evaluating Fever at Time of Transplant

Another function of the infectious disease consultant is the care of candidates who experience acute episodes of infection prior to transplantation, requiring appropriate treatment and potentially mandating removal of the patient from the candidate waiting list and/or delaying the time of transplantation. The input of the infectious disease specialist may be critical in optimizing the care of these episodes and determining when the patient may safely tolerate both liver transplantation and subsequent immunosuppression. If there is clinical or radiographic evidence of lower respiratory tract disease, bacterial peritonitis, or cholangitis, transplantation should be delayed. In children, specific viral infections, even limited to the upper respiratory tract, can be associated with significant morbidity and mortality when they persist or develop in the early postoperative period. These viruses include adenovirus,[52] respiratory syncytial virus,[53] parainfluenza, and influenza virus.[54] Rapid diagnostic assays for these viruses are increasingly available. Evaluation of fever and/or respiratory symptoms in children and adult candidates during the fall and winter months should include these rapid studies.

Evaluation of a fever without a known focus should include a complete blood count with differential white blood cell count, blood culture, urine culture (in children), and viral cultures of buffy coat, throat or nasopharynx, and urine. Chest radiography is also appropriate. If no focus is found and transplantation proceeds, antibiotic prophylaxis should be continued for a minimum of 48 hours while awaiting culture results.

Conclusion

Transplantation leads to a unique form of an acquired immunodeficiency state caused by the critical need for immunosuppressive drugs to ensure allograft survival. In preventing rejection of the new organ, these antirejection drugs disturb various aspects of the immune system and put the recipient at risk for opportunistic infections. Careful screening of the candidate and donor will help identify potential infectious agents before they become a complicating factor.

Pearls and Pitfalls

Pretransplant screening should:
- Identify potential pathogens present in:
  - Candidate
  - Donor
- Allow team to devise appropriate prophylaxis strategies

Screening assays can have false-negative results because of:
- Recent infection without time for seroconversion
- New infection in candidate since time of initial evaluation

To decrease false-negative results, repeat previously negative serology at the time of transplantation.

Screening assays can have false-positive results because of:
- Passive antibody from blood products
- Maternal antibody in child younger than 12 to 18 months of age

---

References

1. Singh N, Dummer JS, Kusne S, et al: Infections with cytomegalovirus and other herpesviruses in 121 liver transplant recipients: Transmission by donated organ and the effect of OKT3 antibodies. J Infect Dis 158:124-131, 1988.
2. Patel R, Snydman DR, Rubin RH, et al: Cytomegalovirus prophylaxis in solid organ transplant recipients. Transplantation 61:1279-1289, 1996.
3. Breinig MK, Zitelli B, Starzl TE, Ho M: Epstein-Barr virus, cytomegalovirus, and other viral infections in children after liver transplantation. J Infect Dis 156:273-279, 1987.
4. Stratta RJ, Shaefer MS, Markin RS, et al: Clinical patterns of cytomegalovirus disease after liver transplantation. Arch Surg 124:1443-1449, 1989.
5. Bowman J, Green M, Scantlebury V. OKT3 and viral disease in pediatric liver transplant recipients. Clin Transplant 5: 294-300, 1991.
6. Stratta RJ, Shaefer MS, Cushing KA, et al: Successful prophylaxis of cytomegalovirus disease after primary CMV exposure in liver transplant recipients. Transplantation 51:90-97, 1991.
7. Saliba F, Arulnaden JL, Gugenheim J, et al: CMV hyperimmune globulin prophylaxis after liver transplantation: A prospective randomized controlled study. Transplant Proc 21: 2260-2262, 1989.
8. Chou SW: Acquisition of donor strains of cytomegalovirus by renal-transplant recipients. N Engl J Med 314:1418-1423, 1986.
9. Razonable RR, Paya CV, Smith TF: Role of the laboratory in diagnosis and management of cytomegalovirus infection in hematopoietic stem cell and solid-organ transplant recipients. J Clin Microbiol 40:746-752, 2002.
10. Gopal MR, Thomson BJ, Fox J, et al: Detection by PCR of HHV-6 and EBV DNA in blood and oropharynx of healthy adults and HIV-seropositives. Lancet 335:1598-1599, 1990.
11. Preiksaitis JK, Diaz-Mitoma F, Mirzayans F, et al: Quantitative oropharyngeal Epstein-Barr virus shedding in renal and cardiac transplant recipients: relationship to immunosuppressive therapy, serologic responses, and the risk of posttransplant lymphoproliferative disorder. J Infect Dis 166:986-994, 1992.
12. Cen H, Breinig MC, Atchison RW, et al: Epstein-Barr virus transmission via the donor organs in solid organ transplantation: Polymerase chain reaction and restriction fragment length polymorphism analysis of IR2, IR3, and IR4. J Virol 65:976-980, 1991.
13. Ho M, Miller G, Atchison RW, et al: Epstein-Barr virus infections and DNA hybridization studies in posttransplantation lymphoma and lymphoproliferative lesions: The role of primary infection. J Infect Dis 152:876-886, 1985.
14. Paya CV, Fung JJ, Nalesnik MA, et al: Epstein-Barr virus-induced posttransplant lymphoproliferative disorders. ASTS/ASTP EBV-PTLD Task Force and The Mayo Clinic Organized International Consensus Development Meeting. Transplantation 68:1517-1525, 1999.
15. Kusne S, Schwartz M, Breinig MK, et al: Herpes simplex virus hepatitis after solid organ transplantation in adults. J Infect Dis 163:1001-1007, 1991.
16. McGregor RS, Zitelli BJ, Urbach AH, et al: Varicella in pediatric orthotopic liver transplant recipients. Pediatrics 83:256-261, 1989.
17. Razonable RR, Paya CV: The impact of human herpesvirus-6 and -7 infection on the outcome of liver transplantation. Liver Transpl 8:651-658, 2002.
18. Yoshikawa T, Ihira M, Suzuki K, et al: Primary human herpesvirus 6 infection in liver transplant recipients. J Pediatr 138:921-925, 2001.
19. Michaels MG, Jenkins FJ: Human herpesvirus 8: Is it time for routine surveillance in pediatric solid organ transplant recipients to prevent the development of Kaposi's sarcoma? Pediatr Transplant 7:1-3, 2003.
20. Rosen HR, Martin P: Viral hepatitis in the liver transplant recipient. Infect Dis Clin North Am 14:761-784, 2000.
21. McGory RW, Ishitani MB, Oliveira WM, et al: Improved outcome of orthotopic liver transplantation for chronic hepatitis B cirrhosis with aggressive passive immunization. Transplantation 61:1358-1364, 1996.

22. Delmonico FL: Cadaver donor screening for infectious agents in solid organ transplantation. Clin Infect Dis 31:781-786, 2000.

23. Wachs ME, Amend WJ, Ascher NL, et al: The risk of transmission of hepatitis B from HBsAg(-), HBcAb(+), HBIgM(-) organ donors. Transplantation 59:230-234, 1995.

24. Dodson SF, Bonham CA, Geller DA, et al: Prevention of de novo hepatitis B infection in recipients of hepatic allografts from anti-HBc positive donors. Transplantation 68:1058-1061, 1999.

25. Gane EJ, Portmann BC, Naoumov NV, et al: Long-term outcome of hepatitis C infection after liver transplantation. N Engl J Med 334:815-820, 1996.

26. Dickson RC, Caldwell SH, Ishitani MB, et al: Clinical and histologic patterns of early graft failure due to recurrent hepatitis C in four patients after liver transplantation. Transplantation 61:701-705, 1996.

27. Tzakis AG, Cooper MH, Dummer JS, et al: Transplantation in HIV+ patients. Transplantation 49:354-358, 1990.

28. Erice A, Rhame FS, Heussner RC, et al: Human immunodeficiency virus infection in patients with solid-organ transplants: Report of five cases and review. Rev Infect Dis 13:537-547, 1991.

29. Simonds RJ, Holmberg SD, Hurwitz RL, et al: Transmission of human immunodeficiency virus type 1 from a seronegative organ and tissue donor. N Engl J Med 326:726-732, 1992.

30. Gow PJ, Pillay D, Mutimer D: Solid organ transplantation in patients with HIV infection. Transplantation 72:177-181, 2001.

31. Guidelines for counseling persons infected with human T-lymphotropic virus type I (HTLV-I) and type II (HTLV-II). Centers for Disease Control and Prevention and the USPHS Working Group. Ann Intern Med 118:448-454, 1993.

32. Tanabe K, Kitani R, Takahashi K, et al: Long-term results in human T-cell leukemia virus type 1-positive renal transplant recipients. Transplant Proc 30:3168-3170, 1998.

33. Update: Investigations of West Nile virus infections in recipients of organ transplantation and blood transfusion. MMWR Morb Mortal Wkly Rep 51:833-836, 2002.

34. Ukah FO, Merhav H, Kramer D, et al: Early outcome of liver transplantation in patients with a history of spontaneous bacterial peritonitis. Transplant Proc 25:1113-1115, 1993

35. Van Thiel DH, Hassanein T, Gurakar A, et al: Liver transplantation after an acute episode of spontaneous bacterial peritonitis. Hepatogastroenterology 43:1584-1588, 1996.

36. Pettitt BJ, Zitelli BJ, Rowe MI. Analysis of patients with biliary atresia coming to liver transplantation. J Pediatr Surg 19:779-785, 1984.

37. Sterneck M, Ferrell LAN, Roberts J, Lake J. Mycobacterial infection after liver transplantation: A report of three cases and review of the literature. Clin Transplant 6:55-61, 1992.

38. Higgins RSD, Kusne S, Reyes J, et al: Mycobacterium tuberculosis after liver transplantation: Management and guidelines for prevention. Clin Transplant 6:81-90, 1992.

39. Naqvi SA, Hussain M, Askari H, et al: Is there a place for prophylaxis against tuberculosis following renal transplantation? Transplant Proc 24:1912, 1992.

40. Malhotra KK, Dash SC, Dhawan IK, et al: Tuberculosis and renal transplantation—observations from an endemic area of tuberculosis. Postgrad Med J 62:359-362, 1986.

41. Qunibi WY, al Sibai MB, Taher S, et al: Mycobacterial infection after renal transplantation—report of 14 cases and review of the literature. QJM 77:1039-1060, 1990.

42. Tuberculosis. In Pickering LK, Baker CJ, Overturf GD, Prober CG (eds): Red Book: 2003 Report of the Committee on Infectious Diseases. Elk Grove Village, IL, Committee on Infectious Diseases, American Academy of Pediatrics, 2003, pp 642-660.

43. Kiuchi T, Tanaka K, Inomata Y, et al: Experience of tacrolimus-based immunosuppression in living-related liver transplantation complicated with graft tuberculosis: Interaction with rifampicin and side effects. Transplant Proc 28:3171-3172, 1996.

44. Lumbreras C, Sanz F, Gonzalez A, et al. Clinical significance of donor-unrecognized bacteremia in the outcome of solid-organ transplant recipients. Clin Infect Dis 33:722-726, 2001.

45. Lopez-Navidad A, Domingo P, Caballero F, et al: Successful transplantation of organs retrieved from donors with bacterial meningitis. Transplantation 64:365-368, 1997.

46. Ko WJ, Chu SH, Lee YH, et al: Successful prevention of syphilis transmission from a multiple organ donor with serological evidence of syphilis. Transplant Proc 30:3667-3668, 1998.

47. Cantarovich F, Vazquez M, Garcia WD, et al: Special infections in organ transplantation in South America. Transplant Proc 24:1902-1908, 1992.

48. Mayes JT, O'Connor BJ, Avery R, et al: Transmission of *Toxoplasma gondii* infection by liver transplantation. Clin Infect Dis 21:511-515, 1995.

49. Blair JE, Logan JL. Coccidioidomycosis in solid organ transplantation. Clin Infect Dis 33:1536-1544, 2001.

50. Wong SY, Allen DM. Transmission of disseminated histoplasmosis via cadaveric renal transplantation: Case report. Clin Infect Dis 14:232-234, 1992.

51. Serody JS, Mill MR, Detterbeck FC, et al: Blastomycosis in transplant recipients: Report of a case and review. Clin Infect Dis 16:54-58, 1993.

52. Michaels MG, Green M, Wald ER, et al: Adenovirus infection in pediatric liver transplant recipients. J Infect Dis 165:170-174, 1992.

53. Pohl C, Green M, Wald ER, Ledesma-Medina J. Respiratory syncytial virus infections in pediatric liver transplant recipients. J Infect Dis 165:166-169, 1992.

54. Apalsch AM, Green M, Ledesma-Medina J, et al: Parainfluenza and influenza virus infections in pediatric organ transplant recipients. Clin Infect Dis 20:394-399, 1995.

Clinical Nurse Coordinator: Nursing Focus on Care of Patients with End-Stage Liver Disease

KELLY WICKER

Goal for the clinical transplant coordinator   439

The referral process   440

Evaluation of patients with end-stage liver
    disease   440
    Outpatient transplant evaluation   442
    Inpatient transplant evaluation   443

Finding the best medical therapy   443

The liver transplant waiting list   445

Transplantation   445

Conclusion   445

Less than 25 years ago, a major nursing medical-surgical textbook stated: "The successful transplantation of organs and tissues as a means of preserving life, correcting deformities, and repairing organic damage has been an age old dream of physicians. In recent years, as a result of scientific advances in both surgery and physiology, that dream seems to be coming true."[1] The "dream" of successful transplantation and the possibilities that exist in assisting these critically ill patients to regain their quality of life have had a direct and immense impact on the field of nursing.

This impact is especially true of the registered nurses who work specifically in the role of clinical nurse coordinator (CNC), also known as transplant coordinator. The following text examines the role of these clinical experts, specifically, pretransplant liver coordinators, who under the direction of a hepatologist or gastroenterologist facilitate the care of patients with end-stage liver disease.

Goal for the Clinical Transplant Coordinator

The goal of the CNC is to successfully guide patients who have no other therapy available besides liver transplantation through a maze of processes that may ultimately lead to liver transplantation. This maze includes the referral process, transplant evaluation, selection as an appropriate candidate for transplantation in a committee setting, financial clearance for transplantation, placement on a waiting list, and follow-up needed to remain on the list. Not only are several steps involved, but multiple health care professionals are also involved at each step. The process can seem to be an overwhelming task to patients and their families. To solve this dilemma, the transplant coordinator must be the primary contact for patients and their caregivers. As the primary contact, the CNC can actively participate in all levels of the patient's care, communicate openly with the patient and other members of the health care team regarding patient care issues, take the opportunity to continually monitor the patient and assess any educational needs, and finally, advocate for the patient because a liver patient can often experience significant deterioration before transplantation.

The Referral Process

Referral for liver transplantation can come from a variety of different sources, including but not limited to a primary care physician, a hepatologist or gastroenterologist, an oncologist, or possibly an insurance case manager. No matter what the source of the referral, it is essential that the CNC obtain accurate and current medical information from the referral source so that decisions on the patient's care can be made in a timely fashion. To do so, a CNC must not only verbally gather baseline information regarding the patient but also obtain medical records that substantiate what has been verbally reported. As with many other areas of nursing, with experience, a CNC will find that one question leads to the next and to the next, thus giving the pretransplant team a good picture of the patient before arrival at the transplant center. Figure 30–1 is the liver transplant referral form that, along with the medical record information, is shared with the hepatologist before initiation of the evaluation. This early communication ensures that the standardized pretransplant evaluation testing and consultations are completed without delay, as well as any additional testing that may be warranted. Additional tests or consultations may be deemed necessary by the hepatologist, depending on the specific liver disease and other factors in the patient's medical history.

One consideration at the time of referral is the medical condition of the patient at that moment. If the patient is presented as a critically ill patient, the urgency of the referral needs to be communicated immediately so that physician-to-physician communication can take place. Often, such communication will prompt urgent financial clearance for transplant evaluation, followed by a hospital-to-hospital transfer in which a medical evaluation can be completed in a matter of just a few hours.

Over the past several years, the United Network for Organ Sharing (UNOS) has been actively pursuing regulatory standards, specifically in the field of liver transplantation, in which the goal is that patients who have the greatest need, defined as the highest probability of death,[2] will be transplanted first. Included in these same guidelines are medical criteria for patients with hepatocellular carcinoma with regard to size and number of tumors.[3] Often, the referring physician is unaware of these guidelines, and it is frequently the role of the CNC to help educate referral sources regarding these regulatory demands during the referral for transplantation.

It is also not uncommon for referring physicians to request a transplant evaluation very early in the patient's disease process. A patient in whom liver disease has been diagnosed but who has normal laboratory values and scans without evidence of malignancy may be too early for transplant listing but will need close follow-up to monitor the disease process. Review of the medical information by the medical staff may lead to consultation and an opportunity for the patient to be closely monitored by a liver specialist without having to undergo a complete transplant evaluation. This is of great benefit to the patient, who may possibly have an opportunity to be treated with other medical therapies and thus be "in the system" in case transplantation is needed in the future. This practice is also of great benefit to the payer source, since unnecessary or too early evaluation for transplantation is a costly practice.

Once the medical information has been obtained, the CNC then works closely with the team of financial experts to obtain clearance to begin the transplant evaluation process. At the same time, the CNC begins to build the relationship with the patient and family by laying the groundwork for open communication. This is easily accomplished by an introductory phone call or correspondence to let the patient know that a referral has been received. Other topics discussed with the patient in these early conversations or correspondence include specific information regarding the medical center, available housing, transportation, and any information that is helpful during the evaluation, such as the availability of radiology films or biopsy slides for review. Once the medical information has been fully reviewed and the payer is financially committed, the transplant evaluation can begin.

Evaluation of Patients with End-Stage Liver Disease

All transplant protocols, including the pretransplant evaluation, should be established in writing and approved by both the hepatology staff and the transplant surgery staff. At the time of transplantation, the two very different worlds of internal medicine and

Liver Transplant Referral Form
REFERRAL SOURCE: Physician: _____

Date: _____
Insurance: _____

DEMOGRAPHICS

Patient name: _____ _____ _____
              (Last)   (First)   (Middle)

Address: _____

         _____ _____ _____
         (City)   (State)   (Zip Code)

Phone #: _____ _____ _____
         (Home)   (Work)   (Cellular)

Sex (M/F): _____   DOB: _____   AGE: _____

Social Security #: _____

INSURANCE

MEDICARE #: _____   MEDICAID #: _____   State: _____

INSURANCE #1: _____

Phone #: _____   DOB of Insured: _____
Insured: _____   Relation to Patient: _____
Insured SS #: _____   ID #: _____
Employer/Group: _____ Group #: _____

INSURANCE #2: _____

Phone #: _____   DOB of Insured: _____
Insured: _____   Relation to Patient: _____
Insured SS #: _____   ID #: _____
Employer/Group: _____ Group #: _____

REFERRAL PHYSICIAN

Name: _____   Specialty: _____

Address: _____

         _____ _____ _____
         (City)   (State)   (Zip Code)

Phone #: _____ _____ _____
         (City)   (FAX)   (Other)

PATIENT HISTORY

Diagnosis: _____   HT: _____   WT: _____

History Of: Yes   No
Encephalopathy?   _____ _____ ; If Yes, Grade: _____
Ascites?   _____ _____ ; Date of Last Paracentesis: _____
                                               Frequency: _____
TIPS?   _____ _____ ; Date: _____
GI Bleed?   _____ _____ ; Date: _____
Hepatorenal Syndrome?   _____ _____ ;
Hepatopulmonary Syndrome?   _____ _____ ;
SBP?   _____ _____ ;
Substance abuse?   _____ _____ ; Type: _____ Date: _____
Currently Hospitalized?   _____ _____
Recent Laboratory Values:

     Date: _____
     INR: _____ , CR _____ , ALB: _____   CURRENT MELD: _____

CLINICAL NOTES _____
_____
_____
_____

FIGURE 30–1

Liver transplant referral form.

surgery meet on a common field, and all players must be satisfied with the information that is known about the patient. This starts with the information obtained during the transplant evaluation.

Figure 30–2 is an example of the standardized evaluation for all patients seen at the Baylor Regional Transplant Institute, whereas Figure 30–3 is an example of supplementary testing and consultations that would be completed in addition to the standardized testing, depending on the diagnosis. These protocols do not hinder the treating hepatologist from obtaining other studies or consultations deemed necessary; however, these guidelines should be followed by the CNC for all patients being evaluated.

Outpatient Transplant Evaluation

For the majority of patients, the transplant evaluation can be completed efficiently in an outpatient setting.

LIVER TRANSPLANT EVALUATION

Consultations

Transplant Surgery

Transplant Coordinator

Transplant Nutrition Specialist

Transplant Social Worker

Transplant Cardiologist
- If patient is >40 years of age, has a history of IV drug use, or an abnormal EKG
- Cardiac echo
- Stress Echo - Bruce protocol and/or thallium

Transplant Psychiatry
- If patient has a history of alcohol and/or drug abuse or if the patient has any psychiatric history

Hepatology

Testing

MRI with liver volumes
Chest radiograph
EKG
Glofil
Hepatic function profile
PT with INR, PTT
Amylase
Iron
Total T3
Ammonia
Alpha fetoprotein
Alpha$_1$-antitrypsin level
Antinuclear antibody
Ceroplasmin
HbsAb
HbeAb
HAVAb-IgM
Urine sodium
PPD skin test

Doppler ultrasound of the abdomen
KUB - abdominal radiograph
Mammogram (for females ≥35 yr)
Basic metabolic profile
CBC with differential
Ferritin
TIBC
TSH
PSA (for males ≥50 yr)
Magnesium
Alpha$_1$-antitrypsin phenotype
Serum protein electrophoresis
Antimitochondrial antibody
Antismooth muscle antibody
HbeAg
HAVAb
Urinalysis
Chain of custody - urine drug screen
ABO - to reconfirm the ABO obtained in the processing profile

Processing Profile, which includes:
ABO, RH, Antibody Screen, Anti-HIV-1, Anti-HIV-2, Anti-HTLV-1, Anti-HBc, HBsAg, Anti-HCV, RPR

FIGURE 30–2

Liver transplant evaluation: consultations and testing.

LIVER TRANSPLANT EVALUATION

Additonal Testing and Consultation: Diagnosis of a Primary Liver Tumor

Transplant oncologist
MUGA
Bone scan

CT scan of chest, abdomen, and pelvis
Skeletal survey
Liver Pancreas Center surgeon w/ assessment of radiofrequency thermal ablation

Additional Testing and Consultation: Diagnosis of Primary Sclerosing Cholangitis

CEA
CA 19-9
Vitamin A
Vitamin D, 1,25 Dihydroxyvitamin D_3

Additional Testing and Consultation: Diagnosis of Primary Biliary Cirrhosis

Vitamin A
Vitamin D, 1,25 Dihydroxyvitamin D_3

Additional Testing and Consultation: Diagnosis of Chronic Hepatitis C with Cirrhosis

HCV RNA - Quantitative (bDNA)

Additional Testing and Consultation: Diagnosis of Chronic Hepatitis B with Cirrhosis

HBV DNA
Hepatitis B Delta

Additional Consultations Based on Medical Need

Transplant Nephrology
Pulmonology
Infectious Disease
Gastroenterology
Neurology
Anesthesiology

FIGURE 30–3

Liver transplant evaluation: additional testing.

In a period of 4 or 5 days, the information needed to determine a patient's candidacy for liver transplantation can be obtained through testing and consultation. At the same time, the educational process intensifies with the patient and the designated support team. To obtain success in both, it is essential that the evaluation be well organized and patient friendly. Because each patient may learn differently, it may be necessary to present the same information in several different formats. Obviously, the stress of chronic liver disease, as well as issues with encephalopathy, can make patients with end-stage liver disease challenging to educate.

For outpatient evaluations, the first person that the patient should have direct contact with is a CNC, who can handle any immediate issues. The Baylor Regional Transplant Institute in Dallas meets with prospective candidates at a liver evaluation orientation each Monday morning. This group orientation provides a general overview of the transplant program and the many steps involved in the evaluation and briefly touches on the regulatory standards set by UNOS, specifically regarding the

Model for End-Stage Liver Disease (MELD)[2] scoring system, acceptance as a candidate, placement on the list, and the transplant surgery.

Immediately after this group meeting, each patient meets with a specific CNC, who again will discuss and reinforce information regarding the transplant process but, more specifically, the evaluation schedule that has been established for that particular patient.

During this initial time with the patient, the CNC also reviews highlights of the patient's medical history to make sure that the medical information obtained from the referring physician is complete. After this review, the patient is also provided the *Patient Manual for Liver Transplantation*. Originally published in 1988, this publication is now undergoing its sixth edition update to reflect the most recent changes in liver transplantation. Written specifically with the pretransplant liver patient in mind, this text discusses all aspects of transplantation from transplant evaluation to the long-term follow-up needed after transplantation.

Whether through group presentations, written literature, or one-on-one meetings, each transplant patient and family will need reinforcement of the information and how it applies to their situation personally. As the transplant evaluation week continues, the CNC has regularly scheduled meetings with the patient to answer any questions that may have come up during the week or to notify the patient that additional tests or consultations have been added to the schedule based on the recommendation of a consulting physician. This time is used to reinforce the patient's basic knowledge of transplantation, and often by the midpoint of the evaluation, the patient and family are ready to begin taking in additional information regarding the transplant experience. Accordingly, additional group meetings are scheduled to continue the educational process and discuss topics such as what to expect at the time of liver transplantation and afterward, living donor liver donation, and transplant financing.

Inpatient Transplant Evaluation

Although the majority of liver transplant evaluations can be completed on an outpatient basis, the CNC must always be prepared for patients who may present at the transplant facility at any time and need an inpatient transplant evaluation. Such patients include those with chronic liver failure in a period of decompensation and patients in acute fulminant liver failure.

The CNC must work closely with the admitting physician, physician consultants, and the nursing staff to ensure that all of the evaluation testing and consultations are completed and communicated in a timely manner. Standardized order sets placed on the nursing units so that the patient can immediately begin the evaluation process at time of admission are key to initiating the evaluation without delay. Intensive care units and medicine floor units must be regularly updated by the transplant team regarding changes in pretransplant protocols, including changes in the evaluation process.

If a patient with chronic liver failure has stabilized and is ready for discharge from the hospital before completion of the evaluation, the patient will need to complete the evaluation on an outpatient basis. Careful review and planning by the CNC can help alleviate duplications in testing once the patient converts to an outpatient evaluation.

Patients who arrive at the facility in acute liver failure may not have the luxury of an extended transplant evaluation. Under the guidance of the transplant hepatologist, the CNC must work diligently to make sure that information deemed necessary for urgent listing is gathered and reviewed within a period of a few hours. Once the patient is placed on the transplant list, the pretransplant CNC must also continue to gather the evaluation information and communicate it to the entire transplant team as the patient waits for the life-saving organ. This information is often critical for the hepatologist as the cause of the acute liver failure is being investigated and needed therapy is being determined while the wait for transplantation continues. This information is also critical to the transplant surgeon as offers are beginning to be received from the local organ procurement organization and posttransplant immunosuppression is being considered.

The educational needs of the patient and family must be individualized as determined during the inpatient transplant evaluation. For the majority of inpatient evaluations, the CNC will have ample opportunity to meet with the patient and the support team to begin the educational process during the hospital admission. Patients who are critically ill may not have the capacity to participate in the pretransplant education. In such cases, it is essential that the CNC work directly with the patient's family or designated support team to provide education and emotional support.

Finding the Best Medical Therapy

The goal of the transplant committee is to recommend the best medical therapy that is available for the patient and, more specifically, to determine whether that therapy is liver transplantation. This multidisciplinary team brings together the expertise of many to make a life-changing decision one patient at a time. The structure of the transplant committee should truly follow the meaning of many disciplines. Members on this committee include physicians from the following disciplines: hepatology, gastroenterology, transplant surgery, general surgery, internal medicine, oncology, and psychiatry. Others included are psychologists, social workers, transplant dietitians, and members from the pretransplant and posttransplant CNC staff, as well as chaplain services. A quorum of members must be present to begin the patient presentation process. This quorum includes the presenting hepatologist, as well as one other hepatologist or gastroenterologist, a transplant surgeon, and a social worker. It is also essential that this committee have close ties with the hospital ethics committee to ensure that any patient situation presenting an ethical dilemma can have immediate response and resolution.

Because of patient confidentiality issues, few visitors are allowed to attend the transplant committee meeting—and then only at the discretion of the chairman. Patients and their family members are not allowed to attend the weekly transplant conference.

The CNC who has assisted the patient through the evaluation process summarizes all essential information obtained during the evaluation. An administrative assistant can gather this information, but the summary must be reviewed before the presentation for accuracy of the medical information. Information to be provided during the presentation includes a history and physical examination that has been completed by the hepatologist, as well as all consultations, radiological examinations, and laboratory values. In nonurgent situations, this summary is ready for the committee meeting within 7 to 10 days from completion of the evaluation.

During the selection process, the patient's primary hepatologist presents the medical information to the committee, along with new therapies that have been initiated, and other pertinent information. Each consulting physician or member of the transplant team who has had an opportunity to assess the patient brings to the table the pros and cons of liver transplantation for this particular patient. At the end of each patient discussion, the group will come to a consensus regarding the appropriateness of liver transplantation. This decision is recorded and becomes a part of the official meeting minutes of the transplant committee.

During the transplant committee meeting, the CNC works diligently to ensure that the members follow all regulatory guidelines, that clinical information is provided as needed to the decision-making team, and that notes are made to update any new data brought forward. New information could be hospitalizations that have occurred since the patient has returned home, medication changes, or additional diagnoses that the clinical team needs to be cognizant of for pretransplant and posttransplant care.

After the committee meeting and within 1 business day, the CNC contacts the patient and referring physician to notify them of the decision regarding the need for transplantation. In certain instances, the hepatologist will discuss this recommendation with the patient and designated support team, and in all cases the hepatologist is available for questions or concerns regarding the committee decision.

The committee recommendation typically falls into one of three separate categories:

1. Accepted as a transplant candidate—this candidate meets the national standards set by UNOS, as well as the inclusion criteria that have been established for the individual transplant program. The transplant evaluation is completed, and the candidate will proceed to the next step.

2. Denied transplantation—this candidate has been found to not be a candidate for liver transplantation. The patient does not meet the national standards set by UNOS or may have a contraindication that has been established by the individual transplant program. An example is a patient who has a MELD score lower than 6 but may be a transplant candidate in the future. Another example would be a patient who has a single tumor larger than 5 cm in total diameter, who would thus not meet the tumor criteria established by UNOS.[4]

3. Deferred—this candidate is still being considered for liver transplantation, but further testing is required based on the results of the evaluation and the recommendations of the transplant committee. The patient will be brought back to the transplant committee with further information at a later date.

No matter what the result of the transplant committee meeting, it is the CNC's role to help the patient and the support system understand the recommendation. Is there a recommendation for other therapies instead of or before transplantation? Can the patient continue to proceed toward placement on the waiting list, and how can that be accomplished? Patients should receive not only verbal notification from the CNC but also written notification from the hepatologist. At the time of this notification, the CNC again assesses the learning needs of the patient and care team and once more is the primary contact for questions or concerns regarding the decision.

For patients who have been selected to continue the process leading to liver transplantation, the CNC again turns to the financial experts to obtain clearance from the payer source so that listing can proceed. Immediately after the committee process and approval of the minutes, the CNC provides this team with the medical information and a letter of medical necessity from the hepatologist in which the need for liver transplantation is justified. This must be expedited through working with the payer case manager or directly with the medical director to obtain financial assurance for transplantation. Payers may have questions regarding the transplant center's protocol, testing results, or as with some payers, the addition of some tests or consultations based on their own established guidelines. Examples of payer-required testing might include dental clearance or additional laboratory tests not required in the transplant center's own protocol. Once again, the CNC is the primary contact for the insurance representative regarding clinical needs and works closely with the case manager to ensure that all questions are satisfactorily answered to facilitate listing.

The Liver Transplant Waiting List

Once financial clearance has been obtained, it is the CNC's responsibility to make sure that the patient is placed on the liver transplant list according to all UNOS requirements. Depending on the amount of time that it has taken to obtain financial clearance, the CNC may need to contact the patient to obtain updated laboratory work to satisfy the requirements of the MELD system.

It is essential to have a system of checks and balances to make sure that all patients are listed correctly and in timely fashion. At all Baylor facilities, the pretransplant CNC fulfills this requirement by completing the listing form seen in Figure 30–4, with direct communication with the posttransplant CNC, who does the listing within the UNET system. This system of checks ensures that hepatologists, transplant surgeons, and the pretransplant and posttransplant coordinator staff members are in agreement that any additional testing recommendations, financial questions, and MELD scoring requirements have been met. Once listed, the patient is notified by the CNC by phone and by mail regarding placement on the transplant waiting list and what the patient's MELD score is.

The phone call notifying the patient of listing is another critical opportunity to educate the patient. A common question by all patients at time of placement is "Where am I at on the list?" Since its inception in 2002, the MELD system has made it more difficult to predict the average amount of time that each patient will be on the waiting list because it can change randomly. Obviously, higher MELD scores would mean shorter waiting list times, but for patients with an average or below-average MELD score, the wait can be long. At this time, the CNC has the opportunity to educate the patient and the care team about the need for continuous monitoring of the listed patient, including immediate reporting of laboratory values that may have been obtained from a physician outside the transplant center, all hospitalizations, or any changes in the medical condition of the patient. This communication can ensure that as a patient deteriorates, the status on the transplant list reflects this change in medical condition.

A protocol to monitor patients while listed must also be established by the hepatology and transplant team. Patients must obtain laboratory values in accordance with their MELD score; however, at all Baylor facilities, patients with lower MELD scores are required to have laboratory values obtained every 3 months instead of yearly as required by UNOS. Ultrasound of the liver and determination of α-fetoprotein levels every 6 months can assist in monitoring patients for the occurrence of hepatocellular carcinoma. Additional testing requirements while on the list should be based on other factors such as cardiac follow-up for patients who also have diabetes or yearly ^{125}I-iothalamate (Glofil) imaging or creatinine clearance for those with renal impairment. These protocols give guidance to the CNC in monitoring listed patients to ensure that the transplant team has the most current information available at time of transplantation.

This continuous monitoring means that the list can change on a daily if not hourly basis, but it ensures that the spirit of the MELD system is realized by truly transplanting the sickest patients first.

Transplantation

At time of transplantation, the pretransplant CNC is notified by the posttransplant CNC of the imminent surgery. Such notification gives both CNCs an opportunity to discuss any known medical changes that would need to be communicated to the transplant surgeon to assist in successful transplantation.

Follow-up with the patient and the care team by the pretransplant CNC before surgery or immediately afterward can assist the patient in the transition from the pretransplant way of life to the posttransplant arena, where the patient will meet another experienced expert in transplantation—the posttransplant CNC.

Conclusion

Liver transplantation has brought a whole new dynamic to the field of nursing in creating the role of the CNC. Knowledge and expertise in the field of hepatology and transplantation, the ability to successfully communicate with both the health care team and the patient, and finally, the skill to assist patients with end-stage liver disease to successfully bridge the many events that occur between referral and transplantation are essential requirements of the pretransplant CNC. As patients are discharged from the hospital and finally the outpatient setting, the CNC knows that each step in the pretransplant process was instrumental in successful transplantation and ultimately in return to the family and community.

Date: _____

Waiting List Placement or Changes

Pre-Coordinator:_____
Post-Coordinator: _____

Patient Name: _____
SS #:_____
Diagnosis: _____
Male/Female:_____
Race:_____
ABO:_____
Height/Weight: _____   _____
Acceptable Donor Weight Range: _____

New List
MELD Update
Make Status 7
Remove from List
Reactivate from Status 7
RRB MELD Upgrade

MELD CALCULATOR

Date of Birth _____
Bilirubin _____
Serum Creatinine _____
INR _____
Dialysis twice with a week prior to creatinine test? (Yes/No)

Regional Review Board: (if applicable)
Requested MELD: _____
Narrative attached (Yes/No)

HCC: HCC form attached: (Yes/No)

Waitlist Notes_____
_____
_____
_____

FIGURE 30–4

Waiting list placement or changes.

Pitfalls and Pearls

- Always listen carefully to your patients and their caregivers—by listening and educating, the CNC can prevent problems in crisis management.
- Standardized protocols are an essential component for quality patient-centered and cost-effective pretransplant care.
- Clinical nurse coordinators are the regulatory experts—know the national guidelines as well as your own center's protocols.
- Always have complete medical and financial clearance before placing the patient on the transplant waiting list.
- Have all critical medical information readily available when the patient's case is being presented to the liver transplant committee or at the time of transplantation.

Pitfalls and Pearls—cont'd

- Always remember that liver transplantation is a life-changing experience and that we all do not handle stress in the same way. Be a patient advocate.
- Find and use your resources—this is a team effort.

References

1. Luckmann J, Sorensen KC: Medical-Surgical Nursing: A Psycho-physiologic Approach. Philadelphia, WB Saunders, 1980, p 167.
2. Organ Distribution: Allocation of Livers. 21 November 2003. p 3-1. 19 July 2004. http://www.unos.org/policiesandbylaws/policies.asp?resources=true.
3. Organ Distribution: Allocation of Livers. 21 November 2003. p 3-10. 19 July 2004. http://www.unos.org/policiesandbylaws/policies.asp?resources=true.
4. Organ Distribution: Allocation of Livers. 21 November 2003. p 3-12. 19 July 2004. http://www.unos.org/policiesandbylaws/policies.asp?resources=true.

Radiologic Evaluation in the Liver Transplant Patient

ANTOINETTE S. GOMES

Pretransplantation evaluation 447
   Computed tomographic imaging 448
   Magnetic resonance imaging 450

Posttransplantation evaluation 452
   Ultrasonography 452

Evaluation of vascular complications after
transplantation 455
   Hepatic artery complications 455
   Portal vein complications 459
   Inferior vena cava and hepatic vein
     complications 461

Evaluation of the Biliary System 461
   Biliary tract complications 462
   Evaluation and management of
     bile leaks 463
   Radiographic diagnosis and management
     of biliary obstruction 464

Summary 468

Diagnostic and interventional radiologic procedures have an important role in liver transplantation. They are used before operation in the selection and presurgical management of candidates and posttransplantation in the follow-up, diagnosis, and treatment of complications.

Pretransplantation Evaluation

Radiological evaluation of the liver transplant patient is usually performed on an outpatient basis. The goal is to determine abnormalities that preclude transplantation along with abnormalities that will affect the operative procedure. Real-time ultrasonography is used routinely to evaluate the liver, the biliary system, and the portal system. Ultrasonography has been found to have a sensitivity rate of 80% to 100% in detecting bile duct obstruction.[1-4] It is also used to evaluate hepatic echo texture. Focal or diffuse heterogeneity may be seen in cases of fatty infiltration, cirrhosis, or tumor. Additionally, ultrasonography is used to exclude occult hepatic carcinoma and to detect adenopathy in the porta hepatis, ascites, or vascular invasion by tumor. Doppler ultrasonography is used to assess the portal vasculature. The patency and size of the extrahepatic portal vein must be ascertained and the patency of the inferior vena cava (IVC) determined, because narrowing or occlusion of either of these vessels alters surgical technique. The hepatic artery and hepatic veins are also evaluated. Patients with thrombosis of the hepatic veins in the Budd-Chiari syndrome may have thrombosis of the IVC and patency of the suprahepatic IVC, which is necessary for liver transplantation to be performed. The extrahepatic portal vein may be absent in patients with biliary atresia, and the IVC may be absent in polysplenia syndrome. If the portal vessels are clearly identified, ultrasonography alone is sufficient.[5,6] However, nonvisualization or equivocal visualization of the portal vein owing to thrombosis of the portal vein with cavernous transformation and large collateral vessels requires arteriography or magnetic resonance angiography (MRA) for accurate assessment.

Computed Tomographic Imaging

Both a computed tomographic scan of the chest, abdomen, and pelvis and a bone scan are indicated for all patients being evaluated for liver transplantation because of a hepatic tumor. The size, number, and location of intrahepatic masses can be seen on a computed tomographic scan. In addition, a computed tomographic scan provides information regarding splenomegaly, varices, ascites, vascular anomalies, and morphological pancreatic anomalies. It also allows evaluation of the entire abdomen for primary tumors, metastases, and abscesses. The preoperative computed tomographic scans provide information regarding liver size and shape from which liver volume can be calculated, facilitating the selection of a donor liver of appropriate size.

Computed tomographic scans are used initially to determine whether a patient with a hepatic tumor is a candidate for partial hepatic resection or requires transplantation.

The detection of focal liver lesions such as hepatocellular carcinoma (HCC) on computed tomography (CT) is based on the attenuation differences in density between normal liver and the lesion. HCCs receive most of their blood supply from the hepatic artery, whereas normal liver parenchyma is supplied mainly through the portal vein. On CT, lesions with arterial-dominant vascularity show brisk enhancement during the arterial phase (20 to 40 seconds after contrast injection) and are better detected in the background of normal liver parenchyma, which remains relatively hypovascular during this phase. During the portal phase (60 to 90 seconds after the actual injection), the liver still receives opacified blood from the arterial system and also receives four times more blood from the portal system. During this phase, hypervascular lesions such as HCC can be isodense relative to normal liver because both enhance similarly.

With older nonhelical CT units, contrast images were acquired during the portal dominant phase. In this phase, hypovascular lesions are well seen but hypervascular lesions are usually missed because they can be isodense relative to the liver parenchyma. Newer, faster helical scanners permit biphasic imaging, with completion of the liver examination, during the arterial-dominant and portal-dominant phases of contrast enhancement. Multirow helical scanners allow a triple-pass CT scan during early arterial, late arterial, and portal venous phases. Studies show that a significant number of additional HCC lesions can be found during the arterial phase compared with the portal or delayed phases.[7]

Currently, most CT protocols include an arterial phase, a portal phase, and an equilibrium phase (10 to 15 minutes) following injection, when most HCC becomes hypovascular relative to the liver parenchyma. Generally, HCCs show brisk hyperenhancement during the arterial phase and rapidly become iso- or hypo-attenuating during the portal phase. In a small number of cases, however, HCC lesions may be hypoenhancing and nearly isodense in the arterial phase and persist as hypoattenuating lesions during the portal phase.

In patients with hepatic cirrhosis, an enhancement pattern consisting of hyperattenuation in the arterial phase and hypoisodensity in the portal phase is virtually diagnostic of HCC (Fig. 31–1A).[8]

Although the majority of nodules in the setting of chronic liver disease are HCC, other lesions may be detected in cirrhotic patients undergoing screening with biphasic helical CT.[9] Hyperenhancing lesions in the arterial phase include small hemangiomas, transient hepatic attenuation differences (THAD), atypical dysplastic nodules, focal nodular hyperplasia, liver cell

---

FIGURE 31–1

A, Portal phase of dual-phase CT scan shows an HCC in a cirrhotic liver. The HCC is seen as a hypointense lesion medially in segment 7 compressing the inferior vena cava (*arrow*). The mass has an area of vascularity surrounding the lesion and central heterogeneity with an area of low density centrally. **B,** MRI axial T2 HASTE images of same patient show an atrophic liver with the HCC seen as a slightly hyperintense lesion at the dome of the liver extending into the cava (*arrow*). The lesion contains high signal centrally. Multiple small, high-T2-signal lesions are scattered throughout the liver and probably represent cysts. **C,** MRI axial T_1 out-of-phase FL2D gradient echo image shows some decrease in central signal indicating fatty-tissue content within the lesion. Fibrous septa are also seen in the lesion. Out-of-phase images typically show a thick black rim called the *chemical shift artifact* at the margin of tissue that contains both water and fat protons. **D,** MRI axial FL2D delayed postgadolinium contrast-enhanced image shows a bright rim representing the hyperintense capsule of the HCC. **E,** MRI HCC and dysplastic nodule. Axial T_1-weighted image shows isointense HCC in the posterior aspect of dome of liver (*arrow*). **F,** In a lower slice there are several other poorly seen nodules; one is a slightly hyperintense lesion (*arrow*). **G,** On T_2-weighted fast spin echo (FSE) sequence the HCC is hyperintense (*arrow*). **H,** The dysplastic nodule shows hypointensity on the T_2-weighted image (*arrow*).

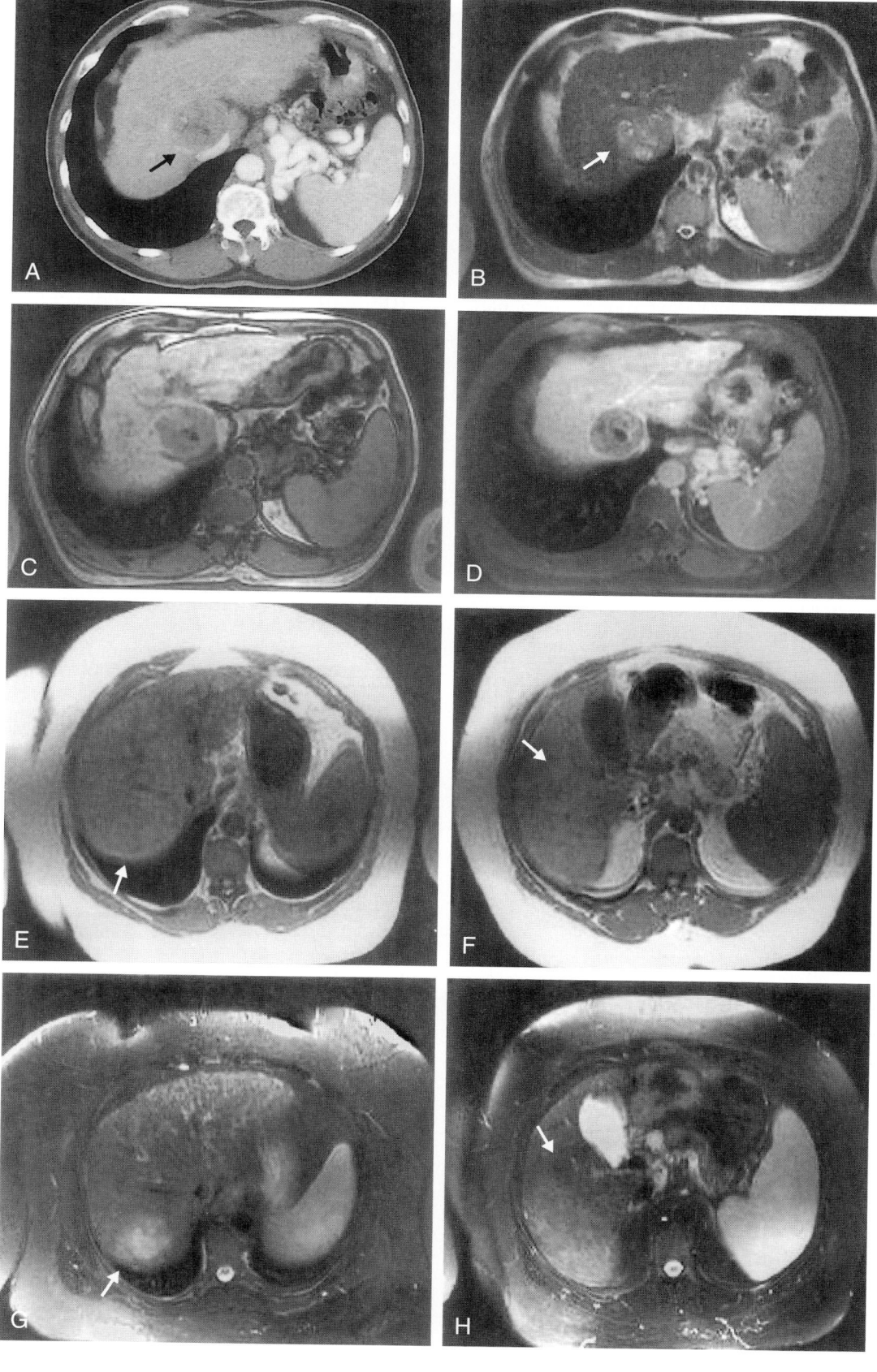

adenoma, and hypervascular metastases. In chronic liver disease, the differential diagnosis of HCC consists largely of hemangioma, THAD, and the rare hypervascular dysplastic nodule. In patients with chronic liver disease, the differential diagnosis of hypodense lesions in the portal or equilibrium phase is hypovascular HCC, peripheral cholangiocarcinoma, dysplastic nodules, and regenerative nodules. Other lesions, such as liver metastases from other primaries, are rare.[10]

Dysplastic nodules are premalignant neoplastic nodules seen in 15% to 25% of cirrhotic livers.[11] They are supplied primarily by the portal vein, but arterial supply can occur. In a series of patients undergoing hepatic transplantation, the sensitivity of helical CT was 39% (9 of 23) with all of the lesions being hypoattenuating.[12]

Large studies are needed to determine the exact sensitivity and specificity of helical CT in the detection of HCC. Lim and colleagues[12] reported a sensitivity of 78% (15 of 21) for helical CT in the detection of HCC. The detection rate for lesions less than 2 cm was 60%, and the detection rate for lesions larger than 2 cm was 82%. In the series of Valls and colleagues[10] helical CT had a sensitivity of 79.5% (39 of 49) and a positive predictive value (PPV) of 86.6% in the detection of HCC. There were six false positive results, largely related to macronodular regenerative nodules and hyperplastic dysplastic nodules.

In the cirrhotic liver, regenerative nodules are formed by regenerative hepatocytes surrounded by fibrotic septa. They can vary from 1 to 3 mm in micronodular cirrhosis to 3 to 15 mm in macronodular cirrhosis. Histologically, they are composed of normal hepatocytes and their blood supply is predominantly portal. Because the blood supply and architecture of regenerative nodules are similar to normal liver parenchyma, visualization of regenerative nodules is difficult. Occasionally they appear as slightly hyperdense lesions on noncontrast studies. More often they appear in the equilibrium phase as tiny hypodense lesions. Although infrequent, large regenerative nodules may present as low-density lesions in the arterial, portal, and equilibrium phases, mimicking hypovascular HCCs.[10]

The detection and staging of HCC is essential in the pretransplant evaluation. Studies support liver transplantation in patients with a solitary HCC that is less than 5 cm or with no more than three tumor nodules (each 3 cm or less in diameter) as long as there is no evidence of vascular invasion and extrahepatic spread. Following these criteria, the reported actuarial survival rate is 75% at 4 or 5 years.[13,14]

Magnetic Resonance Imaging

Magnetic resonance imaging (MRI) is now an alternative technique to CT in transplant imaging. It is used as an alternative in patients who are allergic to iodinated contrast media. It can provide information on focal liver lesions and can clarify CT findings in cases of focal fatty change. It can provide information regarding the biliary tree, and three-dimensional time-of-flight gadolinium-enhanced MRA techniques permit visualization of the arterial and portal venous system. MRI is used to help distinguish dysplastic nodules from HCC. Dysplastic nodules are typically hyperintense on nonenhanced T_1-weighted images and hypoisointense on T_2-weighted images. They are almost never hyperintense on T_2-weighted images.[15]

HCCs are isointense or hyperintense on nonenhanced T_1-weighted images and hyperintense, isointense, or hypointense on T_2-weighted images (see Fig. 31–1B to D). Hyperintensity on T_2-weighted images is characteristic of HCC and is related to a lower degree of histological differentiation. On contrast-enhanced images, most HCCs exhibit diffuse enhancement during the arterial phase, with rapid washout during the portal (venous) phase.[16]

Other typical findings of HCC on MRI include a visible tumor capsule, a mosaic pattern, intratumoral fat deposition, portal or hepatic vein invasion, and arterioportal venous shunting.[17,18] These major findings may be absent in very small tumors, with only the hypervascularity detected.

The HCC capsule, a major morphological finding in HCC, is a fibrous area surrounding the tumor formed by condensation and collagenation of reticulum fibers after the disappearance of hepatocytes from compression of the tumor. It usually is hypointense on unenhanced T_1- and T_2-weighted spin-echo (SE) images, hypointense on unenhanced gradient echo images, and hyperintense on delayed postgadolinium images. The presence of fatty change within the tumor is another primary and characteristic finding in HCC.

Fibrous septa and a mosaic pattern are characteristic of HCC[19] and are well seen, especially after contrast injection.

Magnetic Resonance Imaging Technique

Currently, breath-hold T_1- and T_2-weighted images of the liver are recommended because they avoid the motion artifact commonly seen with conventional longer SE MRI sequences. For T_2-weighted images, breath-hold turbo spin echo (TSE) with long echo train or half-Fourier acquisition single-shot turbo spin-echo (HASTE) sequences are recommended. For T_1-weighted images, breath-hold gradient-echo sequences permit scanning of the entire liver in a single breath-hold and allow dynamic contrast-enhanced images, which allow the entire liver to be imaged in the arterial phase.

Breath-hold chemical shift (in phase and opposed phase) can show fatty infiltration of the liver as well as fat within hepatic nodules.[20] Chemical shift MRI techniques, which are based on the difference in resonance frequency of water and fat protons, is the most reliable MRI technique in detecting intratumoral fat.[21,22] Lesions containing a mixture of fat and water protons exhibit low signal intensity on opposed-phase images because the signal from water cancels the signal from fat. High signal intensity is seen on in-phase images because the signals are summed.

After the T_1 and T_2 unenhanced MRI study, extracellular-type gadolinium chelate contrast agent is injected, and contrast-enhanced images are obtained in the arterial, portal, and equilibrium phases. Images in the arterial phase (15 to 20 seconds after injection) are needed in cirrhotic livers to show hypervascular lesions or small HCCs.

Imaging in the portal venous phase (60 seconds after injection) and the equilibrium phase (90 seconds to 5 minutes after injection) after contrast is important for showing washout of HCC and delayed enhancement of the capsule.

Although MRI has helped solve diagnostic questions in cirrhotic patients, because the development of HCC in chronic liver disease is a progressive process ranging from regenerative nodules to low- or high-grade dysplastic nodules and HCC, the detection and characterization of nodular lesions in cirrhotic livers remains a challenge. With MRI, regenerative nodules may be hypointense on all pulse sequences if they contain iron and may be hyperintense on T_1-weighted images. They do not enhance on the arterial phase postgadolinium and do not show a capsule in delayed-phase images.[20] Iron-containing siderotic regenerative nodules are well shown as low-signal-intensity nodules on MRI and are seen much better than with CT.

Although there is considerable overlap in signal intensity on unenhanced T_1- and T_2-weighted images between dysplastic nodules and HCC, it has been reported that low-grade dysplastic nodules have a tendency to show hypointensity on T_2-weighted images and hyperintensity on T_1-weighted images (see Fig. 31–1E to H). HCC has an iso- or hyperintense pattern on T_1-weighted images and is isointense with partial hyperintensity on T_2-weighted images.[20]

Because of their predominantly portal supply, low-grade dysplastic nodules do not typically capture extracellular contrast in arterial-phase images. Even though it has been shown that 96% of dysplastic nodules have a portal blood supply and 94% of HCCs have an arterial blood supply,[23] the blood supply of dysplastic nodules is controversial and variable.

Because low-grade dysplastic nodules do not have a tumor capsule, they usually are isointense to liver parenchyma on delayed-phase images with no boundary distinction between the nodule and surrounding liver. Currently, although some imaging features on MRI are reported to be characteristic for dysplastic nodules, it remains difficult to diagnose them definitively by any imaging technique. Perhaps selective MRI contrast agents or a molecular marker is needed.[20]

Although some benign hyperenhancing nodules such as small hemangiomas and focal nodular hyperplasia rarely are encountered in cirrhotic patients, the diagnosis of HCC is highly likely when a hypervascular nodule is identified in a cirrhotic liver.[24] In the absence of other major characteristic findings of HCC, the hypervascularity of the nodule in the arterial phase may be the only feature that helps to diagnose small HCC. These small HCCs should be differentiated from the hyperattenuating transitory parenchymal areas detected on the arterial phase of dynamic CT or MRI,[25,26] which are attributed to nonspecific arterioportal shunts caused by cirrhotic changes or produced by iatrogenic vascular injury. A rounded nodular shape and delayed washout favor the diagnosis of HCC. Geographical morphology and isointensity on delayed venous-phase images favor the diagnosis of vascular nontumoral change.

Portal or hepatic venous invasion is characteristic of HCC. On MRI, portal vein tumor thrombus shows as an intravascular mass of intermediate signal on T_1-weighted images. Similar to liver tumor, the intravascular mass enhances in the arterial phase after contrast injection. Gadolinium-enhanced MRA techniques are particularly useful in visualization of the hepatic artery and the portal venous system.[27]

With biphasic contrast-enhanced helical CT or dynamic gadolinium-enhanced MRI, small, 2-cm, hypervascular HCCs can be detected in the arterial phase.[20]

Cholangiography, although not a routine part of the pretransplant evaluation, may be performed in cases of sclerosing cholangitis, which is the third most common indication for liver transplantation. Recent reports suggest that magnetic resonance cholangiography may be useful.[28] The technique is noninvasive and can provide useful images of the biliary tree. The technique does require patient cooperation. Limitations include image degradation by motion artifact and difficulty detecting and assessing severity of strictures. Its sensitivity and specificity are yet to be determined.

Because occult cholangiocarcinoma is found in 10% of the resected liver specimens of patients with primary sclerosing cholangitis,[29] brush biopsy of suspicious narrowed areas should be considered before transplantation. Patients with sclerosing cholangitis must undergo a choledochojejunostomy rather than the usual choledochocholedochostomy.

Arteriography is performed when suspected vascular problems are detected on ultrasound studies or in difficult cases. In many cases MRA techniques can obviate the need for arteriography and venography, because the IVC and hepatic veins are well seen with MRA. The normal portal vein is also well seen (Fig. 31–2). Another angiographic procedure useful in the management of patients awaiting liver transplantation is the transjugular

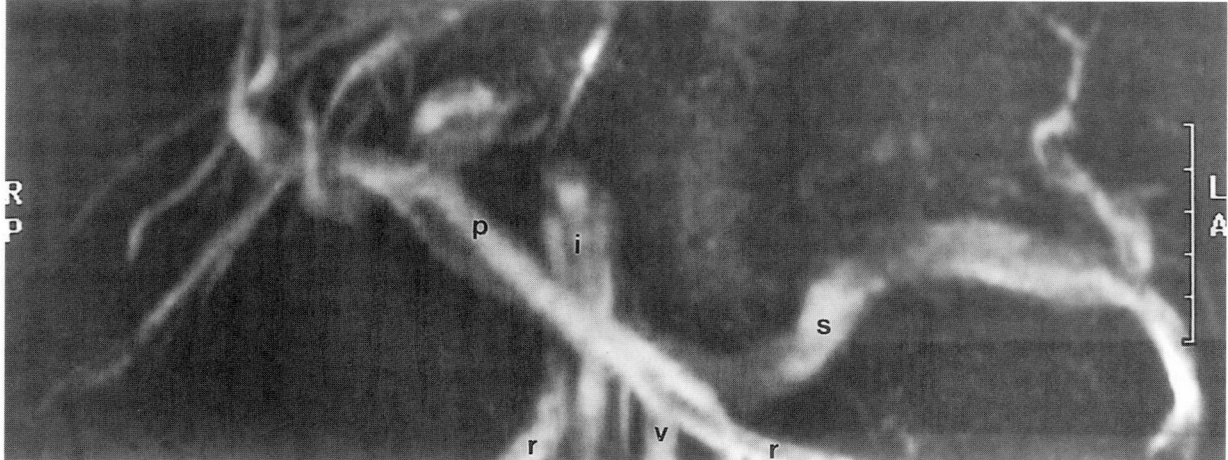

FIGURE 31–2

A magnetic resonance angiogram of a normal portal venous system shows a patent splenic vein (*s*), superior mesenteric vein (*v*), and portal vein (*p*). The inferior vena cava (*i*) and the right and left renal veins (*r*) are also seen.

intrahepatic portosystemic shunt (TIPS) procedure. This procedure, which involves the creation of a tract between a hepatic vein and the portal vein, was first attempted in pigs by Rosch and colleagues[30] and subsequently in humans by Colapinto and colleagues.[31] Early attempts were associated with a high rate of shunt closure, and practical application of the technique awaited the development of metallic stents, which are used to keep the hepatic tract patent.[32] The procedure is performed with jugular vein access for catheterization of a hepatic vein. With fluoroscopic guidance, a specially designed needle-catheter system is used to create a channel from the hepatic vein through the hepatic parenchyma to the portal vein. When the tract has been created, it is dilated with a balloon angioplasty catheter, and a metallic stent is placed in the tract to maintain patency. Various stents are used, most often a Wallstent. The procedure permits effective nonoperative decompression of the portal system. The TIPS procedure has been used successfully to stabilize patients during the period before transplantation. LaBerge and colleagues[33] reported their experience over a 2-year period with 100 patients who underwent a TIPS procedure with the Wallstent prosthesis. Of the 96 patients in whom the procedure was successful, 26 died, 22 underwent liver transplantation, and the remaining 48 survived an average of 7.6 months. Acute variceal bleeding was controlled in 29 of 30 patients, variceal bleeding recurred in 10 patients, and shunt stenosis requiring another intervention developed in 15 patients. New-onset encephalopathy was noted in 14 patients, and worsening of encephalopathy was noted in 3 patients. Liver transplantation was not impeded in any of these cases. When the stents are properly placed well within the liver, with minimal extension into the portal vein or IVC, liver transplantation can be performed in the standard manner. Experience indicates that TIPS is also useful for the treatment of intractable ascites.[34]

Radionuclide imaging studies are rarely performed on donors. Occasionally, single-photon emission computed tomographic (SPECT) liver-spleen scans using technetium (Tc) 99m sulfur colloid are performed to determine the volume of the native liver.[35]

Mammography is performed in women who are 45 years of age or older and have a family history of breast cancer.

Posttransplantation Evaluation

In the immediate postoperative period, chest radiographs are obtained daily to evaluate for atelectasis, pneumonia, diaphragmatic paralysis, and pleural effusions.

Ultrasonography

Ultrasonography has an important role in the postoperative monitoring of the liver transplantation patient. It is routinely used to assess the status of the vascular anastomoses. At most institutions, Doppler ultrasonography is performed at the bedside in the intensive care unit within the first 24 hours after transplantation to assess vascular anastomoses; it is repeated as clinically indicated. The ultrasound examination should include a grayscale of liver homogeneity, bile duct caliber, and the presence of perihepatic and intra-abdominal fluid collections. Perihepatic and intra-abdominal fluid is common in the first postoperative days and gradually disappears.

Focal low-attenuation regions of liver parenchyma may represent infarction and prompt more careful assessment of the hepatic artery branches. The ultrasonography study should include a pulsed and color Doppler evaluation of the hepatic artery as well as the portal vein and IVC. Normal Doppler ultrasonography studies may indicate a nonvascular cause of graft dysfunction.

Each vessel has a characteristic Doppler signal that enables its identification.[36] In adults, the normal hepatic artery is readily recognized on Doppler ultrasonography. A complete examination should include demonstration of flow within the hepatic artery proximal and distal to the anastomosis and in both the right and left hepatic arteries. The normal hepatic artery has a low-impedance waveform pattern with flow demonstrated through diastole (Fig. 31–3). In some cases, a high-impedance pattern with low or absent flow or diastole has been noted early in the postoperative period, with later return to a more normal appearance. This finding is neither an indicator of prognosis nor does it correlate with allograft rejection.[37-39] Abnormal Doppler flow patterns are seen with significant stenoses (Figs. 31–4 and 31–5).

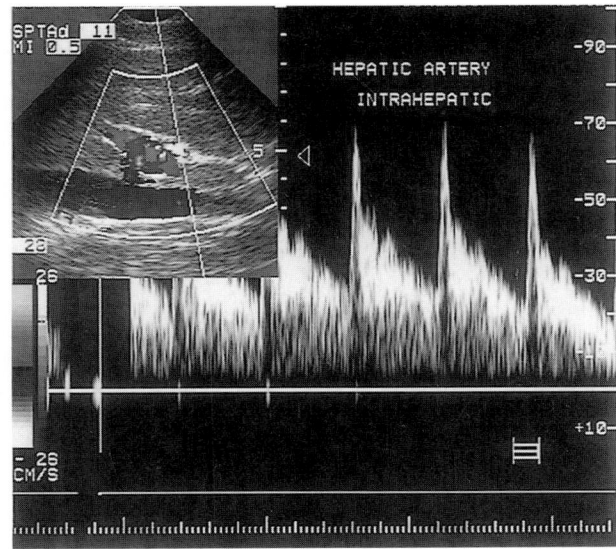

FIGURE 31–3

A Doppler ultrasonography study shows a normal hepatic artery, with its characteristic low-impedance waveform pattern with flow demonstrated throughout diastole.

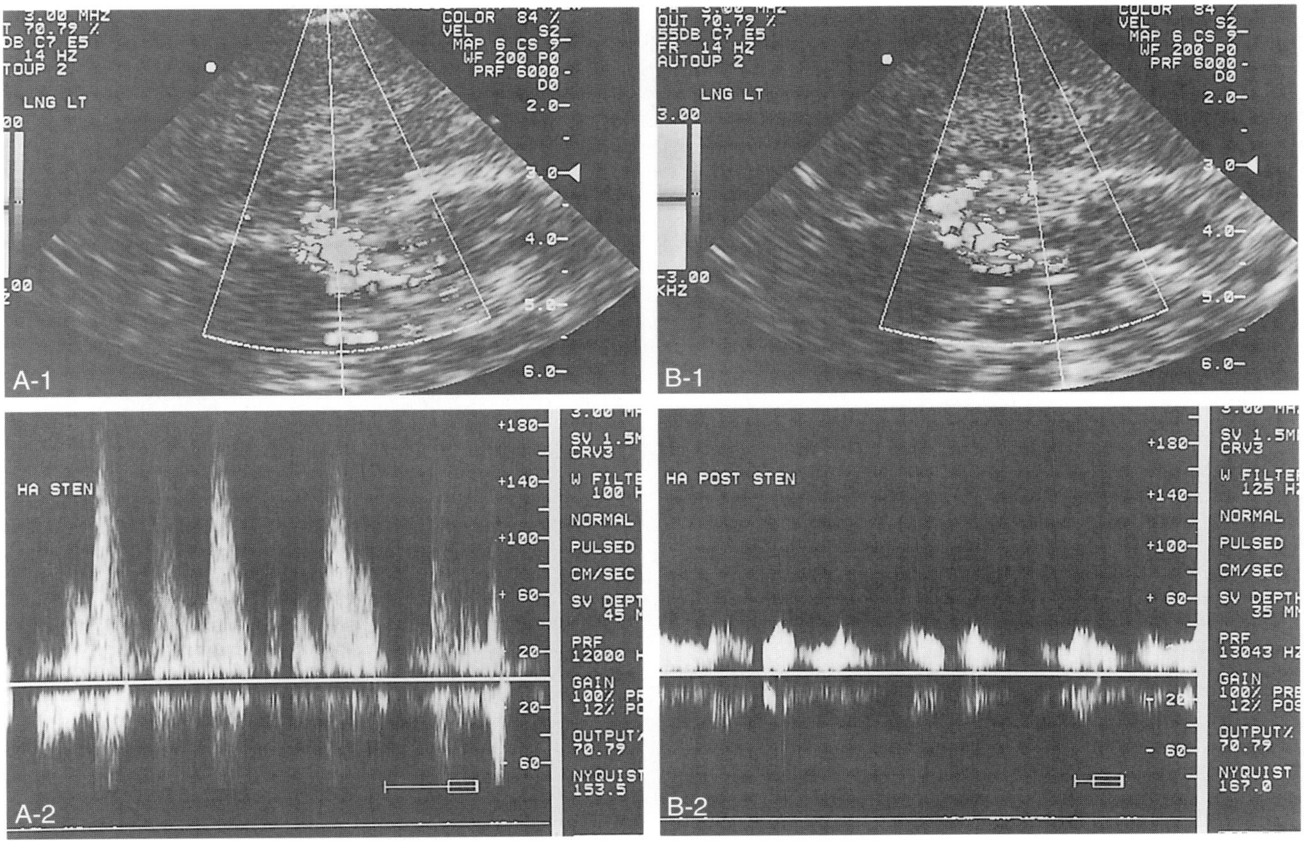

FIGURE 31–4

A Doppler ultrasonography study shows an abnormal hepatic flow pattern in a patient with hepatic artery stenosis. **A,** A Doppler ultrasonography velocity profile at the site of the stenosis shows a high-velocity jet with spectral broadening, indicating turbulence. Aliasing is present, suggesting that the velocities are higher than recorded. **B,** A Doppler ultrasonography study of a vessel distal to the stenosis shows a dampened abnormal waveform with a high diastolic flow.

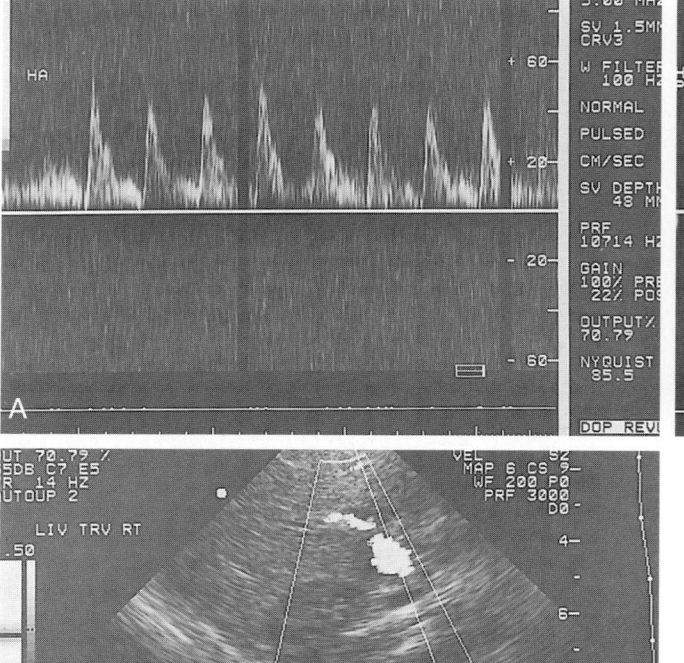

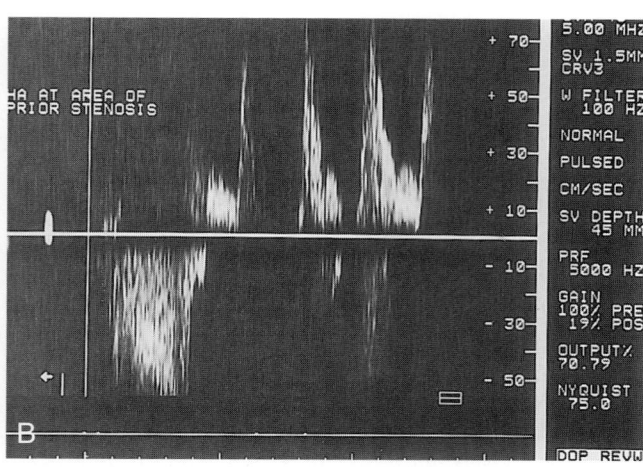

FIGURE 31–5

A Doppler ultrasonography study performed following balloon angioplasty of the stenotic hepatic artery. **A,** The hepatic artery Doppler pattern in the proximal hepatic artery is normal. **B,** At the site of prior stenosis, the flow pattern has a more normal appearance. The loss in diastolic flow may be secondary to a high wall filter.

The normal hepatic vein waveform pattern shows cyclical variations in flow velocity with respiration and reversal of flow with right-sided heart contraction (Fig. 31–6). Complications involving hepatic veins are rare following transplantation.[39] Although a preliminary report suggested that abrupt loss of pulsatility in the hepatic veins may be an early indicator of graft rejection, subsequent studies have not found the hepatic vein waveforms to be useful in the diagnosis of rejection.[39] Nonphasic hepatic vein waveforms can also be observed in normal grafts and in cases of vena cava stenosis.

The IVC is seen best in a parasagittal plane, and findings vary depending on the liver transplant operative technique. In patients with the cava interposition anastomosis, the infrahepatic portion is usually readily identifiable, but the suprahepatic anastomosis may be more difficult to see. Close to the heart, a waveform pattern similar to that of the hepatic veins is seen. With increasing distance from the heart, a dampening of the flow pattern occurs and a continuous wave pattern is seen (Fig. 31–7). A triphasic waveform can be seen in the piggyback anastomosis, reflecting the transmission of pressure changes from the right heart.

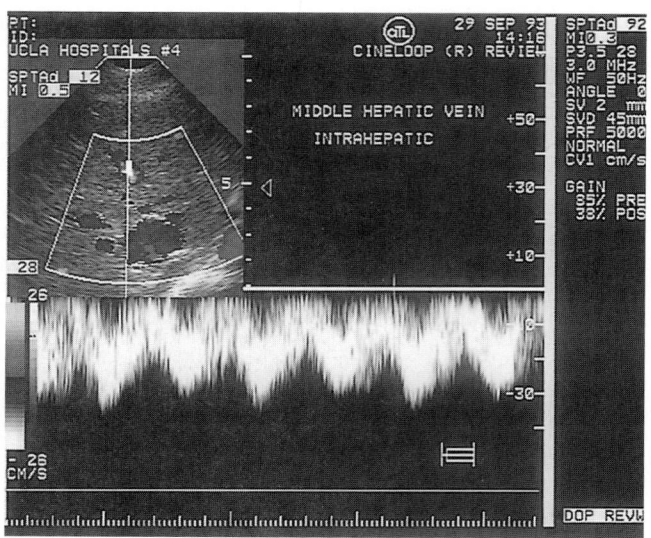

FIGURE 31–6

A Doppler ultrasonography study of a normal hepatic vein shows flow reversal, reflecting the change in pressure in the right side of the heart during contraction.

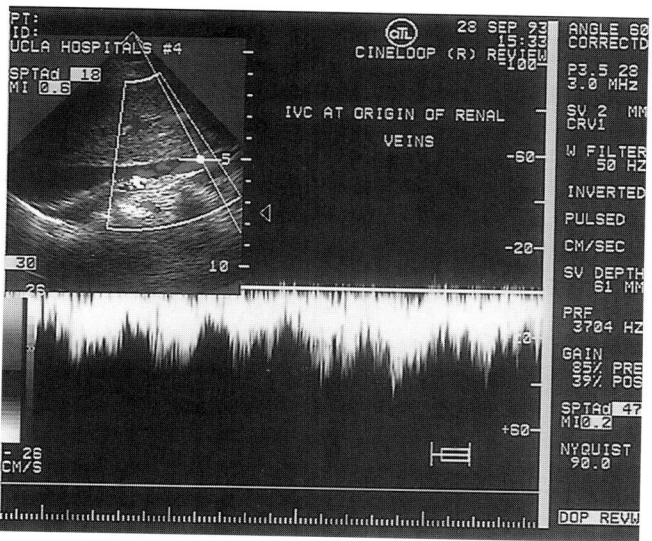

FIGURE 31–7

A normal Doppler ultrasonography study of the IVC shows a cyclical variation of the Doppler waveform pattern.

On an ultrasonography study, the portal vein reveals almost continuous flow, with variation secondary to ventilatory motion (Fig. 31–8).

Radionuclide studies are performed in liver transplant recipients, primarily in the posttransplant period. The radionuclides most frequently used are the technetium Tc-99m iminodiacetic acid (IDA) compounds (hepatoiminodiacetic acid [HIDA] and the derivative diisopropyl iminodiacetic acid [DISIDA]). These compounds are transported from plasma to the hepatocyte

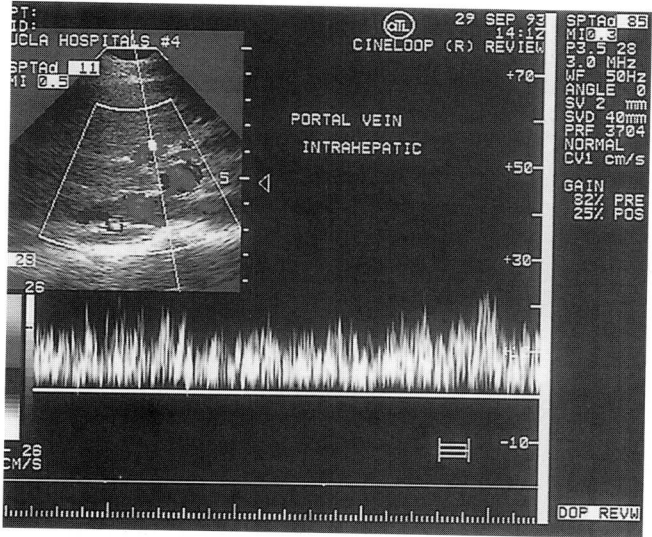

FIGURE 31–8

A normal portal vein Doppler ultrasonography study shows continuous hepatopetal flow.

by the same transport mechanism as that for bilirubin.[40] High levels of bilirubin can competitively inhibit technetium Tc-99m IDA transport and decrease IDA uptake disproportionately to the loss of hepatocyte function. Radionuclide evaluation is used to assess the functional status of the graft and to identify structural complications such as infarcts, abscesses, and bile leaks. In addition to serial radionuclide images, time-activity curves are generated for regions of interest such as over the graft and in the left ventricular blood pool. Measurements of the clearance of IDA compounds from the blood pool graft and their excretion on the gastrointestinal tract permit qualitative and semiquantitative assessment of graft function.

Evaluation of Vascular Complications After Transplantation

Vascular complications after liver transplantation are not uncommon. They present a major threat to allograft and patient survival. Vascular compromise may occur in the immediate transplant period at the hepatic artery, portal vein, or hepatic vein anastomoses.

Hepatic Artery Complications

Complications occurring at the site of arterial revascularization include stenosis, thrombosis, pseudoaneurysm, and hepatic artery rupture. Stenosis of the hepatic artery most commonly occurs at the anastomosis of the donor and recipient arteries (Fig. 31–9). It may also occur adjacent to the anastomosis from a vascular clamp injury. The frequency of hepatic artery stenosis is 11% to 13%.[41-43] Stenosis of the hepatic artery can cause graft ischemia, with resultant deterioration of function and formation of biliary strictures. Progression to thrombosis may result in liver infarction, abscess, or biloma formation. The early clinical signs of vascular occlusion are often nonspecific, and differentiation from other causes of graft dysfunction, such as acute rejection, infection, and prolonged cold or warm preservation ischemic injury, may be difficult.

On HIDA or hepatobiliary IDA radionuclide studies, regions of hepatic infarction are seen as photopenic areas in the graft (Fig. 31–10). In the absence of a hepatic infarction or total absence of graft perfusion, however, these imaging studies may show only nonspecific findings that appear as a decline in functional capacity of the liver with decreased hepatocyte extraction of HIDA and prolonged retention of the agent in the blood pool.[44] The scintigraphic appearances of rejection and infections in the graft (bacterial, viral, or fungal) are essentially

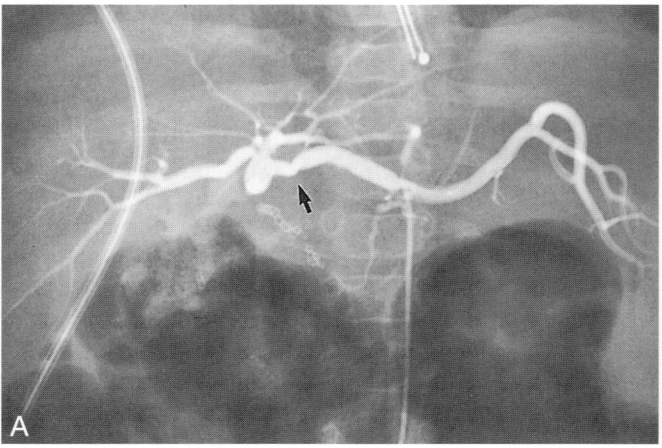
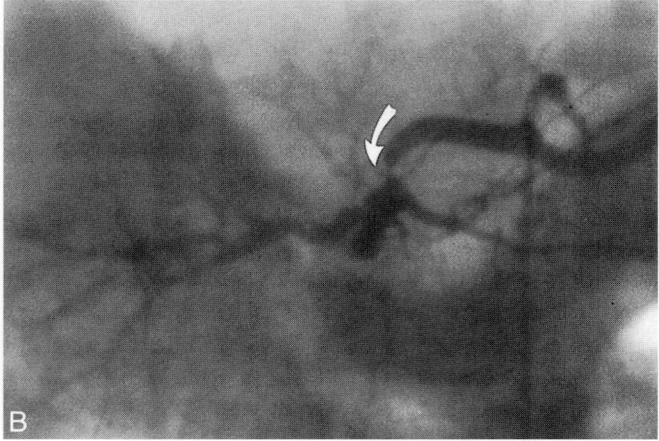

FIGURE 31–9

Hepatic artery stenosis. **A,** Selective celiac artery injection shows an apparent mild stenosis at the anastomosis of the donor and recipient hepatic arteries (*arrow*). **B,** A digital subtraction arteriogram with oblique angulation of the image intensifier shows the stenosis to be severe (*arrow*).

identical, showing high retention of the IDA compound in the blood pool and poor graft uptake. Photopenic regions on the IDA studies may also be seen with abscesses.[45] Indium-111 white blood cell and gallium (Ga)-67 citrate studies are also useful screening procedures for identifying inflammatory processes in the graft.

In suspected hepatic artery obstruction, arteriography should be performed to confirm the ultrasonographic findings. Arteriography should also be used when the clinical findings do not correlate with the ultrasonographic findings. Arteriography is performed via the femoral route with selective catheterization of the celiac

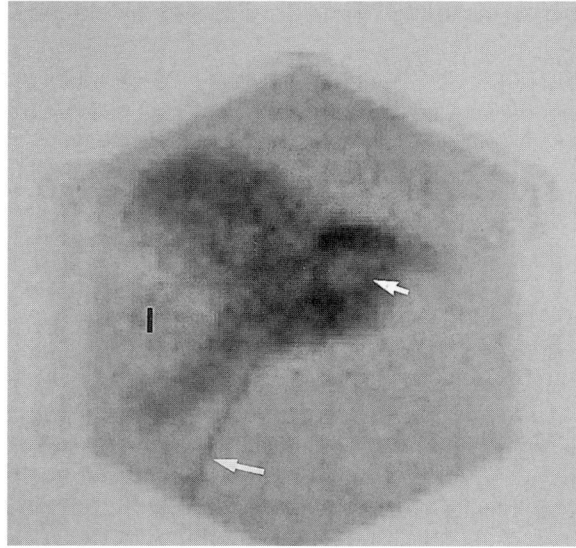
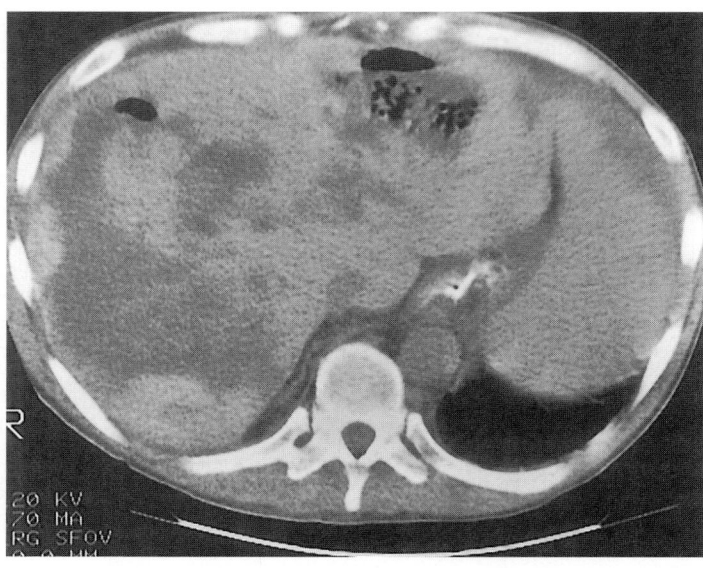

A   B

FIGURE 31–10

Hepatic infarction. **A,** An HIDA scan shows a large photopenic region in the right lobe of the liver that is consistent with a hepatic infarction (*I*) in this patient with severe hepatic artery stenosis. A smaller photopenic region is identified in the left lobe of the liver (*short arrow*). This area could represent another area of infarction, an abscess, or a cyst. The presence of a biliary drainage catheter is visible (*long arrow*). **B,** A computed tomographic scan of the same patient shows multiple low-density lesions in the right lobe of the liver that are consistent with infarcts and correspond to the area of infarction seen on the HIDA study.
A small collection of gas is visible in the right lobe of the liver. It may represent air in a necrotic region or an abscess. In the left lobe, a documented hepatic abscess containing gas is identified. (*A* courtesy of C. Hoh, MD; *B* courtesy of B. Kadell, MD, UCLA Medical Center, Los Angeles, CA.)

axis of the recipient hepatic artery. In pediatric patients, it is particularly important to know the type of anastomosis that was performed to avoid unnecessary injections of contrast material and to reduce study time. Digital subtraction arteriography is usually used in children and is often used in adults.

Once a stenosis is detected angiographically, the treatment indicated depends on the clinical symptoms and liver function. Stenoses occurring in the immediate postoperative period are usually caused by technical problems and generally require operative revision. Stenoses that occur after the anastomosis has healed may be treated by percutaneous transluminal angioplasty (PTA). A small-caliber, low-profile balloon is passed to the site of the stenosis. Several case reports[46,47] describe successful hepatic artery PTA with improvement in liver function following the procedure. At UCLA, the experience is similar. The stenosis recurrence rate is low. Recurrent stenosis was reported by Raby and colleagues[48] in hepatic artery anastomoses at 4 and 6 months in two of three patients; both stenoses responded to another balloon dilation. This technique is a useful method of treating hepatic artery stenosis (Fig. 31–11).

Hepatic artery thrombosis is a serious complication following liver transplantation. The incidence ranges from 3% to 10% in adults and 8% to 19% in children.[49,50] In living donor liver transplantation, the incidence ranges from 0% to 10%.[51] Early thrombosis of the hepatic artery following liver transplantation is more common in pediatric patients because of technical difficulties in the reconstruction and maintenance of flow through the small-caliber anastomoses.[52]

The ultrasonographic diagnosis of hepatic artery thrombosis is made when no arterial Doppler signal is obtained at the hilum and in the right and left intrahepatic branches. Thrombosis usually occurs at the anastomosis. Because a variety of hepatic arterial anastomoses can be performed, knowledge of the type of anastomosis is important for accurate interpretation of the studies (Fig. 31–12). Flint and colleagues[53] reported the correct diagnosis of hepatic artery thrombosis with Doppler ultrasonography in 34 of 37 cases (92%); the diagnoses were confirmed by angiography or surgery. In three instances the results were false-positive, and hepatic arteries that appeared patent with Doppler ultrasonography proved on angiography to be occluded. Hall and colleagues[54] observed false-negative Doppler ultrasonography studies in 4 of 13 cases (30%). These occurred because of mistaken identification of an arterial periportal collateral as the hepatic artery (Fig. 31–13). False-positive results, although uncommon, have also been reported. They may be a result of slow flow within a small but patent vessel, high-grade stenosis, or technical failure.[55]

Once hepatic artery thrombosis occurs, hepatic infarction and biliary ischemia are likely sequelae. It is not uncommon for the thrombosis to remain undetected by ultrasonography. Intrahepatic flow may be detectable

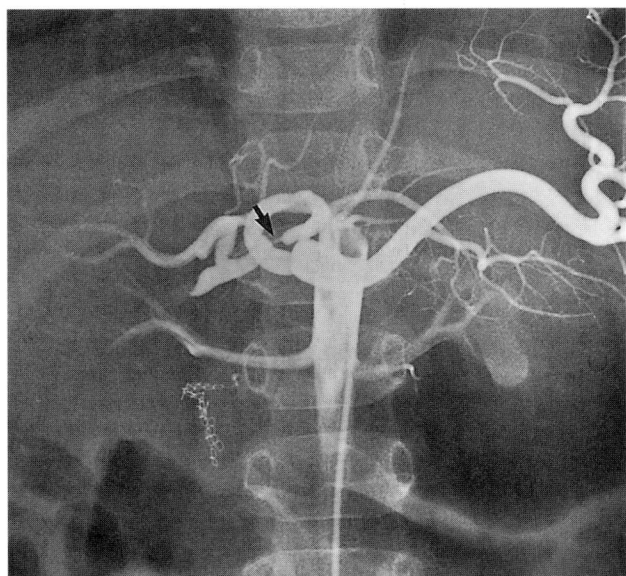

A

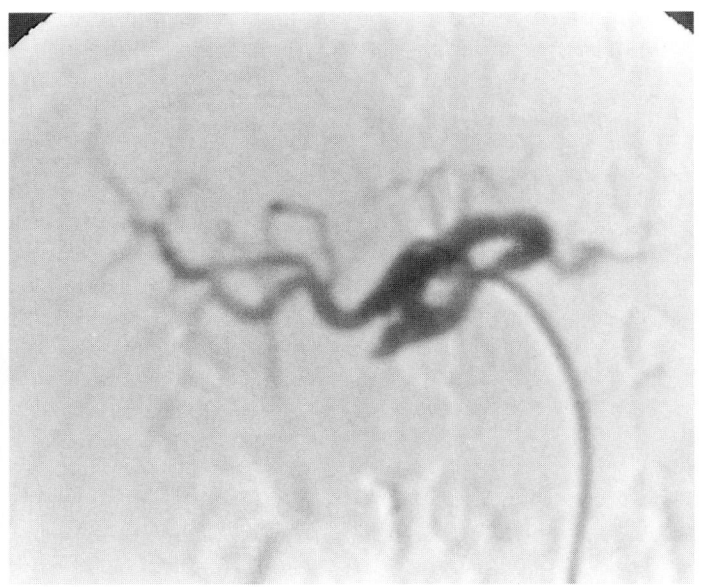

B

FIGURE 31–11

Percutaneous transluminal angioplasty of a stenotic hepatic artery. **A,** The arteriogram shows high-grade stenosis at the hepatic artery anastomosis (*arrow*). **B,** Following balloon angioplasty, residual narrowing persists, but there is a marked improvement in blood flow through the anastomosis.

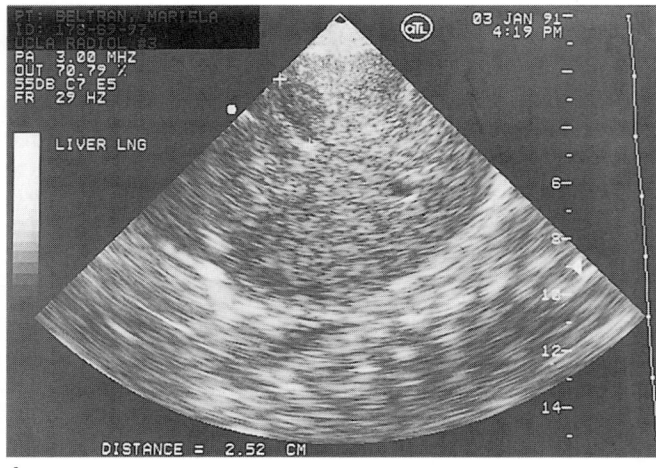
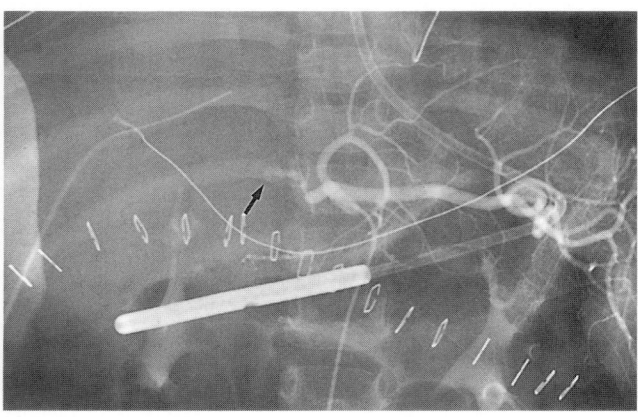

A   B

FIGURE 31–12

Hepatic artery thrombosis. **A,** Flow was not identified in the hepatic artery on Doppler ultrasonography. Real-time ultrasonographic assessment of the liver reveals a heterogenous appearance in the liver parenchyma with multiple discrete areas of low echogenicity, findings consistent with hepatic ischemia or infarction (+). **B,** Celiac axis arteriogram demonstrates occlusion of the hepatic artery proximally (*arrow*).

from the arterial collaterals in the porta hepatis. It is important to avoid this diagnostic error because delay in diagnosis may result in loss of the allograft.

The symptoms of hepatic artery thrombosis are highly variable. When detected early by postoperative ultrasonography, symptoms may be minimal. When detected late, symptoms usually relate to ischemic biliary injury and manifest as recurrent cholangitis, intrahepatic infarction and abscess, bile duct stenosis, or bile leak. Presentation as fulminant hepatic necrosis is uncommon when ultrasonography is used for postoperative monitoring. Early diagnosis may allow emergency surgical thrombectomy or hepatic artery reconstruction, or both, which might prevent or postpone the need for retransplantation, or serve as a bridge until a donor becomes available.[56-58] We attempted thrombolysis of hepatic artery thrombosis in four patients, two with intra-arterial urokinase, and two with intra-arterial recombinant tissue plasminogen activator. The urokinase treatment was unsuccessful. Recanalization has been accomplished with tissue plasminogen activator in several cases (Fig. 31–14). Because thrombolysis with tissue plasminogen activator can entail a risk of bleeding, we recommend that the patient remain in the angiography suite while the infusion is taking place so that extravasation can be detected. Tissue plasminogen activator exerts its thrombolytic effect in 3 to 6 hours. The viability of the liver following thrombolysis is dependent on many factors, and the reestablishment of blood flow does not guarantee graft survival.

False aneurysms of the hepatic artery are uncommon, occurring in less than 2% of patients.[43,57,59-61] Because they may rupture and produce fatal hemorrhage, early diagnosis is necessary. False aneurysms usually occur at the extrahepatic arterial anastomosis. Intrahepatic false aneurysms may occur following a percutaneous liver biopsy or transhepatic biliary drainage. Some false aneurysms are asymptomatic and detectable only on imaging; others may manifest as gastrointestinal bleeding, hemobilia, or hemoperitoneum. On Doppler ultrasonography, they appear as spherical fluid collections showing internal flow.[62]

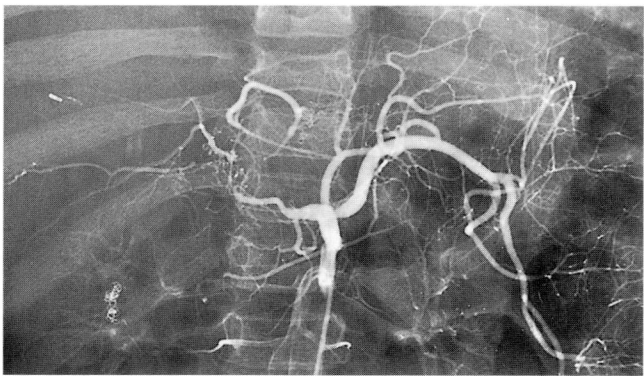

FIGURE 31–13

Severe hepatic artery stenosis. Celiac angiogram shows a severe stenosis of the hepatic artery with numerous collaterals in the porta hepatis. The left hepatic artery is large. Confusion of these collaterals with the main hepatic artery may lead to erroneous interpretation of the ultrasound study and result in the false-positive interpretation that the hepatic artery is patent.

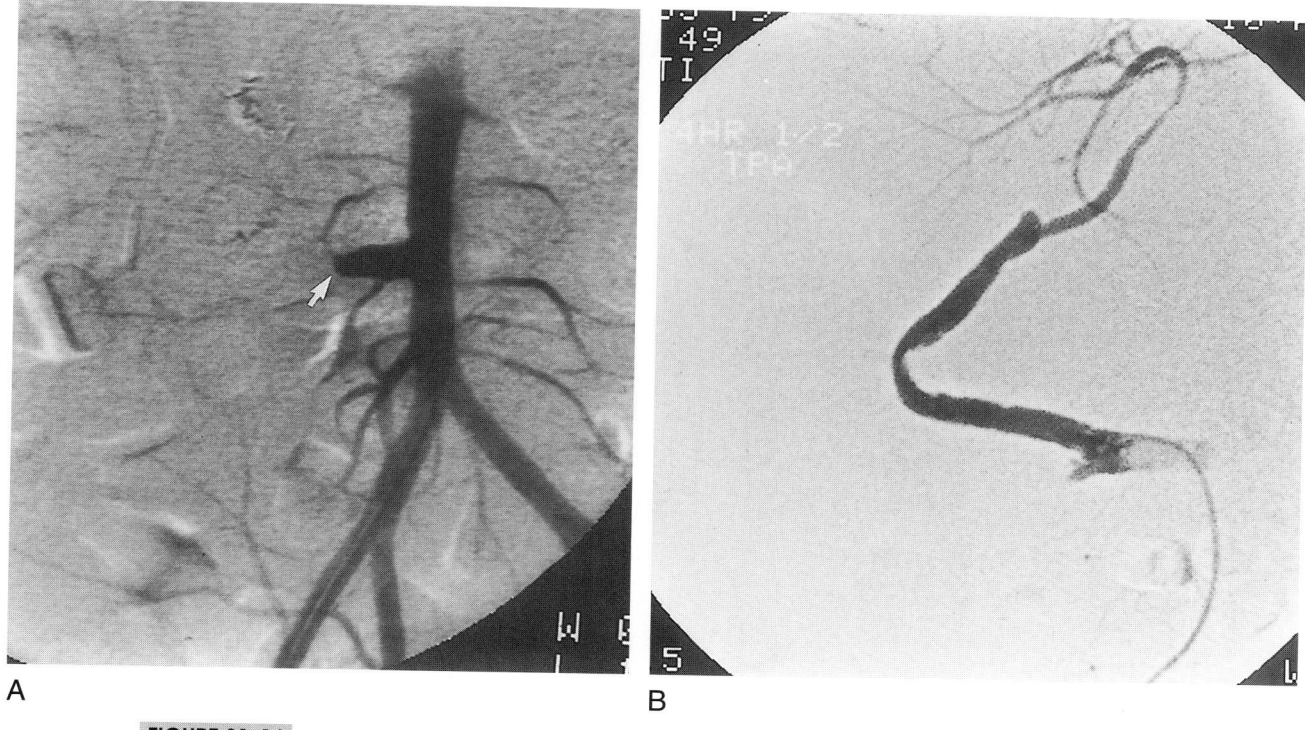

A   B

FIGURE 31–14

Hepatic artery thrombolysis. **A,** A flush aortogram shows the stump of an occluded donor iliac artery graft from the infrarenal aorta to the liver transplant. **B,** Following 4.5 hours of thrombolytic infusion with recombinant tissue plasminogen activator, blood flow in the hepatic artery is restored. A mild irregularity consistent with residual thrombus is seen in the hepatic artery. The patient could not be treated with heparin, because of heparin allergy; reocclusion occurred, necessitating retransplantation.

Intrahepatic aneurysms may be treated with transcatheter embolization. If a catheter cannot be passed to the aneurysm because of allograft tortuosity, direct transhepatic embolization can be performed. Currently, extrahepatic aneurysms are best treated surgically; embolization should be performed only as a lifesaving measure.

Portal Vein Complications

Extrahepatic portal vein complications are uncommon. Portal vein stenosis is rare, and portal vein thrombosis occurs in only 1% to 2.2% of liver transplant recipients.[43,57,59,63] Portal vein stenosis usually occurs in the porta hepatis at the anastomosis of the donor and recipient vessels (Fig. 31–15A). The clinical manifestations of portal vein thrombosis are variable and include graft failure, ascites, varices, and gastrointestinal bleeding. Significant stenosis can usually be detected by duplex and color Doppler ultrasonography.[64,65] In portal vein thrombosis, a real-time echo may demonstrate echogenic thrombus, with Doppler ultrasonography confirming either the absence or the presence of blood flow around a nonoccluding thrombus. Portal vein stenosis is identified on Doppler ultrasonography by the presence of normal proximal flow, a high-velocity jet at the anastomosis, and distal turbulence.

Air in the portal vein has occasionally been detected on Doppler ultrasonography as highly echogenic, nonshadowing particles moving within the portal vein. Although air was reported in one case in association with a gangrenous colon,[66] it may be a transient finding without other serious complication in the first 2 weeks after transplantation.[67]

Three-dimensional time-of-flight gadolinium-enhanced MR angiography is often used in evaluation of portal venous structures because three-dimensional time-of-flight gadolinium-enhanced MRA provides high-quality images of the hepatic artery, hepatic veins, and portal venous system. Varices are well seen.[27] This technique is useful in excluding the presence of portal vein complications posttransplantation (see Fig. 31–15B and C).

In transplant recipients with variceal bleeding and a Doppler study showing no abnormality, arteriography or three-dimensional time-of-flight gadolinium-enhanced MRA should be performed for definitive diagnosis.

Arterial portography is usually performed via a superior mesenteric artery injection with filming in the venous phase. Digital subtraction arteriography is used.

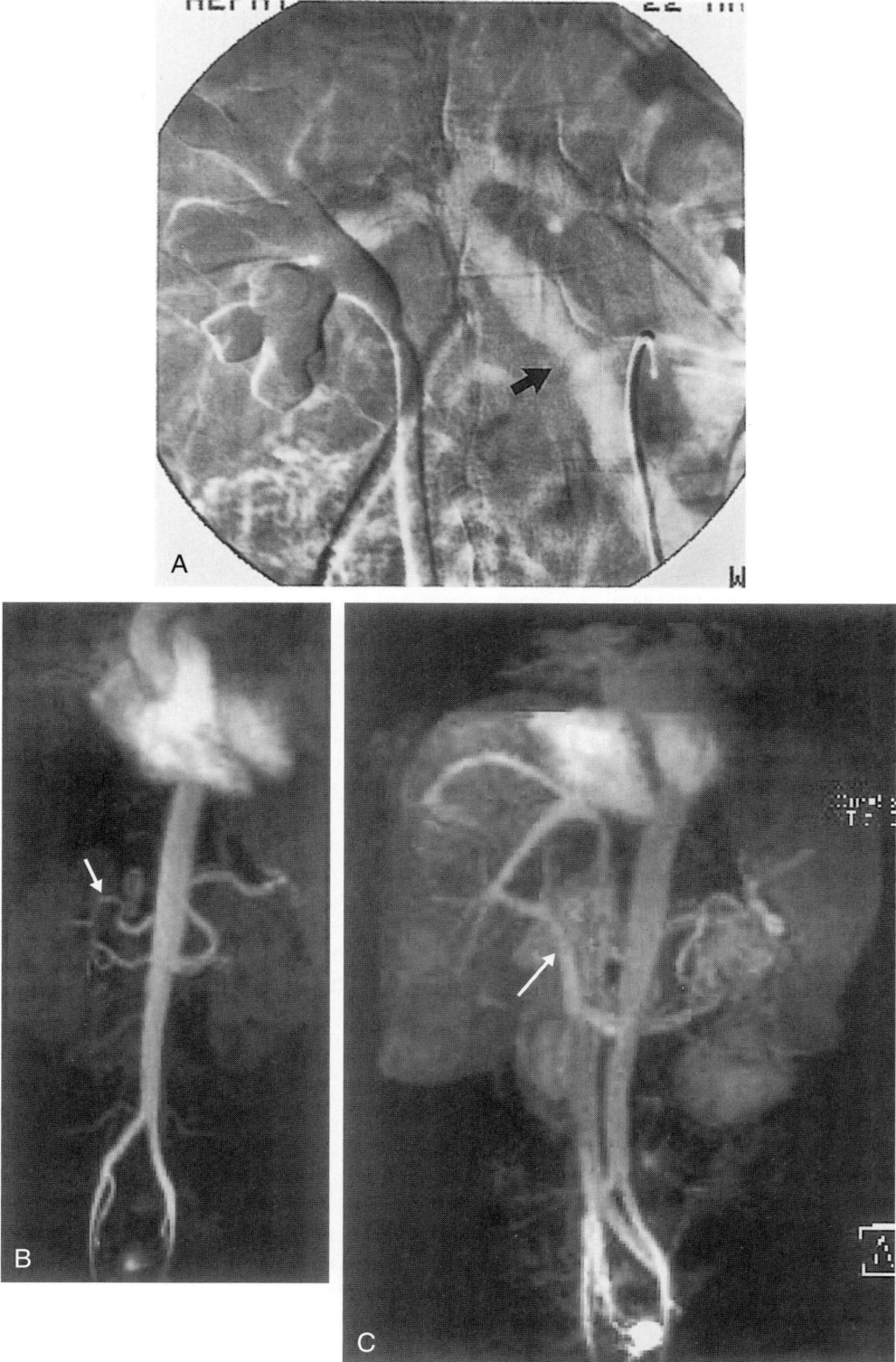

FIGURE 31–15

A, Venous phase of superior mesenteric artery arteriogram shows a normal portal vein anastomosis with mild deformity at the anastomotic site (*arrow*). **B,** Arterial phase of three-dimensional time-of-flight gadolinium-enhanced MRA in a patient after liver transplantation. The celiac axis is seen and the hepatic artery anastomosis (*arrow*) is patent. **C,** Portal phase of three-dimensional time-of-flight gadolinium-enhanced MRA shows a patent portal vein anastomosis (*arrow*). The hepatic veins are well seen and the IVC is patent.

In symptomatic patients, balloon angioplasty is the treatment of choice for portal vein stenosis. The portal vein is entered via a transhepatic puncture; after entry to the portal system is achieved, pressures are measured across the stenosis and balloon angioplasty is performed. A stent may also be placed if angioplasty is insufficient. Raby and colleagues[48] treated three patients with portal hypertension and variceal hemorrhage caused by anastomotic stenosis of the portal vein with PTA. Success was obtained in two patients, both of whom were asymptomatic at 1 year follow-up. Complete portal vein thrombosis has generally required retransplantation if associated hepatic failure develops (Fig. 31–16). Olcott and colleagues[68] described their experience with balloon angioplasty in four patients with portal vein occlusion. Three of the four treated patients died of multiple problems unrelated to the angioplasty. The researchers also described the placement of a metal stent in a patient with portal vein occlusion. This patient died of a brain abscess 1 month later and the stent was patent at autopsy. Zajko and colleagues[42] reported the placement of a Palmaz stent following unsuccessful PTA. However, thrombus developed above the stent and failed to lyse with thrombolytic therapy. Portal vein thrombosis developed, necessitating retransplantation.

Inferior Vena Cava and Hepatic Vein Complications

IVC complications are rare. Raby and colleagues,[48] in a series of more than 600 liver transplantations, found

only 4 cases of IVC anastomotic stenosis. In a large series of more than 2200 transplantations, Zajko and coworkers[42] observed 10 cases of stenosis and 2 cases of thrombosis. The most common site of IVC stenosis of the donor and recipient is at the suprahepatic or infrahepatic anastomosis of the donor and recipient. Rarely, stenoses may occur secondary to extrinsic compression by a hematoma. Infrahepatic stenoses typically produce lower extremity edema, and suprahepatic caval stenoses generally produce obstruction of the hepatic veins, with symptoms similar to those of the Budd-Chiari syndrome. Although most significant caval stenoses can be detected on duplex ultrasonography, and MR angiography may be helpful, contrast venacavography is the most reliable technique for diagnosis (Fig. 31–17). Pressure measurements should be obtained in the inferior vena cava and across the hepatic veins. PTA of suprahepatic and infrahepatic IVC stenosis and of hepatic vein stenosis is now routinely performed.[48,69,70] Recurrence of stenosis has been reported; however, as with venous stenoses in other parts of the body, another dilation can result in long-term patency.[48] Metallic stents can be placed if repeat PTA fails to produce durable results.

Evaluation of the Biliary System

The appearance of the common duct is variable after a choledochocholedochostomy. Size discrepancies between the donor and recipient ducts may be seen (Fig. 31–18). In uncomplicated cases, the size of the ducts tends to remain stable over time; however, a mild increase in the size of the ducts may occur without clinical evidence of obstruction. Diffuse biliary tree changes are often seen in the absence of obstruction or leakage. Attenuation, narrowing, and separation of the intrahepatic ducts may be seen. These are nonspecific findings that are seen with rejection, hepatitis, preservation injury, and infarction.[71]

Although evaluation of the biliary tract is not done routinely in the liver transplant patient unless a problem is suspected, the performance of T-tube cholangiography at some time before the removal of the T-tube is standard care.

T-tubes placed in the recipient bile duct at the time of liver transplantation are removed 2 to 4 months after surgery. Antibiotics are administered before the cholangiography is performed. If the cholangiographic findings reveal no abnormality, the T-tube is removed over a guidewire, and a temporary drain is placed in the tract to avoid leakage of bile into the peritoneum. Because liver transplant patients are given immunosuppressive therapy, there is poor granulation of the T-tube tract. Simple removal of the T-tube using standard techniques can result in bile leakage. At our institution, patients developed bilomas and serious bile peritonitis following

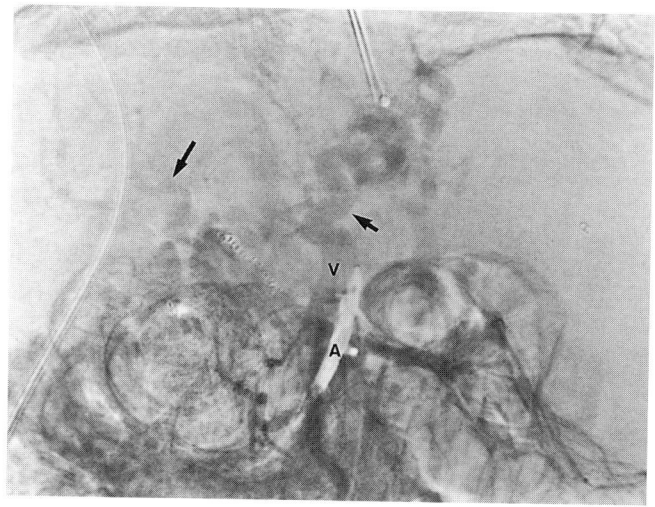

FIGURE 31–16

Portal vein occlusion as seen on a digital subtraction superior mesenteric angiogram in a liver transplant recipient. The portal vein is occluded and there is filling of a dilated coronary vein and varices (*short arrow*). Cavernous transformation of the portal vein is present and there is faint filling of abnormal intrahepatic portal branches (*long arrow*). *A*, superior mesenteric artery incompletely subtracted; *V*, superior mesenteric vein.

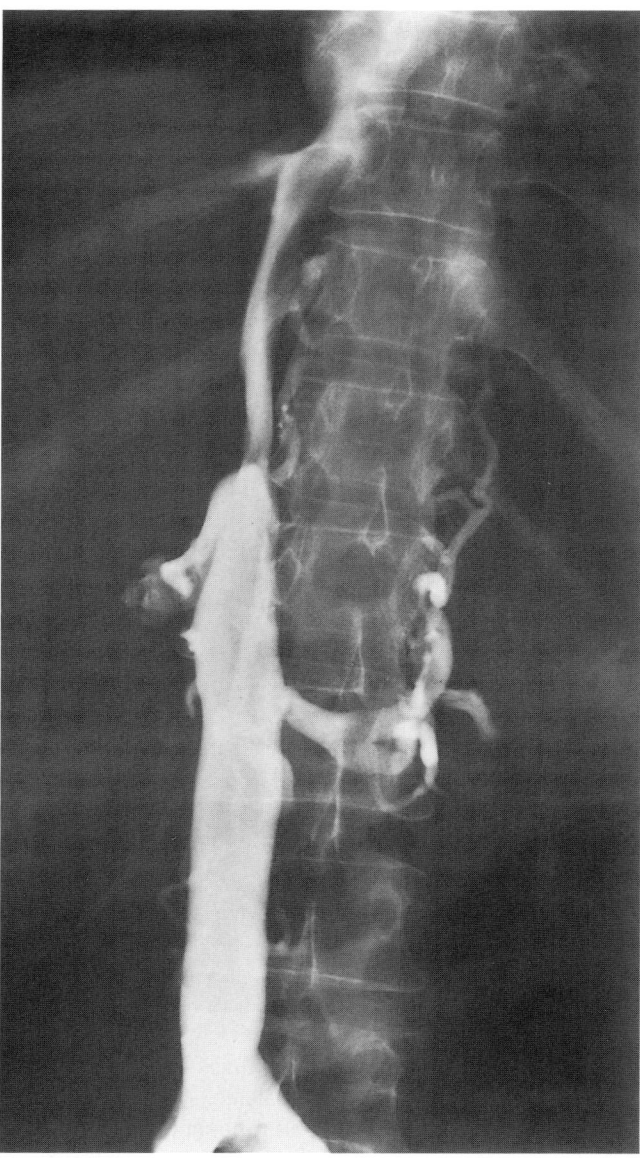

FIGURE 31-17

Inferior venacavogram in a liver transplant recipient with right pleural effusion. The infrahepatic portion of the IVC is attenuated; however, contrast material drained freely into the right atrium, no gradient was detected, and the ultrasonography study was normal.

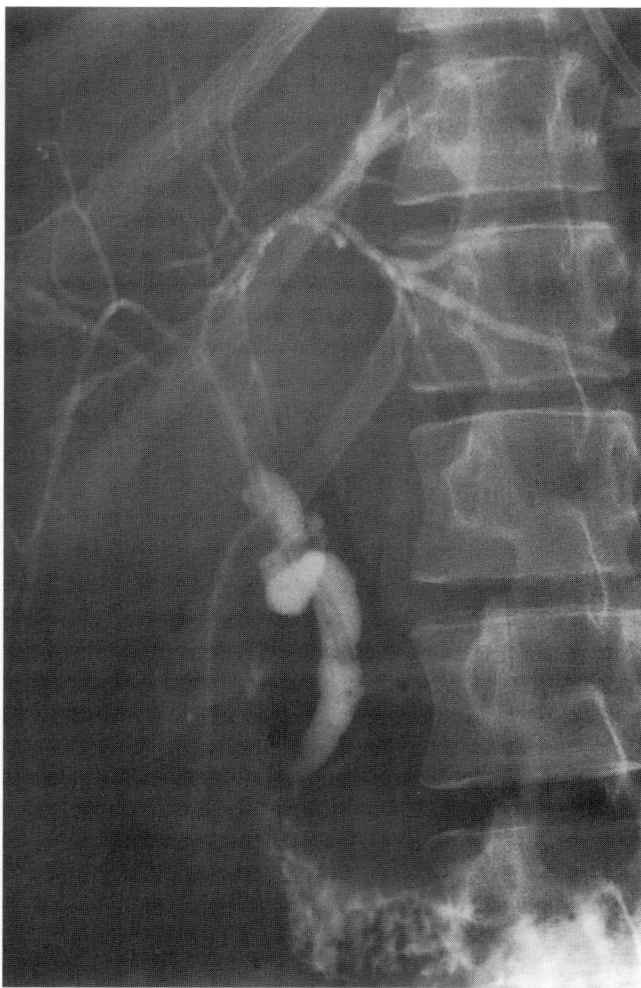

FIGURE 31-18

Normal T-tube cholangiogram in a liver transplant recipient. Note the size discrepancy between the donor and recipient ducts.

Biliary Tract Complications

Biliary tract complications occur in 10% to 13% of liver transplant recipients.[72-74] The biliary complications that can occur include stricture formation, bile leakage with or without biloma formation, intraductal stone or debris formation, diffuse biliary dilatation and dysfunction of the sphincter of Oddi. After rejection, biliary complications are the most common cause of hepatic dysfunction. In many instances, the clinical symptoms associated with biliary complications may be indistinguishable from those associated with a variety of problems, such as rejection, hepatic artery occlusion, primary graft dysfunction, and viral infection. Biliary complications may be the result of primary biliary tract problems or a variety of other posttransplant problems that affect the integrity and function of the biliary tree. The biliary system of the liver transplant is susceptible to ischemic injury. The main source of the blood supply to the normal

simple removal of the T-tube. Therefore, a small-caliber, multiple sidehole, straight catheter is positioned in the T-tube tract. This straight catheter is withdrawn progressively over the course of several days. In the event that access to the tract is lost and the straight catheter cannot be placed, the patient is taken for immediate endoscopic placement of a biliary stent. Because the T-tubes are anchored when placed initially, there are instances in which the tube fractures as it is removed and a portion is retained subcutaneously. Operation is then required for removal of the T-tube fragment.

human common bile duct is from branches of the gastroduodenal artery or a retroportal artery. These branches are divided in the transplant procedure. Because the main source of the blood supply is from below, the donor bile duct is more susceptible to ischemic injury than is the recipient duct. Bile duct ischemia can result in nonanastomotic bile leaks, intrahepatic strictures, and bilomas. Biliary complications usually occur within the first 3 months after transplantation, but they can also occur later. Most bile leaks occur within the first month and most stenoses develop later.[39]

Biliary complications in the liver allograft manifest primarily as biliary obstruction and bile leakage. Reduced bile output from the T-tube or a significant change in bile color may indicate mechanical obstruction of the duct, dislodgement of the T-tube, or liver dysfunction. Obstruction of the T-tube often resolves with simple flushing.

be diagnosed with ultrasonography and computed tomographic scans, on which they appear as hypoechoic or low-attenuation areas. However, with CT and ultrasonography studies, bile collections cannot always be distinguished from other types of collections, such as blood, ascites, pus, or lymph. Fine-needle aspiration biopsy enables determination of fluid composition. Cholangiography is the most frequently used method of diagnosis and provides specific information (Fig. 31–20). Although small anastomotic leaks can be managed conservatively, large leaks at the anastomosis are associated with high morbidity and mortality and require immediate operation. Leaks resulting from dislodgement of the T-tube require immediate exploration (Fig. 31–21) or endoscopic retrograde cholangiopancreatography with nasobiliary stent placement. Leakage of contrast material from the donor biliary tree at nonanastomotic sites is a serious event, possibly indicative of bile duct

Evaluation and Management of Bile Leaks

Most bile leaks occur in the early postoperative period, with the most frequent site of leaking being the T-tube choledochotomy. Leaks may also occur at the site of the biliary anastomosis and at nonanastomotic sites. Small leaks detected on a T-tube cholangiogram usually resolve spontaneously and can be managed conservatively by leaving the T-tube in place for a longer period. Large leaks may appear as leakage from the surgical drain or wound or may cause abdominal pain, distention, fever, and sepsis. Large leaks require reoperation.

Suspected bile leakage can be confirmed with an IDA scan. The demonstration of radiolabeled material[75] outside the bile ducts or in the gastrointestinal system on early or delayed scans is pathognomonic for bile leakage (Fig. 31–19). Bile leaks and collections can also

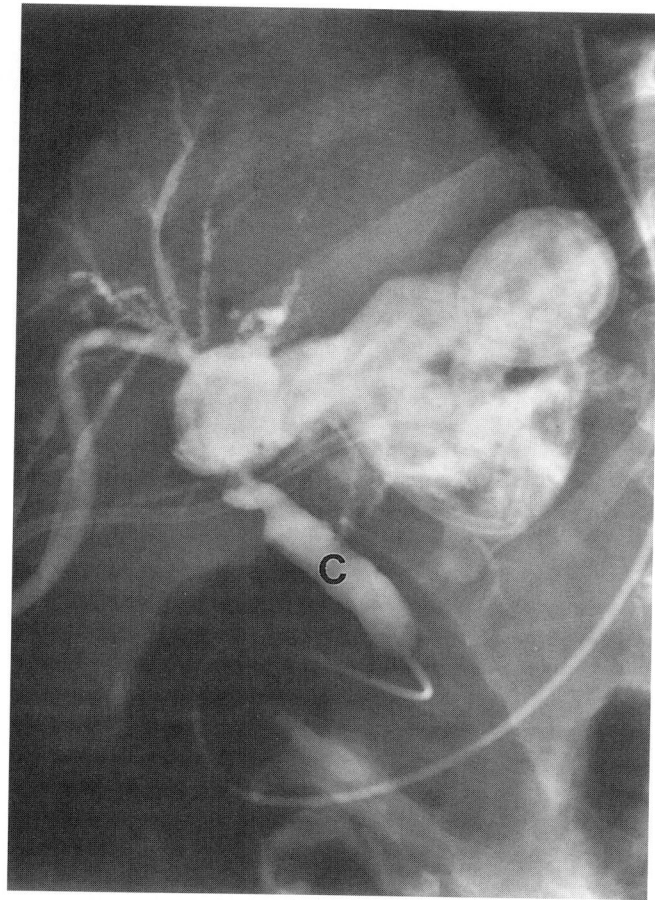

FIGURE 31–20

Biloma. Endoscopic retrograde cholangiopancreatography shows filling of the common bile duct (C) and right biliary ducts. The left biliary ducts are obscured by communication with and opacification of a large biloma. Two drainage catheters are in place, and contrast material is seen draining into the superiorly positioned catheter.

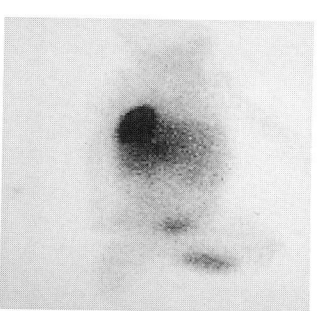
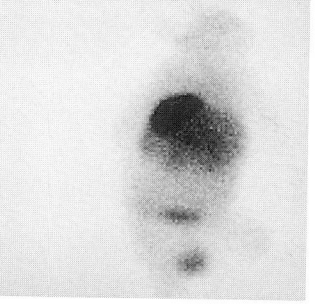

A   B

FIGURE 31–19

AP (**A**) and RAO (**B**) views of a delayed (24 hours) HIDA scan show a subdiaphragmatic collection of radioisotope projected over the dome of the liver, representing a bile leak. (Courtesy of C. Hoh, MD, UCLA Medical Center, Los Angeles, CA.)

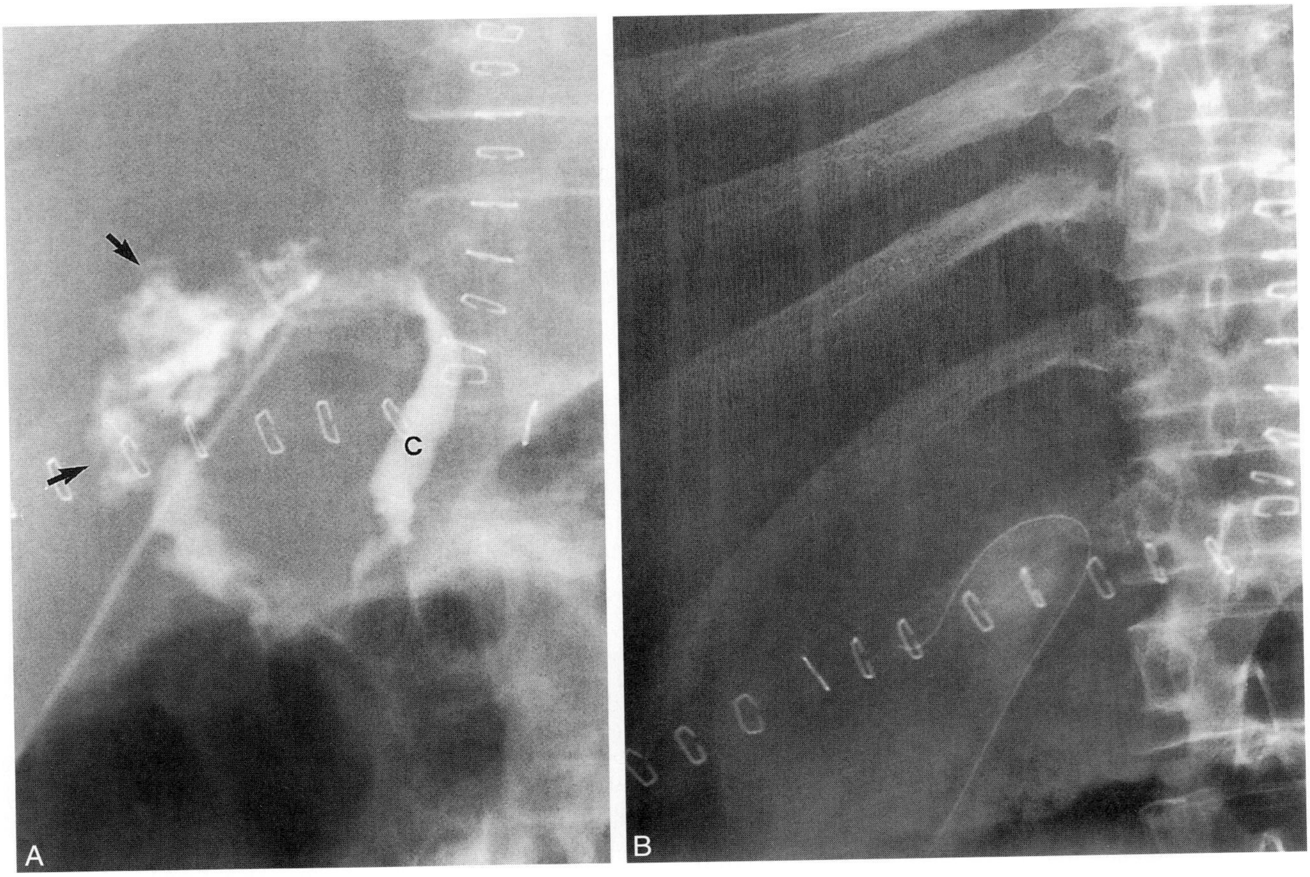

FIGURE 31–21

Dislodged T-tube. **A,** A T-tube cholangiogram shows filling of the common bile duct (C) and free leakage of contrast material from the T-tube into the peritoneal space (*arrows*). **B,** Passage of a guidewire into the T-tube shows that the wire passes freely into the peritoneum, confirming dislodgement of the T-tube.

necrosis secondary to hepatic artery occlusion. Such leaks usually occur in the hilar and parahilar areas; intrahepatic or extrahepatic locations are less common. Bilomas occurring with hepatic artery occlusion are often associated with a poor outcome and require retransplantation.[76]

Radiographic Diagnosis and Management of Biliary Obstruction

The symptoms of biliary obstruction may initially be indistinguishable from a variety of other problems, including rejection, hepatic artery occlusion, primary graft dysfunction, and viral infections. Biliary obstruction may be detected on IDA radionuclide studies if liver function is maintained and uptake of the agent in the intrahepatic ducts is seen with delayed or absent transit to the gastrointestinal tract. Ultrasonography[1,71] and CT may be helpful for diagnosis (Figs. 31–22 to 31–24);

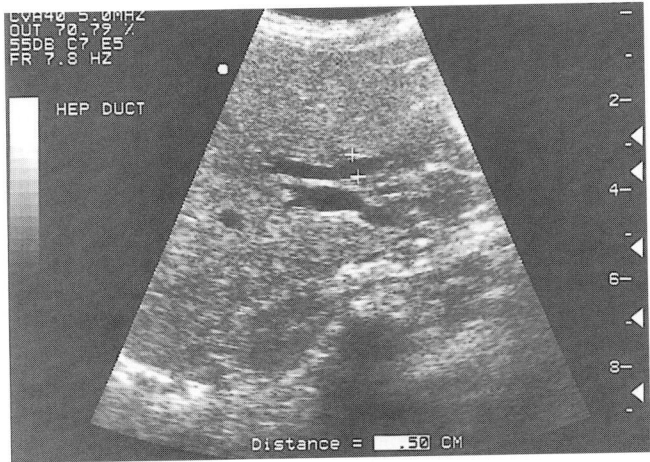

FIGURE 31–22

Biliary dilatation. Ultrasonography study shows dilated bile ducts.

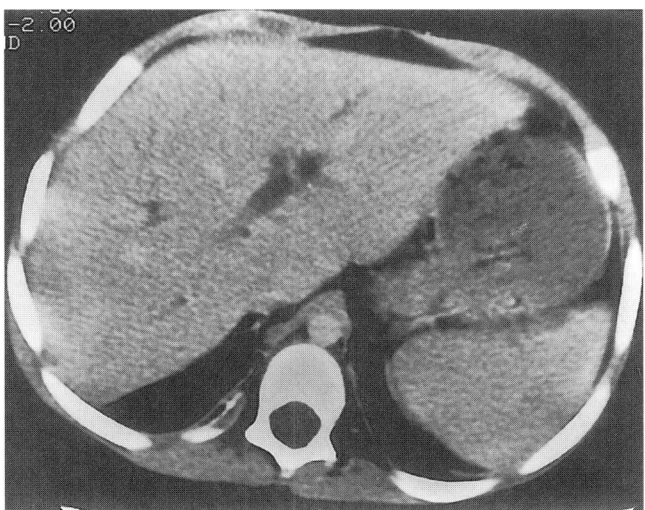

FIGURE 31-23

CT scan shows dilated bile ducts in a child with hepatic artery stenosis. This is the same patient as shown in Figures 31–13 and 31–28.

however, direct cholangiography is usually necessary because the presence of apparently normal ducts on ultrasonography studies does not exclude the possibility of significant biliary obstruction. There is a variable relationship between biliary obstruction and dilatation. Biliary distention after obstruction does not occur simultaneously throughout all branches of the biliary system. The degree of dilatation depends not only on the degree and duration of the obstruction but also on the pliability of both the extrahepatic bile ducts and the parenchymal

supporting skeleton of the intrahepatic ducts. Because prolonged biliary obstruction leads to inflammatory changes and fibrosis of the biliary tract, even long-term obstruction may occur without significant proximal dilatation. Patients with cirrhosis, for example, may have high-grade obstruction with little or no intrahepatic dilatation.[77,78] As in other patients, liver enzyme elevation, particularly alkaline phosphatase elevation, is a more sensitive indicator of biliary obstruction. Cholangiography, either via the T-tube or a percutaneous transhepatic approach, is often necessary for diagnosis. Magnetic resonance cholangiography can also be used to assess biliary duct dilatation. On T-tube cholangiograms, areas of mild narrowing at the anastomosis site are a frequent occurrence, and removal of the T-tube does not usually result in symptoms of obstruction.

Biliary obstruction in the transplant patient can be caused by problems such as stricture, biliary sludge,[79] stones, a retained stent, T-tube dysfunction and, rarely, an allograft cystic duct remnant mucocele and common duct redundancy.

Posttransplant biliary strictures are the most common cause of biliary obstruction and can be classified as anastomotic and nonanastomotic. Those strictures occurring at the biliary anastomosis are attributed to scar formation with retraction and narrowing (Fig. 31–25). Untreated, these may lead to ascending cholangitis with intrahepatic multifocal stricture formation.[28]

Nonanastomotic strictures almost always occur in the donor biliary tree. They may be single but are usually multiple and involve the confluence of the right and left ducts, the common duct, and the intrahepatic ducts (Fig. 31–26). They are usually the result of ischemic duct

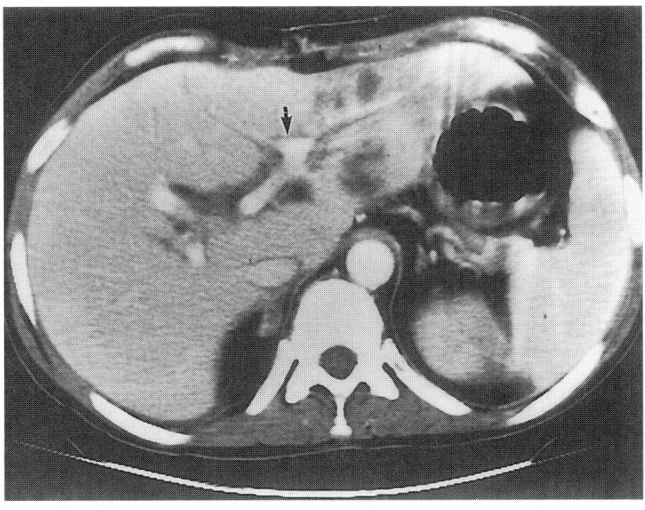

FIGURE 31-24

Computed tomographic scan with good contrast enhancement shows portal vein filled with contrast material *(arrow)*. Immediately adjacent is a low-signal area representing dilated bile ducts.

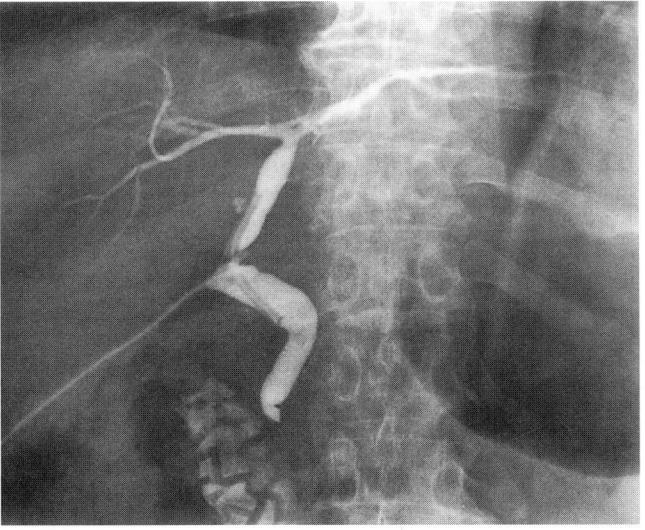

FIGURE 31-25

A T-tube cholangiogram shows an anastomotic stricture in the common bile duct. The stricture was treated successfully with balloon angioplasty.

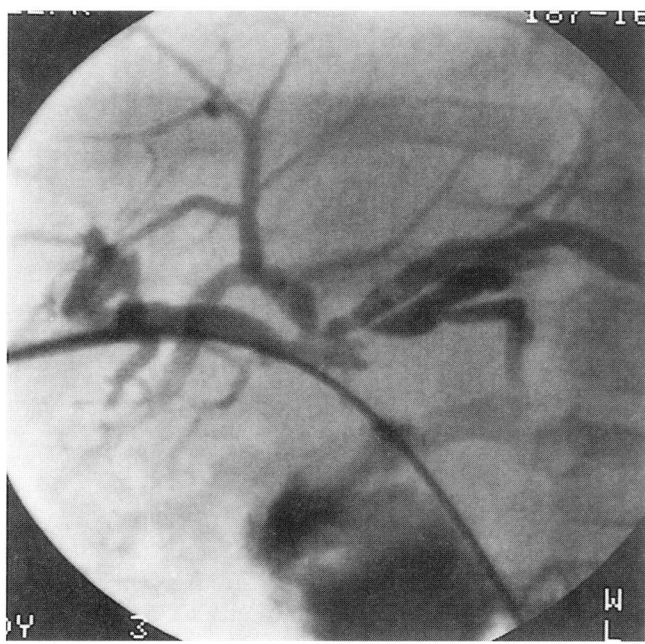

FIGURE 31–26

Nonanastomotic biliary stricture. Typically, nonanastomotic biliary strictures involve both the right and left hepatic ducts and a Roux-en-Y choledochojejunostomy. A transhepatic biliary drainage catheter was placed. This patient had severe hepatic artery stenosis.

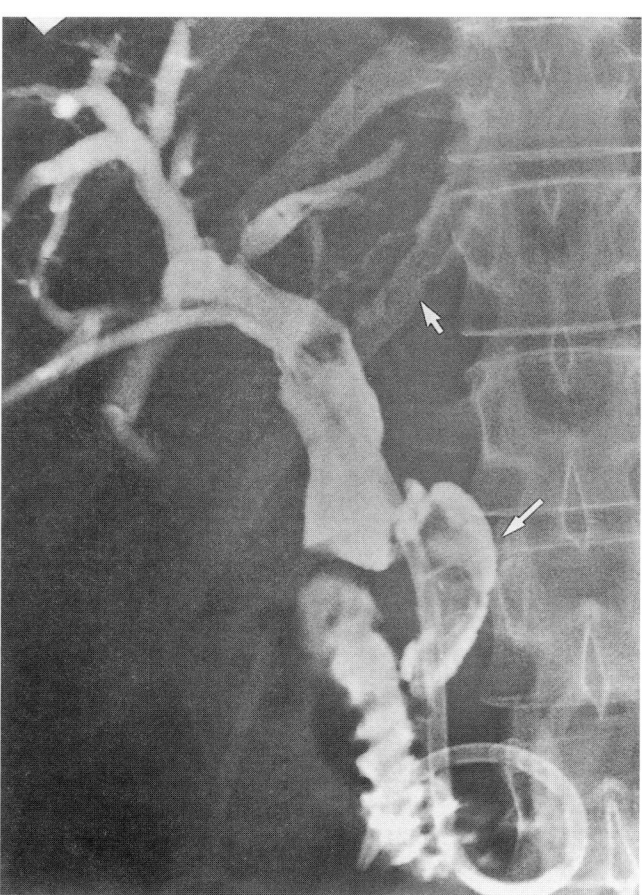

FIGURE 31–27

Biliary sludge. A cholangiogram performed after placement of a transhepatic drainage catheter shows multiple filling defects (*arrows*) in the common bile duct and outlining of the left hepatic duct, which are consistent with the presence of biliary sludge. A mild stricture is seen in a right biliary duct.

injury from hepatic artery obstruction, and the status of the hepatic artery should be assessed in these patients. In some instances, the indwelling straight stents used in patients undergoing a Roux-en-Y choledochojejunostomy may cause obstruction. These stents usually pass out of the anastomosis several weeks after transplantation, but in some instances they become encrusted and cause obstruction. Biliary obstruction also occurs as a result of the presence of masses of inspissated bile or "biliary sludge." This sludge can be seen radiographically on T-tube or transhepatic cholangiograms as amorphous collections of radiopaque material in both the intrahepatic and extrahepatic portions of the donor ducts (Fig. 31–27). Histological examination of the material reveals a composition of sheets of necrotic collagen impregnated with bile pigments.[79] The high necrotic content of the biliary sludge suggests that the primary mechanism, at least in some patients, may be necrosis of the donor bile duct wall and mucosa. This necrosis may be the result of ischemic damage during preservation of the donor liver, ischemia from hepatic artery obstruction following transplantation, superimposed infection, rejection, or a combination of factors. It has also been attributed to alterations in bile composition such as that caused by cyclosporine-induced crystal deposition.[28]

Rarely, recurrent strictures may occur in patients with cholangiocarcinoma. Dilatation of the donor duct may occur. Progressive dilatation of both the donor and

recipient common ducts has been observed in patients who have undergone choledochocholedochostomy biliary reconstruction.[80] The cause is uncertain, but stenosis and dysfunction of the sphincter of Oddi as a result of common bile duct neural denervation have been suggested as causative. By surgically changing the choledochocholedochostomy to a choledochojejunostomy, and thereby bypassing the sphincter of Oddi, clinical and laboratory improvement usually can be achieved.

When transhepatic cholangiography is used to decompress the obstructed biliary system, it is important to be aware that in cases of complete obstruction it may not be possible to cross the obstruction initially. Standard treatment is initial decompression and placement of a temporary drainage catheter. After 48 to 72 hours, when the edema has subsided, it is usually possible to traverse the stricture.

Biliary strictures are best treated with balloon dilation of the stricture (Fig. 31–28). In the series at the author's

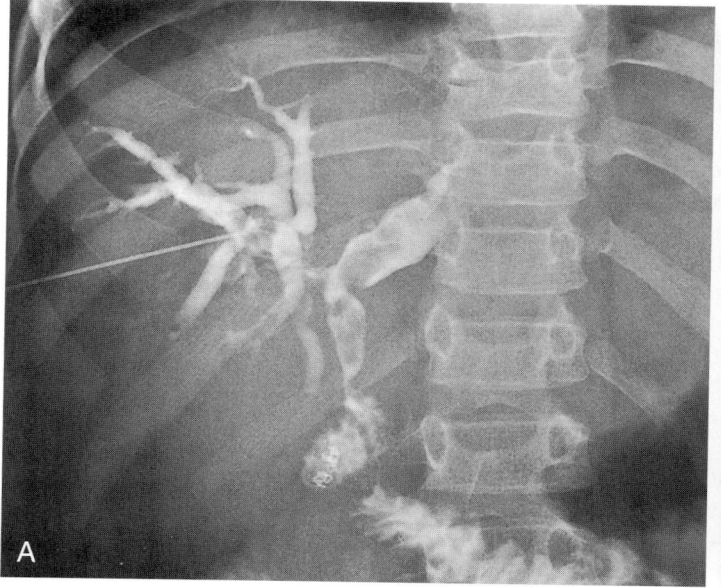

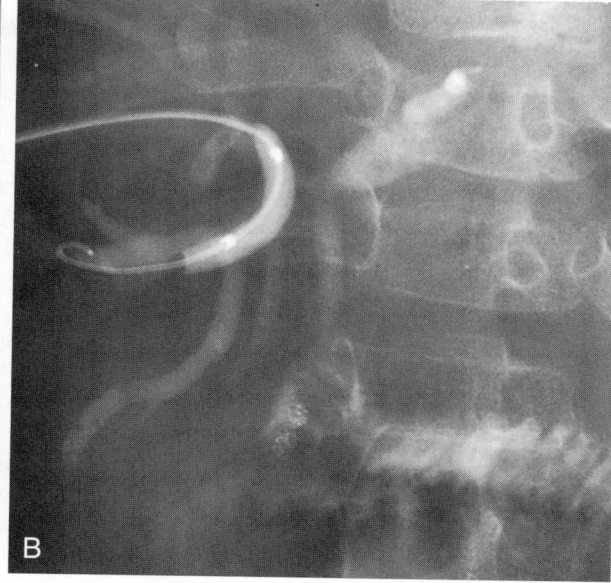

FIGURE 31-28

Biliary stricture dilatation. **A,** A transhepatic cholangiogram in a 6-year-old liver transplant recipient shows biliary dilatation, with biliary strictures in the right and left biliary ducts and at the choledochojejunostomy. **B,** An inflated balloon angioplasty catheter is seen in the right ducts. **C,** A cholangiogram after angioplasty shows residual stricture in the left duct, improved caliber in the right ducts, and relief of the stricture at the choledochojejunostomy. A transhepatic biliary drainage catheter is in place.

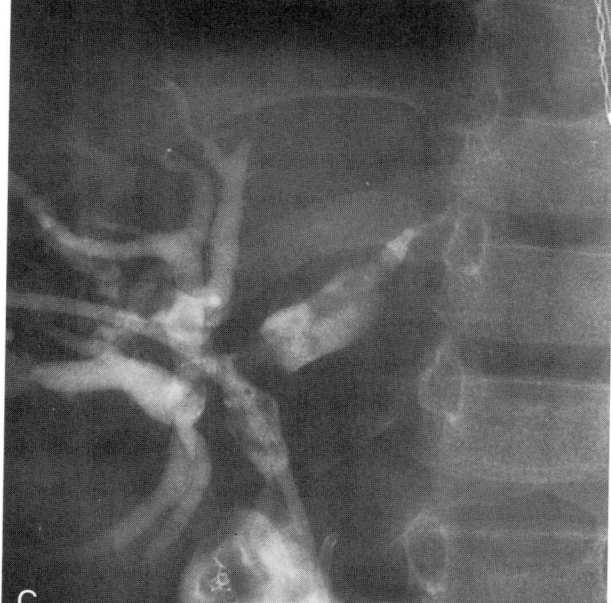

institution, biliary strictures were found in 22 of 106 (21%) patients referred for cholangiography because of hepatic dysfunction. Stricture dilation was accomplished through transhepatic percutaneous puncture. The balloon catheter was passed over a guidewire to the area of obstruction, and dilation was performed. Following dilation, an external biliary drainage catheter was left in place for approximately 2 weeks and then cholangiography was performed again. If the appearance was satisfactory, the tube was removed. If not, additional dilation was performed. It is the practice at the author's institution not to leave these tubes in place for long-term stenting because of the risk of infection. Of the 11 patients

treated with balloon dilation in this series, 4 required more than one dilation and returned in 1 to 2 years for another dilation. Balloon dilation can be an effective method of management for these strictures.[74] Both intrahepatic and extrahepatic strictures can be dilated; however, as expected, the results with multiple strictures may be less satisfactory, especially if the stricture has occurred as a result of ischemia caused by hepatic artery occlusion.[81] Balloon dilation through the T-tube tract is not recommended because of the potential for bile leakage through the T-tube insertion site.

Patients with obstruction caused by the presence of biliary sludge can be managed in several ways. In patients with an indwelling T-tube, a guidewire may be passed through the T-tube and the tip passed up into the biliary tree, where it can be rotated in the occluded ducts to disrupt the material. This method, coupled with gentle irrigation, is effective in producing passage of the material down into the distal duct from which it is cleared. In some instances, however, it is necessary to use a percutaneous transhepatic approach to relieve the obstruction. A balloon occlusion catheter may then be used to clear the occluded ducts gently. Short-term stenting is then performed.

To date, there are only scattered reports of the use of in-dwelling metallic stents in the management of biliary strictures in liver transplant recipients. Although there is experience with the use of metallic stents in other patients with benign biliary strictures,[82,83] there are currently no large series describing the long-term patency rates with these stents. Maccioni and colleagues[82] reported results with metallic stents in 19 nontransplant patients with benign biliary strictures who had failed to respond to repeated balloon angioplasty. In this group, a patency rate of 68.7% was observed at 3 years' follow-up. Mucosal hyperplasia, or inflammatory reactive changes of the ductal wall, or both, were cited as possible causes of late stent obstruction. All patients with complete stent obstruction had multiple intrahepatic strictures, and secondary cholangitis was determined to be a partial contraindication to the use of metallic stents. Maccioni and colleagues recommended stent placement in only those patients who fail to respond to balloon dilation. In the liver transplant series at my institution, the response to a repeated balloon dilation has been satisfactory, and placement of a metallic stent has not been necessary. It is important to note that the metallic stents may become incorporated in the wall of the duct, rendering later surgical removal difficult.

Biliary complications occur in both pediatric and adult liver transplant recipients. Although children, in contradistinction to adults, manifest early collateral arterial growth into the allograft liver, which may maintain viability of the liver, they remain susceptible to ischemic bile duct injury when hepatic artery occlusion occurs. Pediatric complications are managed with the interventional techniques used in adults. The procedures are usually performed under general anesthesia. These interventional techniques play a major role in the maintenance of the allograft and avoidance of additional surgery.

Although the interventional biliary procedures are important aids to the maintenance of the allograft, complications may occur as a result of the intervention. Biliary interventions should be performed under broad-spectrum antibiotic coverage.

A serious complication in these immunosuppressed patients is the development of a biliary vascular communication secondary to placement of a transhepatic biliary drainage catheter. The hemobilia associated with tube placement is poorly tolerated by these patients, so persistent hemobilia through the drainage tube requires prompt correction. Cholangiography should be performed to determine the site of vascular communication, which may be venous or arterial. If a communication with the vascular system is identified by cholangiography, a new transhepatic puncture should be performed at a different entry site, and drainage should be established. At the same sitting, the offending tube should be exchanged for a straight catheter. Embolization should be performed on both sides of the bleeding vessel to isolate the biliary system and the vessel. Absorbable gelatin sponge (Gelfoam) or metallic coils may be used. Embolization of the parenchymal tract should be performed with Gelfoam while the straight catheter is withdrawn. If the bleeding site is not identified on cholangiography, hepatic arteriography should be performed. Hemobilia arising from false aneurysms of the hepatic artery and occurring after transhepatic tube placement has been treated with removal of the tube followed by arteriography and transcatheter embolization. When the bleeding site cannot be identified on arteriography, some physicians recommend that the offending tube be removed and another arteriogram be performed when and if bleeding recurs and the site of arterial injury is determined.[84] The author and colleagues have found that embolization of the bleeding site via the tube tract at the time of removal of the tube avoids the risk of rebleeding and is an effective method in the treatment of most biliary vascular communications.

The transjugular approach is used when liver biopsy is needed in transplant patients who are poor candidates for percutaneous biopsy because of diffuse liver disease, ascites, or coagulopathy. This technique, performed via jugular vein access, minimizes the risk of bleeding.[85]

Summary

Diagnostic and interventional radiological techniques play an important role in the management of biliary complications in the liver transplant recipient. These techniques are often important in the maintenance and survival of the allograft.

Pearls and Pitfalls

- Both dual-phase CT and MRI are used to diagnose HCC. Careful selection of MRI pulse sequences can provide important information regarding the presence of other liver pathology such as regenerative and dysplastic nodules.

Pearls and Pitfalls—cont'd

- Ultrasonography should be routinely used to monitor the post–liver transplant patient to assess the status of the vascular anastomoses.

- The symptoms of hepatic artery thrombosis are highly variable, and false-negative results can be obtained on ultrasonography as a result of misinterpretation of flow signals from collaterals in the porta hepatis.

- Balloon angioplasty is useful for the treatment of vascular obstruction involving the arterial, portal, hepatic vein, and inferior vena cava anastomoses in the liver transplant patient.

- Percutaneous transhepatic cholangiography is useful in the detection of biliary obstruction, and biliary stricture dilation is a routine method of managing postoperative biliary strictures in the liver transplant patient.

References

1. Letourneau JG, Day DL, Ascher NL, et al: Abdominal sonography after hepatic transplantation: Results in 36 patients. AJR Am J Roentgenol 149:299-303, 1987.

2. Lerut J, Tzakis AG, Bron K, et al: Complications of venous reconstruction in human orthotopic liver transplantation. Ann Surg 205:404-414, 1987.

3. Dalen K, Ascher NL, Hunter DW, et al: Imaging of vascular complications after hepatic transplantation. AJR Am J Roentgenol 150:1285-1290, 1988.

4. Taylor KJ, Morse SS, Weltin GG, et al: Liver transplant recipients: Portable duplex US with correlative angiography. Radiology 159:357-363, 1986.

5. Zajko AB, Campbell WL, Bron KM, et al: Diagnostic and interventional radiology in liver transplantation. Gastroenterol Clin North Am 17:105-143, 1988.

6. Longley DG, Skolnick LM, Zajko AB, et al: Duplex Doppler sonography in the evaluation of adult patients before and after liver transplantation. AJR Am J Roentgenol 151:687-696, 1988.

7. Baron RL, Oliver JH, Dodd GD III, et al: Hepatocellular carcinoma: Evaluation with biphasic contract-enhanced helical CT. Radiology 199:505-511, 1996.

8. Lee HM, Lu DSK, Krasny RM, et al: Hepatic lesion characterization in cirrhosis: Significance of arterial hypervascularity on dual-phase helical CT. AJR Am J Roentgenol 169:125-130, 1997.

9. Krinsky GA, Lee VS, Theise ND: Hepatocellular carcinoma and dysplastic nodules in patients with cirrhosis: Prospective diagnosis with MR imaging and explantation correlation. Radiology 219:445-454, 2001.

10. Valls C, Andia E, Roca Y, et al: CT in hepatic cirrhosis and chronic hepatitis. Semin Ultrasound CT MR 23:37-61, 2002.

11. International Working Party: Terminology of nodular hepatocellular lesion. Hepatology 22:983-993, 1995.

12. Lim JH, Kim CK, Lee WJ, et al: Detection of hepatocellular carcinomas and dysplastic nodules in cirrhotic livers: Accuracy of helical CT in transplant patients. AJR Am J Roentgenol 175:693-698, 2000.

13. Mazzaferro V, Regalia E, Doci R, et al: Liver transplantation for the treatment of small hepatocellular carcinomas in patients with cirrhosis. N Engl J Med 334:693-699, 1996.

14. Llovet JM, Bruix J, Fuster J, et al: Liver transplantation for small hepatocellular carcinoma: The tumor-node-metastasis classification does not have prognostic power. Hepatology 27:1572-1577, 1998.

15. Choi BI, Han JK, Kim TK, et al: Dysplastic nodules of the liver: Imaging findings. Abdom Imaging 24:250-257, 1999.

16. Krinsky GA, Lee VS: MR imaging of cirrhotic nodules. Abdom Imaging 25:471-482, 2000.

17. Winter TC, Takayasu K, Muramatsu Y, et al: Early advanced hepatocellular carcinoma: Evaluation of CT and MR appearance with pathologic correlation. Radiology 192:379-387, 1994.

18. Kadoya M, Matsui O, Takashima T, et al: Hepatocellular carcinoma: Correlation of MR imaging and histopathologic findings. Radiology 183:819-825, 1992.

19. Lalonde L, Van Beers B, Jamart J, et al: Capsule and mosaic pattern of hepatocellular carcinoma: Correlation between CT and MR imaging. Gastrointest Radiol 17:241-244, 1992.

20. Martin J, Puig J, Darnell A, Donoso L: Magnetic resonance of focal liver lesions in hepatic cirrhosis and chronic hepatitis. Semin Ultrasound CT MR 214:62-78, 2002.

21. Martin J, Sentis M. Zidan A, et al: Fatty metamorphosis of hepatocellular carcinoma: Detection with chemical-shift gradient-echo MR imaging. Radiology 195:125-130, 1995.

22. Martin J, Sentis M, Puig J, et al: Comparison of in-phase and opposed-phase GRE and conventional SE MR pulse sequences in T_1-weighted imaging of liver lesions. J Comput Assist Tomogr 20:890-897, 1996.

23. Matsui O, Kadoya M, Kameyama T, et al: Benign and malignant nodules in cirrhotic livers: Distinction based on blood supply. Radiology 178:493-497, 1991.

24. Lee HM, Lu DS, Krasny RM et al: Hepatic lesion characterization in cirrhosis: Significance of arterial hypervascularity on dual-phase helical CT. AJR Am J Roentgenol 169:125-130, 1997.

25. Yu JS, Kim KW, Jeong MG, et al: Nontumorous hepatic arterial-portal venous shunts: MR imaging findings. Radiology 217:750-756, 2000.

26. Kim TK, Choi BI, Han JK, et al: Nontumorous arterioportal shunts mimicking hypervascular tumor in cirrhotic liver. Two phase spiral CT findings. Radiology 208:597-603, 1998.

27. Prince MR, Yucel EK, Kaufman JA, et al: Dynamic gadolinium-enhanced three-dimensional abdominal MR arteriography. J Magn Reson Imaging 3:877-881, 1997.

28. Fulcher A, Turner MA: Orthotopic liver transplantation: Evaluation with MR cholangiography. Radiology 211:715-722, 1999.

29. Marsh JW Jr, Iwatsuld S, Makowka L, et al: Orthotopic liver transplantation for primary sclerosing cholangitis. Ann Surg 207:21-25, 1988.

30. Rosch J, Hanafee WN, Snow H: Transjugular portal venography and radiological portosystemic shunt: An experimental study. Radiology 92:1112-1114, 1969.

31. Colapinto RF, Stronell RD, Gildiner M, et al: Formation of an intrahepatic portosystemic shunt using balloon dilatation catheter. Preliminary clinical experience. AJR Am J Roentgenol 140:709-714, 1983.

32. Richter GM, Palmaz JC, Nolge G, et al: The transjugular intrahepatic portosystemic stent-shunt (TIPS): A new nonoperative, transjugular percutaneous procedure. Radiology 29:406-411, 1989.

33. LaBerge JM, Ring EJ, Gordon RL, et al: Creation of transjugular intrahepatic portosystemic shunts with the Wallstent endoprosthesis: Results in 100 patients. Radiology 187:413-420, 1993.

34. Barton RE, Rosch J, Saxton RR, et al: TIPS: Short- and long-term results. A survey of 1750 patients. Semin Interv Radiol 4:364-367, 1995.

35. Mut F, Glickman S, Marciano D, Hawkins RA: Optimum proving protocols for volume determination of the liver and spleen

from SPECT imaging with Tc-99m sulfur colloid. J Nucl Med 29:1768-1775, 1988.

36. Taylor KJW, Burns PN, Woodcock JP, Wells PNT: Blood flow in deep abdominal and pelvic vessels: Ultrasonic pulsed Doppler analysis. Radiology 154:487-493, 1985.

37. Longley DG, Skolnick ML, Sheahan DG: Acute allograft rejection in liver transplant recipients: Lack of correlation with loss of hepatic artery diastolic flow. Radiology 169:417-420, 1988.

38. Marder DM, DeMarino GB, Sumkin JH, Sheahan DG: Liver transplant rejection: Value of the resistive index in Doppler US of hepatic arteries. Radiology 173:127-129, 1989.

39. Garcia-Criado A, Gilabert R, Bargallo X, Bru C: Radiology in liver transplantation. Semin Ultrasound CT MR 23:114-129, 2002.

40. Chervu LR, Nunn AD, Loberg MD: Radiopharmaceuticals for hepatobiliary imaging. Semin Nucl Med 12:5-17, 1982.

41. Wozney P, Zajko AB, Bron KM, et al: Vascular complications after liver transplantation: A 5-year experience. AJR Am J Roentgenol 147:657-663, 1986.

42. Zajko AB, Bron KM, Orons PD: Vascular complications in liver transplant recipients: Angiographic diagnosis and treatment. Semin Interv Radiol 9:270-281, 1992.

43. Bechstein WO, Blumhardt G, Ringe B, et al: Surgical complications in 200 consecutive liver transplants. Transplant Proc 19:3830-3831, 1987.

44. Hawkins RA, Hall T, Gambhir SS, et al: Radionuclide evaluation of liver transplants. Semin Nucl Med 18:199-212, 1988.

45. Brown RKJ, Memsic LDF, Pusey EJ, et al: Hepatic abscess in liver transplantation: Accurate diagnosis and treatment. Clin Nucl Med 11:233-236, 1986.

46. Castaneda F, So SK, Hunter DW, et al: Reversible hepatic transplant ischemia: Case report and review of literature. Cardiovasc Intervent Radiol 13:88-90, 1990.

47. Abad J, Hidalgo EG, Cantarero JM, et al: Hepatic artery anastomotic stenosis after transplantation: Treatment with percutaneous transluminal angioplasty. Radiology 171:661-662, 1989.

48. Raby N, Karani J, Thomas S, et al: Stenoses of vascular anastomoses after hepatic transplantation: Treatment with balloon angioplasty. AJR Am J Roentgenol 157:167-171, 1991.

49. Sheiner PA, Varma CVR, Guarrera JV, et al: Selective revascularization of hepatic artery thrombosis after liver transplantation improves patient and graft survival. Transplantation 64:1295-1299, 1997.

50. Nolten A, Sproat IA: Hepatic artery thrombosis after liver transplantation: Temporal accuracy of diagnosis with duplex US and the syndrome of impending thrombosis. Radiology 198:553-559, 1996.

51. Ohkohchi N, Katoh H, Orii T, et al: Complications and treatment of donors and recipients in living-related liver transplantation. Transplant Proc 30:3218-3220, 1998.

52. Esquivel CO, Konem B, Karrer F, et al: Liver transplantation before 1 year of age. J Pediatr 110:545-548, 1987.

53. Flint EW, Sumkin JH, Zajko AB, Bowen A: Duplex sonography of hepatic artery thrombosis after liver transplantation. AJR Am J Roentgenol 151:481-483, 1988.

54. Hall TE, McDiarmid SV, Grant EG, et al: False negative duplex Doppler studies in children with hepatic artery thrombosis after liver transplantation. AJR Am J Roentgenol 154:573-575, 1990.

55. Segel MC, Zajko AB, Bowen A: Hepatic artery thrombosis after liver transplantation: Radiologic evaluation. AJR Am J Roentgenol 146:137-141, 1986.

56. Langnas AN, Marujo W, Stratta RJ, et al: Hepatic allograft rescue following arterial thrombosis: Role of urgent revascularization. Transplantation 51:8690, 1991.

57. Marujo WC, Langnas AN, Wood RP, et al: Vascular complications following orthotopic liver transplantation: Outcome and the role of urgent revascularization. Transplant Proc 23:1484-1486, 1991.

58. Klintmalm GB, Olson LM, Nery JR, et al: Treatment of hepatic artery thrombosis after liver transplantation with immediate vascular reconstruction: A report of three cases. Transplant Proc 20(Suppl 1):610-612, 1988.

59. Lerut JP, Gordon RD, Iwatsuld S, Starzl TE: Human orthotopic liver transplantation: Surgical aspects in 393 consecutive grafts. Transplant Proc 20:603-606, 1988.

60. Hesselink EJ, Slooff MJH, Schurr KH, et al: Consequences of hepatic artery pathology after orthotopic liver transplantation. Transplant Proc 19:2476-2477, 1987.

61. Merion RM, Burtch GD, Ham JM, et al: The hepatic artery in liver transplantation. Transplantation 48:438-443, 1989.

62. Tobben PJ, Zajko AB, Sumkin JH, et al: Pseudoaneurysms complicating organ transplantation: Roles of CT, duplex sonography, and angiography. Radiology 169:65-70, 1988.

63. Lerut J, Tzakis AG, Bron K, et al: Complications of venous reconstruction in human orthotopic liver transplantation. Ann Surg 205:404-414, 1987.

64. Dalen K, Day DL, Ascher NL, et al: Imaging of vascular complications after hepatic transplantation. AJR Am J Roentgenol 150:1285-1290, 1988.

65. Longley DG, Skolnick ML, Zajko AB, Bron KM: Duplex Doppler sonography in the evaluation of adult patients before and after liver transplantation. AJR Am J Roentgenol 151:687-696, 1988.

66. Taylor KJ, Morse SS, Weltin GG, et al: Liver transplant recipients: Portable duplex US with correlative angiography. Radiology 159:357-363, 1986.

67. Chezmar JL, Nelson RC, Bernardino ME: Portal venous gas after hepatic transplantation: Sonographic detection and clinical significance. AJR Am J Roentgenol 153:1203-1205, 1989.

68. Olcott EW, Ring EJ, Roberts JP, et al: Percutaneous transhepatic portal vein angioplasty and stent placement after liver transplantation: Early experience. J Vasc Interv Radiol 1:17-22, 1990.

69. Zajko AB, Claus D, Clapuyt P, et al: Obstruction to hepatic venous drainage after liver transplantation: Treatment with balloon angioplasty. Radiology 170:763-765, 1989.

70. Rose BS, Van Aman ME, Simon DC, et al: Transluminal balloon angioplasty of infrahepatic caval anastomotic stenosis following liver transplantation: Case report. Cardiovasc Intervent Radiol 11:79-81, 1988.

71. Letourneau JG, Hunter DW, Payne WD, Day DL: Imaging of an intervention for biliary complications after hepatic transplantation. AJR Am J Roentgenol 154:729-733, 1990.

72. Zajko AB, Campbell WL, Bron KM, et al: Diagnostic and interventional radiology in liver transplantation. Gastroenterol Clin North Am 17:105-143, 1988.

73. Gomes AS: Diagnosis and radiologic treatment of binary complications of liver transplantation. Semin Interv Radiol 9:283-289, 1992.

74. Sherman S, Jamidar P, Shaked A, et al: Biliary tract complications after orthotopic liver transplantation. Endoscopic approach to diagnosis and treatment. Transplantation 60:467-470, 1995.

75. Klingensmith WC III, Koep LJ, Fritzberg AR: Bile leak into a hepatic abscess in a liver transplant; Demonstration with 99m Tc-diethyl-iminodiacetic acid. AJR Am J Roentgenol 131:889-891, 1978.

76. Kaplan SB, Zajko AB, Koneru B: Hepatic bilomas due to hepatic artery thrombosis in liver transplant recipients: Percutaneous drainage and clinical outcome. Radiology 174:1031-1035, 1990.

77. Zeman RK, Taylor KJ, Rosenfield AT, et al: Acute experimental biliary obstruction in the dog: Sonographic findings and clinical implications. AJR Am J Roentgenol 136:965-967, 1981.

78. Shawker TH, Jones BL, Girton ME: Distal common bile duct obstruction: An experimental study in monkeys. J Clin Ultrasound 9:77-82, 1981.

79. McMaster P, Herbertson B, Cusick C, et al: Biliary sludging following liver transplantation in man. Transplantation 25:56-62, 1978.

80. Miller WJ, Campbell WL, Zajko AB, et al: Obstructive dilatation of extrahepatic recipient and donor bile ducts complicating orthotopic liver transplantation: Imaging and laboratory findings. AJR Am J Roentgenol 157:29-32, 1991.

81. Ward EM, Kiely MJ, Maus TP, et al: Hilar biliary strictures after liver transplantation: Cholangiography and percutaneous treatment. Radiology 177:259-263, 1990.

82. Maccioni F, Rossi M, Salvatori FM, et al: Metallic stents in benign biliary strictures: Three-year follow-up. Cardiovasc Intervent Radiol 15:360-366, 1992.

83. Coons H: Metallic stents for the treatment of biliary obstruction: A report of 100 cases. Cardiovasc Intervent Radiol 15:367-374, 1992.

84. Zajko AB, Chablani V, Bron KM, Jungreis C: Hemobilia complicating transhepatic catheter drainage in liver transplant recipients: Management with selective embolization. Cardiovasc Intervent Radiol 13:285-288, 1990.

85. Gamble P, Colapinto RF, Stronell RD, et al: Transjugular liver biopsy: A review of 461 biopsies. Radiology 157:589-593, 1985.

Monitoring and Care of the Patient Before Liver Transplantation

PRATIMA SHARMA
HUGO E. VARGAS
JORGE RAKELA

General medical care   473
   Routine examination, prophylaxis, and
      immunization   473
   Treatment of underlying liver diseases   474

Liver-specific complications   476
   Portal hypertension   476
   Spontaneous bacterial peritonitis   479
   Hepatic Encephalopathy   479
   Hepatopulmonary syndrome and other
      pulmonary complications   482
   Hepatic hydrothorax   482
   Pruritus   482
   Osteopenia and osteoporosis   483

Psychosocial Issues and Depression   483

Nutrition   483

The worsening organ availability crisis continues to affect liver transplantation (LT) candidates. According to United Network of Organ Sharing (UNOS), there were 16,963 patients awaiting liver transplantation as of March 14, 2003.[1] The number of deceased donor liver transplants in the year 2002 was 4969.[2] The low number of transplants, coupled with long waiting times, increases the likelihood that candidates will have complications of their liver disease. The transplant hepatologist has to be, by necessity, very skilled in the medical management of candidates awaiting LT.

The aim of this chapter is to delineate the care of patients who await LT. It focuses on clinical issues that do not require hospitalization. It highlights preventive medicine measures as well as disease-specific measures that can maximize the survival of candidates without LT.

General Medical Care

Routine Examination, Prophylaxis, and Immunization

Although the life-threatening complications of end-stage liver disease require a higher degree of care and even life-saving procedures, the general medical care of these patients should not be overlooked. Close follow-up of these patients is a must. The Model for End-Stage Liver Disease (MELD) has emerged as a useful tool that estimates the mortality of patients awaiting LT.[3-6] It was implemented February 26, 2002 by UNOS as criteria for organ allocation in patients with chronic disease awaiting liver transplantation. Although initially developed to predict the survival of patients undergoing transjugular intrahepatic portosystemic shunt (TIPS) procedures,[7] MELD was subsequently validated in patients with decompensated cirrhosis, ambulatory patients with noncholestatic cirrhosis, patients with primary biliary cirrhosis,[3,5] those with alcoholic hepatitis,[8] and an unselected group of cirrhotic patients.[3,5] MELD predicts candidate mortality at different time points with adequate accuracy. For practical purposes, the score is capped at 40, a point at which patients have virtual 100% mortality in 3 months. UNOS has made two adjustments to the MELD to compensate for the increased mortality from advancing disease in patients with small hepatocellular carcinoma (HCC) with long waiting time. The HCC patients who fulfill the so-called Milan criteria[10] get a priority MELD score beyond the degree of hepatic decompensation. Patients with stage T1 HCC (one lesion <2 cm) or stage T2 HCC (one lesion >2 cm but <5 cm or up three lesions not larger than 3 cm) receive a MELD score of 20 (equivalent to 8% 3-month mortality) or 24 (equivalent to 15% 3-month mortality), respectively.

Once patients are listed for LT, MELD maintenance requires regular visits to the transplant clinic (Table 32–1). The frequency with which a patient should be monitored in the clinic is based on the MELD score. MELD scores of 10 warrant visits every 6 months to a year, MELD scores between 11 and 18 warrant visits every 3 months, MELD scores between 19 and 24 warrant monthly visits, and MELD scores of 25 warrant weekly visits. These visits should be used to update the parameters used for MELD scoring and should include assessment of electrolytes, complete blood count, and coagulation profile. As with all cirrhotic patients, assessment of subclinical portosystemic encephalopathy, ascites, and edema are mandatory. If patients have been prescribed β-blockers, blood pressure and pulse measurements should be obtained with the goal of adjusting medications optimally. Screening for HCC should be done with serum α-fetoprotein (AFP) and abdominal ultrasonography. If AFP levels are elevated, triphasic CT or MRI may be more appropriate.[9] Select populations, including those with viral hepatitis B and C, hemochromatosis, and alcoholic liver disease, may warrant a more aggressive schedule because of the elevated risk of HCC.[9]

Vaccinations for hepatitis B virus (HBV) and hepatitis A virus (HAV) have significant value. Vento and associates reported that fulminant hepatitis is associated with hepatitis A superinfection in chronic hepatitis C patients and recommended that these patients be immunized for hepatitis A.[10] Patients who do not have antibodies to the hepatitis B surface antigen should receive a complete vaccination schedule at the beginning of their evaluation. Unfortunately, a number of preliminary studies suggest that the vaccine's effectiveness is less than that in individuals without end-stage liver disease. One study of 21 patients showed only a 29% response rate and suggested that an absolute lymphocyte count of 1300/mm³ was predictive of response.[11] In light of such a low response rate, follow-up antihepatitis B surface antibody levels should be obtained after the second injection. The final injection of the series, given 6 months after the first one, should be given even if the liver transplantation has already been performed.[12] In a study by Kallinowski and associates, the seroprotection rate with an accelerated vaccination schedule (0, 7, and 21 days) is 36% in LT candidates, using 20 μg hepatitis B surface antigen (HbsAg) per dose.[12,13] In addition to hepatitis A and B vaccination, these patients should also receive influenza vaccine yearly and pneumococcal vaccination (0.5 mL intramuscularly) every 5 years.[14] Tuberculin skin testing should be done yearly. Screening for breast, endocervical, colorectal, and prostate cancer should be performed as in other medical patients.[14] A comprehensive ear, nose, and throat evaluation should be done in alcoholics with a history of tobacco use because of their increased nasopharyngeal cancer incidence.

Treatment of Underlying Liver Diseases

In recent years, great strides have been made in improving the management of chronic liver disease. Hepatitis B virus infection (HBV), autoimmune liver disease, and to a lesser extent hepatitis C virus (HCV) have newer treatment approaches that should facilitate management. Whenever possible, treatment of the underlying primary liver disease should be considered; in some instances, clearance of viral infection or bringing disease into remission may resolve aspects of

Table 32–1. FREQUENCY OF VISITS: BASED ON MELD SCORE

MELD Score	Visits
≥25	Weekly
19-24	Monthly
11-18	Three months
≤10	Six months to yearly

hepatic decompensation and make the indication of liver transplantation unnecessary.

Hepatitis B Virus

In HBV-related cirrhosis, antiviral therapy should be considered if HBV replication is present. The most compelling reasons are halting liver disease progression and eliminating viral replication, which leads to decreased disease recurrence in the post-LT period.[15] Inhibition of HBV replication has been shown to be associated with clinical improvement or stabilization of patients.[16] In a study by Fontana and associates reviewing the outcome of lamivudine therapy in 309 patients awaiting LT for chronic hepatitis B, lamivudine did not improve the overall pre-LT survival or LT-free survival.[17] However, their data suggest that a subset of patients with less advanced liver failure may derive clinical benefit from lamivudine treatment, thus delaying the need for LT.[17] There is some evidence that improvement, if not outright regression of cirrhosis, can occur on lamivudine.[18] Lamivudine administration at an oral dose of 100 mg/day is associated with significant suppression of serum HBV DNA, rarely accompanied by alanine transferases flare. Studies of viral clearance kinetics derived from various clinical trials showed that long-term treatment is required to control and eradicate HBV infection.[18-21] Comparison with historical data suggests that a 1-year course of lamivudine monotherapy has similar antiviral efficacy to a 16-week therapy with α-interferon in treatment-naïve patients,[18] and that the combination therapy of α-interferon and lamivudine does not have any evident benefit,[22] although there are several clinical trials evaluating this combination.

Hepatitis C Virus

According to the National Institutes of Health consensus conference of 2002, combination treatment with pegylated α-interferon (PEG-IFN) and ribavirin is clearly indicated in patients with compensated cirrhosis.[23] Although the optimal regimen has yet to be defined for this patient population, overall response rates to a 48-week course of PEG-IFN and ribavirin appear to be in the range of 41% to 44%.[24] Response is much lower for genotype 1–infected patients.

Treatment of decompensated cirrhosis using α-interferon with or without ribavirin has been fraught with serious lethal complications[25] and should not be done outside a clinical trial.[23]

Hemochromatosis

The practice guidelines from the American Association for the Study of Liver Diseases (AASLD) state that all patients with hereditary hemochromatosis (HHC) and evidence of iron overload should be strongly encouraged to undergo regular phlebotomies until iron stores are depleted.[26] Phlebotomies should be continued for life with the frequency of maintenance therapy dependent on serum ferritin level.[26]

Hepatocellular carcinoma accounts for 30% of all deaths in HHC, whereas other complications of cirrhosis account for an additional 20% of deaths in this patient population.[27,28] Consequently, these patients should have regular, aggressive screening for HCC as described earlier.

Primary Biliary Cirrhosis

All patients with primary biliary cirrhosis (PBC) with abnormal liver enzyme levels should be considered for specific therapy.[29] Ursodeoxycholic acid (UDCA) treatment is associated with a marked improvement in serum biochemical markers of cholestasis (bilirubin, alkaline phosphatase, and γ-glutamine transferase).[30] UDCA slows the progression of PBC in treated patients.[31] Unfortunately, this therapy does not lead to the resolution of the disease.[31] The recommended dosage for UDCA is 13 to 15 mg/kg in a divided or single dose.[29,30]

Both decreased osteoblastic activity and increased osteoclastic activity contribute to the development of osteoporosis in PBC patients.[32] The relative risk of osteopenia is 4.4 in PBC patients.[33] Screening and early management of osteoporosis in patients with PBC and primary sclerosing cholangitis should follow current guidelines on the management of osteoporosis associated with chronic liver disease.[34]

Primary Sclerosing Cholangitis

Primary sclerosing cholangitis (PSC), with or without ulcerative colitis, is the most common known predisposing factor for cholangiocarcinoma.[35] Patients with PSC should therefore be regularly screened for this malignancy. The tumor marker CA 19-9 is elevated in up to 85% of patients with cholangiocarcinoma. It has been reported that a CA 19-9 value greater than 100 U/mL has a sensitivity of 75% and specificity of 80% for the detection of cholangiocarcinoma in patients with PSC.[36-38] Despite the availability of this marker, early diagnosis of cholangiocarcinoma is extremely challenging. The hepatologist and therapeutic endoscopist should aggressively address any changes suggestive of new biliary strictures in these patients as they await LT.

In a study published in 1997 by the Mayo Primary Sclerosing Cholangitis–Ursodeoxycholic Acid Study Group, UDCA acid provided no clinical benefit in a group of patients with well-defined cholangitis.[39] A recent study by Stiehl and associates showed that endoscopic opening of a dominant stenosis is effective and appears to be a valuable addition in the long-term treatment of such patients.[40]

The risk for colonic dysplasia or cancer in patients with ulcerative colitis and primary sclerosing cholangitis is 50% after 25 years of colitis.[41-43] Recently, Tung and associates in their retrospective study have shown that the patients who have used UDCA were less likely to develop colonic dysplasia as compared to those who did not receive the agent.[44] Furthermore, these patients should be screened regularly for colon cancer.[45]

Autoimmune Hepatitis

Treatment of autoimmune hepatitis with immunosuppression may not be indicated in patients with inactive cirrhosis, preexisting comorbid conditions, or drug intolerance. AASLD practice guidelines state that treatment regimens should include prednisone (10 mg/day) in combination with azathioprine or higher dose prednisone (20 mg/day) alone.[46] Cyclosporine,[47] 6-mercaptopurine,[48] cyclophosphamide,[49] and mycophenolate mofetil[50] have been used successfully in isolated cases with drug toxicity to prednisone or azathioprine. The treating clinician should understand that individuals with cirrhosis caused by autoimmune hepatitis have a higher frequency of drug-related complications than those without cirrhosis (25% versus 8%).[46]

Liver-Specific Complications

Portal Hypertension

Portal hypertension is the main complication of cirrhosis. This syndrome develops in the majority of patients with cirrhosis and is responsible for most life-threatening complication of cirrhosis, including gastrointestinal bleeding from ruptured gastroesophageal varices, hepatorenal syndrome, and hepatic encephalopathy. The management of these complications in the LT candidate is discussed in detail.

Esophageal Variceal Bleeding

The average lifetime risk of variceal bleeding in patients with cirrhosis who have had no previous bleeding is 30%.[51] Despite significant improvements in the early diagnosis and treatment of esophagogastric variceal hemorrhage, the mortality rate of first variceal hemorrhage remains high.[52] Multivariate analyses of prospective studies indicate that high-risk patients for first variceal bleed are of advanced Child-Pugh class and have large esophageal varices and red wale markings.[53] Other studies show that advanced age, gastric varices, and alcohol-induced cirrhosis increase risk for variceal bleed.[54,55]

Primary Prophylaxis

Pharmacotherapy. Nonselective β-blockers have been shown to reduce the risk of initial variceal bleeding, with a trend toward decreased mortality, and should be considered in all patients with large varices and red markings.[56] β-Blockers decrease portal pressure and collateral flow through a combination of decreased cardiac output and unopposed α-mediated splanchnic vasoconstriction, resulting in decreased effective splanchnic blood flow.[57,58] Propranolol or nadolol can be used and the dose should be titrated weekly to decrease the resting heart rate by 25% but not to less than 55 beats per minute and the systolic blood pressure to no lower than 90 mm Hg.[59]

Hemodynamic studies have shown that the benefit of β-blockers is noted only in patients in whom the hepatic venous pressure gradient is reduced to less than 12 mm Hg or 20% lower than the baseline. The risk reduction with β-blockade averages less than 50% and the maximal benefit is seen in patients with Child's A and B cirrhosis. More than 30% of patients have no decrease in portal pressure despite adequate β-blockade.[60] The addition of long-acting nitrates to nonselective β-blockers has been shown to enhance their hemodynamic effect and reduce the risk of bleeding from esophageal varices and therefore should be considered in patients who do not respond ideally to β-blockers.[61]

Endoscopic Therapy. Endoscopic variceal sclerotherapy has been used in the primary prophylaxis of variceal bleeding. However, poor results compared with pharmacotherapy have led to discontinuation of this modality.[62-64] Sarin and colleagues showed that endoscopic variceal band ligation is safe and more effective than propranolol for the primary prevention of variceal bleeding.[65] Further confirmation of these results is needed before this approach can be routinely recommended. Several multicenter trials are in the planning stage to address this very important clinical question.

TIPS. This approach is associated with a high incidence of hepatic encephalopathy and with costly TIPS malfunction. Despite effectiveness in the arrest of bleeding,[66] TIPS cannot be recommended as a first-line approach to manage variceal bleeding or for primary prophylaxis.[66,67]

Secondary Prophylaxis

Rebleeding is a very common occurrence, with recurrence reported as high as 70% in patients who have had at least one prior bleeding episode. Generally this occurs within 6 weeks of the index episode.[68,69] The use of β-blockers (with and without endoscopic band ligation of varices) is the most accepted approach to manage these patients. There is still debate about the cost-effectiveness of this pharmacological approach combined with endoscopy.[70,71] Conversely, it is not clear whether the addition of nonselective β-blockers to endoscopic therapy enhances benefit.[72]

TIPS remains a valid rescue method for patients in whom pharmacological or endoscopic or combined measures have failed.[67] Despite effective arrest of bleeding, hepatic encephalopathy remains a problem in this set of patients and may lead to the mortality seen in this patient set.

Gastric Variceal Bleeding

No specific measures are available to prevent first bleeding from gastric varices. Most of the current regimens to treat gastric varices are derived from anecdotal evidence or are extrapolated from trials of esophageal varices.[64,73] In a recent randomized controlled trial, endoscopic ablation with cyanoacrylate proved more effective and safer than band ligation in the management of bleeding gastric varices.[74] However, cerebral emboli have been reported with the tissue adhesives, and the interest has therefore been focused on locally administered thrombin, which provides good hemostasis. TIPS is recommended earlier in the management of gastric varices, as the rate of rebleeding after endoscopic treatment is high. TIPS is very effective, with a success rate of 90% for initial hemostasis. The rate of early rebleeding after TIPS is 20% and often the source of such bleeding is nonvariceal, that is, sclerosis or ulcer secondary to banding.[65,66]

Acute Variceal Bleeding

Patients suspected of acute variceal bleeding should be managed in the intensive care setting. General principles of resuscitation should be followed and include protection of airway, insertion of two large-bore intravenous cannulas, blood volume resuscitation with packed erythrocytes, correction of coagulopathy with fresh-frozen plasma, and platelet transfusion if platelet levels are less than 30,000/mm³. Care must be taken not to overexpand the plasma volume, which may increase portal pressure and result in exacerbation of variceal bleeding and ascites.[56,75] Antibiotics should be administered prophylactically, especially in patients with ascites, to prevent spontaneous bacterial peritonitis.[68,76] Emergency endoscopy of the upper gastrointestinal tract can then be performed, and the most appropriate treatment modality should be chosen at that point.

Pharmacotherapy. The drug classes that have been extensively studied in acute variceal bleeding are vasopressin and somatostatin and their analogues. Both somatostatin and vasopressin cause splanchnic vasoconstriction and thereby decrease the portal pressure and the portal blood flow.

Vasopressin and Terlipressin. The efficacy of intravenous vasopressin has been shown in several studies.[64]

Variceal bleeding is arrested but mortality is not reduced.[73] Side effects range from 32% to 64% in various randomized controlled trials, often resulting in cessation of therapy. The most significant complications arise from coronary artery vasoconstriction, leading to myocardial infarction and arrhythmias. Bowel ischemia, cerebrovascular ischemia, and peripheral tissue necrosis have been reported. The severity of complications has led to a virtual discontinuation of this pharmacological regimen.[64] Hyponatremia secondary to antidiuresis has also been reported with vasopressin therapy. To avoid these complications, the combination of vasopressin and nitroglycerin should be used in this clinical setting.

Terlipressin is a longer acting analogue of vasopressin and can be given as bolus infusion every 4 hours. Its efficacy is similar to vasopressin in controlling the acute variceal bleeding and is associated with fewer side effects.[77] The ease of administration has allowed for paramedic administration in the field with arrest of bleeding prior to arrival at the hospital. Unfortunately, terlipressin is not approved for use in the United States.

Somatostatin and Its Analogues. Somatostatin is superior to vasopressin for immediate control of bleeding and has less frequent and less severe side effects than vasopressin, although survival benefit has not been seen with somatostatin.[73] Somatostatin and its analogues can be dosed without concern for arterial vasoconstriction. The complications of vasopressin are virtually never seen with somatostatin use and adjuvant administration of nitroglycerin. Somatostatin is usually given as an initial intravenous bolus of 250 µg followed by a continuous intravenous infusion of 250 to 500 µg per hour. Octreotide is a synthetic analogue of somatostatin. When compared with other vasoactive drugs, octreotide was better than vasopressin and equivalent to terlipressin for controlling bleeding. The side effects were less frequent and less severe with octreotide than with either vasopressin or terlipressin. It is administered intravenously as a continuous infusion of 50 µg per hour for 5 days. The efficacy of octreotide as a single therapy is controversial. Results from a recent meta-analysis suggest that octreotide may improve the results of endoscopic therapy but has no or little effect if used alone.[73]

Endoscopic Therapy. Endoscopic sclerotherapy controls active hemorrhage in 80% to 90% of the patients. However, a skilled endoscopist must be readily available, and the procedure is associated with serious complications in 10% to 20% of patients, with an overall mortality of 2%.[73] The combination of sclerotherapy with somatostatin, octreotide,[78] and vapreotide[79] has been reported to be superior to sclerotherapy alone in terms of control of bleeding and reduction of treatment failures within 5 days.[64] The 6-week survival of the combination of sclerotherapy and drugs was similar to sclerotherapy alone.

Endoscopic band ligation of varices was shown to be better than endoscopic sclerotherapy in controlling the acute bleeding episode and mortality.[80] However, it is limited in the emergency setting because banding may be more challenging during active bleeding. This is felt to be due to reductions in the field of view by as much as 30% when the banding device is attached. The application of emergency tissue adhesive following endoscopic management of esophageal varices is not advantageous over sclerotherapy or band ligation. It was associated with a higher incidence of complications in one study.[80] The choice of procedure depends on the available expertise in the center managing the patient.

Balloon Tamponade. Balloon tamponade is a useful temporary measure to control acute variceal bleeding and to stabilize the patient while more definitive procedures are being planned. Control of bleeding is successful in as many as 80% to 90% of cases, but rebleeding occurs in up to 50% when the balloon or balloons are deflated. Furthermore, significant perforation risk is present, which may lead to high mortality if the balloons are inflated for prolonged periods.[56]

Transjugular Intrahepatic Portosystemic Shunt and Shunt Surgery. In the 10% of patients in whom rebleeding cannot be controlled with two endoscopic therapeutic sessions within 24 hours, either surgery or TIPS should be planned. Shunt surgery should be considered in patients with Child's class A cirrhosis.[56] TIPS could be used in patients with Child's class B or C cirrhosis as a salvage therapy and preferably as a bridge to LT.[66] Worsening of hepatic encephalopathy after the TIPS procedure may impair the outcome.

Ascites

Ascites is the most common major complication of portal hypertension. Although the development of ascites is usually indicative of advanced liver disease, the clinical course of patients with cirrhosis and ascites is highly variable. The initial evaluation of a patient with ascites should include a history, physical evaluation, and abdominal paracentesis with ascitic fluid analysis. Bleeding is sufficiently uncommon to preclude the need for prophylactic fresh-frozen plasma or platelets prior to a diagnostic paracentesis.[81] The initial ascitic fluid analysis should include a cell count and differential and serum:ascites albumin gradient. The culture yield increases to 80% when ascitic fluid with polymorphonuclear count greater than 250 cells/mm³ is inoculated into blood culture bottles at bedside.[82-84]

The mainstay of treatment of patients with ascites includes education regarding dietary sodium restriction (2000 mg/day or 88 mmol/day) and oral diuretic therapy.[85] Fluid loss and weight changes are directly related to sodium balance in patients with portal hypertension–related ascites. Primary emphasis should be placed on sodium restriction and not fluid restriction. The measurement of urinary sodium excretion is a helpful parameter to follow in these patients.[86] The nonurinary sodium loss in afebrile cirrhotic patients is less than 10 mmol/day.[87] One of the goals of treatment is to increase the urinary excretion of sodium so that it is greater than 78 mmol/day (total daily sodium intake – nonurinary sodium excretion).[88]

Chronic hyponatremia is commonly seen in cirrhotic patients and is seldom morbid. Rapid attempts to correct hyponatremia can lead to more complications than can the hyponatremia itself. Severe hyponatremia (serum sodium <120 mmol/L) requires fluid restriction in cirrhotic patients with ascites. **Note**: Rapid correction of hyponatremia of 120 mmol/L or less results in a significant risk of central pontine myelinolysis. These patients need to be treated with utmost care. Cirrhotic patients do not usually have symptoms from hyponatremia until their sodium levels fall to less than 110 mmol/L, or unless the decline in sodium is very rapid. Recently, Gerbes and colleagues showed that VPA-985, an orally active vasopressin V2 receptor antagonist, can correct severe hyponatremia in patients with cirrhosis and ascites.[89]

The usual diuretic therapy consists of single morning doses of oral spironolactone and furosemide, beginning with 100 mg of the former and 40 mg of the latter.[85] Previously, single-agent spironolactone was advocated, but hyperkalemia and the long half-life of this drug have resulted in its use as a single agent only in patients with minimal fluid overload.[90,91] A randomized controlled trial revealed a 2-week interval before the onset of action of single-agent spironolactone.[91] Single-agent furosemide has been shown to be less efficacious than spironolactone in a randomized controlled trial.[92] The dose of both oral diuretics can be increased simultaneously, maintaining the 100 mg:40 mg ratio, with a maximum of 400 mg/day:160mg/day, if weight loss and natriuresis are inadequate on lower doses. In general, this ratio maintains normokalemia. Furosemide can be temporarily withheld in patients presenting with hypokalemia. Single morning dosing tends to increase compliance and is recommended. The antiandrogenic effects of spironolactone such as decreased libido, impotence, and gynecomastia in men require dose reduction or discontinuation of the medicine. Amiloride can be substituted for spironolactone, but it is more expensive and has been shown to be less effective in a randomized controlled trial.[93] The cause of nocturnal muscle cramps is not well understood and may respond to magnesium supplementation or the oral administration of quinine sulfate at a dose of 325 mg in the evening.[94,95]

Dietary sodium restriction and a dual diuretic regimen have been shown to be effective in 90% of patients in the largest, multicenter, randomized controlled trial performed in patients with ascites.[96] Encephalopathy, serum sodium less than 120 mmol/day despite fluid restriction, and serum creatinine greater than 2.0 mg/dL should result in the cessation of diuretic therapy, the reassessment of the situation, and the consideration of second-line options. These patients should be monitored for daily weight, orthostatic symptoms, and serum electrolyte, blood urea nitrogen (BUN), and creatinine levels. Random urine sodium concentration is measured if the weight loss is inadequate. The frequency of follow-up is determined by response to treatment and by patient stability.

Refractory Ascites. Refractory ascites is defined as ascites that is nonresponsive to a sodium-restricted diet and high-dose diuretic treatment in the absence of prostaglandin inhibitors such as nonsteroidal anti-inflammatory drugs.[97] Serial therapeutic paracentesis is effective in controlling ascites, a fact known since the time of the ancient Greeks. Serial therapeutic paracentesis should be performed as needed, approximately every 2 weeks. The postparacentesis albumin infusion is expensive and has not been proved to be necessary for paracentesis of less than 5 L. For larger volume paracentesis, an albumin infusion of 5 to 8 g/L of ascitic fluid removed can be considered.[88]

Peritoneovenous Shunt. LeVeen or Denver shunts were popularized in the 1970s as a physiological treatment of ascites. Shunt placement has been shown in controlled trials to decrease the duration of hospitalization, the number of hospitalizations, and the dose of diuretics.[96,98] However, their poor long-term patency, significant complication profile, and lack of survival advantage compared with medical therapy in controlled trials have led to near abandonment of these devices.[96,98] Shunt-related fibrous adhesions and even fibrous cocoon formation can make subsequent liver transplantation difficult.[99] **Note:** If the shunt is patent, it is *mandatory* to occlude the shunt surgically before entering the abdomen during the transplant procedure to avoid massive air emboli.

Transjugular Intrahepatic Portosystemic Stent. The transjugular intrahepatic portosystemic stent that is placed by an interventional radiologist is physiologically equivalent to the side-to-side portocaval shunt.[100] A randomized controlled trial has reported higher mortality in a TIPS group compared with a medically treated group.[101] The results from the North American Study for the Treatment of Refractory Ascites (NASTRA) showed that TIPS is substantially superior to conventional medical therapy for ascites but does not improve the survival or quality of life.[102]

Spontaneous Bacterial Peritonitis

Spontaneous bacterial peritonitis (SBP) is a particularly important complication because the presence of infection usually removes a patient from consideration for transplantation until the infection is cleared. A diagnostic abdominal paracentesis must be performed and the ascitic fluid analyzed for cell count and bacteria before a confident diagnosis of ascitic fluid infection can be made. The diagnosis is made when there are more than 250 polymorphonuclear (PMN) cells present and/or a positive ascitic fluid bacterial culture without an evident intra-abdominal or surgically correctable source.[103,104] These patients should receive empirical treatment with broad-spectrum antibiotics.[104] Delaying treatment until the ascitic fluid culture grows bacteria may result in the patient's death from overwhelming infection. Cefotaxime, a third-generation cephalosporin, was superior to ampicillin in combination with tobramycin in a controlled trial.[105] A randomized, controlled trial involving 100 patients reported that 5 days of treatment was as efficacious as 10 days of treatment in the treatment of carefully characterized patients with SBP.[106] Patients with fewer than 250 PMN cells in ascitic fluid and signs or symptoms of infection should also receive empirical antibiotic therapy.[88,104] In a randomized, controlled trial, oral ofloxacin has been reported to be as effective as parenteral cefotaxime in the treatment of SBP in patients who are not vomiting and are not in shock.[107] Repeat paracentesis should be performed to document a culture's sterility and decrease in PMN count in patients with SBP; this step is particularly important when clinical improvement is not apparent after the first 3 days of antibiotic therapy.[108]

Short-term inpatient quinolone should be considered in the prevention of bacterial infections in patients with low protein (<1 g/dL) ascites, variceal hemorrhage, and prior SBP. Long-term outpatient antibiotic use probably can be reserved for patients who have survived an SBP infection.[88,108]

Hepatic Encephalopathy

Hepatic encephalopathy may be defined as a disturbance in central nervous system function because of hepatic insufficiency. This broad definition reflects the existence of a spectrum of neuropsychiatric manifestations related to a normal range of pathophysiological mechanisms. These manifestations are present in acute as well as chronic liver failure and are potentially reversible. Short-term memory loss, lack of concentration, sleep cycle reversal, and irritability in the early stages can profoundly affect the activities of daily living; more advanced disease with lethargy, stupor, or coma necessitates hospitalization and may be life-threatening.

Medical management by the primary care giver is of the utmost importance in improving the quality of life, as well as to reverse a potentially life-threatening condition. Most theories explaining the pathogenesis of hepatic encephalopathy accept that nitrogenous substances derived from the gut adversely affect brain function. These compounds gain access to the systemic circulation as a result of decreased hepatic function or portosystemic shunts.[109] Once in the brain tissues, they produce alterations of neurotransmission that affect consciousness and behavior. Abnormalities in glutamatergic, serotoninergic, γ-aminobutyric acidergic (GABAergic), and catecholamine pathways, among others, have been described in experimental hepatic encephalopathy.[109] A large body of work points toward ammonia as a key factor in the pathogenesis of hepatic encephalopathy.[110] In acute and chronic liver disease, increased arterial levels of ammonia are commonly seen. In fulminant liver failure, elevated arterial levels (>200 mg/dL of ammonia) are associated with an increased risk of cerebral herniation.[111] However, correlation of blood levels with mental state in cirrhosis is often inaccurate.

The approach to hepatic encephalopathy has not changed significantly in recent years. The suspicion of hepatic encephalopathy in patients with chronic liver disease should prompt the search for the precipitating factors and the other causes of change in mental status. The common precipitating factors include gastrointestinal bleeding, electrolyte abnormalities, renal failure, infection, recent placement of a TIPS[112] and use of sedatives/hypnotics, development of hepatocellular carcinoma, and constipation. Other less likely causes of altered mental status, such as an intracranial bleed or masses, hypoglycemia, and a postictal state, should also be considered. Hepatic encephalopathy is the diagnosis of exclusion and is mainly clinical. Although hyperammonemia is associated with hepatic encephalopathy, ammonia levels do not correlate with the level of encephalopathy. An electroencephalogram may be helpful in advanced stages to avoid erroneous diagnosis.

Treatment Goals. The treatment goals for hepatic encephalopathy are provision of supportive care, identification and removal of precipitating factors, and reduction of nitrogenous load from the gut. Ultimately, assessment of the need for long-term therapy is very important.[113] Patients presenting with new onset or worsening of hepatic encephalopathy should be evaluated for dehydration, variceal bleeding, spontaneous bacterial peritonitis, and renal insufficiency. Besides these, other causes of acute change in mental status such as intracranial bleeding, a mass, drug toxicity, systemic infection, or aberrant electrolyte levels should be ruled out.

Nutritional Management. The increased catabolic rate of cirrhosis leads to a recommendation of 1 to 1.5 g protein/kg per day.[113] Zinc, a cofactor of urea cycle enzymes, may be deficient in cirrhotic patients, especially if associated with malnutrition. Zinc supplementation improves the activity of the urea cycle in experimental models of cirrhosis.[114] One trial has evaluated the effects of zinc over a short period (up to 1 week), without major improvement.[115] A positive study administered zinc for 3 months, although the study was not randomized.[116] Zinc deficiency precipitated encephalopathy in a well-described patient.[117] Patients with zinc deficiency should receive oral zinc supplements (see Chapter 34, "Management of Portal Hypertensive Hemorrhage in the Era of Liver Transplantation").[113]

Ammonia-Lowering Strategy. Nonabsorbable disaccharides such as lactulose are routinely used to decrease ammonia production in the gut. Lactulose increases the fecal nitrogen excretion by facilitation of the incorporation of ammonia into bacteria as well as by a cathartic effect.[118] Lactulose administered orally reaches the cecum, where it is metabolized by the enteric bacteria, causing a fall in pH.[119] This drop in pH leads to a metabolic shift in bacteria favoring uptake of ammonia. The dose is adjusted to produce two or three soft bowel movements daily.[118] Antibiotics such as neomycin are also useful for lowering blood ammonia, mainly by an effect on ammonia production by intestinal bacteria. However, neomycin therapy is associated with significant toxic side effects.[118]

An alternative strategy for lowering blood ammonia levels is the stimulation of ammonia fixation.[120] Under normal physiological conditions, ammonia is removed by the formation of urea in periportal hepatocytes and by glutamine synthesis in perivenous hepatocytes, skeletal muscle, and brain. In cirrhosis, urea cycle enzymes and glutamine synthetase activity are decreased in the liver. Strategies to stimulate residual urea cycle activities and/or glutamine synthesis have been tried over the last 20 years. One of the most successful agents to be used so far is L-ornithine–L-aspartate (OA). Randomized controlled clinical trials with OA demonstrate significant lowering of ammonia levels and concomitant improvement in psychometric testing.[121]

Benzoate is also effective in reducing blood ammonia levels, both in patients with inherited urea cycle disorders and in cirrhotic patients.[120] In a randomized, controlled clinical trial with sodium benzoate versus lactulose, improvement in neuropsychiatric performance was found to be comparable.[122]

Use of Central Nervous System–Acting Drugs. Several controlled clinical trials have been performed to assess the efficacy of the benzodiazepine receptor antagonist flumazenil in cirrhotic patients with various degrees of severity of hepatic encephalopathy.[120] Spectacular improvements in neuropsychiatric status were recorded in a subset of patients receiving flumazenil.[123,124] However, the possible confounding effects of prior exposure to benzodiazepines and lack of correlation between the clinical response and blood levels of substances have tempered enthusiasm for this approach with benzodiazepine receptor antagonists in these patients.[125]

Renal Insufficiency and Hepatorenal Syndrome

Acute renal failure is thought to be common in patients with cirrhosis,[126] but its exact incidence is variable. Patients with cirrhosis are predisposed to acute renal failure following complications such as variceal bleeding or administration of nephrotoxic drugs such as nonsteroidal anti-inflammatory drugs, antibiotics, and diltiazem. The cause of renal insufficiency could be prerenal, intrarenal, or hepatorenal. The management of renal insufficiency in patients awaiting liver transplantation focuses on prevention of additional injury and optimization of existing renal function. Accurate assessment of baseline renal function is imperative during the initial workup. The serum creatinine measurements may not accurately reflect the underlying renal function because muscle mass is frequently depleted in cirrhotic patients. Glomerular filtration rates using iothalamate are more accurate. Once the baseline renal function is established, additional insults should be avoided. Careful attention must be paid to volume status, which is frequently tenuous in patients with marked ascites on high-dose diuretic therapy. Nonsteroidal anti-inflammatory drugs should be used only with close follow-up because the subsequent decrease in renal prostaglandin may precipitate acute renal failure. Radiographic imaging studies using intravenous contrast dye also need to be approached with caution because of the known risk of renal injury. The use of acetylcysteine together with hydration is the treatment of choice to protect against radiographic contrast media–induced nephropathy.[127] Large-volume paracentesis followed by intravenous albumin infusion decreases the risk of acute renal failure after the paracentesis.[88] The results of albumin use in this clinical setting are better than other volume expanders such as dextran.[128,129]

Moreover, patients with cirrhosis develop a specific acute renal failure called hepatorenal syndrome (HRS). It is a diagnosis of exclusion (Table 32–2). HRS is an ominous complication of end-stage liver disease. Retrospective studies indicate that HRS is present in approximately 17% of patients admitted to the hospital with ascites and in more than 50% of cirrhotics who die of liver failure. The hallmarks of HRS are reversible renal constriction and mild systemic hypotension.[130,131] The kidneys are structurally normal and at least in the early part of the syndrome, tubular function is intact, as reflected by avid sodium retention and oliguria.[130,131]

Table 32–2. DIAGNOSTIC CRITERIA FOR HEPATORENAL SYNDROME ACCORDING TO THE INTERNATIONAL ASCITES CLUB

Major Criteria*

- Low glomerular filtration rate, indicated by serum creatinine level greater than 1.5 mg/dL or 24-hour creatinine clearance less than 40 mL/min
- Absence of shock, ongoing bacterial infection, fluid loss, and current management with nephrotoxic drugs
- No sustained improvement in renal function (decrease in serum creatinine to 1.5 mg/dL or less or increase in creatinine clearance to 40 mL/min or more) following diuretic withdrawal and expansion of plasma volume with 1.5 L of a plasma expander
- Proteinuria less than 500 mg/day and no ultrasonographic evidence of obstructive or parenchymal renal disease

Additional Criteria

- Urine volume less than 500 mL/d
- Urine sodium less than 10 mEq/L
- Urine osmolality greater than plasma osmolality
- Fewer than 50 urine red blood cells per high power field
- Serum sodium concentration less than 130 mEq/L

*Only major criteria are necessary for the diagnosis of hepatorenal syndrome.

From Arroyo V, Gines P, Gerbes AL, et al: Definition and diagnostic criteria of refractory ascites and hepatorenal syndrome in cirrhosis. International Ascites Club. Hepatology 23:164-176, 1996.

The cause of renal vasoconstriction is unknown but may involve both increased vasoconstrictor and decreased vasodilator factors predominantly involved in its pathogenesis.[130,131] Two patterns of HRS are observed in clinical practice: type 1 and type 2. Type 1 HRS is an acute form of HRS in severe liver disease and is progressive. It is associated with poor prognosis, with 80% mortality in 2 weeks. Type 2 HRS occurs in patients with diuretic-resistant ascites. The course of renal failure is slow. It is also associated with poor prognosis, although the survival time is longer than that of patients with type 1 HRS. Table 32–2 summarizes the definition of HRS proposed by the International Ascites Club.[97]

Although the best treatment for HRS is liver transplantation, patients with HRS who undergo the transplantation procedure have more complications and a higher in-hospital mortality rate than those without HRS.[132] It has been suggested that systemic vasoconstrictor therapy may improve renal function in patients with HRS by increasing the effective arterial blood volume.[133] A nonrandomized retrospective study in a large series of patients with HRS suggests that the vasopressin analogue, terlipressin, is effective in the treatment of renal failure.[134] Other nonrandomized studies suggest that vasoconstrictive therapy with noradrenaline[135] or midodrine (combined with octreotide)[136] may improve renal function in these patients. One prospective nonrandomized trial showed that terlipressin reversed the HRS in a high proportion of patients, and the addition of albumin to terlipressin therapy markedly improved the beneficial effect of terlipressin.[137] Conversely, a randomized study in a small series of patients, comparing the molecular adsorbent recirculating system (MARS) (eventually combined with intermittent venovenous hemofiltration) and intermittent venovenous hemofiltration alone, suggested that MARS may improve survival in HRS.[138] Nonrandomized studies suggested that the TIPS may improve renal function with HRS.[39]

Hepatopulmonary Syndrome and Other Pulmonary Complications

The hepatopulmonary syndrome (HPS) is defined as pulmonary gas exchange abnormalities leading to arterial deoxygenation and widespread pulmonary vascular dilatation, which is more commonly associated with cirrhosis.[140,141] Pulmonary features include digital clubbing, cyanosis, dyspnea, platypnea, and orthodeoxia: the last two are defined as dyspnea and arterial deoxygenation induced by upright position and relieved by recumbency.[142]

Transplantation candidates with hypoxemia should be screened for HPS because the syndrome appears to resolve after OLT.[143,144] Resolution of portopulmonary hypertension has been reported only in highly selected patients after LT.[145,146]

A diagnosis of HPS is established when three criteria are fulfilled.[147] First, chronic liver disease, usually complicated by portal hypertension, must be present. Second, arterial hypoxemia, defined by reduced partial pressure of arterial oxygen (Pao_2) or more accurately by an increased alveolar-arterial difference in the partial pressure of oxygen ($[A-a]Do_2$), must be observed. The latter includes determination of the partial pressure of arterial carbon dioxide ($Paco_2$), which is often low in cirrhotic patients as a result of hyperventilation. Last, the intrapulmonary vascular dilatation detected either by two-dimensional contrast echocardiography or macroaggregated albumin lung perfusion scanning must be documented. Efforts have to be made to rule out intrapulmonic shunting.[147]

Pharmacological approaches have been disappointing in providing consistent and reproducible improvement in hypoxemia associated with HPS.[148] The largest clinical trials have involved the open-label use of vascular mediators such as almitrine bismesylate, somatostatin analogues, and garlic preparations.[148-150]

Except for garlic, marked improvement in Pao_2 could not be consistently demonstrated in these studies.[151]

TIPS performed to improve hypoxemia because of HPS remains controversial and cannot be advised without further prospective study.[152,153] Coil embolotherapy to occlude discrete arteriovenous communications in a patient with severe hypoxemia has resulted in significant improvement in Pao_2 in two adults.[154] Embolotherapy is an accepted approach to the management of severe hypoxemia associated with discrete arteriovenous malformation.[155]

HPS is now an indication for LT per pediatric and adult UNOS criteria.[156,157] Pretransplantation risk factors for increased mortality are Pao_2 less than 50 mm Hg and technetium-99m macroaggregated albumin (^{99m}Tc MAA) brain uptake greater than 20%.[144] Complete resolution, even in the setting of severe hypoxemia, is well documented.[144]

Hepatic Hydrothorax

Hepatic hydrothorax is defined as the accumulation of fluid in the pleural space as a consequence of liver disease.[158] The most common symptom is dyspnea without chest pain. It can be detected with chest radiographs in as many as 13% of patients with cirrhosis.[157] Right-sided pleural effusion is seen in 66% of patients with hepatic hydrothorax.[158]

The management options for hepatic hydrothorax include medical management of ascites and therapeutic paracentesis for the control of shortness of breath.[158] Pleurodesis with chemical means such as talc, antibiotics, or chemotherapeutic agents usually fails. TIPS has been used successfully to manage the symptoms of hepatic hydrothorax in the setting of marked ascites.[159,160] Pleural to peritoneal and peritoneal to central venous shunts are associated with complications such as infection, disseminated intravascular coagulation, and failure to resolve effusions.[158] Videothoracoscopy with the repair of presumed diaphragmatic defect has been described in the literature.

Pruritus

Pruritus is a common symptom of chronic cholestatic liver diseases, particularly PBC.[161] First-line treatment is cholestyramine, an anion exchange resin. It should be administered at least 4 hours before or after taking the other medications because it binds many drugs.[162] Side effects include bloating, constipation, and sometimes diarrhea. Second-line treatment is rifampin.[163] The mechanism of action is unclear, but it is effective in controlling pruritus in 50% of patients with PBC.[163]

The dosage is 150 mg twice a day and it is effective within 6 weeks of therapy.[163] The drug should be taken regularly for the effectiveness of treatment. These patients should be monitored closely for the possibility of drug hepatotoxicity.

Several studies have demonstrated the effectiveness of opioid receptor antagonists (nalmefene, naloxone, and naltrexone) in the control of pruritus.[164,165] The major side effects are the symptoms of opioid withdrawal. The treatment should be started slowly, preferably in a hospital setting.

Osteopenia and Osteoporosis

Osteoporosis and fractures are more common in cirrhotics than in the general population in the absence of confounding risk factors such as female sex, cholestasis, and excess alcohol.[166,167] The role of calcium and vitamin D in preventing osteoporosis is unclear. In a cross-sectional study of 55 patients who were taking adequate dietary calcium and vitamin D, or who were given supplementation if levels of these substances were deficient, the mean bone mineral densitometry (BMD) was 8% lower than in age- and sex-matched controls.[168] In another retrospective study in PBC, vitamin D and calcium supplementation did not lead to significant increase in BMD over baseline in the treated group.[169] In the absence of larger studies on the effect of vitamin D supplementation on BMD, it seems reasonable to recommend correction of vitamin D deficiency with an oral daily dose of 800 IU of vitamin D, and 1 to 2 g of elemental calcium supplementation. According to recently published guidelines on the management of osteoporosis associated with chronic liver disease, patients with cirrhosis or severe cholestasis should have a baseline BMD.[34] If the T score is more than −1.5 or between −1.5 and −2.5, no treatment is recommended. These patients should be followed up with BMD every 2 years.[34] The workup for patients with a BMD less than −2.5 should include thyroid function tests and serum calcium, phosphate, estradiol, follicle-stimulating hormone, leuteinizing hormone, testosterone, and sex hormone-binding globulin (SHBG) levels.[34] The optimal duration of therapy has not been established. The current recommendation is that the treatment should be given for a minimum of 5 years and the BMD repeated after 2 years and at the end of treatment.[34] In women, hormone replacement therapy (HRT) with estrogen and progesterone should be offered to premenopausal females. For men, transdermal testosterone can be given to hypogonadal men after a discussion of theoretical risks of hepatocellular carcinoma. The treatment recommendation for patients unable to take HRT/testosterone or who are eugonadal is bisphosphonates. Calcitriol or calcitonin should be considered in patients with osteoporosis who are either intolerant of HRT and bisphosphonates or whose BMD worsens despite either the use of bisphosphonates or treatment of hypogonadism.[34]

Psychosocial Issues and Depression

Cirrhotic patients listed for LT have a poor quality of life and a low level of perceived well-being. They have severe psychopathological distress arising from the fear of waiting for a transplant and the awareness of the scarcity of allografts, the potential for deterioration that will render them unqualified for transplantation, and death. The patients and their families should be encouraged to go to support group meetings to cope with the stress and to talk about their experience. DeBona and colleagues showed that all post-LT patients had improved perceived quality of life as evident by quality-of-life scale scores when compared with the patients listed for LT.[170]

High rates of depression have been demonstrated in patients with advanced liver disease. In one study, the incidence of depression in cirrhotics was as high as 63%.[171] The depressed patients had significantly worse adaptive coping, poorer perceived quality of life, and greater perception of bodily pain suggesting that depression is of considerable clinical consequence and adversely affects well-being and functioning of such patients. End-stage liver disease patients should be routinely screened for depression, and early treatment with a selective serotonin reuptake inhibitor (SSRI) should be instituted.

The majority of cirrhotic patients usually have a history of alcohol abuse and substance abuse. The physicians should reinforce the importance of support groups and abstinence from alcohol and abusive drugs to these patients. Random urine drug screen should be done periodically in these patients (see Chapter 28, "Pretransplant Evaluation: Pulmonary, Cardiac, and Renal").

Nutrition

Malnutrition is one of the most unrecognized problems of patients with end-stage liver disease awaiting LT. The prevalence of malnutrition in liver disease is difficult to assess because of the lack of a standardized diagnosis and classification of malnutrition in this population. Fluid retention and the fact that the plasma levels of most visceral proteins reflect both poor liver function and nutritional reserve complicate nutritional assessment in cirrhosis. Some physicians consider protein calorie malnutrition (PCM) to be the most common complication in patients with cirrhosis.[172] The prevalence of PCM differs according to the cause. It has been described in 20% of the patients with compensated cirrhosis, and the incidence rises to 60% in patients with liver insufficiency.[173] The pathogenesis of malnutrition in cirrhosis is unclear. An interesting hypothesis was proposed by Richardson and associates, who stated that hyperinsulinemia in cirrhosis may cause a preference for carbohydrates, consequently leading to early gastrointestinal satiety and reduction of intake.[174] Another hypothesis is that changes in substrate use with increased lipid oxidation and decreased carbohydrate oxidation, as well as increased energy expenditure, contribute to malnutrition in these patients. Although many patients are in a state of protein catabolism, these metabolic changes could not adequately explain malnutrition.[173] The metabolic changes revert back to normal within a few days after nutritional support is initiated.

Nutritional status is correlated to mortality in the total group of patients with cirrhosis and in Child's A and B patients if analyzed separately. Malnutrition is an independent predictor for the first bleeding episode and the survival of patients with esophageal varices. It is also associated with the presence of refractory ascites. Poor preoperative nutritional status is correlated to postoperative complications and mortality.[173]

Nutritional management of patients with liver disease can be a difficult task. Every effort should be made to prevent any period of prolonged fasting. To improve nitrogen economy and to avoid undue catabolism of muscle protein, patients should be encouraged to eat six to seven meals per day, including one late-night meal. This should prevent depletion of glycogen stores as well as diminish the loss of fat stores and lean body mass. If a patient has a reasonable appetite, 35 to 45 kcal/kg per day should be supplied, including 0.8 to 1 g/kg per day of protein. This may need to be modified for patients with protein intolerance caused by encephalopathy.

Micronutrient deficiency has been observed in 10% to 50% of patients with cirrhosis.[175] Fat-soluble vitamins may be deficient in patients with cholestatic diseases; additionally, a deficiency of water-soluble vitamins, vitamin B_{12}, and folic acid is more frequent in patients with alcoholic cirrhosis. Multivitamin supplements may be considered in these patients. Zinc deficiency is very common in cirrhotics.[175] This might be secondary to higher zinc loss in the urine. Supplementation with zinc has been shown to improve hepatic encephalopathy and with vitamin A improves the sense of taste and thereby may also improve the patient's dietary intake.[115]

Parenteral nutrition should be used as a second-line approach in those who cannot be fed adequately by the oral or enteral route. For the majority of patients, standard amino acids are recommended.[176] Solutions rich in branched-chain amino acids and low in aromatic acids and tryptophan should be used in patients with encephalopathy[177] and with appropriate caution

in those with acute liver failure (see Chapter 34, "Management of Portal Hypertensive Hemorrhage in the Era of Liver Transplantation").[176]

Table 32–3 summarizes what to consider in a systematic review of the patient.

Table 32-3. REVIEW OF THE PATIENT

System	Symptoms and Signs
Central nervous system	Confusion, memory loss, reversal of sleep cycle, altered mental status, narcotics and benzodiazepine use, seizures, mental status changes, asterixis, nystagmus, focal deficits
HEENT	Signs of frequent falls, icterus, pallor, malar flush
Skin and nails	Spider angiomata, pruritus, vasculitis, clubbing, cyanosis
Chest	Cough, dyspnea, platypnea, orthodeoxia
Cardiovascular	Chest pain, palpitations, signs of heart failure
Gastrointestinal	Abdominal pain, hematemesis, melena, constipation, tense ascites
Genitourinary	Signs of urinary tract infection, decreased urinary output, review of medications causing renal insufficiency
Musculoskeletal	Leg cramps, frequent falls, muscle wasting
Constitutional	Fatigue, weight loss, signs of dehydration, fever

HEENT, head, ears, eyes, nose, throat.

Pearls and Pitfalls

- As patients wait on the OLT list, the transplanting physician has more primary care responsibilities. Cirrhotic patients have other medical problems that must be addressed.

- Preventive screening for nonliver cancers is very important. Of particular interest in the OLT candidate pool are oropharyngeal squamous cell, cervical, colon, and skin cancers.

- Regular screening for coronary artery disease should be done in patients with cardiovascular risk factors such as older age, family history of premature coronary artery disease, smoking, diabetes, and history of hyperlipidemia.

- Patients should be monitored for smoking and alcohol cessation. Also, patients should be informed about seat belt use.

Pearls and Pitfalls—cont'd

- A purified protein derivative test should be performed. Tuberculosis can affect OLT candidates.

- Human immunodeficiency virus (HIV) testing and risk factors should be ascertained.

- Vaccination against HAV and HBV is cheap and can be a lifesaver. Advise your patients to get these vaccinations to prevent death from preventable hepatitis.

- Lamivudine therapy slows the rate of decompensation of patients who have HBV-related cirrhosis.

- Sudden discontinuation of oral antivirals against HBV (lamivudine, adefovir) in a patient with advanced liver disease may lead to rapid, life-threatening decompensation.

- If candidates have hemochromatosis, it is very important to decrease iron stores with phlebotomy to prevent cardiac, pancreatic, and pituitary involvement.

- PBC patients should be screened for osteopenia/osteoporosis and treated if the problem is diagnosed.

- Patients with ulcerative colitis and PSC may be at increased risk of colon cancer. Yearly screening should be performed if the patients still have colons.

- If β-blockers are started, baseline pulse decreases should be monitored; these drugs are poorly tolerated, but most frequently are underdosed by clinicians, and the primary care physician may not know what parameters to use.

- If a TIPS is placed, it *must* be followed. Also, ultrasound Doppler studies are usually insensitive to stenosis. If portal hypertension is apparent clinically, a direct angiographic check of TIPS should be instituted. In particular, attention must be paid to the spontaneous improvement of encephalopathy or presence of ascites or varices as clues that TIPS has failed.

- If large-volume paracentesis is performed or ordered, it must be ensured that the patient has orders for postprocedure albumin infusion. This will reduce the incidence of renal failure and hemodynamic compromise.

- Albumin decreases HRS if used while treatment for SBP is ongoing.

Pearls and Pitfalls—cont'd

- The taste of lactulose syrup may lead to poor compliance. The sugar is available in crystal form and many patients improve compliance if on this regimen.

References

1. OPTN/UNOS: Current waiting list for liver transplantation. Available at http://www.optn.org/latestdata/rptdata.asp Accessed March 3, 2003.
2. OPTN/UNOS: Liver transplantation by donor type from 1/1/1988 to 12/31/2002. Available at http://www.optn.org/latestdata/rptdata.asp Accessed March 3, 2003.
3. Kamath PS, Wiesner RH, Malinchoc M, et al: A model to predict survival in patients with end-stage liver disease. Hepatology 33:464-470, 2001.
4. McCaughan GW, Strasser SI: To MELD or not to MELD? Hepatology 34:215-216, 2001.
5. Wiesner RH, McDiarmid SV, Kamath PS, et al: MELD and PELD: Application of survival models to liver allocation. Liver Transpl 7:567-580, 2001.
6. Pagliaro L: MELD: The end of Child-Pugh classification? J Hepatol 36:141-142, 2002.
7. Malinchoc M, Kamath PS, Gordon FD, et al: A model to predict poor survival in patients undergoing transjugular intrahepatic portosystemic shunts. Hepatology 31:864-871, 2000.
8. Sheth M, Riggs M, Patel T: Utility of the Mayo End-Stage Liver Disease (MELD) score in assessing prognosis of patients with alcoholic hepatitis. BMC Gastroenterol 2:2, 2002.
9. Ryder SD: Guidelines for the diagnosis and treatment of hepatocellular carcinoma (HCC) in adults. Gut 52 (Suppl 3):1-8, 2003.
10. Vento S, Garofano T, Renzini C, et al: Fulminant hepatitis associated with hepatitis A virus superinfection in patients with chronic hepatitis C. N Engl J Med 338:286-290, 1998.
11. Berner J, Kadian M, Post J, et al: Prophylactic recombinant hepatitis B vaccine in patients undergoing orthotopic liver transplantation. Transplant Proc 25:1751-1752, 1993.
12. Perrillo RP, Bodicky C, Campbell C, Sanders GE: Response to hepatitis B virus vaccine in subjects with low levels of antibody to hepatitis B surface antigen. N Engl J Med 310:1463, 1984.
13. Kallinowski B, Benz C, Buchholz L, Stremmel W: Accelerated schedule of hepatitis B vaccination in liver transplant candidates. Transplant Proc 30:797-799, 1998.
14. United States Preventive Services Task Force: Guide to Clinical Preventive Services, 2nd ed. Agency for Health Care Research and Quality, Dept. of Health and Human Services, 1996. Available at http://www.ahrq.gov/clinic/uspstfix.htm Accessed April 11, 2003.
15. Perrillo RP, Wright T, Rakela J, et al: A multicenter United States–Canadian trial to assess lamivudine monotherapy before and after liver transplantation for chronic hepatitis B. Hepatology 33:424-432, 2001.
16. Fontana RJ, Hann HW, Perrillo RP, et al: Determinants of early mortality in patients with decompensated chronic hepatitis B treated with antiviral therapy. Gastroenterology 123:719-727, 2002.
17. Fontana RJ, Keeffe EB, Carey W, et al: Effect of lamivudine treatment on survival of 309 North American patients awaiting liver transplantation for chronic hepatitis B. Liver Transpl 8:433-439, 2002.

18. Dienstag JL, Schiff ER, Wright TL, et al: Lamivudine as initial treatment for chronic hepatitis B in the United States. N Engl J Med 341:1256-1263, 1999.

19. Nowak MA, Bonhoeffer S, Hill AM, et al: Viral dynamics in hepatitis B virus infection. Proc Natl Acad Sci U S A 93:4398-4402, 1996.

20. Lai CL, Chien RN, Leung NW, et al: A one-year trial of lamivudine for chronic hepatitis B. Asia Hepatitis Lamivudine Study Group. N Engl J Med 339:61-68, 1998.

21. Liaw YF, Leung NW, Chang TT, et al: Effects of extended lamivudine therapy in Asian patients with chronic hepatitis B. Asia Hepatitis Lamivudine Study Group. Gastroenterology 119:172-180, 2000.

22. Schalm SW, Heathcote J, Cianciara J, et al: Lamivudine and alpha interferon combination treatment of patients with chronic hepatitis B infection: A randomised trial. Gut 46:562-568, 2000.

23. Wright TL: Treatment of patients with hepatitis C and cirrhosis. Hepatology 36:S185-S194, 2002.

24. Fried MW, Shiffman ML, Reddy KR, et al: Peginterferon alfa-2a plus ribavirin for chronic hepatitis C virus infection. N Engl J Med 347:975-982, 2002.

25. Crippin JS: Motion—patients with primary sclerosing cholangitis should undergo early liver transplantation: Arguments against the motion. Can J Gastroenterol 16:700-702, 2002.

26. Tavill AS: Diagnosis and management of hemochromatosis. Hepatology 33:1321-1328, 2001.

27. Adams PC, Deugnier Y, Moirand R, Brissot P: The relationship between iron overload, clinical symptoms, and age in 410 patients with genetic hemochromatosis. Hepatology 25:162-166, 1997.

28. Niederau C, Fischer R, Purschel A, et al: Long-term survival in patients with hereditary hemochromatosis. Gastroenterology 110:1107-1119, 1996.

29. Heathcote EJ: Management of primary biliary cirrhosis. The American Association for the Study of Liver Diseases practice guidelines. Hepatology 31:1005-1013, 2000.

30. Poupon RE, Lindor KD, Cauch-Dudek K, et al: Combined analysis of randomized controlled trials of ursodeoxycholic acid in primary biliary cirrhosis. Gastroenterology 113:884-890, 1997.

31. Lindor KD, Jorgensen RA, Therneau TM, et al: Ursodeoxycholic acid delays the onset of esophageal varices in primary biliary cirrhosis. Mayo Clin Proc 72:1137-1140, 1997.

32. Hodgson SF, Dickson ER, Wahner HW, et al: Bone loss and reduced osteoblast function in primary biliary cirrhosis. Ann Intern Med 103:855-860, 1985.

33. Springer JE, Cole DE, Rubin LA, et al: Vitamin D–receptor genotypes as independent genetic predictors of decreased bone mineral density in primary biliary cirrhosis. Gastroenterology 118:145-151, 2000.

34. Collier JD, Ninkovic M, Compston JE: Guidelines on the management of osteoporosis associated with chronic liver disease. Gut 50 (Suppl 1):1-9, 2002.

35. Chapman RW: Risk factors for biliary tract carcinogenesis. Ann Oncol 10 Suppl 4:308-311, 1999.

36. Ramage JK, Donaghy A, Farrant JM, et al: Serum tumor markers for the diagnosis of cholangiocarcinoma in primary sclerosing cholangitis. Gastroenterology 108:865-869, 1995.

37. Patel AH, Harnois DM, Klee GG, et al: The utility of CA 19-9 in the diagnoses of cholangiocarcinoma in patients without primary sclerosing cholangitis. Am J Gastroenterol 95:204-207, 2000.

38. Hultcrantz R, Olsson R, Danielsson A, et al: A 3-year prospective study on serum tumor markers used for detecting cholangiocarcinoma in patients with primary sclerosing cholangitis. J Hepatol 30:669-673, 1999.

39. Lindor KD: Ursodiol for primary sclerosing cholangitis. Mayo Primary Sclerosing Cholangitis-Ursodeoxycholic Acid Study Group. N Engl J Med 336:691-695, 1997.

40. Stiehl A, Rudolph G, Kloters-Plachky P, et al: Development of dominant bile duct stenoses in patients with primary sclerosing cholangitis treated with ursodeoxycholic acid: Outcome after endoscopic treatment. J Hepatol 36:151-156, 2002.

41. Shetty K, Rybicki L, Brzezinski A, et al: The risk for cancer or dysplasia in ulcerative colitis patients with primary sclerosing cholangitis. Am J Gastroenterol 94:1643-1649, 1999.

42. Brentnall TA, Haggitt RC, Rabinovitch PS, et al: Risk and natural history of colonic neoplasia in patients with primary sclerosing cholangitis and ulcerative colitis. Gastroenterology 110:331-338, 1996.

43. Broome U, Lofberg R, Veress B, Eriksson LS: Primary sclerosing cholangitis and ulcerative colitis: Evidence for increased neoplastic potential. Hepatology 22:1404-1408, 1995.

44. Tung BY, Emond MJ, Haggitt RC, et al: Ursodiol use is associated with lower prevalence of colonic neoplasia in patients with ulcerative colitis and primary sclerosing cholangitis. Ann Intern Med 134:89-95, 2001.

45. Loftus EV Jr, Aguilar HI, Sandborn WJ, et al: Risk of colorectal neoplasia in patients with primary sclerosing cholangitis and ulcerative colitis following orthotopic liver transplantation. Hepatology 27:685-690, 1998.

46. Czaja AJ: Treatment of autoimmune hepatitis. Semin Liver Dis 22:365-378, 2002.

47. Jackson LD, Song E: Cyclosporin in the treatment of corticosteroid-resistant autoimmune chronic active hepatitis. Gut 36:459-461, 1995.

48. Pratt DS, Flavin DP, Kaplan MM: The successful treatment of autoimmune hepatitis with 6-mercaptopurine after failure with azathioprine. Gastroenterology 110:271-274, 1996.

49. Kanzler S, Gerken G, Dienes HP, et al: Cyclophosphamide as alternative immunosuppressive therapy for autoimmune hepatitis—report of three cases. Z Gastroenterol 35:571-578, 1997.

50. Richardson PD, James PD, Ryder SD: Mycophenolate mofetil for maintenance of remission in autoimmune hepatitis in patients resistant to or intolerant of azathioprine. J Hepatol 33:371-375, 2000.

51. Roberts LR, Kamath PS: Pathophysiology and treatment of variceal hemorrhage. Mayo Clin Proc 71:973-983, 1996.

52. Chalasani N, Kahi C, Francois F, et al: Improved patient survival after acute variceal bleeding: A multicenter, cohort study. Am J Gastroenterol 98:653-659, 2003.

53. Beppu K, Inokuchi K, Koyanagi N, et al: Prediction of variceal hemorrhage by esophageal endoscopy. Gastrointest Endosc 27:213-218, 1981.

54. D'Amico G, Luca A: Natural history. Clinical-haemodynamic correlations. Prediction of the risk of bleeding. Baillieres Clin Gastroenterol 11:243-256, 1997.

55. The North Italian Endoscopic Club for the Study and Treatment of Esophageal Varices: Prediction of the first variceal hemorrhage in patients with cirrhosis of the liver and esophageal varices. A prospective multicenter study. N Engl J Med 319:983-989, 1988.

56. Vargas HE, Gerber D, Abu-Elmagd K: Management of portal hypertension–related bleeding. Surg Clin North Am 79:1-22, 1999.

57. Conn HO, Grace ND, Bosch J, et al: Propranolol in the prevention of the first hemorrhage from esophagogastric varices: A multicenter, randomized clinical trial. The Boston-New Haven-Barcelona Portal Hypertension Study Group. Hepatology 13:902-912, 1991.

58. Feu F, Bordas JM, Luca A, et al: Reduction of variceal pressure by propranolol: Comparison of the effects on portal pressure and azygos blood flow in patients with cirrhosis. Hepatology 18:1082-1089, 1993.

59. Poynard T, Cales P, Pasta L, et al: Beta-adrenergic-antagonist drugs in the prevention of gastrointestinal bleeding in patients

with cirrhosis and esophageal varices. An analysis of data and prognostic factors in 589 patients from four randomized clinical trials. Franco-Italian Multicenter Study Group. N Engl J Med 324:1532-1538, 1991.

60. Garcia-Tsao G, Grace ND, Groszmann RJ, et al: Short-term effects of propranolol on portal venous pressure. Hepatology 6:101-106, 1986.

61. Garcia-Pagan JC, Feu F, Bosch J, Rodes J: Propranolol compared with propranolol plus isosorbide-5-mononitrate for portal hypertension in cirrhosis. A randomized controlled study. Ann Intern Med 114:869-873, 1991.

62. Fardy JM, Laupacis A: A meta-analysis of prophylactic endoscopic sclerotherapy for esophageal varices. Am J Gastroenterol 89:1938-1948, 1994.

63. Paquet KJ, Kalk JF, Klein CP, Gad HA: Prophylactic sclerotherapy for esophageal varices in high-risk cirrhotic patients selected by endoscopic and hemodynamic criteria: A randomized, single-center controlled trial. Endoscopy 26:734-740, 1994.

64. D'Amico G, Pagliaro L, Bosch J: The treatment of portal hypertension: A meta-analytic review. Hepatology 22:332-354, 1995.

65. Sarin SK, Lamba GS, Kumar M, et al: Comparison of endoscopic ligation and propranolol for the primary prevention of variceal bleeding. N Engl J Med 340:988-993, 1999.

66. Burroughs AK, Patch D: Transjugular intrahepatic portosystemic shunt. Semin Liver Dis 19:457-473, 1999.

67. Boyer TD, Vargas HE: Interventional imaging of the liver and biliary system: Transjugular intrahepatic portosystemic shunts. In Schiff ER, Sorrell MF, Maddrey WC (eds): Diseases of the Liver. Vol. 1. Philadelphia, Lippincott Williams & Wilkins, 2003, pp 369-382.

68. de Franchis R: Updating consensus in portal hypertension: Report of the Baveno III Consensus Workshop on definitions, methodology and therapeutic strategies in portal hypertension. J Hepatol 33:846-852, 2000.

69. Grace ND, Groszmann RJ, Garcia-Tsao G, et al: Portal hypertension and variceal bleeding: An AASLD single topic symposium. Hepatology 28:868-880, 1998.

70. Patch D, Sabin CA, Goulis J, et al: A randomized, controlled trial of medical therapy versus endoscopic ligation for the prevention of variceal rebleeding in patients with cirrhosis. Gastroenterology 123:1013-1019, 2002.

71. Lo GH, Chen WC, Chen MH, et al: Banding ligation versus nadolol and isosorbide mononitrate for the prevention of esophageal variceal rebleeding. Gastroenterology 123:728-734, 2002.

72. Bosch J, Garcia-Pagan JC: Prevention of variceal rebleeding. Lancet 361:952-954, 2003.

73. D'Amico G, Pagliaro L, Bosch J: Pharmacological treatment of portal hypertension: An evidence-based approach. Semin Liver Dis 19:475-505, 1999.

74. Lo GH, Lai KH, Cheng JS, et al: A prospective, randomized trial of butyl cyanoacrylate injection versus band ligation in the management of bleeding gastric varices. Hepatology 33:1060-1064, 2001.

75. Williams SG, Westaby D: Recent advances in the endoscopic management of variceal bleeding. Gut 36:647-648, 1995.

76. Bernard B, Grange JD, Khac EN, et al: Antibiotic prophylaxis for the prevention of bacterial infections in cirrhotic patients with gastrointestinal bleeding: A meta-analysis. Hepatology 29:1655-1661, 1999.

77. Bosch J, Lebrec D, Jenkins SA: Development of analogues: Successes and failures. Scand J Gastroenterol Suppl 226:3-13, 1998.

78. Besson I, Ingrand P, Person B, et al: Sclerotherapy with or without octreotide for acute variceal bleeding. N Engl J Med 333:555-560, 1995.

79. Cales P, Masliah C, Bernard B, et al: Early administration of vapreotide for variceal bleeding in patients with cirrhosis. French Club for the Study of Portal Hypertension. N Engl J Med 344: 23-28, 2001.

80. de Franchis R, Primignani M: Endoscopic treatments for portal hypertension. Semin Liver Dis 19:439-455, 1999.

81. Runyon BA: Paracentesis of ascitic fluid. A safe procedure. Arch Intern Med 146:2259-2261, 1986.

82. Runyon BA, Canawati HN, Akriviadis EA: Optimization of ascitic fluid culture technique. Gastroenterology 95:1351-1355, 1988.

83. Bobadilla M, Sifuentes J, Garcia-Tsao G: Improved method for bacteriological diagnosis of spontaneous bacterial peritonitis. J Clin Microbiol 27:2145-2147, 1989.

84. Castellote J, Xiol X, Verdaguer R, et al: Comparison of two ascitic fluid culture methods in cirrhotic patients with spontaneous bacterial peritonitis. Am J Gastroenterol 85:1605-1608, 1990.

85. Runyon BA: Care of patients with ascites. N Engl J Med 330: 337-342, 1994.

86. Eisenmenger WJ AE, Blondheim SH, Kunkel HG: The effect of rigid sodium restriction in patients with cirrhosis of the liver and ascites. J Lab Clin Med 34:1029-1038, 1949.

87. Eisenmenger WJ BS, Boniovanni AM, Kunkel HG: Electrolyte studies on patients with cirrhosis of the liver. J Clin Invest 29:1491-1499, 1950.

88. Runyon BA: Management of adult patients with ascites caused by cirrhosis. Hepatology 27:264-272, 1998.

89. Gerbes AL, Gulberg V, Gines P, et al: Therapy of hyponatremia in cirrhosis with a vasopressin receptor antagonist: A randomized double-blind multicenter trial. Gastroenterology 124:933-939, 2003.

90. Sungaila I, Bartle WR, Walker SE, et al: Spironolactone pharmacokinetics and pharmacodynamics in patients with cirrhotic ascites. Gastroenterology 102:1680-1685, 1992.

91. Fogel MR, Sawhney VK, Neal EA, et al: Diuresis in the ascitic patient: A randomized controlled trial of three regimens. J Clin Gastroenterol 3 (Suppl 1):73-80, 1981.

92. Perez-Ayuso RM, Arroyo V, Planas R, et al: Randomized comparative study of efficacy of furosemide versus spironolactone in nonazotemic cirrhosis with ascites. Relationship between the diuretic response and the activity of the renin-aldosterone system. Gastroenterology 84:961-968, 1983.

93. Angeli P, Dalla Pria M, De Bei E, et al: Randomized clinical study of the efficacy of amiloride and potassium canrenoate in nonazotemic cirrhotic patients with ascites. Hepatology 19:72-79, 1994.

94. Jansen PH, Veenhuizen KC, Wesseling AI, et al: Randomised controlled trial of hydroquinine in muscle cramps. Lancet 349:528-532, 1997.

95. Quinine and cramp: Uncertainty efficacy, major risks. Prescrire Int 9:154-157, 2000.

96. Stanley MM, Ochi S, Lee KK, et al: Peritoneovenous shunting as compared with medical treatment in patients with alcoholic cirrhosis and massive ascites. Veterans Administration Cooperative Study on Treatment of Alcoholic Cirrhosis with Ascites. N Engl J Med 321:1632-1638, 1989.

97. Arroyo V, Gines P, Gerbes AL, et al: Definition and diagnostic criteria of refractory ascites and hepatorenal syndrome in cirrhosis. International Ascites Club. Hepatology 23:164-176, 1996.

98. Gines P, Arroyo V, Vargas V, et al: Paracentesis with intravenous infusion of albumin as compared with peritoneovenous shunting in cirrhosis with refractory ascites. N Engl J Med 325:829-835, 1991.

99. Stanley MM, Reyes CV, Greenlee HB, et al: Peritoneal fibrosis in cirrhotics treated with peritoneovenous shunting for ascites. An autopsy study with clinical correlations. Dig Dis Sci 41:571-577, 1996.

100. Ochs A, Rossle M, Haag K, et al: The transjugular intrahepatic portosystemic stent-shunt procedure for refractory ascites. N Engl J Med 332:1192-1197, 1995.

101. Lebrec D, Giuily N, Hadengue A, et al: Transjugular intrahepatic portosystemic shunts: Comparison with paracentesis in patients with cirrhosis and refractory ascites: A randomized trial.

French Group of Clinicians and a Group of Biologists. J Hepatol 25:135-144, 1996.

102. Sanyal AJ, Genning C, Reddy KR, et al: The North American Study for the Treatment of Refractory Ascites. Gastroenterology 124:634-641, 2003.

103. Guarner C, Runyon BA: Spontaneous bacterial peritonitis: Pathogenesis, diagnosis, and management. Gastroenterologist 3:311-328, 1995.

104. Rimola A, Garcia-Tsao G, Navasa M, et al: Diagnosis, treatment and prophylaxis of spontaneous bacterial peritonitis: A consensus document. International Ascites Club. J Hepatol 32:142-153, 2000.

105. Felisart J, Rimola A, Arroyo V, et al: Cefotaxime is more effective than is ampicillin-tobramycin in cirrhotics with severe infections. Hepatology 5:457-462, 1985.

106. Runyon BA, McHutchison JG, Antillon MR, et al: Short-course versus long-course antibiotic treatment of spontaneous bacterial peritonitis. A randomized controlled study of 100 patients. Gastroenterology 100:1737-1742, 1991.

107. Navasa M, Follo A, Llovet JM, et al: Randomized, comparative study of oral ofloxacin versus intravenous cefotaxime in spontaneous bacterial peritonitis. Gastroenterology 111:1011-1017, 1996.

108. Garcia-Tsao G: Current management of the complications of cirrhosis and portal hypertension: Variceal hemorrhage, ascites, and spontaneous bacterial peritonitis. Gastroenterology 120:726-748, 2001.

109. Blei AT: Hepatic Encephalopathy. In Bircher J, Benhamou J-P, McIntyre N, et al (eds): Oxford Textbook of Clinical Hepatology. Oxford, UK, Oxford University Press, 1999, pp 765-786.

110. Norenberg MD: Astrocytic-ammonia interactions in hepatic encephalopathy. Semin Liver Dis 16:245-253, 1996.

111. Clemmesen JO, Larsen FS, Kondrup J, et al: Cerebral herniation in patients with acute liver failure is correlated with arterial ammonia concentration. Hepatology 29:648-653, 1999.

112. Blei AT: Hepatic encephalopathy in the age of TIPS. Hepatology 20:249-252, 1994.

113. Blei AT, Cordoba J: Hepatic encephalopathy. Am J Gastroenterol 96:1968-1976, 2001.

114. Riggio O, Merli M, Capocaccia L, et al: Zinc supplementation reduces blood ammonia and increases liver ornithine trans-carbamylase activity in experimental cirrhosis. Hepatology 16:785-789, 1992.

115. Riggio O, Ariosto F, Merli M, et al: Short-term oral zinc supplementation does not improve chronic hepatic encephalopathy. Results of a double-blind crossover trial. Dig Dis Sci 36:1204-1208, 1991.

116. Marchesini G, Fabbri A, Bianchi G, et al: Zinc supplementation and amino acid–nitrogen metabolism in patients with advanced cirrhosis. Hepatology 23:1084-1092, 1996.

117. Van der Rijt CC, Schalm SW, Schat H, et al: Overt hepatic encephalopathy precipitated by zinc deficiency. Gastroenterology 100:1114-1118, 1991.

118. Cordoba J, Blei AT: Treatment of hepatic encephalopathy. Am J Gastroenterol 92:1429-1439, 1997.

119. Brown RL, Gibson JA, Sladen GE, et al: Effects of lactulose and other laxatives on ileal and colonic pH as measured by a radiotelemetry device. Gut 15:999-1004, 1974.

120. Ferenci P, Herneth A, Steindl P: Newer approaches to therapy of hepatic encephalopathy. Semin Liver Dis 16:329-338, 1996.

121. Kircheis G, Nilius R, Held C, et al: Therapeutic efficacy of L-ornithine-L-aspartate infusions in patients with cirrhosis and hepatic encephalopathy: Results of a placebo-controlled, double-blind study. Hepatology 25:1351-1360, 1997.

122. Sushma S, Dasarathy S, Tandon RK, et al: Sodium benzoate in the treatment of acute hepatic encephalopathy: A double-blind randomized trial. Hepatology 16:138-144, 1992.

123. Gyr K, Meier R, Haussler J, et al: Evaluation of the efficacy and safety of flumazenil in the treatment of portal systemic encephalopathy: A double blind, randomised, placebo controlled multicentre study. Gut 39:319-324, 1996.

124. Pomier-Layrargues G, Giguere JF, Lavoie J, et al: Flumazenil in cirrhotic patients in hepatic coma: A randomized double-blind placebo-controlled crossover trial. Hepatology 19:32-37, 1994.

125. Butterworth RF, Wells J, Pomier Layragues G: Detection of benzodiazepines in hepatic encephalopathy: Reply. Hepatology 2:605, 1995.

126. Arroyo V, Fernandez-Esparrach G, Gines P: Diagnostic approach to the cirrhotic patient with ascites. J Hepatol 25 (Suppl 1): 35-40, 1996.

127. Tepel M, Zidek W: Acetylcysteine and contrast media nephropathy. Curr Opin Nephrol Hypertens 11:503-506, 2002.

128. Gines A, Fernandez-Esparrach G, Monescillo A, et al: Randomized trial comparing albumin, dextran 70, and polygeline in cirrhotic patients with ascites treated by paracentesis. Gastroenterology 111:1002-1010, 1996.

129. Gines P, Tito L, Arroyo V, et al: Randomized comparative study of therapeutic paracentesis with and without intravenous albumin in cirrhosis. Gastroenterology 94:1493-502, 1988.

130. Gines A, Escorsell A, Gines P, et al: Incidence, predictive factors, and prognosis of the hepatorenal syndrome in cirrhosis with ascites. Gastroenterology 105:229-236, 1993.

131. Gines P, Fernandez-Esparrach G, Arroyo V: Ascites and renal functional abnormalities in cirrhosis. Pathogenesis and treatment. Baillieres Clin Gastroenterol 11:365-385, 1997.

132. Bataller R, Gines P, Guevara M, Arroyo V: Hepatorenal syndrome. Semin Liver Dis 17:233-247, 1997.

133. Moreau R: Hepatorenal syndrome in patients with cirrhosis. J Gastroenterol Hepatol 17:739-747, 2002.

134. Moreau R, Durand F, Poynard T, et al: Terlipressin in patients with cirrhosis and type 1 hepatorenal syndrome: A retrospective multicenter study. Gastroenterology 122:923-930, 2002.

135. Duvoux C, Zanditenas D, Hezode C, et al: Effects of noradrenalin and albumin in patients with type I hepatorenal syndrome: A pilot study. Hepatology 36:374-380, 2002.

136. Angeli P, Volpin R, Gerunda G, et al: Reversal of type 1 hepatorenal syndrome with the administration of midodrine and octreotide. Hepatology 29:1690-1697, 1999.

137. Ortega R, Gines P, Uriz J, et al: Terlipressin therapy with and without albumin for patients with hepatorenal syndrome: Results of a prospective, nonrandomized study. Hepatology 36:941-948, 2002.

138. Mitzner SR, Stange J, Klammt S, et al: Improvement of hepatorenal syndrome with extracorporeal albumin dialysis MARS: Results of a prospective, randomized, controlled clinical trial. Liver Transpl 6:277-286, 2000.

139. Brensing KA, Textor J, Strunk H, et al: Transjugular intrahepatic portosystemic stent-shunt for hepatorenal syndrome. Lancet 349:697-698, 1997.

140. Krowka MJ, Cortese DA: Hepatopulmonary syndrome. Current concepts in diagnostic and therapeutic considerations. Chest 105:1528-1537, 1994.

141. Rodriguez-Roisin R, Agusti AG, Roca J: The hepatopulmonary syndrome: New name, old complexities. Thorax 47:897-902, 1992.

142. Lange PA, Stoller JK: The hepatopulmonary syndrome. Ann Intern Med 122:521-529, 1995.

143. Egawa H, Kasahara M, Inomata Y, et al: Long-term outcome of living related liver transplantation for patients with intrapulmonary shunting and strategy for complications. Transplantation 67:712-717, 1999.

144. Krowka MJ, Porayko MK, Plevak DJ, et al: Hepatopulmonary syndrome with progressive hypoxemia as an indication for liver transplantation: Case reports and literature review. Mayo Clin Proc 72:44-53, 1997.

145. Castro M, Krowka MJ, Schroeder DR, et al: Frequency and clinical implications of increased pulmonary artery pressures in liver transplant patients. Mayo Clin Proc 71:543-551, 1996.

146. Ramsay MA, Simpson BR, Nguyen AT, et al: Severe pulmonary hypertension in liver transplant candidates. Liver Transpl Surg 3:494-500, 1997.

147. Krowka MJ: Hepatopulmonary syndrome. In Plevak D SL (ed): Critical Care Issues in Liver Transplantation. The American Association for the Study of Liver Diseases and the International Liver Transplantation Society, 1999, pp 58-65.

148. Herve P, Lebrec D, Brenot F, et al: Pulmonary vascular disorders in portal hypertension. Eur Respir J 11:1153-1166, 1998.

149. Soderman C, Juhlin-Dannfelt A, Lagerstrand L, Eriksson LS: Ventilation-perfusion relationships and central haemodynamics in patients with cirrhosis. Effects of a somatostatin analogue. J Hepatol 21:52-57, 1994.

150. Krowka MJ, Dickson ER, Cortese DA: Hepatopulmonary syndrome. Clinical observations and lack of therapeutic response to somatostatin analogue. Chest 104:515-521, 1993.

151. Abrams GA, Fallon MB: Treatment of hepatopulmonary syndrome with *Allium sativum L.* (garlic): A pilot trial. J Clin Gastroenterol 27:232-235, 1998.

152. Corley DA, Scharschmidt B, Bass N, et al: Lack of efficacy of TIPS for hepatopulmonary syndrome. Gastroenterology 113:728-730, 1997.

153. Riegler JL, Lang KA, Johnson SP, Westerman JH: Transjugular intrahepatic portosystemic shunt improves oxygenation in hepatopulmonary syndrome. Gastroenterology 109:978-983, 1995.

154. Poterucha JJ, Krowka MJ, Dickson ER, et al: Failure of hepatopulmonary syndrome to resolve after liver transplantation and successful treatment with embolotherapy. Hepatology 21:96-100, 1995.

155. Gossage JR, Kanj G: Pulmonary arteriovenous malformations. A state of the art review. Am J Respir Crit Care Med 158:643-661, 1998.

156. Krowka M: Hepatopulmonary syndrome and liver transplantation. Liver Transpl 6:113-115, 2000.

157. Krowka MJ: Hepatopulmonary syndromes. Gut 46:1-4, 2000.

158. Alberts WM, Salem AJ, Solomon DA, Boyce G: Hepatic hydrothorax. Cause and management. Arch Intern Med 151:2383-2388, 1991.

159. Gordon FD, Anastopoulos HT, Crenshaw W, et al: The successful treatment of symptomatic, refractory hepatic hydrothorax with transjugular intrahepatic portosystemic shunt. Hepatology 25:1366-1369, 1997.

160. Strauss RM, Martin LG, Kaufman SL, Boyer TD: Transjugular intrahepatic portal systemic shunt for the management of symptomatic cirrhotic hydrothorax. Am J Gastroenterol 89:1520-1522, 1994.

161. Bergasa NV, Jones EA: Management of the pruritus of cholestasis: Potential role of opiate antagonists. Am J Gastroenterol 86:1404-1412, 1991.

162. Javitt NB: Timing of cholestyramine doses in cholestatic liver disease [letter]. N Engl J Med 1974;290:1328-9.

163. Ghent CN, Carruthers SG: Treatment of pruritus in primary biliary cirrhosis with rifampin. Results of a double-blind, crossover, randomized trial. Gastroenterology 94:488-493, 1988.

164. Wolfhagen FH, Sternieri E, Hop WC, et al: Oral naltrexone treatment for cholestatic pruritus: A double-blind, placebo-controlled study. Gastroenterology 1997;113:1264-1269.

165. Bergasa NV, Schmitt JM, Talbot TL, et al: Open-label trial of oral nalmefene therapy for the pruritus of cholestasis. Hepatology 27:679-684, 1998.

166. Gallego-Rojo FJ, Gonzalez-Calvin JL, Munoz-Torres M, et al: Bone mineral density, serum insulin-like growth factor I, and bone turnover markers in viral cirrhosis. Hepatology 28:695-699, 1998.

167. Chen CC, Wang SS, Jeng FS, Lee SD: Metabolic bone disease of liver cirrhosis: Is it parallel to the clinical severity of cirrhosis? J Gastroenterol Hepatol 11:417-421, 1996.

168. Van Berkum FN, Beukers R, Birkenhager JC, et al: Bone mass in women with primary biliary cirrhosis: The relation with histological stage and use of glucocorticoids. Gastroenterology 99:1134-1139, 1990.

169. Crippin JS, Jorgensen RA, Dickson ER, Lindor KD: Hepatic osteodystrophy in primary biliary cirrhosis: Effects of medical treatment. Am J Gastroenterol 89:47-50, 1994.

170. De Bona M, Ponton P, Ermani M, et al: The impact of liver disease and medical complications on quality of life and psychological distress before and after liver transplantation. J Hepatol 33:609-615, 2000.

171. Singh N, Gayowski T, Wagener MM, Marino IR: Depression in patients with cirrhosis. Impact on outcome. Dig Dis Sci 42:1421-1427, 1997.

172. Charlton MR: Branched chains revisited. Gastroenterology 111:252-255, 1996.

173. Plauth M, Merli M, Kondrup J: Management of hepatic encephalopathy. N Engl J Med 337:1921-1922, 1997.

174. Richardson RA, Davidson HI, Hinds A, et al: Influence of the metabolic sequelae of liver cirrhosis on nutritional intake. Am J Clin Nutr 69:331-337, 1999.

175. Muller MJ: Malnutrition in cirrhosis. J Hepatol 23 (Suppl 1):31-35, 1995.

176. Lochs H, Plauth M: Liver cirrhosis: Rationale and modalities for nutritional support—the European Society of Parenteral and Enteral Nutrition consensus and beyond. Curr Opin Clin Nutr Metab Care 2:345-349, 1999.

177. Mizock BA: Nutritional support in hepatic encephalopathy. Nutrition 15:220-228, 1999.

Nutritional Aspects of Adult Liver Transplantation

JEANETTE HASSE

The role of the liver in nutrient metabolism   491

Malnutrition and liver disease   492

Obesity and liver disease   494

Pretransplant nutrition support   494

Short-term posttransplant nutrition
    management   495
    Nutrient requirements   495
    Nutrition support   496
    Postoperative complications and nutrition
        support   498

Long-term posttransplant nutrition
    management   499
    Obesity   499
    Hyperlipidemia   500
    Hypertension   500
    Diabetes mellitus   501
    Osteoporosis   502
    Long-term nutrition goals   502

Future   503

Summary   503

The Role of the Liver in Nutrient Metabolism

The liver is a key organ in the metabolism of nutrients. The high metabolic activity of the liver accounts for approximately 20% to 30% of oxygen consumption and energy expenditure.[1] Liver dysfunction induces a catabolic state accompanied by increased energy expenditure; elevated serum insulin, glucagon, epinephrine, and cortisol concentrations; and insulin resistance.[1,2] Because the liver is vitally involved in nutrient metabolism (Table 33–1), liver disease causes alterations in protein, calorie, carbohydrate, fat, fluid, vitamin, and mineral needs.

Protein metabolism is altered in patients with end-stage liver disease (ESLD). Protein catabolism and hyperammonemia are enhanced, and synthesis of serum proteins, including albumin, secretory proteins, and clotting factors, is decreased. Derangement of plasma amino acid concentrations occurs.[3] Concentrations of plasma aromatic amino acids (AAAs: phenylalanine, tyrosine, tryptophan) plus methionine and cystine increase, whereas levels of plasma branched-chain amino acids (BCAAs: valine, leucine, isoleucine) decrease. The resulting alteration in the plasma molar BCAA/AAA ratio has been proposed as a causative factor in hepatic encephalopathy.

Liver disease may increase caloric requirements and affect energy substrate metabolism.[1,2,4] The presence of ascites has been shown to elevate resting energy expenditure (REE) in patients with liver cirrhosis.[5]

Table 33-1. ROLE OF THE LIVER IN NUTRIENT METABOLISM

Protein

Synthesis of serum proteins such as albumin

Synthesis of blood-clotting factors

Formation of urea from ammonia

Deamination/transamination of amino acids

Formation of creatine

Oxidation of the amino acids arginine, histidine, lysine, methionine, alanine, tryptophan, and tyrosine

Carbohydrate

Glycogenesis

Gluconeogenesis

Glycogenolysis

Fat

Hydrolysis of triglycerides, cholesterol, and phospholipids to fatty acids and glycerol

Fat storage

Cholesterol synthesis

Ketogenesis

Formation of lipoproteins

Production of bile necessary for digestion of dietary fat

Vitamins

Site of enzymatic steps in the activation of vitamins

    Thiamine (thiamine pyrophosphate)

    Pyridoxine (pyridoxal phosphate)

    Folic acid (tetrahydrofolic acid)

    Vitamin D (25-hydroxycholecalciferol)

Site of synthesis of carrier proteins for vitamins such as A and B_{12}

Vitamin E is transported in lipoproteins synthesized by the liver

Storage site for vitamins A, D, E, K, B_{12}

Minerals

Storage site for copper, iron, zinc

Other studies have found an increase in REE in patients with ESLD only when REE was expressed as energy expenditure per gram of creatinine excreted.[6] This measure represents REE in relation to lean body mass.[6] However, another study corrected REE for urinary creatinine excretion in 40 alcoholic cirrhotic patients and did not find that an increase in metabolic rate was dependent on the severity of the cirrhosis, nutritional status, or existence of alcoholic hepatitis.[7]

Liver failure alters energy metabolism as well. Liver glucose transport is reduced, and peripheral glucose metabolism decreases.[8] The rate of gluconeogenesis is increased, and the body prefers noncarbohydrate fuels such as lipids and amino acids to provide energy.[2,3] Plasma free fatty acids, glycerol, and ketone concentrations increase in cirrhosis, and the body favors fat as a fuel substrate.[3] Gluconeogenic capacity is retained in the early stages of liver failure, but elevated blood glucose levels can develop chronically. In patients with cirrhosis, decreased first-pass hepatic uptake of glucose and reduced insulin-mediated glucose uptake in peripheral tissues increase glucose levels after an oral load.[9] In addition, hyperglycemia occurs as a result of the reduced insulin action.[2,9] Circulating insulin levels may be increased, but insulin sensitivity is reduced.[9] In the late stages of liver disease, liver glycogen stores can become depleted, and gluconeogenic capacity deteriorates. The result is fasting hypoglycemia.

Vitamin and mineral alterations also occur as a result of liver disease. Fat malabsorption is common in patients with cholestatic liver disease and leads to loss of energy and fat-soluble vitamins. Deficiencies in fat-soluble vitamins can also occur as a result of other mechanisms. Low vitamin A levels may occur because of the inability of the liver to synthesize retinol-binding protein. Decreased biliary excretion of 1,25-dihydroxycholecalciferol can result from liver disease. Because vitamin E is transported in lipoproteins, the hyperlipidemias associated with cholestatic liver disease may affect vitamin E status. Vitamin B_6, vitamin B_{12}, thiamine, folate, and niacin levels are often depleted as a result of alcoholism. Minerals excreted via the biliary system, such as manganese and copper, can be affected by an interruption in enterohepatic circulation.[10] Magnesium, phosphorus, and zinc stores are commonly depleted in liver disease secondary to malnutrition, malabsorption, alcoholism, and diuretic use. Finally, mineral bioavailability, tissue distribution, and toxicity can be affected by decreased liver production of their protein carriers.[10]

Malnutrition and Liver Disease

Debility, malnutrition, encephalopathy, and massive ascites have been considered risk factors for liver transplantation. All these factors are nutrition related. Various methods of nutrition assessment have been used to determine nutritional status and risk, including subjective global assessment (SGA), anthropometric measurements, and body cell mass.[11-15] Up to 79% of patients awaiting liver transplantation are malnourished. Figure 33–1 illustrates a malnourished patient awaiting liver transplantation. Malnutrition is associated with increased rates of infection,[11] increased use of blood products,[12] prolonged length of hospital and intensive care unit (ICU) stay,[13] and reduced posttransplant survival.[11,13-15]

With the introduction of Model for End-Stage Liver Disease (MELD) scores, it is possible that patients with high MELD scores (with the exception of those

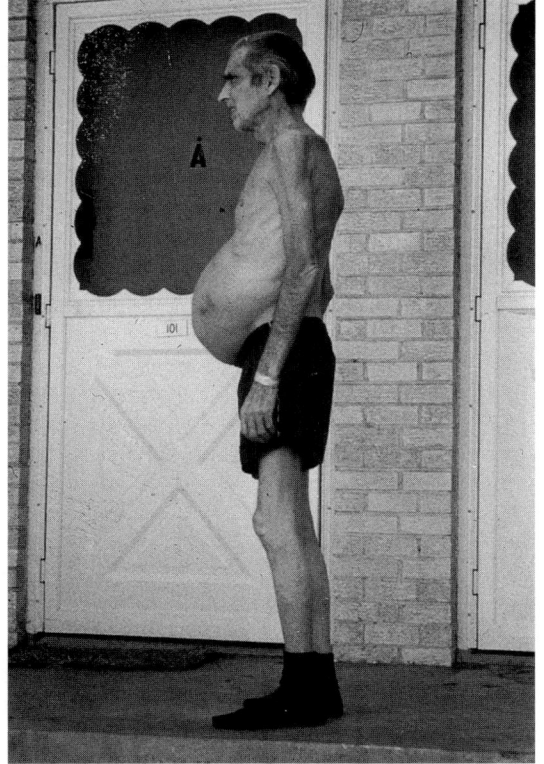

FIGURE 33–1

Severe malnutrition and ascites in a man with end-stage liver disease. (From Hasse JM, Matarese LE: Medical nutrition therapy for liver, biliary system, and exocrine pancreas disorders. In Mahan LK, Escott-Stump S (eds): Krause's Food, Nutrition, and Diet Therapy, 11th ed. Philadelphia, WB Saunders, 2004, p 749.)

with hepatocellular carcinoma) may have an elevated nutrition risk and worsened nutritional status. Abbott and associates demonstrated that grip strength and midarm muscle area were lower in patients with Child-Pugh class B or C scores versus class A. However, the nutritional indicators and Child-Pugh scores did not correlate with 1-year survival.[16]

Because of the prevalence of malnutrition, a registered dietitian should conduct a thorough nutritional assessment of all liver transplant candidates to identify patients at nutritional risk and determine appropriate nutrition therapy. Determining nutritional status in a patient with ESLD can be difficult because common objective nutritional assessment parameters are affected by liver disease (Table 33–2). However, arm muscle circumference and handgrip strength may be important objective markers of body cell mass depletion in patients with ESLD.[17] As an alternative, the SGA method should be considered.[18-20] SGA nutritional ratings are based on a thorough patient history, patient examination, and existing conditions (Table 33–3). SGA has been found to be a valid and reliable tool to assess nutritional status.[18-20]

The incidence of malnutrition in patients with ESLD varies depending on the cause of the liver disease and the parameters used to determine nutritional status. The cause of malnutrition in ESLD is multifactorial. Nutritional depletion can result from a poor diet (in both quantity and quality), anorexia, nausea, vomiting, metabolic aberrations, hypermetabolism, malabsorption, and psychological stress. In addition, the diet restrictions

Table 33–2. FACTORS THAT AFFECT THE INTERPRETATION OF OBJECTIVE NUTRITIONAL ASSESSMENT TESTS IN PATIENTS WITH END-STAGE LIVER DISEASE

Parameter	Factors Affecting Interpretation
Body weight	Affected by edema, ascites, and diuretic use
Anthropometric measurements	Questionable sensitivity, specificity, and reliability
	Multiple sources of error
	Unknown whether skinfold measurements reflect total-body fat
	References do not account for variation in hydration status and skin compressibility
Creatinine-height index	Affected by malnutrition, aging, decreased body mass, and protein intake
	Affected by renal function
	Creatinine is a metabolic end product of creatine synthesized in the liver; therefore, severe liver disease alters creatinine synthesis rates
Nitrogen balance studies	Nitrogen is retained in the body in the form of ammonia
	Hepatorenal syndrome can affect the excretion of nitrogen
3-Methylhistidine excretion	Affected by dietary intake, trauma, infection, and renal function
Visceral protein levels	Synthesis of visceral proteins is decreased
	Affected by hydration status, malabsorption, and renal insufficiency
Immune function tests	Affected by hepatic failure, electrolyte imbalances, infection, and renal insufficiency
Bioelectrical impedance	Invalid with ascites and/or edema

Table 33-3. SUBJECTIVE GLOBAL ASSESSMENT PARAMETERS FOR NUTRITIONAL EVALUATION OF LIVER TRANSPLANTATION CANDIDATES

History

Weight change (consider fluctuations secondary to ascites and edema)

Appetite

Taste changes and early satiety

Dietary recall (calories, protein, sodium)

Persistent gastrointestinal problems (nausea, vomiting, diarrhea, constipation, difficulty chewing or swallowing)

Physical Examination

Muscle wasting

Fat stores

Ascites or edema

Existing Conditions

Disease state and other problems that could influence nutritional status such as hepatic encephalopathy, gastrointestinal bleeding, renal insufficiency, infection

Nutritional Rating (Based on Results of Above Parameters)

Well nourished

Moderately (or suspected of being) malnourished

Severely malnourished

Data from references 18–20.

used to control ESLD symptoms limit food choices and optimal nutrient intake.

Obesity and Liver Disease

At the opposite end of the spectrum, morbid obesity is considered a relative contraindication for liver transplantation. Morbid obesity presents a technical challenge to transplantation surgeons. There are also concerns regarding possible postoperative complications such as wound infections, pulmonary problems, and anesthetic difficulties. Several single-center studies found that wound infections after transplantation were increased in obese as compared with nonobese patients.[21-24] In one study, obese patients also required longer hospitalization, hospital costs were increased, and respiratory failure developed more frequently than in nonobese liver transplant recipients.[24] These single-center studies did not demonstrate adverse mortality associated with obesity.[21-24] However, an analysis using multicenter data from the United Network for Organ Sharing (UNOS) database found reduced survival at 1, 2, and 5 years after transplantation in morbidly obese subjects.[25] Cardiovascular events accounted for reduced 5-year survival rates in severely and morbidly obese patients.[25]

Pretransplant Nutrition Support

Potential benefits of providing nutrition support to a patient include enhanced immunological defense, improved wound healing, and replacement of energy stores. It has been theorized that if nutrition support is provided early enough, it may help maintain quality of life before transplantation, decrease perioperative mortality, and shorten recovery time after transplantation.[26] While transplantation candidates wait to receive a transplant, malnutrition often worsens and thus warrants nutritional intervention. The goal of pretransplant nutrition therapy is to prevent further depletion and possibly replenish lost stores. A summary of pretransplantation nutritional needs is shown in Table 33–4.

Oral dietary supplementation is the first method that should be attempted to replenish energy stores. In a controlled trial of oral supplementation in 51 alcoholic cirrhosis patients, 26 received enhanced calorie and protein supplements and had shortened hospitalization (especially secondary to infections).[27] Nutritional parameters also improved significantly in the supplemented group in comparison to the 25 controls.[27]

LeCornu and colleagues provided oral supplements to 42 malnourished liver transplant candidates and compared outcomes with 40 control patients not drinking supplements.[28] Surprisingly, both groups improved their caloric intake, probably because of the influence of nutrition intervention and counseling. The supplemented group had improved midarm circumference, midarm muscle circumference, and grip strength, but outcomes were not changed.

In another study, malnourished pre–liver transplant patients with a history of encephalopathy were randomized to receive either diet plus a BCAA supplement (n = 24), diet plus a casein supplement (n = 26), or diet alone (n = 12).[29] Each supplement was dosed to provide 0.5 g protein/kg/day. Patients receiving supplements had significantly higher caloric intake than the control group did. Patients receiving the BCAA supplement had a reduced frequency and length of hospitalizations before liver transplantation.

If patients are not able to eat adequate nutrients, enteral tube feeding (TF) is the most desirable alternative. Two studies compared a group of patients with liver disease who were receiving TF and matched groups receiving oral diets.[30,31] Thirty-one patients with alcoholic liver disease were randomized to receive either a regular diet alone or a diet supplemented with casein-based TF.[30] The TF group had greater mean nutrient intake, an improvement in hepatic encephalopathy scores, reduced serum bilirubin, and a shorter antipyrine half-life in comparison to the control group. In a similar

Table 33-4. NUTRITIONAL RECOMMENDATIONS FOR A LIVER TRANSPLANTATION CANDIDATE

Nutrient	Recommendations
Calories	25–35 kcal/kg dry weight for maintenance
	35–40 kcal/kg dry weight for malnourished patient
	130–150% of predicted BEE (calculated with the Harris-Benedict equation)
Protein	0.8–1.0 g/kg dry weight in compensated liver disease
	1.5–2.0 g/kg dry weight in decompensated liver disease
	Consider use of BCAA-enriched formulas for hepatic encephalopathy
Fat	25–40% of calories
	Consider MCT oil when steatorrhea is present
Carbohydrate	High complex and simple carbohydrate
	Carbohydrate should be controlled if glucose intolerance is present
Sodium	2–4 g/day
Fluid	1000–1500 mL/day if hyponatremia is present
Vitamins	Monitor levels and signs of deficiency; supplement to RDI
	Give water-miscible forms of fat-soluble vitamins if steatorrhea is present
Minerals	Monitor levels and signs of deficiency; supplement to RDI
	Serum potassium, magnesium, and phosphorus levels may decrease as a result of diuretic administration or refeeding syndrome
	1200 mg calcium/day; supplement at-risk populations

BCAA, branched-chain amino acid; BEE, basal energy expenditure; MCT, medium-chain triglyceride; RDI, recommended daily intake.

study, 35 cirrhotic patients were randomized to receive either a low-sodium diet or TF.[31] The TF group had significantly higher calorie intake, an improvement in serum albumin levels and Child's score, and a decreased mortality rate when compared with controls. Because these trials did not involve transplant patients, controlled trials are necessary to evaluate the effect of TF on outcomes in patients with ESLD who undergo liver transplantation.

Obtaining access for a feeding tube can be problematic in patients with liver disease. A large-bore nasogastric feeding tube is not a feasible long-term option. A gastrostomy tube is contraindicated in patients with ascites. Therefore, a small-bore, Silastic nasoenteral tube is the best option.

Parenteral nutrition (PN) remains an option only in patients with absent gut function or significant malabsorption. PN is costly and results in a higher incidence of infection and electrolyte imbalance than TF does. PN can also potentially worsen liver function.

Supplementation (either enterally or parenterally) with formulas enriched with BCAAs and depleted in AAAs has been proposed to improve nutritional status without inducing or worsening hepatic encephalopathy. Some studies have supported this theory,[32-34] whereas others have failed to show the same benefit. The use of these formulas remains controversial.

Short-Term Posttransplant Nutrition Management

Nutrient Requirements

The primary nutritional goal in the immediate posttransplant period (generally the first 2 posttransplant months) is to provide adequate nutrition to promote recovery and replenish lost nutritional stores. A posttransplant catabolic state is induced by preoperative malnutrition, stress of the transplant surgery, corticosteroid administration, and in some cases, renal or hepatic dysfunction (or both) and sepsis. Protein catabolism increases markedly immediately after liver transplantation and necessitates a protein intake of 1.3 to 2.0 g/kg dry weight.[35-39] Nitrogen loss is increased after surgery because of surgical stress and the administration of corticosteroids. As much as 3.6 kg skeletal muscle mass may be lost in the first 10 days after liver transplantation.[40] Theoretically, patients treated with steroid-free immunosuppression regimens would lose less nitrogen than would those receiving traditional high-dose corticosteroid regimens.

Serum AAA levels normalize after successful transplantation.[41] However, Tietge and coworkers demonstrated that BCAA levels remain depressed more than

6 months after transplantation. A correlation between elevated BCAA levels and circulating catecholamines led the authors to conclude that insulin hypersecretion and elevations in adrenergic tone contribute to persistent BCAA metabolism in muscle.[41]

Unlike the dramatic rise in protein catabolism, the metabolic rate does not seem to be elevated to the same degree. Delafosse and colleagues[37] measured REE in eight patients on the first 2 days after transplantation. Mean REE was only 36% to 38% above the predicted basal energy expenditure (BEE—Harris Benedict equation). In another study of 11 post–liver transplant patients, REE was only 7% higher than the predicted BEE, but the patient's actual weight was used in the BEE calculation instead of dry weight (which increases BEE).[6] REE measured in 28 liver transplant patients on days 1, 3, 5, 14, and 28 after transplantation was less than 120% of the predicted BEE.[35] Mean REE in 31 liver transplant recipients measured on posttransplant days 2, 5, 7, and 12 was 127% of BEE.[36] Finally, REE peaked at 42% above predicted (with the use of a site-specific prediction equation) in 14 liver transplant patients on day 10 after transplantation (2149 ± 68 kcal or 26.7 kcal/kg).[40]

A mixed-fuel system of both carbohydrate and fat is suggested to provide energy in the postoperative period. Carbohydrate should usually provide about 70% of nonprotein calories after transplantation. Posttransplant hyperglycemia frequently occurs as a result of corticosteroid administration, physiological stress, and recovering liver function. Hyperglycemia may necessitate the use of fat for up to 50% of nonprotein calories to provide adequate calories until glucose control is achieved. Data regarding the most appropriate type of fatty acids for transplant patients are lacking.

Electrolyte alterations are common in the short-term posttransplant period. Sodium is lost via urine, nasogastric aspiration, and abdominal drains. Serum potassium, phosphorus, and magnesium levels may be depleted rapidly in liver transplant recipients secondary to diuretic use and refeeding syndrome. Calcineurin inhibitors can also accelerate magnesium loss. In contrast, cyclosporine, tacrolimus, and renal insufficiency can lead to hyperkalemia and other electrolyte disturbances. Table 33–5 reviews additional nutritional side effects of immunosuppressive medications. Finally, although not specifically defined in liver transplant patients, vitamin and mineral stores need to be replenished, especially in malnourished patients.

Nutrition Support

Three modalities are available to provide nutrition to patients after transplantation—oral diet, enteral TF, and PN. A liquid diet is initiated 1 to 3 days after transplantation, with progression to a general diet. When hyperglycemia persists, a carbohydrate-controlled diet

Table 33–5. NUTRITIONAL SIDE EFFECTS OF IMMUNO-SUPPRESSIVE MEDICATIONS

Immunosuppressive Drug	Potential Nutritional Side Effects
Antilymphocyte serum	Decreased appetite
Azathioprine	Nausea
	Vomiting
	Sore throat
	Altered taste acuity
	Macrocytic anemia
Basiliximab	None reported
Corticosteroids	Catabolism/impaired wound healing
	Hyperglycemia
	Sodium retention
	Electrolyte disturbances
	Hyperphagia
	Increased calciuria
Cyclosporine	Hyperlipidemia
	Hyperglycemia
	Hypomagnesemia
	Hyperkalemia
	Hypertension
Daclizumab	None reported
Muromonab-CD3	Nausea
	Vomiting
	Diarrhea
	Loss of appetite
Sirolimus	Hyperlipidemia
	Gastrointestinal disorders (constipation, diarrhea, nausea, vomiting, dyspepsia)
Tacrolimus	Hyperglycemia
	Hyperkalemia
	Nausea and vomiting
Mycophenolate mofetil	Diarrhea

is recommended. Most transplant recipients initially suffer from anorexia, altered taste, and early satiety. These symptoms hamper patients' ability to eat, and oral nutritional supplements are often indicated.

Enteral TF is the alternative method of choice to provide nutrition after transplantation. Although gastric and colonic ileus is common in the first few days after transplantation, enteral nutrition can be administered successfully via a feeding tube that is inserted during surgery.[36,42-45] Figure 33–2 illustrates a decision tree for initiation of TF after liver transplantation. TF can be started within several hours after transplantation by infusing a moderate-osmolality formula at a low rate. Once the patient begins to eat, the TF can be transitioned to nocturnal feeding to enhance the patient's

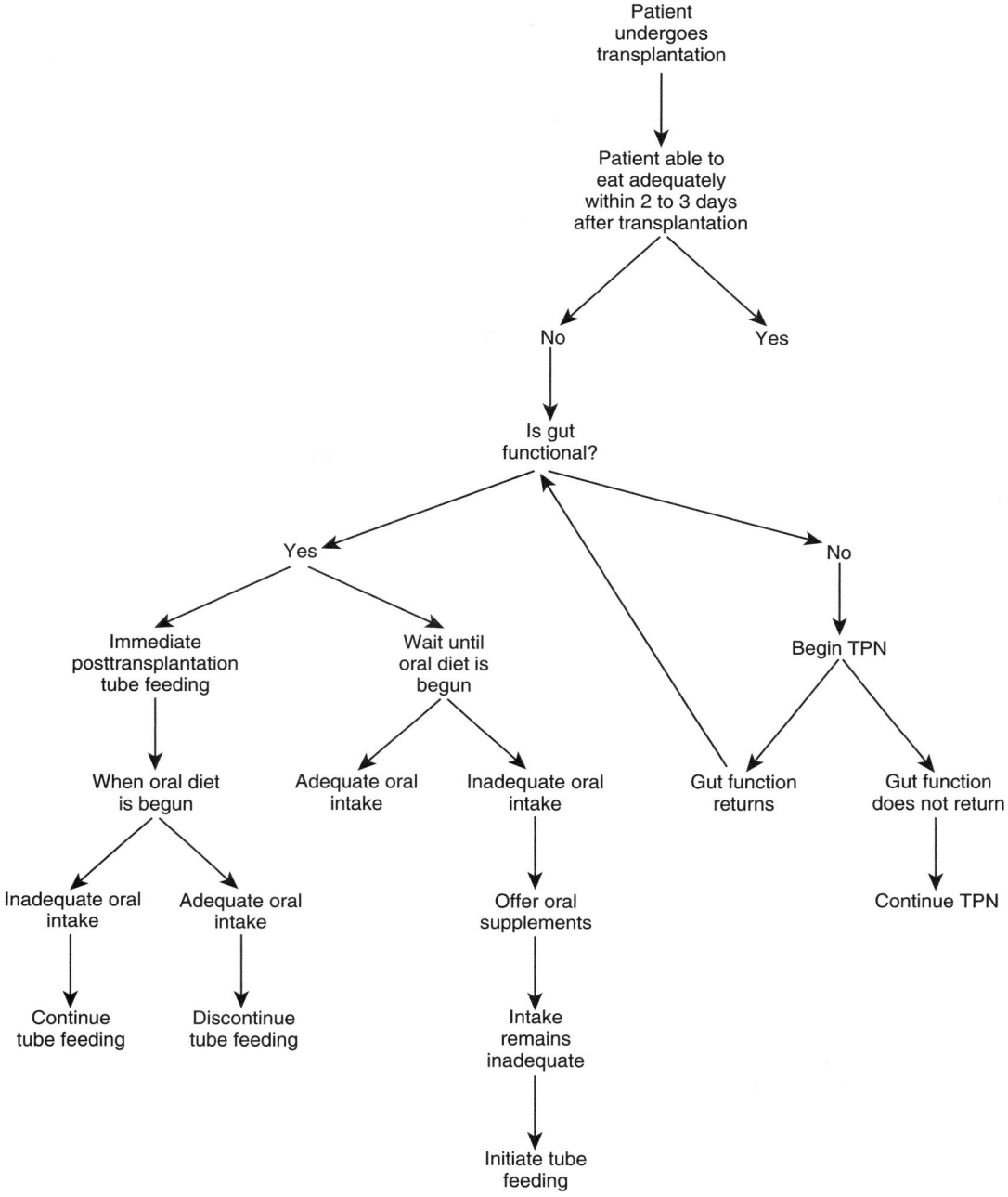

FIGURE 33–2

Nutritional support algorithm for organ transplant recipients. (From Hasse JM, Roberts S: Transplantation. In Rombeau JL, Rolandelli RH (eds): Clinical Nutrition: Parenteral Nutrition, 3rd ed. Philadelphia, WB Saunders, 2001, p 533.)

appetite and allow for increased ambulation during the day. The TF infusion can be discontinued completely once calorie count results confirm the adequacy of a patient's oral intake.

A prospective, randomized study was performed to determine the effects of early posttransplant TF on outcomes of liver transplant recipients.[36] Liver transplant patients were prospectively randomized to receive either an enteral formula via nasointestinal feeding tubes (placed during surgery) within 12 hours after liver transplantation (TF group) or maintenance intravenous fluid until oral diets were initiated (control group). Feeding was well tolerated in the TF group (n = 14). The TF group had significantly greater 12-day cumulative calorie and protein intake than the control group did. The TF patients also had better nitrogen balance on posttransplant day 4 and quicker recovery in grip strength than the control patients did. Viral infections occurred in 17.7% of the control patients versus 0% of the TF patients ($P = .05$). Additionally, there was a trend for other infections to occur more frequently in the control group than in the TF group (bacterial, 29.4% versus 14.3%; overall infections, 47.1% versus 21.4%). This study concluded that early TF after liver transplantation was well tolerated and promoted improvement in patient outcomes.

Wicks and colleagues compared enteral nutrition via a nasojejunal tube (n = 14) with PN (n = 10) in patients after liver transplantation.[42] Intestinal permeability, infection rates, and anthropometric measurements did not differ between groups, nor did the number of days to reach 70% of requirements with oral intake (4 days for TF versus 5 days for PN).

Rayes and associates compared different types of TF in liver transplant patients.[43] Group 1 underwent small bowel decontamination and was fed a standard formula, group 2 received a fiber-containing formula plus *Lactobacillus plantarum* 299, and group 3 received a fiber-containing formula plus heat-killed *L. plantarum* 299. The addition of a probiotic (*L. plantarum 299*) resulted in reduced infection rates. The study design provided patients with TF for 12 days, which is unlikely in a scenario in which patients can meet needs with an oral diet and are discharged from the hospital in less than a week. It does raise an interesting concept of using oral probiotics after transplantation.

A retrospective review of 108 patient fed via a jejunal tube after liver transplantation showed that TF was tolerated.[44] However, complications with this type of tube may be unacceptable for short-term TF (mechanical obstruction of tubes in six, reoperation for infection in six, small bowel obstruction in two, catheter displacement in two, and requirement for surgical removal of the tube in one).[45]

With the shortened hospital stay and frequent occurrence of transplantation in severely compromised patients, the use of home TF after discharge is becoming more frequent. Additional outpatient monitoring of the TF access device, gastrointestinal symptoms, laboratory values (especially electrolytes), and oral intake is required to determine tolerance and continued need for TF. Insurance coverage for home TF can sometimes be difficult to obtain if TF is not the only source of nutrition and will be needed for less than 3 months.

TF is favored over PN, but PN is indicated when a malnourished patient's gut cannot be used for 5 to 7 days. One study evaluated the effect of PN after transplantation surgery.[46] Twenty-eight patients were randomly assigned to one of three groups: (1) no nutrition support, (2) PN (35 kcal/kg/day) with a standard amino acid solution (1.5 g/kg/day), or (3) total PN (35 kcal/kg/day) with a BCAA-enriched amino acid solution (1.5 g/kg/day). PN was administered for 1 week. The PN groups had improved nitrogen balance and a significantly shorter length of stay in the ICU. The BCAA-enriched solution was not found to be superior to the standard amino acid group. These data are difficult to apply in today's practice when TF is available and ICU and hospital stays can be very brief. However, when PN is administered, a concentrated solution containing a mixed-fuel system is generally required. Electrolytes should be monitored carefully and adjusted in the PN accordingly (Table 33–6).

Postoperative Complications and Nutrition Support

Potential postoperative complications include rejection, infection, renal insufficiency, intestinal complications (ileus, diarrhea, ulcers), abdominal bleeding, biliary complications, vascular or splenic complications,

Table 33–6. CONSIDERATIONS FOR A POSTTRANSPLANT TOTAL PARENTERAL NUTRITION REGIMEN

Amino acids	Use standard amino acid solutions
	May use a 15% initial concentration of amino acids when volume must be restricted
Dextrose	Provide 50–70% of nonprotein calories as glucose
	Decrease final glucose concentration or provide insulin when serum glucose > 150 mg/dL
	May use a $D_{70}W$ initial concentration when volume must be restricted
Lipid	Provide 30% of nonprotein calories as lipid
	May provide up to 50% of nonprotein calories as lipid when hyperglycemia is difficult to control
Electrolytes	Monitor and supplement as needed
	Potassium, magnesium, and phosphorus can become depleted rapidly
Vitamins	Administer daily recommended dose (10 mL) of multivitamin supplement
	Provide vitamin K weekly unless provided in the multivitamin supplement
	Can supplement with individual vitamins as needed
Trace elements	Administer daily recommended dose (1 mL) of a standard trace element supplement
	Can supplement with individual trace elements as needed
Medications	Depending on compatibility, may be able to administer medication in TPN (e.g., H_2 blockers)

$D_{70}W$, 70% dextrose in water; TPN, total parenteral nutrition.

pancreatitis, and metabolic complications. The onset of any of these complications or their treatment may necessitate a change in the nutritional care plan for an individual.

Treatment of rejection with additional corticosteroids results in heightened protein catabolism and hyperglycemia. Treatment with a monoclonal antibody may cause anorexia, nausea, vomiting, and diarrhea. Adequate nutrition is required to prevent infection, and treatment of an infection with antibiotics can decrease appetite and cause gastrointestinal upset. Renal insufficiency may require limitation of potassium, phosphorus, sodium, or fluid. Complications requiring surgical treatment or bowel rest, or both, indicate a need for nutrition support. An alteration in bile excretion can affect fat digestion. Finally, metabolic complications may require alterations in nutritional substrates or electrolytes.

Monitoring of nutrition in immediate posttransplant patients should include measurement of weight, laboratory values, and nutrient intake. For patients receiving nutrition support, REE and nitrogen balance studies may be useful.

Long-Term Posttransplant Nutrition Management

Liver transplantation usually results in correction of malnutrition (Fig. 33–3). The goal of long-term posttransplantation nutrition is maintenance. Many liver transplant recipients suffer from problems of "overnutrition" as early as 2 months after transplantation. Common long-term posttransplant nutrition problems include excessive weight gain, hypertension, hyperlipidemia, osteoporosis, and diabetes mellitus (DM). Many of these comorbid conditions contribute to the risk for cardiovascular disease and can adversely affect a patient's medical condition and quality of life.

Obesity

Liver transplant patients lose fat mass after transplantation, but it is usually regained by 90 days.[40] In addition, although many patients lose weight before transplantation as a result of liver disease, obesity is prevalent after liver transplantation and may be associated with a higher incidence of posttransplant liver abnormalities. The cause of posttransplant obesity is multifactorial. Obesity before the onset of liver disease predicts posttransplant obesity. Some patients have a good appetite after recovery and may develop an attitude of "I can eat anything I want." This mind-set is coupled with the false hunger created by the corticosteroids. Patients who experienced pretransplant malabsorption are no longer excreting valuable nutrients. Many patients are forced to adopt a sedentary lifestyle during their illness as a result of uncontrolled fatigue and weakness. After transplantation, they increase their dietary intake but continue a sedentary lifestyle. Finally, once these patients recover, they often resume old eating habits, which may have been the cause of these same problems before the onset of their liver disease.

Patients maintained on a cyclosporine-based immunosuppression regimen tend to have more obesity problems than do patients receiving a tacrolimus-based

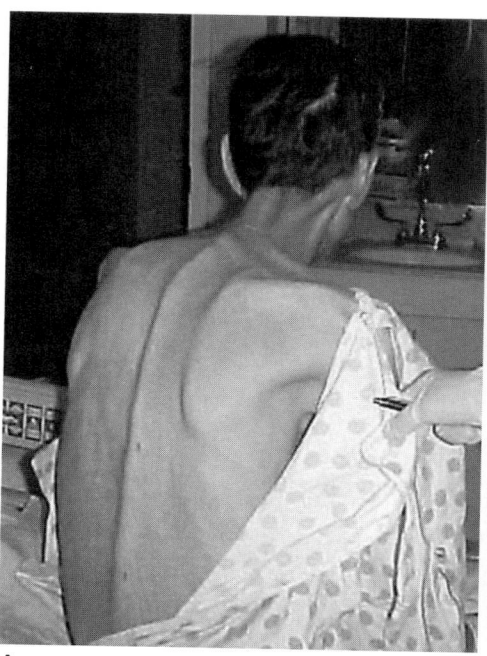
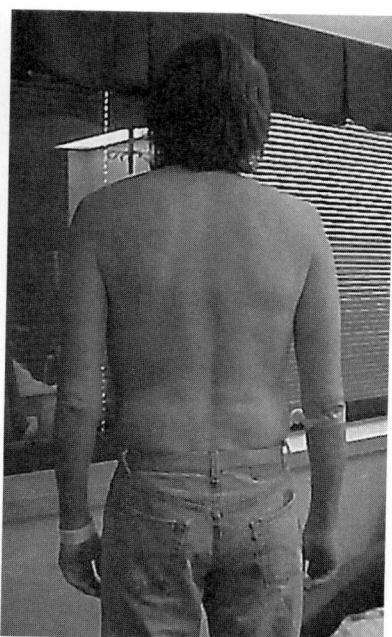

FIGURE 33–3

Correction of malnutrition in a patient who underwent liver transplantation. **A**, Male patient awaiting liver transplantation. **B**, Same patient 1 year after liver transplantation.

A

B

regimen.[47,48] The body mass index 1 year after liver transplantation in the U.S. FK506 trial was lower in the tacrolimus group (25.5 kg/m²) than in the cyclosporine group (27.7 kg/m²); 18.2% of cyclosporine patients were more than 140% of their ideal body weight versus 10.9% in the tacrolimus group.[48] One would theorize that the total dose of corticosteroids contributes to this effect.[48] When corticosteroid therapy was discontinued in 51 liver transplant recipients, weight loss occurred in 88% of the patients.[49] The mean weight loss was 9.5 lb. In another small study of 26 patients, when immunosuppression was switched from cyclosporine to tacrolimus, there was a mean weight loss of 3.3 kg over a 1-month period.[50] Many newer immunosuppressive regimens use lower or no doses of corticosteroids. Theoretically, the risk of excessive weight gain would be decreased. However, overall obesity rates continue to rise in the United States, and this trend is probably reflected in transplant patients as well.

Traditional therapy for posttransplant obesity includes caloric restriction and exercise. No prospective study to date has evaluated the effectiveness of dietary interventions on posttransplant weight. Even though exercise performance (as defined by Vo₂max) improves after liver transplantation,[51] it remains impaired.[51,52]

Other more aggressive therapy available for weight management includes pharmacological and surgical interventions. Orlistat is contraindicated in patients taking cyclosporine because the medication would reduce absorption of cyclosporine. Sibutramine has not been evaluated as a weight loss aid in liver transplant patients. However, precautions for this drug include liver and renal impairment and therefore make one reluctant to prescribe this drug. Bariatric surgery is reserved for individuals with morbid obesity. Two case reports demonstrated weight loss and regression of recurrent nonalcoholic steatohepatitis in morbidly obese liver transplant recipients who underwent Roux-en-Y gastric bypass.[53] This procedure is an extreme measure that should be evaluated cautiously.

Hyperlipidemia

Hyperlipidemia has been reported in liver transplant survivors.[54-57] The prevalence depends on the immunosuppression regimen, the definition of hyperlipidemia, and the time since transplantation. Factors contributing to posttransplant hyperlipidemia include weight gain, corticosteroids, cyclosporine, sirolimus, proteinuria and kidney insufficiency, DM and insulin resistance, and antihypertensive medications (thiazides and β-blockers).[58] The possible causative mechanisms of hyperlipidemia by corticosteroids, cyclosporine, and sirolimus are reviewed in Table 33–7.[58,59] Conversion from cyclosporine to tacrolimus has been shown to reduce hyperlipidemia.[50,60] When hyperlipidemia is refractory to dietary alterations and changes in immunosuppression cannot be made (i.e., reduce or discontinue corticosteroids or sirolimus), 3-hydroxy-3-methylglutaryl-coenzyme A (HMG-CoA) reductase inhibitors are the primary drugs for treatment of hyperlipidemia (Table 33–8).[61]

Hypertension

Calcineurin inhibitors cause sodium retention and increase systemic vascular resistance by means of arterial vasoconstriction.[62] Hypertension occurs more frequently in patients treated with cyclosporine than in those treated with tacrolimus.[47,50,56,57] Although no

Table 33-7. EFFECTS OF IMMUNOSUPPRESSIVE MEDICATIONS ON SERUM LIPID LEVELS

Corticosteroid's effects on cholesterol	Stimulates hepatic lipoprotein production
	Stimulates adipocyte hormone-sensitive lipase and thereby results in the release of stored triglycerides as free fatty acids, which are used for further hepatic lipoprotein synthesis
	Causes insulin-potentiating activity, which may increase the activity of lipoprotein lipase and interfere with LDL-cholesterol receptor function
Corticosteroid's effects on triglycerides	Increases peripheral free fatty acid production
	Increases hepatic lipoprotein synthesis
Cyclosporine's effects on cholesterol	CyA is transported in blood in association with lipoproteins; an abnormal interaction between LDL receptors and their ligands may occur because of the presence of CyA
	May inhibit bile acid production, which may decrease excretion of free cholesterol
Sirolimus' effects on triglycerides	Alters insulin signaling pathway, which reduces lipoprotein lipase and/or increases adipose tissue lipase; this response increases hepatic synthesis of triglycerides and VLDL secretion

CyA, cyclosporine A; LDL, low-density lipoprotein; VLDL, very-low-density lipoprotein.
Data from Perez R: Managing nutrition problems in transplant patients. Nutr Clin Pract 8:28-32, 1993; and Morrisett JD, Abdel-Fattah G, Hoogeveen R, et al: Effects of sirolimus on plasma lipids, lipoprotein levels, and fatty acid metabolism in renal transplant patients. J Lipid Res 43:1170-1180, 2002.

Table 33–8. POTENTIAL ADVERSE EFFECTS OF LIPID-LOWERING AGENTS AND DRUG INTERACTIONS IN TRANSPLANT RECIPIENTS

Class of Lipid-Lowering Agent	Examples	Possible Adverse Effects	Comments
Bile acid resin	Cholestyramine	May prevent absorption of fat-soluble vitamins; poor compliance because of constipation and bloating	May inhibit absorption of cyclosporine and other fat-soluble drugs; space dose by 2 hr with interacting drug; may increase triglyceride concentrations
Nicotinic acid	Nicotinic acid, extended-release formulations	Flushing, pruritus, increase in liver enzymes, increased uric acid concentrations, altered glucose tolerance, exacerbation of peptic ulcer disease	Concomitant cyclosporine and prednisone use may exacerbate adverse effects
Fibric acid derivative	Gemfibrozil	Gallstones, myositis (especially in patients with decreased renal function), nausea, gastrointestinal upset	Increased risk of myositis with concomitant HMG-CoA reductase inhibitors and immunosuppressive drugs
Antioxidant	Probucol	Flatulence, loose stools, prolonged QT interval on electrocardiogram, decreased HDL	May interact with cyclosporine and cause fluctuation in cyclosporine concentrations
HMG-CoA reductase inhibitor	Statin drugs	Abdominal pain, flatulence, increase in transaminase concentration, myositis, sleep disturbances	May increase liver function enzymes; increased risk of myositis with high-dose HMG-CoA reductase inhibitors and/or fibric acid derivatives with cyclosporine

HDL, high-density lipoprotein; HMG-CoA, 3-hydroxy-3-methylglutaryl coenzyme A.
Adapted from Kobashigawa JA, Kasiske BL: Hyperlipidemia in solid organ transplantation. Transplantation 63:331-338, 1997.

clinical trials have substantiated the effectiveness of a sodium-restricted diet in controlling hypertension in transplant recipients, a recommended sodium intake after transplantation is 2 to 4 g/day.

The combination of hypertension, obesity, and hyperlipidemia is a strong risk factor for coronary artery disease. An increase in the frequency of atherosclerosis has been documented in heart and renal transplant patients. The impact of risk factors for cardiovascular disease on liver transplant recipients is not yet known. Single-center studies have found that liver transplant patients have increased cardiovascular risk.[47,56,63] One study suggests that cardiovascular risk in liver transplant patients is higher than that in the general population,[63] whereas another suggests that 5 years after transplantation, the risk is similar to that in the general population.[56]

Hyperhomocysteinemia is another risk factor for cardiovascular disease that may be present in liver transplant patients as a result of cyclosporine therapy[56] and renal dysfunction.[64] Hyperhomocysteinemia responds to folic acid supplementation.[64]

Diabetes Mellitus

There are conflicting data regarding the effect of preexisting DM on transplant outcomes. One small study did not demonstrate an association with pretransplant DM and rates of infection, rejection, or hypertension.[65] Another study showed that preexisting DM was linked with increased cardiovascular, infectious, renal, respiratory, neurological, hematological, musculoskeletal, and malignancy complications after liver transplantation.[66] At least two studies showed reduced 5-year posttransplant survival in patients with preexisting DM,[66,67] but another group did not find that pretransplant DM affected survival.[68] With regard to new-onset posttransplant diabetes, one study showed increased morbidity but not increased mortality in patients in whom posttransplant DM developed,[69] and another study reported decreased 5-year survival in patients with posttransplant DM.[68]

The rate of posttransplant DM is difficult to ascertain because the definition of DM has varied in published reports. Obesity, advanced age, a family history of DM, and ethnicity (Hispanic, African American, Native American) are strong risk factors for the development of DM. Cyclosporine, tacrolimus, and corticosteroids are potential diabetogenic agents. Hepatitis C virus is also associated with increased rates of DM both before and after transplantation.[70,71]

Calcineurin inhibitors decrease insulin secretion, increase insulin resistance, and alter beta cell function.[72] Some studies suggest that tacrolimus may be more diabetogenic than cyclosporine.[48,73,74] Corticosteroids also cause insulin resistance.[72] Other potential effects of steroids on glucose metabolism include decreased insulin receptors and affinity, impaired peripheral glucose uptake in muscle, deactivation of glucose/free fatty acid, and faulty suppression of endogenous insulin production.[72] Serum glucose and glycosylated hemoglobin levels have been reported to decrease in liver transplant patients in whom steroid use was discontinued.[75-77]

Osteoporosis

Chronic liver disease and liver transplantation are associated with bone disease.[78-80] Bone mineral density (BMD) is low before liver transplantation and may decrease after transplantation.[40,78,81,82] Vertebral fractures are common before transplantation, and new vertebral fractures develop in a third of patients 3 months after liver transplantation, although BMD values may not help predict fractures.[78] Studies suggest that femoral neck density may decrease without a decrease in total BMD.[78,82] Subsequently, BMD tends to recover in the lumbar spine after transplantation but not in the femoral neck.[79,81]

Risk factors for posttransplant bone loss include the cause of the liver disease, immunosuppressive medications, vitamin D deficiency, hypogonadism, impaired absorption or inadequate intake of calcium, reduced physical activity, and preexisting bone disease. Floreani and colleagues also correlated body mass index, age, creatinine, and parathyroid hormone with lumbar spine BMD.[79]

Corticosteroids seem to accelerate trabecular bone loss while sparing cortical bone.[83] It is hypothesized that the effect of corticosteroids on bone loss occurs through alterations in the secretion of sex hormones, intestinal calcium absorption, the vitamin D system, and kidney excretion of calcium and phosphate, as well as via direct effects on bone formation and resorption.[83] Cyclosporine produces a high-turnover osteopenia.

Careful monitoring of bone mineral loss and treatment is warranted for liver transplant patients. Calcium and vitamin D intake should be considered, as well as other osteoporosis risk factors such as decreased estrogen levels in women, lack of exercise, and smoking. Theoretically, perioperative therapy with bisphosphonates would seem logical, although this effect has not been seen in all studies.[84,85] Long-term studies are needed to evaluate the reversibility of osteopenia after liver transplantation with and without therapy and the effect of newer immunosuppression regimens (i.e., reduced corticosteroids). Estrogen therapy in postmenopausal women after liver transplantation also appears to be effective in increasing BMD.[86] Calcitonin therapy has not been found to reduce bone loss.[87]

Long-Term Nutrition Goals

Long-term nutrition guidelines focus on preventive measures. Moderate intake of fat, sugar, and salt should be accompanied by exercise. Table 33–9 summarizes posttransplant dietary goals. It must be emphasized that most transplant recipients require ongoing nutritional counseling to incorporate healthy eating practices and a regular exercise program into their lives. Compliance is variable, and it is difficult for the transplant team

Table 33–9. POSTTRANSPLANT NUTRITIONAL GUIDELINES		
Nutrient	**Short-Term Recommendations**	**Long-Term Recommendations**
Calories	120–140% of BEE (30–35 kcal/kg) or measure REE	Maintenance: 120–130% of BEE (25–30 kcal/kg), depending on activity level
Protein	1.3–2 g/kg/day	1 g/kg/day
Carbohydrate	50–60% of calories	Restrict simple sugars
Fat	30% of calories	< 30% of total calories
	Up to 50% of calories with severe hyperglycemia	< 10% of calories as saturated fat
Calcium	1200 mg/day	1000–1500 mg/day (consider the need for estrogen or vitamin D supplements)
Sodium	2–4 g/day	3–4 g/day
Magnesium and phosphorus	Encourage intake of foods high in these nutrients	Encourage intake of foods high in these nutrients
	Supplement as needed	Supplement as needed
Potassium	Supplement or restrict based on serum potassium levels	Supplement or restrict based on serum potassium levels
Other vitamins and minerals	Multivitamin/mineral: supplement to RDI levels	Multivitamin/mineral: supplement to RDI levels
	Avoid herbal preparations	Avoid herbal preparations

BEE, basal energy expenditure; RDI, recommended daily intake; REE, resting energy expenditure.

because it is the patient's decision to either follow or disobey the dietary and exercise guidelines prescribed to them. Patients with a history of obesity are at greatest risk of gaining excess weight, but these long-term complications can develop in all patients and affect their physical and psychological quality of life.

Future

Liver transplantation is a relatively new field of medicine, and transplant nutrition is in its infancy. There are many applications of nutrition in other fields that may one day prove to be helpful in transplantation. For example, could nutrients such as arginine or n-3 fatty acids affect rejection or infection after liver transplantation? Because grapefruit interferes with drug metabolism, are there other foods that may exert harmful effects? What role will complementary medicine have in transplantation? Some herbal products are known to be harmful in transplant recipients[88]; for that reason, despite the surge in interest and production of herbal products, they should be avoided until their safety in liver transplant patients is determined. Will probiotics be found to have benefit in transplant patients? Probiotics have been reported to reduce antibiotic-associated diarrhea, recurrent *Clostridium difficile* infection, and symptoms of inflammatory bowel disease. One study showed benefit in liver transplant patients,[43] but the full spectrum of safety and the benefits of probiotics are not yet known.

Summary

Nutrition is a central issue throughout the transplant process. Malnutrition is common in the pretransplant period, and the nutrition goal is to prevent further depletion. A catabolic state exists in the immediate posttransplant period, so nutrition is administered to replenish stores. The long-term posttransplant period may be the most difficult because patients suffer from chronic "overnutrition" problems; therefore, long-term nutritional guidelines emphasize prevention or minimization of these problems.

Pearls and Pitfalls

Nutrition intervention is required throughout all stages of liver transplantation to achieve optimal short- and long-term outcomes. To practice the best medical nutrition therapy, follow the following points:

Pearls and Pitfalls—cont'd

Do

- Involve a registered dietitian in all phases of the treatment of patients.
- Assess and reassess nutritional status throughout the continuum of transplantation.
- Individualize nutrition recommendations for calories, protein, fat, carbohydrates, vitamins, minerals, fluids, and electrolytes based on nutritional status, current nutrient intake, goals for medical and nutritional therapy, current conditions, and medications.
- Be aware of drug-nutrient interactions.
- Initiate nutrition interventions early (e.g., postoperative tube feeding).
- Achieve tight glucose control.
- Consider changing the immunosuppression regimen if metabolic problems ensue (e.g., hypertension, hyperlipidemia, diabetes).
- Monitor bone density and consider prophylactic treatment in patients at high risk for osteoporosis.

Don't

- Use a "one-size-fits-all" nutrition prescription.
- Initiate protein restriction in pretransplant patients.
- Give directives (such as "lose weight") without providing specific action steps and follow-up.
- Hesitate to provide tube feeding if patients are not able to eat.
- Ignore comorbid conditions (such as diabetes, obesity, hyperlipidemia, or hypertension) that can be treated in part with dietary interventions.

References

1. Müller MJ: Hepatic energy and substrate metabolism: A possible metabolic basis for early nutritional support in cirrhotic patients. Nutrition 14:30-38, 1998.
2. Greco AV, Mingrone G, Benedetti G, et al: Daily energy and substrate metabolism in patients with cirrhosis. Hepatology 27:346-350, 1998.
3. McCullough AJ, Tavill AS: Disordered energy and protein metabolism in liver disease. Semin Liver Dis 11:265-277, 1991.
4. Müller MJ, Böttcher J, Selberg O, et al: Hypermetabolism in clinically stable patients with liver cirrhosis. Am J Clin Nutr 69:1194-1201, 1999.
5. Dolz C, Raurich JM, Ibanez J, et al: Ascites increases the resting energy expenditure in liver cirrhosis. Gastroenterology 100:738-744, 1991.

6. Shanbhogue RLK, Bistrian BR, Jenkins RL, et al: Resting energy expenditure in patients with end-stage liver disease and in normal population. JPEN J Parenter Enteral Nutr 11:305-308, 1987.

7. Pierrugues R, Blanc P, Daures JP, et al: Relationship of resting energy expenditure with liver function and nutritional status in patients with alcoholic cirrhosis. Nutrition 8:22-25, 1992.

8. Merritt WT: Metabolism and liver transplantation: Review of perioperative issues. Liver Transpl 4(Suppl 1):S76-S84, 2000.

9. Merli M, Leonetti, Riggio O, et al: Glucose intolerance and insulin resistance in cirrhosis are normalized after liver transplantation. Hepatology 30:649-654, 1999.

10. McClain CJ, Marsana L, Burk RF, et al: Trace metals in liver disease. Semin Liver Dis 11:321-339, 1991.

11. Harrison J, McKiernan J, Neuberger JM: A prospective study on the effect of recipient nutritional status on outcome in liver transplantation. Transpl Int 10:369-374, 1997.

12. Stephenson GR, Moretti EW, El-Moalem H, et al: Malnutrition in liver transplant patients. Transplantation 72:666-670, 2001.

13. Pikul J, Sharpe MD, Lowndes R, et al: Degree of preoperative malnutrition is predictive of postoperative morbidity and mortality in liver transplant recipients. Transplantation 57:469-472, 1994.

14. Selberg O, Böttcher J, Tusch G, et al: Identification of high- and low-risk patients before liver transplantation: A prospective cohort study of nutritional and metabolic parameters in 150 patients. Hepatology 25:652-657, 1997.

15. Hasse JM, Gonwa TA, Jennings LW, et al: Malnutrition affects liver transplant outcomes [abstract]. Transplantation 66(8):S53, 1998.

16. Abbott WJ, Thomson A, Steadman C, et al: Child-Pugh class, nutritional indicators and early liver transplant outcomes. Hepatogastroenterology 48:823-827, 2001.

17. Figueiredo FA, Dickson ER, Pasha TM, et al: Utility of standard nutritional parameters in detecting body cell mass depletion in patients with end-stage liver disease. Liver Transpl 6:575-581, 2000.

18. Hasse J, Strong S, Gorman MA, et al: Subjective global assessment—an alternative nutritional assessment technique for liver transplant candidates. Nutrition 9:339-343, 1993.

19. Detsky AS, McLaughlin JR, Baker JP, et al: What is subjective global assessment of nutritional status? JPEN J Parenter Enteral Nutr 11:8-13, 1987.

20. Baker JP, Detsky AS, Wesson DE, et al: Nutritional assessment: A comparison of clinical judgement and objective measurements. N Engl J Med 306:969-972, 1982.

21. Testa G, Hasse JM, Jennings LW, et al: Morbid obesity is not an independent risk factor for liver transplantation [abstract]. Transplantation 66(8):S53, 1998.

22. Braunfeld MYY, Chan S, Pregler J, et al: Liver transplantation in the morbidly obese. J Clin Anesth 8:585-590, 1996.

23. Sawyer RG, Pelletier SJ, Pruett TL: Increased early morbidity and mortality with acceptable long-term function in severely obese patients undergoing liver transplantation. Clin Transplant 13(1 Pt 2):126-130, 1999.

24. Nair S, Cohen DB, Cohen C, et al: Postoperative morbidity, mortality, costs, and long-term survival in severely obese patients undergoing orthotopic liver transplantation. Am J Gastroenterol 96:842-845, 2001.

25. Nair S, Verma S, Thuluvath PJ: Obesity and its effect on survival in patients undergoing orthotopic liver transplantation in the United States. Hepatology 35:105-109, 2002.

26. Porayko MK, DiCecco S, O'Keefe SJD: Impact of malnutrition and its therapy on liver transplantation. Semin Liver Dis 11:305-314, 1991.

27. Hirsch S, Bunout D, de la Maza P, et al: Controlled trial on nutrition supplementation in outpatients with symptomatic alcoholic cirrhosis. JPEN J Parenter Enteral Nutr 17:119-124, 1993.

28. LeCornu KA, McKiernan FJ, Kapadia SA, et al: A prospective randomized study of preoperative nutritional supplementation in patients awaiting elective orthotopic liver transplantation. Transplantation 69:1364-1369, 2000.

29. Hasse JM, Crippin JS, Blue LS, et al: Branched-chain amino acid–enriched nutrition supplementation reduces hospitalization in malnourished patients with a history of encephalopathy awaiting liver transplantation [abstract]. JPEN J Parenter Enteral Nutr 21:S16, 1997.

30. Kearns PJ, Young H, Garcia G, et al: Accelerated improvement of alcoholic liver disease with enteral nutrition. Gastroenterology 102:200-205, 1992.

31. Cabre E, Gonzalez-Huix G, Abad-Lacruz A, et al: Effect of total enteral nutrition on the short-term outcome of severely malnourished cirrhotics. A randomized controlled trial. Gastroenterology 98:715-720, 1990.

32. Horst D, Grace ND, Conn HO, et al: Comparison of dietary protein with an oral, branched chain–enriched amino acid supplement in chronic portal-systemic encephalopathy: A randomized controlled trial. Hepatology 4:279-287, 1984.

33. Marchesini G, Dioguardi FS, Bianchi GP, et al: Long-term oral branched-chain amino acid treatment in chronic hepatic encephalopathy: A randomized double-blind casein-controlled trial. J Hepatol 11:92-101, 1990.

34. Egberts EH, Schomerus H, Hamster W, et al: Branched chain amino acids in the treatment of latent portosystemic encephalopathy: A double-blind placebo-controlled crossover study. Gastroenterology 88:887-895, 1985.

35. Plevak DJ, DiCecco SR, Wiesner RH, et al: Nutritional support for liver transplantation: Identifying caloric and protein requirements. Mayo Clin Proc 69:225-230, 1994.

36. Hasse JM, Blue LS, Liepa GU, et al: Early enteral nutrition support in patients undergoing liver transplantation. JPEN J Parenter Enteral Nutr 19:437-443, 1995.

37. Delafosse B, Faure JL, Bouffard Y, et al: Liver transplantation—energy expenditure, nitrogen loss, and substrate oxidation rate in the first two postoperative days. Transplant Proc 21:2453-2454, 1989.

38. Shanbhogue RLK, Bistrian BR, Jenkins RL, et al: Increased protein catabolism without hypermetabolism after human orthotopic liver transplantation. Surgery 101:146-149, 1987.

39. O'Keefe SJ, Williams R, Calne RY: "Catabolic" loss of body protein after human liver transplantation. BMJ 280:1107-1108, 1980.

40. Plank LD, Metzger DJ, McCall JL, et al: Sequential changes in the metabolic response to orthotopic liver transplantation during the first year after surgery. Ann Surg 234:245-255, 2001.

41. Tietge UJF, Bahr JM, Manns MP, et al: Plasma amino acids in cirrhosis and after liver transplantation: Influence of liver function, hepatic hemodynamics and circulating hormones. Clin Transplant 16:9-17, 2002.

42. Wicks C, Somasundaram S, Buarnason I, et al: Comparison of enteral feeding and total parenteral nutrition after liver transplantation. Lancet 344:837-840, 1994.

43. Rayes N, Seehofer D, Hansen S, et al: Early enteral supply of lactobacillus and fiber versus selective bowel decontamination: A controlled trial in liver transplant recipients. Transplantation 74:123-127, 2002.

44. Mehta PL, Alaka KJ, Filo RS, et al: Nutrition support following liver transplantation: A comparison of jejunal versus parenteral routes. Clin Transplant 344:837-840, 1995.

45. Pescovitz MD, Mehta PL, Leapman SB, et al: Tube jejunostomy in liver transplant recipients. Surgery 117:642-647, 1995.

46. Reilly J, Mehta R, Teperman L, et al: Nutritional support after liver transplantation: A randomized prospective study. JPEN J Parenter Enteral Nutr 14:386-391, 1990.

47. Varo E, Padin E, Otero E, et al: Cardiovascular risk factors in liver allograft recipients: Relationship with immunosuppressive therapy. Transplant Proc 34:1553-1554, 2002.

48. Mor E, Facklam D, Hasse J, et al: Weight gain and lipid profile changes in liver transplant recipients: Long-term results of the American FK506 multicenter study. Transplant Proc 27:1126, 1995.
49. Punch JD, Shieck VL, Campbell DA, et al: Corticosteroid withdrawal after liver transplantation. Surgery 118:783-788, 1995.
50. Neal DAJ, Cimson AES, Gibbs P, et al: Beneficial effects of converting liver transplant recipients from cyclosporine to tacrolimus on blood pressure, serum lipids, and weight. Liver Transpl 7:533-539, 2001.
51. Beyer N, Aadahl M, Strange B, et al: Improved physical performance after orthotopic liver transplantation. Liver Transpl Surg 5:301-309, 1999.
52. Stephenson AL, Yoshida EM, Abboud RT, et al: Impaired exercise performance after successful liver transplantation. Transplantation 72:1161-1163, 2001.
53. Duchini A, Brunson ME: Roux-en-Y gastric bypass for recurrent nonalcoholic steatohepatitis in liver transplant recipients with morbid obesity. Transplantation 72:156-171, 2001.
54. Zachoval R, Gerbes AL, Schwandt R, et al: Short-term effects of statin therapy in patients with hyperlipoproteinemia after liver transplantation: Results of a randomized cross-over trial. J Hepatol 35:86-91, 2001.
55. Imagawa DK, Dawson S, Holt CD, et al: Hyperlipidemia after liver transplantation. Natural history and treatment with the hydroxy-methylglutaryl-coenzyme A reductase inhibitor pravastatin. Transplantation 62:934-942, 1996.
56. Fernandez-Miranda C, Sanz M, De La Calle A, et al: Cardiovascular risk factors in 116 patients 5 years or more after liver transplantation. Transpl Int 15:556-562, 2002.
57. Rabkin JM, Corless CL, Rosen HR, et al: Immunosuppression impact on long-term cardiovascular complications after liver transplantation. Am J Surg 183:595-599, 2002.
58. Perez R: Managing nutrition problems in transplant patients. Nutr Clin Pract 8:28-32, 1993.
59. Morrisett JD, Abdel-Fattah G, Hoogeveen R, et al: Effects of sirolimus on plasma lipids, lipoprotein levels, and fatty acid metabolism in renal transplant patients. J Lipid Res 43:1170-1180, 2002.
60. Manzarbeitia C, Reich DJ, Rothstein KD, et al: Tacrolimus conversion improves hyperlipidemia states in stable liver transplant recipients. Liver Transpl 2:93-99, 2001.
61. Kobashigawa JA, Kasiske BL: Hyperlipidemia in solid organ transplantation. Transplantation 63:331-338, 1997.
62. Textor SC, Taler SJ, Canzanello VJ, et al: Posttransplantation hypertension related to calcineurin inhibitors. Liver Transpl 6:521-530, 2000.
63. Johnston SD, Morris JK, Cramb R, et al: Cardiovascular morbidity and mortality after orthotopic liver transplantation. Transplantation 73:901-906, 2002.
64. Herrero JI, Quiroga J, Sangro B, et al: Hyperhomocysteinemia in liver transplant recipients: Prevalence and multivariate analysis of predisposing factors. Liver Transpl 6:614-618, 2000.
65. Blanco JJ, Herrero JI, Quiroga J, et al: Liver transplantation in cirrhotic patients with diabetes mellitus: Midterm results, survival, and adverse events. Liver Transpl 7:226-233, 2001.
66. John PR, Thuluvath PJ: Outcome of liver transplantation in patients with diabetes mellitus: A case-control study. Hepatology 34:889-895, 2001.
67. Yoo HY, Thuluvath PJ: The effect of insulin-dependent diabetes mellitus on outcome of liver transplantation. Transplantation 74:1007-1012, 2002.
68. Steinmuller TH, Stockmann M, Bechstein WO, et al: Liver transplantation and diabetes mellitus. Exp Clin Endocrinol Diabetes 108:401-405, 2000.
69. John PR, Thuluvath PJ: Outcome of patients with new-onset diabetes mellitus after liver transplantation compared with those without diabetes mellitus. Liver Transpl 8:708-713, 2002.
70. Bigam DL, Pennington JJ, Carpentier A, et al: Hepatitis-C related cirrhosis: A predictor of diabetes after liver transplantation. Hepatology 32:87-90, 2000.
71. Baid S, Cosimi AB, Farrell ML, et al: Posttransplant diabetes mellitus in liver transplant recipients: Risk factors, temporal relationship with hepatitis C virus allograft hepatitis, and impact on mortality. Transplantation 72:1066-1072, 2001.
72. Jindal RM: Posttransplant diabetes mellitus—a review. Transplantation 58:1289-1298, 1994.
73. Krentz AJ, Dousset B, Mayer D, et al: Metabolic effects of cyclosporin A and FK 506 in liver transplant recipients. Diabetes 42:1753-1759, 1993.
74. Senninger N, Golling M, Datsis K, et al: Glucose metabolism following liver transplantation and immunosuppression with cyclosporine A or FK 506. Transplant Proc 27:1127-1128, 1995.
75. Stegall MD, Everson GT, Schroter G, et al: Prednisone withdrawal late after adult liver transplantation reduces diabetes, hypertension, and hypercholesterolemia without causing graft loss. Hepatology 25:173-177, 1997.
76. Tchervenkov JI, Tector AJ, Cantarovich M, et al: Maintenance immunosuppression using cyclosporine monotherapy in adult orthotopic liver transplant recipients. Transplant Proc 28:2247-2249, 1996.
77. De Carlis L, Belli LS, Rondinara GF, et al: Early steroid withdrawal in liver transplant patients: Final report of a prospective randomized trial. Transplant Proc 29:539-542, 1997.
78. Ninkovic M, Skingle SJ, Bearcroft PWP, et al: Incidence of vertebral fractures in the first three months after orthotopic liver transplantation. Eur J Gastroenterol Hepatol 12:931-935, 2000.
79. Floreani A, Fries W, Luisetto G, et al: Bone metabolism in orthotopic liver transplantation: A prospective study. Liver Transpl Surg 4:311-319, 1998.
80. Hay JE: Bone disease after liver transplantation. Liver Transplant Surg 1(Suppl 1):55-63, 1995.
81. Hao X, Eichstaedt H: Assessment of serial changes of bone mineral density at lumbar spine and femoral neck before and after liver transplantation. Chin Med J 112:379-381, 1999.
82. Hussaini SH, Oldroyd B, Stewart SP, et al: Regional bone mineral density after orthotopic liver transplantation. Eur J Gastroenterol Hepatol 11:157-163, 199.
83. Katz IA, Epstein S: Posttransplant bone disease. J Bone Miner Res 7:123-126, 1992.
84. Reeves HL, Francis RM, Mana DM, et al: Intravenous bisphosphonate prevents symptomatic osteoporotic vertebral collapse in patients after liver transplantation. Liver Transpl Surg 4:404-409, 1998.
85. Ninkovic M, Love S, Tom BDM, et al: Lack of effect of intravenous pamidronate on fracture incidence and bone mineral density after orthotopic liver transplantation. J Hepatol 37:93-100, 2002.
86. Isoniemi H, Appelberg J, Nilsson C-G, et al: Transdermal oestrogen therapy protects postmenopausal liver transplant women from osteoporosis. A 2-year follow-up study. J Hepatol 34:299-305, 2001.
87. Hay JE, Malinchoc M, Dickson ER: A controlled trial of calcitonin therapy for the prevention of post–liver transplantation atraumatic fractures in patients with primary biliary cirrhosis and primary sclerosing cholangitis. J Hepatol 34:292-298, 2001.
88. Moschella C, Jaber BL: Interaction between cyclosporine and *Hypericum perforatum* (St. John's wort) after organ transplantation. Am J Kidney Dis 38:1105-1107, 2001.

Management of Portal Hypertensive Hemorrhage in the Era of Liver Transplantation

SUNIL K. GEEVARGHESE
JONATHAN R. HIATT
RONALD W. BUSUTTIL

Management algorithm   507
   Resuscitation and medical therapy   508
   Endoscopic diagnosis and therapy   508
   Therapeutic options for continuing
     hemorrhage   508

Portosystemic shunts   509

Transjugular intrahepatic portosystemic
   shunting   509

Surgical shunts   509

Comparison of modalities   509

Summary   510

Variceal bleeding is a major manifestation of advanced portal hypertension, with substantial morbidity and mortality. Portal hypertension caused by severe hepatic parenchymal disease is a cardinal indication for liver replacement. Isolated variceal bleeding is often managed successfully without liver transplantation, and some patients experience bleeding early in the course of transplantation candidacy or at a time when a donor organ is not immediately available.

Mortality from bleeding esophageal and/or gastric varices correlates linearly with hepatic function, measured by Child-Pugh grading; mortality for the index bleed is 5%, 18%, and 68% in grades A, B, and C patients, respectively.[1] Since a number of management options are now available, an algorithmic approach that reflects physiological condition and response to therapy is essential for best results.

Management Algorithm

More than half of patients with esophagogastric varices will never experience bleeding. These patients are managed with avoidance of hepatotoxins and with β-blockers, which reduce portal pressure by constriction of the splanchnic vasculature and reduction of cardiac output. The use of prophylactic interventions has been debated. Surgical shunts have no role, and endoscopic therapies may be of benefit in reducing the risk of bleeding but lack a clear effect on mortality.[2] Some centers use hepatic portal venous pressure for measurement of response to β-blockade and other interventions.

Patients with acute variceal bleeding require emergent resuscitation, medical management, endoscopic diagnosis, and directed therapy. Figure 34–1 summarizes the algorithmic strategy for management of these patients.

Resuscitation and Medical Therapy

Patients are admitted to the intensive care unit for resuscitation, monitoring, and procedures. Endotracheal intubation is often needed for airway protection, especially during endoscopy. Large-bore venous access is secured, usually in a central vein. Clotting defects are corrected with transfusion of fresh-frozen plasma and platelets, taking care to avoid elevating central venous pressure to greater than 10 cm H_2O if possible. Ascites and infection with bacterial or fungal organisms should be identified and treated, as these may complicate and exacerbate bleeding.

A variety of vasoactive and other medications is available for control of variceal hemorrhage, and the current regimen uses octreotide and pantoprazole. Octreotide is a synthetic analogue of somatostatin, which is a splanchnic constrictor and inhibitor of glucagon and other vasodilatory peptides. Pantoprazole suppresses gastric acid secretion by inhibition of the parietal cell hydrogen–potassium–adenosine triphosphate pump.

Endoscopic Diagnosis and Therapy

Emergent esophagogastroduodenoscopy (EGD) is performed for diagnosis and therapy. EGD identifies the presence of varices and excludes other bleeding sources, such as portal gastropathy, gastritis, or ulcer.

Bleeding varices in the esophagus or esophagogastric junction are treated with injection sclerotherapy or variceal band ligation. The latter is more difficult to perform but has lower morbidity than sclerotherapy, which may be complicated by aspiration pneumonia or esophageal ulceration. In capable hands, bleeding is controlled by endoscopic measures in more than 90% of patients, with failure most common in grade C hepatic disease. With bleeding controlled, patients are observed closely, and repeat EGD is performed within the first week after the initial session.

Therapeutic Options for Continuing Hemorrhage

Bleeding that is uncontrolled by endoscopic measures represents a major challenge. Initial control is attempted with balloon tamponade using a Sengstaken-Blakemore tube. The next intervention is usually transjugular intrahepatic portosystemic shunting (TIPS; discussed further on). Liver transplantation is a desirable option, provided that the patient can be stabilized hemodynamically and an organ becomes available.

Recurrent bleeding may occur in patients whose bleeding was controlled initially by medical and endoscopic measures. In grade A or B patients with good liver function, a surgical shunt is performed. Various options are discussed later, but in general terms, the choice of shunt is determined by the portal anatomy and the likelihood and timing of liver transplantation.

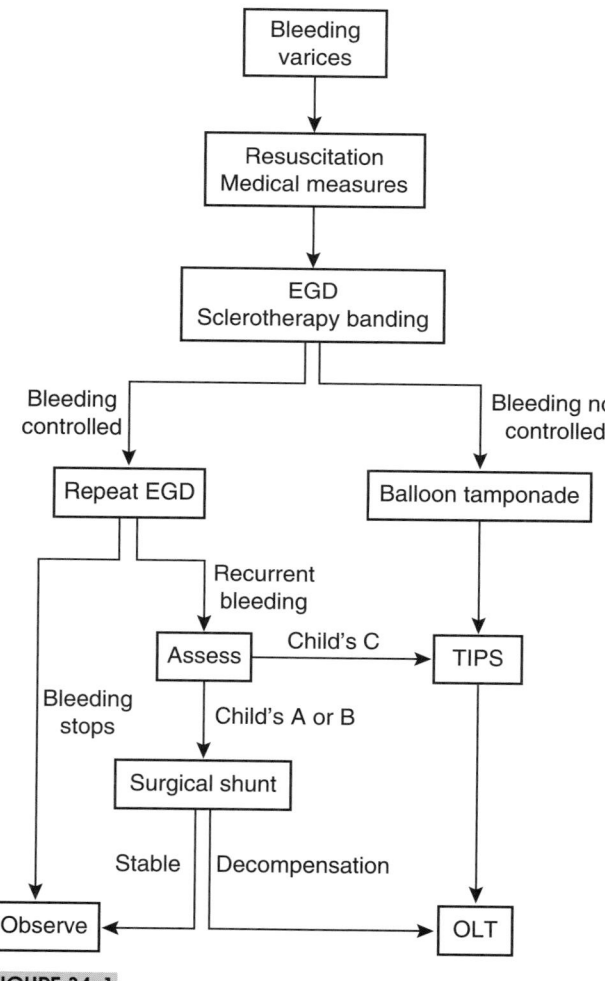

FIGURE 34–1

Algorithm for management of acutely bleeding esophageal varices. EGD, esophagogastroduodenoscopy; OLT, orthotopic liver transplantation; TIPS, transvenous intrahepatic portosystemic shunt.

Portosystemic Shunts

Shunts constructed between portal and systemic circulations are of selective or nonselective types. The latter (portacaval, mesocaval, TIPS) reduce portal pressure and have the advantages of ease of construction and durability, but share the problems of encephalopathy and worsening liver function. Selective shunts, of which distal splenorenal is the most common, provide selective decompression of the portal-azygos system, and thus of the gastroesophageal varices, while preserving nutrient portal inflow to the liver. The use of the distal splenorenal shunt, discussed further on, is limited by its technical difficulty and the eventual loss of selectivity by gradual enlargement of pancreatic collaterals.

Transjugular Intrahepatic Portosystemic Shunting

TIPS has become the first-line therapy for portal hypertension after immediate endoscopic control, despite few controlled studies confirming its benefit. Interventional radiologists perform the procedure, after the patient has been given sedation and local anesthesia, using fluoroscopic and sonographic guidance. A needle is passed from the middle hepatic vein into a portal vein branch, followed by a guidewire that is passed through the needle and into the main portal vein. Next, portal pressure is measured; the tract is dilated with a balloon; portography is performed; and an expandable stent is inserted, sometimes followed by a second stent if needed to reduce the portal pressure gradient to less than 12 mm Hg.

As with any nonselective shunt, hepatic encephalopathy may occur, as may liver failure from diversion of portal flow. The major complications of TIPS include shunt stenosis (33% to 66%), hepatic encephalopathy (15% to 30%), technical failure (5% to 10%), and portal or splenic vein thrombosis, worsening liver function, and chronic hemolysis (less than 5% each).[3]

Surgical Shunts

Distal splenorenal shunt (DSRS) and nonselective shunts have been compared in many studies over the past quarter century.[4-11] The prevailing conclusions from these studies are that rates of survival and recurrent bleeding are similar, but the incidence of postoperative encephalopathy is lower with DSRS. Survival after DSRS in Child's grade A or B is better than that of patients with more severely compromised liver function.[12-14]

Another group of studies comparing DSRS with sclerotherapy has generally supported the concept of sclerotherapy for acute bleeding and DSRS for elective surgical correction of chronic or recurrent bleeding.[12,15-18]

Orloff has been a consistent advocate of emergency side-to-side portacaval shunting for acutely bleeding esophageal varices. In a report of 400 patients, rates of 15-year survival and of recurrent encephalopathy were 57% and 8%, respectively, for the 220 patients treated after 1978.[19] An earlier report described excellent results even with advanced disease: 5-year survival in 64% and postoperative encephalopathy in 18% of 94 Child's C patients.[20]

The mesocaval shunt, or H-graft, has been advocated as a bridge to liver transplantation because it is relatively quick and easy to construct, avoids any dissection in the porta hepatis, and can be simply ligated at the time of transplantation. A randomized prospective comparison of H-graft with small-diameter side-to-side portacaval shunt in good-risk patients found less encephalopathy and better preservation of liver function with the H-graft.[21]

Portal vein thrombosis is an important cause of extrahepatic portal hypertension, particularly in children. Using an inferior mesenteric or internal jugular venous conduit, the Rex procedure reconnects the mesenteric system to the portal system at the Rex recessus, a bridge of liver tissue between segments III and IV.[22] In the first American series of Rex shunts, Bambini described the procedure as superior to DSRS for reasons including restoration of portal flow, normalization of portal venous pressure, and splenic decompression, with relief of secondary thrombocytopenia and leukopenia.[23]

Comparison of Modalities

A number of series have compared TIPS to surgical shunts (Table 34–1).[2,27] Various authors have concluded that surgical shunts are the more durable and cost-effective option for Child's A or B cirrhotics, with TIPS reserved as primary therapy for patients with advanced liver disease awaiting imminent transplantation or with contraindications to an abdominal operation.[24-26,28] Failed TIPS can sometimes be salvaged with DSRS.[29]

Jenkins compared patients with (n = 81) and without (n = 247) DSRS prior to liver transplantation and found no differences in operative time, blood loss, and early mortality following transplantation. Portal vein thrombosis occurred in five DSRS patients. The interval between DSRS and liver transplantation was more than 5 years, demonstrating the utility of the shunt procedure as a temporizing measure.[30]

Cosenza performed a similar study of TIPS prior to liver transplantation. TIPS did not affect operative time or transfusion requirements; portal vein thrombosis occurred in one patient and required thrombectomy at the time of transplantation.[31]

Table 34-1. RESULTS OF TRIALS COMPARING TIPS AND SURGICAL SHUNTS

Author	Procedures	n	Follow-up (mo)	Survival	Rebleeding	Encephalopathy
Henderson[24]	TIPS	200	40	53%	26%	ND
	Surgical	63	36	86%	14%	21%
Helton[25]	TIPS	20	19.5	80%	50%	ND
	PCS/DSRS	20	22.9	90%	0	ND
Rosemurgy[26]	TIPS	29	72	55%	21%	34%
	H-graft	33	80	58%	12%	30%

DSRS, distal splenorenal shunt; ND, no data; PCS, portacaval shunt; TIPS, transjugular intrahepatic portosystemic shunt.

Summary

Portal hypertensive hemorrhage is a major problem in patients with end-stage liver disease. An algorithm for diagnosis and management of acute variceal bleeding is critical for best results. After resuscitation and medical therapy, upper endoscopy is used for diagnosis and initial treatment with injection sclerotherapy or variceal banding. Subsequent management is determined by response to these primary measures. Continuing bleeding is treated first with balloon tamponade. TIPS or surgical shunts provide definitive treatment of continuing or recurrent bleeding. TIPS carries with it the risks of stenosis, occlusion, and worsening encephalopathy. Surgical shunts have the greatest utility in good-risk patients a number of years before liver transplantation.

Pearls and Pitfalls

- The outcome of variceal hemorrhage is primarily related to liver function.
- Sclerotherapy and/or banding is the first line of treatment, along with pharmacological reduction of portal pressure.
- Selective shunting (DSRS) is still indicated in patients with preserved liver function.
- TIPS is indicated for patients in imminent need of liver transplantation.
- Mesocaval shunts should be ligated at the time of liver transplantation.

References

1. Sherlock S, Dooley J: The portal venous system and portal hypertension. In Sherlock S, Dooley J (eds): Diseases of the Liver and Biliary System, 11th ed. Oxford, UK, Blackwell Scientific, 2002, p 173.
2. Rikkers LF: The changing spectrum of treatment for variceal bleeding. Ann Surg 228:536-546, 1998.
3. Sherlock S, Dooley J: The portal venous system and portal hypertension. In Sherlock S, Dooley J (eds): Diseases of the Liver and Biliary System, 11th ed. Oxford, UK, Blackwell Scientific, 2002, p 179.
4. Rikkers L, Rudman D, Galambos J: A randomized controlled trial of distal splenorenal shunts. Ann Surg 188:271-282, 1978.
5. Reichle F, Fahmy W, Golsorkhi M: Prospective comparative clinical trial with distal splenorenal and mesocaval shunts. Am J Surg 137:13-21, 1979.
6. Langer B, Rotstein L, Stone R: A prospective randomized trial of the selective distal splenorenal shunt. Surg Gynecol Obstet 150:45-48, 1980.
7. Conn H, Resnick R, Grace N, et al: Distal splenorenal shunt versus portosystemic shunt: Current status of a controlled trial. Hepatology 1:151–160, 1981.
8. Millikan W, Warren W, Henderson J, et al: The Emory prospective randomized trial: Selective versus nonselective shunt to control variceal bleeding. Ten-year followup. Ann Surg 201:712-722, 1985.
9. Langer B, Taylor B, Mackenzie D, et al: Further report of a prospective randomized trial comparing distal splenorenal shunt with end-to-side portacaval shunt. Gastroenterology 88:424-429, 1985.
10. Harley H, Morgan T, Redeker A, et al: Results of a randomized trial of end-to-side portacaval shunt and distal splenorenal shunt to control variceal bleeding. Gastroenterology 91:802-809, 1986.
11. Raia S, Mies S, Alfieri F: Portal hypertension in mansonic schistosomiasis. World J Surg 15:176–187, 1991.
12. Spina G, Santambrogio R, Opocher E: Distal splenorenal shunt versus endoscopic sclerotherapy in the prevention of variceal rebleeding. Ann Surg 211:178–186, 1990.
13. Pera C, Visa J, Garcia-Valdecasas J, et al: The modified distal splenorenal shunt in the elective treatment of variceal hemorrhage. Hepatogastroenterology 38(Suppl 1):12-15, 1991.
14. Warren W, Millikan W, Henderson J: Ten years of portal hypertension surgery at Emory. Ann Surg 195:530-542, 1982.
15. Warren W, Henderson J, Millikan W, et al: Distal splenorenal shunt versus endoscopic sclerotherapy for long-term management of variceal bleeding. Preliminary report of a prospective, randomized trial. Ann Surg 203:454-462, 1986.
16. Teres J, Baroni R, Bordas M, et al: Randomized trial of portacaval shunt, stapling transection, and endoscopic sclerotherapy in uncontrolled variceal bleeding. J Hepatol 4:159-167, 1987.
17. Rikkers L, Burnett DA, Volentine GD, et al: Shunt surgery versus endoscopic sclerotherapy for long-term treatment of variceal bleeding: Early results of a randomized trial. Ann Surg 206:261-271, 1987.
18. Henderson J, Kutner M, Millikan WJ, et al: Endoscopic variceal sclerosis compared with distal splenorenal shunt to prevent recurrent variceal bleeding in cirrhosis. Ann Intern Med 112:262-269, 1990.

19. Orloff M, Orloff M, Rambotti M, Girard B: Is portal-systemic shunt worthwhile in Child's class C cirrhosis? Ann Surg 216: 256-268, 1992.
20. Orloff MJ, Orloff MS, Orloff SL, et al: Three decades of experience with emergency portacaval shunt for acutely bleeding esophageal varices in 400 unselected patients with cirrhosis of the liver. J Am Coll Surg 180:337-339, 1995.
21. Capussoti L, Vergara V, Polastri R, et al: Liver function and encephalopathy after partial versus direct side-to-side portacaval shunt: A prospective randomized clinical trial. Surgery 127:614-621, 2000.
22. Ates O, Hakguder G, Olguner M, Akgur F: Extrahepatic portal hypertension treated by anastomosing inferior mesenteric vein to left portal vein at Rex recessus. J Pediatr Surg 38:10–11, 2003.
23. Bambini DA, Superina R, Almond PS, et al: Experience with the Rex shunt (mesenterico–left portal bypass) in children with extrahepatic portal hypertension. J Pediatr Surg 35:13-19, 2000.
24. Henderson JM, Nagle A, Curtas S, et al: Surgical shunts and TIPS for variceal decompression in the 1990s. Surgery 128:540-547, 2000.
25. Helton WS, Maves R, Wicks K, Johanson K: Transjugular intrahepatic portasystemic shunt vs surgical shunt in good-risk cirrhotic patients. Arch Surg 136:17-20, 2001.
26. Rosemurgy AS, Zervos EE, Bloomston M, et al: Post-shunt resource consumption favors small-diameter prosthetic H-graft portacaval shunt over TIPS for patients with poor hepatic reserve. Ann Surg 237:820-827, 2003.
27. Seewald S, Mendoza G, Seitz U, et al: Variceal bleeding and portal hypertension: Has there been any progress in the last 12 months? Endoscopy 35:136-144, 2003.
28. Zacks SL, Sandler RS, Biddle AK, et al: Decision-analysis of transjugular intrahepatic portasystemic shunt versus distal splenorenal shunt for portal hypertension. Hepatology 29: 1399-1405, 1999.
29. Selim N, Fendly MJ, Boyer TD, et al: Conversion of failed transjugular intrahepatic portasystemic shunt to distal splenorenal shunt in patients with Child A or B cirrhosis. Ann Surg 227:600-603, 1998.
30. Jenkins RL, Gedaly R, Pomposelli JJ, et al: Distal splenorenal shunt: Role, indications, and utility in the era of liver transplantation. Arch Surg 134:416-420, 1999.
31. Cosenza CA, Hoffman AL, Freidman ML, et al: Transjugular intrahepatic portasystemic shunt: Efficacy for the treatment of portal hypertension and impact on liver transplantation. Am Surg 62:835-839, 1996.

V

Operation

Donor Selection and Management

CONSTANTINO FONDEVILA
RAFIK M. GHOBRIAL

Brain death 516
  Guidelines for determination of
    brain death 516

Confirmatory tests of brain death 516
  Electroencephalography 516
  Evoked cerebral potentials 516
  Doppler sonography 516
  Scintigraphy 517
  Angiography 517

Physiological effects of brain death and
  medical complications 517

Management of brain-dead patients 518
  Medical failures to organ donation 519

Potential organ donor identification
  and consent 520

Deceased donor organ procurement
  process 520

Donor selection 521

Absolute contraindications to organ
  donation 521
  Infectious diseases 521
  Malignancy 521

Extended criteria for organ acceptance 521
  Donor age 521
  Hepatic steatosis 522
  Damaged organs 523
  Bacterial and fungal infections 523
  Viral infections 523

Evaluation of liver donors at time of
  procurement 523

Strategies for increasing the organ pool 524
  Split-liver transplantation 524
  Reuse of grafts and domino transplantation 524
  Living donors 524
  Non–heart-beating donors 525
  Machine perfusion 526

Organ transplantation is a well-accepted therapy for patients with end-stage disease of most major organ systems. However, the applicability of transplantation is greatly limited, essentially because of the scarcity of organ supply. In the European Union and the United States, 10% to 30% of patients on a waiting list for a liver transplant die before obtaining the graft.[1] Sources of organs, excluding xenotransplants, can be (1) living donors, (2) donors who died after cardiorespiratory arrest, and (3) brain-dead donors. Brain-dead donors constitute the greater source of donor organs for transplantation. They have complete and irreversible cessation of cortical and brain stem function and require respiratory and cardiovascular support. To meet the increased need for transplantable organs, the medical staff needs to know how to maintain donors optimally. It has been estimated that 17% to 25% of potential donors are lost because of medical failure while awaiting the formal declaration of brain death.[2] With increased awareness of the problems and needs of the donor and the application of a rational physiological approach, the supply of functional organs for transplantation can be increased.[3] Efforts to maximize donor supply and increase organ donation rates must be accompanied by the provision of humane care to patients and their families.

Brain Death

The term "brain death" was introduced in 1965 after a report of renal transplantation from a heart-beating, but "brain death," donor and was defined formally in 1968 in the report of the Ad Hoc Committee of the Harvard Medical School.[4] The clinical manifestations of brain death encompass complete apnea, brain stem areflexia, and cerebral unresponsiveness, which as a whole indicates complete and irreversible cessation of brain and brain stem function. A patient whose cerebral function is irreversibly lost could be kept functioning by artificial ventilation, intravenous feeding, and other intensive care measures, but treatment of these patients should be terminated after an unequivocal diagnosis of brain death.[5] In 1981, the Report of the Medical Consultants on the Diagnosis of Death to the U.S. President's Commission recommended that the criteria for a diagnosis of brain death should be seen as synonymous with the definition of death of the organism as a whole.[6] Causes of brain death other than trauma consist of subarachnoid hemorrhage, cerebral abscess or tumor, meningitis, encephalitis, and cerebral hypoxia. Several confounding factors must be ruled out, including hypothermia ($<32°C$), shock, drug intoxication, severe metabolic derangement, and the effects of neuromuscular blockade.[7]

Guidelines for Determination of Brain Death

Cessation of life is recognized when evaluation discloses the following[2,6]:

1. Cerebral function, as well as "cerebral responsiveness and receptivity," is absent.
2. Brain stem functions are absent, including pupillary light, corneal, oculocephalic, oculovestibular, oropharyngeal, and respiratory reflexes. To test for apnea, oxygen is delivered by nasal cannula, and failure of respiratory effort at a $Paco_2$ greater than 60 mm Hg indicates apnea. Spinal cord reflexes may persist after death, but true decerebrate or decorticate posturing or seizures are inconsistent with the diagnosis of death.

Irreversibility is recognized when evaluation discloses the following:

1. The cause of coma is established and sufficient to account for the loss of brain function.
2. The possibility of recovery of any brain function is ruled out.
3. Cessation of all brain function persists for an appropriate period of observation or trial therapy;

confirmation of clinical findings by electrocardiography is desirable when objective documentation is needed to substantiate the clinical findings. Complete cessation of circulation to a normothermic adult brain for more than 10 minutes is incompatible with survival of brain tissue, and absent cerebral blood flow, in conjunction with clinical determination of cessation of all brain functions for at least 6 hours, is diagnostic of death.

Confirmatory Tests of Brain Death

Neurophysiological methods to confirm the clinical signs of brain death can be divided into two groups: (1) methods to confirm the loss of bioelectrical activity of the brain (electroencephalography [EEG], evoked cerebral potentials) and (2) methods to demonstrate cerebral circulatory arrest (Doppler sonography, scintigraphy, angiography).[5]

Electroencephalography

EEG is the test most commonly used to confirm the clinical signs of brain death. The electroencephalogram becomes irreversibly isoelectric after more than 8 minutes of complete cerebral anoxia. It should be recorded continuously for at least 30 minutes to demonstrate irreversible bioelectrical silence. Because EEG is very sensitive to drug effects, blood levels of sedative drugs must be tested before EEG examination.[8]

Evoked Cerebral Potentials

Evoked cerebral potentials are elicited by adequate stimulation of peripheral receptors and recorded from the scalp. They are abolished in the presence of clinical signs of brain death. Evoked potential testing is noninvasive and can be performed at the bedside without danger to the patient. The technical expenditure is similar to that of EEG. The advantage of using evoked potentials is virtual independence from the effects of sedative medications, which sets it apart from EEG. EEG is mandatory, however, in patients with primary infratentorial lesions because the activity of the cerebral cortex can survive the loss of brain stem function by a number of hours or days.[5]

Doppler Sonography

Transcranial Doppler sonography demonstrates blood flow in the arteries of the brain base. On cessation of brain perfusion, characteristic flow patterns can be detected that confirm the lack of perfusion of these arteries. Doppler sonography can be performed at the bedside, is inexpensive, and has been reported to be accurate.[9]

Scintigraphy

Cerebral perfusion can be assessed by performing a sequential nuclear medicine brain flow scan with ^{99m}Tc-labeled diethylenetriamine pentaacetic acid (DTPA) or, more reliably, with ^{99m}Tc-labeled hexamethylpropyleneamine oxime (HMPAO).[10] After an intravenous bolus injection of the tracer, lack of uptake of the tracer into the intracranial cavity confirms the loss of cerebral perfusion. This method can be performed at the bedside and therefore does not carry the risks associated with transportation away from the intensive care unit.[5]

Angiography

Four-vessel angiography is the most accurate means of demonstrating cessation of blood flow to the brain.[11] At least two injections, 20 minutes apart, must show no filling of intracranial arteries. Although this method has the advantage of directly confirming cessation of cranial blood flow, it is expensive and requires transportation to the angiographic suite.

Physiological Effects of Brain Death and Medical Complications

The severe physiological derangements induced by the process of the brain dying and by the loss of integrated neurological function produce profound hemodynamic and metabolic abnormalities in brain-dead potential donors (Table 35–1),[12] which can result in loss of valuable organs.[2] The onset of major medical complications is universal after brain death, with at least one complication developing in nearly all brain-dead donors.[12]

The cardiovascular effects of brain death result first from autonomic storm and later from a profound reduction in sympathetic outflow, which results in hemodynamic instability, impaired inotropy and chronotropy, dysrhythmias, and decreased cardiac output.[13] Autonomic instability and hypotension requiring treatment with vasopressors or invasive hemodynamic monitoring occur in 80% to 85% of donors.[14] The increased pulmonary artery pressure associated with the reduction in cardiac output may result in capillary wall disruption and leakage of protein-rich fluid into the pulmonary interstitium and can thus lead to pulmonary edema.[15] Aspiration pneumonitis, pulmonary contusions, neurogenic pulmonary edema, and pneumonia are common complicating factors in patients with significant head injury.

Table 35–1. MAJOR MEDICAL COMPLICATIONS AND CAUSES ENCOUNTERED IN BRAIN-DEAD PATIENTS

Complication	Etiology
Hypotension	Hypovolemia from osmotic agents given to treat high intracranial pressure, poorly treated diabetes insipidus, blood loss, left ventricular dysfunction, decreases in systemic vascular resistance, endocrine disorders
Arrhythmias	Electrolyte imbalances, hypotension with cardiac ischemia, hypothermia, inotropes, myocardial trauma, increased intracranial pressure
Hyponatremia	Alcohol intoxication, hyperglycemia, renal dysfunction, cirrhosis, cardiac failure, adrenal insufficiency, hypothyroidism
Other electrolyte imbalances (hypernatremia, hypomagnesemia, hypokalemia, hypocalcemia, hypophosphatemia)	Diabetes insipidus
Hyperglycemia	Dextrose-containing fluid administration, preexisting diabetes, catecholamine release, inotropic infusions
Hypothermia	Infusion of large amounts of fluid or blood, loss of central temperature regulation, exposure
Coagulopathy	Release of large amounts of tissue fibrinolytic agent from ischemic tissues

Adapted from Karcioglu O, Ayrik C, Erbil B: The brain-dead patient or a flower in the vase? The emergency department approach to the preservation of the organ donor. Eur J Emerg Med 10:52-57, 2003.

Circulatory collapse may also be due to neurogenic or hypovolemic shock. Neurogenic shock is caused by the failure of cerebral mechanisms to maintain effective peripheral vascular resistance. Hypovolemic shock has multiple causes, including therapeutic dehydration to limit cerebral edema before the declaration of brain death, blood loss secondary to trauma, diabetes insipidus, and third-space fluid loss resulting from altered oncotic pressure.

Significant endocrinological changes take place as brain death occurs, mainly secondary to hypothalamic-pituitary dysfunction. The most commonly reported of such manifestations is diabetes insipidus caused by a deficiency of antidiuretic hormone. Dysfunction of the anterior pituitary, which has a blood supply that is different from that of the posterior pituitary and thus may be spared during herniation, may result in a significant reduction in thyroid hormone and cortisol levels. In the absence of normal thyroid hormone levels, inhibition of mitochondria ensues and results in high-energy phosphate depletion, anaerobic metabolism, hemodynamic instability, and deterioration of organ function. Wide variations in body temperature may also result from such central dysregulation.[13] The variety of mechanisms of brain death encountered in the clinical setting explains the variability in the role that endocrine abnormalities play in the status of donors. The physiological derangements determined by the neuroendocrine failure associated with brain death can be successfully reversed by the administration of a combination of thyroxine (T_3), cortisol, and insulin.[2]

Abnormalities in coagulation are common after brain death. Release of thromboplastic, fibrinolytic, and plasminogen-rich substrate from necrotic brain is thought to cause a consumptive coagulopathy with resultant elevation in prothrombin time and thrombocytopenia.[2] Most potential donors require resuscitation with fresh-frozen plasma to treat these abnormalities.

Management of Brain-Dead Patients

As soon as organ donation is considered, emphasis and care shift from protecting the damaged brain toward maintaining organ viability. A brain-dead donor is very fragile and must be managed as carefully and meticulously as other critically ill patients. Once brain death is declared, early referral, resuscitation, and organ retrieval optimize organ viability.

The primary goal of organ donor management is maintenance of an optimal physiological environment for the organs before removal. Hemodynamic stability is fundamental to optimizing organ perfusion. Circulatory collapse must be anticipated and treated promptly.

Aggressive therapy must be directed at restoring and maintaining intravascular volume and effective circulation. Adequate crystalloids or colloids should be given to achieve a blood pressure of 100 mm Hg or a central venous pressure of 4 to 10 cm H_2O. A pulmonary artery catheter can efficiently guide fluid administration, particularly in lung donors.[16] Transfusion of packed red cells is appropriate when the hematocrit is less than 25%. Vasopressors are used when necessary to optimize blood pressure without compromising organ perfusion. Urine output is a key to adequate organ perfusion and should be maintained at greater than 1 mL/kg/hr.

Appropriate oxygenation and acid-base balance are crucial for preserving organ viability. The fraction of inspired oxygen and the respiratory settings should be adjusted to achieve an alveolar oxygen partial pressure greater than 70 mm Hg with 95% oxygen saturation, and a partial pressure of carbon dioxide between 35 and 45 mm Hg is recommended. Optimal pH should range between 7.30 and 7.45. Vigorous pulmonary toilet and minimal positive end-expiratory pressure (5 cm H_2O) are also useful to optimize pulmonary function.

Diabetes insipidus can lead to severe dehydration, hypernatremia, and resultant donor instability if not treated promptly. Treatment with hypotonic solutions and correction of electrolyte abnormalities are mandatory. The use of hormonal resuscitation (HR) has recently been recommended as an integral part of donor management.[1,17] The HR protocol includes methylprednisolone, 15-mg/kg bolus; T_3, 4-μg bolus and then a continuous infusion at 3 μg/hr; arginine vasopressin, 1-U bolus and then a continuous infusion at 0.5 to 4 U/hr; and insulin, 1 U/hr minimum titrated to maintain blood sugar levels at 120 to 180 mg/dL. Selection of donors who are predicted to benefit from HR was outlined at the Crystal City Consensus Conference Report on Maximizing Use of Organs Recovered from the Cadaver Donor.[17] After conventional management to adjust volume status, anemia, and metabolic abnormalities, the conferees recommended that an echocardiogram be obtained to rule out structural abnormalities and document the ejection fraction. If the ejection fraction is less than 45%, a pulmonary artery catheter is placed and HR instituted (Table 35–2).[16,17] The HR resuscitation protocol is able to abrogate some of the deleterious effects of brain death that result in cardiovascular instability and poor organ perfusion and is associated with a 22.5% increase in organs transplanted per donor.[18]

Loss of thermoregulation after brain death can promote the development of arrhythmias and cardiac arrest secondary to untreated hypothermia. Arrhythmias such as asystole or ventricular fibrillation are extremely difficult to treat because the heart is effectively denervated after brain death and becomes resistant to atropine. Prevention and treatment measures for hypothermia should include warming all intravenous fluids and

Table 35–2. RECOMMENDATION FOR CARDIOTHORACIC DONOR MANAGEMENT ACCORDING TO THE CRITICAL PATHWAY FOR THE ORGAN DONOR

1. **Early echocardiogram for all donors.** Insert a PAC to monitor patient management (placement of the PAC is particularly relevant in patients with an EF < 45% or those receiving high-dose inotropes)

   Use aggressive donor resuscitation as outlined below

2. **Electrolytes**

   Maintain Na < 150 mEq/dL

   Maintain K^+ > 4.0

   Correct acidosis with Na bicarbonate and mild to moderate hyperventilation (Pco_2 of 30–35 mm Hg)

3. **Ventilation**—Maintain tidal volume at 10–15 mL/kg

   Keep peak airway pressure < 30 mm Hg

   Maintain mild respiratory alkalosis (Pco_2 of 30–35 mm Hg)

4. Recommend the use of **hormonal resuscitation (HR)** as part of a comprehensive donor management protocol. Key elements:

   Triiodothyronine (T_3): 4-μg bolus; 3-μg/hr continuous infusion

   Arginine vasopressin: 1-U bolus; 0.5- to 4.0-U/hr drip (titrate to an SVR of 800–1200 with a PAC)

   Methylprednisolone: 15-mg/kg bolus (repeat q24h as needed)

   Insulin: drip at a minimum rate of 1 U/hr (titrate blood glucose to 120–180 mg/dL)

   Ventilator: see above

   Volume resuscitation: use of colloid and avoidance of anemia are important in preventing pulmonary edema

     Albumin if PT and PTT are normal

     Fresh-frozen plasma if PT and PTT are abnormal (value ≥ 1.5 × control)

     Packed red blood cells to maintain a PCWP of 8–12 mm Hg and an Hct > 10.0 mg/dL

5. **When patient is stabilized/optimized,** repeat the echocardiogram (an unstable donor has not met 2 or more of the following criteria)

   Mean arterial pressure ≥ 60

   CVP ≤ 12 mm Hg

   PCWP ≤ 12 mm Hg

   SVR of 800–1200 dyne·sec·cm^{-5}

   Cardiac index ≥ 2.5 L/min/m^2

   Left ventricular stroke work index > 15

   Dopamine dosage < 10 μg/kg/min

CVP, central venous pressure; EJ, ejection fraction; Hct, hematocrit; PAC, pulmonary artery catheter; PT, prothrombin time; PTT, partial thromboplastin time; PCWP, pulmonary capillary wedge pressure; SVR, systemic vascular resistance.
From the United Network for Organ Sharing (UNOS), 2001.

blood products, using blankets and heat lamps, and elevating the temperature of the ventilator humidifier and external environment.

Medical Failures to Organ Donation

Once brain death is established, the profound associated pathophysiological damage is of such magnitude that in spite of conventional cardiopulmonary support, as many as 25% of potential donors may suffer loss of perfusion to their organs, thus making them unsuitable for transplantation before the organs be retrieved.[16,19] Rapid and accurate determination of brain death could have a significant impact on the number of actual donors and the number of organs per donor through a decrease in the incidence of medical failure.[13] In addition, aggressive management is necessary to maintain organ function when brain death is declared so that procurement can be undertaken. Such donor management is extremely labor intensive and costly.[20]

The Critical Pathway for the Organ Donor was established to facilitate management and delivery of quality care in an environment where managed care increasingly requires a constraint on resources.[16] It is designed to provide the information necessary to evaluate the functional status of the kidneys, liver, pancreas, heart, and lungs and to determine the management steps that need to be taken to improve and optimize the performance of each organ. Use of this standard donor management algorithm results in a significant increase in organs procured and transplanted without any reduction in quality.[16]

Potential Organ Donor Identification and Consent

Different studies carried out in Europe and the United States have stated that as a general rule, as many as a third of potential donors remain unidentified or poorly managed and another third are lost as a result of family or coroner refusal. Therefore, the actual number of donors is only a third of the potential. It seems that the universal shortage of organ donors is not wholly due to a lack of suitable donors but also to the failure to turn potential donors into actual donors.[21] In the United States, the 1986 Omnibus Reconciliation Act, section 1138, requires that all hospitals participating in Medicare and Medicaid programs refer all potential organ donors to their local organ procurement organization (OPO) and that the families of all potential organ donors become aware of their option to donate. The act is supplemented by required request legislation, which mandates that hospitals ask all families of deceased patients to consider organ donation.[2] Approaching the relatives represents a key point in the process of consent because family refusal remains a serious obstacle to achieving a real increase in donations.[21] By organizing the consent process such that death notification and the consent request are decoupled, the hospital staff and OPO coordinator participate in the consent process, and the request takes place in a private setting, the consent rate can be as high as 74%.[22]

In the early nineties, Spain started an original integrated approach designed to improve donation of deceased donor organs. Three main areas for improvement were identified: potential donor detection, donor management, and approach to the family. A national network of specifically trained, part-time, dedicated and strongly motivated hospital physicians in charge of the whole process of organ donation was created.[23] As a result, rates of procurement of deceased donor organs have experienced a continuous increase over a 10-year period (from 14 to 34 donors per million population) and constitute the highest donor rate by far ever reached by a whole country (Fig. 35–1).[24] In June 2000, the Committee of Experts on the Organizational Aspects of Cooperation in Organ Transplantation (Council of Europe) recommended to its states adoption of the Spanish model for organ donation and acknowledged the continuous formation system developed in Spain.[25] Adoption of such a model has proved to be applicable and successful in other regions such as southern Australia and northern Italy. Depending on the characteristics of the different health systems, the Spanish model can be partially or totally adopted by other countries.[23]

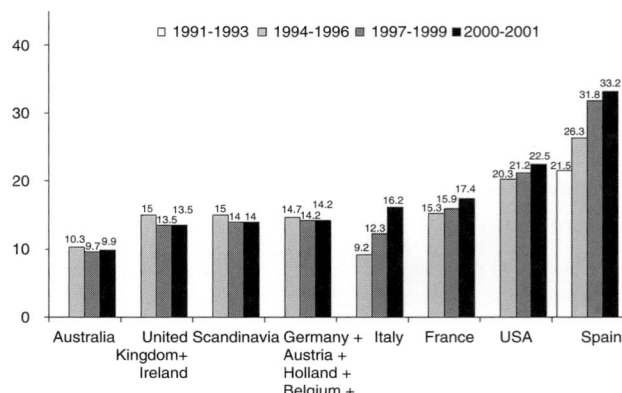

FIGURE 35–1

Annual rate of donation of deceased donor organs per million population (1991–2001). (Adapted from Matesanz R, Miranda B: A decade of continuous improvement in cadaveric organ donation: The Spanish model. J Nephrol 15:22-28, 2002.)

Deceased Donor Organ Procurement Process

Adequate selection and evaluation of deceased donors and organs for transplantation should be performed within the context of satisfactory fulfillment of the previous organ procurement phases: early identification of potential donors, early diagnosis of brain death, and early, close, and strict physiological maintenance of the donor. Procurement of the greatest number of viable organs requires excellence in each of the phases.[26] In the United States, a national network of local OPOs has been developed in response to the need for equitable and efficient coordination of the organ donation and procurement process. These OPOs serve as a link between donor hospitals and transplantation centers and provide a variety of functions to facilitate organ donation, including education of families and health care workers on donation and transplantation, assistance in obtaining the diagnosis of brain death and family consent, donor resuscitation and management, identification of appropriate organ recipients, and coordination of the various surgical recovery teams. A trained coordinator goes to the donor hospital on notification of a possible donor and personally oversees this process.

It is not uncommon for three or four surgical teams to be simultaneously recovering organs from a single donor. A consensus among organ teams must be met to manage all potential donors optimally to ensure the maximum recoverable organs. Recovery teams may request a delay in the timing of surgery so that special studies can be performed to more fully evaluate a particular organ or to better coordinate the timing of donor and recipient procedures. Efforts should be made to accommodate these requests as long as the donor remains stable and no organ is jeopardized.

Donor Selection

Selection of an appropriate donor is crucial to the successful outcome of orthotopic liver transplantation. Donor evaluation criteria include patient age, size, blood type, and medical history, with particular emphasis on substance or alcohol abuse, hepatobiliary disease, infection, and malignancy. The patient's cause of death, length of hospitalization, current liver function studies, and hospital course, including hemodynamic status and pulmonary function, are also analyzed. The goal of donor assessment is to identify donors whose organs have a high likelihood of functioning and to eliminate those that predictably would not function.

Among the most prominent donor characteristics that may influence the development of initial poor function or primary nonfunction in the recipient include increasing age, prolonged ischemia, hypotension and inotropic support, gender mismatch, non–heart-beating donors (NHBDs), and steatosis.[27]

The following characteristics describe an ideal liver donor: 50 years or younger; no hepatobiliary disease; hemodynamic and respiratory stability (systolic blood pressure > 100 mm Hg and central venous pressure > 5 cm H_2O); an acceptable Pao_2 and hemoglobin level; no severe abdominal trauma, systemic infection, or cancer; diuresis greater than 50 mL/hr and normal creatinine; and finally, a dopamine requirement less than 10 µg/kg/min.[28] The critical shortage of deceased donor grafts and the increasing number of recipients awaiting liver transplantation make it extremely difficult to limit organ selection to the use of ideal donors only. The use of donors with extended criteria for organ acceptance has therefore become a necessity in the current era. Furthermore, successful transplantation of donor organs with extended criteria serves to demonstrate that the aforementioned criteria for liver donor selection are not absolute.

Absolute Contraindications to Organ Donation

Infectious Diseases

Absolute contraindications to organ donation include transmissible agents that can cause death of the recipient or a severe disease such as Creutzfeldt-Jakob disease and diseases caused by other prions such as kuru, Gerstmann-Sträussler-Scheinker syndrome, and fatal familial insomnia syndrome.[26] Also contraindicated for acceptance are donor organs with human immunodeficiency virus infection; active, disseminated, and invasive infection by other viruses, microbacteria, or fungi; and systemic infection by methicillin-resistant staphylococci.

Malignancy

The presence of an active malignancy is an absolute contraindication to organ donation. Extracranial cancer that has the capacity to metastasize and has not been cured precludes organ donation. However, low-grade skin cancer, such as basal cell carcinoma and many squamous cell carcinomas, carcinoma in situ (uterine and cervical), and primary brain tumors without extracranial metastases do not exclude organ donation.[29,30]

When considering donors who have only a history (no active disease) of solid-organ neoplasm, the general biological behavior of the tumor type, the histology and stage at the time of diagnosis, and the length of disease-free interval should be considered.[31] Patients with previously treated malignancies can be considered to be cured after a 5-year disease-free interval.[32] The United Network of Organ Sharing (UNOS) report on 488 donors with a past history of cancer resulted in 1276 organ transplants without cancer transmission from the donor to the recipient.[33] However, additional caution must be exercised when considering tumor types such as breast and lung carcinoma, which are known to have the potential for unpredictable behavior, such as late recurrence.[31] Meticulous revision for solitary masses or lymphadenopathy during retrieval is extremely important in donors with malignancies. In the case of an intracranial mass or hemorrhage of unclear cause, performance of a postdonation autopsy before transplantation of the organs is recommended.[31]

Extended Criteria for Organ Acceptance

During 2002, a total of 5329 liver transplantations were performed in the United States. However, the number of patients waiting for a liver has been increasing at greater speed and has reached 17,242. This disproportion enormously decreases the applicability of the procedure, and as a consequence, the number of patients who died while on the waiting list in 2002 was 1752 in the United States (Fig. 35–2).[34] To expand the potential donor pool, clinicians are continually modifying the criteria for an acceptable liver donor and are looking at extended criteria donors to meet the waiting list demands. Although organs from extended criteria donors may not be optimal, they are a viable alternative to dying while waiting for transplantation, and their use needs to be pursued.[28]

Donor Age

The use of donors older than 60 years has made a spectacular major impact on the rate of organ transplantation.

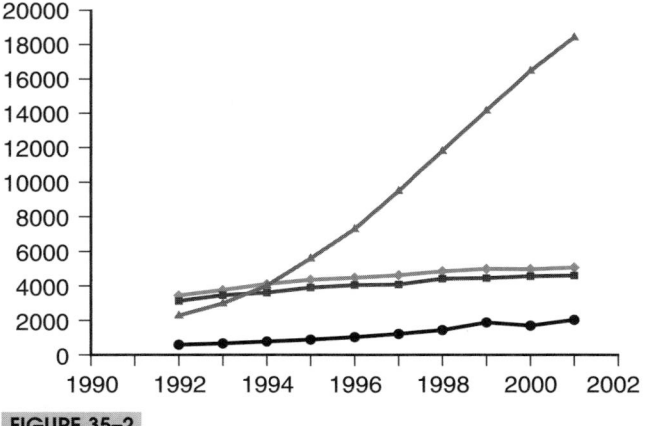

FIGURE 35–2

Shortage of cadaveric organs in the United States. The number of new registrations for liver transplantation (*triangles*) has increased exponentially while the number of available deceased donor livers (*squares*) and the overall number of liver transplantations (*diamonds*) have exhibited modest increases. The number of patient deaths (*circles*) while on the waiting list has linearly increased during the past decade.

In Spain, donors older than 60 years represent more than 30% of the total donor pool, whereas in the United State, they account for only 13.3%.[35] This policy gives rise to a higher number of organs deemed unsuitable for transplantation; specifically, 18% of livers were discarded in Spain in 1999 versus 5.5% in the United States.[35] However, use of these older donors produces an important increase in the number of organs available for transplantation and hence decreases the number of patients on the waiting list.

Among the pitfalls in using older donors for liver transplantation are a higher incidence of generalized chronic severe arterial lesions, as well as a higher incidence of parenchymal lesions such as fatty liver. The pathological conditions of atherosclerotic arterial vessels in older donors, such as the presence of calcified plaques on the hepatic artery, might be the source of severe complications in the liver recipient.[36] The combination of both older donor age and moderate to severe steatosis may also have an adverse impact on early allograft survival.[37] In addition, older donors have a higher prevalence of hypertension and diabetes mellitus. However, preexisting donor hypertension and diabetes mellitus do not exert a negative effect on liver transplant outcome.[26] Another inconvenience in using older donors is related to the higher incidence of unknown cancer, such as kidney and prostate cancer. Some cases of donor-transmitted malignancy stress the importance of meticulous intraoperative examination of the entire operative field by the procuring surgeon, especially in donors of advanced age, to safeguard against transmission of a previously unknown donor malignancy.[38]

At the present time, advanced age is not a barrier to organ donation. The key concept for organ acceptance is the functional and structural state of the organ subject to removal and transplantation.[26] The controversy regarding the upper age limit for liver donation has been overcome since the publication of some reports showing that the course and outcome of liver transplantation are not influenced by donor age.[36,39-41] By limiting cold ischemia time to 8 hours or less, long-term graft function was shown to be equivalent in organs from donors older and younger than 50 years.[42] Analysis of data from the Spanish Registry for Liver Transplantation for the period 1994 to 2000[43] has provided evidence that actuarial graft survival at 1 year after transplantation of livers from deceased donors aged 60 to 90 years is only slightly lower than that after transplantation of livers from 15- to 60-year-old donors, specifically, 80% versus 76% to 72% (60 to 69 and 80 to 89 years old, respectively). At 5 years, the difference in actuarial graft survival between both groups was greater, 66% versus 56% to 51%, respectively, but it is important to underline that recipients of organs from older donors had a higher prevalence of hepatocarcinoma, hepatitis C virus, and relapse of the primary disease.[43]

Hepatic Steatosis

The prevalence of hepatic steatosis in brain-dead adult liver donors ranges from 13% to 26%.[44] Fatty infiltration can be separated into two categories: macrovesicular, when a large vacuole of fat displaces the hepatocyte nuclei, and microvesicular, when the cytoplasm contains many small fatty inclusions. Some studies have shown that primary nonfunction does not develop in donor livers regardless of the severity of microsteatosis, that graft and recipient survival is not influenced by the presence of microsteatosis, and that such microsteatosis is reversible.[45,46] The quantitative evaluation of steatosis is based on the percentage of hepatocytes containing cytoplasmic fat inclusions. Severe steatotic grafts (>60% of hepatocytes have fat vacuoles within the cytoplasm) have been associated with primary nonfunction and should not be used for transplantation until effective protective strategies are identified.[47] However, the outcome of liver grafts with moderate steatosis (30% to 60%) is more variable. Comparable results regarding graft survival in relation to normal livers have been reported, but also increased rates of primary nonfunction (13% versus 3%).[48] With the increased number of patients dying while on the waiting list, livers with moderate steatosis should no longer be rejected for transplantation. These organs should preferably be used when no other significant additional risk factors are present in the donor and recipient.[37,47] Livers with mild steatosis (<30%) do not have worse immediate function or a worse graft survival rate than nonfatty livers do.[44]

Damaged Organs

Acquired and localized parenchymal lesions of the liver, such as simple cysts, hematoma around the organ, or small lacerations, cannot preclude its use for transplantation.[49] Donors with hepatic trauma should not be systematically excluded for liver transplantation. Traumatic parenchymal lesions, even when accompanied by transient hypoperfusion secondary to severe abdominal bleeding treated surgically, are not contraindications to liver procurement if the delay between the first surgical exploration and harvesting is not too long (<72 hours).[50] In a liver with ischemic parenchymal areas or injuries to the hilar structures, vena cava, or suprahepatic veins, transplantation is probably not indicated unless the lesion can be resected or repaired and the organ has sufficient and undamaged parenchyma mass.

Bacterial and Fungal Infections

Bacterial or mycotic infection or colonization can be present in 60% of deceased donor organs and mainly affects the respiratory and urinary tracts such that 15% have pneumonia and 10% have a positive hemoculture.[26] Transmission of bacteria and fungi from the donor to the host culminating in loss of the infected graft or death of the recipient has been widely documented.[51] However, adequate antibiotic treatment of the donor or recipient (or both) prevents infection in the latter. If properly treated, recipients of organs from infected donors have the same incidence of complications and the same rates of patient and graft survival as do recipients of uninfected grafts.[52,53]

Viral Infections

Hepatitis B

A positive result for hepatitis B core antibody (HBcAb) needs to be interpreted with care. The risk of transmission of hepatitis B virus (HBV) by liver transplantation is high, and the donor's negative hepatitis B surface antibody (HBsAb) status does not mitigate the transmission risk.[31]

Organs from IgG/HBsAb-negative and HBcAb-positive donors can transmit HBV infection to HBV-negative liver recipients at a rate of 22% to 100%, but the risk can be dramatically reduced in recipients who have preexisting antibodies to hepatitis B surface antigen (HBsAg) or who were IgG/HBcAb-positive.[54-56] Liver transplantation from IgG/HBsAb-negative and HBcAb-positive donors to recipients with HBV-related cirrhosis does not affect graft or patient survival, but HBV disease is 2.5 times more likely to recur,[57] although recurrence does not develop in recipients who receive preemptive treatment with hepatitis B immune globulin and lamivudine.[58,59] Ideal recipients of livers from HBcAb-positive donors are those undergoing transplantation for HBV-related cirrhosis who are already committed to posttransplantation anti-HBV therapy.

Hepatitis C

Approximately 5% of all potential organ donors in the United States and Europe are positive for antibody to hepatitis C virus (HCV), and half of these donors are RNA HCV positive by polymerase chain reaction.[26] Transplantation of livers from HCV antibody–positive donors into HCV antibody–positive recipients does not seem to increase, in the short or medium term (1 to 5 years), morbidity or mortality in the liver recipient when compared with transplantation of grafts from an HCV antibody–negative donor. Moreover, there has been no difference in either patient survival, graft survival, or the incidence, timing, or severity of recurrent HCV disease.[60,61]

Several studies examining the dynamic interaction of donor and recipient HCV strains after transplantation have found no consistent pattern of viral repopulation.[62] Liver recipients in whom the donor HCV strain becomes predominant can have significantly longer liver disease-free survival than recipients who retain their own HCV strain.[63] Because genotype is predictive of only response to interferon-based therapy and not disease severity, genotype is not an important consideration in the decision to transplant a liver from an HCV antibody–positive donor into an HCV-positive recipient.[31] Analysis of the histological characteristics of the graft before transplantation is advised because only organs with little or no fibrosis and only minimal inflammation should be considered for transplantation.[64]

Evaluation of Liver Donors at Time of Procurement

As discussed in the previous sections, many donor parameters may influence postoperative graft function. A collective review of the literature revealed at least 15 donor variables that may be associated with poor graft survival after transplantation. These variables included donor age (>50 years), sex, race, weight, gender, ABO status, cause of brain death, length of hospital stay (>5 days), pulmonary insufficiency, use of pressors that may cause splanchnic vasoconstriction with liver hypoperfusion, cardiac arrest, serum transaminases, sodium level (>155 mEq/L), cold preservation time, and fat in the liver. A critical analysis of all such donor variables by Strasberg and coworkers[65] divided donor factors into absolute and relative risks. Severe macrosteatosis (>60%) and cold preservation time longer than 30 hours were the main absolute donor risk factors. Relative risk factors were moderate steatosis (30% to 60%), cold preservation time longer than 12 hours, and donor age older than 50 years.[65] Taken together, these data suggest that in the absence of current absolute contraindications, many factors may have a dynamic impact on allograft function. It is therefore doubtful that a single variable may adversely affect graft function alone.

Careful evaluation of the donor's clinical history, as well as careful assessment at the time of procurement, is essential to prevent discarding liver grafts that may function well after transplantation. Patterns of alcohol use and the relevance of elevated liver enzymes must be evaluated carefully at the time of procurement. Elevated transaminase levels are often indicative of reversible liver injury rather than hepatic lesions or chronic hepatic dysfunction. Serial determination of transaminases can be useful to evaluate recovery from a transitory insult. Donors with long hypotensive episodes or heart failure or those with brain death from hypoxia may initially have high levels of transaminases that tend to normalize with adequate donor management. Elevations of γ-glutamyltransferase (GGT) may signal hepatic dysfunction as a result of alcohol abuse or the existence of a steatotic liver. High GGT levels should not exclude liver donation. In such cases, more accurate evaluation of the liver should be undertaken, including preoperative ultrasonography, careful intraoperative examination, and biopsy at the time of procurement. Similarly, bilirubin elevations may be misleading because blood transfusions or hematoma reabsorption in traumatic patients may result in transient hyperbilirubinemia.

It is important to remark that surgical assessment at the time of procurement may be the most important test for assessing the adequacy of a donor liver. Direct examination of the color and consistency of the liver, examination of bile, and in some instances, liver biopsy can provide valuable information before initiation of the recipient intervention.

Strategies for Increasing the Organ Pool

Split-Liver Transplantation

Split-liver transplantation (SLT) is a surgical technique that creates two allografts from one deceased/living donor organ. SLT represents a further step toward more efficient use of deceased donor organs. SLT can eliminate the need for obtaining a graft from a living related donor in adults and children and can produce outcomes that rival those of deceased donor whole organs.[66-68]

In March 2001, the American Society of Transplant Surgeons and the American Society of Transplantation jointly sponsored a conference to explore mechanisms for maximizing the deceased donor organ pool.[69] These committee members concluded that there is adequate experience with splitting of a liver from an adult donor to a child recipient to argue that a split liver should be the first option for donors meeting the appropriate criteria for the split procedure. A national policy for splitting appropriate donor organs into left lateral and extended right grafts whenever possible was recommended.

Reuse of Grafts and Domino Transplantation

Transplanted liver grafts have been successfully reused for transplantation.[70] Moreover, transplant recipients can be living organ donors of their own therapeutically retrieved organs. This procedure is called sequential (domino) liver transplantation. Required preconditions for domino transplantation are that (1) extrahepatic disease must exist, (2) the liver must be fully functional, and (3) the genetic defect in the host should recur with a sufficient latency period.[71]

Familial amyloid polyneuropathy is an autosomal dominant disease that involves a genetic defect in transthyretin, which is predominantly produced by the liver and deposited mainly along nerves, gut, and endocardium. Transplantation is a widely accepted method of treatment for these patients.[72] Their livers can be used to transplant patients 55 to 65 years of age because the latency period for the development of symptoms related to amyloid deposition in the recipient is about 20 years.[73]

Living Donors

Efforts to expand the donor pool have resulted in the introduction of adult living donor liver transplantation (ALDLT) in the United States in 1997. Shortly thereafter, the procedure gained rapid and widespread application. By 2002, more than 1000 ALDLT procedures were performed in the United States.[34] Currently, the deceased donor organ allocation system in the United States, which is based on the ethical principle of prevention of death,[74] favors organ distribution to urgent recipients and thereby reduces the potential for nonurgent patients to receive deceased donor grafts. Justification of ALDLT is therefore based on the critical shortage of adult deceased donor organs and the reduced probability of deceased donor transplantation in nonurgent patients.[75] However, the concentration of all efforts to promote living organ donation in Western countries is not justified unless adequate measures are first adopted to increase deceased donor donation and maximize the number and quality of organs procured from deceased donors.[76]

Potential advantages of living donor liver transplantation have been tempered by the risk of injury or death to a healthy donor. Overall donor morbidity and mortality are a critical issue and the source of much of the controversy that is being debated in medical, surgical, ethical, and public communities.[77,78] Reported complication rates for right lobe liver donors vary widely but are estimated to be approximately 35%, with a surgical mortality rate of approximately 0.3%.[79]

Non–Heart-Beating Donors

NHBDs experience definite cardiac arrest before their organs are recovered. They are thought to be less than optimal for transplantation because of a prolonged warm ischemia time that compromises the viability and posttransplant function of the graft. The most important step when recovering organs from NHBDs is cooling the organs as soon as possible after cessation of circulation, declaration of death, and obtaining consent.[80] Controlled NHBD procedures take place in the operating room after withdrawal of ventilatory support and subsequent cardiac arrest, with a donor surgical team available. Uncontrolled NHBDs sustain circulatory arrest and either fail cardiopulmonary resuscitation (CPR) or arrive dead at the hospital (or both). Obviously, controlled NHBDs provide organs that are comparatively far less prone to ischemic damage and tend to offer superior posttransplant function.

Over the past few years, NHBDs have accounted for approximately 1% of the total number of deceased donors,[34] but it has been estimated that controlled NHBDs have the potential to increase the deceased donor pool 25% to 42%, with at least 1000 controlled NHBD procedures performed each year.[81,82] The OPO's coordinator manages the process of organ donation from controlled NHBDs. Monitoring and resuscitation efforts are similar to those applied to heart-beating deceased donors. Controlled NHBDs do not meet brain death criteria, but their health care teams have determined that further resuscitation efforts are useless. The decision to withdraw life support is made before an OPO coordinator approaches the family to obtain consent for donation. After the declaration of death, initiation of a rapid surgical technique for organ recovery is mandatory.[83] Liver allograft survival from controlled NHBDs has been rising from 50% to 100% at 1-year follow-up periods.[81,83,84]

Safe transplantation from uncontrolled NHBDs depends on maintenance of adequate perfusion to the organs and rapid cooling before organ recovery. The less invasive means of organ perfusion involves postmortem CPR followed by the use of a double-balloon triple-lumen catheter placed in the femoral artery and advanced into the aorta for rapid in situ intravascular cooling.[85] Another possibility after CPR is the use of postmortem cardiopulmonary bypass with external oxygenation and deep hypothermia until organ retrieval is possible (Fig. 35–3).[86] During the past decade, 1-year graft survival from uncontrolled NHBDs has been poor (17% to 41% rates),[83] but recent reports are showing encouraging results with the use of strict policies and selection criteria.[86]

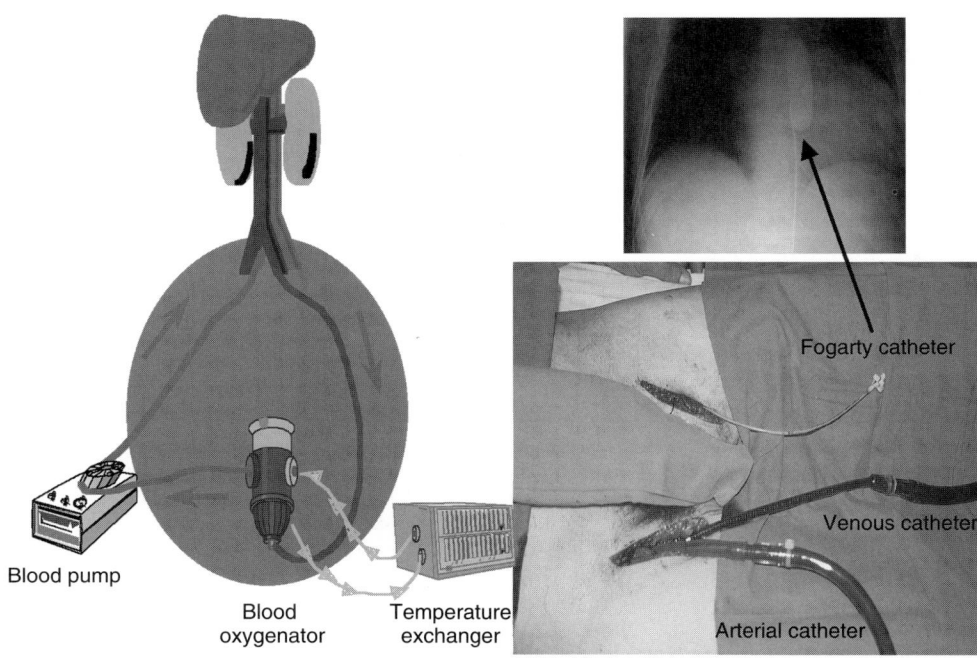

FIGURE 35–3

Maintenance of uncontrolled non–heart-beating donors before organ recovery. Through an incision in the right side of the groin, the femoral vein and artery are cannulated and connected to a cardiopulmonary bypass device with external oxygenation and deep hypothermia. A Fogarty catheter is also placed in the thoracic aorta to avoid chest perfusion. (Pictures and illustration courtesy of Hospital Clinic, Barcelona, Spain.)

Blood pump

Blood oxygenator

Temperature exchanger

Fogarty catheter

Venous catheter

Arterial catheter

In a series from the University of California at Los Angeles, 29 NHBDs (16 uncontrolled and 13 controlled) were used for liver transplantation. In the uncontrolled group, one primary nonfailure occurred in a donor with 75 minutes of warm ischemia time. One-year patient and graft survival rates in this group were 88% and 75%, respectively. In the controlled group, one primary nonfailure was seen in a donor who had 48 minutes of warm ischemia time. Patient and graft survival rates were 85% and 77%. Based on this experience, a warm ischemia time of less than 30 minutes does not adversely affect patient or graft survival (unpublished data).

Machine Perfusion

The reduced ischemic tolerance of extended criteria grafts jeopardizes organ viability during cold storage. Organ machine perfusion has been developed to limit ischemic damage, which can lead to increased expression of selectins, intercellular adhesion molecule 1 (ICAM-1), or major histocompatibility complex molecules. Experimental models have shown that preservation by oxygenated machine perfusion significantly improves parenchymal viability and mitigates the vascular immunogenicity of predamaged donor livers.[87] Future research in warm machine perfusion may provide the ideal form of liver preservation. In renal transplantation, the viability of NHBD kidneys is improved when conventional cold storage is replaced by machine perfusion, and such perfusion has led to a 20% reduction in the incidence of delayed graft function.[88]

Pearls and Pitfalls—cont'd

- The use of partial liver grafts and non–heart-beating donors mandates particular surgical and medical considerations but is an effective way to reduce the waiting list time for some recipients.
- All livers are usable until *proved* otherwise.

Pitfalls

- The shortage of donor organs is increasingly limiting the applicability of liver transplantation.
- The process of brain death induces severe hemodynamic and metabolic abnormalities. The organ function of a donor must be maintained as carefully as other critical cases.
- Failure to provide adequate physiological support to potential donors accounts for at least 25% of lost donor organs.
- The actual number of donors is only a third of the potential. An accurate approach to relatives is a key point in the process of consent.
- Donor characteristics that may influence the development of initial poor function or primary nonfunction in a recipient include increasing age, prolonged ischemia, hypotension and inotropic support, gender mismatch, non–heart-beating donors, and steatosis.

Pearls and Pitfalls

Pearls

- Identification of all potential donors is the first essential step in increasing rates of donation.
- Rapid and accurate determination of brain death and an adequate approach to donor families by trained physicians and medical personnel are the basic steps to successful donation.
- Medical management of suitable donors must be optimized to preserve organ function.
- Currently, the use of extended donor criteria to expand the donor pool is widely accepted. Similar patient and graft survival can be obtained by using extended criteria when adequate management strategies and allocation schemes are adopted.

References

1. Rosengard BR, Feng S, Alfrey EJ, et al: Report of the Crystal City meeting to maximize the use of organs recovered from the cadaver donor. Am J Transplant 2:701-711, 2002.
2. Razek T, Olthoff K, Reilly PM: Issues in potential organ donor management. Surg Clin North Am 80:1021-1032, 2000.
3. Karcioglu O, Ayrik C, Erbil B: The brain-dead patient or a flower in the vase? The emergency department approach to the preservation of the organ donor. Eur J Emerg Med 10:52-57, 2003.
4. A definition of irreversible coma. Report of the Ad Hoc Committee of the Harvard Medical School to Examine the Definition of Brain Death. JAMA 205:337-340, 1968.
5. Haupt WF, Rudolf J: European brain death codes: A comparison of national guidelines. J Neurol 246:432-437, 1999.
6. Guidelines for the determination of death. Report of the medical consultants on the diagnosis of death to the President's Commission for the Study of Ethical Problems in Medicine and Biomedical and Behavioral Research. JAMA 246:2184-2186, 1981.
7. Dobb GJ, Weekes JW: Clinical confirmation of brain death. Anaesth Intensive Care 23:37-43, 1995.
8. Guideline three: Minimum technical standards for EEG recording in suspected cerebral death. American Electroencephalographic Society. J Clin Neurophysiol 11:10-13, 1994.
9. Ropper AH, Kehne SM, Wechsler L: Transcranial Doppler in brain death. Neurology 37:1733-1735, 1987.

10. De la Riva A, Gonzalez FM, Llamas-Elvira JM, et al: Diagnosis of brain death: Superiority of perfusion studies with ^{99m}Tc-HMPAO over conventional radionuclide cerebral angiography. Br J Radiol 65:289-294, 1992.
11. Monsein LH: The imaging of brain death. Anaesth Intensive Care 23:44-50, 1995.
12. Power BM, Van Heerden PV: The physiological changes associated with brain death—current concepts and implications for treatment of the brain dead organ donor. Anaesth Intensive Care 23:26-36, 1995.
13. Jenkins DH, Reilly PM, Schwab CW: Improving the approach to organ donation: A review. World J Surg 23:644-649, 1999.
14. Nygaard CE, Townsend RN, Diamond DL: Organ donor management and organ outcome: A 6-year review from a level I trauma center. J Trauma 30:728-732, 1990.
15. Cooper DK, Novitzky D, Wicomb WN: The pathophysiological effects of brain death on potential donor organs, with particular reference to the heart. Ann R Coll Surg Engl 71:261-266, 1989.
16. Rosendale JD, Chabalewski FL, McBride MA, et al: Increased transplanted organs from the use of a standardized donor management protocol. Am J Transplant 2:761-768, 2002.
17. Zaroff JG, Rosengard BR, Armstrong WF, et al: Consensus conference report: Maximizing use of organs recovered from the cadaver donor: Cardiac recommendations, March 28-29, 2001, Crystal City, Va. Circulation 106:836-841, 2002.
18. Rosendale JD, Kauffman HM, McBride MA, et al: Aggressive pharmacologic donor management results in more transplanted organs. Transplantation 75:482-487, 2003.
19. Mackersie RC, Bronsther OL, Shackford SR: Organ procurement in patients with fatal head injuries. The fate of the potential donor. Ann Surg 213:143-150, 1991.
20. Jenkins DH, Reilly PM, McMahon DJ, et al: Minimizing charges associated with the determination of brain death. Crit Care (Lond) 1:65-70, 1997.
21. Miranda B, Matesanz R: International issues in transplantation. Setting the scene and flagging the most urgent and controversial issues. Ann N Y Acad Sci 862:129-143, 1998.
22. Siminoff LA, Arnold RM, Caplan AL, et al: Public policy governing organ and tissue procurement in the United States. Results from the National Organ and Tissue Procurement Study. Ann Intern Med 123:10-17, 1995.
23. Matesanz R, Miranda B: A decade of continuous improvement in cadaveric organ donation: The Spanish model. J Nephrol 15:22-28, 2002.
24. Miranda B, Vilardell J, Grinyo JM: Optimizing cadaveric organ procurement: The Catalan and Spanish experience. Am J Transplant 3:1189-1196, 2003.
25. Protocol to the Convention on Human Rights and Biomedicine on Transplantation of Organs and Tissues of Human Origin. In Matesanz R, Miranda B (eds): Transplant Newsletter. Madrid, Aula Medica Editores, 2000, pp 1-18. Available at http://www.msc.es/profesional/trasplantes/pdf/NEWSLE_2000.pdf.
26. Lopez-Navidad A, Caballero F: Extended criteria for organ acceptance. Strategies for achieving organ safety and for increasing organ pool. Clin Transplant 17:308-324, 2003.
27. Busuttil RW, Tanaka K: The utility of marginal donors in liver transplantation. Liver Transpl 9:651-663, 2003.
28. Loinaz C, Gonzalez EM: Marginal donors in liver transplantation. Hepatogastroenterology 47:256-263, 2000.
29. Detry O, Honore P, Hans MF, et al: Organ donors with primary central nervous system tumor. Transplantation 70:244-248, 2000.
30. Kauffman HM, McBride MA, Cherikh WS, et al: Transplant tumor registry: Donors with central nervous system tumors 1. Transplantation 73:579-582, 2002.
31. Feng S, Buell JF, Cherikh WS, et al: Organ donors with positive viral serology or malignancy: Risk of disease transmission by transplantation. Transplantation 74:1657-1663, 2002.
32. Kauffman HM, McBride MA, Delmonico FL: First report of the United Network for Organ Sharing Transplant Tumor Registry: Donors with a history of cancer. Transplantation 70:1747-1751, 2000.
33. Myron KH, McBride MA, Cherikh WS, et al: Transplant tumor registry: Donor related malignancies. Transplantation 74:358-362, 2002.
34. 2002 Annual Report of the US Scientific Registry of Transplant Recipients and the Organ Procurement and Transplantation Network: Transplant Data 1989-2002. Available at http://www.optn.org/latestData/rptData.asp. Accessed November 10, 2003.
35. Chang GJ, Mahanty HD, Ascher NL, et al: Expanding the donor pool: Can the Spanish model work in the United States? Am J Transplant 3:1259-1263, 2003.
36. Grazi GL, Cescon M, Ravaioli M, et al: A revised consideration on the use of very aged donors for liver transplantation. Am J Transplant 1:61-68, 2001.
37. Verran D, Kusyk T, Painter D, et al: Clinical experience gained from the use of 120 steatotic donor livers for orthotopic liver transplantation. Liver Transpl 9:500-505, 2003.
38. Lipshutz GS, Baxter-Lowe LA, Nguyen T, et al: Death from donor-transmitted malignancy despite emergency liver retransplantation. Liver Transpl 9:1102-1107, 2003.
39. Emre S, Schwartz ME, Altaca G, et al: Safe use of hepatic allografts from donors older than 70 years. Transplantation 62:62-65, 1996.
40. Grande L, Matus D, Rimola A, et al: Expanded liver donor age over 60 years for hepatic transplantation. Clin Transpl 297-301, 1998.
41. Oh CK, Sanfey HA, Pelletier SJ, et al: Implication of advanced donor age on the outcome of liver transplantation. Clin Transplant 14:386-390, 2000.
42. Yersiz H, Shaked A, Olthoff K, et al: Correlation between donor age and the pattern of liver graft recovery after transplantation. Transplantation 60:790-794, 1995.
43. Cuende N, Grande L, Sanjuan F, et al: Liver transplant with organs from elderly donors: Spanish experience with more than 300 liver donors over 70 years of age. Transplantation 73:1360, 2002.
44. Imber CJ, St Peter SD, Handa A, et al: Hepatic steatosis and its relationship to transplantation. Liver Transpl 8:415-423, 2002.
45. Urena MA, Moreno GE, Romero CJ, et al: An approach to the rational use of steatotic donor livers in liver transplantation. Hepatogastroenterology 46:1164-1173, 1999.
46. Fishbein TM, Fiel MI, Emre S, et al: Use of livers with microvesicular fat safely expands the donor pool. Transplantation 64:248-251, 1997.
47. Selzner M, Clavien PA: Fatty liver in liver transplantation and surgery. Semin Liver Dis 21:105-113, 2001.
48. Strasberg SM, Howard TK, Molmenti EP, et al: Selecting the donor liver: Risk factors for poor function after orthotopic liver transplantation. Hepatology 20:829-838, 1994.
49. Jimenez RC, Moreno GE, Garcia GI, et al: Successful transplantation of a liver graft with a calcified hydatid cyst after back-table resection. Transplantation 60:883-884, 1995.
50. Avolio AW, Agnes S, Chirico AS, et al: Successful transplantation of an injured liver. Transplant Proc 32:131-133, 2000.
51. Gottesdiener KM: Transplanted infections: Donor-to-host transmission with the allograft. Ann Intern Med 110:1001-1016, 1989.
52. Freeman RB, Giatras I, Falagas ME, et al: Outcome of transplantation of organs procured from bacteremic donors. Transplantation 68:1107-1111, 1999.
53. Satoi S, Bramhall SR, Solomon M, et al: The use of liver grafts from donors with bacterial meningitis. Transplantation 72:1108-1113, 2001.
54. Dickson RC, Everhart JE, Lake JR, et al: Transmission of hepatitis B by transplantation of livers from donors positive for antibody to hepatitis B core antigen. The National Institute of Diabetes and

Digestive and Kidney Diseases Liver Transplantation Database. Gastroenterology 113:1668-1674, 1997.

55. Prieto M, Gomez MD, Berenguer M, et al: De novo hepatitis B after liver transplantation from hepatitis B core antibody–positive donors in an area with high prevalence of anti-HBc positivity in the donor population. Liver Transpl 7:51-58, 2001.

56. Muñoz SJ: Use of hepatitis B core antibody–positive donors for liver transplantation. Liver Transpl 8:S82-S87, 2002.

57. Joya-Vazquez PP, Dodson FS, Dvorchik I, et al: Impact of anti-hepatitis Bc–positive grafts on the outcome of liver transplantation for HBV-related cirrhosis. Transplantation 73:1598-1602, 2002.

58. Dodson SF, Bonham CA, Geller DA, et al: Prevention of de novo hepatitis B infection in recipients of hepatic allografts from anti-HBc positive donors. Transplantation 68:1058-1061, 1999.

59. Yu AS, Vierling JM, Colquhoun SD, et al: Transmission of hepatitis B infection from hepatitis B core antibody–positive liver allografts is prevented by lamivudine therapy. Liver Transpl 7:513-517, 2001.

60. Velidedeoglu E, Desai NM, Campos L, et al: The outcome of liver grafts procured from hepatitis C–positive donors. Transplantation 73:582-587, 2002.

61. Saab S, Ghobrial RM, Ibrahim AB, et al: Hepatitis C positive grafts may be used in orthotopic liver transplantation: A matched analysis. Am J Transplant 3:1167-1172, 2003.

62. Laskus T, Wang LF, Rakela J, et al: Dynamic behavior of hepatitis C virus in chronically infected patients receiving liver graft from infected donors. Virology 220:171-176, 1996.

63. Vargas HE, Laskus T, Wang LF, et al: Outcome of liver transplantation in hepatitis C virus–infected patients who received hepatitis C virus–infected grafts. Gastroenterology 117:149-153, 1999.

64. Arenas JI, Vargas HE, Rakela J: The use of hepatitis C–infected grafts in liver transplantation. Liver Transpl 9:S48-S51, 2003.

65. Strasberg SM, Howard TK, Molmenti EP, Hertl M: Selecting donor livers: Risk factors for poor function after orthotopic liver transplantation. Hepatology 20:829-838, 1994.

66. Spada M, Gridelli B, Colledan M, et al: Extensive use of split liver for pediatric liver transplantation: A single-center experience. Liver Transpl 6:415-428, 2000.

67. Deshpande RR, Bowles MJ, Vilca-Melendez H, et al: Results of split liver transplantation in children. Ann Surg 236:248-253, 2002.

68. Yersiz H, Renz JF, Farmer DG, et al: One hundred in situ split-liver transplantations: A single-center experience. Ann Surg 238:496-505, 2003.

69. Emond JC, Freeman RB Jr, Renz JF, et al: Optimizing the use of donated cadaver livers: Analysis and policy development to increase the application of split-liver transplantation. Liver Transpl 8:863-872, 2002.

70. Moreno GE, Gomez R, Gonzalez P, et al: Reuse of liver grafts after early death of the first recipient. World J Surg 20:309-312, 1996.

71. Golling M, Singer R, Weiss G, et al: Sequential (domino) transplantation of the liver in a transthyretin-50 familial amyloid polyneuropathy. Special reference to cardiological diagnosis and complications. Langenbecks Arch Surg 385:21-26, 2000.

72. Suhr OB, Holmgren G, Steen L, et al: Liver transplantation in familial amyloidotic polyneuropathy. Follow-up of the first 20 Swedish patients. Transplantation 60:933-938, 1995.

73. Perdigoto R, Furtado AL, Furtado E, et al: The Coimbra University Hospital experience in liver transplantation in patients with familial amyloidotic polyneuropathy. Transplant Proc 35:1125, 2003.

74. Wiesner RH, McDiarmid SV, Kamath PS, et al: MELD and PELD: Application of survival models to liver allocation. Liver Transpl 7:567-580, 2001.

75. Ghobrial RM, Fondevila C, Busuttil RW: Living donor liver transplantation: The American experience. In Arroyo V, Forns X, Garcia-Pagan JC, Rodes J (eds): Progress in the Treatment of Liver Diseases. Barcelona, Medicina STM Editores, 2003, pp 385-392.

76. Lopez-Navidad A, Caballero F: Organs for transplantation. N Engl J Med 343:1730-1731, 2000.

77. Surman OS: The ethics of partial-liver donation. N Engl J Med 346:1038, 2002.

78. Malago M, Testa G, Marcos A, et al: Ethical considerations and rationale of adult-to-adult living donor liver transplantation. Liver Transpl 7:921-927, 2001.

79. Pomfret EA: Early and late complications in the right-lobe adult living donor. Liver Transpl 9:S45-S49, 2003.

80. Kootstra G, Kievit J, Nederstigt A: Organ donors: Heartbeating and non-heartbeating. World J Surg 26:181-184, 2002.

81. Reich DJ, Munoz SJ, Rothstein KD, et al: Controlled non–heart-beating donor liver transplantation: A successful single center experience, with topic update. Transplantation 70:1159-1166, 2000.

82. Koogler T, Costarino AT Jr: The potential benefits of the pediatric nonheartbeating organ donor. Pediatrics 101:1049-1052, 1998.

83. Casavilla A, Ramirez C, Shapiro R, et al: Experience with liver and kidney allografts from non–heart-beating donors. Transplantation 59:197-203, 1995.

84. D'Alessandro AM, Hoffmann RM, Knechtle SJ, et al: Successful extrarenal transplantation from non–heart-beating donors. Transplantation 59:977-982, 1995.

85. Garcia-Rinaldi R, Lefrak EA, Defore WW, et al: In situ preservation of cadaver kidneys for transplantation: Laboratory observations and clinical application. Ann Surg 182:576-584, 1975.

86. Alvarez J, del Barrio R, Arias J, et al: Non–heart-beating donors from the streets: An increasing donor pool source. Transplantation 70:314-317, 2000.

87. Lauschke H, Olschewski P, Tolba R, et al: Oxygenated machine perfusion mitigates surface antigen expression and improves preservation of predamaged donor livers. Cryobiology 46:53-60, 2003.

88. Wight JP, Chilcott JB, Holmes MW, et al: Pulsatile machine perfusion vs. cold storage of kidneys for transplantation: A rapid and systematic review. Clin Transplant 17:293-307, 2003.

Non–Heart-Beating Donor Liver Transplantation

DAVID J. REICH
COSME Y. MANZARBEITIA

Defining the non–heart-beating donor   530
  Controlled non–heart-beating donors   530
  Uncontrolled non–heart-beating donors   530
  The Maastricht categories   531

Historical perspective   531
  The impact of brain death recognition   531
  Non–heart-beating donor kidney
    transplantation   531
  Controlled non–heart-beating donor
    liver transplantation—early efforts
    by the Madison, Wisconsin, and
    Pittsburgh groups   532

Current results of controlled non–heart-beating
  donor liver transplantation   532
  Madison, Wisconsin, experience   532
  Miami experience   532
  University of Pennsylvania experience   532
  Einstein, Philadelphia, experience   534
  Summary of current results   535

Operative technique for non–heart-beating
  donor liver procurement   536
  Preoperative management (identifying
    potential non–heart-beating donors,
    withdrawing support)   536
  Super-rapid surgical technique   536
  Premortem cannulation technique   537
  Unusual case reports   537

Uncontrolled non–heart-beating donor liver
  transplantation—the Madrid model   538

Potential impact of non–heart-beating donor
  liver transplantation   538
  General estimates   538
  Pediatric non–heart-beating donors   538
  Institute of Medicine efforts   539

Ethical issues (specific to controlled
  non–heart-beating donors)   539
  Basic principles   539
  Controversial ethics topics   540

The role of the organ procurement
  organization   540

Conclusion   541

The non–heart-beating donor (NHBD) has, in some locations, become a major source of transplantable livers, as well as kidneys. In this chapter, the authors seek to categorize the various types of NHBDs, consider the history of NHBD organ transplantation, provide a clinical update of NHBD liver transplantation (LTX) that focuses primarily on the results of controlled NHBD LTX, elaborate on NHBD management protocols and surgical techniques, render estimates of the impact that NHBDs could have on the deceased donor organ pool, discuss the importance of organ procurement organizations (OPOs) and other professional organizations in pursuing successful NHBD programs, and share principles and controversies related to the ethics of NHBD organ procurement. The authors try to provide broad

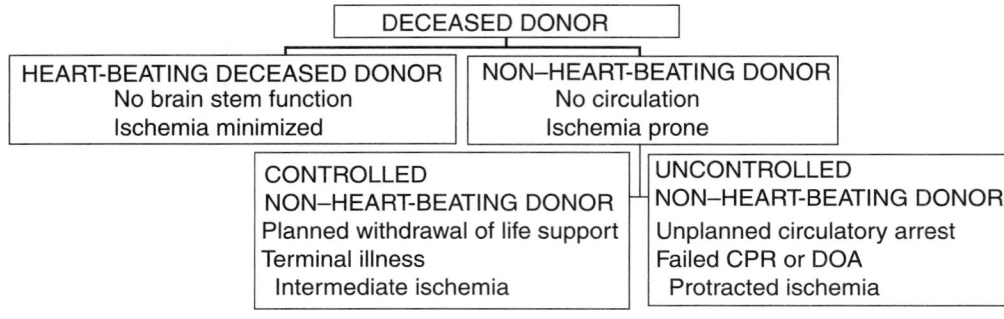

FIGURE 36–1

Definitions of controlled and uncontrolled non–heart-beating donors and heart-beating deceased donors.

coverage of what has been learned by leaders in the field of NHBD organ procurement and transplantation, as well as share our personal experience with controlled NHBD LTX.

Demand is steadily rising for the now highly successful life-saving therapy of LTX. This demand is based on the increased prevalence of end-stage liver disease from the hepatitis C epidemic, widespread access to transplantation care, willingness to perform transplantation in higher-risk candidates, and improved outcomes after LTX. One- and 3-year patient survival rates for primary LTX performed between 1996 and 2001 were 87.1% and 79.7%, respectively.[1] These advances however, are tempered by the worsening shortage of donor organs. As of September 30, 2003, there were 17,679 registrants on the United Network for Organ Sharing (UNOS) national waiting list for LTX, nearly four times the number transplanted during the previous 9 months. This profound disparity has resulted in an increasingly greater number of listed patients succumbing before receiving a new liver. Current mortality rates for patients on the UNOS and Eurotransplant waiting lists are approximately 25% and 20%, respectively.[1,2]

In response, one method of increasing the donor pool is to use expanded criteria donors, or those with organs previously considered less suitable for transplantation. Such donors include older, hepatitis C virus–positive, hepatitis B core antibody–positive, and living donors and those with livers that are steatotic, injured, or reduced in size (split). The NHBD is another type of extended donor, and there is widespread, rapidly growing interest in the field of NHBD organ transplantation.

Defining the Non–Heart-Beating Donor

NHBD death is characterized by simultaneous and irreversible unresponsiveness, apnea, and absence of circulation. In contrast, heart-beating donor death is determined by irreversible cessation of all brain functions.

Organ ischemia is minimized in a brain-dead donor because circulatory arrest typically occurs concurrently with perfusion of preservation solution and rapid core cooling. Thus, the procurement procedure does not implicitly involve circulatory dysfunction. NHBDs are less than ideal because the organs suffer ischemia during the prolonged periods between circulatory dysfunction, circulatory arrest, and subsequent perfusion and cooling. Furthermore, the surgical procedure for NHBD organ recovery is demanding and rushed (Fig. 36–1).

Controlled Non–Heart-Beating Donors

Controlled NHBDs provide organs that are exposed to significantly less ischemic damage and, in general, offer superior posttransplant function when compared with uncontrolled NHBDs (see Fig. 36–1).[3] Controlled NHBDs undergo circulatory arrest after planned withdrawal of life support, most often in the operating room with a donor surgical team readily available. Controlled NHBDs suffer terminal illness, usually a severe neurological injury without the possibility of meaningful recovery or survival. The results of controlled NHBD LTX are excellent, and most of this review focuses on the controlled subgroup of NHBDs.

Uncontrolled Non–Heart-Beating Donors

In contrast, uncontrolled NHBDs sustain circulatory arrest and either fail to respond to cardiopulmonary resuscitation (CPR) or are declared dead on arrival to the hospital (or both). The death of an uncontrolled NHBD is unplanned. Therefore, the organs suffer protracted ischemia before recovery (see Fig. 36–1). Although kidneys may tolerate a short period of the resultant warm ischemia, transplantation of extrarenal organs from uncontrolled NHBDs carries a much greater risk. One-year graft survival rates after uncontrolled NHBD kidney transplantation have been reported to be 79% to 86%, as opposed to 17% to 55% after uncontrolled NHBD LTX.[3-5]

Various postmortem measures have been used to increase the yield of transplantable organs from uncontrolled NHBDs, including CPR, perfusion of preservation solution by femoral vessel cannulation, and core cooling via peritoneal catheterization before organ retrieval.[3] Some protocols involve nonconsensual measures, such as CPR and cardiopulmonary bypass, and are therefore potentially ethically problematic even though organ procurement is aborted if consent for donation is not obtained. Madrid, Spain, has an established uncontrolled NHBD organ procurement program that is based on such nonconsensual initial measures (covered in a later section of this chapter).[5,6]

The Maastricht Categories

In the early 1990s, investigators from Maastricht in The Netherlands described four categories of NHBDs: (1) dead on arrival, (2) unsuccessful resuscitation, (3) awaiting cardiac arrest, and (4) cardiac arrest while brain dead.[7] An NHBD who is dead on arrival is brought to the emergency department after being declared dead in the field. An NHBD who is unsuccessfully resuscitated undergoes a determination that life-saving efforts are useless (such as the Madrid NHBD). An NHBD who is awaiting cardiac arrest has extensive brain damage but does not meet the criteria for brain death, and controlled withdrawal of support is then arranged. Finally, the fourth category includes NHBDs in whom brain death has been diagnosed and who sustain premature and unexpected cardiac arrest before the beginning of the donor operation. All but the third category are considered uncontrolled NHBD situations.

Historical Perspective

The Impact of Brain Death Recognition

During the earliest years of kidney transplantation, starting 50 years ago, organ donation amounted to the removal of kidneys from patients whose hearts had stopped beating. The first human liver and heart transplants, in 1963 and 1967, respectively, were performed with organs recovered from NHBDs. Through the 1960s, determination of death required heartbeat cessation. However, World War II led to the birth of modern critical care, including the use of respirators and CPR. It became possible to reestablish or maintain cardiopulmonary function in severely ill patients, which led neurophysiologists of the 1950s to study irreversible coma. Subsequently, in 1968, the multidisciplinary Ad Hoc Committee of Harvard Medical School to Examine the Definition of Death issued a landmark report that included criteria for the determination of brain death (Harvard Neurologic Definition and Criteria for Death).[8] In 1980, the Uniform Law Commissioners adopted the Uniform Determination of Death Act (UDODA). According to UDODA, "an individual who has sustained either (1) irreversible cessation of circulatory and respiratory functions, or (2) irreversible cessation of all functions of the entire brain, including the brainstem, is dead."[9] UDODA has been endorsed by the major American medical and legal professional associations, and all 50 states have enacted brain death legislation.

During the mid-1970s, the practice of recovering organs from NHBDs was essentially abandoned. Organs recovered from brain-dead donors are considered far more desirable because they are protected from the effects of warm ischemic injury and are less prone to poor graft function. For the following 25 years, virtually all donation was from heart-beating deceased donors (HBDDs) who were declared brain dead or from living donors.

Non–Heart-Beating Donor Kidney Transplantation

The majority of experience with NHBD organs is with kidney transplantation. Controlled NHBD kidney transplantation provides 1-year graft survival rates of 82% to 86%,[3,4] similar to results with uncontrolled NHBD kidneys in Europe and Asia, as well as the results of the following two large reports from the United States that lump together controlled and uncontrolled NHBDs.[10,11]

Using data from the UNOS Kidney Transplant Registry, Cho and colleagues compared early function and 1-year survival of 229 kidney grafts from NHBDs with those of 8718 grafts from HBDDs.[10] Early renal function was better in grafts from HBDDs. Rates of primary nonfunction (PNF) and delayed graft function were significantly higher in the NHBD group than in the HBDD group: 4% versus 1% ($P < .001$) and 48% versus 22% ($P < .001$), respectively. Importantly, however, 1-year graft survival rates were similar, 83% and 86% (P = nonsignificant [NS]), respectively.

Rudich and associates used data from the U.S. Renal Data System to compare graft and patient survival rates in 708 NHBD and 97,990 HBDD renal transplant recipients.[11] Again, NHBD organ recipients had nearly twice the incidence of delayed graft function as HBDD organ recipients did (42% versus 23%). However, 1- and 5-year allograft survival rates were again comparable between groups, 83% versus 87% and 61% versus 65%, respectively. Thus, in spite of temporary problems early after the procedure, renal grafts from NHBDs ultimately function as well as grafts from HBDDs.

Controlled Non–Heart-Beating Donor Liver Transplantation—Early Efforts by the Madison, Wisconsin, and Pittsburgh Groups

NHBD organ transplantation was reintroduced by the University of Pittsburgh transplant program in 1992.[12] The Pittsburgh program and the program in Madison, Wisconsin, were pivotal in initiating controlled NHBD organ transplantation and were the first to describe results of NHBD LTX, both in 1995. The Pittsburgh group reported a 50% patient survival rate in six controlled NHBD liver recipients,[4] and the Madison group reported a 75% 1-year survival rate in four controlled NHBD liver recipients.[13] The Pittsburgh group also reported a 1-year graft survival rate of only 17% after six uncontrolled NHBD LTXs, thus showing that liver allograft function may be adequate after controlled, but not usually after uncontrolled, NHBD LTX. Although not comparable to survival rates after HBDD LTX, those after the early experiences with controlled NHBD LTX were encouraging.

Current Results of Controlled Non–Heart-Beating Donor Liver Transplantation

The 1995 reports from the pioneering teams in Pittsburgh and Madison provided the impetus to further develop the field of controlled NHBD LTX. In 2000, two groups published the first successful series of controlled NHBD LTX; the Madison group updated its earlier experience,[14] and we presented the results of our first eight cases.[15] At a mean follow-up of 18 months, our patient and graft survival rates were 100%; there were no instances of PNF, hepatic artery thrombosis (HAT), or ischemic-type biliary stricture (ITBS), and all patients were doing well. We did note a relatively high incidence of temporary cholestasis and rejection early after LTX. We advocated for increased use of controlled NHBD LTX.

Madison, Wisconsin, Experience

In their 2000 follow-up report, D'Alessandro and coworkers retrospectively compared 19 controlled NHBD LTXs with 364 HBDD LTXs, all performed between 1993 and 1999.[14] There was no difference in 3-year patient survival (73% versus 85%, P = NS), but 3-year graft survival was significantly worse in the NHBD group (54% versus 81%, P = .007). The causes of graft loss were death with function (n = 4), PNF (n = 2), HAT (n = 1), and ITBS (n = 1). It is noteworthy that half the graft losses were due to patient death with normal liver function: malignancy (n = 2), iatrogenic injury (n = 1), and late sepsis (n = 1). NHBD liver recipients had a higher rate of PNF (10.5% versus 1.3%, P = .04), but the two involved patients were among the earliest in the cohort, and in one the cause of PNF was technical in origin. Both groups had a similar incidence of HAT (5.3% versus 10.4%, P = NS) and ITBS (5.3% versus 4.6%, P = NS). The one NHBD recipient with ITBS required retransplantation. Based on these findings, the authors recommended cautious pursuit of NHBD LTX.

Recently, several other reports of large experiences with controlled NHBD LTX have been published.[16-18] The overall results from these studies and from our updated experience are described in Table 36–1.

Miami Experience

The University of Miami group has also spearheaded a successful controlled NHBD program.[16,19] Their 2003 publication demonstrates that controlled NHBD LTX can be successfully performed with the use of older donors. Fukumori and associates retrospectively studied 25 controlled NHBD LTXs performed between 1994 and 2001; 5 donors were 55 years or older (older group, mean age of 63 years), and 20 were younger than 55 years (younger group, mean age of 32 years).[16] One-year patient and graft survival rates were both 80% in older (> 55 years) donors as compared with 75% and 70%, respectively, in younger donors. There was no case of PNF in the older group, but poor early graft function occurred in two patients in the younger group, and one underwent retransplantation. It is possible to extract from the paper overall results for all 25 controlled NHBDs, including 1-year patient and graft survival rates of 76% and 72%, respectively, a PNF rate of 4%, and a HAT rate of 0%. The group did not report their rate of biliary complications.

University of Pennsylvania Experience

The group at the University of Pennsylvania also has a large experience with NHBDs. In 2003, Abt and coauthors published a retrospective analysis of 15 LTXs performed with controlled NHBDs versus 221 HBDD LTX procedures performed at their center.[17] One- and 3-year graft survival rates were similar between groups (72% versus 85% and 72% versus 74%, respectively, P = NS for both). Likewise, 1- and 3-year patient survival rates were similar between groups (79% versus 91% and 79% versus 78%, respectively, P = NS for both). PNF occurred in one NHBD liver recipient (6.7% versus 3.6%, P = NS), but HAT did not develop in any NHBD liver. Of concern, major biliary complications occurred in 33.3% of NHBD recipients versus 9.5% of HBDD recipients (P < .01). ITBS accounted for 66.6% of the

Table 36-1. LARGEST SERIES OF CONTROLLED NON–HEART-BEATING DONOR LIVER TRANSPLANTS

Center	Year	LTXs (n)	F/U (mo)	Total WIT (min)*	True WIT (min)†	Donor Age (yr)	Exclude Older NHBDs?	PNF n (%)	HAT n (%)	Ischemic Biliary Disease n (%)	Graft Survival (1 yr, 3 yr)	Patient Survival (1 yr, 3 yr)
U. Wisconsin, Madison‡	2000	19	31	16	NA	32	Yes§	2 (11%)	1(5%)	1(5%)	NA, 54%	NA, 73%
U. Miami¶	2003	25	40	NA	18**	38	No	1 (4%)	0	NA	72%, NA	76%, NA
U. Pennsylvania††	2003	15	27	20	NA	30	Yes‡‡	1 (7%)	0	5 (33%)	72%, 72%	79%, 79%
Albert Einstein, Philadelphia§§	2004	22	47	21	15¶¶	36	No	0	0	1 (5%)	90%, 66%	90%, 66%

*Interval between withdrawal of support and initiation of perfusion.
†Interval between significant ischemic insult and initiation of perfusion.
‡Data from D'Alessandro et al.[14]
§Exclude NHBDs older than 55 years.[14]
¶Data from Fukumori et al.[16]
**Interval between drop in systolic blood pressure below 35 mm Hg or oxygen saturation below 25% and initiation of perfusion.[16]
††Data from Abt et al.[17]
‡‡Exclude NHBDs older than 45 years.[17]
§§Current review, which is an update of the authors' published experience.[15,18]
¶¶Interval between drop in mean arterial pressure below 50 mm Hg and initiation of perfusion.
F/U, follow-up; HAT, hepatic artery thrombosis; LTXs, liver transplants; NA, not available; NHBD, non–heart-beating donor; PNF, primary nonfunction; WIT, warm ischemia time.

Withdrawal until MAP < 50* Minutes (M ± SD [Range])	MAP < 50* until Declaration Minutes (M ± SD [Range])	Wait Period Minutes	Incision until Flush Minutes (Range)
6 ± 5 (0-16)	5 ± 4 (0-12)	5	2-6

Withdrawal until declaration 12 ± 7 (3-27)

Withdrawal until flush: 21 ± 7 (9-34)

MAP < 50* until Flush: 15 ± 5 (4-22)

FIGURE 36–2

Time intervals between withdrawal of support and initiation of perfusion in controlled non–heart-beating donors who provided liver transplants at Albert Einstein Medical Center, Philadelphia (n = 22). *MAP < 50, a drop in mean arterial pressure below 50 mm Hg, is defined by the authors as marking the development of significant hypotension and the start of the true warm ischemia time.

biliary complications in the NHBD group versus 19.2% in the HBDD group, $P < .01$. Of the five patients in the NHBD group with ITBS or bile cast syndrome, or with both, one underwent retransplantation, one died of cholangitis, and one required multiple interventional procedures. The authors caution that biliary epithelium is particularly prone to ischemia-reperfusion injury and advocate the use of younger NHBDs and minimization of ischemia times.

Einstein, Philadelphia, Experience

We recently provided long-term outcomes for 19 controlled NHBD LTXs performed at our institution through 2002.[18] To date, we have performed 22 controlled NHBD LTXs with grafts procured by our team. Additionally, we transplanted one imported controlled NHBD liver that sustained inadvertent, preflush hepatic arterial transection that resulted in PNF, and retransplantation was successful. Our previous publication includes the case of the imported NHBD liver[18]; the following summary relates only to the other 22 LTX procedures. Controlled NHBDs provided livers for 6% of all LTXs (22/371) that we performed between August 1996 and February 2004. Causes of neurological injury were trauma (n = 10), cerebral vascular accident (n = 6), and anoxia (n = 6). Besides being NHBDs, these donors had other expanded donor characteristics, and few were so-called perfect donors. For example, (1) a third of the donors (7/22) were older than 50 years, with donor age ranging from 11 to 66 years; (2) half the donors (12/22) had received CPR on route to the hospital or in the emergency room (or in both locations); (3) a third of the donors (8/22) were hypotensive and required two vasopressors or more than 10 mg/kg/min dopamine (or both) until the time of withdrawal of support; (4) a third of the donors (7/22) had a terminal alanine aminotransferase (ALT) concentration greater than 100 U/L; and (5) a third of the donors (7/22) had abnormal liver biopsy results in which greater than 10% microvesicular or macrovesicular steatosis (or both) or central necrosis was found.

Details regarding the time intervals between withdrawal of support and initiation of perfusion are depicted in Figure 36–2. The interval between the development of significant hypotension, defined as a drop in mean arterial pressure below 50 mm Hg, and the initiation of perfusion was less than 22 minutes in all cases. The longest interval between cessation of mechanical ventilation and initiation of perfusion was 35 minutes. All donors arrested within 27 minutes of discontinuing ventilation. Perfusion was always initiated within 2 to 6 minutes of incision.

The mean follow-up for the group is 47 ± 27 months; 11 of 22 patients have survived longer than 3 years after LTX, and 17 of 22 are still alive more than 1 year after LTX. Patient and graft survival rates for the 22 NHBD LTXs are the same, and in Figure 36–3 they are compared with the survival rates for the 349 HBDD LTXs that we performed during the same period; there are no significant differences between the NHBD and HBDD curves. As depicted, patient and graft survival rates at 1 and 2 years after NHBD LTX are 90% and 85%, respectively. Six of 22 recipients have died thus far. One death may have been primarily related to the allograft coming from an NHBD. The recipient died of sepsis shortly after retransplantation at 4 months for ITBS. However, this patient also had severe median arcuate ligament syndrome, which was not recognized at the time of the original transplant and very likely caused profound biliary ischemia.[18] The other five deaths seemed to be unrelated to the NHBD allografts and were due to bowel obstruction in the second postoperative month (n = 1), right heart failure 2 years after LTX (n = 1), bladder perforation during cesarean section in the third postoperative year (n = 1), recurrent hepatitis C virus disease in the third year after LTX (n = 1), and allograft damage in the fourth postoperative year as a result of late HAT (n = 1).

No patient suffered PNF or early HAT. There was one instance of reperfusion syndrome and another instance of poor early graft function; both grafts functioned normally within a few days, and the recipients have done well. Notably, temporary transaminitis, temporary cholestasis, or acute cellular rejection developed in a significant number of the recipients. The mean peak ALT concentration was 2688 IU, but ALT quickly normalized in all cases. The mean peak total bilirubin

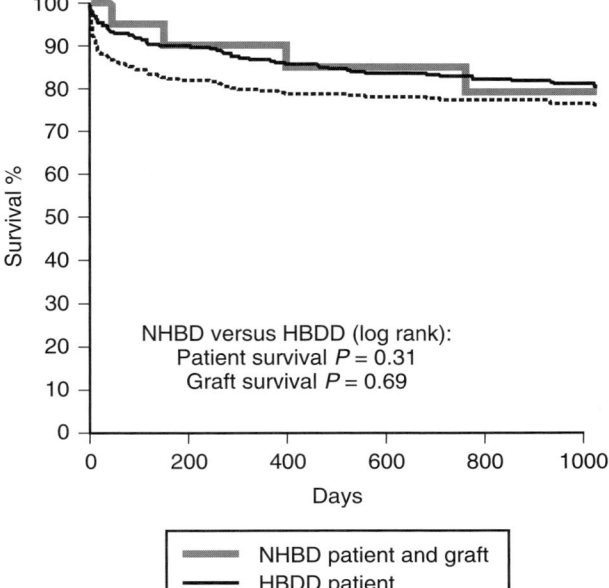

FIGURE 36–3

Patient and graft survival curves after controlled non–heart-beating donor (NHBD) and heart-beating deceased donor (HBDD) liver transplants performed at Albert Einstein Medical Center, Philadelphia. *The NHBD patient and graft survival curves are identical.

was 8 mg/dL, but all cases of hyperbilirubinemia peaked within 3 weeks after LTX and then completely resolved. We hypothesized that NHBD bile canalicular function is particularly prone to ischemia-reperfusion injury, which causes, in stepwise fashion, generation of free radicals, depletion of adenosine triphosphate, disruption of canalicular actin microfilaments, cytoskeletal damage, canalicular dilatation, microvilli loss, reduced bile flow, and consequently, cholestasis.[15,20] Allograft rejection developed within 3 months in 41% of recipients (9/22), but all rejections were successfully treated. This incidence of rejection is much higher than that for HBDD liver allografts. Notably, it has been shown in some cases that when compared with HBDD organs, NHBD organs are less prone to rejection because they are not exposed to the cascade of inflammatory events caused by brain death and subsequent triggering of host immune mechanisms.[21,22] Donor autonomic storm and brain death cause endothelial damage, upregulation of adhesion molecules, slowing of leukocyte traffic, release of proinflammatory lymphokines, expansion of major histocompatibility complex molecules, host T-cell recognition, and thus rejection. However, many of our NHBDs did suffer catastrophic brain injury or exposure to severe hemodynamic instability, or both, and thus they may very well have been exposed to the aforementioned hemodynamic and neuroimmunological cascades.

Based on the gratifying experience just presented, we continue to cautiously liberalize our criteria for using livers from NHBDs with confounding risk factors. We have found that older controlled NHBD livers can function well, similar to the experience of the Miami group,[16] and we do not decline older controlled NHBD livers solely based on donor age, in contrast to the Madison,

Wisconsin, and University of Pennsylvania groups.[14,17] We prefer to have the donor surgery performed by one of our attending surgeons who is experienced in rapid procurement from controlled NHBDs. When deciding on whether to transplant a procured liver, we place great emphasis on assessing the various ischemia time intervals between withdrawal of support and initiation of donor perfusion. We particularly care about the interval between the development of significant hypotension and initiation of perfusion. With all livers that we have decided to use thus far, this interval has been less than 22 minutes; the upper limit might be extended somewhat. Based on the experiences depicted in Table 36–1, no group has routinely used NHBD livers exposed to longer total or true warm ischemia times, and hence the safe limit remains unknown. Although we do not generally use T tubes, it is our practice to place them in NHBD liver recipients to facilitate evaluation of cholestasis, should it occur. We generally maintain NHBD liver recipients on higher levels of immunosuppression during the first posttransplant weeks, although immunosuppression is individualized according to other factors as well.

Summary of Current Results

The combined results depicted in Table 36–1,[14,16-18] which represents the outcomes of 81 controlled NHBD LTXs, may be summarized as follows: controlled NHBD LTX (1) provides excellent short- and long-term patient survival that is comparable to that after HBDD LTX; (2) provides acceptable graft survival—although survival was reduced in the Madison, Wisconsin, cohort of patients,[14] half the graft losses were due to patient death with normal liver function; (3) does not lead to an increased incidence of PNF—although PNF developed in 11% of the Madison patients, these two patients were among the earliest in the cohort, and in one the PNF was technical in origin[14]; (4) does not lead to an increased incidence of HAT; (5) has not led to an increased incidence of ITBS, except in the experience of Abt and colleagues[17]—given that report, the risk of ITBS remains a concern when using NHBD livers, particularly those exposed to longer ischemic times; (6) may, in selective cases, be safely performed with older donors, as shown by the Miami group[16] and the authors,[18] although others advise against this practice[14,17]; and (7) may be safely performed in the face of true and total warm ischemia times up to and perhaps somewhat beyond 20 to 30 minutes and 30 to 45 minutes, respectively.

Operative Technique for Non–Heart-Beating Donor Liver Procurement

Several operative techniques for NHBD hepatectomy have been described.[4,13,15,19] Modifications of the super-rapid technique described by the Pittsburgh group[4] are used by such groups as those at the University of Miami, the University of Pennsylvania, and Albert Einstein Medical Center, Philadelphia.[15-19] In contrast, the Madison, Wisconsin, group uses a premortem cannulation technique.[13,14] The authors' approach to controlled NHBD organ procurement, including a modified super-rapid surgical technique, is described in the following sections, followed by a summary of the alternative, premortem cannulation technique.

Preoperative Management (Identifying Potential Non–Heart-Beating Donors, Withdrawing Support)

The NHBD protocol used by the authors and those at other programs in our OPO is summarized in Table 36–2.[23] NHBD management has been consistent with Institute of Medicine (IOM) guidelines since their availability in 1997.[24] Potential controlled NHBDs are identified by mandatory referral of dying patients to the OPO, pursuant to local state laws.[25] Heparin, but not phentolamine, is administered to the donor, as is done by the Pittsburgh group; the Madison group administers both agents. A preprinted flow sheet, reproduced in Figure 36–4, is filled out in the operating room to document hemodynamic measurements every minute and the times of discontinuation of mechanical ventilation, declaration of death, waiting period, incision, and perfusion. The authors have found that communication between the NHBD surgeon and the nursing staff about conduct

Table 36–2. CONTROLLED NON–HEART-BEATING DONOR PROTOCOL USED BY THE AUTHORS AND OTHER GROUPS SERVED BY THE GIFT OF LIFE DONOR PROGRAM

Donor Eligibility

Medically suitable for donation

Brain death criteria not met

Catastrophic brain injury

No expectation of survival according to donor's physicians

Withdrawal of support requested by donor's surrogate(s)

Consent for donation obtained

Withdrawal of Support

To OR with full life support

Preparation and draping by transplant surgeon

Heparin (some OPOs omit heparin; some OPOs give phentolamine)

Transplant team leaves OR

Donor's care team stops ventilation

Donor's care team declares death (if patient alive after 60 minutes, procurement aborted and patient returned to ward for comfort care)

5-minute wait period after declaration

Transplant team re-enters for super-rapid recovery

Operative Technique

Modified Pittsburgh "super-rapid technique" (some groups in other OPOs prefer the premortem cannulation technique)

Rapid laparotomy and distal aortic cannulation

Preservation fluid flush and ice cooling

Sternal split, IVC vent, and thoracic aortic clamping

Hepatectomy and nephrectomies (with or without pancreatectomy)

Portal flush on back-table

IVC, inferior vena cava; OPO, organ procurement organization; OR, operating room.

of the operation before withdrawal of support facilitates cooperation and speediness of recovery. After procurement, careful assessment of the information on the flow sheet is critical for appraising the ischemic injury. If the patient remains alive 60 minutes after withdrawal of support, organ procurement is aborted and the patient is returned to a ward for continued comfort care. In the rare instances that this occurred in our OPO, the patient always expired within the next few hours.

Super-Rapid Surgical Technique

After death, the distal end of the aorta is cannulated through a midline laparotomy, organ perfusion is initiated, and the abdomen is filled with ice slush. The adult body is perfused with at least 5 L of cold University of

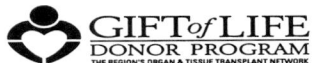

Patient Name_____   UNOS#_____

OPERATING ROOM NON-HEART-BEATING ORGAN DONOR FLOW SHEET

INTRAOPERATIVE MANAGEMENT

Blood Drawn   Date____/____/____   Time____:____   (EST)
Heparin Administered   Date____/____/____   Time____:____   (EST)
Entered OR   Date____/____/____   Time____:____   (EST)
Withdrawal of Support Date____/____/____   Time____:____   (EST)
Pronouncement   Date____/____/____   Time____:____   (EST)
Incision   Date____/____/____   Time____:____   (EST)
Cross-Clamp   Date____/____/____   Time____:____   (EST)

Time From Withdrawal to Pronouncement _____minutes
Time From Pronouncement to Cross-Clamp _____minutes
Total Warm Ischemic Time (withdrawal to cross-clamp) _____minutes
Flush Solution _____   1st Liter in @____:____   Total Flush _____cc
Family Present for Withdrawal ☐ Yes ☐ No   Location of Withdrawal ☐ OR ☐ ICU ☐ PACU ☐ Other_____
Care and Comfort Administered ☐ Yes ☐ No   Was Patient Extubated ☐ Yes ☐ No

START TIME _____ : _____   **HEMODYNAMIC MEASUREMENTS**

	Min 1	Min 2	Min 3	Min 4	Min 5	Min 6	Min 7	Min 8	Min 9	Min 10	Min 11	Min 12	Min 13	Min 14	Min 15	Min 16	Min 17	Min 18	Min 19	Min 20
HR																				
BP																				
RR																				
SPO2																				
	Min 21	Min 22	Min 23	Min 24	Min 25	Min 26	Min 27	Min 28	Min 29	Min 30	Min 31	Min 32	Min 33	Min 34	Min 35	Min 36	Min 37	Min 38	Min 39	Min 40
HR																				
BP																				
RR																				
SPO2																				
	Min 41	Min 42	Min 43	Min 44	Min 45	Min 46	Min 47	Min 48	Min 49	Min 50	Min 51	Min 52	Min 53	Min 54	Min 55	Min 56	Min 57	Min 58	Min 59	Min 60
HR																				
BP																				
RR																				
SPO2																				

Comments: _____

FIGURE 36–4

Gift Of Life Donor Program: non–heart-beating donor operating room flow sheet. (Courtesy of Howard M. Nathan and Richard D. Hasz, Gift of Life Donor Program, Philadelphia.)

Wisconsin (UW) solution containing dexamethasone, 16 mg/L, and insulin, 40 U/L. Immediately after starting the flush, the sternum is divided, the intrapericardial inferior vena cava is vented, and the descending thoracic aorta is cross-clamped. We do not cannulate the portal system in situ. Hepatectomy and then bilateral nephrectomies are performed. The portal system is flushed on the back-table with 1 L of chilled UW solution.

Premortem Cannulation Technique

The group at Madison, Wisconsin, performs consensual, pre-extubation (premortem) femoral vessel cannulation and administers phentolamine in addition to heparin.[13,14] All extrarenal NHBDs are taken to the operating room before withdrawal of life support. Right femoral artery and right femoral vein cannulas are inserted under local anesthesia. After cessation of respiration, lack of a monitored arterial pulse, declaration

of death, and an additional wait time of 5 minutes, cold UW solution is infused into the femoral artery cannula. The femoral vein cannula is opened to gravity to decompress the venous system. Median sternotomy and midline abdominal incisions are made, and the intra-abdominal organs are removed en bloc. Portal flush and organ separation are performed on the back-table.

Unusual Case Reports

Case reports are emerging about the use of unusual controlled NHBD liver allografts. We reported on combined procurement of the liver, pancreas, and kidneys from a controlled NHBD with a large accessory right hepatic artery off the superior mesenteric artery.[26] The right branch was anastomosed to the donor gastroduodenal artery. The liver and pancreas were successfully transplanted into two recipients in Philadelphia and Minneapolis. There were no complications, and both grafts were functioning well at 14 months' follow-up. Adding whole-organ pancreatectomy to hepatectomy during super-rapid recovery carries a significant risk for transecting an aberrant right hepatic artery because there is no opportunity to palpate arterial pulsations in an NHBD. Meticulous in situ dissection in search of a right branch can significantly increase the extraction time. Therefore, the NHBD liver is typically removed with the pancreatic head to avoid injuring an aberrant right hepatic artery. We do not routinely procure NHBD whole pancreases when harvesting NHBD livers unless there is a favorable donor body habitus and other issues are optimal, such as warm ischemia time. Alternatively, the liver and pancreas may be removed en bloc.

Muiesan and coauthors reported the first use of a reduced-size NHBD liver for successful auxiliary right lobe LTX in an 11-year old child with fulminant hepatic failure.[27]

Uncontrolled Non–Heart-Beating Donor Liver Transplantation—The Madrid Model

An organized effort to improve outcomes after uncontrolled NHBD organ transplantation has been in progress in Madrid since 1996.[5,6] This protocol is considered by some to be ethically problematic because it involves nonconsensual postmortem maneuvers to minimize organ ischemia, even though organ procurement is aborted if consent for donation is not eventually obtained. Emergency prehospital care teams evaluate individuals who suffer cardiopulmonary arrest in the "streets" and do not respond to standard resuscitation. After death until the time of organ retrieval, these individuals undergo CPR, followed by either simultaneous chest and abdominal compressions or cardiopulmonary bypass with hypothermic or normothermic extracorporeal circulation and external oxygenation.[5] A patient is considered a potential organ donor if an effective heartbeat is not established in the streets, less than 15 minutes has elapsed between circulatory arrest and initiation of CPR, CPR and intravenous perfusion are administered during transport to the hospital, there are no hemorrhagic injuries to the abdomen or thorax, and less than 2 hours has elapsed from the beginning of initial prehospital assistance to initiation of preservation procedures.[6] The preservation procedures are performed nonconsensually; however, donation is aborted if within 4 hours of the prehospital encounter the next of kin are not contacted or do not consent to organ procurement.[6] This protocol has been used primarily for kidney donation, but there is a recent report on 20 patients who received livers from NHBDs managed in this way.[5] The 1- and 2-year patient survival rates were both 80%, and the corresponding graft survival rates

were both 55%. Overall, there was a high incidence of primary PNF (25%) and ITBS (30%). The risk of PNF or ITBS increased with longer duration of compressions or bypass. Grafts supported by simultaneous compressions fared better than those supported by bypass, but the duration of CPR and bypass was significantly longer than the duration of CPR and simultaneous compressions. No difference was noted in outcomes regardless of whether hypothermic or normothermic bypass was used. The authors recommend uncontrolled NHBD support with compressions alone if consent and harvesting can be arranged within 130 minutes of arrest; otherwise, bypass may be used for additional support, perhaps for up to another 150 minutes.

Potential Impact of Non–Heart-Beating Donor Liver Transplantation

General Estimates

There is increasing interest in pursuing controlled NHBD organ transplantation because NHBDs have the potential to become a significant source of solid organs. Currently, only approximately 3% of deceased donors in the United States are NHBDs.[1] However, it has been estimated that NHBDs could increase the deceased donor pool in the United States by approximately 1000 donors per year, a 25% increase.[25] Indeed, in certain parts of the United States, NHBDs make a major contribution to the local donor pool. For example, the Gift of Life Donor Program, which is the OPO that services the authors' program and other centers in southern New Jersey, eastern Pennsylvania, and Delaware, has developed a highly successful NHBD program (Fig. 36–5) such that last year, 15% of deceased donors in the OPO were NHBDs (51/344).[27] The renewed interest in NHBDs in the United States, particularly liver donors, is focused mostly on controlled NHBDs, who will have life support withdrawn regardless of whether they become organ donors. Some of the reasons that controlled NHBD LTX is gaining acceptance and becoming more widespread involve increasing reluctance to prolong futile treatment and artificial life support of terminally injured and ill patients, increasing use of advance directives and health care proxies, and encouraging data on survival after NHBD organ transplantation.

Pediatric Non–Heart-Beating Donors

Koogler and Costarino[28] retrospectively analyzed the hospital records of children who died in the pediatric intensive care unit at the Children's Hospital of Philadelphia from January 1992 to July 1996. They sought to determine

Gift of Life Donor Program
Non-Heart-Beating Organ Donors
1995 – 2003

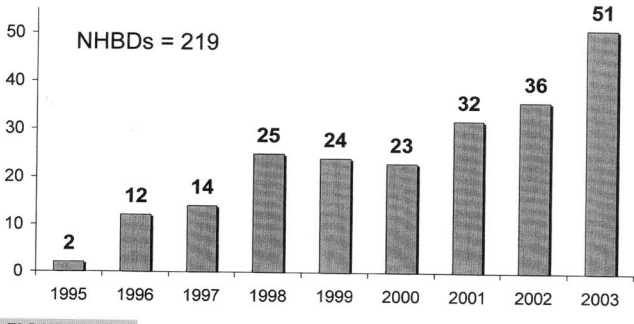

FIGURE 36–5

Gift Of Life Donor Program: non–heart-beating donors 1995 to 2003. (Courtesy of Howard M. Nathan and Richard D. Hasz, Gift of Life Donor Program, Philadelphia.)

the mode of death, organ donation consent rate of potential HBDDs, and the number of children who could have been NHBDs. Of the 319 deaths, 111 had life support withdrawn; after eliminating children who had sepsis, human immunodeficiency virus infection, hepatitis, or extracranial malignancy or took longer than 2 hours after withdrawal of support to die and then applying the consent rate for potential HBDDs (58%), 18 could have qualified as NHBDs. The authors concluded that at their institution, routine use of NHBDs could have increased the number of deceased donors by 42%.

Institute of Medicine Efforts

In 1997, the IOM of the National Academy of Science published its first report on NHBDs.[24] The IOM was commissioned by the Department of Health and Human Services to study the medical and ethical issues that arise when organs are recovered from NHBDs who do not meet the standard criteria for brain death. The study was organized partly in response to a well-publicized, controversial 1997 *60 Minutes* CBS television report that negatively portrayed NHBD initiatives and led to lay skepticism about organ donation in general. The IOM report was based on extensive information collected about the status of the organ supply and demand and about the policies and practices of NHBD organ procurement and transplantation in the United States. The findings revealed considerable variation in practice among both OPOs and hospitals. The IOM team of multidisciplinary experts concluded that policies and practices relating to care of the organ donor should be consistent with regard to fundamental ethical and scientific principles. They recommended guidelines for the practice of NHBD organ procurement. Most importantly, the IOM report concluded that controlled NHBD organ

procurement is effective and ethical, and it encouraged increased use of controlled NHBD organ transplantation.

Initially, the IOM report did not significantly increase the rate of NHBD organ transplantation, so in 1999 a second IOM workshop was held. This workshop led to the second IOM report in 2000, which shares strategies designed to disseminate the recommendations of the first IOM report and facilitate widespread adoption of NHBD protocols.[3] The second report also advocates increased funding for outcomes assessment of NHBD organ transplantation and for research on interventions to decrease ischemic organ injury in NHBDs. The IOM support for using NHBDs, including the IOM reports, has helped bring credibility to the field of NHBD organ transplantation, has increased interest and knowledge about NHBDs, and has assisted in standardizing NHBD protocols.

Ethical Issues (Specific to Controlled Non–Heart-Beating Donors)

Basic Principles

Increased organ donation is a worthy goal, and NHBD organ transplantation holds significant promise as a partial solution to the donor organ dilemma. NHBD organ procurement honors the donor's wishes, brings some comfort to the family, and benefits the recipient. Despite incomplete consensus, most authorities agree that NHBD organ procurement and transplantation are justified and ethically feasible, provided that the following principles are upheld: individuals may not be killed for their organs or killed as a result of removal of their organs (the "dead donor" rule), patients must not be jeopardized to facilitate organ procurement (the goal of organ donation is subordinate to care of the patient), euthanasia is prohibited, informed consent and respect for family wishes must not be violated, interventions for the purpose of expediting organ donation rather than for donor benefit are performed only if they are consensual and do not hasten death or harm the donor, and the autonomous right of patients to refuse treatment must be upheld.[3,12,24,29-33]

It is imperative to ensure that there is no conflict of interest between the duty to provide optimal patient care and the desire to recover organs for transplantation.[30,31,33] Specifically, the rationale for withdrawal of life support and the determination of death must be extricable from the decision to recover organs. Therefore, the patient care and organ donor teams need to be completely separate. Care must be taken to safeguard against conflict of interest, even in the face of an endeavor that entails obligatory haste to minimize warm ischemia times.[33]

Although health care professionals are trained to define concepts such as death in terms of biological principles and to analyze them accordingly, there needs to be sensitivity to the fact that there are multiple nonbiological, culturally defined perceptions of death and the period of suspension between life and death. Among certain groups, such perceptions take precedence over the biologically determined clinical definition of death. For some, deciding on a standard waiting time strictly in terms of minutes—beginning with the declaration of death and ending at the initiation of organ recovery—is too narrow a context in which to operationalize NHBD protocols, whether the wait time is 10 minutes, 5 minutes, or 2 minutes. Professionals dealing with potential NHBDs need to be cognizant of the variety of settings that they work in and mindful of the diverse backgrounds and belief systems that patients and families have.[30]

Controversial Ethics Topics

Several issues related to the ethics of NHBD organ procurement remain sources of considerable debate. Differing views are manifested in the various active NHBD protocols regarding the use of certain medications and interventions in potential NHBDs. There is a commonly accepted code of conduct. A recent American College of Critical Care Medicine position paper generally prohibits medications that expedite death, but it condones medications given to improve the chance of successful donation if they do not harm the patient, as well as medications routinely provided for patient comfort even if they might hasten death.[32] However, there is still controversy on how such guiding principals are to be applied, particularly the use of anticoagulation, vasodilation, narcotic administration, and premortem placement of intravascular cannulas.[31] Another issue that is debated is whether loss of cardiac electrical activity is necessary to define controlled NHBD death. The IOM suggests using this criterion,[3] but waiting for asystole often leads to extensive warm ischemia and can preclude safe transplantation of the liver. Others argue that the absence of heart sounds, pulse, and blood pressure is sufficient for determination of NHBD death, just as it is in patients who are not organ donors.[12] Ultimately, the donor hospital and care team have the responsibility for defining and declaring patient death.

Another important ethical question that has an impact on the warm ischemic time endured by NHBD organs relates to the duration of the waiting period used to ensure irreversible death. Standardized protocols for recovery of organs from NHBDs include a prescribed wait time from the determination of death to organ procurement. Autoresuscitation after 1 minute of pulselessness has not been reported in the literature.[30] However, the wait time is variably defined. For example,

the Maastricht workshop maintains that 10 minutes is required,[29] the IOM proposes 5 minutes,[3] the position paper by the Ethics Committee of the American College of Critical Care Medicine specifies at least 2 minutes and not more than 5 minutes,[32] and the Pittsburgh group waits 2 minutes.[31] The Pittsburgh criterion—the least conservative—is based on the standard that irreversible cessation of cardiopulmonary function is sufficient to certify death and that since the patient or family has refused resuscitation, the patient's clinical state is irreversible. Furthermore, they argue that a period of 2 minutes is routinely used to certify death in nondonor situations and that different criteria should not be used for organ donors.[31] The 5-minute period recommended by the IOM has the added benefit of rendering the NHBD de facto brain dead.[30]

At a time when the transplant community is struggling to increase public support of organ donation, NHBD transplantation must be addressed systematically, scientifically, and sensitively. The harm of failing to do so could outweigh the potential gain in the number of donors. The IOM addressed this issue by attempting to standardize the process with recommended guidelines,[3,24] as did the American College of Critical Care Medicine.[32] Increasingly, there are explicit, readily available, locally approved protocols that consider all stakeholders—the public, law enforcement agencies, the media, and health care practitioners. Such protocols are necessary to avoid skepticism and engender the public's trust. However, NHBD practices and protocols at different centers are still inconsistent, and important issues still require careful clarification.

The Role of the Organ Procurement Organization

Strong OPO initiatives are essential if potential donors, families, and recipients are to benefit from increased access to NHBD transplantation. OPOs must develop NHBD protocols; recruit support at the local and regional hospital levels; provide education to physicians, nurses, and other health care providers; engender enthusiasm not only among the OPO community but also among all transplant team members; and participate in well-designed and well-orchestrated public relations campaigns.[34] Several OPOs serve as examples in this regard, including the Gift of Life Donor Program in Philadelphia,[35] the OPO at the University of Wisconsin in Madison,[13,14] the Center for Organ Recovery and Education in Pittsburgh,[12] and LifeQuest Organ Recovery Services in Gainesville, Florida.[34] For example, the Gift of Life Donor Program, one of the oldest and largest OPOs in the United States, serves a population of approximately 10 million. In 1995, after passage of the routine referral law and recognition of the need to consider expanded criteria donor sources, the OPO implemented an NHBD protocol. From 1995 to 1998, 79 kidneys and 15 livers were successfully transplanted from NHBDs.[25] Hospital policies were developed and refined, and the NHBD program grew quickly (see Fig. 36–5). Through 2003, there have been a total of 185 controlled NHBDs in this OPO.[27]

Ideally, patients who are brain dead or will probably soon become so should donate organs according to brain death protocols, not NHBD protocols. Growing enthusiasm about the option of NHBD organ procurement ought to be tempered by the realization that both the yield of transplantable organs from NHBDs and the outcomes of NHBD organ transplantation are not generally as favorable as those with heart-beating donors. Patients who seem brain dead are usually stable enough to complete brain death protocols. Families infrequently insist on withdrawal of support rather than waiting for brain death if it is imminent, and they are most often willing to permit completion of brain death protocols. When it seems that heart-beating donor organ procurement will be possible, NHBD organ donation should not be viewed as an equally acceptable alternative; even at a time when hospitals are pressed to empty critical care beds, brain death protocols may increasingly be viewed as cumbersome, and transplant professionals strive to expedite organ donation. Besides the ethical slippery slope involved, such strategy would also unnecessarily add a significant extended donor criterion to the organs. NHBDs should be used to truly expand the donor pool, such as in cases in which catastrophic injury has occurred but brain death is not imminent and there is a request for withdrawal of support, in some cases in which a brain-dead or soon to be brain-dead donor is severely unstable, or in uncommon cases in which a family is completely unwilling to wait for completion of the brain death protocol.

Conclusion

NHBD organ transplantation has become highly successful and brings the history of organ donation to full circle. It is important to differentiate controlled from uncontrolled NHBDs; the former account for the majority of NHBDs in the United States, whereas the latter represent the majority elsewhere. In the United States, the number of NHBD organs recovered for transplantation has steadily increased from only 42 in 1993 to 167 in 2001.[1] OPOs and transplant centers across the country are re-evaluating NHBD organ transplantation in response to the escalating organ shortage and because families more frequently request this option in their discussions about removal of life support from patients who suffer devastating trauma or critical, irreversible illness. Although the kidney remains the most commonly

transplanted NHBD organ, in certain OPOs controlled NHBDs contribute a major portion of the transplanted livers.[14,16,25,34,35] Several groups have now published outstanding results after controlled NHBD LTX and have shown that NHBDs safely expand the donor pool for LTX.[13-18]

The accompanying box highlights some pearls and pitfalls related to NHBD LTX. Surgeons who recover organs from NHBDs must be familiar with rapid procurement techniques. Cautious liberalization of criteria for accepting livers from NHBDs with confounding risk factors seems justified, but further study is required to better define the acceptable risks. Discovery of effective cytoprotective agents that could be administered to NHBDs or to NHBD organ recipients (or to both) to protect against ischemic organ injury would further expand the ability to transplant NHBD organs. Given the worldwide resurgence of interest in the various types of NHBD organ transplantation, there is fertile opportunity for this field to continue to mature. Additional refinement of clinical practice and ethics guidelines should facilitate broader approval of NHBD organ transplantation. NHBD LTX has emerged as a successful and critically important clinical endeavor.

Pearls and Pitfalls

Pearls

- Make sure that the OPO has an approved, detailed NHBD protocol and hospital development process in place.

- Discuss the possibility of NHBD LTX with patients during the LTX evaluation so that they are not surprised if asked to provide informed consent later on.

- Have the coordinator fill out a preprinted NHBD flow sheet to document hemodynamic measurements every minute and the times of discontinuation of mechanical ventilation, declaration of death, waiting period, incision, and perfusion. After procurement, careful assessment of information on the flow sheet is critical for appraising the ischemic injury.

- Decrease operating/ischemic time:
  - Before withdrawal of support, communicate with the nursing staff about conduct of the operation, prepare and drape, and set up instruments. Then, exit the operating room but remain gowned and gloved.

Pearls and Pitfalls—cont'd

- Start the aortic flush immediately after cannulation—do not wait until cross clamping or venting. Flush the portal system on the back-table, not in situ.

- Maintain a low threshold for performing a donor liver biopsy to exclude centrilobular necrosis and other predictors of poor graft quality.

- After LTX, do not be surprised by high transaminitis and cholestasis—they are usually self-limited and completely reversible.

- Use T tubes liberally to facilitate (1) evaluation of possible early post-LTX cholestasis and (2) surveillance for ischemic biliary strictures.

- Lean toward heavier immunosuppression early on, even with significant transaminitis and decreased calcineurin inhibitor metabolism, because the ischemically damaged NHBD liver may be more prone to rejection.

Pitfalls

- Confusing uncontrolled NHBDs with controlled NHBDs; in general, livers from the former pose a much higher risk than those from the latter.

- Lack of familiarity with NHBD protocols and relevant ethics principles.

- Inadequate planning and poor communication with the donor coordinator and operating room nurses.

- Involvement in decisions about patient prognosis, withdrawal of support, or determination of death—all are conflicts of interest.

- Pursuing NHBD organ procurement in a patient not likely to die expeditiously after withdrawal of support.

- Adding whole-organ pancreatectomy to hepatectomy during NHBD recovery, unless there is a favorable donor body habitus and a short warm ischemia time. The NHBD liver is typically removed with the pancreatic head to avoid transecting an aberrant right hepatic artery and to minimize extraction time; alternatively, the liver and pancreas may be removed en bloc.

- NHBD LTX after excessive ischemia times:

  - A true warm ischemia time (interval between a significant ischemic insult, such as a drop in mean arterial pressure below 50 mm Hg, and initiation of perfusion) up to and perhaps somewhat beyond 20 to 30 minutes seems safe.

Pearls and Pitfalls—cont'd

- A total warm ischemia time (interval between withdrawal of support and initiation of perfusion) up to and perhaps somewhat beyond 30 to 45 minutes seems safe.

- Keep the cold ischemia time as short as possible.

- Transplanting livers from NHBDs with too many additional extended donor or graft criteria.

- Sending an inexperienced surgical team for NHBD liver procurement or importing an NHBD liver from an unfamiliar team.

Acknowledgment

We thank Khristian Noto, MD, for his dedication and invaluable assistance with data analysis related to the section on our experience at Albert Einstein Medical Center, Philadelphia, and with preparation of the figures and tables.

References

1. Annual Report: URREA; UNOS. 2002 Annual Report of the U.S. Organ Procurement and Transplantation Network and the Scientific Registry of Transplant Recipients: Transplant Data 1992-2001 [Internet]. Rockville, MD, HHS/HRSA/OSP/DOT, 2003 [modified 2003 Feb 18]. Available from http://www.optn.org/ data/ annualReport.asp.
2. Nashan B, Luck R, Becker T, et al: Expansion of the donor pool in liver transplantation: The Hannover experience 1996-2002. Clin Transpl 221-228, 2002.
3. Institute of Medicine, National Academy of Sciences: Non–Heart-Beating Organ Transplantation: Practice and Protocols. Washington, DC, National Academy Press, 2000.
4. Casavilla A, Ramirez C, Shapiro R, et al: Experience with liver and kidney allografts from non–heart-beating donors. Transplantation 59:197-203, 1995.
5. Otero A, Gomez-Gutierrez M, Suarez F, et al: Liver transplantation from Maastricht category 2 non–heart-beating donors. Transplantation 76:1068-1073, 2003.
6. Alvarez J, del Barrio R, Arias J, et al: Non–heart-beating donors from the streets: An increasing donor pool source. Transplantation 70:314-317, 2000.
7. Daemen J-WHC, Koostra G, Wijnen RMH, et al: Nonheart-beating donors: The Maastricht experience. In Terasaki PI, Cecka M (eds): Clinical Transplants 1994. Los Angeles, UCLA Tissue Typing Laboratory, 1994, pp 303-316.
8. A definition of irreversible coma: Report of the Ad Hoc Committee of the Harvard Medical School to Examine the Definition of Brain Death. JAMA 205:337-340, 1968.
9. UDODA—Guidelines for the determination of death: Report of the medical consultants on the diagnosis of death to the President's Commission for the Study of Ethical Problems in Medical and Biomedical and Behavioral Research. JAMA 246:2184-2186, 1981.

10. Cho YW, Terasaki PI, Cecka M, et al: Transplantation of kidneys from donors whose hearts have stopped beating. N Engl J Med 338:221-225, 1998.
11. Rudich SM, Kaplan B, Magee JC, et al: Renal transplantations performed using non–heart-beating organ donors: Going back to the future. Transplantation 74:1715-1720, 2002.
12. DeVita MA, Vukmir R, Snyder JV, et al: Procuring organs from a non–heart-beating cadaver: A case report. Kennedy Institute of Ethics Journal 3:371-385, 1993.
13. D'Alessandro AM, Hoffmann RM, Knechtle SJ, et al: Successful extrarenal transplantation from non–heart-beating donors. Transplantation 59:977-982, 1995.
14. D'Alessandro AM, Hoffmann RM, Knechtle SJ, et al: Liver transplantation from controlled non–heart-beating donors. Surgery 128:579-588, 2000.
15. Reich DJ, Munoz SJ, Rothstein KD, et al: Controlled non–heart-beating donor liver transplantation: A successful single center experience, with topic update. Transplantation 70:1159-1166, 2000.
16. Fukumori T, Kato T, Levi D, et al: Use of older controlled non–heart-beating donors for liver transplantation. Transplantation 75:1171-1174, 2003.
17. Abt PL, Crawford MD, Desai NM, et al: Liver transplantation from controlled and uncontrolled non–heart-beating donors: An increased incidence of biliary complications. Transplantation 75:1659-1663, 2003.
18. Manzarbeitia CY, Ortiz JA, Jeon H, et al: Long-term outcome of controlled non–heart-beating donor liver transplantation. Transplantation 78:211-215, 2004.
19. Olson L, Davi R, Barnhart J, et al: Non–heart-beating cadaver donor hepatectomy: 'The operative procedure.' Clin Transpl 13:98-103, 1999.
20. Cutrin JC, Cantino D, Biasi F, et al: Reperfusion damage to the bile canaliculi in transplanted human liver. Hepatology 24:1053-1057, 1996.
21. Pratschke J, Wilhelm MJ, Kusaka M, et al: Brain death and its influence on donor organ quality and outcome after transplantation. Transplantation 67:343-348, 1999.
22. Pratschke J, Wilhelm MJ, Kusaka M, et al: Accelerated rejection of renal allografts from brain-dead donors. Ann Surg 232:263-271, 2000.
23. Gift of Life Donor Program: Asystolic Cadaveric Organ Recovery Procedures following Patient and/or Family Directed Withdrawal of Life Support. Philadelphia, Gift of Life Donor Program, Inc, 1998.
24. Institute of Medicine, National Academy of Sciences: Non–Heart-Beating Organ Transplantation: Medical and Ethical Issues in Procurement. Washington, DC, National Academy Press, 1997.
25. Edwards JM, Hasz RD, Robertson VM: Non–heart-beating organ donation: Process and Review. AACN Clinical Issues 10:293-300, 1999.
26. Jeon H, Ortiz JA, Manzarbeitia CY, et al: Combined liver and pancreas procurement from a controlled non–heart-beating donor with aberrant hepatic arterial anatomy. Transplantation 74:1636-1639, 2002.
27. Muiesan P, Girlanda R, Baker A, et al: Successful segmental auxiliary liver transplantation from a non–heart-beating donor: Implications for split-liver transplantation. Transplantation 75:1443-1445, 2003.
28. Koogler T, Costarino AT Jr: The potential benefits of the pediatric nonheartbeating organ donor. Pediatrics 101:1049-1052, 1998.
29. Koostra G: The asystolic, or non-heartbeating, donor. Transplantation 63:917-921, 1997.
30. Whetstine L, Bowman K, Hawryluck L: Pro/con ethics debate: Is nonheart-beating organ donation ethically acceptable? Crit Care 6:192-195, 2000.
31. Bell MD: Non–heart beating organ donation: Old procurement strategy—new ethical problems. J Med Ethics 29:176-181, 2003.
32. Recommendations for nonheartbeating organ donation. A position paper by the Ethics Committee, American College of Critical Care Medicine, Society of Critical Care Medicine. Crit Care Med 29:1826-1831, 2002.
33. Arnold RM, Younger SJ: Time is of the essence: The pressing need for comprehensive non–heart-beating cadaveric donation policies. Transplant Proc 27:2913-2921, 1995.
34. Reiner M, Cornell D, Howard RJ: Development of a successful non–heart-beating organ donation program. Prog Transplant 13:225-231, 2003.
35. Gift of Life Donor Program: 2003 Annual Report. Philadelphia, Gift of Life Donor Program, Inc, 2004.

The Donor Operation

JOHN F. RENZ

HASAN YERSIZ

Evaluation of the potential recipient 546

Evaluation of the potential donor 546

The donor operation: Conventional adult
  liver procurement 546
  Preoperative preparation 546
  Preparation for cold perfusion 547
  Organ cold perfusion 550
  Cold dissection 551
  Special circumstances 553
  Back-table preparation of the
    liver allograft 554
  Arterial variations and reconstruction 556
  Pediatric procurement 556

Historically, an operation passed down among fellows, the donor operation remains an integral component of a successful recipient outcome. The expeditious assessment and recovery of deceased-donor organs without surgical injury will always be the central mission of the donor surgeon. The current climate of organ scarcity[1-3] has placed increased demands on the donor surgeon that require reassessment of the skills and experience necessary to perform these procedures routinely while extracting the maximal potential from the existing deceased-donor pool. Transplant programs, with the assistance of organ procurement organizations (OPOs), have responded to the relative plateau in deceased-donor donation by expanding potential donor criteria with respect to age, medical comorbidities, high-risk social behaviors, prolonged hospitalization, known congenital anomalies, and partial brain-death criteria. Donors outside traditional donation criteria, termed expanded criteria (EC) donors,[4-6] currently represent the largest potential expansion of the existing donor pool. Furthermore, procurement agencies desire maximal utility from each existing donor through the procurement of all possible organs with clinical or research potential. These practices increase demands on the donor surgeon for skilled assessment, diagnosis, and management of clinical conditions that are outside the donor organ of interest, in addition to the performance of advanced procurement techniques. The techniques described herein reflect the authors' combined experience of more than 15 years and 3000 procurement procedures. They are widely applicable to a broad patient population and are routinely performed at donor facilities without specialized equipment or staff.

Evaluation of the Potential Recipient

The donor process begins with complete evaluation of the recipient candidate prior to departure for the donor medical facility. The potential recipient is evaluated for medical/surgical history, physiological condition, and size of the abdominal compartment. Pertinent medical/surgical history includes blood group, serum serologic determinations (hepatitis B, hepatitis C, human immunodeficiency virus [HIV], and cytomegalovirus), and intra-abdominal procedures that could affect vascular inflow/outflow.[7,8] The physiological condition of the recipient candidate is assessed with respect to encephalopathy, coagulopathy, hemodynamic stability, pressor requirements, and potential need for additional organs. The goal of this survey is to determine the anticipated needs of the recipient with respect to *immediate* graft function so that the donor organ can be assessed with these data in mind. The potential recipient's abdominal cavity is assessed for capacity; specifically, the potential of previous intra-abdominal operations to reduce overall abdominal capacity through adhesions, decreased intra-abdominal organ mobility, and scarring of the abdominal wall.

Evaluation of the Potential Donor

The authors' combined experience has instilled the highest regard for the suffering of the donor families and the medical professionals who have valiantly cared for them. They have referred *their* patient to us and the family has consented to a procedure that will inevitably delay the grieving process. Procurement teams must recognize these sacrifices and reciprocate through friendly, courteous, and professional conduct at the donor facility. Patient confidentiality must be vigorously upheld, as inadvertent and unknowing contact with the donor's family members during the course of transporting highly recognizable procurement equipment to the operating room is always possible. By the nature of their illness, donors frequently use many components of the hospital, including emergency services, intensive care, radiology, and surgical services. Thus, the donor team is scrutinized from arrival to departure. Arrogant, condescending, or unfriendly actions by a group of individuals who arrive via a high-profile vehicle do immeasurable disservice to the transplant community and belittle the efforts of the donor's health care professionals and family.

Initial donor assessment addresses hemodynamic stability, support services, and vascular access. The current condition of the donor with respect to oxygenation, hemodynamic stability, vasopressor requirements, urine output, and laboratory data, particularly serum electrolytes, is evaluated and optimized. Support equipment and personnel for critical care transport to the operating room are verified. Donor surgeons should participate in transport to the operating room to assist in care and be immediately available in the case of a donor arrest. Lastly, adequate vascular access at sites that will not be affected by the donor operation is verified and secured by the donor surgeon as necessary. The authors' preference is vascular access above the diaphragm with the use of a central line in the setting of vasopressors or hemodynamic instability. Femoral arterial catheters are acceptable with the caveat that information will be lost with interruption of the infrarenal aorta.

As the donor is prepared for surgery, the donor surgeon has the opportunity to review the medical chart to confirm pertinent details of the past medical history, blood type, serum serologic determinations, and appropriate documentation of brain death. Of particular note is a history of liver disease, diabetes, hypertension, or malignancy in addition to previous intra-abdominal surgery. Is there a history of high-risk social or sexual behavior, including alcoholism, substance abuse, sexually transmitted disease, prostitution, and incarceration?

The hospital course of the donor is reviewed, including date of admission, traumatic injuries, performance of surgical procedures, documented infections, vasopressor requirements, cause of death, and period of cardiac arrest with duration of cardiopulmonary resuscitation.[7,8] Lastly, a photocopied chart containing all essential clinical and laboratory data is available for packaging with the allograft.

The Donor Operation: Conventional Adult Liver Procurement

Preoperative Preparation

Donor procurement is performed relatively infrequently at community hospitals. Thus, it is unusual for operating room staff to have experience in organ recovery. Before scrubbing for surgery, the donor surgeon should introduce the procurement team to the operating room staff, provide the nurses and technicians with instructions concerning the procedure, verify that essential equipment and staff are present, and establish a collegial atmosphere. Participation by local staff interested in the procedure should be welcome in an observation role only. If additional procurement teams are in attendance, briefly reviewing your plan and the estimated aortic cross-clamp time will help coordinate their efforts.

Expediency and accuracy are essential to successful organ recovery. Brief operating room times reduce costs, lower operating staff stress, and increase efficiency. The technique described herein is a balance between the initial procurement technique of Starzl,[9] advocating extensive warm dissection, and the later *rapid flush technique*, advocating en bloc evisceration with back-table cold dissection.[10-12] This technique consistently yields aortic cross-clamp times of less than 1 hour, with total procurement times of approximately 2.5 hours, and requires no specialized equipment or staff.

Preparation for Cold Perfusion

Donor position is supine with both arms tucked. The surgical preparation and draping extends from the cricoid cartilage to the mid-thigh to ensure complete access to the thoracic and abdominal cavities. A midline incision from the xiphoid process to the pubis is made with electrocautery, and the abdomen is entered. An extended Balfour self-retaining retractor (spread of greater than 400 mm) with penetrating prongs is used to facilitate exposure, and a complete laparotomy to exclude occult malignancy, assess traumatic organ injury or compromise, and diagnose potential sources of sepsis is performed. Bilateral subcostal incisions may enhance exposure in unique circumstances such as morbid obesity or delayed entry to the thoracic cavity, but we have not found these additional incisions to be routinely necessary.

The liver is assessed for color, texture, parenchyma quality, evidence of ischemia, and size. Evidence of early ischemia or volume overload may be corrected through interaction with the anesthesiologist and the administration of appropriate medical therapy.[7] Frequently, these measures are rewarded with significant improvement in the appearance of the liver prior to aortic cross-clamping. The critical question at this point is: Can this organ, based on the accumulated data, provide the *immediate* metabolic needs of the potential recipient it has been offered to? If so, the recipient team can be notified to prepare the recipient. If not, the OPO coordinator should be notified to offer the organ to another potential recipient. To place an organ that has been declined by the donor surgeon may necessitate discussions with other recipient surgeons to address specific issues in the field. The donor surgeon should be readily available to assist in organ placement.

If preliminary assessment of the liver is acceptable, the skin incision is carried to the suprasternal notch, and the chest is entered via a median sternotomy using a pneumatic saw or Lebsche knife. A Finochietto self-retaining sternal retractor is positioned, and the pericardium is entered through the midline at the diaphragm and extended to above the right atrium. The right side of the chest is opened widely through the parietal pleura, and the pericardial wall is split to the level of the phrenic nerve to complete the thoracic dissection (Fig. 37–1).

The round ligament is divided between heavy silk sutures and the falciform ligament is dissected to the hepatic vein–inferior vena cava confluence. The left coronary and triangular ligaments are released, and the left lateral segment of the liver is elevated and retracted to the donor's right to reveal the gastrohepatic ligament. This is carefully inspected for a replaced/accessory left hepatic artery originating from the left gastric artery. This anatomic variant courses transversely from the left gastric artery on the lesser curvature of the stomach across the gastrohepatic ligament to the umbilical fissure in approximately 15% to 23% of deceased donors and should not be injured during the dissection.[7,13-15] If present, the gastrohepatic ligament is dissected below and above the replaced/accessory left hepatic artery with preservation of approximately 5 mm of adventitia on each side of the artery. Only portions of the gastrohepatic ligament that are translucent should be divided. The dissection proceeds from the lymph nodes overlying the common hepatic artery superiorly to the diaphragm (Fig. 37–2).

Retroperitoneal dissection is initiated with medial rotation of the ascending colon and duodenum en bloc as described by Cattell-Braash.[16] The ascending colon, duodenum, and remaining small bowel are mobilized cephalad out of the incision to the donor's left. The retroperitoneal dissection is carried cephalad to the left renal vein. Identification of the left renal vein signals the cephalad limit, as extensive dissection above the left renal vein risks inadvertent injury of the superior mesenteric artery, left renal artery, left kidney, and pancreas or torsion of the superior mesenteric artery with rotation of the bowel. The final maneuver to liberate the retroperitoneum involves placement of the left index finger through the foramen of Winslow beneath the hilum to expose interstitial and neural tissue lateral to the origin of the superior mesenteric artery (Fig. 37–3). Placing the left index finger beneath the gallbladder and proceeding toward the aorta easily identifies this space. Division of these connective and neural tissues results in full exposure of the entire retroperitoneum, including the infrahepatic vena cava, both renal veins, the superior mesenteric artery, the abdominal aorta, and the inferior mesenteric vein (Fig. 37–4). The inferior mesenteric vein is isolated at the Treitz ligament close to the root of the transverse mesocolon and cannulated to begin a pre-cool perfusion (see Fig. 37–4).[17] The cannula should remain only within the inferior mesenteric vein to prevent inadvertent injury and subsequent thrombosis of the splenic vein. The descending colon is released from its retroperitoneal attachments by opening the white line of Toldt to expose the left kidney.

Donor hypernatremia is an independent predictor of graft dysfunction after transplantation.[18-20] Our protocol is to use a pre-cool solution of 5% dextrose in isotonic saline for donor serum sodium levels less than 160 mEq/dL and

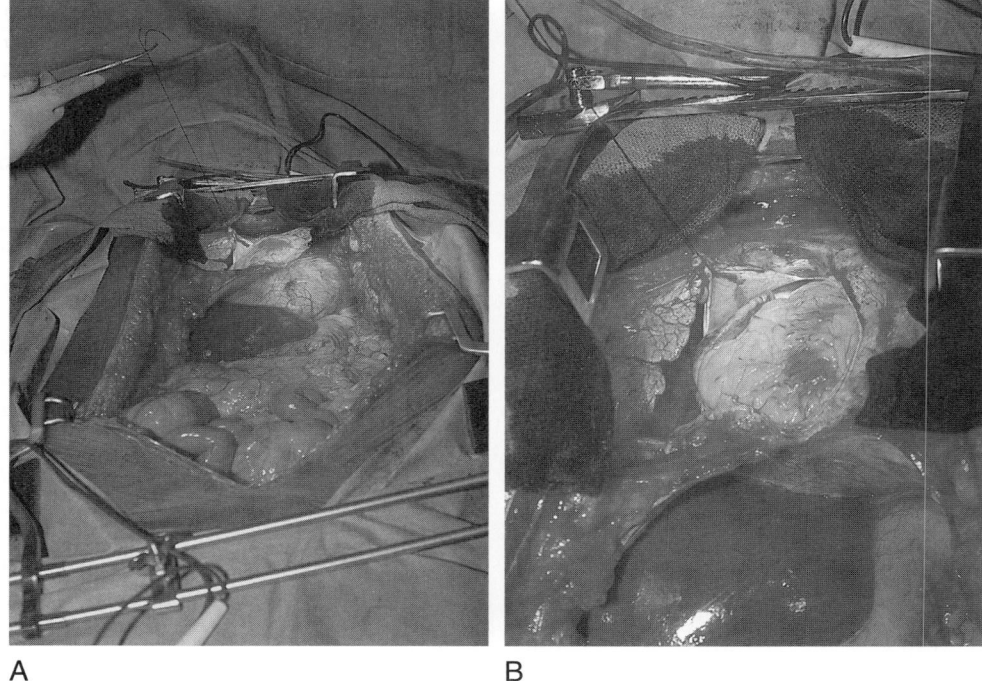

FIGURE 37–1

A, The donor incision extends from the suprasternal notch to the pubic symphysis. The cardiac, thoracic, and abdominal cavities have been entered with the extended Balfour and Finochietto retractors positioned. **B,** The parietal pleura and pericardium of the right side of the chest have been widely opened to facilitate exsanguination into the right chest following cold perfusion.

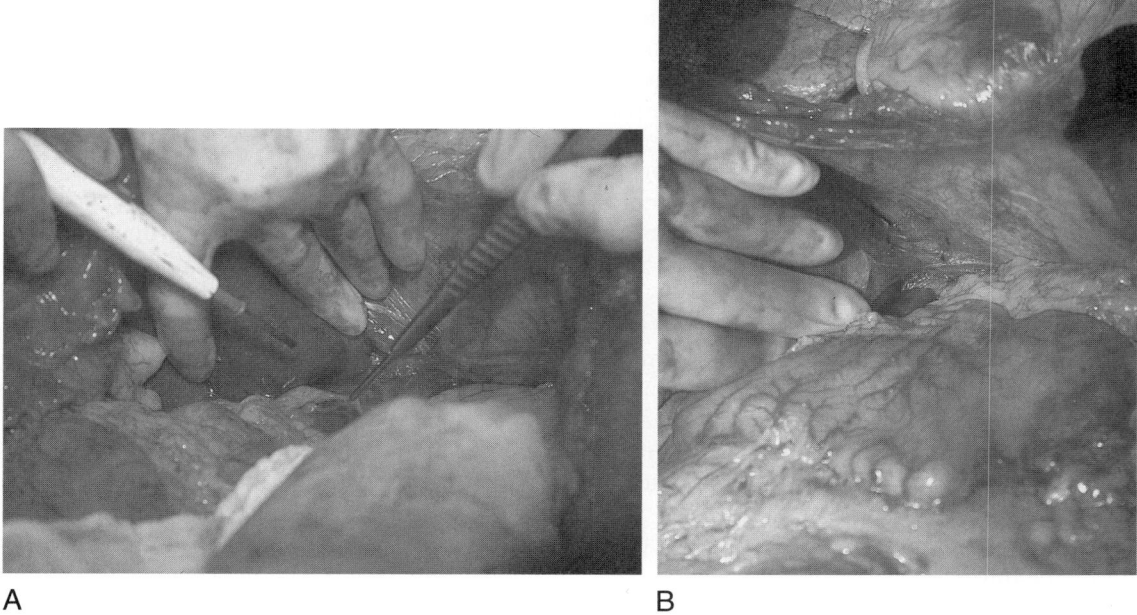

FIGURE 37–2

A, Dissection of the gastrohepatic ligament begins over the caudate lobe. Thin, transparent tissue is divided with electrocautery from the lymph nodes overlying the common hepatic artery to the diaphragm (**B**).

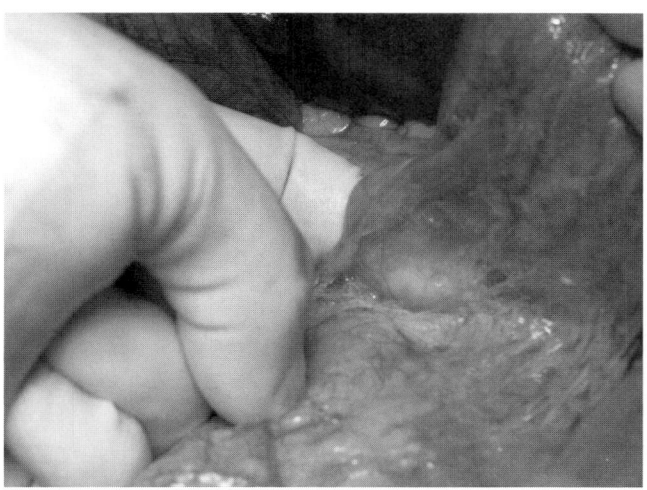

FIGURE 37–3

Placement of the surgeon's index finger below the gallbladder through the foramen of Winslow identifies neural and connective tissue to be divided to facilitate complete exposure of the retroperitoneum and identification of the superior mesenteric artery origin.

5% dextrose in water for donor serum sodium levels greater than 160 mEq/dL. Particular attention is directed toward appropriate resuscitation of the donor during the operative procedure to correct hypernatremia.[6]

The abdominal aorta, below the takeoff of the inferior mesenteric artery, is exposed in preparation for cannulation. The peritoneum and the lymphatic-rich tissue overlying the distal aorta are widely divided at the bifurcation and carried to above the takeoff of the inferior mesenteric artery. The plane of dissection should

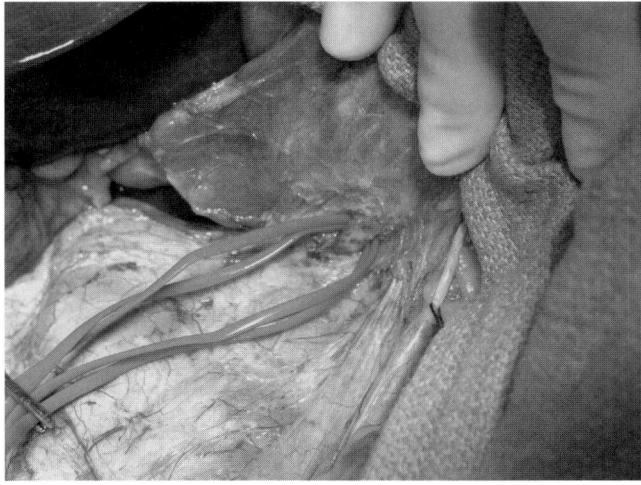

FIGURE 37–4

Complete liberation of the retroperitoneum to the origin of the superior mesenteric artery (enclosed in vessel loops). Complete exposure of the abdominal aorta, inferior vena cava, renal veins, and inferior mesenteric vein (encircled with silk suture) has been achieved.

be slightly lateral toward the inferior vena cava to avoid inadvertent injury of the inferior mesenteric artery origin. The aorta is encircled with two umbilical tapes to complete the dissection—the inferior tape at the level of the aortic bifurcation is held by a Kelly clamp, and the superior tape located just below the inferior mesenteric artery origin is snared with a Rommel tourniquet. Dissection should remain at or below the origin of the inferior mesenteric artery to prevent inadvertent injury to accessory inferior polar renal arteries. If necessary, the inferior mesenteric artery can be divided between silk ligatures to facilitate exposure.

The ascending colon and small bowel are returned to the abdominal cavity, and the hilum is exposed to visualize the common bile duct just above the duodenum (Fig. 37–5). Hilar dissection proceeds from lateral to medial, remaining close to the duodenum. Careful palpation behind the hilum aids the dissection and may identify an early takeoff right hepatic artery or a replaced/accessory right hepatic artery, which is found in approximately 10% to 17% of deceased donor series.[7,13-15] When isolating the common bile duct, it is critical that the dissection not extend into the hilum. It is far better to risk damaging the common bile duct near the duodenum by remaining superficial than to stray into the hilum risking injury to the portal vein or a replaced/accessory right hepatic artery. The distal common bile duct is tied with a 2–0 silk ligature at the duodenal border, and the bile duct is cut sharply above the tie (see Fig. 37–5). The gallbladder is opened and flushed with normal saline until the effluent from the transected common bile duct is clear. The removal of bile from the biliary tree prevents stasis and bile-induced autolysis of biliary epithelium during cold preservation.

Exposure of the supraceliac aorta is the final maneuver prior to cannulation. The left lateral segment is elevated and retracted laterally to expose the diaphragmatic crura. A cruciform incision using electrocautery opens the right crus at the midline while the assistant surgeon retracts the esophagus to the left to expose the aorta (Fig. 37–6). The preaortic fascia is sharply transversed, with the dissection carried anterior and lateral into the chest to increase aorta mobility. A blunt-tipped large right-angle clamp is used to encircle the aorta with an umbilical tape to aid identification and facilitate accurate aortic cross-clamping.

At this point, 30,000 IU of heparin (300 IU/kg) are administered, preferably via a central line, and circulated for at least 3 minutes.[21] Cannulation of the abdominal aorta is initiated with ligation of the distal umbilical tape at the bifurcation. Particular attention to gentle handling of the aorta in the presence of atherosclerotic plaque must be exercised during isolation and cannulation as the aorta in easily injured, which can cause perforation, dissection, or irreparable injury and potential loss of the donor. *Aortic injuries are potentially catastrophic and*

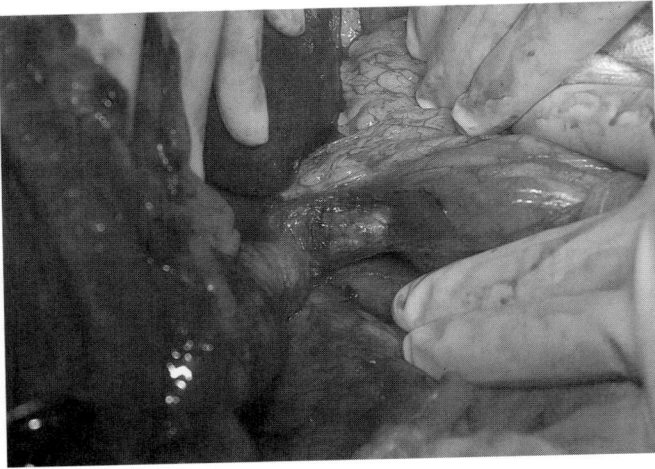
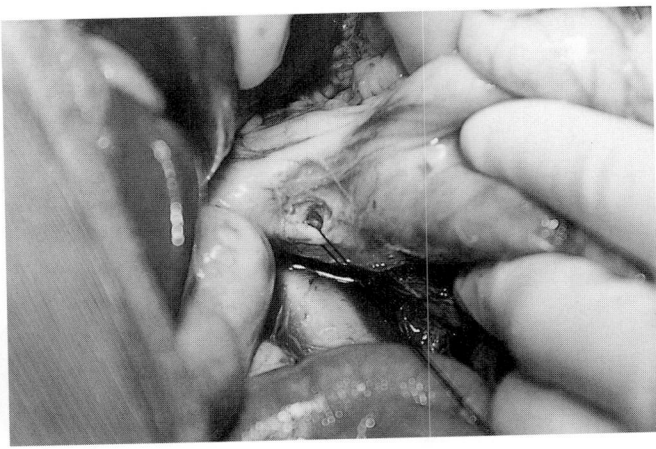

A   B

FIGURE 37–5

Dissection of the hilum. **A,** The common bile duct is isolated along the superior border of the duodenum to preserve length and avoid disruption of vascular supply. **B,** The common bile duct is ligated with a silk ligature prior to proximal division and evacuation of bile from the biliary tree.

must be avoided by attention to detail and gentle manipulation in the presence of atherosclerosis. The surgical assistant then occludes the proximal aorta with a DeBakey forceps just above the cephalad umbilical tape while holding up on the Rommel tourniquet with the nondominant hand. The donor surgeon opens the aorta just above the distal tape ligature and inserts a 22F reinforced cardiac catheter into the aorta. As the catheter is inserted, the aorta is grasped with the surgeon's hand to secure its position and prevent blood loss while the assistant tightens the Rommel tourniquet encircling the aorta. The donor surgeon continues to control the cannula while the assistant loops an umbilical tape around the cannula and Rommel tourniquet to secure them to each other. The cannula tip is positioned

approximately 4 cm above the aortotomy. The donor surgeon verifies with his or her fingertip that the cannula tip is below the takeoff of the superior mesenteric and renal arteries (Fig. 37–7). The OPO coordinator, as well as any other participating recovery teams, is notified that the intra-abdominal dissection is complete and to prepare for cold perfusion.

Organ Cold Perfusion

Successful organ cold perfusion requires the performance of several steps in concert to avert warm ischemia and preserve hepatic function. The objectives are rapid and homogeneous delivery of preservation fluid to the

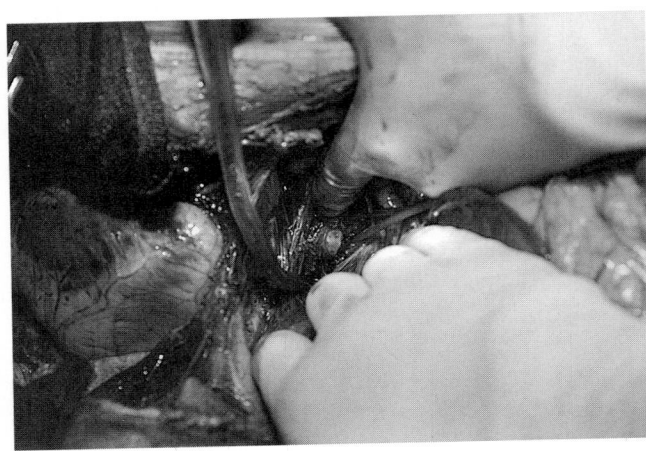

FIGURE 37–6

Isolation of the supraceliac aorta.

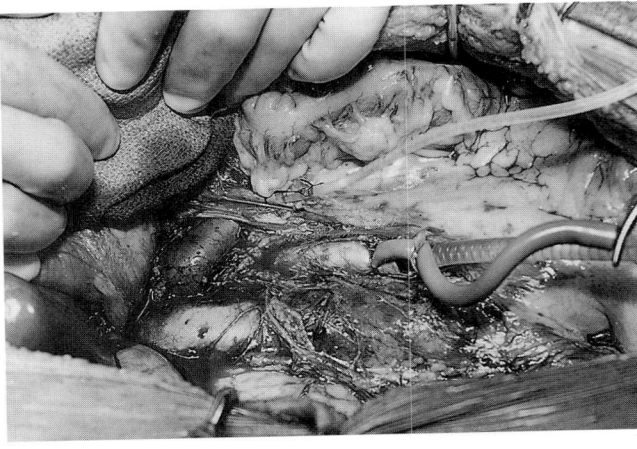

FIGURE 37–7

The abdominal operation is complete with the cannulas for portal vein perfusion *(above)* and aortic perfusion *(below)* in position.

liver such that cooling occurs quickly with uniform exsanguination throughout. This must be achieved without venous hypertension or congestion so that the liver remains soft. Because preservation fluid is delivered principally through arterial supply,[22] it is critical to return the abdominal contents to their natural position to avoid inadvertent torsion, spasm, or occlusion. This point is particularly relevant in the setting of replaced/accessory arterial anatomy that is easily torsed by rotation of the mesenteric root during evisceration.

Cold perfusion will be initiated with aortic cross-clamping. After coordinating the procedure among all recovery teams present and verifying that adequate suction, ice, and preservation fluid are available, the donor surgeon instructs the surgical assistant to *lift the umbilical tape encircling the aorta gently* to facilitate exposure. The donor surgeon's left hand is used to retract the left lateral segment to the right and to place a long, straight vascular clamp across the supraceliac aorta. Cross-clamp time is announced to the room as the surgeon quickly moves to transect the vena cava at the caval-atrial junction, thereby exsanguinating into the donor's right thoracic cavity. A pool-tip suction catheter placed into the vena cava–atria venotomy and directed toward the liver is extremely effective in keeping the chest empty of blood for the thoracic team. The aortic and inferior mesenteric venous cannulas are opened to begin simultaneous cold perfusion while ice is liberally poured into the abdominal cavity to augment rapid viscera cooling. It is important to pack ice gently around the entire liver, including the subdiaphragmatic space, the hilum, and beneath the left lateral segment. This is particularly important as warm blood exsanguinating into the right side of the chest can transmit heat through the diaphragm onto the right lobe of the liver. University of Wisconsin (UW) solution at 4°C (39.2°F) is run through the aortic and inferior mesenteric venous cannulas without pressure. Flow is verified with the perfusionist, and the liver is examined for uniform asanguinity, softness, and temperature to assess cold perfusion. Inadvertent injury of a replaced left hepatic artery during the dissection will be readily apparent by poor perfusion of the left lateral segment.

The authors' experience is based exclusively on the use of UW solution, although promising new technologies in organ preservation are emerging.[23,24] Infusion volumes average 30 to 60 mL/kg, or approximately 2000 to 3000 mL via the aortic cannula and 1000 mL via the inferior mesenteric venous cannula for adults.[7,8] During cold perfusion, the liver is continually assessed, the effluent from the inferior vena cava is examined, and the right side of the diaphragm is felt for cold ice in the subdiaphragmatic space over the right lobe. The liver can occasionally be *vented* or repositioned by bimanual palpation with one hand in the right thoracic cavity and another anteriorly in the abdomen.

Cold Dissection

On completion of cold perfusion, the pericardium and diaphragm are divided by the first assistant, who retracts the esophagus lateral as the surgeon divides each in an anterior-to-posterior direction down to the aorta in the midline. The pericardium is further divided posterior to the inferior vena cava. The donor surgeon grasps the diaphragm between the index and middle fingers and guides the assistant, who cuts the diaphragm posteriorly around the right lobe to the costodiaphragmatic angle, releasing the liver to fall cephalad into the right chest. The liver is covered with ice and a pool-tip suction catheter is placed behind the hilum from right to left and anterior to the aorta to provide a dry field (Fig. 37–8). The duodenum is retracted away from the liver, and the gastroduodenal artery is identified at the level of the superior edge of the duodenum where it is dissected toward the liver until the common hepatic artery is identified. It is critical to clearly verify that the common hepatic artery is proceeding toward the liver and from the celiac trunk before ligating the gastroduodenal artery (Fig. 37–9). Dissection of the proper hepatic artery above the origin of the gastroduodenal artery should be discouraged to maintain adequate blood supply to the common bile duct and avoid inadvertent hepatic arterial injury. If the portal vein is encountered while dissecting the gastroduodenal artery toward the common hepatic artery, this signals a completely replaced arterial system originating from the superior mesenteric artery, which is encountered in approximately 1% of deceased donors.[7,15] Dissection proceeds proximal

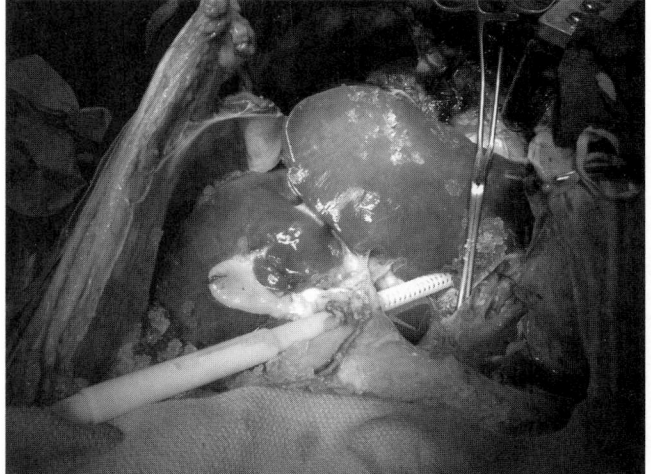

FIGURE 37–8

The diaphragm has been divided to the right costodiaphragmatic angle, releasing the liver superiorly into the chest to expose the hilum. The liver has been covered with ice, and a pool-tip suction catheter has been positioned through the foramen of Winslow to facilitate hilar dissection.

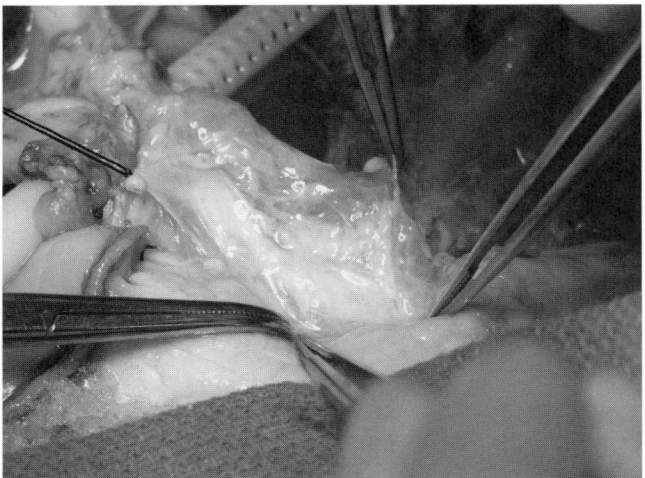

FIGURE 37–9

Arterial dissection. The gastroduodenal artery has been identified at the superior edge of the duodenum and dissected back to verify a common hepatic artery from the celiac trunk prior to division and suture ligation.

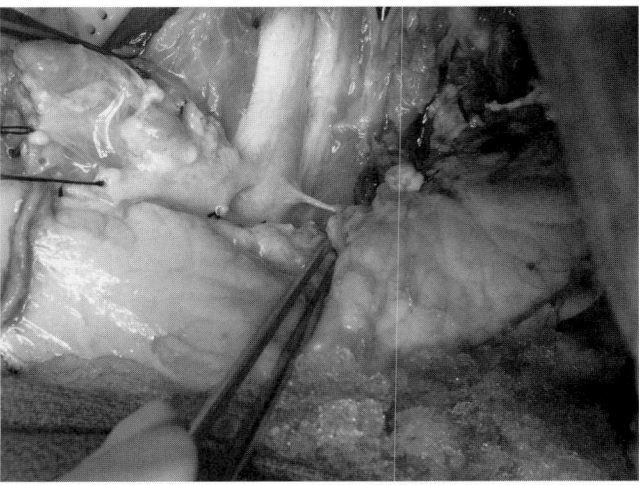

FIGURE 37–11

Completion of the arterial dissection. The origin of the celiac trunk at the aorta is clearly exposed. The distal splenic and gastroduodenal arterial origins have been preserved and ligated.

on the common hepatic artery to encounter the splenic artery (Fig. 37–10), which is verified, ligated, divided, and gently retracted medially. The gastroduodenal and splenic arteries should be ligated as distally as possible from their origins to preserve vessel integrity and length in case either or both are later required for back-table vascular anastomosis. Dissection continues toward the celiac trunk until the aorta is reached (Fig. 37–11).

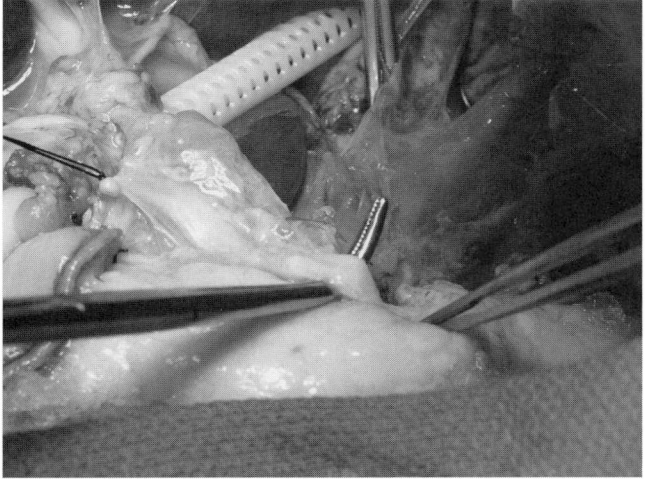

FIGURE 37–10

Identification of the splenic artery. The splenic artery has been isolated distal to its origin from the celiac trunk. The origin is clearly identified before division of the splenic to avoid inadvertent injury to the celiac trunk. The splenic artery is divided as distally as possible from its origin to preserve vessel integrity should vascular reconstruction be required later at the back-table dissection. The ligated gastroduodenal artery is evident.

The fibrous connective tissue, celiac plexus, and diaphragmatic crura encircling the aorta are divided to the left of the aorta as the dissection is carried superiorly to the level of the aortic clamp, where the aorta is divided.

The entire dissection of the common hepatic artery should be on the inferior-lateral border of the vessel (at approximately the 4 o'clock position) to avoid inadvertent injury to the origin of the splenic or left gastric arteries. Throughout the dissection, the left gastric artery origin is not encountered. If a replaced/accessory left hepatic artery has been identified, the lesser omentum, containing the left gastric artery, is completely mobilized off the stomach from the pylorus to the esophagus after transection of the splenic artery. A replaced/accessory left hepatic artery can originate from the left gastric artery, celiac trunk, or directly from the aorta; and the origin frequently will not be apparent during the dissection. Thus, maintaining an inferior-lateral position during dissection of the celiac trunk toward the aorta and remaining along the left lateral border of the aorta will preserve each anatomic variant.

The portal vein is located immediately beneath the origin of the gastroduodenal artery (Fig. 37–12). If the pancreas is not being procured, the dissection proceeds into the head of the pancreas to isolate the junction of the splenic and superior mesenteric veins. The superior mesenteric vein is ligated with the suture preserved long for retraction. The splenic vein is transected open for later cannulation on the back table. If the inferior mesenteric vein joins to form a trifurcated portal vein origin, it too is ligated and divided. Intended pancreas procurement limits portal vein dissection with division immediately distal to the origin of the coronary vein to provide

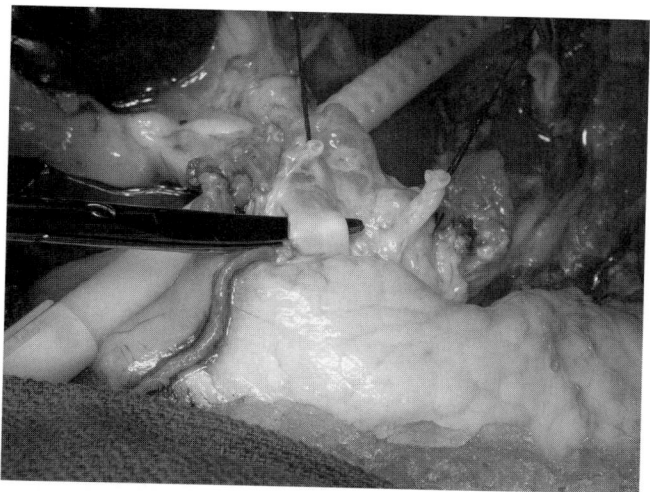

FIGURE 37-12

Identification of the portal vein immediately beneath the gastroduodenal artery.

adequate vein length for both organs. Following division, the portal vein is mobilized to the level of the bile duct ligature with small branches identified and ligated.

A mass of connective and neural tissue containing the common bile duct remains lateral to the portal vein. This must be carefully dissected to exclude a replaced/accessory right hepatic artery originating from the superior mesenteric artery or a low takeoff right hepatic artery originating from the celiac trunk coursing lateral to the portal vein. Inadvertent arterial injury at this level is a significant complication. Carefully, the dissection proceeds through the fibrous tissue of the hilum and the dense neural tissue of the celiac plexus between the celiac trunk and the superior mesenteric artery to expose the anterior surface of the aorta. In the absence of a replaced/accessory right hepatic artery, a small anterior aortotomy is performed between the celiac trunk and the superior mesenteric artery. Renal artery orifices are identified from within the aorta lumen. Under direct vision, the aortotomy is extended obliquely on the left to open the aorta completely. The right luminal wall of the aorta can then be divided to the line of aortic transection under direct vision to yield an aortic patch containing the celiac trunk. If a replaced/accessory right hepatic artery is present, the vessel is followed to the superior mesenteric artery, and the superior mesenteric artery origin is mobilized to the aorta. A low takeoff right hepatic artery from the celiac trunk will also become apparent. The anterior aortotomy is performed immediately distal to the superior mesenteric artery origin with very careful attention to identification of renal artery orifices that are in immediate proximity and may even be cephalad to the superior mesenteric artery origin. Under direct vision and with extreme care, an aortic patch containing both the celiac and superior mesenteric

trunks is created as described previously. The distal superior mesenteric artery is transected immediately beyond the first jejunal branches to ensure adequate vessel length for back-table arterial reconstruction.

The infrahepatic inferior vena cava is transected above the renal veins. Identification of both left and right renal vein origins is recommended because a common mistake involves encroachment on the right renal vein orifice or injury out of concern for preserving sufficient vena cava to the liver. Adequate inferior vena cava length is rarely a technical concern, whereas any encroachment or injury of the right renal vein can significantly affect vascular reconstruction.

The liver is then supported by the surgeon's non-dominant hand by placing the index finger into the inferior vena cava lumen, with the remaining fingers protecting the hilar bundle as remnant diaphragmatic and peritoneal attachments are divided to liberate the organ. The assistant protects the right kidney by retracting caudad while verifying the plane of dissection through the right adrenal gland. The liver is removed and placed in a sterile plastic bag containing 1L of UW solution at 4°C (39.2°F). The bile duct is flushed with 20 mL of cold UW solution prior to packaging and storing in an ice-filled cooler.

Following kidney procurement, the iliac arteries and veins are excised and stored in cold UW solution. These vessels may be required as vascular conduits during the recipient procedure. If atherosclerotic disease prevents use of the iliac arteries, other medium-sized vessels, such as the carotid or superior mesenteric artery, may be used. Premium vessels that are not used should be banked at the recipient hospital by blood type for later use as necessary.

Special Circumstances

The previous description is applicable to a routine adult liver procurement; however, there are frequently variations that must be anticipated. As donor criteria continue to expand, the assessment by the donor team and their ability to adapt technically to a specific donor become increasingly critical. On abdominal exploration, evidence of peritonitis or an undiagnosed neoplasm may be encountered. Unanticipated peritonitis does not exclude procurement; rather, intra-operative culture and immediate Gram stain followed by copious irrigation with normal saline containing a first-generation cephalosporin can be considered adequate treatment. Naturally, the donor hospital should be contacted to obtain definitive culture information, and the recipient should receive broad-spectrum antibiotics until definitive culture information is available.

Discovery of a neoplasm does not necessarily preclude donation. Adenocarcinoma, sarcoma, and stromal tumors of the gastrointestinal tract diagnosed at exploration exclude donation; however, small renal cell carcinomas, early prostate cancer, and biliary tumors require further consideration. Stage A or B prostate cancer and renal cell carcinoma less than 2 cm in diameter with favorable histology (well differentiated) have little metastatic potential and should be used with informed consent. In fact, renal cell cancers of 4 to 5 cm in diameter with favorable histology may be usable in *select* patients (such as those with advanced hepatocellular carcinoma or cholangiocarcinoma) with proper informed consent.

Benign biliary tumors can easily be misinterpreted as malignancy and do not preclude donation. These include biliary hamartoma, biliary cystadenoma, and bile-duct adenoma as well as the pathological phenomenon of focal fatty change.[25] We advocate frozen section at the donor facility *with* procurement and final pathological confirmation at the recipient facility as the default in cases of diagnostic uncertainty or inability to perform experienced pathological evaluation at the donor facility.

The hemodynamically unstable donor and non–heart-beating donor require specific procurement techniques. In each case, the goal is rapid heparin administration, aortic cannulation, cross-clamping, and organ cold perfusion to minimize warm ischemia. A donor arrest during transport is not an uncommon event and is best managed by immediate administration of 30,000 IU heparin, cardiopulmonary resuscitation, and non–heart-beating donor techniques.

Non–heart-beating donor procurements proceed by sharp dissection. The skin is opened with a knife from the xiphoid to the pubis, with the dissection continued sharply into the peritoneal cavity. The Balfour retractor is positioned and a Cattell-Braasch maneuver performed with Metzenbaum scissors to expose the infrarenal aorta. The abdominal aorta is rapidly cannulated, and cold UW flush is initiated. The suprahepatic inferior vena cava is then transected below the right atrium, the pericardium is opened, and the thoracic aorta is cross-clamped in the left side of the chest. The white line of Toldt is opened along the descending colon to expose the left kidney, and ice is liberally applied around the abdominal organs. The inferior mesenteric vein is identified within the mesentery at the Treitz ligament and cannulated for portal perfusion. All further dissection is made cold after completion of cold perfusion.

If the donor had a previous median sternotomy or the donor facility is not equipped for cardiothoracic surgery, access to the thoracic cavity is potentially limited. We do not recommend early median sternotomy in donors who have previously had a sternotomy, as inadvertent cardiac injury can result in potential loss of the donor. In these situations, the donor procurement can be performed entirely within the abdominal cavity through aortic cross-clamping and cold perfusion.

Exsanguination is performed by cannulating the inferior vena cava just above the iliac bifurcation with a 28Fr straight chest tube (or similar large, noncollapsible tubing). Care in isolating the inferior vena cava must be exercised to avoid inadvertent injury to the vessel or right ureter. All other techniques are unchanged. After aortic cross-clamping and during cold perfusion, the diaphragm can be split, the pericardium opened, and the caval-atrial junction divided to facilitate venting of perfusate. Exsanguination through cannulation of the inferior vena cava may also be necessary in the setting of a right lung procurement.

Undiagnosed abdominal aortic aneurysms and severe atherosclerotic disease are frequently encountered, particularly in expanded criteria donors. In this setting, we prefer aortic cannulation via the common iliac (right common iliac is preferable), with careful dissection to avoid the ureter and precise positioning of the catheter tip above the aneurysm or severe atherosclerotic disease at the level of the renal arteries, if at all possible. A severely diseased or difficult-to-access supraceliac aorta should not be manipulated to avoid potential dissection or disruption; rather, the thoracic aorta should be accessed through the central tendon of the left diaphragm or via a left thoracotomy for aortic cross-clamping. An alternative approach of cannulating via the thoracic aorta or aortic arch distal to the left subclavian artery origin has been advocated[26,27]; however, there are several potential disadvantages to attempted thoracic cannulation, including:

- Increased technical difficulty
- The need to transect the aorta completely in the presence of often severe supraceliac atherosclerotic disease
- The potential to shower plaque emboli or create dissection or hematoma *toward* the celiac, superior mesenteric, and renal artery origins

Thus, the authors prefer to approach atherosclerotic disease from the iliac arteries or distal aorta to optimize cold perfusion.

Back-Table Preparation of the Liver Allograft

Back-table preparation typically occurs at the recipient hospital during the recipient hepatectomy and includes detailed inspection for surgical injury, graft preparation, verification of vascular anatomy, and potential arterial reconstruction. The allograft should remain immersed in cold UW solution within the plastic transport bag that is enveloped by ice to avoid inadvertent rewarming. With the anterior liver surface facing the surgeon, the liver's bare area is exposed by complete removal of remnant diaphragm, and the suprahepatic vena cava is

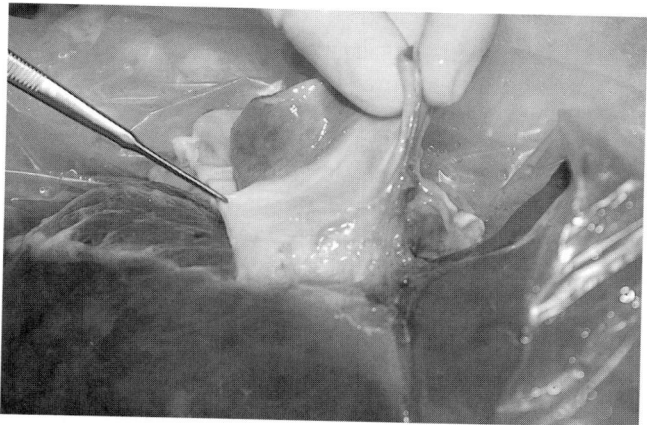

FIGURE 37–13

With the anterior surface of the liver facing the surgeon, diaphragmatic remnants are removed, exposing the bare area, and a plane anterior to the inferior vena cava is established, permitting the fibrous diaphragmatic attachments to be *unwrapped* from the vessel.

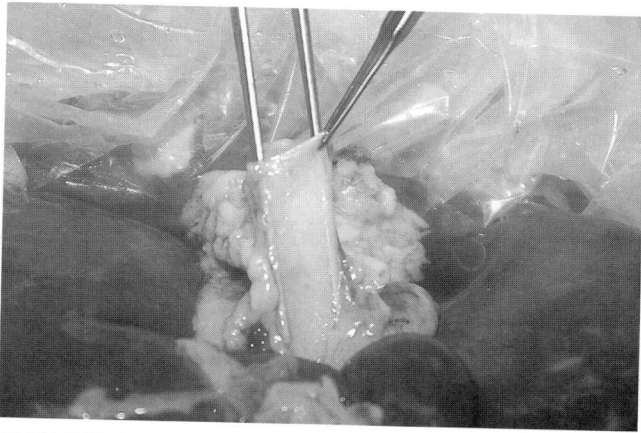

FIGURE 37–15

Isolation of the portal vein.

freed from its diaphragmatic attachments. A plane immediately anterior to the inferior vena cava is established, and the fibrous diaphragmatic remnant encircling the inferior vena cava is divided and *unwrapped* laterally and posteriorly (Fig. 37–13). Phrenic vein orifices are identified and ligated. The graft is repositioned to expose the entire inferior vena cava, which is separated from the surrounding retroperitoneal connective tissue along its entire length. Dissection is performed by spreading and cutting over the midpoint of the posterior inferior vena cava wall before proceeding laterally, with particular attention to avoiding dissection between the inferior vena cava and the caudate lobe. Phrenic veins originating from the inferior vena cava are identified and ligated. The right adrenal remnant is separated from the liver, and the adrenal vein is ligated (Fig. 37–14).

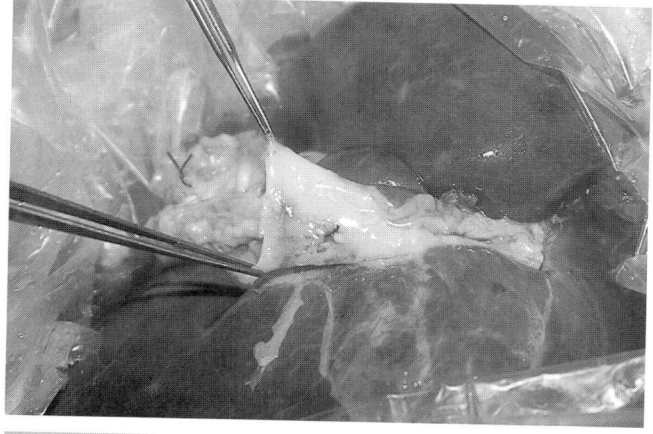

FIGURE 37–14

Dissection of the inferior vena cava with ligation of the right adrenal vein.

If the graft will be implanted by the *piggyback* technique, the inferior vena cava can be oversewn with a running 4–0 polypropylene suture secured by a 0 silk ligature.

Isolation of the portal vein begins with the surgical assistant elevating the portal vein at the 3 and 9 o'clock positions, while the surgeon spreads and cuts the peritoneal tissue along the posterior vessel wall toward the parenchyma to expose the bifurcation (Fig. 37–15). This tissue is principally loose areolae and lymphatics, but it may contain posterior hepatic arterial branches that must be identified and avoided. If encountered, the portal vein can be gently slipped under these branches, en bloc, so that the artery remains anterior during implantation. The dissection proceeds laterally (opposite the hilum) and proximally along the portal vein with small branches identified and ligated. Clear exposure of the bifurcation simplifies orientation during portal vein anastomosis. The portal vein is cannulated to provide for later allograft flush and infused with cold UW solution to verify its integrity.

Arterial dissection begins at the celiac trunk and proceeds distally toward the liver. The surgical assistant holds the aortic patch with one hand and the splenic silk ligature with the other, while the surgeon removes the loose adventitia of the celiac trunk exposing the left gastric and possibly phrenic branches. Each branch must be preserved and followed from its origin to a point of termination to exclude the possibility of an early takeoff vessel proceeding toward the liver. Branches that terminate outside the liver are ligated. The assistant then repositions to support the splenic and gastroduodenal arteries, exposing the common hepatic that is similarly prepared. Dissection of the proper hepatic artery above the takeoff of the gastroduodenal should be avoided because it may compromise the extrahepatic bile duct circulation (Fig. 37–16). The celiac trunk is gently infused with cold UW solution to identify

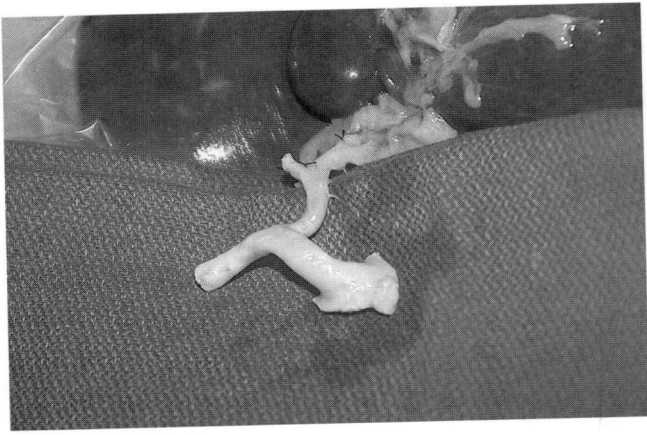

FIGURE 37-16

Back-table arterial dissection. Normal arterial anatomy is shown with an aortic Carrel patch. The splenic and gastroduodenal arterial origins are clearly evident.

small branches in the hilum that require ligation, and the aortic remnant is fashioned into a Carrel patch to complete graft preparation. Arterial variations and reconstruction are discussed later.

Back-table cholecystectomy is optional. The authors prefer cholecystectomy after arterial reperfusion to avoid inadvertent injury of anomalous or replaced right hepatic arterial branches. Cholecystectomy after arterial reperfusion facilitates precise identification of the cystic duct–common hepatic duct junction with complete removal of the cystic duct; a dissection that could be hazardous if performed cold on the back table.

Arterial Variations and Reconstruction

Arterial variations are common, and most are efficiently addressed during the back-table dissection at the recipient institution. Arterial variations may require only careful dissection or reconstruction. Fine vascular instruments and nonabsorbable monofilament suture should be readily available. Injured vessels require similar reconstruction and are included in this discussion.

Arterial variations that require only careful dissection include a replaced/accessory left hepatic artery originating from the left gastric artery and a completely replaced arterial system originating from the superior mesenteric artery. When a replaced/accessory left hepatic artery is identified, the arterial dissection of the celiac trunk remains as described previously through identification of the splenic origin. Following identification and ligature of the splenic origin, the left gastric origin is identified. The assistant then holds the left

gastric origin and the transected distal left gastric remnant to suspend the replaced/accessory left branch within the gastrohepatic ligament. The replaced/accessory left branch is carefully dissected, with the numerous small branches originating from the left gastric branch and servicing the stomach ligated with fine suture. The dissection is carried to within 3 mm of the liver parenchyma to completely define the course of the replaced/accessory left branch. At this point, the distal left gastric artery beyond the origin of the replaced/accessory left branch is transected and ligated to complete arterial preparation.

The goal of arterial reconstruction is to establish a single source of inflow to the allograft. Our preference for arterial inflow is the celiac trunk, followed by the distal superior mesenteric artery, and lastly the splenic artery. The most common arterial variant requiring reconstruction is a replaced/accessory right hepatic artery originating from the superior mesenteric artery. In this situation, the proximal superior mesenteric artery trunk is anastomosed to the distal celiac trunk (Fig. 37–17) using interrupted 7-0 polypropylene suture, and the distal superior mesenteric artery is used for aortic inflow. If a large size discrepancy exists between the superior mesenteric artery trunk and the celiac trunk, the replaced/accessory right hepatic artery can be anastomosed to the splenic or the gastroduodenal origin (interrupted 7-0 polypropylene) and the celiac trunk used for aortic inflow. A replaced/accessory left hepatic artery originating from the aorta also requires reconstruction. For this variant, the replaced/accessory left hepatic artery is separated from the aorta with a Carrel patch and anastomosed to the splenic or to the gastroduodenal origin (Fig. 37–18), depending on vessel diameter.

Inadvertent injury during the procurement or back-table dissection typically involves transection of a replaced left or right hepatic artery within the hilum. These injuries can be primarily repaired, or the remnant transected vessel can be anastomosed to the gastroduodenal or splenic origin, depending on vessel diameter and available length. Arterial conduit is rarely necessary. All anastomoses are performed with interrupted 8-0 polypropylene suture using surgical telescopes with a higher magnification than ×4.5.

Pediatric Procurement

The pediatric donor can be approached exactly as described previously with several minor modifications. The only technical variation is the occurrence of a replaced/accessory left hepatic artery in a small infant or neonatal donor. In this setting, the aorta should be approached through the diaphragm or left chest to prevent inadvertent traction injury. Heparin (500 IU/kg) and aortic flush (50 mL/kg UW solution) are also adjusted by

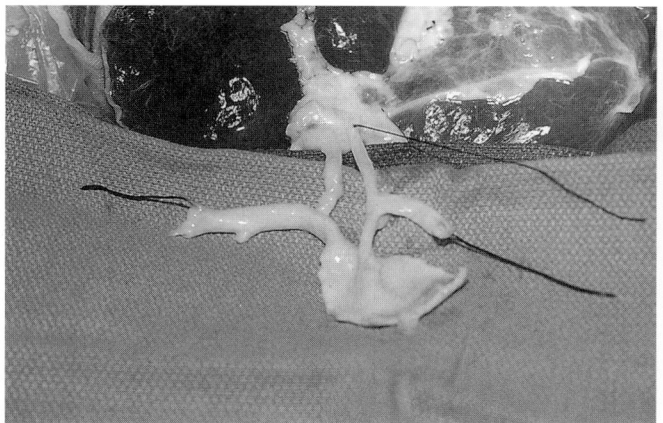

A

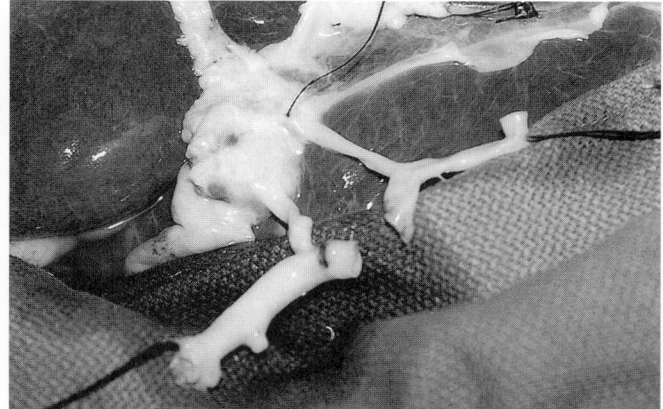

B

FIGURE 37–17

Replaced/accessory right hepatic artery. **A**, The celiac and superior mesenteric arterial trunks are procured on a common patch of aorta. Each arterial branch (jejunal, splenic, left gastric, and gastro-duodenal) is procured long before ligation to maintain vessel integrity for potential vascular reconstruction. **B**, The celiac and superior mesenteric trunks are inked prior to transection to verify orientation. **C**, Vascular reconstruction is completed with the distal superior mesenteric artery as the single inflow source.

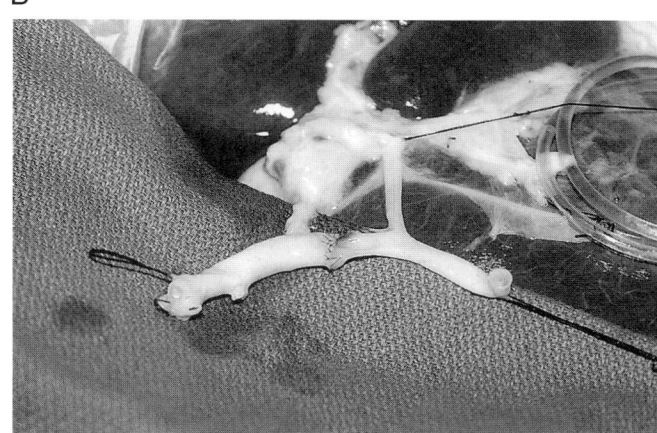

C

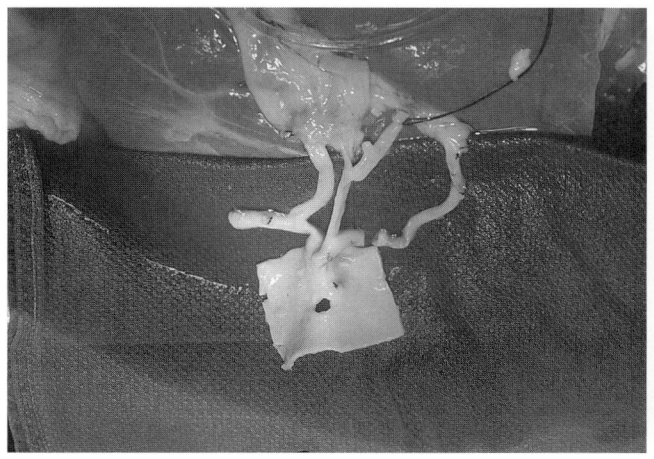

A

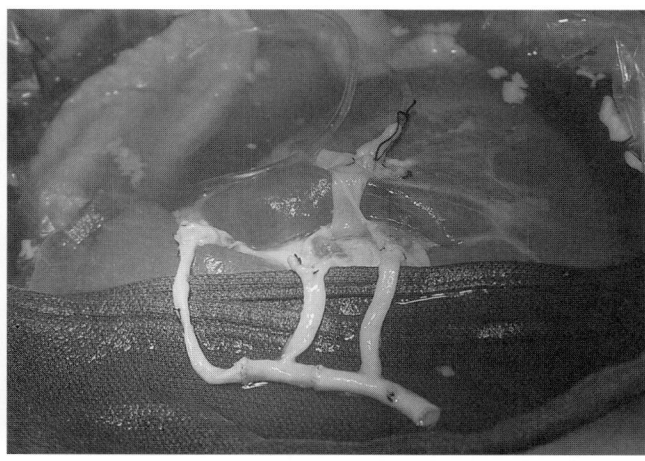

B

FIGURE 37–18

Uncommon arterial variant of replaced/accessory left branch originating from the aorta with a replaced/accessory right branch from the superior mesenteric trunk. **A**, The replaced/accessory left branch originating from the aorta is anastomosed to the splenic origin. **B**, The celiac and superior mesenteric trunks are anastomosed to create a single arterial inflow from the distal superior mesenteric artery.

Continued

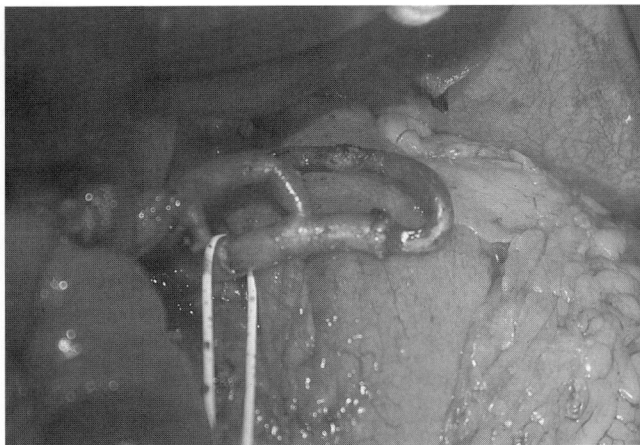

C

FIGURE 37–18, cont'd

C, Arterial reconstruction following reperfusion.

weight in pediatric donors.[7] Lastly, a vascular conduit is frequently required in pediatric recipients; as a result, the authors recommend procurement of iliac and carotid arteries, the thoracic aorta, and saphenous or internal jugular veins, when available, to optimize the availability of a suitable conduit with banking of any unused conduit.

Pearls and Pitfalls

- Always assess the recipient immediately before leaving to perform the donor operation.
- Minimize trauma, handling, and hemorrhage within the donor. If unexpected hemorrhage is encountered, do not attempt repair if the source is not *completely* obvious and accessible; rather, use an assistant to maintain direct pressure while expeditiously proceeding with the donor procedure. The majority of injuries do not affect organ use and are more easily and completely addressed after cold perfusion.
- Avoid traumatic aortic injuries in donors with atherosclerosis. These injuries frequently affect organ use and can quickly result in donor loss.
- Address all vascular anomalies, potential vascular injuries, and vascular reconstructions at the recipient institution where specialized materials and expert assistance are readily available.

References

1. UNOS (United Network for Organ Sharing) online: Available at http://www.UNOS.org.
2. Sheehy E, Conrad S, Brigham L, et al: Estimating the number of potential organ donors in the United States. N Engl J Med 349: 667-674, 2003.
3. Langone A, Helderman J: Disparity between solid-organ supply and demand. N Engl J Med 349:704-706, 2003.
4. Feng S, Buell J, Cherikh W, et al: Organ donors with positive viral serology or malignancy: Risk of disease transmission by transplantation. Transplantation 74:1657-1663, 2002.
5. Angelis M, Cooper J, Freeman R: Impact of donor infections on outcomes of orthotopic liver transplantation. Liver Transpl 9:451-462, 2003.
6. Busuttil R, Tanaka K: The utility of marginal donors in liver transplantation. Liver Transpl 9:651-663, 2003.
7. Emre S, Schwartz M, Miller C: The donor operation. In Busuttil R, Klintmalm G (eds): Transplantation of the Liver. Philadelphia, WB Saunders, 1996, pp 392-404.
8. Kato T, Levi D, Nery J, et al: Operative procedures. In Maddrey W, Schiff E, Sorrell M (eds): Transplantation of the Liver. Philadelphia, Lippincott Williams & Wilkins, 2001, pp 47-64.
9. Starzl TE, Hakala T, Shaw B, et al: A flexible procedure for multiple cadaveric organ procurement. Surg Gynecol Obstet 158:223-230, 1984.
10. Starzl TE, Miller CM, Bronznick B, Makowka L: An improved technique for multiple organ harvesting. Surg Gynecol Obstet 165:343-348, 1987.
11. Miller C, Mazzaferro V, Makowka L, et al: Rapid flush technique for donor hepatectomy: Safety and efficacy of an improved method of liver recovery for transplantation. Transplant Proc 20:948-950, 1988.
12. Nakazato P, Concepcion W, Bry W, et al: Total abdominal evisceration: an en bloc technique for abdominal organ harvesting. Surgery 111:37-47, 1992.
13. Todo S, Makowka L, Tzakis A, et al: Hepatic artery in liver transplantation. Transplant Proc 19:2406-2411, 1987.
14. Healey J, Hodge J: Surgical Anatomy. Philadelphia, BC Decker, 1990.
15. Hiatt J, Gabbay J, Busuttil RW: Surgical anatomy of the hepatic artery in 1000 cases. Ann Surg 220:50-52, 1994.
16. Cattell R, Braasch J: A technique for the exposure of the third and fourth portions of the duodenum. Surg Gynecol Obstet 111:379, 1960.
17. Broelsch C: Removal of cadaver donor liver for adult recipient. In Christoph E, Broelsch MD, Buck T (eds): Atlas of Liver Surgery. New York, Churchill Livingstone, 1993, pp 144-155.
18. Gonzalez F, Rimola A, Grande L, et al: Predictive factors of early postoperative graft function in human liver transplantation. Hepatology 20:565-573, 1994.
19. Figueras J, Busquets J, Grande L, et al: The deleterious effect of donor high plasma sodium and extended preservation in liver transplantation. A multivariate analysis. Transplantation 61: 410-413, 1996.
20. Markmann JF, Markmann JW, Markmann DA, et al: Preoperative factors associated with outcome and their impact on resource use in 1148 consecutive liver transplants. Transplantation 72:1113-1122, 2001.
21. Ismail T, Ferraz-Neto BH, McMaster P: Liver transplantation. In Carter D, Russell R, Pitt H, Bismuth H (eds): Hepatobiliary and Pancreatic Surgery. New York, Chapman & Hall Medical, 1996, pp 62-75.
22. Ascher N, Bolman R, Der S: Multiple organ donation from a cadaver. In Simmons R, Finch M, Ascher N, Najarian J (eds): Manual of Vascular Access, Organ Donation, and Transplantation. New York, Springer-Verlag, 1984, pp 105-143.

23. Nydegger U, Carrel T, Laumonier T, Mohacsi P: New concepts in organ preservation. Transpl Immunol 9:215-225, 2002.

24. McLaren A, Friend P: Trends in organ preservation. Transpl Int 16:701-708, 2003.

25. Meyers W: Neoplasms of the liver. In Sabiston DC Jr (ed): Textbook of Surgery, 7th ed. Philadelphia, WB Saunders, 1991, pp 999-1011.

26. Fukuzawa K, Schwartz M, Katz E, et al: An alternative technique for in situ arterial flushing in elderly liver donors with atherosclerotic occlusive disease. Transplantation 55:445-447, 1993.

27. Molmenti E, Klintmalm G: Procurement of liver, pancreas, and kidneys. In Molmenti E, Klintmalm G (eds): Atlas of Liver Transplantation. Philadelphia, Saunders, 2002, pp 11-33.

Principles of Liver Preservation

STEVEN M. STRASBERG
NAZIA SELZNER
PIERRE-ALAIN CLAVIEN

Principles of organ preservation 561
  Mechanisms of preservation injury 562

Current clinical preservation methods 567
  Clinical liver preservation solutions 567
  Current methods of the use of preservation
    solutions 568

Novel preservation strategies 569
  Preconditioning of the liver 569
  Machine perfusion 569

Liver preservation is a key component of liver transplantation because it allows sharing of deceased donor organs between hospitals at great distances from each other. Initially, organ preservation technology developed in response to the need to preserve kidneys, the first organ to be widely transplanted. With the advent of cyclosporine, liver transplantation became the accepted treatment of end-stage liver disease. The need for improved preservation techniques was immediately evident because Eurocollins solution, the preservation solution then in common use, allowed only a few hours of storage before transplant viability was lost. There are at least two means of preserving organs: cold storage and machine perfusion. The former is the standard technique for liver preservation. In this chapter we describe both, but the majority of the discussion focuses on cold preservation. The goals of this chapter are to describe the mechanisms of injury that lead to early graft dysfunction and the approaches that are used to preserve the liver.

Principles of Organ Preservation

Graft dysfunction occurs in the early postoperative period after liver transplantation and affects every transplanted liver. This injury is usually called "preservation injury." The injury may range from very mild hepatic dysfunction manifested as only slight abnormalities in liver function test values to complete liver failure. The causes of postoperative dysfunction are multifactorial and much broader than the term "preservation" injury implies. Dysfunction of a liver allograft may be due to existing disease in the donor liver or may result from injuries to the liver associated with donor death. Organ damage may also occur during cold preservation or during the period in which vascular connections are being made before reperfusion (rewarming period). All the injuries accumulated in these periods become manifested during reperfusion, and poor perfusion of the organ as a result of hemodynamic problems in the recipient can itself add to injury.

Mechanisms of Preservation Injury

Prepreservation Injury

Prepreservation injury refers to organ damage that was present in the organ or induced before infusion of cold preservation solutions. Three potential sources of this injury are (1) preexisting disease in the liver, (2) injury associated with brain death or events leading to brain death, and (3) injury during organ harvesting.

Preexisting Hepatic Disease. The most common types of preexisting liver injury are steatosis,[1,2] often related to obesity, and hepatitis, often caused by drugs or alcohol. Steatosis aggravates cold preservation injury in hepatocytes[3] and sinusoidal lining cells.[4] The use of drugs or large amounts of alcohol may have been causative in a traumatic death leading to organ donation, and therefore the potential for toxic liver damage must be considered under these circumstances. Diagnosis of preexisting hepatic disease is an integral part of donor organ evaluation. Screening of potential donors by history, physical examination, drug toxicity tests, liver function tests, and liver biopsy eliminates the most obvious cases of preexisting liver injury, but more subtle degrees of injury may be difficult to diagnose, even with biopsy.

Injury Associated with Brain Death or Events Leading to Brain Death. Trauma leading to brain death is often associated with hypotension or hypoxia, which can lead to warm ischemia of the liver. Malnutrition may also contribute to hepatic injury, since some donors have had an intensive care unit stay of many days. During that time, hepatic deglycogenation and potentially other deleterious nutritional effects may occur. Livers that have been depleted of glycogen are less able to tolerate the warm ischemic events that may occur during the rewarming phase or afterward.[5-7] Interestingly, livers from fasted animals function better than those of fed animals, although less well than livers that have been fully glycogenated.[7] Provision of alanine but not pyruvate seems to ameliorate the effects of prolonged fasting.[8] It is possible that more subtle forms of injury exist, possibly associated with brain death, but

recent studies in dogs suggest that brain death per se is a minor or nonexistent component of the overall injury.[9]

Injury during Organ Harvesting. Injury may occur as a result of intraoperative hypotension, which is not rare during organ harvesting. Rarely, injury is due to technical misadventure. One third of donors accepted for transplantation have evidence of prepreservation injury in the form of platelet adhesion to sinusoidal endothelial cells (SECs) on liver biopsy specimens taken at the time of organ harvest.[10] There is a relationship between the degree of this type of injury and organ dysfunction after implantation.[10]

Cold Preservation Injury

Cold preservation is the standard method of organ preservation today. The final temperature achieved in a liver preserved on ice is 1° C.[11] If the liver were to be preserved in cold liquid in a refrigerator, the final temperature would be 4° C. Organs are cooled to reduce metabolic activity and therefore energy demand during a storage period in which they are not being perfused with oxygen and nutrients. Reducing the temperature lowers metabolic activity by 50% for every 10° C of temperature reduction. Consequently, metabolism at 1° C would be expected to be about 5% of normal. However, the effects of temperature on enzymatic activity (and therefore metabolism) are variable. For instance, Na^+,K^+-adenosine triphosphatase (ATPase) and Ca^{2+}-ATPase are completely inhibited at temperatures below 20° C,[12,13] but some proteases retain function at 1° C. The difference in susceptibility of enzymes to lowered temperature accounts for many of the changes that occur in cold-preserved livers.

Initially, it was thought that cold-induced liver injury was due to the so-called classic deleterious effects of cold, which affect all cells. Subsequent studies have indicated that injury to a specific liver cell, the SEC, is the main mechanism of injury. Nonetheless, it is important to recognize the classic effects.

"Classic" Effects of Cold. Although cooling of organs may be necessary to reduce metabolic demand, it introduces a number of "classic" deleterious effects. Metabolism is reduced but not stopped, and thus adenosine triphosphate (ATP) continues to be broken down, albeit at a reduced rate. The only source of new ATP is anaerobic glycolysis, which is inefficient when compared with aerobic glycolysis. In addition, anaerobic glycolysis is associated with intracellular lactic acidosis because lactic acid is the end product of this process. Despite the continuation of ATP generation by anaerobic glycolysis, utilization of ATP exceeds production, and ATP is therefore depleted. Normally, ATP is regenerated from the other phosphorylated nucleotides adenosine diphosphate (ADP) and adenosine monophosphate (AMP), but when there is insufficient energy to do so, ADP and AMP are degraded to adenosine, which can leave the cell. At further stages of the breakdown process, xanthine and hypoxanthine are produced.[14] The enzyme xanthine oxidase is also activated during hypoxic cold preservation. Xanthine and hypoxanthine combine with oxygen in the presence of xanthine oxidase to produce oxygen free radicals. During preservation, molecular oxygen is in short supply, so the reaction is very slow. However, when oxygen is supplied on reperfusion, oxygen free radicals are generated by this mechanism. The free radicals are highly toxic to cell membranes. The severity of the process is accentuated in the presence of Fe^{2+} through the "Fenton" reaction, specifically, $Fe^{2+} + H_2O_2 \rightarrow Fe^{3+} + OH^{\bullet} + OH^-$, in which $OH^{\bullet}$ is the very reactive and damaging hydroxyl free radical.

Temperatures below 20° C are also associated with loss of function of the Na^+,K^+-ATPase pump. This energy-dependent pump moves three sodium molecules from the interior of the cell to the exterior for every two molecules of potassium that it moves in the opposite direction. The result is a high potassium concentration in the cell (about 150 mM) and a low potassium concentration (4 mM) in extracellular fluid; for sodium the opposite ensues (12 mM in intracellular fluid and 140 mM in extracellular fluid). The pump also creates an electrochemical gradient across the cell membrane in which the interior is negative with respect to the exterior. Another effect of the pump is to offset the osmotic effect of impermeant intracellular molecules such as proteins. With loss of the pump there is equilibration of sodium and potassium across the cell membrane and thus loss of the gradient. Impermeant intracellular molecules now exerting an unopposed osmotic effect cause cell swelling. These are the classic effects of cold. Eurocollins and the University of Wisconsin (UW) solutions were formulated to resist these effects, as is explained later.

Sinusoidal Endothelial Cell Injury. The classic effects do not explain why some organs tolerate cold ischemia better than others do or why UW solution is a more effective preservative for the liver than for other organs. Two laboratories, working independently, showed that liver nonparenchymal cells are sensitive to preservation-reperfusion injury.[15,16] Initially, it seemed that Kupffer cell activation was central to the injury[17]; however, it was subsequently found that Kupffer cell activation occurred only on reperfusion and therefore could not be responsible for the critical metabolic alterations that occur as cold storage progresses—metabolic alterations that determine reperfusional events. Imamura and colleagues depleted livers of Kupffer cells without effect on the outcome of cold storage and transplantation in the rat,[18] but this is not true under all conditions.[19]

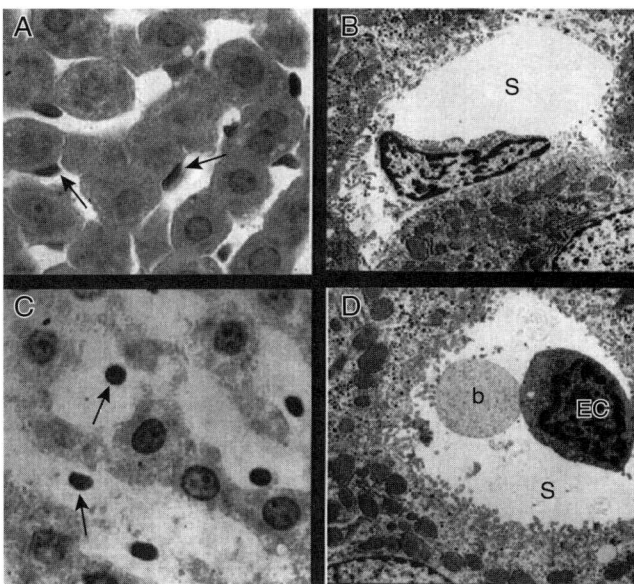

FIGURE 38–1

Light and electron microscopy of normal (**A** and **B**) and cold-preserved (**C** and **D**) sinusoids in the rat. **A**, *Arrows* point to sinusoidal endothelial cell (SEC) nuclei. Note the close approximation to hepatocytes. **B**, Note the cell nucleus and fine cell processes stretching around the wall of the sinusoid (S). Hepatic microvilli are visible in the space of Disse. **C**, Hepatocyte cords are preserved, but SEC nuclei (*arrows*) are rounded and displaced away from the edge of the sinusoid. **D**, Cell processes are drawn up into the rounded cell body (EC). There is no sinusoidal lining or space of Disse. The hepatic microvilli project directly into the lumen of the sinusoid. A microvillus bleb is seen (b).

Our group specifically examined SECs.[15] There is now convincing evidence that the liver injury that occurs at clinically relevant periods of preservation is due to injury to SECs by mechanisms not described by the classic effects of cold (Fig. 38–1).[20,21] Early studies used whole-liver models and provided much useful information. Of particular interest was the observation that proteases were important in genesis of the injury. The importance of proteases was first identified in animal models[22,23] and then confirmed in human allografts by Calmus and associates.[24] One of these important proteases is calpain,[25,26] a calcium-dependent intracellular enzyme (Fig. 38–2). Matrix metalloproteinases (MMP-2 and MMP-9) were implicated when identified in the effluents of rat and human allografts and by the observation of less MMP production when an efficient preservation solution was used than when a poor preservation solution was used (Fig. 38–3).[27] However, whole-organ models are limited because they cannot determine the cell type responsible.

We have examined the effects of cold on isolated hepatic SECs in a series of studies,[13,27-30] as summarized in Figure 38–4. Cold inhibits Ca^{2+}-ATPase,[12] thereby resulting in a slow increase in intracellular calcium levels, probably because of unopposed leakage

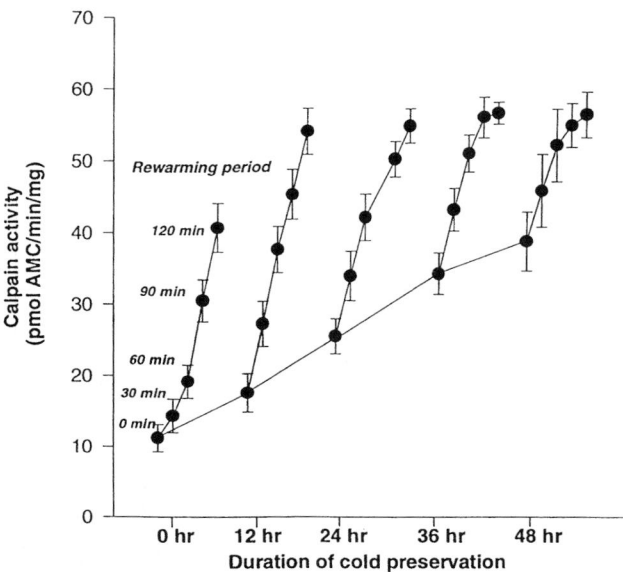

FIGURE 38–2

Calpain activity during cold preservation and rewarming of rat livers. The *solid line* across the bottom of the figure shows calpain activity in rat liver homogenates at different intervals of cold preservation. After each interval there was a sharp increase in activity if livers were rewarmed as shown by the *vertical lines*. (From Kohli V, Gao W, Camargo CA Jr, Clavien PA: Calpain is a mediator of preservation-reperfusion injury in rat liver transplantation. Proc Natl Acad Sci U S A 94:9354-9359, 1997.)

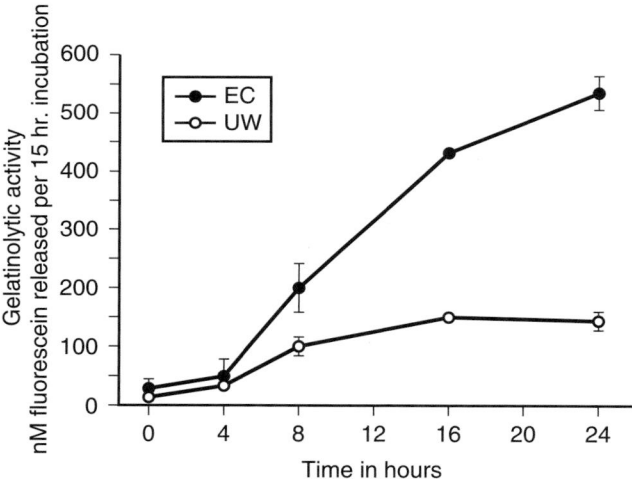

FIGURE 38–3

Results of gelatinolytic assay (activity of the metalloproteinases MMP-2 and MMP-9) of rat liver effluents obtained by washout after various periods of cold storage. The increase was much greater when Eurocollins was the preservative than when University of Wisconsin solution was used as the preservation agent. (From Upadhya AG, Harvey RP, Howard TK, et al: Evidence of a role for matrix metalloproteinases in cold preservation injury of the liver in humans and in the rat. Hepatology 26:922-928, 1997.)

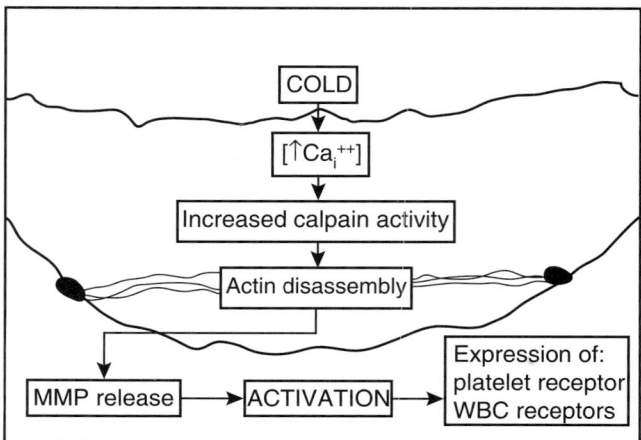

FIGURE 38–4

Schema of the intracellular mechanism of the cold preservation of sinusoidal endothelial cells (SECs). Cold initiates a series of changes in SECs, starting with a slow rise in the intracellular calcium concentration and activation of calpain. A key step is actin disassembly and metalloproteinase secretion. The end result of prolonged preservation is an activated endothelium that traps and activates platelets and leukocytes. (From Upadhya GA, Topp SA, Hotchkiss RS, et al: Effect of cold preservation on intracellular calcium concentration and calpain activity in rat sinusoidal endothelial cells. Hepatology 37:313-323, 2003.)

from intracellular stores. This results in increased calpain activity,[13] which in turn leads to disassembly of actin stress fibers.[13] Actin stress fiber disassembly induces the release of MMPs from SECs.[27] MMP secretion and actin disassembly result in activation of the cell surface, as evidenced by increased expression of von Willebrand factor (vWF) and platelet adhesiveness to the SEC cell surface.[30] Actin stress fiber disassembly is also necessary for the increased white cell adhesion that is seen after reperfusion.[31] The cold-induced injury to SECs can over time convert a resting endothelial cell to one that is highly activated, expressing receptors for normal circulating platelets and leukocytes, and probably able to initiate coagulation on contact with blood. One can imagine that reperfusion of an organ with such highly activated endothelium would produce a picture very much like the hyperacute vascular rejection phenomenon seen with xenografts. It is not surprising that early transplant surgeons occasionally described hyperacute rejection in liver allografts; what they were probably actually observing in some of these cases was the effects of prolonged cold preservation on SECs.

MMP secretion appears to have a central role in the mechanism of SEC activation and cold preservation injury. The events described earlier in rodent models are mimicked in human grafts.[27] As part of these studies it was recognized that lactobionate, the chief ingredient in UW solution, is a potent MMP inhibitor.[29] This helped explain two puzzling observations. Lactobionate was added to the UW formula by Belzer and Southard to reduce cell-swelling, one of the classic effects of cold. As a large impermeant anion, it, unlike chloride, is restricted from entering the cell when the electrochemical gradient dependent on the Na^+,K^+-ATPase pump is lost in the cold. In effect, it balances the osmotic effect of impermeant intracellular molecules and prevents cell swelling. However, when cell swelling is prevented by substituting a different impermeant ion, the altered solution is ineffective in preventing the changes in SECs.[32] In other words, lactobionate possesses other attributes that seem much more important to SEC preservation than prevention of cell swelling. Furthermore, as we shall describe, histidine-tryptophan-ketoglutarate (HTK) solution, whose effectiveness as a preservation solution is similar to that of UW solution, does not contain any ingredients that were intended to suppress the cell-swelling effects of cold. However, its main ingredient, histidine, is also a potent MMP inhibitor. Presumably, cooling of hepatocytes, Kupffer cells, and other hepatic cells has some deleterious effects on their function, but at this time it is not clear that such effects are clinically relevant. It seems that the major mechanism of cold preservation injury is injury to SECs. The major cause of injury to other cells is secondary to the effects of cold preservation injury in SECs.

Rewarming Injury

After the recipient's liver is removed and the donor liver is brought into the operative field, there is a period during which the vascular anastomoses are constructed, usually 30 to 60 minutes. During this time the organ progressively rewarms but is not yet perfused, and therefore it continues to be deprived of oxygen and the ability to produce ATP efficiently by aerobic glycolysis. After 40 minutes, liver core temperature increases from 2° C to almost 20° C[II] with an attendant increase in enzyme activity and metabolic rate (Fig. 38–5). At this temperature there is rapid depletion of any remaining glycogen stores because anaerobic glycolysis is increased to meet metabolic demands.[5,6] It is likely that these temperatures are more deleterious to hepatocytes than to SECs because the former begin to have high energy demands at 20° C. Furthermore, a few minutes at temperature above 20° C is much more injurious than the same duration of hypoxia at a lower temperature. It is important for the transplant surgeon to recognize that the injury caused by rewarming progresses *geometrically* minute by minute. Very long periods of rewarming ischemia (>120 minutes) can probably alone result in organ failure (primary nonfunction); however, shorter periods probably contribute to primary nonfunction in combination with other elements of prepreservation and preservation injury.

The extent to which a donor organ sustains the three types of injury discussed thus far—prepreservation

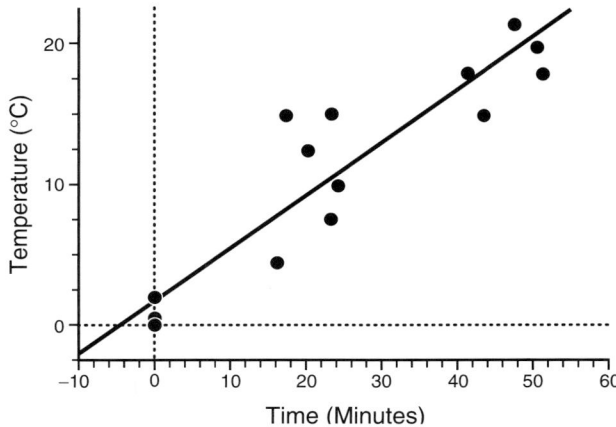

FIGURE 38–5

After 40 minutes, liver core temperature increases from 2° C to almost 20° C with an attendant increase in enzyme activity and metabolic rate. (From Hertl M, Howard TK, Lowell JA, et al: Changes in liver core temperature during preservation and rewarming in human and porcine liver allografts. Liver Transpl Surg 2:111-117, 1996.)

injury, cold preservation injury, and rewarming injury—largely determines how well it functions on reperfusion. For instance, in pure models of cold preservation, the extent of injury on reperfusion is determined entirely by the length of cold preservation. Importantly, no injury is detectable after short periods of preservation; that is, reperfusion of an organ with normal blood at normal blood pressure is not itself a cause of injury. However, when there is preexisting disease in the liver or when periods of cold preservation or rewarming have been prolonged, a series of events may ensue that can lead to organ destruction on reperfusion. This mechanism is supported by the animal studies cited earlier and by histological studies in humans.[33]

Reperfusion Injury

Overview. Injury to the liver after any type of ischemia is manifested clinically on reperfusion when blood flow is restored. In the ideal recipient, normal blood containing unactivated leukocytes and platelets and normal levels of oxygen and inflammatory mediators perfuses the graft. The extent of injury to the graft on reperfusion may vary from almost none to total destruction and depends on the degree to which leukocytes and platelets adhere to endothelium and are activated, the extent to which Kupffer cells are activated, and the extent to which mediators of inflammation from these cellular elements and other sources, including oxygen, are produced. As opposed to the cold storage period, where metabolic events evolve very slowly, events during the reperfusion period take place within seconds or minutes. For instance, the injury induced by very prolonged cold preservation is a vascular phenomenon, very similar to hyperacute rejection, and consists of widespread platelet adhesion, white cell adhesion, and intravascular thrombosis. In the worst cases, blood flow will fall to low levels after minutes of reperfusion, and the organ will cease to function.

Pure recipient factors may also affect outcome in the reperfusion period. For instance, if the recipient is hypotensive during graft reperfusion, the graft may suffer warm ischemia along with the other organs of the recipient. If the recipient's blood contains activated platelets or leukocytes or elevated levels of inflammatory mediators, the injury may be compounded. For instance, in animals, prolonged periods of portal vein clamping may result in the release of endotoxin from the intestine with resultant activation of Kupffer cells on reperfusion, release of tumor necrosis factor-α (TNF-α), and production of a systemic shock–like syndrome.[19,34] We now consider how each of the elements of reperfusing blood may contribute to injury.

Platelets. Activation of the endothelial wall leads to platelet adhesion and activation.[35,36] The mechanism is probably increased expression of vWF on sinusoidal cells.[30,33] Unactivated platelets adhere to vWF when it is fixed to endothelial cells and induce activation of the platelets when they adhere.[30] Platelets are a rich source of transforming growth factor,[37] calpains,[38] and other toxic metabolites. Nitric oxide (NO) production by platelets, in combination with oxygen free radical synthesis on reoxygenation of the ischemic liver, can lead to the formation of peroxynitrite, a highly reactive inducer of apoptosis in endothelial cells.[39]

Leukocytes. After reperfusion, leukocytes rapidly adhere to the sinusoids and contribute significantly to injury.[40-44] The mechanism of adhesion is probably increased expression of intercellular adhesion molecule 1 (ICAM-1), both in warm[45] ischemia and cold preservation.[31,46] Leukocytes release reactive oxygen intermediates by means of the reduced nicotinamide-adenosine dinucleotide phosphate (NADPH)-dependent oxidase system expressed on the cell membrane. Other substances released by neutrophils include proteases and hypochloric acid.[47] Once reperfusion has started, Kupffer cells become activated. Both TNF-α and interleukin-1 (IL-1), released by activated Kupffer cells, can upregulate CD11b expression on leukocytes, which adds to the recruitment of these cells onto sinusoids.[48] Models using the isolated perfused rat liver have revealed that leukocytes and platelets synergistically exacerbate SEC injury by induction of SEC apoptosis and that Kupffer cells are involved in the mechanism of injury mediated by endothelial cells.[49]

Endothelial Cell Apoptosis or Necrosis. Controversy has recently emerged over whether the mechanism of SEC death is necrosis or apoptosis.[50,51] Whereas endothelial cell death after reperfusion of cold-preserved liver has been viewed in the past as coagulative necrosis,[52,53] recent evidence indicates that SEC death occurs through apoptosis.[54,55] Apoptosis represents a pivotal mechanism of reperfusion injury as indicated by the positive correlation between the number of apoptotic cells and graft viability.[54] The importance of apoptosis in hepatic preservation-reperfusion injury has been additionally suggested through the protective effect of antiapoptotic agents added to preservation solutions.[55-57]

Effector Molecules. The mechanisms of reperfusion injury are complex and involve numerous cellular and soluble effectors. Some, such as reactive oxygen species (ROS), TNF-α, increased cytoplasmic calcium concentration, and calpain, are of proven importance. There is less definitive evidence for involvement of many other inflammatory mediators.

Reactive Oxygen Species. A large body of evidence has accumulated on the impact of ROS on reperfusion injury and on Kupffer cells as the major source of ROS formation. Ischemia activates Kupffer cells, which are the main source of vascular ROS during the reperfusion period.[58,59] The injurious effect of ROS after reperfusion of warm and cold ischemic liver has been highlighted in several studies.[60,61] Experimental data indicate that ROS stimulate the secretion of TNF-α and IL-10 by endothelial cells after reperfusion of cold-preserved mouse liver.[62] These cytokines are important mediators of injury. The most convincing hypothesis for the mechanism of ROS-induced cell injury is the destruction of cellular membranes through peroxidation of lipids.[63] The parallel increase in glutathione, myeloperoxidase, and products of lipid peroxidation strongly supports a primary role for this degenerative process. Another possible explanation is that oxidant stress can induce the mitochondrial membrane permeability transition, a central event preceding cell death.[64] Another potential target may be caspases, a family of cysteine proteases important for the initiation and progression of apoptosis.[65] Caspases can be activated by low concentrations of hydrogen peroxide, whereas higher levels inhibit enzymatic activity, presumably because of oxidation of critical sulfhydryl groups. Thus, ROS may induce or inhibit apoptosis, depending on the severity of the oxidative stress. The addition of deferoxamine, an iron chelator, decreased the apoptosis of SECs and hepatocytes after cold preservation, thus suggesting an important role for ROS via the Fenton reaction.[66] NO production may be injurious as noted earlier.[39] In contrast, it has been reported that arginine supplementation and NO synthesis reduce apoptosis and ameliorate transplantation injury in the rat.[67] Addition of the NO donor nitroprusside to UW solution also improved outcome after cold preservation in the rat.[68]

Cytokines. Of the other potential mediators of injury, cytokines are among the most important. Cytokines are produced by liver cells, mainly Kupffer cells and SECs. Numerous candidate molecules have been identified, but TNF-α, IL-1, and IL-6 are viewed as critically important. In 1990, Colletti and coworkers[69] suggested that prolonged ischemic intervals lead to a burst of cytokines, including TNF-α; other groups have subsequently confirmed the finding that TNF-α initiates apoptosis in hepatocytes and SECs.[70-72] Blockage of TNF-α release from Kupffer cells by pentoxifylline prevents upregulation of TNF-α expression and protects the liver against reperfusion injury in models of cold[73-75] and warm ischemia.[72]

Proteases. Several cysteine proteases such as calpain and caspases have been reported to be mediators of preservation-reperfusion injury through modulation of apoptosis[26,57,76] and necrosis.[77] Calpains are a group of cytoplasmic nonlysosomal calcium-dependent cysteine proteases involved in the proteolysis of cytoskeletal and membrane proteins. Calpain activity was found to increase significantly during the period of cold ischemia, with a further rapid increase after reperfusion.[78] The protective effect of calpain inhibition has been reported in cold[13,26,79] and warm ischemic injury.[57,80] Calpain inhibition resulted in decreased tissue injury in both endothelial cells[13,79] and hepatocytes[26] and ultimately provided significant protection of graft function. Other proteases such as caspases have also been involved in the pathogenesis of reperfusion injury. Specific isoforms are involved in the initiation and execution phases of apoptosis. Several groups have demonstrated the protective effect of caspase inhibition during hepatic ischemia and reperfusion in various models of cold and warm ischemia.[55,81]

Other Potential Extracellular and Intracellular Mediators. Preliminary evidence exists for the involvement of endothelin,[82,83] macrophage inflammatory protein-2 (MIP-2), cytokine-induced neutrophil chemoattractant (CINC),[84] and nuclear factor-κB (NF-κB)[85] as leukocyte chemoattractants.

Current Clinical Preservation Methods

Clinical Liver Preservation Solutions

Eurocollins Solution

The first clinically adopted liver preservation solution was Eurocollins solution, the composition of which is given in Table 38–1. It was the standard solution for kidney preservation at the time that liver transplantation became clinically viable with the advent of cyclosporine. Understanding its rationale is still important, although it was a poor preservation solution for the liver and fell out of use, except for emergencies, when UW solution became available. Eurocollins is first an isotonic solution. It is a high-potassium or "intracellular solution," the rationale being that in the absence of sodium, the potassium concentration in and outside the cell in the cold would be high. Consequently, on reperfusion, energy would not be needed to pump sodium out of the cell, thus sparing the recovering cell the need to perform this energy-requiring task. It also contained glucose as an impermeant. Glucose apparently is an effective impermeant for preventing kidney swelling, although it is ineffective in the liver. Phosphate was added as a buffer to prevent intracellular acidosis from lactate accumulation. Eurocollins is an effective solution for periods of preservation of less than 6 hours. Results begin to deteriorate rapidly if livers are preserved for longer periods, and primary nonfunction is nearly universal with preservation periods longer than 12 hours.

Eurocollins, unlike UW solution, is a low-viscosity solution that has been used as a washout solution either purposely to rid the liver and bile ducts of blood more effectively than UW solution does or to reduce the volume of UW solution that must be used during the preservation process for economic reasons or because of a shortage of UW solution. Clinical trials

Table 38–1. COMPOSITION OF COLD STORAGE SOLUTIONS

	Collins	UW
Potassium ion	115.0 mmol/L	125 mmol/L
Sodium ion	10.0 mmol/L	125 mmol/L
Magnesium	30.0 mmol/L	5 mmol/L
Chloride	15.0 mmol/L	0 mmol/L
Bicarbonate	10.0 mmol/L	—
Sulfate	30.0 mmol/L	5 mmol/L
Phosphate	57.5 mmol/L	25 mmol/L
Citrate	—	—
Glucose	140.0 mmol/L	—
Lactobionate	—	100 mmol/L
Raffinose	—	30 mmol/L
Adenosine	—	5 mmol/L
Glutathione	—	3 mmol/L
Allopurinol	—	1 mmol/1
Hydroxyethyl starch	—	50 g/L
mOsm/L	320.0	320
pH	7.0	7.4

Eurocollins solution is similar to Collins solution but with the omission of magnesium sulfate and increased glucose (195 mmol/L).
UW, University of Wisconsin solution.

indicate that this approach does not lead to any deterioration in outcome, provided that Eurocollins solution is replaced with UW solution for the duration of the preservation period.[86,87] In fact, there may be some advantage to this approach in terms of bile duct preservation,[88] and some studies even suggest an improvement in overall liver function.

University of Wisconsin Solution

UW solution was the culmination of work of two investigators, Folkert Belzer and James Southard, the former a surgeon and the latter a basic scientist, working together for many years to understand the classic effects of cold and the means to prevent them.[89,90] The composition of the solution is given in Table 38–1. The clinical impact of their discoveries was immediate and great and matched by few other advances made in surgical laboratories in the 20th century. It remains one of the important enabling steps in clinical liver transplantation. It made organ sharing across large distances such as all of the United States and Canada possible. Organs have even been shared between Europe and North America with the use of this solution. It converted liver transplantation from a rushed emergency procedure to a semielective procedure by extending cold preservation times. Belzer, who died prematurely in 1995, is remembered as a model surgeon-scientist (Fig. 38–6).

The approach taken by Belzer and Southard in formulating the UW solution differed from that in formulating the Collins solution in several respects, although they did adopt the use of an isotonic, high-potassium,

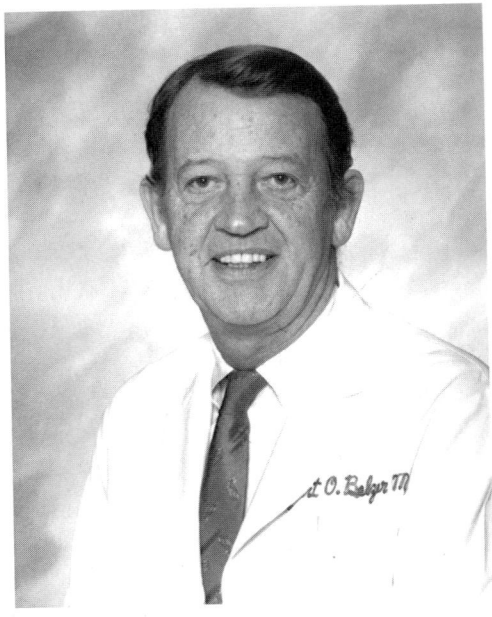

FIGURE 38–6
Folkert Belzer, who with James Southard introduced the revolutionary University of Wisconsin solution.

phosphate-buffered solution as featured in the Collins solution.[90] Glucose was replaced by raffinose and sodium lactobionate as impermeants. Lactobionate is the anion of lactobionic acid, a carboxylic acid based on a disaccharide. Hydroxyethyl starch was added as an oncotic agent to suppress swelling in the extracellular fluid space. Adenosine was used to provide a substrate for ATP resynthesis on reperfusion, and glutathione and allopurinol were added as an oxygen free radical scavenger and inhibitor of xanthine oxidase, respectively. Dexamethasone was included as a membrane stabilizer. In later discussions, Southard suggested that lactobionate might act as an intracellular calcium chelator. However, this seems a somewhat contradictory role for an impermeant, and it is doubtful that lactobionate can chelate down to the micromolar level needed for an intracellular chelator. Although lactobionate is an effective impermeant that prevents cell swelling, we have shown that replacement of it with an equally effective impermeant, choline, does not result in retention of the beneficial effects of UW solution on the liver.[32] Later, we were able to show that lactobionate and glutathione are potent cryptic MMP inhibitors, and it is likely that much of their effect in UW solution can be attributed to this function.[29]

Bretschneider's Solution or HTK Solution

HTK solution was initially designed for cardiac preservation. It was formulated to retard acidosis (histidine), prevent membrane injury (tryptophan), and provide a substrate for energy metabolism (ketoglutarate). This solution was also tested by several groups in liver transplantation and has been shown to be equally effective as UW solution at the usual periods of cold preservation used in human transplantation.[91] It has recently been licensed for use in the United States.

Celsior (Sangstat Medical Corp) is a relatively low-potassium (15 mM) cardiac preservation solution that contains elements of the UW and HTK solutions (lactobionate, histidine). Preliminary studies suggested that it might be effective in liver preservation.[92] It has been tested in the rat transplantation model and found to be inferior to colloid-free UW solution.[93]

The composition of preservation solutions might be improved by the addition of certain ingredients. For instance, preliminary data suggest that deferoxamine[66] and tauroursodeoxycholic acid[94] might improve the function of these solutions.

Current Methods of the Use of Preservation Solutions

The principle of organ preservation is based on flushing and storage of the organ at low temperature with one of the previously cited organ preservation solutions.

The liver is currently preserved primarily in UW solution. This complex solution supports good graft function even after 12 hours of cold preservation time.[95] HTK solution is also in clinical use, especially in Germany. As noted earlier, there seems to be little disadvantage to flushing the liver with other solutions such as Eurocollins solution, provided that they are replaced with UW solution.

Even though the preservation potential of liver cold storage solutions has significantly improved, the rate of graft dysfunction after transplantation has been reported to range between 5% and 20%,[96] although this rate may be currently higher because of the increased use of organs with extended criteria for acceptance.[97] A significant proportion of primary graft dysfunction is attributable to inadequate cold storage, including imperfect storage solutions. Thus, new strategies to increase organ protection during cold preservation are still urgently needed. The development of machine perfusion was intended to improve the results of liver transplantation with respect to the duration and quality of the organs that can be preserved.

Novel Preservation Strategies

Preconditioning of the Liver

Of the many protective strategies that have been shown to be effective against ischemic injury in animal models, very few have been adopted clinically. Ischemic preconditioning has emerged as one of the most effective and easily applicable techniques. Ischemic preconditioning, a brief period of ischemia followed by a short interval of reperfusion before the prolonged ischemic stress,[98-100] is a novel protective approach against ischemic reperfusion injury. Preconditioning effectively prevents reperfusion injury in a normothermic ischemic liver[100] and converts organ injuries incompatible with animal survival to nonlethal injuries.[99] Mechanisms of protection include prevention of apoptosis of SECs and hepatocytes by downregulation of the caspase pathway. Preconditioning is also protective during the period of cold storage of the liver before reperfusion. It reduces endothelial rounding and detachment and matrix MMP activity.[101] Ischemic preconditioning almost completely prevented SEC apoptosis after reperfusion of cold-preserved livers. The protective effect is possibly triggered by a short sublethal burst of oxygen free radicals.[101] Indeed, a mild burst of oxidative stress generated during the process of ischemic preconditioning induces natural defense mechanisms against subsequent lethal injury, as also demonstrated in a model of warm ischemia.[102] A number of other mediators have been identified in the protective pathway of ischemic preconditioning, such as NO and adenosine.[98,103,104] These data suggest that ischemic preconditioning is effective before reperfusion, that is, during the period of ischemia, and not only at the time of reperfusion as suggested by several studies.[103,105,106] Inhibition of tyrosine kinases prevented the beneficial effects of preconditioning in the pig.[107]

Recently, two laboratories have reported beneficial effects on induction of heme oxygenase-1 (HO-1) in rat livers exposed to cold preservation. In one study, rats were pretreated with cobalt protoporphyrin and zinc protoporphyrin, an HO-1 inducer and antagonist, respectively. Cobalt protoporphyrin–pretreated livers had significantly higher portal venous blood flow, increased total bile production, and greater transplant viability than controls did.[108] In another study, heat preconditioning improved the outcome of transplantation in the rat, an effect that was eliminated by tin protoporphyrin, an inhibitor of HO-1 production, and could be reproduced by the administration of cobalt protoporphyrin, a stimulus of HO-1 production.[109]

Machine Perfusion

Extracorporeal machine perfusion systems have been proposed as a tool to stop the process of biodegradation[110,111] and maintain superior tissue preservation. By continuously providing the graft with essential substrates (e.g., glucose, amino acids, nucleotides, oxygen) combined with permanent disposal of toxic metabolites,[112] it is expected that organ viability can be better maintained. Oxygen is the fuel that drives all cellular activity by allowing the cell to efficiently regenerate ATP, the currency of cellular energy. Blood flow is terminated during ischemic preservation, thus eliminating the supply of both oxygen and nutrients. Reducing ATP depletion to a minimum is critical for control of the cascades of ischemic injury. Preventing ATP loss requires perfusion of the liver with an oxygenated solution.[113-115] Perfusion preservation of rat liver has been noted to completely suppress the loss of ATP that occurs in cold storage, even at 48 hours of reperfusion.[114] Other groups have demonstrated that incremental cold ischemia time followed by 45 minutes of ischemic rewarming in rats induces a progressive rise in liver enzymes and a decrease in ATP levels with increasing cold ischemia time.[116] Remarkably, 30 minutes of oxygenated nonsanguineous perfusion before rewarming protects liver function and facilitates recovery of ATP loss to levels comparable to those of nonstored control livers.[116] Similarly, St Peter and colleagues demonstrated that warm oxygenated sanguineous machine perfusion results in recovery of liver function to a viable level after 24 hours of cold preservation whereas simple cold storage (UW solution) for 24 hours renders the liver nonviable.[117,118]

The perfusion systems are based on models of isolated liver perfusion, which have been widely used to study the mechanisms of cold preservation injury. Although this technique has been developed primarily as a tool for temporary extracorporeal liver support in patients with liver failure, it also has potential application in organ preservation or resuscitation before transplantation.[111]

The ideal perfusate for continuous perfusion of an organ has not yet been defined. The perfusate should deliver oxygen to the organ by using an oxygen carrier to obtain the full benefit of perfusion.[119,120] Simple oxygenated buffer solutions require higher flow for adequate oxygen delivery and create degenerative changes in the perfused tissue that are not observed when red blood cells are used as the oxygen carrier.[121,122] In addition to tissue damage, high flow can decrease first-pass hepatic clearance.[123] A hematocrit of 20% has been suggested to provide the optimum combination of hemodynamic and oxygen-carrying capacity.[124] In addition to an oxygen carrier, free radical scavengers, inflammatory mediators, insulin, calcium channel blockers, bile salts, and nutrition have been added to the perfusate to provide a continuous cellular supply. Finally, various other modifications have improved the technique, including oscillating pressure profiles imitating intra-abdominal conditions[125] and simultaneous dialysis of the recirculating perfusate to remove water-soluble toxins and allow regulation of pH and electrolytes,[126,127] as well as the use of normothermic rather than hypothermic perfusion.[117]

The introduction of extracorporeal perfusion systems into clinical routine will depend mainly on the practicability of these still very complicated machines. Currently, continuous perfusion preservation is used for only kidneys and just at a few centers. Despite evidence that machine perfusion provides a higher-quality graft and allows longer preservation periods, standard practice today continues to involve flushing the organ with acellular perfusate or preservation solution and storage at 1° C for the minimum time possible before surgery. A valid argument in favor of this practice is that acceptable results are obtained with a cheaper method of preservation. The demanding and sophisticated handling of perfusion systems may complicate the logistics and significantly increase costs.

Pearls and Pitfalls

Pearls

- Graft injury is manifested on reperfusion but is the result of accumulated graft damage acquired in prepreservation, preservation, and rewarming periods.

Pearls and Pitfalls—cont'd

- Many grafts suffer prepreservation injury, which is detectable by platelet adhesion to the microcirculation, but is not detectable in standard tests of graft evaluation. Therefore, significant degrees of undetected prepreservation injury may exist in a deceased donor graft. This will explain some cases of unexpected poor function.

- Cold preservation injury is mainly due to an effect of cold on the microcirculation. Cold activates the sinusoidal endothelial surface, which makes it adherent for platelets and leukocytes. When fully developed, the effect is similar to the vascular-type hyperacute rejection observed on reperfusion of xenografts.

- During the rewarming period when vascular anastomoses are being made, grafts rewarm at a linear rate going from 1° C to 20° C in 60 minutes. 20° C is a critical temperature at which membrane pumps begin to work. Energy requirements of the cell rise, placing stress on the graft.

Pitfalls

- Primary nonfunction is usually due to multiple risk factors for poor function being combined in one patient. When a known risk factor such as steatosis is present, all other adjustable risk factors such as cold preservation time and rewarming time should be minimized.

- After 60 minutes, a minute of rewarming time has a much greater injurious effect than a minute of rewarming time before 60 minutes has elapsed.

References

1. Markin RS, Wisecarver JL, Radio SJ, et al: Frozen section evaluation of donor livers before transplantation. Transplantation 56:1403-1409, 1993.
2. Briceno J, Marchal T, Padillo J, et al: Influence of marginal donors on liver preservation injury. Transplantation 74:522-526, 2002.
3. Taneja C, Prescott L, Koneru B: Critical preservation injury in rat fatty liver is to hepatocytes, not sinusoidal lining cells. Transplantation 65:167-172, 1998.
4. Fukumori T, Ohkohchi N, Tsukamoto S, Satomi S: The mechanism of injury in a steatotic liver graft during cold preservation. Transplantation 67:195-200, 1999.
5. Cywes R, Greig PD, Sanabria JR, et al: Effect of intraportal glucose infusion on hepatic glycogen content and degradation, and outcome of liver transplantation. Ann Surg 216:235-246, discussion 246-247, 1992.
6. Cywes R, Greig PD, Morgan GR, et al: Rapid donor liver nutritional enhancement in a large animal model. Hepatology 16:1271-1279, 1992.

7. Lindell SL, Hansen T, Rankin M, et al: Donor nutritional status—a determinant of liver preservation injury. Transplantation 61:239-247, 1996.
8. Arnault I, Bao YM, Dimicoli JL, et al: Combined effects of fasting and alanine on liver function recovery after cold ischemia. Transpl Int 15:89-95, 2002.
9. Compagnon P, Wang H, Lindell SL, et al: Brain death does not affect hepatic allograft function and survival after orthotopic transplantation in a canine model. Transplantation 73:1218-1227, 2002.
10. Cywes R, Mullen JB, Stratis MA, et al: Prediction of the outcome of transplantation in man by platelet adherence in donor liver allografts. Evidence of the importance of prepreservation injury. Transplantation 56:316-323, 1993.
11. Hertl M, Howard TK, Lowell JA, et al: Changes in liver core temperature during preservation and rewarming in human and porcine liver allografts. Liver Transpl Surg 2:111-117, 1996.
12. Bigelow DJ, Thomas DD: Rotational dynamics of lipid and the Ca-ATPase in sarcoplasmic reticulum. The molecular basis of activation by diethyl ether. J Biol Chem 262:13449-13456, 1987.
13. Upadhya GA, Topp SA, Hotchkiss RS, et al: Effect of cold preservation on intracellular calcium concentration and calpain activity in rat sinusoidal endothelial cells. Hepatology 37:313-323, 2003.
14. Marzi I, Zhong Z, Lemasters JJ, Thurman RG: Evidence that graft survival is not related to parenchymal cell viability in rat liver transplantation. The importance of nonparenchymal cells. Transplantation 48:463-468, 1989.
15. McKeown CM, Edwards V, Phillips MJ, et al: Sinusoidal lining cell damage: The critical injury in cold preservation of liver allografts in the rat. Transplantation 46:178-191, 1988.
16. Caldwell-Kenkel JC, Thurman RG, Lemasters JJ: Selective loss of nonparenchymal cell viability after cold ischemic storage of rat livers. Transplantation 45:834-837, 1988.
17. Caldwell-Kenkel JC, Currin RT, Tanaka Y, et al: Kupffer cell activation and endothelial cell damage after storage of rat livers: Effects of reperfusion. Hepatology 13:83-95, 1991.
18. Imamura H, Sutto F, Brault A, Huet PM: Role of Kupffer cells in cold ischemia/reperfusion injury of rat liver. Gastroenterology 109:189-197, 1995.
19. Urata K, Brault A, Rocheleau B, Huet PM: Role of Kupffer cells in the survival after rat liver transplantation with long portal vein clamping times. Transpl Int 13:420-427, 2000.
20. Urata K, Imamura H, Brault A, Huet PM: Effects of extended cold preservation and transplantation on the rat liver microcirculation. Hepatology 25:664-671, 1997.
21. Clavien PA, Harvey PR, Strasberg SM: Preservation and reperfusion injuries in liver allografts. An overview and synthesis of current studies. Transplantation 53:957-978, 1992.
22. Takei Y, Marzi I, Kauffman FC, et al: Increase in survival time of liver transplants by protease inhibitors and a calcium channel blocker, nisoldipine. Transplantation 50:14-20, 1990.
23. Clavien PA, Sanabria JR, Upadhaya A, et al: Evidence of the existence of a soluble mediator of cold preservation injury. Transplantation 56:44-53, 1993.
24. Calmus Y, Cynober L, Dousset B, et al: Evidence for the detrimental role of proteolysis during liver preservation in humans. Gastroenterology 108:1510-1516, 1995.
25. Aguilar HI, Steers JL, Wiesner RH, et al: Enhanced liver calpain protease activity is a risk factor for dysfunction of human liver allografts. Transplantation 63:612-614, 1997.
26. Kohli V, Gao W, Camargo CA Jr, Clavien PA: Calpain is a mediator of preservation-reperfusion injury in rat liver transplantation. Proc Natl Acad Sci U S A 94:9354-9359, 1997.
27. Upadhya AG, Harvey RP, Howard TK, et al: Evidence of a role for matrix metalloproteinases in cold preservation injury of the liver in humans and in the rat. Hepatology 26:922-928, 1997.
28. Upadhya GA, Strasberg SM: Evidence that actin disassembly is a requirement for matrix metalloproteinase secretion by sinusoidal

29. Upadhya GA, Strasberg SM: Glutathione, lactobionate, and histidine: Cryptic inhibitors of matrix metalloproteinases contained in University of Wisconsin and histidine/tryptophan/ketoglutarate liver preservation solutions. Hepatology 31:1115-1122, 2000.
30. Upadhya GA, Strasberg SM: Platelet adherence to isolated rat hepatic sinusoidal endothelial cells after cold preservation. Transplantation 73:1764-1770, 2002.
31. Topp SA, Upadhya GA, Strasberg SM: Leukocyte adhesion to cold-preserved rat sinusoidal endothelial cells (SEC): Role of actin disassembly and ICAM-1. Liver Transpl 9:1286-1294, 2003.
32. Holloway CM, Harvey PR, Mullen JB, Strasberg SM: Evidence that cold preservation–induced microcirculatory injury in liver allografts is not mediated by oxygen free radicals or cell swelling in the rat. Transplantation 48:179-188, 1989.
33. Kiuchi T, Oldhafer KJ, Schlitt HJ, et al: Background and prognostic implications of perireperfusion tissue injuries in human liver transplants: A panel histochemical study. Transplantation 66:737-747, 1998.
34. Urata K, Brault A, Huet PM: Effects of portal vein clamping time on rat liver microcirculation following extended cold preservation and transplantation. Transpl Int 12:408-414, 1999.
35. Sindram D, Porte RJ, Hoffman MR, et al: Platelets induce sinusoidal endothelial cell apoptosis upon reperfusion of the cold ischemic rat liver. Gastroenterology 118:183-191, 2000.
36. Cywes R, Packham MA, Tietze L, et al: Role of platelets in hepatic allograft preservation injury in the rat. Hepatology 18:635-647, 1993.
37. Fukuda K, Kojiro M, Chiu JF: Induction of apoptosis by transforming growth factor-beta 1 in the rat hepatoma cell line McA-RH7777: A possible association with tissue transglutaminase expression. Hepatology 18:945-953, 1993.
38. Schoenwaelder SM, Yuan Y, Cooray P, et al: Calpain cleavage of focal adhesion proteins regulates the cytoskeletal attachment of integrin $\alpha IIb\beta 3$ (platelet glycoprotein IIb/IIIa) and the cellular retraction of fibrin clots. J Biol Chem 272:1694-1702, 1997.
39. Gow AJ, Thom SR, Ischiropoulos H: Nitric oxide and peroxynitrite-mediated pulmonary cell death. Am J Physiol 274:L112-L118, 1998.
40. Takei Y, Marzi I, Gao WS, et al: Leukocyte adhesion and cell death following orthotopic liver transplantation in the rat. Transplantation 51:959-965, 1991.
41. Jaeschke H, Farhood A, Smith CW: Neutrophils contribute to ischemia/reperfusion injury in rat liver in vivo. FASEB J 4:3355-3359, 1990.
42. Clavien PA, Morgan GR, Sanabria JR, et al: Effect of cold preservation on lymphocyte adherence in the perfused rat liver. Transplantation 52:412-417, 1991.
43. Clavien PA, Harvey PR, Sanabria JR, et al: Lymphocyte adherence in the reperfused rat liver: Mechanisms and effects. Hepatology 17:131-142, 1993.
44. Jaeschke H, Smith CW: Mechanisms of neutrophil-induced parenchymal cell injury. J Leukoc Biol 61:647-653, 1997.
45. Farhood A, McGuire GM, Manning AM, et al: Intercellular adhesion molecule 1 (ICAM-1) expression and its role in neutrophil-induced ischemia-reperfusion injury in rat liver. J Leukoc Biol 57:368-374, 1995.
46. Rentsch M, Post S, Palma P, et al: Anti–ICAM-1 blockade reduces postsinusoidal WBC adherence following cold ischemia and reperfusion, but does not improve early graft function in rat liver transplantation. J Hepatol 32:821-828, 2000.
47. Weiss SJ: Tissue destruction by neutrophils. N Engl J Med 320:365-376, 1989.
48. Bajt ML, Farhood A, Jaeschke H: Effects of CXC chemokines on neutrophil activation and sequestration in hepatic vasculature. Am J Physiol Gastrointest Liver Physiol 281:G1188-G1195, 2001.

endothelial cells during cold preservation in the rat. Hepatology 30:169-176, 1999.

49. Sindram D, Porte RJ, Hoffman MR, et al: Synergism between platelets and leukocytes in inducing endothelial cell apoptosis in the cold ischemic rat liver: A Kupffer cell–mediated injury. FASEB J 15:1230-1232, 2001.

50. Gujral JS, Bucci TJ, Farhood A, Jaeschke H: Mechanism of cell death during warm hepatic ischemia-reperfusion in rats: Apoptosis or necrosis? Hepatology 33:397-405, 2001.

51. Clavien PA, Rudiger HA, Selzner M: Mechanism of hepatocyte death after ischemia: Apoptosis versus necrosis. Hepatology 33:1555-1557, 2001.

52. Holloway CM, Harvey PR, Strasberg SM: Viability of sinusoidal lining cells in cold-preserved rat liver allografts. Transplantation 49:225-229, 1990.

53. Caldwell-Kenkel JC, Currin RT, Tanaka Y, et al: Reperfusion injury to endothelial cells following cold ischemic storage of rat livers. Hepatology 10:292-299, 1989.

54. Gao W, Bentley RC, Madden JF, Clavien PA: Apoptosis of sinusoidal endothelial cells is a critical mechanism of preservation injury in rat liver transplantation. Hepatology 27:1652-1660, 1998.

55. Natori S, Selzner M, Valentino KL, et al: Apoptosis of sinusoidal endothelial cells occurs during liver preservation injury by a caspase-dependent mechanism. Transplantation 68:89-96, 1999.

56. Bilbao G, Contreras JL, Gomez-Navarro J, et al: Genetic modification of liver grafts with an adenoviral vector encoding the Bcl-2 gene improves organ preservation. Transplantation 67:775-783, 1999.

57. Kohli V, Madden JF, Bentley RC, Clavien PA: Calpain mediates ischemic injury of the liver through modulation of apoptosis and necrosis. Gastroenterology 116:168-178, 1999.

58. Rymsa B, Wang JF, de Groot H: $O_2^{-\bullet}$ release by activated Kupffer cells upon hypoxia-reoxygenation. Am J Physiol 261:G602-G607, 1991.

59. Jaeschke H: Mechanisms of reperfusion injury after warm ischemia of the liver. J Hepatobiliary Pancreat Surg 5:402-408, 1998.

60. Jaeschke H, Farhood A: Neutrophil and Kupffer cell–induced oxidant stress and ischemia-reperfusion injury in rat liver. Am J Physiol 260:G355-G362, 1991.

61. Southard JH, Marsh DC, McAnulty JF, Belzer FO: Oxygen-derived free radical damage in organ preservation: Activity of superoxide dismutase and xanthine oxidase. Surgery 101:566-570, 1987.

62. Le Moine O, Louis H, Demols A, et al: Cold liver ischemia-reperfusion injury critically depends on liver T cells and is improved by donor pretreatment with interleukin 10 in mice. Hepatology 31:1266-1274, 2000.

63. Omar R, Nomikos I, Piccorelli G, et al: Prevention of postischaemic lipid peroxidation and liver cell injury by iron chelation. Gut 30:510-514, 1989.

64. Lemasters JJ: The mitochondrial permeability transition: From biochemical curiosity to pathophysiological mechanism. Gastroenterology 115:783-786, 1998.

65. Cohen GM: Caspases: The executioners of apoptosis. Biochem J 326:1-16, 1997.

66. Kerkweg U, Li T, de Groot H, Rauen U: Cold-induced apoptosis of rat liver cells in University of Wisconsin solution: The central role of chelatable iron. Hepatology 35:560-567, 2002.

67. Yagnik GP, Takahashi Y, Tsoulfas G, et al: Blockade of the L-arginine/NO synthase pathway worsens hepatic apoptosis and liver transplant preservation injury. Hepatology 36:573-581, 2002.

68. Rodriguez JV, Guibert EE, Quintana A, et al: Role of sodium nitroprusside in the improvement of rat liver preservation in University of Wisconsin solution: A study in the isolated perfused liver model. J Surg Res 87:201-208, 1999.

69. Colletti LM, Remick DG, Burtch GD, et al: Role of tumor necrosis factor-alpha in the pathophysiologic alterations after hepatic ischemia/reperfusion injury in the rat. J Clin Invest 85:1936-1943, 1990.

70. Wanner GA, Muller PE, Ertel W, et al: Differential effect of anti–TNF-alpha antibody on proinflammatory cytokine release by Kupffer cells following liver ischemia and reperfusion. Shock 11:391-395, 1999.

71. Peralta C, Fernandez L, Panes J, et al: Preconditioning protects against systemic disorders associated with hepatic ischemia-reperfusion through blockade of tumor necrosis factor–induced P-selectin up-regulation in the rat. Hepatology 33:100-113, 2001.

72. Rudiger HA, Clavien PA: Tumor necrosis factor alpha, but not Fas, mediates hepatocellular apoptosis in the murine ischemic liver. Gastroenterology 122:202-210, 2002.

73. Lemasters JJ, Peng XX, Bachmann S, et al: Dual role of Kupffer cell activation and endothelial cell damage in reperfusion injury to livers stored for transplantation surgery. J Gastroenterol Hepatol 10(Suppl 1):S84-S87, 1995.

74. Nishizawa H, Egawa H, Inomata Y, et al: Efficiency of pentoxifylline in donor pretreatment in rat liver transplantation. J Surg Res 72:170-176, 1997.

75. Vajdova K, Smrekova R, Kukan M, et al: Endotoxin-induced aggravation of preservation-reperfusion injury of rat liver and its modulation. J Hepatol 32:112-120, 2000.

76. Squier MK, Miller AC, Malkinson AM, Cohen JJ: Calpain activation in apoptosis. J Cell Physiol 159:229-237, 1994.

77. Arora AS, de Groen P, Emori Y, Gores GJ: A cascade of degradative hydrolase activity contributes to hepatocyte necrosis during anoxia. Am J Physiol 270:G238-G245, 1996.

78. Croall DE, DeMartino GN: Calcium-activated neutral protease (calpain) system: Structure, function, and regulation. Physiol Rev 71:813-847, 1991.

79. Sindram D, Kohli V, Madden JF, Clavien PA: Calpain inhibition prevents sinusoidal endothelial cell apoptosis in the cold ischemic rat liver. Transplantation 68:136-140, 1999.

80. Wang M, Sakon M, Umeshita K, et al: Prednisolone suppresses ischemia-reperfusion injury of the rat liver by reducing cytokine production and calpain mu activation. J Hepatol 34:278-283, 2001.

81. Kobayashi A, Imamura H, Isobe M, et al: Mac-1 (CD11b/CD18) and intercellular adhesion molecule-1 in ischemia-reperfusion injury of rat liver. Am J Physiol Gastrointest Liver Physiol 281:G577-G585, 2001.

82. Charrueau CA, Carayon A, Thurman RG: Long-term cold liver storage induces endothelin-1 release and a time-dependent increase in portal pressure at reperfusion in the rat. J Gastroenterol 37:717-725, 2002.

83. Kraus T, Golling M, Mehrabi A, et al: Endothelin-1 and big-endothelin concentrations are elevated in liver graft tissue during cold storage and reperfusion. Eur Surg Res 33:1-7, 2001.

84. Kataoka M, Shimizu H, Mitsuhashi N, et al: Effect of cold-ischemia time on C-X-C chemokine expression and neutrophil accumulation in the graft liver after orthotopic liver transplantation in rats. Transplantation 73:1730-1735, 2002.

85. Takahashi Y, Ganster RW, Gambotto A, et al: Role of NF-κB on liver cold ischemia-reperfusion injury. Am J Physiol Gastrointest Liver Physiol 283:G1175-G1184, 2002.

86. Adam R, Astarcioglu I, Raccuia JS, et al: Beneficial effects of Eurocollins as aortic flush for the procurement of human livers. Transplantation 61:705-709, 1996.

87. Cofer JB, Klintmalm GB, Morris CV, et al: A prospective randomized trial between Eurocollins and University of Wisconsin solutions as the initial flush in hepatic allograft procurement. Transplantation 53:995-998, 1992.

88. Pirenne J, Van Gelder F, Coosemans W, et al: Type of donor aortic preservation solution and not cold ischemia time is a major determinant of biliary strictures after liver transplantation. Liver Transpl 7:540-545, 2001.

89. Belzer FO, Southard JH: Organ preservation and transplantation. Prog Clin Biol Res 224:291-303, 1986.

90. Jamieson NV, Sundberg R, Lindell S, et al: A comparison of cold storage solutions for hepatic preservation using the isolated perfused rabbit liver. Cryobiology 25:300-310, 1988.

91. Hatano E, Kiuchi T, Tanaka A, et al: Hepatic preservation with histidine-tryptophan-ketoglutarate solution in living-related and cadaveric liver transplantation. Clin Sci 93:81-88, 1997.

92. Tolba RH, Akbar S, Muller A, et al: Experimental liver preservation with Celsior: A novel alternative to University of Wisconsin and histidine-tryptophan-α-ketoglutarate solutions? Eur Surg Res 32:142-147, 2000.

93. Howden BO, Jablonski P: Liver preservation: A comparison of Celsior to colloid-free University of Wisconsin solution. Transplantation 70:1140-1142, 2000.

94. Falasca L, Tisone G, Palmieri G, et al: Protective role of tauroursodeoxycholate during harvesting and cold storage of human liver: A pilot study in transplant recipients. Transplantation 71:1268-1276, 2001.

95. Belzer FO, D'Alessandro AM, Hoffmann RM, et al: The use of UW solution in clinical transplantation. A 4-year experience. Ann Surg 215:579-583, discussion 584-585, 1992.

96. Strasberg SM, Howard TK, Molmenti EP, Hertl M: Selecting the donor liver: Risk factors for poor function after orthotopic liver transplantation. Hepatology 20:829-838, 1994.

97. Selzner N, Rudiger HA, Graf R, Clavien P-A: Protective strategies against ischemic injury of the liver. Gastroenterology 125:917-936, 2003.

98. Peralta C, Prats N, Xaus C, et al: Protective effect of liver ischemic preconditioning on liver and lung injury induced by hepatic ischemia-reperfusion in the rat. Hepatology 30:1481-1489, 1999.

99. Yadav SS, Sindram D, Perry DK, Clavien PA: Ischemic preconditioning protects the mouse liver by inhibition of apoptosis through a caspase-dependent pathway. Hepatology 30:1223-1231, 1999.

100. Clavien PA, Yadav S, Sindram D, Bentley RC: Protective effects of ischemic preconditioning for liver resection performed under inflow occlusion in humans. Ann Surg 232:155-162, 2000.

101. Sindram D, Rudiger HA, Upadhya AG, et al: Ischemic preconditioning protects against cold ischemic injury through an oxidative stress–dependent mechanism. J Hepatol 36:78-84, 2002.

102. Rudiger HA, Selzner N, Selzner M, Clavien PA: Sublethal oxidative stress protects against ischemic injury in the mouse liver: A new mechanism of ischemic preconditioning [abstract]. Hepatology 34:421A, 2001.

103. Peralta C, Closa D, Hotter G, et al: Liver ischemic preconditioning is mediated by the inhibitory action of nitric oxide on endothelin. Biochem Biophys Res Commun 229:264-270, 1996.

104. Peralta C, Hotter G, Closa D, et al: The protective role of adenosine in inducing nitric oxide synthesis in rat liver ischemia preconditioning is mediated by activation of adenosine A2 receptors. Hepatology 29:126-132, 1999.

105. Sawaya DE Jr, Brown M, Minardi A, et al: The role of ischemic preconditioning in the recruitment of rolling and adherent leukocytes in hepatic venules after ischemia/reperfusion. J Surg Res 85:163-170, 1999.

106. Nilsson B, Friman S, Wallin M, et al: The liver protective effect of ischemic preconditioning may be mediated by adenosine. Transpl Int 13(Suppl 1):S558-S561, 2000.

107. Ricciardi R, Schaffer BK, Kim RD, et al: Protective effects of ischemic preconditioning on the cold-preserved liver are tyrosine kinase dependent. Transplantation 72:406-412, 2001.

108. Kato H, Amersi F, Buelow R, et al: Heme oxygenase-1 overexpression protects rat livers from ischemia/reperfusion injury with extended cold preservation. Am J Transplant 1:121-128, 2001.

109. Redaelli CA, Tian YH, Schaffner T, et al: Extended preservation of rat liver graft by induction of heme oxygenase-1. Hepatology 35:1082-1092, 2002.

110. Adham M, Peyrol S, Chevallier M, et al: The isolated perfused porcine liver: Assessment of viability during and after six hours of perfusion. Transpl Int 10:299-311, 1997.

111. Butler AJ, Rees MA, Wight DG, et al: Successful extracorporeal porcine liver perfusion for 72 hr. Transplantation 73:1212-1218, 2002.

112. Schon MR, Kollmar O, Wolf S, et al: Liver transplantation after organ preservation with normothermic extracorporeal perfusion. Ann Surg 233:114-123, 2001.

113. Lockett CJ, Fuller BJ, Busza AL, Proctor E: Hypothermic perfusion preservation of liver: The role of phosphate in stimulating ATP synthesis studied by ^{31}P NMR. Transpl Int 8:440-445, 1995.

114. Kim JS, Boudjema K, D'Alessandro A, Southard JH: Machine perfusion of the liver: Maintenance of mitochondrial function after 48-hour preservation. Transplant Proc 29:3452-3454, 1997.

115. Lanir A, Clouse ME, Lee RG: Liver preservation for transplant. Evaluation of hepatic energy metabolism by ^{31}P NMR. Transplantation 43:786-790, 1987.

116. Vajdova K, Smrekova R, Mislanova C, et al: Cold-preservation–induced sensitivity of rat hepatocyte function to rewarming injury and its prevention by short-term reperfusion. Hepatology 32:289-296, 2000.

117. St Peter SD, Imber CJ, Lopez I, et al: Extended preservation of non–heart-beating donor livers with normothermic machine perfusion. Br J Surg 89:609-616, 2002.

118. Imber CJ, St Peter SD, Lopez de Cenarruzabeitia I, et al: Advantages of normothermic perfusion over cold storage in liver preservation. Transplantation 73:701-709, 2002.

119. Brettschneider L, Daloze PM, Huguet C: The use of combined preservation techniques for extended storage of orthotopic liver homografts. Surg Gynecol Obstet 126:263, 1968.

120. Gores GJ, Kost LJ, LaRusso NF: The isolated perfused rat liver: Conceptual and practical considerations. Hepatology 6:511-517, 1986.

121. Starnes HF Jr, Tewari A, Flokas K, et al: Effectiveness of a purified human hemoglobin as a blood substitute in the perfused rat liver. Gastroenterology 101:1345-1353, 1991.

122. Motoyama S, Minamiya Y, Saito S, et al: Hydrogen peroxide derived from hepatocytes induces sinusoidal endothelial cell apoptosis in perfused hypoxic rat liver. Gastroenterology 114:153-163, 1998.

123. Pries JM, Staples AB, Hanson RF: The effect of hepatic blood flow on taurocholate extraction by the isolated perfused rat liver. J Lab Clin Med 97:412-417, 1981.

124. Pegg DE, Foreman J, Rolles K: Metabolism during preservation and viability of ischemically injured canine kidneys. Transplantation 38:78-81, 1984.

125. Neuhaus R, Blumhardt G: Applications of an improved model for experimental studies of the liver. Int J Artif Organs 16:729-739, 1993.

126. Schon MR, Puhl G, Frank J, Neuhaus P: Hemodialysis improves results of pig liver perfusion after warm ischemic injury. Transplant Proc 25:3239-3243, 1993.

127. Schon MR, Puhl G, Gerlach J, et al: Hepatocyte isolation from pig livers after warm ischaemic injury. Transpl Int 7(Suppl 1):S159-S162, 1994.

The Recipient Hepatectomy and Grafting

GORAN B. KLINTMALM
RONALD W. BUSUTTIL

Classic technique   576

Portal vein   582

Piggyback technique   583

Hepatic artery   584

Bile duct   585

Summary   587

According to conventional clinical and surgical standards of the early 1960s, removal of a diseased liver and replacing it with a working, undamaged one was a concept that, although visionary and sound, had a low probability of being successfully executed. Only because of the technical brilliance and stubborn perseverance of Thomas E. Starzl did the experiment continue and slowly develop into the refined surgical procedure that we know today. To perform liver replacement in an environment of unsophisticated hemodynamic monitoring, slow turnaround of biochemical and coagulation monitoring profiles, inadequate blood component replacement therapy, and crude surgical instruments that did not even include atraumatic needles is almost beyond comprehension. During the last $1\frac{1}{2}$ years of Starzl's liver transplant program at Colorado General Hospital (1979 to 1980) in Denver, the fastest procedure took $14\frac{1}{2}$ hours, and only cases lasting longer than 20 hours were considered poor from a technical point of view. The preoperative blood order for type and cross-match for 15 U of packed cells was designated for opening the abdomen, during which time the blood bank would have the opportunity to cross-match and supply more blood for the remainder of the case.

Since these pioneering times, innumerable improvements have been made, each one making a small contribution that, as a whole, has transformed today's liver transplant procedure into an evolutionary descendant that barely resembles its ancestor. Of the factors that have done the most to develop liver transplantation from an experimental undertaking to a therapeutic procedure, we first list the development of anesthesia, including central hemodynamic monitoring and coagulation control. We believe that anesthesiologists are the unsung heroes of this operation, and they deserve much credit. Second, the introduction of electrocautery, the argon beam coagulator, and new hemostatic agents created not only a safe technique of controlled coagulation of bleeding areas but also a more sophisticated technique of dissection. Today, the entire dissection is performed with electrocautery in a coagulation mode, most commonly directly by the surgeon or by the assistant cauterizing on the surgeon's dissecting tonsil clamp. Whereas suture ligation was used for all vessels during the recipient hepatectomy, it is now reserved for only major vascular and tissue structures. Third, the introduction of venovenous bypass and its early implementation in the operation have provided a certain equanimity to the conduct of the operation, thereby providing a more suitable atmosphere for the education of liver transplant trainees. A fourth advancement is an adaptable technique of using either the classic orthotopic procedure or the caval-sparing transplant (piggyback). Fifth, the use of modern mechanical retractors permits an unrestricted, nontiring visualization of the field, which allows the procedure to be performed with only two assistants. In Denver, fellows and residents hanging for dear life onto the retractors were rotated every 2 to 4 hours or until they dropped to give the best possible exposure. Nonetheless, most adult patients required a thoracotomy to allow access to the suprahepatic vena cava, a procedure that is now virtually *never* used.

Liver transplantation today is performed principally with two different techniques: the classic technique with vena cava interposition and a piggyback technique[1] that leaves the native cava behind. Venovenous bypass is not mandatory with either one. Until 1983, liver transplantation was performed by what we now call the classic technique, which is when Starzl and coworkers developed the bypass.[2] The bypass maintains cardiovascular stability and normal hemodynamics to a degree that caval-side occlusion is unable to do; it requires fewer intraoperative fluid transfusions and results in a diminished frequency of reperfusion syndrome and a less edematous posttransplant patient. The most important indication for the piggyback technique may be cases in which a small donor liver with a narrow cava is to be transplanted into a large recipient in whom the narrow donor cava causes clinically significant stenosis. Another important advantage of the piggyback technique is in difficult retransplantation, when the vena cava is embedded in an inflamed retroperitoneum.

For a technically adroit surgeon, surgical time and blood loss with the piggyback technique may approach that of the classic technique with the use of venovenous bypass. In a regular transplant procedure using the classic technique, we expect the patient to be anhepatic on bypass for 50 to 60 minutes. Of note, both authors of this chapter routinely use the classic technique in the vast majority of transplants.

Classic Technique

After the patient has been carefully positioned on the table, prepared, and draped, the abdomen is opened via a bilateral subcostal incision with midline extension (Fig. 39–1), so appropriately named the Mercedes incision by Sir Roy Calne. Except for the superficial skin incision, the skin, subcutaneous tissue, and muscle layers are opened with the electrocautery unit. The right-sided incision is extended far enough laterally to allow a horizontal view into the vena cava. The left-sided incision is shorter and extends beyond the lateral border of the rectus. If splenomegaly is present, care should be taken to avoid making this incision very long because the spleen is then easily injured, which could possibly cause serious bleeding and necessitate an otherwise unnecessary splenectomy. The midline incision is extended to the point at which the surgeon has a direct perpendicular view of the suprahepatic vena cava;

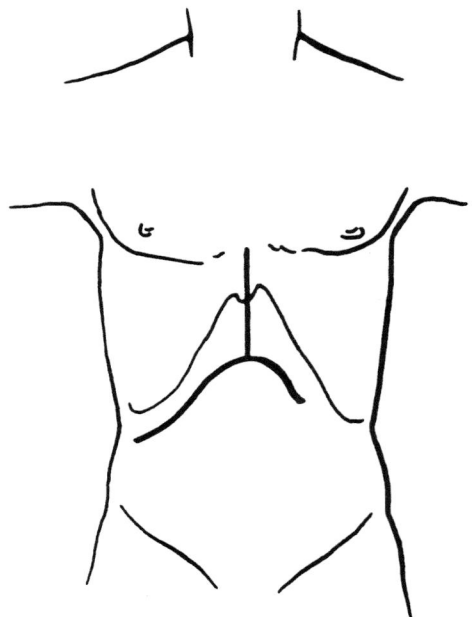

FIGURE 39–1

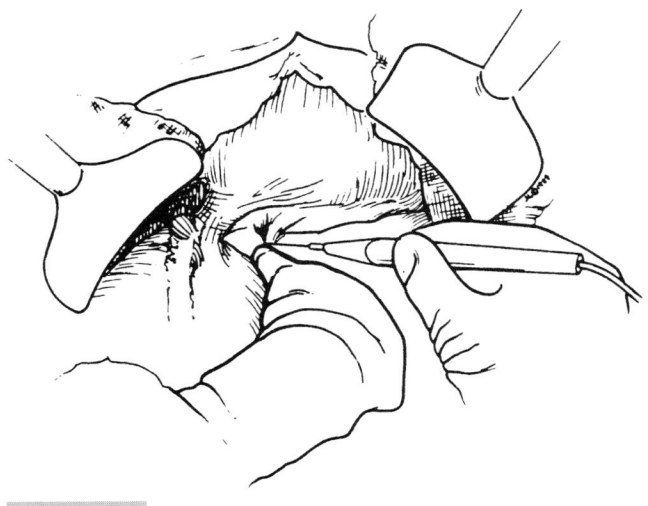

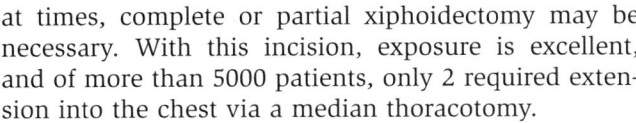

FIGURE 39-2

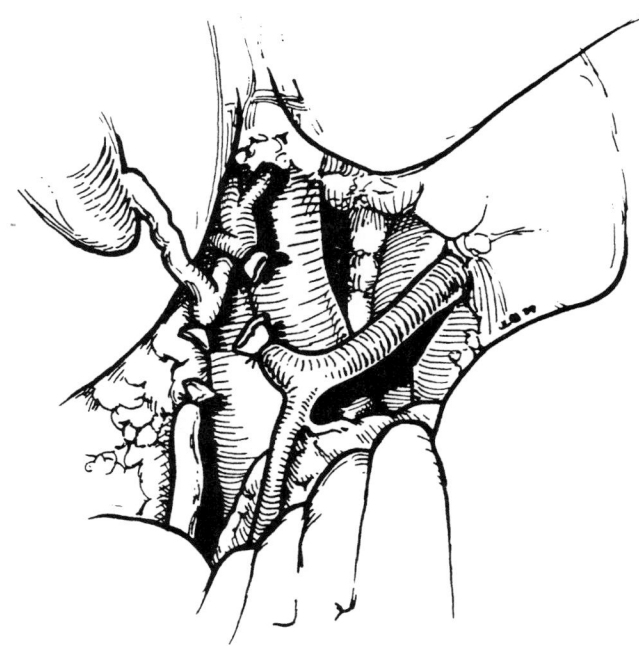

FIGURE 39-3

at times, complete or partial xiphoidectomy may be necessary. With this incision, exposure is excellent, and of more than 5000 patients, only 2 required extension into the chest via a median thoracotomy.

A mechanical retractor is placed with the blades under both costal margins to pull the rib cage laterally and anteriorly to spread the aperture (Fig. 39–2). The falciform ligament is divided, and the tissue with all the collaterals along the falciform ligament and the midline fascia are removed up to the xiphoid, thereby totally preventing further collateral bleeding and obstruction of the field from the tissue mass itself. The fatty tissue below the upper midline extension often contains large collaterals from the umbilical vein that should be controlled with ligatures and entirely removed, which is done without blood loss if the correct tissue plane is found. A ligature placed on the round ligament, when left long and "draped" over the retractor ring, can serve as excellent exposure to the porta hepatis.

The falciform ligament is divided all the way down to the suprahepatic vena cava, and the left triangular ligament is then opened with the cautery. Frequently, collateral veins are present at the very tip of the left lateral segment that require ligature for hemostasis. The left lateral segment is then retracted up out of the wound and to the right. The gastrohepatic ligament is now visualized and requires either cautery division or suture ligation, depending on the extent of the collateral vessels. Obviously, if an accessory left hepatic artery is present, it must be ligated and divided.

The anteroinferior edge of the liver or the ligated round ligament is now lifted up by an assistant to allow an unobstructed view of the porta hepatis (Fig. 39–3).

The dissection is carried down to the hepatic artery, which is then divided above its bifurcation. Before division we find it helpful to isolate the common hepatic and gastroduodenal arteries. This maneuver virtually eliminates initial dissection of the hepatic artery. We then proceed to the right side of the porta hepatis and divide the common duct. Normally, it is unnecessary to divide the cystic duct separately; however, division above the cystic duct entrance can easily be accomplished when necessary to preserve sufficient length of the common duct. In more than 95% of patients with an accessory right hepatic artery, it traverses posterior to the common bile duct and is divided when present. We then complete the dissection around the portal vein. In many cases, the dorsal pancreatic vein drains into the anterior portion of the portal vein and must be divided and ligated.

If adhesions to the liver are present after previous operations or from spontaneous bacterial peritonitis, they are taken down with electrocautery. The tip of the electrocautery is run parallel to the liver surface at all times, never venturing more than 1 mm from the liver surface but never violating the liver capsule. The liver is to be "shaved." In cases in which the liver is encased in adhesions, it is often easier to commence with dissection of the lateral aspects of the right lobe followed by dissection of the stomach and duodenum from segments II and III before venturing into the porta hepatis.

In an uncomplicated case, we now proceed to dissect the right triangular ligament (Fig. 39–4).

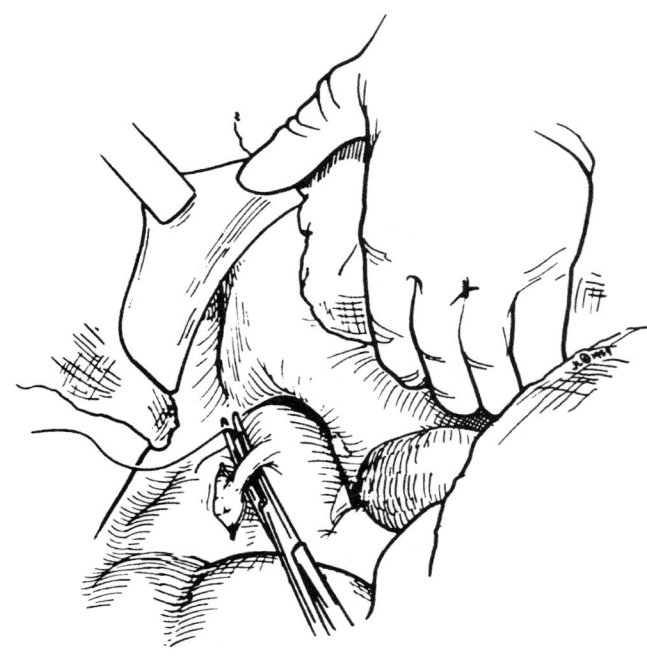

FIGURE 39–4

#96530-015). We use wire-reinforced cannulas, 15-French for the femoral vein. Forced cannulation is contraindicated. The position of the wire is easily checked by palpation of the infrahepatic vena cava. The return cannula is inserted by the anesthesia team into the right intrajugular vein by using a 12-French wire-reinforced cannula (Medtronic, catalog #0J67R2) with a pediatric arterial kit (Argon Medical, catalog #401135B). This cannula is always inserted when the patient has been intubated before preparing the abdomen. An alternative option is to cut down directly on the axillary vein (usually the left) and the left saphenofemoral junction and then insert 20- and 18-French cannulas, respectively.

Once the cannulas have been introduced and secured, we proceed to final dissection of the portal vein. The portal vein is secured with the left hand and cleaned with scissors by simply pushing the tissue away longitudinally along the vein (Fig. 39–5A). The portal vein is then clamped as high in the hilum as possible and divided. Three Munyon (tonsil) clamps are attached to the end of the portal vein and held straight up by the assistants. A surgeon who controls the portal vein with the left hand introduces the 28- to 36-French wire-reinforced cannula (Edwards Lifesciences) with

This dissection is performed completely with cautery, beginning at the lateral inferior aspect and dividing the ligament carefully all the way into the vena cava. If there are technical problems with an unusual amount of collaterals, scarring, and inflammation, this part of the procedure is deferred until after the patient is maintained on total venovenous bypass. With the portal vein transected, the anterior aspect of the infrahepatic inferior vena cava (IVC) is exposed to allow easy circumferential mobilization for placement of a vascular clamp. If the portal vein is not transected at this point, the vena cava is dissected in an inferior-to-superior direction with a dissecting tonsil clamp and cautery. The right adrenal vein is ligated and divided. At this time we allow the right lobe to fall back into the hepatic fossa and expose the left side of the vena cava by retracting the left lateral segment and the caudate lobe to the right. The peritoneal reflection is opened longitudinally along the vena cava with cautery. In most cases, the retrohepatic caval tissue can be taken down with finger dissection. Any resistance to such dissection usually signifies retrohepatic collaterals entering the vena cava, which requires ligation. With this dual-sided approach, the posterior aspect of the retrohepatic cava can be quickly and safely liberated from the retroperitoneum.

At this juncture, the patient is prepared for venovenous bypass by cannulation of the femoral vein. Cannulation is performed via the Seldinger technique in the groin by using a pre-made kit (Medtronic, catalog

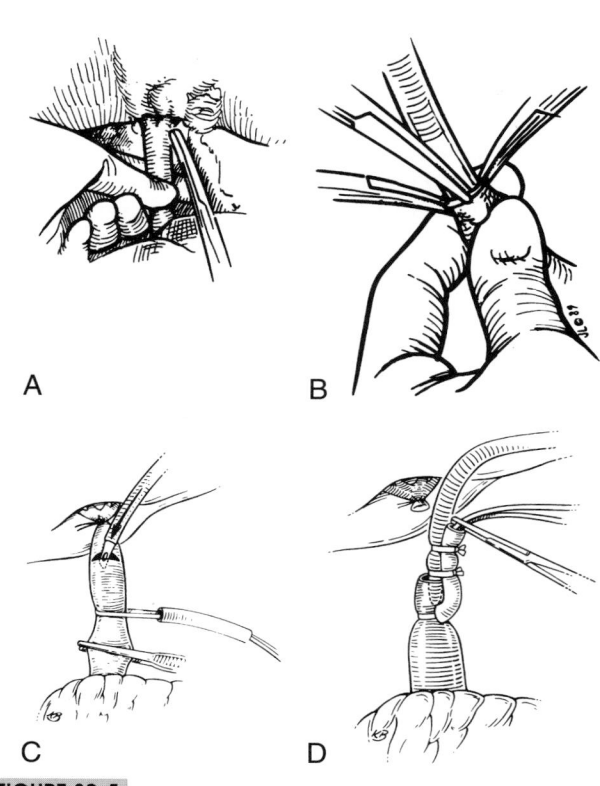

A

B

C

D

FIGURE 39–5

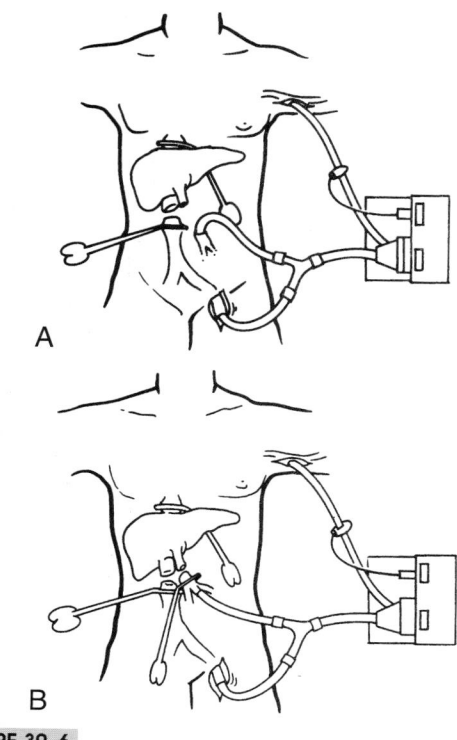

A

B

FIGURE 39–6

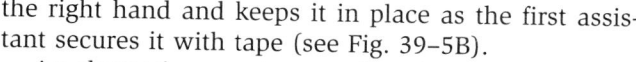

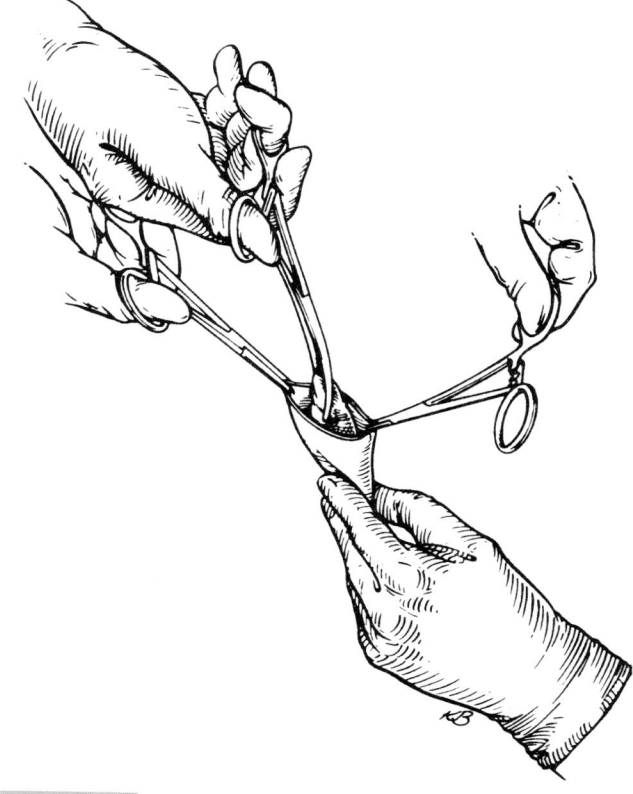

FIGURE 39–7

the right hand and keeps it in place as the first assistant secures it with tape (see Fig. 39–5B).

An alternative way to cannulate the portal vein is to ligate the portal vein up in the hilum and, after placing tape around the portal vein to control the vein where it emerges from the neck of the pancreas, make a transverse cut in the distal end of the portal vein to allow the portal vein cannula to be introduced (see Fig. 39–5C). The cannula is secured with tape and tied down, thereby completing the portal vein cannulation, and the transverse incision of the portal vein is now completed to divide the portal vein in its entirety (see Fig. 39–5D).

Venovenous bypass is now started (Fig. 39–6A). The entire cannulization process for venovenous bypass usually requires 10 minutes.

In cases in which the portal vein is injured or, even more important, when dense adhesions with large collateral veins are surrounding the liver, the inferior mesenteric vein can be used for bypass purposes. For the inferior mesenteric vein a no. 20 cannula is usually sufficient and needs to be introduced only 2 to 3 cm. If it is advanced further, the tip often goes out into the portal vein and makes portal vein clamping very difficult later (see Fig. 39–6B).

In patients with organized portal vein thrombus, a formal thrombendvenectomy can be performed in the majority of situations to remove thrombus all the way down into the superior mesenteric vein under manual

control (Fig. 39–7). In patients with portal vein thrombosis, partial or complete, utmost care should be taken to avoid any further traumatization of the portal vein. In cases in which avoidance of further trauma is impossible, portal vein venous conduits need to be used to ensure portal venous inflow to the liver (Fig. 39–8). Patients with extensive portal vein repairs or conduits are administered low-molecular-weight dextran at 25 mL/hr for 1 or 2 days and then acetylsalicylic acid, 81 mg/day, for 3 months.

Vascular clamps are now placed on the suprahepatic vena cava and the lower infrahepatic vena cava (Fig. 39–9). Care should be taken to place these clamps horizontally and with the liver in its normal anatomical position to prevent rotation of the vessels. The suprahepatic vena cava clamp should be placed on the very edge of the diaphragmatic reflection to avoid phrenic nerve injuries.

We now divide the vena cava while taking care to retain as much of the right and left hepatic veins as possible and pull the veins up by almost cutting into the liver substance (Fig. 39–10). The lower cava is then divided as far proximal as possible. The previously ligated retrocaval tissue is divided and the liver removed.

To achieve hemostasis in the hepatic fossa, the bare area can be reperitonealized, as shown in the inset of

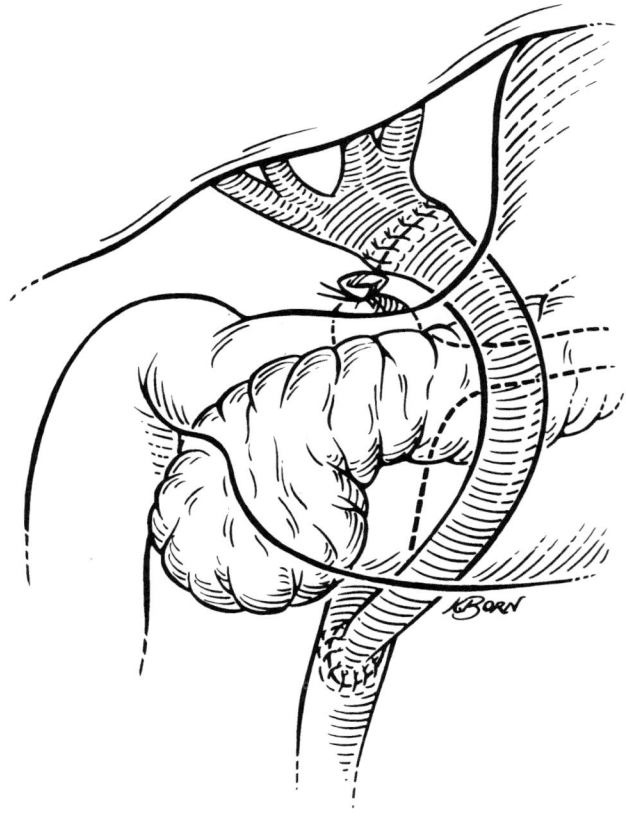

FIGURE 39–8

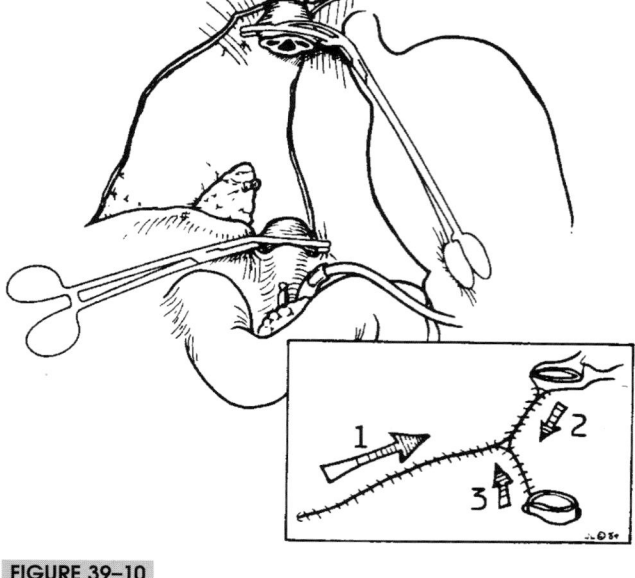

FIGURE 39–10

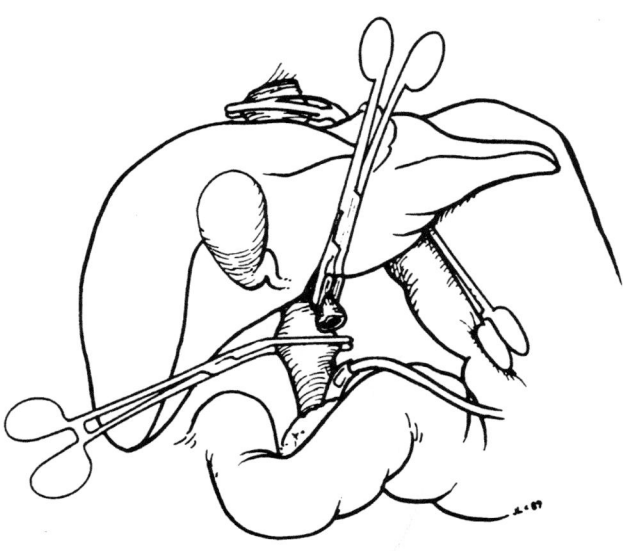

FIGURE 39–9

Figure 39–10. With the use of 3–0 or 2–0 Prolene (monofilament polypropylene suture, Ethicon, Somerville, NJ), the bare area is sutured in the direction of the arrows and back to the starting point, as numbered 1, 2, and 3. Care should be taken to ensure that the needle passes superficially under the bottom of the entire wound to obtain hemostatic control.

In patients with difficult dissections, the vena cava can be clamped above and below the liver before all the right-sided and retrohepatic dissection is performed (Fig. 39–11A). The dissection can now be concluded quickly (see Fig. 39–11B). In such cases, it is often expedient to retain the dorsal side of the vena cava to eliminate the need for elaborate hemostatic control of the retrocaval tissue.

The suprahepatic vena cava is now prepared by opening the right and left hepatic veins into a common cloaca of the IVC (Fig. 39–12). All phrenic vein ostia are oversewn with 4–0 Prolene and the knots placed outside the suprahepatic vena cava cuff. The liver is now brought into the wound. By placing a lap in the hepatic fossa, the liver receives support from below to prevent it from sinking down too far into the wound.

Corner stitches are placed on the two opposing ends (Fig. 39–13A), and a stay suture may be placed in the middle for retraction of the posterior wall. The suprahepatic vena cava anastomosis is performed with 3–0 Prolene; care is taken to ensure perfect intimal adaptation. The dorsal suture is run to the right-sided stay suture and just one bite beyond and anterior to it.

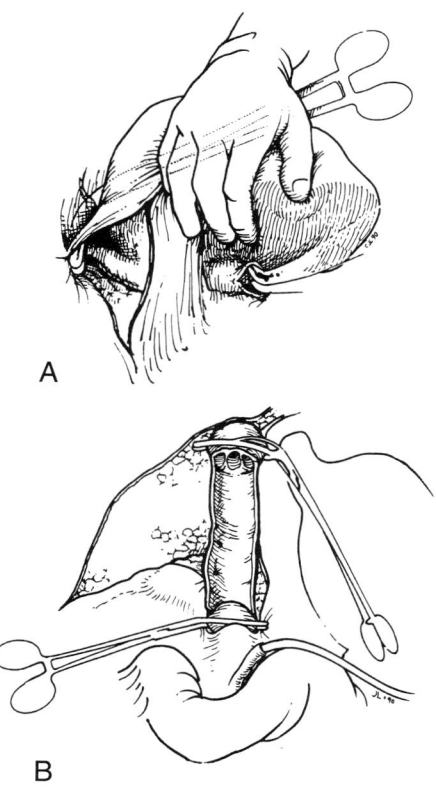

A

B

FIGURE 39–11

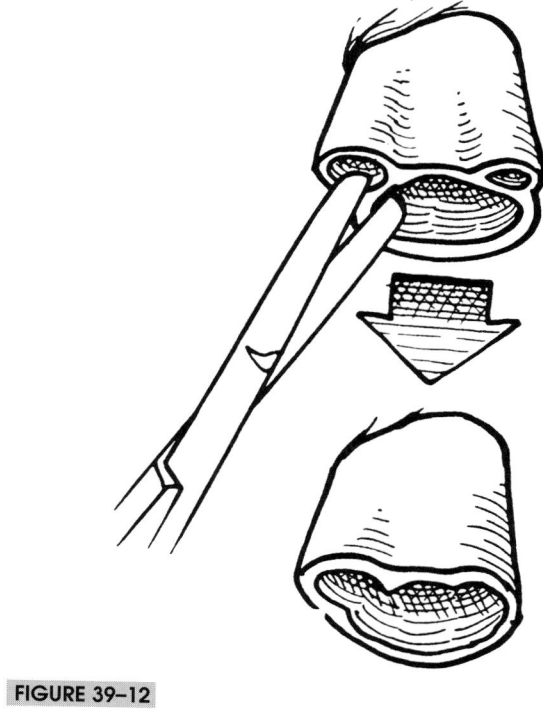

FIGURE 39–12

The midline stay suture is removed, and the front wall closure is completed in a simple running suture fashion.

When the anastomosis is finished, a 1- to 1.5-cm "growth factor" is tied in. The lateral stay suture is tied down securely to prevent the anastomosis from separating as the growth factor is taken up by expansion of the vessel at the time of reperfusion (see Fig. 39–13B).

A portal flush with normal saline or lactated Ringer's solution and 25 g of albumin per liter is run through the portal vein during the completion of the infrahepatic vena cava (Fig. 39–14). Such flushing is needed to empty the graft of air to prevent air emboli, as well as to remove the excessively high concentrations of intravascular potassium left from the preservation solution. When the organ is cooled down for preservation, the sodium-potassium pump is stopped to allow the high concentration of intracellular potassium to leak out into the vascular space. The infrahepatic vena cava is sewn in exactly the same manner as used for the suprahepatic vena cava, usually with 4–0 Prolene, and a 1.5-cm growth factor is included.

Care must be taken to prevent too long a vena cava. Excessive length of vena cava is the main cause of folding, and kinking can cause formidable postoperative

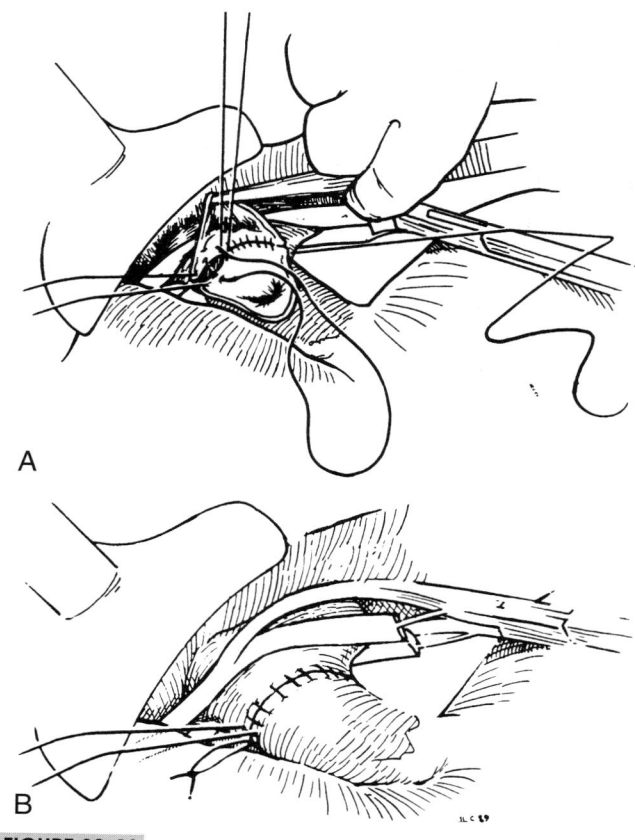

A

B

FIGURE 39–13

problems that require extraordinarily difficult reconstructions at a later stage.

Portal Vein

The portal bypass cannula is now clamped, and only the systemic venovenous bypass is continued. The cannula is removed from the portal vein, and an atraumatic clamp is carefully placed proximally on the portal vein (Fig. 39–15). The donor portal vein is now shortened to the appropriate length. One should not cut the recipient portal vein shorter than 1 cm because length should be conserved in the event that retransplantation becomes necessary. As with the vena cava, this is extraordinarily important to prevent portal vein kinking, folding, and flow obstruction. The portal vein is sutured with running 6–0 Prolene, and the inverting stitch in the back wall also includes a growth factor that is three quarters of the portal vein diameter. If size must be adjusted to either the donor or the recipient portal vein, a fish mouth reconstruction is recommended. There are several methods to reperfuse the liver after portal venous reconstruction: (1) reperfusion through the portal vein with or without vena cava venting, (2) opening of the IVC followed by portal vein reperfusion, and (3) reperfusion through the portal vein and hepatic artery simultaneously. To date, no randomized trial has conferred superiority to any of these methods. Furthermore, a randomized trial conducted at the University of California at Los Angeles (UCLA) has shown that venting through the vena cava before portal vein reperfusion does not result in a lower incidence or decreased severity of reperfusion syndrome. It is our preference to release the portal vein clamp slowly with an eye on the electrocardiogram to monitor the procedure. We usually open the portal vein in stages after any T-wave segment elevations have reversed. Once these elevations have normalized, the portal vein is completely opened. It usually takes three or four partial decompressions before the vein is completely open.

After making sure that there is no significant bleeding from the vena cava, portal vein, or its anastomoses, the systemic bypass is discontinued and the cannula removed from the groin to allow blood in the bypass system to be reinfused into the patient. When the portal vein is unusable, which is extremely rare because of the increased application of thrombendvenectomy, a portal venous conduit is used (see Fig. 39–8). In such cases, arterial reconstruction and reperfusion of the liver are performed before the portal conduit is sewn in. For the portal venous conduit, a donor iliac vein is perfect material. The superior mesenteric vein (SMV) is most commonly used for inflow and is accessed at the base of the colon mesenterium. After the SMV has been

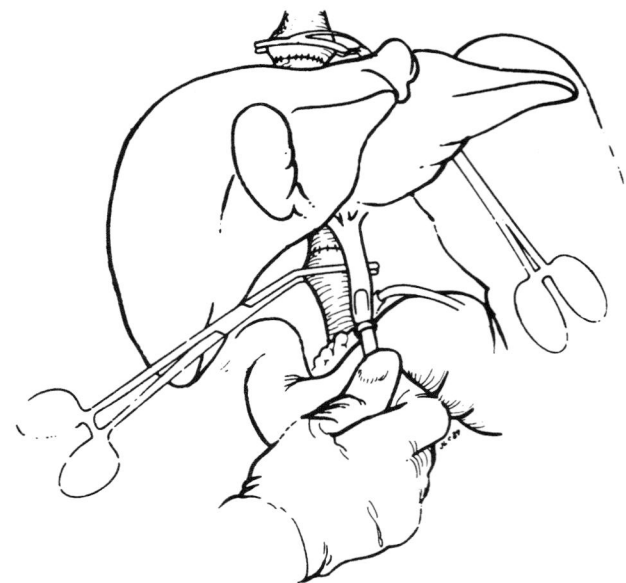

FIGURE 39–14

identified and side-occluded, the venous conduit, which should have already been anastomosed to the donor portal vein and pulled behind the stomach in front of the pancreas through a tunnel in the colon mesenterium toward the SMV, should now be anastomosed with running 6–0 Prolene. It should be pointed out that when the side-occluding clamp on the SMV is released, there *must* be an outflow already established from the venous conduit. Otherwise, the anastomosis line may rupture completely and cause an immediate

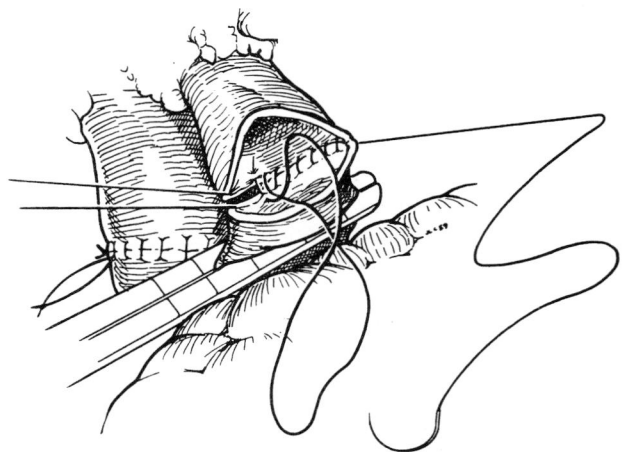

FIGURE 39–15

catastrophe. Sometimes, large collateral veins can be found in the subhepatic area, either along the minor curvature of the stomach or as a collateral to the liver, that can be used for the donor portal vein anastomosis instead of a mesenteric venous conduit.

Piggyback Technique

With the falciform, gastrohepatic, and left and right triangular ligaments taken down, the hepatic hilum is dissected out and the hepatic artery, common duct, and portal vein are divided. If necessary, we proceed to venovenous bypass or perform an end-to-side portocaval shunt. The portal vein is rotated slightly counterclockwise, which makes it reach down comfortably. The anastomosis is sewn with running 5–0 monofilament suture (Fig. 39–16). With the inferior liver surface completely exposed, the dissection is continued in the plane between the cava and the liver. We use titanium surgical clips for small retrohepatic veins (Fig. 39–17). Veins larger than 3 to 4 mm are ligated with silk. Once the liver is removed, all clips and ligatures are secured by 3–0 or 4–0 silk sutures. The right hepatic vein is clamped, divided, and oversewn. The left and middle veins are clamped and divided to allow the liver to be removed from the wound. When dividing the right,

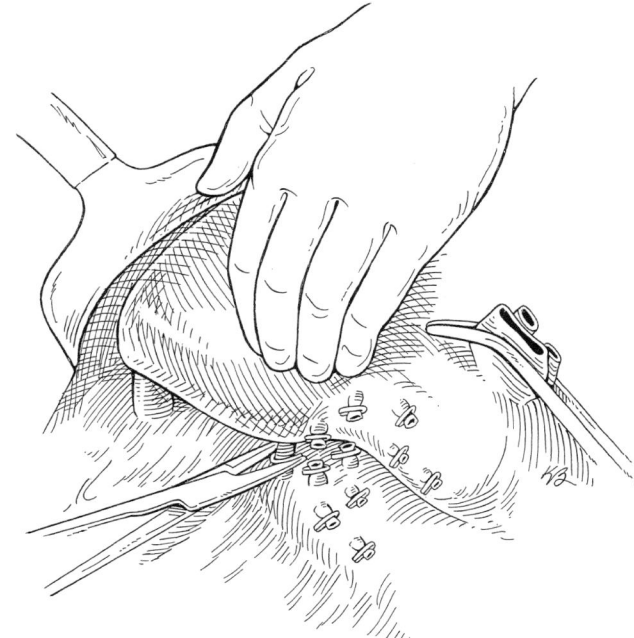

FIGURE 39-17

middle, and left hepatic veins, we divide them as far into the liver as practical. The most expeditious way to clamp the hepatic veins is to side-occlude the vena cava with a Salinsky clamp (Fig. 39–18). Depending on the anatomy, we connect the hepatic veins into a common cloaca and extend the cava incision distally 3 to 4 cm. At this time the donor liver is brought into

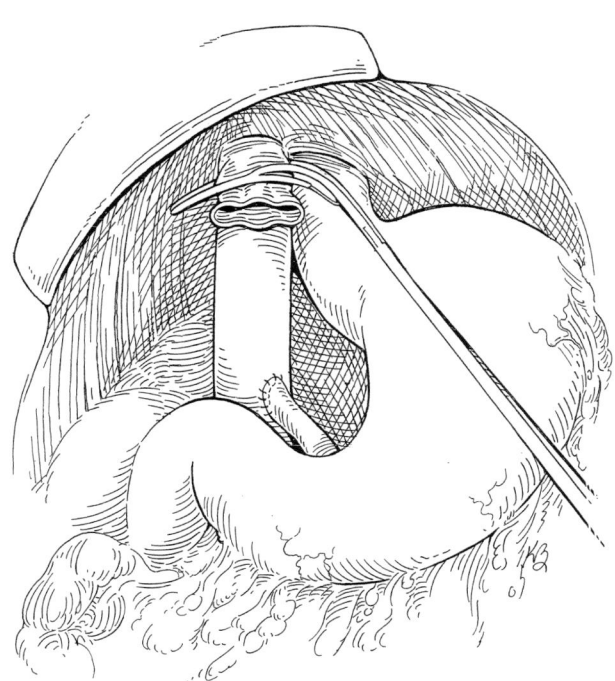

FIGURE 39-16

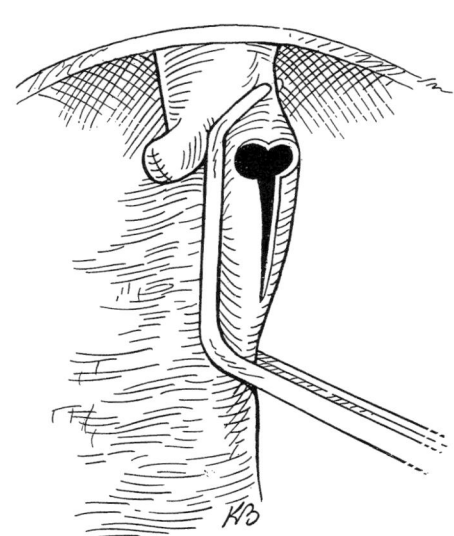

FIGURE 39-18

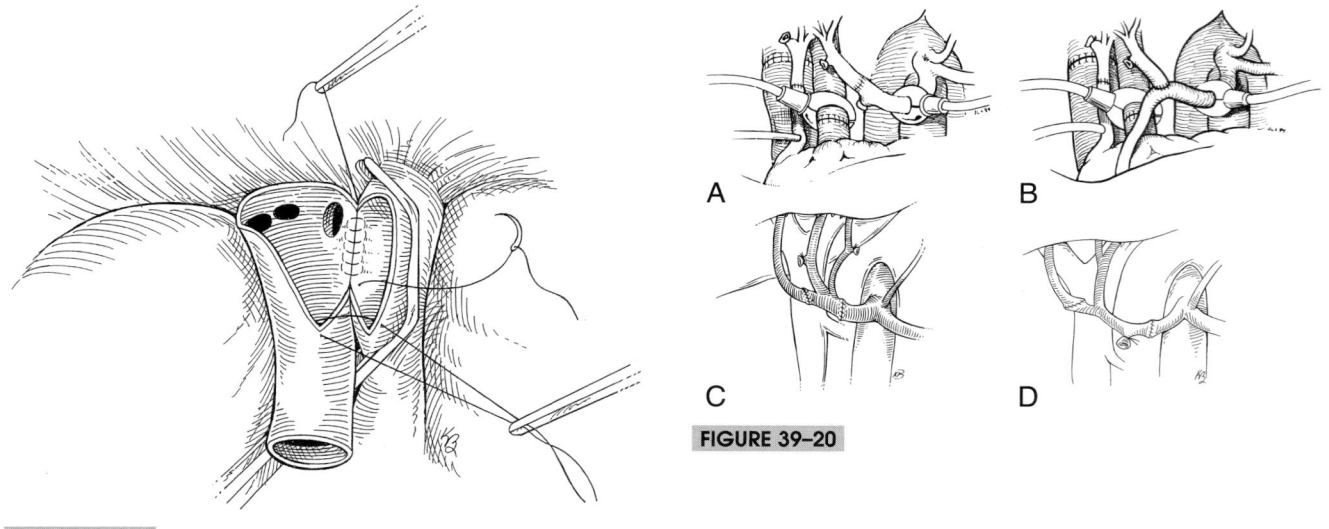

FIGURE 39–19

FIGURE 39–20

the field. The donor cava is cut down longitudinally in the back 3 to 4 cm from the proximal cava to create two corresponding orifices. Great care should be taken to ensure that the anterior wall of the donor cava is long enough to attach to the recipient hepatic veins. If there is any tendency for stretching of the donor hepatic veins in the anastomosis, a Budd-Chiari–type syndrome may result that is very difficult to correct.

The large anastomosis is sewn with 3–0 or 4–0 monofilament suture. It is easily done by placing the right lobe down into the hepatic fossa and lifting the left lobe up to expose the two cavas. A stitch at each end of the anastomosis (cranial, caudal) makes it easy to outline the suture line for completion. We then sew the right side of the anastomosis from the inside in a running fashion and complete it on the left side with an outside approach (Fig. 39–19).

At this point, the portal vein reconstruction is performed in normal fashion (see earlier). For reperfusion, we usually begin by opening the portal vein and flushing air and intravascular high-potassium fluid out of the liver through the open end of the distal portion of the donor cava. The distal end, controlled by two stay sutures, is clamped when the flush seems adequate.

At this time, the recipient cava clamp is opened to establish normal venous return. The distal end of the donor cava is oversewn with running 4–0 monofilament suture.

Hepatic Artery

Successful hepatic artery reconstruction is crucial for graft function, and a variety of methods can be used.

In principle, the type of reconstruction with regard to specific recipient and donor arteries is secondary to achieving excellent inflow and outflow at the first anastomosis. In routine cases, a Carrel patch of donor aorta or the artery is anastomosed end to end to the recipient common hepatic artery or to a branch patch of the bifurcation between the gastroduodenal and the hepatic artery proper (Fig. 39–20A). The arterial anastomosis is sewn with 6–0 or 7–0 Prolene, and a one-half-diameter growth factor is tied in place to provide full expansion of the arterial anastomosis without any constriction. If the gastroduodenal artery is large, as could occur if it is providing significant vascular supply or if stenosis of the celiac artery is present, it is left untouched. The donor celiac artery is then sewn end to side (see Fig. 39–20B). When performing end-to-side anastomoses, no growth factor is tied in. Instead, the corner stay suture is tied, the arteries are unclamped, and after the anastomosis has settled down to a comfortable size, the running suture is tied carefully so that the anastomosis is not pulled up and constricted. In donor livers with an accessory right hepatic artery, the artery is divided, and a Carrel patch is fashioned from the superior mesenteric artery (SMA) and then sewn to the donor splenic artery stump with 6–0 Prolene (see Fig. 39–20C). Today, we tend to complete the reconstruction of the replaced right hepatic artery *after* reperfusion and sew the replaced right hepatic artery end to end to the donor gastroduodenal artery with interrupted 7–0 monofilament sutures (see Fig. 39–20D). The reason for this sequence is to prevent the almost invariable malrotation of the replaced right hepatic artery that can occur if the reconstruction is performed on the back-table.

In some patients, despite a perfect technical result, inflow is inadequate because of compression of the celiac axis by the arcuate ligament. This complication is demonstrated by marked respiratory variation and can be documented by flow measurement. In this situation, the celiac artery must be dissected proximal to the aorta and the arcuate ligament cut. The illustrations (see Fig. 39–20A and B) also show the electrodynamic flow probes (Cliniflow II, Carolina Medical Electronics, King, NC) used to ensure that adequate revascularization has been achieved by measuring flow rates at the end of the procedure.

Arterial reconstruction varies greatly depending on the particular circumstances of each patient. Quite frequently in the case of dual blood supply to the liver from an accessory right hepatic artery and a hepatic artery proper, the accessory right hepatic artery stemming from the SMA is dominant. In such cases, the donor celiac artery is anastomosed to the recipient accessory right hepatic artery. Usually, the donor hepatic artery lies most comfortably when pulled over in front of the portal vein down to the right side for the anastomosis (Fig. 39–21A). When the recipient hepatic artery is insufficient, the donor celiac artery can be anastomosed directly to the supraceliac recipient aorta. This approach to the aorta is more commonly performed for pediatric transplants than for adult transplants (see Fig. 39–21B). When there is no acceptable common hepatic artery or right hepatic artery to which the donor celiac artery can be anastomosed, a donor iliac artery conduit is used. This procedure is performed by exposing the infrarenal aorta just above the inferior mesenteric artery. After the aorta is side-occluded, the iliac arterial conduit is sewn end to side with 5–0 Prolene. The conduit is then tunneled through the transverse mesocolon and pulled behind the stomach in front of the pancreas and up toward the liver hilum, where it is anastomosed end to end to the donor celiac artery with 6–0 Prolene. By sewing the arterial conduit to the aorta before it is attached to the donor celiac artery, the conduit is completely mobile and access for completion of the anastomosis is made easier (see Fig. 39–21C). When extensive scarring is found around the stomach or the pancreas, it is sometimes advantageous to curve the arterial conduit lateral to the pancreas after first mobilizing the duodenum. The attachment to the aorta is the same as for the shorter conduit, but after the aortal anastomosis is completed, the arterial conduit is pulled laterally—with care taken to not traumatize the pancreas—and up toward the hepatic hilum behind the duodenum (see Fig. 39–21D).

Bile Duct

After the gallbladder is removed, the common duct is shortened proximal to the cystic duct. Usually, a lap is placed superior to the liver to push the liver down to approximate the donor and recipient ducts better (Fig. 39–22). It is important to prevent redundancy of the bile duct because redundancy is an important cause of biliary obstruction in the postoperative period. The donor cystic duct, if allowed to remain to preserve common duct length, has to empty freely into the remaining common duct to prevent the development of cytoclesis, which can compress the duct and cause biliary obstruction and serious long-term consequences. If the cystic duct does not empty into the common duct, it has to be excised. The biliary anastomosis is sewn with interrupted or running 6–0 monofilament absorbable suture, PDS (polydioxanone, Ethicon, Somerville, NJ), or Maxon (polyglyconate, Davis & Geck, American Cyanamid Company, Wayne, NJ). Over the past 2 years, the UCLA group has been using a running technique for the biliary anastomosis with successful results. We have not used a T tube since 1997. For the first year we experienced some leaks; however, our current biliary complication rate is half of what it was previously with T tubes. A great advantage is the disappearance of duct obstruction from sphincter spasm and leaks when the T tube is pulled. If a T tube is used, it is brought out of the bile duct with a purse-string suture, as shown in Figure 39–22.

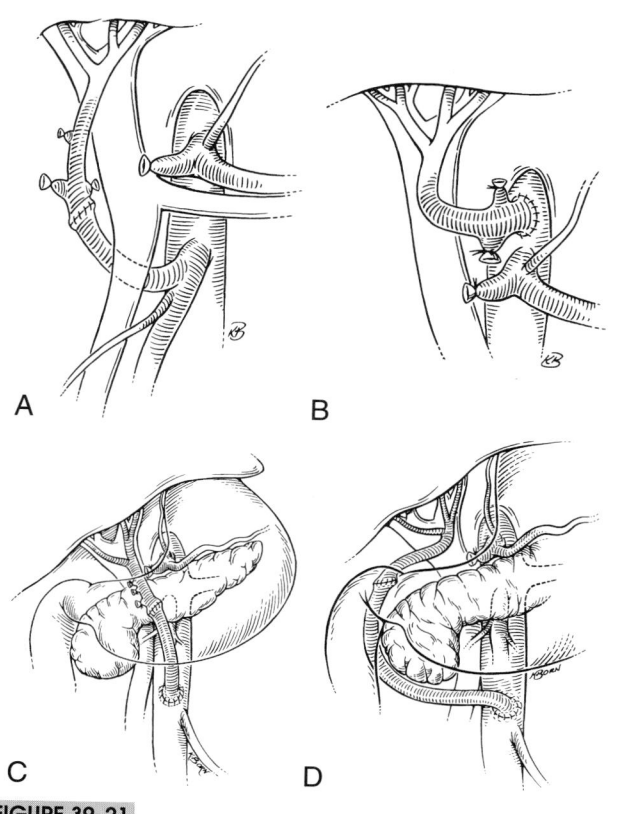

A

B

C

D

FIGURE 39–21

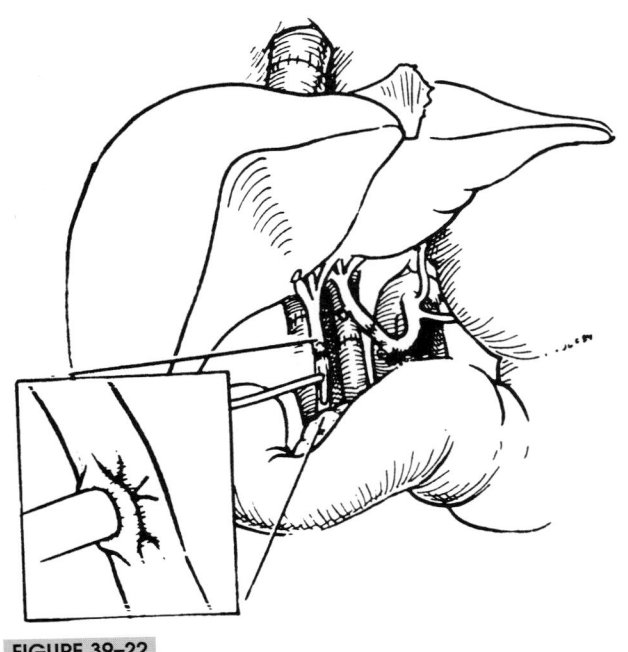

FIGURE 39–22

If there is any discrepancy in bile duct size (Fig. 39–23A) or if both donor and recipient ducts are of normal or small size, we prefer to side-cut the small one; if equal in size, we cut both sides (see Fig. 39–23B). With equally sized normal or small ducts, the side-cut is performed to compensate for the tissue that is effectively lost in the suture line and prevent a stricturing effect of the suture line. If one of the ducts,

usually the recipient, is excessively large, which is frequently seen in patients with previous cholecystectomies, a part of the large duct is closed with running or interrupted 6–0 Prolene suture; the duct opening is left large enough to accommodate the donor duct, which is then sewn in the usual fashion with interrupted 6–0 PDS suture (see Fig. 39–23C).

In patients with very small donor common ducts or with extraordinarily large biliary collateral veins, we prefer to perform a choledochojejunostomy. In patients with a thrombosed portal vein or Budd-Chiari syndrome, the huge venous collaterals that parallel the bile duct can cause excessive blood loss and make performance of the choledochocholedochostomy difficult because collateral veins can completely encase the common duct. Using a stapler, we divide the jejunum approximately 20 to 30 cm distal to the ligaments of Treitz and then construct a 40-cm defunctionalized Roux-en-Y limb (Fig. 39–24). The jejunostomy is sewn in two layers with Vicryl (polyglactin, Ethicon, Somerville, NJ) and silk, and the distal end of the stapled Roux-en-Y is oversewn with an extra layer of silk. In patients with sclerosing cholangitis, the Roux-en-Y is always brought retrocolic to permit colectomy in the later stage if necessary. We do not use biliary drains any more in patients with choledochojejunostomies, just as with T tubes. However, on occasion, when there is an indication for a biliary drain, we use a baby feeding tube. A very small hole is made distally on the antimesenteric side of the Roux-en-Y limb, and an infant feeding tube with a cut distal end is introduced from a separate hole proximal on the Roux-en-Y; the

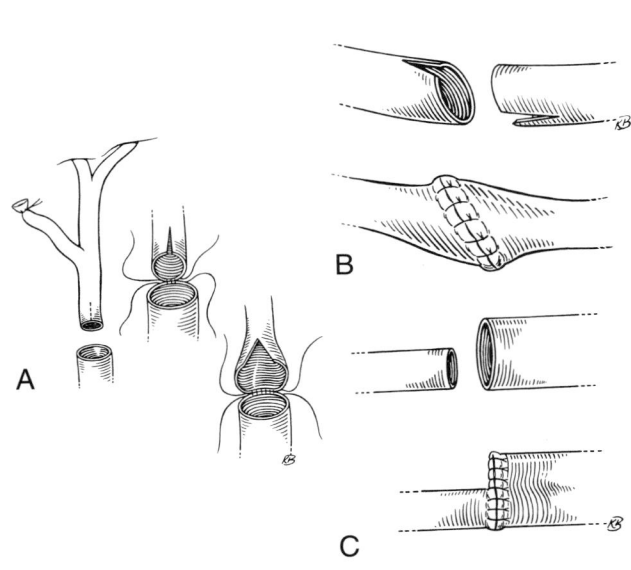

FIGURE 39–23

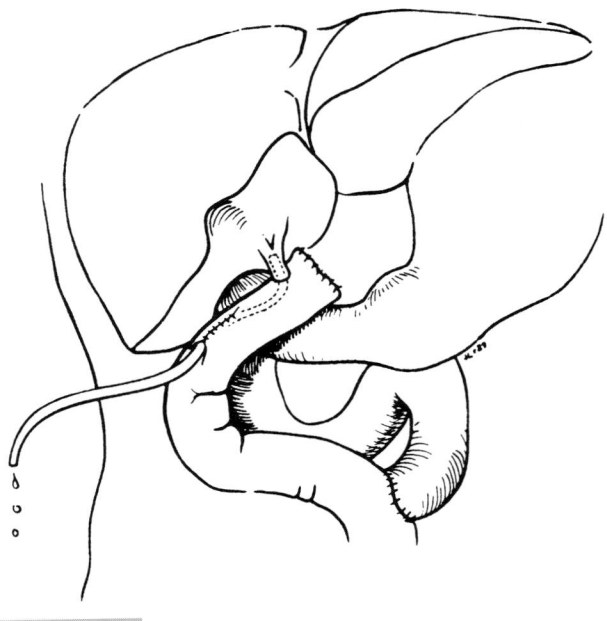

FIGURE 39–24

tube is tunneled in the submucosa before it goes intraluminal and into the bowel lumen and then passes through the anastomosis into the donor common duct. The choledochojejunostomy is sewn with interrupted 5-0 PDS. We noticed that in a few patients the use of 6-0 PDS resulted in early dehiscence by absorption of the suture. The feeding tube is secured in the anastomosis by a single chrome-cut stitch into the bowel mucosa wall and through the catheter to prevent it from coming out before the abdomen is even closed.

After the catheter has been brought out through the bowel lumen, a tunnel is created by oversewing the serosa via a Witzel technique for approximately 5 cm to prevent any leakage. The feeding tube is then brought out through a separate incision in the abdominal wall. The feeding tube is removed after 4 to 6 weeks. We have not experienced any leaks after having removed the feeding tube from the choledochojejunostomy. By placing the stent, we have good access and control of the bile duct in the postoperative period. An alternative to the external stent is an internal one created by placement of a small Silastic catheter, which is allowed to pass spontaneously into the bowel lumen.

Abdominal drains, which were once routine, are now used selectively. The Baylor group has noted fewer problems with fluid balance and serum albumin and no difference in wound infections in the absence of drains. Postoperative ascites is seen no more commonly now than previously.

Summary

The procedures as explained provide only the initial guidelines for the recipient hepatectomy and implantation of the graft. The secret of this operation, as for all surgery, is to have complete mastery of the anatomy to avoid wandering into places or structures where one is not supposed to be. Even the most minute, careless move can have a devastating impact on the outcome of liver transplantation. Nothing supplants experience and technical expertise for the final result. One cannot overemphasize the need for precise atraumatic dissection conducted with dispatch. A ponderous, hesitant technique invariably results in greater bleeding and more complications.

References

1. Tzakis A, Todo S, Starzl TE: Orthotopic liver transplantation with preservation of the inferior vena cava. Ann Surg 210:649-652, 1989.
2. Denmark SW, Shaw BW Jr, Starzl TE, Griffith BP: Veno-venous bypass without systemic anticoagulation in canine and human liver transplantation. Surg Forum 34:380-382, 1983.

Anesthesia for Liver Transplantation

MICHAEL A. E. RAMSAY

Preoperative assessment   590
   Central nervous system   590
   Cardiovascular system   591
   Pulmonary system   592
   Pulmonary hypertension   592
   Hepatopulmonary syndrome   594
   Renal function   594
   Hepatorenal syndrome   595
   Coagulation disorders   595
   Metabolic disorders   596
   Portal hypertension   597

Fulminant hepatic failure   597

Anesthesia care   598
   Donor management   598
   Recipient care   598

Intraoperative anesthesia   599
   Rapid infusion devices   599
   Thermal homeostasis   600

Anesthetic techniques   601

Three phases of orthotopic liver
   transplantation   601
   Preanhepatic phase   601
   Anhepatic phase   601
   Venovenous bypass   602
   Neohepatic phase   602

Fluid management   603

Postoperative care   603

Pediatric aspects   604

Liver transplantation is a very successful and effective treatment for many different disorders of the liver. Improved techniques in surgery, anesthetic management, donor organ procurement, preservation, immunosuppression, and perioperative care have resulted in many centers reporting a 1-year survival rate of nearly 90%. Increasing survival rates have led to the performance of a greater number of liver transplants and to broadened indications for transplantation. Lack of suitable donors is the current rate-limiting factor; however, increasing numbers of marginal donors are now being harvested and transplanted successfully. Many harvested liver grafts are surgically divided to supply two recipients. The impact on the anesthesiologist and the operating room team is that this surgery is again becoming an emergent procedure that keeps the cold ischemia time of the donor organ to a minimum. This timing causes the surgery to be performed frequently in the middle of the night when support teams may not be readily available. To meet the demand for organs and to address cultural reasons for the lack of a deceased donor organ supply, living donor procedures are increasing. The number of living donors providing right or left lobes of their livers for adult or pediatric recipients has escalated, which may complicate the logistics of the procedures because two anesthesia teams may need to be available at the same time. This scenario requires significant preparation and resources by the perioperative team.[1] The major disorders leading to transplantation are end-stage chronic liver disease, acute fulminant liver failure, primary liver malignancy, and certain liver-based metabolic disorders such as Wilson's disease and α_1-antitrypsin deficiency. In the latter category, the donor liver not only replaces a damaged organ but also provides a source for the missing enzyme or protein. The contraindications include active extrahepatic infections and extrahepatic malignancy. Transplantation for viral hepatitis, alcoholic liver disease, and neoplasm remains controversial because the original disease frequently recurs unless adjunct therapy is provided.[2-4]

The introduction of the MELD (Model for End-stage Liver Disease) scoring system and PELD (Pediatric [model] for End-stage Liver Disease) for the pediatric population has allowed organs to be transplanted based on medical urgency with a goal of reducing waiting list mortality.[5] The MELD score is based on three laboratory results: bilirubin and creatinine concentrations and INR (international normalized ratio). These laboratory values are predictive of 3-month mortality. These critically ill patients, often with multiple-organ failure and severe metabolic and coagulation disorders, present a significant challenge to the anesthesiologist.

The concept of a team approach to the care of the liver transplantation patient is an important factor in the development of a successful program. This approach starts with the preoperative selection and preparation of the patients and includes all facets of the perioperative care. Good communication among surgeon, hepatologist, pulmonologist, cardiologist, nephrologist, and anesthesiologist provides the basis for an optimal care team and a successful program.

Preoperative Assessment

Anesthesia management of the liver transplant recipient may involve taking into consideration a severely debilitated patient with multiple organ system malfunctions. There may be alterations in physiology and pharmacology, a severe coagulopathy, encephalopathy, cardiomyopathy, respiratory failure, massive abdominal ascites and pleural effusions, renal dysfunction, and severely deranged serum electrolytes, together with an emergent situation. The patient may have been admitted from home, having been evaluated months prior to the time the donor organ becomes available. The clinical status may have changed significantly from the time of initial evaluation until admission to hospital for the liver transplantation. An acute deterioration in the status of the patient may advance the patient on the waiting list to obtain the next available organ. Consequently, a careful preoperative assessment is necessary.

Significant portopulmonary hypertension may have developed in the months spent waiting the availability of an organ. The patient may have been admitted in fulminant liver failure and be in the intensive care unit (ICU). He or she may be comatose and require dialysis,

mechanical ventilation, and intracranial pressure (ICP) monitoring. The pathophysiology of end-stage liver disease may affect all major organ systems.

Central Nervous System

Cirrhosis of the liver is associated with varying degrees of encephalopathy. Mild encephalopathy has been found in up to 84% of patients with chronic liver failure.[6] Spectral electroencephalogram (EEG) analysis provides reliable quantitative information in the evaluation of subclinical encephalopathy.[7] The intraoperative use of the EEG can guide the management of anesthesia in this set of patients, who may be very sensitive to anesthetic agents. The pathogenesis of hepatic encephalopathy has been associated with increased gamma-aminobutyric acid (GABA) neurotransmission in the brain.[8] This GABA neurotransmission may be potentiated by benzodiazepine drugs such as diazepam; therefore, this group of agents should be avoided in patients with encephalopathy because hepatic coma may be precipitated.[9] The reversal agent flumazenil may improve the mental status of the hepatic encephalopathy patient.[10,11]

The patient in fulminant hepatic failure may develop deep coma, severe brain edema, and a marked increase in ICP. The anesthetic management of the comatose patient with raised ICP is greatly facilitated by the presence of an ICP monitor. However, because of the risk of bleeding in this patient population, many neurosurgeons defer placement of the monitor. An aggressive correction of the coagulopathy is required prior to the placement of a monitoring device. Recombinant activated factor VII temporarily corrects the coagulopathy of liver failure and allows the placement of an ICP monitor.[12] As the encephalopathy becomes worse and the patient becomes slowly obtunded, early intervention to maintain and secure the airway and oxygenation is indicated. Cerebral edema is best monitored and controlled by the direct measurement of ICP.[13] Intraoperative periods of increased risk are when hemodynamic instability occurs and at the time of the new graft reperfusion. Very small changes in hemodynamics may cause major changes in cerebral perfusion pressure. The aim of anesthetic management is to keep the intracranial pressure less than 20 mm Hg, the cerebral perfusion pressure more than 50 mm Hg, and the mean arterial pressure more than 60 mm Hg. At reperfusion of the new liver graft, a significant infusion of acid and vasodilating agents may enter the circulation, together with an increase in cardiac output, resulting in an acute elevation in ICP. The infusion of a bolus of sodium pentothal or propofol at this time may counter the effect.[13]

Hyperventilation may be helpful by causing hypocapnia, resulting in cerebral vasoconstriction; however, this technique is controversial. Maintaining cerebral perfusion pressure is critical at this time. The use of cerebral function monitors that display the cortical electrical activity of the brain may be helpful adjuncts in management. The prevention of volume overload and the increase in central venous pressure can be facilitated by the early introduction of continuous venovenous hemodialysis. Other measures that can help protect the brain include osmotic diuretics and barbiturate coma.

Cardiovascular System

The cardiovascular system must be carefully evaluated. It has been recognized for more than 50 years that a high cardiac output state with extremely low systemic vascular resistance (SVR) typically is present with liver cirrhosis.[14] This state can make the assessment of ventricular function difficult to interpret accurately. A reduced afterload can allow a ventricle that is functioning poorly to appear to be functioning well. This is important to know because severe cardiomyopathy may be associated with liver cirrhosis.[15] Cardiomyopathy has been reported to exist to some degree in all patients with liver cirrhosis.[16] Cardiomyopathy may result in impaired contractility, especially under stress conditions. It also presents as a blunted responsiveness to β-adrenergic receptor agonists because of diminished β-receptor function that may be exacerbated by the chronic use of β-receptor blocking agents. The cardiomyopathy may be further compromised in the alcoholic patient by the presence of an alcoholic cardiomyopathy.[16]

Cirrhotic cardiomyopathy is characterized by an increased cardiac output, attenuated response to inotropic stimuli, mild chamber dilatation, and repolarization changes. If cardiomyopathy is suspected, a dobutamine stress echocardiogram should be performed to assess ventricular function. Any patient who presents for liver transplantation and is found to have a low cardiac index and elevated filling pressures must be closely examined for the presence of a cardiomyopathy. However, the most common cause of a low cardiac index in the immediate preoperative period is hypovolemia.

Because the upper age limit for liver transplantation is being extended in most centers and is now based on physiological age as opposed to chronological age, careful screening for coronary artery disease (CAD) is necessary because the prevalence of this disease increases with age.[17] In the past, it was thought that there was reduced CAD in cirrhotic patients.[18-20] However, recent data demonstrate a significant incidence of severe CAD in up to 16% of liver transplant candidates older than 50 years.[21] The presence of CAD in the patient undergoing liver transplantation is greater than in the general population and has been reported to increase the mortality rate to 50% and the morbidity rate to 81%.[22,23] Therefore, there should be close

screening of at-risk liver transplant candidates for CAD and a low threshold for performing a dobutamine stress echocardiogram.[24] If ischemia is producible, a coronary arteriogram should be obtained. If the coronary arterial obstructive lesions can be dilated and a stent placed, liver transplantation may be an acceptable-risk procedure.[25]

Occasionally, angioplasty is not a viable option, and the decision must be made as to whether coronary artery bypass grafting or liver transplantation should be performed first or if they should be performed together.[26] Cardiac surgery in the patient with severe liver dysfunction may result in an exacerbation of the preexisting coagulopathy and potentially a decrease in liver blood flow, precipitating fulminant liver failure. Conversely, the unavoidable major hemodynamic changes that may occur during liver transplantation make this option very hazardous if it is undertaken first. This therapeutic dilemma requires close consultation among the cardiologist, anesthesiologist, and surgeon. The role of coronary artery bypass surgery is a risk-benefit decision that will depend on the severity of the liver disease.[27] The at-risk patient should receive a dobutamine stress echocardiogram test so that CAD, ventricular function, and valvular function can be assessed and to determine if the pulmonary artery pressures are normal or elevated. Plotkin and colleagues demonstrated that the dobutamine stress echocardiogram had a sensitivity of 100%, a specificity of 90%, a positive predictive value of 100%, and a negative predictive value of 100% when evaluating liver transplant candidates with cardiac risk factors.[28] These data support the use of the dobutamine stress echocardiogram as a screening tool for CAD in those liver transplant patients when indicated by the guidelines of the American College of Cardiology and the American Heart Association.[29] The data supporting the administration of perioperative β-blockers to patients undergoing surgery with a risk of coronary ischemia is compelling and should be applied to liver transplant recipients who meet the criteria.[30]

The monitoring of the cardiovascular system should include intra-arterial and central venous pressure sensors. The role of the pulmonary artery catheter is controversial, but it can detect previously undiagnosed pulmonary hypertension and cardiomyopathy and may be used to guide the administration of vasopressors and volume in the face of hypotension. The differentiation among hypovolemia, low SVR, and poor ventricular function can be critical. The transesophageal echocardiogram (TEE) offers a comprehensive assessment of volume status, together with left and right ventricular function. In patients with pulmonary hypertension who are undergoing liver transplantation, the TEE can provide essential information on right ventricular function. On the rare occasion when pulmonary emboli occur, the TEE can be critical in early diagnosis and management.

Pulmonary System

Ventilation may be restricted by massive abdominal ascites compressing the diaphragm and by large bilateral pleural effusions. The mortality of patients with end-stage liver disease who develop adult respiratory distress syndrome is reported to be 100% unless transplantation is performed.[31] Circulating endotoxins may be pathogenic by initiating an inflammatory cascade, causing a panendothelial injury. These patients present with diffuse bilateral pulmonary infiltrates and poor pulmonary compliance. This clinical picture of adult respiratory distress syndrome is thought to be the result of a sepsis syndrome and not active sepsis, which would be a contraindication to transplantation. Successful resolution of adult respiratory distress syndrome has followed orthotopic liver transplantation.[32]

Pulmonary Hypertension

Pulmonary hypertension is defined as a resting mean pulmonary artery pressure (mPAP) greater than 25 mm Hg, a pulmonary artery occlusion pressure (PAOP) of less than 15 mm Hg, and a pulmonary vascular resistance (PVR) of greater than 240 dynes·s·cm^{-5} (some authorities define a PVR of more than 120 dynes·s·cm^{-5} as pathological). Pulmonary hypertension may be further divided into mild (mPAP 25 to 35 mm Hg), moderate (mPAP >35 and <45 mm Hg), and severe pulmonary hypertension (mPAP >45 mm Hg), and when associated with portal hypertension it is termed *portopulmonary hypertension* (POPH). Mild pulmonary hypertension is found in approximately 20% of patients with cirrhosis and is usually caused by an increased cardiac output, a low SVR, an increased blood volume, and an elevated PAOP. Therefore, it is not POPH and requires different therapy. True POPH is found in 3.1% to 4.7% of patients with cirrhosis. If untreated, POPH carries a high mortality.[33-37]

The pathological changes in the microvasculature of the lung in patients with POPH include plexogenic arteriopathy, medial hyperplasia, thrombosis, and eventually fibrosis. Concomitant with these changes, vascular dilatations and shunt formation may occur.[38] The overall effect of these changes may be to balance the physiological outcome until a single pathology predominates. The resistive changes may progress, even after liver transplantation, unless pulmonary vasodilator therapy is continued until vascular remodeling has taken place.[37] Shunt formations do resolve after transplantation, which may reveal the underlying POPH.

Moderate and severe pulmonary hypertension places the liver transplantation patient at increased risk of perioperative morbidity and mortality. The data available to date indicate a perioperative mortality of greater than 70% if liver transplantation is carried out with a mPAP of 45 mm Hg or above. There is no increase in mortality risk if the mPAP is 35 mm Hg or less.[36,39] The management of the patient with mPAP more than 35 mm Hg requires careful assessment. Preoperative treatment with pulmonary vasodilators such as epoprostenol may bring the mPAP down to 35 mm Hg. Patients with an mPAP more than 45 mm Hg may benefit from a "test of reversal" using pulmonary vasodilators such as inhaled nitric oxide, prostacyclin (PGI$_2$), or other therapy.[40,41] A cardiac assessment by echocardiogram of right and left ventricular function is essential.

It may take many months of treatment with intravenous epoprostenol to reverse or stabilize the pulmonary artery pressures.[41-43] The endothelin receptor antagonist bosentan may be administered orally and is another effective pulmonary vasodilator but is associated with an elevation of liver enzyme levels.[44] Reassessment of the patient at frequent intervals by echocardiography can provide information about the progress of therapy as well as the condition of the right ventricle. Conditioning of the right ventricle over time may occur and a widely dilated chamber may develop into a hypertrophied and well-contracting ventricle. If this occurs, the patient might tolerate liver transplantation with a higher mPAP.[45]

If pulmonary hypertension is diagnosed on the operating room table just before starting surgery, a decision has to made whether to proceed or defer the procedure. This decision needs to be made rapidly because another recipient may need to be admitted. The decision to proceed should be based on the level of the mPAP and SVR, the reversibility of the mPAP and SVR, and the condition of the right ventricle as evaluated by TEE.[46] It must include a careful rechecking of the hemodynamic data to ensure its accuracy and the elimination of other diagnoses such as fluid overload, cardiomyopathy, and respiratory acidosis. The reversibility of mPAP can be rapidly tested by the administration of inhaled nitric oxide or other pulmonary vasodilator. The function of the right ventricle may be evaluated by TEE surveillance while a 1-L fluid bolus and a dobutamine infusion are administered. If the mPAP reduces to less than 40 mm Hg, the PVR is less than 240 dynes·s·cm^{-5}, and the right ventricular function is not severely impaired, a reasonable expectation exists that surgery can proceed safely. Inhaled nitric oxide may assist in the management of transient acute rises in pulmonary artery pressures associated with reperfusion of the new graft.[47] Figure 40–1 shows a decision tree for diagnosing pulmonary hypertension at the start of surgery. The risks of continuing with liver transplantation in patients with moderate or severe pulmonary hypertension are right ventricular dysfunction leading to congestion and acute failure of the new liver graft, or right ventricular failure and a high risk of mortality.

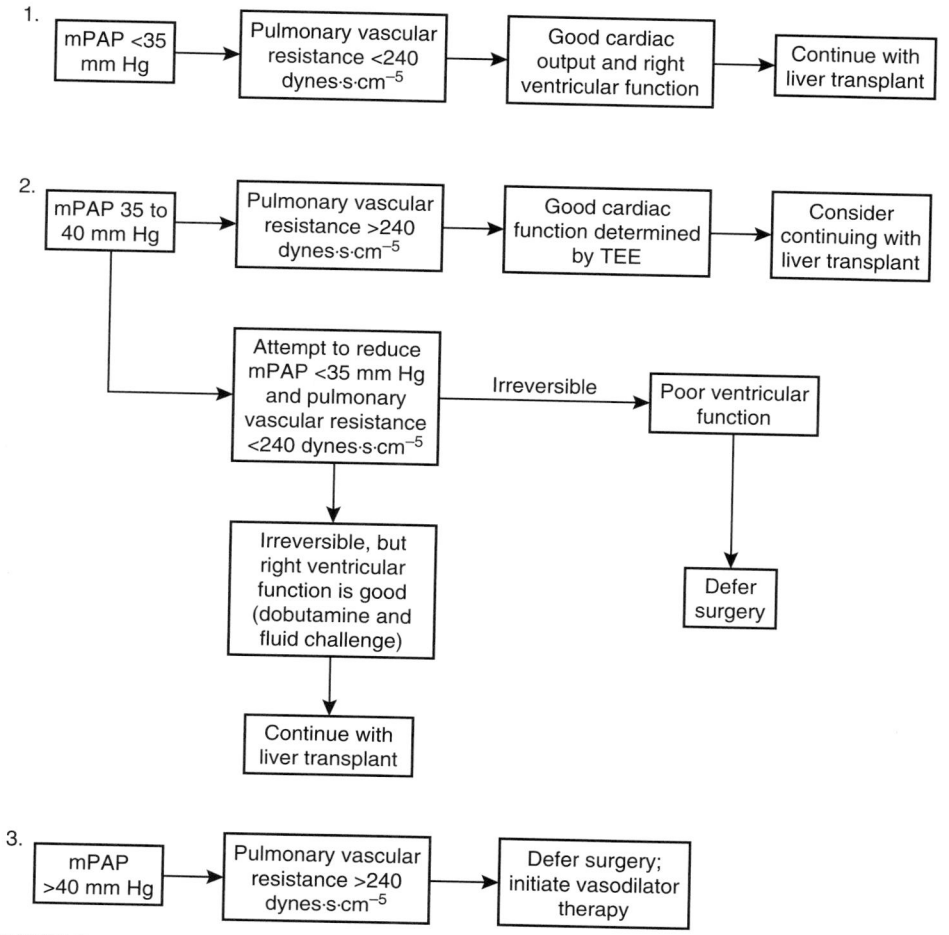

FIGURE 40–1

Management of pulmonary hypertension diagnosed at induction of anesthesia for liver transplantation. (From Ramsay M: Liver transplantation considerations and outcomes for the portopulmonary hypertension patient. Adv Pulmon Hypertens 2:9-18, 2004. Reprinted by permission of *Advances in Pulmonary Hypertension*, the official journal of the Pulmonary Hypertension Association.[46])

Management of pulmonary hypertension diagnosed at induction of anesthesia for liver transplantation is as follows:

1. If mPAP is less than 35 mm Hg, PVR is less than 240 dynes·s·cm^{-5}, and there is good cardiac function, continue with the liver transplantation.

2. If mPAP is 35 to 40 mm Hg, PVR is less than 240 dynes·s·cm^{-5}, and there is good cardiac function as determined by TEE, attempt to reduce mPAP to less than 35 mm Hg and PVR to less than 240 dynes·s·cm^{-5} and proceed with liver transplantation. If irreversible, but right ventricular function is good (dobutamine and fluid challenge), proceed with liver transplantation. If right ventricular function is poor, defer surgery.

3. If mPAP is more than 40 mm Hg and PVR is more than 240 dynes·s·cm^{-5}, defer transplantation and initiate vasodilator therapy.

An increase in cardiac output is frequently seen (5% to 18% of patients) after reperfusion of the new graft. If there is a significant resistance to pulmonary blood flow, the laws of physics dictate that the pressure must increase. Occasionally (3.7% of patients) an increase in cardiac output of more than 100% of baseline may be seen (Fig. 40–2).[45]

This resistance can cause the development of systemic pulmonary artery pressures in patients with preexisting pulmonary hypertension, which can lead to right ventricular failure. Because this massive increase in cardiac output is unpredictable, it is prudent to reduce pulmonary hypertension to a mild (>35 mm Hg) level before undertaking liver transplantation. Postoperatively, epoprostenol infusion therapy may need to continue for as long as 18 months before complete reversal of the pretransplant pulmonary hypertension occurs.[41] If the epoprostenol is not continued, pathological changes in the pulmonary vasculature

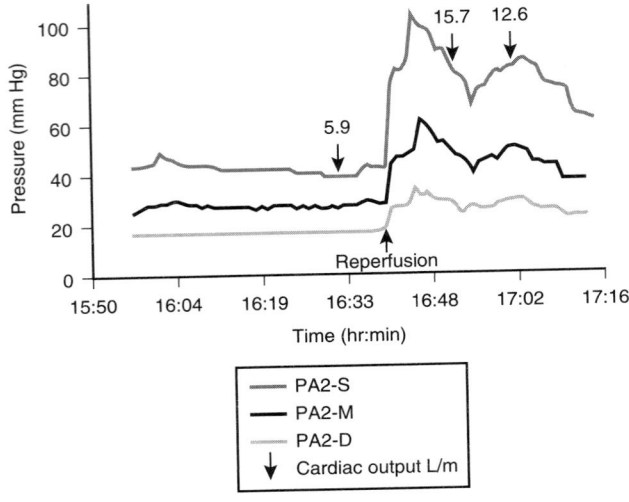

FIGURE 40–2

Reperfusion of liver graft in a patient with pulmonary hypertension. (From Ramsay M: Liver transplantation considerations and outcomes for the portopulmonary hypertension patient. Adv Pulmon Hypertens 2:9-18, 2004. Reprinted by permission of *Advances in Pulmonary Hypertension*, the official journal of the Pulmonary Hypertension Association.[46])

may progress in the majority (>70%) of patients, with eventual demise caused by right ventricular failure.[37]

Hepatopulmonary Syndrome

Hepatopulmonary syndrome (HPS) may be found in up to 47% of patients with liver disease, if contrast-enhanced echocardiography is used to look for it. Hypoxia will be found in approximately 17% of these patients. The criteria for diagnosis include a partial pressure alveolar oxygen (Pao_2) of less than 70 mm Hg or an arterial-alveolar gradient more than 20 mm Hg while breathing room air, caused by pulmonary vascular dilatation, in a patient with liver disease.[48-50] Numerous other causes of hypoxia exist in patients with liver disease. These causes include atelectasis caused by pleural effusions or massive ascites, pneumonia, decreased hypoxic pulmonary vasoconstrictive response, adult respiratory distress syndrome, alveolar hypoventilation, and diffusion abnormalities.

The resulting ventilation-perfusion mismatch may cause hypoxia. The pulmonary vascular dilatation in HPS may be inferred by delayed (more than three cardiac cycles), positive, contrast-enhanced echocardiography or a more than 5% extrapulmonary uptake of technetium-labeled macroaggregated albumin after a perfusion scan. The vasodilations may take the form of dilated precapillary and capillary vessels or direct arteriovenous communications. The former occur diffusely throughout the lung, and the latter appear as discrete vascular shunts. Both pathologies may occur together. If the capillary

changes predominate, it is classified as type 1 HPS, and if the discrete shunts are the major influence, it is termed type 2 HPS. With type 1 HPS, the hypoxia will respond to increased concentrations of inspired oxygen because the physiological problem caused by the capillary dilatations is a reduced transit time for the red cells passing the alveoli. An increase in the alveolar Pao_2 will increase the passage of oxygen across the alveolar membrane to the red cells. Type 2 HPS, however, is a pure anatomical shunting of blood away from the alveoli; thus increasing the inspired oxygen will not correct the hypoxia. Coil embolization by interventional radiology may improve oxygenation in type 2 HPS. The symptoms and signs of HPS include cyanosis, digital clubbing, orthodeoxia, platypnea, shortness of breath, and hypoxemia. The disease's natural history results in a mortality of 18% at 1 year after diagnosis and 41% at 2.5 years after diagnosis. Liver transplantation can cause a complete resolution of type 1 HPS within 15 months of the procedure.[50-52] Type 2 HPS may require further intervention. The mortality associated with liver transplantation and HPS is related to the Pao_2 at the time of surgery. A 29% mortality rate is reported within 90 days postoperatively in patients with a Pao_2 of less than 50 mm Hg.[53] If transplantation is performed with a Pao_2 of more than 50 mm Hg, the mortality rate is less than 4%. The intraoperative risks include the passage of air and other emboli across from the right-side circulation to the systemic side, with the potential for cerebral insult.[54]

The development of HPS is considered an indication for liver transplantation because HPS will reverse after transplantation. Portopulmonary hypertension is not an indication for transplantation because the reversal after transplantation is not established.[55] The resolution of HPS can unmask POPH.[56]

Renal Function

An adequate volume of urine production is critical to the management of the liver transplant patient. Volume overload, if allowed to occur, results in congestion and eventual failure of the graft. Good urine output enables proper management of volume changes associated with the correction of coagulopathy. Satisfactory renal function assists in maintaining electrolyte and acid-base homeostasis. Acute elevations in serum potassium may occur from the rapid transfusion of blood products and from the reperfusion of the new liver graft. The role of monitors of cardiac output and volume state can be essential for optimizing renal perfusion and preventing congestion of the new liver graft. The TEE can provide good information on the cardiac chamber sizes and supplement information provided by the pulmonary artery catheter.

Patients with liver failure frequently have renal dysfunction. It may be the result of prerenal azotemia or intrinsic renal disease. Prerenal azotemia may be the result of chronic hypovolemia caused by long-term diuretic use and can be treated by volume expansion. Liver disease is also associated with increased renin-angiotensin activity and increased antidiuretic hormone activity, leading to sodium and water retention that is often accompanied by a decreased effective plasma volume. Water retention is greater than sodium retention, resulting in hyponatremia.[57] Secondary aldosteronism also occurs, making hypokalemia and total body potassium depletion common.

Hepatorenal Syndrome

Renal dysfunction may also present as hepatorenal syndrome (HRS), in which there is no parenchymal damage, but there is profound hypoperfusion of the kidney caused by vasoconstriction. HRS diagnosis is based on the absence of primary renal disease, proteinuria, hypovolemia, and renal hypoperfusion. It is characterized by normal urinary sediment, low urinary sodium (<10 mEq/L), azotemia, and oliguria. It is important that hypovolemia be ruled out. HRS is reversible with liver transplantation but may progress to acute tubular necrosis that is not reversible and could be treated by a combined liver-kidney transplant. Increased sympathetic tone in the renal vasculature plays an important role in the development of this syndrome. Adequate volume replacement is essential in these patients.[58]

Endogenous production of creatinine is reduced with end-stage liver disease, and therefore serum creatinine may not reflect the severity of the renal dysfunction. The patient's prerenal status must be closely assessed, as reduced plasma volume may exist from chronic use of diuretics. Aggressive rehydration may be necessary to provide and maintain an effective intravascular volume and prevent renal hypoperfusion. Perioperative oliguria should be treated initially as prerenal in origin and a fluid challenge administered. Using diuretics and a renal dose infusion of dopamine, together with a mannitol infusion, may optimize urine output in the patient with HRS. A dopamine infusion, however, is not protective of the kidney in this clinical situation.[59] The role of an infusion of fenoldopam, a dopamine-1 receptor agonist, shows great promise, not only in renal protection but also by improving mesenteric perfusion and new liver graft vascular perfusion.[60] Another therapeutic approach that is being examined is the administration of atrial natriuretic peptide, a potent renal vasodilator. Anaritide, an atrial natriuretic peptide substitute analogue, is currently undergoing clinical trial. A completely different approach that is also being examined is the role of splanchnic vasoconstriction in improving HRS. Vasopressin analogues terlipressin and ornipressin are undergoing clinical trial.[61]

If the patient is unresponsive to therapy, early institution of intraoperative continuous venovenous hemodialysis should be considered. It can easily be accomplished in the operating room and greatly facilitates fluid and electrolyte management. If it is not available, all units of banked blood should be washed prior to infusion to reduce the potassium load. The cell-saver blood salvage system can be used to do this directly in the operating room. The cell-saver system can also be used to "hemodialyze" the patient by drawing off blood through a large-bore central catheter, washing it in the cell saver, and retransfusing it back to the patient. In this manner, volume and potassium can be removed and the patient undergoes hemoconcentration.

Coagulation Disorders

The patient with liver disease may develop major coagulation abnormalities. Frequently, splenomegaly, nutritional deficiencies, and variceal bleeding coexist and result in an associated thrombocytopenia and anemia. The liver is not only responsible for producing many coagulation factors—I, II, V, VII, VIII, IX, X, XI, XII, and XIII—but also for synthesizing coagulation inhibitors, fibrinolytic proteins, and their inhibitors. It also clears all activated coagulation and fibrinolytic enzymes.

Thus the liver functions as an important modulator of the coagulation balance, preventing hyper- or hypocoagulation and fibrinolysis. An alteration in this fine-tuning by the presence of liver disease can result in coagulopathy caused by hypocoagulation, excessive fibrinolysis, or a hypercoaguable state, resulting in thrombosis or disseminated intravascular coagulation (DIC).[62] Metabolic and pharmacological events may also affect the clotting mechanism. Citrate toxicity from transfusion of blood and blood products may cause a profound reduction in ionized calcium levels. Heparin, both endogenous and exogenous, may not be cleared, which may result in decreased coagulation. Normothermia is essential in maintaining the integrity of the coagulation system. Table 40–1 lists the types of factors synthesized.

The severity of the coagulopathy is related to the extent of the liver disease; therefore prolongation of the prothrombin time is a guide to the state of liver function. When the disease is more severe, dysfibrinogenemia develops and the fibrinolytic system is activated.[62] Activated proteins such as tissue plasminogen activator

Table 40–1. LIVER COAGULATION FACTOR SYNTHESIS	
Procoagulant factors	II, VII, IX, X, V, VIII, XI, fibrinogen
Anticoagulant factors	Antithrombin, protein C, protein S
Fibrinolytic factors	Plasminogen, plasminogen activator inhibitor 1, α_2-antiplasmin
Others	Thrombopoietin, protein Z

(t-PA) are not cleared easily by the diseased liver.[63] This hyperfibrinolytic state can be monitored in the laboratory by elevated fibrin split products, D-dimers, and reduced euglobulin-lysis time. The thrombelastogram (TEG) reveals the typical spindle trace of fibrinolysis.

The differentiation between fibrinolysis and DIC by laboratory tests is difficult because of an overlap in the results. The TEG is an essential monitoring tool in liver transplantation management because it provides a visual display of the dynamic function of clot formation and deformation so that differentiation between fibrinolysis and DIC can be made. Thrombocytopenia frequently occurs as a result of splenomegaly and a reduction in thrombopoietin, folic acid deficiency, and excessive platelet consumption, especially if DIC is present.

The empirical or prophylactic treatment of fibrinolysis during liver transplantation has been recommended as the result of a multicenter, randomized, double-blind, placebo-controlled trial. Patients undergoing liver transplantation were enrolled in a study that compared the intraoperative administration of "high-dose" aprotinin (2×10^6 kallikrein-inhibiting units [KIU] as a loading dose over 20 minutes during the start of anesthesia, followed by a continuous infusion of 1×10^6 KIU), "regular dose" aprotinin (2×10^6 KIU as a loading dose over 20 minutes during the start of anesthesia, followed by a continuous infusion of 0.5×10^6 KIU), or placebo. The outcome of this study demonstrated that the intraoperative use of aprotinin in adult patients undergoing liver transplantation significantly reduced blood transfusion requirements, and the authors recommended that aprotinin be used in patients without any known contraindications.[64] A further study demonstrated a minor anticoagulant effect of aprotinin and no evidence of a procoagulant effect.[65]

In programs where the routine transfusion of blood or blood products is excessive, aprotinin may be cost-effective therapy, but the indeterminable risk of thrombosis exists if a hypercoagulable state or DIC exists. The differentiation between severe fibrinolysis and DIC is not easy, and case reports exist of massive thrombosis and thromboembolism—venous, arterial, and intracardiac—associated with the use of aprotinin during liver transplantation.[66,67] The state of coagulation should be monitored both by laboratory testing and TEG. The TEG allows the state of coagulation in whole blood to be monitored and can provide early indication of the presence and severity of fibrinolysis.[68]

The treatment of coagulation defects should be based on sound information and a review of the surgical field. The only therapies that need to take place in the absence of significant bleeding are the correction of a reduced ionized calcium level by the administration of calcium chloride, the use of antifibrinolytic agents if lysis is detected, and protamine administration to reverse the presence of heparin. Maintenance of body temperature is also necessary for effective coagulation. The reduction of other clotting factors causing a prolonged prothrombin time or partial thromboplastin time, hypofibrinogenemia, or thrombocytopenia, need not be treated if surgical bleeding is not a problem. These parameters slowly become corrected as the new graft develops optimal function and splenic hypertension is relieved. The use of blood products to treat on the basis of laboratory data without good clinical judgment is not justified.

Metabolic Disorders

Derangements in acid-base homeostasis and electrolyte balances are common in the patient presenting for liver transplantation. Respiratory acidosis may be the result of an altered level of consciousness caused by encephalopathy or cerebral edema and should be managed by early intervention with endotracheal intubation and mechanical ventilation to prevent further brain swelling. Metabolic acidosis may be seen when there is renal dysfunction or hypotension. It is usually caused by lactic acid accumulation. Therapy with sodium bicarbonate may be individualized, depending on current hemodynamics, presence of hyperkalemia, and serum sodium levels. The presence of a well-functioning graft will result in metabolism of lactic acid and correction of the acidosis, as well as development of a metabolic alkalosis if there has been aggressive bicarbonate treatment.

Glucose-insulin metabolism becomes deranged in severe liver disease, and hypoglycemia may be seen in the severely ill patient before transplantation. Blood glucose levels tend to increase during liver transplantation, as glucose is provided with units of banked blood, and glycogenolysis in the new graft can significantly increase glucose levels. Close control of blood glucose levels perioperatively may improve outcomes.[69]

Hyponatremia is not infrequently seen in patients with end-stage liver disease. The cause may be multifactorial—for example, the result of aggressive diuretic therapy, especially the administration of spironolactone, together with the inability of the kidney to excrete free water. Mild hyponatremia (serum Na^+ >125 mEq/L) may be well tolerated, but lower levels of sodium may be associated with cerebral edema and central pontine myelinosis, particularly if the serum Na^+ is allowed to increase rapidly during the perioperative period. The management of hyperkalemia can become a significant problem during liver transplantation. Patients may present with high serum K^+ levels as a result of renal insufficiency, the use of potassium-sparing diuretics, and the presence of metabolic acidosis. Hyperkalemia may be compounded intraoperatively by the administration of blood and blood products that contain significant concentrations of potassium, especially the more aged units. At the time of new graft reperfusion a significant influx of potassium into the circulation may occur and can be sufficiently severe to cause a cardiac standstill. Control of hyperkalemia includes the maintenance of good diuresis, the judicious use of calcium chloride, sodium bicarbonate, and insulin, together with glucose. If these measures are inadequate, the institution of continuous venovenous hemodialysis should be considered. Preoperative plans must be made to handle potential fluid overload and hyperkalemic situations in patients with impaired kidney function.

Portal Hypertension

Portal hypertension may be severe in cirrhotic patients, and this severity may be ameliorated before transplantation by surgical placement of a portosystemic shunt or by the interventional radiologist in the percutaneous placement of a transjugular intrahepatic portosystemic shunt.[70] This latter procedure may be performed under general anesthesia or monitored anesthesia care. Adequate monitoring and timely access to laboratory and blood bank services are essential and must be available in the radiology department. Creation of a portosystemic shunt may precipitate hepatic encephalopathy. Esophageal varices are common and may present an increased risk of bleeding with the placement of a nasogastric tube or a transesophageal echocardiograph probe.

Fulminant Hepatic Failure

Fulminant liver failure results from severe hepatocellular injury and necrosis. It occurs in 3% to 6% of patients with severe liver disease. Hepatic encephalopathy develops early, together with deep jaundice. Laboratory findings include hyperbilirubinemia, marked elevation of the serum aminotransferase concentration, hypoglycemia, hyperammonemia, and hypoalbuminemia. Severe coagulopathy develops because there is impaired liver synthesis of coagulation factors; a prolongation of the prothrombin time is a sensitive index of hepatocyte dysfunction. Depressed liver gluconeogenesis results in increased anaerobic metabolism and generation of lactic acid, creating a severe metabolic lactic acidosis. A variceal hemorrhage into the gastrointestinal tract causes increases in serum ammonia because the liver is unable to incorporate ammonia into urea and worsens the encephalopathy.

Because some patients in fulminant liver failure recover, guidelines for the selection of patients for orthotopic liver transplantation were developed so that transplantation can occur before grade IV coma sets in.[71,72] Criteria for going ahead with orthotopic liver transplantation include any three of the following variables: younger than 10 years or older than 40 years of age, non-A, non-B hepatitis, halothane hepatitis, idiosyncratic drug reaction, jaundice for at least 7 days before the onset of encephalopathy, prothrombin time greater than 50 seconds, and serum bilirubin level greater than 300 mmol/L. Arterial ketone body ratio is a predictor of prognosis in fulminant liver failure.[73]

Most patients who progress to grade IV encephalopathy experience cerebral edema, which is optimally managed with direct monitoring of ICP. Perioperative use of direct ICP monitoring, with the ability to drain cerebrospinal fluid, may reduce morbidity and mortality rates associated with liver transplantation and cerebral edema.[13] As ICP increases, systemic hypertension and decerebrate posturing may be seen. Once the patient develops grade III (stupor) or grade IV (coma) encephalopathy, airway control and ventilation are indicated because there is a risk of pulmonary aspiration. Elevation of the patient's head 25 degrees and maintenance of cerebral perfusion pressure by supporting systemic arterial blood pressure, reducing central venous pressure, and avoiding agitation are essential. The role of ICP monitoring is controversial but helpful if it can be obtained so that the cerebral perfusion pressure can be accurately monitored and maintained above 50 mm Hg.[74]

In patients for whom death is imminent and for whom a donor liver has not become available, total hepatectomy has been performed to eliminate the toxic effects of a necrotic liver. The liver is removed, and a portacaval shunt is performed to decompress the portal system. The inferior vena cava is left intact and the hepatic veins are ligated. Patients have been shown to improve with less metabolic acidosis and a reduced need for vasoactive drugs and have undergone transplantation successfully up to 72 hours after becoming anhepatic.[75]

Apart from cerebral edema, which is the major cause of death in fulminant liver failure, major gastrointestinal hemorrhage, bacterial infection, kidney failure, circulatory collapse, hypoglycemia, and severe acidosis may all be fatal. To maintain normoglycemia, an infusion of 10% glucose may be necessary. Severe metabolic acidosis, a function of tissue hypoxia and lactic acidosis, is often impossible to reverse even with bicarbonate infusions. Blood pressure may be maintained with epinephrine or norepinephrine infusions but may be at the expense of tissue perfusion and may make lactic acidosis worse. This effect may be mitigated by the addition of an infusion of epoprostenol as a microcirculatory vasodilator.[76] Vasopressin and terlipressin have been shown to reduce mortality related to variceal bleeding.[77] However, they may be associated with cerebral hyperemia in patients with severe encephalopathy.[78]

The clinical manifestations of fulminant hepatic failure are profound jaundice, encephalopathy, cerebral edema, coagulopathy, and multiple organ system failure. The cerebral edema becomes irreversible if treatment cannot control an intracranial pressure of more than 25 mm Hg or a cerebral perfusion pressure of less than 50 mm Hg. Perioperative goals are to maintain cerebral circulation, systemic hemodynamics, acid-base balance, and metabolic/electrolyte homeostasis. Introducing bioartificial liver support systems and the use of xenografts as a bridge to transplantation have improved survivability.

Anesthesia Care

Donor Management

Because the demand for donor organs continues to increase, it is imperative to salvage even marginal organs. The anesthesiologist has an important role to play in this care because hemodynamic heterogeneity in donors is common.[79] Intensive management of the donor, using all the monitoring sensors and laboratory facilities that are used on living patients, is well justified and provides optimal organs to the donor pool. Invasive monitoring, including pulmonary artery catheterization, may optimize donor management. Normal blood pressure alone does not indicate adequate organ perfusion. By ensuring an acceptable cardiac output and SVR, organ perfusion may be optimized and vasopressor administration minimized. With increasing experience, it has been found that no arbitrary maximal vasopressor dose exists as long as hemodynamics are maintained.[80] Crystalloid infusions should be used as fluid replacement unless the hematocrit is less than 21%, at which time the use of erythrocyte infusions is indicated.

Recipient Care

Pharmacokinetics and Pharmacodynamics

The most important contributor to the plasma protein binding of drugs is albumin. In chronic liver disease, as hypoalbuminemia develops, there are fewer drug-binding sites available; therefore, free drug concentration increases, resulting in enhanced distribution and higher concentration at the site of action. This effect may be offset by increased clearance of the drug.

In the liver, the sinusoids provide a large surface area where drugs can diffuse into the hepatocytes. The intrinsic clearance and extraction of a drug depends on the number of enzyme systems present and the rate at which they perform. During development of portosystemic shunts, liver blood flow may decrease. Drug metabolism is reduced as effective liver blood flow decreases and microsomal activity is depressed. A close relationship exists between liver blood flow and metabolic rate for those drugs with a high intrinsic clearance and extraction ratio (e.g., propofol, lidocaine, and fentanyl). Those drugs that have low intrinsic clearance and extraction are unaffected by liver blood flow (e.g., diazepam and phenobarbital).

The enzyme complex cytochrome P450 system plays a major role in drug metabolism. Each distinct P450 protein is the product of a unique gene. Each gene appears to be independently regulated and selectively inducible.[81] Agents such as phenobarbital and alcohol can cause induction to function at a much higher level of activity, so other unrelated drugs are metabolized at a much greater rate (e.g., thiopentone, diazepam, pancuronium). Acute viral hepatitis, alcoholic cirrhosis, and pericentral cirrhosis are associated with a 30% to 50% decrease in P450 levels in contrast to chronic hepatitis and primary biliary cirrhosis, which generally spare this system.[82] Consequently, the response of the patient to anesthetic drugs may be unpredictable and the use of cerebral function monitors during surgery may be helpful. The effects of disturbed liver function on drug disposition may be contradictory. Clearance may be increased because of induction of the cytochrome P450 enzyme complex but decreased as a result of reduced liver blood flow, reduced hepatocellular mass, deranged liver metabolism, or decreased level of plasma enzymes such as cholinesterase. The effect of reduced portal extraction is to reduce "first-pass" metabolism of orally administered drugs, leading to greater bioavailability.

Different disease entities present with different combinations of these disturbances, and each patient presents with an individual pattern of dysfunction. Some derangements will have opposing effects that tend to be self-canceling, whereas others may be additive. Therefore, drug actions should be carefully monitored with titration of drug to effect.

Morphine has a normal clearance in cirrhotic patients, and it is probable that there is extrahepatic glucuronidation of morphine that it is likely to be metabolized at all degrees of liver insufficiency. Meperidine shows a marked reduction in clearance. Fentanyl and sufentanil show no changes in clearance or protein binding in cirrhosis.[83]

Muscle relaxants show a varied response to liver dysfunction. Succinylcholine action is prolonged as plasma cholinesterase levels are reduced. Pancuronium has a 50% increase in volume of distribution, causing lowered plasma concentrations; however, it also has decreased clearance, which causes an increase in elimination half-life of approximately 3 to 5 hours. Vecuronium and rocuronium are dependent on liver excretion and therefore have an increased elimination half-life with liver disease. They can be used as pharmacodynamic probes to assess new graft primary function.[84,85]

Atracurium is degraded normally with end-stage liver disease; however, laudanosine, a principal metabolite and central nervous system stimulant, is dependent on the liver for clearance.

Cardiovascular drugs should generally be administered in reduced doses. Lidocaine and procainamide, β-blockers, calcium channel blockers, and metoclopramide all have reduced clearance in cirrhotic patients.

Monitoring

Liver transplantation is likely to cause massive fluid shifts, blood loss, hemodynamic instability, coagulation disorders, electrolyte and acid-base disorders, and difficulties in maintaining body temperature. Consequently, careful monitoring and the availability of measures to maintain hemostasis, normothermia, and normovolemia are essential. Adequate assistance is necessary, as is the access to "point of service" laboratory equipment or the presence of a "stat laboratory," so that very current data are obtained. Rapid analyses of basic electrolytes, glucose, arterial blood gases, ionized calcium and magnesium levels, as well as hemostasis profiles—hematocrit, prothrombin time, partial thromboplastin time, fibrinogen, platelet count, thrombin clot time, fibrin split products, and D-dimers—are required.

Hemodynamic monitoring consists of a multichannel electrocardiogram, direct arterial blood pressure, central venous pressure and, often, pulmonary artery pressures with cardiac output determinations and hemodynamic profiles. The transesophageal echocardiogram can be helpful in the management of cardiac function, volume status, and monitoring for the presence of intracardiac emboli. Heparin is not added to the flush solution of monitoring catheters because the small amounts of heparin may not be metabolized by the liver and can affect coagulation.

Pulmonary status is monitored by end-tidal carbon dioxide analysis, pulse oximetry, serial arterial blood gas measurements, and compliance assessments. End-tidal nitrogen and carbon dioxide monitoring by mass spectrometry can aid in the diagnosis of air emboli and in the assessment of adequate ventilation.

Cerebral function monitoring may provide useful data in assessing depth of anesthesia and cerebral well-being. These patient populations have varied responses to anesthetic drugs and are more susceptible to unexpected levels of anesthesia. Reperfusion of the liver graft can produce temporary isoelectric cerebral activity. Available monitors include the BIS Monitor (Aspect Medical Systems, Newton, MA) and the PSA 4000 (Physiometrix, Inc., N. Billerica, MA).

The thrombelastograph (Haemoscope Co., Skokie, IL) provides a graphic display of viscoelastic clot strength, allowing a "virtual" assessment of the quality of coagulation. The TEG is set up near the anesthesiologist so that it can be repeatedly reviewed throughout the different stages of the operation. A 0.36-mL sample of blood is placed in a small, rotating cup. As clot forms, fibrin strands develop between the cup and a rod, which is lowered into the cup and connected to a recorder via an amplification system. The motion of the cup is transferred to the rod, and the recorder makes a characteristic trace. The TEG tracing can be described by reporting measured parameters (Fig. 40–3). Reaction time is the time from the start until the amplitude of the trace is 2 mm. The K value is the time from the end of reaction time to the point at which amplitude is 20 mm. The α-angle is formed by the tangential slope of the graft from the initial point of divergence. It is possible to observe fibrinolysis by observing the maximal amplitude decrease more rapidly than normal. The graph, calculated parameters, and normal ranges may be displayed on a computer screen.

Intraoperative Anesthesia

Adequate venous access must be obtained so that massive rapid transfusions may be administered if necessary. Large bore peripheral and central venous catheters may be placed in the upper part of the body because fluid given through lower body venous catheters may be lost in the surgical field or obstructed in passage to the heart. A radial arterial catheter is inserted for continuous blood pressure monitoring and access for arterial blood gas measurement. Following induction of anesthesia, a subclavian triple lumen catheter is placed, which may be useful postoperatively as well as intraoperatively. Two catheters are placed percutaneously in the right internal jugular vein; one, a 12-French catheter, is used for rapid volume replacement and as the return limb of a venovenous bypass circuit. The other internal jugular catheter is used as a pulmonary artery catheter introducer. A pulmonary artery catheter, although not used in all centers, may prove valuable in diagnosing pulmonary hypertension and managing hemodynamic instability. All fluids should pass through warming devices to assist in temperature maintenance. A rapid infusion system may be necessary for those times when massive blood loss occurs.

Rapid Infusion Devices

Infusion of large volumes of warmed blood and blood products at high flow rates may be required if blood loss is rapid and severe. Available units include the Level 1 rapid infusion (SIMS Level 1, Inc., Rockland, MA) system Model H1025 and the Belmont instrument fluid management system Model FMS 2000 (Belmont

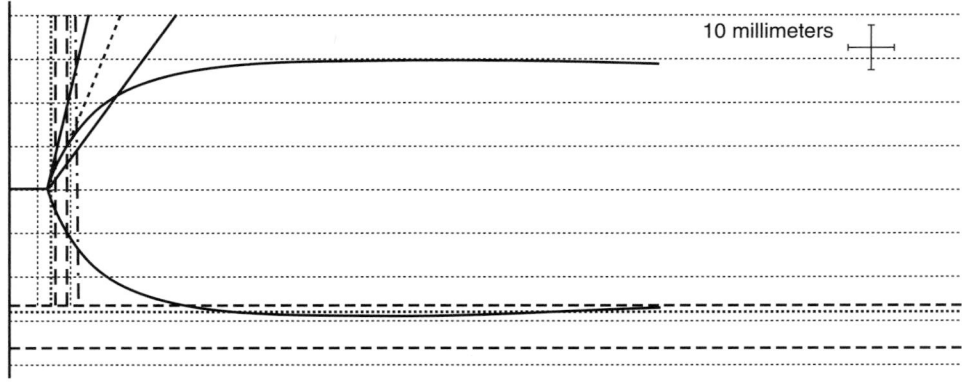

TEG value descriptions:

Reaction time (min)	(4–8)	5.8
Kinetics (speed) (min)	(1–4)	2.2
Angle (°)	(47–74)	61.3
Maximum amplitude (mm)	(55–73)	56.5
Predicted maximum amplitude	(6.0K–13.2K)	0.0
Tensile clot strength (d/sc)	(0–15)	6.5K
Estimated percent lysis (%)	(–3–3)	0.0
Clot build speed (mm)	(0–8)	56.2
Coagulation index	N/A	–0.8
Lysis after 30 min (%)	N/A	0.0

FIGURE 40–3

Thromboelastograph of a patient undergoing liver transplantation.

Instrument Corp., Billerica, MA). A recent comparison between the Level 1 and the Belmont systems demonstrated similar warming capabilities, but more rapid flow rates were achieved by the Level 1, and better air detection and air elimination were achieved by the Belmont system.[86] When these devices are used, cardiac filling pressures must be observed closely because volume overload can occur rapidly. Banked blood units contain increasingly high levels of potassium as they age so that a dangerously high level of serum potassium may occur with resulting cardiac arrest if these units are transfused rapidly.

The older units of banked blood may be washed before use, which can be achieved easily in the operating room by a red cell saving device. In a dire emergency, the cell saver can be connected directly to the rapid infusion device reservoir so that salvaged blood can be transfused directly back into the patient. Blood salvage systems help reduce the demand on the blood bank. A system that washes the red cells before retransfusion, such as the cell saver, is preferable. The cell saver may be used safely in all patients except those with malignant tumors in whom the risk is uncertain. With routine use of the cell saver, there is no risk of trace heparinization of the patient if the blood is aspirated with 20,000 units of heparin/L saline, and no risk of infection has been demonstrated.[87] Alternatively, salvaged blood may be anticoagulated with an infusion of adenosine-citrate-dextrose at 6 mL/min. The cell saver may also be used for exchange autotransfusion in patients who present with elevated blood levels of ammonia, lactate, and potassium as a result of hepatorenal failure.

Thermal Homeostasis

Thermal homeostasis is essential during liver transplantation. Major heat loss occurs after induction of anesthesia, when the patient is exposed and prepared, during the anhepatic phase, and at the time of reperfusion, when the cold, preserved organ is placed in circulation. Hypothermia affects all organ systems and causes reversible platelet dysfunction that could potentiate or cause coagulopathy. There is a generalized slowing of the cardiac conduction system and a decrease in the ventricular fibrillation threshold. These effects on the heart are especially important at the time of reperfusion, when bradycardia and ventricular ectopy are not uncommon. Coronary vasospasm, presumed secondary to placing the cold graft beneath the diaphragm near the heart, has been observed.[88] Routine methods of thermal regulation include maintaining an ambient room temperature as warm as tolerable; using thermal drapes for the lower extremities and head, fluid-warming devices, and a heated humidifier; and placing a forced-air warming device over the upper and lower extremities. If venovenous bypass is used, a heater placed in the circuit can effectively maintain body temperature.

Anesthetic Techniques

A modified rapid-sequence induction technique is used in the majority of patients. Preoxygenation is followed by the administration of propofol (1.5 mg/kg). Intubation is assisted by muscle relaxation by vecuronium (0.2 mg/kg), and cricoid pressure is applied until the airway is secured. Anesthesia is maintained with isoflurane in an air-oxygen mixture, supplemented with fentanyl and vecuronium. Isoflurane provides an optimal relationship between liver oxygen supply and demand; however, in this extensive procedure, this may be only a theoretical consideration.

The use of muscle relaxants that are metabolized by the liver, such as vecuronium or rocuronium, should be accompanied by monitoring of neuromuscular blockade with a nerve stimulator.

Ventilation is set to provide a high tidal volume and low rate. At least 5 cm of positive end-expiratory pressure are added to help maintain adequate alveolar ventilation, particularly of the lower lobes, and to reduce the risk of venous air embolism from the liver bed. Positioning and padding the patient require particular care. Arms should be tucked by the patient's side and well padded. Padding should be checked meticulously at all pressure points because of the potential length of the surgery. Extra padding should be available to protect the arms from surgical retractors.

A high incidence of brachial plexus neuropathy in posttransplantation liver patients and living related donors has been reported despite excellent padding. The cause appears to be multifactorial, including cyclosporine-induced neuropathy and the surgical retraction of the costal margin to gain exposure of the liver, compressing the thoracic outlet in those patients with narrowed outlets.

A nasogastric tube is placed atraumatically and the stomach is kept decompressed. An enteric feeding tube is placed for postoperative hyperalimentation.

Three Phases of Orthotopic Liver Transplantation

The anesthetic management of the operation can be considered with respect to three phases: preanhepatic, anhepatic, and neohepatic. The preanhepatic phase includes dissection and isolation of infra- and suprahepatic vena cava, exposure of the porta hepatis and hilar structures of the liver, and preparation for venovenous bypass when used. The anhepatic phase begins with isolation of the liver and extends until the time of reperfusion of the donor liver. The neohepatic phase begins at reperfusion and lasts until the end of the procedure.

Preanhepatic Phase

During the preanhepatic phase, both overt and covert blood losses can occur, particularly in patients with portal hypertension. Massive volumes of ascitic fluid may be drained, and volume shifts need to be anticipated and corrected. Heavy bleeding may be encountered at any time, and readiness to transfuse massively at any time must be maintained. At the start of the case, 3 units of packed red cells and 3 units of fresh-frozen plasma should be cross-matched. If excessive bleeding is encountered, additional products can be ordered. During the preanhepatic phase, before venovenous bypass, only correction of preexisting coagulopathies accompanied by clinically significant bleeding and an abnormal TEG should be attempted. Platelet counts as low as 20,000/mm^3 may be well tolerated in some patients without transfusion. The use of citrate-rich blood products may result in the development of reduced levels of ionized calcium and ionized magnesium levels. These electrolytes should be monitored closely and replaced as necessary. Hypotension may occur secondary to surgical manipulation in addition to hypovolemia and blood loss. Potential compression of major vessels during dissection can lead to a reduction in venous return. Vigilance regarding the surgical field can allow proper diagnosis. The hepatic artery is ligated followed by the portal vein, and the anhepatic stage is entered.

Anhepatic Phase

The suprahepatic and infrahepatic IVC are clamped and the liver is removed. During the anhepatic phase, in preparation for the new graft entering circulation, a large dose of corticosteroids is given. The steroids prevent macrophages from releasing interleukin-1, thereby initiating immunosuppression.

The anhepatic phase has variable considerations depending on the use of venovenous bypass. Patients without venovenous bypass can be expected to have a major decrease in venous return at the time of clamping the IVC unless there is a well-developed intact shunt system from long-standing portal hypertension or a "piggyback" technique that is used when the vena cava is only partially occluded. This decrease in venous return can be treated with volume and vasopressors.

The decrease in cardiac output combined with obstruction of the IVC may lead to a decrease in kidney perfusion, and oliguria is not uncommon. The use of venovenous bypass counters these effects to some degree.

Venovenous Bypass

There are centers that do not routinely use venovenous bypass because of concerns regarding potential complications, such as air embolism, thromboembolism, and increased surgical time. Many transplant centers, however, do use venovenous bypass routinely during the anhepatic phase to improve venous return and reduce congestion of the intestines, improve renal perfusion, and delay the development of metabolic acidosis. In patients with severe portal hypertension, venovenous bypass may be set up earlier in the procedure to decompress the portal system and to reduce blood loss.

The femoral vein and portal vein are cannulated. Blood is drained from these catheters, run through a centrifugal constrained vortex pump, and returned to the patient by way of the internal jugular vein. This process may be safely completed without heparin or heparin-bonded tubing, provided that flow rate on bypass is kept at greater than 1000 mL/min. Air entrainment may occur if the draining venous cannulas are not tightly tied into their respective veins; therefore, there is an advantage to using a system that includes an air detector. The venovenous circuit may be heated to maintain body temperature effectively. Demonstration of a decreased right ventricular end-diastolic volume is an indication that venovenous bypass is not as efficient as a patent IVC at maintaining venous reurn.[89] Markers of kidney perfusion, however, are preserved with the use of venovenous bypass.[90] The liver is extracted and meticulous hemostasis is obtained. The argon beam coagulator is very effective in aiding hemostasis, but application of the beam to the underside of the diaphragm can cause cardiac arrhythmias, even ventricular tachycardia. After completion of the caval anastomoses, portal bypass is discontinued, and the portal vein is anastomosed. The reduction in venous return may require volume loading at this time. At the completion of this anastomosis, venovenous bypass is discontinued and the suprahepatic and infrahepatic IVC and portal vein are opened, reperfusing the new graft. Venovenous bypass is then discontinued.

Alternatively, if bypass is not used, the hepatic vein pedicle is parachuted down onto the vena cava, the portal vein is anastomosed, and reperfusion occurs.

During the lower vena caval anastomosis, the liver is flushed with cold normal saline through the portal vein. This process of irrigation flushes the preservation solution, metabolites, and air from the donor liver. After the portal anastomosis is completed, the clamps are removed from the inferior vena cava, and the portal vein clamp is slowly removed while closely monitoring the hemodynamic state. Reperfusion of the graft liver via the portal vein marks the beginning of the neohepatic phase.

Neohepatic Phase

The initial period of the neohepatic phase is a critical time marked by the potential development of reperfusion syndrome, which is characterized by hypotension, bradycardia, and arrhythmias; rarely seen are circulatory collapse and ventricular fibrillation. Pulmonary artery pressures are also observed to increase, and right ventricular dysfunction has been observed.[91] The cause appears to be the sudden circulatory influx of a cold, acidic, hyperkalemic volume into the right atrium.

Minor reperfusion syndromes require no treatment; major episodes may require vasopressors and occasionally resuscitation. Hypocalcemia contributes to cardiac dysfunction; therefore, ionized calcium is normalized before reperfusion. Calcium should be given with caution to the hypokalemic patient because it can precipitate arrhythmias in this setting. The portal vein clamp should be released slowly because this method decreases the bolus effect and lessens the likelihood of a severe reperfusion syndrome. Careful observation of pulmonary artery temperature, T-wave amplitude on the echocardiogram, pulmonary artery pressure, and systemic blood pressure as the portal vein is unclamped can guide the speed of unclamping of the portal vein. Alternatively, the suprahepatic vena cava can remain clamped and the infrahepatic anastomosis left partially open so that the initial blood perfusing the liver by way of the portal vein is shed into the wound. The suprahepatic vena cava is then opened, and the infrahepatic vena cava anastomosis is completed. This technique of nonsystemic reperfusion of the transplanted liver reduces significantly the incidence of reperfusion syndrome.[92]

Bolus doses of epinephrine have been used effectively to treat reperfusion syndrome. Large doses of norepinephrine have also been used effectively in some cases of severe cardiovascular collapse. Norepinephrine may provide better support of SVR and perfusion of vital organs, particularly if cardiac massage is required. The effects of reperfusion syndrome and treatment modalities to overcome it on the donor liver are not well elucidated. Successful subsequent liver function, however, has been observed in all of the situations just described. Reperfusion is associated with an increase in cardiac output, a reduction in SVR, a decline in systemic blood pressure, and an increase in pulmonary artery pressure. Low-dose vasopressor support may be required early in the neohepatic stage.

Some livers appear marginal at reperfusion. Free radical formation is considered contributory to this problem.

The addition of allopurinol to the University of Wisconsin preservation solution may be part of the reason for its efficacy, because allopurinol can prevent the release of some free radicals by inhibiting the conversion of xanthine dehydrogenase to xanthine oxidase. Mannitol, also infused at the time of reperfusion, can act as a free radical scavenger. Other free radical scavengers, such as superoxide dismutase and catalase, may be considered. Prostaglandin E$_1$ (PGE$_1$) has been reported to improve the survival of livers that appeared marginal at reperfusion.[93] The effect of PGE$_1$ on vascular endothelium may enhance perfusion of the graft both generally and in areas of "no reflow."

The anesthesiologist must take care after reperfusion not to cause volume overload in the patient. Congestion of the liver graft can seriously impair graft function.

Surgically, the remainder of stage three involves the hepatic artery anastomosis and biliary anastomosis. The hepatic artery is reconstructed by an end-to-end anastomosis. Hepatic artery flow is a critical factor in determining survival of the graft. Blood flow in the hepatic artery and portal vein is measured using an electromagnetic flow probe. If the hepatic arterial flow is inadequate (<400 mL/min), improvement is sought by using various maneuvers such as injection of papaverine directly into the vessel. Hepatic arterial flow in a graft liver is pressure dependent; therefore, systemic pressure should be maintained at this time. If flow remains inadequate, the hepatic artery may be reconstructed by an aortohepatic graft using vessels obtained from the donor. In these cases, the anesthesiologist must anticipate the effects of either partial or total clamping of the aorta.

The biliary anastomosis is performed either as a direct end-to-end connection or as a choledochojejunostomy via Roux-en-Y limb. During this phase, the anesthesiologist's major concerns are rewarming and correction of coagulopathy. Heparin effect and fibrinolysis may be observed after reperfusion and can be treated with protamine and aminocaproic acid, respectively. Antifibrinolytic therapy should be guided by TEG data because this appears to be the most sensitive monitor of fibrinolysis. Cryoprecipitate, fresh-frozen plasma, or platelets may also be needed to correct a coagulopathy at this time.

Signs of a good functioning graft include good hepatic arterial flow, early bile formation, increasing body temperature, improvement in coagulation status, correction of acidosis, a decrease in potassium, and an increase in carbon dioxide production.

Fluid Management

The most common cause of a low cardiac output at the start of liver transplantation is hypovolemia. Good volume replacement is required for adequate tissue perfusion, and more especially for adequate renal perfusion. A nonlactate balanced electrolyte solution can be used as maintenance fluid. This solution will not exacerbate lactic acidosis in patients with little or no liver function. Fluid administration is guided by hemodynamic monitoring and urine output. In the absence of diuretics or kidney failure, a urine output of 0.5 to 1 mL/kg/hr or greater is a good indicator of adequate fluid load and cardiovascular function. If the patient becomes oliguric, a fluid challenge is most often the first option indicated.

Continued oliguria after adequate fluid administration, as evidenced by monitoring of filling pressures or cardiac volume, may indicate a need to optimize cardiac performance (cardiac output) through pharmacological measures, or it may respond to diuretics such as furosemide or mannitol. Intraoperative continuous venovenous hemodialysis is useful in liver transplant recipients with impaired renal function who require ongoing transfusions to treat a coagulopathy. In these patients, the volume of products necessary to correct the coagulopathy may lead to fluid overload together with hyperkalemia. Continuous venovenous hemodialysis can prevent and treat this situation.

Postoperative Care

After liver transplantation, patients are transferred to the intensive care unit for postoperative care. If the operation has been uneventful and the graft is functioning well, routine monitoring of vital signs, fluid balance, coagulation, and liver function is all that is required. Patients are ventilated until they fully recover from anesthesia and are then extubated. This may be performed safely in many patients at the end of the procedure on the operating room table or on arrival in the intensive care unit.[94]

Primary nonfunction of the graft as a result of injury or acute rejection is demonstrated by failure of the coagulation system to normalize and marked elevation in liver enzymes followed by encephalopathy. The hepatic artery is studied by Doppler ultrasonography to ensure that it has remained patent. If no flow is detected, the patient undergoes emergent re-exploration and the hepatic artery is reconstructed. This early intervention can salvage the graft and prevent the need for retransplantation.

Patients with preoperative hepatorenal syndrome can be expected to have a reasonable recovery of kidney function after a successful liver transplantation. The introduction of cyclosporine, although improving the survival of liver grafts, has increased the incidence of kidney dysfunction. Careful correlation of cyclosporine dosage with kidney function must be undertaken in the immediate postoperative period.

The major cause of death after transplantation is infection.[95] Consequently, an aggressive prophylactic regimen against both bacterial and fungal organisms should be instituted.

Sepsis and retransplantation are major risk factors for the development of adult respiratory distress syndrome.[96] Associated with infection and graft failure, multiple organ system failure is an important factor contributing to death.

Postoperative hemorrhage may be the result of surgical bleeding or a coagulopathy. Early intervention is warranted so that large blood clots or collections do not accumulate and result in ongoing coagulopathy or in a nidus for infection or fibrinolysis.

Hypertension is seen in more than 50% of posttransplantation patients and requires treatment with α-adrenergic blockers, calcium channel blockers, angiotensin-converting enzyme inhibitors, and diuretics. The risk of a cerebrovascular accident is increased in the early postoperative period because some degree of bleeding tendency exists.

Postoperative pain control is an important part of postoperative care, and pain medication should not be withheld because of fear that the new graft may not be functioning fully. However, the drug doses should be kept small until the degree of liver function can be assessed. The patient-controlled analgesia pumps provide a good system of intravenous narcotic in small boluses delivered on patient command. This system of on-demand provision of narcotic allows for the titration of an effective and safe dose of analgesic regardless of the level of liver function.

Pediatric Aspects

Children with end-stage liver disease experience a nutritional deficit and growth retardation. Because children with reduced nutritional reserves are less able to handle the demands of liver transplantation, nutritional support should be part of the pretransplant protocol. The anesthesia technique is similar to that in adults, but in many smaller children the information provided by a pulmonary artery catheter is not of great help. It is better to use volume catheters for venous access and to measure central venous pressure as a guide to fluid management.

Venovenous bypass is not used in children and infants because they generally tolerate explantation well provided that volume replacement has been adequate. A "piggyback" technique allows some venous return through the vena cava.

Temperature control is essential and can be provided by good fluid warming and forced air warming devices.

Occasionally in children, and very rarely in adults, abdominal wall closure may be impossible because of the large size of the donor liver. This may be remedied by either downsizing the liver by resection of a lobe or creating a silo on the abdominal wall so that a temporary closure can be made.

Pearls and Pitfalls

- Treat the patient, not the laboratory data.
- Carefully assess right ventricular function.
- A congested graft will not function.
- Maintain normothermia.
- Tightly control blood glucose, serum potassium, and ionized calcium levels.
- The thrombelastograph is the key "virtual" monitor of the coagulation system.
- Ensure adequate vascular access.
- Maintain excellent urine output.
- Be vigilant in identifying the rare patient who is hypercoagulable.
- Administer antifibrinolytic agents to treat identified fibrinolysis only.

References

1. Brown RS, Russo MW, Lai M, et al: A survey of liver transplantation from living adult donors in the United States. N Engl J Med 348:818-825, 2003.
2. Van Thiel DH, Carr B, Iwatsuki S, et al: Liver transplantation for alcoholic liver disease, viral hepatitis, and hepatic neoplasms. Transplant Proc 23:1917-1921, 1991.
3. Stone MJ, Klintmalm GB, Porter D, et al: Neoadjuvant chemotherapy and liver transplantation for hepatocellular carcinoma: A pilot study in 20 patients. Gastroenterology 104:196-202. 1993.
4. Davis GL: Chronic hepatitis C and liver transplantation. Rev Gastroenterol Disord 4:7-17, 2004.
5. Weisner RH, McDiarmid SV, Kamath PS, et al: MELD and PELD: Application of survival models to liver allocation. Liver Transpl 7:567-580, 2001.
6. Moore JW, Dunk AA, Crawford JR, et al: Neuropsychological deficits and morphological MRI brain scan abnormalities in apparently healthy nonencephalopathic patients with cirrhosis. A controlled study. J Hepatol 9:319-325, 1989.
7. Ciancio A, Marchet A, Saracco G, et al: Spectral electroencephalogram analysis in hepatic encephalopathy and liver transplantation. Liver Transpl 8:630-635, 2002.
8. Bakti G, Fisch HU, Karlaganis G, et al: Mechanics of the excessive sedative response of cirrhosis to benzodiazepines: Model experiments with triazolam. Hepatology 7:629-638, 1987.
9. Basile AS, Hughes RD, Harrison PM, et al: Elevated brain concentrations of 1,4-benzodiazepines in fulminant hepatic failure. N Engl J Med 325:473-478, 1991.
10. Dursun M, Caliskan M, Canoruc F, et al: The efficacy of flumazenil in subclinical to mild hepatic encephalopathic ambulatory patients. A prospective, randomized, double-blind, placebo-controlled study. Swiss Med Wkly 133:118-123, 2003.

11. Barbaro G, Di Lorenzo G, Soldini M, et al: Flumazenil for hepatic encephalopathy grade III and IVa in patients with cirrhosis: An Italian multicenter double-blind, placebo-controlled, cross-over study. Hepatology 29:1338-1339, 1998.
12. Shami VM, Caldwell SH, Hespenheide EE, et al: Recombinant activated factor VII for coagulopathy in fulminant hepatic failure compared with conventional therapy. Liver Transpl 9:138-143, 2003.
13. Brajtbord D, Parks RIP, Ramsay MAE, et al: Management of acute elevations of intracranial pressure during hepatic transplantation. Anesthesiology 70:139-141, 1989.
14. Kowalski HJ, Abelmann WH: The cardiac output at rest in Laennec's cirrhosis. J Clin Invest 32:1025-1033, 1953.
15. Liu H, Song D, Lee SS: Cirrhotic cardiomyopathy. Gastroenterol Clin Biol 26:842-847, 2002.
16. Lee SS: Cardiac abnormalities in liver cirrhosis. West J Med 151:530-535, 1989.
17. Kannel WB: Coronary heart disease risk factors in the elderly. Am J Geriatr Cardiol 11:101-107, 2002.
18. Hall EM, Olsen AY, Davis FE: Portal cirrhosis—clinical and pathologic review of 782 cases from 16,600 necropsies. Am J Pathol 29: 993-1023, 1953.
19. Creed DL, Baird WF, Fisher ER: The severity of aortic arteriosclerosis in certain diseases. Am J Med Sci 230:385-391, 1955.
20. Grant WC, Wasserman F, Rodensky PL, et al: The incidence of myocardial infarction in portal cirrhosis. Ann Intern Med 51:774-779, 1959.
21. Carey WD, Dumot JA, Pimentel RR, et al: The prevalence of coronary artery disease in liver transplant candidates over age 50. Transplantation 59:859-864, 1995.
22. Johnston SD, Morris SK, Cramb R, et al: Cardiovascular morbidity and mortality after orthotopic liver transplantation. Transplantation 73:901-906, 2002.
23. Plotkin JS, Scott VL, Pinna A, et al: Morbidity and mortality in patients with coronary artery disease undergoing orthotopic liver transplantation. Liver Transpl Surg 2:426-430, 1996.
24. Plotkin JS, Johnson LB, Rustgi VK, et al: Coronary artery disease and liver transplantation: The state of the art. Liver Transpl 6: S53-S56, 2000.
25. Plevak DJ: Stress echocardiography identifies coronary artery disease in liver transplant candidates. Liver Transpl Surg 4:337-339, 1998.
26. Morris JJ, Hellman CL, Gawey BJ, et al: Three patients requiring both coronary artery bypass and orthotopic liver transplantation. J Cardiothorac Vasc Anesth 9:322-332, 1995.
27. Plotkin JS, Johnson LB, Rustgi VK, et al: Dobutamine stress echocardiograph for orthotopic liver transplantation evaluation. Transplantation 71:818, 2001.
28. Eagle KA, Berger PB, Calkins H, et al: ACC/AHA guideline update for perioperative cardiovascular evaluation for non-cardiac surgery: Executive summary: A report of the American College of Cardiology/American Heart Association Task Force on Practice Guidelines. Circulation 105:1257-1267, 2002.
29. Poldermans D, Boersma E, Bax JJ, et al: The effect of bisoprolol on perioperative mortality and myocardial infarction in high-risk patients undergoing vascular surgery. Dutch Echocardiographic Cardiac Risk Evaluation Applying Stress Echocardiography Study Group. N Engl J Med 341:1789-1794, 1999.
30. Keefe BG, Valantine H, Keefe EB: Detection and treatment of coronary artery disease in liver transplant candidates. Liver Transpl 7:755-761, 2001.
31. Matuschak GM, Rinaldo JE, Pinsky MR, et al: Effects of end-stage liver failure on the incidence and resolution of the adult respiratory distress syndrome. J Crit Care 2:162-173, 1987.
32. Doyle HR, Marino IR, Miro A, et al: Adult respiratory distress syndrome secondary to end stage liver disease—successful outcome following liver transplantation. Transplantation 55:292-296, 1993.
33. Mandell MS: Critical care issues: Portopulmonary hypertension. Liver Transpl 6:S36-S43, 2000.
34. Krowka MJ: Pulmonary hypertension, (high) risk of orthotopic liver transplantation, and some lessons from "primary" pulmonary hypertension [editorial]. Liver Transpl 8:389-390, 2002.
35. Colle IO, Moreau R, Godinho E, et al: Diagnosis of portopulmonary hypertension in candidates for liver transplantation: A prospective study. Hepatology 37:401-409, 2003.
36. Krowka MJ, Plevak DJ, Findlay JY, et al: Pulmonary hemodynamics and perioperative cardiopulmonary-related mortality in patients with portopulmonary hypertension undergoing liver transplantation. Liver Transpl 6:443-450, 2000.
37. Ramsay MA, Simpson BR, Nguyen AT, et al: Severe pulmonary hypertension in liver transplant candidates. Liver Transpl Surg 3:494-500, 1997.
38. Krowka MJ, Edwards WD: A spectrum of pulmonary vascular pathology in portopulmonary hypertension. Liver Transpl 6:241-242, 2000.
39. Ramsay MA: Perioperative mortality in patients with portopulmonary hypertension undergoing liver transplantation. Liver Transpl 6:451-452, 2000.
40. Schroeder RA, Rafii AA, Plotkin JS, et al: Use of aerosolized inhaled epoprostenol in the treatment of portopulmonary hypertension. Transplantation 70:548-550, 2000.
41. Molmenti EP, Ramsay M, Ramsay K, et al: Epoprostenol and nitric oxide therapy for severe pulmonary hypertension in liver transplantation. Transplant Proc 33:1332, 2001.
42. Krowka MJ, Frantz RP, McGoon MD, et al: Improvement in pulmonary hemodynamics during intravenous epoprostenol (prostacyclin): A study of 15 patients with moderate to severe portopulmonary hypertension. Hepatology 30:641-648, 1999.
43. Tan HP, Markowitz JS, Montgomery RA, et al: Liver transplantation in patients with severe portopulmonary hypertension treated with preoperative chronic intravenous epoprostenol. Liver Transpl 7:745-749, 2001.
44. Suleman N, Frost AE: Transition from epoprostenol and treprostinil to the oral endothelin receptor antagonist bosentan in patients with pulmonary hypertension. Chest 126:808-815, 2004.
45. Ramsay MAE, Clark RD, Tai S: Liver transplantation in a patient with persistent portopulmonary hypertension. Liver Transpl 9:C39, 2003.
46. Ramsay MAE: Liver transplant considerations and outcomes for the portopulmonary hypertension patient. Adv Pulm Hypertens 3:9-18, 2004.
47. Ramsay MAE, Spikes C, East CA, et al: The perioperative management of portopulmonary hypertension with nitric oxide and epoprostenol. Anesthesiology 90:299-301, 1999.
48. Krowka MJ: Hepatopulmonary syndrome and liver transplantation. Liver Transpl 6:113-115, 2000.
49. Martinez GP, Barbera JA, Visa J, et al: Hepatopulmonary syndrome in candidates for liver transplantation. J Hepatol 34:651-657, 2001.
50. Krowka MJ: Hepatopulmonary syndrome and portopulmonary hypertension. Curr Treat Options Cardiovasc Med 4:267-273, 2002.
51. Collisson EA, Nourmand H, Fraiman MH, et al: Retrospective analysis of the results of liver transplantation for adults with severe hepatopulmonary syndrome. Liver Transpl 8:925-931, 2002.
52. Arguedas MR, Abrams GA, Krowka MJ, et al: Prospective evaluation of outcomes and predictors of mortality in patients with hepatopulmonary syndrome undergoing liver transplantation. Hepatology 37:192-197, 2003.
53. Taille C, Cadranel J, Bellocq A, et al: Liver transplantation for hepatopulmonary syndrome: A ten-year experience in Paris, France. Transplantation 75:1482-1489, 2003.
54. Abrams GA, Rose K, Fallon MB, et al: Hepatopulmonary syndrome and venous emboli causing intracerebral hemorrhages after liver transplantation: A case report. Transplantation 68:1809-1811, 1999.

55. Hoeper MM, Krowka MJ, Strassburg CP: Portopulmonary hypertension and hepatopulmonary syndrome. Lancet 364:26-27, 2004.

56. Kaspar MD, Ramsay MA, Shuey CB, et al: Severe pulmonary hypertension and amelioration of hepatopulmonary syndrome after liver transplantation. Liver Transpl Surg 4:177-179, 1998.

57. Arroyo V, Gines P, Jimenez W, Rodes J: Ascites, renal failure, and electrolyte disorders in cirrhosis: Pathogenesis, diagnosis, and treatment. In McIntyre N, Benhamou JP, Bircher J, et al. (eds): Oxford Textbook of Clinical Hepatology. Oxford, England, Oxford Medical, 1991, pp 429-469.

58. Gunning TC, Brown MC, Swygert TH, et al: Perioperative renal function in patients undergoing orthotopic liver transplantation. Transplantation 51:422-427, 1991.

59. Swygert TH, Roberts LC, Valek TR, et al: Effect of intraoperative low-dose dopamine on renal function in liver transplant recipients. Anesthesiology 75:571-576, 1991.

60. Carey RM, Siragy HM, Ragsdale NV, et al: Dopamine-1 and dopamine-2 mechanisms in the control of renal function. Am J Hypertens 3:59S-63S, 1990.

61. Gines P, Guevara M, Arroyo V, Rodes J: Hepatorenal syndrome. Lancet 362:1819-1827, 2003.

62. Hambleton J, Leung LL, Levi M: Coagulation: Consultative hemostasis. Hematology (Am Soc Hematol Educ Program) 335-352, 2002.

63. Hersch SL, Kunelis T, Francis RB: The pathogenesis of accelerated fibrinolysis in liver cirrhosis: A critical role for tissue plasminogen activator inhibitor. Blood 69:1315-1319, 1987.

64. Porte RJ, Molenaar IQ, Begliomini B, et al: Aprotinin and transfusion requirements in orthotopic liver transplantation: A multicentre randomized double-blind study. EMSALT Study Group. Lancet 355:1303-1309, 2000.

65. Molenaar IQ, Legnani C, Groenland TH, et al: Aprotinin in orthotopic liver transplantation: Evidence for a prohemostatic, but not a prothrombotic effect. Liver Transpl 7:896-903, 2001.

66. Ramsay M, Randall H: Intravascular thrombosis and thromboembolism during liver transplantation: Antifibrinolytic therapy implicated? Liver Transpl 10:310-314, 2004.

67. Fitzsimons MG, Peterfreund RA, Raines DE: Aprotinin administration and pulmonary thromboembolism during orthotopic liver transplantation: Report of two cases. Anesth Analg 92:1418-1421, 2001.

68. Kang YG, Martin DJ, Marquez J, et al: Intraoperative changes in blood coagulation and thrombelastographic monitoring in liver transplantation. Anesth Analg 64:888-896, 1985.

69. Furnary AP, Gao G, Grunkemeier GL, et al: Continuous insulin infusion reduces mortality in patients undergoing coronary artery bypass grafting. J Thorac Cardiovasc Surg 125:985-987, 2003.

70. Conn HO: Transjugular intrahepatic portal-systemic shunts: "The state of the art." Hepatology 17:148-158, 1993.

71. O'Grady JG, Alexander GJM, Hayllar KM, et al: Early indicators of prognosis in fulminant hepatic failure. Gastroenterology 97:439-445, 1989.

72. de Knegt RJ, Schalm SW: Fulminant hepatic failure: To transplant or not to transplant. Neth J Med 38:131-141, 1991.

73. Saibara T, Onishi S, Gone J, et al: Arterial ketone body ratio as a possible indicator for liver transplantations in fulminant hepatic failure. Transplantation 51:782-786, 1991.

74. Ellis A, Wendon J: Circulatory, respiratory, cerebral, and renal derangements in acute liver failure: Pathophysiology and management. Semin Liver Dis 16:379-388, 1996.

75. Husberg BS, Goldstein RM, Klintmalm GB, et al: A totally failing liver may be more harmful than no liver at all: Three cases of total hepatic devascularization in preparation for emergency liver transplantation. Transplant Proc 23:1533-1535, 1991.

76. Bihari D, Gimson AE, Waterson M, et al: Tissue hypoxia during fulminant hepatic failure. Crit Care Med 13:1034-1039, 1985.

77. Abraldes JG, Dell'Era A, Bosch J: Medical management of variceal bleeding in patients with cirrhosis. Can J Gastroenterol 8:109-113, 2004.

78. Shawcross DL, Davies NA, Mookerjee RP, et al: Worsening of cerebral hyperemia by the administration of terlipressin in acute liver failure with severe encephalopathy. Hepatology 39:471-475, 2004.

79. Duke PK, Ramsay MAE, Paulsen AW, et al: Intraoperative hemodynamic heterogeneity of brain dead organ donors. Transplant Proc 23:2485-2486, 1991.

80. Mor E, Klintmalm GB, Gonwa TA, et al: Use of marginal donors for liver transplantation: A retrospective study of 365 liver donors. Transplantation 53:383-386, 1992.

81. Watkins PB: Role of cytochromes P450 in drug metabolisms and hepatotoxicity. Semin Liver Dis 10:235-250, 1990.

82. Farrell GC, Cooksley WGE, Powell LW: Drug metabolism in liver disease: Activity of hepatic microsomal metabolizing enzymes. Clin Pharmacol Ther 26:483-492, 1979.

83. Chauvin M, Ferrier, C, Haberer JP, et al: Sufentanil pharmacokinetics in patients with cirrhosis. Anesth Analg 68:1-4, 1989.

84. Lukin CL, Hein HAT, Swygert TH, et al: Duration of vecuronium induced neuromuscular blockade as a predictor of liver allograft dysfunction. Anesth Analg 80:526-533, 1995.

85. Marcel RJ, Ramsay MAE, Hein HAT: Duration of rocuronium induced neuromuscular block during liver transplantation: A predictor of primary allograft function. Anesth Analg 84:870-874, 1997.

86. Comunale ME: A laboratory evaluation of the Level 1 Rapid Infuser (H1025) and the Belmont Instrument Fluid Management System (FMS 2000) for rapid transfusion. Anesth Analg 97:1064-1069, 2003.

87. Brajtbord D, Paulsen AW, Ramsay MAE, et al: Potential problems with auto-transfusion during hepatic transplantation. Transplant Proc 21:2347-2348, 1989.

88. Ramsay MAE, Takaoka F, Brown M, et al: Coronary artery vasospasm following placement of a cold liver graft during orthotopic liver transplantation. Anesth Analg 69:854-855, 1989.

89. De Wolf AM, Begliomini B, Gasior TA: Right ventricular function during orthotopic liver transplantation. Anesth Analg 76:562-568, 1993.

90. Gunning TC, Brown MC, Swygert TH, et al: Perioperative renal function in patients undergoing orthotopic liver transplantation. Transplantation 51:422-427, 1991.

91. Lichtor JL: Ventricular dysfunction does occur during liver transplantation. Transplant Proc 23:1924-1926, 1991.

92. Brems JJ, Triff H, McHutchinson J, et al: Systemic versus nonsystemic reperfusion of the transplanted liver. Transplantation 55:527-529, 1993.

93. Greig PD, Woolf GM, Abecassis M, et al: Prostaglandin E, for primary nonfunction following liver transplantation. Transplant Proc 21:3360-3361, 1989.

94. Mandell MS, Lezotte D, Kam I, et al: Reduced use of intensive care after liver transplantation: Influence of early extubation. Liver Transpl 8:676-681, 2002.

95. Park GR, Gomez-Arnau J, Lindop MJ, et al: Mortality during intensive care after orthotopic liver transplantation. Anaesthesia 44:959-963, 1989.

96. Takaoka F, Brown MR, Paulsen AW, et al: Adult respiratory distress syndrome following orthotopic liver transplantation. Clin Transpl 3:294-299, 1989.

VI

Split and Living Donor Transplantation

41

Split-Liver Transplantation for the Pediatric and Adult Recipient

JEAN de VILLE de GOYET
XAVIER ROGIERS
JEAN-BERNARD OTTE

Definition and history   609

Needs for the expansion of the
   donor pool   610

Liver mass requirement   610

Selection of the donor   610

Selection of the recipient   611

Outcome of the other organs recovered during
   in situ split-liver procurement   611

Logistical aspects   611
   Both transplantations in one center   612
   Transplantations in different centers   612

Allocation policies   613
   Anatomic constraints   613
   Parenchymal constraints   614
   Vascular constraints   615

Surgical techniques of splitting   616
   Left lateral segment/extended right lobe
      using the suprahilar approach   616
   Left lateral segment/extended right lobe
      with division of the hilar plate (transhilar
      approach)   618
   Full-right/full-left splitting for transplantation
      in two adults   623

Definition and History

The term *splitting* means the division of the liver parenchyma and its vascular and biliary structures in order to prepare two grafts fit for transplantation into two individuals. Originally, this innovative development aimed at generating size-matched liver grafts for children without reducing the donor organ pool for adult recipients.

The splitting of a deceased donor liver graft can be achieved in two ways. In the ex situ technique, the donor organ is retrieved and core cooled; thereafter, it is split on the back table in an ice bath solution. In the in situ technique, the splitting is performed in the heart-beating donor during a standard multiorgan procurement.

Whether performed in situ or ex situ, the splitting techniques generate left grafts of limited size if the transection is made at the level of the falciform ligament (portal fissure) or on the left side of the middle hepatic vein, across segment IV. They generate a left lateral segment (plus or minus part of segment IV) adapted to the size of a pediatric recipient and an extended right lobe of appropriate size for an adult recipient. To allow safe transplantation of two adults, the transection line must be displaced to the right side of the middle hepatic vein (main fissure) in order to generate two grafts of appropriate size ("full right/full left").

The first four cases of ex situ split transplantation were performed in 1988: three in Europe[1-3] and one in Chicago.[4] Five of the eight recipients were at high risk. Three patients (two children—one in Chicago and one in Brussels—and one adult in Hannover) survived and are currently alive, 16 years later.

Implementation of this innovative technique expanded faster in Europe than in the United States. Between 1988 and 2000, 202 recipients of split grafts prepared ex situ were reported by five European centers,[5-9] with similar numbers of adult and pediatric recipients. The percentage of high-risk recipients ranged between 12% and 75%. Overall patient survival rates ranged between 75% and 93%; overall graft survival rates ranged between 67% and 83%. The incidence of surgical complications (bleeding, vascular, and biliary) was high. During the same time interval, 64 recipients (83% of whom were children) were reported by four U.S. centers.[10-13] The technique was mostly restricted to high-risk recipients and pediatric centers. Overall patient and graft survival rates were similar to the results obtained in Europe, except for a higher rate of primary nonfunction. With increasing experience, better selection of donors, shortening of the ischemic time, exclusion of high-risk recipients, and refinement of techniques, results progressively reached those obtained with full-size liver transplantation, except for a persisting higher rate of biliary complications.

The in situ liver splitting was pioneered by X. Rogiers,[14] soon followed by the UCLA group.[15] Patient and graft survival rates were outstanding: 93% and 92% and 79% and 86%, respectively. The minimal incidence of surgical complications was remarkable. The reduced frequency of biliary complications is of particular interest, although surprising, because the technique of in situ splitting between a left lateral segment and an extended right lobe is the same as that for the procurement of a left lateral segment from a living donor, which still entails a higher rate of biliary complications than in full-size liver transplantation. Interestingly, the Bergamo[16] group reported a 21% incidence of biliary strictures and a 12% incidence of bile leaks in recipients of the left in situ split graft.

Altogether, it may be concluded that ex situ and in situ liver splitting deliver similarly good results in experienced hands.[17-19] Paramount is the center's experience for obtaining results that match those achieved with whole-liver transplantation. The multivariate analysis of 577 split procedures, compared with 21,240 full-sized liver transplants collected by the European Liver Transplant Registry (ELTR)[20] indicated that in split-liver transplantation, the risk ratio decreased from 2.25 to 1.32 if more than 20 procedures had been done in the center, with no increased risk, as compared with whole-liver transplantation in centers that had done more than 30 procedures.

Needs for the Expansion of the Donor Pool

In the past, a very high death rate (>20%) on the waiting list was common for children needing a liver transplant. Both split and living related liver transplants have contributed to considerably reducing their mortality while waiting for a transplant. In contrast, the organ shortage is currently focused on adult recipients who are listed in increasing numbers. Adult mortality while waiting for a transplant remains in excess of 10% to 20%. This explains the fast expansion of adult-to-adult living donor liver transplantation. How much this situation will be alleviated by the expansion of the full right/full left split-liver transplantation[21,22] is unpredictable because of the limited number of potential adult recipients with a low body weight, allowing a safe graft size–to–body weight (GRBW) ratio, and the increasing proportion of older and expanded criteria donors, not allowing safe splitting.

Liver Mass Requirement

Data from living donor liver transplantations indicate that to be successful, the GRBW ratio must be greater than 0.8% to 1% (normal: 2% to 2.5%) or that graft weight must be greater than 30% to 40% of the standard liver volume. However, caution is needed when extrapolating those data to deceased donor liver transplantation and even more so in ex situ splitting (a lengthy procedure that results in long ischemic intervals and manipulation of the ischemic graft during bench work, with potential rewarming that compounds the deleterious effects of ischemia alone). Paramount is the necessity to reduce ischemic intervals as much as possible, which requires that the transplantations be done in parallel when the two split grafts are implanted in the same hospital.

Because the full right and left lobes represent plus or minus 60% and 40%, respectively, of the liver volume, the following rule of thumb can be proposed: the weight of the recipients of the right and left split grafts should be a maximum 100% and 66%, respectively, of the donor weight to provide them with a GRBW of 1.2%. If these requirements can be fulfilled easily with a left lateral segment allocated to a child and a right extended lobe allocated to an adult, the allocation of full-left/full-right split grafts must be restricted to adult recipients of relatively small size.

Selection of the Donor

Criteria for donor selection should be stringent. An upper age limit is common sense but somehow arbitrary: The donor should be younger than age 40 to 50 years, both for ensuring graft quality and limiting the age difference between donor and recipients; the upper age limit should be even lower when one recipient is a child. Although the Bergamo group reported[16,23] that a donor age of more than 50 years did not affect the 3-year patient and graft survival, using livers procured from donors older than 40 to 50 years is controversial in young children and infants. Indeed, a 3-year follow-up is too short to assert that older donor age will not affect the very long-term (>30 years) survival that should be the aim in pediatric recipients. The analysis of the United Network of Organ Sharing (UNOS) data (1992 to 1997)[24] showed a significantly ($P<.001$) higher 3-year graft survival rate in children who had received the graft from pediatric-age donors, compared with donors older than 18 years of age (81% versus 63%). Hemodynamic stability is essential, with no need for high inotropic support. Liver values should be close to normal, steatosis should be absent or minimal, and the stay in the intensive treatment unit (ITU) should be short (<2 to 5 days). Finally, livers from donors who weigh less than 40 kg (88 lb) should not be split (to minimize technical complications), and full-right/full-left splitting ought be limited to large-size donors.

Selection of the Recipient

Patient selection undoubtedly plays an important role in graft and patient outcome. Early series of split-liver transplantation included a large proportion of high-risk patients, which had a negative impact on results. Unstable chronic patients (UNOS status 2A) who do worse with small-for-size grafts should be excluded, whereas patients with fulminant liver failure should be cautiously accepted. This caution is based on the common observation that the sicker the patient, the larger the liver mass required.

Outcome of the Other Organs Recovered During In Situ Split-Liver Procurement

The concern that in situ splitting might have a detrimental effect on the outcome of other organs procured at the same time, because of increased surgical time and blood loss, has not been confirmed, neither in initial reports[14,15] nor in subsequent reports.[25] Indeed, only optimal and stable donors are selected and surgery is performed as carefully as in living donors. However, splitting of the liver should be initiated only after standard steps of abdominal organ procurement have been completed, including supraceliac and infrarenal aortic dissection, so that if a donor becomes unstable, splitting

can be aborted, with rapid progression to aortic cannulation, cross-clamping, and organ cold perfusion.[26]

Logistical Aspects

Split-liver transplantation requires the coordination of one donor operation, a splitting procedure, and two liver transplantations. In addition, early recognition of adequate donors, recipient selection, short cold ischemia times, and optimal transmission in case of sharing between centers are of vital importance for success. Because of these factors, split-liver programs are dependent on experienced transplant coordinators and optimized logistical procedures.

The requirements to allow optimal functioning of a split-liver center, performing both recipient operations in the one institution, are high. Two operation rooms, including experienced anesthesia and nursing staffs, should be available at all times. Also needed are two surgical teams, each headed by a liver transplant surgeon who has extensive experience with the transplantation of these technically variant grafts.

The choice of the recipients is of great importance. Early experiences demonstrate clearly worse results in recipients with advanced disease. Also, it is important to avoid recipients in whom the duration of the operation is not predictable (e.g., portal vein thrombosis, multiple previous abdominal operations). The relationship of the graft weight to the recipient weight is crucial. In children, one has to be careful not to end up with a graft that is too big. Sometimes it is useful to have two children (one infant <10 kg and one child >10 kg), present in the recipient center and to decide which child is to undergo transplantation after seeing the left lateral lobe of the donor liver. Conversely, in adults, to avoid a small-for-size syndrome, one has to be careful to have a sufficient liver volume.

In this technique, in contrast to the situation in living donation, one does not have the opportunity to measure the potential grafts by volumetry beforehand. Table 41–1 shows a simple rule of thumb one can use to choose the recipients of an adult split liver.

The main goal of the logistics is to maintain ischemia times as short as possible, within the optimal limits for deceased donor transplantation (i.e., less than 10 to 12 hours).

Table 41–1. ESTIMATED RECIPIENT WEIGHT RANGES FOR SPLIT GRAFTS OF AN ADULT LIVER DONOR

Graft	Recipient Weight
Segments II, III	<40 kg (88.2 lb)
Segments I, II, III, IV	40-60 kg (88.2-132.3 lb)
Segments V, VI, VII, VIII	60-80 kg (132.3-176.4 lb)
Segments IV, V, VI, VII, VIII	>60 kg (132.3 lb)

Two factors will affect the logistics:

1. Are the split grafts transplanted in one center or are they shared between two centers?
2. Are we dealing with in situ splitting or ex situ splitting?

Both Transplantations in One Center

When both transplantations take place in one, we are dealing with unidirectional organization. Normally this is possible only in centers that have the capability of performing two liver transplantations simultaneously. Strategically, it is important to avoid simultaneous anesthesia inductions and simultaneous reperfusion of both grafts in order to have senior anesthesiological staff at the critical times for both patients. Therefore, in both in situ and ex situ split-liver transplantation, a certain time lag will be sought in starting the implantation. In any case, two experienced surgical teams are needed. Examples for the organization of in situ and ex situ splitting and transplantation are shown in Figures 41–1 and 41–2. With in situ splitting, the organization can be optimized by early removal and transportation of the left graft, giving the opportunity of starting the recipient procedure earlier, while the right liver and other organs still have to be procured.

Transplantations in Different Centers

Although the workload on the recipient centers is less in this case, the logistics are considerably more complicated. It must be emphasized that communication between splitting and recipient surgeons is vitally important. Decisions have to be made about the way to split the vessels. In addition, the quality and volume (weight) of the grafts have to be communicated.

Depending on the mode of splitting, the organization will be different. In ex situ splitting, the organization will be triangular, requiring great attention to keep ischemia times within the limits (Fig. 41–3). Also, communication between the surgeons regarding the mode of hemostasis at the cut section may be needed.

When performing in situ splitting, the organization is considerably easier. It is V-shaped, avoiding loss of time with the transportation of the graft to the first recipient center before ending the splitting procedure in the procurement center (Fig. 41–4). No further benching is needed at any of the recipient centers.

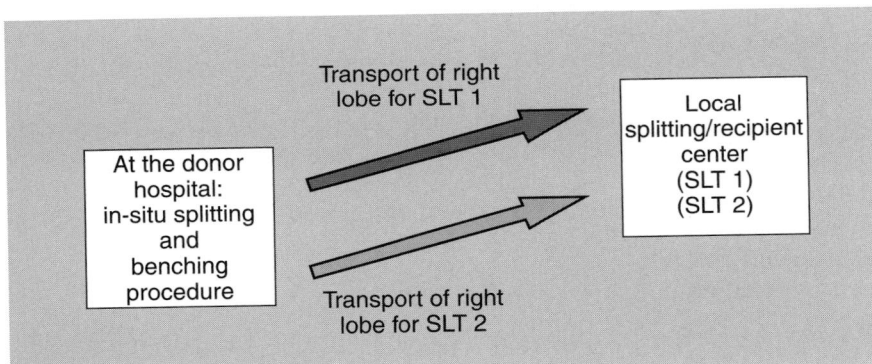

A

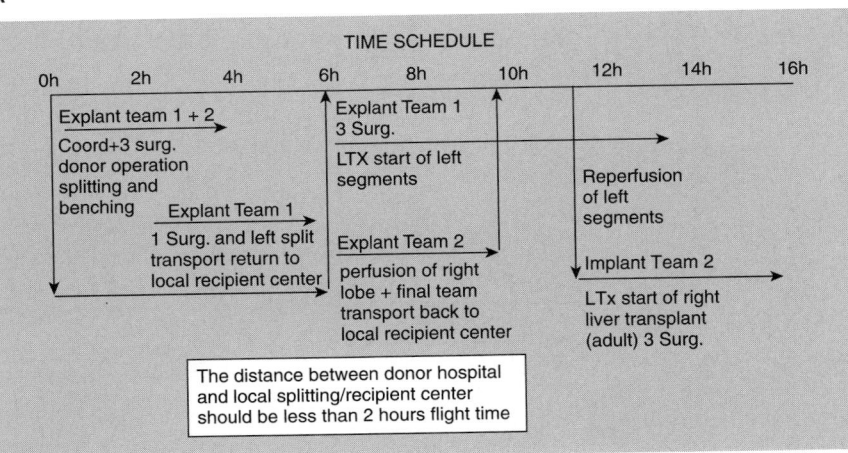

B

FIGURE 41–1

In situ splitting with transplantation in one center. **A,** Organization; **B,** timing. (From Rogiers X, Bismuth H, Busuttil RW, et al. (eds): Split Liver Transplantation: Theoretical and Practical Aspects. Darmstadt, Hessen, Germany: Steinkopff-Verlag, 2002, p 22.)

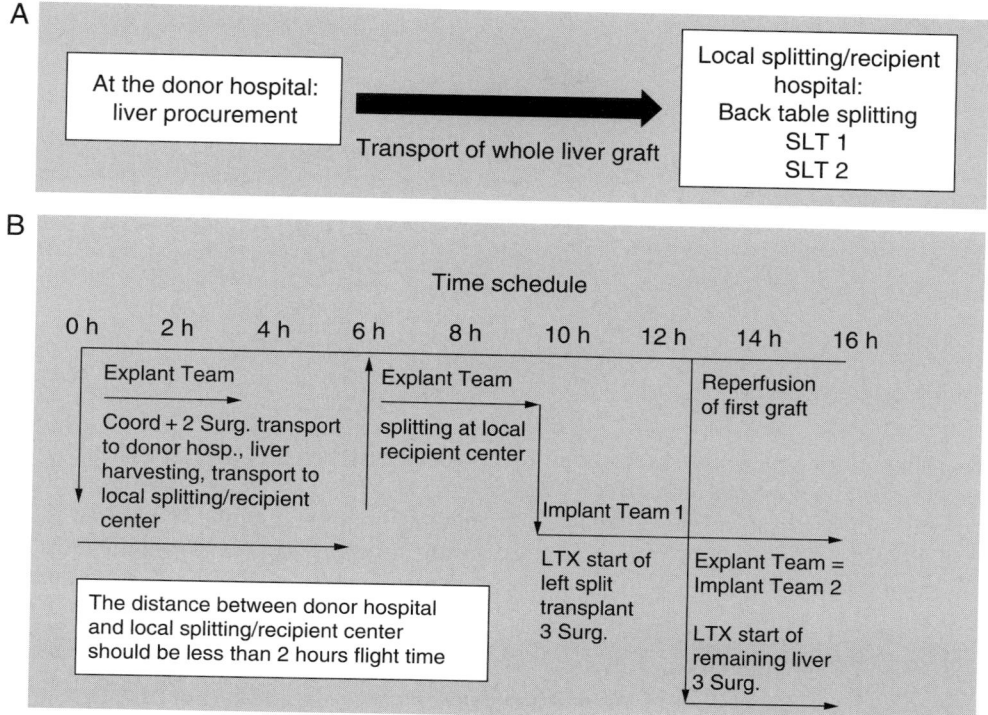

FIGURE 41-2

Ex situ splitting with transplantation in one center. **A,** Organization; **B,** timing.
(From Rogiers X, Bismuth H, Busuttil RW, et al: Split Liver Transplantation: Theoretical and Practical Aspects. Darmstadt, Hessen, Germany: Steinkopff-Verlag, 2002, p 23.)

Allocation Policies

Rules for split-graft allocation require adaptation in order to allow their optimal use. A system should be organized within organ procurement and allocation agencies that takes into account size matches, liver anatomy, and liver volume. Finding matching pairs of recipients requires cooperation between centers and flexible allocation rules. Although 20% to 25% of all potential donors are fulfilling the conditions for a safe liver splitting,[27] only a few percent of the donor livers are split, both in Europe[20] and in North America.[19]

Anatomic Constraints

At least in theory, every liver can be divided into two halves; however, some divisions may lead to complex (and high-risk) vascular reconstructions.[28,29] Practically, the feasibility of liver division is somewhat constrained by variations of anatomy. Ideally, each liver graft should be provided with a single arterial and venous inflow, ready for straight implantation into the recipient. The latter can be achieved in at least 90% of cases (Fig. 41-5A and B).

Because liver anatomy is highly variable, assessment is mandatory before the parenchymal division is started.

FIGURE 41-3

Ex situ splitting with transplantation in two centers. (From Rogiers X, Bismuth H, Busuttil RW, et al. (eds): Split Liver Transplantation: Theoretical and Practical Aspects. Darmstadt, Hessen, Germany: Steinkopff-Verlag, 2002, p 23.)

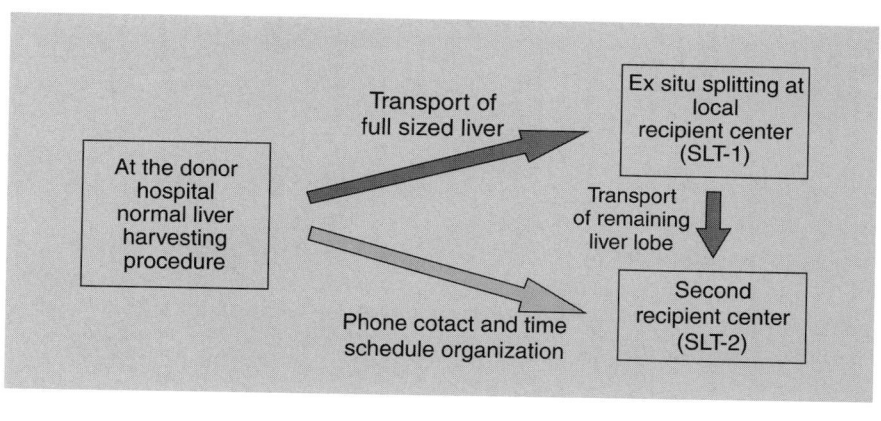

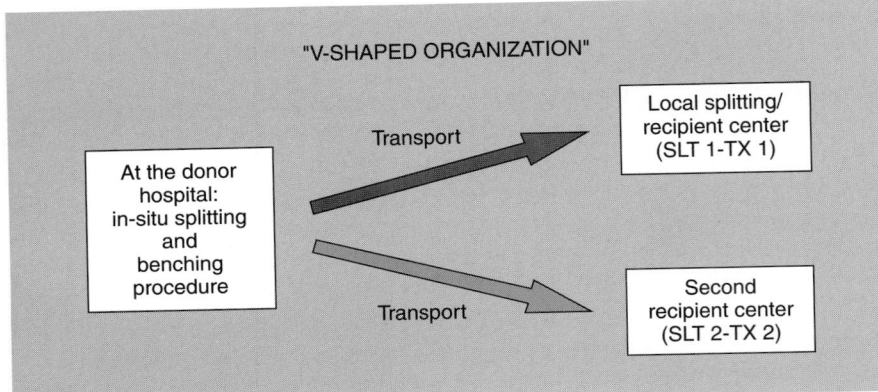

FIGURE 41–4

In situ splitting with transplantation in two centers. (From Rogiers X, Bismuth H, Busuttil RW, et al. (eds): Split Liver Transplantation: Theoretical and Practical Aspects. Darmstadt, Hessen, Germany: Steinkopff-Verlag, 2002, p 23.)

In ex situ splitting, bench angiography can be done to image the hepatic arterial supply precisely,[7,19,30] but currently most teams simply explore liver graft vasculature by surgical dissection.[6,27] Cholangiogram is still recommended by most teams.[8,19,27,30]

Parenchymal Constraints

Relevant parenchymal anomalies (liver lobe agenesis, situs inversus) are very rare. The most obvious constraint is the asymmetrical parenchymal mass distribution that

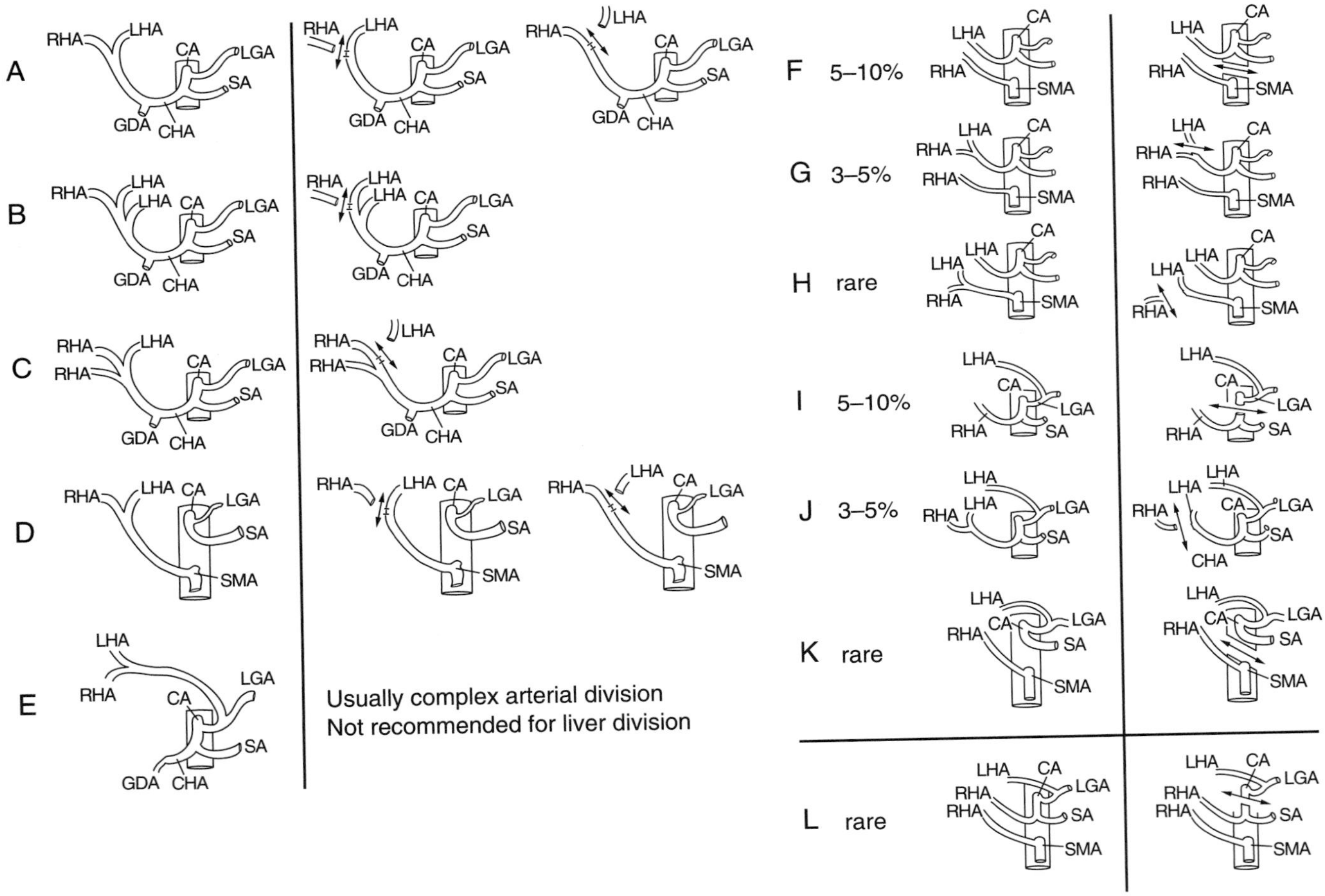

Usually complex arterial division
Not recommended for liver division

FIGURE 41–5

A to E, Variations of hepatic artery anatomy with supply from a single main trunk (75% of livers). **A, B,** and **C,** from the common hepatic artery (CHA) (80%); **D,** from the superior mesenteric artery (SMA) (4% to 5%); **E,** from the left gastric artery (LGA) (0.5%). Possible division modes are shown in the column on the right. **F to L,** Variations of hepatic artery anatomy with supply from two (**F to K**) or three (**L**) main trunks (25% of livers). Possible division mode(s) are shown in the column on the right. RHA and LHA, right and left hepatic artery; CA, celiac axis; GDA, gastroduodenal artery.

leads to preparation of a larger right liver graft and a smaller left liver graft and limits the allocation of both halves to recipients of adequate size.

Dividing the liver parenchyma must follow strictly the guidelines for anatomical resections, thus preserving adequate vascular supply and (biliary and venous) drainage of both halves. Because their vascular supply and outflow can be partly or completely, damaged, resecting segment I (caudate lobe) and segment IV (left medial segment) may be considered when they are not part of the left split graft.[6,30-33]

Vascular Constraints

Vena Cava

The inferior vena cava is usually kept with one liver half, with the contralateral outflow being adequately reconstructed. Usually the left outflow is relatively simple to reconstruct (left or left plus median hepatic veins)[34] when the vena cava is kept with the right graft; this allows preserving all accessory and caudate hepatic veins for draining the right graft.

Alternatively, and in case of complex outflow on both sides, the vena cava can be split into two (right and left) halves; this may be necessary when segments I and IV are kept with the left graft.[35]

Hepatic Veins

Hepatic veins present many variations of their branching anatomy, but many anastomotic arcades have been described. The former was not considered a potential contraindication for splitting until small-for-size split liver grafts were used. It then appeared that much attention had to be given to keep, or reconstruct, an optimal graft venous outflow, thus ensuring good post-transplantation graft recovery and function.[32,36-38] Only main hepatic venous tributaries must be considered for reconstruction (usually large branches of the median hepatic vein or large accessory veins draining the right or caudate lobe) that can be easily done using venous allografts from the same donor.[37,39,40]

Hepatic Artery

Overall, a simple division of "right/left" arterial supply can be carried out in more than 90% of livers, preparing the graft for a single arterial anastomosis in the recipient.[29,39]

Principle

Arterial supply variations are the main constraint for liver division. Although a technical solution can be found in most cases, complex vascular reconstruction should be avoided because it increases the risk of vascular complications. Providing each graft with a single feeding artery is possible in most livers (see Fig. 41–5A and B). Typically, the celiac axis is kept with one half and the other split graft is supplied by either the left or the right hepatic artery. The choice of retaining the celiac axis, preferably with the right or left liver graft, should vary according to the arterial supply type and the anatomy of the recipient; this approach seems more logical than always allocating the main arterial trunk to one side, either the right or the left graft. It has often been proposed that the left graft be prepared with the celiac axis, but using the left hepatic artery only for the left graft (as done for living related donor liver transplants) provides similar results if adequate (microvascular) implantation techniques are used.[41]

Hepatic Artery Anatomy Reminder (see Fig. 41–5A and B) [28,29,32,33]

Approximately 70% of livers are fed by a single main arterial trunk (95% from the celiac axis, 4% from the superior mesenteric artery). In the majority of cases, the main arterial trunk branches into one right and one left hepatic artery or into two left and one right hepatic arteries (20% of cases) or, rarely, the opposite. In most cases, the left side of the liver (segments II, III, and IV) is fed by the left arterial branches and the right artery feeds the right side of the liver (segments V to VIII). Thus simply dividing the right, or a single left, hepatic artery provides an easy "right/left" split.

Liver supply can be by both a right hepatic artery from the superior mesenteric artery and a branch from the celiac axis (15%). In 80% of the latter cases, the right hepatic artery feeds the whole right side of the liver (replaced type), and the celiac axis feeds the left side of the liver. A similar, but reverse, condition is found when the whole left side of the liver is fed by a replaced left hepatic artery arising from the left gastric artery (10% of livers). The latter anatomy variations can be called "natural split," and the splitting is simple.

Rarely, a branch of a left artery can feed one (or more) right liver segments, or a branch of the right artery feeds a left segment (segment IV in most cases).[32] In the latter cases, a "left lateral segment/extended right lobe" split can be considered, but division should be avoided in the other cases.

In 2% to 3% of livers, very rare other anomalies, or a combination of the previously described variations, can be seen and may contraindicate splitting. In 0.5% of all livers, a single artery arising from the left gastric artery feeds the whole liver and usually has a complex division mode. These difficult variants should not be considered for splitting unless performed by very experienced and skilled surgeons.

Portal Vein

Division of the bifurcation can provide a single right and left vein ostium in most cases. Mobilizing the left portal vein and keeping the portal trunk with the right graft is the easiest option. Congenital anomalies are exceptional (absence of the extrahepatic portion of the left portal vein—0.1%). They must be recognized but do not contraindicate splitting by experienced surgeons.[40,42]

Bile Ducts

Bile duct anatomic variations are common, and detailed biliary imaging is recommended.[29,32,43,44] Variations can be summarized as follows. A single common right or left duct is observed in 53% and 88% of cases, respectively. A complex confluence of the bile ducts (tri- or quadrifurcation) is seen in one third of livers, with a possible shift of one sectorial right bile duct to the left (25%) or down along the common hepatic duct (45%). The left duct branches into one duct for segment IV and one duct for segments II and III in 80% of cases.

Because of these common variations on the right side and also taking into account the vascular supply mode of the biliary tract, it is recommended that the left bile duct be divided and the common hepatic duct kept with the right split graft. In the majority of cases, this division mode results in a single ostium for the left bile duct. In the case of "left lateral segment/extended right lobe" split, the division is done more distally on the left duct, which may result in opening two segmental ducts.[32,43]

Surgical Techniques of Splitting

Left Lateral Segment/Extended Right Lobe Using the Suprahilar Approach

Principle and Technique

Typically, the object of a "left lateral segment/extended right lobe" split is to provide a right liver graft, with the vena cava attached, for an adult recipient and a left lateral segment (segments II and III) graft for a child. The liver is divided in the line of the falciform ligament (anterior aspect) and of the ligamentum venosum (posterior aspect) (Fig. 41-6). Initially, segment IV in this situation was resected, as it is normally vascularized from the left. In practice, this has no clinical significance and thus resection,[6,8,19] or not,[12,17] of segment IV depends on the team's own preference. Retention of segment IV with the right side reduces the cut surface area and may reduce bleeding.

The standard procedure is to retain the left hepatic vein and the left bile duct with the left lateral segment split graft. The left hepatic vein is divided at its junction with the vena cava and median hepatic vein; the orifice created is oversewn while paying attention to

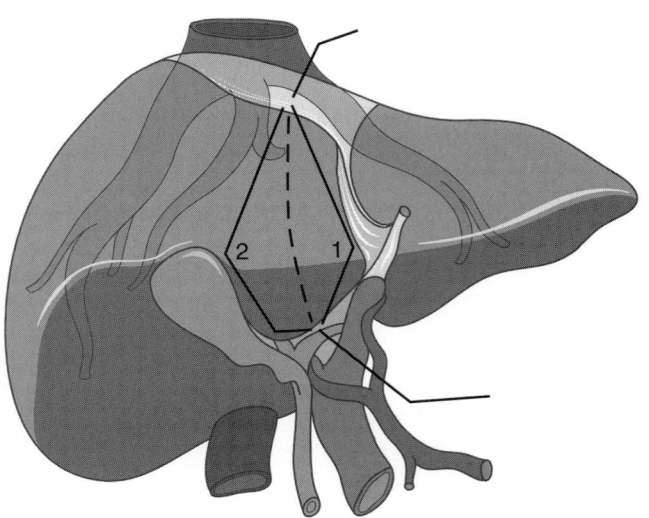

FIGURE 41–6

Transection surface lines for simple liver division and preparing left lateral segment graft using extrahilar approach (*line 1*). The latter line can be slightly shifted to the right to retain a small portion of segment IV (*dotted line*) or even more (*line 2*), but keeping the median hepatic vein with the right graft in all cases.

preserve good patency of the median hepatic vein; in a few cases, a venous patch is useful.

The division of the artery is done in accordance with the anatomy,[17,41] retaining the celiac axis with the left graft in cases of variation of the left artery. Either the portal trunk or the left portal vein can be kept with the left half, our preference being the latter option because the left portal vein is longer than the right and can easily be mobilized from the liver.

The suprahilar approach for dividing the liver along the falciform ligament is simply a straight transparenchymal division of segment IV pedicles. These pedicles can be divided as they arise from the umbilical plate[45] or more distally within the parenchyma when some portion of segment IV is retained (see the discussion later in this chapter) (see Fig. 41-6).

Of course, doing this definitively divides the vascular and biliary supply to segment IV, but it avoids dissecting the left portal vein within the umbilical fissure and the blind sharp division of the umbilical plate with the risk of inadvertently damaging a bile duct or part of the left arterial supply. It has the advantage of allowing the surgeon to increase the volume of the left split graft easily, when appropriate for the recipient, by retaining a variable amount of viable segment IV; this is simply done, without changing the technique, by moving the parenchymal division line toward the right and dividing through the substance of segment IV. It allows a much better tuning of the liver graft mass according to the recipient weight, as compared with the transhilar approach.

Application for In Situ or Ex Situ Division

The technique can be used in situ or ex situ. In situ division would be performed as for transparenchymal liver resection, using ultrasonographic dissection and bipolar diathermy. Early division of the left bile duct is usually done when parenchymal division is half completed because it facilitates dividing further. When the left hepatic vein is freed, the liver can be flushed with preservation solution, en bloc, and then both halves procured. Alternatively, the left liver graft can be procured and flushed before completing the procurement.

Ex situ division, as in usual bench surgery, is done under slush ice. After usual examination of the gross macroscopic aspect and standard graft preparation, the arterial supply is carefully skeletonized to reveal the precise anatomy. Cholangiography is then performed to delineate the biliary anatomy, which allows a more precise division to obtain a single left biliary ostium. Arteriography may be useful if the arterial anatomy seems abnormal on initial inspection.[7,19,30]

Implantation of Grafts

Right Graft. The right graft consists of segments V, VI, VII, VIII, and the whole, or part, of segments I and IV. Of segment I, the left portion (caudate process) may be removed before implantation to facilitate access to the suprahepatic caval anastomosis. This right graft is usually procured with the vena cava attached, with the portal trunk and the common hepatic duct, and with a variable arterial supply (commonly, either the celiac axis or the right hepatic artery). This allows a straightforward implantation in an adult recipient using the conventional techniques. Routine use of a T-tube or biliary internal stent has been proposed to reduce the risk of bile leakage.[17,46]

Left Lateral Segment Graft. The graft is typically provided with the left hepatic vein, the left portal vein, and the left bile duct (sometimes two biliary ostia). The recipient vena cava must be retained for piggyback-type implantation (Fig. 41–7). Attention must be given to

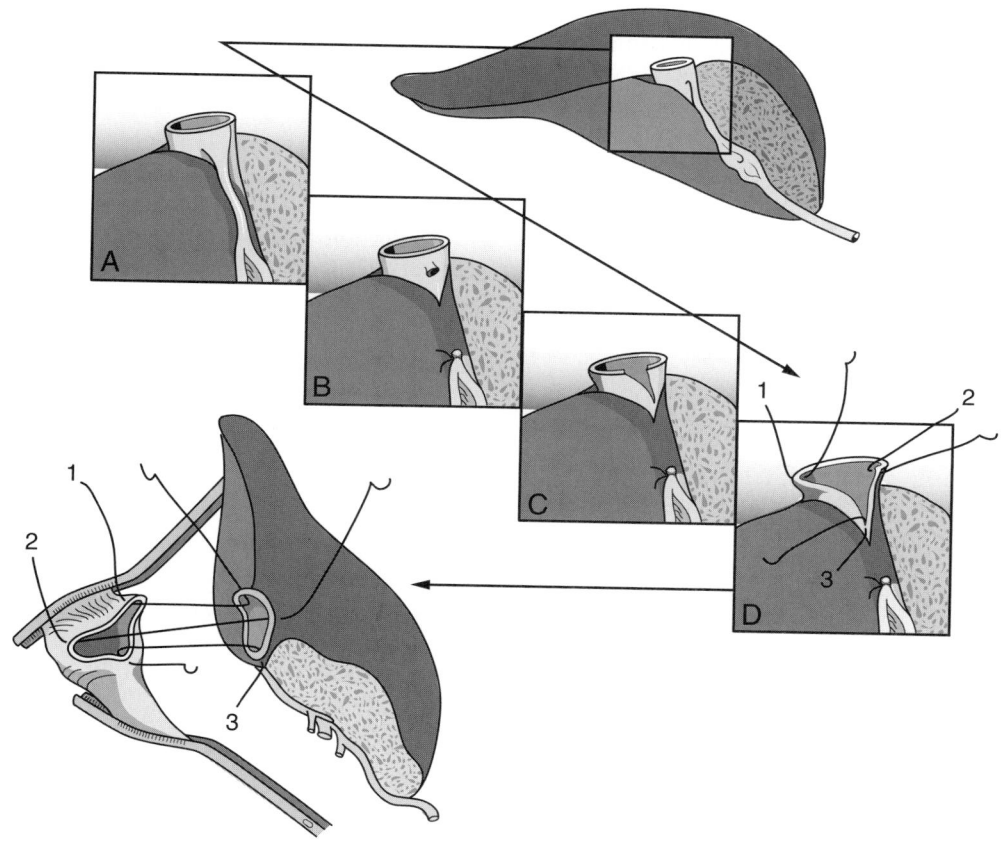

FIGURE 41–7

Schematic view of the hepatic vein reconstruction for left lateral segment graft implantation. **A,** Posterolateral view showing the preparation of the left hepatic vein ostium (LHV). **B,** Division of the Arantius ligament and freeing of the posterior aspect of the LHV. **C,** Posterior sagittal split of LHV. **D,** Preparation of the triangular anastomosis onto the vena cava (ostia of the three recipient hepatic veins). (From de Ville de Goyet J: Surgical techniques and management. In Tejani AH, Fine RN, Harmon WE (eds): Pediatric Solid Organ Transplantation. Malden, MA, Blackwell Science, 2000, p 274.)

achieve a large triangular anastomosis[47] and a correct graft positioning with anchoring to the diaphragm at the end of the operation to avoid outflow problems.[48]

Minor anatomic variations of venous outflow are not uncommon and are not difficult to deal with. Double-barrel-type ostium is corrected by simple plasty, the need for a formal reconstruction (venous jump graft) being rare.[34,43,49,50]

Portal vein reconstruction can be done by direct anastomosis between the recipient portal vein bifurcation and the donor left portal vein. When the recipient portal vein is hypoplastic, our preference is to first implant a venous graft from the same donor onto the splenomesenteric confluence or the superior mesenteric vein during the anhepatic phase in order to shorten the portal reconstruction time.

Reconstruction of the artery may vary according to the graft arterial supply type. Experience with both split livers and living donor grafts shows no disadvantage in using grafts procured with a small left hepatic artery provided that microsurgical expertise is available for performing the anastomosis; excellent results have been reported.[41]

The left bile duct reconstruction is, as is common in children, done to a Roux-en-Y jejunal loop. This makes it easy to perform two separate anastomoses when division leads to sectioning of two bile ducts. It is recommended that the Roux loop be positioned to end in the reverse way (blind end toward right) to avoid kinking of the loop when the liver graft is in the final position at closing the abdomen (Fig. 41–8).

Ex Situ Splitting Results

Technique-related risks are (1) possible preservation injury related to prolongation of bench surgery and ischemic time, (2) risk of biliary leakage or hemorrhage from the cut surface, and (3) increased morbidity in recipients in poor condition at transplantation. Compared with in situ splitting, the advantages are (1) decreased logistic demand in the donor center because ex situ splitting can be performed "at home" after conventional procurement in the donor hospital and (2) easier full anatomic assessment of the liver graft (including angio- and cholangiography) before any decision about splitting is made.

Inevitably, there is a learning curve and an initial increase in incidence of technical complications (Table 41–2). In the first large series published by the European Split Liver Registry,[51] portal vein thrombosis, hepatic artery thrombosis, biliary complications, and retransplantation rates were 4%, 11.5%, 18.7%, and 18.7%, respectively. Importantly, the report from the European Split Liver Registry showed that the clinical condition of the recipients at transplantation must be taken into account to compare split series fairly with

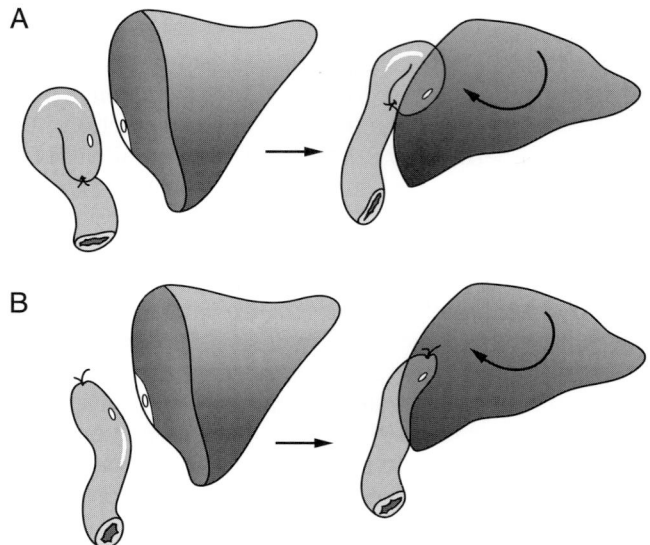

FIGURE 41–8

Positioning of Roux-en-Y loop for biliojejunal anastomosis. The conventional position (**A**) can advantageously be replaced by a straight positioning with the end of the loop looking toward the right and the diaphragm (**B**). The latter position avoids kinking of the loop and stasis in the blind end.

other (nonsplit) transplant series; similar results were obtained in comparable groups in regard to age and clinical condition.

Since then it has been confirmed by many centers and by UNOS data that in more elective conditions and with increased experience, results of split transplants match those of conventional transplants with, for series after 1995, 1-year patient survival rates of approximately 90%[5,6,12,13,30,46,51-54] or even higher in pediatric series.[17-19] Table 41–2 provides a detailed review of complication rates and outcomes in reported series of ex situ split-liver transplants.

Left Lateral Segment/ Extended Right Lobe with Division of the Hilar Plate (Transhilar Approach)

Principle

This technique consists of dissecting the extrahepatic structures first, as far as possible. The advantage is having more chances of conserving the artery of segment IV and of obtaining a slightly longer left portal vein. In view of the very lateral transection of the bile duct, a cholangiogram is not needed unless one wants to detect the rare case of very distal confluence of segment II and segment III bile ducts. The price for this is a slightly longer dissection.

Table 41-2. EX SITU SPLIT-LIVER TRANSPLANTATION: WORLD EXPERIENCE

Reference	Author	Year	Patients (N)	Adults (N)	Children (N)	High Risk (%)	Biliary Complications (%)	HAT (%)	PVT (%)	PNF (%)	Patient Survival Total (%)	Adults	Children	Graft Survival Total (%)	Adults	Children
1	Pichlmayr	1988	2	2	0	0	0	0	0	0	50	50		50	50	50
2	Bismuth	1989	2	2	0	100	0	0	0	0	0	0	0	0	0	0
3	Otte	1990	4	1	3	75	0	0	0	0	50	0	66	50	0	66
4	Emond	1990	18	5	13	38	27	6	6	24	67	40	63	50	40	53
10	Broelsch	1990	30	4	21	40	27	na	na	na	60	25	66	43	20	48
11	Langnas	1992	10	1	9	73	20	7	0	17	69	na	na	67	na	na
7	Houssin	1993	16	6	10	50	25	13	25	0	75	83	70	69	83	60
30	Otte	1994	29	11	18	27	17	10	0	10	79	na	na	69	na	na
51	de Ville de Goyet	1995	96	39	54	33	22	12	4	4	71	81	71	64	59	66
52	Slooff	1995	15	na	na	na	na	na	na	na	73	na	na	67	na	na
12	Kalayoglu	1996	12	5	7	8	17	8	0	0	92	100	85	75	80	71
31	Rogiers	1996	12	5	7	44	15	15	0	0	75	57	100	66	42	100
5	Azoulay	1996	27	26	1	14	22	15	0	4	79	80	100	78	76	100
13	Dunn	1997	12	0	12	50	0	0	0	0	75		75	66		66
6	Rela	1998	41	15	26	12	15	3	0	0	90	93	89	88	93	84
8	Mirza	1998	24	10	14	58	8	8	0	16	78	80	78	68	na	na
55	Chardot	1999	15	0	15	31	25	12	19	0	66		66	62		62
19	Reyes	2000	25	13	12	66	8	12	0	na	74	69	66	61	61	50
18	Deshpande	2002	80	0	80	20	9	5	1	0	89		89	86		86
17	Noujaim pre-1998	2003	29	10	19	38	28	14	0	34	72	na	na	59	na	na
17	Noujaim post-1998	2003	60	24	36	25	20	3	0	3	85	na	na	78	na	na

HAT, hepatic artery thrombosis; na, data not available; PNF, primary nonfunction; PVT, portal vein thrombosis.

Procedure

The first step of the procedure is careful observation of the liver. Good general quality and homogeneous perfusion of the liver should be present. In case of significant steatosis (>15% to 20%), splitting should not be performed. When splitting ex situ, the perfusion with preservation solution must be adequate and homogeneous. Next the volumes of the extended right lobe and the left lateral segment are estimated and a prospective decision is made about which recipients are to undergo transplantation.

The peritoneum over the left half of the hepatoduodenal ligament is opened. The right half of the hepatoduodenal ligament is left intact. The left portal vein and left hepatic artery are carefully dissected free up to the point at which one is sure that they serve only the left lateral segment.

Next the portal branches to segment IV are transected. This is most conveniently performed by following the umbilical ligament. An eventual bridge of liver tissue anteriorly to Rex recessus (the vertical segment of the left portal vein) is transected. Following the right side of the umbilical ligament and of Rex recessus, the fine peritoneal layer is opened. The small portal branches to segment IV are now readily visible and can be isolated and transected between clips. Care has to be taken to preserve the small artery to segment IV, which usually runs exactly between these branches and the hilar plate. After having completed this step, the left hilar plate lays open (Fig. 41–9). One or two portal vein branches to segment I may have to be severed between clips in order to provide for enough length of the left portal vein and to avoid injury to it during later transection of the left hilar plate. In ex situ splitting, the left or right hepatic artery and left or right portal vein can be transected at this moment. The decision as to which side of the vessels to transect is made on the basis of the actual anatomy of the vessels and the specific requirements of the recipients.

The next step consists of isolating the left hepatic vein. In the in situ technique, a vessel loop is put around it; in the ex situ technique, it is transected immediately. If a patch of inferior vena cava is taken with it, it may be necessary to repair the defect in the inferior vena cava with a venous patch in order to avoid stenosis. In very rare cases, the segment III vein may drain directly into the middle hepatic vein. In such cases, one may have to transect it during the parenchymal transection and reconstruct it with a venous interposition graft. In any case, great care has to be taken not to impede the venous outflow of segment IV because this uniformly leads to necrosis of the segment.

The parenchymal transection is very different between the in situ and ex situ techniques. The line of transection is exactly on the line of insertion of the falciform ligament.

In the ex situ technique, the parenchyma is simply transected using a sharp blade. The goal is to have a quick transection with a very even transection plane. At the end of the transection, only the hilar plates connect the two grafts. This is also transected using the sharp knife. The hilar plate on the right side is carefully oversewn with 6-0 polydioxanone suture (PDS). On both transection surfaces, the visible blood vessel stumps are oversewn. Further hemostasis with simple stitches and coagulation is made at the time of implantation (Table 41–3).

In the in situ technique, the transection of the parenchyma, on the same transection line, can be performed with a variety of techniques from traditional liver surgery. After transecting about one third of the surface, the left hilar plate can be controlled with a clamp and transected sharply. Hemostasis of the transected

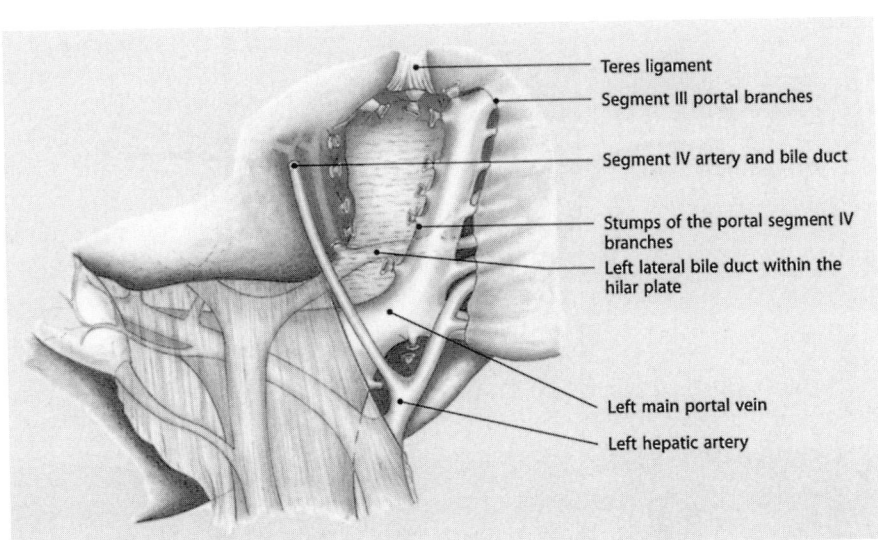

Teres ligament
Segment III portal branches

Segment IV artery and bile duct

Stumps of the portal segment IV branches
Left lateral bile duct within the hilar plate

Left main portal vein
Left hepatic artery

FIGURE 41–9

Dissection of the left hilar plate. (From Rogiers X, Bismuth H, Busuttil RW, et al. (eds): Split Liver Transplantation: Theoretical and Practical Aspects. Darmstadt, Hessen, Germany, Steinkopff-Verlag, 2002, p 51.)

Table 41-3. EXTENDED RIGHT/LEFT LATERAL SEGMENT SPLITTING WITH TRANSECTION OF THE HILAR PLATE: EX SITU
1. Inspect the liver
2. Dissect left hepatic artery and portal vein
3. Transect segment IV branches along Rex recessus
4. Isolate left hepatic vein
5. Transect blood vessels
6. Transect parenchyma
7. Transect hilar plate
8. Suture blood vessels on section surface
9. Suture blood vessel stumps and right-side hilar plate
10. Weigh, document anatomy, provide grafts

Table 41-4. EXTENDED RIGHT/LEFT LATERAL SEGMENT SPLITTING WITH TRANSECTION OF THE HILAR PLATE: IN SITU
1. Inspect the liver
2. Dissect left hepatic artery and portal vein
3. Transect segment IV branches along Rex recessus
4. Isolate left hepatic vein
5. Transect parenchyma
6. Transect hilar plate
7. Oversew right hilar plate stump
8. Explant left graft separately or together with right graft (perfuse left graft on back table)
9. Perfuse organ donor with preservation solution and procure
10. Transect blood vessels and sew stumps
11. Weigh, document anatomy, provide grafts

hilar plate, if done at all, should be performed only with fine stitches. At this point the lateral limb of the vessel loop around the left hepatic vein can be passed through the arterial and portal bifurcation. From this point on the vessel loop serves as a guide to lead the transection line in the angle between the left and the middle hepatic veins (Fig. 41–10). Once the transection is complete, both grafts can be observed in perfused status, and complete hemostasis of the transection surface can be obtained. Now the surgeon has a choice of two strategic options. The surgeon can clamp the vessels to the left graft, remove it, and flush the left graft on the back table. The right graft is then removed with the other organs. This allows the transplantation of the left

graft to start earlier. Alternatively, the surgeon can perfuse both grafts in situ with the other organs. After removal of the liver, only the blood vessels have to be transected to obtain two separate grafts (Table 41–4).

It is usual practice to weigh the grafts and describe their exact anatomy at the end of the procedure. Adequate donor blood vessels should be provided for eventual interposition grafts.

Table 41–5 details the reported world experience with in situ split-liver transplantation.

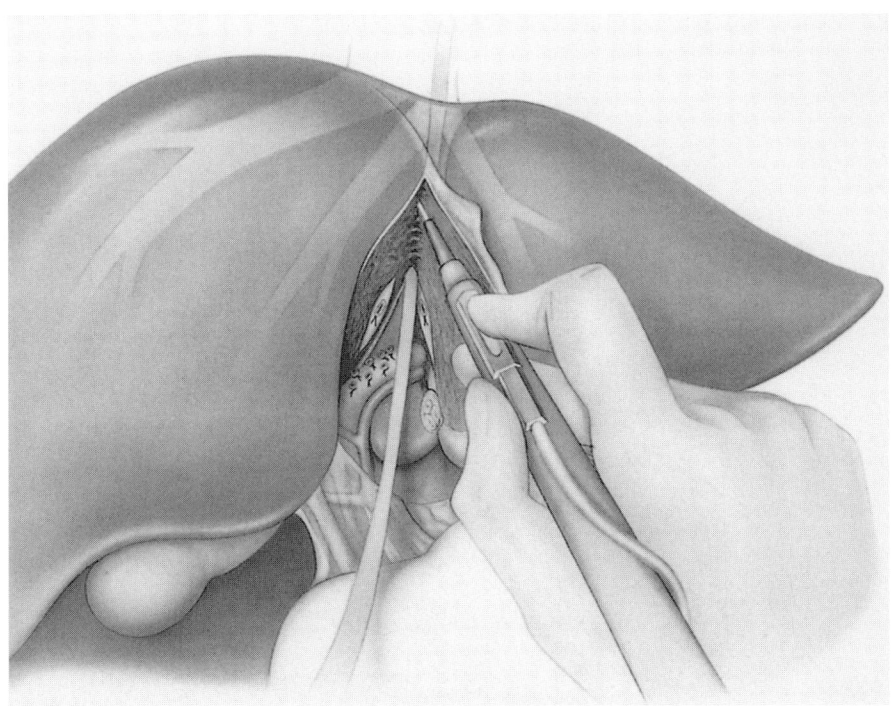

FIGURE 41–10

Vessel loop technique for finding the right plane. (From Rogiers X, Bismuth H, Busuttil RW, et al. (eds): Split Liver Transplantation: Theoretical and Practical Aspects. Darmstadt, Hessen, Germany: Steinkopff-Verlag, 2002, p 94.)

Table 41-5. IN SITU SPLIT-LIVER TRANSPLANTATION: WORLD EXPERIENCE

Reference	Author	Year	Patients (N)	Adults (N)	Children (N)	High Risk (%)	Biliary Complications (%)	HAT (%)	PVT (%)	PNF (%)	Patient Survival Total (%)	Patient Survival Adults	Patient Survival Children	Graft Survival Total (%)	Graft Survival Adults	Graft Survival Children
31	Rogiers	1996	14	7	7	35	0	0	0	0	93	100	85	78	85	71
15	Goss	1997	28	14	12	58	14	0	0	11	92	85	100	86	78	91
54	Busuttil	1999	65	na	na	66	3	3	1	8	90	85	96	80	86	75
56	Ghobrial	2000	102	51	51	49	na	2	2	8	81	83	78	75	na	na
19	Reyes	2000	29	na	na	na	3	3	0	7	96	93	100	81	79	83
Personal communication	Rogiers	2002	128	63	65	66	3	3	1	8	90	85	97	80	86	75
16	Gridelli	2003	90	0	90	28	33	7	6	1	90	90	90	80	—	80
—	—	—	—	Right split	Left split	—	—	Right split: 4 / Left split: 9	Right split: 8 / Left split: 3	Right split: 18 / Left split: 8	—	Right split 78% / Left split 75%	—	—	Right split 69% / Left split 64%	—
62	Yersiz	2003	71 (57ad, 14 ch)	71 (57ad, 14 ch)	90 ch	—	Right split: 10 / Left split: 9				—			—		
—	—	—	—	—	—	—	—	—	—	—	—	—	—	—	—

HAT, hepatic artery thrombosis; na, data not available; PNF, primary nonfunction; PVT, portal vein thrombosis.
Data from Yersiz H, Renz JF, Farmer DG, et al: One hundred in situ split-liver transplantations: A single-center experience. Ann Surg 238:496–505, 2003.

Full-Right/Full-Left Splitting for Transplantation in Two Adults

To apply splitting of the liver for two adults, one has to face the issue of minimal graft size. Although this issue was first addressed in living donor liver transplantation, it is important to recognize that more liver tissue is needed in deceased donor liver transplantation than in living donor transplantation. This is because of the worse condition of deceased donor livers in general and also because of the additional ischemia-reperfusion damage related to longer ischemia times in comparison with living donation. In a recipient in relatively good condition, a graft weight in excess of 0.8% to 1% of the recipient's body weight is generally safe. This usually cannot be reached for both adult recipients by using the classic split-liver techniques. Consequently, techniques derived from adult living donation have been adapted for deceased donor liver splitting. These techniques allow the splitting of the liver along the line of Cantlie (on the right side of the median hepatic vein), resulting in a full right hemiliver (segments V, VI, VII, and VIII) and a full left hemiliver (segments I, II, III, and IV). Even when using this plane for splitting the liver, graft volumes are usually close to the critical range. Therefore the choice of an excellent liver donor and avoiding poor recipients (in analogy to living donation) is vitally important. The use of the in situ technique to reduce further ischemic damage and allow the evaluation of the grafts before their implantation is vital when there is an extra risk factor in either donor or recipients.

The splitting technique is essentially the same as that of right lobe living donation. The problems regarding venous drainage, biliary vascularization, vascular anomalies, and small-for-size syndrome are the same. Some differences apply, however. Because the vena cava of the donor can be procured with the graft, one can split the vena cava (Fig. 41-11),[21] providing large venous cuffs, including the minor hepatic veins on both grafts. These are helpful in allowing an easy implantation (Fig. 41-12). They also guarantee a better venous outflow of the caudate lobe, thus preserving valuable functional graft volume for the most critical left graft. The splitting of the blood vessels and the bile duct can be performed on the back table, allowing the optimal compromise between the existing anatomy and the requirement of the recipients.

The present series of full-right/full-left splits is still very small. This is a result of several factors that limit the spread of this variant such as (1) the requirement of an excellent donor and acceptable recipients (size and condition), (2) the technical difficulty of the procedure, which has not reached the level of standardization of normal splitting, and (3) the difficulty of sharing these complex grafts between different centers.

Nevertheless, it is important to note that the feasibility of the procedure has been demonstrated in different centers throughout the world with good results (Table 41-6).

Acknowledgment

The authors warmly thank Mrs. Cathy Vuylsteke for her efficient secretarial assistance.

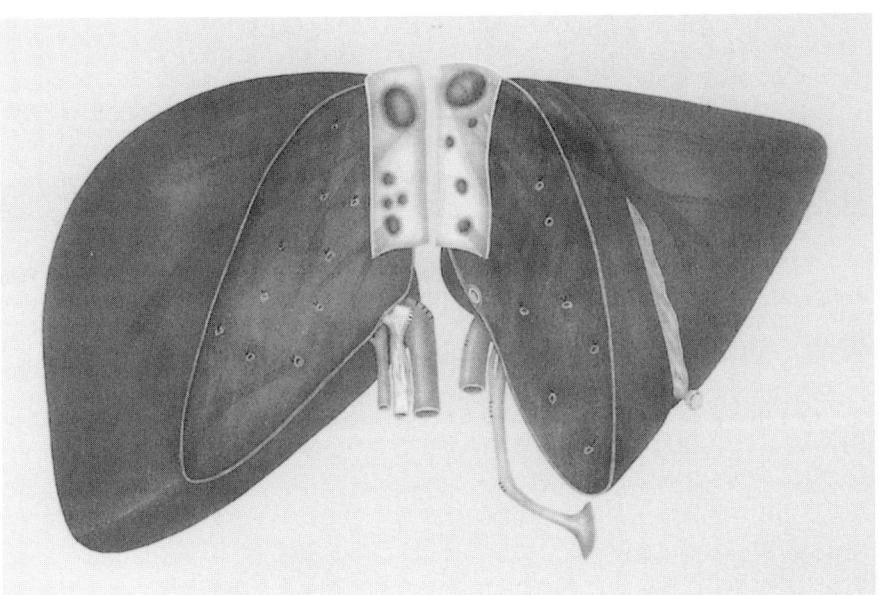

FIGURE 41-11

Splitting of the inferior vena cava. (From Rogiers X, Bismuth H, Busuttil RW, et al. (eds): Split Liver Transplantation: Theoretical and Practical Aspects. Darmstadt, Hessen, Germany, Steinkopff-Verlag, 2002, p 57.)

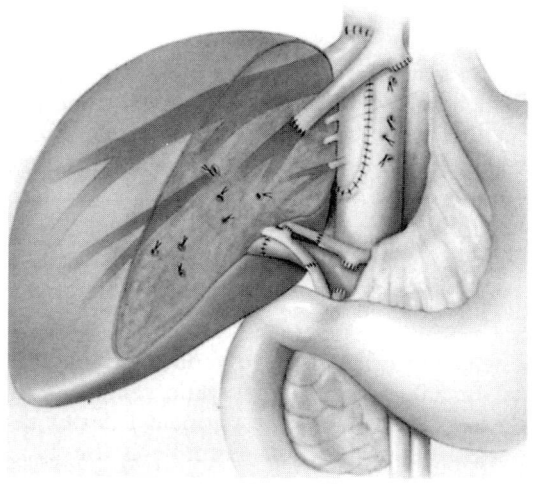

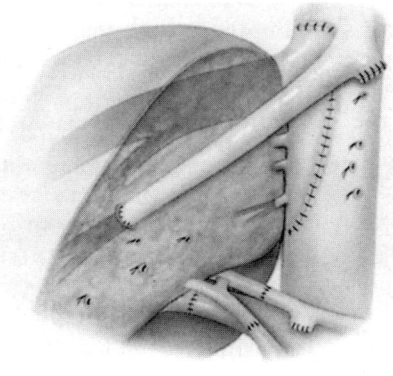
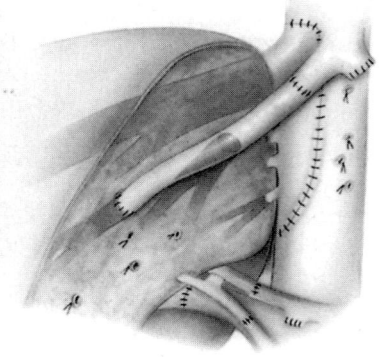

FIGURE 41–12

Implantation of the right graft: venous implantation and eventual reconstructions. (From Rogiers X, Bismuth H, Busuttil RW, et al. (eds): Split Liver Transplantation: Theoretical and Practical Aspects. Darmstadt, Hessen, Germany, Steinkopff-Verlag, 2002, p 58.)

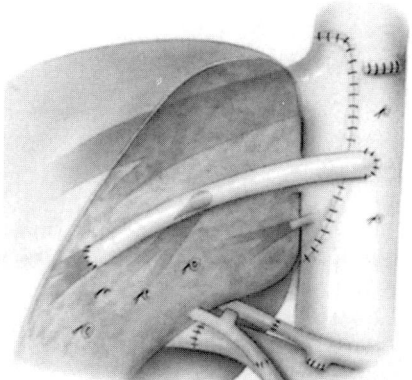
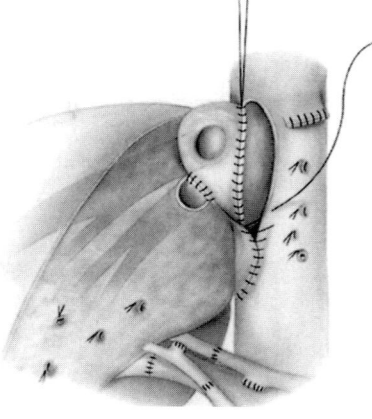

Table 41–6. FULL-RIGHT/FULL-LEFT SPLIT-LIVER TRANSPLANTATION IN TWO ADULT RECIPIENTS: WORLD EXPERIENCE

Reference	Author	Year	Patients (N)	Biliary Complications (%)	HAT (%)	PVT (%)	PNF (%)	Patient Survival			Graft Survival		
								Total (%)	Left	Right	Total (%)	Left	Right
61	Sommacale	2000	2	0	0	0	0	100	100	100	100	100	100
58	Colledan	2000	6	0	16	0	33	83	66	100	66	66	66
22	Humar	2001	12	25	16	0	0	83	5/6	83	83	83	83
59	Azoulay	2001	34	22	6	0	8	82	88	76	76	76	76
60	Andorno	2001	8	0	12	0	12	75	75	75	62	75	50
57	Kilic	2001	8	12	0	0	0	100	100	100	100	100	100
Personal communication	Rogiers	2003	24	na	na	na	na	86	84	90	86	84	90

HAT, hepatic artery thrombosis; na, data not available; PNF, primary nonfunction; PVT, portal vein thrombosis.

Pearls and Pitfalls

- Splitting of the liver can be performed ex situ or in situ; both techniques deliver similarly good results in experienced hands.
- In situ liver splitting can be performed in the local procurement center by an experienced surgeon.
- In situ liver splitting offers the potential advantages of a perfect hemostasis, proper identification of the vascular and biliary structures, and the shortening of ischemia time, which allows an exchange between transplant centers.
- In situ splitting has no detrimental effects on the other organs procured at the same time.
- Split-liver transplants help to reduce the mortality of children on waiting lists.
- Rule of thumb: the weight of the recipients' right and the split grafts should be a maximum 100% and 60%, respectively, of the donor weight to provide both recipients with a graft-to-body-weight ratio of 1.2%.
- Safe splitting of the liver for two adult recipients is feasible by splitting the liver on the right side of the median hepatic vein, resulting in a full right hemiliver (segments V to VIII) and a full left hemiliver (segments I to IV).
- Further expansion of the split-liver transplantation requires motivation, expertise, and optimized logistical procedures in transplant centers.
- Caution is needed when extrapolating data regarding the liver mass requirement from living liver transplantation to deceased donor split-liver transplantation; even greater caution is needed in ex situ splitting (because of prolonged ischemia). The graft-to–body weight ratio should be greater than or equal to 1.2% and the graft weight should be greater than or equal to 40% of the standard liver volume.
- The splitting procedures require a precise knowledge of the liver anatomy and sufficient expertise with major liver resections.
- How far the mortality of adult patients on waiting lists can be reduced by the expansion of the full-right/full-left split-liver transplantation is hardly predictable because of the limited number of adult recipients with a low body weight and the increasing proportion of older and marginal donors in whom a safe splitting is not possible.

Pearls and Pitfalls—cont'd

- Unstable chronic patients (UNOS status 2A) and patients with fulminant liver failure who do worse with small-for-size grafts should be excluded from a split-liver program.
- Less than optimal liver donor grafts should *not* be split. Less than optimal liver donors include donors older than age 40 to 50 years and donors with hemodynamic instability, steatosis, elevated liver values, or long intensive treatment unit stay (>5 days).

References

1. Pichlmayr R, Ringe B, Gubernatis G, et al: Transplantation of one donor liver to two recipients (splitting transplantation). A new method for further development of segmental liver transplantation. Langenbecks Arch Chir 373:127-130, 1988.
2. Bismuth H, Morino M, Castaing D, et al: Emergency orthotopic liver transplantation in two patients using one donor liver. Br J Surg 76:722-724, 1989.
3. Otte JB, de Ville de Goyet J, Alberti D, et al: The concept and technique of the split liver in clinical transplantation. Surgery 107:605-612, 1990.
4. Emond JC, Whitington PF, Thistlethwaite JR, et al: Transplantation of two patients with one liver. Analysis of a preliminary experience with "split-liver" grafting. Ann Surg 212:14-22, 1990.
5. Azoulay D, Astarcioglu I, Bismuth H, et al: Split-liver transplantation. The Paul Brousse policy. Ann Surg 224:737-746, 1996.
6. Rela M, Vougas V, Muisan P, et al: Split liver transplantation. King's College Hospital experience. Ann Surg 227:282-288, 1998.
7. Houssin D, Boillot O, Soubrane O, et al: Controlled liver splitting for transplantation in two recipients: Technique, results and perspectives. Br J Surg 80:75-80, 1993.
8. Mirza D, Achilleos OA, Pirenne J, et al: Encouraging results of split-liver transplantation. Br J Surg 85:494-497, 1998.
9. de Ville de Goyet J, Hausleithner V, Reding R, et al: Impact of innovative techniques on the waiting list and results in pediatric liver transplantation. Transplantation 56:1130-1136, 1993.
10. Broelsch CE, Emond JC, Whitington PF, et al: Application of reduced-size liver transplants as split grafts, auxiliary orthotopic grafts, and living related segmental transplants. Ann Surg 212:368-375, 1990.
11. Langnas AN, Marujo WC, Inagaki M, et al: The results of reduced-size liver transplantation, including split livers, in patients with end-stage liver disease. Transplantation 53:387-391, 1992.
12. Kalayoglu M, D'Alessandro AM, Knechtle SJ, et al: Preliminary experience with split liver transplantation. J Am Coll Surg 182:381-387, 1996.
13. Dunn DC, Haynes JH, Nicolette LA, et al: Split liver transplantation benefits the recipient of the leftover liver. J Pediatr Surg 32:252-255, 1997.
14. Rogiers X, Malago M, Gawad K, et al: In situ splitting of cadaveric livers. The ultimate expansion of a limited donor pool. Ann Surg 224:331-339, 1996.

15. Goss JA, Yersiz H, Shackleton CR, et al: In situ splitting of the cadaveric liver for transplantation. Transplantation 64:871-877, 1997.
16. Gridelli B, Spada M, Petz W, et al: Split-liver transplantation eliminates the need for living-donor liver transplantation in children with end-stage cholestatic liver disease. Transplantation 75:1197-1203, 2003.
17. Noujaim HM, Gunson B, Mirza DF, et al: Worth continuing doing ex vivo liver graft splitting in an in situ division era? A single center detailed study. Am J Transplantation 3:318-323, 2003.
18. Deshpande RR, Bowles MJ, Vilca-Melandez H, et al: Results of split liver transplantation in children. Ann Surg 236:248-253, 2002.
19. Reyes J, Gerber D, Maziaregos GV, et al: Split-liver transplantation: A comparison of ex-vivo and in situ techniques. J Pediatr Surg 35:283-290, 2000.
20. Adam R, Cailliez V, Majno P, et al: Normalised intrinsic mortality risk in liver transplantation: European Liver Transplant Registry study. Lancet 356:621-627, 2000.
21. Gundlach M, Broering D, Topps S, et al: Split-cava technique: Liver splitting for two adult recipients. Liver Transpl 6:703-706, 2000.
22. Humar A, Ramcharan T, Sielaff T, et al: Split liver transplantation for two adult recipients: An initial experience. Am J Transplantation 1:366-372, 2001.
23. Petz W, Spada M, Sonzogni A, et al: Pediatric split liver transplantation using elderly donors. Transplant Proc 33:1361-1363, 2001.
24. McDiarmid SV, Davies DB, Edwards EB: Improved graft survival of pediatric liver recipients transplanted with pediatric-aged liver donors. Transplantation 70:1283-1291, 2000.
25. Ramcharan T, Glessing B, Lake JR, et al: Outcome of other organs recovered during in situ split-liver procurements. Liver Transpl 7:853-857, 2001.
26. Yersiz H, Renz JF, Hisatake G, et al: Technical and logistical considerations of in situ split-liver transplantation for two adults: Part I. Creation of left segment II, III, IV and right segment I, V-VIII grafts. Liver Transpl 7:1077-1080, 2001.
27. Azoulay D, Marin-Hargreaves G, Castaing D, Bismuth H: Ex situ splitting of the liver. The versatile Paul Brousse technique. Arch Surg 136:956-961, 2001.
28. Couinaud C: Surgical anatomy of the liver revisited. Paris: Personal Edition, 1989.
29. Couinaud C, Houssin D: Controlled partition of the liver for transplantation. Anatomical limitations. Paris: Personal Edition, 1991.
30. Otte JB: Is it right to develop living related liver transplantation? Do reduced and split livers not suffice to cover the needs? Transpl Int 8:447-491, 1994.
31. Rogiers X, Malago M, Gawad K, et al: One year experience with extended application and modified techniques of split liver transplantation. Transplantation 61:1059-1061, 1996.
32. Onishi H, Kawarada Y, Das BC, et al: Surgical anatomy of the medial segment (S4) of the liver with special reference to bile ducts and vessels. Hepatogastroenterology 47:143-150, 2000.
33. Rat P, Paris P, Friedman S, Favre JP: Split-liver orthotopic liver transplantation: How to divide the portal pedicle. Surgery 112:522-526, 1992.
34. Noujaim HM, Mirza DF, Mayer DA, de Ville de Goyet J: Hepatic vein reconstruction in ex situ split-liver transplantation. Transplantation 74:1018-1021, 2002.
35. Marcos A: Split-liver transplantation for adult recipients. Liver Transpl 6:707-709, 2000.
36. Lee SG, Park KM, Hwang S, et al: Congestion of right liver graft in living donor liver transplantation. Transplantation 71:812-817, 2001.
37. Marcos A, Ham JM, Fisher RA, et al: Surgical management of anatomical variations of the right lobe in living donor liver transplantation. Ann Surg 231:824-831, 2000.
38. Ghobrial RM, Hsieh C-B, Lerner S, et al: Technical challenge of hepatic venous outflow reconstruction in right lobe adult living donor liver transplantation. Liver Transpl 7:551-555, 2001.
39. Renz JF, Reichert PR, Emond JC: Hepatic arterial anatomy as applied to living-donor and split-liver transplantation. Liver Transpl 6:367-369, 2000.
40. Mitchell A, Mirza DF, de Ville de Goyet J, Buckels JAC: Absence of the left portal vein: a difficulty for reduction of liver grafts? Transplantation 69:1731-1732, 2000.
41. Noujaim HM, Gunson B, Mirza DF, et al: Ex-situ preparation of left split grafts with left vascular pedicle only: Is it safe? A comparative single center study. Transplantation 71:1386-1390, 2002.
42. Lerut J, Ciccarelli O, Danse E, et al: Left lobe living related liver transplantation in the absence of an extrahepatic left portal vein. Transplantation 74:278-279, 2002.
43. Reichert PR, Renz JF, d'Albuquerque LAC, et al: Surgical anatomy of the left lateral segment as applied to living-related and split-liver transplantation—a clinico-pathologic study. Ann Surg 232:658-664, 2000.
44. Yoshida J, Chijiiwa K, Yamaguchi K, et al: Practical classification of the branching types of the biliary tree: An analysis of 1,904 consecutive direct cholangiograms. J Am Coll Surg 182:37-40, 1996.
45. Launois B, Jamieson GG: The importance of Glisson's capsule and its sheaths in the intrahepatic approach to resection of the liver. Surg Gynecol Obstet 174:7-10, 1992.
46. Rela M, Heaton N: Split liver transplantation. Br J Surg 85:881-883, 1998.
47. Emond JC, Heffron TG, Whitington PF, Broelsch CE: Reconstruction of the hepatic vein in reduced size hepatic transplantation. Surg Gynecol Obstet 176:11-17, 1993.
48. Mazariegos GV, Garrido V, Jaskowski-Phillips S, et al: Management of hepatic venous obstruction after split-liver transplantation. Pediatr Transplant 4:322-327, 2000.
49. Egawa H, Inomata Y, Uemoto S, et al: Hepatic vein reconstruction in 152 living-related donor liver transplantation patients. Surgery 121:250-257, 1997.
50. Genzone A, Al-Shurafa H, Mondello R, et al: In situ splitting of a liver with middle hepatic vein anomaly. Liver Transpl 7:826-828, 2001.
51. de Ville de Goyet J: Split liver transplantation in Europe, 1988 to 1993. Transplantation 59:1371-1376, 1995.
52. Slooff MJH: Reduced size liver transplantation, split liver transplantation, and living related liver transplantation in relation to the donor organ shortage. Transpl Int 8:65-68, 1995.
53. Broering DC, Topp S, Schaefer U, et al: Split liver transplantation and risk to the adult recipient: Analysis using matched pairs. J Am Coll Surg 195:648-657, 2002.
54. Busuttil RW, Goss JA: Split liver transplantation. Ann Surg 229:313-321, 1999.
55. Chardot C, Branchereau S, de Dreusy O, et al: Pediatric liver transplantation with a split graft: Experience at Bicêtre. Eur J Pediatr Surg 9:146-152, 1999.
56. Ghobrial RM, Yersiz H, Farmer DG, et al: Predictors of survival after in vivo split liver transplantation: Analysis of 110 consecutive patients. Ann Surg 232:312-323, 2000.
57. Kilic M, Seu P, Stribling RJ, et al: In situ splitting of the cadaveric liver for two adult recipients. Transplantation 72:1853-1858, 2001.
58. Colledan M, Segalin A, Andorno E, et al: Modified splitting technique for liver transplantation in adult-sized recipients. Technique and preliminary results. Acta Chir Belg 100:289-291, 2000.

59. Azoulay D, Castaing D, Adam R, et al: Split liver transplantation for two adult recipients: Feasibility and long-term outcomes. Ann Surg 233:565-574, 2001.

60. Andorno E, Genzone A, Morelli N, et al: One liver for two adults: In situ split liver transplantation for two adult recipients. Transplant Proc 33:1420-1422, 2001.

61. Sommacale D, Farges O, Ettorre GM, et al: In situ split liver transplantation for two adult recipients. Transplantation 69:707-708, 2000.

62. Yersiz H, Renz JF, Farmer DG, et al: One hundred in situ split-liver transplantations: A single-center experience. Ann Surg 238:496-505, 2003.

Living Related Liver Transplantation in Pediatric Recipients

KOICHI TANAKA
YUKIHIRO INOMATA

History and significance of pediatric living
 related liver transplantation 629

Ethical issues and informed consent 630

Indications 632

Donor evaluation 632
 Current status of donor evaluation in pediatric
  living related liver transplantation 632
 Disease transmission and donor selection 634
 Significance of HLA matching in living related
  liver transplantation 634
 Size and anatomy of the donor liver 635

Technical considerations 636
 Donor surgery 636
 Recipient procedure 637
 Vascular reconstruction 638
 Bile duct reconstruction 641

Surgical complications and treatment
 of recipients 641
 Early complications 641
 Late complications 642
 Repeat living related liver transplantation
  in pediatric recipients 643

Immunosuppression 643
 Tolerance 643
 ABO incompatibility in pediatric living related
  liver transplantation 643

Living related liver transplantation (LRLT) has been extended to adult recipients, but it was initially developed for pediatric patients with hepatic failure. This chapter covers the brief history of LRLT, controversial ethical issues associated with LRLT and informed consent, the process of donor evaluation and selection, technical considerations, immunological tolerance, and ABO-incompatible matching in pediatric LRLT. LRLT is based on the sacrifice of a donor who seeks no compensation except a chance for the recipient to live. Members of the transplant team should recognize this profoundly altruistic emotion, and every effort must be concentrated on respect for such love and self-sacrifice.

History and Significance of Pediatric Living Related Liver Transplantation

The first LRLT in the world was performed in Brazil by Raia in December 1988, but the recipient did not survive long.[1] The first successful LRLT was reported by Strong and colleagues in 1990.[2] The recipient was a Japanese boy who received a left lateral segment from his mother. Unfortunately, chronic rejection developed a year later, and the patient underwent retransplantation with a liver from a deceased donor. He has been doing well since then. In 2003, this boy graduated from junior high school with excellent academic achievement. In 1989, Nagasue and coworkers performed the first LRLT in Japan on a boy with biliary atresia.[3] In the United States, Broelsch and associates started an LRLT program in Chicago in 1989 and reported the cumulative result of 20 cases in 1990.[4] Encouraged by these results, Dr. Ozawa in Kyoto and Dr. Makuuchi in Matsumoto started LRLT programs in Japan.[5,6]

In the first experiences with LRLT, the target subjects were pediatric patients. LRLT was developed as a technical innovation to overcome the shortage of size-matched deceased liver donors. Before the development of LRLT, reduction of an adult graft for use in a pediatric patient was attempted. In this procedure, a large part of the graft was discarded and thus did not help adult patients, who accounted for the majority of patients on the waiting list. As the next step, an innovative technique of splitting an adult graft was developed and has become increasingly sophisticated.[7] Despite the development of these techniques, there was still a shortage of organs. Subsequently, however, LRLT was started. Pediatric recipients were the first targets of LRLT for two reasons: parents can be most easily selected as potential donors with the fewest ethical problems, and donor safety can be more easily preserved by leaving the larger right lobe of the donor intact after harvesting the left side of the liver. The left lobe is usually sufficient for the metabolic demands of a pediatric recipient. LRLT was a significant advance in countries in which deceased donor organs are rarely available. Split-liver transplantation from deceased donors, if sufficiently available, can reduce the number of pediatric patients waiting for organ donation without decreasing the persistently inadequate donor pool for adult patients. So theoretically, this procedure should be the first choice for pediatric liver transplantation in countries in which deceased donor livers can be retrieved easily, as reported by the Rogiers group.[8] However, splitting of deceased donor livers is still limited because of their marginal condition and the greater reluctance of centers to establish split-liver programs in the United States than in Europe, although such programs have started to expand.[9] Alternatively, the development and clinical application of LRLT could successfully reduce mortality on the waiting list as reported by both Essen and Brussels.[10] Multimodal procedures, including the splitting technique and LRLT, should henceforth be considered as means of enlarging the overall donor pool for not only pediatric patients but also all recipients. At least in pediatric recipients, LRLT already has a solid foundation and is much more advantageous than deceased donor transplantation because it confers relatively small risk to the donor and produces a better-quality graft under elective surgery after meticulous conditioning of both the donor and recipients.

In selected institutions, an adult liver surgeon in one hospital and a pediatric transplant surgeon in a children's hospital are both involved in LRLT for the pediatric recipient[11]; such combined participation is one means of respecting specialization on both sides.

Ethical Issues and Informed Consent

LRLT involves surgery on a living, healthy human, and this issue has been ethically controversial for a long time, especially in countries in which deceased donors are reasonably available.[12] However, in Asian countries, LRLT was easily accepted and has developed into the main liver transplantation technique performed because the concept of brain death is not well established in this region.[13] The LRLT process depends on the availability of deceased donor transplantation (Fig. 42–1). If deceased donor transplantation is well established and common, the number of recipients needing LRLT may be limited. In contrast, if deceased donors are not available, most recipients desire LRLT if an appropriate donor is available.

In pediatric LRLT, the donor is usually one of the parents, a situation that affords the best matching of the donor and recipient with the least ethical conflict. Preserving the life of their child may be very gratifying for parents. However, in some instances, social pressure may oblige the parents to become donors. During the informed consent process, other means to avoid being a living donor should always be mentioned after all the risks and benefits of LRLT have been explained to the family in complete detail. In rare cases, siblings or parents younger than 18 years may be included as donor candidates for pediatric LRLT. In such cases, not only their emotional response to being a living donor but also their competence to understand the LRLT process and donor risk should be carefully evaluated during the initial stages of the LRLT process. Grandparents may be also included among the donor candidates, and in such cases, extra risk to an elderly donor should be included in the informed consent discussion after meticulous evaluation of the health of the donor candidate. When the donor is a more distant relative, such as an uncle or aunt, voluntary willingness should be carefully ascertained. Donor candidates should be interviewed independently in the absence of the recipient and family members of the recipient. If the parents are divorced, the parent living with the child is usually selected as the donor; however, the noncustodial parent may be included as a donor candidate if so desired.

During the informed consent process, the discussion of donor risk should include the possibility of donor mortality.[12] In a review of 1508 LRLTs in Asia, the incidence of complications after donor surgery was 9.3%

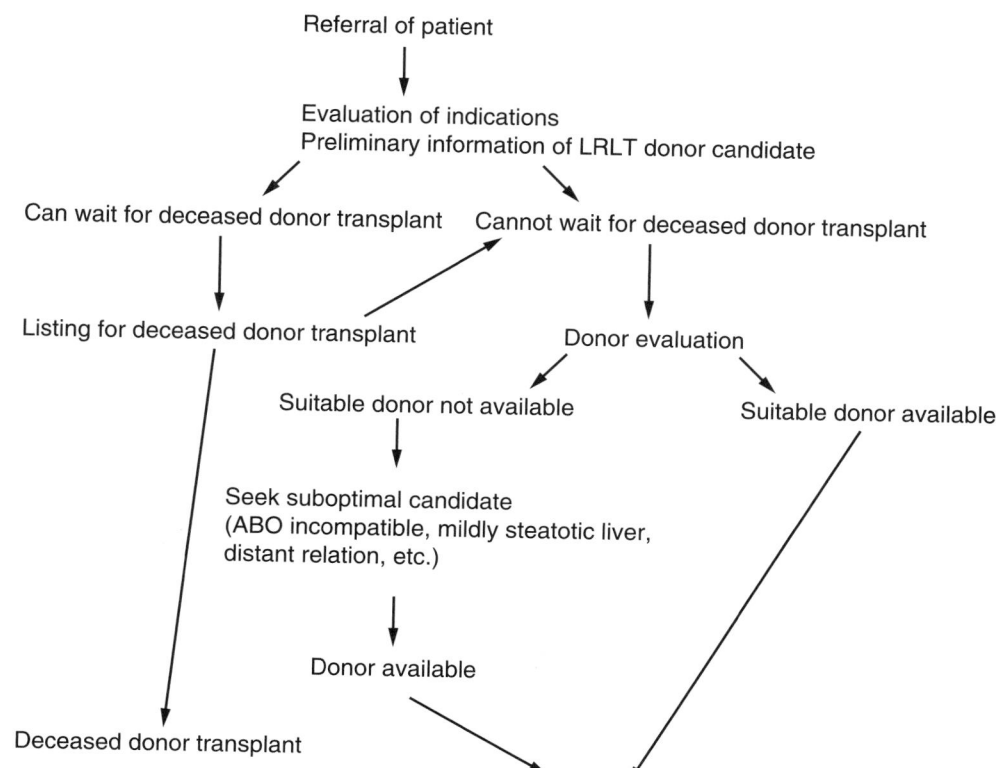

FIGURE 42–1

Process involved in living related liver transplantation in Japan. The availability of deceased donors in Japan is very limited, and most patients belong to the group that cannot wait for deceased donor transplantation.

for left lateral segmentectomy and 7.5% for left lobectomy (Tables 42–1 and 42–2).[14] Unlike adult LRLT, postdonation liver failure is considered unlikely in the donor, but events such as pulmonary embolism may nevertheless result in death of the donor.[15] The incidence of bile leakage from the residual medial segment is higher after left lateral segmentectomy than after whole left lobectomy. Adhesion of the gastric wall to

Table 42–1. COMPLICATIONS OF DONORS AFTER LIVING RELATED LIVER TRANSPLANTATION IN ASIAN CENTERS

Complication	Lateral Segmentectomy (n = 605)	Left Lobectomy (n = 334)
Bile leakage	33	8
Hyperbilirubinemia	2	0
Small bowel obstruction	5	1
Biliary stricture	1	0
Pulmonary embolism	0	1
Pancreatitis	1	0
Bleeding duodenal ulcer	1	0
Gastric perforation	0	1
Wound infection	9	10
Gastric outlet obstruction	4	3
Pneumonia	0	1
Total (%)	56 (9.3)	25 (7.5)

Modified from Lo CM: Complications and long-term outcome of living liver donors: A survey of 1508 in five Asian centers. Transplantation 75:S12-S15, 2003.

Table 42–2. COMPLICATIONS OF LIVING RELATED LIVER TRANSPLANTATION DONORS AFTER LEFT LOBE OR LEFT LATERAL SEGMENT HARVESTING AT KYOTO UNIVERSITY (N = 438)

Bile duct	
Bile leakage: 31	
Abdominal cavity	
Small bowel obstruction: 6 (adhesiolysis in 2)	
Peptic ulcer: 6	
Intra-abdominal abscess: 2	
Cholecystitis: 1	
Peritonitis: 1	
Drain tube dislodgment: 1	
Extra-abdominal organs	
Pulmonary embolism: 2	
Granulocytopenia: 2	
Atelectasis: 1	
Pneumonia: 1	
Depression: 1	
Total: 55 (12.5%)	

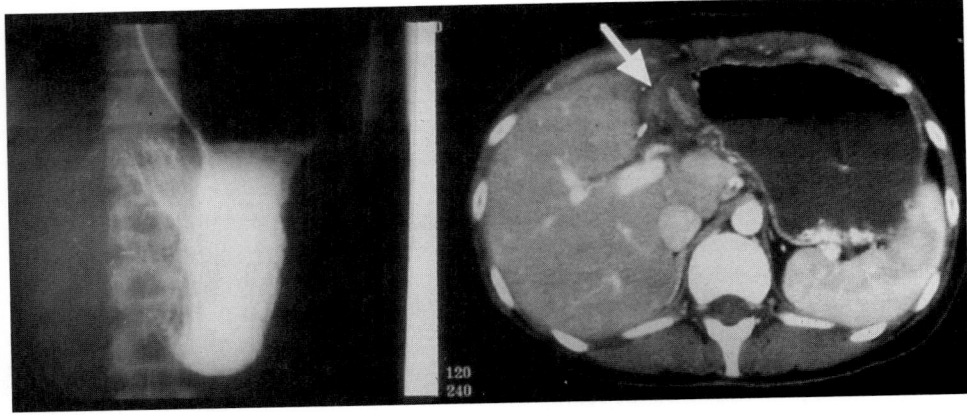

FIGURE 42–2

Adhesion of the gastric wall to the cut surface of liver after left lateral segmentectomy in pediatric living related liver transplantation. **Left**, Gastric stasis as a result of outlet obstruction. **Right**, Computed tomography shows the hairpin curve of the gastric outlet at the adhesion site (*arrow*).

the cut surface of the liver also occurs more frequently after left-sided hepatectomy than after right lobectomy. Such adhesion causes gastric stasis (Fig. 42–2). Donor candidates should be advised of all possible donor risks.

Even though the recipients are children, they have the right to select the treatment option according to their age and ability. Family members or physicians and coordinators must explain the treatment before the procedure. During puberty or adolescence, LRLT is sometimes difficult for patients to accept. They may be distressed to live with the sacrifice being made by their parent or relative. They may experience considerable anxiety about the operation and the future if not completely informed. Their anxiety should be relieved after a patient, thorough explanation. The goal that all family members can enjoy and participate in the happy healthy life of the patient should be presented as the motivation for LRLT.

Indications

Indications for LRLT are basically no different from those for deceased donor transplantation. However, in LRLT, the organ is donated to a specified recipient and not shared by other candidates. Therefore, the indication is not affected by the problem of organ allocation as it is in deceased donor transplantation. Contraindications to deceased donor transplantation are not necessarily the same for LRLT. For example, livers with malignant disease such as hepatoblastoma, which is large and invasive, may be considered to have low priority in deceased donor transplantation. However, if there is a possibility of total excision, including local invasion without distant metastasis, such a case should be considered for LRLT with the full understanding of the potential donor, recipient, and other relatives about the potential risks of surgery, tumor recurrence, and donor surgery.[16]

Donor Evaluation

Current Status of Donor Evaluation in Pediatric Living Related Liver Transplantation

Donor evaluation in LRLT is necessary for the safety of the donor and recipient (Table 42–3). Suitable donors can be selected on the basis of two perspectives: (1) donors with normal liver function and normal anatomy and (2) donors without any systemic diseases or abnormalities. In Japan, criteria for donor selection are determined in each institution with approval of the institution's review board (Table 42–4). As the initial phase, preliminary conditions such as age, relationship to the recipient, ABO blood matching, and history of any diseases can be identified during basic screening. After full consent has been given, the medical tests start. If multiple candidates are available, conventional studies are performed at the initial screening. Such studies include a blood count, coagulation profile, blood chemistry for hepatic and renal function, serology for hepatitis C and B virus, serological tests for syphilis and human immunodeficiency virus, electrocardiography, chest radiography, and ultrasonography of the liver. If the candidates live far from the hospital, this screening can be performed by a local physician. After preliminary examination, the results are presented as a tool for selecting the final candidate.

The age of the donor should ideally be between 20 and 60 years of age. Younger candidates should be evaluated for their competence in making a voluntary decision. Candidates older than 60 years are judged on an individual basis in terms of cardiopulmonary and neurological function.

Postoperative pulmonary embolism is a genuine threat to the donor. Smoking, routine use of birth control pills, or serious obesity should be considered a possible risk factor for this complication. However, the possibility

Table 42-3. DONOR WORKUP

Confirmation of voluntary willingness to donate after a full explanation of the risks and benefits

Confirmation of cooperative and supportive willingness of the donor candidate's intimate relatives/spouse

Medical history

No major current diseases or drug therapy

No history of malignancies (confirmation of "cure" if positive)

No history of transmittable diseases (confirmation of a nontransmittable state if positive)

Blood tests

Complete blood count; biochemistry, including renal and hepatic function; coagulation profile (prothrombin time, activated partial thromboplastin time, fibrinogen, antithrombin III, bleeding time)

Serology of hepatitis A, B, C; serology for sexually transmitted diseases, human immunodeficiency virus and human T-lymphotrophic virus 1, cytomegalovirus, Epstein-Barr virus

Tumor markers (α-fetoprotein, carcinoembryonic antigen, CA 19-9, CA 125)

ABO blood group, preformed irregular antibodies

HLA typing

Electroencephalogram

Chest and abdominal plain radiographs

Spirogram or arterial blood gas analysis

Abdominal ultrasonography of the hepatic parenchyma and vasculature, evaluation of other abdominal organs

Abdominal computed tomography (assessment of hepatic parenchyma, three-dimensional reconstruction of blood vessels, and estimation of graft volume)

Needle biopsy of the liver if steatosis is reasonably suspected

Table 42-4. FACTORS INVOLVED IN DONOR SELECTION FOR LIVING RELATED LIVER TRANSPLANTATION (KYOTO UNIVERSITY)*

Age: 20-60

Relatives: parents, siblings, offspring, spouses, grandparents, uncles, and aunts

ABO matching: compatible or identical (incompatible is not completely excluded)

HLA matching: a homozygous haploidentical donor is not recommended

Health of the donor

History and present condition of any systemic diseases

Longer than 1 month after child delivery

Assessment of the present disease (consult a specialist)

Blood chemistry (liver and kidney), complete blood count, coagulation profile

Electrocardiogram and ultrasonic cardiogram (UCG), chest and abdominal plain radiographs

Arterial blood gas analysis and ventilatory function if older than 50 years

Serious obesity (body mass index > 30)

Neurological evaluation if older than 60 years

Evaluation by the recipient coordinator and psychiatrist

Disease transmission

Infection: positive hepatitis viruses, human immunodeficiency virus, serological test for syphilis

Malignancy

Tumor markers (carcinoembryonic antigen, α-fetoprotein, CA 19-9, CA 125)

Endoscopy of the upper and lower gastrointestinal tract if older than 40 years

No residual tumor after the treatment of any previous malignant disease (consult with a specialist)

Metabolic diseases: loading test, liver biopsy for assessment of target enzyme activity

Graft evaluation

Doppler and conventional ultrasound: fatty liver, space-occupying lesion (SOL)

Three-dimensional computed tomography: fatty liver, architecture of vessels

Three dimensional computed tomographic cholangiography: branching pattern

Needle biopsy (if steatosis or other pathology is suspected on ultrasound, computed tomography, or blood chemistry)

More than 30% of the fatty infiltration should be excluded and treated by diet

Computed tomographic volumetry: expected graft volume > 1%, < 5% of body weight

*Patients with values out of the range in each criterion are evaluated on an individual basis.

of diet and correction of the habit is one of the advantages of living donor transplantation. A body mass index greater than 30 should be corrected, or an alternative donor should be selected out of concern for the donor's safety.

ABO blood typing should be compatible, although incompatible matching is not absolutely excluded in countries in which deceased donor transplantation is not available. The second line of screening is endoscopy of the upper gastrointestinal tract and colon, blood tests to check for tumor markers (α-fetoprotein, carcinoembryonic antigen), respiratory function tests, echocardiography, and an imaging study of the liver. The imaging study of the donor liver is very important to ensure safe surgical procedures in both the donor and recipient. For this purpose, three-dimensional computed tomography (CT) angiography is a suitable modality because it is less invasive and provides considerable information.[17] Conventional catheter angiography is being used less and less frequently because it is invasive for the donor. Magnetic resonance imaging may present the same information as enhanced CT does, but sometimes the images are not as clear as those obtained with CT.[18] It is very important to assess the potential volume of the graft in adult transplantation. However, in pediatric cases, the graft is usually the whole left lobe or the left lateral segment. Small-for-size problems are rare, but in small infants, large-for-size problems are more important. Specifically, the size of the potential graft estimated on computed tomographic scan should be compared with the diameter of the peritoneal cavity of the recipient. Preoperative three-dimensional cholangiography is also important for both adult and pediatric cases.

Fatty liver is a common contraindication to donation, with fatty infiltration of more than 25% to 35% being a criterion for exclusion.[14] Noninvasive studies such as ultrasonography and CT can identify a severely fatty liver.[19] In our institution, the averaged plain CT value of the liver measured at multiple spots is compared with that of the spleen. If the ratio is lower than 1, which means that the liver has less density than the spleen does, fatty infiltration is more than 30%.[20] However, an exact diagnosis of the degree of fatty infiltration depends on preoperative liver biopsy. Needle biopsy under ultrasound guidance is safe, although it is not routinely recommended in all cases. If any pathology is suspected on imaging studies, needle biopsy is recommended to exclude severe fatty liver or other pathological lesions. Accurate diagnosis of nonalcoholic steatohepatitis, which may be suspected from hepatic profile and imaging studies, depends on the pathological findings by needle biopsy.

Disease Transmission and Donor Selection

In pediatric LRLT, inherited diseases such as metabolic disorders and Alagille syndrome are not as rare as the indication. If a parent is selected as the donor, the potential donor may have a heritable genetic factor or a subclinical manifestation of disease. A metabolic loading test or measurement of the target enzyme in a liver specimen taken by needle biopsy may be helpful as a tool for excluding such a patient from becoming a donor candidate.[21] In the case of Alagille syndrome, the pathological diagnosis of paucity of the intrahepatic bile ducts should be considered and investigated in the potential donor. However, adults with subclinical Alagille syndrome may have only mild elevation of biliary tract–related enzymes without any sign of cholestasis.[22]

Ruling out infectious diseases or malignancy is not specific for determining acceptability for LRLT. Nonetheless, if there is a patient with a disease such as tuberculosis or hepatitis in the family of the patient, the

Table 42–5. DONOR CONTRAINDICATIONS
Infectious diseases
Hepatitis B surface antigen, hepatitis C virus antibody, human immunodeficiency virus positive
Active infection with any pathogen
Uncured malignancy
Major systemic or organ diseases inappropriate for hepatectomy
Liver abnormality or dysfunction
Steatosis greater than 30%
Rare variant of vascular anatomy that may make harvesting dangerous
Subclinical phenotype of the inheritable diseases of the recipient
Metabolic diseases
Alagille syndrome
One-way mismatch in HLA typing

possibility of latent or previous subclinical infection of the donor candidates is high. Very careful examination of the donor candidates is necessary in such a situation. Contraindications to donor selection are summarized in Table 42–5.

Significance of HLA Matching in Living Related Liver Transplantation

As in the case of deceased donor transplantation, HLA matching has not been considered a significant tool to date for donor selection in LRLT. In pediatric LRLT, the donor is usually one of the parents, which means that the recipient has haploidentical HLA typing. Sugawara and coauthors reported that zero HLA mismatching was associated with a low incidence of acute rejection in 58 pediatric LRLT cases.[23] Part of this advantage may be related to the better HLA matching in LRLT. However, a study of HLA matching in the largest series of pediatric LRLT by Kasahara and colleagues showed poor correlation of HLA matching and the incidence of rejection.[24] The zero-mismatch group had a tendency toward a lower incidence of steroid-resistant rejection and a lower level of tacrolimus maintenance 5 years after LRLT and a higher rate of withdrawal of immunosuppression, although there was no significant difference. Longer follow-up and further accumulation of experience may be necessary to clarify the role of HLA matching in LRLT. A merit of pre-LRLT HLA matching is the predictability of possible graft-versus-host disease (GVHD). After liver transplantation, GVHD is generally a rare complication. In LRLT from parent to offspring, the donor may have homozygous HLA typing and the recipient, heterozygous typing. In such a case involving a so-called one-way mismatch, the incidence of GVHD has been reported to be high in organ transplantation, including liver transplantation.[25] Before LRLT, the potential for matching a homozygous donor with a heterozygous recipient in HLA typing should be identified, and in such cases it is better to use an alternative donor.

Size and Anatomy of the Donor Liver

In most pediatric LRLT, graft options consist of the full left lobe, including the middle hepatic vein (segments II, III, and IV); the left lateral segment with a part of segment IV, but without the middle hepatic vein; and the left lateral segment (segments II and III). Selection of the graft is based on graft volume in relation to the recipient's body size. The relative size of the standard liver volume is used as an index.[26] We use the ratio of graft weight to recipient body weight: graft weight (g)/recipient's body weight (g) × 100 (%).[27] If this ratio is within 1% to 3%, the graft size is considered adequate. Generally, the left lobe is used in a recipient with a body weight between 20 and 40 kg, whereas the left lateral segment or the left lateral segment plus a portion of segment IV is used for smaller recipients. When a slightly larger graft than the left lobe is necessary, the left half of the caudate lobe can be added.[28] In preoperative volumetry, the volume of the potential graft is estimated in cubic centimeters. The specific gravity of the hepatic graft is considered to be 1. Therefore, volume is calculated in the same manner as weight. If the potential graft is 200 g and the recipient's body weight is 10 kg, the ratio is 2%. The smallest unit in conventional LRLT is the left lateral segment. If the ratio of graft weight to recipient body weight is more than 5%, poor perfusion of the graft may cause unsatisfactory primary function. In general, the mother may be more suitable than the father in infantile cases because of her possibly smaller liver. Of course, after information is provided about the risks of the large-for-size problem, the final decision is made by the family. If only a large donor liver is available, reduction of the left lateral segment is necessary. Monosegment transplantation using segment III, as discussed later in this chapter, is a solution in such a case. Regarding size matching, the size of the graft should be compared with the size of the recipient's peritoneal cavity on computed tomographic images. If the anteroposterior diameter of the potential graft is 2 cm or longer than the anteroposterior diameter of the recipient's peritoneal cavity, primary closure is expected to be difficult. In such a case, skin closure or prosthesis closure can be used, but this technique may cause more trouble than simple closure.

The anatomy of the left lobe of the donor is an important factor in LRLT in pediatric recipients. The structures that should receive attention are vessels and bile ducts. In left lateral segmentectomy, the hepatic vein from segments II and III may become separated on entry into the inferior vena cava (IVC). In left lobectomy, the left and middle hepatic veins may also separately drain into the IVC. Consideration of such possibilities is necessary when developing a strategy for hepatic vein reconstruction. Regarding the anatomy of the portal vein, P2 and P3 may branch separately from the main portal trunk and form a trifurcation with the right portal trunk (Fig. 42–3). If this branching is located at an extraparenchymal site, it is not difficult to transect these two branches separately. However, if the branching is thought to be intrahepatic, it is very difficult to safely perform a transection. A left-sided gallbladder is frequently associated with this variation of the portal vein.[29] If available, an alternative donor should be chosen. On evaluation of the donor artery, an aberrant left hepatic artery arising from the left gastric artery is not very rare. This artery is in the lesser

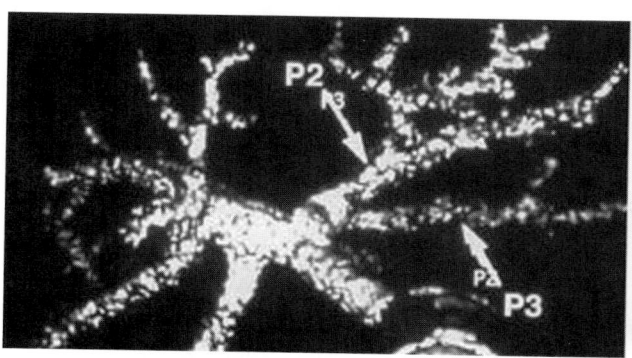
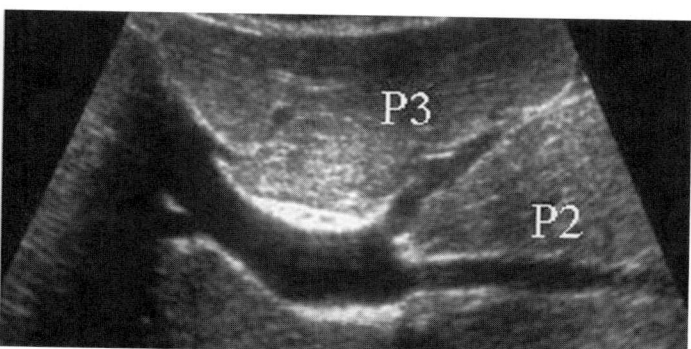

FIGURE 42–3

Variation of the portal vein to the left lateral segment. The portal vein to segment III (P3) and segment II (P2) is branching separately. If this lateral segment is taken as the graft, the graft will have two orifices in the portal stump. **Left,** Three-dimensional computed tomography. **Right,** Ultrasonography.

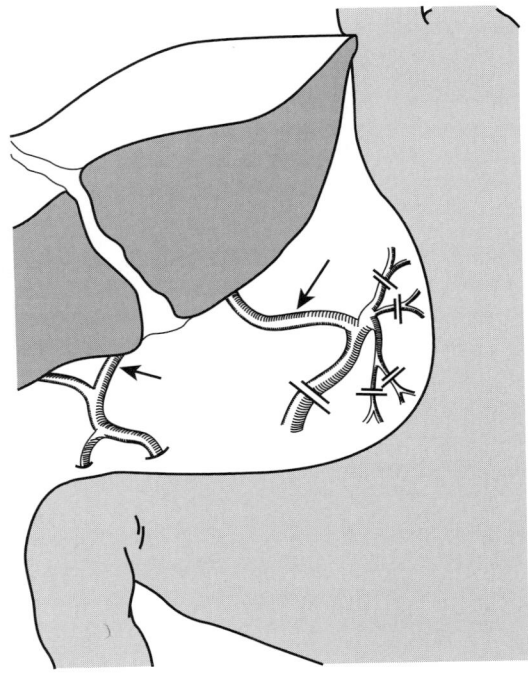

FIGURE 42–4

Aberrant hepatic artery supplying the left lateral segment (*long arrow*) originating from the left gastric artery. If the main left hepatic artery (*small arrow*) is small, this aberrant artery may be large. For reconstruction in the recipient, this artery should be kept long by transecting as indicated by the *double line*.

omentum, and attention should be paid to preserving as long a vessel as possible because a longer vessel can be used as the reconstruction vessel (Fig. 42–4). When considering left lobectomy, the size and distribution of the middle hepatic artery should be assessed. For evaluation of bile duct anatomy, three-dimensional reconstruction CT is very useful. Preoperative assessment by such imaging facilitates better understanding of the intraoperative cholangiogram.

Technical Considerations

Donor Surgery

Left Lateral Segmentectomy and Left Lobectomy

The abdomen is opened through an inverted T incision. The horizontal incision can be very short in left lateral segmentectomy. After transection of the falciform ligament, intraoperative Doppler ultrasound is performed to confirm the anatomy of the hepatic and portal veins. The Arantius duct is transected just at the entrance to the left hepatic vein. The most cranial portion of the caudate lobe is dissected from the left wall of the IVC. After dissection of this area, the hepatic porta is approached.

The left hepatic artery is dissected proximally to the point at which it branches from the common hepatic artery. If the middle hepatic artery is supplying the left lateral segment, it should also be dissected. The bifurcation of the left hepatic duct is not necessarily identified in the left lateral segment. Instead, the wall of the left hepatic duct is identified just on the surface of the left portal vein, usually through the space between the middle and left hepatic arteries (Fig. 42–5). Small hemoclips are applied here as markers for the transection site on the intraoperative cholangiogram. A 24-gauge intravenous catheter is inserted directly into the common bile duct and used for the cholangiogram in left lateral segmentectomy. The common bile duct on the duodenal side and the neck of the gallbladder are clamped with small bulldog clamps. In left lobectomy, cholangiography is performed through the cystic duct because the gallbladder is resected. Since branches may overlap on the film, fluoroscopic images may be more helpful for identification of each duct if the operating table is tilted while the operator is watching the x-ray images. The left portal vein is identified but can be encircled later after transection of the left duct.

In our institution, parenchymal transection is performed without clamping the hepatic pedicle. Makuuchi recommends a Pringle procedure for donor hepatectomy.[30] The line of transection is 0.5 to 1 cm to the right along the falciform ligament in left lateral segmentectomy and along the right side of the traced route of the middle hepatic vein in left lobectomy. The parenchymal transection is performed with the Cavitron ultrasonic aspirator (CUSA) held by the surgeon and a bipolar electrocautery with a water-dripping system held by the first assistant.[31] The bile duct is sharply transected at the marked site under the guidance of intraoperative cholangiography. The stump on the donor side is closed with 6–0 running suture, whereas the graft side is left open. After transection, the

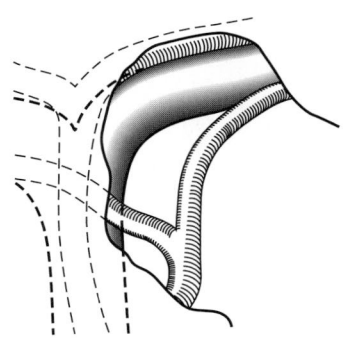

FIGURE 42–5

Identification of the left hepatic duct in left lateral segmentectomy. Between the left and middle hepatic arteries on the ventral surface of the left portal vein, a wall of the left hepatic duct can be identified. Tracing the hepatic duct from the bifurcation of the hepatic ducts is not necessary.

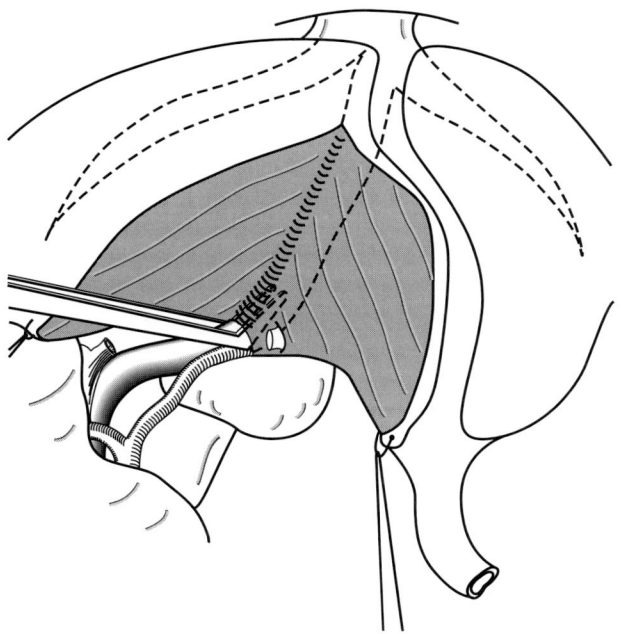

FIGURE 42–6

Parenchymal transection in left lateral segmentectomy. After transection of the left hepatic duct, the left portal vein is encircled. If curved DeBakey forceps are inserted between the lateral segment and the caudate lobe and pulled up ventrally, a crest of parenchyma is fashioned. With this procedure, the direction of transection is clearly shown, and the operating field is made shallow. The operator holds the forceps in the left hand and uses the right hand to manipulate the Cavitron ultrasonic aspirator (CUSA).

left portal vein can easily be encircled. Once the portal vein is encircled, curved DeBakey forceps are inserted under the left lateral segment along the fissure between the segment and the caudate lobe. After the segment is pulled up with the forceps, the transection line is easily identified and resembles a crest in a valley (Fig. 42–6).

Once the parenchymal transection is completed, heparin sodium (1000 units) is injected intravenously just before harvesting. Usually, in situ perfusion of the graft is possible in left lobe resection because the left portal trunk is long enough for insertion of the perfusion catheter. First, the hepatic artery is transected. After clamping the portal vein at the bifurcation, a perfusion catheter is then inserted into the left portal vein before transecting the portal vein. Clamping of the left hepatic vein or the common trunk of the middle and left hepatic veins is followed by transection of the vein or veins, and portal perfusion of the graft is started immediately. To facilitate reconstruction in the recipient, there should be only one orifice in the hepatic vein. To make a single orifice, transection of the Arantius duct and the left phrenic vein is helpful for deeper clamping of the common trunk of the left and middle hepatic veins in left lobectomy.[32] After confirming that the color of the perfusate from the hepatic venous stump has lightened, the graft is removed from

the peritoneal cavity and transferred to a basin filled with preservation solution. The weight of the graft is measured. In situations in which the cold preservation time should be kept as short as possible, as in a donor with hepatic steatosis, the graft should remain vascularized in the body of the donor after parenchymal transection until the recipient side is ready.

Recently, laparoscopic left lateral segmentectomy has been reported in pediatric LRLT.[33] This technique requires a combination of special skills in both transplant surgery and endoscopic surgery. Developing a specialized team for the operation is the best way to perform such an advanced technique.

When a vein graft is expected to be necessary during the recipient procedure, the ovarian or inferior mesenteric vein is harvested from the donor.

Monosegment Transplantation

In small babies, it is difficult to keep the graft-recipient body weight ratio less than 5%. If the recipient has a large peritoneal cavity, which is common when ascites is massive, a large graft can be accommodated easily. However, from the perspective of graft perfusion, it is better to keep the ratio less than 5%. When the ratio is larger than 5%, monosegmental transplantation can be performed. The left lateral segment is cut down in situ before the hepatic pedicle is transected in the body of the donor. Segment II or III is used with reduction of the other tissue.[34] If the graft is still large, the caudal portion of the reduced graft can be further resected (Fig. 42–7).

Recipient Procedure

Recipient surgery consists of total hepatectomy and reconstruction. In patients with biliary atresia, which is the most common indication for pediatric LRLT, one or more techniques such as the Kasai procedure have usually been performed previously. The bowel is firmly attached to the anterior margin and lower surface of the liver. Numerous collaterals are passing through these adhesions. Meticulous adhesiolysis by electrocautery is useful to shorten the duration of surgery and decrease blood loss. Possible burn of the bowel can be prevented by the assistant intermittently flushing cold water over the bowel. The Roux-en-Y limb fashioned at the Kasai operation should be kept as long and intact as possible. Hepatic arteries are transected as distal as possible to facilitate selection of a vessel of appropriate diameter for reconstruction. Usually, the wall of the hepatic artery is very fragile in small babies with biliary atresia. To prevent intimal dissection of the artery, holding, ligating, and cutting should be done gently. After transection of the hepatic arteries, the portal vein is

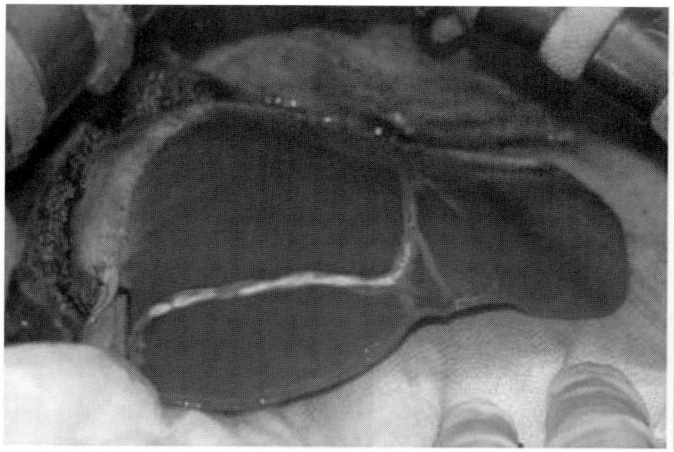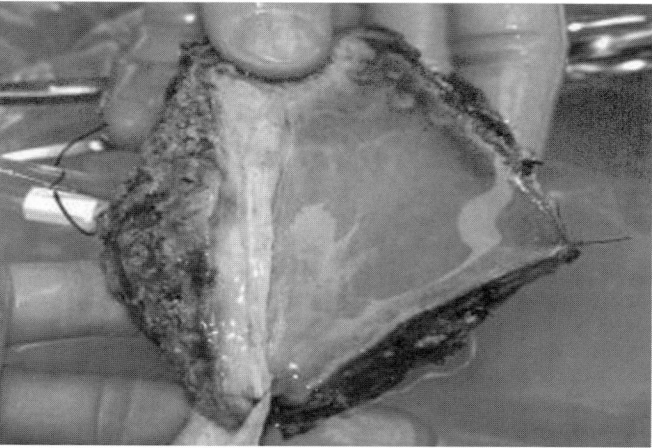

FIGURE 42–7

Reduced left lateral segment transplanted from the mother to her 3.5-kg 1-month-old boy. In this case, the left lateral segment was 200 g, and the transplanted graft was 140 g. **Left**, Marking the reduction on the surface of the left lateral segment. **Right**, After reduction, the graft weighs 140 g.

dissected and preserved untransected until the last phase of the hepatectomy. In LRLT, hepatectomy is performed with the IVC left intact. In patients without cirrhotic changes in the livers, as in those with metabolic diseases or fulminant hepatic failure, it is not difficult to dissect the retrohepatic space while preserving the IVC, even if the hepatic pedicle is not transected. This technique can reduce the clamping time of the portal vein as much as possible. However, in the case of cirrhosis, as in biliary atresia, transection of the hepatic hilum before dissection of the retrohepatic space makes hepatectomy very easy. In such a case, cutting the portal vein in the early phase of the hepatectomy does not usually cause severe congestion of the bowel because of the presence of so many preformed collateral vessels. In general, venovenous bypass or a temporary portosystemic shunt is not necessary in pediatric LRLT, regardless of the indication. After transection of the short hepatic veins, a blunt dissector can easily be passed through the avascular space just to the left of the right hepatic vein to encircle the root of the right hepatic vein (Fig. 42–8). Transection of the right hepatic vein followed by transection of the middle and left hepatic veins completes the hepatectomy.

Vascular Reconstruction

The two basic principles of vascular reconstruction are a "larger anastomosis and abundant flow."

Hepatic Vein

In LRLT, the retrohepatic IVC of the recipient is always preserved, and the graft's hepatic vein is anastomosed to the IVC in an end-to-side fashion. Typically, the left hepatic vein or the common trunk of the left or middle hepatic vein is anastomosed to the recipient side in left lateral segment or left lobe LRLT, respectively. When the hepatic vein has two orifices on the graft side, either reconstruction to make one hole or creation of two separate anastomoses between the two orifices is selected.[34] Anastomosis of a single hepatic vein is simple and safe. If two separate anastomoses are necessary, stumps of the middle hepatic vein and left hepatic vein or stumps of the right hepatic vein and trunk of the middle/left hepatic vein can be used on the recipient side.

When the trunk of the middle and left hepatic vein on the recipient side is used for anastomosis, the orifice is enlarged to a dimension adjusted for the size of the graft's hepatic vein by incising the IVC wall on the right side of the common trunk (Fig. 42–9). This procedure

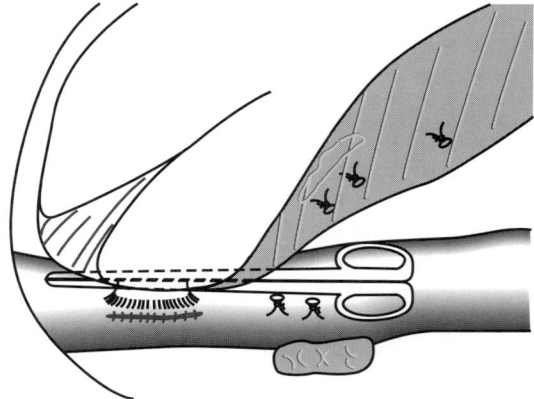

FIGURE 42–8

The final phase of dissection of the retrohepatic space in a recipient. A blunt dissector can be passed through the avascular space just to the left of the right hepatic vein to ensure safe encircling of the root of this vein.

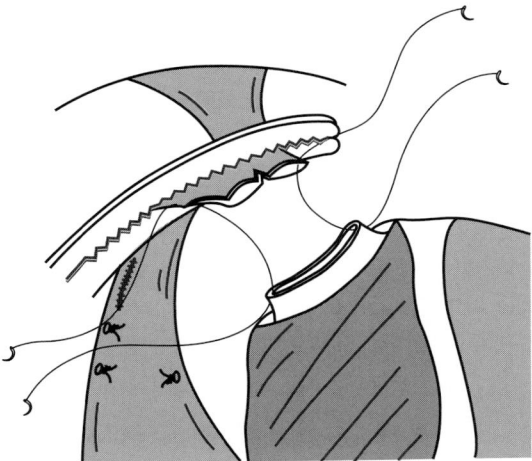

short. In patients with biliary atresia, the retrohepatic IVC may be incorporated into the severely hypertropic hepatic parenchyma. In patients with situs inversus or polysplenia syndrome, the retrohepatic IVC may be completely absent. In such cases, the hepatic vein of the graft is anastomosed in an end-to-end fashion with complete clamping of the suprahepatic IVC (Fig. 42–10). Venovenous bypass is also not usually necessary in these cases because of good collaterals.

Portal Vein

In pediatric LRLT, portal vein reconstruction is one of the crucial elements for success. In cases of biliary atresia, the portal vein of the recipient is commonly sclerotic and hypoplastic. In such cases, some augmentation of the portal vein is necessary to secure abundant flow.[38] The presence of hepatofugal flow in the portal vein before transplantation indicates a greater possibility that augmentation will be needed. Many methods have been used for such procedures, including donor autologous or homologous grafts. Usually, the segment of portal vein distal to the confluence of the superior mesenteric and splenic veins is replaced by an interposition graft or augmented with a patch graft. Another important point in reconstruction of the portal vein is alignment of the axis of anastomosis. For this purpose, we use curved forceps inserted into the graft's portal vein to determine the direction (Fig. 42–11). The axis of the recipient's side is oriented by placement of the clamp. The anastomosis is usually created with a two–stay suture technique. If the calibers are very different, a four–stay suture technique is

FIGURE 42–9

Hepatic venous anastomosis using the stump of the middle and left hepatic veins. The right edge of the middle hepatic vein is incised to enlarge the orifice to a dimension in keeping with the size of the graft hepatic vein. This technique fixes the graft to the wall of the inferior vena cava itself and is helpful in preventing rotation of the graft.

fits the graft directly to the wall of the IVC and is helpful in preventing rotation of the graft around the axis made by the hepatic vein pedicle.[35] Triangular anastomosis is recommended by Emond and coworkers for creation of a large anastomosis with good fixation of the graft to the IVC wall.[36] End-to-end anastomosis after reconstruction of the recipient's hepatic venous stump is reported to be an easy and safe method by Makuuchi and Sugawara.[37] To prevent restriction of outflow secondary to torsion on the graft, the vascular pedicle should be

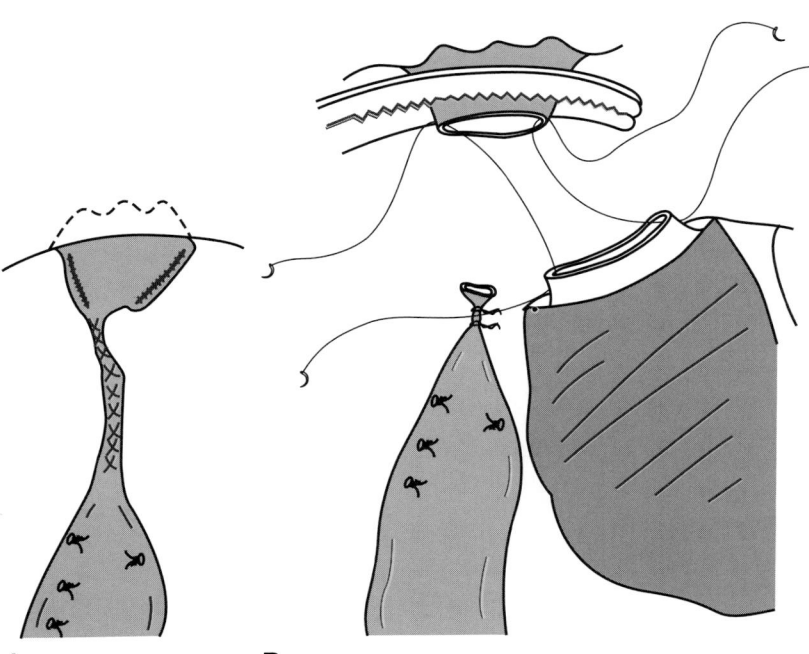

FIGURE 42–10

End-to-end anastomosis of the hepatic vein in a patient with a hypoplastic retrohepatic inferior vena cava (IVC). **A**, Before transection of the IVC. **B**, End-to-end anastomosis.

A   B

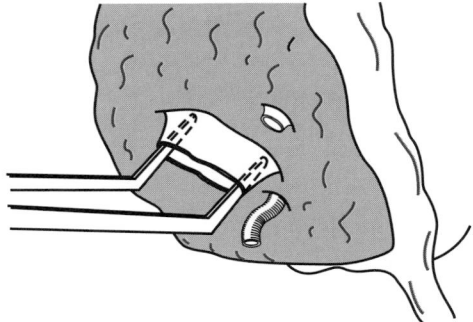

FIGURE 42–11

To clarify the direction of the graft-side portal vein, curved forceps are inserted while closed and then opened while pulling out a little. This technique can be used to determine the horizontal direction of the graft portal vein, even if it is quite short.

recommended. When the diameter is larger than 10 mm, creation of an anastomosis with running 6–0 monofilament suture is easy and fast. If the diameter is smaller, partly or completely interrupted suture is recommended.

Hepatic Artery

Microsurgical technique is recommended for reconstruction of the hepatic artery in pediatric LRLT. Such technique could reduce the incidence of hepatic arterial thrombosis.[39] In pediatric LRLT, establishing an adequate surgical field for reconstruction of the hepatic artery is difficult when the graft is relatively large because the graft covers the surgical field. Holding the graft with a malleable blade fixed to the head arch is very useful for ensuring adequate exposure of the surgical field (Fig. 42–12). Generally, the diameter of the hepatic artery in a cirrhotic recipient is large enough, and its size is compatible with the arterial size of a

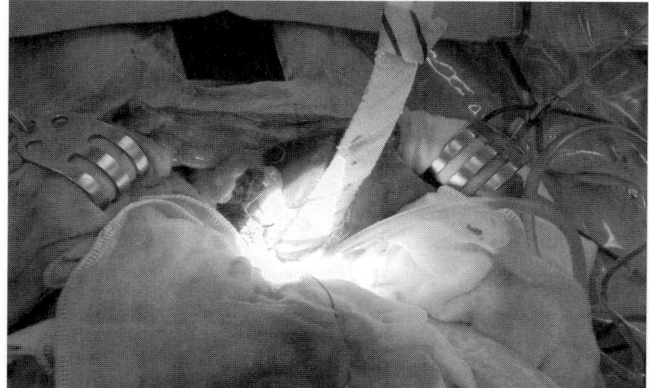

FIGURE 42–12

Establishing an operative field for microsurgical reconstruction of a hepatic artery in a small child undergoing living related liver transplantation. Gentle, but secure, fixation of the graft after reperfusion through the portal vein is necessary for good field exposure.

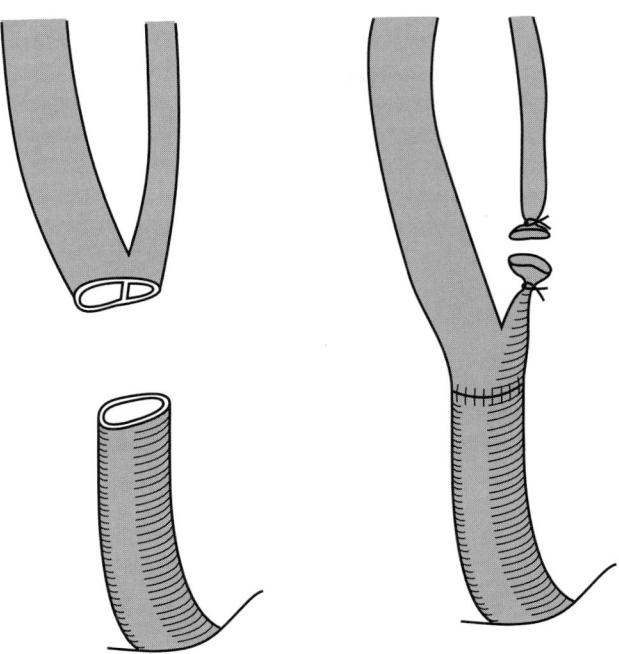

FIGURE 42–13

Anastomosis of the artery in the case of bifurcation just distal to the stump on the graft side. The branch is transected, and the dominant artery is first anastomosed to the recipient side. Usually, good backflow is obtained from the other stump, which indicates that a second anastomosis is not necessary.

graft from an adult donor. However, in noncirrhotic cases, the size discrepancy is usually large. The branch patch technique and tapering can be used to adjust the size. End-to-side anastomosis should be avoided because of the high incidence of hepatic arterial thrombosis as a result of turbulence. If the artery on the graft side bifurcates near the anastomosis, it may also cause turbulence after anastomosis. In such cases, the branching artery is transected, and the dominant artery is anastomosed first (Fig. 42–13). If two or more arteries are present, the most dominant one is anastomosed first. Then backflow from the others is checked. If backflow is good and pulsatile, the other artery or arteries can be safely ligated. If backflow is not sufficient, additional anastomosis is necessary. When multiple anastomoses are expected from the findings during the donor operation, at least two orifices should be prepared during hepatectomy of the recipient. The suture material is 8–0 or 9–0 nonabsorbable monofilament, and as little tension as possible is placed on the anastomosis. If the recipient side has some tension, the gastroduodenal artery can be divided to elongate the stump on the recipient side. As an alternative to the proper or common hepatic artery, the stump of the splenic or gastroduodenal artery can be used. In cases requiring an interposition graft, a segment of autologous inferior mesentery artery or radial artery can be harvested and used.

Bile Duct Reconstruction

In biliary atresia, the bile duct of the graft is anastomosed to the previously existing or newly made Roux-en-Y limb. Regarding bile duct reconstruction, there are still many controversial issues, such as the suture material, use of an inside or outside knot, continuous or interrupted sutures, and so on. If the bile duct of the recipient can be used in those with metabolic diseases or fulminant hepatic failure, duct-to-duct anastomosis is possible in pediatric as well as adult cases. In infants, the bile duct on the recipient side is very fragile and thin. The blood supply to the distal tip of the recipient's bile duct should be carefully preserved without dissecting the connective tissue around the common bile duct.

Surgical Complications and Treatment of Recipients

Early Complications

Early surgical complications specific for pediatric LRLT are problems related to large-for-size grafts, small vessels for reconstruction, and gastrointestinal tract injury, especially after a failed Kasai procedure for biliary atresia (Table 42–6). Primary nonfunction is quite rare in LRLT.

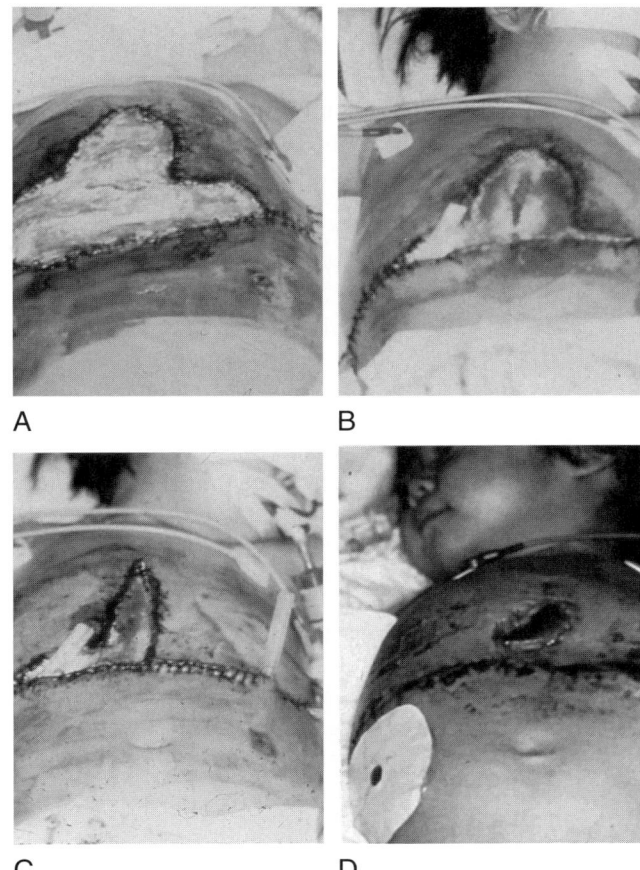

A   B

C   D

FIGURE 42–14

Closure of the abdominal cavity after transplantation of a large graft. The abdomen could be closed without a prosthesis by performing serial operations over the period of a month. **A,** Just after surgery; **B,** after 7 days; **C,** after 14 days; **D,** after 1 month.

Table 42–6. RECIPIENT COMPLICATIONS IN PEDIATRIC LIVING RELATED LIVER TRANSPLANTATION
Early
Hemorrhage (intra-abdominal and intestinal)
Vascular complications
Hepatic arterial thrombosis
Hepatic vein stenosis or torsion
Portal vein stenosis
Gastrointestinal complications
Bowel perforation
Anastomotic leakage
Poor perfusion of the graft ("large-for-size" problem)
Late
Vascular complications
Portal vein stenosis
Hepatic vein stenosis
Biliary complications
Biliary stricture at the anastomotic site

When the graft is relatively large, portal vein inflow may be partly or completely interrupted as a result of the high pressure on the graft after closure of the abdominal wall. Skin closure is performed or artificial mesh is applied in these cases (Fig. 42–14). Artificial mesh or a prosthesis is not strongly recommended because it may add a source of postoperative infection. Skin closure may be safer. Trial closure and monitoring of flow by Doppler ultrasound may be helpful in choosing between primary and secondary abdominal closure.

After the routine use of microsurgical techniques was introduced, the incidence of hepatic arterial thrombosis was 2.4% (8/332) in a large series of LRLT.[40] In a recent report comparing pediatric and adult LRLT, the incidence of hepatic arterial thrombosis in pediatric patients was 0% as opposed to 4% in adults.[41] The most dangerous arterial injury is intimal dissection on the graft or the recipient side (or on both). If intimal dehiscence occurs on the recipient side, the artery must be traced proximally to obtain an intact wall and good forward flow for safe construction of an anastomosis.

The basic principle in treating hepatic arterial thrombosis in LRLT is reanastomosis to salvage the original graft. Early detection of hepatic arterial thrombosis is essential for successful re-reconstruction. Doppler ultrasonography is performed at least three times a day during the first 7 days and two times daily during the subsequent 7 days. If the signal is detectable but shows poor flow, anticoagulant therapy is increased, and administration of systemic urokinase (60,000 IU/6 hr as a continuous intravenous infusion) is mandatory. Emergency angiography and arterial infusion of a thrombolytic agent such as urokinase may be implemented. Complete disappearance of the arterial signal within the first 10 days necessitates urgent reanastomosis, even though there are no signs of hepatic necrosis on imaging studies or biochemical analysis. Angiography before repeat surgery is skipped to save time. At repeat surgery, quick disruption of the anastomosis should be performed to stop progression of the thrombosis. Good backflow from the graft-side artery after irrigation with a fine soft catheter (24 or 28 gauge) is an encouraging sign for possible success of the reanastomosis. When no arterial signal is detected on Doppler 10 days after LRLT and no signs of hepatic necrosis are apparent, close observation without any intervention can be performed. In such cases—and even in cases in which the reanastomosis was not successful—the graft may survive by portal perfusion and later rearterialization by spontaneously formed collaterals.[42] This route is through the diaphragmatic artery or the mesenteric artery of the Roux-en-Y limb. Even in these "spontaneously recovered" cases, intrahepatic or extrahepatic biliary stricture may subsequently occur several months later.

Biliary complications are more common after LRLT than after whole-liver transplantation. Such complications are not specific for pediatric LRLT. Bile leakage from the hepaticojejunostomy in the immediate early postoperative period may be fatal as a result of peritonitis and sepsis. Early diversion of the limb to prevent reflux of amylase-rich bowel contents is recommended (Fig. 42–15). Bowel injury during vigorous adhesiolysis is also a common complication of pediatric LRLT after a failed Kasai procedure for biliary atresia. Fasting and drainage are not usually sufficient to control infection. Exteriorization of the perforation site may be necessary.

Late Complications

Late complications after pediatric LRLT include hepatic vein stenosis, portal vein stenosis, and biliary stricture (see Table 42–6). These complications are not specific for pediatric LRLT and are relatively common, as in deceased donor partial-liver transplantation.

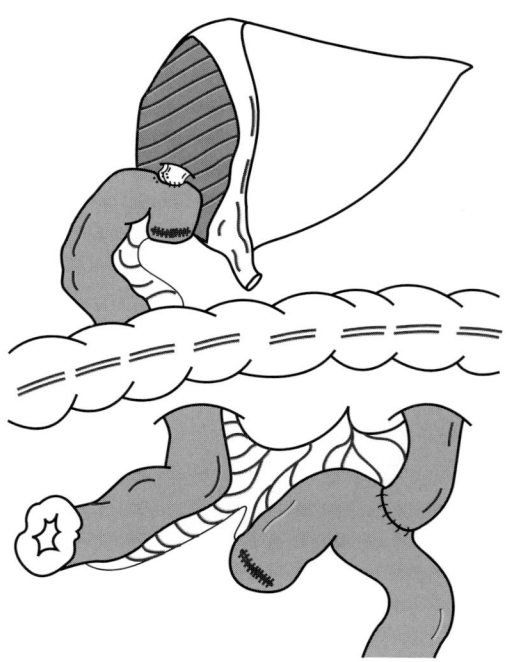

FIGURE 42–15
Diversion of the Roux-en-Y limb in the event of anastomotic dehiscence of the hepaticojejunostomy. The stoma can be taken down after healing of the leakage.

Torsion or compression of the hepatic venous cuff by the enlarging liver may cause hepatic vein stenosis after several months or a few years. A long cuff may be associated with a higher incidence of such complications. The symptoms of hepatic vein stenosis are ascites, a low albumin level, and a decreased platelet count. Doppler ultrasound shows a dilated hepatic vein with low flow velocity inside the liver and jet flow at the confluence to the IVC. In catheter angiography, imaging with contrast dye enhancement and pressure study through the anastomotic site can confirm the diagnosis. The catheter is inserted via the transhepatic route (normograde) or the IVC route (retrograde). Balloon dilatation has been highly successful. Repeated dilatation may be necessary, and placement of an expandable metallic stent is required in these cases. For possible retransplantation in patients with hepatic fibrosis secondary to graft congestion despite conservative procedures, the location of the stent should be chosen cautiously and in a manner that does not interfere with any reoperation if such becomes necessary.[43,44]

On occasion, portal stenosis is a late complication after pediatric LRLT. Portal vein thrombosis is usually associated with stenosis. Reconstruction using the venous conduit is reported to be associated with a higher incidence of stenosis, although there is no definite evidence.[43]

The symptoms are those of portal hypertension—ascites and thrombocytopenia. Doppler ultrasonography can be used to diagnose stenosis by detection of narrowing of the lumen, poststenotic dilatation, and a jet flow with damping of the flow velocity. If the thrombus is already formed, the lumen cannot be detected by B-mode ultrasonography. If portal flow in the liver is detectable by ultrasound, percutaneous transhepatic portography is the first choice for diagnosis and treatment. A catheter inserted transhepatically is passed through the stenosis or thrombus to the proximal side, and contrast dye flushed from the catheter can show the lesion. Balloon dilatation is the first line of treatment of the hepatic vein.[43] If it successful, surgical thrombectomy plus re-reconstruction is clinically feasible, although it is not easy. Even though portal flow is not detected in the liver, initially the patient may not have any symptoms. However, symptoms of a portosystemic shunt or portal hypertension become prominent later. In such cases with difficult re-reconstruction, retransplantation is indicated.

Late-onset biliary stenosis does not present any specific problems in pediatric LRLT. Because the original anastomosis is mainly a hepaticojejunostomy, intervention through endoscopic retrograde cholangiopancreatography is not possible. Usually, percutaneous transhepatic cholangiodrainage (PTCD) under ultrasound guidance is first selected. Balloon dilatation through this route is commonly used. If not effective after repeated trials, stenting is also possible. Revision after long-term follow-up is not very difficult. If balloon dilatation is not easy or not very effective, it is better to proceed to reanastomosis than to risk any incidental complications caused by interventional procedures.

Repeat Living Related Liver Transplantation in Pediatric Recipients

In the initial experience with LRLT, there was hesitancy about performing repeat LRLT (re-LRLT) after failure of LRLT. It is generally difficult to find another proper donor because the selection range is limited within the closed family. Of course, if a deceased donor is available, it is reasonable to list the patient as an urgent case. Discussing the possibility of re-LRLT when the availability of a deceased donor is not expected may place great pressure on the family. However, if they are not told all of the options, the recipient may progress along the worst course before the family recognizes the necessity for retransplantation. The possibility of re-LRLT should be included as one of the general issues in the informed consent in the initial LRLT. If the recipient is a child, the range of selection of a second donor is wider than for adults. Parents, grandparents younger than 65 years, and uncles or aunts can be included as candidates.

The most common indication for re-LRLT is chronic rejection (Table 42–7). Recurrence of the original disease is rare after pediatric LRLT. However, in the Kyoto experience, young children undergoing LRLT for fulminant hepatic failure have a higher incidence of further massive hepatic necrosis requiring re-LRLT, although it is difficult to differentiate from severe rejection.[45] Naturally, re-LRLT presents greater technical difficulty than the initial procedure does. The overall survival rate after re-LRLT in Kyoto is less than 40%. Early retransplantation is performed if the recipient's condition is poor, and the result is worse than when it is done after a long period (see Table 42–7).

Immunosuppression

Tolerance

After liver transplantation, complete weaning of immunosuppression has been reported to be possible in select cases. In pediatric LRLT, immunosuppression could initially be reduced or the patient weaned because of complications or noncompliance. After confirmation of the possibility of complete withdrawal in such incidental cases, protocols for weaning were developed.[46] During the protocol trial, 25% of the post-LRLT pediatric recipients enrolled in the study could be completely weaned off immunosuppressants for a median of more than 21.9 months.[47] The tentative protocol for weaning is shown in Figure 42–16, and criteria for use of the protocol are listed in Table 42–8. Predicting the possibility of acquiring tolerance is not yet possible.

ABO Incompatibility in Pediatric Living Related Liver Transplantation

ABO-incompatible matching cannot be avoided in countries in which LRLT is the main method of liver transplantation. The outcome after LRLT depends on the age of the recipient. In the pediatric group younger than 1 year, the posttransplant survival rate is comparable to that of the equivalent ABO-matched group of adults.[40] In the experience at Kyoto University, the outcome of ABO-incompatible LRLT in infantile patients is almost the same as that of ABO-compatible LRLT in the same age group (unpublished data). Therefore, in recipients younger than 1 year, the immunosuppression regimen after ABO-incompatible matching is similar to that after compatible matching, except for a procedure to decrease the anti-AB antibody titer before transplantation, such as blood or plasma exchange. In pediatric recipients older than 7 years, innovations in immunosuppression, including intraportal infusion, may be effective, as in adult cases.[48]

Table 42-7. REPEAT LIVING RELATED LIVER TRANSPLANTATION IN PEDIATRIC RECIPIENTS (KYOTO UNIVERSITY 1990–2003)

Age at re-LRLT	Original Indication	Indication for re-LRLT	1st Donor	2nd Donor	Time after 1st LRLT (yr.mo.day)	Outcome
11	BA	SFS	Mother	Father	0.0.2	Dead
9 mo	FHF	Massive necrosis	Grandfather	Grandmother	0.0.24	Alive
8	BA	Massive necrosis	Father	Mother*	0.1.0	Dead
1	FHF	Massive necrosis	Mother	Father	0.1.0	Dead
1	FHF	Massive necrosis	Mother	Father*	0.1.0	Dead
2	BA	CR	Father	Mother	0.1.0	Alive
12	BA	Massive necrosis	Mother	Father	0.2.0	Dead
2	BA	CR	Father	Mother	0.3.0	Dead
1	BA		Mother	Grandmother	0.3.0	Dead
1	BA	CR	Mother	Father*	0.4.0	Dead
5	Alagille syndrome	Cholestasis	Mother	Grandfather	0.6.0	Dead
4	Glycogen storage disease	CR	Mother	Father*	0.6.0	Dead
3	BA	CR	Mother	Father*	1.0.0	Alive
2	BA	HV stenosis	Father	Mother	1.0.0	Dead
4	BA	CR	Mother	Father	1.4.0	Alive
3	BA	CR	Father	Grandmother	2.6.0	re-re-LRLT
9	LC	CR	Father	Mother	3.0.0	Alive
15	BA	CR	Father	Mother	3.1.0	Dead
17	BA	CR	Mother	Domino	4.0.0	Dead
6	BA	Cholangitis	Mother	Father	4.7.0	Alive
16	BA	Massive necrosis	Mother	Aunt	5.8.0	Alive
15	BA	CR	Father	Mother*	5.8.0	Dead
7	BA	HV stenosis	Mother	Father*	6.0.0	Alive
9	BA	FHF	Father	Mother	8.7.0	Dead
11	BA	CR	Mother	Father	11.5.0	Alive

*ABO-incompatible donor.
BA, biliary atresia; CR, chronic rejection; FHF, fulminant hepatic failure; HV, hepatic vein; LC, liver cirrhosis; SFS, small for size.

WEANING PROTOCOL OF TACROLIMUS

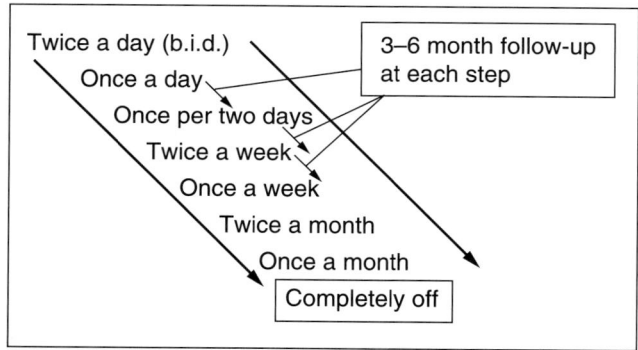

Twice a day (b.i.d.)
Once a day
Once per two days
Twice a week
Once a week
Twice a month
Once a month
Completely off

3–6 month follow-up at each step

FIGURE 42-16

Protocol for weaning from tacrolimus immunosuppression.

Table 42-8. CRITERIA FOR PROTOCOL WEANING

Longer than 2 years after liver transplantation

Normal liver function

No episode of rejection during the previous year

Evidence of medical compliance

Cooperative local physician for follow-up

Pearls and Pitfalls

Pearls

- Obtain informed consent detailing the risk to the donor, including mortality, before performance of LDLT.
- Minimal handling of the vascular pedicle and the graft itself is necessary in both the donor and recipient operations.
- A flat and straight line should be used for transection of hepatic parenchyma in the donor operation.
- The Arantius duct should be completely transected at its confluence with the left hepatic vein when harvesting the left lobe from the donor.
- The bowel should be cooled by flushing of water during enterolysis by electrocautery.
- Good flow through the portal vein should be confirmed before the graft is inserted.
- In any vascular reconstruction, a stoma as large as possible with flow as abundant as possible is strongly recommended.
- Interrupted suture is recommended in patients with a small portal vein.
- A microsurgical technique of hepatic arterial reconstruction should be used.
- Reconstruction of the dominant artery may be sufficient without reconstructing other arteries in patients with multiple arterial supply to the graft.
- If possible, a duct-to-duct anastomosis is safe and also useful in pediatric LDLT.
- Blood flow should be confirmed by Doppler ultrasonography just after closure of the abdomen and before exiting the operation room.
- A regular (bimonthly) checkup of the grafted liver by Doppler ultrasonography should be performed in the posttransplant outpatient clinic for early detection of vascular and biliary anastomotic stenosis.
- Lifelong follow-up is necessary, especially for pediatric LDLT.

Pitfalls

- Ignorance of the subclinical phenotype in a donor candidate with inheritable diseases such metabolic disorders, Alagille syndrome, or Caroli's disease.
- In HLA matching, a graft from a homozygous donor to a heterozygous recipient.

Pearls and Pitfalls—cont'd

- Unrepaired physical injury in the bowel of the recipient.
- Graft larger than 5% of the recipient's body weight.
- Hesitation regarding portal vein augmentation before insertion of the graft in recipients with sclerotic or thrombotic changes in the portal vein.
- End-to-side anastomosis of the artery may result in a higher incidence of hepatic artery thrombosis.
- In patients in whom hepatic artery thrombosis occurs within 10 days of the operation, waiting until an increase in transaminases occurs will make saving the graft hopeless.
- Bilioenteric dehiscence or intestinal perforation after transplantation requires a more aggressive surgical intervention than simple drainage and fasting.

Acknowledgment

The authors would like to thank Hideaki Okajima, MD, for his help in preparation of the figures.

References

1. Raia S, Nery JR, Mies S: Liver transplantation from live donors. Lancet 2:497, 1989.
2. Strong RW, Lynch SV, Ong TH, et al: Successful liver transplantation from a living donor to her son. N Engl J Med 322:1505-1507, 1990.
3. Nagasue N, Kohno H, Matsuo S, et al: Segmental (partial) liver transplantation from a living donor. Transplant Proc 24:1958-1959, 1992.
4. Broelsch CE, Emond JC, Whitington PF, et al: Application of reduced-size liver transplants as split grafts, auxiliary orthotopic grafts, and living related segmental transplants. Ann Surg 212:368-375, 1990.
5. Ozawa K, Uemoto S, Tanaka K, et al: An appraisal of pediatric liver transplantation from living relatives. Initial clinical experiences in 20 pediatric liver transplantations from living relatives as donors. Ann Surg 216:547-553, 1992.
6. Makuuchi M, Kawarazaki H, Iwanaka T, et al: Living related liver transplantation. Surg Today 22:297-300, 1992.
7. Testa G, Malago M, Broelsch CE: From living related to in-situ split liver transplantation: How to reduce waiting-list mortality. Pediatr Transplant 5:16-20, 2001.
8. Broering DC, Mueller L, Ganschow R, et al: Is there still a need for living-related liver transplantation in children? Ann Surg 234:713-721, 2001.
9. Emond JC, Freeman RB, Renz JF, et al: Optimizing the use of donated cadaveric livers: Analysis and policy development to increase the application of split-liver transplantation. Liver Transpl 8:863-872, 2002.

10. Otte JB: History of pediatric liver transplantation. Where are we coming from? Where do we stand? Pediatr Transplant 6:378-387, 2002.

11. Revillon Y, Michel JL, Lacaille F, et al: Living-related liver transplantation in children: The Parisian' strategy to safely increase organ availability. J Pediatr Surg 34:851-853, 1999.

12. Surman OS: The ethics of partial-liver donation. N Engl J Med 346:1038, 2002.

13. de Villa VH, Lo CM, Chen CL: Ethics and rationale of living-donor liver transplantation in Asia. Transplantation 75:S2-S5, 2003.

14. Lo CM: Complications and long-term outcome of living liver donors: A survey of 1508 in five Asian centers. Transplantation 75:S12-S15, 2003.

15. Sterneck MR, Fischer L, Nischwitz U: Selection of the living liver donor. Transplantation 60:667-671, 1995.

16. Chardot C, Saint Martin C, Gilles A, et al: Living-related liver transplantation and vena cava reconstruction after total hepatectomy including the vena cava for hepatoblastoma. Transplantation 73:90-92, 2002.

17. Kanazawa A, Hirohashi K, Tanaka H, et al: Usefulness of three-dimensional computed tomography in a living-donor extended right lobe liver transplantation. Liver Transpl 8:1076-1079, 2002.

18. Cheng YF, Chen CL, Huang TL, et al: Single imaging modality evaluation of living donors in liver transplantation: Magnetic resonance imaging. Transplantation 72:1527-1533, 2001.

19. Jacobs JE, Birnbaum BA, Shapiro MA, et al: Diagnostic criteria for fatty infiltration of the liver on contrast-enhanced helical CT. AJR Am J Roentgenol 171:659-664, 1998.

20. Hayashi M, Fujii K, Kiuchi T, et al: Effects of fatty infiltration of the graft on the outcome of living-related liver transplantation. Transplant Proc 31:403, 1999.

21. Kasahara M, Kiuchi T, Uryuhara K: Treatment of ornithine transcarbamylase deficiency in girls by auxiliary liver transplantation: Conceptual changes in a living-donor program. J Pediatr Surg 33:1753-1756, 1998.

22. Gurkan A, Emre S, Fishbein TM, et al: Unsuspected bile duct paucity in donors for living-related liver transplantation: Two case reports. Transplantation 67:416-418, 1999.

23. Sugawara Y, Mizuta K, Kawarasaki H: Risk factors for acute rejection in pediatric living related liver transplantation: The impact of HLA matching. Liver Transpl 7:769-773, 2001.

24. Kasahara M, Kiuchi T, Uryuhara K, et al: Role of HLA compatibility in pediatric living-related liver transplantation. Transplantation 74:1175-1180, 2002.

25. Kiuchi T, Harada H, Matsukawa H, et al: One-way donor-recipient HLA-matching as a risk factor for graft-versus-host disease in living-related liver transplantation. Transpl Int 11(Suppl 1):S383-S384, 1998.

26. Urata K, Kawasaki S, Matsunami H, et al: Calculation of child and adult standard liver volume for liver transplantation. Hepatology 21:1317-1321, 1995.

27. Kiuchi T, Kasahara M, Uryuhara K, et al: Impact of graft size mismatching on graft prognosis in liver transplantation from living donors. Transplantation 67:321-327, 1999.

28. Miyagawa S, Hashikura Y, Miwa S, et al: Concomitant caudate lobe resection as an option for donor hepatectomy in adult living related liver transplantation. Transplantation 66:661-663, 1998.

29. Asonuma K, Shapiro AM, Inomata Y, et al: Living related liver transplantation from donors with the left-sided gallbladder/portal vein anomaly. Transplantation 68:1610-1612, 1999.

30. Imamura H, Takayama T, Sugawara Y, et al: Pringle's manoeuvre in living donors. Lancet 360:2049-2050, 2002.

31. Yamaoka Y, Ozawa K, Tanaka A, et al: New devices for harvesting the hepatic graft from the living donor. Transplantation 52:157-160, 1991.

32. Kubota K, Makuuchi M, Takayama T, et al: Successful hepatic vein reconstruction in 42 consecutive living related liver transplantations. Surgery 128:48-53, 2000.

33. Cherqui D, Soubrane O, Husson E, et al: Laparoscopic living donor hepatectomy for liver transplantation in children. Lancet 359:392-396, 2002.

34. de Santibanes E, McCormack L, Mattera J, et al: Partial left lateral segment transplant from a living donor. Liver Transpl 6:108-112, 2000.

35. Egawa H, Inomata Y, Uemoto S, et al: Hepatic vein reconstruction in 152 living-related donor liver transplantation patients. Surgery 121:250-257, 1997.

36. Emond JC, Heffron TG, Whitington PF, et al: Reconstruction of the hepatic vein in reduced size hepatic transplantation. Surg Gynecol Obstet 176:11-17, 1993.

37. Makuuchi M, Sugawara Y: Living-donor liver transplantation using the left liver, with special reference to vein reconstruction. Transplantation 75:S23-S24, 2003.

38. Marwan IK, Fawzy AT, Egawa H, et al: Innovative techniques and results of portal vein reconstruction in living-related liver transplantation. Surgery 125:265-270, 1999.

39. Reding R, de Goyet J de V, Delbeke I, et al: Pediatric liver transplantation with cadaveric or living related donors: Comparative results in 90 elective recipients of primary grafts. J Pediatr 134:280-286, 1999.

40. Kiuchi T, Inomata Y, Uemoto S, et al: Living-donor liver transplantation in Kyoto, 1997. In Cecka JM, Terasaki PI (eds): Clinical Transplants 1997. Los Angeles, UCLA Tissue Typing Laboratory, 1998, pp 191-198.

41. Goldstein MJ, Salame E, Kapur S, et al: Analysis of failure in living donor liver transplantation: Differential outcomes in children and adults. World J Surg 27:356-364, 2003.

42. Sugawara Y, Ohtsuka H, Kaneko J, et al: Spontaneous revascularization of arterial thrombosis after living donor liver transplantation. Abdom Imaging 27:546-548, 2002.

43. Buell JF, Funaki B, Cronin DC, et al: Long-term venous complications after full-size and segmental pediatric liver transplantation. Ann Surg 236:658-666, 2002.

44. Ko GY, Sung KB, Yoon HK, et al: Endovascular treatment of hepatic venous outflow obstruction after living-donor liver transplantation. J Vasc Interv Radiol 13:591-599, 2002.

45. Uemoto S, Inomata Y, Sakurai T, et al: Living donor liver transplantation for fulminant hepatic failure. Transplantation 70:152-157, 2000.

46. Takatsuki M, Uemoto S, Inomata Y, et al: Weaning of immunosuppression in living donor liver transplant recipients. Transplantation 72:449-454, 2001.

47. Oike F, Yokoi A, Nishimura E, et al: Complete withdrawal of immunosuppression in living donor liver transplantation. Transplant Proc 34:1521, 2002.

48. Tanabe M, Shimazu M, Wakabayashi G, al. Intraportal infusion therapy as a novel approach to adult ABO-incompatible liver transplantation. Transplantation 73:1959-1961, 2002.

Split-Liver Transplantation for Two Adults

DANIEL AZOULAY
MASSIMO DEL GAUDIO
PAULA ANDREANI
HENRI BISMUTH

History   647

Ex situ split-liver transplantation technique   648

In situ split-liver transplantation technique   648

Selection of donors   648

Technique   649
  Split-liver graft preparation   649
  Split-liver graft implantation   650
  Postoperative care   651

Paul-Brousse results   651

Literature results   651

Conclusion   651

The number of patients waiting for a liver transplant is increasing faster than the number of organs available, with waiting list mortality rates of 8% to 15% in many centers.[1,2] Split-liver transplantation is the best solution to increase the number of organs from the existing pool of deceased donors. In recent series, patient and graft survival rates are similar to those of whole-organ transplantation,[3-7] and systematically applying the splitting technique can reduce the waiting time for both pediatric and adult lists.[3,5] Split-liver procedures that divide a deceased donor organ into a small left graft for a child and a larger right graft for an adult have reduced the graft shortage for children[8] and could even eliminate the need for elective living donors in this population.[9,10] Currently, however, the majority of patients on the liver transplant waiting list are adults, and more than 90% of deaths while on the waiting list occur in adults.[11] Our group demonstrated that producing grafts for two adults is technically feasible and has increased the number of recipients by 62% in comparison to whole-liver transplantation. In addition, rates of arterial (6%) and biliary (22%) complications are similar to those in published data for conventional transplantation in an adult and a child.[12]

History

In 1988, R. Pichlmayr and colleagues were the first to report transplantation of one donor liver into two recipients.[13] H. Bismuth and colleagues were the first to transplant two adult patients with one liver.[14] The initiation of adult living donor liver transplantation, which has resulted in successful transplantation of either the left or right lobe of the liver into an adult recipient, has prompted interest in the development of a similar split-liver technique for deceased donors. In theory, both lobes of the liver should provide sufficient tissue mass in the respective recipients until full regeneration has been achieved. After the 1989 report of split-liver transplantation in two adults by Bismuth and colleagues,[14] the first report in the new era came from Colledan and coworkers in 1999.[15] They performed a transection as done in right hepatectomy in living donor liver transplantation, but left the middle hepatic vein with the left liver.

Ex Situ Split-Liver Transplantation Technique

In the ex situ split-liver technique, the whole organ is retrieved and preserved with University of Wisconsin (UW) solution according to standard techniques of multiple organ procurement. Grafts are prepared at the recipient transplant center in an ice bath of UW solution. Predissection cholangiography and arteriography to more precisely delineate the anatomy are performed in some centers, as in ours[3,16]; others have not found this step necessary.[5,17] In reality, with increasing experience, our group also tends to not perform arteriography and cholangiography anymore. Indeed, a metal cannula is used to gently probe the hepatic artery and bile duct to facilitate detection of any aberrant anatomy. Dissection of the portal triad is performed to separate the branches of the hepatic artery, portal vein, and right and left hepatic ducts. Although the ex situ split, as just described, is the most widely used method for transplantation of two patients with one liver, there are drawbacks to this approach. Long ischemic times during protracted back-table dissection, hepatic artery thrombosis, and biliary tract complications were the most common problems.[18,19] Extended cold ischemic times and the required dissection and manipulation of the graft compound the deleterious effects of ischemia alone. During the separation process into right and left grafts, some allograft rewarming occurs; even if slight, it has been found to be associated with increased susceptibility to hepatic ischemia reperfusion injury.[20] The collective impact of prolonged ischemia and rewarming during the ex situ split results in graft injury, which predisposes to a high incidence of poor function unless the organ is placed in a very favorable environment. In a nonurgent patient, unfavorable operative and recipient factors can be minimized, thus decreasing the incidence of poor graft function, as shown by Rela and associates.[5] The ex situ technique may be relegated to elective cases, particularly in adult recipients.

In Situ Split-Liver Transplantation Technique

A modification of the ex situ splitting technique is in situ splitting, an extension of the techniques established for living related donor procurement that is practiced in heart-beating deceased donors. The first description of in situ liver splitting was published by Rogiers and coauthors[21] in 1995; they reported a lower rate of biliary complications, intra-abdominal hemorrhage, and nonfunction of the right graft in comparison to other series in which ex situ splitting techniques were used.

Complete hemostasis on the cut surface can be achieved before harvesting the liver.[4,18,21] The shorter duration of the back-table preparation makes sharing between centers possible. A major problem with ex situ splitting is the extended cold ischemic time in comparison to conventional liver transplantation as a result of the long benching procedure. Some centers have become expert in minimizing the extent of back-table ischemia,[3] but in general, this cold ischemia could lead to an increased rate of primary dysfunction and nonfunction.[22,23] In situ splitting potentially eliminates this problem completely and results in normal ischemic times for the right graft and potentially shorter than normal times for the left graft. The subsequent excellent primary function of in situ split livers allows safe transplantation of higher-risk patients. Because the cut surface is perfused and bile leaks are better detected, biliary complications are fewer than with ex situ splitting.

Disadvantages of in situ splitting, when compared with the ex situ technique, include the longer duration of the explant procedure, the more technically demanding operative procedure, and the more difficult implantation of the left segment, which resembles a living donor procedure. The additional time needed for the procedure during explantation is 1.5 to 2 hours, and the hospital at which the donor operation is performed needs to give approval. In addition, the other explant teams must be informed of the delay.

Selection of Donors

The optimal donor for a split-liver procedure in our opinion is one who is younger than 55 years with body weight greater than 70 kg, stable hemodynamics, normal liver function test results, and no macroscopic aspect of liver steatosis at harvesting.[12] The anatomical feasibility of dividing the liver is confirmed on the back-table with arteriography and cholangiography.[3] For donors with familial amyloid polyneuropathy (FAP), arteriography is performed in the usual pretransplant workup and cholangiography during surgery.[12,24] In our

FAP domino donors (the explanted native liver of a patient with FAP is split in situ, and the explanted hemilivers are transplanted into two recipients), an in situ split procedure was performed.[24] Selection of donors for in situ splitting is not only a logistical problem[8,25] but also depends on hemodynamic stability of the donor, which can be achieved by optimization of electrolytes, diuresis, ventilation, and circulation. The ratio of graft weight to body weight was lowered, and splitting to benefit two adults has begun to be performed in selected centers.[15,26] It must be kept in mind that this ratio should remain above 1.0% in deceased donors.[27] Other authors work with the ratio of graft weight to ideal weight, which is the graft weight of the transplanted organ divided by the ideal liver weight of the recipient. Determination of ideal liver weight can be accomplished with several formulas.[28] At present, this is the safety margin to minimize initial dysfunction from insufficient liver mass. The excellent results obtained with smaller grafts from living donors (0.8% graft weight–recipient body weight ratio) should not be interpreted as permission to test this limit.[28] The minimal mass of a deceased donor segment will necessarily be greater. Without exception, organs from living donors are in pristine condition, and their ability to meet the metabolic demands of the recipient and regenerate is almost certainly superior.

Technique

Split-Liver Graft Preparation

The liver is harvested by means of the en bloc rapid technique of Starzl and colleagues[29] with both aortic and portal infusion of UW preservation solution. At procurement, arterial (aortic bifurcation or carotid arteries) and venous (proximal inferior vena cava [IVC] with both iliac veins) grafts are systematically harvested. The in situ splitting technique has produced excellent results, particularly regarding biliary complications.[4,6-8,30,31] We have performed in situ splitting of the liver[12] and have found indisputably easier hemostasis of the raw surfaces of the grafts and a shorter ischemia time than with ex situ splitting. However, we have also experienced the major disadvantage of this procedure, namely, prolonged operating time in the donor (by an additional 2 to 3 hours), which is not always feasible because of hemodynamic instability of the donor or reluctance of the other procurement teams to permit this delay. Rather than viewing in situ and ex situ splitting as opposing techniques, both should be developed according to their logistical possibilities, since both may lead to comparably good results as long as optimal technique and choice of donors and recipients are ensured.

Assessment of the Feasibility of the Split

The back-table procedure is performed in an operating room in which the temperature is set to 10° C. On the back-table, the liver is immersed in UW solution in its plastic carrying bag and placed in a smooth metal bucket filled with ice. The temperature of the preservation fluid is checked regularly. Should the temperature rise above 4° C, ice is added to the bucket. Towels moistened with chilled preservation solution are placed on the surface of the liver for additional topical cooling and to minimize the amount of surface exposed to air. During the initial stage of dissection, the liver is flushed with an additional 1 L of UW solution (500 mL through both the artery and portal vein) and prepared as a standard whole graft.[29] The gallbladder is removed and the cystic duct is ligated to avoid subsequent leakage of contrast medium during cholangiography. The presence of a portal bifurcation is checked by inserting a blunt metallic probe into the portal trunk (absence of the portal bifurcation, which is found in 1% of cases, is the only absolute contraindication to splitting the liver).[32,33] The liver is weighed and returned to the back-table, where it is placed flat in the anatomical position, with its inferior face downward. A radiopaque marker is placed for identification of the left side of the liver while the liver is still wrapped in an ice-cold towel.

Cholangiography is performed by injection of pure contrast medium (Radioselectan 76%; Schering SA, Lys-les-lannoy, France) through an 8-French Silastic cannula (Sherwood Medical, Evry, France) inserted in the distal end of the bile duct. Radiographs are printed out for immediate analysis of the biliary configuration of the graft. The anatomy of the left side is studied for the possibility of a right branch arising from the left hepatic duct. Contrast medium is rinsed out of the biliary tree with UW solution. This is useful in identification of biliary structures at the hilum.

If splitting of the liver is still intended, arteriography is performed to more precisely identify the anatomy of the arterial supply to the liver. Depending on the individual anatomy, contrast medium is injected through the celiac trunk or any other artery present (or through both). The contrast medium is rinsed out of the arterial tree with chilled UW solution, and the liver is rapidly returned to the chilled preservation solution. The intrahepatic distribution of the glissonian pedicle is then fully characterized, and the level of transection of the hepatic parenchyma can be decided.

Separation of Vessels and Bile Ducts

The main bile duct will always remain with the right graft because variations at the confluence of the bile ducts are much more frequent on the right side, the right bile duct is much shorter than the left duct (and sometimes nonexistent), and the arterial vasculature of

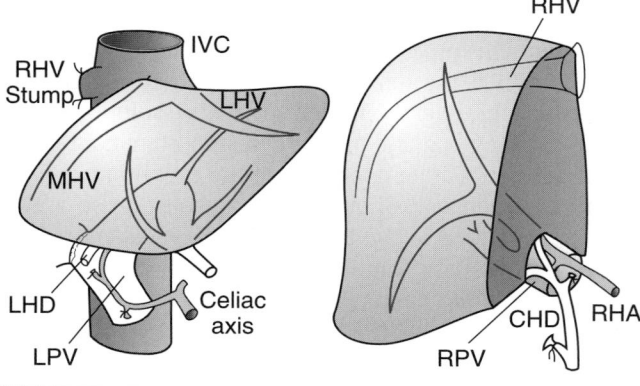

FIGURE 43–1

Right and left lobes of the liver from a splitting procedure for two adult recipients. CHD, common hepatic duct; IVC, inferior vena cava; LHD, left hepatic duct; LHV, left hepatic vein; LPV, left portal vein; MHV, middle hepatic vein; RHA, right hepatic artery; RHV, right hepatic vein; RPV, right portal vein.

the main bile duct depends chiefly on the right branch of the hepatic artery.[34,35] The left or right portal vein is cut at its origin on the portal trunk. The orifice in the portal trunk is closed with 7–0 monofilament running suture (Teflex; Peters France, Bobigny, France). When the left branch of the portal vein is cut at its root in the portal vein, the one to three tiny first branchings arising from the first 1 cm of the left branch of the portal vein are severed between ligatures. Such mobilization allows coaxial anastomosis of the left branch of the graft's portal vein to the native portal vein, thus avoiding any angulation phenomenon. The artery is cut, and the celiac trunk is usually left with the left graft because the right branch is larger than the left one (Fig. 43–1). Through an intraparenchymal suprahilar approach, the hilar plate is now brought down and a blunt metallic probe inserted to identify the bifurcation of the left branch. The hilar plate is cut straight with a scalpel slightly toward the left side to maintain continuity between the right and main hepatic ducts. The biliary structures are, in effect, cut blindly within the hilar plate. Minimal dissection avoids possible damage to the biliary arterial supply. The spigelian lobe is partially resected, with ligation of the portal branches originating from the posterior aspect of the portal bifurcation and ligation of the spigelian hepatic veins draining into the IVC. Such ligation facilitates implantation of the right graft in continuity with the IVC on the native IVC when this structure is preserved.[36] The resection encompasses the caudatus process on the left and extends as far as the right side of the IVC. The anatomy of the termination of the main hepatic veins in the suprahepatic IVC is then inspected visually and with a probe. The middle hepatic vein is kept on the left in continuity with the common trunk of the left and middle hepatic veins (see Fig. 43–1).

The IVC may be included in either of the grafts. When the IVC is to be resected in one of the future recipients (for example, for oncological reasons), the graft to be transplanted in this recipient retains the IVC.

Separation of the Grafts

Parenchymal transection is performed to the right of the middle hepatic vein, the whole of segment IV then being included in the left graft. Rubber tape is firmly applied to mark the proposed line of transection on the surface of the capsule of Glisson. The line is drawn at the right of the middle hepatic vein under ultrasonographic guidance. With the left hand acting as a block, both the right and left portions tend to fall apart on each side, and the liver is cut sharply with a knife along the transecting line previously marked. The two grafts are progressively cut apart. It is very important that the parenchyma be cut sharply in a single even plane and that a flat surface be left so that hemostasis may be achieved most efficiently.

Parenchymal transection may be performed with an ultrasonic dissector and clips or ligatures (or both). In our experience, the ultrasonic dissector leaves tiny fragile vessels that are difficult to ligate. Clips, whether resorbable or not, have a high propensity to be twisted off during the implantation procedure because of manipulation of the graft. With the procedure just described, as refined at our institution, control of hemorrhage at the raw surface of the grafts appears to no longer be a problem.[37] The use of a scalpel to cut the liver allows one to work on a plane at which every individual cut vessel can be easily individualized and precisely closed. The cut liver offers a certain thickness that allows stitches to be firmly applied. First, every individual tiny vessel seen on the cut surface is closed with a 4–0 silk stitch (Peters France). Running sutures may be used to close small hepatic vein branches that may have been cut longitudinally by the scalpel. During this phase, care is taken to avoid liver rewarming by applying wet towels over the graft with only the cut surface left exposed. Two surgeons, each working on a graft, treat both surfaces at the same time. When no remaining vessels can be seen to be unoccluded at the liver surface, arterial, portal, biliary, and hepatic venous leaks are searched for by injection of UW solution through the corresponding hilar or caval elements. Additional stitches are used when necessary. Second, fibrin glue is applied to the treated cut surfaces.

Split-Liver Graft Implantation

The technique is selected as indicated for each split graft–patient couple,[13,14,16,38] with percutaneous venovenous bypass instituted as needed.[39] The implantation technique is adapted as necessary with regard to preservation of the native vena cava,[36,40] creation of arterial or venous grafts,[41-43] or prevention of kinking of the venous anastomosis.[44] First-order arteries are anastomosed with 2.5× magnifying loupes, and second-order arteries are anastomosed under a microscope.[45,46]

Postoperative Care

Graft perfusion is checked by Doppler ultrasound daily in the intensive care unit and then weekly until discharge from the hospital. Patients whose partial thromboplastin time is less than 1.3 times control or whose platelet count is more than 30,000/µL receive anticoagulation with heparin (target partial thromboplastin time, 1.5 to 2.0 times control). Heparin is discontinued on discharge from the hospital, and aspirin (250 mg/day) is started.

Paul-Brousse Results

In our study,[12] 34 adults underwent split-liver transplantation with grafts from optimal donors prepared by ex situ splitting (n = 30) or in situ splitting (n = 4); the control group consisted of whole-liver grafts (n = 88). We did not find any difference in graft survival between whole-liver grafts and right split grafts, but survival of left split grafts was significantly lower at 2 years (43%) when compared with whole-liver grafts (85%; P = .003). There was no significant difference in inpatient survival rates whether patients received whole-liver grafts or right or left split-liver grafts at 1 year (87.7%, 74.2%, 87.5%) or at 2 years (85%, 74.2%, 64%). The principal pretransplantation factors influencing patient survival were graft steatosis and the hospital status of the recipient. The two most important factors affecting graft survival were graft steatosis and a graft-to-recipient body weight ratio less than 1%. We had expected that the loss of functional parenchyma from cold ischemia[47] would be additive with small graft size as a cause of primary nonfunction or anastomotic failure. However, we avoided transplantation of organs with very long cold ischemia times, so the lack of an observable effect of cold ischemia time in our series is not unexpected. The much shorter cold ischemia time in the in situ split procedures in the FAP patients, however, suggests that deceased donor livers should also be split in situ. Recipients had a higher risk of death (relative risk of 3.6%, 95% confidence interval of 1.3 to 10.4) if they were in the hospital (either in an intensive care unit or in a regular hospital bed) than when at home. An elective transplantation procedure in a patient normally at home appears to be a better

indication, with the risk of death being 3.6 times less than after urgent transplantation in an inpatient. The rate of arterial complications in our series is 6%, within the range of the present state of the art (the reported rate of arterial occlusion after whole-liver transplantation in adults and in children and after the split-liver procedure is 0% to 6%,[48-50] 3.2% to 16.7%,[48,49,51-55] and 0% to 15%,[3-5,17,30,56] respectively). The application of microsurgical techniques to the split-liver procedure should optimize the results, as reported for living related liver transplantation.[30] Venous outflow obstruction in left split grafts did not occur when the venoplasty technique was used.[44] Biliary complications occurred in 22% of patients in this series. Published rates range from 12.5% to 19.5% in adults,[51,57,58] from 5% to 22% in children,[48,52,54,55,58] and from 0% to 25% in recent series of split-liver transplantation.[3-5,17,30,56] There are two types of biliary complications. The more benign are leaks from the raw surface, which usually resolve with percutaneous drainage; however, problems concerning the biliary anastomosis are more troublesome, especially stenosis. In our study, three complications all occurred in a left split graft, in a choledochojejunostomy, and were relieved by percutaneous balloon dilatation and temporary stenting. The application of microsurgical techniques to biliary reconstruction could reduce the incidence of biliary complications, but there are other approaches. Dissection of the left hepatic duct and hilar plate can be minimized to avoid devascularization. Stenting of the anastomosis has been reported in living related liver transplantation.[59] Constructing the anastomosis on a Roux-en-Y loop on the right side takes advantage of the healthier vascular supply of the intrahepatic right duct.

Literature Results

Table 43–1 gives the results of larger series in which the split-liver technique provided two large grafts for adult transplantation. Only series with more than three split procedures are mentioned.

Conclusion

We have shown that split-liver procedures for two adults are technically feasible and can provide outcomes equivalent to those after whole-liver transplantation.[12] The recipient of a right split graft is not penalized in terms of graft survival, patient survival, or complications. Conversely, for left split-graft recipients, rigid selection criteria must be adopted to avoid primary liver nonfunction or poor graft survival results. In our series,[12] split-liver transplantation yielded a 62% net increase in adult transplant recipients. Toso and

Table 43-1. RECENT SERIES OF SPLIT-LIVER TRANSPLANTATION FOR TWO ADULT RECIPIENTS

Author, Location	No. of Cases	Patient Survival (%)		Graft Survival (%)	
		r s5-s8	l s1-s4	r s5-s8	l s1-s4
Zamir, Philadelphia	3R, 3L	100	43.4	100	43.4
Kilic, Houston	4R, 4L	100	100	100	100
Azoulay, Paris	17R, 17L	74.2	87.5	74.2	75
Andorno, Genoa	4R, 4L	75	75	50	75
Broering, Hamburg	6R, 6L	93	93	85	85
Humar, Minnesota	5R, 5L	80	80	80	80
Koenigsrainer, Innsbruck	4R, 4L	100	75	100	75

associates[60] adopted very strict selection criteria for donors and showed that graft availability increased by 8% to 23% for two adult recipients. The liver should definitely be considered a paired organ as often as possible, and the goal of clinical application of the split-liver technique in two adults has to be, as reported by Bismuth and coauthors in 1989,[14] to address the problem of organ shortage in this population, which accounts for more than 90% of the deaths in patients on the waiting list.[11]

References

1. Keeffe EB: Liver transplantation at the millennium. Past, present, and future. Clin Liver Dis 4:241-255, 2000.
2. United Network for Organ Sharing: Annual Report 2000. Available at http://www.unos.org/data.
3. Azoulay D, Astarcioglu I, Bismuth H, et al: Split liver transplantation: The Paul Brousse policy. Ann Surg 224:737-748, 1996.
4. Rogiers X, Malagò M, Gawad K, et al: In situ splitting of cadaveric livers: The ultimate expansion of a limited donor pool. Ann Surg 224:331-341, 1996.
5. Rela M, Vougas V, Muiesan P, et al: Split liver transplantation: King's College Hospital Experience. Ann Surg 227:282-288, 1998.
6. Spada M, Colledan M, Segalin A, et al: Extensive use of split liver for pediatric liver transplantation: A single centre experience [abstract]. Hepatology 30:221A, 1999.
7. Ghobrial RM: In situ splitting of the donor liver. Paper presented at the Living Donor and Split Liver Transplantation Symposium, September 22-24, 1999, Pittsburgh.
8. Busuttil RW, Goss JA: Split liver transplantation. Ann Surg 229:313-321, 1999.
9. Marcos A: Right lobe living donor liver transplantation: A review. Liver Transpl 6:3-20, 2000.
10. Azoulay D, Bismuth H: Living donor liver transplantation. Present and future alternatives [in French]. Gastroenterol Clin Biol 24:782-790, 2000.
11. Smith CME: Annual Report of the US Scientific Registry of Transplant Recipients and the Organ Procurement and Transplantation Network—Transplant Data: 1988-1996. Rockville, MD, Division of Transplantation, Bureau of Health Resources and Services Administration, US Department of Health and Human Services, 1997.
12. Azoulay D, Castaing D, Adam R, et al: Split-liver transplantation for two adult recipients: Feasibility and long-term outcomes. Ann Surg 233:565-574, 2001.
13. Pichlmayr R, Ringe B, Gubernatis G, et al: Transplantation einer Spenderleber auf zwei Empfanger (splitting-transplantation): Eine neue Methode in der Weiterentwicklung der Lebersegment-transplantation. Langenbecks Arch Chir 373:127-130, 1988.
14. Bismuth H, Morino M, Castaing D, et al: Emergency orthotopic liver transplantation in two patients using one donor liver. Br J Surg 76:722-724, 1989.
15. Colledan M, Andorno E, Valente U, et al: A new splitting technique for liver grafts [letter]. Lancet 353:1763, 1999.
16. Otte JB, de Ville de Goyet J, Alberti D, et al: The concept and technique of the split liver in clinical transplantation. Surgery 107:605-612, 1990.
17. Kalayoglu M, D'Alessandro A, Knechtle SJ, et al: Preliminary experience with split liver transplantation. J Am Coll Surg 182:381-387, 1996.
18. Broelsch CE, Emond JC, Whitington PF, et al: Liver transplantation in children from living related donors: Surgical techniques and results. Ann Surg 214:428-438, 1991.
19. De Ville de Goyet J: Split liver transplantation in Europe—1988 to 1993. Transplantation 59:1371-1376, 1995.
20. Hertl M, Howard TK, Lowell JA, et al: Changes in liver core temperature during preservation and rewarming in human and porcine liver allografts. Liver Transpl Surg 2:111-117, 1996.
21. Rogiers X, Malago M, Habib N, et al: In situ splitting of the liver in the heart beating cadaveric donor for transplantation in two recipients. Transplantation 55:835-840, 1995.
22. Furukawa H, Todo S, Imventarza O, et al: Effect of cold ischemia time on the early outcome of human hepatic allografts preserved with UW solution. Transplantation 51:1000-1004, 1991.
23. Furukawa H, Todo S, Imventarza O, et al: Cold ischemia time vs outcome of human liver transplantation using UW solution. Transplant Proc 23:1550-1551, 1991.
24. Azoulay D, Castaing D, Adam R, et al: Transplantation of three adult patients with one cadaveric graft: Wait or innovate? Liver Transpl Surg 6:239-240, 2000.
25. Karbe T, Rogiers M, Malago M, et al: Technical procedures and logistics of split-liver transplantation. Transplant Proc 27:1179, 1995.
26. Andorno E, Genzone A, Morelli N, et al: One liver for two adults: In situ split liver transplantation for two adult recipients. Transplant Proc 33:1420-1422, 2001.
27. Kiuchi T, Kasahara M, Uryuhara K, et al: Impact of graft size mismatching on graft prognosis in liver transplantation from living donors. Transplantation 67:321-327, 1999.
28. Lo C, Fan S, Liu C, et al: Minimum graft size for successful living donor liver transplantation. Transplantation 68:1112-1116, 1999.
29. Starzl TE, Miller C, Broznick B, Makowka L: An improved technique for multiple organ harvesting. Surg Gynecol Obstet 165:343-348, 1987.

30. Goss JA, Yersiz H, Shackleton CR, et al: In situ splitting of the cadaveric liver for transplantation. Transplantation 64:871-877, 1997.
31. Rogiers X, Topp S, Broering DC: Split liver transplantation: Split in-situ or ex-situ? Curr Opin Transpl 5:57-63, 2000.
32. Couinaud C: Le Foie: Etudes Anatomiques et Chirurgicales. Paris, Masson, 1957.
33. Couinad C, Houssin D: Analysis of the anatomical difficulties of bipartition. In Couinad C, Houssin D (eds): Controlled Partition of the Liver for Transplantation: Anatomical Limitation, vol 1. Paris, C. Couinad, 1991, pp 10-43.
34. Stapleton GN, Hickman R, Terablanche J: Blood supply of the right and left hepatic ducts. Br J Surg 82:817-818, 1995.
35. Padbury R, Azoulay D: Anatomy of the biliary tracts. In Taouli J (ed): Surgery of the Biliary Tract. London, Churchill Livingstone, 1993, pp 35-92.
36. Lerut J, de Ville de Goyet J, Donataccio M, et al: Piggyback transplantation with side-to-side cavocavostomy is an ideal technique for right split liver allograft implantation. J Am Coll Surg 179:573-576, 1994.
37. Azoulay D, Marin-Hargreaves G, Castaing D, et al: Ex-situ splitting of the liver. The versatile Paul Brousse technique. Arch Surg 136:956-961, 2001.
38. Emond JC, Whitington PF, Thistlethwaite JR, et al: Transplantation of two patients with one liver. Analysis of preliminary experience with "split liver" grafting. Ann Surg 21:14-22, 1990.
39. Ozaki CF, Langnas AN, Bynon JS, et al: A percutaneous method for venovenous bypass in liver transplantation. Transplantation 57:472-473, 1994
40. Calne RY, William R: Transplantation in man. I. Observations on technique and organization in five cases. BMJ 4:535-540, 1968.
41. Shaw BW Jr, Iwatsuki S, Starzl TE: Alternative methods of hepatic graft arterialization. Surg Gynecol Obstet 159:490-493, 1984.
42. Shaw BW Jr, Iwatsuki S, Bron K, et al: Portal vein grafts in hepatic transplantation. Surg Gynecol Obstet 161:67-68, 1985.
43. Shaw BW, Wood RP, Stratta RJ, et al: Management of arterial anomalies encountered in split-liver transplantation. Transplant Proc 22:420-422, 1990.
44. Emond JC, Heffon TG, Whitington PF, et al: Reconstruction of the hepatic vein in reduced-size hepatic transplantation. Surg Gynecol Obstet 176:11-17, 1993.
45. Mori K, Nagata I, Yamagata S, et al: The introduction of microvascular surgery to hepatic artery reconstruction in living donor liver transplantation: Its surgical advantages compared to conventional procedures. Transplantation 54:263-268, 1992.
46. Inomoto T, Nishizawa F, Sasaki H, et al: Experience with 120 microsurgical reconstructions of hepatic artery in living related liver transplantation. Surgery 119:20-26, 1996.
47. Adam R, Castaing D, Bismuth H: Transplantation of small donor livers in adult recipients. Transplant Proc 25:1105-1106, 1993.
48. Busuttil RW, Seu PH, Millis JM, et al: Liver transplantation in children. Ann Surg 213:48-53, 1991.
49. Langnas AN, Marujo W, Stratta RJ, et al: Vascular complications after orthotopic liver transplantation. Am J Surg 161:76-83, 1991.
50. Mor E, Schwartz ME, Sheiner PA, et al: Prolonged preservation in University of Wisconsin solution associated with hepatic artery thrombosis after orthotopic liver transplantation. Am J Surg 161:76-83, 1991.
51. Szapakowski JL, Cox K, Nakazato P, et al: Liver transplantation: Experience with 100 cases. West J Med 155:494-501, 1991.
52. Houssin D, Soubrane O, Boillot O, et al: Orthotopic liver transplantation with a reduced-size graft: An ideal compromise in pediatrics? Surgery 111:532-542, 1992.
53. Lomas DJ, Britton PD, Farman P, et al: Duplex Doppler ultrasound for the detection of vascular occlusion following liver transplantation in children. Clin Radiol 46:38-42, 1992.
54. Valayer J, Gauthier F, Yandza T, et al: Chirurgie de la transplantation hepatique chez l'enfant. Pediatrie 48:139-141, 1993.
55. De Ville de Goyet J, Hausleithner V, Reding R, et al: Impact of innovative techniques on the waiting list and results in pediatric liver transplantation. Transplantation 5:1130-1136, 1993.
56. Mirza DF, Achilleos O, Pirenne J, et al: Encouraging results of split-liver transplantation. Br J Surg 85:494-497, 1998.
57. Stratta RJ, Wood RP, Langnas AN, et al: Diagnosis and treatment of biliary tract complications after orthotopic liver transplantation. Surgery 106:675-684, 1989.
58. Greif F, Bronsther OL, Van Thiel DH, et al: The incidence, timing and management of biliary tract complications after orthotopic liver transplantation. Surgery 106:675-684, 1989.
59. Tanaka K, Uemoto S, Tokunaga Y, et al: Surgical techniques and innovations in living related liver transplantation. Ann Surg 217:82-91, 1993.
60. Toso C, Ris F, Mentha G, et al: Potential impact of in situ liver splitting on the number of available grafts. Transplantation 74:222-226, 2002.

Donor and Recipient Evaluation and Selection for Adult-to-Adult Right Hepatic Lobe Liver Transplantation

JAMES F. TROTTER
PAUL H. HAYASHI
IGAL KAM

Advantages and disadvantages of living donor liver transplantation   656

Recipient evaluation and selection   658

Donor evaluation and selection   659

Special considerations for living donor liver transplantation   664
Anatomic considerations   664
Patients outside the general criteria for transplantation   666
Hepatitis C   667
Hepatitis B core antibody–positive donor   668
Acute liver failure (UNOS status 1)   668
"Nondirected" or "Good Samaritan" donation   668
Syngeneic living donor liver transplantation   669

The future   669

Adult-to-adult right hepatic lobe living donor liver transplantation (LDLT) has recently emerged as a viable treatment option for selected patients with end-stage liver disease.[1-11] The rapid growth of the procedure over the past 5 years is due to the early favorable outcomes, as well as the critical shortage of deceased donor organs (Fig. 44–1). In 1998, only 86 LDLTs were performed, or 1.7% of all liver transplants in the United States.[12] By 2001, the number of LDLTs surpassed 500 (Fig. 44–2), or approximately 10% of all liver transplants. However, in the past 2 years the number of LDLTs has decreased. Only 359 LDLTs were performed in the United States from July 2001 to June 2002, and the number of cases for 2003 was 321, which represents a 38% reduction in volume since 2001. The national reduction in LDLTs is a result of careful re-examination of the procedure after a widely publicized donor death in 2002. As a result, transplant physicians are taking a more cautious approach toward living donation to ensure favorable outcomes in both donors and recipients. In this context, the process of evaluation and selection of potential donors and recipients has

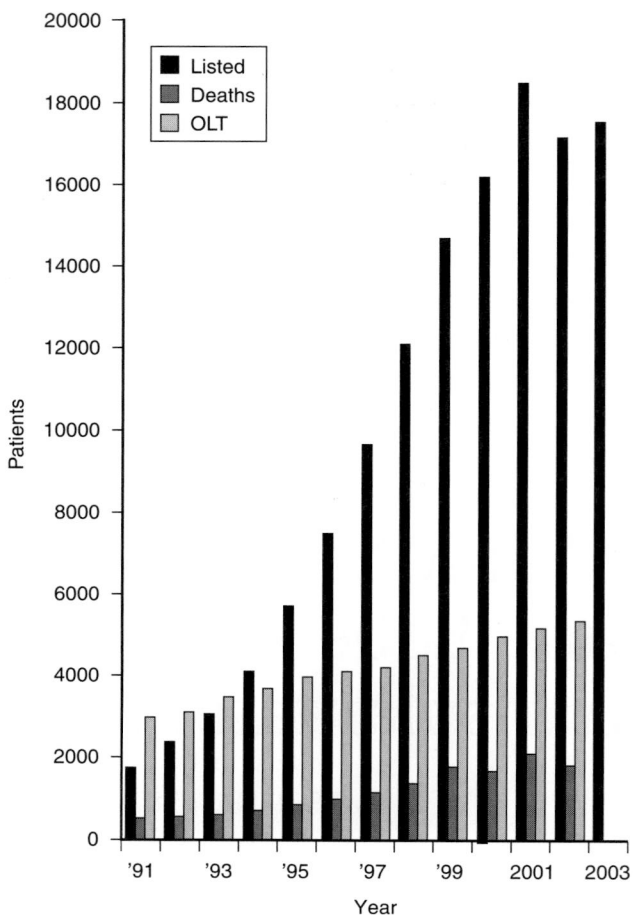

FIGURE 44-1

U.S. liver transplant list. Deaths, the number of patients dying each year while on the liver transplant list; Listed, number of liver transplant waiting list registrants at the end of the calendar year; OLT, orthotopic liver transplants performed each year. (Data from the United Network of Organ Sharing transplantation database. Available at http://www.unos.org/Data/.)

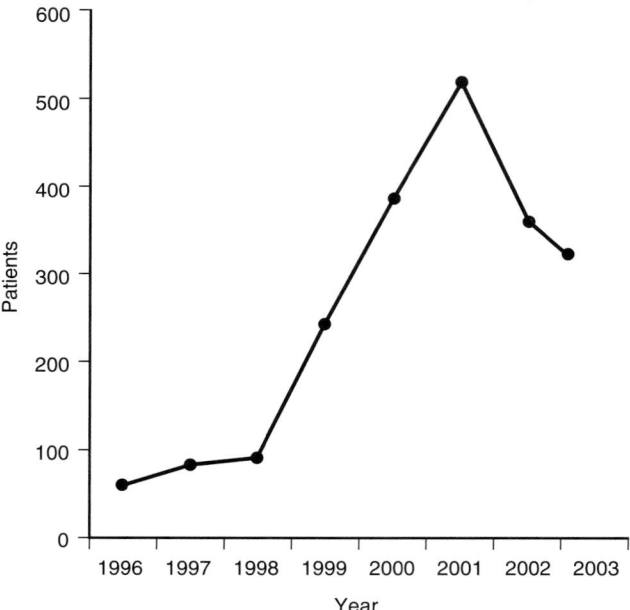

FIGURE 44-2

Number of patients in the United States who received living donor liver transplants by year. (Data from the United Network of Organ Sharing transplantation database. Available at http://www.unos.org/Data/.)

liver transplantation list die each year. Patients with a living donor can undergo LDLT within hours to weeks after identification of a suitable donor. As a result, waiting list mortality may be lower in patients undergoing LDLT. Patients without a living donor, however, are relegated to deceased donor liver transplantation and therefore have an increased risk of decompensation

taken on even greater importance. This chapter describes the current evaluation and selection of donors and recipients for LDLT.[13-22]

Advantages and Disadvantages of Living Donor Liver Transplantation

Selection of donors and recipients for LDLT is based on an understanding of the advantages and disadvantages of the procedure (Fig. 44-3). The most important advantage of LDLT is the significant reduction in waiting time before transplantation. Expedited transplantation with a living donor allows the surgery to occur before severe clinical decompensation, which could jeopardize a successful outcome or lead to death of the patient on the waiting list. Approximately 10% of patients on the

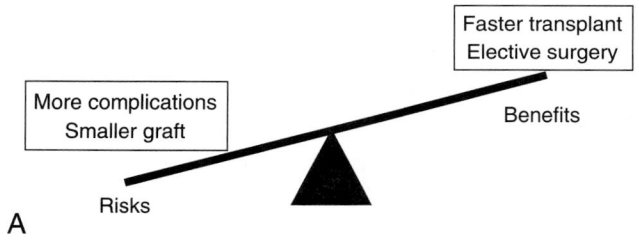

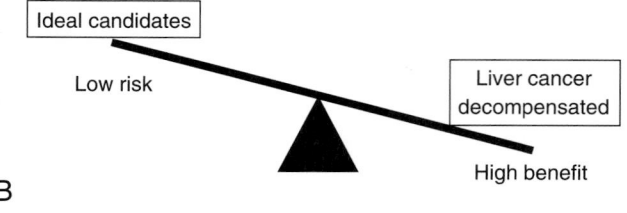

FIGURE 44-3

A and **B**, Risks and benefits of living donor liver transplantation.

or death on the transplant list as they wait for an organ from a deceased donor. At our center, the median waiting time for LDLT recipients from 1999 until 2002 was two thirds less than that for recipients of deceased donor organs (before implementation of the Model for End-Stage Liver Disease [MELD] score). However, no published data have demonstrated a reduction in waiting list mortality in LDLT recipients in comparison to recipients of deceased donor livers.

Another advantage of LDLT is that the surgery may be scheduled for days, weeks, or even months before the procedure; in deceased donor liver transplantation, in contrast, surgery is performed on an "on-call" basis. The elective nature of LDLT may allow recipients to receive medical treatment to stabilize or improve their underlying medical condition before transplantation so that they are in the best medical condition at the time of surgery. For example, hepatitis C may be treated for several weeks or months with interferon and ribavirin to achieve viral eradication, which may prevent posttransplant recurrence of hepatitis C. In addition, patients with sepsis can undergo antibiotic therapy for several days to eliminate the bacterial infection before the anticipated day of surgery.

An additional advantage of LDLT is that the cold ischemic time is significantly less than with deceased donor liver transplantation. For most LDLT recipients, the cold ischemic time is approximately 1 hour versus 6 to 12 hours for conventional transplantation. Because a prolonged cold ischemic time is associated with graft loss and postoperative complications, the shorter cold ischemic time in LDLT recipients may result in fewer postoperative problems.[23-26] However, any benefit from a reduction in cold ischemia time is only theoretical, and no data currently show that the reduced cold ischemia time with LDLT provides any benefit over deceased donor liver transplantation. Besides minimal cold ischemia time, a graft from a living donor may be of higher intrinsic quality than a deceased donor organ. A living donor graft is obtained from a healthy person who, by definition, has no underlying medical problems. A deceased donor, in contrast, is critically ill and frequently maintained on life support for several days in the intensive care unit (ICU). In addition, a living donor is able to undergo more extensive testing than a deceased donor is, including abdominal imaging to rule out intrahepatic lesions and vascular anomalies. Finally, a living donor is typically younger than a deceased donor. Advanced donor age is a risk factor for patient and graft loss after deceased donor liver transplantation and is one of the most important causes of a poor outcome in hepatitis C–positive recipients of deceased donor organs.

There are also disadvantages associated with LDLT, the greatest of which is the risk of death and complications in the living donor. The actual risk to the donor (including donor death) is unknown because of the

Table 44–1. COMPLICATIONS OF PARTIAL-LIVER DONATION IN 449 LIVE DONORS*

Type of Complication	Number of Donors (%)
Death	1 (0.2)
Need for rehospitalization	38 (8.5)
Bile stricture or leak	27 (6.0)
Nonautologous blood transfusion	22 (4.9)
Need for reoperation	20 (4.5)
Major postoperative infection	5 (1.1)
Other	10 (2.2)
Total	65 (14.5)

*Some donors had more than one complication.
From Brown RS Jr, Russo MW, Lai M, et al: A survey of liver transplantation from living adult donors in the United States. N Engl J Med 348:818-825, 2003. Available at http://content.nejm.org/content/vol348/issue9/.

absence of a comprehensive database to record outcomes in living donors. However, two recent surveys of liver transplant centers in the United States (Table 44–1) and Asia provide some insight.[27,28] The overall complication rate in living donors was between 15% and 28%. Biliary problems such as bile leak or stricture were the most common complications and occurred in 6% of cases. Between 0.5% and 4.9% of donors required a nonautologous blood transfusion. Of note, complication rates were higher in U.S. centers that performed fewer LDLTs, an observation that reflects a learning curve previously reported by single centers.[10,27] The actual risk of donor death after donor hepatectomy is unknown, but data from single-center reports and survey data estimate a rate of 1 in 300.[27-31] However, the actual risk of donor death may be higher as a result of the absence of a comprehensive record of all donor deaths. Because of the measurable risk that donors incur with the donor surgery, only recipients with a reasonable chance of a favorable outcome should be considered for LDLT (see discussion of this topic later).

Another important disadvantage of LDLT is that the right hepatic lobe graft is generally a third smaller than a whole deceased donor liver. For sick patients, the smaller graft size may not provide adequate hepatic function after transplantation. A study from Germany reported that posttransplant mortality in critically ill LDLT recipients (United Network of Organ Sharing [UNOS] status 2A) is threefold higher than that in recipients of deceased donor livers.[32,33] These findings have been corroborated by data from the Scientific Registry of Transplant Recipients, which measured LDLT recipient survival relative to the severity of illness at the time of transplantation. This analysis showed that the risk-adjusted mortality rate for LDLT recipients is 23% higher than that in recipients of deceased donor livers.[12] Another study reported outcomes in LDLT recipients relative to their severity of illness at the time of transplantation and found that sicker patients fared better with a larger LDLT graft.[34] Small graft size (graft-recipient body weight [GRBW] ratio of 0.6%) did not have a negative impact on survival in Child's class A recipients. However, LDLT recipients with more advanced liver disease (Child's class B and C) had significantly poorer graft survival (33% graft survival rate) when the GRBW ratio was less than 0.85% than when it was greater than 0.85% (74% graft survival rate). LDLT recipients also have more biliary complications than recipients of deceased donor livers do.[35-39] A study from our center found that the incidence of biliary complications was more than twofold higher in LDLT recipients (44%) than in recipients of deceased donor livers (13%, $P < .05$).[38] Another study also reported that the incidence of biliary complications was more than twofold higher in LDLT recipients (58%) than in recipients of deceased donor organs (25%, $P < .002$).[39] There are two reasons why LDLT recipients have an increased incidence of biliary complications. LDLT recipients are at increased risk of leaks from the cut surface of the right hepatic graft. In addition, LDLT recipients frequently have more than one bile duct anastomosis, which increases the risk of biliary strictures at the anastomotic site.

The advantages and disadvantages of LDLT must be carefully weighed in the evaluation and selection of recipients for the procedure. Critically ill patients (ICU bound and requiring mechanical ventilation) are generally poor candidates for LDLT because of the increased risk of death after transplantation in comparison to deceased donor transplantation. Moreover, recipients who are significantly debilitated may not tolerate the additional surgery that may be required to repair biliary complications. Therefore, the best candidates for LDLT are patients with low surgical risk and an urgent medical need for expedited transplantation.

Recipient Evaluation and Selection

The initial step in the evaluation of a recipient for LDLT is to list the patient for deceased donor transplantation. Potential LDLT recipients must first be listed for deceased donor transplantation for three reasons. Obviously, to undergo LDLT, the patient must be physiologically fit for transplantation. In addition, the patient should qualify for deceased donor transplantation, which could be necessary if the LDLT graft fails and retransplantation with a whole deceased donor organ is required. Approximately 10% of LDLT recipients require retransplantation. Finally, all third-party payers require listing for deceased donor transplantation before evaluating and approving a patient for LDLT.

In our experience, LDLT is recognized as an approved therapy by all major insurance carriers. Therefore, denial of coverage for LDLT is almost never an impediment to performing the procedure. However, in most cases, approval for LDLT generally requires a separate application to the insurance carrier after approval for deceased donor transplantation.

Many patients listed for deceased donor transplantation are not suitable for LDLT. Patients listed for deceased donor transplantation may be considered for LDLT if they are deemed "medically eligible" and "surgically suitable" for the procedure. As discussed earlier, to be considered "medically eligible" for LDLT, the patient must have an urgency for transplantation and, in the judgment of the transplant team, must have a significant risk of dying before the anticipated deceased donor transplantation. Selected patients with non–life-threatening complications (pruritus, fatigue) may be considered for LDLT on a case-by-case basis. The ultimate decision to perform LDLT on a specific patient rests with the judgment and experience of the physicians at the transplant center. The MELD score is a valuable selection criterion for LDLT recipients. However, clinical judgment is as important or more important than the MELD score in recipient selection. The risk of 90-day mortality associated with a MELD score higher than 18 is greater than 10%.[40] Therefore, for patients with a MELD score higher than 18, the 90-day mortality without transplantation (> 10%) exceeds the 1-year mortality after LDLT (10%). As a result, all patients with a MELD score higher than 18 should be considered potential candidates for LDLT. However, some patients with a MELD score less than 18 may also have a medical urgency for transplantation. Typically, these patients experience life-threatening symptoms that have no bearing on their MELD score, such as cachexia, recurrent encephalopathy, or recurrent infections. For sick patients with a low MELD score (< 18), the chances of imminent deceased donor transplantation are low at most transplant centers. As a result, expedited transplantation with a live donor may be their best treatment option. When compared with patients who have viral hepatitis, those with cholestatic liver disease (primary biliary cirrhosis and sclerosing cholangitis) are more likely to have significantly decompensated liver disease with a low MELD score. Data from the Scientific Registry of Transplant Recipients indicate that LDLT recipients have lower MELD scores at the time of transplantation than their deceased donor counterparts.[12] Between February 2002 and June 2002, the median MELD score for LDLT recipients was 15, as opposed to 23 for recipients of deceased donor livers, and a greater proportion of LDLT recipients (71%) than recipients of deceased donor livers (48%) received transplants, with a MELD score less than 20.

Although all patients with MELD scores higher than 18 should be considered medically eligible for LDLT, clinicians have questioned whether there is an upper limit for the MELD score above which LDLT should not be performed. As noted earlier, critically ill patients (listed as status 2A under the old UNOS allocation system) are generally poor candidates for LDLT because of poor outcomes. However, there are very few data documenting outcomes with LDLT under the new MELD allocation system. A preliminary analysis from our center assessed the predictive value of pretransplant MELD score on posttransplantation survival.[41] We found that there was no difference in patient or graft survival associated with the MELD score, even for patients with very high MELD scores (MELD score > 30). However, LDLT recipients with a MELD score higher than 18 spent nearly twofold more days in the hospital during the first 3 months after transplantation than did those with a MELD score of 18 or lower. Even though this study is limited by the relatively small number of patients, these data suggest that LDLT may be successfully performed even in patients with very high MELD scores (> 30). However, we anticipate that with larger numbers of LDLT and greater statistical power, a decreased survival rate will become apparent for LDLT recipients with MELD scores higher than 30. In our experience, we have found that in patients with chronic liver disease, the following factors are associated with poor outcome after LDLT independent of the MELD score: mechanical ventilation, hemodialysis, and a very low Karnofsky score. One or more of these factors in patients with chronic liver disease is a strong relative contraindication for LDLT. To summarize the use of MELD scores in the selection of LDLT recipients, (1) we have not found a specific MELD score above or below which LDLT should be contraindicated. In general, when a patient has a MELD score higher than 18, obvious features of decompensation (ascites, jaundice, encephalopathy, variceal bleeding) are frequently present, and these patients should routinely be considered medically eligible for LDLT. (2) However, a substantial minority of patients listed for deceased donor transplantation with MELD scores less than 18 have significant features of decompensation associated with a high risk of waiting list mortality and warrant consideration of LDLT. Using the selection criteria described earlier, we have found that at our center, approximately 25% of the patients listed for liver transplantation are "medically eligible" (have an identified medical urgency for transplantation).

At a few LDLT centers, all patients listed for liver transplantation are considered eligible for LDLT regardless of the presence of a medical urgency for transplantation. Proponents of this approach argue that performing LDLT in a patient with stable liver disease reduces the risk of death or decompensation while on the transplant list and gives the recipient the best possible chance of a successful transplantation. In fact, data from UNOS indicate that a substantial number of LDLT recipients have stable liver disease at the time of transplantation. Thirty-seven percent of LDLT recipients in the United States are status 3 (chronic liver disease with < 10 Child-Pugh points) at the time of surgery.[12] However, the risk of complications and death in the living donor should always be considered heavily when contemplating LDLT in stable patients with chronic liver disease. In addition, the risk of recurrent disease in the recipient, especially those with hepatitis C, should also be carefully considered.

Once the recipient has been determined to be "medically eligible" for LDLT, the surgical team must determine whether the recipient is "surgically suitable" for the procedure. There are no absolute exclusion criteria for LDLT, and the decision to perform LDLT on a specific patient must be based on the skill, experience, and judgment of the transplant physician or physicians and the surgeon in charge. In general, medical or surgical issues that could significantly jeopardize the success of the LDLT disqualify the patient for LDLT. Medical and surgical contraindications for LDLT are listed in Table 44–2. Common medical problems that may preclude LDLT are conditions that increase the risk of posttransplant complications and death, including morbid obesity, significant deconditioning, advanced age, previous major abdominal surgery, and poorly controlled diabetes mellitus. Although the presence of one of these conditions may not preclude successful deceased donor liver transplantation, a combination of multiple risk factors may significantly jeopardize the likelihood of successful LDLT.

Of the 25% of listed patients who are considered "medically eligible" for LDLT (presence of medical urgency for LDLT), many patients have one or more comorbid conditions that significantly jeopardize the potential success of the transplantation. In fact, only half the patients who are deemed "medically eligible" for LDLT are found to be "surgically suitable."[19] Consequently, approximately 12.5% of patients listed for deceased donor transplantation are eligible to accept volunteers for evaluation for donor surgery (Fig. 44–4). Specific issues related to recipient evaluation and selection are discussed later.

Donor Evaluation and Selection

Once a recipient is accepted as a suitable candidate for LDLT, the recipient may accept volunteers for donor evaluation. The specific evaluation process for potential donors varies between LDLT centers. The purpose of the donor evaluation is twofold: (1) to ensure donor safety and (2) to determine whether the donor can

Table 44-2. CONTRAINDICATIONS TO LIVING DONOR LIVER TRANSPLANTATION

	Absolute Contraindications	Relative Contraindications
Medical	Unsuitable for deceased donor liver transplantation	No previous relationship to donor
	ICU bound and requiring mechanical ventilation and hemodialysis with chronic liver disease (old UNOS status 2A)	Stable hepatitis C cirrhosis
		Severe deconditioning
		Obesity
		Poorly controlled diabetes
		Age > 65 yr
		Lack of financial approval
		Significant lung, heart, renal disease (except hepatopulmonary syndrome)
		Stable cirrhosis (old UNOS status 3)
Surgical		Anomalous hepatic biliary anatomy
		Portal vein thrombosis
		Budd-Chiari syndrome
		Previous major abdominal surgery
		Morbid obesity

UNOS, United Network of Organ Sharing.

yield a suitable graft for transplantation. Currently, there are no guidelines by which the recipient may solicit potential donors. However, one of the basic criteria for a potential donor is that the donor have a significant long-term relationship with the recipient. Public advertisement for potential donors through the general media (television, radio, newspaper) or through church or community bulletins is inappropriate because in such cases, the advertisement is directed at individuals who do not have a significant long-term relationship with the donor. Once a potential donor has been identified, the donor must directly contact the transplant center to initiate the donor evaluation. In general, the

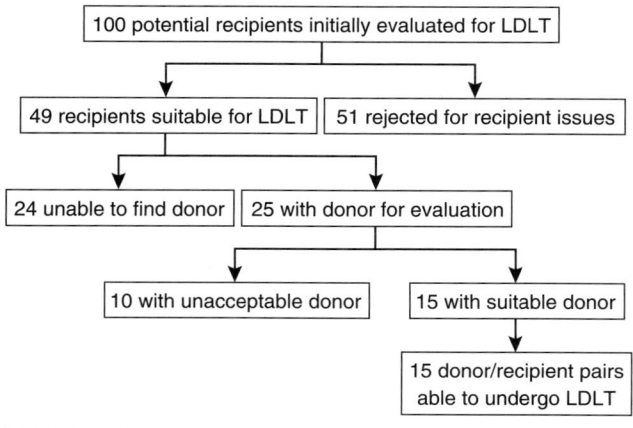

FIGURE 44-4

Outcomes of 100 patients evaluated for living donor liver transplantation.[19]

potential donor should initiate contact with the transplant center to start the donor evaluation because requiring the potential donor to do so forces the individual to take an active step (in calling the transplant center) toward donation. If the transplant center makes the initial contact with the potential donor, the likelihood of evaluating individuals with minimal interest in donating may be higher. After the donor has contacted the transplant center, evaluation of the potential donor proceeds in a stepwise fashion so that unsuitable donors may be excluded as early as possible in the evaluation process. Table 44-3 outlines the three specific phases of donor evaluation used at our center. Phase 1 is designed to determine whether the potential donor meets all the appropriate inclusion criteria for donation: appropriate blood type, age, body size, and relationship to the recipient. However, at our center, only 50% of patients who are considered suitable candidates for LDLT have a potential donor available for evaluation.[19] The reasons why a patient is unable to identify a potential donor for evaluation are frequently multifactorial and complex. The most common reasons are absence of family members or friends between the ages of 18 and 55, estrangement from family or friends, or a potential donor with an obvious medical problem, morbid obesity, or active substance abuse. Rarely, patients eligible for LDLT refuse to allow any donors to be evaluated because of concern related to the donor surgery. In our experience, less than 5% of patients decline LDLT for this reason.

At our center, an experienced registered nurse performs phase 1 of the donor evaluation by confirming

Table 44-3. PHASES OF RECIPIENT AND DONOR EVALUATION

Phase 1

RECIPIENT

Listed for deceased donor transplantation with a defined medical urgency for transplantation

Financial clearance for living donor liver transplantation

Absence of significant contraindications (see Table 44-2)

DONOR

Age ≥ 18 and ≤ 55

Identical or compatible blood type with the recipient

Absence of significant medical or psychiatric problems and previous abdominal surgery

Demonstrable, significant long-term relationship with the recipient

Normal liver function test results, serum electrolytes, and complete blood count with differential cell count; negative hepatitis B surface antigen, hepatitis B core antibody, and hepatitis C antibody

Phase 2

Complete medical history and physical examination of the potential donor Laboratory studies:

  Serum ferritin, iron, transferrin, ceruloplasmin

  α_1-Antitrypsin level and phenotype

  Rapid plasmin reagin

  Cytomegalovirus antibody (IgG), Epstein-Barr virus antibody (IgG)

  Antinuclear antibody

  Human immunodeficiency virus antibody

  Toxicology/substance abuse screen

  Urinalysis

  Blood oxygen saturation

  Chest radiograph

  Electrocardiogram

  Surgical evaluation of the donor

  Anesthesia preoperative evaluation

  Magnetic resonance imaging of the liver, biliary system, and hepatic vasculature

Phase 3

Other tests or consultations to clarify problems uncovered during phase 2*:

  Endoscopic retrograde cholangiopancreatography

  Hepatic angiogram

  Liver biopsy

  Echocardiogram

  Stress echocardiogram

*Some centers obtain these tests as part of the routine donor evaluation.

that the potential donor is between 18 and 55 years of age and has a significant long-term relationship with the recipient, an identical or compatible blood type with the recipient, and no significant medical problems. In addition, height, weight, and a brief medical, psychosocial, and surgical history are documented along with current medications. Serum electrolytes, blood count with differential, liver function tests, blood type, and hepatitis serology are obtained. At our center, we have found that body size compatibility between the donor and recipient is an important preliminary consideration in the donor evaluation. We require that the donor and recipient be within approximately 30% body size of each other. Potential donors whose body size is less than 70% of the recipient are rarely able to provide an adequate graft for the larger recipient, especially if the recipient has significantly decompensated liver disease. Other centers use a specific formula to determine the liver mass required for the recipient.[42,43] Cirrhotic patients who are physically large have great difficulty identifying suitable potential donors for evaluation. In fact, LDLT recipients are physically smaller than recipients of deceased donor livers. The percentage of LDLT recipients versus deceased donor liver recipients with a body mass index (BMI) higher than 31 is 13.0% versus 20.4%, and for those with a BMI of 26 to 30, the percentage is 21.4% versus 25.1%.[12] At our center, the largest LDLT recipient weighed 104 kg at the time of surgery.

After phase 1 (preliminary evaluation) data are obtained, the potential donor is presented to the transplant team to decide whether to proceed with phase 2 (comprehensive donor evaluation). Before proceeding to the comprehensive donor evaluation, the data from phase 1 are reviewed, and any specific issues related to the donor and recipient that may require special attention are considered. For instance, if the donor is positive for hepatitis B core antibody (HBcAb), a donor liver biopsy is required in the donor evaluation. Potential donors with a remote or poorly defined history of a medical problem, such as depression or a thrombotic tendency, require consultation with the appropriate specialist during the donor evaluation. Phase 2 consists of further radiological and serological testing, as well as a complete medical history, physical examination, and psychosocial, surgical, and preoperative anesthesia evaluations. At 50% of LDLT centers, the donor history and physical examination are performed by a physician not affiliated with the liver transplantation team.[27] Separation of the evaluating physician and the transplantation team may help reduce the inherent conflict of interest that transplant physicians may have in the donor evaluation.[44] At other centers, a physician member of the transplant team evaluates the donor, although this physician is not attending the recipient. Phase 3 of the evaluation is performed to clarify any abnormalities or issues discovered during phase 2. The survey by

Brown and colleagues describes the percentage of donor candidates who undergo invasive procedures during the donor evaluation.[27] Most centers perform liver biopsy on selected donors (with risk factors for histological abnormalities). Arteriography is not generally part of the standard evaluation, and half the centers routinely require endoscopic retrograde cholangiopancreatography (ERCP) to define the donor's biliary anatomy.

Psychosocial evaluation of the donor is an important component of the overall evaluation process.[45-53] The primary goals of psychosocial evaluation of the potential donor are to (1) educate the potential donor regarding the psychosocial impact of the donor surgery and recovery, (2) identify potential psychological or psychiatric issues that preclude donation, and (3) ensure that the donor is able to consent for the operation without coercion by the recipient, the recipient's family, or the transplant team. The type of psychosocial evaluation performed at each center depends on the composition of the transplant team and local expertise. In the United States, 95% of programs include a social worker, 86% a psychiatrist, and 17% an ethicist as part of the donor evaluation.[27] At our center, a social worker familiar with LDLT evaluates all potential donors. Although psychiatric evaluation is not mandatory, potential donors with any identified psychological or psychiatric issues are formally evaluated by a psychiatrist. The donor must recognize that undergoing donor surgery has many important long-term implications.[46] The average time required to return to work after donor hepatectomy is 10 weeks. Although the costs directly related to donor evaluation and surgery are paid by the recipient's insurance carrier, the indirect costs of donation must be borne by the donor. The mean indirect costs of donor evaluation not covered by insurance (travel, lodging, lost wages) are $3600. In addition, 70% of donors report long-term mild abdominal symptoms after donor surgery. During the donor evaluation, it may become apparent that the donor is being coerced, either intentionally or unintentionally, by the recipient or the recipient's family. If the transplant team or the potential donor feel uncomfortable with regard to coercion, the donor should not undergo the surgery. The transplant team should make special considerations so that the potential donor may freely decide to withdraw consent for donation at any time during the donor evaluation. The potential donor may be reluctant to withdraw consent for donation if disclosure of this decision is made to the recipient. Therefore, as a rule, the transplant team should not reveal the indication for donor rejection to the recipient or recipient's family. In cases in which the donor withdraws consent for surgery, the interests of the donor are best served by providing the donor with a medical indication for rejection that the donor may reveal to the recipient, if required.

The donor must be given sufficient time to carefully consider all the information gained during the evaluation process so that an informed decision can be made regarding the choice for donation. In some cases, the pressure on the transplant team and the donor to proceed with LDLT is intense because of the severity of the recipient's illness. However, the integrity of the evaluation process, including donor rights and privacy, must be maintained above all other interests.

The spectrum of psychological and psychiatric complications in donors after LDLT is not known. However, psychiatric problems are not uncommon after donation. Psychiatric disorders listed in the Diagnostic and Statistical Manual of Mental Disorders—Fourth Edition (DSM-IV), including major depression, posttraumatic stress disorder, dysthymia, and psychosis, may develop in up to 61% of LDLT donors after donation.[52] However, long-term follow-up of donors from center to center is generally very limited. Beavers and coauthors reported practice patterns of long-term follow-up in LDLT donors in the United States.[47] Beyond 1 year after donor surgery, only 25% of centers had scheduled clinic visits with the donor, only 14% required blood chemistry studies, and only one program administered a follow-up survey of donors. Conversely, many donors have communicated to us that they would prefer to have a scheduled follow-up assessment after the donor surgery. Because of the relatively common occurrence of post-LDLT psychiatric problems in donors and their desire to undergo scheduled follow-up, transplant physicians would be advised to consider long-term donor follow-up. By doing so, the full extent of posttransplant psychiatric problems could be identified. In addition, transplant physicians may recognize risk factors for psychiatric or psychological complications so that these problems may be avoided in future donors. More important, donors with psychological or psychiatric problems related to donation could be identified and treated.

An important recent development in the donor evaluation process is the recommendation for a "donor advocate." Currently, the Ad Hoc UNOS Committee on Living Donor Liver Transplantation, the Secretary of the Health and Human Services Advisory Committee of Organ Transplantation (ACOT), and the New York State Health Board all recommend that each LDLT center provide a "donor advocate" for each person evaluated for LDLT donation.[54-56] The requirement for a "donor advocate" was created largely after careful examination of the donor evaluation process following the widely publicized donor death that occurred in New York early in 2002. The primary role of the "donor advocate" is to "represent and advise the donor so as to ensure that the [appropriate] elements and ethical principles are applied to the practice of live donor transplantation."[55] The donor advocate's primary obligation is to "help [the] donor understand the process, the procedure and risks and benefits of live organ donation; and to protect and promote the interests and well-being of the donor." The "donor advocate" does not have the right to exclude the potential donor from undergoing the donor surgery because by law, this decision ultimately rests with the donor. However, the "donor advocate" may help the potential donor consider the risks of donor surgery independent of the deliberations of the transplant team.

Hepatic imaging is a key component of the donor evaluation. The type of imaging (computed tomography [CT] or magnetic resonance imaging [MRI]) performed at each center is largely based on local experience, expertise, and preference.[57-66] There is no evidence that one modality is superior to the other. At our center, each potential donor undergoes MRI (of the hepatic parenchyma), magnetic resonance cholangiopancreatography (MRCP), and magnetic resonance angiography (MRA) of the hepatic venous and arterial anatomy. The hepatic vasculature and biliary anatomy must be defined to ensure that the donor can undergo the hepatectomy safely and provide an adequate graft for the recipient. In addition, abdominal imaging will identify intrahepatic lesions, such as large hepatic cysts or hemangiomas, that could complicate or preclude successful hepatectomy. The volume of the right hepatic graft is determined by abdominal CT or MRI. As noted earlier, some centers use formulas to assist in the prediction of whether the donor has adequate hepatic mass.[42,43] Two formulas are used to assess the adequacy of graft size for the recipient's needs: (1) the GRBW ratio and (2) graft weight as a percentage of standard liver mass. Both are equally useful, with the lower limits of graft acceptability being 0.8% to 1.0% for GRBW and 40% to 50% of standard liver mass. However, as previously discussed, there may be a wider range of acceptability, depending on the severity of illness in the recipient.

Liver biopsy is a useful tool in the evaluation of a potential donor. However, the role of liver biopsy in donor evaluation varies from center to center. All donors undergo biopsy at 14% of centers, selected donors at 60%, and none of the donors at 26%.[27] Liver biopsy can define histological liver damage and establish the presence and extent of hepatic steatosis. One potential problem in performing liver biopsy in all potential donors is the discovery of minimal histological abnormalities. A recent preliminary study reported that 73% of all potential donors had minimal histological abnormalities (isolated granuloma, minimal portal inflammation, or < 10% steatosis) on liver biopsy.[67] The value of minimal histological abnormalities in the determination of donor suitability is unclear and requires further investigation. In some cases, donors with minimal histological abnormalities may be able to donate successfully with minor long-term risk.

Obesity (BMI > 28 kg/m²) in potential donors is an increasingly common problem because the prevalence of obesity is rising in the United States.[68] In general, obese individuals are poor donor candidates because most have hepatic steatosis. A recent study showed that hepatic steatosis (> 10% steatosis) was present in more than 75% of patients with a BMI higher than 28 kg/m².[69,70] Because hepatic steatosis is associated with poor graft function after transplantation, most centers exclude donors who have greater than 10% steatosis on liver biopsy. (However, no data in LDLT recipients have shown worse outcomes relative to the presence or extent of hepatic steatosis.) The likelihood of accepting an obese individual for donation is small because the majority have significant hepatic steatosis. If an obese donor is considered for donor surgery, a liver biopsy is mandatory to rule out the presence of hepatic steatosis. Because steatosis can occur in persons with a normal or mildly elevated BMI, the argument for liver biopsy in all potential donors has been made. In one study, protocol liver biopsies were performed on 100 consecutive potential donors, and 1 (1.5%) of 67 potential donors with a BMI of 28 or less had 30% steatosis.[71,72] However, there are no data regarding outcomes after LDLT with the use of steatotic grafts. The argument against mandatory liver biopsy in all potential donors stems from the small mortality risk (1 in 11,000) and pain associated with the procedure.[72] Another reason that obesity is a general exclusion criterion for donors relates to the increased risk of complications with the donor surgery. Studies have shown that the risk of bleeding and postoperative complications is higher after abdominal surgery in obese patients.[73-76] In addition, the incidence of comorbid conditions (hypertension, hypercholesterolemia, diabetes) that could increase the risk of postoperative complications after donor hepatectomy is higher in obese individuals.[77] Body fat topography is important to consider in an overweight or minimally obese potential donor. Hepatic steatosis is more prevalent in patients with a high waist-to-hip circumference ratio (an "apple" distribution), as opposed to those with a low ratio (a "pear" distribution).[78] Therefore, patients with abdominal fat are more likely to have hepatic steatosis than when excess fat is present in the hips and thighs. As a result, potential donors who are minimally overweight with a "pear" distribution of fat may be able to donate more often than patients with excess abdominal fat. There are no data on outcomes of overweight or obese LDLT donors after donor hepatectomy. However, using obesity as a relative exclusion criterion for donation seems to be a prudent decision.

Regional demographic variations in the prevalence of obesity may have a significant impact on the availability of donors for LDLT.[79] The prevalence of obesity varies across the United States, with the highest rates in the southeast and north-central United States. As a result, transplant centers in these regions may have more difficulty identifying suitable donors for LDLT. Conversely, the availability of donors for LDLT may be higher in the Rocky Mountain west, where the prevalence of obesity is the lowest in the United States. The state with the lowest prevalence of obesity is Colorado.

Ethnicity may also have an impact on the availability of donors for LDLT. Hispanic patients are more likely to have an LDLT donor than other ethnicities are. In the United States, 24% more Hispanics undergo LDLT (16.8%) than deceased donor transplantation (13.6%).[12] At our center, the percentage of Hispanics undergoing LDLT (30%) is twice the percentage of those undergoing deceased donor transplantation (15%). Another center has reported similar results.[80] The likelihood of having a potential living donor was significantly higher in Hispanics than in non-Hispanics (odds ratio of 3.1, $P = .001$). The reasons for this ethnic disparity in LDLT are unknown. However, Hispanic patients typically have larger families and may therefore have a greater number of potential donors for evaluation. Minority groups may also believe that they have less access to deceased donor organs than whites do. Therefore, minorities may view living donation as a better treatment option than deceased donor transplantation. In addition, Hispanic families may have stronger familial connections that could result in a greater tendency to donate than in other groups. Regional variations in the distribution of Hispanics may have a substantial impact on the live donor pool available to transplant centers.[81] The western portion of the United States has the greatest proportion of Hispanics, 24.3% of the population. The six states with the greatest proportion of Hispanics are Texas (32%), California (32%), New Mexico (42%), Arizona (25%), Nevada (19%), and Colorado (17%). Transplant centers in these states may have a larger pool of LDLT donors.

The financial cost of evaluating LDLT donors deserves special mention. There are obvious reasons why the cost of LDLT donation could be different from that of deceased donor transplantation. The complex nature of evaluating living donors could potentially increase the cost of LDLT over conventional transplantation. In addition, postsurgical complications in a living donor could increase the cost. We recently reported a cost analysis of LDLT and deceased donor transplantation.[82] This analysis included the cost of recipient pretransplant care, transplant admission, and posttransplant care, as well as all costs related to donor evaluation, including donors who were rejected for evaluation. We found that all costs associated with the acquisition of a graft from a living donor were virtually identical to the acquisition costs for a deceased donor graft (23.5 cost units for LDLT versus 23.3 cost units for a deceased donor graft, $P = NS$). The cost breakdown

for the different phases of the living donor evaluation and hepatectomy is as follows (expressed as a percentage of the total cost): donor evaluation, 13%; donor hepatectomy, 74%; postoperative care for 365 days after hepatectomy, 7%; and "failed donors" (rejected for donation after evaluation), 6%.

Special Considerations for Living Donor Liver Transplantation

Anatomic Considerations

Donor

From a surgical standpoint, parenchymal, biliary, and vascular anomalies that could complicate or preclude successful donor hepatectomy must be identified during the donor and recipient evaluation.[83] Although many donors undergoing evaluation do not have conventional biliary, venous, and arterial anatomy, most anatomical abnormalities do not preclude successful hepatectomy by an experienced surgical team. The decision to proceed with hepatectomy in a donor with anatomical anomalies is based on the judgment and experience of the surgeon. In all cases, the safety of the donor should be considered the paramount concern.

Common parenchymal abnormalities found during routine imaging of the potential donor include hepatic cysts, hemangiomas, and other benign hepatic tumors. Donors with single, small (< 1 cm) benign lesions may successfully undergo donor hepatectomy. However, as the lesion or lesions increase in size and number, the safety of donor hepatectomy and the quality of the donor graft may be compromised, and the donor may be judged unsuitable for donation. The size of the right hepatic graft can be estimated by abdominal imaging. As noted earlier, specific formulas can be used to estimate whether the right lobe is large enough for the recipient.[42,43] In general, a GRBW ratio higher than 0.8% is desirable. In practice, however, we rarely use this calculation for determination of a potential donor's suitability for LDLT because other recipient factors are of equal importance. The degree of portal hypertension and the severity of illness in the recipient are critical factors in the determination of whether the right hepatic lobe is sufficiently large for a given recipient. Recipients with severe portal hypertension or clinical decompensation (or with both) require larger grafts than do less sick patients, who may do well with a small right hepatic lobe graft. The donor surgeon must also consider the size of the remnant (left) hepatic lobe. Donors with a diminutive left hepatic lobe may have insufficient hepatic mass after donor right hepatectomy. However, the exact size of remnant liver mass that is required by the donor after hepatectomy is unknown. To our knowledge, there are no data that provide a rational basis for estimating the required size of the remnant hepatic mass. However, we estimate that the donor requires greater than 0.4% (remnant hepatic mass/body mass × 100%) to ensure adequate hepatic function after right donor hepatectomy. Therefore, the average 70-kg donor would require a left hepatic lobe size of 280 g or larger. In our experience, a small fraction of potential donors (approximately 2%) undergoing evaluation have a diminutive left hepatic lobe that would preclude the safety of donor right hepatectomy.

Although abnormalities of the biliary tract are common, they rarely preclude the donor from donation.[14,83-85] However, biliary leaks are the most frequent complication after donor hepatectomy.[27] The most important issue in preventing biliary complications in the donor is to clearly identify the biliary anatomy. Preoperative imaging with MRCP or CT is very useful; nonetheless, we perform intraoperative cholangiography on all of our donors and believe that this diagnostic modality is the best for defining the donor's biliary anatomy. However, up to 50% of centers require preoperative ERCP for all donor candidates.[27] Proper definition of the biliary anatomy prevents excessive hilar dissection and transection of critical donor biliary ducts, which may lead to increased complications in the donor. In addition, careful preoperative definition of the biliary anatomy identifies anatomical variations in the donor, which are quite frequent, as reported by Nakamura and coauthors.[85] In 120 right hepatic lobe living donors, 61% had a single duct orifice and a single anastomosis and the remaining 39% had two or three duct orifices. Biliary complications in the recipient were higher in patients who had two ducts and one anastomosis with ductoplasty than in those with either a double anastomosis or a single anastomosis without ductoplasty.

Abnormalities in the donor portal vein are uncommon and rarely exclude donor candidates from donation. Nakamura and colleagues reported that only one donor (in 120 LDLTs) was rejected on the basis of preoperative assessment of portal venous anatomy.[85] In their series, 92% of donors had conventional portal venous anatomy and the remaining 8% had one of four types of variants. Common abnormalities in the portal venous system include trifurcation in the donor portal vein and anomalous branches from the right portal vein, both of which result in two portal vein orifices in the right hepatic graft.[83,85,86] The hepatic venous anatomy is well defined with CT angiography or MRA. The approach to hepatic venous reconstruction varies widely from center to center. Many experienced LDLT surgeons have learned that adequate venous drainage requires inclusion of the middle hepatic vein branches from segments V and VIII with the right lobe graft. During donor hepatectomy, accessory hepatic veins smaller than 1 cm are ligated, whereas large veins are preserved with the donor graft. The donor right hepatic vein is anastomosed to the recipient right hepatic vein, whose orifice is extended down the anterior surface of the vena cava to match the right hepatic vein orifice on the donor graft. In almost all cases there is only one right hepatic vein. In only 1% to 2% of cases two right hepatic veins may be present, whereas 30% to 40% of donors have significant accessory hepatic veins (> 5 mm).[83,85]

Variations in the hepatic artery are not uncommon, but rarely the reason for donor rejection. Nakamura and coworkers found conventional anatomy in 87% of their cases.[85] The right hepatic artery originated from the superior mesenteric artery in 13%. Marcos and coauthors reported that 59% of 95 right lobe donors had conventional anatomy. The two most common variants were a replaced right hepatic artery (14%) and "unique aberrant anatomy" (11%).[87] Patients with multiple arteries supplying the right hepatic artery or with crossing arteries from the left hepatic artery to the right hepatic artery (or with both) may be rejected for donation. In our experience, many of these patients also have concomitant anatomical variations in the portal venous and biliary anatomy that increase the complexity of the surgery and thus increase the risk of complications in the donor and recipient.

Recipient

The most common anatomical problems in the recipient that may increase the complexity of the LDLT operation are in the hepatic and portal venous anatomy. There are virtually no biliary or parenchymal anomalies in the recipient that increase the complexity of the LDLT operation. The most common hepatic venous problem is hepatic vein thrombosis (Budd-Chiari syndrome). Although LDLT may be successfully performed in a patient with Budd-Chiari syndrome,[88,89] the complexity of the recipient surgery is greater and the risk of postoperative thrombotic complications in the recipient may be higher because most patients have an underlying thrombotic disorder. As a result, Budd-Chiari syndrome is a relative contraindication for LDLT. Portal vein thrombosis is present in 5% to 10% of liver transplant recipients. The approach to a potential LDLT recipient with portal vein thrombosis varies from center to center.[90] Portal vein thrombosis in the recipient was an absolute contraindication at 11% of centers, a relative contraindication in 51%, and not a contraindication at 38% of centers. We have routinely performed successful LDLT in recipients with portal vein thrombosis, but we require the availability of a venous graft from a recently deceased donor to perform the LDLT. As a result, LDLT recipients with portal vein thrombosis may have the date of LDLT delayed until a venous graft is available from a deceased donor with a compatible blood type. A misplaced transjugular intra-hepatic portosystemic shunt (TIPS) stent (adjacent to the confluence of the superior mesenteric and splenic vein) may present a similar problem regarding the availability of a venous graft for successful LDLT. Therefore, we have found that careful documentation of the anatomical placement of TIPS stents (by abdominal computed tomographic imaging) is critical in the evaluation of LDLT recipients, especially in recipients who have undergone TIPS procedures outside our center.

Patients Outside the General Criteria for Transplantation

In general, LDLT should not be considered in patients who do not meet the recognized criteria for deceased donor transplantation. However, two types of patients require special consideration. Selected patients with extensive-stage hepatocellular carcinoma (HCC) may be considered for LDLT on a case-by-case basis. UNOS has specific criteria for liver transplantation in patients with limited-stage HCC. Patients who fulfill the following criteria receive a MELD score of 20 or 24, depending on their TMN stage, and an additional 10% increment each 90 days thereafter: one lesion 5 cm or smaller or three or fewer lesions, each being 3 cm or smaller. As a result, patients with limited-stage HCC are given a high priority for liver transplantation. However, patients with HCC that exceeds these criteria are not awarded any additional MELD points because the extent of their carcinoma is so great that their predicted posttransplant survival is too low to justify the use of a deceased donor organ. Consequently, these patients have virtually no chance of receiving a deceased donor liver and are relegated to palliative care in which their expected survival is usually less than 1 year. The prospect of LDLT in these desperate patients offers a marginal chance for curative surgery. However, after transplantation, the likelihood of recurrent HCC, which is uniformly fatal, is usually greater than 50%.

Recent data have described the outcomes in (primarily deceased donor) liver transplant recipients with HCC exceeding UNOS criteria. A retrospective analysis of tumor burden (based on histological examination of the explanted liver) found acceptable survival data in patients with a single lesion 6.5 cm or smaller or up to three lesions with the largest one being 4.5 cm or smaller and the sum of tumor diameters no more than 8 cm. Patients fulfilling these "extended" criteria had 1- and 5-year survival rates of 90% and 75.2%, respectively.[91] A prospective study examining 43 transplant patients who had HCC lesions smaller than 5 cm yielded 5-year survival and recurrence-free survival rates of 44% and 48%, respectively.[92] In this study, tumors between 5 and 7 cm were associated with a

55% 5-year survival rate. The approach to a potential LDLT recipient with HCC lesions exceeding UNOS criteria must be cautious. Selected patients may undergo successful LDLT. However, transplant physicians, recipients, and donors must recognize the high statistical risk of posttransplant recurrence of HCC, which is rapidly fatal in virtually all cases. Donor risk is a critical consideration when the recipient has a marginal anticipated outcome. Physicians and the lay public have disparate views on this subject. A survey of patients in a general medical clinic found that the median recipient 1-year survival rate that respondents would require before consenting for donation was only 55%.[93] This survey hypothetically indicates that the lay public (i.e., donors) might routinely agree to donate even though the anticipated recipient mortality rate would be as high as 45%. Conversely, transplant surgeons asked the same question would require a median 1-year survival rate of 79%.[94] Therefore, many potential donors may be willing to donate for recipients with marginal outcomes, even though the transplant surgeon may view the operation as futile. The utility of LDLT in this group of desperate patients awaits the results of further studies with long-term outcome data in donors and recipients.

Another group of patients who functionally lie outside the general criteria for transplantation are those with (1) chronic liver disease, including an intrahepatic mass or masses; (2) a low MELD score; and/or (3) symptoms that have a significant impact on quality of life but are not life-threatening. Common examples include patients with pruritus caused by cholestatic liver disease, fatigue from viral hepatitis, symptomatic benign hepatic masses (hemangioma,[95] hemangioendothelioma,[96] hepatic cystic disease[97-99]), pulmonary vascular disease,[100,101] and hepatic metabolic diseases (see discussion later).[102-123] Because of their low MELD scores, these patients usually have little to no chance for imminent deceased donor transplantation. In addition, most of these patients have well-preserved hepatic function, and their MELD score rarely progresses. Although additional MELD points may be obtained through the regional review board, most of these patients are rejected. As a result, the prospects for deceased donor transplantation for many of these patients are usually remote, and LDLT offers their only real opportunity for transplantation. At our center, we have successfully treated a small number of these patients with LDLT. However, the utility of LDLT for this indication in an individual patient must be considered on a case-by-case basis.

Patients with metabolic diseases of the liver are ideal candidates for LDLT because their MELD score is often too low for deceased donor transplantation and the underlying metabolic disease may be completely cured with liver replacement.[102-105] Two types of hepatic metabolic disease of the liver may be successfully treated with LDLT: diseases that cause liver damage

Table 44-4. METABOLIC DISEASES TREATED BY LIVING DONOR LIVER TRANSPLANTATION

Disease	Reference
Alagille syndrome	103–107
Byler's disease	107, 108
Citrullinemia	109–111
Crigler-Najjar syndrome	112, 113
Familial amyloidosis	114, 115
Familial hypercholesterolemia	116
Glycogen storage disease	117
Hemophilia	118, 119
Hyperoxaluria	104, 108, 120
Tyrosinemia	121
Urea cycle enzyme deficiencies	122, 123

(tyrosinemia, glycogen storage disease) and diseases that cause systemic complications with minimal or no hepatic manifestations (familial amyloidosis, familial hypercholesterolemia, hyperoxaluria). Each of these diseases has been successfully treated with LDLT (Table 44-4).[102-123] However, since these disorders are typically autosomal recessive, many of the potential donors may be heterozygotes for the disorder ("carriers"). The safety of using "carriers" of autosomal genetic disorders as donors for LDLT is a subject of debate.[102,103] Familial amyloidosis is a unique disorder in transplantation in that the liver produces a protein (amyloid) that causes systemic disease but the affected liver is histologically normal. Patients afflicted with familial amyloidosis are cured by liver transplantation and may, in turn, donate their liver to a recipient in a "domino transplantation."[114,115] Because the liver from a patient with amyloidosis is histologically normal and the systemic effects of amyloidosis require decades to develop, the recipient of the affected liver may live many years without systemic manifestations of amyloidosis. Typically, recipients of these affected livers are older to minimize their lifetime risk of amyloidosis.

Hepatitis C

Hepatitis C requires special consideration in LDLT recipients. Preliminary data from three separate reports suggest that recurrent hepatitis in LDLT recipients develops earlier and is more aggressive than in recipients of deceased donor livers.[124-126] Each of these studies is limited by small numbers of patients, absence of protocol liver biopsy, and relatively short follow-up (less than 1 year) relative to the natural history of post-transplantation hepatitis C. Ghobrial and coworkers reported that the incidence of hepatitis in nine LDLT recipients was more than twofold higher than in comparative recipients of deceased donor livers.[124] Another report found that the incidence of severe recurrent hepatitis was 50% higher in LDLT recipients (18% versus 12%) than in recipients of deceased donor livers and that the hepatitis recurred earlier.[125] Combined data from our center and Mt. Sinai in 41 hepatitis C virus (HCV)-infected LDLT recipients found that histological evidence of recurrent hepatitis C occurred earlier and that alanine aminotransferase levels were significantly elevated in comparison to deceased donor controls.[126] At our center, graft failure as a result of recurrent hepatitis C developed in 15% of the LDLT recipients who were HCV RNA positive at the time of transplantation. The Scientific Registry of Transplant Recipients has recorded patient and graft loss rates for all LDLTs performed in the United States between 1998 and 2001, adjusted for comorbidity, age, and urgency for transplantation.[12] The relative rate of graft loss was 2.0-fold higher for HCV-infected LDLT recipients than for HCV-infected recipients of deceased donor livers, and the mortality rate was 1.7-fold higher. The relative risk of graft and patient loss was 1.9- and 2.1-fold higher in HCV-infected LDLT recipients than in non–HCV-infected LDLT patients, $P = .08$. However, one study found that HCV-infected LDLT recipients had no worse outcomes than deceased donor liver recipients did. Shiffman and colleagues performed protocol liver biopsies in patients at their center and reported no difference in portal inflammation or portal fibrosis scores in HCV-infected LDLT recipients and recipients of deceased donor livers at a mean follow-up interval of 2.8 years after transplantation.[127]

In summary, the data suggesting that LDLT recipients with hepatitis C have worse outcomes than recipients of deceased donor livers do are inconclusive. Despite the absence of definitive data, we believe that this information must be weighed carefully in the selection of recipients for the procedure. At our center, we have sufficient concern about the severity of recurrent hepatitis C in LDLT recipients that we reserve LDLT in HCV-infected patients to those with clear life-threatening symptoms. Routine performance of LDLT in stable cirrhotics with HCV may be unwise because of the potential for severe recurrence of hepatitis C in more than 15% of LDLT recipients after transplantation. Outcome in HCV-infected patients is a critical issue because of the large proportion of recipients undergoing LDLT with hepatitis C and the preliminary evidence that outcomes may be worse. Definitive data on the relative severity of recurrence of hepatitis C after LDLT await longer follow-up intervals and the inclusion of more patients. If hepatitis C is more severe and recurs earlier in LDLT recipients, the mechanism responsible for the accelerated disease is unclear, but it could be a result of intense hepatic regeneration in the right hepatic lobe graft or increased immunological matching in LDLT donors and recipients.[128]

Hepatitis B Core Antibody–Positive Donor

Although individuals who are hepatitis B surface antigen positive are excluded from donation, selected patients with HBcAb (and hepatitis B surface antigen negative) may be evaluated for donation. There are two important considerations in the evaluation of an HBcAB-positive donor. First, the donor must be able to yield a suitable graft. The presence of HBcAb indicates previous exposure to hepatitis B. Even though the patient is hepatitis B surface antigen negative and does not have an active infection, some patients with previous hepatitis B virus (HBV) exposure have chronic liver damage from the earlier hepatitis B infection. Therefore, at our center, liver biopsy is mandatory in a donor who is HBcAB positive and hepatitis B surface antigen negative. Biopsy can determine whether the donor has underlying liver fibrosis, which would preclude successful donation. Donor outcome data in this subset of patients are limited, but one group from Korea reported no significant differences in hospital stay, postdonation liver chemistry values, and transfusion requirements in 34 HBcAb-positive and 52 HBcAb-negative right lobe donors.[129] Interestingly, this group did not perform predonation liver biopsies, but used indocyanine green testing instead. Wedge biopsy findings at the time of donor hepatectomy were no different from those in the HBcAb-negative donor group.

Another important issue in HBcAB-positive donors is viral transmission to the recipient. In deceased donor transplantation, there is a measurable risk of HBV transmission despite hepatitis B surface antigen negativity. The presumed means of transmission is minute quantities of inactive HBV harbored in the liver. Transplantation of a liver (or liver lobe) from an HBcAb-positive donor can lead to viral reactivation in the immunosuppressed recipient. Up to 80% of recipients of livers from deceased donors who are HBcAB positive and hepatitis B surface antigen negative acquire hepatitis B without administration of prophylaxis to the recipient.[130-132] To prevent viral transmission from donor to recipient, the recipient should receive standard hepatitis B prophylaxis with hepatitis B immune globulin. The addition of lamivudine may be added to the posttransplant prophylactic regimen. There are reports of successful LDLT from an HBcAb-positive donor after hepatitis B immune globulin prophylaxis has been administered to the recipient.[133] Most of these reports originate from areas where hepatitis B is endemic, and the prevalence of HBcAb in the donor pool can exceed 50%.[134]

The elective nature of LDLT also raises the possibility of hepatitis B vaccination of the recipient once an HBcAb-positive donor has been identified. This strategy was successful in Taiwan, where 15 of 16 recipients seroconverted before LDLT from an HBcAb-positive donor.[134] Moreover, the same group reported using lamivudine as monoprophylaxis without evidence of de novo hepatitis B in the recipient, presumably because the recipients could make their own protective antibody.[134,135] It should be noted that the Asian recipients have a much higher likelihood of previous HBV exposure and may therefore respond more frequently and strongly to HBV vaccination because of amnestic mechanisms. Application of such prophylactic measures in areas with less endemic hepatitis B should be done with caution.

Acute Liver Failure (UNOS Status 1)

Several studies have reported successful LDLT in acute liver failure.[136-142] Patients with acute liver failure are clinically very unstable and typically have a very short window for transplantation (a few hours to days) from the time of listing until death. In this setting, LDLT offers a potential important advantage in that the surgery can be performed within hours after identification of a suitable donor. However, there are potential problems with LDLT in the setting of acute hepatic failure. Most important, the donor has a very limited time to undergo evaluation and may not have sufficient time to adequately consider the decision to donate. The donor must make the decision while the family member suffers a critical illness that is rapidly progressive. In addition, the transplant team is under pressure to perform a comprehensive, careful donor evaluation over a very short time interval. Because of concern regarding LDLT in the setting of acute liver failure, some centers have elected to exclude fulminant liver failure as an indication for LDLT.[143,144] The utility of LDLT in fulminant liver failure depends in part on the availability of deceased donor organs. In the United States, where deceased donor organs are scarce but usually available for status 1 patients, the overall impact of LDLT will probably be minimal. Between July 2001 and June 2002, only 5% of LDLTs were performed for acute liver failure. A national survey of U.S. transplant centers reported acute liver failure as the indication for LDLT in only 2.2% of recipients.[47] However, in Asia, where virtually all liver transplantation is performed with living donors, LDLT will probably remain the only viable treatment option for these critically ill patients.

"Nondirected" or "Good Samaritan" Donation

"Nondirected" donors or "Good Samaritan" donors are individuals without a significant long-term relationship with a potential recipient. The actual number of "nondirected" LDLTs in the United States is unknown, but probably less than 10. A recent national survey of U.S. liver transplant centers recorded just three such cases between 1997 and 2000.[27] However, there are considerable ethical concerns regarding the routine evaluation of nondirected living donors for LDLT. The primary concern with nondirected donors is related to (1) their motivation to accept a measurable level of risk to their health for a stranger and (2) their ability to comprehend and consent to accept the risk associated with the donor hepatectomy. Although nondirected donation has been accepted practice in renal transplantation for many years for carefully selected donors and has some justifying ethical basis,[145,146] the relative risk of death and complications for an LDLT donor is several-fold higher than in kidney donation, and the long-term complications in liver donors are unknown. As a result, most LDLT centers will not evaluate nondirected donors for LDLT. If an individual is being considered as a nondirected liver donor, the psychological state and motivations for donation must be evaluated very carefully. For the foreseeable future, the role of nondirected donors in LDLT will probably remain trivial. However, when these cases are considered, they may become the subject of significant media attention and ethical discussions.[147]

Syngeneic Living Donor Liver Transplantation

LDLT offers a rare "experiment of nature" when immunological twins serve as a donor-recipient pair. A recipient who receives a graft from an immunological twin may not require immunosuppression after transplantation. Two reports of LDLT in identical twins have appeared in the literature.[148,149] In these three cases, the recipients successfully underwent transplantation with little or no immunosuppression. A similar scenario may arise in bone marrow transplant recipients (whose immune system is reconstituted by bone marrow from the donor) who are cured of their hematological disorder, but chronic liver disease develops. In this unique clinical setting, if the bone marrow donor is able to serve as a living liver donor for the bone marrow recipient, immunosuppression may not be required after LDLT. To our knowledge, there have been no such cases reported in the literature

The Future

Just a few years ago, there was widespread optimism surrounding LDLT, and some physicians predicted that half of all liver transplants would be performed with a living donor. However, over the past 2 years, most centers have adopted a more conservative approach to this procedure, in large part because of widespread recognition of the substantial risk incurred by the donor. As a result, the total number of LDLTs performed in the United States decreased 30% from 2001 to 2002 and will decrease this year by 10% more. This year (2003) only approximately 5% of all liver transplantations will be performed with a living donor.

However, LDLT remains a viable treatment option for carefully selected patients who require liver transplantation. We anticipate that in the future, only a small number of transplant centers will continue to perform the majority of LDLTs in this country. Recent data suggest that many centers may choose to not routinely offer the procedure to their patients. A survey published in 2003 found that only 42 of 84 responding centers (50%)[47] reported that they have performed LDLT and that only half the liver transplant surgeons believed that their programs need to offer adult LDLT to remain competitive.[94] In fact, some liver transplant programs may not be well suited to perform LDLT. Several important components are required for a transplant center to have a long-term, successful LDLT program. (1) The transplant surgeons, transplant physicians, and hospital administration must be fully committed to the procedure. The donor/recipient evaluation, transplant procedure, and postsurgical care of the donor and recipient are far more complex than with deceased donor transplantation. Therefore, an LDLT program with a successful, long-term record must have a dedicated, efficient multidisciplinary team to deal with the surgical, medical, and social complexities inherent in LDLT donors and recipients. The hospital must dedicate additional resources for increased demands for operating room time and space, as well as additional personnel to evaluate donors and secure insurance coverage for LDLT recipients. In addition, the hospital may need to be financially responsible for covering the expense of complications in uninsured donors. (2) A large number of patients must be listed for transplantation to provide enough candidates with a medical urgency for LDLT. Current UNOS statistics indicate that only about 15% of all listed patients have a MELD score higher than 18. As noted earlier, very few patients with a MELD score lower than 18 require urgent transplantation from a living donor. Approximately half of the 15% of listed patients (7.5%) who are medically eligible for LDLT will be rejected because they are not surgically suitable as a result of the presence one or more comorbid conditions, and about half these patients (3.75%) will not have a suitable donor. Consequently, only about 4% of patient listed for liver transplantation will be able to undergo LDLT. For transplant centers with a small number of listed patients (< 100), the number of patients ultimately able to undergo LDLT may be too small (four or fewer patients per year) to sustain a viable LDLT program. Currently, 40 of 98 U.S. liver transplant center programs (41%) have fewer than 100 patients. Based on this calculation, these programs would probably perform fewer than five LDLTs per year. As a result, these small centers probably would not be able to sustain a long-term, viable LDLT program with so few LDLT patients. (There may be notable exceptions to this rule, namely, at transplant centers in which the severity of illness of the listed patients is significantly higher than the national list and the proportion of patients medically eligible for LDLT may be significantly higher.) (3) The transplant center must have a critical shortage of deceased donor organs. Although almost all liver transplant centers in the United States have a critical shortage of deceased donor organs, a very small number of centers are able to transplant patients with deceased donor organs at a rate far greater than the national average. As a result, LDLT may have a more limited role at these selected centers.

The role of LDLT as a viable treatment option for patients with chronic liver disease ultimately depends on the success of the procedure. To assess the efficacy of LDLT, the National Institutes of Health has funded the LDLT Cohort Study to measure outcomes of LDLT recipients in comparison to recipients of deceased donor livers. This study will measure the following outcomes: (1) technical success of LDLT versus deceased donor transplantation; (2) long-term graft and patient loss, including patient mortality in candidates for deceased donor livers while on the waiting list; (3) outcomes relative to HCV, immunosuppression, and regeneration in LDLT recipients; and (4) donor complications and quality of life. These critical end points will help determine the most appropriate candidates for this innovative procedure.

Pearls

- The best donors are generally identified very early in the evaluation process. There is a "law of diminishing returns" in evaluating a large number of potential donors.
- When more than one potential donor is available, the donor evaluations should be performed in serial fashion and not in parallel. Each donor should be fully evaluated, and if rejected, the next donor should begin the evaluation process.
- The vast majority of unsuitable donors may be rejected very early in the donor evaluation process (phase 1).

Pearls—cont'd

- By using the criteria outlined in this chapter, the expected annual number of LDLTs performed at a transplant center will probably not exceed 5% of the number of patients listed for transplantation.
- Only begin an LDLT program with a liver surgeon who has vast experience in liver transplantation and hepatobiliary surgery. In addition, the hospital, surgeons, and physicians must be dedicated and committed to performing a minimum of 20 cases.
- In our experience, we have found that in patients with chronic liver disease, the following factors are associated with a poor outcome after LDLT independent of the MELD score: mechanical ventilation, hemodialysis, and a very low Karnofsky score. One or more of these factors in patients with chronic liver disease represent a strong relative contraindication for LDLT.
- To summarize the use of MELD scores in the selection of LDLT recipients, (1) we have not found a specific MELD score above or below which LDLT should be contraindicated. In general, when a patient has a MELD score higher than 18, obvious features of decompensation (ascites, jaundice, encephalopathy, variceal bleeding) are frequently present, and these patients should routinely be considered medically eligible for LDLT. (2) However, a substantial minority of patients listed for deceased donor transplantation with MELD scores lower than 18 have significant features of decompensation associated with waiting list mortality that warrant consideration of LDLT.

References

1. Trotter JF, Wachs M, Everson GT, Kam I: Adult-to-adult transplantation of the right hepatic lobe from a living donor. N Engl J Med 346:1074-1082, 2002.
2. Chen CL, Fan ST, Lee SG, et al: Living-donor liver transplantation: 12 years experience in Asia. Transplantation 75(Suppl):S6-S11, 2003.
3. Renz JF, Busuttil RW: Adult-to-adult living donor liver transplantation: A critical analysis. Semin Liver Dis 20:411-424, 2000.
4. Marcos A, Fisher RA, Ham JM, et al: Right lobe living donor liver transplantation. Transplantation 68:798-803, 1999.
5. Marcos A: Right lobe living donor liver transplantation: A review. Liver Transpl 6:3-20, 2000.

6. Schiano TD, Kim-Schluger L, Gondolesi G, Miller CM: Adult living donor liver transplantation: The hepatologist's perspective. Hepatology. 33:3-9, 2001.

7. Pomfret EA, Pomposelli JJ, Jenkins RL: Live donor liver transplantation. J Hepatol 34:613-624, 2001.

8. Ghobrial RM, Saab S, Lassman C, et al: Donor and recipients outcomes in right lobe living donor liver transplantation. Liver Transpl 8:901-909, 2002.

9. Miller CM, Gondolesi GE, Florman S, et al: One hundred nine living donor liver transplants in adults and children: A single-center experience. Ann Surg 234:301-311, 2001.

10. Bak T, Wachs M, Trotter J, et al: Adult-to-adult living donor liver transplantation using right-lobe grafts: Results and lessons learned from a single-center experience. Liver Transpl 7:680-686, 2001.

11. Williams RS, Alisa AA, Karani JB, et al: Adult-to-adult living donor liver transplant: UK experience. Eur J Gastroenterol Hepatol 15:7-14, 2003.

12. Annual report of the Scientific Registry of Transplant Recipients and the Organ Procurement and Transplantation Network: Transplant data, 2003, Richmond, VA, United Network for Organ Sharing (accessed June 2003 at http://www.ustransplant.org).

13. Trotter JF: Selection of donors and recipients for living donor liver transplantation. Liver Transpl 6:S52-S58, 2000.

14. Chen YS, Cheng YF, De Villa VH, et al: Evaluation of living liver donors. Transplantation 75:S16-S19, 2003.

15. Schwartz M: Candidate selection criteria for living donor liver transplantation. Mt Sinai J Med 70:171-173, 2003.

16. Pascher A, Sauer IM, Walter M, et al: Donor evaluation, donor risks, donor outcome, and donor quality-of-life in adult-to-adult living donor liver transplantation. Liver Transpl 8:829-837, 2002.

17. Pomfret EA, Pomposelli JJ, Lewis WD, et al: Live donor adult liver transplantation using right lobe grafts: Donor evaluation and surgical outcome. Arch Surg 136:425-433, 2001.

18. Marcos A, Fisher RA, Ham JM, et al: Selection and outcome of living donors for adult to adult liver transplantation. Transplantation 69:2410-2415, 2000.

19. Trotter JF, Wachs M, Trouillot T, et al: Evaluation of 100 patients for living donor liver transplantation. Liver Transpl 6:290-295, 2000.

20. Baker A, Dhawan A, Devlin J, et al: Assessment of potential donors for living related liver transplantation. Br J Surg 86:200-205, 1999.

21. Renz JF, Mudge CL, Heyman MB, et al: Donor selection limits use of living-related liver transplantation. Hepatology 22:1122-1126, 1995.

22. Sterneck MR, Fischer L, Nischwitz U, et al: Selection of the living liver donor. Transplantation 60:667-671, 1995.

23. Nuno J, Cuervas-Mons V, Vicente E, et al: Prolonged graft cold ischemia: A risk factor for early bacterial and fungal infection in liver transplant recipients. Transplant Proc 27:2323-2325, 1995.

24. Strasberg SM, Howard TK, Molmenti EP, Hertl M: Selecting the donor liver: Risk factors for poor function after orthotopic liver transplantation. Hepatology 20:829-838, 1994.

25. Adam R, Bismuth H, Diamond T, et al: Effect of extended cold ischaemia with UW solution on graft function after liver transplantation. Lancet 340:1373-1376, 1992.

26. Sanchez-Urdazpal L, Gores GJ, Ward EM, et al: Ischemic-type biliary complications after orthotopic liver transplantation. Hepatology 16:49-53, 1992.

27. Brown RS Jr, Russo MW, Lai M, et al: A survey of liver transplantation from living adult donors in the United States. N Engl J Med 348:818-825, 2003.

28. Lo CM: Complications and long-term outcomes of living liver donors: A survey of 1508 cases in five Asian centers. Transplantation 75:S12-S15, 2003.

29. Marcos A: Right lobe living donor liver transplantation. Liver Transpl 6:S59-S63, 2000.

30. Broelsch CE, Malago M, Testa G, Valentin-Gamazo C: Living donor liver transplantation in adult: Outcome in Europe. Liver Transpl 6:S64-S65, 2000.

31. Todo S, Furukawa H, Jin MB, Shimamura T: Living donor liver transplantation in adults: Outcome in Japan. Liver Transpl 6:S66-S72, 2000.

32. Testa G, Malago M, Nadalin S, et al: Right-liver living donor transplantation for decompensated end-stage liver disease. Liver Transpl 8:340-346, 2002.

33. Kam I: Adult-adult right hepatic lobe living donor liver transplantation for status 2A patients: Too little, too late. Liver Transpl 8:347-349, 2002.

34. Ben-Haim M, Emre S, Fishbein TM, et al: Critical graft size in adult-to-adult living donor liver transplantation: Impact of the recipient's disease. Liver Transpl 7:948-953, 2001.

35. Icoz G, Kilic M, Zeytunlu M, et al: Biliary reconstructions and complications encountered in 50 consecutive right-lobe living donor liver transplantations. Liver Transpl 9:575-580, 2003.

36. Fan ST, Lo CM, Liu CL, et al: Biliary reconstruction and complications of right lobe live liver donor liver transplantation. Ann Surg 236:676-683, 2002.

37. Testa G, Malago M, Valentin-Gamazo C, et al: Biliary anastomosis in living related liver transplantation using the right liver lobe: Techniques and complications. Liver Transpl 6:710-714, 2000.

38. Kugelmas M, Nichols M, Trotter JF, et al: Management of biliary complications after adult-adult right lobe live-donor liver transplantation [abstract]. Hepatology 36:305A, 2002.

39. Shah J, Ahmad N, Shetty K, et al: Endoscopic management of biliary complications after adult living donor transplantation. Am J Gastroenterol 99:1291-1295, 2004.

40. Wiesner R, Edwards E, Freeman R, et al: Model for end-stage liver disease (MELD) and allocation of donor livers. Gastroenterology 124:91-96, 2003.

41. Hayashi PH, Forman L, Steinberg T, et al: Model for end-stage liver disease (MELD) does not predict patient or graft survival in living donor liver transplant recipients. Liver Transpl 9:737-740, 2003.

42. Urata K, Kawasaki S, Matsunami H, et al: Calculation of child and adult standard liver volume for liver transplantation. Hepatology 21:1317-1321, 1995.

43. Heinemann A, Wischhusen F, Puschel K, Rogiers X: Standard liver volume in the Caucasian population. Liver Transpl Surg 5:366-368, 1999.

44. Shaw BW: Where monsters hide. Liver Transpl 7:928-932, 2001.

45. Walter M, Bronner E, Pascher A, et al: Psychosocial outcome of living donors after living donor liver transplantation: A pilot study. Clin Transplant 16:339-344, 2002.

46. Trotter JF, Talamantes M, McClure M, et al: Right hepatic lobe donation for living donor liver transplantation: Impact on donor quality of life. Liver Transpl 7:485-493, 2001.

47. Beavers KL, Cassara JE, Shrestha R: Practice patterns for long-term follow-up of adult-to-adult right lobectomy donors at US transplantation centers. Liver Transpl 9:645-648, 2003.

48. Fukunishi I, Sugawara Y, Takayama T, et al: Association between pretransplant psychological assessments and posttransplant psychiatric disorders in living-related transplantation. Psychosomatics 43:49-54, 2002.

49. Kim-Schluger L, Florman SS, Schiano T, et al: Quality of life after lobectomy for adult liver transplantation. Transplantation 73:1593-1597, 2002.

50. Goldman LS: Liver transplantation using living donors. Preliminary donor psychiatric outcomes. Psychosomatics 34:235-240, 1993.

51. Fukunishi I, Sugawara Y, Takayama T, et al: Psychiatric problems in living-related liver transplantation (III): Pretransplant psychological assessment in living-related transplantation. Transplant Proc 34:2628-2629, 2002.

52. Fukunishi I, Sugawara Y, Takayama T, et al: Psychiatric problems in living-related liver transplantation (I): Incidence rate of psychiatric disorders in living-related transplantation. Transplant Proc 34:2630-2631, 2002.

53. Fukunishi I, Sugawara Y, Takayama T, et al: Psychiatric problems in living-related liver transplantation (II): The association between paradoxical psychiatric syndrome and guilt feelings in adult recipients after living donor liver transplantation. Transplant Proc 34:2632-2633, 2002.

54. Ad Hoc UNOS Committee on Living Donor Liver Transplantation, 2003.

55. Ascher N: Secretary's Advisory Committee on Organ Transplantation, 2002.

56. New York State Health Department: New York State Committee on Quality Improvement in Living Liver Donation, 2002.

57. Hiroshige S, Shimada M, Harada N, et al: Accurate preoperative estimation of liver-graft volumetry using three-dimensional computed tomography. Transplantation 75:1561-1564, 2003.

58. Kanazawa A, Hirohashi K, Tanaka H, et al: Usefulness of three-dimensional computed tomography in a living-donor extended right lobe liver transplantation. Liver Transpl 8:1076-1079, 2002.

59. Schroeder T, Nadalin S, Stattaus J, et al: Potential living liver donors: Evaluation with an all-in-one protocol with multi-detector row CT. Radiology 224:586-591, 2002.

60. Schroeder T, Malago M, Debatin JF, et al: Multidetector computed tomographic cholangiography in the evaluation of potential living liver donors. Transplantation 73:1972-1973, 2002.

61. Goyen M, Barkhausen J, Debatin JF, et al: Right-lobe living related liver transplantation: Evaluation of a comprehensive magnetic resonance imaging protocol for assessing potential donors. Liver Transpl 8:241-250, 2002.

62. Hiroshige S, Nishizaki T, Soejima Y, et al: Beneficial effects of 3-dimensional visualization on hepatic vein reconstruction in living donor liver transplantation using right lobe graft. Transplantation 72:1993-1996, 2001.

63. Cheng YF, Chen CL, Huang TL, et al: Single imaging modality evaluation of living donors in liver transplantation: Magnetic resonance imaging. Transplantation 72:1527-1533, 2001.

64. Bogetti JD, Herts BR, Sands MJ, et al: Accuracy and utility of 3-dimensional computed tomography in evaluating donors for adult living related liver transplantation. Liver Transpl 7:687-692, 2001.

65. Fulcher AS, Szucs RA, Bassignani MJ, Marcos A: Right lobe living donor liver transplantation: Preoperative evaluation of the donor with MRI imaging. AJR Am J Roentgenol 176:1483-1491, 2001.

66. Kamel IR, Raptopoulos V, Pomfret EA, et al: Living adult right lobe liver transplantation: Imaging before surgery with multidetector multiphase CT. AJR Am J Roentgenol 175:1141-1143, 2000.

67. Tran T, Changstri C, Peterson A, et al: Living donor liver transplantation: The majority of donors have histologic abnormalities on liver biopsy [abstract]. Gastroenterology 124:A692, 2003.

68. Mokdad AH, Ford ES, Bowman BA, et al: Prevalence of obesity, diabetes, and obesity related health risk factors, 2001. JAMA 289:76-79, 2003.

69. Rinella ME, Alonso E, Rao S, et al: Body mass index as a predictor of hepatic steatosis in living liver donors. Liver Transpl 7:409-414, 2001.

70. Trotter JF: Thin chance for fat people (to become living donors). Liver Transpl 7:415-417, 2001.

71. Ryan CK, Johnson LA, Germin BI, Marcos A: One hundred hepatic biopsies in the workup of living donors for right lobe liver transplantation. Liver Transpl 8:1114-1122, 2002.

72. Rinella ME, Abecassis MM: Liver biopsy in living donors. Liver Transpl 8:1123-1125, 2002.

73. Makela JT, Kiviniemi H, Juvonen T, Laitinen S:. Factors influencing wound dehiscence after midline laparotomy. Am J Surg 170:387-390, 1995.

74. Israelsson LA, Jonsson T: Overweight and healing of midline incisions: The importance of suture technique. Eur J Surg 163:175-180, 1997.

75. Nair S, Cohen DB, Cohen MP, et al: Postoperative morbidity, mortality, costs, and long-term survival in severely obese patients undergoing orthotopic liver transplantation. Am J Gastroenterol 96:842-845, 2001.

76. Sawyer RG, Pelletier SJ, Pruett TL: Increased early morbidity and mortality with acceptable long-term function in severely obese patients undergoing liver transplantation. Clin Transplant 13:126-130, 1999.

77. Allison DB, Saunders SE: Obesity in North America. Med Clin North Am 84:305-332, 2000.

78. Kral JG, Schaffner F, Pierson RN, Wang J: Body fat topography as an independent predictor of fatty liver. Metabolism 42:548-551, 1993.

79. http://www.cdc.gov/nccdphp/dnpa/obesity/trend/obesity_diabetes_states.htm (accessed June 2003).

80. Rudow DL, Russo MW, Hafliger S, et al: Clinical and ethnic differences in candidates listed for liver transplantation with and without potential living donors. Liver Transpl 9:254-259, 2003.

81. http://www.census.gov/prod/2001pubs/c2kbr01-3.pdf (accessed June 2003).

82. Trotter JF, Mackenzie S, Wachs M, et al: Comprehensive cost comparison of adult-adult right hepatic lobe living-donor liver transplantation with cadaveric transplantation. Transplantation 75:473-476, 2003.

83. Marcos A, Ham JM, Fisher RA, et al: Surgical management of anatomical variations of the right lobe in living donor liver transplantation. Ann Surg 231:824-831, 2000.

84. Cheng YF, Huang TL, Chen CL, et al: Variations of the intrahepatic bile ducts: Application in living related liver transplantation and splitting liver transplantation. Clin Transplant 11:337-340, 1997.

85. Nakamura T, Tanaka K, Kiuchi T, et al: Anatomical variations and surgical strategies in right lobe living donor liver transplantation: Lessons from 120 cases. Transplantation 73:1896-1903, 2002.

86. Lee SG, Hwang S, Kim KH, et al: Approach to anatomic variations of the graft portal vein in right lobe living-donor liver transplantation. Transplantation 75:S28-S32, 2003.

87. Marcos A, Killackey M, Orloff MS, et al: Hepatic arterial reconstruction in 95 adult right lobe living donor liver transplants: Evolution of anastomotic technique. Liver Transpl 9:570-574, 2003.

88. Yasutomi M, Egawa H, Kobayashi Y, et al: Living donor liver transplantation for Budd-Chiari syndrome with inferior vena cava obstruction and associated antiphospholipid antibody syndrome. J Pediatr Surg 36:659-662, 2001.

89. Saing H, Fan ST, Tam PK, et al: Surgical complications and outcome of pediatric liver transplantation in Hong Kong. J Pediatr Surg 37:1673-1677, 2002.

90. Kadry Z, Selzner N, Handschin A, et al: Living donor liver transplantation in patients with portal vein thrombosis: A survey and review of technical issues. Transplantation 74:696-701, 2002.

91. Yao FY, Ferrell L, Bass NM, et al: Liver transplantation for hepatocellular carcinoma: Expansion of the tumor size limits does not adversely impact survival. Hepatology 33:1394-1403, 2001.

92. Roayaie S, Frischer JS, Emre SH, et al: Long-term results with multimodal adjuvant therapy and liver transplantation for the treatment of hepatocellular carcinoma larger than 5 centimeters. Ann Surg 235:533-539, 2002.

93. Cotler SJ, McNutt R, Patil R, et al: Adult living donor liver transplantation: Preferences about donation outside the medical community. Liver Transpl 7:335-340, 2001.

94. Cotler SJ, Cotler S, Gambera M, et al: Adult living donor liver transplantation: Perspectives from 100 liver transplant surgeons. Liver Transpl 9:637-644, 2003.

95. Kumashiro Y, Kasahara M, Nomoto K, et al: Living donor liver transplantation for giant hepatic hemangioma with Kasabach-Merritt syndrome with a posterior segment graft. Liver Transpl 8:721-724, 2002.

96. Azoulay D, Castaing D, Adam R, et al: Adult to adult living-related liver transplantation. The Paul-Brousse Hospital preliminary experience. Gastroenterol Clin Biol 25:773-780, 2001.

97. Takegoshi K, Tanaka K, Nomura H, et al: Successful living donor liver transplantation for polycystic liver in a patient with autosomal-dominant polycystic kidney disease. J Clin Gastroenterol 33:229-231, 2001.

98. Nakamura M, Fuchinoue S, Nakajima I, et al: Three cases of sequential liver-kidney transplantation from living-related donors. Nephrol Dial Transplant 16:166-168, 2001.

99. Koyama I, Fuchinoue S, Urashima Y, et al: Living related liver transplantation for polycystic liver disease. Transpl Int 15: 578-580, 2002.

100. Kikuchi H, Ohkohchi N, Orri T, Satomi S: Living-related liver transplantation in patients with pulmonary vascular disease. Transplant Proc 32:2177-2178, 2000.

101. Ho MC, Hu RH, Ni YH, et al: Liver transplantation in a patient with pulmonary hypertension. Transplant Proc 32:2179-2181, 2000.

102. Florman S, Shneider B: Living-related liver transplantation in inherited metabolic liver disease: Feasibility and cautions. J Pediatr Gastroenterol Nutr 33:520-521, 2001.

103. Shneider BL: Pediatric liver transplantation in metabolic disease: Clinical decision making. Pediatr Transplant 6:25-29, 2002.

104. Kayler LK, Merion RM, Lee S, et al: Long-term survival after liver transplantation in children with metabolic disorders. Pediatr Transplant 6:295-300, 2002.

105. Burdelski M, Rogiers X: Liver transplantation in metabolic disorders. Acta Gastroenterol Belg 62:300-305, 1999.

106. Haberal M, Arda IS, Karakayali H, et al: Successful heterotopic segmental liver transplantation from a live donor to a patient with Alagille syndrome. J Pediatr Surg 36:667-671, 2001.

107. Revillon Y, Michel JL, Lacaille F, et al: Living-related liver transplantation in children: The 'Parisian' strategy to safely increase organ availability. J Pediatr Surg 34:851-853, 1999.

108. Negita M, Nour B, Sebastian A, et al: Living related liver transplantation in Oklahoma. J Okla State Med Assoc 90:89-93, 1997.

109. Kasahara M, Ohwada S, Takeichi T, et al: Living-related liver transplantation for type II citrullinemia using a graft from a heterozygote donor. Transplantation 71:157-159, 2001.

110. Ban K, Sugiyama N, Sugiyama K, et al: A pediatric patient with classical citrullinemia who underwent liver-related partial liver transplantation. Transplantation 71:1495-1497, 2001.

111. Yazaki M, Ikeda S, Takei Y, et al: Complete neurological recovery of an adult patient with type II citrullinemia after living related partial liver transplantation. Transplantation 62:1679-1684, 1996.

112. van der Veere CN, Sinaasappel M, McDonagh AF, et al: Current therapy for Crigler-Najjar syndrome type 1: Report of a world registry. Hepatology 24:311-315, 1996.

113. Al Shurafa H, Wali S, Chehab MS, et al: Living-related liver transplantation for Crigler-Najjar syndrome in Saudi Arabia. Clin Transplant 16:222-226, 2002.

114. Nishizaki T, Kishikawa K, Yoshizumi T, et al: Domino liver transplantation from a living related donor. Transplantation 70:1236-1239, 2000.

115. Stangou AJ, Heaton ND, Rela M, et al: Domino hepatic transplantation using the liver from a patient with familial amyloid polyneuropathy. Transplantation 65:1496-1498, 1998.

116. Shirahata Y, Ohkohchi N, Kawagishi N, et al: Living-donor liver transplantation for homozygous familial hypercholesterolemia from a donor with heterozygous hypercholesterolemia. Transpl Int 16:276-279, 2003.

117. Lui PP, de Villa VH, Chen YS, et al: Outcome of living donor liver transplantation for glycogen storage disease. Transplant Proc 35:366-368, 2003.

118. Sugawara Y, Ohkubo T, Makuuchi M, et al: Living-donor liver transplantation in an HIV-positive patient with hemophilia. Transplantation 74:1655-1656, 2002.

119. Horita K, Matsunami H, Shimizu Y, et al: Treatment of a patient with hemophilia A and hepatitis C virus–related cirrhosis by living-related liver transplantation from an obligate carrier donor. Transplantation 73:1909-1912, 2002.

120. Gruessner RW: Preemptive liver transplantation from a living related donor for primary hyperoxaluria type I. N Engl J Med 338:1924, 1998.

121. Mohan N, McKiernan P, Preece MA, et al: Indications and outcome of liver transplantation in tyrosinemia type I. Eur J Pediatr 158:S49-S54, 1999.

122. Nagasaka H, Yorifuji T, Egawa H, et al: Successful living-donor liver transplantation from an asymptomatic carrier mother in ornithine transcarbamylase deficiency. J Pediatr 138:432-434, 2001.

123. Kiuchi T, Edamoto Y, Kaibori M, et al: Auxiliary liver transplantation for urea-cycle enzyme deficiencies: Lessons from three cases. Transplant Proc 31:528-529, 1999.

124. Ghobrial RM, Amersi F, Farmer DG, et al: Rapid and severe early HCV recurrence following adult living donor liver transplantation [abstract]. Am J Transplant 2:163A, 2002.

125. Gaglio PJ, Malireddy S, Russo M, et al: Hepatitis C recurrence in recipients of grafts from living vs. cadaveric liver donors [abstract]. Hepatology 36:265A, 2002.

126. Trotter JF, Schiano T, Wachs M, et al: Preliminary report: Hepatitis C occurs earlier and is more severe in living donor liver transplant recipients [abstract]. Am J Transplant 1:316A, 2001.

127. Shiffman ML, Risher RA, Stravitz T, et al: Histologic analysis of recurrent hepatitis C virus infection following living donor and cadaveric liver transplantation [abstract]. Am J Transplant 3:203A, 2003.

128. Baltz A, Trotter JF: Living donor liver transplantation and hepatitis C. Clin Liver Dis 7:651-665, 2003.

129. Hwang S, Moon DB, Lee SG, et al: Safety of anti–hepatitis B core antibody–positive donors for living-donor liver transplantation. Transplantation 75:S45-S48, 2003.

130. Dodson F, Issa S, Araya V, et al: Infectivity of hepatic allografts with antibodies to hepatitis B. Transplantation 64:1582-1584, 1997.

131. Wachs M, Amend WJ, Ascher NL, et al: The risk of transmission of hepatitis B from HBsAg(-), HBcAb(+), HBIgM(-) organ donors. Transplantation 59:230-234, 1995.

132. Dickson RC, Everhart JE, Lake JR, et al: Transmission of hepatitis B by transplantation of livers from donors positive for antibody to hepatitis B core antigen. The National Institute of Diabetes and Digestive and Kidney Disease Liver Transplantation Database. Gastroenterology 113:1668-1674, 1997.

133. Uemoto S, Sugiyama K, Marusawa H, et al: Transmission of hepatitis B virus from hepatitis B core antibody–positive donors in living related liver transplants. Transplantation 65:494-499, 1998.

134. Chen YS, Wang CC, de Villa VH, et al: Prevention of de novo hepatitis B virus infection in living donor liver transplantation using hepatitis B core antibody positive donors. Clin Transplant 16:405-409, 2002.

135. de Villa VH, Chen YS, Chen CL: Hepatitis B core antibody–positive grafts: Recipient's risk. Transplantation 75:S49-S53, 2003.

136. Liu CL, Fan ST, Lo CM, et al: Right-lobe live donor liver transplantation improves survival of patients with acute liver failure. Br J Surg 89:317-322, 2002.

137. Nishizaki T, Hiroshige S, Ikegami T, et al: Living-donor liver transplantation for fulminant hepatic failure in adult patients with a left-lobe graft. Surgery 131:S182-S189, 2002.

138. Uemoto S, Inomata Y, Sakurai T, et al: Living donor liver transplantation for fulminant hepatic failure. Transplantation 70:152-157, 2000.

139. Marcos A, Ham JM, Fisher RA, et al: Emergency adult to adult living donor liver transplantation for fulminant hepatic failure. Transplantation 69:2202-2205, 2000.

140. Miwa S, Hashikura Y, Mita A, et al: Living-related liver transplantation for patients with fulminant and subfulminant hepatic failure. Hepatology 30:1521-1526, 1999.

141. Lo CM, Fan ST, Liu CL, et al: Applicability of living donor liver transplantation to high-urgency patients. Transplantation 67:73-77, 1999.

142. Liu CL, Fan ST, Lo CM, Wong J: Living-donor liver transplantation for high-urgency situations. Transplantation 75:S33-S36, 2003.

143. Marino IR, Doyle HR: Living donor in urgent cases: Ethical hazard. Liver Transpl 8:859-860, 2002.

144. Abouna GJ: Emergency adult to adult living donor liver transplantation for fulminant hepatic failure—is it justifiable? Transplantation 71:1498-1500, 2001.

145. Matas AJ, Garvey CA, Jacobs CL, Kahn JP: Nondirected donation of kidneys from living donors. N Engl J Med 343:433-436, 2000.

146. Levinsky NG: Organ donation by unrelated donors. N Engl J Med 343:430-432, 2000.

147. Ross LF: Media appeals for directed altruistic living liver donations: Lessons from Camilo Sandoval Ewen. Perspect Biol Med 45:329-337, 2002.

148. Liu LU, Schiano TD, Min AD, et al: Syngeneic living-donor liver transplantation without the use of immunosuppression. Gastroenterology 123:1341-1345, 2002.

149. Sugawara Y, Ohtsuka H, Kaneko J, et al: Successful treatment of hepatitis C virus after liver transplantation from an identical twin. Transplantation 73:1850-1851, 2002.

Adult Living Donor Hepatectomy and Recipient Operation

SANDER S. FLORMAN
CHARLES M. MILLER

Adult living donor liver transplantation 676
　Patient evaluation 676
　Graft selection 681
　Actual and functional graft size 682

Adult living donor operations 682
　Perioperative considerations 682
　General operative techniques 683
　Cholecystectomy and cholangiography 683
　Right lobectomy 683
　Left lobectomy 687
　Graft removal 688
　Additional operative considerations 689
　Back-table procedure 689
　Postoperative management 689

Adult living donor liver recipient procedure 690
　Perioperative considerations 690
　Hepatectomy 690
　Anhepatic strategies 690
　Graft implantation 691
　Venous congestion 694
　Biliary reconstruction 695
　Postoperative management 696

Summary 697

In 1967, Thomas Starzl and colleagues performed the first deceased donor human liver transplants with prolonged survival in Denver.[1] Over the next 20 years, liver transplantation became a clinical reality as significant advances were made in surgical techniques, immunosuppression, and organ preservation.[2,3] Virtually from the beginning, the demand for organs has far exceeded the supply, and as a result, surgeons have searched for innovative strategies to bridge the gap.

In 1988, Pichlmayr and coworkers transplanted partial-liver grafts from a single deceased donor into one adult and one pediatric patient.[4] That same year, Bismuth and associates transplanted partial-liver grafts from a single deceased donor into two adult recipients.[5] As our understanding of segmental liver anatomy improved, reduced-size transplantation and split-liver transplantation have become more common. With the extreme shortage of deceased donor organs and an ever-increasing demand for transplantation, however, there remains a drastic need for alternative sources of livers.[6] In an attempt to meet this need, surgeons have turned to marginal or so-called extended criteria deceased donors and, more recently, to living liver donors.

The roots of solid-organ transplantation are firmly grounded in living donation. In the 1950s, some of the first kidney transplants were performed with living donors.[7,8] Living donors have more recently also been used for lung, pancreas, and intestinal transplantation.[9,10] The techniques for segmental living donor liver transplantation were first successfully developed by

Broelsch and associates in dogs.[11] Raia and colleagues first attempted living donor liver transplantation in pediatric patients in 1988 and again in 1989.[12] In 1989, Strong and coworkers performed the first successful living donor liver transplantation in a 17-month-old with biliary atresia by using a left lateral segment graft from his mother.[13] Shortly after these reports, Broelsch and associates, who not only pioneered the surgical techniques but also established an ethical context for this new procedure,[14] reported successful human living donor liver transplantation.[15,16] The chief motivation for these procedures was the high mortality rate in pediatric patients on the waiting list because of the scarcity of small donors.[17] With living donor liver transplantation, mortality in pediatric liver transplant candidates has been dramatically reduced.[18]

The success of pediatric living donor liver transplantation provided an impetus to perform more extensive donor resections for transplantation in larger recipients. The Japanese, in particular, aggressively pursued this option for their adult patients because societal beliefs precluded the use of deceased donors until very recently.[19,20] In 1993, Hashikura and colleagues performed the first successful transplantation of an adult recipient with a left lobe graft from a living donor.[21] The 53-year-old patient with primary biliary cirrhosis received this transplant from her 25-year-old son.

In the United States, with mortality rates higher than 10% in adults on the liver transplant waiting list and far too few organs from deceased donors to meet the demand, many programs have aggressively pursued living donation for their adult recipients.[22] Initially, only left lobectomies were performed. The risk to left lobe donors is relatively small given that healthy adults should tolerate a 40% resection without hepatic decompensation. Unfortunately, some recipients, particularly those with advanced portal hypertension, seemed to require more liver mass than a left lobe could provide and thus suffered from varying degrees of liver insufficiency.[23] This syndrome, which has become known as small-for-size syndrome, led many centers to begin to use right lobe resections in living donors to increase the actual mass of the graft and allow wider application of these life-saving procedures.

Yamaoka and coauthors reported the first successful transplantation using the right lobe from a living donor in 1993.[24] The donor was the mother of a 9-year-old child with biliary atresia who was found at exploration to have complex left lobe arterial anatomy, and an intraoperative decision was made to use the right lobe. In 1996, Lo and associates performed the first successful transplantation of a right lobe graft from a living donor to an adult recipient.[25] The recipient was a 28-year-old man with Wilson's disease who received the transplant from his 30-year-old brother. At Mount Sinai, we began adult living donor liver transplantation

in 1998 with the use of left lobes, but despite early success, the results overall were suboptimal.[26] As a result, we and others turned to right lobe transplantation to obtain larger grafts for our adult recipients. The first right lobe living donor liver transplantation in the United States was reported in 1998.[27] In the late 1990s and early 2000s, the number of adult living donor liver transplants performed increased dramatically throughout the world. The right lobe graft was a natural means by which actual graft size could be significantly increased, thereby avoiding small-for-size syndrome. Right lobectomy, however, is associated with significantly more donor morbidity.[25,28,29]

Even though enthusiasm for adult living donor liver transplantation persists, there is also apprehension because of the reported need for transplantation in donors, as well as the death of donors.[30] Although no formal national or international registries currently exist, it is estimated that more than 4000 living donor liver transplants have been performed worldwide.[22,31-33] Roughly half of these transplants have been performed in adult recipients.

The living donor hepatectomy and recipient operations are technically advanced and require significant experience in both whole-organ liver transplantation and hepatobiliary surgery. Some states, such as New York, have even established minimum criteria for surgeons to be qualified to perform these procedures.[34] In this chapter, we review the adult living liver donor and liver transplant recipient operations.

Adult Living Donor Liver Transplantation

Patient Evaluation

Successful living donor liver transplantation is dependent on careful selection of both the donor and recipient. Donor safety is paramount, and by definition, donors are healthy people with no significant medical illness who voluntarily and altruistically offer to subject themselves to potentially life-threatening surgery. There is an absolute responsibility to protect the donor preoperatively, intraoperatively, and postoperatively. Many important factors must be evaluated when determining the suitability of both the donor and recipient for their respective procedures. Living donation is not an option for every recipient, and not every recipient has a potential living donor. The evaluation for living donation is discussed in detail in Chapter 44.

Anatomical variations are common in the liver—they are the rule rather than the exception. The vast majority, however, are not contraindications to donation and can be managed safely.[32,35,36] To best ensure donor safety, it is imperative that surgeons have a thorough understanding of common hilar anatomy, as well as the anatomy of a specific donor. The most common anatomical relationship of the hilar structures is shown in Figure 45–1. The surgical importance of hepatic anatomical variations as they apply to living donor transplantation is briefly reviewed.

Portal Venous Anatomy

The extrahepatic portal vein lies in the most dorsal, or posterior, aspect of the liver hilum. Generally, the extrahepatic portal vein has very constant anatomy, with its bifurcation lying to the right and a longer extrahepatic left portal vein. The transverse portion of the left portal vein runs to the ligamentum venosum, whereas the umbilical portion runs up into the umbilical fissure.[37,38] It is therefore much easier to gain sufficient extrahepatic left portal length than right portal length.

A simple classification scheme of portal venous anatomy with particular relevance for right lobe liver donation is shown in Figure 45–2; this classification is

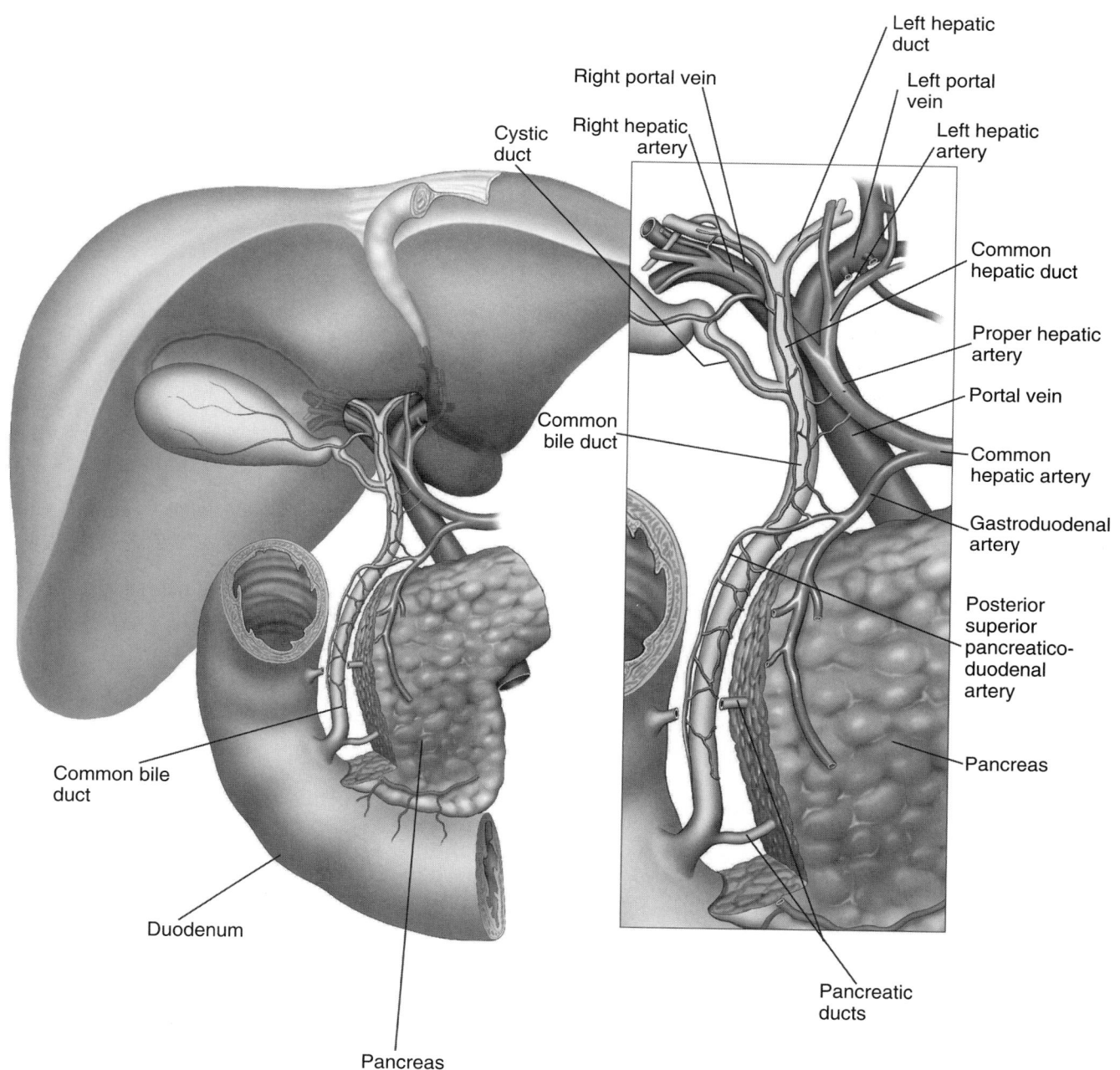

FIGURE 45–1

Standard hilar anatomy. (Redrawn from Imamura H, Makuuchi M, Sakamoto Y, et al: Anatomical keys and pitfalls in living donor liver transplantation. J Hepatobiliary Pancreat Surg 7:380-394, 2000.)

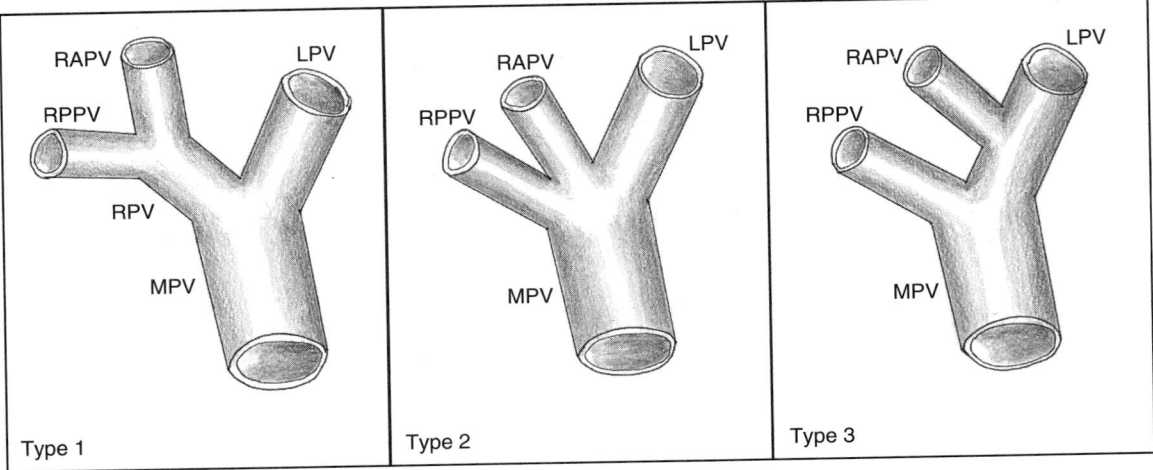

FIGURE 45–2

Portal vein anatomy based on variations in the right anterior portal vein. LPV, left portal vein; MPV, main portal vein; RAPV, right anterior portal vein; RPPV, right posterior portal vein; RPV, right portal vein. (From Varotti G, Gondolesi GE, Goldman J, et al: Anatomic variations in right liver living donors. J Am Coll Surg 198:577-582, 2004.)

based on variations in anatomy of the anterior segment of the portal vein.[39-41] The intrahepatic branching pattern of the portal vein may be variable. The vast majority of patients (75% to 90%), however, have standard anatomy.[35,40,42,43] Nearly 10% of donors have a trifurcation in the portal venous anatomy that may require (type 3) reconstruction of separate anterior and posterior right portal veins.[35,36,38,42] An important observation has been made that variations in biliary anatomy are most often associated with variations in portal venous anatomy.[41]

The type 3 variation, or so-called double portal vein, is not a contraindication to donation but does require proper identification and, in many cases, more technically advanced reconstruction. Potential donors with multiple intraparenchymal portal branches to the anterior segment should, however, be declined. In our experience in the evaluation of more than 550 potential donors, 2 were declined specifically because of their aberrant portal venous anatomy. In one, the left portal vein coursed through the medial aspect of the right lobe and thus precluded donation. In the other, the portal branch to segment IV arose from a separate anterior right portal vein, thereby precluding right lobe donation because portal flow to the medial aspect of the remnant left lobe would be compromised. Intrahepatic left portal venous anomalies rarely preclude left lobe donation.

Hepatic Arterial Anatomy

It has long been known that the arterial supply of the liver is highly variable.[39] In 1928, Adachi reported the arterial anatomy in more than 200 dissections.[44]

Based on Adachi's work and nearly 500 cadaveric dissections performed by Browne[45] and Michels[46] in 1940, it is known that the arterial anatomy is standard (i.e., single right and left hepatic arteries from a common hepatic artery as a branch of the celiac artery originating from the aorta) in 50% of people. The rest of the population has accessory or replaced arteries or anomalous origins of these arteries (or any combination of these variations). The basic variations in hepatic arterial anatomy are shown in Figure 45–3.

The more common variations include an accessory or replaced left hepatic artery originating from the left gastric artery (25%), as well as an accessory or replaced right hepatic artery originating from the superior mesenteric artery (17%). In our own series of nearly 500 deceased donors procured for transplantation, a third did not have the standard arterial anatomy, nearly 20% had a left branch, and about 15% had a right branch.[47] Soin and coauthors reported similar findings in more than 500 deceased donors.[48] These arterial variations are important to recognize when evaluating living donors for partial hepatectomy.

With right lobe grafts, most commonly there is a single right hepatic artery that lies anterior to the right portal vein and, more importantly, just posterior to the common hepatic duct. In our experience, more than 95% of right lobe grafts had a single right hepatic artery.[42] In 10% of individuals, the right hepatic artery courses anterior to the common bile duct. The right hepatic artery may divide early into separate anterior and posterior right hepatic arteries. In such cases, it may still be possible to have a single right hepatic artery proximally. If, however, the arterial supply to

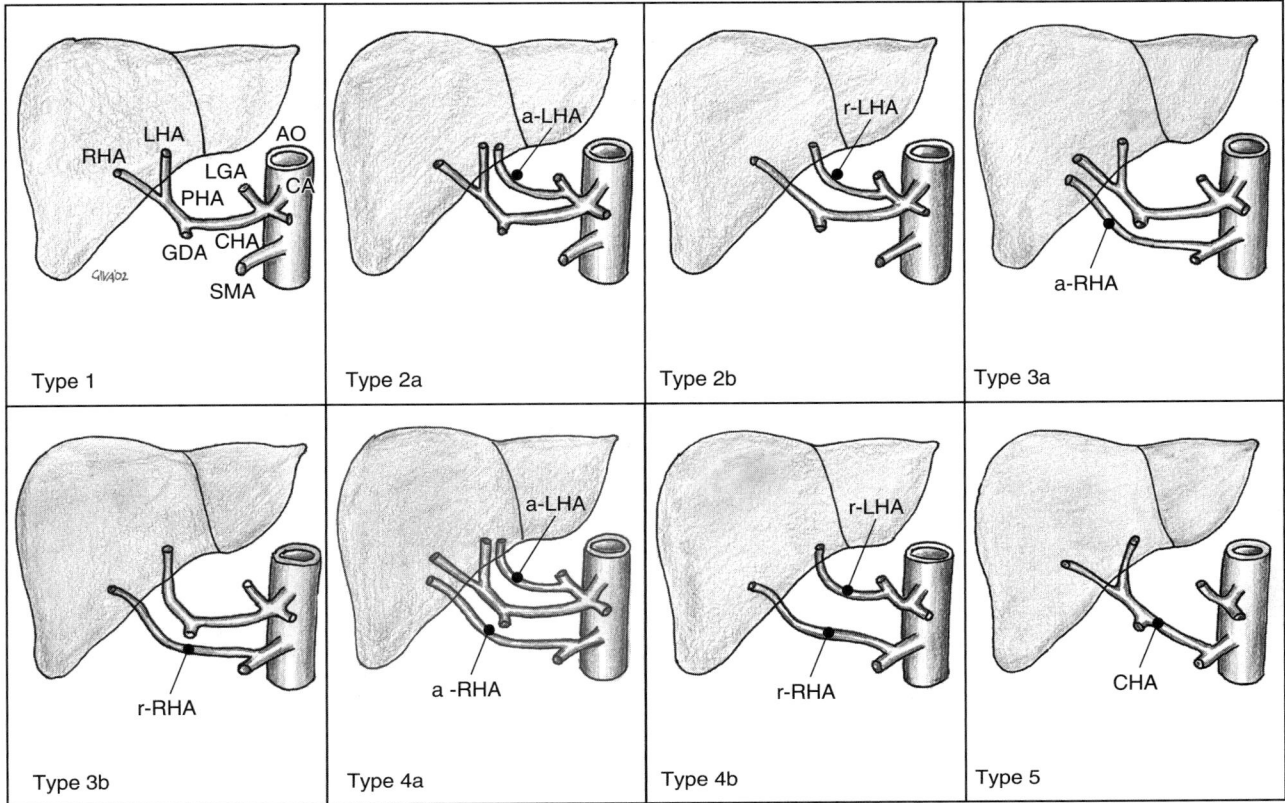

FIGURE 45–3

Hepatic artery anatomy. a, accessory; AO, aorta; CHA, common hepatic artery; GDA, gastroduodenal artery; LGA, left gastric artery; LHA, left hepatic artery; PHA, proper hepatic artery; r, replaced; RHA, right hepatic artery; SA, splenic artery; SMA, superior mesenteric artery. (From Varotti G, Gondolesi GE, Goldman J, et al: Anatomic variations in right liver living donors. J Am Coll Surg 198:577-582, 2004.)

segment IV of the left lobe arises from the anterior right hepatic artery, it may be necessary to divide this artery separately to preserve inflow to segment IV. Such division may create two separate right lobe arteries. In addition, in patients with an accessory right hepatic artery branch, two separate arterial anastomoses may be necessary.

Although an arterial variant rarely precludes right lobe donation, this is not necessarily true for left lobe donation. The arterial supply to the left lobe may be highly complex, and there is a significantly higher likelihood of multiple arteries to contend with, specifically because of the variability of the arterial supply to segment IV.[49] In 20% of individuals, the arterial supply to segment IV, often referred to as the middle hepatic artery, originates from the right hepatic artery.[50]

Hepatic Venous Anatomy

It is important to assess the anatomical relationship of the hepatic veins as they enter the vena cava. This relationship can have important implications for identifying the correct transection point in the donor, as well as for graft outflow reconstruction in the recipient. Commonly, the right hepatic vein enters the vena cava separately from the left and middle hepatic veins, which enter together as a common trunk. Such anatomy potentially makes division of the left and middle hepatic veins, when necessary for extended right lobe grafts or left lateral segment grafts, more difficult.

The intrahepatic venous anatomy can be highly variable (Fig. 45–4).[51] There is considerable overlap between the veins that drain specific anatomical segments, and such overlap usually allows for interruption of single venous tributaries without affecting the drainage of an entire segment. Unfortunately, this is not always the case, and frequently, a significant anterior segment venous tributary from the right lobe to the middle hepatic vein requires reconstruction. It is difficult to predict exactly which tributaries are significant and which are nonessential. Significant accessory hepatic venous tributaries are identified in roughly 50% of right lobe cases.[26,35]

Some surgeons have advocated a variety of alternative transection planes for the donor right lobectomy.[52-55]

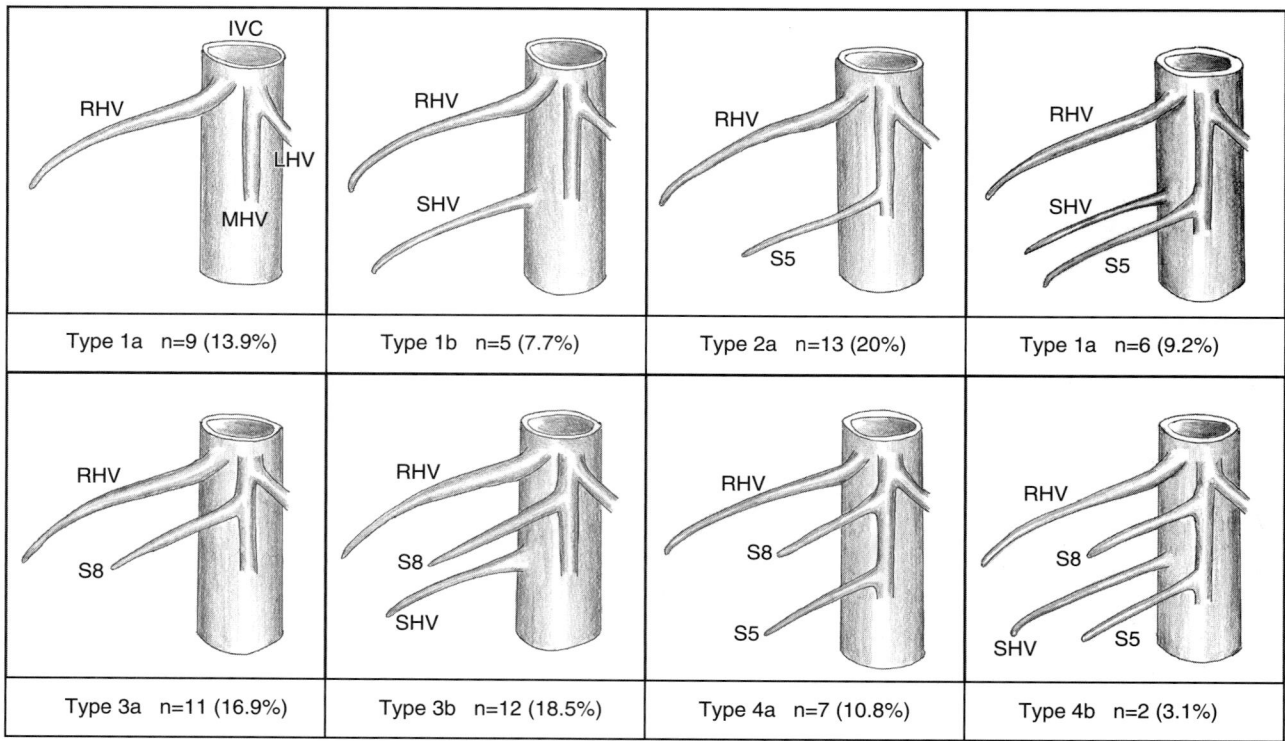

FIGURE 45–4

Hepatic venous anatomy. IRHV, inferior right hepatic vein(s); IVC, inferior vena cava; LHV, left hepatic vein; MHV, middle hepatic vein; RHV, right hepatic vein; S5, segment V; S8, segment VIII. (From Varotti G, Gondolesi GE, Goldman J, et al: Anatomic variations in right liver living donors. J Am Coll Surg 198: 577-582, 2004.)

Some of these approaches have been purported to obviate the need for venous reimplantation. In essence, all these approaches are modifications of extended right lobectomy techniques. By taking portions or most of the middle hepatic vein with the graft, the need for venous tributary reconstruction becomes less necessary. These procedures are performed by using a parenchymal transection plane slightly further to the left of the gallbladder fossa and on the left border of the middle hepatic vein, thereby incorporating varying portions of the distal middle hepatic vein with the right lobe graft.

The main argument for including portions or the entire middle hepatic vein with the right lobe graft is to optimize venous drainage of the anterior segments (i.e., V and VIII). Inclusion of the distal middle hepatic vein improves segment V drainage but not that of segment VIII. Whether the right lobe resection should be extended to include the donor's middle hepatic vein is highly controversial. We and others have not included the middle hepatic vein with right lobe resections in the belief that such inclusion may compromise donor safety.[56,57] Because the middle hepatic vein is resected with the left lobe, venous drainage is rarely a problem for living donor left lobectomy.

Biliary Anatomy

The biliary anatomy is the most variable anatomical factor in living donor procedures.[58] Intraoperative cholangiography is invaluable as a means of defining a "road map" of the biliary anatomy and for identifying the exact site of division. Although magnetic resonance imaging (MRI) now permits highly advanced imaging of the biliary tree for living donors,[59] intraoperative cholangiography remains the gold standard. Just a few millimeters can be the difference between one biliary reconstruction in the recipient and five! Even more important, a millimeter in the wrong direction could have lifelong crippling consequences for the donor.

Preoperatively, MRI can generally provide reliable and accurate biliary anatomy and obviate the need for invasive imaging with endoscopic retrograde cholangiopancreatography (ERCP), which itself can cause significant morbidity and even mortality. Based on the MRI scans, a preliminary operative approach can be planned. As a result of the high variability in biliary anatomy, subtle differences in anatomy can have significant implications for reconstruction in recipients. It is imperative for the surgeon to have detailed understanding of an individual donor's biliary anatomy.

The right lobe biliary anatomy can have significant variations (Fig. 45–5).[39] Roughly two thirds of donors have "normal" or "standard" biliary anatomy,[35,39,42] with the right anterior and posterior hepatic ducts joining together to form the right hepatic duct. When the right hepatic duct is absent, there are several configurations that are commonly encountered (see Fig. 45–5). The periductal blood supply arises from branches of the posterior superior pancreaticoduodenal artery, the right hepatic artery, and the hepatic hilum (see Fig. 45–1 inset).[38,60,61] Left lobe biliary anatomy is equally as variable, particularly that of the medial left lobe.[39] When performing a left lobectomy, it is imperative to identify any posterior right duct that drains into the left hepatic duct, a common anomaly.

Graft Selection

The choice of the appropriate donor resection for a specific recipient is complex. There is a fine balance between protecting the donor by performing the smallest resection possible and, at the same time, providing the recipient with adequate liver mass and the best chance for survival. Volumetric calculations are important and have been shown to accurately predict the probability of hepatic dysfunction after liver resection.[62] There are, however, other important anatomical and physiological considerations in graft selection.

Modern imaging technology makes it possible to assess steatosis in the potential donor's liver.[63] When steatosis is present, most centers require liver biopsy to determine the degree and type (macrosteatosis or microsteatosis). Some surgeons accept otherwise healthy donors with steatosis and correct the liver volume by subtracting the percentage of steatosis from the estimated liver volume.[64] We do not accept donors with a significant degree of steatosis regardless of the adequacy of the recalculated liver volume. Instead, we have recommended weight loss and aggressive hypercholesterolemia management or a search for a more suitable donor.

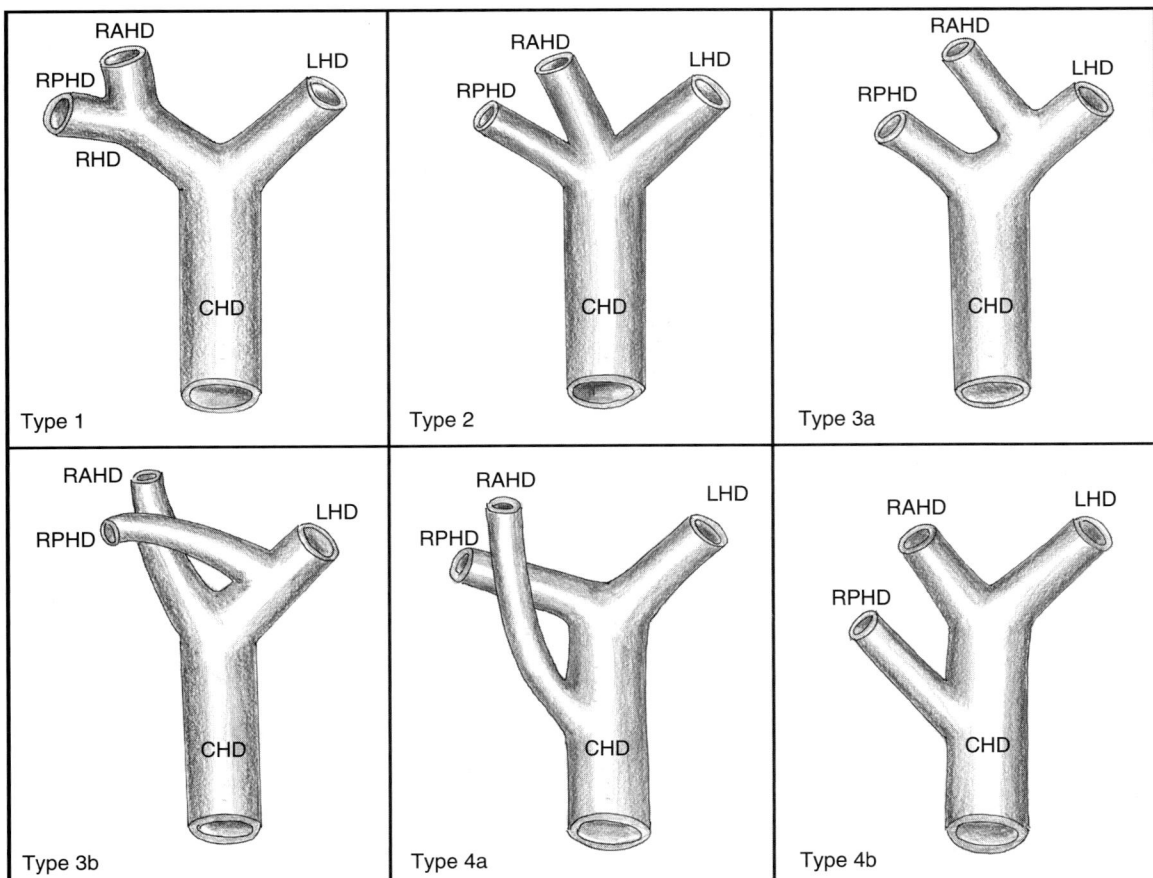

FIGURE 45–5

Variations in biliary anatomy of the right lobe. CHD, common hepatic duct; LHD, left hepatic duct; RAHD, right anterior hepatic duct; RHD, right hepatic duct; RPHD, right posterior hepatic duct. (From Varotti G, Gondolesi GE, Goldman J, et al: Anatomic variations in right liver living donors. J Am Coll Surg 198:577-582, 2004.)

Donor safety must take precedence. Therefore, the smallest resection that provides adequate actual and functional mass for the recipient should be selected. Occasionally, the caudate lobe has been included with the left lobe to increase the actual mass of the graft and to best protect the vascularity of the proximal left hepatic duct.[65,66] Although the average caudate lobe is relatively small and only minimally increases the size of the graft,[67] particular attention must be paid to the venous drainage of the caudate lobe.[68] Right lobectomy clearly has an advantage over left lobectomy in that actual graft mass is increased.[28] The benefit of including the middle hepatic vein is solely to optimize anterior segment venous drainage, which maximizes functional mass while not significantly increasing the actual mass of the graft.[53]

Actual and Functional Graft Size

Of extreme importance for successful transplantation of partial-liver grafts is accurate preoperative determination of donor graft adequacy for a specific recipient. Many donor and recipient factors are involved in this determination,[56,69-76] the most important of which are graft volume and recipient size. With these two variables, a simple calculation known as the graft-recipient weight ratio (GRWR) can be made to determine the adequacy of the actual graft size. The GRWR equals the graft weight divided by the recipient's body weight. The generally accepted safe minimum graft volume is at least 40% to 50% of the recipient's ideal liver volume, or a GRWR higher than 0.8%. The ideal liver volume can be estimated with several formulas.[77,78] Successful liver transplantation from living donors has been reported, however, when grafts with estimated liver volumes of less than 25% of the recipient's ideal liver volume have been used.[73]

When the GRWR is too low to support the needs of a given recipient, small-for-size syndrome occurs. Small-for-size syndrome is clinically characterized by early graft dysfunction, including protracted cholestasis, coagulopathy, renal dysfunction, and possibly sepsis.[23] Although small-for-size syndrome can occur with grafts of any size, the incidence is far greater if the graft size is less than 35% to 40% of the recipient's estimated liver volume, or an estimated GRWR of less than 0.8%.[28,79]

The size of the liver graft necessary to support the recipient is known as the functional graft size. Functional graft size is a composite function of actual graft size modified by factors of recipient performance status and hyperdynamic circulation (i.e., portal inflow). Small-for-size syndrome may also develop when the calculated GRWR seems adequate but the functional graft size is inadequate. This discrepancy occurs because these calculations do not take into consideration

important variables such as the recipient's degree of portal hypertension or disease severity.

Thus, regardless of the GRWR, the more important determinant of graft function is the functional graft size, which is largely influenced by portal hemodynamics and is, to a large degree, dependent on the recipient's cardiac index.[69] Early graft venous congestion can also produce a functional small-for-size syndrome.[69,80,81] Understanding actual and functional graft size is important in determining donor suitability for a specific recipient and in choosing which graft, left or right lobe, to procure from the donor.

From experience with left lobe grafts, we and others have found that in patients with little or no portal hypertension and stable disease, grafts with an actual size less than 40% of ideal liver volume (and a GRWR less than 0.8%) provide adequate functional mass. However, when these grafts were used in sicker patients with significantly greater hyperdynamic portal flow, the grafts swelled and could not sustain life.[23,26,69,70,73] Portal hemodynamics in partial-liver transplantation should not be underestimated. The role of sinusoidal shear stress, or the effect of high portal velocity on grafts of varying size, is a critical determinant of graft function, small-for-size syndrome, and overall success.[69,71,76,82-84]

Similarly, early in our experience with right lobe grafts, we found that suboptimal venous outflow can result in graft damage and poor function. When suboptimal venous outflow occurs with severe portal hypertension, even grafts in recipients with a GRWR greater than 0.8% may function poorly.[69] Poor venous outflow causes a Budd-Chiari syndrome of the anterior segment, which in turn results in portal overflow to the posterior segment.[80] This unrelieved portal hypertension causes a functional small-for-size syndrome clinically. Because of the well-known reciprocal relationship between portal venous and hepatic arterial flow, secondary hepatic artery thrombosis and biliary complications may occur.[71,83]

Adult Living Donor Operations

Perioperative Considerations

A variety of approaches can be used to prepare the donor for surgery in the immediate preoperative period. The day before surgery, the donor is instructed to have only liquids and nothing by mouth after midnight. An enema is prescribed as bowel preparation that night. In some programs, donors are given a full bowel preparation.[85] The donor is optimally admitted the day before surgery to ensure that no acute illness or problems have developed. The transplant team and the anesthesiologists see the donor in the holding area and review the donor's chart one last time. An epidural catheter with patient-controlled analgesia should be placed for postoperative pain control, although postoperative pain management may vary between centers.

Before induction of general anesthesia, bilateral compression devices are placed on the lower extremities to prevent deep venous thrombosis. After induction of general endotracheal anesthesia, a Foley catheter is inserted and the patient's abdomen is prepared and draped in the usual sterile fashion. Prophylactic antibiotics are administered. In our practice, standard antibiosis is a second-generation cephalosporin or, in the case of penicillin allergy, clindamycin and aztreonam. An internal jugular central venous catheter is inserted, and central venous pressure (CVP) is transduced. The patient is positioned on the operating room table so that the retractor system can be optimally placed. A nasogastric tube is placed at this time. An autologous blood transfusion system (e.g., Cell Saver) is used in every case. Donors may also have recently donated autologous blood available.

General Operative Techniques

A right subcostal incision with a long midline extension is used in all cases. A bilateral subcostal incision with midline extension is intentionally avoided to prevent the morbidity of cruciate necrosis and incisional hernias. On entering the peritoneal cavity, the ligamentum teres is divided and purposefully left long so that after right lobectomies, it may be reaffixed to the anterior abdominal wall at the end of the procedure. This technique helps ensure that the remnant liver does not undergo torsion. In left lobectomy cases, the ligamentum teres is also left long so that it can be reaffixed to the anterior abdominal wall in the recipient after graft implantation.

The falciform ligament is divided and the suprahepatic vena cava is exposed. In right lobe cases, the right hepatic vein will be exposed anteriorly at this time as it enters the vena cava. The triangular space between the right hepatic vein, middle hepatic vein, and the anterior surface of the liver is developed down to the level of the vena cava. In left lobe cases, the left and middle hepatic veins are exposed anteriorly, and the same triangular space is developed. As a rule and when safely possible, structures on the remnant side should not be dissected and tissue planes should not be violated in living donor surgery.

A brief but thorough evaluation of the peritoneal cavity should be performed. The liver should be assessed for size, anatomy, and abnormalities (e.g., lesions, steatosis, congestion). The intestines should be evaluated for masses or other abnormalities. In females, the ovaries and uterus should be palpated. On rare occasion, an unsuspected finding precludes donation. This situation occurred in our experience when the donor liver was found to be severely congested as a result of acute cocaine use.[26] In another case, the mother of a child with Alagille syndrome was unexpectedly found to have bile duct paucity herself.[86]

A brief evaluation of the liver with intraoperative ultrasonography may be performed. A systematic examination is performed with B-mode ultrasound in real time with a 5- or a 7-MHz probe. The hepatic veins are individually traced to their insertion into the vena cava. The line of parenchymal transection is verified and can generally be determined by identifying the right border of the middle hepatic vein and the inferior vena cava in the same longitudinal plane.[53]

For right lobectomies, particular attention is paid to the relationship of the right and middle hepatic veins as they near the vena cava. Significant accessory hepatic veins draining the right lobe, either directly into the vena cava (i.e., segment VI or VII) or directly into the middle hepatic vein (i.e., segment V or VIII), are identified. Additionally, the portal vein confluence is identified and the segmental branching patterns are evaluated, especially branches to the medial aspect of the left lobe (i.e., segment IV). For left lobectomies, the middle hepatic vein should be fully evaluated. In addition, the left portal vein should be assessed, particularly branches supplying the medial aspect of the left lobe (i.e., segment IV).

Cholecystectomy and Cholangiography

After these initial steps, cholecystectomy and cystic duct cannulation are performed for cholangiography. The biliary anatomy is clearly visualized via fluoroscopy at multiple angles to best discern the anatomical relationships and to make a more informed operative plan. When necessary, a noncrushing clamp can be placed across the distal end of the common bile duct to enhance the flow of dye into the intrahepatic branches. A perfectly clear understanding of the individual donor's biliary anatomy is critical for success in both the donor and recipient. The catheter is left in place for a completion cholangiogram just before abdominal closure.

Right Lobectomy

Mobilization

After cholangiography is completed, attention is directed to mobilization of the liver from its lateral attachments so that the liver can be shifted up toward the donor's left side. The left triangular and gastrohepatic ligaments are left intact so that the remnant left lobe will not be excessively mobile. This approach partially exposes the right lateral aspect of the retrohepatic inferior vena cava.

With the right lobe fully mobilized from its lateral, posterior, and inferior peritoneal attachments, attention is directed to the retrohepatic vena cava. Inferior right hepatic veins that are identified on preoperative imaging to run deep into segments VI or VII are preserved for reimplantation in the recipient. Smaller tributaries are identified, ligated, and divided, and the retrohepatic inferior vena cava is exposed (Fig. 45–6). By defining and dividing the posterior caval ligament, which often contains a small vessel, the uppermost portion of the retrohepatic vena cava and the right hepatic vein are fully exposed. Anteriorly, the window between the right and middle hepatic veins is developed to facilitate full exposure and vascular control of the right hepatic vein.

Hilar Dissection

Attention is next directed to the hilum of the liver. The dissection begins by lowering the hilar plate just to the left of the gallbladder fossa. The right hepatic artery, just to the right of the common hepatic bile duct, is fully defined and carefully dissected free (Fig. 45–7). Manipulation of the artery itself is purposefully minimized. Particular attention is paid to identifying and preserving any segment IV arterial branches that may arise proximally.

Next, the right portal vein is identified posterior to the right hepatic artery and only on the right side of the common bile duct. The right portal vein should initially

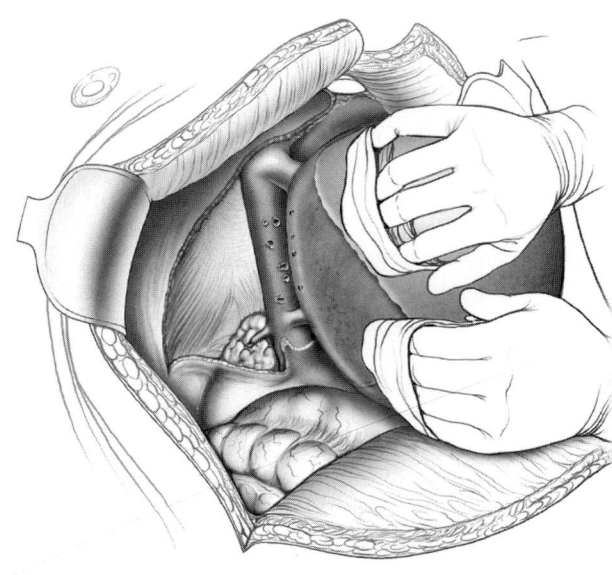

FIGURE 45–6

The lateral attachments are divided, and the right lobe is mobilized to the left. The right hepatic vein and the retrohepatic inferior vena cava are exposed, and small venous tributaries are ligated and divided.

be approached laterally and then be fully dissected circumferentially. Small caudate branches from the right portal vein are ligated and divided, but this does not adversely affect viability of the caudate lobe.[38]

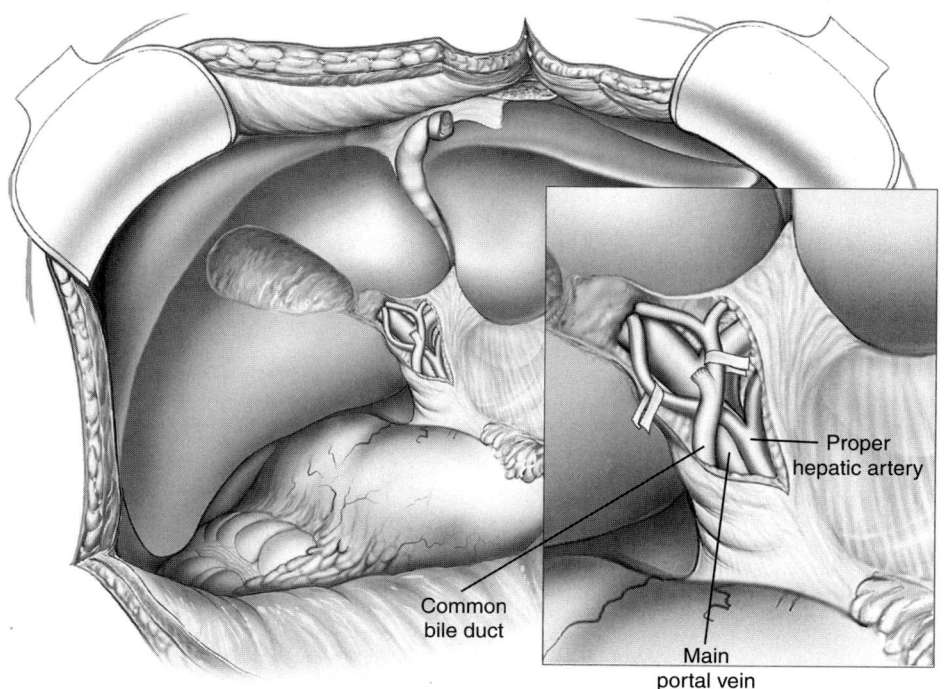

Common bile duct

Proper hepatic artery

Main portal vein

FIGURE 45–7

The gastroduodenal ligament is opened, and the main hilar structures are exposed at the level of the hilar plate.

The confluence of the right portal vein, left portal vein, and main portal vein should be exposed and clearly identified during this dissection.

Throughout the hilar dissection, extreme care should be exercised around the common bile duct to avoid devascularization. With the hilar plate lowered and mobilized anteriorly and posteriorly just above the caudate lobe, the entire plate is bluntly encircled just within the hepatic parenchyma. When exactly in the procedure the bile duct is transected varies from surgeon to surgeon. In general, we have divided the bile duct after completion of the hilar dissection to facilitate placement of an umbilical tape during the parenchymal transection (see later) and to maintain the correct transection plane. Others have advocated waiting until the parenchymal transection is nearly complete.[87]

Bile Duct Transection

By intraoperative cholangiography and direct visualization, an experienced hepatobiliary surgeon should be able to clearly define the biliary anatomy and perform a safe and accurate transection of the donor bile duct. Technically, it is imperative that the periductal blood supply be preserved as best as possible. The hepatic duct bifurcation receives blood via a periductal plexus fed by arterial branches from the left hepatic, right hepatic, caudate, and gastroduodenal arteries; as a consequence of the donor operation, the blood supply to the cut edge of the donor right hepatic duct of the graft depends entirely on the right hepatic artery.[88] Minimal manipulation of periductal tissue, avoidance of electrocautery, and sharp transection of the duct are important principles. Local ischemia of the cut edge of the donor duct is probably an important etiologic factor in the development of both biliary leaks and strictures.

The bile duct is transected after completing the hilar dissection and before starting the parenchymal division. Once the duct has been partially transected, it may be possible to change course slightly to best ensure transection in the common portion of the right hepatic duct in patients with an early bifurcation of the anterior and posterior branches. A margin of 2 mm or so of the right hepatic duct should be left to provide ample room to close the duct without compromising the donor's hepatic duct confluence. With an adequate stump, it is safe and more secure to suture the hepatic duct stump in longitudinal fashion.

After transection of the bile duct, there is often a modest amount of bleeding, which is good. Hemostasis should be achieved with fine periductal sutures, both on the donated side and on the remnant side of the liver. The remnant side should be probed to ensure that the point of duct transection has not compromised the donor's common hepatic duct or, in the case of right lobectomy, the donor's left hepatic duct. It is far better to recognize this complication intraoperatively than to discover it postoperatively. Donors have required T tubes or even Roux-en-Y hepaticojejunostomies as a result of encroachment on the common hepatic duct. The open duct or ducts on the side of the donor should be oversewn, and a careful search along the hilar plate for small, missed transected ducts should be done repeatedly throughout the remainder of the procedure.

Inspection of the hilar plate of the graft should allow the surgeon to make an accurate assessment of what reconstructions will be necessary in the recipient. When the procedures are performed simultaneously, this information should be relayed to the recipient surgical team as soon as possible so that when appropriate and possible, the recipient's native biliary tree may be preserved and used in the reconstruction after graft implantation.

Parenchymal Transection

Establishing the proper line for parenchymal transection is essential to successful liver splitting. Just a few millimeters can make a significant difference, and it is imperative to preserve the base of segment V and VIII venous tributaries as they enter the middle hepatic vein. Working in a plane several millimeters to the right can leave one with multiple unreconstructable tributaries. For donor right lobectomy, there has been considerable debate over the exact plane of transection. The central issue in this debate is less about parenchymal mass and more about whether to include the entire middle hepatic vein with the graft. When the middle hepatic vein is not included in the graft, the correct plane should be directly on the right border of the middle hepatic vein (Fig. 45–8). To begin, it is useful to transiently clamp the right hepatic artery and right portal vein to observe and score a line of demarcation.

The parenchymal transection is performed with electrocautery for the first 3 to 5 mm of parenchyma. Further dissection is performed by using a combination of the Cavitron ultrasonic surgical aspirator (CUSA), clamp-crush technique, and electrocautery. Portal structures, biliary radicals, and small venous tributaries are, whenever possible, individually identified and ligated with surgical clips or fine sutures, or with both. At the level of the hilar plate, care must be taken with the parenchyma immediately surrounding the bile ducts because electrocautery may injure the bile duct or its blood supply (or both).

To facilitate maintaining the correct parenchymal transection plane, we routinely pass an umbilical tape between the right and middle hepatic veins (anteriorly) and then behind the posterior aspect of the right lobe along the anterior wall of the inferior vena cava. The tape is then brought out at the level of the hilum behind the hilar plate (Fig. 45–9). This technique is useful to keep the vasculature down, out of the way,

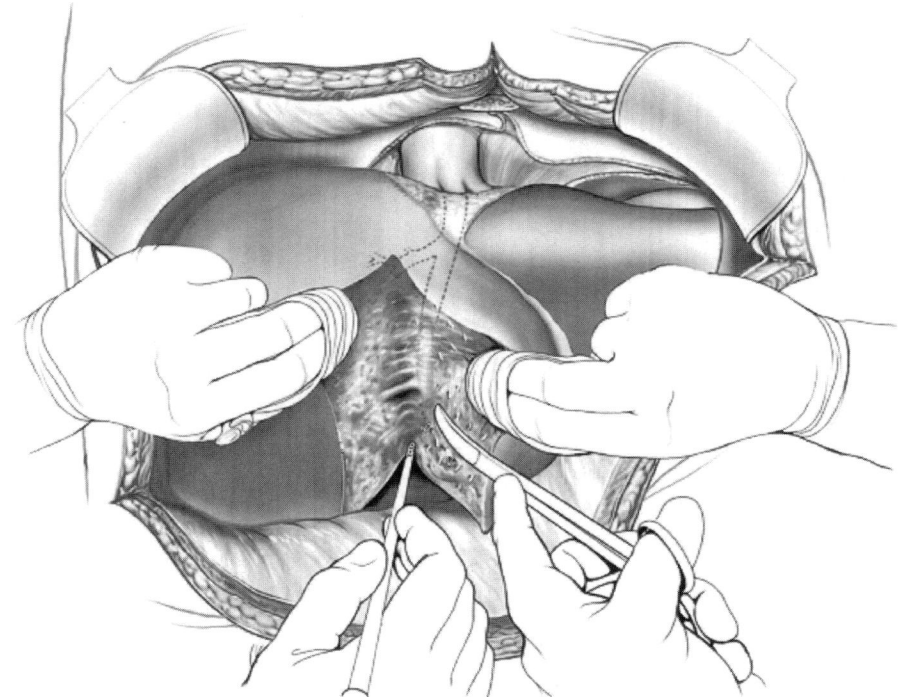

FIGURE 45-8

The parenchymal transection proceeds in a plane directly along the right border of the middle hepatic vein. (From Miller CM, Gondolesi GE, Florman S, et al: One hundred nine living donor liver transplants in adults and children: A single-center experience. Ann Surg 234:301-312, 2001.)

and the parenchyma that needs to be transected up in the field. Once the parenchymal transection is complete, the right lobe is attached to the remnant left lobe only by the vasculature.

Regardless of the technique, certain general principles are important. The patient is placed in a slight Trendelenburg position, about 15 degrees, and low CVP (2 to 4 mm Hg) is maintained during the transection to avoid excessive blood loss and to reduce the potential for air embolization.[89] CVP can be maintained by a variety of techniques, including adjustments in the inhaled anesthetic agents, as well as diuretics and rationing of intravenous fluids. It is imperative that the anesthesia team be experienced in these techniques and have expert understanding of the specific considerations with hepatic resections.

Many surgeons avoid even temporary inflow occlusion (i.e., Pringle's maneuver) during the parenchymal transection in the belief that transient warm ischemia may be detrimental to the donor remnant liver, as well as the donated segment.[75] Successful use of inflow occlusion has, however, been reported in living donors without adverse effect on the donor or the graft.[90,91] It is very useful to decrease blood loss. Furthermore, there is now evidence that intermittent inflow occlusion may in fact be beneficial in terms of outcomes and may have a preconditioning effect on the liver.[90,92,93]

Segments V and VIII venous tributaries draining into the middle hepatic vein are meticulously dissected free and preserved for possible reimplantation in the recipient to provide optimal venous drainage. Reconstructions can be completed in a variety of ways with a variety of conduits. Recently procured deceased donor artery or vein grafts, or both, preferably of compatible blood type, are optimal conduits. When unavailable, the donor inferior mesenteric vein and the recipient inferior mesenteric or saphenous vein are reasonable substitutes. In one case we even used a large, recannulated recipient umbilical vein as a conduit. Finally, a variety of prosthetic grafts are available but should be used only when autogenous grafts are not available or adequate.

An adept surgeon must have a fluid understanding of hepatic hemodynamics for real success with partial-liver grafts. Intraoperative ultrasonography can provide invaluable information for surgeons. A variety of intra-operative techniques can be used to determine the adequacy of graft venous drainage. The anterior segments of the right lobe (i.e., V and VIII) are at greatest risk. Grafts with obvious impairment may have demarcated congested areas.[94] After parenchymal transection, the right hepatic artery should be temporarily occluded so that segmental portal flow can be evaluated.[80,95] Persistent hepatopedal flow with temporary arterial occlusion suggests the presence of adequate intrahepatic venous collaterals for drainage without reconstruction. This simple test is invaluable in cases in which the importance of a segmental venous tributary is in question, and it remains the best measure of significance.

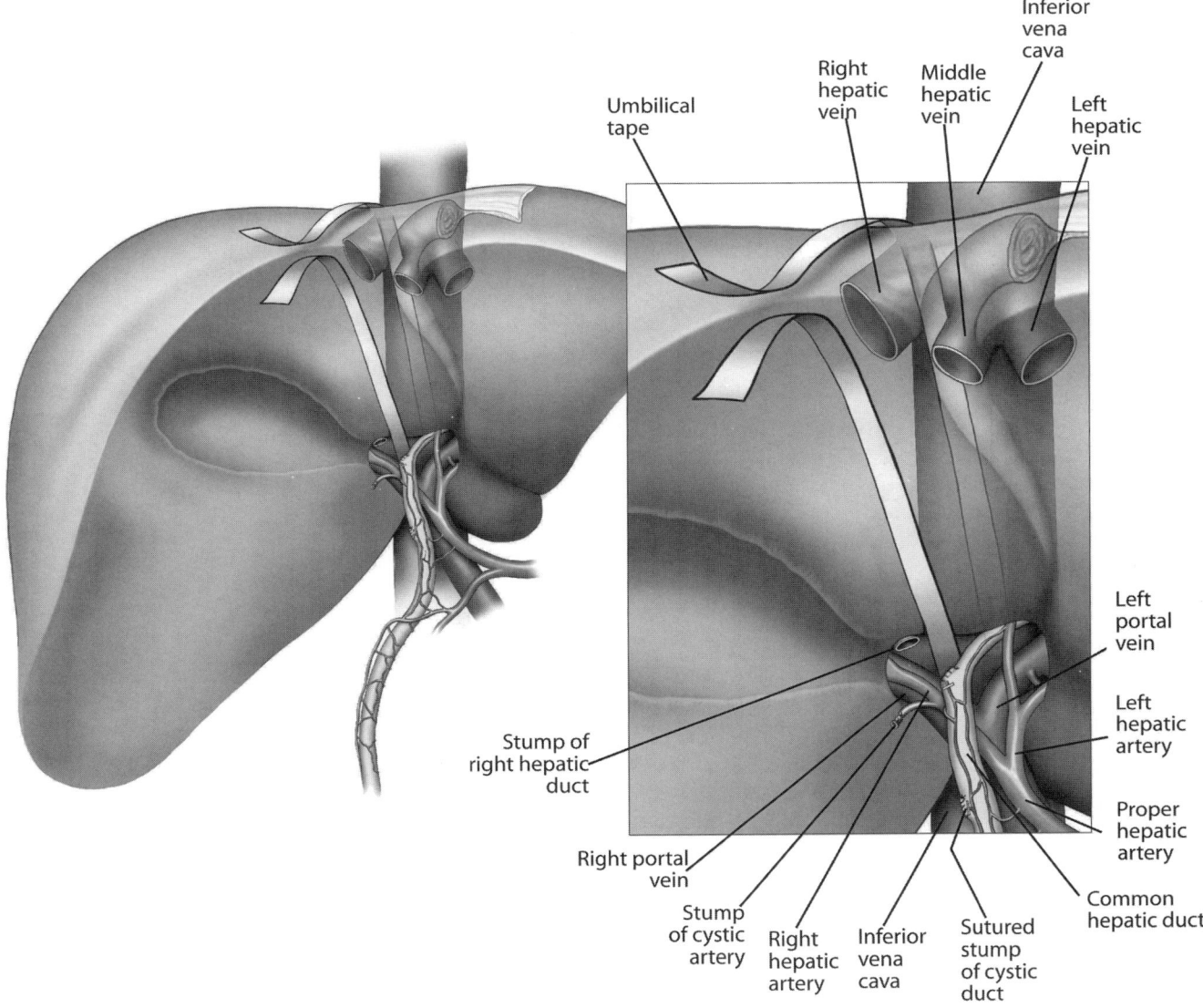

FIGURE 45–9

Umbilical tape is passed between the right and middle hepatic veins, along the retrohepatic inferior vena cava, and brought up between the right and left portal veins and hepatic arteries to assist in the parenchymal transection.

Left Lobectomy

The basic surgical techniques for left lobectomy are similar to those for right lobectomy as described. The following are technical points for donor left lobectomy that vary from those of right lobectomy.

Mobilization

After initial exploration, cholecystectomy and intraoperative cholangiography are performed. The gastrohepatic ligament is then divided while carefully identifying and preserving any accessory or replaced left hepatic artery from the left gastric artery within this ligament. The left triangular ligament is also divided, and the junction of the left hepatic vein with the suprahepatic vena cava is defined.

Hilar Dissection

The hilar dissection is begun on the medial aspect of the left side of the hilum, and the left hepatic artery is isolated. Care is taken to identify separate segment IV arterial branches that may be present. Additionally, any accessory or replaced left hepatic arteries are identified in the hepatogastric ligament. These arteries are branches of the left gastric artery, and when isolating these vessels, small branches to the stomach should be ligated and divided.

The left portal vein is identified medial and posterior to the left hepatic artery and dissected circumferentially. A significant length of extrahepatic left portal vein should be easily isolated. In most cases the caudate lobe should be included, and drainage of the caudate lobe should be optimized by preserving for reconstruction the largest vein that drains directly into the vena cava.[96] Couinaud reported that nearly 70% of caudate lobes have a single, dominant vein directly draining the caudate lobe into the vena cava.[97]

Retrohepatic Dissection

The peritoneum directly overlying the infrahepatic vena cava is opened anteriorly and extended cephalad along the left lateral aspect of the retrohepatic vena cava up to the level of the insertion of the left hepatic vein into the vena cava. The entire left lobe and caudate lobe can then be retracted further laterally to expose any left lobe veins draining directly into the vena cava (Fig. 45–10). The left and middle hepatic veins are isolated as they enter the vena cava.

Bile Duct Transection

Of major concern with left lobe donation is the vascular integrity of the biliary tree of segment IV. This portion of the left lobe biliary tree may have significant arterial supply from the right hepatic artery,[88] and therefore the arterial supply to segment IV should be meticulously preserved. This is also the basis for which accessory medial left lobe arteries are reconstructed by some centers whenever present.[98] The left hepatic duct should be transected sharply. Care must be taken to avoid injuring a right posterior hepatic duct that arises from the left hepatic duct, a well-known anomaly.

Parenchymal Transection

The principles and the line of parenchymal transection are similar for right and left lobectomies (see earlier)—along the right border of the middle hepatic vein.

Graft Removal

After the parenchymal transection is completed, hemostasis is achieved. Electrocautery, direct suture ligation, hemostatic agents (e.g., Surgicel, Gel-foam, thrombin), and argon beam coagulation are the mainstays of establishing hemostasis. The argon beam coagulator (Valley Lab, Boulder, CO) is particularly useful for controlling small vessel oozing. Hemostasis is critical because the best way to identify open bile ducts is in a completely dry operative field. Communication with the recipient operating room, when cases are occurring simultaneously, is critical for success. Knowledge of potential reconstructions can be important for planning recipient caval clamp placement, preparing interposition grafts, and deciding on the use of venovenous bypass.

At the appropriate time, the hepatic artery is ligated proximally and divided. Next, the portal vein is ligated

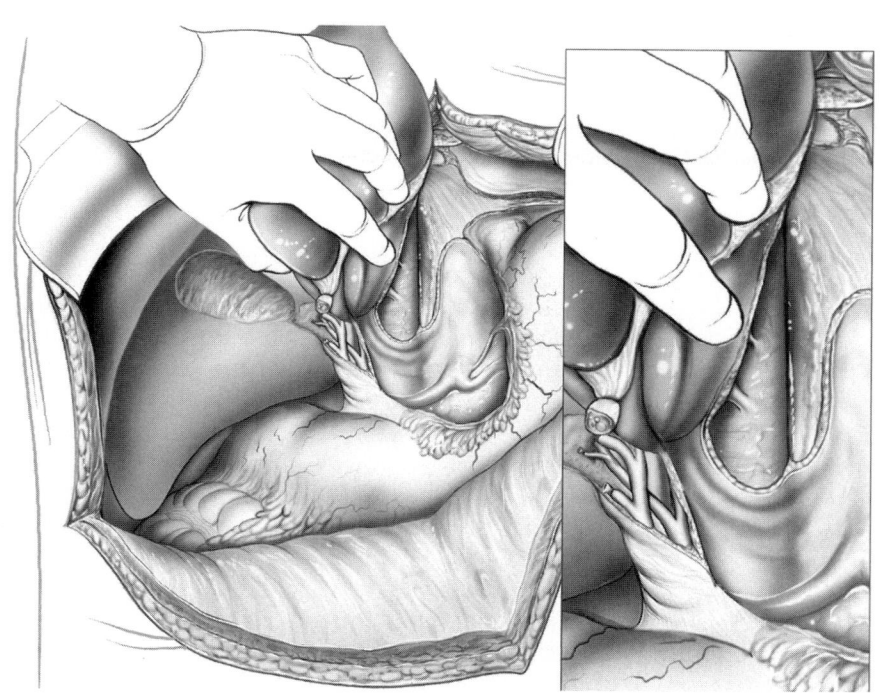

FIGURE 45–10

With the left triangular ligament divided, the left lobe is retracted to the right and the retrohepatic inferior vena cava is exposed.

and divided, with care taken to avoid compromise of the donor's main portal vein. When the right portal vein is absent and the right anterior portal vein branch arises directly from the left portal vein, the right anterior and posterior portal veins are transected separately. Proper placement of the portal clamp is critical because angulation of the clamp may cause encroachment when the stump of the portal vein is oversewn, which could lead to stenosis or even thrombosis. By clamping the portal vein vertically, as opposed to the traditional horizontal clamp placement, the diameter of the portal vein is increased.[99]

In right lobe cases, preserved accessory venous tributaries are clamped and divided, and a clamp is placed tangentially on the inferior vena cava around the orifice of the right hepatic vein, which is subsequently divided. In left lobe cases, the caval clamp is placed tangentially around the confluence of the left and middle hepatic veins, which are subsequently divided. Although some surgeons administer systemic heparin to the donor before clamping and dividing the vasculature, we have not found such administration to be necessary.

Additional Operative Considerations

After removal of the graft from the donor, there are additional technical considerations. The stump of the hepatic vein or veins is oversewn with monofilament suture. The main portal trunk and remaining left or right portal vein should be inspected to ensure hemostasis and the absence of any compromise that might be of hemodynamic significance. Hemostasis of the remnant liver must be absolute to best determine the presence of small bile leaks. The cut edge of the liver, as well as the hilar plate, should be evaluated for bile staining. Gently placing a clean laparotomy pad against the cut edge and hilar plate of the liver is a good technique to identify small open biliary radicals, which should be ligated with suture.

Completion cholangiography is performed to ensure that there is no narrowing of the donor's bile duct and to identify occult bile leaks that may be corrected at this time. In addition, completion ultrasonography is performed to ensure that venous drainage of the remnant segments is not compromised and that portal and arterial flow is good. The falciform ligament is reapproximated to the anterior abdominal wall to prevent torsion of the left lobe remnant, which can be a disastrous complication.[100] A closed suction drain is placed alongside the cut edge of the liver and brought out through the anterior abdominal wall.

Rarely, a donor will require blood transfusion in addition to the autologous blood that may previously have been given. In our experience, only two right lobe donors required such a transfusion.[26] Brown and coauthors reported a nearly 5% incidence in 449 adult-to-adult living donors in the United States,[101] whereas Lo reported a 0.5% incidence in more than 1500 living donors (all graft types) in Asia for transfusion from the blood bank.[102]

Back-Table Procedure

Before the graft is removed from the donor, the back-table should be inspected by a member of the surgical team for the appropriate cannulas, instruments, solutions, ice, and so forth. Once removed, the partial graft is immediately brought to the back-table for flushing with preservative solution. The graft is submerged in chilled heparinized solution and flushed through the stump of the portal vein. The flushing continues until the effluent from the hepatic vein or veins is clear, which usually requires 500 to 1000 mL for a right lobe graft. After this flushing, the hepatic artery may be flushed with another 50 to 100 mL of solution, with care taken to avoid injuring the intima of this small vessel. A biopsy specimen is taken and sent for histological and microbiological studies.

Significant venous tributaries of the middle hepatic vein are reconstructed at this time. In some cases, portal venous or hepatic arterial reconstructions (or both) are performed on the back-table. Finally, the graft is weighed, submersed in preservative solution, packed in ice, and taken to the recipient operating room. In general, left lobe grafts are more likely to require hepatic arterial reconstructions and right lobe grafts are more likely to require portal venous reconstructions.

Postoperative Management

Certain aspects of postoperative care after living donor lobectomy merit special emphasis. Living donors are a unique group of patients because they are healthy individuals who would otherwise not be hospitalized or having an operation. As a result, their postoperative expectations differ drastically from those of other patients. In particular, their pain threshold is generally much lower, and they do not easily assume the classic sick role because they have previously been healthy.[103] Pain management issues should ideally be discussed with living donors preoperatively. It has been our preference to have an epidural placed immediately preoperatively.

Donors should be monitored closely during their immediate postoperative course for signs of hepatic insufficiency. Frequent laboratory studies, including liver function tests, creatinine, and prothrombin time, are important. The nasogastric tube placed intraoperatively should remain in place until the return of bowel function (i.e., passage of flatus). Lower extremity sequential compression devices should remain in place until patients are ambulatory. Acid-blocking agents are administered until hepatic function is restored, and they are discontinued before resuming an oral diet. Incentive spirometry is encouraged to prevent atelectasis. Prophylactic antibiotics, begun immediately preoperatively, are continued for 24 to 48 hours postoperatively. Stool softeners should be prescribed liberally because general anesthesia, intraoperative manipulation of the intestines, and narcotics all contribute to the high likelihood of constipation postoperatively. Donors should be encouraged to ambulate early postoperatively. The financial pressures that exist to expedite a patient's discharge should not apply to living donors. These special patients should be ambulatory, tolerate a regular diet, and have full return of bowel function before discharge.

Adult Living Donor Liver Recipient Procedure

Perioperative Considerations

General patient evaluation, selection, and management are discussed in Chapter 44. Significant emphasis must be placed on determining recipient factors that can influence graft function, particularly the degree of portal hypertension and the severity of illness.

Ideally, the recipient is brought to the operating room at the same time as the donor to allow ischemia time to be minimized. The only exception is recipients with tumors, particularly those greater than stage T1. In these cases, because of the risk of extrahepatic tumor spread, the recipient is explored before the donor procedure begins. At exploration through a limited right subcostal incision, the porta hepatis is palpated, and any suspicious nodes undergo biopsy and are sent for frozen section diagnosis. Once extrahepatic disease is excluded, the procedure proceeds and the incision is extended to a full bilateral subcostal incision with midline extension. At the same time, the donor surgeons are notified to begin. All recipients with tumors, as well as their donors, should understand explicitly that if extrahepatic tumor is identified, the transplantation is aborted.

Hepatectomy

In general, hepatectomy for the recipient of a partial-liver graft is similar to that for a whole-organ transplant with caval preservation (a.k.a., piggyback).[104,105] There are, however, several important considerations that do not necessarily apply to the standard transplant hepatectomy. The main technical principle is to preserve

implantation options by maintaining the length and integrity of all hilar structures. The right and left hepatic arteries should be individually ligated as high in the hilum as possible. When accessory or replaced arteries are present, they too should be left long. Similarly, at the appropriate time in the procedure, the right and left portal veins should be isolated as high as possible and individually ligated.

Furthermore, and perhaps most difficult technically, the right and left hepatic ducts, as well as the cystic duct, should be divided individually while preserving their supraduodenal blood supply (see Fig. 45–1). Makuuchi has even made an effort to preserve the entire hilar plate with eight separate biliary orifices to fully maximize options.[106] The vascular integrity of the native bile ducts should be preserved by avoiding unnecessary dissection of the tissues immediately surrounding the ducts.

When the arterial, venous, and biliary structures are preserved, a variety of options remain when the partial graft is implanted. After completion of the hilar dissection, the lateral attachments of the liver are divided and the right lobe is mobilized. Caval preservation is imperative, although there are reports of caval replacement in unusual circumstances.[107] All short hepatic venous tributaries are ligated. The right, middle, and left hepatic veins are isolated. Additionally, vascular control of the vena cava is established both above and below the level of the hepatic veins.

An important aspect of living donor liver transplantation is assessment of recipient splanchnic flow at the beginning of the recipient hepatectomy, as well as throughout the transplant procedure. This assessment may include an evaluation of the cardiac index and continuous measurement of portal pressure via a catheter placed through the inferior mesenteric vein into the base of the portal vein. With continuous measurement, the utility of pharmacological or surgical inflow modification (or both) can be assessed and altered.

Anhepatic Strategies

A variety of techniques have been described for dealing with recipient portal inflow once the diseased liver is removed. Venovenous bypass has been used by different centers in all cases, selectively, and only in rare circumstances. The arguments for using bypass in all cases are mainly prevention of intestinal edema and preservation of recipient hemodynamic stability. In our experience, we began using bypass after performing nearly 40 adult living donor transplants and then used it selectively.

Bypass is not, however, without risks, including air embolism, fibrinolysis, hemolysis, platelet trapping, hypothermia, and brachial plexopathies.[79,108-113] Fan reports that recipients of living donor right lobe grafts in whom venovenous bypass was used had worse outcomes with higher mortality and worse postoperative hepatic and renal function.[79] The majority of appropriately managed recipients tolerate portal clamping without hemodynamic instability. Most graft implantations require less than 60 minutes to perform, although multiple reconstructions may require additional time. It has therefore become our preference to use venovenous bypass only when absolutely necessary.

It is important during the anhepatic phase to accurately assess portal inflow. As previously discussed, even large grafts with a very high GRWR may be severely adversely affected by excessive inflow.[69] Graft function is intimately related to both inflow and outflow. Normal hepatic parenchymal inflow is approximately 1.2 mL/g/min.[114] For partial grafts in cirrhotic recipients, inflow should be maintained at less than 2.6 mL/g/min and ideally at less than 2 mL/g/min.[115] When inflow is excessive, parenchymal portal overflow and shear stress create a phenomenon that may cause graft dysfunction and functional small-for-size syndrome.[69,76,116]

To prevent portal overflow, a variety of surgical and pharmacological techniques are potentially useful. Octreotide, a somatostatin analogue known to decrease mesenteric flow, may provide a temporary decrease in portal flow. In our experience, however, its effects have been brief and erratic, and it rarely provides durable improvement. Temporary portocaval shunting at the time of native hepatectomy may be performed. Because the liver graft begins to accommodate virtually instantaneously to the higher portal inflow of the recipient,[82] temporary shunts may be useful in select cases, depending on the degree of portal hypertension.

Creation of a permanent shunt for inflow modification may have a role in certain cases. A variety of shunts have been used for this purpose, including mesocaval, portocaval, and splenorenal shunts.[69,117] In addition, successful splenic artery ligation has been reported to decrease portal inflow.[71] Optimal hemodynamic manipulation and management of the partial-liver graft remain elusive. Clearly, however, portal inflow and hepatic venous outflow are important determinants of graft function. As our understanding of these issues improves, it may eventually become possible to use smaller grafts, which are associated with lower donor morbidity. The determination of which grafts require inflow modification and which type of modification to use is multifactorial. Intraoperative measurement of portal flow provides a means to assess the effectiveness of any pharmacological or surgical interventions.

Graft Implantation

Caval Drainage

One of the more important technical aspects of partial-graft implantation is caval drainage. The same technical principles developed for implantation of left lateral segments and left lobes in pediatric patients are important for success in the transplantation of partial grafts in adults.[118] It is imperative that these grafts have optimal outflow. In this respect, not only is the anastomosis important, but the ultimate positioning of the graft can also play an important role in outflow, both immediately and during the first 2 to 3 weeks of maximum liver regeneration. The graft should be placed in an orthotopic position, and care should be taken to consider the final position of the graft once the abdomen is closed. This principle cannot be overemphasized because relatively small changes in graft positioning can have a dramatic impact on venous drainage.

Located posteriorly and inferiorly along the medial aspect of the right lobe graft is the caval groove, or indentation, where the donor's vena cava ran. This groove is an important landmark and should be used for orientation and alignment of the right lobe graft with the recipient's vena cava. The anastomotic site of the donor right hepatic vein is positioned on the recipient vena cava to maintain this alignment. The orifice of the recipient's right hepatic vein is maximally extended onto the vena cava caudally and to the left to provide optimal graft outflow (Fig. 45–11). It is important to realize that regeneration causes the right lobe graft to axially rotate from right to left. Additionally, the right hepatic vein of the graft should be short, even flush with the graft, to ensure that twisting cannot compromise venous outflow.

After completion of the right hepatic vein anastomoses, significant venous tributaries are reconstructed. The orifice of the recipient's middle hepatic vein provides a favorable position for drainage of segment V or VIII interposition grafts (Fig. 45–12). Occasionally, a composite reconstruction is necessary, particularly when multiple reconstructions need to be performed. Significant segment VI (i.e., the inferior right hepatic) veins can be anastomosed directly to the recipient vena cava, usually without any need for an interposition graft (see Fig. 45–12). It is often best to complete these caval implantations before anastomosis of the main right hepatic vein.

Left lobe graft implantation has significantly different considerations. The left lobe must be held in the appropriate anatomical position during implantation. Ultimately, the ligamentum teres is reaffixed to the anterior abdominal wall, thereby holding the graft in place (Fig. 45–13). The temporary use of a tissue expander has even been reported as a means to maintain the position of small left lobes and to slowly obliterate the dead space in the right upper quadrant.[119] Alignment of the hepatic venous anastomosis, as well as the portal venous anastomosis, may be technically more challenging than that for the right lobe graft. The confluence of the left and middle hepatic veins of the

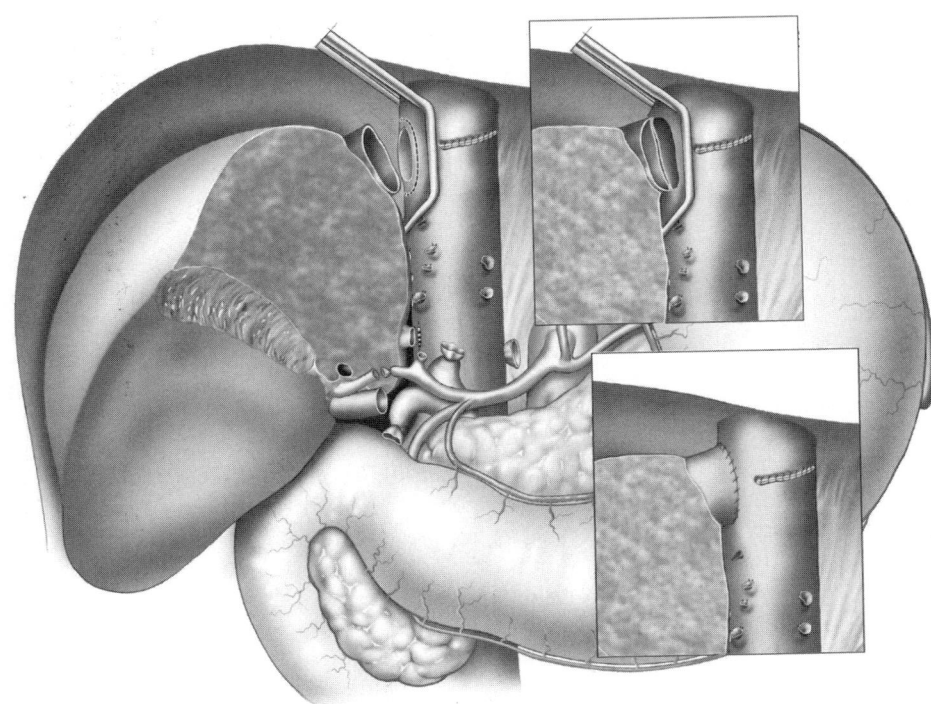

FIGURE 45–11

The right hepatic vein orifice of the recipient is opened caudally to optimize venous drainage of the right lobe graft.

graft is anastomosed to the anterior wall of the vena cava where the orifices of the recipient's left and middle hepatic veins have been joined and, when necessary, opened to the right or caudally to maximize venous outflow. Because the left lobe graft contains the middle hepatic vein, venous outflow is generally excellent.

When the caudate lobe is included with the left lobe graft, venous drainage of the caudate lobe should be considered. In these cases, the most significant (i.e., largest diameter) short hepatic venous tributary from the caudate lobe is directly reconstructed to the vena cava to optimize caudate drainage.[65,96] Poor caudate

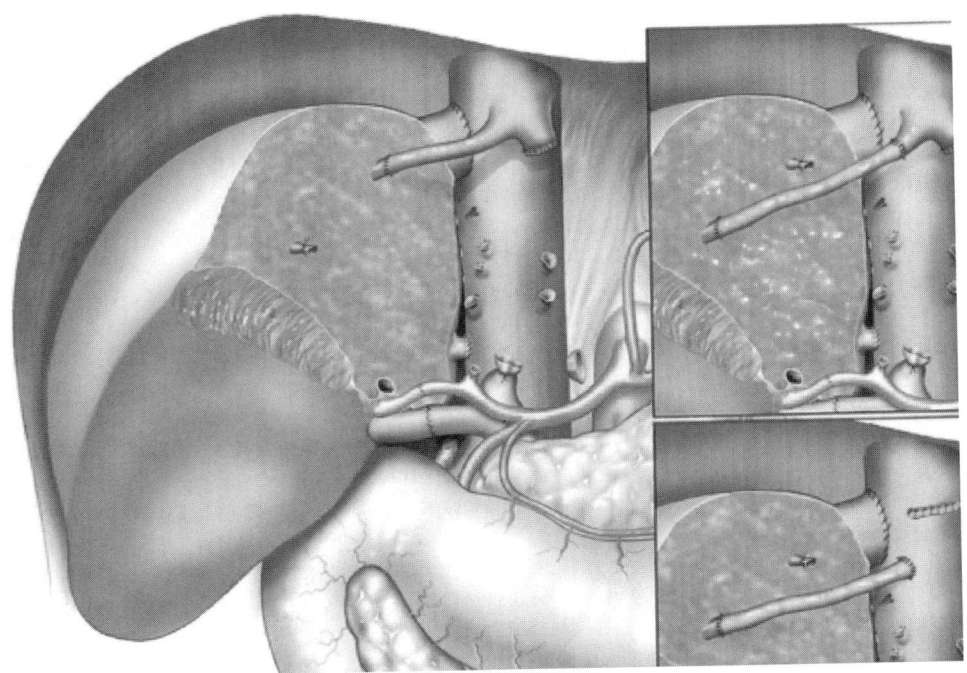

FIGURE 45–12

Venous reconstruction of significant segment V and VIII tributaries to the middle hepatic vein stump and directly to the inferior vena cava, as well as reconstruction of the segment VI tributary directly to the vena cava. (From Miller CM, Gondolesi GE, Florman S, et al: One hundred nine living donor liver transplants in adults and children: A single-center experience. Ann Surg 234: 301-312, 2001.)

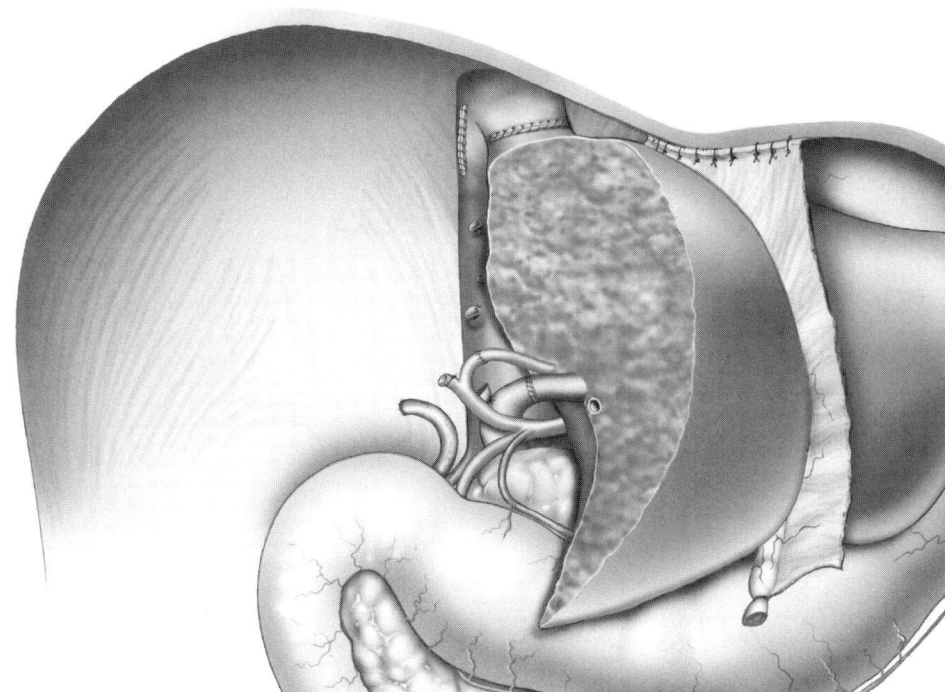

FIGURE 45–13

With the vascular anastomoses complete, the ligamentum teres of the graft is reapproximated to the anterior abdominal wall of the recipient.

regeneration has been reported when this reconstruction has not been performed.[67]

Portal Venous Reconstruction

In the majority of right lobe cases, a single portal reconstruction is typically performed between the donor right portal vein and the recipient main portal vein. Occasionally, the recipient's right portal vein is a better size match or is aligned in an anatomically more favorable position than the main portal vein (or both). These anastomoses are generally performed in running fashion with 6–0 Prolene sutures and incorporation of a "growth factor."[120]

Infrequently, the right lobe graft has separate right anterior and posterior portal veins that require reconstruction and anastomosis. There are several options to deal with this reconstruction. It is still possible to create a single portal orifice in most cases by performing venoplasty of the anterior and posterior branches to make a single lumen for the anastomosis.[38,42] When not achievable, it may be possible to anastomose the native right and left portal veins directly to the right lobe graft's posterior and anterior branches, respectively. The alignment with this reconstruction, however, is never quite perfect.

To correct rotational misalignment, it is better to resect the bifurcation of the recipient's portal vein and then attach this Y-graft to the liver graft's anterior and posterior portal veins on the back-table.[43] Similarly, a bifurcated iliac vein graft from a recent deceased donor may be used. The external and internal iliac vein limbs of the graft should be fashioned in a manner that circumvents redundancy or twisting (or both) of the anterior and posterior right portal veins. In the recipient, the common iliac portion of the vein graft can be anastomosed to the main portal vein at a convenient place.

Left lobe cases almost always require only a single portal reconstruction between the graft left portal vein and the recipient's left or main portal vein. Alignment is critical and should take into account future left-to-right graft rotation as a result of regeneration, particularly when performing the portal venous reconstruction. It is better for the left lobe graft portal anastomosis to be a little long, but not redundant. When too short, there can be significant problems as the graft regenerates and rotates.

Recipients with portal vein thrombosis, once thought to be an absolute contraindication to the already technically challenging living donor procedure, have been successfully transplanted with partial grafts from living donors.[121] Although these cases are more challenging and associated with worse overall results, they are not absolutely contraindicated.[122,123] Similar to whole-organ deceased donor transplantation, either endovenectomy or mesenteric interposition grafts are necessary. Patients who require caval transposition or arterialization of the portal vein, or both, are at significantly higher risk for morbidity and mortality and are, perhaps, inappropriate candidates for living donor partial-graft transplantation.

Arterial Reconstruction

The technical aspects of arterial reconstruction are important and critical for success. The donor vessel is thin and small, often only 2 to 5 mm in diameter, and relatively short in length as well.[124] These small anastomoses are generally performed in an interrupted fashion with 7-0 or 8-0 Prolene sutures and the use of surgical loupe magnification or the operating microscope. In many Japanese centers, a separate microsurgical team performs the microscopic reconstruction. With microsurgical techniques, extremely small arteries can be anastomosed with excellent patency. Arguably, however, the most important determinant for successful reconstruction with partial-liver grafts is having options. When done well, the proper hepatic artery of the recipient has been dissected distally past the level of the bifurcation to right and left hepatic arteries.

In some cases, multiple donor hepatic arteries may be present. Whether all accessory vessels require reconstruction remains debatable.[98,124-126] There are, however, guidelines to help determine which vessels require reconstruction and which can simply be ligated. It should be assumed until proved otherwise that all hepatic arteries, including replaced and accessory arteries, are essential because hepatic arteries are end-vessels that supply specific areas of the liver. There may, however, be hilar or intrahepatic communications (or both) that provide collateral arterial supply to specific areas of the liver. These collaterals may be present normally but are not demonstrable with arteriography unless they are actively functioning as collaterals.[127] In cases with demonstrable collateral flow, it may be justifiable to ligate a smaller artery with redundant supply rather than perform a technically difficult and perhaps unnecessary reconstruction.

Because of the highly variable arterial supply to segment IV, left lobe grafts are more likely to require arterial reconstruction with more than one hepatic artery. This factor makes preoperative assessment of the arterial anatomy even more important for planned left lobectomy cases. Reconstruction should be performed whenever there is questionable compensatory collateral arterial circulation. Initially, when more than one artery is present, the artery with the largest diameter should be reconstructed first and attention then directed to the degree of pulsatile arterial flow that comes retrograde through the unreconstructed artery. If there is good pulsatile backflow, reconstruction of the smaller artery may not be necessary. Intraoperative Doppler ultrasound can be used to confirm arterial flow patterns to all segments of the liver graft to corroborate this decision. What impact this may or may not have on the arterial blood supply to segmental bile ducts is unclear.[98]

The majority of arterial reconstructions in right lobe cases can be performed to the recipient's right or proper hepatic artery. In some cases, it may be necessary to dissect the common hepatic artery more proximally, toward the aorta. The gastroduodenal artery can then be ligated and divided to release the hepatic artery and allow it more mobility and length to reach the hilum of the graft. It also allows for the anastomosis to be performed over a temporary stent inserted through the orifice of the gastroduodenal artery.[128] In addition, interposition grafts (e.g., saphenous vein, iliac vein, inferior mesenteric vein, inferior epigastric artery) can be used to provide length or to perform multiple arterial reconstructions. Occasionally, an aortic graft is necessary for the arterial reconstruction.

Although rarely necessary, there are several ways to manage reconstruction of multiple hepatic arteries in the right lobe recipient. Direct anastomosis of the two donor vessels to the right and left hepatic arteries of the recipient has been our standard approach. These anastomoses are technically more demanding because of the small caliber of the vessels and also because of their anatomical relationship to the portal vein. An alternative reconstruction has been described whereby the recipient's native proper hepatic artery is removed and, on the back-table under optimal conditions, anastomosed as a Y-graft to the two arteries of the graft. At implantation, a technically much easier anastomosis is fashioned between the autologous proper hepatic artery (now with the right lobe graft) and the native common hepatic artery at the origin of the gastroduodenal artery.[129] This approach has two potential downsides. First, it requires two anastomoses. Second, by removing the artery from the recipient, the native bile duct may be devascularized, thereby possibly committing the surgeon to performing a Roux-en-Y biliary reconstruction. In addition to these techniques, interposition grafts may be used in a variety of creative reconstructions, depending on the individual recipient's arterial anatomy.

Venous Congestion

One of the dreaded intraoperative complications of transplantation with a partial graft is venous congestion. Acutely, fresh transplants tolerate venous congestion poorly. With whole-organ liver transplantation, venous congestion is seen strictly as a technical complication of outflow at the level of the vena cava or at the confluence of the hepatic veins if the graft is implanted in piggyback fashion. When using partial grafts, however, congestion may result from portal flooding and appears identical to outflow restriction. It is crucial to determine and correct the proximate cause of congestion because either may doom the graft and recipient to small-for-size syndrome. With right lobe grafts, the anterior segments (i.e., V and VIII) are at considerable risk for congestion because they may have significant venous tributaries that once drained into the middle hepatic vein.[130]

When congestion is identified intraoperatively, there are several important considerations and potential interventions. The right hepatic vein–caval anastomosis should be assessed to ensure the absence of actual or functional obstruction to flow. Obstruction generally causes congestion of the entire right lobe graft. In addition, all venous reconstructions should be similarly assessed. Technical problems with the drainage of segmental venous tributaries often cause only segmental congestion. Intraoperative Doppler ultrasound to evaluate the hepatic veins for triphasic flow is useful in these situations.

Considerable literature now exists on the importance of venous drainage for partial-liver grafts, particularly right lobe grafts.[26,54,80,95,131] Venous congestion in the immediate postoperative period can be devastating for the partial-liver graft and even life-threatening for the recipient. Adequate venous drainage is essential for both liver function and regeneration. Inadequate segmental venous drainage directly reduces segmental portal flow and results in poor segmental regeneration. Even when grafts grossly appear well drained (i.e., not congested), regeneration may be impaired when venous drainage is not optimal,[131] hence the importance of segmental venous tributary reconstruction for partial grafts.

Biliary Reconstruction

Biliary reconstructions were once considered the "Achilles' heel" of deceased donor liver transplantation.[132] This is even more true for partial grafts, which often have multiple segmental ducts that require individual reconstruction. These segmental ducts are small, generally only 2 to 5 mm in diameter, and are cut flush with the hilar plate of the graft. These reconstructions are technically more demanding than the choledochocholedochostomy or Roux-en-Y hepaticojejunostomy of the standard whole-organ deceased donor transplant procedure. As a result, the incidence of biliary complications, including leaks and strictures, is considerably higher with living donor partial grafts.

In our experience, 60% of right lobe grafts required reconstruction of multiple ducts.[133] Bile leaks generally occurred early, with an incidence of approximately 20%. Biliary strictures usually occurred late, also with an incidence of approximately 20%.[133] In other large series, the overall incidence of biliary complications has varied considerably, with a range up to 60%.[57,134-136] It is critical that the biliary reconstruction be technically perfect and performed with the same skill as that for graft implantation. In some centers, a separate and rested microsurgical team performs the biliary reconstruction.

The standard biliary reconstruction with partial-liver grafts was originally the Roux-en-Y hepaticojejunostomy with or without stenting (Fig. 45–14). When fashioning the Roux-en-Y limb, it is imperative to remember to close the jejunal mesenteric defect as well as the transverse colonic mesenteric defect to prevent internal herniation. In preparing the Roux-en-Y limb for hepaticojejunostomy, we have used a serosa-splitting technique and tacked the mucosa to the serosa with fine, absorbable sutures.

More recently, with improved surgical techniques and preservation of the supraduodenal blood supply to the common hepatic duct, successful biliary reconstruction using the native bile duct or ducts with and without a T tube in both right and left lobe grafts has become standard.[133,137-141] To facilitate this approach, the recipient's hilar plate should be included en bloc with the common hepatic duct. The potential advantages of using the recipient bile duct for the reconstruction are that no enteric anastomoses are necessary, T-tube cholangiography and ERCP are then possible, and a functional sphincter of Oddi decreases the incidence of cholangitis.

Initially, duct-to-duct reconstruction was performed only in cases with a single donor duct. More recently, there have been reports of use of the recipient right and left hepatic ducts, as well as the cystic duct, when multiple anastomoses are required. Both duct-to-duct and Roux-en-Y reconstructions have been used in the same patient. An alternative option for reconstruction is end-to-side anastomosis of the bile ducts of the graft to the recipient's native common bile duct.[142] Several centers, including our own, have reported that the incidence of biliary complications increases with multiple reconstructions.[133,135,143] In our experience with nearly 100 right lobe grafts, slightly more than half were reconstructed with a Roux-en-Y limb, approximately 40% with a native duct-to-duct anastomosis, and the rest with a combination of both reconstructions.[133]

Regardless of which type of reconstruction is ultimately performed, certain principles apply to all biliary reconstructions. Preservation of the periductal blood supply and venous drainage is critical to success. Periductal parenchymal tissue is preserved with minimal manipulation and the avoidance of electrocautery. In addition, care is taken to avoid dissection between the distal right hepatic artery and the right hepatic duct. Sutures should not be placed too close together when performing the anastomosis because of the potential for ischemia. Creation of the jejunal opening

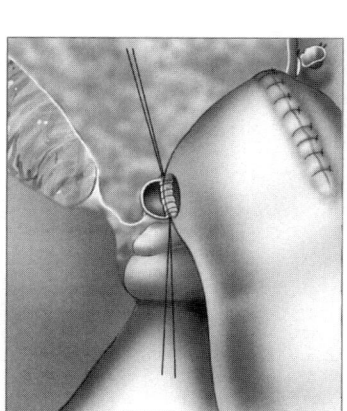

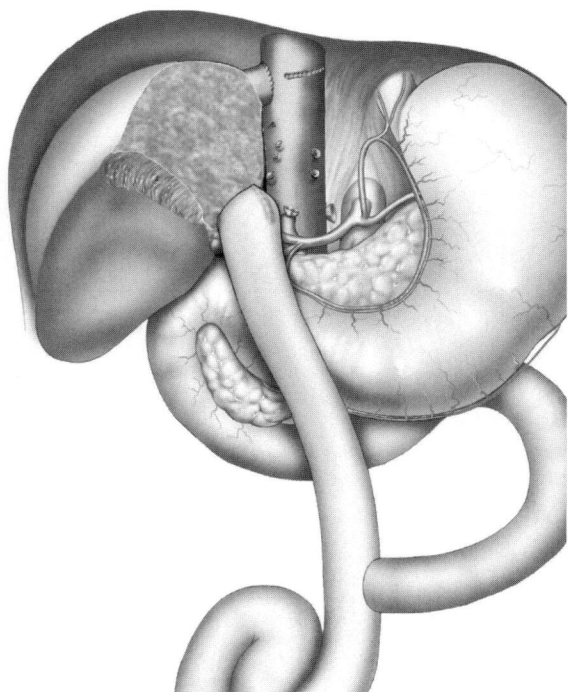

FIGURE 45–14

Roux-en-Y hepaticojejunostomy to a right lobe graft.

in reconstructions with hepaticojejunostomies should be done meticulously. Fan stresses the importance of making the jejunal opening the same size as the duct, without stretching the opening, which may lead to local tissue ischemia.[79]

Multiple ducts in close proximity and sharing a common wall should be syndactylized, or joined together, so that a single anastomosis can be performed. In these cases, the shared septum of the adjacent ducts may be divided vertically and then combined with fine absorbable sutures to create a single, large orifice for the anastomosis (Fig. 45–15).[143] When the shared medial wall of two adjoining ducts is simply sutured together, unnecessary tension is created on the lateral walls of both ducts, and the combined lumen size is smaller than when combined via the aforementioned technique. It is imperative to be sure that all ducts are identified in both the donor and the recipient. On rare occasion, a very small duct is identified in the recipient that was not identified in the donor, or vice versa. Some very small ducts may even be oversewn and not reconstructed.

In addition to meticulous preservation of the biliary microcirculation of both the recipient and, in duct-to-duct reconstructions, the donor, biliary decompression is an important component of successful reconstruction of these small segmental ducts. Decompression is achieved with either a small stent (e.g., a 5-French pediatric feeding tube) for Roux-en-Y reconstructions or T tubes for duct-to-duct reconstructions. Stents may be completely internal or may be brought out through the native duct, such as a T tube, or through the Roux-en-Y limb itself. Stents have also been successfully brought out through the native cystic duct stump in some duct-to-duct reconstructions.[140]

All biliary anastomoses should be fashioned tension free and, at their completion, should be checked for leakage. Closed suction drains are placed in the dependent vicinity of all biliary anastomoses, as well as the cut edge of the graft. Some surgeons advocate the use of a dye test (e.g., indocyanine green, methylene blue) to detect leakage at the completion of the biliary reconstructions.[79,144] Routine completion cholangiography should be performed when a T tube or externalized stent is placed. Leaks are best identified and corrected at the time of transplantation.

Postoperative Management

Postoperative management of a living donor recipient is similar to that of a deceased donor liver recipient. In the immediate postoperative period, close invasive cardiac monitoring is essential to avoid excessive CVP, which may cause graft congestion and dysfunction. Cardiac parameters maintained in the operating room when the graft appeared well perfused and not congested should be the ideal for each individual patient. There should be a very low threshold for return to the operating room if the patient has signs that the graft is not functioning well. Very small bile

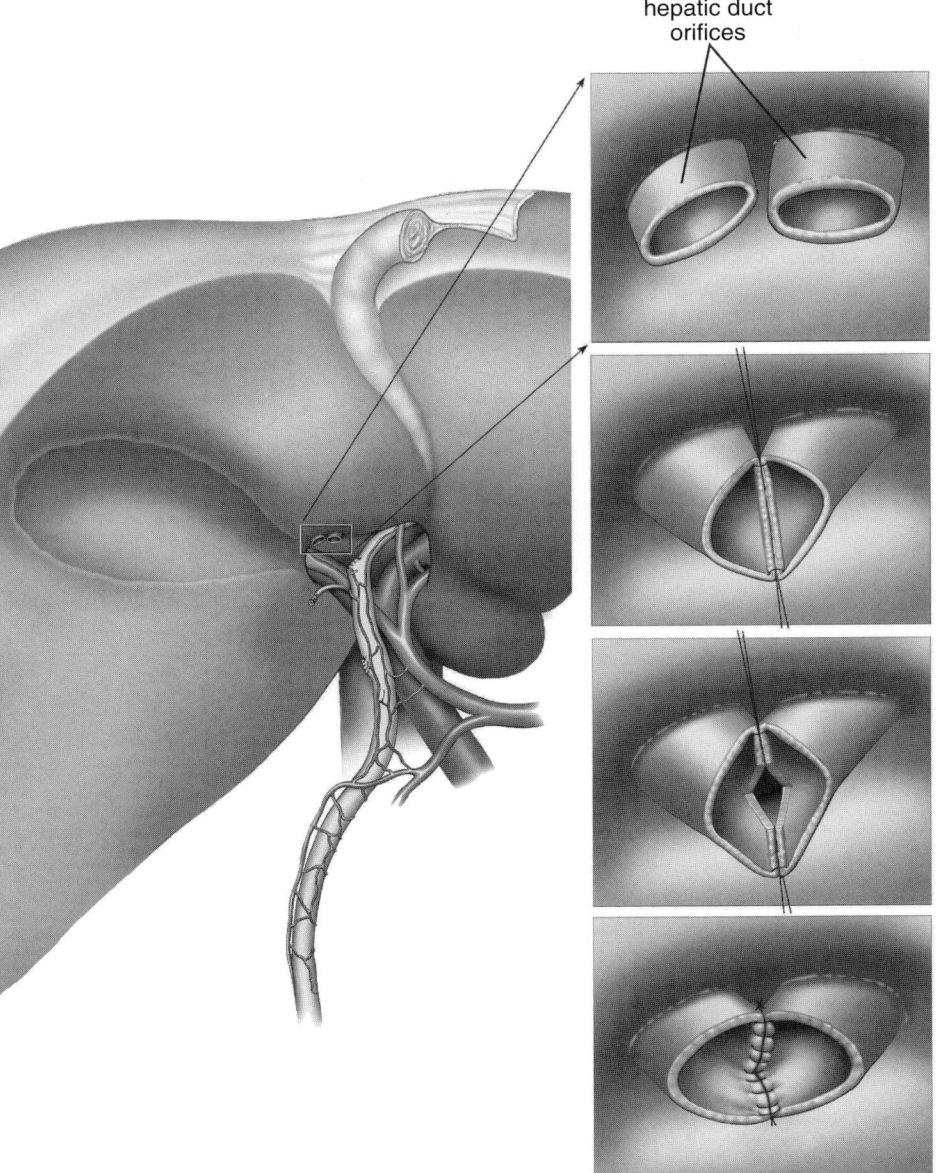

Adjacent right
hepatic duct
orifices

FIGURE 45–15

Schematic depiction demonstrating the approximation of two adjacent right hepatic duct orifices to form a single orifice. The newly created septum should be divided vertically and sutured transversely to create a large opening. Simply joining the medial wall creates tension and narrowing of the lumen. (Redrawn from Fan ST, Lo CM, Liu CL, et al: Biliary reconstruction and complications of right lobe live donor liver transplantation. Ann Surg 236:676-683, 2002.)

leaks are occasionally managed nonoperatively; however, most are best corrected surgically when identified early postoperatively.

Summary

Living donor liver transplantation for adult recipients is now a clinical reality, and the number of cases, as well as the number of centers performing these cases, has dramatically increased over the last 2 years. Initially only left lobes were taken from donors for transplantation. Because left lobes are often marginally sized grafts for adult recipients, surgeons have moved more and more toward using the right lobe. The larger right lobe resection is, however, associated with higher morbidity than left lobectomy is.

The left lobe is anatomically inherently better suited for optimal venous drainage because it includes the middle hepatic vein. The right lobe, in contrast, although providing approximately 40% to 50% more actual mass, is potentially poorly designed for venous drainage, particularly in individuals with significant venous tributaries that drain directly into the middle hepatic vein, which is not generally included. Conversely, right lobe arterial anatomy is generally straightforward, whereas the left lobe frequently has a separate segment IV arterial supply.

Our current understanding of portal venous inflow and its significance with regard to graft function suggests that inflow may be at least as important a factor for successful transplantation as outflow. Optimizing both inflow and outflow is likely to lead to the greatest success with living donor liver transplantation. Improving our understanding of the pathophysiological mechanisms of portal overflow, shear stress, and small-for-size syndrome is critical to our future success with these procedures. The concepts of actual and functional graft size requirements are still in their infancy. More accurate definitions of these terms and more widespread application will determine the future successes and failures of partial–liver graft transplantation.

Until alternative sources of organs for liver replacement are identified, living donors will remain an important means by which this life-saving procedure can be offered. Only through the altruistic volunteerism of the living donor is this possible. It is our primary responsibility to protect these individuals and demand the highest standards for their care. Continued technical innovations will make this procedure even safer for both donors and their recipients. Because there will always be risk associated with these procedures, surgeons should continue to strive to perfect these procedures as well as patient management.

Acknowledgment

The authors wish to thank Nancy Ehrlich Lapid for her editorial assistance and dedication. The authors also thank Giovanni Varotti, MD and Hugh Thomas for their expert illustrations.

Pearls and Pitfalls

Donor Procedure

- Donor safety is paramount and takes precedence over any recipient considerations. There is no substitute for careful preoperative assessment and planning.

- Although hepatic anatomic variations are exceedingly common, few are absolute contraindications to donation.

- Unlike surgeons who are performing tumor resections, surgeons operating on living donors must preserve the integrity of the anatomical structures not only in the donor but also in the resected portion that is to be transplanted.

Pearls and Pitfalls—cont'd

- Biliary anatomy is the most variable anatomical factor, and variations are often associated with variations in portal venous anatomy. The right posterior hepatic duct may drain into the left hepatic duct, a common anomaly that is important to remember in both right and left lobe donation.

- In 10% of individuals, the right hepatic artery passes anterior to the common bile duct. In 20% of individuals, the arterial supply to the medial aspect of the left lobe (i.e., segment IV), often referred to as the middle hepatic artery, originates from the right hepatic artery.

- The relationship of the hepatic veins as they enter the vena cava is important because it can have important implications for identifying the correct transection point in the donor, as well as for performing graft outflow reconstruction in the recipient.

- The benefit of including the middle hepatic vein with the right lobe graft is solely to optimize anterior segment venous drainage, which maximizes functional graft size while not significantly affecting actual graft size.

- Meticulous care should be taken around the bile duct, and dissection should be avoided between the distal end of the right hepatic artery and the right hepatic duct. Minimal manipulation of periductal tissue, avoidance of electrocautery, and sharp transection of the duct are important principles.

- During parenchymal transection, placing the patient in the Trendelenburg position, maintaining low central venous pressure, and using intermittent occlusion of inflow all help decrease blood loss.

- After parenchymal transection, persistent segmental hepatopedal flow with temporary arterial occlusion suggests the presence of adequate intrahepatic venous collaterals.

- The portal clamp should be placed vertically, as opposed to the traditional horizontal placement, because such placement increases the diameter of the portal vein and helps avoid stenosis.

- Hemostasis is critical to avoid unnecessary blood loss and also to best identify small open bile ducts.

Pearls and Pitfalls—cont'd

Recipient Procedure

- Successful transplantation with a partial graft is highly dependent on careful donor selection for a specific recipient and includes an accurate assessment of actual and, perhaps more important, functional graft size.

- Functional graft size is a composite of actual graft size modified by factors of recipient performance status and portal hemodynamics.

- When portal inflow is excessive, parenchymal portal overflow and shear stress create a phenomenon that may cause graft dysfunction and small-for-size syndrome.

- The most important technical principle is to preserve implantation options by maintaining the length and integrity of all hilar structures.

- Acutely, venous congestion is tolerated very poorly by a partial graft, and therefore, optimizing venous outflow and portal inflow is an important principle for success. Although graft venous outflow must be optimized to avoid congestion, inflow may be an even greater determinant of graft function.

- The caval groove, or the indentation where the donor's vena cava ran, is an important landmark that should be used to orient and align the right lobe graft with the recipient's vena cava.

- When significant segment VI veins require reimplantation, it is technically easier to complete these before anastomosis of the main right hepatic vein.

- Graft alignment is important and should take into consideration the future rotation (left to right for left lobe grafts and right to left for right lobe grafts) that occurs as a result of regeneration, particularly when performing the portal venous reconstruction.

- Decompression and maintenance of vascular integrity of the bile ducts are critical factors for successful biliary reconstructions; they remain the Achilles' heel of living donor transplantation.

- In general, left lobe grafts are more likely to require hepatic arterial reconstruction and right lobe grafts are more likely to require portal venous reconstruction.

- Intraoperative pharmacological and even surgical inflow modifications are viable therapeutic options.

References

1. Starzl TE, Groth CG, Brettschneider L, et al: Orthotopic homotransplantation of the human liver. Ann Surg 168:392-415, 1968.
2. Starzl TE: Liver transplantation. Gastroenterology 112:228-291, 1997.
3. Groth CG, Brent LB, Calne RY, et al: Historic landmarks in clinical transplantation: Conclusions from the consensus conference at the University of California, Los Angeles. World J Surg 24:834-843, 2000.
4. Pichlmayr R, Ringe B, Gubernatis G: Transplantation einer Spenderleber auf zwei Empfanger: Eine neue Methode in der Weiterentwicklung der lebersegment Transplantation. Langenbecks Arch Chir 373:127, 1989.
5. Bismuth H, Morino M, Castaing D, et al: Emergency orthotopic liver transplantation in two patients using one liver. Br J Surg 76:722, 1989.
6. Otte JB: Is it right to develop living related liver transplantation? Do reduced and split livers not suffice to cover the needs? Transpl Int 8:69-73, 1995.
7. Michon L, Hamburger J, Oeconomos N, et al: Une tentative de transplantation renale chez l'homme: Aspects medicaux et biologiques. Presse Med 61:1419, 1953.
8. Murray JE, Merrill JP, Harrison JH: Renal homotransplantation in identical twins. Surg Forum 6:432, 1955.
9. Cohen RG, Starnes VA: Living donor lung transplantation. World J Surg 25:244-250, 2001.
10. Magreiter R: Living-donor pancreas and small-bowel transplantation. Langenbecks Arch Surg 384:544-549, 1999.
11. Cherqui D, Emond JC, Pietrabissa A, et al: Segmental liver transplantation from living donors. Report of the technique and preliminary results in dogs. HPB Surg 2:189-202, 1990.
12. Raia S, Nery JR, Mies S: Liver transplantation from live donors. Lancet 2:497, 1989.
13. Strong RW, Lynch SV, Ong TH, et al: Successful liver transplantation from a living donor to her son. N Engl J Med 322:1505-1507, 1990.
14. Singer PA, Siegler M, Whitington PF, et al: Ethics of liver transplantation with living donors. N Engl J Med 321:620-622, 1989.
15. Broelsch CE, Emond JC, Whitington PF, et al: Application of reduced-size liver transplants as split grafts, auxiliary orthotopic grafts, and living related segmental transplants. Ann Surg 212:368-375, 1990.
16. Broelsch CE, Whitington PF, Emond JC, et al: Liver transplantation in children from living related donors. Surgical techniques and results. Ann Surg 214:428-437, 1991.
17. Otte JB: History of pediatric liver transplantation. Where are we coming from? Where do we stand? Pediatr Transplant 6:378-387, 2002.
18. Testa G, Malago M, Broelsch CE: From living related to in-situ split liver transplantation: How to reduce waiting-list mortality. Pediatr Transplant 5:16-20, 2001.
19. Otte JB: The availability of all technical modalities for pediatric liver transplant programs. Pediatr Transplant 5:1-4, 2001.
20. Kawasaki S, Hashikura Y, Ikegami T, et al: First case of cadaveric liver transplantation in Japan. J Hepatobiliary Pancreat Surg 6:387-390, 1999.
21. Hashikura Y, Makuuchi M, Kawasaki S, et al: Successful living-related partial liver transplantation to an adult patient. Lancet 343:1233-1234, 1994.
22. United Network for Organ Sharing (UNOS): http://www.unos.org (accessed July 2003).
23. Emond J, Renz JF, Ferrel LD, et al: Functional analysis of grafts from living donors. Implications for the treatment of older recipients. Ann Surg 224:544-554, 1996.

24. Yamaoka Y, Washida M, Honda K, et al: Liver transplantation using a right lobe graft from a living related donor. Transplantation 57:1127-1130, 1994.

25. Lo CM, Fan ST, Liu CL, et al: Extending the limit on the size of adult recipient in living donor liver transplantation using extended right lobe graft. Transplantation 63:1524-1528, 1997.

26. Miller CM, Gondolesi G, Florman S, et al: 109 living donor liver transplants in children and adults: A single center experience. Ann Surg 234:301-312, 2001.

27. Wachs ME, Bak TE, Karrer FM, et al: Adult living donor liver transplantation using a right hepatic lobe. Transplantation 66:1313-1316, 1998.

28. Sugawara Y, Makuuchi M, Takayama T, et al: Small-for-size grafts in living-related liver transplantation. J Am Coll Surg 192:510-513, 2001.

29. Salame E, Goldstein MJ, Kinkhabwala M, et al: Analysis of donor risk in living-donor hepatectomy: The impact of resection type on clinical outcome. Am J Transplant 2:780-788, 2002.

30. Surman OS: The ethics of partial-liver donation. N Engl J Med 346:1038, 2002.

31. Hashikura Y, Kawasaki S, Miyagawa S, et al: Recent advance in living donor liver transplantation. World J Surg 26:243-246, 2002.

32. Chisuwa H, Hashikura Y, Mita A, et al: Living liver donation: Preoperative assessment, anatomic considerations, and long-term outcome. Transplantation 75:1670-1676, 2003.

33. Otte JB: Analyses and commentaries: Donor complications and outcomes in live-liver transplantation. Transplantation 75:1625-1626, 2003.

34. New York State Committee on Quality Improvement in Living Liver Donation: A report to New York State Transplant Council and New York State Department of Health, 2002.

35. Nakamura T, Tanaka K, Kiuchi T, et al: Anatomical variations and surgical strategies in right lobe living donor liver transplantation: Lessons from 120 cases. Transplantation 73:1896-1903, 2002.

36. Marcos A, Ham JM, Fisher RA, et al: Surgical management of anatomical variations of the right lobe in living donor liver transplantation. Ann Surg 231:824-831, 2000.

37. Kawasaki S, Makuuchi M, Miyagawa S, et al: Extended lateral segmentectomy using intraoperative ultrasound to obtain a partial liver graft. Am J Surg 171:286-288, 1996.

38. Imamura H, Makuuchi M, Sakamoto Y, et al: Anatomical keys and pitfalls in living donor liver transplantation. J Hepatobiliary Pancreat Surg 7:380-394, 2000.

39. Kawarada Y, Das BC, Taoka H: Anatomy of the hepatic hilar area: The plate system. J Hepatobiliary Pancreat Surg 7:580-586, 2000.

40. Couinaud C: Controlled Hepatectomies and Exposure of the Intrahepatic Bile Ducts. Anatomical and Technical Study. Paris, C Couinaud, 1981 (ISBN 2-903672-00-8).

41. Kida H, Uchimura M, Okamoto K: Intrahepatic architecture of bile and portal vein [in Japanese]. Tan to Sui [J Biliary Tract and Pancreas] 8:1-7, 1987.

42. Varotti G, Gondolesi G, Goldman J, et al: Anatomic variations in right liver living donors. J Am Coll Surg 198:577-582, 2004.

43. Marcos A, Orloff M, Mieles L, et al: Reconstruction of double hepatic arterial and portal venous branches for right-lobe living donor liver transplantation. Liver Transpl 7:673-679, 2001.

44. Adachi B: Das Arteriensystem der Japaner. Bd I 440 and Bd II 353, 1928, Maruzen, Kyoto.

45. Browne EZ: Variations in origin and course of the hepatic artery and its branches. Surgery 8:424, 1940.

46. Michels NA: Newer anatomy of the liver and its variant blood supply and collateral circulation. Am J Surg 112:337-347, 1940.

47. Emre S, Schwartz ME, Miller CM: The donor operation. In Busuttil RW, Klintmalm GB (eds): Transplantation of the Liver. Philadelphia, WB Saunders, 1996, pp 392-404.

48. Soin AS, Friend PJ, Rasmussen A, et al: Donor arterial variations in liver transplantation: Management and outcome of 527 consecutive grafts. Br J Surg 83:637-641, 1996.

49. Couinaud C: A "scandal": Segment IV and liver transplantation. J Chir 130:443-446, 1993.

50. Hiatt JR, Gabbay J, Busuttil RW: Surgical anatomy of the hepatic arteries in 1000 cases. Ann Surg 220:50-52, 1994.

51. Nakamura S, Tsuzuki T: Surgical anatomy of the hepatic veins and the inferior vena cava. Surg Gynecol Obstet 152:43-50, 1981.

52. Cattral MS, Greig PD, Muradali D, et al: Reconstruction of middle hepatic vein of a living-donor right lobe liver graft with recipient left portal vein. Transplantation 71:1864-1866, 2001.

53. Fan S-T, Lo C-M, Liu C-L: Technical refinement in adult-to-adult living donor liver transplantation using right lobe graft. Ann Surg 231:126-131, 2000.

54. Lee SG, Park KM, Hwang S, et al: Adult-to-adult living donor liver transplantation at the Asan Medical Center, Korea. Asian J Surg 25:277-284, 2002.

55. Marcos A, Orloff M, Mieles L, et al: Functional venous anatomy for right-lobe grafting and techniques to optimize outflow. Liver Transpl 7:845-852, 2001.

56. Marcos A: Right lobe living donor liver transplantation: A review. Liver Transpl 6:3-20, 2000.

57. Bak T, Wachs M, Trotter J, et al: Adult-to-adult living donor liver transplantation using right lobe grafts: Results and lessons learned from a single-center experience. Liver Transpl 7:680-686, 2001.

58. Huang T, Cheng Y, Chen C, et al: Variants of the bile ducts: Clinical application in the potential donor in living-related hepatic transplantation. Transplant Proc 28:1669-1670, 1996.

59. Goldman J, Florman S, Varotti G, et al: Non-invasive preoperative evaluation of biliary anatomy in right lobe living donors with mangafodipir trisodium–enhanced MR cholangiography. Transplant Proc 35:1421-1422, 2003.

60. Healey JE, Schroy PC: Anatomy of the biliary ducts within the human liver: Analysis of the prevailing pattern of branchings and the major variations of the biliary ducts. Arch Surg 66:599-616, 1953.

61. Parke WW, Michels NA, Ghosh GH: Blood supply of the common bile duct. Surg Gynecol Obstet 117:47-55, 1963.

62. Shoup M, Gonen M, D'Angelica M, et al: Volumetric analysis predicts hepatic dysfunction in patients undergoing major liver resection. J Gastrointest Surg 7:325-331, 2003.

63. Kamel IR, Kruskal JB, Raptopoulos V: Imaging for right lobe living donor liver transplantation. Semin Liver Dis 21:271-282, 2001.

64. Marcos A, Fisher RA, Ham JM, et al: Liver regeneration and function in donor and recipient after right lobe adult to adult living donor liver transplantation. Transplantation 69:1375-1379, 2000.

65. Takayama T, Makuuchi M, Kubota K, et al: Living-related transplantation of left liver plus caudate lobe. J Am Coll Surg 190:635-638, 2000.

66. Miyagawa S, Hashikura Y, Miwa S, et al: Concomitant caudate lobe resection as an option for donor hepatectomy in adult living-related liver transplantation. Transplantation 66:661-663, 1998.

67. Ikegami T, Nishizaki T, Yanaga K, et al: Changes in the caudate lobe that is transplanted with extended left lobe liver graft from living donors. Surgery 129:86-90, 2001.

68. Makuuchi M, Sugawara Y: Living-donor liver transplantation using the left liver, with special reference to vein reconstruction. Transplantation 75:S23-S24, 2003.

69. Miller CM, Masetti M, Cautero N, et al: The impact of cardiac index and inflow modification on acceptable graft size in living donor liver transplantation. Am J Transplant 3(Suppl 5):204, 2003.

70. Ben-Haim M, Emre S, Fishbein TM, et al: Critical graft size in adult-to-adult living donor liver transplantation: Impact of the recipient's disease. Liver Transpl 7:948-953, 2001.

71. Troisi R, Cammu G, Militerno G, et al: Modulation of portal graft inflow: A necessity in adult living-donor liver transplantation? Ann Surg 237:429-436, 2003.

72. Kuichi T, Kasahara M, Uryuhara K, et al: Impact of graft size mismatching on graft prognosis in liver transplantation from living donors. Transplantation 67:321-327, 1999.

73. Lo CM, Fan ST, Liu CL, et al: Minimum graft size for successful living donor liver transplantation. Transplantation 68:1112-1116, 1999.

74. Ozawa K: Living Related Liver Transplantation: An Assessment of Graft Viability Based on Redox Theory. Geneva, Kager, 1994.

75. Lo CM, Fan ST, Liu CL, et al: Adult-to-adult living donor liver transplantation using extended right lobe grafts. Ann Surg 226:261-270, 1997.

76. Schmucker DL, Curtis JC: A correlated study of the fine structure and physiology of the perfused rat liver. Lab Invest 30:201-212, 1974.

77. Urata K, Kawasaki S, Matsunami H, et al: Calculation of child and adult standard liver volume for liver transplantation. Hepatology 21:1317-1321, 1995.

78. Gondolesi, G, Yoshizumi T, Bodian C, et al: Accurate method for clinical assessment of right lobe liver weight in adult living-related liver transplant. Transplant Proc 36:14-29-1433, 2004.

79. Fan ST: Adult-to-Adult Live Donor Liver Transplantation Using Right Lobe Graft [doctoral thesis]. Hong Kong, University of Hong Kong, 2002.

80. Sano K, Makuuchi M, Miki K, et al: Evaluation of hepatic venous congestion: Proposed indication criteria for hepatic vein reconstruction. Ann Surg 236:241-247, 2002.

81. Lee S, Park K, Hwang S, et al: Congestion of right liver graft in living donor liver transplantation. Transplantation 71:812-817, 2001.

82. Gondolesi G, Florman S, Matsumoto C, et al: Venous hemodynamics in living donor right lobe liver transplantation. Liver Transpl 8:809-813, 2002.

83. Marcos A, Olzinski AT, Ham JM, et al: The interrelationship between portal and arterial blood flow after adult to adult living donor liver transplantation. Transplantation 70:1697-1703, 2000.

84. Shimada M, Shiotani S, Ninomiya M, et al: Characteristics of liver grafts in living-donor adult liver transplantation. Arch Surg 137:1174-1179, 2002.

85. Broelsch CE: Personal communication, 2002.

86. Gurkan A, Emre S, Fishbein TM, et al: Unsuspected bile duct paucity in donors for living-related liver transplantation: Two case reports. Transplantation 67:416-418, 1999.

87. Marcos A, Fisher RA, Ham JM, et al: Right lobe living donor liver transplantation. Transplantation 68:798-803, 1999.

88. Stapleton GN, Hickman R, Terblanche J: Blood supply of the right and left hepatic ducts. Br J Surg 85:202-207, 1998.

89. Cunningham JD, Fong Y, Shriver C, et al: One hundred consecutive hepatic resections. Blood loss, transfusion, and operative technique. Arch Surg 129:1050-1056, 1994.

90. Imamura H, Takayama T, Sugawara Y, et al: Pringle's manoeuvre in living donors. Lancet 360:2049-2050, 2002.

91. Makuuchi M, Kawasaki S, Noguchi T, et al: Donor hepatectomy for living related partial liver transplantation. Surgery 113:395-402, 1993.

92. Clavien PA, Yadav S, Sindram D, et al: Protective effects of ischemic preconditioning for liver resection performed under inflow occlusion in humans. Ann Surg 232:155-162, 2000.

93. Miller CM, Masetti M, Cautero N, et al: Intermittent inflow occlusion in living liver donors: Impact on safety and remnant function. Liver Transpl 10:244-247, 2004.

94. Cui D, Kiuchi T, Egawa H, et al: Microcirculatory changes in right lobe grafts in living-donor liver transplantation: A near-infrared spectrometry study. Transplantation 72:291-295, 2001.

95. Cescon M, Sugawara Y, Sano K, et al: Right liver graft without middle hepatic vein reconstruction from a living donor. Transplantation 73:1164-1166, 2002.

96. Sugawara Y, Makuuchi M, Kaneko J, et al: New venoplasty technique for the left liver plus caudate lobe in living donor liver transplantation. Liver Transpl 8:76-77, 2002.

97. Couinaud C: The paracaval segments of the liver. J Hepatobiliary Pancreat Surg 2:145-151, 1994.

98. Suehiro T, Ninomiya M, Shiotani S, et al: Hepatic artery reconstruction and biliary stricture formation after living donor adult liver transplantation using left lobes. Liver Transpl 8:495-499, 2002.

99. Yanaga K, Kamohara Y, Takatsuki M, et al: Vertical portal vein clamping in right hepatic lobectomy for live donation or neoplasm. Liver Transpl 8:565-567, 2002.

100. Pitre J, Panis Y, Belghiti J: Left hepatic vein kinking after right hepatectomy: A rare cause of acute Budd-Chiari syndrome. Br J Surg 79:7948-7949, 1992.

101. Brown RS, Russo MW, Lai M, et al: A survey of liver transplantation from living adult donors in the United States. N Engl J Med 348:818-825, 2003.

102. Lo CM: Complications and long-term outcome of living liver donors: A survey of 1,508 cases in five Asian centers. Transplantation 75:S12-S15, 2003.

103. Schluger LK, Florman S, Schiano T, et al: Quality of life after lobectomy for adult liver transplantation. Transplantation 73:1593-1597, 2002.

104. Lerut J, de Ville de Goyet J, Donataccio M, et al: Piggyback transplantation with side-to-side cavocavostomy is an ideal technique for right split liver allograft implantation. J Am Coll Surg 179:573-576, 1994.

105. Tzakis A, Todo S, Starzl TE: Orthotopic liver transplantation with preservation of the inferior vena cava. Ann Surg 210:649-652, 1989.

106. Makuuchi M: Personal communication, 2002.

107. Chardot C, Saint Martin C, Gilles A, et al: Living-related liver transplantation and vena cava reconstruction after total hepatectomy including the vena cava for hepatoblastoma. Transplantation 73:90-92, 2002.

108. Arcari M, Phillips SD, Gibbs P, et al: An investigation into the risk of air embolus during veno-venous bypass in orthotopic liver transplantation. Transplantation 68:150-152, 1999.

109. Scholz T, Solberg R, Okkenhaug C, et al: Veno-venous bypass in liver transplantation: Heparin-coated perfusion circuits reduce the activation of humoral defense systems in an in vitro model. Perfusion 16:285-292, 2001.

110. Eleborg L, Sallander S, Tollemar J: Minimal hemolytic effect of veno-venous bypass during liver transplantation. Transpl Int 4:157-160, 1991.

111. van der Hulst VP, Henny CP, Moulijn AC, et al: Veno-venous bypass without heparinization using a centrifugal pump: A blind comparison of a heparin bonded circuit versus a non heparin bonded circuit. J Cardiovasc Surg (Torino) 30:118-123, 1989.

112. Neelakanta G, Colquhoun S, Csete M, et al: Efficacy and safety of heat exchanger added to venovenous bypass circuit during orthotopic liver transplantation. Liver Transpl Surg 4:506-509, 1998.

113. Neelakanta G, Csete M, Busuttil RW: Arteriovenous obstruction of arm due to venovenous bypass during liver transplantation. J Clin Anesth 9:507-509, 1997.

114. Campra JL, Reynolds TB: The hepatic circulation. In Arias IM, Jakoby WB, Popper H, et al (eds): The Liver: Biology and Pathobiology, 2nd ed. New York, Raven Press, 1988, pp 911-930.

115. Furukawa H, Shimamura H, Jin IMB, et al: What is the limit of graft size for successful living donor liver transplantation in adults? Transplant Proc 33:1322, 2001.

116. Sato Y, Tsukada K, Hatakeyama K: Role of shear stress and immune responses in liver regeneration after a partial hepatectomy. Surg Today 29:1-9, 1999.

117. Smyrniotis VE, Kostopanagiotou G, Theodoraki K, et al: Effect of mesocaval shunt on survival of small-for-size liver grafts: Experimental study in pigs. Transplantation 75:1737-1760, 2003.

118. Emond JC, Heffron TG, Whitington PF, et al: Reconstruction of the hepatic vein in reduced size hepatic transplantation. Surg Gynecol Obstet 176:11-17, 1993.

119. Inomata Y, Tanaka K, Egawa H, et al: Application of a tissue expander for stabilizing graft position in living-related liver transplantation. Clin Transplant 11:56-59, 1997.

120. Starzl TE, Iwatsuki S, Shaw BW Jr: A growth factor in fine vascular anastomoses. Surg Gynecol Obstet 159:164-165, 1984.

121. Kadry Z, Selzner N, Handschin A, et al: Living donor liver transplantation in patients with portal vein thrombosis: A survey and review of technical issues. Transplantation 74:696-701, 2002.

122. Yerdel MA, Gunsen B, Mirza D, et al: Portal vein thrombosis in adults undergoing liver transplantation: Risk factors, screening, management and outcome. Transplantation 69:1873-1881, 2000.

123. Stieber AC, Zetti G, Todo S, et al: The spectrum of portal vein thrombosis in liver transplantation. Ann Surg 213:199-206, 1991.

124. Sakamoto Y, Takayama T, Nakatsuka T, et al: Advantage of using living donors with aberrant hepatic artery for partial liver graft arterialization. Transplantation 74:518-521, 2002.

125. Ikegami T, Kawasaki S, Matsunami H, et al: Should all hepatic arterial branches be reconstructed in living-related liver transplantation? Surgery 119:431-436, 1996.

126. Tanaka K, Uemoto S, Tokunaga Y, et al: Surgical techniques and innovations in living-related liver transplantation. Ann Surg 217:82-91, 1993.

127. Redman HC, Reuter SR: Arterial collaterals in the liver hilus. Radiology 94:575-579, 1970.

128. Pinna AD: Personal communication, 2003.

129. Marcos A, Killackey M, Orloff MS, et al: Hepatic arterial reconstruction in 95 adult right lobe living donor liver transplants: Evolution of anastomotic technique. Liver Transpl 9:570-574, 2003.

130. Settmacher U, Nussler NC, Glanemann M, et al: Venous complications after orthotopic liver transplantation. Clin Transplant 14:235-241, 2000.

131. Maema A, Imamura H, Takayama T, et al: Impaired volume regeneration of split livers with partial venous disruption: A latent problem in partial liver transplantation. Transplantation 73:765-769, 2002.

132. Calne RY: A new technique for biliary drainage in orthotopic liver transplantation utilizing the gall bladder as a pedicle graft conduit between the donor and recipient common bile ducts. Ann Surg 184:605-609, 1976.

133. Gondolesi GE, Varotti G, Florman SS, et al: Biliary complications in 96 consecutive right lobe living donor transplant recipients. Transplantation 77:1842-1848, 2004.

134. Schindel D, Dunn S, Casas A, et al: Characterization and treatment of biliary anastomotic stricture after segmental liver transplantation. J Pediatr Surg 35:940-942, 2000.

135. Testa G, Malago M, Valentin-Gamazo C, et al: Biliary anastomosis in living related liver transplantation using the right liver lobe: Techniques and complications. Liver Transpl 6:710-714, 2000.

136. Marcos A, Ham JM, Fisher RA, et al: Single-center analysis of the first 40 adult-to-adult living donor liver transplants using the right lobe. Liver Transpl 6:296-301, 2000.

137. Azoulay D, Marin-Hargreaves G, Castaing D, et al: Duct-to-duct biliary anastomosis in living related liver transplantation. Arch Surg 136:1197-1200, 2001.

138. Shokouth-Amiri MH, Grewal HP, Vera SR, et al: Duct-to-duct biliary reconstruction in right lobe adult live donor liver transplantation. Ann Coll Surg 192:798-803, 2001.

139. Sugawara Y, Makuuchi M, Sano K, et al: Duct-to-duct biliary reconstruction in living-related liver transplantation. Transplantation 73:1348-1350, 2002.

140. Ishiko T, Egawa H, Kasahara M, et al: Duct-to-duct biliary reconstruction in living donor liver transplantation utilizing right lobe graft. Ann Surg 236:235-240, 2002.

141. Soejima Y, Shimada M, Suehiro T, et al: Feasibility of duct-to-duct biliary reconstruction in left-lobe adult-living-donor liver transplantation. Transplantation 75:557-559, 2003.

142. Malago M, Testa G, Hertl M, et al: Biliary reconstruction following right adult living donor liver transplantation end-to-end or end-to-side duct-to-duct anastomosis. Langenbecks Arch Surg 387:37-44, 2002.

143. Fan S-T, Lo C-M, Liu C-L, et al: Biliary reconstruction and complications of right lobe live donor liver transplantation. Ann Surg 236:676-683, 2002.

144. Ikegami T, Nishizaki T, Kishikawa K, et al: Biliary reconstruction in living donor liver transplantation with dye injection leakage test and without stent use. Hepatogastroenterology 48:1582-1584, 2001.

Imaging Techniques for Living Donor Transplantation

PIYAPORN LIMANOND
STEVEN S. RAMAN
DAVID S. K. LU

Surgical techniques   703

Imaging techniques   704
   Multidetector computed tomography and
    computed tomography angiography   704
   Magnetic resonance
    cholangiopancreatography   704
   Magnetic resonance angiography   704
   Computed tomographic
    cholangiography   704

Image interpretation   704
   Computed tomographic segmental volume
    analysis   704
   Quantification of the degree of
    macrovesicular steatosis   705
   Relevant hepatic pathology   707
   Evaluation of hepatic vascular anatomy   707
   Biliary anatomy evaluation   710

Comprehensive magnetic resonance
   imaging   711

Comprehensive computed tomography   711

Summary   711

For adult-to-adult living related liver transplantation (LRLT), preoperative imaging plays an important role in donor selection and surgical planning to maximize the success and minimize the risks of postoperative complications in both donor and recipient.[1,2] Roles of preoperative imaging assessment of potential living related donors include accurate identification of the hepatic segmental volumes, exclusion of hepatic pathologies (e.g., macrovesicular steatosis, incidental liver masses), and guiding surgical planning for vascular and biliary anastomoses. Those livers with inadequate volume, detectable pathology, or anatomic variations, which may necessitate complex vascular or biliary reconstruction, may not be selected for LRLT.

Surgical Techniques

In most institutions in the United States, the donor operation consists of cholecystectomy followed by right hepatectomy, which includes Couinaud segments 5, 6, 7, and 8, right hepatic artery, right portal vein, and right hepatic vein. Detailed surgical technique is beyond the scope of this chapter and is discussed elsewhere. In brief, the plane of right lobe resection in the donor is identified intraoperatively by sonography, using the line just lateral to the middle hepatic vein and extending inferiorly to the bifurcation of right and left portal veins. Right lobe vascular structures (right hepatic artery, right portal vein, right hepatic vein) and biliary drainage are identified and preserved. After harvesting, the donor right lobe is placed in the University of Wisconsin solution until transplantation time. All vascular and biliary anastomoses are subsequently created in the recipient.[3]

Imaging Techniques

A variety of imaging techniques may be used for preoperative imaging. Traditionally, liver imaging and segmental volume quantification are assessed by computed tomography (CT), vascular mapping achieved by conventional angiography, and biliary anatomy by intraoperative cholangiogram. With the introduction of multidetector computed tomography (MDCT) scanners that can produce high-quality CT angiography, most institutions are relying on computed tomography angiography (CTA), thus obviating the need for invasive angiography. For biliary anatomy, magnetic resonance cholangiopancreatography (MRCP) remains the predominant noninvasive technique for preoperative ductal mapping. At UCLA (University of California, Los Angeles), we perform hepatic MDCT to assess the adequacy of segmental liver volumes, quantify the degree of macrovesicular steatosis, and exclude incidental liver masses; we use hepatic CTA to delineate arterial, portal venous, and hepatic venous anatomy. For the purpose of preoperative mapping of biliary anatomy, MRCP is performed.

Multidetector Computed Tomography and Computed Tomography Angiography

Hepatic MDCT and CTA can be performed on any commercial MDCT scanner. After contiguous nonenhanced axial images of the liver, intravenous iodinated contrast is power injected at a rate of 4 to 5 mL per second, and after an optimal time delay (determined by automatic triggering software, or by a prior timing run sequence, using a small dose of contrast), a volumetric data set is acquired with ultrathin slice thickness (0.5 to 1.25 mm) at peak arterial enhancement. Venous phase imaging is obtained at approximately 60 to 70 seconds' delay after injection, usually with thicker slice thickness (1 to 3 mm). From these acquisitions, three-dimensional hepatic arteriograms and portal and hepatic venograms are rendered on a three-dimensional workstation with commercially available angiographic software.

Magnetic Resonance Cholangiopancreatography

MRCP is performed on a 1.5 Tesla magnetic resonance (MR) magnet. A phased array torso coil is used.

MRCP images are obtained by using breath-hold, heavily T2-weighted, half-Fourier rapid acquisition with relaxation enhancement (T2-weighted half-Fourier RARE) sequence. This technique is performed either in axial/coronal planes with contiguous thin sections (3 to 5 mm) or rotating (coronal and off-coronal) slabs of variable thickness (3, 5, 7, and 10 cm). We use the vertical axis of the common hepatic duct as a center for rotation in coronal/off-coronal thick slabs.

Magnetic Resonance Angiography

MR angiography is an evolving technique now accepted for assessment of a variety of vascular conditions such as aortoiliac disease, carotid stenosis, and aneurysm detection. A three-dimensional gradient echo sequence is usually used, with multiple sequential acquisitions following intravenous gadolinium contrast administration. In addition, subtraction arteriograms and venograms can be generated. Similar techniques can be applied to the hepatic vasculature, with good depiction of the major hepatic artery branches and venous anatomy. However, because the source images are usually thicker than in multidetector CTA, and acquisition times are longer, giving rise to more motion blurring, the smaller vessels, such as small accessory right or left hepatic arteries and segment IV artery, may not be reliably defined. Nevertheless, improving MR technology is expected to eventually overcome these shortcomings.

Computed Tomographic Cholangiography

Preliminary data using intravenously administered biliary contrast agents coupled with volumetric MDCT acquisition and three-dimensional rendering demonstrate excellent depiction of the bile ducts.[4] However, these contrast agents have a relatively high rate of adverse side effects, and these agents are not widely available. Also, opacified bile ducts may interfere with CTA if they are to be performed at the same setting.

Image Interpretation

Computed Tomographic Segmental Volume Analysis

The adequacy of the right lobe volume is essential to sustain metabolic function in the recipient. The graft size–to–body weight ratio (GRBW) should be at least 0.8% to 1%.[5] A sufficient left lobe volume (at least 0.8% to 1% of donor body weight) is also required to ensure adequate reserve for the donor. Reliably predicting these values is crucial to ensure adequate postoperative liver function in both donor and recipient.

Sonographic and MR techniques for hepatic volumetric analysis are reliable, although they can be hindered by potential misregistration in patients who are unable to breath-hold. At our institution, all potential donors undergo CT for hepatic volumetric analysis. Analysis is performed on any three-dimensional workstation with volumetric software package. In one technique, the borders of the left lobe (segments II, III, and IV and caudate lobe) (Fig. 46–1A) and the right lobe (segments V, VI, VII, and VIII) (Fig. 46–1B) are independently outlined manually on selected axial images with electronic cursors, and the software then interpolates the margins for the slices in between, and total volume is calculated. Another technique requires manual outlining of the lobes on each axial image. This can easily be accomplished if 10-mm thick slices are used. The relevant areas (square centimeters) on each cross-sectional slice are then summed and multiplied by 1 cm (the slice thickness) to give the total volume in cubic centimeters. CT volumetric analysis is a reliable and accurate method of estimating liver volume with a maximum deviation from the true volume of 10%.[6]

Quantification of the Degree of Macrovesicular Steatosis

Preoperative evaluation of hepatic steatosis, especially the macrovesicular subtype, is critical for donor selection.[7,8] Severe macrovesicular steatosis (>60%) in the donor liver is associated with a greater than 60% risk of primary nonfunction after transplantation. Moderate degrees of macrovesicular steatosis (30% to 60%) in donor liver may also result in decreased hepatocyte regeneration and higher rates of graft nonfunction, dysfunction, and ischemic injury.[9,10] Although preoperative hepatic core biopsy is currently the standard method for accurate quantitation and characterization of macrovesicular steatosis, it is invasive, carries risk, and contributes to overall cost and morbidity. CT may help decrease the need for biopsies in donors with moderate (>30%) or severe (>60%) macrovesicular steatosis, considered unacceptable for donation.

At our institution, we have developed the liver attenuation index (LAI), a simple, prospective CT-based grading system to predict the degree of hepatic macrovesicular steatosis. The LAI is derived from unenhanced computed tomographic scan as the difference between mean hepatic CT and mean splenic CT attenuation:

$$LAI = MHA - MSA$$

where MHA is mean hepatic attenuation and MSA is mean splenic attenuation.

Although muscle may be used, we have found that splenic measurement is a more reliable internal control for CT attenuation measurement. From our preliminary study in 42 potential living related donors,[11] the LAI derived from the unenhanced computed tomographic scan correlated well with the percentage of macrovesicular steatosis from biopsy. An LAI greater than 5 Hounsfield units (HU) reliably predicted donor livers without significant histological macrovesicular steatosis (≤5% steatosis) (Fig. 46–2). An LAI between −10 HU

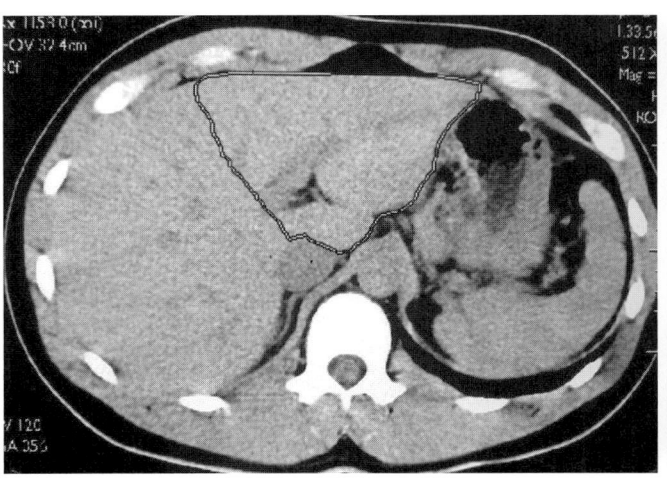
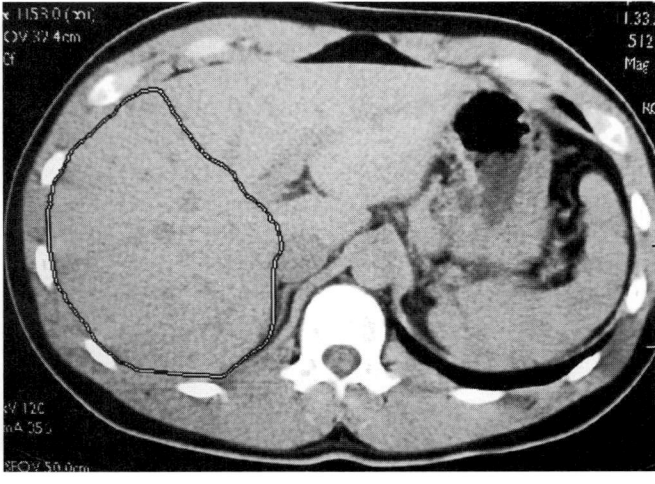

A   B

FIGURE 46–1

Volumetric hepatic lobar analysis performed manually on a GE workstation. The borders of the left (**A**) and right (**B**) hepatic lobes were outlined manually on unenhanced hepatic computed tomographic scan and the relevant computer-generated lobar volumes were integrated on a workstation.

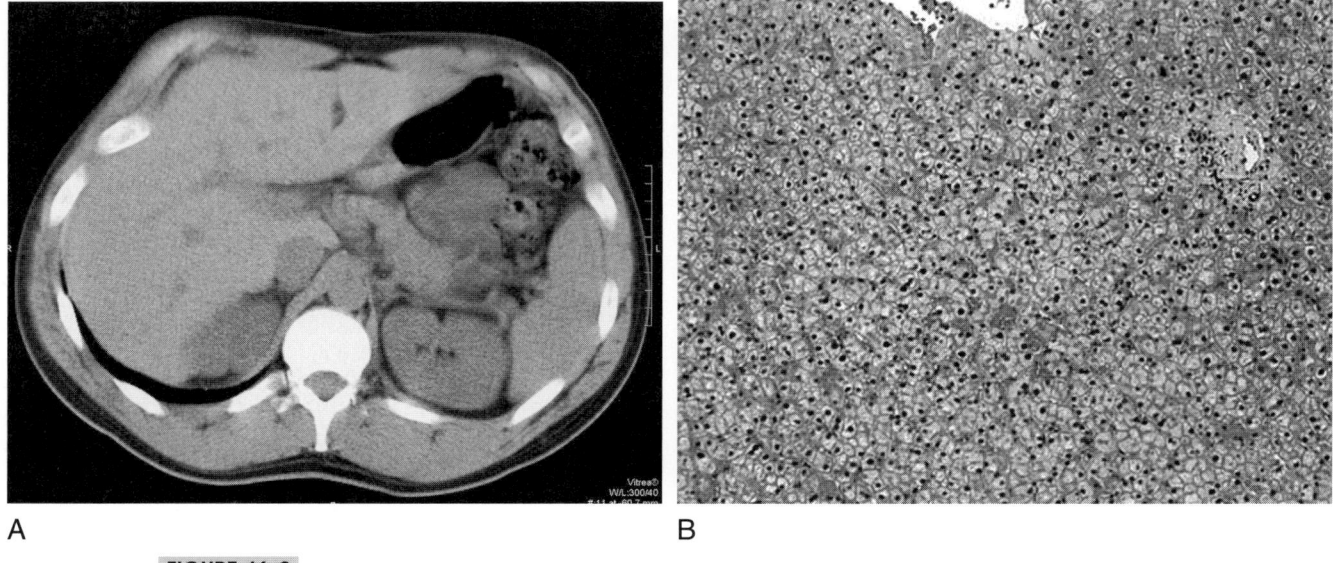

A   B

FIGURE 46–2

A, Noncontrast axial CT image of a 30-year-old male potential liver donor demonstrates a liver with normal attenuation. The LAI is 9.3 HU, representing normal liver without significant macrovesicular steatosis. **B,** Corresponding histology (H&E ×100) shows no detectable macrovesicular steatosis.

and 5 HU predicted mild to moderate macrovesicular steatosis (6% to 30%), which was a relative contraindication for transplantation (Fig. 46–3). An LAI less than –10 HU reliably predicted donor livers with moderate to severe macrovesicular steatosis (more than 30%) and were considered unacceptable for LRLT (Fig. 46–4). Using linear regression analysis, the degree of histological macrovesicular steatosis correlated well with CT LAI, achieving a high degree of correlation (r = 0.92) (Fig. 46–5). Although other methods have also been

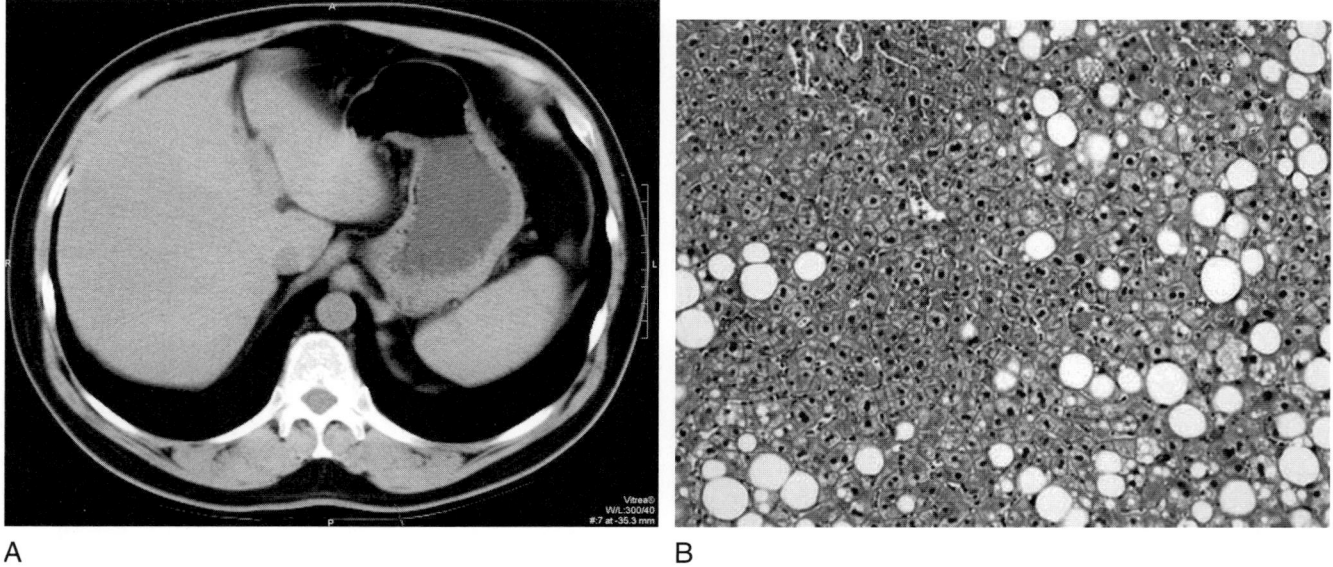

A   B

FIGURE 46–3

A, Noncontrast axial CT image of a 44-year-old male potential liver donor demonstrates a liver with diffuse decreased hepatic attenuation. The LAI is 3.8 HU, representing 6% to 30% steatosis. **B,** Corresponding histology (H&E ×100) shows moderate steatosis (30%).

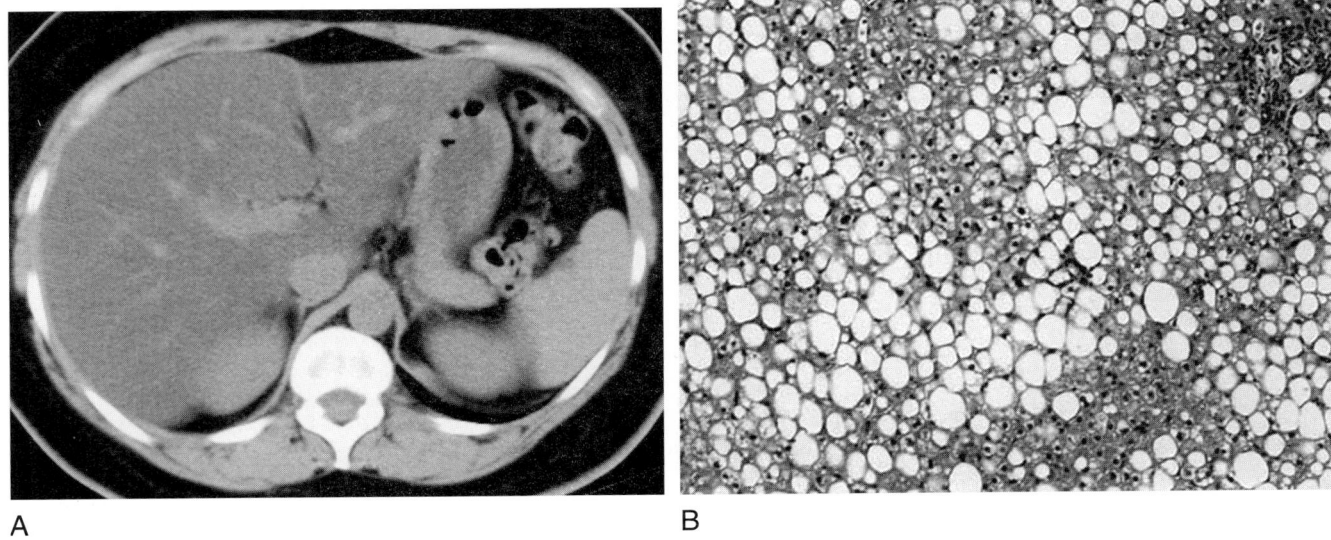

A   B

FIGURE 46-4

A, Noncontrast axial CT image of a 43-year-old female potential donor demonstrates a liver with markedly decreased attenuation. The LAI is −47.4 HU, representing greater than 30% macrovesicular steatosis. **B,** Corresponding histology (H&E ×100) shows severe macrovesicular steatosis (80%).

described to quantitate macrovesicular steatosis,[12] we find the LAI measurement to be a simple and reliable technique.

Use of CT LAI or other attenuation-based fat quantitation techniques may help decrease the need for preoperative liver biopsy because those donors with fatty livers do not need to undergo this invasive procedure. In contrast, in donors with a normal LAI, biopsy is still required to detect otherwise undetectable underlying diffuse liver disease. In our study population, we found that unenhanced and multiphasic-enhanced CT failed to detect some cases of noncirrhotic diffuse hepatic parenchymal disease (apparent only on biopsy) in donors thought to be otherwise healthy. Also, coexisting hemochromatosis may mask the degree of macrovesicular steatosis by elevation of CT attenuation value. Consequently, a core liver biopsy should be performed in every donor with normal hepatic CT LAI to exclude radiologically occult liver diseases.

Relevant Hepatic Pathology

The computed tomographic scan also plays a significant role in the detection of incidental focal liver lesions and of some diffuse hepatic diseases (cirrhosis) that may preclude an individual from being a donor (Fig. 46–6).

Evaluation of Hepatic Vascular Anatomy

Hepatic Arterial Anatomy

Anatomic variations of the branching pattern and origin of the hepatic arteries are common. Michel's original series,[13] published in 1966, defined the normal hepatic arterial anatomy in only 55% of 200 cadavers. Subsequent study[14] in 1000 patients who underwent liver harvesting demonstrated an incidence of normal

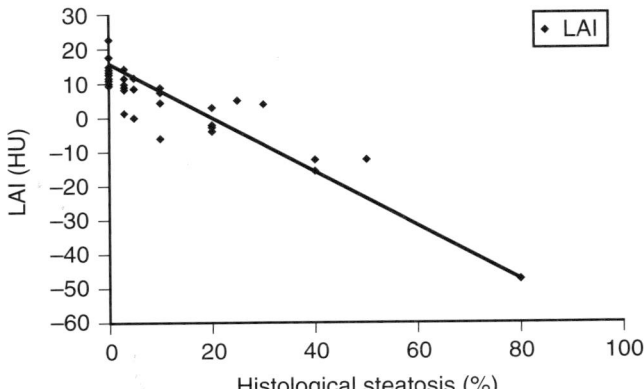

LAI VS HISTOLOGICAL STEATOSIS

FIGURE 46-5

A graph demonstrates the high degree of correlation between the LAI (*y axis*) as a function of histological percentage of macrovesicular steatosis (*x axis*) across a range of values.

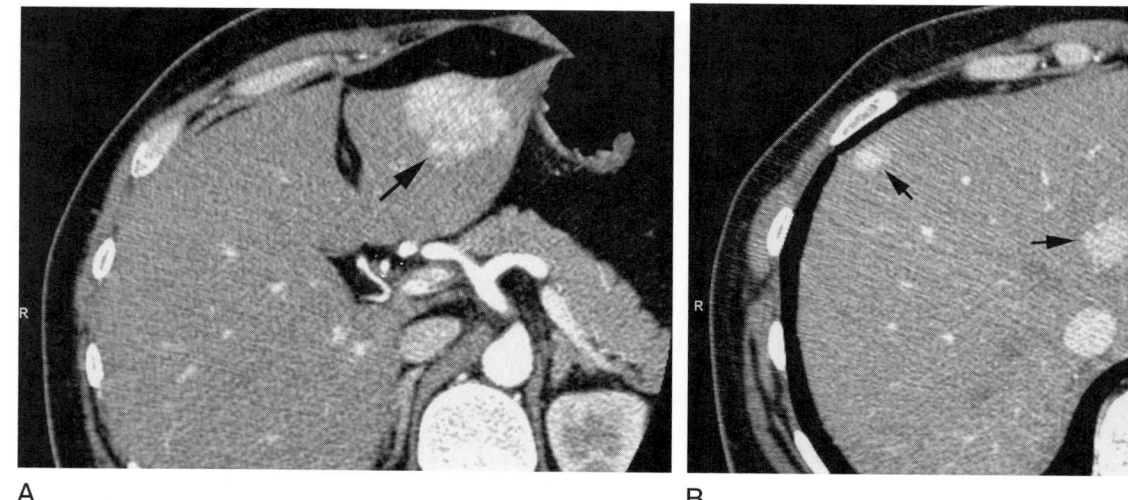

FIGURE 46–6

A and **B,** Three incidental liver masses (*arrows*) were shown on hepatic MDCT of a 42-year-old female potential liver donor. This incidental finding eliminated her chance to be a donor.

hepatic arterial pattern in 75.7%. These hepatic arterial variants are as follows:

Type 1: Normal; proper hepatic artery arises from the common hepatic artery and divides distally to form the left and right hepatic arteries (75.7%) (Fig. 46–7)

Type 2: Replaced or accessory left hepatic artery arising from left gastric artery (9.7%) (Fig. 46–8)

Type 3: Replaced or accessory right hepatic artery arising from the superior mesenteric artery (10.6%) (Fig. 46–9)

Type 4: Replaced or accessory left hepatic artery plus replaced or accessory right hepatic artery (2.3%)

Type 5: Common hepatic artery arising from superior mesenteric artery (1.5%)

Type 6: Common hepatic artery arising from aorta (0.2%)

All arteries supplying the right lobe, either normal (see Fig. 46–7) or of aberrant origin (see Fig. 46–9), require preservation and microvascular anastomoses to prevent postoperative ischemia in the recipient. Another important vessel to delineate is artery to segment IV.[15] This small vessel could have a normal origin (left hepatic artery) or aberrant origin (right hepatic artery), or both (Fig. 46–10). Preservation of segment IV artery

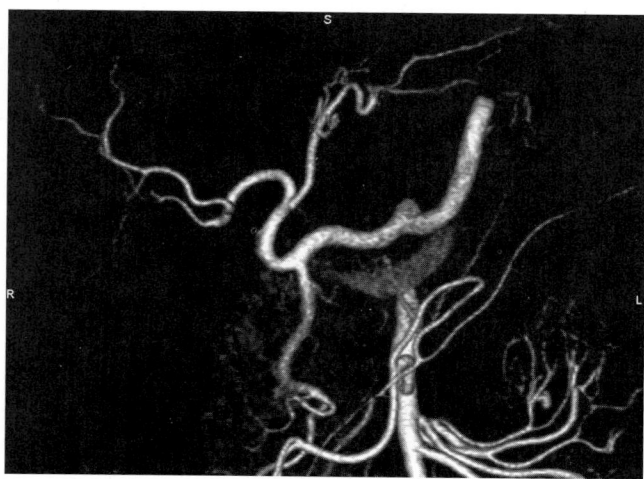

FIGURE 46–7

Three-dimensional volume-rendered CTA in a 52-year-old male potential liver donor demonstrates normal hepatic arterial anatomy.

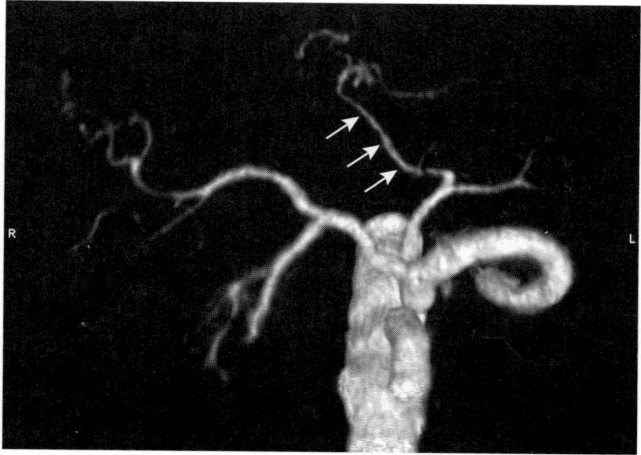

FIGURE 46–8

Three-dimensional volume-rendered CTA in a potential donor demonstrates a replaced left hepatic artery (*white arrows*) from the left gastric artery.

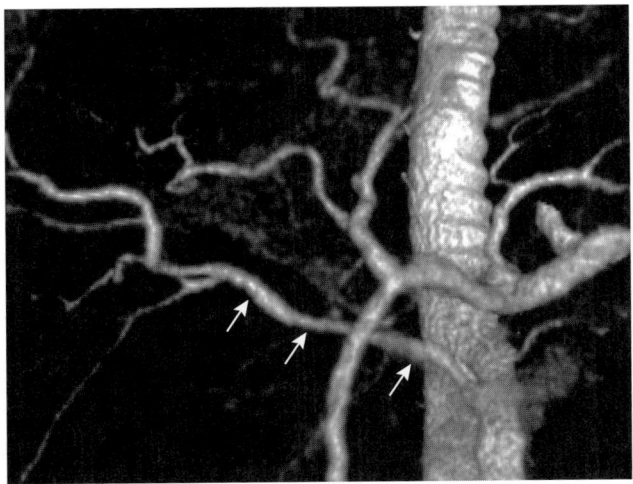

FIGURE 46–9

Three-dimensional volume-rendered CTA in a 30-year-old male potential liver donor demonstrates a big accessory right hepatic artery (*white arrows*) from the superior mesenteric artery.

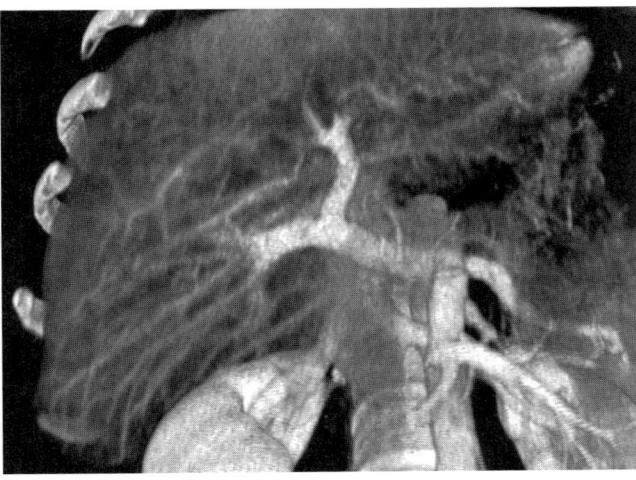

FIGURE 46–11

Normal portal bifurcation of a 37-year-old male potential liver donor is demonstrated on volume-rendered three-dimensional CT portography.

in the donor is essential to ensure adequate regeneration of the remaining left lobe. In the case of a segment IV artery arising from the right hepatic artery, the division of the right hepatic artery needs to be distal to the origin of segment IV artery. Hence the preoperative evaluation of the arterial anatomy is crucial to either donor selection or operative planning.

Although potential donors at our institution underwent conventional catheter angiography in the past, this has increasingly been replaced by noninvasive CT arteriography, which has proved to be excellent for demonstrating even small variants, correlating closely with conventional catheter angiography and operative findings.[16,17]

Portal Venous Anatomy

Variant portal venous anatomy is much less common than in hepatic arteries, being reported in only 20% of cases.[15] However, knowledge of portal venous anatomy preoperatively is essential. In a donor with normal portal bifurcation (Fig. 46–11), only single anastomosis is required in the recipient. Some portal variations include trifurcation (confluence of right posterior, right anterior, and left anterior to the main portal vein) (Fig. 46–12),

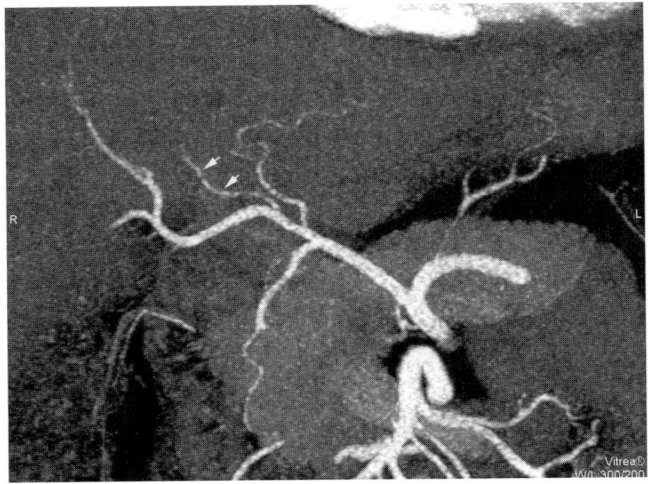

FIGURE 46–10

Three-dimensional CTA of a potential donor demonstrates an aberrant origin of segment IV (*white arrows*) artery from the right hepatic artery.

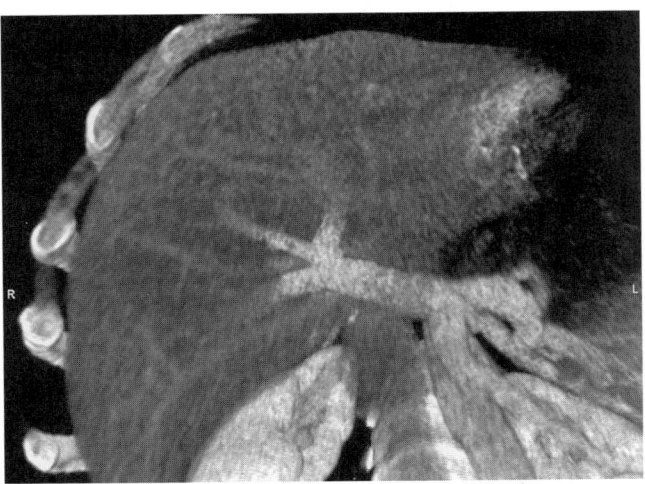

FIGURE 46–12

Trifurcation of the portal vein in a 44-year-old male potential liver donor is shown on volume-rendered three-dimensional CT portography.

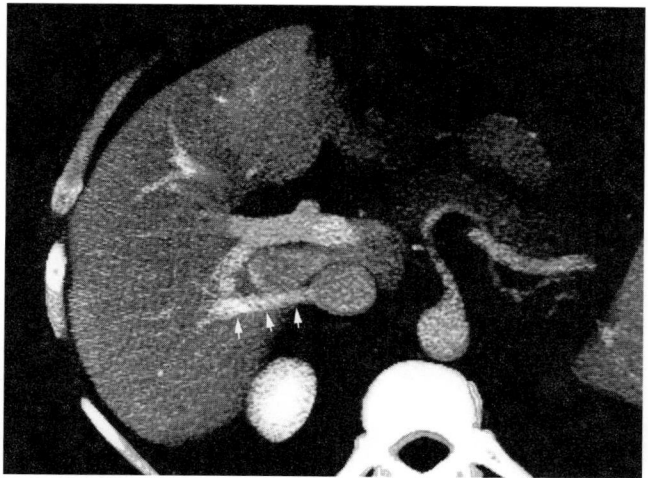

FIGURE 46–13

A significant inferior hepatic vein (IHV) (*white arrows*) draining the posteroinferior portion of the right lobe into the IVC on axial computed tomographic hepatic venography.

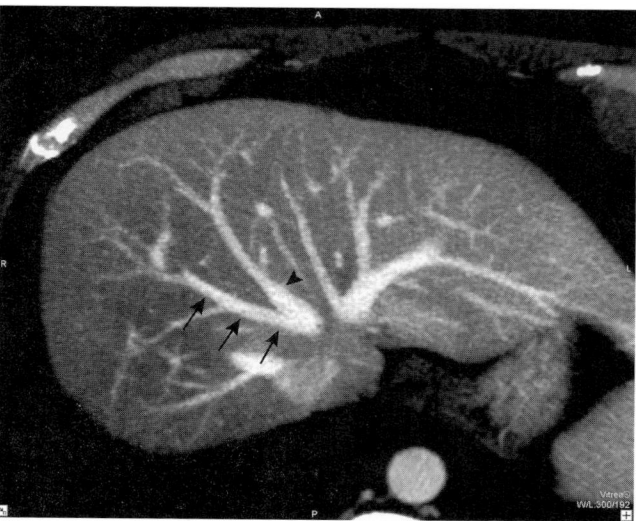

FIGURE 46–14

A significant aberrant segment VIII vein (*arrows*) draining a portion of the right lobe into the middle hepatic vein (*arrowhead*) on axial computed tomographic hepatic venography.

right anterior originating from left portal vein, and left anterior originating from right anterior portal vein. These variations require two separate anastomoses in the recipient.

Hepatic Venous Anatomy

The accessory inferior right hepatic vein draining the posteroinferior portion of the right lobe (Fig. 46–13) is reported in 68% of cases.[15] This aberrant vein requires special attention if it is larger than 5 mm and should be preserved during surgery to prevent the risk of graft malfunction. Also, a large aberrant segment VIII vein draining significant portions of the anterior right lobe into the middle hepatic vein (Fig. 46–14) must be identified preoperatively if it is larger than 5 mm. Additional anastomoses of these major hepatic veins must be performed to ensure the proper hepatic drainage in the recipient after transplantation.

Biliary Anatomy Evaluation

Anatomic variants of the biliary system are well recognized and important to identify preoperatively for optimal donor selection and to avoid biliary leaks. Huang and colleagues[18] classified the variants of right lobe ductal drainage into five types. These included normal bifurcation in 62.6% of the normal population, trifurcation variant (confluence of the right posterior, right anterior, and left anterior to the common hepatic duct) in 19%, aberrant drainage of the right posterior duct into the left main duct in 11%, low-lying drainage of the right posterior duct into the common hepatic duct in

5.8%, and into the cystic duct in 1.6%. Normal biliary bifurcation (Fig. 46–15) of donor liver requires only single biliary reconstruction (choledochocholedochostomy or hepaticojejunostomy) in the recipient. In donor livers with aberrant drainage of right lobe ducts (Figs. 46–16 and 46–17), two separate biliary anastomoses at transplant are essential to prevent postoperative biliary leakage and long-term segmental atrophy in the recipient graft. Preoperative mapping of donor biliary anatomy is therefore mandatory for guiding surgical planning.

Although endoscopic retrograde cholangiopancreatography (ERCP) is well accepted as a gold standard for

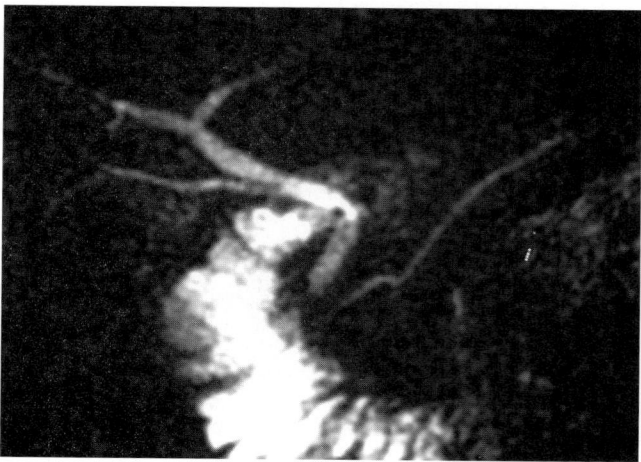

FIGURE 46–15

Normal biliary anatomy on an MRCP of a 46-year-old male potential liver donor.

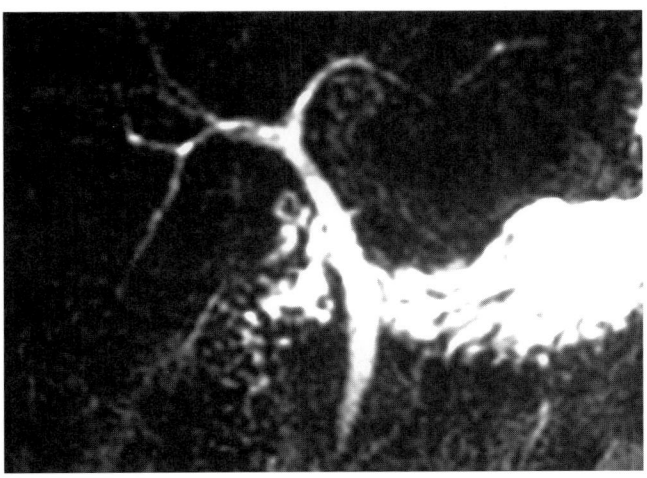

FIGURE 46-16

Trifurcation variant of biliary system (confluence of right posterior, right anterior, and left duct to the common hepatic duct) on an MRCP of a 49-year-old female potential liver donor.

evaluation of the biliary anatomy, it can be technically challenging and may result in significant complications (5.5% risk of pancreatitis; 3% to 5% risk of perforation),[19] which is considered an invasive technique for otherwise healthy donors. At our institution, we use noninvasive MRCP for preoperative mapping of biliary anatomy in living related liver donors. Overall, 96.3% of our MRCPs[20] show sufficient information for preoperative mapping of biliary anatomy. By using intraoperative cholangiography as a study of reference, our preoperative MRCP had an 88.5% accuracy in the detection of biliary variants in 26 living related donors. New MRCP techniques using MR contrast agents secreted into the bile ducts (e.g., mangafodipir trisodium [MnDPDP][21]

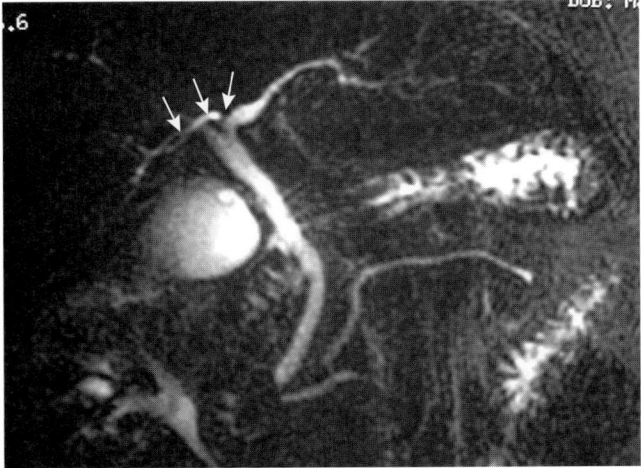

FIGURE 46-17

Aberrant drainage of right posterior duct (*white arrows*) into the left main duct on an MRCP of a 52-year-old female potential liver donor.

and gadolinium benzylopropionic tetracetate [Gd-BOPTA][22]) are in progress. Preliminary data show even more accuracy over conventional MRCP, and contrast-enhanced MRCP is very promising in improving preoperative mapping of biliary anatomy in living related donors.

Comprehensive Magnetic Resonance Imaging

Magnetic resonance imaging (MRI) has the capability to provide all imaging needs in the assessment of the potential liver donor. Other than MRCP, MRI of liver and MR angiography could be performed in lieu of CT and CTA. MRI of the liver is certainly adequate for exclusion of incidental pathology, and fatty deposition could be identified by chemical shift techniques. However, correlation of chemical shift with fat content will need to be quantified. Segmental liver volumes could be calculated from axial MR images in the same way they are calculated by CT. For vascular anatomy, the larger hepatic vessels are usually well depicted, but the smaller accessory branches and detailed branching of smaller arteries such as segment IV artery may not be sufficiently delineated. Thus CTA remains the test of choice for vascular anatomy. Nevertheless, with future improvements in MR angiography, MRI has the potential to evaluate comprehensively the potential living related liver donor.

Comprehensive Computed Tomography

As is apparent from the previous discussion, CT is optimal for the assessment of all relevant information except for delineation of biliary anatomy, hence the additional need for MRCP. Nevertheless, improvements in biliary contrast agents in the future, and other technical advances in CT that allow widespread use of CT cholangiography, may ultimately permit all-in-one CT in the evaluation of living related liver donors.

Summary

Living related liver transplantation is a major surgical undertaking with significant risks to the healthy donor, and imaging plays a vitally important role in donor selection and preoperative planning. Segmental volume calculation, exclusion of hepatic pathology, delineation of arterial, portal, and hepatic venous anatomy, and biliary anatomy are all important tasks that can be performed by non-invasive CT or MRI, or both. Currently we advocate CT with CT angiography, and MRCP, to leverage the optimal strengths of CT and MRI, although in the future, it may be feasible to perform either comprehensive MRI or comprehensive CT for all imaging needs.

Pearls and Pitfalls

- Noninvasive imaging by either CT or MRI can be used for donor selection.
- CTA is currently the best noninvasive imaging method for detailed evaluation of small segmental hepatic arteries.
- CTA is excellent in depicting variant portal venous and hepatic venous anatomy.
- CT fat density calculation can obviate liver biopsy in some patients if gross fatty infiltration is found.
- Three-dimensional quantification of segmental liver volume requires knowledge of precise segmental boundaries on imaging.
- Normal CT density, although excluding significant fatty liver, still does not preclude the possibility of other diffuse disease, and biopsy is still indicated in these patients.
- MR angiography, although excellent for mapping larger vessels, including main right and left arteries, is challenged in depiction of the smaller segmental arteries such as segment IV artery.
- Conventional MRCP, although fairly good in biliary mapping, is not always adequate if the ducts are delicate; currently, biliary contrast-enhanced MRCP is better.
- Although comprehensive imaging is possible using either CT alone or MR alone, currently, the best angiographic depiction is by CTA and the best biliary depiction is by MRCP.

References

1. Renz JF, Busuttil RW: Adult-to-adult living-donor liver transplantation: A critical analysis. Semin Liver Dis 20:411-424, 2000.
2. Wachs ME, Bak TE, Karrer FM, et al: Adult living donor liver transplantation using a right hepatic lobe. Transplantation 66:1313-1316, 1998.
3. Bassignani MJ, Fulcher AS, Szucs RA, et al: Use of imaging for living donor liver transplantation. Radiographics 21:39-52, 2001.
4. Schroeder T, Malago M, Debatin JF, et al: Multidetector computed tomographic cholangiography in the evaluation of potential living liver donors. Transplantation 73:1972-1973, 2002.
5. Kiuchi T, Kasahara M, Uryuhara K, et al: Impact of graft size mismatching on graft prognosis in liver transplantation from living donors. Transplantation 67:321-327, 1999.
6. Schiano TD, Bodian C, Schwartz M, et al: Accuracy and significance of computed tomographic scan assessment of hepatic volume in patients undergoing liver transplantation. Transplantation 69:545-550, 2000.
7. Selzner M, Clavien PA: Fatty liver in liver transplantation and surgery. Semin Liver Dis 21:105-113, 2001.
8. Cheng YF, Chen CL, Lai CY, et al: Assessment of donor fatty livers for liver transplantation. Transplantation 71:1221-1225, 2001.
9. Ploeg RJ, D'Alessandro AM, Knechtle SJ, et al: Risk factors for primary dysfunction after liver transplantation—a multivariate analysis. Transplantation 55:807-813, 1993.
10. Hiyashi M, Fujii K, Kiuchi T, et al: Effects of fatty infiltration of the graft on the outcome of living-related liver transplantation. Transplant Proc 31:403, 1999.
11. Limanond P, Raman SS, Lassman C, et al: Macrovesicular hepatic steatosis in living related liver donors: Correlation between CT and histologic findings. Radiology 230:276-280, 2004.
12. Raptopoulos V, Karellas A, Bernstein J, et al: Value of dual-energy CT in differentiating focal fatty infiltration of the liver from low-density masses. AJR Am J Roentgenol 157:721-725, 1991.
13. Michel NA: Newer anatomy of the liver and its variant blood supply and collateral circulation. Am J Surg 112:337-347, 1966.
14. Hiatt JR, Gabbay J, Busuttil RW: Surgical anatomy of the hepatic arteries in 1000 cases. Ann Surg 220:50-52, 1994.
15. Kamel IR, Kruskal JB, Raptopoulos V: Imaging for right lobe living donor liver transplantation. Semin Liver Dis 21:271-282, 2001.
16. Lu DS, Limanond P, Raman SS, et al: Accuracy of CT angiography in mapping of hepatic vascular anatomy in adult to adult living related liver transplant donors [abstract for Radiological Society of North America 2002 annual meeting]. Radiology (Suppl), 2002.
17. Winter TC 3rd, Nghiem HV, Freeny PC, et al: Hepatic arterial anatomy: Demonstration of normal supply and vascular variants with three-dimensional CT angiography. Radiographics 15:771-780, 1995.
18. Huang TL, Cheng YF, Chen CL, et al: Variants of the bile ducts: Clinical application in the potential donor of living-related hepatic transplantation. Transplant Proc 28:1669-1670, 1996.
19. Cohen SA, Siegel JH, Kasmin FE: Complications of diagnostic and therapeutic ERCP. Abdom Imaging 21:385-394, 1996.
20. Limanond P, Raman SS, Ghobhrial M, et al: Accuracy of MRCP in preoperative mapping of biliary anatomy in adult to adult living related liver transplant donors [abstract for Radiological Society of North America 2002 annual meeting]. Radiology (Suppl), 2002.
21. Kapoor V, Peterson MS, Baron RL, et al: Intrahepatic biliary anatomy of living adult liver donors: Correlation of mangafodipir trisodium–enhanced MR cholangiography and intraoperative cholangiography. AJR Am J Roentgenol 179:1281-1286, 2002.
22. Goyen M, Barkhausen J, Debatin JF, et al: Right-lobe living related liver transplantation: Evaluation of a comprehensive magnetic resonance imaging protocol for assessing potential donors. Liver Transpl 8:241-250, 2002.

Outcomes of Living Donor Liver Transplantation

JOHN F. RENZ
CINDY J. KIN
BOB H. SAGGI
JEAN C. EMOND

Historical background   714

Donor outcomes   715
    Pediatric LDLT donor outcomes   715
    Adult-to-adult LDLT donor outcomes   716

Pediatric LDLT recipient outcomes   717

Adult LDLT recipient outcomes   718
    North America   718
    Europe   719
    Asia   719

Discussion   720

Living donor liver transplantation (LDLT) procedures are remarkable technical achievements designed to increase the organ supply for children and adults. Justification of living donation originates from the increasing wait list morbidity and mortality in transplant candidates. LDLT has been performed in children and adults throughout the world, with more than 1000 European, 1600 North American, and 2000 Asian living donor procedures reported.[1] Successful application of LDLT mandates specific medical and surgical considerations for the donor and recipient to circumvent complications unique to the transplantation of partial-liver allografts.

The rapid evolution of surgical strategies to increase the organ supply has occurred in less than a decade and has spawned new areas of discovery that affect liver transplantation as well as hepatobiliary surgery.[2] Such advancements include medical management of recipients with "small-for-size" allografts,[3,4] treatment of complications unique to partial-allograft transplantation,[2,5-9] liver regeneration in donors and recipients,[10,11] and post-donation donor management.[12-17]

As the application of LDLT increases, the inevitable donor morbidity and mortality that accompany these procedures have stimulated a continuing ethical debate. This chapter details the historical background and summarizes current donor and recipient outcomes of LDLT in children and adults.

Historical Background

Transplantation of a partial-liver allograft was theoretically proposed for children by Smith in 1969[18] and first successfully performed by Raia and colleagues in 1989.[19] LDLT in children originated as a response to the disparity in pediatric wait list times that resulted in wait list mortality exceeding 25%.[20,21] Strong was the first to perform pediatric living donor liver transplantation (pLDLT) with long-term success,[22] and Broelsch reported the first clinical series of pLDLT in which recipient and allograft survival equaled that of deceased donor whole organs.[23] Through the 1990s, pLDLT was applied throughout the world with excellent results and has become accepted therapy for children with end-stage liver disease. The success of pLDLT, coupled with dramatic increases in adult wait list times and morbidity, has provided a powerful stimulus to extend the use of LDLT to adult recipients.[24,25]

Successful application of adult-to-adult living donor liver transplantation (aLDLT) mandates unique surgical and medical considerations. The principal surgical challenges include the procurement of an allograft with sufficient liver volume to meet the metabolic needs of the recipient; positioning of the allograft to optimize vascular inflow, venous outflow, and biliary drainage; and appreciation of anatomic variations that necessitate complex biliary or vascular reconstruction.[26]

Several types of allografts are available for aLDLT, and the specific choice of an allograft predisposes the recipient and donor to a unique set of potential complications. Potential complications that require attention include biliary complications, bleeding of the cut liver surface, acute and chronic hepatic venous outflow obstruction, hepatic arterial complications, and poor synthetic function secondary to insufficient hepatic residual volume in the donor or insufficient transplanted allograft volume to fulfill the recipient's metabolic demands.

The anatomic classification of the liver described by Couinaud[27] and refined by Bismuth[28] has been universally accepted by the transplant communities in Europe, Asia, and North America as the reference system for describing allografts created by LDLT. The four anatomic allografts used for LDLT (Fig. 47–1) include the right liver lobe (Couinaud segments V to VIII), the left liver lobe (Couinaud segments II to IV), the left lateral segment (Couinaud segments II and III), and the extended right liver or "trisegment" allograft (Couinaud segments IV to VIII).

Although all four allografts have been successfully applied to select adult recipients,[29,30] the right lobe allograft, which accounts for greater than 60% of the donor's total liver mass, is the most commonly used allograft for aLDLT worldwide. Right lobe allografts typically provide liver mass that permit donors of equal or slightly smaller size to donate. Use of a right lobe allograft was

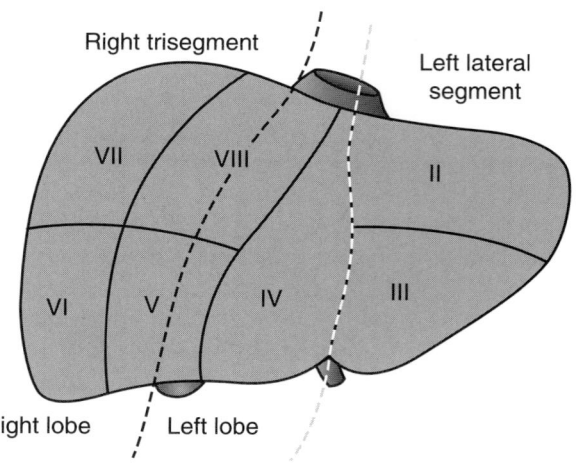

FIGURE 47–1

Surgical division of the liver. Surgical division of the liver along Cantlie's line (*hatched*) yields left (segments I to IV) and right (segments V to VIII) lobes that can be used in adult-to-adult living donor liver transplantation. Division along the falciform ligament (*white line*) yields the pediatric left lateral segment allograft (segments II and III) or the adult extended right lobe allograft (segments IV to VIII).

initially described by Habib and Tanaka of Kyoto, who were attempting to harvest a left lobe for LDLT when anatomic considerations favored a right lobectomy.[31] Wachs and associates from the University of Colorado were the first in North America to describe LDLT with a right lobe allograft.[32]

The left lobe allograft (Couinaud segments II to IV) accounts for approximately 35% of the total liver volume and typically provides 300- to 500-cc allografts. These allografts are commonly used for smaller adults or older adolescents with recipient weights of approximately 50 kg.

Transplantation of the left lateral segment (Couinaud segments II and III) to children and smaller adult recipients has been performed in the setting of large donor-to-recipient size disparity. The volume of the left lateral segment typically accounts for approximately 20% of the standard liver volume and yields a 200- to 300-cc allograft. In the authors' experience, the upper limit of recipient weight for living donation of left lateral segment allografts has been less than 40 kg. These parameters clearly limit the applicability of left lateral segment allografts to a small subgroup of adult recipients.

The least commonly applied aLDLT allograft is the extended right lobe derived from Couinaud segments IV to VIII.[33,34] Extended right lobe allografts account for greater than 70% of the standard liver volume and permit relatively small donors to donate to larger recipients. Retrospective analysis of donor risk in which extended right lobectomy was compared with left lobectomy found that the former was associated with increased transient liver dysfunction with prolonged cholestasis and the development of biliary strictures.[34] Although extended right donor lobectomy has been refined to reduce the incidence of complications,[35] the potential risk to the donor of performing greater than a three-fourths hepatectomy cannot currently justify widespread use of this technique.

"Small-for-size syndrome" is characterized by synthetic dysfunction, transaminitis typically two to four times the upper limit of normal, and prolonged cholestasis.[3] Synthetic function typically improves within 72 hours of transplantation as the allograft undergoes rapid hypertrophy, whereas cholestasis generally improves over the course of weeks to months. The occurrence of only these symptoms without the need for augmentation of synthetic function predicts a reversible situation that will improve as the allograft undergoes regeneration; however, the appearance of encephalopathy, hypoglycemia, metabolic acidosis, or continued augmentation of synthetic function beyond 48 hours heralds irreversible allograft failure that should prompt evaluation for retransplantation. Small-for-size syndrome in a donor requires immediate and careful assessment.

Biopsy of small-for-size allografts reveals a pattern of diffuse ischemic injury characterized by hepatocyte ballooning, steatosis, centrilobular necrosis, and parenchymal cholestasis that may be misinterpreted as preservation injury.[3] As the allograft regenerates, normalization of biopsy specimens typically occurs within 2 weeks, except for the presence of cholestasis, which usually persists for longer than a month. Although radiological data from Kawasaki[10] and Nakagami[11] and their colleagues demonstrate that the majority of volume regeneration occurs within 7 days of LDLT, small-for-size allografts should be considered highly vulnerable to insult with an increased risk for significant sequelae from complications or additional metabolic stress in the immediate postoperative period.

No formal registry of aLDLT has been successfully implemented despite widespread calls for its creation.[36-40] The National Institutes of Health (NIH) has supported a multicenter study on aLDLT[41]; however, these data have not matured, and accurate data on the performance of aLDLT exist only as individual reports in the literature. The following text summarizes the English literature from Asia, Europe, and North America through September 2004.

Donor Outcomes

Pediatric LDLT Donor Outcomes

More than a decade of experience has accumulated on the performance of pLDLT, and reports from multiple centers describe excellent donor outcomes.[14,15,17,42] Donor length of stay is typically less than 10 days, average donor blood loss is approximately 400 to 800 mL, and the need for heterologous blood transfusion is uncommon. Grewal[17] and Yamaoka[42] and their associates have each reported outcomes of 100 pLDLT donors with the aforementioned findings. Their data have been mirrored by smaller studies in North America[12] and Europe.[43] The overall incidence of complications ranges from 15% to 40% (Table 47–1), with roughly half classified as serious (requiring either a surgical or interventional procedure or increased hospital stay) and half classified as nonserious.

Serious complications cited by more than one transplant center include biliary leak or stricture, pulmonary embolism, cholestasis, and hernia. Biliary complications were the most commonly reported source of donor morbidity, with an overall incidence of 5% to 10%.[15,17,42] Leakage of bile prolonged donor hospitalization and was most frequently treated by percutaneous drainage; however, reoperation for repair of biliary leaks has also been performed. There are no data in the literature on long-term sequelae from biliary complications.

Hernia occurs in approximately 5% of pLDLT donors. In the authors' experience, the use of a midline incision during performance of the procedure has decreased the observed incidence of hernia. Intra-abdominal abscesses have been reported but are rare.[46]

A nonserious complication frequently noted is postdonation dyspepsia or altered gastric motility. The left vagal trunk sends branches from the stomach to the hepatic hilum through the gastrohepatic ligament. In pLDLT, this ligament is divided during the dissection, and the stomach and diaphragm are retracted. Thus, a real possibility exists for vagal trunk or branch injury. Indeed, two reports[15,16] document dyspepsia/gastritis in previously healthy donors. In the authors' series of more than 100 pLDLT procedures, the observed incidence is approximately 11%, with the majority of donors treated successfully with H_2 antagonists.

An anonymous survey soliciting donor opinions of pLDLT revealed overall satisfaction with the process.[47] Donor attitudes toward the role of pLDLT were

Table 47–1. DONOR COMPLICATIONS OF PEDIATRIC LIVING DONOR LIVER TRANSPLANTATION

Author	Year	N	Follow-up (yr)	Complication (%)
Lo[44]	2003	605	5	9
Grewal[17]	1998	100	3	34
Ohkohchi[15]	1998	25	3	40
Haberal[45]	1998	19	5	15
Yamaoka[42]	1995	100	2	15
Malago[43]	1994	36	2	19

overwhelmingly positive. Endorsement of the procedure was acknowledged by donors regardless of allograft outcome or the presence of a postdonation complication. Eighty-eight percent of donors thought that the role of LDLT should be "increased" and should not be reserved solely for "emergency situations." No donors believed that pLDLT should be abandoned or that they were "forced" to donate. All donors were satisfied with the information provided to them before donation.

Donor physical symptoms, including pain and the appearance of the surgical wound, were common concerns. Thirty-seven percent of donors reported postoperative pain that was "greater than anticipated," whereas 25% reported a surgical wound that was "larger than anticipated." However, complete return to predonation activities, including employment, was observed in all donors, and donor perception of time to "complete recovery" was reported as less than 1 month (25%), 1 to 3 months (50%), 3 to 6 months (12%), and longer than 12 months (12%). No changes in sexual function or menstruation were reported after donation, and five of six donors who attempted to have another child successfully procreated.

Donor deaths have occurred during the performance of pLDLT, although the precise number of donor deaths to date is speculative.[43,48] The estimated number of pLDLT procedures performed in North America and Europe exceeds 1500, with an even greater number performed in Asia. At least two deaths in pLDLT donors have been reported: one in North America and one in Europe. The cause of death in both donors was pulmonary embolism. Of note, each occurred in overweight females with a smoking history. To date, there are no reports of pLDLT donor death in Asia.[44] These data yield an approximately 0.1% incidence of donor mortality in Western countries, which is the figure generally estimated by most pLDLT transplant programs.

Adult-to-Adult LDLT Donor Outcomes

Although excellent donor outcomes have been reported after pLDLT, these results may not be directly applicable to aLDLT because of the vastly different surgical procedure and the wider spectrum of donor candidates. Direct technical comparisons are invalid because procurement of a right lobe, extended right lobe, or left lobe allograft is substantially more difficult than procurement of a left lateral segment allograft. Furthermore, most pLDLT donor candidates are parents, which narrows the population with respect to age and relationship. aLDLT includes a more heterogeneous donor population with variable age, health, physical characteristics, and emotional attachment to the potential recipient.

Donor candidates may range from a teenage child of the potential recipient to an older spouse, sibling, or friend. The available data on liver regeneration and physiology after donation, derived principally from pLDLT, are not directly applicable to such a wide population.

aLDLT is practiced throughout the world, including Asia, North America, South America, and Europe. The total number of right lobe aLDLT procedures performed worldwide has been estimated to currently exceed 2000 according to data from the September 2004 International Symposium of Living Donor Transplantation. With this experience, aLDLT donor outcome data are emerging. The incidence and severity of aLDLT donor complications are higher than those reported for pediatric donation.[38] The donor undergoes a more extensive and prolonged operation and donates a much larger fraction of hepatic parenchyma, thereby resulting in less metabolic reserve to maintain homeostasis or recover from a complication.

The lack of a formal registry impedes verifiable donor outcome data on aLDLT. Unfortunately, data on long-term donor outcomes are very limited.[49-51] Furthermore, a survey of U.S. transplant centers' practice patterns of long-term follow-up for aLDLT donors indicates widespread variation. During the first year, 68% have an established formal follow-up protocol; however, follow-up longer than 1 year was typically "as needed," with appointments initiated by the donor.[52] Although multiple reports indicate an average hospital stay of less than 7 days and performance of living donation without the need for nonautologous blood transfusion,[29,32,53] serious donor complications and death are possible. Complications related to anesthesia, performance of surgery, the surgical technique, postoperative recovery, the metabolic stress of liver regeneration, and impaired wound healing, as well as the psychosocial impact of major surgery and recovery, have become evident with the increasing clinical experience of aLDLT.[54] Marcos and coauthors and Todo reported no significant donor complications in early series of 40 and 27 right lobe allografts, respectively,[53,55] whereas Testa and associates reported an overall complication rate of greater than 50% in the performance of 30 right lobe allografts.[56] An American Society of Transplant Surgeons (ASTS) survey of 30 North American transplant centers that performed 208 aLDLT procedures identified an overall donor complication rate of 10%.[57] The most common donor complication was postoperative biliary leakage, which was typically treated by percutaneous drainage. Additional complications included pressure sores, incisional hernia, pulmonary embolism, pneumonia, and pleural effusions. Approximately 5% of donors required heterologous blood transfusion, and 3% required reoperation for complications related to donation. Abortion of the living donor procedure because of intraoperative findings or donor events has been reported. These data

Table 47-2. DONOR COMPLICATIONS OF ADULT-TO-ADULT LIVING DONOR LIVER TRANSPLANTATION

Author	Year	N	Follow-up (yr)	Complication (%)
Lo[59]	2004	100	2	27
Walter[60]	2003	28	2	18
Ito[61]	2003	200	2	37
Boillot[62]	2003	88	4	46
Umeshita[63]	2003	25	5	19
Malago[64]	2003	74	3	40

were mirrored by a later survey of 433 aLDLT procedures by Brown and colleagues.[58] However, individual center reports of donor complications are higher and range from 18% to 46% (Table 47-2). This discrepancy demonstrates the inherent limitations of retrospective surveys and underscores the limitations of existing data in the absence of a verifiable data collection instrument. The available data on donor complications are summarized in Table 47-3. Additional serious donor complications multiply reported include portal vein thrombosis, neurapraxia, pleural effusion, ascites, and pneumonia.

A donor outcome survey from five Asian centers that included 334 left lobe and 561 right lobe aLDLT procedures was reported by Lo.[65] Right lobe donors experienced a 28% overall complication rate, as opposed to a rate of 7% in left lobe allograft donors and 9% in left lateral segment donors. Complications included cholestasis (7%), bile leak (6%), biliary stricture (1%), portal vein thrombosis (0.5%), intra-abdominal bleeding (0.5%), and pulmonary embolism (0.5%). No hospital mortality occurred, but there was a late donor death 3 years after donation. Long-term follow-up information was available from only 15% of the donor population.[65]

Extended right lobe donors experience significant complications. In an early series, Lo and coauthors reported a donor survival rate of 100%; however, significant donor complications included infection, prolonged cholestasis, bile leak, and late biliary stricture.[34]

Table 47-3. COMPLICATIONS REPORTED AFTER ADULT-TO-ADULT LIVING DONOR LIVER TRANSPLANTATION: SERIES DATA

Complication	Incidence (%)
Overall	15–50
Biliary leak	8–15
Rehospitalization	≈8
Small for size	≈5
Reoperation	≈5
Biliary stricture	≈3

Although the technique has been refined to reduce the complication rate,[35] the potential risks to donors by removing more than three fourths of their livers mandates limitation of this technique to highly select circumstances.

Although the precise number of donor deaths to date is speculative,[48,66,67] donor mortality is much more frequent in aLDLT. Tragically, donors have required emergency liver transplantation for hepatic insufficiency. Donor deaths have been reported in North America,[57,68,69] Europe,[62,64] and Asia.[70] The lack of precise morbidity and mortality data will be addressed by the NIH-sponsored study,[41] as well as by the development of Japanese and European registries; however, these data are not currently available. Based on existing data, a reasonable estimate of the incidence of donor mortality is 0.4%.[57,67,71]

Pediatric LDLT Recipient Outcomes

In the initial series of pLDLT, Broelsch and colleagues reported recipient and allograft survival to be equal to that after transplantation of deceased donor whole organs.[23] Through the 1990s, pLDLT was broadly applied to infants throughout the world with excellent results.[72-74] Implementation of pLDLT resulted in significant decreases in wait list morbidity and mortality in pediatric transplant centers.[75,76] Improved results and technical innovations followed as the technique became accepted therapy for children with end-stage liver disease.[5-7] Presently, pLDLT provides more than half of infant organs at pediatric referral centers.[72,73,75]

The theoretical advantages of "timing" liver transplantation to avoid patient deterioration while awaiting a deceased donor allograft, decreasing hospital stay by earlier transplantation, and providing "optimum" allografts that have received intense medical screening with minimal ischemic times were realized.[72,73,75,76] Timed application of pLDLT restores growth and development and thereby optimizes recipient quality of life.[77] Furthermore, pLDLT has been demonstrated to provide satisfactory outcomes in the retransplantation of children.[78] In 2004, Roberts and coworkers analyzed pediatric outcomes of living donor, deceased donor whole-organ, and deceased donor partial-liver allografts from the database of the U.S. Scientific Registry of Transplant Recipients (SRTR). The data clearly indicate that pLDLT outcomes meet or exceed those of deceased donor whole-organ and partial-liver allografts in children younger than 2 years.[79] LDLT in larger children with metabolic needs that cannot be supplied by a left lateral segment allograft require either a left or a right lobe allograft and have complications similar to those observed in adult recipients.

Adult LDLT Recipient Outcomes

Makuuchi and colleagues were the first to report successful aLDLT with a left lobe allograft,[29] and Miller and associates of Mt. Sinai Medical Center in New York reported the largest North American series.[30] Although complications and allograft survival in left lobe recipients have paralleled those of right lobe recipients, transplantation of left lobe allografts is technically more difficult than right lobe allografts. Technical challenges of left lobe allografts include greater anatomic variance, smaller transplanted volumes, and increased difficulty in precise anatomic allograft positioning as a result of the left-to-right orientation of hilar structures.

North America

Of the 5125 liver transplants reported by the SRTR in 2003, aLDLT procedures accounted for 253.[80] The performance of aLDLT peaked at 408 procedures in 2001.[80] SRTR data are limited to the performance of a procedure, and they neither identify the type of allograft used nor explore outcomes; however, the right lobe allograft (Couinaud segments V to VIII) was used in most procedures. In North America, the average adult body habitus excludes the use of left lobe allografts, which are typically restricted to recipients with a body mass less than 60 kg. In an initial series of 40 right lobe allografts, Marcos and coauthors reported an 80% recipient survival rate in their first 20 recipients, which improved to 95% in the second group of 20 recipients.[53] Bak and coworkers of the University of Colorado reported an 85% recipient survival rate in an initial series of 20 right lobe allografts.[81] Multiple detailed reviews have followed.[82-85] Individual center reports from the literature are summarized in Table 47–4.

The ASTS initiated the earliest attempt to create a registry identifying outcomes of aLDLT in North America. A data-protected survey was distributed to all transplant centers in the United States and Canada that contribute to the SRTR. The overall response rate exceeded 88%, and 30 North American liver transplant centers were identified that had performed a total of 208 aLDLT procedures.[57] Twenty-eight (13%) aLDLT recipient deaths were reported: 14 (7%) were related to allograft dysfunction, 10 (5%) were unrelated to allograft function, and 4 (2%) were undetermined. Causes of recipient death not attributed to allograft function included intracranial hemorrhage, myocardial infarction, hemolytic-uremic syndrome, recurrent hepatitis C, graft-versus-host disease, multiple myeloma, recurrent hepatoma, recidivism, and aspergillosis 6 months after aLDLT.

Sixty-three complications were reported, for an overall complication rate of 30%.[57] The three most frequent complications were biliary, vascular, and primary allograft nonfunction. Thirty-seven biliary complications were reported (incidence of 18%), including parenchymal bile leak, biliary anastomotic leak, and biliary anastomotic stricture. Vascular complications, including aneurysm, anastomotic stricture, and hepatic arterial thrombosis, resulted in the loss of four allografts, for an overall incidence of 6%. Ten allografts (5%) were lost because of primary nonfunction. Additional surgical complications included Roux-en-Y limb leak, duodenal ulcer requiring surgery, and Roux-en-Y limb dehiscence, each in one patient. The incidence of complications did not correlate with the annual number of deceased donor whole-organ transplants performed by an individual center, but it did improve in centers that had greater experience with aLDLT, thus reflecting a "learning curve" effect.[35,53,59,81] The overall incidence of allograft failure, including primary nonfunction and recipient death as a result of allograft failure or complications, was 12%. These data are in agreement with the 10% incidence of allograft failure reported by Broelsch and

Table 47–4. LIVING DONOR LIVER TRANSPLANTATION IN THE UNITED STATES: RIGHT LOBE ALLOGRAFTS

Center	Author	Year	N	Recip (%)	Graft (%)	Comp (%)
New York[86]	Miller	2003	99	92	88	38
Los Angeles[87]	Ghobrial	2002	20	95	85	39
New York[88]	Fishbein	2001	50	87	80	32
Denver[81]	Bak	2001	41	93	88	> 34
New York[89]	Goldstein	2001	20	75	55	30
Chapel Hill[68]	Fair	2001	14	93	78	N/A
Memphis[90]	Grewal	2001	11	91	88	63
Rochester[53]	Marcos	2000	40	88	85	47
Richmond[91]	Marcos	1999	25	88	88	52

Comp, incidence of complications; Graft, graft 1-year survival rate; Recip, recipient 1-year survival rate.

colleagues[92] and notably better than the 19% incidence of allograft loss reported by Inomata and coworkers.[93]

Brown and associates conducted a later survey of U.S. transplant programs and reported data on 433 aLDLT procedures.[58] Centers that performed aLDLT were more likely to have larger deceased donor volumes and experience in pediatric transplantation. Although recipient and allograft survival were not reported, the reported incidence of biliary and vascular complications was 23% and 8%, respectively.

Fishbein and coworkers performed an analysis of the impact of aLDLT on transplant volume and demographics in United Network for Organ Sharing (UNOS) region 9 (New York).[88] The state of New York shares a single waiting list but has five programs offering aLDLT. During the period August 1998 through November 2000, the volume of deceased donor allografts was unchanged, whereas the proportion of living donor allografts increased from 2.2% of the total transplants performed to 28%, for a net increase of 118 aLDLT procedures.[88] Overall actuarial 1-year recipient and allograft survival rates were 84% and 78%, respectively, thus demonstrating a learning curve effect. Notably, the incidence of emergency retransplantation as a UNOS status 1 category for allograft primary nonfunction was 7.8% for aLDLT allografts versus 10.8% for deceased donor allografts. The authors concluded that aLDLT increased the capacity for transplantation in stable patients awaiting transplantation with no increased incidence of primary nonfunction; however, aLDLT did not have a significant impact on wait list mortality.[88]

Europe

aLDLT was first performed in Europe by Broelsch and colleagues in 1998.[94] These authors later summarized European aLDLT outcomes by reporting the activity of 11 centers in eight countries that performed 105 pediatric and 123 adult living donor procedures. Of the 123 aLDLT procedures, 111 were right lobe allografts.[94] The reporting period spanned 1996 through 2000, during which 2055 adult transplant procedures were performed, with aLDLT representing approximately 6% of the total. Crude recipient and allograft survival rates were 86% and 83%, respectively, with an observed 14.6% incidence of recipient biliary complications. Other recipient complications were not reported; however, Broelsch and coauthors did report one European donor death and an overall 30% incidence of donor complications, subclassified as "minor" (14%) and "major" (17%).[64,94] These data are in agreement with the literature from individual centers (Table 47–5).

Asia

The evolution of aLDLT has been notably different in Asia, where religious, cultural, and political ideologies have created significant obstacles to deceased donor organ donation.[100] The reported annual incidence of deceased donor liver donation remains as low as 0.5 per million population[101] despite legislation for deceased donor organ retrieval.[102,103] Transplant programs throughout Asia extended LDLT to adults as a matter of necessity. To date, successful aLDLT series have been reported in China, Taiwan, Hong Kong, Japan, and Korea (Table 47–6). Shinshu University in Japan performed the first successful aLDLT procedure with a left lobe allograft in 1993.[29] Inomata and colleagues of Kyoto, Japan, reported a 77% survival rate in an initial series of 26 right lobe allografts,[93] whereas Todo and associates of Hokkaido University reported an 80% actual allograft survival rate in an initial series of 21 right lobe allografts.[100] Regional summary data that mirror individual center data have been published[111-113] (see Table 47–6).

Unlike the dearth of left lobe allograft data from Western transplant centers, extensive data are available on left as well as right lobe allografts in Asia. These data demonstrate outcomes similar to those derived from the limited Western data, namely, a higher incidence of small-for-size syndrome, graft failure, and recipient

Table 47–5. LIVING DONOR LIVER TRANSPLANTATION IN EUROPE

Center	Author	Year	N	Recip (%)	Graft (%)	Comp (%)
France[95]	Boillot	2003	88	92	85	32
Essen[64]	Malago	2003	74	79	75	30
Moscow[96]	Gautier	2003	35	100	97	37
Bornova[97]	Tokat	2001	20	75	75	75
Paris[98]	Azoulay	2001	7	100	85	42
Barcelona[99]	Garcia-Valdecasas	2001	7	71	71	42
Essen[92]	Malago	2001	43	75	63	N/A

Comp, incidence of complications; Graft, graft 1-year survival rate; Recip, recipient 1-year survival rate.

Table 47–6. LIVING DONOR LIVER TRANSPLANTATION IN ASIA

Center	Author	Year	N	Recip (%)	Graft (%)	Comp (%)
Hong Kong[59]	Lo	2004	100	92	90	38
New Delhi[104]	Rajasekar	2003	10	100	60	30
Tokyo[105]	Hirata	2002	90	92	N/A	> 20
Seoul[106]	Lee	2001	157	87	87	25
Matsumoto[107]	Hashikura	2001	38	85	N/A	16
Sapporo[108]	Furukawa	2001	14	85	N/A	14
Okayama[109]	Inagaki	2001	10	N/A	N/A	40
Tokyo[110]	Kawasaki	1998	13	84	84	8

complications (both biliary and vascular) in left lobe allograft recipients than in right lobe recipients.[30,114-116] The University of Hong Kong Medical Center introduced the use of extended right lobe allografts in 1996 in an attempt to overcome the inadequate allograft volume and positional problems encountered with the smaller left lobe allografts. Lo and coauthors reported the first series of seven aLDLT procedures performed with extended right lobe allografts in patients with acute or fulminant hepatic failure (FHF).[34] This study reported recipient and allograft survival rates of 86%, which was significantly better than left lobe allograft outcomes; however, the incidence of recipient complications exceeded 30%. Recipient complications included sepsis and hemorrhage from segment IV necrosis, hepatic vein thrombosis, anastomotic biliary leaks, and pancreatitis. After making several technical modifications, a revised series of 22 patients undergoing aLDLT with extended right lobe allografts demonstrated excellent recipient results with low donor morbidity.[35]

Discussion

The existing organ shortage has propelled the widespread application of LDLT to adults and children. Application of these techniques mandates technical, medical, ethical, and logistic considerations that can be expeditiously addressed through the creation of a national or international database. Regional registries have been established and are collecting data, but conclusions are premature. Presently, most centers performing LDLT restrict this option to patients who meet a center's minimum listing criteria for deceased donor liver transplantation. Guidelines governing donor and recipient selection, the application of aLDLT, and post-donation donor health must be established. aLDLT provides the greatest benefit to patients with early signs of liver failure and is poorly tolerated by patients suffering from acute decompensation of chronic liver disease who are in poor health and have exceedingly high

metabolic demands. These patients are physiologically tenuous and immediately require the maximum liver volume available. For this indication, superior results are achieved with whole-organ deceased donor liver transplantation.

FHF is a clinical situation in which aLDLT may be applicable. Although few data exist on aLDLT recipient outcomes for FHF,[117,118] the success of auxiliary allografts in patients with FHF secondary to acetaminophen and *Amanita phylloides* toxicity suggests that adequate metabolic function for recovery is supplied by partial-liver allografts in these two subgroups of FHF patients.[119,120] The use of aLDLT for posttransplant primary allograft nonfunction or hepatic artery thrombosis represents a more difficult medical decision that favors whole-organ deceased donor transplantation. To date, data on aLDLT in these settings are anecdotal, and future analysis will probably demonstrate that outcomes are dependent on the cause of the liver failure. Protocols can be expedited for donor identification, consent, and preparation if requested by the family, although this situation is certainly less than ideal.

Long-term donor complications in pLDLT are uncommon, but potentially serious complications are well documented. Present data suggest overall donor satisfaction with pLDLT; however, detailed long-term follow-up with respect to medical condition, quality of life, and donor satisfaction with the procedure has not been widely performed and should be a priority.

The risk for donor complications in the performance of aLDLT is higher as the donor remnant becomes smaller because of its greatly reduced metabolic reserve. Preliminary data indicate an increased incidence of morbidity and mortality. Presently, no data are available to predict long-term liver function after living donation. Although authors have attempted to interpolate long-term donor outcomes from hepatectomy data, accurate long-term outcome data will be generated only through the creation of a national or international database.

Adult-to-adult living donation will not be the final solution to the current organ shortage. In fact, overall performance of aLDLT in the United States has steadily declined since 2001. The cause of this decline is probably multifactorial and includes clinical concerns of increased recurrence of hepatitis C and hepatocellular carcinoma in aLDLT recipients, two donor deaths, an improved organ allocation system, and better recipient and donor selection in transplant centers.[121-126] Limited data indicate that these procedures are applicable to only 10% to 30% of the current recipient pool[57,127,128]; however, similarly pessimistic early projections of the use of pLDLT were exceeded as the transplant community gained experience in the procedure. Increased data collection will begin to uncover the ultimate role of aLDLT in meeting organ demand. Early selection of patients will optimize results, build experience, and inspire public confidence that may permit future expansion of indications.

Pearls and Pitfalls

- LDLT is a significant surgical achievement by the transplant community, but its ultimate acceptance and role in the field of liver transplantation have yet to be defined.

- Successful application of LDLT mandates specific medical and surgical considerations for the donor and recipient because transplantation of partial-liver allografts predisposes to unique complications.

- Donor complications, including death and the need for emergency liver transplantation, have occurred and need to be formally incorporated into the education of potential donors.

- Outcomes of pLDLT equal or exceed outcomes of whole-organ and deceased donor partial-liver transplantation in infants.

- Outcomes of aLDLT are excellent in select patient populations—notably, recipients with early disease and adequate physiological reserve. Application of aLDLT to patients with advanced cirrhosis or in the setting of fulminant hepatic failure (excluding acetaminophen and *Amanita phylloides* toxicity) has yielded inferior results when compared with deceased donor whole-organ transplantation.

References

1. Tokat Y: Impact of living donor organ transplantation on transplant programs. Paper presented at the International Symposium on Living Donor Organ Transplantation, 2004, Essen, Germany.
2. Emond JC, Renz JF: Surgical anatomy of the liver and its application to hepatobiliary surgery and transplantation. Semin Liver Dis 14:158-168, 1994.
3. Emond JC, Renz JF, Ferrell LD, et al: Functional analysis of grafts from living donors. Implications for the treatment of older recipients. Ann Surg 224:544-552, discussion 552-554, 1996.
4. Kiuchi T, Kasahara M, Uryuhara K, et al: Impact of graft size mismatching on graft prognosis in liver transplantation from living donors. Transplantation 67:321-327, 1999.
5. Tanaka K, Uemoto S, Tokunaga Y, et al: Surgical techniques and innovations in living related liver transplantation. Ann Surg 217:82-91, 1993.
6. Ozaki C, Katz SM, Monsour HP Jr, Wood RP: Vascular reconstruction in living-related liver transplantation. Transplant Proc 26:167-168, 1994.
7. Kuang AA, Rosenthal P, Roberts JP, et al: Decreased mortality from technical failure improves results in pediatric liver transplantation. Arch Surg 131:887-892, discussion 892-893, 1996.
8. Heffron TG, Emond JC, Whitington PF, et al: Biliary complications in pediatric liver transplantation. A comparison of reduced-size and whole grafts. Transplantation 53:391-395, 1992.
9. Reichert PR, Renz JF, Rosenthal P, et al: Biliary complications of reduced-organ liver transplantation. Liver Transpl Surg 4:343-349, 1998.
10. Kawasaki S, Makuuchi M, Ishizone S, et al: Liver regeneration in recipients and donors after transplantation. Lancet 339:580-581, 1992.
11. Nakagami M, Morimoto T, Itoh K, et al: Patterns of restoration of remnant liver volume after graft harvesting in donors for living related liver transplantation. Transplant Proc 30:195-199, 1998.
12. Renz JF, Mudge CL, Heyman MB, et al: Donor selection limits use of living-related liver transplantation. Hepatology 22:1122-1126, 1995.
13. Sterneck M, Nischwitz U, Fischer L, et al: Evaluation and morbidity of the living liver donor in pediatric liver transplantation. Transplant Proc 27:1164-1165, 1995.
14. Morimoto T, Tanaka A, Ikai I, et al: Donor safety in living related liver transplantation. Transplant Proc 27:1166-1169, 1995.
15. Ohkohchi N, Katoh H, Orii T, et al: Complications and treatments of donors and recipients in living-related liver transplantation. Transplant Proc 30:3218-3220, 1998.
16. Tojimbara T, Fuchinoue S, Nakajima I, et al: Analysis of postoperative liver function of donors in living-related liver transplantation: Comparison of the type of donor hepatectomy. Transplantation 66:1035-1039, 1998.
17. Grewal H, Thistlethwaite JR Jr, Loss GE, et al: Complications in 100 living-liver donors. Ann Surg 228:214-219, 1998.
18. Smith B: Segmental liver transplantation from a living donor. J Pediatr Surg 4:126-132, 1969.
19. Raia S, Nery J, Mies S: Liver transplantation from live donors. Lancet 2:497, 1989.
20. Zitelli BJ, Gartner JC, Malatack JJ, et al: Pediatric liver transplantation: Patient evaluation and selection, infectious complications, and life-style after transplantation. Transplant Proc 19:3309-3316, 1987.
21. Broelsch CE, Emond JC, Thistlethwaite JR, et al: Liver transplantation with reduced-size donor organs. Transplantation 45:519-524, 1988.
22. Strong RW, Lynch SV, Ong TH, et al: Successful liver transplantation from a living donor to her son. N Engl J Med 322:1505-1507, 1990.
23. Broelsch CE, Whitington PF, Emond JC, et al: Liver transplantation in children from living related donors. Surgical techniques and results. Ann Surg 214:428-437, discussion 437-439, 1991.
24. Harper A, Taranto S, Edwards E: The OPTN waiting list, 1988-2001. Clin Transpl 79-92, 2002.
25. Brown R, Rush SH, Rosen HR, et al: Liver and intestine transplantation. Am J Transplant 4(Suppl 9):81-92, 2004.
26. Renz J, Yersiz H, Farmer DG, et al: Changing faces of liver transplantation: Partial-liver grafts for adults. J Hepatobiliary Pancreat Surg 10:31-44, 2003.

27. Couinaud C: Le Foie. Etudes Anatomiques et Chirurgicales. Paris, Masson, 1957.

28. Bismuth H: Surgical anatomy and anatomical surgery of the liver. World J Surg 6:3-9, 1982.

29. Makuuchi M, Kawasaki S, Noguchi T, et al: Donor hepatectomy for living related partial liver transplantation. Surgery 113:395-402, 1993.

30. Miller CM, Gondolesi GE, Florman S, et al: One hundred nine living donor liver transplants in adults and children: A single-center experience. Ann Surg 234:301-311, discussion 311-312, 2001.

31. Habib N, Tanaka K: Living-related liver transplantation in adult recipients: A hypothesis. Clin Transplant 9:31-34, 1995.

32. Wachs ME, Bak TE, Karrer FM, et al: Adult living donor liver transplantation using a right hepatic lobe. Transplantation 66:1313-1316, 1998.

33. Lo CM, Fan ST, Lo RJ, et al: Extending the limit on the size of adult recipient in living donor liver transplantation using extended right lobe graft. Transplantation 63:1524-1528, 1997.

34. Lo CM, Fan ST, Liu CL, et al: Adult-to-adult living donor liver transplantation using extended right lobe grafts. Ann Surg 226:261-269, 1997.

35. Fan S, Lo C, Liu C: Technical refinement in adult-to-adult living donor liver transplantation using right lobe graft. Ann Surg 231:126-131, 2000.

36. American Society of Transplant Surgeons' position paper on adult-to-adult living donor liver transplantation. Liver Transpl 6:815-817, 2000.

37. Shapiro R, Adams M: Ethical issues surrounding adult-to-adult living donor liver transplantation. Liver Transpl 6(Suppl 2):77-80, 2000.

38. Cronin DN, Millis J, Siegler M: Transplantation of liver grafts from living donors into adults—too much, too soon. N Engl J Med 344:1633-1637, 2001.

39. Malago M, Testa G, Marcos A, et al: Ethical considerations and rationale of adult-to-adult living donor liver transplantation. Liver Transpl 7:921-927, 2001.

40. Caplan A: Proceed with caution: Live living donation of lobes of liver for transplantation. Liver Transpl 7:494-495, 2001.

41. National Institutes of Health. http://www.nih-a2all.org, 2004.

42. Yamaoka Y, Morimoto T, Inamoto T, et al: Safety of the donor in living-related liver transplantation—an analysis of 100 parental donors. Transplantation 59:224-226, 1995.

43. Malago M, Rogiers X, Burdelski M, Broelsch CE: Living related liver transplantation: 36 cases at the University of Hamburg. Transplant Proc 26:3620-3621, 1994.

44. Lo C: Complications and long-term outcome of living liver donors: A survey of 1508 cases in five Asian centers. Transplantation 75:S12-S15, 2003.

45. Haberal M, Bilgin N, Karakayah H, et al: Long-term follow-up of living-related partial liver donors. Transplant Proc 30:708-709, 1998.

46. Kawagishi N, Ohkohchi N, Fujimori K, et al: Safety of the donor operation in living-related liver transplantation: Analysis of 22 donors. Transplant Proc 30:3279-3280, 1998.

47. Diaz G, Renz JF, Mudge C, et al: Donor health assessment after living-donor liver transplantation. Ann Surg 236:120-126, 2002.

48. Strong RW: Whither living donor liver transplantation? Liver Transpl Surg 5:536-538, 1999.

49. Trotter JF, Talamantes M, McClure M, et al: Right hepatic lobe donation for living donor liver transplantation: Impact on donor quality of life. Liver Transpl 7:485-493, 2001.

50. Beavers K, Sandler RS, Fair JH, et al: The living donor experience: Donor health assessment and outcomes after living donor liver transplantation. Liver Transpl 7:943-947, 2001.

51. Beavers K, Sandler R, Shrestha R: Donor morbidity associated with right lobectomy for living donor liver transplantation to adult recipients: A systematic review. Liver Transpl 8:110-117, 2002.

52. Beavers K, Cassara J, Shrestha R: Practice patterns for long-term follow-up of adult-to-adult right lobectomy donors at US transplantation centers. Liver Transpl 9:645-648, 2003.

53. Marcos A, Ham JM, Fisher RA, et al: Single-center analysis of the first 40 adult-to-adult living donor liver transplants using the right lobe. Liver Transpl 6:296-301, 2000.

54. Walter M, Papachristou C, Fliege H, et al: Psychosocial stress of living donors after living donor liver transplantation. Transplant Proc 34:3291-3292, 2002.

55. Todo S: Adult-to-adult living donor liver transplantation: The Japanese experience. In Controversies in Transplantation. Breckenridge, CO, University of Colorado, 2000.

56. Testa G, Malago M, Broelsch CE: Living-donor liver transplantation in adults. Langenbecks Arch Surg 384:536-543, 1999.

57. Renz JF, Busuttil RW: Adult-to-adult living-donor liver transplantation: A critical analysis. Semin Liver Dis 20:411-424, 2000.

58. Brown RS Jr, Russo MW, Lai M, et al: A survey of liver transplantation from living adult donors in the United States. N Engl J Med 348:818-825, 2003.

59. Lo C, Fan ST, Liu CL, et al: Lessons learned from one hundred right lobe living donor liver transplants. Ann Surg 240:151-158, 2004.

60. Walter M, Dammann G, Papachristou C, et al: Quality of life of living donors before and after living donor liver transplantation. Transplant Proc 35:2961-2963, 2003.

61. Ito T, Kiuchi T, Egawa H, et al: Surgery-related morbidity in living donors of right-lobe liver graft: Lessons from the first 200 cases. Transplantation 76:158-163, 2003.

62. Boillot O, Belshiti J, Azoulay D, et al: Initial French experience in adult-to-adult living donor liver transplantation. Transplant Proc 35:962-963, 2003.

63. Umeshita K, Fujiwara K, Kiyosawa K, et al: Operative morbidity of living liver donors in Japan. Lancet 362:687-690, 2003.

64. Malago M, Testa G, Frilling A, et al: Right living donor liver transplantation: An option for adult patients: Single institution experience with 74 patients. Ann Surg 238:853-862, discussion 862-863, 2003.

65. Lo C: Complications and long-term outcome of living liver donors: A survey of 1508 cases in five Asian centers. Transplantation 75:S12-S15, 2003.

66. Shaw B: Where monsters hide. Liver Transpl 7:928-932, 2001.

67. Trotter J, Wachs M, Everson GT, Kam I: Adult-to-adult transplantation of the right hepatic lobe from a living donor. N Engl J Med 346:1074-1082, 2002.

68. Fair JH, Johnson MW, Gerber D, et al: Adult-to-adult living donor liver transplantation using right lobe: Single center experience. Paper presented at The Joint American Transplant Meeting, 2001, Chicago, IL.

69. Emre S: Living donor liver transplantation: A critical review. Transplant Proc 33:3456-3457, 2001.

70. Akabayashi A, Slingsby B, Fujita M: The first donor death after living-related liver transplantation in Japan. Transplantation 77:634, 2004.

71. Renz J, Roberts J: Long-term complications of living donor liver transplantation. Liver Transpl 6(Suppl 2):573-576, 2000.

72. Emond JC, Heffron TG, Kortz ED, et al: Improved results of living-related liver transplantation with routine application in a pediatric program. Transplantation 55:835-840, 1993.

73. Otte JB, de Ville de Goyet J, Reding R, et al: Living related donor liver transplantation in children: The Brussels experience. Transplant Proc 28:2378-2379, 1996.

74. Tanaka K, Uemoto S, Tokunaga Y, et al: Liver transplantation in children from living-related donors. Transplant Proc 25:1084-1086, 1993.

75. Ryckman FC, Flake AW, Fisher RA, et al: Segmental orthotopic hepatic transplantation as a means to improve patient survival and diminish waiting-list mortality. J Pediatr Surg 26:422-427, discussion 427-428, 1991.

76. Sindhi R, Rosendale R, Mundy D, et al: Impact of segmental grafts on pediatric liver transplantation—a review of the United Network for Organ Sharing Scientific Registry data (1990-1996). J Pediatr Surg 34:107-110, discussion 110-111, 1999.

77. Renz JF, de Roos M, Rosenthal P, et al: Posttransplantation growth in pediatric liver recipients. Liver Transpl 7:1040-1055, 2001.

78. Ogura Y, Kaihara S, Haga H, et al: Outcomes for pediatric liver retransplantation from living donors. Transplantation 76:943-948, 2003.

79. Roberts J, Hulbert-Shearon TE, Merion RM, et al: Influence of graft type on outcomes after pediatric liver transplantation. Am J Transplant 4:373-377, 2004.

80. United Network for Organ Sharing. http://www.UNOS.org, 2004.

81. Bak T, Wachs M, Trotter J, et al: Adult-to-adult living donor liver transplantation using right-lobe grafts: Results and lessons learned from a single-center experience. Liver Transpl 7:680-686, 2001.

82. Humar A: Donor and recipient outcomes after adult living donor liver transplantation. Liver Transpl 9(10 Suppl 2):S42-S44, 2003.

83. Pomfret E: Early and late complications in the right-lobe adult living donor. Liver Transpl 9(10 Suppl 2):S45-S49, 2003.

84. Russo M, Brown R: Adult living donor liver transplantation. Am J Transplant 4:458-465, 2004.

85. Abt P, Mange KC, Olthoff KM, et al: Allograft survival following adult-to-adult living donor liver transplantation. Am J Transplant 4:1302-1307, 2004.

86. Miller C: Living donor liver transplantation. Transplant Proc 35:964-965, 2003.

87. Ghobrial R, Saab S, Lassman C, et al: Donor and recipient outcomes in right lobe adult living donor liver transplantation. Liver Transpl 8:901-909, 2002.

88. Fishbein T, Gondolesi G, Matsumoto C, et al: Analysis of 50 consecutive right lobe liver transplants from living donors. Paper presented at the Joint Meeting of the International Liver Transplantation Society, the European Liver Transplantation Association, and the Liver Intensive Care Group of Europe, 2001, Berlin.

89. Goldstein MJ, Salame E, Kinkhabwala M, et al: Analysis of failure in living donor liver transplantation: Differential outcomes in children and adults. World J Surg 27:356-364, 2003.

90. Grewal H, Shokouh-Amiri MH, Vera S, et al: Surgical technique for right lobe adult living donor liver transplantation without venovenous bypass or portocaval shunting and with duct-to-duct biliary reconstruction. Ann Surg 233:502-508, 2001.

91. Marcos A, Fisher RA, Ham JM, et al: Right lobe living donor liver transplantation. Transplantation 68:798-803, 1999.

92. Malago M, Testa G, Valentin-Gamazo C, et al: Living donor liver transplantation at the University of Essen. Paper presented at the Joint Meeting of the International Liver Transplantation Society, the European Liver Transplantation Association, and the Liver Intensive Care Group of Europe, 2001, Berlin.

93. Inomata Y, Uemoto S, Asonuma K, et al: Right lobe graft in living donor liver transplantation. Transplantation 69:258-264, 2000.

94. Broelsch CE, Malago M, Testa G, Valentin Gamazo C: Living donor liver transplantation in adults: Outcome in Europe. Liver Transpl 6(6 Suppl 2):S64-S65, 2000.

95. Boillot O, Belshiti J, Azoulay D, et al: Initial French experience in adult-to-adult living donor liver transplantation. Transplant Proc 35:962-963, 2003.

96. Gautier S: Living donor liver transplantation in Russia. Transplant Proc 35:957, 2003.

97. Tokat Y, Yuzer Y, Karasu Z, et al: New frontiers: Adult to adult living donor liver transplantation, single center experience from Turkey. Transplant Proc 33:3458-3460, 2001.

98. Azoulay D, Castaing D, Adam R, et al: [Adult to adult living-related liver transplantation. The Paul-Brousse Hospital preliminary experience.] Gastroenterol Clin Biol 25:773-780, 2001.

99. Garcia-Valdecasas J, Fuster J, Grande L, et al: Adult living donor liver transplantation. Paper presented at the Joint Meeting of the International Liver Transplantation Society, the European Liver Transplantation Association, and the Liver Intensive Care Group of Europe, 2001, Berlin.

100. Todo S, Furukawa H, Jin MB, Shimamura T: Living donor liver transplantation in adults: Outcome in Japan. Liver Transpl 6 (6 Suppl 2):S66-S72, 2000.

101. de Villa VH, Chen CL, Chen YS, et al: Split liver transplantation in Asia. Transplant Proc 33:1502-1503, 2001.

102. Watts J: Concept of brain death to be accepted in South Korea. Lancet 352:1996, 1998.

103. Gutierrez E: Japan's House of Representatives passes brain-death bill. Lancet 349:1304, 1997.

104. Rajasekar M, Vijayarajakumari D, Goyal R, Sewkani AS: Adult-to-adult living donor right lobe liver transplantation: The first series in India. Transplant Proc 35:70-71, 2003.

105. Hirata M, Sugawara Y, Makuuchi M: Living-donor liver transplantation at Tokyo University. Clin Transpl 215-219, 2002.

106. Lee SG, Park KM, Lee YJ, et al: 157 adult-to-adult living donor liver transplantation. Transplant Proc 33:1323-1325, 2001.

107. Hashikura Y, Kawasaki S, Terada M, et al: Long-term results of living-related donor liver graft transplantation: A single-center analysis of 110 transplants. Transplantation 72:95-99, 2001.

108. Furukawa H, Shimamura T, Ishikawa H, et al: What is the limit of graft size for successful living donor liver transplantation in adults? Transplant Proc 33:1322, 2001.

109. Inagaki M, Yagi T, Sadamori H, et al: Analysis of donor complications in living donor liver transplantation. Transplant Proc 33:1386-1387, 2001.

110. Kawasaki S, Makuuchi M, Matsunami H, et al: Living related liver transplantation in adults. Ann Surg 227:269-274, 1998.

111. Chen CL, Fan ST, Lee SG, et al: Living-donor liver transplantation: 12 years of experience in Asia. Transplantation 75(3 Suppl): S6-S11, 2003.

112. Chen C: Living donor liver transplantation: Experience from Asian countries. Paper presented at the International Symposium on Living Donor Organ Transplantation, 2004, Essen, Germany.

113. Sugawara Y, Makuuchi M: Advances in adult living donor liver transplantation: A review based on reports from the 10th anniversary of the adult-to-adult living donor liver transplantation meeting in Tokyo. Liver Transpl 10:715-720, 2004.

114. Strong R, Fawcett J, Lynch S: Living-donor and split-liver transplantation in adults: Right versus left-sided grafts. J Hepatobiliary Pancreat Surg 10:5-10, 2003.

115. Soejima Y, Shimada M, Suehiro T, et al: Outcome analysis in adult-to-adult living donor liver transplantation using the left lobe. Liver Transpl 9:581-586, 2003.

116. Sugawara Y, Makuuchi M, Kaneko J, et al: Living-donor liver transplantation in adults: Tokyo University experience. J Hepatobiliary Pancreat Surg 10:1-4, 2003.

117. Kato T, Nery JR, Morcos JJ, et al: Successful living related liver transplantation in an adult with fulminant hepatic failure. Transplantation 64:415-417, 1997.

118. Bak T, Everson G, Wachs M, et al: Living-donor liver transplantation for adults with fulminant hepatic failure: An underutilized resource? Liver Transpl 5:C45, 1999.

119. Sudan D, Shaw BW Jr, Fox IJ, Langnas AN: Long-term follow-up of auxiliary orthotopic liver transplantation for the treatment of fulminant hepatic failure. Surgery 122:771-777, discussion 777-778, 1997.

120. van Hoek B, de Boer J, Boudjema K, et al: Auxiliary versus orthotopic liver transplantation for acute liver failure. J Hepatol 30:699-705, 1999.

121. Russo M, Galanko J, Beavers K, et al: Patient and graft survival in hepatitis C recipients after adult living donor liver transplantation in the United States. Liver Transpl 10:340-346, 2004.

122. Gaglio P, Malireddy S, Levitt BS, et al: Increased risk of cholestatic hepatitis C in recipients of grafts from living versus cadaveric liver donors. Liver Transpl 9:1028-1035, 2003.

123. Shiffman M, Stravitz RT, Contos MJ, et al: Histologic recurrence of chronic hepatitis C virus in patients after living donor and deceased donor liver transplantation. Liver Transpl 10:1248-1255, 2004.

124. Todo S, Furukawa H: Living donor liver transplantation for adult patients with hepatocellular carcinoma. Ann Surg 240:451-461, 2004.

125. Lo CM, Fan ST, Liu CL, et al: The role and limitation of living donor liver transplantation for hepatocellular carcinoma. Liver Transpl 10:440-447, 2004.

126. Ohkubo T, Sugawara Y, Imamura H, et al: Early recurrence of hepatocellular carcinoma after living donor liver transplantation. Hepatogastroenterology 51:237-238, 2004.

127. Trotter JF: Selection of donors and recipients for living donor liver transplantation. Liver Transpl 6(6 Suppl 2):S52-S58, 2000.

128. Valentin-Gamazo C, Malago M, Karliova M, et al: Experience after the evaluation of 700 potential donors for living donor liver transplantation in a single center. Liver Transpl 10:1087-1096, 2004.

Ethics of Living Donor Liver Transplantation

DAVID C. CRONIN II
MARK SIEGLER

Using living donor organs: historical review   726
  Use of living donors in kidney
    transplantation   726
  Use of living donors in liver
    transplantation   728

**Ethical guidelines for the use of living liver
donors of right lobes**   729
  Patient selection   730
  Risk/benefit assessment of the donor and
    recipient   732
  Informed consent   734
  Experience and capacity of the
    transplantation team and climate
    of the institution   734

Special ethical concerns   735
  Double equipoise for donors and
    recipients   735
  Research on adult living donor liver
    transplantation   735
  Financial incentives   736
  Regulation of innovative surgery   736

Conclusion   737

Because liver transplantation has become the standard of care for many types of end-stage liver disease, the number of patients awaiting this life-saving therapy has increased greatly (Fig. 48–1). As stated in the annual report of the United Network for Organ Sharing (UNOS), as of August 2002 there were 18,505 registrants listed and waiting for liver transplantation. Over the preceding 5-year period (1997 to 2001), the number of livers recovered from deceased donors increased only 11.4%, whereas the number listed increased 96%. Therefore, the disparity between those in need of liver transplantation and those who receive a liver for transplantation continues to widen (Fig. 48–2). One illustration of the impact of this disparity between organ supply and demand is the progressive and significant increase in time spent waiting for a liver transplant. Across all blood groups, the median time spent listed and awaiting transplantation has steadily increased (Fig. 48–3).

Endeavors to increase the supply of transplantable solid organs from deceased donors have included increased efforts in public education and awareness of organ donation; improved efforts at organ procurement, including mandatory request; expansion of what is considered an acceptable organ for transplantation; and discussions about incentives (financial and other) for donation. None has succeeded because the number of deceased donors has increased only marginally in the last decade (Fig. 48–4). For this reason,

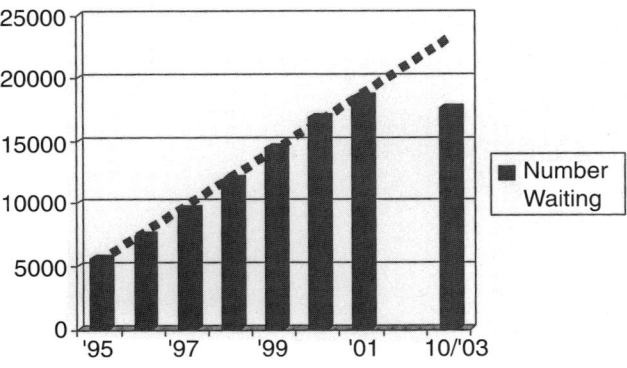

FIGURE 48–1

Number of registrants listed with UNOS who are awaiting liver transplantation. (Data from University Renal Research and Education Association [URREA] and United Network for Organ Sharing [UNOS]: 2002 Annual Report of the U.S. Organ Procurement and Transplantation Network [OPTN] and the Scientific Registry of Transplant Recipients [SRTR]: Transplant Data 1992-2001. Rockville, MD: Organ Procurement and Transplantation Network [OPTN], 2003. Modified 2003 Feb 18; cited 2003 June 27. Available from http://www.optn.org/data/annualReport.asp; and OPTN data as of October 24, 2003.)

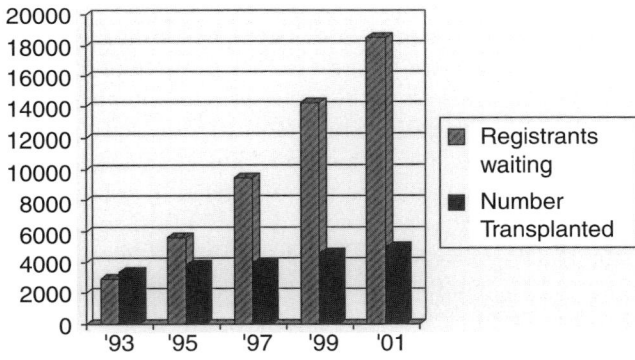

FIGURE 48–2

Disparity between the number of patients listed and waiting for liver transplantation and the number of liver transplants performed, liver transplant activity in the United States, and the number of registrants and the number of transplants performed from all organ sources (living and deceased donors). (Data from University Renal Research and Education Association [URREA] and United Network for Organ Sharing [UNOS]: 2002 Annual Report of the U.S. Organ Procurement and Transplantation Network [OPTN] and the Scientific Registry of Transplant Recipients [SRTR]: Transplant Data 1992-2001. Rockville, MD: Organ Procurement and Transplantation Network [OPTN], 2003. Modified 2003 Feb 18; cited 2003 June 27. Available from http://www.optn.org/data/annualReport.asp.)

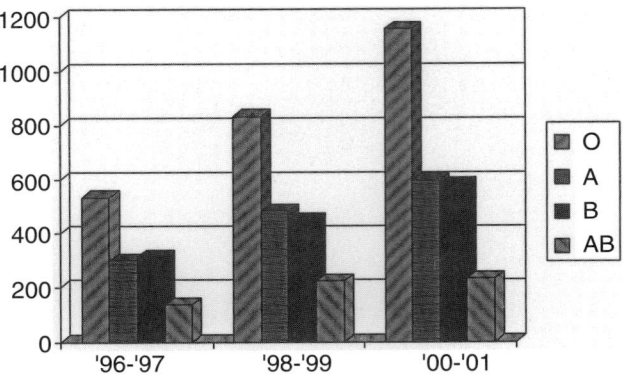

FIGURE 48–3

Median waiting time for liver transplantation by blood group. (Data from University Renal Research and Education Association [URREA] and United Network for Organ Sharing [UNOS]: 2002 Annual Report of the U.S. Organ Procurement and Transplantation Network [OPTN] and the Scientific Registry of Transplant Recipients [SRTR]: Transplant Data 1992-2001. Rockville, MD: Organ Procurement and Transplantation Network [OPTN], 2003. Modified 2003 Feb 18; cited 2003 June 27. Available from http://www.optn.org/data/annualReport.asp.)

living liver donors have been used increasingly as donors (Fig. 48–5). The effort to increase the number of transplantable liver grafts by the use of living donors, within ethical guidelines, is the subject of this chapter.

Using Living Donor Organs: Historical Review

Use of Living Donors in Kidney Transplantation

The first series of solid-organ transplantations in humans began in 1951 with a succession of failed attempts at kidney transplantation. Interestingly, although many of the

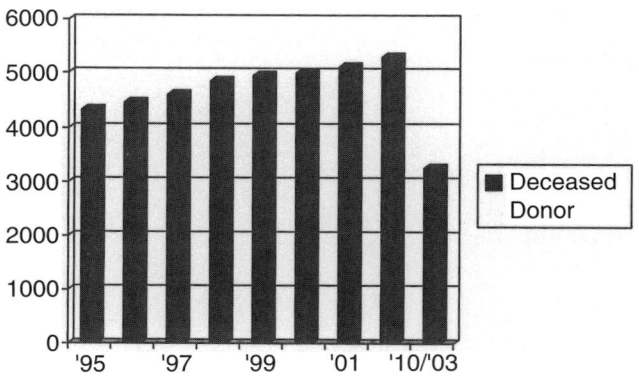

FIGURE 48–4

Number of deceased liver donors. (Data from University Renal Research and Education Association [URREA] and United Network for Organ Sharing [UNOS]: 2002 Annual Report of the U.S. Organ Procurement and Transplantation Network [OPTN] and the Scientific Registry of Transplant Recipients [SRTR]: Transplant Data 1992-2001. Rockville, MD: Organ Procurement and Transplantation Network [OPTN], 2003. Modified 2003 Feb 18; cited 2003 June 27. Available from http://www.optn.org/data/annualReport.asp; and OPTN data as of October 24, 2003.)

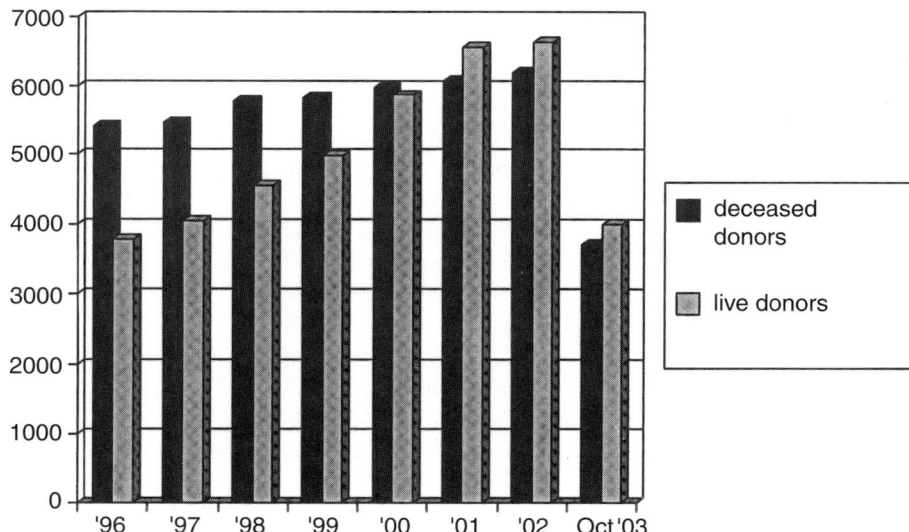

FIGURE 48–5

U.S. organ donor characteristics. Numbers represent the total of all organs procured for transplantation. (Data from University Renal Research and Education Association [URREA] and United Network for Organ Sharing [UNOS]: 2002 Annual Report of the U.S. Organ Procurement and Transplantation Network [OPTN] and the Scientific Registry of Transplant Recipients [SRTR]: Transplant Data 1992-2001. Rockville, MD: Organ Procurement and Transplantation Network [OPTN], 2003. Modified 2003 Feb 18; cited 2003 June 27. Available from http://www.optn.org/data/annualReport.asp; and OPTN data as of October 24, 2003.)

kidneys originally used for transplantation were from deceased donors, a small number of kidneys in this early series were from living donors. Even though the surgical techniques required for successful kidney transplantation had improved, understanding of the immunological barriers to transplantation remained in its infancy, and transplant surgeons were unable to stop the process of rejection, which ultimately destroyed the transplanted graft. It was into this environment in the mid-1950s of failed efforts at kidney transplantation that the use of living kidney donors emerged as an ethically controversial clinical approach.

The first successful organ transplant was performed in 1954 when a healthy volunteer donor provided a kidney for his identical twin. That transplant procedure used improved surgical techniques developed by Drs. Joseph Murray and Francis Moore, but the sustained function of the graft was due to the genetic similarity between the donor and recipient. For the first time, the immunological barrier to transplantation had been bypassed by the use of identical twins as a donor and recipient pair. Since the use of the first healthy volunteer organ donor in 1954, the medical community has walked a fine line struggling to balance the interests of the recipient and the donor, as well as the interests of the surgeon, the medical team, and society. The crucial ethical question has always been whether it is acceptable to use a healthy living donor for the sole purpose of providing an organ for another. Dr. Moore put the point succinctly: "Is it morally right and ethically acceptable to injure one person to help another?"[1]

In general and with some noteworthy objections,[2] the public and the medical community have thus far answered this question in the affirmative, especially by their willingness to accept the practice of using living donors. In fact, since 1954 more than 50,000 kidney transplants have been performed with living donors in the United States. The year 2001 marks the first time in the history of organ transplantation that more living donors than deceased donors were used as a source of organs for transplantation (see Fig. 48–5). From 1997 to 2001, there was a 60% increase in living organ donation, with only a 10% increase in deceased donors.[3] However, not all living organ donations are attended by the same donor risks and recipient benefits, and the increased activity within the live donor pool is not universally applicable to all organs donated.

In the first living donor kidney transplant between identical twins, the ethical justification was based on a risk/benefit calculation that considered that the donor's physical risk was offset by the potential emotional harm associated with losing a twin brother whose life might be saved by the donor's gift. However, as medical technology progressed and improved, dialysis therapy soon offered an alternative means of preventing death from renal failure. Additionally, our knowledge of the immunological events responsible for acute cellular rejection rapidly increased the development of immunosuppressive drugs to allow successful transplantation in genetically nonidentical individuals.

Currently, regardless of the donor source, kidney transplantation is viewed as the best treatment of end-stage renal disease. When compared with dialysis, it has been shown to improve quality of life and length of life and to decrease the cost associated with end-stage renal disease, and it is thus the preferred treatment. Living donors of kidneys have a low risk of mortality and morbidity. In fact, the current application of minimally invasive surgical techniques used for procurement of the kidney has further decreased donor risk and resulted in a dramatic increase in donor rates throughout the United States.

For kidney transplantation, living donors have become the preferred source in many centers and the only source of transplantable organs in some countries. As the waiting list continues to expand and waiting time continues to lengthen, living kidney donors represent an additional source of transplantable organs. Furthermore, living donor kidney transplants demonstrate better and longer function than deceased donor kidney transplants do. This observed improvement in function and durability of a living donor graft is in part ascribed to better health of the living donor organ, a decrease in cold ischemia time, earlier transplantation of the recipient patient, and in some cases, an immunological advantage among closely matched donor and recipient pairs.

Use of Living Donors in Liver Transplantation

Living Donors in Pediatric Liver Transplantation

In contrast to renal transplantation, where dialysis is now a life-saving alternative, use of a living donor in pediatric liver transplantation was justified on the basis of a more urgent situation: without a liver transplant, patients would die. The most frequent cause of end-stage liver disease in children is biliary atresia,[4] and the majority of children with this disease require liver transplantation before 2 years of age.[5] Since very few babies or small children die of head trauma or brain death, circumstances in which they could be a source of a donor liver, there is a large gap between pediatric patients in need of liver transplantation and the availability of pediatric donors. In the 1980s, this situation resulted in reported mortality rates of 20% to 30% in infants and children awaiting transplants at the leading transplantation centers.[6] In many parts of the world, especially Asia, where for various reasons organ transplantation from brain-dead donors was severely restricted,[7] most children with biliary atresia died.

By the mid-1980s, innovative surgical techniques such as reduced-size[8] and split-liver deceased donor grafts lowered, but did not eliminate, waiting list mortality in infants and children.[6,9-11] Although these innovative approaches benefitted children, such approaches were criticized on two points: (1) reduced-size grafts may have exacerbated adult waiting list mortality by "stealing" a graft from potential adult recipients, and (2) the split-liver procedure resulted in lower graft survival than that achieved with a full-sized graft.[12]

Thus, in the late 1980s, several groups began to consider the use of living adult donors to supply liver grafts to children. Early case reports from Brazil[13] and Australia[14] described using the procedure to overcome the unavailability of deceased donor organs. These case reports, including the first successful living donor operation by Dr. Strong in a Japanese family for whom deceased donor organs were not available, provided a foundation for investigating the role of adult-to-child living donor liver transplantation. A team from the University of Chicago published a paper that discussed both the clinical need for living donor liver transplantation and the ethical justification for performing an investigational review board (IRB)-approved, single-center, prospective protocol study of 20 pediatric living donor liver transplantations (PLDLTs).[15] The excellent results of the first 20 donor-recipient pairs published in 1991[16] served as the basis for expansion of the technique to many of the leading liver surgery programs in the United States,[17,18] Europe,[19] and Asia.[20-25]

The pediatric operative procedure has undergone substantial modification since the first cases.[17,26] During the University of Chicago's protocol series, left lobectomy was quickly abandoned after three cases in favor of left lateral segmentectomy as a graft source for infants and children because of the high incidence of surgical complications experienced with the former procedure.[16] Further technical modifications have included avoiding the use of vascular conduits, using microscopic arterial anastomotic techniques,[20,26-28] and extending recipient indications for living donor transplantation.[18,29] Presently, the surgical procedure for transplantation in small and large pediatric patients—left lateral segmentectomy or left lobectomy from living donors as a source of grafts—has become a standard procedure with widely accepted indications.

It is estimated that more than 2000 pediatric transplants from living donors have been performed worldwide. The operation is relatively safe for both the recipient and donor, although two donor deaths have been reported.[30,31] The relatively low complication rate and lack of long-term sequelae in donors continue to make this procedure a clinically and ethically acceptable source of organs for transplantation in selected recipients.[32,33] The overall 1-year survival rate for pediatric recipients of living donor grafts is approximately 80%.[22] Center-specific data from our own institution demonstrate 1-year survival rates in excess of 90%.[17] Additionally, pediatric recipients of living donor grafts have significantly improved survival when compared with recipients of deceased donor full-size, reduced-size, or split grafts. Currently, in properly selected cases, adult-to-child living donor liver transplantation has become a standard of care in many developed countries, including the United States, Japan, South Korea, Germany, Belgium, and France.

In summary, two broad issues of surgical innovation have been addressed by the development and maturation of PLDLT: (1) it meets a demonstrated need by saving lives with a safe and predictable operation, and (2) it was introduced to the surgical community after intensive scrutiny of its clinical and ethical justification. The principal impetus for development of the living donor program was the high mortality in small pediatric patients awaiting liver transplantation in many countries. After a few initial case reports, the process by which the procedure was introduced involved publishing a peer-reviewed article 3 months before performing the first operation and announcing to the public and professional communities our intention to perform a protocol study of 20 cases. The protocol outlined a process for informed donor consent, including the assignment of a donor advocate to safeguard the donor from coercion. The team performing the protocol study had extensive experience in innovative liver surgery and transplantation, and the results of the protocol study were excellent and were published immediately.[16] Based on published results in which donor safety and recipient benefit were demonstrated, other leading surgical teams around the world began performing the PLDLT procedure. After almost 10 years of experience and more than 2000 cases worldwide, it is clear that the pediatric living donor operation remains relatively safe for donors and provides recipients with long-term survival benefits. As a consequence, PLDLT is now a clinically and ethically acceptable procedure.

Living Donors in Adult Liver Transplantation

The first adult-to-adult living donor liver transplantation (ALDLT) was performed at the University of Chicago in 1991 with the use of a left lobe graft; the donor did well, but the recipient died after the transplant.[34] The Kyoto group published the first successful case in which a living donor right lobe graft was transplanted into a 9-year-old recipient.[27] Use of the right lobe was necessary because of abnormal arterial anatomy supplying the left lobe. Lo and coauthors reported the first ALDLT with an extended right lobe graft (segments IV to VIII and the middle hepatic vein) in 1997.[35] The first successful ALDLT in the United States was reported by the Colorado group in 1998.[36] Recently, however, Howard reports to have performed the first right lobe ALDLT in the United States.[37] After the initial case reports, a number of centers on three continents began performing ALDLT with right lobe and extended right lobe grafts and reported their experiences.[35,38-40]

This method of introducing an innovative surgical procedure, through isolated case reports and small series, has been associated with many problems, some of which continue today. The early and later experiences reported a high complication rate in donors[41-43] and recipients.[44,45] Many of these complications were secondary to anatomical variability in the draining hepatic veins and biliary system, difficult vascular reconstruction, and mismatches between the metabolic and hemodynamic demands of the recipient because of transplantation of an insufficient hepatic mass from the donor.[45,46] The minimal amount of hepatic mass

required for successful transplantation into a particular recipient continues to be poorly defined. In addition to both recipient and donor complications associated with this new and innovative procedure, the indications for which it should be applied were poorly defined. Some programs viewed the living donor option as a means of transplantation in recipients who were excluded from receiving a deceased donor organ because of a contraindication (e.g., large hepatocellular carcinoma). At its inception, the use of living donors had a broad application. Some programs used living donors as an opportunity to provide transplants for the sickest patients on their waiting list, others used living donors to provide transplants for healthy patients on their waiting list, and some programs quickly moved to use strangers as donors for adult liver transplantation. For all these reasons, the ALDLT procedure remains an "innovative" form of surgery and should be controlled by standards that apply to innovative or experimental surgery.

In contrast to the measured manner in which PLDLT was introduced by the transplant community, only after a reported protocol series proved its efficacy and safety, ALDLT was disseminated rapidly without a comparable protocol study. As a consequence, many key components of ALDLT remain unclear. First, there is a lack of standard technique defining the extent of resection required to obtain an appropriate graft. In addition, it is not entirely clear how much residual liver must be left in the donor to assume safe recovery. Presently, the indications are not clearly defined for whom ALDLT rather than a deceased donor transplant should be performed (except in areas where deceased donors do not exist). Absent such indications, it is often difficult to justify the use of living donors in particular cases. Additionally, the procedure has been undertaken with variable IRB review. Furthermore, the proliferation of centers performing ALDLT is alarming. A review of data obtained by the UNOS registry demonstrates the rapid growth of this innovative surgical procedure.[3] A recent survey found that more than 42 centers had performed at least 449 such transplants in the United States alone.[42] Over the past 5 years the number of adult donors used for ALDLT has exceeded the number used over the past 11 years since the initiation of PLDLT (Fig. 48-6).

Ethical Guidelines for the Use of Living Liver Donors of Right Lobes

To allocate scarce solid organs obtained from deceased donors to an expanding pool of potential recipients, guidelines have been established that meet clinical and ethical standards. In contrast to the clear and formal

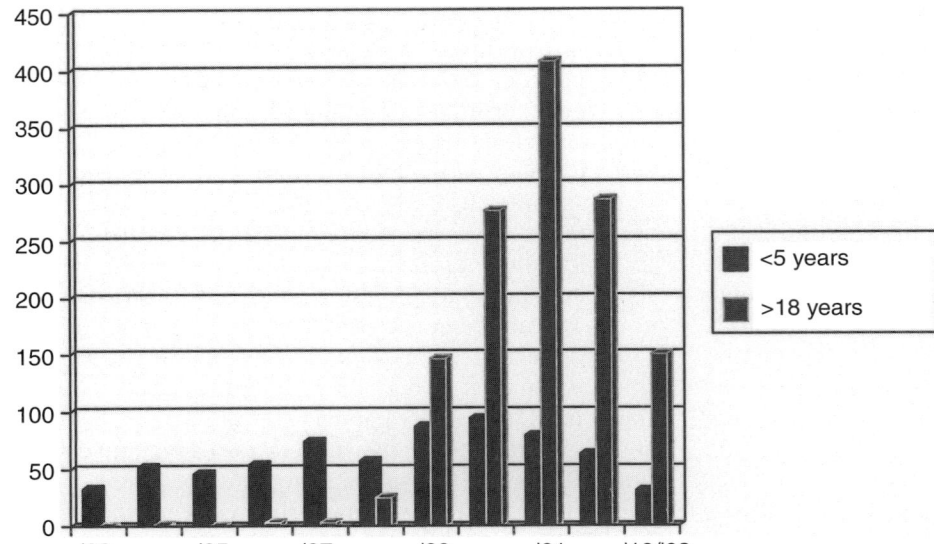

FIGURE 48–6

Recipients of living donor liver transplants 1992 to 2001 as report by UNOS. Recipients are divided according to age at the time of transplantation (all patients 5 years or younger, patients 18 years or older). (Data from University Renal Research and Education Association [URREA] and United Network for Organ Sharing [UNOS]: 2002 Annual Report of the U.S. Organ Procurement and Transplantation Network [OPTN] and the Scientific Registry of Transplant Recipients [SRTR]: Transplant Data 1992-2001. Rockville, MD: Organ Procurement and Transplantation Network [OPTN], 2003. Modified 2003 Feb 18; cited 2003 June 27. Available from http://www.optn.org/data/annualReport.asp; and OPTN data as of October 24, 2003.)

guidelines used to allocate solid organs from deceased donors, allocation of organs from living donors is less rigid and more idiosyncratic. As a result, the ethical justification for using living donors for solid-organ transplantation is less well established.

For several reasons, the ethical justification for use of a living donor kidney transplant differs from that in liver transplantation. First, living donor kidney transplantation has a very low donor mortality rate (probably less than 1 in 3000) and is rarely associated with prolonged morbidity. Furthermore, recipients of living donor kidneys are not exposed to any additional risk imposed by use of the living donor graft. In fact, recipients benefit from living donor organs in that patient and graft survival exceeds that associated with deceased donor organ transplants, and the use of a living donor may enable the recipient to avoid dialysis and its associated morbidity. Thus, the ethical justification for a living donor kidney transplant is based on very low risk to the donor and very great benefit to the recipient.

When contrasted with living donor kidney transplantation, living donor liver transplantation has a different risk-benefit ratio for both the donor and recipient. Overall (see later), a liver donor is exposed to a greater risk of mortality than a kidney donor is during the donation process, especially right lobe donors. Among living liver donors, those donating a left lateral segment have a greater risk of mortality than kidney donors do, but less of a mortality risk than donors of a full right lobe. Donor morbidity is also significantly greater in both incidence and magnitude in right lobe donors than in donors of a left lateral segment. Furthermore, when compared with a standard, full-sized deceased donor graft, adult recipients of living donor liver grafts may not derive added benefit or even equivalent benefit from a living donor graft. Recipient benefit from the living donor transplant may be modified significantly by the health status of the recipient at the time of transplantation, the indication for the transplantation, the type of transplant performed (right lobe, extended right lobe, or left lobe), the "quality" of the donor liver segment that is transplanted, and most important, the total hepatic mass transplanted. Finally and less well documented, performance of living donor liver transplantation, especially right lobes, requires great clinical experience and technical skill, and thus the benefits to the recipient and protection of the donor may vary according to the quality and experience of the surgical team and the "field strength" of the institution.[47] For all these reasons, the superiority of receiving living donor transplantation rather than deceased donor transplantation is not as well established for ALDLT as it is for living donor kidney transplantation or PLDLT.

Therefore, the ethical and medical justifications that support acceptance of living donor kidney transplantation and PLDLT, both of which have a highly favorable benefit-risk ratio, are not at this time established for ALDLT. The following sections consider the ethics of ALDLT with reference to (1) patient selection, (2) risk/benefit assessment of the donor and recipient, (3) informed consent, (4) the experience and capacity of the surgical team, and (5) financial considerations relating to ALDLT.

Patient Selection

Recipient selection

Not every patient with end-stage liver disease is an appropriate candidate or will benefit from liver transplantation. To assist in the rational allocation of this scare resource, UNOS has established indications and contraindications for potential recipients of liver transplants. In addition, under the current allocation scheme of the sickest first, limits have been placed so that the clearly high-risk (poor expected posttransplant survival) patients do not have an advantage.[48] In contrast to the formal rules that guide allocation of deceased donor livers, allocation of a living donor liver is less well regulated. Individual programs, surgeons, and patients are left to make decisions of appropriate recipient selection, often with little oversight. Although this discretionary process is not inherently wrong, it does leave room for abuse and poor decision-making that may place the donor and recipient at high risk for little potential benefit.

For example, it is now understood that patients with severe portal hypertension and significant physiological decompensation have poor outcomes after ALDLT. This fact was recognized retrospectively after a significant number of living donors were placed at risk for questionable recipient benefit.[44,49,50] Furthermore, using a living donor as a source of transplantable organs in situations in which a contraindication for deceased donor organ transplantation exists is difficult to justify. For instance, patients with a large hepatocellular carcinoma and end-stage liver disease are excluded from deceased donor liver transplantation because of the size of the tumor and the high likelihood of recurrence. This policy seeks to improve the utility of the scarce resource available for transplantation and avoid transplantation in situations in which the expected outcome is poor. Some programs have used the living donor option to offer transplantation to recipients with large cancers. This undertaking is flawed on two levels: (1) it is difficult to justify using a living donor for a transplant situation that society deems so unlikely to benefit the recipient that a deceased donor is prohibited, and (2) recipients in whom the transplant fails are added to the deceased donor transplant waiting list and compete with other patients even when their initial disease was a contraindication to transplantation. Although these situations are difficult to negotiate and the nontransplant option usually results in death of the intended recipient, the urgency of the situation and the limited options for treatment of a terminal illness are not in themselves sufficient reasons to circumvent rules that would apply to deceased donor organs or to expose the donor to the risk of donating when there is little potential benefit for the recipient.

In some situations, however the living donor option may be appropriately justified. In the current system of regional distribution of deceased donor livers, a wide disparity in waiting times exists between regions and centers. In situations in which the waiting time is disproportionately long—because of blood type (see Fig. 48–3)

or geographic location or because of patient disease (e.g., those with small hepatocellular carcinomas and an expected prolonged waiting time for transplantation)—use of a living donor may be justifiable. Additionally, in some circumstances, use of a living donor can be immediately life-saving, such as transplantation in a patient with fulminant hepatic failure.

Overall, selection of a recipient for living donor transplants must optimize the expected recipient benefit. The graft-to-recipient weight ratio should be sufficiently large to provide enough hepatic mass and avoid small-for-size syndrome. A living donor should not be used for a salvage operation in situations in which 1-year patient mortality is greater than 20%. Living liver donors should not be used for non–UNOS-approved transplants. In fact, living donors should be used only for UNOS-approved transplantation and thus only for those with a physiological Model for End-Stage Liver Disease (MELD) score of less than 25 or greater than 15. In isolation (without regard to blood type, regional allocation, waiting times, etc.), this range appears to be a reasonable place to begin study and application of living donors. Patients with a MELD score lower than 15 may experience a greater mortality risk associated with living donor transplantation than they would if they waited for a full-sized deceased donor organ. At the other extreme, patients with a MELD score higher than 25 may need a larger hepatic mass than can safely be provided by a living donor or are too debilitated to tolerate the increased morbidity associated with receipt of a living donor graft.

Donor Selection

Living donors for adult liver transplantation differ from the donors used for pediatric liver transplantation in two important ways: (1) the relationship between the donor and recipient and (2) the risk to the donor.

Donor-Recipient Relationships. Many individuals who serve as donors for a pediatric recipient are first- or second-degree relatives of the intended recipient. In fact, the majority of donors are parents of the sick children. In the ALDLT situation, although many of the donors are also first-degree relatives (children) of the recipient, there is a great range of relationships between the intended donor and recipient, including blood relationships, emotional relationships, and even strangers. Acceptance of stranger donors in the performance of kidney transplantation has been well documented.[51] Volunteer donors, including strangers, have occasionally come forward, but most programs have discounted these patients as psychologically unsound.[52] However, because of the increasing shortage of organs, the charitable donation of a stranger after careful evaluation is now becoming a more common occurrence. In the practice of kidney transplantation, the relative risk of mortality and morbidity in the donor is sufficiently low.[53] Extension to the situation of adult living liver donation has occurred on an infrequent basis. We believe that the higher incidence of complications and mortality risk associated with right hepatic lobe donation and the fact that the procedure is nonstandardized and innovative should limit acceptance of strangers for this undertaking. As the stakes increase for donor complications and the risk of death, the program and physicians must bear increased responsibility and not expose healthy volunteers to the increased risk associated with their desire to provide a transplantable solid organ.

Donor Risk. The donor risk associated with the act of liver donation is substantially greater for donors of a right or extended right or full left lobe than for those donating either a kidney or a left lateral hepatic segment.[54] For liver donors, the risk associated with the donation is not just limited to the amount of hepatic mass removed and the amount left in the donor. It also relates to the increased complexity of the operation, the impact of abnormal vascular and biliary anatomy, and the heretofore undefined long-term health impact that hepatic resection may have on the donor.

Consequently, strict donor selection criteria that seek to absolutely minimize donor risk should be developed.[55] Only individuals in excellent general health and without any liver abnormalities (including nonalcoholic steatohepatitis) should be considered as potential candidates. The evaluation should be sufficiently complete to determine the size, anatomy, and health of the donor liver. The operative strategy should be planned so that sufficient hepatic mass is left for the donor. If leaving sufficient donor mass does not provide adequate mass for the recipient, the donor operation should not be performed. Donor safety is paramount and mandatory.

Risk/Benefit Assessment of the Donor and Recipient

Donor Risk

True donor morbidity and risk of mortality are difficult to quantify because of the lack of required reporting, lack of standard donor selection criteria and standardized donor and recipient operations, and variability in the quality and experience of the surgeon and transplant program. The magnitude of the hepatic resection is substantially greater when providing a liver graft for an adult recipient as opposed to an infant. Estimates of the incidence of donor mortality of 0.3% to 1% have been quoted (Table 48–1).[42,56,57] Donor morbidity has an equally large range of occurrence, 15% to 67%.[41,58] Unlike the adult-to-pediatric living donor operation, the seriousness of these complications results in reoperation, liver transplantation of the donor, infection, biliary tract complications, and wound complications. Although regeneration does occur in the remaining liver in the donor and the transplanted graft, the liver does not regenerate to 100% of its predonation mass.[59] Consequently, the regenerative capacity and long-term health consequences of such a resection are unknown.

Table 48–1. DONOR RISK AND RECIPIENT RISK/BENEFIT RELATIONSHIP

	Kidney	Liver for Pediatric Patient (Left Lateral)	Liver for Adult (Right Lobe)
Donor Risk			
Death (probability)	< 0.02%	< 0.1%	0.3–1.0% ?
Morbidity (incidence)	10%	15%	10–67% ?
Recipient Benefit (Potential) with LDT			
LDT versus waiting list mortality	↓↓↓	↓↓↓	↓↑ ?
LDT versus deceased donor graft (posttransplant)	↑↑↑	↑↑	↓↑ ?
Alternatives to LDT			
Transplant	Deceased donor	Deceased donor	Deceased donor
		Split liver	Split liver
		Reduced size	Expanded criteria donor
Medical support	Dialysis	None	None
Graft survival versus deceased donor graft	↑↑↑	↑↑	↓↑ ?
Recipient Risk (Potential) with LDT			
Transplant-associated risk: living donor versus deceased donor graft	↔	↓↔	↑↑

LDT, living donor transplantation.

Donor Benefit

Under the current practice of living donation, the donor benefit is restricted to that of psychological benefit. Many donors have a higher sense of self-esteem and contribution to the saving of another's life. As discussed in a subsequent section, financial compensation may in the future become another benefit.

Recipient Risk

When compared with standard deceased donor transplantation, ALDLT recipients have different risks associated with the transplant. First, hepatocyte mass is less with a right lobe transplant than with a full-sized deceased donor transplant. Although the risk of primary nonfunction is higher in the deceased donor group, primary nonfunction also occurs in the living donor group. Second, the smaller hepatocyte mass is more susceptible to hyperperfusion syndrome as a cause of graft dysfunction or loss.[60] Third, the technical requirements of performing and maintaining a successful living donor transplant are significantly greater than those required to successfully complete and maintain a deceased donor transplant or those encountered in living donation for pediatric recipients.[61] Fourth, it appears that the diminished hepatocyte mass may have a negative impact on the recurrence of some diseases for which the transplantation was indicated.[62] For these reasons, livers from adult living donors should at this time be considered "marginal grafts."

Unlike pediatric recipients, who are cured by liver transplantation, the majority of adult transplant recipients suffer end-stage liver disease caused by or associated with potentially recurrent disease (hepatitis C and hepatocellular cancer). The prospect of recurrent disease and the increased risk of technical complications, in some cases, serve to limit the durability of the transplanted graft.[63] Limited durability is also a factor in terms of life expectancy. Adult recipients have a higher incidence of recurrent disease and comorbidity and lower patient and graft survival than pediatric recipients do.[45]

Because of the increased mortality risk for the donor, the increased morbidity associated with donation, and the uncertainty of the impact that the donation will have on the future health of the donor, a more rigid calculation must be made to justify the use of ALDLT.

Recipient Benefit

The principal benefit to a recipient is that waiting time for a liver transplant is substantially reduced. In fact, it is possible that some recipients of living donor liver transplantation undergo transplantation too early. Much has been made of the rapidly increasing number of patients added to the waiting list for liver transplantation, but few data exist that differentiate between those who are true candidates for transplantation and those listed without any expectation of receiving a transplant. Justification of ALDLT based on this disparity, therefore, is flawed. Unlike the situation in pediatric liver transplantation, where there is an absolute lack of size-appropriate donors, adult recipients do have alternative donor options. Currently, allocation of deceased donor organs is based on a system that provides organs to the sickest first. The MELD score has been demonstrated to accurately predict pretransplant mortality,[48] but it does not predict posttransplant mortality when living donor liver transplantation is used.[64] The MELD score helps define when the risk of undergoing liver transplantation is safer for the recipient than continued waiting on the list. The difficulty rests in the uncertainty of finding a deceased donor liver when the patient's MELD score is sufficiently high that continued waiting is more risky than immediate (but not emergency) transplantation. It is this uncertainty that encourages the use of living donors.

Several other clinical situations in adult liver transplantation may benefit from ALDLT. Patients who experience a disproportionately long waiting time resulting in severe decompensation or exclusion from transplant candidacy may benefit from an appropriately timed living donor transplant. Examples of these groups may be found in blood groups O and A (see Fig. 48–3) or in certain U.S. regions of allocation.[65] Until recent modification of the MELD score to benefit recipients with hepatocellular carcinoma, patients with hepatocellular carcinoma improved their chance of transplantation by having a living donor.[66] This patient group had a finite period before tumor growth often excluded them from transplantation. Now this cohort receives weighting in the MELD system to account for the tumor growth rate.[67] At present, some have advocated use of a living donor for patients who have been excluded from UNOS indications because of large tumors.[63] Other situations such as recipients small in stature or those with acute hepatic necrosis may also benefit from the living donor option.

In summary, there appears to be significantly higher donor morbidity and mortality associated with living donation to adult recipients. Despite more than 1000 such donations, few centers have shared all their complications through peer-reviewed publications. More importantly, most of the donor deaths have not been reviewed in such a format. The long-term consequences associated with such a large hepatic resection remain to be defined.

For adult recipients undergoing living donor liver transplantation, the indications, contraindications, timing of surgery, and volume of hepatic mass needed are still poorly defined. Additionally, no risk-adjusted analysis has been conducted to clearly define which recipients may be harmed and which may benefit from this operation.

Informed Consent

Patient preferences are essential to the ethical analysis of clinical issues, including organ transplantation. Specific clinical indications often lead to medical recommendations by the physician for a treatment plan. The patient has control over the decision-making and may choose to accept or reject the treatment plan. This ability to control decisions is often referred to as patient autonomy. Patient autonomy requires that the patient have decisional capacity and be informed of the risks and benefits of the treatment plan and other treatment options. Patient decisions are often influenced by ethical, legal, religious, and cultural factors unique to the individual patient. The interaction and negotiation between the physician and the patient form the basis of the doctor-patient relationship.

The concept of autonomy is fundamental to the process of informed consent. With few exceptions (e.g., hepatic coma or pediatric recipients), patients with end-stage liver disease should be allowed to participate in the process of informed consent leading to the performance of liver transplantation. Importantly, the consent process should include not only information about performance of the transplant surgery but also information about the effect of the surgery on life after transplantation and the requirements for close follow-up and lifelong compliance with immunosuppression therapy. In the case of living donor liver transplantation, where the risks are greater than with other living donations, the recipient should be informed of the donor risks and be allowed the final decision of rejecting the option of living liver donation. This concept of declining the donation is important to honor. In contrast to the experience in living liver donation from an adult to a child, adult-to-adult donation may have different psychosocial motivations. Consequently, the psychological burden placed on the potential adult recipient feeling responsible for the outcome of the donor's operation may be too great to accept.

For several important reasons, potential living liver donors should also be provided informed consent separate from the consent for the recipient. First, these donors do not have a medical indication for the donation, but are placing their life at risk to benefit another. Second, for reasons stated, ALDLT is innovative or experimental surgery and thus requires a high level of informed consent by donors to an experiment. Specifically, we cannot tell donors about their short- or long-term risks, both medical and psychological. Therefore, it is incumbent on the physician to clearly identify why a living liver donation is required or preferred based on the recipient's specific medical needs. Third, donor preference may differ from the consent of the intended recipient. Many donors make the decision to donate before their medical evaluation or provision of information regarding the risks and benefits of the donor procedure.[68] It is here that autonomy alone is insufficient to justify the act of donation.[69] Rather, the surgeon has an obligation to not accept living donors whose comorbid conditions put them at high risk for surgical complications or death.

Even in the practice of living donor kidney transplantation, which is less risky and more universally accepted, not all donors are accepted on the basis of their perceived right to donate. Acceptance of liver donors must be based on the premise that the transplant is more likely than not to be successful and be of significant benefit to the recipient. In addition to being provided with informed consent, living donors should be able to demonstrate an informed understanding of the potential consequences of their donation. In a situation in which the medical community, transplant community, and society participate, donor autonomy is necessary but not sufficient to validate the act of donation.

At this time, since the ALDLT operative procedure is not standardized and the outcomes are not entirely known, we must conclude that informed consent for both donors and recipients is less than informed and that the consent procedure should be similar to that for innovative procedures (which are reviewed by IRBs).

Experience and Capacity of the Transplantation Team and Climate of the Institution

Dr. Francis Moore referred to the capacity of the transplant team as field strength and the motivations that fuel the performance of innovative surgery as the climate of the institution. As defined by Moore, field strength refers to the competency of the team in performance of the entire transplant undertaking[47] and includes performance of the operation, as well as preoperative assessment and postoperative care of the patient.

Undergoing resection of the right lobe of the liver is associated with a fixed and not yet fully defined risk of death and postoperative complications. This fixed risk can be minimized only by ensuring the quality and competency of the team involved in care of the donor. Unfortunately, the rapid dissemination and performance of this operation in many institutions without previous experience in innovative liver surgery and the care of such patients are cause for concern. Therefore, it seems reasonable that the caliber and quality of the health care team and the institution be at a level high enough to limit the possibility of adding to the donor risk. Recently, Malago and colleagues outlined criteria defining requirements needed by the surgeon, the team, and the institution performing ALDLT.[70] With the occurrence of a widely publicized donor death at a New York hospital, the New York State Department of Health has drafted a similar document outlining minimum standards for staff and institutions wishing to perform ALDLT in New York.[71] Finally, minimum standards have been defined for UNOS Certification of Live Liver Donor Transplant Programs.[72]

Although these documents set forth the minimum requirements believed necessary for safe performance of living donor liver transplantation, they do not address the "ethical climate of the institution." As defined by Moore, this concept refers to the ethical conduct of the surgeons and the institutions performing living donor liver transplantation.[47] Specifically, how does one ensure that the operation is necessary and appropriate, that appropriate selection and matching of donor and recipient pairs have occurred, and that patients are protected from conflict of interest on the part of the surgeon, the institution, and other parties involved in living donor transplantation? Although difficult to measure and more difficult to regulate, it is critical that the operation being performed primarily serve the needs of the recipient and donor and not the academic, financial, or professional interests of the surgeon or the marketing and financial interests of the institution.

In our view, since ALDLT is a complex and risky procedure for donors (see the next section), it should never be used as an alternative to deceased donor liver transplantation in countries that have a functioning deceased donor procurement system (the way, for example, that living donor kidney transplants are), except when there is a compelling need that justifies subjecting the donor to a high risk of surgical morbidity and mortality. Thus far, many programs performing this procedure have not made clear the clinical circumstances in which ALDLT should be used and can be justified.

Special Ethical Concerns

Double Equipoise for Donors and Recipients

In the performance of an ethically based clinical trial investigating two therapies, a degree of uncertainty must exist between the two treatment groups. This uncertainty is referred to as equipoise.[73] A state of equipoise is essential because assignment of a patient to an inferior therapy would be unethical. As such, a clinical trial serves to compare the risks and benefits between two therapies as they affect an individual patient. In the performance of liver transplantation, there are, of course, recipient risks and benefits associated with the therapy. However, in the performance of adult-to-adult liver transplantation, the balance of the risk and benefit is interdependent and shared between the recipient and donor. There are donor risks associated with the donor operation. In addition, the recipient risk/benefit is largely dependent on clinical status at the time of the transplant, the specific liver disease, and the quality and volume of the donor

liver segment. In the case of ALDLT, donor risk must be balanced against recipient benefit, a situation that we refer to as double equipoise.[57]

The risk of morbidity and mortality in the donor is relatively constant and relates to recipient need only in terms of the volume of liver that will be removed from the donor. The potential benefit for recipients varies according to their clinical status at the time of transplantation and their specific liver disease. We use the concept of double equipoise to describe the balance between potential benefits and risks for both donors and recipients. If donor risk is relatively constant, the double-equipoise assessment asks whether the recipient's potential benefit is sufficient for the surgeon to permit the potential donor to take the fixed risk. In certain situations, the use of a graft from a living donor cannot be justified ethically. For example, it would be unethical to transplant a graft from an informed, enthusiastic volunteer living donor into a moribund recipient who had only hours to live. Similarly, it would be unethical to expose a donor to any risk for a recipient with widely metastatic carcinoma and a prognosis of less than a few months with or without a liver transplant, even if both the donor and the recipient were willing to proceed.

At this stage in the development of ALDLT, where many short-term and long-term donor risks are not known and surgical teams of varying competency are performing this complex operation, it may be prudent to restrict ALDLT to situations in which the recipient has a high likelihood of a long-term benefit based on published data. The community of liver transplantation programs should take the initiative to define situations when double equipoise allows us to proceed ethically (or not proceed) with ALDLT.

Research on Adult Living Donor Liver Transplantation

Use of the right hepatic lobe from a living donor for transplantation into an adult recipient began only in 1996. Since that time, more than 1500 procedures have been performed worldwide. Despite this rapid growth and global dissemination, many aspects of this operation remain unsettled, including donor and recipient selection criteria, the correct donor operation, the correct recipient operation, establishing the risks to recipients and the relative risks of living donation versus the use of deceased donor livers, establishing the risks to donors in both the short and the long term, physical and psychological aspects, and other issues. Because of the lack of information and lack of standardization of the procedure, ALDLT must be considered an innovative or experimental procedure. As such, it should continue to be reported to IRBs, and its informed consent procedures should be scrutinized and also monitored by the IRB. Because the operation is innovative and experimental, it is very important that good clinical research continue to be conducted to clarify and help answer some of the issues that remain unsettled.

However, ALDLT patients should not be enrolled in experimental protocols that are designed to answer questions not intended to improve the technical aspects of the living liver donor operation (improving donor and recipient selection, operative techniques, volume questions, and outcomes) directly related to this innovative, nonstandardized and dangerous operation. For example, we should not use living donor liver operations to study new combinations of immunosuppressive drugs (or tolerance-inducing agents) or to assess whether human immunodeficiency virus–infected patients will experience increased viral replication after liver transplantation. Such studies should be confined to transplants performed with organs from deceased donors so that living donors are not placed at risk for an operation whose risks are not yet established. The basic principle should be "Do not experiment on an experiment." In this case, since ALDLT remains an innovative experiment, research should not be conducted with living donors except to improve the operation itself.

Financial Incentives

Recently, there has been a resurgence of discussions concerning both financial and nonfinancial incentives for organ donation.[74] Most of the proposed incentive plans have confined themselves to deceased donor organs. In many of the proposals, financial and nonfinancial incentives will be delivered to the family, estate, or loved one of the deceased organ donor. Additional discussions have included the actual buying and selling of organs in a market and commodification of organs.[75] In the case of organs procured from living liver donors, in addition to being illegal (PL 98-507-NOTA 1984), it should be clearly stated that financial incentive for donation should not be offered either directly or indirectly. In the case of living donors for pediatric recipients, these are most commonly directed donations, and the donor has a direct and tangible interest in the well-being of the recipient. In the case of ALDLT, most donations are directed, no compensation is needed, and directed donation should not be financially rewarded. Furthermore, in situations in which donor risk is high and the procedure can still be considered experimental, it would be unethical to enter into the market of buying and selling of organs.

Regulation of Innovative Surgery

The field of surgery has minimal regulatory standards and oversight committees. Unlike the pharmaceutical industry, there is nothing like the Food and Drug Administration for surgery. Consequently, the ethical conduct of surgical innovation depends on the ethics of the innovators and local oversight by peers and colleagues. Most innovative procedures in surgery are derived from an urgent clinical need that is unmet by current therapeutic options and is undertaken to benefit the individual patient on whom it is being performed. Further application of the innovative technique to other patients may occur and is usually associated with refinement of the innovation. Once the innovation has been technically standardized, its indications understood, and the innovation shown to provide measurable improvement, it usually becomes adopted and disseminated. If the innovation is unsuccessful, it is generally abandoned. This model has worked well for more than 200 years of surgical innovation. Society at large has benefitted from the brave patients and pioneering work of surgeons who have advanced the practice of surgery. Surgical innovation and advances in technology have resulted in a wave of minimally invasive surgical techniques (laparoscopic cholecystectomy, nephrectomy, bowel surgery), improved survival from many diseases (kidney transplantation, coronary artery bypass), decreased morbidity and mortality (appendectomy), and broader application of surgical options for a wider patient population. In the field of liver transplantation specifically, surgical innovation has improved the safety of liver transplantation, increased recipient survival and decreased morbidity, and expanded the therapy to a broader population of patients. Surgical innovation has also been used to help address the shortage of organs by using split-liver transplantation, reduced-size liver transplantation, and expanded criteria (marginal) donor organs. What must be acknowledged, however, is that these innovations were developed, investigated, and refined in a patient population that stood to benefit from their success. In the realm of living donor surgery, the donor does not stand to gain substantial benefit from participating in the innovative experiment. Therefore, the surgical community, institution, and individual surgeon have a duty to conduct the research with a higher than usual standard of responsibility and accountability. Real and potential conflicts of interest need to be acknowledged, and the rights of the donor must be protected throughout the process.

Responsibility for reporting complications and deaths is an imperative in any new innovative procedure. The safety of experimental subjects and living donors should be of the highest priority. Information learned from the self-sacrifice and complications of others should be shared and used to prevent the suffering and loss of those who follow. It is unconscionable to think that donors have died[76] and that the involved transplant programs may not be reporting these or other complications that could benefit future donors and the entire transplant community.

Conclusion

Since 1954 when the first healthy volunteer donor provided a kidney to an identical twin brother, the medical community and society have wrestled with the conflicting interests of the recipient and the donor. The central ethical question remains the same today as in 1954: is it ever ethical to perform surgery on a healthy individual (the donor) to benefit another person (the recipient)? Justification for the first living donor transplant was based on a desperate case: the diagnosis of end-stage renal disease was universally fatal, and of the small number of kidney transplants performed, no patients survived more than a few months because of limited understanding of the immune system and lack of effective immunosuppression agents. In those early living donor operations, donor risks and morbidity were unknown, but were thought to be similar to those of nephrectomy performed for medical indications. Long-term donor risk was similarly unknown. The potential recipient benefit was tremendous and life-saving. The living donor operation provided a means to save the recipient's life, advance the science of transplantation, and avoid the destructive forces of the immune system. The first successful living donor kidney transplant established transplantation as an acceptable therapeutic option. With improvements in immunosuppression, better understanding of the immune system, and development of organ preservation techniques, the use of deceased donor kidneys was possible with acceptable success. Coincident with improvements in immunosuppression and transplantation were improvements in dialysis therapy. Together, these medical modalities increased the number of people who qualified for kidney transplantation. Until recently, living donor kidney transplantation was an option only for patients who had an appropriately matched and healthy genetically or emotionally related donor. Recent application of laparoscopic techniques has allowed more individuals to become living donors than ever before in history (see Fig. 48–5). Additionally, with the exceedingly low potential for donor mortality and low short-lived morbidity, donor acceptance has been extended beyond genetically and emotionally related individuals to include friends and altruistic or stranger donors.

The first series of living donors for pediatric liver transplantation was undertaken under similar desperate conditions. Many infants in need of liver transplantation were unable to receive a size-appropriate graft. This lack of transplantable organs resulted in a waiting list mortality that approached 40%. However, unlike the experience of living donor kidney transplantation, a prospective protocol study was performed to evaluate this type of living donor surgery. The Chicago protocol[15] serves as an ethically based model for the development of innovative techniques in surgery. Success of that protocol has resulted in worldwide application of adult-to-pediatric living donor liver transplantation as a clinically and ethically acceptable treatment option for infants with liver disease.[77] Additionally, recipients of living donor grafts obtained superior results when compared with those who received a deceased donor graft. Application of living donor liver therapy has also expanded to include emotional and genetically related donors and, in some circumstance, altruistic donors. Acceptance of these unrelated donors is justified because of the low donor morbidity and mortality and the exceptional benefit derived by the recipient of such a graft.

Despite the rapid growth and wide dissemination of ALDLT, fundamental questions still remain to be answered. Does the same ethical justification exist for ALDLT that served to validate the use of living donors for kidney and pediatric liver transplantation? Does the "desperate case" scenario exist for adult patients with end-stage liver disease?

Geographically, there seems to be some justification for ALDLT. In Asia, where living donation is the primary source of organs for transplantation, a desperate case does exist. Without the use of living donors, candidates for liver transplantation will not survive. Even in the United States, because waiting times vary dramatically between and within different regions, some areas may benefit from the availability of living donors. In the United States, however, a more stringent justification is required because of the availability of deceased donors. Currently, deceased donor organs are allocated to the sickest first, patients determined to be in the greatest need. On this basis, those who are most in need (shortest life expectancy) of potentially life-saving liver transplantation are brought to the top of the list. Unfortunately, not all patients receive an organ for transplantation in time. In this group of patients with advanced physical deterioration, it appears that the sickest do not greatly benefit from living donor transplantation. Alternatively, in patients who are not desperately ill, transplantation of an organ from a living donor too early in their disease process may expose the patient to an inappropriately high risk from transplantation with a living donor graft.

Patients with certain medical conditions or with certain blood types might also benefit from the use of a living donor. For example, patients with blood type O have a significantly increased waiting time for organs when compared with those who are type B or AB. Patients with metabolic disease and hepatocellular cancer are another subgroup of patients who might justifiably benefit from living donor liver transplantation. With respect to patients with hepatocellular cancer, the recent modification to the MELD system has diminished the advantage given to patients with hepatocellular cancer waiting for deceased donor organs. Patients with small lesions might benefit from earlier transplantation at a time when they are in good physiological condition and their tumor is small. We cannot, however, find justification for the use of living donors under circumstances that are contraindicated for receipt of a deceased donor graft. This situation is made even more unacceptable when recipients of a living donor liver transplant for a condition previously excluding them from the deceased donor pool suffer a complication (hepatic artery thrombosis) that qualifies them as status I for deceased donor allocation. Similarly, there should be a minimum expected durability of the transplant when using a living donor. Transplantation in patients with tumors too large to qualify for deceased donor allocation is suspect because of the inability to predict which patients will be free of tumor recurrence.

Use of living donors should be based on donor safety and protection and be reserved for situations of maximally beneficial donor outcome. Therefore, donors should not be used for indications that result in only short-term gains for the recipient, donors should not be used just because they are available and convenient, and donation should be performed in an institution and by a surgical team that has demonstrated expertise in all facets of selection, surgery, and postoperative care. Recent recommendations that outline minimal standards have been long overdue. Institutions that seek to offer and benefit from living donation should assume the responsibility of long-term follow-up of the donor and recipient pair, and a national registry for donors and recipients must be started.

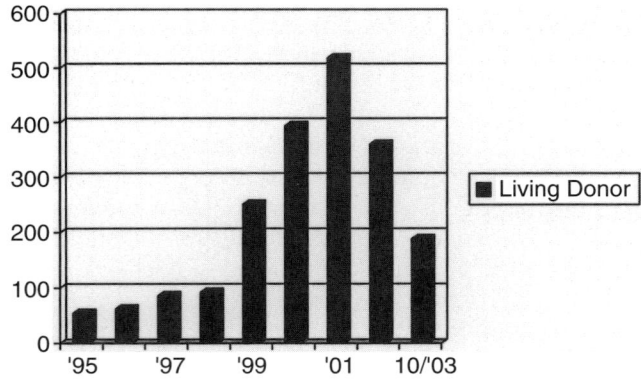

FIGURE 48–7

All recipients of living donor liver transplants. (Data from University Renal Research and Education Association [URREA] and United Network for Organ Sharing [UNOS]: 2002 Annual Report of the U.S. Organ Procurement and Transplantation Network [OPTN] and the Scientific Registry of Transplant Recipients [SRTR]: Transplant Data 1992-2001. Rockville, MD: Organ Procurement and Transplantation Network [OPTN], 2003. Modified 2003 Feb 18; cited 2003 June 27. Available from http://www.optn.org/data/annualReport.asp; and OPTN data as of October 24, 2003.)

No doubt, ALDLT will continue to be offered and performed by many surgeons and transplant centers. However, protection of donor safety cannot be stressed enough as an ethical defense for this procedure. The disparity between the number of patients waiting for transplantation and the lack of deceased donors is not by itself sufficient justification for using living donors. The disparity in supply and demand will always continue. If more organs are acquired for transplantation and the procedure continues to improve, the indications will be broadened and the disparity will therefore continue. Nor is the provision of informed consent and respect for donor autonomy sufficient to justify the donation. As we stated, informed consent is difficult to negotiate when meaningful data on many aspects of the procedure are lacking. Additionally, donors may be exploited or coerced by the nature of the recipient's terminal illness. This subtle pressure may partially explain why many donors have decided to become donors (and rarely change their mind) even before being evaluated by the transplant team.

Although many in the transplant community disagree on whether the adult-to-adult living donor procedure remains experimental or is now the standard of care, what is very clear is that the public and the profession will not tolerate donor deaths. One very public donor death resulted in temporary suspension of the program, governmental investigation and oversight, and regulatory responses from various agencies. This death was also associated with a dramatic decrease in the number of ALDLT procedures performed in the United States (Fig. 48–7).

End-stage liver disease is a tragic and terrible illness that usually results in premature death of the patient unless a liver transplant is received in the appropriate time. The risk of recipient death, however, does not justify surgeons departing from the sacred and fundamental tenet of medicine, to "do no harm." In the context of ALDLT, this means that protection of the donor is the surgeon's highest ethical responsibility.

References

1. Moore FD: Transplant. The Give and Take of Tissue Transplantation. New York, Simon & Schuster, 1972.
2. Starzl TE: The Puzzle People. Memoirs of a Transplant Surgeon. Pittsburgh, University of Pittsburgh Press, 1992.
3. 2001 OPTN/SRTR Annual Report 1991-2000. HHS/HRSA/OSP/DOT; UNOS; URREA. Vol. 1, 2001.
4. Burdelski M, Nolkemper D, Ganschow R, et al: Liver transplantation in children: Long-term outcome and quality of life. Eur J Pediatr 158(Suppl 2):S34-S42, 1999.
5. Amersi F, Farmer DG, Busuttil RW: Fifteen-year experience with adult and pediatric liver transplantation at the University of California, Los Angeles. Clin Transpl 255-261, 1998.
6. Emond JC, Whitington PF, Thistlethwaite JR, et al: Reduced-size orthotopic liver transplantation: Use in the management of children with chronic liver disease. Hepatology 10:867-872, 1989.

7. Gutierrez E: Japan's House of Representatives passes brain-death bill. Lancet 349:1304, 1997.

8. Bismuth H, Houssin D: Reduced-sized orthotopic liver graft in hepatic transplantation in children. Surgery 95:367-370, 1984.

9. Broelsch CE, Emond JC, Thistlethwaite JR, et al: Liver transplantation, including the concept of reduced-size liver transplants in children. Ann Surg 208:410-420, 1988.

10. Broelsch CE, Emond JC, Thistlethwaite JR, et al: Liver transplantation with reduced-size donor organs. Transplantation 45:519-524, 1988.

11. Emond JC, Whitington PF, Broelsch CE: Overview of reduced-size liver transplantation. Clin Transplant 5:168-173, 1991.

12. Emond JC, Whitington PF, Thistlethwaite JR, et al: Transplantation of two patients with one liver. Analysis of a preliminary experience with 'split-liver' grafting. Ann Surg 212:14-22, 1990.

13. Raia S, Nery JR, Mies S: Liver transplantation from live donors [letter]. Lancet 2:497, 1989.

14. Strong RW, Lynch SV, Ong TH, et al: Successful liver transplantation from a living donor to her son. N Engl J Med 322:1505-1507, 1990.

15. Singer PA, Siegler M, Whitington PF, et al: Ethics of liver transplantation with living donors [see comments]. N Engl J Med 321:620-622, 1989.

16. Broelsch CE, Whitington PF, Emond JC, et al: Liver transplantation in children from living related donors. Surgical techniques and results. Ann Surg 214:428-437, 1991.

17. Millis JM, Cronin DC, Brady LM, et al: Primary living-donor liver transplantation at the University of Chicago: Technical aspects of the first 104 recipients. Ann Surg 232:104-111, 2000.

18. Emre S, Schwartz ME, Shneider B, et al: Living related liver transplantation for acute liver failure in children. Liver Transpl Surg 5:161-165, 1999.

19. Rogiers X, Burdelski M, Broelsch CE: Liver transplantation from living donors. Br J Surg 81:1251-1253, 1994.

20. Tanaka K, Uemoto S, Tokunaga Y, et al: Living related liver transplantation in children. Am J Surg 168:41-48, 1994.

21. Fan ST, Lo CM, Chan KL, et al: Liver transplantation—perspective from Hong Kong. Hepatogastroenterology 43:893-897, 1996.

22. Chen CL, Chen YS, Liu PP, et al: Living related donor liver transplantation. J Gastroenterol Hepatol 12:S342-S345, 1997.

23. Kiuchi T, Inomata Y, Uemoto S, et al: Living-donor liver transplantation in Kyoto, 1997. Clin Transpl 191-198, 1997.

24. Harihara Y, Makuuchi M, Kawarasaki H, et al: Initial experience with living-related liver transplantation at the University of Tokyo. Transplant Proc 30:129-131, 1998.

25. Inomata Y, Tanaka K, Uemoto S, et al: Living donor liver transplantation: An 8-year experience with 379 consecutive cases. Transplant Proc 31:381, 1999.

26. Millis JM, Alonso EM, Piper JB, et al: Liver transplantation at the University of Chicago. Clin Transpl 187-197, 1995.

27. Mori K, Nagata I, Yamagata S, et al: The introduction of microvascular surgery to hepatic artery reconstruction in living-donor liver transplantation—its surgical advantages compared with conventional procedures. Transplantation 54:263-268, 1992.

28. Furuta S, Ikegami T, Nakazawa Y, et al: Hepatic artery reconstruction in living donor liver transplantation from the microsurgeon's point of view. Liver Transpl Surg 3:388-393, 1997.

29. Hashimoto T, Suzuki T, Shimizu Y, et al: ABO-incompatible living related liver transplantation for fulminant hepatitis: Report of a successful pediatric case with long-term follow-up. Transplant Proc 30:3510-3512, 1998.

30. Kitai T, Higashiyama H, Tanada Y, et al: Pulmonary embolism in a donor of living-related liver transplantation: Estimation of donor's operative risk. Surgery 120:570-573, 1996.

31. Sterneck M, Nischwitz L, Fischer L, et al: Evaluation and morbidity of the living donor in pediatric liver transplantation. Transplant Proc 27:1164-1165, 1995.

32. Yamaoka Y, Morimoto T, Inamot T, et al: Safety of the donor in living-related liver transplantation—an analysis of 100 parental donors. Transplantation 59:224-226, 1995.

33. Grewal HP, Thistlewaite JR Jr, Loss GE, et al: Complications in 100 living-liver donors. Ann Surg 228:214-219, 1998.

34. Piper JB, Whitington PF, Woodle ES, et al: Pediatric liver transplantation at the University of Chicago Hospitals. Clin Transpl 179-189, 1992.

35. Lo CM, Fan ST, Liu CL, et al: Adult-to-adult living donor liver transplantation using extended right lobe grafts. Ann Surg 226:261-269, 1997.

36. Wachs ME, Bak TE, Karrer FM, et al: Adult living donor liver transplantation using a right hepatic lobe. Transplantation 66:1313-1316, 1998.

37. Howard TK: Transplantation of the right hepatic lobe. N Engl J Med 347:615-618, author reply 615-618, 2002.

38. Testa G, Malago M, Broelsch CE: Living-donor liver transplantation in adults. Langenbecks Arch Surg 384:536-543, 1999.

39. Marcos A, Fisher RA, Ham JM, et al: Right lobe living donor transplantation. Transplantation 68:798-803, 1999.

40. Inomata Y, Uemoto S, Asonuma K, Egawa H: Right lobe graft in living donor liver transplantation. Transplantation 69:258-264, 2000.

41. Pomfret EA, Pomposelli JJ, Lewis WD, et al: Live donor adult liver transplantation using right lobe grafts: Donor evaluation and surgical outcome. Arch Surg 136:425-433, 2001.

42. Brown RS Jr, Russo MW, Lai M, et al: A survey of liver transplantation from living adult donors in the United States. N Engl J Med 348:818-825, 2003.

43. Lo CM: Complications and long-term outcome of living liver donors: A survey of 1,508 cases in five Asian centers. Transplantation 75:S12-S15, 2003.

44. Testa G, Malago M, Nadalin S, et al: Right-liver living donor transplantation for decompensated end-stage liver disease. Liver Transpl 8:340-346, 2002.

45. Goldstein MJ, Salame E, Kapur S, et al: Analysis of failure in living donor liver transplantation: Differential outcomes in children and adults. World J Surg 27:356-364, 2003.

46. Lo CM, Liu CL, Fan ST: Portal hyperperfusion injury as the cause of primary nonfunction in a small-for-size liver graft—successful treatment with splenic artery ligation. Liver Transpl 9:626-628, 2003.

47. Moore FD: Three ethical revolutions: Ancient assumptions remodeled under pressure of transplantation. Transplant Proc 20:1061-1067, 1988.

48. Freeman RB Jr, Wiesner RH, Harper A, et al: The new liver allocation system: Moving toward evidence-based transplantation policy. Liver Transpl 8:851-858, 2002.

49. Emond JC, Renz JF, Ferrell LD, et al: Functional analysis of grafts from living donors. Implications for the treatment of older recipients. Ann Surg 224:544-554, 1996.

50. Kiuchi T, Kasahara M, Uryuhara K, et al: Impact of graft size mismatching on graft prognosis in liver transplantation from living donors. Transplantation 67:321-327, 1999.

51. Spital A: Public attitudes toward kidney donation by friends and altruistic strangers in the United States. Transplantation 71:1061-1064, 2001.

52. Henderson AJ, Landolt MA, McDonald MF, et al: The living anonymous kidney donor: Lunatic or saint? Am J Transplant 3:203-213, 2003.

53. Matas AJ, Bartlett ST, Leichtman AB, Delmonico FL: Morbidity and mortality after living kidney donation, 1999-2001: Survey of United States transplant centers. Am J Transplant 3:830-834, 2003.

54. Schwartz M: Candidate selection criteria for living donor liver transplantation. Mt Sinai J Med 70:171-173, 2003.

55. Chisuwa H, Hashikura Y, Mita A, et al: Living liver donation: Preoperative assessment, anatomic considerations, and long-term outcome. Transplantation 75:1670-1676, 2003.

56. Surman OS: The ethics of partial-liver donation. N Engl J Med 346:1038, 2002.

57. Cronin DC 2nd, Millis JM, Siegler M: Transplantation of liver grafts from living donors into adults—too much, too soon. N Engl J Med 344:1633-1637, 2001.

58. Ito T, Kiuchi T, Egawa H, et al: Surgery-related morbidity in living donors of right-lobe liver graft: Lessons from the first 200 cases. Transplantation 76:158-163, 2003.

59. Marcos A, Fisher RA, Ham JM, et al: Liver regeneration and function in donor and recipient after right lobe adult to adult living donor liver transplantation. Transplantation 69:1375-1379, 2000.

60. Man K, Fan ST, Lo CM, et al: Graft injury in relation to graft size in right lobe live donor liver transplantation: A study of hepatic sinusoidal injury in correlation with portal hemodynamics and intragraft gene expression. Ann Surg 237:256-264, 2003.

61. Salame E, Goldstein MJ, Kinkhabwala M, et al: Analysis of donor risk in living-donor hepatectomy: The impact of resection type on clinical outcome. Am J Transplant 2:780-788, 2002.

62. Baltz AC, Trotter JF: Living donor liver transplantation and hepatitis C. Clin Liver Dis 7:651-665, viii, 2003.

63. Kaihara S, Kiuchi T, Ueda M, et al: Living-donor liver transplantation for hepatocellular carcinoma. Transplantation 75:S37-S40, 2003.

64. Hayashi PH, Forman L, Steinberg T, et al: Model for End-Stage Liver Disease score does not predict patient or graft survival in living donor liver transplant recipients. Liver Transpl 9:737-740, 2003.

65. Schaffer RL, Kulkarni S, Harper A, et al: The sickest first? Disparities with model for end-stage liver disease–based organ allocation: One region's experience. Liver Transpl 9:1211-1215, 2003.

66. Cheng SJ, Pratt DS, Freeman RB Jr, et al: Living-donor versus cadaveric liver transplantation for non-resectable small hepatocellular carcinoma and compensated cirrhosis: A decision analysis. Transplantation 72:861-868, 2001.

67. Yao FY, Bass NM, Nikolai B, et al: A follow-up analysis of the pattern and predictors of dropout from the waiting list for liver transplantation in patients with hepatocellular carcinoma: Implications for the current organ allocation policy. Liver Transpl 9:684-692, 2003.

68. Crowley-Matoka M, Siegler M, Cronin DC: Long-term quality of life issues among adult-to-pediatric living liver donors: A qualitative exploration. Am J Transplant 4:744-750, 2004.

69. Siegler M, Lantos JD: Commentary: Ethical justification for living liver donation. Cambridge Q Healthcare Ethics 4:320-325, 1992.

70. Malago M, Testa G, Marcos A, et al: Ethical considerations and rationale of adult-to-adult living donor liver transplantation. Liver Transpl 7:921-927, 2001.

71. New York State Committee on Quality Improvement in Living Liver Donation. Vol 2003. New York, New York State Transplant Council and New York State Department of Health, 2002, pp 1-44.

72. Bylaws, Appendix B IV, Section B: OPTN/UNOS, 2003.

73. Freedman B: Equipoise and the ethics of clinical research. N Engl J Med 317:141-145, 1987.

74. Delmonico FL, Arnold R, Scheper-Hughes N, et al: Ethical incentives—not payment—for organ donation. N Engl J Med 346:2002-2005, 2002.

75. Joralemon D: Shifting ethics: Debating the incentive question in organ transplantation. J Med Ethics 27:30-35, 2001.

76. Strong RW: Whither living donor liver transplantation? Liver Transpl Surg 5:536-538, 1999.

77. Singer PA, Siegler M, Lantos JD, et al: The ethical assessment of innovative therapies: Liver transplantation using living donors. Theor Med 11:87-94, 1990.

VII

Unusual Operative Problems

Portal Vein Thrombosis and Other Venous Anomalies in Liver Transplantation

NIRAJ M. DESAI
KIM M. OLTHOFF

Portal vein thrombosis   743
  Incidence and diagnostic imaging   743
  Operative strategy   745
  Outcomes in recipients with portal vein
    thrombosis   747
  Portal vein thrombosis after
    transplantation   748

Prior portosystemic shunts   748
  Surgical shunts   748
  Transjugular intrahepatic portosystemic
    shunts   749

Anomalies of the inferior vena cava   750
  Preexisting vena cava anomalies   750
  Variations in vena cava reconstruction   750
  Vena cava anomalies after
    transplantation   751

Summary   751

Among the unusual operative problems found in liver transplantation today, venous anomalies are a relatively frequent finding. These abnormalities include acute and chronic portal vein thrombosis (PVT), the presence of a prior portosystemic shunt, total portosplenomesenteric venous thrombosis, and anomalies of the inferior vena cava. These situations usually require relatively straightforward solutions; however, more creative approaches are sometimes necessary to allow successful transplantation. This chapter addresses venous anomalies and complicating factors that may be encountered in the course of liver transplantation and operative approaches to these often challenging problems.

Portal Vein Thrombosis

Incidence and Diagnostic Imaging

The presence of PVT was once considered an absolute contraindication to orthotopic liver transplantation (OLT) because of the technical difficulties encountered during the transplant procedure and the high rate of patient mortality.[1] The technical difficulties included excessive hemorrhaging and an inability to establish adequate portal blood flow with resulting allograft nonfunction. However, as greater experience was obtained and improved surgical techniques were implemented, recipients with PVT were able to undergo successful transplantation, albeit with an increased level of surgical complexity and higher perioperative morbidity and mortality.[2-5] Today, transplantation in the face of PVT is accomplished using the operative techniques of thrombectomy of the native vessel,[2] extensive thrombendvenectomy up to the splenomesenteric confluence,[6] venous conduits from the superior mesenteric vein (SMV),[7] and use of alternative sources of portal inflow such as the inferior vena cava (IVC).[8] Although results have improved significantly, these recipients should still be considered "high risk" and referred to experienced transplant surgeons and centers.[5,6,9,10]

The incidence of PVT in patients undergoing OLT ranges from 2.1% to 26% in large reported series.[2,5,6,9-14] Risk factors implicated in the development of PVT vary depending on the report. In one large series, the implicated risk factors included older age, cryptogenic cirrhosis, and Laënnec's cirrhosis.[6] Other authors have additionally implicated male sex, Child-Pugh class C liver disease, autoimmune hepatitis, hypercoagulable state, hepatocellular carcinoma, prior splenectomy, and prior portosystemic shunting.[15,16] In our experience at the University of Pennsylvania, the incidence of PVT was 39 of 422 recipients (9%) for the period 1996 through 2000, which is similar to other contemporary and older reports (Table 49–1). There was evidence in our series that the incidence of PVT increased over the time course of the study, and this increase was paralleled by longer waiting times to transplantation. With the implementation of the Model for End-stage Liver Disease (MELD) scoring system in the United States for assigning deceased donor allografts, it remains to be seen whether the incidence of PVT at the time of transplantation will change.

Preoperative knowledge of portal vein disease is imperative and greatly facilitates operative strategy. As part of the evaluation process, most candidates for liver transplantation undergo color-flow Doppler ultrasonography to assess vascular patency or the presence of partial or complete PVT, or both. This modality is sensitive and specific, even in the setting of prior shunt surgery.[3,9] If PVT is suspected, patients should undergo further imaging with magnetic resonance (MR) angiography or helical computed tomography (CT) to confirm the finding and to delineate the anatomical extent of PVT. This further cross-sectional imaging also serves to screen the patient for hepatocellular carcinoma. Both modalities are extremely accurate in the detection of venous anomalies, and complex three-dimensional reconstructions of the portal venous system are possible with either MR angiography or CT.[13,17-19] Published studies demonstrate equivalent or superior results of both MR and CT angiography as compared with digital subtraction angiography for imaging the portal venous system.[20,21] The choice between MR angiography and CT depends largely on local radiological expertise, as well as the requirement for iodinated contrast for CT imaging that often limits its utility in patients with concomitant renal insufficiency. In addition, MR angiography may have a distinct advantage over CT in identifying and characterizing liver masses, if present. For these reasons, MR angiography is the preferred imaging modality for our patients undergoing liver transplantation evaluation. There is the occasional patient with PVT in whom adequate imaging of the portal system cannot be obtained with noninvasive modalities, and a selective visceral arteriogram with portal phase venography is needed to map the portal venous system adequately. With current noninvasive imaging technology, this situation is extremely rare.

Table 49–1. INCIDENCE AND MANAGEMENT OF PORTAL VEIN THROMBOSIS IN REPRESENTATIVE LIVER TRANSPLANTATION SERIES

Center, Year, and Reference	Incidence of Portal Vein Thrombosis	Thrombectomy or Other Method (n)	Venous Conduit (n)
Pittsburgh 1991[2]	34/1585 (2.1%)	18	14
Nebraska 1992[11]	16/495 (3.2%)	12	4
UCLA 1996[5]	70/1423 (4.9%)	61	9
Birmingham, UK 2000[9]	63/779 (8.1%)	57	6
Valencia, Spain 2001[10]	62/391 (16%)	62	0
Pittsburgh 2001[13]	39/379 (10%)	23	12
University of Pennsylvania 2001 (unpublished data)	39/422 (9%)	39	0
Lyon, France 2002[14]	38/468 (8.1%)	38	0
Dallas 2002[6]	85/1546 (5.5%)	85	0

*Figures represent number of patients with PVT/total number of patients undergoing transplantation (percent of total with PVT).
UCLA, University of California at Los Angeles.

Operative Strategy

The presence and extent of PVT should be determined before OLT whenever possible. Preoperative studies may demonstrate partial thrombosis, a simple segmental thrombus amenable to thrombectomy, cavernous transformation of the portal vein, or complete portosplenomesenteric venous thrombosis. Knowledge of PVT preoperatively can help with the selection of an appropriate deceased donor organ and in obtaining appropriate venous conduits at the time of procurement, especially if pancreas and small intestine teams are also in need of additional vessels. The anesthesiologist and transfusion services should also be alerted that blood loss could be greater than normal so that appropriate lines are placed and enough blood is available. In addition, the most experienced members of the surgical team can be notified so that they are present for the critical portions of the operation. Advanced planning is especially useful if preoperative studies demonstrate the thrombus to extend beyond the confluence of the SMV and splenic vein. This information can save considerable operative time and blood loss at the time of transplantation by avoiding prolonged attempts at portal vein thrombectomy and proximal dissection. Instead, other strategies to obtain portal inflow can be attempted, as discussed subsequently.

The status of the portal vein and the extent of thrombosis are determined during dissection of the porta hepatis. Careful dissection of the portal vein proximally toward the splenomesenteric venous junction may reveal a soft vessel with a patent lumen behind the head of the pancreas. Prior to any attempts to restore blood flow in the portal vein, complete control of inflow and outflow should be obtained. Inflow control is usually manual with a hand or forceps, whereas outflow control is achieved by ligation of the distal portal vein high in the hilum of the liver, ideally above the bifurcation of the left and right portal veins. If only fresh thrombus is present, a thrombectomy of the portal vein should be attempted carefully by inserting large Fogarty balloon catheters through a transverse incision in the portal vein. However, if organized thrombus is encountered, thrombendvenectomy is required to restore portal venous blood flow.

Several techniques for thrombendvenectomy have been described. Our method is to first secure the edges of the portal vein using stay sutures (e.g., 5–0 Prolene) or fine-tip clamps. The thrombectomy is then performed using a carotid endarterectomy spatula to separate the thrombus from the vessel wall while simultaneously everting the vessel. The thrombus can be clamped with a tonsil clamp and carefully manipulated with gentle but firm traction while it is separated from the vessel wall. Consecutive tonsil clamps are placed as the thrombus is gently freed toward the splenomesenteric junction and carefully pulled out once it is completely dislodged from the wall of the portal vein (Fig. 49–1A).[5,14] An alternative method involves clamping the thrombus with a tonsil clamp and rotating it while simultaneously pushing it toward the splenomesenteric junction and then pulling out the thrombus once it is free from the vein wall (see Fig. 49–1B).[6] With either method, the distal tip of the thrombus should have a feathered edge, and brisk blood flow should be seen from the portal vein. If brisk flow is not observed, a thrombectomy catheter is inserted carefully and swept along the vein to identify more distant thrombus or narrowing. After a straightforward thrombectomy, a portal bypass cannula usually can be inserted if venovenous bypass is being used. However, following thrombendvenectomy the portal vein is sometimes thin and fragile and the use of a portal cannula is not possible.[6] Because these patients usually have extensive collaterals as a result of PVT, they will often be able to tolerate systemic bypass only (if vena cava clamping is planned). If decompression of the portal system is required and the portal vein cannot be used, the inferior mesenteric vein can be cannulated for bypass and the transplant procedure can then proceed.[5] In instances following thrombectomy in which portal hypertension is problematic and the use of venous bypass is not planned, some surgeons create a temporary portocaval shunt that is dismantled prior to performing the portal anastomosis.

When thrombosis extends a significant distance beyond the splenomesenteric venous junction, the approach just described may not be sufficient. These cases will require a venous conduit between the SMV and the donor portal vein, which is accomplished using donor iliac vein or vena cava. Use of venous conduits, which was first described by Shaw and colleagues,[7] avoids extensive dissection of the proximal portal vein, which can be extremely difficult and hazardous, causing pancreatic trauma and excessive bleeding.[5] When a venous graft is found to be necessary, a portion of the SMV below the transverse mesocolon and to the right of the superior mesenteric artery at the root of the small bowel mesentery is exposed. A segment of SMV approximately 3 to 4 cm long is isolated where the vessel is found to be soft and patent, which may require a fairly distal dissection in mesentery that can be quite thickened. This segment of SMV is then occluded with a gentle side-biting vascular clamp, and a previously prepared vein graft is anastomosed to the SMV in a sharply angled end-to-side fashion (Fig. 49–2).[11,22-24] The degree of angulation is important in order to avoid kinking of the graft, and this angle will depend somewhat on the thickness of the mesentery overlying the SMV. The vein graft is then brought through a tunnel in the transverse mesocolon. Although the literature describes a course anterior to the pancreas and behind the distal antrum and pylorus, this is often extremely difficult and hazardous in patients with portal hypertension. We now

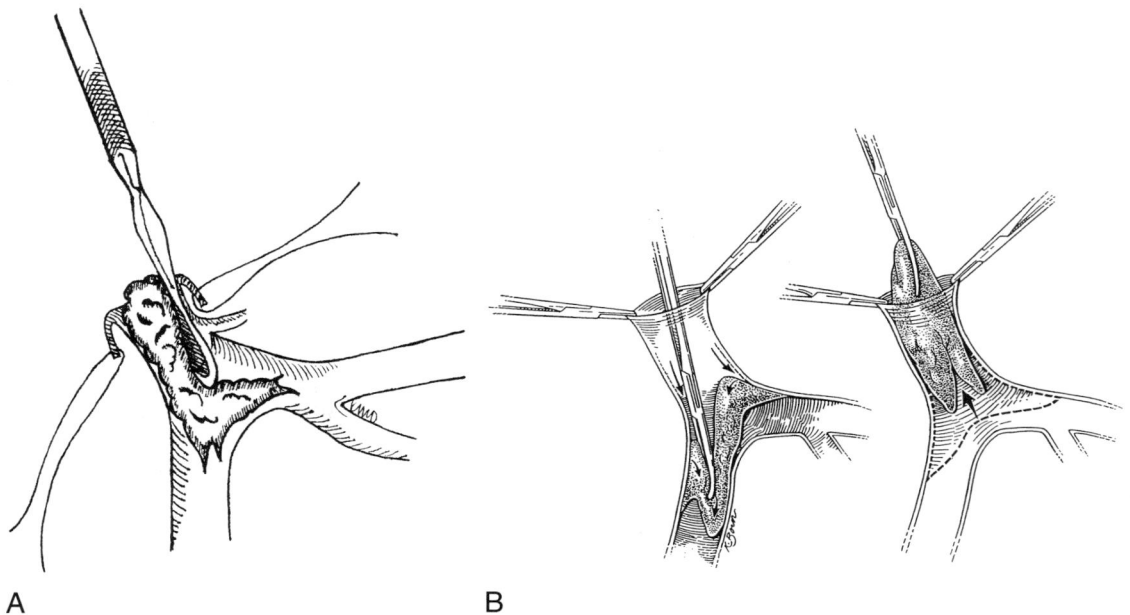

A   B

FIGURE 49-1

Approaches for portal vein thrombendvenectomy. **A,** Eversion thrombectomy of portal vein thrombus using endarterectomy technique. **B,** An alternative method in which the clot is dislodged by pushing it into the vein with a circular maneuver and after the clot is dislodged by this circular and inward motion, it is pulled out. (**A,** From Stieber AC, Zetti G, Todo S, et al: The spectrum of portal vein thrombosis in liver transplantation. Ann Surg 213:199-206, 1991, Figure 6. **B,** From Molmenti EP, Roodhouse TW, Molmenti H, et al: Thrombendvenectomy for organized portal vein thrombosis at the time of liver transplantation. Ann Surg 235:292-296, 2002.)

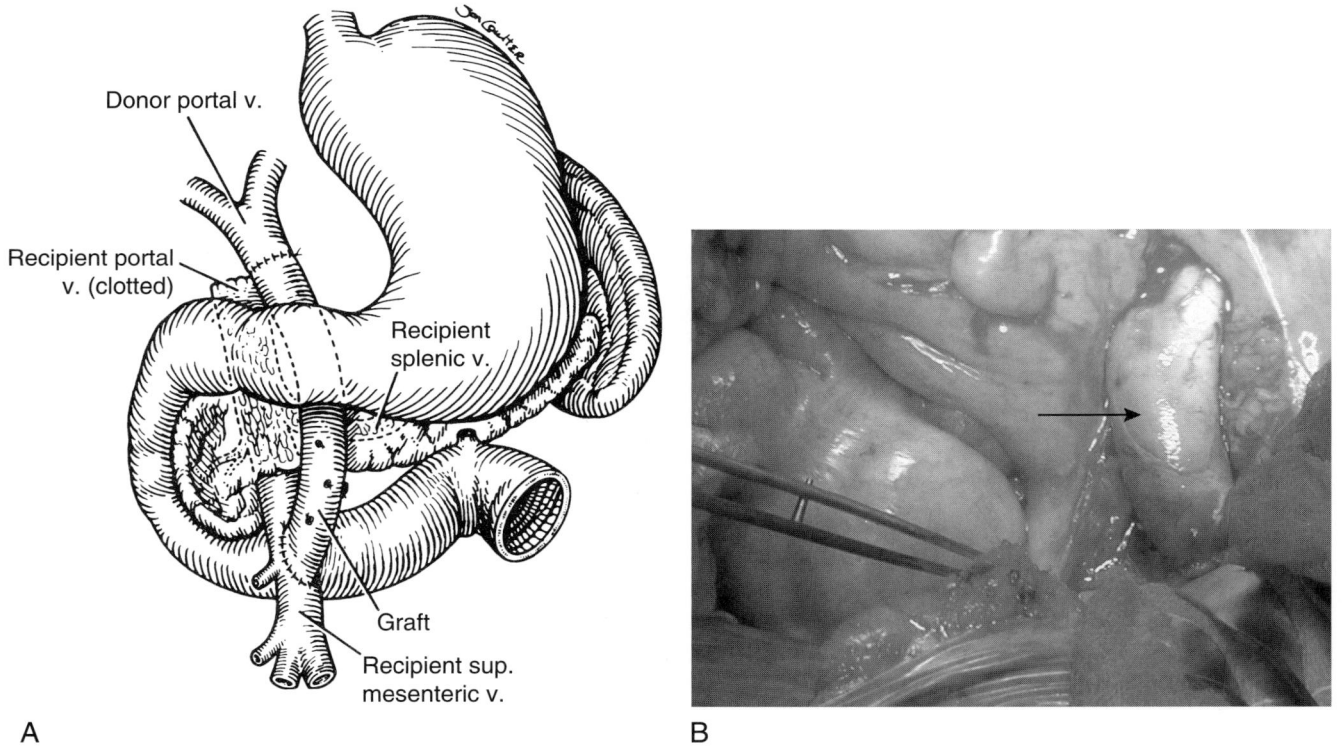

A   B

FIGURE 49-2

A, Schematic of a venous conduit from the infrapancreatic SMV to the donor portal vein via a retropyloric course. **B,** Intraoperative photograph of an iliac vein graft (*arrow*) from SMV to portal vein, illustrating the retrocolic and antepyloric approach we now use. (**A,** From Stieber AC, Zetti G, Todo S, et al: The spectrum of portal vein thrombosis in liver transplantation. Ann Surg 213:199-206, 1991, Figure 12.)

bring the graft in a retrocolic antepyloric position, still allowing a gentle curve of the graft, and a much safer approach. Retropancreatic position of the vein graft has also been reported.[24,25]

Even in the rare instance in which diffuse thrombosis of the entire portal system is present, revascularization of the liver allograft can be accomplished. The initial solution proposed for this complex, but extremely rare, problem was the use of a large coronary vein, collateral vein, or gastroepiploic vein for portal inflow in either an end-to-end or end-to-side fashion. Great caution should be used when controlling and suturing these alternative inflow vessels because they are extremely thin-walled and can tear easily.[2,11,15] In complex pediatric retransplantation cases with extensive portal thrombosis, the mesentery of the Roux-en-Y limb from the previous transplant may contain a large collateral vein that can be used for portal inflow. Alternatively, a large collateral vein in the small intestine mesentery can provide portal inflow.

An alternative approach to complete portosplenomesenteric venous occlusion has been the use of cavoportal hemitransposition, a technique in which the IVC is used for portal inflow to the allograft. Starzl and colleagues extensively studied complete cavoportal transposition in dogs to determine the effect of systemic venous inflow on liver function and histology and found that liver function and histology remained normal when systemic venous blood was used as portal inflow into the liver.[26] The use of this technique in clinical liver transplantation was originally reported by four centers in nine patients[8]; since then several other groups have also reported their experience.[27-31] Cavoportal hemitransposition entails performing an anastomosis between the allograft portal vein and the suprarenal recipient IVC in an end-to-side or end-to-end manner (Fig. 49–3). When the portal vein will not easily reach the IVC, an interposition vein graft is necessary. Blood flow through the IVC is diverted toward the new liver by either ligating the IVC with a clip or by formally dividing it, thus creating a functional end-to-end anastomosis. One caveat to this procedure is the persistence of portal hypertension and the ongoing risk of bleeding from gastroesophageal varices and hypertensive gastropathy, which occurred in 37% of reported cases.[31] These bleeding problems have been treated by splenectomy, gastric devascularization, splenic artery embolization, or endoscopic intervention. This high rate of posttransplant bleeding has caused some to advocate routine splenectomy and gastric devascularization when cavoportal hemitransposition is performed,[8,29] although this is certainly debatable. In addition, persistent ascites and lower extremity edema can result after this procedure; however, these problems improve with time and are treated by avoiding fluid overload and the judicious use of diuretic therapy until resolution occurs.[29]

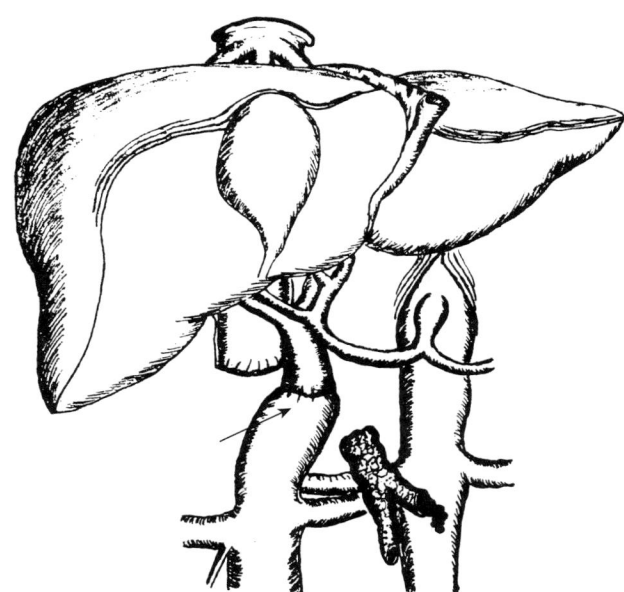

FIGURE 49–3

Cavoportal hemitransposition for complete portosplenomesenteric venous occlusion. The suprarenal vena cava is interrupted and an anastomosis is performed between the inferior vena cava and the donor portal vein (*arrow*) in an end-to-end fashion. (From Tzakis AG, Kirkegaard P, Pinna AD, et al: Liver transplantation with cavoportal hemitransposition in the presence of diffuse portal vein thrombosis. Transplantation 65:619-624, 1998.)

Outcomes in Recipients with Portal Vein Thrombosis

The results in recipients undergoing liver transplantation with PVT were initially reported to be worse than the outcomes in other patients. Early series reported patient survival rates between 57% and 81%, usually with less than 1 year of follow-up.[2,3,11,15] Nonetheless, two large reports that are more recent indicate improved outcomes in recipients with PVT. In 1423 patients at the University of California at Los Angeles, 70 patients (4.9%) were found to have PVT. One-year actuarial patient survival was only 66% in the first 35 of these recipients (versus 82% in contemporaneous controls); however, the 1-year survival in the second group of 35 recipients with PVT increased to 82% (versus 85% in controls).[5] In another large series of 1546 liver recipients at Baylor University Medical Center in Dallas, 85 patients (5.5%) had PVT and these patients had identical 1-year graft (80%) and patient (85%) survival rates as controls. Of additional importance was the finding that patient survival at 3 and 6 years following transplantation was nearly identical between recipients with and without PVT.[6] These excellent results have not been universal, with other centers reporting significantly worse outcomes in recipients with PVT, especially in those with extension into the splanchnic veins. Certainly outcomes in recipients with PVT have dramatically improved compared with the early experience in liver transplantation when PVT was considered a contraindication to transplantation.[1] The question of whether PVT is an independent risk factor for worse patient outcome should be answered as more data are acquired.

The morbidity of liver transplantation in the setting of PVT has also been examined. Several studies demonstrate a higher transfusion requirement and a higher incidence of renal failure and graft nonfunction in patients with PVT.[2,3,5,9,10,15] In recipients in whom cavoportal hemitransposition has been performed, the outcomes are worse when compared with those in non-PVT recipients.[8,29,31] The mortality rate has exceeded 30%, the portal vein patency rate is only 65%, and there is very high morbidity as a result of persistent portal hypertension, as mentioned previously. Of course the individuals who have required this procedure have complete portosplenomesenteric venous occlusion and are not comparable to recipients with less extensive PVT that is amenable to thrombendvenectomy or a venous conduit procedure.

Studies demonstrate that the technical complexities of PVT can be overcome with generally excellent results. There are increased risks associated with transplantation in these patients that should be understood by the surgical team. Steps to decrease complications include detailed knowledge of the degree of thrombosis preoperatively to assist with operative planning, minimization of risk factors associated with poor graft function such as cold ischemia time and the use of a marginal donor, and the availability of suitable venous conduits in case they are necessary. Attention to detail, knowledge of the various options available, and flexibility at the time of OLT are mandatory to obtain favorable results.

Portal Vein Thrombosis After Transplantation

The patency of the portal vein is of concern following transplantation in the setting of PVT. Early studies demonstrated a lower rate of postoperative portal vein patency in PVT patients,[9,15] but the reported patency rates in more recent studies has been between 95% and 100%.[5,6] Strategies have been proposed to monitor for and to help prevent recurrent PVT following transplantation. Most centers will use color-flow Doppler ultrasonography to monitor the patency of the portal vein in recipients with PVT on the day following surgery and at varying intervals thereafter. These recipients are also often treated with a continuous infusion of low-molecular-weight dextran (20 to 30 mL per hour in adults) as an antiplatelet agent to prevent recurrent PVT.

When appropriate, a daily 81-mg aspirin is substituted for the dextran for 3 months postoperatively.[6] Of course the use of any anticoagulation in the immediate posttransplant period should be done cautiously with close monitoring of the recipient because the patient is often naturally anticoagulated and thrombocytopenic for a short time after transplantation.

Early posttransplant PVT can present with liver failure, ascites, intestinal congestion, and gastrointestinal bleeding.[25] Mortality is extremely high in this group of patients. Although immediate operative thrombectomy can allow for successful salvage of the liver allograft,[15] patients may require emergent retransplantation.[25] Early PVT can also be approached by interventional methods, either by percutaneous or transjugular approaches to the portal venous system and the use of thrombolysis, mechanical fragmentation, systemic anticoagulation, and stenting. These techniques have been used successfully in recipients who developed PVT between 2 and 4 weeks after transplantation when operative revision would be difficult.[32-34] Patients who develop late recurrent PVT generally present with preserved liver function and have been managed more conservatively with anticoagulation therapy. This group of patients may develop complications of portal hypertension. Consideration should be made for performing a distal splenorenal shunt (or other portosystemic shunt) in patients with late PVT and preserved hepatic function but refractory portal hypertension.

Postoperative portal vein complications can be particularly problematic in pediatric recipients weighing less than 10 kg undergoing OLT. The incidence of posttransplant PVT has been between 1% and 14.7% in large pediatric liver transplant series, with this problem being especially prevalent in infants and children with biliary atresia.[35-38] The increased incidence of thrombosis in biliary atresia is likely multifactorial, with small recipient size, prior Kasai surgery, and native portal vein atresia all being contributing factors.[36] The outcome in pediatric recipients who develop PVT after transplantation is poor despite aggressive attempts at allograft salvage. Preventive strategies with anticoagulation are used by many groups and include the use of aspirin, low-molecular-weight dextran, dipyridamole, and heparin.[35-38]

Prior Portosystemic Shunts

Surgical Shunts

The two major types of open operative procedures intended for decompression of portal hypertension are nonselective and selective surgical shunts. The nonselective category includes the portocaval and mesocaval shunts, whereas the distal splenorenal shunt is the main type of selective shunt that is performed.

Each shunt has its own advantages and disadvantages in terms of efficacy of portal decompression and subsequent liver transplantation. The portal vein may become small and sclerotic after operative shunting; thus, preoperative imaging to determine patency and size is extremely important to help operative planning.[3] Shunt patency should also be evaluated because an open, nonselective shunt can be maintained during the operative procedure for portal decompression, thus avoiding the need for portal venous bypass or a temporary portocaval shunt.

The portocaval shunt is almost always successful in controlling bleeding from portal hypertension and has a low rate of thrombosis. However, this shunt requires extensive dissection within the liver hilus, thus making subsequent liver transplantation more difficult.[3,39,40] Both end-to-side and side-to-side portocaval shunts require dismantling during the transplant procedure and greatly increase the complexity of the portal anastomosis. To facilitate dismantling of the shunt, control of the IVC and the portal vein should be obtained both above and below the level of the shunt before removal of the explant. During the anhepatic phase, the shunt provides decompression of the portal system through the vena cava, allowing for an IVC cannula alone if venovenous bypass is used. The remainder of the hepatectomy and the suprahepatic IVC anastomosis are completed with the shunt intact. At this point the portal vein is occluded proximally and a vascular clamp is used to occlude the IVC side of the shunt. The shunt is then sharply dismantled, the involved portion of the distal portal vein is transected, and the IVC is repaired using a lateral venorrhaphy, thus preserving adequate length and width of the IVC. The infrahepatic IVC (for a bicaval anastomosis) and portal anastomoses are then performed in the usual fashion. The portal anastomosis may require a venous extension graft if a significant length of portal vein is lost following shunt ligation. If inadequate donor portal vein length is anticipated, a donor iliac vein extension graft can be sewn to the donor portal vein during back table preparation, thus reducing liver warm ischemia time.[39]

The mesocaval shunt, another nonselective shunt, has the advantage in potential transplant recipients of avoiding adhesions in the porta hepatis because the field of dissection is inferior to the transverse colon. Thus the technical difficulty of performing a liver transplantation in a patient with a prior mesocaval shunt is not as high. The shunt can be used for portal decompression during the transplant procedure, and the graft requires simple ligation after reperfusion of the new liver.[39,40]

Selective shunts, of which the distal splenorenal shunt is most common, are often performed in well-compensated cirrhotic patients who have intractable variceal bleeding. Again, the porta hepatis is not disturbed during this operation and subsequent transplantation

is simpler than in patients with a prior portocaval shunt.[39,40] The distal splenorenal shunt usually does not require ligation at the end of the transplant operation unless portal flow to the new liver is deemed inadequate by Doppler flow probes (usually less than 1 L per minute).[39] If the shunt requires dismantling, a splenectomy is typically performed and the shunt ligated. When a splenorenal shunt is large and the majority of portal blood travels through the shunt, an alternative method of portal reconstruction is to use the left renal vein as the source of portal inflow to the liver allograft. The left renal vein is disconnected from the vena cava and an end-to-end anastomosis between the portal vein and the left renal vein is performed.[27,41]

In terms of outcomes, early reports of liver transplantation in patients who had undergone prior surgical shunt procedures demonstrated that patients with portocaval shunts had higher intraoperative blood loss, increased incidence of primary nonfunction, and longer hospitalization.[3,39] In another series, the overall survival of patients with prior portocaval shunts was 52% at 9 years as compared with 87% at 9 years in patients who had undergone mesocaval or distal splenorenal shunts.[40]

The number of liver transplant recipients with a prior surgical shunt has declined over time as a result of the increased use of the transjugular intrahepatic portosystemic shunt (TIPS). Several groups have directly compared surgical shunting to TIPS for patients with variceal bleeding caused by portal hypertension. In Child-Pugh class A and B patients, studies demonstrate a higher patency rate, better control of refractory bleeding, and a lower overall mortality rate for surgical shunts than for TIPS.[42,43] Surprisingly, very few of the patients who underwent a surgical shunt procedure eventually required transplantation. Although these authors do not advocate surgical shunts in patients with advanced cirrhosis who are awaiting liver transplantation, they do favor surgical shunts for cirrhotic patients with well-preserved liver function.[42,43] Further studies correlating the MELD score of patients undergoing surgical shunting with outcomes may help to discern which patients are good shunt candidates versus those who are likely to need a liver transplant.

Transjugular Intrahepatic Portosystemic Shunts

Several studies have examined the impact of prior TIPS on liver transplantation, both in terms of operative parameters and of patient outcomes.[44-48] Some studies suggest that TIPS may serve as a safe bridge to transplantation, stabilizing a potential liver recipient and allowing him or her to undergo the transplant procedure at a lower level of acuity.[46,47] In addition, some authors suggest that TIPS would facilitate the transplant procedure by reducing the amount of bleeding caused by portal hypertension.[44] Although TIPS does facilitate the management of patients awaiting liver transplantation, especially in terms of ascites management and control of variceal bleeding,[44] well-controlled studies do not support the use of TIPS for facilitating the transplant procedure itself.[48,49] The largest of these studies was an analysis of a multicenter liver transplant database that did not demonstrate a reduction in operative time, transfusion requirement, or outcome in patients with prior TIPS as compared with controls.[49]

Transplantation in the setting of a prior TIPS can be complex as a consequence of migration or placement of the shunt outside the liver in either the cephalad or caudad direction. These situations, although infrequent, can result in unforeseen technical challenges. One situation encountered is placement or migration of the stent too far caudad in the portal vein. This problem requires complete removal of the stent from the recipient portal vein and may require clamping below the stent and transection across the stent, followed by careful extraction of the remaining stent.[46,50,51] If stent removal cannot be performed safely, a venous extension graft to the SMV should be considered.[50,51] Cephalad placement or migration of TIPS is potentially a more complicated problem and it is discussed later.

Anomalies of the Inferior Vena Cava

Preexisting Vena Cava Anomalies

Liver recipients may have preexisting abnormalities of the IVC, but these anomalies are rare and generally do not preclude liver transplantation. They are divided into those seen in adults and those seen in children. The major preexisting IVC anomaly seen in adults is that of hepatic venous thrombosis and IVC compression or thrombosis in patients with Budd-Chiari syndrome.[25] This condition and the operative strategies used during OLT are discussed elsewhere in this book. In addition, the increasing use of TIPS in adults awaiting transplantation has led to instances in which the stent crosses into the IVC, either because of technical issues at the time of TIPS placement or because of stent migration. Attempting to fully remove the TIPS is recommended and usually possible with careful dissection and clamping techniques. Removal may require dissection onto the SMV and splenic veins, or dissection along the suprahepatic IVC into the pericardium. However, incorporation of the TIPS into the vessel wall or extension of the TIPS beyond the suprahepatic IVC

clamp may prevent complete removal in rare cases. In these instances, alternative approaches have been described, such as performing the suprahepatic IVC anastomosis within the pericardial space, open cardiotomy for complete removal of the TIPS,[52] or transecting the TIPS and incorporating the stent containing vessel wall into the suprahepatic IVC anastomosis.[53] In addition, one group has described the use of interventional radiology techniques to retrieve a newly placed TIPS extension that migrated into the left pulmonary artery during the liver transplant procedure.[54]

IVC anomalies are more common in the pediatric population and are usually congenital and associated with biliary atresia. These anomalies include absence of the retrohepatic IVC, interrupted retrohepatic IVC, direct drainage of the hepatic veins into the right atrium or the azygous system, and direct drainage of innominate veins into the IVC.[25,55] These anomalies may be known preoperatively from imaging studies or discovered intraoperatively. The reported incidence of IVC anomalies has been between 3.7% and 8.5% of pediatric liver transplant patients, with most cases occurring in children with biliary atresia. Transplantation in these challenging recipients is possible, with an important principle being to achieve low-resistance venous drainage for the liver allograft. In most instances in which the IVC is abnormal, anastomosis can be performed between the donor suprahepatic IVC (or the hepatic vein) and the common orifice (cloaca) of the hepatic veins in the recipient. However, in some rare instances, a direct anastomosis of the liver to the right atrium may be necessary in order to achieve adequate venous drainage of the graft.

Variations in Vena Cava Reconstruction

The original description of the vena cava reconstruction for OLT was the bicaval anastomosis in which the recipient IVC is resected and replaced by that of the allograft, thus requiring both a suprahepatic and infrahepatic IVC anastomosis.[49] The major variant to this is the "piggyback" technique, in which the recipient IVC is preserved and a single anastomosis is performed between the allograft suprahepatic IVC and the confluence of the recipient hepatic veins.[56] The relative merits of each procedure have been greatly debated and are discussed elsewhere in this book. Alternatives to these two predominant techniques have been described and are important to know for cases in which vena cava problems are encountered during the transplant procedure.

A method using a side-to-side cavocaval anastomosis for OLT has been reported by several European groups with excellent results. The Brussels group advocates the cavocaval anastomosis as their preferred method of IVC anastomosis, and they have been able to use this technique in 98% of primary OLT cases and 90% of retransplantation cases.[57] This technique is generally useful in vena cava–preserving OLT when either the cuff of recipient hepatic veins is inadequate (too short or too friable) to be used for a "piggyback" anastomosis[58] or when the recipient vena cava is significantly narrowed during the course of the hepatectomy procedure.

An additional technique of IVC anastomosis has been the use of an infrahepatic vena cavocavostomy. This technique has been useful in "piggyback" OLT for rare instances when the venous outflow of the liver allograft is obstructed following reperfusion and graft congestion and swelling occur. A second anastomosis using an infrahepatic vena cavocavostomy technique can be performed to provide additional allograft venous outflow with resulting decompression of the liver.[59,60]

Although transplantation surgeons rarely use these techniques, knowledge of these alternatives is worthwhile when dealing with difficult situations involving the vena cava during OLT. Retransplantation is one situation in which alternative techniques to the bicaval anastomosis are especially useful. In this setting, knowledge of the type of IVC reconstruction used for the first transplant is important and the surgeon can save a great deal of operative time and blood loss if previous planes of dissection are known. Using an alternative method of vena cava reconstruction may simplify the complexity of the procedure.

Vena Cava Anomalies After Transplantation

Significant stenosis or thrombosis of the IVC after OLT is a rare phenomenon, mostly a result of the large caliber of this vessel; however, complications such as compression, kinking, or twisting of the IVC do occasionally occur and can lead to significant pathologic conditions.[25,53,55,61] Diagnosis of IVC stenosis can be difficult because signs or symptoms associated with IVC disease are often attributed to other causes. Suprahepatic IVC stenosis can present with hepatomegaly, liver dysfunction, ascites, edema, and centrilobular congestion on biopsy, whereas infrahepatic IVC disease (in recipients in whom a bicaval anastomosis is performed) can present with ascites, hematuria, renal failure, and lower body edema. Doppler ultrasonography is a good screening tool for postoperative vena cava problems. If there is suspicion of vena cava abnormalities by ultrasonography, findings should be confirmed by contrast venography,

which also provides an opportunity for intervention and correction.

A review from the University of Pittsburgh found the incidence of significant postoperative IVC disease to be very low. Twelve of 2379 recipients (0.5%) had a vena cava anomaly after OLT, with 11 patients found to have moderate or severe IVC stenosis and only 1 patient found to have IVC thrombosis.[61] In this series, Doppler ultrasonography was 100% sensitive for infrahepatic IVC stenosis and 50% sensitive for suprahepatic IVC stenosis. Contrast venography was used to confirm ultrasonographic findings in all of these patients. Of note, the threshold for a clinically significant anastomotic stenosis was a pressure gradient of 8 cm of water or greater. The approach used by these authors was to observe mild or moderate infrahepatic IVC stenosis and to revise severe infrahepatic IVC stenosis operatively. For instances of severe suprahepatic IVC stenosis, the authors advocated treatment with either multiple sessions of balloon angioplasty until the pressure gradient fell to less than 8 cm of water or operative revision, recognizing that this procedure can be difficult and may require direct anastomosis of the suprahepatic vena cava to the right atrium.[61] With the advances in interventional techniques since the publication of this series, we believe that almost all instances of both infrahepatic and suprahepatic caval stenosis can be managed initially by angioplasty and possible stenting (Fig. 49–4). A follow-up venogram should be obtained in 4 to 6 weeks to ensure that restenosis has not occurred. Operative revisions should be reserved for cases in which interventional techniques have failed or for cases in which a technical complication that can be corrected has been identified early after OLT.

Summary

Anomalies of the venous system in liver transplantation are relatively infrequent; however, they represent an important challenge for the transplantation surgeon and can still be associated with significant morbidity and mortality if the surgeon is not prepared with an operative plan and technical armamentarium. In the past, many of these findings were considered a contraindication to performing liver transplantation. However, technical expertise, accumulation of experience, and creative use of various options for both portal vein and IVC reconstruction have allowed excellent results. There are several important points and caveats, which are listed under "Pearls and Pitfalls." When patients with venous anomalies are approached with the knowledge discussed there, virtually every recipient can undergo successful liver transplantation with acceptable morbidity and mortality risks.

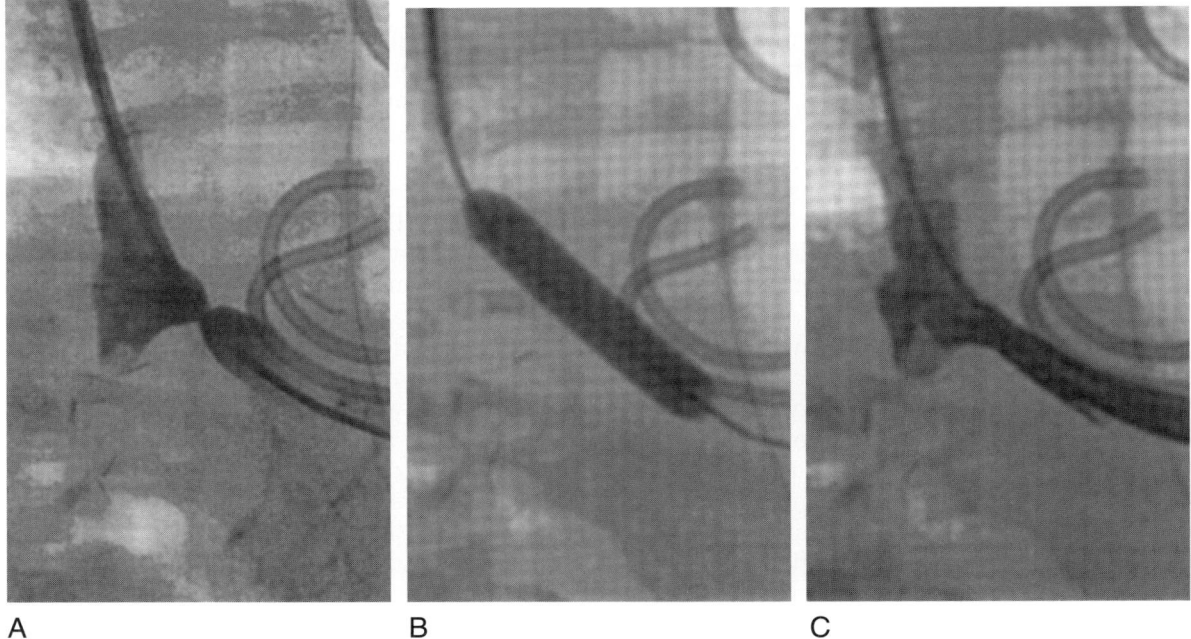

A   B   C

FIGURE 49–4

A, Venogram of hepatic venous outflow obstruction. Venogram demonstrates a stenosis at the hepatic vein anastomosis in a partial liver graft recipient. **B,** Balloon angioplasty of the lesion is performed with resolution of the stenosis (**C**).

Pearls and Pitfalls

- With careful planning, meticulous technique, and creative thinking, a vein can almost always be found for inflow and outflow of a new liver graft.

- In patients with known portal venous thrombosis, preoperative imaging using advanced three-dimensional reconstruction techniques (CT, MR angiography) can be extremely helpful in providing a roadmap of highest detail. Occasionally, venography may add further information that cannot be ascertained from noninvasive studies.

- Advanced planning by the transplant surgical team as a group (e.g., at an imaging conference) can help avoid uncertainty and delay during the operative procedure. This advanced preparation allows for the development of a best approach to the identified venous anomaly as well as a back-up plan.

- Having two experienced surgeons and a well-prepared anesthesiologist available during these

Pearls and Pitfalls—cont'd

cases can decrease blood loss and operative time and can limit complications.

- The availability of donor venous conduits is essential; however, if these are not available, the recipient's internal jugular vein is a possible alternative.

- Despite thorough imaging, unexpected portal vein thrombosis may be encountered. This situation should be suspected when the dissection in the porta hepatis is bloodier than normal and extensive collateralization is present. Identifying unknown thrombosis early during the hepatectomy allows additional time for the anesthesia and blood bank teams to prepare and also allows time to call for additional experienced assistance if necessary.

- Flexibility and a working knowledge of the reconstruction options available are perhaps the most important caveats, especially when an unexpected venous anomaly is encountered during the transplant procedure.

References

1. Van Thiel DH, Schade R, Starzl TE, et al: Liver transplantation in adults. Hepatology ...7-640, 1982.
2. Stieber AC, Zetti G, ...S, et al: The spectrum of portal vein thrombosis in liver ...plantation. Ann Surg 213:199-206, 1991.
3. Shaked A, Busu... W: Liver transplantation in patients with portal vein thro... and central portacaval shunts. Ann Surg 214:696-702, ...
4. Busuttil RW... d A, Millis JM, et al: One thousand liver transplants: ...ns learned. Ann Surg 219:490-499, 1994.
5. Seu P, ...n CR, Shaked A, et al: Improved results of liver transp... in patients with portal vein thrombosis. Arch Sur... 845, 1996.
6. M...P, Roodhouse TW, Molmenti H, et al: Thrombend...Sur...for organized portal vein thrombosis at the time of ...splantation. Ann Surg 235:292-296, 2002.
7. ...W, Iwatsuki S, Bron K, Starzl TE: Portal vein grafts in ... transplantation. Surg Gynecol Obstet 161:66-68, 1985.
8. ...s AG, Kirkegaard P, Pinna AD, et al: Liver transplantation ... cavoportal hemitransposition in the presence of diffuse por... vein thrombosis. Transplantation 65:619-624, 1998.
9. ...erdel MA, Gunson B, Mirza D, et al: Portal vein thrombosis in adults undergoing liver transplantation: Risk factors, screening, management, and outcome. Transplantation 69:1873-1881, 2000.
10. Manzanet G, Sanjuan F, Orbis P, et al: Liver transplantation in patients with portal vein thrombosis. Liver Transpl 7:125-131, 2001.
11. Langnas AN, Marujo WC, Stratta RJ, et al: A selective approach to preexisting portal vein thrombosis in patients undergoing liver transplantation. Am J Surg 163:132-136, 1992.
12. Gayowski TJ, Marino IR, Doyle HR, et al: A high incidence of portal vein thrombosis in veterans undergoing liver transplantation. J Surg Res 60:333-338, 1996.
13. Brancatelli G, Federle MP, Pealer K, Geller DA: Portal venous thrombosis or sclerosis in liver transplantation candidates: Preoperative CT findings and correlation with surgical procedure. Radiology 220:321-328, 2001.
14. Dumortier J, Czyglik O, Poncet G, et al: Eversion thrombectomy for portal vein thrombosis during liver transplantation. Am J Transplant 2:934-938, 2002.
15. Davidson BR, Gibson M, Dick R, et al: Incidence, risk factors, management, and outcome of portal vein abnormalities at orthotopic liver transplantation. Transplantation 57:1174-1177, 1994.
16. Sobhonslidsuk A, Reddy KR: Portal vein thrombosis: A concise review. Am J Gastroenterol 97:535-541, 2002.
17. Ward J, Spencer JA, Guthrie JA, Robinson PJ: Liver transplantation: Dynamic contrast-enhanced magnetic resonance imaging of the hepatic vasculature. Clin Radiol 51:191-197, 1996.
18. Smith PA, Klein AS, Heath DG, et al: Dual-phase spiral CT angiography with volumetric 3D rendering for preoperative liver transplant evaluation: Preliminary observations. J Comput Assist Tomogr 22:868-874, 1998.
19. Eubank WB, Wherry KL, Maki JH, et al: Preoperative evaluation of patients awaiting liver transplantation: Comparison of multiphasic contrast-enhanced 3D magnetic resonance to helical computed tomography examinations. J Magn Reson Imaging 16:565-575, 2002.
20. Kopka L, Rodenwaldt J, Vosshenrich R, et al: Hepatic blood supply: Comparison of optimized dual phase contrast-enhanced three-dimensional MR angiography and digital subtraction angiography. Radiology 211:51-58, 1999.
21. Boeve WJ, Kok T, Haagsma EB, et al: Superior diagnostic strength of combined contrast enhanced MR-angiography and MR-imaging compared to intra-arterial DSA in liver transplantation candidates. Magn Reson Imaging 19:609-622, 2001.
22. Sheil AGR, Thompson JF, Stephen MS, et al: Meso-portal graft for thrombosed portal vein in liver transplantation. Clin Transplant 1:18-20, 1987.
23. Tzakis A, Todo S, Stieber A, Starzl TE: Venous jump grafts for liver transplantation in patients with portal vein thrombosis. Transplantation 48:530-531, 1989.
24. Kirsch JP, Howard TK, Klintmalm GB, et al: Problematic vascular reconstruction in liver transplantation. Part II. Portovenous conduits. Surgery 107:544-548, 1990.
25. Lerut J, Tzakis AG, Bron K, et al: Complications of venous reconstruction in human orthotopic liver transplantation. Ann Surg 205:404-414, 1987.
26. Meyer WH, Starzl TE: The reverse portacaval shunt. Surgery 45:531-534, 1959.
27. Azoulay D, Hargreaves GM, Castaing D, Bismuth H: Caval inflow to the graft: A successful way to overcome diffuse portal system thrombosis in liver transplantation. J Am Coll Surg 190:493-496, 2000.
28. Varma CR, Mistry BM, Glockner JF, et al: Cavoportal hemitransposition in liver transplantation. Transplantation 72:960-963, 2001.
29. Pinna AD, Nery J, Kato T, et al: Liver transplant with portocaval hemitransposition: Experience at the University of Miami. Transplant Proc 33:1329-1330, 2001.
30. Olausson M, Norrby J, Mjornstedt L, et al: Liver transplantation using cavoportal hemitransposition—a life-saving procedure in the presence of extensive portal vein thrombosis. Transplant Proc 33:1327-1328, 2001.
31. Gerunda GE, Merenda R, Neri D, et al: Cavoportal hemitransposition: A successful way to overcome the problem of total porto-splenomesenteric thrombosis in liver transplantation. Liver Transpl 8:72-75, 2002.
32. Cherukuri R, Haskal ZJ, Naji A, Shaked A: Percutaneous thrombolysis and stent placement for the treatment of portal vein thrombosis after liver transplantation: Long-term follow-up. Transplantation 65:1124-1126, 1998.
33. Ciccarelli O, Goffette P, Laterre PF, et al: Transjugular intrahepatic portosystemic shunt approach and local thrombolysis for treatment of early posttransplant portal vein thrombosis. Transplantation 72:159-161, 2001.
34. Baccarani U, Gasparini D, Risalti A, et al: Percutaneous mechanical fragmentation and stent placement for the treatment of early posttransplantation portal vein thrombosis. Transplantation 72:1572-1574, 2001.
35. Cacciarelli TV, Esquivel CO, Moore DH, et al: Factors affecting survival after orthotopic liver transplantation in infants. Transplantation 64:242-248, 1997.
36. Chardot C, Herrera JM, Debray D, et al: Portal vein complications after liver transplantation for biliary atresia. Liver Transpl Surg 3:351-358, 1997.
37. Goss JA, Shackleton CR, McDiarmid SV, et al: Long-term results of pediatric liver transplantation: An analysis of 569 transplants. Ann Surg 228:411-420, 1998.
38. Sieders E, Peeters PM, TenVergert EM, et al: Early vascular complications after pediatric liver transplantation. Liver Transpl 6:326-332, 2000.
39. Brems JJ, Hiat JR, Klien AS, et al: Effect of a prior portasystemic shunt on subsequent liver transplantation. Ann Surg 209:51-56, 1989.
40. Mazzaferro V, Todo S, Tzakis AG, et al: Liver transplantation in patients with previous portasystemic shunt. Am J Surg 160:111-116, 1990.
41. Kato T, Levi DM, DeFaria W, et al: Liver transplantation with renoportal anastomosis after distal splenorenal shunt. Arch Surg 135:1401-1404, 2000.
42. Henderson JM, Nagle A, Curtas S, et al: Surgical shunts and tips for variceal decompression in the 1990s. Surgery 128:540-547, 2000.

43. Rosemurgy AS, Serafini FM, Zweibel BR, et al: Transjugular intra-hepatic portosystemic shunt vs. small-diameter prosthetic H-graft portacaval shunt: Extended follow-up of an expanded random-ized prospective trial. J Gastrointest Surg 4:589-597, 2000.
44. Freeman RB Jr, FitzMaurice SE, Greenfield AE, et al: Is the trans-jugular intrahepatic portocaval shunt procedure beneficial for liver transplant recipients? Transplantation 58:297-300, 1994.
45. Somberg KA, Lombardero MS, Lawlor SM, et al: A controlled analysis of the transjugular intrahepatic portosystemic shunt in liver transplant recipients. Transplantation 63:1074-1079, 1997.
46. Chui AKK, Rao ARN, Waugh RC, et al: Liver transplantation in patients with transjugular intrahepatic portosystemic shunts. Aust N Z J Surg 70:493-495, 2000.
47. Castellani P, Campan P, Bernardini D, et al: Is transjugular intra-hepatic portosystemic shunt really deleterious for liver trans-plantation issue? A monocentric study on 86 liver transplanted patients. Transplant Proc 33:3468-3469, 2001.
48. Tripathi D, Therapondos G, Redhead DN, et al: Transjugular intrahepatic portosystemic stent-shunt and its effects on ortho-topic liver transplantation. Eur J Gastroenterol Hepatol 14:827-832, 2002.
49. Starzl TE, Marchioro TL, Von Kaulla KN, et al: Homotransplan-tation of the liver in humans. Surg Gynecol Obstet 117:658-676, 1963.
50. Clavien PA, Selzner M, Tuttle-Newhall JE, et al: Liver transplan-tation complicated by misplaced TIPS in the portal vein. Ann Surg 227:440-445, 1998.
51. Farney AC, Gamboa P, Payne WD, Gruessner WG: Donor iliac vein interposition during liver transplantation in a patient with a migrated transjugular intrahepatic portosystemic shunt. Transplantation 65:572-574, 1998.
52. Te HS, Jeevanandam V, Millis JM, et al: Open cardiotomy for removal of migrating transjugular intrahepatic portosystemic shunt stent combined with liver transplantation. Transplantation 71:1000-1003, 2001.
53. Meyer C, Odeh M, Herrera JJ, et al: Orthotopic liver transplanta-tion with a suprahepatic vena caval anastomosis over a trans-jugular intrahepatic portosystemic shunt. J Am Coll Surg 187:217-220, 1998.
54. Rumi MN, Schumann R, Freeman RB, et al: Acute transjugular intrahepatic portosystemic shunt migration into pulmonary artery during liver transplantation. Transplantation 67:1492-1494, 1999.
55. Boillot O, Sarfati PO, Bringier J, et al: Orthotopic liver transplan-tation and pathology of the inferior vena cava. Transplant Proc 22:1567-1568, 1990.
56. Calne RY, Williams R: Liver transplantation in man. I. Observations on technique and organization in five cases. Br Med J 4:535-540, 1968.
57. Lerut J, Ciccarelli O, Roggen F, et al: Cavocaval adult liver trans-plantation and retransplantation without venovenous bypass and without portocaval shunting: A prospective feasibility study in adult liver transplantation. Transplantation 75:1740-1745, 2003.
58. Nishida S, Pinna A, Verzaro R, et al: Domino liver transplanta-tion with end-to-side infrahepatic vena cavocavostomy. J Am Coll Surg 192:237-240, 2001.
59. Merenda R, Gerunda GE, Neri D, et al: Infrahepatic terminolat-eral cavo-cavostomy as a rescue technique in complicated "mod-ified" piggyback liver transplantation. J Am Coll Surg 185:576-579, 1997.
60. Stieber AC, Gordon RD, Bassi N: A simple solution to a technical complication in "piggyback" liver transplantation. Transplantation 64:654-655, 1997.
61. Merhav H, Bronsther O, Pinna A, et al: Significant stenosis of the vena cava following liver transplantation—a six year experience. Transplantation 56:1541-1545, 1993.

Liver Transplantation and Situs Inversus

DOUGLAS G. FARMER
RONALD W. BUSUTTIL

Background   755

Embryology   756

Experience with situs inversus   757

Technical aspects   759

Conclusion   763

Although outcomes after liver transplantation (LT) have enjoyed unprecedented success, particularly in children, anatomic anomalies increase the complexity of the procedure. Situs inversus (SI) is associated with aberrant intra-abdominal anatomy, as well as vascular anomalies. At one time, patients with SI were not considered candidates for LT because of the high risk associated with these associated anomalies. Today, with advances in surgical techniques and experience gained, patients with liver disease and SI undergo successful LT. This chapter reviews the biological basis for anomalies of orientation, the experience with LT for SI, and recommendations for evaluation and operative management of these rare cases.

Background

SI, a condition characterized by mirror-image orientation of the viscera relative to the midline, was first described by Aristotle[1] and is estimated to occur in less than 0.1% of the population.[2-6] The cause of SI is unknown. An acquired cause resulting from an in utero insult that interrupts the normal process of differentiation and orientation has been postulated in view of the frequent association between abnormal situs and other rare congenital defects.[7,8] However, evidence for causative agents is scant.[9,10] Alternatively, evidence favoring a congenital/genetic cause derives from animal studies,[1,11] as well as familial genetic studies indicating an autosomal or X-linked recessive mode of inheritance.[1,11-14] It is possible that both mechanisms contribute to the development of abnormal situs in various situations, but further investigation is required.

The association between congenital malformations and SI is common. Several syndromes associated with abnormal situs have been described, including polysplenia syndrome,[1,15-17] asplenia or Ivemark's syndrome,[15,18,19] and Kartagener's syndrome.[20] Congenital heart disease is found in up to 60% of these patients.[3,19,21] Vascular anomalies such as an interrupted inferior vena cava (I-IVC) and preduodenal portal vein (PD-PV) have been reported in as many as 20% and 42% of patients, respectively.[3-18] Aberrant hepatic arterial anatomy also has a higher frequency in patients with abnormal situs.[22-24] Biliary atresia (BA) is commonly found in patients with abnormal situs (Fig. 50–1).[3,25,26] Whether a relationship exists between the development of BA and abnormal situs remains to be seen. Still, BA remains the most common indication for LT in children with[22,27-31] and without[22-24,32-37] abnormal situs.

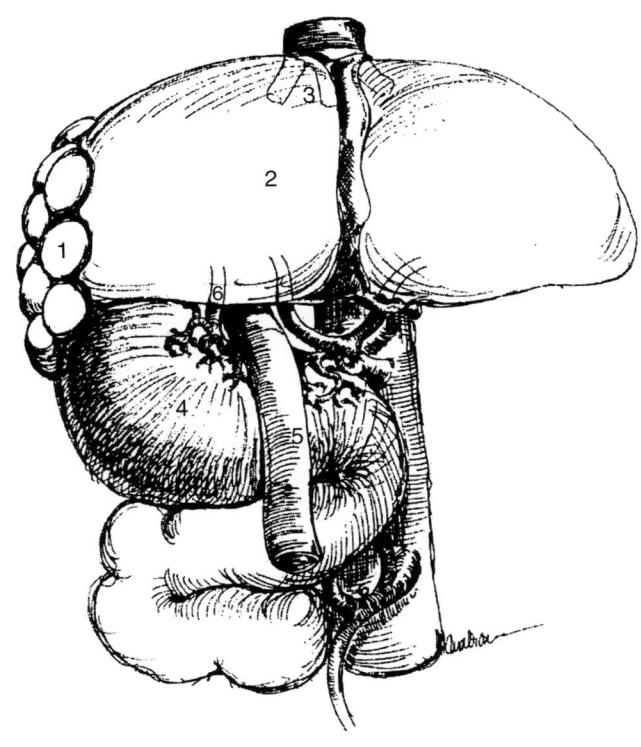

Embryology

For purposes of this chapter, situs solitus describes a normal visceral and vascular orientation relative to the midline, situs inversus describes a mirror-image orientation of the normal visceral and vascular anatomy, and situs ambiguus or heterotaxia describes an abnormal orientation of viscera and vasculature that does not correspond to either of the other two states. Polysplenia syndrome is a condition of abnormal spleen formation and related cardiac anomalies and may also have PD-PV, I-IVC, and BA. For further details, the reader is referred to a more comprehensive review.[15]

The differentiation and rotation critical to the development of sidedness and organogenesis begin early in embryogenesis and are briefly reviewed herein. During the fourth gestational week, the distal end of the foregut undergoes differential rates of growth and clockwise rotation to produce the visceral orientation found in situs solitus.[38,39] Concomitantly, development of the liver begins with extension of the liver bud into the septum transversum, followed by rapid proliferation and anastomosis with the vitelline venous system.[38,39] By the ninth week, the liver is a symmetrical organ that accounts for approximately 10% of embryonic weight.[39,40] The lobar asymmetry seen in a normal adult liver has been postulated to result from asymmetrical hepatic venous flow during embryogenesis.[40] Persistence of the transverse liver, a common anomaly in abnormal situs, has been postulated to result from failure of a pattern of asymmetrical venous flow to develop.[18] However, the mechanism by which abnormal liver anatomy develops remains unknown.

Development of the portal vein occurs during the fifth to seventh embryonic weeks. At this stage, the duodenum is intimately associated with the right, left, and communicating branches of the vitelline veins.[38,39,41] Normally, the middle or dorsal communicating branch persists whereas the cephalic and caudal branches atrophy, and the portal vein is left in a retroduodenal (i.e., normal) position.[40,41] Variant atrophy of the communicating branches presumably results in preduodenal positioning (Fig. 50–2).[41]

Development of the IVC results from a complex process of differential atrophy and fusion of the primitive venous system, including the right vitelline, subcardinal, and supracardinal veins.[38] I-IVC presumably results from anomalous atrophy of this primitive system with persistence of the azygos or hemiazygos systems in the abdominal compartment.[38,39]

It is apparent that many of the anomalies commonly associated with abnormal situs probably originate during embryonic weeks 4 to 10. Theoretically, any disturbance in the programmed sequence of rotation and organogenesis during this period may result in vascular

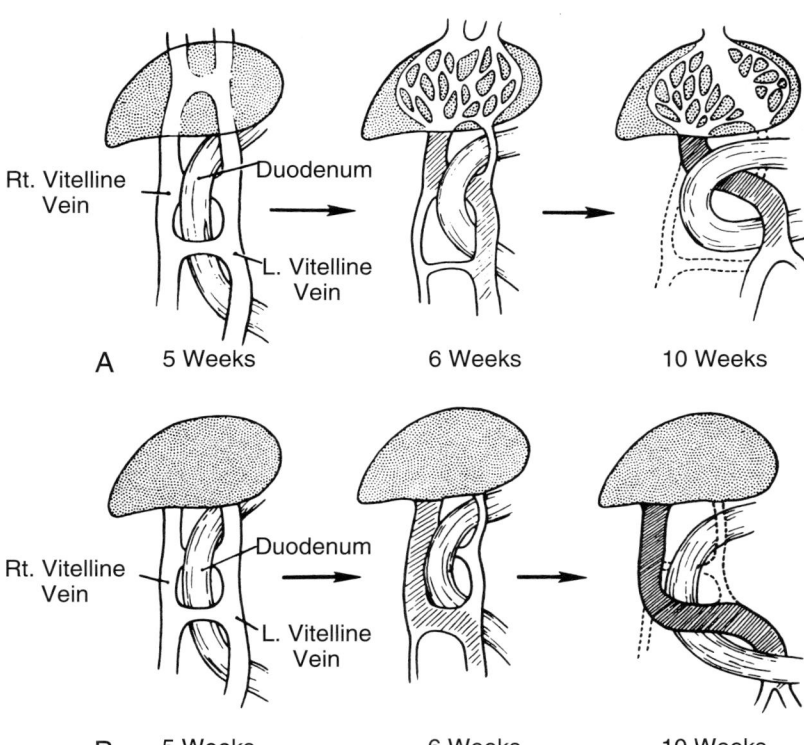

FIGURE 50–2

Proposed mechanism for the development of a pre-duodenal portal vein. **A,** Normal (retroduodenal) development of the duodenum relative to the right, left, and communicating branches of the vitelline vein. **B,** Differential atrophy of the communicating branches of the vitelline vein produces preduodenal positioning. See text for details. (From Bower RJ, Ternberg JL: Preduodenal portal vein. J Pediatr Surg 7:579-584, 1972.)

and visceral anomalies.[40] Whether these anomalies result from a genetic mechanism or an environmental insult in utero is a matter of debate. Regardless, the constellation of defects associated with abnormal situs renders surgical intervention technically challenging.

Experience with Situs Inversus

Although the technical aspects of orthotopic LT are well established,[42-46] complex congenital and developmental abnormalities involving the abdominal viscera can lead to radical changes in these techniques and greatly increase the complexity of the procedure. This situation is borne out in the first report of LT in patients with abnormal situs. Lilly and Starzl[24] performed LT in three patients with heterotaxia and associated anomalies, including I-IVC, PD-PV, aberrant hepatic artery, polysplenia, and intestinal malrotation. Significant technical problems were encountered, and no patient survived more than 11 days. The authors concluded that the triad of vascular malformations seen in these patients should preclude consideration for LT, thus effectively establishing SI as a contraindication to LT.

Since publication of this initial report, refinements in technique and greater experience with orthotopic LT have led to reconsideration of these conclusions.

Table 50–1 outlines the published experience with SI and LT,[22,35,37,47-54] and Table 50–2 presents our own experience.[26,36,55] Collectively, 31 patients with SI have undergone LT, the majority of whom were younger than 5 years (20/30 = 67%) and female (15/21 = 71%) and had BA (27/31 = 87%). Commonly associated anomalies included PD-PV (19/30 = 63%), aberrant hepatic artery (13/26 = 50%), and I-IVC (18/30 = 60%). Segmental grafts were used for nine of these patients. Technical complications included primary nonfunction (n = 2), hepatic artery thrombosis (n = 1), and biliary factors (n = 4). Twenty-seven recipients (87%) were reported alive 1 to 65 months after LT. The four deaths occurred after attempted retransplantation for chronic rejection (n = 2) and infection (n = 2).

Table 50–3 outlines the published experience with liver transplantation for heterotaxia, including the first three cases described previously.[17,22-24,50,51] Note that the last patient in the experience of the University of California at Los Angeles in Table 50–2 was a BA recipient with heterotaxia; the series in Table 50–3 are presented as groups of patients, not individually. Collectively, 18 patients with varying degrees of heterotaxia and associated vascular anomalies have been described. Polysplenia syndrome with or without intestinal malrotation and BA was present in the majority. Common vascular anomalies included an aberrant hepatic artery (50% to 100%), PD-PV (50% to 100%),

Table 50-1. PUBLISHED EXPERIENCE FOR LIVER TRANSPLANTATION IN SITUS INVERSUS

Ref	Age (yr)	Sex	Dx	Hepatic Arterial Anomaly	Venous Anomaly	Technical Complications	Outcome
35	4.8	F	BA	No	PDPV, L-IVC	None	A, 7 mo
37	3.7	F	BA	Unk	PDPV	None	D, 9.5 mo
37	7.5	F	BA	No	L-IVC	None	A, 10 mo
22	3	M	BA	Yes	PDPV, I-IVC	None	D, 2 mo
22	0.6	Unk	BA	Yes	L-IVC	None	A, 5 mo
47	17	F	CHF	No	None	None	A, 6 mo
48	45	F	ETOH	Yes	L-IVC	None	A, 18 mo
53	1.9	M	BA	No	I-IVC	None	A, 45 mo
53	7	F	BA	No	PDPV	None	A, 30 mo
52			BA				A
54	9.2	Unk	BA	Unk	PDPV, I-IVC	Biliary Strx	A, 60 mo
54	11	Unk	BA	No	L-IVC	HAT	A, 44 mo
54	0.6	Unk	BA	Yes	PDPV, L-IVC	None	A, 42 mo
54	2.6	Unk	BA	Unk	PDPV, I-IVC	None	A, 26 mo
54	2.5	Unk	BA	Yes	PDPV, I-IVC	None	A, 22 mo
54	0.9	Unk	BA	Unk	PDPV, I-IVC	PNF	A, 13 mo
54	11.9	Unk	BA	No	I-IVC	None	A, 14 mo
54	35	Unk	CC	No	None	Bile leak	A, 7 mo
50	3	F	BA	Yes	PDPV, L-IVC	None	A, 48 mo
51	6	M	BA	No	I-IVC	None	A, 42 mo
49	2.9	M	BA	No	L-IVC	None	A, 20 mo

A, alive; BA, biliary atresia; Biliary Strx, biliary stricture; CC, cryptogenic cirrhosis; CHF, congenital hepatic fibrosis; D, dead; Dx, diagnosis; ETOH, alcohol; HAT, hepatic artery thrombosis; I-IVC, interrupted inferior vena cava; L-IVC, left-sided inferior vena cava; PDPV, preduodenal portal vein; PNF, primary nonfunction; Unk, unknown.

Table 50-2. PATIENTS UNDERGOING TRANSPLANTATION WITH SITUS INVERSUS AT THE UNIVERSITY OF CALIFORNIA AT LOS ANGELES

Ref	Age (yr)	Sex	Dx	Hepatic Arterial Anomaly	Venous Anomaly	Technical Complications	Outcome
36, 55	5.4	F	BA	None	PDPV	None	A, > 100 mo
55	2.1	F	BA	None	PDPV, I-IVC	None	A, 57 mo
55	1.8	F	BA	Yes	PDPV, I-IVC	Bile leak	A, > 100 mo
—	37.5	M	HCV	None	L-IVC	None	A, 50 mo
55	0.7	F	BA	Yes	PDPV, I-IVC	None	A, > 100 mo
55	4.6	F	BA	Yes	PDPV, I-IVC	None	A, > 100 mo
55	1.1	F	BA	Yes	PDPV, I-IVC	None	D, 1.4 mo
—	0.5	M	BA	Yes	PDPV, I-IVC	None	D, 3.1 mo
—	0.4	F	BA	Yes	PDPV, I-IVC	PNF	A, 49 mo
26	0.9	F	BA	Yes	PDPV, I-IVC	Bile Strx	A, 53 mo
—	0.4	M	BA	Yes	PDPV, I-IVC	None	A, 18 mo

A, alive; BA, biliary atresia; Bile Strx, biliary stricture; D, dead; Dx, diagnosis; HCV, hepatitis C virus; I-IVC, interrupted inferior vena cava; L-IVC, left-sided inferior vena cava; PDPV, preduodenal portal vein; PNF, primary nonfunction.

Table 50–3. PUBLISHED EXPERIENCE WITH LIVER TRANSPLANTATION IN HETEROTAXIA

Ref	N	Mean Age (yr)	Sex (M/F)	Hepatic Arterial Anomaly (%)	PDPV (%)	HPV (%)	I-IVC (%)	Technical Complications	Outcome (A/D)
24	3	2.3	0:3	100	100	0	100	Duodenal devascularization (1), SH-IVC obstruction (1), HAT (1), PVT (1)	0:3
23	2	4.0	0:2	50	50	0	100	HAT (1), PVT (1)	0:2
22	10	2.0	Unk	60	70	70	90	HAT (3), PNF (1), biliary stenosis (1), hemorrhage (1)	6:4
50	1	3.0	0:1	Unk	100	0	100	HAT (1)	1:0
51	1	3.0	0:1	0	100	100	—	Graft dysfunction (1)	0:1

A, alive; D, dead; HAT, hepatic artery thrombosis; HPV, hypoplastic portal vein; I-IVC, interrupted inferior vena cava; PDPV, preduodenal portal vein; PNF, primary nonfunction; PVT, portal vein thrombosis; SH-IVC, suprahepatic inferior vena cava; Unk, unknown.

a hypoplastic retroduodenal portal vein (0% to 70%), and I-IVC (90% to 100%). A segmental graft was used for one recipient. Significant technical complications were encountered in almost all these patients, including hepatic artery thrombosis (n = 6), portal vein thrombosis (n = 2), poor graft function/primary nonfunction (n = 2), and others (n = 4). Not surprisingly, the overall survival rate was 39% (7/18).

In another study,[56] three patients with polysplenia syndrome underwent LT. It is unclear from the manuscript whether SI was present or absent. All were pediatric patients with BA. Segmental grafts were used for two of these recipients. All three patients were reported alive 11 months to 7 years after LT. Because of the unclear presence of SI, none of these patients are included in any of the aforementioned tables.

Technical Aspects

One of the most important technical aspects of LT in patients with abnormal situs remains flexibility. Although a standard surgical technique probably does not exist, the ability to apply any of a number of reconstructive techniques to the procedure is essential. In this section, a review with recommendations for preoperative assessment, intraoperative conduct, and postoperative management is undertaken.

Evaluation of patients with abnormal situs should not differ radically from that of other patients. In general, assessment of the severity of liver disease is standard. The usual radiographic assessment at our institution includes plain chest films, abdominal computed tomography, and duplex ultrasound of the liver. These investigations should provide adequate information regarding the presence of dextrocardia, location of the suprahepatic IVC, the presence of I-IVC, and the presence of PD-PV. In unusual circumstances, specialized testing such as angiography can be obtained. Special focus

should be given to identifying and treating potential congenital cardiac or pulmonary conditions that may have an impact on intraoperative and postoperative management.

Careful selection of potential donors cannot be overemphasized. Size matching is essential for successful transplantation. In general, the use of a smaller donor allows maximum flexibility when whole organs are transplanted. Specifically, the size and depth of the right hepatic lobe is important because the anatomic right lobe of a donor with situs solitus will need to overlie either the right-sided stomach or the vertebral column (or both) in a recipient with SI. A donor-to-recipient weight ratio less than 1 is optimal and recommended for whole-organ donors. Standard donor liver procurement techniques are suitable, and vascular conduits must be used.[46,57,58] The combination of donor size matching and use of vascular conduits allows flexibility during the recipient operation.

Recently, the use of segmental donor grafts, particularly left lateral segments, has become more frequent.[59,60] For an SI recipient, these options not only facilitate shorter waiting times and optimize allograft quality but also allow for easier placement/orientation in the abdominal cavity. Because there is no right lobe, the size considerations noted earlier do not apply. Successful transplantation using segmental donors for SI recipients has been reported,[22,26,51] and the surgical reconstruction is shown in Figure 50–3.[26]

Placement and orientation of the liver allograft in the recipient are some of the most important considerations for successful engraftment. Conceptually, the major obstacle is placement of a situs solitus graft into an SI recipient. Relevant anatomic considerations include a left-sided or midline native liver, a left-sided IVC, variable location of the suprahepatic IVC, and the size and location of the spleen. In general, the location of the suprahepatic IVC or hepatic veins will dictate the position of the graft. This is obviously dependent on

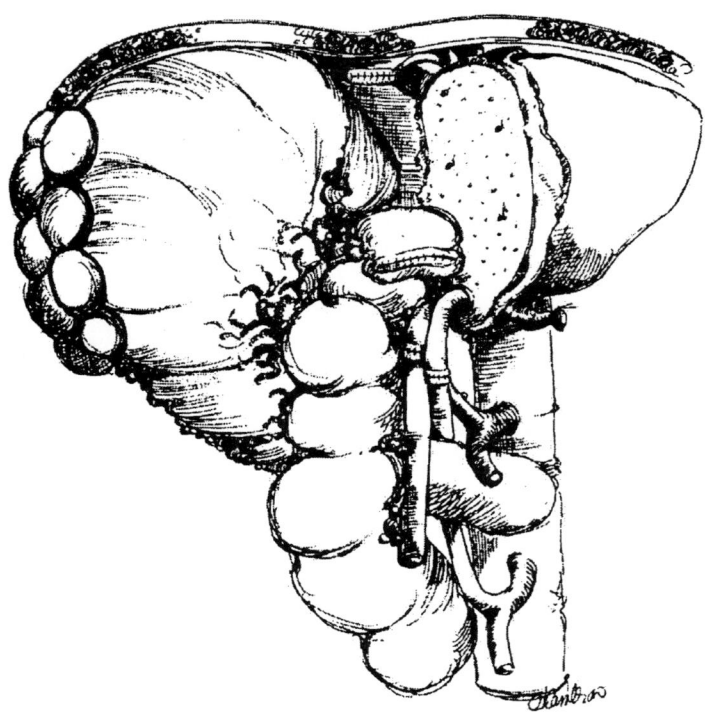

FIGURE 50–3

Diagram delineating the positioning and anatomic relationship of a transplanted left lateral segment graft in a recipient with situs inversus. Depicted are (1) multiple spleens, (2) a right-sided stomach with malrotation of the intestine, (3) arterial inflow off the superior mesenteric artery, (4) venous inflow off the preduodenal portal vein, (5) venous outflow via a cloaca of hepatic veins with the right hepatic vein oversewn in this diagram, and (6) Roux-en-Y choledochojejunostomy. (From Maggard MA, Goss JA, Swenson KL, et al: Liver transplantation in polysplenia syndrome: Use of a living-related donor. Transplantation 68:1206-1209, 1999. © 1999, The Williams & Wilkins Company, Baltimore.)

the location of the right atrium, thus emphasizing the importance of levocardia or dextrocardia. In patients with dextrocardia and a left-sided IVC, the right lobe of the donor liver will occupy the midline where space is limited by the vertebral bodies and stomach. No totally satisfactory solution has been found; however, in most instances, the liver graft has been placed in the situs solitus position with a midline shift so that the anatomic right lobe of the graft overlies the recipient's right upper quadrant (Fig. 50–4).[22,23,35-37,47]

Other alternatives have been reported. Raynor and colleagues have advocated rotating a situs solitus donor

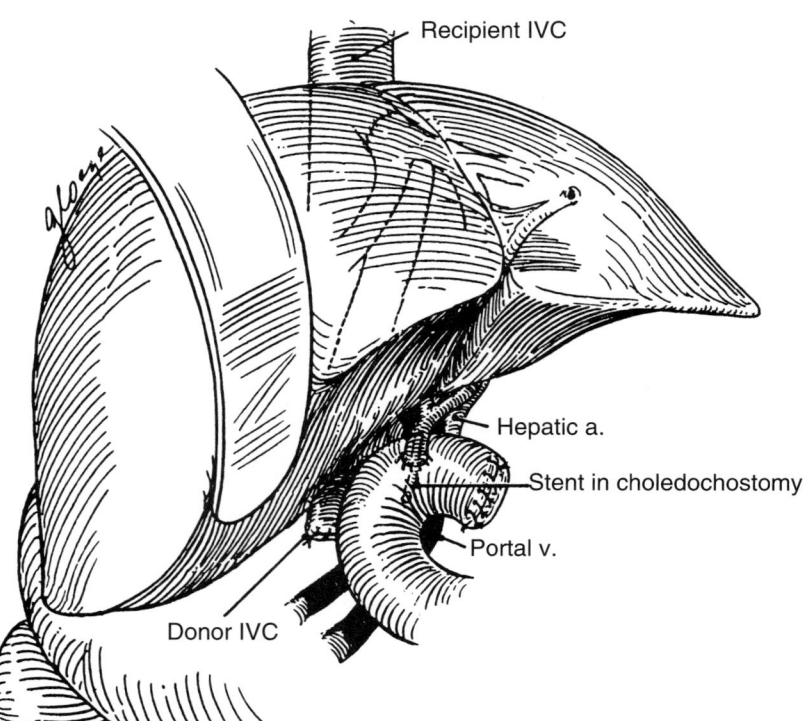

FIGURE 50–4

Midline positioning of the donor situs solitus graft in a patient with situs inversus. Note that the donor anatomic right lobe is overlying the patient's left-sided stomach, the donor hepatic veins are sutured into the infradiaphragmatic inferior vena cava (IVC) via an end-to-side technique, and the infrahepatic IVC is oversewn. (From Klein AS, Brems JJ, Ashizawa T, Busuttil RW: Orthotopic liver transplantation in a patient with biliary atresia and abdominal situs inversus. Surg Rounds 11(10):37-48, 1988.)

graft 180 degrees around its vertical axis and placing it in the left upper quadrant.[35] Klintmalm and associates described a 90-degree rotation of the graft in which the anatomic left lobe lies toward the left iliac fossa and the anatomic right IVC is oversewn (Fig. 50–5).[48] Several groups have successfully used a reduced-size graft consisting of the donor's anatomic left lobe placed into the left upper quadrant.[22,26,52,54] Todo and coworkers used an auxiliary liver transplant placed in the right lateral aspect of the abdomen of a technically complex patient (Fig. 50–6).[37] Although these options have been technically successful in a limited number of patients and offer an alternative for graft placement, the vast majority of recipients with abnormal situs have been well served by either a whole-organ or segmental donor allograft.

The suprahepatic IVC anastomosis is generally facilitated through the creation of a common cloaca between the recipient hepatic veins. As in all cases of LT, adequate size matching and outflow are important.

A direct anastomosis to the vena cava can be used in select circumstances. Anastomosis directly to the right atrium, although not reported in any of the abnormal situs patients, is possible.

Infrahepatic IVC reconstruction can differ with abnormal situs but is not a major barrier to engraftment. Because the infrahepatic IVC is absent in most cases, the donor infrahepatic IVC, when present in whole grafts, must be oversewn (see Fig. 50–3).[22-24,36,37] This technique has not adversely affected graft function when used in patients with situs solitus[61] or in any of the reports on recipients with abnormal situs. In the case in which the recipient has an intact retrohepatic IVC, excision plus replacement with the donor IVC is an option as has been reported by Raynor and coauthors[35] and Falchetti and colleagues.[22]

The chief consideration in the portal reconstruction of patients with heterotaxia undergoing LT is the size and location of the native portal vein. The general

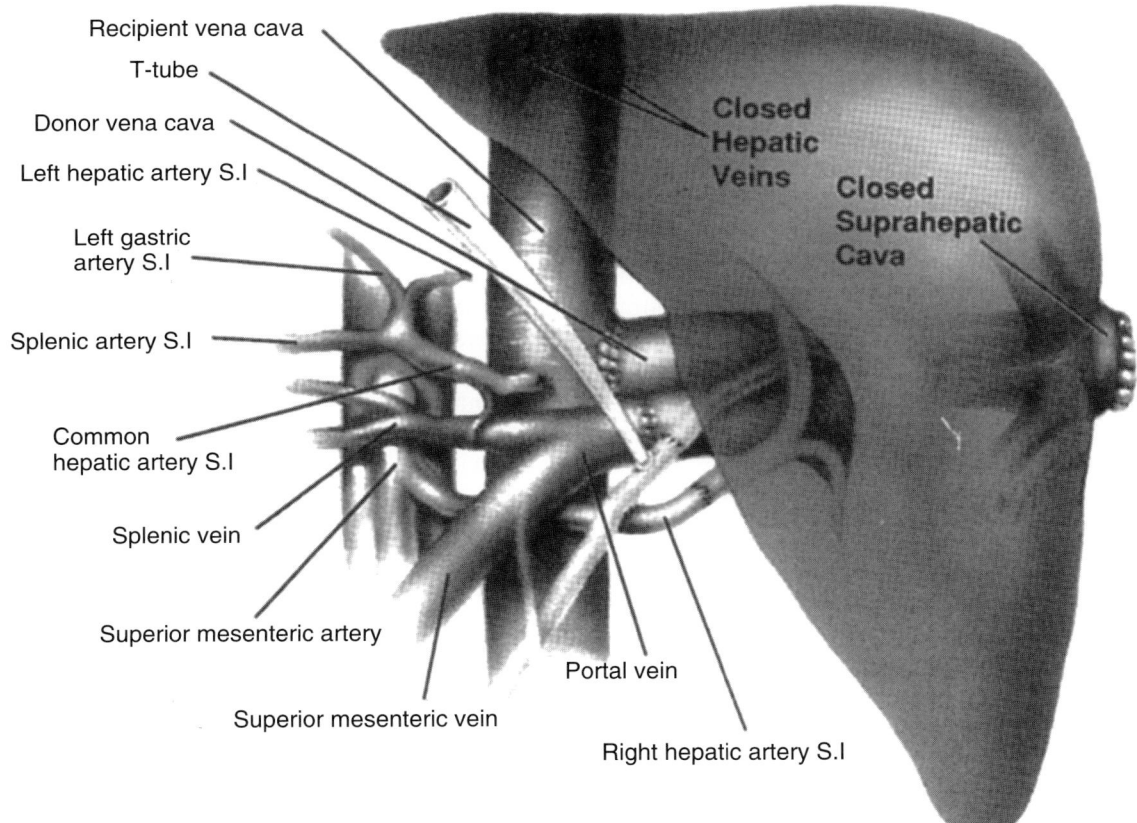

FIGURE 50–5

An alternative option for positioning of a situs solitus donor liver graft in a patient with situs inversus is depicted. In this instance, the native liver has been removed and the donor liver positioned with its anatomic right lobe in the recipient's left upper quadrant. The suprahepatic vena cava outflow is oversewn, and the infrahepatic vena cava now becomes the outflow for the graft and is sutured to the recipient left-sided vena cava. Portal venous inflow is from the recipient mesenteric circulation, and hepatic arterial inflow is established from the aorta. (From Klintmalm GB, Bell MS, Husberg BS, et al: Liver transplant in complete situs inversus: A case report. Surgery 114:102-106, 1993.)

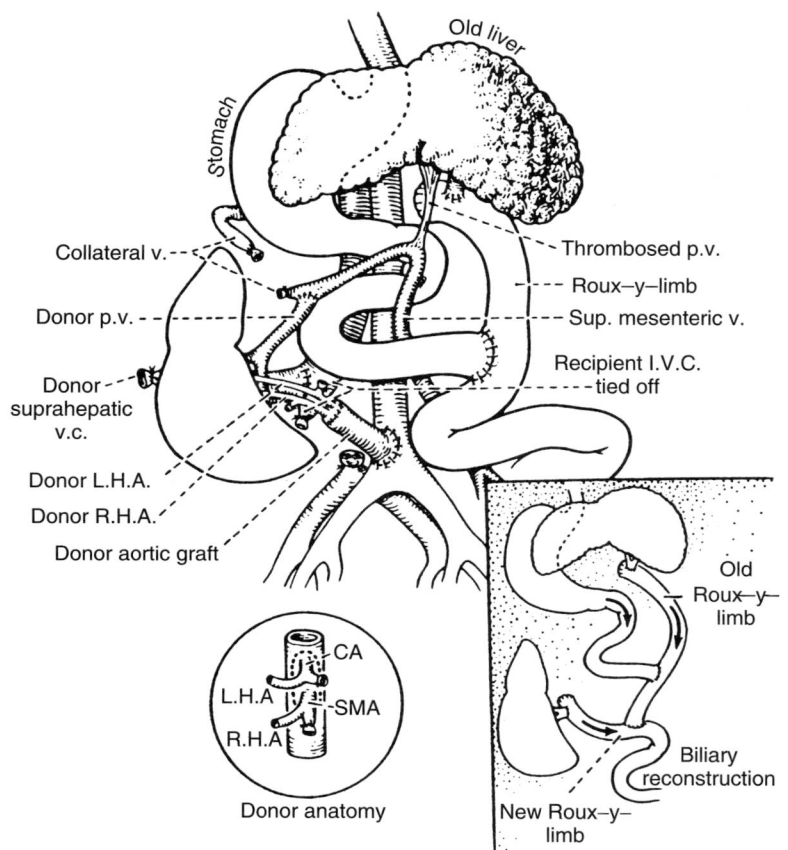

FIGURE 50–6

The use of auxiliary liver transplant techniques for a patient with situs inversus is depicted. In this case, auxiliary positioning was chosen because of the presence of portal vein thrombosis, as well as the other associated vascular anomalies associated with situs inversus. The cirrhotic liver is left in position, and decompression of the mesenteric circulation is achieved through a venous conduit from the superior mesenteric vein. The inset demonstrates the biliary reconstruction using a Roux-en-Y choledochojejunostomy. (From Todo S, Hall R, Tzakis A, Starzl TE: Liver transplantation in patients with situs inversus. Clin Transplant 4:5-8, 1990.)

surgical experience with PD-PV has demonstrated that recognition of its presence is essential to preventing surgical complications.[40] Otherwise, as long as the vein is of sufficient size and flow, standard direct portal-portal anastomoses have been applied during LT without significant technical complications.[22,35-37,47] However, one intraoperative death in a patient with heterotaxia was attributed to hemorrhage related to portal hypertension, coagulopathy, and difficult PD-PV dissection.[22]

Hypoplastic portal vein has been defined and described in patients with abnormal situs, including seven such patients in the series by Falchetti and associates.[22,61] Obtaining adequate portal venous inflow is essential for successful LT. The key principle for hypoplastic portal veins, either preduodenal or retro-duodenal, is to dissect the vein more proximaly until a vein with adequate diameter is obtained. Frequently, use of the splenomesenteric junction is required for inflow. Should this maneuver not prove adequate, the use of jump grafts directly off the splenic or mesenteric veins is another option. The last resort is to provide inflow off the infrarenal or perirenal IVC as dictated by the recipient anatomy.

Preexisting thrombosis of the portal vein can complicate the technical reconstruction during orthotopic LT.[61,62] One case has been reported in the literature of a patient with SI and BA who concomitantly had portal vein thrombosis.[37] An auxiliary liver transplant was performed as a result of a combination of technical problems potentially associated with orthotopic positioning (see Fig. 50–5). In theory, however, portal vein thrombosis should not preclude orthotopic placement of the liver graft in patients with abnormal situs, and it can be handled in a manner similar to that of situs solitus patients with portal vein thrombosis and liver disease.[61-63]

The basic principles of arterialization of the liver allograft apply to patients with heterotaxia. It is essential to obtain adequate inflow from an artery of suitable caliber and flow. Use of the branch patch technique, direct supraceliac aortic anastomosis, and supraceliac aortic conduits has minimized arterial complications after orthotopic LT.[64-66] In patients with abnormal situs undergoing LT (see Table 50–3), there have been several episodes of hepatic artery thrombosis reported,[22-24] with most of these patients having aberrant arterial anatomy. In cases in which aberrant arterial anatomy is associated with poor inflow, the use of direct anastomoses to the aorta or aortic conduits is strongly recommended because of the excellent results reported.[22,35,37,47]

Biliary reconstructive techniques in recipients with heterotaxia should not differ radically from those used in situs solitus recipients. Factors important in biliary reconstruction are the associated high incidence of BA and the small caliber of the common bile duct. As a consequence, choledochocholedochostomy is rarely used to achieve biliary continuity in these patients. A review of the literature reveals that choledochojejunostomy was used in the vast majority of patients with SI undergoing LT (see Fig. 50–3).[22,35-37] Several biliary complications have been reported in the literature after LT for SI. However, these complications—leaks and strictures—are not unique to this patient population.

Postoperative management of these patients does not differ significantly from that required for other patients undergoing LT. The medical teams need to be made aware of the unique anatomy of these patients. This is particularly important for postoperative radiographic and invasive studies such as liver biopsy.

Conclusion

SI, a condition first described by Aristotle, remains a subject of continued investigation. Although the embryogenesis of situs solitus has been described, the cause of abnormal situs remains unknown. SI is known to be associated with several cardiac and noncardiac congenital malformations, including BA.

The pioneering work of Lilly and Starzl in 1974 first indicated the potential of LT for the treatment of patients with SI and liver disease.[24] At that time, technical considerations limited the success of the procedure. Currently, 31 patients with SI and 18 patients with heterotaxia have undergone LT as reported in the English language literature. Successful outcomes have been seen in up to 87%. The results from published series indicate that the technical challenges presented by patients with abnormal situs are great but that successful engraftment is possible if the following principles are used:

1. Standard preoperative evaluation of patients with abnormal situs is essential for operative planning, as well as for identification of associated conditions.

2. Donor selection should attempt to procure a smaller graft to allow maximum flexibility during placement. The use of segmental grafts should be considered in cases in which a smaller donor is not available.

3. The location of the suprahepatic IVC should dictate placement of the liver graft.

4. Oversewing the infrahepatic IVC is frequently necessary and does not impair function.

5. Awareness of associated arterial and portal venous anomalies is crucial for successful grafting.

Pearls and Pitfalls

- Situs inversus and situs ambiguus are infrequent congenital malformations of unknown cause that can commonly be associated with biliary atresia.

- Published experience indicates that 31 patients with situs inversus and 18 patients with situs ambiguus have undergone liver transplantation worldwide.

- Extensive preoperative workup is not necessary, but preoperative planning based on standard evaluation testing is imperative.

- The use of size-matched liver allografts is essential.

- Orthotopic positioning of the allograft liver is possible in most cases, although the location of suprahepatic venous outflow dictates graft positioning.

- The liberal use of vascular conduits is essential for optimal engraftment.

References

1. Brassett C, Ellis H: Transposition of the viscera: A review. Clin Anat 4:139-147, 1991.
2. Blegen HM: Surgery in situs inversus. Ann Surg 129:244-259, 1949.
3. Ruben GD, Templeton JM Jr, Ziegler MM: Situs inversus: The complex inducing neonatal intestinal obstruction. J Pediatr Surg 18:751-756, 1983.
4. Mayo CW, Rice RG: Situs inversus totalis: A statistical review of data on seventy-six cases with special reference to disease of the biliary tract. Arch Surg 58:724-730, 1949.
5. Wood GO, Blalock A: Situs inversus totalis and disease of the biliary tract: Survey of the literature and report of a case. Arch Surg 40:885-896, 1940.
6. Fonkalsrud EW, Tompkins R, Clatworthy HW Jr: Abdominal manifestations of situs inversus in infants and children. Arch Surg 92:791-795, 1966.
7. Davenport M, Savage M, Mowat AP, Howard ER: Biliary atresia splenic malformation syndrome: An etiologic and prognostic subgroup. Surgery 113:662-668, 1993.
8. Miyamoto M, Kajimoto T: Associated anomalies in biliary atresia and its related disorders. In Proceedings of an International Symposium, Sendai, Japan, May 24 and 25, 1983. Amersterdam, Excerpta Medica, 1983, pp 13-19.
9. Dimmick JE, Bove KE, McAdams AJ: Extrahepatic biliary atresia and the polysplenia syndrome. J Pediatr 86:644-645, 1975.
10. Fujinaga M, Baden JM: Evidence for an adrenergic mechanism in the control of body asymmetry. Dev Biol 143:203-205, 1991.
11. Arnold GL, Bixler D, Girod D: Probable autosomal recessive inheritance of polysplenia, situs inversus and cardiac defects in an Amish family. Am J Med Genet 16:35-42, 1983.
12. Niikawa N, Kohsaka S, Mizumoto M, et al: Familial clustering of situs inversus totalis, and asplenia and polysplenia syndromes. Am J Med Genet 16:43-47, 1983.

13. Gershoni-Baruch R, Gottfried E, Pery M, et al: Immotile cilia syndrome including polysplenia, situs inversus, and extrahepatic biliary atresia. Am J Med Genet 33:390-393, 1989.
14. Hutchins GM, Moore GW, Lipford EH, et al: Asplenia and polysplenia malformation complexes explained by abnormal embryonic body curvature. Pathol Res Pract 177:60-76, 1983.
15. Winer-Muram HT, Tonkin IL: The spectrum of heterotaxic syndromes. Radiol Clin North Am 27:1147-1170, 1989.
16. Chandra RS: Biliary atresia and other structural anomalies in the congenital polysplenia syndrome. J Pediatr 85:649-655, 1974.
17. Karrer FM, Hall RJ, Lilly JR: Biliary atresia and the polysplenia syndrome. J Pediatr Surg 26:524-527, 1991.
18. Campbell M, Deuchar DC: Absent inferior vena cava, symmetrical liver, splenic agenesis, and situs inversus, and their embryology. Br Heart J 29:268-275, 1967.
19. Ivemark B: Implications of agenesis of the spleen on the pathogenesis of conotruncus anomalies in childhood. Acta Pediatr 44:1-110, 1955.
20. Kartagener M: Zur Pathogenese der Bronkiektasien, Bronkiektasien bei Situs viscerum inversus. Beitr Klin Tuberk 83:489-501, 1933.
21. Merklin RJ, Varano NR: Situs inversus and cardiac defects: A study of 111 cases of reversed asymmetry. J Thorac Cardiovasc Surg 45:334-342, 1963.
22. Falchetti D, de Carvalho FB, Clapuyt P, et al: Liver transplantation in children with biliary atresia and polysplenia syndrome. J Pediatr Surg 26:528-531, 1991.
23. Hoffman MA, Celli S, Ninkov P, et al: Orthotopic transplantation of the liver in children with biliary atresia and polysplenia syndrome: Report of two cases. J Pediatr Surg 24:1020-1022, 1989.
24. Lilly JR, Starzl TE: Liver transplantation in children with biliary atresia and vascular anomalies. J Pediatr Surg 9:707-714, 1974.
25. Silveira TR, Salzano FM, Howard ER, Mowat AP: Congenital structural abnormalities in biliary atresia: Evidence for etiopathogenic heterogeneity and therapeutic implications. Acta Paediatr Scand 80:1192-1199, 1991.
26. Maggard MA, Goss JA, Swenson KL, et al: Liver transplantation in polysplenia syndrome: Use of a living-related donor. Transplantation 68:1206-1209, 1999.
27. Ryckman F, Fisher R, Pedersen S, et al: Improved survival in biliary atresia patients in the present era of liver transplantation. J Pediatr Surg 28:382-385, 1993.
28. Wood RP, Langnas AN, Stratta RJ, et al: Optimal therapy for patients with biliary atresia: Portoenterostomy ("Kasai" procedures) versus primary transplantation. J Pediatr Surg 25:153-160, 1990.
29. Busuttil RW, Seu P, Millis JM, et al: Liver transplantation in children. Ann Surg 213:48-57, 1991.
30. Goss JA, Shackleton CR, McDiarmid SV, et al: Long-term results of pediatric liver transplantation: An analysis of 569 transplants. Ann Surg 228:411-420, 1998.
31. Goss JA, Shackleton CR, Swenson K, et al: Orthotopic liver transplantation for congenital biliary atresia. An 11-year, single-center experience. Ann Surg 224:276-284, 1996.
32. Starzl TE, Esquivel C, Gordon R, Todo S: Pediatric liver transplantation. Transplant Proc 19:3230-3235, 1987.
33. Jain A, Mazariegos G, Kashyap R, et al: Pediatric liver transplantation. A single center experience spanning 20 years. Transplantation 73:941-947, 2002.
34. Iwatsuki S, Shaw BW Jr, Starzl TE: Liver transplantation for biliary atresia. World J Surg 8:51-56, 1984.
35. Raynor SC, Wood RP, Spanta AD, Shaw BW Jr: Liver transplantation in a patient with abdominal situs inversus. Transplantation 45:661-663, 1988.
36. Klein A, Brems JJ, Ashizawa T, Busuttil RW: Orthotopic liver transplantation in a patient with biliary atresia and situs inversus. Surg Rounds 11:37-48, 1988.
37. Todo S, Hall R, Tzakis A, Starzl TE: Liver transplantation in patients with situs inversus. Clin Transplant 4:5-8, 1990.
38. Arey LR: Developmental Anatomy: A Textbook and Laboratory Manual of Embryology. Philadelphia, WB Saunders, 1974, pp 245-262.
39. Moore KL, Persaud TVN: The Developing Human: Clinically Oriented Embryology, 5th ed. Philadelphia, WB Saunders, 1993.
40. Lilly JR, Chandra RS: Surgical hazards of co-existing anomalies in biliary atresia. Surg Gynecol Obstet 139:49-54, 1974.
41. Bower RJ, Ternberg JL: Preduodenal portal vein. J Pediatr Surg 7:579-584, 1972.
42. Bismuth H, Castaing D, Ericzon BG, et al: Hepatic transplantation in Europe. First report of the European Liver Transplant Registry. Lancet 2:674-676, 1987. Erratum in Lancet 2:1414, 1987.
43. Busuttil RW, Colonna JO 2nd, Hiatt JR, et al: The first 100 liver transplants at UCLA. Ann Surg 206:387-402, 1987.
44. Anselmo DM, Baquerizo A, Geevarghese S, et al: Liver transplantation at Dumont-UCLA Transplant Center: An experience with over 3,000 cases. Clin Transpl 179-186, 2001.
45. Iwatsuki S, Starzl TE, Todo S, et al: Experience in 1,000 liver transplants under cyclosporine-steroid therapy: A survival report. Transplant Proc 20(1 Suppl 1):498-504, 1988.
46. Starzl TE, Iwatsuki S, Esquivel CO, et al: Refinements in the surgical technique of liver transplantation. Semin Liver Dis 5:349-356, 1985.
47. Barone GW, Henry ML, Elkhammas EA, et al: Orthotopic liver transplantation with abdominal situs inversus and dextrocardia. Am Surg 58:651-653, 1992.
48. Klintmalm GB, Bell MS, Husberg BS, et al: Liver transplant in complete situs inversus: A case report. Surgery 114:102-106, 1993.
49. Sugawara Y, Makuuchi M, Takayama T, et al: Liver transplantation from situs inversus to situs inversus. Liver Transpl 7:829-830, 2001.
50. Mattei P, Wise B, Schwarz K, et al: Orthotopic liver transplantation in patients with biliary atresia and situs inversus. Pediatr Surg Int 14:104-110, 1998.
51. Braun F, Rodeck B, Lorf T, et al: Situs inversus of donor or recipient in liver transplantation. Transpl Int 11:212-215, 1998.
52. Kawamoto S, Strong RW, Lynch SV, et al: Liver transplantation in the presence of situs inversus totalis: Application of reduced-size graft. Liver Transpl Surg 1:23-25, 1995.
53. Colomb K, Mizrahi S, Downes T, et al: Liver transplantation in patients with situs inversus. Transpl Int 6:158-160, 1993.
54. Watson CJ, Rasmussen A, Jamieson NV, et al: Liver transplantation in patients with situs inversus. Br J Surg 82:242-245, 1995.
55. Farmer DG, Shaked A, Olthoff KM, et al: Evaluation, operative management, and outcome after liver transplantation in children with biliary atresia and situs inversus. Ann Surg 222:47-50, 1995.
56. Vazquez J, Lopez Gutierrez JC, Gamez M, et al: Biliary atresia and the polysplenia syndrome: Its impact on final outcome. J Pediatr Surg 30:485-487, 1995.
57. Hiatt JR, Quinones-Baldrich WJ, Ramming KP, Busuttil RW: Liver harvest for orthotopic liver transplantation. Surg Rounds 9:17-28, 1986.
58. Starzl TE, Hakala TR, Shaw BW Jr, et al: A flexible procedure for multiple cadaveric organ procurement. Surg Gynecol Obstet 158:223-230, 1984.
59. Hirata M, Sugawara Y, Makuuchi M: Living-donor liver transplantation at Tokyo University. Clin Transpl 215-219, 2002.
60. Yersiz H, Renz JF, Farmer DG, et al: One hundred in situ split-liver transplantations: A single-center experience. Ann Surg 238:496-505, 2003.
61. Lerut J, Tzakis AG, Bron K, et al: Complications of venous reconstruction in human orthotopic liver transplantation. Ann Surg 205:404-414, 1987.
62. Blumhardt G, Ringe B, Lauchart W, et al: Vascular problems in liver transplantation. Transplant Proc 19:2412, 1987.

63. Shaw BW Jr, Iwatsuki S, Bron K, Starzl TE: Portal vein grafts in hepatic transplantation. Surg Gynecol Obstet 161:66-68, 1985.

64. Brems JJ, Millis JM, Hiatt JR, et al: Hepatic artery reconstruction during liver transplantation. Transplantation 47:403-406, 1989.

65. Quinones-Baldrich WJ, Memsic L, Ramming K, et al: Branch patch for arterialization of hepatic grafts. Surg Gynecol Obstet 162:488-490, 1986.

66. Shaked AA, Takiff H, Busuttil RW: The use of the supraceliac aorta for hepatic arterial revascularization in transplantation of the liver. Surg Gynecol Obstet 173:198-202, 1991.

Retransplantation

SUSAN M. LERNER
JAMES MARKMANN
ODED JURIM
RONALD W. BUSUTTIL

Incidence   768

Indications   768

Results of retransplantation   771

Timing of retransplantation   771

Causes of death   771

Selection of patients for retransplantation   772

Technical considerations   773

Summary   774

The dramatic success of organ transplantation in the last 20 years has led to a growing imbalance in the number of patients awaiting transplantation and the number of organs available for that purpose. As a result, the process of prioritizing individual patients for organ allocation is constantly a source of debate. Nowhere is this issue more pressing than in discussion of the appropriate allocation of livers to patients with a failed first graft. During 2002, 1779 patients died while awaiting a first liver; at the same time, 437 patients underwent retransplantation with deceased donor organs.[1]

Despite the success over the last decade in liver transplantation, patients who have received a first transplant can still experience graft failure and thus require retransplantation. Retransplants account for approximately 8% to 10% of all transplants performed in the United States per year.[1] Although advances in immunosuppression have resulted in prolonged graft and patient survival, virtually all liver diseases that necessitate orthotopic liver transplantation can recur. When disease recurs, graft failure can ensue, often necessitating retransplantation.[2] Several approaches to salvaging failing grafts have been used, including complicated revascularization techniques and the use of prostaglandins or highly potent immunosuppressants. Unfortunately, in the absence of effective methods of extracorporeal support, hepatic retransplantation provides the only available option for patients in whom an existing graft has failed, regardless of the cause.

Placing a second or even a third liver graft into a patient poses clinical, financial, and ethical challenges. From a technical point of view, retransplantation varies from primary liver transplantation in several significant ways. Revascularization of the graft can be complex, particularly if thrombosis is the cause of the graft failure. The surgeon must procure vascular grafts for retransplantation and is occasionally required to take creative approaches to arterializing the organ. Given the development of adhesions, the recipient hepatectomy can be fraught with potential pitfalls, and the surgeon must pay particular attention during dissection of the liver and porta hepatis. Finally, this group of recipients, when compared with recipients of primary transplants, tend to be more critically ill at the time of retransplantation. Moreover, they are fully immunosuppressed. These factors combine to affect patient and graft survival rates for retransplantation. A review of the Organ Procurement Transplant Network data registry reveals a 3-year survival rate of 59.5% versus 79.7% for primary liver transplant patients.[1]

With increased health care costs and a finite number of available donors, serious financial and ethical issues are brought to bear regarding this procedure as well. Hospital charges are significantly higher and the length of stay is longer for patients undergoing retransplantation.[3] Moreover, there is an obligatory net loss from the donor organ pool that affects all other patients listed, particularly those waiting for a first transplant. Patients who have not yet received a primary transplant tend to have a greater chance for survival and thus, in monetary terms, organs for these patients would appear to be a more economical use of limited resources.[4] Because of these clinical, financial, and ethical concerns, it has become imperative to study retransplantation to not only determine predictors of survival but also develop potential models to maximize the chances of overall patient survival.

Incidence

The overall reported rate of retransplantation varies between 7% and 23%,[3-13] as illustrated in Table 51-1. These rates have not remained constant over time. The University of Pittsburgh examined rates of retransplantation and causes of liver failure in patients who received retransplants over various periods. The time periods were set arbitrarily and covered 18 years of clinical activity: era A accounted for all liver transplants (n = 478) between 1981 and 1985, era B covered transplants (n = 1382) between 1986 and 1990, and era C included transplants (n = 2140) that took place between 1991 and 1998. The overall rate of retransplantation declined significantly in the three time periods, starting at 33.4% in era A, decreasing to 23.7% in era B, and further decreasing to 13.4% in era C.[6] This decline

Table 51-1. INCIDENCE OF RETRANSPLANTATION

Author, Era, No. Cases	Retransplantation (%)
Powelson,[4] 1983–1991, 73	11
Azoulay,[3] 1986–2000, 139	12
De Carlis,[5] 1986–2000, 41	8.1
Kashyap,[6] 1991–1998, NA	13.4
Meneu Diaz,[12] 1986–1997, 122	12.6
Jimenez,[8] 1986–1999, 41	11.5
Dudek,[9] 1989–2001, 6	7.0
Lerut,[10] 1984–1997, 54	14.5
Kumar,[11] 1981–1997, 72	9.1
Wong,[13] 1987–1994, 70	23
Markmann,[22] 1984–1996, 356	17

probably reflects advances made in the field of transplantation in general. Immunosuppression improved, technical skills advanced, and effective antiviral therapy was instituted. Multiple grafts, beyond the first retransplant, were also occasionally given to a single patient.

When compared with the adult population, pediatric patients have higher retransplantation rates. These rates are generally quoted to be between 15% and 29%.[16-20] Two specific considerations that pertain primarily to children—reduced-size grafts and hepatic artery thrombosis (HAT)—are predisposing factors for the higher incidence of retransplantation in this population. Similar to the adult situation, new advances have tempered these rates of retransplantation. For instance, new microsurgical techniques of arterial reconstruction have decreased the incidence of HAT in children.[21]

Indications

Currently, the most common causes of hepatic graft loss and subsequent retransplantation are primary nonfunction (PNF), HAT, and chronic rejection. Recurrence of primary disease is the next most common cause. Less frequent indications for retransplantation are acute rejection, biliary complications, portal vein thrombosis, hyperacute rejection, and posttransplantation lymphoproliferative disease (Fig. 51-1).[6,22]

However, just as the overall rate of retransplantation has changed over time, so have its indications. In a series of 114 patients who underwent retransplantation in Hanover, Germany, the major causes of retransplantation during the early 1980s were acute rejection and chronic rejection, each with an incidence of 27%.[23] By the late 1980s, acute rejection and chronic rejection were no longer the dominant diagnoses associated with retransplantation. In a series of 356 retransplant operations performed at the University of California at Los Angeles (UCLA) from 1984 to 1996, PNF was the

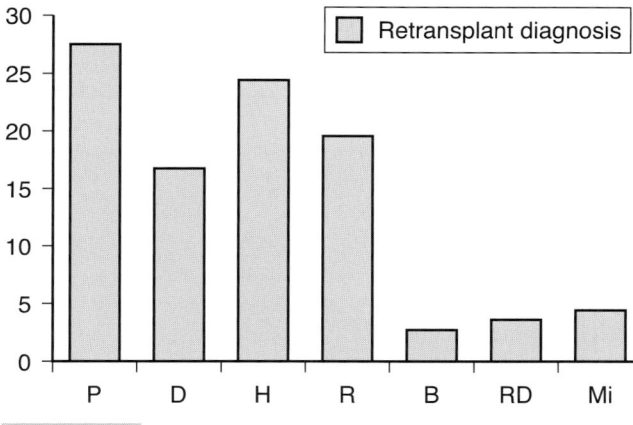

FIGURE 51–1

Diagnoses in patients undergoing retransplantation. B, biliary; D, delayed nonfunction; H, hepatic artery thrombosis; Mi, miscellaneous; P, primary nonfunction; R, rejection; RD, recurrent disease. (From Markmann JF, Markowitz JS, Yersiz H, et al: Long-term survival after retransplantation of the liver. Ann Surg 226:408-420, 1997.)

predominant cause of graft failure and occurred in 27.9% of all retransplantation cases.[22] The University of Pittsburgh identified this same trend. According to data from Pittsburgh's retrospective study of retransplantation over the last 19 years, the rate of retransplantation for rejection at that institution has declined from 13.2% to 1%. The rate of retransplantation for HAT also declined from 8.1% to 3.8%. Conversely, the rate of retransplantation for PNF increased from 4.6% to 6.0%.[6]

These trends in disease patterns are attributable in part to the improvement in donor organ preservation and immunosuppression. Unfortunately, there has not been a similar decline in rates of retransplantation for other disease processes.[15,22] HAT, for example, despite a low general incidence of 3% to 9%, remains a life-threatening problem once it occurs. Often, a patient in whom HAT is diagnosed has precious few options except for retransplantation and will have a hospital course characterized by markedly increased morbidity and mortality. Strange and colleagues reviewed 7000 liver transplant cases performed in 15 transplant centers. The overall incidence of HAT was less than 5%, but the patients' mortality rate, once HAT was diagnosed, was as high as 55%, and the retransplantation rate reached 80%.[24] Fibrinolysis during angiography, surgical thrombectomy, and immediate vascular reconstruction have all been used, alone or together, in treating HAT. These approaches have had varying success rates, and in some circumstances patients have been able to avoid retransplantation, with such an option instead reserved for patients with a nonfunctioning or deteriorating liver graft.[24]

A diagnosis of PNF is a diagnosis of exclusion that is made if a graft never shows evidence of initial function and the failure cannot be attributed to technical or other causes. The more stringent definition of PNF, used for allocation of a second organ, defines such graft dysfunction as occurring in the first week after transplantation and leading to either retransplantation or eventual patient demise. The current practice of using "marginal" or extended criteria livers as a way to mitigate the organ pool shortage has increased the risk of PNF.[25] Such organs are procured from higher-risk donors based on demographic, clinical, laboratory, or histological data. When transplant centers first began using extended criteria grafts, desperate high-risk patients were usually the recipients. Not surprisingly, placement of an extended criteria graft in the most critically ill of patients was often associated with dismal graft and patient survival. More recently, however, these grafts have been used in relatively healthier recipients and have resulted in improved clinical outcomes. Nevertheless, these extended criteria organs still occasionally fail to work, and the practice of using extended criteria liver grafts probably also accounts for the increased rate of retransplantation for PNF.[25] As seen in the review from the University of Pittsburgh, the higher rate of PNF has been associated with an increase in organs procured from donors older than 50 years, which expanded from 1.5% of all organs used in era A (1981 to 1985) to 3.3% of organs used in era B (1986 to 1990) and 22.5% of the total in era C (1991 to 1998).[6] From an ethical perspective, the practice of retransplantation may indirectly enlarge the total donor pool by providing a safety net if the extended criteria organ does not function.

More controversial than the use of extended criteria organs is retransplantation for recurrent hepatitis B or hepatitis C. Chronic hepatitis B is a common cause of advanced liver disease; the disease affects an estimated 1.25 million people in the United States and more than 300 million people worldwide. Liver transplantation is the treatment of choice for patients in whom decompensated liver disease develops, but it was historically limited by high rates of hepatitis B virus (HBV) reinfection and decreased patient survival. In addition, recurrent hepatitis B resulted in rapidly progressive hepatic deterioration and extremely high mortality rates. However, with the advent of hepatitis B immune globulin (HBIG) and effective antiviral agents such as lamivudine, recurrence of hepatitis B has been significantly reduced. Patient and graft survival in patients with hepatitis B is now equivalent to that seen in those with other indications for orthotopic liver transplantation, and these patients now represent a smaller percentage of those needing retransplantation.[26-29] A recent retrospective study from UCLA analyzed 166 patients who underwent transplantation from 1984 to 2001 for end-stage liver disease secondary to chronic HBV infection. Of the 23 patients needing a second transplant, only 6 required retransplantation for recurrent hepatitis B. Of these six, only one occurred in the group that had received combination prophylaxis. The other patients with recurrent hepatitis B had received their initial transplant when such treatment was not yet available or when only monotherapy with either HBIG or lamivudine was used. The median time to retransplantation for recurrent hepatitis B was 30.5 months.[26] The actual incidence of hepatitis B recurrence in recipients treated with combination prophylaxis at UCLA was 2.8%.[26] Although significant benefit has been attributed to combination therapy, the optimal dosing schedule and regimen have not yet been established, and logistic and economic factors, as well as potential induction of viral resistance, continue to plague the practice of transplantation for hepatitis B.

Hepatitis C, in contrast, remains a more difficult disease to eradicate. End-stage liver disease secondary to hepatitis C has become the most common indication for transplantation. Recurrence of hepatitis C after transplantation is nearly universal and may lead to graft loss requiring retransplantation.[30-35] Unlike hepatitis B, no therapy has been conclusively shown to alter recurrence or progression of hepatitis C,[30] but the natural history of posttransplant hepatitis C virus infection is more indolent than that of recurrent HBV infection. Graft failure develops in less than 10% of patients with recurrence of hepatitis C.[35] Among recurrent hepatitis C patients with graft failure, the majority of second transplants are performed for causes other than recurrent viral disease,[31] a situation analogous to that of recurrent hepatitis B patients. Moreover, when retransplant survival rates are compared, there is little difference between patients whose cause is recurrent hepatitis C and those with other causes. Retransplantation should therefore be considered an important option in the treatment of recurrent hepatitis C, but a careful selection process should be undertaken before decompensation.[25,33]

Recurrence of any primary liver disease is actually responsible for only a small percentage of patients undergoing retransplantation. In the UCLA series, recurrent disease accounted for just 3.6% (Fig. 51–2).[22] Even when responsible for specific disease processes, recurrent disease, other than in historical hepatitis B studies, plays a minor role in retransplantation. Alcoholic liver disease (ALD), for example, is the second most common cause of liver failure leading to transplantation. Multiple studies have looked at recidivism rates and recurrent disease. ALD recipients use alcohol after their transplantation at a rate similar to that of non-ALD recipients, but those with ALD may consume more alcohol when drinking.[36] In addition, earlier arguments suggesting that alcohol recidivism would lead to poor compliance with immunosuppressive regimens, thus leading to premature graft loss, have also been proved to be false.[37] In all, this group of patients seems to be at no more increased risk for retransplantation than the general transplant population.

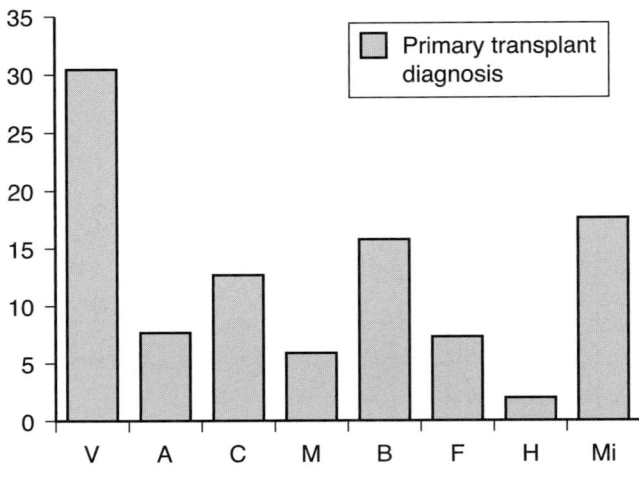

FIGURE 51–2

Frequency of retransplantation according to pretransplantation disease. A, alcohol abuse; B, biliary atresia; C, cholestatic disease; F, fulminant failure; H, hepatocellular cancer; M, metabolic; Mi, miscellaneous; V, viral hepatitis. (From Markmann JF, Markowitz JS, Yersiz H, et al: Long-term survival after retransplantation of the liver. Ann Surg 226:408-420, 1997.)

A diagnosis of recurrent autoimmune hepatitis (AIH) has also been believed to predispose a patient to retransplantation. Currently, liver transplantation for AIH is highly successful, and it accounts for approximately 6% of all liver transplantation procedures in the United States. However, according to a review by Reich and associates, there is a high risk of rejection and severe recurrent AIH. In their series, 32 patients underwent transplantation for AIH alone from 1988 to 1995. Among the 24 recipients with long-term follow-up, recurrence developed in 6 of the 18 patients transplanted for chronic disease, but not a single one of the six patients in whom fulminant AIH was diagnosed at the time of transplantation. Furthermore, of the six in whom recurrent AIH did develop, only three required retransplantation, with subsequent re-recurrence developing in two. It would thus appear that recurrent AIH necessitating retransplantation is the only identifiable risk factor for recurrence.[38]

Although initially controversial, recurrence of primary biliary cirrhosis (PBC) and primary sclerosing cholangitis (PSC) has been reported by several centers. A study from the Mayo Clinic reports evidence of recurrent PSC in 24 of 120 (20%) transplanted patients, either by histological or cholangiographic criteria. The mean time to a diagnosis of recurrent disease was 421 days, and two of the patients ultimately required retransplantation.[39] Recurrence of PBC is also possible, but the rate is uncertain. Currently, PBC recurrence seems to have little impact on long-term graft function and survival, but with longer follow-up, additional problems may be detected.[40]

Results of Retransplantation

Early studies in liver transplantation showed significantly worse patient and graft survival rates after retransplantation than after primary transplantation (68.5% versus 49%).[23,41] During the next decade, the general results of liver transplantation improved, and many centers are now reporting 1-year survival rates greater than 75%.[1] More specifically, similar trends can be seen with retransplantation, although these outcomes remain significantly worse than those of first-time recipients. In a retrospective study at UCLA, a total of 356 retransplants in 299 patients performed from 1984 to 1996 were analyzed. Survival rates of retransplanted patients at 1, 5, and 10 years were 62%, 47%, and 45%, respectively. This survival is significantly less than that seen in patients undergoing primary hepatic transplantation at the same center during the same period (83%, 74%, and 68%) (Fig. 51–3).[22] A similar differential has been demonstrated at other centers.[3,6,10-12,15,42]

Although a retransplant recipient has a poorer prognosis than a first-time recipient does, several recent studies have indicated that these outcomes can be reliably predicted and even modeled. Several clinical criteria, including timing of the retransplant, can predict the mortality of patients after retransplantation.[13,15,22,25,42]

Timing of Retransplantation

The timing of retransplantation has an important role in both patient and graft outcome.[4,15,22] Patients who received retransplants more than 30 days after their initial transplant fared better than did those who received retransplants between 8 and 30 days after receiving their first one, and survival in patients transplanted within 1 week of the primary transplant was nearly equivalent to that seen in the chronic group.[22] The respective 1-year survival rate for these patients in the UCLA series was 64% for the group retransplanted longer than 30 days after the first transplant versus 58% for those retransplanted less than 8 days after the

primary transplant and 42% for those retransplanted between 8 and 30 days after initial grafting.[22] This finding emphasizes the need for early recognition of patients who require retransplantation, especially those who require second grafts for PNF or HAT.

Other studies make the distinction in timing in more general terms, as urgent versus elective retransplantation. In these studies, the elective group, often corresponding to those retransplanted many months after the primary transplant, had survival curves indistinguishable from those of the single-transplant group. The urgent group, probably corresponding to those in need of a retransplant within the first 30 days after surgery, had worse survival. Moreover, their primary graft failure is more likely to be secondary to PNF, and these patients were more likely to incur higher hospital charges and longer length of stay.[3] Although the operations performed in the urgent group may be easier from a technical point of view, the poor clinical condition before retransplantation ultimately predisposes the recipient to higher mortality rates.[5]

Causes of Death

The development of sepsis and multiorgan failure accounts for the majority of deaths in retransplanted patients. In addition, the largest proportion of deaths occur in the first 4 weeks after transplantation.[11,13,15,22,42] The incidence of death secondary to sepsis in the UCLA series was significantly higher in retransplanted patients than in those receiving just one graft (60.7% versus 29%).[22] In retransplanted patients for whom sepsis was the primary cause of death, there was a striking incidence of fungal infection, nearly 50%.[22] A high incidence of graft loss in retransplanted patients as a result of sepsis has also been reported by others.[5,8,15,42] This increased incidence of sepsis may reflect the higher cumulative dose of immunosuppression in retransplanted patients. Collectively, these studies suggest that interventional strategies should be designed to reduce immunosuppression or initiate more effective antimicrobial prophylaxis for

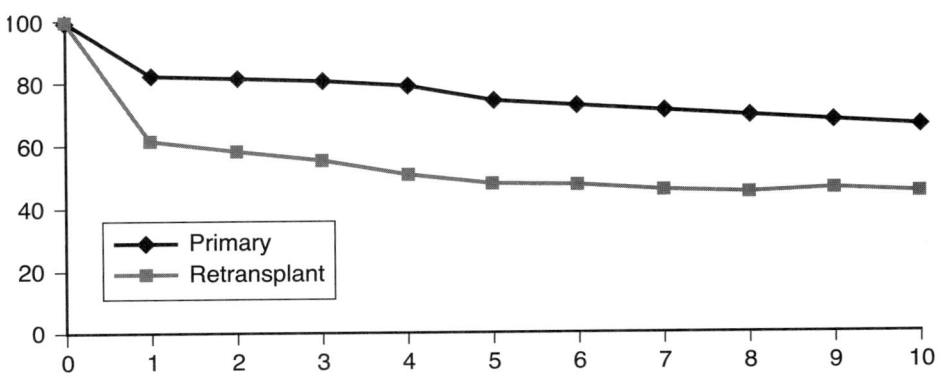

FIGURE 51–3

Results of retransplantation—percent survival versus years after transplantation. (From Markmann JF, Markowitz JS, Yersiz H, et al: Long-term survival after retransplantation of the liver. Ann Surg 226:408-420, 1997.)

patients undergoing retransplantation.[5,22] Whether the apparent "over-immunosuppression" of retransplanted patients is also reflected in lower rejection rates remains to be determined. Less frequent causes of death in retransplant patients include technical problems such as arterial and portal vein thrombosis, brain damage and intracerebral hemorrhage, recurrent cholangiocarcinoma, intraoperative mortality, and persistent liver failure.[11,13]

Selection of Patients for Retransplantation

The only therapeutic option for patients with a failing liver allograft is retransplantation. All the studies demonstrate quite conclusively, however, that patient and graft survival is worse after retransplantation than after primary grafting.[22] These poorer outcomes have prompted many to question the appropriateness of hepatic retransplantation on both economic and ethical grounds. Conversely, prohibiting retransplantation would raise its own ethical questions regarding patient abandonment. Moreover, since retransplantation functions as a backup option when extended criteria donors are used, eliminating retransplants would inhibit these much needed efforts to expand the organ pool.[15]

In an attempt to optimize the use of valuable organs, many have sought to develop a model that might accurately predict outcome and survival in patients undergoing liver retransplantation. A multivariate analysis was performed at UCLA on a cohort of patients to determine independent risk factors predictive of poor patient survival after retransplantation. Donor cold ischemia time longer than 12 hours, preoperative mechanical ventilator requirement, age older than 18 years, preoperative serum creatinine greater than 1.6 mg/dL, and preoperative serum total bilirubin higher than 13 mg/dL were all independently predictive of a poor outcome.[22] Similar findings have been described from research out of the University of Pittsburgh. They identified three other significant factors: donor age, donor gender, and type of primary immunosuppression.[15] A recent study at Mount Sinai Medical Center also looked at predictors of mortality in retransplanted patients and found that recipient age older than 50 years, preoperative creatinine greater than 2 mg/dL, and the use of intraoperative blood products had a significant impact on survival in patients requiring late retransplantation more than 6 months after primary transplantation.[42]

The critical shortage of donor organs and the increasing waiting periods before transplantation have prompted many to not only investigate preoperative factors predictive of a poor outcome but also define a mathematical model that adequately predicts survival after retransplantation. By analyzing the UCLA data, a mathematical model based on five noninvasive and readily available clinical parameters was created. A complex Cox regression equation was simplified into what has been called the UCLA Risk Classification System. This system groups patients into five classes based on a 5-point scoring system. A single point is received for each of the following parameters: age older than 18 years, organ cold ischemia time longer than 12 hours, preoperative mechanical ventilator requirement, total bilirubin greater than 13 mg/dL, and creatinine greater than 1.6 mg/dL. Patients scoring a 4 or 5 out of a possible 5 points had a 1-year survival rate of approximately 27% when using the UCLA patient database. Survival of patients scoring 4 or 5 was significantly less than the 67% 1-year survival rate seen in patients with a risk class of 3 or less (Fig. 51–4). When applied retrospectively to three other databases (UCLA, Baylor University Medical Center, and the United Network for Organ Sharing registry), this risk classification system adequately discriminated high-risk/low-survival patients. By using this type of model as part of the selection process, survival after retransplantation should theoretically improve, as well as the efficiency of organ utilization.[43]

A final approach to improving the outcome of retransplantation is modification of the underlying cause of graft failure. An aggressive approach to HAT consisting of early detection and revascularization can reduce the need for retransplantation. If a second graft is still required, the operation should be performed before the patient deteriorates significantly. For cases of PNF, the most common cause of early retransplantation, it is hoped that work currently under way may decrease the incidence of this diagnosis. Improving organ preservation, devising better methods to predict graft viability, and developing salvage therapy regimens for

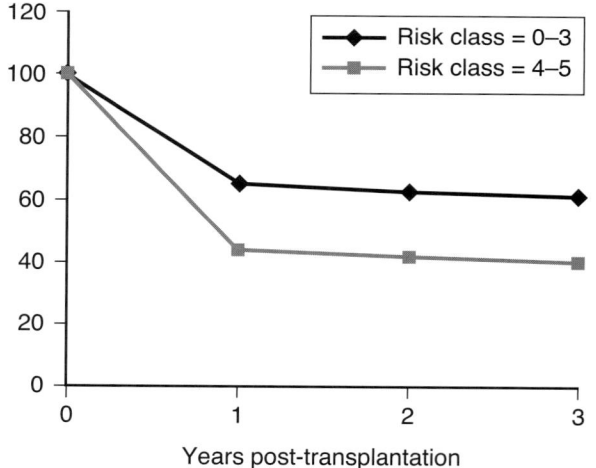

FIGURE 51–4

Survival by risk score—survival versus years after transplantation. (From Markmann JF, Gornbein J, Markowitz JS, et al: A simple model to estimate survival after retransplantation of the liver. Transplantation 67:422-430, 1999.)

extended criteria grafts, such as prostaglandin use, all may help decrease the need for retransplantation.

Technical Considerations

The difficulty of the recipient hepatectomy may vary significantly, depending on the interval between the primary transplantation and subsequent transplants. The abdomen is opened via the previous bilateral subcostal incision. A mechanical retractor is placed with blades under both costal margins to pull the ribs laterally and anteriorly and spread the aperture. Early reoperations require significantly less dissection, and the degree of portal hypertension is significantly less than in conventional liver transplantation. However, when performing late retransplantation, the surgeon may be faced with dense adhesions and scar tissue that can tax even the most experienced surgical team. Blunt dissection should be avoided; judicious use of electrocautery with sharp dissection along tissue planes may prevent injury to vital structures and minimize blood loss.

The adhesions of the liver to the anterior abdominal wall and diaphragm are divided, and the suprahepatic vena cava is identified. Meticulous dissection of the porta hepatis must be performed because it is often very difficult to identify vascular structures. If too much scarring or collateral vessel formation has occurred, it may be necessary to place the patient on venovenous bypass before completing dissection of the right triangular ligament. In either case, venovenous bypass is performed by first cannulating the saphenous and axillary veins and then the portal vein. If the portal vein cannot be used for venovenous bypass, it may be necessary to use the inferior mesenteric vein. In addition, using the piggyback technique can sometimes facilitate retransplantation.

An important technical modification is leaving the upper vena cava anastomosis intact so that when removing the old graft, a cuff of its suprahepatic vena cava remains in place to allow enough length for the new anastomosis. The suprahepatic vena cava is prepared by opening the right and left hepatic veins into a common cloaca of the inferior vena cava. Corner stitches are placed on the two opposing ends. The anastomosis is created with care to ensure perfect intimal approximation. The new row of sutures should incorporate at least part of the original vena cava cuff to prevent bleeding at the anastomosis (Fig. 51–5). The infrahepatic vena cava and portal vein should be divided close to the liver with the old anastomosis left intact. Generally, there is no need to use these portions of the previous graft vessels, but occasionally, when extra length is required, such use may become necessary. These anastomoses are usually fashioned with two running sutures.

Before completion of the portal anastomosis, a portal flush of the donor liver is performed with normal saline

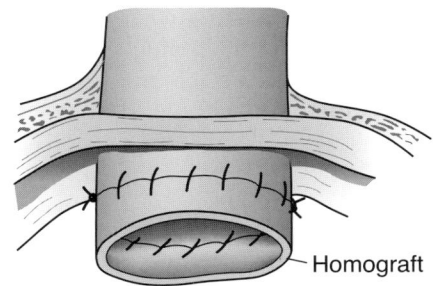

Homograft

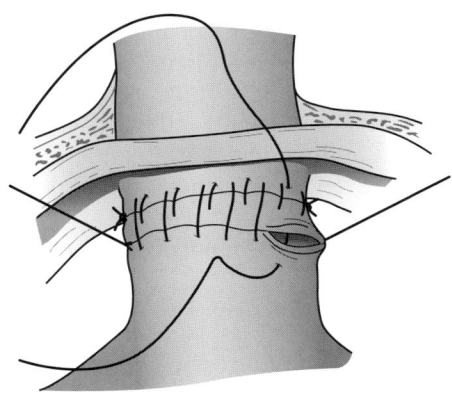

Donor liver

FIGURE 51–5

Suprahepatic vena cava anastomosis in retransplantation.

or lactated Ringer's solution with 25 g of albumin per liter. This flush removes any residual air, thus eliminating potential air emboli, and clears the graft of excessively high concentrations of intravascular potassium from the preservation solution. The final length and lay of the vena cava and portal vein are critical as well. Excessive length can cause folding or kinking of these important vessels and lead to flow obstruction, whereas too short a length places strain on the anastomosis.

The graft hepatic artery is never reused. There are several reports in which necrosis of the vessel led to arterial thrombosis or rupture. Because one of the most common indications for retransplantation is HAT, an alternative method of arterial reconstruction (i.e., a supraceliac or infrarenal aortic graft) should be considered, as dictated by the anatomic situation. Thus, the importance of routine procurement of vascular grafts along with the donor liver is re-emphasized in cases of retransplantation.

The viability of the recipient bile duct should also be carefully assessed before performing biliary reconstruction. Parts of the previous graft bile duct should not be reused in the new anastomosis. When the quality of the recipient bile duct is questionable or when a duct-to-duct anastomosis cannot be constructed without tension, a Roux-en-Y choledochojejunostomy is mandatory.

If a Roux-en-Y loop was used in the previous transplantation, its blind end, including the site of the first anastomosis, should be resected and closed, and a new choledochoenterostomy should be performed at another point along the loop.

Summary

Retransplantation is still the only alternative for patients with failing liver grafts. The most common causes of liver graft loss are PNF, HAT, and chronic rejection. The leading cause of retransplantation in children is HAT.

Along with improvement in the results of primary grafting, a comparable trend is noted in retransplantation outcomes. The multicenter 1-year survival rate after retransplantation is currently about 70%. Certain clinical criteria and models have been found to predict the outcome of retransplantation. The most important factors appear to be preoperative organ system failure, as indicated by ventilator dependence and renal dysfunction. Donor cold ischemia time, recipient age, and preoperative bilirubin are also key factors in outcome prediction. Intervals between transplants of less than 1 week or longer than 30 days have been shown to be associated with improved survival. The overall impact of retransplantation on the survival of all patients awaiting liver transplantation and the cost-effectiveness of this procedure are issues of debate. For that reason, mathematical models based on key predictive factors are being developed. It is hoped that such models will identify the subset of patients awaiting retransplantation who will have survival and graft outcomes similar to those who have received their first graft.

Several technical considerations are unique to retransplantation. Vascular grafts should be routinely procured along with the donor liver and then used liberally during arterial reconstruction. The recipient hepatectomy should be modified to include meticulous dissection and other precautions according to the patient's history, clinical status, and particular anatomic issues. Finally, the recipient bile duct should be carefully assessed before deciding on the type of biliary anastomosis.

Despite the ethical and economic considerations, retransplantation is the only option for transplant patients whose grafts fail. Given these desperate situations, as well as the use of this operation as a salvage option for those with extended criteria livers, retransplants cannot and should not be abandoned. However, these decisions should proceed with some discretion. Retransplantation in subgroups of patients with little chance of a successful outcome should probably be avoided. Various models have been developed to identify factors that influence survival and are therefore useful for identifying patients at high risk for a poor outcome after retransplantation of the liver.

These models should provide valuable information on which to base sound clinical judgment in the selection of candidates suitable and appropriate for retransplantation.

Pearls and Pitfalls

- The only therapeutic option for patients with a failing liver allograft is retransplantation.

- Retransplants account for approximately 8% to 10% of all liver transplants performed in the United States per year.

- Survival of retransplanted patients is significantly less than that of primary liver transplant patients—59.5% at 3 years versus 79.7%.

- The most common causes of hepatic graft loss and subsequent retransplantation are primary nonfunction, hepatic artery thrombosis, and chronic rejection.

- When compared with the adult population, pediatric patients have higher retransplantation rates, approximately 15% to 29%. Two specific considerations that pertain primarily to children—reduced-size grafts and hepatic artery thrombosis—are predisposing factors for the higher incidence of retransplantation in this population.

- With the exception of viral diseases, recurrence of primary liver disease is responsible for only a small percentage of patients undergoing retransplantation, less than 4%.

- With the advent of hepatitis B immune globulin and effective antiviral agents such as lamivudine, recurrence of hepatitis B has been significantly reduced, and these patients now represent a smaller percentage of those needing retransplantation.

- Recurrence of hepatitis C after transplantation is nearly universal and may lead to graft loss requiring retransplantation in approximately 10% of those who originally underwent transplantation for hepatitis C.

- Although a retransplant recipient has a poorer prognosis than a first-time recipient does, several studies indicate that these outcomes can be reliably predicted and even modeled. Outcome criteria include timing of the retransplant, preoperative organ system failure as indicated by ventilator dependence and renal dysfunction, preoperative bilirubin, donor cold ischemia time, and recipient age.

References

1. Based on OPTN data as of May 30, 2003.
2. Rosen H: Disease recurrence following liver transplantation. Clin Liver Dis 4:675-689, 2000.
3. Azoulay D, Linhares M, Huguet E, et al: Decision for retransplantation of the liver: An experience- and cost-based analysis. Ann Surg 236:713-721, 2002.
4. Powelson J, Cosimi A, Lewis W, et al: Hepatic retransplantation in New England—a regional experience and survival model. Transplantation 55:802-806, 1993.
5. De Carlis L, Slim A, Giacomoni A, et al: Liver retransplantation: Indications and results over a 15-year experience. Transplant Proc 33:1411-1413, 2001.
6. Kashyap R, Jain A, Reyes J, et al: Causes of retransplantation after primary liver transplantation in 4000 consecutive patients: 2 to 19 years follow-up. Transplant Proc 33:1486-1487, 2001.
7. Meneu Diaz J, Moreno Gonzalez E, Vicente E, et al: Early mortality in liver retransplantation: A multivariate analysis of risk factors. Transplant Proc 34:301-302, 2002.
8. Jimenez M, Turrion V, Alvira L, et al: Indications and results of retransplantation after a series of 406 liver transplantations. Transplant Proc 34:262-263, 2002.
9. Dudek K, Nyckowski P, Zieniewicz K, et al: Liver retransplantation: Indications and results. Transplant Proc 34:638-639, 2002.
10. Lerut J, Laterre P, Roggen F, et al: Adult hepatic retransplantation. UCLA experience. Acta Gastroenterol Belg 62:261-266, 1999.
11. Kumar N, Wall W, Grant D, et al: Liver retransplantation. Transplant Proc 31:541-542, 1999.
12. Meneu Diaz J, Vicente E, Moreno Gonzalez E, et al: Indications for liver retransplantation: 1087 orthotopic liver transplantations between 1986 and 1997. Transplant Proc 34:306, 2002.
13. Wong T, Devlin J, Rolando N, et al: Clinical characteristics affecting the outcome of liver retransplantation. Transplantation 61:878-881, 1997.
14. Sanchez-Bueno F, Acosta F, Ramirez P, et al: Incidence and survival rate of hepatic retransplantation in a series of 300 orthotopic liver transplants. Transplant Proc 32:2671-2672, 2000.
15. Doyle H, Morelli F, McMichael J, et al: Hepatic retransplantation—an analysis of risk factors associated with outcome. Transplantation 61:1499-1505, 1996.
16. Achilleos O, Mirza D, Talbot D, et al: Outcome of liver transplantation in children. Liver Transpl Surg 5:401-406, 1999.
17. Newell K, Alonso E, Millis J, et al: Retransplantation for failed hepatic allografts in children. Transplant Proc 29:442-443, 1997.
18. Newell K, Millis J, Bruce D, et al: An analysis of hepatic retransplantation in children. Transplantation 65:1172-1177, 1998.
19. Hamada H, Valayer J, Gauthier F, et al: Liver retransplantation in children. J Pediatr Surg 30:705-708, 1995.
20. Deshpande R, Rela M, Girlanda R, et al: Long-term outcome of liver retransplantation in children. Transplantation 74:1124-1130, 2002.
21. Shakleton C, Goss J, Swenson K, et al: The impact of microsurgical hepatic arterial reconstruction on the outcome of liver transplantation for congenital biliary atresia. Am J Surg 173:431-435, 1997.
22. Markmann J, Markowitz J, Yersiz H, et al: Long-term survival after retransplantation of the liver. Ann Surg 226:408-420, 1997.
23. Fangmann J, Ringe B, Hauss J, Pichlmayr R: Hepatic retransplantation: The Hanover experience of two decades. Transplant Proc 25:1077, 1993.
24. Stange B, Glanemann M, Nuessler N, et al: Hepatic artery thrombosis after adult liver transplantation. Liver Transpl 9:612-620, 2003.
25. Biggins S, Beldecos A, Rabkin J, Rosen H: Retransplantation for hepatic allograft failure: Prognostic modeling and ethical considerations. Liver Transpl 8:313-322, 2002.
26. Anselmo D, Ghobrial R, Jung L, et al: New era of liver transplantation for hepatitis B: A 17-year single-center experience. Ann Surg 235:611-620, 2002.
27. Ishitani M, McGory R, Dickson R, et al: Successful retransplantation for recurrent posttransplant hepatitis B virus infection in the primary allograft. Transplant Proc 28:1714-1716, 1996.
28. Ishitani M, McGory R, Dickson R, et al: Retransplantation of patients with severe posttransplant hepatitis B in the first allograft. Transplantation 64:410-414, 1997.
29. Roche B, Samuel D, Feray C, et al: Retransplantation of the liver for recurrent hepatitis B virus infection—the Paul Brousse experience. Liver Transpl Surg 5:166-174, 1999.
30. Rosen H: Retransplantation for hepatitis C: Implications of different policies. Liver Transpl 6:S41-S46, 2000.
31. Ghobrial R: Retransplantation for recurrent hepatitis C. Liver Transpl 8:S38-S43, 2002.
32. Berenguer M, Prieto M, Palau A, et al: Severe recurrent hepatitis C after liver retransplantation for hepatitis C virus–related graft cirrhosis. Liver Transpl 9:228-235, 2003.
33. Ghobrial R, Farmer D, Baquerizo A, et al: Orthotopic liver transplantation for hepatitis C: Outcome, effect of immunosuppression, and causes of retransplantation during an 8-year single-center experience. Ann Surg 229:824-833, 1999.
34. Ghobrial R, Colquhoun S, Rosen H, et al: Retransplantation for recurrent hepatitis C following tacrolimus or cyclosporine immunosuppression. Transplant Proc 30:1740-1741, 1998.
35. Rosen H, Martin P: Hepatitis C infection in patients undergoing liver retransplantation. Transplantation 66:1612-1616, 1998.
36. Bravata D, Olkin I, Barnato A, et al: Employment and alcohol use after liver transplantation for alcoholic and nonalcoholic liver disease: A systematic review. Liver Transpl 7:191-203, 2001.
37. Pageaux G, Michel J, Coste V, et al: Alcoholic cirrhosis is a good indication for liver transplantation, even for cases of recidivism. Gut 45:421-426, 1999.
38. Reich D, Fiel I, Guarrera J, et al: Liver transplantation for autoimmune hepatitis. Hepatology 32:693-700, 2000.
39. Graziadei I, Wiesner R, Batts K, et al: Recurrence of primary sclerosing cholangitis following liver transplantation. Hepatology 29:1050-1056, 1999.
40. Neuberger J: Recurrent primary biliary cirrhosis. Liver Transpl 9:539-546, 2003.
41. Shaw B, Gordon R, Iwatsuki S: Hepatic retransplantation. Transplant Proc 17:264, 1985.
42. Facciuto M, Heidt D, Guarrera J, et al: Retransplantation for late liver graft failure: Predictors of mortality. Liver Transpl 6:174-179, 2000.
43. Markmann J, Gornbein J, Markowitz J, et al: A simple model to estimate survival after retransplantation of the liver. Transplantation 67:422-430, 1999.

Clinical Management of the Necrotic Liver During Transplantation

ERNESTO P. MOLMENTI
PAUL J. SCHEEL, Jr

Auxiliary liver transplantation   778

Liver-assist devices   778

Primary nonfunction   779
    Presentation   779
    Diagnosis   779
    Treatment   779

Vascular thromboses   779

Hepatic artery thrombosis   780
    Presentation   780
    Diagnosis   780
    Microscopic findings   780
    Risk factors   780
    Treatment   780

Portal vein thrombosis   781
    Presentation   781
    Diagnosis   781
    Treatment   781

Inferior vena cava thrombosis   781
    Presentation   781
    Diagnosis   781
    Treatment   781

Hepatic vein thrombosis   781
    Presentation   781
    Diagnosis   781
    Treatment   782

Other causes   782
    Compartment syndrome of the abdomen
        leading to hepatic infarction   782
    Hepatic infarction associated with
        compression of the hilar vessels   782
    Hepatic infarction associated with
        embolization of thrombi   783

Emergency hepatectomy   783
    Indications   783
    Technique   783

The presence of a necrotic liver is a serious condition that requires the highest degree of attention in order to prevent the patient's demise. Although the ultimate treatment for a completely necrotic liver is replacement, clinical skills come into play in the diagnosis of such a terminal event. Furthermore, it is imperative to identify and appropriately address those cases in which there is a potential for recovery. Knowledge of the underlying cause of liver dysfunction, status of the patient, and medical and surgical skills necessary for temporary as well as ultimate treatments provide a combination that will result in the most favorable of all possible outcomes.

Infarction is usually associated with a sudden increase in liver function test values and sepsis.

Clinical manifestations include but are not limited to fever, various degrees of hemodynamic compromise, and leukocytosis.[1] Data seem to indicate that factors associated with necrosis in a liver lead to hepatic encephalopathy and multiple organ failure.[2] Areas of hepatic infarction are seen as regions of low density in computed tomographic scans.[1] Ultrasonographic evaluation may also be used for evaluation, but it is operator dependent and lacks the definition obtained with computed tomographic imaging.[1] The extent of infarction is associated with prognosis.[1] Discrete and localized areas of infarction may be treated conservatively in the initial period, with intravenous antibiotics and percutaneous drainage of the necrotic abscess cavities. Alternatively, the infarcted site can be surgically resected.[1] Infarcted areas usually evolve into liquefactive necrosis with subsequent formation of abscess cavities.[1] Frequently, a honeymoon of apparent hemodynamic stability is observed immediately after the occurrence of the infarction prior to the full-blown septic picture. It is up to the clinical skills of the treating physician to make the most appropriate use of this interval, which may range from hours to days. When clinical conditions permit, retransplantation is the treatment for massive hepatic necrosis with no possibility of recovery.[1]

When an emergency hepatectomy is required, it is interesting to see that patients immediately improve in hemodynamic status, with a drastically decreased need for vasopressor support and improved encephalopathy, once the necrotic liver is removed. This improvement allows for a brief period during which every possible maneuver must be undertaken to procure a replacement allograft.

Auxiliary Liver Transplantation

An auxiliary heterotopic liver transplant was used in the first reported successful recovery of native liver function after acute liver failure.[3] This was subsequently modified and the auxiliary allograft placed orthotopically.[4] The latter technique provided added advantages, such as a decreased incidence of primary nonfunction (PNF) and portal vein thrombosis.[5] Auxiliary partial orthotopic liver transplantation (APOLT) has been reported for cases of massive hepatic necrosis. In one reported case, a man with fulminant viral hepatitis developed 95% hepatic necrosis. After having undergone a left lobectomy, he received a left lobe allograft from his father. Regeneration of the native liver was monitored by means of sequential biopsy specimens. Hepatocyte differentiation was observed at approximately 1 month after APOLT in the ductular hepatocytes. By 14 months after APOLT, the necrotic native liver had evolved from massive necrosis into full recovery.[6]

Another report of a 4-year-old boy with hepatitis A subacute liver failure mentions the use of an orthotopic reduced adult liver graft. The native liver, found to be 90% necrotic at the time, recovered normal histological morphology within 3 months. The allograft was subsequently removed and immunosuppression discontinued.[7]

Liver-Assist Devices

Extracorporeal devices to treat acute failure of the kidneys, heart, and lungs have rapidly progressed from design to generalized clinical use over a brief period. These devices, which are now in clinical use, enable physicians to maintain patients while awaiting recovery of a specific organ or eventual transplantation. Unfortunately, the design and clinical implementation of an artificial liver device to support the failing liver have remained elusive. The difficulty in developing this device primarily results from the complex metabolic and synthetic functions of the liver. There are currently four liver-assist devices in various stages of clinical trials in the United States.

The HepatAssist is an extracorporeal device that uses preserved primary porcine hepatocytes that are grown on collagen-coated dextrin beads. These hepatocytes are positioned between hollow fiber membranes that are perfused with isolated patient plasma. Unlike other devices, the HepatAssist pretreats the plasma with a charcoal column to adsorb toxins prior to contact with the bioreactor. In preliminary trials using this device, 10 patients with fulminant hepatic failure who were awaiting orthotopic liver transplants and who were encephalopathic either stabilized or improved their Glasgow Coma Scale score while on the device.[8] There were no apparent infectious complications as a result of using porcine hepatocytes.

The ELAD system uses a similar hollow fiber cartridge with human hepatocytes from the C3A cell line that have been seeded and grown within the extraluminal space. A Phase I trial using this device has shown it to be safe, and the authors were able to show that the cells within the cartridges were metabolically active. All of the patients in this particular trial underwent successful orthotopic liver transplantation.[9] Future multicenter randomized trials are planned.

The BELS device, developed by Gurlach and colleagues, uses either primary human hepatocytes or porcine hepatocytes that are embedded in a collagen matrix between the hollow fibers.[10] No human trials have been reported using this device.

The BLSS device is also in early stages of human trials. This device uses a high density of porcine hepatocytes and, unlike the other three systems, uses whole blood instead of plasma to perfuse the hollow fiber cartridge.[11]

Each of these systems requires a large burden of either porcine or human hepatocytes, ranging from 50 to 800 g of tissue. Porcine systems have the theoretical concern regarding transmission of porcine-specific viruses, that is, porcine endogenous retrovirus (PERV), and the induction of antibodies directed against the porcine tissue. During early clinical trials, significant stimulation of the human immune system has not been documented nor has there been any detectible PERV in human blood detected by polymerase chain reaction (PCR) techniques. Other challenges and questions that need to be resolved include the accurate dosing and duration of therapy and whether continuous intermittent therapy is more efficacious.

Primary Nonfunction

It is estimated that PNF occurs in approximately 6% of all liver transplantations. This condition encompasses all those cases of allografts unable to sustain life in the early postoperative period. Initial poor primary function has an estimated incidence of 15%.[12-14] As opposed to the former case, an allograft in this category is able to maintain life but also exhibits a major degree of hepatic injury.[14] Various biochemical and physiological parameters have been suggested for the classification of these entities. PNF is characterized by the combination of poor bile production, hypoglycemia, coagulopathy, alterations in mental status, renal dysfunction, markedly elevated transaminase levels, and shock.[14]

Presentation

Primary nonfunction is usually suspected at the time of reperfusion, when the allograft function can first be evaluated. Factors such as poor quality and quantity of bile production, abnormal tissue color, uncontrollable oozing despite replacement with blood products, marked edema, persistently low core body temperature, low urine output, hemodynamic instability, and glucose, potassium, and lactate abnormalities are early indicators of abnormal liver function. Biochemical results (especially in reference to liver function tests), alterations in mental status, hemodynamic instability, low urinary output, acidosis, hypothermia, hypoglycemia, hyperkalemia, respiratory insufficiency, high lactate, and hyperbilirubinemia within the first 12 to 24 hours after transplantation provide additional guidelines.[1,15]

Diagnosis

Duplex ultrasonography is a rapid and noninvasive surveillance method. We routinely obtain such a study on the first postoperative day to evaluate the status of the allograft. Of special interest is the resistive index (RI), defined as the difference between peak systolic (PS) and end-diastolic (ED) hepatic artery velocities, divided by the peak systolic velocity [RI = (PS − ED)/PS]. Normal RI for the hepatic artery is usually 0.6 to 0.9 (or 60% to 90% if using percent values). A low RI in the setting of allograft dysfunction is a worrisome finding. It could be suggestive of hepatic artery thrombosis, hepatic artery stenosis, or hepatic necrosis with loss of vascular tone in the allograft.[1] Because of the severe coagulopathy unresponsive to blood products that is usually present in these cases, a transjugular liver biopsy specimen is obtained. Microscopic examination frequently reveals necrosis in the presence of patent vasculature.[1]

Treatment

In cases of poor initial function mimicking PNF, improvement tends to be observed by the third postoperative day.[1] The classic approach to PNF has been retransplantation. However, with a diminishing availability of allografts, the search for alternative methods has increased. Plasmapheresis has been advocated for treatment of PNF. Plasmapheresis had been previously used as a supplement in cases of ABO-incompatible liver allografts, resistant rejection, and hepatic coma associated with fulminant liver failure.[16-19] In a series of seven patients with PNF, five were treated successfully with two to five sessions of plasmapheresis. In these cases, the plasma volume was replaced with fresh-frozen plasma (FFP), or alternatively with 50% FFP and 50% albumin. Prolonged cholestasis was observed after treatment. The exact mechanism of action of plasmapheresis has not been clearly elucidated.[12,13,19]

Vascular Thromboses

Many times, hepatic ischemia is associated with vascular pathologies. It is usually manifested by elevations in liver function test results.[1] Hepatic artery thromboses or strictures are usually suggested by a low RI (<0.50 or <50%) on duplex sonography. Portal vein thromboses or strictures produce abnormal color Doppler and spectral studies. Confirmation of the diagnosis is by means of angiography.[1] Alternatively, at centers with a high degree of experience with computed tomography (CT), confirmation can be established by such imaging modalities. Portal vein, hepatic vein, and inferior vena cava (IVC) thromboses are infrequent. Not so, hepatic artery thrombosis.[1,20,21] Hepatic artery thrombosis is usually encountered in the posttransplant period. Portal vein thrombosis can also be encountered before transplantation. Cirrhotic livers are more susceptible to portal vein thrombosis. Portal vein thrombosis in a noncirrhotic liver is rare.[21]

Hepatic Artery Thrombosis

Presentation

Hepatic artery thrombosis may present with fulminant hepatic necrosis and sepsis. Early signs of graft dysfunction include elevated lactate levels, poor bile production, hemodynamic instability, and elevated and increasing liver function test results.[21]

In the immediate postoperative period, hepatic artery thrombosis (HAT) usually presents with a sudden abrupt elevation of liver function test results. If not corrected immediately, it usually progresses to hepatic infarction, necrosis, and overwhelming sepsis.[1]

Diagnosis

Initial screening is by means of duplex Doppler examination.[1] Confirmation is by means of angiography.[1]

Microscopic Findings

Severe injury after reperfusion manifests histologically as coagulative necrosis and neutrophilic exudation. When mild, such changes resemble those of the normal regenerative response after transplantation. In severe cases in which the patient recovers, periportal fibrosis may be encountered together with cholangiolar proliferation.[21] Microscopic evaluation of the failing necrotic liver is of paramount importance. Although needle biopsy may have limited value in establishing the precise pathogenesis of the liver dysfunction, it will reveal the degree of injury of the area of tissue sampled and will be of use in excluding other pathologies. In some cases, hilar necrosis may be encountered despite a relatively unimpressive peripheral biopsy.[21]

Risk Factors

Pediatric patients seem to be at high risk for HAT, especially children of small size and low weight, when compared with adults. Rejection and prolonged cold ischemia time have been postulated as putative agents. Other variables have been suggested, although there is not complete agreement.[20]

Treatment

Treatment depends on presentation and findings, which in turn are usually associated with the degree of necrosis. Hepatic ischemia requires immediate correction.

In the early postoperative period, thrombosis of the hepatic artery is a surgical emergency that requires immediate and aggressive correction.[1] In patients with fulminant sepsis and gas gangrene of the allograft, initial maneuvers should be geared toward stabilization of the patient and rapid administration of broad-spectrum antibiotics while en route to perform an emergency hepatectomy with preservation of the retrohepatic inferior vena cava. Once the allograft is removed, a portocaval shunt is constructed and a search for a new liver is actively undertaken. Until one is obtained, the patient is maintained under close observance in an intensive care unit or kept in the operating room with close supervision. In such instances of anhepatia, continuous infusion of replacement blood products and administration of vasoactive substances are required to maintain baseline hemodynamic stability.[20]

In cases of HAT in which there is partial involvement of the liver, an attempt at revascularization is warranted. There is usually a 24- to 48-hour window in which hepatic artery thrombectomy may be undertaken with satisfactory results in patients who are stable enough throughout that period.[1] Such cases are most frequently encountered in the immediate postoperative period, although rare instances of delayed presentation after transplantation are sometimes observed. Hemodynamic resuscitation and administration of broad-spectrum antibiotics are instituted. After having explored the site of thrombosis, a decision regarding the most appropriate type of reconstruction should be made. Thrombectomy of the transplanted artery is undertaken first. Technical complications can be corrected, and the original anastomosis reconstructed if there is adequate inflow via the native hepatic artery. In patients with poor or questionable inflow, an arterial interposition graft can be placed from the aorta (usually with an infrarenal takeoff) to the hepatic artery. Based on our experience, we believe that the latter approach may be beneficial because there is no splanchnic vasoconstriction associated with the hemodynamic instability usually encountered in cases of HAT. The iliac artery from the donor or a synthetic arterial graft is used in the reconstruction. We routinely maintain the patient on low-molecular-weight dextran for 24 to 48 hours and a daily aspirin thereafter.[1,20]

Rapid intervention helps to decrease the potential risk of morbidity, mortality, and graft loss. Although biliary strictures may be encountered after thrombectomy, revascularization aids in the healing of hepatic infarcts. This transforms the emergency from one requiring immediate retransplantation to a non–life-threatening one. If thrombosis of a major branch of the hepatic artery occurs, thrombectomy is recommended except in cases of proven collateral circulation or when the area of infarction is very limited.[1] It is estimated that 50% to 75% of patients with HAT will eventually require retransplantation.[20]

Portal Vein Thrombosis

Portal vein thrombosis is a rare complication. In the immediate postoperative period it is usually associated with technical complications. Other factors leading to portal vein thrombosis include twists, kinks, endothelial injuries, reconstructions, peritoneal bands, and mass effect from external compression.[1]

Presentation

Portal vein thrombosis usually presents with gastrointestinal bleeding, ascites, encephalopathy, sepsis, and intestinal congestion or infarction. Sudden and catastrophic liver failure is encountered in cases of hepatic necrosis.[21] In our experience, thrombosis of the portal vein has a higher incidence in cases with intraoperative portal flows of less than 1 L per minute and with hepatic artery RIs of less than 0.65 in the first postoperative day.[1]

Diagnosis

Initial diagnosis is by means of duplex ultrasonography examination, subsequently confirmed by angiography.[1] It should be kept in mind, however, that in some cases of very early portal vein thromboses in the immediate postoperative period, by the time ultrasonography or angiography is done to verify the diagnosis, the thrombosis may have already dissolved as a result of the intense fibrinolysis caused by the necrosis.

Posttransplant portal vein thrombosis associated with allograft failure shows widespread coagulative necrosis on histological examination.[21]

Treatment

As in other instances, resuscitation of the recipient is the initial maneuver in order to optimize hemodynamic parameters. Institution of intravenous antibiotics is also recommended. Surgical correction with thrombectomy is recommended in cases of acute thrombosis. In instances of long-standing thrombosis, anticoagulation, percutaneous approaches, and infusion of thrombolytic agents are viable considerations.[1] Such an approach is warranted to minimize allograft damage.

Inferior Vena Cava Thrombosis

Inferior vena cava thrombosis is a rare complication. It can be associated with technical complications, vascular injuries, mass effect, or recurrent Budd-Chiari syndrome.[1]

Presentation

According to the site of thrombosis, presentation includes graft congestion with dysfunction and potential necrosis, intestinal edema, ascites, lower extremity edema, and renal dysfunction.[1]

Diagnosis

Diagnosis is usually suggested by duplex ultrasonography and confirmed by angiography.

Treatment

In hemodynamically significant cases, as well as in cases with allograft compromise, an urgent approach is required. Reoperation with thrombectomy or thrombolysis with percutaneous angioplasty is an option. When the venous anastomosis is involved, revision of the anastomosis, stenting, or a shunting procedure may be required.[1] Reoperations on the upper caval anastomosis pose one of the most technically challenging cases. Identification of potential hypercoagulable states should also be investigated. In cases of fulminant hepatic necrosis, retransplantation is warranted provided that the patient can tolerate the procedure.

Hepatic Vein Thrombosis

Hepatic vein thrombosis is an infrequent finding and is usually associated with technical factors when encountered in the early postoperative period. It is seen more frequently in left lateral segment transplants. It may also be seen when the venous outflow of the liver is restricted, such as in piggyback livers with narrow entrances into the recipient inferior vena cava. An underlying hematological hypercoagulable state should be investigated.[1]

Presentation

The resulting physiological finding is reminiscent of a de novo Budd-Chiari syndrome.[1,22]

Diagnosis

Diagnosis is usually by means of duplex ultrasonography; confirmation is by means of angiography.[1] Radiological imaging studies may show an area of hepatic infarction corresponding to the parenchymal zone drained by the involved hepatic vein.

Treatment

As in other cases, hemodynamic stability and control of underlying or potentially septic events should be addressed immediately. Treatment is dependent on the degree of parenchymal damage. In cases of massive necrosis, retransplantation may be necessary. In cases of partial involvement, an attempt at percutaneous thrombectomy, dilation, stenting, or a combination, may be warranted depending on the individual patient's conditions and status.[1] Treatment also involves identification of potential predisposing factors such as hypercoagulable states. In this respect, it should be kept in mind that the donor liver could also be associated with a hematological dyscrasia not previously present in the recipient and undetected in the donor prior to procurement.[1]

Other Causes

Compartment Syndrome of the Abdomen Leading to Hepatic Infarction

Hepatic ischemia and necrosis can also be associated with tight closures of the abdominal wall (especially in cases of allografts that are too big for the recipient) that lead to an abdominal compartment syndrome.[1]

Presentation

Cases of hepatic infarction associated with tight abdominal closure tend to occur in the immediate postoperative period. The presentation is nonspecific, with signs of liver injury or failure, or both, depending on the severity of the case.

Diagnosis

Diagnosis of compartment syndrome requires a high degree of suspicion, coupled with some knowledge of the events during the surgery. It should be suspected when the abdominal wall closure was difficult, the donor was much larger in size than the recipient, there was prominent hepatic congestion, or when fluid accumulated within the peritoneal cavity. These are among some of the most frequent causes. Abdominal compartment syndrome per se is diagnosed in routine ways, such as measurement of urinary bladder pressures. CT shows a tight fit of the allograft associated with areas of ischemia and necrosis. Ultrasonography shows similar findings.

Treatment

Treatment of hepatic infarction associated with abdominal compartment syndrome requires immediate intervention,

prior to the confirmation of the diagnosis. An exploratory laparotomy is warranted based solely on suspicion. Releasing the intra-abdominal pressure will prevent further damage but will not relieve the injury already sustained. Once the abdomen has been reopened, Tru-Cut liver biopsies at multiple sites may help determine the degree of injury. When timely treatment is performed, recovery is possible. In very severe cases associated with massive hepatic necrosis and hemodynamic instability, retransplantation is necessary. When closing the abdomen, an expanding device, such as a temporary prosthetic material, should be used. Alternatively, the skin can be reapproximated, leaving the fascia unclosed. Although appealing, closing the skin alone in cases of hepatic dysfunction can be associated with bleeding from the raw surfaces of the abdominal muscle wall and fascia.

Hepatic Infarction Associated with Compression of the Hilar Vessels

Hepatic infarction in association with compression of the hilar vessels is usually associated with expanding hematomas that impinge on the hepatic vessels and lead to hypoperfusion.[1] Initially, the vessels are usually patent, but flow is gradually diminished by increasing external compression.

Presentation

In cases of an expanding hematoma that compresses the porta hepatis, the elevation in liver function test results may be gradual up to the point of significant hemodynamic compromise, at which point there is a spectacular increase. Imaging studies usually reveal the presence of a hematoma in the region of the hilum of the liver.

Diagnosis

Diagnosis is by documenting the presence of an expanding hematoma with imaging modalities. Ultrasonographic examination is usually the most frequently used study, because it can be repeated without major inconvenience to the patient. Alterations in the flow of the portal vessels can be observed. Abnormal portal vein flow waves or changes in the arterial flow patterns are encountered.

Treatment

Treatment in such cases is immediate correction.[1] Evacuation of the hematoma is required. We prefer to perform a laparotomy so that the underlying cause can be investigated. Usually a lavage is performed and the bleeding site repaired. Alternatively, percutaneous drainage can be accomplished. In such cases, care should be taken not to injure any further structures during the procedure. Because percutaneous drainage will only relieve the hematoma, monitoring of continuous bleeding at the site should be instituted. Evacuating the collection will prevent further damage but will not relieve the injury already sustained. Liver biopsy specimens will reveal an estimate of the degree of injury. When the damage is limited, improvement in liver function as documented by biochemical and hemodynamic parameters is almost immediate. When damage is severe, hemodynamic support may be necessary. Rarely, the damage is so severe that retransplantation is required.

Hepatic Infarction Associated with Embolization of Thrombi

We have encountered hepatic infarction in association with embolization of thrombi when complete or partial thrombosis of liver vessels was observed prior to or at the time of transplantation.

Presentation

Presentation is usually in the immediate postoperative period. Ultrasonography may reveal heterogeneous areas of hepatic parenchyma. The vessels may be patent or may show clot within them. As time goes on, the areas of infarction will progress to necrosis. Although initially the recipient of the allograft may show no signs of decompensation, sepsis may evolve rapidly.

Diagnosis

Knowledge of the events that took place during surgery together with clinical, imaging, and biochemical data, will lead to the diagnosis. Transplantations that required intraoperative manipulation of thrombi, in which abnormalities of the liver parenchyma are detected in the immediate postoperative course, should always raise the question of necrosis associated with emboli. On occasion, continued showering of emboli may lead to further areas of infarction and necrosis.

Treatment

Retransplantation is usually required in cases of significant necrosis. The transplant team may be initially under the impression of a benign evolution because sepsis may not be manifested immediately. However, once established, sepsis may progress to death in a matter of hours or days. It may be prudent to proceed with retransplantation during the early period while the recipient is still stable. When septic manifestations are present, and the transplant surgeon is deciding whether to proceed with retransplantation, he or she should ensure that the liver constitutes the most likely source of the septic event.

Emergency Hepatectomy

Indications

Emergency hepatectomy constitutes the ultimate effort in the treatment of the necrotic liver. It is impossible to establish a set of guidelines for its timing. Those of us who have performed it successfully rely on observation of the evolution of the clinical settings. Each instance should be considered carefully and decisions made according to each specific case. Prior to embarking on an emergency hepatectomy, the potential risks and benefits should be thoroughly evaluated by the transplant team and the patient's family.

Emergency hepatectomy constitutes a desperate temporizing maneuver, not a curative measure. Its purpose is to free the body of toxic products produced by a necrotic organ. Often, the hemodynamic status immediately improves once the patient's necrotic liver is removed, with a drastically decreased need for vasopressor support and improved encephalopathy. This transient period of diminished physiological instability is obtained from a relentless and unstoppable ongoing multisystem organ failure. During this time, blood products, fluids, vasopressors, and other agents should be administered continuously to compensate for the hemodynamic changes associated with the absence of the liver. Concomitant with this, efforts should be under way to obtain a replacement allograft. Although this grace period is variable in length, results are less discouraging when it is kept to a minimum. Anhepatia of 48 hours and longer has been anecdotally mentioned. Prior to implantation of the allograft (in cases when one becomes available), central nervous system herniation should be ruled out. As in all liver transplants, the potential recipient should exhibit a minimal hemodynamic function that would warrant the use of an allograft.

Technique

Starting at the time of laparotomy, hemostasis should be carefully addressed. The absence of the liver implies that almost none of the coagulation factors will be synthesized. The approach may vary according to each case, and variations in the technique should be undertaken by the surgeon in order to optimize the procedure. We routinely address the hepatic hilum first. The hepatic artery is identified and dissected beyond its bifurcation, as close to the liver parenchyma as possible.

The branches are then tied and transected. The biliary duct is addressed next. We routinely transect it at the site of the anastomosis performed during the initial implantation. Preservation of donor duct has the almost certain fate of ischemia associated with devascularization. The portal vein is fully exposed by this time. Its right and left branches are dissected up to the hepatic parenchyma. They are tied and transected as close to the liver as possible in order to maximize its length. The retrohepatic inferior vena cava is then addressed. Bridging veins between the liver and inferior vena cava are tied (or clipped) and transected. Such a maneuver should free the liver up to the hepatic veins. The hepatic veins are subsequently dissected. They are addressed in the order that gives more comfort to the surgeon. A clamp is placed at each vein and the liver removed. The veins are then oversewn, preserving the IVC intact to allow continued return of blood from the lower extremities to the heart. Careful hemostasis should be achieved, because in the absence of the liver there is a marked deficiency of clotting factors. A portocaval shunt is then constructed. To do so, the surgeon may anastomose a branch of the portal vein, or the portal vein itself, to the inferior vena cava. This permits decompression of the enteric blood into the systemic circulation (Fig. 52–1). The anhepatic patient may be kept in the operating room or in an intensive care unit setting until retransplantation.

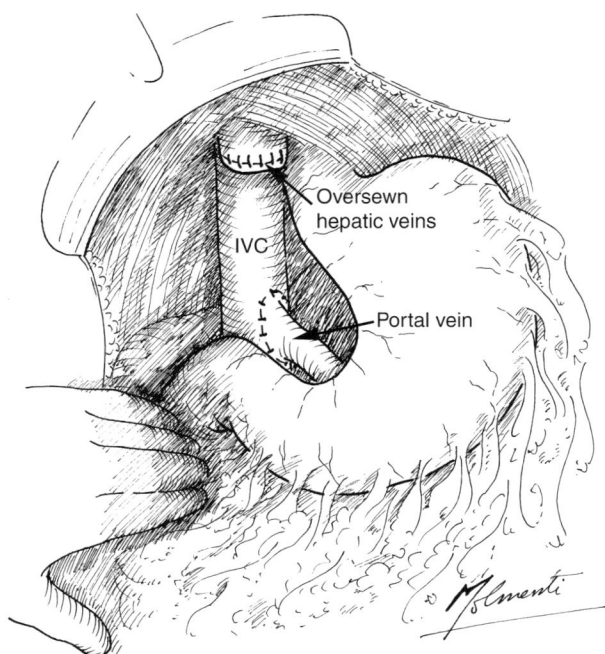

FIGURE 52–1

View of the abdominal cavity in a case of emergency hepatectomy with portocaval shunt. Note that the hepatic veins have been oversewn.

Pearls and Pitfalls

- The ultimate treatment for a completely necrotic liver is replacement.
- Identify and appropriately address those cases in which there is potential for recovery.
- Infarction is usually associated with a sudden increase in liver function tests and sepsis.
- The extent of infarction is associated with prognosis.
- A honeymoon of apparent hemodynamic stability is frequently observed. Make use of it!
- Emergency hepatectomy is usually associated with an immediate short-lasting hemodynamic improvement. This improvement allows for a brief period during which every possible maneuver must be undertaken in order to procure a replacement allograft.

References

1. Molmenti EP, Klintmalm GB: Atlas of Liver Transplantation. Philadelphia, WB Saunders, 2002.
2. Shi Q: On bioartificial liver assist system: Theoretical exploration and strategies for further development. Artif Cells Blood Substit Immobil Biotechnol 28:535-546, 2000.
3. Metselaar HJ, Hesselink EJ, de Rave S, et al: Recovery of failing liver after auxiliary heterotopic transplantation [letter]. Lancet 335:1156, 1990.
4. Gubernatis G, Pichlmayr R, Kemnitz J, et al: Auxiliary partial liver transplantation (APOLT) for fulminant hepatic failure: First successful case report. World J Surg 15:660-665, 1991.
5. van Hoek B, de Boer D, Boudjema K, et al: Auxiliary versus orthotopic liver transplantation for acute liver failure. J Hepatol 30:699-705, 1999.
6. Fujita M, Furukawa H, Hattori M, et al: Sequential observation of liver cell regeneration after massive hepatic necrosis in auxiliary partial orthotopic liver transplantation. Mod Pathol 13:152-157, 2000.
7. Boudjema K, Jaeck D, Simeoni U, et al: Temporary auxiliary liver transplantation for subacute liver failure in a child. Lancet 42:778-779, 1993.
8. DiDica S, Ichai P, Feray C, et al: Neurological improvement during bio-artificial liver sessions in patients with acute liver failure awaiting transplantation. Transplantation 73:257-264, 2002.
9. Millis J, Cronin D, Johnson R, et al: Initial experience with the modified extracorporeal liver assist device for patients with fulminant hepatic failure: System modification and clinical impact. Transplantation 74:1735-1746, 2002.
10. Gerlach JC, Lemmers, Schor M, et al: Experimental evaluation of a hybrid liver support system. Transplant Proc 29:852, 1997.
11. Mazariegos GV, Kramer DJ, Lopez RC, et al: Safety observations in phase I clinical evaluation of the Excorp Bioartificial Liver Support System after the first four patients. ASAIO J 47:471-475, 2001.
12. Mandal AK, King KE, Humphreys SL, et al: Plasmapheresis: An effective therapy for primary allograft nonfunction after liver transplantation. Transplantation 70:216-220, 2000.

13. Ploeg RJ, D'Alessandro AM, Knechtle SJ, et al: Risk factors for primary dysfunction after liver transplantation-A multivariate analysis. Transplantation 55:807-813, 1993.

14. Strasberg SM, Howard TK, Molmenti EP, et al: Evaluation of the donor liver—risk factors for poor function. Hepatology 20:829-838, 1994.

15. Colquhoun SD, Busuttil RW: Graft failure: Cause, recognition, and treatment. In Busuttil RW, Klintmalm GK: Transplantation of the Liver. Philadelphia, Saunders, 1996, pp 607-616.

16. Evrard HM, Miller C, Schwartz M, et al: Resistant hepatic allograft rejection successfully treated with cyclophosphamide and plasmapheresis. Transplantation 50:702-704, 1990.

17. Mor E, Skerrett D, Manzarbeitia C, et al: Successful use of an enhanced immunosuppressive protocol with plasmapheresis for ABO-incompatible mismatched grafts in liver transplant recipients. Transplantation 59:986-990, 1995.

18. Buckner CD, Clift RA, Volwiler W, et al: Plasma exchange in patients with fulminant hepatic failure. Arch Intern Med 132:487-492, 1973.

19. Skerrett D, Mor E, Curtiss S, et al: Plasmapheresis in primary dysfunction of hepatic transplants. J Clin Apheresis 11:10-13, 1996.

20. Imagawa DK, Busuttil RW: Technical problems: Vascular. In Busuttil RW, Klintmalm GK: Transplantation of the Liver. Philadelphia, Saunders, 1996, pp 626-632.

21. Demetris AJ, Tsamandas AC, Delaney CP, et al: Pathology of liver transplantation. In Busuttil RW, Klintmalm GK: Transplantation of the Liver. Philadelphia, Saunders, 1996, pp 681-723.

22. Klein AS, Molmenti EP: Surgical treatment of Budd-Chiari syndrome. Liver Transpl 9:891-896, 2003.

53

Transplantation of the Liver with Digestive Organs

TOMOAKI KATO
ANDREAS G. TZAKIS

Indications for combined liver and small
  bowel transplantation 788
  Intestinal and liver failure 788
  Indications for liver and small bowel
    transplantation in children 789
  Indications for liver and small bowel
    transplantation in adults 789
  Selection of graft type 790

Preoperative evaluation 790

Surgical technique 791
  Donor selection and harvesting
    of grafts 791
  Transplantation of the liver and
    intestine 791
  Transplantation of the liver and intestine
    with the pancreaticoduodenal
    complex 792
  Multivisceral transplantation 793

Postoperative care 794
  Immunosuppression 794
  Monitoring 794
  Nutrition 795

Postoperative complications 795
  Rejection 795
  Technical complications 796
  Infection 796
  Posttransplant lymphoproliferative
    disease 797
  Graft-versus-host disease 797

Outcomes 797

Related procedures 798
  Abdominal wall transplantation 798
  Intestinal autotransplantation 800

Transplantation of the liver together with the gastrointestinal (GI) tract was primarily performed to treat patients with liver failure resulting from long-term use of parenteral nutrition (PN). For this type of liver failure, the liver must be transplanted with the small bowel because the original problem requiring PN is intestinal failure. The first successful transplantation of the liver together with the GI organs was performed by Grant and colleagues,[1] who transplanted a combined liver and bowel graft into an adult with short-gut syndrome and antithrombin III deficiency. The idea of combining liver transplantation with small bowel transplantation in this case was to use the liver not only to correct a coagulation abnormality but also to protect against small bowel graft rejection. Starzl and associates[2] and Williams and coworkers[3] published their first experiences with transplanting multiple viscera in 1989. Starzl and associates transplanted multiple abdominal viscera, including the stomach, pancreas, liver, small bowel, and colon; Williams and coworkers transplanted these same organs but without the colon. The longest survival period in these two early series did not exceed 1 year, but the attempts proved that the procedure was feasible with then-existing technology. After these initial attempts, efforts were made to improve outcome by introducing new immunosuppressive drugs, modifying the surgical technique, and improving postoperative monitoring. As a result of improved outcome, combined transplantation of the liver and digestive organs has been performed more frequently in recent years. In managing the composite abdominal organ graft, the main focus must be on the small bowel because acute rejection of the small bowel is the most difficult problem to treat. Therefore, transplantation of the liver with digestive organs has been classified as a subcategory of intestinal transplantation. As cases have accumulated, indications and types of grafts used for intestinal transplantation have been better defined. Grafts used in intestinal transplantation are classified into one of three different types:

1. Isolated intestinal transplantation for patients with intestinal failure who do not have liver failure

2. Combined liver and intestinal transplantation for patients with liver and intestinal failure but a normal stomach and pancreas (the pancreaticoduodenal complex is added to the graft for recipients of transplants from small pediatric donors)

3. Multivisceral transplantation (transplantation of the stomach, pancreas, liver, and intestine) for patients with liver and intestinal failure whose stomach, pancreas, or both must be replaced.

Intestinal failure alone is treated with isolated small bowel transplantation. The idea of including the liver for its protective effect against bowel rejection has been abandoned because the protective effect of the liver on human small bowel grafts has not been proved and inclusion of the liver increases the complexity of the transplant procedure. In addition, isolated small bowel transplantation has a safety valve in that the patient can resume PN if the small bowel graft fails. Therefore, the liver is included only for patients with irreversible liver damage. In recent years, the technique of including part or all of the pancreas together with the duodenum and the liver and intestine has been introduced (see later). This technique is mainly used for technical reasons because separation of the pancreaticoduodenal complex from the multivisceral organ block can cause kinking of the portal vein or injury to the minute vessels around the head of the pancreas, particularly in grafts from small pediatric donors.[4-6]

In this chapter we describe the indications for composite abdominal organ transplantation, the surgical technique, care of the patient, and recent outcomes of the procedure. We also briefly describe two novel surgical procedures developed as the result of our experience with these forms of transplantation: abdominal wall transplantation and intestinal autotransplantation.

Composite liver, stomach, and pancreas transplantation has been performed for upper abdominal malignancy[7]; however, because this procedure is no longer routinely performed, we do not discuss it in this chapter.

Indications for Combined Liver and Small Bowel Transplantation

Intestinal and Liver Failure

Intestinal failure is defined as "the inability of the intestine to maintain nutrition and/or positive fluid and electrolyte balance without parenteral support." Therefore, patients with intestinal failure will be receiving chronic PN. Two types of problems render the intestine incapable of handling nutrition or fluid. One is anatomic loss of the absorptive surface area of the intestine, known as short-gut syndrome; the other is functional abnormality of the intestine. Short-gut syndrome is typically caused by massive resection of the intestine or by a congenital condition such as jejunal atresia, gastroschisis, or necrotizing enterocolitis. Functional abnormality of the intestine is the result of relatively rare conditions such as chronic pseudo-obstruction syndrome, megacystis-microcolon syndrome, or microvillus inclusion disease.

A small proportion of patients who are chronically dependent on PN could experience liver disease as a complication of PN.[8-10] However, the precise pathogenesis of PN-induced liver disease is unclear. Patients who are treated with PN from a very early age,[8] those with frequent bacterial infection,[9,10] those with a long-standing diverting stoma,[11] and patients who do not tolerate caloric intake from the gut[11] are more susceptible to liver disease. Early cholestatic liver disease is known to be reversible.[12] When the bowel adapts and patients are weaned off PN, liver parameters could become normal. When liver disease reaches the level of cirrhosis, it is considered irreversible. Nonetheless, even patients with very deep jaundice and a relatively firm liver can experience an amazing recovery of liver function. Histopathological changes in these patients are not well described; however, once the cause is eliminated, hepatic fibrosis could regress, even from the stage of cirrhosis.[13-15] When the underlying cause of the liver damage is removed as patients are taken off PN, it may be advisable to delay transplantation as long as the liver disease is well compensated.

In contrast, when patients chronically dependent on PN experience symptoms of portal hypertension such as GI bleeding, these patients must be evaluated for combined liver and GI transplantation as soon as possible. Because the waiting time for a combined transplant is rather long, waiting list mortality rates are relatively high for this population.[16] Ideally, patients with permanent PN dependency should be referred to the transplant center as soon as liver disease is detected.

In exceptional cases, patients with PN-induced liver disease can also be considered for isolated liver transplantation.[17] Such patients are those who are almost off PN or already off PN but have experienced substantial liver disease while on PN. Isolated liver transplantation can be considered when these patients begin to show symptoms of decompensation. These patients must be carefully selected because surgical changes in the abdomen may cause feeding intolerance and a return to PN. Biliary reconstruction in these cases should avoid the creation of Roux-en-Y anastomoses because they decrease the functional absorptive area. For small children who are not suitable for duct-to-duct anastomosis, choledochoduodenostomy may be required.

Indications for Liver and Small Bowel Transplantation in Children

Common causes of liver and intestinal failure in children are listed in Table 53–1. Short-gut syndrome is usually congenital or results from massive surgical resection of the bowel in the neonatal period for conditions such as gastroschisis,[18,19] necrotizing enterocolitis,[20-22] intestinal atresia,[23] and Hirschsprung's disease.[24] Other less common causes include functional abnormalities such as megacystis-microcolon syndrome[25,26] and microvillus inclusion disease.[27,28] Liver disease does not develop in most PN-dependent patients; however, liver failure may be accelerated in some patients.[29] These patients

frequently require replacement of their liver within the first year of life. They are typically first seen with deep jaundice, an enlarged, firm liver, and a gigantic spleen. In our program, the median age of patients who undergo combined transplantation is younger than 18 months. As the liver disease progresses, patients often experience GI bleeding, commonly from varices around the gastrostomy site. Once the patient has end-stage liver disease, any systemic infection can trigger decompensation. Because these patients are at risk for central line–associated sepsis, careful follow-up for any symptoms of infection is important.

Indications for Liver and Small Bowel Transplantation in Adults

Indications for composite abdominal organ transplantation in adults are very different from those in children (Table 53–2). The most common cause of short-gut syndrome in adults is mesenteric vascular thrombosis. Some of these cases of thrombosis are due to a known cause of hypercoagulability, such as protein C or antithrombin III deficiency, but for many the cause is uncertain. The thrombosis frequently occurs after abdominal surgery. Other causes of short-gut syndrome are Gardner's syndrome/desmoid tumor, trauma, and Crohn's disease. Functional abnormalities are relatively rare in adults, but some are due to chronic intestinal pseudo-obstruction syndrome. Patients with large desmoid tumors at the root of the mesentery can be considered candidates for transplantation before resection of the tumor if the development of short-gut syndrome appears imminent. Recently in our program, patients with tumors at the root of the mesentery have been considered candidates for upper abdominal

Table 53–1. INDICATIONS FOR INTESTINAL TRANSPLANTATION IN CHILDREN

Disease	%
Volvulus	17
Gastroschisis	21
Necrotizing enterocolitis	12
Intestinal atresia	8
Short gut—other	3
Microvillus inclusion disease	6
Malabsorption—other	4
Pseudo-obstruction	9
Aganglionosis/Hirschsprung's disease	7
Motility—other	1
Tumor	1
Retransplantation	8
Other	4

From the Intestinal Transplant Registry, May 2003.

Table 53–2. INDICATIONS FOR INTESTINAL TRANSPLANTATION IN ADULTS

Disease	%
Ischemia	23
Crohn's disease	14
Trauma	10
Volvulus	7
Other	7
Motility	8
Desmoid tumor	9
Gardner's syndrome/familial polyposis	3
Other tumor	4
Retransplantation	6
Other	5

From the Intestinal Transplant Registry, May 2003.

eviscertion and reimplantation of the native bowel segment after it has been freed from tumor at the back-table (ex vivo resection and intestinal autotransplantation, see later).

Selection of Graft Type

To prepare a composite liver and intestine graft, the pancreas and duodenum must be separated from the organ block. Avoiding such separation by retaining the donor pancreas, either in part or as a whole, in the organ block has several advantages, particularly when the donor is a very small child (liver, intestine, and pancreas transplantation, see later). In recent years, this technique has become a more commonly used method of pediatric liver and intestine transplantation at major transplant centers in North America.[4-6] With this procedure, recipients receive additional pancreas from the donor.

Multivisceral transplantation is usually indicated for patients with liver and intestinal failure whose pancreas and stomach must be replaced. Such patients are those with severe gastric dysmotility (e.g., chronic pseudo-obstruction), trauma to the stomach, severe adhesions of the upper part of the abdomen, or pancreatitis. However, the difference between multivisceral transplantation and liver-intestine-pancreas transplantation is only removal of the native foregut and addition of the donor stomach (Figs. 53–1 and 53–2). Children with chronic PN dependency often have a tube gastrostomy and a dilated stomach. The spleen can be gigantic in these patients with liver failure. By removing the native stomach, pancreas, and spleen of such patients, we can create a very large space. In our program, we have recently begun using multivisceral transplantation for very small children with a dilated stomach and severe splenomegaly, even if the stomach is not involved in the disease process. Multivisceral transplantation may have additional advantages over liver, intestine, and pancreas transplantation because it is orthotopic, it preserves the entire vascular network of the abdominal viscera, and it allows a simpler vascular reconstruction (drainage of the native portal system is unnecessary). A potential problem in expanding the use of multivisceral transplantation to treat these children lies in the gastric and pancreatic function of the graft and the upper GI reconstruction. Our past experience with multivisceral transplantation has shown that motility of the transplanted stomach and function of the transplanted pancreas seem to be normal. In a few cases, we have seen stricture or reflux at the esophagogastric anastomosis. Although the incidence of these problems is relatively low, in an attempt to avoid them we began using a gastrogastric anastomosis by preserving a small rim of the native stomach (see later).

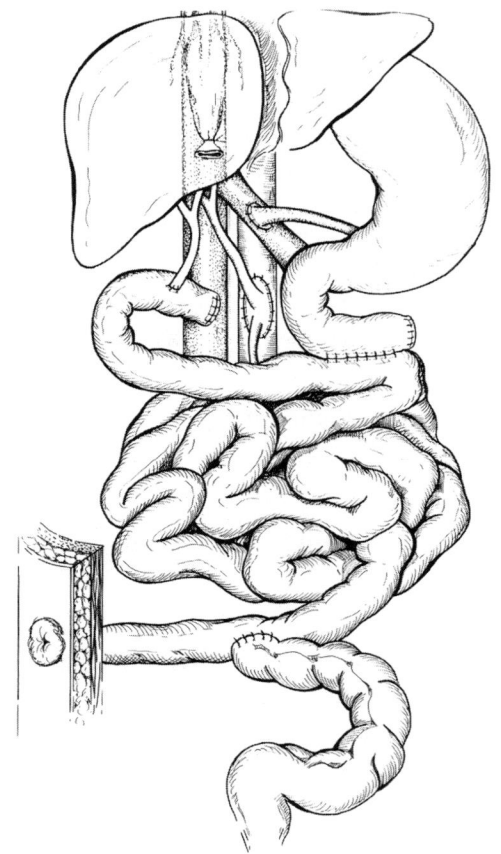

FIGURE 53–1

Transplantation of the liver and intestine (composite).

Recently, we have begun including the spleen in the multivisceral graft as well. So far, there have been no obvious complications related to the grafted spleen (unpublished observation).

Preoperative Evaluation

Preoperative evaluation of candidates for combined liver and GI transplantation includes obtaining precise information about the remaining GI tract and the status of central venous access, in addition to the standard workup for liver transplantation. The information about the remaining GI tract is usually well documented by the referring physician; however, to obtain exact anatomic information, a barium upper GI study and a barium enema may be necessary, particularly in patients with an extensive history of previous abdominal surgery.

Patients with a long-term history of PN could suffer multiple deep vein thromboses. Precise information about central line access is crucial if these patients have been maintained on PN for a prolonged period or have a history of frequent line infections. When all conventional

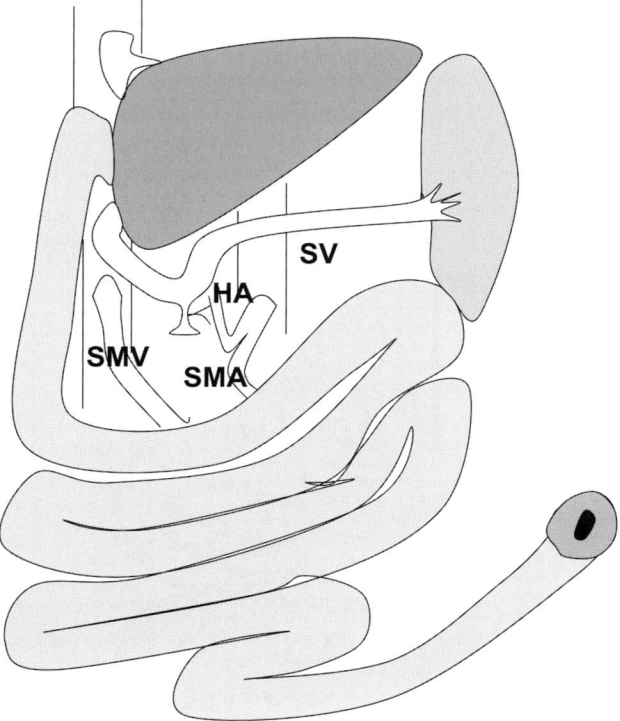

FIGURE 53–2

Noncomposite liver and intestine transplant. HA, hepatic artery; SMA, superior mesenteric artery; SMV, superior mesenteric vein; SV, splenic vein.

access to major veins is lost, cutdown of an intercostal vein, insertion of a catheter into the azygos vein via thoracoscopy, or direct insertion of the catheter into the inferior vena cava (IVC) by puncture of a lumbar vein may be considered.

Long-term PN-dependent patients could also have chronic renal insufficiency. Patients with substantial renal impairment may be considered for simultaneous kidney transplantation because the nephrotoxicity of immunosuppression drugs may lead to renal failure after transplantation and dialysis access is limited in these patients.

Surgical Technique

Donor Selection and Harvesting of Grafts

Donors for combined liver and GI grafts are selected on the basis of ABO blood group and body size. Although a few instances of successful use of ABO-compatible but non–ABO-identical donors have been reported,[30] this procedure has not been widely performed because of fear that it will cause complications such as serious hemolysis as a result of the relatively large hematopoietic

component of the graft. The donor should be smaller than the recipient. Donors with half the recipient's body weight can be a perfect size match because the recipient's abdominal cavity is contracted as a result of the short bowel. Cytotoxic cross-match has not been a criterion for donor selection. To date, no report has suggested an impact of cytotoxic cross-match on the outcome of recipients of composite liver and GI grafts, despite a report from our own institution suggesting its relationship to vascular rejection of the intestinal component of the graft.[31]

A composite liver and GI graft is normally harvested via an en bloc technique.[32] All the abdominal organs can be harvested en bloc and separated at the back-table according to the patient's need. Our standard technique of en bloc harvesting starts with mobilization of the right hemicolon and the duodenum until the anterior surface of the vena cava and aorta are exposed. The spleen and pancreas are then mobilized from the left side, thereby dissecting the avascular plane of the retroperitoneum. After being flushed with cold University of Wisconsin solution, the esophagus is transected above the diaphragm and the colon is separated at the level of the sigmoid colon. The colon could be separated from the stomach before the cold flush. The thoracic aorta is divided in the chest, and the abdominal side of the aorta is divided between the superior mesenteric artery (SMA) and the renal arteries. As much as possible of the donor's thoracic aorta should be harvested because it can be used as a conduit for arterial reconstruction.

Transplantation of the Liver and Intestine

The minimal organs to be transplanted in patients with liver and intestinal failure are the liver and the small bowel. Traditionally, this type of transplantation has been performed en bloc, thus retaining the continuity of the portal vein. When the liver and small bowel graft is prepared, the stomach, pancreas, and duodenum are removed from the organ block at the back-table. The native portal system can be anastomosed to the splenic vein of the donor, or it could be drained into the systemic circulation via an end-to-side portocaval shunt (see Fig. 53–1). This technique requires biliary reconstruction and has not been used frequently in recent years. Alternatively, grafts containing the liver, intestine, and pancreaticoduodenal complex (described in the next section) can be used.

The liver and small bowel can be grafted separately as well (see Fig. 53–2). When the organs are separated, the liver and bowel can be reduced easily without the necessity of preserving the root of the mesentery or the portal vein. The total size of the organ can be reduced much more than possible with the en bloc reduced liver

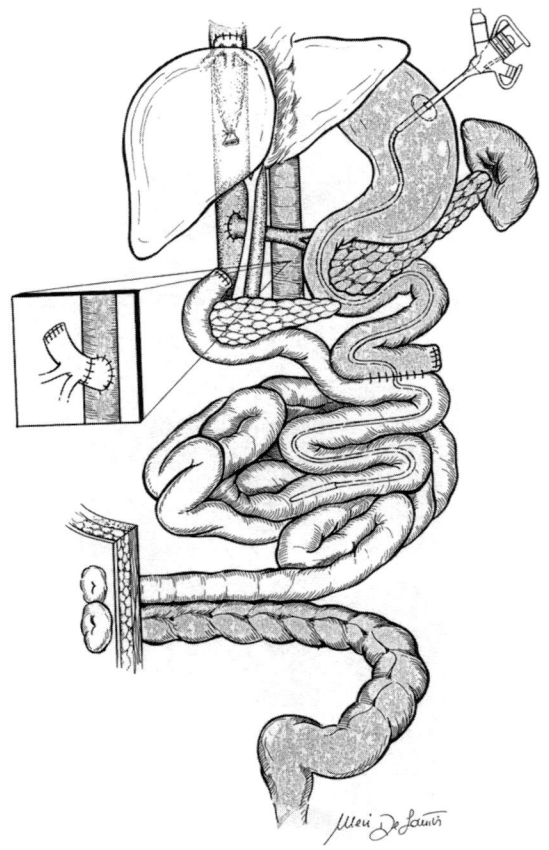

FIGURE 53-3

Transplantation of the liver and intestine with the pancreaticoduodenal complex.

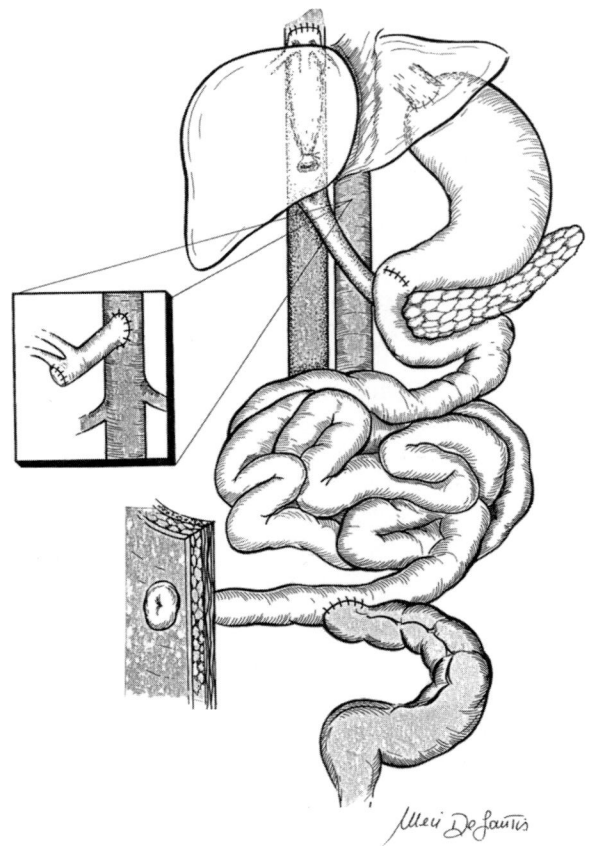

FIGURE 53-4

Multivisceral transplantation.

and bowel graft. We have performed separate grafting in five cases.[33] The whole liver was used in two cases and the left lateral segment in three. The portal vein is reconstructed to the native portal vein taking flow only from the stomach, pancreas, and spleen. The bowel component of the graft can be transplanted as for isolated bowel transplantation. The superior mesenteric vein (SMV) of the donor's small bowel is anastomosed to the IVC or the native SMV. The arterial anastomosis is fashioned with a Y-graft onto the infrarenal aorta for both the liver and intestine grafts. With this method, the liver and bowel grafts are completely separated. Such separation allows us to change one component of the graft while leaving the other untouched. In one of our cases, graft injury of unknown cause (possibly atypical rejection) developed in the small bowel, and graft enterectomy was required. We transplanted an intestinal graft from another donor but left the liver component of the original graft untouched. In another of our cases, primary graft nonfunction developed in the liver component of the graft. Another liver graft from an adult donor (split technique) was immediately transplanted,

but the intestine from the primary pediatric donor was left untouched. Both recipients are still alive and well at 30 and 16 months' follow-up. The downside of grafting the organs separately is prolonged operative time, but the technique can theoretically be applied to a living donor procedure.

Transplantation of the Liver and Intestine with the Pancreaticoduodenal Complex

Langnas and coworkers were the first to perform liver and small bowel transplantation with preservation of the pancreaticoduodenal complex.[6] The original technique preserved a small rim of the pancreas with the duodenum. This technique was particularly useful with small pediatric donors because injury to the small vessels at the head of the pancreas could be avoided and biliary reconstruction was unnecessary (Fig. 53-3). The technique was then adopted by other large centers in the United States[5] and expanded to include the entire pancreas because of the risk of a pancreatic fistula when the pancreas was divided.[4] This form of transplantation is usually classified as a modification of liver and intestine transplantation (despite the fact that it includes multiple viscera) because the purpose of including the pancreas is not to replace the native pancreas but to address technical concerns.

When the pancreas is divided, the native portal vein could be connected to the stump of the splenic vein. When the entire pancreas is preserved, the native portal flow is drained into the vena cava via a portocaval shunt. The graft's duodenal stump is closed, and reconstruction of the GI tract involves connecting the recipient duodenum or jejunum to the side of the graft's jejunum (see Fig. 53–3). The lower GI reconstruction can be a side-to-end ileocolostomy with a terminal ileostomy (see Fig. 53–4), a Mikulicz ileocolostomy (see Fig. 53–3), or an ileocolostomy with a loop ileostomy.

Including the colon in the graft has been abandoned because of findings of a previous study.[34] However, patients who received a graft containing a small portion of the colon with the ileocecal valve produced very well-formed stools after the transplant procedure. Including the colon may be reconsidered for patients with a short native colon. In treating a few recent patients with very short native colons, we left a small portion of the colon (essentially only the cecum) with an intact ileocecal valve in the graft; there have been no serious problems to date.

Multivisceral Transplantation

Multivisceral transplantation is usually defined as en bloc transplantation of the stomach, pancreas, intestine, and liver (Fig. 53–4). The donor organs replace the native stomach, pancreas, and spleen in this form of transplantation. When multivisceral transplantation is performed in a patient with serious portal hypertension and collateralized adhesions, a "quick devascularization" technique is useful. After entering the abdomen and before dissecting any other structure, we mobilize the spleen and pancreas from the retroperitoneum and expose the left side of the roots of the celiac artery and SMA. Even in patients who have undergone multiple abdominal operations, it is relatively easy to enter the retroperitoneal plane without causing blood loss. After the esophagus has been transected and the stomach has been retracted downward, the roots of the celiac artery and SMA can be clamped en mass. This procedure dramatically decreases oozing in the surgical field. As soon as the vascular pedicle has been mass-clamped, the entire abdominal viscera lose blood circulation and go into what is essentially an anhepatic condition. For patients with relatively fewer adhesions and less intense

portal hypertension, preserving a small piece of the cardia of the stomach is useful because it prevents reflux disease by preserving the native gastroesophageal junction and makes GI reconstruction easier by allowing a gastrogastric anastomosis rather than an esophagogastric anastomosis, which requires anastomosis in a deeper plane. So that a small rim of stomach can be retained, an ascending branch of the left gastric artery must be preserved together with the celiac axis.

The hepatectomy should be performed in piggyback fashion with continuity of the vena cava because venous access for venovenous bypass is limited in these patients, who have a history of long-term use of PN. Once the upper part of the abdomen has been exenterated, the lower portion of the abdomen can be easily dissected. After the colon has been divided, all the abdominal organs are removed en bloc.

Arterial inflow to the multivisceral grafts can come from the infrarenal aorta or the suprarenal aorta. It is important that the surgeon determine the best anatomic alignment on the basis of the recipient's and donor's anatomy. We usually insert an interpositional graft of thoracic aorta from the donor before bringing the organ block to the surgical field because direct anastomosis to the aorta while holding a large cluster of organs can be very difficult. The aorta or a large aortic patch that includes the celiac artery and the SMA of the donor organ cluster is then anastomosed to this interpositional graft. Venous outflow is reconstructed by anastomosing the suprahepatic vena cava to the joined orifice of the native hepatic veins, just as is done in the usual piggyback technique for liver transplantation.

The organs are then flushed with blood through the donor infrahepatic vena cava after the arterial clamp has been opened. Because of the large size of the organ cluster, hyperkalemic cardiac arrest can occur at the time of reperfusion if the organs are not well flushed.

Upper GI reconstruction entails esophagogastrostomy or gastrogastrostomy, depending on the division line of the native stomach. When the small rim of the native stomach is left with the ascending branch of the left gastric artery, gastrogastric anastomosis provides a very easy and wide connection. It preserves the native gastroesophageal junction and prevents potential complications of esophagogastric anastomosis such as reflux or stricture. When preservation of the native gastroesophageal junction is not technically possible or the patient has a history of reflux disease, esophagogastrostomy is required. We have been performing this anastomosis in a hand-sewn fashion. In our experience, serious reflux disease developed in one case and stricture in two cases in which this anastomosis was used. The strictures were successfully treated by balloon dilatation, and the reflux was surgically corrected, with satisfactory outcomes to date. Pyloroplasty is performed to facilitate gastric emptying because of denervation of the stomach.

Postoperative Care

Postoperative care of patients who have received combined liver and GI transplants is very different from that of patients who have received isolated liver transplants. Acute rejection of the small bowel can progress very rapidly, and advanced stages of rejection are associated with a very high mortality rate.[35,36] Therefore, patients require a high level of immunosuppression, and as a consequence, they are at increased risk for infectious complications. Currently, an immunomodulatory approach rather than pure intensification of immunosuppression is being studied in centers in the United States. The preliminary data are encouraging, but a longer follow-up period is needed.

Immunosuppression

The care of recipients of grafts that include the small intestine has always been challenging because of the serious consequences of intestinal graft rejection. For these patients, unlike those who receive isolated liver transplants, steroids and calcineurin inhibitors such as tacrolimus (Prograf) or cyclosporine (Neoral) alone are not sufficient to control bowel rejection. Various immunosuppressive agents have been used in intestinal transplantation. Table 53-3 summarizes the immunosuppressants used at our institution for recipients of intestinal grafts. At the beginning of our program we tried OKT3 and cyclophosphamide for induction, with no substantial improvement in outcome. These regimens were abandoned because of their strong side effects. We then used no induction with triple immunosuppression consisting of tacrolimus, steroids, and mycophenolate mofetil, but this combination also failed to improve the outcome. The use of daclizumab (Zenapax) seemed to stabilize the situation. However, this improvement in

outcome is not solely attributable to improvement in immunosuppression because patient selection, surgical technique, and postoperative monitoring of recipients also improved as our experience accumulated.

Other transplant centers similarly use a conventional immunosuppressive approach. Induction with an interleukin-2 receptor antagonist such as daclizumab or basiliximab (Simulect) together with tacrolimus and steroids seems to provide adequate coverage against intestinal rejection.[37] Using sirolimus (Rapamune) together with a tacrolimus-based regimen is also reported to improve outcomes.[38]

Recently, an antilymphocyte preparation with rabbit antithymocyte globulin (Thymoglobulin), or alemtuzumab (Campath 1H) has been used at large transplant centers in North America in an attempt to induce tolerance. At our own institution, we have used Campath 1H since 2000. Campath 1H is a humanized monoclonal anti-CD52 antibody that can rapidly deplete T lymphocytes completely and B lymphocytes and monocytes to a lesser degree. It was first used to treat patients in the field of oncology. Campath 1H was initially used for recipients of kidney transplants by Calne and colleagues at the University of Cambridge.[39] These researchers showed that kidney recipients who underwent Campath 1H induction could be treated with low-dose cyclosporine monotherapy. In our preliminary report of 12 adult recipients of intestinal and multivisceral grafts, Campath 1H combined with tacrolimus seemed to provide adequate control of small bowel allograft rejection without increasing the likelihood of opportunistic infection.[40]

Monitoring

Because bowel rejection can progress rapidly and in advanced stages is associated with very high mortality rates, monitoring of the bowel allograft is a very important issue in the management of intestinal transplants. The anatomic nature of intestinal grafts makes monitoring more challenging. The results of biopsy of the stoma are often misleading because of surgical damage to the tissue in the area. Thus far, the sole means of performing biopsy of the bowel allograft is endoscopy, but only a very limited portion of the entire graft can be accessed by endoscopy. To enhance endoscopic surveillance, we introduced the use of zoom endoscopy in 1999.[41] With the use of magnification, changes in intestinal mucosa can be observed in greater detail.

Common symptoms of rejection are fever and increased output from the stoma. At a more advanced stage of rejection, bloody discharge from the stoma or sloughing of tissue in the stomal discharge can be observed. Stomal output can also be decreased because of ileus caused by the rejection. However, at an early

Year	Induction	Maintenance
1994–1995	OKT3 or cyclophosphamide	Tacrolimus + steroids
1996–1997	No induction	Tacrolimus + steroids + MMF
1998–2001	Daclizumab	Tacrolimus + steroids
2001–2005	Campath 1H or daclizumab	Tacrolimus or tacrolimus + steroids

Table 53–3. IMMUNOSUPPRESSION REGIMENS AT THE UNIVERSITY OF MIAMI

MMF, mycophenolate mofetil.

Table 53-4. PROTOCOL ENDOSCOPY SCHEDULE

Postoperative Period	Frequency
First 2 weeks	Every 2–4 days
3–8 weeks	Weekly
2–6 months until stoma closure	Monthly
During the course of rejection	Every 2–4 days

stage of rejection, all the aforementioned symptoms may be absent. Because bowel rejection can progress rapidly to an advanced stage, the bowel graft may no longer be salvageable once these symptoms are obvious. In an attempt to detect rejection in its early stage, most centers are now performing surveillance endoscopy and biopsy as part of the treatment protocol. Our surveillance schedule is shown in Table 53–4.

Because the bowel allograft is a long, hollow organ and because biopsy can be performed on only a small portion of the entire graft, it is ideal to have a serum marker for bowel graft rejection. A recent study at our center suggested that the serum citrulline concentration can be used as such a marker.[42]

In cases of isolated liver transplantation, increase in a liver chemical profile suggests that liver biopsy is necessary. However, in cases of combined liver and bowel transplantation, increased transaminase levels do not necessarily indicate the need for liver biopsy because isolated liver rejection occurs very rarely in recipients of composite grafts. Increases in transaminase activity can occur in conjunction with bowel rejection or other infectious processes rather than liver rejection per se. Biopsy of the liver would not provide much information relevant to patient care.

Nutrition

Nutritional management after liver and GI transplantation is an important issue. In the past, we began feeding patients as soon as we saw output from the stoma because general surgical experience had indicated that early feeding could prevent bacterial translocation or villus atrophy. We have encountered what appears to be necrotizing enterocolitis in two patients.[43] Both exhibited symptoms of acute abdominal distention and pneumatosis intestinalis at about the seventh postoperative day after a perfect recovery from the surgical procedure. Both patients were maintained on full feeding with no total parental nutrition (TPN) at the time. The precise pathogenesis of necrotizing enterocolitis is unknown, but it appears to occur when a baby's enteral feeding is increased. Since encountering these episodes, we have been more conservative in starting feeding.

We do not usually initiate feeding for a week so that the graft can recover from the ischemic damage.

Feedings could consist of a complete elemental formula (amino acid formula) or a formula with protein hydrolysates. Each individual graft tolerates feeding differently; some may tolerate volume better than osmolarity, whereas some may tolerate osmolarity better than volume. Management of feeding must be adjusted to fit each patient's needs. In general, we start feeding at half strength and increase the volume to about half the required volume. At that point, we stop increasing the volume and concentrate on increasing the formula to full strength in a few days. Once the formula is at full strength, we again begin to increase the volume until the required volume is reached. Some patients show significant feeding intolerance and require special modification of the formula.

The reason for high stomal output is still unknown. Loss of signal from the autonomic nervous system, decreased water reabsorption capacity, and hypermotility are believed to contribute to the problem to various degrees. The high-output problem seems to last for a long time, but the graft will finally adjust and the problem will disappear. Loperamide, diphenoxylate with atropine (Lomotil), and paregoric are commonly used to control output while patients are in the high-output phase. Octreotide can also be used to treat patients with high output.

Postoperative Complications

Rejection

Acute rejection of small bowel allografts has been a challenge in the management of combined liver and GI transplants. With conventional immunosuppression, the incidence of mild rejection exceeds 80% and that of severe rejection is around 10% to 30%.[37,44-46] Severe rejection, defined as exfoliation of the surface epithelium, is associated with a very high mortality rate.[35,36] Once the rejection progresses to a severe stage, recovery is very difficult.

Histologically, acute cellular rejection of an intestinal allograft starts with edema, blunting of the villi, a mild degree of mixed cellular infiltrates, and crypt cell apoptosis. Symptoms of moderate rejection include more blunting of villi with more intense infiltrates, damage in more than 50% of crypts, and the presence of confluent apoptosis in a crypt or crypt abscesses. When the rejection progresses further, surface epithelium is lost, and a massive mixed cellular infiltrate with crypt necrosis (or disappearance of crypt cells) is seen. The tissue may appear to be granulation tissue.

In views through a zoom endoscope, a mild degree of rejection appears as background erythema and mild blunting of villi. The space between villi seems to be expanded. Intravillous hemorrhage can also be seen in the early stage of rejection. At more advanced stages of rejection, the villi seem to be shortened and their length appears irregular; in addition, erythema in the background and within villi is increased, as is mucosal friability. In severe stages of rejection, the surface epithelium is sloughed off and the graft appears denuded and hemorrhagic (mucosal exfoliation). Villi are lost and the surface is flattened.

A steroid bolus and OKT3 have been used to treat rejection. Because intestinal rejection can progress very rapidly, we do not hesitate to start OKT3 if the rejection is not adequately responding to steroid boluses. Rapamycin can be added to boost baseline immunosuppression after refractory rejection. The response rate to OKT3 is quite good for mild to moderate rejection but very poor for severe exfoliative rejection.[35,36]

Vascular rejection of a small bowel allograft is an evolving concept in this field of transplantation.[31] This unusual type of rejection typically causes intravillous hemorrhage without increased cellular infiltrates in the lamina propria. Endoscopy reveals that the graft appears inflamed with increased erythema within villi. The picture of vascular rejection and cellular rejection is mixed when the rejection progresses further; at the most advanced stage of rejection the same exfoliation of the mucosa would occur. Vascular rejection seems to correlate with a positive cytotoxic cross-match. First-line treatment of vascular rejection would be steroids, but second-line treatment may be OKT3. Intravenous immune globulin may be used. However, the effectiveness of these treatments for vascular rejection remains unknown.

The incidence and natural course of chronic rejection of bowel allografts have not been well documented. In our experience, chronic rejection appears to correlate with the development of arteriopathy and fibrosis of the graft, just as with other solid-organ transplants. Clinical symptoms could include feeding intolerance, malabsorption, or the formation of a stricture or strictures in the bowel graft. It is not easy to assess this process with mucosal biopsy; however, submucosal fibrosis may be associated with chronic rejection.[47] Endoscopically, the mucosal surface could appear normal but the lumen will not distend with increased fibrosis. No effective therapy has been reported.

Liver rejection is rare in association with combined liver and GI transplantation. Most of the time the elevation in transaminase activity or bilirubin concentration is the result of causes other than liver rejection. Biopsy of the liver in such situations would not provide much information. Some of the increased hepatic enzyme activity seems to take a very benign course with no substantial clinical relevance. Rejection of other organs in a multivisceral graft is also very rare.

Technical Complications

Some of the technical complications that can occur after combined liver and GI transplantation could be fatal. A relatively high degree of contamination is associated with this procedure and can at times cause infectious pseudoaneurysm or rupture of an arterial anastomosis. The consequences of this complication are almost always fatal. Long-term antibiotic use before the transplant procedure, abdominal contamination caused by entering the bowel during the surgical procedure, or postsurgical peritonitis may contribute to this complication.

A leak at the GI anastomosis could also be a fatal complication of this procedure because of the high level of immunosuppression required. It is important that the surgical team maintain a high level of intensity throughout the procedure. When the operative time is prolonged, having a second surgical team perform the GI reconstruction may be advisable.

Infection

As a consequence of the relatively high level of immunosuppression, infectious complications are the most common cause of death in recipients of composite abdominal organ transplants. A wide variety of organisms can cause disease with different levels of seriousness. Viral infection can lead to serious consequences, particularly in children.

Adenovirus enteritis can complicate bowel transplantation[48-50]; its symptoms can mimic those of rejection because the two conditions could have a similar clinical course. Once damage to the graft reaches a certain level, differentiating adenovirus enteritis from rejection is difficult, even with pathological assessment. A diagnosis of adenovirus infection could be made by polymerase chain reaction (PCR) of tissue, immunoperoxidase staining, or culture of tissue or stomal output. However, these tests are not always readily available or may take a long time. In such circumstances, endoscopy of the native organ can help differentiate the process of infectious disease from that of rejection. Endoscopic surveillance of the anastomotic suture line is particularly useful. Clear demarcation between a very inflamed graft and a normal-appearing native bowel is a strong indication of rejection, whereas the presence of similar pathological indicators on the native organ may suggest an infectious disease process.

Other unusual infectious processes seen in bowel grafts are mycobacterial enterocolitis,[51] *Cryptosporidium* infection,[52] and herpes simplex enterocolitis.[53] Necrotizing fasciitis could be a complication of composite abdominal organ transplantation because of the relatively contaminated nature of the surgical procedure.[54]

Posttransplant Lymphoproliferative Disease

Posttransplant lymphoproliferative disease (PTLD) complicates this form of transplantation relatively more frequently than other forms of transplantation (reported incidence of 5% to 20%).[37,45,46] The diagnosis of PTLD is made by biopsy of the tissue. The use of various forms of Epstein-Barr virus (EBV) PCR appears to be informative. Common sites of disease are the GI tract and the mesenteric lymph nodes, but it could occur in any location. Symptoms vary widely from patient to patient and include fever of unknown origin, malaise, diarrhea, symptoms of upper respiratory infection, hepatosplenomegaly, abdominal distention, and peripheral lymphadenopathy, but in some cases symptoms are completely lacking. If PTLD is suspected, we routinely perform surveillance computed tomography and GI biopsy. When patients have palpable lymph nodes, biopsy should be performed. Tonsillectomy can also help with the diagnosis in pediatric patients.

Biopsy of the GI tract (the stomach, duodenum, and colonic mucosa) can provide useful information for the diagnosis of PTLD. PTLD lesions in the GI tract typically cause a diffuse nodular appearance in the mucosa, but even when the endoscopic appearance is normal, biopsy may still show an abnormally increased level of lymphoplasmacytic infiltrates. If the infiltrating cells test positive for EBV by in situ hybridization (EBER stain), the condition should be considered to be PTLD. It is important to note that surveillance biopsies do not necessarily target the primary lesion. For example, the main lesion may be in the abdominal lymph nodes, but the extent of the disease may be seen in the GI biopsy specimen. Therefore, the early appearance of tissue retrieved by GI biopsy may not actually show the early stage of the disease but, instead, may show only the tip of the iceberg.

The most important treatment of PTLD is stopping the immunosuppressive regimen. Most cases of PTLD respond to cessation of the immunosuppressive agent. However, in bowel transplantation, complete cessation may induce rejection and complicate the situation. We recently began using anti-CD20 antibody (rituximab) as first-line therapy for PTLD.[55] Rituximab could be used in a prolonged course, thus increasing the treatment response rate. Conventional chemotherapy is not recommended as first-line treatment of PTLD because it could suppress the immune system.

Graft-versus-Host Disease

Graft-versus-host disease (GVHD) is one of the most feared complications in association with this form of transplantation because the bowel contains a large amount of lymphoid tissue. In recent experience with liver and GI transplantation, GVHD is a relatively rare complication. Once GVHD occurs, however, it could be very persistent and eventually fatal, as is the case in transplantation of other solid organs. GVHD is treated with a steroid bolus and increased immunosuppression; however, an increase in immunosuppression could increase the risk for infection and could thus be fatal.

Outcomes

The history of small bowel transplantation is still relatively short. Cumulative worldwide experience has amounted to just 989 cases in the most updated information from the Intestinal Transplant Registry (D. Grant, University of Toronto, personal communication, May 2003). Of these cases, 556 included liver transplantation. The results of liver and GI transplantation are improving but are still far behind the outcomes of conventional liver transplantation. Since 2001, patient survival rates after liver and small bowel transplantation have been 59.0% at 1 year and 51.3% at 2 years; graft survival rates in the same periods have been 56.5% and 46.5% (Kaplan-Meier method). In contrast, patient survival rates after multivisceral transplantation have been 63.5% at 1 year and 63.5% at 2 years; graft survival rates at the same time periods have been 63.5% and 63.5%.

At the University of Miami, we have performed 32 liver and intestine transplant procedures and 81 multivisceral transplant procedures. More multivisceral transplant procedures have been performed than in the past since we expanded their use to small children who would benefit from the creation of more space by means of multivisceral transplantation (see earlier). The results of multivisceral transplant procedures in children in our program have improved substantially in recent years (Fig. 53–5). One-year patient and graft survival rates were both higher than 90% in the most recent series.

The causes of death after liver and GI transplantation at our institution are listed in Table 53–5. The primary causes are rejection and infection associated with immunosuppressive therapy. Technical failure could also be a relatively frequent cause of death after this form of transplantation.

Our recent study analyzing the outcome of 70 children who received small bowel transplants for short-gut syndrome at our center between 1994 and 2002[29] showed that factors substantially affecting patient survival were age of the patient at the time of transplantation and pretransplant clinical stability of the patient. Our study included 25 cases of liver and small bowel transplantation and 23 cases of multivisceral transplantation. It appears that when grafts that include the

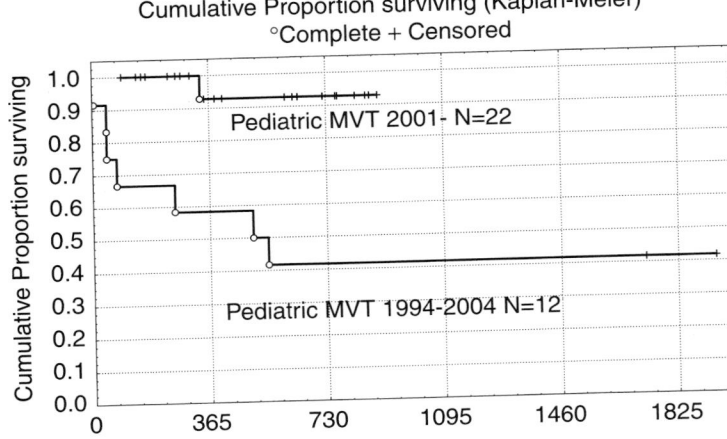

FIGURE 53–5

Survival of pediatric multivisceral transplant (MVT) recipients at the University of Miami (Kaplan-Meier method). (Recipients of Campath 1H induction are not included.)

small bowel are used to treat children, the results of the transplant procedure improve when the patient's condition is stable enough so that the procedure can be delayed until the child is older. In contrast, in the same analysis we found that a substantial proportion of patients died while on the waiting list, predominantly as a result of GI bleeding. The indication for intestinal transplantation in young children was primarily liver involvement (75% of recipients who received transplants at younger than 1 year experienced liver failure). This finding suggests that there is a subgroup of patients in whom liver failure develops at an early age and that these patients require urgent transplantation as a life-saving option. On the basis of this analysis, we proposed an algorithm for patient referral to a transplant center (Fig. 53–6). If infants or neonates with short-bowel syndrome also have liver disease, they should be referred to a transplant center to be evaluated for combined liver and GI transplantation. If they do not have liver disease, they should be monitored carefully and provided with TPN and a bowel adaptation protocol. During the follow-up period, if liver disease or a recurrent line infection develops, thus depleting the

line access site, the patient should be referred to a transplant center. If no liver disease develops and the patient's condition remains stable with TPN, we try to wait until they reach the age of 3 years for bowel adaptation. If the bowel does not adapt and permanent TPN dependency becomes a reality, patients should be referred to a transplant center for determination of the indication and timing for transplantation of a bowel graft that does not include the liver.

Related Procedures

Abdominal Wall Transplantation

A contracted abdominal cavity is one of the biggest problems associated with transplantation in patients with short-gut syndrome. As mentioned earlier ("Donor Selection and Harvesting of Grafts"), for recipients with a small, contracted abdomen, the ideal donor could

Table 53-5. CAUSE OF DEATH OF LIVER AND GASTROINTESTINAL TRANSPLANT RECIPIENTS	
Causes of Death	**N**
Sepsis/multisystem organ failure	19
Rejection	11
Pneumonia	4
Aortic disruption/aortoenteric fistula	3
Pancreatitis	2
Necrotizing fasciitis	2
Aspergillosis	2

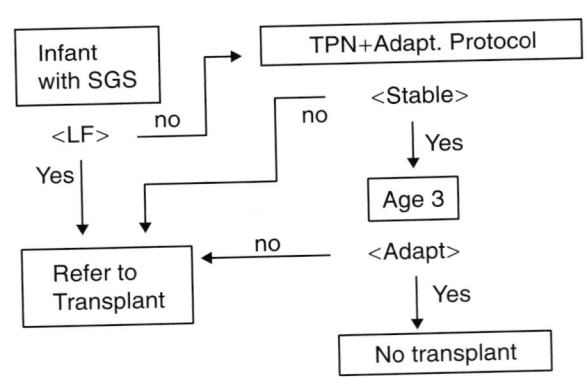

FIGURE 53–6

Proposed algorithm for children with short-gut syndrome (SGS). LF, liver failure; TPN, total parenteral nutrition.

have half the body size of the recipient. Furthermore, when patients have either a substantial abdominal wall defect caused by multiple enterocutaneous fistulas or multiple stomas as a result of numerous surgeries, closure of the abdomen is practically impossible after liver and GI transplantation. We recently implemented the use of full-thickness abdominal wall allografts (including skin, muscle, and peritoneum) to compensate for the abdominal wall defect.[56] To date, we have performed abdominal wall transplantation in 9 patients with abdominal wall defects who received intestinal transplants.

For this procedure, the donor abdominal wall (with bilateral inferior epigastric arteries and veins and with continuity of the iliac vessels) is harvested from deceased donors. The vessels are connected to the common iliac artery and vein or to the aorta or the IVC in an end-to-side fashion (Fig. 53–7). The abdominal wall graft can be harvested from the same donor from whom the visceral organ graft was taken, or it can be harvested from a different donor. When an abdominal wall graft from a different donor is used, transplantation of the abdominal wall can be performed as a separate procedure a few days to a week after transplantation of the visceral organs (the abdomen should be closed with synthetic mesh while the patient is waiting for an abdominal wall transplant). The advantage of using a different donor is that we can select a larger donor to provide a larger abdominal wall graft and a smaller donor to provide the visceral organs. It is also beneficial to perform abdominal wall transplantation a few days after the visceral organ transplantation because the patient will have less edema and closure of the abdomen will be easier.

Table 53–6. DEMOGRAPHIC CHARACTERISTICS AND OUTCOME OF ABDOMINAL WALL TRANSPLANT RECIPIENTS

Age	Sex	Diagnosis	Transplant Type	Patient Status (Month of Follow-up)
53	F	Midgut strangulation	MV	Alive (30)
1	F	Gastroschisis	MV	Died
2	M	Hirschsprung's disease	MV	Alive
21	M	Blunt trauma	ISB	Alive (19)
41	M	Desmoid tumor	ISB	Died
6	F	Midgut volvulus	MV	Died
15	M	Blunt trauma	ISB	Alive (11)
19	M	Penetrating trauma	ISB	Died
19	F	Desmoid tumor	MV	Alive (4)

ISB, isolated small bowel; MV, multivisceral.

Table 53–6 summarizes the demographic characteristics and outcomes of our nine patients. Five of the nine underwent multivisceral transplantation. Four were children and five were adults. Five of the nine are currently alive, four of them with an intact abdominal wall. Two patients died during the early postoperative course, one at 5 months postoperatively as a result of sepsis, and one at 7 months as a result of anoxic brain injury. Three of four patients had an intact abdominal wall graft at death. Three patients experienced rejection of the abdominal wall graft that was manifested as erythema, a maculopapular rash of the grafted skin, or both.[57]

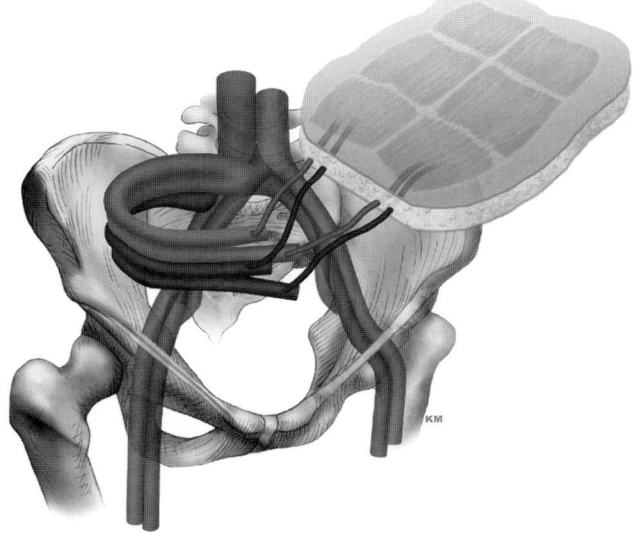

A

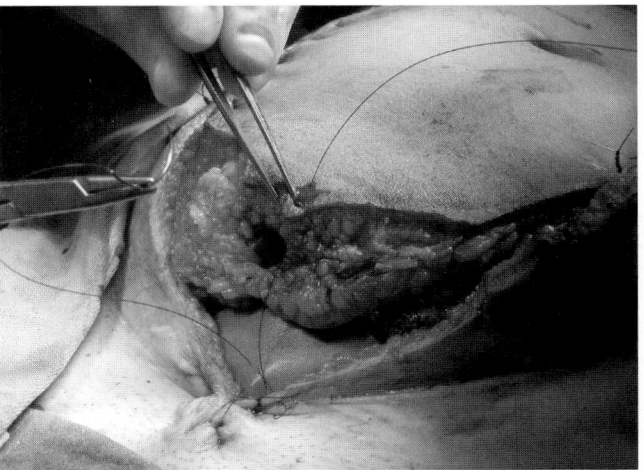

B

FIGURE 53–7

Implantation of an abdominal wall graft.

All episodes of abdominal wall rejection reversed with treatment.

Intestinal Autotransplantation

Certain types of tumors (e.g., desmoid tumor) that extensively involve the small bowel mesentery have generally been treated with small bowel transplantation if the development of short-bowel syndrome is imminent because of resection of the tumor.[58] However, when the mesenteric mass is confined to the root of the mesentery but most of the small bowel at the periphery of the mesentery is free of tumor, part or all of the small bowel could be reimplanted after resection of the tumor. This procedure, intestinal autotransplantation, involves en bloc removal of the tumor together with the small bowel, the head of the pancreas or the entire pancreas, the duodenum, and part of the colon. The tumor is resected ex vivo, and the tumor-free segment of the bowel is reimplanted. This procedure was developed to treat patients with a mass confined to the area around the root of the mesentery.[59,60]

We have performed eight intestinal autotransplantation procedures. All the masses were located at the root of the mesentery; some directly involved the head of the pancreas and the duodenum. The head of the pancreas, the duodenum, and part of the colon were excised together with the tumor because the SMA had to be divided at its takeoff from the aorta. The entire pancreas and the spleen were excised when preservation of the splenic artery was impossible. After en bloc removal of the mass together with the small bowel, part of the colon, the duodenum, and part of the pancreas (or the entire organ), the organ block was flushed at the back-table with cold preservation solution. The tumor-free segment of the bowel was then separated at the back-table in a bloodless field. The small bowel autograft was implanted by using the same technique as performed for isolated small bowel transplantation.

Pearls and Pitfalls

Pearls
- The composition of the graft should be individualized to the patient's needs.
- A relatively smaller size donor may make the best size match for the recipient because the recipient's abdominal cavity is often contracted as a result of a short gut.
- Be flexible in designing arterial reconstruction. Take into consideration graft size and recipient anatomy.

Pearls and Pitfalls—cont'd

- The "quick devascularization technique" is useful when performing multivisceral transplantation in patients with advanced portal hypertension.
- The best "treatment" of rejection is early recognition, and to that end, endoscopic surveillance with protocol mucosal biopsies is imperative.

Pitfalls
- The clinical signs and symptoms of rejection are nonspecific and appear late. Do not wait until tomorrow to perform a biopsy. Biopsy today!
- Rejection can progress rapidly and can be devastating. Use OKT3 early!
- Mucosal biopsy near the stoma can yield misleading information. Endoscopically directed biopsies are far superior.
- Severe enteritis at times mimics bowel rejection. However, remember that regardless of its severity, rejection is limited to the graft. A biopsy specimen from some portion of the native intestine may help distinguish rejection from enteritis.

References

1. Grant D, Wall W, Mimeault R, et al: Successful small-bowel/liver transplantation. Lancet 335:181-184, 1990.
2. Starzl TE, Rowe MI, Todo S, et al: Transplantation of multiple abdominal viscera. JAMA 261:1449-1457, 1989.
3. Williams JW, Sankary HN, Foster PF, et al: Splanchnic transplantation. An approach to the infant dependent on parenteral nutrition who develops irreversible liver disease. JAMA 261:1458-1462, 1989.
4. Kato T, Romero R, Verzaro R, et al: Inclusion of entire pancreas in the composite liver and intestinal graft in pediatric intestinal transplantation. Pediatr Transplant 3:210-214, 1999.
5. Bueno J, Abu-Elmagd K, Mazariegos G, et al: Composite liver–small bowel allografts with preservation of donor duodenum and hepatic biliary system in children. J Pediatr Surg 35:291-295, discussion 295-296, 2000.
6. Sudan DL, Iyer KR, Deroover A, et al: A new technique for combined liver/small intestinal transplantation. Transplantation 72:1846-1848, 2001.
7. Tzakis AG, Todo S, Madariaga J, et al: Upper-abdominal exenteration in transplantation for extensive malignancies of the upper abdomen—an update. Transplantation 51:727-728, 1991.
8. Sondheimer JM, Asturias E, Cadnapaphornchai M: Infection and cholestasis in neonates with intestinal resection and long-term parenteral nutrition. J Pediatr Gastroenterol Nutr 27:131-137, 1998.
9. Meehan JJ, Georgeson KE: Prevention of liver failure in parenteral nutrition–dependent children with short bowel syndrome. J Pediatr Surg 32:473-475, 1997.
10. Kubota A, Yonekura T, Hoki M, et al: Total parenteral nutrition–associated intrahepatic cholestasis in infants: 25 years' experience. J Pediatr Surg 35:1049-1051, 2000.

11. Andorsky DJ, Lund DP, Lillehei CW, et al: Nutritional and other postoperative management of neonates with short bowel syndrome correlates with clinical outcomes. J Pediatr 139:27-33, 2001.

12. Grosfeld JL, Rescorla FJ, West KW: Short bowel syndrome in infancy and childhood. Analysis of survival in 60 patients. Am J Surg 151:41-46, 1986.

13. Jackson CC, Wu Y, Chenren S, et al: Bile decompression in children with histopathological evidence of pre-existing liver cirrhosis. Am Surg 68:816-819, 2002.

14. Hammel P, Couvelard A, O'Toole D, et al: Regression of liver fibrosis after biliary drainage in patients with chronic pancreatitis and stenosis of the common bile duct. N Engl J Med 344:418-423, 2001.

15. Bonis PA, Friedman SL, Kaplan MM: Is liver fibrosis reversible? N Engl J Med 344:452-454, 2001.

16. Fryer J, Pellar S, Ormond D, et al: Mortality in candidates waiting for combined liver-intestine transplants exceeds that for other candidates waiting for liver transplants. Liver Transpl 9:748-753, 2003.

17. Horslen SP, Sudan DL, Iyer KR, et al: Isolated liver transplantation in infants with end-stage liver disease associated with short bowel syndrome. Ann Surg 235:435-439, 2002.

18. Driver CP, Bruce J, Bianchi A, et al: The contemporary outcome of gastroschisis. J Pediatr Surg 35:1719-1723, 2000.

19. Molik KA, Gingalewski CA, West KW, et al: Gastroschisis: A plea for risk categorization. J Pediatr Surg 36:51-55, 2001.

20. Ladd AP, Rescorla FJ, West KW, et al: Long-term follow-up after bowel resection for necrotizing enterocolitis: Factors affecting outcome. J Pediatr Surg 33:967-972, 1998.

21. Grosfeld JL, Cheu H, Schlatter M, et al: Changing trends in necrotizing enterocolitis. Experience with 302 cases in two decades. Ann Surg 214:300-306, discussion 306-307, 1991.

22. Horwitz JR, Lally KP, Cheu HW, et al: Complications after surgical intervention for necrotizing enterocolitis: A multicenter review. J Pediatr Surg 30:994-998, discussion 998-999, 1995.

23. Sato S, Nishijima E, Muraji T, et al: Jejunoileal atresia: A 27-year experience. J Pediatr Surg 33:1633-1635, 1998.

24. Festen S, Brevoord JC, Goldhoorn GA, et al: Excellent long-term outcome for survivors of apple peel atresia. J Pediatr Surg 37:61-65, 2002.

25. Granata C, Puri P: Megacystis-microcolon-intestinal hypoperistalsis syndrome. J Pediatr Gastroenterol Nutr 25:12-19, 1997.

26. Masetti M, Rodriguez MM, Thompson JF, et al: Multivisceral transplantation for megacystis microcolon intestinal hypoperistalsis syndrome. Transplantation 68:228-232, 1999.

27. Bunn SK, Beath SV, McKeirnan PJ, et al: Treatment of microvillus inclusion disease by intestinal transplantation. J Pediatr Gastroenterol Nutr 31:176-180, 2000.

28. Oliva MM, Perman JA, Saavedra JM, et al: Successful intestinal transplantation for microvillus inclusion disease. Gastroenterology 106:771-774, 1994.

29. Kato T, Mittal N, Nishida S, et al: The role of intestinal transplantation in the management of babies with extensive gut resections. J Pediatr Surg 38:145-149, 2003.

30. Sindhi R, Landmark J, Shaw BW Jr, et al: Combined liver/small bowel transplantation using a blood group compatible but non-identical donor. Transplantation 61:1782-1783, 1996.

31. Ruiz P, Garcia M, Pappas P, et al: Mucosal vascular alterations in isolated small-bowel allografts: Relationship to humoral sensitization. Am J Transplant 3:43-49, 2003.

32. Casavilla A, Selby R, Abu-Elmagd K, et al: Logistics and technique for combined hepatic-intestinal retrieval. Ann Surg 216:605-609, 1992.

33. Kato T, Tzakis AG: Noncomposite simultaneous liver and intestinal transplantation. Transplantation 78:485, author reply 485-486, 2004.

34. Todo S, Reyes J, Furukawa H, et al: Outcome analysis of 71 clinical intestinal transplantations. Ann Surg 222:270-280, discussion 280-282, 1995.

35. Ishii T, Mazariegos GV, Bueno J, et al: Exfoliative rejection after intestinal transplantation in children. Pediatr Transplant 7:185-191, 2003.

36. Kato T, Berho M, Weppler D, et al: Is severe rejection an indication for retransplantation? Transplant Proc 32:1201, 2000.

37. Farmer DG, McDiarmid SV, Yersiz H, et al: Outcome after intestinal transplantation: Results from one center's 9-year experience. Arch Surg 136:1027-1031, discussion 1031-1032, 2001.

38. Fishbein TM, Florman S, Gondolesi G, et al: Intestinal transplantation before and after the introduction of sirolimus. Transplantation 73:1538-1542, 2002.

39. Calne R, Moffatt SD, Friend PJ, et al: Campath IH allows low-dose cyclosporine monotherapy in 31 cadaveric renal allograft recipients. Transplantation 68:1613-1616, 1999.

40. Tzakis AG, Kato T, Nishida S, et al: Preliminary experience with campath 1H (C1H) in intestinal and liver transplantation. Transplantation 75:1227-1231, 2003.

41. Kato T, O'Brien CB, Nishida S, et al: The first case report of the use of a zoom videoendoscope for the evaluation of small bowel graft mucosa in a human after intestinal transplantation. Gastrointest Endosc 50:257-261, 1999.

42. Pappas PA, Saudubray JM, Tzakis AG, et al: Serum citrulline and rejection in small bowel transplantation: A preliminary report. Transplantation 72:1212-1216, 2001.

43. Khan FA, Kato T, Berho M, et al: Graft failure secondary to necrotizing enterocolitis in multi-visceral transplantation recipients: Two case reports. Pediatr Transplant 4:215-220, 2000.

44. Fishbein TM, Gondolesi GE, Kaufman SS: Intestinal transplantation for gut failure. Gastroenterology 124:1615-1628, 2003.

45. Pinna AD, Weppler D, Nery J, et al: Intestinal transplantation at the University of Miami—five years of experience. Transplant Proc 32:1226-1227, 2000.

46. Abu-Elmagd K, Reyes J, Bond G, et al: Clinical intestinal transplantation: A decade of experience at a single center. Ann Surg 234:404-416, discussion 416-417, 2001.

47. Perez MT, Garcia M, Weppler D, et al: Temporal relationships between acute cellular rejection features and increased mucosal fibrosis in the early posttransplant period of human small intestinal allografts. Transplantation 73:555-559, 2002.

48. Berho M, Torroella M, Viciana A, et al: Adenovirus enterocolitis in human small bowel transplants. Pediatr Transplant 2:277-282, 1998.

49. McLaughlin GE, Delis S, Kashimawo L, et al: Adenovirus infection in pediatric liver and intestinal transplant recipients: Utility of DNA detection by PCR. Am J Transplant 3:224-228, 2003.

50. Pinchoff RJ, Kaufman SS, Magid MS, et al: Adenovirus infection in pediatric small bowel transplantation recipients. Transplantation 76:183-189, 2003.

51. Kato T, Dowdy L, Weppler D, et al: Non-tuberculous mycobacterial–associated enterocolitis in intestinal transplantation. Transplant Proc 30:2537-2538, 1998.

52. Delis SG, Tector J, Kato T, et al: Diagnosis and treatment of *Cryptosporidium* infection in intestinal transplant recipients. Transplant Proc 34:951-952, 2002.

53. Delis S, Kato T, Ruiz P, et al: Herpes simplex colitis in a child with combined liver and small bowel transplant. Pediatr Transplant 5:374-377, 2001.

54. Kobayashi S, Kato T, Nishida S, et al: Necrotizing fasciitis following liver and small intestine transplantation. Pediatr Transplant 6:344-347, 2002.

55. Berney T, Delis S, Kato T, et al: Successful treatment of post-transplant lymphoproliferative disease with prolonged rituximab treatment in intestinal transplant recipients. Transplantation 74:1000-1006, 2002.

56. Levi DM, Tzakis AG, Kato T, et al: Transplantation of the abdominal wall. Lancet 361:2173-2176, 2003.

57. Bejarano PA, Levi D, Nassiri M, et al: The pathology of full-thickness cadaver skin transplant for large abdominal defects: A proposed grading system for skin allograft acute rejection. Am J Surg Pathol 28:670-675, 2004.
58. Kaufman SS, Atkinson JB, Bianchi A, et al: Indications for pediatric intestinal transplantation: A position paper of the American Society of Transplantation. Pediatr Transplant 5:80-87, 2001.
59. Tzakis AG, De Faria W, Angelis M, et al: Partial abdominal exenteration, ex vivo resection of a large mesenteric fibroma, and successful orthotopic intestinal autotransplantation. Surgery 128:486-489, 2000.
60. Tzakis AG, Tryphonopoulos P, De Faria W, et al: Partial abdominal evisceration, ex vivo resection, and intestinal autotransplantation for the treatment of pathologic lesions of the root of the mesentery. J Am Coll Surg 197:770-776, 2003.

Combined Liver-Kidney Transplantation

EDMUND Q. SANCHEZ
GORAN B. KLINTMALM

Statistics   804

Immunological aspects   804
  Cross-matching   804
  Immunosuppression   805

Pathophysiology   806
  Primary hyperoxaluria   806
  Polycystic disease   807
  Hepatitic C–related glomerulonephritis   807
  Other causes of end-stage renal disease   807

Indications for liver-kidney transplantation   808
  Abdominal imaging   808
  Cardiac clearance   808
  Special considerations   808
  Pulmonary hypertension   809

Technique   809
  Liver transplantation   809
  Kidney transplantation   810
  Intraoperative management   810
  Postoperative management   810

Survival and rejection rates   811

Conclusion   811

Single-organ transplantation was originally thought to be a major undertaking. In the days when the first solid-organ transplants were being performed, one would not have dreamed that double- or even triple-organ transplants could be performed. In the current era, double-organ transplantation is becoming more frequent. In fact, with certain combinations of organs such as the kidney and pancreas, graft and patient survival rates can be improved with double-organ transplantation. Until recently, renal failure was a contraindication to liver transplantation, but combined transplantation is currently the answer for selected recipients.

The first combined liver-kidney transplantation (LKTx) was performed on December 28, 1983, and subsequently reported by Margreiter and colleagues in 1984.[1] The patient was a 32-year-old man who had previously undergone renal transplantation for chronic glomerulonephritis in 1977. Subsequently, chronic rejection developed, and he was also suffering from end-stage liver disease because of hepatitis B virus infection. Unlike the index case, end-stage liver disease is known to be associated with concurrent or subsequent renal dysfunction and renal failure (however, as described, the converse may happen). Hepatorenal syndrome is a prime example[2] of the physiological relationship between the liver and kidney that is clinically relevant. However, hepatorenal syndrome is a *reversible* condition with liver transplantation alone.[3,4]

More likely in the adult population, chronic irreversible renal dysfunction as a result of many other causes is seen in those with end-stage liver disease. For example, hepatitis C, which is the most common liver disease requiring transplantation in the United States, has been found to have irreversible extrahepatic manifestation in the kidneys. Therefore, it seems natural that LKTx has become an operation that is being performed with increasing frequency since the mid-1980s.

As previously mentioned, chronic irreversible renal failure was formerly a contraindication to liver transplantation. The combination of end-stage liver disease and end-stage renal disease is now treated by LKTx, with excellent results in both the adult and pediatric population. LKTx in this chapter refers to transplantation of the liver and kidney simultaneously from the same donor, as opposed to sequential liver-kidney transplantation, in which the liver is transplanted initially and, subsequently, end-stage renal disease develops and requires a kidney transplant at a later time. The renal allograft will most likely be from a separate donor, unless both organs come from the same living donor.

Liver transplantation has now entered an era in which patients with extended (longer than 10 year) survival are common. Therefore, chronic exposure to the nephrotoxic side effects of calcineurin inhibitors becomes significantly more clinically relevant. In both the adult and pediatric populations, the development of chronic renal failure and end-stage renal disease is a major factor that affects long-term quality of life and hinders survival. Liver transplantation is therefore paying a price for its success. A solution to this problem is sequential kidney transplantation after liver transplantation; however, this too is fraught with inherent complications.

From 1988 to 2002 there have been 1228 combined LKTx procedures, 113 of them being pediatric recipients in the United States.[5] The incidence of the operation appears to be rising over the years, and in some United Network for Organ Sharing (UNOS) regions the number of LKTx procedures has increased drastically. Reasons for the increasing number of these combined organ transplants are many, and the decision to perform them depends on institutional policy and may be a result of institution of the Model for End-Stage Liver Disease (MELD) scoring system for liver allocation. The MELD system, sicker patient populations, and differences that exist in kidney transplant policies between institutions may offer possible explanations for the increasing number of LKTx procedures. Increased creatinine in recipients at the top of institutional lists may represent either chronic irreversible renal failure or reversible acute renal failure. At initial evaluation there is often some difficulty determining the recipient's renal status, and as a result, LKTx may be performed for acute renal failure, although it did not appear to be the case in the workup.

Liver transplantation with its attendant and inherent risks, coupled with simultaneous or sequential kidney transplantation, is quite an immunological and surgical undertaking. Therefore, the exact indications, the disease processes involved, the patient's expected outcome, the immunosuppression regimen, and graft survival and outcome data should be evaluated thoroughly before one undertakes the procedure.

Statistics

According to data obtained from UNOS, 16,959 liver and 53,821 kidney transplant candidates are listed as of March 2003. Of the potential recipients of LKTx, liver transplant candidates account for only a small subset. Because there is no special list for LKTx candidates, they are included in the liver transplant list. Therefore, as with all organs, candidates should be well selected because of the scarcity of available organs.

The median waiting time for liver transplant recipients is now influenced by MELD scores.[6] Waiting times by ABO blood type have increased over the years as a result of the increasing number of patients on the waiting list (Table 54–1). Potential recipients are now subject to the development of clinically apparent nephropathy because of the lengthening waiting periods, which is perhaps one of the many reasons why the number of LKTx procedures appears to be on an upward trend (Fig. 54–1).

Immunological Aspects

Cross-matching

LKTx can be performed safely in patients with a positive T- and B-cell cross-match. The transplanted liver was thought to confer a protective effect on the transplanted kidney[7,8] by inducing tolerance, even in presensitized recipients.[9,10] The Pittsburgh group was the first to report that positive antibody cross-matching in the liver transplant was not a significant factor in determining success[11]; in addition, they demonstrated acceptable results in LKTx.[12,13] However, not all centers have produced the same results.[14]

Table 54–1. MEDIAN WAITING LIST TIME (IN DAYS) BY ABO BLOOD TYPE

ABO	1996–1997	1998–1999	2000–2001
O	534	835	1114
A	297	485	602
B	313	450	603
AB	135	220	232

Data from the United Network for Organ Sharing.

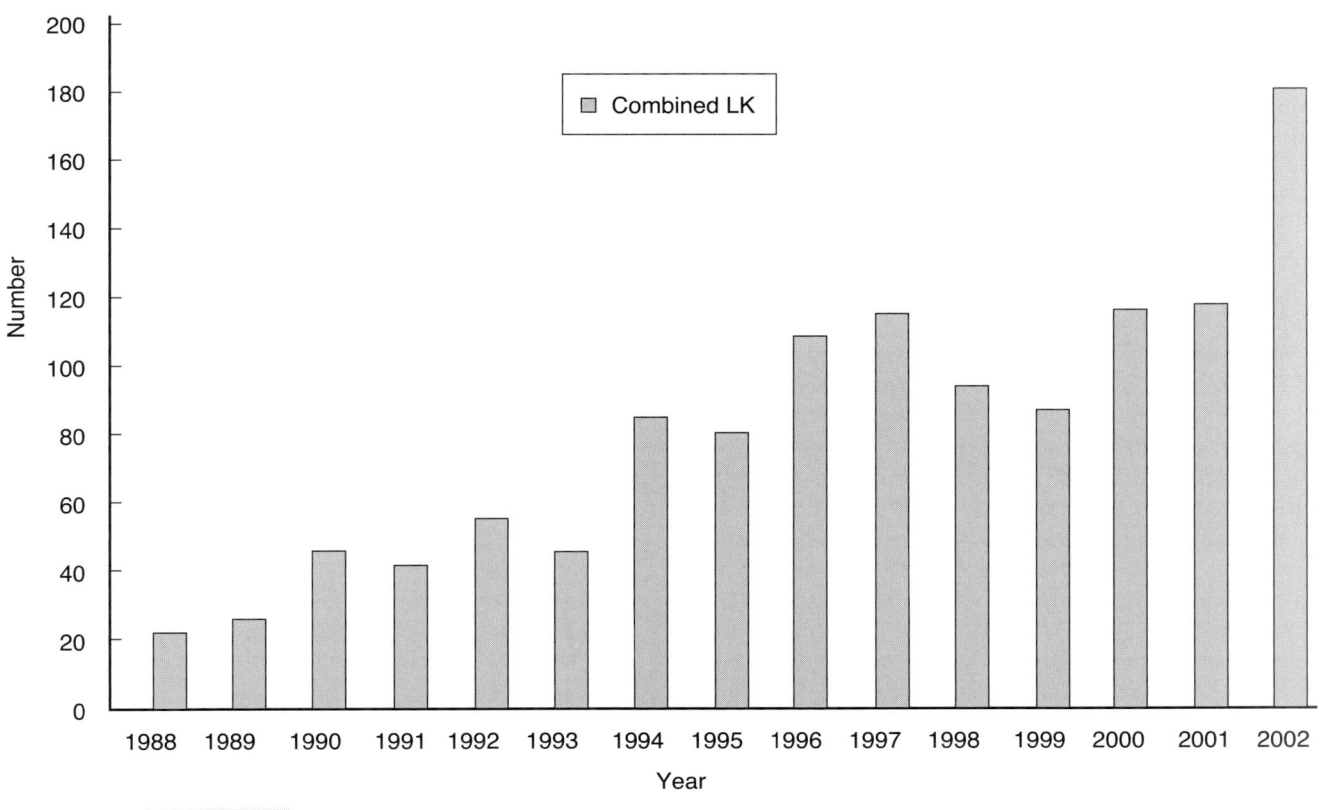

FIGURE 54-1

Number of combined liver-kidney transplants per year, 1988 to 2002. (Data from the Organ Procurement and Transplantation Network.)

Patient survival is not improved with LKTx, but rates of acute rejection of the renal allograft are decreased, an observation demonstrating a protective effect of the liver transplant. The exact mechanism is not known, but a possible explanation is that the liver transplant allograft contains larger numbers of passenger leukocytes that make it possible to induce microchimerism (and subsequent tolerance).[15] Additionally, the large size of the liver allograft makes it possible to absorb circulating antibodies, which has been shown by Fung,[10] Morrissey,[16] and their colleagues to occur within the first hour of transplantation. Such absorption may induce a tolerizing effect as a result of direct antigen shedding.[17] Additional mechanisms that have been proposed are induction of apoptosis[18] in the specific alloreactive T lymphocytes or induction of suppressor cells.[19] In any event, long-term renal allograft survival in sensitized patients is similar to that in cross-match–negative recipients.

Another protective effect is seen in animal models in which pancreatic islet allografts were transplanted into recipients that had received a liver transplant.[20] This effect is thought to be due to an immune process that involves upregulation of FAS ligand expression and apoptosis of lymphocytes infiltrating the islet graft.

Additionally, other combined-organ transplants demonstrate protective effects on the renal allograft. For instance, in combined heart-kidney transplantation, renal allograft survival rates were not significantly different from those of LKTx 8 years after transplantation (63.5% versus 61.1% , P = NS).[21] This similarity in survival is possibly due to another mechanism, since the heart is not a large solid organ like the liver. Finally, combined kidney-pancreas transplantation also results in improved long-term renal allograft survival and a reduction in acute rejection episodes.

Immunosuppression

Standard immunosuppression for LKTx at our institution involves the use of tacrolimus, mycophenolate mofetil, and steroid. Our institution does not routinely use induction agents in LKTx. However, in patients with evidence of delayed graft function of the kidney transplant, one could opt to use antibody and delay the introduction of calcineurin inhibitors to provide maximal renal sparing. In those with severe delayed graft function or acute tubular necrosis (ATN), the use of rapamycin is attractive. Rapamycin, a macrocyclic lactone structurally similar to tacrolimus, is an immuno-suppressive agent that inhibits m-TOR. The salient features of this agent are that it is an effective immuno-suppressive agent but has very little nephrotoxicity. Care should be taken when administering rapamycin with cyclosporine or tacrolimus because of the synergism that occurs, especially with regard to nephrotoxicity.

Acute cellular rejection episodes can be treated with intravenous methylprednisolone recycle. The rate of acute cellular rejection in the renal allograft is lower; however, the acute cellular rejection rate of the liver transplant is not lowered by the renal allograft. Dosing of Solu-Medrol is dependent on the institution. In cases of steroid-resistant rejection, the use of antibody therapy is typically the next step in treatment.

The long-term effect of calcineurin inhibitor on renal function in liver transplant recipients is well known, as is the nephrotoxicity of calcineurin inhibitor on renal allografts. However, the effect of the long-term use of calcineurin inhibitor in LKTx recipients has not been investigated in large studies. Kidney allografts transplanted in conjunction with a liver demonstrate fewer episodes of acute cellular rejection and typically have excellent function initially after transplantation. Perhaps this population could use somewhat lower doses of calcineurin inhibitor in the long term to minimize effects on the renal allograft. Fuchinoue's group[22] demonstrated successful steroid withdrawal in patients after LKTx, thus suggesting that less immuno-suppression is possible in this group.

Pathophysiology

Liver and kidney disease can coexist, as seen in hepatorenal syndrome and the development of acute renal failure after liver transplantation. However, the course of renal failure in hepatorenal syndrome after liver transplantation is characterized by nearly complete return of renal function postoperatively. Only a small proportion (5%) progress to end-stage renal disease.[2] Acute renal failure postoperatively, however, is not so predictable. Persistence of acute renal failure after liver transplantation has been shown to be associated with a definite increase in mortality.[23]

LKTx is undertaken in cases in which renal function in a patient with end-stage liver disease is not thought to be recoverable. The following disease processes account for the majority of combined-organ transplants: primary hyperoxaluria type I, adult polycystic liver and kidney disease, metabolic disorders, glomerulonephritis, tubular and interstitial disorders, hypertensive nephrosclerosis, and diabetic nephropathy, as well as various other causes (Table 54–2). Primary hyperoxaluria, adult polycystic disease, and hepatitis C glomerulonephritis are discussed

in detail in the following sections. Comments about other disease processes are also presented.

Primary Hyperoxaluria

Primary hyperoxaluria type I is a hepatic-based inborn error of metabolism, but extrahepatic manifestations provide the impetus for liver transplantation. The enzyme responsible for the derangements was not reported until 1986.[24] In type I disease, the hepatic enzyme alanine-glyoxylate transaminase is deficient or mistargeted from peroxisomes to mitochondria, with resulting increased production of oxalate by the liver. Oxalate is cleared primarily through renal excretion, so

Table 54–2. DIFFERENTIAL DIAGNOSIS OF CAUSES OF RENAL FAILURE IN PATIENTS WITH END-STAGE LIVER DISEASE
Idiopathic
Postinflammatory crescentic glomerulonephritis
Membranous glomerulonephritis
Mesangiocapillary glomerulonephritis
IgA nephropathy
Focal glomerulosclerosis
Chronic pyelonephritis
Reflux nephropathy
Polycystic kidneys
Nephritis
Diabetic nephropathy
Oxalate nephropathy
Amyloidosis
Gout
Progressive systemic sclerosis
Hemolytic-uremic syndrome
Acute tubular necrosis
Sickle cell anemia
Alport's syndrome
Malignant hypertension
Retransplant/graft failure
Membranous nephropathy
Analgesic nephropathy
Radiation nephritis
Cyclosporine toxicity
Renal artery thrombosis
Wegener's granulomatosis
Sarcoidosis
Nephrolithiasis
Drug related

marked hyperoxaluria ensues. There are no known pathways for oxalate degradation, and therefore oxalate combines with calcium to create calcium oxalate deposits, mainly as renal stones and eventually as nephrocalcinosis. In the long term, oxalate is deposited in bones, blood vessels, myocardium, and other organs. Eventually, renal failure develops, and systemic oxalosis is associated with high morbidity and mortality.

The clinical course is quite slow. Frequently, a progressive slow decline in renal function along with obstructive uropathy and urinary tract infections is typical. The median age of patients with end-stage renal disease is 25 years, and 80% of such patients require renal replacement therapy by their third decade.[25] The patient survival rate 1 year after transplantation is 91.8%. The 1-year renal allograft survival rate is 76%, with a liver graft survival rate of 84%. (Organ Procurement and Transplantation Network [OPTN] data). Renal allograft survival has been shown to be significantly better with LKTx than with kidney transplantation alone (76% versus 47.9%) at 8 years' follow-up.[26] Additionally, there has been a case report of reversal of oxalosis cardiomyopathy after LKTx.[27]

The type II variant is less common. It is also characterized by hyperoxaluria and urolithiasis, but less frequently by renal failure. This variant is caused by a defect in the glyoxylate/hydroxypyruvate reductase enzyme.

Inadequate treatment of hyperoxaluria-induced renal failure by renal replacement therapy and rapid recurrence of renal failure in renal transplant recipients have led to significant mortality. In fact, the National Institutes of Health has declared that this disease is unsuitable for treatment by renal transplantation.[28] Discovery of the enzyme deficiency in the liver was a major breakthrough in treatment of this disease. Presently, LKTx is widely accepted as treatment of type I disease. In type II disease, the enzyme defect has now been linked to organs other than the liver,[29,30] and thus treatment of type II disease has been limited to kidney transplantation alone, which has produced acceptable results.

Polycystic Disease

Adult polycystic kidney disease is an autosomal dominant disorder that affects nearly 1 in every 1000 people. The disorder has nearly 100% penetrance in patients surviving into the seventh to eighth decades of life. The genetic marker is located on chromosome 16, and the disease is caused by mutation in the *PKD1* and *PKD2* genes. Renal function is typically maintained until the fourth or fifth decades of life.

Patients with adult polycystic kidney disease also tend to have other congenital cysts. Roughly 40% have one or several liver cysts (polycystic liver disease) that are usually asymptomatic. Cysts can frequently appear in the spleen, pancreas, and lungs. Intracranial berry aneurysms in the circle of Willis are present in 10% to 30% of patients, with subarachnoid hemorrhage resulting in death in 10% of these patients. Mitral valve prolapse occurs as well. Death is typically due to three causes: (1) renal failure, (2) hypertension-related disease (cardiac disease, berry aneurysm), and (3) unrelated conditions. Combined transplantation for this indication has resulted in 1-year patient survival rates of 87.1% and 1-year renal and liver graft survival rates of 84.3%.

Finally, autosomal dominant polycystic liver disease is a distinct entity from autosomal dominant polycystic kidney disease. The gene has been localized to the chromosome 19p13.2-13.1 region. *PRKCSH* gene mutations lead to loss of function in "protein kinase C substrate 80 K-H" or the "noncatalytic beta subunit of glucosidase II."[31] Apparently, expression of the polycystic condition is dependent on a two-hit mechanism.

Hepatitis C–Related Glomerulonephritis

Hepatitis C end-stage liver disease is perhaps the most frequent reason now for liver transplantation at many centers. In addition to liver disease, it has been associated with glomerulonephritis. Type I membranoproliferative glomerulonephritis is more frequent in this population. Additionally, mixed cryoglobulinemia with or without membranoproliferative glomerulonephritis and nephrotic syndrome may occur with hepatitis C infection/reactivation after transplantation. Renal function may deteriorate with progressive end-stage liver disease. Again, if the patient is suffering from chronic irreversible renal disease at the time of evaluation, consideration must be given to performance of LKTx.

Cantarell and coauthors[32] described a series of four patients, two of whom were maintained on hemodialysis and underwent LKTx. In contrast to those treated by liver transplantation alone, proteinuria or renal dysfunction did not develop in the LKTx patients. Not much is known about posttransplant recurrence of hepatitis C and glomerulonephritis in the renal allograft.

Other Causes of End-Stage Renal Disease

Pretransplant chronic renal failure or end-stage renal disease requiring hemodialysis (or both) occurs in a small proportion of liver transplant candidates. Renal failure before liver transplantation has been reported to be a significant predictor of infection, continued renal failure, and death.[33]

Other metabolic/genetic diseases that may be remedied by LKTx include glycogen storage disease type I,[34] sickle cell anemia,[35-37] familial hemolytic-uremic syndrome,[38] amyloidosis, Wilson's disease,[39] hemochromatosis,[40] and α_1-antitrypsin deficiency.[41]

Post–liver transplant renal failure deserves special mention. The incidence of chronic renal failure and end-stage renal disease can approach 20% at greater than 10 years after liver transplantation. Frequently, this renal failure is due to calcineurin inhibitor toxicity, as well as other nephropathies and glomerulopathies. The survival rate of liver transplant recipients who initiate hemodialysis is 28% 6 years after renal replacement therapy. Liver transplant recipients who are approved by kidney transplant committees should undergo kidney transplantation. Patient survival after sequential liver-kidney transplantation is lower than that in those who undergo kidney transplantation alone, but it is nearly identical to the survival of liver recipients matched chronologically.[42]

Indications for Liver-Kidney Transplantation

Patients with documented end-stage liver disease, as well as irreversible renal failure, are candidates for combined transplantation. Indications for LKTx are highly dependent on the institution. The selection process at our and other institutions consists of approval by both a liver transplant selection committee and a kidney transplant selection committee. Additionally, sequential kidney transplantation after liver transplantation also requires approval by the kidney transplant selection committee.

Potential LKTx recipients must meet highly stringent criteria to optimize survival. Medically, a patient at our institution with liver disease must have end-stage liver disease and a minimum Child-Turcotte-Pugh score of 7 to meet the criteria for enrollment on the liver transplant list. Additionally, the patient must be evaluated by a nephrologist and irreversible end-stage renal failure must be diagnosed. This combination will then advance the patient toward evaluation as a LKTx candidate.

As with single-graft transplantation, medical clearance otherwise consists of abdominal radiologic imaging, cardiac clearance, pulmonary clearance (if indicated), renal assessment, and other evaluations based on patient history. The following sections consist of a brief summary of the testing that should occur as part of the evaluation.

Abdominal Imaging

Abdominal imaging is mandatory in the evaluation for liver transplantation. Doppler ultrasonography is performed first and is extremely useful as a screening study. The evaluating surgeon must pay attention to patency of the hepatic vasculature, detection of possible hepatic masses or tumors, and imaging of the abdominal organs, as well as other key characteristics. Additionally, ultrasonography can detect whether suspicious lesions are present in the liver or surrounding structures. Frequently, ultrasound is followed by computed tomography or magnetic resonance imaging of the abdomen to validate the ultrasonographic findings. Moreover, interval follow-up ultrasound may be indicated to monitor patency of the hepatic vasculature if particular issues require such follow-up.

Magnetic resonance angiography and venography can also be used for imaging of pertinent surgical issues such as aberrant hepatic arterial anatomy (arcuate ligament syndrome, replaced right hepatic artery, etc.) and portal anatomy (portal vein patency/thrombosis). Such imaging is particularly useful if a candidate has marginal renal function and cannot tolerate the use of ionic contrast agents because of the risk of nephrotoxicity. The use of ionic contrast agents could mean the difference in needing hemodialysis before the transplant procedure is performed. When ultrasound and magnetic resonance imaging demonstrate different findings, confirmation by selective mesenteric arteriography with a portal venous phase is undertaken if specific anatomic issues are present that may decide a patient's candidacy (e.g., complete portal system thrombosis).

Cardiac Clearance

The minimum cardiac workup consists of 12-lead electrocardiography and transthoracic two-dimensional echocardiography. Cardiac catheterization (both right and left) and cardiac muscle biopsy should be performed in clinically indicated situations as directed by the cardiologist. Once again, contrast agent nephrotoxicity is of concern. Therefore, if a potential candidate who is not yet undergoing hemodialysis does not appear to be a suitable candidate because of other medical issues, cardiac catheterization should not be pursued to preserve what remaining renal function may exist.

Special Considerations

Patients with systemic diseases such as amyloidosis, sarcoidosis, hemochromatosis, Wilson's disease, primary hyperoxaluria, and other conditions may need particular attention paid to organs other than the liver and kidney, in particular the heart. The other organ systems can be affected to a degree that may make the patient unsuitable for LKTx.

Pulmonary Hypertension

If elevated pulmonary artery systolic pressure (typically > 45 mm Hg) is detected in patients with end-stage renal failure by two-dimensional echocardiography, referral is made for right heart catheterization to determine the cause of the pulmonary hypertension. Occasionally, volume overload may cause a degree of pulmonary hypertension or contribute to it. When dry weight/diuresis has been maximized, repeat evaluation should be performed. Additionally, other issues to consider are type I or II hepatopulmonary syndrome and congestive heart failure not responsive to aggressive medical management.

Technique

Once the institution's selection committee has cleared a suitable recipient, the patient is placed on the waiting list when the appropriate MELD score has been attained. Once a suitable donor is available and the patient is the next candidate, the patient is examined preoperatively and suitability for transplantation determined at that time.

The liver transplant precedes the kidney transplant. The kidney transplant portion of the operation can be omitted if the recipient is too hemodynamically unstable for the additional procedure.

Liver Transplantation

The liver transplant is performed in an orthotopic fashion. This procedure has been well described, and various modifications have been made. The use of venovenous bypass for this combined procedure is the method of choice at our institution; however, similar results can be obtained without the use of venovenous bypass.

Additionally, the caval interposition or piggyback methods can be used and do not affect the kidney transplant procedure. The choice of incision is perhaps an important aspect of the procedure, and a variety of skin incisions can be used for the liver transplant. The "Mercedes" incision provides the most exposure, although smaller incisions may offer the same degree of exposure in different patients. A very important factor when selecting the location for the liver transplant incision is to consider where the kidney transplant incision will be made. Incorrect placement of skin incisions may lead to abdominal skin necrosis as a result of the vascular compromise that can occur with transection of the inferior epigastric bundle and the superior epigastric bundle. Such complications can occur with both the liver and kidney transplant incisions. Additionally, overlapping incisions will compromise the vascular integrity of the skin and potentially lead to skin necrosis.

Polycystic Disease

Some special technical considerations must be borne in mind when performing a liver transplant in polycystic patients. First, the liver is markedly enlarged, and the hilar anatomic relationships may be distorted. Typically, these structures are stretched and displaced anteriorly because of expansion of the liver in an anterior and caudad direction. Great care should be taken when dissecting the hilar structures.

In addition, these recipients may have other organs (besides polycystic kidneys) affected by the polycystic transformation. Rarely, the recipient kidneys need to be removed before transplantation. Patients may have pancreatic, mesenteric, and ovarian cysts that require removal to rule out malignancy and generate more space for implantation of the donor allograft or allografts.

Of special note also is the association of polycystic disease with aneurysm of intracranial vessels. Therefore, as with all liver transplant recipients, maintenance of normotension is of utmost importance after transplantation.

Primary Hyperoxaluria

The liver transplant procedure may be performed by two different methods. The first is the standard orthotopic liver transplantation. The alternative method is to perform an orthotopic left lateral auxiliary transplantation. This method involves transplantation of segments II and III in an orthotopic fashion after performing a left lateral hepatic lobectomy for the recipient operation. Anastomoses to the left hepatic vein, the left proper hepatic artery, the left portal vein branch, and the left biliary duct (via either a Roux-en-Y choledochojejunostomy or hepaticojejunostomy) may then be fashioned. Although it is a technically more challenging procedure, an important benefit in performing it in this fashion is its potential for use in the rare circumstance in which a left hepatic lobectomy is the safest procedure that the patient may tolerate because of previous surgical procedures in the right side of the abdomen.

The procedure of choice remains the standard orthotopic liver transplantation with complete hepatectomy. Auxiliary liver transplantation in primary hyperoxaluria is not usually effective because oxalate overproduction, not decreased catabolism, will continue in any remaining liver tissue.[43] Along the same lines, gene therapy techniques would require transfection of a significant proportion of hepatocytes (75%) to counteract the increased synthesis of oxalate in neighboring nontransfected cells.[44] Perhaps if enough liver volume were transplanted to overcome the effect of the remaining recipient liver, a partial-graft transplantation may be a more viable alternative. Quantifying exactly how much liver is needed to offset the effect of the remaining recipient liver is essential to the success of partial-liver transplantation in this setting.

Kidney Transplantation

The kidney transplant procedure is performed after completion of the liver transplant procedure. Because the procedure can be performed in patients with a positive cross-match (as described earlier), one does not need to wait for the results of cross-matching before initiating the kidney transplant procedure. The kidney transplant is performed in a retroperitoneal pocket established through a separate incision. Again, the incision must be placed in a fashion that minimizes potential ischemic complications in the anterior abdominal wall. One of the most important points to remember is to spare the inferior epigastric bundle so that the vascular integrity of the anterior abdominal wall is not compromised. Typically, there is no compromise in available space once the liver transplant is completed. The native kidneys are left intact, and the renal transplant is performed in standard fashion.

Intraoperative Management

The intraoperative management issues associated with liver transplantation are well known. Liver transplantation must be undertaken by an experienced team of anesthesiologists, surgeons, and operating room staff that is very familiar with the instruments and protocols of transplantation.

The use of intraoperative hemodialysis is of utmost importance in patients undergoing liver transplantation who are anuric. Because of the tremendous amount of fluid shift and blood products and crystalloid administered, a means of controlling intravascular volume must be in place before initiating the kidney transplant procedure. Acute volume overload, especially during reperfusion of the liver transplant, has proved to be fatal. Volume overload in this setting can cause acute myocardial infarction, severe pulmonary edema (with resulting hypoxia and an inability to ventilate) with subsequent acute right-sided heart failure, and even liver allograft dysfunction as a result of passive congestion. Intraoperative hemodialysis can be performed through any existing hemodialysis access or via a percutaneously placed catheter designed for hemodialysis.

Venovenous bypass in these recipients is initiated according to surgeon preference and should be considered on a case-by-case basis. Its benefit in liver transplantation has been debated, and liver transplant institutions vary greatly in the use of venovenous bypass. However, in combined transplantation, the surgeon must have a lower threshold for the use of bypass. Some relative indications for its use are transplant procedures in unstable patients, elderly patients, those who have undergone multiple abdominal operations before transplantation, and patients with rare blood types.

Postoperative Management

Management of LKTx recipients after transplantation is typically much like that of patients who undergo liver transplantation alone. The primary goals in the initial 24- to 72-hour period are to keep the recipient's central venous pressure low enough to minimize passive congestion in the newly transplanted liver so that the ongoing preservation injury is minimized and to protect the patient from volume excess and, subsequently, protect the lungs from pulmonary edema. These objectives are easily achieved with a functioning renal allograft. If the renal allograft is in high-output diuresis, maintenance of adequate central venous pressure is not usually difficult. In cases of nonoliguric ATN, supplemental diuretics may be needed to increase urine output so that the patient's intravascular volume is lowered. However, difficulty arises if the renal allograft does not respond to diuretic challenge, is experiencing delayed graft function, or is oliguric/anuric.

A functioning renal allograft after LKTx will most likely be in either high-output ATN or nonoliguric ATN. High-output ATN associated with a diminished or declining central venous pressure (signifying hypovolemia) and hypotension should be treated with aggressive fluid resuscitation to maintain blood pressure and urine output. Again, one must be extremely cautious to avoid fluid overload and passive congestion of the liver allograft and lungs. Fluid resuscitation can frequently be maintained with an increase in maintenance intravenous fluids; however, if inadequate, an alternative resuscitation regimen involving hourly urine output replacement is beneficial.

Delayed graft function or oliguric/anuric ATN poses a significant potential problem for postoperative management of intravascular volume in LKTx. Typically, in this scenario, continuous hemodialysis with ultrafiltration is performed until the kidney is functioning or fluid status is maintained. In this situation, delayed introduction of calcineurin inhibitors may be of benefit until renal function is adequate. In fact, only 2 of 53 patients in our experience did not demonstrate immediate renal function. Therefore, if immediate renal allograft function is not observed, technical problems must be actively ruled out as soon as possible. In kidney transplantation alone, rates of delayed graft function approach 20%. The reason for the difference in delayed graft function rates after LKTx is not certain.

Survival and Rejection Rates

Patient survival after LKTx has been reported in multiple series.[45-60] At Baylor University Medical Center, we performed 51 LKTx procedures from 1988 to 2003. Survival rates of LKTx recipients were 86% at 1 year, 79% at 2 years, and 64.7% at 5 years. Renal allograft survival rates were 83% at 1 year, 76.5% at 2 years, and 62.1% at 5 years. Liver allograft survival rates were 82.9% at 1 year, 76.4% at 2 years, and 62.1% at 5 years.

Reported 1-year patient survival rates range from 67% to 100%. Extended results at 2 and 5 years are reported to be 67% to 95% and 48% to 93%, respectively. These survival rates from the literature extend back to the early 1990s and may therefore be misleading. In U.S. centers, OPTN results from 1997 to 2001 demonstrate 1-year survival rates comparable to those reported in these studies. The 1-year patient survival rate ranged from 74.4% to 87.1%, depending on the primary diagnosis. The 1-year liver allograft survival rate from the same database ranged from 84.3% to 91.8%, whereas the renal allograft survival rate was 67% to 84%, depending on the primary diagnosis. Overall, long-term patient and renal allograft survival rates are not significantly different. Opelz and coworkers[21] reported that after 8 years of follow-up, renal allograft survival after LKTx was not significantly different from that after kidney transplantation alone. However, it appears that if the data are censored for death with a functioning graft, the rate of renal allograft loss in LKTx recipients is very low (9.7% in 8 years). This finding strongly suggests that the rate of immunological renal allograft loss is very low in LKTx recipients.

Liver allograft rejection rates after LKTx remain the same as for liver transplantation alone, as has been described in the previously cited reviews. Furthermore, as mentioned earlier, renal allograft rejection rates after LKTx are lower[61] than after kidney transplantation alone, as well as after sequential liver transplantation and then kidney transplantation.[62] Again, these lower rates are due to the "protective" effect created by the liver allograft (as described previously).

Conclusion

The increased number of combined simultaneous allograft transplantation procedures is a result of the marked technical and medical advancements made in transplantation. LKTx has been shown to be effective in appropriately identified patients suffering from concomitant end-stage liver and kidney disease. The liver provides a unique protective environment for the renal allograft, as demonstrated by the reduction in acute cellular rejection episodes and decline in graft loss for immunological reasons—even in the face of positive cross-matches.

There are many possible indications and combinations of indications for LKTx, and graft and patient survival are somewhat dependent on the diagnosis. Hepatitis C is the leading cause of liver transplantation at many centers; however, recurrence is quite rapid in most cases. Transplantation for correction of polycystic and metabolic diseases is often associated with the best graft and patient survival rates.

Perioperative management issues are extremely important in this subset of patients. Additional support consisting of continuous hemodialysis and ultrafiltration, as well as venovenous bypass, should be strongly considered when performing a combined transplant procedure. Meticulous fluid and volume management after transplantation must be ensured to minimize postoperative allograft injury. Nephrotoxic immunosuppression must also be minimized in patients with delayed renal allograft function.

Although no data have definitely shown that combined transplantation is associated with extended liver and renal allograft survival when compared with solitary-organ transplantation, the procedure has proved to be life-saving in patients in whom transplantation was thought to be contraindicated in the past.

Pearls and Pitfalls

Pearls

- Combined liver-kidney transplantation must be performed in medically suitable recipients.
- Liver-kidney transplants can be performed in patients with positive cross-matches, even in presensitized recipients, so one should not wait for cross-matches to be completed.
- Skin incisions for the combined liver-kidney transplant must be placed in a manner to minimize the chance of skin/abdominal wall necrosis.
- The use of continuous venovenous hemodialysis intraoperatively during the liver transplant phase of the operation is extremely beneficial in managing fluid balance in the operating room.

Pitfalls

- Renal status must be confirmed to be an irreversible process affecting the kidney, although at times it is extremely difficult to do so.
- Delayed renal allograft function may occur and lead to volume overload and its sequelae. In this case, immediate hemodialysis or continuous hemodialysis may be indicated.

References

1. Margreiter R, Kramer R, Huber C, et al: Combined liver and kidney transplantation. Lancet 1:1077, 1984.
2. Cardenas A, Uriz J, Gines P, Arroyo V: Hepatorenal syndrome. Liver Transpl 6(4 Suppl 1):S63-S71, 2000.
3. Iwatsuki S, Corman J, Popovtzer M, et al: Recovery from hepatorenal syndrome after successful orthotopic liver transplantation. Surg Forum 24:348-350, 1973.
4. Iwatsuki S, Popovtzer MM, Corman JL, et al: Recovery from "hepatorenal syndrome" after orthotopic liver transplantation. N Engl J Med 289:1155-1159, 1973.
5. UNOS website www.optn.org.
6. Wiesner RH, McDiarmid SV, Kamath PS, et al: MELD and PELD: Application of survival models to liver allocation. Liver Transpl 7:567-580, 2001.
7. Margareiter R, Kornberger R, Koller J, et al: Can a liver graft from the same donor protect a kidney from rejection? Transplant Proc 20:522, 1988.
8. Rasmussen A, Davies H, Jamieson N, et al: Combined transplantation of liver and kidney from the same donor protects the kidney from rejection and improves kidney graft survival. Transplantation 59:919, 1995.
9. Kamada N, Davies HS, Roser B: Reversal of transplantation immunity by liver grafting. Nature 292:840-842, 1981.
10. Simpson K, Bunch D, Amemiya H, et al: Humoral antibodies and coagulation mechanisms in the accelerated or hyperacute rejection of renal homografts in sensitized canine recipients. Surgery 68:77-85, 1970.
11. Iwatsuki S, Iwaki Y, Kano T, et al: Successful liver transplantation from crossmatch-positive donors. Transplant Proc 13:286-288, 1981.
12. Fung J, Griffin R, Duquesnoy R, et al: Successful sequential liver-kidney transplantation in a patient with preformed lymphocytotoxic antibodies. Transplant Proc 19:767-768, 1987.
13. Fung J, Makowka L, Tzakis A, et al: Combined liver-kidney transplantation: Analysis of patients with preformed lymphocytotoxic antibodies. Transplant Proc 20:88-91, 1988.
14. Katz SM, Kimball PM, Ozaki C, et al: Positive pretransplant crossmatches predict early graft loss in liver allograft recipients. Transplantation 57:616-620, 1994.
15. Starzl T, Demitris A, Murase N, et al: Cell migration, chimerism, and graft acceptance. Lancet 339:1579, 1992.
16. Morrissey P, Gordon F, Shaffer D, et al: Combined liver-kidney transplantation in patients with cirrhosis and renal failure: Effect of a positive cross match and benefits of combined transplantation. Liver Transpl Surg 4:363-369, 1998.
17. Davis H, Pollard S, Calne R: Soluble HLA antigens in the circulation of liver graft recipients. Transplantation 47:524-527, 1989.
18. Zavazava N, Kronke M: Soluble HLA class I molecules induce apoptosis in alloreactive cytotoxic lymphocytes. Nat Med 2:1005, 1996.
19. Graeb C, Scherer M, Knechtle S, et al: Immunologic suppression mediated by genetically modified hepatocytes expressing secreted allo MHC class I molecules. Hum Immunol 59:415, 1998.
20. Wang XY, Sun J, Wang C, et al: Effect of liver transplantation on islet allografts. Transplantation 71:102-111, 2001.
21. Opelz G, Margreiter R, Dohler B: Prolongation of long-term kidney graft survival by a simultaneous liver transplant: The liver does it and the heart does it too. Transplantation 74:1390-1394, 2002.
22. Fuchinoue S, Sawada T, Tsuji K, et al: Kidney transplantation after liver transplantation from the same donor: Four cases of successful steroid withdrawal. Transplantation 73:948-952, 2002.
23. Markmann J, Markmann J, Markmann D, et al: Perioperative factors associated with outcome and their impact on resource use in 1148 consecutive primary liver transplants. Transplantation 72:1113-1122, 2001.
24. Danpure CJ: Peroxisomal alanine: glyoxylate aminotransferase deficiency in primary hyperoxaluria type I. FEBS Lett 201:20-24, 1986.
25. Cochat P, Deloraine A, Rotily M, et al: Epidemiology of primary hyperoxaluria type I. Nephrol Dial Transplant 10(Suppl 8):S3-S7, 1995.
26. Cibrik DM, Kaplan B, Arndorfer JA, Meier-Kriesche H: Renal allograft survival in patients with oxalosis. Transplantation 74:707-710, 2002.
27. Detry O, Honore P, DeRoover A, et al: Reversal of oxalosis cardiomyopathy after combined liver and kidney transplantation. Transpl Int 15:50-52, 2002.
28. Wilson RE: A report from the ACS/NIH renal transplant registry. Renal transplantation in congenital and metabolic disease. JAMA 232:148-153, 1975.
29. Williams HE, Smith LH: Hyperoxaluria in L-glyceric aciduria: Possible pathogenic mechanism. Science 171:390-391, 1971.
30. Giafi CF, Rumsby G: Kinetic analysis and tissue distribution of human D-glycerate dehydrogenase/glyoxylate reductase and its relevance to the diagnosis of primary hyperoxaluria type 2. Ann Clin Biochem 35:104-109, 1998.
31. Li A, Davila S, Furu L, et al: Mutations in the PRKCSH cause isolated autosomal dominant polycystic liver disease. Am J Hum Genet 72:691-703, 2003.
32. Cantarell MC, Charco R, Capdevila L, et al: Outcome of hepatitis C virus–associated membranoproliferative glomerulonephritis after liver transplantation. Transplantation 68:1131, 1999.
33. Fraley DS, Burr R, Bernardini J, et al: Impact of acute renal failure on mortality in end-stage liver disease with or without transplantation. Kidney Int 54:518-524, 1998.
34. Labrune P: Glycogen storage disease type I: Indications for liver and/or kidney transplantation. Eur J Pediatr 161(Suppl 1): S53-S55, 2002.
35. Emre S, Kitibayashi K, Schwartz M, et al: Liver transplantation in a patient with acute liver failure due to sickle cell intrahepatic cholestasis. Transplantation 69:675-676, 2000.
36. Ross A, Graeme-Cook F, Cosimi A, Chung R: Combined liver and kidney transplantation in a patient with sickle cell disease. Transplantation 73:605-608, 2002.
37. Lang T, Berquist WE, So S, et al: Liver transplantation in a child with sickle cell anemia. Transplantation 59:1490, 1995.
38. Remuzzi G, Ruggenenti P, Codazzi D, et al: Combined kidney and liver transplantation for familial hemolytic uraemic syndrome. Lancet 359:1671-1672, 2002.
39. Rakela J, Kurtz SB, McCarthy JT, et al: Fulminant Wilson's disease treated with postdilution hemofiltration and orthotopic liver transplantation. Gastroenterology 90:2004-2007, 1986.
40. Rela M, Muiesan P, Heaton ND, et al: Orthotopic liver transplantation for hepatic-based metabolic disorders. Transpl Int 8:41-44, 1995.
41. Loreno M, Boccagni P, Rigotti P, et al: Combined liver kidney transplantation in a 15 year old boy with alpha 1 antitrypsin deficiency. J Hepatol 36:565-568, 2002.
42. Gonwa TA, Mai M, Melton L, et al: End stage renal disease (ESRD) after orthotopic liver transplantation (OLTX) using calcineurin-based immunotherapy. Transplantation 72:1934-1939, 2001.
43. Danpure C: Scientific Rationale for Hepatorenal Transplantation in Primary Hyperoxaluria Type I. Amsterdam, Excerpta Medica, 1991.
44. Danpure C: Primary hyperoxaluria. In Scriver C, Beaudet A, Sly W, Valle D (eds): The Metabolic and Molecular Bases of Inherited Disease, 8th ed. New York, McGraw-Hill, 2001, pp 3323-3367.
45. Jeyarajah D, Gonwa T, McBride M, et al: Hepatorenal syndrome: Combined liver kidney transplants versus isolated liver transplant. Transplantation 64:1760-1765, 1997.

46. Bartosh S, Alonso E, Whitington P: Renal outcomes in pediatric liver transplantation. Clin Transplant 11:354-360, 1997.
47. Hiesse C, Samuel D, Bensadoun H: Combined liver and kidney transplantation in patients with chronic nephritis associated with end stage liver disease. Nephrol Dial Transplant 10(Suppl 6): S129-S133, 1995.
48. Benedetti E, Pirenne J, Troppmann C, et al: Combined liver and kidney transplantation. Transpl Int 9:486-491, 1996.
49. Kliem V, Ringe B, Frei U, Pichlmayr R: Single center experience of combined liver and kidney transplantation. Clin Transplant 9:39-44, 1995.
50. Larue J, Hiesse C, Samuel D, et al: Long term results of combined kidney and liver transplantation at one center. Transplant Proc 29:2365-2366, 1997.
51. Lang M, Neumann U, Bechstein W, et al: Long term outcome of 27 patients after combined liver kidney transplantation [abstract]. Proceedings of the XVIII International Congress of the Transplantation Society. August 27-Sept 1, 2000. Rome, Italy. Transplant Proc 33:A345, 2001.
52. Lang M, Kahl A, Bechstein W, et al: Combined liver kidney transplantation: Long term follow up in 18 patients. Transpl Int 11(Suppl 1):S155-S159, 1998.
53. Fung J, Makowka L, Tzakis A, et al: Combined liver-kidney transplantation: Analysis of patients with preformed lympho-cytotoxic antibodies. Transplant Proc 20:88-91, 1988.
54. Vogel W, Steiner E, Kornberger R, et al: Preliminary results with combined hepatorenal allografting. Transplantation 45:491-492, 1988.
55. Gil-Vernet S, Prieto C, Grino J, et al: Combined liver kidney transplantation. Transplant Proc 24:128-129, 1992.
56. Shaked A, Thompson M, Wilkinson A, et al: The role of combined liver/kidney transplantation in end stage hepatorenal disease. Am Surg 59:606-609, 1993.
57. Soriano S, Castillo D, Perez R, et al: Long term results of combined kidney and liver transplantation in patients with nephropathy associated with liver disease. Transplant Proc 31:2306-2307, 1999.
58. Torregrosa J, Inigo P, Navasa M, et al: Combined liver kidney transplantation: Our experience. Transplant Proc 31:2308, 1999.
59. Greweal H, Brady L, Cronin D, et al: Combined liver and kidney transplantation in children. Transplantation 70:100-105, 2000.
60. Goldstein R, Solomon H, Holman M, et al: Liver transplantation, 1990: A Dallas perspective. Clin Transpl 4:123-132, 1990.
61. Margreiter R, Konigsrainer A, Spechtenhauser B, et al: Our experience with combined liver kidney transplantation: An update. Transplant Proc 34:2491-2492, 2002.
62. Mejia A, Iyer K, Mercer D, et al: Results of combined liver kidney and kidney after liver transplantation [abstract 829]. American Transplant Congress 2003. Washington D.C. Am J Transplant 3(Suppl 5):365, 2003.

Auxiliary Liver Transplantation

CARLOS MARGARIT

Surgical techniques 816

Heterotopic auxiliary liver transplantation 817
  Advantages and disadvantages 817

Auxiliary partial orthotopic liver
  transplantation 818

Heterotopic auxiliary liver transplantation with
  portal vein arterialization 818

Auxiliary liver transplantation for fulminant
  hepatic failure 821
  Selection criteria 821
  Criteria to decide on the auxiliary liver
    transplantation technique 822

Postoperative course and graft function 822
  Withdrawal of immunosuppression
    and graft removal 823

Experience in auxiliary liver transplantation for
  fulminant liver failure 824

Auxiliary liver transplantation for inborn errors
  of metabolism 826

Auxiliary liver transplantation for small-for-size
  living donor graft liver transplantation 826

Auxiliary liver transplantation for chronic
  liver failure 827

The concept of auxiliary liver transplantation (ALT) is that a new donor liver is implanted without complete removal of the native diseased liver. Thus, the patient is left with two livers, the graft and the native. The auxiliary liver graft can be placed in two positions: the heterotopic position in which the liver is implanted in the right paracolic gutter, caudal to the native liver, and the orthotopic position, whereby a portion of the native liver is resected and a partial graft is implanted in the vacated resection site.

In the early days of liver transplantation (LT), the rationale for using heterotopic auxiliary liver transplantation (HALT) was the difficulty and danger of removing the liver of patients suffering from end-stage liver cirrhosis with portal hypertension, massive ascites, and coagulation disorders. Significant blood loss and hemodynamic instability during hepatectomy with inferior vena cava resection were common events leading to high perioperative mortality. At that time, deceased donor liver grafts were obtained after cardiac arrest of the donor because brain death had not been legally accepted; moreover, the immunosuppression available was not very efficient and, consequently, severe ischemic-reperfusion injury and refractory graft rejection were common complications leading to graft failure and patient death, as retransplantation was almost impossible. Leaving the native liver in place with its residual function was an attractive concept in cases of transplant failure. The initial reports of experimental liver transplantation by Welch[1] and Goodrich[2] used the heterotopic auxiliary approach, following the technique used in heterotopic kidney transplantation, the most commonly performed organ transplantation. Absolon[3] and Fortner[4] and their colleagues reported the first cases of heterotopic liver transplantation in chronic liver disease. Although the problems of native hepatectomy were obviated, it soon became evident that the disadvantages of this option arose from the abnormal or unfavorable hemodynamic status of the auxiliary graft. Technical complications were common: insufficient venous outflow and portal vein thrombosis led to graft dysfunction and failure.[5] Finally, the diseased liver remnant was a source of serious problems that compromised the outcome of the patient, such as development of hepatocellular carcinoma or cholangitis and liver abscess.[6] Advances both in surgical techniques, such as venovenous bypass or piggyback technique, and intraoperative management of coagulation disorders and hemodynamic problems have rendered recipient hepatectomy a safe procedure.[7] Therefore, orthotopic liver transplantation (OLT) soon became the standard technical option in LT, leading to a loss of interest in the ALT technique.[8]

In the past decade, interest in ALT as an option in the treatment of fulminant liver failure (FLF) and some metabolic diseases has been renewed.[9,10] The capacity of the liver to regenerate after near-complete necrosis is remarkable. The hepatocytes remaining are able to proliferate and achieve ad integrum restitution of the liver. However, the time required for regeneration to take place can be weeks or months. In the meantime, the patient suffering acute liver failure will die if a procedure to support liver function is not instituted. Extracorporeal liver-assist devices do not currently constitute a good option for longtime liver support; patients can be maintained alive for only hours or a few days until a liver graft becomes available or the patient recovers.[11] Transplant of an auxiliary graft is the only option to substitute the function of the native liver, which is left in place to provide an opportunity for recovery. However, this very attractive option for the treatment of FLF poses many unresolved or unanswered queries,[12,13] such as what the indications are for this procedure and what the best techniques are—orthotopic or heterotopic. To date, no evidence has emerged that ALT is better than OLT; therefore, OLT continues to be the gold standard for the treatment of FLF. However, with loss of the native liver there is no potential for liver regeneration, and the patient is committed to lifelong risks of immunological rejection and immunosuppression.

A further indication for ALT has been small-for-size living donor LT. Several cases had been reported before donation of the right lobe for adult living donor LT became generally accepted.[14] Resection of the left lobe was considered less dangerous for the living donor than resection of the right lobe, which accounts for 60% of liver parenchyma. Frequently, the left lobe, and sometimes even the right lobe, provides insufficient liver mass for an adult. In these cases, the recipient may present the small-for-size syndrome characterized by jaundice, ascites, and other signs of liver failure. A two-step treatment is planned: first, a left hepatectomy is performed in the recipient, and the left lobe of the living donor is transplanted orthotopically. Once the graft has regenerated, the remaining right lobe of the recipient is removed in a second operation.

Implantation of an auxiliary liver graft has also been proposed for the treatment of certain metabolic diseases.[15] The native liver in such cases is anatomically and functionally completely normal; the donor liver provides a gene or enzyme that is missing or altered in the recipient. The advantage of auxiliary transplantation is that in cases of graft failure from primary nonfunction, rejection, or technical failures, the patient survives thanks to the function of the native liver. However, for success of the transplant, long-time immunosuppression is required and the shared portal venous flow should be directed to the graft, which otherwise will atrophy. ALT in these cases leaves the door open for future gene therapy of the metabolic defect.

Auxiliary LT is technically more difficult than OLT. Postoperative management is more complicated, as diagnosis of graft dysfunction by laboratory tests is misleading owing to the presence of the native liver, which contributes to abnormal liver function tests. Toxic liver syndrome complicates postoperative management of the critically ill patient with FLF. For all these reasons, the role of ALT is not completely established in the armamentarium of LT and the treatment of FLF.

Surgical Techniques

Original laboratory experiments on auxiliary liver transplantation adopted the heterotopic model with a whole or partial liver. The donor portal vein was anastomosed to the iliac vein of the recipient; therefore, portal vein inflow originated from the systemic venous circulation. Graft atrophy was a common event with this model. The classic experiments of Marchioro and associates[16] in 1965 provided a physiological explanation for the graft atrophy. They showed portal vein inflow from the splenopancreatic and intestinal venous beds to be an important requirement for long-term heterotopic auxiliary graft survival. Hepatotropic substances from the portal vein were not fully identified but included insulin and glucagon. The experimental work of Van der Hyde and associates,[17] with a model of heterotopic liver grafts without portal venous inflow and with or without impairment of the native liver by ligation of the bile duct and portocaval shunt, showed the importance of functional competition between both livers, the native and the grafted. In the model of impaired or "disadvantaged" native liver, the graft without portal vein inflow did not atrophy. Those authors concluded that atrophy was dependent on which liver was more advantaged from a physiological standpoint and that portal blood flow to the graft is not an absolute requirement in preventing atrophy. The hypothesis was that by providing a "handicap" to the healthy host liver, the heterotopic graft would be in a more favorable situation to compete. Other experiments and clinical situations, such as cavoportal transposition in cases of diffuse portal vein thrombosis[18] or portal vein arterialization,[19] suggest that it is not the quality but rather the quantity of the blood that is important for graft function.[20]

In 1991, Gubernatis and associates[21] reported the first successful case of auxiliary partial orthotopic liver transplantation (APOLT). Since then, this technique has gained more acceptance because it overcomes the considerable disadvantages of HALT, such as the outflow problem and lack of room in the abdomen for two livers. In 1995, Erhard and associates[22] described the first cases of HALT for FLF with portal vein arterialization (PVA). The rationale was that the liver can function normally with complete arterialized inflow and that high-pressure inflow can overcome the venous outflow problem originated by high pressure in the hepatic veins of the heterotopic graft. The native liver, in contrast, is left untouched with no portal vein diversion, thereby affording the best chance of rapid regeneration.

Heterotopic Auxiliary Liver Transplantation

The first successful surgeries using the HALT technique were performed by Fortner and associates[4]; however, review of all 47 cases performed prior to 1980 showed that only two patients survived longer than 1 year. Terpstra modified the surgical technique after careful study of the experimental models.[23] A whole or partial graft is placed in the right paracolic gutter after mobilization of the right colon. The suprarenal inferior vena cava (IVC) and infrarenal aorta are exposed and the hepatic hilum dissected to achieve good control of the portal vein, as for portocaval shunt surgery. Implantation of the graft begins with an end-to-side anastomosis between the suprahepatic donor IVC and recipient IVC; this anastomosis is placed as near as possible to the diaphragm where venous pressure is lower. The second anastomosis is an end-to-side anastomosis between the graft and recipient portal veins. After graft revascularization with portal blood, the anastomosis between the donor celiac trunk and the recipient aorta is fashioned. Finally, a choledochojejunostomy to a Roux-en-Y loop of jejunum is performed (Fig. 55–1). Expansion of the abdominal cavity with a Silastic or Gore-Tex sheet is commonly required in patients transplanted for FLF, as there is no abdominal distention by chronic ascites.

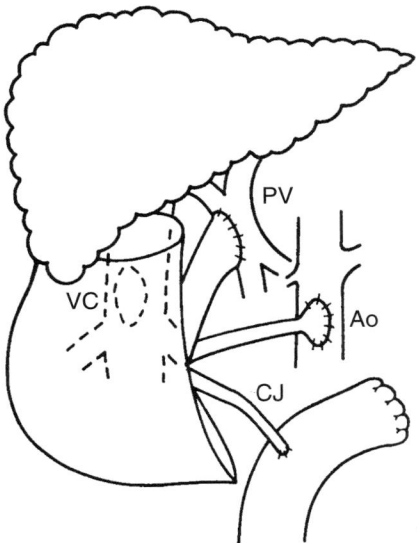

FIGURE 55–1

Schematic representation of a heterotopic auxiliary liver transplant following the technique described by O.T. Terpstra. Ao, aorta; CJ, choledochojejunostomy; PV, portal vein; VC, vena cava.

Advantages and Disadvantages

Native hepatectomy, the most difficult phase of OLT in Child-Pugh C patients with severe portal hypertension, coagulopathy, previous surgery, and so on is avoided. However, recipient hepatectomy is currently performed even in difficult cases, with minimal blood loss and hemodynamic stability by means of venovenous bypass or piggyback procedure with or without temporary portocaval shunt.[7] Moreover, the dissection required to place the heterotopic graft in these cirrhotic patients can also be difficult and bloody. Leaving the native liver in place has the potential advantage of allowing liver regeneration in cases of FLF; when regeneration occurs, immunosuppression can be stopped and the graft removed if necessary. However, leaving the native necrotic liver has potential disadvantages in FLF because hemodynamic instability and cerebral edema may persist because of the toxic liver syndrome. In patients who undergo transplantation for chronic liver failure, the risk of development of hepatocellular carcinoma (HCC) is high, particularly in hepatitis B and C viral cirrhosis. Moreover, infection of the graft by these viruses could be more severe, as the hepatic reservoir of the viruses is not removed. The great concern with this technique lies in the abnormal hemodynamic situation of the graft with high outflow pressure and portal vein flow diversion, and the risks of graft dysfunction and portal vein thrombosis are high.

The results with HALT for FLF are not good owing to the technical problems implied by portal vein thrombosis and graft dysfunction; thus, this option is not recommended by the majority of authors who prefer the orthotopic approach.[24]

Auxiliary Partial Orthotopic Liver Transplantation

Since Gubernatis and associates[21,41] described APOLT in 1991, it has become the technique of choice for ALT. A partial graft is used, although sometimes a small whole graft from a pediatric donor has been transplanted orthotopically as an auxiliary graft. Donor liver should be of very good quality because a partial graft has to maintain liver function. Donor liver can be split in situ for transplantation of both parts into two recipients or it can be harvested and divided ex situ as a bench procedure. The arterial pedicle of the auxiliary graft should be as long as possible and donor iliac vessels must be harvested. The decision as to which part of the liver will be resected—the right lobe, left lobe, or left lateral segment—depends on the quality of the graft, donor-recipient body weight ratio (DRBWR), and the clinical status of the patient. Right hepatectomy and transplantation of the right lobe is performed when the recipient is an adult, DRBWR is low, or toxic liver syndrome is present. In children or low-weight adults with high DRBWR and without toxic liver syndrome, transplantation of the left lobe is recommended. Recipient hepatectomy is a demanding operation in the context of a critically ill patient with coagulation disorders and hemodynamic instability. Bloodless transection of the liver can be achieved under total vascular isolation by cross-clamping the hepatic hilum and hepatic veins. After resection of the lobe, the supraceliac or infrarenal aorta is dissected and a donor iliac artery conduit is anastomosed end-to-side to the aorta. Implantation of the auxiliary graft will start with anastomosis of the corresponding hepatic veins of the donor and recipient, and the donor portal vein is then anastomosed end-to-side to the recipient portal vein. The liver can then be perfused with portal vein blood or the iliac conduit anastomosed to the celiac trunk of the donor and complete revascularization performed. Finally, a hepatico-jejunum Roux-en-Y is fashioned (Figs. 55–2 and 55–3). In general, no space problem in the abdomen for the two grafts is observed and regular closure without prosthetic material can be performed.

The orthotopic position of the graft favors excellent venous outflow; therefore, the graft has good hemodynamic location. Portal venous blood flow diversion to the graft occurs spontaneously in cases of FLF; however, in cases of inborn errors of metabolism the liver is normal without higher resistance to venous flow, and partial or total occlusion of the portal vein of the native liver is necessary to ensure adequate portal blood supply to the graft. When no regeneration of the native

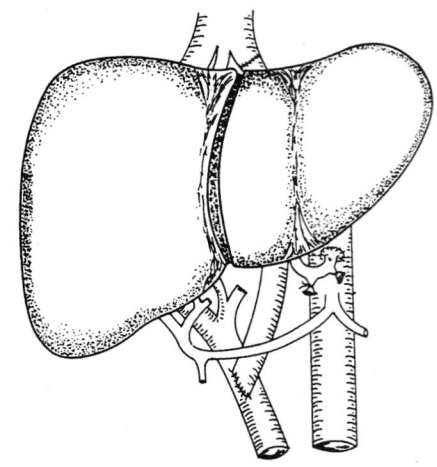

FIGURE 55–2

Schematic representation of a left lobe auxiliary orthotopic liver transplant (APOLT) following the technique described by Gubernatis and associates.

liver occurs, native liver atrophy and graft hypertrophy are present; if regeneration takes place, growth of the native liver is observed and the graft can be left to atrophy by withdrawing immunosuppression or it can be removed. Removal of the graft is a much more complicated operation in APOLT than in HALT.

APOLT is a difficult operation, requiring a right or left hepatectomy in a critically ill patient, and a partial graft of sufficient size and excellent quality must be used to support liver function. The potential for complications, including hemorrhage, bile leaks, collections, sepsis, and graft dysfunction, is high. Native liver regeneration can be jeopardized by resection of part of the liver and absence of portal vein flow to the native liver.

APOLT is the technique of choice in ALT, with results far better than those of HALT. Patient and graft survival are similar to those of OLT. However, an increased number of complications such as portal vein thrombosis, graft dysfunction, and biliary complications still occur compared with OLT.[25-28]

Heterotopic Auxiliary Liver Transplantation with Portal Vein Arterialization

The heterotopic graft is placed in the right paracolic gutter following the HALT technique, but a donor common iliac artery with its bifurcation is placed as a conduit between the infrarenal aorta and the portal vein and celiac trunk or hepatic artery of the donor in each of its branches. A whole or partial liver is used depending on size and quality (Fig. 55–4). The graft is perfused

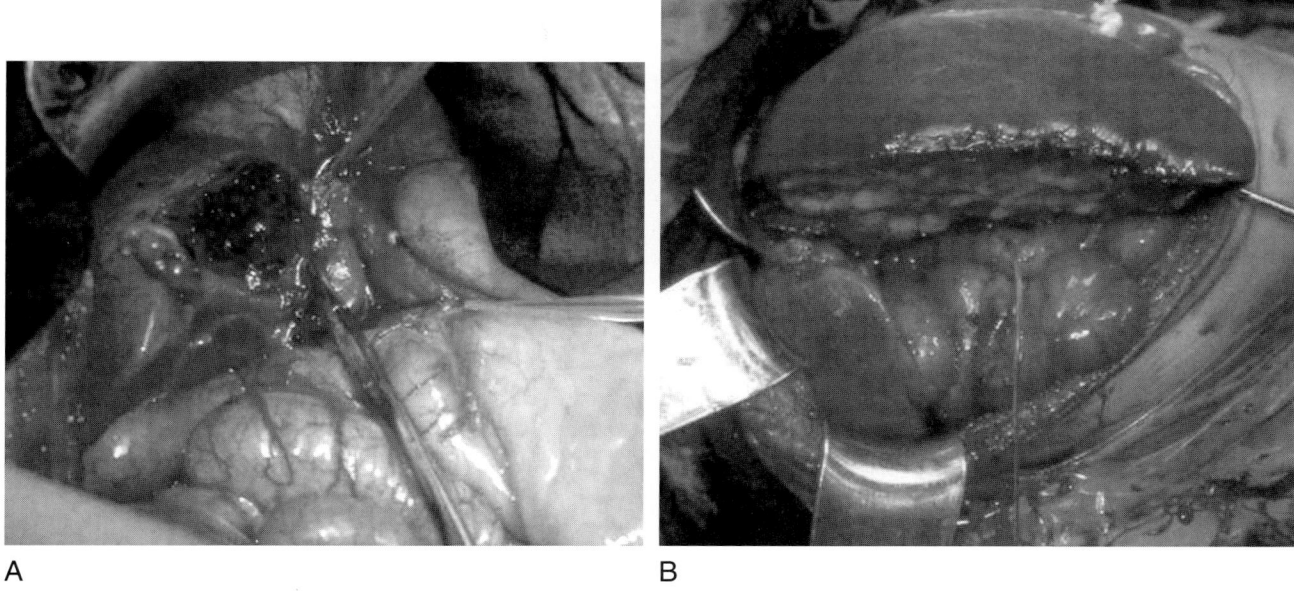

A   B

FIGURE 55–3

Operative photographs of a left APOLT in a 5-year-old boy with fulminant liver failure. **A,** Left lateral segmental (segments II and III) resection of the native liver to accommodate the left liver graft. **B,** Left liver lobe transplanted in auxiliary orthotopic position.

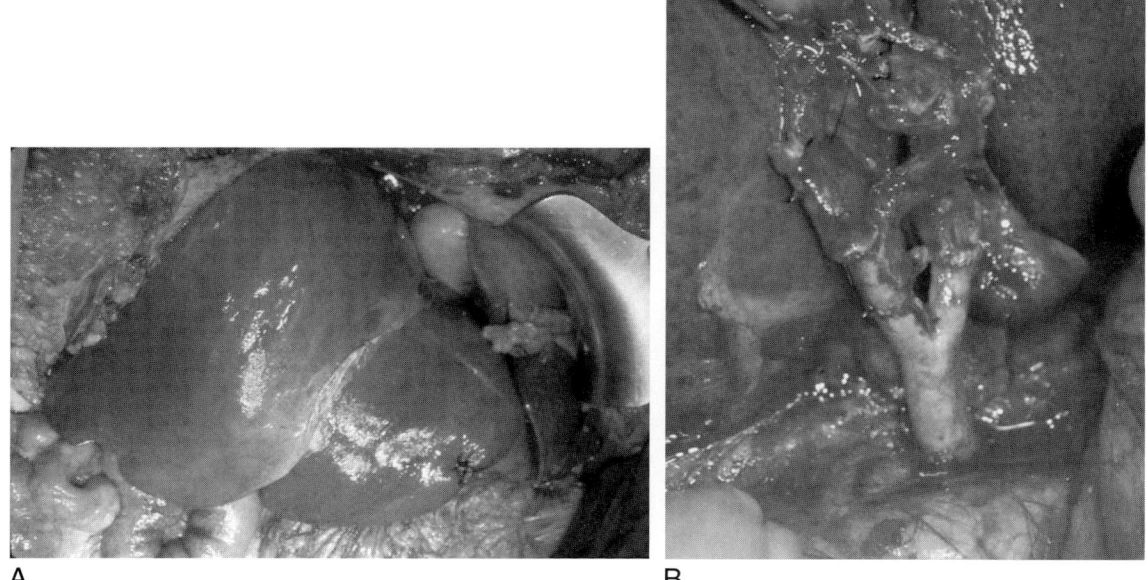

A   B

FIGURE 55–4

Operative photographs of a heterotopic auxiliary graft with portal vein arterialization for fulminant liver failure in a 52-year-old woman with seronegative hepatitis. **A,** The atrophied native liver and the heterotopic graft. **B,** Donor iliac conduit between the aorta and portal vein and celiac trunk of the graft.

only with arterial high-pressure blood from the aorta. The aim of this option is to leave the hepatic hilum undisturbed with no diversion of portal venous blood flow; therefore chances of rapid regeneration are optimal.[29,30] Expansion of the abdominal cavity is usually required by placement of prosthetic material. This is an easy and rapid operation: minimal dissection is required, the vascular anastomoses are straightforward and in cases of native liver regeneration, explantation of the graft is also easy. If no regeneration occurs, the situation is complicated by the fact that portal hypertension and ascites persist, thereby complicating the outcome of the patient. Autotransplantation of the graft to the orthotopic position or retransplantation with a second graft in orthotopic position are the potential solutions to this problem.

Arterialization of the liver is a well-known phenomenon occurring in the evolution of the cirrhotic liver. A progressive decrease in portal venous flow because of an increase in intrahepatic flow resistance and, at the same time, a compensatory increase in arterial flow are observed. Orthotopic liver transplantation with portal vein arterialization has been described as an alternative technique in cases of diffuse thrombosis of the splanchnic veins, and a further alternative is cavoportal hemitransposition.[18] The limited experience with long-term follow-up of these grafts with PVA shows that liver architecture is conserved and liver function is normal.[19] We performed hemodynamic studies in one auxiliary heterotopic graft with PVA. High pressure of 25 mm Hg was observed in hepatic veins, wedge hepatic venous pressure was 32 mm Hg, and hepatic venous pressure gradient was 8 mm Hg, corresponding to normal sinusoidal pressure. Presinusoidal pressure corresponding to mean arterial pressure was 91 mm Hg. This high inflow pressure that superseded the high outflow pressure would explain the good hemodynamic status of the heterotopic graft with PVA compared with the heterotopic graft with low inflow pressure from portal venous inflow.[30]

In summary, ALT presents the following problems (Table 55–1):

- *Problems of space* for two livers in the abdominal cavity can create high intra-abdominal pressure with hemodynamic consequences such as renal impairment, compression of the graft with decreased perfusion, impaired venous return, and elevation of the diaphragm causing respiratory failure.

- *Functional competition* for portal venous flow between the native and grafted livers exists in cases of HALT for metabolic diseases when the native liver is normal; in these cases portal flow has to be directed toward the graft. In cases of end-stage liver cirrhosis or acute liver failure, increased resistance is observed in the native liver because the portal flow and diversion of portal venous flow to the graft is spontaneous.

- *Venous outflow.* Under normal conditions in humans, the pressure gradient between liver sinusoids and hepatic veins measures 2 mm Hg, and pressure in hepatic veins is low and close to the intrathoracic pressure and is affected by the respiratory cycle. In the recumbent position, pressure in the inferior vena cava increases a few millimeters of mercury caudally toward the iliac vein. In the orthostatic position, pressure in the IVC is affected by gravity and each centimeter below the level of the right atrium yields a pressure increase of 0.77 mm Hg. When the heterotopic liver graft is anastomosed to the infrarenal IVC, pressure in hepatic veins in the upright position is 10 to 15 mm Hg higher than under physiological conditions, thus jeopardizing sinusoidal blood flow.

- *Toxic liver syndrome.* Hemodynamic instability and cerebral edema are common complications of acute or fulminant liver failure. The pathogenesis of these complications remains controversial: they can be produced by liver failure or release of

Table 55–1. PROBLEMS OF AUXILIARY LIVER TRANSPLANTATION IN DIFFERENT TECHNIQUES

Technique	Recipient Hepatectomy	Toxic Liver Syndrome	Hemodynamic Status of the Graft	Portal Venous Flow Diversion	Conditions for Native Liver Regeneration	Problem of Space
OLT	Total	No	Excellent	No	No	No
APOLT	Partial		Excellent	Yes	Yes	No
Right lobe	60%	Mild		Yes	Suboptimal	
Left lobe	40%	Moderate			Intermediate	
HALT	No	Severe	Deficient	Yes	Yes, suboptimal	Yes
HALT with PVA	No	Severe	Good	No	Yes, excellent	Yes

APOLT, auxiliary partial orthotopic liver transplantation; HALT, heterotopic auxiliary liver transplantation; OLT, orthotopic liver transplantation; PVA, portal vein arterialization.

toxins and cytokines from the necrotic liver, or both.[31,32] Liver transplantation in a two-step procedure reported by Ringe and associates[31] showed the beneficial effect of native liver hepatectomy on the control of toxic liver syndrome.

- *Regeneration of the native liver.* In theory, the best possibilities for native liver regeneration would be for the liver to remain untouched, without hepatectomy and portal vein flow diversion. Conversely, hepatectomy is known to be an important stimulus for regeneration.

Auxiliary Liver Transplantation for Fulminant Hepatic Failure

The aim of ALT in patients with FLF is to provide temporary liver support to allow the native liver to regenerate. Once sufficient regeneration occurs and native liver function is normal, immunosuppression is withdrawn and the graft can either be left to atrophy or removed. The patient is no longer condemned to the hazards of life-long risks of rejection and immunosuppression. If insufficient regeneration of the native liver occurs after ALT, immunosuppression can be maintained and the graft will give permanent support, no longer being "auxiliary."

OLT is currently the gold standard for the treatment of FLF; 1-year survival reaches 60% to 70%, whereas spontaneous survival without LT is approximately 10% to 30%. Patients surviving the procedure must be treated for life with immunosuppression, with potentially life-threatening side effects such as infections, lymphomas and de novo tumors. There is also the potential for chronic rejection and graft loss, drug toxicity resulting in renal failure, arterial hypertension, diabetes, hyperlipidemias, and increased cardiovascular risk. These risks are difficult for patients to accept, as they are often young and healthy before the FLF episode.

FLF is defined as acute liver necrosis complicated by encephalopathy within 3 months after the onset of jaundice. FLF is classified, according to timing of presentation of encephalopathy, as hyperacute form, when encephalopathy appears before the 8th day; acute form, when it appears before the 28th day; and subacute, when it appears between 5 and 12 weeks. The decision for LT in FLF is based on well-accepted criteria reported by the Clichy[33] or King's College[34] groups. Mortality without LT is approximately 90%. Transient improvement can be achieved with artificial devices such as MARS (molecular adsorbent recirculating system) hemodiafiltration or artificial liver; however, these methods cannot consistently substitute liver function for long enough to allow the native liver to recover. For now they can only form a bridge to LT.

The first and imperative objective of ALT, as well as of OLT, is that the patient recover from liver failure and survive. Therefore, ALT should offer the same results in terms of patient and graft survival as OLT to justify its application. Moreover, the number of patients reaching the ultimate goal of ALT, that is, survival without sequelae and full recovery of native liver function with no need for immunosuppression should be high enough to justify the greater complexity of the procedure and the postoperative course.[13]

Selection Criteria

Criteria for deciding to perform ALT instead of OLT are not well established. The key issue is the identification of factors for accurate prediction of complete native liver regeneration (Table 55–2). The following factors should be taken into account:

- *Age of the patient.* ALT should be reserved for young patients. Livers of patients older than 45 to 50 years of age have fewer possibilities of regeneration because the incidence of fibrosis or steatosis is higher. Complete native liver regeneration achieved in 78% of patients younger than age 40 years and only 25% of those older than age 40 years was reported by Van Hoek and associates[24] from the European Registry of ALT (EURALT). Moreover, older patients do not tolerate a complicated postoperative course well and the risks of chronic immunosuppression are lower.

- *Cause of FLF.* Liver failure because of acute hepatitis A or B or toxic hepatitis induced by drugs such as paracetamol, ecstasy, tuberculostatic drugs, or *Amanita phalloides* poisoning has a greater chance of recovery once the virus or toxic drugs have been eliminated than does liver failure of unknown cause or that caused by hepatitis C virus. The treatment of FLF caused by metabolic or inborn errors of metabolism must be OLT because

Table 55–2. CRITERIA FOR PERFORMING AUXILIARY LIVER TRANSPLANTATION IN FULMINANT LIVER FAILURE

Age younger than 40 years

Hyperacute or acute form of acute liver failure (interval jaundice/encephalopathy < 4 weeks)

Cause of acute liver failure: hepatitis A or B, drugs, *Amanita phalloides* poisoning

No cerebral edema or severe toxic liver syndrome

No fibrosis or cirrhosis on frozen-section biopsy at operation

Good donor liver

Possibility of noncompliance

the patient can recover from liver failure and the metabolic problem be cured.

- *Type of presentation of FLF.* The hyperacute form of FLF is a dramatic presentation and indication for LT. However, rapid and extensive liver necrosis can be followed by regeneration from the few hepatocytes left alive. Subacute or subfulminant liver failure is a slower process in which it takes weeks for the liver failure to appear. During that time, the liver is not able to recover; consequently, the possibilities of liver regeneration after ALT are scant.

- *Clinical status of the patient.* If the patient presents with toxic liver syndrome characterized by hemodynamic instability, high vasoactive drug requirements, multiorgan failure, respiratory and renal failure and cerebral edema, the best procedure is OLT because it is rapid, simpler, and completely removes the necrotic liver cause of this syndrome.

- *Histology of the native liver at the time of LT.* Liver biopsy is mandatory before the decision to perform ALT is made. No relationship exists between the extent of liver cell necrosis at biopsy and the possibility of regeneration.[35] However, the presence of fibrosis, macroscopic regenerative nodules within a small, necrotic liver, or signs of chronic liver disease predict abnormal regeneration and potential evolution to chronic liver disease; in such cases the verdict should be to perform OLT.

- *Donor liver.* APOLT must always be performed with a good donor because only a part of the liver or a small whole liver will be transplanted. Whole-liver OLT or HALT with PVA are the best options when a suboptimal donor has to be accepted. ALT could constitute a good option when ABO blood group–incompatible grafts are transplanted because the risks of graft failure are greater, and it may be that when the liver graft fails, the native liver has already regenerated and retransplantation is not required.

- *Patient characteristics.* ALT is a good option in patients with the potential danger of noncompliance, such as those with psychiatric disorders, those who have made previous suicide attempts, drug abusers, adolescents, illegal immigrants, and those with lack of social or economic support.

Criteria to Decide on the Auxiliary Liver Transplantation Technique

APOLT is the best choice in stable patients without toxic liver syndrome or cerebral edema and when the donor liver is of good quality. These patients will tolerate native-liver partial hepatectomy, a partial liver graft will be implanted orthotopically in a favorable hemodynamic position, and there will be no space problems. Two types of APOLT can be performed—right and left.

- Right APOLT: The advantages of right hepatectomy and right graft implantation are that there will be less toxic liver syndrome, because 60% of the liver is removed, and better postoperative liver function, because more functional liver parenchyma is transplanted. Disadvantages include more difficult hepatectomy and fewer possibilities of rapid regeneration because the patient is left with less than 40% of the native liver and without portal perfusion because all portal venous flow is diverted to the graft.

- Left APOLT: Left hepatectomy or left lateral segmentectomy and implantation of a left lobe liver graft will leave the patient with more necrotic liver in place and a smaller sized graft. The postoperative course may be more complicated, with more toxic liver syndrome and less function of the graft; however, the possibility of regeneration is greater.

HALT can be performed in young, stable patients without toxic liver syndrome or cerebral edema and with maximum possibilities of regeneration, and toxic or hepatitis A or B as the origin of FLF. When the available graft is suboptimal, ABO-incompatible, or of small size, HALT is also a good option. Whenever HALT is indicated, we prefer to perform HALT with PVA to improve graft hemodynamics and leave the native liver in an optimal situation to regenerate.

Postoperative Course and Graft Function

Recovery may be slower, and the postoperative management of ALT patients is commonly more difficult than that of OLT patients. Toxic liver syndrome persists to a greater or lesser degree owing to the presence of the remaining necrotic native liver. Portal hypertension and ascites production continues, particularly when the portal venous system is not decompressed as in HALT with PVA. The presence of two grafts, ascites, intestinal edema, and ileus may produce high abdominal pressure and, consequently, prolongation of the need for mechanical ventilation, renal failure, and hemodialysis requirements. Monitoring of graft function is also more difficult owing to the presence of two livers. Alterations in liver function tests originating from the necrotic native liver can hinder the diagnosis of ischemia-preservation injury or acute rejection. Liver graft biopsy should be performed with ultrasound guidance to distinguish the graft from the native liver. Hemorrhage can complicate a liver biopsy in grafts with PVA and high-pressure inflow. As rejection is a frequent event in patients who undergo transplantation for FLF and the diagnosis of rejection is difficult and many patients have renal failure, immunosuppression regimens should combine calcineurin inhibitors, mycophenolate mofetil, steroids, and anti–interleukin 2 receptor (IL-2R) monoclonal antibodies.

Daily Doppler ultrasound examination during the first week and weekly abdominal computed tomographic scans are performed to check the size, vascular patency, and flow direction of both livers.

Native liver regeneration is the specific goal of ALT. Assessment of the degree of regeneration and function of the native liver and its differentiation from the function of the graft is not easy. Biochemical liver function tests do not permit differentiation between the metabolic activity of each liver. Radiological assessment is helpful, and serial Doppler ultrasound and computed tomographic scans may show normalization of parenchymal characteristics and increase in volume as signs of native liver regeneration (Fig. 55–5). Sequential radionuclide hepatobiliary scintigraphy with quantitative analysis provides a useful noninvasive technique for assessing differential graft and native liver functions and can be readily repeated.[36] Serial technetium-99m IDA (iminodiacetic acid) scans clearly demonstrated an increase in hepatocyte extraction (uptake) and biliary excretion (elimination) of tracer by the native liver that correlated

with histological regeneration (Fig. 55–6). Sequential biopsy specimens of the native liver and the auxiliary graft are invaluable in assessing their histological evolution and normalization of liver histology (Fig. 55–7).

Withdrawal of Immunosuppression and Graft Removal

The decision to withdraw immunosuppression should be made once the native liver has completely regenerated. The graft can be left to atrophy or can be removed. Graft removal is usually indicated for grafts in a heterotopic position because it is easier and, at the same time, prosthetic material used to expand the abdominal cavity can be removed. Graft removal in the orthotopic position is much more difficult and is not recommended unless problems with the graft arise. In the EURALT study, the auxiliary graft was removed in 60% of patients alive at 1 year without immunosuppression, whereas in 40% of patients alive at 1 year it was left to atrophy.[24,28] Immunosuppression can be progressively tapered to induce a chronic rejection process that will lead to slow atrophy and fibrosis of the graft or it can be abruptly stopped, which is likely to produce an acute and symptomatic rejection requiring graft removal.

The possibility of immunosuppression withdrawal in long-term OLT survivors would make the rationale

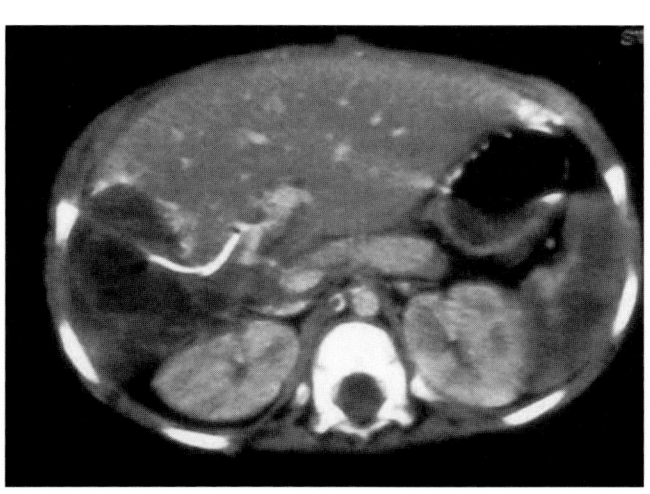

A

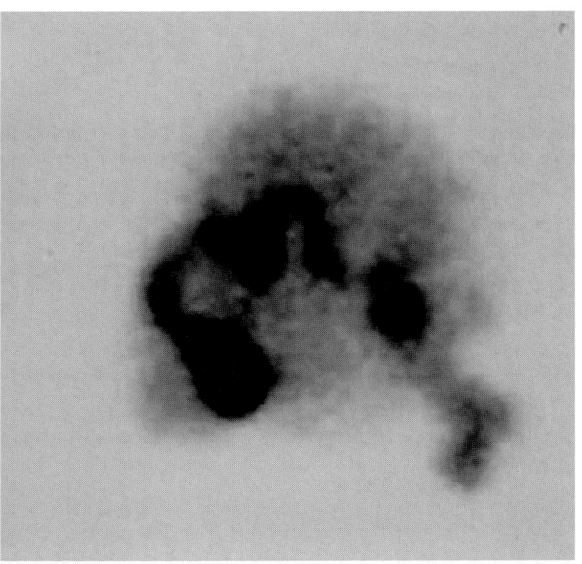

B

FIGURE 55–5

Absence of native liver regeneration 6 months after left APOLT in a 5-year-old boy. **A,** Computed tomographic scan shows atrophy of native liver and a normal left lobe graft. **B,** Radioisotope scan with no uptake and elimination of the tracer by the native liver and normal uptake and elimination to the loop of jejunum by the graft.

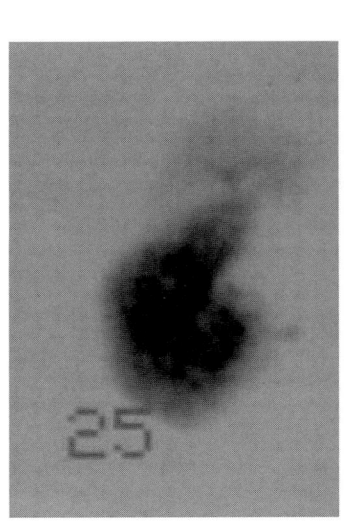
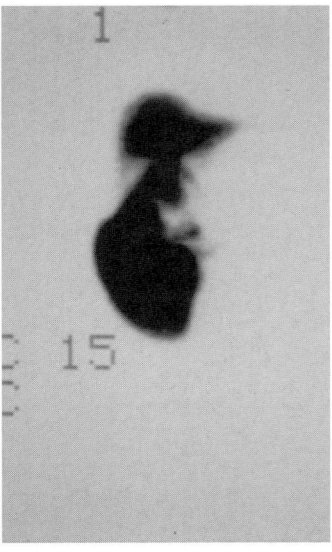

A   B

FIGURE 55–6

Radioisotope scanning (technetium-99m IDA tracer) of native liver and transplanted liver (**A**) 1 week after HALT with PVA, with minimal uptake and no elimination of the tracer by the native liver, and a good functional heterotopic liver graft and (**B**) 3 months after HALT, with good uptake and elimination of the tracer by the regenerated native liver.

for APOLT obsolete.[37] The goal of APOLT is rarely achieved and, in addition, the price to be paid in terms of complications is high.

Recurrence of the original disease was a concern in cases of FLF from acute hepatitis B treated with ALT, as the native infected liver is left behind. However, experience has shown that there is clearance of the virus in acute hepatitis B and patients who recover do not develop chronic HBV infection, as occurs after OLT. These patients should be treated with lamivudine and hepatitis B immune globulin during the time they are on immunosuppression.

Experience in Auxiliary Liver Transplantation for Fulminant Liver Failure

The European experience with ALT in FLF was presented in 1996[28] and 1999.[24] Forty-seven patients from 12 centers were compared with a control group of 384 patients who underwent OLT for FLF. One-year patient survival was 61% for OLT and 62% for ALT (71% APOLT and 33% HALT). Incidence of primary nonfunction (PNF) was higher after HALT (25%) than after either APOLT

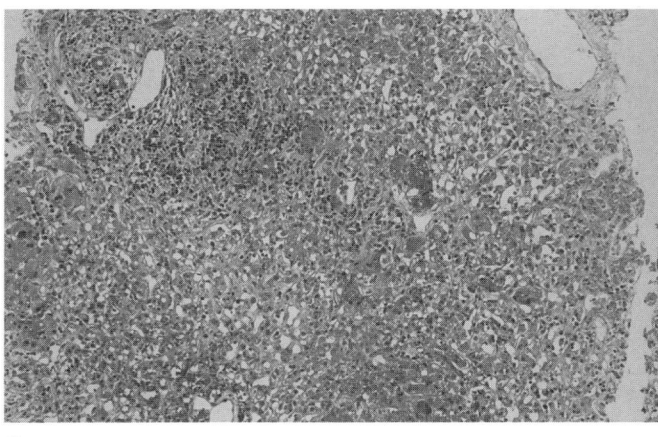
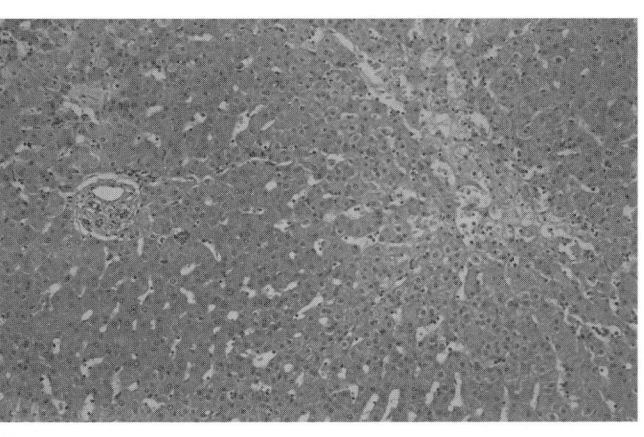

A   B

FIGURE 55–7

Histology of the native liver (**A**) specimen taken during the transplant. Acute toxic hepatitis with submassive necrosis, eosinophilic infiltration of portal triad and hepatocellular necrosis in areas II and III are seen (trichromic, original magnification ×100). **B**, Specimen of the regenerating liver 3 months after HALT with PVA. Regeneration of hepatic parenchyma, minimal residual lesions of perivenular necrosis, and no fibrosis or inflammation in portal triad are seen (hematoxylin and eosin, original magnification ×100).

(8.5%) or OLT (5.5%). Portal vein thrombosis was more frequent after HALT (42%) and APOLT (14%) than after OLT (0.5%); 65% of the patients surviving more than 1 year were free of immunosuppression. Three factors were important for prediction of native liver regeneration: age younger than 40 years, viral hepatitis, or paracetamol overdose and hyperacute course, all of which are acknowledged indicators of relatively favorable outcome in patients with FLF (Table 55–3).

Boudjema and associates[11] presented 18 APOLT (12 right and 6 left) in 17 patients, with patient survival of 65%. Native liver regeneration was seen in 65% of 11 living patients; however, only 5 of the survivors were able to stop immunosuppression therapy.

Sudan and associates[38] treated seven patients with APOLT; four are alive and regeneration was observed in six of seven patients. However, a high incidence of reoperations and two cases of aplastic anemia were reported.

Pereira and associates[40] from King's College Hospital London presented seven cases of APOLT for FLF: two left APOLT and five right. They observed slow improvement in graft function, high frequency of bacterial infections, and a long period of mechanical ventilation. Three were alive, but only two achieved complete native liver regeneration and immunosuppression withdrawal. The other four died from sepsis.

The experience at Paul Brousse Hospital[13] with 12 APOLT (8 received a right lobe and 4 received a left lobe) was compared with 24 OLT cases. Cold ischemia time (CIT) and duration of the procedure were longer in the APOLT group than in the OLT group. More biliary complications, infections, and need for retransplantation were observed in the APOLT group, although similar 1-year patient survival (66%) was achieved in both groups. Brain death from neurological sequelae was significantly more frequent after APOLT. Only 3 of 12 (25%) had native liver regeneration and only 2 of 12 (17%) had full success with APOLT (patient survival, liver regeneration, and withdrawal of immunosuppression), but one of these two had neurological sequelae. They conclude that APOLT should have a limited place in the treatment of ALF owing to risks of technical complications and neurological sequelae.

Durand and associates[39] from Beaujon Paris presented six patients with FHF from acute hepatitis B infection. Left APOLT was performed in two and right APOLT in four. Only one patient died, from systemic aspergillosis, the other five were still alive, four with a follow-up of longer than 1 year. An 83% patient

Table 55–3. EXPERIENCE WITH AUXILIARY LIVER TRANSPLANTATION FOR FULMINANT LIVER FAILURE

Author	No. Patients	ALT Technique	1-3-Y Patient Survival	1-3-Y Graft Survival	Native Liver Regeneration (Percent of Patients)	OLT No. Patients	1-3-Y Patient Survival	1-3-Y Graft Survival	P
Chenard-Neu 1996[28]	30	APOLT, 24 patients; HALT, 6 patients	71%-63%	60%	68%	384	61%	52%	ns
Sudan 1997[38]	7	APOLT	57%-57%	57%-57%	86%	11	82%-74%		ns
Pereira 1997[40]	7	APOLT	57%	57%	33%				
ELTR 2001		ALT	52%	42%			69%	62%	.03, .01
Azoulay 2001[13]	12	APOLT	66%	39%	25%	24	66%	66%	ns
Erhard 1998[29]	6	HALT, 6 patients, 4 with PVA	50%		100%				
Van Hoek 1999[24]	47	APOLT, 35 patients; HALT 12 patients	62%	53%		384	61	52	
Boudjema 2002[11]	18	APOLT	65%		65%				
Durand 2002[39]	6	APOLT	83%		80%				
Liver transplantation registry		APOLT	52%		42%		69%	62%	.01

ALT, auxiliary liver transplantation; APOLT, auxiliary partial orthotopic liver transplantation; HALT, heterotopic auxiliary liver transplantation; OLT, orthotopic liver transplantation; PVA, portal vein arterialization.

survival rate and an 80% native liver regeneration were achieved and without recurrence of hepatitis B. A short course of ganciclovir during the postoperative period and anti–hepatitis B surface (HBs) immunoglobulin for 15 to 27 months after transplantion were administered. Durand and associates concluded that the remnant part of the native liver does not compromise immunization against HBV.

Auxiliary Liver Transplantation for Inborn Errors of Metabolism

Some liver-based metabolic disorders do not cause cirrhosis but do cause severe or life-threatening extrahepatic complications. Crigler-Najjar syndrome type 1 (CNS1), which is characterized by an unconjugated hyperbilirubinemia because of complete lack of hepatic bilirubin uridine diphosphate-glucuronyltransferase activity, can result in kernicterus and neurological injury. Experimental studies show that only 2% of normal hepatocytes are required for adequate bilirubin conjugation; thus, the idea that APOLT may provide an alternative option in CNS1 patients is attractive. The largest experience of ALT for CNS1 comes from King's College Hospital in London.[42] Surgeons at the hospital have performed seven APOLT procedures in six patients, all of whom had been receiving daily phototherapy since birth. Five of the six patients are alive, with normal serum bilirubin levels and without phototherapy. One patient died of diffuse lymphoma involving the central nervous system after retransplantation for technical problems.

Some cases of ALT for propionicacidemia and urea cycle defects such as ornithine transcarbamoylase deficiency have been reported.[43,44] ALT has potential for the management of homozygous familial hypercholesterolemia, disorders of fatty acid metabolism, and hemophilia, metabolic diseases that do not structurally damage the liver or produce abnormal proteins or enzymes that damage other target organs, as is the case in familial amyloid polyneuropathy[45] or primary hyperoxaluria type 1.

The rationale for ALT is that it is possible to provide sufficient liver mass to correct the underlying metabolic disorder while retaining the majority of the native liver. The advantage of ALT is that should the graft fail, it can be removed without endangering the life of the patient. In addition, gene therapy can be used in the future and the need for life-long immunosuppression avoided.[46]

The specific circumstances of ALT for metabolic diseases are the problem of graft atrophy caused by poor portal venous flow. Portal venous flow is diverted to the normal native liver where resistance to blood flow is lower than in the graft. At least 70% narrowing of the native portal vein is necessary to divert the flow to the graft, although Japanese authors prefer to completely divert portal venous flow to the graft to prevent long-term graft atrophy.[47] Relapse of the metabolic defect following an episode of rejection in patients with ALT has been reported to be due to graft dysfunction secondary to rejection and portal flow diversion.[42] Diagnosis of rejection is difficult in these patients with ALT and is sometimes made following relapse of the disease.

Long-term success will be defined as the ability to withdraw immunosuppression either following gene therapy or with development of tolerance. It is possible that advances in ability to induce tolerance will make auxiliary grafting redundant.

Auxiliary Liver Transplantation for Small-for-Size Living Donor Graft Liver Transplantation

Living donor liver transplantation (LDLT) is increasingly performed in all countries. In some countries such as Japan, brain-dead donors are not yet available, although a new law permitting organ retrieval from a cadaver with the consent of the family came into force in 1997. LDLT is the only real option for patients with liver failure in these countries, and sometimes a small liver graft from a living donor is the only possibility available. Patients receiving small grafts from living donors are in danger of developing the so-called small-for-size syndrome. The Kyoto group reported patient survival of 85% when graft–recipient body weight ratio (GRBW) was more than 1 and only 50% when GRBW was less than 0.8 in elective and ABO-compatible transplantation.[48]

Thus, the concept of ALT for small-for-size syndrome is that part of the native liver is kept in place to support graft function until sufficient regeneration occurs.[14,48] A second-stage native hepatectomy is then performed. The technique is as follows: A left hepatectomy is performed in the recipient and the left part of the graft is implanted. Portal flow to the native liver is interrupted to secure sufficient blood flow to the graft. To facilitate second-stage native hepatectomy, the short hepatic veins are ligated and the right hepatic vein identified. After graft regeneration has occurred, native right lobe hepatectomy is performed, usually 1 month later.[49] With the advent of right lobe transplantation for adults, the indications for this technique are minimal. However, it may constitute a better alternative to the use of two donors for performing transplantation in one patient, as reported by Korean authors.

Auxiliary Liver Transplantation for Chronic Liver Failure

ALT was developed in the 1970s as an alternative to OLT for Child-Pugh C patients. At that time, in patients with portal hypertension, coagulopathy, muscle wasting, and cachexia, recipient hepatectomy constituted a major undertaking. Perioperative mortality was high as a consequence of significant blood loss and hemodynamic alterations during the surgical procedure. However, the results obtained with ALT were far from favorable, patient survival was poor, and the disadvantage of leaving the cirrhotic liver in place with its potential for carcinogenesis became evident with the appearance of hepatocellular carcinoma in the few long-term survivors.

Advances in surgical techniques and perioperative anesthetic management have made OLT a standard procedure.[7,8] ALT for chronic liver disease is justified only in exceptional cases of very difficult hepatectomy owing to adhesions from previous surgery or portal vein thrombosis, or anatomic anomalies such as situs inversus. There are some reports of ALT associated with intestinal transplantation in cases of intestinal failure and total parenteral nutrition–associated liver disease. In these cases, the auxiliary liver graft supports liver function, has a tolerogenic effect with the intestinal graft, and may offer the native liver a possibility of regenerating once total parenteral nutrition is withdrawn.

Figure 55–8 shows a decision tree that graphically presents the process of choosing between OLT and the various forms of ALT.

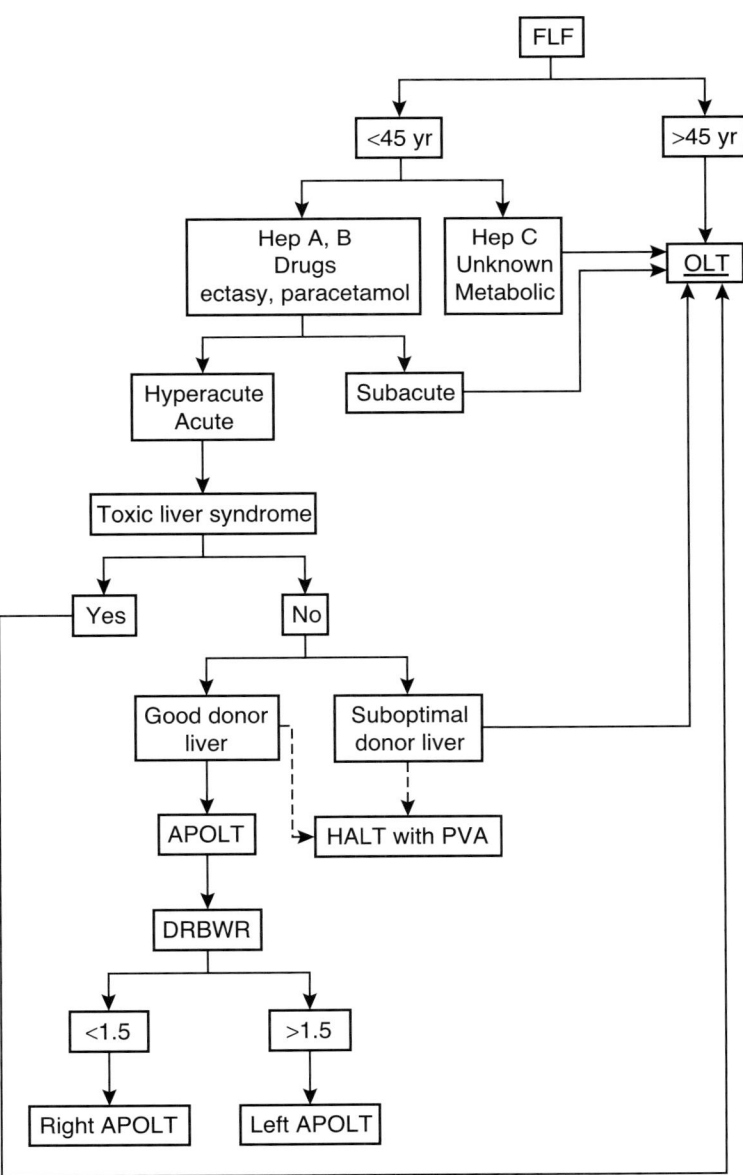

FIGURE 55–8

Decision tree: Choosing between OLT and the various forms of ALT in patients with fulminant liver failure (FLF). APOLT, auxiliary partial orthotopic liver transplantation; DRBWR, donor-recipient body weight ratio; HALT, heterotopic auxiliary liver transplant; OLT, orthotopic liver transplantation; PVA, portal vein arterialization.

Pearls and Pitfalls

- In FLF, transplantation of an auxiliary graft is the only option available to substitute the function of the native liver that is left in place to provide an opportunity for recovery.
- ALT is indicated in patients younger than 40 years of age, with acute or hyperacute form of FLF, without toxic liver syndrome, no fibrosis on liver biopsy. and a good donor liver available.
- APOLT is the technique of choice in FLF, with results far better than those of HALT. Patient and graft survival are similar to those of OLT.
- Once regeneration of the native liver occurs, immunosuppression is withdrawn. The patient is no longer condemned to the hazards of lifelong risks of rejection and immunosuppression.
- HALT with PVA leaves the hepatic hilum undisturbed with no diversion of portal vein flow; therefore chances of rapid regeneration are optimal. However, this technical option is indicated only with maximum possibilities of regeneration.
- ALT has little place in the treatment of metabolic disorders, chronic liver failure, and living donor liver transplantation. No evidence has emerged to date in the treatment of FLF that ALT is better than OLT. Therefore OLT continues to be the gold standard of treatment.
- APOLT is a more complex operation than OLT in a critically ill patient. There is an increased number of complications and the postoperative course is more complex.
- In HALT, the graft is in an abnormal hemodynamic situation with high outflow pressure and portal vein flow diversion; consequently, the risks of graft dysfunction and portal vein thrombosis are high.
- Leaving the native necrotic liver has potential disadvantages in FLF because hemodynamic instability and cerebral edema may persist as a consequence of the toxic liver syndrome.
- Although regeneration occurs in 60% of cases, few patients achieve all the benefits of ALT—survival without sequelae and full recovery of the native liver with no need for immunosuppression.

References

1. Welch CS: A note on transplantation of the whole liver in dogs. Transplant Bull 2:55-68, 1955.
2. Goodrich E, Welch HF, Nelson JA, et al: Homotransplantation of the canine liver. Surgery 39:244-251, 1956.
3. Absolon AB, Hagihara PF, Griffen WO, et al: Experimental and clinical heterotopic liver homotransplantation. Int Rev Hepatol 15:1481-1487, 1965.
4. Fortner JG, Beatie EJ, Shiu MH, et al: Orthotopic and heterotopic liver homografts in man. Ann Surg 172:23-32, 1970.
5. Terpstra OT, Schalm SW, Weimar W, et al: Auxiliary partial liver transplantation for end-stage chronic liver disease. N Engl J Med 319:1507-1511, 1988.
6. Shaked AA, Busuttil RW: Auxiliary liver transplantation: A negative viewpoint. Hepatology 12:173-175, 1990.
7. Belghiti J, Noun R, Sauvanet A, et al: Transplantation for fulminant and subfulminant hepatic failure with preservation of portal and caval flow. Br J Surg 82:986-989, 1995.
8. Bismuth H, Samuel D: Orthotopic liver transplantation in fulminant and subfulminant hepatitis. The Paul Brousse experience. Ann Surg 222:109-119, 1995.
9. Moritz MJ, Jarrell BE, Armenti V, et al: Heterotopic liver transplantation for fulminant hepatic failure—a bridge to recovery. Transplantation 50:524-526, 1990.
10. Boudjema K, Jaeck D, Simeoni U: Temporary auxiliary liver transplantation for subacute liver failure in a child. Lancet 342:778-779, 1993.
11. Boudjema K, Bachellier P, Wolf P, et al: Auxiliary liver transplantation and bioartificial bridging procedures in treatment of acute liver failure. World J Surg 26:264-274, 2002.
12. Shaw BW Jr: Auxiliary liver transplantation for acute liver failure. Liver Transpl Surg 1:194-200, 1995.
13. Azoulay D, Samuel D, Ichai PH, et al: Auxiliary partial orthotopic versus standard orthotopic whole liver transplantation for acute liver failure. Ann Surg 234:723-731, 2001.
14. Yabe S, Egawa H, Inomata Y, et al: Auxiliary partial orthotopic liver transplantation from living donors. Transplantation 66:484-488, 1998.
15. Whitington PF, Emond JC, Heffron T, et al: Short reports: Orthotopic auxiliary liver transplantation for Crigler-Najjar syndrome type I. Lancet 342:779-780, 1993.
16. Marchioro TL, Porter KA, Dickinson TC, et al: Physiologic requirements for auxiliary liver homotransplantation. Surg Gynecol Obstet 121:17-31, 1965.
17. Van der Hyde MN, Schalm I: Auxiliary liver graft without portal blood: Experimental autotransplantation of the liver lobes. Br J Surg 55:111-115, 1968.
18. Tzakis AG, Kirkegaard P, Pinna AD, et al: Liver transplantation with cavoportal hemitransposition in the presence of diffuse portal vein thrombosis. Transplantation 65:619-624, 1998.
19. Charco R, Margarit C, Lopez-Talavera JC, et al: Outcome and hepatic hemodynamics in liver transplant patients with portal vein arterialization. Am J Transplant 1:146-151, 2001.
20. Fisher B, Russ C, Updegraff H, et al: Effect of increased hepatic blood flow upon liver regeneration. Arch Surg 69:263-271, 1954.
21. Gubernatis G, Pichlmayr R, Kemnitz J,et al: Auxiliary partial liver transplantation (APOLT) for fulminant hepatic failure: First successful case report. World J Surg 15:660-666, 1991.
22. Erhard J, Lange R, Giebler R, et al: Arterialization of the portal vein in orthotopic and auxiliary liver transplantation: A report of three cases. Transplantation 60:877-879, 1995.
23. Terpstra OT: Auxiliary liver grafting: A new concept in liver transplantation. Lancet 342:758-759, 1993.
24. Van Hoek B, de Boer J, Boudjema K, et al, on behalf of the EURALT Study Group: Auxiliary versus orthotopic liver transplantation for acute liver failure. J Hepatol 30:699-705, 1999.
25. Terpstra OT, Reuvers CB, Schalm SW, et al: An auxiliary heterotopic liver transplantation. Transplantation 45:1003-1007, 1988.
26. Bismuth H, Azoulay D, Samuel D, et al: Auxiliary partial orthotopic liver transplantation for fulminant hepatitis. The Paul Brousse experience. Ann Surg 224:712-726, 1996.

27. Boudjema K, Cherqui D, Jaeck D, et al: Auxiliary liver transplantation for fulminant and subfulminant hepatic failure. Transplantation 59:218-223, 1995.
28. Chenard-Neu MP, Boudjema K, Bernau J, et al: Auxiliary liver transplantation: Regeneration of the native liver and outcome in 30 patients with fulminant hepatic failure. A multicenter European study. Hepatology 23:1119-1127, 1996.
29. Erhard J, Lange R, Rauen U, et al: Auxiliary liver transplantation with arterialization of the portal vein for acute liver failure. Transplant Int 11:266-271, 1998.
30. Margarit C, Bilbao I, Charco R, et al: Auxiliary heterotopic liver transplantation with portal vein arterialization for fulminant hepatic failure. Liver Transpl 6:805-809, 2000.
31. Ringe B, Lubbe N, Kuse E, et al: Total hepatectomy and liver transplantation as two-stage procedure. Ann Surg 218:3-9, 1994.
32. Rozga J, Podesta L, Lepage E, et al: Control of cerebral oedema by total hepatectomy and extracorporeal liver support in fulminant hepatic failure. Lancet 342:898-899, 1993.
33. Bernau J, Samuel D, Durand F, et al: Criteria for emergency liver transplantation in patients with acute viral hepatitis and factor V below 50% of normal: A prospective study. Hepatology 14:49A, 1991.
34. O'Grady JG, Alexander GJM, Hayllar KM, et al: Early indicators of prognosis in fulminant hepatic failure. Gastroenterology 97:439-444, 1989.
35. Hanau C, Muñoz SJ, Rubin R: Histopathological heterogeneity in fulminant hepatic failure. Hepatology 21:345-351, 1995.
36. Buyck D, Bonnin F, Bernau J, et al: Auxiliary liver transplantation in patients with fulminant hepatic failure: Hepatobiliary scintigraphic follow-up. Eur J Nucl Med 24:138-142, 1997.
37. Mazariegos GV, Reyes J, Marino IR: Weaning of immunosuppression in liver transplant recipients. Transplantation 63: 243-249, 1997.
38. Sudan DL, Shaw BW Jr, Fox IJ, et al: Long-term follow-up of auxiliary liver transplantation for the treatment of fulminant hepatic failure. Surgery 122:771-778, 1997.
39. Durand F, Belghiti J, Handra-Luca A, et al: Auxiliary liver transplantation for fulminant hepatitis B: Results from a series of six patients with special emphasis on regeneration and recurrence of hepatitis B. Liver Transpl 8:701-707, 2002.
40. Pereira SP, McCArthy M, Ellis AJ, et al: Auxiliary partial orthotopic liver transplantation for acute liver failure. J Hepatol 26:1010-1017, 1997
41. Oldhafer KJ, Gubernatis G, Schlitt HJ, et al: Auxiliary partial orthotopic liver transplantation for acute liver failure: The Hannover experience. Clin Transpl 8:181-187, 1994.
42. Rela M, Muiesan P, Vilca-Melendez H, et al: Auxiliary partial orthotopic liver transplantation for Crigler-Najjar syndrome type 1. Ann Surg 229:565-569, 1999.
43. Kiuchi T, Edamoto Y, Kaibori M, et al: Auxiliary liver transplantation for urea-cycle enzyme deficiencies: Lessons from three cases. Transplant Proc 31:528-529, 1999.
44. Uemoto S, Yabe S, Inomata Y, et al: Coexistence of a graft with the preserved native liver in auxiliary partial orthotopic liver transplantation from a living donor for ornithine transcarbamylase deficiency. Transplantation 63:1026-1028, 1997.
45. Ikegami T, Kawasaki S, Ohno Y, et al: Temporary auxiliary liver transplantation from a living donor to an adult recipient with familial amyloid polyneuropathy. Transplantation 73:628-630, 2002.
46. Tada K, Chowdhury NR, Neufeld D, et al: Long-term reduction of serum bilirubin levels in Gunn rats by retroviral gene transfer in vivo. Liver Transpl Surg 4:78-88, 1998.
47. Nagashima I, Bergmann L, Schweizer R: How can we share the portal blood inflow in auxiliary partial heterotopic liver transplantation without portal hypertension? Surgery 116:101-106, 1994.
48. Kiuchi T, Kasahara M, Uryuhara K, et al: Impact of graft size mismatching on graft prognosis in liver transplantation from living donors. Transplantation 67:321-327, 1999.
49. Kaibori M, Uemoto S, Fujita S, et al: Native hepatectomy after auxiliary partial orthotopic liver transplantation. Transpl Int 12:383-386, 1999.

VIII

Postoperative Care

56

Postoperative Intensive Care Unit Management: Adult Liver Transplant Recipients

HENRY B. RANDALL
GORAN B. KLINTMALM

Immediate arrival at the intensive care unit   833

Assessment of organ function   835
  Cardiac function   835
  Respiratory function   835
  Neurological assessment   836
  Renal assessment   836

Assessment of graft function   838
  Preservation injury and shock liver   838
  Primary nonfunction   838
  Fatty liver   839
  Hepatic infarction   839
  Hyperacute rejection   840

Technical complications   840
  Postoperative hemorrhage   840
  Vascular complications   841
  Biliary problems   843

Medical considerations and complications   845
  Neurological complications   845
  Cardiovascular complications   846
  Respiratory complications   846
  Infectious complications   848
  Nutrition   848

Summary   848

Since the inception of liver transplantation in the United States, postoperative care of liver transplant recipients has continued to evolve rapidly. Significant changes have come about since the first edition of this book was introduced in 1996. Increasingly, more scientific study, including controlled clinical multicenter trials, is reaching the published literature, and a multidisciplinary approach has become standard practice in most liver transplant programs. A better understanding of pathophysiology specifically related to end-stage liver disease has brought about novel therapeutic approaches to problems arising after orthotopic liver transplantation. Furthermore, more intensivists and other specialists have become involved in the postoperative care of liver transplant recipients. Variables such as pretransplant diagnosis, degree of debility before transplantation, comorbid diseases, and operative complexity appear to have a significant influence on the rapidity at which patients progress through their early postoperative recovery phase.

Immediate Arrival at the Intensive Care Unit

Initial postoperative assessment of a liver transplant patient actually begins in the operating room but in large part takes place once the patient has arrived at the intensive care unit (ICU). Immediately after completion of the transplant operation, most patients recover in the ICU and a small number in a recovery room setting. Reports show that, occasionally, uncomplicated patients can bypass the ICU and be discharged to the transplant floor after an appropriate period of extremely close observation.[1-4] However, the majority of liver transplant recipients are sent to the ICU, where both the anesthesiologist and surgeon are available to give pertinent details of the operation to the receiving ICU team. The intensive care team usually consists of nurses, respiratory therapists, residents, transplant and hepatology fellows, the staff hepatologist, and the transplant surgeon, with or without a separate intensivist. For a liver transplant patient with an uncomplicated operation, the anticipated stay in the ICU should be less than 24 hours before being transferred to the inpatient setting. In some centers in an elective liver transplant situation, the patient is awakened in the operating room soon after the incision is dressed, and if the extubation criteria are fulfilled, the patient is extubated.[4] It should be advised that not all patients are candidates for early extubation and that each case should be judged on its own merits. On arrival at the ICU, vital signs are recorded and hemodynamic monitoring is performed (Table 56–1): heart rate, respiratory rate and ventilator settings, arterial blood pressure, cardiac output, 12-lead electrocardiogram, core body temperature, oxygen saturation, and central venous pressure (CVP). In some cases, mixed venous oxygen saturation is measured. All fluids being infused are recorded, including any remaining CellSaver blood, in addition to measurement of nasogastric drain output, urine output, and biliary drainage (if tubes are used). Since use of the biliary drain has fallen out of favor in

Table 56-2. INTENSIVE CARE UNIT LABORATORY TESTS

Complete blood count	White blood cell count, hemoglobin,hematocrit, platelet count, differential
Arterial blood gases	pH, Pco_2, Po_2, HCO_3^-, saturation, base deficit, base excess
Coagulation profile	Prothrombin time, partial prothrombin time, international normalized ratio, fibrinogen
Complete metabolic panel	Sodium, potassium, chloride, CO_2, blood urea nitrogen, creatinine, glucose, aspartate transaminase, alanine transaminase, alkaline phosphatase, total bilirubin, calcium, magnesium, phosphorus, serum lactic acid

many institutions, observation of the quantity and quality of bile present in the operative field after reperfusion is an important issue.

If intra-abdominal drains are used, the quantity and character of ascites are determined, whether clear or bloody. If an intracranial pressure monitor was placed preoperatively, cerebral perfusion pressure readings are calculated and recorded. Immediate laboratory tests ordered include arterial blood gases, serum electrolytes, serum glucose, coagulation profile (mainly serum prothrombin time), liver enzymes, hemoglobin and hematocrit, and platelet counts (Table 56–2). A chest radiograph is taken to confirm placement of lines and endotracheal tube position and ensure that pneumothorax has not occurred. Determination of serum lactate or lactic acid is helpful to assess the liver's ability to metabolize acids, as well as verify the presence of effective cardiac output and perfusion of systemic tissue. Every effort should be made to maintain normothermia (core body temperature >37° C), which in some cases may require the use of an external heating device. Maintenance of euthermia assists in preventing or treating fibrinolysis and keeps any new or ongoing coagulopathy from developing or worsening. In theory, such practice should help decrease the use of blood products such as packed red cells, fresh-frozen plasma, platelets, and antifibrinolytic agents (i.e., ε-aminocaproic acid and aprotinin). As described in a recently submitted report by our institution, we have seen severe arterial and venous thrombosis and death after the use of aprotinin.[5] It is a well-established fact that as larger volumes of blood products are used intraoperatively, complications after transplantation increase dramatically,[6-9] including renal failure, respiratory problems, infectious complications, and cardiac complications. An immediate neurological assessment is made and consists of evaluation of the general level of consciousness and sensory and motor function, along with spinal reflexes. Neurological changes or abnormalities are fairly common in the

Table 56-1. MONITORING CARDIAC FUNCTION WITH A SWAN-GANZ CATHETER

Heart rate

Mean arterial pressure

Cardiac output

Cardiac index

Stroke volume

Stroke volume index

Central venous pressure

Systemic vascular resistance

Systemic vascular resistance index

Pulmonary vascular resistance

Pulmonary vascular resistance index

Pulmonary arterial pressure (mean)

Pulmonary artery pressure (diastolic)

postoperative period and include nerve palsy as a result of compression injury, laryngeal nerve injury from intubation, radial and ulnar nerve injury from improper padding and the use of self-retaining retractors, and femoral nerve injury as a result of the use of venovenous bypass cannulas.

The marginal liver metabolism of anesthetic agents can contribute to delayed emergence from surgery, as well as residual hepatic encephalopathy.[3] Most recipients experience some degree of psychosis or neurological dysfunction after transplantation. Problems range from anxiety, depression, and sleep deprivation to frank hallucinations and delusional states, but most of these problems resolve with no intervention. Encephalopathy can be a result of metabolic derangements or an anoxic event. Postoperative seizures of new onset are not uncommon after liver transplantation and often develop after the initiation of calcineurin inhibitor therapy, especially tacrolimus, as well as after the administration of high-dose corticosteroids. For a liver recipient with fulminant hepatic failure, it is of particular importance that neurological function be assessed frequently and thoroughly. Cerebral perfusion pressure is monitored if a device such a bolt or other apparatus has been placed. We delay the start of calcineurin inhibitors and instead begin immunosuppression with agents that do not have any neurological side effects, such as monoclonal or polyclonal antibodies (OKT3 or thymoglobulin). As an aside, in a patient undergoing antibody induction, rejection can still occur within the first week to 10 days after transplantation. If the patient is admitted to the ICU while intubated and after reversal of the paralytic agents, the ventilator settings are adjusted according to the patient's respiratory status and arterial blood gases. Pulse oximetry monitors are placed on the extremities but can be unduly influenced if the recipient is deeply jaundiced. Warm extremities can play a profound role in determining whether perfusion is deemed adequate by sensing devices. In patients with cold extremities and less than ideal perfusion, the ear lobe may be a more sensitive site for determining the adequacy of perfusion.

Assessment of Organ Function

Cardiac Function

In the ICU, patients are monitored by frequent laboratory tests and hemodynamic assessment. To assist in hemodynamic monitoring and infusion of large volumes of fluid, central venous access is necessary. Centers that use the venovenous bypass (VVBP) technique during liver transplantation place a percutaneous internal jugular vein catheter and a femoral vein catheter or, less

frequently, place a catheter by cut-down technique in the axillary vein for VVBP. However, use of this extracorporeal circuit appears to have decreased. Use of a different surgical technique (piggyback technique) and experience avoid the need for complete vena cava cross-clamping when the donor liver is implanted and may decrease the need for VVBP in the future. Once hemodynamic stability has been achieved, a triple-lumen catheter replaces the percutaneous internal jugular bypass cannula. Continuous hemodynamic monitoring is performed with a Swan-Ganz catheter placed through a Cordis introducer system, and a second catheter with at least an 8.5-French caliber is routinely used. The Swan-Ganz catheter allows continuous measurement of cardiac output and instantaneous calculation of systemic vascular resistance (SVR), stroke volume, and stroke work. Because most liver transplant patients have such a short stay in the ICU, monitoring indices such as mixed venous monitoring are usually superfluous but may be of use in patients with an anticipated prolonged stay. Arterial catheters are used to draw blood for routine laboratory tests and to monitor systemic arterial pressure because peripheral sphygmomanometer-type cuffs are generally inadequate for accurately measuring systemic blood pressure, especially in situations in which the patient is hypotensive and hypovolemic. Medications, vital signs, daily weight, hematological parameters, serum chemistry values, and fluid output are recorded on the patient's bedside wall chart.

Respiratory Function

Postoperatively, the patient is usually weaned from mechanical ventilation once it has been firmly established that all postoperative factors have been accurately assessed.[2] Factors such as renal dysfunction, altered mental status, significant fluid shifts, ascites, obesity, hemorrhage, atelectasis, pain, muscle wasting, pleural effusions, and diaphragmatic dysfunction play a large role in determining the need for long-term ventilatory support. Several recent studies have evaluated the ability to "fast-track" liver transplant recipients and have found that a select group of liver recipients can safely be extubated either in the operative suite or within 3 hours or less of reaching the ICU.[2,3] However, most patients are extubated in the ICU once it has been determined that hemodynamic stability has been achieved. At our institution, weaning parameters include a satisfactory cough and gag reflex, return of muscle tone, and the parameters presented in Table 56–3.

For a patient who has not met the weaning and extubation criteria, the next factor that needs to be assessed is how long the patient will actually require intubation and mechanical ventilation. Numerous factors besides

Table 56-3. PARAMETERS FOR EXTUBATION

Awake, alert, good muscle strength/tone	
Respiratory rate	< 30 breaths per minute
Tidal volume	> 5 mL/kg
Arterial P_{O_2}	> 70 mm Hg
F_{IO_2}	< 0.4
Minute ventilation	< 10 L/min
Methacholine inhalational challenge	> –25 cm H_2O
Peak inspiratory pressure	> 52 to 30 cm H_2O
Compliance	> 30 mL/cm

not meeting the aforementioned criteria could prevent weaning, including diaphragmatic paralysis of the right hemidiaphragm, an inability to clear secretions, malnourishment, abdominal distention, and metabolic acidosis. When it is necessary to mechanically ventilate someone for more than 1 week, a percutaneously placed tracheostomy performed at the bedside is an ideal choice to clear airway secretions and reduce the resistance that accompanies the use of standard long endotracheal tubes.[10] In patients with obesity, difficult or unusual airways, or sleep apnea, it might be necessary or prudent to administer biphasic or continuous positive airway pressure nightly to maintain an open airway and reduce the risk for urgent intubation. Obese patients should be kept in a 30- to 45-degree position to reduce abdominal pressure on the diaphragm and facilitate breathing. These patients should be extubated as soon as possible or they tend to stay intubated for extended periods (e.g., 10 to 14 days) for simple mechanical ventilation.

Neurological Assessment

Pain Management

It has been firmly established that the most reliable, most common, and most well validated measure of pain intensity is a visual or verbal analog scale ranging from 0 to 10. However, there are differences in how pain is perceived. For instance, it is reported that older patients experience less pain.[11,12] Immunosuppressive agents, namely steroids, blunt the response to pain,[13] cultural differences exist,[14] and gender differences related to the pain experience vary widely. Significant issues regarding past substance abuse also influence how pain is controlled after transplantation. Control of pain with analgesics is a challenge for the ICU team. Adequate pain control allows the patient to be more cooperative and less agitated, permits smooth extubation, and decreases systemic blood pressure.[15]

However, a delicate balance does exist between narcotic use and oversedation, particularly when the liver has marginal function. In most patients the need for narcotic medication is minimal, except those with an antecedent history of drug abuse. For the occasional patient, patient-controlled analgesia can be instituted. Narcotic use is sometimes supplemented with intravenous diphenhydramine to hasten weaning from narcotics. Anesthesia providers typically use short-acting agents such as fentanyl, which provides adequate analgesia and does not interfere with liver function. Nonsteroidal anti-inflammatory drugs are seldom if ever used because of a decrease in renal flow and gastrointestinal effects (e.g., nausea, gastritis). Few controlled trials have been performed to determine what pain control method is best for a liver transplant patient. Some centers may routinely use patient-controlled analgesia, whereas administration of intravenous narcotics by the ICU nursing staff is adequate in most centers.

Renal Assessment

As liver transplantation has grown over the past 2 decades, renal dysfunction has emerged as a major cause of morbidity and mortality before and after transplantation. Posttransplant survival has been shown to be directly correlated with pretransplant renal function. When assessing a cirrhotic patient for suitability for transplantation, one must also look for both intrinsic and extrinsic causes of renal disease. Hepatorenal syndrome (HRS) (an extrinsic cause) is a major cause of renal dysfunction in a significant number of patients who undergo transplantation. In those in whom HRS is diagnosed, return of renal function after transplantation is to be expected.[16,17] However, if an intrinsic cause of renal dysfunction has occurred, careful evaluation by a nephrologist may reveal the need for a combined kidney and liver transplant.[18] At our institution, a pretransplant true glomerular filtration rate (^{125}I-iodothalamate) is determined for evaluation of baseline renal function.[19,20] Since the Model for End-Stage Liver Disease (MELD) system was put in place (February 2001) as a measure of how urgently a transplant may be needed, renal impairment is now part of the algorithm for determining such need. The prevailing thought is that if renal dysfunction is caused by HRS, return of renal function can be expected within 2 to 6 weeks after transplantation. Nearly 50% of patients with HRS can expect to receive some form of dialysis (continuous venovenous hemodialysis [CVVH] or hemodialysis) before or soon after transplantation. If dialysis is required, the ICU stay will be prolonged, and a higher incidence of complications is expected in these patients as well. Acute tubular necrosis (ATN) can result from intraoperative perfusion problems, especially in patients with marginal renal function from the outset. ATN is as common as HRS as an indication for pretransplant dialysis. Postoperatively, intravascular hypovolemia is another common cause of renal insufficiency, as well as drug-induced nephrotoxicity.

Care must be taken with fluid administration and medication dosages to avoid dialysis in the immediate postoperative period. If the patient is found to have profound fluid overload in the face of ATN or HRS, CVVH or conventional hemodialysis may be a necessity. We routinely use CVVH because it is more effective in controlling fluid balance during the first several days after transplantation. Later, if necessary, we may opt for conventional hemodialysis.[20]

Electrolyte Abnormalities

Sodium. Hyponatremia is often seen in liver transplant patients with fluid retention. The choice of which posttransplant fluids to administer in the ICU should be based on the serum sodium level. If the serum sodium concentration is less than 125 mEq/L, normal saline (0.9%) should be the fluid of choice. Conversely, if serum sodium is greater than 135 mEq/L, half-normal saline (0.45%) would be a wise choice. Should there ever exist a point at which the serum sodium level is higher than 150 mEq/L, it is best that correction proceed at a very slow pace. Rapid correction can result in a condition known as central pontine myelinolysis and could in fact lead to permanent brain injury by demyelinating white matter in the brain.

Potassium. Correction of potassium is an ongoing process in transplant patients. In the operating room, all preservation solution should get flushed out of the liver before or while the allograft is being sewn in. Patients arriving in the ICU with vigorous urine output can be expected to have a low serum potassium level and therefore need early replacement. In most cases, potassium supplementation is administered by the intravenous route, but it can be given orally via a nasogastric tube. Correction of hypokalemia can be blunted if serum magnesium is also low,[6] which of course requires intravenous magnesium as well. Hyperkalemia after transplantation occurs in patients with renal dysfunction or renal failure and requires urgent treatment with pharmacological agents or early dialysis. Correction of an underlying metabolic acidosis or administration of oral or rectal sodium polystyrene sulfonate (Kayexalate) usually corrects this abnormality. If severe enough to cause electrocardiographic changes, intravenous calcium to stabilize cardiac membranes, intravenous insulin, and glucose can be given to decrease serum potassium levels.

Magnesium. Magnesium is the essential ion in the adenosine triphosphatase complex. Commonly, patients have a low serum magnesium level or hypomagnesemia as a result of postoperative blood loss and the use a of loop diuretics. Other causes include massive blood transfusion requirements from excessive intraoperative blood loss. Normally, the serum level is around 1.5 to 2.0 mEq/L. Clinical symptoms of hypomagnesemia include muscle aches, twitching, cramps, and cardiac arrhythmias. Hypomagnesemia is commonly seen in association with hypokalemia and hypocalcemia. Correction is achieved simply by repletion of the low levels by magnesium salt infusion and oral maintenance therapy with magnesium-containing complexes (e.g., magnesium oxide).

Calcium. Calcium is a highly regulated and ubiquitous cation that is essential for homeostasis. Normocalcemia, like normomagnesemia, should be maintained throughout the perioperative period. Similar to magnesium, calcium exists in extracellular plasma in a free ionized state, as well as bound to other molecules. The normal range of bound calcium is between 8.5 and 10 mg/dL. Changes in serum albumin levels significantly alter total calcium levels, since most of it is bound to serum protein albumin (80%). The most commonly used mathematical formula to determine calcium levels with disparate albumin concentrations is to decrease calcium by 0.8 mg/dL for every 1.0-mg decrease in albumin. Calcium concentrations are regulated by parathyroid hormone, calcitonin, and vitamin D acting on the end-targets bone, kidney, and the gastrointestinal tract. Calcium increases through an interplay between bone resorption, renal production of vitamin D, and an increase in intestinal absorption of calcium and phosphate. Patients with renal dysfunction may have a difficult time reabsorbing calcium and phosphate. Malnourished patients with vitamin D deficiency and critically ill patients can also show evidence of hypocalcemia. Steroids can alter uptake of calcium in the gastrointestinal tract, increase renal excretion, and inhibit osteoclast-activating factor.

In the immediate posttransplant period, gastrointestinal absorption is also deranged and thus calcium uptake via the gastrointestinal tract is altered. Most patients suffer from hypocalcemia as opposed to hypercalcemia unless they are given large doses of thiazide diuretics, antacids, and digoxin or lithium. Low levels are detected by measuring serum total and ionized Ca^{2+} levels. Early symptoms of hypocalcemia include perioral numbness, paresthesias, muscle cramps, and mild mental status changes such as irritability. If the hypocalcemia becomes more severe, manifestations such as neuromuscular and cardiac signs (Chvostek's and Trousseau's signs), mental status changes, seizures, tetany, hypotension, and acute cardiac failure can become evident.

Mild hypocalcemia is managed by administering intravenous calcium as the gluconate salt (calcium gluconate, 10%), or for more urgent treatment of severe hypocalcemia, calcium chloride (200 mg to 1000 mg) is administered via a central venous line.

Assessment of Graft Function

Observation of allograft function is initiated in the operating room at the time of graft reperfusion and includes assessment of the quantity and quality of bile production. Graft edema, any unusual or discolored appearance of the allograft, abnormal CO_2 production, inadequacy of urine output, inability of patients to raise their core temperature, hemodynamic instability, and abnormalities in glucose, potassium, and lactic acid all signal inadequate allograft function. The surgical team should report an assessment of graft function on delivery of the patient to the ICU. The degree of liver parenchymal injury is demonstrated by the elevation in serum aspartate transaminase (AST) and alanine transaminase (ALT) levels. The prothrombin time reflects the synthetic activity of the liver graft. Doppler ultrasonography is a dominant part of the postoperative evaluation in most centers and is used when warranted by clinical indicators in other transplant centers. The resistive index (RI) is an important clinical tool that is used to assess vascular patency, graft function, or graft dysfunction. It is routinely determined on the first postoperative day and when necessary thereafter. RI = (peak systolic velocity (PS) − end-diastolic velocity)/PS for hepatic arteries, and normal is 0.6 to 0.9 (60% to 90%). Low RIs (i.e., <60%) are seen in patients with hepatic artery thrombosis (HAT) or stenosis or in those with massive hepatic necrosis when vascular tone has been lost. A very low RI (i.e., <30%) in the face of sharply elevated liver transaminases coupled with an inability to synthesize prothrombin (international normalized ratio [INR] >2.0) usually portends a poor outcome because it suggests primary nonfunction (PNF) of the liver. These patients require strict observation and should get relisted for retransplantation. Conversely, high RIs (i.e., 90% to 100%) are generally seen in the setting of graft edema, preservation injury, and in some cases, acute cellular rejection. We should mention that findings on ultrasonography should be regarded as a screening examination only and are best served by confirmation with angiography. If there is evidence of rejection or massive necrosis, a tissue diagnosis obtained by biopsy is recommended.

Preservation Injury and Shock Liver

The normal evolution of preservation injury is exactly like that of shock liver. The initial transaminase elevation peaks in 1 to 2 days and then begins to resolve, followed by a cholestatic picture with increases in alkaline phosphate and γ-glutamyltransferase beginning on or about postoperative day 3 to 5. In severe cases bilirubin also becomes elevated. The cholestasis peaks 7 to 12 days postoperatively and then slowly improves. The prothrombin time or the INR should improve throughout this time without fresh-frozen plasma. To a varying degree, some preservation injury should be anticipated in all livers. The level of injury is ascertained by allograft function after reperfusion of the graft and the level of transaminase elevation. The actual significance of the increase in transaminase is arguable; however, most believe that an AST level greater than 2500 IU/L is suggestive of significant injury and that an AST greater than 5000 IU/L suggests severe preservation injury and may even be predictive of PNF.[20-23] Patient recovery is therefore delayed in this instance, and general supportive therapy is highly recommended. Infusion of prostaglandin and prostacyclin may be helpful because of their cytoprotective effects. In uncontrolled studies, these agents have led to recovery in allografts suspected of having PNF. The worse the preservation injury, the more prone the liver is to episodes of rejection.[24-26] A liver graft with significant preservation injury is extremely sensitive to venous hyperperfusion. A CVP higher than 12 to 14 cm H_2O must be treated vigorously with diuresis. If urine output exceeding 250 to 300 mL/hr cannot be generated, urgent institution of continuous hemofiltration can result in revival of the injured allograft.

Primary Nonfunction

PNF is an extreme form of preservation injury, and its presence prevents recovery of graft function and delays or prevents recovery of the patient as well. This syndrome is treatable only by retransplantation. PNF is manifested by hepatic coma, renal dysfunction (oliguria), coagulopathy (prothrombin time >20 seconds despite infusion of fresh-frozen plasma), jaundice, and hypoglycemia. Duplex ultrasound examination and angiography are important in ruling out treatable vascular causes of graft dysfunction. The incidence of PNF is reported to be only about 5%. Intraoperatively, the hallmark of poor graft function is no bile production or watery bile production and generalized "oozing" as a result of the coagulopathy and lysis of all cut surfaces. This is seen even with ongoing correction of the coagulopathy by the anesthesia team. The patient is fully supported during this period while a search for a second liver is under way. In patients who are extremely unstable, total hepatectomy and a portocaval shunt have been shown to be helpful in providing stability by removing the necrotic allograft. Percutaneous biopsy is virtually impossible in the postoperative period; however, a transjugular biopsy of the liver reveals histological evidence of massive zonal necrosis, a mixed inflammatory infiltrate, and ballooning hepatocytes. Ultrasonography reveals a very low RI of 0.1 to 0.2, which indicates loss of vascular tone. Radiological studies show no evidence of vascular thrombosis. The cause of PNF is usually attributed to several factors, such as donor macrosteatosis as opposed to microsteatosis, advanced donor age, prolonged donor hospitalization, protracted cold and warm ischemia times, and prolonged and uncorrected hypernatremia.[22,27,28] The mechanism of hypernatremia-induced liver dysfunction is unclear, but the prevailing thought is that an increase in hepatocellular osmolality is the cause of hepatocyte death and graft dysfunction.

Fatty Liver

The term fatty liver is used to describe livers in which more than 5% of their wet weight consists of lipids.[29,30] Fatty livers are associated with diabetes, nutrition, obesity, dyslipidemia, and alcoholism. Classification is according to the percentage of hepatocyte involvement: mild (<30%), moderate (30% to 60%), and severe (>60%).[31] The changes associated with a fatty liver are recognized in about 25% of brain-dead donors. After cold storage and reperfusion, fatty liver reperfusion–ischemia injury is heralded by an elevation in serum transaminases, impaired regeneration, and even PNF.

Livers from morbidly obese donors have been of particular concern at many transplant centers. However, it has been shown that fatty livers (<30% macrosteatosis) from obese patients fare as well as or better (equivalent patient and graft survival rates) than nonsteatotic livers from similar donors.[82] Several centers have conducted elegant studies with a number of agents, such as prostaglandin E, interleukin-6, heat shock protein, and other free radical inhibitors, and have shown significant promise in livers with more

than 30% macrosteatosis.[32-37] Despite the absence of distinct cutoff values for the use of fatty livers in transplantation, most centers use a value of 30% macrosteatosis if the cold ischemia time is anticipated to be longer than 6 hours and 40% if the ischemia time is kept less than 6 hours. Note that microscopic examination of a hematoxylin-eosin–stained frozen section is used to judge steatosis. It is imperative that a fat stain not be used because it severely overdiagnoses steatosis. However, in the case of an extremely sick patient who is in need of urgent transplantation, these guidelines may be relaxed. Often, a significant elevation in transaminases is to be anticipated, and supportive therapy is required. Prostaglandin infusion, which has shown some cytoprotective effect on sinusoidal endothelial cells and on ischemia–reperfusion injury, has been useful in this setting.[23,38] Clinically, PNF is a syndrome characterized by failure of the liver to function on revascularization. The diagnosis can be made by the presence of low or no bile production, persistent or worsening coagulopathy, markedly elevated liver enzymes (AST >10,000 IU), prolonged prothrombin time and INR, uncorrectable metabolic acidosis, need for CVVH or hemodialysis, and hepatic coma despite a patent hepatic artery and portal vein. The patient is reassessed for immediate retransplantation and is supported in the ICU until a new graft can be found.

Hepatic Infarction

Hepatic infarction is a very serious postoperative complication that is usually manifested as a sudden sharp increase in transaminases (Table 56–4); it occurs as a result of vascular occlusion followed by ischemia and infarction. Hepatic infarction is diagnosed with the aid of Doppler ultrasound to confirm vascular occlusion and confirmed with the use of computed tomography (CT) (Fig. 56–1). If the segment of

Table 56–4. CHANGES IN LABORATORY VALUES IN HEPATIC DISORDERS

Hepatic Dysfunction	Total Bilirubin	Alkaline Phosphatase	AST	ALT	GGT	PT	INR
Preservation injury	↑	↑			↑		
Shock liver	↑↑↑	↑↑	↑↑↑	↑↑↑	↑↑↑	↑	↑
Primary nonfunction	↑↑	↑↑	↑↑↑	↑↑↑	↑↑↑	↑	↑
Hepatic artery thrombosis	↑↑	↑↑	↑↑↑	↑↑↑	↑↑	↑↑	↑↑
Hepatic artery stenosis	↑	↑	↑	↑	↑		
Portal vein thrombosis			↑↑↑	↑↑↑			
Biliary leak	↑↑		→	→		↑	↑
Biliary stenosis	↑↑	↑	→	→	↑		

ALT, alanine transaminase; AST, aspartate transaminase; GGT, γ-glutamyltransferase; INR, international normalized ratio; PT, prothrombin time.

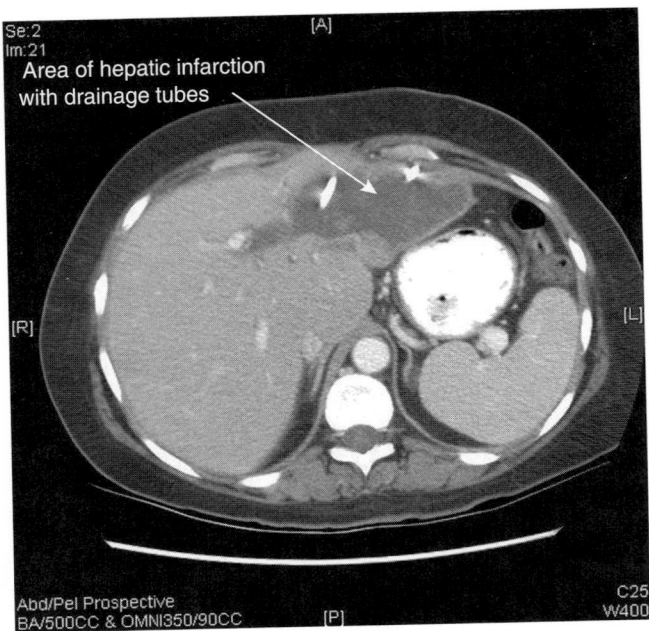

Se:2
Im:21
Area of hepatic infarction with drainage tubes
[A]
[R]
[L]
Abd/Pel Prospective
BA/500CC & OMNI350/90CC
[P]
C25
W400

FIGURE 56–1

Computed tomographic scan of a hepatic infarct with indwelling drainage tubes.

liver infarction is relatively small, the impact on graft function may be minimal. One can expect to see a marked elevation in transaminases with infarction. An abscess as a direct result of hepatic infarction should prompt the clinician to maintain antibiotic coverage with or without antifungal therapy for a prolonged period. In patients with a focal change that is large and significant enough to cause sepsis, either percutaneous drainage in the interventional radiology suite or surgical resection may be warranted.

Hyperacute Rejection

Although reported in the early days of transplantation, hyperacute rejection is rarely seen in the current era of transplantation, and there is no known treatment. Immediately postoperatively, clinical signs and symptoms of hyperacute rejection include profound coagulopathy, uncorrectable acidosis, fibrinolysis, elevated liver enzymes, hepatic coma, and a prolongation in the prothrombin time; the suspected diagnosis is usually PNF. For accurate diagnosis, a liver biopsy is essential. The biopsy reveals hemorrhagic necrosis and congestion within the sinusoids of the graft. Laboratory studies demonstrate an antibody (IgM) and complement-mediated response. The use of immunofluorescence is helpful in the diagnosis. Hyperacute rejection has been known to occur in the face of ABO-incompatible grafts and can be reproduced in experimental animal models.[39] Features that suggest hyperacute rejection are migration

of myocytes within small arterioles and edema of the vasculature wall. The older antibody staining techniques tended to produce poor results, but the newer generations of antibody and molecular stains are much better in diagnosing hyperacute rejection. Checking for the presence of endothelial cell antibodies (anti-TY-2) by flow cytometry, ensuring ABO compatibility, checking the T- and B-cell cross-matching, and determining the pretransplant and posttransplant panel reactive antibody level all appear to be useful diagnostic tools. Of note is that when livers with a positive cross-match are transplanted, hyperacute rejection is not known to occur.[40-42] The most plausible theory is that the liver absorbs the antibody, thereby inhibiting the attack, a phenomenon used when performing combined liver-kidney transplants. Kidney transplantation can be performed after liver transplantation with a positive pretransplant cross-match. Success with this practice has led many to believe that hyperacute rejection is not a true phenomenon but merely a form of PNF. We subscribe to a contrary theory, namely, that PNF may actually be a form of rejection that over time is controlled by the immune system. It is likely that if immunological markers are used to identify immune complexes or endothelial cell antigens, evidence of rejection may be uncovered.

Technical Complications

Postoperative Hemorrhage

On arrival at the ICU, clinical parameters such as arterial blood pressure, heart rate, and CVP are obtained. The most common cause of postoperative hypotension is intra-abdominal bleeding. The coagulation profile is checked along with a complete blood count and chemistry panel. Prolongation of the prothrombin time and partial prothrombin time, a persistently low platelet count, a drop in serum hematocrit and blood pressure, an increase in pulse pressure, and decreased mixed venous O_2 saturation if a mixed venous saturation monitor is used should raise suspicion of postoperative hemorrhage. Other indicators of ongoing intra-abdominal bleeding include an increasing abdominal girth and a decrease in urine output. If drains are in place, large volumes of frank bleeding from the drains will be evident. In patients with a prolonged ischemic time or those with a significant amount of macrosteatosis in the liver (>30%), a tendency toward bleeding and fibrinolysis can be expected. Hemodynamic instability is the sine qua non of ongoing blood loss and demands immediate return to the operating room. Previously, it was reported that an estimated 10% to 15% of posttransplant recipients required a reoperation to control early postoperative bleeding.[43] Today, current improvement in anesthesia care and postoperative treatment of coagulopathy in the ICU have reduced the incidence to roughly 5%. In approximately 50% of patients, no specific site of bleeding is found, and the blood loss can often be attributed to many other factors.[44] Hyperacute rejection, a phenomenon rarely seen these days, initiates a cascade of coagulation problems manifested by severe coagulopathy and can be a cause of significant postoperative bleeding. Fortunately, most bleeding is found at the site of an anastomosis, and reinforcing the site of bleeding generally corrects the problem. In a small number of cases the anastomosis itself has to be redone. When assessing a patient with posttransplant hemorrhage, we have used the guidelines of hemodynamic instability and blood loss of more than 6 U in 24 hours to determine the timing of reoperation. Clinical parameters such as an increased heart rate, low blood pressure, low CVP, and elevated SVR, when taken together, all herald ongoing bleeding. If the patient is cold and coagulopathic, it may be prudent to wait until clot lysis has subsided and stabile clot formation is occurring before subjecting the patient to a trip back to the operating room and thereby worsening the already established coagulopathy. In the United States and many European countries, aprotinin has been advocated as a means of reducing blood transfusions and limiting thrombolysis and fibrinolysis. However, several reports have found an association between aprotinin and severe and extensive vascular thrombosis.[45-47] At Baylor, we prefer to use ε-aminocaproic acid to control fibrinolysis. In most cases, prerenal failure as a result of ongoing blood loss is often improved once the blood loss has been firmly controlled and the abdomen has been opened to counteract the effect of increased intra-abdominal pressure on renal blood flow. It is our firm policy to perform intra-abdominal lavage with large volumes of double antibiotic solution and amphotericin B for prophylaxis against intra-abdominal infections. It is often prudent to consider early re-exploration for repeat intra-abdominal lavage in 24 to 48 hours to prevent abscess formation and decrease the likelihood of death from sepsis. These patients can also be monitored by CT to determine whether intra-abdominal fluid collections are present before elective exploration.

Vascular Complications

Vascular complications provide the surgeon with an array of technical challenges when they occur. Most of these complications are life-threatening or require retransplantation if not found early and corrected expeditiously.

Hepatic Artery Thrombosis

As the newly implanted liver is beginning to correct the coagulation defects that have been ongoing for the

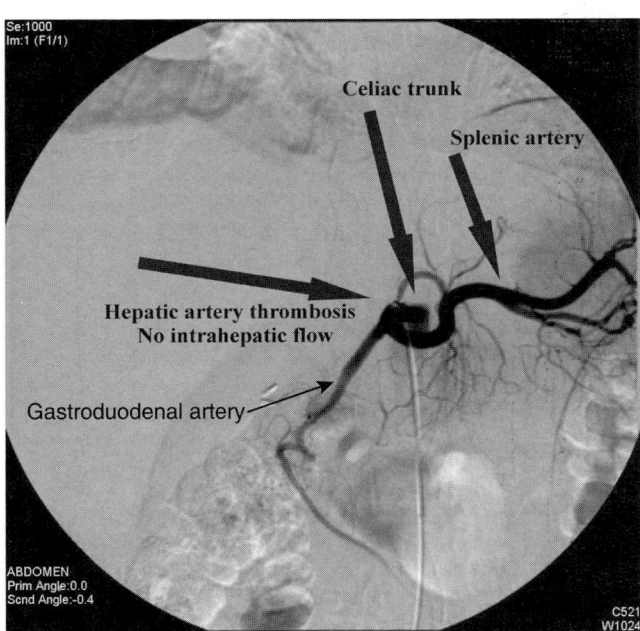

FIGURE 56–2

Angiogram demonstrating hepatic artery thrombosis. The celiac trunk is shown with splenic flow and no evidence of hepatic arterial flow.

duration of the inherent liver disease, blood products such as fresh-frozen plasma, platelets, vitamin K, and cryoprecipitate are administered; a transient hypercoagulable state often becomes apparent and is manifested in the form of vascular thrombosis. HAT (Fig. 56–2) can occur early after transplantation or in the late postoperative period and can be a devastating complication.[48-51] HAT is manifested by a sudden elevation in liver enzymes, prolongation of the prothrombin time, and an abrupt change in mental status (see Table 56–4). Left unattended, HAT will lead to parenchymal infarction, necrosis, and sepsis. Because the arterial tree is the sole blood supply to the biliary system, biliary strictures result in HAT. Short-term manifestations of HAT include parenchymal abscesses, sepsis, recurrent bacteremia, and biliary strictures. HAT occurs with a high degree of frequency in pediatric liver transplants,[52-54] split-liver transplants,[52,55-57] and living donor liver transplants.[54-60] The estimated frequency of occurrence in pediatric liver transplants is 15% to 20% in most centers and 5% to 10% in adults.[52,60] If arterial extension grafts are used, the incidence of HAT is also affected. In children, the use of an extension graft is associated with a 70% incidence of HAT. Routine use of Doppler ultrasonography allows the surgical team to prepare for immediate exploration because once the diagnosis has been made, immediate surgical attention is required. However, the arterial angiogram is the "gold" standard for diagnosis if a Doppler signal is not detectable. One should remember that false-positive and false-negative findings are not unusual with Doppler examination.

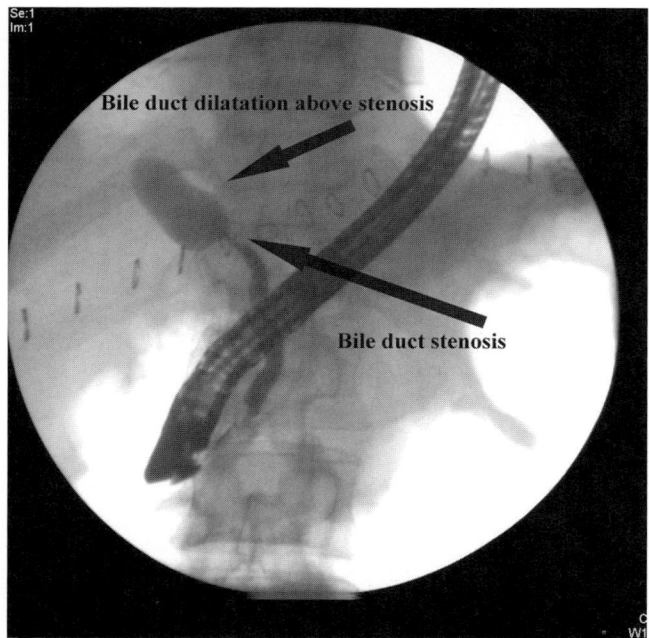

Bile duct dilatation above stenosis

Bile duct stenosis

FIGURE 56–3

Endoscopic retrograde cholangiopancreatography demonstrating severe stenosis or stricture of the common bile duct. Above the stenosis is a dilated duct.

Hepatic Artery Stenosis

Early stenosis of the hepatic artery is rarely if ever recognized if diagnostic Doppler ultrasound is not routinely performed. Stenosis is often secondary to anastomotic narrowing and kinking or twisting of the artery after reconstruction. Allograft arteriopathy is also a cause of hepatic artery stenosis. Elevation in total bilirubin is a manifestation of hepatic artery stenosis (see Table 56–4). However, a Doppler study showing increased flow velocity (>200 cm/sec) across the anastomosis will alert the surgeon to an imminent problem. A low resistive index (RI <50% or <0.50) can be found in the main, right, or left hepatic artery (Fig. 56–3). Resection of the area of stenosis and primary reanastomosis should be carried out immediately. In some cases, interposition with donor artery, a vein graft, or a saphenous vein patch may become necessary. Left unattended, half may experience obstruction and thrombosis. Angioplasty for stenosis is not as productive as primary resection and reanastomosis. Lesions amenable to surgery should be corrected in the operating room if at all possible.

Arcuate Ligament Syndrome

Arcuate ligament syndrome is a disorder in which the celiac axis becomes narrowed because of the existence of fibrous bands across the crus of the diaphragm. At our institution, we have encountered this condition

not infrequently. The diagnosis is based on early recognition of high-velocity flow in the celiac artery at end-expiration by Doppler ultrasound. The hepatic artery RI is low (<50%). Confirmation with a hepatic artery angiogram is necessary. Treatment is surgical and requires an aortic interposition graft. Busuttil and coauthors reported a 60% success rate with division of the fibrous bands that are compressing the celiac trunk and common hepatic artery at the diaphragm[61]; however, recurrence was seen frequently. Preoperative workups have begun to demonstrate increased recognition of arcuate ligament syndrome. After magnetic resonance angiography, a CT angiogram with celiac artery reconstruction is obtained. Detection of the syndrome allows us to prepare patients for an aortohepatic artery conduit at the time of transplantation to avoid an unnecessary reoperation and the complications associated with decreased blood flow through the hepatic artery, mainly parenchymal injury and biliary tract injury. As with standard hepatic artery anastomosis, the conduit is subject to stenosis and thrombosis as well. We typically initiate antiplatelet therapy with dextran for 24 hours, followed by oral antiplatelet agents. We have begun to use enteric-coated aspirin, 81 mg daily for life, when patients can tolerate an oral diet (day 3 to 5 postoperatively), with or without clopidogrel, 75 mg daily for 1 month.

Portal Vein Thrombosis

Portal vein thrombosis is a rare complication. In the immediate postoperative period it is usually the result of technical complications. If diagnosed preoperatively, a thrombosed portal vein warrants an attempt at eversion thrombectomy/venectomy. When reconstructing the portal vein, endothelial injury often occurs, and migrating thrombus may lead to complete thrombosis. Other factors such as a twist in the vein, external compression, anastomotic strictures, venous reconstructions (venous "jump" grafts), and excessive length of the veins leading to kinking and rejection have all been implicated. If portal vein thrombosis is suspected, laboratory studies usually show a marked elevation in liver enzyme levels (see Table 56–4). Clinical manifestations of thrombosis may include variceal hemorrhage, venous intestinal congestion, intestinal ischemia, necrosis, ascites, or any combination of these complications. Doppler studies reveal low-flow states or no evidence of venous flow. Intraoperative flow of less than 1L/min portends a potential for portal venous thrombosis. Postoperatively, hepatic arterial flow with an RI of 65% or less should raise suspicions of portal vein thrombosis. Techniques used to reestablish flow include thrombectomy/embolectomy and the use of thrombolytic and anticoagulant agents, but reconstruction of the portal vein with a venous graft may be required.

Portal Vein Stenosis

Technical misadventures appear to be the leading cause of portal vein stenosis, which occurs in only 1% to 3% of liver transplant recipients. Tight anastomoses, kinking or twisting of the vein, and extrinsic compression are the main causes. Doppler studies are used as a screening test, and tripling of portal velocity is a tip-off. Angiography is the confirmatory test of choice and shows a pressure gradient across the anastomosis. Typically, growth factor left on the suture at the site of anastomosis will prevent this complication from occurring. In severe cases, portal hypertension may occur.[62,63] Treatment usually involves revising the anastomosis in the early postoperative period; such revision entails resection and primary anastomosis. Should significant hepatic necrosis occur, retransplantation might be required. Interventional radiology has proved invaluable in preventing reoperation in selected cases. Selective angiography and percutaneous transhepatic angioplasty with or without the use of stents could be useful in some cases.

Hepatic Vein Thrombosis

When hepatic vein thrombosis occurs, it is usually the result of a technical problem unless Budd-Chiari syndrome or a hypercoagulable state is evident. These conditions have a tendency to develop most often with left lateral segment grafts, as can be seen with living donor liver transplants and with split-liver transplants in infants.

Recurrent Budd-Chiari syndrome has the potential to be a life-threatening condition, but we have never seen it in the first postoperative week, and thus heparin is not needed. Anticoagulation should be avoided, just as after all adult liver transplants in the immediate postoperative period, because it is extremely dangerous. Patients with Budd-Chiari syndrome require treatment of the underlying hematological process, which is polycythemia rubra vera in more than 90%. Our institution favors the use of hydroxyurea and aspirin as a long-term treatment regimen[64]; it is begun when the patient can tolerate oral medication, usually 3 to 5 days postoperatively. We have found that this combination works exceptionally well and prevents long-term anticoagulation and the complications associated with anticoagulation. If thrombosis is suspected, Doppler ultrasound is typically helpful and is supplemented by venography. Should it be necessary, percutaneous angioplasty with stenting could be a useful adjunctive procedure. In severe cases, retransplantation may need to be a consideration.

Caval Stenosis

Another serious technical problem is constriction at the anastomotic suture line of the upper cava. Clinically, what is seen with caval stenosis are ascites, lower extremity edema, and renal and intestinal congestion, similar to severe preservation injury. Severe liver dysfunction as a result of graft outflow obstruction, edema, and congestion in the liver usually accompanies caval stenosis. On Doppler ultrasound, a threefold to fourfold increase in velocity is hemodynamically significant and should prompt follow-up with angiography (venocavogram) and pressure gradient measurements. A pressure gradient of 10 mm Hg or greater and a fixed stenosis are confirmatory. Interventional radiology can sometimes be used to achieve caval dilatation and leave expandable stents in place. If the stenosis cannot be dilated, revision of the anastomosis is warranted. Surgical techniques include dissection along the cava laterally and cephalad, and opening of the diaphragm along either side of the cava and may even be required. Caval patch venoplasty or bypass is another option to consider. In "piggyback" livers, stretching of the hepatic veins can lead to very difficult reconstruction, and a patch may be required to relieve the situation. In the largest single report of caval stenosis associated with the piggyback technique, the reported morbidity was 2.5% with a mortality rate of 0.5%. Most of the complications related to caval stenosis were associated with the use of two hepatic vein ostia as opposed to using the confluence of the three ostia. The incidence of caval stenosis in conventional-type transplantation with maintenance of a retrohepatic cava is reported to range from 1% to 3%. In the age of living donor transplantation, a new era of caval stenosis is being realized, and it remains to be seen what the impact of caval stenosis will be in the long term. Certainly, such stenosis can be treated in similar fashion, with angioplasty and stent placement.[65,66]

Biliary Problems

Biliary complications at the inception of the transplant era were considered the "Achilles' heel of liver transplantation" by Sir Roy Calne and continue to plague liver transplant surgeons throughout the world. Biliary problems can occur any time after transplantation and vary in their origin. Common laboratory values that indicate biliary tract problems are elevated and rising concentrations of alkaline phosphatase, γ-glutamyltransferase, and bilirubin. Typical pathological problems in the biliary tree include inflammation, infection, hepatic artery thrombosis, and any complications resulting from manipulation of the biliary tree.

Preservation injury universally causes elevation of canalicular enzymes in the early postoperative phase of recovery. Canalicular enzyme elevations related to acute rejection are rarely seen before postoperative day 5. Ultrasound examination on the first postoperative day is the first line of defense against biliary pathology by excluding a vascular cause of the biliary problems. However, ultrasound is rarely of help in judging the biliary tree because an increase in diameter of the bile ducts is masked by accompanying sludge with the same echogenicity as liver parenchyma. Fluid collections are noted and may indicate a bile leak or, in the worst-case scenario, complete disruption of a common bile duct. A biliary leak is usually suspected by an unrelenting increase in bilirubin together with a much more modest increase in other canalicular enzymes. The transaminases, in contrast, are rarely affected. A biliary stricture results in a slower increase in bilirubin but a higher concentration of canalicular enzymes. Note that a liver biopsy shows a picture of cholangitis in both instances, as well as in patients with a leak. Arterial pathology is an important factor in bile duct complications. If hepatic artery thrombosis is suspected, arteriography followed by rapid surgical exploration should be undertaken.

Bile Leaks

Bile duct leaks are commonly a result of technical complications associated with hepatic artery misadventures. They occur in roughly 6% to 10% of patients. Ischemia and necrosis often follow hepatic artery stenosis or HAT or occur simply because of an inadequate arterial supply to the end of the donor common bile duct. In the early phase of recovery from the transplant operation, surgical intervention is usually required, as opposed to manipulations via the duodenum or by the percutaneous route. Leaks occur at the sites of anastomosis, drainage tube insertion sites, and nonanastomotic sites. During the days of routine T-tube use, the leakage rate was reported to have been as high as 40%,[67] mostly as a result of T-tube removal. Biliary leaks from the cut surface of a liver are common if a split-liver or living donor transplant has been performed. In this case, drains placed around the liver reveal bile staining or bile-stained ascites that is apparent through the patient's chevron incision. Large volumes of bile staining generally indicate a significant problem and should prompt the surgeon to consider surgical exploration. If no abdominal drains are used, a leak is manifested as an isolated increase in bilirubin despite normalizing transaminase and canalicular enzyme levels. Left unchecked, a large bile leak can quickly turn into an abscess, infection, and sepsis. However, it is not uncommon to see completely asymptomatic leaks. In the case of bile peritonitis or an infected biloma, continued perioperative antibiotic coverage is prudent, as is the use of antifungal agents to prevent sepsis. Bilomas that are seen on ultrasound can be drained percutaneously without returning the patient to the operating room, as long as adequate drainage is performed.

In the case of bile duct disruption, all necrotic and devitalized tissue is débrided and resected until healthy bleeding tissue is encountered. Should total disruption of the bile duct occur and healthy tissue be difficult to obtain, it is wise to perform a Roux-en-Y choledochojejunostomy. If a choledochojejunostomy is the original anastomosis, revision of the bile duct anastomosis with the use of a stent is considered. We perform anastomoses with absorbable suture in all cases. However, in an infected field, we use nonabsorbable monofilament suture such as Prolene for the bile duct reconstruction. For reduced-sized grafts, splits, and living donor grafts, bile duct leaks require special attention to detail. Small bile duct leaks from a cut surface with distal obstruction will continue to leak. They require decompression of the obstruction and oversewing of the cut liver edge. If the patient has been stable for several days before the leak forms, a stent can be placed via the oral-gastric route into the bile duct to reduce outflow resistance and thereby reduce leakage on the cut surface.

Bile Duct Strictures

Early strictures of the bile duct are usually the result of a "purse-string" effect of the anastomosis or hepatic arterial flow complications (Fig. 56–4; see also Fig. 56–3). The symptoms impart a cholestatic picture with an unexplained, unrelenting increase in bilirubin and canalicular enzyme levels. Edema of the duct is also seen and may be the culprit in this early phase.

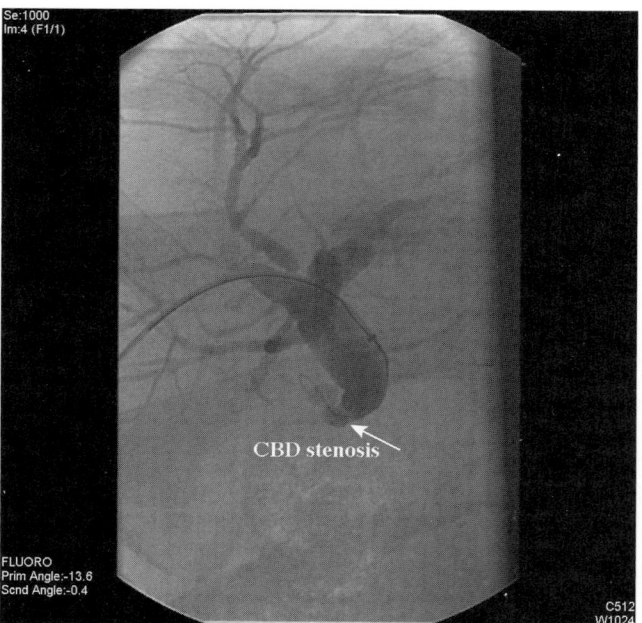

FIGURE 56–4

Percutaneous transhepatic cholangiogram showing the dilated common bile duct of a Roux-en-Y choledochojejunostomy. The guidewire is unable to traverse the area of narrowing.

Severe strictures require surgical repair because endoscopic and percutaneous techniques are generally inadequate to relieve the strictures. However, it is not unheard of for interventional radiologists to place stents or in/out drains across surgical anastomoses. Medium- to low-grade strictures can easily be treated with an internal or percutaneous technique. Should these techniques fail to relieve the stricture, surgical revision becomes a necessity. Strictures that fail to respond to endoscopic or radiographic manipulation (or to both) or cannot be corrected by primary revision thus need conversion to a Roux-en-Y choledochojejunostomy. Strictures that are the result of HAT and subsequent ischemia are often best treated with long-term stents. However, these complications are usually seen later in the patient's course.

Medical Considerations and Complications

Neurological Complications

In some patients, neurological problems after liver transplantation develop as a continuum of the pretransplant mental status changes that occur as a result of hepatic encephalopathy. In others, the mental status changes are a result of previous hepatic encephalopathy, sleep deprivation, ICU psychosis, and immunosuppression. Manifestations of neurological complications consist of seizures, visual or auditory hallucinations, coma, inability to awaken, and headaches. Correction of all altered electrolytes, use of supplemental oxygen as needed, and administration of glucose-containing intravenous fluids are measures undertaken in an effort to lessen the likelihood of seizures. Lumbar puncture may be necessary to rule out central nervous system infections, although the yield is usually very low. Electroencephalography (EEG), contrast CT of the brain, or magnetic resonance imaging (MRI) can also be of diagnostic assistance. In our experience, calcineurin inhibitors are by far the most common cause of early postoperative neurological complications. MRI and CT evidence of calcineurin inhibitor neurotoxicity is detectable. Lesions are typically located in the occipital region of the brain and tend to be fairly symmetrical, confluent, and centralized in the subcortical white matter. Radiographic studies show these lesions to be localized to the corpus callosum, pons, cerebellum, and temporal, parietal, and frontal lobes as well. In years past, the use of cyclosporine in conjunction with low magnesium levels was a large contributor to seizure activity. The same phenomenon is seen even more commonly with tacrolimus; both agents have a significant neurotoxic side effect profile associated with their use. In addition, both agents, along with steroids, have been known to lower the seizure threshold.

Sleep deprivation, which is not usually an immediate problem for a fresh liver transplant patient, may become somewhat of a problem beginning 3 to 4 days postoperatively. To ensure that each patient gets adequate sleep at our center, we give hypnotic agents such as zolpidem in 5- to 10-mg doses and diazepam, 2 to 5 mg, at bedtime. Patients recover from sleep deprivation without many sequelae in most cases. Haloperidol is used in cases of pseudopsychosis. Other centers have anecdotal experience with frank psychotic states from the use of haloperidol and do not use such agents.

Central Pontine Myelinolysis

Central pontine myelinolysis is an extremely serious cause of central nervous system injury. It has been written about with some regularity[68] and is typically seen after rapid changes in serum sodium and profound hyponatremia. At Baylor University, we have set the lower limit of surgically acceptable pretransplant serum Na^+ at 128 mEq/L for patients whose condition is not an emergency. This limit is set in an effort to prevent the likelihood of central pontine myelinolysis occurring during significant fluid shifts while the patient is anesthetized. We have found it impossible to prevent rapid correction of hyponatremia during surgery. Thus, the only means to prevent central pontine myelinolysis is to avoid transplantation in patients with such a problem if their status tolerates additional waiting time. The neurological and mental result of rapid sodium correction cannot be assessed until the patient is awake from anesthesia.

Delirium

Delirium is a common postoperative finding in patients after transplantation. Various manifestations of changes in mental status are seen, including acute delirium, seizures, anxiety, depression, psychosis, and hallucinations. Encephalopathy is a common and serious complication that results from metabolic or anoxic causes. Intraoperative events can lead to the postoperative changes seen on emergence from anesthesia (e.g., air embolism and migration of venous clots). We treat these problems symptomatically with anxiolytics such as benzodiazepines.

Seizures

Seizures are not particularly uncommon in the postoperative period and are often seen in patients with acute intracranial hemorrhage. Control of seizure activity should be immediate administration of benzodiazepines while the cause of the seizure is quickly ascertained. Calcineurin inhibitors are commonly found to be the offending agent. Additional possible causes of seizures include other medications such as high-dose steroids, derangement of the serum electrolytes Ca^{2+} and Mg^{2+}, abnormal serum blood gas values, hypoglycemia, hypocholesterolemia, infections, mass lesions, cerebral infarction, and hemorrhage.

Calcineurin inhibitors, high-dose corticosteroids, and hypomagnesemia are associated with a lower threshold for induction of seizure activity. Calcineurin inhibitor toxicity accounts for about 40% of the seizure activity seen in liver transplant patients. Clinical examination along with elevated serum levels is diagnostic. Neurotoxicity tends to occur more frequently with tacrolimus in the elderly than with cyclosporine. Switching from one calcineurin inhibitor to the other is often adequate treatment, along with withholding a dose or two. Treatment of the seizure is the first maneuver. Normally, diazepam is sufficient to control an acute event. Sometimes, however, phenytoin or barbiturates is required to interrupt the seizure activity. Rarely is antiepileptic medication needed on a long-term basis. Because of interference with drug metabolism, such drugs are not administered unless repeat seizure activity occurs. Should both agents cause seizure activity, the immunosuppressive agents sirolimus and mycophenolate mofetil should be initiated. EEG may provide some useful data and is performed at the patient's bedside. Metabolic derangements should be ruled out, and EEG will often show a slowing of waves that is consistent with metabolic causes.

Cardiovascular Complications

Arrhythmias

Many arrhythmias can occur after liver transplantation. Atrial fibrillation as a result of fluid overload and inotropic drug therapy (dopamine and epinephrine) are the most likely causes. Therapeutic options include treating the underlying cause, such as correction of electrolyte imbalances (low K^+ and Mg^{2+}), and limiting the use of agents that are potentially arrhythmogenic. Phenylephrine, which increases blood pressure through α-adrenergic receptors, is sometimes preferable to dopamine and epinephrine. If the patient is hemodynamically stable, control of the rate with pharmacological agents (β-blockers) should be carried out. If the patient is hemodynamically unstable, synchronized electrical cardioversion is performed. Antiarrhythmics should be considered in an effort to enhance sinus rhythm.

Hypertension

The correlation between postoperative hypertension and intracranial bleeding is very strong. Thus, we do not allow and vigorously treat systolic blood pressure higher than 160 mm Hg and diastolic pressure higher than 100 mm Hg. We treat all systolic pressure greater than 140 mm Hg and diastolic pressure of 90 mm Hg. Hypertension is very common in liver transplant recipients and begins almost immediately after the transplant; it is to be expected in almost 80% of liver transplant patients.[69,70] The cause is arterial hypertension and is multifactorial in nature, and postoperative problems such as an antecedent history of hypertension, pain, low systemic blood pressure, renal insufficiency, hypoventilation, and fluid overload are all thought to play a role in systemic hypertension. Pretransplant medications such as β-blockers and clonidine can cause rebound hypertension. These medications are best reinstituted as soon as possible in the immediate postoperative period. Drugs that can be substituted for β-blockers are labetalol and clonidine, which can be used in sublingual form to maintain the heart rate below 90 beats per minute and systolic blood pressure below 140 mm Hg. For systemic hypertension caused by pain, adequate use of an analgesic is generally sufficient to reduce systemic blood pressure to an acceptable level (usually <140 mm Hg). The direct effects of immunosuppressive agents on vascular endothelium are thought to play a role in systemic hypertension, and cyclosporine has been shown to affect blood pressure by its direct effect on the kidneys. The use of calcium channel blockers such as nifedipine and amlodipine has shown great promise in reducing blood pressure.

Cerebrovascular Accidents

Systemic hypertension is a treatable cause of cerebrovascular accidents, and liver transplant patients are particularly susceptible. An incidence of cerebrovascular accidents in the immediate posttransplant period of 31% has been reported.[71] It is strongly recommended that hypertension be treated so that a systolic blood pressure of 140 mm Hg or less and a diastolic blood pressure of 80 mm Hg or less are maintained. Other treatable causes of systemic hypertension include volume overload (fluid restriction, aggressive diuresis, or both are appropriate therapy), coagulation abnormalities, and pain (analgesics).[72] It has been discovered that most causes of cerebrovascular accidents are not attributable to coagulation defects but to infectious conditions, so careful pretransplant screening and prudent use of lumbar puncture and CT can be useful diagnostic tools.

Respiratory Complications

Pulmonary Edema and Fluid Overload

In general, all liver transplant patients are fluid-overloaded by the end of surgery. Usually, patients need to receive intravenous fluids during surgery and the immediate posttransplant period. Careful documentation of the fluids administered and output is essential in all patients in the ICU. However, body weight is a more reliable factor to monitor than simply measuring input and output. Fluid is deposited everywhere, most of all in the splanchnic bed, and third-space fluid is mobilized back into the circulatory system on the fourth to fifth postoperative day. Because of a variety of factors, such as calcineurin nephrotoxicity, pretransplant incipient HRS, subclinical ATN from intraoperative hypoperfusion, low colloidal osmotic pressure, and high intra-abdominal pressure, the kidneys may be unable to respond to the mobilized third-space fluid. In this situation, the only place that the fluid can go is into the lungs. Patients who do not receive adequate diuretic therapy to counteract the perioperative injuries that the kidney experiences may be prone to sudden pulmonary edema and fluid overload. A full third of all ICU readmissions are caused by "pulmonary edema or acute respiratory distress syndrome," which is directly related to the inability of the kidneys to respond to the fluid mobilized from the third space.[73-75] Our practice is to initiate aggressive diuretic therapy in all patients on the first postoperative day. If kidney function (creatinine and blood urea nitrogen) increases as a result of prerenal factors, we accept this increase as long as urine output is vigorous (i.e., >150 mL/ hr). This increase in creatinine and blood urea nitrogen is benign and totally reversible. Commonly used diuretics include furosemide, bumetanide, chlorothiazide, and metolazone. Both furosemide and bumetanide can be administered by continuous intravenous infusion as well. For the most part we start bumetanide at 4 mg every 8 hours together with chlorothiazide, 500 mg every 12 hours. If the patient shows a tendency for metabolic alkalosis, or a CO_2 of 25 mEq/L or higher, we switch from chlorothiazide to acetazolamide, 250 to 500 mg every 12 hours. If initiated early, metabolic alkalosis is rarely a problem. If the patient shows little or no response to intermittent diuretics, a diuretic infusion drip is instituted; again, both furosemide and bumetanide can be administered by continuous intravenous infusion as well. The threshold for the use of CVVH or conventional dialysis should remain low for any patient who cannot undergo diuresis by the intravenous route. The goal for most patients is a CVP of 4 to 8 cm H_2O. It is our policy to institute CVVH if CVP exceeds 14 cm H_2O in the early postoperative period. Elevated CVP is injurious to the liver and may precipitate PNF, especially in an extended criteria donor liver. Not infrequently, one sees a patient whose urine output is dropping to 50 mL/hr or less in the early postoperative phase. The patient usually has peripheral edema and a noticeable weight gain, often 4 kg or more over preoperative weight. CVP may be anywhere from 4 to 10 cm H_2O, systolic pressure from 100 to 120 mm Hg, and hematocrit from 29% to 32%.

The diagnostic information here lies in SVR. If SVR is 900 to 1200, the patient is in fact intravascularly hypovolemic. Transfusion of blood products (peripheral red blood cells) in 2-U increments results in unchanged CVP (4 to 10 cm H_2O) and hematocrit (29% to 32%), a slight increase in blood pressure (120 to 130 mm Hg), and normalization of SVR (500 to 700) with a response to diuretics. The next day will demonstrate a loss of weight (third-space fluid) and a decrease in any fluid overload. If SVR was normal to begin with or low, the oliguria has other explanations such as drug nephrotoxicity, hypotension, or sepsis.

Pulmonary Hypertension

Formerly, pulmonary hypertension was considered an absolute contraindication to liver transplantation. Pulmonary hypertension is diagnosed by detection of increased pulmonary artery pressure on a right-sided heart catheterization study or by a positive bubble study demonstrating a right-to-left shunt of greater than 5% in the pulmonary vasculature. During the operative phase, right-sided heart failure would develop at the time of reperfusion, with death quickly following. Recently, extensive experience using the drug epoprostenol (5 ng/kg/hr) has allowed patients who formerly were refused transplantation to enjoy results similar to those without pulmonary hypertension.[76] Use of this agent has allowed patients with a mean pulmonary artery pressure of 35 mm Hg or less to be transplanted without concern for immediate right-sided heart failure. It has been shown that weaning patients too early from epoprostenol renders them insensitive to the drug and makes them susceptible to increased pulmonary artery pressure in the postoperative period and therefore at risk for late-onset right heart failure. Pulmonary artery pressure with a sustainable mean greater than 35 mm Hg remains an absolute contraindication to transplantation. At our center, if a patient with known pulmonary hypertension is brought in for transplantation, a backup patient is sought. The primary patient is admitted to the ICU for placement of a Swan-Ganz catheter to measure pulmonary artery pressure. If the patient has a mean pressure higher than 35 mm Hg, epoprostenol is administered, and the backup patient is prepared for the transplant operation expeditiously. This practice serves two purposes: it maintains the sterility of the operative suite and avoids the cost/charges of taking the patient to the operating room. Furthermore, this maneuver helps keep the cold ischemia time to a minimum, which is important, more so for the expanded criteria donor livers that are so often used in light of the current situation of limited organ availability. Inhaled nitric oxide has also been used with some success. Postoperatively, patients must be kept as dry as possible.

They must be subjected to forceful diuresis to help keep pulmonary arterial pressure under control. Use of hemofiltration should be considered immediately if the diuresis is insufficient to keep the patient dry. We try to keep CVP in the 0- to 4-cm H_2O range. If the patient is treated with epoprostenol, it must not be interrupted because the patient may become unresponsive to the drug when it is restarted.

Hepatopulmonary Syndrome

Hepatopulmonary syndrome (HPS) is a condition that affects approximately 1% to 2% of cirrhotics.[77,78] It is diagnosed by right heart catheterization or "bubble" echocardiography. Shunt fractions for HPS are on the order of 30% when technetium Tc 99m macroaggregated albumin is used. Clinical manifestations of HPS include hypoxemia that responds to supplemental oxygen. In fact, the ICU team may find it difficult to extubate some liver recipients. The condition is reversed in 60% to 90% after transplantation. Supplemental oxygen is continued for some 6 to 12 months after transplantation. Mortality is 16% at 3 months and 38% at the 1-year mark. It is also imperative to keep a patient with HPS dry. Diuresis and hemofiltration must be forcefully maintained to allow extubation and prevent reintubation.

Infectious Complications

Bacterial infections diagnosed during the first postoperative week usually correspond to pretransplant infections that may or may have not been diagnosed. Preoperative and intraoperative cultures are imperative for timely diagnosis of infections. Infectious complications follow an orderly trend; unless a minor infectious process exists in the preoperative phase, bacterial infections such as pneumonia (25%) and wound infections (10%) dominate in the first week. Infection of the biliary tree commonly leads to gram-negative bacteremia. Gram-negative bacteremia is likewise common in diabetic patients and those with poor nutritional status. In patients with prolonged ICU stay and poor graft function, the mortality rate is higher. Viral infections and opportunistic infections are uncommon during the usual 24- to 48-hour ICU stay in uncomplicated liver transplantation. However, in complicated liver transplant recipients and those with a protracted ICU stay, prophylactic antibiotics and antibiotic treatment of active infections are important measures. Biliary tract infections are notorious for creating some of the most difficult to treat infections. The use of antifungal agents with fungicidal activity as opposed to fungistatic activity is preferred. At Baylor, we prefer the agents liposomal amphotericin B (AmBisome) and caspofungin (Cancidas) for this particular reason. After 1 month, viral infections with cytomegalovirus, Epstein-Barr virus, varicella-zoster virus, and adenovirus become important. When a patient is very sick, namely, is in the ICU or was admitted to the hospital before transplantation and is prone to postoperative fungal infections, prophylaxis with amphotericin B, 10 mg/day, is administered until discharge or for a maximum of 10 days. At this dose, side effects are rarely, if ever, seen. The reported incidence of postoperative fungal infections in primary liver transplant recipients is about 10%.[79]

Nutrition

A newly transplanted patient is a challenge for the liver transplant team, including the nutritional staff. Moderate to severe protein-calorie malnutrition can be seen in 70% to 80% of patients awaiting transplantation.[80] Immediate concerns are to prevent catabolism and support the anabolic state, replenish depleted nutrient stores, correct electrolyte abnormalities, and treat elevated serum glucose levels. The calories generally required are 20% to as high as 50% above basal needs.[81] Corticosteroids stimulate catabolism, which offsets the increased calories, and promote wound healing; protein requirements should be around 1.5 g/kg of dry weight. All patients in our center receive a nasojejunal feeding tube during surgery, and feeding is started after arrival at the ICU. Other centers begin early oral feeding on the first or second postoperative day. Some centers even resort to total parenteral nutrition (TPN) after transplantation. However, it is rare that a patient is placed on TPN postoperatively because of the risk of line sepsis and because feeding the bowel tends to preserve gut mucosal integrity with minimization of bacterial translocation and bacterial overgrowth. Studies have shown a decreased risk for infection in patients receiving enteric feeding instead of using TPN as the primary source of nutritional support.[83] We typically start with a high-nitrogen enteral formula ($\approx$1200 kcal/L, 55 to 60 g protein/L) at 10 to 20 mL/hr. Tube feeding is increased every 12 hours as tolerated until feeding goals are met. Once gastrointestinal tract function has returned, a regular diet is started unless the patient is diabetic, in which case an American Diabetes Association diet is initiated. Nutritional supplements with high protein and calorie value are made available to the patient as well. On occasion when necessary, tube feeding is cycled at nighttime and then discontinued once 75% of the nutritional needs have been met.

Summary

Postoperative care of liver transplant patients has evolved dramatically over the past 10 years and continues to be one of the most exciting, challenging, and complex areas outside the surgical arena. Since transplant recipients have been incorporated into ICUs where our medical colleagues are now afforded the opportunity to work with them, many advances have been realized. The multidisciplinary approach to postoperative care provides patients with the best clinical care and research possible. As more and more ICUs incorporate posttransplant care into the formal training of their fellowship programs, and as more of our own liver transplant surgical fellows gain greater experience, the level of care provided to these complex patients will grow exponentially. Randomized and formal clinical intensive care trials will soon become a standard practice as the years progress.

Pearls and Pitfalls

- Neurological status or calcineurin neurotoxicity cannot be accurately assessed until the patient is awake.
- Urine output is more important than serum creatinine or BUN.
- Prerenal azotemia is reversible and no justification for failing to institute diuresis in a patient.
- "Adequate" urine output is 150 mL/hr or greater.
- Alkalosis is a powerful renal vasoconstrictor that can be treated.
- Keep the lungs dry at all costs, even if hemofiltration is required.
- Patients are always, without exception, edematous from third-space fluid—even when hypovolemic.
- The only blood volume expander that truly works is blood transfusion.

References

1. Mandell MS, Lezotte D, Kam I, Zamudio S: Reduced use of intensive care after liver transplantation: Influence of early extubation. Liver Transpl 8:676-681, 2002.
2. Biancofiore G, Romanelli A, Bindi M, et al: Very early tracheal extubation without predetermined criteria in a liver transplant recipient population. Liver Transpl 7:777-782, 2001.
3. Mandell S, Lockrem J, Kelley S: Immediate tracheal extubation after liver transplantation: Experience of two transplant centers. Anesth Analg 84:249-253, 1997.
4. Wong D, Cheng D, Kustra R, et al: Risk factors of delayed extubation, prolonged length of stay in the intensive care unit, and mortality in patients undergoing coronary artery bypass graft with fast-track cardiac anesthesia: A new cardiac risk score. Anesthesiology 91:936-950, 1999.
5. Ramsay M, Randall H, Burton E: Intravascular thrombosis and thromboembolism during liver transplantation: Antifibrinolytic therapy implicated? Liver Transpl 10:310-314, 2004.
6. Raj D, Abreo K, Zibari G: Metabolic alkalosis after orthotopic liver transplantation. Am J Transplant 3:1566-1569, 2003.
7. Baliga P, Merion RM, Turcotte JG, et al: Preoperative assessment in liver transplantation. Surgery 112:704-711, 1992.
8. Deschenes M, Belle SH, Krom RA, et al: Early allograft dysfunction after liver transplantation. Transplantation 66:302-310, 1998.
9. Paramesh AS, Roayaie S, Doan Y, et al: Post–liver transplant acute renal failure: Factors predicting development of end-stage renal disease. Clin Transplant 18:94-99, 2004.
10. Petros S: Percutaneous tracheostomy. Crit Care (Lond) 3(2): R5-R10, 1999.
11. Lasch K, Carr D: Pain assessment in seriously ill patients: Its importance and need for technical improvement. Crit Care Med 24:1943-1944, 1996.
12. Melzack R: The McGill Pain Questionnaire: Major properties and scoring methods. Pain 8:143-154, 1975.
13. Ferrell BA: Pain management in elderly people. J Am Geriatr Soc 39:64-73, 1991.
14. Zborowski M: Cultural components in response to pain. J Social Issues 8:16-30, 1952.
15. Daut RL, Cleeland CS, Flannery RC: Development of the Wisconsin Brief Pain Questionnaire to assess pain in cancer and other diseases. Pain 17:197-210, 1983.
16. Iwatsuki S, Popovtzer MM, Corman JL, et al: Recovery from "hepatorenal syndrome" after orthotopic liver transplantation. N Engl J Med 289:1155-1159, 1973.
17. Gonwa TA, Morris CA, Goldstein RM, et al: Long-term survival and renal function following liver transplantation in patients with and without hepatorenal syndrome: Experience with 300 patients. Transplantation 51:428-430, 1991.
18. Davis CL, Gonwa TA, Wilkinson AH: Identification of patients best suited for combined liver-kidney transplantation: Part II. Liver Transpl 8:193-211, 2002.
19. Israelit AH, Long DL, White MG, Hall AR: Measurement of glomerular filtration rate utilizing a simple subcutaneous injection of ^{125}I-iothalamate. Kidney Int 4:346-349, 1973.
20. Gonwa T, Jennings L, Mai M, et al: Estimation of glomerular filtration rates before and after orthotopic liver transplantation: Evaluation of current equations. Liver Transpl 10:301-309, 2004.
21. Jaeschke H: Preservation injury, mechanisms, preservation and consequences. J Hepatol 25:774-780, 1996.
22. Serracino-Inglott F, Habib NA, Mathie RT: Hepatic ischemia-reperfusion injury. Am J Surg 181:160-166, 2001.
23. Blizer M, Gerbes AL: Preservation injury of the liver: Mechanisms and novel therapeutic strategies. J Hepatol 32:508-515, 2000.
24. Katz E, Mor E, Schwartz ME, et al: Preservation injury in clinical liver transplantation. Incidence and effect on rejection and survival. Clin Transpl 8:492-496, 1994.
25. Bao YM, Adam R, Farges O, et al: Impact of preservation-induced liver injury on the risk of rejection of rat and human liver grafts. Transplant Proc 27:2502-2503, 1995.
26. Howard TK, Klintmalm GB, Cofer JB, et al: The influence of preservation injury on rejection in the hepatic transplant recipient. Transplantation 49:103-107, 1990.
27. Marino IR, Doyle HR, Aldrighetti L, et al: Effect of donor age and sex on the outcome of liver transplantation. Hepatology 22:1754-1762, 1995.
28. Seaberg EC, Belle SH, Beringer KC, et al: Long-term patient and retransplantation-free survival by selected recipient and donor characteristics: An update from the Pitt-UNOS liver transplant registry. In Cecka JM, Terasaki PI (eds): Clinical Transplants 1997. Los Angeles, UCLA Tissue Typing Laboratory, 1997, pp 15-28.

29. Fishbein TM, Fiel MI, Emre S, et al: Use of liver with microvesicular fat safely expands the donor pool. Transplantation 64:248-251, 1997.

30. Mor E, Klintmalm GB, Gonwa TA, et al: The use of marginal donors for liver transplantation. Transplantation 52:383-386, 1992.

31. Verran D, Kusyk T, Painter D, et al: Clinical experience gained from the use of 120 steatotic donor livers for orthotopic liver transplantation. Liver Transpl 9:500-505, 2003.

32. Greig PD, Woolf GM, Sinclair SB, et al: Treatment of primary liver graft nonfunction with prostaglandin E_1. Transplant Proc 29:2381-2384, 1997.

33. Klein AS, Cofer JB, Pruett TL, et al: Prostaglandin E_1 administration following orthotopic liver transplantation: A randomized prospective multicenter trial. Gastroenterology 111:710-715, 1996.

34. Selzner M, Graf R, Clavien PA: IL-6: A magic potion for liver transplantation? Gastroenterology 125:256-259, 2003.

35. Mokuno Y, Berthiaume F, Tompkins RG, et al: Technique for expanding the donor pool: Heat shock preconditioning in a rat fatty liver model. Liver Transpl 10:264-272, 2004.

36. Arnault I, Bao YM, Sebagh M, et al: Beneficial effect of pentoxifylline on microvesicular steatotic livers submitted to a prolonged cold ischemia. Transplantation 76:77-83, 2003.

37. Natori S, Higuchi H, Contreras P, et al: The caspase inhibitor IDN-6556 prevents caspase activation and apoptosis in sinusoidal endothelial cells during liver preservation injury. Liver Transpl 9:278-284, 2003.

38. Peltekian KM, Makowka L, Williams R, et al: Prostaglandins in liver failure and transplantation: Regeneration, immunomodulation, and cytoprotection. Liver Transpl Surg 2:171-184, 1996.

39. Imagawa DK, Noguchi K, Iwaki Y, et al: Hyperacute rejection following ABO-incompatible orthotopic liver transplantation—a case report. Transplantation 54:1114-1117, 1992.

40. Mor E, Skerrett D, Manzarbeitia C, et al: Successful use of an enhanced immunosuppressive protocol with plasmapheresis for ABO-incompatible mismatched grafts in liver transplant recipients. Transplantation 59:986-990, 1995.

41. Gugenheim J, Samuel D, Reynes M, et al: Liver transplantation across ABO blood group barriers. Lancet 336:519-523, 1990.

42. Lo CM, Shaked A, Busuttil RW: Risk factors for liver transplantation across the ABO barrier. Transplantation 58:543-547, 1994.

43. Lebeau G, Yanaga K, Marsh JW, et al: Analysis of surgical complications after 397 hepatic transplantations. Surg Gynecol Obstet 170:123-147, 1989.

44. Everson GT: A hepatologist's perspective on the management of coagulation disorders prior to liver transplantation. Liver Transpl Surg 3:646-653, 1997.

45. Alvarez JM, Chandraratan H, Newman MA, et al: Case 3-1999. Intraoperative coronary thrombosis in association with low-dose aprotinin therapy. J Cardiothorac Vasc Anesth 13:623-628, 1999.

46. Gitter R, Alivizators P, Capehart J, et al: Aprotinin and aortic cannula thrombosis. J Cardiovasc Surg 112:537-538, 1996.

47. Bohrer H, Fleischer F, Lang J, et al: Early formation of thrombi on pulmonary artery catheters in cardiac surgical patients receiving high-dose aprotinin. J Cardiovasc Anesth 4:222-225, 1990.

48. Tzakis AG, Gordon RD, Shaw BW, et al: Clinical presentation of hepatic artery thrombosis after liver transplantation in the cyclosporine era. Transplantation 40:667-671, 1985.

49. Vivarelli M, La Barba G, Legnani C, et al: Repeated graft loss caused by recurrent hepatic artery thrombosis after liver transplantation. Liver Transpl 9:612-620, 2003.

50. Gunsar R, Rolando N, Pastacaldi S, et al: Late hepatic artery thrombosis after orthotopic liver transplantation. Liver Transpl 9:604-611, 2003.

51. Garcia-Criado A, Gilabert R, Nicolau C, et al: Early detection of hepatic artery thrombosis after liver transplantation by Doppler ultrasonography: Prognostic implications. J Ultrasound Med 20:51-58, 2001.

52. Stringer MD, Marshall MM, Muiesan P, et al: Survival and outcome after hepatic artery thrombosis complicating pediatric liver transplantation. J Pediatr Surg 36:888-891, 2001.

53. Tan KC, Yandza T, de Hemptinne B, et al: Hepatic artery thrombosis in pediatric liver transplantation. J Pediatr Surg 23:927-930, 1988.

54. Mazzaferro V, Esquivel CO, Makowka L, et al: Hepatic artery thrombosis after pediatric liver transplantation—a medical or surgical event? Transplantation 47:971-977, 1989.

55. Busuttil RW, Goss JA: Split liver transplantation. Ann Surg 229:313-321, 1999.

56. Superina RA, Strasberg SM, Greig PD, Langer B: Early experience with reduced-size liver transplants. J Pediatr Surg 25:1157, 1990.

57. Langnas AN, Marujo WC, Inagaki M, et al: The results of reduced-size liver transplantation, including split livers, in patients with end-stage liver disease. Transplantation 40:667-671, 1992.

58. Marcos A, Killackey M, Orloff MS, et al: Hepatic arterial reconstruction in 95 adult right lobe living donor liver transplants: Evolution of anastomotic technique. Liver Transpl 9:570-574, 2003.

59. Mori K, Nagata I, Yamagata S, et al: The introduction of microvascular surgery to hepatic artery reconstruction in living-donor liver transplantation—its surgical advantages compared with conventional procedures. Transplantation 71:767-772, 2001.

60. Testa G, Massimo M, Silvio N, et al: Complications and outcomes in adult living donor liver transplantation. Curr Opin Organ Transplant 6:367-370, 2001.

61. Jurim O, Shaked A, Kiai K, et al: Celiac compression syndrome and liver transplantation. Ann Surg 218:10-20, 1993.

62. Scantlebury VP, Zajko AB, Esquivel CO, et al: Successful reconstruction of late portal vein stenosis after hepatic transplantation. Arch Surg 124:945-946, 1989.

63. Gonzolez-Tutor A, Abascal F, Cerezai L, et al: Transjugular approach to treat portal vein stenosis after liver transplantation—a case report. Angiology 51:511-514, 2000.

64. Melear JM, Goldstein RM, Levy MF, et al: Hematologic aspects of liver transplantation for Budd-Chiari syndrome with special reference to myeloproliferative disorders. Transplantation 74:1090-1095, 2002.

65. Weeks SM, Gerber DA, Jacques PF, et al: Primary Gianturco stent placement for inferior vena cava abnormalities following liver transplantation. J Vasc Interv Radiol 11(2 Pt 1):177-187, 2000.

66. Zulke C, Berger H, Anthuber M, et al: Detection of suprahepatic caval stenosis following liver transplantation and treatment via balloon-expandable intravascular stent. Transpl Int 8:330-332, 1995.

67. Stratta RJ: Diagnosis and treatment of biliary complications after orthotopic liver transplantation. Surgery 106:676-684, 1989.

68. Buis CI, Wijdicks EF: Serial magnetic resonance imaging of central pontine myelinolysis. Liver Transpl 8:643-645, 2002.

69. Taler SJ, Textor SC, Canzanello VJ, et al: Hypertension after liver transplantation: A predictive role for pretreatment hemodynamics and effects of isradipine on the systemic and renal circulations. Am J Hypertens 13:231-239, 2000.

70. Semhoun-Ducloux S, Ducloux D, Bresson-Hadni S, et al: Systemic hypertension and renal function in long-term liver transplant recipients of cyclosporine. Transplant Proc 32:449-452, 2000.

71. Neal DA, Tom BD, Luan J, et al: Is there disparity between risk and incidence of cardiovascular disease after liver transplant? Transplantation 77:93-99, 2004.

72. Bronster DJ, Gousse R, Fassas A, et al: Anticardiolipin antibody–associated stroke after liver transplantation. Transplantation 63:908-909, 1997.

73. Soubani AO, Rohrer RJ: Pulmonary complications of liver transplantation. Clin Pulm Med 5:69-80, 1998.

74. Aduen JF, Stapelfeldt WH, Johnson MM, et al: Clinical relevance of time onset, duration and type of pulmonary edema after liver transplantation. Intensive Care Med 28:376, 2003.

75. Yost CS, Matthay MA, Gropper MA: Etiology of acute pulmonary edema during liver transplantation: A series of cases with analysis of the edema fluid. Chest 119:219-223, 2001.

76. Rubin LJ: Pulmonary hypertension. N Engl J Med 336:111-117, 1997.

77. Arguedas MR, Abrams GA, Krowka MJ, Fallon MB: Prospective evaluation of outcomes and predictors of mortality in patients with hepatopulmonary syndrome undergoing liver transplantation. Hepatology 37:192-197, 2003.

78. Collison EA, Nourmand H, Fraiman MH, et al: Retrospective analysis of the results of liver transplantation for adults with severe hepatopulmonary syndrome. Liver Transpl 8:925-931, 2002.

79. Razonable RR: Infections in solid organ transplant recipients. Highlights of the 40th Annual Meeting of Infectious Diseases Society of America 3(2):1-7, 2002.

80. Hasse JM: Nutrition implications of liver transplantation. Henry Ford Hosp Med J 38:235-240, 1990.

81. Harrison J, McKiernan J, Neuberger JM: A prospective study on the effect of recipient nutritional status on outcome of liver transplantation. Transpl Int 10:369-374, 1997.

82. Selzner M, Clavien PA: Fatty liver in liver transplantation and surgery. Semin Liver Dis 21:105-113, 2001.

57

Postoperative Intensive Care Management in Children

RICK HARRISON

Neurological care   854

Respiratory care   856

Cardiovascular care   857

Fluids and electrolytes   858

Gastrointestinal care   858

Liver management   859

Hematological care   860

Infectious diseases   861

Psychosocial issues   862

Conclusion   862

The transition from the operating room after transplantation to the pediatric intensive care unit (ICU) and the subsequent 48 hours are a critical time for success of the procedure. During this time period, there is great potential for life-threatening problems to occur, and they must be anticipated and, it is hoped, prevented. This is a time of significant risk for morbidity and mortality; one series reported more than a third of post-transplantation deaths to occur during the first 7 days postoperatively,[1] and another found that 75% of deaths occurred in the ICU early postoperatively.[2,3] Clinically significant changes in the patient's condition must be recognized promptly and appropriate interventions taken without delay. This requires a multidisciplinary team effort with well-defined responsibilities of care and clear communication between caregivers. The immediate postoperative care is a joint effort of the transplantation surgeon, intensivist, hepatologist, and the specially trained pediatric intensive care nursing staff.

The time of patient transfer and care from the operating room to the ICU is one of potential instability, and preparation and communication are key to prevent deterioration during this period. Before the patient's arrival, the bed space must be ready, with all necessary equipment immediately available. This requires communication between the operating room and nursing staff receiving the patient to delineate the expected time of arrival, arterial and venous catheters in place, ongoing infusion of any medications, and any anticipated

853

special needs of the patient. With this knowledge, the room can be prepared with all necessary equipment ready to be attached to the patient. Infusion pumps can be labeled for any medications and continuous drips mixed at concentrations appropriate for the age and dose required. An appropriate ventilator should be set up with a best estimate of needed ventilatory settings and adjustments made as necessary after the patient's arrival.

When the patient arrives from the operating room accompanied by the surgeon and anesthesiologist, there must be a smooth transition to the ICU. This transition is facilitated by having two nurses with clearly defined responsibilities assigned to receive the patient. Ventilatory status and hemodynamic stability must be assessed before changing over any monitoring equipment or drug infusions because changes may have occurred en route from the operating room to the ICU. After relative stability is ascertained, all monitoring is switched to the ICU monitors, and all infusions are changed over as necessary. After changeover is accomplished, a full report is given to the ICU physician and nursing staff. This report is greatly facilitated by having a standard reporting form to ensure that appropriate information is transferred in an organized, concise manner.

Necessary information includes patient information such as name, age, weight, and underlying condition requiring transplantation. Some details of the surgical procedure should be provided, such as whether the graft was ABO matched or unmatched and whole or reduced size and the type of vascular and biliary anastomoses performed. Fluids infused during the surgical case need to be itemized, including actual quantities of various blood products received. Blood loss may be estimated, although the amount lost is best determined from requirements for replacement rather than from direct observations of losses. Urine output should be reported for the duration of the procedure, with emphasis on the recent trend. Medications given in the operating room should be detailed and recent or continuing medications highlighted because they may alter initial assessment in the ICU. Most recent ventilatory requirements, as well as the most recent measurements of arterial blood gas, should be reported to the intensivist and respiratory therapist. Intraoperative laboratory values are reported, with particular attention paid to the most recent values and any parameter that has required ongoing correction or that currently requires correction. Finally, output from the surgically placed drains is recorded with some note on the character of the drainage. In addition, any special or unique intraoperative problems should be discussed and any special concerns of the surgeon or anesthesiologist communicated to the pediatric intensivist managing the patient postoperatively. Postoperative orders should be written at or before the patient's arrival in the ICU. A preprinted order sheet greatly facilitates this process,

ensures that all necessary orders are included initially, and helps prevent the need for clarification later. Dosage calculations should be included on the order sheet to minimize errors with the realization that some standard medication doses may need to be altered on the basis of the patient's physiological state.

Neurological Care

Neurological events are an important cause of morbidity and mortality in the early postoperative period; a significant proportion of deaths occur in the first several postoperative days as a result of cerebral edema and herniation.[4] In one study, all postoperative deaths were found to be associated with neuropathological findings on postmortem examination,[4] thus suggesting that neurological alterations were present even in patients not dying of a neurological cause. Initial postoperative assessment after transplantation requires knowledge of both the patient's preoperative neurological condition and the presence of any drugs that might alter the neurological status of the patient. Medications given during the surgical procedure will have been reported by the anesthesiologist, but it may be difficult to predict the duration of action of some of these agents in the altered physiological state of the patient. If the patient is not moving spontaneously, the presence of neuromuscular blocking agents must be assessed with the use of a nerve stimulator. The presence of all four responses to train-of-four stimulation indicates that less than 75% of the receptors are blocked and that neuromuscular blocking agents are not significantly affecting clinical assessment.[5] The pharmacodynamics of analgesic agents is also altered in transplantation patients, and a more prolonged effect may be seen. Nevertheless, a patient without significant preoperative liver encephalopathy should be waking within a few hours of returning to the ICU.

Assessment of the patient's neurological status must include the level of consciousness, cranial nerve function, motor function, sensation, and reflexes. New cranial nerve findings, abnormal posturing, or significant asymmetry in the examination mandates an urgent computed tomographic scan of the brain to evaluate the possibility of intracranial hemorrhage. The computed tomographic scan must also be evaluated for diffuse findings consistent with increased intracranial pressure (ICP), such as loss of the sulci cerebri and interhemispheric and sylvian fissures and diminution in the body of the lateral ventricle. A further rise in ICP results in complete loss of the sulci and fissures, as well as loss of the chiasmatic, quadrigeminal, and interpeduncular cisterns. Finally, with severe increases in ICP, there will be complete loss of all perimesencephalic cisterns.[6]

If computed tomography reveals the presence of central nervous system hemorrhage, neurosurgical consultation and correction of any underlying coagulopathy are required. If increased ICP is present, as manifested by examination or computed tomographic scan, consideration should be given to ICP monitoring. Clinical findings of increased ICP include decreased mental status, increased muscle tone and deep tendon reflexes, hyperventilation, and dilation of pupils with a sluggish response to light. With a further increase, the patient postures, initially decorticate and then decerebrate, and later the pupils become fixed and dilated from compression of the third cranial nerves.

Several options are available to monitor ICP. Blei and colleagues performed a survey to examine complications of ICP monitoring in liver transplantation candidates (262 patients). The use of epidural monitors as opposed to subdural or parenchymal monitoring appears to have a lower complication rate, with an infection rate of less than 1% and a 3% incidence of hemorrhage.[7] Intraparenchymal monitors have been associated with a 13% complication rate from hemorrhage and a 4% infection rate, whereas subdural monitors have had an 18% incidence of hemorrhage with 5% of monitored patients dying of intracranial bleeding.[7] A more recent study involving subdural ICP monitors in similar patients reported only 3 episodes of subdural bleeding in 161 patients and only 1 death from intracranial hemorrhage.[8] Management of increased ICP should be directed at maintaining adequate cerebral perfusion pressure, which is the difference between mean arterial pressure and ICP.

The absolute value of adequate cerebral perfusion pressure varies from patient to patient but appears to be the value at which ICP spikes are minimized and below which ICP increases. Attainment of this goal often requires maintenance of mean arterial pressure above normal for age, which many postoperative patients maintain spontaneously. Intravascular volume must be adequately preserved, and hypovolemia should not be allowed to occur because it will adversely affect cerebral perfusion pressure. Thus, a hypovolemic or euvolemic patient should not be fluid restricted. The use of hyperventilation in patients with increased ICP is controversial. Although hyperventilation does initially lower ICP, its effect is relatively transitory and may make segments of the brain ischemic and thus result in further brain injury and swelling. Most centers have discontinued the use of hyperventilation for raised ICP and maintain the partial pressure of arterial carbon dioxide between 35 and 40 mm Hg. Mannitol may be useful for treating increased ICP by decreasing blood viscosity and the water content of the brain.[9,10] Care must be exercised, however, because posttransplantation patients are often hyperosmolar initially, and mannitol should not be used if osmolality is greater than 315 mOsm/kg. An alternative means of raising serum osmolality is to use hypertonic saline to raise the serum sodium level, and this technique is increasingly being used to treat raised ICP. A recent randomized controlled study in adults with acute liver failure and grade 3 or 4 encephalopathy demonstrated decreased intracranial hypertension in the group in whom hypertonic saline was given to maintain serum sodium at 145 to 155 mmol/L.[11] Moderate hypothermia with temperatures as low as 32° C has been used with some evidence of efficacy in patients with acute liver failure and intracranial hypertension unresponsive to other medical therapies.[12]

For a patient not under the effect of neuromuscular blockade, analgesic and sedative medications should be withheld until the patient begins to wake because the duration of intraoperative analgesic and sedative agents may be quite prolonged. When the patient wakes, narcotics should be administered to provide analgesia; intermittent dosing of morphine sulfate at 0.05 to 0.1 mg/kg per dose is usually adequate, although the dosing interval will be highly variable and titration will be necessary. Orthotopic liver transplant recipients typically require less analgesia than comparable hepatic resection patients do.[13] Although benzodiazepines have become the sedative drug of choice in the pediatric ICU, caution must be exercised in their use in postoperative transplantation patients because those with liver encephalopathy have an endogenous substance with benzodiazepine activity and use of the benzodiazepine antagonist flumazenil has been shown to improve liver encephalopathy transiently.[14,15] For this reason, benzodiazepines should be avoided in an encephalopathic patient.

Seizures occur in approximately 8% of children after liver transplantation.[1] Although hypoglycemia is an unusual cause of early posttransplantation seizures because patients are nearly always hyperglycemic, the glucose level must be assessed immediately and treated if low. Electrolytes, including magnesium, should be measured and abnormalities corrected. Hypomagnesemia was previously a significant cause of seizures. Seizures often correlate with high tacrolimus or cyclosporine levels, and thus levels should be monitored and the dosage reduced if possible. Any seizure without a discernible cause and all focal seizures necessitate a computed tomographic scan to evaluate the possibility of central nervous system bleeding. The seizure episode itself may be treated with lorazepam initially if the patient is not encephalopathic, and then loading doses of phenytoin may be administered. Phenytoin increases cyclosporine and tacrolimus metabolism by stimulating the liver cytochrome P450 system; therefore, gabapentin is often used as an alternative anticonvulsant in patients requiring ongoing therapy. In the absence of structural lesions on the computed tomographic scan and with no subsequent seizures, anticonvulsant therapy may be discontinued 2 weeks after the seizure. Structural lesions require a longer duration of treatment.

Respiratory Care

Nearly all liver transplantation patients return to the ICU endotracheally intubated and maintained on positive pressure ventilation. Occasionally, an older child who was previously in excellent health other than the underlying liver disease may be extubated in the operating room, but such is the exception rather than the rule.[16] All intubated patients are continuously observed via end-tidal carbon dioxide monitoring, pulse oximetry, and intermittent arterial blood gas analysis, in addition to the standard ventilator monitoring and alarm systems.

No evidence supports the superiority of any specific mode of ventilation in children. If there is a significant leak around the endotracheal tube, which is common with the uncuffed tubes often used in children, a pressure-limited mode of ventilation often provides more consistent tidal volumes. Either an assist control or a synchronized intermittent mandatory ventilation mode may be used. Compliance should be monitored closely because it may be significantly altered by changes in abdominal distention.

The ventilatory rate is chosen to provide adequate minute ventilation as manifested by the partial pressure of carbon dioxide, with the initial set rate approximating the patient's physiological respiratory rate. To increase the small functional residual capacity commonly seen with these patients' abdominal distention, positive end-expiratory pressure (PEEP) of 4 cm H_2O is initially used. PEEP is titrated upward if adequate oxygenation cannot be achieved at a fractional inspired oxygen concentration (FIO_2) of 0.60 or less. The FIO_2 is initially chosen to provide an oxygen saturation of greater than 0.95 as measured by pulse oximetry, with the FIO_2 being weaned as tolerated.

In a relatively stable postoperative patient, it is typically possible to extubate the patient within the first 12 hours. Several factors may make such extubation impossible in selected patients (Table 57–1). Persistent paralysis or a depressed respiratory drive secondary to encephalopathy or excessive sedation precludes rapid extubation. Reversal of paralytic agents and narcotics is not usually required, and these agents are allowed to wear off as they are metabolized by the body. Fluid overload may delay extubation as a result of both pulmonary edema and pleural effusions, which are typically on the right. The effusion is generally a transudate through the traumatized diaphragm from ascitic fluid in the abdomen. Aggressive diuresis is usually efficacious for both pulmonary edema and

Table 57-1. CAUSES OF PROLONGED VENTILATION
Decreased Capacity
Neuromuscular blockade
Oversedation
Diaphragmatic dysfunction
Malnutrition
Metabolic derangements
Fatigue
Increased Workload
Decreased compliance
Pleural effusion
Atelectasis
Increased carbon dioxide production
Infection
Small airway

pleural effusions. Placement of chest tubes is avoided in view of the often dilated chest wall vasculature and the coagulopathy generally present in the immediate postoperative period.

The metabolic alkalosis commonly seen in the immediate postoperative period leads to a compensatory respiratory acidosis. Although the resultant high partial pressure of carbon dioxide is not in itself a contraindication to extubation, the hypoventilation often causes or exacerbates atelectasis and results in an increasing oxygen requirement, which makes successful extubation less likely. For this reason, a base excess greater than +7 is often treated with acetazolamide. Occasionally, with severe metabolic alkalosis, 0.2 N hydrochloric acid is initiated at 0.5 mL/kg/hr and titrated as necessary on the basis of serial serum bicarbonate levels. Other metabolic abnormalities such as hypophosphatemia, hypomagnesemia, hypocalcemia, and hypokalemia may lead to respiratory muscle dysfunction and an inability to wean from the ventilator.[17,18]

A small infant often presents a challenge to wean from the ventilator. These patients have variable and fluctuating degrees of abdominal distention from ascites, edematous bowel, and large liver grafts. This combination results in a decrease in effective pulmonary compliance and highly variable delivered tidal volumes with the pressure-limited ventilation typically used. Peak inspiratory pressure may need to be frequently altered, and successful extubation may need to await improvement of the abdominal distention.

An infant who is otherwise doing well but fails to wean from the ventilator probably has either abnormal mechanics of breathing or an infection. In infants with chronic ascites and abdominal distention, a short, broad chest develops, with decreased diaphragmatic motion often leading to atelectasis. Aggressive chest physiotherapy may be helpful to open collapsed areas of lung, but bronchoscopy may be necessary to re-expand the atelectatic lung if the patient is unable to wean from the ventilator. Diaphragmatic paralysis from phrenic nerve injury or direct injury to the diaphragm itself will delay extubation in a small infant. Diaphragmatic motion under conditions of spontaneous respiratory effort needs to be examined with either ultrasonography or fluoroscopy to look for paradoxical diaphragmatic movement. Rarely, plication of the diaphragm to prevent paradoxical motion is necessary to facilitate successful extubation. Another cause of failure to wean from the ventilator is an inappropriately small endotracheal tube, which significantly increases resistance to airflow and thus increases the work of breathing. This problem requires either changing to a larger endotracheal tube or extubating from higher levels of ventilatory support.

A very ill, malnourished infant may not have adequate strength to wean from the ventilator, and a period of ventilatory support followed by a gradual defined weaning program will thus be required. To constantly try to wean such a patient before improvement in nutritional status only exhausts the patient, uses precious calories, and delays extubation. Increasing periods of "sprinting" are often used to wean such patients, although there is no documentation of the superiority of such a weaning technique over a gradual reduction in the intermittent mandatory ventilation rate. Nutritional support should provide sufficient, but not excessive, calories with adequate noncarbohydrate calories to avoid an increased respiratory quotient with the resulting high carbon dioxide load. A small child who continues to require ventilatory support despite correction of these factors may have a pulmonary infection. Infants with an increased alveolar-arterial oxygen gradient, fever, diffuse interstitial infiltrates on chest roentgenograms, and inflammatory cells on sputum Gram stain in the absence of a bacterial process often have a viral pneumonitis. Viral cultures and antigen detection studies should be performed on an endotracheal sputum sample. Management is generally limited to good supportive care, minimization of immunosuppressive agents as tolerated, and time. Symptomatic adenoviral pneumonia has a significant mortality rate in this population.[19]

Reliable guidelines for the timing of extubation in pediatric patients do not exist. Application of the rapid, shallow breathing index, which is useful in the adult population, would incorrectly predict failure of a normal infant to tolerate extubation.[20] A maximum negative inspiratory force greater than 45 cm H_2O and a crying vital capacity greater than 15 mL/kg were predictive of successful discontinuation of positive pressure ventilation in one group of infants undergoing ventilation postoperatively.[21] Randolph and coworkers compared a pressure support method of ventilatory weaning with a volume support method and found no difference.[22] Of note is the readiness-to-extubate criteria used for that comparison trial. This extubation readiness test consisted of a maximal FIO_2 of 0.50, maximal PEEP of 5 cm H_2O, and if the patient then maintained an oxygen saturation of 95% or higher by pulse oximetry (SpO_2), changing the ventilatory mode to pressure support ventilation at a minimal level based on endotracheal tube size. If the patient tolerated a 2-hour trial with acceptable SpO_2, tidal volume, and respiratory rate, extubation was performed. This extubation readiness test is increasingly being used in clinical practice.

Cardiovascular Care

All patients are monitored with an electrocardiogram, invasive and noninvasive blood pressure devices, and central venous pressure recordings. Occasionally, a patient requires placement of a pulmonary artery catheter for an ongoing shock state, often sepsis, but this is unusual. Patients are frequently started on low-dose dopamine for kidney perfusion, although the efficacy of this therapy is unproven[23] and it may actually be deleterious.[24] No other catecholamines are systematically used. A minimum systolic blood pressure of 90 to 100 mm Hg is maintained in all patients in the immediate postoperative period for adequate graft perfusion; fluid support and occasionally inotropic agents are used to maintain these perfusion pressures. Vasopressor agents are avoided and used only if the patient remains in shock despite vigorous fluid support and is inappropriately vasodilated. These patients are invariably septic and are treated in the same manner as other septic patients. The typical postoperative patient is not hypotensive but is actually hypertensive; more than 70% of pediatric patients require therapeutic intervention for their hypertension.[19] The cause of the hypertension appears to be multifactorial, with fluid overload, cyclosporine, tacrolimus, steroids, and elevated renin levels implicated.[25-28] Attention to adequate analgesia and appropriate diuresis for hypervolemia is sufficient therapy for many patients who are hypertensive. In the absence of clinically significant bleeding and without severe coagulopathy, some degree of moderate hypertension is tolerated. Systolic pressures up to 140 mm Hg and diastolic pressures up to 90 mm Hg are not treated in all but the smallest patients for the first several days postoperatively. If other pharmacological intervention is deemed necessary, nifedipine in a low dose may be used. In an unstable patient, a nicardipine infusion may be titrated to optimize blood pressure control. One should err on the side of underdosing initially and increase the dosage as necessary to minimize the chance of acutely making the patient hypotensive and perhaps increasing the risk of hepatic artery thrombosis.

Fluids and Electrolytes

Patients usually return to the ICU in a state of total-body fluid overload. They may be intravascularly hypovolemic, euvolemic, or hypervolemic, and initial postoperative fluid management depends on the patient's intravascular fluid status on arrival at the ICU. Monitoring includes the heart rate, central venous pressure, and blood pressure, as well as hourly urine output, and clinically, the adequacy of perfusion as manifested by capillary refill time is observed. Generally, fluids, including medicines, are initially restricted to approximately 60% to 80% of maintenance requirements. If the patient has significant third spacing of fluids, fluid infusions need to be increased. Because most patients are in a state of total-body sodium overload and are hyperglycemic, a solution of 5% dextrose in water and 0.25 N saline is used to provide relatively small amounts of glucose and sodium. Fluid losses from abdominal drains must be monitored and may need to be replaced if excessive. Fluid management should be reevaluated every 3 to 4 hours, with attention directed to intravascular volume status as manifested by hemodynamic monitoring, including central venous pressure and blood pressure, as well as urine output and perfusion. Patients are typically maintained on renal-dose dopamine, 2 to 4 µg/kg/min, immediately postoperatively to optimize both kidney and liver perfusion and to increase urine output,[29,30] although the efficacy of this practice has been questioned.[23,24] Urine output should be monitored hourly with an indwelling drainage catheter and urine output maintained at more than 1 to 2 mL/kg/hr. If urine output diminishes to below this level, the adequacy of intravascular volume needs to be reassessed and any hypovolemia corrected. If blood pressure, intravascular volume, and perfusion are all satisfactory and urine output remains low, diuretics are used to improve output. Typically, furosemide, 1 to 2 mg/kg, is given, followed by a furosemide infusion of 0.2 to 0.4 mg/kg/hr titrated to maintain adequate urine flow. The continuous infusion results in increased urine output without the large swings in volume status often seen with intermittent bolus therapy.[31,32] If urine output still fails to improve, fluids must be restricted and electrolytes, especially potassium, monitored closely.

When it is apparent that kidney failure is present, dialysis should be initiated early to avoid life-threatening electrolyte, fluid, and acid-base imbalances. Continuous venovenous hemofiltration with or without dialysis has proved effective and avoids the large fluid and osmotic shifts often seen with hemodialysis.[33]

Electrolyte abnormalities are common in the early postoperative period (Table 57–2). Most patients experience total-body sodium overload and thus are kept relatively sodium restricted. If hyponatremia is present, it is typically from free-water overload and is best

Table 57–2. POSTOPERATIVE ELECTROLYTE ABNORMALITIES

Abnormality	Correction
Hyponatremia	Restrict fluids
Hypokalemia	KCl, 0.5 mEq/kg over 2-hr period
Hypocalcemia	$CaCl_2$, 20 mg/kg over 1-hr period
Hypomagnesemia	$MgSO_4$, 50 mg/kg every 6 hr × 4
Hypophosphatemia	Na_2PO_4, 0.33 mmol/kg over 6-hr period

$CaCl_2$, calcium chloride; KCl, potassium chloride; $MgSO_4$, magnesium sulfate; Na_2PO_4, sodium phosphate.

treated by fluid restriction rather than additional sodium. Hypokalemia is also common and is treated initially with intravenous infusions of concentrated potassium chloride, 0.5 mEq/kg, infused intravenously over a 2-hour period. Once good kidney function is apparent, potassium may be added to the maintenance fluids and, especially if diuretics are being used, may need to be given in a relatively high concentration. Hypocalcemia is common postoperatively and is related to calcium binding by the citrate in transfused blood products. Ionized calcium levels should be monitored rather than total calcium because there is relatively poor correlation between the two and the ionized form is the biologically active state. Calcium supplementation should be given as a 20-mg/kg calcium chloride dose until liver function has improved. Hypophosphatemia is a common finding and, if severe, may delay weaning from mechanical ventilation. Patients are typically hypophosphatemic from a combination of poor nutritional status, high parathyroid hormone levels, and increased phosphate excretion secondary to steroids. Hypophosphatemia is corrected with an intravenous infusion of sodium phosphate, 0.33 mmol/kg given over a 6-hour period.[34] Although magnesium levels are often normal immediately postoperatively, with initiation of one of the calcineurin inhibitors, tacrolimus or cyclosporine, hypomagnesemia is common, and seizures may result if magnesium stores are not repleted. Serum magnesium levels should be measured daily, and intravenous magnesium sulfate, 50 mg/kg every 6 hours for 18 to 24 hours, should be given for hypomagnesemia. In addition, magnesium-containing antacids are used when gastric pH buffering is required.

Gastrointestinal Care

Immediately after transplantation, patients are at risk for ulceration of both the stomach and duodenum secondary to stress and steroid therapy. An H_2 receptor antagonist such as famotidine is administered to all patients at moderately high doses. Famotidine is used preferentially because it does not appear to inhibit the metabolism of other drugs, as cimetidine and ranitidine do. Intermittent therapy is used the first day, with continuous infusion in total parenteral nutrition used thereafter when fluid needs are more easily predictable. Although H_2 receptor blocking agents may cause a dose-dependent transient elevation in liver enzymes, the incidence of drug-induced hepatitis is quite low.[28,29] Gastric pH is monitored at regular intervals, and antacids are administered if the pH falls below 4. If significant gastrointestinal bleeding occurs, especially in the absence of coagulopathy, upper endoscopy should be performed. Should no bleeding site be noted in the esophagus, stomach, or duodenum, the most likely source of bleeding is from the Roux-en-Y jejunostomy surgical site. If bleeding is significant without a source seen on upper or lower endoscopy, surgical exploration is often necessary. A technetium 99m pertechnetate–labeled red cell scan may be helpful in localizing the source of bleeding, although with brisk bleeding the time required for the scan is problematic, and urgent surgical intervention may be more expeditious.

Many patients with liver failure are malnourished preoperatively, and some are unable to tolerate significant enteral nutrition for several days after transplantation. Evaluation of energy expenditure and nitrogen balance within the first 2 postoperative days has revealed a hypermetabolic state with energy expenditure 1.37 times that predicted and a hypercatabolic state as manifested by a negative nitrogen balance of 22 g/day.[30] To provide early nutritional support, parenteral nutrition is initiated on the first postoperative day. Dextrose is typically started at a 10% to 15% concentration and increased by 5% daily with an amino acid concentration selected to provide age-appropriate daily amounts of protein (Table 57–3). If liver function is adequate, standard amino acids are used; branched-chain amino acids are administered if graft function is questionable. Most patients have a relatively normal serum glucose level by 24 hours postoperatively and tolerate the glucose load without requiring insulin infusion.[35] Fat emulsion is initiated at 1 g/kg/day and increased as tolerated, with trough triglyceride levels kept at less than 200 mg/dL and fat calories at less than 60% of total nonprotein calories. Enteral nutrition is initiated as soon as possible after intestinal function has recovered.

Table 57-3. PROTEIN REQUIREMENTS

Age	Protein
Birth–6 mo	2–2.5 g/kg
7–12 mo	2.0 g/kg
1–12 yr	1.5–2.0 g/kg
Adult	1.0–1.5 g/kg

Liver Management

The most common liver complications seen in the immediate posttransplant period are vascular occlusion, biliary leaks, and primary nonfunction. These complications may all be life-threatening, may require retransplantation, and must be considered in all postoperative patients who are not improving as expected. The SPLIT registry of 1092 pediatric first liver transplants since 1995 shows that the leading causes of graft failure within 30 days are postoperative vascular complications (43%) and primary graft dysfunction (26%).[36]

Primary nonfunction was shown to be a leading cause of early graft failure in the pediatric population and may require urgent retransplantation.[37,38] Liver function is assessed postoperatively by measuring liver transaminases and bilirubin and by performing clotting studies, especially the prothrombin time. Laboratory values obtained immediately postoperatively are more a function of liver harvesting and preservation, the extent of intraoperative blood loss, and clotting factor replacement in the operating room than a function of initial graft function. The laboratory tests are repeated 12 hours postoperatively, at which time values are more indicative of liver function. The prothrombin time especially is a sensitive indication of function because the biological half-life of factor VII is only 4 to 6 hours and, without adequate liver synthesis, plasma concentrations fall rapidly.[39] Clinically, neurological status is a relatively sensitive indicator of liver function, with prolonged encephalopathy or coma signifying decreased metabolic function of the liver. If liver function does not show rapid improvement with decreasing transaminases, decreasing international normalized ratio (INR), and clearing of encephalopathy, emergency retransplantation must be considered.

Vascular occlusion, either the hepatic artery or portal vein, is the major cause of graft dysfunction in the pediatric population in the early postoperative period. The rate of hepatic artery thrombosis has decreased significantly over time. In one large series[40] the rate has decreased from more than 12% to 4%, and a rate of 1.7% was reported in a series of living related transplants performed with microsurgical reconstruction.[41] Hepatic artery thrombosis can occur in one of three clinical manifestations: fulminant liver failure, biliary leak, or intermittent fever as a late finding in minimally symptomatic or asymptomatic patients. Hepatic artery thrombosis in the first 48 hours is typically manifested as fulminant liver necrosis with a very rapid course of deterioration. Transaminase values rise abruptly, often into the thousands, the prothrombin time is prolonged, and the patient becomes encephalopathic.

A diagnosis of hepatic artery thrombosis is suggested by the absence of arterial Doppler signals by duplex Doppler sonography of the hepatic artery. This technique has been 100% sensitive in the pediatric population in some studies but provided false-negative results in another.[40-42] The false-negative examinations were believed to be secondary to the presence of collateral arterial supply to the liver; because collaterals are not likely to be present immediately after transplantation, the incidence of duplex sonography indicating a patent hepatic artery when it is thrombosed should be approaching zero. Hepatic artery thrombosis early in the postoperative period is an emergency. At angiography, intra-arterial tissue plasminogen activator can be infused to lyse clots, restore hepatic arterial flow, and thus avoid the need for retransplantation. Other investigators have advocated emergency surgical re-exploration and thrombectomy, with examination of the anastomosis and reanastomosis if indicated.[42,43] In a single-center study of 31 instances of hepatic artery thrombosis, 18 required retransplantation. All 13 patients not undergoing retransplantation survived, including 9 treated conservatively without early surgical intervention.[44]

Risk factors for hepatic artery thrombosis include the size of the hepatic artery, the type of arterial reconstruction, and the number of times that the anastomosis was intraoperatively performed to achieve satisfactory results (Table 57–4).[45] Nonsurgical risk factors include the use of fresh-frozen plasma intraoperatively and lack of anticoagulant administration.[45] In the adult population, a postoperative hematocrit greater than 44% was an independent risk factor for hepatic artery thrombosis.[46]

In an effort to decrease the incidence of hepatic artery thrombosis, postoperative care should include no correction of coagulopathy in the absence of clinical bleeding and an INR of less than 2.5. Anticoagulation in the form of low-molecular-weight dextran at 0.5 mL/kg/hr and heparin is initiated when the INR is less than 1.8 and there is no clinically significant bleeding. The hematocrit is kept below 30% unless severe hypoxemia necessitates increased oxygen-carrying capacity. Despite these interventions, hepatic artery thrombosis remains a significant cause of graft failure and retransplantation in the early postoperative period.

The development of biliary obstruction and leaks is another cause of early postoperative deterioration,

Table 57–4. RISK FACTORS FOR HEPATIC ARTERY THROMBOSIS
Size of the hepatic artery
Type of arterial reconstruction
Number of anastomotic attempts
Use of fresh-frozen plasma
No anticoagulation
Hematocrit > 44%

although these complications typically occur more than 5 days postoperatively.[37,47-49] The SPLIT registry has revealed a biliary tract complication rate of 14%.[36] Clinically, the patient is often febrile, with right upper quadrant pain or tenderness and bilious drainage from abdominal drains. Laboratory examination reveals leukocytosis, increasing serum bilirubin and alkaline phosphatase levels, and increased bilirubin in abdominal drainage greater than serum levels in the presence of a leak. Ultrasonographic examination reveals a biliary collection in the case of a leak and biliary dilation proximal to the site of any obstruction. Cholangiography or hepatobiliary scintigraphy demonstrates leakage of contrast or radionuclide into the subhepatic space. Delayed views may be necessary to differentiate intraluminal accumulation from an intraperitoneal leak.[50] A symptomatic bile leak requires surgical exploration and repair. At the time of surgery, the hepatic artery needs to be examined for patency because hepatic artery thrombosis is a common cause of biliary tree infarction and leak.

Although rejection is a major cause of graft dysfunction postoperatively, it is not typically a problem in the first several days postoperatively. Hyperacute rejection, although seen with other organ transplants, rarely occurs after liver transplantation.[51] Postoperative immunosuppressive regimens are discussed elsewhere.

Hematological Care

Postoperative bleeding can be a major source of morbidity and mortality, especially when liver function is slow to improve after transplantation. Significant intra-abdominal bleeding requiring surgical intervention is more common after transplantation with reduced-size grafts.[37]

Initially postoperatively, the hematocrit is measured every 2 to 4 hours. The hematocrit is kept greater than 20% to provide adequate oxygen-carrying capacity and less than 30% to potentially decrease the risk of hepatic artery thrombosis. Output from the abdominal drains is quantified every hour initially, and a hematocrit is spun on the drainage if it appears sanguineous. Platelet counts are often low for the first few days after transplantation, but platelets are not transfused for platelet counts greater than 20,000/mm^3 in the absence of significant bleeding. Coagulopathy is not corrected unless the patient is bleeding significantly with a prothrombin time greater than 18 seconds. Because the use of fresh-frozen plasma has been associated with hepatic artery thrombosis,[45] coagulation parameters are not normalized in a small, bleeding infant; surgical re-exploration is undertaken early. Routine anticoagulation was previously discussed with respect to hepatic artery thrombosis.

Infectious Diseases

Infections are a significant source of morbidity and mortality in the postoperative period and are the leading cause of death in the SPLIT registry, in which they account for more than 28% of the mortality.[36,47,52-54] Within the first week after transplantation, bacteria are the most common pathogen, with the abdomen and blood stream being the most frequently infected sites.[53] A majority of these infections followed an operative or postoperative intra-abdominal complication. Forty-four percent of postoperative infections occurred within the first 2 weeks; 78% were bacterial, 19% were fungal, and 3% were viral in origin. The most prevalent bacterial pathogens in the postoperative period in pediatric patients are listed in Table 57–5. The vast majority of fungal infections are from *Candida albicans*, with the abdomen being the most common primary source.

In an effort to decrease postoperative infectious complications, a wide variety of perioperative antibiotic regimens of variable duration have been used after liver transplantation. The optimal choice of prophylactic antibiotics and duration of therapy remain unclear. In addition, the use of selective decontamination of the digestive tract is now being performed at some centers.

The use of a short course of nonabsorbable polymyxin B, tobramycin, and amphotericin B enterally and by oropharyngeal swab has been shown to decrease the incidence of aerobic gram-negative infections, as well as colonization of the pharynx and stool. There was, however, no difference in hospital or ICU length of stay or in mortality when compared with a concurrent control group.[55] Selective decontamination of the digestive tract with the use of enteral gentamicin, polymyxin B, and nystatin suspension was shown to decrease bacterial infections in the early postoperative period but did not change the rate of fungal infections or infection-related mortality.[56] The optimal surgical prophylaxis remains uncertain and should be guided by local infection patterns and antibiotic sensitivities.

Fever in the early postoperative course is highly suggestive of infection, and when leukocytosis is also present, empirical antibiotic coverage should be initiated after appropriate material for culture is obtained, including sputum, blood, urine, and peritoneal fluid. The combination of vancomycin and ceftazidime provides good coverage for the typical bacterial pathogens and is reasonable empirical coverage pending culture and sensitivity results.

Fungal infections are also a significant problem in the early postoperative period, with *C. albicans* being the most common fungus isolated.[52,57] A majority of patients with fungal infection have more than one site involved; more than 30% have more than three sites of infection.[58] Disseminated disease is the most common manifestation, with peritonitis, pneumonitis, and fungemia also relatively frequent infections. Risk factors for fungal infection include antibiotic therapy, vascular complications, intra-abdominal complications, reintubation, steroid use, and retransplantation.[52,57,58] Although a Roux-en-Y choledochojejunostomy is a risk factor for fungal infection in the adult population, children do not have a higher incidence of fungal infections than adults do.[58] The use of fluconazole prophylaxis after liver transplantation has been shown to decrease superficial and invasive fungal infections and decrease deaths from fungal infection, although no change in overall mortality was noted.[59] In view of the significant incidence of unsuspected fungal infections found at postmortem examination after liver transplantation, it is often necessary to begin antifungal therapy before fungal infection has been demonstrated. When a vascular or other type of intra-abdominal complication occurs postoperatively, prophylactic antifungal coverage is typically started because a significant proportion of this population will have an invasive fungal infection.

Although viruses do not usually cause infection in the first postoperative week, they are a significant pathogen later in the postoperative course; cytomegalovirus (CMV) is the most common viral infection noted, with an incidence rate as high as 85%.[52,60] CMV infection is a major cause of morbidity and mortality; one pediatric series reported that two thirds of all posttransplantation deaths were associated with severe CMV infection.

The incidence of CMV infection is variable and depends on the serological status of both the recipient and the donor. The patient at highest risk is a seronegative recipient who receives a graft from a seropositive donor. The lowest incidence of infection occurs when both the recipient and donor are seronegative; seropositive recipients are at intermediate risk.[61,62] Various regimens of prophylaxis have been proposed, including the use of acyclovir, ganciclovir, and

Table 57–5. MICROBIOLOGY OF PEDIATRIC POSTOPERATIVE INFECTIONS

Bacteria	%
Enterococcus species	17
Escherichia coli	14
Coagulase-negative *Staphylococcus*	14
Other aerobic gram-negative bacilli	13
Pseudomonas aeruginosa	11
Staphylococcus aureus	10
Enterobacter species	10
Anaerobes	6
Other	5

intravenous immunoglobulin, or various combinations.[52,62-64] No specific regimen has been shown to be clearly superior to others, although most prophylaxis regimens do lower the incidence and severity of CMV infection. In view of the much higher cost and no proven higher efficacy, the use of intravenous immune globulin for CMV prophylaxis is not recommended.[65] Seronegative donors receiving a seronegative graft should be given only seronegative blood products and probably do not require prophylaxis. For all other patients, a regimen of acyclovir, ganciclovir, or both is advocated.

Psychosocial Issues

Children with end-stage liver disease undergoing transplantation are faced with the stresses inherent in such an undertaking. They must be previously prepared for the ICU environment to which they will awaken postoperatively. This is ideally done shortly after deciding to list the child for transplantation and again in the immediate preoperative period. Postoperatively, having familiar toys at the bedside as well as a parent with the child is helpful in providing comfort.

The informational needs of the family must also be addressed while the patient is in the ICU. Families find the ICU phase of the transplantation the most stressful and have some difficulty assimilating information provided at this time.[66] Parents have, however, expressed a need to know primarily whether the newly transplanted liver is working, as well as the reasons for various invasive tubes, especially those related to ventilatory support.[67] Parents should be given ample opportunity to ask questions of the medical and ancillary staff, with answers provided at an appropriate level of comprehension.

Conclusion

The first several days after liver transplantation are critical to successful outcome of the procedure. A multidisciplinary approach is required, along with effective communication among all caregivers. With attentive, anticipatory care, many potential problems can be averted and new problems detected early and treated appropriately. New developments in surgical technique, anesthetic management, and postoperative care continue to improve outcomes after liver transplantation; long-term survival rates of 88%, 85%, and 85% at 1, 3, and 5 years, respectively, have been reported from a single center,[40] and the SPLIT registry has reported survival rates of 86% and 83% at 1 and 3 years, respectively. The first 48 hours is a time of many changes and, it is hoped, will begin the journey toward full recovery of these infants and children.

Pearls and Pitfalls

- Delayed awakening postoperatively suggests graft dysfunction.
- Avoid benzodiazepines.
- Analgesic requirements are less than expected.
- Extubate even though tachypneic if not in distress.
- Hypomagnesemia is common and may cause seizures.
- Allow coagulopathy if bleeding is minimal.
- Monitor abdominal drains for biliary leaks.

References

1. Atkinson PR, Ross BC, Williams S, et al: Long-term results of pediatric liver transplantation in a combined pediatric and adult transplant program. CMAJ 166:1663-1671, 2002.
2. Ganichow R, Wolkemper D, Helmke K, et al: Intensive care management after pediatric liver transplantation: A single-center experience. Pediatr Transplant 4:273-279, 2000.
3. Armandans L, Lazaro JL, Hidalgo E, et al: Predictive factors for early mortality following liver transplantation. Clin Transplant 17:401-411, 2003.
4. Hall WA, Martinez AI: Neuropathology of pediatric liver transplantation. Pediatr Neurosci 15:269, 1989.
5. Ching-Muh L: Train-of-4 quantitation of competitive neuromuscular block. Anesth Analg 54:649, 1975.
6. Tasker RC, Matther DJ, Kendall B: Computed tomography in the assessment of raised intracranial pressure in non-traumatic coma. Neuropediatrics 21:91, 1990.
7. Blei AT, Sigurdur O, Webster S, et al: Complications of intracranial pressure monitoring in fulminant hepatic failure. Lancet 341:157, 1993.
8. Jalan R: Intracranial hypertension in acute liver failure: Pathophysiological basis of rational management. Semin Liver Dis 23:271-282, 2003.
9. Muizelaar JP, Wei EP, Konlos HA, et al: Mannitol causes compensatory cerebral vasoconstriction and vasodilation in response to blood viscosity changes. J Neurosurg 59:822, 1983.
10. Muizelaar JP, Lutz HA, Becker DP: Effect of mannitol on ICP and CBF and correlation with pressure autoregulation in severely head-injured patients. J Neurosurg 61:700, 1984.
11. Murphy N, Uziner G, Benel W, et al: The effect of hypertonic sodium chloride on intracranial pressure in patients with acute liver failure. Hepatology 39:464-470, 2004.
12. Jalan R, Davies NA, Damink SW: Hypothermia for the management of intracranial hypertension in acute liver failure. Metab Brain Dis 17:327-344, 2003.
13. Moretti EW, Robertson KM, Tuttle-Newhall JE, et al: Orthotopic liver transplant patients require less postoperative morphine than do patients undergoing hepatic resection. J Clin Anesth 14:416-420, 2002.
14. Jones EA, Skilnick P, Gammal SH, et al: The γ-aminobutyric acid A (GABA$_A$) receptor complex and hepatic encephalopathy. Ann Intern Med 110:532, 1989.
15. Mullen KD, Szauter KM, Kaminsky-Russ K: "Endogenous" benzodiazepine activity in body fluids of patients with hepatic encephalopathy. Lancet 336:81, 1990.

16. Ulukaya S, Arikan C, Aydogdu S, et al: Immediate tracheal extubation of pediatric liver transplant recipients in the operating room. Pediatr Transplant 7(Suppl):381-384, 2003.

17. Aubier M, Murciano D, Lecocguic Y, et al: Effect of hypophosphatemia on diaphragmatic contractility in patients with acute respiratory failure. N Engl J Med 313:420, 1985.

18. Aubier M, Trippenbach T, Roussos C: Respiratory muscle fatigue during cardiogenic shock. J Appl Physiol 151:499, 1981.

19. Michaels MG, Green M, Wald ER, et al: Adenovirus infection in pediatric liver transplant patients. J Infect Dis 165:170, 1992.

20. Yang KL, Tobin MJ: A prospective study of indexes predicting the outcome of trials of weaning from mechanical ventilation. N Engl J Med 324:1445, 1991.

21. Shimada Y, Yoshiya I, Tanaka K, et al: Crying vital capacity and maximal inspiratory pressure as clinical indicators of readiness for weaning of infants less than a year of age. Anesthesiology 51:456, 1979.

22. Randolph AG, Wypij D, Venkataraman ST, et al: Effect of mechanical ventilator weaning protocols on respiratory outcomes in infants and children. JAMA 288:2561-2568, 2002.

23. Debaveye YA, Vanden Berghe GH: Is there still a place for dopamine in the modern intensive care unit? Anesth Analg 98:461-468, 2004.

24. Kellum JA, Decker JM: Use of dopamine in acute renal failure: A meta-analysis. Crit Care Med 29:1526-1531, 2001.

25. Lustig S, Stem N, Eggena P, et al: Effect of cyclosporine on blood pressure and renin-aldosterone axis in rats. Am J Physiol 253:H1596, 1987.

26. Lawless S, Ellis D, Thompson A, et al: Mechanisms of hypertension during and after orthotopic liver transplantation in children. J Pediatr 115:372, 1989.

27. Weidle PJ, Vlasses PH: Systemic hypertension associated with cyclosporine: A review. Drug Intell Clin Pharm 22:443-451, 1988.

28. Noble-Jamieson G, Barnes NO, Thiru S, et al: Severe hypertension after liver transplantation in α_1-antitrypsin deficiency. Arch Dis Child 65:1217, 1990.

29. Hasselgren P, Biber B, Fomander J: Improved blood flow and protein synthesis in the postischemic liver following infusion of dopamine. J Surg Res 34:44, 1983.

30. Lee MR: Dopamine and the kidney. Clin Sci 62:439, 1982.

31. van Meyel JJM, Smits P, Russel FGM, et al: Diuretic efficiency of furosemide during continuous administration versus bolus injection in healthy volunteers. Clin Pharmacol Ther 51:440, 1992.

32. Singh NC, Kisson N, Mofada SA, et al: Comparison of continuous versus intermittent furosemide administration in postoperative pediatric cardiac patients. Crit Care Med 20:17-21, 1992.

33. Reynolds HN, Borg V, Belzerg H, et al: Efficacy of continuous arteriovenous hemofiltration with dialysis in patients with renal failure. Crit Care Med 19:1387, 1991.

34. Perkin RM, Levin DL: Common fluid and electrolyte problems in the pediatric intensive care unit. Pediatr Clin North Am 27:657, 1980.

35. Plevak DJ, Southorn PA, Narr BJ, et al: Intensive-care unit experience in the Mayo liver transplantation program: The first 100 cases. Mayo Clin Proc 64:433, 1989.

36. McDiarmid SV: Current status of liver transplantation in children. Pediatr Clin North Am 50:1335-1374, 2003.

37. Bilik R, Yellen M, Superina RA: Surgical complications in children after liver transplantation. J Pediatr Surg 27:1371, 1992.

38. Reding R, Feyaerts A, de Ville de Goyet J, et al: Early graft loss after liver transplantation: Etiology, chronology, and prognosis. Transplant Proc 23:1487, 1991.

39. Roloff JS: Disseminated intravascular coagulation and other acquired bleeding disorders. In Levin DL, Morris FC (eds): Essentials of Pediatric Intensive Care. St Louis, Quality Medical Publishing, 1990.

40. Goss JA, Shackleton CR, McDiarmid SV, et al: Long-term results of pediatric liver transplantation: An analysis of 569 transplants. Ann Surg 228:411-420, 1998.

41. Inomoto T, Nishizawa F, Sasaki H, et al: Experience of 120 microsurgical reconstructions of hepatic artery in living related liver transplantation. Surgery 119:20-26, 1996.

42. Langnas AN, Marujo W, Stratta RI, et al: Hepatic allograft rescue following arterial thrombosis. Transplantation 51:86, 1991.

43. Klintmalm GB, Olson LM, Nery JR, et al: Treatment of hepatic artery thrombosis after liver transplantation with immediate vascular reconstruction: A report of three cases. Transplant Proc 20:610, 1988.

44. Stringer MO, Marshall MM, Mulesan P, et al: Survival and outcome after hepatic artery thrombosis complicating pediatric liver transplantation. J Pediatr Surg 36:888-891, 2001.

45. Mazzaferro V, Esquivel CO, Makowka L, et al: Factors responsible for hepatic artery thrombosis after pediatric liver transplantation. Transplant Proc 21:2466, 1989.

46. Buckels JAC, Tisone G, Gunson BK, et al: Low hematocrit reduces hepatic artery thrombosis after liver transplantation. Transplant Proc 21:2460, 1989.

47. Busuttil RW, Seu P, Millis JM, et al: Liver transplantation in children. Ann Surg 213:48, 1991.

48. Yandza T, Anteur F, Gauthier F, et al: Reoperative procedures following pediatric liver transplantation. Transplant Proc 24:1963, 1992.

49. Letourneau JG, Casteneda-Zuniga WR: The role of radiology in the diagnosis and treatment of biliary complications after liver transplantation. Cardiovasc Intervent Radiol 113:278, 1990.

50. Letourneau JG, Hunter DW, Payne WO, et al: Imaging of and intervention for biliary complications after hepatic transplantation. AJR Am J Roentgenol 154:729, 1990.

51. Starzl TE, Ishikawa CW, Putoam KA, et al: Progress in and deterrents to orthotopic liver transplantation, with special reference to survival, resistance to hyperacute rejection, and biliary duct reconstruction. Transplant Proc 6:129, 1974.

52. George OL, Arnow PM, Fox A, et al: Patterns of infection after pediatric liver transplantation. Am J Dis Child 146: 924, 1992.

53. Andrews WS, Wanek E, Fyock B, et al: Pediatric liver transplantation: A 3-year experience. J Pediatr Surg 24:77, 1989.

54. Saint-Vil D, Luks FI, Lebel P, et al: Infectious complications of pediatric liver transplantation. J Pediatr Surg 26:908, 1991.

55. Smith SO, Jackson RJ, Hannakan CJ, et al: Selective decontamination in pediatric liver transplants. Transplantation 55:1306, 1993.

56. Emre S, Sebastian A, Chodoff L, et al: Selective decontamination of the digestive tract helps prevent bacterial infections in the early postoperative period after liver transplant. Mt Sinai J Med 66:310-313, 1999.

57. Castaldo P, Stratta RJ, Wood RP, et al: Fungal disease in liver transplant recipients: A multivariate analysis of risk factors. Transplant Proc 23(1Pt 2):1517, 1991.

58. Castaldo R, Stratta RJ, Wood P, et al: Clinical spectrum of fungal infections after orthotopic liver transplantation. Arch Surg 126:149, 1991.

59. Winston DJ, Pakrasi A, Busuttil RW: Prophylactic fluconazole in liver transplant recipients—a randomized, double-blind, placebo controlled trial. Ann Intern Med 131:729-737, 1999.

60. Barkholt LM, Ericzon BO, Ehrnst A, et al: Cytomegalovirus infections in liver transplant patients: Incidence and outcome. Transplant Proc 22:235, 1990.

61. Dussaix E, Wood C: Cytomegalovirus infection in pediatric liver recipients. Transplantation 48:272, 1989.

62. King SM, Petric M, Superina R, et al: Cytomegalovirus infections in pediatric liver transplantation. Am J Dis Child 144:1307, 1990.

63. Ruskin JO, Wood RP, Bailey MR, et al: Comparative trial of oral clotrimazole and nystatin for oropharyngeal candidiasis prophylaxis in orthotopic liver transplant patients. Oral Surg Oral Med Oral Pathol 74:567-571, 1992.

64. Arnow PM, Furmaga K, Flaherty JP, et al: Microbiological efficacy and pharmacokinetics of prophylactic antibiotics in liver transplant patients. Antimicrob Agents Chemother 36:2125, 1992.

65. Pan SH, Rosenthal P, Howard TK, et al: Evaluation of three cytomegalovirus infection prophylactic regimens in liver transplant recipients. Transplant Proc 24:1466, 1992.

66. Weichler NK: Assessment of the information needs of mothers of children after liver transplantation. Transplant Proc 20:598, 1988.

67. Weichler N, Hakos L: Information needs of primary care givers in pediatric liver transplantation. Transplant Proc 21:3562, 1989.

58

Postoperative Management Beyond the Intensive Care Unit: Adults

EDMUND Q. SANCHEZ
GORAN B. KLINTMALM

Inpatient convalescence 866
  Monitoring graft function 866

Common posttransplant clinical problems 873
  Hypertension 873
  Renal dysfunction 873
  Glucose intolerance 874
  Headaches 874
  Diarrhea 875
  Patient rehabilitation 875

Outpatient care 876
  Immunizations 877
  Antibiotic prophylaxis for procedures 877
  Pregnancy 877

The recent era of liver transplantation before and including inception of the Model of End-Stage Liver Disease (MELD) in the United States has been one of increased clinical complexity in liver transplant recipients. Frequently, patients in this era and in the future will have coexisting conditions that may or may not improve after successful liver transplantation. For example, patients with pure hepatorenal syndrome frequently have improved renal function after liver transplantation. These patients will be able to be weaned from renal replacement therapies. Alternatively, patients with intrinsic renal insufficiency (glomerulonephritis, diabetic nephropathy, hypertensive nephropathy) will not improve with liver transplantation and may even worsen after it. In addition, patients in hepatic coma may have improved levels of consciousness after successful transplantation performed in timely fashion. Successful liver transplantation is dependent on engraftment in the recipient, which by and large becomes evident within 48 to 72 hours postoperatively. A prothrombin time (PT) of less than 20 seconds and aspartate transaminase (AST) and alanine transaminase (ALT) levels that have peaked at less than 2000 IU/L and are decreasing are hallmarks of that process. If these improvements are not seen, primary nonfunction must be a strong consideration, and the decision to relist that patient must be made quickly.

Usually, uncomplicated patients are ready to be transferred out of the intensive care unit on the first or second posttransplant day. For others, it will obviously take somewhat longer. Some complicating events after transplantation, such as primary nonfunction, need for reoperation/retransplantation, respiratory failure, renal failure, infection, and others, have a serious impact on mortality and morbidity, not to mention the degree of medical care required. Although patients confined to the intensive care unit before transplantation are frequently able to be transferred to the general hospital transplant unit before the end of the first week after transplantation,[1] patients' progress from intensive care to the general hospital unit and, ultimately, to discharge from the hospital follows a variable timeline. Care of liver transplant recipients should be multidisciplinary in nature to maximize success. The key points in post–liver transplant management (both inpatient and outpatient) are highlighted in this chapter.

Inpatient Convalescence

Monitoring Graft Function

Laboratory Monitoring

The two principal hepatic functions that can be closely monitored in the immediate postoperative period are hepatocellular activity and secretory function. A third (equally important) role of the liver, that of the reticuloendothelial system, is not ignored but is much more difficult to assess by common clinical measures. Much of the surveillance of proper engraftment, then, is aimed at discerning the adequacy of hepatocyte function, biliary flow, and vascular inflow. Directed studies are used on a routine basis within the first 1 to 2 weeks after transplantation to proactively detect potential problems. The key in liver transplantation is to address a problem before it becomes apparent clinically. Frequently, major problems are heralded by minor changes in serum laboratory values and can be avoided if acted on in an aggressive fashion.

Normalization of hepatic physiology is most practically assessed by daily performance of liver function tests (total and direct bilirubin, AST, ALT, alkaline phosphatase, γ-glutamyl transpeptidase). A normalizing PT is a particularly sensitive index of successful engraftment. Ammonia levels may occasionally be helpful, but such assessment is seldom required on a daily basis. Normalization of serum ammonia is extremely rapid, even in the presence of moderate preservation injury. Likewise, the serum albumin content is a good index of synthetic function, but in the immediate posttransplant period, this value is too influenced by fluid shifts and existing exudative states to be of any predictive value in determining graft function.

Transaminases (AST, ALT) have normally peaked by the first 24 to 48 hours after transplantation and reach values two to four times normal, on average, by the end of the first posttransplant week. Secondary, less pronounced rises in AST and ALT in the first few posttransplant days are almost always a manifestation of preservation injury in the allograft or early acute cellular rejection.[2]

Alkaline phosphatase and γ-glutamyl transpeptidase levels are laboratory values critical to assessment of proper bile flow, especially at the canalicular level. These levels bear little relevance to immediate graft function and are usually normal or near normal in the immediate posttransplant period, even in patients with severe preservation injury. The usual pattern of these serum enzymes consists of an increase near the end of the first week. Such elevations may be modest or severe and, together with a rising bilirubin level, are indicative of early acute cellular rejection or acute arterial insufficiency. An increase in alkaline phosphatase and γ-glutamyl transpeptidase with no increase or even a decrease in total bilirubin is a pattern typical of preservation injury (i.e., shock liver). Although the clinical course (presence or absence of fever, tachycardia, elevated AST and ALT) may suggest a diagnosis, arterial insufficiency is evaluated with the use of Doppler (and if needed, arteriography), and the "gold standard" of differentiation between acute rejection and preservation injury is core liver biopsy.[3] Some liver transplant centers have chosen to include core liver biopsy 1 week after transplantation as a routine part of their treatment protocol, regardless of biochemical function at the time. However, liver biopsies performed too early after liver transplantation often reflect changes related to preservation injury and are therefore not advised. The findings of severe preservation injury obscure the presence of early developing acute cellular rejection and do not add to the diagnostic value of liver biopsy. Timing of liver biopsy is critical, especially within the first 5 to 10 days after liver transplantation.

Other laboratory values guide therapy during the first weeks after transplantation. Hematological indexes (white cell count, differential, hemoglobin, hematocrit, platelet count) reveal valuable clues to problems such as bone marrow suppression, ongoing or new hemorrhage, or infection. Persistent hypersplenism, ongoing platelet adherence to the liver's vascular endothelium, drug side effects, and allograft rejection may be important factors in reducing platelet numbers. One should also keep in mind the possibility of graft-versus-host disease (GVHD) as a cause of bone marrow suppression early in the posttransplant course (true GVHD is rarely seen earlier than 3 weeks after transplantation; the usual time is closer to 6 weeks after transplantation). Electrolyte profiling, including assessment of serum sodium, potassium, bicarbonate, and chloride, is

Table 58-1. COMMONLY OBTAINED DAILY LABORATORY STUDIES IN THE EARLY POSTTRANSPLANTATION PERIOD

Electrolyte	Hepatic
Sodium	Bilirubin
Potassium	AST
Chloride	ALT
Bicarbonate	Alkaline phosphatase
	γ-Glutamyl transpeptidase
	Albumin (as needed)
	Ammonia (as needed)
	Prothrombin time (after normalization, may check as needed)
Metabolic	**Hematological**
Calcium	White blood count and differential
Magnesium	Hemoglobin
Phosphorus	Hematocrit
Uric acid	Platelet count
Glucose	
Cholesterol/lipid panel*	
Renal	
Blood urea nitrogen	
Creatinine	
Immunosuppression	
FK506 level	
Cyclosporine level	
Rapamycin level (twice weekly)	
Mycophenolate levels[†]	

*While taking rapamycin.
[†]As indicated.
ALT, alanine transaminase; AST, aspartate transaminase,

necessary to prevent or correct abnormal concentrations of these ions. Likewise, hyperuricemia, hypomagnesemia, and hypophosphatemia are commonly seen in these patients and mandate frequent monitoring. Serum glucose levels are determined daily and perhaps several times each day in some cases. Table 58–1 presents commonly obtained laboratory values during inpatient convalescence of liver transplant recipients.

Although laboratory studies are often part of the routine postsurgical care for most major intra-abdominal procedures, liver transplant recipients are subject to specific tests that directly assess the surgical anastomoses. Doppler-augmented ultrasound examination, available at the bedside if necessary, provides accurate (91% sensitivity and 99.1% specificity[4]), reproducible visual and flow images throughout all major vessels of the liver and can assess the patency of the major intrahepatic and extrahepatic vessels.[5,6] This examination, when performed in the early postoperative period (i.e., posttransplant day 1), can detect technical anastomotic problems when they are most easily corrected. The flow characteristics of the hepatic artery can give insight into allograft function. An edematous liver, whether from high central venous pressure or severe preservation injury, will not usually allow much (if any) forward diastolic flow in the hepatic artery. A system with very high resistance may even lead to flow reversal in diastole. In this case, resistive indices of 0.9 to 1.00 are often demonstrated immediately postoperatively. Two important factors can lead to high resistive indices: (1) older liver donors and (2) extended preservation times. However, these factors do not have an impact on long-term graft or patient survival in the absence of a true arterial abnormality.[7] In our practice, we treat absent or reversed diastolic flow with the rheological agent dextran 40 (Rheomacrodex), 10 to 25 mL/hr intravenously, depending on renal function, until such time as daily serial ultrasound examinations show normal diastolic flow.[8] It should be kept in mind, when reviewing the Doppler waveform, that increases in systolic acceleration time (>0.08), abnormalities in systolic peak morphology, and abnormal resistive indices often signify arterial compromise.[4] Performance of hepatic arteriography must be based on clinical suspicion if an ultrasonographic abnormality such as pulsus parvus et tardus, high-velocity jets, or nonvisualization of the hepatic artery is present.

Additionally, arterial reconstructions or the use of aortic conduits to revascularize the donor liver necessitates the use of dextran 40 immediately after transplantation, followed by lifelong administration of an antiplatelet agent (aspirin, clopidogrel [Plavix], etc.) to maximize prevention of arterial thrombosis. The presence of multiple arterial anastomoses was found to be a significant risk factor for hepatic artery thrombosis in a large series of 683 adult liver transplants.[9] We recently (in our practice) instituted the use of aspirin or clopidogrel as a preventive measure in all of our liver transplant recipients regardless of arterial anatomy. Moreover, the use of sirolimus has increased in our practice in patients with arterial abnormalities because of its antiproliferative properties.[10] The resistive indices of aortic conduits are frequently between 0.5 and 0.6, values somewhat lower than in those without a conduit.

Hepatic artery thrombosis after adult liver transplantation, now a rare complication, has significant consequences.[11] Therefore, Doppler ultrasound is a critical component of the transplant physician's arsenal of screening and diagnostic tools. Liberal use of this examination is encouraged in patients demonstrating laboratory abnormalities early or late after transplantation. Diminishing resistive indices in long-term liver transplant patients also deserve special attention (arteriography) to rule out impending hepatic artery thrombosis.

Patient: _____   Transplant: _____   Recipient Diagnosis: _____   Donor Blood Group: _____ / Age: _____

Date of Transplant: _____   Chart Number: _____   Blood Group: _____ Crossmatch + / −   HLA: _____

HLA/PRA: _____   Ischemia Time: _____ Donor Viral: CMV + / − / ND

Transplant Procedure: ☐ LTX ☐ L/K ☐ KTX ☐ K/P ☐ PAK ☐ ISLETS ☐ _____   Birthdate: _____ Pre-TX Glofil: _____   Liver Size: Whole / L. Lobe / L. L.S. / LRD

Status 1 _____ / MELD / PELD _____   Allergies: _____

Location: ☐ ICU ☐ Hosp ☐ Home

YEAR		☐ BUMC ☐ BAS ☐ CMC		IMMUNOSUPPRESSION		MEDICATION	PHYSIOLOGY				
DATE	PROCEDURES / COMMENTS		I.S. LEVEL	MAIN. PRED	REJECT RX		OUTPUT 24 HR. URINE	HT. cm.	WT. Kg.	BLOOD PRESSURE MAX	TEMP. MAX

FIGURE 58–1

Wall chart for tracking posttransplantation data.

(*Continued*)

In addition, any residual intra-abdominal hematoma or intrahepatic mass can be detected with ultrasound. However, any large intra-abdominal collection that is seen on ultrasound (that is not ascites) may be followed by a hepatoiminodiacetic acid (HIDA) scan to exclude a bile leak or a computed tomographic scan to rule out an abscess, as clinically indicated.

When either choledochocholedochostomy or choledochojejunostomy is used for biliary reconstruction, an indwelling biliary catheter provides an easy, convenient way to assess anastomotic integrity. Near the end of the first posttransplant week, a tube cholangiogram confirms anastomotic patency, absence of extravasation, and prompt flow into the intestine. This early evaluation allows tube clamping with a clear conscience or, conversely, prompts further diagnostic or therapeutic maneuvers to address difficulties. T-tube clamping is especially important for proper absorption in cyclosporine-treated patients, most of whom are receiving their drug enterally.[12] The use of T tubes has, however, become much less frequent in recent years.[13] Nevertheless, they minimize leaks associated with ampullary dysfunction.[14] T-tube–free anastomoses do not adversely affect anastomotic integrity and eliminate the bile leaks that may result from T-tube removal.[15] The diagnosis of biliary tract abnormalities is best made with either percutaneous transhepatic cholangiography (PTC) or endoscopic retrograde cholangiopancreatography (ERCP). Doppler ultrasonography is rarely a useful test to diagnose biliary strictures/leaks immediately after transplantation. PTC is associated with a minimal incidence of pancreatitis when compared with ERCP (up to 30%)[16] and is the diagnostic test of choice in patients who have a Roux-en-Y choledochojejunostomy as their biliary reconstruction. In patients without a Roux-en-Y reconstruction and in whom the biliary tree cannot be accessed by percutaneous methods, ERCP is used.

Nonanastomotic strictures deserve special mention here as well. They may occur early or late in the posttransplant course. Some causes include ischemia–reperfusion injury, bacterial cholangitis, acute cellular rejection, viral infection (cytomegalovirus [CMV] in particular),[17] small-for-size graft, hepatotoxic medications,

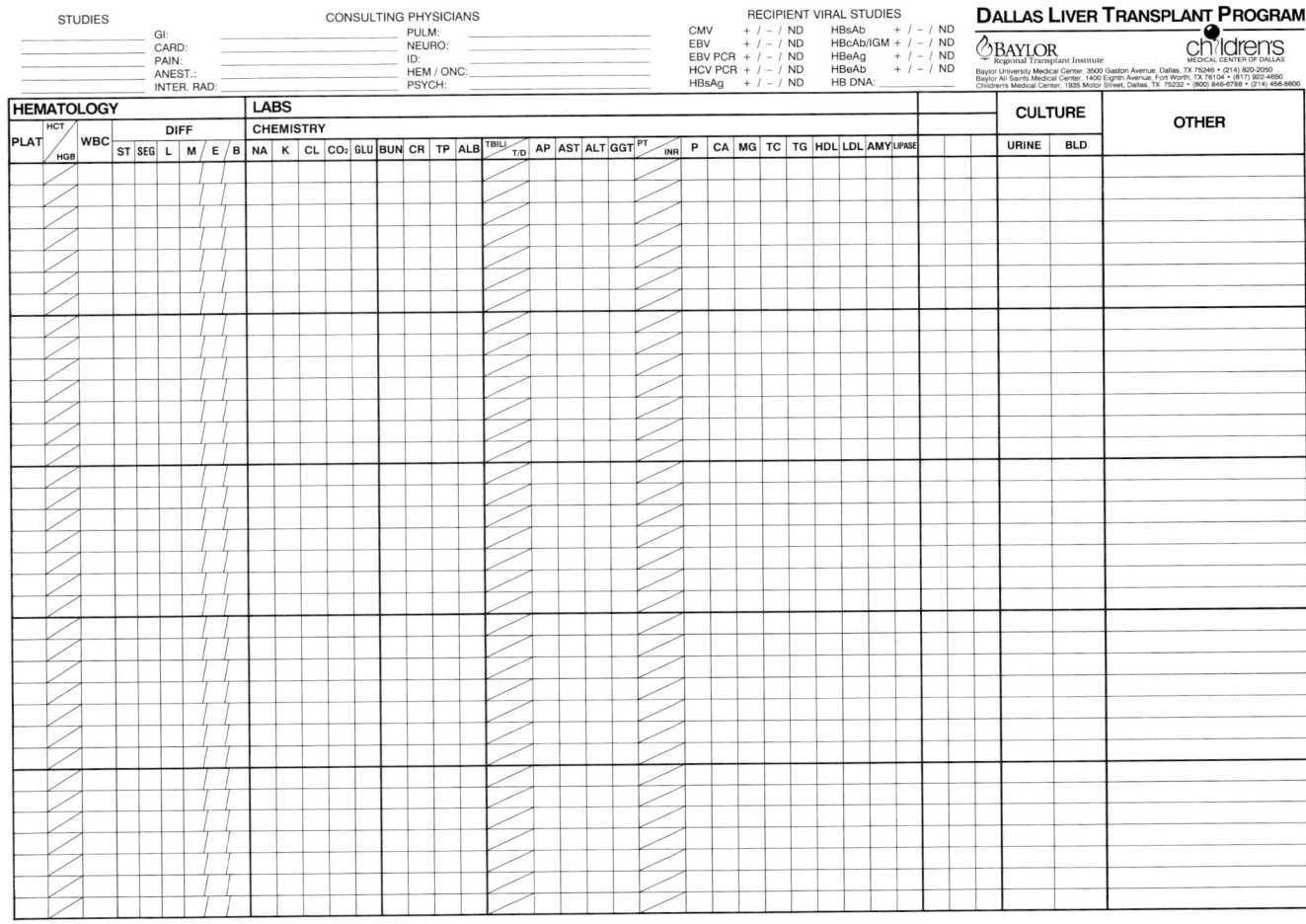

FIGURE 58–1, cont'd

hepatic artery thrombosis, and ABO incompatibility (more so in the long term).[18,19] The diagnosis of nonanastomotic biliary strictures is made also by ERCP or PTC.

Clinical Documentation—The Wall Chart

A very concise, practical way of tracking posttransplantation data is the bedside flow sheet, which when updated daily, allows centralization of what is often a voluminous amount of information (Fig. 58–1). Moreover, modern information systems technology has invaded the bedside. Electronic versions of posttransplant clinical databases offer a means of record keeping on laptop computers linked to servers (and data backup/redundancy) by wireless radiofrequency transmission. However, these systems do not allow an overview of all data on a patient over a certain period in one glance as a wall chart does.

A wall chart will have all the tests and results of the transplanted individual documented on it. These wall charts are standardized per institution and typically contain daily laboratory results, microbiological culture results, pathology findings, and radiographic results, as well as documentation of key events in the patient's course (e.g., reoperations, liver biopsies, changes in immunosuppression regimens). Wall charts allow rapid tracking of the multitude of study results performed, in addition to allowing all individuals participating in the patient's care to visualize and devise medical care plans without much confusion.

Once a transplant patient is discharged from the hospital and, subsequently, the transplant center's care, the information obtained from primary care physicians is documented on the wall chart as well. The data collected are vital to the transplant center to allow continuous reevaluation of protocols and maintenance of other various database functions (research, patient tracking, demographic evaluation, etc.). Continuous updating of wall charts is of utmost importance.

Allograft Dysfunction

When biochemical measures of liver function worsen or fail to improve during the early posttransplant

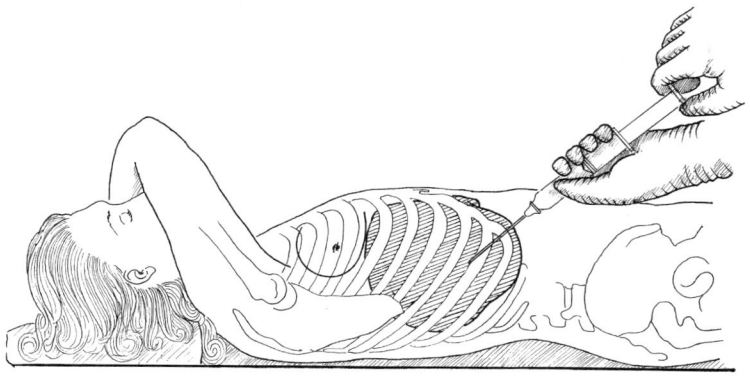

FIGURE 58–2

Liver biopsy. The lower third of the hepatic span is identified by percussion. The biopsy needle is inserted along the midaxillary line, on top of the rib. (From Molmenti EP, Klintmalm GB: Atlas of Liver Transplantation. Philadelphia, WB Saunders, 2002, p 143.)

period, a systematic approach to the diagnosis of allograft dysfunction is best. The single most useful test is core liver biopsy, which usually reveals the presence of acute cellular rejection or preservation injury. Preservation injury in the first week is primarily manifested by the presence of polymorphonuclear leukocytes around the bile ductules (mimicking cholangitis). Secondary and later changes associated with preservation injury can include centrilobular degeneration or hepatocyte loss and bile plugs or inspissated bile within the hepatic parenchyma.

Liver Biopsy

Liver biopsy after liver transplantation can be performed at the patient's bedside with great success. Immediate posttransplant requirements for bedside liver biopsy include adequate platelet counts (>30,000/mm^3) and near-normal PT (<18 seconds) or INR (<1.8). If platelet counts are low or coagulation times are elevated (as seen in liver dysfunction), platelets or fresh-frozen plasma (or both) must be transfused to minimize bleeding complications. In healed, established liver transplants, we do not require platelet counts or PT/INR for a liver biopsy. We have not found them useful because the liver is well scarred in and the risk for abdominal bleeding from the biopsy puncture is minimal (unless patients are taking anticoagulants) in established liver transplants. Rarely, bedside biopsy is not successful, and therefore ultrasound-guided liver biopsy may be used in these instances.

The technique for bedside liver biopsy is quite simple. Patients are placed supine with their right hand behind their head to widen the intercostal spaces. Percussion determines the liver span. The puncture is made in the middle of the liver span (usually between the fifth and seventh intercostal spaces) to be safely below the pleural cavity. The biopsy needle is inserted along the upper edge of the rib, almost scraping it, to avoid injury to the intercostal artery, vein, or nerve (located at the lower edge of the rib). A single deliberate

pass of the needle in a dorsocranial direction is generally required to obtain liver parenchyma (Fig. 58–2).

The protocol that we follow after liver biopsy includes positioning the patient on the right side for 1 hour. Vital signs are monitored every 15 minutes. Hypotension, tachycardia, and severe abdominal pain may develop, in which case bleeding (subcapsular, intraparenchymal, or rarely intra-abdominal) may be present. Liver transplants progressively get scarred in as length of time from transplantation increases, and therefore the likelihood of free intra-abdominal bleeding is low.

The most dangerous bleeding is that occurring into the pleural cavity. An acute onset of dyspnea may herald pneumothorax or possibly hemothorax. Injury to the intercostal or diaphragmatic vessels is responsible for significant bleeding. The workup needed in each of these cases (regardless of clinical stability) includes an emergency determination of the patient's hematocrit (or hemoglobin) and a chest radiograph. The presence of a small pleural effusion (e.g., a developing hemothorax) or a drop in the patient's hematocrit/hemoglobin, or both, should be acted on in an emergency fashion. The patient must have good intravenous access for resuscitation if hemodynamic instability does occur because more than 500 mL of blood can rapidly be discharged into the pleural cavity. Frequently, these symptoms are minor and self-limited; however, hemorrhage after liver biopsy may be significant and should not be overlooked. Bleeding after liver biopsy is possibly a life-threatening complication of this procedure and must be treated urgently and aggressively. Treatments include blood transfusions, placement of a thoracostomy tube, and possibly surgical intervention.

Other complications after liver biopsy include subcutaneous hematoma, bile leak, a hepatic artery–to–portal vein fistula, bowel perforation, renal injury, and rarely death.

A liver biopsy may also reveal zones of ischemia, which is usually suggestive of hepatic artery stenosis or thrombosis. Centrilobular congestion can signal venous outflow stenosis and mandates evaluation of the suprahepatic vena cava anastomosis by either ultrasonography or direct intraluminal pressure measurements (performed radiographically). Centrilobular ischemia, when not associated with vascular insufficiency, may reflect drug toxicity. Administration of hepatotoxic agents such as trimethoprim-sulfamethoxazole and other antibiotics, furosemide, and azathioprine should then be discontinued. Individual medications with known drug toxicity must be systematically discontinued if drug toxicity is high on the differential diagnosis.

Bile duct proliferation is histologically indicative of biliary obstruction, although it is not likely to be noted in the immediate posttransplant period. Its finding should be followed by cholangiography, either with the indwelling T tube or via ERCP or PTC.

Marked, rapid rises in serum transaminase levels in the first few posttransplant days are sometimes seen. The differential diagnosis includes acute vascular insufficiency (hepatic artery thrombosis or, less likely, portal vein thrombosis) as a result of a technical complication. Another cause of a rapid increase in transaminases can be hemolysis, which even in the presence of an ABO-identical or ABO-compatible allograft is believed to be antibody mediated. Some centers such as ours may proceed with multiple sessions of plasmapheresis in the acute posttransplant period when cell lysis is documented in the recipient.

Immunosuppression

The need to suppress allograft rejection in transplant recipients of all organs separates them from other postsurgical patients, even those who may have had technically very complex procedures. Hence, a key feature of postoperative management of a liver transplant patient is the regulation of immunosuppressant drugs. In general, whether the primary agent is cyclosporine or tacrolimus, daily determination of drug levels is indispensable for proper patient management. Currently, tacrolimus dosing is based on 12-hour trough levels; cyclosporine can be dosed according to 12-hour levels, but C2 monitoring[20,21] has been shown to be quite effective in the management of cyclosporine. Additionally, the use of sirolimus has increased in liver transplantation. The half-life of sirolimus is quite long (57 to 62 hours), so once-daily dosing is sufficient and determination of daily trough levels is not effective in the management of this drug. Our center monitors sirolimus levels twice weekly until the level is within the acceptable range (5 to 10 ng/mL). Recently, the use of everolimus (RAD 001) has been authorized, mainly in cardiac transplantation, but its use in liver transplantation has yet to become widespread. Unlike sirolimus, it has a shorter half-life of 16 to 19 hours.

Additionally, area under the curve (AUC) determination of mycophenolate mofetil (MMF), as well as mycophenolic acid levels, has been shown to be clinically useful. An enteric-coated form of mycophenolic acid (the active metabolite in mycophenolate mofetil) is now available, and its use is associated with fewer side effects and thus less need to make dose changes.

The use of specific immunosuppressive agents and strategies is reviewed in detail in Chapter 72, "Rejection after Transplantation." All contemporary regimens are based on cyclosporine or tacrolimus and include varying doses of steroid. Antilymphocyte preparations, whether polyclonal or monoclonal, are generally reserved for steroid-resistant rejection; nonetheless, some transplant centers do induce immunosuppression with antilymphocyte preparations. With their use, adequate immunosuppression is observed along with nearly complete obliteration of the lymphocyte count in the differential obtained daily during the course of antilymphocyte therapy. However, if the patient's course is not responding to treatment or if the lymphocyte differential is not adequately suppressed, further confirmation of lymphocyte suppression may be confirmed by CD3 counts. Mycophenolate mofetil, sirolimus, and azathioprine, among other various agents, are also commonly used, although with great center-specific variation.

Infections

Infections of all types are perhaps the single most important threat to the life or well-being of a liver transplant recipient. Their true incidence and impact on mortality are difficult to assess for several reasons. Positive cultures, a prerequisite to the accurate diagnosis of infection, do not help distinguish uninfected but colonized patients. The classic clinical signs (fever, tachycardia, leukocytosis, increased number of immature neutrophils) may be only partially apparent or not at all present in immunosuppressed patients. Bacterial peritonitis, for example, may be far advanced despite a soft, nontender abdomen. Furthermore, although infection may be the most apparent cause of death in a given clinical setting, the true cause of a patient's death (e.g., bile leak, hepatic artery thrombosis, primary nonfunction of the allograft, persistent acute rejection, and chronic rejection to name a few) often temporally precedes the infection. Rare is a hospitalized patient who succumbs to a prolonged chronic illness such as liver failure (before or after transplantation) uninfected.

Successful management of infection begins with prophylaxis. Intravenous antibiotics are commonly administered before the operation. Although a multitude of antibacterial agents are likely to be quite efficacious, coverage should be provided for skin organisms (*Staphylococcus aureus, Staphylococcus epidermidis*), as well as for enteric organisms likely to be encountered on division of the small intestine or the common bile duct. Many transplant centers now provide prophylaxis against candidal perioperative infection through oral agents (i.e., fluconazole or itraconazole),[22] systemic amphotericin, or peritoneal irrigation with amphotericin at the time of abdominal closure.[23] Evidence substantiates colonization of a liver transplant candidate's gut when *Candida* is present.[24] Our preference is for low-dose amphotericin B intravenously (10 mg/day) for 10 perioperative days in all patients whose gut flora has been altered by lactulose, neomycin, or hospitalization. We do not use selective gut decontamination because its efficacy remains unproven, although its expense is well documented.[25] Finally, antifungal prophylaxis and treatment have significantly diminished the incidence of post–liver transplant fungal infection and should be used as part of the posttransplant protocol. The routine use of antifungal agents, as well as other factors involved in liver transplantation (decreased blood transfusion, cold ischemia time, length of operation, rate of retransplantation), has played a role in the reduction in invasive fungal infections seen over the past few years.[26]

Prudent clinical management of a liver transplant recipient includes a low threshold for the use of empirical antibiotic therapy. Fever, leukocytosis, and suspected infection (pulmonary, urinary, or wound) should probably prompt serious consideration of broad-spectrum antibiotic coverage (gram-positive cocci and gram-negative rods), especially after appropriate material for culture has been procured. Antibiotic therapy is, of course, tailored to the offending organisms on the basis of antimicrobial susceptibility results. Opportunistic infections should also be considered, although current prophylactic regimens are quite effective. Infection with antibiotic-resistant microorganisms is being seen with increased frequency as well, thus making antibiotic selection very important. Individual hospital data are extremely important in managing the use of antibiotics in transplant patients.

Antiviral therapy is also central to proper infection control in liver transplantation. In recent years, a variety of prophylactic regimens against CMV have been studied. Centers vary broadly in approach, with some advocating prophylaxis of the increasing[27] numbers of high-risk patients (CMV-negative recipient of a CMV-positive donor, patients hospitalized before transplantation) and others recommending universal prophylaxis. Likewise, several agents, alone or in combination, have been proposed and have shown efficacy, including intravenous ganciclovir,[28] oral ganciclovir or valganciclovir, oral or intravenous acyclovir (in high or low dose), and CMV hyperimmune globulin (Cytogam) (pooled sera with a high anti-CMV antibody titer). Our preference, for reasons of efficacy, low cost, minimal toxicity, and ease of administration, is intravenous ganciclovir. In all patients, ganciclovir is administered at a dose of 5 mg/kg/day immediately after transplantation (or with the onset of rejection) and continued for 14 days or until hospital discharge. The dose is reduced to 2.5 mg/kg/day when the patient's serum creatinine level is greater than 2.0 mg/dL. Initially, our protocol called for oral acyclovir for 14 days at a dose of 400 mg four times daily after the ganciclovir therapy. Currently, after discharge from the hospital, no antiviral prevention is given. Because of the lack of significant benefit with acyclovir, its use was discontinued. Additional evidence now demonstrates oral ganciclovir to be superior to acyclovir.[29] Clinical evidence of CMV infection (biopsy proven, CMV detected by polymerase chain reaction) warrants treatment with intravenous ganciclovir (for 2 to 4 weeks) with conversion to oral valganciclovir for completion of therapy.

CMV infection in liver transplant recipients, once an important cause of mortality, has now essentially become a concern regarding morbidity. Despite occasional reports of CMV hepatitis as a potential trigger of chronic rejection, this entity and its cousin CMV pneumonitis now respond extraordinarily well to ganciclovir therapy. In large series, the presence of CMV infection, although adding to hospital cost and length of stay, has no impact on mortality statistics.[30]

Nutrition

Frequently, patients with end-stage liver disease awaiting transplantation suffer the ravages of nutritional failure. Unable to synthesize protein and with insufficient calorie intake, a pretransplant patient is often cachectic and weak, with minimal muscle mass. Other nutrition-related complications of end-stage liver disease include osteopenia, altered glucose metabolism, and nutrient malabsorption. Osteopenia occurs most frequently in patients with alcoholic liver disease, cholestatic liver disease, or conditions such as autoimmune hepatitis when corticosteroids have been prescribed. Altered glucose metabolism can be manifested as diabetes mellitus or fasting hypoglycemia as a result of the reduced gluconeogenic capability of the diseased liver. Nutrient loss occurs via steatorrhea (primarily in patients with cholestatic liver disease) and protein loss via paracentesis. Pretransplant nutritional depletion places posttransplant patients at higher risk for prolonged ventilatory support, increased intensive care and hospital length of stay, and tracheostomy and may also increase mortality.[31-34]

In the surgical literature, emphasis is being placed on proper nutrition as an important therapeutic strategy in both the critically and chronically ill populations. Moreover, the lower morbidity and lower cost of enteral nutrition are shifting the focus away from parenteral nutrition toward tube feeding whenever possible. Studies have shown that early posttransplant enteral nutrition via a nasoduodenal tube is cost-effective, efficient, and well tolerated.[35,36] Tube feeding can supplement or replace oral or parenteral nutrition support and may contribute to a decrease in early viral infections in liver recipients.[36] At least one study has shown that the addition of probiotics to tube feeding reduces infection rates more than tube feeding alone does.[37] Ongoing studies are assessing the impact of pretransplantation nutritional supplementation on the posttransplant outcome of the recipient. A more detailed discussion of nutritional considerations can be found in Chapter 35, "Donor Selection and Management."

Common Posttransplant Clinical Problems

Hypertension

Both cyclosporine and tacrolimus induce systemic arterial hypertension as a side effect (Table 58–2).[38] Whereas the mechanism of cyclosporine-induced hypertension may well be linked to higher sympathetic tone or acquired renal insufficiency, that of tacrolimus remains obscure.[39] Because both drugs increase calcineurin intracellular activity to a similar extent (although through two very different drug receptors), their toxicity profiles may be linked. Indeed, clinical experience reveals the remarkably similar toxic side effects of these agents.[36]

Liver transplant recipients, of course, may also experience hypertension from the mineralocorticoid effect of their steroid immunosuppressants, from genetic predisposition, or as a result of obesity. Their medication-induced risk only adds to that found in the general population.

Strategies for treating posttransplant hypertension vary. We treat all patients in an aggressive fashion if their blood pressure exceeds 160/100 mm Hg. However, in patients who require chronic therapy, we aim to keep their blood pressure less than 140/90 mm Hg. The first line of therapy is to ensure the appropriateness of a patient's tacrolimus or cyclosporine dose by means of sampled trough blood levels.[38] Systolic or diastolic hypertension in the absence of toxic immunosuppressant levels warrants pharmacological therapy. Our preference is for agents that do not interfere with cyclosporine or tacrolimus metabolism and the cytochrome P450 pathway. One drug that interferes with this pathway is diltiazem. It inhibits CYP3A, P-glycoprotein, and tacrolimus metabolism in a predictable fashion.[40] Patients who respond to sublingual nifedipine (Procardia) are good candidates for the sustained-release Procardia XL, which is administered only once or twice a day. When a second agent is required, we generally add a selective β-receptor antagonist such as atenolol. More recently, we have also begun using transdermal preparations of the α-receptor agonist clonidine (Catapres-TTS), which are dose metered and quite convenient from a patient compliance standpoint. Amlodipine besylate (Norvasc) is another commonly used medication that is quite effective; however, its use must be adjusted according to liver function.

Control of hypertension is of utmost importance in liver transplant recipients, especially long-term control. In a study of 181 liver transplant recipients,[41] a significant increase in risk factors for cardiovascular disease (myocardial infarction and stroke) was found when compared with the general population. Hypertension was seen in 77% of these patients, and the risk for coronary heart disease was calculated to be 11.5% 1 year after transplantation versus 7% in the general population. By minimizing the contributory risk factors for cardiovascular disease, long-term patient survival can be optimized.

Renal Dysfunction

Profound depression of the glomerular filtration rate (GFR) is often noted in liver transplant recipients once cyclosporine or tacrolimus treatment is begun (see Table 58–2). Neither drug seems less (or more) nephrotoxic than the other.[42] As measured by iodothalamate clearance, the GFR reaches a minimum several weeks to months after transplantation and then recovers somewhat. Usually, a plateau in GFR is reached by the end of the first posttransplant year; its value is approximately two thirds of the pretransplant GFR.[43] This side effect is, in the case of cyclosporine, also believed to be mediated by increased sympathetic tone.[44] Hyperkalemia and hyperuricemia are two common metabolic consequences seen in these patients.

Therapeutic intervention for renal insufficiency begins with exclusion of tacrolimus or cyclosporine toxicity. Evaluation of the patient should also center on intravascular volume status, pump status (adequacy of

Table 58–2. COMMON CLINICAL PROBLEMS AFTER LIVER TRANSPLANTATION
Hypertension
Renal dysfunction
Glucose intolerance
Headaches
Diarrhea
Physical debility

cardiac output), and the use of other nephrotoxic agents (e.g., aminoglycosides). In a patient who is truly believed to be toxic from cyclosporine or tacrolimus (despite therapeutic blood levels), the dose of these agents can be cautiously lowered to reach a target level in the low therapeutic range. In our patients, cyclosporine levels are allowed to be 150 to 300 ng/mL (12-hour trough, whole blood monoclonal assay) in patients whose GFR reaches 40 mL/min or less. We add mycophenolate mofetil or sirolimus to the immunosuppressive regimen of all these patients.

The success of liver transplantation has been tremendous over the past decade, as reflected by ever-increasing patient and graft survival times. With longer patient survival, the long-term effects on renal function are now being realized. Severe renal insufficiency is seen with increasing frequency (8% to 28% of patients) as the length of time from liver transplantation increases.[45-47] Often, these patients suffer the combined insults of pretransplant renal disease and chronic posttransplant cyclosporine and tacrolimus toxicity. A few of them will eventually require kidney transplantation. Interestingly enough, patients with hepatorenal syndrome who receive a liver transplant only (instead of a liver plus kidney transplant) achieve the same measured long-term GFR as do patients without hepatorenal syndrome.[48] Alternative immunosuppression regimens (calcineurin inhibitor minimization or withdrawal)[49-51] are now the focus to aid in preservation of renal function in the long term after liver transplantation.

Glucose Intolerance

Elevations in serum glucose levels after liver transplantation are a common event (see Table 58–2). High-dose steroids in the early posttransplant period, along with steroid treatment of rejection, may predispose recipients to glucose intolerance and insulin resistance.[52] Cyclosporine may also be contributory to the diabetic state inasmuch as experimental evidence suggests that it induces pancreatic islet cell toxicity and decreased insulin secretion.[53,54] The pretransplant cirrhotic state may itself contribute to diabetes, perhaps both by impaired insulin secretion and by hepatic insulin resistance.[55] In fact, some pretransplantation diabetics can be freed of all hyperglycemic agents after successful liver transplantation.[1] Earlier data on tacrolimus-treated patients did not demonstrate significant differences; however, recent evaluations have shown otherwise. The reported incidence of new-onset diabetes during the past decade was significantly higher in non–renal transplant patients receiving tacrolimus than in those receiving cyclosporine (11.1% versus 6.2%) in a recent meta-analysis.[56] Hepatitis C is also a possible risk factor for new-onset diabetes after liver transplantation.[57]

Regardless of the cause, high blood glucose levels in liver transplant recipients are always treated. Initial control can be achieved by the use of a sliding-scale regular insulin regimen. A few patients, especially if diabetic before transplantation, require a continuous intravenous infusion of insulin for early control. Some patients, in contrast, may do very well with oral hypoglycemic agents. The mainstay of successful therapy is individualization of the regimen to reflect each patient's needs.

Frequent as it is, posttransplant hyperglycemia is usually short lived. The rate of induced diabetes is low. Less than 10% of pretransplant nondiabetics require oral or parenteral hyperglycemic agents 6 months after their operation.[1,57]

Headaches

Mild or severe headaches can be a common symptom in an adult liver transplant recipient (see Table 58–2). Unfortunately, such complaints are also vague and relatively nonspecific. Addressing them can require a delicate balance of clinical acumen and suspicion of disease.

Several specific conditions can lead to headaches and warrant special mention. The toxicity of the immunosuppressants cyclosporine and tacrolimus can commonly be manifested as headaches.[38] The correlation between severe neurotoxicity (confusion, coma, hallucinations, seizures) and high whole blood and plasma tacrolimus levels is good. Mild neurotoxicity (including headaches) can and does occur even when tacrolimus levels are well within the therapeutic range. Calcineurin inhibitor–induced headaches are very common and frequently have a migraine-like character. We now prefer the use of Midrin (acetaminophen-dichloralphenazone, isometheptene mucate) or sumatriptan (Imitrex) for the treatment of these headaches because other routine medications (e.g., acetaminophen [Tylenol]) used for headaches are frequently ineffective. One approach to persistent headaches should be consideration of tacrolimus or cyclosporine dose reduction despite the presence of therapeutic levels.

Headaches can also be a manifestation of hypertension and, as such, can herald impending cerebrovascular accidents. Meningitis is always a concern in immunosuppressed patients and should be part of the differential diagnosis of headaches, although more so in case of unexplained fever. These patients are particularly susceptible to opportunistic infections, especially with *Cryptococcus*, herpesviruses, and *Nocardia* (see Chapter 64, "Infections after Liver Transplantation"). Our approach to patients with severe new headaches or unrelenting (chronic) headaches includes evaluation of tacrolimus or cyclosporine levels. Continued suspicion leads to a head computed tomographic scan, which if negative, results in sampling of spinal fluid for evidence of meningitis. Few persistent headaches remain an unsolved clinical entity.

Diarrhea

Frequent loose stools are another common clinical problem after liver transplantation (see Table 58–2). They may be an expected manifestation of the postsurgical state and should normalize within the first 1 to 2 weeks after transplantation. The role of (even transient) augmented portal hypertension during surgery is unclear. Altered gut flora, either from chronic lactulose use before transplantation or from broad-spectrum antibiotics given perioperatively, can certainly lead to pseudomembranous enterocolitis from *Clostridium difficile* exotoxin. Excessive use of magnesium-containing antacids, a common ulcer-preventing medication, can likewise lead to diarrhea. Antilymphocyte preparations, especially monoclonal antibodies, have frequent watery stools as a well-described side effect. Also to be considered is the exacerbation of ulcerative colitis that is so often present before transplantation in patients with primary sclerosing cholangitis.

Immunosuppressive drugs causing diarrhea (mycophenolate mofetil, rapamycin, tacrolimus, cyclosporine) have all been reported to cause gastrointestinal side effects. Agents such as mycophenolate mofetil[58] and rapamycin have a higher propensity to cause diarrhea than cyclosporine or tacrolimus does. Drug levels should be determined, and if toxic, the dose must be reduced. Drug-related diarrhea frequently improves within 72 hours of dose change.

Other medications have been reported to cause diarrhea in post–liver transplant patients. One in particular is angiotensin-converting enzyme (ACE) inhibitor. It can be associated with visceral angioedema, which has been reported with the onset of diarrhea. The typical scenario, hypertension caused by calcineurin inhibitor use, is treated by an ACE inhibitor. On initiation of the ACE inhibitor, abdominal pain, nausea, vomiting, and diarrhea occur. Follow-up computed tomography demonstrates small bowel edema and ascites.[59] Additionally, chemotherapeutic agents such as CPT-11, which may be used in the treatment of hepatocellular carcinoma, have been observed to cause diarrhea as well.[60] Another cause of posttransplant diarrhea may be GVHD. The constellation of fever, skin rash, diarrhea, and pancytopenia develops 2 to 6 weeks after transplantation.[61] This entity is difficult to distinguish from CMV or drug reaction early in the course. A definitive diagnosis is made by confirming donor lymphoid chimerism. The outcome is frequently poor, and treatment strategies range from treatment with antibody to a reduction in immunosuppression.

Regardless of the cause (except in GVHD), treatment of posttransplant diarrhea is initially supportive. Offending medications are removed or altered when possible. Stool specimens are obtained for pathogen culture and identification of *C. difficile* toxin. Fluid and electrolyte losses through the gut lumen are replaced intravenously when necessary. Finally, colonoscopy with biopsy is reserved for patients who do not respond to simple diagnostic and therapeutic maneuvers or for whom a viral infection (e.g., CMV colitis) is suspected. Early posttransplant exacerbations of ulcerative colitis are infrequent.

Common as it is, posttransplant diarrhea is a clinical problem that is most often easily and quickly solved. Two items of note should be remembered with regard to immunosuppression levels during episodes of diarrhea. First, trough levels of cyclosporine are decreased with diarrhea. However, tacrolimus levels have been shown to increase with episodes of diarrhea, and therefore dose adjustments must be made.[62]

Patient Rehabilitation

In principle, patients are discharged from the inpatient service once they are medically stable and able to care for themselves (see Table 58–2). Generally, patients spend less than 2 to 3 weeks (median, 7 days; mean, 11 days) as inpatients after liver transplantation.[1] Concern for self-care is an important issue. Many end-stage liver disease sufferers lose muscle mass, strength, appetite, nutritional status, and conditioning. Although all these deficiencies are corrected with successful transplantation, return to normal can be slow. Stable patients lacking physical strength may benefit from aggressive care at an inpatient rehabilitation hospital. Moreover, physical therapy should be considered in all liver transplant recipients as well.

Functional status as assessed by the Karnofsky Performance Status Scale (see Chapter 81, "Long-Term Functional Recovery and Quality of Life: Childhood, Adulthood, Employment, Pregnancy, and Family Planning") is almost always low before transplantation. Measurements of this widely used scale of physical and psychosocial performance reveal these patients to need occasional assistance, at best, solely to be able to care for themselves. Functional status is brought back to normal by the first year after transplantation and is sustained long term.[63]

Psychological or psychiatric intervention can be necessary in the posttransplant period. High-dose steroids, for instance, may precipitate a psychotic break. These episodes are sometimes manifested by agitation, confabulations, delusions, ideations, mania, and hostile behavior. Often, potent psychotropic agents such as haloperidol are necessary for patient cooperation. One should exercise great caution, however, when prescribing haloperidol for a patient with impaired liver function. The drug can rapidly accumulate and precipitate emprosthotonos or an oculogyric crisis, even at "standard" doses. We recommend a low initial dose (1 to 2 mg) orally and small incremental increases. Residua from intensive care unit psychosis, hepatic encephalopathy, and old age can also contribute to mental status changes after transplantation, as can a mechanical event such as intracranial bleeding. Finally, neurotoxicity from cyclosporine and tacrolimus can be expressed as mental status changes.[38]

Patients and their families can also experience psychological stress and anxiety after successful transplantation.[64] Relief at having obtained a transplant and surviving such a major operation gives way to anxiety over potential rejection, other complications, and long-term survival. Some patients have great difficulty assimilating back into society, overcoming obstacles to employment, and obtaining health insurance because of their previous liver transplantation.[65] These challenges and many others highlight the need for social workers to be integral members of the liver transplant team.

Before discharge from the hospital, liver transplant recipients should have basic knowledge of their medication dose and schedules. Certain commonsense precautions when living as an immunosuppressed patient should also be reviewed (Table 58–3). Follow-up clinic visits, laboratory blood tests, and outpatient treatment are emphasized. Without proper attention to some of these important details, the well-being of these patients can be jeopardized.

Outpatient Care

A medically stable liver transplant recipient is discharged from the hospital sometime during the second to third week after transplantation. Stable patients still too weak or deconditioned to care for themselves are probably best discharged from the acute care setting to a rehabilitation hospital. There, intensive physical therapy can progress under specialized supervision to maximize the return to independent self-care.

The level of scrutiny brought to bear on an outpatient adult liver transplant recipient may vary widely from center to center. In general, however, regardless of whether the patient is monitored by a personal physician or directly by the transplant center, certain guidelines apply. Because the vast majority of first acute rejections occur within the first 3 weeks after transplantation and because CMV infection is diagnosed within 4 to 6 weeks after transplantation, liver function tests and complete blood counts should be monitored biweekly.[66] Cyclosporine or tacrolimus levels may also need frequent adjustments, and monitoring of renal function is important as well. Some centers such as ours check laboratory test results twice a week and also see patients in the clinic two times weekly. Prudence may be exercised in patients who demonstrate stability and continued recovery, and visits and laboratory tests may be spaced out further. Very few patients encounter significant acute rejection or infection beyond the third month after transplantation and are usually discharged from our center by then. This period not only allows the transplant team control over the most fragile posttransplant days but also ensures a stable patient for the referring or follow-up physician.

Removal of T tubes also follows center-specific protocols, and they are usually removed on an outpatient basis during the 10th postoperative week. Patients who experience peritoneal signs consistent with bile leakage are admitted to the hospital for bowel rest and intravenous antibiotics. Persistent leaks, as proved by hepatobiliary scan, are treated either with endoscopically placed biliary stents or with open oversewing of the T-tube tract.[67] No attempt is made at surgery to expose the common bile duct proper.

The final discharge of patients from the transplant center is an excellent opportunity to reinforce key aspects of patient education, the medication regimen, and treatment compliance. This time can also be used to emphasize the importance of communication with the transplant center regarding unexpected or unfamiliar clinical situations that may occur in the future. Here also is an opportunity to arm the patient with information about the expected course, follow-up, and common characteristics of the immunosuppressant medications (especially tacrolimus or cyclosporine) with which many follow-up physicians may be unfamiliar. Telephone and electronic means by which the transplant center can be reached are reiterated.

Table 58–3. SUGGESTED PRECAUTIONS FOR IMMUNOSUPPRESSED PATIENTS

Know the signs and symptoms of infection and rejection.

Frequently wash hands with antimicrobial soap.

Avoid large crowds and poorly ventilated areas.

Avoid individuals who are ill.

Ensure antibiotic prophylaxis for dental cleaning, dental work, and invasive procedures.

Always use sunscreen with a sun protection factor of 15 or greater.

Women should have a yearly Papanicolaou smear.

Contraception must be used after transplantation.

A diaphragm or condoms (or both) with spermicide is the recommended means of contraception.

Pregnancy is not recommended for female transplant patients.

Immunizations

The vast majority of adults who come to liver transplantation have received all of their routine (i.e., childhood) immunizations. In general, then, the need for posttransplant vaccinations is limited, but pertinent.

As a matter of convention, live attenuated virus immunizations are contraindicated. Although the risk of disease development from these preparations is theoretical and has never been proved, that risk is not taken. Examples of live attenuated vaccines are smallpox, yellow fever, measles, mumps, rubella, and oral polio. The only published data on immune-deficient patients and live attenuated vaccines (i.e., in human immunodeficiency virus–infected children) did not show them to have experienced disease from the vaccine. Permitted vaccines are those for influenza, *Pneumococcus*, hepatitis B, and the diphtheria-tetanus booster (not the initial diphtheria-tetanus inoculation).

No information has been published regarding the risks and benefits of yearly influenza vaccinations against the predominant epitopes of the season. The Centers for Disease Control and Prevention, however, recommends these immunizations for the elderly and the very young. We have left that decision to the primary physician and the patient.

Although liver transplant recipients may not fall into high-risk groups for hepatitis B exposure (anyone likely to come in contact with human blood or secretions), we recommend that they be vaccinated after transplantation with either killed virus or recombinant virus if they have not already received these vaccines while waiting for the transplant. Pretransplant immunization is preferable because patients' ability to respond to the vaccine is much better while not immunosuppressed. Although the risk of infection is undefined and may be low, vaccination against hepatitis B in these patients seems prudent.

Antibiotic Prophylaxis for Procedures

Once a liver transplant recipient progresses well beyond 3 months, the patient may elect to undergo procedures that were delayed because of their end-stage liver disease. These procedures may involve dental work, joint surgery, back surgery, and other elective procedures. The transplant center is frequently notified, and inquiries regarding antibiotic prophylaxis and immunosuppressive management are made.

Dental prophylaxis follows that of the American Heart Association guideline for antibiotic use in patients with valve abnormalities. Higher-risk patients (those who have recurring infections with very low levels of immunosuppression) may need a more prolonged course of antibiotics that encompasses the entire periprocedural period (before, during, and after the procedure).

Surgical prophylaxis should be specific to the procedure. The duration of the antibiotic course should encompass the perioperative phase as well. Indwelling drains, open wounds, and synthetic material all warrant extended use of antibiotics. Patients who are not progressing well after an elective procedure should have their antibiotic coverage broadened until infectious causes are ruled out.

Pregnancy

Although pregnancy is discouraged after liver transplantation, there are now increasing numbers of patients who have delivered children successfully. Frequently, transplant centers do advise that if a woman is going to attempt to become pregnant after liver transplantation, she must wait 1 year after the transplant date. Additionally, males intending to father a child are also advised to wait 1 year after transplantation. Of course, this is a high-risk pregnancy from start to finish, and the expertise of the transplant center is required, along with an obstetrical program that has experience with such a pregnancy.

Immunosuppressive agents that have been taken with successful pregnancies include cyclosporine, tacrolimus, azathioprine, and steroids. Less assurance can be given with newer agents such as sirolimus and mycophenolate mofetil. The use of mycophenolate mofetil has not been advocated because of its teratogenic effects in animals. To date, no controlled studies in humans have substantiated or refuted the animal findings.

Jain and colleagues[68] have documented 13 years' experience with tacrolimus and pregnancy. In that experience, low-birth-weight babies and preterm labor were persistent problems. However, 37 mothers delivered 49 babies in their series. Only one death was reported in a mother who had an aortic graft that clotted because of the gravid uterus. Twelve mothers demonstrated an elevation in their liver enzymes, which was remedied by increasing immunosuppression.

The National Transplantation Pregnancy Registry follows the pregnancies of solid-organ transplant recipients. Based on its analysis and data, no specific graft or newborn outcome differences have been noted between different calcineurin inhibitor regimens. Extensive data published on azathioprine- and cyclosporine-treated recipients suggest that despite a pattern of prematurity among the newborn, there has not been an increase in the incidence or pattern of specific malformations noted in the newborns. Of course, sporadic cases of rejection, graft dysfunction, and graft deterioration have occurred, but no specific patterns of occurrence. Birth defect patterns have not appeared to be specific to any particular regimen as yet.[69]

Breast-feeding is discouraged because of infant exposure to the immunosuppressive agents and their metabolites. To date, there are no data on these infants and the impact of exposure to immunosuppressive agents on them later in life. There is potential harm to the infants and the development of their immune system and overall growth.

Pearls and Pitfalls

Pearls

- Liver transplantation is truly a multidisciplinary specialty. Successful liver transplantation can occur only with such an approach.
- A combination of experience in interpreting radiographic studies, pathological conditions, and laboratory studies allows the transplant team to make appropriate treatment plans (i.e., recognize preservation injury versus early acute cellular rejection).
- Biliary reconstruction involving T-tube stenting is associated with complications. The diagnosis of biliary abnormalities is best done with PTC or ERCP (although there is a risk of ERCP-associated pancreatitis).
- Clinical charting of the patients' posttransplant course is best accomplished through the use of a series of wall charts.
- Fungal prophylaxis and early treatment are vital to minimizing the incidence of severe fungal infections.
- Early administration of nutrition is vital to posttransplant patients.
- Detailed knowledge and understanding of the side effects of immunosuppression (hypertension, diabetes mellitus, renal dysfunction, etc.) are vital in the management of posttransplant patients.

Pitfalls

- Success of the transplant team depends on the multidisciplinary experience and knowledge of individuals involved in posttransplant care. No single individual or specialty can truly handle the complexity of this special patient population.
- Misinterpretation of liver function tests may lead to inaccurate diagnosis early in the posttransplant course (i.e., preservation injury versus early acute cellular rejection).
- The use of ERCP can be associated with up to a 30% incidence of pancreatitis.

Pearls and Pitfalls—cont'd

- Medications used to treat some of the associated side effects caused by calcineurin inhibitors may cause interactions leading to variability in calcineurin inhibitor blood levels, thereby making immunosuppressant management difficult.

References

1. Levy MF, Goldstein RM, Husberg BS, et al: Baylor update: Outcome analysis in liver transplantation. In Terasaki P, Cecka R (eds): Clinical Transplants 1993. Los Angeles, UCLA Tissue Typing Laboratory, 1993, pp 161-173.
2. Howard TK, Klintmalm GB, Cofer JB, et al: The influence of preservation injury on rejection in the hepatic transplant recipient. Transplantation 49:103-107, 1990.
3. Mor E, Solomon H, Gibbs JF, et al: Acute cellular rejection following liver transplantation: Clinical pathologic features and effect on outcome. Semin Liver Dis 12:28-40, 1992.
4. Vit A, De Candia A, Como G, et al: Doppler evaluation of arterial complications of adult orthotopic liver transplantation. J Clin Ultrasound 31:339-345, 2003.
5. Sayage LH, Husberg BS, Klintmalm GB, et al: Vascular complications in adult liver transplant patients: The value of postoperative Doppler ultrasound screening and the surgical management of hepatic arterial thrombosis. Clin Transpl 3: 344-348, 1989.
6. Huang DZ, Le GR, Zhang QP, et al: The value of color Doppler ultrasonography in monitoring normal orthotopic liver transplantation and postoperative complications. Hepatobiliary Pancreat Dis Int 2:54-58, 2003.
7. Garcia-Criado A, Gilabert R, Salmeron JM, et al: Significance of and contributing factors for a high resistive index on Doppler sonography of the hepatic artery immediately after surgery: Prognostic implications for liver transplant recipients. AJR Am J Roentgenol 181:831-838, 2003.
8. Meire HB, Farrant P: Liver transplantation: Ultrasound in gastroenterology. Clin Diagn Ultrasound 29:93-125, 1994.
9. Soliman T, Bodingbauer M, Langer F, et al: The role of complex hepatic artery reconstruction in orthotopic liver transplantation. Liver Transpl 9:970-975, 2003.
10. Trotter JF: Sirolimus in liver transplantation. Transplant Proc 35(Suppl):193S-200S, 2003.
11. Stange BJ, Glanemann M, Nuessler NC, et al: Hepatic artery thrombosis after adult liver transplantation. Liver Transpl 9: 612-620, 2003.
12. Kahan BD: Cyclosporine. N Engl J Med 321:1725-1738, 1989.
13. Scatton O, Meunier B, Cherqui D, et al: Randomized trial of choledochocholedochostomy with or without a T tube in orthotopic liver transplantation. Ann Surg 233:432-437, 2001.
14. Gopal DV, Pfau PR, Lucey MR: Endoscopic management of biliary complications after orthotopic liver transplantation. Curr Treat Options Gastroenterol 6:509-515, 2003.
15. Sanchez E, Ueno T, Martin A, et al: T-tube free biliary anastomosis in liver transplantation is safe. Poster presented at the American Society of Transplant Surgeons 4th Annual State of the Art Winter Symposium, Scottsdale, AZ, January 2004.
16. Lella F, Bagnolo F, Colombo E, Bonassi U: A simple way of avoiding post-ERCP pancreatitis. Gastrointest Endosc 59:830-834, 2004.

17. Halme L, Hockerstedt K, Lautenschlager I: Cytomegalovirus infection and development of biliary complications after liver transplantation. Transplantation 75:1853-1858, 2003.

18. Ben-Ari Z, Pappo O, Mor E: Intrahepatic cholestasis after liver transplantation. Liver Transpl 9:1005-1018, 2003.

19. Guichelaar MM, Benson JT, Malinchoc M, et al: Risk factors for and clinical course of non-anastomotic biliary strictures after liver transplantation. Am J Transplant 3:885-890, 2003.

20. Johnston A, Chusney G, Schutz E, et al: Monitoring cyclosporin in blood: Between-assay differences at trough and 2 hours post-dose (C2). Ther Drug Monit 25:167-173, 2003.

21. Baraldo M, Risaliti A, Bresadola F, et al: Circadian variations in cyclosporine C2 concentrations during the first 2 weeks after liver transplantation. Transplant Proc 35:1449-1451, 2003.

22. Winston DJ, Busuttil RW: Randomized controlled trial of oral itraconazole solution versus intravenous/oral fluconazole for prevention of fungal infections in liver transplant recipients. Transplantation 74:688-695, 2002.

23. Mora NP, Cofer JB, Solomon H, et al: Analysis of severe infections (INF) after 180 consecutive liver transplants: The impact of amphotericin B prophylaxis for reducing the incidence and severity of fungal infections. Transplant Proc 23:1528-1530, 1991.

24. Wiesner RH, Hermans PE, Rakela J, et al: Selective bowel decontamination to decrease gram-negative aerobic bacterial and Candida colonization and prevent infection after orthotopic liver transplantation. Transplantation 45:570-574, 1988.

25. Bion JF, Badger I, Crosby HA, et al: Selective decontamination of the digestive tract reduces gram-negative pulmonary colonization but not systemic endotoxemia in patients undergoing elective liver transplantation. Crit Care Med 22:40-49, 1994.

26. Singh N, Wagener MM, Marino IR, et al: Trends in invasive fungal infections in liver transplant recipients: Correlation with evolution in transplantation practices. Transplantation 73:63-67, 2002.

27. Singh N, Wannstedt C, Keyes L, et al: Impact of evolving trends in recipient and donor characteristics on cytomegalovirus infection in liver transplant recipients. Transplantation 77:106-110, 2004.

28. Winston DJ, Busuttil RW: Randomized controlled trial of sequential intravenous and oral ganciclovir versus prolonged intravenous ganciclovir for long-term prophylaxis of cytomegalovirus disease in high-risk cytomegalovirus-seronegative liver transplant recipients with cytomegalovirus-seropositive donors. Transplantation 77:305-308, 2004.

29. Winston DJ, Busuttil RW: Randomized controlled trial of oral ganciclovir versus oral acyclovir after induction with intravenous ganciclovir for long-term prophylaxis of cytomegalovirus disease in cytomegalovirus-seropositive liver transplant recipients. Transplantation 75:229-233, 2003.

30. Levy MF, Crippin JS, Gonwa TA, et al: Cytomegalovirus infections in liver transplant recipients: Morbidity in the DHPG era [abstract]. Hepatology 16:282A, 1992.

31. Lautz HU, Selberg O, Körber J, et al: Protein-calorie malnutrition in liver cirrhosis. Clin Invest 70:478-486, 1992.

32. Harrison J, McKiernan J, Neuberger JM: A prospective study on the effect of recipient nutritional status on outcome in liver transplantation. Transpl Int 10:369-374, 1997.

33. Pikul J, Sharpe MD, Lowndes R, Ghent CN: Degree of preoperative malnutrition is predictive of postoperative morbidity and mortality in liver transplant recipients. Transplantation 57:469-472, 1994.

34. Hasse JM, Gonwa TA, Jennings LW, et al: Malnutrition affects liver transplant outcomes [abstract]. Transplantation 66:S53, 1998.

35. Wicks C, Somasundaram S, Bjarnason I, et al: Comparison of enteral feeding and total parenteral nutrition after liver transplantation. Lancet 344:837-840, 1994.

36. Hasse JM, Blue LS, Liepa GU, et al: Early enteral nutrition support in patients undergoing liver transplantation. JPEN J Parenter Enteral Nutr 19:437-443, 1995.

37. Rayes N, Seehofer D, Hansen S, et al: Early enteral supply of Lactobacillus and fiber versus selective bowel decontamination: A controlled trial in liver transplant recipients. Transplantation 74:123-127, 2002.

38. Backman L, Nicar M, Levy MF, et al: FK506 trough levels in whole blood and plasma in liver transplant recipients. Correlation with clinical events and side effects. Transplantation 57:519-525, 1994.

39. High KP: The antimicrobial activities of cyclosporine, FK506, and rapamycin. Transplantation 57:1689-1700, 1994.

40. Hebert MF, Lam AY: Diltiazem increases tacrolimus concentrations. Ann Pharmacother 33:680-682, 1999.

41. Neal DA, Tom BD, Luan J, et al: Is there disparity between risk and incidence of cardiovascular disease after liver transplant? Transplantation 77:93-99, 2004.

42. McDiarmid SV, Colonna JO 2nd, Shaked A, et al: A comparison of renal function in cyclosporine- and FK506-treated patients after primary orthotopic liver transplantation. Transplantation 56:847-853, 1993.

43. Poplawski S, Gonwa T, Goldstein R, et al: Long term nephrotoxicity in liver transplantation. Transplant Proc 21:2469-2471, 1989.

44. Scherrer U, Vissing SF, Morgan BJ, et al: Cyclosporine-induced sympathetic activation and hypertension after heart transplantation. N Engl J Med 323:693-699, 1990.

45. Gonwa TA, Mai ML, Melton LB, et al: End-stage renal disease (ESRD) after orthotopic liver transplantation (OLTX) using calcineurin-based immunotherapy: Risk of development and treatment. Transplantation 72:1934-1939, 2001.

46. Gayowski T, Singh N, Keyes L, et al: Late-onset renal failure after liver transplantation: Role of posttransplant alcohol use. Transplantation 69:383-388, 2000.

47. Fisher NC, Nightingale PG, Gunson BK, et al: Chronic renal failure following liver transplantation: A retrospective analysis. Transplantation 66:59-66, 1998.

48. Gonwa TA, Morris CA, Goldstein RM, et al: Long-term survival and renal function following liver transplantation in patients with and without hepatorenal syndrome—experience in 300 patients. Transplantation 51:428-430, 1991.

49. Gonwa TA: Treatment of renal dysfunction after orthotopic liver transplantation: Options and outcomes. Liver Transpl 9:778-779, 2003.

50. Nair S, Eason J, Loss G: Sirolimus monotherapy in nephrotoxicity due to calcineurin inhibitors in liver transplant recipients. Liver Transpl 9:126-129, 2003.

51. Cotterell AH, Fisher RA, King AL, et al: Calcineurin inhibitor–induced chronic nephrotoxicity in liver transplant patients is reversible using rapamycin as the primary immunosuppressive agent. Clin Transplant 16(Suppl 7):49-51, 2002.

52. Luzi L, Secchi A, Facchini F, et al: Reduction of insulin resistance by combined kidney-pancreas transplantation in type 1 (insulin-dependent) diabetic patients. Diabetologia 33:549-556, 1990.

53. Yale JF, Roy RD, Grose M, et al: Effects of cyclosporine on glucose tolerance in the rat. Diabetes 34:1309-1313, 1985.

54. Robertson RP: Cyclosporine-induced inhibition of insulin secretion in isolated rat islets and HIT cells. Diabetes 35:1016-1019, 1986.

55. Petrides AS, Vogt C, Schulze-Berge D, et al: Pathogenesis of glucose intolerance and diabetes mellitus in cirrhosis. Hepatology 19:616-627, 1994.

56. Heisel O, Heisel R, Balshaw R, et al: New onset diabetes mellitus in patients receiving calcineurin inhibitors: A systematic review and meta-analysis. Am J Transplant 4:583-595, 2004.

57. Khalili M, Lim JW, Bass N, et al: New onset diabetes mellitus after liver transplantation: The critical role of hepatitis C infection. Liver Transpl 10:349-355, 2004.

58. Maes BD, Dalle I, Geboes K, et al: Erosive enterocolitis in mycophenolate mofetil–treated renal-transplant recipients with persistent afebrile diarrhea. Transplantation 75:665-672, 2003.

59. Rosenberg EI, Mishra G, Abdelmalek MF: Angiotensin-converting enzyme inhibitor–induced isolated visceral angioedema in a liver transplant recipient. Transplantation 75:730-732, 2003.

60. Gornet JM, Lokiec F, Duclos-Vallee JC, et al: Severe CPT-11–induced diarrhea in presence of FK-506 following liver transplantation for hepatocellular carcinoma. Anticancer Res 21:4203-4206, 2001.

61. Smith DM, Agura E, Netto G, et al: Liver transplant–associated graft-versus-host disease. Transplantation 75:118-126, 2003.

62. Hochleitner BW, Bosmuller C, Nehoda H, et al: Increased tacrolimus levels during diarrhea. Transpl Int 14:230-233, 2001.

63. Levy MF, Jennings L, Abouljoud MS, et al: Quality of life improvements at one, two, and five years after liver transplantation. Transplantation 59:515-518, 1995.

64. Chappell S: Anxiety in liver transplant patients. Paper presented at the Third International Transplant Nurses Society Symposium and General Assembly, San Francisco, February 1994.

65. Gutkind L: Life after transplantation. Transplant Proc 20 (Suppl 1):1092-1099, 1988.

66. Goldstein RM, Solomon H, Holman MJ, et al: Liver transplantation, 1990: A Dallas perspective. In Terasaki PL (ed): Clinical Transplants 1990. Los Angeles, UCLA Tissue Typing Laboratory, 1991, pp 123-133.

67. Osorio RW, Freise CE, Stock PG, et al: Nonoperative management of biliary leaks after orthotopic liver transplantation. Transplantation 55:1074-1077, 1993.

68. Jain AB, Reyes J, Marcos A, et al: Pregnancy after liver transplantation with tacrolimus immunosuppression: A single center's experience update at 13 years. Transplantation 76:827-832, 2003.

69. Armenti VT, Radomski JS, Moritz MJ, et al: Report from the National Transplantation Pregnancy Registry (NTPR): Outcomes of pregnancy after transplantation. Clin Transpl 121-130, 2002.

Postoperative Care of Pediatric Liver Transplant Recipients

STEVEN J. LOBRITTO
JEAN C. EMOND

Preoperative factors affecting
posttransplant care   882
　Chronic cholestatic liver disease   882
　Fulminant liver failure   882
　Metabolic liver disease   882
　Retransplantation   882

Operative factors affecting posttransplant
care   883

Initial postoperative intensive care
unit care   883

Postoperative orders   883

Postoperative indicators of graft function   885

Hemodynamic indicators   885

Postoperative indicators of surgical
complications   886

Postoperative laboratory indicators   886

Postoperative ascites   886

Postoperative fever   887

Postoperative nutritional management   887

The typical postoperative course   887

Improvements in surgical technique and anesthesia over the past decade have simplified the postoperative care of the pediatric liver transplant recipient, with rapid transition out of the intensive care unit (ICU) and early discharge home becoming the rule.[1-4] As with all major operations, the postoperative care of the potential pediatric liver transplant recipient really begins with judicious management in the preoperative period. Preoperative care to address the complications of liver insufficiency, the management of portal hypertension, the optimization of nutritional state, the suppression of infectious complications, and the correction of metabolic derangements has been shown to decrease both the morbidity and mortality associated with the transplant operation.[5-12] With the widespread use of living related liver transplantation (LRLT), it is possible to choose the optimal time for operative intervention and minimize pretransplant morbidity.[13] The preoperative care challenges are predictive of the needs and postoperative issues of the liver recipient. Therefore, the optimal care of the pediatric liver transplant recipient must be a coordinated effort with efficient communication between the medical and surgical members of the transplant team. The medical-surgical blended team model of preoperative and postoperative management affords the patient the best result, combining the skills and expertise of both disciplines.[14]

Preoperative Factors Affecting Posttransplant Care

Chronic Cholestatic Liver Disease

All liver transplant recipients are not equal. The majority of pediatric liver transplantations are still performed to address liver insufficiency from disorders of chronic cholestasis.[15] Patients with biliary cirrhosis have special nutritional requirements, with particular detail to fat malabsorption and overall calorie delivery.[16] In addition, cirrhotic patients may undergo a liver transplantation procedure with profound synthetic dysfunction and hypersplenism, putting them at greater risk of intraoperative blood loss because of coagulation defects and thrombocytopenia. Patients with advanced portal hypertension may undergo decompensation in the preoperative period, having their liver transplant performed in the setting of uncontrolled ascites, relative hypoxia, renal insufficiency, electrolyte disarray, or recent gastrointestinal hemorrhage. In addition, these patients are immunosuppressed by their underlying disorders and are at risk of infectious complications postoperatively.

Besides the problems common to any chronic cholestatic cirrhosis, there are special considerations with implications for postoperative management, depending on the specific underlying disorder. For example, the pediatric patient with biliary atresia has usually had prior abdominal surgery, increasing the risk of operative blood loss and inadvertent enterotomies during the surgical dissection at the time of liver transplantation. In addition, patients with biliary atresia may have other associated anomalies, such as cardiac disease and gastrointestinal malrotation.[17,18] Some syndromic cholestatic disorders are associated with pulmonary hypertension. Patients with progressive familial intrahepatic cholestasis have defects in intestinal function, leading to difficulties with severe diarrhea in the postoperative period, which compromises the delivery of nutritional support and medications.[19,20] Similarly, patients with primary sclerosing cholangitis may have underlying bowel disease, infectious complications, and chronic dependency on pain medications; each has implications for management after transplantation.[21] Another example is the patient with chronic cholestasis in the setting of long-term dependency on parenteral nutrition who may have significant underlying pulmonary disease and marginal gastrointestinal absorptive capacity.[22,23] It is only with this thorough knowledge of the preoperative condition of the patient that the optimal postoperative care can be rendered.

Fulminant Liver Failure

The next major category of pediatric patients requiring liver transplantation are those with acute liver failure.[24,25]

The cause of liver failure varies in this group and may be associated with other major organ injury as well. This heterogeneous group of patients differs in prior medical comorbid disorders that may have specific implications for postoperative management. Patients in this group are at specific risk of severe encephalopathy and life-threatening cerebral edema. The pre- and postoperative management of fluids, electrolytes, blood pressure, and cerebral perfusion pressure must be judicious to permit patient survival with or without liver transplantation.[24] The perioperative management of these patients often necessitates the placement of an intracranial pressure monitoring device for optimal delivery of care.[26] The risks of bleeding from the device placement and of infection are balanced by the improved ability to monitor and manage cerebral hypertension to ensure the best possible transplant outcome.[27] The risk of cerebral hypertension unfortunately does not end immediately after successful liver transplantation and can persist into the second and third postoperative day.[28] These patients often have severe coagulation anomalies, placing them at increased risk of intraoperative bleeding. In addition, these patients have an increased risk of sepsis and should be monitored closely in the postoperative period with empirical antibiotic coverage to improve outcomes.[9]

Metabolic Liver Disease

The third general group of patients undergoing pediatric liver transplantation includes those with metabolic liver disease, such as urea cycle defects, glycogen storage disease, neonatal hemochromatosis, tyrosinemia, Crigler-Najjar type 1, α_1-antitrypsin deficiency, and Wilson's disease.[3,29-35] Patients in this category may have had specific medication and dietary restrictions before liver transplant that need to be adjusted in the postoperative period. Some of these patients require urgent neonatal liver transplantation that further complicates the postoperative care because of technical complications and immature physiology.[36] Some of the patients with metabolic disease have associated organ injuries such as brain and lung involvement that will affect postoperative tolerance to medications and other care issues. Portal hypertension can be absent in these patients, and some are at risk for postoperative hepatocellular carcinoma.[37]

Retransplantation

The last general group of patients with specific considerations in the postoperative period includes those undergoing repeat liver transplantation. The patient in need of a second liver transplant is at increased risk of perioperative issues, including increased blood loss, inadvertent bowel injury, poor wound healing, and severe acute cellular rejection.[38] These patients may have significant altered renal function from prior medication exposure affecting their postoperative management. The outcomes in such patients will also depend on the degree of liver insufficiency entering retransplantation, the nutritional status of the patient, and the presence of associated biliary or vascular injuries. The choice of medications to prevent rejection will often be more aggressive than during the first transplant. The presence of infections such as cytomegalovirus (CMV) and posttransplant lymphoproliferative disease should be monitored with vigilance.

Operative Factors Affecting Posttransplant Care

It is crucial that information regarding intraoperative events is passed from the anesthesia and surgical teams to the ICU personnel and the hepatology team. Although some surgical teams manage every aspect of postoperative care, we advocate an integrated multidisciplinary postoperative care team, because the surgical team may be involved in other operations or may be physically taxed after operating through the night. Parameters such as blood loss, plasma infused, hourly urine output, endotracheal tube size and position, medications infused, intraoperative vital signs, intraoperative laboratory results, warm and cold ischemia times, types of vascular access, and monitoring modalities are presented by the anesthesia team. The surgical team must report the type of graft, the donor attributes, the color and texture of the graft following reperfusion, the details regarding biliary and vascular anastomoses, any bowel injuries or spillage, the number and type of drains, and the type of wound closure. This communication will permit the postoperative management team to predict likely needs and expected complications from intraoperative findings and events.

The type of graft used has important implications for the postoperative management. As the nationwide shortage of pediatric deceased donor liver grafts continues, the transplant surgeon is forced to use technical variant grafts, such as split right or left lobes, or living donor liver grafts.[13,39-43] In many centers, partial grafts account for the majority of pediatric liver transplant procedures performed. These partial liver transplants can have complicated vascular and biliary anastomoses, creating postoperative problems with graft perfusion and biliary outflow.[44-48] In addition, partial liver grafts with a cut edge can predispose to biliary leaks and postoperative infection.[46] The outcomes of these types of transplants seem to correlate with the experience of the operative team and should be confined to centers of excellence.

Initial Postoperative Intensive Care Unit Care

After the operative team has communicated the course and findings to both the intensivist and the hepatology team, the continuity of the patient's care is ensured. We favor the use of standard protocol postoperative orders and care algorithms. The initial management of the patient includes transferring portable monitoring devices to those of the ICU, reestablishing lines and infusions, and reestablishing mechanical ventilation. A rapid yet thorough assessment is made to evaluate adequacy of ventilation, hemodynamic stability, vascular access, and monitoring modalities. The patient's fluid status is assessed by vital signs, central venous pressure (CVP) monitoring, capillary refill, and weight comparison with preoperative values. A set of metabolic and hematological admission laboratory tests are obtained to assess the need for electrolyte and fluid adjustments, further blood products, acid-base balance, adequacy of oxygenation and ventilation, and overall liver function. Chest and abdominal radiographs are obtained to check line, drain, and endotracheal tube placement. We favor a single abdominal sonogram with Doppler within 12 hours to assess vascular patency and to exclude large intraabdominal collections. Others have reported more frequent sonographic surveillance.[49]

Postoperative Orders

Transplant teams commonly use standardized order sets with weight-based dosing to minimize medication errors and omissions.[3,50,51] The typical postoperative orders include the following (Table 59–1):

1. Intravenous (IV) fluids are administered to provide the necessary intravascular volume to ensure adequate graft and vital organ perfusion. Typically, a buffered resuscitation fluid such as lactated Ringer's is delivered at 1.5 to 2 times the calculated weight-based maintenance rate. The fluid rate is adjusted to optimize organ perfusion as estimated by a CVP between 4 and 10 mm Hg, and urine output is monitored closely. The acid-base balance and serum electrolytes are used to make adjustments in fluid constituents. Particular attention is given to the presence of hyperkalemia and metabolic acidosis, two early clues to graft vascular insufficiency or major dysfunction. In patients at risk for cerebral edema, the delivery of fluid requires a balance between maintaining adequate intravascular volume and avoiding increasing intracranial pressure. Diuretics such as furosemide and renal-dose dopamine are often administered to stimulate renal function after

Table 59–1. POSTOPERATIVE ORDERS

Intravenous fluids—lactated Ringer's solution at 1.5 to 2 times weight-based maintenance rate

Acid suppression with IV histamine blockers followed by an enteral proton pump inhibitor

Antibacterial agents—enterics, *Staphylococcal* species, and enterococcus

CMV prophylaxis—IV ganciclovir for 7 days followed by high-dose acyclovir

Fungal prophylaxis—oral nystatin

Aspirin—vascular thrombosis prophylaxis

Immunosuppressive agents

  Steroids

  Antimetabolites (azathioprine or mycophenolate mofetil)

  Calcineurin blocker (cyclosporine or tacrolimus)

  Monoclonal IL-2 receptor antagonists (daclizumab or basiliximab)

  Antilymphocyte globulin (antithymocyte globulin or muromonab/CD3)

  Sirolimus

Narcotic pain medication (fentanyl or morphine) and sedation (short-acting anxiolytics)

Laboratory monitoring parameters

Mechanical ventilation and weaning parameters

Renal-dose dopamine and diuretics

caval cross-clamping. Cirrhotic patients are sodium avid and commonly retain fluids necessarily for weeks following liver transplantation.[52] Such patients often require diuretics during this period of adaptation.

2. Acid suppression with IV histamine blockers followed by an enteral proton pump inhibitor is administered to decrease the risk of superficial gastric ulceration and gastrointestinal bleeding. If mycophenolate mofetil (MMF) is included in the immunosuppression regimen, proton pump inhibitors are maintained to prevent drug-induced intestinal injury.

3. Standard perioperative antibacterial agents are administered to provide coverage for both gram-negative and gram-positive organisms with particular attention to staphylococcal species and enterococcus.[53] Patients with prior bacterial infection, those with delayed wound closure, and patients with intraoperative gut injury or spillage continue to receive antibiotics for longer periods as appropriate. These patients are at risk for antibiotic-resistant infections. Prophylactic antibiotic exposure should be limited to prevent the emergence of resistant organisms such as methicillin-resistant *Staphylococcus aureus* and vancomycin-resistant enterococcal species. Other prophylactic antimicrobials are administered to prevent opportunistic infections. We provide CMV prophylaxis to all recipients, with a combination of IV ganciclovir for 7 days followed by either oral ganciclovir or high-dose acyclovir delivered for the first 3 months following liver transplantation. Recipients at particular risk for CMV include those that are CMV-naïve and have a donor with prior CMV exposure.[54] The peak incidence of CMV infection that affects the graft or the gut is at about 6 weeks. *Pneumocystis* prophylaxis is achieved with trimethoprim-sulfamethoxazole administered three times per week for the first year after transplantation. Fungal prophylaxis is usually achieved with oral nystatin administered during the period of steroid administration. Patients receiving long-term preoperative antibiotics, those with fulminant hepatic failure, patients with biliary leaks, or those with documented invasive fungal infection are treated with long-term fluconazole with careful attention to calcineurin drug levels.

4. Aspirin is administered for the first postoperative month for vascular thrombosis prophylaxis, although this practice has never been studied rigorously.[55] This is not universally accepted at all centers nor is the administration of heparin, dextrans, or prostacyclin.[56,57]

5. Immunosuppressive agents are administered to prevent acute cellular rejection. Most centers use some combination of steroids, antimetabolites (azathioprine or MMF), and a calcineurin blocker (cyclosporine or tacrolimus).[58] Some centers are attempting steroid-free protocols that involve some combination of one of the monoclonal interleukin (IL)-2 receptor antagonists (daclizumab or basiliximab) or antilymphocyte globulin (antithymocyte globulin or muromonab-CD3) with conventional agents.[59,60] For patients with renal insufficiency, calcineurin inhibitors may be delayed by intention, and these globulin-mediated immunosuppressant agents may provide a bridge until improved renal function permits conventional agents. Sirolimus has also been used in renal protective protocols but has limited use in the immediate postoperative period, as it has been associated with hepatic artery thrombosis and impedes wound healing.[61] Because of their inherent neurotoxicity, it is our center's practice not to use either calcineurin-blocking agent until the recipient shows signs of neurological recovery after liver transplantation. This neurotoxicity, characterized by demyelinization of both gray

and white matter, may lead to seizures that are exacerbated by concurrent hypomagnesemia.[62,63]

6. Although occasional patients may be extubated in the operating room, most patients remain on mechanical ventilation during the operative day. Patients without prior lung disease with a well-functioning graft are usually extubated on the first postoperative day as sedation is withdrawn. Patients with delayed graft function should receive mechanical ventilation until signs of improved graft function and mentation occur. Patients with preexisting lung disease, preoperative sedation, or prolonged preoperative ventilator dependency are weaned and extubated as tolerated. Common factors delaying timely extubation include poorly positioned endotracheal tubes, atelectasis, transient diaphragmatic dysmotility, right reactive pleural effusion, fluid overload, and excess sedation. Infants are particularly susceptible to gastric dilatation, and well functioning gastric decompression tubes are essential during positive-pressure ventilation.

7. Narcotic pain medication (fentanyl or morphine) and sedation (short-acting anxiolytics) are essential to the management of the pediatric liver transplant recipient. Most sedation can be discontinued, permitting extubation as discussed earlier. Narcotics are usually required for the first 3 to 4 postoperative days with conversion to nonnarcotic analgesics thereafter. Prolonged narcotic use has been associated with delayed return of gut function and ineffective ventilation and should be avoided.

8. Laboratory monitoring parameters are used to assess graft function, metabolic balance, and adequacy of ventilatory support. Drug levels are monitored after the first 2 postoperative days.

Postoperative Indicators of Graft Function

On transport to the ICU, the patient is monitored for indicators of graft function. The earliest predictor of graft function is the appearance and consistency of the liver after reperfusion in the operative suite.[64] Bile production is commonly observed during the operation as well. Hemodynamic stability with diuresis, good acid-base balance, and signs of neurological recovery are all clinical indicators of good graft function. In patients with elevated intracranial pressure at the time of transplantation, return of neurological function may lag behind other signs of stable graft function. Intracranial pressure monitoring is essential in comatose patients.[28] Abnormalities in coagulation are common in the first

24 to 48 hours after transplantation. We expect to see progressive improvement in coagulation times without the use of plasma infusions. We do not routinely correct abnormalities in coagulation in the absence of bleeding, although supplemental vitamin K should be considered in recipients with chronic cholestatic disease as the indication for liver transplantation. Serum bilirubin levels are a poor initial indicator, as these values are diluted by volume shifts intraoperatively and may actually rise postoperatively despite excellent graft function. Unexpected rises in serum bilirubin may indicate graft congestion, a bile leak, sepsis, drug toxicity, hemolysis, intraperitoneal bleeding, or small-for-size syndrome with reperfusion injury.

Primary nonfunction of the implanted liver has become a rare event in recent years. The surgical team may report a liver with poor color and firm texture at the time of reperfusion. Hemodynamic instability, oliguria, acidosis, persistent coagulopathy, and failure to recover neurological function are signs of graft nonfunction. The grafts at greatest risk are those with advanced steatosis, grafts from elderly donors, and grafts with prolonged ischemic insult, which are rarely used in children.[65,66] Damaged or ischemic livers release aminotransferases, so laboratory results that demonstrate rising hepatic enzyme levels necessitate emergent liver imaging to detect acute arterial thrombosis, which is correctable. We now advocate angiography with thrombolysis and stent placement instead of open revision. Image-guided therapy is more precise for rescuing the hepatic artery, because most early thromboses are caused by intimal flaps rather than anastomotic problems.[49,55] Immediate relisting for urgent retransplantation is indicated.

Hemodynamic Indicators

The postoperative hemodynamics of the recipient are monitored in a number of ways, including routine vital signs by intraarterial catheterization, CVP monitoring, urine output, skin perfusion, and acid-base balance. Pulmonary arterial catheters are rarely used in children. Postoperative hypertension is commonly observed and is likely the result of volume shifts, medications, and discomfort. The preoperative cirrhotic physiology is often indistinguishable from sepsis; it is characterized by low systemic vascular resistance, wide pulse pressure, relative hypotension, and supernormal cardiac output. Asymptomatic bradycardia is a common observation in the early postoperative period and rarely requires intervention. Possible causes include excessive intravascular volume, normalization of preoperative vasodilatory tone, vagal stimulation or injury during transplantation, medications, venous access position, and mechanical ventilation.[67] Antihypertensive agents that do not lower heart rate may therefore be needed in the perioperative period.

Postoperative Indicators of Surgical Complications

Surgical complications can usually be recognized early in the postoperative course while the patient is still in the ICU setting. Early reoperation for bleeding is no longer common but is required in the setting of ongoing blood loss. Postoperative bleeding may be a function of diffuse coagulopathy or a focal bleeding vessel. Management of this postoperative complication is similar in approach to that practiced in nontransplantation abdominal surgery. Initial management consists of correction of clotting anomalies and appropriate volume and blood product resuscitation, with surgery reserved for severe or persistent bleeding.

Early bile leaks are readily detected by bile drainage from the abdominal drains. Because bile leaks may resolve spontaneously, we do not recommend routine immediate surgical exploration. An abdominal sonogram should be performed to exclude an undrained intra-abdominal collection.[68,69] If an intestinal perforation is suspected, reoperation is essential.[70] Anastomotic biliary leaks may have a delayed presentation, as edema may initially mask this event. Perforation of the bowel may also present after the first few days, as steroids and narcotics mask symptoms. Chylous ascites may represent transient disruption of lymphatics but may be an indication of a bowel perforation.[71] Early analysis of ascites for cell count, bilirubin, amylase, and triglycerides often suggests a cause for the finding and will help guide medical and/or surgical intervention. Appropriate drainage of collections and empirical antibacterial and antifungal agents appear prudent.

Postoperative Laboratory Indicators

Elevated aminotransferase levels after pediatric liver transplantation is a common event (Table 59–2). The differential diagnosis for this observation is reperfusion injury, infection, vascular thrombosis, pressure necrosis, medications, and thermal surface injury. Acute cellular rejection in the first few days after liver transplantation is unusual, with the peak incidence around 1 week to 10 days after operation.[3,58] Abdominal ultrasonography with vascular Doppler analysis is essential to evaluate the patency of all hepatic vessels. If the sonogram is inconclusive, more invasive studies, including hepatic angiography or surgical exploration, are indicated.

Table 59–2. DIFFERENTIAL DIAGNOSIS OF POSTOPERATIVE LABORATORY ABNORMALITIES
Elevated aminotransferases
Reperfusion injury
Infection
Vascular thrombosis
Pressure necrosis
Medication reaction
Thermal surface injury
Rejection
Elevated cholestatic enzymes and bilirubin
Reperfusion injury
Biliary leaks
Medication reaction
Infection
Graft congestion
Biliary obstruction
Rejection

Early vascular thrombosis after liver transplantation is a medical emergency that may result in graft loss or severe necrosis. Some patients have been reported to have severe acidosis and hyperkalemia, leading to cardiac arrhythmias.[72,73] Unfortunately, even if the graft can be salvaged after correction of a vascular obstruction, focal or diffuse biliary injury may occur, requiring eventual graft replacement.

Abnormal elevations in cholestatic enzymes, alkaline phosphatase, γ-glutamyltranspeptidase, and bilirubin levels are commonly observed in the posttransplant period (see Table 59–2). These elevations may indicate reperfusion injury, biliary leaks, drug reactions, infection, graft congestion, biliary obstruction, or rejection. In patients with chronic preoperative cholestasis, the serum bilirubin level drops dramatically after transplantation as compared with preoperative values as a result of volume shifts and serum dilution. These values rise in the first few postoperative days as tissue bilirubin is mobilized and intravascular volume normalizes. Imaging is of limited value to assess rises in cholestatic enzyme levels, and liver biopsy is often required to determine the cause in persistent cases.[68,69]

Postoperative Ascites

Ascites after liver transplant surgery is quite common. High drainage output is a direct function of mismatch in overall intake and output of fluids. A cirrhotic renal physiology favors salt and water retention and persists for weeks after liver replacement therapy, predisposing the patient to ascites formation.[52] Patients receiving small-for-size grafts have relative congestion from hyperperfusion and are prone to ascites formation. Relative mismatch of donor and recipient vascular size may also contribute to ascites in the posttransplant period.[44] Chylous ascites was mentioned earlier and may be related to lymphatic disruption or bowel perforation.[71] Bilious ascites always merits investigation to exclude leaks, collections, and bowel disruptions.[74,75] The management of ascites in the postoperative period depends on the underlying cause. The general approach is to limit fluid intake, mobilize fluids with diuretics, and replace protein losses with salt-poor albumin products. Chylous ascites is confirmed by lipid measurements and responds rapidly to fat-restricted diets. Although uncommon, hepatic outflow obstruction can occur, particularly in partial grafts. Hepatic venography with pressure measurements may be indicated for persistent transudative ascites.

Postoperative Fever

Fever in the postoperative period is common. The cause of fever varies with the time from transplantation and is a nonspecific finding. Early fevers are usually the result of pulmonary atelectasis, responding to chest physical therapy, incentive spirometry, and early mobilization from bed. A careful search must be made to exclude bacterial infections, especially in patients with multiple intravenous catheters and drains (Table 59–3). The blood,

sputum, and urine should be cultured to pinpoint infection. The wound should be carefully examined to exclude cellulitis or infected collections. The volume and nature of ascites drainage should be assessed with careful analysis to exclude peritonitis, bile leaks, and bowel perforations. Extremities should be examined to exclude underlying thrombosis in patients with indwelling catheters and in those chronically immobilized. Liver test results should be reviewed to exclude acute cellular rejection and vascular insufficiency. A liver biopsy may need to be performed after sonographic imaging does not clarify the cause of fevers in patients with liver test result anomalies. The skin should be examined for rashes, and the patient's medication list should be reviewed and minimized to exclude drug-induced fevers. The febrile patient with diarrhea should have full stool studies performed, including analysis for CMV infection and *Clostridium difficile*. Empirical therapy with metronidazole should be considered in patients at greatest risk, especially if diarrhea is bloody. Patients with delayed wound closure and a Gore-Tex skin patch should continue to receive antibiotics until wound closure. Common posttransplant infections involve staphylococcal species, enterococci, candidal species, rotavirus, CMV, and respiratory syncytial virus.[6,7,53,76,77]

Postoperative Nutritional Management

Nutritional support is often an important issue in the pretransplantation period. Although the need for specialty formulas may no longer be necessary after successful liver transplantation, certainly the outcomes are affected by continued efforts at nutritional repletion.[11,78,79] Luckily, steroids stimulate excessive oral intake, and the hypermetabolic state improves after transplantation to permit assimilation of calories. In fact, after a period of catch-up growth, parents should be warned to avoid excess calories, as obesity is not uncommon after successful liver transplantation, and this negatively affects overall health. Dietary counseling by the nutritional support staff is crucial to ensuring proper care during this transition period.

The Typical Postoperative Course

The general course for an uncomplicated pediatric liver transplantation is an ICU stay of 24 to 48 hours with termination of mechanical ventilation within 12 to 24 hours of transplantation. Patients are weaned off dopamine after successful extubation, and IV fluids are

Table 59–3. PATTERNS OF INFECTION AFTER LIVER TRANSPLANTATION

Early Infections (Within First 3 Weeks)

Usually involve the urine, blood, wound, or abdomen

Usual organisms

  Gram-negative enterics

  Staphylococcus species

  Enterococcus species

  Candida species

  Clostridium difficile

Late Infections (4 Weeks and Later)

Usually involve the blood, intestine, lungs, or graft

Usual organisms

  Cytomegalovirus

  Epstein-Barr virus

  Adenovirus

  Respiratory syncytial virus

  Rotavirus

  Clostridium difficile

reduced to maintenance rates after 24 hours. Enteral medications are generally started immediately after transplantation as tolerated. Oral feeds are usually started around 6 to 12 hours after extubation and advanced as tolerated to a regular diet within 24 to 48 hours. Most medications are delivered enterally, with the exception of antibiotics, initial steroids, and ganciclovir. The patients receive physical therapy, feeding therapy, and pulmonary therapy to stimulate early ambulation and mobilization from bed to avoid unnecessary postoperative complications. Patients remain in private rooms without isolation during their initial hospitalization. Recipients and their families are educated about medication administration and side effects. After stable liver function test results and medication levels are achieved, when the patients can enterally nourish and hydrate themselves, and when they are comfortable and mobile enough to function, they are discharged to home with weekly outpatient follow-up. The median length of stay should be about 7 to 10 days for uncomplicated transplant procedures. Laboratory test results are checked on a weekly basis and more frequently if indicated. Sutures are removed 3 weeks after transplantation. Growth and development are monitored closely in the outpatient setting. Medications are tapered according to center protocol, with most patients on monotherapy by 1 year after transplantation. Investigations for fever and abnormal liver test results are performed as outlined earlier. Live vaccines are prohibited until the patient is on monotherapy for at least 6 months. All care is coordinated among the transplant team, the family, and the patient's primary care physician. Late complications such as biliary strictures and posttransplant lymphoproliferative disorder are always assessed at each encounter and with periodic laboratory analysis.

Pearls and Pitfalls

Know your patient's pretransplant state to anticipate postoperative needs.
- Keep communication between members of the care team open.
- Acidosis is an ominous perioperative sign.
- Unexplained liver test elevations early suggest a vascular occlusion.
- Avoid unnecessary renal-toxic medications, including aminoglycosides and nonsteroidal antiinflammatory agents.
- Posttransplant patients can have acetaminophen if needed.
- Avoid fluid overload after liver transplantation.

Pearls and Pitfalls—cont'd

- Approximately 10% of pediatric liver transplant patients require early postoperative exploration.
- Just because some immunosuppression is good, does not mean that more is better.
- Know your drug-drug interactions.
- Late bile duct obstructions can present insidiously and are frequently missed by noninvasive studies.
- Patients do not always do what you tell them to do.
- Liver transplantation is not an experiment, but it does remain a high-risk sport.

References

1. Emond JC: What's new in transplantation. J Am Coll Surg 194:636-641, 2002.
2. Emre S: Living-donor liver transplantation in children. Pediatr Transplant 6:43-46, 2002.
3. Rand EB, Olthoff KM: Overview of pediatric liver transplantation. Gastroenterol Clin North Am 32:913-929, 2003.
4. McDiarmid SV: Management of the pediatric liver transplant patient. Liver Transpl 7:S77-S86, 2001.
5. Lichtor JL, Emond J, Chung MR, et al: Pediatric orthotopic liver transplantation: Multifactorial predictions of blood loss. Anesthesiology 68:607-611, 1988.
6. Their M, Holmberg C, Lautenschlager I, et al: Infections in pediatric kidney and liver transplant patients after perioperative hospitalization. Transplantation 69:1617-1623, 2000.
7. Bouchut JC, Stamm D, Boillot O, et al: Postoperative infectious complications in paediatric liver transplantation: A study of 48 transplants. Paediatr Anaesth 11:93-98, 2001.
8. Balistreri WF: Transplantation for childhood liver disease: An overview. Liver Transpl Surg 4:S18-S23, 1998.
9. Alonso MH, Ryckman FC: Current concepts in pediatric liver transplant. Semin Liver Dis 18:295-307, 1998.
10. Hasegawa T, Fukui Y, Tanano H, et al: Factors influencing the outcome of liver transplantation for biliary atresia. J Pediatr Surg 32:1548-1551, 1997.
11. McDiarmid SV: Risk factors and outcomes after pediatric liver transplantation. Liver Transpl Surg 2:44-56, 1996.
12. Quak SH: Pre-liver transplantation management of children. Ann Acad Med Singapore 20:534-539, 1991.
13. Emond JC: Living donor liver transplantation in children: What to recommend? Am J Transplant 4:293-294, 2004.
14. Ganschow R, Nolkemper D, Helmke K, et al: Intensive care management after pediatric liver transplantation: A single-center experience. Pediatr Transplant 4:273-279, 2000.
15. Whitington PF, Emond JC, Black DD, et al: Indications for liver transplantation in pediatric patients. Clin Transplant 5:155-160, 1991.
16. Cohran VC, Heubi JE: Treatment of pediatric cholestatic liver disease. Curr Treat Options Gastroenterol 6:403-415, 2003.
17. Carmi R, Magee CA, Neill CA, et al: Extrahepatic biliary atresia and associated anomalies: Etiological heterogeneity suggested by distinctive patterns of associations. Am J Med Genet 45:683-693, 1993.
18. Kataria R, Kataria A, Gupta D: Spectrum of congenital anomalies associated with biliary atresia. Indian J Pediatr 63:651-654, 1996.

19. Chen F, Ananthanarayanan M, Emre S, et al: Progressive familial intrahepatic cholestasis, type 1, is associated with decreased farnesoid X receptor activity. Gastroenterology 126:756-764, 2004.

20. van Mil SW, Klomp LW, Bull LN, et al: FIC1 disease: A spectrum of intrahepatic cholestatic disorders. Semin Liver Dis 21:535-544, 2001.

21. Narumi S, Roberts JP, Emond JC, et al: Liver transplantation for sclerosing cholangitis. Hepatology 22:451-457, 1995.

22. Garcia S, Ruza F, Gonzalez M, et al: Evolution and complications in the immediate postoperative period after pediatric liver transplantation: Our experience with 176 transplantations. Transplant Proc 31:1691-695, 1999.

23. Kelly DA: Nutritional factors affecting growth before and after liver transplantation. Pediatr Transplant 1:80-84, 1997.

24. Ascher NL, Lake JR, Emond JC, et al: Liver transplantation for fulminant hepatic failure. Arch Surg 128:677-682, 1993.

25. Daas M, Plevak DJ, Wijdicks EF, et al: Acute liver failure: Results of a 5-year clinical protocol. Liver Transpl Surg 1:210-219, 1995.

26. Jalan R: Intracranial hypertension in acute liver failure: Pathophysiological basis of rational management. Semin Liver Dis 23:271-282, 2003.

27. Blei AT, Olafsson S, Webster S, et al: Complications of intracranial pressure monitoring in fulminant hepatic failure. Lancet 341:157-158, 1993.

28. Keays R, Potter D, O'Grady J, et al: Intracranial and cerebral perfusion pressure changes before, during, and immediately after orthotopic liver transplantation for fulminant hepatic failure. QJM 79:425-433, 1991.

29. Matern D, Starzl TE, Arnaout W, et al: Liver transplantation for glycogen storage disease types I, III, and IV. Eur J Pediatr 158:S43-S48, 1999.

30. Whitington PF, Alonso EM, Boyle JT, et al: Liver transplantation for the treatment of urea cycle disorders. J Inherit Metab Dis 21:112-118, 1998.

31. Peeters PM, Sieders E, De Jong KP, et al: Comparison of outcome after pediatric liver transplantation for metabolic diseases and biliary atresia. Eur J Pediatr Surg 11:28-35, 2001.

32. Ghishan FK, Greene HL: Liver disease in children with PiZZ alpha 1-antitrypsin deficiency. Hepatology 8:307-310, 1988.

33. Bertolani MF, Pellegrino AM, Summa C, et al: [Tyrosinosis. A difficult diagnosis of late infancy]. Minerva Pediatr 42:1-7, 1990.

34. Hasegawa T, Tzakis AG, Todo S, et al: Orthotopic liver transplantation for ornithine transcarbamylase deficiency with hyperammonemic encephalopathy. J Pediatr Surg 30:863-865, 1995.

35. Muiesan P, Rela M, Kane P, et al: Liver transplantation for neonatal haemochromatosis. Arch Dis Child Fetal Neonatal Ed 73:F178-180, 1995.

36. Durand P, Debray D, Mandel R, et al: Acute liver failure in infancy: A 14-year experience of a pediatric liver transplantation center. J Pediatr 139:871-876, 2001.

37. Kim SZ, Kupke KG, Ierardi-Curto L, et al: Hepatocellular carcinoma despite long-term survival in chronic tyrosinaemia I. J Inherit Metab Dis 23:791-804, 2000.

38. Deshpande RR, Rela M, Girlanda R, et al: Long-term outcome of liver retransplantation in children. Transplantation 74:1124-1130, 2002.

39. Broelsch CE, Emond JC, Whitington PF, et al: Application of reduced-size liver transplants as split grafts, auxiliary orthotopic grafts, and living related segmental transplants. Ann Surg 212:368-375, 1990.

40. Emond JC: Clinical application of liver-related liver transplantation. Gastroenterol Clin North Am 22:301-315, 1993.

41. Guarrera JV, Emond JC: Advances in segmental liver transplantation: Can we solve the donor shortage? Transplant Proc 33:3451-3455, 2001.

42. Renz JF, Yersiz H, Reichert PR, et al: Split-liver transplantation: A review. Am J Transplant 3:1323-1335, 2003.

43. Renz JF, Emond JC, Yersiz H, et al: Split-liver transplantation in the United States: Outcomes of a national survey. Ann Surg 239:172-181, 2004.

44. Emond JC, Heffron TG, Whitington PF, et al: Reconstruction of the hepatic vein in reduced size hepatic transplantation. Surg Gynecol Obstet 176:11-17, 1993.

45. Emond JC: Liver transplantation in children: Advances in patient selection, technique, and immunosuppression. Zhonghua Min Guo Xiao Er Ke Yi 38:249-254, 1997.

46. Reichert PR, Renz JF, Rosenthal P, et al: Biliary complications of reduced-organ liver transplantation. Liver Transpl Surg 4:343-349, 1998.

47. Renz JF, Reichert PR, Emond JC: Biliary anatomy as applied to pediatric living donor and split-liver transplantation. Liver Transpl 6:801-804, 2000.

48. Stevens LH, Emond JC, Piper JB, et al: Hepatic artery thrombosis in infants. A comparison of whole livers, reduced-size grafts, and grafts from living-related donors. Transplantation 53:396-399, 1992.

49. Dalgic A, Dalgic B, Demirogullari B, et al: Clinical approach to graft hepatic artery thrombosis following living related liver transplantation. Pediatr Transplant 7:149-52, 2003.

50. Emond JC, Rosenthal P, Roberts JP, et al: Living related donor liver transplantation: The UCSF experience. Transplant Proc 28:2375-2377, 1996.

51. Jain A, Mazariegos G, Kashyap R, et al: Pediatric liver transplantation in 808 consecutive children: 20-years experience from a single center. Transplant Proc 34:1955-1957, 2002.

52. McCormick PA, McIntyre N: Pathogenesis and management of ascites in chronic liver disease. Br J Hosp Med 47:738-744, 1992.

53. George DL, Arnow PM, Fox A, et al: Patterns of infection after pediatric liver transplantation. Am J Dis Child 146:924-929, 1992.

54. Couchoud C, Cucherat M, Haugh M, et al: Cytomegalovirus prophylaxis with antiviral agents in solid organ transplantation: A meta-analysis. Transplantation 65:641-647, 1998.

55. Heffron TG, Pillen T, Welch D, et al: Hepatic artery thrombosis in pediatric liver transplantation. Transplant Proc 35:1447-1448, 2003.

56. Wolf DC, Freni MA, Boccagni P, et al: Low-dose aspirin therapy is associated with few side effects but does not prevent hepatic artery thrombosis in liver transplant recipients. Liver Transpl Surg 3:598-603, 1997.

57. Mazzaferro V, Esquivel CO, Makowka L, et al: Hepatic artery thrombosis after pediatric liver transplantation—a medical or surgical event? Transplantation 47:971-977, 1989.

58. Renz JF, Lightdale J, Mudge C, et al: Mycophenolate mofetil, microemulsion cyclosporine, and prednisone as primary immunosuppression for pediatric liver transplant recipients. Liver Transpl Surg 5:136-43, 1999.

59. Reding R, Gras J, Sokal E, et al: Steroid-free liver transplantation in children. Lancet 362:2068-2070, 2003.

60. Eason JD, Nair S, Cohen AJ, et al: Steroid-free liver transplantation using rabbit antithymocyte globulin and early tacrolimus monotherapy. Transplantation 75:1396-1399, 2003.

61. Trotter JF: Sirolimus in liver transplantation. Transplant Proc 35(3 Suppl):193S-200S, 2003.

62. McDiarmid SV: Liver transplantation. The pediatric challenge. Clin Liver Dis 4:879-927, 2000.

63. Ghaus N, Bohlega S, Rezeig M: Neurological complications in liver transplantation. J Neurol 248:1042-1048, 2001.

64. Sano K, Makuuchi M, Takayama T, et al: Technical dilemma in living-donor or split-liver transplant. Hepatogastroenterology 47:1208-1209, 2000.

65. Maring JK, Klompmaker IJ, Zwaveling JH, et al: Poor initial graft function after orthotopic liver transplantation: Can it be predicted and does it affect outcome? An analysis of 125 adult primary transplantations. Clin Transplant 11:373-379, 1997.

66. Hwang S, Lee SG, Lee YJ, et al: A case of primary non-function following adult-to-adult living donor liver transplantation. Hepatogastroenterology 49:1412-1414, 2002.

67. McDonnell N, Ames WA, Potter D: Bradycardia in children less than two years of age during liver transplantation. Transpl Int 11:237-238, 1998.

68. Peh WC, Olliff SP: The role of the radiologist in liver transplantation. Ann Acad Med Singapore 22:688-695, 1993.

69. Griffith JF, John PR: Imaging of biliary complications following paediatric liver transplantation. Pediatr Radiol 26:388-394, 1996.

70. Renz JF, Rosenthal P, Roberts JP, et al: Planned exploration of pediatric liver transplant recipients reduces posttransplant morbidity and lowers length of hospitalization. Arch Surg 132:950-956, 1997.

71. Gaglio PJ, Leevy CB, Koneru B: Peri-operative chylous ascites. J Med 27:369-376, 1996.

72. Kaku R, Matsumi M, Fujii H, et al: [A case of severe acute hyperkalemia during pre-anhepatic stage in living-related liver transplantation]. Masui 51:1003-1006, 2002.

73. Acosta F, Sansano T, Contreras RF, et al: Changes in serum potassium during reperfusion in liver transplantation. Transplant Proc 31:2382-2383, 1999.

74. Egawa H, Inomata Y, Uemoto S, et al: Biliary anastomotic complications in 400 living related liver transplantations. World J Surg 25:1300-1307, 2001.

75. Egawa H, Uemoto S, Inomata Y, et al: Biliary complications in pediatric living related liver transplantation. Surgery 124:901-910, 1998.

76. George DL, Arnow PM, Fox AS, et al: Bacterial infection as a complication of liver transplantation: Epidemiology and risk factors. Rev Infect Dis 13:387-396, 1991.

77. Gladdy RA, Richardson SE, Davies HD, et al: Candida infection in pediatric liver transplant recipients. Liver Transpl Surg 5:16-24, 1999.

78. Amii LA, Moss RL: Nutritional support of the pediatric surgical patient. Curr Opin Pediatr 11:237-240, 1999.

79. Hade AM, Shine AM, Kennedy NP, et al: Both under-nutrition and obesity increase morbidity following liver transplantation. Ir Med J 96:140-142, 2003.

Renal Failure in Adult Liver Transplant Recipients

PHUONG-THU T. PHAM
PHUONG-CHI T. PHAM
ALAN H. WILKINSON

Assessment of renal function in end-stage liver disease patients awaiting liver transplantation 892

Causes of renal failure before orthotopic liver transplantation 892
  Renal failure as an entity independent of the cause of end-stage liver disease 892
  Renal failure as part of the disease entity associated with end-stage liver disease 895
  Renal failure as a consequence of end-stage liver disease 895

Electrolyte abnormalities and intraoperative hemodynamic changes in end-stage liver disease patients undergoing orthotopic liver transplantation 900
  Fluid and electrolyte abnormalities 900
  Acid-base disturbances 902
  Intraoperative risk factors for the development of acute renal dysfunction in end-stage liver disease patients undergoing orthotopic liver transplantation 903

Factors affecting posttransplant renal function 903
  Cyclosporine and tacrolimus nephrotoxicity 904
  Drug interactions 905

Impact of acute renal failure or renal insufficiency on patient and allograft outcome in orthotopic liver transplantation 906

Combined kidney-liver transplantation 907
  Indications 907
  Early experience 907
  Disease-specific indications 908

Outcome in patients with hepatorenal syndrome after liver-alone transplantation 909

Summary 910

Orthotopic liver transplantation (OLT) is a well-established definitive treatment for patients with chronic advanced cirrhosis or acute fulminant hepatic failure and a viable therapeutic option for those with primary resectable hepatic malignancies with or without cirrhosis. Over the past 4 to 5 years, an average of 4945 such transplants were performed in the United States annually.[1] Whereas the demand for liver transplantation has steadily increased, the supply of deceased donor organs has remained relatively constant. As a result, an increasing percentage of wait-listed patients either died or suffered various complications while awaiting transplantation. The pretransplant evaluation process therefore requires careful and continued assessment of the patient's pulmonary, cardiac, and renal function. This chapter describes a systematic approach to the evaluation of renal dysfunction and electrolyte and acid-base disturbances complicating the course of advanced liver disease, the pathogenic mechanisms and current recommendations for treatment of hepatorenal syndrome (HRS), and the indications for combined liver-kidney transplantation (CLKT). Renal dysfunction of diverse causes continues to be an important source of morbidity and mortality in both the immediate and long-term postoperative period. The potential intraoperative and perioperative factors contributing to postoperative renal failure, the long-term consequences of renal insufficiency after transplantation, and the impact of renal insufficiency on ultimate allograft and patient survival are also reviewed.

Assessment of Renal Function in End-Stage Liver Disease Patients Awaiting Liver Transplantation

Early recognition of renal dysfunction in patients with end-stage liver disease (ESLD) can be challenging inasmuch as assessment of renal function based on the serum creatinine level or estimation of the glomerular filtration rate (GFR) by creatinine-based equations (e.g., the Cockcroft-Gault formula) has been shown to overestimate the true GFR to variable degrees in this patient population. Reduced muscle mass, a protein-poor diet, severe hyperbilirubinemia, and diminished hepatic biosynthesis of creatine, a substrate for skeletal muscle production of creatinine, can all contribute to a falsely low serum creatinine level. In addition, volume overload from aggressive fluid administration in hypotensive patients may cause a dilutional effect that normalizes the measured serum creatinine concentration.[2] Similar to patients with chronic kidney disease of other causes, cirrhotic patients with renal insufficiency have a relatively increased ratio of tubular creatinine secretion to filtration when compared with those who have normal renal function. Consequently, serum creatinine is falsely low in the setting of renal impairment, and assessment of renal function with creatinine-based equations leads to overestimation of GFR. In a study to assess renal function in cirrhotic patients, Carego and colleagues found that patients with inulin clearance less than 80 mL/min had significantly greater fractions of creatinine excreted through tubular secretion than did cirrhotic patients with normal renal function (0.53 ± 0.39 versus 0.28 ± 0.22, respectively, $P < .05$).[3] Using inulin clearance as the gold standard for evaluation of GFR, the authors demonstrated that the serum creatinine level, predicted

GFR (based on the Cockcroft-Gault formula), and creatinine clearance had a sensitivity of 18.5%, 51%, and 74%, respectively, in detecting renal failure in 55 consecutive stable cirrhotic patients. Papadakis and Arieff reported a mean 200% overestimation of GFR by creatinine clearance in 13 cirrhotic patients with reduced GFR.[4] It has been suggested that more severe renal impairment may have accounted for a greater difference between creatinine clearance and inulin clearance in the series of Papadakis and Arieff than in that of Carego and coworkers. Independent investigators have shown that the discrepancy between creatinine and inulin clearance is greater in patients with impaired than in those with normal renal function.[5] Ideally, the GFR in ESLD patients should be measured by inulin clearance or by studies using radioisotopes such as ^{125}I-iothalamate or chromium 51-ethylenediaminetetraacetic acid (^{51}Cr-EDTA).

The second challenge in the management of renal failure in ESLD patients is diagnosing the cause of the renal dysfunction. Besides the subset of patients with simultaneous kidney-liver diseases, almost all ESLD patients are commonly exposed to therapies and clinical circumstances that place them at high risk for renal failure. ESLD patients are frequently exposed to multiple renal insults, including invasive diagnostic procedures, multiple imaging studies requiring nephrotoxic dyes, nephrotoxic medications, urinary tract manipulations causing recurrent urinary tract infection and obstruction, and therapies leading to volume depletion and subsequent prerenal renal failure.[2] The differential diagnosis of renal failure in ESLD patients is not infrequently made more complicated by the potential development of the well-described entity HRS. Despite the challenge involved, determination of the cause of renal failure is necessary for short-term management, determination of prognosis and long-term survival, and evaluation for CLKT.

Causes of Renal Failure before Orthotopic Liver Transplantation

Renal Failure As an Entity Independent of the Cause of End-Stage Liver Disease

Similar to patients without liver disease, the causes of renal failure in ESLD patients can be classified as prerenal, intrinsic renal, and postrenal renal failure. The initial evaluation should include a complete history and thorough chart review focusing on the recent use of nephrotoxic medications, imaging studies using contrast agents, excessive use of diuretics or large-volume paracentesis, and evidence of renal or gastrointestinal fluid loss. Physical examination should focus on volume status; sources of fluid loss, including insensible

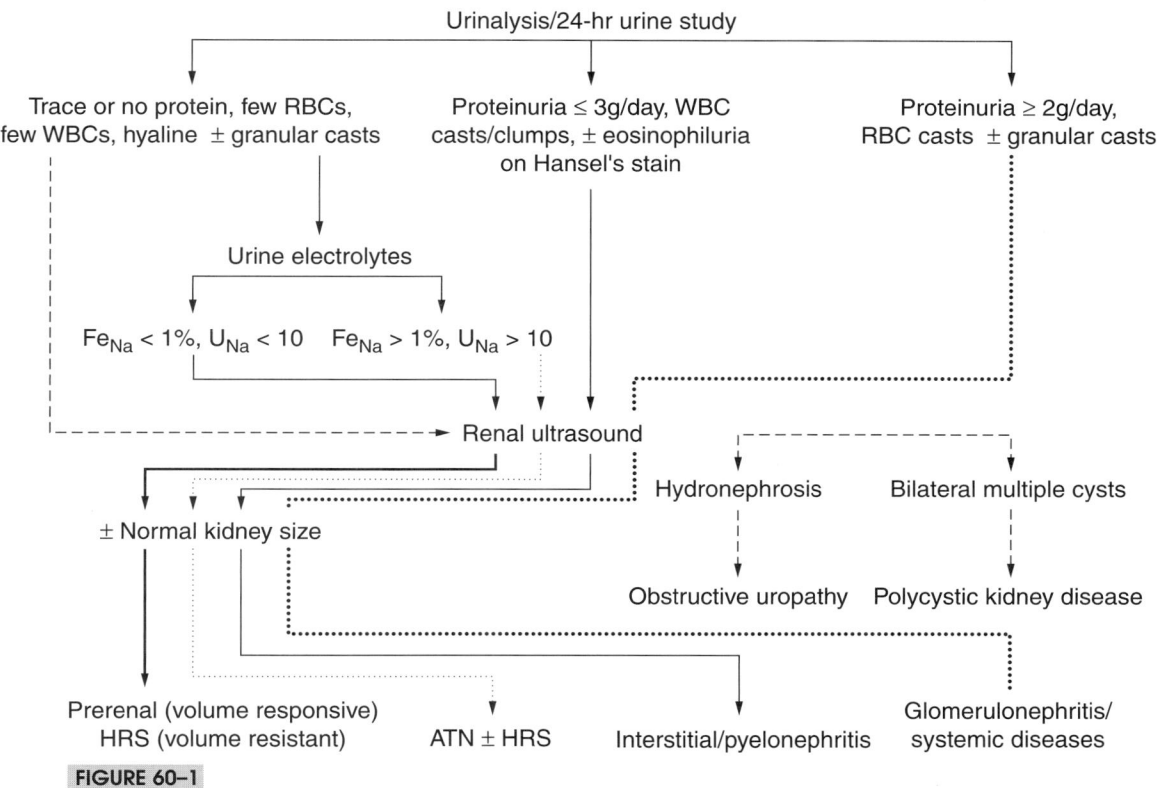

FIGURE 60-1

Overview of renal failure workup in patients with end-stage liver disease. ATN, acute tubular necrosis; HRS, hepatorenal syndrome; RBCs, red blood cells; WBCs, white blood cells. (Adapted from Pham PT, Pham PC, Wilkinson AH: The kidney in liver transplantation. Clin Liver Dis 4:567-590, 2000.)

fluid loss; possible urinary tract obstruction; and Foley catheter patency. Laboratory studies should include routine urinalysis, urine electrolytes, a urine eosinophil count, a complete serum electrolyte panel, and renal ultrasound (Fig. 60–1).[2] Although prerenal and postrenal renal failure can often be diagnosed on clinical grounds or imaging studies, or both, intrinsic renal failure can be difficult to diagnose clinically. A kidney biopsy may be recommended when the renal diagnosis is obscure or the degree of irreversibility of renal failure cannot be determined from clinical and laboratory evidence. For patients in whom severe coagulopathy makes percutaneous core needle biopsy unsafe, either a transjugular venous approach or an open kidney biopsy may be considered.

Prerenal Renal Failure

Prerenal renal failure in ESLD patients is frequently multifactorial and may be due to true volume depletion, drug-associated preglomerular-type renal dysfunction, or decreased effective arterial blood volume and sustained hypotension (or any combination of these processes). Examples of true volume depletion include variceal bleeding, decreased food or fluid intake because of early satiety from distended ascites, excessive use of diuretics, and diarrhea caused by lactulose. Commonly used drugs that may potentially precipitate acute preglomerular-type renal dysfunction include contrast dye, nonsteroidal anti-inflammatory drugs (NSAIDs) and selective cyclo-oxygenase-2 (COX-2) inhibitors, angiotensin-converting enzyme inhibitors, and angiotensin receptor blockers.[2,6] Decreased effective arterial blood volume and decreased arterial pressure may be seen in severe sepsis or HRS. The proposed pathogenic mechanism or mechanisms of HRS and its treatment options are discussed in a later section.

Intrinsic Renal Failure

Intrinsic causes of acute renal failure (ARF) may be classified according to the primary site of injury, including the tubules, interstitium, glomerulus, and small intrarenal vessels. Although data on the incidence of the different types of acute intrinsic renal failure in ESLD patients are limited, small-vessel vascular causes of ARF are uncommon. The United Network for Organ Sharing (UNOS) Organ Procurement and Transplantation Network (OPTN) database revealed that over a 4-year period from May 1, 1999, to March 31, 2003, only 1 of

595 combined kidney-liver transplants (0.17%) was performed for the renal diagnosis of hemolytic-uremic syndrome and 1 for progressive systemic sclerosis (0.17%) (Table 60–1). Interestingly however, hypertensive nephrosclerosis accounted for 4.20% (25 of 595) and malignant hypertension for an additional 0.67% (4 of 595) of combined kidney-liver transplantations (CKLTs) performed.

Acute injury to the renal tubules leading to acute tubular necrosis (ATN) may be ischemic or toxic in origin. The former is frequently due to sustained prerenal renal failure and the latter to the use of nephrotoxic drugs such as amphotericin B or aminoglycoside antibiotics. In a multivariate logistic regression analysis, Hampel and associates have shown that in hospitalized cirrhotic patients, aminoglycoside treatment was a strong risk factor for renal dysfunction, independent of the severity of liver disease or peritonitis.[7] However, in critically ill patients such as those with septic shock, ATN is commonly due to a combination of ischemic injury and the use of nephrotoxins.

ARF caused by acute interstitial nephritis is often due to drug-induced hypersensitivity reactions. Potential and common offending agents include sulfa drugs, oxacillin, nafcillin, ciprofloxacin, levofloxacin, cephalosporins, NSAIDs, and diuretics, including hydrochlorothiazide, furosemide, triamterene, and ethacrynic acid. The UNOS database revealed that between May 1, 1999, and March 31, 2003, 4 of 595 (0.67%) CKLTs were performed for the renal diagnosis of drug-related interstitial nephritis (see Table 60–1).

The incidence of glomerulonephritis causing ARF or chronic kidney disease in ESLD is unknown. In a series of 55 patients with liver cirrhosis and coagulopathy who underwent successful transjugular renal biopsy for evaluation of serum creatinine levels higher than 130 μmol/L or proteinuria greater than 0.5 g/day, glomerular lesions were identified in 41 out of 55 patients (74.5%), interstitial lesions in 7 (12.7%), end-stage renal failure in 2 (3.6%), and normal biopsy findings in 5 (9.09%).[8] In a small series consisting of 28 patients with both liver disease and renal abnormalities who underwent successful transjugular renal biopsy (with or without simultaneous liver biopsy), glomerular pathology was found in 15 of 28 (53.6%), tubular pathology in 6 of 28 (21.4%), end-stage renal failure in 2 of 28 (7.1%), nonspecific changes in 1 of 28 (3.6%), and normal renal biopsy findings in 4 of 28 (14.3%). The glomerular lesions included membranoproliferative glomerulonephritis in 5, nephrosclerosis in 3, diabetic nephropathy in 2, IgA nephropathy in 2, minimal change disease in 2, and early glomerulosclerosis in 1.[9] For CLKT recipients, the glomerular diagnoses reported to UNOS in order of decreasing frequency included diabetic nephropathy, unspecified chronic glomerulonephritis, membranous glomerulonephropathy, IgA nephropathy, mesangiocapillary glomerulonephritis type 1, idiopathic or postinfectious glomerulonephritis, chronic glomerulosclerosis, and focal glomerulosclerosis (see Table 60–1).

Postrenal Renal Failure

Postrenal renal failure is not commonly recognized in ESLD patients (see Table 60–1). Despite its low incidence, obstructive uropathy develops in ESLD patients at a frequency that is at least similar to that in the general population, and it may be functional or anatomic in nature. The former can be caused by a neurogenic bladder or anticholinergic drugs, whereas the latter may be due to recurrent urinary tract instrumentation with associated blood clots, kidney stones, prostatic hypertrophy,

Table 60–1. NUMBER OF TRANSPLANTS PERFORMED FROM 05/01/1999 TO 03/31/2003 BY KIDNEY PRIMARY DIAGNOSIS ACCORDING TO THE UNOS DATABASE

Kidney Primary Diagnosis	No. of Transplants	% of Transplants
Retransplant/graft failure	70	11.76
Polycystic kidneys	44	7.39
Type 2 IDDM/adult onset	39	6.55
Cyclosporine nephrotoxicity	37	6.22
Hypertensive nephrosclerosis	25	4.20
Type 2 NIDDM/adult onset	24	4.03
Chronic GN, unspecified	18	3.03
Membranous GN/nephropathy	16	2.69
Oxalate nephropathy	16	2.69
Analgesic nephropathy	15	2.52
IgA nephropathy	10	1.68
Malignant hypertension	9	1.51
Acute tubular necrosis	9	1.51
Type 1 IDDM/juvenile onset	7	1.18
Idiopathic/postinfectious GN	4	0.67
Mesangiocapillary GN, type 1	4	0.67
Drug-related interstitial nephritis	4	0.67
Chronic glomerulosclerosis, unspecified	3	0.50
Focal glomerulosclerosis	2	0.34
Acquired obstructive uropathy	1	0.17
Progressive systemic sclerosis	1	0.17
Hemolytic-uremic syndrome	1	0.17
Miscellaneous	31	5.23
Kidney diagnosis not reported	205	34.45
Total	595	100.00

GN, glomerulonephritis; IDDM, insulin-dependent diabetes mellitus; NIDDM, non-insulin-dependent diabetes mellitus; UNOS, United Network for Organ Sharing.

or even papillary necrosis.[2] Bladder catheterization and renal ultrasound are readily available and should be performed in all patients with ARF. Prompt diagnosis and management of obstructive uropathy are of prognostic significance, since the likelihood for recovery of renal function decreases with the duration of obstruction.

Renal Failure as Part of the Disease Entity Associated with End-Stage Liver Disease

Renal failure may be a manifestation of the same systemic disease responsible for the liver disease, or it may develop as a direct complication of the disease affecting the liver. In addition, there are different glomerulopathies that are secondarily associated with specific types of liver disease through either immunological or undetermined causes. Broad categories of conditions or diseases affecting both the liver and kidney include infections, toxins, collagen vascular diseases, generalized vascular dysfunction, adult polycystic kidney disease, congenital diseases, neoplasms, and metabolic disorders.[2] Other disease processes that may involve both the liver and kidney include hemochromatosis, ulcerative colitis, and toxemia of pregnancy. Table 60–2 lists the diseases or conditions known to affect both the liver and kidney that are commonly encountered in candidates for OLT and CKLT. For a more extensive review of the glomerular and interstitial diseases associated with liver disease, readers are referred to an article by Davis and colleagues.[10]

Renal Failure as a Consequence of End-Stage Liver Disease

Hepatorenal Syndrome

Also known as functional renal failure secondary to ESLD, HRS was first described by Austin Flint in 1863 in a clinical analysis of 46 cases.[11] In a 1993 study, Gines and coauthors estimated the incidence of HRS in non-azotemic cirrhotic patients with ascites to be 18% at 1 year and 39% at 5 years.[12] Although its pathogenesis is complex, HRS has long been recognized to be reversible with a well-functioning orthotopic liver transplant. Depending on the duration and severity of HRS, however, the reversibility of HRS after liver transplantation is usually delayed and incomplete.

Definition, Clinical Features, and Diagnosis

HRS can be qualitatively defined as impaired renal function that occurs in patients with chronic advanced or acute liver failure secondary to intense renal vasoconstriction and concomitant extrarenal arterial vasodilation.[2] Over the years, diagnosing HRS has been a challenge for clinicians because it has traditionally

Table 60–2. DISEASES OR CONDITIONS COMMONLY ENCOUNTERED IN ORTHOTOPIC LIVER TRANSPLANT AND COMBINED KIDNEY-LIVER TRANSPLANT CANDIDATES THAT ARE KNOWN TO AFFECT BOTH THE LIVER AND KIDNEY

Chronic Liver Cirrhosis	Associated Renal Disease
Parenchymal Liver Disease	
Hepatitis B	MGN, MPGN, PAN
Hepatitis C	MPGN, MGN, fibrillary GN, immunotactoid GN, IgA nephropathy, postinfectious GN
Alcoholic cirrhosis	IgA nephropathy, hepatic sclerosis
Autoimmune hepatitis	Immune complex GN, RTA
Primary Cholestatic Disease	
Primary biliary cirrhosis	MGN, ANCA-positive vasculitis, RTA
Cryptogenic cirrhosis	IgA nephropathy, hepatic sclerosis
Vascular Disease	
Budd-Chiari syndrome	Metastatic renal cell carcinoma
Acute Fulminant Hepatic Failure	
Viral hepatitis (HBV, HCV)	
Drug induced (acetaminophen, halothane)	
Metabolic liver disease (Reye's syndrome)	
Inborn Error of Metabolism	
Glycogen storage disease type 1	Focal glomerulosclerosis
α_1-Antitrypsin deficiency	MPGN, anti-GBM disease
Wilson's disease	Fanconi syndrome
Miscellaneous	
Polycystic liver disease	Polycystic kidney disease
Primary hyperoxaluria type I	Interstitial fibrosis

ANCA, antineutrophil cytoplasmic antibody; GBM, glomerular basement membrane; GN, glomerulonephritis; HBV, hepatitis B virus; HCV, hepatitis C virus; MGN, membranous glomerulonephritis; MPGN, membranoproliferative glomerulonephritis; PAN, polyarteritis nodosa; RTA, renal tubular acidosis.

been classified as a diagnosis of exclusion. In 1990, the International Ascites Club (IAC) met in Florence, Italy, to focus on research involving the mechanisms of circulatory and renal dysfunction in liver disease and the pathogenesis and treatment of ascites, HRS, and spontaneous bacterial peritonitis. Representing the spectrum of clinical practice from North America to Europe, the IAC set forth major and minor diagnostic criteria for the diagnosis of HRS that are now widely accepted (Table 60–3).

Based on the IAC definition, HRS "is a clinical condition that occurs in patients with chronic liver disease, advanced hepatic failure, and portal hypertension

Table 60-3. CRITERIA PROPOSED BY THE INTERNATIONAL ASCITES CLUB FOR THE DIAGNOSIS OF HEPATORENAL SYNDROME

Major Criteria

Chronic or acute liver disease with advanced hepatic failure and portal hypertension

Low glomerular filtration rate (serum creatinine > 1.5 mg/dL or 24-hr creatinine clearance < 40 mL/min)

Absence of shock, ongoing bacterial infection, current or recent treatment with nephrotoxic drugs, excessive gastrointestinal or renal fluid losses

No sustained improvement in renal function after diuretic withdrawal and plasma volume expansion with 1.5 L isotonic saline

Proteinuria < 500 mg/dL and no ultrasonographic evidence of obstructive uropathy or parenchymal disease

Minor Criteria

Urine volume < 500 mL/day

Urine sodium < 10 mEq/L

Urine osmolality > plasma osmolality

Urine red blood cells < 50 per high-power field

Serum sodium concentration < 130 mEq/L

Table 60-5. PREDICTIVE VALUE OF DIFFERENT VARIABLES FOR HEPATORENAL SYNDROME

Positive Predictive Value	Negative Predictive Value
Previous episodes of ascites	Age, gender
Liver size*	Etiology: EtOH versus non-EtOH
Poor nutritional status	Abstinence (EtOH)
GFR < 88 mL/min, BUN >15 mg/dL, S_{Cr} >0.9 mg/dL	Previous episodes of GIB, encephalopathy
$S(Na^+)$ < 133 mmol/L,* (K^+) >4 mEq/L	Splenomegaly
U Na^+ excretion	Hepatic stigmata
P_{osm} < 279 mOsm/L	AST, ALT, GGT, bilirubin, albumin
U_{osm} > 553 mOsm/kg	PT, platelet count, WBC
PRA > 3.5 ng/mL/hr*	Urine volume, K^+ excretion
MAP < 85 mm Hg	Child-Pugh score
Free H_2O clearance	Treatment of ascites during 1st hospitalization
Plasma norepinephrine > 544 pg/mL	Protein concentration in ascitic fluid
Esophageal varices	

*Variables that are independent predictors of the development of hepatorenal syndrome on multivariate analysis.

ALT, alanine transaminase; AST, aspartate transaminase; BUN, blood urea nitrogen; EtOH, ethanol; GFR, glomerular filtration rate; GGT, γ-glutamyltransferase; GIB, gastrointestinal bleeding; MAP, mean arterial pressure; PRA, plasma renin activity; PT, prothrombin time; S_{Cr}, serum creatinine; U Na^+, urinary sodium; WBC, white blood cell count.

Adapted from Gines A, Escorsell A, Gines P, et al: Incidence, predictive factors, and prognosis of the hepatorenal syndrome in cirrhosis with ascites. Gastroenterology 105:229-236, 1993.

characterized by impaired renal function and marked abnormalities in the arterial circulation and activity of the endogenous vasoactive systems. In the kidney there is marked renal vasoconstriction that results in a low GFR. In the extrarenal circulation there is predominance of arterial vasodilation that results in reduction of total systemic vascular resistance and arterial hypotension."[13]

To aid in successful multicenter trials, the IAC further classified HRS into types I and II (Table 60-4). Whereas the former includes patients with rapidly progressive renal failure and doubling of serum creatinine to a level greater than 2.5 mg/dL or a reduction in creatinine clearance of greater than 50% within 2 weeks, the latter includes patients with a more moderate or stable reduction in renal function. With advanced liver disease, however, type II HRS may evolve into type I.

A range of variables have been suggested to have positive or negative predictive value for the development of HRS (Table 60-5). In a multivariate analysis, Gines and coworkers have shown that independent predictors of the development of HRS include absence of hepatomegaly,

Table 60-4. SUBTYPES OF HEPATORENAL SYNDROME

Type I	Type II
Doubling of initial serum creatinine to > 2.5 mg/dL or a 50% reduction in initial creatine clearance to < 20 mL/min within 2 wk	Moderate and stable reduction in glomerular filtration rate
	Renal failure does not have a rapidly progressive course

serum sodium concentration less than 133 mEq/L, and plasma renin activity higher than 3.5 ng/mL/hr.[12] An increased resistive index of the renal arcuate and interlobar arteries of greater than 0.7 by Doppler ultrasound has also been suggested to have a positive predictive value for the development of HRS.[14] Interestingly, whereas Gines and colleagues found that neither the cause of liver failure nor the Child-Pugh score had a positive predictive value, Platt and coauthors reported that two major determinants of the Child-Pugh score, total bilirubin ($P <.05$) and prothrombin time ($P <.05$), are independent predictive indicators for HRS.[14]

Pathogenesis

The pathogenesis of ascites formation and HRS is not clearly understood. Nevertheless, three major hypotheses have been proposed, including the "overflow," the "underfilling," and the "peripheral arterial vasodilatation" hypotheses.

The overflow hypothesis is based on a primary increase in portal vascular resistance in which intrahepatic mechanoreceptors sense decreased hepatocyte perfusion and activate a hepatorenal reflex that causes severe renovasoconstriction with associated water and sodium retention, increased circulating blood volume, and, eventually, overflow of fluid into the peritoneal cavity.[15] The underfilling hypothesis suggests that accumulation of blood in the splanchnic circulation and increased splanchnic lymph production are primary defects contributing to decreased effective intravascular volume and associated stimulation of the renin-angiotensin system.[16] The theory of peripheral arterial vasodilatation proposes a primary fall in peripheral vascular resistance with resulting arterial underfilling and associated hyperdynamic circulation and compensatory activation of various vasoconstrictor systems, including renal vasoconstriction with sodium and water retention.[17] Although peripheral vascular resistance may be further decreased and renal vasoconstriction further increased with relatively normal renal function in the compensated state, severe renal vasoconstriction with excess sodium and water retention in the decompensated state results in ascites formation and the development of HRS. Even though the last hypothesis is more popular, all three hypotheses have been challenged by experts in the field.

Management

Survival after the development of HRS (type I) without renal replacement therapy or OLT is generally 2 to 3 weeks.[14,18] Ideally, OLT is the treatment of choice for patients with HRS and ESLD; however, because of the limited supply of deceased donor organs, management of HRS in OLT candidates is restricted to preventive measures and supportive care. The following discussion gives an overview of the literature on the different treatment modalities currently available for ESLD patients with HRS, as well as suggested preventive measures for HRS.

Because HRS is often exacerbated or precipitated by therapies directed at the complications of cirrhosis, any such therapy must be closely monitored. Well-described precipitating factors include large-volume paracentesis without plasma expansion[19,20] and spontaneous bacterial peritonitis. In general, albumin is more effective than artificial plasma expanders in prevention of the circulatory dysfunction associated with large-volume paracentesis. However, not all investigators agree that plasma expansion is necessary during large-volume paracentesis or that paracentesis can precipitate HRS.[2] Gines and colleagues suggested that artificial plasma expanders such as dextran-70 and polygeline are equally effective as albumin when less than 4000 mL of ascitic fluid is removed whereas albumin is more effective than other plasma expanders when larger-volume paracentesis (i.e., >4000 mL) is performed.[21] Recent studies suggest that the risk for development of HRS in the setting of spontaneous bacterial peritonitis may be reduced by the

administration of albumin along with antibiotic therapy[20] whereas in severe alcoholic hepatitis, the incidence of HRS may be lowered by pentoxifylline treatment.[20] Other suggested precipitating factors include intravascular volume depletion secondary to diuretic therapy or lactulose and gastrointestinal bleeding. However, whether the cause of renal failure in patients with gastrointestinal bleeding is due to ATN secondary to hypovolemic shock or due to HRS per se remains a diagnostic challenge. Regardless of the precipitating factors, the use of drugs that can compromise renal perfusion should be avoided, particularly in patients whose preservation of adequate renal perfusion is predominantly "prostaglandin dependent." Implicated drugs include angiotensin-converting enzyme inhibitors, angiotensin receptor blockers, NSAIDs, and selective COX-2 inhibitors. Finally, the use of nephrotoxic drugs should be carefully weighed against the risk for development of ARF. It has been suggested that the risk for aminoglycoside nephrotoxicity is 10-fold higher in cirrhotic patients than in the general population.[22]

Nontransplant management of HRS in OLT candidates has included the use of a transjugular intrahepatic portosystemic shunt (TIPS), vasoactive agents, and the molecular adsorbent recirculating system (MARS). The choice of therapy may be dictated by the severity of liver failure and the availability of different treatment modalities.

TIPS placement has been designed to divert portal blood flow to the hepatic vein, thereby redistributing splanchnic and portal blood centrally and effectively improving both variceal bleeding and renal perfusion.[23] Clinically, TIPS has been shown to increase urinary sodium excretion[24-26] and, in some studies,[26] has led to improvement in renal function and a reduction in the de novo development of HRS or conversion from type II to type I.[27] In selected patients with type I HRS, a median survival of 2 to 4 months has been achieved with this procedure.[20] Limitations of TIPS placement, however, include worsening of liver function and hepatic encephalopathy.[23] For these reasons, TIPS is generally reserved for patients with Child-Pugh class B or early C status.

For patients with more advanced liver disease, treatment with vasoactive agents has resulted in different degrees of success. A variety of vasoactive agents have been used in the treatment of HRS and include renal vasodilators such as saralasin, dopamine, misoprostol, and endothelin-A antagonists or splanchnic vasoconstrictors such as octapressin, ornipressin, terlipressin, and octreotide (or various combinations of these drugs) (Table 60–6).

The use of saralasin, an angiotensinogen antagonist, has been shown to only worsen systemic hypotension without improving renal function.[28] Similar to saralasin, "renal-dose dopamine" has been shown to be of no

Table 60–6. VASOACTIVE MEDICAL TREATMENT

Renal Vasodilators	Splanchnic Vasoconstrictors
Saralasin	Octapressin
Dopamine	Ornipressin
Misoprostol	Terlipressin
Endothelin-A antagonist	Midodrine + octreotide

benefit in patients with HRS.[29] Misoprostol, a synthetic prostaglandin E_1 analogue, has also been used in an attempt to reverse renal vasoconstriction in HRS. Although low doses of misoprostol are vasodilatory, natriuretic, and diuretic, a literature review has revealed that none of the five studies that investigated misoprostol for HRS seem to indicate a substantial benefit.[30-33] Improvement in renal function occurred in one study in which volume expansion was also used. Because endothelin-1 has been proposed to play a role in both renal and hepatic vasoconstriction in HRS, the use of endothelin antagonists has also been suggested to ameliorate HRS. In a small study involving three patients, Soper and coauthors reported dose-dependent renal improvement during treatment with the endothelin-A antagonist BQ123. No deleterious systemic hemodynamic changes were observed during the study, but all three patients subsequently died.[34] Table 60–7 summarizes the mechanism of actions of various renal vasodilators and the outcome associated with their use.

The rationale for the use of splanchnic vasoconstrictors is the reduction in splanchnic organ blood flow and resultant reduction in portal blood flow and pressure. The splanchnic vasoconstrictors octapressin, ornipressin, and terlipressin are vasopressin synthetic analogues with decreased antidiuretic properties. Octapressin, when infused at low doses (0.002 to 0.004 U/min), produced an increase in renal blood flow with an associated decrease in renal vascular resistance. At higher doses, however, renal vascular resistance increased significantly,

Table 60–7. RENAL VASODILATORS

Drug	Mechanisms	Outcome
Saralasin	Angiotensinogen antagonist	Hypotension
		No improvement
Dopamine	↑ Renal perfusion	↑ Complications
	↓ Na^+ reabsorption	No benefit
Misoprostol	Synthetic prostaglandin E_1	No benefit (4/5 studies)
BQ123	Endothelin-A antagonist	Improvement in 3 patients

and changes in renal blood flow diminished. In an earlier study involving 11 patients, only 4 of 5 patients who had a systemic improvement in blood pressure greater than 5 mm Hg had improvement in renal perfusion. The drug appeared to work only for hypotensive patients who responded with increased blood pressure. Despite temporary improvement in renal hemodynamics and function, all patients eventually died.[35]

Ornipressin has been shown to confer minimal improvement in renal function with or without the addition of dopamine, unless the medication was administered as a continuous and prolonged infusion. Its use, however, is not currently recommended because of a high rate of complications, including intestinal and tongue infarctions and arrhythmias.[36-38]

Unlike ornipressin, terlipressin has a longer biological half-life, which allows for administration as a bolus every 4 hours. In 1998, Hadengue and coworkers first reported success in 10 patients who had improvement in renal function and diuresis after low-dose administration of terlipressin at 1 mg every 12 hours over a 48-hour period.[39] Subsequent studies using different protocols, including variations in dosage and duration of terlipressin infusion and the addition of albumin, have resulted in similar favorable outcomes (Table 60–8).[39-45] Unlike previous vasopressin analogues, side effects of terlipressin have been reported to be minimal and reversible with dose reduction or discontinuation of terlipressin. More recently, a randomized placebo-controlled clinical trial similarly confirmed that terlipressin administered at 1 mg intravenously at 12-hour intervals over a study period of 15 days significantly improved renal function and systemic hemodynamics and was associated with a trend toward better clinical outcome.[46] Another experimental approach to the use of terlipressin is the addition of albumin infusion. Although inconclusive, the data available appear to suggest that the addition of albumin may be beneficial in terms of better response rates and a greater reduction in serum creatinine.[41-43] Anecdotal reports suggest that HRS patients may also benefit from other therapies, including norepinephrine plus albumin,[47] N-acetylcysteine,[48] and the combination of octreotide, midodrine, and albumin.[49] In a recent randomized, double-blind, placebo-controlled, crossover study, octreotide alone was shown to be ineffective in treating HRS.[50]

In patients with complete renal failure, various renal replacement therapies, including intermittent hemodialysis (HD), continuous renal replacement therapy (CRRT), and MARS, may be performed as a bridge to liver transplantation. The choice of intermittent HD versus CRRT is often based on the clinical condition of the patient. In patients with severe liver disease and significant hypotension, intermittent HD may worsen their hemodynamic status. In addition, in fulminant hepatic failure patients, who are at greater risk for increased

Table 60–8. SUMMARY OF RESULTS OF STUDIES USING TERLIPRESSIN IN PATIENTS WITH HEPATORENAL SYNDROME

Study	Study Design	Improvement in Renal Function, %:n	Survival, %:n (f-u)	OLT, %:n
Hadengue	Terlipressin, 2 mg qd × 2 days	100:9	N/A	N/A
	2nd washout, 2nd without drug			
	Double blind, controlled cross-over			
Duhamel	Terlipressin, 4–6 mg qd	50:6	33:4 (1 mo)	17:2
	Prospective open			
Uriz	Terlipressin, 3–12 mg qd × 5–15 days	100:9	23:3 (12 mo)	33:3
	+ Albumin, 1 g/kg → 20–40 g qd			
	Prospective open			
Mulkay	Terlipressin, 2–6 mg qd	100:12	25:3 (3 mo)	25:3
	Prospective open			
Ortega	Terlipressin, 3–12 mg qd × 15 days	86:18	66:14 (1 mo)	14:3
	13 pts + albumin		38:8 (3 mo)	24:5
	Prospective open			
Alessandria	Terlipressin, 6 mg qd × 7 days	73:8	N/A	N/A
	Prospective open			
Halimi	Terlipressin, 4 mg qd × 7 days	72:13	11:2 (> 24 mo)	
	Multicenter retrospective			
Solanki	Terlipressin, 1 mg q12h × 15 days	100:12	100:12 (15 days)	
	Randomized controlled single-blind (one pt with type I and one with type II HRS survived beyond 2 yr)			

%, percentage of patients studied; f-u, follow-up period; HRS, hepatorenal syndrome; n, number of patients studied; N/A, not available.

intracranial pressure, worsening of hemodynamic stability, and a rapid change in serum osmolality, intermittent HD may increase cerebral hypoxia and cerebral edema with a subsequent rise in intracranial pressure.[51] Slow continuous correction of volumes and solutes with CRRT (preferably in the form of continuous venovenous hemodialysis [CVVHD]) in these patients is preferred for better maintenance of cardiovascular and cerebral stability. Although peritoneal dialysis may offer similar hemodynamic advantages as CRRT, effective solute clearance in hypotensive patients may be reduced because of the associated reduction in capillary blood flow. More recently, it has been suggested that MARS might offer a survival advantage over dialysis therapy in type I HRS patients awaiting liver transplantation. MARS is based on the concept that kidney dialysis removes only water-soluble toxins whereas the liver removes albumin-bound toxins. In Teraklin's MARS system, blood is cleansed in an extracorporeal circuit designed as a combination of both kidney and "liver dialysis." For this reason, in addition to conventional kidney dialysis, MARS uses human albumin in a second closed-loop circuit to cleanse the blood of albumin-bound toxins, hence mimicking the detoxification function of the liver. Additional toxins that may be dialyzed by Teraklin's MARS system include bilirubin, bile acids, phenols, mercaptans, dioxin-like substances, tryptophan, ammonia, copper, and iron. Thus far, the MARS system has shown promising results. A recent review based on experience from the International MARS Registry involving 176 patients revealed improved survival accompanied by significant improvement in hepatic encephalopathy, mean arterial pressure, serum bilirubin level, creatinine, urea, albumin, international normalized ratio, ammonia, and Model for End-Stage Liver Disease (MELD) score.[52,53] A prospective, controlled randomized study involving 13 patients specifically with type I HRS and an average Child-Pugh score of 12.4 ± 1 revealed a survival rate of 38.5% at 7 days and 25% at 30 days in 8 patients treated with MARS and hemodiafiltration versus 0% at 7 days in 5 patients treated with conventional hemodiafiltration.[53] Although not yet widely available, MARS may prove to be a viable option for patients with the most advanced liver failure.

The various therapeutic options currently available for ESLD patients with HRS are shown in Figure 60–2.

Increasing Child-Pugh/MELD score

Hepatorenal syndrome: therapuetic options:

- TIPS:
  - If relatively preserved liver function
  - Improves renal function, sodium excretion
  - ? improves survival
- Vasopressors:
  - Terlipressin > midodrine + octreotide + albumin, ?N-acetylcysteine, ?ET-A antagonist
  - May prolong short-term survival as bridging to transplant
  - May be better in combination with albumin
- MARS

FIGURE 60–2

Therapeutic options in the management of hepatorenal syndrome in order of increasing Child-Pugh/MELD score. Options are center dependent. MARS, molecular adsorbent recirculating system; MELD, Model for End-Stage Liver Disease; TIPS, transjugular intrahepatic shunt.

Electrolyte Abnormalities and Intraoperative Hemodynamic Changes in End-Stage Liver Disease Patients Undergoing Orthotopic Liver Transplantation

Electrolyte and acid-base disturbances often complicate the course of advanced liver disease. In patients who undergo OLT, unique hemodynamic, electrolyte, and acid-base imbalances occur during the surgical procedure. For the purpose of analysis, OLT is traditionally divided into three distinct phases: phase I, or the preanhepatic phase, begins with the introduction of anesthesia and concludes with occlusion of blood flow to the patient's diseased liver (anhepatic time); phase II, or the anhepatic phase, begins at initiation of the anhepatic state and terminates with reperfusion of the donor liver by the patient's circulating blood; and phase III, or the postanhepatic or reperfusion phase, begins at the time of reperfusion and continues until the end of the surgical procedure. The following section discusses the electrolyte and acid-base disturbances and the intraoperative hemodynamic changes in ESLD patients undergoing OLT.

Fluid and Electrolyte Abnormalities

Sodium

Patients awaiting liver transplantation frequently suffer from hyponatremia because of decreased renal free-water clearance from various causes and infusions of multiple medicated hypotonic solutions. After successful liver transplantation, increases in serum sodium concentration may occur over a matter of hours,[54] presumably in association with infusion of blood products high in sodium content, amelioration of the syndrome of inappropriate antidiuretic hormone secretion, and eventual improvement in renal function. The rapid autocorrection of hyponatremia seen in OLT patients has been reported by several authors to be associated with development of the osmotic demyelination syndrome.[55-59] Nevertheless, it should be noted that other factors, including a history of alcoholism, malnutrition, hypoxia, and hepatic encephalopathy, may be contributory, since the association between the rate of sodium correction and neurological complications in OLT patients is not uniformly observed.[60-61]

Potassium

Before liver transplantation, most patients are mildly to moderately hypokalemic, frequently as a result of malnutrition and the excessive use of laxatives and diuretics. Potassium levels may be altered at different phases of liver transplantation as dictated by infusion of large volumes of blood products and noncolloidal crystalline and alterations in acid-base status, renal function, endogenous insulin secretion, and hemodynamic and thermodynamic stability. Generally, during the first two phases of liver transplantation (I and II), the potassium concentration remains stable. However, if the donor liver potassium-rich perfusate is allowed to enter the circulation at the end of the anhepatic phase, a transient rise in potassium concentration may occur. The high potassium concentration in the donor liver perfusate is partially due to extracellular potassium leakage resulting from cold-temperature (4° C) inhibition of the hepatocyte sodium-potassium pump during liver preservation. This potassium rise, however, reverses within 10 to 15 minutes, presumably because of re-entry of potassium into cells on reperfusion and rewarming. In contrast, if the donor liver perfusate is discarded, significant potassium loss may occur and can result in a significant fall in potassium concentration. Another contributing factor to hypokalemia at the end of the anhepatic or reperfusion stage is the increased production of bicarbonate, improvement in metabolic acidosis, and eventual increased intracellular potassium shift. Other sources of potassium loss include volume expansion–induced polyuria and its associated obligatory potassium loss, as well as nasogastric, biliary, and ascitic drainage. In a series reported from the Mayo Clinic, 58% of patients required potassium supplementation to maintain normal concentrations.

Although hypokalemia is common, hyperkalemia may also occur in the setting of renal failure, especially in patients who receive large blood volume transfusions and cyclosporine. In cases of concomitant severe hyperkalemia and oliguria or anuria, initiation of dialysis may be required.

Calcium

Total and ionized calcium concentrations in patients with ESLD are typically reduced as a result of malnutrition, malabsorption, vitamin D deficiency, hypomagnesemia-associated hypoparathyroidism, or diuretic-induced renal calcium wasting (or any combination of these causes).[62] Although hypocalcemia occurs more frequently in ESLD patients, hypercalcemia may also occur. Hypercalcemia in patients with advanced liver disease associated with mild to moderate renal failure independent of hyperparathyroidism and hypervitaminosis has been described.[63] In addition, patients with hepatocellular carcinoma may have hypercalcemia secondary to the production of parathyroid-related peptides by tumor cells.[64] In our experience, this form of hypercalcemia is generally resistant to medical therapy, including plicamycin, calcitonin, and etidronate disodium. Removal of the tumor by hepatectomy is the most effective treatment if liver transplantation is an option.

During the three phases of liver transplantation, calcium metabolism can be further disrupted and hence requires vigilant monitoring and management. During the preanhepatic phase, when large-volume replacement with citrate-containing blood products is used to compensate for the massive blood loss resulting from the underlying portal hypertension, coagulopathy, and thrombocytopenia, ionized calcium can be significantly lowered as a result of rapid chelation with citrate. Although each 1.0 mmol of citrate theoretically chelates 0.6 mmol of calcium, full replacement of the calculated calcium deficit is not recommended because of potential overcorrection and development of severe hypercalcemia. Instead, regular intraoperative monitoring with ionized calcium–specific electrodes is performed, and calcium replacement is administered accordingly to maintain a normal ionized calcium range.

During the anhepatic phase, ionized calcium levels may fall to a nadir of 0.6 mmol/L because of a maximum increase in citrate up to 100-fold in comparison to preoperative levels despite calcium supplementation. Other factors that may adversely lower ionized calcium levels include a hemodilutional factor induced by the use of venovenous bypass (VVB) and the release of donor liver perfusate into the recipient's circulation at the end of the anhepatic phase or the start of the reperfusion phase. Current practice at many centers, however, no longer allows the donor liver perfusion fluid to be infused into the recipient, thereby effectively reducing further acid-base and electrolyte imbalances.

In the postanhepatic phase, when the donor liver establishes function and begins to metabolize citrate to bicarbonate, calcium ions are released. In effect, the metabolic acidosis and hypocalcemia are slowly corrected. In cases in which oversupplementation of calcium and large quantities of citrate-containing blood products have been given during the previous phases of transplantation, metabolic alkalosis and hypercalcemia may develop. In the presence of adequate renal function, these abnormalities can be corrected within 36 to 48 hours with volume expansion and diuretic-induced polyuria. Otherwise, dialysis against a lower bicarbonate and calcium dialysate may be performed. Patients with hypercalcemia and concomitant renal failure and secondary hyperparathyroidism have been reported to be at increased risk for metastatic calcifications.[65,66]

Magnesium

Hypomagnesemia is common in patients with liver disease and is mainly due to malnutrition and chronic use of diuretics. During OLT, significant decreases in ionized magnesium concentration occur during dissection and the anhepatic phase[67,68] in association with increasing citrate levels induced by the transfusion of citrate-rich blood products. Within 2 hours after graft reperfusion, serum citrate levels gradually return toward baseline values, and improvement in hypomagnesemia follows.[68] Since magnesium is an important cofactor involved in the maintenance of cardiovascular homeostasis and neurological stability, any acute changes in magnesium levels must be detected and treated promptly. Nevertheless, caution must be exercised to avoid overnormalization of magnesium levels during the anhepatic phase in anticipation of the partial correction of hypomagnesemia with citrate clearance after graft reperfusion. In the postoperative period, hypomagnesemia may again be exacerbated by the use of calcineurin inhibitors[69] and diuretics.

Phosphate

Phosphate levels in patients with ESLD are typically normal or low. Even with concomitant renal failure, normophosphatemia or hypophosphatemia is not uncommon, particularly in inpatients, because of strict dietary modification, aggressive dialysis, and the use of phosphate binders. After successful liver transplantation, hypophosphatemia may be exacerbated by both volume expansion– and diuretic-induced polyuria. An increase in parathyroid hormone secretion induced by hypocalcemia during the perioperative period or renal failure secondary to HRS may further enhance renal phosphate wasting with renal function improvement. Medications, including the use of antacids in the past and calcineurin inhibitors, may also play a role in promoting renal phosphate wasting. Hypophosphatemia must be promptly diagnosed and managed to facilitate recovery, as well as avoid rhabdomyolysis and cardio-pulmonary catastrophes.

Acid-Base Disturbances

Patients with ESLD typically have mixed acid-base disorders, including respiratory alkalosis, metabolic alkalosis, or metabolic acidosis (or any combination of the three). Respiratory acidosis rarely occurs, but it may develop in association with severe respiratory muscle fatigue caused by massive ascites or pleural effusions; by severe electrolyte abnormalities such as hypophosphatemia, hypomagnesemia, and hypokalemia; or by depressed respiratory drive secondary to sedatives and narcotics. Table 60–9 lists the various causes of the acid-base disorders seen in ESLD patients. Respiratory alkalosis may be observed in 20% to 50% of patients with advanced liver disease with or without ascites.[70,71] Although not universally accepted, respiratory alkalosis in the setting of advanced liver disease has been attributed to enhanced stimulation of the central nervous system by the increased levels of progesterone and estradiol as a result of decreased hepatic clearance.[71,72] Metabolic alkalosis has been reported to occur in approximately 15% of relatively stable liver patients, mainly as a consequence of medical intervention, including the use of loop diuretics and nasogastric suction. Although metabolic acidosis may similarly be due to various medical interventions, including the excessive use of potassium-sparing diuretics and laxatives, it may also occur in association with lactic acidosis. The presence of metabolic acidosis generally portends an ominous prognosis.[70]

During liver transplantation, however, the development of acidosis is not unusual and commonly results from the transfusion of large volumes of citrate-containing blood products, worsening of both types A and B lactic acidosis, and in some cases, infusion of donor liver acidic perfusate. As a result, sodium bicarbonate infusion is often required to maintain normal pH during the operation.

At the completion of liver engraftment and recovery of various liver functions, including conversion of citrate to bicarbonate and metabolism of lactic acid, the existing metabolic acidosis is eventually corrected and, in some cases, overcorrected to result in metabolic alkalosis. Other factors contributing to the development of metabolic alkalosis postoperatively include continuous nasogastric suction, continuing use of diuretics, and the hyperaldosteronism state associated with the postoperative period. Caution must therefore be exercised to avoid excessive alkalinization intraoperatively. Postoperatively, care must be taken to avoid the development of respiratory alkalosis with mechanical ventilation and subsequent compounded alkalemia. In patients with significant alkalemia or pH higher than 7.45, relative carbon dioxide retention should be allowed because

Table 60–9. ACID-BASE DISORDERS IN PATIENTS WITH END-STAGE LIVER DISEASE*

Acid-Base Disorder	Origin
Respiratory alkalosis	Hypoxemia
	Hyperammonemia
	Increased plasma progesterone levels
	Hyponatremia
	Intracellular acidosis
	Physical stimuli: anxiety, pain, fever
Metabolic alkalosis	Chloride sensitive
	Diuretics
	GI loss (vomiting, GI bleeding)
	Reduced oral intake/inadequate fluid administration
	Chloride resistant
	Hypoalbuminemia
	Hypokalemia
Metabolic acidosis	Increased anion gap
	Lactic acidosis
	Concomitant renal failure
	Sepsis
	Normal anion gap
	Renal tubular acidosis
	Potassium-sparing diuretics
	Autoimmune liver disease
	Ethanol-induced chronic liver disease
	Diarrhea
	Lactulose
	Antibiotics
	Hyperalimentation
Respiratory acidosis	Respiratory muscle fatigue
	Massive ascites
	Pleural effusions
	Severe electrolyte abnormalities
	Hypophosphatemia
	Hypomagnesemia
	Hypokalemia
	Hypocalcemia
	Depressed respiratory drive
	Sedatives
	Narcotics
	Severe hepatic encephalopathy

*In order of decreasing prevalence.
Adapted from Pham PT, Pham PC, Wilkinson AH: The kidney in liver transplantation. Clin Liver Dis 4:567-590, 2000.

severe alkalemia is not generally well tolerated. In patients requiring dialysis, the dialysate bicarbonate content should be minimized. Persistent pH elevation above 7.5 with evidence of hemodynamic instability requires the infusion of 150 mM hydrochloric acid to reduce the pH to below 7.5. Nevertheless, it should be cautioned that there is a theoretical, although not proven, concern that hydrochloric acid infusion may raise pulmonary artery pressure[73] and exacerbate any underlying pulmonary hypertension in some transplant recipients and adversely affect liver graft function.

Intraoperative Risk Factors for the Development of Acute Renal Dysfunction in End-Stage Liver Disease Patients Undergoing Orthotopic Liver Transplantation

Cross-clamping of the portal vein and inferior vena cava during the anhepatic phase (phase II) interrupts venous return from the lower extremities and splanchnic bed and thereby results in decreased cardiac output and blood pressure, increased systemic vascular resistance, and reduced perfusion to vital organs. The latter may lead to renal hypoperfusion and potentially to ischemic renal injury. Although VVB has been shown to improve or restore normal hemodynamic physiology during the anhepatic phase, the use of VVB has not been consistently shown to decrease the incidence of perioperative or early postoperative renal failure.[74-77] In a retrospective study consisting of 87 recipients of OLT, Shaw and colleagues have shown that the use VVB was associated with a lower serum creatinine level at postoperative day 3 and a decreased requirement for postoperative dialysis.[74] In contrast, in a more recent prospective controlled trial involving 77 recipients of OLT randomized to receive VVB support (group I) versus no VVB (group II), the degree of renal dysfunction (assessed by inulin clearance) measured at different perioperative periods (anesthesia induction, hepatectomy, anhepatic phase, biliary anastomosis, and 24 hours after surgery) was not significantly different between the two groups at all time points, except for the anhepatic phase, in which more marked renal function impairment occurred in group II patients (no VVB). Nonetheless, renal function on the seventh postoperative day and the need for HD/hemofiltration during the first week were similar in both groups. Deterioration in renal function occurred in both groups, and renal impairment persisted in a subset of patients during the early postoperative period. Multivariate analysis revealed that low mean arterial pressure at induction of anesthesia was an independent risk factor for early postoperative severe renal failure (inulin clearance < 10 mL/min/1.73 m² at the 24th postoperative hour).[78] Although large prospective

clinical trials are lacking, it is conceivable that intraoperative risk factors for the development of perioperative and early postoperative ARF in orthotopic transplantation of the liver are similar to those in the nontransplant setting. These factors may include an anesthesia-induced decrease in effective blood volume, preexisting cardiovascular disease or severe cardiomyopathy, prolonged episode of hemodynamic instability or hypotension, severe intravascular volume depletion, use of drugs that can adversely affect intrarenal hemodynamics, older age, preexisting renal insufficiency, and diabetes mellitus. In this respect, hemodynamic instability associated with a prolonged anhepatic phase and major bleeding during hepatectomy can potentially predispose recipients of OLT to postoperative ARF. Limited studies suggest that selective use of VVB may be beneficial in patients who demonstrated hemodynamic instability during inferior vena cava cross-clamping trials.

Factors Affecting Posttransplant Renal Function

Postoperative ARF occurs in 17% to 95% of patients undergoing OLT. The difference in the incidence reported may be due in part to the wide disparity in the criteria used to define "acute renal failure." Nonetheless, commonly suggested causes of postoperative ARF include ATN secondary to an ischemic or toxic insult to the kidneys, preexisting HRS, and drug-induced interstitial nephritis.[79-81] The former may include prolonged hypotension, sepsis or septic shock, sustained prerenal renal failure, and the use of nephrotoxic drugs. ARF or declining renal function associated with the use of cyclosporine or tacrolimus in the posttransplant period has been well described and is discussed in more detail later. Preoperative renal dysfunction, delayed liver graft function or primary graft nonfunction, and higher serum bilirubin levels have also been variably shown to predispose OLT recipients to postoperative ARF.[81-83] Potential intraoperative risk factors were discussed previously.

Chronic renal insufficiency or chronic kidney disease has been reported to occur in 4% to more than 80% of OLT recipients.[79,84,85] The wide range in reported incidence may be partly due to differences in the criteria used to define chronic renal failure, as well as differences in the duration of follow-up. Commonly suggested causes or risk factors for the development of progressive chronic kidney disease or end-stage renal disease (ESRD) in long-term survivors of OLT include calcineurin inhibitor nephrotoxicity, pre-OLT HRS, preexisting renal insufficiency, and diabetes mellitus.[81,83,85,86] Postoperative ARF, requirement for dialysis in the preoperative or posttransplant period (or both), hepatitis C infection, and older age have also been variably shown to be associated with an increased risk for the development of chronic kidney disease.[86-89]

In a study conducted by Fisher and associates, severe chronic renal failure developed in 4% of patients surviving 1 year or more. Progression to ESRD occurred in nearly half these patients. In almost all patients who underwent renal biopsy, the histological findings were suggestive of cyclosporine toxicity. Specific pathological changes included vascular obliteration, tubular atrophy, interstitial scarring, and glomerular sclerosis.[84]

In a retrospective study consisting of 834 recipients of liver-alone transplantation performed between June 1985 and the end of 1999, chronic severe renal dysfunction during the study period occurred in 10.3% of patients, more than 50% of whom had ESRD (severe renal dysfunction was defined as serum creatinine >2.5 mg/dL or ESRD requiring dialysis or transplantation). At 10-year follow-up, the total incidence of severe renal dysfunction rose to 14.4%, with more than 50% of these patients having ESRD (7.9%). The presumptive renal diagnoses of those in whom ESRD developed were calcineurin inhibitor toxicity (73.3%), nonrecovered HRS (6.66%), focal segmental glomerulosclerosis (6.66%), progression of underlying renal disease (11.1%), and ATN/amphotericin toxicity (2.22%). For those who survived 13 years beyond OLT, severe renal dysfunction developed in 18.1%.[87] It is likely that the incidence of ESRD both in native kidneys (in OLT recipients) and renal allografts (in CKLT recipients) increases with time after transplantation.

Cyclosporine and Tacrolimus Nephrotoxicity

Although biochemically distinct, cyclosporine and tacrolimus are two potent immunosuppressive agents with similar mechanisms of action, as well as similar clinical and pathological patterns of nephrotoxicity. The various clinical and histological manifestations of cyclosporine and tacrolimus toxicity may include the frequently occurring functional decrease in renal blood flow and GFR and the infrequently occurring thrombotic microangiopathy.[90] Cyclosporine and, to a lesser extent, tacrolimus have been shown to cause acute, dose-related reversible afferent arteriolar vasoconstriction and "preglomerular-type" renal dysfunction. In liver transplant recipients, the fall in GFR occurs immediately after the introduction of cyclosporine, and this effect is exaggerated when the calcineurin inhibitor is administered intravenously. Cyclosporine toxicity usually resolves within 24 to 48 hours after dose reduction, whereas tacrolimus toxicity may take longer to resolve. Nephrotoxicity may also develop at apparently low levels of both drugs, and indeed, some degree of toxicity may be intrinsic to their use.[90] In contrast to the acute

dose-related reversible decrease in GFR, prolonged use of calcineurin inhibitors can cause chronic interstitial fibrosis and irreversible chronic kidney disease. It has been suggested that calcineurin inhibitor–induced interstitial fibrosis involves angiotensin-dependent upregulation of profibrotic molecules, such as transforming growth factor-β, endothelin-1, and osteopontin, whereas matrix degradation is inhibited—the latter through inhibition of matrix metalloproteinase activity.[91,92] Intense and prolonged vasoconstriction of the renal microcirculation has also been suggested to be a contributing factor.[91]

Clinical studies comparing the chronic nephrotoxic effects of cyclosporine and tacrolimus in organ transplant recipients have yielded variable and conflicting results. Early reports by Fisher and coauthors revealed a similar incidence of severe chronic renal failure in OLT patients receiving tacrolimus or cyclosporine during the same study period.[84] Creatinine levels at 4 years were comparable in both groups. In agreement with Fisher and colleagues, Platz and coworkers found a similar incidence of late renal insufficiency in cyclosporine- and tacrolimus-treated patients.[85] In contrast to the findings reported by Fisher and Platz and their colleagues, a number of studies suggest that renal function is better preserved with tacrolimus than with cyclosporine. In a retrospective study conducted to determine long-term renal function in OLT recipients receiving either cyclosporine- or tacrolimus-based immunosuppression at discharge, Pham and associates[93] have shown that at 5-year follow-up, nondiabetic OLT recipients treated with tacrolimus had better kidney function than did those receiving cyclosporine for the period reviewed ($P < .01$). Similar analysis for diabetics revealed a comparable trend, but statistical significance was not achieved (data obtained from the UNOS database between 4/1/1994 and 12/31/1997). In a recent large population-based cohort study involving more than 32,000 recipients of OLT reported to the Scientific Registry of Transplant Recipients, the risk for chronic renal failure (defined as GFR <29 mL/min or the development of ESRD) associated with the use of calcineurin inhibitors was also found to be higher in patients treated with cyclosporine than in those treated with tacrolimus (relative risk, 1.25; $P < .001$). Interestingly, this difference was not seen in patients with other types of solid-organ transplants.[88] Recently, some but not all studies suggest that in long-term OLT recipients, Neoral cyclosporine monitoring using the 2-hour postdose (C2) technique preserves renal function without increasing the risk of rejection.[94-96] Whether short-term or sustained long-term improvement in renal function can be achieved in OLT recipients receiving Neoral and the C2 technique for dosing determination remains to be determined.

Modification of nephrotoxic immunosuppressive regimens to avoid postoperative ARF or chronic renal failure, or both, has met with variable results.

Despite the lack of a well-defined protocol to prevent or minimize cyclosporine or tacrolimus nephrotoxicity, a number of centers advocate the use of a calcineurin inhibitor–sparing protocol adjusted for the degree of renal dysfunction. Gonwa and coworkers had previously suggested that cyclosporine be withheld in recipients with HRS or in those with moderate to severe renal dysfunction (GFR <30 mL/min) and, in its place, azathioprine be used along with steroids. Induction therapy with an antilymphocyte preparation was used only in cases of prolonged renal dysfunction.[97] With the advent of the monoclonal antibody anti–interleukin-2 (IL-2) receptor antagonists (basiliximab and daclizumab), mycophenolate mofetil, and sirolimus, independent investigators have developed various immunosuppressive protocols that avoid the nephrotoxic side effects associated with calcineurin inhibitor therapy while providing adequate immunosuppression. In a small series consisting of 11 adult transplant recipients (7 heart, 2 liver, 2 heart-kidney transplants) with established acute renal dysfunction (defined as an increase in serum creatinine to >25% of baseline), withholding cyclosporine in conjunction with the use of basiliximab or daclizumab resulted in an improvement in renal function without an increased risk for acute rejection.[98]

In a small series consisting of 19 adults, long-term (>1 year) OLT recipients with renal dysfunction (defined as creatinine clearance decreased >25% in comparison to the first month after transplantation), Cantarovich and colleagues have shown that the introduction of mycophenolate mofetil followed by tapering of cyclosporine to a very low dose (25 mg twice a day) resulted in a significant improvement in renal function. At 1-year follow-up, serum creatinine decreased from 141 ± 24 to 105 ± 22 μmol/L, P = .002, and the GFR increased from 40 ± 13 to 64 ± 18 mL/min, P = .002. However, acute rejection occurred in 29% of the subjects studied, thus suggesting that this strategy may be associated with a risk for acute rejection.[99] In contrast to the results reported by Cantarovich and associates, Neau-Cransac and coworkers failed to demonstrate any significant improvement in renal function in OLT recipients with biopsy-proven chronic calcineurin inhibitor nephrotoxicity despite withdrawal of cyclosporine or tacrolimus and institution of either mycophenolate mofetil or azathioprine. Nonetheless, there was no increase in the incidence of graft rejection.[100]

Sirolimus is a new and potent immunosuppressant with a mechanism of action and a side effect profile distinct from that of calcineurin inhibitors. When used as base therapy without a calcineurin inhibitor, sirolimus has been shown to be devoid of nephrotoxicity. In a retrospective study consisting of 16 long-term (>3 years) OLT recipients with different degrees of renal insufficiency (ranging from mild [creatinine clearance >70 mL/min] to severe [creatinine clearance of 20 to 40 mL/min]), conversion from cyclosporine or tacrolimus to sirolimus-based immunosuppression resulted in variable improvement in renal function and no rejection at 6-month follow-up.[101]

Because of the lack of large prospective controlled trials and the mixed results obtained from small series of patients, manipulation of immunosuppressive therapy to avoid nephrotoxicity should best be tailored to each patient. In patients with HRS, mycophenolate mofetil in conjunction with low-dose tacrolimus and standard steroid therapy appears to be safe and effective (unpublished observation). Although the use of IL-2 receptor blocker induction therapy in a calcineurin inhibitor–sparing protocol has been reported to result in improvement in renal function without an increased risk for rejection, there have been anecdotal reports suggesting that IL-2 receptor blockers in combination with mycophenolate mofetil or rapamycin increase the risk for viral reactivation or the development of more severe hepatitis C recurrence (or both) after liver transplantation.[102,103] Interestingly an increased incidence of hepatitis C viral reactivation associated with IL-2 receptor blockers has also been observed at our center, thus re-emphasizing that modification of immunosuppressive therapy should be individualized. Although early studies suggest that mycophenolate mofetil may have a ribavirin-like antiviral effect and may provide synergism when used with interferon alfa, its use in the posttransplant period has not been consistently shown to be beneficial or deleterious. Studies on the association between an increased incidence or severity of HCV recurrence (or both) and the use of polyclonal antilymphocyte preparations or anti-OKT3 monoclonal antibody (or the use of both) have also resulted in contradictory results.[104] In the authors' opinion, these agents should be reserved for patients with delayed graft function and for the treatment of acute rejection. Their routine use in a calcineurin inhibitor–sparing protocol as prophylactic therapy is not recommended. In patients with chronic renal insufficiency who have unrelenting renal failure despite drastic dose reduction or withdrawal of calcineurin inhibitors, the options available to prevent further decline in renal function remain contentious. Although angiotensin-converting enzyme inhibitors or angiotensin receptor blockers, or both, have been suggested to retard the progression of interstitial fibrosis, the role of these agents in halting or alleviating the progression of chronic calcineurin inhibitor nephrotoxicity remains to be determined.[91]

Drug Interactions

Well-substantiated potentiation of renal impairment has been described when amphotericin, aminoglycosides, NSAIDs, angiotensin-converting enzyme inhibitors, angiotensin receptor antagonists, or any combination of these agents is used in patients receiving calcineurin inhibitor therapy. More recently, exacerbation of nephrotoxicity has been observed in renal transplant patients receiving sirolimus and cyclosporine combination therapy. Two phase III clinical trials (The Global and U.S. Rapamune Study Group) have shown that concomitant administration of cyclosporine and sirolimus potentiates cyclosporine-induced nephrotoxicity.[105,106] Substantial evidence suggests that cyclosporine exposure is increased by a pharmacokinetic interaction with sirolimus. In rat animal models, sirolimus has also been shown to increase partitioning into renal tissue to a greater extent than it increases whole blood concentrations.[107] When combination therapy is used, a reduction in therapeutic cyclosporine levels is desirable, particularly when there is an unexplained rise in the serum creatinine level. The pharmacological interaction between sirolimus and tacrolimus has been less rigorously studied. Coadministration of tacrolimus and sirolimus has been shown to result in reduced exposure to tacrolimus at sirolimus doses higher than 2 mg/day.[108] However, in renal transplant recipients, cases of acute renal allograft failure after sirolimus-tacrolimus therapy have been reported.[109] Caution should be exercised when combination immunosuppressive agents are used.

Impact of Acute Renal Failure or Renal Insufficiency on Patient and Allograft Outcome in Orthotopic Liver Transplantation

Studies on the impact of ARF or renal insufficiency on patient and allograft outcome have yielded variable and conflicting results. This section provides an overview of the literature on the clinical implications of ARF/renal insufficiency on patient and allograft survival in OLT. Based on the literature, the authors' view of the possible impact of renal insufficiency on survival in patients undergoing OLT is discussed.

Early studies by Cuerva-Mons and colleagues showed that a preoperative serum creatinine level of either less than or greater than 1.72 mg/dL accurately predicted survival or death in 79% of cases.[110] Similarly, a strong correlation between preoperative renal dysfunction and postoperative patient survival was later demonstrated by Rimola and coworkers.[111] In their series of 102 patients, 26 (25%) had renal impairment at the time of OLT. The causes of renal failure were HRS in 21 patients, ATN in 3 patients, and unclassified in 2 patients. After OLT, 68 patients (67%) experienced renal dysfunction. Twenty-five patients died during the observation period (range,

4 to 167 days). Renal failure was a major contributory cause of death in 13 (52%). Multivariate risk factor analysis identified serious postoperative infection, graft failure, and preoperative renal function to be independent predictors of mortality.

In contrast to the results reported by Cuerva-Mons and Rimola and their colleagues, Gonwa and coworkers found no difference in graft and patient survival up to 5 years in non-HRS OLT recipients with different levels of pretransplant renal dysfunction.[97] In a large retrospective study, the same group of investigators demonstrated that the development of ARF requiring renal replacement therapy postoperatively was associated with a significantly lower 1-year survival rate regardless of the treatment modality than when renal replacement therapy was started preoperatively (41% versus 73.6%, respectively, $P = .03$).[112] Further analysis revealed that mortality was highest in patients with ARF requiring postoperative CVVHD. The 90-day mortality in those who required HD both before and after OLT versus those who required CVVHD both before and after versus those who required CVVHD only postoperatively was 25% versus 27.7% versus 50%, respectively ($P = NS$ between groups). Sepsis, primary graft nonfunction, and hepatic artery thrombosis were commonly observed in patients after the development of postoperative ARF requiring renal replacement therapy.

Fraley and associates have previously shown that both pre- and post-OLT ARF was associated with increased mortality. When ARF was stratified by pre- and post-OLT status and by subgroups who required HD versus CRRT versus no dialysis, the highest mortality rates were seen in patients with postoperative ARF requiring CRRT (primarily in the form of CVVHD), a finding similar to that of Gonwa and colleagues (mortality in patients with ARF before OLT, no dialysis versus HD versus CRRT: 0% versus 10% versus 44%, respectively; mortality in patients with ARF after OLT: 15% versus 22% versus 67%, respectively). The authors further demonstrated that the number of comorbid conditions, most notably sepsis, encephalopathy, respiratory failure, and disseminated intravascular coagulation, correlated best with a worse outcome.[113]

An association between postoperative ARF requiring renal replacement therapy and increased morbidity and mortality was also demonstrated by Gainza and associates.[114] In their series of 259 consecutive liver transplantations performed in 251 patients, 4 of whom underwent CLKT, the mortality rate of patients requiring renal replacement therapy was 52.1% versus 6.77% in the total population studied ($P < .00001$). A higher Child-Pugh score and previous renal insufficiency were identified as strong risk factors for the development of postoperative ARF. Other risk factors included the use of calcineurin inhibitors, sepsis, liver dysfunction, and the use of nephrotoxic antimicrobials, among others.

In conclusion, although the literature on the impact of renal insufficiency on patient and allograft survival is inconsistent, commonly identified factors predicting a worse outcome appear to be renal failure associated with sepsis and renal failure requiring renal replacement therapy, particularly in those who require CRRT (frequently performed because of hemodynamic instability associated with sepsis as a major comorbid condition) in the postoperative period.

Combined Kidney-Liver Transplantation

Indications

The number of CKLTs performed annually has steadily increased over the past $1\frac{1}{2}$ decades. For OLT candidates with simultaneous end-stage kidney failure, CKLT is a well-established effective therapeutic option for virtually all suitable candidates. However, there have been no well-defined guidelines to determine whether a kidney transplant should be offered to OLT candidates who have chronic kidney disease or prolonged HRS or ATN while awaiting a liver transplant. Accurate assessment of the degree of renal dysfunction may be difficult in the former, and predicting the extent of renal function recovery in the latter may be equally challenging. In contrast, in diseases that involve both the liver and the kidney, such as polycystic kidney and liver disease and primary hyperoxaluria type I, CKLT is not necessarily performed because of end-stage failure of both organs. With the ever-increasing disparity between demand and supply of deceased donor organs, CKLT must be used judiciously. This section reviews data from the UNOS database on the renal indications for CKLT, the literature on the indications for CKLT, and the authors' opinion on identification of candidates who are best suited for double-organ transplantation.

Between January 1988 and April 30, 1999, the most common renal indications for CKLT reported to the UNOS OPTN scientific registry database were polycystic kidney disease (7.3%), oxalate nephropathy (6.3%), unspecified chronic glomerulonephritis (5.2%), cyclosporine nephrotoxicity (4.3%), and kidney retransplant/graft failure (3.6%).[2]

More recent UNOS OPTN data collected between May 1, 1999, and March 31, 2003, indicate that polycystic kidney disease remains a common renal diagnosis in recipients of CKLT (7.39%). During that time period, however, CKLT was performed with increasing frequency in patients with renal failure as a result of diabetic nephropathy (type 2 diabetes mellitus, adult onset) and cyclosporine nephrotoxicity (10.58% and 6.22%, respectively). It is conceivable that early or unrecognized diabetic nephropathy or cyclosporine nephrotoxicity,

or both, progressed with time after transplantation and that the incidence of severe chronic kidney disease increased over time in long-term survivors of OLT.

With the introduction of the MELD score for the allocation of OLT in February 2002, an abrupt increase of greater than 50% in the number of CKLT procedures was observed at the University of California at Los Angeles (UCLA) kidney and liver transplant program during an 8-month study period from March 2002 to October 1, 2002 (average number of CKLTs performed before and after adoption of the MELD score: four to six versus eight, respectively).

Analysis of the UNOS database revealed a nearly 84% increase in the number of CKLT procedures performed between February 27, 2002, and June 30, 2003, when compared with the immediate previous 16-month period (between November 1, 2000, and February 26, 2002). During a 16-month period, the total number of CKLTs performed before and after adoption of the MELD score was 161 versus 287, respectively. Because the MELD score–based allocation of OLT prioritizes patients with renal dysfunction, the prevalence of various renal indications for double-organ transplantation has also changed over time. During the period studied, CKLT was increasingly performed for the renal diagnosis of cyclosporine nephrotoxicity (before and after the MELD era: 1.86% versus 6.97%, respectively [UNOS database as of June 2003]).

Early Experience

The first successful CLKT was reported in 1984 by Margreiter and coauthors and was performed in a patient with a failed renal transplant because of chronic rejection and ESLD secondary to chronic hepatitis B.[115] Since then, more than 1300 such transplants have been performed in the United States alone (UNOS OPTN database as of June 2003). The procedures were initially performed in patients with simultaneous end-stage failure of both organs who were maintained on chronic HD; however, preemptive kidney transplantation immediately after OLT was later considered an option for patients with severe chronic kidney disease in anticipation of further worsening of renal failure in the posttransplant period with the introduction of cyclosporine or tacrolimus. In 1988, Gonwa and colleagues reported the results of CKLT in their first series of seven patients at 6 weeks' to 32 months' follow-up.[116] Of these seven patients, two were predialysis with a severely depressed GFR of 14 and 14.5 mL/min. Six of seven patients (85.7%) were alive with functioning grafts at the latest follow-up. The authors further reported that 1-year patient survival in the combined-organ transplant series was identical to that of the liver-alone transplantation series during the same period. In an updated series consisting of 29 CLKTs from the same group of investigators, 2-year patient and liver graft survival rates were 78.6% and 62.7%, respectively. Corresponding 5-year survival rates were 48.1% and 41.2%, respectively.[117] In 1995, Hiesse and associates compared and contrasted the results of CLKT and liver transplantation alone in patients with unrecognized chronic kidney disease before liver transplantation.[118] In the first group, nine patients with biopsy-proven severe nephropathy underwent CLKT. The kidney biopsies were performed because of the presence of unexplained renal dysfunction or significant proteinuria discovered during preoperative evaluation for OLT. All patients received OLT, followed immediately by kidney transplantation. There were no deaths or cases of renal failure in the postoperative period. All patients had immediate renal allograft function with normalization of renal function and proteinuria within the first postoperative month. An acute rejection episode of the liver occurred in one patient, and acute kidney rejection was suspected on clinical grounds in another patient. Renal function remained within normal range, and no chronic rejection was documented in any of the patients during follow-up ranging from 6 months to 4 years. In contrast to the favorable outcomes of patients who received CLKT for ESLD and severe nephropathy, Hiesse and collegues found increased morbidity and mortality in nine liver-alone transplant recipients who had chronic kidney disease that was unrecognized in the pretransplant period. Renal abnormalities were found at various time points during the patients' follow-up (1 month to 5 years), but in the majority of cases (six of nine), the diagnoses were made within the first year after transplantation. Renal biopsy demonstrated mesangiocapillary glomerulonephritis in five patients, interstitial nephritis in two, advanced end-stage kidney fibrosis in one, and focal segmental glomerulosclerosis with mesangial IgA deposits in one. Retrospective analysis of the pretransplant and immediate posttransplant course revealed elevated serum creatinine before transplantation in three patients. Emergency OLT had to be performed without accurate renal assessment. Six other patients had serum creatinine within the normal range. True GFR was not measured. Proteinuria was absent in three patients, and urinalysis was not performed in the other six. Postoperative ARF occurred in four patients, in whom it was necessary to delay the introduction of tacrolimus or cyclosporine. Two patients had rebound rejection because of inadequate immunosuppression. Four patients died shortly after the renal diagnosis. The causes of death were sepsis in three and stroke in one. Two other patients had rapidly deteriorating renal function requiring initiation of HD. One patient had severe graft dysfunction caused by chronic rejection and subsequently underwent CLKT. One-, 2-, and 3-year patient survival rates were 78%, 65%, and 52%, respectively.

From their experience, Heisse and associates concluded that CLKT is a therapeutic option in patients with ESLD associated with advanced kidney disease. The procedure avoids added complications caused by renal failure or nephritic syndrome, especially since nephrotoxic immunosuppressive drugs are mandatory in OLT. Several centers worldwide have now reported excellent patient and allograft outcomes in patients who underwent CLKT for various renal indications. Of note, CKLT is not necessarily performed because of end-stage failure of both organs. Jeyarajah and colleagues suggested that CLKT might be a reasonable option for patients with symptomatic polycystic liver disease and renal failure caused by polycystic kidney disease.[119] Similar to polycystic liver disease, the indication for liver transplantation in patients with primary hyperoxaluria type I is not ESLD per se. The rationale for double-organ transplantation in patients with polycystic liver and kidney disease and in patients with oxalate nephropathy secondary to primary hyperoxaluria type I is discussed in the following sections.

Disease-Specific Indications

Polycystic Kidney and Liver Disease

Hepatic cysts are a common extrarenal manifestation of adult polycystic kidney disease and can result in massive hepatomegaly. In patients with ESRD caused by polycystic kidney disease, simultaneous liver and kidney transplantation has been suggested as a viable therapeutic option for those with debilitating symptoms associated with massive hepatomegaly, such as intractable abdominal pain or distention, early satiety, dyspnea, or limited mobility (or any combination of these symptoms). Although percutaneous cyst aspiration, cyst unroofing, extensive fenestration, and extensive fenestration combined with hepatic resection have been reported to be effective in relieving symptoms in selected cases, these procedures have been shown to be associated with significant morbidity and mortality and with high recurrence rates, particularly in those with severe polycystic liver disease.[120-122] At the Dumont-UCLA Liver Transplant Center, candidates for CKLT are selected on the basis of severe limitations in daily activities, the extent and pattern of hepatic cysts, the degree of hepatic and renal dysfunction, and the presence of hepatic cysts not amenable to or refractory to other surgical interventions. In appropriately selected candidates, excellent long-term results and minimal morbidity and mortality have been achieved.[123]

Primary Hyperoxaluria Type I

Similar to polycystic liver disease, the indication for liver transplantation in patients with primary hyperoxaluria type I is not ESLD per se. Lack of the liver-specific peroxisomal enzyme alanine-glyoxylate aminotransferase (AGT) in patients with type I primary hyperoxaluria results in decreased transamination of glyoxylate to glycine and increased production of oxalate and glycolate. Because oxalate is eliminated unaltered by renal excretion, isolated renal transplantation can result in rapid deposition of oxalate in the allograft and subsequent renal stone formation, nephrocalcinosis, and early allograft failure. Liver transplantation corrects the underlying hepatic-based metabolic disorder, and the effectiveness of CKLT in patients with primary hyperoxaluria has been well established. Both early and recent experience in Europe favors double-organ transplantation over isolated kidney transplantation for patients with renal failure secondary to primary hyperoxaluria type I.[124,125] However, analysis of data obtained from three North American sources, including the U.S. Renal Data System, UNOS, and the North American Pediatric Renal Transplantation Cooperative Study, suggest that kidney-alone transplantation offers better patient survival than either CKLT or no transplant does.[126] Recent results of European studies (1984 to 1997) reveal 2- and 5-year CKLT patient survival rates of 80% and 72%, respectively, and renal graft survival rates of 78% and 62%, respectively.[125] Analysis of the U.S. experience showed 2- and 5-year CKLT patient survival rates of 79% and 55%, respectively, and an isolated kidney graft survival rate of 55% at 5 years. The cumulative mortality rate after 10 years was 23% for European and 31% for U.S. series.[126] The reason or reasons for the seemingly better patient survival in the European series are not known. There have been no well-defined clinical characteristics or laboratory parameters (or both) to accurately predict the outcome of the different surgical options. Nonetheless, in the authors' opinion, preemptive kidney-alone transplantation appears to be a viable option for "pyridoxine-responsive" patients or for those who have a living donor kidney, whereas CKLT may offer better patient or graft survival, or both, in patients with prolonged renal failure who are awaiting a deceased donor renal transplant or in those with a previous failed renal transplant. UNOS OPTN data revealed that the percentage of CKLTs performed for the renal diagnosis of oxalate nephropathy decreased from 6.3% to 2.69% between the period January 1, 1988, to January 5, 1999, and the period June 1, 1999, to March 31, 2003, respectively.

Rationale for Isolated Kidney Transplantation versus Combined Kidney-Liver Transplantation for Primary Hyperoxaluria Type I

Pyridoxal phosphate is an essential cofactor for aminotransferases such as AGT, and pharmacological doses of pyridoxine have been shown to significantly reduce hyperoxaluria in a subset of patients with primary hyperoxaluria type I, particularly those with residual functional AGT activity.[127] In this respect, it is not unreasonable to perform isolated kidney transplantation in pyridoxine-responsive patients (pyridoxine responsiveness is defined as >30% reduction in urinary oxalate excretion from baseline).[127] Preventive measures in the perioperative period should include pyridoxine therapy to decrease oxalate production and excretion, high fluid intake, and administration of drugs that increase urinary calcium oxalate solubility (discussed later).

Preemptive kidney-alone transplantation (GFR of 20 to 30 mL/min) when a living donor kidney is available may limit progressive systemic oxalosis and avoid rapid recurrence of oxalate deposition in the allograft. Once the patient reaches end-stage renal failure, neither high-flux HD nor peritoneal dialysis is able to keep pace with the endogenous production rate of oxalate. Intensified HD, with five to six 5-hour sessions weekly, has been advocated until renal transplantation is performed.[127] In a small series involving six infants with end-stage renal failure secondary to primary hyperoxaluria type I and advanced systemic oxalosis, combined HD and peritoneal dialysis have resulted in lower posttransplant urinary oxalate and more rapid clearance of oxalate stores than in those who received pretransplant HD alone.[128] Despite its theoretical advantage, the role of combined dialysis treatment in alleviating systemic oxalosis—and hence in the prevention of early graft loss from recurrent urolithiasis, nephrolithiasis, or nephrocalcinosis—remains to be defined.

Posttransplant management of isolated kidney transplant or CKLT recipients is directed at increasing urinary calcium oxalate solubility. Although OLT is able to provide the missing AGT enzyme in its normal cellular and subcellular locations,[129] both plasma oxalate levels and plasma calcium oxalate saturation, as well as urinary oxalate, may remain elevated for several months or even years after CKLT.[127,130] High fluid intake (>2.5 L/m² surface area per day) to keep the urinary oxalate concentration less than 0.5 to 0.8 nmol/L, administration of drugs that decrease or inhibit stone formation (orthophosphate, potassium or sodium citrate, and magnesium), and avoidance of food high in oxalate content (spinach, rhubarb, and tea) are the mainstays of therapy.[127] Additional preventive measures include aggressive perioperative dialysis to reduce oxalate stores.

Outcome in Patients with Hepatorenal Syndrome after Liver-Alone Transplantation

The functional nature of HRS was first suggested in 1969 by Koppel and colleagues, who noted reversal of renal dysfunction after transplantation of deceased donor kidneys from patients with HRS into patients with a normal liver.[131] This reversal was later confirmed in 1973 by Iwatsuki and associates, who demonstrated recovery from HRS after OLT.[132] There is now ample literature documenting the potential for recovery or improvement of renal dysfunction caused by HRS after OLT. Hence, liver-only transplantation rather than CKLT should be considered in patients with ESLD and associated HRS. Management of HRS in the pretransplant period was previously described. Management of HRS in the posttransplant period includes dialysis support and judicious use of calcineurin inhibitors or a calcineurin inhibitor–sparing protocol at the discretion of the transplant physician. When compared with non-HRS patients, those with HRS have been shown to be more likely to require dialysis in the pretransplant and posttransplant periods.[132,133] Early reports from our center revealed that in patients with HRS, modification of the immunosuppressive protocol resulted in a 20% decrease in the requirement for postoperative dialysis.[133] After successful OLT, renal function invariably improved over time, although at long-term follow-up, renal function in patients with HRS remained inferior to that of non-HRS patients.[132,133] In a retrospective study consisting of 834 recipients of OLT who survived 6 months after transplantation, Gonwa and colleagues showed that patients with HRS, particularly those requiring dialysis in the first 3 months after transplantation, had the greatest risk for chronic renal failure (defined as sustained serum creatinine >2.5 mg/dL) and ESRD. In those with HRS, chronic renal failure developed in 7.9% and ESRD in 11.4% at 13 years' follow-up versus 4.4% and 4.4%, respectively, in those without HRS ($P = .04$).[134]

In a large retrospective study conducted to evaluate the incidence of chronic renal failure in recipients of nonrenal transplants that included intestine, liver, heart, and heart-lung transplants, the 5-year risk for chronic renal failure (defined as GFR <29 mL/min/1.73 m^2 body surface area or ESRD) has been shown to vary from 6.9% in recipients of heart-lung transplants to 21.3% in recipients of intestinal transplants.[88] Hence, despite a higher incidence of chronic renal failure/ESRD in OLT recipients with HRS than in those without HRS, it should be noted that the 7.9% risk for chronic renal failure and the 11.4% risk for ESRD at 13 years were less than or comparable to the risk for chronic renal failure in recipients of other nonrenal solid-organ transplants, thus re-emphasizing that patients with renal dysfunction secondary to HRS should receive a liver-only transplant; however, when patients with presumed HRS or ATN require dialysis for more than 4 to 6 weeks before transplantation, renal cortical fibrosis may develop and renal function may not recover. Under these circumstances, simultaneous liver-kidney transplantation is recommended. Despite the lack of well-defined clinical criteria to determine the potential for recovery

of renal function in patients who remain dialysis dependent for a prolonged period, evaluation of renal cortical blood flow by means of renal Doppler ultrasound, renal scan, or gadolinium-enhanced magnetic resonance imaging (or any combination of these studies) may be a helpful adjunct to clinical assessment. A marked decrease or absence of cortical blood flow suggests irreversible renal failure, and CKLT should be considered.

Summary

Early recognition and determination of the cause of renal dysfunction in ESLD patients can be difficult because of the potential interplay among various factors and the wide array of differential diagnoses. Nonetheless, a systematic approach can assist clinicians in identifying common and potentially reversible causes of ARF. Distinguishing patients with functional renal failure such as HRS from those with advanced irreversible disease can have important prognostic and therapeutic implications. Isolated liver transplantation is the treatment of choice for the former, whereas CKLT may be an option for the latter. With the ever-increasing disparity between demand and supply of deceased donor organs, CKLT should be used judiciously. Renal biopsy may resolve any diagnostic dilemmas. In patients with coagulopathy, transjugular renal biopsy has been suggested to be relatively safe. Despite considerable progress in supportive medical measures and advances in immunosuppressive therapy, management of renal complications after OLT remains a challenge for physicians caring for transplant patients. Modification of nephrotoxic immunosuppressive regimens to avoid postoperative ARF or halt the progression of established chronic kidney disease, or both, has met with variable results. The advent of IL-2 receptor blockers, mycophenolate mofetil, and more recently, sirolimus has allowed transplant physicians to develop various immunosuppressive strategies that provide adequate immunosuppression while avoiding the nephrotoxic effect of calcineurin inhibitors. In patients with ESLD secondary to hepatitis C, anecdotal reports suggest that the use of these newer immunosuppressive agents may increase the risk for viral reactivation or more severe recurrence of hepatitis C (or both) after liver transplantation. Still, the use of mycophenolate mofetil in OLT recipients with hepatitis C has not been consistently shown to be beneficial or harmful. Polyclonal antilymphocyte preparations or anti-OKT3 monoclonal antibody, or both, should be reserved for patients with delayed graft function and for the treatment of acute rejection, and manipulation of immunosuppressive therapy to avoid nephrotoxicity should be individualized. Data on the impact of renal dysfunction on patient and allograft outcome are inconsistent. Nonetheless, the authors' literature review suggests that renal failure associated with sepsis and renal failure requiring CRRT are the most commonly identified factors predicting a worse outcome. Despite a higher incidence of chronic renal failure/ESRD in patients with HRS than in their non-HRS counterparts, it should be noted that in most patients with HRS, renal function recovers to an acceptable level and these patients should receive a liver-only transplant. However, in patients with HRS requiring prolonged dialysis (>4 to 6 weeks), irreversible renal failure may develop, and CKLT is justifiable. Although timely referral of patients for OLT may potentially avoid severe renal complications and obviate the need for double-organ transplantation, the growing shortage of donor organs is emerging as an obstacle to early transplantation despite the current effort to expand the donor pool by using donor organs with extended criteria, split-liver transplants, and living donor transplants. Non-nephrotoxic immunosuppressive strategies are clearly needed.

Pearls and Pitfalls

- In ESLD patients, assessment of renal function based on the serum creatinine level may significantly overestimate the true GFR.

- Similar to patients without liver disease, causes of renal failure in ESLD patients can be classified as prerenal, intrinsic, and postrenal renal failure. A systematic approach to identify potential causes of acute renal failure or underlying renal insufficiency must be done before the diagnosis of HRS.

- It is crucial to distinguish patients with functional renal failure or HRS from those with advanced irreversible renal disease. Isolated liver transplantation is the treatment of choice for the former, whereas combined kidney-liver transplantation may be a therapeutic option for the latter.

- A kidney biopsy may be recommended when the renal diagnosis is obscure or the degree of irreversibility of renal failure cannot be determined from clinical and laboratory evidence.

- Management of HRS in orthotopic liver transplant candidates is restricted to preventive measures and supportive care. Because HRS is often exacerbated or precipitated by therapies directed at complications of cirrhosis, any such therapy has to be closely monitored.

Pearls and Pitfalls—cont'd

- Bridging therapies for orthotopic liver transplant candidates with HRS include the use of a transjugular intrahepatic shunt, vasoactive agents, and molecular adsorbent recirculating system. The choice of therapy may be dictated by the severity of liver failure, the availability of different treatment modalities, and center experience.

- Modification of nephrotoxic immunosuppressive regimens to avoid postoperative acute renal failure or chronic renal failure (or both) must be tailored to each patient.

- Careful selection of candidates for combined kidney-liver transplantation avoids added renal-related complications after orthotopic liver transplantation.

References

1. United Network for Organ Sharing and Organ Procurement Transplantation Network (UNOS OPTN) database as of January 2, 2004.
2. Pham PT, Pham PC, Wilkinson AH: The kidney in liver transplantation. Clin Liver Dis 4:567-590, 2000.
3. Carego L, Menon F, Angeli P, et al: Limitations of serum creatinine level and creatinine clearance as filtration markers in cirrhosis. Arch Intern Med 154:201-205, 1994.
4. Papadakis MA, Arieff AI: Unpredictability of clinical evaluation of renal function in cirrhosis. Am J Med 82:945-952, 1987.
5. Sherman DS, Fish DN, Teitelbaum I: Assessing renal function in cirrhotic patients: Problems and pitfalls. Am J Kidney Dis 41:269-278, 2003.
6. Guevara M, Abecasis R, Jimenez W, et al: Effect of celecoxib on renal function in cirrhotic patients with ascites. A pilot study. J Hepatol 36(Suppl 1):203, 2002.
7. Hampel H, Bynum GD, Zamora E, et al: Risk factors for the development of renal dysfunction in hospitalized patients with cirrhosis. Am J Gastroenterol 96:2206-2210, 2001.
8. Jouet P, Meyrier A, Mal F, et al: Transjugular renal biopsy in the treatment of patients with cirrhosis and renal abnormalities. Hepatology 24:1143-1147, 1996.
9. Sam R, Leehey DJ, Picken MM, et al: Transjugular renal biopsy in patients with liver disease. Am J Kidney Dis 37:1141-1151, 2001.
10. Davis CL, Gonwa TA, Wilkinson AH: Pathophysiology of renal disease associated with liver disorders: Implications for liver transplantation. Part I. Liver Transpl 8:91-109, 2002.
11. Flint A: Clinical report on hydroperitoneum, based on an analysis of forty-six cases. Am J Med Sci 45:306, 1863.
12. Gines A, Escorsell A, Gines P, et al: Incidence, predictive factors, and prognosis of the hepatorenal syndrome in cirrhosis with ascites. Gastroenterology 105:229-236, 1993.
13. Arroyo V, Gines P, Gerbes AL, et al: Definition and diagnostic criteria of refractory ascites and hepatorenal syndrome in cirrhosis. Hepatology 23:164-176, 1996.
14. Platt JF, Ellis JH, Rubin JM, et al: Renal duplex Doppler ultrasonography: A noninvasive predictor of kidney dysfunction and hepatorenal failure in liver disease. Hepatology 20:362-369, 1994.

15. Lieberman FL: Functional renal failure in cirrhosis. Gastroenterology 58:108-110, 1970.
16. Witte CL, Witte MH, Dumont AE: Lymph imbalance in the genesis and perpetuation of the ascites syndrome in hepatic cirrhosis. Gastroenterology 78:1059-1068, 1980.
17. Schrier RW, Arroyo V, Bernardi M, et al: Peripheral arterial vasodilatation hypothesis: A proposal for the initiation of renal sodium and water retention in cirrhosis. Hepatology 8:1151-1157, 1988.
18. Epstein M: Hepatorenal syndrome: Emerging perspective. Semin Nephrol 17:563, 1997.
19. Gines P, Arroyo V, Rhodes J : Renal complications. In Schiff ER, Sorrell MR, Maddrey WL (eds): Schiff's Diseases of the Liver, 8th ed. Philadelphia, Lippincott-Raven, 1999, p 453.
20. Gines P, Guevara M, Arroyo V, et al: Hepatorenal syndrome. Lancet 362:1819-1827, 2003.
21. Gines A, Fernandez-Esparrach G, Monescillo A, et al: Randomized trial comparing albumin, dextran-70 and polygelin in cirrhotic patients with ascites treated by paracentesis. Gastroenterology 111:1002, 1996.
22. Aguillon D, Seguin P, Malledant Y: Syndrome hepatorenal: De la physiopathologie au traitement. Ann Fr Anesth Reanim 22:30-38, 2003.
23. Rossle M, Haag K, Ochs A, et al: The transjugular intrahepatic portosystemic stent-shunt procedure for variceal bleeding. N Engl J Med 330:165-171, 1994.
24. Lebrec D, Giuily N, Hadengue A, et al: Transjugular intrahepatic portosystemic shunts: Comparison with paracentesis in patients with cirrhosis and refractory ascites: A randomized trial. J Hepatol 25:135-144, 1996.
25. Sanyal AJ, Genning C, Reddy KR, et al: The North American study for the treatment of refractory ascites. Gastroenterology 124:634-641, 2003.
26. Rossle M, Ochs A, Gulberg V, et al: A comparison of paracentesis and transjugular intrahepatic portosystemic shunting in patients with ascites. N Engl J Med 342:1701-1707, 2000.
27. Gines P, Uriz J, Calahorra B, et al: Transjugular intrahepatic portosystemic shunting versus paracentesis plus albumin for refractory ascites in cirrhosis. Gastroenterology 123:1839-1847, 2002.
28. Schroeder ET, Anderson GH, Goldman SH, et al: Effect of blockade of angiotensin II on blood pressure, renin and aldosterone in cirrhosis. Kidney Int 9:511-519, 1976.
29. Bennett WM, Keeffe E, Melnyk C, et al: Response to dopamine hydrochloride in the hepatorenal syndrome. Arch Intern Med 135:964-967, 1975.
30. Fevery J, Van Cutsem E, Nevens F, et al: Reversal of hepatorenal syndrome in four patients by peroral misoprostol (prostaglandin E$_1$ analogue) and albumin administration. J Hepatol 11:153-158, 1990.
31. Gines A, Salmeron JM, Gines P, et al: Oral misoprostol or intravenous prostaglandin E$_2$ does not improve renal function in patients with cirrhosis and ascites with hyponatremia or renal failure. J Hepatol 17:220-226, 1994.
32. Wong F, Massie D, Hsu P, et al: Dose-dependent effects of oral misoprostol on renal function in alcoholic cirrhosis. Gastroenterology 106:658-663, 1994.
33. Kramer L, Hori WH: Hepatorenal syndrome. Semin Nephrol 22:290-301, 2002.
34. Soper CP, Latif AB, Bending MR: Amelioration of hepatorenal syndrome with selective endothelin-A antagonist [letter]. Lancet 347:1842-1843, 1996.
35. Kew MC, Varma RR, Sampson DJ, et al: The effect of octapressin on renal and intrarenal blood flow in cirrhosis of the liver. Gut 13:293-296, 1973.
36. Lenz K, Hortnagl H, Druml W, et al: Ornipressin in the treatment of functional renal failure in decompensated liver cirrhosis. Gastroenterology 101:1060-1067, 1991.
37. Gulberg V, Bilzer M, Gerbes AL: Long-term therapy and retreatment of hepatorenal syndrome type I with ornipressin and dopamine. Hepatology 30:870-875, 1999.
38. Guevara M, Gines P, Fernandez-Esparrach G, et al: Reversibility of hepatorenal syndrome by prolonged administration of ornipressin and plasma volume expansion. Hepatology 27:35-41, 1998.
39. Hadengue A, Gadano A, Moreau R, et al: Beneficial effects of the 2-day administration of terlipressin in patients with cirrhosis and hepatorenal syndrome. J Hepatol 29:565-570, 1998.
40. Duhamel C, Mauillon J, Berkelmans I, et al: Hepatorenal syndrome in cirrhotic patients: Terlipressin is a safe and efficient treatment [letter]. Am J Gastroenterol 95:2984-2985, 2000.
41. Uriz J, Gines P, Cardenas A, et al: Terlipressin plus albumin infusion: An effective and safe therapy of hepatorenal syndrome. J Hepatol 33:43-48, 2000.
42. Mulkay JP, Louis H, Donckier V: Long-term terlipressin administration improves renal function failure in cirrhotic patients with type I hepatorenal syndrome: A pilot study. Acta Gastroenterol Belg 64:15-19, 2001.
43. Ortega R, Gines P, Uriz J, et al: Terlipressin therapy with and without albumin for patients with hepatorenal syndrome: Results of a prospective, nonrandomized study. Hepatology 36:941-948, 2002.
44. Alessandria C, Venon WD, Marzano A, et al: Renal failure in cirrhotic patients: Role of terlipressin in clinical approach to hepatorenal syndrome type 2. Eur J Gastroenterol Hepatol 14:1363-1368, 2002.
45. Halimi C, Bonnard P, Bernard B, et al: Effect of terlipressin (Glypressin) on hepatorenal syndrome in cirrhotic patients: Results of a multicenter pilot study. Eur J Gastroenterol Hepatol 14:153-158, 2002.
46. Solanki P, Chawla A, Garg R, et al: Treatment of hepatorenal syndrome. Beneficial effects of terlipressin in hepatorenal syndrome: A prospective, randomized placebo-controlled clinical trial. J Gastroenterol Hepatol 18:152-156, 2003.
47. Duvoux C, Zanditenas D, Hezode C, et al: Effects of noradrenalin and albumin in patients with type I hepatorenal syndrome: A pilot study. Hepatology 36:374-380, 2002.
48. Holt S, Goodier D, Marley R, et al: Improvement in renal function in hepatorenal syndrome with N-acetylcysteine. Lancet 353:294-295, 1999.
49. Angeli P, Volpin R, Gerunda G, et al: Reversal of type I hepatorenal syndrome with the administration of midodrine and octreotide. Hepatology 29:1690-1697, 1999.
50. Pomier-Layrargues G, Paquin SC, Hassoun Z, et al: Octreotide in hepatorenal syndrome: A randomized, double-blind, placebo-controlled, crossover study. Hepatology 38:238-243, 2003.
51. Davenport A: Is there a role for continuous renal replacement therapies in patients with liver and renal failure? Kidney Int 56(Suppl 72):S62-S66, 1999.
52. Steiner C, Mitzner S: Experiences with MARS liver support therapy in liver failure: Analysis of 176 patients of the International MARS Registry. Liver 22(Suppl 2):20-25, 2002.
53. Mitzner SR, Stange J, Klammt S, et al: Improvement of hepatorenal syndrome with extracorporeal albumin dialysis MARS: Results of a prospective, randomized, controlled clinical trial. Liver Transpl 6:277-286, 2000.
54. Rettke SR, Janossy TA, Chantigian RC, et al. Hemodynamic and metabolic changes in hepatic transplantation. Mayo Clin Proc 64:232-240, 1989.
55. Estol CJ, Faris AA, Martinez AJ, Ahdab-Barmada M: Central pontine myelinolysis after liver transplantation. Neurology 39:493-498, 1989.
56. Wszolek ZK, McComb RD, Pfeiffer RF, et al: Pontine and extrapontine myelinolysis following liver transplantation. Relationship to serum sodium. Transplantation 48:1006-1012, 1989.
57. Boon AP, Carey MP, Adams DH, et al: Central pontine myelinolysis in liver transplantation. J Clin Pathol 44:909-914, 1991.

58. Singh N, Yu VL, Gayowski T: Central nervous system lesions in adult liver transplant recipients: Clinical review with implications for management. Medicine (Baltimore) 73:110-118, 1994.

59. Abbasoglu O, Goldstein RM, Vodapally MS, et al: Liver transplantation in hyponatremic patients with emphasis on central pontine myelinolysis. Clin Transplant 12:263-269, 1998.

60. Murdoch M, Chang M, McVicar J: Central pontine myelinolysis after liver transplantation: A case report. Transpl Int 8:399-402, 1995.

61. Wijdicks EF, Blue PR, Steers JL, Wiesner RH: Central pontine myelinolysis with stupor alone after orthotopic liver transplantation. Liver Transpl Surg 2:14-16, 1996.

62. Pitts TO, Van Thiel DH: Disorders of divalent ions and vitamin D metabolism in chronic alcoholism. Recent Dev Alcohol 4:357-377, 1986.

63. Gerhardt A, Greenberg A, Reilly JJ, Van Thiel DH: Hypercalcemia. A complication of advanced chronic liver disease. Arch Intern Med 147:274-277, 1987.

64. Sealy MM: Severe hypercalcemia due to a parathyroid-type hormone secreting tumour of the liver treated by hepatic transplantation. Anaesthesia 40:170-177, 1985.

65. Munoz SJ, Nagelberg SB, Green PJ, et al: Ectopic soft tissue calcium deposition following liver transplantation. Hepatology 8:476-483, 1988.

66. Wachtel MS, Dhettry U, Arkin CF: Tissue calcification after orthotopic liver transplantation. An autopsy study. Arch Pathol Lab Med 116:930-933, 1992.

67. Bennett MW, Webster NR, Sadek SA: Alterations in plasma magnesium concentrations during liver transplantation. Transplantation 56:859-561, 1993.

68. Scott VL, De Wolf AM, Kang Y, et al: Ionized hypomagnesemia in patients undergoing orthotopic liver transplantation: A complication of citrate intoxication. Liver Transpl Surg 2:343-347, 1996.

69. McDiarmid SV, Colonna JO 2nd, Shaked A, et al: A comparison of renal function in cyclosporine- and FK-506–treated patients after primary orthotopic liver transplantation. Transplantation 56:847-853, 1993.

70. Prytz H, Thomsen AC: Acid-base status in liver cirrhosis. Disturbances in stable, terminal and portal-caval shunted patients. Scand J Gastroenterol 11:249-256, 1976.

71. Fernandez OJJ, Moya FA, Rodriguez LA, et al: Study of arterial blood gases in liver cirrhosis with and without ascites [in Spanish]. Rev Esp Enferm Dig 88:197-201, 1996.

72. Lustik SJ, Chhibber AK, Kolano JW, et al: The hyperventilation of cirrhosis: Progesterone and estradiol effects. Hepatology 25:55-58, 1997.

73. Shirer HW, Erichson DF, Orr JA: Cardiorespiratory responses to HCl vs lactic acid infusion. J Appl Physiol 65:534-540, 1988.

74. Shaw BW Jr, Martin DJ, Marquez JM, et al: Advantages of venous bypass during orthotopic transplantation of the liver. Semin Liver Dis 5:344-348, 1985.

75. Shaw BW Jr, Martin DJ, Marquez JM, et al: Venous bypass in clinical liver transplantation. Ann Surg 200:524-534, 1984.

76. Wall WJ, Grant DR, Duff JH, et al: Liver transplantation without venous bypass. Surgery 43:56-61, 1995.

77. Veroli P, Hage C, Ecoffrey C: Does adult liver transplantation without venovenous bypass result in renal failure? Anesth Analg 75:489-494, 1992.

78. Grande L, Rimola A, Cugat E, et al: Effect of venovenous bypass on postoperative renal function in liver transplantation: Results of a randomized, controlled trial. Hepatology 23:1418-1428, 1996.

79. McCauley J, Van Thiel DH, Starzl TE, et al: Acute and chronic renal failure in liver transplantation. Nephron 55:121, 1990.

80. Fraley DS, Burr R, Bernardi J, et al: Impact of acute renal failure on mortality in end-stage liver disease with or without transplantation. Kidney Int 54:518, 1998.

81. Davis CL, Gonwa TA, Wilkinson AH: Identification of patients best suited for combined liver-kidney transplantation: Part II. Liver Transpl 8:193-211, 2002.

82. Lima EQ, Zanetta DM, Castro I, et al: Risk factors for development of acute renal failure after liver transplantation. Ren Fail 25:553-560, 2003.

83. Pawarode A, Fine DM, Thuluvath PJ: Independent risk factors and natural history of renal dysfunction in liver transplant recipients. Liver Transpl 9:741-747, 2003.

84. Fisher NC, Nightingale PG, Gunson BK, et al: Chronic renal failure following liver transplantation. Transplantation 66:59-66, 1998.

85. Platz KP, Mueller AR, Blumhardt G, et al: Nephrotoxicity following orthotopic liver transplantation. A comparison between cyclosporine and FK506. Transplantation 58:170-178, 1994.

86. Velidedeoglu E, Desai CNM, Campos L, et al: Predictors of late kidney dysfunction post–liver transplantation. Transplant Proc 34:3315-3316, 2002.

87. Gonwa TA, Mai ML, Melton LB, et al: End-stage renal disease (ESRD) after orthotopic liver transplantation (OLTX) using calcineurin-based immunotherapy. Transplantation 72:1934-1939, 2001.

88. Ojo AO, Held PJ, Port FK, et al: Chronic renal failure after transplantation of a nonrenal organ. N Engl J Med 349:931-940, 2003.

89. Gayowski T, Singh N, Keyes L, et al: Late-onset renal failure after liver transplantation: Role of posttransplant alcohol use. Transplantation 3:383-388, 2000.

90. Pham PT, Nast C, Pham PC, et al: Diagnosis and therapy of graft dysfunction. In Sayegh MH, Pereira BJG, Blake P (eds): Chronic Kidney Disease: Dialysis and Transplantation, 2nd ed. Philadelphia, WB Saunders (in press).

91. Davis CL, Gonwa TA, Wilkinson AH: Pathophysiology of renal disease associated with liver disorders: Implications for liver transplantation. Part I. Liver Transpl 8:91-109, 2002.

92. Danovitch GM: Immunosuppressive medications and protocols for kidney transplantation. In Danovitch GM (ed): Handbook of Kidney Transplantation, 3rd ed. Philadelphia, Lippincott Williams & Wilkins, 2001, pp 62-110.

93. Pham PT, Wilkinson AH, Danovitch GM, Pham PC: The effect of cyclosporine versus tacrolimus on long-term renal function in liver transplant recipients. Paper presented at the Annual Meeting of the American Society of Nephrology, San Diego, CA, November 17, 2003.

94. Cantarovich M, Barkun JS, Tchervenkov JI, et al: Comparisons of Neoral dose monitoring with cyclosporine trough levels versus 2-hr postdose levels in stable liver transplant patients. Transplantation 66:1621-1627, 1998 .

95. Teisseyre J, Markiewicz, Drewniak T, et al: Switching cyclosporine blood concentration monitoring from C0 to C2 in children late after liver transplantation. Transplant Proc 35:2287-2288, 2003.

96. Sterneck M, Zadeh KM, Groteluschen R, et al: Clinical use of C2 monitoring in long-term liver transplant recipients. Transplant Proc 34:3304-3306, 2002.

97. Gonwa TA, Klintmalm GB, Levy M, et al: Impact of pretransplant renal function on survival after liver transplantation. Transplantation 59:361, 1995.

98. Cantarovich M, Metrakos P, Giannetti N, et al: Anti-CD25 monoclonal antibody coverage allows CNI "holiday" in solid organ transplant patients with acute renal dysfunction. Transplantation 73:1169-1172, 2002.

99. Cantarovich M, Tzimas GN, Barkun J, et al: Efficacy of mycophenolate mofetil combined with very low-dose cyclosporine microemulsion in long-term liver-transplant patients with renal dysfunction. Transplantation 15:98-102, 2003.

100. Neau-Cransac M, Morel D, Bernard P-H, et al: Renal failure after liver transplantation: Outcome after calcineurin inhibitor withdrawal. Clin Transplant 16:368-373, 2002.

101. Nair S, Eason J, Loss G: Sirolimus monotherapy in nephrotoxicity due to calcineurin inhibitors in liver transplant recipients. Liver Transpl 9:126-129, 2003.
102. Nelson DR, Soldevila-Pico C, Red A, et al: Anti–interleukin-2-receptor therapy in combination with mycophenolate mofetil is associated with more severe hepatitis C recurrence after liver transplantation. Liver Transpl 7:1064-1070, 2001.
103. Everson TE: Impact of immunosuppressive therapy on recurrence of hepatitis C. Liver Transpl 8:S19-S27, 2002.
104. Lucey MR: Induction immunosuppression in hepatitis C virus–infected liver transplant recipients. Liver Transpl 8(Suppl 1):S44-S46, 2002.
105. Kahan BD, for The Rapamune US Study Group: Efficacy of sirolimus compared with azathioprine for reduction of acute renal allograft rejection: A randomized multicentre study. Lancet 356:194-202, 2000.
106. MacDonald AS, for The Rapamune Global Study Group: A worldwide, phase III, randomized, controlled, safety and efficacy study of a sirolimus/cyclosporine regimen for prevention of acute rejection in recipients of primary mismatched renal allografts. Transplantation 71:271-280, 2001.
107. Podder H, Stepkowski SM, Napoli KL, et al: Pharmacokinetic interactions augment toxicities of sirolimus/cyclosporine combinations. J Am Soc Nephrol 12:1059-1071, 2001.
108. Undre NA: Pharmacokinetics of tacrolimus-based combination therapies. Nephrol Dial Transplant 18:S12-S15, 2003.
109. Lawsin L, Light JA: Severe acute renal failure after exposure to sirolimus-tacrolimus in two living donor kidney recipients. Transplantation 75:157-160, 2003.
110. Cuervas-Mons V, Millan I, Gavaler JS, et al: Prognostic value of preoperatively obtained clinical and laboratory data in predicting survival following orthotopic liver transplantation. Hepatology 6:922-927, 1986.
111. Rimola A, Gavaler JS, Schade RR, et al: Effects of renal impairment on liver transplantation. Gastroenterology 93:148, 1987.
112. Gonwa TA, Mai ML, Melton LB, et al: Renal replacement therapy and orthotopic liver transplantation: The role of continuous veno-venous hemodialysis. Transplantation 71:1424-1428, 2001.
113. Fraley DS, Burr R, Bernardi J, et al: Impact of acute renal failure on mortality in end-stage liver disease with or without transplantation. Kidney Int 54:518-524, 1998.
114. Gainza FJ, Valdivieso A, Quintanilla N, et al: Evaluation of acute renal failure in the liver transplantation perioperative period: Incidence and impact. Transplant Proc 34:250-251, 2002.
115. Margreiter R, Kramar R, Huber C, et al: Combined liver and kidney transplant. Lancet 1:1077-1078, 1995.
116. Gonwa TA, Nery JR, Husburg BS, et al: Simultaneous liver and renal transplantation in man. Transplantation 46:690, 1988.
117. Jeyarajah DR, McBride M, Klintman GB, et al: Combined liver-kidney transplantation: What are the indications? Transplantation 64:1091, 1997.
118. Hiesse C, Samuel D, Bensadoun H, et al: Combined liver and kidney transplantation in patients with chronic nephritis associated with end-stage liver disease. Nephrol Dial Transplant (Suppl 6):129, 1995.
119. Jeyarajah DR, Gonwa TA, Testa G, et al: Liver and kidney transplantation for polycystic disease. Transplantation 66:529-544, 1998.
120. Newman KD, Torres VE, Rakela J, Nagorney DM: Treatment of highly symptomatic polycystic liver disease. Ann Surg 212:30-37, 1990.
121. Turnage RH, Eckhauser FE, Knol JA, Thompson NW: Therapeutic dilemma in patients with symptomatic polycystic liver disease. Am Surg 4:365-372, 1988.
122. Soravia C, Mentha G, Giostra E, et al: Surgery for adult polycystic liver disease. Surgery 117:272-275, 1995.
123. Swenson K, Seu P, Kinkhabwala M, et al: Liver transplantation for adult polycystic liver disease. Hepatology 28:412-415, 1998.
124. Cochat P, Gaulier JM, Koch Nogueira PC, et al: Combined liver-kidney transplantation in primary hyperoxaluria type I. Eur J Pediatr 158(Suppl 2)S75-S80, 1999.
125. Jamieson NV: The results of combined liver/kidney transplantation for primary hyperoxaluria (PH1) 1984-1997: The European PH I transplant registry report. J Nephrol 11(Suppl):S36-S41, 1998.
126. Saborio P, Scheinman JI: Transplantation for primary hyperoxaluria in the United States. Kidney Int 56:1094-1100, 1999.
127. Leumann E, Hoppe B: The primary hyperoxalurias. J Am Soc Nephrol 12:1986-1993, 2001.
128. Millan MT, Berquist WE, So SK, et al: One hundred percent patient and kidney allograft survival with simultaneous liver and kidney transplantation in infants with primary hyperoxaluria: A single center experience. Transplantation 76:1458-1463, 2003.
129. Danpure CJ: Scientific rationale for hepato-renal transplantation in primary hyperoxaluria type 1. Transplant Clin Immunol 22:91-98, 1991.
130. Leumann E, Hoppe B: What is new in primary hyperoxaluria? Nephrol Dial Transplant 14:2556-2558, 1999.
131. Koppel MH, Coburn JW, Mims MM, et al: Transplantation of cadaveric kidney from patients with hepatorenal syndrome. Evidence for the functional nature of renal failure in patients with advanced liver disease. N Engl J Med 280:1367, 1969.
132. Iwatsuki S, Popovtzer MM, Corman JL, et al: Recovery from "hepatorenal syndrome" after orthotopic liver transplantation. N Engl J Med 289:1155, 1973.
133. Seu P, Wilkinson AH, Shaked A: The hepatorenal syndrome in liver transplant recipients. Am Surg 57:806, 1991.
134. Gonwa TA, Klintman GB, Levy M, et al: Impact of pretransplant renal function on survival after liver transplantation. Transplantation 59:361, 1995.

Graft Failure: Etiology, Recognition, and Treatment

NICHOLAS N. NISSEN
STEVEN D. COLQUHOUN

Definition   915

Incidence   916

Challenge   916

Diagnosis   917

Etiology   917
  Donor-related factors   918
  Procurement-related factors   922
  Recipient-related factors   922
  Predictors of primary nonfunction and
    initial poor function   922

Treatment   923
  Avoidance   923
  Graft hepatectomy   924
  Retransplantation   924
  Specific treatment of primary
    nonfunction   924
  Liver assist devices   925
  Blocking ischemia/reperfusion injury   925
  Small-for-size syndrome   925

Conclusions/summary   925

Although there have been many dramatic advances in the field of liver transplantation in the past 10 years, the problems of overcoming graft dysfunction and failure have been less gratifying. Despite better understanding of the associations, risks, and probable mechanisms of graft failure, truly effective interventions have remained more elusive.

The increasing shortage of organs for transplantation has forced the use of allografts with even more expanded criteria for selection, as well as allocation to progressively more decompensated recipients, thereby resulting in increasingly fewer organs for retransplantation.[1] It has also led to the use of living donor transplantation, which has brought its own set of issues related to graft function. These facts have now made the problem of graft dysfunction and failure more important than ever.

The objective of this chapter is to comprehensively review the issues relevant to early functioning of allografts so that when feasible, risk factors can be prevented, dysfunction recognized, and appropriate measures taken to avoid poor outcomes.

Definition

"A diagnosis of PNF [primary nonfunction] is made by exclusion, when early graft failure develops and no significant causal factor can be identified."[2]

Table 61-1. DESCRIPTORS OF GRAFT DYSFUNCTION AFTER LIVER TRANSPLANTATION

Primary nonfunction

Initial poor function

Delayed graft function

Initial graft nonfunction

Poor early graft function

Initial graft nonfunction

Table 61-2. DIAGNOSIS OF PRIMARY NONFUNCTION—PROPOSED UNOS CRITERIA (ADULT)

≤10 days

AST ≥ 5000 U/L *and*

INR ≥ 3.0 (regardless of FFP) *or*

Presence of acidosis (pH ≤ 7.3) or lactate concentration ≥ 2× normal

AST, aspartate transaminase; FFP, fresh-frozen plasma; INR, international normalized ratio; UNOS, United Network for Organ Sharing.

The topic of this chapter is early cryptogenic graft dysfunction or failure, exclusive of any identifiable technical problems such as hepatic artery or portal vein thrombosis. Clinically, this type of graft failure can occur anywhere on a continuum from an ambiguous and potentially reversible dysfunction to an unqualified absence of function. This wide range of manifestations has led to several frustrating aspects of this problem. First is the lack of any exact definitions, and the second follows in that there is no universally accepted terminology (Table 61–1). Third is the seeming unpredictability of its occurrence and, finally, the unpredictability of its course. Indeed, because dysfunctional grafts may improve with time, the outcome of a particular allograft can be known with certainty only in retrospect. Obviously, once an organ is retransplanted, its course can no longer be followed, thus leading to a potentially diagnostic self-fulfilling prophecy. With such vague and subjective definitions, it should be no surprise that there is significant inconsistency in the literature. In this respect, graft dysfunction can be compared with pornography: easy to recognize, but difficult to define.

The term "primary nonfunction" (PNF) is perhaps best defined as graft failure soon after revascularization with no discernible cause that leads to either retransplantation or death of the patient. All other circumstances of early cryptogenic graft dysfunction then define "initial poor function" (IPF). Although risk factors can be identified in the majority of patients with PNF or IPF, such factors can also be present when a graft functions normally.

Even though most would agree that PNF and IPF become manifested within the first 24 to 72 hours after transplantation, current organ allocation policy of the United Network for Organ Sharing (UNOS) specifies that the diagnosis of PNF be restricted to 7 days or less from the time of transplantation.[3] Interestingly, current UNOS policy offers no objective criteria or any other clinical parameters or guidelines for the definition of PNF. However, there has recently been an effort within UNOS to better define PNF for organ allocation to both adult and pediatric recipients. These definitions include both a present time limit of 10 days or less and some clinically relevant parameters of graft function (Table 61–2).

With the increasing use of allografts from living donors, a new type of early graft dysfunction has been recognized. Small-for-size syndrome (SFSS) is early graft dysfunction occurring in the setting of a small-for-size (SFS) allograft. Although SFSS has been described extensively in the context of living donor liver transplantation, it has relevance for whole-organ and reduced-size deceased donor grafts as well.

Incidence

In a report covering the first 1000 liver transplants performed at the University of California at Los Angeles, the incidence of PNF was 4%.[4] In a more recent update of 3000 transplants from the same institution, PNF was responsible for 38.5% of all retransplants performed.[5] In another large single-center review of 4000 consecutive transplants performed over a 17-year period, PNF remained one of the two most common causes of retransplantation.[6] In that study, the rate of PNF was also surprisingly constant over the years—ranging from 4.6% in the earliest era to 7% in the middle era and finally 6% most recently. Generally, the reported incidence of both IPF and PNF is expectedly quite variable given the rather vague diagnostic criteria that exist. Overall, the incidence of PNF ranges from 0.6% to as high as 22%. Most centers continue to report an incidence ranging from 2% to 10%, with an average of about 6%, and a higher rate of IPF in the range of 15% to 30%.[7-10] Programs with more aggressive use of donors with expanded criteria for selection may experience higher rates, although PNF can occur even in the most optimal circumstances.[11] It is also conceivable that PNF could be significantly underreported. Early postoperative deaths attributed to sepsis, neurological injury, multiorgan system failure, or other causes could be the indirect effect of a nonfunctioning graft.

Challenge

The challenges that IPF, PNF, and SFSS present are of major significance to the liver transplant community.

With the ongoing shortage of organs, increased effort has been directed at using "expanded criteria" deceased donors, as well as living donors, thus increasing the risk of encountering one of the aforementioned entities.[12]

Diagnosis

Most clinicians, when faced with a patient with early graft dysfunction, use a composite of clinical, laboratory, and sometimes histological findings to diagnose IPF and PNF. The diagnosis of PNF is generally made within 72 hours after transplantation, when either death or retransplantation intervenes. The signs and symptoms may be recognized as early as during the transplant operation itself. Worsening coagulopathy soon after reperfusion can be an early ominous sign. Persistent lactic acidosis or hemodynamic instability, or both, also imply graft nonfunction. In the most severe circumstance, the compromised allograft appears to perpetuate the acidosis and hemodynamic instability, and the only alternative may be to render the patient anhepatic while looking for another organ. Fortunately, the scenario of total graft nonfunction is charitably rare, and a variety of more subtle clinical findings usually reflect the degree of dysfunction.

Bile production during the transplant procedure itself is an excellent prognostic sign, and the bile flow rate has been reported in many studies to be one of the most useful predictors of postoperative function. Bile production may reflect the recovery of adenosine triphosphate (ATP) synthesis in the graft. Anecdotally, the color of the bile may be equally important, with a golden brown color held as the ideal. Similarly, reversal of acidosis and improving renal function are signs of good function. The absence of these findings may signify IPF or PNF.

Laboratory values can also contribute to the diagnosis of PNF. Serum transaminases in the tens of thousands or levels that are steadily increasing imply severe organ damage and unlikely recovery. Rosen and coauthors reported that a peak aspartate transaminase (AST) level higher than 5000 U/L resulted in a PNF rate of 41%, as opposed to a rate of 10% in those with peak AST levels of 2000 to 5000.[13] Others have identified an initial AST level higher than 2000 or levels that are slow to resolve as being predictive of PNF.[10,14] Elevated alanine transaminase (ALT) levels and prothrombin times may have a similar predictive value. Persistent lactic acidosis, hypoglycemia, hyperkalemia, increasing hyperbilirubinemia, and persistent severe hypoprothrombinemia are all obvious signs of poor function. Rather than an absolute value of any test, it is always the trends in values that are of greatest importance.

Other bedside findings indicative of graft function include the patient's mental status, urinary output, and pulmonary status. Multiorgan system failure is the inevitable result in the absence of a working liver. The best correlation with poor outcome does not appear to be the failure of any particular individual organ system, but rather the absolute number of organ systems involved.

Five specific criteria as used at Johns Hopkins have been advocated in the evaluation of IPF: (1) ongoing injury/rising serum transaminase levels, (2) poor synthetic function/elevated international normalized ratio (INR) despite continuous administration of fresh-frozen plasma (FFP), (3) "minimal" bile production (no comment on color), (4) impaired metabolic clearance/hyperammonemia, and (5) patent vascular anastomoses by Doppler ultrasound.[15] Most patients with poor, but reversible, function begin to improve by the third posttransplant day, whereas those with PNF will continue to worsen.[16]

It is essential that with any evidence of graft dysfunction, vascular or other technical abnormalities be considered and excluded. Again by definition, IPF and PNF exclude hepatic artery, portal vein, or hepatic venous outflow abnormalities, as well as other systemic processes such as abdominal compartment syndrome and elevated right heart pressure. Although vascular abnormalities can usually be excluded by noninvasive studies, surgical exploration is often the most expeditious manner in which to exclude a wide variety of vascular and mechanical factors and allow "hands-on" assessment and safe biopsy of the graft.

All definitions of PNF remain subjective in that the clinical decision for retransplantation is operator dependent. Efforts to more clearly define PNF and IPF would facilitate management of graft dysfunction by allowing more controlled discussion, reporting, interventions, and organ allocation policies.

Etiology

A number of studies over the years have attempted to analyze a multitude of donor and recipient variables to determine the cause of graft failure. An exhaustive list of factors implicated in PNF/IPF is provided in Table 61–3.[10,17-20] Knowledge as well as avoidance of combinations of these risk factors is probably the best strategy for preventing both IPF and PNF.[9] The underlying mechanisms leading to graft dysfunction in each of these risk categories are also likely to have considerable overlap.

For purposes of discussion, factors influencing graft function can be chronologically categorized within the transplant process as being related to (1) the donor, (2) procurement, and (3) the recipient. Currently, the most globally important issues linked with graft failure include donor age, donor steatosis, SFSS in the living donor setting, and the cellular and molecular events of

Table 61–3. RISK FACTORS FOR PRIMARY NONFUNCTION AND INITIAL POOR FUNCTION

Donor

Age older than 65 yr

Steatosis in > 30% of graft volume

Peak sodium > 155 mEq/L

Use of high-dose or multiple pressors

Prolonged intensive care unit stay

Prolonged interval between brain death and organ procurement

Procurement

Cold ischemic time > 12 hr

Non–heart-beating donor

Recipient

Retransplantation

Severely ill/high MELD score

Use of high-dose or multiple pressors

Renal failure

MELD, Model for End-Stage Liver Disease.

ischemia and subsequent reperfusion. The last is of such significance that it warrants its own chapter in this text and will therefore not be considered in detail here.

Donor-Related Factors

A recent single-center review of 400 liver transplants identified several variables to be independently associated with allograft dysfunction, including the use of high-dose inotropes, donor age, steatosis, duration of cold ischemia, and prolonged intensive care unit (ICU) stay before procurement.[21] Numerous previous studies have also directly linked steatosis, age, and prolonged cold ischemia time to IPF and PNF.

Age

Although Hans Popper himself once reported that "the liver knows no senescent change"[22] and although no hepatic disorders are known to be restricted to old age, a number of alterations have now been appreciated to occur in the liver with aging. Even though gross and histological changes may be minimal, functional alterations do appear to take place. Liver weight and volume tend to diminish with age, and hepatic blood flow is reduced.[23] Underlying atherosclerotic disease of the aorta and mesenteric vessels may also alter organ perfusion during procurement. These and other age-related changes that are insignificant during life might be magnified by the extremes of the transplant process.

Data on outcomes of liver transplants from older deceased donors are conflicting. Even the definition of "older" varies from more than 30 years to more than 70.[24] Several studies have suggested that donor age older than 60 or 65 is an independent risk factor for graft dysfunction,[17,24a] whereas others have reported an increased risk for delayed graft function but no change in patient survival or PNF when older donors are used.[25] Still others have reported no increase in PNF or IPF in recipients of livers from older donors.[24,26–28] Even the use of select organs from donors 80 years or older has been reported to have good results with no early graft dysfunction.[28,29]

Despite the lack of consensus, it is clear that the use of livers from older donors has increased over the last 15 years.[1] According to the most recent data from the Organ Procurement and Transplantation Network/Scientific Registry of Transplant Recipients, the percentage of donors 50 years or older has increased from 17.3% in 1992 to 30.1% in 2001,[30] whereas the use of donors 65 years and older has risen from 2.5% to more than 9% between 1992 and 1999.

Even with the many conflicting reports, a number of studies as well as empirical sense have suggested an increased incidence of graft dysfunction in organs procured from "older" donors.[10,12] Although a specific mechanism is not known, donor age should be considered a risk factor for both IPF and PNF. Finally, it is important to remember that other confounding factors may influence donor age–related outcome data. For example, if prejudice against older donors leads to their use more often in extreme circumstances when recipients cannot wait for a "better" organ, the severity of the recipient's illness may also influence the incidence of IPF and PNF.

Steatosis

A fatty liver is defined as one in which lipid (primarily triglyceride) accounts for more than 5% of the weight of the liver. Macrovesicular steatosis, in which the vacuole occupies the majority of the hepatocyte cytoplasm and displaces the nucleus peripherally, is most common. This type of steatosis is associated with alcohol abuse, diabetes, hyperlipidemia, obesity, and the use of certain drugs. Microvesicular steatosis is characterized by vacuoles that are smaller than the cell nucleus and have a centrilobular distribution. This type of steatosis is found in pathological conditions often associated with mitochondrial injury, such as Reye's syndrome, acute viral or drug injury, chronic total parenteral nutrition, sepsis, and some genetic metabolic disorders.[31]

The incidence of hepatic steatosis in the general population is variably reported as being between 6.3% and 24%.[32,33] In an autopsy study of more than 500 traffic accident victims, fatty liver changes had an overall incidence of 24% and were correlated with age: 1% in those younger than 20 years, 18% in those 20 to 40 years old, and 39% in those older than 60 years.[34] Deceased donors may present additional risk factors, including both exposure to hyperalimentation and prolonged starvation. In fact, brain death itself appears to predispose to steatosis in the absence of other risk factors. The prevalence of steatosis in deceased donors ranges by report from 13% to 26%.[8,35]

An association between fatty infiltration and PNF has long been appreciated in clinical liver transplantation.[36] D'Allesandro and colleagues looked at the predictive value of donor liver biopsy and generally found that those with macrosteatosis had a higher rate of PNF.[8] In a large multivariate analysis of risk factors for graft dysfunction, Ploeg and associates found that fatty changes in the donor liver were independently associated with both IPF and PNF.[10] In another study, Adam and coauthors reported that organs with 30% or greater steatosis had a PNF rate of 13%, as opposed to only 2.5% in those that were nonfatty.[33] Higher rates of PNF have been reported with increasing degrees of steatosis.

In contrast to these reports, an analysis of UNOS data on more than 22,000 liver transplants between 1987 and 2001 found no correlation between donor body mass index (BMI) or graft steatosis and early retransplantation rates.[37] Along with a number of other inherent limitations in a study of this nature, these data undoubtedly reflect the selection bias of the common clinical practice of discarding severely steatotic allografts; in fact, the group of donors with BMI greater than 35 was comparatively small. However, transcending smaller single-center anecdotal reports, it does suggest that certainly not all fatty organs fail. Several other single-center studies have also reported that select fatty grafts can be used with acceptable outcomes. Finally, it is interesting to note that the use of fatty livers in the living donor setting does not appear to be associated with the same incidence of graft dysfunction. Allografts with up to 50% macrovesicular steatosis have been used with acceptable function and patient outcome.[38,39] In addition, at least one report has shown successful use of donor organs with 30% to 60% or greater microvesicular steatosis; the reported 5% incidence of PNF and 10% incidence of IPF were not higher than rates for nonfatty grafts.[40]

Inconsistency regarding the relevance of allograft steatosis is probably due in part to the subjective nature of estimating the extent of fatty change. Most assessments are made clinically by gross appearance of an organ. Liver biopsy performed at the time of procurement has limited utility because of sampling error and the inaccuracy of frozen section analysis, although it may be useful in providing some objective information to off-site transplant teams. A generally accepted scheme classifies macrovesicular steatosis as mild (<30% of liver volume), moderate (30% to 60%), and severe (>60%). Although grafts with mild steatosis generally do well, moderate steatosis is associated with an increased risk for IPF and PNF. Grafts with severe steatosis should be avoided.[32] As with many other donor factors, graft steatosis alone is unlikely to determine the outcome of liver transplantation. Except in the case of severe steatosis, many fatty grafts can be used successfully if careful attention is paid to contributory donor variables, recipient selection, and limitation of ischemic time.

The mechanisms underlying the increased sensitivity of steatotic grafts to transplantation remain incompletely understood. The importance of this area of research is obvious in the context of an expanding donor organ shortage and increasing incidence of donor obesity. In perhaps the first report to document an association between PNF and steatosis, Todo and coworkers described the failure of two allografts with severe diffuse macrovesicular steatosis and no other histological or clinical abnormalities. They observed early histological changes, including extracellular fatty droplets associated with sinusoidal disruption and occlusion.[36] These authors speculated that the resulting microcirculatory changes could result in ischemia and events leading to necrosis. Numerous interrelated mechanisms have subsequently been proposed to account for the changes in steatotic grafts. Some of these mechanisms include an increased sensitivity to microcirculatory disruption, dysfunctional mitochondria/ATP production, and impaired apoptosis ultimately leading to impaired hepatocellular regeneration.[32,41,42] Other changes that have been found to occur include Kupffer cell activation and release of mediators that further diminish sinusoidal blood flow and lead to the generation of oxygen free radicals. The role of oxidative stress per se in the development of IPF and PNF is, however, extremely complex and defies oversimplification.[43]

Our understanding of the mechanisms associated with IPF/PNF in steatotic grafts has progressed from an association through observation of histological changes to events at an intracellular level in the study of ischemia/reperfusion injury. Indeed, the best evidence of progress in this field is the devotion of an entire chapter of this text to this topic. Clearly, further studies will be required to elucidate the full details. At the very least, it certainly does appear that steatosis exacerbates the mechanisms of injury related to ischemia/reperfusion.

"Small-for-Size" Syndrome

Even before the era of living donor liver transplantation, it was known that use of an allograft of inadequate size for a given recipient could result in graft dysfunction or failure. With the increasing importance of adult-to-adult living donor transplantation, the importance of relative graft-to-recipient size has become more evident.

When Emond and colleagues explored the feasibility of living donor adult-to-adult transplantation, they found that graft size strongly correlated with function in the recipient. This group was perhaps the first to use the term "small for size" when describing a pattern of dysfunction that occurred when allograft volume was less than 50% of the recipient's expected liver volume.[44] Since then, many others have described SFSS, and it appears to be as much a challenge as IPF and PNF in the deceased donor realm.[11,45]

Currently, the best definition of SFSS is that of early graft dysfunction occurring in the setting of an SFS allograft and the absence of any technical problems. The currently accepted limit of graft size for living donors is 40% to 50% or greater of the calculated ideal liver weight or, alternatively, 0.8% to 1% of the graft-to-recipient weight ratio.[46] As a rule of thumb, the liver is approximately 2% to 3% of body weight in healthy individuals,[47] but there is considerable individual variability in the size of a given segment.[48] An SFS graft is now generally accepted to be that with a graft-to-recipient weight ratio less than 0.8% to 1.0% or less than 30% to 50% of the standard estimated liver volume.[45,47,49]

As with IPF/PNF, the occurrence of SFSS is far from predictable, and many SFS grafts have been used successfully. Like IPF/PNF, SFSS can also demonstrate the same spectrum of severity.[11] Most commonly seen are delayed synthetic function, poor bile production, prolonged cholestasis, and susceptibility to a variety of other complications, including sepsis and overall diminished graft survival.[49] It is likely that a number of both graft- and recipient-related factors are important in determining when SFSS will occur. It also now seems likely that not only anatomic graft size but also functional size can be of relevance. The latter may be influenced by some of the same parameters associated with IPF/PNF, such as age and steatosis.

As with whole organs, a number of issues other than graft size have been associated with SFSS, including the severity and chronicity of the recipient's illness (i.e., greater "metabolic debt"), the donor's age or other latent disease, and technical issues such as duration of ischemia and adequacy of venous drainage.[49] In a large series of 276 cases of living donor transplantation, Kiuchi and colleagues found significantly lower graft survival overall and many more complications in general when grafts had a volume less than 1% of the recipient's body weight.[48] Indeed, when allografts were "extra small" (<0.8%) and "small" (<1.0%), actuarial survival rates were only 42% and 74%, respectively, as compared with a 92% survival rate in those that were "medium" (≥1.0% to ≤3.0%). Although not all were lost to IPF or PNF, a syndrome of delayed bilirubin clearance and synthetic function has been described that appeared to predispose to other surgical or septic complications (or to both). Ben-Haim and coworkers found that "small grafts in sicker patients have an additive negative impact on early graft survival." In this study, the overall incidence of SFSS was 12.5%, but it was observed exclusively in recipients with Child's B and C status. In that group the incidence of SFSS was 83% (five of six) when small grafts were used, which led to death or retransplantation in 80% (four of five).[46] The incidence reported in the living donor literature ranges from 2.9% to 12.5%.[46,50]

Early on, Emond and associates speculated on a mechanism of SFSS that included portal hyperperfusion and an overwhelmed metabolic capacity of the small graft.[44] Many others now agree, and the prevailing theory for a mechanism of SFSS is that of portal hyperperfusion with injury resulting from portal pressure exceeding sinusoidal compliance. The relatively high volume of gut-derived substrates or toxins, or both, may also contribute by overwhelming the metabolic capacity of the small graft.[44,48] Serial biopsy specimens from affected organs appear to have histological changes consistent with ischemia, including ballooning, steatosis, centrilobular necrosis, and cholestasis.[44] Clinical support for the theory of portal hyperperfusion can be found in a number of studies. Using electromagnetic probes, Troisi and colleagues measured right portal vein and right hepatic artery flow in living donors and then their recipients.[51] By comparison, recipient portal flow was always at least three times greater than that in the donor. SFSS was primarily noted in recipients with exceptionally high portal flow. However, no cases of SFSS were encountered when various measures were taken to reduce flow to the graft (e.g., splenic artery ligation, portocaval shunt, and portal vein banding), in contrast to a control group in which the incidence was 27%. Ito and coworkers[52] actually measured portal venous pressure with an indwelling catheter in patients after living donor transplantation. They found a strong correlation between elevated portal venous pressure, small grafts (<0.8% of recipient body weight), and poor patient survival. Those with small grafts treated by splenic artery ligation fared significantly better.[52] Finally, in a recent, albeit anecdotal report, Lo and coauthors observed dramatic clinical improvement and avoided seemingly inevitable retransplantation by reducing portal flow and pressure via splenic artery ligation.[2]

Animal data derived from the use of small grafts have also supported the concept of portal hyperperfusion in SFSS. In a rat transplant model, Man and colleagues found both significantly higher portal venous pressure and hepatic microcirculatory blood flow in SFS grafts than in whole organs. After 24 hours, light and electron microscopic features of SFS grafts showed striking sinusoidal congestion, mitochondrial swelling, and collapse of the space of Disse.[53] Insights into the molecular mechanisms of this process have also been explored. Microarray analysis of gene expression has shown early expression and overexpression of a host of genes related to vasoconstriction, some adhesion molecules, and factors related to the acute phase response. This finding implies a dual mechanism of early mechanical injury to sinusoids with a subsequent ischemia/reperfusion-type injury.[54]

The current understanding of SFSS represents an example of the evolution in understanding and management of previously cryptogenic graft dysfunction. Although the cellular mechanisms that are disrupted in SFSS have yet to be defined, clinical appreciation and empirical management of this phenomenon have paralleled the expanding field of living donor liver transplantation. Similar effort into uncovering the mechanisms of cryptogenic graft dysfunction after deceased donor transplantation may ultimately lead to successful augmentation of the expanded criteria donor organ pool.

Other Donor-Related Issues

Hemodynamic Stability. Hypotension is a well-described cause of shock liver. As such, it seems intuitive that prolonged hypotension or cardiac arrest in the deceased donor may add to the risk for graft dysfunction. The use of multiple or high-dose vasopressors has in fact been identified as a risk factor for early graft dysfunction.[18,55] Vasopressors are well known to cause splanchnic vasoconstriction, which may add to the "harvest injury" frequently invoked when an organ fails to function. However, hypoxia, hypotension, and cardiac arrest are often surprisingly well tolerated by the liver, and grafts from such donors may still show excellent function.[7] Previous cardiac arrest with successful resuscitation has been hypothesized to induce a form of protective ischemic preconditioning that may partly protect the graft during the transplant process. The use of high-dose or multiple pressors is clearly a risk factor for PNF and IPF, but by itself should not preclude use of an organ. This is in contrast to the biochemical evidence of recalcitrant shock liver, which should be considered a high-risk donor organ.

Additional Donor Factors. Several metabolic, electrolyte, and genetic factors have been identified in deceased donors that may contribute to the risk for graft dysfunction. Although some of these findings are largely anecdotal, others, such as hypernatremia, have repeatedly been implicated in graft failure and warrant close consideration. Unfortunately, the relative risk contribution of these factors alone or in combination is difficult to predict.

A number of studies suggest that donor hypernatremia can affect graft function.[56] Diabetes insipidus and poor fluid management in potential donors are the most common cause of this condition. Totuska and

colleagues looked at peak donor serum sodium as well as corrected sodium at the time of procurement.[57] They found a significant correlation between uncorrected hypernatremia (>155 mEq/L) and both IPF and PNF. The incidence of PNF was 18.5% in the uncorrected hypernatremia group versus 3.4% in those with normal sodium levels. When serum sodium is corrected before procurement, the increase in PNF is no longer found. Although the exact mechanism is not known with certainty, it is postulated that hypernatremia leads to increased intracellular osmolality, with the subsequent cellular edema incurred at reperfusion leading to graft dysfunction.

Lengthy hospitalization or a prolonged interval from the insult resulting in brain death to the time of procurement has also been noted empirically to be a factor associated with IPF/PNF. No studies to date have definitively shown a correlation between this parameter and poor graft function. Several factors, including glycogen depletion, inflammatory mediators of the systemic inflammatory response cascade, and the progressive microcirculatory dysfunction of brain death, may contribute to the increased susceptibility of these organs to poor graft function after transplantation.

Immunological factors related to both donor race and gender have been questioned as possible contributors to graft dysfunction. In a retrospective review of UNOS data from 1992 through 2000, Rustgi and associates[58] found that gender mismatch was associated with a 6.9% increased likelihood of graft failure, with the worst outcome seen in male recipients of grafts from females. Regarding race, the only noteworthy combination was that of a significant increase in the risk for graft failure when white recipients received organs from black donors.[58]

Brain death itself has obvious systemic implications, with major changes in a number of hormones, myocardial dysfunction, and alterations in central control of vascular tone. Diminished serum antidiuretic hormone levels lead to the development of diabetes insipidus, dehydration, and hypernatremia. Low levels of tri-iodothyronine also occur with central nervous system injury and can have profound effects on donor hemodynamics. Successful procurement of organs for transplantation can occur only within a narrow window of opportunity, after which global deterioration of the donor is inevitable. A number of studies have looked at the systemic manifestations of brain death and its implications on the liver. In animal models, specific compromise of hepatic sinusoidal perfusion has been documented along with other changes in leukocyte/endothelial interactions.[59] Such observations appear to be the harbinger of what will subsequently be the manifestations of ischemia/reperfusion-related injury.

Preexisting donor conditions such as hepatitis, genetic defects, and errors in metabolism or coagulation have also been reported to contribute to posttransplant graft failure.[55] Certain drugs taken by donors before brain death, such as seizure medications or warfarin (Coumadin), could also conceivably contribute to graft dysfunction. Komokata and coauthors reported a case of PNF after the use of an organ from a donor intoxicated with methamphetamines.[60] Donor hypertension has also been linked to PNF. There is at least one report in which PNF occurred in two normotensive recipients of organs from donors with long-standing hypertension. Assessment of the failed grafts revealed marked narrowing of the medium and large intrahepatic arteries; thus it was postulated that relative arterial ischemia was primarily responsible for the PNF.[61]

Procurement-Related Factors

Several different aspects of the preservation process may simultaneously affect organ function. These aspects are generally divided into two categories: those occurring during the ischemic or anoxic period, which begins at the moment of in situ donor perfusion, and those related to reperfusion injury when blood flow is reestablished during the recipient procedure.

The advent of University of Wisconsin (UW) preservation solution revolutionized organ procurement by increasing the effective duration of organ storage. At the same time, UW solution has significantly lowered the incidence of PNF.[62] Nonetheless, the interval of cold ischemia remains extremely important. Cold preservation slows, but does not prevent cellular metabolic processes. It is clear that the length of time that an organ is exposed to storage affects outcome and the incidence of PNF. Furukawa and coinvestigators reviewed the storage times for close to 600 human allografts and found an almost direct correlation between increasing cold ischemia time and increasing incidence of PNF.[63] Clearly, the susceptibility of grafts to ischemic time varies with the quality of the graft. Although total ischemic times of less than 12 to 16 hours may be well tolerated by a perfect donor organ, an expanded criteria organ is best handled by minimizing ischemic time in any way possible.

Livers obtained from non–heart-beating donors (NHBDs) appear to be at higher risk for PNF and IPF than do those from brain-dead donors. Abt and colleagues recently reviewed UNOS data on 144 NHBD livers and found the incidence of PNF to be approximately twice that of heart-beating donors (12% versus 6%).[64] Similarly, retransplantation rates were higher in recipients of NHBD grafts (14% versus 8%). This study found a trend toward decreased survival in recipients of NHBD grafts as well. This observation is not surprising because NHBD organs face a period of obligate warm ischemia while cardiac function ceases. This donor pool may become increasingly important as the donor organ shortage grows, but clearly, these organs should be considered at jeopardy for PNF and appropriate measures taken by procurement and recipient teams to minimize compounding risk factors.

Recipient-Related Factors

Several recipient factors may have a direct impact on the risk for PNF or IPF. The most widely accepted contributing factor is the severity of the recipient illness. An expanded criteria allograft may be expected to function well in a relatively stable recipient or one with a short duration of disease such as fulminant hepatic failure. However, the same graft may perform quite poorly in an extremely ill recipient with a high "metabolic debt." Few studies have quantified this finding, yet it is widely accepted to be empirically true.[46] This parallels the observation in living donor transplantation that SFS grafts fare poorly in severely ill recipients. Occasionally, an individual with PNF will again exhibit PNF in a second graft after retransplantation, thus suggesting a definite "hostile" recipient environment.

Hemodynamically unstable recipients also appear to be at higher risk for PNF and IPF. Most patients requiring significant vasopressors are excluded from transplantation because of concerns related to intraoperative death or postoperative graft failure. Occasionally, however, particularly in patients with fulminant hepatic failure or PNF, transplantation may proceed and the allograft is placed into an immediately hostile environment. Failure to rapidly wean from pressors risks excessive graft injury and may result in PNF or IPF, particularly in a less than perfect allograft.

Rejection is not likely to contribute significantly to early graft dysfunction after liver transplantation. Classic hyperacute rejection, as defined in renal transplantation, is the result of preformed antibodies causing microvascular occlusion. The liver has long been held to be privileged in its resistance to antibody-mediated injury. Although other immune-mediated events may contribute to early graft injury, the existence of true hyperacute rejection in hepatic allografts remains unlikely. Additionally, the time course for acute cellular hepatic rejection is clearly beyond the period defining PNF. However, a correlation has recently been noted between SFSS and positive cross-matching in living donor recipients.[65]

Predictors of Primary Nonfunction and Initial Poor Function

Development of a system to predict graft function or failure would obviously be of benefit. Although severe graft failure is rare and relatively easy to identify, assessing a partially functioning graft is more difficult.

Early identification of grafts that will never fully recover would allow earlier retransplantation while sparing unnecessary retransplantation in those predicted to have full graft recovery.

Over the past several years, a number of scoring systems that can be applied to either the donor or the recipient have been devised to predict graft function or failure.[66] As others before, Briceno and coworkers[67] recently attempted to develop a predictive scoring system based on donor parameters that may have a negative impact on organ quality, including donor age (>60 years), length of ICU stay (>4 days), cold ischemia time (>3 hours), episodes of hypotension (<60 mm Hg for more than 1 hour), elevated bilirubin (>2), elevated enzymes (ALT > 170, AST > 140), pressor requirements, and the presence of hypernatremia. Unfortunately, as in the past, this system did not reliably predict PNF or delayed graft function. Heise and colleagues[68] recently proposed a scoring system designed to analyze posttransplant recipient variables.[68] Similar to several other recipient-based systems (Ploeg and associates[10]), this system analyzed transaminase levels, prothrombin activity, and bile production, but added repeated measurements on posttransplant days 1, 3, 7, and 14. These scoring systems have not been evaluated prospectively and should not replace clinical judgment in determining the need for retransplantation.

Other miscellaneous tests have been used to diagnose or predict graft failure. In at least one study, bile cytology consisting of high cellularity has been noted in patients ultimately found to need retransplantation.[69] Unfortunately, this would seem to be an unlikely and cumbersome test for general clinical use. Donor liver biopsies have also been used with some success in an attempt to predict graft function. Extremely abnormal biopsy findings did correlate with graft dysfunction; however, PNF also occurred when specimens were found to be normal.[8] Near-infrared spectroscopy of in vivo grafts has been used in animals to predict graft function.[70] Although intriguing, this again would appear to have extremely limited practical application. Studies looking at functional measures to predict outcome have also been tested. Gao and colleagues recently looked at clearance of the neuromuscular blocking agent rocuronium during the transplant procedure.[71] In patients receiving grafts that ultimately functioned well, they found a predictable decrease in rocuronium after reperfusion, whereas levels increased in those in whom the grafts ultimately failed. Although this measure could be of some use during surgery to predict early graft function, it is extremely unlikely to be more useful than the much simpler clinical observation.

Despite attempts to develop objective pretransplant indices that are predictive of PNF, the most valuable assessment of a donor liver continues to be evaluation by the surgeon at the time of organ procurement.

The appearance and feel of the organ to an experienced surgeon are still probably the best indicators of outcome. Nevertheless, even an organ judged to be "perfect" and transplanted in a technically uncompromised procedure can still be subject to IPF or PNF. In a graft that appears steatotic or otherwise abnormal, core biopsy with frozen section analysis may offer some information on the percentage of macrosteatosis. Such analysis may also provide some objective information if the organ is offered to an off-site surgeon.

A number of functional tests have been developed that have endeavored to assess donor organ function before transplantation. Unfortunately, no test yet devised has been able to predict either IPF or PNF with clinically relevant accuracy.[9] A great number of laboratory tests are currently under investigation as predictors of hepatic allograft function. Among these parameters are allograft hydrogen clearance rates as an assessment of microcirculation, hepatic tissue oxygenation at the time of reperfusion, plasma coagulation factor levels after reperfusion, histopathology of the donor gallbladder, platelet adherence within the graft, posttransplant thrombocytopenia, amino acid and lactate levels, lecithin-cholesterol acyltransferase levels, lidocaine metabolism rates, and magnetic resonance spectroscopy to estimate hepatic energy content.

Treatment

Avoidance

Prevention of PNF largely amounts to avoidance of grafts that are thought to carry inordinate risk by the recipient surgical team. Severely fatty allografts are routinely not used, and organs from other "high-risk" donors are used at the discretion of the recipient surgical team. Pretreatment of steatotic grafts with agents to prevent leukocyte-mediated damage on revascularization has been described and carries future potential for widespread application in organ procurement. Careful donor management, however, can ameliorate some risk factors. Educating organ procurement personnel and ICU teams in fluid management and diabetes insipidus can minimize hypernatremia. Obviously, the recipient surgical team should make every effort to avoid adding risk factors such as prolonged ischemic times to an expanded criteria graft. Additionally, recipient selection plays an important role when contemplating the use of an expanded criteria organ. Hemodynamically unstable or otherwise moribund patients are unlikely to survive the added insult of a struggling graft, whereas a patient with more physiological reserve may be better able to tolerate a period of graft recovery.

Other than avoiding known risks and associations, especially combinations of these factors, prevention of an entity with an unknown cause is by definition difficult. Once a transplant is performed, with the exception of retransplantation, the available options are extremely limited. With any other intervention at this juncture there can be only arbitrary distinction between what is preventive and what is therapeutic. Once PNF becomes a concern, the initiation and timing of treatment are critical. Without prompt recognition and treatment, multiorgan system failure, cerebral edema with brain stem herniation, and death will occur.

Graft Hepatectomy

In cases in which early graft nonfunction is associated with severe hemodynamic or pulmonary instability, it may be necessary to perform hepatectomy and temporary portocaval shunting. Although this measure is obviously drastic, it can result in temporary stabilization in a patient on the verge of cardiopulmonary collapse. Oldhafer and coauthors[72] reported on 20 patients treated in this manner with two-stage hepatectomy and retransplantation for graft nonfunction. Of 16 patients transplanted between 7 and 72 hours later, 7 survived to discharge for an overall survival rate of 35%.[72] Although rendering a patient anhepatic represents the most drastic temporizing measure in the management of PNF, this option should clearly be kept in the repertoire of the transplant surgeon.

Retransplantation

The most definitive treatment of PNF remains retransplantation. Retransplantation is itself a risk factor for graft failure, which may result from a variety of factors ranging from recipient instability to lower-quality donors, but if performed before multisystem organ failure is established, the outcomes are acceptable. If retransplantation is necessary, it should be undertaken as soon as possible after the initial transplant because delays even beyond 7 days add considerable risk of intraoperative complications, sepsis, and multisystem organ failure. Until more is known about PNF and its preventability or reversibility, retransplantation will continue to remain the mainstay of treatment.

Specific Treatment of Primary Nonfunction

N-Acetylcysteine

N-acetylcysteine (NAC) is a glutathione precursor that acts by replenishing intrahepatic stores of the endogenous antioxidant glutathione. For many years the primary clinical use of NAC has been to provide a protective effect against the metabolic hepatocellular injury of acetaminophen overdose. NAC has also been shown to improve hemodynamics and oxygen transport in patients with fulminant hepatic failure of various causes. In animal models, NAC has shown a protective effect against ischemia/reperfusion-type liver injury.[73,74] NAC has had mixed results when studied as an adjunct to liver transplantation in humans. Thies and colleagues[74] concluded that NAC has protective effects on transplanted livers and that NAC may lower some parameters of graft dysfunction and improve hepatic artery and portal vein flow after transplantation. In contrast, in a study by Stieb and associates,[73] no benefit of intravenous NAC over placebo could be demonstrated in posttransplant graft function. Currently, NAC is not used routinely after liver transplantation in most programs. Further confirmation of the value of NAC is required before its routine use after liver transplantation can be recommended.

Prostaglandins

At least two prostaglandins have now been reported to have a beneficial effect in the treatment of PNF. Prostaglandin E_1 (PGE_1) and prostacyclin (PGI_2) have both been hypothesized to improve hepatic function after transplantation by mechanisms that include vasodilatation, lysosomal membrane stabilization, inhibition of platelet aggregation, and increased splanchnic blood flow.[45] Both human and animal studies have reported improved hepatic blood flow with prostaglandin therapy, but whether this improved flow translates into improved outcomes after liver transplantation is less clear. Several studies have suggested improvement in PNF rates or outcomes in patients treated with prostaglandins. To date, the most definitive study has been a well-designed, prospective randomized placebo-controlled trial using prostaglandins prophylactically in 160 consecutive liver transplant patients. In this study, Henley and coworkers[74a] found no significant difference in the incidence or outcome of PNF in placebo- and PGE_1-treated groups. Interestingly, PGE_1 may have had some other beneficial immunological, hemodynamic, or hematological effects and was found to be cost-effective and to lower length of hospital stay. Currently, there is not enough evidence to advocate the widespread use of PGE_1 in patients at risk for PNF. Select use of prostaglandins in patients with PNF or IPF might be considered when impaired splanchnic perfusion is suspected.

Plasmapheresis

Plasmapheresis has been used in an effort to improve function in patients with IPF/PNF. Circulating toxins or preformed antibodies could conceivably be removed by this therapy. Skerrett and associates[75] looked at the effectiveness of plasmapheresis in a group of 18 patients in whom primary dysfunction was diagnosed after orthotopic liver transplantation, but no significant effect was found on graft survival. These investigators were able to document significant reductions in serum tumor necrosis factor and interleukin-6 with plasmapheresis, which could be of importance because these and other cytokines may play a role in the etiology of graft dysfunction. Mandal and colleagues[15] have also looked at the role of plasmapheresis in the treatment of PNF. They used daily plasmapheresis consisting of one plasma volume replacement with FFP. The number of treatments varied according to patient recovery but ranged from two to five sessions. In this small group of five patients, all showed improvement temporally related to the treatment. One of the five died with a pulmonary embolus for an overall survival rate of 80%.[15] Unfortunately, because controls are impossible, all such reports remain anecdotal, and the true effect of the treatment is unclear.

Liver Assist Devices

Several reports have described the use of a variety of liver assist devices to treat patients with initial graft nonfunction after transplantation. For purposes of interventional reports such as these, PNF is defined as graft dysfunction severe enough to warrant relisting for transplantation. Two devices of note include the nonbiological molecular adsorbent recirculating system (MARS) and the biological porcine hepatocyte–based system.[14]

The MARS liver assist system has been used to treat PNF in a small number of cases. In the report of a registry of MARS cases, Novelli and coauthors described four of nine cases of PNF in which the graft recovered after implementation of MARS.[14] MARS has also been reported to decrease neurological dysfunction and improve cerebral blood flow in patients with fulminant hepatic failure or PNF.

Demetriou and colleagues[76] recently reported the largest randomized trial to date of treatment with a liver assist device.[76] In this study, 171 patients with fulminant hepatic failure or PNF were randomized over a 3-year period to treatment or observation. The subgroup of 24 patients with PNF is the largest group of PNF patients treated with liver support therapy in the literature. Unfortunately, no subgroup analysis of these patients was provided. Overall, use of the HepatAssist device in this study was reported to have an impact on survival only in the fulminant hepatic failure subgroup. Detailed analysis of the group of patients with PNF is anticipated.

These studies and other small case series do not provide compelling evidence for the routine use of liver assist technology in patients with PNF or IPF. Although it is possible that these devices may "bridge" a patient in some way, there is no evidence that their use will hasten or augment hepatic recovery after transplantation. However, in patients with PNF and cerebral edema or severe encephalopathy, these devices may provide a useful treatment option.

Blocking Ischemia/Reperfusion Injury

A number of other promising interventions loom on the horizon and are nearing clinical application. Most of these interventions are aimed at circumventing the cascade of events associated with ischemia/reperfusion injury. Migration of leukocytes into the vascular endothelium of the allograft appears to be an early step in ischemia/reperfusion injury. Inhibition of the adhesion molecules that aid in the recruitment of these cells has shown promising results in animal models of steatosis.[77]

Small-for-Size Syndrome

Three measures should be considered in attempts to prevent SFSS. First, the use of SFS grafts should be avoided if possible. Second, portal hyperperfusion of an SFS graft should be avoided, either by creation of a temporary portocaval shunt or by using portal vein banding or splenic artery ligation to limit portal vein inflow. Third, if they must be used, SFS grafts should be transplanted only in relatively well-compensated patients.[2,49] In living donor or split-liver transplantation, it is also vital to ensure adequate venous drainage to prevent undue damage to the allograft by venous congestion.[2]

Conclusions/Summary

Accurate assessment of early graft function after liver transplantation has become vitally important in an era in which donor organ shortages and changes in organ allocation policies have forced many centers to use expanded criteria grafts and perform transplantation in marginal recipients. Although life-threatening complications of graft dysfunction clearly mandate retransplantation, the definition, treatment, and even terminology of less severe graft dysfunction have eluded consensus.

A better understanding of the factors that lead to compromised early graft function after transplantation is clearly needed. Key areas of active research include identifying mechanisms and treatment of ischemia/reperfusion injury, extending the use of expanded criteria organs, refining the ability to predict graft salvage after transplantation, and preventing and treating SFSS. In addition, the transplant community must agree on definitions of graft dysfunction, PNF, and IPF, particularly as they relate to organ allocation policies. These definitions must in some way encompass and reflect the clinical judgment of experienced transplant physicians inasmuch as bedside evaluation of graft function continues to be an integral part of liver transplantation.

Clinical Pearls

Assessment of Early Function of Hepatic Allografts

- Return to normal body temperature ("warm up")
- Normal mental status ("wake up")
- Return of vascular tone and freedom from vasopressors ("tighten up")
- Good renal function ("open up")
- Resolution of metabolic acidosis
- Production of bile
- Noncoagulopathic status

Evaluation of Poor Graft Function

- Rapidly exclude hepatic artery or portal vein thrombosis
  - Doppler ultrasound of the liver
  - Contrast angiography
  - Early surgical exploration
- Exclude mechanical or systemic factors
  - Abdominal compartment syndrome
  - Hepatic vein obstruction: elevated positive end-expiratory pressure and elevated central venous pressure
  - Hypovolemia/pressors
- Consider early surgical exploration
  - Provides "hands on" assessment
  - Allows safe biopsy
  - Definitively excludes vascular/mechanical causes

Management of Primary Nonfunction/Initial Poor Function

- Prevention
  - Donor and recipient selection
  - Minimization of ischemic time
- Consider graft hepatectomy and portocaval shunts for catastrophic hemodynamic or pulmonary collapse

---

Clinical Pearls—cont'd

- Consider early retransplantation for life-threatening dysfunction (hemodynamic instability, refractory coagulopathy, cerebral edema) or signs of irreparable graft dysfunction (marked enzyme elevation, severe cholestasis, persistent coagulopathy)
- Eliminate contributing mechanical factors
- Avoid small-for-size syndrome
  - Use adequate-sized grafts
  - Consider measuring portal venous pressure
  - Ensure adequate venous drainage

References

1. Busuttil RW, Tanaka K: The utility of marginal donors in liver transplantation. Liver Transpl 9:651-663, 2003.
2. Lo CM, Liu CL, Fan ST: Portal hyperperfusion injury as the cause of primary nonfunction in a small-for-size liver graft—successful treatment with splenic artery ligation. Liver Transpl 9:626-628, 2003.
3. United Network of Organ Sharing. www.UNOS.org, 2003.
4. Busuttil RW, Shaked A, Millis JM, et al: One thousand liver transplants. The lessons learned. Ann Surg 219:490-497, discussion 498-499, 1994.
5. Anselmo DM, Baquerizo A, Geerarghese S, et al: Liver transplantation at Dumont-UCLA Transplant Center: An experience with over 3,000 cases. Clin Transpl 179-186, 2001.
6. Jain A, Reyes J, Kashyap R, et al: Long-term survival after liver transplantation in 4,000 consecutive patients at a single center. Ann Surg 232:490-500, 2000.
7. Greig PD, Woolf GM, Sinclair SB, et al: Treatment of primary liver graft nonfunction with prostaglandin E$_1$. Transplantation 48:447-453, 1989.
8. D'Alessandro AM, Kalayoglu M, Sollinger HW, et al: The predictive value of donor liver biopsies for the development of primary nonfunction after orthotopic liver transplantation. Transplantation 51:157-163, 1991.
9. Strasberg SM, Howard TK, Molmenti EP, Hertl M: Selecting the donor liver: Risk factors for poor function after orthotopic liver transplantation. Hepatology 20:829-838, 1994.
10. Ploeg RJ, D'Alessandro AM, Knechtle SJ, et al: Risk factors for primary dysfunction after liver transplantation—a multivariate analysis. Transplantation 55:807-813, 1993.
11. Hwang S, Lee SG, Lee YJ, et al: A case of primary non-function following adult-to-adult living donor liver transplantation. Hepatogastroenterology 49:1412-1414, 2002.
12. Mor E, Klintmalm GB, Gonwa TA, et al: The use of marginal donors for liver transplantation. A retrospective study of 365 liver donors. Transplantation 53:383-386, 1992.
13. Rosen HR, Martin P, Goss J, et al: Significance of early aminotransferase elevation after liver transplantation. Transplantation 65:68-72, 1998.
14. Novelli G, Rossi M, Pretagostini R, et al: MARS (Molecular Adsorbent Recirculating System): Experience in 34 cases of acute liver failure. Liver 22(Suppl 2):43-47, 2002.
15. Mandal AK, King KE, Humphreys SL, et al: Plasmapheresis: An effective therapy for primary allograft nonfunction after liver transplantation. Transplantation 70:216-220, 2000.

16. Grande L, Rimola A, Garcia-Valdecasas JC, et al: Recovery of liver graft after initial poor function. Transplantation 53:228-230, 1992.
17. Rull R, Vidal O, Momblan D, et al: Evaluation of potential liver donors: Limits imposed by donor variables in liver transplantation. Liver Transpl 9:389-393, 2003.
18. Makowka L, Gordon RD, Todo S, et al: Analysis of donor criteria for the prediction of outcome in clinical liver transplantation. Transplant Proc 19:2378-2382, 1987.
19. Fernandez-Merino FJ, Nuno-Garza J, Lopez-Hervas P, et al: Impact of donor, recipient, and graft features on the development of primary dysfunction in liver transplants. Transplant Proc 35:1793-1794, 2003.
20. Zamboni F, Franchello A, David E, et al: Effect of macrovesicular steatosis and other donor and recipient characteristics on the outcome of liver transplantation. Clin Transplant 15:53-57, 2001.
21. Briceno J, Marchal T, Padillo J, et al: Influence of marginal donors on liver preservation injury. Transplantation 74:522-526, 2002.
22. Popper H: Relations between liver and aging. Semin Liver Dis 5:221-227, 1985.
23. Wynne HA, Cope LH, Mutch E, et al: The effect of age upon liver volume and apparent liver blood flow in healthy man. Hepatology 9:297-301, 1989.
24. Busquets J, Xiol X, Figueras J, et al: The impact of donor age on liver transplantation: Influence of donor age on early liver function and on subsequent patient and graft survival. Transplantation 71:1765-1771, 2001.
24a. Tisone G, Manzia TM, Zazza S, et al: Marginal donors in liver transplantation. Transplant Proc 36:525-526, 2004.
25. Yersiz H, Shaked A, Olthoff K, et al: Correlation between donor age and the pattern of liver graft recovery after transplantation. Transplantation 60:790-794, 1995.
26. Grazi GL, Cescon M, Ravaioli M, et al: A revised consideration on the use of very aged donors for liver transplantation. Am J Transplant 1:61-68, 2001.
27. Deschenes M, Forbes C, Tchervenkov J, et al: Use of older donor livers is associated with more extensive ischemic damage on intraoperative biopsies during liver transplantation. Liver Transpl Surg 5:357-361, 1999.
28. Cuende N, Grande L, Sanjuan R, Cuervas-Mons V: Liver transplant with organs from elderly donors: Spanish experience with more than 300 liver donors over 70 years of age. Transplantation 73:1360, 2002.
29. Cescon M, Grazi GL, Ercolani G, et al: Long-term survival of recipients of liver grafts from donors older than 80 years: Is it achievable? Liver Transpl 9:1174-1180, 2003.
30. 2002 Annual Report. The U.S. Organ Procurement and Transplantation Network and The Scientific Registry of Transplant Recipients Transplant Data 1992-2001, 2002.
31. Imber CJ, St Peter DS, Handa A, Friend RJ: Hepatic steatosis and its relationship to transplantation. Liver Transpl 8:415-423, 2002.
32. Selzner M, Clavien PA: Fatty liver in liver transplantation and surgery. Semin Liver Dis 21:105-113, 2001.
33. Adam R, Reynes M, Johann M, et al: The outcome of steatotic grafts in liver transplantation. Transplant Proc 23:1538-1540, 1991.
34. Hilden M, Christofferson P, Juhl E, Dalgaard JB: Liver histology in a 'normal' population—examinations of 503 consecutive fatal traffic casualties. Scand J Gastroenterol 12:593-597, 1977.
35. Garcia Urena MA, Colina Ruiz-Delgado F, Moreno Gonzalez E, et al: Hepatic steatosis in liver transplant donors: Common feature of donor population? World J Surg 22:837-844, 1998.
36. Todo S, Demetris AJ, Makowka L, et al: Primary nonfunction of hepatic allografts with preexisting fatty infiltration. Transplantation 47:903-905, 1989.
37. Yoo HY, Molmenti E, Thuluvath PJ: The effect of donor body mass index on primary graft nonfunction, retransplantation rate, and early graft and patient survival after liver transplantation. Liver Transpl 9:72-78, 2003.
38. Soejima Y, Shimada M, Suehiro T, et al: Use of steatotic graft in living-donor liver transplantation. Transplantation 76:344-348, 2003.
39. Ryan CK, Johnson LA, Germin BI, Marcos A: One hundred consecutive hepatic biopsies in the workup of living donors for right lobe liver transplantation. Liver Transpl 8:1114-1122, 2002.
40. Fishbein TM, Fiel MI, Emre S, et al: Use of livers with microvesicular fat safely expands the donor pool. Transplantation 64:248-251, 1997.
41. Clavien PA, Selzner M: Hepatic steatosis and transplantation. Liver Transpl 8:980, 2002.
42. Fukumori T, Ohkohchi N, Tsukamoto S, Satomi S: The mechanism of injury in a steatotic liver graft during cold preservation. Transplantation 67:195-200, 1999.
43. Ardite E, Ramos C, Rimola A, et al: Hepatocellular oxidative stress and initial graft injury in human liver transplantation. J Hepatol 31:921-927, 1999.
44. Emond JC, Renz JF, Ferrell LD, et al: Functional analysis of grafts from living donors. Implications for the treatment of older recipients. Ann Surg 224:544-552, discussion 552-554, 1996.
45. Lo CM, Fan ST, Liu CL, et al: Minimum graft size for successful living donor liver transplantation. Transplantation 68:1112-1116, 1999.
46. Ben-Haim M, Emre S, Fishbein TM, et al: Critical graft size in adult-to-adult living donor liver transplantation: Impact of the recipient's disease. Liver Transpl 7:948-953, 2001.
47. Urata K, Kawasaki S, Matsunami H, et al: Calculation of child and adult standard liver volume for liver transplantation. Hepatology 21:1317-1321, 1995.
48. Kiuchi T, Kasahara M, Uryuhara K, et al: Impact of graft size mismatching on graft prognosis in liver transplantation from living donors. Transplantation 67:321-327, 1999.
49. Kiuchi T, Tanaka K, Ito T, et al: Small-for-size graft in living donor liver transplantation: How far should we go? Liver Transpl 9(9):S29-S35, 2003.
50. Farmer DG, Yersiz H, Ghobrial RM, et al: Early graft function after pediatric liver transplantation: Comparison between in situ split liver grafts and living-related liver grafts. Transplantation 72:1795-1802, 2001.
51. Troisi R, de Hemptinne B: Clinical relevance of adapting portal vein flow in living donor liver transplantation in adult patients. Liver Transpl 9(9):S36-S41, 2003.
52. Ito T, Kiuchi T, Yamamoto H, et al: Changes in portal venous pressure in the early phase after living-donor liver transplantation: Pathogenesis and clinical implications. Transplantation 75:1313-1317, 2003.
53. Man K, Lo CM, Ng IO, et al: Liver transplantation in rats using small-for-size grafts: A study of hemodynamic and morphological changes. Arch Surg 136:280-285, 2001.
54. Man K, Lo CM, Lee Tk, et al: Intragraft gene expression profiles by cDNA microarray in small-for-size liver grafts. Liver Transpl 9:425-432, 2003.
55. Starzl TE, Demetris AJ, Van Theil D: Liver transplantation. N Engl J Med 321:1014-1022, 1989.
56. Figueras J, Busquets J, Grande L, et al: The deleterious effect of donor high plasma sodium and extended preservation in liver transplantation. A multivariate analysis. Transplantation 61:410-413, 1996.
57. Totsuka E, Dodson F, Urakami A, et al: Influence of high donor serum sodium levels on early postoperative graft function in human liver transplantation: Effect of correction of donor hypernatremia. Liver Transpl Surg 5:421-428, 1999.
58. Rustgi VK, Marino G, Halpern MT, et al: Role of gender and race mismatch and graft failure in patients undergoing liver transplantation. Liver Transpl 8:514-518, 2002.

59. Okamoto S, Corso CO, Nolte D, et al: Impact of brain death on hormonal homeostasis and hepatic microcirculation of transplant organ donors. Transpl Int 11(Suppl 1):S404-S407, 1998.

60. Komokata T, Nishida S, Ganz S, et al: The impact of donor chemical overdose on the outcome of liver transplantation. Transplantation 76:705-708, 2003.

61. Wisecaver JL, Radio SJ, Shaw BW Jr, et al: Intrahepatic arteriopathy associated with primary nonfunction of liver allografts. Hum Pathol 25:960-963, 1994.

62. D'Alessandro AM, Kalayoglu M, Sollinger HW, et al: Current status of organ preservation with University of Wisconsin solution. Arch Pathol Lab Med 115:306-310, 1991.

63. Furukawa H, Todo S, Imventarza O, et al: Effect of cold ischemia time on the early outcome of human hepatic allografts preserved with UW solution. Transplantation 51:1000-1004, 1991.

64. Abt PL, Desai NM, Crawford MD, et al: Survival following liver transplantation from non–heart-beating donors. Ann Surg 239:87-92, 2004.

65. Suh KS, Kim SB, Chang SH, et al: Significance of positive cytotoxic cross-match in adult-to-adult living donor liver transplantation using small graft volume. Liver Transpl 8:1109-1113, 2002.

66. Moreno Sanz C, Jiminez Romero C, Moreno Gonzalez E, et al: Primary dysfunction after liver transplantation. Is it possible to predict this complication? Rev Esp Enferm Dig 91:401-419, 1999.

67. Briceno J, Solorzano G, Pera C: A proposal for scoring marginal liver grafts. Transpl Int 13(Suppl 1):S249-S252, 2000.

68. Heise M, Settmacher U, Pfitzmann R, et al: A survival-based scoring-system for initial graft function following orthotopic liver transplantation. Transpl Int 16:794-800, 2003.

69. Carrasco L, Sanchez-Bueno F, Sola J, et al: Use of bile cytology for early diagnosis of complications in orthotopic liver transplantation. Cytopathology 9:406-414, 1998.

70. Fan XH, Asahara T, Ohdan H, et al: Nondestructive and real-time evaluation of liver viability in brain dead donor for liver transplantation using near-infrared spectroscopy. Transpl Int 13 (Suppl 1):S272-S277, 2000.

71. Gao L, Ramzan I, Baker B: Rocuronium plasma concentrations during three phases of liver transplantation: Relationship with early postoperative graft liver function. Br J Anaesth 88:764-770, 2002.

72. Oldhafer KJ, Bornscheuer A, Fruhauf NR, et al: Rescue hepatectomy for initial graft non-function after liver transplantation. Transplantation 67:1024-1028, 1999.

73. Steib A, Freys G, Collin F, et al: Does N-acetylcysteine improve hemodynamics and graft function in liver transplantation? Liver Transpl Surg 4:152-157, 1998.

74. Thies JC, Teklote J, Clauer U, et al: The efficacy of N-acetylcysteine as a hepatoprotective agent in liver transplantation. Transpl Int 11(Suppl 1):S390-S392, 1998.

74a. Henley KS, Lucey MR, Normolle DP, et al: A double-blind, randomized, placebo-controlled trial of prostaglandin E1 in liver transplantation. Hepatology 21:366-372, 1995.

75. Skerrett D, Mor E, Curtiss S, Mohandas K: Plasmapheresis in primary dysfunction of hepatic transplants. J Clin Apheresis 11:10-13, 1996.

76. Demetriou AA, Brown RS Jr, Busuttil RW, et al: Prospective, randomized, multicenter, controlled trial of a bioartificial liver in treating acute liver failure. Ann Surg 239:660-667, discussion 667-670, 2004.

77. Amersi F, Farmer DG, Shaw GD, et al: P-selectin glycoprotein ligand-1(rPSGL-Ig)-mediated blockade of CD62 selectin molecules protects rat steatotic liver grafts from ischemia/reperfusion injury. Am J Transplant 2:600-608, 2002.

Technical Problems: Biliary

PETER NEUHAUS
ANDREAS PASCHER

Epidemiology 930

Pathophysiology 932

Clinical presentation 934

Diagnostic workup 934
 Serum chemical markers 934
 Abdominal ultrasonography 934
 Graft biopsy 934
 Cholangiography 934
 Computed tomography 935
 Hepatobiliary scintigraphy 935
 Magnetic resonance cholangiography/
  cholangiopancreatography 935

Specific biliary complications 936
 Bile leaks 936
 Early bile leaks 936
 Late bile leaks 937
 Bile collection/biliary abscesses 937
 Biliary strictures 937
 Anastomotic strictures 939
 Nonanastomotic strictures 939
 Ampullary dysfunction 940
 Biliary stones, sludge, and casts 941
 Complications related to bilioenteric
  anastomosis 942
 Mucocele 942
 Hemobilia 942

Treatment 942
 Bile leaks 943
 Bile collection/biliary abscesses 944
 Anastomotic strictures 944
 Nonanastomotic strictures 944

Ampullary dysfunction 947
Biliary stones, sludge, and casts 947
Mucocele 947
Hemobilia 947

Complications involving the biliary tract after orthotopic liver transplantation (OLT) have been a common problem since the early beginning of OLT.[1] As a consequence of the limited deceased donor pool, more OLTs are performed using alternative techniques such as living donor liver transplantation and split-liver transplantation. Approximately 5% of OLTs are currently conducted as adult-to-adult right lobe liver transplantations.[2] These emerging methods have altered the incidence and characteristics of biliary complications. The most common biliary complications are biliary leaks and strictures. However, there is a wide range of potential biliary complications that can occur after liver transplantation (Table 62–1). Their incidence varies according to the type of graft, type of donor (deceased donor versus living donor), and the type of biliary anastomosis performed. According to the time of onset after OLT, biliary complications may be divided into early and late complications. Approximately two thirds of all biliary complications occur as early complications within the first 3 months after OLT and are a significant source of morbidity and mortality.[3]

Early diagnosis and adequate treatment of biliary complications are pivotal for reducing biliary-related morbidity and mortality and for ensuring graft and

Table 62–1. SPECIFIC BILIARY COMPLICATIONS

Biliary leakage

    Anastomotic leakage

        Bile duct anastomosis

        Bilioenteric anastomosis

    Nonanastomotic leakage

        T-tube related

        Bile duct necrosis

        Cystic duct leakage

        Cut surface of reduced grafts

Bile collection/biliary abscess

Biliary obstruction

    Extrahepatic obstruction

        Anastomotic stricture

        Nonanastomotic stricture

    Intrahepatic stricture

    Papillary dyskinesia

Cholangitis

Sludge, stones, and casts

Mucocele

Biliary complications related to bilioenteric anastomosis

    Anastomotic leakage

    Intestinal perforation

    Gastrointestinal bleeding

    Cholangitis

    Blind loop syndrome

    Calcineurin inhibitor malabsorption

Biliary complications related to percutaneous biopsy

    Bilioportal or biliovenous fistula

    Arteriobiliary fistula

patient survival after OLT. The diagnosis and management of biliary complications has changed fundamentally since the early days of liver transplantation with the establishment of new diagnostic methods such as magnetic resonance cholangiography. Treatment modalities have changed over the years toward a primarily nonoperative, endoscopy-based strategy, leaving the surgical intervention for lesions that otherwise are not curable.

Epidemiology

Biliary complications have been reported to occur in 6% to 34% of all deceased donor full-size OLTs,[3-12] with large series reporting a relatively constant rate of approximately 10% to 15% (Table 62–2). Apart from the integrity of the hepatic artery anastomosis, the type of biliary reconstruction is a major determinant in the subsequent risk of biliary complications after OLT and influences the nature, timing, and management of biliary complications.

The two most common forms of biliary reconstruction are choledochocholedochostomy (CC) and choledochojejunostomy (CJ), usually with a Roux-en-Y loop. There is no consensus on the optimal biliary reconstruction, and considerable variability exists among transplant centers.[4,13] Apart from the personal preference of the surgeon, the choice is influenced by multiple factors, such as the underlying liver disease, the size of donor and recipient bile ducts, and prior transplant or other biliary surgery. More than three quarters of deceased donor full-size OLTs in adults are performed as CC; only 10% of pediatric cases are CC. This method is preferred because it is technically easier to perform and incorporates the well-vascularized recipient common bile duct. It preserves the sphincter of Oddi, which serves as a natural barrier to reflux of enteric contents into the biliary tree,[14] thus theoretically decreasing the risk of ascending cholangitis. It may be performed end-to-end or side-to-side,[10,15,16] and either with or without a T tube. A recent prospective, randomized trial of end-to-end versus side-to-side CC revealed no significant difference in biliary complications.[17] Many centers prefer the routine use of a T tube, because it partially bridges the biliary anastomosis and allows early postoperative assessment of bile quality and cholangiographic anatomy. Moreover, it may reduce the incidence of anastomotic stricture formation.[18]

Internal stents have been used in some patients, but were reported to be associated with a high rate of serious complications, including obstruction, migration, and erosion with hemobilia.[19] CC without the use of a T tube has been advocated by several groups to avoid postoperative bile leaks related to removal of the T tube. Nonrandomized studies suggest a similar overall risk of biliary complications in patients who underwent transplantation with or without a T tube.[4,12] Reports indicate that the risk of bile leak after OLT and the necessity for radiological or endoscopic procedures[20] is lower in patients not receiving a T tube. However, the risk of anastomotic stricture may be higher without the use of a T tube.[20] Two prospective, randomized trials examined the impact of T tube use after OLT. Only one stricture was seen in the 30 patients receiving CC with a T tube; however, 6 of 30 patients (20%) who had CC without a T tube developed strictures and 3 eventually required conversion to CJ.[21] The largest prospective randomized study compared 90 patients with or without a T tube. The authors found a significant increase of biliary complications in the T tube group (33%) as compared with patients who received transplantation without a T tube (15.5%). Of the complications in the T tube group, 60% were related to the T tube, with cholangitis being the most prominent complication.[22] Shimoda and associates performed an analysis of

Table 62-2. BILIARY COMPLICATIONS AFTER DECEASED DONOR FULL-SIZE AND SPLIT-LIVER TRANSPLANTATION

Author and Ref.	Year	Center	No. of OLT	Biliary Complications (%)		
				Overall	Leakages	Strictures
Deceased Donor Full-Size OLT						
Lerut et al.[6]	1987	Pittsburgh	393	13	11	5
Colonna et al.[9]	1992	Los Angeles	738	–	8	3
Neuhaus et al.[10]	1994	Berlin	300	9	0.3	3
Grief et al.[3]	1994	Pittsburgh	1792	12	–	–
Grande et al.[11]	1999	Barcelona	500	14	–	–
Verran et al.[12]	1997	Ontario	502	13.5	1.6	6.6
Split-liver Transplantation						
EX SITU						
Emond et al.[28]	1990	Chicago	18	27	–	–
Broelsch et al.[29]	1990	Chicago	30	27	–	–
Otte et al.[30]	1995	Brussels	29	17	–	–
De Ville et al.[31]	1995	Europe	98	23.5	7	13.3
Azoulay et al.[32]	1996	Paris	27	22	–	–
Deshpande et al.[34]	2002	London	80	8.7	6.3	2.5
IN SITU						
Rogiers et al.[33]	1996	Hamburg	14	0	0	0
Goss et al.[36]	1998	Los Angeles	36	15	–	–
Busuttil et al.[37]	1999	Los Angeles	78	2.8	–	–

cost-effectiveness regarding the use of T tubes in OLT.[23] The application of T tubes resulted in significantly higher complication rates (32.9% versus 15.5% without the T tube); however, complication-related costs were not significantly higher.

CJ is usually indicated for patients with diseased extrahepatic bile ducts (primary sclerosing cholangitis, cholangiocarcinoma, biliary atresia); prior biliary surgery; size disparities between donor and recipient ducts; reduced-size, split-, and living donor grafts (Fig. 62–1); retransplantation; or when the blood supply to the distal donor bile duct is suboptimal.[19] CJ is the most common anastomosis used in pediatric liver transplant patients because of the small size or absence of bile ducts in this patient population. Problems and potential complications unique to Roux-en-Y CJ include increased surgical time, stricture, or leakage of the CJ, bleeding at the jejunojejunostomy, bowel ischemia, Roux limb torsion, intestinal perforation, delayed mixing of bile with intestinal contents, altered cyclosporine absorption, and cholangitis induced by reflux of intestinal pathogens.[24-26] In addition, creation of a CJ restricts endoscopic evaluation of the biliary system, occasionally requiring a percutaneous transhepatic cholangiogram (PTC). Because magnetic resonance cholangiography (MRC) has emerged as a sensitive, noninvasive diagnostic tool, CJ-related diagnostic problems are likely to decrease.

The spectrum of biliary complications has changed over the past decade as a result of the establishment of split-liver transplantation and reduced-size liver transplantation. The incidence of biliary complications in reduced-size liver transplantation was reported to be as high as 24%[27]; however, approximately 50% of complications related to cut surface leakages. The initial experience with ex situ split-liver transplantation for infants and children resulted in an average biliary complication rate of 24% to 27% (see Table 62–2).[28-32] Meanwhile, complication rates for ex situ split OLTs have been markedly reduced.[33,34] In situ split OLT was reported to result in lower complication rates in the biliary system of approximately 0% to 15%, reflecting the better anatomic orientation during the in situ splitting process (see Table 62–2).[35-37] In pediatric recipients, a biliary complication rate of 8.7% to 15% was reported.[38,39] A further modification is currently being seen with the growing acceptance of adult-to-adult living donor liver transplantation (Table 62–3).[40-46] The incidence of biliary leaks and strictures was reported to be as high as 30% in the early phase (see Table 62–3), and may be attributed to initial difficulties in defining the dissection plane around the right hepatic duct and complex reconstructions including several orifices (Fig. 62–2; see also Fig. 62–1). A similar development has taken place in pediatric living donor OLT.[43,46-51]

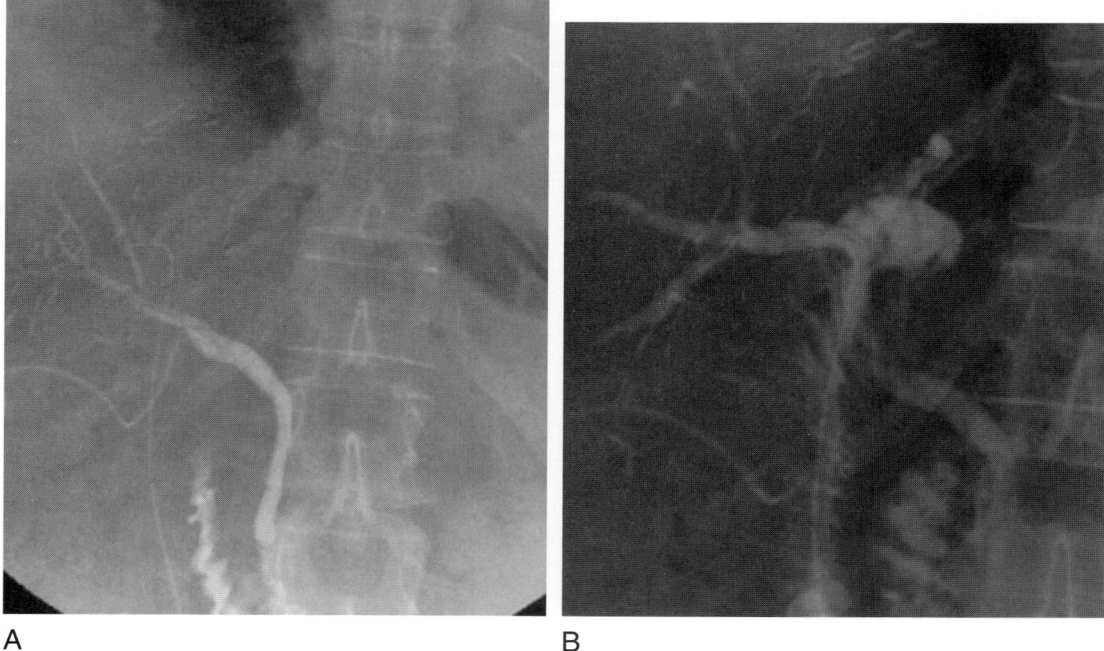

A   B

FIGURE 62–1

Complex biliary reconstruction using a combination of duct-to-duct and bilioenteric anastomosis in a patient who received a right hepatic lobe from a living donor. **A**, Duct-to-duct reconstruction of two orifices of the right lobe graft with the ductus choledochus of the recipient. The image was performed on the fifth postoperative day depicting a regular biliary anastomosis. **B**, In a second step, contrast medium was given via the transintestinal internal drain stenting a bilioenteric anastomosis that was established for draining a separate orifice. The residual contrast medium applied via the T-tube is still visible in the background.

According to a survey of liver transplantation from living adult donors in the United States, the overall biliary complication rate is approximately 22%.[2] However, with the learning curve being overcome, complication rates related to biliary reconstruction are expected to decrease. Published single-center reports indicate that a biliary complication rate of 8% to 14% has been achieved in living donor liver transplantation (see Table 62–3).

Pathophysiology

In early bile leaks and anastomotic strictures, surgical and technical reasons, such as suture-related insufficiencies or stenoses or T-tube dislodgement, should be ruled out. However, in a relevant number of cases the reasons are not that obvious. Further technical factors predisposing for early bile leaks must be considered: Patients with acute hepatic artery thrombosis (HAT) after transplantation are at risk for ischemic strictures unless the vascular flow is immediately reconstituted or adequate collateral blood flow exists.[52-55] Hence, routine Doppler ultrasound is recommended in the first days after OLT. This is particularly relevant in technically demanding types of OLT, such as pediatric OLT, split OLT, and living donor liver transplantation. Additionally, low-flow phenomena in the hepatic artery unrelated to the anastomosis may occur in the case of a preexisting splenic artery steal syndrome or stenosis of the celiac axis. Both phenomena should be subject to examination during the evaluation process of a potential recipient. Splenic artery steal syndrome may be treated sufficiently by interventional radiological methods that reduce blood flow through the splenic artery. Intermittent celiac axis stenosis may be caused by the arcuate ligament impairing patency of the axis during inspiration; a persistent stenosis may be congenital or related to arteriosclerosis. In the latter case, an arterial jump graft is advised, and intermittent stenosis can be avoided by incision of the arcuate ligament. Further technical reasons may be related to the delicate vascular supply of the bile duct. In particular, excess dissection of periductal tissue during organ procurement that impairs the vascular supply of the donor's bile duct and the use of electrocautery for biliary duct bleeding control in both donor and recipient may contribute. Additionally, excess tension on the ductal

Table 62–3. BILIARY COMPLICATIONS AFTER LIVING DONOR LIVER TRANSPLANTATION

Author and Ref.	Year	Center	No. of OLT	Biliary Complications (%)		
				Overall	Leakages	Strictures
Adult Living Donor Liver Transplantation						
Right Lobe						
Marcos et al.[40]	2000	USA	275	18	–	–
Broelsch et al.[41]	2000	Europe	123	14.6	–	–
Testa et al.[47]	2000	Essen	30	26.6	26.6	3.3
Fan et al.[45]	2002	Hong Kong	74	26	6.6	20
Sugawara et al.[109]	2002	Tokyo	25	8	0	8
Chen et al.[46]	2003	Asia	766	17.8	7.3	10.5
Brown et al.[2]	2003	USA	449	22	–	–
Settmacher et al.[51]	2003	Berlin	50	14	12	4
Various Type of Grafts (Right Lobe, Left Lobe)						
Todo et al.[42]	2000	Japan	308	32	8.1	5.2
Miller et al.[43]	2001	New York	59	–	23.7	6.8
Lee et al.[44]	2001	Seoul	157	–	5.1	5.7
Pediatric Living Donor Liver Transplantation						
Cronin et al.[48]	1997	Chicago	91	38	9.9	29
Egawa et al.[49]	1998	Kyoto	205	13.9	9.3	5.4
Egawa et al.[50]	2001	Kyoto	346	≈18	–	–
Miller et al.[43]	2001	New York	50	–	6	12
Chen et al.[46]	2003	Asia	742	15	9	6

anastomosis[56,57] and active bleeding from the cut ends of the bile duct prior to anastomosis are risk factors for biliary complications.

Although the exact mechanisms of bile duct injury unrelated to technical reasons sometimes remain elusive, the damage is believed to result from several contributing factors, including ischemic and immunological injury, preservation injury as a consequence of prolonged ischemia,[58] and infection.[5] Busquets and associates[59] reported the usefulness of postreperfusion biopsies in predicting bile duct complications. They correlated the extent of neutrophilic infiltrates indicative of preservation injury with biliary complications. Several other associated conditions were identified, including ABO incompatibility, cytomegalovirus infection, age, cross-match, chronic ductopenic rejection, and patients with a pretransplantation diagnosis of primary sclerosing cholangitis.[9,60] Both the bile duct and the vascular endothelium were shown to be vulnerable to the damaging effects of humoral and cellular immune mechanisms.[61] Both mechanisms can result in bile duct cell death and stricturing, either directly or as a result of a compromised vascular supply, and they can ultimately lead to ischemic cholangitis.[19]

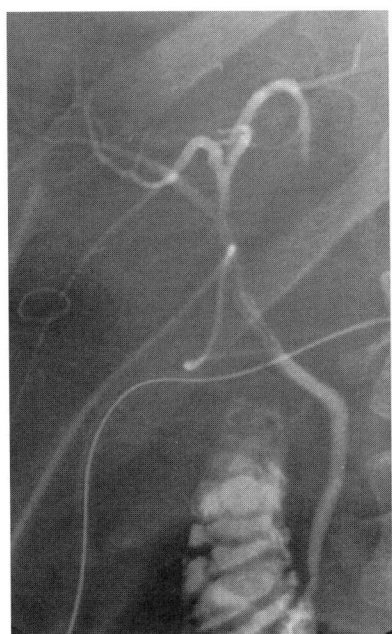

FIGURE 62–2

Radiopaque contrast via T tube showing regular biliary anatomy after transplantation of a deceased donor full-size graft.

Whether the use of certain immunosuppressive drugs, such as antiproliferative immunosuppressants, will influence the incidence of biliary complications remains to be investigated.

Clinical Presentation

Patients with biliary complications may present with a variety of complaints. Complaints such as right upper quadrant abdominal pain, anorexia, abdominal distention, singultus, paralytic ileus, and right shoulder pain are typically associated with biliary tract disorders, but are not specific or could be absent. Pain, a leading complaint, can be totally absent in liver transplantation patients as a result of hepatic denervation. Fever may accompany biliary leakage or cholangitis, but it usually indicates infections of various kinds.[62] Jaundice, acholic stools, no bile drainage through the T tube, bilious ascites, or respiratory complaints caused by pleural effusion or elevation of the right side of the diaphragm are usually late symptoms and signs. In all these cases, a comprehensive examination is indicated. However, patients with biliary complications may remain asymptomatic for an extended period because abdominal symptoms may be masked by corticosteroid use. Bile leaks should also be considered in asymptomatic patients with unexplained elevations in serum bilirubin, unexplained fluctuations in cyclosporine levels, bilious ascites, or intraperitoneal fluid collections on imaging studies.

Diagnostic Workup

Serum Chemical Markers

The first clue of a posttransplantation biliary complication may be an asymptomatic rise in liver enzyme levels. γ-Glutamyltransferase was assessed to be the most effective indicator of biliary complications in the early period after OLT (first 30 days).[63] Total bilirubin elevation was most sensitive between days 30 and 90 after transplantation. The extent of early aminotransferase elevation as a marker for ischemia-reperfusion injury was found to correlate independently with graft and patient survival, but not with biliary complications, chronic rejection, or long-term graft quality.[64]

Abdominal Ultrasonography

The subsequent diagnostic workup has been repeatedly reviewed in an attempt to reach the most accurate strategy.[65-67] Transabdominal ultrasonography (TAUS) as a noninvasive means of evaluating complications in

transplant patients is often the first step. However, there is a common belief that TAUS cannot be considered reliable for the early detection of biliary complications because it lacks sufficient sensitivity to detect small but clinically important obstructions, generalized ductal changes, and leaks.[68] Zemel and associates[69] observed that sonograms were abnormal in only 22 of 41 patients (54%) with cholangiographically defined abnormalities. In contrast, Hussaini and colleagues[70] reported an overall sensitivity of 77%, and a specificity of 67%, with positive and negative predictive values of 26% and 95%, respectively, when adjusted to an endoscopically assessed complication rate of 12.8% in the given patient population. Having a certain variability of experience with TAUS, a cautious approach seems advisable, suggesting that the absence of bile duct dilatation on sonography should not preclude further evaluation in clinically suspicious cases.[71] Additionally, the use of TAUS with simultaneous Doppler evaluation of hepatic artery patency is of paramount importance for the exclusion of hepatic artery stenosis.[72] Hepatic angiography may be indicated if Doppler signals suggest hepatic vascular obstruction, but evidence of biliary ischemia based on other data can be an indication for angiography regardless of the ultrasound findings.[73]

Graft Biopsy

In many cases a liver biopsy will be performed prior to cholangiography to exclude rejection and ischemia and other differential diagnoses of elevated liver enzyme levels. However, despite the description of distinct histological findings of extrahepatic cholestasis caused by extrahepatic obstruction, the liver biopsy can miss an extrahepatic obstruction by portal inflammation being misinterpreted as rejection,[74] thus confusing the primary diagnosis and leading to the misdiagnosis of rejection.[75] Campbell and colleagues[76] found that cholangitis was the only biopsy feature significantly associated with a documented stricture.

Cholangiography

A more definitive assessment of biliary complications can be made by means of direct cholangiography via T tube, PTC, or endoscopic retrograde cholangiography (ERC), which can also be used as an access for therapeutic purposes.[77,78] Cholangiography via T tube ERC is, if pertinent and possible, the gold standard and considered to be the most effective and accurate method for identifying early posttransplant biliary complications.[79,80] A routine cholangiography is conducted before clamping the T tube and after about 6 weeks to 3 months, prior to T tube removal; doing so will detect bile leaks, T-tube migration, rarification of the intrahepatic biliary tree, edema of the anastomotic site or early strictures, and papillary dysfunction. Commonly, a transient increase in the levels of liver enzymes 1 to 2 days following T-tube clamping will occur.

In the absence of a T tube, visualization of the biliary system is possible only when invasive procedures such as PTC and ERC are used, which are themselves associated with complications in 3.4% of PTC and 7% of ERC procedures.[81] In patients with bilioenteric anastomoses, PTC is generally required for minimal invasive therapeutic intervention.

Routine use of ERC after OLT in asymptomatic patients with abnormal liver enzyme levels was not found to be useful. Conversely, liver biopsy results were usually abnormal in this subset of patients and biopsy should therefore be the initial invasive procedure.[82] Sensitivity, specificity, and positive and negative predictive values for successful ERC in detecting early biliary complications in patients with unsplinted CC were reported to be 80%, 98%, 89%, and 97%, respectively, whereas those for predicting the overall rate of biliary complications were 53%, 98%, 89%, and 89%, respectively. Although highly specific and moderately sensitive in detecting early biliary complications, ERC performed routinely has low sensitivity in predicting the overall risk for biliary complications.[83]

Computed Tomography

Computed tomography (CT) is the method of choice for detecting and assessing intra-abdominal fluid collections such as biloma while simultaneously enabling an investigation of the vascular supply of the graft. Progress was made in describing vascular and biliary anatomy by using three-dimensional helical CT for the assessment of living donors.[84,85] It can provide valuable information, particularly for patients with indeterminate TAUS results or patients in whom TAUS is difficult. However, its value to screen for biliary obstruction or leaks still awaits evaluation in imaging studies.[86] CT has its established place in the detection and interventional treatment of intra-abdominal fluid collections. Because CT requires less cooperation by the patient as compared with magnetic resonance cholangiography (MRC), CT is of special importance in the early posttransplant phase and for the early assessment of intensive care unit (ICU) patients.

Hepatobiliary Scintigraphy

Hepatobiliary scintigraphy (HBS) has also been used to screen for T-tube–related bile duct leaks and other early biliary complications.[87] The reported sensitivity and specificity of HBS in detecting biliary leakage after transplantation were only 50% and 79%, respectively, and the corresponding figures for biliary strictures were 62% and 64%, respectively.[88] The usefulness of HBS was recently studied in the diagnosis of biliary complications after adult-to-adult living donor OLT.[89] Sensitivity and specificity for biliary obstruction were 93% and 88%, respectively, in a cohort of 54 patients with clinical complaints or abnormal liver function test results. The sensitivity and specificity were 100% each for bile leakages.

Magnetic Resonance Cholangiography/ Cholangiopancreatography

MRC has been proposed as a reliable noninvasive screening method in patients with biliary and pancreatic disease and biliary complications after OLT.[90-92] MRC was successfully used to delineate the anatomy and morphology of bile ducts in living-related pediatric OLTs, thus guiding the interventional radiological or surgical treatment of biliary complications.[93] Several studies suggested that MRC may be a useful noninvasive diagnostic tool for the follow-up of recipients of liver transplantation.[94-97] MRC is also useful in detecting bile leaks. However, formal comparative studies with other imaging modalities have not yet been published.[81,98] Because the biliary tract is inaccessible by ERC in patients with bilioenteric anastomosis, MRC would appear particularly attractive in these patients.[99]

Boraschi and associates[81] prospectively compared MRC and ERC and clinical history in 113 recipients of liver transplantation with suspected biliary complications. The overall accuracy of MRC for various complications including strictures, bilomas with leaks, choledocholithiasis, and ampullary stenosis was 93%. The sensitivity and specificity were more than 90%, and the positive predictive value was reported to be 86%. The authors concluded that MRC is a feasible imaging modality for biliary tract evaluation when there is low or nonspecific suspicion of biliary tract disease or when ERC and PTC are unsuccessful. Additionally, a comprehensive assessment of concomitant vascular, parenchymal, and extrahepatic complications was described by using dynamic interpolated three-dimensional MR imaging.[100] However, three main restrictions were defined: (1) MRC tends to overestimate biliary strictures at the anastomotic site, (2) MRC cannot usually distinguish circumscribed perianastomotic ascitic fluid from biloma, and (3) the precision of its measurement of the length of nonanastomotic strictures, particularly those involving the hepatic bifurcation and right or left hepatic ducts, is restricted.

Specific Biliary Complications

Biliary complications after OLT constitute an important source of acute and chronic injury that can lead to loss of the graft and the patient. Proper care of the graft prior to transplantation and accurate surgical technique are important features to avoid posttransplant biliary complications. The prompt recognition and management of these complications ensures complete and definitive treatment in many cases.

Based on the vast experience of the University of Pittsburgh's transplantation program, approximately one third of the biliary complications were diagnosed within 1 month of surgery, and 80% of complications were diagnosed within 6 months.[3] A variety of posttransplant biliary complications exist, but the most common are leaks and strictures. Leaks occur predominantly in the early posttransplant period (within 1 month of surgery). Stricture formation typically develops gradually over several months to years, depending on the degree of the insult. The annual incidence of biliary complications was reported to be less than 4% after the first posttransplant year.[5]

Bile Leaks

Bile leaks are common after OLT and may complicate 1% to 25% of OLT procedures performed.[4,5] They can be divided into early and late bile leaks. The definition of the term *early* varies in the literature, defining a period of 1 to 3 months after OLT.[56] Thus, reported complication rates may vary considerably, too. However, the incidence of biliary problems is highest in the first few months after transplantation. It declines to very low incidences after the first posttransplantation year, but occasionally biliary problems appear after several years. Early complications comprise mainly bile leaks and anastomotic strictures. Early leaks are often caused by local ischemia or technical mishap, such as suturing technique that produced insufficiency. The incidence of early postoperative bile leaks is reportedly unrelated to the type of biliary reconstruction.[57]

Early Bile Leaks

Leaks may originate from the anastomosis (Fig. 62–3); either the donor or recipient cystic duct stump; the cut surface in the case of a reduced-size graft, split graft, or a graft from a living donor; or the T-tube exit site if a T tube is used. After CC, bile leaks that are not related to T-tube removal usually present within the first 30 days after OLT.[3,8] Most leaks have technical causes.

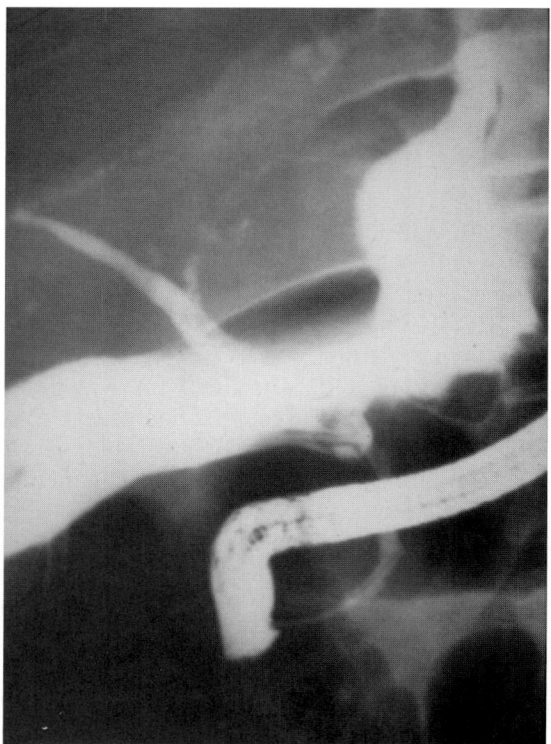

FIGURE 62–3

Anastomotic leakage after deceased donor full-size liver transplantation. ERC displayed a broad anastomotic leakage resulting in a release of radiopaque contrast into the subhepatic space.

Anastomotic leaks are caused primarily by ischemic necrosis at the end of the bile duct (most commonly the donor duct) or a technically unsatisfactory anastomosis. Nonanastomotic (non–T-tube-related) leaks often result from vascular insufficiency. Therefore, the possibility of hepatic artery thrombosis or other compromises to the arterial perfusion must be excluded.[56] Cut surface leaks can occur as a result of insufficient suturing or aberration of the resection plane, resulting in unsatisfactorily drained segments. Bile leakage from any source can be serious; however, leaks from the anastomosis are the most hazardous. Anastomotic leaks can be visualized with a T-tube cholangiogram and managed conservatively by leaving the T tube open to divert bile flow. A repeat cholangiogram every 1 to 2 weeks will eventually confirm healing of the bile duct. Although ERC/PTC may be successful in some cases, many cases require surgical revision.[101]

Bile leaks after CJ are less frequent and occur early in the post-OLT period. The involvement of the intestinal loop presumably contributes to an increased chance of intra-abdominal abscess formation and sepsis. Regional sepsis and poor postoperative infection control can result in recurrent biliary leaks. Insufficiency can be diagnosed with hepatobiliary scintigraphy, MRC, and in selected patients with PTC[5,88]; most of this latter set of patients eventually require surgical revision of the bilioenteric anastomosis.[102,103]

Leaks from other nonanastomotic sites, such as around T tubes or from the cut surface, are less likely to endanger the graft or the patient. The majority of early bile leaks after OLT are related to elective or inadvertent T-tube removal and occur at the T-tube insertion site. Bile leaks may complicate up to 33% of all T tube removals, depending on the diagnostic criteria used.[8,104,105] The incidence of late bile duct leak was reported to be 7%, with a mean time to presentation of 118 days after transplantation despite prolonged T tube placement.[19] Early T-tube insertion site leaks may reflect relative downstream obstruction or papillary dysfunction. They usually respond to unclamping of the T tube, placement of a PTC-guided drainage (PTCD), or endoscopic sphincterotomy or stenting.[103,106] The incidence may be lowered by tunneling the T drain through the mesocolon on its way outside the abdominal cavity. There is no clear correlation between either progressive duct dilation or graft ischemia time and the subsequent development of bile leak after T tube removal. An impact of T-tube removal earlier than the usual period of 6 weeks to 3 months has not yet been confirmed.[105] The frequent occurrence of T-tube–related leaks has prompted many transplant centers to abandon the routine placement of T tubes.[17,21,22] Other centers have proposed a modified technique of T-tube removal, using the T tube itself as a counterdrain under fluoroscopic guidance.[107]

The incidence of cut surface leaks in living donor liver transplantation varies considerably, ranging from 0% to 22%.[45,47,51,108,109] The actual incidence of cut surface leaks for the various types of reduced-size OLT is difficult to assess, because most reports on biliary leaks are not subdivided into cut surface leaks and other types of biliary leaks.

A rare, but grave, complication in the early postoperative period is diffuse biliary necrosis secondary to acute arterial thrombosis or blood group incompatibility between donor and recipient. The presentation is usually a combination of massive bile leakage, sepsis, cholestasis, and associated complications such as pleural effusion.

Late Bile Leaks

Late bile leaks are infrequent events. They are sometimes caused by recurrence or persistence of early complications or they can be due to delayed removal of T-tubes, transhepatic anastomotic stents, or biliary stent migration and perforation.[110] Leakages secondary to late hepatic artery thrombosis were also reported and correlated significantly with donor age.[111] Chronic biliary problems are particularly difficult to treat

when thrombosis of the hepatic artery is part of the cause. Despite recurrent cholangitis and cholestasis secondary to ischemic injury of the biliary tree, synthetic graft function may still be good. Hence, nondefinitive, temporary measures may often be considered until definitive treatment by retransplantation is necessary.

Bile Collection/Biliary Abscesses

Any biliary leakage can lead to extravasation of bile into the intrahepatic parenchyma or free abdominal cavity, resulting in a biloma (Fig. 62–4). The worst scenario is severe bile duct necrosis with subsequent bile duct rupture. Undetected or clinically inapparent bilomas predispose to a number of serious and insidious complications. Bilomas may be superinfected by ascending pathogens, leading to intra-abdominal abscesses and sepsis. One of the most feared secondary complications is erosion of the hepatic artery with massive and often deleterious bleeding. Emergency surgery is required; however, it is often too late to rescue the patient. Other rare but serious complications could be biliothoracic and biliopulmonary fistula and pleural empyema. The typical site of abdominothoracic fistula is the former insertion of the coronary ligament into the diaphragm, from which the recipient's diseased liver had been separated surgically.

Biliary Strictures

Bile duct strictures are the most frequent cause of delayed biliary complications and usually occur later than bile leaks.[3,19] However, they do also occur in the early phase and then are mainly anastomotic strictures because of technical error, whereas later appearing strictures are often the result of vascular insufficiency and fibrotic healing.[4,5,57] Biliary strictures complicate approximately 3% to 14% of all OLTs performed[3,4,7] and account for up to 40% of all biliary complications. Biliary strictures can occur with either type of biliary reconstruction. At least two large series report strictures to be more common with Roux-en-Y CJ reconstruction.[3,72] The incidence of late anastomotic strictures may rise in the future because more complex biliary reconstructions of often two or more small-caliber bile ducts are necessary in split-liver and living donor liver transplantation.[51,47,109]

It is useful to classify late strictures as anastomotic and nonanastomotic. The latter are subclassified as hilar or intrahepatic, reflecting differences in cause and responses to treatment.

Stricture formation is most commonly detected by an increase of γ-glutamyltransferase, alkaline phosphatase,

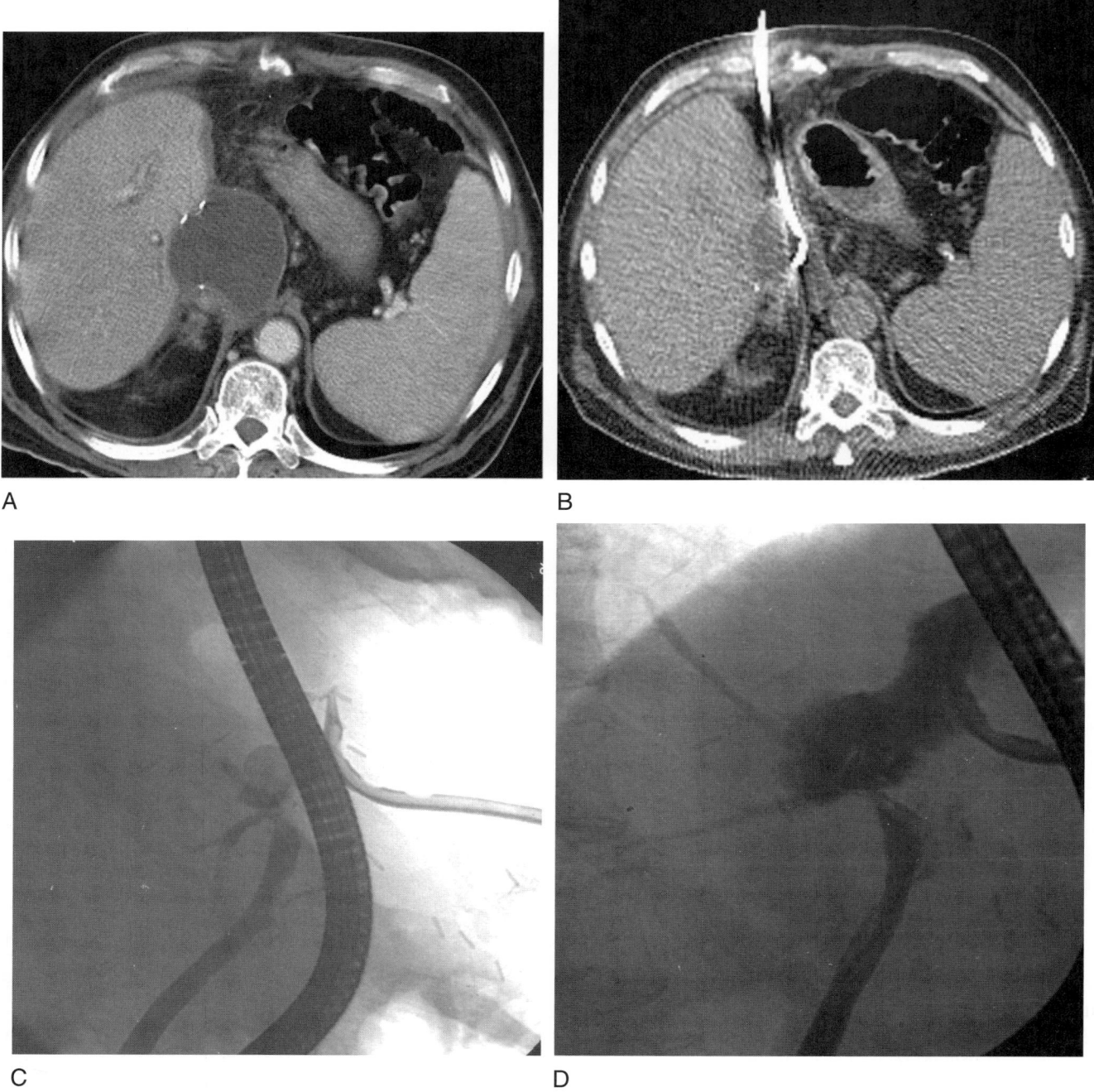

FIGURE 62–4

Computed tomography displaying a biloma at the cut edge of a right lobe graft before (**A**) and after (**B**) CT-guided transcutaneous drainage. ERC was performed after placement of the transcutaneous drain to localize the leak. It turned out to be an anastomotic leak after duct-to-duct anastomosis of two separate orifices with the recipient choledochus (**C**). ERC clearly displayed that contrast medium was drained via the transcutaneous drain (**D**).

and total bilirubin. However, strictures often remain undetected until hepatic dysfunction or infection become apparent. They should also be considered in any recipient of transplantation who presents with histological findings suggestive of biliary obstruction and cholangitis. Unfortunately, dilatation of the intra- or extrahepatic biliary tree in imaging studies is nonspecific and is common in the absence of biochemical abnormalities or cholangiographic evidence of biliary obstruction.[4,112]

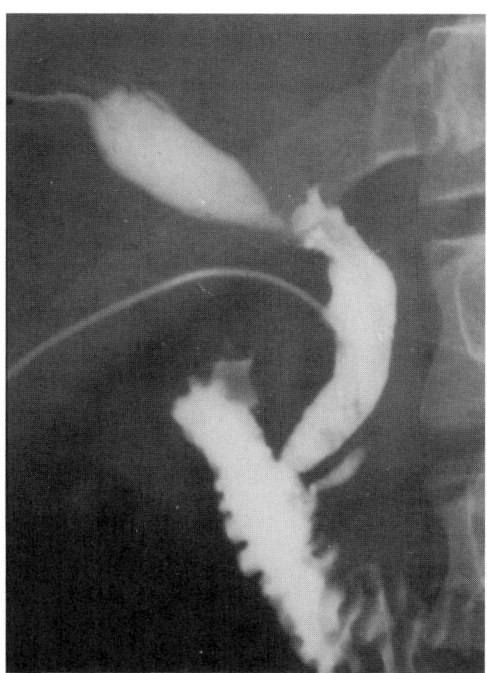

FIGURE 62–5

Early anastomotic stricture with a T tube in situ was used to produce this image. The proximal end of the T-tube is flexed distal to the stenosis, thus not fulfilling its function. An ERC and balloon dilatation with subsequent placement of an internal stent was performed afterward.

Anastomotic Strictures

Early anastomotic strictures (Fig. 62–5) are predominantly caused by technical failure. A transient narrowing at the duct-to-duct anastomosis caused by edema or inflammation may typically occur within the first 4 to 8 weeks after transplantation. Delayed anastomotic strictures are believed to originate from a combination of surgical technique, local tissue ischemia, and fibrotic healing.[19] They tend to be isolated to a short segment of the common duct and typically are not evident until after removal of the T tube. Three prospective trials on the usefulness of T tubes did not support the hypothesis that patients without T tubes are at higher risk for stricture formation.[17,21,22] Anastomotic strictures were reported to be more common after bilioenteric anastomosis than after duct-to-duct anastomosis.[72] Because of the direct bilioenteric connection, signs and symptoms of cholangitis may be more common at presentation.

Nonanastomotic Strictures

Nonanastomotic strictures are frequently hilar in location but may be diffusely intrahepatic. These strictures are often complex and in multiple locations and may be associated with the formation of biliary casts or stones.

Hepatic artery stenosis and thrombosis are well-recognized complications of OLT and well-known risk factors for the development of biliary strictures.[113-115] Approximately 50% of patients who present with nonanastomotic strictures have hepatic artery thrombosis.[4,72,116] Thus, the assessment of arterial blood supply to the graft is an integral part of differential diagnosis for nonanastomotic strictures. Extensive anatomic studies showed that the blood supply of the supraduodenal bile duct is mainly provided by the posterior superior pancreaticoduodenal artery. Branches to the bile duct that originate from this vessel are transected during both donor and recipient operations.[117,118] The remaining blood supply to the donor bile duct, mainly from branches of the hepatic artery and branches running caudally from the hepatic hilum, is thus delicate and susceptible to ischemic injury.[119] In 2% to 20% of patients, pathological changes of the biliary tree develop and are localized proximal to the anastomotic site and occur in the presence of an obviously normal vascular situation.[9,10,120-123] Because they resemble the biliary tract changes observed in cases of ischemic biliary damage[54,124] they have been referred to as ischemic-type biliary complications[120] or ischemic-type biliary lesions (ITBLs).[10] They are subclassified as intrahepatic lesions (Fig. 62–6), as extrahepatic lesions (Fig. 62–7B), or both intra- and extrahepatic ITBLs (see Fig. 62–7A).[125]

The appearance of these lesions suggests that microcirculatory problems may play a role in their development, but their exact pathogenesis remains speculative. An increased frequency of such lesions has been

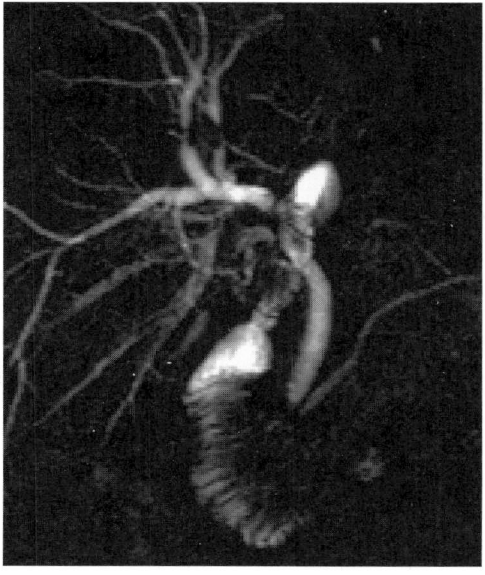

FIGURE 62–6

Magnetic resonance cholangiography displaying two nonanastomotic, isolated intrahepatic stenoses as an example for a circumscribed intrahepatic ischemic-type biliary lesion.

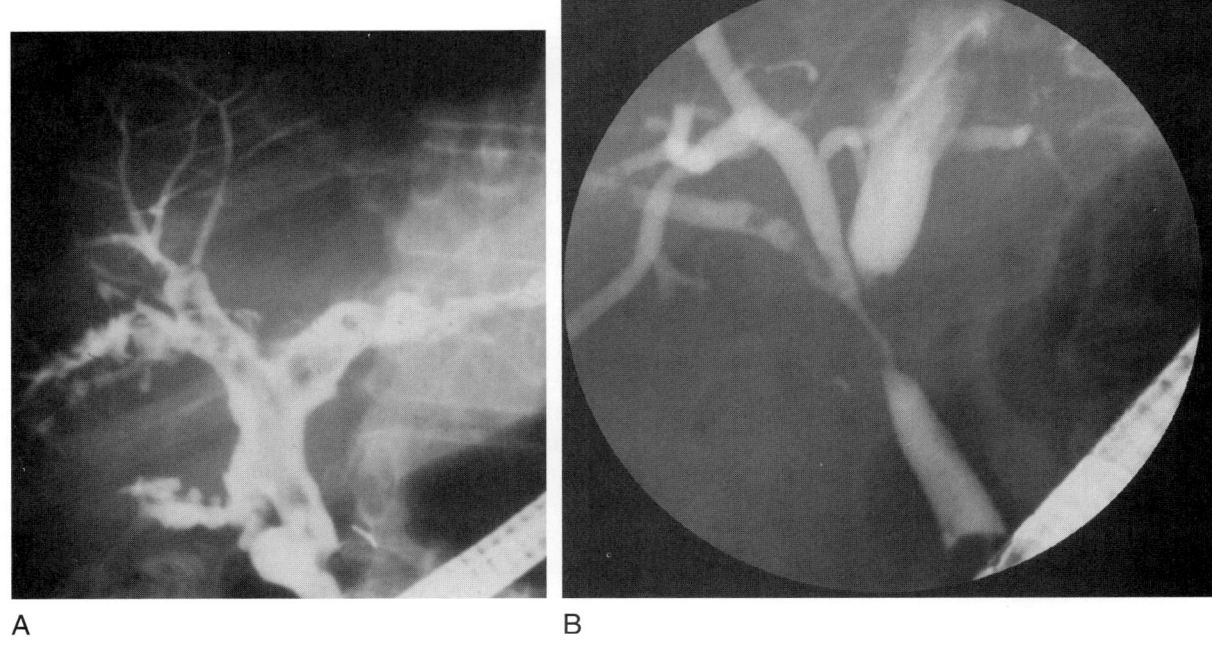

A   B

FIGURE 62–7

A, Multiple intra- and extrahepatic nonanastomotic strictures (ischemia-type biliary lesion [ITBL]). The biliary tree is filled with debris and subtotally destroyed. There are only a few parts of the liver, predominantly in segments VII and VIII, in which a regular biliary anatomy has remained. **B,** Stricture of common hepatic duct and bifurcation (ITBL).

described in patients with prolonged cold ischemic times[9,54,120,121,126-128] or with delayed rearterialization of the graft.[129] Thus, ischemia-reperfusion injury may be a factor. The injury may be a direct effect of cold ischemia on the biliary epithelium or damage to the biliary tree microvasculature.[130]

The main role of microcirculatory impairment is supported by a recent study hypothesizing that insufficient perfusion of biliary arterial vessels might be responsible for the ITBL phenomenon. Arterial back-table pressure perfusion to achieve reliable perfusion of the biliary tract capillary system, which may be impaired by the high viscosity of the University of Wisconsin's solution, was conducted in a controlled study. One hundred thirty-one grafts, which were preserved by in situ standard perfusion, including portal perfusion, were compared with 59 procedures in which additional arterial back-table perfusion was performed. The ITBL rate in the arterial perfusion group was significantly lower (1 of 59) when compared with the standard procedure (21 of 131). Within the first 3 days, peak aspartate aminotransferase (AST) and alanine aminotransferase (ALT) levels were significantly lower in the arterial perfusion group. The authors advocated additional arterial back-table perfusion as the standard technique in liver procurement.[131] Additionally, multivariate analysis identified donor age as determinant of the incidence of ITBL. However, immunological

factors could also contribute to its development by secondary changes in the small arterioles supplying the bile ducts in the absence of gross vascular pathology.[132,133] An increased risk of nonanastomotic strictures is seen in patients with chronic ductopenic rejection,[134] in patients with concomitant cytomegalovirus (CMV) infection, and in those who receive an ABO blood type mismatched graft.[132,135] This process is postulated to involve a combination of vascular disruption and direct biliary injury, because ABO blood group antigens are expressed on both bile duct epithelium and vascular endothelial cells. CMV infection may increase alloantigen expression, making the biliary tree more susceptible to an immunological attack.[136]

Finally, several studies provided convincing evidence that a primary sclerosing cholangitis can recur after OLT, with an incidence of 5% to 20% and interval to diagnosis of at least 1 year after OLT,[137-139] resulting in predominantly intrahepatic, nonanastomotic strictures.

Ampullary Dysfunction

A mild dilatation of both donor and recipient bile duct is a commonly described phenomenon after OLT and is usually not accompanied by symptoms or biochemical abnormalities.[112] In 2% to 5% of all patients who undergo liver transplantation, significant dilatation in

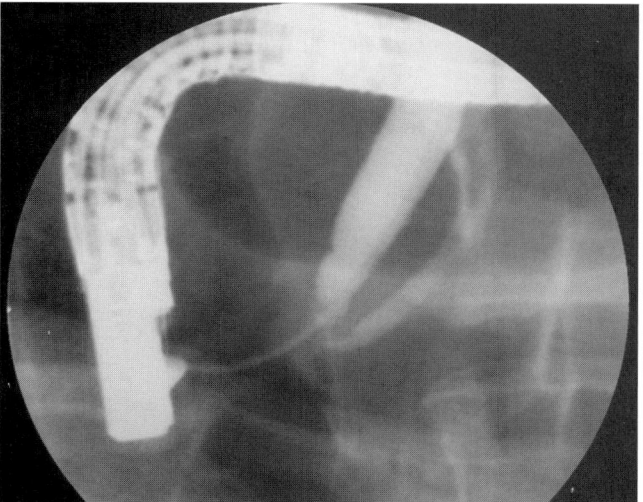

FIGURE 62–8

Ampullary dysfunction with the typical sign of choledochopancreatic reflux of radiopaque contrast during ERCP.

association with biochemical abnormalities occurs in the absence of cholangiographic evidence of obstruction.[3,4,10,72,140] Usually no associated clinical symptoms occur.[141] This entity is referred to as ampullary or sphincter of Oddi dysfunction, or papillary dyskinesia. It was postulated to be caused by operative denervation of the sphincter of Oddi,[140] resulting in abnormal

ampullary relaxation. However, further risk factors are assumed, but not clearly defined. The average time to onset was reported to be 35 weeks; however, early onset may occur after just several days following OLT. The diagnosis is supported by improvements in liver test results with T-tube unclamping, by delayed drainage of contrast medium (more than 15 minutes) after cholangiography, delayed biliary emptying demonstrated by hepatobiliary scintigraphy, and by sphincter or T-tube manometry. Endoscopic retrograde cholangiopancreatography (ERCP) shows the typical sign of biliopancreatic reflux of contrast medium (Fig. 62–8). Bile duct pressures measured through the T tube were found to be elevated following OLT when compared with that following cholecystectomy, but returned to normal within 3 to 4 months.[142] Sphincter of Oddi manometry in a small cohort of patients with suspected ampullary dysfunction after OLT[143] revealed elevated mean basal sphincter pressures and abnormal responses to cholecystokinin infusion in four of five patients, whereas one patient had a low basal sphincter pressure and absent phasic activity.

Biliary Stones, Sludge, and Casts

Biliary stones and sludge can occur at any time following OLT (Fig. 62–9) but are predominantly seen as late

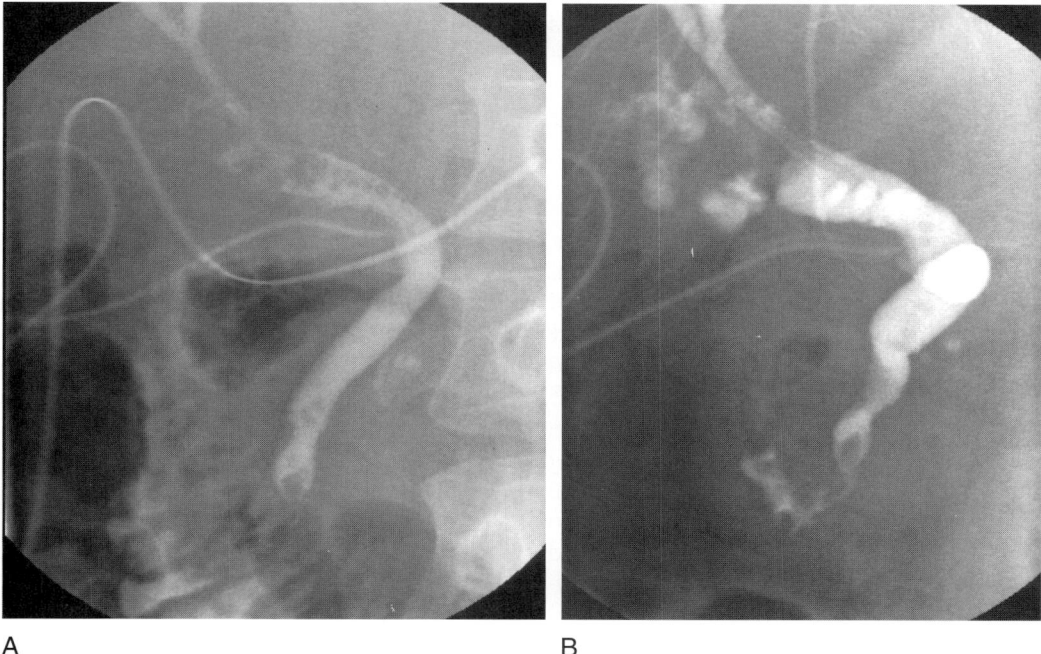

A   B

FIGURE 62–9

A, Multiple biliary stones causing extrahepatic cholestasis 3 weeks after liver transplantation. The biliary system is visualized by contrast medium administered via the T tube. **B,** Recurrent preampullary biliary stone 1 week after ERC with stone removal.

complications occurring later than 3 months after OLT. Occasionally, an aggregation of extensive casts termed a staghorn calculus has been described.[4] Biliary strictures predispose to additional sludge and stone formation and may be seen in up to 90% of patients with bile stones.[144,145] Biliary sludge is commonly associated with either anastomotic or nonanastomotic biliary strictures. In addition to biliary obstruction, kinking of the bile duct, mucosal damage, ischemia, infection, foreign bodies (T tube, stents), cholesterol supersaturation of the bile acid, and depletion of the bile acid pool because of external drainage via T tube were discussed as further causes of stones and sludge.[144,146,147] There also seems to be a lithogenic effect by calcineurin inhibitors, which are thought to contribute by inhibiting bile secretion and promoting functional biliary stasis.[148-150] Whether the type of biliary reconstruction influences the risk of bile stone formation has not yet been studied in detail.

Complications Related to Bilioenteric Anastomosis

Bilioenteric anastomosis in terms of an end-to-side CJ is a rare type of biliary drainage in deceased donor full-size OLT and preferred in recipients suffering from primary or secondary biliary tract disease, such as primary sclerosing cholangitis and cholangiocarcinoma. Additionally, the Roux-en-Y CJ is frequently used as biliary drainage during retransplantations, with size disparities between donor and recipient ducts, when a critical blood supply to the distal donor bile duct is foreseeable,[19] and for surgical treatment of biliary strictures inadequately treated endoscopically.[123] Furthermore, it is the most common anastomosis used in pediatric liver transplant patients, because of the small size or absence of bile ducts in this patient population. It has gained importance for living donor liver transplantation (see Fig. 62–1) and split OLT because complex reconstruction of several small bile ducts has to be performed frequently. Primary bilioenteric anastomosis is necessary to prevent a higher incidence of biliary leakages and strictures, which have to be cured by CJ secondarily.[47,51] Some centers regularly use an internal stent to maintain the patency of the biliary enteric anastomosis during the immediate postoperative weeks.[5] These internal stents may drain the biliary system by one of two percutaneous drainages: They are either inserted transenterically and exit the biliary tree transhepatically or they are placed transenterically with a free end proximal to the anastomosis.

Potential problems related to the bilioenteric anastomosis include bowel ischemia, perforation, and torsion; enteric anastomotic bleeding; delayed mixing of bile with intestinal contents; altered cyclosporine absorption; blind loop syndrome; and biliary colonization/infection from intestinal microbial reflux.[24]

Mucocele

Defective drainage of mucus produced by the lining cells of the cystic duct remnant into the bile duct may lead in rare cases to the formation of a mucocele,[151] eventually leading to extrinsic compression of the common duct. A mucocele must be differentiated from other circumscribed perihilar fluid collections, including hepatic artery pseudoaneurysm, biloma, loculated ascites, abscess, liquefied hematoma, tumor, adenopathy, and a fluid-filled Roux-en-Y loop of jejunum.

Hemobilia

Hemobilia is a rare complication (approximately 0.1%) after OLT. It is usually related to percutaneous liver biopsy or PTC by creating an arteriobiliary fistula.[4,152-154] The converse phenomenon, bilhemia, can be observed under similar circumstances when a bilioportal or biliovenous fistula is accidentally created. Such fistulas usually vanish spontaneously. Facultative clinical symptoms may be right upper quadrant pain, jaundice, and gastrointestinal bleeding.[152] Apart from massive loss of blood, transpapillary gastrointestinal bleeding, and formation of clots, biliary obstructions are the most prominent potential immediate consequences. In rare cases in which hemobilia was associated with underlying biliary strictures, multiple intrahepatic stones have formed above the level of obstruction.[153]

Treatment

The management of biliary complications after OLT requires a multidisciplinary approach involving transplant surgeons, endoscopists, and interventional radiologists. Because biliary complications after OLT are a heterogenous entity with multifactorial causes, a therapeutic strategy has to meet these requirements. Conservative, interventional, or endoscopic treatment options have to be weighed against surgical reintervention. Although T-tube–related leaks are an indication for endoscopic treatment,[155] complex hilar or intrahepatic strictures caused by ITBL may be treated temporarily or long-term by ERC and stenting,[125] but eventually require surgical repair using a Roux-en-Y CJ,[123] with excellent 5-year survival rates of 71%,[156] or even retransplantation. In many centers, however, early and large anastomotic leakages are indications for immediate reoperation.[4,5,56] Generally speaking, endoscopic treatment has gained an increasing role in the treatment of biliary complications after OLT. Our own experience has clearly demonstrated that a majority of complications could be resolved by endoscopic treatment.[125] In many cases, diagnostic ERC or PTC may be followed immediately by therapeutic measures aimed at definitive restoration of bile flow in the biliary tract by balloon dilation of strictures and removal of debris and stones. They may thus provide curative treatment, ease the patient's complaints, or bridge the time until definitive treatment is decided. However, an essential guideline in the use of ERC is to recognize its limitations. Particularly in the patient with diffuse intrahepatic strictures (see Fig. 62–7A) and underlying hepatic artery thrombosis, the goals of endoscopic therapy must be clearly delineated prior to the procedure. There are no valid data confirming a higher risk of endoscopic treatment regarding cholangitis or bleeding complications as long as the routine precautionary measures are kept. Although prophylactic antibiotic therapy is frequently recommended, there are no consistent data proving a higher risk of cholangitis or bacteriemia when compared without antibiotic prophylaxis. Moreover, despite the theoretical long-term risk of cholangitis from exposure of the biliary tree to enteric contents, this complication of sphincterotomy has not been commonly reported. With longitudinal follow-up and continued improvement in the survival of liver transplant patients, more complete data on the long-term consequences of biliary complications and the long-term efficacy of endoscopic therapy will become available.

Bile Leaks

The commonly recommended approach to extra-anastomotic leakages is ERC with stenting of the bile leak using plastic internal stents. The advocated intervals until re-ERC and stent removal range from 4 weeks to 3 months.[4,5,57,125]

Leaks at the T-tube insertion site may be treated conservatively and symptomatically over a limited period of 24 hours.[4] From one third to one half of such leaks were reported to close spontaneously within 24 hours.[8,105] If signs and symptoms persist, further intervention is indicated. Ampullary dysfunction may be the underlying cause. Recommended approaches comprise conservative, endoscopic, and surgical approaches.[13] Accumulated experience shows that in most cases nonsurgical management is effective.[56] Biliary tract stenting with or without endoscopic sphincterotomy can be applied successfully in more than 90% of biliary tract leaks.[19,24,56,102,157] Endoscopic sphincterotomy alone has also been reported to be effective in treating post-OLT bile leaks.[158] Some centers advocate endoscopic placement of nasobiliary catheters proximal to the leak,[104] which was reported to ensure closure of bile leak in almost all patients within 14 days.[80,159,160] Recurrent leaks were demonstrated to be less frequent with the use of nasobiliary drainage when compared with biliary stents.[161] Some centers prefer to use internal plastic stents, which are placed by endoscopy and remain in place for 2 weeks[74] to several months.[125] Others prefer to place plastic biliary stents across the T-tube insertion site and the biliary anastomosis, which remain there for approximately 1 to 2 months.[4] However, this procedure does require a second endoscopic procedure for stent removal.[80,162,163] Associated fluid collections are drained percutaneously under sonography or CT guidance (see Fig. 62–4C), or are surgically drained if infected or symptomatic.

Anastomotic leakages (see Figs. 62–3 and 62–4), particularly in the case of duct-to-duct anastomosis, can also be successfully managed without surgery if they are small and localized. Endoscopic or percutaneous stenting can resolve minor leaks in the absence of significant right upper quadrant peritonitis or systemic sepsis (Fig. 62–10). However, if the anastomosis is seriously disrupted or biliary extravasation is major (see Fig. 62–3), reoperation with revision is the safest approach.[56]

A therapeutic percutaneous (PTC) approach to Roux-en-Y CJ anastomotic leaks with placement of an internal-external drain is feasible. It should be accompanied by percutaneous drainage of fluid collections, biloma, or abscesses.[164] However, in many cases, operative management with primary repair or refashioning of the anastomosis is required[57] after intra-abdominal infection has resolved.[7] Conversely, an endoscopic approach to such anastomotic leaks is often not feasible because of the Roux-en-Y construction.

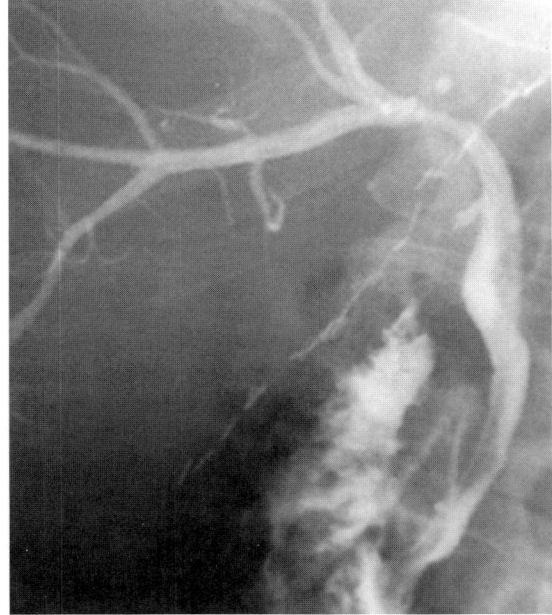

FIGURE 62–10

ERC image displaying a Yamakawa stent placement for an anastomotic leakage after right lobe living donor liver transplantation.

Cut surface leaks may be located and treated by ERC and sphincterotomy, thus reducing the intraductal pressure. Associated biloma can be treated by percutaneous, sonography-guided, or CT-guided drainages.[51,164]

Surgical intervention is required if conservative management fails, if the anastomosis is seriously disrupted or biliary extravasation is major, and often when there is evidence of hepatic artery thrombosis. In most cases periductal infection makes direct reinstitution of duct-to-duct anastomosis impossible. Conversion to a bilioenteric anastomosis, which allows wide débridement of necrotic and infected tissue is advocated.[5,12,65] Primary repair of duct-to-duct anastomotic leaks has been reported in technically ideal situations.[101]

Late bile leaks are a rare event and usually resolve spontaneously. If symptoms persist, endoscopic management is the therapy of choice with which to proceed.[57] Late biliary leaks may be accompanied by strictures caused by chronic inflammatory reactions in the surrounding tissue, finally necessitating surgical intervention.

Bile Collection/Biliary Abscesses

Treating biloma requires diagnosis and treatment of the underlying leakage as well as intervention regarding the threat of abscesses and sepsis caused by bacterial superinfection of the biloma. Drainage by an indwelling catheter that can be placed using sonography or computed tomographic guidance is adequate and sufficient in most cases (see Fig. 62–4).[164] If necessary, this should be accompanied by antibiotics and further symptomatic therapy. Intrahepatic bile leaks communicating with the biliary system may resolve spontaneously or may respond adequately to sphincterotomy. The role of ERC in patients presenting with this clinical scenario is diagnostic[24,102] and therapeutic by defining and eventually treating the underlying leakage. Surgical repair of the biliary tree is required[165] in case of insufficient endoscopic therapy of the underlying biliary leakage or secondary complications.

Anastomotic Strictures

Nonoperative endoscopic treatment should be preferred. Although early experience with endoscopic therapy for anastomotic strictures revealed a significant rate of failures requiring surgical intervention,[57,121,166] more recent studies support the primacy of ERC with stenting.[116,159,167] Reports indicate long-term success in more than 70% of patients.[168] One series reported 15 patients with anastomotic strictures. These patients were treated with long-term stenting of the common bile duct for 1 year and were followed up for more than 12 months after stent removal.[167] All patients displayed short-term success. In 67% of patients (10/15) who completed the 1-year treatment, the anastomosis was kept patent more than 1 year after stent removal. In a series of 30 patients suffering from anastomotic strictures, short-term successful treatment with regard to reduction of cholestasis by balloon dilation and stenting was demonstrated in 26 patients. None of the patients required surgical revision.[169] Because a 30% to 40% relapse rate was reported, requiring repeat dilations,[169] there is a concern about the long-term effect of balloon dilation and temporary stent placement for late-appearing anastomotic strictures (usually after 3 months).[125,170] However, several reports stressed the necessity of long-term endoscopic stenting of anastomotic strictures with intercurrent endoscopic reassessment.[123] Up to 75% of patients diagnosed with anastomotic strictures were stent-free 18 months after initial ERC,[4] using the combination of endoscopic balloon dilation and stenting of anastomotic strictures. Others reported 1-year patency rates of 67%.[116] With these treatment modalities, patient and graft survival rates similar to the ones of an uncomplicated control population after OLT were achieved. The use of self-expanding metal stents in the management of anastomotic strictures after OLT is controversial because of the high rate of stent occlusion and the obvious difficulties in the case of surgical conversion to CJ.[106,171] In one study, percutaneous transhepatic balloon dilation of anastomotic strictures had a 66% long-term success rate.[113] Considering the discomfort of the presence of an indwelling transhepatic drainage catheter between dilations, ERC treatment for anastomotic strictures of choledochocholedochostomies may be more convenient and appropriate. A case in favor of the transhepatic procedure can be made for strictures with a significant amount of debris because the stent can be flushed daily with sterile saline to ameliorate biliary obstruction and can be opened to dependent drainage.[19]

Surgical revision and creation of a Roux-en-Y CJ is indicated if endoscopic treatment has failed.[4,5,19,12,56] In some cases, reestablishment of a CC is possible (Fig. 62–11).

Initial management of strictures affecting CJs usually involves PTC with balloon dilation. Some centers prefer to leave percutaneous biliary drains across the stricture, maintaining the patency of the anastomosis and allowing easy access to the stricture for repeated treatment.[19] Some centers use self-expanding metal stents.[170,171] Persistent Roux-en-Y CJ strictures often require surgical revision.

Nonanastomotic Strictures

Nonanastomotic strictures are commonly classified as having a less favorable prognosis and being less responsive to conservative endoscopic or interventional

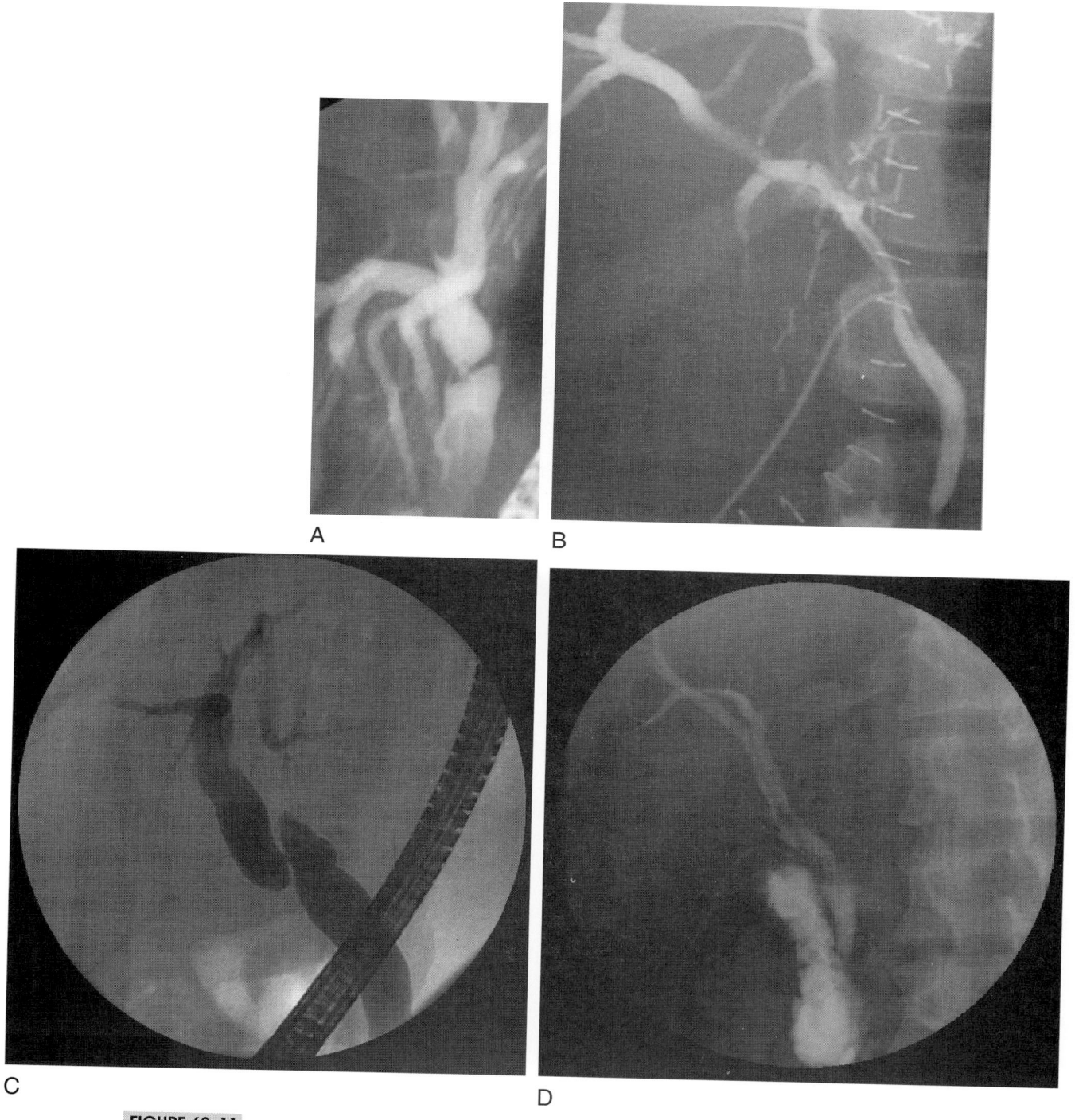

FIGURE 62–11

A, Early anastomotic stenosis after right lobe living donor OLT. **B,** Biliary tract of the same patient after surgical revision and placement of a T tube. ERC failed to dilate the anastomosis. **C,** Late anastomotic stricture 1 year after deceased donor OLT. **D,** Biliary tract of the patient in **C** after surgical revision and placement of a T tube.

therapy[5] than anastomotic strictures. Despite this dismal outcome, these changes have primarily been treated using interventional endoscopic or transhepatic techniques.[9,120,125,172] However, frequent reinterventions and

long-term antibiotic treatment are required in many patients when compared with patients with anastomotic strictures. Moreover, patients have a higher prevalence of concomitant choledocholithiasis and biliary casts, and successful endoscopic therapy takes longer.[4] Although 15 of 16 patients were able to undergo dilation in a series of patients with hilar strictures, only 4 patients had no stricture recurrence with a follow-up of 12 to 30 months.[172] A subsequent study of dilation and stenting of hilar and intrahepatic strictures achieved a success rate of only 28.6%, compared with a 75% success rate with anastomotic strictures.[116] Percutaneous balloon dilation and stenting or use of external-internal drainages over a prolonged period can also be effective in certain cases[9,120,128] but may not be as well tolerated as endoscopic therapy. In contrast, a recent study showed controversial results. In a cohort of 260 patients who underwent liver transplantation, 13 patients developed biliary strictures, 8 of which were anastomotic strictures. The median number of ERC procedures required was three. The success rate for endoscopic treatment of anastomotic strictures by balloon dilation and stenting was 50%, whereas nonanastomotic strictures responded to endoscopic therapy in 80%.[155] In selected cases, double or triple parallel stenting may be successful (Fig. 62–12).

Factors associated with a greater probability of successful treatment were strictures developing within 3 months after transplantation and the absence of ductopenic rejection, CMV infection, or hepatic artery thrombosis. Patients with progressively worsening cholestatic and clinical symptoms or persistent severe infection of the biliary tree, or both, as well as those with potential development of secondary biliary cirrhosis, or those who either are not amenable to or do not respond to nonsurgical therapy may require

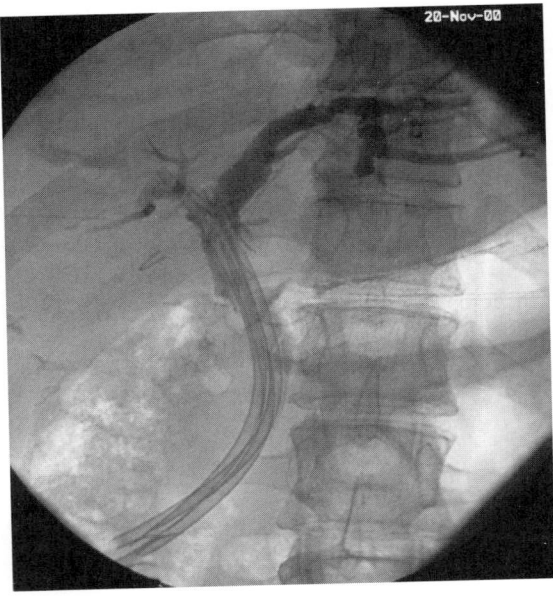

FIGURE 62–12

Triple parallel stenting for an extrahepatic, nonanastomotic bile duct stenosis.

retransplantation.[120,128] Early reports suggested that despite attempts at nonsurgical intervention, 25% to 50% of patients with nonanastomotic strictures die or undergo retransplantation for these complications.[8,9,120,128,172] Advances in endoscopic and percutaneous therapy of biliary strictures have improved these outcomes so that the overall patient survival does not differ from transplant recipients without stricture[116,120] as long as the indication for retransplantation occurs in a timely fashion. In particular, patients with suspected recurrence of primary sclerosing cholangitis should be considered for retransplantation in due time.

A 1999 report by Schlitt and associates[123] stressed the value of surgical reconstruction for hilar strictures. According to Ward and associates,[172] hilar strictures appeared a median of 10 weeks after OLT. Strictures that appeared within the first 3 months were more amenable to endoscopic measures than those that developed later. They almost invariably needed surgical intervention. Until recently, reports on the surgical reconstruction of bile duct complications after transplantation included only a few patients suffering from ITBL with stenosis and sludge.[3,173-175] Schlitt and associates[123] evaluated the feasibility, complication rate, and results of a reconstructive surgical approach that included resection of the hepatic bifurcation for the treatment of 17 patients with ITBL unrelated to vascular problems after OLT. All patients treated in this study either already had undergone several endoscopic interventions or the biliary tree could not be approached adequately either after primary hepaticojejunostomy or because of extensive stenosis. Important findings were that stenotic or sclerotic lesions always involved the bifurcation of the bile duct, whereas the extrahepatic ducts frequently were not stenotic but showed sclerotic changes. In most patients there was a discrepancy between the intraoperative finding of a normal intrahepatic biliary system and the ERC findings, suggesting that the presence of intrahepatic intraductal sludge or debris may have appeared as irregularities of the biliary wall on ERC. Surgical reconstruction in 14 patients was accomplished by resection of the bifurcation and hepaticojejunostomy. In 3 patients with more extensive biliary destruction, portoenterostomy with or without peripheral hepatojejunostomy was performed. Only 1 patient who underwent an additional peripheral hepatojejunostomy showed considerable improvement for about 18 months. The other 2 patients required rapid retransplantation. Thus, clinical symptoms and biochemical parameters normalized or improved significantly in 15 of 17 patients (88%) included in the study. Langnas and associates have also reported portoenterostomy for reconstruction of the biliary tract after liver transplantation.[176] Morbidity and reintervention rates in their series were high, but the series included patients with arterial thrombosis. Because of the restricted availability of donor organs and the increased risk of a retransplantation, the option of retransplantation should be reserved for patients in whom no adequate surgical reconstruction can be accomplished.

Ampullary Dysfunction

Because bile duct pressure (and presumably sphincter of Oddi pressure) reportedly decreases to normal values by 3 to 4 months after OLT,[142] transpapillary stenting or endoscopic sphincterotomy,[177] or both, should be considered as an initial approach. In a small series of patients, endoscopic sphincterotomy and stent placement were successful in 80% to 100% of patients.[141,155] Conversion to CJ, which was the traditional management,[140] should be reserved for patients in whom endoscopic sphincterotomy is ineffective.[3]

Biliary Stones, Sludge, and Casts

Several studies reported success rates of endoscopic sphincterotomy and stone extraction in 88% to 91% of patients.[4,155] Percutaneous therapy and oral dissolution therapy have also been described.[175] Biliary casts are more difficult to extract endoscopically than are discrete stones. Endoscopic extraction may be tried, but even repeated interventions usually do not result in complete and permanent clearance of the biliary tree (see Fig. 62–9). For casts that are particularly difficult to extract, surgical extraction, conversion to Roux-en-Y CJ or retransplantation may be required.[155]

Mucocele

The therapy of choice is surgical excision or drainage of the cystic duct remnant by enteric anastomosis.[19]

Hemobilia

Treatment of hemobilia and associated biliary obstruction requires both hemostasis and treatment of the biliary obstruction. Angiographic embolization of hepatic artery pseudoaneurysms is indicated for hemostasis.[4] Biliary obstruction can be managed with percutaneous drainage, endoscopic thrombus extraction and, in unusual cases, surgical intervention.[152,153] Nasobiliary drainage has the advantage of allowing irrigation of blood and clots as well as an assessment for continued bleeding.

Acknowledgments

Radiological and endoscopic illustrations were in part supplied by H. Abou-Rebey, MD, and R. Hintze, MD, Department of Internal Medicine, Division of Gastroenterology and Hepatology, Charité, Campus Virchow, Berlin, and E. Lopez-Haenninen, MD, Department of Radiology, Charité, Campus Virchow, Berlin.

Pearls and Pitfalls

- Excessive preparation or application of monopolar coagulation near the recipient and donor bile duct during explantation and transplantation may lead to impaired vascular supply to both donor and recipient bile duct. It is considered to be a major cause of insufficient healing of biliary anastomoses and biliary leaks. Moreover, it may cause excessive scarring around the anastomosis, representing one of the precursors of anastomotic stricture.

- The arterial supply of the biliary tree is essential to the integrity of biliary drainage of the graft. Therefore, the arterial supply to bile duct, that is, the epicholedochal plexus, which is supplied by three arteries, should be preserved. Vessels arise from arteries at the upper and lower ends of the duct and travel longitudinally with it.[117] Approximately two thirds of the blood supply arises from vessels below, whereas the remainder originates from the right hepatic artery above and direct branches off the hepatic artery as it crosses near the duct. The donor duct should be divided high enough to ensure that its length is adequately supplied by the axial supply from above, and mobilization of the duct from the periductular tissues should be kept at a minimum. The knowledge of arterial bile duct supply also has enormous implications for split OLT and living donor OLT.[118]

- The intrahepatic biliary tree of the transplanted liver is critically dependent on patency of the hepatic artery. Although arterial thrombosis may result in global graft ischemia and profoundly disturbed graft dysfunction, or even graft failure, sometimes the only indication of a thrombosed artery is a biliary leak or stricture. Confirmation of hepatic artery patency is essential when biliary problems develop and is especially important if the proximal or intrahepatic biliary tree is the site of the abnormality.

- Back-table perfusion of the bile duct may clear the donor biliary system from sludge and detritus, thus avoiding early intrinsic obstruction.

Pearls and Pitfalls—cont'd

- Ischemic-type biliary lesions lead to considerable morbidity after OLT. The exact pathogenesis is still unknown. However, a recent study hypothesized that insufficient perfusion of biliary arterial vessels might be responsible for ITBLs. Arterial back-table pressure perfusion to achieve reliable perfusion of the biliary tract capillary system, which may be impaired by the high viscosity of the University of Wisconsin's solution, was conducted in a controlled study. One hundred thirty-one grafts, which were preserved by in situ standard perfusion, including portal perfusion, were compared with 59 procedures in which additional arterial back-table perfusion was performed. The ITBL rate in the arterial perfusion group was significantly lower (1 of 59) than in the standard procedure group (21 of 131). Additionally, peak AST and ALT levels within the first 3 days were significantly lower in the arterial perfusion group. The authors advocated additional arterial back-table perfusion as the standard technique in liver procurement.[131]

- Early enteral supply of probiotic treatment and fiber versus selective bowel decontamination significantly lowered the incidence of cholangitis, pneumonia, and other infectious episodes in a controlled trial at our institution. Additionally, there was a trend toward lower duration of antibiotic therapy, intensive care unit stay, and hospital stay.[178]

- Anomalies of the bile ducts necessitating modification of surgical strategy in living donor hepatectomy are more common than those of the portal vein; however, they are less frequent than surgically relevant anomalies of the hepatic artery.[117] Intraoperative cholangiography is strongly recommended to identify biliary anatomy and help define the adequate transection plane.[179]

- Side-to-side CC using running sutures has the advantage of a broad coaptation of small bile ducts with a low incidence of stenosis and very low probability of developing early anastomotic leaks.[10] Moreover, mechanical trauma to the edges and traction on the suture are more likely to cause necrosis and leakage in an end-to-end than in a side-to-side situation.

References

1. Calne RY: A new technique for biliary drainage in orthotopic liver transplantation using the gallbladder as a pedicle graft conduit between the donor and recipient common bile ducts. Ann Surg 184:605-609, 1976.
2. Brown RS, Russo MW, Lai M, et al: A survey of liver transplantation from living adult donors in the United States. N Engl J Med 348:818-825, 2003.
3. Grief F, Bronsther OL, VanThiel DH, et al: The incidence, timing and management of biliary tract complications after orthotopic liver transplantation. Ann Surg 219:40-45, 1994.
4. Tung BY, Kimmey MB: Biliary complications of orthotopic liver transplantation. Dig Dis 17:133-144, 1999.
5. Jagganath S, Kaloo AN: Biliary complications after liver transplantation. Curr Treat Opin Gastroenterol 5:101-112, 2002.
6. Lerut J, Gordon RD, Iwatsuki S, et al: Biliary tract complications in human orthotopic liver transplantation. Transplantation 43:47-51, 1987.
7. Klien AS, Savader S, Burdick JP, et al: Reduction of morbidity and mortality from biliary complications after liver transplantation. Hepatology 14:818-823, 1991.
8. O'Connor TP, Lewis D, Jenkins RL: Biliary tract complications after liver transplantation. Arch Surg 130:312-317, 1995.
9. Colonna JO, Shaked A, Gomes AS, et al: Biliary strictures complicating liver transplantation. Incidence, pathogenesis, management, and outcome. Ann Surg 216:344-350, 1992.
10. Neuhaus P, Blumhardt G, Bechstein WO, et al: Technique and results of biliary reconstruction using side-to-side choledochocholedochostomy in 300 orthotopic liver transplants. Ann Surg 219:426-434, 1994.
11. Grande L, Pérez-Castilla A, Matus D, et al: Routine use of the T-tube in the biliary reconstruction of liver transplantation: Is it worthwhile? Transplant Proc 31:2396-2397, 1999.
12. Verran DJ, Asfar SK, Ghent CN, et al: Biliary reconstruction without T-tubes or stents in liver transplantation: Report of 502 consecutive cases. Liver Transpl Surg 3:365-373, 1997.
13. Vallera RA, Cotton PB, Clavien PA: Biliary reconstruction for liver transplantation and management of biliary complications: Overview and surgery of current practices in the United States. Liver Transpl Surg 1:143-152, 1998.
14. Sung JY, Costerton JW, Shaffer EA: Defense system in the biliary tract against bacterial infection. Dig Dis Sci 37:689-696, 1992.
15. Keck H, Langrehr JM, Blumhardt G, et al: Incidence of biliary complications following side-to-side choledochocholedochostomy after liver transplantation. Transplant Proc 26:3544-3545, 1994.
16. Rabkin JM, Orloff SL, Reed MH, et al: Biliary tract complications of side-to-side without T-tube versus end-to-end with or without T-tube choledochocholedochostomy in liver transplant recipients. Transplantation 65:193-199, 1998.
17. Davidson BR, Rai R, Kurzawinski TR, et al: Prospective randomized trial of end-to-end versus side-to-side biliary reconstruction after orthotopic liver transplantation. Br J Surg 86:447-452, 1999.
18. Shaked A: Use of T-tube in liver transplantation. Liver Transpl Surg 3 Suppl:22-23, 1997.
19. Porayko MK, Kondo M, Steers JL: Liver transplantation: Late complications of the biliary tract and their management. Semin Liver Dis 15:139-155, 1995.
20. Randall HB, Wachs ME, Somberg KA, et al: The use of the T-tube after orthotopic liver transplantation. Transplantation 61:258-261, 1996.
21. Vougas V, Rela M, Gane E, et al: A prospective randomized trial of bile duct reconstruction at liver transplantation: T-tube or no T-tube? Transpl Int 9:392-395, 1996.
22. Scatton O, Meunier B, Cherqui D, et al: Randomized trial of choledochocholedochostomy with or without a T-tube in orthotopic liver transplantation. Ann Surg 233:432-437, 2001.

23. Shimoda M, Saab S, Morrisey M, et al: A cost-effectiveness analysis of biliary anastomosis with or without T-tube after orthotopic liver transplantation. Am J Transplant 1:157-161, 2001.
24. Van Thiel DH, Fagiuoli S, Wright HI, et al: Biliary complications of liver transplantation. Gastrointest Endosc 39:455-460, 1993.
25. Bubak ME, Porayko MK, Krom RAF, et al: Complications of liver biopsy in liver transplant patients: Increased sepsis associated with choledochojejunostomy. Hepatology 14:1063-1065, 1991.
26. Galati JS, Monsour HP, Donovan JP, et al: The nature of complications following liver biopsy in transplant patients with Roux-en-Y choledochojejunostomy. Hepatology 20:651-653, 1994.
27. Reichert PR, Renz JF, Rosenthal P, et al: Biliary complications of reduced-organ liver transplantation. Liver Transpl Surg 4:343-349, 1998.
28. Emond JC, Whitington PF, Thistlewaite JR, et al: Transplantation of two patients with one liver: Analysis of a preliminary experience with "split-liver" grafting. Ann Surg 212:14-22, 1990.
29. Broelsch CE, Emond JC, Whitington PF, et al: Application of reduced-size liver transplants as split grafts, auxiliary orthotopic grafts and living related segmental transplants. Ann Surg 214:368-377, 1990.
30. Otte JB: Is it right to develop living related liver transplantation: Do reduced and split livers not suffice to cover the needs? Transpl Int 8:69-73, 1995.
31. De Ville de Goyet J: Split liver transplantation in Europe—1988 to 1993. Transplantation 59:1371-1376, 1995.
32. Azoulay D, Astarcioglu I, Bismuth H, et al: Split liver transplantation: The Paul Brousse policy. Ann Surg 224:737-748, 1996.
33. Rogiers X, Malagó M, Gawad K, et al: One year of experience with extended application and modified techniques of split liver transplantation. Transplantation 61:1059-1061, 1996.
34. Deshpande RR, Bowles M, Vilca-Melendez H, et al: Results of split liver transplantation in children. Ann Surg 236:248-253, 2002.
35. Rogiers X, Malagó M, Gawad K, et al: In situ splitting of cadaveric livers. Ann Surg 224:331-341, 1996.
36. Goss JA, Shackleton CR, McDiarmid SV, et al: Long-term results of pediatric liver transplantation: An analysis of 569 transplants. Ann Surg 228:411-420, 1998.
37. Busuttil RW, Goss JA: Split liver transplantation. Ann Surg 229:313-321, 1999.
38. Group SR: Studies of pediatric transplantation (SPLIT): Year 2000 outcomes. Transplantation 72:463-476, 2001.
39. Heffron T, Emond J, Whitington P, et al: Biliary complications in pediatric liver transplantation. Transplantation 53:391-395, 1992.
40. Marcos A: Right lobe living donor liver transplantation. Liver Transpl 6 (Suppl 2):S59-S63, 2000.
41. Broelsch CE, Testa G, Malagó M, et al: Living donor liver transplantation in adults: Outcome in Europe. Liver Transpl 6 (Suppl 2):S64-S65, 2000.
42. Todo S, Furukawa H, Jin MB, et al: Living donor liver transplantation in adults: Outcome in Japan. Liver Transpl 6 (Suppl 2):S66-S72, 2000.
43. Miller CM, Gondolesi GE, Florman S, et al: One hundred nine living donor liver transplants in adults and children: A single center experience. Ann Surg 234:301-312, 2001.
44. Lee SG, Park KM, Lee YJ, et al: 157 adult-to-adult living donor liver transplantations. Transplant Proc 33:1323-1325, 2001.
45. Fan ST, Lo CM, Liu CL, et al: Biliary reconstruction and complications of right lobe live donor liver transplantation. Ann Surg 236:676-683, 2002.
46. Chen CL, Fan ST, Lee SG, et al: Living donor liver transplantation: 12 years of experience in Asia. Transplantation 75:S6-S11, 2003.
47. Testa G, Malagó M, Valentin-Gamazo C, et al: Biliary anastomosis in living related liver transplantation using the right liver lobe: Techniques and complications. Liver Transpl 6:710-714, 2000.

48. Cronin D, Alonso E, Piper J, et al: Biliary complications in living donor liver transplantation. Transplant Proc 29:419-420, 1997.
49. Egawa H, Uemoto S, Inomata Y, et al: Biliary complications in pediatric living-related liver transplantation. Surgery 124:901-910, 1998.
50. Egawa H, Inomata Y, Uemoto S, et al: Biliary anastomotic complications in 400 living-related liver transplantations. World J Surg 25:1300-1307, 2001.
51. Settmacher U, Steinmueller Th, Schmidt SC, et al: Technique of bile duct reconstruction and management of biliary complications in right lobe living donor liver transplantation. Clin Transpl 17:37-42, 2003.
52. Langnas AN, Marujo W, Stratta RJ, et al: Hepatic allograft rescue following arterial thrombosis. Transplantation 15:86-90, 1991.
53. Vorwerk D, Gunther RW, Klever P, et al: Angioplasty and stent placement for treatment of hepatic artery thrombosis following liver transplantation. J Vasc Interv Radiol 5:309-314, 1994.
54. Sanchez-Urdazpal L, Gores GJ, Ward EM, et al: Ischemic-type biliary complications after orthotopic liver transplantation. Hepatology 16:49-53, 1992.
55. Sheiner PA, Varma CV, Guarrera JV, et al: Selective revascularization of hepatic artery thrombosis after liver transplantation improves patient and graft survival. Transplantation 64:1295-1299, 1997.
56. Moser MA, Wall WJ: Management of biliary problems after liver transplantation. Liver Transpl 7(11 Suppl):S46-S52, 2001.
57. Testa G, Malago M, Broelsch CE: Complications of biliary tract in liver transplantation. World J Surg 25:1296-1299, 2001.
58. Kakizoe S, Yanaga K, Starzl TE, et al: Evaluation of protocol before transplantation and after reperfusion biopsies from human orthotopic liver allografts: Considerations of preservation and early immunological injury. Hepatology 11:932-941, 1990.
59. Busquets J, Figueras J, Serrano T, et al. Postreperfusion biopsies are useful in predicting complications after liver transplantation. Liver Transpl 7:432-435, 2001.
60. Sebagh M, Farges O, Kalil A, et al: Sclerosing cholangitis following human orthotopic liver transplantation. Am J Surg Pathol 19:81-90, 1995.
61. Lo CM, Snaked A, Busuttil RW, et al: Risk factors for liver transplantation across the ABO barrier. Transplantation 58:543-547, 1994.
62. Singh N, Chang FY, Gayowski T, et al: Fever in liver transplant recipients in the intensive care unit. Clin Transplant 13:504-511, 1999.
63. Dunham DP, Aran PP: Receiver operating characteristic analysis for biliary complications in liver transplantation. Liver Transpl Surg 3:374-378, 1997.
64. Rosen HR, Martin P, Goss J, et al: Significance of early aminotransferase elevation after liver transplantation. Transplantation 65:68-72, 1998.
65. Holbert BL, Campbell WL, Skolnick ML: Evaluation of the transplanted liver and postoperative complications. Radiol Clin North Am 33:521-540, 1995.
66. Bowen AD, Hungate RG, Kaye RD, et al: Imaging in liver transplantation. Radiol Clin North Am 34:757-778, 1996.
67. Keogan MT, McDermott VG, Price SK, et al: The role of imaging in the diagnosis and management of biliary complications after liver transplantation. AJR Am J Roentgenol 173:215-219, 1999.
68. Kok T, Van der Sluis A, Klein JP, et al: Ultrasound and cholangiography for the diagnosis of biliary complications after orthotopic liver transplantation: A comparative study. J Clin Ultrasound 24:103-115, 1996.
69. Zemel G, Zajko AB, Skolnick ML, et al: The role of sonography and transhepatic cholangiography in the diagnosis of biliary complications after liver transplantation. AJR Am J Roentgenol 151:943-946, 1988.
70. Hussaini SH, Sheridan MB, Davies M: The predictive value of transabdominal ultrasonography in the diagnosis of biliary tract complications after orthotopic liver transplantation. Gut 45:900-903, 1999.

71. Campbell WL, Sheng R, Zajko AB, et al: Intrahepatic biliary strictures after liver transplantation. Radiology 191:735-740, 1994.

72. Colonna JO: Technical problems: Biliary. In Busuttil R, Klintmalm G (eds): Transplantation of the Liver, 1st ed. Philadelphia, WB Saunders; 1996, pp 617-625.

73. McDiarmid SV, Hall TR, Grant EG, et al: Failure of duplex sonography to diagnose hepatic artery thrombosis in a high risk group of pediatric liver transplant recipients. J Pediatr Surg 26:710-713, 1991.

74. Ostroff JW: Posttransplant biliary problems. Gastrointest Endosc Clin N Am 11:163-183, 2001.

75. Ludwig J, Batts KP, MacCarty RL: Ischemic cholangitis in hepatic allografts. Mayo Clin Proc 67:519-526, 1992.

76. Campbell WL, Sheng R, Zajko AB, et al: Intrahepatic biliary strictures after liver transplantation. Radiology 191:735-740, 1994.

77. Keogan MT, McDermott VG, Price SK, et al: The role of imaging in the diagnosis and management of biliary complications after liver transplantation. AJR Am J Roentgenol 173:215-219, 1999.

78. Letourneau JG, Castaneda-Zuniga WR: The role of radiology in the diagnosis and treatment of biliary complications after liver transplantation. Cardiovasc Intervent Radiol 13:278-282, 1990.

79. O'Connor HJ, Vickers CR, Buckels JA, et al: Role of endoscopic retrograde cholangiopancreatography after orthotopic liver transplantation. Gut 32:419-423, 1991.

80. Sherman S, Jamidar P, Shaked A, et al: Biliary tract complications after orthotopic liver transplantation. Endoscopic approach to diagnosis and therapy. Transplantation 60:467-470, 1995.

81. Boraschi P, Braccini G, Gigoni R, et al: Detection of biliary complications after orthotopic liver transplantation with MR cholangiography. Magn Reson Imaging 19:1097-1105, 2001.

82. Eckhoff DE, Baron TH, Blackard WG, et al: Role of ERCP in asymptomatic orthotopic liver transplant patients with abnormal liver enzymes. Am J Gastroenterol 95:141-144, 2000.

83. Shah R, Dooley J, Agarwal R, et al: Routine endoscopic retrograde cholangiography in the detection of early biliary complications after liver transplantation. Liver Transpl 8:491-494, 2002.

84. Quiroga S, Sebastia MC, Margarit C, et al: Complications of orthotopic liver transplantation: Spectrum of findings with helical CT. Radiographics 21:1085-1102, 2001.

85. Cheng YF, Lee TY, Chen CL, et al: Three-dimensional helical computed tomographic cholangiography: Application to living related hepatic transplantation. Clin Transplant 11:209-213, 1997.

86. Dinkel HP, Gassel HJ, Knupffer J, et al: New noninvasive procedure of diagnosing bile leaks: Spiral CT cholangiography. Dtsch Med Wochenschr 124:21-23, 1999.

87. Banzo I, Blanco I, Gutierrez-Mendiguchia C, et al: Hepatobiliary scintigraphy for the diagnosis of bile leaks produced after T-tube removal in orthotopic liver transplantation. Nucl Med Commun 19:229-236, 1998.

88. Kurzawinski TR, Selves L, Farouk M, et al: Prospective study of hepatobiliary scintigraphy and endoscopic cholangiography for the detection of early biliary complications after orthotopic liver transplantation. Br J Surg 84:620-623, 1997.

89. Kim JS, Moon DH, Lee SG, et al: The usefulness of hepatobiliary scintigraphy in the diagnosis of complications after adult-to-adult living donor liver transplantation. Eur J Nucl Med Mol Imaging 29:473-479, 2002.

90. Becker CD, Grossholz M, Mentha G, et al: MR cholangiopancreatography: Technique, potential indications, and diagnostic features of benign, postoperative, and malignant conditions. Eur Radiol 7:865-874, 1997.

91. Reinhold C, Bret PM: Current status of MR cholangiopancreatography. AJR Am J Roentgenol 166:1285-1295, 1996.

92. Soto JA, Barish MA, Yucel EK, et al: MR cholangiopancreatography: Findings on 3D fast spin-echo imaging. AJR Am J Roentgenol 165:1397-1401, 1995.

93. Laor T, Hoffer FA, Vacanti JP, et al: MR cholangiography in children after liver transplantation from living related donors. AJR Am J Roentgenol 170:683-687, 1998.

94. Laghi A, Pavone P, Catalano C, et al: MR cholangiography of late biliary complications after liver transplantation. AJR Am J Roentgenol 172:1541-1546, 1999.

95. Fulcher AS, Turner MA: Orthotopic liver transplantation: Evaluation with MR cholangiography. Radiology 211:715-722, 1999.

96. Meersschaut V, Mortele KJ, Troisi R, et al: Value of MR cholangiography in the evaluation of postoperative biliary complications following orthotopic liver transplantation. Eur Radiol 10:1576-1581, 2000.

97. Norton KI, Lee JS, Kogan D, et al: The role of magnetic resonance cholangiography in the management of children and young adults after liver transplantation. Pediatr Transplant 5:410-418, 2001.

98. Vitellas KM, El-Dieb A, Vaswani K, et al: Detection of bile duct leaks using MR cholangiography with mangafodipir trisodium (Teslascan). J Comput Assist Tomogr 25:102-105, 2000.

99. Ott R, Greess H, Aichinger U, et al: Clinical value of MRC in the follow-up of liver transplant patients with a choledochojejunostomy. Abdom Imaging 27:336-343, 2002.

100. Pariphande PV, Lee VS, Morgan GR, et al: Vascular and extravascular complications of liver transplantation: Comprehensive evaluation with three-dimensional contrast-enhanced volumetric MR imaging and MR cholangiopancreatography. AJR Am J Roentgenol 177:1101-1107, 2001.

101. Sheng R, Sammon JK, Zajko AB, et al: Bile leak after hepatic transplantation: Cholangiographic features, prevalence, and clinical outcome. Radiology 192:413-416, 1994.

102. Stratta RJ, Wood RP, Langnas AN, et al: Diagnosis and treatment of biliary tract complications after orthotopic liver transplantation. Surgery 106:675-684, 1989.

103. Osorio RW, Freise CE, Stock PG, et al: Nonoperative management of biliary leaks after orthotopic liver transplantation. Transplantation 55:1074-1077, 1993.

104. Ostroff JW, Roberts JP, Gordon RL, et al: The management of T-tube leaks in orthotopic liver transplant recipients with endoscopically placed nasobiliary catheters. Transplantation 49:922-924, 1990.

105. Shuhart MC, Kowdley KV, McVicar JP, et al: Predictors of bile leaks after T-tube removal in orthotopic liver transplant recipients. Liver Transpl Surg 4:62-70, 1998.

106. Donovan J: Nonsurgical management of biliary tract disease after liver transplantation. Gastroenterol Clin North Am 22:317-336, 1993.

107. Urbani L, Campatelli A, Romagnoli J, et al: T-tube removal after liver transplantation: A new technique that reduces biliary complications. Transplantation 74:410-413, 2002.

108. Bak T, Wachs M, Trotter J, et al: Adult-to-adult living donor liver transplantation using right lobe grafts: Results and lessons learned from a single-center experience. Liver Transpl 7:680-686, 2001.

109. Sugawara Y, Makuuchi M, Sano K, et al: Duct-to-duct biliary reconstruction in living-related liver transplantation. Transplantation 73:1348-1350, 2002.

110. Esterl RM Jr, St Laurent M, Bay MK, et al: Endoscopic biliary stent migration with small bowel perforation in a liver transplant recipient. J Clin Gastroenterol 24:106-110, 1997.

111. Margarit C, Hidalgo E, Lázaro JL, et al: Biliary complications secondary to late hepatic artery thrombosis in adult liver transplant patients. Transpl Int 11(Suppl 1):S251-S254, 1998.

112. Campbell WL, Foster RG, Miller WJ, et al: Changes in extrahepatic bile duct caliber in liver transplant recipients without evidence of biliary obstruction. AJR Am J Roentgenol 158:997-1000, 1992.

113. Zajko AB, Campbell WL, Logsdon GA, et al: Biliary complications in liver allografts after hepatic artery occlusion: A $6^1/_2$-year study. Transplant Proc 20:607-609, 1988.

114. Orons PD, Sheng R, Zajko AB: Hepatic artery stenosis in liver transplant recipients: Prevalence and cholangiographic appearance of associated biliary complications. AJR Am J Roentgenol 165:1145-1149, 1995.

115. Abbasoglu O, Levy MF, Vodapally MS, et al: Hepatic artery stenosis after liver transplantation—incidence, presentation, treatment, and long-term outcome. Transplantation 63:250-255, 1997.

116. Rizk RS, McVicar JP, Edmond MJ, et al: Endoscopic management of biliary strictures in liver transplant recipients: Effect on patient and graft survival. Gastrointest Endosc 47:128-135, 1998.

117. Imamura I, Makuuchi M, Sakamoto Y, et al: Anatomical keys and pitfalls in living donor liver transplantation. J Hepatobiliary Pancreat Surg 7:380-394, 2000.

118. Deshpande RR, Heaton ND, Rela M: Surgical anatomy of segmental liver transplantation. Br J Surg 89:1078-1088, 2002.

119. Northover J, Terblanche J: Bile duct blood supply. Its importance in human liver transplantation. Transplantation 26:67-69, 1978.

120. Sanchez-Urdazpal L, Batts KP, Gores GJ, et al: Diagnostic features and clinical outcome of ischemic-type biliary complications after liver transplantation. Hepatology 17:605-609, 1993.

121. Theilmann L, Küppers B, Kadmon M, et al: Biliary tract strictures after orthotopic liver transplantation: Diagnosis and management. Endoscopy 26:517-522, 1994.

122. Fisher A, Miller CM: Ischemic-type biliary strictures in liver allografts: The Achilles heel revisited? Hepatology 21:589-591, 1995.

123. Schlitt HJ, Meier PN, Nashan B, et al: Reconstructive surgery for ischemic-type lesions at the bile duct bifurcation after liver transplantation. Ann Surg 229:137-145, 1999.

124. Sebagh M, Farges O, Kalil A, et al: Sclerosing cholangitis following human orthotopic liver transplantation. Am J Surg 19:81-90, 1995.

125. Hintze RE, Adler A, Veltzke W, et al: Endoscopic management of biliary complications after orthotopic liver transplantation. Hepatogastroenterology 44:258-262, 1997.

126. Moreno-Gonzalez E, Alvarado A, Gomez R, et al: Cold ischemia time and biliary complications in liver transplantation. Transplant Proc 26:3546, 1994.

127. Mor E, Schwartz ME, Sheiner PA, et al: Prolonged preservation in University of Wisconsin solution associated with hepatic artery thrombosis after orthotopic liver transplantation. Transplantation 56:1399-1402, 1993.

128. Li S, Stratta RJ, Langnas AN, et al: Diffuse biliary tract injury after orthotopic liver transplantation. Am J Surg 164:536-540, 1992.

129. Sankary HN, McChesney L, Frye E, et al: A simple modification in operative technique can reduce the incidence of nonanastomotic biliary strictures after orthotopic liver transplantation. Hepatology 21:63-69, 1995.

130. Scotte M, Dousset B, Calmus Y, et al: The influence of cold ischemia time on biliary complications following liver transplantation. J Hepatol 21:340-346, 1994.

131. Moench C, Moench K, Lohse AW, et al: Prevention of ischemic-type biliary lesions by arterial back-table pressure perfusion. Liver Transpl 9:285-289, 2003.

132. Sanchez-Urdazpal L, Batts KP, Gores GJ, et al: Increased bile duct complications in liver transplantations across the ABO barrier. Ann Surg 218:152-158, 1993.

133. Oguma S, Belle S, Starzl TE, et al: A histometric analysis of chronically rejected human liver allografts: Insights into mechanisms of bile duct loss: Direct and indirect immunological factors. Hepatology 9:204-209, 1989.

134. Ludwig J, Wiesner RH, Batts KP, et al: Acute vanishing bile duct syndrome (acute irreversible rejection) after orthotopic liver transplantation. Hepatology 7:476-483, 1987.

135. Lo CM, Shaked A, Busuttil RW: Risk factors for liver transplantation across the ABO barrier. Transplantation 58:543-547, 1994.

136. Waldman WJ, Knight DA, Adams PW: In vitro induction of endothelial HLA class II antigen expression by cytomegalovirus activated CD4+ T-cells. Transplantation 56:1504-1512, 1993.

137. Graziadei IW: Recurrence of primary sclerosing cholangitis after liver transplantation. Liver Transpl 8:575-581, 2002.

138. Graziadei IW, Wiesner RH, Marottta PJ, et al: Long-term results of patients undergoing liver transplantation for primary sclerosing cholangitis. Hepatology 30:1121-1127, 1999.

139. Goss JA, Shackleton CR, Farmer DG, et al: Orthotopic liver transplantation for primary sclerosing cholangitis. A 12-year single center experience. Ann Surg 225:472-483, 1997.

140. Stieber AC, Ambrosino G, Kahn D, et al: An unusual complication of choledochocholedochostomy in orthotopic liver transplantation. Transplant Proc 20:619-621, 1988.

141. Clavien PA, Camargo CA, Bailile L, et al: Sphincter of Oddi dysfunction after liver transplantation. Dig Dis Sci 40:73-74, 1995.

142. Thune A, Friman S, Persson H, et al: Raised pressure in the bile ducts after orthotopic liver transplantation. Transpl Int 7:243-246, 1994.

143. Douzdjian V, Abecassis MM, Johlin FC: Sphincter of Oddi dysfunction following liver transplantation. Dig Dis Sci 39:253-256, 1994.

144. Starzl TE, Putnam CW, Hansbrough JF, et al: Biliary complications after liver transplantation: With special reference to the biliary cast syndrome and techniques of secondary duct repair. Surgery 81:212-221, 1997.

145. Sheng R, Ramirez CB, Zajko AB, et al: Biliary stones and sludge in liver transplant patients: A 13-year experience. Radiology 198:243-247, 1996.

146. Waldram R, Williams R, Calne RY: Bile composition and bile cast formation after transplantation of the liver in man. Transplantation 19:382-387, 1975.

147. Farouk M, Branum GD, Walters CR, et al: Bile compositional changes and cholesterol stone formation following orthotopic liver transplantation. Transplantation 52:727-730, 1991.

148. Rotolo FS, Branum GD, Bowers BA, et al: Effect of cyclosporine on bile secretion in rats. Am J Surg 151:35-40, 1986.

149. Le Thai B, Dumont M, Michel A, et al: Cholestatic effect of cyclosporine in the rat. Transplantation 46:510-512, 1988.

150. Cao S, Cox K, So SSK, et al: Potential effect of cyclosporin A in formation of cholesterol gallstones in pediatric liver transplant recipients. Dig Dis Sci 42:1409-1415, 1997.

151. Ostroff JW: Post-transplant biliary problems. Gastrointest Endosc Clin N Am 11:163-183, 2001.

152. Manzarbeitia C, Jonsson J, Rustgi V, et al: Management of hemobilia after liver biopsy in liver transplant recipients. Transplantation 56:1545-1547, 1993.

153. Pitre J, Dousset B, Massault P, et al: Multiple intrahepatic stones caused by hemobilia in liver transplant recipients. Surgery 121:352-354, 1997.

154. Lang M, Neumann U, Mueller AR, et al: Complications of percutaneous liver biopsy in patients after liver transplantation. Z Gastroenterol 37:205-208, 1999.

155. Pfau PR, Kochman ML, Lewis JD, et al: Endoscopic management of postoperative biliary complications in orthotopic liver transplantation. Gastrointest Endosc 52:55-63, 2000.

156. Gomez R, Moreno E, Castellon C, et al: Choledochocholedochostomy conversion to hepaticojejunostomy due to biliary obstruction in liver transplantation. World J Surg 25:1308-1312, 2001.

157. Johnston TD, Gates R, Reddy KS, et al: Nonoperative management of bile leaks following liver transplantation. Clin Transplant 14:365-369, 2000.

158. Wolfsen HC, Porayko MK, Hughes RH, et al: Role of endoscopic retrograde cholangiopancreatography after orthotopic liver transplantation. Am J Gastroenterol 87:955-960, 1992.

159. Bourgeois N, Deviere J, Yeaton P, et al: Diagnostic and therapeutic endoscopic retrograde cholangiography after liver transplantation. Gastrointest Endosc 42:527-534, 1995.

160. Sherman S, Shaked A, Cryer HM, et al: Endoscopic management of biliary fistulas complicating liver transplantation and other hepatobiliary operations. Ann Surg 218:167-175, 1993.

161. Saab S, Martin P, Soliman GY, et al: Endoscopic management of biliary leaks after T-tube removal in liver transplant recipients: Nasobiliary drainage versus biliary stenting. Liver Transpl 6:627-632, 2000.

162. Catalano MF, Van Dam J, Sivak MV Jr: Endoscopic retrograde cholangiopancreatography in the orthotopic liver transplant patient. Endoscopy 27:584-588, 1995.

163. Clark J, Uzer M: Endoscopic stent placement in the treatment of bile leaks occurring after orthotopic liver transplantation [abstract]. Gastroenterology 108:A412, 1995.

164. Johnston TD, Gates R, Reddy KS, et al: Nonoperative management of bile leaks following liver transplantation. Clin Transplant 14:365-369, 2000.

165. Kaplan SB, Zajko AB, Koneru B: Hepatic bilomas due to hepatic artery thrombosis in liver transplant recipients: Percutaneous drainage and clinical outcome. Radiology 174:1031-1035, 1990.

166. Mosca S, Guiseppe M, Guardascione MA, et al: Late biliary tract complications after orthotopic liver transplantation: Diagnostic and therapeutic role of endoscopic retrograde cholangiopancreatography. J Gastroenterol Hepatol 15:654-660, 2000.

167. Rossi AF, Grosso C, Zanasi G, et al: Long-term efficacy of endoscopic stenting in patients with stricture of the biliary anastomosis after orthotopic liver transplantation. Endoscopy 30:360-366, 1998.

168. Schwartz DA, Pettersen BT, Poterucha JJ, et al: Endoscopic therapy of anastomotic bile duct strictures occurring after liver transplantation. Gastrointest Endosc 51:169-174, 2000.

169. Mahajani RV, Cotler SJ, Uzer MF: Efficacy of endoscopic management of anastomotic biliary strictures after liver transplantation. Endoscopy 32:943-949, 2000.

170. Lake JR: Long-term management of biliary tract complications. Liver Transpl Surg 1:45-54, 1995.

171. Petersen BD, Maxfield SR, Ivancev K, et al: Biliary strictures in hepatic transplantation: Treatment with self-expanding Z stents. J Vasc Interv Radiol 7:221-228, 1996.

172. Ward EM, Kiely MJ, Maus TP, et al: Hilar biliary strictures after liver transplantation: Cholangiography and percutaneous treatment. Radiology 177:259-263, 1990.

173. Starzl TE, Putnam CW, Hansbrough JF, et al: Biliary complications after liver transplantation with special reference to the biliary cast syndrome and techniques of secondary duct repair. Surgery 81:212-221, 1977.

174. Kuo PC, Lewis WD, Stokes K, et al: A comparison of operation, endoscopic retrograde cholangiopancreatography, and percutaneous transhepatic cholangiography in biliary complications after hepatic transplantation. J Am Coll Surg 179:177-181, 1994.

175. Barton P, Steininger R, Maier A, et al: Biliary sludge after liver transplantation: 2. Treatment with interventional techniques versus surgery and/or oral chemolysis. AJR Am J Roentgenol 164:865-869, 1995.

176. Langnas AN, Stratta RJ, Wood RP, et al: The role of intrahepatic cholangiojejunostomy in liver transplant recipients after extensive destruction of the extrahepatic biliary system. Surgery 112:712-718, 1992.

177. Douzdjian V, Abecassis MM, Johlin FC: Sphincter of Oddi dysfunction following liver transplantation. Dig Dis Sci 39:253-256, 1994.

178. Rayes N, Seehofer D, Hansen S, et al: Early enteral supply of lactobacillus and fiber versus selective bowel decontamination: A controlled trial in liver transplant recipients. Transplantation 74:123-127, 2002.

179. Makuuchi M, Kawasaki S, Noguchi T, et al: Donor hepatectomy for living related partial liver transplantation. Surgery 113:395-402, 1993.

Arterial Complications After Liver Transplantation

SHERILYN A. GORDON
IAN C. CARMODY

Arcuate ligament syndrome   953

Steal syndrome   954

Hepatic artery thrombosis   954
  Clinical features   955
  Diagnosis   955
  Management   956
  Recurrent hepatic artery thrombosis   957

Pediatric hepatic artery thrombosis   957
  Risk factors   957
  Prevention   957

Hepatic artery stenosis   958

Hepatic artery pseudoaneurysms   958

Hepatic artery rupture   959

Conclusion   959

Despite refinements in surgical technique and immunosuppression, arterial complications continue to be a major source of morbidity and mortality after orthotopic liver transplantation (OLT). Although the liver allograft maintains a dual blood supply, arterial reconstruction is frequently accomplished by ligation of the recipient collateral circulation, including the gastroduodenal artery, which renders the celiac trunk the sole arterial blood supply to the transplanted liver. This process presents a unique opportunity for pathological clinical entities such as arcuate ligament syndrome, steal syndrome, hepatic artery thrombosis and stenosis, hepatic artery pseudoaneurysm, and hepatic artery rupture to arise and compromise graft viability and patient survival. Early diagnosis with prompt intervention is mandatory; frequently, urgent or emergency retransplantation is required. The authors of preceding chapters have reviewed pertinent arterial anatomy; in this chapter we focus on diagnosis and treatment of these conditions.

Arcuate Ligament Syndrome

The median arcuate ligament is formed by fusion of the diaphragmatic crura on either side of the aortic hiatus posterior to the origin of the celiac axis. During embryogenesis, the celiac trunk migrates caudally, thereby resulting in a variable origin from the level of

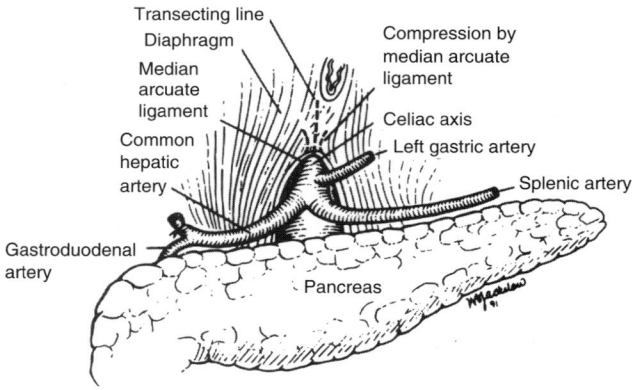

FIGURE 63-1

Arcuate ligament syndrome. The origin of the celiac axis is compressed by the median arcuate ligament. Compression is released by transecting the ligament. (From Fukuzawa K, Schwartz ME, Katz E, et al: The arcuate ligament syndrome in liver transplantation. Transplantation 56:223-224, 1993. © 1993, The Williams & Wilkins Company, Baltimore.)

the 11th thoracic vertebra to the 1st lumbar vertebra. Consequently, a high celiac axis takeoff relative to the median arcuate ligament may result in arterial compression (Fig. 63–1).[1,2] Szilagyi and colleagues[3] and Lindner and Kemprud[4] have demonstrated a variable degree of celiac axis compression in 10% to 50% of patients during deep expiration; this compression has been noted to be accompanied by compensation of hepatic artery blood via retrograde flow through the pancreaticoduodenal system.[5]

Hepatic arterial reconstruction with ligation of collateral flow, which is required for OLT, presents an opportunity to study the relationship of the median arcuate ligament and hepatic artery circulation. Arcuate ligament syndrome in association with OLT was reported simultaneously by the University of California at Los Angeles and Mount Sinai transplant centers in 1993.[1,2] The incidence varied from 1.6% to 10%. Intraoperative measurement of donor hepatic arterial blood flow demonstrated a spectrum ranging from significant reduction to complete disruption of flow during the expiratory phase of the respiratory cycle. Restoration of normal flow was obtained by dividing the muscular and fibrous tissue bands on the superior aspect of the supraceliac aorta. When arcuate ligament release did not appear to achieve a satisfactory effect, aortoceliac grafting was used for reconstruction. In neither series was hepatic artery thrombosis or stenosis diagnosed postoperatively.

Despite these favorable results, the clinical significance of this anatomic phenomenon remains controversial. In addition to surgical division of the median arcuate ligament or reconstruction via aortoceliac grafting, retrograde trans-splenic celiac dilation has been attempted by several authors,[6] with varying degrees of success.

Steal Syndrome

First described by Manner and coauthors in reporting hepatic allograft hypoperfusion in two transplant recipients with visceral anatomic abnormalities,[7] arterial steal syndrome is an entity now used to characterize a marked diversion of blood flow from the hepatic allograft to the often enlarged, hyperperfused spleen via the splenic artery. The result is hepatic hypoperfusion with an attendant clinical manifestation of elevated liver function enzymes, allograft dysfunction, and cholestasis.

The incidence of steal syndrome is 3% to 5%[8,9]; if left untreated, it represents a significant potential risk for postoperative morbidity and graft loss. Although duplex Doppler ultrasonography and angiography are effective in making the diagnosis postoperatively, a high level of suspicion should be maintained intraoperatively at the time of OLT to ensure the best chance for good patient and graft outcome. Intraoperative Doppler is useful in confirming the diagnosis. Therapeutic operative maneuvers include splenectomy or splenic artery or gastroduodenal artery ligation. If the diagnosis is made postoperatively and the patient's symptoms are mild, some authors advocate a percutaneous approach with coiling or banding of the splenic artery under fluoroscopic guidance.[8] A worrisome complication of this approach is misdirection of the catheter with inadvertent thrombosis of the hepatic artery. If the patient's symptoms are advanced, urgent exploration is warranted so that the allograft can be evaluated. Splenectomy or splenic artery ligation can be accomplished at this time.

With early diagnosis and remediation, patient and graft outcomes are excellent; however, without intervention, the recipient remains at high risk for ischemic biliary complications, including cholangitis, sepsis, and ultimately, graft loss.

Hepatic Artery Thrombosis

Hepatic artery thrombosis (HAT) is the most common vascular complication after OLT[10,11] and the most common technical complication requiring retransplantation.[12] The impact of dearterialization of the liver allograft was first emphasized in a 1985 review of 309 OLT recipients by Tzakis and associates.[13] They noted a 7% incidence of HAT with an overall mortality of 50%. Of those 50%, nearly a third (27.3%) expired even after definitive therapy with retransplantation was instituted. The incidence of HAT and, to a lesser degree, the morbidity and mortality attributable to HAT have decreased in recent years. Contemporary reviews demonstrate the incidence to be 1.6% to 4% in adult recipients[14,15] and 12% to 30% in pediatric recipients.[16,17] Depending on the interval after OLT, symptoms at initial evaluation, and the mode of therapy, mortality rates now range from 11%[18] to 35%[19] for adults. Unfortunately, HAT still carries an overall mortality of nearly 40% in the pediatric population.[17] Reasons for the relative decrease in the incidence of HAT and improvement in outcomes are multifactorial. Of significance are improved microvascular technique, optimization of postoperative anticoagulation, refinement in radiological modalities allowing for expeditious diagnosis, and increasingly effective antibiotic therapy. Notwithstanding these improvements, significant morbidity and mortality from HAT after OLT persist.

Clinical Features

Acute, subacute, or chronic symptoms develop in patients with HAT, with the type of symptoms generally dependent on the time interval between OLT and the development of HAT (Table 63–1). To facilitate a comparison of patient populations and risk for morbidity and mortality between centers, many authors broadly classify HAT into one of two categories: early or late (delayed). The exact definition depends on the author. Although many investigators have defined late HAT as that occurring after 4 weeks, others use 6 months as a time point to delineate the two.[14,20] For the purposes of this discussion, HAT occurring more than 4 weeks after OLT is classified as late.

The most dramatic manifestation is fulminant hepatic ischemic necrosis, which occurs in 33% of patients with HAT.[15] Patients often demonstrate rapid onset of hepatic decompensation with sepsis, fever, altered mental status, hypotension, and coagulopathy. Laboratory values are significant for transaminitis, leukocytosis, and altered coagulation profile. Blood cultures may show multiple enteric organisms, and radiographs may demonstrate gas within the liver parenchyma (Fig. 63–2).

Another 33% of patients present subacutely either in the early or late period with progressive symptoms related to ischemic bile duct injury. Although adequate

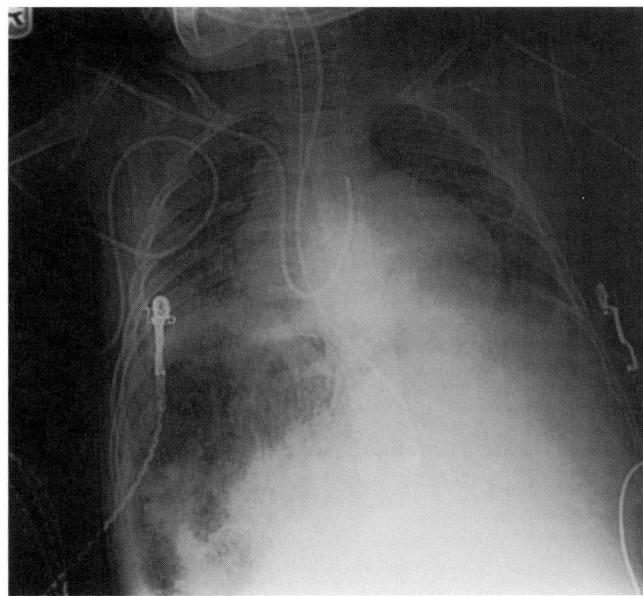

FIGURE 63–2

Gas gangrene of the liver. The patient had signs of hepatic decompensation, along with fever and hypotension.

vascular collateralization may have occurred to prevent extensive hepatocyte necrosis, it has been demonstrated that collateralization may be insufficient to prevent ischemic bile duct injury.[21] Interruption of the singular blood supply to the biliary anastomosis may be manifested as transaminitis, leukocytosis, cholangitis, or sepsis syndrome with microscopic or macroscopic hepatic abscesses seen pathologically or radiographically. Symptoms may progress from an initial period of indolent postoperative fever of unknown origin to relapsing bacteremia, acute cholangitis, and subsequently, intrahepatic biliary necrosis.

The remaining third of HAT patients may remain mildly symptomatic or asymptomatic. The diagnosis is usually made serendipitously while evaluating the patient for an unrelated condition or for transient mild transaminitis to rule out problems such as acute cellular rejection, hepatitis, or recurrence of primary disease. The significance of the lack of (specific) symptoms is unclear; however, serious morbidity may develop over time if HAT is left untreated.

Diagnosis

Although the diagnosis of HAT is often suspected postoperatively, only through imaging studies or operative exploration, or both, can the diagnosis be confirmed. Most centers use duplex Doppler examination for screening purposes. It is difficult to ascertain the accuracy of ultrasound for HAT because not every patient is subjected to the test with the highest

Table 63-1. FEATURES OF HEPATIC ARTERY THROMBOSIS

Early	Late
Fulminant hepatic necrosis	Fever
Transaminitis	Transaminitis
Biliary stricture	Relapsing bacteremia
Primary nonfunction	Cholangitis
Fever	Bile leak
	Hepatic abscess
	Failure to thrive
	Asymptomatic

sensitivity—operative exploration. Factors such as operator dependency and collateralization with a consequent reduction in the resistive index decrease the sensitivity (60% to 90%) and specificity (64% to 97%) of this examination.[22,23] Moreover, routine protocol ultrasound has not been definitively found to reduce the incidence of HAT or shorten the time to diagnosis,[24] although anecdotally some cases have been diagnosed early in asymptomatic patients. The radiographic gold standard for the diagnosis of HAT is selective celiac angiography. With the recent availability of multiphase, multislice, computed tomography (CT) angiography with multidetector reconstruction at certain institutions, the sensitivity of this examination approaches that of conventional angiography (Fig. 63–3).[25] Decreased invasiveness and contrast injection result in fewer vascular and renal complications when compared with angiography. Finally, gadolinium-enhanced magnetic resonance angiography (MRA) is an increasingly more often used noninvasive option for patients capable of breath holding. Sadick and colleagues report 95% concordance between MRA and operative findings in patients suspected of having mesenteric vascular disease.[26]

Management

Operative

Treatment of HAT is dependent on the clinical status of the patient. There are three subsets of HAT patients who have been demonstrated to benefit from operative management.

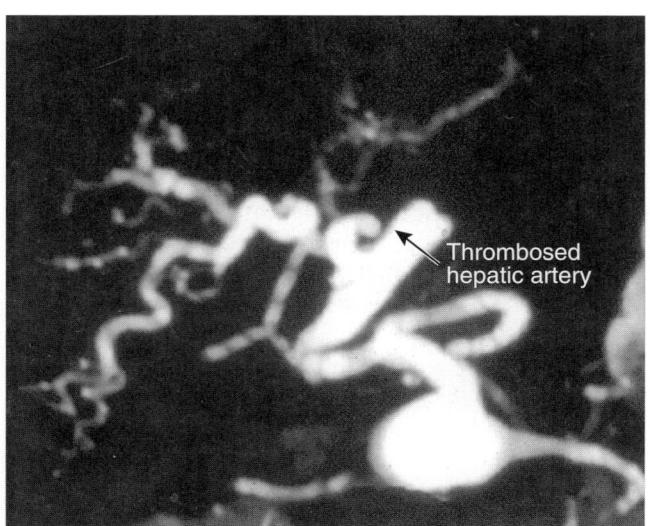

FIGURE 63–3

Reconstructed computed tomographic angiogram demonstrating hepatic artery thrombus in an orthotopic liver transplant recipient.

Patients in fulminant hepatic failure with early HAT require resuscitation, broad-spectrum antibiotics, and expeditious retransplantation. In the United States, acute HAT within the first week after OLT is an absolute indication for relisting a recipient as a status 1 candidate. In cases in which a recipient is rapidly decompensating and a replacement graft is not immediately available, anhepatic maneuvers such as allograft hepatectomy with supportive venovenous bypass or end-to-side portacaval shunting with preservation of the retrohepatic inferior vena cava[14,15] have been applied at our center with success.

The metabolic demands of a patient in fulminant liver failure as a result of HAT mandates that the choice of replacement graft be maximally optimized. Reduced-size and extended criteria grafts should be used judiciously to minimize potential morbidity and maximize survival.

Recipients with early HAT who are asymptomatic or mildly symptomatic are candidates for graft salvage with operative exploration and arterial reconstruction. The choice of technique for hepatic arterial revascularization is critical. If inflow from the recipient celiac axis is adequate, thrombectomy with revision of the offending segment, whether it is the hepatic artery anastomosis or reconstructed, replaced graft vasculature, is an option. Revision may require adhesiolysis and foreshortening of a segment of donor artery to prevent kinking and recurrent HAT. If celiac inflow is inadequate, our preference is to use the supraceliac aorta. In adults, a primary end-to-side anastomosis or interposition iliac artery graft is used. In infants, an interposition graft is necessary. The exploration is not complete until the surgeon is satisfied with the arterial Doppler signal and the adequacy of venous outflow. Consideration may be given to resecting ischemic or necrotic portions of the graft. In addition, we routinely perform biopsy on grossly normal liver.

Patients in whom late HAT develops but who have biliary sepsis as a consequence are also best served by retransplantation. Nonoperative techniques address the vascular complication but do not reverse the potentially lethal infectious complications seen in these recipients. These patients may require percutaneous abscess drainage or even partial hepatectomy as a temporizing measure to control ischemic necrosis and biliary sepsis while awaiting retransplantation.

The use of thrombolytic agents at the time of thrombectomy, with or without continuous hepatic artery infusion postoperatively, has been described; however, there are insufficient data to allow evaluation of its efficacy.[19]

Nonoperative

Few authors advocate wide application of nonoperative management of minimally symptomatic HAT lesions, whether early or late. As the shortage of deceased donor organs persists, however, nonoperative management in appropriate candidates may have to be given added consideration.

Catheter-directed thrombolysis with or without angioplasty or stenting (or both) by an experienced interventional radiologist in lieu of surgery has been effective in some patients with HAT and minimal symptoms. Acute and intermediate lesions have the best response rate. Chronic lesions have been demonstrated to exhibit an initial response; however, long-term patency rates are suboptimal.[27]

Many centers offering nonoperative therapy administer lytic agents such as tissue plasminogen activator via a celiac artery catheter left in situ for approximately 48 hours. A repeat angiogram to ensure patency is often performed before catheter removal. The patient then receives systemic anticoagulation such as intravenous heparin or low-molecular-weight dextran throughout the hospitalization. The duration and dose of systemic anticoagulation are dependent on the patient's propensity for the development of recurrent HAT. Life-threatening intraprocedure or postprocedure hemorrhage remains a significant complication of the thrombolytic approach.

It is of interest to note that the recent development of stents capable of continuous delivery of local antithrombotic or antiproliferative gene therapy may result in increased efficacy and durability of nonoperative HAT management in the future.

Finally, expectant management based on the development of symptoms is proposed for select cases of silent late HAT in which it is presumed that neovascularization has provided arterial inflow and obviates the need for urgent intervention.[25]

Recurrent Hepatic Artery Thrombosis

The outcome after surgery for HAT and the propensity for recurrence depend on the time span before diagnosis, the age of the patient, and the cause of the thrombosis. In a small series reported by Vivarelli and coauthors, recurrent HAT developed at an incidence of 17%.[28] Experience has shown that its occurrence mandates an evaluation for nontechnical causes of HAT such as inherited or acquired hypercoagulable disorders or immunologically mediated or infectious thrombi (or both) before embarking on a third transplant.

Pediatric Hepatic Artery Thrombosis

Because of the increased incidence of HAT, the pediatric population deserves special mention. As previously stated, graft and patient salvage is more likely

in adults than in children. Indeed, Tan and associates report that HAT is the leading cause of death in pediatric recipients in the postcyclosporine era.[17] They also note an increased risk in recipients younger than 3 years or those weighing less than 15 kg, as well as with livers obtained from donors weighing less than 15 kg. Similarly, Langnas and colleagues reported a higher risk in recipients weighing less than 10 kg.[11] Ciciarelli and coworkers reported nine cases of HAT in a cohort of 73 recipients all younger than 12 months, thus reiterating that HAT is the most frequent obstacle to a successful outcome after pediatric OLT.[29] It is thought that pediatric recipients are candidates at high risk for HAT because of small-caliber hepatic arteries—Mazzaferro and associates suggest that 3 mm or less represents a significant threshold for an increased incidence of HAT.[30] In addition, pediatric patients demonstrate greater fluctuations in hematocrit postoperatively than adults do, as well as higher concentrations of coagulation factors such as protein C.[16,31] For these reasons, continuous intravenous heparin is encouraged in the postoperative management of these patients.

Risk Factors

Although several risk factors for the development of HAT have been identified, in the majority of cases, the cause of HAT has not been definitively determined at the time of reoperation. The impact of mechanical risk factors has been better delineated than that of medical factors; the effects of the latter group remain controversial and more difficult to demonstrate (Table 63–2).

Prevention

Based on the known risk factors noted in Table 63–2, recommendations for adherence to the following techniques aimed at prevention of HAT can be made, particularly for high-risk recipients. Of utmost significance is that the surgeons be cognizant of donor and recipient anatomy to avoid vascular injury. In addition, one should ensure (1) gentle handling of vessels at procurement with the minimal number of anastomoses should reconstruction be necessary,[30] (2) early dissection and isolation of the recipient hepatic artery at recipient hepatectomy with the use of the branch patch technique at the junction of the gastroduodenal and common hepatic arteries for anastamosis,[33] (3) appropriate size matching of vessels, and (4) avoidance of intimal injury, particularly when extraction of thrombus is required. Revision of arterial anastomoses in cases of excessive length and kinking, as well as the use of conduit, should be done only when absolutely necessary.[30]

Table 63-2. RISK FACTORS FOR HEPATIC ARTERY THROMBOSIS

Technical	Medical
HA < 3 mm[30]	Previous HAT
Recipient < 10 kg[32]	Polycythemia/acquired or inherited hyper-coagulable state[11,35]
HA anastomosis other than common HA/branch patch technique[33]	ABO incompatibility[36]
Multiple anastomotic attempts[34]	Multiple ACR episodes[37]
Anomalous HA anatomy (donor or recipient) with reconstruction[34]	CMV infection[38]
HA angulation	Hypotension/vasopressor requirement
Intimal flap	Increased CIT[39]
Aggressive HA clamping	Intra-abdominal infection
	PNF[40]

ACR, acute cellular rejection; CIT, cold ischemia time; CMV, cytomegalovirus; HA, hepatic artery; PNF, primary nonfunction.

Finally, the surgeon should take care to minimize the intraoperative and postoperative administration of blood products[30] and avoid antifibrinolytic agents such as aminocaproic acid and aprotinin[41] when possible. The use of systemic anticoagulation has been demonstrated to be of particular benefit in the pediatric population as discussed earlier. Of note, in reference to maximizing microvascular technique, the Kyoto group has reported no cases of HAT with the use of 10× to 20× operating microscopes instead of surgical loupes.[42]

In conclusion, early diagnosis of HAT is essential for acceptable graft and patient survival. A high level of suspicion based on known risk factors is necessary to make a timely diagnosis because prompt retransplantation, particularly in decompensated recipients, is required to avoid mortality. Overall, 50% to 75% of these patients will require retransplantation (Fig. 63-4).[1,10] Meticulous surgical technique and attention to the nontechnical factors contributing to HAT help minimize the morbidity and mortality associated with this complication.

Hepatic Artery Stenosis

Stenosis of the hepatic artery after OLT usually occurs at the anastomosis and may result from operative trauma, anastomotic narrowing, increased resistance to hepatic artery blood flow during rejection,[43] or microvascular injury associated with cold preservation.

The incidence is difficult to ascertain in that many cases are thought to progress to complete HAT by the time that clinical symptoms warrant evaluation. Early clinical manifestations may include an insidious form of biliary dysfunction or graft failure related to diminution in hepatic blood flow progressing to cholangitis and ischemic infarcts.

The diagnosis can be made noninvasively via duplex Doppler. Calculation of resistive indices ([peak systolic flow − end diastolic flow]/peak systolic flow) and systolic acceleration time and the use of electromagnetic blood flow measurement are modalities available to assist in determining the precise rate of blood flow. Anastomoses with blood flow less than 200 mL/min mandate revision. As with HAT, the celiac angiogram remains the diagnostic gold standard.

Treatment options include operative revision of the stenotic hepatic artery (an option best suited for patients with advanced symptoms or long-segment lesions) or interventionally guided techniques, including balloon angioplasty. Mondragon and Raby and their colleagues independently reported a series of seven and three patients, respectively, whose angiographically confirmed stenotic lesions were treated by angioplasty. Patients without advanced symptoms (five of seven and three of three) at the time of intervention responded to percutaneous therapy with improvement in graft function and did not require operative intervention.[43,44]

The goal of therapy is to prevent progression to complete occlusion as a result of diminished blood flow and consequently avert associated ischemic biliary strictures and allograft loss.

Hepatic Artery Pseudoaneurysms

Pseudoaneurysms are rarely reported after OLT, and thus their incidence is difficult to determine.[45] They may be a result of traumatic or infectious processes.

Patients may present with gastrointestinal bleeding, hemobilia, or both conditions. Diagnosis requires a high index of suspicion and can be achieved with duplex Doppler or CT; however, as Tobben and colleagues note in their review of 11 post-OLT patients with pseudoaneurysm, angiography provides the sensitivity and specificity necessary for definitive diagnosis.[46]

Treatment options are limited: deliberate hepatic artery ligation with its high potential for graft ischemia and biliary complications offers the only chance for avoiding the complication of hepatic artery rupture (HAR) with potentially fatal hemorrhage. Immediate grafting plus revascularization reconstitutes the blood

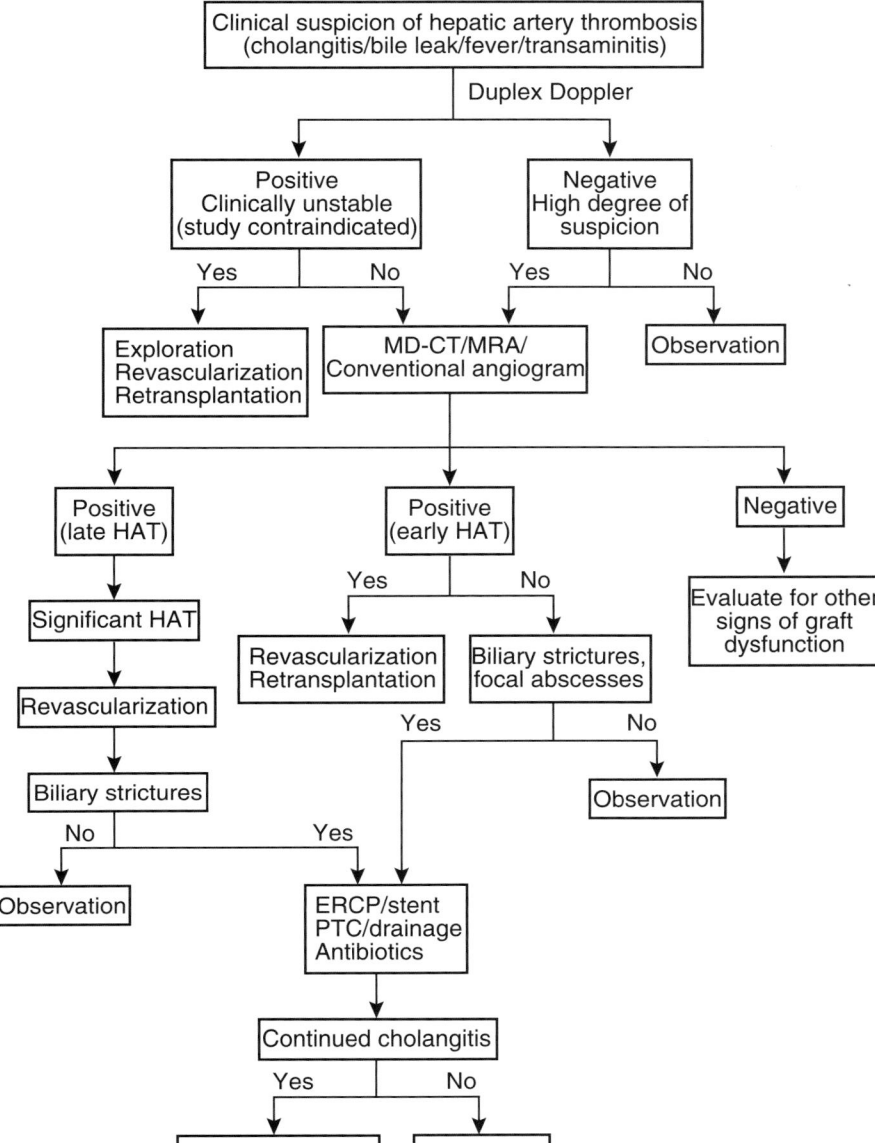

FIGURE 63–4

Algorithm for the diagnosis and treatment of early and late hepatic artery thrombosis (HAT). ERCP, endoscopic retrograde cholangiopancreatography; MD-CT, multidetector computed tomography; MRA, magnetic resonance angiography; PTC, percutaneous transhepatic cholangiography.

supply, but it also maintains the risk of infectious vascular rupture if the aneurysm is mycotic in nature.

Hepatic Artery Rupture

Also an infrequently reported but lethal complication, HAR is thought to result from a combination of technical failure and infection. The typical manifestation is that of septic shock. As noted by Langnas and coworkers, the origin of HAR-associated infections is probably direct intraperitoneal contamination; 75% of patients monitored for HAR in their review underwent choledochojejunostomy at the time of OLT.[11] Therapy consists of resuscitation, broad-spectrum antibiotics, and expeditious operative exploration. Surgical options again include ligation or reconstruction of the hepatic arterial supply with the use of an uninfected donor or recipient vessel (or both).[11,33]

Conclusion

Arterial complications after OLT remain a formidable challenge because of the high risk of subsequent graft loss and patient morbidity and mortality. Diagnosis and management of the chief complications—arcuate ligament syndrome, steal syndrome, HAT, hepatic artery stenosis, pseudoaneurysm, and HAR—require that clinicians be familiar with the risk factors, symptoms, diagnostic modalities, and treatment options available to treat patients in the urgent or emergency fashion that they often require.

References

1. Jurim O, Shaked A, Kiai K, et al: Celiac compression syndrome and liver transplantation. Ann Surg 218:10-12, 1993.
2. Fukuzawa K, Schwartz ME, Katz E, et al: The arcuate ligament syndrome in liver transplantation. Transplantation 56:223-224, 1993.
3. Szilagyi DE, Rian RL, Elliot JP, et al: The celiac artery compression syndrome: Does it exist? Surgery 72:849-863, 1972.
4. Lindner HH, Kemprud E: A clinicoanatomic study of the arcuate ligament of the diaphragm. Arch Surg 103:600-605, 1971.
5. Reuter SR: Accentuation of celiac compression by the median arcuate ligament of the diaphragm during deep expiration. Radiology 98:561-564, 1971.
6. Stoney RJ, Lusby RJ: Surgery of celiac and mesenteric arteries. In Hainovici H (ed): Vascular Surgery Principles and Techniques. New York, Appleton, 1984, pp 813-825.
7. Manner M, Otto G, Senninger N, et al: Arterial steal: An unusual case for hepatic hypoperfusion after liver transplantation. Transpl Int 4:122-124, 1991.
8. Nussler N, Settnacher U, Haase R: Diagnosis and treatment of arterial steal syndromes in liver transplant recipients. Liver Transpl 9:596-202, 2003.
9. Geissler I, Lamesch P, Witzigmann H, et al: Splenohepatic arterial steal syndrome in liver transplantation: Clinical features and management. Transpl Int 15:139-141, 2002.
10. Wozney P, Zajko AB, Bron KM, et al: Vascular complications after liver transplantation: A 5-year experience. AJR Am J Roentgenol 147:657-663, 1986.
11. Langnas A, Marujo W, Stratta R, et al: Vascular complications after orthotopic liver transplantation. Am J Surg 161:76-83, 1991.
12. Yanaga K, Lebeau G, Marsh W, et al: Hepatic artery reconstruction for hepatic artery thrombosis after orthotopic liver transplantation. Arch Surg 125:628-631, 1990.
13. Tzakis AG, Gordon RD, Shaw BW, et al: Clinical presentation of hepatic artery thrombosis after liver transplantation in the cyclosporine era. Transplantation 40:667-671, 1985.
14. Drazan K, Shaked A, Olthoff KM, et al: Etiology and management of symptomatic adult hepatic artery thrombosis after orthotopic liver transplantation. Am Surg 62:237-240, 1996.
15. Shaked A, McDiarmid SV, Harrison RE, et al: Hepatic artery thrombosis resulting in gas gangrene of the transplanted liver. Surgery 111:462-465, 1992.
16. Hashikura Y, Kawasaki S, Okumura N, et al: Prevention of hepatic artery thrombosis in pediatric liver transplantation. Transplantation 60:1109-1112, 1995.
17. Tan KC, Yandza T, de Hemptinne B, et al: Hepatic artery thrombosis in pediatric liver transplantation. J Pediatr Surg 23:927-930, 1988.
18. Cavallari A, Vivarelli M, Bellusci R, et al: Treatment of vascular complications following liver transplantation: Multidisciplinary approach. Hepatogastroenterology 48:179-183, 2001.
19. Pinna AD, Smith CV, Furukawa H, et al: Urgent revascularization of liver allografts after hepatic artery thrombosis. Transplantation 62:1584-1587, 1997.
20. Bhattacharjya S, Gunson B, Mirza D, et al: Delayed hepatic artery thrombosis in adult liver transplantation—a 12-year experience. Transplantation 71:1592-1596, 2001.
21. Northover J, Terblanche J: Bile duct blood supply; its importance in human liver transplantation. Transplantation 26:67-69, 1978.
22. Hall T, McDiarmid S, Grant E, et al: False-negative duplex Doppler studies in children with hepatic artery thrombosis after liver transplantation. AJR Am J Roentgenol 154:573-575, 1990.
23. Dodd G, Memel D, Zajko A, et al: Hepatic artery stenosis and thrombosis in transplant recipients: Doppler diagnosis with resistive index and systolic acceleration time. Radiology 192:657-661, 1994.
24. McDiarmid SV, Hall TR, Grant EG: Failure of duplex sonography to diagnose hepatic artery thrombosis in a high-risk group of pediatric liver transplant recipients. Transplant Proc 22:1529-1530, 1990.
25. Fleischmann D: Multiple detector-row CT angiography of the renal and mesenteric vessels. Eur J Radiol 45(Suppl 1):S79-S87, 2003.
26. Sadick M, Diehl SJ, Lehmann KJ, et al: Evaluation of breath-hold contrast-enhanced 3D magnetic resonance angiography technique for imaging visceral abdominal arteries and veins. Invest Radiol 5:111-117, 2000.
27. Figueras J, Busquets J, Dominguez J, et al: Intra-arterial thrombolysis in the treatment of acute hepatic artery thrombosis after liver transplantation. Transplantation 59:1356-1357, 1995.
28. Vivarelli M, LaBarba G, Legnani C, et al: Repeated graft loss caused by recurrent hepatic artery thrombosis after liver transplantation. Liver Transpl 9:629-631, 2003.
29. Ciciarelli TV, Esquivel CO, Moore DH, et al: Factors affecting survival after orthotopic liver transplantation in infants. Transplantation 64:242-248, 1997.
30. Mazzaferro V, Esquivel CO, Makowka L, et al: Hepatic artery thrombosis after pediatric liver transplantation—a medical or surgical event? Transplantation 47:971-977, 1989.
31. Harper P, Luddington R, Carrell, R, et al: Protein C deficiency and portal thrombosis in liver transplantation in children. Lancet 2:924-927, 1988.
32. Nakazato PZ, Cox KL, Concepcion W, et al: Revascularization technique for reduced-size liver transplantation for infants weighing less than 10 kg. J Pediatr Surg 28:923-926, 1993.
33. Merion R, Burtch G, Ham J, et al: The hepatic artery in liver transplantation. Transplantation 45:438-443, 1989.
34. Lallier M, Dickens S, Dubois J, et al: Vascular complications after pediatric liver transplantation. J Pediatr Surg 30:1122-1126, 1995.
35. Velasco F, Villalba R, Fernandez M, et al: Diminished anticoagulant and fibrinolytic activity following liver transplantation. Transplantation 53:1256-1261, 1992.
36. Hatano E, Terajima H, Yabe S, et al: Hepatic artery thrombosis in living related liver transplantation. Transplantation 64:1443-1446, 1997.
37. Samuel D, Gillet D, Castaing D, et al: Portal and arterial thrombosis in liver transplantation: A frequent event in severe rejection. Transplant Proc 21:2225-2227, 1989.
38. Madalosso C, Souza N, Ilstrup D, et al: Cytomegalovirus and its association with hepatic artery thrombosis after liver transplantation. Transplantation 66:294-297, 1998.
39. Mor E, Schwartz ME, Sheiner PA, et al: Prolonged preservation in University of Wisconsin solution associated with hepatic artery thrombosis after orthotopic liver transplantation. Transplantation 56:1399-1402, 1993.
40. Soliman T, Bodingbauer M, Langer F, et al: The role of complex hepatic artery reconstruction in orthotopic liver transplantation. Liver Transpl 9:970-975, 2003.
41. Sopher M, Braunfeld M, Shackleton C, et al: Fatal pulmonary embolism during liver transplantation. Anesthesiology 87:429-432, 1997.
42. Inomoto T, Nishizawa F, Sasaki H, et al: Experiences of 120 microsurgical reconstructions of hepatic artery in living related transplantation. Surgery 119:20-26, 1996.

43. Mondragon R, Karani J, Heaton N, et al: The use of percutaneous transluminal angioplasty in hepatic artery stenosis after transplantation. Transplantation 57:228-231, 1994.

44. Raby N, Karani J, Thomas S, et al: Stenosis of vascular anastomoses after hepatic transplantation: Treatment with balloon angioplasty. Am J Radiol 157:167-171, 1991.

45. Leonardi LS, Soares C Jr, Boin IF, et al: Hemobilia after mycotic hepatic artery pseudoaneurysm after liver transplantation. Transplant Proc 33:2580-2582, 2001.

46. Tobben PJ, Zajko AB, Sumkin JH, et al: Pseudoaneurysms complicating organ transplantation: Roles of CT, duplex sonography, and angiography. Radiology 169:65-70, 1988.

Infections After Liver Transplantation

CURTIS D. HOLT
DREW J. WINSTON

Pretransplant screening: recipient and donor   964

General screening   964

Serological testing   964
  Human immunodeficiency virus   964
  Epstein-Barr virus   965
  Hepatitis B and C   965
  Cytomegalovirus   965
  Cryptococcosis, coccidioidomycosis, and histoplasmosis   965
  Other pathogens   965

Donor- and allograft-transmitted infections   965

Time of occurrence of posttransplant infections   966

Risk factors for infections   966
  Pretransplant period   967
  Intraoperative period   967
  Posttransplant period   968

Bacterial infections   968
  Treatment of bacterial infection   971

Fungal infections   972
  Spectrum of fungal pathogens, clinical features, and diagnosis   972
  Management of fungal infections   975
  Fungal prophylaxis   975
  Treatment of fungal infections   977

Viral infections   978
  Cytomegalovirus   978
  Herpes simplex virus   980
  Varicella-zoster virus   981
  Epstein-Barr virus   981
  Other human herpesviruses   981
  Adenovirus   982
  Papovaviruses   982
  Influenza virus types A and B, parainfluenza virus, and respiratory syncytial virus   982
  Parvovirus   982
  Human immunodeficiency virus   982
  Hepatitis B and C virus   983

Protozoan infections   984

Prophylaxis of infection   984

Summary and conclusions   986

Despite the remarkable advances in orthotopic liver transplantation (OLT), infection can be a major and often life-threatening complication, with approximately two thirds of OLT patients experiencing one episode of serious infection. The spectrum and manifestations of these infections are broad and variable and often reflect the fact that a patient awaiting liver transplantation is a unique host who is usually in an impaired state of health before transplantation, undergoes a technically complex operation, and then requires lifelong immunosuppressive therapy, which may be intensified as a result of rejection. For these reasons, if an infectious process is not identified early enough, it can rapidly escalate to a serious disseminated disease leading to death. Conversely, recognition of infection can be problematic because symptoms of infection may mimic rejection and it is sometimes difficult to distinguish between true infection and mere colonization.

Sixty percent to 80% of all liver transplant patients experience infection. The average number of infections per infected patient ranges between 1.5 and 2.5.[1-4] Historically, infections contribute to more than half of the reported episodes of mortality after liver transplantation. In one series, infections were associated with 89% of all deaths, even after the availability of cyclosporine.[1] In a more recent report, the incidence of infection-related mortality was noted to be higher than 50% before 1980, 25% to 35% in the 1980s, and less than 10% in the 1990s.[5] These reports are indicative of a high-risk subpopulation of patients who suffer multiple infectious episodes that are often lethal. Thus, the incidence of infectious complications in OLT recipients is generally greater than that reported in other solid-organ transplant (SOT) recipients. With the new millennium, the Model for End-Stage Liver Disease (MELD) has been used to prioritize candidates for OLT.[6] Patients with the highest MELD scores generally receive organs first. However, this practice may lead to a greater risk for infectious complications in the posttransplant setting. This chapter provides an overview of the time course, risk factors, clinical features, diagnosis, and management of infectious complications in OLT.

Pretransplant Screening: Recipient and Donor

Before OLT, several factors may predispose an OLT candidate to infection after surgery. Of these factors, identification of latent infections that may be reactivated in the presence of postoperative immunosuppression and recognition of active infection that may require therapy or preclude OLT are most significant.[5] Latent infections or infectious exposure in the pretransplant period can lead to reappraisal of transplant candidacy or alterations in standard posttransplant management. Untreated or unrecognized infections in the recipient can become clinically apparent in the posttransplant period. Any infection, such as pneumonia, or smoldering intra-abdominal, hepatobiliary, or genitourinary tract infection, can be reactivated or exacerbated in the immediate postoperative period during induction of immunosuppression or later, depending on the overall net state of immunosuppression.[5,7]

General Screening

Evaluation of patients for infectious disease should include a meticulous history of antibiotic allergies, dental assessment, preoperative urine culture, and a chest radiograph to exclude active pneumonic processes and identify evidence of previous granulomatous disease.[5,7] The risk of latent infection with tuberculosis or a geographically related endemic mycosis should be determined by eliciting a travel and residency history because old "healed" granulomatous lesions, such as tuberculosis, histoplasmosis, or coccidioidomycosis, can become reactivated in the posttransplant setting under conditions of routine immunosuppression or after treatment of rejection. A purified protein derivative (PPD) skin test with appropriate controls (i.e., mumps, Candida, and tetanus) should be applied. However, the higher incidence of cutaneous anergy in patients with end-stage liver disease can lead to false-negative results. The American Thoracic Society recommendations for isoniazid prophylaxis include most SOT recipients. However, the potential for isoniazid-induced hepatotoxicity and its confusion with graft rejection or dysfunction may prohibit routine prophylaxis in OLT recipients. At UCLA, we do not recommend isoniazid for OLT candidates in response to a positive tuberculin skin test unless conversion has been recently documented or significant abnormalities consistent with previous tuberculosis are present on chest radiography. Generally, patients who previously completed a full treatment course for active tuberculosis do not require additional antituberculous therapy after liver transplantation.[5] However, early diagnosis and treatment are essential in organ transplant recipients.[8,9]

Serological Testing

Preoperative serological testing should include the following: human immunodeficiency virus (HIV) antibody by enzyme immunoassay, with confirmation by Western blot analysis if warranted; Epstein-Barr virus (EBV) antibody; hepatitis B virus (HBV) surface antibody, surface antigen, and core IgG and IgM antibody; hepatitis C virus (HCV) antibody or RNA detection assay as warranted; herpes simplex virus (HSV) antibodies; varicella-zoster virus (VZV) antibody; cytomegalovirus (CMV) antibody, and specific endemic mycosis antibody tests when applicable (e.g., anticoccidioidal antibody detection in any patient with exposure to an endemic area).

Human Immunodeficiency Virus

All potential OLT recipients should be tested for HIV antibody regardless of risk factors. HIV-positive patients meeting specified criteria now undergo transplantation at some centers, but long-term outcomes of these patients have not been established.[10-12] All potential transplant donors, both living and deceased, should be tested for HIV regardless of risk factors. Many centers reject livers from high-risk donors for fear of failure to detect antibody during the "window" after acute infection. Although transmission of HIV by infected organs has been described, these screening precautions have reduced the risk for infection to a negligible degree in the modern transplant era.[10-12]

Epstein-Barr Virus

Both EBV-seronegative recipients of grafts from EBV-seropositive donors and EBV-seropositive recipients may be at increased risk for posttransplant lymphoproliferative disorder (PTLD), particularly if they receive prolonged or repeated courses of antilymphocytic therapy or are pediatric allograft recipients.[13-16] In high-risk patients, the quantitative EBV viral load can be assayed by polymerase chain reaction (PCR) after increasing the net state of immunosuppression or when clinically indicated.

Hepatitis B and C

Historically, recurrent disease developed in most patients undergoing OLT for hepatitis B or hepatitis C.[17-26] Current prophylaxis with hepatitis B immune globulin and antiviral agents has minimized recurrence of hepatitis B and improved patient and allograft survival rates similar to those of patients transplanted without hepatitis B.[27,28] In contrast, recurrence of hepatitis C is universal, and strategies are still being developed to minimize disease recurrence and progression during the posttransplant period (see Chapter 10).[26,29-31] Detection of HBV and HCV in both transplant donors and recipients has improved with newer laboratory methods designed to detect viral-specific antibody, antigens, and nucleic acids. In fact, hepatitis B core antibody–positive donors are used under stringent protocols with antiviral prophylaxis (i.e., lamivudine and HBIg) in several liver transplant centers.[27,28] HCV-positive donors are rarely used because of a lack of effective preventive therapies.[32]

Cytomegalovirus

Prior to the availability of effective prophylaxis, CMV had been the most common viral pathogen after OLT. CMV infection may vary in severity from asymptomatic infection to multiorgan involvement and death.[33-39]

The incidence of CMV seropositivity increases with age such that most adult patients have detectable IgG antibody to CMV. Primary CMV infection is more severe than reactivated infection after transplantation. Thus, seronegative patients should be considered candidates for prophylaxis at the time of OLT or after posttransplant exposure. The clinical significance of the CMV antibody status of the donor and recipient is discussed later in this chapter.

Cryptococcus, Coccidioidomycosis, and Histoplasmosis

Detection of *Cryptococcus neoformans* by the presence of antigen, *Coccidioides immitis* antibody by complement fixation or immunodiffusion, or *Histoplasma capsulatum* antibody by immunodiffusion during transplant evaluation should alert the clinician to the possibility of reactivation of disease after transplantation.[40-42] Reactivation can occur during routine immunosuppression or after augmented immunosuppression for rejection. Patients who have resided in geographical areas at risk for coccidioidomycosis or histoplasmosis should be tested for antibody before transplantation, and if antibody positive or if there is radiological evidence of residual disease, they should receive prophylactic azole antifungal therapy.

Other Pathogens

Spontaneous bacterial peritonitis, cholangitis, respiratory tract infection, and nosocomial fungal infection are frequently encountered infections in candidates for OLT. With the exception of invasive *Candida* or *Aspergillus* infection and overwhelming pneumonia, these infections do not preclude successful transplantation as long as adequate treatment is given and clinical improvement is documented before transplantation.

Donor- and Allograft-Transmitted Infections

It is frequently difficult to differentiate between a pure donor allograft source of infection, exogenous infection, and reactivation of latent disease. The following agents have been implicated with reasonable certainty as being transmissible with the donor allograft: HIV, CMV, HBV, HCV, and *H. capsulatum*.[44] Probable transmission has been reported with herpes simplex virus (HSV); aerobic gram-positive and gram-negative bacteria; anaerobes; atypical mycobacteria; and EBV. Serious consequences of such transmission include infectious disruption of the vascular anastomoses, formation of mycotic aneurysms, infective endocarditis, and sepsis. The incidence of true donor-transmitted infection can be reduced by scrupulous screening and epidemiological evaluation, as discussed in Chapter 29, "Pretransplantation Infectious Disease Screening for Transplantation: Candidates and Donors."

Time of Occurrence of Posttransplant Infections

Of all infections, 50% to 60% are bacterial, 20% to 40% are viral, 5% to 15% are fungal. Less than 10% are due to parasites such as *Toxoplasma*.[5,7,38] The type, severity, and incidence of observed infections often depend on prophylactic practices. Since there is some standardization of immunosuppressive regimens among liver transplant centers, a timetable for determining when postoperative infections are most likely to occur has been developed. (Fig. 64–1) Knowledge of this timetable may allow the clinician to form a differential diagnosis, develop methods of monitoring for infection, and

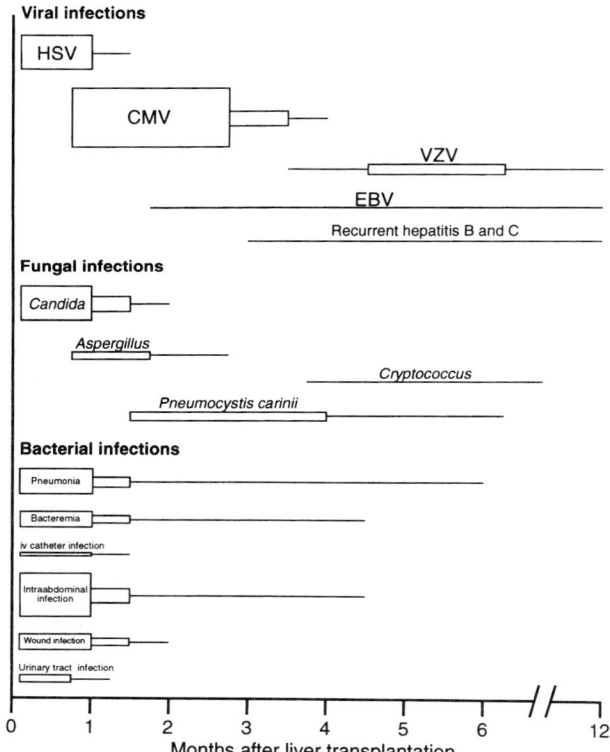

FIGURE 64–1

Common infections by time after liver transplantation. CMV, cytomegalovirus; EBV, Epstein-Barr virus; HSV, herpes simplex virus; IV, intravenous; VZV, varicella-zoster virus.

implement pharmacoeconomically effective management strategies.

Generally, there are three timeframes during which liver transplant recipients may develop infection: the first postoperative month, between 1 and 6 months after transplantation, and beyond the 6-month postoperative period.[5,7] Notably, most infections occur in the first 2 months after liver transplantation.[5,7,38,45-47] a time that corresponds to the period of most episodes of rejection and greatest immunosuppression.

In the first month after transplantation, infections are associated with either pretransplant conditions or postoperative complications (see later).[5,7,38] Most bacterial as well as several fungal infections are observed during this period. Of interest, the onset of fungal infection in OLT recipients occurs earlier than in other SOT recipients.[38,45-47] Of these fungal infections, greater than 90% are nosocomial candidal infections of wounds, intra-abdominal organs, or intravascular catheters.[45-47]

After this early period, reactivated or primary CMV infections occur and peak around the sixth week after transplantation.[5,7,38] HSV viral reactivation occurs earlier, whereas EBV infection may have a delayed onset. *Pneumocystis carinii* pneumonia (PCP) and toxoplasmosis occur late in the first 6 months after transplantation and very rarely beyond this period.[5,7,38,48,49]

Infections beyond the sixth month after transplantation are uncommon and occur primarily in patients with chronic rejection, those who require repeat transplantation, or patients that are being maintained on higher doses of immunosuppression.[5,7,38] Furthermore, the majority of these infections are similar to those found in nontransplanted patients, such as community-acquired infections (viral respiratory tract infections or bacterial pneumonia), or they may represent reactivation of viral infection from pathogens such as VZV. Ultimately, events that affect the net state of immunosuppression, prolonged hospitalization, retransplantation, renal and respiratory failure, new-onset medical illness, and new nosocomial or environmental exposure may alter the anticipated time course for infections in OLT recipients.

Risk Factors for Infections

The overall state of health of the patient and the urgency of the transplantation may affect the type and severity of postoperative infections. Specific risk factors for infection in OLT recipients include underlying medical conditions, environmental exposures (occurring in the community and hospital), technical complications of the transplant surgery, and the overall net state of immunosuppression (pharmacological and disease state related) (Table 64–1).[1-5,7,38] Knowledge of these risk factors may allow identification of OLT recipients at greatest risk for infection and the implementation of

Table 64-1. RISK FACTORS FOR INFECTION IN LIVER TRANSPLANTATION

Pretransplant	Transplant	Posttransplant
UNDERLYING MEDICAL CONDITION	**SURGERY**	**POSTOPERATIVE MANAGEMENT**
Corticosteroid therapy	Prolonged procedure	Indwelling vascular or bladder catheters
Poor nutritional status	Increased transfusion requirement	Prolonged intubation
Chronic lung disease	Graft ischemia or injury	Prolonged antibiotic administration
Diabetes mellitus	Intra-abdominal bleeding	Repeat laparotomy
	Bowel leak	Repeat transplantation
	Choledochojejunostomy	
COLONIZATION	**DONOR GRAFT**	**HOSPITAL FLORA**
Preoperative antibiotics	Cytomegalovirus	Resistant bacteria
Duration of hospitalization (especially in ICU)	Hepatitis viruses	*Aspergillus*
	Human Immunodeficiency virus	*Legionella*
LATENT INFECTION IN RECIPIENT		**IMMUNOSUPPRESSION**
Cytomegalovirus		Cyclosporine
Herpes simplex virus		Tacrolimus
Varicella-zoster virus		Azathioprine
Hepatitis viruses		Mycophenolate mofetil
Endemic mycosis (*Coccidioides, Histoplasma*)		Corticosteroids
Pneumocystis		Muromonab CD3 (OKT3)
Tuberculosis		Thymoglobulin
		Sirolimus

appropriate prophylactic and therapeutic strategies. Pretransplant, intraoperative, and posttransplant risk factors are reviewed in the following sections.

Pretransplant Period

The overall health of the recipient and the urgency of the transplantation may affect the severity of pretransplant infections.[1,5,7,38] Previous medical conditions, chronic underlying diseases, renal failure (hemodialysis), fulminant hepatic failure, mechanical ventilation, malnutrition, a high MELD score, and diabetes mellitus are examples of pretransplant factors that may predispose allograft recipients to infection (see Table 64-1).[1-6,38]

Infections in the pretransplant setting are also associated with several environmental factors, of which both recent and remote exposure is noteworthy.[7,38] Potential bacterial environmental pathogens include *Pseudomonas* species and *Legionella*, which may contaminate water supplies, and *Listeria* and *Salmonella*, which have been associated with food-related epidemics.[7,38] Significant community-related fungal exposure includes endemic mycoses (*C. immitis, Blastomyces dermatitidis,* and *H. capsulatum*), and *C. neoformans*.[7,38,50,51]

Exposure to nosocomial fungal pathogens such as *Aspergillus* and *Candida* is also concerning.[5,7,38,50,51] With respect to *Aspergillus* infection, an association with hospital construction or water has been described. Furthermore, domiciliary and nondomiciliary patterns are possible. Domiciliary exposure occurs in the room or ward where the patient is housed, whereas nondomiciliary exposure occurs when the patient travels for a procedure and is exposed en route or at the destination site (radiological suite, operating room, catheterization, or laboratory). Additional risk factors for these pathogens include central venous or bladder catheterization (or both), extended use of systemic antibiotics, colonization by a fungal pathogen, total parenteral nutrition, and contaminated air conditioning or filtering systems.[7,38]

Intraoperative Period

Equally important are factors pertaining to the surgical procedure.[5,7,38] For example, disruption of the integrity of the gastrointestinal tract by surgery or anastomotic leaks creates an avenue for infections by endogenous flora. Any technical complication that leads to devitalized tissue, vascular thrombosis, or accumulation of fluid may also enhance the risk of infection. Additionally, vascular access devices and drainage catheters present a risk for infection in an OLT recipient because these devices disrupt the physical barrier to infection and produce portals of entry for endogenous and nosocomial flora. The transplanted liver may also become a focus of infection as a result of vascular-related ischemia or rejection. Infections are also more common in OLT recipients who require a high number of intraoperative blood products, retransplantation or re-exploration, prolonged operative time, or a choledochojejunostomy compared to a choledochocholedochostomy.[5,7,38] Transfusion-associated infections (caused by CMV, hepatitis viruses, HIV, and others) may also occur in OLT recipients receiving large amounts of blood products.[5,38]

Posttransplant Period

Retransplantation, reintubation or prolonged ventilatory support, renal failure, prolonged use of antimicrobial agents, colonization with resistant hospital flora, and the net state of immunosuppression play a critical role in the development of infections in the posttransplant setting.[5] The net state of immunosuppression has been reviewed by others and is considered to be a function of the dosage, duration, and temporal sequence of immunosuppressive therapy, any underlying immune deficiency, integrity of the mucocutaneous barriers, metabolic conditions, and infection with immunomodulating viruses.[7,38]

Immunosuppressive agents continue to have the greatest impact on host susceptibility to infection. Various strategies are used to prevent rejection and depend on the center, the type of transplant performed, and the relative immunological risks for development of rejection. Based on these factors, agents such as cyclosporine, tacrolimus, corticosteroids, azathioprine, and mycophenolate mofetil with or without T-cell–depleting agents have been implemented in various combinations to reduce the risk of rejection. Cyclosporine and tacrolimus reduce interleukin-2 (IL-2) production, which subsequently inhibits mixed lymphocytic reactions and preferentially impairs immune reactions against the allograft. The overall incidence of infectious complications with cyclosporine or tacrolimus appears to be similar.[52-55]

Pulses of corticosteroids and various antilymphocytic globulins administered for the treatment of rejection increase the risk for infection. Corticosteroids affect all aspects of immunity, and high doses have been associated with fungal but not CMV infection in solid-organ recipients.[56-58] Azathioprine and mycophenolate have antilymphoproliferative activity, but they can also cause neutropenia, which may predispose to a wide range of infectious complications. The use of mycophenolate has not been clearly established to increase the risk for

infections after OLT.[59] T-cell–depleting agents such as the monoclonal agent muromonab-CD3 or the polyclonal agent thymoglobulin are some of the most potent immunosuppressive agents currently available. Historically, muromonab-CD3 has been associated with a definite increase in infectious complications, primarily those caused by CMV, EBV, and HCV.[5,7,38,60,61] The impact of thymoglobulin on infection in OLT recipients remains to be elucidated.[62]

IL-2 receptor monoclonal antibody preparations (e.g., basiliximab, daclizumab) are also used for the prophylaxis of acute organ rejection in conjunction with tacrolimus (or cyclosporine), with or without mycophenolate and corticosteroids. Although initial trials with these agents in renal transplant patients failed to demonstrated an increased incidence of infection, it remains to be seen whether this observation will continue in liver allograft recipients, especially when these agents are used in combination with other immunosuppressive drugs.[63-65]

Sirolimus, a newer immunosuppressive agent for the prevention of rejection in renal allografts, differs from cyclosporine and tacrolimus in its mechanism of action.[66] Whereas cyclosporine and tacrolimus act by blocking calcineurin and inhibiting T-cell–dependent growth factors such as IL-2 at the level of gene transcription through a Ca^{2+}-dependent signal, sirolimus appears to inhibit growth factor–dependent proliferation of hematopoietic cells at a later stage of the cell cycle through a Ca^{+2}-independent signal.[66] In initial studies, sirolimus has demonstrated efficacy equal to that of cyclosporine in maintaining heart and renal allografts.[66] Although the drug has not been approved for use in OLT recipients, it is still used in these patients in certain clinical situations. In a study of renal allograft recipients, the incidence and severity of infections were somewhat greater with sirolimus than cyclosporine, although the number of patients experiencing infections was similar between the two groups.[67] The risk of *P. carinii* infection may be greater in OLT patients receiving sirolimus; thus, long-term prophylaxis with trimethoprim-sulfamethoxazole (TMP-SMX) is recommended.[68,69] More experience is required with sirolimus alone or in combination with other available immunosuppressive agents to further evaluate any possible association with infections in OLT recipients.

Bacterial Infections

The overall rates of bacterial infection after OLT range between 33% and 68%, with an associated mortality ranging between 13 to 77%.[1,2,5,70-82] The large variability in the reported percentages of OLT patients with bacterial infections from different institutions may be attributed to several factors: (1) differences in definition and documentation of infection and duration of follow-up; (2) differences in the type and severity of underlying disease and the number of transplants; (3) differences in the type and duration of antimicrobial agents used for bowel decontamination, systemic prophylaxis, and treatment of infections; (4) surgical technique; (5) duration of intensive care unit stay; (6) immunosuppressive strategies; and (7) different infection control measures (i.e., isolation of patients with resistant organisms, hand washing, glove and gown requirements). Specific risk factors for bacterial infection in OLT recipients include transplant surgery longer than 12 hours, pretransplant bilirubin concentration greater than 12 mg/dL, increased duration of antibiotic therapy (>5 days) during the immediate postoperative period, increased number of red cell (>25 U) or fresh-frozen plasma (>30 U) transfusions, and multiple abdominal operations.[1,5,38,70]

Common bacterial pathogens include gram-positive organisms (*Staphylococcus aureus*, coagulase-negative staphylococci, *Enterococcus fecalis*, and *Enterococcus faecium*) and gram-negative organisms (Enterobacteriaceae and *Pseudomonas aeruginosa*) (Table 64–2).[1,5,38,83] In a study of bacteremic OLT recipients, aerobic gram-negative bacilli constituted 49% of all pathogens found in blood cultures. More recent data have suggested that an epidemiological shift toward a higher incidence of gram-positive–related infections is occurring in OLT recipients. Of the episodes of early-onset bacteremia in one liver transplant center, 70.7% were caused by gram-positive pathogens.[79] Coagulase-negative staphylococci accounted for 37.8% of all bacteremias, whereas methicillin-resistant *S. aureus* (MRSA) represented only 4.2% of these cases. Others have reported a higher incidence of MRSA in OLT recipients, up to 23%.[74] Common sites of infection with MRSA include vascular catheters (39%), wounds (18%), the abdomen (18%), and the lungs (13%).[74] Crude mortality rates of up to 21% have been seen in these patients, with the highest rates occurring in those with bacteremic MRSA pneumonia or abdominal infections.[74] CMV seronegativity

and primary CMV infection were significant risk factors associated with the development of MRSA infection.[74] Some centers now recommend screening for MRSA in high-risk patients being assessed for OLT. Unfortunately, elimination of *S. aureus* nasal carriage in OLT candidates with such agents as mupirocin has not been successful in preventing postoperative *S. aureus* infection.[84] Furthermore, emergence of glycopeptide-intermediate *S. aureus* (GISA) has also been reported in liver transplant recipients.[85]

Infection or colonization by vancomycin-resistant *E. faecium* (VRE) has been reported in liver transplant recipients and has been associated with increased morbidity and mortality.[38,80-82,86,87] The most common site of VRE infection is the abdomen, followed by blood stream, wound, and intravascular catheters.[80-82,86,87] OLT patients infected with VRE generally have received more preoperative antibiotics, are more likely to have received vancomycin preoperatively, and have been hospitalized in the intensive care unit.[86,87] Additional characteristics in OLT recipients infected with VRE included repeat laparotomy after OLT, pulmonary or renal failure, coinfection with other microbial pathogens, and biliary complications.[80-82] Invasive infection with VRE has been associated with poor outcomes in OLT recipients, with mortality ranging from 60% to 82%; polymicrobial sepsis was the most common cause of death in several reports.[80-82,86-88] Pretransplant VRE colonization has been reported in OLT candidates, and these patients represent a substantial reservoir for continued nosocomial VRE transmission. Measures aimed at reducing VRE colonization in critically ill individuals with high MELD scores or new transplant recipients should be pursued, since the risk of morbidity and mortality is greater in these patients.[80] Agents available for the treatment of VRE infections are quinupristin-dalfopristin, linezolid, and more recently, daptomycin.[89-91]

Infections caused by multidrug-resistant gram-negative pathogens, especially *P. aeruginosa* and

Table 64–2. COMMON BACTERIAL PATHOGENS IN LIVER TRANSPLANT RECIPIENTS

Bacteremia	Pneumonia	Intra-abdominal	Wound	Urinary Tract
Enterobacteriaceae	Enterobacteriaceae	Enterobacteriaceae	Polymicrobial	Enterobacteriaceae
Pseudomonas aeruginosa	*Pseudomonas aeruginosa*	Polymicrobial	*Staphylococcus aureus*	*Pseudomonas aeruginosa*
Coagulase-negative *Staphylococcus*	*Staphylococcus aureus*	*Enterococcus*	Enterobacteriaceae	*Enterococcus*
Staphylococcus aureus		Anaerobes (*Bacteroides* spp.)	*Pseudomonas aeruginosa*	
Enterococcus		*Staphylococcus aureus*	*Streptococcus*	
Anaerobes (*Bacteroides* spp.)				

Klebsiella-Enterobacter species, have been documented in OLT recipients.[92-96] At some transplant centers gram-negative bacilli with transferable resistance to extended-spectrum cephalosporins have been reported with increased frequency among liver transplant recipients.[93] Most of these strains, predominantly *Klebsiella pneumoniae* and *Enterobacter* species, are generally resistant to all β-lactam antimicrobials except carbapenems.

Anaerobic pathogens are less prevalent in OLT recipients.[4,38,97-101] Similarly, *Nocardia, Legionella* and *Listeria* are uncommon but potentially significant pathogens.[102-108] In one series, *Nocardia* was reported in 7 of 191 patients (3.7%) over a period of 3.5 years with a 35% mortality rate.[83] Specific risk factors for *Nocardia* infection include early rejection, enhanced immunosuppression, neutropenia, and uremia. *Nocardia* infections are most commonly manifested as acute or subacute pneumonia, but hematogenous spread to the brain, skin and subcutaneous tissue, bone, and eye has also been reported. Infection by *Legionella* species is reported in less than 5% of transplant patients but can develop within 3 to 12 weeks postoperatively with a mortality rate of 29%.[104-107] Specific risk factors for *Legionella* infection include excessive corticosteroid use, prolonged postoperative intubation, and contaminated hospital water supply despite superheating and hyperchlorination.[104-107] Signs and symptoms of *Legionella pneumophila* infection include a nonproductive cough, temperature-pulse dissociation, elevated hepatic enzymes, diarrhea, hyponatremia, myalgia, and confusion. Radiographic findings consist of alveolar or interstitial infiltrates, frank cavities, pleural effusions, and lobar consolidation. Infections caused by *Listeria* species are often associated with a reduction of T-cell–mediated macrophage activation and have infrequently been reported in OLT recipients.[108] *Listeria monocytogenes* infection is most commonly manifested as meningoencephalitis, brain abscess, or bacteremia. Patients with cirrhosis may also have spontaneous bacterial peritonitis. *L. monocytogenes* infection typically occurs 6 or more months after transplantation. This late onset may be related to the routine use of TMP-SMX for PCP prophylaxis, since TMP-SMX also provides excellent coverage against *Listeria*. A substantial proportion of sporadic cases of listeriosis are associated with the ingestion of processed meat; patients should be instructed to eat only properly cooked meat and pasteurized dairy products.

A majority of bacterial infections occurring after OLT are similar to those observed following major abdominal surgery and include intra-abdominal infection, pneumonia, wound infection, urinary tract infection, intravascular catheter infection, and primary bacteremia.[38,70-73,109,110] Intra-abdominal infections account for the majority of localized bacterial infections and have been reported in 30% to 50% of OLT patients. These infections include peritonitis, hepatic and extrahepatic abscesses, and cholangitis. Complications associated with the biliary anastomosis, biliary obstruction, and the presence of a splinting T tube are unique factors that may predispose patients to intra-abdominal infection.[23,38,111] These complications may introduce bacteria into bile, allow them to multiply, and then reduce clearance of colonizing bacteria from the biliary tree. Of interest, in the immediate postoperative period, patients who undergo choledochocholedochostomy do not routinely have bacteria present in their bile. The primarily complication observed in these patients appears to be obstruction at the anastomosis, whereas in patients who require a Roux-en-Y choledochojejunostomy, reflux of bacterial organisms may occur.[111,112] The incidence of intra-abdominal infections is greater in OLT recipients who require Roux-en-Y choledochojejunostomy and undergo retransplantation than in patients who receive one transplant and undergo choledochocholedochostomy.[1,38] Other intra-abdominal infections may result from the accumulation of infected intra-abdominal fluid, although many fluid collections in the surgical bed are sterile. Aspiration plus culture of fluid collections is frequently required in OLT recipients who exhibit persistent fever and fever of unknown origin.

OLT recipients may be predisposed to nosocomial bacterial pneumonia as a result of encephalopathy, aspiration, and prolonged intubation. Common nosocomial pathogens causing pneumonia include aerobic gram-negative bacilli (*Klebsiella-Enterobacter* spp. and *P. aeruginosa*) and *S. aureus*. During the immediate posttransplant period, any evidence of pneumonia mandates an extensive and urgent evaluation to identify potential pathogens because mortality rates from nosocomial pneumonia can be as high as 40%.[1,38,94] OLT recipients are also at risk for community-acquired bacterial pneumonia, which usually occurs many months after transplantation.[7,38] *Mycoplasma, Streptococcus pneumoniae, Haemophilus influenza*, and *S. aureus* often cause such infections. Chest radiography is used to confirm the presence of pneumonia, but interpretation of the findings may be complicated by the almost universal presence of right-sided pleural effusion and right lower lobe atelectasis after surgery. Infection of the pleural space or empyema is extremely rare.

Bacterial infections of the central nervous system (CNS) in liver transplant recipients are very uncommon, but have high mortality (44% to 77%).[96] Aggressive workup (lumbar puncture, magnetic resonance imaging [MRI] or computed tomography [CT], diagnostic needle aspiration, and biopsy of brain mass) and appropriate treatment are needed in a patient with fever and abnormal neurological findings to minimize mortality.

Both asymptomatic and symptomatic bacterial infection of the urinary tract may also occur, usually as a result of indwelling catheters.

Systemic bacterial infections or bacteremias have been observed in up to 27% of OLT recipients, with mortality rates ranging between 13% and 36%.[1,38,70,74,76,94] Bacteremia has been known to result from several portals of entry, including the abdomen, wounds, infected intravascular catheters, biliary obstruction or leakage, loculated abdominal fluid, hepatic artery thrombosis, and hepatic infarction. In approximately a third of patients with bacteremia, no apparent source can be identified.[1,38,70,74,76,94] Pulmonary sources of bacteremia in OLT recipients are less common and seen in only 10% to 16% of patients with bacteremia. They are often associated with aspiration or endotracheal intubation.[1,38,71,113,114]

Bacterial infections in OLT recipients may be difficult to diagnose because the usual signs and symptoms of infection may be masked or absent as a result of the patient's net state of immunosuppression. Additionally, allograft rejection, preservation injury, and graft ischemia can have clinical manifestations similar to those of infection. Specific diagnostic techniques involve noninvasive measures (cultures of blood, urine, sputum, wounds, bile, and drains) and invasive measures (angiography and liver biopsy) to distinguish infectious complications from ischemia or rejection of the allograft.[115] A presumptive diagnosis of an abdominal or liver abscess can be made by CT or ultrasonography and confirmed by radiographically guided fine-needle aspiration. Specimens that can be used to identify the specific cause of posttransplant pneumonia include sputum, tracheal aspirates (in patients maintained on a ventilator), or bronchoalveolar lavage fluid. Although cultures of sputum and tracheal aspirates can readily be obtained, the results are often difficult to interpret with regard to bacterial colonization versus actual infection. Several unique laboratory tests are available for the diagnosis of *Legionella* infection, including serum antibody determination, use of immunofluorescent antigen detection or a DNA probe on pulmonary secretions, and urine antigen detection.[16,17]

Treatment of Bacterial Infection

Implementation of antibacterial therapy can be considered under the following categories: (1) *surgical prophylaxis*: antimicrobial agents used to prevent a commonly encountered infection in the immediate postoperative period; (2) *empirical therapy*: antimicrobials initiated without identification of the infecting pathogen; and (3) *specific therapy*: antimicrobials administered to treat a documented pathogen.[7,38]

Surgical Prophylaxis

Generally, prophylactic antibiotics should be directed against skin pathogens (e.g., staphylococci, streptococci) and intra-abdominal pathogens (*enteric gram-negative bacteria*). Ampicillin-sulbactam, cefoxitin, cefotetan, or vancomycin plus an aminoglycoside (penicillin-allergic patient) can be used for prophylaxis and should be discontinued after 24 hours to reduce the risk for superinfection with resistant bacterial organisms. The use of third- or fourth-generation cephalosporins, extended-spectrum quinolones, or extended-spectrum β-lactam plus β-lactamase inhibitor combinations for prophylaxis is discouraged due to concerns related to cost and the emergence of resistant organisms which may compromise the effectiveness of these antibiotics for treatment of established infections.

Empirical Therapy

For OLT recipients with suspected bacterial sepsis, a number of antimicrobials can be selected for empirical treatment. Empirical therapy should be guided by the suspected anatomic site of infection, the probable bacterial flora and institution-specific susceptibility patterns, any previously administered antimicrobial therapy, the time since transplantation, the severity of renal and hepatic dysfunction, and the net state of immunosuppression. Initial empirical therapy should be broad spectrum.[116] Agents commonly used for empirical therapy include third- and fourth-generation cephalosporins (ceftizoxime, ceftazidime, cefepime), a β-lactam plus β-lactamase inhibitor combination (piperacillin-tazobactam), quinolones (ciprofloxacin and levofloxacin), vancomycin, and metronidazole. If possible, the aminoglycosides are avoided due to concerns over nephrotoxicity in OLT recipients also on cyclosporine or tacrolimus. The carbapenems (imipenem, meropenem), streptogramins (quinupristin-dalfopristin), oxazolidinones (linezolid), and lipopeptides (daptomycin) are reserved for treatment of documented infections caused by resistant organisms. After a specific pathogen is isolated and sensitivities are available, a narrow-spectrum agent should be substituted whenever possible.

Specific Therapy

After isolation of a specific organism, drug therapy is guided by the results of sensitivity tests and possible drug interactions between antimicrobial drugs and immunosuppressive agents. (Table 64–3).

As previously mentioned, certain resistant nosocomial gram-negative bacteria may be isolated from liver allograft recipients, and warrant special attention.[38,92,94] Organisms such as *Enterobacter cloacae* may be resistant

Table 64-3. ANTIMICROBIAL DRUG INTERACTIONS WITH TACROLIMUS/CYCLOSPORINE/SIROLIMUS

Pharmacokinetic Drug Interactions

DRUGS THAT INCREASE TAC/CSA/SIR CONCENTRATIONS	DRUGS THAT DECREASE TAC/CSA/SIR CONCENTRATIONS
Antibacterial Agents	
Erythromycin, clarithromycin, roxithromycin (not azithromycin)	Rifampin
Clindamycin	Caspofungin (20% reduction in tacrolimus; ? effect on sirolimus);
Tetracyclines (minor inhibition of metabolism)	
Quinupristin-dalfopristin (inhibits metabolism)	
Antifungal Agents	
Fluconazole	
Itraconazole	
Voriconazole, posaconazole (less than other azole antifungals)	

Pharmacodynamic Drug Interactions

Enhanced Nephrotoxicity

Aminoglycosides (gentamicin, tobramycin, amikacin)

Trimethoprim-sulfamethoxazole (trimethoprim may interfere with the tubular secretion of creatinine or interfere with the assay for serum creatinine; it does not reduce the glomerular filtration rate)

Amphotericin B

Adefovir dipivoxil

Enhanced Neurotoxicity

imipenem-cilastatin

Antiviral agents (acyclovir, ganciclovir, lamivudine)

Other Interactions

The caspofungin area under the curve concentration is increased 35% when coadministered with cyclosporin; concomitant administration of caspofungin with cyclosporine may cause hepatic dysfunction

Selected cephalosporins with N-methylthiotetrazole side chain and metronidazole (potential disulfiram-like reaction with alcohol in intravenous preparations of cyclosporine/tacrolimus)

to third-generation cephalosporins; effective therapies for this pathogen include imipenem, ciprofloxacin, and piperacillin-tazobactam. Aminoglycosides, although generally active against *E. cloacae* and most other gram-negative bacteria, should be used judiciously in liver allograft recipients because of the risk for increased nephrotoxicity with calcineurin blockers (tacrolimus, cyclosporine). When *P. aeruginosa* is suspected or cultured, combination therapy using an antipseudomonal penicillin (piperacillin) or ceftazidime plus an aminoglycoside is recommended for possible synergistic bactericidal activity. The streptogramins (quinupristin-dalfopristin), oxazolidinones (linezolid), and lipopeptides (daptomycin) are reserved for OLT recipients with documented infections caused by *Enterococcus* resistant or only intermediately sensitive to vancomycin.

Fungal Infections

Liver transplant recipients have a higher incidence of fungal infection than other SOT recipients. In several large historical series, the incidence of fungal infection ranges between 20% and 50%.[2,7,38,45-48,117-121] However, in recent studies using antifungal prophylaxis or pre-emptive therapy, the incidence may be as low as 4% and is approximately 10% overall. Mortality rates have ranged between 38% and 40% in OLT recipients with invasive fungal infections.[2,7,38,45-48,117-124] It has been suggested that the liver transplant surgery, by disrupting the normal integrity of the biliary tract and small bowel, promotes translocation of fungal organisms colonizing the gastrointestinal tract. The majority of risk factors for fungal infection in OLT recipients have been reviewed earlier. More than 90% of fungal infections occur within the first 2 months after OLT.[124]

Spectrum of Fungal Pathogens, Clinical Features, and Diagnosis

Candida species cause about 80% of all invasive fungal infections in SOT recipients.[47,48,50,51,117-121] Candida infections in liver recipients are associated with

C. albicans (78%), *C. tropicalis* (8%), *C. glabrata* (7%), *C. parapsilosis* (5%), and *C. lusitaniae* (1%).[38,117,119-121,125-128] Recent data suggest that improvements in surgical technique and more conservative immunosuppression have reduced the incidence of fungal infection in OLT recipients and that non-*albicans* species are becoming more common, especially in patients who have received previous antifungal therapy. *Aspergillus* accounts for approximately 15% of all fungal infections, with *A. fumigatus* being most common; *A. flavus*, *A. niger*, and *A. terreus* are less common pathogens.[129-133] Additionally, sporadic fungal infections may be caused by *Cryptococcus*, endemic mycosis (coccidioidomycosis, histoplasmosis, blastomycosis), *Mucor* or emerging fungal pathogens such as *Trichosporon*, *Scedosporium*, and *Fusarium*.[40-42,48,50,51,117-121,134-136] When compared with bacterial and viral infections, fungal infections in liver transplant recipients are associated with much greater mortality (50% to 75%, but up to 100% in OLT recipients infected with *Aspergillus*). Table 64–4 summarizes the fungal pathogens seen in OLT recipients.

Candidiasis

The clinical features of candidiasis in liver transplant recipients can take several forms: local invasive infection, dissemination with involvement of several sites, and candidemia without evidence of tissue invasion. Candidal syndromes include mucocutaneous infection, wound infection, esophagitis, abdominal infection (visceral involvement in the liver/spleen, cholangitis, peritonitis, abdominal abscesses), candiduria, catheter-associated infection, and candidemia. Clinically, the features of candidiasis in liver allograft recipients differ from those in other SOT recipients by the preponderance of abdominal infections.[119,121] The onset of candidiasis may be sudden with fever, chills, and malaise, or it may be insidious. A septic shock syndrome may accompany disseminated candidiasis or candidemia.

A high index of suspicion is required for the timely diagnosis of invasive *Candida* infection. The diagnosis of deeply invasive or disseminated candidiasis may be difficult and often requires multiple blood cultures, invasive biopsy with histological examination, or radiological procedures. Isolation of *Candida* from blood cultures has improved through use of the lysis-centrifugation system.[137-140] Recently, several tests have been evaluated for detecting various *Candida* antigens in serum and urine. Detection of mannan or other proteins in serum by latex agglutination, enzyme immunosorbent assay, or radioimmunosorbent assay has been performed. Nucleic acid detection by PCR is also being used to diagnose *Candida* infection. However, the accuracy of these tests in OLT recipients needs to be further established before they are used routinely.[140] The use of surveillance cultures for predicting invasive candidiasis has also been reported. Although isolation of *Candida* from multiple body sites or fluids raises suspicion of invasive disease, results should be interpreted with caution because not all colonized patients experience candidiasis. Nevertheless, the presence of *Candida* in multiple surveillance culture sites in a patient who is febrile despite antibacterial therapy may be sufficient to initiate empirical systemic antifungal therapy.

Aspergillosis

Invasive aspergillosis is often a fatal complication after liver transplantation despite currently available therapies. *Aspergillus* species account for approximately 10% to 20% of all fungal infections in liver transplant recipients, with *A. fumigatus* being the predominant species in OLT recipients.[38,117,119,121,129-133] Additional species such as *A. flavus*, *A. terreus*, and *A. niger* have also been observed. *Aspergillus* spores are ubiquitous. *Aspergillus* can be a nosocomial pathogen causing contamination of hospital air, especially during periods of hospital construction or renovation. The organism can be found in ventilation systems and hospital water. Once *Aspergillus* spores are inhaled, *Aspergillus* colonizes the respiratory tract of immunocompromised hosts. As the use of immunosuppressive agents is intensified, a reduction in macrophage and immunosurveillance activity is

Table 64-4. COMMON FUNGAL PATHOGENS IN ORTHOTOPIC LIVER TRANSPLANT RECIPIENTS

Fungemia	Pulmonary Disease	Urinary Tract	Central Nervous System	Skin/Subcutaneous
Candida	*Aspergillus*	*Candida*	*Aspergillus*	*Candida*
Fusarium	*Cryptococcus*		*Pseudallescheria boydii*	Dermatophytes
Cryptococcus	*Pseudallescheria boydii*		*Cryptococcus*	*Aspergillus*
Trichosporum	*Histoplasma capsulatum*		*Coccidioides immitis*	*Fusarium*
	Coccidioides immitis		Zygomycoses (*Rhizopus, Mucor, Cunninghamella, Apophysomyces, Absidia*)	*Pseudallescheria boydii*
				Dematiaceous fungi
				Zygomycoses (*Rhizopus, Mucor*)

thought to occur and lead to invasive disease. Detection of *Aspergillus* from one or more sites has been predictive of significant infection and a poor prognosis.[121,129,130] The reported incidence of aspergillosis after OLT varies among transplant centers, depending on local institutional factors and diagnostic criteria. Although an incidence as high as 22% has been reported from Italy, others have reported an incidence between 1.5% and 4% when more specific criteria for diagnosis are used.[124,131] Aspergillosis primarily occurs within the first 2 to 6 weeks after transplantation (median time to onset of 1.2 months).[5,7,38,117,119-121,129-131] Occasionally, *Aspergillus* infection may be diagnosed in OLT recipients beyond the third month, usually related to chronic graft failure, increased immunosuppression, or repeat transplantation. Additional factors associated with *Aspergillus* infection include renal failure requiring dialysis and antirejection therapy.

In liver transplant recipients, clinical manifestations of *Aspergillus* infection include localized invasive pulmonary disease, necrotizing pneumonia, sinusitis, wound infections, and disseminated disease with CNS involvement (brain abscess).[5,38,117,121,129-131] Of importance, the features of the most common manifestation, acute pulmonary aspergillosis, can be quite variable. Fever and sputum production are not always present. The initial findings may be indolent and manifested solely as a slowly developing pneumonia on chest radiographs. Many patients have pulmonary infiltrates and fever that fail to respond to antibacterial therapy. Others may have wedge-shaped infiltrates and symptoms of pulmonary infarction. Hemoptysis is often a clue to the diagnosis. Exsanguinating pulmonary hemorrhage may occasionally occur in OLT recipients.

CNS infection by *Aspergillus* is usually manifested as single or multiple brain abscesses and very rarely as meningitis. CNS disease is usually part of disseminated infection. The initial manifestation may be a stroke as a result of vascular involvement causing thrombosis or hemorrhage.

Infection of surgical wounds by *Aspergillus* occurs in 6% to 20% of OLT recipients with *Aspergillus* infection.[119,141] An uncommon soft tissue infection caused by *Aspergillus* in OLT recipients occurs 3 or more months after transplantation and is characterized by violaceous cutaneous nodules. In contrast to the other forms of aspergillosis, the prognosis of this infection is favorable after excision and treatment with antifungal drug therapy.

The diagnosis of invasive aspergillosis can be made by culture, nucleic acid detection, antigen detection, histopathology, or radiological examination.[137-143] *Aspergillus* infection is usually confirmed by finding characteristic septate hyphae in tissue obtained by biopsy or by identification of the pathogen in a culture of the same tissue. However, many recipients are not able to undergo invasive diagnostic procedures because

of underlying coagulopathy or overall poor medical condition. Although isolation of *Aspergillus* by culture of sputum or bronchoscopically obtained material may represent only colonization, a positive respiratory tract culture should alert one to the possibility of invasive disease.[141] If the patient has clinical findings on the chest radiograph or chest CT compatible with *Aspergillus* pneumonia, antifungal therapy should be initiated (see later). Similarly, detection of multiple mass lesions in the brain on CT or MRI in a patient with pneumonia and a positive respiratory tract culture is usually enough to initiate therapy for disseminated infection with CNS involvement.

Unfortunately, almost all *Aspergillus* infections of the CNS are fatal unless there is an isolated single abscess that can be surgically drained.[5,117,121,129] CNS infections usually appear as one or more low-density, nonenhancing mass lesions on head CT in a patient with acute neurological deterioration. The introduction of the second-generation triazole voriconazole may improve the outcome of OLT recipients with CNS infection. Blood cultures are rarely positive for *Aspergillus*. Thus, negative cultures do not exclude invasive disease.

Difficulty in establishing the diagnosis of invasive disease has led to efforts to develop serological testing for *Aspergillus* antibodies or circulating fungal antigens (e.g., *Aspergillus* galactomannan), as well as PCR.[137-139,142,143] However, these tests have generally lacked the sensitivity and specificity for routine clinical use. A sensitivity of 50% to 90% plus a specificity of 81% to 93% for the diagnosis of invasive *Aspergillus* infection has been reported with the galactomannan assay.[137-139,142,143] A potential benefit of this test is the ability to detect antigen before the appearance of clinical or radiological signs of invasive disease.

Cryptococcosis

The overall incidence of cryptococcal infection is 2.4% (range, 0.3% to 6%) in liver transplant recipients.[38,117,134,144-146] Cryptococcal infection may present as either a fungemia or pneumonia within the first month after OLT or as a meningitis beyond 3 months after transplantation. Early postoperative manifestations of cryptococcal infection are seen in OLT recipients with far-advanced end-stage liver disease before transplantation.[146] Overall mortality as a result of cryptococcal infection in SOT recipients is 42%.[5,7,38,117,134,145,146] Of interest, tacrolimus is thought to possess some inherent antifungal activity and perhaps reduce the risk of cryptococcal infection in OLT recipients receiving this agent.

Endemic Mycosis

Although infections caused by endemic mycosis are infrequently reported in transplant recipients, cases of coccidioidomycosis, blastomycosis, and histoplasmosis have been documented.[5,7,38,42,50,51,117]

C. immitis is a dimorphic fungus endemic to the southwestern United States and northern Mexico. Characteristically, pulmonary disease is the primary manifestation of infection, with systemic disease resulting from early dissemination to bone, joints, skin, and meninges. Coccidioidomycosis in SOT recipients has been reported, either from reactivation or from newly acquired disease.[50,51,140,141] Of interest, we reported seven cases of coccidioidomycosis in liver transplant recipients after the 1994 Northridge earthquake and a subsequent prolonged seasonal drought.[135] In these recipients, coccidioidomycosis occurred 1 month to 5 years after transplantation, and had a 50% mortality rate despite systemic antifungal therapy.[135]

B. dermatitidis is a dimorphic fungus endemic to the Ohio and Mississippi River Valleys and the upper midwestern United States in areas bordering the Great Lakes and southern Canadian region. Blastomycosis has been reported in renal, heart, and liver allograft recipients.[38,50,51] Clinical manifestations in OLT recipients include progressive respiratory involvement with nodular, lobar, or cavitary pneumonia, and disseminated infection involving the skin (pyogranulomatous lesions), meninges, and retina. Reactivation of disease has occurred during immunosuppressive therapy from 1 month to longer than 4 years after transplantation.

H. capsulatum is a dimorphic fungus endemic to the Ohio and Mississippi River Valleys. Cases of histoplasmosis in OLT recipients have been reported between 3 months and 19 years after transplant and represent either reactivation of latent lesions or new exposure in *Histoplasma*-endemic zones.[38,42,50,51,117,119] Patients receiving treatment for rejection are at increased risk. Pulmonary disease is the most common presentation, although necrotizing myofasciitis, meningitis, gastrointestinal involvement with perforation, and portal vein obstruction may occur. Donor-derived histoplasmosis in liver allografts has been reported and generally results in disseminated disease leading to graft loss and rarely death. These cases strongly support the requirement for performing a thorough donor exposure review, especially in zones of endemic mycosis.

Emerging Fungal Pathogens

Infections caused by emerging fungal pathogens in SOT recipients have recently been reported.[38,50,51,147,148] Some of these pathogens include *Acremonium* spp., *Beauveria* spp., *Chrysosporium* spp., *Fusarium* spp., *Geotrichum* spp., *Paecilomyces* spp., *Penicillium marneffei*, *Pseudallescheria boydii* (sexual state; *Scedosporium apiospermum* reflects the asexual state of *P. boydii*), *Trichoderma* spp., *Rhizopus oryzae*, and *Mucor* spp. These pathogens may pose significant challenges in

liver transplant recipients because of lack of effective therapy. Finally, zygomycosis is a rare but highly invasive fungal infection that develops in OLT recipients.[147] The rhinocerebral form can occur in up to 57% of cases, the pulmonary, cutaneous and disseminated forms develop in another 39% of cases, and gastrointestinal and renal forms account for the remaining infections. One hundred percent mortality has been associated with the disseminated form, whereas only 50% is seen with the rhinocerebral form. The median time of occurrence is 2 months after OLT (range, 5 days to 8 years), with specific risk factors including diabetes and the use of corticosteroids to treat acute allograft rejection.

Management of Fungal Infections

To reduce the morbidity and mortality associated with fungal infections in OLT recipients, several treatment strategies have been attempted. Initially, the development of any serious fungal infection in a transplant recipient demands a critical evaluation of the immunosuppressive regimen. The corticosteroid dose should be minimized, blood levels of cyclosporine and tacrolimus should be kept in the low therapeutic range, and adjunctive agents can often be temporarily discontinued. Failure of clinical response to an antifungal regimen may require discontinuation of immunosuppression, even at the cost of abandoning the graft. Additional strategies include the administration of antifungal agents for both prevention (prophylaxis) and treatment of infection. These approaches are discussed in the following sections.

Fungal Prophylaxis

Among solid organ transplant recipients, patients undergoing liver transplantation are at greatest risk for the development of invasive fungal infection. Thus, several trials have been performed to assess the impact of antifungal prophylaxis. Agents used for antifungal prophylaxis have included clotrimazole, nystatin, conventional amphotericin B, lipid-based formulations of amphotericin B, and the azoles (fluconazole, itraconazole, and voriconazole).[5,47]

Caspofungin, an echinocandin antifungal, may also be effective, but no trials have evaluated this drug for prophylaxis in SOT recipients.

Triazoles

Fluconazole, itraconazole, and voriconazole exert their antifungal effects by inhibiting ergosterol, the principal sterol in the fungal cell membrane.[149-151] Ergosterol synthesis is interrupted through azole inhibition of

C-14 α-demethylase, an enzyme dependent on cytochrome P450. This leads to defective cell membranes with altered permeability. Because this inhibitory effect is not selective for fungal cytochrome P450, human cytochrome P450 isoenzymes are also altered, thus leading to changes in the metabolic rate of various endogenous and exogenous substances, including cyclosporine and tacrolimus.

The spectrum of activity of fluconazole includes *Candida* species (but not *C. glabrata* or *C. krusei)*, *Cryptococcus neoformans* and dimorphic fungi (*C. immitis, B. dermatitidis*). Molds and filamentous fungi such as *Aspergillus, Rhizopus, Fusarium,* and *Scedosporium,* are not usually susceptible to fluconazole.[149-151] These pathogens are of concern because their frequency is increasing in immunocompromised hosts. Fluconazole can be administered intravenously but also has excellent oral bioavailability and is well tolerated.

Itraconazole has a spectrum of activity which includes *Aspergillus* as well as *Candida.*[50,51,149-151] Although itraconazole capsules have erratic bioavailability dependent upon gastric acidity, the oral itraconazole solution containing hydroxypropyl-β-cyclodextrin is much better absorbed and has been shown to have adequate bioavailability in liver transplant recipients for effective prophylaxis. Except for gastrointestinal side effects (nausea, vomiting, abdominal pain), oral itraconazole is well tolerated.

Several controlled trials evaluating fluconazole, oral itraconazole solution, or lipid-based amphotericin B for prophylaxis have been reported in OLT recipients (Table 64–5).[152-157] Results from large randomized, controlled trials of fluconazole versus placebo (or itraconazole versus fluconazole) conducted at our institution indicate that the incidence of both superficial and systemic fungal infection may be reduced and that both have utility as prophylactic antifungal agents.[153,155] Other researchers have also published the benefit of itraconazole (versus placebo) in reducing fungal infection in OLT recipients.[156] Voriconazole is a second-generation triazole with increased activity for *Aspergillus,* *Candida, Scedosporium,* and *Fusarium.* Voriconazole has demonstrated clinical efficacy in the treatment of invasive aspergillosis and *Scedosporium* and *Fusarium* infections.[150,158] The drug is available in an intravenous and oral dosage form, has an exceptional pharmacokinetic profile, and is hepatically metabolized. Currently, no prophylactic trials with voriconazole have been conducted in OLT recipients, but its potential use in this capacity is attractive.

Fluconazole, itraconazole, and voriconazole inhibit cytochrome P450 isoenzymes and have clinically significant drug interactions with calcineurin immunosuppressive agents (see Table 64–3).[159-162] These agents may increase the concentration of tacrolimus or cyclosporine and enhance the risk of toxicity. When fluconazole, itraconazole, and voriconazole are discontinued, a decrease in calcineurin blocker concentrations leading to rejection can occur. *Thus, close monitoring of blood concentrations and the dosing of cyclosporine and tacrolimus is necessary when initiating or discontinuing azole therapy. Of note, administration of voriconazole is contraindicated in OLT recipients treated with sirolimus* because of an 11-fold increase in sirolimus concentration after the administration of voriconazole.[163] Further descriptions of interactions between azole drugs and immunosuppressive agents have been reviewed elsewhere and are summarized in Table 64–3.[159-162]

Echinocandins

The echinocandin antifungal agents, caspofungin and micafungin, inhibit the synthesis of 1,3β-D-glucan in the fungal cell wall.[164-166] Caspofungin and micafungin have been used effectively for candidiasis and invasive aspergillosis refractory to other antifungal drugs.[166] The echinocandins have activity against species of *Candida* that are resistant to fluconazole and other azoles, but are not active against *Cryptococcus.*[164-166] Both caspofungin and micafungin are currently available only in an intravenous formulation and are generally

Table 64–5. RANDOMIZED CONTROLLED TRIALS OF FUNGAL PROPHYLAXIS IN LIVER TRANSPLANT RECIPIENTS

Author	Regimen	Incidence of Fungal Infection
Lumbreras[152]	Fluconazole, 100 mg/day PO, versus nystatin, 1 mU qid × 28 days	2/67 (3%) versus 6/67 (9%)
Winston[153]	Fluconazole, 400 mg/day IV/PO, versus placebo qd × 10 wk	10/108 (9%) versus 45/104 (43%)
Winston[155]	Fluconazole, 400 mg/day IV/PO, versus itraconazole solution, 200 mg q12h PO × 10 wk	4/91 (4%) versus 9/97 (9%)
Sharpe[156]	Itraconazole solution, 5-mg/kg loading dose PO, then 2.5 mg/kg PO bid, versus placebo until POD 56, discharge, or endpoint	1/25 (4%) versus 6/37 (16%)
Tollemar[157]	AmBisome, 1 mg/kg IV qd, versus placebo until POD 5	0/40 (0%) versus 6/37 (16%)

well-tolerated. Although initial studies suggested an increased risk for hepatotoxicity when caspofungin is used concomitantly with cyclosporine, subsequent clinical experience suggests that the drug can be safely used with cyclosporine.[164-166] A randomized, controlled trial has shown that micafungin is more effective than fluconazole for antifungal prophylaxis in stem cell transplant patients. However, there have been no trials evaluating the prophylactic efficacy of the echinocandins in liver transplant recipients.

Amphotericin

Amphotericin B binds to sterols and causes pore formation in the fungal cytoplasmic membrane, thereby facilitating leakage of intracellular potassium and other molecules by disrupting osmotic integrity and leading to impaired viability of fungal cells.[167,168]

The spectrum of activity of amphotericin B includes most pathogenic yeasts (*Candida* spp., *Cryptococcus neoformans*), dimorphic fungi (*Blastomyces, Histoplasma, C. immitis, Paracoccidioides*), and mold or filamentous fungi (*Aspergillus* spp., *Mucor, Rhizopus*). Fungi such as *Trichosporon*, some *Penicillium* species, and *Pseudallescheria* are generally considered less sensitive or resistant to amphotericin B.[167,168] The most common adverse effects of amphotericin B are infusion-related reactions, nephrotoxicity, and electrolyte imbalances. Of note, lipid-based formulations of amphotericin B have been produced which are as efficacious as conventional amphotericin B, but less toxic. Currently, three formulations are commercially available (AmBisome, Abelcet, and Amphotec).[169-177]

Limited data are available regarding the use of prophylactic amphotericin B in OLT recipients. Low-dose amphotericin B deoxycholate (0.1 to 0.2 mg/kg/day) did not prevent *Aspergillus* infection and was associated with significant toxicity in OLT recipients.[5] In one trial using lipid amphotericin, Singh and colleagues demonstrated a significant reduction in invasive fungal infections in high-risk OLT recipients (dialysis dependant) receiving 5 mg/kg/day of a lipid formulation of amphotericin B in comparison to a historical control.[173] Another study described the use of low-dose prophylactic liposomal amphotericin B versus placebo in 85 OLT recipients.[157] Patients received 1 mg/kg/day for 5 days. Among 40 AmBisome-treated patients, no invasive *Candida* infection was reported during the first month versus five invasive *Candida* infections in the 37 control patients (*P* <.05). These lipid-based formulations of amphotericin B are expensive. Future prophylactic studies comparing lipid-based amphotericin B products with triazoles (fluconazole, itraconazole, or voriconazole), or the echinocandins (caspofungin or micafungin) are needed to determine their relative therapeutic benefit, toxicity, drug interactions, and cost-effectiveness for prophylaxis of fungal infections in OLT recipients.

Treatment of Fungal Infections

Management of invasive mycosis in OLT recipients depends on rapid recognition of infection (diagnosis), appropriate modification of immunosuppressive therapy, surgical interventions (débridement, removal of infected catheters, drainage of fluid collections), and timely administration of antifungal agents. The choice of antifungal agent is often based on antifungal spectrum and toxicity of the drug, the potential for drug interactions with immunosuppressive agents, and cost. Historically, amphotericin B had been the antifungal agent of choice for the treatment of most systemic fungal infections in OLT recipients. However, concern over nephrotoxicity when amphotericin B is used with tacrolimus or cyclosporine has lead to the more frequent use of newer, less toxic agents.

Candidiasis

Candidiasis in OLT recipients can be treated with amphotericin B deoxycholate, 0.6 to 1.0 mg/kg/day.[5] In seriously ill patients, a stepwise increase in the amphotericin B dose is not recommended. Patients should receive the full therapeutic dose immediately after a test dose of 1 mg. A total dose of at least 1 g of amphotericin B is usually given for documented invasive candidiasis, whereas patients receiving empirical therapy for suspected, but undocumented infection may require less if they clinically improve. Renal toxicity is a common adverse effect associated with amphotericin B in OLT recipients who are also receiving tacrolimus or cyclosporine. In patients who are intolerant of this formulation or have underlying renal dysfunction, lipid-based amphotericin B products may be used, as well as fluconazole, caspofungin, or micafungin (for susceptible pathogens). For non-*albicans* species of *Candida*, agents such as caspofungin, micafungin, and voriconazole may be useful alternatives to fluconazole or amphotericin B. Potential drug interactions with these agents and immunosuppressive drugs should be closely monitored to avoid adverse effects.

Aspergillosis

Treatment of invasive aspergillosis in OLT recipients with amphotericin B deoxycholate (1.0 to 1.5 mg/kg/day) has generally been unsatisfactory.[5] While underlying host factors are largely responsible for these poor results, several investigators have suggested that lipid-based preparations of amphotericin B may be more effective.[157]

In a recent randomized, controlled, trial, voriconazole was more effective than amphotericin B deoxycholate for initial therapy of invasive aspergillosis.[178] Itraconazole has been used primarily as follow-up therapy in patients with aspergillosis responding to amphotericin. Caspofungin is approved for salvage therapy of invasive aspergillosis failing to respond to other antifungal drugs but has not been formally evaluated for primary therapy.[165,166]

Based on in vitro and animal studies showing synergy between an echinocandin (caspofungin or micafungin) active on the fungal cell wall and an azole (voriconazole or itraconazole) or amphotericin B active on the fungal cell membrane, there may be a potential role for combination antifungal therapy for treatment of more severe cases of aspergillosis. However, the clinical efficacy of combination therapy relative to monotherapy needs further study. [179]

Viral Infections

Viral infections are a major problem in allograft recipients, particularly 1 to 6 months after transplantation (see Fig. 64–1). Clinical disease may occur later, especially after intensification of immunosuppression or physiological insults that increase the net state of immunosuppression.

Cytomegalovirus

Historically, CMV was the most common viral pathogen found after liver transplantation, with an estimated incidence of 30% to 78%, depending on the serological status of the donor and recipient. Symptomatic CMV infection or CMV disease was reported in about 20% to 30% of all OLT patients.[2,33-35,39,180-189] The incidences of infection and disease are also dramatically influenced by the use of prophylaxis and the net state of immunosuppression.

CMV infection can be either a primary infection or reactivation of a previously latent infection. The highest incidence of primary infection is among CMV-seronegative liver transplant patients who receive a liver from a CMV-seropositive donor. These patients also have a higher incidence of symptomatic CMV disease than CMV-seropositive patients. The donor liver and blood transfusions are the sources for primary infection. In CMV- seropositive transplant recipients, preexisting latent CMV infection is usually reactivated, and the incidence of infection and disease is intermediate between that of the CMV-negative/CMV-negative donor- recipient group and the CMV-positive/CMV-negative donor-recipient group.

Most CMV infections occur between 3 and 8 weeks after transplantation, with a peak incidence during the fifth posttransplant week.[33-35,39,186-189] Late CMV disease, occurring beyond the eighth week after transplantation, can be seen in patients who require retransplantation or who are treated for rejection. In addition to the CMV serological status of both the donor and recipient, the type and extent of immunosuppression and rejection therapy may have an impact on the incidence of CMV disease. Treatment of rejection with antilymphocytic globulin, muromonab-CD3, or thymoglobulin especially increases the incidence of CMV disease.[1,39,185,190] Modalities that reduce allograft rejection may have an effect on the incidence and severity of CMV disease. Of note, a randomized study comparing cyclosporine with tacrolimus showed an increased requirement for additional immunosuppression in the cyclosporine group along with a trend for more frequent symptomatic CMV infections.[190] Studies using mycophenolate mofetil have also demonstrated trends toward an increase in the incidence of CMV infection in renal allograft, but not OLT recipients. CMV infection has likewise been associated with chronic rejection in some studies but not others.[35,39,180,182,191,192]

The clinical manifestations of CMV infection in liver transplant patients are variable. Many patients have asymptomatic infection detectable only by performing routine surveillance tests for viral DNA or antigen. Direct clinical effects of CMV infection include fever, malaise, anorexia, myalgia, and arthralgia. Hematological abnormalities, namely, atypical lymphocytosis, neutropenia, and thrombocytopenia, and elevation of liver function test values may also occur in OLT recipients.

CMV hepatitis is the most common type of symptomatic CMV disease in liver transplant patients and accounts for about half of all cases of CMV disease. The clinical and laboratory findings of CMV hepatitis are often indistinguishable from those of acute rejection. A liver biopsy is required to make the distinction. Liver biopsy specimens from liver transplant recipients with CMV hepatitis usually have histological evidence of CMV infection (intranuclear inclusions, neutrophil or mononuclear cell aggregates surrounding necrotic debris). In contrast, viral cultures of liver tissue are frequently negative. CMV DNA probes may also enhance detection of CMV in the liver. The prognosis of uncomplicated CMV hepatitis is excellent. Ganciclovir therapy is given to most patients, although some patients with CMV hepatitis may recover without any therapy.[33] The prognosis is worse when CMV hepatitis follows resistant allograft rejection or ischemia or is associated with disseminated CMV disease.

CMV pneumonia occurs less frequently but is reported in as many as a third of patients with CMV disease, frequently in association with viremia or hepatitis. Pneumonitis is the most serious sequela of CMV infection and is manifested by dyspnea, hypoxemia, and interstitial infiltrates.

CMV infection of the gastrointestinal tract also occurs and is probably overlooked in many patients who have nonspecific gastrointestinal symptoms. CMV upper and lower gastrointestinal disease is manifested as esophagitis, duodenitis, or colitis. Diagnostic endoscopy can reveal solitary or multiple ulcerations and hemorrhage; biopsy material should be examined by immunohistochemical or cytological methods for CMV antigens or inclusion bodies, respectively. Other types of CMV disease, including CMV retinitis, are very rare after liver transplantation.

The indirect effects of CMV are associated with immunomodulatory derangements (such as reduced helper-to-suppressor T-cell ratio) that can lead to opportunistic bacterial or fungal superinfections, allograft injury or rejection, and the development of PTLD. CMV may incite proinflammatory cytokines (e.g., tumor necrosis factor), which can bind to latently infected cells, and generate nuclear transcription factors that initiate CMV replication.[5,7,35,38,117] CMV infection induces endothelial cell antibodies and the in vitro expression of HLA class I and class II antigens, which may also be risk factors for both acute and chronic rejection (vanishing bile duct syndrome), although these associations have been disputed in the literature.[5]

Diagnosis

CMV can be isolated from culture of various clinical specimens, and a monoclonal antibody against early viral antigens can be used to detect the early presence of CMV in conventional cell or shell vial culture. Enzyme immunoassay or other serological assays can detect CMV IgM or IgG in a previously seronegative patient, although some transplant recipients may fail to mount an antibody response to their infections.[7,38,193-197] Thus, serologic tests cannot be relied upon for the diagnosis of active CMV infection.

CMV DNA assays involve a signal-amplified hybridization assay for detection and quantitation of CMV DNA in peripheral white blood cells.[194,195] The CMV antigenemia assay detects the presence of CMV antigens in white blood cells.[198,199] After effective treatment of symptomatic CMV disease, CMV DNA may persist despite the disappearance of antigenemia.

Management

The availability of effective agents for CMV prophylaxis and treatment has greatly diminished the morbidity and mortality associated with CMV infection after transplantation. Treatment of active CMV disease is usually initiated with intravenous ganciclovir. There are limited data on the efficacy of oral valganciclovir for treatment of CMV disease in transplant recipients.[199-201] Oral valganciclovir may be an option for patients who initially improve on intravenous ganciclovir but then require continued maintenance therapy or prophylaxis against recurrent disease. Frequent monitoring for signs and symptoms of CMV disease is warranted after a treatment course of ganciclovir in liver transplant recipients with ongoing risk factors for CMV disease. CMV DNA and antigen tests of the blood are commonly used to monitor patients during and after treatment for CMV disease.[200,201] The most common adverse effects of ganciclovir are granulocytopenia and thrombocytopenia.[200,201]

Most cases of CMV disease respond to ganciclovir monotherapy. Some transplant physicians add CMV hyperimmune globulin or polyvalent intravenous immune globulin to ganciclovir if the patient has CMV pneumonia or fails to improve on ganciclovir alone.[200,202] Foscarnet and cidofovir have been used to treat the infrequent patient who has infection caused by a ganciclovir-resistant strain of CMV or who cannot tolerate ganciclovir due to toxicity. Both foscarnet and cidofovir have nephrotoxicity.[200,203-205]

Prophylaxis

Several prophylactic strategies have been used to reduce CMV infection and disease in liver allograft recipients.[180-182,184,200,206] By recognizing the CMV serological status of the donor and recipient before transplantation and by assessing the net state of immunosuppression, CMV prophylactic strategies can be optimized to limit the incidence of CMV disease.

CMV prophylaxis regimens used in transplant recipients include monotherapy with antiviral agents such as acyclovir, ganciclovir, and valganciclovir; monotherapy with CMV immune globulin; or a combination of antiviral agents and CMV immune globulin (Table 64-6).[184,206-223] Currently, most liver transplantation centers use a ganciclovir-based regimen for either routine prophylaxis or as part of a preemptive treatment approach.

In a randomized comparison of intravenous ganciclovir and high-dose acyclovir, long-term therapy with ganciclovir over the first 100 days after transplant was superior to acyclovir in preventing CMV in OLT recipients.[212] Subsequent to this trial, a prophylactic regimen of 2 weeks of intravenous ganciclovir followed by an additional 12 weeks of oral ganciclovir (3 g/day) was superior to a regimen of intravenous ganciclovir followed by oral acyclovir (3200 mg/day) until postoperative day 100.[218] Ultimately, this ganciclovir-based regimen almost completely eliminated CMV disease without the emergence of ganciclovir resistance. In a third randomized, controlled trial comparing sequential intravenous and oral ganciclovir with prolonged intravenous ganciclovir for long-term prophylaxis of CMV

Table 64-6. RANDOMIZED CONTROLLED TRIALS OF CYTOMEGALOVIRUS PROPHYLAXIS IN LIVER TRANSPLANT RECIPIENTS

Author	Regimen	CMV Infection	CMV Disease
Saliba[208]	IV acyclovir, 500 mg/m² q8h × 10 days, then PO acyclovir, 800 mg qid, versus observation	11/60 (18%) versus 22/60 (37%)	4/60 (7%) versus 13/60 (22%)
Snydman[210]	CMVIG, 150 mg/kg q2-4wk × 120 days, versus placebo	39/69 (57%) versus 44/72 (61%)	13/69 (19%) versus 22/72 (31%)
Martin[211]	IV ganciclovir, 5 mg/kg q12h × 14 days, then PO acyclovir, 800 mg qid × 76 days, versus acyclovir, 800 mg PO qid × 90 days	17/69 (25%) versus 42/71 (59%)	7/69 (10%) versus 19/71 (27%)
Winston[212]	IV ganciclovir, 6 mg/kg/day × 30 days, then IV ganciclovir, 6 mg/kg/day (Monday–Friday) × 70 days, versus IV acyclovir, 10 mg/kg/day from POD 1 to discharge, then PO acyclovir, 800 mg qid from discharge until POD 100	6/124 (5%) versus 48/126 (38%)	1/126 (0.8%) versus 12/126 (10%)
Gane[216]	PO ganciclovir, 1000 mg tid until POD 98, versus placebo	37/150 (25%) versus 79/154 (51%)	7/150 (5%) versus 29/154 (19%)
Winston[218*]	IV ganciclovir, 6 mg/kg/day on POD 1-14, then PO ganciclovir, 1000 mg tid, or PO acyclovir, 800 mg qid from POD 15–100	Not reported	1/110 (0.9%) versus 8/109 (7%)
Winston[219†]	IV ganciclovir, 6 mg/kg/day from POD 1-14, then PO ganciclovir, 1000 mg/day, or IV ganciclovir, 6 mg/kg/day Monday–Friday from POD 15–100	Not reported	3/32 (9%) versus 4/32 (13%)

*Cytomegalovirus-seropositive transplant recipients only.
†CMV-seronegative transplant recipients with CMV-seropositive donors.
CMVIG, cytomegalovirus immune globulin; POD, post-operative day.

disease in high-risk OLT patients, CMV disease occurred in 3 of 32 patients (9.3%) receiving oral ganciclovir and in 4 of 32 patients (12.5%) receiving intravenous ganciclovir within the first 100 days after transplantation (P >0.2).[219] There were no deaths from CMV in either study group. These results support the use of induction with 14 days of intravenous ganciclovir followed by long-term oral ganciclovir in high-risk CMV-seronegative liver transplant recipients with CMV-seropositive donors.

Others have shown that oral ganciclovir (3 g/day) compared to placebo provides effective CMV prophylaxis (4.8% versus 18.9% incidence of CMV disease, respectively) in CMV-seropositive liver transplant recipients.[216] Similarly, 900 mg of oral valganciclovir (a valine ester prodrug of ganciclovir with 60% bioavailability[220]) was compared with oral ganciclovir (3000 mg/day) for prophylaxis during the initial 100 days after transplant in CMV-seronegative SOT recipients receiving organs from CMV-seropositive donors.[221] This study demonstrated that oral valganciclovir (900 mg/day) was as effective as oral ganciclovir (3 g/day) for prevention of CMV in high-risk SOT recipients (17.2% versus 18.4% incidence of CMV disease at 1 year, respectively) and was well tolerated.[220,221]

Another effective approach to prevention of CMV disease is preemptive therapy or initiation of ganciclovir in an asymptomatic patient with a positive surveillance test result (culture, antigenemia, PCR) predictive of CMV disease. This strategy is designed to restrict prophylaxis to high-risk OLT patients and subsequently reduce drug costs and drug-induced toxicity. Preemptive therapy has been very successful in low-risk CMV-seropositive transplant recipients but has been studied in only a limited number of CMV-seronegative recipients with CMV-seropositive donors.[224-231]

Patients who are treated with OKT3 or polyclonal antibodies also have a high incidence of symptomatic CMV disease. Preemptive intravenous ganciclovir therapy (6 mg/kg/day) administered during antibody treatment can reduce the incidence of CMV disease.[232] Liver transplant recipients who require multiple treatments for rejection may also require additional courses of CMV prophylaxis to diminish the occurrence of CMV disease. Intravenous ganciclovir, followed by oral ganciclovir (3 g/day), or oral valganciclovir (900 mg/day), has been used in this setting. Patients should be assessed clinically regarding their risk for reactivation of CMV as a function of their cumulative net state of immunosuppression.

Herpes Simplex Virus

The majority of patients who undergo liver transplantation are seropositive for HSV. Without antiviral prophylaxis, reactivated HSV infection develops in as many as 40% of these patients, usually during the initial 3 weeks after transplantation.[5,38,187,233-235] Occasionally, infection occurs many months later. HSV infection usually involves mucosal surfaces. In 5% of patients with HSV infection, the disease is manifested as esophagitis or hepatitis.

Fatal disseminated HSV infection with visceral involvement very rarely occurs.[233-235] The diagnosis of HSV infection is confirmed by isolation of the virus in culture. Both acyclovir and ganciclovir are active against HSV in vitro, and both can prevent HSV infection. Acyclovir, valacyclovir, and famciclovir are used for treatment of HSV infection.

Varicella-Zoster Virus

Primary or de novo varicella can be a serious complication after liver transplantation and can cause a severe hemorrhagic rash and multiple organ failure.[38,233,235-237] In contrast, herpes zoster infection, which occurs in 5% to 10% of liver transplant recipients seropositive for VZV antibody, is usually a localized cutaneous disease that rarely disseminates.[38,240,242-244] Acyclovir, valacyclovir, and famciclovir can be used for treatment of herpes zoster and varicella. Intravenous acyclovir (10 mg/kg every 8 hours if kidney function is normal) is frequently recommended for the initial treatment of varicella or herpes zoster virus in transplant patients. After improvement, therapy may be changed to high-dose oral acyclovir or valacyclovir. Disseminated VZV, usually as a result of primary VZV infection, is rare but may cause pneumonia, encephalitis, disseminated intravascular coagulation, and graft dysfunction. If a seronegative patient is inadvertently exposed to a person with varicella or herpes zoster virus, prophylactic zoster immune globulin should be administered.

Epstein-Barr Virus

On the basis of results of serological tests before and after transplantation, primary or reactivated EBV infection occurs in up to 25% of liver transplant patients. The timing of the infection can be quite variable, but the majority of patients are affected within the first 6 months after transplantation.[13-16,238-241] In most patients, the infection is asymptomatic. However, seronegative patients who experience primary infection are at greater risk for symptomatic EBV disease. Fever, lymphadenopathy, pharyngitis, splenomegaly, and atypical lymphocytosis are common features of the disease. Atypical findings such as a prolonged mononucleosis-like illness lasting several weeks, pneumonia, and encephalitis have also been observed.[70,71] Hepatitis with mild elevation of liver enzymes may likewise occur.

EBV is a B-cell lymphotropic virus capable of inducing proliferative changes leading to frank lymphoma, especially when immune surveillance is overly impaired by muromonab-CD3 or thymoglobulin. Such EBV-associated post-transplant lymphoproliferative disorders (PTLDs) are serious complications that can evolve from polyclonal reactive lymphoid hyperplasias to monoclonal large cell lymphomas. In one center's long-term experience of 4000 liver transplants, 170 (4.3%) experienced PTLD. The incidence was significantly higher in children than in adults (9.7% versus 2.9%, respectively), with a similar incidence in patients receiving cyclosporine or tacrolimus. The 1-year patient survival rate in OLT recipients without PTLD was 85%, whereas the actuarial survival rate in patients with PTLD was estimated at 45%.[241]

The presence of the EBV genome in lymphoid tissue has been demonstrated by DNA hybridization techniques and quantitative PCR and can be helpful in distinguishing PTLD from lymphocytic infiltrates of rejection. Longitudinal monitoring of the EBV load in peripheral blood has been used for the prediction, diagnosis, and therapeutic management of PTLD.[13,38] Treatment of EBV syndromes consists of reduction of immunosuppression.[38,242] Although acyclovir, adefovir, cidofovir, ganciclovir, or monoclonal antibodies (e.g., rituximab) have been used to treat PTLD in OLT patients, their efficacy remains uncertain.[242-245]

Other Human Herpesviruses

Human herpes virus (HHV) types 6, 7, and 8 are ubiquitous and may be isolated from liver transplant recipients and other immunocompromised patients.[38,246-255] HHV-6 and HHV-7 can cause persistent infection in their hosts. Reactivation of HHV-6 within the early posttransplant period (first 2 to 4 weeks) may occur in 31% to 55% of SOT recipients.[247-250] Symptomatic disease due to HHV-6 is uncommon, but HHV-6 has been associated with febrile syndromes, skin rash, pneumonia, encephalitis, and bone marrow suppression.[247-250] Others have reported that HHV-6 has immunomodulating effects and may increase the risk for early fibrosis on recurrence of hepatitis C in OLT recipients with HCV.[247-250] Ganciclovir prophylaxis appears to reduce the rate of HHV-6 infection.

Infection with HHV-7 may also occur in the early posttransplant period (3 to 10 weeks after transplantation).[246,248,249] However, disease related to HHV-7 has not been well documented in OLT recipients.

Transmission of HHV-8 from liver donors to recipients may occur. Infection with HHV-8 has been associated with the development of symptomatic Kaposi's sarcoma (KS) after liver transplantation.[38,249,251-255] KS is one of the earliest posttransplant malignancies to occur in SOT recipients, with a mean onset of 22 months compared to 32 months for lymphomas, and 69 months for epithelial malignancies. OLT recipients appear to have the highest incidence of KS among SOT recipients.[38,249,251-255] The diagnosis of KS is supported by morphological study and by the presence of HHV-8 DNA sequences in involved tissue. Although the skin is the most common site of infection, visceral lesions may develop in up to 40% of SOT recipients, including gastrointestinal, pulmonary, bladder, and laryngeal involvement. Management strategies include reduction of immunosuppression, treatment with antiviral agents (acyclovir, adefovir, cidofovir, foscarnet, ganciclovir, or penciclovir) or cytotoxic chemotherapy.

Adenovirus

In SOT recipients, adenovirus infections may occur between 15 and 130 days after transplantation and have been associated with the use of corticosteroids and muromonab-CD3.[256-259] A diagnosis can be made with immunohistochemistry methodology or culture. After liver transplantation, the spectrum of disease includes asymptomatic shedding (urine, respiratory secretions, or stool), hepatitis, hemorrhagic cystitis, gastroenteritis, or pneumonia.[256-259] Effective antiviral therapy is unproven. Reduction in immunosuppression may be beneficial in certain patients.

Papovaviruses

The BK and JC viruses (BKV and JCV) belong to the human papovavirus family. Reactivation of virus can occur (primarily reported in kidney allograft recipients) and has been implicated as a cause of ureteral stricture, progressive multifocal leukoencephalopathy, and interstitial nephritis.[260-262] Other clinical findings include respiratory tract disease and hemorrhagic cystitis. Differentiation among the viral inclusions of BKV, JCV, CMV, HSV, and adenovirus can be difficult. Specific in situ hybridization and PCR techniques can demonstrate papovavirus. Viral culture is rarely used in the clinical setting. Although vidarabine and cidofovir have been used to treat papovavirus infections, effective treatment still needs to be established.[260,261] Thus, reduction of immunosuppression offers the best therapeutic option.

Influenza Virus Types A and B, Parainfluenza Virus, and Respiratory Syncytial Virus

Community-acquired respiratory viral disease in liver transplant recipients is usually manifested as upper respiratory tract symptoms that progress to systemic symptoms such as high fever, myalgia, arthralgia, anorexia, and mucosal inflammation.[263] The spectrum of illness includes mild upper respiratory illness, bronchiolitis, and pneumonia with respiratory failure.

The diagnosis of respiratory viral illness is facilitated by rapid detection of virus-laden upper respiratory cells (e.g., nasopharyngeal washing, bronchoalveolar fluid) by virus-specific fluorescent-labeled antibody probes. Progressive viral infection can lead to fatal pneumonia or death from superinfection with bacterial pathogens such as *S. aureus*, *Streptococcus* species, or nosocomial gram-negative bacilli.

SOT recipients have been reported to be more susceptible to influenza virus. In a study of influenza viral infection in SOT recipients at the University of Pittsburgh Medical Center, 30 cases of influenza were diagnosed in SOT recipients (influenza A, n = 22; influenza B, n = 8).[263] These patients included five liver transplant recipients. The incidence of influenza viral infection was 2.8 cases per 1000 person-years in liver transplant patients. Symptoms were reported in all patients and included malaise, myalgia/arthralgia, fever, cough, and shortness of breath. Secondary bacterial pneumonia also occurred. Immunization with influenza vaccine may be ineffective in immunosuppressed patients because of their reduced antibody response. Treatment of influenza A has included early administration of amantadine or rimantadine. However, neither agent is effective against influenza B. Newer agents, such as oseltamivir and zanamivir, are neuraminidase inhibitors that if started within 30 to 36 hours after the onset of symptoms, can shorten the duration of illness and decrease some upper respiratory complications. Respiratory syncytial virus (RSV) pneumonitis may respond to aerosolized ribavirin delivered in a controlled, contained administration system over a 24-hour period.[264-266]

Parvovirus

In transplant recipients, parvovirus infection is an occasional cause of refractory severe anemia, pancytopenia, and thrombotic microangiopathy.[267,268] Infection is recognized by detection of typical giant proerythroblasts in bone marrow, followed by confirmation with PCR assay. In one report, chronic transfusion-dependent anemia developed in an adult liver transplant recipient with parvovirus B19 infection within a month after OLT.[267] Treatment with intravenous immune globulin may be effective.

Human Immunodeficiency Virus

HIV infection can be transmitted by an infected liver donor or by blood transfusion.[10,269] Routine screening of organ and blood donors for HIV antibodies has been performed since 1985 and has resulted in a reduced risk of infection. However, false-negative results of the enzyme-linked immunosorbent assay may occur, especially during the initial postinfectious period. This can lead to transmission of HIV infection from a presumably seronegative donor.[270] Addition of the p24 antigen detection assay increases the sensitivity of HIV screening.

Historically, patients with life-threatening end-stage organ failure who are infected with HIV were not considered for OLT.[271-276] Generally, these patients were excluded from OLT because of the poor prognosis associated with HIV, the subsequent development of acquired immunodeficiency syndrome (AIDS), and the fact that other patients needing liver transplants were expected to live much longer. However, current regimens using highly active antiretroviral therapy (HAART) have led to significant improvement in morbidity and mortality in HIV-infected patients.[10-13,273,274,276] Therefore, some HIV-infected patients with end-stage organ disease are being considered for OLT. Criteria for transplantation are not universally established in HIV-infected patients. A detectable preoperative HIV load of more than 400 copies/mL and a $CD4^+$ cell count of less than 200 cells/mL have constituted exclusion criteria at many transplant centers, but not others.[10-13,273,274,276] A recent series suggests that HIV-positive patients who may benefit most from SOT include those who have no HCV coinfection, are able to tolerate HAART, and have undetectable HIV RNA with immune reconstitution.[10-13] Ongoing studies may further address some of the critical clinical and ethical issues associated with transplantation in the HIV-infected patient population.

Hepatitis B and C Virus

The posttransplant risk for viral hepatitis in a liver transplant recipient can be related to acquisition of infection from an infected organ, a blood donor, or recurrence of infection existing before transplantation. Fortunately, most patients who undergo transplantation for liver disease associated with chronic HBV infection can be managed with long-term administration of hepatitis B immune globulin and the antiviral lamivudine.[17-23,27,28] The combination of these agents prevents recurrence in the majority of OLT recipients. However, hepatitis B immune globulin is expensive, and YMDD escape mutants have been seen with the use of lamivudine. Fortunately, adefovir dipivoxil and tenofovir are useful in treating HBV infection and the YMDD escape mutants. A comprehensive review of hepatitis B and liver transplantation is found in Chapter 8.

HCV is a single-stranded, 50-nm RNA virus that infects more than 100 million people worldwide.[277,278] In the United States, cirrhosis will develop in 25% of HCV-infected people, with annual mortality rates in these patients approaching 5%.[277] Furthermore, only 15% to 30% of patients infected with HCV fully recover, and

the remaining 70% to 85% remain chronically infected and are at risk for cirrhosis, end-stage liver disease, or hepatocellular carcinoma.[278,279] Ultimately, end-stage liver disease associated with chronic HCV infection has become the predominant indication (estimated at 35% to 45%) for liver transplantation in the United States.

Partly because of the absence of pharmacological agents that prevent recurrent infection, recurrent HCV infection has become one of the greatest threats to liver allograft recipients.[26,31] Recurrent HCV infection, as defined by viremia following OLT, is nearly universal, with graft hepatitis developing in 50% to 80% of OLT patients and cirrhosis developing in up to 20% of patients within 5 years after transplantation.[26,280-282] While some earlier studies have suggested that graft and patient survival for the first decade after transplantation is unaffected by HCV serostatus before transplantation, more recent data have shown reduced survival at 5 years after initial OLT in HCV-positive versus HCV-negative patients (56.7% and 65.6%, respectively).[280-285] Additionally, early recurrence of HCV in the liver is a poor predictor of long-term survival.

The clinical manifestations of HCV disease after OLT are similar to those observed before transplantation and include early fibrosing cholestatic hepatitis (occurring within 1 to 3 months and associated with high mortality) and end-stage cirrhotic liver disease. In addition to liver disease, HCV-infected patients are at increased risk for diabetes, lipid disorders, lymphoproliferative disease, and glomerular disease.[286-288] However, the progression to cirrhosis is much more rapid in HCV-infected OLT patients than in immunocompetent individuals. Eventually, many patients with recurrent HCV will require a second liver transplant to survive. However, the outcome with a second transplant is suboptimal because of recurrent HCV. Thus the indications for retransplantation in this patient population remain controversial.[281,289,290]

Recurrence of hepatitis C has been related to several factors, including pretransplant viral factors (viral load, genotype), host factors (Child-Pugh score, race, recipient age), and posttransplant factors such as immunosuppression.[31,65,291-305] With respect to immunosuppression (excluding corticosteroids), global immunosuppressive exposure—not exposure to a single agent—is probably associated with recurrence of hepatitis C. Although the choice of calcineurin blockers has not clearly been shown to have an impact on histological recurrence of hepatitis C, cumulative exposure to corticosteroids has been associated with enhanced viremia, more severe histological recurrence, and higher mortality rates.[295,296,299] Treatment of acute rejection and development of steroid-resistant rejection have also diminished patient survival in OLT recipients with HCV.[294,298,299] Other agents such as mycophenolate mofetil[300-302] and the newer IL-2 receptor antagonists (basiliximab and daclizumab[65,303,305]) require additional randomized prospective trials to fully comprehend their impact on hepatitis C recurrence in OLT recipients.

The general goals of HCV therapy in the liver transplant setting are to prevent the development of HCV-related graft failure and to minimize mortality. Currently, three potential alternative or complementary approaches can be used to manage an HCV-infected OLT recipient: (1) preemptive antiviral therapy in a patient on the waiting list before receiving an organ, (2) antiviral therapy given immediately after the transplant before the occurrence of histological damage, and (3) antiviral treatment of recurrent HCV in patients who have evidence of fibrosis progression after OLT. Given the limited efficacy, poor tolerability, and cost of current management options of HCV infection (e.g., interferon, ribavirin, interferon plus ribavirin, or pegylated interferons alone or in combination with ribavirin), additional drug therapies need to be evaluated. Chapter 10 reviews HCV infection in OLT recipients in detail.

Protozoan Infections

P. carinii has usually been considered a protozoan because of its morphological properties, but it has been reclassified as a fungus based on DNA homology. *P. carinii* pneumonia most often occurs 2 to 6 months after transplantation and is a direct result of the net state of immunosuppression.[5,38,306-308] It is typically manifested as fever, nonproductive cough, arterial-alveolar mismatching, and diffuse interstitial infiltration or focal air space consolidation. Bronchoalveolar lavage with transbronchial biopsy is a highly sensitive method of identifying pulmonary disease. The incidence of *P. carinii* pneumonia in liver transplant patients not receiving prophylaxis is 5% to 10%.[5,38,306-308] This disease has been eliminated in most transplant centers by the use of routine prophylaxis.

First-line treatment is with TMP-SMX.[5,38,306-308] Although corticosteroids have been shown to be beneficial in patients with AIDS and moderate to severe *P. carinii* pneumonia, they are of unproven efficacy in transplant patients. We currently do not recommend the use of corticosteroids for treatment of *P. carinii* pneumonia in transplant patients. If patients cannot tolerate TMP-SMX, second-line agents include intravenous pentamidine or dapsone-trimethoprim. Mild to moderate *P. carinii* pneumonia can be treated with atovaquone (750 mg orally three times daily for 21 days) in patients intolerant of TMP-SMX. Prophylactic agents, in order of efficacy, include TMP-SMX, bimonthly intravenous or aerosolized pentamidine, dapsone, and atovaquone.[309-312]

Toxoplasma gondii is a ubiquitous human pathogen that often causes asymptomatic latent infection in normal hosts. Reactivation of latent infection may occur after immunosuppression. Primary infection may also be acquired from a donor organ. Toxoplasmosis is relatively common in heart transplant recipients because *T. gondii* cysts may often be present in the myocardium. In liver transplant patients, toxoplasmosis is very rare. Only a few cases have been reported and were manifested by encephalitis, focal lesions in the brain, or pneumonia.[313-318] The diagnosis is established by microscopic examination of lesions for characteristic organisms. Serological tests are not always reliable. Pyrimethamine plus sulfadiazine or clindamycin are used for treatment.

Prophylaxis of Infection

Despite a paucity of controlled, randomized clinical trials demonstrating a benefit of perioperative antibacterial prophylaxis in liver transplant recipients, most transplant centers use intravenous antibiotics and, in some cases, oral agents as well for prevention of bacterial infections. The antibiotics chosen for prophylaxis are directed against organisms commonly found in the gastrointestinal flora (Enterobacteriaceae, anaerobes, group D streptococci) plus staphylococci. Intravenous cefoxitin, ceftizoxime, ampicillin-sulbactam, and cefotaxime plus ampicillin have all been used successfully. At the University of California at Los Angeles (UCLA), we observed in a randomized, controlled study that ampicillin-sulbactam is as effective as a broad-spectrum combination of cefotaxime plus ampicillin for prophylaxis. Furthermore, we did not find any advantage to extending the duration of intravenous antibiotic prophylaxis beyond 24 hours.

For decontamination of the gastrointestinal tract both before and after surgery, several oral regimens have been used with mixed results.[319-325] A recent meta-analysis supports a beneficial effect of selective bowel decontamination on gram-negative infection after liver transplantation; however, the risk of antimicrobial resistance must be considered.[319] At UCLA, we administer oral erythromycin, neomycin, and nystatin preoperatively to all patients beginning when a donor is located. No oral antibiotics are given postoperatively. In contrast, other liver transplant centers have used polymyxin, gentamicin, and nystatin or polymyxin, tobramycin, and nystatin starting preoperatively and continuing for several weeks postoperatively.[323,324] Similarly, based on favorable results in neutropenic patients, both oral norfloxacin and oral ciprofloxacin have been given for selective decontamination of the gastrointestinal tract.[325]

Because of the high frequency and severity of fungal infections in liver transplant patients, oral prophylaxis with nystatin, clotrimazole, or amphotericin B and intravenous prophylaxis with low-dose amphotericin B have been attempted. However, the efficacy of these antifungal agents for prophylaxis has never been clearly established. The efficacy of two azole antifungal agents, fluconazole and itraconazole, for prevention of invasive and superficial *Candida* infection has been demonstrated in double-blind, placebo-controlled trials. Fluconazole and itraconazole had similar efficacy for prevention of fungal infections in a comparative study of liver transplant patients, although gastrointestinal side effects were more frequent with the itraconazole. Due to the erratic bioavailability of oral itraconazole capsules, either oral itraconazole solution or intravenous itraconazole should be used. We currently administer prophylactic fluconazole to all UCLA liver transplant recipients at high-risk for invasive fungal infection. For patients colonized with *Aspergillus* or have other specific risk factors for invasive aspergillosis, a lipid formulation of amphotericin, itraconazole, or voriconazole can be used for antifungal prophylaxis.

Several regimens and strategies for prevention of CMV infection and symptomatic CMV disease have been evaluated in liver transplant recipients (see Table 64–6). Prophylactic CMV immune globulin has no substantial effect on the incidence of CMV infection in liver transplant patients but is associated with a reduction in CMV disease. Similar to the experience in kidney transplant patients, high-dose acyclovir appears to reduce the incidence of both CMV infection and CMV disease when compared with patients receiving no prophylaxis.[186] However, in a randomized trial, intravenous ganciclovir was shown to be more effective than high-dose acyclovir for prevention of both CMV infection and CMV disease, especially when ganciclovir is administered throughout the entire high-risk period for CMV disease or until day 100 after liver transplantation. Intravenous ganciclovir followed by oral ganciclovir or oral valganciclovir has emerged as a common prophylactic regimen in many OLT centers. Early preemptive therapy with ganciclovir of asymptomatic patients shedding CMV can also prevent subsequent CMV disease. Preemptive ganciclovir is more effective in CMV-seropositive patients than CMV-seronegative patients with CMV-seropositive donors.[229-231] Since CMV infections have developed after prolonged prophylaxis or preemptive therapy with ganciclovir, patients need to be continuously monitored for infection. Both prophylactic ganciclovir (valganciclovir) and acyclovir (valacyclovir) prevent HSV infection.

P. carinii pneumonia in liver transplant patients can be prevented by using TMP-SMX. At UCLA, TMP-SMX is given to all patients at a dosage of one double-strength tablet (160 mg of trimethoprim) daily or three times daily on any 2 consecutive days of each week. *P. carinii* prophylaxis is continued for 1 year after transplantation or longer if the patient is receiving additional immunosuppressive therapy for rejection. For patients unable to tolerate TMP-SMX, intravenous pentamidine (4 mg/kg every 2 weeks) or oral dapsone (100 mg/day) is used. Since we have observed breakthrough cases of *P. carinii* infection in liver transplant patients taking prophylactic dapsone only twice weekly, we recommend that prophylactic dapsone be given daily. Oral atovaquone (750 mg twice daily) has also been used as a second-line prophylactic agent in a limited number of transplant patients. Table 64–7 summarizes

Table 64–7. ANTIMICROBIAL PROPHYLAXIS FOR UCLA LIVER TRANSPLANT RECIPIENTS

Bacterial

Neomycin, 1.0 g orally q1h × 4 doses, plus erythromycin, 1.0 g orally q1h × 4 doses, before surgery

Ampicillin-sulbactam, 3 g IV, starting before transplantation surgery and continuing q6h until 24 hr after surgery is completed; if the patient has penicillin allergy manifested by rash, use ceftizoxime, 2.0 g IV q8h, plus vancomycin, 1 gram IV q12h, starting before surgery and continuing until 24 hr after surgery; if the patient has penicillin allergy manifested by anaphylaxis, use gentamicin, 1.5 mg/kg IV q8h, plus vancomycin, 1 gram IV q12h, starting before surgery and continuing until 24 hr after surgery

For cholangiogram or T-tube manipulation, ampicillin-sulbactam, 3 g IV q6h × 2 doses; if the patient has penicillin allergy, use ceftizoxime, 2.0 g IV q8h × 2 doses, plus vancomycin, 1 gram IV q12h × 2 doses, or gentamicin, 1.5 mg/kg IV q8h × 2 doses, plus vancomycin, 1 gram IV q12h × 2 doses

Fungal

Fluconazole, 400 mg IV or orally qd* starting before transplantation surgery and continuing until day 42 after transplantation in patients at high risk for fungal infection

Pneumocystis carinii

Trimethoprim-sulfamethoxazole (160 and 800 mg, respectively) orally or IV tid on Saturdays and Sundays only (or one double-strength tablet orally qd*) until 1 yr after transplantation; continue beyond 1 yr in patients requiring additional immunosuppression for rejection; if the patient has sulfa allergy, use pentamidine, 4 mg/kg IV q2wk, or dapsone, 100 mg orally qd

Viral

Ganciclovir, 6 mg/kg IV qd* from day 1 after transplantation to day of discharge; after discharge, change to ganciclovir 1 gram PO tid or valganciclovir, 900 mg orally qd

*Drug dosages may require adjustment in patients with kidney failure.

current prophylactic regimens used in liver transplant patients at UCLA.

Summary and Conclusions

Multiple host and external factors place liver transplant patients at increased risk for infection. To minimize morbidity and mortality from infection after liver transplantation, it is important to identify patients at greatest risk for serious infection as a consequence of these factors. Before transplantation, acutely ill patients with advanced liver disease frequently have been hospitalized for prolonged periods and are already colonized or infected with potentially pathogenic organisms. Patients with intraoperative complications at the time of initial transplant surgery or who require repeat transplantation because of graft failure have an increased risk for infection. After transplantation, prolonged hospitalization in the intensive care unit and treatment of multiple episodes of rejection with corticosteroids, OKT3, thymoglobulin, and other immunosuppressive agents raise the risk for opportunistic infection. Careful infectious disease surveillance of these high-risk patients and prompt initiation of appropriate prophylactic and therapeutic anti-infective strategies can decrease the morbidity and mortality from infection in OLT recipients.

Despite a lack of published controlled clinical trials showing a clear benefit for perioperative antibiotic prophylaxis in liver transplant patients, it is reasonable to provide patients with intravenous antibiotic prophylaxis with a β-lactam drug directed against the gastrointestinal flora for 24 hours after transplant surgery. Based on limited data, selective decontamination of the gastrointestinal tract with oral antimicrobial agents does not appear to provide additional protection against bacterial infection. In contrast, except for infrequent bacterial infections caused by multiresistant organisms (*Enterobacter, P. aeruginosa, Enterococcus faecium*), most bacterial infections in liver transplant patients can be treated effectively with one or more of the many currently available antibacterial drugs. Newer agents such as quinupristin-dalfopristin, linezolid, and daptomycin have added to the antibacterial armamentarium used against gram-positive pathogens in OLT recipients.

It is hoped that additional data from trials using new second-generation azoles (voriconazole, posaconazole) and the echinocandins (caspofungin, micafungin) will provide the indications for additional antifungal prophylactic and therapeutic regimens. The development of novel antifungal agents for treating emerging resistant fungal pathogens is a constant need. *P. carinii* can be eliminated as a significant pathogen in liver transplant patients by prophylactic TMP-SMX.

Ganciclovir administered either as prophylaxis or preemptive therapy can prevent most CMV and HSV infections in liver transplant patients. Introduction of the valine ester form of ganciclovir, oral valganciclovir, has provided the opportunity to give patients effective prophylaxis and treatment without the need for prolonged intravenous access.

Effective prevention of recurrent HBV after liver transplantation has been achieved with hepatitis B immune globulin and lamivudine. Similar effective agents for prevention of HCV, the most common indication for liver transplantation, would greatly improve the outcome of transplantation for many patients. Thus, research aimed at developing more effective agents against HCV should continue to receive the highest priority.

References

1. Kusne S, Dummer JS, Singh N, et al: Infections after liver transplantation: An analysis of 101 consecutive cases. Medicine (Baltimore) 67:132-143, 1988.
2. Colonna JO, Winston DJ, Brill JE, et al: Infectious complications in liver transplantation. Arch Surg 23:360-364, 1988.
3. Ascher NL, Stock PG, Bumgardner GL, et al: Infection and rejection of primary hepatic transplant in 93 consecutive patients treated with triple immunosuppressive therapy. Surg Gynecol Obstet 167:474-484, 1988.
4. Paya CV, Hermans PE, Washington JA, et al: Incidence, distribution, and outcome of episodes of infection in 100 orthotopic liver transplantations. Mayo Clin Proc 64:555-564, 1989.
5. Winston DJ, Emmanouilides C, Busuttil RW: Infection in liver transplant recipients. Clin Infect Dis 21:2077-2091, 1995.
6. Freeman RB, Wiesner RH, Roberts JP, et al: Improving liver allocation: MELD and PELD. Am J Transplant 9(Suppl):114-131, 2004.
7. Fishman JA, Rubin RH: Infection in organ-transplant recipients. N Engl J Med 338:1741-1751, 1998.
8. Singh N, Patterson DL: *Mycobacterium tuberculosis* infection in solid-organ transplant recipients: Impact and implications for management. Clin Infect Dis 27:1266-1277, 1998.
9. Torre-Cisneros J, Caston JJ, Moreno J, et al: Tuberculosis in the transplant candidate: Importance of early diagnosis and treatment. Transplantation 77:1376-1380, 2004.
10. Halpern SD, Ubel PA, Caplan AL: Solid organ transplantation in HIV-infected patients. N Engl J Med 347:284, 2002.
11. Fishman JA: Transplantation of patients infected with human immunodeficiency virus: No longer experimental but not yet routine. J Infect Dis 188:1405, 2003.
12. Roland ME, Stock PG: Review of solid organ transplantation in HIV-infected patients. Transplantation 75:425, 2003.
13. Green M, Webber S: Posttransplantation lymphoproliferative disorders. Pediatr Clin North Am 50:1471-1491, 2003.
14. Orentas RJ, Schauer DW Jr, Ellis FW, et al: Monitoring and modulation of Epstein-Barr virus loads in pediatric transplant patients. Pediatr Transplant 7:305-314, 2003.
15. Randhawa PS, Markin RS, Starzl TE, Demetris AJ: Epstein-Barr virus–associated syndromes in immunosuppressed liver transplant recipients: Clinical profile and recognition on routine allograft biopsy. Am J Surg Pathol 14:538-547, 1990.
16. Montone KT, Friedman H, Hodinka RL, et al: In situ hybridization for Epstein-Barr virus NotI repeats in posttransplant lymphoproliferative disorder. Mod Pathol 5:292-302, 1992.

17. Lucey MR, Graham DM, Martin P, et al: Recurrence of hepatitis B and delta hepatitis after orthotopic liver transplantation. Gut 33:1390-1396, 1992.
18. Demetris AJ, Jaffe R, Sheahan DG: Recurrent hepatitis B in liver allograft recipients. Am J Pathol 125:161-172, 1986.
19. Lykavieris P, Fabre M, Yvart J, Alvarez F: HBV infection in pediatric liver transplantation. J Pediatr Gastroenterol Nutr 16:321-327, 1993.
20. Feray C, Zignego AL, Samuel D, et al: Persistent hepatitis B virus infection of mononuclear blood cells without concomitant liver infection: The liver transplantation model. Transplantation 49:1155-1158, 1990.
21. Todo S, Demetris AJ, Van Thiel D, et al: Orthotopic liver transplantation for patients with hepatitis B virus–related liver disease. Hepatology 13:619-626, 1991.
22. Samuel D, Muller R, Alexander G, et al: Liver transplantation in European patients with the hepatitis B surface antigen. N Engl J Med 329:1842-1847, 1993.
23. Rimoldi P, Belli LS, Rondinara GF, et al: Recurrent HBV/HDV infections under different immunoprophylaxis protocols. Transplant Proc 25:2675-2676, 1993.
24. Ferrell LD, Wright TL, Roberts J, et al: Hepatitis C viral infection in liver transplant recipients. Hepatology 16:865-876, 1992.
25. Wright TL: Liver transplantation for chronic hepatitis C viral infection. Gastroenterol Clin North Am 22:231-242, 1993.
26. Gane EJ, Portmann BC, Naoumov NV, et al: Long-term outcome of hepatitis C infection after liver transplantation. N Engl J Med 334:815-820, 1996.
27. Anselmo DM, Ghobrial RM, Jung LC, et al: New era of liver transplantation for hepatitis B: A 17-year single-center experience. Ann Surg 235:611-619, 2002.
28. Han SH, Ofman J, Holt C, et al: An efficacy and cost-effectiveness analysis of combination hepatitis B immune globulin and lamivudine to prevent recurrent hepatitis B after orthotopic liver transplantation compared with hepatitis B immune globulin monotherapy. Liver Transpl 6:741-748, 2000.
29. Ghobrial RM:. Treatment for recurrent hepatitis C. Minerva Chir 58:693-703, 2003.
30. Terrault NA: Prophylactic and preemptive therapies for hepatitis C virus–infected patients undergoing liver transplantation. Liver Transpl 9:S95-S100, 2003.
31. Rosen HR: Hepatitis C in the liver transplant recipient: Current understanding and treatment. Microbes Infect 4:1253-1258, 2002.
32. Saab S, Chang AJ, Comulada S, et al: Outcomes of hepatitis C– and hepatitis B core antibody–positive grafts in orthotopic liver transplantation. Liver Transpl 9:1053-1061, 2003.
33. Paya CV, Hermans PE, Wiesner RH, et al: Cytomegalovirus hepatitis in liver transplantation: Prospective analysis of 93 consecutive orthotopic liver transplantations. J Infect Dis 160:752-758, 1989.
34. Sayage LH, Gonwa TA, Goldstein RM, et al: Cytomegalovirus infection in orthotopic liver transplantation. Transpl Int 2:96-101, 1989.
35. Rubin RH: The direct and indirect effects of infection in liver transplantation: Pathogenesis, impact, and clinical management. Curr Clin Top Infect Dis 22:125-154, 2002.
36. Singh N: Infectious diseases in the liver transplant recipient. Semin Gastrointest Dis 9:136-146, 1998.
37. Kanj SS, Sharara AI, Clavien PA, Hamilton JD: Cytomegalovirus infection following liver transplantation: Review of the literature. Clin Infect Dis 22:537-549, 1996.
38. Patel R, Paya CV: Infections in solid-organ transplant recipients. Clin Microbiol Rev 10:86-124, 1997.
39. Patel R, Snydman DR, Rubin RH, et al: Cytomegalovirus prophylaxis in solid organ transplant recipients. Transplantation 61:1279-1289, 1996.
40. Vilchez RA, Fung J, Kusne S: Cryptococcosis in organ transplant recipients: An overview. Am J Transplant 2:575-580, 2002.
41. Blair JE, Logan JL: Coccidioidomycosis in solid organ transplantation. Clin Infect Dis 33:1536-1544, 2001.
42. Vinayek R, Balan V, Pinna A, et al: Disseminated histoplasmosis in a patient after orthotopic liver transplantation. Clin Transplant 12:274-277, 1998.
43. Singh N, Husain S, De Vera M, et al: *Cryptococcus neoformans* infection in patients with cirrhosis, including liver transplant candidates. Medicine (Baltimore) 83:188-192, 2004.
44. Angelis M, Cooper JT, Freeman RB: Impact of donor infections on outcome of orthotopic liver transplantation. Liver Transpl 9:451-462, 2003.
45. Hibbard PL, Rubin RH: Clinical aspects of fungal infections in organ transplant recipients. Clin Infect Dis 19(Suppl 1):S33, 1994.
46. Hadley S, Karchmer AW: Fungal infections in solid organ transplant recipients. Infect Dis Clin North Am 9:1045, 1995.
47. Singh N: Fungal infections in the recipients of solid organ transplantation. Infect Dis Clin North Am 17:1, 2003.
48. Hagerty JA, Ortiz J, Reich D, Manzarbeitia C: Fungal infections in solid organ transplant patients. Surg Infect 4:263-271, 2003.
49. Fishman JA: Prevention of infection caused by *Pneumocystis carinii* in transplant recipients. Clin Infect Dis 33:1397-1405, 2001.
50. Kubak BM, Pegues DA, Holt CD, et al: Changing patterns of fungal infection in transplantation. Curr Opin Organ Transplant 5:176, 2000.
51. Walsh TJ, Groll AH: Emerging fungal pathogens: Evolving challenges to immunocompromised patients for the twenty first century. Transpl Infect Dis 1:247, 1999.
52. Canadian Multicenter Transplant Study Group: A randomized clinical trial of cyclosporine in cadaveric renal transplantation. N Engl J Med 309:809-815, 1983.
53. European FK506 Multicenter Study Group: Randomised trial comparing tacrolimus (FK506) and cyclosporine in prevention of liver allograft rejection. Lancet 344:423-428, 1994.
54. Singh N, Gayowski T, Wagener MM, et al: Invasive fungal infections in liver transplant recipients receiving tacrolimus as the primary immunosuppressive agent. Clin Infect Dis 24:179-184, 1997.
55. Singh N, Gayowski T, Wagener M, et al: Pulmonary infections in liver transplant recipients receiving tacrolimus. Changing pattern of microbial etiologies. Transplantation 61:396-401, 1996.
56. Rifkind D, Marchioro T, Schneck T, Hill RB Jr: Systemic fungal infection complicating renal transplantation and immunosuppression therapy. Am J Med 43:28-38, 1967.
57. Stratta RJ: Clinical patterns of cytomegalovirus infection after solid-organ transplantation. Transplant Proc 25:15-21, 1993.
58. Wiesner RH, Marin E, Porayko MK, et al: Advances in the diagnosis, treatment, and prevention of cytomegalovirus infections after liver transplantation. Gastroenterol Clin North Am 22:351-366, 1993.
59. Paterson DL, Singh N, Panebianco A, et al: Infectious complications occurring in liver transplant recipients receiving mycophenolate mofetil. Transplantation 66:593-598, 1998.
60. Peterson PK, Balfour HH, Fryd DS, et al: Risk factors in the development of cytomegalovirus-related pneumonia in renal transplant recipients. J Infect Dis 148:1121, 1983.
61. Rosen HR, Shackleton CR, Higa L, et al: Use of OKT3 is associated with early and severe recurrence of hepatitis C after liver transplantation. Am J Gastroenterol 92:1453-1457, 1997.
62. Eason JD, Blazek J, Mason A, et al: Steroid-free immunosuppression through thymoglobulin induction in liver transplantation. Transplant Proc 33:1470-1471, 2001.
63. Nelson DR, Soldevila-Pico C, Reed A, et al: Anti–interleukin-2 receptor therapy in combination with mycophenolate mofetil is associated with more severe hepatitis C recurrence after liver transplantation. Liver Transpl 7:1064-1070, 2001.

64. Calmus Y, Scheele JR, Gonzalez-Pinto I, et al: Immunoprophylaxis with basiliximab, a chimeric anti–interleukin-2 receptor monoclonal antibody, in combination with azathioprine-containing triple therapy in liver transplant recipients. Liver Transpl 8:123-131, 2002.

65. Heffron TG, Smallwood GA, Pillen T, et al: Liver transplant induction trial of daclizumab to spare calcineurin inhibition. Transplant Proc 34:1514, 2002.

66. Ingle GR, Sievers TM, Holt CD: Sirolimus: Continuing the evolution of transplant immunosuppression. Ann Pharmacother 34:1044-1055, 2000.

67. Groth CG, Backman L, Morales JM, et al: Sirolimus based therapy in human renal transplantation; similar efficacy and different toxicity compared with cyclosporine. Transplantation 67:1036-1042, 1999.

68. Fisher A, Seguel JM, de la Torre AN, et al: Effect of sirolimus on infection incidence in liver transplant recipients. Liver Transpl 10:193-198, 2004.

69. Husain S, Singh N: The impact of novel immunosuppressive agents on infections in organ transplant recipients and the interactions of these agents with antimicrobials. Clin Infect Dis 35:53-61, 2002.

70. George DL, Arnow PM, Fox AS, et al: Bacterial infection as a complication of liver transplantation: Epidemiology and risk factors. Rev Infect Dis 13:387-396, 1991.

71. Barkholt L, Ericzon BG, Tollemar J, et al: Infections in human liver recipients: Different patterns early and late after transplantation. Transpl Int 6:77-84, 1993.

72. Wagener MM, Yu VL: Bacteremia in transplant recipients: A prospective study of demographics, etiologic agents, risk factors, and outcomes. Am J Infect Control 20:239-247, 1992.

73. Lumbreras C, Lizasoain M, Moreno E, et al: Major bacterial infections following liver transplantation: A prospective study. Hepatogastroenterology 39:362-365, 1992.

74. Singh N, Patterson DL, Gayowski T, et al: Predicting bacteremia and bacteremic mortality in liver transplant patients. Liver Transpl 6:54-61, 2000.

75. Singh N, Gayowski T, Wagener MM, et al: Bloodstream infections in liver transplant recipients receiving tacrolimus. Clin Transplant 11:275-281, 1997.

76. Singh N, Gayowski T, Wagener MM, et al: Predictors and outcome of early versus late-onset major bacterial infections in liver transplant recipients receiving tacrolimus (FK506) as primary immunosuppression. Eur J Clin Microbiol Infect Dis 16:821-826, 1997.

77. Said A, Safdar N, Lucey MR, et al: Infected bilomas in liver transplant recipients, incidence, risk factors and implications for prevention. Am J Transplant 4:574-582, 2004.

78. Desai D, Desai N, Nightingale P, et al: Carriage of methicillin-resistant Staphylococcus aureus is associated with an increased risk of infection after liver transplantation. Liver Transpl 9:754-759, 2003.

79. Torre-Cisneros J, Herrero C, Canas E, et al: High mortality related with Staphylococcus aureus bacteremia after liver transplantation. Eur J Clin Microbiol Infect Dis 21:385-388, 2002.

80. Hagen EA, Lautenbach E, Olthoff K, Blumberg EA: Low prevalence of colonization with vancomycin-resistant Enterococcus in patients awaiting liver transplantation. Am J Transplant 3:902-905, 2003.

81. Bakir M, Bova JL, Newell KA, et al: Epidemiology and clinical consequences of vancomycin-resistant enterococci in liver transplant patients. Transplantation 72:1032-1037, 2001.

82. Orloff SL, Busch AM, Olyaei AJ, et al: Vancomycin-resistant Enterococcus in liver transplant patients. Am J Surg 177:418-422, 1999.

83. Kubak BK, Holt CD: Bacterial infections in the transplant patients. Ochsner Clin Rep 11:1-15, 1999.

84. Paterson DL, Rihs JD, Squier C, et al: Lack of efficacy of mupirocin in the prevention of infections with Staphylococcus aureus in liver transplant recipients and candidates. Transplantation 75:194-198, 2003.

85. Bert F, Clarissou J, Durand F, et al: Prevalence, molecular epidemiology, and clinical significance of heterogeneous glycopeptide-intermediate Staphylococcus aureus in liver transplant recipients. J Clin Microbiol 4:5147-152, 2003.

86. Papanicolaou GA, Meyers BR, Meyers J, et al: Nosocomial infections with vancomycin-resistant Enterococcus faecium in liver transplant recipients: Risk factors for acquisition and mortality. Clin Infect Dis 23:760-766, 1996.

87. Luber AD, Jacobs RA, Jordan M, et al: Relative importance of oral versus intravenous vancomycin exposure in the development of vancomycin-resistant enterococci. J Infect Dis 173:1292-1294, 1996.

88. Edmond MB, Ober JF, Dawson JD, et al: Vancomycin-resistant enterococcal bacteremia: Natural history and attributable mortality. Clin Infect Dis 23:1234-1239, 1996.

89. Winston DJ, Emmanouilides C, Kroeber A, et al: Quinupristin/dalfopristin therapy for infections due to vancomycin-resistant Enterococcus faecium. Clin Infect Dis 30:790-797, 2000.

90. Odakowska-Jedynak U, Paczek L, Krawczyk M, et al: Resistance of gram-positive pathogens to antibiotics is a therapeutic challenge after liver transplantation: Clinical experience in one center with linezolid. Transplant Proc 35:2304-2306, 2003.

91. Kauffman CA: Therapeutic and preventative options for the management of vancomycin-resistant enterococcal infections. J Antimicrob Chemother 51(Suppl 3):23-30, 2003.

92. Gouvea EF, Branco RC, Monteiro RC, et al: Outcome of infections caused by multiple drug-resistant bacteria in liver transplant recipients. Transplant Proc 36:958-960, 2004.

93. Paterson DL, Singh N, Rihs JD, et al: Control of an outbreak of infection due to extended-spectrum beta-lactamase–producing Escherichia coli in a liver transplantation unit. Clin Infect Dis 33:126-128, 2001.

94. Singh N, Wagener MM, Obman A, et al: Bacteremias in liver transplant recipients: Shift toward gram-negative bacteria as predominant pathogens. Liver Transpl 10:844-849, 2004.

95. Singh N, Gayowski T, Rihs JD, et al: Evolving trends in multiple-antibiotic–resistant bacteria in liver transplant recipients: A longitudinal study of antimicrobial susceptibility patterns. Liver Transpl 7:22-26, 2001.

96. Wade J, Rolando N, Williams R: The significance of aerobic gram-negative bacilli in clinical specimens following orthotopic liver transplantation. Liver Transpl Surg 4:51-57, 1998.

97. Clark NM, Chenoweth CE: Aeromonas infection of the hepatobiliary system: Report of 15 cases and review of the literature. Clin Infect Dis 37:506-513, 2003.

98. Lykavieris P, Fabre M, Pariente D, et al: Clostridium difficile colitis associated with inflammatory pseudotumor in a liver transplant recipient. Pediatr Transplant 7:76-79, 2003.

99. Keven K, Basu A, Re L, et al: Clostridium difficile colitis in patients after kidney and pancreas-kidney transplantation. Transpl Infect Dis 6:10-14, 2004.

100. Munoz P, Palomo J, Yanez J, Bouza E: Clinical microbiological case: A heart transplant recipient with diarrhea and abdominal pain. Recurring C. difficile infection. Clin Microbiol Infect 7:451-452, 458-459, 2001.

101. Bartlett JG: Antibiotic-associated diarrhea. N Engl J Med 346:334-339, 2002.

102. Forbes GM, Harvey FA, Philpott-Howard JN, et al: Nocardiosis in liver transplantation: Variation in presentation, diagnosis and therapy. J Infect 20:11-19, 1990.

103. Weinberger M, Eid A, Schreiber L, et al: Disseminated Nocardia transvalensis infection resembling pulmonary infarction in a liver transplant recipient. Eur J Clin Microbiol Infect Dis 14:337-341, 1995.

104. Ampel NM, Wing EJ: *Legionella* infection in transplant patients. Semin Respir Infect 5:30-37, 1990.
105. Ernst A, Gordon FD, Hayek J, et al: Lung abscess complicating *Legionella micdadei* pneumonia in an adult liver transplant recipient: Case report and review. Transplantation 65:130-134, 1998.
106. Seu P, Winson DJ, Olthoff KM, et al: Legionnaires' disease in liver transplant recipients. Infect Dis Clin Pract 2:109-113, 1993.
107. Tokunaga Y, Conception W, Berquist WE, et al: Graft involvement by *Legionella* in a liver transplant recipient. Arch Surg 127:475-477, 1992.
108. Rettally CA, Speeg KV: Infection with *Listeria monocytogenes* following orthotopic liver transplantation: Case report and review of the literature. Transplant Proc 35:1485-1487, 2003.
109. Lumbreras C, Lizasoain M, Moreno E, et al: Major bacterial infections following liver transplantation: A prospective study. Hepatogastroenterology 39:362-365, 1992.
110. Arnow PM: Infections following orthotopic liver transplantation. HPB Surg 3:221-233, 1991.
111. Brayman KL, Stephanian E, Matas AJ, et al: Analysis of infectious complications occurring after solid-organ transplantation. Arch Surg 127:38-48, 1992.
112. Bubak ME, Porayko MK, Krom RA, Wiesner RH: Complications of liver biopsy in liver transplant patients: Increased sepsis associated with choledochojejunostomy. Hepatology 14:1063-1065, 1991.
113. Pirat A, Ozgur S, Torgay A, et al: Risk factors for postoperative respiratory complications in adult liver transplant recipients. Transplant Proc 36:218-220, 2004.
114. Mennel LA, Maki D: Bacterial pneumonia in solid organ transplantation. Semin Respir Infect 5:10-29, 1990.
115. Markin RS, Stratta RJ, Woods GL: Infection after liver transplantation. Am J Surg Pathol 14(Suppl 1):64-78, 1990.
116. Philpott-Howard J, Burroughs A, Fisher N, et al: Piperacillin-tazobactam versus ciprofloxacin plus amoxicillin in the treatment of infective episodes after liver transplantation. J Antimicrob Chemother 52:993-1000, 2003.
117. Fung JJ: Fungal infection in liver transplantation. Transpl Infect Dis 4(Suppl 3):18-23, 2002.
118. Fishman JA: Overview: Fungal infections in the transplant patients. Transpl Infect Dis 4(Suppl 3):3, 2002.
119. Singh N, Wagener NM, Gayowski T: Trends in invasive fungal infections in liver transplant recipients: Correlation with evolution in transplant practices. Transplantation 73:63-67, 2002.
120. Castaldo P, Stratta RJ, Wood RP, et al: Clinical spectrum of fungal infections after orthotopic liver transplantation. Arch Surg 126:149-156, 1991.
121. Paya CV: Fungal infections in solid-organ transplantation. Clin Infect Dis 16:677-688, 1993.
122. Rabkin JM, Oroloff SL, Corless CL, et al: Association of fungal infection and increased mortality in liver transplant recipients. Am J Surg 179:426-430, 2000.
123. Husain S, Tollemar J, Dominguez EA, et al: Changes in the spectrum and risk factors for invasive candidiasis in liver transplant recipients: Prospective, multicenter, case-controlled study. Transplantation 75:2023-2029, 2003.
124. Viviani MA, Tortorano AM, Malaspina C, et al: Surveillance and treatment of liver transplant recipients for candidiasis and aspergillosis. Eur J Epidemiol 8:433-436, 1992.
125. Patel R, Poertela D, Badley A, et al: Risk factors of invasive candida and non-candida fungal infections after liver transplantation. Transplantation 62:926, 1996.
126. Samaranayake YH, Samaranayake LP: *Candida krusei*: Biology, epidemiology, pathogenicity and clinical manifestations of an emerging pathogen. J Med Microbiol 41:295, 1994.
127. Fortun J, Lopez-San Roman A, Velasco JJ, et al: Selection of *Candida glabrata* with reduced susceptibility to azoles in four liver transplant recipients with invasive candidiasis. Eur J Clin Microbiol Infect Dis 16:314, 1997.
128. Nieto-Rodriguez JA, Kusne S, Manez R, et al: Factors associated with the development of candidemia and candidemia-related death among liver transplant recipients. Ann Surg 223:70-76, 1996.
129. Singh N, Arnow PM, Bonham A, et al: Invasive aspergillosis in liver transplant recipients in the 1990s. Transplantation 64:716, 1997.
130. Brown RS Jr, Lake JR, Katzman BA, et al: Incidence and significance of *Aspergillus* cultures following liver and kidney transplantation. Transplantation 61:666-669, 1996.
131. Singh N, Avery RK, Munoz P, et al: Trends in risk profiles for and mortality associated with invasive aspergillosis among liver transplant recipients. Clin Infect Dis 36:46-52, 2003.
132. Fortun J, Martin-Davila P, Moreno S, et al: Risk factors for invasive aspergillosis in liver transplant recipients. Liver Transpl 8:1065-1070, 2002.
133. Husain S, Alexander BD, Munoz P, et al: Opportunistic mycelial fungal infections in organ transplant recipients: Emerging importance of non-*Aspergillus* mycelial fungi. Clin Infect Dis 37:221-229, 2003.
134. Husain S, Wagener MN, Singh N: *Cryptococcus neoformans* infection in organ transplant recipients: Variables influencing clinical characteristics and outcome. Emerg Infect Dis 7:375-381, 2001.
135. Holt CD, Winston DJ, Kubak BK, et al: Coccidioidomycosis in liver transplantation. Clin Infect Dis 24:216, 1997.
136. Welty FK, McLeod GX, Ezratty C, et al: *Pseudallescheria boydii* endocarditis of the pulmonic valve in a liver transplant recipient. Clin Infect Dis 15:858-860, 1992.
137. Alexander BD: Diagnosis of fungal infection: New technologies for the mycology laboratory. Transpl Infect Dis 4(Suppl 3):32-37, 2002.
138. Patterson TF: Approaches to fungal diagnosis in transplantation. Transpl Infect Dis 1:262-272, 1999.
139. Verweij PE, Meis JF: Microbiological diagnosis of invasive fungal infections in transplant recipients. Transpl Infect Dis 2:80, 2000.
140. Walsh T, Pizzo PA: Laboratory diagnosis of candidiasis. In Bodry GP (ed): Candidiasis. New York, Raven Press, 1992, pp 109-135.
141. Kusne S, Torre-Cisneros J, Manez R, et al: Factors associated with invasive lung aspergillosis and the significance of positive *Aspergillus* culture after liver transplantation. J Infect Dis 166:1379-1383, 1992.
142. Wheat JJ: Rapid diagnosis of invasive aspergillosis by antigen detection. Transpl Infect Dis 5:158-166, 2003.
143. Kwak EJ, Husain S, Obman A, et al: Efficacy of galactomannan antigen in the Platelia *Aspergillus* enzyme immunoassay for diagnosis of invasive aspergillosis in liver transplant recipients. J Clin Microbiol 42:435-438, 2004.
144. Mueller NJ, Fishman JA: Asymptomatic pulmonary cryptococcosis in solid organ transplantation: Report of four cases and review of the literature. Transpl Infect Dis 5:140-143, 2003.
145. Singh N, Gayowski T, Wagener MM, et al: Clinical spectrum of invasive cryptococcosis in liver transplant recipients receiving tacrolimus. Clin Transplant 11:66-70, 1997.
146. Wu G, Vilchez RA, Eidelman B, et al: Cryptococcal meningitis: An analysis among 5,521 consecutive organ transplant recipients. Transpl Infect Dis 4:183-188, 2002.
147. Singh N, Gayowski T, Singh J, Yu VL: Invasive gastrointestinal zygomycosis in a liver transplant recipient: Case report and review of zygomycosis in solid-organ transplant recipients. Clin Infect Dis 20:617-620, 1995.
148. Castiglioni B, Sutton DA, Rinaldi MG, et al: *Pseudallescheria boydii* (Anamorph *Scedosporium apiospermum*). Infection in solid organ transplant recipients in a tertiary medical center and review of the literature. Medicine (Baltimore) 81:333-348, 2002.

149. Baily EM, Krakovsky DJ, Rybak M: The triazole antifungal agents: A review of itraconazole and fluconazole. Pharmacotherapy 10:146, 1990.

150. Wong-Beringer A, Kriengkauykiat J: Systemic antifungal therapy: New options, new challenges. Pharmacotherapy 23:1441, 2003.

151. Bodey GP: Azole antifungal agents. J Infect Dis 14(Suppl 1): S161-S169, 1992.

152. Lumbreras C, Cuervas-Mons V, Jara P, et al: Randomized trial of fluconazole versus nystatin for the prophylaxis of *Candida* infection following liver transplantation. J Infect Dis 174:583, 1996.

153. Winston DJ, Pakrasi A, Busuttil RW: Fluconazole prophylaxis of fungal infections in liver transplant recipients: Results of a placebo-controlled, double blind trial. Ann Intern Med 131:729, 1999.

154. Patel R: Prophylactic fluconazole in liver transplant recipients: A randomized, double-blind, placebo-controlled trial. Liver Transpl 6:376, 2000.

155. Winston DJ, Busuttil RW: Randomized controlled trial of oral itraconazole solution versus intravenous/oral fluconazole for prevention of fungal infections in liver transplant recipients. Transplantation 74:688, 2002.

156. Sharpe MD, Ghent C, Grant D, et al: Efficacy and safety of itraconazole prophylaxis for fungal infections after orthotopic liver transplantation: A prospective, double-blind study. Transplantation 76:977, 2003.

157. Tollemar J, Hockerstedt K, Ericzon BG, et al: Liposomal amphotericin B prevents invasive fungal infections in liver transplant recipients. Transplantation 59:45, 1995.

158. Pearson MM, Rogers PD, Cleary JD, et al: Voriconazole: A new triazole antifungal agent. Ann Pharmacother 37:420, 2003.

159. Albengres E, Lelouet H, Tillement JP: Systemic antifungal agents: Drug interactions of clinical significance. Drug Saf 18:83, 1998.

160. Mignat G: Clinically significant drug interactions with new immunosuppressive agents. Drug Saf 16:267, 1997.

161. Christians U, Jacobson W, Benet LZ, et al: Mechanisms of clinically relevant drug interactions associated with tacrolimus. Clin Pharmacokinet 41:813, 2002.

162. Campana C, Regazzi MB, Buggia I, et al: Clinically significant drug interactions with cyclosporine. Clin Pharmacokinet 30:141, 1996.

163. Voriconazole (prescribing information).

164. Denning DW: Echinocandin antifungal drugs. Lancet 362:1142, 2003.

165. Johnson MD, Perfect JR: Caspofungin: First approved agent in a new class of antifungals. Exp Opin Pharmacother 4:807, 2003.

166. Caspofungin (prescribing information).

167. Gallis HA, Drew RH, Pickard WW: Amphotericin B: 30 years of clinical experience. Rev Infect Dis 12:308, 1990.

168. Kucers A, Crowe S, Grayson ML, Hoy J: The Use of Antibiotics, 5th ed. Butterworth-Heinemann, 1997, pp 1245-1294.

169. Herbrecht R, Natarajan-Ame S, Nivoix Y, et al: The lipid formulations of amphotericin B. Exp Opin Pharmacother 4:1277, 2003.

170. Wong-Beringer A, Jacobs RA, Guglielmo BJ: Lipid formulations of amphotericin B: Clinical efficacy and toxicities. Clin Infect Dis 27:603, 1998.

171. Janknegt R, DeMarie S, Bakker-Woudenberg AJM, Crommelin JA: Liposomal and lipid formulations of amphotericin B. Drugs 23:279, 1992.

172. Singhal S, Ellis RW, Jones SG, et al: Targeted prophylaxis with amphotericin B lipid complex in liver transplantation. Liver Transpl 6:588-595, 2000.

173. Singh N, Patterson DL, Gayowski T, et al: Preemptive prophylaxis with a lipid preparation of amphotericin B for invasive fungal infections in liver transplant recipients requiring renal replacement therapy. Transplantation 71:910-913, 2001.

174. Fisher NC, Singhal S, Miller SJ, et al: Fungal infection and liposomal amphotericin B (AmBisome) therapy in liver transplantation: A 2 year review. J Antimicrob Chemother 43:597-600, 1999.

175. Linden P, Williams P, Chan KM: Efficacy and safety of amphotericin B lipid complex injection (ABLC) in solid-organ transplant recipients with invasive fungal infections. Clin Transplant 14(4 Pt 1):329-339, 2000.

176. Lorf T, Braun D, Ruchel R, et al: Systemic mycoses during prophylactical use of liposomal amphotericin B (Ambisome) after liver transplantation. Mycoses 42:47-53, 1999.

177. Fortun J, Martin-Davila P, Moreno S, et al: Prevention of invasive fungal infections in liver transplant recipients: The role of prophylaxis with lipid formulations of amphotericin B in high-risk patients. J Antimicrob Chemother 52:813, 2003.

178. Herbrecht R, Denning DW, Patterson TF, et al: Voriconazole versus amphotericin B for primary therapy of invasive aspergillosis. N Engl J Med 347:408-415, 2002.

179. Tsiodras S, Zafiropoulou R, Giotakis J, et al: Deep sinus aspergillosis in a liver transplant recipient successfully treated with a combination of caspofungin and voriconazole. Transpl Infect Dis 6:37-40, 2004.

180. van der Bij W, Speich R: Management of cytomegalovirus infection and disease after solid-organ transplantation. Clin Infect Dis 33(Suppl 1):S32-S37, 2001.

181. Paya CV: Prevention of cytomegalovirus disease in recipients of solid-organ transplants. Clin Infect Dis 32:596-603, 2001.

182. Hibberd PL, Snydman DR: Cytomegalovirus infection in organ transplant recipients. Infect Dis Clin North Am 9:863-877, 1995.

183. Singh N, Wannstedt C, Keyes L, et al: Impact of evolving trends in recipient and donor characteristics on cytomegalovirus infection in liver transplant recipients. Transplantation 77:106-110, 2004.

184. Singhal S, Khan OA, Bramble RA, et al: Cytomegalovirus disease following liver transplantation: An analysis of prophylaxis strategies. J Infect 47:104-109, 2003.

185. Kusne S, Shapiro R, Fung J: Prevention and treatment of cytomegalovirus infection in organ transplant recipients. Transpl Infect Dis 1:187-203, 1999.

186. Stratta RJ, Shaefer MS, Markin RS, et al: Clinical patterns of cytomegalovirus disease after liver transplantation. Arch Surg 124:1443-1450, 1989.

187. Singh N, Dummer JS, Kusne S, et al: Infections with cytomegalovirus and other herpesviruses in 121 liver transplant recipients: Transmission by donated organ and the effect of OKT3 antibodies. J Infect Dis 158:124-131, 1988.

188. Sido B, Hoffman WJ, Otto G, et al: Cytomegalovirus infection of the liver graft early after transplantation: Incidence and clinical relevance. Transplant Proc 25:2671-2672, 1993.

189. Bronsther O, Makowka L, Jaffe R, et al: Occurrence of cytomegalovirus hepatitis in liver transplant patients. J Med Virol 24:423-434, 1988.

190. Alessiani M, Kusne S, Fung JJ, et al: CMV infection in liver transplantation under cyclosporine or FK506 immunosuppression. Transplant Proc 23:3035-3037, 1991.

191. O'Grady JG, Alexander GJ, Sutherland S, et al: Cytomegalovirus infection and donor/recipient HLA antigens: Interdependent co-factors in pathogenesis of vanishing bile-duct syndrome after liver transplantation. Lancet 2:302-305, 1988.

192. Paya CV, Wiesner RH, Hermans PE, et al: Lack of association between cytomegalovirus infection, HLA matching and the vanishing bile duct syndrome after liver transplantation. Hepatology 16:66-70, 1992.

193. Pancholi P, Wu F, Della-Latta P: Rapid detection of cytomegalovirus infection in transplant patients. Exp Rev Mol Diagn 4:231-242, 2004.

194. Schroeder R, Michelon T, Fagundes I, et al: Comparison between RFLP-PCR and antigenemia for pp65 antigen for diagnosis of cytomegalovirus disease after kidney transplantation. Transplant Proc 36:891-893, 2004.

195. Abecassis MM, Koffron AJ, Kaplan B, et al: The role of PCR in the diagnosis and management of CMV in solid organ recipients: What is the predictive value for the development of disease and should PCR be used to guide antiviral therapy? Transplantation 63:275-279, 1997.

196. Paya CV, Smith TF, Ludwig J: Rapid shell vial culture and tissue histology compared with serology for the rapid diagnosis of cytomegalovirus infection in liver transplantation. Mayo Clin Proc 64:670-675, 1989.

197. Norris S, Kosar Y, Donaldson N: Cytomegalovirus infection after liver transplantation: Viral load as a guide to treating clinical infection. Transplantation 74:527-531, 2002.

198. Piiparinen H, Hockerstedt K, Gronhagen-Riska C, et al: Comparison of plasma polymerase chain reaction and pp65-antigenemia assay in the quantification of cytomegalovirus in liver and kidney transplant patients. J Clin Virol 22:111-116, 2001.

199. Pereyra F, Rubin RH: Prevention and treatment of cytomegalovirus infection in solid organ transplant recipients. Curr Opin Infect Dis 17:357-361, 2004.

200. McGavin JK, Goa KL: Ganciclovir: An update of its use in the prevention of cytomegalovirus infection and disease in transplant recipients. Drugs 61:1153-1183, 2001.

201. Scott JC, Partovi N, Ensom MH: Ganciclovir in solid organ transplant recipients: Is there a role for clinical pharmacokinetic monitoring? Ther Drug Monit 26:68-77, 2004.

202. Snydman DR: Historical overview of the use of cytomegalovirus hyperimmune globulin in organ transplantation. Transpl Infect Dis 3(Suppl 2):6-13, 2001.

203. Mylonakis E, Kallas WM, Fishman JA, et al: Combination antiviral therapy for ganciclovir-resistant cytomegalovirus infection in solid-organ transplant recipients. Clin Infect Dis 34:1337-1341, 2002.

204. Isada CM, Yen-Lieberman B, Lurain NS, et al: Clinical characteristics of 13 solid organ transplant recipients with ganciclovir-resistant cytomegalovirus infection. Transpl Infect Dis 4:189-194, 2002.

205. Limaye AP: Ganciclovir-resistant cytomegalovirus in organ transplant recipients. Clin Infect Dis 35:866-872, 2002.

206. Sia IG, Patel R: New strategies for prevention and therapy of cytomegalovirus infection and disease in solid-organ transplant recipients. Clin Microbiol Rev 13:83-121, 2000.

207. Stratta RJ, Shaefer MS, Cushing KA, et al: Successful prophylaxis of cytomegalovirus disease after primary CMV exposure in liver transplant recipients. Transplantation 51:90-97, 1991.

208. Saliba F, Eyraud D, Samuel D, et al: Randomized controlled trial of acyclovir for the prevention of cytomegalovirus infection and disease in liver transplant recipients. Transplant Proc 25:1444-1445, 1993.

209. Singh N, Yu VL, Mieles L, et al: High-dose acyclovir compared with short-course preemptive ganciclovir therapy to prevent cytomegalovirus disease in liver transplant recipients: A randomized trial. Ann Intern Med 120:375-381, 1994.

210. Snydman DR, Werner BG, Dougherty NN, et al: Cytomegalovirus immune globulin prophylaxis in liver transplantation: A randomized, double-blind, placebo-controlled trial. Ann Intern Med 119:984-991, 1993.

211. Martin M, Manez R, Linden P, et al: A prospective randomized trial comparing sequential ganciclovir–high dose acyclovir to high dose acyclovir for prevention of cytomegalovirus disease in adult liver transplant recipients. Transplantation 58:779-785, 1994.

212. Winston DJ, Wirin D, Shaked A, Busuttil RW: Randomised comparison of ganciclovir and high-dose acyclovir for long-term cytomegalovirus prophylaxis in liver-transplant recipients. Lancet 346:69-74, 1995.

213. Green M, Kaufmann M, Wilson J, Reyes J: Comparison of intravenous ganciclovir followed by oral acyclovir with intravenous ganciclovir alone for prevention of cytomegalovirus and Epstein-Barr virus disease after liver transplantation in children. Clin Infect Dis 25:1344-1349, 1997.

214. King SM, Superina R, Andrews W, et al: Randomized comparison of ganciclovir plus intravenous immune globulin (IVIG) with IVIG alone for prevention of primary cytomegalovirus disease in children receiving liver transplants. Clin Infect Dis 25:1173-1179, 1997.

215. Gavalda J, de Otero J, Murio E, et al: Two grams daily of oral acyclovir reduces the incidence of cytomegalovirus disease in CMV-seropositive liver transplant recipients. Transpl Int 10:462-465, 1997.

216. Gane E, Saliba F, Valdecasas GJ, et al: Randomised trial of efficacy and safety of oral ganciclovir in the prevention of cytomegalovirus disease in liver-transplant recipients. The Oral Ganciclovir International Transplantation Study Group. Lancet 350:1729-1733, 1997.

217. Badley AD, Seaberg EC, Porayko MK, et al: Prophylaxis of cytomegalovirus infection in liver transplantation: A randomized trial comparing a combination of ganciclovir and acyclovir to acyclovir. NIDDK Liver Transplantation Database. Transplantation 64:66-73, 1997.

218. Winston DJ, Busuttil RW: Randomized controlled trial of oral ganciclovir versus oral acyclovir after induction with intravenous ganciclovir for long-term prophylaxis of cytomegalovirus disease in cytomegalovirus-seropositive liver transplant recipients. Transplantation 75:229-233, 2003.

219. Winston DJ, Busuttil RW: Randomized controlled trial of sequential intravenous and oral ganciclovir versus prolonged intravenous ganciclovir for long-term prophylaxis of cytomegalovirus disease in high-risk cytomegalovirus-seronegative liver transplant recipients with cytomegalovirus-seropositive donors. Transplantation 77:305-308, 2004.

220. Pescovitz MD, Rabkin J, Merion RM, et al: Valganciclovir results in improved oral absorption of ganciclovir in liver transplant recipients. Antimicrob Agents Chemother 44:2811-2815, 2000.

221. Paya C, Humar A, Dominguez E, et al: Efficacy and safety of valganciclovir vs. oral ganciclovir for prevention of cytomegalovirus disease in solid organ transplant recipients. Am J Transplant 4:611-620, 2004.

222. Boivin G, Goyette N, Gilbert C, et al: Absence of cytomegalovirus-resistance mutations after valganciclovir prophylaxis, in a prospective multicenter study of solid-organ transplant recipients. J Infect Dis 189:1615-1618, 2004.

223. Akalin E, Sehgal V, Ames S, et al: Cytomegalovirus disease in high-risk transplant recipients despite ganciclovir or valganciclovir prophylaxis. Am J Transplant 3:731-735, 2003.

224. Pescovitz MD: Formulary considerations for drugs used to prevent cytomegalovirus disease. Am J Health Syst Pharm 60(23 Suppl 8): S17-S21, 2003.

225. Sommerville KT: Cost advantages of oral drug therapy for managing cytomegalovirus disease. Am J Health Syst Pharm 60(23 Suppl 8):S9-S12, 2003.

226. Das A: Cytomegalovirus infection in solid organ transplantation: Economic implications. Pharmacoeconomics 21:467-475, 2003.

227. Daly JS, Kopasz A, Anandakrishnan R, et al: Preemptive strategy for ganciclovir administration against cytomegalovirus in liver transplantation recipients. Am J Transplant 2:955-958, 2002.

228. Paya CV, Wilson JA, Espy MJ, et al: Preemptive use of oral ganciclovir to prevent cytomegalovirus infection in liver transplant patients: A randomized, placebo-controlled trial. J Infect Dis 185:854-860, 2002.

229. Torre-Cisneros J, Madueno JA, Herrero C, et al: Pre-emptive oral ganciclovir can reduce the risk of cytomegalovirus disease in liver transplant recipients. Clin Microbiol Infect 8:773-780, 2002.

230. Singh N, Paterson DL, Gayowski T, et al: Cytomegalovirus antigenemia directed pre-emptive prophylaxis with oral versus I.V. ganciclovir for the prevention of cytomegalovirus disease in liver transplant recipients: A randomized, controlled trial. Transplantation 70:717-722, 2000.

231. Rayes N, Seehofer D, Schmidt CA, et al: Prospective randomized trial to assess the value of preemptive oral therapy for CMV infection following liver transplantation. Transplantation 72:881-885, 2001.

232. Seu P, Winston DJ, Holt CD, et al: Long-term ganciclovir prophylaxis for successful prevention of primary cytomegalovirus (CMV) disease in CMV-seronegative liver transplant recipients with CMV-seropositive donors. Transplantation 64:1614-1617, 1997.

233. Yoshikawa T: Significance of human herpesviruses to transplant recipients. Curr Opin Infect Dis 16:601-606, 2003.

234. Ljungman P: Prophylaxis against herpesvirus infections in transplant recipients. Drugs 61:187-196, 2001.

235. Haagsma EB, Klompmaker IJ, Grond J, et al: Herpes virus infections after orthotopic liver transplantation. Transplant Proc 19:4054-4056, 1987.

236. Gourishankar S, McDermid JC, Jhangri GS, Preiksaitis JK: Herpes zoster infection following solid organ transplantation: Incidence, risk factors and outcomes in the current immunosuppressive era. Am J Transplant 4:108-115, 2004.

237. Pacini-Edelstein SJ, Mehra M, Ament ME, et al: Varicella in pediatric liver transplant patients: A retrospective analysis of treatment and outcome. J Pediatr Gastroenterol Nutr 37:183-186, 2003.

238. Holmes RD, Sokol RJ: Epstein-Barr virus and post-transplant lymphoproliferative disease. Pediatr Transplant 6:456-464, 2002.

239. Duvoux C, Pageaux GP, Vanlemmens C, et al: Risk factors for lymphoproliferative disorders after liver transplantation in adults: An analysis of 480 patients. Transplantation 74:1103-1109, 2002.

240. Fellner MD, Durand K, Correa M, et al: A semiquantitative PCR method (SQ-PCR) to measure Epstein-Barr virus (EBV) load: Its application in transplant patients. J Clin Virol 3:323-330, 2003.

241. Jain A, Nalesnik M, Reyes J, et al: Posttransplant lymphoproliferative disorders in liver transplantation: A 20-year experience. Ann Surg 236:429-436, 2002.

242. Hurwitz M, Desai DM, Cox KL, et al: Complete immunosuppressive withdrawal as a uniform approach to post-transplant lymphoproliferative disease in pediatric liver transplantation. Pediatr Transplant 8:267-272, 2004.

243. Razonable RR, Paya CV: Herpesvirus infections in transplant recipients: Current challenges in the clinical management of cytomegalovirus and Epstein-Barr virus infections. Herpes 10:60-65, 2003.

244. Ganne V, Siddiqi N, Kamaplath B, et al: Humanized anti-CD20 monoclonal antibody (rituximab) treatment for post-transplant lymphoproliferative disorder. Clin Transplant 17:417-422, 2003.

245. Yedibela S, Reck T, Niedobitek G, et al: Anti-CD20 monoclonal antibody treatment of Epstein-Barr virus–induced intrahepatic lymphoproliferative disorder following liver transplantation. Transpl Int 16:197-201, 2003.

246. Razonable RR, Paya CV: The impact of human herpesvirus-6 and -7 infection on the outcome of liver transplantation. Liver Transpl 8:651-658, 2002.

247. Singh N, Husain S, Carrigan DR, et al: Impact of human herpesvirus-6 on the frequency and severity of recurrent hepatitis C virus hepatitis in liver transplant recipients. Clin Transplant 16:92-96, 2002.

248. Emery VC: Human herpesviruses 6 and 7 in solid organ transplant recipients. Clin Infect Dis 32:1357-1360, 2001.

249. Singh N: Human herpesviruses-6, -7 and -8 in organ transplant recipients. Clin Microbiol Infect 6:453-459, 2000.

250. Rogers J, Rohal S, Carrigan DR, et al: Human herpesvirus-6 in liver transplant recipients: Role in pathogenesis of fungal infections, neurologic complications, and outcome. Transplantation 69:2566-2573, 2000.

251. Marcelin AG, Roque-Afonso AM, Hurtova M, et al: Fatal disseminated Kaposi's sarcoma following human herpesvirus 8 primary infections in liver-transplant recipients. Liver Transpl 10:295-300, 2004.

252. Garcia-Sesma A, Jimenez C, Loinaz C, et al: Kaposi's visceral sarcoma in liver transplant recipients. Transplant Proc 35:1898-1899, 2003.

253. Allen UD: Human herpesvirus type 8 infections among solid organ transplant recipients. Pediatr Transplant 6:187-192, 2002.

254. Pozo F, Tenorio A, de la Mata M, et al: Persistent human herpesvirus 8 viremia before Kaposi's sarcoma development in a liver transplant recipient. Transplantation 70:395-397, 2000.

255. Colina F, Lopez-Rios F, Lumbreras C, et al: Kaposi's sarcoma developing in a liver graft. Transplantation 61:1779-1781, 1996.

256. McGrath D, Falagas ME, Freeman R, et al: Adenovirus infection in adult orthotopic liver transplant recipients: Incidence and clinical significance. J Infect Dis 177:459-462, 1998.

257. Saad RS, Demetris AJ, Lee RG, et al: Adenovirus hepatitis in the adult allograft liver. Transplantation 64:1483-1485, 1997.

258. Michaels MG, Green M, Wald ER, Starzl TE: Adenovirus infection in pediatric liver transplant recipients. J Infect Dis 165:170-174, 1992.

259. Koneru B, Jaffe R, Esquivel CO, et al: Adenoviral infections in pediatric liver transplant recipients. JAMA 258:489-492, 1987.

260. Boubenider S, Hiesse C, Marchand S, et al: Post-transplantation polyomavirus infections. J Nephrol 12:24-29, 1999.

261. Mylonakis E, Goes N, Rubin RH, et al: BK virus in solid organ transplant recipients: An emerging syndrome. Transplantation 72:1587-1592, 2001.

262. Bronster DJ, Lidov MW, Wolfe D, et al: Progressive multifocal leukoencephalopathy after orthotopic liver transplantation. Liver Transpl Surg 1:371-372, 1995.

263. Vilchez RA, McCurry K, Dauber J, et al: Influenza virus infection in adult solid organ transplant recipients. Am J Transplant 2:287-291, 2002.

264. Krinzman S, Basgoz N, Kradin R, et al: Respiratory syncytial virus–associated infections in adult recipients of solid organ transplants. J Heart Lung Transplant 17:202-210, 1998.

265. Singhal S, Muir DA, Ratcliffe DA, et al: Respiratory viruses in adult liver transplant recipients. Transplantation 68:981-984, 1999.

266. Pohl C, Green M, Wald ER, Ledesma-Medina J: Respiratory syncytial virus infections in pediatric liver transplant recipients. J Infect Dis 165:166-169, 1992.

267. Ndimbie OK, Frezza E, Jordan JA, et al: Parvovirus B19 in anemic liver transplant recipients. Clin Diagn Lab Immunol 3:756-760, 1996.

268. Chang FY, Singh N, Gayowski T, Marino IR: Parvovirus B19 infection in a liver transplant recipient: Case report and review in organ transplant recipients. Clin Transplant 10:243-247, 1996.

269. Dummer JS, Erb S, Breinig MK, et al: Infection with human immunodeficiency virus in the Pittsburgh transplant population: A study of 583 donors and 1043 recipients, 1981-1986. Transplantation 47:134-140, 1989.

270. Simonds RJ, Holmberg SD, Hurwitz RL, et al: Transmission of human immunodeficiency virus type 1 from a seronegative organ and tissue donor. N Engl J Med 326:726-732, 1992.

271. Roland ME, Adey D, Carlson LL, Terrault NA: Kidney and liver transplantation in HIV-infected patients: Case presentations and review. AIDS Patient Care STDs 17:501-507, 2003.

272. Roland ME, Lo B, Braff J, Stock PG: Key clinical, ethical, and policy issues in the evaluation of the safety and effectiveness of solid organ transplantation in HIV-infected patients. Arch Intern Med 163:1773-1778, 2003.

273. Kuo PC, Stock R: Transplantation in the HIV+ patient. Am J Transplant 1:13-17, 2001.

274. Gow PJ, Pillay D, Mutimer D: Solid organ transplantation in patients with HIV infection. Transplantation 72:177-181, 2001.

275. Jacobson SK, Calne RY, Wreghitt TG: Outcome of HIV infection in transplant patient on cyclosporin. Lancet 337:794, 1991.

276. Samuel D, Duclos Vallee JC, Teicher E, Vittecoq D: Liver transplantation in patients with HIV infection. J Hepatol 39:3-6, 2003.

277. Alter MJ, Kruszon-Moran D, Nainan OV, et al: The prevalence of hepatitis C virus infection in the United States, 1988 through 1994. N Engl J Med 341:556-562, 1999.

278. Flamm SL: Chronic hepatitis C infection. JAMA 289:2413-2417, 2003.

279. Wong JB, McQuillan GM, McHutchison JG, Poynard T: Estimating future hepatitis C morbidity, mortality, and costs in the United States. Am J Public Health 90:1562-1569, 2000.

280. Berunguer M: Natural history of recurrent hepatitis C. Liver Transpl 8(Suppl 1):S14-S18, 2002.

281. Charlton M, Seaberg E, Wiesner R, et al: Predictors of patient and graft survival following liver transplantation for hepatitis C. Hepatology 28:823-830, 1998.

282. Berenguer M, Ferrell L, Watson J, et al: HCV-related fibrosis progression following liver transplantation: Increase in recent years. J Hepatol 32:673-684, 2000.

283. Johnson MW, Washburn WK, Freeman RB, et al: Hepatitis C viral infection in liver transplantation. Arch Surg 131:284-291, 1996.

284. Berenguer M, Prieto M, Palau A, et al: Severe recurrent hepatitis C after liver retransplantation for hepatitis C virus–related graft cirrhosis. Liver Transpl 9:228-235, 2003.

285. Forman LM, Lewis JD, Berlin JA, et al: The association between hepatitis C infection and survival after orthotopic liver transplantation. Gastroenterology 122:889-896, 2002.

286. McLaughlin K, Wajsaub S, Marotta P, et al: Increased risk for posttransplant lymphoproliferative disease in recipients of liver transplants with hepatitis C. Liver Transpl 6:570-574, 2000.

287. Abrahamian GA, Cosimi AB, Farrell ML, et al: Prevalence of hepatitis C virus–associated mixed cryoglobulinemia after liver transplantation. Liver Transpl 6:185-190, 2000.

288. Khalili M, Lim JW, Bass N, et al: New onset diabetes mellitus after liver transplantation: The critical role of hepatitis C infection. Liver Transpl 10:349-355, 2004.

289. Ghobrial RM, Steadman R, Gombein J, et al: A 10-year experience of liver transplantation for hepatitis C: Analysis of factors determining outcome in over 500 patients. Ann Surg 234:384-393, 2001.

290. Rosen HR: Retransplantation for hepatitis C: Implications of different policies. Liver Transpl 6(Suppl 2):S41-S46, 2000.

291. Pelletier SJ, Raymond DP, Crabtree TD, et al: Pretransplantation hepatitis C virus quasispecies may be predictive of outcome after liver transplantation. Hepatology 32:375-381, 2000.

292. Dimartino V, Saurini F, Samuel D, et al: Long-term longitudinal study of intrahepatic hepatitis C virus replication after liver transplantation. Hepatology 26:1343-1350, 1997.

293. Charlton M: The impact of advancing donor age on histologic recurrence of hepatitis C infection: The perils of ignored maternal advice. Liver Transpl 9:535-537, 2003.

294. Sheiner PA, Schwartz ME, Mor E, et al: Severe or multiple rejection episodes are associated with early recurrence of hepatitis C after orthotopic liver transplantation. Hepatology 21:30-34, 1995.

295. Berenguer M, Lopez-Labrador FX, Greenberg HB, et al: Hepatitis C virus and the host: An imbalance induced by immunosuppression? Hepatology 32:433-435, 2000.

296. Wiesner RH: A long-term comparison of tacrolimus (FK506) versus cyclosporine in liver transplantation: A report of the United States FK506 Study Group. Transplantation 66:493, 1998.

297. Mueller AR, Platz K, Willimski C, et al: Influence of immunosuppression on patient survival after liver transplantation for hepatitis C. Transplant Proc 33:1347-1349, 2001.

298. Charlton M, Seaberg E: Impact of immunosuppression and acute rejection on recurrence of hepatitis C: Results of the National Institute of Diabetes and Digestive and Kidney Diseases Liver Transplantation Database. Liver Transpl Surg 5(Suppl 1):S107, 1999.

299. Papatheodoridis GV, Davies S, Dhillon AP, et al: The role of different immunosuppression in the long-term histological outcome of HCV reinfection after liver transplantation for HCV cirrhosis. Transplantation 72:412, 2001.

300. Jain A, Kashyap R, Demetris AJ, et al: A prospective randomized trial of mycophenolate mofetil in liver transplant recipients with hepatitis C. Liver Transpl 8:40, 2002.

301. Fasola CG, Netto GJ, Christensen LL, et al: Delay of hepatitis C recurrence in liver transplant recipients: Impact of mycophenolate mofetil on transplant recipients with severe acute rejection or with renal dysfunction. Transplant Proc 34:1561, 2002.

302. Smallwood GA, Davis L, Martinez E, et al: Mycophenolate's influence in the treatment of recurrent hepatitis C following liver transplantation. Transplant Proc 34:1559, 2002.

303. Neuhaus P, Clavien PA, Kittur D, et al: Improved treatment response with basiliximab immunoprophylaxis after liver transplantation: Results from a double-blind randomized placebo-controlled trial. Liver Transpl 8:132, 2002.

304. Calmus Y, Scheele JR, Gonzalez-Pinto I, et al: Immunoprophylaxis with basiliximab, a chimeric anti–interleukin-2 receptor monoclonal antibody, in combination with azathioprine-containing triple therapy in liver transplant recipients. Liver Transpl 8:123-131, 2002.

305. Nelson DR, Soldevila-Pico C, Reed A, et al: Anti–interleukin-2 receptor therapy in combination with mycophenolate mofetil is associated with more severe hepatitis C recurrence after liver transplantation. Liver Transpl 7:1064-1070, 2001.

306. Hayes MJ, Torzillo PJ, Sheil AG, et al: *Pneumocystis carinii* pneumonia after liver transplantation in adults. Clin Transplant 8:499-503, 1994.

307. Colombo JL, Sammut PH, Langnas AN, Shaw BW: The spectrum of *Pneumocystis carinii* infection after liver transplantation in children. Transplantation 54:621-624, 1992.

308. Gluck T, Geerdes-Fenge HF, Straub RH, et al: *Pneumocystis carinii* pneumonia as a complication of immunosuppressive therapy. Infection 28:227-230, 2000.

309. Meyers B, Borrego F, Papanicolaou G, et al: *Pneumocystis carinii* pneumonia prophylaxis with atovaquone in trimethoprim-sulfamethoxazole–intolerant orthotopic liver transplant patients: A preliminary study. Liver Transpl 7:750-751, 2001.

310. Torre-Cisneros J, de la Mata M, Lopez-Cillero P, et al: Effectiveness of daily low-dose cotrimoxazole prophylaxis for *Pneumocystis carinii* pneumonia in liver transplantation—an open clinical trial. Transplantation 62:1519-1521, 1996.

311. Saukkonen K, Garland R, Koziel H: Aerosolized pentamidine as alternative primary prophylaxis against *Pneumocystis carinii* pneumonia in adult hepatic and renal transplant recipients. Chest 109:1250-1255, 1996.

312. Gordon SM, LaRosa SP, Kalmadi S, et al: Should prophylaxis for *Pneumocystis carinii* pneumonia in solid organ transplant recipients ever be discontinued? Clin Infect Dis 28:240-246, 1999.

313. Barcan LA, Dallurzo ML, Clara LO, et al: *Toxoplasma gondii* pneumonia in liver transplantation: Survival after a severe case of reactivation. Transpl Infect Dis 4:93-96, 2002.

314. Patel R: Disseminated toxoplasmosis after liver transplantation. Clin Infect Dis 29:705-706, 1999.

315. Lappalainen M, Jokiranta TS, Halme L: Disseminated toxoplasmosis after liver transplantation: Case report and review. Clin Infect Dis 27:1327-1328, 1998.

316. Salt A, Sutehall G, Sargaison M, et al: Viral and *Toxoplasma gondii* infections in children after liver transplantation. J Clin Pathol 43:63-67, 1990.

317. Wreghitt TG: Viral and *Toxoplasma gondii* infections. In Came R (ed): Liver Transplantation, 2nd ed. London, Grune & Stratton, 1987, pp 365-383.

318. Kusne S, Dummer JS, Ho M, et al: Self-limited *Toxoplasma* parasitemia after liver transplantation. Transplantation 44:457-458, 1987.

319. Safdar N, Said A, Lucey MR: The role of selective digestive decontamination for reducing infection in patients undergoing liver transplantation: A systematic review and meta-analysis. Liver Transpl 10:817-827, 2004.

320. Hellinger WC, Yao JD, Alvarez S, et al: A randomized, prospective, double-blinded evaluation of selective bowel decontamination in liver transplantation. Transplantation 73:1904-1909, 2002.

321. Arnow PM, Carandang GC, Zabner R, Irwin ME: Randomized controlled trial of selective bowel decontamination for prevention of infections following liver transplantation. Clin Infect Dis 22:997-1003, 1996.

322. Arnow PM: Prevention of bacterial infection in the transplant recipient. The role of selective bowel decontamination. Infect Dis Clin North Am 9:849-862, 1995.

323. Wiesner RH, Hermans PE, Rakela J, et al: Selective bowel decontamination to decrease gram-negative aerobic bacterial and *Candida* colonization and prevent infection after orthotopic liver transplantation. Transplantation 45:570-574, 1988.

324. Rossaint R, Raakow R, Lewandowski K, et al: Strategy for prevention of infection after orthotopic liver transplantation. Transplant Proc 23:1965-1966, 1991.

325. Gorensek MJ, Carey WD, Washington JA, et al: Selective bowel decontamination with quinolones and nystatin reduces gram-negative and fungal infections in orthotopic liver transplant recipients. Clev Clin J Med 60:139-144, 1993.

Late Complications of Liver Transplantation and Recurrence of Disease

MICHAEL R. CHARLTON
K. V. NARAYANAN MENON

Late complications of liver transplantation 995
Diabetes mellitus 995
Hyperuricemia and gout 996
Bone disease 996
Hyperlipidemia 997
Coronary artery disease 998
Hypertension 998
Renal dysfunction 998
Obesity 999
Malignancies 999
Allograft rejection 999
Vascular and biliary complications 1000

Recurrence of disease 1000
Hepatitis C 1000
Hepatitis B 1005
Autoimmune and cholestatic
liver disease 1009
Nonalcoholic steatohepatitis
and obesity 1010

According to a prospective study of data from the Liver Transplant Database carried out by the National Institutes of Health, 10-year patient survival rates for deceased donor, orthotopic liver transplantation in adults are currently approximately 50% to 60%, depending on the primary indication. As technical complications after liver transplantation and allograft rejection continue to diminish in frequency, the focus on causes of long-term patient and graft loss has increased. Improved short- and medium-term outcomes reflect advances in patient selection (most of the early recipients had metastatic liver disease), immunosuppression (<2% of livers are currently lost to chronic rejection), surgical technique, and expertise in related fields (e.g., intensive care, anesthesia, infectious diseases). This chapter focuses on the causes and management of long-term complications and recurrence of disease after liver transplantation.

Late Complications of Liver Transplantation

Diabetes Mellitus

Background and Etiology

The reported prevalence of diabetes mellitus in liver transplant recipients ranges from about 4.5% to 53%.[1-6]

When posttransplant diabetes mellitus is defined strictly by the use of insulin beyond the first postoperative month but within 30 days of discharge, the prevalence is about 5.2%.[5] Corticosteroids, cyclosporine, tacrolimus, azathioprine, and mycophenolic acid all have hyperglycemic effects through mechanisms that include corticosteroid-induced insulin resistance and, possibly, calcineurin inhibitor (CNI) toxicity to beta cells. The prevalence of insulin use falls progressively from 26% at 1 year to 9% at 2 years and 1% at 3 years after transplantation.[5]

Management

Management of posttransplant diabetes in the long term is similar to that in the nontransplant setting—diet and lifestyle modification, exercise, weight reduction, and insulin. Oral hypoglycemic agents, including thiazolidenediones, are increasingly being used but have poorly defined immunosuppressive interaction and hepatotoxicity profiles. All oral hypoglycemic agents should be considered to be potentially hepatotoxic. Transplant-specific strategies include prednisone-tapering and CNI-sparing protocols.[7-10] Hepatitis C has been putatively reported to be a risk factor for the development of diabetes mellitus,[4,11,12] although improved glycemic control has not been shown after treatment of hepatitis C virus (HCV) infection.

The impact of diabetes mellitus on long-term outcomes of liver transplant recipients is not definitively known, but the United Network for Organ Sharing (UNOS) database suggests an association of diabetes mellitus with attenuated patient and graft survival. As in the nontransplant setting, posttransplant diabetes has been variably associated with an increased risk for infection and renal impairment.

Hyperuricemia and Gout

Background and Etiology

Hyperuricemia is a recognized complication of transplantation[13,14] that occurs in approximately 50% of all solid organ recipients.[15] Clinically overt gout develops in 6% to 28% of cyclosporine-treated transplant recipients (liver recipients less frequently than cardiac and renal recipients).[13,14,16] Risk factors for the development of posttransplant gout include male gender and elevated serum uric acid. Renal dysfunction caused by CNIs can impair the ability of kidneys to excrete uric acid. Alternatively, hyperuricemia caused by CNIs can result in renal dysfunction. Hyperuricemia occurs in more than 40% of liver transplant recipients.[17]

Management

Acute attacks of gout can be managed with courses of nonsteroidal anti-inflammatory drugs or corticosteroids, or with both. Colchicine is poorly tolerated and may decrease absorption of immunosuppressive agents through gastrointestinal side effects or cause prerenal insufficiency secondary to diarrhea (or both). Long-term prevention of recurrence with allopurinol is generally safe, provided that the interaction between allopurinol and azathioprine is taken into account.

Bone Disease

Background and Etiology

The most common form of bone disease in liver transplant recipients is osteoporosis, defined as a bone mineral density T-score of −2.5 in the spine or hip (or both), with or without one or more fractures. Avascular necrosis of the hips and osteomalacia are also prevalent after liver transplantation. Osteopenia, osteoporosis, or both are observed in 10% to 60% of liver transplant recipients.[18]

The incidence of osteoporosis is increased in patients with cirrhosis, especially those with cholestatic liver disease.[19] Liver transplantation results in rapid bone loss within the first 3 to 6 months.[18-22] After this period, however, there appears to be an improvement in bone mineral density; such improvement can occur for up to 2 years after liver transplantation.[23] The most important complication of osteoporosis after liver transplantation is bone fracture. Patients with cholestatic liver disease have the greatest incidence of pathological fractures (43% of patients with primary biliary cirrhosis [PBC] and 31% of patients with primary sclerosing cholangitis [PSC] versus only 4% of patients with chronic active hepatitis).[24]

The pathophysiology of bone disease in patients with chronic liver disease and after liver transplantation is not well understood. A number of factors, however, are thought to contribute to posttransplant osteoporosis (Fig. 65–1), including the use of glucocorticoid therapy (resulting in increased urinary calcium loss and diminished intestinal absorption), secondary hypoparathyroidism, hypogonadism, and vitamin D deficiency.

Osteoporosis is characterized by reduced bone mass and destruction of bone architecture leading to decreased bone strength and a propensity for fracturing. Bone fractures can be associated with a high level of morbidity and increased mortality. The most common site of pathological fractures in liver transplant recipients is the vertebral body. Other sites include the pelvis, hips, ribs, and wrists. Early studies reported a fracture rate of about 25% to 35% within the first 6 months after transplantation.[18,20,21,25] In a single-center study, new vertebral fractures developed within the first 3 months postoperatively in 27% of patients undergoing liver transplantation between 1993 and 1995. In a subsequent study by the same authors, the incidence of fractures in patients undergoing liver transplantation between 1995 and 1998 was only 5%.[26]

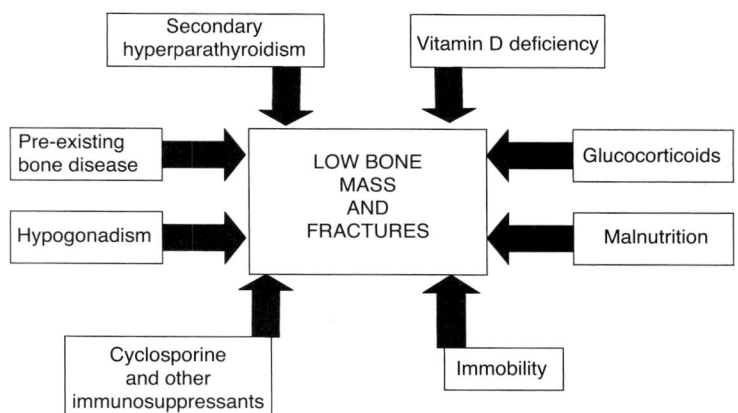

FIGURE 65–1

Factors contributing to bone demineralization after liver transplantation are shown. Corticosteroids are probably the most important contributing factor.

The apparent decrease in incidence is probably due to a combination of events: decreased use of corticosteroids, with most patients being weaned off corticosteroid therapy by the end of the first postoperative year; increased prescribing of antiresorptive agents in the pretransplant phase; and decreased proportion of liver transplant recipients with cholestatic liver disease versus other chronic liver diseases.

Management

Management of osteoporosis in a posttransplant recipient involves optimization of bone health before transplantation and management of bone loss after liver transplantation. All liver transplant recipients, especially those with cholestatic liver disease, should undergo periodic bone densitometry and spinal radiography to screen for osteoporosis. Vitamin D deficiency should be sought and corrected, with follow-up measurements of serum 25-hydroxyvitamin D to ensure that adequate doses of vitamin D have been given. Pharmacological and antiresorptive agents include calcitonin, cyclical etidronate, calcium and sodium fluoride, and the bisphosphonates pamidronate and alendronate.

Although calcitonin is not effective in the treatment of posttransplant osteoporosis, newer antiresorptive agents have been shown to prevent and reverse osteoporosis in the posttransplant setting. Patients at high risk for bone fractures (T-score less than −2.5 or patients with a previous fracture, or both) should be considered for antiresorptive therapy (e.g., alendronate).

Hyperlipidemia

Background and Etiology

Hypercholesterolemia is found in 16% to 43% of liver transplant recipients. About 40% have hypertriglyceridemia.[27-29] Contributing factors are likely to include increased dietary intake of saturated fats secondary to corticosteroid-induced appetite stimulation and corticosteroid-induced increase in low-density lipoprotein (LDL) production. CNIs reduce cholesterol secretion into bile and increase LDL production. There is evidence that hyperlipidemia occurs more frequently with cyclosporine than with tacrolimus. Hyperlipidemia is a specific side effect of sirolimus. Pretransplant serum cholesterol levels have also been found to be an independent predictor of posttransplant hypercholesterolemia on multivariate analysis in one study.[30]

Management

Although an excess of cardiovascular disease has not been definitively demonstrated in liver transplant recipients, cardiovascular disease is the second most common cause of late posttransplant mortality. Management of hyperlipidemia may therefore be important in the long-term management of liver transplant recipients and generally parallels that of nontransplant patients. Initial steps should include an exercise program in conjunction with dietary measures, including a low-fat diet and avoidance of alcohol. 3-Hydroxy-3-methylglutaryl-coenzyme A (HMG-CoA) reductase inhibitors are generally safe and effective in reducing LDL, raising high-density lipoprotein (HDL), and lowering cholesterol and triglyceride levels.[31] Potential adverse effects of the statins include hepatotoxicity, myositis, and rhabdomyolysis. Gemfibrozil and other fibric acid derivatives are effective in treating hypertriglyceridemia but may increase the likelihood of myositis when given with HMG-CoA reductase inhibitors. Bile acid–binding resins such as cholestyramine may reduce absorption of immunosuppressive agents, particularly CNIs, and thereby result in reduced serum levels. Nicotinic acid is generally avoided because of the potential for hepatotoxicity and its relatively poor efficacy when compared with the statins.

In addition to direct pharmacotherapy, altered immunosuppressive prescribing should also be considered. Reduction of CNIs and steroid withdrawal may improve lipid profiles. Conversion from cyclosporine- to tacrolimus-based immunosuppression has also been reported to improve dyslipidemia.

Coronary Artery Disease

With increasing long-term survival in patients undergoing liver transplantation, coronary artery disease has become an important determinant of survival. Cardiovascular risk factors are increasingly common in patients after liver transplantation,[29] including an increase in the incidence of obesity, diabetes mellitus, and hyperlipidemia. The high prevalence of cardiovascular risk factors after liver transplantation might be expected to translate to an increased incidence of cardiovascular diseases in the long term. Romero and colleagues[32] found cardiovascular complications in 4.9% of patients, none of whom had previous cardiovascular disease. The mean time to appearance of these complications after orthotopic liver transplantation was 2.6 years. When compared with an age-matched population not undergoing transplantation, the relative risk of ischemic cardiac events in liver transplant recipients has been reported to be 3.07 (95% confidence interval, 1.98 to 4.53) and the relative risk of cardiovascular death to be 2.56 (95% confidence interval, 1.52 to 4.05).[32]

Management of coronary artery disease in liver transplant recipients mirrors that in nontransplant patients and should focus on risk factor modification as described in the sections on diabetes, obesity, hypertension, and hyperlipidemia.

Hypertension

Background and Etiology

Hypertension occurs in approximately 75% of patients after liver transplantation.[33,34] Contributing factors include immunosuppression and weight gain. Cyclosporine-based immunosuppression is associated with an increased incidence of hypertension when compared with tacrolimus-based regimens.[33] The mechanism of cyclosporine-associated hypertension has been investigated in great detail. Cyclosporine causes renal venous restriction and sodium retention by activating afferent and efferent renal nodes.[35] Cyclosporine can also cause sympathetic activation and hypertension, as seen in heart transplant recipients.[36] Tapering of steroids in liver transplant recipients has been shown to have a beneficial effect on patients with hypertension and can even lead to withdrawal of antihypertensive medication.[37]

Management and Prognosis

Management of hypertension in patients should include pharmacological and nonpharmacological therapies. Weight loss, salt restriction, and regular exercise may help decrease blood pressure in posttransplant recipients. Steroid withdrawal should be considered if appropriate.[9,37] Antihypertensive therapy after liver transplantation requires recognition of the hazards of changing arterial pressure during calcineurin use and the potential for altering CNI levels (e.g., increasing absorption of CNIs with nifedipine). Preferential use of vasodilating drugs, particularly dihydropyridine calcium channel blocking agents, is recommended because of their potent vasodilating properties.[34] Increased systemic vascular resistance and renovasoconstriction are hallmarks of CNI-associated hypertension. Effective blood pressure control can be achieved in more than 85% of recipients with CNI-associated hypertension. The utility of diuretics in the management of post–liver transplant systemic hypertension is limited by the potential for exacerbating hyperuricemia and by the tendency of diuretics to elevate serum creatinine through volume contraction.

Renal Dysfunction

Background and Etiology

Renal dysfunction is an increasingly prevalent long-term complication of liver transplantation. End-stage renal disease occurs in 4.2% to 9.5% of liver transplant recipients after the 10th postoperative year.[38,39] The development of severe posttransplant renal dysfunction is associated with significantly decreased patient survival.[39] Additionally, liver transplant recipients who undergo kidney transplantation have shorter survival than do patients with renal failure who undergo primary kidney transplantation. Perhaps more important, however, liver transplant recipients treated by hemodialysis have a survival rate that is about a third of that in those who undergo kidney transplantation.[39] Risk factors for the development of renal failure after liver transplantation include the use of CNIs (including associated hypertension), the presence of renal dysfunction before transplantation, and a variety of renal abnormalities present in patients with chronic liver disease, including glomerulonephritis, glomerulosclerosis, and IgA nephropathy.

Management

Management of renal dysfunction after liver transplantation is multifaceted. The cornerstones of such management are as follows:

1. Reducing or avoiding the use of CNIs

2. Managing risk factors such as hypertension and diabetes

Approaches to these issues have been dealt with in greater detail in a separate chapter.

Obesity

Background and Etiology

Obesity after liver transplantation is rapidly becoming an important issue. Weight gain in patients who are obese (body mass index > 30 kg/m^2) before transplantation is much greater than that in nonobese recipients.[15,16] The reported prevalence of posttransplant obesity ranges from 17% to as high as 42%.[33,40,41] In a prospective analysis of data from the National Institute of Diabetes, Digestive, and Kidney Disease (NIDDK) Liver Transplant Database, 32% of patients who were not obese before transplantation became obese within 2 years of transplantation.[41] Independent posttransplant predictors of obesity were rejection and a higher cumulative prednisone dose. However, it was noted that despite marked weight gain after liver transplantation, the prevalence of obesity at 2 years was only slightly greater than that in the general U.S. population.[41]

Management

Achieving sustained weight loss in any setting is an elusive goal. Withdrawal of corticosteroids has been associated with weight loss in transplant recipients. In a study by Punch and associates, discontinuing corticosteroids in 51 patients after at least 1 year following liver transplantation resulted in weight loss in 88% of patients (average weight loss of 9.5 lb).[42] Diet and exercise programs are, of course, cornerstones of management but are typically not adhered to. Pharmacotherapy for obesity, such as with sibutramine or orlistat (or with both), is not recommended because of potential reductions in CNI absorption. Conversion from cyclosporine to tacrolimus has been reported to be associated with weight reduction.[32] The safety and efficacy of bariatric surgery after liver transplantation are not known, although success has been reported.[43]

Malignancies

Background and Etiology

Improved posttransplant patient and graft survival has, as might be expected, been associated with an increased prevalence and incidence of posttransplant malignancies.[44,45] Malignancies are a major cause of late death in liver transplant recipients.[44,46] There is irrefutable evidence of an increased incidence of skin, cervical, and lymphoid tumors after liver transplantation.[47] The incidence of oropharyngeal, esophageal, lung, throat, and tongue cancer may also be increased.[45] Risk factors for the development of cancer are thought to be alcoholic liver disease, increasing age, and possibly the intensity of immunosuppression. Skin cancer eventually develops in more than 40% of liver transplant recipients, and posttransplant lymphoproliferative disease develops in about 10%. Approximately 25% of the deaths occurring more than 2 years after transplantation are caused by nonlymphoid de novo malignancy.[45] The incidence, risk factors for, and treatment of malignancies after liver transplantation are dealt with in greater detail in a separate chapter.

Allograft Rejection

The incidence of acute cellular and chronic rejection continues to decline with the advent of new immunosuppressive agents. Acute cellular rejection as a cause of late allograft dysfunction is becoming less common (Table 65–1). Approximately 20% of recipients experience acute cellular rejection beyond the

Table 65-1. CAUSES OF LATE HEPATIC ALLOGRAFT DYSFUNCTION

Category	Cause
Rejection	Late acute and chronic (ductopenic) rejection
Vascular	Hepatic artery, portal vein, hepatic vein occlusion
Biliary complications	Strictures (anastomotic, nonanastomotic) Stones
Recurrent disease	Hepatitis B and C (recurrent or de novo) Autoimmune liver diseases (PBC, PSC, AIH) Nonalcoholic steatohepatitis Alcoholic liver disease
Infections	Bacterial cholangitis Fungal Nonhepatotropic viral, e.g., CMV, Ebstein-Barr
Malignancy	Lymphoproliferative disease/lymphoma Recurrent or de novo primary cancer (hepatocellular carcinoma and cholangiocarcinoma) Metastatic disease
Drug-induced	As for the nontransplant setting

AIH, autoimmune hepatitis; CMV, cytomegalovirus; PBC, primary biliary cirrhosis; PSC, primary sclerosing cholangitis.

first postoperative month.[48] Precipitating factors include a reduction or withdrawal of immunosuppression, poor absorption of medications, and noncompliance.[48] Risk factors for late-onset acute cellular rejection include age younger than 30 years and previous autoimmune hepatitis or fulminant hepatic failure as the cause of transplantation. Tacrolimus-based regimens are associated with lower rates of late rejection than cyclosporine-based regimens are.[48,49] With less rigorous follow-up, the diagnosis of late rejection is often delayed, and it is more often resistant to corticosteroid therapy.[50]

Chronic ductopenic rejection occurs in less than 4% of recipients.[50] One or more episodes of corticosteroid-resistant acute cellular rejection usually predate the onset of ductopenic rejection. Liver biopsy findings include cholestasis and the disappearance of interlobular and septal bile ducts in more than 50% of portal tracts examined.[51] In patients managed with cyclosporine, a switch to tacrolimus in the early stages of chronic ductopenic rejection may lead to biochemical and histological improvement.

Allograft rejection is dealt with thoroughly elsewhere in this textbook.

Vascular and Biliary Complications

Vascular and biliary complications after liver transplantation are reviewed extensively in dedicated chapters.

Recurrence of Disease

Hepatitis C

Liver disease secondary to HCV infection continues to be the most common indication for liver transplantation worldwide. Although the impact of HCV infection on allograft histology varies substantially,[52-58] allograft failure secondary to recurrence of HCV infection is the most common cause of death and retransplantation in recipients with HCV infection.[59]

Dynamics of Posttransplant Hepatitis C Virus Infection

Timing of Reinfection. Although the interval between liver transplantation and clinical allograft infection varies, negative-strand HCV RNA, the best indicator of HCV replication, has been detected in the first week after liver transplantation.[60,61]

A recent, detailed report of the impact of liver transplantation on HCV kinetics found HCV RNA concentrations decreased by a mean of approximately 0.5 $\log_{10}$ IU/mL in the anhepatic phase of transplantation,[62] with a calculated elimination half-life of about 2 hours. These results are similar to those obtained with a plasma apheresis model.[63] Based on these results, the daily production rate of HCV was estimated to be 11.6 $\log_{10}$ to 13.0 $\log_{10}$ viral particles in patients with chronic HCV infection. The magnitude of the decrease in viremia levels in the anhepatic phase has been reported to vary significantly with transfusion requirements during surgery.[62]

After reperfusion, HCV RNA levels typically decrease at an exponential rate that *exceeds* the decrease that occurs during the anhepatic phase. Although the mechanism of this early posttransplant decrease in viremia has not been determined, it seems likely that HCV binding to or uptake by hepatocytes, or both, are contributing factors. It is reasonable to assume that allograft infection occurs immediately after transplantation, thus leaving a very narrow potential window for initiation of passive immunoprophylaxis. Early posttransplant kinetics does not seem to vary with pretransplant HCV RNA concentrations, genotype, or deceased versus living donor donation.[62]

The first substantial report of HCV medium and late posttransplant kinetics was presented by Gane and coworkers.[64] Others have followed.[62,65-67] The sum of these studies suggests that serum levels of HCV RNA typically increase rapidly from week 2 after transplantation and peak by the fourth postoperative month. HCV RNA levels 1 year after transplantation are 10- to 20-fold greater than pretransplant levels. The timing of peak HCV RNA levels is similar to the mean incubation period after HCV infection in nonimmunocompromised hosts (approximately 8 weeks).[68] Although correlation of pretransplant and posttransplant HCV RNA levels has been inconsistent,[61] a high pretransplant viral load (>1 $\log_{10}$ MEq/mL, a level previously correlated with increased mortality and graft loss[59]) has been significantly associated with higher mean posttransplant HCV RNA levels.[67] Tissue HCV RNA levels are, on average, 50- to 100-fold greater than serum levels and correlate strongly with serum levels.[67,69] The relationship between posttransplant viral kinetics and the severity of recurrence of hepatitis C remains unclear. Sreekumar and colleagues[67] found that the HCV RNA level 4 months after liver transplantation was a sensitive and specific predictor of the subsequent histological activity index (HAI) and stage of fibrosis. In addition, high HAI scores (>3) 4 months after liver transplantation have been associated with higher subsequent fibrosis stage.[67] These findings are consistent with previous reports of an association between viral load 1 year after transplantation and subsequent fibrosis stage[66] and an association between higher HCV RNA levels and hepatocellular injury in nonimmunocompromised hosts.[70] The association of higher levels of viremia with a more

FIGURE 65-2

A composite of posttransplant viral kinetics is shown in which the results from several studies are incorporated.[62,64,67] The x-axis time scale is nonlinear as a result of early and late kinetics. Hepatitis C virus (HCV) levels (shown in IU/mL) fall significantly during the anhepatic phase of liver transplantation, fall more steeply after reperfusion, and continue to fall during the first 12 to 24 hours after transplantation. Serum HCV RNA levels typically increase rapidly from week 2 after transplantation and peak by the fourth postoperative month. HCV RNA levels 1 year after transplantation are 10- to 20-fold greater than pretransplant levels.

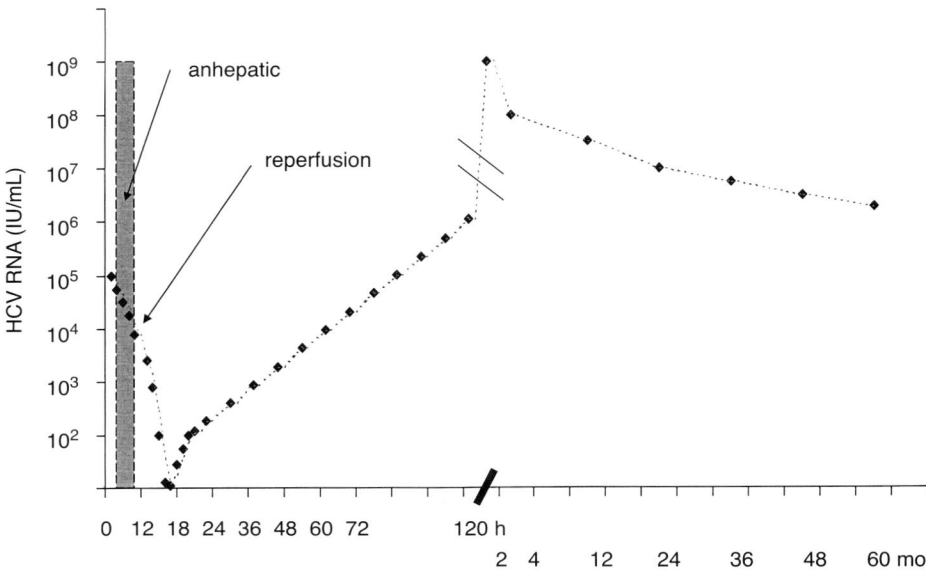

rapidly progressive histological course suggests a cytopathic mechanism of HCV-induced allograft injury, perhaps related to immunosuppression-mediated attenuation of viral clearance. Figure 65-2 shows a composite representation of the typical posttransplant viral kinetics.

Impact of Immunosuppression on Viremia and Recurrence

Corticosteroid treatment of acute cellular rejection is associated with large increases in HCV RNA levels. In the nontransplant setting, corticosteroids are known to increase levels of HCV viremia[71,72] and to be associated with more severe patterns of histological injury.[73] It is thus not altogether surprising that corticosteroids should also affect posttransplant HCV RNA levels and histological recurrence. Pulsed intravenous methylprednisolone therapy is associated with transient 4- to 100-fold increases in HCV RNA levels, and these levels increase steeply (between 2 and 20 times) during episodes of acute lobular hepatitis and decrease with improved graft function.[64] HCV RNA levels do not appear to vary with the choice of CNI. Although no studies have focused on the posttransplant setting, an independent impact of cyclosporine administration on HCV levels was assessed in patients with chronic HCV infection. Kakumu and coworkers observed no changes in HCV viremia after 3 months of cyclosporine administration.[74]

The impact of other immunosuppressive agents on viral kinetics, including mycophenolate mofetil, interleukin-2 receptor antibodies, OKT3, and sirolimus, is unknown.

Although the relevance of studies of posttransplant HCV kinetics to the timing of initiation of antiviral therapy remains to be determined, the correlation between early levels of viremia and subsequent allograft injury suggests that initiation of antiviral therapy early in the posttransplant course might be desirable. In addition, similar to posttransplant hepatitis B virus (HBV) infection, the window for initiation of potential passive immunity measures appears to be limited to the very early postoperative period, perhaps the anhepatic phase.

Donor and Recipient Risk Factor Modification

Acute lobular hepatitis develops in approximately 75% of recipients with hepatitis C in the first 6 months after liver transplantation.[53,64,75,76] By the fifth postoperative year, histological evidence of chronic allograft injury secondary to hepatitis C will develop in more than 80% of HCV-infected liver transplant recipients,[53] with cirrhosis developing in up to 30%.[67,77] An accelerated course of liver injury (cholestatic hepatitis C) with subsequent rapid allograft failure is seen in a small proportion of patients (4% to 7%).[78-80] The course of HCV reinfection is thus greatly accelerated in liver transplant recipients when compared with those who are immune competent. Identification and modification of factors associated with more severe recurrence of HCV infection are likely to be a component of any strategy aimed at improving outcomes.

Although the basis for the observed variability in severity of recurrence of HCV infection is poorly understood, a number of potentially modifiable risk factors have been identified. Table 65-2 summarizes these factors.

Viral Factors. Viral factors that may influence disease severity include HCV genotype and quasispecies.

Table 65–2. RISK FACTORS FOR MORE SEVERE RECURRENCE OF HEPATITIS C

Factor	Strength of Evidence
Pretransplant	
Donor age	+++
Living donor	++
Donor/recipient HLA matching	+
Genotype 1B	+
Operative	
Cold ischemic time	+
Donor genetic factors	+
Posttransplant—Recipient	
Age	+++ (patient/graft survival)
Nonwhite	+++ (patient survival)
Severity of illness	+++ (patient/graft survival)
Virological Variables	
Pretransplant viral load	+++
Posttransplant viral load	+++
Immunosuppression	
OKT3, corticosteroids	+++
Time to recurrence	+++
Cytomegalovirus infection	+++

To date, the reported impact of HCV genotype on posttransplant outcomes has been too inconsistent to influence clinical decision-making.[59,81,82] Posttransplant tracking of the emergence of HCV quasispecies has, in small studies, suggested a strong correlation between genetic diversification in the viral envelope region and asymptomatic or mild disease patterns. In contrast, mutations in the HVR1 area have been associated with a low likelihood of viral clearance, the development of acute hepatitis C, lack of response to antiviral therapy, and a higher likelihood for the development of hepatocellular cancer.[83-85] Viral factors lack sufficient sensitivity and specificity to be used in determining the eligibility of patients for liver transplantation or identifying candidates for preemptive antiviral therapy.

Recipient Factors. Several recipient variables have also been associated with more severe recurrence, including recipient age and recipient race, particularly nonwhite (African American, Asian).[59,77] HLA compatibility between donor and recipient has likewise been associated with more severe hepatitis C recurrence,[86] although the association of HLA matching and the severity of recurrence of hepatitis C was not confirmed in a subsequent study.[87]

Donor Factors. Donor factors associated with a negative outcome in HCV-infected liver transplant recipients include (1) donor age, (2) donor fat content, (3) ischemic time, and (4) the use of living donors. These factors are potentially modifiable. Three articles have highlighted an association of advancing donor age with more rapid histological progression of hepatitis C recurrence.[88-90] Donor age older than 50 years seems to be consistently associated with more rapid progression of fibrosis and allograft failure.

Prolonged warm ischemia time[91] and the use of living donors have also been associated with increased severity of recurrence and overall decreased patient and graft survival.[92,93] These observations may be related to the greater susceptibility of regenerating hepatocytes to HCV infection or greater production and activity (or both).

Clinical Factors. A number of potentially modifiable posttransplant factors have also been associated with increased severity of hepatitis C recurrence and poorer patient and graft survival. The impact of immunosuppression on levels of viremia has already been discussed. A strong correlation between rejection episodes that were treated with bolus corticosteroids and increased severity of histological recurrence of hepatitis C has been well documented.[54,94] A relationship between treated rejection and attenuated patient survival in recipients with hepatitis C was confirmed by analysis of data from the NIDDK Liver Transplant Database.[94] When compared with patients not treated for rejection, those treated for acute cellular rejection were independently associated with increased mortality (relative risk, 2.9; $P < .03$). Although the basis of such increased mortality risk remains unclear, the two most common causes of death in HCV-infected recipients were non-HCV infections and allograft failure secondary to hepatitis C recurrence.

The independent effect of T-lymphocyte–depleting agents, such as OKT3 and antithymocyte globulin, on the severity of recurrence has been difficult to determine because of the inherent overlap between antilymphocyte treatment, rejection, and cumulative steroid exposure. Regardless of the mechanism, being treated with T-cell–depleting agents is a significant risk factor for both more rapid development and more severe histological recurrence of hepatitis C and is associated with a fivefold or greater increased risk of mortality or graft loss, or both.[94,95]

Finally, cytomegalovirus (CMV) infection has been strongly associated with increased severity of recurrence.[89,96] This observation suggests that targeted prophylaxis against CMV might reduce the impact of CMV infection on posttransplant outcomes in HCV-infected liver transplant recipients. Further data are clearly needed with regard to the interaction between immunosuppressive agents and clinical factors because such interaction affects the overall impact of hepatitis C recurrence. As noted previously, the development of animal models to study these relationships will greatly facilitate future progress in this area.

Antiviral Therapy for Posttransplant Hepatitis C Virus Infection

No well-controlled, large clinical trials have been conducted to determine the optimal approach to treatment of recurrent HCV infection after liver transplantation. Most published studies have been small, lack controls, have short periods of follow-up, and are devoid of histological analysis. Furthermore, most of the published studies are largely incomparable because of differences in the definition of recurrent hepatitis C; the timing of administration of anti-HCV therapy relative to transplantation; the drugs, doses, and regimens used; and the study endpoints assessed (i.e., biochemical, virological, and histological endpoints have not all been consistently investigated). A review of the published experience with antiviral therapy in the transplant setting follows.

Pretransplant Antiviral Therapy. The NIDDK-sponsored Liver Transplant Database group observed that patients with higher pre–liver transplant HCV RNA titers experienced mortality and graft loss approximately 30% more frequently than did recipients with lower pretransplant HCV RNA titers,[59] a finding confirmed in a subsequent multicenter study that included European recipients.[77] In light of this finding, a pilot study of the tolerability and efficacy of pretransplant antiviral therapy was conducted.[97] Only a small number of UNOS status 2b HCV-infected patients met treatment initiation criteria and were given interferon (IFN) alfa, either as monotherapy or in combination with ribavirin. Although the frequency of viral response was comparable to that reported in other cohorts of patients with cirrhosis, treatment was poorly tolerated; serious adverse events, including systemic infections, occurred commonly. Similar results were obtained in a single-center study incorporating pretransplant antiviral therapy.[98] Thus, the routine use of immediate pretransplant antiviral therapy in patients with Child's B/C cirrhosis is not recommended. In contrast, patients with compensated cirrhosis should be considered for antiviral therapy before transplantation.

Posttransplant Interferon Alfa Monotherapy. The published experience with nonpegylated IFN monotherapy in the treatment of posttransplant HCV infection has also been disappointing. Wright and colleagues achieved transient decreases in HCV RNA, but no impact on histology with IFN alfa alone.[99] In a larger study, Sheiner and coworkers found that IFN administered prophylactically early in the posttransplant course decreased the frequency of histological recurrence of hepatitis C,[100] although none of the recipients achieved a virological response in this study.

Posttransplant Ribavirin Monotherapy. Four reports of the safety and efficacy of ribavirin monotherapy in the treatment of posttransplant HCV infection have been published. In the first study,[101] 6 months of treatment with ribavirin was associated with a reduction in either lobular or periportal inflammation in all seven participants and a reduction in periportal fibrosis in one patient. HCV RNA remained detectable in serum from all patients at the end of this study. In the second report,[102] ribavirin monotherapy was associated with hemolysis in all treated patients, with serum hemoglobin levels decreasing to less than 10 g/dL in 50% of patients. Total leukocyte and lymphocyte counts also decreased significantly during ribavirin treatment. Although necroinflammatory activity improved, there were no virological responders and no improvement in fibrosis stage in this study. The results of two pilot studies of ribavirin monotherapy were similarly disappointing and showed actual worsening of inflammation and fibrosis scores in patients receiving 12 to 17 months of treatment.[103,104] Bizollon and colleagues showed that the use of ribavirin alone as maintenance monotherapy may be effective in preventing re-emergence of hepatitis C after transplantation and that it was associated with an improvement in histological scores when given after 6 months of combination IFN/ribavirin therapy.[105]

Posttransplant Combination Therapy with Nonpegylated Interferon and Ribavirin. Combination therapy with IFN and ribavirin in the nontransplant setting has produced a greater than twofold increase in both end-of-treatment and sustained virological responses when compared with standard IFN monotherapy.[106,107] Four European studies found end-of-treatment virological response rates of 25% to 50% after combination therapy, with approximately 15% of recipients failing to tolerate therapy.[108-112] In the largest report to date, the virological relapse rate was greater than 50% 6 months after cessation of combination therapy.[112] Three of the European studies found histological improvement in virological responders. The North American experience has been less impressive. The University of Miami reported, in abstract form, an end-of-treatment virological response rate of 12%, with histological improvement in a further 12%.[105] Another North American center found an approximate 25% end-of-treatment virological response rate to combination therapy.[113] The differences in efficacy in the European and North American studies may reflect a fundamental difference in study design: treatment was initiated on a prophylactic basis in two of the four European studies (regardless of biochemical or histological profile) versus initiation of treatment after documentation of histological/biochemical recurrence in the North American studies.

The efficacy of IFN plus ribavirin combination therapy in the treatment of posttransplant HCV infection appears to be reduced in recipients with more advanced recurrence.[114] Reversal of fibrosing cholestatic posttransplant HCV infection, although reported, appears to be unusual.[115] The high prevalence of anemia, thrombocytopenia, leukopenia, and renal insufficiency contributes to the high reported dose reduction and treatment cessation of both IFN and ribavirin during the posttransplant period. Based on the cumulative published experience to date, dose reduction/cessation of ribavirin alone can be expected in approximately 50% of recipients during ribavirin therapy, thus limiting the efficacy of combination therapy. Early initiation of erythropoietin has been reported in small studies to facilitate increased tolerability of ribavirin.[116] Dose adjustments of ribavirin for renal insufficiency are imperative in the posttransplant setting.

Posttransplant Pegylated Interferon Alfa Therapy. Three studies using pegylated IFN (PEG-IFN) alfa have been reported to date—two with monotherapy and one with combination therapy. PEG-IFN alfa-2a monotherapy at a dose of 90 µg/wk, initiated 6 to 60 months after transplantation (n = 65), achieved HCV RNA negativity in 35% of patients after 48 weeks of treatment and a sustained virological response in 19% of patients.[117] No episodes of rejection were reported. In a separate study (n = 54), only 11% of recipients lost HCV RNA after 48 weeks of PEG-IFN alfa-2a treatment when initiated prophylactically in the first 3 weeks after transplantation.[118] None of the untreated controls lost HCV RNA in either of these monotherapy studies. Histological follow-up is pending.

There are two detailed reports of the efficacy, as measured by sustained HCV RNA negativity, of PEG-IFN alfa-2b and ribavirin combination therapy for the treatment of histologically established recurrent HCV infection. With the use of 0.5 µg/kg/wk PEG-IFN alfa-2b and 400 to 600 mg/day of ribavirin (combined n = 61), the sustained virological response rates were 25% and 36%. The higher sustained virological response rate was obtained with the 600-mg/day ribavirin dose. Dose reduction frequencies of PEG-IFN with or without ribavirin of greater than 80% can be expected if standard doses are used. Given the superior efficacy of PEG-IFN over standard IFN in the nontransplant setting, future protocols for liver transplant recipients are likely to incorporate combination therapy with PEG-IFN and ribavirin, although at lower doses than those used in the nontransplant setting. Because reduced doses of PEG-IFN (135 µg/wk of PEG-IFN alfa-2a and 0.5 µg/kg/wk of PEG-IFN alfa-2b) are not associated with reduced efficacy in the nontransplant setting, it seems reasonable to start liver transplant recipients at these lower doses. Ribavirin dosing is much more difficult. Although ribavirin levels are likely to be more important than doses and are certainly the major determinant of toxicity, dose adjustments of ribavirin according to levels seems logical. Unfortunately, the optimal level of ribavirin necessary to achieve maximal efficacy while reducing toxicity is unknown. The relative importance of tissue versus serum ribavirin levels is also unknown. Because ribavirin is primarily renally excreted and has a half-life of about 300 hours, the potential for dose-dependent toxicity is substantial in the posttransplant setting.

Summary

Figure 65–3 shows the mean reported virological response rates and frequencies of dose reduction and cessation for standard IFN and ribavirin, for PEG-IFN monotherapy, and for PEG-IFN plus ribavirin. The figure represents crude means calculated from full manuscripts and presentations at scientific meetings. Although combination therapy with PEG-IFN plus

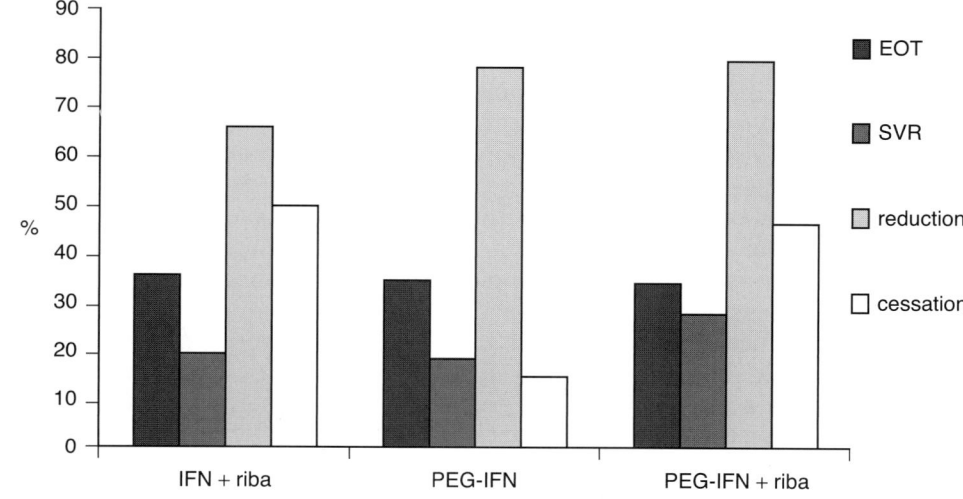

FIGURE 65–3

Comparative mean end-of-treatment (EOT) and sustained virological responses (SVR) for standard and pegylated interferon (PEG-IFN) therapy are shown. The frequency of dose reduction and cessation of therapy is also shown. Values are means derived from the pooled results of published studies (manuscripts and presentations at the 2002 Annual Meeting of the American Association for the Study of Liver Diseases). N refers to the total number of treated patients in all studies combined. riba, ribavirin.

ribavirin appears to have the greatest efficacy, toxicity is also greater, with approximately 50% of recipients requiring cessation of antiviral therapy with this regimen, more than half of which is secondary to ribavirin-associated anemia.

Optimal timing for the initiation of post–liver transplant antiviral therapy is not known (i.e., early in the posttransplant course as prophylaxis or after histologically established recurrence). Although published data suggest that posttransplant HCV infection may be most amenable to therapy when initiated on a prophylactic basis early in the posttransplant course, a direct comparison of the safety and efficacy of antiviral therapy initiated prophylactically versus after hepatitis C is evident histologically has not been performed.

Interferon and the Risk of Rejection in Liver Transplant Recipients. Of the handful of studies describing the outcome of standard IFN therapy for recurrent hepatitis C in liver transplant recipients, two have suggested that IFN treatment may increase the risk for organ rejection. In a study by Sheiner and colleagues, chronic rejection occurred in 5 of the 14 treated patients versus 1 of 32 untreated recipients and led to retransplantation in 3.[100] In a study by Vargas and associates, severe acute rejection developed in one of seven treated patients and chronic rejection developed in another.[119] IFN monotherapy was not associated with an increased risk for rejection in three other studies. Only one case of possible rejection was reported in the 18 patients treated by Wright and coinvestigators.[99] None of the larger more recent studies of combination therapy with IFN and ribavirin have reported an increased frequency or severity of rejection.[112,113,115,120] Some have reported remarkably low rates of rejection during combination therapy (e.g., 0/44 patients, 1/33 patients[121]). Preliminary data from a randomized study of PEG-IFN alfa-2a (40 kD) versus no treatment in patients with established recurrent hepatitis C show no episodes of late acute cellular rejection to date (n = 28).

On balance, there is no compelling evidence that IFN therapy is associated with an increased frequency or severity of rejection in liver transplant recipients.

Hepatitis C Immune Globulin. Hepatitis B immune globulin (HBIG) has moved HBV-infected patients from the ranks of the untransplantable to ideal candidates for liver transplantation. The hope has long been that hepatitis C immune globulin (HCIG) will similarly ameliorate the impact of recurrence of HCV infection. Feray and colleagues demonstrated that HBIG containing anti-HCV reduced HCV reinfection in HBV/HCV-coinfected liver transplant recipients and conferred limited protection against de novo HCV infection.[122] However, a randomized controlled study of HCIG in the prevention of posttransplant HCV infection (n = 26) found no benefit in terms of posttransplant clinical reinfection rate or HCV RNA levels.[123] The availability, cost, and concerns about potential infectivity of pooled HCIG are likely to limit the impact of this therapy even if ultimately proved efficacious. A new monoclonal immune globulin directed at the envelope protein E2 and developed in the trimeric mouse model is currently in phase II trials. No preliminary results have been published to date for this preparation.

Hepatitis B

Background and Epidemiology

More than 350 million people worldwide are estimated to be infected with HBV, 75% of whom are Asian. Liver disease associated with HBV infection is an indication for liver transplantation in approximately 5% of recipients in North America and Europe.[124,125] Despite the introduction of efficacious prophylactic vaccines, the prevalence of liver disease secondary to hepatitis B has not yet declined in North America. The prevalence of chronic HBV infection varies widely by race, from 32 cases per 100,000 for white males to 1740 cases per 100,000 for people of African descent and 2286 per 100,000 for people of Asian descent in the United States.[126] The plateau of prevalence of infection is due principally to chronic HBV infection in immigrants from parts of the world where HBV infection is endemic.[127] Because immigration patterns seem to be set to continue, end-stage liver disease secondary to HBV infection is also likely to continue at a similar frequency in at least the medium term in Western transplant centers as well as in Asia.

Outcomes after liver transplantation for chronic HBV infection vary tremendously by era. Analysis of the NIDDK Liver Transplant Database showed that recipients with HBV infection had the poorest patient and graft survival rates.[59] The graft survival rate at 10 years is 33% and the patient survival rate is 48% in recipients with HBV infection, as opposed to 10-year patient survival rates of 67% and 81% and graft survival rates of 60% and 68% for hepatitis C and cholestatic liver disease, respectively.[59] This difference in patient and graft survival was also apparent in the short and medium term after transplantation. The excess mortality and graft loss in patients with HBV infection was due largely to recurrence of disease, with a relatively high prevalence of fibrosing cholestatic hepatitis B–associated liver injury. The development of HBIG and the nucleoside analogue lamivudine has transformed the posttransplant course of patients with HBV infection.[128] Less than 10 years ago, posttransplant outcomes in recipients with HBV infection were so poor that government and third-party payers were unprepared to underwrite liver transplantation for this indication. Currently, liver failure secondary to HBV infection is one of the premier indications for liver transplantation, with outcomes similar or superior to those for all other indications.

Clinically, posttransplant HBV infection can occur in two principal forms: as reinfection of the allograft (true recurrence) and de novo (e.g., as a result of transmission in blood products or from the allograft). Posttransplant recurrence of HBV infection is most common in patients who are replicative before transplantation as measured by the presence of HBV DNA (by either hybridization assays or polymerase chain reaction [PCR]) or HBV e antigen.[129] The frequency of recurrence is lower in patients with fulminant HBV infection, in those coinfected with hepatitis delta virus, and in patients with no detectable HBV e antigen or HBV DNA.[129] Up until the mid-1990s it was thought that donors with isolated hepatitis B core antibody positivity posed little or no risk of transmission of HBV infection to the recipient. The frequency of de novo HBV infection in recipients of allografts from donors who are isolated hepatitis B core antibody positive is on the order of 50%.[130] The risk of transmission of hepatitis B through transfusion of blood products is 1 in 200,000 per unit of screened packed red blood cells. The overall rate of transmission of de novo HBV infection after liver transplantation has been reduced to less than 1% by the advent of routine screening for hepatitis B immunity and the use of prophylactic hepatitis B vaccination before transplantation.[130] All potential liver transplant recipients should be screened for hepatitis B surface antibody and should be vaccinated when surface antibody is not detected. The risk for posttransplant HBV infection is close to zero in patients who have detectable hepatitis B surface antibody before transplantation. Without immunoprophylaxis, clinical recurrence of hepatitis B will develop in 75% of patients with chronic HBV infection who have replicative disease at the time of transplantation.[128,129] The frequency is reduced to approximately 10% 2 years after transplantation when HBIG is administered.[129,131-133] The rate of clinical posttransplant HBV infection is less than 10% in patients undergoing liver transplantation for fulminant HBV infection, approximately 15% in patients coinfected with hepatitis delta virus, and less than 30% in patients who are HBV DNA negative but surface antigen positive at the time of transplantation.[129,132,133]

Clinically, recurrence of hepatitis B can become manifested almost anytime after the first postoperative month, with the great majority of recurrence having occurred by the 18th postoperative month.[129,132,133] The picture is similar to nontransplant HBV infection with a broad range of biochemical findings. The most severe form of recurrence of HBV infection, fibrosing cholestatic hepatitis, occurs in approximately 5% of HBV-infected recipients. It is associated with progressive cholestasis and fibrosis with rapid allograft failure. Histologically, it is characterized by periportal and perisinusoidal fibrosis, hepatocyte ballooning with apoptotic bodies, histologic evidence of cholestasis, and relatively few inflammatory cells. These findings are associated with very high titers of HBV and with immunohistochemical stains showing intense expression of viral antigens. Although the mechanism of posttransplant recurrence of HBV infection is incompletely understood, it is typically associated with higher HBV levels than seen in the nontransplant setting, which suggests a prominent cytopathic mechanism of injury. It is also possible, however, that increased abundance of viral antigens leads to greater HBV-directed proliferative responses by CD4-positive T cells. Given the relationship between increased immunosuppression and greater frequency and severity of recurrence of hepatitis B, a cytopathic mechanism of posttransplant hepatitis B recurrence and progressive liver injury seems more likely.

Prophylaxis of Recurrence

Publication of the European Concerted Action on Viral Hepatitis (EUROHEP) study of passive immunoprophylaxis with hepatitis B surface antigen immune globulin in 1993 dramatically changed the management and outcomes of transplantation for HBV-infected patients.[129] Recurrence of hepatitis B peaks and plateaus 36 months after transplantation. Approximately half the episodes of recurrence have occurred clinically by the sixth postoperative month. Although the principle of HBIG-based prophylaxis of hepatitis B recurrence is well established, the optimal regimen is not known.[129,132,133] The benefit of HBIG prophylaxis is greatest when it is provided in the long term and at higher doses. HBV DNA can be detected in peripheral blood mononuclear cells and lymph nodes indefinitely after liver transplantation, thus suggesting that posttransplant prophylaxis is suppressive and does not eradicate HBV infection.[134] Even with long-term high-dose HBIG prophylaxis, breakthrough reinfection will occur in 10% to 20% of recipients.[128] A suggested management algorithm to ameliorate posttransplant recurrence of hepatitis B is provided in Figure 65–4 and Table 65–3 (HBIG plus oral antiviral therapy). Based on published data,[129,132,133] the following regimen is likely to be efficacious:

1. 10,000 IU of HBIG intravenously during the anhepatic phase
2. 10,000 IU daily for the first week and on day 14
3. Subsequent dosing to maintain anti–hepatitis B surface antigen (HBsAg) antibody levels greater than 500 IU/L for the first 6 postoperative months and then greater than 250 IU/L.

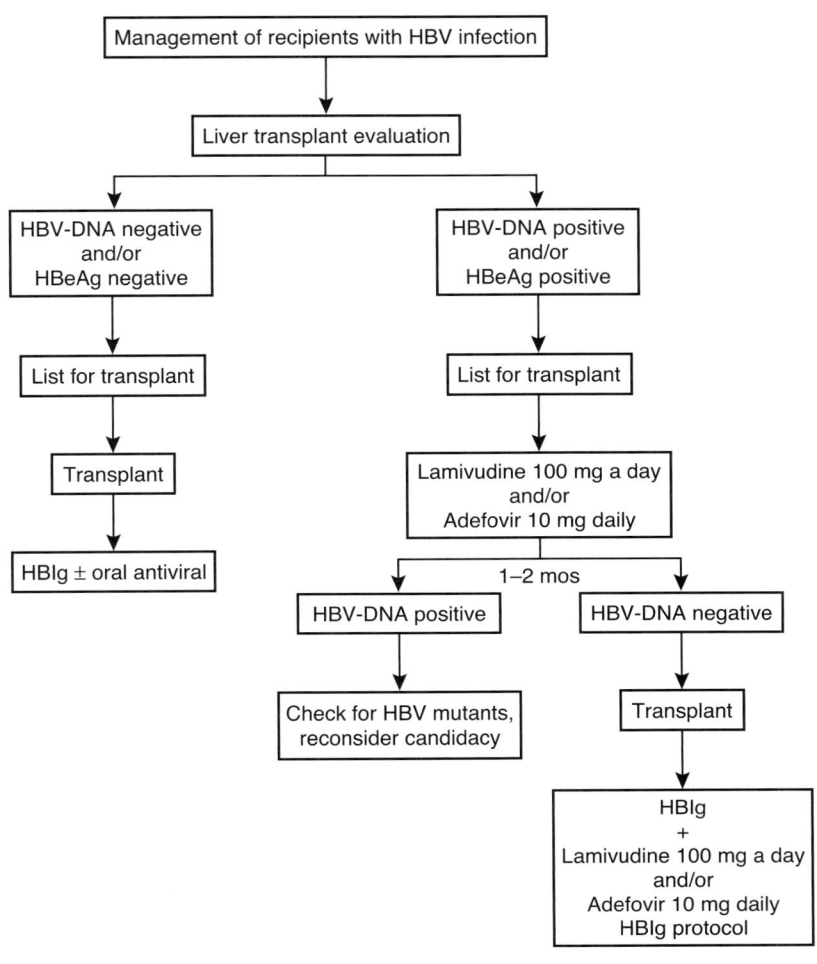

FIGURE 65–4

A suggested algorithm for the prevention of recurrence of hepatitis B after liver transplantation is shown. Many variations have been reported in small series. HBIg, hepatitis B immune globulin.

Table 65-3. SAMPLE HEPATITIS B IMMUNE GLOBULIN PROTOCOL	
HBIG, 10,000 IU per intravenous dose administered at the following time points and during the anhepatic phase:	
Days 1, 2, 3, 4, 5, 6	
Day 14	
Months 1, 2, 3, 4, 5, 6—maintain HBIG level at >500 IU/L	
>6 mo—maintain HBIG level at >250 IU/L	
HBIG level	
Days 1–7	Daily
Days 8–14	M, W, F
Days 14–28	M, Th
Month 2	Weekly
Months 3–6	Twice monthly
>6 mo	Monthly
HBsAg	Days 7, 21
HBeAg	Monthly for 2–12 mo
HBV DNA	If positive, check DNA studies and identify mutation

An alternative strategy is to administer 10,000 IU per month regardless of anti-HBsAg levels. Even short periods of subtherapeutic levels of anti-HBsAg can be associated with viral breakthrough.[133] The cost of HBIG therapy varies widely with the HBIG preparation and frequency of administration but can easily exceed the cost of liver transplantation over a 5-year period.

Breakthrough of HBV infection in patients who have been receiving and maintaining adequate levels of HBIG is commonly associated with a mutation in the surface gene region of the HBV genome.[135,136] This region includes the "a" determinant, which is thought to be a principal epitope in antibody binding. The most commonly reported mutation in the "a" determinant associated with breakthrough of HBV infection during HBIG prophylaxis is a substitution of glycine for arginine at amino acid position 145. Once breakthrough has occurred with HBIG therapy, resistance to HBIG suppression of detectable levels of e antigen in HBV DNA is the rule.[136,137] This is generally the case despite reversion to wild-type virus. HBsAg mutations generally persist even with continuation of HBIG.[137]

In summary, passive immunoprophylaxis with HBIG has had a dramatic impact on the frequency of recurrence and outcomes after liver transplantation for end-stage liver disease associated with HBV infection. Passive immunoprophylaxis is, however, limited substantially by an overall approximate 10% lack of efficacy despite target dosing, high cost, and the requirement for indefinite treatment.

Oral Antiviral Agents. The approval of lamivudine and adefovir for the treatment of chronic HBV infection has added important new options to posttransplant prophylaxis for recurrence of hepatitis B. Lamivudine is a nucleoside analogue. Adefovir dipivoxil is a monophosphorylated nucleotide derivative with activity against wild-type HBV as well as lamivudine-resistant mutant variants. Dosing needs to be adjusted for renal function with both agents. In patients with normal renal function, lamivudine is administered at 100 mg once daily and adefovir at 10 mg daily. Costs of either therapy currently range from $10 to $20 per day. Ease of administration and cost are thus major advantages of oral antiviral agents. Optimal use of lamivudine and adefovir is still being evaluated. The principle of reducing HBV DNA levels before transplantation is, however, well established.[138] In patients with cirrhosis who are listed for liver transplantation and do not have strong relative or absolute contraindications to receiving oral antiviral therapy with lamivudine (or adefovir), dosing should be initiated once the chronicity of HBV infection has been established.[131,138-141] Although both drugs are currently approved as monotherapy for chronic HBV infection, it is likely that combination therapy will emerge as more effective in long-term suppression. Both lamivudine and adefovir are associated with the emergence of resistant viral mutants. For lamivudine, the most common resistant mutation is the YMDD mutation.[137] This mutation occurs in the polymerase region of the HBV genome. It is thought that this mutation decreases the affinity of polymerase for nucleotides in general and thus also for the nucleoside analogue lamivudine. The YMDD mutation is most commonly associated with the substitution of either valine or isoleucine for methionine at residue 552 in domain C of the polymerase gene. There is a strongly synergistic effect when this mutation occurs in conjunction with the L528M mutation.[137] The risk of lamivudine resistance is approximately 20% per year.[138] Strains resistant to lamivudine are also resistant to famciclovir.

The frequency of resistant mutations to adefovir dipivoxil is much lower. Based on the registration studies for adefovir dipivoxil, resistance can be expected in approximately 2% of patients per year of therapy.[142] The most commonly identified adefovir-resistant mutation is the N236T variant; this mutation is not cross-resistant to lamivudine.[143] Serum HBV DNA loss can be expected in approximately 20% of patients receiving adefovir dipivoxil versus 44% of patients receiving lamivudine for 1 year.[142] The goal of pretransplant therapy is to suppress HBV DNA levels. Ideally this will be to the point of loss of HBV DNA or e antigen (or both). Whether a 1 $\log_{10}$ or greater decline in HBV DNA levels will also be associated with satisfactory posttransplant outcomes is not currently known. After liver transplantation, lamivudine monotherapy was initially reported to be associated with posttransplant patient and graft survival rates similar to those achieved with the use of HBIG monotherapy.[144] The current trend is for combination oral antiviral and HBIG posttransplant immunoprophylaxis.[145] Several regimens of HBIG in low or high doses of short- and long-term duration in combination with lamivudine have been evaluated in small studies. An early report included 10 patients who were positive for HBV DNA before transplantation and received high-dose HBIG with oral lamivudine after transplantation.[146] All 10 of these patients were negative for hepatitis B surface antigen and HBV DNA by PCR 1 year after transplantation. In a subsequent study using lamivudine with low-dose intramuscular HBIG (400 to 800 IU daily the first week after transplantation and then monthly), 31 of 32 patients remained hepatitis B surface antigen negative 18 months after transplantation.[143] In an even lower dosing schedule, 10 patients who were HBV DNA negative at the time of transplantation received a single dose of intravenous HBIG followed by intramuscular injections every 3 weeks.[147] With a mean follow-up of more than 15 months, virological and histological recurrence of HBV infection developed in only 1 of the 10 patients in this study. Although the studies point to a need for lower dosing of HBIG in conjunction with oral antiviral therapy, no long-term randomized controlled studies have compared regimens to determine optimal combination dosing and frequency. The availability of two effective oral antiviral agents and multiple antiviral drugs in late stages of development (entecavir, emtricitabine) and others in earlier stages of development will mean a continually changing landscape for hepatitis B posttransplant prophylaxis. Short courses of HBIG followed by oral antiviral therapy without HBIG are currently under evaluation and seem likely to emerge as the optimal approach to prophylaxis of recurrence.

Active Prophylaxis. A proportion of hepatitis B surface antibody negative recipients respond to vaccination with hepatitis B surface antigen. Fourteen of 17 patients in whom 10 IU/L or greater of hepatitis B surface antibody developed and who received 18 months or more of HBIG therapy were able to discontinue HBIG.[148] These results could not be confirmed in a subsequent study.[149] Because patients with chronic HBV infection have generally had no shortage of exposure to hepatitis B surface antigen before transplantation, it seems unlikely that this strategy will succeed after transplantation without some immunomodulatory therapy. Studies of a vaccine based on core antigen with a toll-like receptor adjuvant are currently under way.

Treatment of Recurrence of Hepatitis B— Breakthrough and Resistance

Once hepatitis B has recurred clinically in association with the reappearance of HBV DNA and e antigen, continued HBIG therapy has little utility.[133] Recurrence of HBV infection is associated with high levels of HBV DNA.[150] Patients with lamivudine-resistant mutations, including the previously described YMDD mutation, as well as the YIDD and YVDD mutations, have also been described.[137] Median time to breakthrough is approximately 12 months for patients taking lamivudine, with a reported range of 6 months to 5 years after transplantation.[145] For patients who are receiving prophylaxis with HBIG monotherapy at the time of breakthrough/recurrence, initiation of oral antiviral therapy with lamivudine or adefovir, or with both, is recommended. Treatment should be continuous. In patients in whom resistance to lamivudine develops, adefovir should be considered (10 mg/day).[142] Any theoretical benefit to continuing lamivudine in this setting (the YMDD mutant occurs in HBV polymerase, thus theoretically inhibiting viral replication), although reported,[151] has not been proved. Rapid allograft failure after the emergence of lamivudine resistance is well described.[152,153] The role of adjuvant IFN therapy in the posttransplant setting is not well described. In the setting of HCV infection, posttransplant IFN therapy with PEG-IFN alfa-2a or alfa-2b (or both) has not been importantly associated with an increased risk of acute cellular rejection. The likelihood is that the same will be true for HBV-infected recipients. Although many centers treat chronic HBV infection in the nontransplant setting with a combination of adefovir or lamivudine with PEG-IFN, this combination of therapy has not been tested in the posttransplant setting. For patients with recurrence resistant to both adefovir and lamivudine, IFN treatment should be considered. Famciclovir[154,155] and ganciclovir[156] are only weakly active in the treatment of posttransplant HBV infection. Resistance to lamivudine and HBIG persists despite discontinuation of these agents.[137] Compassionate use of emtricitabine, tenofovir, or entecavir might be considered in the setting of lamivudine and adefovir resistance with recurrence. Entecavir is a carboxylic analogue of guanosine with activity against HBV.[157] A cornerstone of management of hepatitis B recurrence is minimization of immunosuppression. This should include CNIs, although a proviral effect of tacrolimus or cyclosporine has not definitively been demonstrated. Corticosteroids are proviral because of a steroid-responsive promoter region in the HBV genome.

Famciclovir resistance has also been reported. It most commonly occurs in the B domain of HBV polymerase.[137] Because lamivudine resistance can also occur through mutation in the B domain of polymerase, cross-resistance may develop. Lamivudine-resistant strains, up to this point in time, are susceptible to adefovir.

Autoimmune and Cholestatic Liver Disease

Autoimmune liver diseases, including PBC, PSC, and autoimmune hepatitis, are known to recur after liver transplantation. Previously considered a controversial topic, recurrence of PBC after liver transplantation has now been demonstrated to be as high as 15% at 3 years and 30% at 10 years with prospective follow-up.[158,159] Serum anti-mitochondrial antibody status is independent of recurrence risk. When strict histological criteria are applied, a conservative estimate of the rate of recurrent PBC based on a rigorous prospective analysis is 17% within the first 5 postoperative years.[160] When criteria for histological recurrence are expanded (to include moderate lymphocytic cholangitis with lymphoplasmacytic portal infiltrates), the recurrence rate of PBC increases to 26%.[160]

Reduction of immunosuppression or tapering of corticosteroids and tacrolimus-based[161] regimens has been suggested as potential risk factors for recurrent PBC. Others have found no difference attributed to the choice of CNI.[162] No information is available regarding the efficacy of ursodeoxycholic acid (UDCA) therapy in halting disease progression from early-stage recurrent PBC. Because of the probable benefit in the nontransplant setting and an excellent safety profile, UDCA is frequently prescribed if recurrence of PBC is suspected (15 mg/kg/day).

An increasing body of evidence suggests that PSC is a recurrent disease after liver transplantation in select patients. In 120 PSC patients undergoing liver transplantation at the Mayo Clinic, evidence of recurrent PSC using strict criteria was found in 24 (20%) individuals.[163,164] Cholangiography was diagnostic for recurrent PSC in 92% of cases, whereas 46% of liver biopsy specimens were compatible with recurrence. The identification of sustained elevations in serum alkaline phosphatase levels (>2 times the upper limit of normal) at least 2 years after liver transplantation may be associated with an increased risk for disease recurrence. Although overall survival of patients with recurrence of PSC is not statistically significantly lower than that of patients without recurrence, graft failure rates are increased.[165] As in the nontransplant setting, there is no proven pharmacotherapy for recurrence of PSC. Treatment is limited to endoscopic and percutaneous management of strictures as indicated clinically.

Recurrent autoimmune hepatitis develops in approximately 20% of patients with the original hepatic disease within 5 years of liver transplantation.[166] Diagnostic criteria used in the nontransplant setting are also used for establishing clinical disease after transplantation. Risk factors include reduced immunosuppression, corticosteroid withdrawal, and the HLA-DR3 and HLA-DR4 alleles. Most patients are asymptomatic, with liver biochemical profiles resembling those of acute cellular rejection. Liver biopsy is required for diagnostic confirmation. De novo autoimmune hepatitis has also been observed in patients who received transplants for idiopathic fulminant hepatic failure or other autoimmune liver disease such as PBC and PSC. Recurrence is typically responsive to increased immunosuppression with corticosteroids or azathioprine/mycophenolate (or both). Histological follow-up is important.

Nonalcoholic Steatohepatitis and Obesity

Background and Etiology

The UNOS database has not recorded the frequency of nonalcoholic fatty liver disease (NAFLD)/nonalcoholic steatohepatitis (NASH) as an indication for liver transplantation until recently, and data capture has been sporadic. Similarly, the NIDDK Liver Transplant Database did not list NASH or fatty liver disease as a specific indication or primary cause of liver disease. Thus there are no national figures to indicate the frequency of liver disease associated with NASH as an indication for liver transplantation, nor the frequency

or impact of recurrence. It has been reported that 2.7% of liver transplants at the Mayo Clinic were carried out for decompensated cirrhosis secondary to NASH.[167] In the 5 years between January 1, 1998, and December 30, 2003, 439 patients with decompensated liver disease have undergone liver transplantation at our center. Twenty-eight of these patients (6.4%) had histological and clinical evidence of NASH as the primary cause of liver disease. The frequency of NASH as an indication for liver transplantation, at our center at least, has thus more than doubled in 5 years.

The national increase in the prevalence of obesity may have important implications for the medical community as a whole. Figure 65–5 shows Centers for Disease Control and Prevention data regarding changes in the frequency of new HCV infections and the prevalence of obesity between 1982 and 2000. Between January 1, 1998, and December 30, 2003, a total of 22,676 liver transplants were carried out in adults in the United States according to UNOS (www.unos.org.data). If we extrapolate the Mayo Clinic experience nationally, the number of people undergoing liver transplantation for NASH is on the order of 1.0 per million U.S. residents per year (based on 6.4% of 22,676 adult liver transplants being carried out for NASH and assuming a mean U.S. population in 1998 to 2003 of 280 million—http://www.census.gov/population/www/projections). Based on the known increases in the prevalence of obesity in the United States[168] (see Fig. 65–5), the frequency of liver transplantation for NASH will increase to 2.2 to 4.0 cases per million U.S. residents per year in 10 to 15 years. The higher estimate reflects known increases in the severity of NAFLD with the degree of obesity. Steatohepatitis is found in 3% of lean, approximately 20% of obese, and almost half of morbidly obese people.[169,170] Of severely obese patients with diabetes, 100% have at least mild steatosis, half have steatohepatitis, and about 20% have cirrhosis.[171]

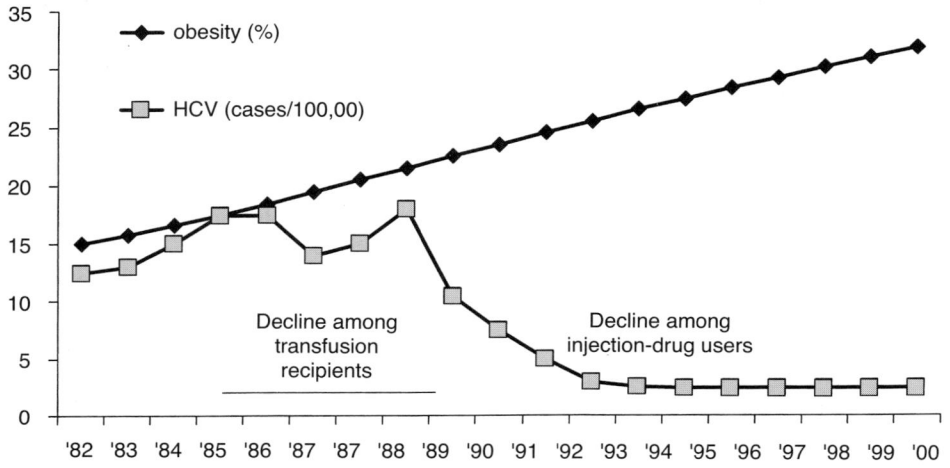

FIGURE 65–5

Centers for Disease Control and Prevention (http://www.census.gov/population/www/projections) data for changes in the incidence of new hepatitis C virus infection and the prevalence of obesity in the United States are shown.

thiazolidenediones on NASH.[183,184] Unfortunately, although pioglitazone produces histological and biochemical improvement in patients with NASH, it is associated with a significant increase in body mass index and has been linked to hepatotoxicity.[184] Because PPAR-γ agonists are adipogenic by nature, weight gain is likely to be a class effect of the thiazolidenediones and may well negate any histological benefit. Combined PPAR-γ/α agonists appear to be beneficial in animal models of steatohepatitis,[185] but they may be limited by the finding of excess morbidity and mortality associated with PPAR-α agonists in large cohort studies.

Pearls and Pitfalls

Gout

- If azathioprine and allopurinol must be prescribed together, reduce azathioprine dosing by approximately 50% and monitor the complete blood count for signs of aplasia.

Osteoporosis

- Consider annual bone densitometry to screen for osteoporosis after liver transplantation, particularly in women, patients requiring maintenance corticosteroids, and those whose original liver disease was cholestatic.
- Antiresorptive agents such as alendronate and pamidronate are effective in the treatment of posttransplant osteoporosis.

Dyslipidemia

- Remember the potential role of immunosuppression in posttransplant dyslipidemia—cyclosporine (and to a lesser extent, tacrolimus), sirolimus, and corticosteroids may all be causative.
- HMG-CoA reductase inhibitors are generally safe and free of drug-drug interactions in the posttransplant setting. Consider HMG-CoA reductase inhibitor hepatotoxicity for temporally related elevations in liver biochemical markers (this uncommon side effect typically reverses on discontinuation of HMG-CoA reductase inhibitor).

Hypertension

- Consider ambulatory blood pressure monitoring that includes an overnight period of observation when screening for posttransplant hypertension. Loss of the nocturnal decrease in systemic blood pressure is an important early manifestation of posttransplant hypertension.

Pearls and Pitfalls—cont'd

- Vasodilating drugs, particularly dihydropyridine calcium channel blocking agents, are frequently effective in the treatment of posttransplant hypertension associated with calcineurin inhibition.

Hepatitis C

- HCV infection of the allograft occurs immediately after liver transplantation and may affect posttransplant histology as early as the first postoperative week.
- Consider protocol-based liver biopsies in recipients with posttransplant HCV infection.
- Avoid steroid bolus treatment of mild (Banff A1) acute cellular rejection in recipients with HCV infection.
- T-cell–depleting therapies are associated with high rates of patient mortality and graft loss in recipients with HCV infection.
- Consider CMV prophylaxis in all recipients with HCV infection, with the exception of cases in which CMV IgG was negative in the donor and recipient.
- Adjust ribavirin dosing for renal insufficiency and consider dose escalation schedules for ribavirin when treating recurrence of HCV.
- Consider initiation of erythrocyte-stimulating therapies such as erythropoietin or darbepoetin if the hemoglobin level falls below 12 g/dL.

Hepatitis B

- Posttransplant recurrence of HBV infection is most common in patients who are replicative before transplantation.
- Consider suppressive therapy for HBV in patients awaiting liver transplantation.
- All potential liver transplant recipients should be screened for hepatitis B surface antibody and should receive vaccination when surface antibody is not detected.
- Adefovir dipivoxil is effective in suppression of the majority of lamivudine-resistant strains of HBV.
- Clinically important posttransplant HBV infection frequently develops in allografts from donors with isolated anti-HBc.
- Once breakthrough has occurred during HBIG therapy, resistance to HBIG suppression of detectable levels of e antigen in HBV DNA is the rule even if reversion to the wild type occurs.

Pearls and Pitfalls—cont'd

- Treatment with short courses of HBIG followed by oral antiviral therapy without HBIG is currently under evaluation and seems likely to emerge as the optimal approach to prophylaxis of recurrence.

References

1. Wahlstrom HE, Cooper J, Gores G, et al: Survival after liver transplantation in diabetics. Transplant Proc 23:1564-1566, 1991.
2. Stegall MD, Everson G, Schroter G, et al: Metabolic complications after liver transplantation. Diabetes, hypercholesterolemia, hypertension, and obesity. Transplantation 60:1057-1060, 1995.
3. Shields PL, Tang H, Neuberger JM, et al: Poor outcome in patients with diabetes mellitus undergoing liver transplantation. Transplantation 68:530-535, 1999.
4. Marroni CA, Hoppe L, Diehl JL, et al: Diabetes mellitus and liver transplantation in adults. Transplant Proc 31:3046, 1999.
5. Navasa M, Bustamante J, Marroni C, et al: Diabetes mellitus after liver transplantation: Prevalence and predictive factors. J Hepatol 25:64-71, 1996.
6. Blanco JJ, Herrero JI, Quiroga J, et al: Liver transplantation in cirrhotic patients with diabetes mellitus: Midterm results, survival, and adverse events. Liver Transpl 7:226-233, 2001.
7. Padbury RT, Gunson BK, Dousset B, et al: Steroid withdrawal from long-term immunosuppression in liver allograft recipients. Transplantation 55:789-794, 1993.
8. Fraser GM, Grammoustianos K, Reddy J, et al: Long-term immunosuppression without corticosteroids after orthotopic liver transplantation: A positive therapeutic aim. Liver Transpl Surg 2:411-417, 1996.
9. Stegall MD, Everson GT, Schroter G, et al: Prednisone withdrawal late after adult liver transplantation reduces diabetes, hypertension, and hypercholesterolemia without causing graft loss. Hepatology 25:173-177, 1997.
10. Romani F, Belli LS, De Carlis L, et al: Cyclosporin monotherapy (after 3 months) in liver transplant patients: A prospective randomized trial. Transplant Proc 26:2683-2685, 1994.
11. Knobler H, Stagnaro-Green A, Wallenstein S, et al: Higher incidence of diabetes in liver transplant recipients with hepatitis C. J Clin Gastroenterol 26:30-33, 1998.
12. Bigam DL, Pennington JJ, Carpentier A, et al: Hepatitis C–related cirrhosis: A predictor of diabetes after liver transplantation. Hepatology 32:87-90, 2000.
13. Burack DA, Griffith BP, Thompson ME, Kahl LE: Hyperuricemia and gout among heart transplant recipients receiving cyclosporine. Am J Med 92:141-146, 1992.
14. Lin HY, Rocher LL, McQuillan MA, et al: Cyclosporine-induced hyperuricemia and gout. N Engl J Med 321:287-292, 1989.
15. Neal DA, Tom BD, Gimson AE, et al: Hyperuricemia, gout, and renal function after liver transplantation. Transplantation 72:1689-1691, 2001.
16. Delaney V, Sumrani N, Daskalakis P, et al: Hyperuricemia and gout in renal allograft recipients. Transplant Proc 24:1773-1774, 1992.
17. Eastell R, Dickson ER, Hodgson SF, et al: Rates of vertebral bone loss before and after liver transplantation in women with primary biliary cirrhosis. Hepatology 14:296-300, 1991.
18. Monegal A, Navasa M, Guanabens N, et al: Bone disease after liver transplantation: A long-term prospective study of bone mass changes, hormonal status and histomorphometric characteristics. Osteoporos Int 12:484-492, 2001.
19. McDonald JA, Dunstan CR, Dilworth P, et al: Bone loss after liver transplantation. Hepatology 14:613-619, 1991.
20. Hussaini SH, Oldroyd B, Stewart SP, et al: Regional bone mineral density after orthotopic liver transplantation. Eur J Gastroenterol Hepatol 11:157-163, 1999.
21. Abdelhadi M, Eriksson SA, Ljusk ES, et al: Bone mineral status in end-stage liver disease and the effect of liver transplantation. Scand J Gastroenterol 30:1210-1215, 1995.
22. Floreani A, Fries W, Luisetto G, et al: Bone metabolism in orthotopic liver transplantation: A prospective study. Liver Transpl Surg 4:311-319, 1998.
23. Meys E, Fontanges E, Fourcade N, et al: Bone loss after orthotopic liver transplantation. Am J Med 97:445-450, 1994.
24. Porayko MK, Wiesner RH, Hay JE, et al: Bone disease in liver transplant recipients: Incidence, timing, and risk factors. Transplant Proc 23:1462-1465, 1991.
25. Navasa M, Monegal A, Guanabens N, et al: Bone fractures in liver transplant patients. Br J Rheumatol 33:52-55, 1994.
26. Ninkovic M, Skingle SJ, Bearcroft PW, et al: Incidence of vertebral fractures in the first three months after orthotopic liver transplantation. Eur J Gastroenterol Hepatol 12:931-935, 2000.
27. Charco R, Cantarell C, Vargas V, et al: Serum cholesterol changes in long-term survivors of liver transplantation: A comparison between cyclosporine and tacrolimus therapy. Liver Transpl Surg 5:204-208, 1999.
28. Abouljoud MS, Levy MF, Klintmalm GB: Hyperlipidemia after liver transplantation: Long-term results of the FK506/Cyclosporine A US Multicenter trial. US Multicenter Study Group. Transplant Proc 27:1121-1123, 1995.
29. Munoz SJ: Hyperlipidemia and other coronary risk factors after orthotopic liver transplantation: Pathogenesis, diagnosis, and management. Liver Transpl Surg 1(5 Suppl 1):29-38, 1995.
30. Gisbert C, Prieto M, Berenguer M, et al: Hyperlipidemia in liver transplant recipients: Prevalence and risk factors. Liver Transpl Surg 3:416-422, 1997.
31. Imagawa DK, Dawson S III, Holt CD, et al: Hyperlipidemia after liver transplantation: Natural history and treatment with the hydroxy-methylglutaryl-coenzyme A reductase inhibitor pravastatin. Transplantation 62:934-942, 1996.
32. Romero M, Parera A, Salcedo M, et al: Cardiovascular risk factors and late cardiovascular disease in liver transplantation. Transplant Proc 31:2364-2365, 1999.
33. Canzanello VJ, Schwartz L, Taler SJ, et al: Evolution of cardiovascular risk after liver transplantation: A comparison of cyclosporine A and tacrolimus (FK506). Liver Transpl Surg 3:1-9, 1997.
34. Textor SC, Taler SJ, Canzanello VJ, et al: Posttransplantation hypertension related to calcineurin inhibitors. Liver Transpl 6:521-530, 2000.
35. Moss NG, Powell SL, Falk RJ: Intravenous cyclosporine activates afferent and efferent renal nerves and causes sodium retention in innervated kidneys in rats. Proc Natl Acad Sci U S A 82:8222-8226, 1985.
36. Scherrer U, Vissing SF, Morgan BJ, et al: Cyclosporine-induced sympathetic activation and hypertension after heart transplantation. N Engl J Med 323:693-699, 1990.
37. Everson GT, Trouillot T, Wachs M, et al: Early steroid withdrawal in liver transplantation is safe and beneficial. Liver Transpl Surg 5(4 Suppl 1):S48-S57, 1999.
38. Jain A, Reyes J, Kashyap R, et al: What have we learned about primary liver transplantation under tacrolimus immunosuppression? Long-term follow-up of the first 1000 patients. Ann Surg 230:441-448, 1999.
39. Gonwa TA, Mai ML, Melton LB, et al: End-stage renal disease (ESRD) after orthotopic liver transplantation (OLTX) using

recipients with established recurrent hepatitis C: Preliminary results of a randomized multicenter trial. Hepatology 34:406A, 2001.

118. Manzarbeitia C, Teperman L, Chalasani N, et al: 40 kDA Peginterferon alfa-2a (Pegasys) as a prophylaxis against hepatitis C infection recurrence after liver transplantation (LT): Preliminary results of a randomized multicenter trial. Hepatology 34:406A, 2001.

119. Vargas HE, Rosati MJ, Douglas DD, et al: Combination pegylated interferon alpha-2b and ribavirin in transplant patients with recurrent hepatitis C infection: A preliminary report. Hepatology 34:407A, 2001.

120. Willner IR, Chavin KD, Rogers J, et al: Combination interferon-ribavirin is ineffective and poorly tolerated by liver transplant recipients with genotype 1 recurrent hepatitis C. Hepatology 32:290A, 2000.

121. de Vera ME, Smallwood GA, Rosado K, et al: Interferon-alpha and ribavirin for the treatment of recurrent hepatitis C after liver transplantation. Transplantation 71:678-686, 2001.

122. Feray C, Gigou M, Samuel D, et al: Incidence of hepatitis C in patients receiving different preparations of hepatitis B immunoglobulins after liver transplantation. Ann Intern Med 128:810-816, 1998.

123. Willems B, Ede M, Marotta P, et al: Anti-HCV human immunoglobulin for the prevention of graft infection in HCV-related liver transplantation—a pilot study. J Hepatol 36:32, 2002.

124. Roche B, Samuel D, Gigou M, et al: De novo and apparent de novo hepatitis B virus infection after liver transplantation. J Hepatol 26:517-526, 1997.

125. Belle SH, Beringer KC, Detre KM: An update of liver transplantation in the United States: Recipient characteristics and outcome. In Cecka JM, Terasaki PI (eds): Clinical Transplants 1995. Los Angeles, UCLA Tissue Typing Laboratory, 1996.

126. Maynard JE: Hepatitis B: Global importance and need for control. Vaccine 8(Suppl):S18-S20, discussion S21-S23, 1990.

127. Kim WR, Benson JT, Therneau TM, et al: Changing epidemiology of hepatitis B in a U.S. community. Hepatology 39:811-816, 2004.

128. Shouval D, Samuel D: Hepatitis B immune globulin to prevent hepatitis B virus graft reinfection following liver transplantation: A concise review. Hepatology 32:1189-1195, 2000.

129. Samuel D, Muller R, Alexander G, et al: Liver transplantation in European patients with the hepatitis B surface antigen. N Engl J Med 329:1842-1847, 1993.

130. Dickson RC, Everhart JE, Lake JR, et al: Transmission of hepatitis B by transplantation of livers from donors positive for antibody to hepatitis B core antigen. The National Institute of Diabetes and Digestive and Kidney Diseases Liver Transplantation Database. Gastroenterology 113:1668-1674, 1997.

131. Teo EK, Han SH, Terrault N, et al: Liver transplantation in patients with hepatitis B virus infection: Outcome in Asian versus white patients. Hepatology 34:126-132, 2001.

132. Muller R, Samuel D, Fassati LR, et al: 'EUROHEP' consensus report on the management of liver transplantation for hepatitis B virus infection. European Concerted Action on Viral Hepatitis. J Hepatol 21:1140-1143, 1994.

133. Terrault NA, Zhou S, Combs C, et al: Prophylaxis in liver transplant recipients using a fixed dosing schedule of hepatitis B immunoglobulin. Hepatology 24:1327-1333, 1996.

134. Feray C, Zignego AL, Samuel D, et al: Persistent hepatitis B virus infection of mononuclear blood cells without concomitant liver infection. The liver transplantation model. Transplantation 49:1155-1158, 1990.

135. Carman WF, Trautwein C, van Deursen FJ, et al: Hepatitis B virus envelope variation after transplantation with and without

136. Protzer-Knolle U, Naumann U, Bartenschlager R, et al: Hepatitis B virus with antigenically altered hepatitis B surface antigen is selected by high-dose hepatitis B immune globulin after liver transplantation. Hepatology 27:254-263, 1998.

137. Germer JJ, Charlton MR, Ishitani MB, et al: Characterization of hepatitis B virus surface antigen and polymerase mutations in liver transplant recipients pre- and post-transplant. Am J Transplant 3:743-753, 2003.

138. Perrillo RP, Wright T, Rakela J, et al: A multicenter United States–Canadian trial to assess lamivudine monotherapy before and after liver transplantation for chronic hepatitis B. Hepatology 33:424-432, 2001.

139. Rosenau J, Bahr MJ, Tillmann HL, et al: Lamivudine and low-dose hepatitis B immune globulin for prophylaxis of hepatitis B reinfection after liver transplantation: Possible role of mutations in the YMDD motif prior to transplantation as a risk factor for reinfection. J Hepatol 34:895-902, 2001.

140. Yoshida EM, Erb SR, Partovi N, et al: Liver transplantation for chronic hepatitis B infection with the use of combination lamivudine and low-dose hepatitis B immune globulin. Liver Transpl Surg 5:520-525, 1999.

141. Angus PW, McCaughan GW, Gane EJ, et al: Combination low-dose hepatitis B immune globulin and lamivudine therapy provides effective prophylaxis against posttransplantation hepatitis B. Liver Transpl 6:429-433, 2000.

142. Schiff ER, Lai CL, Hadziyannis S, et al: Adefovir dipivoxil therapy for lamivudine-resistant hepatitis B in pre– and post–liver transplantation patients. Hepatology 38:1419-1427, 2003.

143. Angus P, Vaughan R, Xiong S, et al: Resistance to adefovir dipivoxil therapy associated with the selection of a novel mutation in the HBV polymerase. Gastroenterology 125:292-297, 2003.

144. Grellier L, Mutimer D, Ahmed M, et al: Lamivudine prophylaxis against reinfection in liver transplantation for hepatitis B cirrhosis [erratum appears in Lancet 1997 Feb 1 349(9048):364]. Lancet 348:1212-1215, 1996.

145. Papatheodoridis GV, Sevastianos V, Burroughs AK: Prevention of and treatment for hepatitis B virus infection after liver transplantation in the nucleoside analogues era. Am J Transplant 3:250-258, 2003.

146. Markowitz JS, Martin P, Conrad AJ, et al: Prophylaxis against hepatitis B recurrence following liver transplantation using combination lamivudine and hepatitis B immune globulin. Hepatology 28:585-589, 1998.

147. Yao FY, Osorio RW, Roberts JP, et al: Intramuscular hepatitis B immune globulin combined with lamivudine for prophylaxis against hepatitis B recurrence after liver transplantation. Liver Transpl Surg 5:491-496, 1999.

148. Sanchez-Fueyo A, Rimola A, Grande L, et al: Hepatitis B immunoglobulin discontinuation followed by hepatitis B virus vaccination: A new strategy in the prophylaxis of hepatitis B virus recurrence after liver transplantation. Hepatology 31:496-501, 2000.

149. Angelico M, Di Paolo D, Trinito MO, et al: Failure of a reinforced triple course of hepatitis B vaccination in patients transplanted for HBV-related cirrhosis. Hepatology 35:176-181, 2002.

150. Davies SE, Portmann BC, O'Grady JG, et al: Hepatic histological findings after transplantation for chronic hepatitis B virus infection, including a unique pattern of fibrosing cholestatic hepatitis. Hepatology 13:150-157, 1991.

151. Ling R, Mutimer D, Ahmed M, et al: Selection of mutations in the hepatitis B virus polymerase during therapy of transplant recipients with lamivudine. Hepatology 24:711-713, 1996.

152. Mutimer D, Dusheiko G, Barrett C, et al: Lamivudine without HBIg for prevention of graft reinfection by hepatitis B: Long-term follow-up. Transplantation 70:809-815, 2000.

153. Lo CM, Cheung ST, Lai CL, et al: Liver transplantation in Asian patients with chronic hepatitis B using lamivudine prophylaxis. Ann Surg 233:276-281, 2001.

154. Rayes N, Seehofer D, Hopf U, et al: Comparison of famciclovir and lamivudine in the long-term treatment of hepatitis B infection after liver transplantation. Transplantation 71:96-101, 2001.

155. Singh N, Gayowski T, Wannstedt CF, et al: Pretransplant famciclovir as prophylaxis for hepatitis B virus recurrence after liver transplantation. Transplantation 63:1415-1419, 1997.

156. Gish RG, Lau JY, Brooks L, et al: Ganciclovir treatment of hepatitis B virus infection in liver transplant recipients. Hepatology 23:1-7, 1996.

157. de Man RA, Wolters LM, Nevens F, et al: Safety and efficacy of oral entecavir given for 28 days in patients with chronic hepatitis B virus infection. Hepatology 34:578-582, 2001.

158. Balan V, Batts KP, Porayko MK, et al: Histological evidence for recurrence of primary biliary cirrhosis after liver transplantation. Hepatology 18:1392-1398, 1993.

159. Hubscher SG, Elias E, Buckels JA, et al: Primary biliary cirrhosis. Histological evidence of disease recurrence after liver transplantation. J Hepatol 18:173-184, 1993.

160. Sylvestre PB, Batts KP, Burgart LJ, et al: Recurrence of primary biliary cirrhosis after liver transplantation: Histologic estimate of incidence and natural history. Liver Transpl 9:1086-1093, 2003.

161. Dmitrewski J, Hubscher SG, Mayer AD, Neuberger JM: Recurrence of primary biliary cirrhosis in the liver allograft: The effect of immunosuppression. J Hepatol 24:253-257, 1996.

162. Levitsky J, Hart J, Cohen SM, Te HS: The effect of immunosuppressive regimens on the recurrence of primary biliary cirrhosis after liver transplantation. Liver Transpl 9:733-736, 2003.

163. Graziadei IW, Wiesner RH, Batts KP, et al: Recurrence of primary sclerosing cholangitis following liver transplantation. Hepatology 29:1050-1056, 1999.

164. Graziadei IW, Wiesner RH, Marotta PJ, et al: Long-term results of patients undergoing liver transplantation for primary sclerosing cholangitis. Hepatology 30:1121-1127, 1999.

165. Guichelaar MM, Benson JT, Malinchoc M, et al: Risk factors for and clinical course of non-anastomotic biliary strictures after liver transplantation. Am J Transplant 3:885-890, 2003.

166. Gonzalez-Koch A, Czaja AJ, Carpenter HA, et al: Recurrent autoimmune hepatitis after orthotopic liver transplantation. Liver Transpl 7:302-310, 2001.

167. Charlton M, Kasparova P, Weston S, et al: Frequency of non-alcoholic steatohepatitis as a cause of advanced liver disease. Liver Transpl 7:608-614, 2001.

168. Kuczmarski RJ, Carroll MD, Flegal KM, Troiano RP: Varying body mass index cutoff points to describe overweight prevalence among U.S. adults: NHANES III (1988 to 1994). Obes Res 5:542-548, 1997.

169. Wanless IR, Lentz JS: Fatty liver hepatitis (steatohepatitis) and obesity: An autopsy study with analysis of risk factors. Hepatology 12:1106-1110, 1990.

170. Silverman JF, O'Brien KF, Long S, et al: Liver pathology in morbidly obese patients with and without diabetes. Am J Gastroenterol 85:1349-1355, 1990.

171. Silverman JF, Pories WJ, Caro JF: Liver pathology in diabetes mellitus and morbid obesity. Clinical, pathological, and biochemical considerations. Pathol Annu 24:275-302, 1989.

172. Kim WR, Poterucha JJ, Porayko MK, et al: Recurrence of non-alcoholic steatohepatitis following liver transplantation. Transplantation 62:1802-1805, 1996.

173. Maor-Kendler Y, Batts KP, Burgart LJ, et al: Comparative allograft histology after liver transplantation for cryptogenic cirrhosis, alcohol, hepatitis C, and cholestatic liver diseases. Transplantation 70:292-297, 2000.

174. Vajro P, Fontanella A, Perna C, et al: Persistent hyperaminotransferasemia resolving after weight reduction in obese children. J Pediatr 125:239-241, 1994.

175. Coche G, Gottrand F, Sevenet F, Ducrocq C: [Hepatic steatosis in obesity in children] [in French]. J Radiol 72:235-237, 1991.

176. Drenick EJ, Simmons F, Murphy JF: Effect on hepatic morphology of treatment of obesity by fasting, reducing diets and small-bowel bypass. N Engl J Med 282:829-834, 1970.

177. Seeff LB, Zimmerman HI: Relationship between pancreatic and hepatic disease. In Popper H, Schaffner F (eds): Progress in Liver Disease, 5th ed. New York, Grune & Stratton, 1976, p 595.

178. Lin HZ, Yang SQ, Chuckaree C, et al: Metformin reverses fatty liver disease in obese, leptin-deficient mice. Nat Med 6:998-1003, 2000.

179. Laurin J, Lindor KD, Crippin JS, et al: Ursodeoxycholic acid or clofibrate in the treatment of non–alcohol-induced steatohepatitis: A pilot study. Hepatology 23:1464-1467, 1996.

180. Basaranoglu M, Acbay O, Sonsuz A: A controlled trial of gemfibrozil in the treatment of patients with nonalcoholic steatohepatitis. J Hepatol 31:384, 1999.

181. Lavine JE: Vitamin E treatment of nonalcoholic steatohepatitis in children: A pilot study. J Pediatr 136:734-738, 2000.

182. Abdelmalek MF, Angulo P, Jorgensen RA, et al: Betaine, a promising new agent for patients with nonalcoholic steatohepatitis: Results of a pilot study. Am J Gastroenterol 96:2711-2717, 2001.

183. Neuschwander-Tetri BA, Brunt EM, Wehmeier KR, et al: Interim results of a pilot study demonstrating the early effects of the PPAR-gamma ligand rosiglitazone on insulin sensitivity, aminotransferases, hepatic steatosis and body weight in patients with non-alcoholic steatohepatitis. J Hepatol 38:434-440, 2003.

184. Promrat K, Lutchman G, Uwaifo GI, et al: A pilot study of pioglitazone treatment for nonalcoholic steatohepatitis. Hepatology 39:188-196, 2004.

185. Ye JM, Iglesias MA, Watson DG, et al: PPARα/γ ragaglitazar eliminates fatty liver and enhances insulin action in fat-fed rats in the absence of hepatomegaly. Am J Physiol Endocrinol Metab 284:E531-E540, 2003.

flumazenil[13] has led to the application of functional neuroimaging techniques to identifying abnormalities of endogenous benzodiazepine-like compounds in the brain. Slowly a characteristic "snapshot" has emerged of abnormal regional brain chemistry in encephalopathy, with evidence that clinically effective lactulose therapy and successful transplantation are associated with statistically significant normalizing trends.[14,15]

In addition to cognitive problems, patients with advanced liver disease suffer from a wide range of associated neuropsychiatric symptoms, including extrapyramidal and other movement disorders,[16,17] mood and anxiety disorders,[18] sexual dysfunction and other neuroendocrine-derived problems,[19] and a wide range of circadian and sleep physiological disturbances.[20,21]

Profiles of Neuropsychological Outcome

In 1984, Tarter and colleagues[22] published the first neuropsychological testing profiles of liver transplantation survivors. They studied 10 young (mean age: 27.8 years) 3-year survivors of liver transplantation and compared them with a slightly older control group of patients with Crohn's disease; they found no differences between the groups or in relation to population-based norms. Pretransplantation neuropsychological status was not reported. The authors cautioned that it remained uncertain whether pretransplantation impairments would be entirely reversed after surgery in old or more ill recipients.

In 1988, Tarter and his group[23] extended their evaluations of Pittsburgh transplant recipients to include more global quality-of-life assessments. These evaluations contained expanded neuropsychological testing of a transplantation population whose demographical features are not described. Trends toward normalization after transplantation were again documented, although this time with characteristic persistent deficits in visuospatial domains.

In 1989, Wolcott and associates[24] reported postoperative results from a larger series of liver transplantation patients at the University of California, Los Angeles with a mean age of 43.6 years. Although the investigators noted trends toward generally improved quality of life similar to those found in Tarter's studies, "moderate" focal cognitive dysfunction was more common. Disturbingly, the group of patients tested more than 12 months after liver transplantation showed poorer cognitive function than a comparator group tested less than 1 year after transplantation, suggesting possible cumulative toxicity related to immunosuppressive agents or other end-organ problems affecting brain function.

In 1990, Tarter's group reported on outcomes in a transplant recipient group much more clinically akin to typical patients seen in the late 1990s and the new century: those with baseline "subclinical encephalopathy" (defined as neuropsychological testing abnormalities in the absence of clinically manifested hepatic encephalopathy).[25] Against a background trend of improvements in neuropsychological functioning after transplantation, these recipients showed focal persistent deficits in visuospatial and short-term memory functions compared with chronically medically ill and healthy age-matched controls. The authors cited atrophic structural brain changes not reversed by orthotopic liver transplantation (OLT) as possible anatomic substrates for the persistent deficits; also introduced was the possibility that iatrogenic factors, particularly immunosuppressants, contribute to persistent deficits.

Recognizing a broadening candidate pool that would more frequently include alcoholics and the importance of understanding neuropsychological outcome in carefully selected alcoholic recipients, Arria and associates,[26] in 1991, reported on a series of 13 alcoholic transplant recipients from the University of Pittsburgh program. The alcoholic group improved after transplantation in all measured neuropsychological domains (psychomotor function, visuopractic domains, and perceptual speed) except memory, in which no significant improvement occurred. In the absence of episodes of recurrent encephalopathy, alcoholic liver disease did not independently predict adverse neuropsychological outcomes. These findings significantly supported the argument that persons with end-stage alcohol-related liver disease should not be denied access to transplantation because of concern for a lack of cognitive recovery different from other groups of transplant candidates and, along with similar surgical and medical findings, paved the way for liberalizing selection criteria to include these patients.

In 1992, Tarter and colleagues[27] showed that severity of pretransplantation encephalopathy accounted for up to 20% of the variances in improvement in quality of life after OLT.

In their truly encyclopedic 2000 review of 144 studies on quality of life in organ transplantation, Dew and colleagues[28] identify 25 studies that specifically describe liver recipients. Against a background trend of universal global improvements in quality of life after transplantation in all solid organ recipient groups, liver patients tended as a group to fare in the middle range in specific quality-of-life domains: physical functioning, mental/cognitive status, and social functioning. The extent to which cognitive status after transplantation accounts for overall quality-of-life variance remains unknown.

It can now be asserted that the available neuropsychological outcome data for OLT survivors, including those with alcoholic liver disease, show generally improved neuropsychological test performance compared with before transplantation, but with varying degrees of persistent deficits in visuopractic, psychomotor, and memory functions. Caution must still prevail in extrapolating these findings to clinical work, however. As was the case with the initial edition of this book, most of the available neuropsychological outcome studies are products of one large center (the University of Pittsburgh). It is possible, therefore, that patient selection criteria, medical and surgical management variables, or other factors could make these patient groups different from liver transplant patient populations as a whole. Indeed, most of the available studies excluded participants who had clinically overt hepatic encephalopathy or significant medical illness other than their primary liver disease, and whose mean age was greater than 50 years.

Clinicians working in liver transplantation programs today recognize that multiple medical illnesses, age older than 50 years, and multiple episodes of hepatic encephalopathy are common. Sadly, little has been added to the neuropsychological outcomes literature in the years since the first publication of this book.[29]

Perhaps the most important caveat relates to the methodological necessity that patients who die or have postoperative complications sufficient to preclude "standard" outpatient clinical follow-up will never appear in the neuropsychological outcomes data. This skewed sampling issue masks the fact that at most transplant centers, perioperative neuropsychiatric complications of transplantation are highly prevalent in patients with catastrophic outcomes.[17,26] For example, the University of Toronto group reported that 33% of all deaths in the 3 months after transplantation were accounted for by severe neuropsychiatric complications of OLT, such as pontine myelinolysis, extended delirium, and neurological death.[30,31] Although most clinicians working today would view the Toronto figures as an overestimate of the contemporary prevalence of severe neuropsychiatric complications, it remains correct to point out that these critical undesirable outcomes go unreported in the neuropsychological literature. This "blind spot" underscores the importance of the following discussion of acute clinical neuropsychiatric syndromes in liver transplant recipients.

Delirium and Disorders of Consciousness

In light of the reported prevalence rate of 20% to 30% for clinically evident encephalopathy in prospectively studied liver transplantation candidates,[1] it is not surprising that acute organic mental disorders are common in the immediate postoperative period. Of the "organic brain syndromes" reported to occur in up to 33% of all liver transplant patients postoperatively,[28,30-32] delirium,

an organic mental disorder characterized by global brain dysfunction,[33] is the most common. Rarely can the multiple delirium-causing variables routinely associated with OLT be teased apart; preoperative clinical or subclinical encephalopathy, general anesthesia, lengthy surgery, volume and electrolyte shifts associated with reperfusion, loading with immunosuppressants, postoperative opioids, early graft function or dysfunction, fever, coagulopathy, infection, days of disrupted sleep-wake cycle, and other factors are commonly present simultaneously.[34] Despite pretransplantation agreements or monitoring for abstinence, withdrawal states from alcohol, benzodiazepines, opioids, and other substances also must be considered.

A large literature convincingly associates cyclosporine, tacrolimus, and other elements of the transplantation pharmacopeia with postoperative delirium and neurotoxicity.[30-33,35-42] Among transplantation patients, liver recipients seem most susceptible to these adverse events[33-36,43] with large centers originally reporting some degree of cyclosporine or tacrolimus neurotoxicity in 25% to 35% of patients in the perioperative phase.[29-31,41] The first signs of immunosuppressant neurotoxicity may be seen in the intensive care unit, where, after an early lucid period, patients may become lethargic, confused, and require reintubation despite previously adequate ventilatory status.[30,44,45] A specific timeline cannot be defined, however, and neurotoxicity may be present at almost any stage of or after transplantation immunosuppression.[40,46,47] A wide range of symptoms, including seizures, cortical blindness, aphasia, dysarthria, paresthesias, neuropathy, hallucinations, delusions, mania-like symptoms, and agitation, may emerge.[33,46,48] Obtundation, deeper coma, status epilepticus, and neurological death rarely follow.[40] Diffuse white matter changes have been reported with computed tomographic and magnetic resonance imaging (MRI) study, often accompanied by abnormal electroencephalographic findings.[49-51] What were once empirical strategies for improving these symptoms, such as cyclosporine/tacrolimus dose reduction or holidays, or switching from one primary immunosuppressant to another (e.g., from cyclosporine to tacrolimus, or vice versa), are often associated with symptom improvement and are now supported as rational clinical maneuvers by clinical trials data.[52-54]

Many theories have been offered to explain mechanisms of the neurotoxicity of the primary immunosuppressive agents cyclosporine and tacrolimus. Tables 66–1 and 66–2 summarize these theories, wherein metabolic confounders, specific pharmacological properties, and neuropathological studies are described.[55-59] A contemporary summary of the many effects of the calcineurin inhibitors cyclosporine and tacrolimus is found in the DiMartini and Trzepacz review.[45]

hypomania,[33] and major depressive episodes[32,33,35,41,42,44-47] in liver transplantation patients. Many of these reports describe symptom onset temporally linked to the initiation of posttransplantation calcineurin-inhibitor immune suppression, with symptom amelioration or remission after dose changes, drug holidays, empirical switching, and other strategies.

The UCLA program has observed de novo psychotic mania as part of the clinical presentation of late-onset (>6 months after transplantation) secondary mood symptoms apparently induced by calcineurin-inhibitor immune suppression. Because mania and depression have also been linked to high-dose steroid treatment[60,61,88] or its cessation, temporal observations are critical in inferring etiological connections between symptoms and particular elements of the immunosuppressive regimen. Our clinical experience suggests that dose changes, or changes in end-organ function that are associated with changes in serum levels of calcineurin inhibitors, can often be linked to the induction of mood symptoms.

As noted earlier in this chapter, early optimism that there might be less likelihood of neuropsychiatric symptoms associated with tacrolimus compared with cyclosporine has been tempered by both prospective trials data and clinical experience.

Both new-onset and preexisting anxiety disorders can also become symptomatic after liver transplantation. Panic symptoms and generalized anxiety have been most common in our program's experience. At the UCLA program we have also seen apparently new-onset obsessive-compulsive disorder with ego-alien intrusive thoughts and ritualizing. We look carefully for associations with immunosuppressive dose changes, especially when we see patients with clear de novo symptoms, in the same manner described in the preceding discussion of mood symptoms. When these disorders persist despite all possible attention to immunosuppressive dosing and other metabolic variables, they respond well to standard cognitive-behavioral and psychopharmacological treatment.

A small number of case reports describe transient paranoid psychoses in the absence of other symptoms of delirium in liver recipients.[40,46] These psychotic states have been variably attributed to cyclosporine,[40,46] tacrolimus,[76] antibacterial agents and antifungal agents or the cytokines associated with infection,[45,80] sleep deprivation, and "stress reactions" to the transplantation setting.

Modest progress has been made in determining the relative safety of using contemporary antidepressants/antianxiety agents in solid-organ recipients. It is likely that all of the selective serotonin reuptake inhibitor (SSRI)-class agents (fluoxetine, paroxetine, sertraline, citalopram, escitalopram), the serotonin-norepinephrine reuptake inhibitor (SNRI) venlafaxine, and the noradrenergic and specific serotonergic antidepressant (NaSSA) mirtazapine can be used in liver transplantation recipients without excessive concern regarding pharmacokinetic interactions that might alter immunosuppressant steady-state blood levels.[89] Except under special circumstances, the antidepressant agent nefazodone (Serzone) should be avoided in liver transplantation recipients: as a uniquely potent inhibitor of P4503A3/4 (the isozyme family predominantly responsible for the metabolism of both cyclosporine and tacrolimus), nefazodone is associated with precipitous elevations in calcineurin-inhibitor blood levels and clinical toxicity[90] and, as an independent matter, is associated with direct hepatotoxicity in patients without preexisting liver disease.[91]

Movement Disorders

Gross tremor is a common problem in liver transplant recipients. High serum calcineurin inhibitor levels are often associated with extreme symptoms, although tremor occurs in many patients with normal/low normal levels. OKT3 has also been reported to cause or exacerbate tremor.[62] The chronic brain effects of alcohol abuse/dependence may predispose patients to tremor after liver transplantation.[17] Other potentiating factors include hypomagnesemia or hypocalcemia[40,41] and coadministration of other drugs that may elevate calcineurin-inhibitor levels, such as erythromycin, oral contraceptives, methylprednisolone, azole antifungals, cimetidine, verapamil, nefazodone, and other potent inhibitors of P4503A3/4.[45,90] Many patients experience fasciculations or myoclonic jerks, symptoms that are frequently worse at night and may interrupt sleep. No controlled data exist to guide treatment of these symptoms in transplant patients. When calcineurin-inhibitor dose manipulations and attention to pharmacokinetic interactions are not sufficient, we have successfully managed tremor and myoclonus empirically with clonazepam and gabapentin.

More severe and disabling syndromes of cerebellar dysfunction, characterized by ataxia, nystagmus, weakness, and dysarthria, have also been described.[40-42,47] These symptoms have been portrayed as acute neurotoxic states that generally improve or clear entirely despite uncertain causes. Transient limb paresis, hemiplegia, and spasticity have also been reported.[31,33,92]

A symptom complex of akinetic mutism or "locked-in syndrome," orofacial dyskinesias, pseudobulbar palsy, and MRI-confirmed central pontine myelinolysis has been described in liver transplant recipients from a number of different centers.[46,50,92-95] This dramatic syndrome has been convincingly linked to calcineurin inhibitors (both cyclosporine and tacrolimus), and has been reported to clear with dose decrements, drug holidays, and empirical switching.[46,51-54,64,76] Residual dysarthria and aphasia have been reported after the resolution of the florid primary symptoms, an observation echoed by our program's experience.[41,46] The risk of recurrence after rechallenge with the primary immunosuppressant agents remains unclear, in part because transplant teams have become quite facile at the pragmatic maneuver of switching. Lucey's prescient observation that some calcineurin-inhibitor neurotoxicity may occur as a function of allograft genotypic P4503A3/4 "poor metabolizer" status[96] was followed by a tremendous growth in knowledge regarding the mechanisms of pharmacokinetic drug interactions.

Other Constitutional Symptoms

Impaired taste and smell sensations are common complaints after liver transplantation. Hypersensitivity to olfactory input is also frequently reported. Hyper- and hypoacusis are also noted. Incontinence[33] and male and female sexual dysfunction have also been reported, although liver transplantation often is associated with the restoration of reproductive endocrine function.[97] Related matters, such as depression, body image adjustment, self-esteem, and relationship issues, are also critically important to postoperative sexual functioning.

Close attention to posttransplantation recovery also reveals that some patients endure persistent fatigue, neuropsychologically demonstrable psychomotor and visuospatial deficits,[98] and general malaise after liver transplantation, all in the absence of conventionally defined mood disorder or demonstrable metabolic abnormality. Whether this represents the chronic brain consequences of liver disease or some new "equilibrium" state potentiated by the central nervous system effects of calcineurin-inhibitors remains unknown. Psychostimulants (methylphenidate, dextroamphetamine, and the novel agent modafinil) have been empirically useful.[72,99]

Summary

As liver transplantation has evolved from "a desperate treatment for desperate patients" to a more commonly performed procedure, greater attention has been paid to the neuropsychiatric consequences of liver disease and its treatment. Increasingly sophisticated functional neuroimaging techniques confirm that neuropsychological impairments of late-stage liver disease generally improve after transplantation. Yet careful clinical observations continue to describe a complex variety of neuropsychiatric symptom patterns, many of which may be understood as complications of the broad spectrum of effects of necessary immunosuppressants. Despite the fact that these clinical problems transiently affect a significant minority of patients after transplantation, overall high rates of satisfaction with quality of life are the rule.

Pearls and Pitfalls

Pre- or Posttransplant Confusion/ Disorientation/Intensive Care Unit Insomnia

- Suspect acute metabolic abnormality
- Induce normal sleep-wake cycle with sedating, atypical antipsychotics or butyrophenones and judicious doses of opioids
- Avoid empirical treatment with benzodiazepines, which may worsen delirium

New-Onset Mood, Anxiety, or Cognitive Problems in Newly Transplanted Patients

- Suspect calcineurin-inhibitor toxicity
- Attempt to achieve lowest effective serum levels
- Do not ignore these symptoms; they lengthen hospital stay and adversely affect rehabilitation and convalescence

Lethargy/Somnolence in Hepatic Encephalopathy When Clinical Discussion is Necessary with the Patient

- Flumazenil challenge
- Episodic short-interval intravenous push flumazenil dosing will be necessary to maintain wakefulness; N.B., can provoke seizure activity
- Avoid iatrogenic benzodiazepine administration

References

1. Trzepacz PT, Brenner R, Van Thiel D: A psychiatric study of 247 liver transplantation candidates. Psychosomatics 30:147-153, 1989.
2. Trzepacz PT, Tarter R, Shad A, et al: SPECT scan and cognitive findings in subclinical hepatic encephalopathy: Alcoholic and non-alcoholic cirrhosis. Presented at the meeting of the Academy of Psychosomatic Medicine, Atlanta, GA, October, 1991.
3. Trzepacz PT, Brenner RP, Coffman G, et al: Delirium in liver transplantation candidates: Discriminant analysis of multiple test variables. Biol Psychiatry 24:3-14, 1988.
4. Rehnstrom S, Simert F, Hansson JA, et al: Chronic hepatic encephalopathy: A psychometrical study. Scand J Gastroenterol 12:305-311, 1977.

Postoperative Neurological Disorders and Prognosis

EDWIN C. AMOS III

Alteration in mental status   1029

Seizures   1030

Vascular events occurring after liver transplantation   1031

Disorders of white matter or leukoencephalopathy   1031

Central nervous system infections   1032

Neurotoxic effects of medication   1033

Peripheral neuropathy in orthotopic liver transplantation   1033

Movement disorders in orthotopic liver transplantation   1033

Neuropathology of orthotopic liver transplantation   1034

Evaluation of postoperative neurological disorders and functional outcome in orthotopic liver transplantation   1034

Since the first orthotopic liver transplant was performed almost 37 years ago, advances in surgical technique and postoperative immunosuppressive regimens have allowed this to become a widely practiced therapeutic intervention for end-stage liver disease.[1] The neurological complications and disorders that arise after transplantation are common and complex in their clinical presentation.[2-5] It has been estimated that between 8% and 47% of all patients undergoing orthotopic liver transplantation (OLT) experience some form of postoperative neurological disorder.[6-11] These neurological complications range from encephalopathy to seizure activity, stroke, infections, secondary central nervous system malignancies, and death. The majority of disturbances in neurological function occur in the first 3 months after transplantation. Diagnosis and evaluation of these neurological phenomena are complex and require a high index of clinical suspicion for successful diagnosis and treatment. Table 67–1 outlines the most common neurological disorders in the postoperative OLT patient.

Alteration in Mental Status

Postoperative alteration in mental status has been described in more than 80% of patients undergoing OLT.[12] The patient's pretransplantation level of impairment in mental status related to liver encephalopathy is often associated with the degree of impairment in the

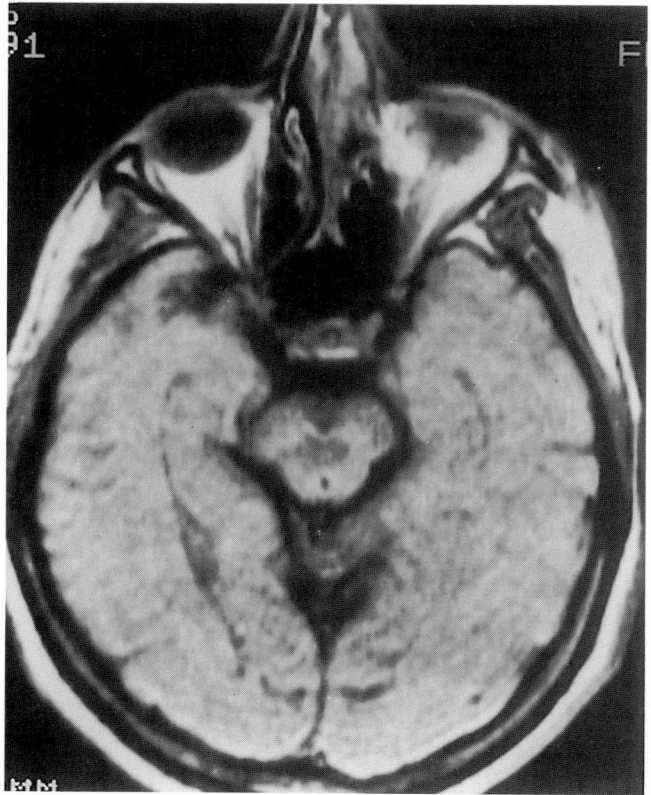

FIGURE 67–2

Central pontine myelinolysis is evident after OLT. Note again the low signal intensity in the pons on this T1-weighted axial magnetic resonance image.

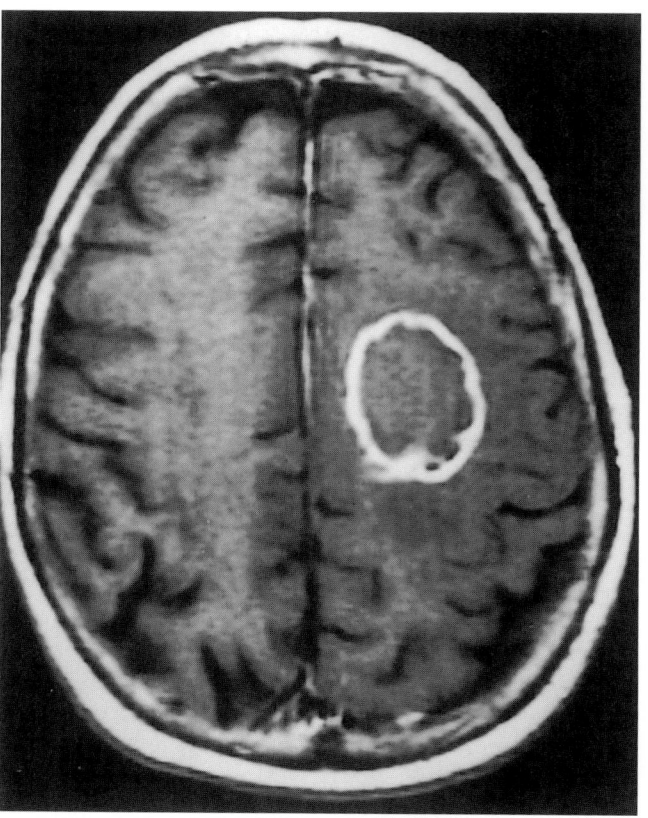

FIGURE 67–3

Brain abscess is evident in a patient after OLT. This is a gadolinium-enhanced, T1-weighted axial magnetic resonance image.

Central Nervous System Infections

Infections of the central nervous system may present insidiously in immunocompromised patients, for example those undergoing OLT. Cases of fungal, bacterial, and viral meningoencephalitis have been described with pathogens such as *Aspergillus, Candida,* cytomegalovirus, and others.[20,21] Clinical presentation may be subtle, especially in the presence of other factors causing alteration in mental status, but may be heralded by seizure activity, fever, or focal motor deficits. The latter findings may suggest intracranial disease such as abscess (Fig. 67-3) or hemorrhage, which may result from these infectious processes. Systemic infections—for example, pulmonary and others such as endocarditis—may spread to the central nervous system, causing neurological dysfunction.

Aspergillus infection of the central nervous system remains an important cause of morbidity and mortality in posttransplantation patients. This opportunistic fungal infection commonly involves the central nervous system and tends to invade the blood vessels, causing subsequent ischemic and hemorrhagic infarction and abscess formation. Mycotic aneurysm has been noted as a cause of subarachnoid hemorrhage. Depending on the location of the abscess or vascular lesion, focal motor changes, hemianopia, and even third cranial nerve palsy have been described.[22] Central nervous system aspergillosis is especially common after intense antirejection therapy requiring high doses of immunosuppressive agents. The most common finding of disseminated central nervous system aspergillosis is that of alteration in mental status with little or no meningism present. In general, the prognosis for transplantation patients with central nervous system aspergillosis is poor, a fact that indicates the often delayed diagnosis of this pathogen. Certainly, central nervous system involvement with *Aspergillus* should be suspected in patients in whom pulmonary infiltrates and focal neurological signs or seizures develop. Early diagnosis and treatment require high clinical suspicion and aggressive intervention.

Other conditions associated with postoperative liver transplantations have included recurrence of hepatitis B and C, herpes simplex, human immunodeficiency virus, and one case of cerebrophaeohyphomycosis.[23]

Neurotoxic Effects of Medication

As previously noted, the neurotoxic effects of medications such as cyclosporine, tacrolimus, and others are prevalent in patients undergoing OLT. It is of interest that the oral formulation of cyclosporine has been found to reduce the severity of neurotoxicity observed in liver transplant patients significantly.[10]

In addition to tremor, headache, and seizures, as well as mental status alterations, focal and diffuse leukoencephalopathy (Fig. 67–4) has been described as a sequela of cyclosporine administration. Other less common side effects described in the literature include complex visual hallucinations, cortical blindness, a cerebellar syndrome, extrapyramidal syndrome, and akinetic mutism, tremors, and ataxia.[8,16,18,19,24-27] Many of these problems are related to initial intravenous use of cyclosporine and may be eliminated with reduction in dosage.

Tacrolimus will produce neurological disorders similar to those seen with the administration of cyclosporine, but more frequently. These include seizures, cortical blindness, and leukoencephalopathy, which is also reversible with a decrease or a discontinuation of the medication.[28-30] OKT3, often used in the treatment of severe rejection, may cause headache, which is sometimes refractory to analgesic medication. A pattern of aseptic meningitis with sterile spinal fluid pleocytosis has been reported. After discontinuation of the monoclonal antibody, resolution of the meningitis occurs.[4] Hypocholesterolemia and hypomagnesemia have been noted to be more prevalent in patients receiving tacrolimus.[8]

Corticosteroids, a mainstay of immunosuppression, may cause changes in mood such as depression, dysphoria, or even euphoria. Frank psychosis has been reported along with insomnia, headache, vertigo, and even convulsions. Chronic steroid-induced myopathy may also be seen in patients receiving these medications over long periods.

Azathioprine is also used in OLT patients and may cause seizure activity on occasion. It should also be noted that in general, immunosuppressive agents, when used chronically, may cause a condition known as *progressive multifocal leukoencephalopathy,* which is a viral disease related to the polyomavirus (JC virus) and has also been reported in patients immunosuppressed during treatment of malignancy or in patients with acquired immunodeficiency syndrome (AIDS).

Peripheral Neuropathy in Orthotopic Liver Transplantation

Peripheral neuropathy, including cranial nerve lesions, distal lower extremity neuropathy, brachial plexopathy, polyneuropathy, and mononeuropathy, has been reported in patients undergoing OLT. Causes are multifactorial and include chronic toxic medication administration such as cyclosporine and tacrolimus, as well as periviral processes including a chronic postinfectious demyelinating polyradiculoneuropathy-type syndrome (Guillain-Barré syndrome). Mononeuropathy multiplex has been reported in patients with chronic viral hepatitis and infections due to cytomegalovirus and human immunodeficiency virus.

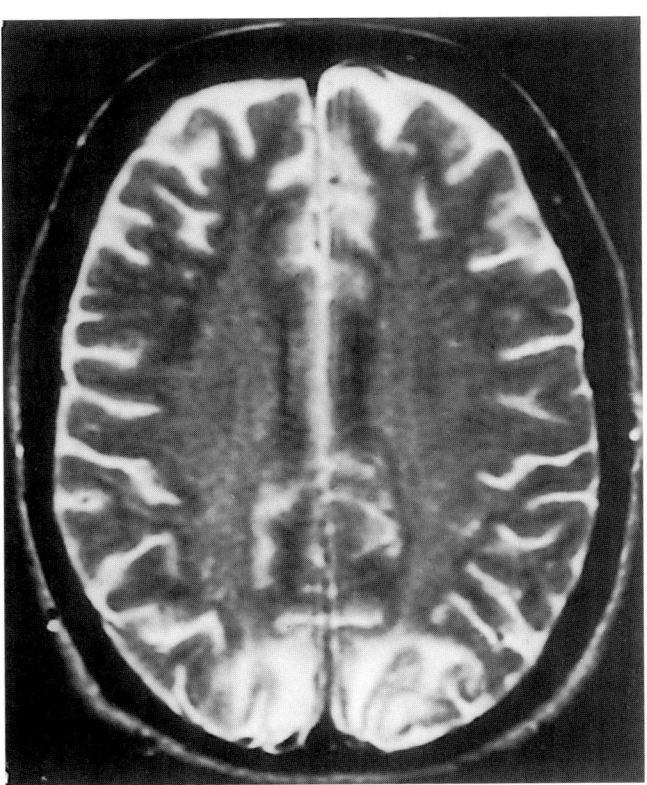

FIGURE 67–4

Diffuse leukoencephalopathy in a patient after OLT. The condition resulted from the administration of cyclosporine. Note the diffuse and focal posterior high signal in the white matter tracts on this T2-weighted axial magnetic resonance image.

Movement Disorders in Orthotopic Liver Transplantation

Tremor is the most common movement disorder described as a side effect of generalized encephalopathic state as well as that of medications such as cyclosporine, tacrolimus, and steroids. A cerebellar syndrome has been described as has an extrapyramidal syndrome

24. Bird GLA, Meadows J, Goka J, et al: Cyclosporin-associated akinetic mutism and extrapyramidal syndrome after liver transplantation. J Neural Neurosurg Psychiatry 53:1068-1071, 1990.

25. Cilio MR, Danhaive O, Gadisseux JF, et al: Unusual cyclosporin-related neurological complications in recipients of liver transplants. Arch Dis Child 68:405-407, 1993.

26. Gottrand F, Largilliere C, Farriaux JP: Cyclosporine neurotoxicity [letter]. N Engl J Med 324:1744-1745, 1991.

27. Lucey MR, Kolars JC, Merion RM, et al: Cyclosporin toxicity at therapeutic blood levels and cytochrome P-450 IIIA. Lancet 335:11-15, 1990.

28. Eidelman BH, Abu-Elmagd K, Wilson J, et al: Neurologic complications of FK506. Transplant Proc 23:3175-3178, 1991.

29. Freise CE, Rowley H, Lake J, et al: Similar clinical presentation of neurotoxicity following FK506 and cyclosporine in a liver transplant recipient. Transplant Proc 23:3173-3174, 1991.

30. Lopez OL, Martinez AJ, Torre-Cisneros J: Neuropathologic findings in liver transplantation: A comparative study of cyclosporine and FK506. Transplant Proc 23:3181-3182, 1991.

31. Ferreiro JA, Rober MA, Townsend J, Vinters HV: Neuropathologic findings after liver transplantation. Acta Neuropathol 84:1-14, 1992.

32. Hall WA, Martinez AJ: Neuropathology of pediatric liver transplantation. Pediatr Neurosci 15:269-275, 1989.

33. Lidofsky SB, Bas NM, Prager MC, et al: Intracranial pressure monitoring and liver transplantation for fulminant hepatic failure. Hepatology 16:1-7, 1992.

34. Keays R, Potter D, O'Grady J, et al: Intracranial and cerebral perfusion pressure changes before, during, and immediately after orthotopic liver transplantation for fulminant hepatic failure. Q J Med 79:425-433, 1991.

Role of the Posttransplant Coordinator

GREGG KUNDER

Considerations in the posttransplant clinical coordinator care process 1037

Transition of patient care to the outpatient environment 1039

Coordination of patient care immediately after discharge 1040

Coordination of long-term outpatient care 1042

Future trends for the posttransplant coordinator 1046

The posttransplant clinical coordinator (PTCC) is an integral part of the patient management team. The PTCC is involved in the continuum of patient care that begins postoperatively in the hospital and continues to coordinate this care in the outpatient setting. Throughout this continuum there are many forces that define the PTCC's responsibilities, knowledge requirements, and resource needs related to the coordination of patient care. This chapter briefly discusses these concepts.

Considerations in the Posttransplant Clinical Coordinator Care Process

Liver transplant programs throughout the world differ greatly in patient volume, resources, and management styles. The PTCC's role in patient care is defined by many factors that differ from one program to the next. One important factor in the PTCC's role is the division of tasks throughout the continuum of patient care. In programs with high patient volume and an adequate number of nurses, the skill mix of the PTCC can be highly specialized. The PTCC can focus on either inpatient care or outpatient care. Coordinators may specialize only in patient education, outpatient surgical clinics, or outpatient hepatology clinics. In smaller programs, the PTCC may be responsible for both inpatient and

during the hospitalization phase and a concise discharge summary should be provided to the patient's health care providers. Community health care providers should be given the opportunity to clarify issues and should understand whom to contact for further information regarding the patient's care. Community health care providers frequently require teaching by members of the transplant team to keep them informed of the ever-changing spectrum of transplant medicine and recipient care.

Coordination of Patient Care Immediately after Discharge

The most intense focus of patient care immediately after discharge occurs in the transplant center's outpatient clinics. The PTCC is often responsible for assessing the patient, coordinating ongoing care, and facilitating treatment of identified problems. The frequency of blood studies and clinic visits is dependent on patient progress and the policies of the transplant center. Before the transition of patient care from the surgical team to the hepatologist, the PTCC must assess the patient for any unresolved surgical issues (Table 68–4). Should unresolved surgical issues be identified, the patient should remain under the care of the surgical team.

The PTCC is frequently responsible for ordering and monitoring the results of patient blood studies. Table 68–5 lists common baseline blood studies, as well as specific studies based on the patient's original liver disease. Initially, these blood studies are performed in the transplant center's clinics. As time from transplantation increases, all or some of these blood studies can become the responsibility of community providers. The PTCC is responsible for ensuring that blood studies are performed correctly and expediently.

After discharge, patients should be encouraged to reestablish their relationship with their primary care physician. Traditionally, the PTCC is the first line of communication between the transplant center and the primary care physician. Primary care physicians may require education from the PTCC regarding care of the transplant recipient. The PTCC can reinforce to the

Table 68-4. ISSUES THAT PRECLUDE DISCHARGE FROM SURGICAL MANAGEMENT

Abnormal graft function that requires frequent clinical assessment and laboratory studies

Severe untoward side effects from immunosuppressive medications

Unhealed open wounds

Presence of drains or tubes, with the exception of T tubes

Active infection

Excessive fluid imbalance

Failure to thrive

Table 68-5. BLOOD STUDY REQUIREMENTS FOR ROUTINE SURVEILLANCE AND DISEASE MANAGEMENT

Routine blood studies for all patients	Hemoglobin, hematocrit, white blood cell and platelet count (a manual differential should be performed for any white blood cell count less than 3000/mm^3) Comprehensive metabolic chemistry panel ALT (SGPT) Cholesterol Phosphorus Immunosuppressant trough level Magnesium
Patients with hyperglycemia	Glycosylated hemoglobin every 3 mo
Patients receiving HBV prophylaxis	Before HBIG administration: Hepatitis B surface antigen Anti–hepatitis B surface antibody Hepatitis B DNA every 3 mo
Patients receiving HCV antiviral agents	Hepatitis C RNA quantitation every 3 mo minimum
Patients with a history of HCC	AFP every 3 mo
Patients with a history of PSC or ulcerative colitis	CEA every 3 mo
Patients with a history of PBC or CCA	CA 19-9 every 3 mo
Patients taking warfarin or who have been relisted for liver transplantation	PT/INR according to dosing or MELD requirements
Patients with hemochromatosis	Every 3 mo: Total iron-binding capacity Ferritin Transferrin AFP
Patients with a history of substance abuse	Random toxicology screens

AFP, alpha-fetoprotein; ALT, alanine transaminase; CAHC, chronic active hepatitis C; CCA, cholangiocarcinoma; CEA, carcinoembryonic antigen; HBIG, hepatitis B immune globulin; HBV, hepatitis B virus; HCC, hepatocellular carcinoma; HCV, hepatitis C virus; INR, international normalized ratio; MELD, Model for End-Stage Liver Disease; PBC, primary biliary cirrhosis; PSC, primary sclerosing cholangitis; PT, prothrombin time; SGPT, serum glutamic pyruvic transaminase.

Table 68-6. CRITICAL INDICATORS THAT REQUIRE THE PRIMARY CARE PHYSICIAN TO CONTACT THE TRANSPLANT CENTER
Unexplained, sustained fever of 38° C with or without associated leukocytosis
Uncontrollable hypertension or persistently elevated blood pressure associated with symptoms
Central nervous system infections
Signs or symptoms of drug toxicity, such as seizures, severe tremors, or headaches
Pneumonitis or complicated pneumonia
Vomiting or diarrhea lasting longer than 24 hr
Gastrointestinal bleeding or acute abdominal pain
Acute or chronic increase in serum creatinine
Persistent leukopenia or unexplained leukocytosis
Acute or chronic unexplained lymph node or tonsillar enlargement
Any sign or symptom of serious infection, graft rejection, or malignant disease
Emergency admission or transfer to the transplant center
Elective admission for
Incisional hernia repair
Removal of wound seromas
Revision of the biliary anastomosis
Any other abdominal surgical procedure
Addition, subtraction, or dose change of any medication

Table 68-7. EMERGENCY OR URGENT SIGNS AND SYMPTOMS THAT REQUIRE IMMEDIATE INTERVENTION BY THE POSTTRANSPLANT CLINICAL COORDINATOR
Sustained fever of 38° C with or without symptoms
Uncontrolled hypertension with diastolic pressure greater than 110 mm Hg
New onset or worsening of neurological complaints, altered mental status, or decreased level of consciousness
Shortness of breath with or without a productive cough
Acute or chronic increase in serum creatinine greater than 3.0 mg/dL or serum potassium greater than 6.5 mmol/L
Acute peripheral edema unresponsive to diuretic therapy
Vomiting or inability to keep medications down for longer than 24 hr
Diarrhea lasting longer than 3 days
Gastrointestinal bleeding
Profuse wound drainage from an incision or drain entry site
Acute abdominal pain
Absolute neutrophil count less than 800/mm^3
Acute or worsening jaundice, pruritus, clay-colored stools, or tea-colored urine
Acute opening of a previously closed wound
Any sign or symptom of infection or rejection
Magnesium less than 1.0 mg/dL
Hematocrit less than 26% and/or signs and symptoms of symptomatic anemia
Chest pain
Dislodgement or manipulation of the T tube or other surgical drain or tube

primary care physician the importance of communicating changes in patient status that require immediate consideration by the transplant center (Table 68-6).[2]

Outpatients may come to the emergency department with a wide variety of problems, including graft rejection, infection, graft vascular complications, biliary complications, adverse medication side effects, fluid and electrolyte imbalance, fever, transhepatic tube (T tube) leaks, and wound problems.[3] The PTCC must have criteria to follow in deciding when to advise a patient to seek emergency department care (Table 68-7).

Wound care is an essential part of patient care immediately after transplantation. Patients seen in outpatient clinics are undergoing the proliferative and regenerative stages of primary wound closure. Maximal tensile strength of the wound is achieved within 6 to 8 weeks after the last incision. The PTCC can identify patients at risk for delayed wound healing and infection and institute interventions to remedy the identified problems (Table 68-8). Should wound infection be identified, treatment should be followed by assessment for wound complications such as fistulas, sinus tracts, and sepsis (see Table 68-8). The surgical team should be contacted to assess and treat wound complications. Secondary wound closure is necessary if wound opening

occurs after removal of the incision staples. The wound heals by contraction and epithelialization. Tissue granulation appears within 4 to 6 days after wound opening. The PTCC must instruct the patient to change the wound dressing according to the surgeon's orders.[4]

During assessment of the patient the PTCC will commonly encounter complaints of abdominal pain. Incision pain is common up to 12 weeks after transplantation. Manipulation of nerves close to the diaphragm can cause referred pain to the midback area. As nerves and tissues heal, numbness, burning, stabbing pain, aching, and "pins and needles" have all been described by patients. Pain that is atypical or out of proportion to the patient's incision should prompt the PTCC to facilitate a surgeon's assessment of the patient. Abdominal pain can be indicative of rejection, infection, and a multitude of other abdominal pathologies, many of which can quickly become detrimental complications.

Patients receiving intravenous therapy at home will be discharged with a peripheral intravenous central catheter line or a central venous access line. Care of these lines should comply with the protocol of the

Table 68–10. KEY POINTS REGARDING COMPLICATIONS IN THE IMMEDIATE POSTTRANSPLANT PERIOD

Incisional Hernias

Instruct the patient to contact the transplant center immediately for vomiting, increased hernia size, inability to reduce the hernia, or increased pain

Small Bowel Obstruction

Manifestations of small bowel obstruction can include cramping (colic), abdominal pain, vomiting, abdominal distention, hypovolemia, or a radiograph demonstrating a distended bowel proximal to the obstruction with air-fluid levels

Bypass Seroma

Seromas are reabsorbed over time without incident. Drained seromas commonly recur. Instruct the patient to contact the transplant center for any signs of neurovascular deterioration in the affected limb. Seromas lasting longer than 3 months may require surgical exploration and lymphocele repair. Residual numbness, paresthesia, and weakness lasting longer than 3 months should prompt neurological referral

Pleural Effusions

A right-sided pleural effusion is a normal physical finding. The pleural effusion may last for life and does not indicate a need for therapy unless dyspnea, fever, pleuritic chest pain, or increasing size is discovered

Thromboembolic Events

Unilateral lower extremity swelling, pain, low-grade fever, and cramping in the calf on dorsiflexion of the foot require investigation to rule out deep vein thrombosis. Pulmonary emboli can be signaled by complaints of dyspnea, fever, and chest pain. The posttransplant clinical coordinator (PTCC) should facilitate emergency care for these symptoms. Instruct patients taking warfarin to convert their trimethoprim-sulfamethoxazole dosing to a daily dose instead of a weekend dose to ensure steady-state serum warfarin levels and prothrombin times

Hepatic Artery Thrombosis (HAT)

When the clinical history does not support rejection and acute elevations in liver function test values occur with fever and/or new onset of abdominal pain, HAT, dilated biliary ducts, biliary stricture, and abdominal fluid collections should be suspected. Patients with HAT are at high risk for biliary strictures and abscess formation. Subhepatic abscesses may require image-guided drainage, external drain placement, and antibiotic therapy

Extrahepatic Biliary Strictures

Strictures may be manifested as graft dysfunction and may or may not be detected by ultrasound. Balloon dilatation or stenting across strictures that occur below the hilum can be performed via endoscopic retrograde cholangiopancreatography (ERCP), T-tube cholangiography, or percutaneous transhepatic cholangiography. ERCP cannot be performed in patients with a Roux-en-Y choledochojejunostomy biliary anastomosis. The PTCC should be alert to the type of biliary anastomosis present to ensure that appropriate interventions are implemented. The PTCC should also ensure that the patient receives adequate antibiotic prophylaxis before any manipulation of the biliary tract

Pancreatitis

The PTCC should be alert for signs or symptoms of pancreatitis after manipulation of the biliary tract, especially after ERCP

Cholangitis

The PTCC should always suspect cholangitis in patients with biliary stricture and fever. Symptoms of cholangitis include right upper quadrant pain, fever, and jaundice (Charcot's triad). If hypotension and/or altered mental status are also noted, Reynold's syndrome is present. Cholangitis can be life-threatening and requires urgent hospitalization for intravenous antibiotic therapy

Intrahepatic Biliary Strictures

Causes include ischemia, prolonged preservation time, ABO mismatch, and chronic (ductopenic) rejection. Intrahepatic biliary strictures are not amenable to endoscopic or radiological intervention, are progressive, and often require retransplantation. Progressive hepatic dysfunction is the typical course

Graft-versus-Host-Disease (GVHD)

GVHD is a rare and catastrophic complication of organ transplantation. Signs and symptoms occur 3 to 4 months after transplantation and include low-grade fever, neutropenia, alopecia, diarrhea, weight loss, enteric ileus, hemolytic anemia, and erythematous maculopapular rash, particularly involving the ears and distal portions of the extremities. The PTCC should immediately alert the transplant team to any patient suspected of contracting GVHD

Acute rejection can occur at any time after transplantation. Pharmacological agents are used to block the immunological cascade responsible for acute rejection. The PTCC should be familiar with the mechanism of action, dosing, side effects, drug interactions, and methods of monitoring the effectiveness of all these antirejection medications. The PTCC is an important resource to the community health care provider and the patient for information about these medications and their interactions with other pharmacological agents.

The patient should have a clear understanding of the potential harm that these interactions can produce and should be instructed to contact the PTCC before any medication change, addition, or deletion.

Infection is a leading cause of death in transplant patients. Studies indicate that up to 80% of transplant patients will have one to two infections in the first year after transplantation. Infections are 50% to 60% bacterial, 20% to 40% viral, and 5% to 15% fungal.[6] Ensuring adequate prophylaxis against bacterial infections is an important responsibility of the PTCC. The PTCC must ensure that antibiotic prophylaxis is instituted before any surgical procedure, biliary study, or dental procedure.

The most effective method of preventing bacterial infections is eliminating the patient's exposure to bacterial pathogens. The PTCC can facilitate this goal by educating the patient about how to avoid bacterial pathogens through techniques such as proper hand washing, personal hygiene, and maintenance of a clean home environment. Exposure to certain bacteria can be avoided by lifestyle modification. *Legionella* is a gram-negative rickettsial organism that is spread via aerosolized water. Table 68–11 lists interventions that should be taught to the patient before discharge to reduce the risk of *Legionella* exposure.

Exposure to tuberculosis without disease progression is common in the general public and has become more prevalent in large urban centers with large immigrant populations. Experience with immunocompromised individuals indicates that activation of the disease can occur many years after exposure. Recipients with positive skin tests and negative chest x-rays may benefit from receiving antituberculosis therapy. The PTCC should identify patients with positive skin tests and confer with the appropriate team member regarding the need for antituberculosis therapy after transplantation.

Prophylaxis against fungal infection can be provided through the use of intravenous or oral antifungal agents (or both) for 6 to 10 weeks after transplantation. Patients considered to be at high risk for fungal infections have the characteristics listed in Table 68–12. It is imperative that the PTCC be aware of when a patient terminates fungal prophylaxis because discontinuation of most of

these agents can cause a sudden decrease in immunosuppression levels and precipitate a rejection episode. Table 68–13 lists preventive interventions that the PTCC should explain to the recipient to prevent infection with *Coccidioides*, *Aspergillus*, *Cryptococcus*, and *Histoplasma*.

Antiviral medications in oral and intravenous form are prescribed to recipients for up to 100 days after transplantation to prevent cytomegalovirus (CMV), Epstein-Barr virus (EBV), and herpes simplex virus (HSV) infections. Prophylaxis is more extensive for patients at high risk for the development of CMV infection. Risk factors for CMV infection are listed in Table 68–14. Recipients who are naïve to chickenpox infection and are exposed should be instructed to receive varicella-zoster immune globulin (VZIG) within 24 to 48 hours of exposure. VZIG is available in most community emergency departments. The PTCC should instruct recipients to avoid all live virus vaccinations. Recipients should

Table 68-12. PATIENT RISK FACTORS FOR THE DEVELOPMENT OF FUNGAL INFECTIONS

Patients transplanted with high MELD scores
Prolonged ventilator time
Recipient of 20 or more units of blood products
Previous infection or colonization with a fungal pathogen
History of bacterial peritonitis

MELD, Model for End-Stage Liver Disease.

Table 68-13. PATIENT INSTRUCTIONS FOR PREVENTION OF FUNGAL INFECTIONS

Coccidioidomycosis Prophylaxis

Avoid exposure to soil and dust in areas where this pathogen is endemic
Be aware that the presence of spores in the air dramatically increases after earthquakes
Avoid contact with infected mammals with open skin sores

Aspergillosis and Cryptococcosis Prophylaxis

Avoid construction or renovation areas, changing of carpets, and cleaning of air vents (if unavoidable, use dust barriers, air filters, positive airflow, and window sealing)
Avoid hay, vegetation, soil exposure, dust, and mold
Do not garden without gloves and a protective mask
Do not empty water dishes under houseplants; water should be drained by family members immediately after watering

Histoplasmosis Prophylaxis

Do not keep birds as pets in the house
Avoid contact with birds raised outside the home, such as chickens, turkeys, and birds bred for sale as pets

Table 68-11. PATIENT INSTRUCTIONS FOR *LEGIONELLA* PROPHYLAXIS

Clean produce thoroughly if purchased in a market that uses mist machines
Maintain hot tubs in sanitary condition
Avoid cooling towers
Avoid sump pumps
Avoid ultrasonic misting devices
Avoid tap water from nonchlorinated systems

Table 68-14. RISK FACTORS FOR CYTOMEGALOVIRUS INFECTION
Recipient serology is negative; donor serology is positive
Recipient serology is positive; donor serology is positive
High steroid doses
OKT3, polyclonal or monoclonal antibody treatment of the recipient
Therapy for acute rejection
Multiple organs transplanted
Hyperglycemia
Previous cytomegalovirus infection
High level of immune suppression
Liver retransplantation

also avoid the body fluids of recently vaccinated individuals, including children, because live virus can be shed in body fluids for up to 3 months after vaccination. Children generally receive live virus vaccinations at 2, 4, 6, and 15 months and at years 4 through 6. Live virus vaccinations include smallpox, yellow fever, measles, mumps, rubella, varicella, oral polio, and the initial diphtheria-tetanus-pertussis series. Should smallpox vaccinations resume for the general public, the patient must be instructed to avoid this vaccination, as well as contact with the vaccination scab on newly vaccinated persons. No research has been conducted to determine the danger that a recently vaccinated host poses to the transplant recipient. The PTCC should instruct the recipient to check the vaccination requirements for cruise ships and overseas travel packages because these requirements can include live virus vaccination.

Hepatitis B prophylaxis with hepatitis B immune globulin (HBIG) and lamivudine has been shown to be safe and effective in liver transplant recipients. This regimen is most effective when the recipient is hepatitis B DNA and hepatitis Be antigen negative before transplantation. Prophylaxis should be initiated during the anhepatic phase of the transplant operation. Coordination of HBIG administration and monitoring of anti–hepatitis B surface antigen antibody levels and hepatitis B surface antigen serology are often the responsibility of the PTCC. The PTCC must ensure that prophylactic target levels of antibody are maintained and must also assist in treating the side effects of intravenous HBIG administration in the community setting.

Protozoan prophylaxis includes avoiding environmental sources of these pathogens and providing pharmaceutical protection against *Pneumocystis carinii* pneumonia (PCP). PCP prophylaxis can consist of oral, intravenous, or inhaled agents taken for 1 year after transplantation. The PTCC should instruct the recipient to avoid cat feces, litter boxes, and raw or undercooked animal flesh to prevent infection with *Toxoplasma*.

To avoid *Cryptosporidium* infection, the recipient should be instructed to drink water only from chlorinated systems, distilled bottled water, or water that has been passed through filters that are capable of filtering out protozoan pathogens. Reports of *Cryptosporidium* infection in immunocompromised individuals from nondistilled bottled water and public chlorinated water systems deserve close attention and may necessitate future changes in drinking water recommendations to the transplant recipient.

When infection does occur in the transplant recipient, it must be recognized and treated quickly. It is important for the PTCC to know when the recipient is most prone to specific infections. Most bacterial infections, *Candida* infections, and reactivation of HSV infection occur within the first month after transplantation. CMV reactivation and aspergillosis usually occur at weeks 4 through 10. EBV and varicella-zoster infections occur at months 4 through 6. PCP and toxoplasmosis also develop within the first 6 months after transplantation. Recurrent hepatitis B or C, cryptococcal pneumonia, and meningitis can begin to occur during the fourth through sixth months after transplantation. The incidence of infections decreases 6 to 12 months after transplantation, but when they do occur, they are often associated with graft dysfunction or high-dose immunosuppression.[6] Serious opportunistic infections rarely develop in patients 1 year after transplantation, but these patients are susceptible to common community-acquired infections, including pneumonia from *Streptococcus pneumoniae* and *Haemophilus influenzae*. Annual influenza vaccines and the *Pneumococcus* vaccine can be safely used as prophylaxis against these organisms beginning 1 year after transplantation. Hepatitis A and B vaccine and tetanus boosters are also permissible 1 year after transplantation.

Intra-abdominal infections and pneumonia are the most common bacterial infections in the early posttransplant period. Pneumonia, urinary tract infections, and viral syndromes are common causes of late posttransplant fever. The possibility of resistant organisms should be considered in liver transplant recipients because of their history of multiple antibiotic treatments and frequent hospitalizations. Febrile episodes above 38° C that last longer than 24 hours should prompt the PTCC to pursue examination of the patient by a physician. Table 68–15 lists the classic causes of fever in newly discharged patients. Emergency physicians and community health care providers will often contact the PTCC for the transplant center's procedures for a fever workup. Table 68–16 outlines a fever workup that the PTCC can discuss with the inquiring physician.

The PTCC is often responsible for advising patients about "over-the-counter" (OTC) medications. Because many OTC medications can interact with medications

Table 68–15. CAUSES OF FEVER IN NEWLY TRANSPLANTED PATIENTS

Atelectasis

Wound infection

Urinary tract infection

Deep vein thrombosis

Pulmonary emboli

Central line or drain sepsis

commonly taken by transplant recipients, it is important for the PTCC to give patients correct and concise information. Table 68–17 gives examples of patient instructions for OTC medication use.[7,8]

Long-term patient care issues are caused by the side effects of immunosuppressive agents, the original liver disease, and the quality of graft function. The issues are numerous and vary in degree of severity from one recipient to the next. Treatment of these issues requires communication and cooperation between the transplant team and community health care providers. Many community physicians are hesitant to treat complaints in transplant patients because they lack experience with this patient population. The PTCC is instrumental in coordinating this treatment and must possess skill in communicating information on patient issues, treatments, and treatment outcomes to transplant team physicians and community health care providers. Table 68–18 lists common immunosuppression side effects and other long-term posttransplant issues that the PTCC must consider when coordinating treatment of the recipient.[9-15]

It is important for the PTCC to ensure that needed interventions specific to the recipient's pretransplant disease be considered during the course of long-term posttransplant care. Many preoperative disease pathologies can affect the health of the liver graft and therefore require monitoring regimens, preventive interventions, and treatment modalities for management of these conditions. Table 68–19 describes these considerations.

Transplant recipients exhibit higher rates of malignancy than the general public does. The PTCC is a key educator in interventions that the patient must institute to monitor for and reduce the incidence of cancer. Table 68–20 lists patient risk factors for the development of hepatocellular carcinoma (HCC) and the interventions that the PTCC should institute to provide adequate tumor surveillance for patients at high risk. Table 68–21 lists interventions that should be taught to the patient to reduce risk for the development of cancer.

Guiding the patient swiftly back into normal activities of daily living takes on high priority for the PTCC. Simple modifications in the patient's daily behavior can mean the difference between a fulfilling and higher quality of life and a life filled with inconveniences and continued illness. Table 68–22 lists key points that the PTCC must consider when educating patients about issues concerning activities of daily living.[16-18]

Future Trends for the Posttransplant Coordinator

The hepatitis C virus (HCV) epidemic in the United States is a force that will have a great impact on liver transplantation. The PTCC will be required to coordinate current and new antiviral therapies for HCV graft infection. HCV-associated cirrhosis is the principal indication for liver transplantation in the United States and is expected to outpace all other causes for many more years. The use of combination ribavirin and various interferon agents in this growing patient population will present many challenges to the PTCC. Many of the side effects of antiviral agents used to treat HCV infection, such as neutropenia, anemia, and thrombocytopenia, are identical to those caused by immunosuppressive agents.

Table 68–16. FEVER WORKUP

General Fever Workup	Additional Workup Based on Symptoms or History
CBC	Acute phase serum samples for EBV, CMV, HSV, coccidiomycosis, hepatitis
Chest films and KUB (if indicated)	Stool for O&P, enteric pathogens, and *Clostridium difficile*
Sputum for Gram stain and culture	Pelvic examination
Urinalysis and urine culture	Skin tests for TB and coccidioidomycosis
Culture of any existing drains, wounds, or indwelling lines	*Legionella* titers with DNA probe Abdominal ultrasound and/or CT to rule out fluid collections
Liver function studies	Lumbar puncture, including a cryptococcal examination
Blood cultures	Transhepatic cholangiogram or ERCP

CBC, complete blood count; CMV, cytomegalovirus; CT, computed tomography; EBV, Epstein-Barr virus; ERCP, endoscopic retrograde cholangiopancreatography; HSV, herpes simplex virus; KUB, kidney, ureter, bladder; O&P, ova and parasites; TB, tuberculosis.

Table 68-17. PATIENT INSTRUCTIONS FOR USE OF OVER-THE-COUNTER MEDICATIONS

Headache, fever, body aches	Always take your temperature with a thermometer. If your temperature is 100.5° F or higher, contact the transplant center before taking any medicine Take two regular-strength plain Tylenol (acetaminophen) tablets every 6 hours as needed. Allow the Tylenol to wear off and recheck your temperature with a thermometer between doses. Do not take aspirin, Motrin (ibuprofen), Aleve or Naprosyn (naproxen), Orudis (ketoprofen), or any other nonsteroidal anti-inflammatory or aspirin compound
Sneezing, runny nose	Take plain Chlor-Trimeton (chlorpheniramine), plain Dimetapp (brompheniramine), or plain Benadryl (diphenhydramine); the latter medication causes drowsiness
Nasal or sinus congestion	Take 6-hour Afrin nasal spray or 6-hour Neo-Synephrine nasal spray Do not use nasal sprays for longer than 3 days. If your symptoms last longer than 3 days, call the transplant center
Cough	If your chest is congested and you are coughing up phlegm, take a plain cough syrup such as Robitussin. If you have no chest congestion and you have a dry hacking cough without phlegm, take a plain cough syrup with an expectorant such as Robitussin-DM. Do not take cough syrups with other additives such as decongestants or acetaminophen
Sore throat	Take a throat lozenge or spray according to the package directions
Warning	Carefully read the label of all over-the-counter medications. Many medications are combinations of drugs that may harm you. Always try to buy the medication in its plain form. Avoid Contac, Actifed, Tavist, and any other medicines that contain pseudoephedrine or phenylpropanolamine unless told to do so by the transplant center. Avoid medications that contain aspirin or nonsteroidal anti-inflammatory agents; medications containing acetaminophen are safe. Zinc lozenges, vitamin C, Oscillococcinum, echinacea, and goldenseal are safe to use but may not be effective. Not all herbal remedies may be safe for you; if you have a question, call your transplant center. If your symptoms do not improve in a few days or become worse, contact your transplant center
Upset stomach, heartburn, nausea, vomiting	You may try Pepto-Bismol, but you must take it 2 hours before or 2 hours after you take your immunosuppression medications. You may try TUMS for heartburn. Avoid Maalox and Mylanta. You may also try Zantac or Pepcid; avoid Tagamet You must contact your transplant center for nausea or vomiting that has prevented you from taking your medications for longer than 24 hours. Vomiting blood or coffee ground material is an emergency that requires immediate attention. If you vomit within 1 hour after taking your medication, you must repeat the doses and take them again. If you vomit more than 1 hour after taking your medications, you do not need to repeat taking them. If you continue to have heartburn for more than 3 days, you must contact your transplant center
Diarrhea	We must obtain your stool specimen before you may take medicine for diarrhea, especially if you have a fever or are nauseated. Contact the transplant center before taking any medicine for diarrhea Pepto-Bismol, Kaopectate, or Metamucil must be taken 2 hours before or 2 hours after taking your immunosuppression medicines. Imodium A-D should not be used for more than 2 days unless otherwise instructed by your transplant center If your stools appear bloody or black and tarry, you must urgently contact the transplant center. Iron supplements and several other medications will turn your stool black. Small amounts of bright red blood may be caused by hemorrhoids
Constipation	Take Colace once or twice daily. You may also try the following: Peri-Colace, as directed on the label Dulcolax (bisacodyl) suppositories (use for no longer than 7 days) Glycerin suppositories, as directed on the label Fleet enema (use no more than twice in 3 days). You may try Metamucil as directed but must take it 2 hours before or 2 hours after your immune suppression medicine If constipation continues, contact your transplant center. If constipation is accompanied by nausea, severe bloating, or pain, this could indicate a serious problem that must be taken care of immediately
Gas	Take Gas-X (simethicone); avoid Beano, Maalox, and Mylanta

Treatment of antiviral side effects exacerbated by the side effects of immunosuppressive agents requires the use of more time, labor, and financially intensive treatments such as erythropoietin and granulocyte colony-stimulating factor. The development of hepatitis C immune globulin will require the PTCC to become proficient in coordinating the administration of this new treatment, as well as concomitant monitoring of serum antibody levels and serology markers. The development of antiretroviral agents effective against HCV that are similar to those

Table 68–18. KEY POINTS ON SIDE EFFECTS OF IMMUNOSUPPRESSIVE MEDICATIONS AND COMMON OUTPATIENT ISSUES

Central Pontine Myelinolysis

Akinetic mutism, orofacial dyskinesias, and pseudobulbar palsy are the result of a rare cytochrome P450 III-A isoenzyme abnormality in the allograft liver. These symptoms usually resolve after switching the primary immunosuppressant to another agent and allowing for a washout period between medication changes

Chronic Fatigue

Usually associated with poor graft function. Carnitine deficiency may be a contributing factor. Carnitine deficiency is linked to graft dysfunction and renal insufficiency

Chronic Headaches

Deleterious effects on cerebral arterial autoregulation caused by immunosuppressive medications are thought to be the cause. Hypertension and toxic levels of immune suppression should always be ruled out

Chronic Pain

Osteoporosis, arthritis, residual neuralgias, and chronic headache are the most common causes. Patient education should focus on the use of topical analgesics, heat and cold application to peripheral pain sites, massage, physical therapy, and psychological therapy

Chronic Rejection

Risk factors include previous graft loss because of chronic rejection, underlying primary sclerosing cholangitis, primary biliary cirrhosis or autoimmune hepatitis; low-level immunosuppression (common with a history of hepatitis C virus infection or malignancy); late or recurrent episodes of rejection; and cytomegalovirus infections

Constipation

Over-the-counter medications usually correct this complaint. If these fail to work, lactulose can be used safely. Query overuse of narcotics and dehydration

Decreased Gastric Motility

Instruct the patient to eat small, frequent meals. The use of metoclopramide for longer than 8 weeks can produce a cumulative sedating effect

Depression

Highly underdiagnosed in transplant patients. The posttransplant clinical coordinator should know the hallmark symptoms (at least 5 or more of the following symptoms in a 1-week period; 1 of the symptoms must include depressed mood or loss of interest):

Depressed mood

Loss of interest or pleasure in normal activities

Insomnia

Psychomotor agitation or retardation

Fatigue

Feelings of worthlessness or guilt

Poor concentration

Recurrent thoughts of death or suicide

Diarrhea

This complaint is common in the immediate postoperative period. *Clostridium difficile* should always be suspected. Lactase is the last enzyme to be upregulated after a sustained fasting period (such as with orthotopic liver transplantation)

Fluid Retention

Patient teaching should be directed toward compliance with a low-sodium diet. Reinforce the dangers of self-medication with diuretics and the importance of serial blood studies when diuretic dose changes are frequent

Gastroesophageal Reflux Disease

Lifestyle modification should be reinforced. The patient should eat smaller meals and low-fat foods and avoid caffeine, tobacco, chocolate, peppermint, spearmint, and carbonated beverages. Instruct the patient to wear loose-fitting clothing, raise the head of the bed, and not to eat 2 or 3 hours before sleeping

Hemorrhoids

A residual consequence of portal hypertension. Patient instructions should include the use of a high-fiber diet, stool softeners, anal hygiene, and the use of sitz baths and topical ointments

Table 68–18. KEY POINTS ON SIDE EFFECTS OF IMMUNOSUPPRESSIVE MEDICATIONS AND COMMON OUTPATIENT ISSUES—cont'd

Hyperglycemia

Teaching should emphasize the importance of diet, self-testing, and dosing compliance. Maintenance of optimal weight, exercise, and activity is just as important as medications. Annual dilated eye examinations, flu shots, microalbuminuria screens, dental visits, and foot care should also be emphasized

Hyperlipidemia

Lifestyle modification should be emphasized. Patients should increase activity, maintain optimal weight, and comply with a low-fat diet containing no more than 300 mg of cholesterol per day

Hypertension

Always rule out toxic levels of immunosuppressants. Calcium channel blockers will increase drug levels of immunosuppressive medications. Emphasize patient teaching aimed at stress reduction, weight loss, sodium restriction, and exercise

Hyperuricemia

The patient should be instructed to contact the transplant center before instituting any therapy. Many medications used to treat this condition can have dangerous side effects when combined with immunosuppressants. Instruct the patient that nonsteroidal anti-inflammatory medications, including new-generation cyclooxygenase-2 inhibitors and aspirin, must be avoided

Hypomagnesemia

Instruct the patient to report diarrhea. Magnesium is available in different forms, including oxide, maleate, bound to protein, and in a sulfate solution. Absorption and side effects are different for each patient and depend on the form used. Try different forms until the desired result is achieved

Insomnia

Instructions for improvement of sleep hygiene should include the following:

Decrease or eliminate the use of caffeine after noon

Do not use tobacco near bedtime

Avoid vigorous exercise within 3 to 4 hours of bedtime

Establish a regular schedule for going to bed and getting up

Avoid daytime naps

Keep the bedroom at a comfortable temperature and minimize noise and light

Use of over-the-counter drugs is generally safe (Nytol, Sominex, Benadryl, or Unisom)

Use of prescription drugs should be limited to 6 to 8 weeks of therapy

Psychological approaches to treatment have greater safety and better long-term efficacy

Muscle Cramps

Electrolyte imbalances (especially in calcium and magnesium) should be ruled out. Quinine sulfate may be helpful if no metabolic or neurological cause can be identified

Osteoporosis and Osteoarthritis

Long-term steroid use, hyperglycemia, and cholestatic disease are contributing factors. Physical therapy is an important treatment modality that is often overlooked. Instruct the patient to avoid nonsteroidal anti-inflammatory medications, including new-generation cyclooxygenase-2 inhibitors and aspirin

Renal Insufficiency

The posttransplant clinical coordinator should be vigilant in ensuring that serum creatinine values are not increasing without intervention

Tremors

Low-dose β-blockers and oral magnesium supplementation can be helpful. Patients should be instructed to perform stretching exercises daily

---

developed to treat human immunodeficiency virus infection will probably lead to side effects similar to those produced by immunosuppressive agents, such as diabetes, renal insufficiency, hypertension, and hyperlipidemia. Should this scenario became fact, the PTCC will be required to allocate additional effort to coordinate the treatment of these side effects.

With the increase in the incidence of HCV infection in the United States a concomitant increase in the incidence of HCC can be anticipated. Posttransplant treatment of

Table 68-19. KEY POINTS FOR DISEASE-SPECIFIC CONSIDERATIONS

Autoimmune Hepatitis

Concomitant nonhepatic autoimmune disorders are often associated with autoimmune hepatitis. The PTCC should be alert for signs and symptoms of thyroiditis, Raynaud's disease, rheumatoid arthritis, and Sjögren's syndrome

Gilbert's Syndrome

One percent to 2% of all grafts carry a benign genetic metabolic defect that causes Gilbert's syndrome. Elevations in unconjugated bilirubin and jaundice can occur in response to increased life stressors. The PTCC can help facilitate stress reduction education in this patient population

Hemochromatosis

Hemochromatosis can affect other body systems. The PTCC should be aware that this disease can cause hyperglycemia, cardiomyopathy, renal insufficiency, and increased skin pigmentation. Serial testing of iron parameters should continue after transplantation. The PTCC should ensure that the patient and family have undergone genetic testing and counseling

Substance Abuse

A substance abuse personality is not cured by transplantation. The PTCC should facilitate anonymous and sound psychosocial support. Random toxicology screens should continue after transplantation

PTCC, posttransplant clinical coordinator.

recipients who demonstrate HCC on explant pathology includes chemotherapy and surveillance imaging studies with serial serum tumor markers. Adjuvant chemotherapy for HCC causes side effects similar to those caused by immunosuppressive agents, such as renal insufficiency, anemia, and leukopenia.

The increase in the HCV-infected patient population can only portend that the PTCC will need to develop greater expertise and effort in the coordination of treatment of HCV infection, prophylaxis of HCV infection of the graft (when treatment is developed), posttransplant treatment of HCC, and treatment of the side effects caused by these therapies.

Many centers continue to pursue adult living related donor (LRD) programs. Should LRD programs produce time-proven successful recipient and safe donor outcomes, this treatment option will become more common in liver transplant centers. Institution of LRD programs will require the PTCC to coordinate care for the donor. Care of LRDs will consist of routine postoperative follow-up for 6 to 12 weeks after the procedure. Care of the recipient of an LRD organ is identical to that for a recipient of a deceased donor organ. The investigational nature of the LRD liver transplant procedure intimates that the PTCC will also be involved in research to define long-term outcomes for both the recipient and donor.

With institution of the Model for End-stage Liver Disease (MELD) system of liver allocation in the United States in February 2002, "post-MELD" transplant recipients have a higher degree of renal insufficiency than their "pre-MELD" counterparts do and are more likely to have a history of HCC. Pretransplant patients with HCC or renal insufficiency are more apt to receive transplants because of their higher MELD scores. The impact of patients with a history of HCC has already been discussed. The increase in the degree of renal insufficiency in the recipient population will translate into an increase in the number of recipients with combined liver and kidney transplants. The PTCC will require expertise in coordinating care for this dual-organ transplant patient subgroup.

As small bowel transplant outcome and patient survival improve, the number of combined liver and small bowel transplant patients can be expected to increase. Liver and small bowel transplant patients differ from liver transplant patients in areas of patient follow-up, infection prophylaxis, treatment of rejection, rejection

Table 68-20. RISK FACTORS FOR THE DEVELOPMENT OF HCC AND ROUTINE HCC SURVEILLANCE

Risk Factors for the Development of HCC	Tumor Surveillance in Patients with a History of Primary Liver Malignancies
Liver cirrhosis	Surveillance CT scans of the chest, abdomen, and pelvis, with and without contrast, at months 3, 6, and 12 after transplantation, then annually. Serum AFP and/or CA19-9 studies every 3 months
Chronic active hepatitis C	
Chronic active hepatitis B	
Alcohol abuse	
Hemochromatosis	
α_1-Antitrypsin deficiency	
HCC on explant pathology	

AFP, alpha-fetoprotein; CT, computed tomography; HCC, hepatocellular carcinoma.

Table 68-21. PATIENT EDUCATION FOR CANCER PREVENTION

Undergo melanoma screening annually

Apply sunscreen with an SPF of 15 or greater before sun exposure

Decrease direct sun exposure as much as possible through the use of protective clothing and shelter

Annual breast examinations, mammograms, and Pap smears are recommended for women

Annual testicular examinations, digital rectal examinations, prostate examinations, and serum PSA are recommended for men

Obtain an annual fecal occult blood test

Undergo colonoscopy annually if you have a history of PSC and/or ulcerative colitis; request a serum CEA determination every 3 months

Request a serum CA19-9 test every 3 months if you have a history of PBC

Do not smoke tobacco and avoid second-hand smoke exposure

Increase your dietary intake of fruits and vegetables

CEA, carcinoembryonic antigen; PBC, primary biliary cirrhosis; PSA, prostate-specific antigen; PSC, primary sclerosing cholangitis; SPF, sun protective factor.

prophylaxis, and nutritional support.[19] The differences in treatment will require additional skills and knowledge on the part of the PTCC.

The impact of the hepatitis C epidemic, adult LRD programs, and the MELD system of liver allocation will produce additional stressors that will shape the future of the PTCC's role within the liver transplant team. The increase in the complexity of patient care in conjunction with decreasing budget and support resources will challenge the PTCC's ability to deliver the exemplary patient care needed for successful patient outcomes. To meet these challenges, the PTCC will need to develop a greater knowledge base and a broader skill mix and will be required to institute strategies that counteract the stressors affecting their role within the transplant team.

Table 68-22. KEY POINTS IN PATIENT EDUCATION REGARDING ACTIVITIES OF DAILY LIVING

Acne

Patient education should include washing oily areas of skin several times a day. Avoid scrubbing. Use a soap that removes oil but does not dry out the skin. Avoid moisturizing soaps and antibacterial soaps. Do not squeeze or pick pimples. Use acne preparations containing benzoyl peroxide. Topical antibiotics, Retin-A (tretinoin), Accutane (isotretinoin), or Azelex (azelaic acid) can be used under dermatological supervision

Alopecia and Hirsutism

The PTCC should instruct patients with alopecia to avoid chlorine, sun exposure, and perming, dyeing, tinting, or bleaching of the hair; patients should be encouraged to use a conditioner after shampooing. Patients with hirsutism may bleach facial hair or remove unwanted hair by waxing, trimming, or shaving. Hair removal by laser is a safe alternative

Disability and Returning to Work

Patients with normal graft function should be encouraged to return to work. The PTCC should instruct the patient to avoid jobs that require heavy lifting or exposure to known hepatotoxic agents and infectious organisms. The PTCC should be cognizant of several issues related to disability and returning to work:

Hiring discrimination against the transplant recipient and the legal protection available to the patient

The patient's self-imposed barriers to re-employment and the interventions needed to address these barriers

The economic consequences of not returning to work, loss of insurance or disability coverage, and the strategies needed to prevent these consequences

Exercise and Activity

The PTCC should emphasize that brisk walking is the preferred method of aerobic exercise. Only low-level aerobic exercise should be performed during high-dose steroid use. Driving should not be resumed until after the fourth postoperative week. Upper body weight training should be done while sitting on a bench or chair to relieve abdominal strain. Abdominal exercises should be avoided during the first 6 months after transplantation. Stretching and conditioning should be a part of the exercise regimen

Continued

Table 68-22. KEY POINTS IN PATIENT EDUCATION REGARDING ACTIVITIES OF DAILY LIVING—cont'd

Gingival Hyperplasia

Patient instructions should include brushing and flossing twice daily. A soft nylon toothbrush should be used. Peroxide-based mouthwashes are helpful when gums bleed. Dental visits should be at a minimum of twice a year. Gum massage with water picks or electric toothbrushes reduce and strengthen gum tissue. Mouth breathing should be avoided. Excessive gum tissue may be removed surgically. Laser removal of excess tissue is an alternative treatment option

Noncompliance

Specific constructive interventions that the PTCC may institute for noncompliance are as follows:

Try to understand the patient's perspective

Identify the patient's goal of treatment

Share control and responsibility for treatment with the patient

Educate the patient so that informed decisions can be made

Involve patients in their treatment as much as possible

Negotiate a behavioral contract with the patient

Consult a psychiatrist or psychologist for assistance in patient management or determination of decision-making capacity

Be patient but persistent

Do not tolerate verbal abuse

Contact law enforcement if physical abuse is threatened or occurs

Consider transfer of care to another facility

Nutrition

A low-sodium diet should be explained to the patient. Raw or undercooked meat, fish, poultry, and eggs should be avoided. Water should be consumed only from a chlorinated system or from a system using bacterial filters. Grapefruit should not be consumed. Interventions for maintaining optimal weight should be discussed. Patients should avoid foods containing fat substitutes. Vitamins should not contain more than 5000 IU of vitamin A, 400 IU of vitamin E, or 800 IU of vitamin D. Patients with hemochromatosis should not take iron supplements. Patients taking warfarin should avoid foods high in vitamin K. Herbs and other homeopathic remedies should generally be avoided because they may interact with the patient's medications

Pregnancy, Sex, and Contraception

Pregnancy is possible and successful but should be avoided in the first 12 months after transplantation. A high-risk obstetrician must monitor patients who become pregnant. Sex should not resume until after the fourth postoperative week. The PTCC should educate the patient and significant other regarding safe sex practices if indicated. The PTCC should ensure that the patient understands the dangers of oral contraception and intrauterine devices. Barrier contraceptives are safe alternatives

Smoking

The PTCC should discourage smoking of tobacco because of its inherent health risks. Marijuana leaves may harbor live fungus such as *Aspergillus*

References

1. Pakrasi A: Life after Transplantation—Taking Care of Your New Liver, ed 1. Los Angeles, Dumont-UCLA Transplant Center, 1997, pp 4-8.
2. Kunder GD: The Role of the Transplant Center: Primary Care Physician Management of the Adult Liver Transplant Recipient, ed 1. Los Angeles, Dumont-UCLA Transplant Center, 2000, pp 15-17.
3. Savitsky EA, Uner AB, Votey SR: Evaluation of orthotopic liver transplant recipients presenting to the emergency department. Ann Emerg Med 31:507-515, 1998.
4. Blackbourne LH, Minasi J, Newburg D, et al: Wounds, Drains and Tubes: Surgical Recall, ed 1. Baltimore, Williams & Wilkins, 1994, pp 23-24.
5. Gomes AS: Diagnosis and radiologic treatment of biliary complications of liver transplantation. Semin Interv Radiol 9:283-289, 1992.
6. Winston DJ, Emmanouilides C, Busuttil RW: Infections in liver transplant recipients. Clin Infect Dis 21:1077-1091, 1995.
7. Randolph S, Scholz K: Self-care guidelines: Finding a common ground. J Transpl Coord 9:156-160, 1999.
8. Ellingson T, Wipke-Tevis D, Messina C, et al: The use of over-the-counter medications by transplant recipients: A guideline. J Transpl Coord 9:17-24, 1999.
9. Edwards SS: The "noncompliant" transplant patient: A persistent ethical dilemma. J Transpl Coord 9:202-208, 1999.
10. Simon JM: Chronic pain syndrome: Nursing assessment and intervention. Rehabil Nurs 21:10-13, 1996.
11. Pittman JR, Bross MH: Diagnosis and management of gout. Am Fam Physician 59:1799-1806, 1999.
12. Castell DO, Brunton SA, Earnest DL: GERD: Management algorithms for the primary care physician and the specialist. Pract Gastroenterol 22:18-44, 1998.
13. Eddy M, Walbroehl GS: Insomnia. Am Fam Physician 59:1911-1916, 1999.

14. Brickman AL, Yount SE: Noncompliance in end-stage renal disease: A threat to quality of care and cost containment. J Clin Psychol Med Settings 3:399-410, 1996.

15. Wells KB, Stewart A, Hays RD, et al: The functioning and well-being of depressed patients: Results from the Medical Outcome Study. JAMA 262:914-919, 1989.

16. Thomas DJ: Returning to work after liver transplant: Experiencing the roadblocks. J Transpl Coord 6:134-138, 1996.

17. Grassinger M, Schonder K: Managing side effects of immuno-suppressant medications. Lifetimes 4:13-20, 1999.

18. Seraj A: Nutrition and Liver Transplant Disease, ed 1. Los Angeles, Dumont-UCLA Transplant Center 1998, pp 1-8.

19. Kunder GD: Combined Liver Small Bowel Transplant: Outpatient Case Manager Guidelines for the Care of the Adult Liver Transplant Recipient, ed 2. Los Angeles, Dumont-UCLA Transplant Center, 2001, pp 38-44.

Liver Transplant Pathology

IX

Histological Patterns of Rejection and Other Causes of Liver Dysfunction

A. J. DEMETRIS
MIKE NALESNIK
PARMJEET RANDHAWA
TONG WU
MARIDA MINERVINI
CHI LAI
ZHENGBIN LU

Historical perspective   1058

Background experience and information helpful in specimen evaluation   1058

Special considerations for specific specimens   1059
Pretransplant biopsies   1059
Native hepatectomy specimens   1059
Failed allografts   1060
Posttransplant allograft needle biopsies   1060

Evaluation of the donor liver   1060
Frozen sections of deceased donor livers   1060
"Back-table biopsies" of deceased donor livers   1065
Biopsy evaluation of living donor livers   1065

General immunological concepts that affect biopsy pathology   1065
Phases of the immunological response   1065
Antigenic and tissue targets of rejection   1068
Role of direct and indirect antigen presentation   1069

Determination of causes of graft dysfunction after transplantation   1071

"Preservation" or ischemic injury and primary dysfunction   1071
Vascular complications   1073
Bile duct complications   1076
Rejection   1077
Graft-versus-host disease   1089
Bacterial and fungal infections   1089
Viral infections   1090

Recurrent diseases and diseases induced by transplantation   1100
Postinfantile giant cell hepatitis   1105
Primary biliary cirrhosis   1105
Recurrent and new-onset "autoimmune" hepatitis   1107
Recurrent primary sclerosing cholangitis   1109
Toxic and metabolic diseases   1110

Long-term changes not readily explained by recurrent disease   1111

Liver allograft pathology associated with systemic diseases   1111
Septicemia   1111
Adverse drug reactions and toxic injury   1112

Historical Perspective

Many of the unique aspects of hepatic transplant histopathology were first described in experimental animals by Brock[1] and Dammin[2] and their colleagues, who worked with the pioneering surgeons in this field. Dr. Thomas Starzl and coauthors reported the first human liver transplant operation in 1963,[3] but nearly 2 decades elapsed before the development of cyclosporine made routine long-term survival achievable.[4] Readers interested in a more detailed history of the development of liver transplantation are referred elsewhere.[5]

Pathologists describing much of the original work in liver transplant pathology were those supporting the major programs. These investigators included Hank Fennell based in Denver[6,7] and Kendrick Porter at St. Mary's Hospital in London,[8,9] both of whom supported Starzl's program in Denver. Porter also played a significant role in pioneering kidney transplant pathology, which preceded the development of liver transplantation. Bernard Portmann and associates[10,11] and Derek Wight[12,13] provided pathology support for the Cambridge–King's College program initiated by Sir Roy Calne.[14] More recent contributors to the field have become too numerous to mention by name.

The format for this chapter includes a description of the various causes of allograft dysfunction that have histopathological manifestations. Included in each description are a brief introduction and overview of pathophysiological concepts, followed by clinical features and correlations, histopathological findings, and a histopathological differential diagnosis. This approach reflects the reliance of transplant pathology on pathophysiological concepts and clinicopathological correlations. Reliance strictly on morphological findings is discouraged because new variables, such as new immunosuppressive drugs and regimens, are frequently introduced into patient management and these changes can influence the histopathological findings. Portions of this chapter were recently included in a surgical pathology textbook on gastrointestinal and liver pathology[15] and updated for the current text.

Background Experience and Information Helpful in Specimen Evaluation

Proficiency in the clinical aspects of liver allograft pathology requires (1) a sound working knowledge of hepatic pathology and pathophysiology (probably the most important); (2) an understanding of transplantation immunology and familiarity with interpretation of immunological tests and immunofluorescence or immunoperoxidase staining for antibody-mediated rejection; (3) familiarity with the terminology, surgical approaches, and clinical management problems; (4) and an ability to recognize a wide variety of opportunistic infections and immunosuppression-related malignancies.

Interpretation of pathology specimens obtained after transplantation requires knowledge of the original disease, time after transplantation, operative approach, recipient immunological profile (e.g., cross-match results), and the presence of known technical complications such as anastomotic strictures or long cold ischemic times. The donor and recipient are matched for size and ABO blood groups. Cross-match tests are commonly performed, but uncommonly taken into account when triaging organs, except for living donors.[16] These variables greatly influence the susceptibility to certain complications and consequently affect the histopathological differential diagnosis.

Most necroinflammatory diseases and leading indications for liver replacement recur in the allograft after transplantation (see Table 69–1 and "Recurrent Diseases and Diseases Induced by Transplantation"). Technically demanding operative approaches and those that deviate from reconstruction of normal anatomy increase the risk for complications. Orthotopic liver transplantation from a deceased donor after donor cholecystectomy via end-to-end anastomoses of the portal vein, hepatic artery, bile duct, and vena cava between the donor and recipient structures is the "standard" operation.[5] There are numerous surgical variations, which are explained best in surgical texts,[17] and some of these variations predispose to complications. For example, hepatic vein outflow obstruction is increased with the use of a nonstandard hepatic vein–vena cava anastomosis, such as in the "piggyback" approach.[5] The risk for hepatic artery thrombosis is increased in small-caliber vessels from pediatric donors and recipients and when vascular interposition arterial grafts are used. Operative manipulation of the donor liver before transplantation, such as "split" livers or reduced-size livers, and the use of living donors generally increase the risk for vascular and biliary tract complications and cause compensatory hyperplasia after transplantation. Consequently, these grafts frequently show baseline changes, including ductular reaction and nodular regenerative hyperplasia, that in part represent adaptive responses to the operation and physiological demands of the recipient.

Clinicians are encouraged to submit directed clinical questions on the surgical pathology requisition along with the tissue specimens, but compliance with the request is usually a problem. Therefore, we rely primarily on electronic medical records and our in-house information portal software (EDIT[18]) for pertinent clinical and laboratory information while signing out cases and on weekly clinicopathological conferences for quality assurance purposes. Any relevant previous biopsy specimens

Table 69-1. INDICATIONS FOR LIVER TRANSPLANTATION, INCLUDING DECEASED (N = 5350) AND LIVING (N = 321) DONORS IN THE UNITED STATES DURING 2003

	N	%
Acute hepatic necrosis	397	7
Alcoholic cirrhosis	833	15
Metabolic diseases	192	3
Primary liver malignancy	445	8
Primary biliary cirrhosis	209	4
Primary sclerosing cholangitis	305	5
Biliary/cholestatic, other	343	6
Cirrhosis: viral, autoimmune, drug, cryptogenic	2379	42
Other	568	10
Total	5671	100

Data obtained from the United Network for Organ Sharing website http://www.OPTN.org.

should be reviewed with the current one. This practice not only establishes a "baseline" for each allograft but also greatly assists in interpretation of the effect of therapy or disease progression, or both. Conducting the initial histological review without clinical information minimizes bias, but the final interpretation *must be* based on complete clinicopathological correlation.

Special Consideration for Specific Specimens

Pretransplant Biopsies

Familiarity with liver disorders that commonly recur after transplantation (see "Recurrent Diseases and Diseases Induced by Transplantation") and those that significantly increase the risk for hepatocellular carcinoma assists in recipient selection and determination of the need for adjuvant therapy before or after transplantation. Patients with fulminant hepatic failure may be referred for transplantation without a firm diagnosis or thorough workup. In such cases, pathologists may be requested to evaluate frozen sections or "rapidly processed" slides (or both) of the native liver obtained via transjugular biopsy.[19-21] The etiological and prognostic significance of microscopic findings may be used to assess the potential for specific treatment and the reversibility and stage of the process. All these factors influence the need for transplantation.

Biopsy findings are particularly helpful when a specific and potentially treatable or reversible acute insult is identified. Removal or control of such insults in some cases can lead to regeneration of the native liver and avoidance of transplantation. Examples include

herpes simplex hepatitis,[22] ischemic injury, and acetaminophen toxicity. Reference to a standard liver pathology text for further specific information is suggested.[23] It must be emphasized, however, that histopathological findings are only one laboratory result and should be combined with other clinical and laboratory data. The recipient surgeon is ultimately responsible for the final and very difficult decision to proceed with or delay transplantation. The decision is usually made after collating all the relevant clinical and laboratory information and advice or opinions of various specialists.

Native Hepatectomy Specimens

Accurate diagnosis of the original disease is dependent on a thorough pretransplant workup accomplished by careful correlation between the clinical history, laboratory results, and histopathological findings. Accurate diagnosis of the original disease forms one of the cornerstones of an academic database in liver transplantation pathology.[18] Because disease recurrence is a major problem in long-term survivors, it is not uncommon to revisit slides from native hepatectomy specimens to determine whether unexplained findings in allograft biopsy specimens resemble those of the original disease.

Native livers removed at the time of transplantation often become available for pathological examination outside normal working hours (between 2 and 5 AM). Immediate tissue processing may be required for proper preservation of the tissue for cell culture or for RNA or protein isolation. This requires special arrangements for an "on-call" tissue triage team that includes at least one member trained in gross liver pathology. If the tissue or any derivatives are to be used for research, previous informed consent of the patient may be required at most centers in the United States.

Gross examination of native hepatectomy specimens should be performed according to a predefined protocol.[24] First, the liver is weighed and its external surface examined. The gallbladder, if present, is opened longitudinally starting at the fundus. The incision is extended up through the common bile duct and the right and left hepatic ducts into the hepatic parenchyma. The hepatic artery and portal vein are then identified in the hilum and opened longitudinally, starting at the resection line and extending up into the parenchyma. Any thrombi, vegetations, calculi, strictures, fibrosis, or tumors are noted. Next, the hepatic vein or veins or the vena cava, if present, is identified and dissected back into the hepatic parenchyma.

The liver is then serially sectioned in a horizontal plane at 1.0-cm intervals to yield slices similar to those observed on a computed axial tomography scan. In our experience, small, clinically undetected hepatocellular carcinoma is the most common unexpected gross finding.

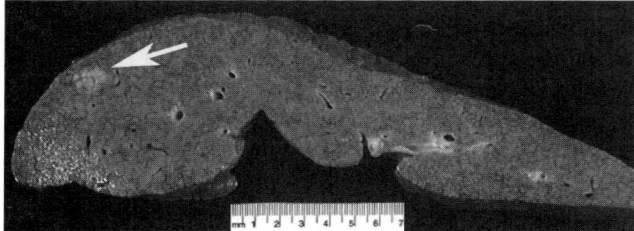

FIGURE 69–1

Slice of a native hepatectomy specimen from a patient with hepatitis C virus–induced cirrhosis. Note the 2.0-cm nodule that is more pale than the surrounding cirrhotic liver. This nodule was sampled for microscopic examination, and the sections showed moderately well differentiated hepatocellular carcinoma.

Therefore, it is *extremely important* to slice the entire liver thinly (1 cm more or less). Any nodule that distinguishes itself from the surrounding cirrhotic parenchyma by virtue of size or color should be sampled (Fig. 69–1). The location of any other intrahepatic defects is recorded and the lesions sampled. Microscopic sections other than those from suspicious nodules or obvious anatomical defects are taken according to a protocol. Routine sections should include the right and left hepatic lobes, resection margins of the hepatic artery, the portal and hepatic veins and bile duct, and a deep hilar section. Bulk frozen, optimum cold temperature compound–embedded and bulk formalin-fixed tissue is saved from each case in an "in-house" tissue bank. We routinely store digital photographs of most native hepatectomy specimens.

Failed Allografts

Causes of liver allograft failure depend on the time after transplantation. Most failures within the first several weeks after transplantation are usually related to "preservation" injury or primary nonfunction, vascular thrombosis, and patient death.[25-30] Acute cellular rejection is relatively uncommon as a cause of early graft failure unless immunosuppressive therapy was deliberately withdrawn; antibody-mediated rejection is also an uncommon cause of early graft failure, except in ABO-incompatible organs.[28,29,31,32] Late graft failures (> 1 year) are usually attributable to delayed manifestations of technical complications such as vascular thrombosis or to biliary sludge syndrome, recurrent disease, and patient death, often as a result of complications from immunosuppression.[28,29,32,33] Chronic rejection is relatively uncommon as a cause of late graft failure; the incidence of chronic rejection is decreasing and most cases generally occur within the first year after transplantation.[28,29,32,34,35]

The primary goal of gross and microscopic examination of failed allograft hepatectomy specimens is precise identification of the cause of the graft failure. This requires review of previous biopsy specimens and correlation with the clinical course. The gross examination of the failed allograft is the same as that used for native hepatectomy specimens.[24] However, special attention is paid to the inspection and dissection of hilar structures, including the anastomoses, which may require the assistance of the operative surgeon. The location of any thrombi and the relationship to any suture lines, vascular injuries, or other obvious defects such as intramural dissections, intraluminal mural flaps, or aneurysms should be noted. Necrosis of hilar structures, especially the bile duct wall with leakage of bile into the hilar connective tissue and superimposed bacterial and fungal infection, is quite common in allografts with arterial thrombosis.[24,26,36-38] Microscopic sections are taken by the same protocol used in native livers.

Posttransplant Allograft Needle Biopsies

Posttransplant allograft needle biopsy samples are obtained to determine the cause of graft dysfunction or to examine the immunological or architectural status of the allograft (or both). Proper triage of the tissue specimen depends on the clinical differential diagnosis, which in turn depends on the time after transplantation. Most diagnostically important histopathological studies can be completed on routinely processed, formalin-fixed, paraffin-embedded sections. Immunofluorescence staining to exclude antibody-mediated rejection requires fresh-frozen tissue. We routinely prepare only two hematoxylin and eosin (H&E)-stained slides from each biopsy specimen, each of which contains a ribbon of sections. Trichrome, iron, periodic acid–Schiff/D, and any other special histochemical or immunohistochemical stains are ordered on indication only after reviewing the H&E findings. Our sign-out station is equipped with a multiheaded microscope and a computer for access to the electronic medical records and laboratory results. We routinely complete a histological examination protocol for all liver allograft biopsy specimens and code the histopathological diagnosis. Following this algorithm prospectively populates a robust database that can be used for research purposes.[18]

Evaluation of the Donor Liver

Frozen Sections of Deceased Donor Livers

Uncertainty about the quality of the donor organ frequently prompts requests for frozen section evaluation of donor livers.[21,39-48] The uncertainty can be triggered by the macroscopic appearance, preexisting donor disease,

Table 69-2. PITFALLS TO AVOID IN PREPARATION AND INTERPRETATION OF FROZEN SECTIONS OF DECEASED DONOR LIVERS

Pitfall	Artifact/Consequence	Safeguards to Avoid Pitfall
Mishandling of donor liver with steatosis: prolonged storage in preservative solution or placement on dry paper towel	Fat leaches out of tissue, and severity of steatosis can be underestimated, thereby resulting in inappropriate use of donor organ	Grossly inspect donor liver, obtain fresh biopsy, and immediately freeze; avoid immersion in preservation solution altogether. Transport tissue to frozen section room on *paper towel moistened with preservation solution* and cut deep into block before selecting a section for staining
Storage of biopsy in "physiological" saline	Hepatocytes often appear crenated/necrotic, thereby leading to overestimation of hepatocyte injury	See above; preferred method is to avoid immersion of biopsy in preservation solution altogether
Difficulty cutting frozen section	Suspect fatty or necrotic liver; misinterpretation of findings and inappropriate use or disqualification of donor organ	Follow above procedure and ask for another biopsy. Perform needle biopsies at 45-degree angle with cryostat blade
Difficulty estimating early subtle ischemic hepatocyte injury because of tissue storage (see above), preparation, or staining	Ischemic injury may be overestimated or missed altogether; misinterpretation of findings and inappropriate use or disqualification of donor organ	Cut 6–8 serial sections and stain each for increasing length of time in eosin. In one or two sections staining will be optimal to distinguish between ischemically damaged and healthy hepatocytes. Correlate findings with serial liver injury tests in donor before harvesting

Adapted from Demetris A, Crawford J, Nalesnik M, et al: Transplantation pathology of the liver. In Odze R, Goldblum J, Crawford JM (eds): Surgical Pathology of the GI Tract, Liver, Biliary Tract, and Pancreas. Philadelphia, WB Saunders, 2004, pp 909-966.

the clinical history, or circumstances surrounding donor death or the harvesting procedure. The following guidelines were developed over the last 2 decades at the University of Pittsburgh Medical Center (UPMC); using this approach avoids a number of pitfalls (Table 69–2).

The biopsy should be freshly obtained, preferably in the presence of the pathologist. The pathologist should grossly inspect the donor liver and assist in choosing the biopsy site. We routinely obtain a 1.0-cm² wedge from the right lobe and a 2.0-cm needle core from the anterior inferior edge of both lobes. Subcapsular wedge biopsies frequently overestimate the severity of fibrosis of a donor liver with preexisting chronic hepatitis. If there is any question about the heterogeneity of a particular gross finding, several biopsy specimens are obtained from different areas of the liver. Direct biopsy sampling of localized defects is intuitive.

The liver tissue should be transported to the frozen section area on a nonabsorptive surface or a paper towel moistened with preservation fluid such as the University of Wisconsin solution. Immersion in saline or preservation fluid for more than a few minutes should be avoided. Instead, the sample should be immediately frozen and examined. The histopathological findings should then be correlated with the complete donor history and laboratory values before a diagnosis or opinion is given.

Clinical history and biopsy findings that *absolutely disqualify* donor organs for transplantation include a number of serologically diagnosed infections (e.g., human immunodeficiency virus); history of a recent extra–central nervous system (CNS) malignancy; sepsis; a manipulated CNS malignancy (e.g., biopsy, operation, shunt); and donor liver biopsy specimens showing widespread necrosis/apoptosis usually involving more than 50% of the parenchyma, a malignant neoplasm in the donor liver, or severe *macro*vesicular steatosis involving 50% or more of the hepatocyte volume.[21,39-50]

Several clinical parameters and histopathological findings are *relative contraindications* and render a donor an "expanded criteria" donor. Such donor organs are generally considered suboptimal, but they are not disqualified because many show excellent postoperative function. Unfortunately, the ability to predict postoperative function in an individual donor organ with expanded criteria for transplantation is sorely in need of improvement. Factors that place donors in the expanded criteria category include older age (> 60 years); long cold ischemic time (> 13 to 15 hours); donor hemodynamic instability or cardiac arrest before harvesting; use of vasopressors; hypernatremia; obesity; hepatitis B virus (HBV) or hepatitis C virus (HCV) infection or antibody to hepatitis B core antigen (anti-HBc) positivity; a grossly fatty liver; or the presence of a liver mass, fibrosis, or other focal lesion (Table 69–3).[50-61]

In general, the greater the number of factors that place a donor in the expanded criteria category, the more likely that graft dysfunction or failure will occur

Table 69-3. CLINICOPATHOLOGIC ANALYSIS OF EXPANDED CRITERIA DECEASED DONORS (SEE TEXT)

Clinical History/Circumstances	Histopathological Findings	Comments
Biopsy Findings May Not Be Helpful		
Older donor age (> 60 yr)	Centrilobular lipofuscin, centrilobular sinusoidal widening/hepatocyte atrophy, and hepatocyte anisonucleosis	Older donor livers do not generally function as well as those from younger donors and require longer recovery time. However, individual cases vary, and dysfunction/recovery potential cannot be predicted from biopsy findings
Non–heart-beating donor	Harvesting should occur shortly after cessation of the heartbeat, and often there are no histopathological changes. However, changes vary according to the relationship of the ischemic period to harvesting. Findings very widely from nonspecific to widespread coagulative necrosis (the organ should be discarded).	Depending on the circumstances of ischemia and harvesting, pathology may or may not be helpful (see text). Non–heart-beating donor livers generally have a higher rate of complications and failure than traditional donor livers do.
Prolonged donor intensive care unit stay (> 3-4 days)	Reactive hepatitis with mononuclear portal inflammation and mild ductular reaction simulating chronic hepatitis	Biopsy findings cannot predict dysfunction
History of extra-CNS malignancy	Not applicable unless a liver mass is detected; donor liver biopsy should not be used as a screening tool	Generally disqualifies an organ donor depending on circumstances and histological type of tumor
CNS malignancy	Not applicable unless a liver mass is detected; donor liver biopsy should not be used as a screening tool	Donor not disqualified unless the CNS lesion was manipulated (biopsy, operation) and the blood-brain barrier was breached
Donor hypernatremia	No consistent histopathological findings	Biopsy findings generally not helpful
Biopsy Findings Usually Helpful		
Donor obesity or grossly fatty donor liver	> 50% macrovesicular steatosis usually disqualifies an organ; 10%-50% macrovesicular steatosis usually associated with suboptimal posttransplant function; microvesicular steatosis often associated with a period of warm ischemia, but does not reliably predict posttransplant function	Biopsy specimen should be freshly obtained and immediately frozen to prevent artifacts that can underestimate the severity of the steatosis (see text and Table 69-2)

Masses and other focal lesions	Benign and malignant tumors, granulomas, and areas of fibrosis	Malignant tumors and hepatic adenomas disqualify the donor. Focal nodular hyperplasia and bile duct adenomas can be resected and the livers used; a liver with old infectious granulomas can generally be used, but an infection workup and treatment may be needed after transplant (see text)
Chronic viral hepatitis types B or C or anti-HBc–positive donors	Low-grade chronic hepatitis (mHAI ≤ 4) and low fibrous stage (≤ 2) most common; livers with more severe inflammation and fibrosis generally eliminated on gross examination. Anti-HBc–positive donors may not show any significant pathology (see text). Subcapsular biopsy can overestimate the severity of fibrosis	HBV- or HCV-positive donors with low-grade chronic hepatitis, but negative for bridging fibrosis, are triaged to HBV- and HCV-positive recipients, respectively, after informed consent. Anti-HBc–positive donors can transmit HBV infection to naïve recipients (see text)
Donor hemodynamic instability, hypotensive episodes, use of vasopressors	Varying degrees of ischemic hepatocellular injury, including cytoaggregation, microvesicular steatosis, apoptosis, and zonal coagulative necrosis	Changes can be quite subtle (see Table 69-2); correlation with serial liver injury tests in donor before harvesting is helpful
Severe donor atherosclerosis	Variable, but moderate (> 50%) narrowing of intrahepatic branches of hepatic artery by fibrointimal hyperplasia should render liver highly suspect	Significant sampling problem exists; severity of atherosclerosis in donor aorta and other organs useful for comparison in borderline cases

Anti-HBc, antibody to hepatitis B core antigen; CNS, central nervous system; HBV, hepatitis B virus; HCV, hepatitis C virus; mHAI, mean hepatitis activity index.
Adapted from Demetris A, Crawford J, Nalesnik M, et al: Transplantation pathology of the liver. In Odze R, Goldblum J, Crawford JM (eds): Surgical Pathology of the GI Tract, Liver, Biliary Tract, and Pancreas. Philadelphia, WB Saunders, 2004, pp 909-966.

after transplantation.[50-62] For example, the combination of a 68-year-old donor liver, a long cold ischemic time (>15 hours), hepatic artery atherosclerosis, and 30% macrovesicular steatosis is very likely to disqualify the donor liver. In the absence of histopathological findings that might have an impact on organ function or recovery, the pathologist is unable to predict the adequacy of organ function after transplantation based on frozen section light microscopic evaluation before the operation.

Histopathological findings may or may not be helpful in the evaluation of an expanded criteria donor (see Table 69–3).[21,39-48] Biopsy findings represent just one laboratory result used by the recipient surgeon, who is ultimately responsible for the decision to use or dispose of the donor organ. The pathologist can offer an opinion about the suitability of the organ but should not be placed in the position of being the final arbiter.

Donor macrovesicular steatosis is one of the most common reasons for obtaining a frozen section. This is not surprising given the prevalence of obesity in the United States. At UPMC, the severity of steatosis is *roughly estimated* on H&E-stained slides alone; in our experience, fat stains are not necessary. Our cutoff for donor disqualification is *macrovesicular* steatosis involving roughly 50% or more of the hepatocyte volume based on low-power microscopic examination (Fig. 69–2A). More precise measurement of steatosis is not generally required. Posttransplant dysfunction associated with donor macrovesicular steatosis is proportional to its severity. Even livers with less than 50% macrovesicular steatosis are at increased risk for dysfunction early after transplantation, but graft failure is not common.[21,39-50] *Microvesicular* steatosis, in contrast, is often found after a short period of warm ischemia and other insults. In our experience, microvesicular steatosis does not usually adversely affect the clinical course after transplantation.

Because recurrent HCV infection is universal after liver transplantation and, in general, hepatitis C is an indolent disease, many centers use HCV-positive donors. At UPMC, we routinely screen such donors by frozen section histology at the time of harvesting. Only donor livers that show mild or less inflammation and no evidence of bridging fibrosis on needle biopsy samples are used after informed consent by the recipient. Formal evaluation of the policy to use HCV-positive donors shows that the rate of recurrent hepatitis and serious disease after transplantation is not affected by the HCV status of the donor.[63] Thus, minimally diseased HCV-positive donor organs that would otherwise have been discarded can be used to prolong the life of a recipient with end-stage HCV-induced liver failure, with graft and patient survival rates similar to those of HCV-negative donors.[63-65]

Non–heart-beating donors or donors who have experienced complete cardiac arrest or "downtime" are also frequently a source of donor frozen sections. If the

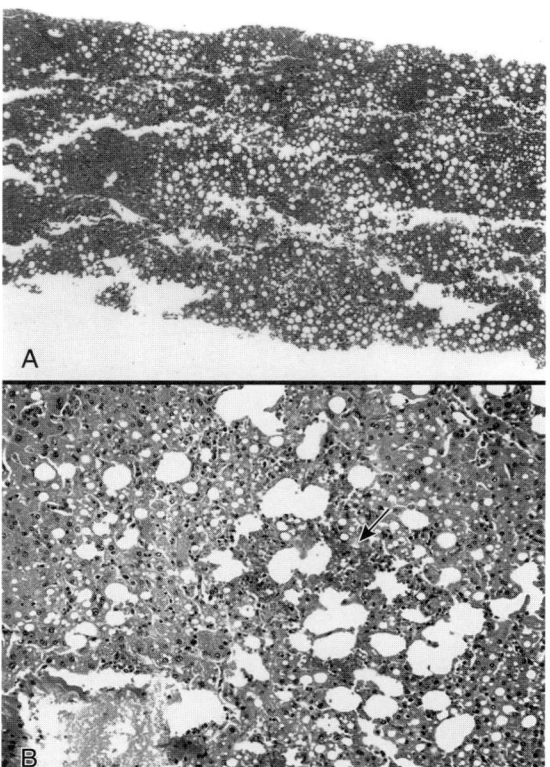

FIGURE 69–2

A, Low-power image of a core needle biopsy specimen from a donor liver with 50% macrovesicular steatosis. The severity of the macrovesicular steatosis is estimated by using H&E-stained slides alone. **B**, Postreperfusion biopsy specimens from livers with greater than 50% macrovesicular steatosis show coalescence of large fat globules, which impairs sinusoidal blood flow and causes local congestion, fibrin deposition, and neutrophilic inflammation (*arrow*). These findings are associated with a clinical syndrome of fibrinolysis, pulmonary edema, and coagulopathy, usually manifested as wound site bleeding. The fat globules will eventually resolve over a period of several weeks if liver function is adequate.

cardiac arrest or "downtime" occurred within 1 hour or less before or during harvesting, the histopathological findings are probably not going to be helpful in assessing the damage. If however, the period of transient ischemia occurred several hours or more before harvesting, biopsy evaluation can frequently be of assistance. In such cases, the biopsy findings should be correlated with serial liver injury test results. If the liver injury tests show a downward trend or have returned to normal or near-normal, regenerative changes are the usual findings. In contrast, if the liver injury test results were significantly elevated and still rising at the time of harvesting, coagulative necrosis of variable severity is the usual finding.

Livers from anti-HBc–positive donors might be considered in the expanded criteria category because they can transmit HBV to recipients, especially those with no previous exposure to HBV.[66-68] However, biopsy evaluation of such livers does not usually provide any useful information because the majority do not show any specific features of HBV-induced liver disease.

"Back-Table Biopsies" of Deceased Donor Livers

In the absence of gross abnormalities, biopsies are usually performed on donor organs on the "back-table" before implantation, and the specimens are routinely processed for viewing the next day.[40] Rarely, unrecognized donor disease may slip past all of the fail-safe points before implantation, only to be detected after the organ has been placed into the recipient. α_1-Antitrypsin deficiency,[24] hemochromatosis,[69,70] and low-grade chronic hepatitis[63-65] have been detected in this manner.

Biopsy Evaluation of Living Donor Livers

Living donors are needed to supplement the significant shortage of deceased donors. A maximum mass of about 70% to 80% of liver volume can be safely removed from healthy living donors, but hyperdynamic portal circulation in the recipient limits the minimal mass of liver that can be safely transplanted to about 1% of body mass or about 30% of the expected liver volume.[71-76] Exceeding either limitation usually leads to an increased rate of complications, the most feared being catastrophic liver failure when the donor liver is "too small for size," discussed in greater detail later.[71-76] Therefore, the left lobe can often be used for adult-to-pediatric transplants, but adult-to-adult living donor transplantation generally requires right lobe donation,[74,77-79] which is a major operation with mortality roughly estimated at about 2 in 700.[80]

A thorough evaluation minimizes the risk of liver donation. Such evaluation includes stepwise medical and surgical screening for any major medical diseases, obesity, previous major abdominal surgery, infectious diseases that could be transmitted to the recipient, psychosocial instability, and any liver abnormality that might put the donor or recipient at risk.[80] Abnormalities detected during the workup can disqualify a potential donor or signal the need for a liver biopsy.

We routinely subject all living donors to biopsy evaluation, although this practice is not mandatory. Ryan and Marcos and their colleagues[81] reported on biopsy findings in 100 consecutive living donors and found that the body mass index was not as accurate as liver biopsy in determining the severity of hepatic steatosis. In addition, three patients were disqualified because of occult liver disease, such as low-grade chronic hepatitis, portal fibrosis, and unclassified vascular abnormalities. Our results have been similar: we have detected unsuspected macrovesicular steatosis and have disqualified

livers with greater than 30% macrovesicular steatosis, as well as one additional patient with occult steatohepatitis and bridging fibrosis.

General Immunological Concepts That Affect Biopsy Pathology

Phases of the Immunological Response

The purpose of this brief transplant immunology overview is to provide a framework for understanding the evolution of the immunological interface between the recipient immune system and the liver allograft. This will help explain why certain histopathological findings are more or less common during certain time periods.

Rejection is the primary immunological concern after transplantation and occurs because of a genetic disparity between the donor and recipient. It is manifested as an immunological reaction elicited by foreign donor cells that behave as antigens in the recipient. Various inductive, effector, and regulatory immunological pathways participate in the reaction, and like other immune responses, the alloresponse demonstrates both specificity and memory. A previous encounter with the same antigen or antigens because of pregnancy, blood transfusion, or organ transplantation can result in a "presensitized" state. Such patients can harbor preformed antidonor antibodies. Reexposure to that same antigen can result in antibody-mediated rejection and provoke a more rapid and vigorous cellular response, much like a vaccination.

Livers are composed of hepatocytes and bile duct, endothelial, smooth muscle, fibroblast, and a variety of hematolymphoid cells. The hematolymphoid cells are derived from bone marrow and intrahepatic stem cell precursors and consist of various types of T and B lymphocytes, Kupffer cells, and various types of dendritic cells, natural killer cells, natural killer T cells, and conventional tissue macrophages. The hematolymphoid cells continuously traffic into and out of the liver via the blood and lymphatics. Completion of the liver allograft vascular anastomoses reestablishes the hematogenous migratory routes, and the donor hematolymphoid populations, or "passenger leukocytes" or donor antigens, migrate throughout the body of the recipient. Most of the donor cells/antigens lodge in the recipient spleen and other central lymphoid tissues, where they precipitate an exuberant immune reaction.[82-84] Revascularization of the donor liver also enables recipient hematolymphoid cells to enter the allograft.[82,83]

Donor dendritic cells are potentially the most immunogenic/antigenic donor passenger leukocytes.[85-87] However, they represent only a small fraction of the total passenger leukocyte pool.[84] Most liver-based dendritic cells exist in a relatively immature or nonantigenic state[87] until cytokines induced by local injury (e.g., preservation injury, necrosis) stimulate differentiation or maturation.[87] Dendritic cell maturation greatly increases antigenicity. Numerous donor B cells and fragments of donor cells migrate to the recipient B-cell follicles in the spleen and lymph nodes within hours after liver transplantation.[84] Donor T cells and a small population of dendritic cells migrate to T-cell–dependent areas in the recipient hematolymphoid tissue.[84]

Mixing of donor and recipient cells within the recipient lymphoid tissue stimulates a bidirectional immune response. *Direct stimulation* refers to the ability of viable mature donor dendritic cells to directly stimulate recipient lymphocytes, and vice versa (Fig. 69–3). In addition, donor and recipient antigens from nonviable donor and recipient cells can be engulfed by allogeneic antigen-presenting cells (APCs) and *indirectly* presented to syngeneic lymphocytes. This bidirectional immune response results in donor and recipient lymphocyte blastogenesis, cytokine and chemokine secretion, and proliferation.[82,83] The reaction occurring in the recipient lymphoid tissues is known as "*central*" sensitization.

Sensitized lymphocytes begin to accumulate in the allograft usually after 3 to 4 days, where they undergo further activation and proliferation, and effector

pathways develop. The immune reaction in the allograft is known as "*peripheral*" sensitization, and pathologists recognize this reaction as acute rejection.[82,83] Recent studies suggest that central sensitization is more important than peripheral sensitization because absence of the former greatly reduces the severity of acute rejection.[88] Regardless, both central and peripheral sensitization reactions are strongest early after transplantation because of the one-time large wave of donor cells (antigen) migrating into the recipient lymphoid tissue. Therefore, the need for immunosuppression is greatest during the first several months after transplantation. Thereafter, donor hematolymphoid cells in the allograft are largely replenished by recipient cells from the bone marrow, thus making the allograft less immunogenic. Consequently, the immunosuppression can be lowered and, in some patients, discontinued altogether.

The two preceding paragraphs outline the most important immunological events for the pathologist to remember and explain the characteristic timing of causes of allograft dysfunction after transplantation (Table 69–4). Acute rejection is most common and severe during the first several months after transplantation and coincides with the central immune reaction precipitated by the massive migration of donor leukocytes into recipient lymphoid tissues. Consequently, high doses and blood levels of immunosuppression are generally required to

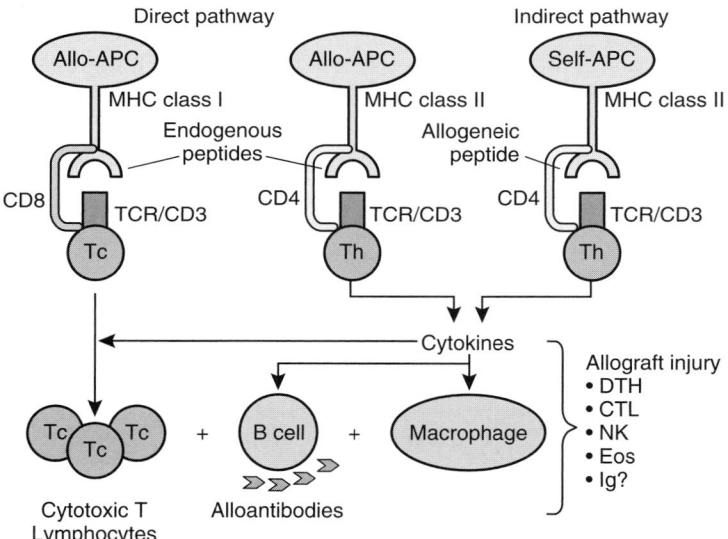

FIGURE 69–3

Diagram illustrating the two pathways of recipient immune system stimulation by donor tissues. In the direct pathway, illustrated on the left side of the diagram, intact viable donor allogeneic antigen-presenting cells (APCs) *directly* interact with and stimulate recipient T lymphocytes. In the *indirect* pathway illustrated on the right side of the diagram, antigens (peptides) from disrupted donor cells are engulfed by recipient antigen-presenting cells and then presented to recipient T lymphocytes in a major histocompatibility complex (MHC)-restricted fashion. Stimulation by either of these pathways leads to T-lymphocyte activation and secretion of cytokines and maturation factors, which in turn triggers cytotoxic T-lymphocyte and B-lymphocyte maturation and effector functions that can damage the allograft. (From Vierling JM: Immunology of acute and chronic hepatic allograft rejection. Liver Transpl Surg 5[4 Suppl 1]:S1-S20, 1999.)

Table 69-4. APPROXIMATE TIMING OF COMMON ALLOGRAFT SYNDROMES

Syndrome	Clinical Associations/Observations	Peak Time Period
"Preservation" injury	Older, hemodynamically unstable, and hypernatremic donors Long cold (> 14 hr) or warm (> 120 min) ischemic time Reconstruction of vascular anastomoses Poor bile production	Can be recognized in postreperfusion biopsies and might persist for several months, depending on the severity of injury
Rejection		
Antibody-mediated rejection	ABO-incompatible donor; high-titer (> 1:32) lymphocytotoxic cross-match	Immediately after reperfusion and persisting for several weeks
Acute cellular rejection	Younger "healthier" females, inadequately immunosuppressed recipients, and those with autoimmune disorders	Three days to 6 wk; later onset usually associated with inadequate immunosuppression or coexistent viral infection
Chronic rejection	Moderate/severe or persistent episodes of acute rejection; noncompliant and inadequately immunosuppressed patients (e.g., infections, tumors, PTLD)	Bimodal distribution; early peak during first year and later increase in noncompliant and inadequately immunosuppressed patients
Mechanical Problems		
Hepatic artery thrombosis	Pediatric (small-caliber) vessels; donor and/or recipient atherosclerosis; suboptimal or difficult arterial anastomosis; large difference in vessel caliber across anastomosis	Bimodal distribution; early peak between 0 and 4 wk and later peak between 18 and 36 mo (see text)
Biliary tract obstruction or strictures	Arterial insufficiency or thrombosis; difficult biliary anastomosis; original disease of PSC	Variable
Venous outflow obstruction	Difficult "piggyback" hepatic vein reconstruction; cardiac failure	Usually during first several weeks
Infections		
"Opportunistic" viral and fungal infections (e.g., CMV, HSV, VZV, EBV, *Candida*, *Aspergillus*)	Seropositive donors to seronegative recipients (often pediatric); overimmunosuppressed recipients	0–8 wk, much less common thereafter except for EBV-related PTLD and other EBV-related tumors (see text)
Recurrent Diseases		
Recurrent or new onset of viral or autoimmune hepatitis (e.g., HBV, HCV)	Original disease HBV, HCV, or autoimmune hepatitis	Usually first becomes apparent 4–6 wk after transplantation and persists thereafter, but earlier onset (within 2 wk) in aggressive cases
PBC and PSC	Original disease PBC or PSC; donor-recipient HLA-DR matching for PBC patients, weaning of immunosuppression	Usually first becomes apparent more than 6 mo after transplantation; incidence of PSC increases with time after transplantation
Alcohol abuse	High per day alcohol intake before transplantation; noncompliance with treatment protocols; γ-GTP/ALP ratio > 1.4	Usually > 6 mo
Nonalcoholic steatohepatitis	Original disease NASH or cryptogenic cirrhosis; persistent risk factors for NASH	Usually > 3–4 wk

ALP, alkaline phosphatase; CMV, cytomegalovirus; EBV, Epstein-Barr virus; γ-GTP, γ-glutamyl transpeptidase; HBV, hepatitis B virus; HCV, hepatitis C virus; HSV, herpes simplex virus; NASH, nonalcoholic steatohepatitis; PBC, primary biliary cirrhosis; PSC, primary sclerosing cholangitis; PTLD, posttransplant lymphoproliferative disorder; VZV, varicella-zoster virus.

Adapted from Demetris A, Crawford J, Nalesnik M, et al: Transplantation pathology of the liver. In Odze R, Goldblum J, Crawford JM (eds): Surgical Pathology of the GI Tract, Liver, Biliary Tract, and Pancreas. Philadelphia, WB Saunders, 2004, pp 909-966.

protect the allograft from damage. Shortly thereafter at 6 to 8 weeks after transplantation, "opportunistic" infections appear as a result of the high levels of immunosuppression needed to control acute rejection. Subsequently, immunosuppression can usually be significantly lowered for long-term patient management.[89-95] However, decreasing the immunosuppression occasionally unleashes immunological mechanisms responsible for return of either rejection or recurrence of the original disease, especially in patients with immune-dysregulated syndromes such as primary biliary cirrhosis (PBC), primary sclerosing cholangitis (PSC), and autoimmune hepatitis.

The effector phase of acute rejection begins when the peripheral and central sensitization reactions cause maturation of helper and cytotoxic T lymphocytes, release of cytokines and chemokines, and synthesis and secretion of antibodies directed at donor antigens (Fig. 69–4).[96] Inflammatory mediators such as cytokines and chemokines upregulate major histocompatibility complex (MHC), adhesion, and costimulatory molecules within the rejecting liver. These molecules then help recruit and retain inflammatory cells within the allograft and make it more susceptible to immunological attack. Readers interested in greater detail about specific effector mechanisms are referred to an excellent review.[96]

Antigenic and Tissue Targets of Rejection

The most important antigenic targets of the effector phase are those encoded by MHC and major ABO blood group antigens, which are expressed on the portal microvasculature, portal and central veins, and hepatic artery endothelium and bile ducts.[96,97] Other vascular- and tissue-specific antigen systems are also involved, particularly late after transplantation when the allograft has already been damaged by the initial rejection response. Antigen expression by various cell types within the allograft is a dynamic process influenced by many factors (e.g., drugs, cytokines). For example, bile ducts can express class II MHC antigens when perturbed by any type of inflammation,[98-100] and class I antigen expression is increased on hepatocytes[101] after transplantation (Table 69–5). Although changes in the expression of MHC antigens have been detected in liver allografts in association with certain graft syndromes, none appear to be specific or clinically useful.[26,98-100,102]

There are several possible nonexclusionary explanations for the preferential destruction of bile ducts,[103] including (1) the presence of a basement membrane, which could potentially play a role in migration,

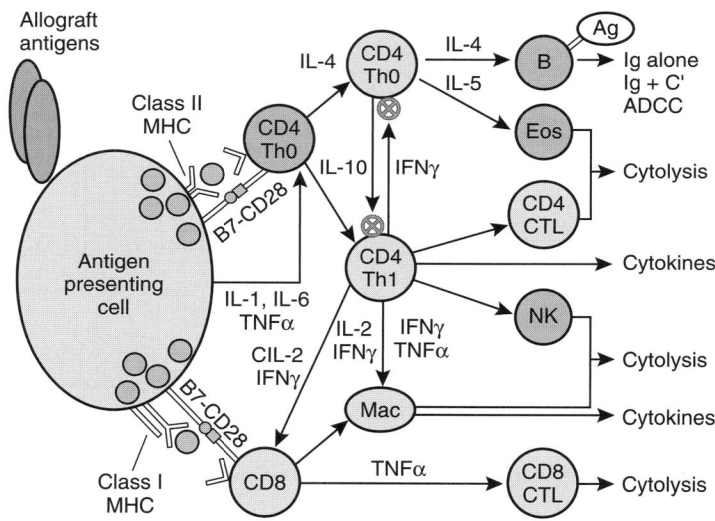

FIGURE 69–4

Diagram illustrating the important molecules and pathways involved in T-lymphocyte activation (*left side*) and differentiation of effector cells and pathways (*right side*). The interaction between antigen-presenting cells and T lymphocytes requires "two signals": one signal is delivered by the major histocompatibility molecule and the other by "costimulatory" molecules such as B7-CD28. These interactions trigger T-lymphocyte activation, which in turn causes maturation or differentiation of effector cells. Interferon-γ production by T lymphocytes fosters the development of T_H1-type CD4 T lymphocytes, which in turn assist in the maturation and activation of cytotoxic T lymphocytes and natural killer cells, as well as activation of macrophages, all of which can damage the allograft. Interleukin-4 production fosters the development of T_H2-type CD4 T lymphocytes, which in turn can cause maturation of B cells to produce alloantibodies and interleukin-5 for eosinophil maturation. Strong T_H1-type responses are usually seen with severe acute rejection episodes, which can be the precursor phase for chronic rejection. (From Vierling JM: Immunology of acute and chronic hepatic allograft rejection. Liver Transpl Surg 5[4 Suppl 1]:S1-S20, 1999.)

Table 69–5. HEPATIC EXPRESSION OF MAJOR HISTOCOMPATIBILITY COMPLEX MOLECULES, ADHESION MOLECULES, AND TISSUE-SPECIFIC ANTIGENS IN NORMAL AND REJECTING LIVERS

	Class I MHC	Class II MHC	CD58 (LFA-3)	CD54 and CD102 (ICAM-1, 2)	CD62E (ELAM-1)	CD62	CD106 (VCAM-1)	Tissue-Specific Antigens
Normal liver								
Hepatocyte	+	−	−	−/−	−	−	−	Yes
BEC	+	−	−	−/−	−	−	−	Yes
Kupffer cell	+	+	+	+/−	−	−	−	Unlikely
Artery	+	−	−	−/++	−	−	−	Unlikely
Sinusoid	+	−	−	+/+	−	−	−	Possible
Portal vein	+	−	+	−/−	±	±	−	Unlikely
Acute cellular rejection								
Hepatocyte	++	+	+	+/−	−	−	−	Yes
BEC	++	+++	+	+/−	−	−	−	Yes
Kupffer cell	++	++	+	+/−	−	−	+	Unlikely
Artery	+	±	+	±/++	±	+	+	Unlikely
Sinusoid	+	+	+	++/+	−	−	−	Possible
Portal vein	+	±	+	+/+	+	+	+	Unlikely
Ductopenic rejection								
Hepatocyte	++	+	+	+/−	−	−	−	Yes
BEC	++	+++	+	+/−	−	−	−	Yes
Kupffer cell	++	++	+	+/−	−	−	+	Unlikely
Artery	+	±	+	+/++	+	++	+	Unlikely
Sinusoid	+	+	+	+++/+	−	−	±	Possible
Portal vein	+	±	++	+/+	++	++	++	Unlikely

BEC, biliary epithelial cell; MHC, major histocompatibility complex.
From Vierling JM: Immunology of acute and chronic hepatic allograft rejection. Liver Transpl Surg 5(4 Suppl 1):S1-S20, 1999.

positioning, and costimulation of T cells; (2) an immunologically active antigenic profile of biliary epithelial cells that is significantly different from that of other parenchymal cells, including class I and II MHC and various adhesion and costimulatory molecules (Table 69–6); and (3) the presence of nearby APCs and lymphatics that facilitate the functional role of these conduits in processing environmental antigen for local presentation and traffic to the regional lymph nodes.[103]

Recent studies indicate that activated endothelial cells participate in allograft rejection in three major ways[96]: (1) selective recruitment of CD4+ T-cell subsets; (2) costimulation of T cells; and (3) involvement in the signaling pathways for CD40, CD40L, Fas, and Fas ligand (FasL). Antigen activation of T cells leads to effector cell differentiation and expression of a memory cell phenotype. In addition, damage and activation of the endothelium disrupt intimal hemostasis, which in turn triggers the proliferation of intimal myofibroblasts and eventually leads to the arterial manifestations of chronic rejection discussed later.[104,105]

Role of Direct and Indirect Antigen Presentation

Several lines of evidence support the contention that direct allorecognition is involved in acute rejection,[106-108] including (1) the high frequency of precursor T cells recognizing allogeneic MHC molecules directly; (2) marked amelioration or absence of acute rejection, but persistence of chronic rejection, in allografts depleted of donor APCs before transplantation; (3) enhancement of acute rejection by pretreatment of donors with agents that increase the number of donor APCs; and (4) the ability of T-cell lines specific for direct recognition of allogeneic MHC molecules to induce acute rejection in immunocompromised hosts.

The high precursor frequency and strength of the reaction explain the brisk polyclonal activation of T lymphocytes, secretion of cytokines and chemokines, and subsequent upregulation of various costimulatory and adhesion molecules on surrounding tissues. This is followed by maturation of cytotoxic T lymphocytes,

Table 69–6. MOLECULES EXPRESSED ON BILIARY EPITHELIAL CELLS AND THEIR LIGANDS FROM NORMAL OR DISEASED LIVERS THAT ARE IMPORTANT IN IMMUNE REACTIONS

BEC Adhesion or Signaling Molecule	Ligand	Functions
Class I MHC (A, B)	CD8 and TCR complex	Antigen presentation to CD8+ T lymphocytes for effective immunity to intracellular pathogens
Class II MHC (DR, DP, DQ)	CD4 and TCR complex	Antigen presentation to CD4+ T lymphocytes for amplification of immune responses and proliferation of reactive cells
LFA-3 (CD58)	CD2 (LFA-2)	Adhesion between activated T cells and cytotoxic targets or antigen-presenting cells; may assist in signaling for cytotoxic and helper activity of T cells
VLA-2, 3, and 6	Laminin, collagen, fibronectin, invasin	Mediates adhesion to extracellular matrix and inflammatory cells that express matrix-like surface proteins. Can assist the entry of bacteria into cells via invasin
ICAM-1 (CD54)	LFA-1, Mac-1	Facilitates low-frequency or low-avidity binding between class II MHC/TCR; facilitates NK recognition of targets; ? comitogen for T cells; receptor for rhinovirus and *Plasmodium falciparum*
NCAM (CD56)	NCAM, heparan sulfate, receptors on NK cells	Mediates cellular interactions in development of nervous system; may play role in NK recognition of alloantigenic targets
sialyl Lew^x	E-selectin, ELAM-1, P-selectin, CD62	Mediates binding to selectins, which are a family of adhesive receptors found on leukocytes (L), platelets (P), and endothelial cells (E)
CD51	RGD sequence in ECM	Recognizes and binds to RGD sequence in the ECM proteins vitronectin, von Willebrand factor, fibrinogen, and thrombospondin
BB1/B7	CD28	Costimulation of T cells via the CD3/TCR complex

BEC, biliary epithelial cell; ECM, extracellular matrix; ELAM, endothelial cell leukocyte adhesion molecule; ICAM, intercellular adhesion molecule; LFA, lymphocyte function–associated antigen; MHC, major histocompatibility complex; NCAM, nerve cell adhesion molecule; NK, natural killer cell; TCR, T-cell receptor; VLA, very late activation antigen.
From Demetris AJ: Immunopathology of the human biliary tree. In Sirica AE, Longnecker DS (eds): Biliary and Pancreatic Ductal Epithelia. Pathobiology and Pathophysiology. New York, Marcel Dekker, 1997, pp 127-180.

expansion and maturation of B cells, and recruitment of macrophages, eosinophils, neutrophils, and other effector cells, all of which have the potential to damage the organ.[96,109-111] The robust nature of the direct presentation pathway explains the frequency of clinical symptoms and the potential for rapid allograft failure.

Direct allostimulation has also been associated with a predominance of T_H1 activation, as evidenced by the type of cytokines (interleukin-2 [IL-2], interferon-γ [IFN-γ], tumor necrosis factor-α [TNF-α], granulocyte-macrophage colony-stimulating factor [GM-CSF], IL-3) and chemokines[112-115] produced in the allograft. Monitoring the severity of this reaction and controlling it with immunosuppression are the mainstays of patient management during the first several months after transplantation. Fortunately, the direct allostimulation pathway is highly sensitive to increased immunosuppression, and acute rejection is controllable in the majority of patients.[106,116,117]

Recognizing the morphological correlates of potentially irreversible damage that can eventually cause graft failure provides the conceptual basis for the histopathological grading of acute rejection.[118] Recipients in whom moderate or severe acute rejection develops usually (1) show a strong T_H1-type response in the allograft,[92,119-121] (2) require more immunosuppression to control the reaction,[122] and (3) are at increased risk for graft failure from acute rejection and the development of chronic rejection.[123-126] In fact, most cases of chronic rejection directly evolve from inadequately controlled acute rejection.[127] Strong T_H1 activation during acute rejection fosters the activation and differentiation of macrophages and recipient dendritic cells, which have been highly implicated in virtually all aspects of chronic rejection. Included are indirect allopresentation, tissue injury, upregulation of adhesion molecules, alterations in blood flow, and release of fibrogenic growth factors.[128-139]

Donor passenger leukocytes that migrate into the recipient were thought to be rapidly destroyed within days or weeks after transplantation. However, we have conclusively shown that donor cells can persist in some recipients for decades[83,140-146] and mediate or precipitate graft-versus-host, sensitizing, or tolerogenic immune reactions.[147-151] These reactions enable some lucky patients to be completely withdrawn from immunosuppression.[89-91,94]

Indirect antigen presentation is receiving increasing attention for its importance in both acute and chronic rejection. Supportive evidence[107,108,117,152-154] includes (1) ongoing immunological injury in the allograft despite disappearance of donor APCs,[155] (2) influx of activated recipient macrophages,[155] (3) the important role of allo-antibodies in chronic rejection (covered in detail later) mediated by B cells serving as APCs for CD4$^+$ T cells generating these antibodies, (4) susceptibility of allo-grafts that have been depleted of donor APCs before transplantation to chronic rejection; (5) and a high incidence of CD4$^+$ T-cell responses to donor MHC allopeptides via indirect recognition in patients with chronic rejection.[152,153] Indeed, allografts that exhibit persistent acute rejection[107,153] and those that evolve toward chronic rejection[107,152,153] show increased indi-rect alloantigen presentation and diminished direct presentation.[106]

The indirect alloresponse is initially oligoclonal and involves only a few dominant antigen peptides pre-sented by donor MHC class II DR determi-nants.[107,117,152,153] However, with persistent or severe injury, "epitope spreading" can occur. This refers to the presentation of cryptic or "self" autoantigens shared by the donor and recipient, including tissue-specific anti-gens or "autoantigens."[107,117,152,153,156-158] In addition, the indirect pathway is less sensitive to immunosuppres-sive blockade. These observations help explain the overlap of some forms of rejection with recurrent "autoimmune" disease and the comparatively poor response of late-onset versus early-onset rejection to increased immunosuppression.[18,122,125,126,159-162]

Determination of Causes of Graft Dysfunction after Transplantation

"Preservation" or Ischemic Injury and Primary Dysfunction

The term "preservation" or harvesting injury refers to damage that causes dysfunction immediately after trans-plantation, but not readily explainable on the basis of a technical or vascular insult, immunological factor, adverse drug reaction or infection, or toxin exposure. Insults that contribute to preservation injury include donor and recipient hypotension and other causes of warm ischemia, cold ischemia during organ preserva-tion, and reperfusion injury. Cold ischemia and warm ischemia are the most important.

Pathophysiology

Ischemic injury that occurs while the organ is at body temperature, but inadequately perfused with blood, is referred to as "warm ischemia." It can occur before or during harvesting and during rewarming after implan-tation. Warm ischemia is thought to preferentially damage hepatocytes and is not usually a clinical problem if kept under 90 to 120 minutes.[163-165] "Cold ischemia" occurs during storage in preservation fluid and ice bath immersion and preferentially damages sinusoidal endothelial cells.[40,166] General guidelines suggest that the cold ischemic time should be kept below 15 hours for organs preserved in University of Wisconsin solu-tion, if possible. Although longer cold ischemic times can be tolerated, the outcome in individual cases is unpre-dictable because of increased rates of dysfunction, post-transplant complications, and allograft failure.[55,167-170]

During cold preservation, hypothermia reduces the metabolic rate and prolongs the time that anoxic cells can retain essential metabolic functions.[166] However, the ischemic insult still causes loss of mitochondrial respiration and, consequently, depletion of adenosine triphosphate. This is followed by deterioration of energy-dependent metabolic pathways and transport processes[166] and activation of various proteinases, including matrix metalloproteinases, that induce lifting of sinusoidal endothelial cells from the underlying matrix. Loss of sinusoidal microvascular integrity and function along with subsequent interference with hepatic blood flow after revascularization is thought to be the major determinant of graft viability.[40,166,171,172] However, damage to hepatocytes and biliary epithelial cells and the interaction between parenchymal and nonparenchymal cells are receiving increased attention as important determinants of graft function (reviewed elsewhere[173]). Donor livers with preexisting steatosis show an increased susceptibility to both warm and cold ischemic injury.[173-175]

Complete revascularization and reperfusion with blood cause Kupffer cell activation mediated by priming with TNF-α from the intestines.[166,171,172] The hypoxia and subsequent reoxygenation lead to activation of complement components. Activated Kupffer cells release reactive oxygen species that induce a network of cytokines, which in turn contribute to granulocyte accumulation within the sinusoids[166,171,172] and can sec-ondarily contribute to the damage by release of reactive oxygen species and proteases. All these processes lead to an imbalance of vasoconstrictors over vasodilators—a major determinant contributing to microcirculatory failure. Therefore, agents that favor vasodilatation, such as endothelin antagonists, can lessen reperfusion injury, whereas those that favor vasoconstriction can worsen it.[166]

Bile duct cells are also susceptible to ischemic injury during cold preservation, as well as processes that occur after reperfusion injury, including the toxic action of hydrophobic bile salts.[173] The biliary tree is flushed during cold preservation, but residual bile remains and damages biliary epithelial cells. Long cold ischemic times are associated with an increased number of biliary epithelial cells shed into bile after transplantation.[176] Failure of biliary epithelial cells to heal after sloughing probably explains the increased incidence of biliary sludge syndrome in expanded criteria, non–heart-beating donors and in those with long cold ischemic times.[167] This causes the prolonged cholestatic phase of the preservation-reperfusion dysfunction syndrome.

Clinical Features

Poor bile production and persistent elevation of serum lactate after complete revascularization are the most reliable early signs of severe preservation injury[177-179]; serum alanine transaminase (ALT) and aspartate transaminase (AST) levels greater than 2500 IU/mL during the first few days after transplantation also usually signal severe damage.[40,180,181] Transaminases normalize rapidly after the first few days[171-173] unless the allograft fails or is damaged by another insult. If the graft survives the initial damage, a prolonged cholestatic phase usually begins with elevations in total serum bilirubin and γ-glutamyl transpeptidase (γ-GTP).[24,40,171-173,182-185] The general trend is toward gradual improvement, but resolution of the abnormal bilirubin values and restoration of the normal architecture may require several months.[24,40,182-185]

Reperfusion of a donor liver with preexisting macrovesicular steatosis results in a characteristic intraoperative syndrome manifested as fibrinolysis and wound site bleeding. "Oozing" from disrupted vessels makes it difficult to achieve hemostasis.[44,49,186] Recovery of recipients who were critically ill before transplantation can be even more complicated and protracted if they receive an expanded criteria donor liver.

Histopathological Findings

Even though cold ischemic injury preferentially damages sinusoidal endothelial cells, routine light microscopic examination of either frozen or permanent sections before transplantation *cannot* accurately assess the damage or predict allograft function after transplantation. Electron microscopy is required to assess the endothelial damage, but routine application is impractical.[40,180,181,187] Light microscopic examination of biopsy samples obtained *after reperfusion* is more informative.

The changes associated with preservation injury in specimens obtained after reperfusion can be divided into those associated with damage and those signifying subsequent repair reactions.[24,40,180-185,187] Biopsy samples obtained within hours of complete revascularization (so-called reperfusion biopsies) show only the damage and can predict poor allograft function during the first few postoperative weeks with reasonable accuracy.[24,40,180-185,187] Indicators of severe preservation injury in reperfusion biopsies include zonal or confluent coagulative necrosis, particularly if it is periportal or bridging, and severe neutrophilic infiltration. The subcapsular parenchyma is especially vulnerable[188]; a needle biopsy sample taken from this area may show more severe pathology than present in the deeper parenchyma and thus overestimate the damage.[188] Perivenular neutrophilia without necrosis as a result of operative manipulation (so called surgical hepatitis) is not a sign of severe injury.

Repair responses usually begin by 2 to 3 days after transplantation and are proportional to the severity of the insult. Mild hepatocellular injury, such as microvesicular steatosis, hepatocellular cytoaggregation (i.e., rounding up of hepatocyte cytoplasm with detachment from adjacent hepatocytes), and hepatocellular swelling,[24,40,180-185,187,189] is rapidly reversible. Reparative responses in such cases are usually limited to hepatocellular mitosis, thickening of the plates, and nuclear enlargement. Mild centrilobular hepatocellular swelling and hepatocanalicular cholestasis may persist for several weeks (Fig. 69–5A). The response to more severe injury depends on the location and severity of hepatocyte necrosis. Mild centrilobular hepatocyte necrosis usually triggers mitosis in neighboring viable zone 2 hepatocytes, which rapidly proliferate and restore the normal architecture. Periportal and bridging necrosis with architectural collapse triggers cholangiolar proliferation,[24,40,182-185] which can link adjacent portal tracts and distort the architecture. More severe injury is also usually accompanied by centrilobular hepatocellular swelling and hepatocanalicular and cholangiolar cholestasis (see Fig. 69–5B).[24,40,180-185,187] These changes generally persist for 1 or 2 months or more. This period corresponds to the prolonged cholestatic phase of the clinical preservation-reperfusion injury syndrome. If the graft recovers, the normal lobular architecture will eventually be restored if biliary strictures do not develop because of the biliary sludge syndrome.

Reperfusion of a donor liver with preexisting macrovesicular steatosis (see earlier) results in lysis of fat-containing hepatocytes, which releases lipid droplets into the sinusoids (see Fig. 69–2B). The lipid-water interface in the blood causes the lipid droplets to coalescence into large fat globules that clog sinusoidal blood flow and trigger nearby fibrin deposition, neutrophilia, and red blood cell congestion.[49] The large fat globules have been given the colorful label "lipopeliosis."[190] Their presence in posttransplant biopsy specimens can be confidently traced back to macrovesicular steatosis in the donor, even if no pretransplant or back-table biopsy specimen was obtained. If the liver recovers, the large fat globules will eventually resolve over a period of several weeks.

Differential Diagnosis

The histopathological differential diagnosis includes sepsis, biliary obstruction, antibody-mediated rejection, and cholestatic hepatitis. Recognition of acute rejection

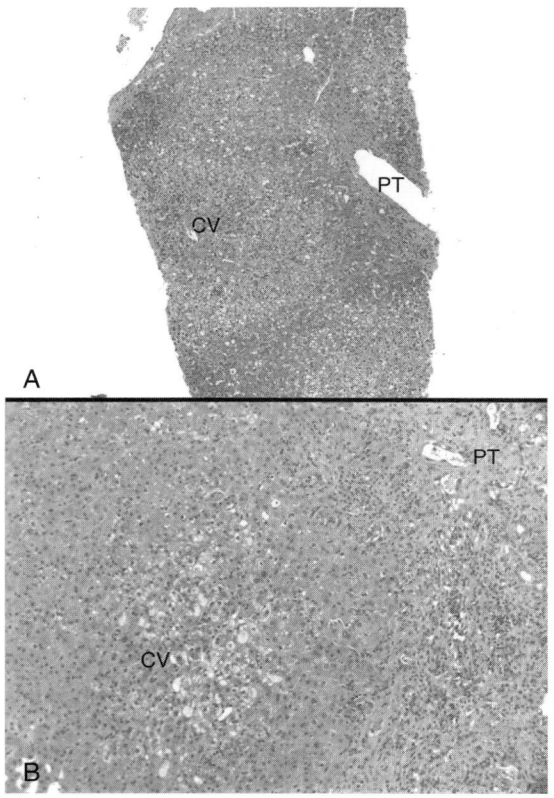

FIGURE 69–5

A, Example of mild preservation injury characterized by mild centrilobular hepatocyte swelling and hepatocanalicular cholestasis. Note the absence of portal and periportal inflammation and cholangiolar proliferation. **B,** Severe preservation injury is characterized by centrilobular hepatocyte swelling and hepatocanalicular cholestasis, as well as prominent cholangiolar proliferation, cholangiolar cholestasis, and mild acute cholangiolitis. CV, central vein; PT, portal tract.

superimposed on preservation injury is an additional problem. Distinguishing between sepsis, preservation injury, and antibody-mediated rejection on the basis of histopathology alone can be extremely difficult. The pathophysiological mechanisms of injury are very similar and include sinusoidal endothelial cell injury with poor microvascular flow, arterial vasospasm, and coagulative necrosis. The injury is followed by a prolonged cholestatic phase characterized by hepatocyte swelling and cholangiolar proliferation.

In such cases, considerable reliance is placed on the clinical history for guidance in further analysis and interpretation. Donor age, cold and warm ischemic times, operative difficulties, the clinical profile, and blood culture and cross-match results often help determine the type of additional testing (e.g., immunofluorescent or C4d staining) that might assist in distinguishing among the aforementioned possibilities. In most instances, however, preservation injury and technical problems prove to be the culprit early after transplantation.

Distinguishing between preservation injury and obstruction/cholangitis can be accomplished by closely examining "true" bile ducts contained within the portal tract connective tissue and comparing the "true" bile ducts with "cholangioles" located at the interface zone. In biliary obstruction/cholangitis, the usual findings are periductal lamellar edema surrounding the true bile ducts, accompanied by neutrophils within the lumen or infiltrating between biliary epithelial cells. In contrast, periductal edema and acute cholan*gitis* are not usually seen in preservation injury. Instead there is "acute cholang*iolitis,*" or acute inflammation surrounding the cholangioles. Both disorders can show marked centrilobular hepatocanalicular and cholangiolar cholestasis and intralobular neutrophil clusters. Fortunately, a T-tube stent is usually kept in place for the first several months after transplantation, when this difficulty most frequently arises. This stent helps prevent biliary obstruction and provides ready access for monitoring of bile flow and biliary tract patency.

Differentiation between preservation injury and cholestatic hepatitis is based on the clinical history and time after transplantation. Cholestatic hepatitis has been reported only in patients infected with HBV or HCV, is unusual before 2 to 3 weeks after transplantation, and generally worsens with time unless the patient is specifically treated with decreased immunosuppression or antiviral therapy, or both. In contrast, preservation injury begins immediately after transplantation and generally improves with time after transplantation.

Acute rejection superimposed on preservation injury is recognized by the appearance of mild to moderate mixed portal inflammation containing blastic lymphocytes, and especially eosinophils, combined with infiltration and damage to the true bile ducts. Mononuclear inflammation of the portal and central veins provides additional support for the diagnosis of acute rejection.

Finally, apoptotic bodies or coagulative necrosis in a biopsy specimen obtained more than several days after transplantation should not be attributed to preservation injury.[173] Only 4 to 6 hours is required for a normal hepatocyte to undergo the entire apoptotic cycle; therefore, their presence generally signifies an additional, usually ischemic, insult.

Vascular Complications

Vascular complications are the most common major technical problem leading to serious allograft damage and failure. Most are manifested during the first several months after transplantation and are usually related to the anastomosis, manipulation of the vascular tree, pre-existing vascular disease, metabolic or physiological abnormalities that predispose to thrombosis, or a combination of these factors. Examples include anastomotic narrowing and other irregularities such as intimal flaps, intimal or medial tears (or both), dramatic reductions in caliber across a suture line, and the creation of "kinks" or abnormal tortuosity.[177-179,191] Potential problems are compounded by preexisting atherosclerotic disease and any factors that increase the technical difficulty of completing the vascular anastomosis, such as small-caliber vessels in pediatric recipients or abnormal anatomy (e.g., piggyback venal caval anastomosis). Finally, physiological or metabolic abnormalities that decrease hepatic blood flow or predispose to thrombosis, such as clotting abnormalities, rejection, infections, and cardiac failure, also increase the risk of complications, especially at sites of abnormal anatomy.[192]

Vascular interposition grafts, or small (most often iliac) arterial or venous segments used to link the donor and recipient arteries or veins, respectively, are a "double-edged sword." They are a convenient "plumbing" solution, but also a source of problems. Vascular grafts increase the number of anastomoses required for vascular reconstruction,[5] and grafts cryopreserved or stored in preservation fluid for 1 to several days before implantation may be marginally viable at the time of placement. Consequently, they can serve as a thrombogenic or atherogenic stimulus or nidus of infection.[193]

In general, sonography is used to evaluate vascular flow because it is the most useful noninvasive screening tool for vascular complications.[194] Though accurate in most instances, in our experience, invasive or magnetic resonance angiography should be pursued when there is strong clinical or pathological evidence of ischemia, vascular obstruction, or otherwise unexplained biliary tract complications.

Hepatic Artery Thrombosis

Pathophysiology. The hepatic arterial tree is the most frequent source of vascular complications after liver transplantation and a major cause of allograft dysfunction and failure.[177-179,191] Unlike native livers, an allograft is devoid of collateral arterial circulation, at least early after transplantation. This deficiency increases susceptibility to ischemic injury.

The pathophysiological consequences of inadequate arterial flow are related primarily to ischemia of structures supplied by the hepatic artery: the extrahepatic and intrahepatic bile ducts, hilar and portal tract connective tissue, and lymph nodes.[195] Damage to these structures eventually leads to biliary tract strictures, cholangitic abscesses, and the biliary sludge syndrome, complications lumped together under the phrase "ischemic cholangitis."[24,196]

A second wave of technically related arterial thromboses occurs between 1 and 3 years after transplantation.[29,32,197] A less than perfect anastomosis often causes turbulent arterial flow immediately downstream from the suture line, which eventually leads to arterial

narrowing and thrombosis. In addition, fibrointimal hyperplasia frequently develops in arterial interposition vascular grafts more quickly than in the native or the allograft arterial vasculature, thereby predisposing to thrombosis and subsequent complications.[24,38,191,196,198]

Clinical Features. Symptoms, when present, are usually related to hepatic infarcts, abscesses, and impaired bile flow and include right upper abdominal pain/discomfort, intermittent fever, bacteremia/fungemia, bile peritonitis, and jaundice.[177-179,191,199] Occasionally, fulminant hepatic failure can be seen if large areas of the liver are infarcted. If sufficient collaterals have developed, the patient may be asymptomatic.

Histopathological Findings. The histological changes are quite varied, and the structures most commonly affected, the hilum and large bile ducts, are not routinely sampled. Therefore, needle biopsies are subject to more sampling error than the usual evaluation and are thus an unreliable method for establishing the diagnosis of hepatic artery thrombosis.[24,38,200] Peripheral needle biopsy specimens can have a completely normal appearance, frank coagulative necrosis or marked centrilobular hepatocyte swelling, cholangiolar proliferation with or without bile plugs, and acute cholangiolitis.[24,38,201] In some cases, spotty acidophilic necrosis of hepatocytes or so-called ischemic hepatitis can mimic acute viral hepatitis.[24,38,201] These sampling problems should be remembered when surgeons, encouraged by a grossly and microscopically "viable" appearance at the capsular surface, attempt to "salvage" an allograft by arterial thrombectomy[202,203] only to be disappointed later by allograft failure from necrosis of the bile ducts (Fig. 69–6).

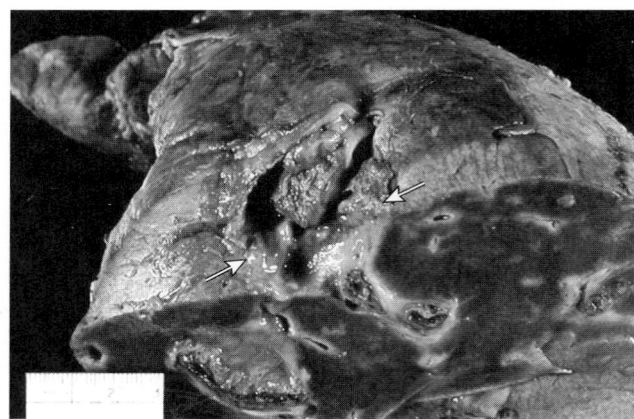

FIGURE 69–6

Gross image of a section of a failed liver allograft with hepatic artery thrombosis. Note the perihilar necrosis (highlighted by *arrows*) and leakage of bile into the surrounding connective tissue. Note also that the subcapsular hepatic parenchyma is more viable than the perihilar region.

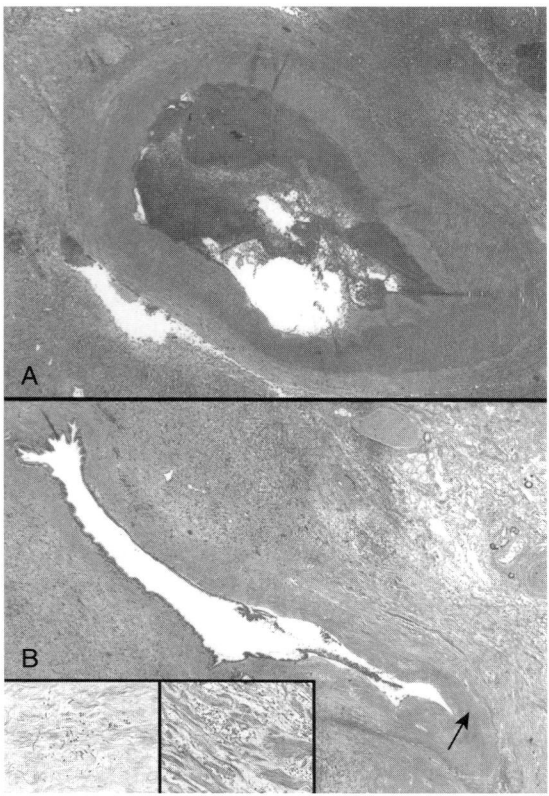

FIGURE 69-7

A, A cross section of the hepatic artery at the liver hilum shows acute thrombosis. **B**, Cross section of the common hepatic duct in the hilum of the same liver. Note the necrosis of the bile duct wall with leakage of bile into the surrounding connective tissue (*arrow*). The *insets* show the area highlighted by the *arrow* at higher magnification and illustrate the presence of fungi (*left inset*) and colonies of coccoid bacteria (*right inset*).

Examination of failed allografts with hepatic artery thrombosis often shows transmural necrosis of the hilar bile ducts with leakage of bile into the surrounding connective tissue (Fig. 69–7). The necrotic tissue is not infrequently colonized with bacterial and fungal colonies, and special staining for microorganisms should be carried out routinely.

Differential Diagnosis. Hepatic artery narrowing or thrombosis can mimic almost every other cause of allograft dysfunction, including biliary tract obstruction and cholangitis, acute and chronic rejection, and acute and chronic viral hepatitis. The biopsy specimen may even be unremarkable, either because vascular collaterals have developed and the thrombosis is inconsequential or because necrosis of the hilar bile ducts has occurred but changes secondary to biliary sludging have not yet developed in the periphery. More frequent findings include biliary tract obstruction or strictures.[24,38,191,196] The relationship between arterial thrombosis and

biliary tract complications is so common that examination of hepatic arterial patency is standard practice when biliary tract complications are encountered.[196]

Portal Vein Thrombosis

Pathophysiology. Portal vein thrombosis, strictures, and poor flow because of persistent collateral circulation or hypotension are uncommon early after transplantation.[177-179,191,204] However, the portal vein is a major source of blood flow, and when suboptimal flow or complete occlusion does occur, it is usually clinically significant. The incidence of complications is increased when cryopreserved venous interposition grafts are used.[205] Cirrhotic allografts are more susceptible to portal vein thrombosis than noncirrhotic allografts are.

Clinical Features. Complete portal vein thrombosis of a noncirrhotic allograft can result in fulminant hepatic failure, or signs and symptoms of portal hypertension with massive ascites and edema can develop. If the thrombus is nonocclusive, relapsing fever and miliary seeding of the liver with bacteria may be encountered. Symptoms of portal vein thrombosis in a cirrhotic allograft are the same as those in a native liver with cirrhosis: variceal hemorrhage, splenomegaly, and ascites.

Histopathological Findings. The histopathological findings can be quite varied and depend on the severity of portal vein flow compromise and time after transplantation. Complete obstruction early after transplantation is often associated with massive coagulative necrosis. Suboptimal portal flow because of strictures, kinks, or persistent collateral circulation can cause zonal (often periportal or midzonal) coagulative necrosis, hepatocyte atrophy or small cell changes, unexplained zonal or panlobular steatosis, or nodular regenerative hyperplasia–like changes. Bacterial or fungal infection of a partial portal vein thrombus can lead to miliary seeding of the liver with small abscesses.

Differential Diagnosis. Unexplained zonal ischemic or hepatocellular changes, like those described earlier, should raise the possibility of compromised portal vein blood flow, which can be evaluated by ultrasound or angiography. Portal vein complications uncommonly show inflammation, and particular attention should be paid to the size and shape of the portal vein branches and their relationship to the parenchyma.

Hepatic Vein and Vena Cava Complications

Pathophysiology. Hepatic vein and vena cava complications are relatively uncommon. When they do occur, the clinical history usually includes a description of difficulties in reconstructing the venous outflow tract or the use of alternative anastomoses such as the "piggyback" approach.[5] Clinically significant vena caval stenosis or thrombosis is associated with characteristic histopathological changes.

Clinical Features. The clinical manifestations of severe stenosis or thrombosis resemble the Budd-Chiari syndrome and include hepatic enlargement, tenderness, and ascites and edema. Less severe stenosis might initially result only in histopathological manifestations or an increase in the portal vein–vena cava pressure gradient.

Histopathological Findings. Typical acute findings include centrilobular congestion and hemorrhage that extends into the surrounding perivenular sinusoids. The congestion and hemorrhage are often associated with hepatocyte necrosis and dropout, and red blood cells can usually be observed within the lumen of at least some hepatic venules. Chronic outflow stenosis or obstruction can cause perivenular fibrosis and occasional central-to-central bridging if the stenosis is not repaired (Fig. 69–8). Nodular regenerative hyperplasia is another complication of chronic outflow obstruction.

Differential Diagnosis. Centrilobular or perivenular congestion, hemorrhage, and hepatocyte necrosis can be caused by mechanical outflow obstruction and immune-mediated injury such as acute and chronic rejection, adverse drug reactions, and viral and autoimmune hepatitis. The key feature used to distinguish between mechanical and immune-mediated causes of perivenular congestion is perivenular mononuclear inflammation in the latter. However, inflammation can be transient in "immune-mediated" injury. If immune-mediated injury is not recognized until a later stage when only perivenular fibrosis and congestion are present, it can be indistinguishable from mechanical or toxic causes.[206]

Review of previous biopsies, the clinical history, and ancillary histopathological findings can provide information useful in making the distinction between immunological and mechanical causes. For example, previous biopsy specimens may show centrilobular-based acute rejection, which was successfully treated, but perivenular fibrosis and congestion subsequently developed. Alternatively, the surgeons may acknowledge a difficult vena caval anastomosis and a probable cause for concern. In addition, most central veins are involved when there is a mechanical problem, adverse drug reaction, or rejection. In contrast, perivenular involvement is usually patchy in viral or autoimmune hepatitis. The focus of any coexistent portal necroinflammatory activity can provide additional information useful in distinguishing between these possibilities: inflammatory damage to bile ducts and portal veins suggests coexistent rejection, whereas prominent interface activity indicates coexistent viral or autoimmune hepatitis. It will still be difficult to determine the underlying cause in some patients. In such cases, review of the original disease, operative anatomy, previous rejection history, and venous flow and pressure studies may be needed to finally determine the nature of the underlying problem.

Bile Duct Complications

Pathophysiology

The two most common factors underlying biliary tract complications are ischemic injury and iatrogenically introduced abnormal anatomy, both of which predispose to mucosal damage and inadequate drainage or inordinate reflux.[207] The damage can lead to anastomotic dehiscence, transmural necrosis and bile leakage, cholangitic abscesses, ascending cholangitis, anastomotic or intrahepatic strictures, bile casts, obstruction, or biliary-vascular fistulas.[38,208,209]

There are several other causes of biliary tract ischemia other than frank arterial thrombosis or narrowing, including prolonged cold ischemia[167] and preformed anti-donor antibodies (anti-MHC or ABO blood group).[210-213] The latter can cause arterial vasospasm and immunological damage to the artery and peribiliary arterial plexus.[212,214] Biliary tract complications are also more common after living donor[213,215-217] and split-liver transplant operations.[218] In patients whose original disease was primary sclerosing cholangitis (PSC), the possibility of recurrent disease should be entertained[219-221] once all other causes of biliary tract complications have been reasonably excluded.

Clinical Features

The biliary tract is usually reconstructed by performing either a duct-to-duct or a choledochojejunal anastomosis. The former is temporarily stented with a suitably sized T tube and Silastic stent. Minor biliary tract problems such as strictures and stones are the most common

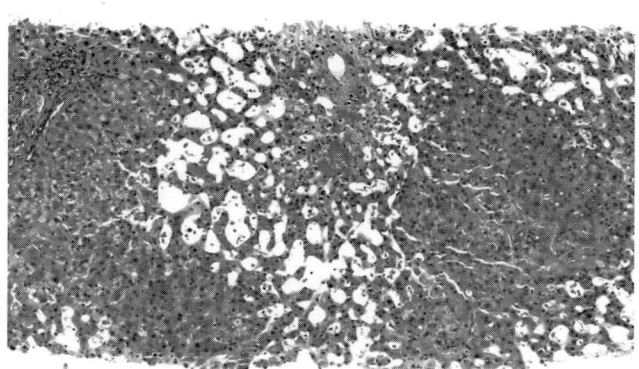

FIGURE 69–8

Chronic venous outflow obstruction or strictures can cause centrilobular congestion and sinusoidal dilatation with centrilobular hepatocyte atrophy, which can eventually lead to perivenular fibrosis as shown in this image.

and usually first suspected in recipients with selective elevation of γ-GTP and alkaline phosphatase on routine liver injury testing. Actual clinical symptoms are less frequently seen. Biliary imaging studies are used to confirm the diagnosis.[38,208,209] When the T tube is still in place early after transplantation, cholangiography is routinely preformed before clamping (1 week), at the time of T-tube removal (3 months), and when indicated in patients with clinical or biochemical evidence suggestive of biliary obstruction.

Major biliary tract complications such as complete obstruction, cholangitic abscesses, and ascending cholangitis are often manifested by fever, jaundice, upper right quadrant pain, and intermittent bacteremia. These complications usually require surgical correction unless there is uncorrectable intrahepatic biliary tract disease.

Histopathological Findings

The histopathological changes associated with biliary tract complications are the same as those encountered in native livers.[37,38,222] Most complications are recognized by detection of predominantly neutrophilic portal inflammation, periductal edema, and intraepithelial and intraluminal neutrophils within the true bile ducts. Mild ductular proliferation, centrilobular hepatocanalicular cholestasis, and small clusters of neutrophils throughout the lobules are also commonly seen. Chronic biliary tract strictures can be associated with chronic portal inflammation, biliary epithelial cell senescence, and patchy small bile duct loss. This constellation of findings can closely mimic chronic rejection, discussed later.

Red blood cells in the lumen of bile ducts or, conversely, bile concretions surrounded by foreign body giant cells in blood vessels are abnormal and signal the presence of a biliary-vascular fistula.[24] Prompt surgical intervention is often needed when either finding is encountered. Periductal hemorrhage surrounding a small interlobular bile duct is not an uncommon finding when a biopsy specimen is obtained within a day after transhepatic cholangiography.[223] Such patients are usually asymptomatic, and the findings generally resolve without intervention.

Differential Diagnosis

The histopathological differential diagnosis depends on the time after transplantation. Biliary obstruction/cholangitis can be difficult to distinguish from preservation injury and acute rejection within the first several weeks, particularly if the patient was treated with increased immunosuppression before the biopsy specimen was obtained.[224,225] Distinguishing between preservation injury and biliary obstruction was discussed earlier (see "Preservation or Ischemic Injury and Primary Dysfunction").

The most important features for distinguishing between acute rejection and biliary obstruction/cholan-*gitis* are the composition of the portal inflammation, the presence of a ductular reaction, the cytological appearance of the biliary epithelial cells, and the presence of perivenular and subendothelial mononuclear inflammation. Neutrophils generally predominate in biliary obstruction/cholangitis, whereas biliary epithelial cells usually retain a relatively normal nuclear-to-cytoplasmic ratio and perivenular mononuclear inflammation is absent. In acute rejection, the portal inflammation is composed of lymphocytes, plasma cells, and eosinophils, the latter of which may be quite striking or may actually predominate when patients are treated with "steroid-sparing" immunosuppressive regimens.[226,227] In addition, in rejection the biliary epithelial cells show distinct reactive changes such as an increased nuclear-cytoplasmic ratio.[24,225,228] Perivenular and subendothelial inflammation further distinguishes acute rejection from acute cholangitis/obstruction.

More than 6 months after transplantation, biliary obstruction or strictures can mimic acute and chronic rejection, viral hepatitis, and recurrent autoimmune disorders. Chronic intermittent biliary obstruction or cholangitis, as seen in patients with biliary sludge syndrome, can be associated with a mixed or even predominantly mononuclear portal infiltrate and biliary epithelial cell senescence changes.[229] Portal fibrosis with mild duct proliferation, mild portal neutrophilic or eosinophilic inflammation, and mild centrilobular cholestasis are features that should suggest obstructive cholangiopathy. A clinical and laboratory clue that biliary tract pathology is masquerading as acute rejection is that more than 6 months has elapsed after transplantation and the patient has adequate immunosuppressive drug levels with preferential elevation of γ-GTP and alkaline phosphatase.[220] Late-onset acute rejection is unusual in this circumstance.

Chronic obstructive cholangiopathy can also mimic chronic viral hepatitis. The presence of cholan*gitis* rather than acute cholan*giolitis* and the finding of lobular disarray, which is seen in viral hepatitis but not in cholangiopathy, are useful distinguishing features. The profile of liver injury test elevations is also usually helpful. Exclusion of viral pathogens by adjuvant testing procedures can be used to rule out viral infection. It should be remembered, however, that at times biliary tract problems might be first suspected on biopsy, but cholangiography (magnetic resonance cholangiopancreatography, endoscopic retrograde cholangiopancreatography [duct to duct], or percutaneous transhepatic cholangiography) is needed to confirm the diagnosis.

Rejection

Although all patients are potentially at risk for rejection, the incidence and severity of rejection are greater in certain patient populations and under certain circumstances. In general, younger, "healthier" (e.g., Child's type A, lack of renal failure, good muscle mass), black, and female recipients and patients with disorders of immune regulation (PBC, PSC, autoimmune hepatitis) before transplantation have a higher incidence and severity of acute and chronic rejection.[35,122-126,230-233] Responsiveness to the allograft is also enhanced by earlier exposure to the same or similar alloantigens via blood transfusions or previous transplants or pregnancies. Inadequate immunosuppression is also a major risk factor.

Rejection in liver allografts is categorized into "antibody mediated," acute (cellular), and chronic.[234] Antibody-mediated rejection usually occurs within the first several weeks after transplantation and is mediated primarily by antibodies. Acute (cellular) rejection can occur anytime after transplantation, but it is most common during the first month and is mediated primarily by cell-mediated immune mechanisms. Chronic rejection usually develops directly from severe or persistent and unresolved acute rejection and is probably mediated by a combination of both antibodies and cell-mediated mechanisms. Late-onset antibody-mediated rejection in liver allografts is in need of further study. Each is discussed in greater detail in the following sections.

Antibody-Mediated Rejection

Antidonor antibodies can be "preformed," or present in the recipient before transplantation, or can develop afterward in response to the allograft.[31] Antidonor antibodies can cause damage or failure, enhance survival, or have no effect on the allograft.[31] Their ability to cause rejection or damage is covered here.

Liver allografts are much less susceptible to antibody-mediated rejection from preformed lymphocytotoxic antibodies than other solid-organ allografts are.[24,214,235-239] Therefore, cross-match results do not routinely influence the triage of donor organs. However, crossing ABO blood group barriers is still generally avoided[211,240-242] because doing so leads to a high incidence ($\approx 60\%$) of antibody-mediated rejection in unconditioned recipients.[211,240-242] Some groups still perform ABO-incompatible liver transplantation with reasonable results in candidates with fulminant hepatic failure or pediatric recipients, where the need can be more urgent and the donor pool is limited. If ABO-incompatible recipients are preconditioned by splenectomy, cytoreductive therapy, or plasmapheresis (or any combination of these measures),[243] graft failure from acute antibody-mediated rejection can generally be avoided. However, such patients are still at risk for late complications of antibody-mediated rejection, such as infarcts and ischemic cholangitis.[196,198,244]

Living donor liver allografts seem to be more susceptible to antibody-mediated rejection than whole-liver deceased donor allografts are,[16] probably because of further strain on already precarious blood flow in living donor allografts early after transplantation.

Pathophysiology. The consequences of antidonor antibodies depend on the class, titer, timing of the antibody response, and the density and distribution of target antigens in the organ.[31,214] Isoagglutinins[211,240-242] and anti-MHC lymphocytotoxic antibodies,[212,245-250] which are directed at antigens expressed on endothelial cells, are the most dangerous and can cause accelerated liver allograft injury and failure, but rarely in a hyperacute fashion. Binding of antibodies to the graft vasculature results in complement fixation, endothelial damage, deposition of platelet-fibrin thrombi, and initiation of the clotting and fibrinolytic cascades. Subsequent microvascular thrombosis, arterial vasospasm, and coagulopathy act in concert to impair blood flow and cause hemorrhagic necrosis.

Relatively high-titer antibodies are needed to overcome the natural resistance of liver allografts to antibody-mediated rejection. This resistance is attributable to (1) secretion of soluble MHC class I antigens by the donor liver that bind to and neutralize the antibodies; (2) Kupffer cell phagocytosis of subsequent immune complexes and activated platelet aggregates[235,236,251-253]; (3) the dual afferent hepatic blood supply; (4) the unique hepatic sinusoidal microvasculature, which is devoid of a conventional basement membrane (reviewed elsewhere[31,254]); and (5) possibly a homologous source of complement.[255,256]

In general, isoagglutinins cause significantly more injury than lymphocytotoxic antibodies do, which do not routinely cause early allograft damage unless they are present in high titer (> 1:32) and of the IgG class.[212,245-250,257] However, the relative risk should be kept in perspective. Positive cross-match results are encountered in 8% to 12% of recipients, and only 30% have relatively high titers. Thus, the patient population at risk for severe antibody-mediated rejection is fairly small.[248,250,257,258] Consequently, it may be overlooked as a cause of dysfunction or failure if it occurs only once or twice per year in programs that carry out fewer than 100 cases per year.

Clinical Features. Early allograft dysfunction from preformed antidonor antibodies is usually manifested over a period of hours to days rather than minutes to hours as seen in kidney allografts.[210,211,240,242,259] The first signs of serious injury often develop in the operating room after complete revascularization. The liver might reperfuse uniformly and produce bile initially, but then become hard and swollen before bile flow slows or stops altogether. Difficulty in achieving hemostasis and an inordinate need for platelets and blood component replacement therapy signal the initiation of an intrahepatic consumptive coagulopathy.[31,212,214,240] However, the intraoperative events are rarely serious enough to abort the procedure or undertake immediate retransplantation. Instead, a relentless rise in liver injury test values during the first several posttransplant days and other signs of impending hepatic failure signal the onset of severe antibody-mediated rejection.[210,211,240,259] In cases of suspected antibody-mediated rejection, hepatic angiograms are often used to exclude arterial thrombosis. The presence of segmental narrowing or a "sausage link" appearance[210,211,240,246,259] and diffuse luminal narrowing with poor peripheral circulation are changes suggestive of immunologically mediated arterial vasospasm. In severe cases, this is accompanied by marked increases in serum transaminases and other systemic signs of synthetic and functional hepatic failure.[210,211,240,246,259]

More frequent manifestations of antibody-mediated rejection include a persistent rise in serum bilirubin during the first week after transplantation accompanied by refractory thrombocytopenia, low complement activity, and a biopsy specimen showing changes similar to those described for "preservation" injury or biliary obstruction.[257] These findings are usually followed by the onset of acute (cellular) rejection and the need for increased immunosuppression.[212,214,260] Ischemic biliary necrosis later manifested as biliary sludge, obstructive cholangiopathy, and small bile duct loss are other late manifestations of early antibody-mediated arterial injury, vasospasm, and thrombosis.[212,214,260-262]

Histopathological Findings. The histopathological findings depend on the timing of the biopsy and the presensitized state. Biopsies of ABO-incompatible organs obtained within 2 to 6 hours after reperfusion show prominent red blood cell and focal neutrophil sludging in the sinusoids, focal platelet-fibrin thrombi in the portal and central veins, and acidophilic hepatocyte necrosis.[210,211,240,259] These changes can progress within 1 to 2 days to large areas of confluent coagulative hepatocyte necrosis, prominent sinusoidal and venous congestion, and hemorrhage into the portal tract connective tissue. Portal veins often show circumferential fibrin deposition. Arteries occasionally show neutrophilic or necrotizing arteritis (or both), but more common findings are endothelial cell hypertrophy and evidence of arterial vasospasm, such as mural myocyte vacuolization, wrinkling of the elastic lamina, and thickening of the wall with narrowing of the lumen.

Mild portal neutrophilia usually appears at 2 to 3 days, along with focal cholangiolar proliferation. The histological features up to this point are quite difficult to separate from those of preservation injury, except if convincing immune deposits are detected. Thereafter, progressive hemorrhagic infarction of the organ can occur in ABO-incompatible organs.[210,211,240,259]

Antibody-mediated injury in patients harboring preformed lymphocytotoxic antibodies is generally less florid, but rare cases mimic ABO-incompatible allografts.

Reperfusion biopsy specimens more often contain platelet aggregates in the portal and/or central veins than cross-match negative controls do, but red blood cell congestion is not usually a significant finding.[212,260] Spotty acidophilic necrosis of hepatocytes and centrilobular hepatocellular swelling, accompanied by cholangiolar proliferation and hepatocanalicular cholestasis, often appear during the first week after transplantation. Inflammatory or necrotizing arteritis is rare.[212,260]

The gross appearance of failed ABO-incompatible grafts at the time of retransplantation is similar to that of other organ allografts undergoing "hyperacute" rejection: they are enlarged, cyanotic, and mottled with areas of necrosis.[210,240] Rupture of the capsule is occasionally seen. Hepatic artery or portal vein thrombosis is not uncommon. Hilar changes include congestion of the peribiliary vascular plexus, partially organized thrombi in arterial branches, and focal mural necrosis of large septal bile ducts.[212,260] Long-term sequelae of an early antibody-mediated insult can include biliary sludge and strictures with obstructive cholangiopathy, as well as obliterative arteriopathy and loss of small bile ducts, or chronic rejection.

Immune deposits are ephemeral in antibody-mediated rejection. Even in allografts known to be affected, deposits are generally detectable only in postreperfusion biopsy specimens and for a few days after transplantation. Thereafter, immune deposits become patchy in distribution and may be difficult to distinguish from background staining. In our experience, the immunofluorescence findings can be used to support the diagnosis of antibody-mediated rejection, but by themselves are uncommonly diagnostic. IgM and C1q alone frequently become lodged in necrotic arterial walls, regardless of the cause of damage, and therefore should not be interpreted as evidence of antibody-mediated rejection. Portal capillary staining for C4d, which is a reliable marker of antibody-mediated rejection in kidney allografts,[263,264] has been detected in liver allografts with primarily cell-mediated rejection.[265] This finding suggests that antibody-mediated injury also contributes to liver allograft damage in "cell-mediated" rejection. However, more work on the significance of C4d deposits in liver allografts is needed. In florid cases of antibody-mediated rejection, there are focal deposits of IgG or IgM (or both) and C3 and C4 in perihilar arteries, portal veins, and the peribiliary plexus, along with diffuse sinusoidal staining. These deposits do not contain α_2-macroglobulin or other macromolecules.

Differential Diagnosis. Severe antibody-mediated rejection in an ABO-incompatible organ is difficult to distinguish from hemorrhagic liver necrosis caused by severe hypotension, sepsis, or vascular thrombosis.[210,212,240,266,267] The distinction is often based on the results of clinicopathological correlation and immunofluorescence analysis rather than the routine histopathological findings.

Knowing that the allograft is ABO blood group incompatible, recognizing the injury described earlier, and correlating the findings with the clinical course often provide enough information to confidently distinguish between these entities.

Antibody-mediated rejection is difficult to differentiate from preservation injury in ABO-compatible organs, although knowing the presensitization state and posttransplant clinical profile will prompt further appropriate testing (see "Clinical Features"). The typical clinical profile of patients in whom antibody-mediated rejection develops shortly after transplantation includes a high titer of pretransplant antidonor antibodies, followed by persistent hyperbilirubinemia and refractory and otherwise unexplained thrombocytopenia and low complement levels despite a short cold ischemic time.[257]

Acute Rejection

Acute (cellular) rejection has been defined as "inflammation of the allograft, elicited by a genetic disparity between the donor and recipient, primarily affecting interlobular bile ducts and vascular endothelia, including portal and hepatic veins and occasionally the hepatic artery and its branches."[234] Most episodes occur within 30 days after transplantation and are precipitated by mass migration of donor cells into recipient lymphoid tissues.[82,83] These early acute rejection episodes are usually controlled easily by increased immunosuppression and rarely lead to allograft failure.[18,122,125,268]

Risk factors for the development of acute rejection within the first several months depend on the immunosuppressive regimen but generally include younger recipient age; "healthier" recipients (e.g., normal serum creatinine, lower pretransplant Model for End-Stage Liver Disease [MELD] score); donor/recipient HLA-DR mismatch; patients with immune-dysregulated syndromes, such as PSC, autoimmune hepatitis, and PBC; long cold ischemic time; and increased donor age.[122,125,232] Late-onset acute rejection occurring more than 1 year after transplantation is often associated with inadequate immunosuppression, may be more difficult to control, and more frequently leads to allograft failure.[18,126,159,161]

Pathophysiology. Recognition of the allograft as foreign through central and peripheral sensitization, discussed earlier, triggers a cascade of events that change the microenvironment of the allograft. Local secretion of cytokines and chemokines alters the expression of various MHC, adhesion, and costimulatory molecules on various cell populations within the liver (see Fig. 69–4 and Table 69–5). This results in the retention of more inflammatory cells within the graft, especially in the portal tracts and perivenular tissue. The biliary epithelia of small bile ducts and the endothelia of the portal and central veins and the hepatic artery branches (in severe rejection) are preferentially targeted for injury.

Various immunological effector mechanisms contribute to graft injury during acute rejection. Antibody- and complement-mediated injury, cytolytic T-cell lympholysis (Fas-FasL interactions), and effector molecules and cytokines released from various inflammatory cells (e.g., TNF, eosinophil cationic protein, reactive oxygen species) can directly injure bile ducts[269] and endothelial cells, which in turn can interfere with blood flow and indirectly lead to ischemic injury.[96] The exuberance of inflammation and the severity of damage are used to histologically grade acute rejection. The most feared consequence of acute rejection is rapid allograft failure, which usually occurs because of immunologically mediated microcirculatory failure and poor arterial flow or thrombosis. The second most feared, but relatively uncommon complication of acute rejection is the development of fibrosis and chronic rejection.[127]

Clinical Features. Acute rejection generally first occurs between 5 and 30 days after transplantation, although earlier or later occurrence can be seen in presensitized patients or in those who receive less than optimal baseline immunosuppression. Clinical findings are often absent in early or mild acute rejection, although in late or severe cases, fever as well as enlargement, cyanosis, and tenderness of the allograft frequently occurs. Bile draining from the T tube often becomes thin and pale, and flow is decreased. Ascites develops occasionally because of increased intrahepatic pressure, liver swelling, and enhanced production of lymphatic fluid.[270]

Liver dysfunction is usually manifested as concomitant nonselective elevations in some or all of the standard liver injury tests, including total bilirubin, ALT, AST, γ-GTP, and alkaline phosphatase.[270] Peripheral blood leukocytosis and eosinophilia are also frequently present.[226,227,271] Biochemical tests of peripheral blood often show elevation in various interleukin levels or their receptors, neopterin, amyloid A protein, and antidonor class I MHC antibodies.[26,254,272-274] Unfortunately, all the clinical and laboratory findings lack sensitivity or specificity. The diagnosis is suspected on clinical grounds and confirmed by examination of a core needle biopsy specimen, which has become the "gold standard" method of establishing the diagnosis.

The decision to increase immunosuppressive therapy is usually based on a combination of clinical and histopathological parameters. Patients with indeterminate and mild acute rejection *without* significant liver function abnormalities are not generally treated with increased immunosuppression, and this approach does not appear to put the patient at risk for later complications.[18,268,275,276] Patients with mild acute rejection who show significant liver function abnormalities and those with moderate or severe acute rejection are usually treated with increased immunosuppression because of a small, but definite increased risk for graft loss and the development of chronic rejection.[18,277,278]

Histopathological Findings and Grading. There is little controversy regarding the histopathology of acute rejection, and most groups report similar, if not identical findings.* Acute rejection is characterized by (1) predominantly mononuclear, but mixed portal inflammation containing blastic or activated lymphocytes, neutrophils, and eosinophils; (2) subendothelial inflammation of portal or terminal hepatic venules (or both); and (3) bile duct inflammation and damage.[270] *Minimal diagnostic criteria needed to establish the diagnosis of acute rejection include at least two of the aforementioned histopathological findings.* The diagnosis is strengthened if greater than 50% of the ducts or central veins are damaged or if unequivocal endotheliitis of the portal or terminal hepatic vein branches can be identified.[270] Histopathological findings associated with severe injury (and used for histopathological grading) include perivenular inflammation, centrilobular necrosis, arteritis, and inflammatory bridging.[18,118]

The composition and location of inflammation are important features used to recognize acute rejection and are dependent on the immunosuppressive protocol. Blastic and smaller mononuclear cells are usually the majority population, but eosinophils are often conspicuous and can predominate in patients treated with "steroid-sparing" immunosuppressive regimens (Fig. 69–9).[226,227] Mononuclear cells tunnel beneath the portal and central vein endothelium (Figs. 69–9 and 69–10), a process referred to as "endotheliitis" or "endothelialitis." This much-publicized feature of acute rejection can be seen with other causes of allograft dysfunction and should not be relied on too heavily, particularly if it is only a focal finding.

Immunophenotypic analysis of acute rejection infiltrates shows a predominance of T lymphocytes dominated by the CD8[+] subset in the portal tracts, particularly in damaged bile ducts.[99,288-290] Minority populations of B cells, macrophages, and other leukocytes are also present,[99,100,102,288,291] including occasional donor and recipient dendritic cells. In general, immunohistochemical analysis of the portal infiltrate is not clinically useful, except when distinguishing between acute rejection (T cell predominant) and a posttransplant lymphoproliferative disorder (PTLD) (B cell predominant; also see "Differential Diagnosis").

Inflammatory damage to small bile ducts is manifested by the presence of lymphocytes inside the basement membrane in association with biliary epithelial cell alterations such as paranuclear vacuolization, an increased nuclear-to-cytoplasmic ratio, mitoses, nucleoli, occasional apoptotic bodies, and cytoplasmic eosinophilia. There is also decreased expression of bcl-2 in the biliary epithelial cells during acute rejection.[292] Luminal disruption with breaks in the basement membrane signifies severe bile duct damage. Peribiliary granulomas are not a feature of either acute or chronic rejection; in our experience, their presence is indicative of a non–rejection-related cause of duct injury (e.g., recurrent PBC).

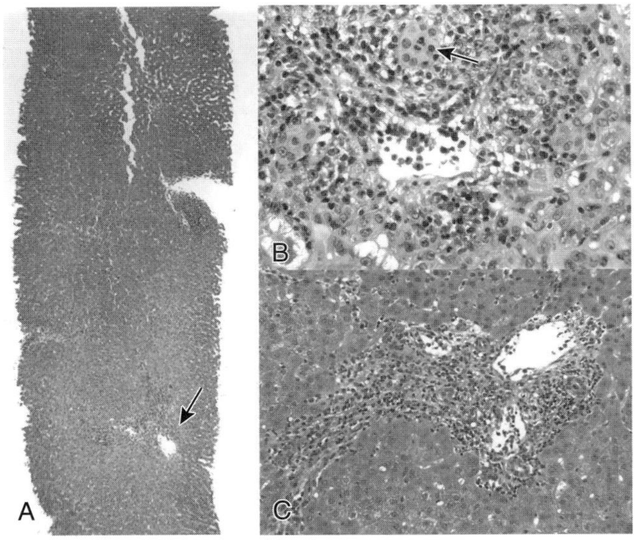

FIGURE 69–9

Mild acute cellular rejection. **A**, Note that the portal tracts are mildly expanded because of a predominantly mononuclear, but mixed portal inflammation. **B**, This high magnification of a portal tract shows the typical "rejection infiltrate." It is composed of blastic and smaller lymphocytes, eosinophils, macrophages, and occasional plasma cells. Note also the presence of lymphocytes inside the basement membrane of the small bile duct (*arrow*) and the subendothelial localization of lymphocytes in a small portal vein branch. The portal tract highlighted by the *arrow* in **A** is shown at higher magnification in **C**. Note the subendothelial infiltration of the portal vein and the inflammation and damage in small bile ducts.

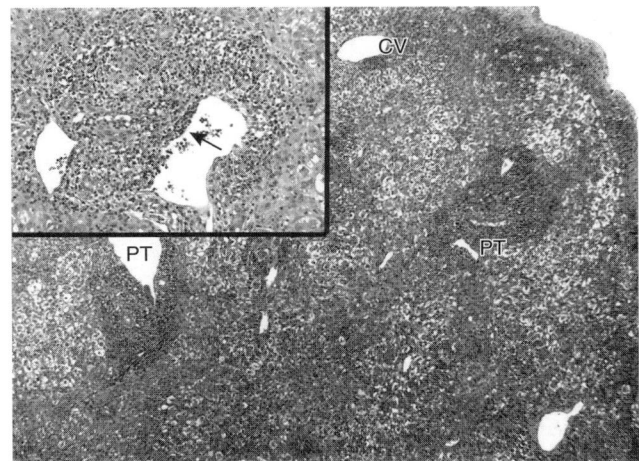

FIGURE 69–10

Moderate acute cellular rejection. Note that virtually all the portal tracts are markedly expanded by a predominantly mononuclear, but mixed inflammation. CV, central vein; PT, portal tract. Note also the absence of centrilobular inflammation and hepatocyte necrosis and dropout. The *inset* shown at the upper left corner of the image illustrates the composition of the typical "rejection infiltrate" and subendothelial localization of lymphocytes in a small portal vein branch (*arrow*).

---

*See references 8, 9, 11-13, 24, 36, 224, 225, 273, 274, 279-287.

Small portal tract arteries and arterioles are difficult to locate during acute rejection. Endothelial swelling and mural hypertrophy are most commonly observed when the arteries are found. Inflammatory or necrotizing arteritis is an important feature used to recognize and grade severe acute rejection (Fig. 69–11), but the vessels most commonly affected are located in the hilum and are not usually accessible by needle biopsy. However, histopathological recognition of arteritis in peripheral needle biopsy specimens is poorly reproducible.[293] Therefore, arteritis is not generally included in grading schema unless it is unequivocally identified in an artery branch containing an internal elastic lamina.

Lobular findings include mild Kupffer cell hypertrophy and a slight increase in inflammatory cells in the sinusoids. Infiltration of the sinusoids and connective tissue surrounding the central vein by cells similar to the portal tract infiltrate, or so-called central venulitis, can be seen in up to 30% of acute rejection episodes. In severe acute rejection, zonal centrilobular congestion, hemorrhage, and hepatocyte necrosis and dropout accompany the perivenular inflammation (see Fig. 69–11).

Occasionally, acute rejection can be manifested as predominantly or exclusively perivenular inflammation.[294-296] This form of acute rejection is usually associated with perivenular hepatocyte necrosis and dropout,

hemorrhage, and pigmented macrophages (Fig. 69–12) and in severe cases can lead to perivenular fibrosis and a Budd-Chiari or veno-occlusive–like clinical syndrome.[18,206,297-299] In fact, early acute rejection can be missed clinically and histologically, only to be manifested later as ascites associated with bland perivenular fibrosis.[18,206,297-299]

Several well-known systems have been used to grade acute rejection,[8,36,277,281-287,300-303] but the Banff schema represents the consensus opinion of a group of recognized expert liver transplant pathologists, hepatologists, and surgeons from many of the major hepatic transplant centers in North America, Europe, and Asia.[118] It incorporates concepts from these earlier systems that satisfied requirements for simplicity, reproducibility, scientific correctness, and clinical utility.[8,36,277,281-287,300-303] The earliest and one of the most influential systems was derived from fundamental observations by K.A. Porter, who did much of the pioneering work in liver transplantation pathology.[8] He recognized that the combination of typical portal tract changes associated with rejection, along with

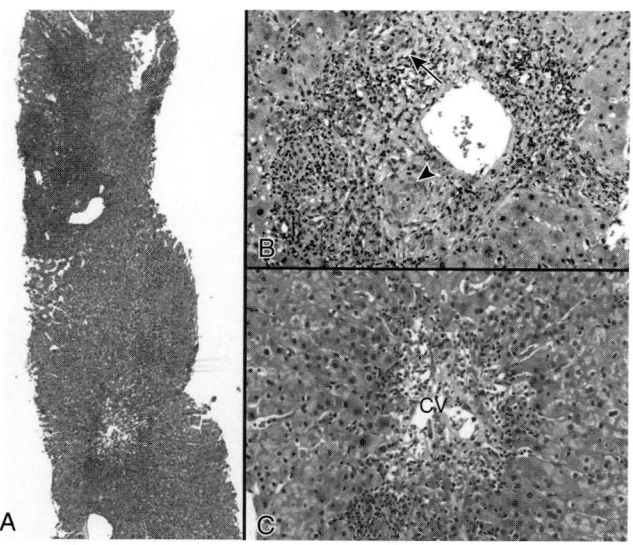

FIGURE 69–11

Severe acute cellular rejection. **A,** Note the severe expansion of the portal tracts because of inflammation with focal portal-to-portal bridging. Note also the perivenular inflammation and hepatocyte necrosis and dropout. **B,** A higher magnification of an atypical portal tract shows inflammation and damage to small bile ducts (*arrow*). In addition, note the fibrinoid necrosis of a small hepatic artery branch (*arrowhead*). **C,** A higher magnification of the centrilobular area shows perivenular inflammation, congestion, and hepatocyte necrosis and dropout. This lesion, when combined with typical rejection-related findings in the portal tracts, is diagnostic of severe acute cellular rejection. CV, central vein.

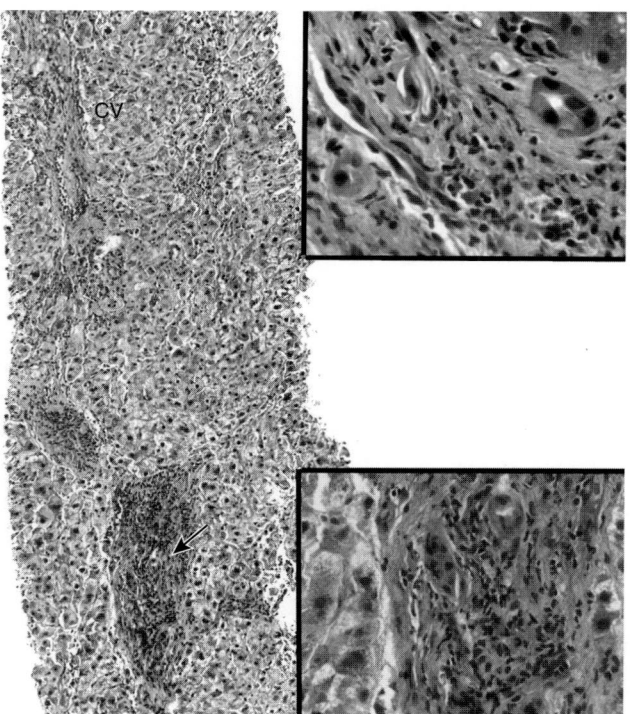

FIGURE 69–12

Early chronic rejection is characterized by mild portal inflammation (*arrow*) in association with ongoing bile duct damage and senescence-related changes in the biliary epithelium. Note the mild perivenular fibrosis. The upper right and lower right *insets* show the senescence-related changes in biliary epithelial cells, which are typical of early chronic rejection. Note the eosinophilic transformation of the biliary epithelial cytoplasm, which is frequently associated with uneven nuclear spacing and ducts only partially lined by biliary epithelial cells. CV, central vein.

Table 69-7. BANFF GRADING OF ACUTE LIVER ALLOGRAFT REJECTION

Global Assessment*	Criteria
Indeterminate	Portal inflammatory infiltrate that fails to meet criteria for the diagnosis of acute rejection (see text)
Mild	Rejection infiltrate in a minority of the triads that is generally mild and confined within the portal spaces
Moderate	Rejection infiltrate expanding most or all of the triads
Severe	As above for moderate, with spillover into the periportal areas and moderate to severe perivenular inflammation that extends into the hepatic parenchyma and is associated with perivenular hepatocyte necrosis

*Global assessment of the rejection grade made on a review of the biopsy specimen and after the diagnosis of rejection has been established. A verbal description of mild, moderate, or severe acute rejection could also be labeled as grade I, II, and III, respectively.
From Banff schema for grading liver allograft rejection: An international consensus document. Hepatology 25:658-663, 1997.

centrilobular inflammation and hepatocyte necrosis and dropout, was a poor prognostic feature that can be used to identify severe acute rejection (see Fig. 69–11).[8] This constellation of findings was first described in untreated canine liver allograft recipients by Brock[1] and Dammin[2] and their colleagues.

The Banff schema (Tables 69-7 and 69-8) includes the descriptive grades indeterminate, mild, moderate, and severe and a semiquantitative rejection activity index (RAI).[118] The latter component, adopted from the European grading system,[277] is the conceptual equivalent of the hepatitis activity index.[304] The RAI scores the prevalence and severity of three separate features on a scale of 0 to 3: portal inflammation, bile duct damage, and subendothelial inflammation. These components are then added together for a total RAI score.

In general, the higher the total RAI score, the more severe the rejection episode[18] and the more likely is graft failure from acute rejection and the development of chronic rejection.[18,118,277,278,302,305] In the Banff schema, the total RAI score for indeterminate acute rejection usually ranges between 1 and 2. Mild acute rejection biopsy specimens score between 3 and 4, moderate between 5 and 6, and those with severe acute rejection usually attain a total RAI score of greater than 6. Although the maximum possible total is 9, biopsy specimens are rarely scored this high.[18] Instead, most episodes of acute rejection are mild, have a total RAI score less than 6, respond to increased immunosuppression, and do not lead to significant fibrosis, bile duct loss, or arteriopathy in subsequent or follow-up biopsies.[18]

Additional immunosuppression should not be given before a biopsy specimen is obtained because histopathological interpretation is made more difficult. Treatment with increased immunosuppression may cause some of the infiltrate to subside within 24 hours; subendothelial infiltration of the veins is one of the first findings affected. In addition, centrilobular hepatocyte swelling and hepatocanalicular cholestasis may also appear after treatment. However, it usually takes 7 to 10 days after treatment for the changes to completely resolve.

Differential Diagnosis. The differential diagnosis for acute rejection depends on the time after transplantation. Acute rejection can be distinguished from preservation injury and acute cholangitis during the first several months by several key features, as discussed earlier.

Acute rejection can be particularly difficult to differentiate from recurrence of viral hepatitis B or C between 3 and 10 weeks after liver transplantation. Acute rejection and recurrent viral hepatitis show predominantly mononuclear portal inflammation, bile duct damage, and Kupffer cell hypertrophy with variable acidophilic necrosis of hepatocytes. Distinction is achieved by closely examining the severity and prevalence of the bile duct damage, interface activity, lobular changes, and perivenular inflammation and hepatocyte dropout. In acute rejection, inflammatory bile duct damage and perivenular inflammation, if present, usually involve a majority of the ducts and central veins. In contrast, bile ducts are only occasionally damaged in recurrent viral hepatitis, and perivenular inflammation, if present, involves a minority of the central veins. Conversely, interface activity involves most of the portal tracts, and the lobular changes are more severe and conspicuous in recurrent hepatitis. More than 10 weeks after transplantation, distinguishing between chronic viral or autoimmune hepatitis and rejection is not usually a problem and is based on these same features.

More than 6 months after transplantation, acute rejection must also be distinguished from chronic biliary tract strictures, PTLD, and recurrent viral or autoimmune hepatitis. Chronic biliary tract strictures can produce histopathological findings in peripheral core needle biopsy specimens that are virtually indistinguishable from those of acute rejection. In such cases, it is helpful to remember that acute rejection occurring more than 6 months after transplantation is unusual in patients with adequate immunosuppression. Therefore, simply checking blood levels of baseline immunosuppressive drugs and the liver injury test profile often provides sufficient data to suggest a cholangiogram before increasing immunosuppressive therapy.

Table 69–8. ACUTE REJECTION ACTIVITY INDEX

Category	Criteria	Score
Portal inflammation	Mostly lymphocytic inflammation involving, but not noticeably expanding, a minority of the triads	1
	Expansion of most or all of the triads by a mixed infiltrate containing lymphocytes with occasional blasts, neutrophils, and eosinophils	2
	Marked expansion of most or all of the triads by a mixed infiltrate containing numerous blasts and eosinophils with inflammatory spillover into the periportal parenchyma	3
Bile duct inflammation damage	A minority of the ducts are cuffed and infiltrated by inflammatory cells and show only mild reactive changes such as an increased nuclear-to-cytoplasmic ratio of the epithelial cells	1
	Most or all of the ducts infiltrated by inflammatory cells. More than an occasional duct shows degenerative changes such as nuclear pleomorphism, disordered polarity, and cytoplasmic vacuolization of the epithelium	2
	As above for the 2nd criterion, with most or all of the ducts showing degenerative changes or focal luminal disruption	3
Venous endothelial inflammation	Subendothelial lymphocytic infiltration involving some, but not a majority, of the portal and/or hepatic venules	1
	Subendothelial infiltration involving most or all of the portal and/or hepatic venules	2
	As above for the 2nd criterion, with moderate or severe perivenular inflammation that extends into the perivenular parenchyma and is associated with perivenular hepatocyte necrosis	3

Note: The total score equals the sum of the components. Criteria that can be used to score liver allograft biopsy specimens with acute rejection were defined by the World Gastroenterology Consensus Document.
From Banff schema for grading liver allograft rejection: An international consensus document. Hepatology 25:658-663, 1997.

Subtle histopathological clues that favor chronic biliary strictures over acute rejection include sinusoidal clusters of neutrophils, periportal deposition of elemental copper, centrilobular hepatocanalicular cholestasis, and lamellar periductal edema involving any of the sampled bile ducts. Distinguishing viral or autoimmune hepatitis from rejection in specimens obtained more than 6 months after transplantation is based on the same guidelines proposed at earlier time points.

Chronic Rejection

Chronic rejection has been defined as an immunological injury to the liver allograft that usually evolves from severe or persistent acute rejection and results in potentially irreversible damage to the bile ducts, arteries, and veins.[124,127,270,306-309] It currently affects less than 3% of liver allograft recipients by 5 years after transplantation, which is a dramatic decrease since the 1980s, when the incidence was 15% to 20%.[310] The decline is probably attributable to better recognition and control of acute and the early phases of chronic rejection, combined with the unique immunological properties of liver allografts and the remarkable ability of the liver to regenerate without fibrosis.[140,230,306-308,311-315] Nevertheless, chronic rejection has not been entirely eliminated and is still an important cause of late liver allograft dysfunction and failure.[25,170,197,220,316,317]

The term "chronic" technically implies a time parameter, but none is intended[270] because chronic rejection often occurs within several months after transplantation and allograft failure typically occurs within the first year after transplantation.[124,306,308,318,319] In contrast to other vascularized allografts, the incidence of chronic rejection in the liver does not appear to increase with time after transplantation.[124,319,320] There is, however, a small group of patients with late-onset chronic rejection. These patients usually suffer from complications of overimmunosuppression, and the baseline drugs are often decreased or discontinued altogether because of immunosuppression-related complications.[124] Older terms for chronic rejection such as "vanishing bile duct syndrome" or "ductopenic rejection" are fading from use because bile duct loss is now recognized as just one histopathological feature of chronic rejection.[127,270]

Risk factors have usually been divided into two general categories. The first and most important are "alloantigen-dependent," immunological, or rejection-related factors. Among these risk factors, the number and severity of acute rejection episodes are the most significant,[18,124,299,308] regardless of the immunosuppressive regimen. In cyclosporine-treated cohorts, late-onset acute rejection episodes,[126,231,306,321] younger recipient age,[306,308] male-to-female sex mismatch, a primary diagnosis of autoimmune hepatitis or biliary disease,[308] baseline immunosuppression,[231,314,322] interactions between HLA-DR3, TNF-2 status, and cytomegalovirus (CMV) infection,[323] and nonwhite recipient race[123,306,324] have all been associated with an increased risk for chronic rejection. The role of histocompatibility differences is still controversial,[261,306,324-328] as is the effect of CMV infection.[122,123,231,306,320,323,327-329]

Many of the matching factors just described for cyclosporine-treated patients were not a significant risk factor for chronic rejection in a large tacrolimus-treated cohort, but the influence of the number and severity of acute rejection episodes was similar.[124] Non–alloantigen-dependent or "nonimmunological" risk factors that contribute to the development of chronic rejection include donor age older than 40 years.[124] Older donor organs have also been found to have a higher incidence of acute rejection.[122]

Pathophysiology. Because chronic rejection primarily evolves from severe or multiple recurrent and uncontrolled acute rejection episodes,[18,124,299,308] many of the immunological mechanisms of injury discussed for acute rejection are likely to be relevant to chronic rejection. Instead of hepatocyte and biliary epithelial cell proliferation and architecturally correct repair, bile ducts are destroyed, perivenular and portal fibrosis develops, and arteries narrow.[127,298]

The bile duct damage and loss in chronic rejection are due to a combination of direct immunological damage by the effector mechanisms of rejection and indirect ischemic damage because of obliterative arteriopathy, small artery/arteriolar loss, and destruction of the peribiliary capillary plexus.[330-332] The cumulative damage results in enhanced biliary epithelial cell senescence[229] manifested as distinct cytological changes recognizable on routine light microscopy and enhanced expression of nuclear p21 without Ki-67 labeling.[229] These changes precede bile duct loss.[127,308] Any factors that can lessen the damage associated with acute rejection, such as treatment with increased immunosuppression, or that foster nonfibrogenic repair reactions have the potential to lessen the impact of chronic rejection.

There is increased hepatocyte expression of Fas, FasL, and CD40 associated with dropout of centrilobular hepatocytes during chronic rejection.[333] It is thought that CD40 activation induces apoptosis via Fas because ligation of CD40 upregulates hepatocyte FasL expression.

Paul[158] summarized the various hypotheses used to explain the pathogenic mechanisms leading from immunological tissue injury to the development of chronic rejection in renal allografts. These hypotheses can be extrapolated to the liver and are useful in conceptualizing approaches to therapeutic intervention. Fundamental to all of them is acceptance of the premise that *chronic rejection develops as a pathogenic "response to injury," similar to atherosclerosis.*[105,129,334] The basic algorithm is as follows:

Severe or persistent immunological injury →
Disruption of normal structure → Fibrogenic repair response → Parenchymal fibrosis, loss of bile ducts, and obliterative arteriopathy

Because livers usually recover completely without fibrosis from acute transient immunological insults such as acute hepatitis, persistent immunological damage is usually needed for the development of chronic rejection.

The *immunolymphatic theory* of chronic rejection contends that freedom from chronic rejection requires robust tolerance, and because tolerance is a biological function of the immune system, the presence of the donor immune system (hematopoietic chimerism) is required.[155] An important component of the donor immune system is the various APCs that reside within the allograft and migrate to recipient lymphoid tissues.[155,335] They help maintain tolerance to the organ[155] and enable the organ to respond to environmental antigenic challenges.[155] Destruction of these cells by severe or persistent immunological injury has several consequences. It eliminates the possibility for robust tolerance, but also disrupts the egress of lymphatic cells and fluid that normally accumulate in the interstitium of the allograft. Such disruption compromises the normal response to environmental challenges such as infection. It also predisposes to the development of obliterative arteriopathy and interstitial fibrosis because cytokine- and growth factor–rich fluid stagnates in the allograft. Thus, normal physiology (i.e., production and reabsorption of lymph) is transformed into a driving force of tissue pathology.

The *cytokine excess theory* suggests that chronic rejection develops because of excessive scar formation in response to the tissue injury.[158] Evidence supporting this contention includes the correlation between high intragraft transforming growth factor-β (TGF-β) production and increased risk for late graft failure.[121,133,336-342] Although most studies have focused on TGF-β because of its role in fibrogenesis, additional mediators will become the focus of study as their role in organ repair reactions becomes clarified.

The *loss of supporting architecture theory*[158] is based on the concept that repair processes, such as epithelial cell regeneration after injury, are dependent on the three-dimensional stromal framework, including the basement membrane. Destruction of the supporting architecture by severe injury compromises repair responses. Parenchymal cells that would normally migrate and divide to repair a defect might undergo apoptosis. The net effect is a tendency for the development of excessive scarring of the allograft in response to injury.

The *premature senescence theory*[158,322] suggests that the excessive fibrosis associated with chronic rejection might be the result of accelerated aging of allograft parenchymal and endothelial cells. Such aging occurs as a consequence of exposure to multiple stressors, such as organ harvesting, implantation, and rejection episodes, that subject these cell populations to ischemia, oxidative damage, and increased demand for cell division. Over time, parenchymal and endothelial

Table 69-9. FEATURES OF EARLY AND LATE CHRONIC LIVER ALLOGRAFT REJECTION

Structure	Early CR	Late CR
Small bile ducts (< 60 μm)	Bile duct loss in < 50% of portal tracts Degenerative change involving a majority of ducts: eosinophilic transformation of cytoplasm, nuclear hyperchromasia, uneven nuclear spacing, ducts only partially lined by biliary epithelial cells	Loss in ≥ 50% of portal tracts Degenerative changes in remaining bile ducts
Terminal hepatic venules and zone 3 hepatocytes	Intimal/luminal inflammation Lytic zone 3 necrosis and inflammation Mild perivenular fibrosis	Focal obliteration Variable inflammation Severe perivenular fibrosis, defined as central-to-central bridging fibrosis
Portal tract hepatic arterioles	Occasional loss involving < 25% of portal tracts	Loss involving > 25% of portal tracts
Other	So-called transition hepatitis with spotty necrosis of hepatocytes	Sinusoidal foam cell accumulation; marked cholestasis
Large perihilar bile ducts	Inflammation damage and focal foam cell deposition	Mural fibrosis

Adapted from Demetris A, Adams D, Bellamy C, et al: Update of the International Banff Schema for Liver Allograft Rejection: Working recommendations for the histopathologic staging and reporting of chronic rejection. An International Panel. Hepatology 31:792-799, 2000.

cells reach their Hayflick limit,[343,344] and similar to normal aged organs, allografts display a propensity to heal by fibrosis. This hypothesis is partially supported by studies showing that bile duct loss in chronic rejection is preceded by a period of biliary epithelial cell replicative senescence,[229] described later. However, rather than senescence induced by Hayflick limitations, the inability of the biliary epithelium and hepatocytes to proliferate and repair may be related to a toxic microenvironment, which is treatable. Cytokines and growth factors, such as TGF-β, as well as the baseline immunosuppressive agent, can inhibit hepatocyte and biliary epithelial cell regeneration.[229]

All the hypotheses just presented are likely to be valid to some extent and highlight mechanisms that contribute to various aspects of chronic rejection. Common to all is a central theme of severe or persistent tissue injury and abnormal repair. Regardless of the specific mechanism or mechanisms contributing to its development, it seems clear that limiting the severity or persistence (or both) of the immunological injury will be the most effective way of preventing chronic rejection.[158]

Clinical Features. A clinical diagnosis of chronic rejection is usually suspected after progressive cholestasis and an increase in canalicular enzymes that is unresponsive to antirejection treatment develop in a patient with a history of acute rejection.[270] Chronic rejection typically occurs in three clinical settings: (1) the end stage of unresolved acute rejection, (2) after multiple episodes of acute rejection,* and (3) indolent evolution without preceding clinically recognized episodes of

acute rejection.† The first two scenarios are by far the most common and usually occur within the first year after transplantation. The last situation is relatively uncommon and may simply reflect inadequate monitoring. Late-onset chronic rejection occurring more than 1 year after transplantation is typically seen in inadequately immunosuppressed patients, either because of noncompliance or because immunosuppression had to be lowered as a result of infectious, neoplastic, or toxic complications of overimmunosuppression.[124]

Unresolved or indolent rejection may become apparent only because of a persistent elevation in liver injury test values. If clinical symptoms are present, they usually resemble those of acute rejection until the allograft dysfunction becomes severe enough to cause jaundice. Biliary sludging or the appearance of biliary strictures, hepatic infarcts, and finally loss of hepatic synthetic function, which can be manifested as coagulopathy and malnutrition, are other late findings presaging allograft failure.[270]

Standard liver injury tests in patients with chronic rejection usually show a progressive cholestatic pattern manifested as preferential elevation of γ-GTP and alkaline phosphatase.[220,270,348] Transition from acute to chronic rejection may be marked by a persistent elevation in ALT and total bilirubin that presage allograft failure.[124,294,308]

Histopathological Findings and Staging. The portal tracts and perivenular regions are primarily affected by chronic rejection, and changes in these areas are divided into "early" and "late" stages (Table 69-9).

---

*See references 7,11, 124, 270, 281, 298, 299, 306-309, 318, 330, 345, 346.

†See references 7, 11, 124, 270, 281, 298, 299, 306-309, 318, 330, 345-347.

Portal tract alterations in early chronic rejection include mild lymphocytic cholangitis, which leads to biliary epithelial cell senescence changes (see Fig. 69–12), eventually followed by loss of small bile ducts in the later stages (Figs. 69–13 and 69–14). When compared with acute rejection, the portal inflammation in chronic rejection is usually less severe and contains primarily lymphocytes and plasma cells. Mast cells are increased in some cases.[349] Eosinophils are much less common than in acute rejection.

Distinct histopathological changes of biliary epithelial cell senescence[229] presage bile duct loss.[294,307,312,350] These changes include eosinophilic transformation of the biliary epithelial cytoplasm, uneven nuclear spacing, syncytia formation, nuclear enlargement and hyperchromasia resembling cytological dysplasia (see Fig. 69–12), and ducts only partially lined by biliary epithelial cells. The senescent biliary epithelial cells stain positive for p21[WAF1/Cip1] (but not for Ki-67), an inhibitor of cell cycle progression that becomes upregulated in cells under severe stress or showing replicative senescence.[229] Late-stage chronic rejection is manifested as bile duct and arteriolar loss, the severity of which is determined by quantitative morphometry.

In a normal liver, Crawford and colleagues[351] defined a portal tract as "a focus within the parenchyma containing connective tissue (by Masson trichrome stain) and at least two luminal structures embedded in the connective tissue mesenchyme, each with a continuous connective tissue circumference." Using this definition, 93% ± 6% and 91% ± 7% of portal tracts contain bile ducts and hepatic artery branches, respectively.[351]

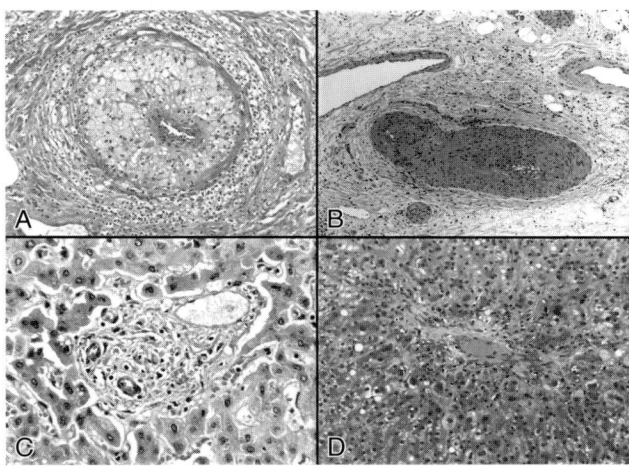

FIGURE 69–14

Specific features of late chronic rejection. **A**, Prominent foam cell arteriopathy is often seen with late chronic rejection and most frequently affects first- and second-order branches of the hepatic artery in the liver hilum. **B**, However, the foam cells can be replaced by intimal myofibroblasts that narrow the lumen, as shown in this example. **C**, Late chronic rejection is also characterized by bile duct loss affecting more than 50% of the portal tracts. Bile duct loss is recognized by comparing hepatic artery branches with bile ducts. More than 85% to 90% of hepatic artery branches should be accompanied by a bile duct of similar size. The presence of artery branches without bile ducts, as seen in this photomicrograph, is diagnostic of bile duct loss. **D**, Severe perivenular fibrosis with areas of focal central-to-central bridging is also frequently seen in late chronic rejection. It is often accompanied by severe centrilobular hepatocanalicular cholestasis and clusters of intralobular foam cells that are related to the cholestasis.

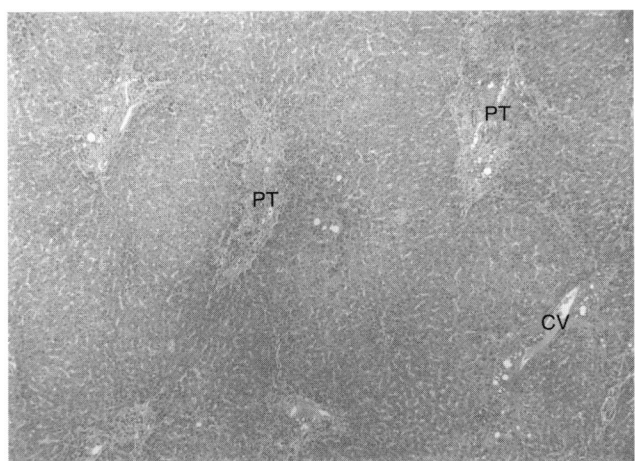

FIGURE 69–13

Late chronic rejection is characterized by little portal inflammation in conjunction with bile duct loss affecting more than 50% of the portal tracts and moderate or severe perivenular fibrosis. Note that well-developed cirrhosis is not seen, which is typical of most cases of late chronic rejection, although occasionally a micronodular pattern of cirrhosis can develop. CV, central vein; PT, portal tract.

Somewhat lower figures were cited by others using larger tissue samples.[330] If 2 SD from normal is used as a cutoff, bile duct loss is considered present when less than 80% of the portal tracts contain bile ducts; arterial loss is considered present when less than 77% of the portal tracts contain hepatic artery branches.

Because chronic rejection can result in loss of both bile duct and hepatic artery branches,[330-332] strict application of the aforementioned definition, which requires two of three normal portal profiles (bile duct, hepatic artery, and portal vein), is not possible in some cases. When both bile duct and arterial loss is seen, recognition and quantification of the portal tracts ultimately depend on the subjective interpretation of the pathologist. Recognition of portal tracts in such cases should be based primarily on the location (cholestasis in chronic rejection is centrilobular), shape, and internal structure of the connective tissue mesenchyme. If both bile ducts and arteries are destroyed, we recommend that determination of bile duct and arterial loss be based on a count of the total number of portal tracts with and without bile ducts and arteries and compared with expected values from normal livers. Despite the destruction of bile ducts, a ductular reaction[103,352,353] at the interface zone is unusual in chronic rejection, unless the liver is recovering from chronic rejection. In such cases, a ductular reaction at the interface zone usually precedes the regrowth of bile ducts.[306-308]

The early phase of chronic rejection in the terminal hepatic venules and surrounding perivenular parenchyma is characterized by subendothelial and perivenular mononuclear inflammation.[127,299] This inflammation is accompanied by perivenular hepatocyte dropout and an accumulation of pigment-laden macrophages and mild perivenular fibrosis.[124,298,299,308] Spotty acidophilic necrosis of hepatocytes, or so-called transitional hepatitis, may occur during the evolution from early to late stages of chronic rejection.[309]

Late chronic rejection is characterized by severe (bridging) perivenular fibrosis with at least focal central-to-central or central-to-portal bridging and occasional obliteration of terminal hepatic venules (see Figs. 69–13 and 69–14).[124,298,308] However, well-developed cirrhosis from chronic rejection is unusual[301] until the very late stages when venous obliteration leads to areas of parenchyma extinction.[298] True "regenerative" nodules are uncommon, perhaps because the combination of venous and arterial obliteration blunts any regenerative response.[195]

Other common findings in late chronic rejection include perivenular hepatocyte ballooning and dropout, centrilobular hepatocanalicular cholestasis, nodular regenerative hyperplasia–like changes, and intrasinusoidal foam cell clusters.* The clusters of foamy macrophages probably represent a nonspecific response to cholestasis and therefore, alone, are not diagnostic of chronic rejection.

The final diagnosis of chronic rejection should be based on various combinations of clinical, radiological, laboratory, and histopathological findings. In a biopsy specimen, the minimal diagnostic criteria for chronic rejection are (1) senescent changes affecting a majority of the bile ducts, with or without bile duct loss; (2) convincing foam cell obliterative arteriopathy; or (3) bile duct loss affecting more than 50% of the portal tracts.[127]

The diagnosis of chronic rejection is easier to establish in an explanted *failed allograft* because the characteristic sequential changes that develop in the branches of the hepatic arterial tree can be appreciated. Arteriopathy is usually seen in at least some of the muscular arteries in the hilum,† except in cases solely characterized by bile duct loss or perivenular fibrosis (or both).

Sequential changes in the hepatic arterial tree include a progressive accumulation of foamy macrophages that trigger the proliferation of donor-derived subintimal myofibroblasts (see Fig. 69–14).[354] The entire wall can be completely replaced by foam cells or completely obliterated in severely affected arteries and result in arterial thrombosis and subsequent necrosis of the large bile ducts. These changes are followed by thinning of the media as the arteries attempt to dilate and compensate for the reduced arterial flow. Eventually, the foam cells are replaced by intimal myofibroblasts.

Other alterations in the major hilar bile ducts include focal sloughing of the epithelium, papillary intraluminal hyperplasia, mural fibrosis, and acute and chronic inflammation.[355] Foamy macrophages may also be seen around bile ducts and veins in the connective tissue.

As with the grading of acute liver allograft rejection, the *staging of chronic rejection* (see Table 69–9) assumes that the diagnosis has already been correctly established.[127] *Early chronic rejection* implies that significant potential exists for recovery if the insult can be controlled or removed. *Late chronic rejection* suggests that potential for recovery is limited and that perhaps retransplantation should be considered. However, more study is needed in this area because it is not well established that all patients sequentially proceed in an orderly fashion from the early to the late stage of chronic rejection. Some patients appear to persist in the acute/early stage for months or years, whereas severe fibrosis and late changes rapidly develop in others. In addition, some patients show predominantly or exclusively either bile duct loss or foam cell arteriopathy alone, but usually both features are found together.[127,330,346,351]

The decision to proceed with retransplantation should be based on both clinical and histopathological parameters, such as a progressive decline in synthetic function, superimposed hepatic artery thrombosis, and bile duct necrosis or biliary sludging. The important practical implication of staging of chronic rejection is that the biopsy findings do not absolutely define a point of no return; they provide information about the likelihood of reversal. Thus, the decision to continue medical therapy or proceed with retransplantation should be based on a complete clinicopathological evaluation.

Differential Diagnosis. Considerable significance is placed on damage and loss of small bile ducts and perivenular fibrosis because arteries with pathognomonic changes are rarely present in needle biopsy specimens.[127] However, a similar pattern of duct injury and ductopenia can be a result of non–rejection-related complications such as obstructive cholangiopathy (including recurrent PSC), hepatic artery strictures or thrombosis, adverse drug reactions, and CMV infection.[99,294,348] Non–rejection-related causes of ductal injury and loss or perivenular fibrosis, which histopathologically appear similar to chronic rejection, should be reasonably excluded in cases of chronic rejection identified by biliary epithelial

---

*See references 7, 11, 12, 270, 281, 306, 319, 320, 330, 331, 345.
†See references 7, 8, 11, 12, 270, 281, 306, 319, 320, 330, 331, 345.

senescence or loss or perivenular fibrosis alone. Bile duct loss in some portal tracts accompanied by a ductular reaction in other portal tracts should raise suspicion of a biliary tract stricture. Cholangiography or angiography, or both, may be required in some cases to distinguish between chronic rejection and biliary obstruction.[294] In other cases, isolated ductopenia involving less than 50% of the portal tracts can be seen without significant elevations in liver injury test values.[124,308,356] Whether these uncommon cases are an early phase of chronic rejection is uncertain. Selective hepatic angiography showing pruning of the intrahepatic arteries with poor peripheral filling and segmental narrowing can also be used to support the diagnosis of chronic rejection.[270,305,319,357,358]

Isolated perivenular fibrosis can be caused by mechanical outflow obstruction, adverse drug reactions,[359] and all the nonrejection causes of veno-occlusive disease and Budd-Chiari syndrome in native livers.[360]

The safest approach to the diagnosis of chronic rejection in any setting is to review previous biopsy findings and closely correlate the histopathological findings with the clinical course. The usual scenario is a history of severe or unresolved acute rejection preceding the development of histological findings interpreted as chronic rejection.

Graft-versus-Host Disease

Pathophysiology

Acute graft-versus-host disease (GVHD) can occur after liver transplantation as a result of the large component of immunocompetent mature donor T cells in the passenger leukocyte pool[361-364] combined with a weakened recipient immune system.[365] Donor T cells respond to recipient MHC-bearing cells in the immature epithelial cell populations in the basal layers of the skin, gastrointestinal tract, liver, and lung. GVHD can further suppress recipient immunity and predispose to both bacterial and viral infection. In addition, donor B cells can produce antirecipient antibodies that cause lysis of recipient red blood and hematolymphoid cells.[177-179,366] GVHD can be particularly severe in children who receive a liver from parents who are homozygous at all HLA loci.[150]

Clinical Features

Patients in whom GVHD develops are usually seen in the first 6 months after transplantation with a fever, rash, and diarrhea.[143,151,367,368] We have also observed cases that occurred as long as 5 years after combined liver and small intestinal transplantation (unpublished observation). In mismatched ABO-compatible cases, GVHD disease can take the form of red blood cell hemolysis and pancytopenia.[366] A diagnosis of GVHD is confirmed by detailed analysis of a tissue biopsy specimen, usually taken from the skin or gastrointestinal tract.[369,370]

Histopathological Findings

The histopathological findings of GVHD in nonhepatic tissue are identical to those described for GVHD after bone marrow transplantation; the liver allograft is not susceptible to GVHD. In the skin, a mild, mixed lymphocytic and eosinophilic infiltrate appears in the upper reticular and papillary dermis. It is typically associated with lymphocytic exocytosis, spongiosis, and acidophilic necrosis of individual keratinocytes. Epithelial cells surrounded by lymphocytes, or "satellitosis," is a helpful feature. In the intestines, there is usually no increase in inflammatory cells above those already present. Instead, apoptosis of crypt epithelial cells without viral inclusions is the typical finding. Severe GVHD in the intestine is manifested as crypt abscesses with focal crypt destruction and, ultimately, as areas of mucosal necrosis and sloughing. Severe GVHD in the skin is characterized by bullae and epidermal sloughing.

Differential Diagnosis

The two most common syndromes mimicking acute GVHD in the skin are adverse drug reactions and viral exanthems.[369] In the gastrointestinal tract, GVHD is most similar to CMV or other causes of viral enteritis. Differentiation of GVHD from these entities by routine histopathological findings alone is extremely difficult, if not impossible. In addition to a detailed clinical history that includes a list of medications, possible allergies, and other infections, stains for CMV antigens, the use of anti-MHC monoclonal antibodies, or in situ hybridization for the X and Y chromosomes to distinguish between donor and recipient cells is needed in most cases.[143] The presence of an occasional donor cell in the skin or gastrointestinal tract is usual because of the hematolymphoid trafficking after transplantation and is not diagnostic of GVHD. The presence of many donor cells, preferentially distributed to the areas of tissue damage, confirms a diagnosis of GVHD.

Bacterial and Fungal Infections

Serious "opportunistic" fungal and viral infections generally occur within the first 2 months after transplantation.[371] Late-onset infections occurring after 6 months tend to be bacterial in origin. Early after transplantation the more serious opportunistic infections are attributable to the high levels of immunosuppression used to prevent rejection and stress from the operation. Although a high index of suspicion should always be maintained, clinical histories that should further arouse suspicion of an infection include fever, anastomotic or wound dehiscence, retransplantation, persistent abdominal pain, and vascular thrombosis. The following discussion is limited to infections involving the allograft.

Bacterial and fungal infections most commonly arise in nonviable tissue, which should be routinely subjected to special stains for bacteria and fungi. Although inflammation and granulomas are always good markers of potential infection, they may or may not be present because of immunosuppression. Histopathological changes associated with common bacterial or fungal infections are well known to most surgical pathologists and will not be discussed. However, a familiarity with less common bacterial, superficial and deep fungal, and viral infections is suggested.

Viral Infections

Viral hepatitis types B and C are leading indications for liver transplantation worldwide. Because reinfection of the allograft is nearly universal in those with active viral replication before transplantation and because blood products are screened, HBV and HCV infections are largely restricted to those who had these viruses before transplantation. However, new cases that develop after transplantation are not rare.[372] The manifestations and evolution of hepatitis B and C in liver allografts are similar to those seen in the general population, except that viral replication is enhanced and subsequent disease is usually more aggressive in allograft recipients. Markedly enhanced levels of viral replication can also lead to atypical clinical and histopathological manifestations, described later.

The immunosuppression needed to prevent rejection also renders liver allograft recipients vulnerable to hepatitis caused by "opportunistic" hepatitis viruses such as CMV, Epstein-Barr virus (EBV), herpes simplex virus (HSV) or varicella-zoster virus (VZV), and adenovirus. These viruses do not usually cause acute hepatitis in the general population. None of these "opportunistic" viruses cause chronic hepatitis that leads to fibrosis. Most liver allograft recipients, like the majority of the general population, have been infected and latently carry these opportunistic viruses. The exception is pediatric recipients and the minority of adults who have not been previously exposed. The CMV, EBV, HSV, and VZV disease that usually develops in these "naïve" patient populations after transplantation is more severe than in those with preexisting immunity. The onset of clinical disease is generally associated with enhanced viral replication, and therefore peripheral blood monitoring for viral antigens or nucleic acids is used to guide preemptive lowering of immunosuppression or treatment with specific antiviral agents.[373]

"Opportunistic" Hepatitis Viruses

Cytomegalovirus Hepatitis

Pathophysiology. CMV is the most commonly encountered opportunistic viral infection in liver allograft recipients, but effective prophylactic and preemptive therapy has greatly lessened the incidence and impact of symptomatic disease.[374-376] When symptomatic infection or disease does develop, it usually does so between 3 and 8 weeks after transplantation toward the end of or shortly after a cycle of increased immunosuppressive therapy used to treat acute rejection.[374,377] Disease may be the result of recrudescence in a carrier or be acquired by naïve recipients via transmission through blood products or the donor organ. Seronegative recipients who receive seropositive donor organs are at the greatest risk for the development of symptomatic disease.[378-387] Viral infection and latency in granulocytes or endothelial cells[388] and monocytes may explain the early appearance of viral antigens in sinusoidal cells.[378] CMV infection is thought to be a risk factor for hepatic artery thrombosis,[192,389,390] especially in pediatric patients, and for chronic rejection[123,231,233,323,329,391] and, possibly, aggressive hepatitis C recurrence.[392,393]

Clinical Features. Signs and symptoms of active CMV infection include fever, diarrhea and gastrointestinal ulcers, leukopenia, and low-grade hepatitis with modestly elevated liver injury test values.[378-387] Any organ system can be involved, depending on the extent of viral dissemination. Respiratory insufficiency and retinitis occur when the disease is severe. Occasionally, CMV can produce a syndrome that mimics EBV-associated PTLD, including mild liver function abnormalities, lymphadenopathy, fever, and atypical lymphocytosis.[378-387]

Histopathological Findings. The histopathological manifestations of active CMV infection depend, in part, on the immune status of the host. Any cell type of the liver may be infected in heavily immunosuppressed and untreated naïve allograft recipients. Large eosinophilic intranuclear inclusions surrounded by a clear halo and, occasionally, small basophilic or amphophilic cytoplasmic inclusions develop in the CMV-infected cells. Despite widespread CMV infestation of the liver allograft, submassive or massive necrosis from CMV alone has never been reported.[24,378-387]

In the occasional patient in whom active disease develops, CMV hepatitis is usually characterized by spotty lobular necrosis, Kupffer cell hypertrophy, and mild lobular disarray. Hepatocytes near the necrotic cells may contain nuclear or cytoplasmic inclusions, or both (Fig. 69–15), and are often surrounded by neutrophils (microabscess) or clusters of macrophages and lymphocytes (microgranulomas). In these days of prophylactic or preemptive therapy, well-formed intranuclear inclusions are rarely seen; instead, the

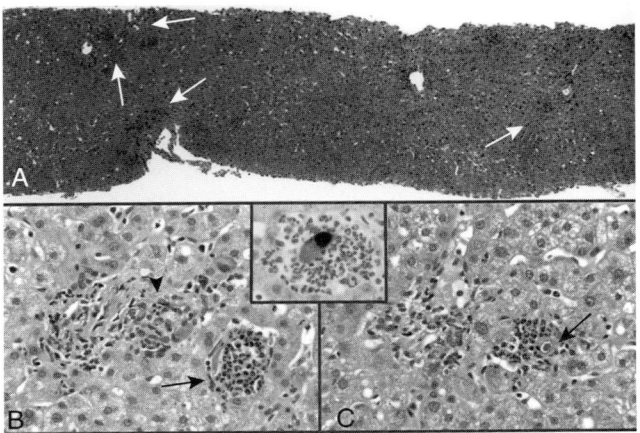

FIGURE 69-15

A, Cytomegalovirus (CMV) hepatitis is characterized by mild patchy portal and lobular inflammation that forms small microgranulomas or microabscesses (*arrows*). **B**, The microgranulomas (*arrow*) and microabscesses (*arrowhead*) are shown at higher magnification. **C**, Cells in and around the microabscesses frequently have characteristic CMV intranuclear eosinophilic inclusions surrounded by a clear halo. Immunoperoxidase staining for CMV antigens is confirmatory (*inset* in the middle of the panel).

intranuclear inclusions are often fragmented. Mild plasmacytic and lymphocytic portal inflammation in conjunction with bile duct cell infiltration and damage may also be seen and can mimic or actually be associated with acute or chronic rejection. Bile duct loss has also been associated with persistent CMV infection of the allograft.[327,329,391,394-399]

On occasion, the characteristic parenchymal alterations just described may be seen, but without clear evidence of cytomegaly or nuclear or cytoplasmic CMV inclusions. In such cases, immunoperoxidase staining for early viral antigens or in situ hybridization can be used to detect the infected cells.[380,388,400] In addition, "activated" or rapidly dividing tissues such as young granulation tissue, proliferating cholangioles seen in ischemically damaged livers, edges of infarcts, abscesses, or other intraparenchymal defects are fertile soil for CMV growth.[24] When such tissue is encountered, a more careful search for CMV is warranted.

Differential Diagnosis. When no viral inclusions are detected, CMV hepatitis can be difficult to distinguish from early recurrence of hepatitis B or C and, on occasion, EBV hepatitis. When inclusions are seen, CMV can still be difficult to distinguish from HSV infection because both can cause multinucleation and intranuclear eosinophilic inclusions. However, CMV-infected cells also show small basophilic or amphophilic cytoplasmic inclusions, which are not seen in HSV infection. In addition, the circumscribed zones of coagulative necrosis characteristic of HSV are not generally encountered with CMV.

In the absence of inclusions, subtle clues that can be used to distinguish between CMV and early acute HBV or HCV infection include less lobular disarray and hepatocyte swelling in CMV infection. Conversely, microabscesses or microgranulomas are not generally seen in HBV or HCV infection. The final diagnosis, however, often relies on adjuvant techniques such as immunoperoxidase staining for viral antigens (CMV, HBV) or in situ hybridization for viral nucleic acids (EBV) and correlation with the clinical profile.

Cases of CMV hepatitis resembling EBV hepatitis show mild lymphoplasmacytic portal and lobular inflammation. Blastic and atypical lymphocytes may or may not be present. Microgranulomas are usually seen in the lobules, although characteristic CMV inclusions are absent. The use of deeper cuts into the block, immunoperoxidase stains for EBV and CMV viral antigens, and in situ hybridization for EBV nucleic acids is generally required to establish the final diagnosis.[401-403]

A difficult challenge is determining whether the liver injury is due to residual CMV hepatitis or the onset of acute or chronic rejection because of low immunosuppression levels used to treat the viral infection. This difficulty occurs because CMV hepatitis most commonly develops in patients who have recently completed an augmented immunosuppressive regimen for rejection and are therefore at risk for rejection and CMV infection. Further complicating the issue are reports by O'Grady and associates and others showing an association between CMV infection and chronic rejection.[327,391,394-398] Others have not seen this association.[328] Difficulties arise in the pathological interpretation of specimens in which obvious CMV inclusions are not detected, but staining for viral antigens is positive and other histopathological findings typically seen with acute rejection or loss of bile ducts are also present. In our experience, the presence of CMV inclusions or antigens is generally given priority, and the immunosuppressive therapy is lightened and ganciclovir is given. Follow-up biopsy after 1 to 2 weeks, if liver function abnormalities persist, is used to monitor therapy. Unfortunately, bile duct loss may develop in such patients, but long-term follow-up can show apparent regrowth of lost ducts.

Herpes Simplex and Varicella-Zoster Viral Hepatitis. Subtypes of HSV (types I and II) and VZV have been identified as causes of liver allograft hepatitis.[24,37,38,404] Onset can occur as early as 3 days after transplantation or anytime thereafter. Clinical findings include fever, vesicular rashes, fatigue, and body pain, combined with elevated liver injury test values. If HSV hepatitis goes unrecognized, it can rapidly lead to submassive or massive hepatic necrosis, hypotension, disseminated intravascular coagulation, and metabolic acidosis.[404] Fulminant cases occur more often in patients without evidence of previous antibody-mediated immunity. Early recognition

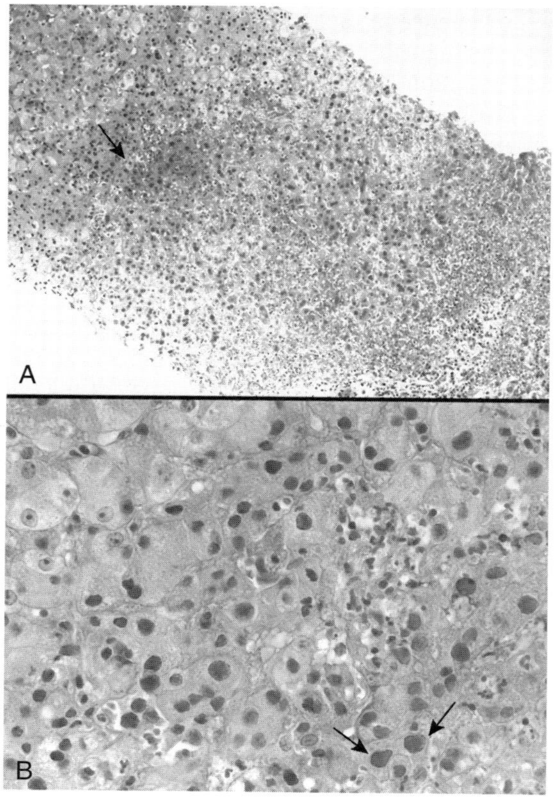

FIGURE 69–16

Herpes hepatitis is characterized by large areas of coagulative-type necrosis that show no respect for or relationship to the lobular architecture. **A,** The center of the necrotic lesions usually contains ghosts of hepatocytes and cellular debris along with neutrophils. More viable cells at the interface between the area of necrosis and viable hepatic parenchyma usually have characteristic inclusion bodies (*arrow*). **B,** Area highlighted by the *arrow* in **A** shown at higher magnification. Note the hepatocytes with characteristic ground-glass nuclei (*arrows*).

by needle biopsy sampling is particularly crucial because effective pharmacological therapy is available.

Histopathological Findings. Two histopathological patterns of HSV hepatitis have been identified,[404] localized and diffuse. Separation of the two patterns may be related to swiftness in establishing the diagnosis, the level of immune competence, and evidence of previous immunity. Common to both patterns are circumscribed areas of coagulative-type necrosis showing no respect for the lobular architecture.[24,37,38,404] Ghosts of hepatocytes, intermixed with neutrophils and nuclear debris, are seen in the center of the lesions. More viable hepatocytes at the periphery may be slightly enlarged and contain "smudgy," ground-glass nuclei or characteristic Cowdry type A eosinophilic inclusions (Fig. 69–16).

We have not been able to reliably distinguish HSV from VZV on H&E-stained slides alone. Multinucleate cells are occasionally present but, not infrequently, changes diagnostic of HSV or VZV are absent on H&E slides. In such cases, immunoperoxidase stains for HSV

or VZV antigens (or both) can be confirmatory. Some antibody preparations used to detect HSV subtypes show considerable cross-reactivity, thus making it difficult to separate type I from type II HSV by immunohistochemistry. Cross-reactivity between VZV and HSV with the use of monoclonal antibodies has not been a problem in our experience.

Differential Diagnosis. If a histopathological diagnosis of HSV or VZV hepatitis is even considered, regardless of whether the diagnosis is confirmed, clinical physicians should be notified immediately. Necrotic HSV hepatitis lesions can be very difficult to distinguish from the edge of an infarct or area of ischemic necrosis. The most reliable finding is an inclusion body, but unequivocal HSV inclusions may not be present. Frequently, only cells with smudged nuclear chromatin are seen. In such cases, it is our policy to overdiagnose HSV hepatitis because without administration of the highly effective acyclovir treatment, HSV and VZV hepatitis can rapidly cause liver failure and death.

It is difficult on occasion to distinguish HSV/VZV hepatitis from CMV hepatitis. HSV is associated with large areas of coagulative-type necrosis, whereas alone, CMV rarely causes significant hepatocyte necrosis. In addition, CMV hepatitis can be characterized by both nuclear and cytoplasmic inclusions, whereas HSV inclusions are exclusively nuclear.

Epstein-Barr Virus

Pathophysiology. EBV lies dormant in B lymphocytes and some epithelial cells once the immune system effectively controls viral replication after a primary infection. EBV infection "immortalizes" B lymphocytes in vitro. In vivo, control of the virus is maintained by T-cell immune surveillance, which keeps viral replication and B-cell proliferation in check.[405-407] However, potent immunosuppressive therapy depresses immune surveillance and leads to enhanced viral replication and the various disease manifestations listed in the next section. A more detailed discussion of the pathophysiology of the interaction of EBV and liver allograft recipients is beyond the scope of this chapter. Interested readers are referred to several excellent reviews.[405-407]

Clinical Features. Diverse clinicopathological manifestations of active EBV infection can occur after transplantation. In nearly 1% to 2% of adults with preexisting immunity, persistent or recurrent disease (EBV) will develop after transplantation and can be manifested as hepatitis, gastroenteritis, PTLDs (including B-cell disorders,[402,403,405,408-411] Hodgkin's disease,[405,412] and T-cell lesions[413]), and smooth muscle stromal tumors.[414,415] The incidence and severity of EBV-related diseases are magnified in pediatric patients and adults who were seronegative before transplantation and receive a seropositive donor organ.[402,403,405-411]

Other risk factors for serious EBV-associated disease, including PTLDs, are the use of heavy immunosuppression, underlying Langerhans cell histiocytosis,[416] and CMV disease.[417] The risk of PTLD developing late in the posttransplant course does not appear to be influenced by the type of immunosuppressive agents used, but by the total immunosuppression.[418]

The systemic viral syndrome associated with EBV often resembles classic infectious mononucleosis. Fever, lymphadenitis, pharyngitis, and jaundice[402,403,405-411] are typical findings. Atypical signs and symptoms include jaw pain, arthralgia, joint space effusions, diarrhea, encephalitis, pneumonitis, mediastinal lymphadenopathy, and ascites.[402,403,405-411] Laboratory investigation generally shows an elevation in hepatocellular liver enzymes, and circulating atypical lymphocytes and pancytopenia are noted on occasion.[402,403,405-411] Monitoring of peripheral blood for EBV nucleic acids is used to guide preemptive reductions in immunosuppression before more serious manifestations occur.[373,419]

Unresolved or recurrent EBV syndromes (or both) most often culminate in a PTLD.[406,420-422] PTLDs can involve any site in the body, but the lymph nodes, hepatic allograft, and gastrointestinal tract are the most common sites. Signs and symptoms attributable to a mass lesion at the site of PTLD involvement are common. Withdrawal or a dramatic reduction in immunosuppression, a maneuver that restores immune regulation or surveillance, combined with the addition of antiviral agents such as acyclovir is the first line of therapy, regardless of the clinical or histopathological features or clonality.[405-407] If unsuccessful, supplemental treatment with anti-CD20 antibodies or conventional chemotherapy should be considered.[405,423]

Histopathological Findings. The histopathological features of EBV-associated disorders in the allograft range from nonspecific portal and sinusoidal lymphocytosis (classic EBV hepatitis) to malignant-appearing PTLDs.[401-403,405,408-411,423,424] Rare EBV-containing cells can also be detected in rejection and other disorders in patients with increased levels of viral replication.[401]

EBV hepatitis usually shows mild portal and sinusoidal mononuclear infiltrates composed of small or mildly atypical lymphocytes. "Lining up" of lymphocytes in the sinusoids is a conspicuous finding that should suggest an EBV-related disorder and can be confirmed by in situ hybridization for EBV RNA (EBER). Lobular changes include focal hepatocellular swelling, mild acidophilic necrosis of hepatocytes, and mild lobular disarray.[402,403,408-411] Regenerative activity, including double-layered plates, pseudoacinar formation, and mitotic figures, is common.

Patients with less effective control of viral replication evolve toward a PTLD, which is recognized by atypical lymphoplasmacytoid cells. In early cases, atypical cells

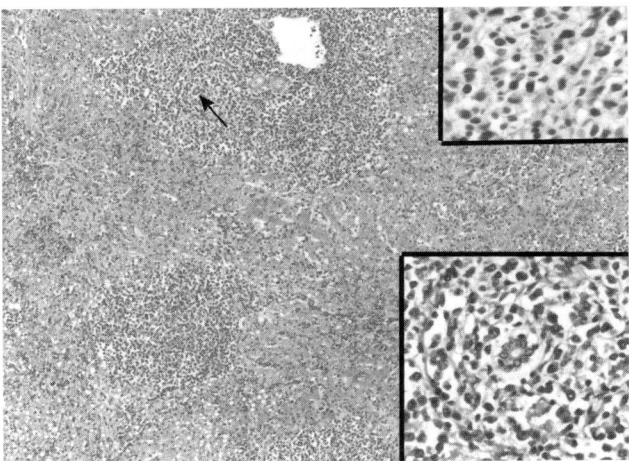

FIGURE 69–17

Posttransplant lymphoproliferative disorder (PTLD) is usually characterized by map-like enlargement of the portal tracts because of a relatively monomorphic population of lymphoid cells, many of which show features of plasmacytoid differentiation. Despite the rather striking portal inflammation, there is usually only minimal bile duct inflammation and damage (*arrow* and *lower right inset*). Most PTLDs are associated with Epstein-Barr virus, which can be detected by in situ hybridization for EBER RNA (*upper right inset*).

are intermixed with small and blastic lymphocytes, plasmacytoid lymphocytes, and plasma cells.[402,403,408-411] In late or well-developed lesions, the atypical cells predominate. Similar to acute rejection, subendothelial localization of lymphocytes can be seen in the portal or central veins in cases of PTLD or EBV hepatitis. Frank PTLD is manifested as a map-like enlargement of the portal tracts as a result of sheets of monomorphic atypical immunoblastic cells (Fig. 69–17) that obscure the normal architectural landmarks.[402,403,408-411] Smaller aggregates composed of similar cells can be seen in the sinusoids, and focal areas of necrosis may be detected. Cytologically, a PTLD infiltrate resembles an immunoblastic lymphoma, and occasionally, Reed-Sternberg–like cells can be seen. A diagnosis of EBV-related PTLD is confirmed by in situ hybridization for the EBER sequence. The reader is referred elsewhere for a detailed discussion of the extrahepatic manifestation of PTLD in lymph nodes and other tissues.[405,423]

Cases of suspected PTLD should be routinely stained for κ and λ light chains, CD20 (to determine possible responsiveness to anti-CD20 antibodies),[406] EBV antigens, and EBER. If enough fresh tissue is available, a portion is also submitted for flow cytometry and molecular analysis for more detailed phenotypic characterization and immunoglobulin gene rearrangements, respectively.

Differential Diagnosis. EBV hepatitis should be distinguished from acute rejection, nonspecific "reactive hepatitis," and acute hepatitis caused by HCV or CMV.[402,403,408-411] Hepatitis C and EBV hepatitis can demonstrate sinusoidal lymphocytosis, but EBV hepatitis generally has at least some cytologically atypical cells. In contrast, hepatitis C usually evokes a response of small, round, inactive-appearing lymphocytes in the sinusoids and portal tracts.[402,403,408-411] When compared with acute rejection, the portal infiltrate in EBV-related disorders is less pleomorphic and consists primarily of activated and immunoblastic mononuclear cells, many of which show features of plasmacytic differentiation, whereas eosinophils and neutrophils are much less common. The severity and prevalence of duct damage in EBV-related disorders are less than in acute rejection.[402,403,408-411] Patients with EBV-related disorders are prone to bile duct loss because of decreased immunosuppression.

Adjuvant techniques to identify EBV antigens or nucleic acids, or both, are used to ascertain the diagnosis of EBV-related disorders.[402,403,408-411] Therefore, availability of the EBER probe technology is a necessity for interpreting allograft biopsies (see Fig. 69–17). However, EBER probe results have to be interpreted with caution.[425] Rare EBER-positive lymphocytes are not uncommon in the general population and are found with increased frequency in allograft recipients. The significance of rare EBER-positive cells in biopsy specimens is open to debate,[425] but clustering of such cells into aggregates or the presence of EBER-positive cells in tissues showing other histopathological features of EBV-associated disease is indicative of enhanced EBV replication. Such patients are at increased risk for PTLDs, and more frequent peripheral blood monitoring for EBV antigens or nucleic acids and cautious immunosuppression management are warranted.

EBV-negative PTLDs are being increasingly recognized and account for up to 31% of PTLDs in some series.[426]

Adenoviral Hepatitis

Pathophysiology. Adenoviral-associated diseases, including hepatitis, are largely limited to the pediatric population,[427-429] although occasional cases have been reported in adults.[430] The difference is probably related to protective immunity before transplantation. Viral subtypes 1, 2, and 5 have been isolated from the lung, gastrointestinal tract, and liver in patients with fever, respiratory distress, diarrhea, and liver dysfunction.[427-429,431] Disease onset usually occurs between 1 and 10 weeks after transplantation, and biopsy histopathology is used to ascertain the diagnosis. Hepatitis is most often caused by viral subtype 5, but subtypes 2, 11, and 16 have been associated with hepatitis in the general population and could be expected to infect and cause disease in liver allografts recipients.[427-429]

Histopathological Findings. Adenoviral hepatitis is distinctive histopathologically, but some experience is required to establish the diagnosis with certainty.

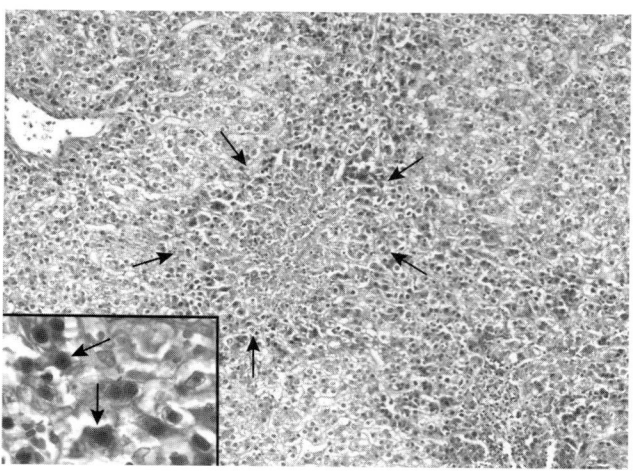

FIGURE 69–18

Adenoviral hepatitis is characterized by pox-like areas of hepatocyte necrosis (outlined by the *arrows*) that are often infiltrated by macrophages. Hepatocytes at the interface between areas of necrosis or lesions and the hepatic parenchyma usually contain the characteristic inclusion bodies shown at higher magnification in the *lower left inset.* Note the smudged appearance of the infected hepatocyte nuclei and the eosinophilic inclusions that push the chromatin to the periphery of the nucleus.

The most characteristic findings are "pox-like" areas of necrosis or granulomas consisting of a central core of necrotic hepatocytes or macrophages that are spread randomly throughout the parenchyma.[427-430] Adenoviral nuclear inclusions are often found in hepatocytes near the edge of the necrotic zones or in granulomas (or in both) (Fig. 69–18). Diagnostic eosinophilic intranuclear inclusions push the chromatin toward the nuclear membrane and impart a muffin-shaped appearance to the nucleus. Immunohistochemical stains are confirmatory.

Differential Diagnosis. Adenoviral hepatitis should be distinguished from other causes of focal hepatic necrosis and hepatic granulomas such as infarcts and deep fungal or mycobacterial infections. Other infections can be excluded by microbiological cultures of the biopsy specimen and negative special stains for granuloma-causing organisms. The macrophage-rich granulomas associated with adenovirus hepatitis are much larger than the "microgranulomas" of CMV, which often contain neutrophils. Multinucleated giant cells are rare in adenoviral hepatitis. In contrast, CMV causes cytomegaly and produces either eosinophilic intranuclear inclusions surrounded by a clear halo or basophilic or amphophilic small *cytoplasmic* inclusions. Adenovirus does not cause cytomegaly, the nucleus assumes a "smudgy" appearance, and there are no cytoplasmic inclusions. The hepatocyte necrosis associated with adenovirus is generally less than that seen with HSV or VZV hepatitis, although isolated cases can appear quite similar. In such cases, reliance on immunoperoxidase stains for specific viral antigens is needed.

Hepatitis Virus Infections (A, B, C, and D)

Hepatitis A. Hepatitis A virus has not been identified as a cause of allograft dysfunction or failure, but Fagan and colleagues[432] documented reinfection of a liver allograft in a recipient who required transplantation for hepatitis A virus–induced fulminant hepatic failure. Extrahepatic reservoirs of the virus were thought to account for reinfection of the allografted liver, but allograft dysfunction was not encountered.

Hepatitis B and Delta. HBV infection, with or without hepatitis delta virus (HDV) coinfection, is largely restricted to patients whose original liver disease was caused by this virus.[10,433-441] Most patients who have evidence of viral replication before transplantation (i.e., hepatitis B early antigen [HBeAg] seropositivity or HBV DNA positivity) will reinfect their allograft. Reinfection and recurrent disease are less predictable in patients who had HBV-induced fulminant liver failure or in those with chronic liver disease who had become anti-HBe positive and serum HBV DNA and HBeAg negative before transplantation[10,433-441]; approximately 10% to 25% of these patients will not "reinfect" the allograft, nor will HBV disease develop. Despite blood product screening, a small number of patients without previous HBV disease will acquire HBV infection during or after transplantation.[372,442] Livers from anti-HBc–positive donors are one possible source of infection because they can transmit HBV to recipients, especially those with no previous exposure to HBV.[66-68]

Several treatment modalities, including hepatitis B immune globulin (polyclonal and monoclonal), active vaccination with hepatitis B surface antigen (HBsAg), IFN alfa, and antiviral drugs such as foscarnet, ganciclovir, famciclovir, and lamivudine,[443] cannot prevent *reinfection* of the allograft, but the antiviral drugs and hepatitis B immune globulin are particularly effective in preventing recurrent *disease*.[443-459] The high cost of long-term drug therapy and the emergence of viral mutants that escape pharmacological control are major problems.[458-461]

Pathophysiology. HBV is generally considered to be noncytopathic, and liver damage is mediated primarily by immunological mechanisms in nonimmunosuppressed adult hosts. Marinos and coworkers[462] suggested that the same concepts apply to the majority of liver allograft recipients. They propose that HBV viral peptides are presented to circulating recipient T helper cells in association with HLA class II molecules by host APCs that repopulate the allograft after transplantation.[8,100] Recognition of viral antigens by primed T helper cells leads to expansion and activation of antigen-specific T_H1-type CD4$^+$ lymphocytes, which release IFN-γ, a potent activator of monocytes/macrophages. Activation of monocytes/macrophages results in the production of proinflammatory cytokines and chemokines, especially TNF-α. These two cytokines (IFN-γ and TNF-α) cause damage by (1) recruiting and activating nonspecific inflammatory cells; (2) upregulating TNF receptor expression, thereby making hepatocytes more vulnerable to the cytolytic and apoptotic actions of TNF-α; (3) exerting a direct cytotoxic effect on the HBsAg-expressing hepatocytes; and (4) inducing local mediators of tissue injury such as nitric oxide. All these mechanisms can operate independent of HLA matching between the host and donor and the immunosuppression.[462]

Massive viral replication can directly lead to liver injury with little or no hepatic inflammation in a minority of patients. Most of these patients are overimmunosuppressed, which suggests that under these special circumstances, the virus may be directly cytopathic.[434-437,463,464]

Clinical Features. Most cases of recurrent hepatitis B are first manifested about 6 to 8 weeks after transplantation as mild elevations in liver injury test values. Nausea, vomiting, jaundice, and hepatic failure signal more severe recurrent disease. The clinical spectrum of disease is similar to that of viral hepatitis seen in nonimmunosuppressed patients.[10,433-441] Needle biopsy evaluation confirms the diagnosis.

Histopathological Findings. The histopathological appearance of HBV infection in hepatic allografts is similar to that seen in nonallograft livers,[10,433-439,441,463,464] but antiviral therapy can effectively control viral replication and significantly limit tissue pathology. Chronic disease will eventually develop in untreated or inadequately treated patients and those harboring resistant viral mutants. There is a typical progression from acute to chronic hepatitis, and cirrhosis can develop with striking rapidity.[10,433-439,441,463,464] Occasional patients show histopathological resolution of disease activity after a bout of acute hepatitis, and rare patients actually exert immunological "control" of the virus after transplantation.

For those in whom disease develops, the "acute" phase usually begins within 4 to 6 weeks after transplantation, coincident with the expression of HBcAg in the cytoplasm of occasional hepatocytes.[433,434] Core antigen spreads throughout the liver and surface antigen appears,[10,433-439,441,463,464] followed by lobular necroinflammatory activity, Kupffer cell hypertrophy, lobular disarray, and varying amounts of portal inflammation. Bridging or even submassive necrosis can develop in a small percentage, particularly if immunosuppression is decreased or withdrawn.[433]

Evolution into chronic hepatitis is characterized by lymphoplasmacytic portal inflammation associated with interface activity of varying severity in conjunction with cholangiolar proliferation or a ductular reaction. Bile ducts and portal veins are relatively spared in chronic hepatitis. Lobular findings include ground-glass hepatocytes or sanded nuclei that stain positively for HBcAg and HBsAg, respectively, accompanied by lobular disarray, Kupffer cell hypertrophy, and lobular necroinflammatory activity.

A unique pattern of liver injury associated with HBV, fibrosing cholestatic hepatitis (FCH), is not usually encountered in the general population and is related to massive viral replication associated with immunosuppression and MHC nonidentity between the liver and recipient.[434-437,463,464] FCH can also occur with the emergence of viral mutants. Usual findings include marked hepatocyte swelling, lobular disarray, and cholestasis combined with a prominent ductular reaction, but little or no portal or lobular inflammation. These cases are usually associated with massive hepatocellular expression of HBcAg or HBsAg, or both, in degenerating hepatocytes that show swelling, steatosis, or necrosis. Progression to portal and periportal sinusoidal fibrosis and lobular collapse can occur without a significant inflammatory component,[434-437,463,464] which has led several groups to suggest that HBV is directly cytopathic under these special circumstances.[434-437,463,464]

Delta agent coinfection may complicate reinfection of the allograft by HBV, as in the general population, and follow-up of these patients has yielded conflicting results of more and less severe disease.[439,441,465-467] There are also conflicting reports about the cytopathic effect of HDV after transplantation and its relationship to HBV replication. David and colleagues[468] noted that HDV infection can be associated with nonreplicative HBV infection and hepatitic lesions similar to those described in FCH, but without HBcAg expression in the liver. In contrast, active HBV replication in HBV- plus HDV-positive recipients produced necroinflammatory activity similar to that seen in hepatitis B and D in patients from the general population.[468]

Differential Diagnosis. Distinguishing acute hepatitis B from other causes of acute hepatitis is usually achieved with the aid of special studies to detect viral antigens or nucleic acids (or both) in blood or tissue or antibody reactions to the virus. Acute rejection and acute hepatitis can also be confused with each other.[433,434] The lobule is the focus of injury in acute hepatitis, and findings include spotty hepatocyte necrosis, disarray, and necroinflammatory activity. In contrast, the immune damage in acute rejection is primarily directed at the portal structures, including the portal vein and bile ducts.[433,434]

Late-onset acute and chronic rejection can also be difficult to distinguish from chronic hepatitis (see "Acute Rejection," "Differential Diagnosis"). Prominent interface activity, damage to a minority of bile ducts, and lobular disarray and necroinflammatory activity are not common features of acute rejection and point toward hepatitis, whereas damage to a majority of bile ducts and bile duct loss are not features of hepatitis and signal rejection. It is not possible to distinguish between acute rejection and chronic hepatitis in occasional cases, and in others both rejection and hepatitis are present.[220,294,469,470] Infection of the allograft by HBV does not equate with HBV disease or exclude rejection.[434] Either core or surface antigen may be detected by immunohistochemistry in allografts that otherwise have all the features of acute or chronic rejection.[434] When both hepatitis and rejection are present, it has been suggested that patients be treated with immunosuppression when histopathological criteria for rejection are prevalent and clearly present; such cases are usually graded as moderate rejection according to the Banff schema.[470]

Hepatitis C Virus. Chronic HCV-induced cirrhosis is the most common indication for liver transplantation in many programs.[471,472] At most large centers it accounts for about 30% of all patients undergoing hepatic replacement.[314,473-475] Reinfection of the liver allograft with HCV after transplantation in conjunction with subsequent systemic viremia is practically a universal occurrence that probably occurs within hours after transplantation.[476,477] Fortunately, screening of blood products for HCV has led to a low incidence of de novo infection, on the order of 0.84% in some studies[478,479] but as high as 10% to 20% in others.[372,480]

Recurrent infection leads to recurrent hepatitis in the majority of recipients and recapitulation of the same sequence of events that originally led to liver transplantation, only at an accelerated pace. However, recurrent disease evolves slowly enough in the majority of recipients to justify hepatic replacement.[473] Nonetheless, very aggressive disease develops in a small percentage of allograft recipients after transplantation.[481] New and more effective antiviral drugs are needed to break this disheartening cycle of infection, hepatitis, fibrosis, and cirrhosis.

Even if newer antiviral agents can effectively cure HCV infection before transplantation, HCV-induced cirrhosis requiring liver transplantation will continue to be a major problem for the foreseeable future. The incidence of infection in the general population ranges from 1% to 3% in low-incidence areas to 25% to 30% in high-risk countries or regions. Understanding the issues related to HCV recurrence and disease severity and progression will be essential for optimal patient management. There are excellent reviews of virtually all aspects of liver transplantation for HCV-induced cirrhosis in the November 2003 issue of *Liver Transplantation,* including consensus reports by the

First International Liver Transplantation Society Expert Panel Consensus Conference on HCV.

HCV infections in liver allograft recipients reflect the distribution of HCV genotypes before transplantation, with type 1b predominating in European centers[482,483] and, in a North American site,[484] accounting for 25% to 60% of patients. Type 1a is also common.[484]

Pathophysiology. The pathogenesis of HCV infection in the allograft is similar to that in native livers, except that allograft recipients have a greater viral burden because of the baseline immunosuppression needed to control rejection.[485-488] Consequently, a greater percentage of allograft recipients experience aggressive disease (reviewed elsewhere[471,472,489]).[481] The already enhanced viral burden in allograft recipients plateaus at 1 month after transplantation and peaks at the time of onset of acute hepatitis, between 1 and 4 months after transplantation. This phase is associated with T-cell infiltration and Fas-mediated hepatocyte apoptosis,[490] which is manifested as lobular hepatitis, described later.[487,488] Chronic hepatic HCV seems to be associated with the activation of T_H1-type inflammatory, profibrotic, and proapoptotic pathways.[487,488]

Various pretransplant and posttransplant, donor and recipient, and virological factors appear to increase the risk for more severe disease after transplantation. These factors include older donor age, living donors (controversial), HLA compatibility (controversial), the year of transplantation (worse in recent years),[491] race (worse in blacks),[491] the degree of pretransplantation viremia (worse with high levels),[491,492] the presence of more pathogenic HCV genotypes (worse with type 1 genotypes), CMV coinfection, and more rapid onset of recurrent disease after transplantation (see later), the integrity of the cellular immune response, quasispecies homogeneity (worse with viral diversity),[493] and treatment of rejection and total immunosuppression, especially corticosteroids and antibody induction therapy (more immunosuppression, worse outcome).[472,491,494-498]

Increased immunosuppression to control episodes of acute rejection has been associated with an increased incidence, earlier onset, and more severe recurrent acute or chronic HCV-induced disease in the liver allograft. Immunosuppressive agents associated with a higher incidence of HCV infection include IL-2 receptor antibodies,[497] corticosteroids,[494-496] azathioprine, OKT3, and "total" immunosuppression.[494,495] For example, treatment of rejection with corticosteroids can increase serum HCV RNA from 4- to 100-fold. There does not appear to be a significant difference between the calcineurin inhibitors cyclosporine and tacrolimus.[472,487]

Some studies show that HCV genotypes are not associated with specific clinical courses of recurrent HCV infection,[478,492,499] but many of them report an earlier onset or increased incidence of disease, higher viremia, or increased severity of hepatitis (or any combination) in patients infected with type 1 viruses.[482-485,500-502] Even studies in which the disease appears to be more severe in those with type 1b virus report no significant differences in patient or graft survival by genotype. In addition, no specific qualitative histopathological features can be used to distinguish between the several different viral genotypes on the basis of routine histopathology alone.

When an HCV-positive donor liver is implanted into an HCV-positive recipient, Laskus and associates[503] showed that within a few months after transplantation, either the donor (57%) or the recipient (43%) strain predominated. Subtype 1b and type 1 (1a + 1b) appeared to have a replicative advantage because they became the predominant strains in all recipient-donor pairs in which they were present. This finding is consistent with several studies that have shown a more aggressive course associated with genotype 1b and higher levels of viremia.[504,505] Interestingly, patients retaining their own strain were found to have significantly more active liver disease than were those infected by the donor strain.[503] This may be related to the existence of primed lymphocytes within the body of HCV-positive recipients.

Cholestatic hepatitis C seems to be a disease characterized by direct HCV cytopathic injury in the setting of extreme virus levels, an intrahepatic T helper subtype 2 cell (T_H2)-like response, and lack of a specific HCV-directed response.[506]

Clinical Features. The early phase of recurrent HCV disease is often asymptomatic and detectable only by an elevation in liver injury test results, manifested primarily by persistent elevation of the liver injury test values (especially ALT and AST) to four to eight times the normal levels. Liver injury test values may increase further at the first histological signs of hepatitis, usually between 3 and 6 weeks after transplantation, but an earlier onset within 10 to 14 days has also been observed. Fatigue, nausea, jaundice and other typical signs of acute hepatitis are less frequent. Fulminant liver failure is uncommon and occurs only in patients with massive viral replication and FCH.[476,479,507-509] Needle biopsy evaluation is used to confirm the diagnosis.[476,479,508-510]

Severe clinical recurrent HCV infection can be manifested as FCH and is characterized clinically by malaise, jaundice, and a cholestatic liver injury test profile that often evolves subacutely over a period of weeks to months. The key to early recognition relies on suspicion by both the clinical physician and the pathologist. HCV levels in peripheral blood are usually higher than 50 million IU/mL.[470] The international panel[472] suggested the following criteria for the diagnosis of FCH after liver replacement: (1) longer than 1 month after transplantation (usually ≤ 6 months); (2) serum bilirubin level higher than 6 mg/dL; (3) serum alkaline phosphatase and γ-glutamyl transferase levels greater than five times the upper limits of normal; (4) characteristic histological state with ballooning of hepatocytes predominantly in the perivenular zone (not necrosis or fallout), a paucity of inflammation, and variable degrees of cholangiolar proliferation without bile duct loss; (5) very high serum HCV RNA levels; and (6) absence of surgical biliary complications (normal cholangiogram) and evidence of hepatic artery thrombosis.

By 5 years after transplantation, approximately 5% to 20% of patients have cirrhosis caused by recurrent hepatitis.[481,493,511,512]

Histopathological Findings. HCV infection in the liver allograft is very similar to that seen in the general population, and the histopathological features that can be reliably used to first detect disease activity generally appear within 3 to 6 weeks; in some cases, recurrence can be detected as early as 10 to 14 days. Evolution of the disease usually follows a predictable sequence through predominantly lobular and portal phases,[38,473,510,513] although atypical evolution can occur.

The acute or lobular-predominant phase typically includes lobular disarray, Kupffer cell hypertrophy, spotty acidophilic hepatocyte necrosis, mild sinusoidal lymphocytosis, variable mononuclear portal inflammation, and periportal and midzonal macrovesicular steatosis. Lymphocytes invading the basement membrane and reactive changes in the biliary epithelium can be seen focally, but these changes are neither severe nor widespread. Some studies show that acute lobular hepatitis is often accompanied by a steep increase in HCV RNA levels and the appearance of core and NS4 antigens in the graft,[504,514] whereas others show no strong relationship between the level of viremia and the degree of hepatic damage.[486] Lobular changes usually start to wane, portal inflammation increases, and interface activity, including an accompanying ductular reaction, begins to distort the architecture during the transition from acute to chronic hepatitis.

The chronic phase generally begins between 4 and 12 months after transplantation. The predominant features include portal inflammation and periportal hepatitis with varying degrees of interface activity, lobular disarray, and necroinflammatory activity. Inflammatory bile duct damage can be seen, but it is not usually severe or widespread and there is no bile duct loss (Fig. 69–19). Subendothelial inflammation or inflammation around the connective tissue sheath of the central vein (or both), known in the liver as "central venulitis," can be seen in an occasional vessel, but similar to the duct damage, it is neither severe nor widespread in recurrent hepatitis C.

Severe disease is associated with two histopathological patterns: (1) aggressive conventional hepatitis with

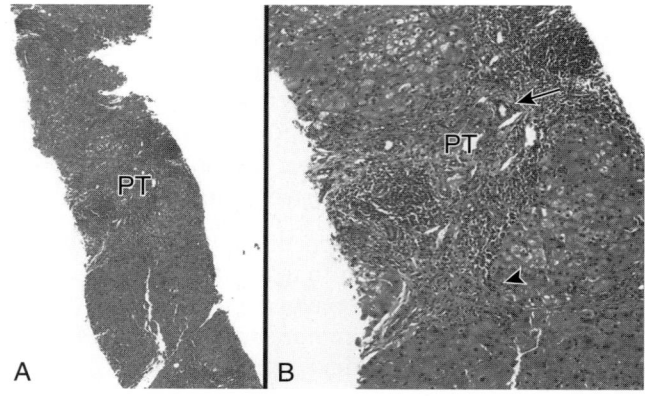

FIGURE 69–19

A, The histopathological appearance of recurrent chronic hepatitis C is very similar to that seen in native livers. It is characterized by variable chronic portal inflammation that is often arranged in nodular aggregates. **B,** A higher magnification of the portal tract (PT) shows the nodular aggregates of lymphocytes, relative sparing of the bile ducts (*arrow*), and preferential involvement of the interface zone (*arrowhead*).

prominent interface activity and rapid progression of fibrosis and (2) FCH. FCH is an atypical manifestation of HCV (Fig. 69–20) characterized by extensive centrilobular hepatocyte swelling and degeneration, cholestasis, spotty acidophilic hepatocyte necrosis, and Kupffer cell hypertrophy, combined with portal tract expansion because of ductular proliferation, fibrosis, and a mild mixed or even neutrophilic-predominant portal infiltrate.[510,515]

Several studies have specifically examined the effect of viral genotype and titer on quantitative and qualitative aspects of the histopathology of recurrent HCV infection. Most studies show a strong correlation between HCV-related FCH and massive viral replication, with HCV titers typically greater than 40 to 50 million IU/mL.[470] In the more common conventional hepatitis C, some studies showed no correlation between viral titers and the severity of liver damage,[516] whereas others showed that HCV RNA levels were higher during the lobular phase of the infection and that progression to the chronic phase with interface activity was associated with a highly significant decrease in liver HCV RNA (discussed earlier). These data suggest that progression to chronic active disease is associated with a host immune response to the virus that is marked by aberrant intrahepatic expression of molecules involved in antigen recognition, intercellular and vascular adhesion, and recruitment and activation of cytotoxic T lymphocytes.[516] In fact, higher levels of viral replication during the lobular phase[505] might precipitate a stronger response because they are an independent predictor of progression to chronic active disease.[505] Other studies have shown that ballooning degeneration and cholestasis at initial evaluation[517,518] are associated with the subsequent development of allograft cirrhosis.[517,518] In one study there was no

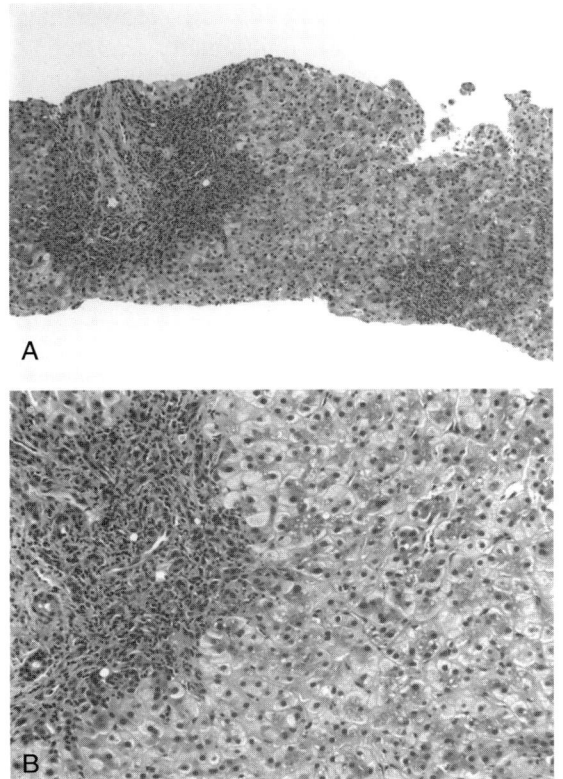

FIGURE 69-20

A, Fibrosing cholestatic hepatitis C virus–induced hepatitis is characterized by hepatocellular swelling and hepatocanalicular cholestasis combined with variable, but usually mild, portal inflammation and a prominent ductular reaction at the interface zone. **B**, A higher magnification of the interface zone shows the hepatocellular swelling, hepatocanalicular cholestasis, and prominent ductular reaction combined with mild portal inflammation that is often associated with acute pericholangiolitis.

significant difference in the histopathology of recurrent versus de novo disease, whereas in another, de novo infection more often led to significant disease.[510]

Differential Diagnosis. Distinguishing the various phases of hepatitis C from other causes of allograft dysfunction is one of the most common and difficult problems encountered by the pathologist. The differential diagnosis includes acute and chronic rejection, recurrent non-HCV viral hepatitis (e.g., HBV, CMV, EBV), recurrent autoimmune hepatitis, recurrent PBC, and recurrent PSC, as well as bile duct obstruction.[220,508,510] Exclusion of chronic HCV liver disease is based on negative reverse transcriptase polymerase chain reaction (RT-PCR) results for HCV on liver tissue. HBV is identified on the basis of viral antigens, which are present and detected in serum or with immunoperoxidase staining of tissue specimens.

Cholestatic hepatitis can be difficult to distinguish from bile duct obstruction and hepatic artery thrombosis. Portal edema and portal, rather than periportal neutrophilia are common in duct obstruction and acute cholangitis. In contrast, cholangiolar proliferation and acute cholangiolitis without portal edema are more characteristic of cholestatic hepatitis. In addition, lobular disarray and marked hepatocellular swelling are more typical in viral hepatitis in contrast to duct obstruction.

Acute rejection may be extremely difficult to differentiate from chronic hepatitis C, mostly because both can show portal inflammation and bile duct damage. However, in acute or chronic rejection, bile duct damage or biliary epithelial senescence involves a majority of bile ducts, whereas a minority of bile ducts are damaged in hepatitis C.[220] In addition, the combination of centrilobular inflammation, fibrosis, and hepatocellular dropout involving a majority of the central veins is more typical of rejection.[220,294] Conversely, Saxena and colleagues[519] showed that acidophilic bodies within the lobules are significantly more numerous in recurrent hepatitis C than in acute rejection. This differential is also discussed under "Acute Rejection."

We recently and prospectively assessed our ability to distinguish between hepatitis C and acute and chronic rejection primarily by histopathology, along with the clinical course and viral titers.[470] The result was that recurrent HCV infection can be reliably and accurately distinguished from acute and chronic rejection by using the aforementioned criteria. However, there was a very low rate of errors, and all were in the same direction: recurrent HCV infection was overdiagnosed as rejection. As a consequence, we recommended that significant and unequivocal histopathological evidence of rejection be present before making the diagnosis of acute rejection in the context of recurrent hepatitis C. Such biopsies are usually graded as "moderate" acute rejection according to the Banff schema.

The time after transplantation is very useful in distinguishing acute rejection from recurrent HCV infection. During the first several weeks after transplantation, HCV is an uncommon cause of allograft dysfunction, although in isolated cases the typical sequence of changes described earlier can begin in only 10 to 14 days. Most cases of recurrent hepatitis C begin between 3 and 8 weeks after transplantation. In contrast, the majority of acute rejection episodes occur within the first 30 days, with a median of 8 days.[122]

Acute or chronic rejection (or both) and recurrent hepatitis C can occur together, thus making it difficult in some cases to determine the more important cause of allograft injury. In such cases, the pathologist should first determine whether acute rejection is present. The key features used to identify acute rejection are (1) the prevalence and severity of mononuclear inflammatory bile duct damage and (2) the prevalence and severity of central vein inflammation. If either of these features involves a majority of the bile ducts or central veins, acute rejection is present. Conversely, key features used to identify HCV infection are the prevalence and severity of (1) interface activity and (2) ductular reaction, both of which are minimal or absent in rejection. The presence of prevalent or prominent type I or II ductular reactions[103] is strong evidence of a non–rejection-related cause of allograft dysfunction. The risk of treating acute rejection with increased immunosuppression in the context of recurrent hepatitis C should be based on thorough clinicopathological correlations that take into consideration the severity of findings (mild rejection may not require treatment), viral titers (avoid immunosuppressive treatment with high viral titers), and the liver injury test profile.

Differentiation of hepatitis C from hepatitis B, autoimmune hepatitis, drug-induced hepatitis, PBC, and obstructive cholangiopathy is based on a complete clinical, biochemical, serological, and histopathological profile. For example, the distinction between recurrent or de novo autoimmune hepatitis and hepatitis C is largely based on the clinical profile and the results of laboratory tests other than the liver biopsy, such as autoantibodies (e.g., antinuclear antibodies, anti–smooth muscle antibody, liver-kidney microsomal antibody). No specific histopathological features can reliably be used to distinguish between autoimmune and HCV-induced hepatitis in an individual case. However, similar to native livers, it has been our experience that autoimmune disease is characterized by more plasma cell–rich inflammation and less steatosis and portal lymphoid nodules than recurrent HCV disease is.

Distinguishing between HCV disease and recurrent PBC can be quite difficult in some cases because portal granulomas can be seen in allograft recipients with HCV.[520] In addition, patients with PBC before transplantation can be infected with HBV or HCV. Because de novo PBC after liver transplantation is rare, simply knowing the original disease greatly facilitates sorting through the various histopathological diagnostic possibilities. In cases in which difficulties are encountered, the key histopathological clue in distinguishing between the two disorders turns on recognition of the "biliary gestalt" that typically evolves in specimens with recurrent PBC, but not in HCV, including a prominent ductular reaction at the interface zone combined with small bile duct loss and periportal edema (halo sign), periportal lysosomal pigment and copper/protein deposition, and only mild lobular changes.[220,356,521-524] The penultimate diagnostic lesion for recurrent PBC is non-suppurative destructive cholangitis (florid duct lesion).

Obstructive cholangiopathy is not usually difficult to distinguish from chronic hepatitis C, although on occasion, incomplete biliary tract obstruction or strictures can be associated with a predominantly mononuclear portal tract infiltrate and interface activity that can resemble chronic hepatitis.

Several groups have reported a higher incidence of chronic rejection in HCV-positive recipients.[475,525,526] There are several possible nonexclusionary explanations

for this association. First, it is well known that viral infections can cause an inflammatory microenvironment within an allograft, which in turn can upregulate adhesion, costimulatory, and MHC antigens.[527,528] All these factors acting in concert can precipitate a rejection response. Partial MHC class I compatibility between the donor and recipient might permit an MHC-restricted T-cell–mediated response to viral infection at the same time as an allogeneic response.[527,528] In addition, the ability to properly respond to infectious and environmental antigenic challenges may be compromised in allografts and lead to a vicious cycle alternating between rejection and an infectious immune reaction.[310] These scenarios are made even more likely if there is a concomitant reduction in immunosuppression or the addition of an immune stimulator such as IFN alfa,[529,530] both of which can be used to treat the viral infection. Chronic rejection developing in the context of HCV infection is diagnosed by the same criteria used to diagnose chronic rejection in livers not also infected with HCV (see "Chronic Rejection").

Infection with Multiple Viruses. Huang and coworkers[531] described the evolution of hepatitis in liver allograft recipients with HBV and HCV coinfection. They found two major histopathological patterns: one with predominant features of HCV and the other with those of HBV. Although the study was limited by a small number of patients, it appeared that the presence of HCV might actually improve the clinical outcome of HBV patients when compared with the expected outcome of persistent HBV infection alone.[531] In contrast, others have found that HBV-related disease more frequently dominates the posttransplant course and, in doing so, adversely affects patient and allograft survival.[532]

Coinfection with the hepatitis G virus does not appear to influence either the clinical or pathological course of recurrent or de novo hepatitis C in liver allograft recipients.[533,534] This is probably related to the fact that the hepatitis G virus does not replicate in the liver,[535] at least in patients with hepatitis C and G virus coinfection.

Recurrent Diseases and Diseases Induced by Transplantation

Recurrent native liver diseases can be categorized as (1) infectious (e.g., viral hepatitis A, B, C, D), (2) dysregulated immunity (autoimmune hepatitis, PBC, PSC, and overlap syndromes), (3) primary hepatic malignancies (hepatocellular and bile duct carcinoma or cholangiocarcinoma), (4) toxic (e.g., alcohol, adverse drug reactions, drug overdoses), and (5) metabolic disorders (Tables 69–10 to 69–13).

Table 69-10. RECURRENCE OF THE ORIGINAL DISEASE AFTER LIVER TRANSPLANTATION

Original Disease	Incidence of Recurrence (at ≈ 5 yr)	Comments	References
Viral Hepatitis			
HAV	< 5%	Preexisting anti-HAV titers decline after OLTx, but recurrent or new-onset HAV is rare after OLTx	432, 536, 537
HBV/HDV	Variable	Rate of recurrence depends on viral status at time of OLTx: especially high (100%) in HBV DNA– or HBeAg-positive recipients. Natural course of recurrent disease significantly improved by treatment with various antiviral agents. Good long-term survival and histological findings if viral replication kept in check. Long-term problems include cost of therapy and emergence of viral mutants	434, 438, 443, 447, 450, 458, 538–543
HCV	Nearly 100%*	Reinfection nearly universal and high incidence of recurrent chronic hepatitis. Risk factors for rapidly progressive recurrent disease include transplantation in recent years, advanced donor age, high immunosuppression, high viral load (before or early after transplantation), early recurrence within several weeks or months after transplantation, and ballooning and cholestasis in liver biopsy specimens early after transplantation. Cirrhosis will develop in 5%–30% with recurrence within 5 yr	64, 512, 513, 544–552
Disorders of Immune Regulation			
Autoimmune hepatitis	25%–42%*	Risk factors for recurrence in some studies include HLA-DR3+ and DR4+ recipients, patients with high-grade inflammation in native liver, steroid withdrawal and weaning from other immunosuppressives, and young age. A more aggressive form of recurrent disease may also develop in children	553–558
PBC	20%–90%*	Recurrence risk increased by immunosuppression regimen (tacrolimus > cyclosporine), steroid withdrawal and weaning from other immunosuppressives, and HLA-DR matching (Dvorchik, unpublished observation)	220, 356, 521, 559–563
PSC	≈30%*	Incidence appears to increase with time after transplantation, but specific risk factors for recurrence are difficult to identify. Recurrent disease has little impact on patient or graft survival up to 5–7 yr after transplantation	219, 220, 564–571
Toxic Diseases			
Alcoholic	13%–50%	Rate of recidivism difficult to precisely document, and coexisting diseases (e.g., hepatitis C, hemochromatosis, α_1-antitrypsin heterozygotes, head and neck cancers) are frequently present. Severe relapse can lead to graft loss or patient death, but recurrent alcoholic liver disease is not a significant problem for the majority of alcoholics for up to 6 yr after transplantation	572–576
NASH	25%–100%*	Problem of increasing significance and incidence; depends on whether NASH or cryptogenic cirrhosis was the original diagnosis	577–579
Malignancies			
HCC	See comments	Factors associated with a lower rate of recurrence include size (single tumor < 5 cm or 3 tumors each < 3 cm), stage (≤ T2), histological grade (well differentiated), vascular invasion (absence), and lymph node metastasis (absence) Multiparameter modeling systems used to predict recurrence after OLTx and thus eligibility for OLTx	580–589
Bile duct/CC	See comments	Prognosis is generally poor, but patients with peripheral cholangiocarcinoma and those with early-stage hilar tumors (stage 0–II) without lymph node metastasis and with negative resection margins can show reasonable (≈40%) 5-yr survival	590–593

*The incidence depends on the definition and whether protocol biopsy specimens were obtained.
CC, cholangiocarcinoma; HAV, hepatitis A virus; HBeAg, hepatitis B early antigen; HBV, hepatitis B virus; HCC, hepatocellular carcinoma; HCV, hepatitis C virus; HDV, hepatitis delta virus; NASH, nonalcoholic steatohepatitis; OLTx, orthotopic liver transplantation; PBC, primary biliary cirrhosis; PSC, primary sclerosing cholangitis.
Adapted from Demetris A, Crawford J, Nalesnik M, et al: Transplantation pathology of the liver. In Odze R, Goldblum J, Crawford JM (eds): Surgical Pathology of the GI Tract, Liver, Biliary Tract, and Pancreas. Philadelphia, WB Saunders, 2004, pp 909-966.

Table 69-11. METABOLIC DISEASE TREATED BY LIVER TRANSPLANTATION WHEN THE PRIMARY DEFECT LIES WITHIN THE LIVER AND IS ASSOCIATED WITH LIVER DISEASE (SEE TEXT)

Disease	Explanation of Disease and Alternative Treatment	Associated Liver Disease	Correction of Metabolic Defect	References
α_1-Antitrypsin deficiency	Mutation in protease inhibitor synthesized in liver leads to defective transport from endoplasmic reticulum because of protein misfolding No alternative treatments	Cirrhosis	Partial, patients are biochemically chimeric because protease inhibitor is produced by other cells, but no evidence of recurrent liver disease	594–598
Wilson's disease	Autosomal recessive gene mapped to chromosome 13q14-q21.1, which codes for abnormal copper-transporting ATPase; leads to increased biliary copper excretion, decreased copper binding to ceruloplasmin, and copper accumulation in tissues Alternative therapy: pharmacological therapy available to reduce copper absorption and stimulate endogenous proteins that block copper toxicity (zinc) or chelating agents to remove copper from body	Fulminant hepatic failure and/or cirrhosis	Yes, although correction is partial, it results in phenotypic cure; OLTx usually indicated now in patients with liver failure	594, 599–605
Tyrosinemia	Fumarylacetoacetate hydrolase deficiency leads to accumulation of toxic intermediates that cause hepatocyte and DNA damage leading to cirrhosis and liver tumors Alternative therapy: pharmacological, NTBC, which lessens need for liver replacement	Cirrhosis, hepatoma	Nearly complete	606–608
Type I and Ib glycogen storage disease	Glucose-6-phosphatase deficiency leads to storage products in liver that cause fibrosis Alternative therapy: nocturnal nasogastric infusion of glucose or orally administered cornstarch	Glycogen storage, fibrosis, tumors	Yes, but may not cure associated renal disease	609, 610
Type III glycogen storage disease	Autosomal recessive deficiency of amylo-1,6-glucosidase, 4-α-glucan transferase enzyme (AGL or glycogen debranching enzyme) leads to storage products in liver that cause fibrosis	Liver fibrosis, adenomas	Incomplete, extrahepatic manifestations may progress	610
Type IV glycogen storage disease	Amylo-1:4,1:6-transglucosidase (branching enzyme) defect. Amylopectin accumulation leads to liver fibrosis/cirrhosis	Cirrhosis	Incomplete, extrahepatic manifestations may or may not improve, depending on variant of disease	594, 601, 610
Inborn errors of bile acid synthesis	Defective bile acid synthesis (see Kaylor et al.[611] for listing of specific enzyme defects) that leads to cholestasis and liver injury Alternative treatment with bile acids (cholic acid)	Cholestasis and liver failure	Yes	611

ATPase, adenosine triphosphatase; NTBC, 2-(2-nitro-4-trifluoromethylbenzoyl)cyclohexane-1-3-dione; OLTx, orthotopic liver transplantation.
Adapted from Demetris A, Crawford J, Nalesnik M, et al: Transplantation pathology of the liver. In Odze R, Goldblum J, Crawford JM (eds): Surgical Pathology of the GI Tract, Liver, Biliary Tract, and Pancreas. Philadelphia, WB Saunders, 2004, pp 909-966.

Table 69-12. METABOLIC DISEASE TREATED BY LIVER TRANSPLANTATION WHEN THE PRIMARY DEFECT LIES INSIDE THE LIVER, BUT THE LIVER IS OFTEN NORMAL OR NEAR NORMAL (SEE TEXT)

Disease	Explanation of Disease and Alternative Treatment	Associated Liver Disease	Correction of Metabolic Defect	References
Familial amyloid polyneuropathy (FAP)	Defective transthyretin (prealbumin) molecule accumulates as amyloid in extrahepatic (endoneurial and gastrointestinal and intracardiac) organs No alternative therapy	Mild liver abnormalities with amyloid deposits in portal tracts and nerve trunks; use of FAP-affected liver is controversial[613-615]	Nearly complete; extrahepatic amyloid deposits may not resolve, but natural history of disease is improved	612–621
Crigler-Najjar syndrome	Glucuronyl transferase deficiency leads to unconjugated hyperbilirubinemia and neuronal injury Alternative therapy: pharmacological and phototherapy	None	Yes	622, 623
Type I hyperoxaluria	Peroxisomal alanine-glyoxylate aminotransferase deficiency leads to deposition of calcium oxalate crystals in tissue, especially the kidneys Alternative therapy: pharmacological (pyridoxine, crystalline inhibitors) and high fluid intake	None	Yes, but may or may not prevent or reverse kidney disease, which is major limiting factor	611, 624–626
Urea cycle enzyme deficiencies	X-linked recessive disorders; biosynthesis of urea dependent on 6 enzymes, all of which are located in the liver Alternative therapy: pharmacological	None	Yes	611, 624
Protein C deficiency	Defective protein C synthesis resulting in predisposition to thrombosis Alternative therapy: oral anticoagulation and blood component therapy; replacement gene therapy anticipated	None	Yes	627
Familial hypercholesterolemia	Low-density lipoprotein receptor deficiency; low-density lipoprotein overproduction leads to accelerated atherosclerosis Alternative therapy: pharmacological	None	Incomplete	624, 628–631
Hemophilia A	Factor VIII deficiency leads to bleeding tendency Alternative therapy: recombinant protein or gene therapy	None; cirrhosis occurs as a complication of hepatitis virus infection	Yes	624, 632–634
Hemophilia B	Factor IX deficiency leads to bleeding tendency Alternative therapy: recombinant protein or gene therapy	None; cirrhosis occurs as complication of hepatitis virus infection	Yes	624, 635

Adapted from Demetris A, Crawford J, Nalesnik M, et al: Transplantation pathology of the liver. In Odze R, Goldblum J, Crawford JM (eds): Surgical Pathology of the GI Tract, Liver, Biliary Tract, and Pancreas. Philadelphia, WB Saunders, 2004, pp 909-966.

Table 69–13. METABOLIC DISEASE TREATED BY LIVER TRANSPLANTATION WHEN THE PRIMARY DEFECT LIES OUTSIDE THE LIVER (SEE TEXT)

Disease	Explanation of Disease	Associated Liver Disease	Correction of Metabolic Defect	References
Hemochromatosis or inadvertent transplantation of donor with hemochromatosis	Autosomal recessive disorder associated with point mutation C282Y in *HFE* gene that results in increased iron absorption from intestine and abnormal storage in hepatocytes, which causes liver injury and fibrosis. All patients with iron overload may not have the same metabolic defect; therefore, disease development not fully understood. Alternative therapy: chelating agents and phlebotomy	Cirrhosis	Recurrent disease does not seem to be a significant problem. Possible that both intestinal and hepatic iron-handling defects may be required for full disease expression. Inadvertant transplantation of donor liver with hemochromatosis results in rapid loss of iron stores after transplantation	69, 636–640 Reviewed in 637, 639
Niemann-Pick disease	Defect in *NPC1* gene resulting in sphingomyelinase deficiency leads to dysregulation of cholesterol trafficking	None	Not known	624, 641
Sea-blue histiocyte syndrome	Unknown, neurovisceral lipochrome storage	Cirrhosis	No	642
Erythropoietic protoporphyria	Hepatic ferrochelatase deficiency, overproduction of protoporphyrin by erythropoietic tissues. Alternative therapy: heme preparations and supportive	Cirrhosis	Incomplete; orthotopic liver transplantation considered palliative	643–647
Cystinosis	Lysosomal storage disorder mapped to chromosome 17p. Defect apparently lies in impaired ATPase cystine transport across lysosomal membranes and accumulation of cystine crystals in lysosomes. Alternative therapy: pharmacological	Does not generally cause liver disease; intrahepatic crystal deposits in liver with perivenular fibrosis and recurrent disease in the allograft developed in one patient[624]	No	624
Cystic fibrosis	Autosomal recessive mutations in chloride channel gene, cystic fibrosis transmembrane conductance regulator (*CFTR*), result in inspissated secretions in lung and liver. Alternative therapy: supportive, nutritional, and antibiotic	Biliary fibrosis/cirrhosis	Cures liver disease, and if liver transplant is performed early, lung function can improve	648–650

Adapted from Demetris A, Crawford J, Nalesnik M, et al: Transplantation pathology of the liver. In Odze R, Goldblum J, Crawford JM (eds): Surgical Pathology of the GI Tract, Liver, Biliary Tract, and Pancreas. Philadelphia, WB Saunders, 2004, pp 909-966.

Recurrence of infectious diseases is common[177-179,612]; in virtually all patients with active HBV or HCV infection before transplantation, the new liver will become reinfected, and at least some degree of chronic hepatitis will develop in the allograft. In general, recurrent hepatitis C is more virulent than the disease before transplantation because of the immunosuppression and enhanced viral replication. However, effective antiviral therapy has significantly reduced the impact of recurrent HBV infection. Details regarding the incidence and severity of recurrent viral hepatitis and the clinical and histopathological manifestations are presented in the respective sections on those disorders.

Disorders of immune regulation, including PBC, autoimmune hepatitis, and PSC, also commonly recur after liver transplantation. By 5 years after transplantation, some evidence of recurrent disease will develop in roughly 25% to 50% of patients with PBC, PSC, or autoimmune hepatitis. Recurrent disease is often less severe than the same disease before transplantation.[356,521-523,553,651-654] However, for this particular category of diseases, establishing the diagnosis

can be problematic. Various
...stopathological, and radi-
... establish the diagnosis before
... somewhat nonspecific after
...xample, there are several causes
... strictures besides recurrent PSC,
... present before transplantation
...ransplantation, albeit at lower titer,
...e of clinical or histopathological
... disease. Consequently, we routinely
...ase after liver transplantation into
...," and "possible" categories and
...cording to sensitivity and speci-

...ease at the time of transplanta-
...patients with primary hepatic
...replacement and to prioritize
...lantation.[580,655-657] Microscopic
...werful predictor of recurrence
...oma, as are multiple liver
...verall tumor burden (see Table
..., early-stage hepatocellular carcinoma
...lar invasion is generally cured by liver
...tion. Bile duct carcinoma and cholangiocar-
...have a poor prognosis after liver transplantation
...ause most cases are discovered only after significant
local tissue invasion has occurred.

Toxic insults and adverse drug reactions do not recur
after transplantation unless the patient is again exposed
to the same agent, which is obviously a problem with
alcoholics.

Jaffe[624] placed the various metabolic diseases that lead
to liver transplantation into three categories: (1) the liver
is the prime site of the defect, and involvement leads to
end-stage liver disease (see Table 69–11); (2) the liver
is the site of the defect, but the predominant effects are
systemic and not hepatotoxic (see Table 69–12); and
(3) the defect lies outside the liver, and the effects on the
liver are secondary (see Table 69–13). The first group of
patients are prime candidates for liver replacement: the
cirrhotic liver is replaced by a genetically and structurally
normal one that cures the disease. Examples include
type 1 tyrosinemia, α_1-antitrypsin deficiency, Wilson's
disease, neonatal hemochromatosis, and types 1, 3, and
4 glycogen storage disease.[624] The liver may be structurally normal or near normal in the second group, but
the goal is to alleviate the systemic disease burden of
abnormal liver physiology. Examples include familial amyloid polyneuropathy, type 1 oxalosis, urea cycle defects
and hyperammonemia syndromes, familial hypercholesterolemia, and hepatic clotting factor disorders.[624]
In the third group, the liver is susceptible to recurrent
disease because the metabolic disorder persists, but a
survival advantage and improved quality of life justify
liver replacement.[658] Examples include lysosomal storage diseases such as Niemann-Pick disease, Gaucher's
disease, cystinosis, and erythropoietic protoporphyria.

Diseases of uncertain cause, such as sarcoidosis,[658]
idiopathic granulomatous hepatitis,[220] and Budd-Chiari
syndrome,[177-179] also recur after liver replacement.

Postinfantile Giant Cell Hepatitis

Postinfantile giant cell hepatitis is a diagnosis of exclusion in patients showing multinucleated giant cell
transformation of hepatocytes on liver biopsy. It also
recurs after liver replacement.[659-663] By definition,
affected patients are negative for HBV, HCV, CMV,
EBV, or HSV infection and have a negative history for
exposure to hepatotoxic drugs.[664] A subgroup of these
patients have evidence of autoimmunity.[663-666]
Ultrastructural evidence of hepatocytes with paramyxovirus particles has been detected in some native
livers,[667,668] but not in allograft recipients.[663]

The incidence of recurrence is difficult to determine
precisely because the incidence of postinfantile giant cell
hepatitis is not known in the general population or in
those awaiting liver transplantation. In our small series,
recurrent disease developed in five of seven patients
between 1 and 21 months after transplantation.[663] The
high incidence of recurrence and therapeutic response to
ribavirin[660,662] seem to reinforce speculation of an infectious cause, but we could *not* ultrastructurally identify
paramyxovirus particles or any other putative infectious
agents in the liver allograft.[663]

The histopathological diagnosis of recurrent or new-
onset postinfantile giant cell hepatitis rests on identification of giant cell transformation of hepatocytes
combined with a "hepatitic" background histology.
Lobular findings are predominant and include disarray,
inflammation, Kupffer cell hypertrophy, spotty
acidophilic necrosis of hepatocytes, and hepatocyte
ballooning. Giant cell transformation of hepatocytes
should be defined as six or more nuclei per hepatocyte,
and six or more hepatocytes per lobule should be
involved in more than an occasional lobule. Less
extensive giant cell transformation can also be seen
in HBV and HCV infection and during recovery from
prolonged preservation injury in older donors (unpublished observation). If giant cell transformation is seen
on liver allograft biopsy, re-review of native hepatectomy
slides is warranted to determine whether recurrent
disease is a possibility.

Primary Biliary Cirrhosis

Pathophysiology

PBC is a common indication for liver transplantation
at some large centers and recurs in about
recipients by 5 years after transplantation
69–10).[220,356,521-523,553,651-654] New-onset PBC
although the author (A.J.D.) has observed

convincing, but unreported case in a patient with coexistent HCV infection. The broad range in the incidence of recurrent disease can be attributed to certainty of the pretransplant and posttransplant diagnosis, immunosuppressive agents and management policies, use of protocol biopsies, length of posttransplant follow-up, and other factors influencing biliary tract physiology after transplantation.[220,356,521-523,553,651-654]

Van de Water and colleagues[559] showed that immunohistochemical evidence of altered expression of the immunodominant mitochondrial autoantigen of PBC (E2 component of the pyruvate dehydrogenase complex) developed in 28 of 38 (74%) patients with PBC sometimes within days after transplantation. However, in only eight of these patients did routine histopathological and clinical evidence of recurrent PBC develop. Other studies were unable to confirm this finding.[669,670] Centers that conduct protocol biopsies tend to report a higher incidence of recurrent disease than do centers that perform biopsies only on indication.

PBC is often classified as an "autoimmune" disease because autoantibodies (antimitochondrial, antinuclear pore antibodies gp-210 and Sp-100) are a defining feature along with characteristic histopathology. However, evidence supporting the contention of autoimmunity can be challenged because PBC in native livers does not respond favorably to increased immunosuppression and there is no universal association with HLA types, as with autoimmune hepatitis. Patients ̣ated with potent immunosuppressive agents, such ̣acrolimus, have a higher incidence and earlier onset ̣ecurrent PBC than do patients maintained on ̣porine.[560,561] Recurrent PBC is also more common ̣ving related liver transplantation[671] and after ̣vithdrawal.[89,90,672]

̣atures

̣ of recurrent PBC are usually detected more ̣ after transplantation and as lymphocytic ̣us cholangitis on routine or protocol ̣s. Most patients with early recurrent ̣ptomatic, but some come to clinical ̣f a preferential increase in routinely ̣hosphatase and γ-GTP or pruritus. ̣acute febrile onset associated with ̣test values, combined with a ̣itic histology, within 2 months ̣ublished observation).

̣lation, recurrent PBC in the ̣nd short- and intermediate- ̣val rates are not adversely ̣t PBC can be progres- ̣l disease, and jaundice, ̣nd portal hypertension

The diagnosis is establisḥ biopsy specimens of the ạ antibodies are of little additioṇ sis of recurrent PBC because tḥ the majority of patients after tṛ [523,553,651-654] The effect of treatment ̣ acid[673,674] on recurrent disease in allẹ systematically investigated, but the ̣ the results will be similar to those seeṇ

Histopathological Findings

Needle biopsy of the allograft is needed to ẹ diagnosis of recurrent PBC with certạ histopathological manifestations are identical ̣ seen in native livers,[220,356,522-524,651-653] and the ̣ nomonic lesion for recurrent PBC is the floriḍ lesion, or noninfectious granulomatous cholaṇ (Fig. 69–21). Although portal granulomas have ḅ identified in patients with HCV infection,[520] this obseṛ vation is not common in our experience, and the graṇ ulomas in HCV infection are rarely associated with ̣ significant ductal damage.

Diagnostic florid duct lesions are not always present, but prominent patchy lymphocytic cholangitis accompanied by portal lymphoid nodules containing

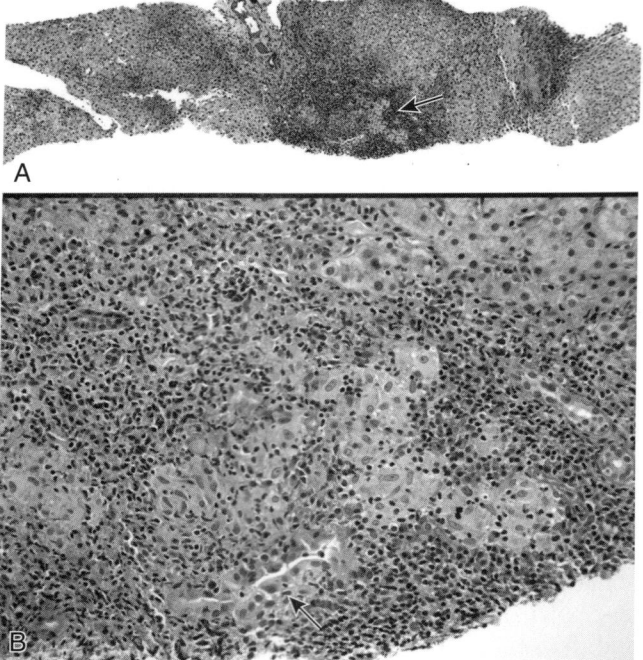

FIGURE 69–21

The histopathological appearance of recurrent primary biliary cirrhosis is very similar to that seen in native livers and is characterized by granulomatous destructive duct lesions (florid duct lesions) as shown here, which is needed to establish the diagnosis with certainty in allograft livers.

...inal centers and an interface ductular reaction ...findings strongly suggestive of recurrent disease. ...ular findings are nonspecific and usually include ...ld spotty necrosis, Kupffer cell hypertrophy, a slight ...crease in sinusoidal lymphocytes, mild nodular ...egenerative hyperplasia changes, and Kupffer cell ...granulomas. "Biliary" fibrosis develops as recurrent disease progresses and is characterized by a ductular reaction at the interface zone, cholestasis, and deposition of copper and copper-associated proteins in periportal hepatocytes. These findings provide strongly supportive evidence of recurrent PBC if other causes of biliary tract pathology have been reasonably excluded.

In the absence of pathognomonic or strongly suggestive findings, the histopathological diagnosis of recurrent PBC can be problematic. For example, "possible" recurrent PBC might be first manifested as an unexplained chronic hepatitis,[220,356] either because the duct damage was missed on biopsy or because the recurrent disease was manifested as autoimmune hepatitis.[675] In addition, the findings of recurrent PBC can overlap with those of recurrent autoimmune hepatitis,[356] and plasma cell–rich periportal hepatitis early after transplantation has been suggested as an early marker predictive of PBC recurrence.[676]

Differential Diagnosis

Recurrent PBC should be distinguished from acute and chronic rejection; biliary tract obstruction and strictures; chronic viral, autoimmune, or idiopathic hepatitis; and adverse drug reactions. The key to establishing the diagnosis of recurrent PBC with certainty is identification of granulomatous duct destruction, or florid duct lesions, in the proper context. The proper context includes PBC as an original disease, persistence of anti-mitochondrial antibodies, and exclusion of mechanical biliary tract problems and other causes of portal granulomas (e.g., fungal or acid-fast bacterial infections and HCV). Prominent focal lymphocytic cholangitis accompanied by portal lymphoid nodules containing germinal centers and an interface ductular reaction is strongly suggestive, but not absolutely diagnostic of recurrent PBC.

In cases without diagnostic findings, the development of a "biliary gestalt" points toward recurrent PBC and distinguishes such cases from other nonbiliary causes of chronic allograft dysfunction. The most helpful findings in this context include a ductular reaction at the interface zone, periportal "clearing" or edema, cholestasis, accumulation of copper or copper-associated protein in periportal hepatocytes, and patchy small bile duct loss. It is assumed that there is no evidence of large bile duct obstruction or strictures.

A ductular reaction is typical of recurrent PBC and is the key feature used to distinguish it from acute or chronic rejection, which lack a persistent ductular reaction and therefore do not lead to biliary fibrosis. In addition, the portal inflammation and rejection-associated lymphocytic cholangitis usually involve a majority of portal tracts and preferentially involve small bile ducts (<20 μm in largest diameter), whereas PBC-associated portal inflammation and lymphocytic cholangitis are typically patchy and preferentially involve medium-sized bile ducts (>40 to 50 μm in shortest diameter). Chronic hepatitis does not lead to a "biliary gestalt" over time.

In occasional patients with PBC, "autoimmune" hepatitis develops after liver transplantation[675,677] and is thought to represent a "switch" of autoimmune activity from biliary epithelial cells (PBC) to periportal hepatocytes (autoimmune hepatitis). Alternatively, it might represent new-onset autoimmune hepatitis or an alternative form of rejection.[678] A "biliary gestalt" may not develop in these patients, and they need to be distinguished from those with other causes of chronic hepatitis, such as HBV or HCV infection, and adverse drug reactions.

Recurrent and New-Onset "Autoimmune" Hepatitis

Pathophysiology

The diagnosis of autoimmune hepatitis in a native liver is based on a combination of clinical, pathological, and serological findings, combined with the exclusion of other causes of chronic liver injury.[679] The diagnosis of autoimmune hepatitis after transplantation is even more problematic because of a conceptual and pathophysiological overlap with rejection and other late post-transplant complications.[678,680-682] Further complicating the issue are the observations that autoantibodies present before transplantation often persist after transplantation, albeit usually at lower titer, and that autoantibodies can develop in patients with chronic rejection.[554,683-685] Even relatively strict criteria for the diagnosis of autoimmune hepatitis,[679] such as those proposed by the international scoring system for native livers, may not be appropriate for allograft livers.[681] Manns and Bahr[682] suggested that the diagnosis of recurrent autoimmune hepatitis should fulfill even more stringent criteria: sustained elevated serum transaminase levels, autoantibodies in significant titer, elevated serum immunoglobulins, compatible liver histology, corticosteroid dependency, and exclusion of other causes of graft dysfunction such as HCV infection.

At a minimum, the diagnosis of autoimmune hepatitis in an allograft should be based on chronic "hepatitis" histopathology in a liver biopsy specimen, accompanied by persistent elevation of liver injury test values, negative RT-PCR for HBV and HCV infection, and no other evidence for a cause of chronic hepatitis.[678] Regardless of the difficulties in establishing the diagnosis, there is convincing evidence from a number of centers that recurrent autoimmune hepatitis develops in roughly 30% of recipients by 5 years after transplantation. It is usually first manifested more than 1 year after transplantation.[90,220,522,553-558,564,654,663,672,683-691]

Risk factors for the development of recurrent autoimmune hepatitis include suboptimal immunosuppression,[90,522,684,688] HLA-DR3– and HLA-DR4–positive recipients,[553,558,692] the type of autoimmune disease (greater recurrence incidence with type I versus type II[678]), severe inflammation in the native liver before transplantation,[557] and the duration of follow-up.[678] Children appear to be at increased risk for new-onset or de novo autoimmune hepatitis after transplantation.[555,689,693-695] This observation is probably attributable to the immaturity of the pediatric immune system, including an active thymus susceptible to damage from calcineurin-inhibiting immunosuppressive drugs and subsequent premature release of autoreactive clones into the periphery.[696]

Rejection reactions, especially chronic rejection, also trigger "autoimmune" effector pathways.[156,697,698] This is most likely attributable to the phenomenon of "epitope spreading."[107,153] Severe or chronic injury from severe or persistent acute rejection can uncover new "altered-self" antigenic determinants in the damaged tissue that are processed and indirectly presented to the recipient immune system. This mechanism could cause various donor MHC and tissue-specific or autoantigen reactive clones to appear in the recipient T-cell repertoire.[107,153]

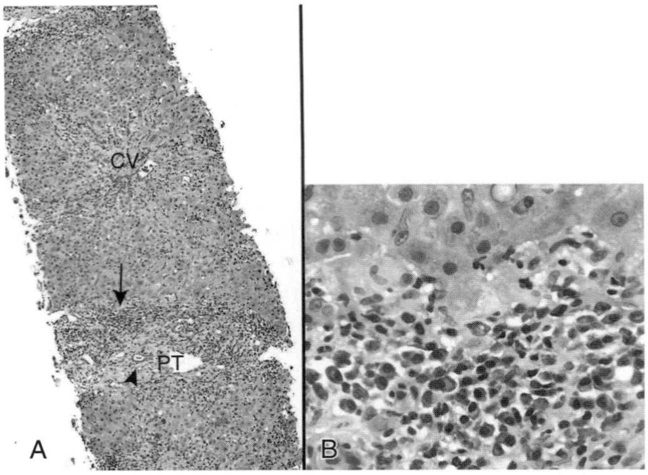

Clinical Features

Most cases of recurrent autoimmune hepatitis first come to clinical attention because of increased liver injury test results manifested primarily as elevated ALT and AST. This often occurs during lowering of immunosuppression. Because of the propensity for the development of rejection and recurrent disease, patients with autoimmune hepatitis are generally treated with higher levels of immunosuppression after transplantation and more often fail attempts at weaning from immunosuppression.[681] More severe recurrent or fulminant autoimmune hepatitis is rare because of baseline immune suppression, but evolution toward cirrhosis has been reported with recurrent disease.[681] The possibility of a diagnosis of autoimmune hepatitis is based on findings in a core needle biopsy. However, the diagnosis is confirmed only with the aid of serological (e.g., autoantibodies, serum immune globulin levels, HLA type) and molecular biological tests to verify autoimmune reactions and exclude other causes of allograft dysfunction.

Histopathological Findings

Autoimmune hepatitis cannot be reliably distinguished from other causes of acute or chronic hepatitis by

FIGURE 69–22

A, The histopathological appearance of recurrent or new-onset "autoimmune" hepatitis is very similar to that seen in native livers. It is characterized by moderate portal inflammation, prominent interface activity (*arrow*), relative sparing of the bile ducts (*arrowhead*), and perivenular accumulation of inflammation. CV, central vein; PT, portal tract. **B**, A higher magnification of the interface zone highlighted by the *arrow* in **A** shows that the portal and periportal inflammation is rich in plasma cells, typical of autoimmune hepatitis

histopathology alone, but there is often a set of characteristic features, including prominent interface activity mediated by moderate to severe portal and periportal mononuclear inflammation containing a conspicuous percentage of plasma cells (Fig. 69–22). This is frequently accompanied by lobular hepatitis and marked regenerative activity with pseudorosetting of hepatocytes, which can precede the development of full-blown recurrent disease.[557] Not infrequently, mononuclear inflammation will accumulate around the central veins in association with perivenular hepatocyte necrosis and dropout. This latter feature closely resembles the so-called central venulitis of acute rejection, but recurrent autoimmune hepatitis has minimal bile duct damage and more prominent interface activity.

Differential Diagnosis

Once the "chronic hepatitis" histology is recognized, complete clinicopathological and serological correlation is needed to establish a diagnosis of recurrent or new-onset autoimmune hepatitis with certainty. Most importantly, there must be persistent elevations in liver injury test values, and other causes of chronic hepatitis, such as HBV and HCV infection, recurrent PBC or PSC, chronic obstructive cholangiopathy, adverse drug reactions, and acute rejection, must be reasonably excluded. Distinguishing autoimmune hepatitis from acute and chronic rejection involves the use of the same guidelines as those used to distinguish rejection from viral hepatitis (see "Hepatitis C Virus").

Recurrent Primary Sclerosing Cholangitis

Pathophysiology

PSC is a disease of unknown cause that often arises in patients with coexistent ulcerative colitis. It recurs in about 20% to 30% of patients by 5 years after transplantation.[219,220,565,699-704] The presence of known hilar bile duct cancer before transplantation significantly degrades survival after transplantation.[565,700] Coexistent ulcerative colitis generally worsens after transplantation,[703,705] and the risk for development of colon cancer and death is substantial.[702] However, the cancer risk is not any greater than that in nonallograft patients with a long history of ulcerative colitis.[705] Patients with PSC are also at greater risk for acute, chronic, and steroid-resistant rejection.[565,701,702,704]

Establishing the diagnosis of recurrent PSC can be quite difficult because many other insults, such as ischemic injury from prolonged preservation or transplantation of organs from non–heart-beating donors, imperfect biliary anastomoses, inadequate hepatic arterial flow, and antibody-mediated rejection, can also cause nonanastomotic intrahepatic biliary strictures that mimic recurrent PSC.[219,220,565,699-703] Graziadei and colleagues[566,704] restrictively defined recurrent PSC in terms of both positive and negative criteria. The definition included a confirmed diagnosis of PSC before transplantation and cholangiographically confirmed biliary strictures occurring more than 90 days after transplantation or biopsy findings showing fibrous cholangitis or fibro-obliterative lesions with or without ductopenia, biliary fibrosis, or biliary cirrhosis, all in the absence of hepatic artery thrombosis/stenosis, established chronic (ductopenic) rejection, anastomotic strictures alone, nonanastomotic strictures occurring before posttransplant day 90, and ABO incompatibility between the donor and recipient. Regardless of these difficulties, otherwise unexplained nonanastomotic intrahepatic biliary strictures occur with greater frequency after transplantation in patients who had PSC before liver replacement.[219,220,565,699-704]

Clinical Features

Recurrent PSC is usually first manifested more than 1 year after transplantation and, in our experience, appears to increase with time after transplantation.[219,220,565,699-704] Nonanastomotic intrahepatic strictures developing *before* 90 days after transplantation are not usually attributable to recurrent disease. Instead, the early stage of recurrent disease generally first comes to clinical attention more than 1 year after transplantation because of selective elevation of alkaline phosphatase and γ-GTP. Recurrent disease usually progresses over a period of years. Symptoms of ascending cholangitis and biliary cirrhosis can develop, but up to 5 years after transplantation patient and allograft survival is not adversely influenced.[565,700-704] Cholangiographic findings helpful in distinguishing recurrent disease from other causes of biliary strictures include mural irregularity, diverticulum-like outpouchings, and an overall appearance resembling PSC in the native liver.[567]

Histopathological Findings

The histopathological findings of recurrent PSC are identical to those described for native livers with sclerosing cholangitis and similar to other causes of biliary tract obstruction or strictures.[222] Early stages are characterized by mild nonspecific acute and chronic "pericholangitis," often accompanied by a very mild type I ductular reaction involving a variable percentage of the portal tracts. A "biliary gestalt" develops as the disease progresses, including irregular fibrous expansion of most portal tracts accompanied by variable portal edema and a ductular reaction. In established cases, periductal lamellar edema or fibrous cholangitis, intraepithelial or intraluminal neutrophils, pigmented macrophages in the portal connective tissue, and periportal deposition of golden pigment and copper and copper-associated protein signal chronically impaired bile flow. This leads to further expansion of the portal tracts by proliferating ductules and surrounding myofibroblasts that progressively distort the architecture. Focal small bile duct loss can also be seen. Superimposed acute cholangitis can lead to marked portal periductal and intraductal neutrophilia. As in other biliary diseases, the spatial relationship between the expanded portal tracts and the central veins remains intact until very late in the disease.

Lobular findings early in recurrent disease include Kupffer cell hypertrophy, lobular neutrophil clusters, and mild nodular regenerative hyperplasia changes with thickening of the periportal plates and slight displacement of the central veins. Later stages are characterized by the development of biliary cirrhosis, cholestasis, intralobular foam cell clusters, marked deposition of copper and copper-associated protein, and Mallory's hyaline at the edge of the nodules.

Differential Diagnosis

An important first step in recognizing recurrent PSC and distinguishing it from other causes of chronic allograft dysfunction is recognition of the early stages of a "biliary gestalt," described earlier. This impression can be reinforced by preferential elevation of γ-GTP and alkaline phosphatase. Clinicopathological correlation is needed to determine whether the changes can be attributed to recurrent PSC or other causes of biliary tract obstruction or strictures.

Harrison and associates[219] suggested that the presence of classic "fibro-obliterative duct lesions" might be restricted to liver allograft recipients who had PSC before transplantation. However, fibro-obliterative duct lesions can develop in patients with ischemic cholangitis and in those with chronic reflux cholangiopathy.[207,706] In our experience, a diagnosis of recurrent PSC is best based on a combination of clinical, histopathological, and radiographic findings.

Toxic and Metabolic Diseases

Recurrent Alcoholic and Nonalcoholic Steatohepatitis

Pathophysiology. Alcoholic liver disease is a leading indication for liver transplantation at many large centers,[568,572,707,708] but nonalcoholic steatohepatitis (NASH) is a problem of increasing significance and is recognized as a major contributor to "cryptogenic" cirrhosis.[709,710] Both alcoholic liver disease and NASH recur after liver replacement or develop as new diseases. Pretransplant screening programs attempt to identify patients who are likely to return to drinking in excess and those with persistent risk factors for NASH, such as obesity, diabetes, and an insulin resistance syndrome.[710] However, recurrent alcohol abuse and NASH can directly cause allograft dysfunction, and alcohol can indirectly contribute to allograft dysfunction because of noncompliance with immunosuppression.[572,573]

Estimates of the incidence of recurrent alcohol use/abuse after transplantation range from 15% to 50% by 5 years after transplantation.[574,711,712] Many of the risk factors for NASH persist or develop as a complication of treatment after transplantation and thereby predispose to disease recurrence or new-onset disease.[710]

Most alcoholics do relatively well after transplantation, and recurrent disease has a relatively small impact on long-term patient and allograft survival.[564,572,574,575,711-713] A minority experience a rapid downhill course after transplantation because of alcohol recidivism, and aggressive recurrent disease develops in a small fraction of patients with NASH.[714-716]

Clinical Features. Recurrent alcohol use/abuse, alcoholic liver disease, and NASH are usually detected on routine follow-up liver biopsies or because of elevation of routinely obtained liver injury tests.[572] Other indicators of recurrent alcoholism include missed medical appointments,[576] inappropriate social behavior,[220] and noncompliance with immunosuppression.[572,573,717] A high γ-GTP–to–alkaline phosphatase ratio identifies potential alcoholic liver disease recurrence.[220,572]

Histopathological Findings. The histopathology of alcoholic steatohepatitis and NASH in a liver allograft is identical to that seen in the general population. Steatosis is the defining feature of both. The steatosis is mixed macrovesicular and microvesicular and involves primarily the centrilobular hepatocytes in recurrent alcoholic liver disease.[220,572-574,714,716,718] The centrilobular distribution of fat is usually not as striking in recurrent or new-onset NASH. So-called foamy degeneration of centrilobular hepatocytes can develop in alcoholic steatohepatitis[220] and can progress to fully developed alcoholic hepatitis with Mallory's hyaline, ballooning degeneration of hepatocytes, and associated lobular inflammation. Persistent or recurrent alcoholic steatohepatitis and NASH can lead to perivenular and subsinusoidal fibrosis. Occasional patients with alcoholic relapse show only increased iron deposition in periportal hepatocytes and occasional reticular endothelial cells without steatosis.[220]

Changes associated with coexistent viral hepatitis (especially hepatitis C) or biliary obstruction frequently complicate recurrent alcoholic liver disease. Liver fibrosis and architectural distortion develop more quickly in patients with coexistent disorders.[572,714]

Differential Diagnosis. Establishing the diagnosis of steatohepatitis is not usually difficult, but determining the underlying cause can be problematic. All the disorders known to cause steatohepatitis in the general population can occur in liver allograft recipients, and some causes are unique to allografts. Included are the well-known causes such as obesity, poorly controlled diabetes, insulin resistance, intestinal bypass surgery, malabsorption, hyperlipidemia, and toxicities of several drugs.[23] HCV genotype 3 has been reported as a cause of severe steatosis, although coexistent alcoholic liver disease was a complicating factor in this report.[719] Steatohepatitis can also develop because of nausea-induced rapid weight loss and the portal vein "steal" syndrome, in which nutrient-rich portal blood bypasses the liver and elicits centrilobular steatosis.

A thorough clinicopathological correlation, including the original disease or diseases, a detailed clinical history, blood alcohol levels, the ratio of γ-GTP to alkaline phosphatase, and a list of medications, should be used to distinguish among the multiple potential causes of steatohepatitis.

Idiopathic Posttransplant Hepatitis

Hubscher[678] coined the diagnosis of "idiopathic posttransplant hepatitis" to describe a group of patients who have no clinical or serological evidence of viral hepatitis, autoimmunity, or adverse drug reactions but show mononuclear portal inflammation with variable interface activity on liver allograft biopsies. By definition, bile duct damage and venous endothelial inflammation are not conspicuous. Cases with inflammatory changes in zone 3 and foci of confluent perivenular necrosis[678] were also placed in this category, but others might characterize such cases as centrilobular-based acute rejection, which responds to increased immuno-suppression.[294-296,350,720] Another small subgroup probably represents recurrent or new-onset autoimmune hepatitis.[678]

Aside from these minor controversies, most programs that routinely survey long-term survivors by liver biopsy will first encounter idiopathic posttransplant hepatitis[220,316,557,695,721,722] more than 6 months after transplantation in asymptomatic patients, although minor elevations in liver injury test results are not uncommon.[220,316,557,695,721,722] In approximately 5% of patients monitored for a minimum of 10 years, progressive fibrosis will develop and result in established cirrhosis.[678]

The differential diagnosis for idiopathic posttransplant hepatitis is the same as that for HBV or HCV infection or autoimmune hepatitis, which have been previously described.

Long-Term Changes Not Readily Explained by Recurrent Disease

Several studies[220,356,721,723,724] examined the structural integrity and causes of dysfunction in recipients surviving from 1 to 19 years after liver transplantation. Despite differences in the recipient pool, immunosuppressive management policies, and study designs, causes of allograft dysfunction were similar.[220,356,721,723,724] All showed a relatively low incidence of acute and chronic rejection that varied from 4% to 38%, which supported the contention that liver allografts are immunologically privileged.[146] Recurrence of the original disease, especially viral hepatitis, was a leading cause of dysfunction, and obstructive cholangiopathy was also surprisingly common. Pappo and coworkers[220] emphasized that awareness of the original disease, recent change in immunosuppressive management policies, and review of previous biopsies, the clinical profile, and the results of any therapeutic or diagnostic tests or intervention should be incorporated with the biopsy findings to correctly identify the cause of late allograft dysfunction. They also emphasized that interpretation of liver allograft biopsies obtained from long-term survivors is often more difficult than interpretation of specimens obtained early after transplantation.[220]

Changes in long-surviving allografts that cannot be attributed to recurrence of a specific disease include mild lymphocytic portal inflammation without significant duct damage, venulitis, or interface activity; portal arterial and arteriolar thickening and hyalinization; and nodular regenerative hyperplasia (NRH)–like changes, characterized on one end of the spectrum by

thickening of the plates and pseudorosette formation and on the other end by fully developed NRH.[220] The arterial changes are probably attributable to a combination of hypertension and diabetes as complications of the immunosuppression.[220] Full-blown NRH with the development of portal hypertension has also been seen in recipients who did not have the disease before transplantation.[725]

Because more centers may attempt drug withdrawal trials in the near future, obtaining protocol biopsy specimens before stopping or reducing immunosuppression is encouraged.[93,143,726] Such biopsies provide an important baseline for changes that can develop after drug withdrawal.

Liver Allograft Pathology Associated with Systemic Diseases

Septicemia

Sepsis and intra-abdominal infections are frequent occurrences during the first 1 to 2 months after liver transplantation and, alone, can be the main insult responsible for allograft dysfunction. The usual clinical signs and symptoms of infection, such as fever and an elevated white blood cell count, are accompanied by liver dysfunction primarily manifested as hyperbilirubinemia. The underlying mechanism of liver dysfunction in this setting may be related to endotoxemia and cytokine release from Kupffer cells.

Histopathological Findings

The histopathological changes associated with sepsis are identical to those seen in nonallograft livers and include cholangiolar proliferation with bile plugging, acute cholangiolitis usually without cholangitis, and hepatocanalicular cholestasis. Megakaryocytes can be seen occasionally within the sinusoids,[23,24,38] along with Kupffer cell hypertrophy, small clusters of sinusoidal neutrophils, and extramedullary hematopoiesis.[727] The histopathological differential diagnosis includes preservation injury, bile duct obstruction or strictures, and antibody-mediated rejection.[23,24,38]

Differential Diagnosis

Blood or peritoneal fluid cultures that test positive for bacteria or fungi confirm the diagnosis of sepsis or intra-abdominal infection. The diagnosis of preservation injury is substantiated by review of the early posttransplant clinical course and previous biopsies, if available. A positive pretransplant cross-match, low platelet counts and hypocomplementemia after transplantation, and IgG, C3, and C4 deposits in the liver biopsy specimen favor a diagnosis of the antibody-mediated rejection. It may be impossible to distinguish among these possibilities on the basis of a single biopsy in some cases. In general, dysfunction attributable to sepsis improves with appropriate antimicrobial therapy, whereas preservation injury spontaneously improves without specific therapeutic intervention. In contrast, the histopathological changes and allograft dysfunction usually worsen over a period of 1 to 2 weeks, and acute (cellular) rejection occurs if antibody-mediated rejection is the cause of dysfunction.

Adverse Drug Reactions and Toxic Injury

The clinical manifestations and histopathological changes associated with adverse drug reactions are beyond the scope of this chapter. As a general rule, morphological manifestations associated with a particular agent are the same as those described for nonallografted livers. The exception may be drugs that induce an immunological response or cases in which altered self-antigens may precipitate or drive the reaction. Such reactions could be blunted or become even less common because of the potent immunosuppression. The use of azathioprine as an immunosuppressant in liver allograft recipients has been associated with the development of centrilobular necrosis and central vein and sinusoidal fibrosis in the short term,[728] and NRH has been seen with long-term use.[725]

Acknowledgment

The editorial assistance of Mrs. Linda Askren is acknowledged and greatly appreciated. We are also grateful to our surgical colleagues and mentors who have provided the specimens and environment to study them.

References

1. Starzl T, Kaupp H, Brock D, Linman J: Studies on the rejection of the transplanted homologous dog liver. Surg Gynecol Obstet 112:135, 1961.
2. McBride R, Wheeler H, Smith L, et al: Homotransplantation of the canine liver as an orthotopic vascularized graft. Am J Pathol 41:501, 1962.
3. Starzl TE, Marchioro TL, Von Kaulla KN, et al: Homotransplantation of the liver in humans. Surg Gynecol Obstet 117:659-676, 1963.
4. Starzl TE, Klintmalm GB, Porter KA, et al: Liver transplantation with use of cyclosporin A and prednisone. N Engl J Med 305:266-269, 1981.
5. Starzl TE: History of liver and other splanchnic organ transplantation. In Busuttil R, Klintmalm G (eds): Transplantation of the Liver. Philadelphia, WB Saunders, 1996, pp 3-22.
6. Fennell RH Jr, Roddy HJ: Liver transplantation: The pathologist's perspective. Pathol Annu 14:155-182, 1979.
7. Fennell RH Jr: Ductular damage in liver transplant rejection: Its similarity to that of primary biliary cirrhosis and graft-versus-host disease. Pathol Annu 16:289-294, 1981.
8. Porter KA: Pathology of liver transplantation. Transplant Rev 2:129-170, 1969.
9. Porter KA: Pathology of the orthotopic homograft and heterograft. In Starzl TE (ed): Experience in Hepatic Transplantation. Philadelphia, WB Saunders, 1969, p 422.
10. Portmann B, O'Grady J, Williams R: Disease recurrence following orthotopic liver transplantation. Transplant Proc 18(Suppl 4):136-141, 1986.
11. Portmann B, Neuberger J, Williams R: Intrahepatic bile duct lesions. In Calne R (ed): Liver Transplantation: The Cambridge–Kings College Hospital Experience. New York, Grune & Stratton, 1983, pp 279-287.
12. Wight D: Pathology of rejection. In Calne R (ed): Liver Transplantation: The Cambridge–King's College Hospital Experience. New York, Grune & Stratton, 1983, pp 247-277.
13. Wight D: The morphology of rejection of liver transplants. In Transplant Immunology, Clinical and Experimental. Oxford, Oxford University Press, 1984, pp 385-435.
14. Calne R, Williams R: Liver transplantation. Curr Probl Surg 16:3-44, 1979.
15. Demetris A, Crawford J, Nalesnik M, et al: Transplantation pathology of the liver. In Odze R, Goldblum J, Crawford JM (eds): Surgical Pathology of the GI Tract, Liver, Biliary Tract, and Pancreas. Philadelphia, WB Saunders, 2004, pp 909-966.
16. Takakura K, Kiuchi T, Kasahara M, et al: Clinical implications of flow cytometry crossmatch with T or B cells in living donor liver transplantation. Clin Transplant 15:309-316, 2001.
17. Klintmalm G, Busuttil R: Transplantation of the Liver. Philadelphia, WB Saunders, 1996.
18. Demetris AJ, Ruppert K, Dvorchik I, et al: Real-time monitoring of acute liver-allograft rejection using the Banff schema. Transplantation 74:1290-1296, 2002.
19. McAfee JH, Keeffe EB, Lee RG, Rosch J: Transjugular liver biopsy. Hepatology 15:726-732, 1992.
20. Donaldson BW, Gopinath R, Wanless IR, et al: The role of transjugular liver biopsy in fulminant liver failure: Relation to other prognostic indicators. Hepatology 18:1370-1376, 1993.
21. Kakizoe S, Yanaga K, Starzl TE, Demetris AJ: Frozen section of liver biopsy for the evaluation of liver allografts. Transplant Proc 22:416-417, 1990.
22. Pinna AD, Rakela J, Demetris AJ, Fung JJ: Five cases of fulminant hepatitis due to herpes simplex virus in adults. Dig Dis Sci 47:750-754, 2002.
23. Lee R: Acute hepatitis. In Diagnostic Liver Pathology. St Louis, Mosby–Year Book, 1994, pp 23-66.
24. Demetris AJ, Jaffe R, Starzl TE: A review of adult and pediatric post-transplant liver pathology. Pathol Annu 22:347-386, 1987.
25. Quiroga J, Colina I, Demetris AJ, et al: Cause and timing of first allograft failure in orthotopic liver transplantation: A study of 177 consecutive patients. Hepatology 14:1054-1062, 1991.
26. Wight D: Pathology of liver transplantation. In Wight D (ed): Liver, Biliary Tract and Exocrine Pancreas. London, Churchill Livingstone, 1994, pp 543-596.
27. Hamada H, Valayer J, Gauthier F, et al: Liver retransplantation in children. J Pediatr Surg 30:705-708, 1995.
28. Jain A, Reyes J, Kashyap R, et al: Long-term survival after liver transplantation in 4,000 consecutive patients at a single center. Ann Surg 232:490-500, 2000.
29. Kashyap R, Jain A, Reyes J, et al: Causes of retransplantation after primary liver transplantation in 4000 consecutive patients: 2 to 19 years follow-up. Transplant Proc 33:1486-1487, 2001.
30. Sieders E, Peeters PM, TenVergert EM, et al: Graft loss after pediatric liver transplantation. Ann Surg 235:125-132, 2002.

31. Demetris AJ, Murase N, Nakamura K, et al: Immunopathology of antibodies as effectors of orthotopic liver allograft rejection. Semin Liver Dis 12:51-59, 1992.
32. Kashyap R, Jain A, Reyes J, et al: Causes of death after liver transplantation in 4000 consecutive patients: 2 to 19 year follow-up. Transplant Proc 33:1482-1483, 2001.
33. Rabkin JM, de La Melena V, Orloff SL, et al: Late mortality after orthotopic liver transplantation. Am J Surg 181:475-479, 2001.
34. Ludwig J, Hashimoto E, Porayko MK, Therneau TM: Failed allografts and causes of death after orthotopic liver transplantation from 1985 to 1995: Decreasing prevalence of irreversible hepatic allograft rejection. Liver Transpl Surg 2:185-191, 1996.
35. Jain A, Demetris AJ, Kashyap R, et al: Does tacrolimus offer virtual freedom from chronic rejection after primary liver transplantation? Risk and prognostic factors in 1,048 liver transplantations with a mean follow-up of 6 years. Liver Transpl 7:623-630, 2001.
36. Portmann B, Wight DGD: Pathology of liver transplantation. In Calne R (ed): Liver Transplantation, 2nd ed. London, Grune & Stratton, 1987, pp 435-470.
37. Demetris AJ: The pathology of liver transplantation. Prog Liver Dis 9:687-709, 1990.
38. Demetris A, Kakizoe S, Oguma S: Pathology of liver transplantation. In Williams JW (ed): Hepatic Transplantation. Philadelphia, WB Saunders, 1990, pp 61-111.
39. Yanaga K, Kakizoe S, Ikeda T, et al: Procurement of liver allografts from non–heart beating donors. Transplant Proc 22:275-278, 1990.
40. Kakizoe S, Yanaga K, Starzl TE, Demetris AJ: Evaluation of protocol before transplantation and after reperfusion biopsies from human orthotopic liver allografts: Considerations of preservation and early immunological injury. Hepatology 11:932-941, 1990.
41. Adams R, Reynes M, Johann M, et al: The outcome of steatotic grafts in liver transplantation. Transplant Proc 23:1538-1540, 1991.
42. D'Alessandro AM, Kalayoglu M, Sollinger HW, et al: The predictive value of donor liver biopsies for the development of primary nonfunction after orthotopic liver transplantation. Transplantation 51:157-163, 1991.
43. Mor E, Klintmalm GB, Gonwa TA, et al: The use of marginal donors for liver transplantation. A retrospective study of 365 liver donors. Transplantation 53:383-386, 1992.
44. Markin RS, Wisecarver JL, Radio SJ, et al: Frozen section evaluation of donor livers before transplantation. Transplantation 56:1403-1409, 1993.
45. Portmann B, Slapak GI, Gane E, Williams R: Pathology and biopsy diagnosis of the transplanted liver. Verh Dtsch Ges Pathol 79:277-290, 1995.
46. Deschenes M, Forbes C, Tchervenkov J, et al: Use of older donor livers is associated with more extensive ischemic damage on intraoperative biopsies during liver transplantation. Liver Transpl Surg 5:357-361, 1999.
47. Crowley H, Lewis WD, Gordon F, et al: Steatosis in donor and transplant liver biopsies. Hum Pathol 31:1209-1213, 2000.
48. Vera-Sempere F, Vicente JL, Prieto M, et al: [Frozen section biopsy in the assessment of organs for transplantation.] Med Clin (Barc) 114:81-84, 2000.
49. Todo S, Demetris AJ, Makowka L, et al: Primary nonfunction of hepatic allografts with preexisting fatty infiltration. Transplantation 47:903-905, 1989.
50. Zamboni F, Franchello A, David E, et al: Effect of macrovesicular steatosis and other donor and recipient characteristics on the outcome of liver transplantation. Clin Transplant 15:53-57, 2001.
51. Agnes S, Avolio AW, Magalini SC, et al: Marginal donors for patients on regular waiting lists for liver transplantation. Transpl Int 9(Suppl 1):S469-S471, 1996.
52. Alexander JW, Vaughn WK, Carey MA: The use of marginal donors for organ transplantation: The older and younger donors. Transplant Proc 23:905-909, 1991.
53. Alexander JW, Zola JC: Expanding the donor pool: Use of marginal donors for solid organ transplantation. Clin Transplant 10:1-19, 1996.
54. Briceno J, Lopez-Cillero P, Rufian S, et al: Impact of marginal quality donors on the outcome of liver transplantation. Transplant Proc 29:477-480, 1997.
55. Briceno J, Solorzano G, Pera C: A proposal for scoring marginal liver grafts. Transpl Int 13(Suppl 1):S249-S252, 2000.
56. De Carlis L, Colella G, Sansalone CV, et al: Marginal donors in liver transplantation: The role of donor age. Transplant Proc 31:397-400, 1999.
57. De Carlis L, Sansalone CV, Rondinara GF, et al: Is the use of marginal donors justified in liver transplantation? Analysis of results and proposal of modern criteria. Transpl Int 9(Suppl 1):S414-S417, 1996.
58. Loinaz C, Gonzalez EM: Marginal donors in liver transplantation. Hepatogastroenterology 47:256-263, 2000.
59. Matesanz R, Miranda B: "Marginal quality" donor livers: Not so marginal. Clin Transplant 9:492, 1995.
60. Melendez HV, Heaton ND: Understanding "marginal" liver grafts. Transplantation 68:469-471, 1999.
61. Trotter JF: Expanding the donor pool for liver transplantation. Curr Gastroenterol Rep 2:46-54, 2000.
62. Alexander JW, Vaughn WK: The use of "marginal" donors for organ transplantation. The influence of donor age on outcome. Transplantation 51:135-141, 1991.
63. Testa G, Goldstein RM, Netto G, et al: Long-term outcome of patients transplanted with livers from hepatitis C–positive donors. Transplantation 65:925-929, 1998.
64. Vargas HE, Laskus T, Wang LF, et al: Outcome of liver transplantation in hepatitis C virus–infected patients who received hepatitis C virus–infected grafts. Gastroenterology 117:149-153, 1999.
65. Velidedeoglu E, Desai NM, Campos L, et al: The outcome of liver grafts procured from hepatitis C–positive donors. Transplantation 73:582-587, 2002.
66. Douglas DD, Rakela J, Wright TL, et al: The clinical course of transplantation-associated de novo hepatitis B infection in the liver transplant recipient. Liver Transpl Surg 3:105-111, 1997.
67. Dodson SF, Issa S, Araya V, et al: Infectivity of hepatic allografts with antibodies to hepatitis B virus. Transplantation 64:1582-1584, 1997.
68. Uemoto S, Sugiyama K, Marusawa H, et al: Transmission of hepatitis B virus from hepatitis B core antibody–positive donors in living related liver transplants. Transplantation 65:494-499, 1998.
69. Adams PC, Ghent CN, Grant DR, et al: Transplantation of a donor liver with haemochromatosis: Evidence against an inherited intrahepatic defect. Gut 32:1082-1083, 1991.
70. Adams PC, Jeffrey G, Alanen K, et al: Transplantation of haemochromatosis liver and intestine into a normal recipient. Gut 45:783, 1999.
71. Ben-Haim M, Emre S, Fishbein TM, et al: Critical graft size in adult-to-adult living donor liver transplantation: Impact of the recipient's disease. Liver Transpl 7:948-953, 2001.
72. Kiuchi T, Kasahara M, Uryuhara K, et al: Impact of graft size mismatching on graft prognosis in liver transplantation from living donors. Transplantation 67:321-327, 1999.
73. Lee SG, Hwang S, Lee YJ, et al: Regeneration of graft liver in adult-to-adult living donor liver transplantation using a left lobe graft. J Korean Med Sci 13:350-354, 1998.
74. Lee SG, Park KM, Hwang S, et al: Adult-to-adult living donor liver transplantation at the Asan Medical Center, Korea. Asian J Surg 25:277-284, 2002.
75. Lo CM, Fan ST, Chan JK, et al: Minimum graft volume for successful adult-to-adult living donor liver transplantation for fulminant hepatic failure. Transplantation 62:696-698, 1996.

76. Nishizaki T, Ikegami T, Hiroshige S, et al: Small graft for living donor liver transplantation. Ann Surg 233:575-580, 2001.

77. Inomata Y, Uemoto S, Asonuma K, Egawa H: Right lobe graft in living donor liver transplantation. Transplantation 69:258-264, 2000.

78. Marcos A, Fisher RA, Ham JM, et al: Selection and outcome of living donors for adult to adult right lobe transplantation. Transplantation 69:2410-2415, 2000.

79. Shimada M, Shiotani S, Ninomiya M, et al: Characteristics of liver grafts in living-donor adult liver transplantation: Comparison between right- and left-lobe grafts. Arch Surg 137:1174-1179, 2002.

80. Trotter JF, Wachs M, Everson GT, Kam I: Adult-to-adult transplantation of the right hepatic lobe from a living donor. N Engl J Med 346:1074-1082, 2002.

81. Ryan CK, Johnson LA, Germin BI, Marcos A: One hundred consecutive hepatic biopsies in the workup of living donors for right lobe liver transplantation. Liver Transpl 8:1114-1122, 2002.

82. Demetris AJ, Qian S, Sun H, et al: Early events in liver allograft rejection. Delineation of sites of simultaneous intragraft and recipient lymphoid tissue sensitization. Am J Pathol 138:609-618, 1991.

83. Demetris AJ, Murase N, Fujisaki S, et al: Hematolymphoid cell trafficking, microchimerism, and GVH reactions after liver, bone marrow, and heart transplantation. Transplant Proc 25:3337-3344, 1993.

84. Okuda T, Ishikawa T, Azhipa O, et al: Early passenger leukocyte migration and acute immune reactions in the rat recipient spleen during liver engraftment: With particular emphasis on donor major histocompatibility complex class II+ cells. Transplantation 74:103-111, 2002.

85. Steinman RM, Cohn ZA: Identification of a novel cell type in peripheral lymphoid organs of mice. I. Morphology, quantitation, tissue distribution. J Exp Med 137:1142-1162, 1973.

86. Steinman RM, Cohn ZA: Identification of a novel cell type in peripheral lymphoid organs of mice. II. Functional properties in vitro. J Exp Med 139:380-397, 1974.

87. Demetris AJ, Murase N, Fung JJ: Dendritic cells in rejection and acceptance of solid organ allografts. In Lotze MT, Thomson A (eds): Dendritic Cells, 2nd ed. San Diego, CA, Academic Press, 2001, pp 439-458.

88. Lakkis FG, Arakelov A, Konieczny BT, Inoue Y: Immunologic 'ignorance' of vascularized organ transplants in the absence of secondary lymphoid tissue. Nat Med 6:686-688, 2000.

89. Ramos HC, Reyes J, Abu-Elmagd K, et al: Weaning of immunosuppression in long-term liver transplant recipients. Transplantation 59:212-217, 1995.

90. Mazariegos GV, Reyes J, Marino IR, et al: Weaning of immunosuppression in liver transplant recipients. Transplantation 63:243-249, 1997.

91. Takatsuki M, Uemoto S, Inomata Y, et al: Weaning of immunosuppression in living donor liver transplant recipients. Transplantation 72:449-454, 2001.

92. Takatsuki M, Uemoto S, Inomata Y, et al: Analysis of alloreactivity and intragraft cytokine profiles in living donor liver transplant recipients with graft acceptance. Transpl Immunol 8:279-286, 2001.

93. Padbury RT, Gunson BK, Dousset B, et al: Steroid withdrawal from long-term immunosuppression in liver allograft recipients. Transplantation 55:789-794, 1993.

94. Devlin J, Doherty D, Thomson L, et al: Defining the outcome of immunosuppression withdrawal after liver transplantation. Hepatology 27:926-933, 1998.

95. Wong T, Nouri-Aria KT, Devlin J, et al: Tolerance and latent cellular rejection in long-term liver transplant recipients. Hepatology 28:443-449, 1998.

96. Vierling JM: Immunology of acute and chronic hepatic allograft rejection. Liver Transpl Surg 5(4 Suppl 1):S1-S20, 1999.

97. Rouger PH, Poupon R, Gane P, et al: Expression of blood group antigens including HLA markers in human adult liver. Tissue Antigens 27:78-86, 1986.

98. Takacs L, Szende B, Monostori E, et al: Expression of HLA-DR antigens on bile duct cells of rejected liver transplant. Lancet 2:1500, 1983.

99. Demetris AJ, Lasky S, Van Thiel DH, et al: Induction of DR/IA antigens in human liver allografts. An immunocytochemical and clinicopathologic analysis of twenty failed grafts. Transplantation 40:504-509, 1985.

100. Gouw AS, Houthoff HJ, Huitema S, et al: Expression of major histocompatibility complex antigens and replacement of donor cells by recipient ones in human liver grafts. Transplantation 43:291-296, 1987.

101. So SK, Platt JL, Ascher NL, Snover DC: Increased expression of class I major histocompatibility complex antigens on hepatocytes in rejecting human liver allografts. Transplantation 43:79-85, 1987.

102. Steinhoff G, Behrend M, Wonigeit K: Expression of adhesion molecules on lymphocytes/monocytes and hepatocytes in human liver grafts. Hum Immunol 28:123-127, 1990.

103. Demetris AJ: Immunopathology of the human biliary tree. In Sirica AE, Longnecker DS (eds): Biliary and Pancreatic Ductal Epithelia. Pathobiology and Pathophysiology. New York, Marcel Dekker, 1997, pp 127-180.

104. Demetris AJ, Murase N, Lee RG, et al: Chronic rejection. A general overview of histopathology and pathophysiology with emphasis on liver, heart, and intestinal allografts. Ann Transplant 2:27-44, 1997.

105. Ross R: Rous-Whipple Award Lecture. Atherosclerosis: A defense mechanism gone awry. Am J Pathol 143:987-1002, 1993.

106. Hornick PI, Mason PD, Yacoub MH, et al: Assessment of the contribution that direct allorecognition makes to the progression of chronic cardiac transplant rejection in humans. Circulation 97:1257-1263, 1998.

107. Suciu-Foca N, Harris PE, Cortesini R: Intramolecular and intermolecular spreading during the course of organ allograft rejection. Immunol Rev 164:241-246, 1998.

108. Shirwan H: Chronic allograft rejection. Transplantation 68:715-726, 1999.

109. Suthanthiran M, Strom TB: Mechanisms and management of acute renal allograft rejection. Surg Clin North Am 78:77-94, 1998.

110. Douillard P, Cuturi MC, Brouard S, et al: T cell receptor repertoire usage in allotransplantation: An overview. Transplantation 68:913-921, 1999.

111. Pattison JM, Krensky AM: New insights into mechanisms of allograft rejection. Am J Med Sci 313:257-263, 1997.

112. Zhai Y, Ghobrial RM, Busuttil RW, Kupiec-Weglinski JW: Th1 and Th2 cytokines in organ transplantation: Paradigm lost? Crit Rev Immunol 19:155-172, 1999.

113. Li XC, Zand MS, Li Y, et al: On histocompatibility barriers, Th1 to Th2 immune deviation, and the nature of the allograft responses. J Immunol 161:2241-2247, 1998.

114. Romagnani S, Parronchi P, D'Elios MM, et al: An update on human Th1 and Th2 cells. Int Arch Allergy Immunol 113:153-156, 1997.

115. Strom TB, Roy-Chaudhury P, Manfro R, et al: The Th1/Th2 paradigm and the allograft response. Curr Opin Immunol 8:688-693, 1996.

116. Hornick P, Lechler R: Direct and indirect pathways of alloantigen recognition: Relevance to acute and chronic allograft rejection [editorial]. Nephrol Dial Transplant 12:1806-1810, 1997.

117. Benichou G: Direct and indirect antigen recognition: The pathways to allograft immune rejection. Front Biosci 4:D476-D480, 1999.

118. Banff schema for grading liver allograft rejection: An international consensus document. Hepatology 25:658-663, 1997.

119. Ganschow R, Broering DC, Nolkemper D, et al: Th2 cytokine profile in infants predisposes to improved graft acceptance after liver transplantation. Transplantation 72:929-934, 2001.

120. Minguela A, Torio A, Marin L, et al: Implication of Th1, Th2, and Th3 cytokines in liver graft acceptance. Transplant Proc 31:519-520, 1999.

121. Hayashi M, Martinez OM, Garcia-Kennedy R, et al: Expression of cytokines and immune mediators during chronic liver allograft rejection. Transplantation 60:1533-1538, 1995.

122. Wiesner RH, Demetris AJ, Belle SH, et al: Acute hepatic allograft rejection: Incidence, risk factors, and impact on outcome. Hepatology 28:638-645, 1998.

123. Gupta P, Hart J, Cronin D, et al: Risk factors for chronic rejection after pediatric liver transplantation. Transplantation 72: 1098-1102, 2001.

124. Blakolmer K, Jain A, Ruppert K, et al: Chronic liver allograft rejection in a population treated primarily with tacrolimus as baseline immunosuppression: Long-term follow-up and evaluation of features for histopathological staging. Transplantation 69:2330-2336, 2000.

125. Neuberger J: Incidence, timing, and risk factors for acute and chronic rejection. Liver Transpl Surg 5(4 Suppl 1):S30-S36, 1999.

126. Anand AC, Hubscher SG, Gunson BK, et al: Timing, significance, and prognosis of late acute liver allograft rejection. Transplantation 60:1098-1103, 1995.

127. Demetris A, Adams D, Bellamy C, et al: Update of the International Banff Schema for Liver Allograft Rejection: Working recommendations for the histopathologic staging and reporting of chronic rejection. An International Panel. Hepatology 31:792-799, 2000.

128. Nadeau KC, Azuma H, Tilney NL: Sequential cytokine dynamics in chronic rejection of rat renal allografts: Roles for cytokines RANTES and MCP-1. Proc Natl Acad Sci U S A 92:8729-8733, 1995.

129. Oguma S, Banner B, Zerbe T, et al: Participation of dendritic cells in vascular lesions of chronic rejection of human allografts. Lancet 2:933-936, 1988.

130. Adams DH, Russell ME, Hancock WW, et al: Chronic rejection in experimental cardiac transplantation: Studies in the Lewis-F344 model. Immunol Rev 134:5-19, 1993.

131. Russell ME, Wallace AF, Hancock WW, et al: Upregulation of cytokines associated with macrophage activation in the Lewis-to-F344 rat transplantation model of chronic cardiac rejection. Transplantation 59:572-578, 1995.

132. Utans U, Arceci RJ, Yamashita Y, Russell ME: Cloning and characterization of allograft inflammatory factor-1: A novel macrophage factor identified in rat cardiac allografts with chronic rejection. J Clin Invest 95:2954-2962, 1995.

133. Demirci G, Nashan B, Pichlmayr R: Fibrosis in chronic rejection of human liver allografts: Expression patterns of transforming growth factor-TGFβ1 and TGF-β3. Transplantation 62:1776-1783, 1996.

134. Kajiwara I, Kawamura K, Takebayashi S: An analysis of monocyte/macrophage subsets and granulocyte-macrophage colony-stimulating factor expression in renal allograft biopsies. Nephron 73:536-543, 1996.

135. Kouwenhoven EA, Stein-Oakley AN, Maguire JA, et al: Increased expression of basic fibroblast growth factor during chronic rejection in intestinal transplants is associated with macrophage infiltrates. Transpl Int 12:42-49, 1999.

136. Nagano H, Nadeau KC, Kusaka M, et al: Infection-associated macrophage activation accelerates chronic renal allograft rejection in rats. Transplantation 64:1602-1605, 1997.

137. Kallio EA, Koskinen PK, Aavik E, et al: Role of platelet-derived growth factor in obliterative bronchiolitis (chronic rejection) in the rat. Am J Respir Crit Care Med 160:1324-1332, 1999.

138. Kallio EA, Koskinen PK, Aavik E, et al: Role of nitric oxide in experimental obliterative bronchiolitis (chronic rejection) in the rat. J Clin Invest 100:2984-2994, 1997.

139. Hamano K, Ito H, Shirasawa B, et al: Correlations among expression of intercellular adhesion molecule 1, cellular infiltration, and coronary arteriosclerosis during chronic rejection using the rat heart transplantation model. Eur Surg Res 30:235-242, 1998.

140. Starzl TE, Demetris AJ, Murase N, et al: Cell migration, chimerism, and graft acceptance. Lancet 339:1579-1582, 1992.

141. Starzl TE, Demetris AJ, Trucco M, et al: Systemic chimerism in human female recipients of male livers. Lancet 340:876-877, 1992.

142. Starzl TE, Demetris AJ, Trucco M, et al: Chimerism and donor-specific nonreactivity 27 to 29 years after kidney allotransplantation. Transplantation 55:1272-1277, 1993.

143. Starzl TE, Demetris AJ, Trucco M, et al: Cell migration and chimerism after whole-organ transplantation: The basis of graft acceptance. Hepatology 17:1127-1152, 1993.

144. Starzl TE, Demetris AJ, Trucco M, et al: Chimerism after liver transplantation for type IV glycogen storage disease and type 1 Gaucher's disease. N Engl J Med 328:745-749, 1993.

145. Demetris AJ, Murase N, Rao AS, Starzl TE: The role of passenger leukocytes in rejection and "tolerance" after solid organ transplantation: A potential explanation of a paradox. In Touraine JL, Traeger J, Betuel H, et al (eds): Rejection and Tolerance. Dordrecht, Netherlands, Kluwer, 1994, pp 325-392.

146. Demetris AJ, Murase N, Delaney CP, et al: The liver allograft, chronic (ductopenic) rejection, and microchimerism: What can they teach us? Transplant Proc 27:67-70, 1995.

147. Dunn SP, Krueger LJ, Butani L, Punnett H: Late onset of severe graft-versus-host disease in a pediatric liver transplant recipient. Transplantation 71:1483-1485, 2001.

148. Starzl TE, Murase N, Demetris A, et al: The mystique of hepatic tolerogenicity. Semin Liver Dis 20:497-510, 2000.

149. Reyes J, Todo S, Green M, et al: Graft-versus-host disease after liver and small bowel transplantation in a child. Clin Transplant 11:345-348, 1997.

150. Whitington PF, Rubin CM, Alonso EM, et al: Complete lymphoid chimerism and chronic graft-versus-host disease in an infant recipient of a hepatic allograft from an HLA-homozygous parental living donor. Transplantation 62:1516-1519, 1996.

151. Burdick JF, Vogelsang GB, Smith WJ, et al: Severe graft-versus-host disease in a liver-transplant recipient. N Engl J Med 318: 689-691, 1988.

152. Vella JP, Spadafora-Ferreira M, Murphy B, et al: Indirect allorecognition of major histocompatibility complex allopeptides in human renal transplant recipients with chronic graft dysfunction. Transplantation 64:795-800, 1997.

153. Ciubotariu R, Liu Z, Colovai AI, et al: Persistent allopeptide reactivity and epitope spreading in chronic rejection of organ allografts. J Clin Invest 101:398-405, 1998.

154. Bradley JA: Indirect T cell recognition in allograft rejection. Int Rev Immunol 13:245-255, 1996.

155. Demetris AJ, Murase N, Ye Q, et al: Analysis of chronic rejection and obliterative arteriopathy. Possible contributions of donor antigen-presenting cells and lymphatic disruption. Am J Pathol 150:563-578, 1997.

156. Dubel L, Farges O, Johanet C, et al: High incidence of antitissue antibodies in patients experiencing chronic liver allograft rejection. Transplantation 65:1072-1075, 1998.

157. Paul LC, Muralidharan J, Muzaffar SA, et al: Antibodies against mesangial cells and their secretory products in chronic renal allograft rejection in the rat. Am J Pathol 152:1209-1223, 1998.

158. Paul LC: Chronic allograft nephropathy: An update. Kidney Int 56:783-793, 1999.

159. D'Antiga L, Dhawan A, Portmann B, et al: Late cellular rejection in paediatric liver transplantation: Aetiology and outcome. Transplantation 73:80-84, 2002.

160. Wiesner RH, Batts KP, Krom RA: Evolving concepts in the diagnosis, pathogenesis, and treatment of chronic hepatic allograft rejection. Liver Transpl Surg 5:388-400, 1999.

161. Yoshida EM, Shackleton CR, Erb SR, et al: Late acute rejection occurring in liver allograft recipients. Can J Gastroenterol 10:376-380, 1996.

162. Cakaloglu Y, Devlin J, O'Grady J, et al: Importance of concomitant viral infection during late acute liver allograft rejection. Transplantation 59:40-45, 1995.

163. Piratvisuth T, Tredger JM, Hayllar KA, Williams R: Contribution of true cold and rewarming ischemia times to factors determining outcome after orthotopic liver transplantation. Liver Transpl Surg 1:296-301, 1995.

164. Takada Y, Taniguchi H, Fukunaga K, et al: Prolonged hepatic warm ischemia in non–heart-beating donors: Protective effects of FK506 and a platelet activating factor antagonist in porcine liver transplantation. Surgery 123:692-698, 1998.

165. Kootstra G, Kievit J, Nederstigt A: Organ donors: Heartbeating and non-heartbeating. World J Surg 26:181-184, 2002.

166. Bilzer M, Gerbes AL: Preservation injury of the liver: Mechanisms and novel therapeutic strategies. J Hepatol 32:508-515, 2000.

167. McDonald V, Matalon TA, Patel SK, et al: Biliary strictures in hepatic transplantation. J Vasc Interv Radiol 2:533-538, 1991.

168. Ploeg RJ, D'Alessandro AM, Knechtle SJ, et al: Risk factors for primary dysfunction after liver transplantation—a multivariate analysis. Transplantation 55:807-813, 1993.

169. Strasberg SM, Howard TK, Molmenti EP, Hertl M: Selecting the donor liver: Risk factors for poor function after orthotopic liver transplantation. Hepatology 20:829-838, 1994.

170. Porte RJ, Ploeg RJ, Hansen B, et al: Long-term graft survival after liver transplantation in the UW era: Late effects of cold ischemia and primary dysfunction. European Multicentre Study Group. Transpl Int 11(Suppl 1):S164-S167, 1998.

171. Lichtman SN, Lemasters JJ: Role of cytokines and cytokine-producing cells in reperfusion injury to the liver. Semin Liver Dis 19:171-187, 1999.

172. Lemasters JJ, Thurman RG: Reperfusion injury after liver preservation for transplantation. Annu Rev Pharmacol Toxicol 37:327-338, 1997.

173. Kukan M, Haddad PS: Role of hepatocytes and bile duct cells in preservation-reperfusion injury of liver grafts. Liver Transpl 7:381-400, 2001.

174. Teramoto K, Bowers JL, Khettry U, et al: A rat fatty liver transplant model. Transplantation 55:737-741, 1993.

175. Hayashi M, Tokunaga Y, Fujita T, et al: The effects of cold preservation on steatotic graft viability in rat liver transplantation. Transplantation 56:282-287, 1993.

176. Carrasco L, Sanchez-Bueno F, Sola J, et al: Effects of cold ischemia time on the graft after orthotopic liver transplantation. A bile cytological study. Transplantation 61:393-396, 1996.

177. Starzl TE, Demetris AJ: Liver transplantation: A 31-year perspective. Part I. Curr Probl Surg 27:55-116, 1990.

178. Starzl TE, Demetris AJ: Liver transplantation: A 31-year perspective. Part II. Curr Probl Surg 27:123-178, 1990.

179. Starzl TE, Demetris AJ: Liver transplantation: A 31-year perspective. Part III. Curr Probl Surg 27:187-240, 1990.

180. Gaffey MJ, Boyd JC, Traweek ST, et al: Predictive value of intraoperative biopsies and liver function tests for preservation injury in orthotopic liver transplantation. Hepatology 25:184-189, 1997.

181. Kiuchi T, Oldhafer KJ, Schlitt HJ, et al: Background and prognostic implications of perireperfusion tissue injuries in human liver transplants: A panel histochemical study. Transplantation 66:737-747, 1998.

182. Ray RA, Lewin KJ, Colonna J, et al: The role of liver biopsy in evaluating acute allograft dysfunction following liver transplantation: A clinical histologic correlation of 34 liver transplants. Hum Pathol 19:835-848, 1988.

183. Tillery W, Demetris J, Watkins D, et al: Pathologic recognition of preservation injury in hepatic allografts with six months follow-up. Transplant Proc 21:1330-1331, 1989.

184. Goldstein NS, Hart J, Lewin KJ: Diffuse hepatocyte ballooning in liver biopsies from orthotopic liver transplant patients. Histopathology 18:331-338, 1991.

185. Ng IO, Burroughs AK, Rolles K, et al: Hepatocellular ballooning after liver transplantation: A light and electronmicroscopic study with clinicopathological correlation. Histopathology 18:323-330, 1991.

186. D'Alessandro AM, Kalayoglu M, Sollinger HW, et al: The predictive value of donor liver biopsies on the development of primary nonfunction after orthotopic liver transplantation. Transplant Proc 23:1536-1537, 1991.

187. Carles J, Fawaz R, Neaud V, et al: Ultrastructure of human liver grafts preserved with UW solution. Comparison between patients with low and high postoperative transaminases levels. J Submicrosc Cytol Pathol 26:67-73, 1994.

188. Russo PA, Yunis EJ: Subcapsular hepatic necrosis in orthotopic liver allografts. Hepatology 6:708-713, 1986.

189. Neil DA, Hubscher SG: Are parenchymal changes in early post-transplant biopsies related to preservation-reperfusion injury or rejection? Transplantation 71:1566-1572, 2001.

190. Ferrell L, Bass N, Roberts J, Ascher N: Lipopeliosis: Fat induced sinusoidal dilatation in transplanted liver mimicking peliosis hepatis. J Clin Pathol 45:1109-1110, 1992.

191. Lerut JP, Gordon RD, Tzakis AG, et al: The hepatic artery in orthotopic liver transplantation. Helv Chir Acta 55:367-378, 1988.

192. Pastacaldi S, Teixeira R, Montalto P, et al: Hepatic artery thrombosis after orthotopic liver transplantation: A review of nonsurgical causes. Liver Transpl 7:75-81, 2001.

193. Martinez JA, Rigamonti W, Rahier J, et al: Preserved vascular homograft for revascularization of pediatric liver transplant: A clinical, histological, and bacteriological study. Transplantation 68:672-677, 1999.

194. Hussain HK, Nghiem HV: Imaging of hepatic transplantation. Clin Liver Dis 6:247-270, viii-ix, 2002.

195. Wanless I: Physioanatomic considerations. In Schiff ER, Sorrell MF, Maddrey WC (eds): Diseases of the Liver, 8th ed. Philadelphia, Lippincott Williams & Wilkins, 1999, pp 3-37.

196. Ludwig J, Batts KP, MacCarty RL: Ischemic cholangitis in hepatic allografts. Mayo Clin Proc 67:519-526, 1992.

197. Backman L, Gibbs J, Levy M, et al: Causes of late graft loss after liver transplantation. Transplantation 55:1078-1082, 1993.

198. Batts KP: Ischemic cholangitis. Mayo Clin Proc 73:380-385, 1998.

199. Koneru B, Tzakis AG, Bowman J III, et al: Postoperative surgical complications. Gastroenterol Clin North Am 17:71-91, 1988.

200. Esquivel CO, Jaffe R, Gordon RD, et al: Liver rejection and its differentiation from other causes of graft dysfunction. Semin Liver Dis 5:369-374, 1985.

201. Sedivy R, Gollackner B, Casati B, et al: Apoptotic hepatocytes in rejection and vascular occlusion in liver allograft specimens. Histopathology 32:503-507, 1998.

202. Pinna AD, Smith CV, Furukawa H, et al: Urgent revascularization of liver allografts after early hepatic artery thrombosis. Transplantation 62:1584-1587, 1996.

203. Langnas AN, Marujo W, Stratta RJ, et al: Hepatic allograft rescue following arterial thrombosis. Role of urgent revascularization. Transplantation 51:86-90, 1991.

204. Lerut J, Tzakis AG, Bron K, et al: Complications of venous reconstruction in human orthotopic liver transplantation. Ann Surg 205:404-414, 1987.

205. Kuang AA, Renz JF, Ferrell LD, et al: Failure patterns of cryopreserved vein grafts in liver transplantation. Transplantation 62:742-747, 1996.

206. Sebagh M, Debette M, Samuel D, et al: "Silent" presentation of veno-occlusive disease after liver transplantation as part of the process of cellular rejection with endothelial predilection. Hepatology 30:1144-1150, 1999.

207. Hartman GG, Gordon R, Lerut J, et al: Intrahepatic bile duct strictures in a liver allograft recipient mimicking recurrent primary sclerosing cholangitis. Follow-up of a case report. Transpl Int 4:191-192, 1991.

208. Sanchez-Urdazpal L, Gores GJ, Ward EM, et al: Diagnostic features and clinical outcome of ischemic-type biliary complications after liver transplantation. Hepatology 17:605-609, 1993.

209. Lerut J, Gordon RD, Iwatsuki S, et al: Biliary tract complications in human orthotopic liver transplantation. Transplantation 43:47-51, 1987.

210. Demetris AJ, Jaffe R, Tzakis A, et al: Antibody mediated rejection of human liver allografts: Transplantation across ABO blood group barriers. Transplant Proc 21:2217-2220, 1989.

211. Gugenheim J, Samuel D, Reynes M, Bismuth H: Liver transplantation across ABO blood group barriers. Lancet 336:519-523, 1990.

212. Demetris AJ, Nakamura K, Yagihashi A, et al: A clinicopathological study of human liver allograft recipients harboring preformed IgG lymphocytotoxic antibodies. Hepatology 16:671-681, 1992.

213. Egawa H, Uemoto S, Inomata Y, et al: Biliary complications in pediatric living related liver transplantation. Surgery 124:901-910, 1998.

214. Furuya T, Murase N, Nakamura K, et al: Preformed lymphocytotoxic antibodies: The effects of class, titer and specificity on liver vs. heart allografts. Hepatology 16:1415-1422, 1992.

215. Ayata G, Pomfret E, Pomposelli JJ, et al: Adult-to-adult live donor liver transplantation: A short-term clinicopathologic study. Hum Pathol 32:814-822, 2001.

216. Testa G, Malago M, Broelseh CE: Complications of biliary tract in liver transplantation. World J Surg 25:1296-1299, 2001.

217. Cheng YF, Chen YS, Huang TL, et al: Biliary complications in living related liver transplantation. Chang Gung Med J 24:174-180, 2001.

218. Amersi F, Farmer DG, Busuttil RW: Fifteen-year experience with adult and pediatric liver transplantation at the University of California, Los Angeles. Clin Transpl 255-261, 1998.

219. Harrison RF, Davies MH, Neuberger JM, Hubscher SG: Fibrous and obliterative cholangitis in liver allografts: Evidence of recurrent primary sclerosing cholangitis? Hepatology 20:356-361, 1994.

220. Pappo O, Ramos H, Starzl TE, et al: Structural integrity and identification of causes of liver allograft dysfunction occurring more than 5 years after transplantation. Am J Surg Pathol 19:192-206, 1995.

221. Wiesner RH, Porayko MK, Hay JE, et al: Liver transplantation for primary sclerosing cholangitis: Impact of risk factors on outcome. Liver Transpl Surg 2(5 Suppl 1):99-108, 1996.

222. Desmet VJ: Cholestasis: Extrahepatic obstruction and secondary biliary cirrhosis. In MacSween RNM, Anthony PP, Scheuer PJ, et al (eds): Pathology of the Liver, 3rd ed. Edinburgh, Churchill Livingstone, 1994, pp 425-476.

223. Hartshorne N, Hartman G, Markin RS, et al: Bile duct hemorrhage: A biopsy finding after cholangiography or biliary tree manipulation. Liver 12:137-139, 1992.

224. Demetris AJ, Lasky S, Van Thiel DH, et al: Pathology of hepatic transplantation: A review of 62 adult allograft recipients immunosuppressed with a cyclosporine/steroid regimen. Am J Pathol 118:151-161, 1985.

225. Snover DC, Sibley RK, Freese DK, et al: Orthotopic liver transplantation: A pathological study of 63 serial liver biopsies from 17 patients with special reference to the diagnostic features and natural history of rejection. Hepatology 4:1212-1222, 1984.

226. Foster PF, Sankary HN, Hart M, et al: Blood and graft eosinophilia as predictors of rejection in human liver transplantation. Transplantation 47:72-74, 1989.

227. Nagral A, Ben-Ari Z, Dhillon AP, Burroughs AK: Eosinophils in acute cellular rejection in liver allografts. Liver Transpl Surg 4:355-362, 1998.

228. Sankary H, Foster P, Hart M, et al: An analysis of the determinants of hepatic allograft rejection using stepwise logistic regression. Transplantation 47:74-77, 1989.

229. Lunz JG 3rd, Contrucci S, Ruppert K, et al: Replicative senescence of biliary epithelial cells precedes bile duct loss in chronic liver allograft rejection: Increased expression of p21(WAF1/Cip1) as a disease marker and the influence of immunosuppressive drugs. Am J Pathol 158:1379-1390, 2001.

230. Wiesner RH, Ludwig J, van Hoek B, Krom RA: Current concepts in cell-mediated hepatic allograft rejection leading to ductopenia and liver failure. Hepatology 14:721-729, 1991.

231. Candinas D, Gunson BK, Nightingale P, et al: Sex mismatch as a risk factor for chronic rejection of liver allografts. Lancet 346:1117-1121, 1995.

232. Bathgate AJ, Hynd P, Sommerville D, Hayes PC: The prediction of acute cellular rejection in orthotopic liver transplantation. Liver Transpl Surg 5:475-479, 1999.

233. Milkiewicz P, Gunson B, Saksena S, et al: Increased incidence of chronic rejection in adult patients transplanted for autoimmune hepatitis: Assessment of risk factors. Transplantation 70:477-480, 2000.

234. Terminology of chronic hepatitis, hepatic allograft rejection, and nodular lesions of the liver: Summary of recommendations developed by an international working party, supported by the World Congresses of Gastroenterology, Los Angeles, 1994. Am J Gastroenterol 89(8 Suppl):S177-S181, 1994.

235. Gugenheim J, Le Thai B, Rouger P, et al: Relationship between the liver and lymphocytotoxic alloantibodies in inbred rats. Specific absorption by nonparenchymal liver cells. Transplantation 45:474-478, 1988.

236. Houssin D, Bellon B, Brunaud MD, et al: Interactions between liver allografts and lymphocytotoxic alloantibodies in inbred rats. Hepatology 6:994-998, 1986.

237. Iwatsuki S, Iwaki Y, Kano T, et al: Successful liver transplantation from crossmatch-positive donors. Transplant Proc 13:286-288, 1981.

238. Starzl TE, Ishikawa M, Putnam CW, et al: Progress in and deterrents to orthotopic liver transplantation, with special reference to survival, resistance to hyperacute rejection, and biliary duct reconstruction. Transplant Proc 6(4 Suppl 1):129-139, 1974.

239. Andres GA, Ansell ID, Halgrimson CG, et al: Immunopathological studies of orthotopic human liver allografts. Lancet 1:275-280, 1972.

240. Demetris AJ, Jaffe R, Tzakis A, et al: Antibody-mediated rejection of human orthotopic liver allografts. A study of liver transplantation across ABO blood group barriers. Am J Pathol 132:489-502, 1988.

241. Gordon RD, Iwatsuki S, Esquivel CO, et al: Liver transplantation across ABO blood groups. Surgery 100:342-348, 1986.

242. Rego J, Prevost F, Rumeau JL, et al: Hyperacute rejection after ABO-incompatible orthotopic liver transplantation. Transplant Proc 19:4589-4590, 1987.

243. Fischel RJ, Ascher NL, Payne WD, et al: Pediatric liver transplantation across ABO blood group barriers. Transplant Proc 21:2221-2222, 1989.

244. Demetris AJ: Ischemic cholangitis. Mayo Clin Proc 67:601-602, 1992.

245. Hanto DW, Snover DC, Sibley RK, et al: Hyperacute rejection of a human orthotopic liver allograft in a presensitized recipient. Clin Transpl 1:304-310, 1987.

246. Bird G, Friend P, Donaldson P, et al: Hyperacute rejection in liver transplantation: A case report. Transplant Proc 21:3742-3774, 1989.

247. Starzl TE, Demetris AJ, Todo S: Evidence of hyperacute rejection of human liver grafts: The case of the canary kidneys. Clin Transpl 3:37-45, 1989.

248. Takaya S, Duquesnoy R, Iwaki Y, et al: Positive crossmatch in primary human liver allografts under cyclosporine or FK 506 therapy. Transplant Proc 23:396-399, 1991.

249. Karruppan S, Ericzon BG, Moller E: Relevance of a positive crossmatch in liver transplantation. Transplant Int 4:18-25, 1991.

250. Takaya S, Iwaki Y, Starzl TE: Liver transplantation in positive cytotoxic crossmatch cases using FK506, high-dose steroids, and prostaglandin E1. Transplantation 54:927-929, 1992.

251. Gugenheim J, Charpentier B, Gigou M, et al: Delayed rejection of heart allografts after extracorporeal donor-specific liver hemoperfusion. Role of Kupffer cells. Transplantation 45:628-632, 1988.

252. Houssin D, Gugenheim J, Bellon B, et al: Absence of hyperacute rejection of liver allografts in hypersensitized rats. Transplant Proc 17:293-295, 1985.

253. Orosz CG, Zinn NE, Sirinek LP, Ferguson RM: Delayed rejection of heart allografts in hypersensitized rats by extracorporeal donor-specific liver hemoperfusion. Transplantation 41:398-404, 1986.

254. Demetris AJ, Markus BH: Immunopathology of liver transplantation. Crit Rev Immunol 9:67-92, 1989.

255. Starzl TE, Valdivia LA, Murase N, et al: The biological basis of and strategies for clinical xenotransplantation. Immunol Rev 141:213-244, 1994.

256. Valdivia LA, Fung JJ, Demetris AJ, et al: Donor species complement after liver xenotransplantation. The mechanism of protection from hyperacute rejection. Transplantation 57:918-922, 1994.

257. Manez R, Kelly RH, Kobayashi M, et al: Immunoglobulin G lymphocytotoxic antibodies in clinical liver transplantation: Studies toward further defining their significance. Hepatology 21:1345-1352, 1995.

258. Takaya S, Iwatsuki S, Noguchi T, et al: The influence of liver dysfunction on cyclosporine pharmacokinetics—a comparison between 70 per cent hepatectomy and complete bile duct ligation in dogs. Jpn J Surg 19:49-56, 1989.

259. Woodle ES, Perdrizet GA, Brunt EM, et al: FK 506: Reversal of humorally mediated rejection following ABO-incompatible liver transplantation. Transplant Proc 23:2992-2993, 1991.

260. Nakamura K, Murase N, Becich MJ, et al: Liver allograft rejection in sensitized recipients. Observations in a clinically relevant small animal model. Am J Pathol 142:1383-1391, 1993.

261. Batts KP, Moore SB, Perkins JD, et al: Influence of positive lymphocyte crossmatch and HLA mismatching on vanishing bile duct syndrome in human liver allografts. Transplantation 45:376-379, 1988.

262. Sanchez-Urdazpal L, Sterioff S, Janes C, et al: Increased bile duct complications in ABO incompatible liver transplant recipients. Transplant Proc 23:1440-1441, 1991.

263. Feucht HE, Felber E, Gokel MJ, et al: Vascular deposition of complement-split products in kidney allografts with cell-mediated rejection. Clin Exp Immunol 86:464-470, 1991.

264. Collins AB, Schneeberger EE, Pascual MA, et al: Complement activation in acute humoral renal allograft rejection: Diagnostic significance of C4d deposits in peritubular capillaries. J Am Soc Nephrol 10:2208-2214, 1999.

265. Krukemeyer MG, Moeller J, Morawietz L, et al: Description of B lymphocytes and plasma cells, complement, and chemokines/receptors in acute liver allograft rejection. Transplantation 78:65-70, 2004.

266. Hubscher SG, Adams DH, Buckels JA, et al: Massive haemorrhagic necrosis of the liver after liver transplantation. J Clin Pathol 42:360-370, 1989.

267. Gubernatis G, Kemnitz J, Bornscheuer A, et al: Potential various appearances of hyperacute rejection in human liver transplantation. Langenbecks Arch Chir 374:240-244, 1989.

268. Seiler CA, Renner EL, Czerniak A, et al: Early acute cellular rejection: No effect on late hepatic allograft function in man. Transpl Int 12:195-201, 1999.

269. Nawaz S, Fennell RH: Apoptosis of bile duct epithelial cells in hepatic allograft rejection. Histopathology 25:137-142, 1994.

270. Terminology for hepatic allograft rejection. International Working Party. Hepatology 22:648-654, 1995.

271. Foster PF, Bhattacharyya A, Sankary HN, et al: Eosinophil cationic protein's role in human hepatic allograft rejection. Hepatology 13:1117-1125, 1991.

272. Lee R: Transplantation. In Lee R (ed): Diagnostic Liver Pathology, 1st ed. St Louis, Mosby–Year Book, 1994, pp 379-404.

273. Ludwig J: Histopathology of the liver following transplantation. In Maddrey WC (ed): Transplantation of the Liver. New York, Elsevier, 1988, pp 191-218.

274. Hubscher SG: Pathology of liver allograft rejection. Transpl Immunol 2:118-123, 1994.

275. Dousset B, Hubscher SG, Padbury RT, et al: Acute liver allograft rejection—is treatment always necessary? Transplantation 55:529-534, 1993.

276. Dousset B, Conti F, Cherruau B, et al: Is acute rejection deleterious to long-term liver allograft function? J Hepatol 29:660-668, 1998.

277. Hubscher S: Diagnosis and grading of liver allograft rejection: A European perspective. Transplant Proc 28:504-507, 1996.

278. Batts K: Liver allograft rejection: Current status of classification and grading. Transplant Proc 28:453-456, 1996.

279. Wight D: Pathology of rejection. In Calne R (ed): Liver Transplantation, 2nd ed. London, Grune & Stratton, 1987, pp 385-435.

280. Eggink HF, Hofstee N, Gips CH, et al: Histopathology of serial graft biopsies from liver transplant recipients. Am J Pathol 114:18-31, 1984.

281. Vierling JM, Fennell RH Jr: Histopathology of early and late human hepatic allograft rejection: Evidence of progressive destruction of interlobular bile ducts. Hepatology 5:1076-1082, 1985.

282. Williams JW, Peters TG, Vera SR, et al: Biopsy-directed immunosuppression following hepatic transplantation in man. Transplantation 39:589-596, 1985.

283. Williams JW, Foster PF, Sankary HN: Role of liver allograft biopsy in patient management. Semin Liver Dis 12:60-72, 1992.

284. Hubscher SG, Clements D, Elias E, McMaster P: Biopsy findings in cases of rejection of liver allograft. J Clin Pathol 38:1366-1373, 1985.

285. Snover DC, Freese DK, Sharp HL, et al: Liver allograft rejection. An analysis of the use of biopsy in determining outcome of rejection. Am J Surg Pathol 11:1-10, 1987.

286. Kemnitz J, Ringe B, Cohnert TR, et al: Bile duct injury as a part of diagnostic criteria for liver allograft rejection. Hum Pathol 20:132-143, 1989.

287. Demetris AJ, Qian SG, Sun H, Fung JJ: Liver allograft rejection: An overview of morphologic findings. Am J Surg Pathol 14(Suppl 1):49-63, 1990.

288. McCaughan GW, Davies JS, Waugh JA, et al: A quantitative analysis of T lymphocyte populations in human liver allografts undergoing rejection: The use of monoclonal antibodies and double immunolabeling. Hepatology 12:1305-1313, 1990.

289. Ibrahim S, Dawson DV, Killenberg PG, Sanfilippo F: The pattern and phenotype of T-cell infiltration associated with human liver allograft rejection. Hum Pathol 24:1365-1370, 1993.

290. Kolbeck PC, Wood RP, Markin RS: The immunopathology and clinical relevance of lymphocyte cultures in liver transplantation. Mod Pathol 6:307-312, 1993.

291. Perkins JD, Rakela J, Sterioff S, et al: Immunohistologic pattern of the portal T-lymphocyte infiltration in hepatic allograft rejection. Mayo Clin Proc 64:565-569, 1989.

292. Gapany C, Zhao M, Zimmermann A: The apoptosis protector, bcl-2 protein, is downregulated in bile duct epithelial cells of human liver allografts. J Hepatol 26:535-542, 1997.

293. Demetris AJ, Belle SH, Hart J, et al: Intraobserver and interobserver variation in the histopathological assessment of liver allograft rejection. The Liver Transplantation Database (LTD) Investigators. Hepatology 14:751-755, 1991.

294. Demetris AJ, Fung JJ, Todo S, et al: Conversion of liver allograft recipients from cyclosporine to FK506 immunosuppressive therapy—a clinicopathologic study of 96 patients. Transplantation 53:1056-1062, 1992.

295. Tsamandas AC, Jain AB, Felekouras ES, et al: Central venulitis in the allograft liver: A clinicopathologic study. Transplantation 64:252-257, 1997.

296. Krasinskas AM, Ruchelli ED, Rand EB, et al: Central venulitis in pediatric liver allografts. Hepatology 33:1141-1147, 2001.

297. Ludwig J, Gross JB Jr, Perkins JD, Moore SB: Persistent centrilobular necroses in hepatic allografts. Hum Pathol 21:656-661, 1990.

298. Nakazawa Y, Jonsson JR, Walker NI, et al: Fibrous obliterative lesions of veins contribute to progressive fibrosis in chronic liver allograft rejection. Hepatology 32:1240-1247, 2000.

299. Neil DA, Hubscher SG: Histologic and biochemical changes during the evolution of chronic rejection of liver allografts. Hepatology 35:639-651, 2002.

300. Snover DC, Freese DK, Bloomer JR, et al: An analysis of histological prognostic features of liver allograft rejection based on 270 serial biopsies. Transplant Proc 19:2457-2458, 1987.

301. Kemnitz J, Gubernatis G, Bunzendahl H, et al: Criteria for the histopathological classification of liver allograft rejection and their clinical relevance. Transplant Proc 21:2208-2210, 1989.

302. Demetris AJ, Seaberg EC, Batts KP, et al: Reliability and predictive value of the National Institute of Diabetes and Digestive and Kidney Diseases Liver Transplantation Database nomenclature and grading system for cellular rejection of liver allografts. Hepatology 21:408-416, 1995.

303. Datta Gupta S, Hudson M, Burroughs AK, et al: Grading of cellular rejection after orthotopic liver transplantation. Hepatology 21:46-57, 1995.

304. Ishak K, Baptista A, Bianchi L, et al: Histological grading and staging of chronic hepatitis. J Hepatol 22:696-699, 1995.

305. Ludwig J: Classification and terminology of hepatic allograft rejection: Whither bound? Mayo Clin Proc 64:676-679, 1989.

306. Freese DK, Snover DC, Sharp HL, et al: Chronic rejection after liver transplantation: A study of clinical, histopathological and immunological features. Hepatology 13:882-891, 1991.

307. Hubscher SG, Buckels JA, Elias E, et al: Vanishing bile-duct syndrome following liver transplantation—is it reversible? Transplantation 51:1004-1010, 1991.

308. Blakolmer K, Seaberg EC, Batts K, et al: Analysis of the reversibility of chronic liver allograft rejection implications for a staging schema. Am J Surg Pathol 23:1328-1339, 1999.

309. Quaglia AF, Del Vecchio Blanco G, Greaves R, et al: Development of ductopaenic liver allograft rejection includes a "hepatitic" phase prior to duct loss. J Hepatol 33:773-780, 2000.

310. Demetris AJ, Murase N, Lee RG, et al: Chronic rejection. A general overview of histopathology and pathophysiology with emphasis on liver, heart and intestinal allografts. Ann Transplant 2:27-44, 1997.

311. Starzl TE, Todo S, Fung J, et al: FK 506 for liver, kidney, and pancreas transplantation. Lancet 2:1000-1004, 1989.

312. Demetris AJ, Fung JJ, Todo S, et al: Pathologic observations in human allograft recipients treated with FK 506. Transplant Proc 22:25-34, 1990.

313. Pirsch JD, Kalayoglu M, Hafez GR, et al: Evidence that the vanishing bile duct syndrome is vanishing. Transplantation 49:1015-1018, 1990.

314. Ascher NL, Lake JR, Emond J, Roberts J: Liver transplantation for hepatitis C virus–related cirrhosis. Hepatology 20:24S-27S, 1994.

315. Sher LS, Cosenza CA, Michel J, et al: Efficacy of tacrolimus as rescue therapy for chronic rejection in orthotopic liver transplantation: A report of the U.S. Multicenter Liver Study Group. Transplantation 64:258-263, 1997.

316. Slapak GI, Saxena R, Portmann B, et al: Graft and systemic disease in long-term survivors of liver transplantation. Hepatology 25:195-202, 1997.

317. Starzl TE, Marchioro TL, Porter KA: Experimental and clinical observations after homotransplantation of the whole liver. Rev Int Hepatol 15:1447-1480, 1965.

318. Ludwig J, Wiesner RH, Batts KP, et al: The acute vanishing bile duct syndrome (acute irreversible rejection) after orthotopic liver transplantation. Hepatology 7:476-483, 1987.

319. Lowes JR, Hubscher SG, Neuberger JM: Chronic rejection of the liver allograft. Gastroenterol Clin North Am 22:401-420, 1993.

320. Hoek BV, Wiesner R, Krom R, et al: Severe ductopenic rejection following liver transplantation: Incidence, time of onset, risk factors, treatment and outcome. Semin Liver Dis 12:41-50, 1992.

321. Farges O, Nocci Kalil A, Sebagh M, et al: Low incidence of chronic rejection in patients experiencing histological acute rejection without simultaneous impairment in liver function tests. Transplant Proc 27:1142-1143, 1995.

322. Halloran PF, Melk A, Barth C: Rethinking chronic allograft nephropathy: The concept of accelerated senescence. J Am Soc Nephrol 10:167-181, 1999.

323. Evans PC, Smith S, Hirschfield G, et al: Recipient HLA-DR3, tumour necrosis factor-α promoter allele-2 (tumour necrosis factor-2) and cytomegalovirus infection are interrelated risk factors for chronic rejection of liver grafts. J Hepatol 34:711-715, 2001.

324. Devlin JJ, O'Grady JG, Tan KC, et al: Ethnic variations in patient and graft survival after liver transplantation. Identification of a new risk factor for chronic allograft rejection. Transplantation 56:1381-1384, 1993.

325. Donaldson PT, Alexander GJ, O'Grady J, et al: Evidence for an immune response to HLA class I antigens in the vanishing–bile duct syndrome after liver transplantation. Lancet 1:945-951, 1987.

326. Donaldson PT, Thomson LJ, Heads A, et al: IgG donor-specific crossmatches are not associated with graft rejection or poor graft survival after liver transplantation. An assessment by cytotoxicity and flow cytometry. Transplantation 60:1016-1023, 1995.

327. Manez R, White LT, Linden P, et al: The influence of HLA matching on cytomegalovirus hepatitis and chronic rejection after liver transplantation. Transplantation 55:1067-1071, 1993.

328. Paya CV, Wiesner RH, Hermans PE, et al: Lack of association between cytomegalovirus infection, HLA matching and the vanishing bile duct syndrome after liver transplantation. Hepatology 16:66-70, 1992.

329. Lautenschlager I, Hockerstedt K, Jalanko H, et al: Persistent cytomegalovirus in liver allografts with chronic rejection. Hepatology 25:190-194, 1997.

330. Oguma S, Belle S, Starzl TE, Demetris AJ: A histometric analysis of chronically rejected human liver allografts: Insights into the mechanisms of bile duct loss: Direct immunologic and ischemic factors. Hepatology 9:204-209, 1989.

331. Oguma S, Zerbe T, Banner B, et al: Chronic liver allograft rejection and obliterative arteriopathy: Possible pathogenic mechanisms. Transplant Proc 21:2203-2207, 1989.

332. Matsumoto Y, McCaughan GW, Painter DM, Bishop GA: Evidence that portal tract microvascular destruction precedes bile duct loss in human liver allograft rejection. Transplantation 56:69-75, 1993.

333. Afford SC, Randhawa S, Eliopoulos AG, et al: CD40 activation induces apoptosis in cultured human hepatocytes via induction of cell surface Fas ligand expression and amplifies Fas-mediated hepatocyte death during allograft rejection. J Exp Med 189:441-446, 1999.

334. Ross R: The pathogenesis of atherosclerosis: A perspective for the 1990s. Nature 362:801-809, 1993.

335. Murase N, Ichikawa N, Ye Q, et al: Dendritic cells/chimerism/alleviation of chronic allograft rejection. J Leukoc Biol 66:297-300, 1999.

336. Cohen AH, Nast CC: TGF-β in renal allograft rejection. Miner Electrolyte Metab 24:197-201, 1998.

337. Campistol JM, Inigo P, Jimenez W, et al: Losartan decreases plasma levels of TGF-β1 in transplant patients with chronic allograft nephropathy. Kidney Int 56:714-719, 1999.

338. Cuhaci B, Kumar MS, Bloom RD, et al: Transforming growth factor-β levels in human allograft chronic fibrosis correlate with rate of decline in renal function. Transplantation 68:785-790, 1999.

339. El-Gamel A, Sim E, Hasleton P, et al: Transforming growth factor beta (TGF-β) and obliterative bronchiolitis following pulmonary transplantation. J Heart Lung Transplant 18:828-837, 1999.

340. Freedman BI, Yu H, Spray BJ, et al: Genetic linkage analysis of growth factor loci and end-stage renal disease in African Americans. Kidney Int 51:819-825, 1997.

341. Horvath LZ, Friess H, Schilling M, et al: Altered expression of transforming growth factor-beta S in chronic renal rejection. Kidney Int 50:489-498, 1996.

342. Suthanthiran M, Khanna A, Cukran D, et al: Transforming growth factor-β1 hyperexpression in African American end-stage renal disease patients. Kidney Int 53:639-644, 1998.

343. Hayflick L: A brief history of the mortality and immortality of cultured cells. Keio J Med 47:174-182, 1998.

344. Hayflick L: How and why we age. Exp Gerontol 33:639-653, 1998.

345. Grond J, Gouw AS, Poppema S, et al: Chronic rejection in liver transplants: A histopathologic analysis of failed grafts and antecedent serial biopsies. Transplant Proc 18:128-135, 1986.

346. Wight DA: Chronic liver transplant rejection: Definition and diagnosis. Transplant Proc 28:465-467, 1996.

347. Neil DA, Adams DH, Gunson B, Hubscher SG: Is chronic rejection of liver transplants different from graft arteriosclerosis of kidney and heart transplants? Transplant Proc 29:2539-2540, 1997.

348. Demetris AJ, Seaberg EC, Batts KP, et al: Chronic liver allograft rejection: A National Institute of Diabetes and Digestive and Kidney Diseases interinstitutional study analyzing the reliability of current criteria and proposal of an expanded definition. National Institute of Diabetes and Digestive and Kidney Diseases Liver Transplantation Database. Am J Surg Pathol 22:28-39, 1998.

349. O'Keeffe C, Baird AW, Nolan N, McCormick PA: Mast cell hyperplasia in chronic rejection after liver transplantation. Liver Transpl 8:50-57, 2002.

350. Demetris AJ, Fung JJ, Todo S, et al: FK 506 used as rescue therapy for human liver allograft recipients. Transplant Proc 23:3005-3006, 1991.

351. Crawford AR, Lin XZ, Crawford JM: The normal adult human liver biopsy: A quantitative reference standard. Hepatology 28:323-331, 1998.

352. Popper H, Kent G, Stein R: Ductular cell reaction in the liver in hepatic injury. J Mt Sinai Hosp 24:551-556, 1957.

353. Popper H: The relation of mesenchymal cell products to hepatic epithelial systems. Prog Liver Dis 9:27-38, 1990.

354. Demetris AJ, Zerbe T, Banner B: Morphology of solid organ allograft arteriopathy: Identification of proliferating intimal cell populations. Transplant Proc 21:3667-3669, 1989.

355. Demetris AJ, Markus BH, Burnham J, et al: Antibody deposition in liver allografts with chronic rejection. Transplant Proc 19(4 Suppl 5):121-125, 1987.

356. Hubscher SG, Elias E, Buckels JA, et al: Primary biliary cirrhosis. Histological evidence of disease recurrence after liver transplantation. J Hepatol 18:173-184, 1993.

357. White RM, Zajko AB, Demetris AJ, et al: Liver transplant rejection: Angiographic findings in 35 patients. AJR Am J Roentgenol 148:1095-1098, 1987.

358. Devlin J, Page AC, O'Grady J, et al: Angiographically determined arteriopathy in liver graft dysfunction and survival. J Hepatol 18:68-73, 1993.

359. Dhillon AP, Burroughs AK, Hudson M, et al: Hepatic venular stenosis after orthotopic liver transplantation. Hepatology 19:106-111, 1994.

360. MacSween RN, Burt AD, Portmann B, et al (eds): Pathology of the Liver, 4th ed. Philadelphia, Churchill Livingstone, 2002, p 982.

361. Fung J, Zeevi A, Demetris AJ, et al: Origin of lymph node derived lymphocytes in human hepatic allografts. Clin Transpl 3:316-324, 1989.

362. Navarro F, Portales P, Pageaux JP, et al: Activated sub-populations of lymphocytes and natural killer cells in normal liver and liver grafts before transplantation. Liver 18:259-263, 1998.

363. Pruvot FR, Navarro F, Janin A, et al: Characterization, quantification, and localization of passenger T lymphocytes and NK cells in human liver before transplantation. Transpl Int 8:273-279, 1995.

364. Schlitt HJ, Raddatz G, Steinhoff G, et al: Passenger lymphocytes in human liver allografts and their potential role after transplantation. Transplantation 56:951-955, 1993.

365. Simonsen M: Graft versus host reactions: Their natural history, and applicability as tools of research. Prog Allergy 6:349-467, 1962.

366. Ramsey G, Nusbacher J, Starzl TE, Lindsay GD: Isohemagglutinins of graft origin after ABO-unmatched liver transplantation. N Engl J Med 311:1167-1170, 1984.

367. Collins RH Jr, Anastasi J, Terstappen LW, et al: Brief report: Donor-derived long-term multilineage hematopoiesis in a liver-transplant recipient. N Engl J Med 328:762-765, 1993.

368. Roberts JP, Ascher NL, Lake J, et al: Graft vs. host disease after liver transplantation in humans: A report of four cases. Hepatology 14:274-281, 1991.

369. Hymes SR, Farmer ER, Lewis PG, et al: Cutaneous graft-versus-host reaction: Prognostic features seen by light microscopy. J Am Acad Dermatol 12:468-474, 1985.

370. Sale GE, Shulman HM, McDonald GB, Thomas ED: Gastrointestinal graft-versus-host disease in man. A clinicopathologic study of the rectal biopsy. Am J Surg Pathol 3:291-299, 1979.

371. Kusne S, Dummer JS, Singh N, et al: Infections after liver transplantation. An analysis of 101 consecutive cases. Medicine (Baltimore) 67:132-143, 1988.

372. Cavallari A, De Raffele E, Bellusci R, et al: De novo hepatitis B and C viral infection after liver transplantation. World J Surg 21:78-84, 1997.

373. Bai X, Rogers BB, Harkins PC, et al: Predictive value of quantitative PCR-based viral burden analysis for eight human herpesviruses in pediatric solid organ transplant patients. J Mol Diagn 2:191-201, 2000.

374. Badley AD, Seaberg EC, Porayko MK, et al: Prophylaxis of cytomegalovirus infection in liver transplantation: A randomized trial comparing a combination of ganciclovir and acyclovir to acyclovir. NIDDK Liver Transplantation Database. Transplantation 64:66-73, 1997.

375. Barkholt L, Lewensohn-Fuchs I, Ericzon BG, et al: High-dose acyclovir prophylaxis reduces cytomegalovirus disease in liver transplant patients. Transpl Infect Dis 1:89-97, 1999.
376. McGavin JK, Goa KL: Ganciclovir: An update of its use in the prevention of cytomegalovirus infection and disease in transplant recipients. Drugs 61:1153-1183, 2001.
377. Portela D, Patel R, Larson-Keller JJ, et al: OKT3 treatment for allograft rejection is a risk factor for cytomegalovirus disease in liver transplantation. J Infect Dis 171:1014-1018, 1995.
378. Theise ND, Conn M, Thung SN: Localization of cytomegalovirus antigens in liver allografts over time. Hum Pathol 24:103-108, 1993.
379. Paya CV, Hermans PE, Wiesner RH, et al: Cytomegalovirus hepatitis in liver transplantation: Prospective analysis of 93 consecutive orthotopic liver transplantations. J Infect Dis 160:752-758, 1989.
380. Paya CV, Holley KE, Wiesner RH, et al: Early diagnosis of cytomegalovirus hepatitis in liver transplant recipients: Role of immunostaining, DNA hybridization and culture of hepatic tissue. Hepatology 12:119-126, 1990.
381. Bronsther O, Makowka L, Jaffe R, et al: Occurrence of cytomegalovirus hepatitis in liver transplant patients. J Med Virol 24:423-434, 1988.
382. Snover DC, Hutton S, Balfour HH Jr, Bloomer JR: Cytomegalovirus infection of the liver in transplant recipients. J Clin Gastroenterol 9:659-665, 1987.
383. Gorensek MJ, Carey WD, Vogt D, Goormastic M: A multivariate analysis of risk factors for cytomegalovirus infection in liver-transplant recipients. Gastroenterology 98:1326-1332, 1990.
384. Sayage LH, Gonwa TA, Goldstein RM, et al: Cytomegalovirus infection in orthotopic liver transplantation. Transpl Int 2:96-101, 1989.
385. Stratta RJ, Shaefer MS, Markin RS, et al: Clinical patterns of cytomegalovirus disease after liver transplantation. Arch Surg 124:1443-1449, 1989.
386. Stratta RJ, Shaeffer MS, Markin RS, et al: Cytomegalovirus infection and disease after liver transplantation. An overview. Dig Dis Sci 37:673-688, 1992.
387. Wiesner RH, Marin E, Porayko MK, et al: Advances in the diagnosis, treatment, and prevention of cytomegalovirus infections after liver transplantation. Gastroenterol Clin North Am 22:351-366, 1993.
388. Toorkey CB, Carrigan DR: Immunohistochemical detection of an immediate early antigen of human cytomegalovirus in normal tissues. J Infect Dis 160:741-751, 1989.
389. Madalosso C, de Souza NF Jr, Ilstrup DM, et al: Cytomegalovirus and its association with hepatic artery thrombosis after liver transplantation. Transplantation 66:294-297, 1998.
390. Oh CK, Pelletier SJ, Sawyer RG, et al: Uni- and multi-variate analysis of risk factors for early and late hepatic artery thrombosis after liver transplantation. Transplantation 71:767-772, 2001.
391. O'Grady JG, Alexander GJ, Sutherland S, et al: Cytomegalovirus infection and donor/recipient HLA antigens: Interdependent co-factors in pathogenesis of vanishing bile-duct syndrome after liver transplantation. Lancet 2:302-305, 1988.
392. Rosen HR, Chou S, Corless CL, et al: Cytomegalovirus viremia: Risk factor for allograft cirrhosis after liver transplantation for hepatitis C. Transplantation 64:721-726, 1997.
393. Teixeira R, Pastacaldi S, Davies S, et al: The influence of cytomegalovirus viraemia on the outcome of recurrent hepatitis C after liver transplantation. Transplantation 70:1454-1458, 2000.
394. Arnold JC, Portmann BC, O'Grady JG, et al: Cytomegalovirus infection persists in the liver graft in the vanishing bile duct syndrome. Hepatology 16:285-292, 1992.
395. Manez R, White LT, Kusne S, et al: Association between donor-recipient HLA-DR compatibility and cytomegalovirus hepatitis and chronic rejection in liver transplantation. Transplant Proc 25:908-909, 1993.
396. Arnold JC, Gmelin K, Otto G, et al: Effect of cytomegalovirus infection on expression of HLA-antigens in liver allografts. Transplant Proc 23:442-443, 1991.
397. Arnold JC, O'Grady JG, Otto G, et al: CMV reinfection/reactivation after liver transplantation. Transplant Proc 23:2632-2633, 1991.
398. Wright TL: Cytomegalovirus infection and vanishing bile duct syndrome: Culprit or innocent bystander? Hepatology 16:494-496, 1992.
399. Lautenschlager I, Nashan B, Schlitt HJ, et al: Early intragraft inflammatory events of liver allografts leading to chronic rejection. Transpl Int 8:446-451, 1995.
400. Colina F, Juca NT, Moreno E, et al: Histological diagnosis of cytomegalovirus hepatitis in liver allografts. J Clin Pathol 48:351-357, 1995.
401. Randhawa P, Blakolmer K, Kashyap R, et al: Allograft liver biopsy in patients with Epstein-Barr virus–associated posttransplant lymphoproliferative disease. Am J Surg Pathol 25:324-330, 2001.
402. Randhawa PS, Jaffe R, Demetris AJ, et al: Expression of Epstein-Barr virus–encoded small RNA (by the EBER-1 gene) in liver specimens from transplant recipients with post-transplantation lymphoproliferative disease. N Engl J Med 327:1710-1714, 1992.
403. Randhawa PS, Jaffe R, Demetris AJ, et al: The systemic distribution of Epstein-Barr virus genomes in fatal post-transplantation lymphoproliferative disorders. An in situ hybridization study. Am J Pathol 138:1027-1033, 1991.
404. Kusne S, Schwartz M, Breinig MK, et al: Herpes simplex virus hepatitis after solid organ transplantation in adults. J Infect Dis 163:1001-1007, 1991.
405. Nalesnik MA, Jaffe R, Starzl TE, et al: The pathology of post-transplant lymphoproliferative disorders occurring in the setting of cyclosporine A–prednisone immunosuppression. Am J Pathol 133:173-192, 1988.
406. Nalesnik MA: Clinicopathologic characteristics of post-transplant lymphoproliferative disorders. Recent Results Cancer Res 159: 9-18, 2002.
407. Nalesnik MA: The diverse pathology of post-transplant lymphoproliferative disorders: The importance of a standardized approach. Transpl Infect Dis 3:88-96, 2001.
408. Randhawa PS, Markin RS, Starzl TE, Demetris AJ: Epstein-Barr virus–associated syndromes in immunosuppressed liver transplant recipients. Clinical profile and recognition on routine allograft biopsy. Am J Surg Pathol 14:538-547, 1990.
409. Alshak NS, Jiminez AM, Gedebou M, et al: Epstein-Barr virus infection in liver transplantation patients: Correlation of histopathology and semiquantitative Epstein-Barr virus-DNA recovery using polymerase chain reaction. Hum Pathol 24: 1306-1312, 1993.
410. Telenti A, Smith TF, Ludwig J, et al: Epstein-Barr virus and persistent graft dysfunction after liver transplantation. Hepatology 14:282-286, 1991.
411. Markin RS, Wood RP, Shaw BW Jr, et al: Immunohistologic identification of Epstein-Barr virus–induced hepatitis reactivation after OKT-3 therapy following orthotopic liver transplant. Am J Gastroenterol 85:1014-1018, 1990.
412. Bierman PJ, Vose JM, Langnas AN, et al: Hodgkin's disease following solid organ transplantation. Ann Oncol 7:265-270, 1996.
413. Sivaraman P, Lye WC: Epstein-Barr virus–associated T-cell lymphoma in solid organ transplant recipients. Biomed Pharmacother 55:366-368, 2001.
414. Brichard B, Smets F, Sokal E, et al: Unusual evolution of an Epstein-Barr virus–associated leiomyosarcoma occurring after liver transplantation. Pediatr Transplant 5:365-369, 2001.
415. Lee ES, Locker J, Nalesnik M, et al: The association of Epstein-Barr virus with smooth-muscle tumors occurring after organ transplantation. N Engl J Med 332:19-25, 1995.

416. Newell KA, Alonso EM, Whitington PF, et al: Posttransplant lymphoproliferative disease in pediatric liver transplantation. Interplay between primary Epstein-Barr virus infection and immunosuppression. Transplantation 62:370-375, 1996.

417. Manez R, Breinig MC, Linden P, et al: Posttransplant lymphoproliferative disease in primary Epstein-Barr virus infection after liver transplantation: The role of cytomegalovirus disease. J Infect Dis 176:1462-1467, 1997.

418. Cockfield SM: Identifying the patient at risk for post-transplant lymphoproliferative disorder. Transpl Infect Dis 3:70-78, 2001.

419. Matsukura T, Yokoi A, Egawa H, et al: Significance of serial real-time PCR monitoring of EBV genome load in living donor liver transplantation. Clin Transplant 16:107-112, 2002.

420. Tanner JE, Alfieri C: The Epstein-Barr virus and post-transplant lymphoproliferative disease: Interplay of immunosuppression, EBV, and the immune system in disease pathogenesis. Transpl Infect Dis 3:60-69, 2001.

421. Green M: Management of Epstein-Barr virus–induced post-transplant lymphoproliferative disease in recipients of solid organ transplantation. Am J Transplant 1:103-108, 2001.

422. Cao S, Cox K, Esquivel CO, et al: Posttransplant lymphoproliferative disorders and gastrointestinal manifestations of Epstein-Barr virus infection in children following liver transplantation. Transplantation 66:851-856, 1998.

423. Nalesnik MA, Makowka L, Starzl TE: The diagnosis and treatment of posttransplant lymphoproliferative disorders. Curr Probl Surg 25:367-472, 1988.

424. Collins MH, Montone KT, Leahey AM, et al: Autopsy pathology of pediatric posttransplant lymphoproliferative disorder. Pediatrics 107:E89, 2001.

425. Hubscher SG, Williams A, Davison SM, et al: Epstein-Barr virus in inflammatory diseases of the liver and liver allografts: An in situ hybridization study. Hepatology 20:899-907, 1994.

426. Muti G, Cantoni S, Oreste P, et al: Post-transplant lymphoproliferative disorders: Improved outcome after clinico-pathologically tailored treatment. Haematologica 87:67-77, 2002.

427. Koneru B, Jaffe R, Esquivel CO, et al: Adenoviral infections in pediatric liver transplant recipients. JAMA 258:489-492, 1987.

428. Michaels MG, Green M, Wald ER, Starzl TE: Adenovirus infection in pediatric liver transplant recipients. J Infect Dis 165:170-174, 1992.

429. Varki NM, Bhuta S, Drake T, Porter DD: Adenovirus hepatitis in two successive liver transplants in a child. Arch Pathol Lab Med 114:106-109, 1990.

430. Saad RS, Demetris AJ, Lee RG, et al: Adenovirus hepatitis in the adult allograft liver. Transplantation 64:1483-1485, 1997.

431. McGrath D, Falagas ME, Freeman R, et al: Adenovirus infection in adult orthotopic liver transplant recipients: Incidence and clinical significance. J Infect Dis 177:459-462, 1998.

432. Fagan E, Yousef G, Brahm J, et al: Persistence of hepatitis A virus in fulminant hepatitis and after liver transplantation. J Med Virol 30:131-136, 1990.

433. Demetris AJ, Jaffe R, Sheahan DG, et al: Recurrent hepatitis B in liver allograft recipients. Differentiation between viral hepatitis B and rejection. Am J Pathol 125:161-172, 1986.

434. Demetris AJ, Todo S, Van Thiel DH, et al: Evolution of hepatitis B virus liver disease after hepatic replacement. Practical and theoretical considerations. Am J Pathol 137:667-676, 1990.

435. O'Grady JG, Smith HM, Davies SE, et al: Hepatitis B virus reinfection after orthotopic liver transplantation. Serological and clinical implications. J Hepatol 14:104-111, 1992.

436. Davies SE, Portmann BC, O'Grady JG, et al: Hepatic histological findings after transplantation for chronic hepatitis B virus infection, including a unique pattern of fibrosing cholestatic hepatitis. Hepatology 13:150-157, 1991.

437. Mason AL, Wick M, White HM, et al: Increased hepatocyte expression of hepatitis B virus transcription in patients with features of fibrosing cholestatic hepatitis. Gastroenterology 105:237-244, 1993.

438. Todo S, Demetris AJ, Van Thiel D, et al: Orthotopic liver transplantation for patients with hepatitis B virus–related liver disease. Hepatology 13:619-626, 1991.

439. Samuel D, Bismuth H: Liver transplantation for hepatitis B. Gastroenterol Clin North Am 22:271-283, 1993.

440. Lauchart W, Muller R, Pichlmayr R: Long-term immunoprophylaxis of hepatitis B virus reinfection in recipients of human liver allografts. Transplant Proc 19:4051-4053, 1987.

441. Rizzetto M, Macagno S, Chiaberge E, et al: Liver transplantation in hepatitis delta virus disease. Lancet 2:469-471, 1987.

442. Prieto M, Gomez MD, Berenguer M, et al: De novo hepatitis B after liver transplantation from hepatitis B core antibody–positive donors in an area with high prevalence of anti-HBc positivity in the donor population. Liver Transpl 7:51-58, 2001.

443. Vargas HE, Dodson FS, Rakela J: A concise update on the status of liver transplantation for hepatitis B virus: The challenges in 2002. Liver Transpl 8:2-9, 2002.

444. Muller R, Gubernatis G, Farle M, et al: Liver transplantation in HBs antigen (HBsAg) carriers. Prevention of hepatitis B virus (HBV) recurrence by passive immunization. J Hepatol 13:90-96, 1991.

445. Konig V, Hopf U, Neuhaus P, et al: Long-term follow-up of hepatitis B virus–infected recipients after orthotopic liver transplantation. Transplantation 58:553-559, 1994.

446. Tchervenkov JI, Tector AJ, Barkun JS, et al: Recurrence-free long-term survival after liver transplantation for hepatitis B using interferon-alpha pretransplant and hepatitis B immune globulin posttransplant. Ann Surg 226:356-365, 1997.

447. Angus PW: Review: Hepatitis B and liver transplantation. J Gastroenterol Hepatol 12:217-223, 1997.

448. Roche B, Samuel D, Feray C, et al: Retransplantation of the liver for recurrent hepatitis B virus infection: The Paul Brousse experience. Liver Transpl Surg 5:166-174, 1999.

449. Cane PA, Mutimer D, Ratcliffe D, et al: Analysis of hepatitis B virus quasispecies changes during emergence and reversion of lamivudine resistance in liver transplantation. Antiviral Ther 4:7-14, 1999.

450. Rayes N, Seehofer D, Bechstein WO, et al: Long-term results of famciclovir for recurrent or de novo hepatitis B virus infection after liver transplantation. Clin Transplant 13:447-452, 1999.

451. Roche B, Samuel D, Gigou M, et al: Long-term ganciclovir therapy for hepatitis B virus infection after liver transplantation. J Hepatol 31:584-592, 1999.

452. Mutimer D, Pillay D, Shields P, et al: Outcome of lamivudine resistant hepatitis B virus infection in the liver transplant recipient. Gut 46:107-113, 2000.

453. Seehofer D, Rayes N, Neuhaus R, et al: Antiviral combination therapy for lamivudine-resistant hepatitis B reinfection after liver transplantation. Transpl Int 13(Suppl 1):S359-S362, 2000.

454. Gutfreund KS, Williams M, George R, et al: Genotypic succession of mutations of the hepatitis B virus polymerase associated with lamivudine resistance. J Hepatol 33:469-475, 2000.

455. Seehofer D, Rayes N, Steinmuller T, et al: Occurrence and clinical outcome of lamivudine-resistant hepatitis B infection after liver transplantation. Liver Transpl 7:976-982, 2001.

456. Walsh KM, Woodall T, Lamy P, et al: Successful treatment with adefovir dipivoxil in a patient with fibrosing cholestatic hepatitis and lamivudine resistant hepatitis B virus. Gut 49:436-440, 2001.

457. Castells L, Esteban R: Hepatitis B vaccination in liver transplant candidates. Eur J Gastroenterol Hepatol 13:359-361, 2001.

458. Ben-Ari Z, Mor E, Shapira Z, Tur-Kaspa R: Long-term experience with lamivudine therapy for hepatitis B virus infection after liver transplantation. Liver Transpl 7:113-117, 2001.

459. Bock CT, Tillmann HL, Torresi J, et al: Selection of hepatitis B virus polymerase mutants with enhanced replication by

lamivudine treatment after liver transplantation. Gastroenterology 122:264-273, 2002.

460. Pramoolsinsup C: Management of viral hepatitis B. J Gastroenterol Hepatol 17(Suppl):S125-S145, 2002.

461. Santantonio T, Gunther S, Sterneck M, et al: Liver graft infection by HBV S-gene mutants in transplant patients receiving long-term HBIg prophylaxis. Hepatogastroenterology 46:1848-1854, 1999.

462. Marinos G, Rossol S, Carucci P, et al: Immunopathogenesis of hepatitis B virus recurrence after liver transplantation. Transplantation 69:559-568, 2000.

463. Phillips MJ, Cameron R, Flowers MA, et al: Post-transplant recurrent hepatitis B viral liver disease. Viral-burden, steatoviral, and fibroviral hepatitis B. Am J Pathol 140:1295-1308, 1992.

464. Benner KG, Lee RG, Keeffe EB, et al: Fibrosing cytolytic liver failure secondary to recurrent hepatitis B after liver transplantation. Gastroenterology 103:1307-1312, 1992.

465. Zignego AL, Dubois F, Samuel D, et al: Serum hepatitis delta virus RNA in patients with delta hepatitis and in liver graft recipients. J Hepatol 11:102-110, 1990.

466. Reynes M, Zignego L, Samuel D, et al: Graft hepatitis delta virus reinfection after orthotopic liver transplantation in HDV cirrhosis. Transplant Proc 21:2424-2425, 1989.

467. Ottobrelli A, Marzano A, Smedile A, et al: Patterns of hepatitis delta virus reinfection and disease in liver transplantation. Gastroenterology 101:1649-1655, 1991.

468. David E, Rahier J, Pucci A, et al: Recurrence of hepatitis D (delta) in liver transplants: Histopathological aspects. Gastroenterology 104:1122-1128, 1993.

469. Snover DC: Problems in the interpretation of liver biopsies after liver transplantation. Am J Surg Pathol 13(Suppl 1):31-38, 1989.

470. Demetris AJ, Eghtesad B, Marcos A, et al: Recurrent hepatitis C in liver allografts: Prospective assessment of diagnostic accuracy, identification of pitfalls, and observations about pathogenesis. Am J Surg Pathol 28:658-669, 2004.

471. Bernard PH, Le Bail B, Rullier A, et al: Recurrence and accelerated progression of hepatitis C following liver transplantation. Semin Liver Dis 20:533-538, 2000.

472. Wiesner RH, Sorrell M, Villamil F: Report of the first International Liver Transplantation Society expert panel consensus conference on liver transplantation and hepatitis C. Liver Transpl 9:S1-S9, 2003.

473. Randhawa PS, Demetris AJ: Hepatitis C virus infection in liver allografts. Pathol Annu 30:203-226, 1995.

474. Fishman JA, Rubin RH, Koziel MJ, Periera BJ: Hepatitis C virus and organ transplantation. Transplantation 62:147-154, 1996.

475. Lumbreras C, Colina F, Loinaz C, et al: Clinical, virological, and histologic evolution of hepatitis C virus infection in liver transplant recipients. Clin Infect Dis 26:48-55, 1998.

476. Feray C, Samuel D, Thiers V, et al: Reinfection of liver graft by hepatitis C virus after liver transplantation. J Clin Invest 89:1361-1365, 1992.

477. Weinstein JS, Poterucha JJ, Zein N, et al: Epidemiology and natural history of hepatitis C infections in liver transplant recipients. J Hepatol 22(1 Suppl):154-159, 1995.

478. Arnold JC, Kraus T, Otto G, et al: Recurrent hepatitis C virus infection after liver transplantation. Transplant Proc 24:2646-2647, 1992.

479. Mateo R, Demetris A, Sico E, et al: Early detection of de novo hepatitis C infection in patients after liver transplantation by reverse transcriptase polymerase chain reaction. Surgery 114:442-448, 1993.

480. Marzano A, Smedile A, Abate M, et al: Hepatitis type C after orthotopic liver transplantation: Reinfection and disease recurrence. J Hepatol 21:961-965, 1994.

481. Sanchez-Fueyo A, Restrepo JC, Quinto L, et al: Impact of the recurrence of hepatitis C virus infection after liver transplantation on the long-term viability of the graft. Transplantation 73:56-63, 2002.

482. Belli LS, Silini E, Alberti A, et al: Hepatitis C virus genotypes, hepatitis, and hepatitis C virus recurrence after liver transplantation. Liver Transpl Surg 2:200-205, 1996.

483. Feray C, Gigou M, Samuel D, et al: Influence of the genotypes of hepatitis C virus on the severity of recurrent liver disease after liver transplantation. Gastroenterology 108:1088-1096, 1995.

484. Gayowski T, Singh N, Marino IR, et al: Hepatitis C virus genotypes in liver transplant recipients: Impact on posttransplant recurrence, infections, response to interferon-alpha therapy and outcome. Transplantation 64:422-426, 1997.

485. Gane EJ, Portmann BC, Naoumov NV, et al: Long-term outcome of hepatitis C infection after liver transplantation. N Engl J Med 334:815-820, 1996.

486. Chazouilleres O, Kim M, Combs C, et al: Quantitation of hepatitis C virus RNA in liver transplant recipients. Gastroenterology 106:994-999, 1994.

487. McCaughan GW, Zekry A: Impact of immunosuppression on immunopathogenesis of liver damage in hepatitis C virus–infected recipients following liver transplantation. Liver Transpl 9:S21-S27, 2003.

488. Rosen HR: Hepatitis C virus in the human liver transplantation model. Clin Liver Dis 7:107-125, 2003.

489. Charlton M: Natural history of hepatitis C and outcomes following liver transplantation. Clin Liver Dis 7:585-602, 2003.

490. Crespo J, Rivero M, Mayorga M, et al: Involvement of the Fas system in hepatitis C virus recurrence after liver transplantation. Liver Transpl 6:562-569, 2000.

491. Berenguer M, Ferrell L, Watson J, et al: HCV-related fibrosis progression following liver transplantation: Increase in recent years. J Hepatol 32:673-684, 2000.

492. Charlton M, Seaberg E, Wiesner R, et al: Predictors of patient and graft survival following liver transplantation for hepatitis C. Hepatology 28:823-830, 1998.

493. Burroughs AK: Posttransplantation prevention and treatment of recurrent hepatitis C. Liver Transpl 6(6 Suppl 2):S35-S40, 2000.

494. Sheiner PA, Schwartz ME, Mor E, et al: Severe or multiple rejection episodes are associated with early recurrence of hepatitis C after orthotopic liver transplantation. Hepatology 21:30-34, 1995.

495. Singh N, Gayowski T, Ndimbie OK, et al: Recurrent hepatitis C virus hepatitis in liver transplant recipients receiving tacrolimus: Association with rejection and increased immunosuppression after transplantation. Surgery 119:452-456, 1996.

496. Berenguer M, Prieto M, Cordoba J, et al: Early development of chronic active hepatitis in recurrent hepatitis C virus infection after liver transplantation: Association with treatment of rejection. J Hepatol 28:756-763, 1998.

497. Boker KH, Dalley G, Bahr MJ, et al: Long-term outcome of hepatitis C virus infection after liver transplantation. Hepatology 25:203-210, 1997.

498. Ahmed A, Keeffe EB: Hepatitis C virus and liver transplantation. Clin Liver Dis 5:1073-1090, 2001.

499. Zhou S, Terrault NA, Ferrell L, et al: Severity of liver disease in liver transplantation recipients with hepatitis C virus infection: Relationship to genotype and level of viremia. Hepatology 24:1041-1046, 1996.

500. Caccamo L, Gridelli B, Sampietro M, et al: Hepatitis C virus genotypes and reinfection of the graft during long-term follow-up in 35 liver transplant recipients. Transpl Int 9(Suppl 1):S204-S209, 1996.

501. Gordon FD, Poterucha JJ, Germer J, et al: Relationship between hepatitis C genotype and severity of recurrent hepatitis C after liver transplantation. Transplantation 63:1419-1423, 1997.

502. Gigou M, Roque-Afonso AM, Falissard B, et al: Genetic clustering of hepatitis C virus strains and severity of recurrent hepatitis after liver transplantation. J Virol 75:11292-11297, 2001.

503. Laskus T, Wang LF, Rakela J, et al: Dynamic behavior of hepatitis C virus in chronically infected patients receiving liver graft from infected donors. Virology 220:171-176, 1996.

504. Gane EJ, Naoumov NV, Qian KP, et al: A longitudinal analysis of hepatitis C virus replication following liver transplantation. Gastroenterology 110:167-177, 1996.

505. Di Martino V, Saurini F, Samuel D, et al: Long-term longitudinal study of intrahepatic hepatitis C virus replication after liver transplantation. Hepatology 26:1343-1350, 1997.

506. Zekry A, Bishop GA, Bowen DG, et al: Intrahepatic cytokine profiles associated with posttransplantation hepatitis C virus–related liver injury. Liver Transpl 8:292-301, 2002.

507. Wright TL, Donegan E, Hsu HH, et al: Recurrent and acquired hepatitis C viral infection in liver transplant recipients. Gastroenterology 103:317-322, 1992.

508. Thung SN, Shim KS, Shieh YS, et al: Hepatitis C in liver allografts. Arch Pathol Lab Med 117:145-149, 1993.

509. Wright TL: Liver transplantation for chronic hepatitis C viral infection. Gastroenterol Clin North Am 22:231-242, 1993.

510. Ferrell LD, Wright TL, Roberts J, et al: Hepatitis C viral infection in liver transplant recipients. Hepatology 16:865-876, 1992.

511. Paik SW, Tan HP, Klein AS, et al: Outcome of orthotopic liver transplantation in patients with hepatitis C. Dig Dis Sci 47:450-455, 2002.

512. Berenguer M: Natural history of recurrent hepatitis C. Liver Transpl 8(10 Suppl 1):S14-S18, 2002.

513. Greenson JK, Svoboda-Newman SM, Merion RM, Frank TS: Histologic progression of recurrent hepatitis C in liver transplant allografts. Am J Surg Pathol 20:731-738, 1996.

514. Charlton M: Liver biopsy, viral kinetics, and the impact of viremia on severity of hepatitis C virus recurrence. Liver Transpl 9:S58-S62, 2003.

515. Tsamandas AC, Furukawa H, Abu-Elmagd K, et al: Liver allograft pathology in liver/small bowel or multivisceral recipients. Mod Pathol 9:767-773, 1996.

516. Asanza CG, Garcia-Monzon C, Clemente G, et al: Immunohistochemical evidence of immunopathogenetic mechanisms in chronic hepatitis C recurrence after liver transplantation. Hepatology 26:755-763, 1997.

517. Rosen HR, Gretch DR, Oehlke M, et al: Timing and severity of initial hepatitis C recurrence as predictors of long-term liver allograft injury. Transplantation 65:1178-1182, 1998.

518. Rosen HR, Martin P: Hepatitis C infection in patients undergoing liver retransplantation. Transplantation 66:1612-1616, 1998.

519. Saxena R, Crawford JM, Navarro VJ, et al: Utilization of acidophil bodies in the diagnosis of recurrent hepatitis C infection after orthotopic liver transplantation. Mod Pathol 15:897-903, 2002.

520. Farges O, Bismuth H, Sebagh M, Reynes M: Granulomatous destruction of bile ducts after liver transplantation: Primary biliary cirrhosis recurrence or hepatitis C virus infection? Hepatology 21:1765-1767, 1995.

521. Neuberger J, Portmann B, Macdougall BR, et al: Recurrence of primary biliary cirrhosis after liver transplantation. N Engl J Med 306:1-4, 1982.

522. Neuberger J, Portmann B, Calne R, Williams R: Recurrence of autoimmune chronic active hepatitis following orthotopic liver grafting. Transplantation 37:363-365, 1984.

523. Balan V, Batts KP, Porayko MK, et al: Histological evidence for recurrence of primary biliary cirrhosis after liver transplantation. Hepatology 18:1392-1398, 1993.

524. Ferrell LD, Brixko C, Lake J, Bass J: The specificity of portal-based granulomas in recurrent primary biliary cirrhosis after liver transplantation [abstract]. Mod Pathol 7:131A, 1994.

525. Charco R, Vargas V, Allende H, et al: Is hepatitis C virus recurrence a risk factor for chronic liver allograft rejection? Transpl Int 9(Suppl 1):S195-S197, 1996.

526. Hoffmann RM, Gunther C, Diepolder HM, et al: Hepatitis C virus infection as a possible risk factor for ductopenic rejection (vanishing bile duct syndrome) after liver transplantation. Transpl Int 8:353-359, 1995.

527. Markus BH, Duquesnoy RJ, Gordon RD, et al: Histocompatibility and liver transplant outcome. Does HLA exert a dualistic effect? Transplantation 46:372-377, 1988.

528. Ontanon J, Muro M, Garcia-Alonso AM, et al: Effect of partial HLA class I match on acute rejection in viral pre-infected human liver allograft recipients. Transplantation 65:1047-1053, 1998.

529. Jain A, Demetris AJ, Manez R, et al: Incidence and severity of acute allograft rejection in liver transplant recipients treated with alfa interferon. Liver Transpl Surg 4:197-203, 1998.

530. Dousset B, Conti F, Houssin D, Calmus Y: Acute vanishing bile duct syndrome after interferon therapy for recurrent HCV infection in liver-transplant recipients. N Engl J Med 330:1160-1161, 1994.

531. Huang EJ, Wright TL, Lake JR, et al: Hepatitis B and C coinfections and persistent hepatitis B infections: Clinical outcome and liver pathology after transplantation. Hepatology 23:396-404, 1996.

532. Loda M, Fiorentino M, Meckler J, et al: Hepatitis C virus reinfection in orthotopic liver transplant patients with or without concomitant hepatitis B infection. Diagn Mol Pathol 5:81-87, 1996.

533. Vargas HE, Laskus T, Radkowski M, et al: Hepatitis G virus coinfection in hepatitis C virus–infected liver transplant recipients. Transplantation 64:786-788, 1997.

534. Vargas HE, Wang LF, Laskus T, et al: Distribution of infecting hepatitis C virus genotypes in end-stage liver disease patients at a large American transplantation center. J Infect Dis 175:448-450, 1997.

535. Laskus T, Radkowski M, Wang LF, et al: Lack of evidence for hepatitis G virus replication in the livers of patients coinfected with hepatitis C and G viruses. J Virol 71:7804-7806, 1997.

536. Gane E, Sallie R, Saleh M, et al: Clinical recurrence of hepatitis A following liver transplantation for acute liver failure. J Med Virol 45:35-39, 1995.

537. McCaughan GW, Torzillo PJ: Hepatitis A, liver transplants and indigenous communities. Med J Aust 172:6-7, 2000.

538. Steinmuller T, Seehofer D, Rayes N, et al: Increasing applicability of liver transplantation for patients with hepatitis B–related liver disease. Hepatology 35:1528-1535, 2002.

539. Neumann UP, Langrehr JM, Naumann U, et al: Impact of HLA-compatibilities in patients undergoing liver transplantation for HBV-cirrhosis. Clin Transplant 16:122-129, 2002.

540. Hasegawa K, Hashimoto E, Kanai N, et al: Living-related partial liver transplantation for decompensated hepatitis B without reactivation of hepatitis B in the following 30 months. J Gastroenterol 36:637-642, 2001.

541. Al Faraidy K, Yoshida EM, Davis JE, et al: Alteration of the dismal natural history of fibrosing cholestatic hepatitis secondary to hepatitis B virus with the use of lamivudine. Transplantation 64:926-928, 1997.

542. Samuel D, Zignego AL, Reynes M, et al: Long-term clinical and virological outcome after liver transplantation for cirrhosis caused by chronic delta hepatitis. Hepatology 21:333-339, 1995.

543. Holt CD, Millis JM, Busuttil RW: Role of liver transplantation in patients with hepatitis B infection. Clin Transplant 9:269-276, 1995.

544. Willems M, Metselaar HJ, Tilanus HW, et al: Liver transplantation and hepatitis C. Transpl Int 15:61-72, 2002.

545. Pruthi J, Medkiff KA, Esrason KT, et al: Analysis of causes of death in liver transplant recipients who survived more than 3 years. Liver Transpl 7:811-815, 2001.

546. Teixeira R, Papatheodoridis GV, Burroughs AK: Management of recurrent hepatitis C after liver transplantation. J Viral Hepat 8:159-168, 2001.
547. Rosen HR, Martin P: Hepatitis B and C in the liver transplant recipient. Semin Liver Dis 20:465-480, 2000.
548. Rosen HR: Retransplantation for hepatitis C: Implications of different policies. Liver Transpl 6(6 Suppl 2):S41-S46, 2000.
549. Teixeira R, Pastacaldi S, Papatheodoridis GV, Burroughs AK: Recurrent hepatitis C after liver transplantation. J Med Virol 61:443-454, 2000.
550. Terrault NA: Hepatitis C virus and liver transplantation. Semin Gastrointest Dis 11:96-114, 2000.
551. Vierling JM, Villamil FG, Rojter SE, et al: Morbidity and mortality of recurrent hepatitis C infection after orthotopic liver transplantation. J Viral Hepat 4(Suppl 1):117-124, 1997.
552. Johnson MW, Washburn WK, Freeman RB, et al: Hepatitis C viral infection in liver transplantation. Arch Surg 131:284-291, 1996.
553. Wright HL, Bou-Abboud CF, Hassanein T, et al: Disease recurrence and rejection following liver transplantation for autoimmune chronic active liver disease. Transplantation 53:136-139, 1992.
554. Ratziu V, Samuel D, Sebagh M, et al: Long-term follow-up after liver transplantation for autoimmune hepatitis: Evidence of recurrence of primary disease. J Hepatol 30:131-141, 1999.
555. Birnbaum AH, Benkov KJ, Pittman NS, et al: Recurrence of autoimmune hepatitis in children after liver transplantation. J Pediatr Gastroenterol Nutr 25:20-25, 1997.
556. Milkiewicz P, Hubscher SG, Skiba G, et al: Recurrence of autoimmune hepatitis after liver transplantation. Transplantation 68:253-256, 1999.
557. Ayata G, Gordon FD, Lewis WD, et al: Liver transplantation for autoimmune hepatitis: A long-term pathologic study. Hepatology 32:185-192, 2000.
558. Gonzalez-Koch A, Czaja AJ, Carpenter HA, et al: Recurrent autoimmune hepatitis after orthotopic liver transplantation. Liver Transpl 7:302-310, 2001.
559. Van de Water J, Gerson LB, Ferrell LD, et al: Immunohistochemical evidence of disease recurrence after liver transplantation for primary biliary cirrhosis. Hepatology 24:1079-1084, 1996.
560. Dmitrewski J, Hubscher SG, Mayer AD, Neuberger JM: Recurrence of primary biliary cirrhosis in the liver allograft: The effect of immunosuppression. J Hepatol 24:253-257, 1996.
561. Liermann Garcia RF, Evangelista Garcia C, McMaster P, Neuberger J: Transplantation for primary biliary cirrhosis: Retrospective analysis of 400 patients in a single center. Hepatology 33:22-27, 2001.
562. Neuberger J: Recurrent primary biliary cirrhosis. Liver Transpl 7:596-599, 2001.
563. Wong PY, Portmann B, O'Grady JG, et al: Recurrence of primary biliary cirrhosis after liver transplantation following FK506-based immunosuppression. J Hepatol 17:284-287, 1993.
564. Yusoff IF, House AK, De Boer WB, et al: Disease recurrence after liver transplantation in Western Australia. J Gastroenterol Hepatol 17:203-207, 2002.
565. Graziadei IW, Wiesner RH, Marotta PJ, et al: Long-term results of patients undergoing liver transplantation for primary sclerosing cholangitis. Hepatology 30:1121-1127, 1999.
566. Graziadei IW, Wiesner RH, Batts KP, et al: Recurrence of primary sclerosing cholangitis following liver transplantation. Hepatology 29:1050-1056, 1999.
567. Sheng R, Campbell WL, Zajko AB, Baron RL: Cholangiographic features of biliary strictures after liver transplantation for primary sclerosing cholangitis: Evidence of recurrent disease. AJR Am J Roentgenol 166:1109-1113, 1996.
568. Renz JF, Ascher NL: Liver transplantation for nonviral, nonmalignant diseases: Problem of recurrence. World J Surg 26:247-256, 2002.
569. Rai RM, Boitnott J, Klein AS, Thuluvath PJ: Features of recurrent primary sclerosing cholangitis in two consecutive liver allografts after liver transplantation. J Clin Gastroenterol 32:151-154, 2001.
570. Kubota T, Thomson A, Clouston AD, et al: Clinicopathologic findings of recurrent primary sclerosing cholangitis after orthotopic liver transplantation. J Hepatobiliary Pancreat Surg 6:377-381, 1999.
571. Sekido H, Takeda K, Morioka D, et al: Liver transplantation for primary sclerosing cholangitis. J Hepatobiliary Pancreat Surg 6:373-376, 1999.
572. Bellamy CO, DiMartini AM, Ruppert K, et al: Liver transplantation for alcoholic cirrhosis: Long term follow-up and impact of disease recurrence. Transplantation 72:619-626, 2001.
573. Lucey MR, Carr K, Beresford TP, et al: Alcohol use after liver transplantation in alcoholics: A clinical cohort follow-up study. Hepatology 25:1223-1227, 1997.
574. Burra P, Mioni D, Cecchetto A, et al: Histological features after liver transplantation in alcoholic cirrhotics. J Hepatol 34:716-722, 2001.
575. Pageaux GP, Michel J, Coste V, et al: Alcoholic cirrhosis is a good indication for liver transplantation, even for cases of recidivism. Gut 45:421-426, 1999.
576. Abosh D, Rosser B, Kaita K, et al: Outcomes following liver transplantation for patients with alcohol- versus nonalcohol-induced liver disease. Can J Gastroenterol 14:851-855, 2000.
577. Kim WR, Poterucha JJ, Porayko MK, et al: Recurrence of non-alcoholic steatohepatitis following liver transplantation. Transplantation 62:1802-1805, 1996.
578. Contos MJ, Cales W, Sterling RK, et al: Development of non-alcoholic fatty liver disease after orthotopic liver transplantation for cryptogenic cirrhosis. Liver Transpl 7:363-373, 2001.
579. Charlton M, Kasparova P, Weston S, et al: Frequency of non-alcoholic steatohepatitis as a cause of advanced liver disease. Liver Transpl 7:608-614, 2001.
580. Iwatsuki S, Starzl TE: Role of liver transplantation in the treatment of hepatocellular carcinoma. Semin Surg Oncol 9:337-340, 1993.
581. Wong LL: Current status of liver transplantation for hepatocellular cancer. Am J Surg 183:309-316, 2002.
582. Figueras J, Ibanez L, Ramos E, et al: Selection criteria for liver transplantation in early-stage hepatocellular carcinoma with cirrhosis: Results of a multicenter study. Liver Transpl 7:877-883, 2001.
583. Frilling A, Malago M, Broelsch CE: Current status of liver transplantation for treatment of hepatocellular carcinoma. Dig Dis 19:333-337, 2001.
584. Iwatsuki S, Dvorchik I, Marsh JW, et al: Liver transplantation for hepatocellular carcinoma: A proposal of a prognostic scoring system. J Am Coll Surg 191:389-394, 2000.
585. Klintmalm GB: Liver transplantation for hepatocellular carcinoma: A registry report of the impact of tumor characteristics on outcome. Ann Surg 228:479-490, 1998.
586. Marsh JW, Casavilla A, Iwatsuki S, et al: Predicting the risk of tumor recurrence following transplantation for hepatocellular carcinoma. Hepatology 26:1689-1691, 1997.
587. McPeake JR, O'Grady JG, Zaman S, et al: Liver transplantation for primary hepatocellular carcinoma: Tumor size and number determine outcome. J Hepatol 18:226-234, 1993.
588. Starzl TE, Porter KA, Putnam CW, et al: Orthotopic liver transplantation in ninety-three patients. Surg Gynecol Obstet 142:487-505, 1976.
589. Tamura S, Kato T, Berho M, et al: Impact of histological grade of hepatocellular carcinoma on the outcome of liver transplantation. Arch Surg 136:25-30, 2001.
590. Casavilla FA, Marsh JW, Iwatsuki S, et al: Hepatic resection and transplantation for peripheral cholangiocarcinoma. J Am Coll Surg 185:429-436, 1997.

591. Iwatsuki S, Todo S, Marsh JW, et al: Treatment of hilar cholangiocarcinoma (Klatskin tumors) with hepatic resection or transplantation. J Am Coll Surg 187:358-364, 1998.

592. Meyer CG, Penn I, James L: Liver transplantation for cholangiocarcinoma: Results in 207 patients. Transplantation 69:1633-1637, 2000.

593. Weimann A, Varnholt H, Schlitt HJ, et al: Retrospective analysis of prognostic factors after liver resection and transplantation for cholangiocellular carcinoma. Br J Surg 87:1182-1187, 2000.

594. Starzl T: Surgery for metabolic liver disease. In McDermott WV (ed): Surgery of the Liver. Boston, Blackwell, 1986, pp 127-136.

595. Putnam CW, Porter KA, Peters RL, et al: Liver replacement for alpha1-antitrypsin deficiency. Surgery 81:258-261, 1977.

596. Hood JM, Koep LJ, Peters RL, et al: Liver transplantation for advanced liver disease with alpha-1-antitrypsin deficiency. N Engl J Med 302:272-275, 1980.

597. Esquivel CO, Vicente E, Van Thiel D, et al: Orthotopic liver transplantation for alpha-1-antitrypsin deficiency: An experience in 29 children and ten adults. Transplant Proc 19:3798-3802, 1987.

598. Vennarecci G, Gunson BK, Ismail T, et al: Transplantation for end stage liver disease related to alpha 1 antitrypsin. Transplantation 61:1488-1495, 1996.

599. DuBois RS, Rodgerson DO, Martineau G, et al: Orthotopic liver transplantation for Wilson's disease. Lancet 1:505-508, 1971.

600. Groth CG, Dubois RS, Corman J, et al: Metabolic effects of hepatic replacement in Wilson's disease. Transplant Proc 5:829-833, 1973.

601. Zitelli BJ, Malatack JJ, Gartner JC, et al: Orthotopic liver transplantation in children with hepatic-based metabolic disease. Transplant Proc 15:1284-1287, 1983.

602. Esquivel CO, Marino IR, Fioravanti V, Van Thiel DH: Liver transplantation for metabolic disease of the liver. Gastroenterol Clin North Am 17:167-175, 1988.

603. Sokol RJ, Francis PD, Gold SH, et al: Orthotopic liver transplantation for acute fulminant Wilson disease. J Pediatr 107:549-552, 1985.

604. Polson RJ, Rolles K, Calne RY, et al: Reversal of severe neurological manifestations of Wilson's disease following orthotopic liver transplantation. Q J Med 64:685-691, 1987.

605. Schilsky ML: Diagnosis and treatment of Wilson's disease. Pediatr Transplant 6:15-19, 2002.

606. Fisch RO, McCabe ER, Doeden D, et al: Homotransplantation of the liver in a patient with hepatoma and hereditary tyrosinemia. J Pediatr 93:592-596, 1978.

607. Starzl TE, Zitelli BJ, Shaw BW Jr, et al: Changing concepts: Liver replacement for hereditary tyrosinemia and hepatoma. J Pediatr 106:604-606, 1985.

608. Van Thiel DH, Gartner LM, Thorp FK, et al: Resolution of the clinical features of tyrosinemia following orthotopic liver transplantation for hepatoma. J Hepatol 3:42-48, 1986.

609. Malatack JJ, Finegold DN, Iwatsuki S, et al: Liver transplantation for type I glycogen storage disease. Lancet 1:1073-1075, 1983.

610. Matern D, Starzl TE, Arnaout W, et al: Liver transplantation for glycogen storage disease types I, III, and IV. Eur J Pediatr 158(Suppl 2):S43-S48, 1999.

611. Kayler LK, Merion RM, Lee S, et al: Long-term survival after liver transplantation in children with metabolic disorders. Pediatr Transplant 6:295-300, 2002.

612. Lewis WD, Skinner M, Simms RW, et al: Orthotopic liver transplantation for familial amyloidotic polyneuropathy. Clin Transplant 8:107-110, 1994.

613. Figueras J, Pares D, Munar-Ques M, et al: Experience with domino or sequential liver transplantation in familial patients with amyloid polyneuropathy. Transplant Proc 34:307-308, 2002.

614. Shaz BH, Lewis WD, Skinner M, Khettry U: Livers from patients with apolipoprotein A-I amyloidosis are not suitable as "domino" donors. Mod Pathol 14:577-580, 2001.

615. Nishizaki T, Kishikawa K, Yoshizumi T, et al: Domino liver transplantation from a living related donor. Transplantation 70:1236-1239, 2000.

616. de Carvalho M, Conceicao I, Bentes C, Luis ML: Long-term quantitative evaluation of liver transplantation in familial amyloid polyneuropathy (Portuguese V30M). Amyloid 9:126-133, 2002.

617. Suhr OB, Ericzon BG, Friman S: Long-term follow-up of survival of liver transplant recipients with familial amyloid polyneuropathy (Portuguese type). Liver Transpl 8:787-794, 2002.

618. Ikeda S, Nakazato M, Ando Y, Sobue G: Familial transthyretin-type amyloid polyneuropathy in Japan: Clinical and genetic heterogeneity. Neurology 58:1001-1007, 2002.

619. Bittencourt PL, Couto CA, Farias AQ, et al: Results of liver transplantation for familial amyloid polyneuropathy type I in Brazil. Liver Transpl 8:34-39, 2002.

620. Kawasaki S, Makuuchi M, Matsunami H, et al: Living related liver transplantation in adults. Ann Surg 227:269-274, 1998.

621. Ericzon BG, Suhr O, Broome U, et al: Liver transplantation halts the progress of familial amyloidotic polyneuropathy. Transplant Proc 27:1233, 1995.

622. Wolff H, Otto G, Giest H: Liver transplantation in Crigler-Najjar syndrome. A case report. Transplantation 42:84, 1986.

623. Kaufman SS, Wood RP, Shaw BW Jr, et al: Orthotopic liver transplantation for type I Crigler-Najjar syndrome. Hepatology 6:1259-1262, 1986.

624. Jaffe R: Liver transplant pathology in pediatric metabolic disorders. Pediatr Dev Pathol 1:102-117, 1998.

625. Watts RW, Calne RY, Rolles K, et al: Successful treatment of primary hyperoxaluria type I by combined hepatic and renal transplantation. Lancet 2:474-475, 1987.

626. Shneider BL: Pediatric liver transplantation in metabolic disease: Clinical decision making. Pediatr Transplant 6:25-29, 2002.

627. Casella JF, Lewis JH, Bontempo FA, et al: Successful treatment of homozygous protein C deficiency by hepatic transplantation. Lancet 1:435-438, 1988.

628. Starzl TE, Bilheimer DW, Bahnson HT, et al: Heart-liver transplantation in a patient with familial hypercholesterolaemia. Lancet 1:1382-1383, 1984.

629. Bilheimer DW, Goldstein JL, Grundy SM, et al: Liver transplantation to provide low-density-lipoprotein receptors and lower plasma cholesterol in a child with homozygous familial hypercholesterolemia. N Engl J Med 311:1658-1664, 1984.

630. Hoeg JM, Starzl TE, Brewer HB Jr: Liver transplantation for treatment of cardiovascular disease: Comparison with medication and plasma exchange in homozygous familial hypercholesterolemia. Am J Cardiol 59:705-707, 1987.

631. Mora NP, Cienfuegos JA, Ardaiz J, et al: Special operative events in the first case of liver grafting after heart transplantation. Surgery 103:264-267, 1988.

632. Lewis JH, Bontempo FA, Spero JA, et al: Liver transplantation in a hemophiliac. N Engl J Med 312:1189-1190, 1985.

633. Bontempo FA, Lewis JH, Gorenc TJ, et al: Liver transplantation in hemophilia A. Blood 69:1721-1724, 1987.

634. Gibas A, Dienstag JL, Schafer AI, et al: Cure of hemophilia A by orthotopic liver transplantation. Gastroenterology 95:192-194, 1988.

635. Merion RM, Delius RE, Campbell DA Jr, Turcotte JG: Orthotopic liver transplantation totally corrects factor IX deficiency in hemophilia B. Surgery 104:929-931, 1988.

636. Parolin MB, Batts KP, Wiesner RH, et al: Liver allograft iron accumulation in patients with and without pretransplantation hepatic hemosiderosis. Liver Transpl 8:331-339, 2002.

637. Brandhagen DJ: Liver transplantation for hereditary hemochromatosis. Liver Transpl 7:663-672, 2001.

638. Halme L, Helio T, Makinen J, et al: HFE haemochromatosis gene mutations in liver transplant patients. Scand J Gastroenterol 36:881-885, 2001.

639. Brandhagen DJ, Alvarez W, Therneau TM, et al: Iron overload in cirrhosis-HFE genotypes and outcome after liver transplantation. Hepatology 31:456-460, 2000.

640. Wigg AJ, Harley H, Casey G: Heterozygous recipient and donor HFE mutations associated with a hereditary haemochromatosis phenotype after liver transplantation. Gut 52:433-435, 2003.

641. Daloze P, Delvin EE, Glorieux FH, et al: Replacement therapy for inherited enzyme deficiency: Liver orthotopic transplantation in Niemann-Pick disease type A. Am J Med Genet 1:229-239, 1977.

642. Gartner JC Jr, Bergman I, Malatack JJ, et al: Progression of neuro-visceral storage disease with supranuclear ophthalmoplegia following orthotopic liver transplantation. Pediatrics 77:104-106, 1986.

643. Samuel D, Boboc B, Bernuau J, et al: Liver transplantation for protoporphyria. Evidence for the predominant role of the erythropoietic tissue in protoporphyrin overproduction. Gastroenterology 95:816-819, 1988.

644. Polson RJ, Lim CK, Rolles K, et al: The effect of liver transplantation in a 13-year-old boy with erythropoietic protoporphyria. Transplantation 46:386-389, 1988.

645. Meerman L, Haagsma EB, Gouw AS, et al: Long-term follow-up after liver transplantation for erythropoietic protoporphyria. Eur J Gastroenterol Hepatol 11:431-438, 1999.

646. de Torres I, Demetris AJ, Randhawa PS: Recurrent hepatic allograft injury in erythropoietic protoporphyria. Transplantation 61:1412-1413, 1996.

647. Dellon ES, Szczepiorkowski ZM, Dzik WH, et al: Treatment of recurrent allograft dysfunction with intravenous hematin after liver transplantation for erythropoietic protoporphyria. Transplantation 73:911-915, 2002.

648. Cox KL, Ward RE, Furgiuele TL, et al: Orthotopic liver transplantation in patients with cystic fibrosis. Pediatrics 80:571-574, 1987.

649. Mieles LA, Orenstein D, Teperman L, et al: Liver transplantation in cystic fibrosis. Lancet 1:1073, 1989.

650. Milkiewicz P, Skiba G, Kelly D, et al: Transplantation for cystic fibrosis: Outcome following early liver transplantation. J Gastroenterol Hepatol 17:208-213, 2002.

651. Polson RJ, Portmann B, Neuberger J, et al: Evidence for disease recurrence after liver transplantation for primary biliary cirrhosis. Clinical and histologic follow-up studies. Gastroenterology 97:715-725, 1989.

652. Esquivel CO, Van Thiel DH, Demetris AJ, et al: Transplantation for primary biliary cirrhosis. Gastroenterology 94:1207-1216, 1988.

653. Demetris AJ, Markus BH, Esquivel C, et al: Pathologic analysis of liver transplantation for primary biliary cirrhosis. Hepatology 8:939-947, 1988.

654. Sanchez-Urdazpal L, Czaja AJ, van Hoek B, et al: Prognostic features and role of liver transplantation in severe cortico-steroid-treated autoimmune chronic active hepatitis. Hepatology 15:215-221, 1992.

655. Iwatsuki S, Gordon RD, Shaw BW Jr, Starzl TE: Role of liver transplantation in cancer therapy. Ann Surg 202:401-407, 1985.

656. Iwatsuki S, Starzl TE, Sheahan DG, et al: Hepatic resection versus transplantation for hepatocellular carcinoma. Ann Surg 214:221-228, 1991.

657. Wang VS, Saab S: Liver transplantation in the era of model for end-stage liver disease. Liver Int 24:1-8, 2004.

658. Hunt J, Gordon FD, Jenkins RL, et al: Sarcoidosis with selective involvement of a second liver allograft: Report of a case and review of the literature. Mod Pathol 12:325-328, 1999.

659. Nair S, Baisden B, Boitnott J, et al: Recurrent, progressive giant cell hepatitis in two consecutive liver allografts in a middle-aged woman. J Clin Gastroenterol 32:454-456, 2001.

660. Hassoun Z, N'Guyen B, Cote J, et al: A case of giant cell hepatitis recurring after liver transplantation and treated with ribavirin. Can J Gastroenterol 14:729-731, 2000.

661. Lerut JP, Claeys N, Ciccarelli O, et al: Recurrent postinfantile syncytial giant cell hepatitis after orthotopic liver transplantation. Transpl Int 11:320-322, 1998.

662. Durand F, Degott C, Sauvanet A, et al: Subfulminant syncytial giant cell hepatitis: Recurrence after liver transplantation treated with ribavirin. J Hepatol 26:722-726, 1997.

663. Pappo O, Yunis E, Jordan JA, et al: Recurrent and de novo giant cell hepatitis after orthotopic liver transplantation. Am J Surg Pathol 18:804-813, 1994.

664. Johnson SJ, Mathew J, MacSween RN, et al: Post-infantile giant cell hepatitis: Histological and immunohistochemical study. J Clin Pathol 47:1022-1027, 1994.

665. Ben-Ari Z, Broida E, Monselise Y, et al: Syncytial giant-cell hepatitis due to autoimmune hepatitis type II (LKM1+) presenting as subfulminant hepatitis. Am J Gastroenterol 95:799-801, 2000.

666. Melendez HV, Rela M, Baker AJ, et al: Liver transplant for giant cell hepatitis with autoimmune haemolytic anaemia. Arch Dis Child 77:249-251, 1997.

667. Hicks J, Barrish J, Zhu SH: Neonatal syncytial giant cell hepatitis with paramyxoviral-like inclusions. Ultrastruct Pathol 25:65-71, 2001.

668. Phillips MJ, Blendis LM, Poucell S, et al: Syncytial giant-cell hepatitis. Sporadic hepatitis with distinctive pathological features, a severe clinical course, and paramyxoviral features. N Engl J Med 324:455-460, 1991.

669. Neuberger J, Wallace L, Joplin R, Hubscher S: Hepatic distribution of E2 component of pyruvate dehydrogenase complex after transplantation. Hepatology 22:798-801, 1995.

670. Neuberger J: Liver transplantation for primary biliary cirrhosis. Autoimmun Rev 2:1-7, 2003.

671. Hashimoto E, Shimada M, Noguchi S, et al: Disease recurrence after living liver transplantation for primary biliary cirrhosis: A clinical and histological follow-up study. Liver Transpl 7:588-595, 2001.

672. Jaeckel E, Tillmann HL, Manns MP: Liver transplantation and autoimmunity. Acta Gastroenterol Belg 62:323-329, 1999.

673. Neuberger J: Recurrent primary biliary cirrhosis. Baillieres Best Pract Res Clin Gastroenterol 14:669-680, 2000.

674. Paumgartner G, Beuers U: Ursodeoxycholic acid in cholestatic liver disease: Mechanisms of action and therapeutic use revisited. Hepatology 36:525-531, 2002.

675. Jones DE, James OF, Portmann B, et al: Development of autoimmune hepatitis following liver transplantation for primary biliary cirrhosis. Hepatology 30:53-57, 1999.

676. Sebagh M, Farges O, Dubel L, et al: Histological features predictive of recurrence of primary biliary cirrhosis after liver transplantation. Transplantation 65:1328-1333, 1998.

677. Khettry U, Anand N, Faul PN, et al: Liver transplantation for primary biliary cirrhosis: A long-term pathologic study. Liver Transpl 9:87-96, 2003.

678. Hubscher SG: Recurrent autoimmune hepatitis after liver transplantation: Diagnostic criteria, risk factors, and outcome. Liver Transpl 7:285-291, 2001.

679. Alvarez F, Berg PA, Bianchi FB, et al: International Autoimmune Hepatitis Group Report: Review of criteria for diagnosis of autoimmune hepatitis. J Hepatol 31:929-938, 1999.

680. Demetris AJ, Murase N, Delaney CP: Overlap between allo- and autoimmunity in the rat and human evidence for important contributions for dendritic and regulatory cells. Graft 6:21-32, 2003.

681. Neuberger J: Transplantation for autoimmune hepatitis. Semin Liver Dis 22:379-386, 2002.

682. Manns MP, Bahr MJ: Recurrent autoimmune hepatitis after liver transplantation—when non-self becomes self. Hepatology 32:868-870, 2000.

683. Ahmed M, Mutimer D, Hathaway M, et al: Liver transplantation for autoimmune hepatitis: A 12-year experience. Transplant Proc 29:496, 1997.

684. Prados E, Cuervas-Mons V, de la Mata M, et al: Outcome of autoimmune hepatitis after liver transplantation. Transplantation 66:1645-1650, 1998.

685. Reich DJ, Fiel I, Guarrera JV, et al: Liver transplantation for autoimmune hepatitis. Hepatology 32:693-700, 2000.

686. Devlin J, Donaldson P, Portmann B, et al: Recurrence of autoimmune hepatitis following liver transplantation. Liver Transpl Surg 1:162-165, 1995.

687. Neuberger J: Recurrence of primary biliary cirrhosis, primary sclerosing cholangitis, and autoimmune hepatitis. Liver Transpl Surg 1(5 Suppl 1):109-115, 1995.

688. Sempoux C, Horsmans Y, Lerut J, et al: Acute lobular hepatitis as the first manifestation of recurrent autoimmune hepatitis after orthotopic liver transplantation. Liver 17:311-315, 1997.

689. Faust TW: Recurrent primary biliary cirrhosis, primary sclerosing cholangitis, and autoimmune hepatitis after transplantation. Semin Liver Dis 20:481-495, 2000.

690. Heneghan MA, Portmann BC, Norris SM, et al: Graft dysfunction mimicking autoimmune hepatitis following liver transplantation in adults. Hepatology 34:464-470, 2001.

691. Molmenti EP, Netto GJ, Murray NG, et al: Incidence and recurrence of autoimmune/alloimmune hepatitis in liver transplant recipients. Liver Transpl 8:519-526, 2002.

692. Salcedo M, Vaquero J, Banares R, et al: Response to steroids in de novo autoimmune hepatitis after liver transplantation. Hepatology 35:349-356, 2002.

693. McDiarmid SV: Liver transplantation. The pediatric challenge. Clin Liver Dis 4:879-927, 2000.

694. Gupta P, Hart J, Millis JM, et al: De novo hepatitis with autoimmune antibodies and atypical histology: A rare cause of late graft dysfunction after pediatric liver transplantation. Transplantation 71:664-668, 2001.

695. Hernandez HM, Kovarik P, Whitington PF, Alonso EM: Autoimmune hepatitis as a late complication of liver transplantation. J Pediatr Gastroenterol Nutr 32:131-136, 2001.

696. Czaja AJ: Autoimmune hepatitis after liver transplantation and other lessons of self-intolerance. Liver Transpl 8:505-513, 2002.

697. Duclos-Vallee JC, Johanet C, Bach JF, Yamamoto AM: Auto-antibodies associated with acute rejection after liver transplantation for type-2 autoimmune hepatitis. J Hepatol 33:163-166, 2000.

698. Graze PR, Gale RP: Chronic graft versus host disease: A syndrome of disordered immunity. Am J Med 66:611-620, 1979.

699. Faust TW: Recurrent primary biliary cirrhosis, primary sclerosing cholangitis, and autoimmune hepatitis after transplantation. Liver Transpl 7(11 Suppl 1):S99-S108, 2001.

700. Goss JA, Shackleton CR, Farmer DG, et al: Orthotopic liver transplantation for primary sclerosing cholangitis. A 12-year single center experience. Ann Surg 225:472-481, 1997.

701. Jeyarajah DR, Netto GJ, Lee SP, et al: Recurrent primary sclerosing cholangitis after orthotopic liver transplantation: Is chronic rejection part of the disease process? Transplantation 66:1300-1306, 1998.

702. Narumi S, Roberts JP, Emond JC, et al: Liver transplantation for sclerosing cholangitis. Hepatology 22:451-457, 1995.

703. Gow PJ, Chapman RW: Liver transplantation for primary sclerosing cholangitis. Liver 20:97-103, 2000.

704. Graziadei IW: Recurrence of primary sclerosing cholangitis after liver transplantation. Liver Transpl 8:575-581, 2002.

705. Dvorchik I, Subotin M, Demetris AJ, et al: Effect of liver transplantation on inflammatory bowel disease in patients with primary sclerosing cholangitis. Hepatology 35:380-384, 2002.

706. Lerut J, Demetris AJ, Stieber AC, et al: Intrahepatic bile duct strictures after human orthotopic liver transplantation.

707. Platz KP, Mueller AR, Spree E, et al: Liver transplantation for alcoholic cirrhosis. Transpl Int 13(Suppl 1):S127-S130, 2000.

708. Bjoro K, Friman S, Hockerstedt K, et al: Liver transplantation in the Nordic countries, 1982-1998: Changes of indications and improving results. Scand J Gastroenterol 34:714-722, 1999.

709. Ayata G, Gordon FD, Lewis WD, et al: Cryptogenic cirrhosis: Clinicopathologic findings at and after liver transplantation. Hum Pathol 33:1098-1104, 2002.

710. Burke A, Lucey MR: Non-alcoholic fatty liver disease, non-alcoholic steatohepatitis and orthotopic liver transplantation. Am J Transplant 4:686-693, 2004.

711. Osorio RW, Ascher NL, Avery M, et al: Predicting recidivism after orthotopic liver transplantation for alcoholic liver disease. Hepatology 20:105-110, 1994.

712. Berlakovich GA, Steininger R, Herbst F, et al: Efficacy of liver transplantation for alcoholic cirrhosis with respect to recidivism and compliance. Transplantation 58:560-565, 1994.

713. Cohen C, Benjamin M: Alcoholics and liver transplantation. The Ethics and Social Impact Committee of the Transplant and Health Policy Center. JAMA 265:1299-1301, 1991.

714. Conjeevaram HS, Hart J, Lissoos TW, et al: Rapidly progressive liver injury and fatal alcoholic hepatitis occurring after liver transplantation in alcoholic patients. Transplantation 67:1562-1568, 1999.

715. Molloy RM, Komorowski R, Varma RR: Recurrent nonalcoholic steatohepatitis and cirrhosis after liver transplantation. Liver Transpl Surg 3:177-178, 1997.

716. Tang H, Boulton R, Gunson B, et al: Patterns of alcohol consumption after liver transplantation. Gut 43:140-145, 1998.

717. Gish RG, Lee A, Brooks L, et al: Long-term follow-up of patients diagnosed with alcohol dependence or alcohol abuse who were evaluated for liver transplantation. Liver Transpl 7:581-587, 2001.

718. Lee RG: Recurrence of alcoholic liver disease after liver transplantation. Liver Transpl Surg 3:292-295, 1997.

719. Gordon FD, Pomfret EA, Pomposelli JJ, et al: Severe steatosis as the initial histologic manifestation of recurrent hepatitis C genotype 3. Hum Pathol 35:636-638, 2004.

720. Khettry U, Backer A, Ayata G, et al: Centrilobular histopathologic changes in liver transplant biopsies. Hum Pathol 33:270-276, 2002.

721. Nakhleh RE, Schwarzenberg SJ, Bloomer J, et al: The pathology of liver allografts surviving longer than one year. Hepatology 11:465-470, 1990.

722. Berenguer M, Rayon JM, Prieto M, et al: Are posttransplantation protocol liver biopsies useful in the long term? Liver Transpl 7:790-796, 2001.

723. Starzl TE, Koep LJ, Halgrimson CG, et al: Fifteen years of clinical liver transplantation. Gastroenterology 77:375-388, 1979.

724. Starzl TE, Iwatsuki S, Van Thiel DH, et al: Evolution of liver transplantation. Hepatology 2:614-636, 1982.

725. Gane E, Portmann B, Saxena R, et al: Nodular regenerative hyperplasia of the liver graft after liver transplantation. Hepatology 20:88-94, 1994.

726. Reyes J, Zeevi A, Ramos H, et al: Frequent achievement of a drug-free state after orthotopic liver transplantation. Transplant Proc 25:3315-3319, 1993.

727. Tsamandas AC, Jain AB, Raikow RB, et al: Extramedullary hematopoiesis in the allograft liver. Mod Pathol 8:671-674, 1995.

728. Sterneck M, Wiesner R, Ascher N, et al: Azathioprine hepatotoxicity after liver transplantation. Hepatology 14:806-810, 1991.

Pathology of Recurrence of Non-Neoplastic Disease After Liver Transplantation

CHARLES R. LASSMAN

Hepatitis C   1129
  Histology of recurrent hepatitis C   1130
  Recurrent hepatitis C versus acute
    rejection   1130
  Grading of hepatitis C and acute
    rejection   1135
  Hepatitis C versus preservation injury
    and bile duct obstruction   1135
  Histology and polymerase chain reaction
    for hepatitis C virus RNA   1135
  Fibrosis   1136
  Recurrent hepatitis C versus chronic
    rejection   1136
  Fibrosing cholestatic hepatitis   1137
  Epstein-Barr virus infection versus recurrent
    hepatitis C   1137
  Hepatitis C–positive donors   1137
  Hepatitis C in living donor
    transplantation   1137
  Treatment of hepatitis C in the
    transplant liver   1137

Recurrent hepatitis B   1138

Recurrent autoimmune hepatitis   1139
  Autoimmune hepatitis versus chronic
    rejection   1140

Recurrent primary biliary cirrhosis   1140
  Primary biliary cirrhosis versus chronic
    rejection   1141

Recurrent primary sclerosing cholangitis   1141
  Recurrent primary sclerosing cholangitis versus
    acute rejection   1143
  Recurrent primary sclerosing cholangitis versus
    chronic rejection   1143

Recurrent alcoholic liver disease and
  nonalcoholic steatohepatitis   1143
  Grading and staging of steatohepatitis   1145

Liver transplantation has enjoyed tremendous success, in part because of the unique immunological properties of the liver and in part because of the development of new pharmaceutical agents to treat rejection and infection. Fortunately, liver allografts are infrequently lost to rejection or opportunistic infection. Recurrent disease, however, remains a serious problem and is a frequent cause of graft dysfunction and loss.

Hepatitis C

Hepatitis C, unfortunately, recurs in nearly all allografts.[1-7] The severity of recurrence and the progression of fibrosis to cirrhosis are variable, and neither can be reliably predicted without biopsy.[8-10] In most patients, viral RNA can be detected in peripheral blood[11-14] by polymerase chain reaction (PCR) as early as a few days after transplantation.[15] Histological recurrence is usually evident in biopsy specimens at 2 to 3 months but can be seen as early as 1 week after transplantation in patients with high pretransplant viral loads.[9,16,17] Biopsies are therefore frequently performed at a time when both recurrent hepatitis C and acute rejection (AR) are likely. Progression of hepatitis C to cirrhosis is more rapid in patients who have been treated for multiple episodes of AR.[18,19] Therefore, the primary reason to perform a liver biopsy has been to distinguish recurrent disease from AR and thereby avoid unnecessary immunosuppression. Furthermore, as increasingly successful treatment of hepatitis C has been implemented, biopsies are also performed to confirm histological injury from hepatitis C before beginning antiviral treatment, as well as later to assess the efficacy of treatment.[5,20-27]

Although the diagnosis of recurrent hepatitis C and AR in the early posttransplant period is relatively straightforward, such distinction becomes more difficult with the transition to chronic hepatitis. Indeed, because most patients have histological evidence of recurrent disease within a few months, the differential diagnosis is not simply hepatitis C versus rejection, but instead is hepatitis C versus hepatitis C and AR.

Histology of Recurrent Hepatitis C

The histological features of hepatitis C in a transplanted liver are much like those in a native liver with a few exceptions. Early in the course of recurrence, the initial histological picture resembles that of acute hepatitis with a predominance of lobular activity. Later, there is a transition to predominantly portal infiltrates and interface hepatitis typical of chronic hepatitis C.[8-10]

The earliest histological feature of recurrent hepatitis C may be steatosis; however, this finding is not specific or sensitive.[10,28,29] In most patients, scattered apoptotic hepatocytes are the first histological sign of recurrent hepatitis C, and although more specific than steatosis, this finding can also be seen in non–hepatitis C virus (HCV)-infected grafts, particularly in the first few weeks after transplantation. Lobular activity (Fig. 70–1) in most patients consists of small clusters of lymphocytes, apoptotic hepatocytes, patchy ballooning change, or any combination of these findings. Aggregates of hypertrophic Kupffer cells are often present. Alternatively, there may be an extensive sinusoidal lymphocytic infiltrate with only rare apoptotic hepatocytes.[16] In some biopsy specimens, ballooning change, as seen in acute hepatitis in the native liver, is extensive but not zonal. Zone III ballooning change should raise the differential diagnosis of ischemic injury and trigger a workup for vascular compromise. Portal infiltrates are often but not

always present, are generally mild, and may be associated with mild interface activity.

With time, most biopsy specimens in patients with recurrent hepatitis C demonstrate portal lymphoid aggregates with varying degrees of interface activity. These aggregates are characterized by extension of lymphocytes across the limiting plate in association with apoptotic or degenerative-appearing hepatocytes (Fig. 70–2).[8,16,30] Most specimens demonstrate minimal or mild activity; however, in our experience, marked activity or bridging necrosis is more commonly seen in allografts than in native livers. Bile duct infiltration by lymphocytes is frequently seen but is generally mild and without significant epithelial injury. Ductular reaction at the interface often results from interface activity and may complicate the assessment of biliary obstruction in these patients (see later).

Recurrent Hepatitis C versus Acute Rejection

There is extensive overlap between the features of recurrent hepatitis C and AR (Table 70–1). Differentiation from AR is based on identifying features of AR not seen in hepatitis C and features of hepatitis C not seen in AR. The diagnosis of AR is based on three findings[31] (see Chapter 69): (1) mixed portal inflammatory infiltrates; (2) infiltration of bile ducts by lymphocytes, with epithelial cell injury in the form of pyknosis and vacuolization; and most important, (3) portal and central vein endotheliitis and, in very severe cases, arteriolar endotheliitis.

Portal Inflammatory Infiltrates. In hepatitis C the infiltrates are predominantly lymphocytic and often nodular. In AR, the infiltrates are mixed and composed of lymphocytes, eosinophils, and neutrophils. Furthermore, in AR the infiltrates are diffuse, not nodular as is typical of hepatitis C. Eosinophils are occasionally seen in native liver biopsy specimens from patients with hepatitis C but are only rarely prominent, so their presence is helpful in establishing a diagnosis of AR. Likewise, the presence of neutrophils favors a diagnosis of AR; however, because they frequently accompany the ductular reaction of chronic interface hepatitis and are usually present in bile duct obstruction (BDO) and cholangitis, they are not as helpful as eosinophils in distinguishing between recurrent hepatitis C and AR.

Bile Duct Injury/Infiltration. Bile duct infiltration in AR is quite variable and ranges from mild to extensive. Bile duct infiltration may also be seen in hepatitis C; however, it is generally mild and not accompanied by significant epithelial injury, pyknosis, or vacuolization. Therefore, when bile duct infiltration by lymphocytes is

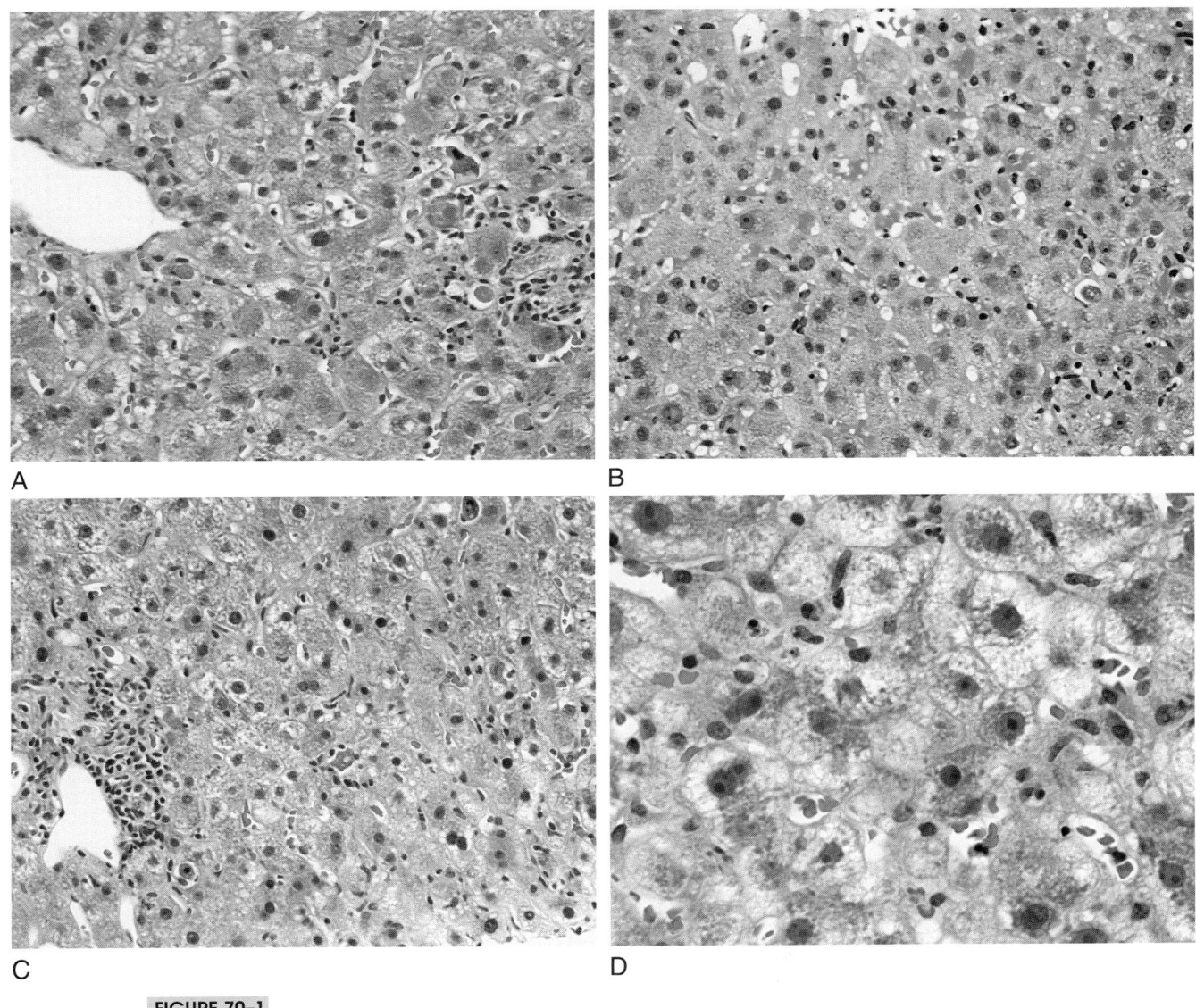

FIGURE 70-1

Recurrent hepatitis C, early phase, predominantly lobular hepatitis with small clusters of lymphocytes and apoptotic hepatocytes (**A**) (hematoxylin-eosin stain [H&E] ×200), sinusoidal lymphocytes (**B**) (H&E ×200), mild portal infiltrates and interface activity (**C**) (H&E ×200), and mild ballooning change (**D**) (H&E ×400).

mild, it is not helpful in distinguishing AR from hepatitis C. When it is moderate to marked and accompanied by significant epithelial cell injury, it favors AR.

Endotheliitis. Endotheliitis is the most helpful feature in differentiating hepatitis C from AR. However, if endotheliitis is defined too loosely, it can be found in a wide variety of conditions and cannot be used as effectively when differentiating AR from other processes. In hepatitis C as well as other inflammatory conditions, portal lymphocytes abut portal vein endothelial cells and may be adherent to the luminal surface of endothelial cells. True endotheliitis, in contrast, is characterized by swollen, damaged-appearing endothelial cells

separated from the underlying basement membrane by subendothelial lymphocytes and is virtually never present in native liver biopsy specimens with hepatitis C. When the endothelium is seemingly "lifted off" the basement membrane by lymphocytes, one can be relatively certain that one is dealing with AR (Fig. 70–3).

Central Vein Endotheliitis. Because lymphoid infiltrates in patients with hepatitis C may obscure portal structures and thus render their examination difficult, the finding of central vein endotheliitis can be very helpful in establishing a diagnosis of AR. Central vein endotheliitis may be accompanied by perivenular hepatocellular necrosis or dropout; however, hepatitis C occasionally

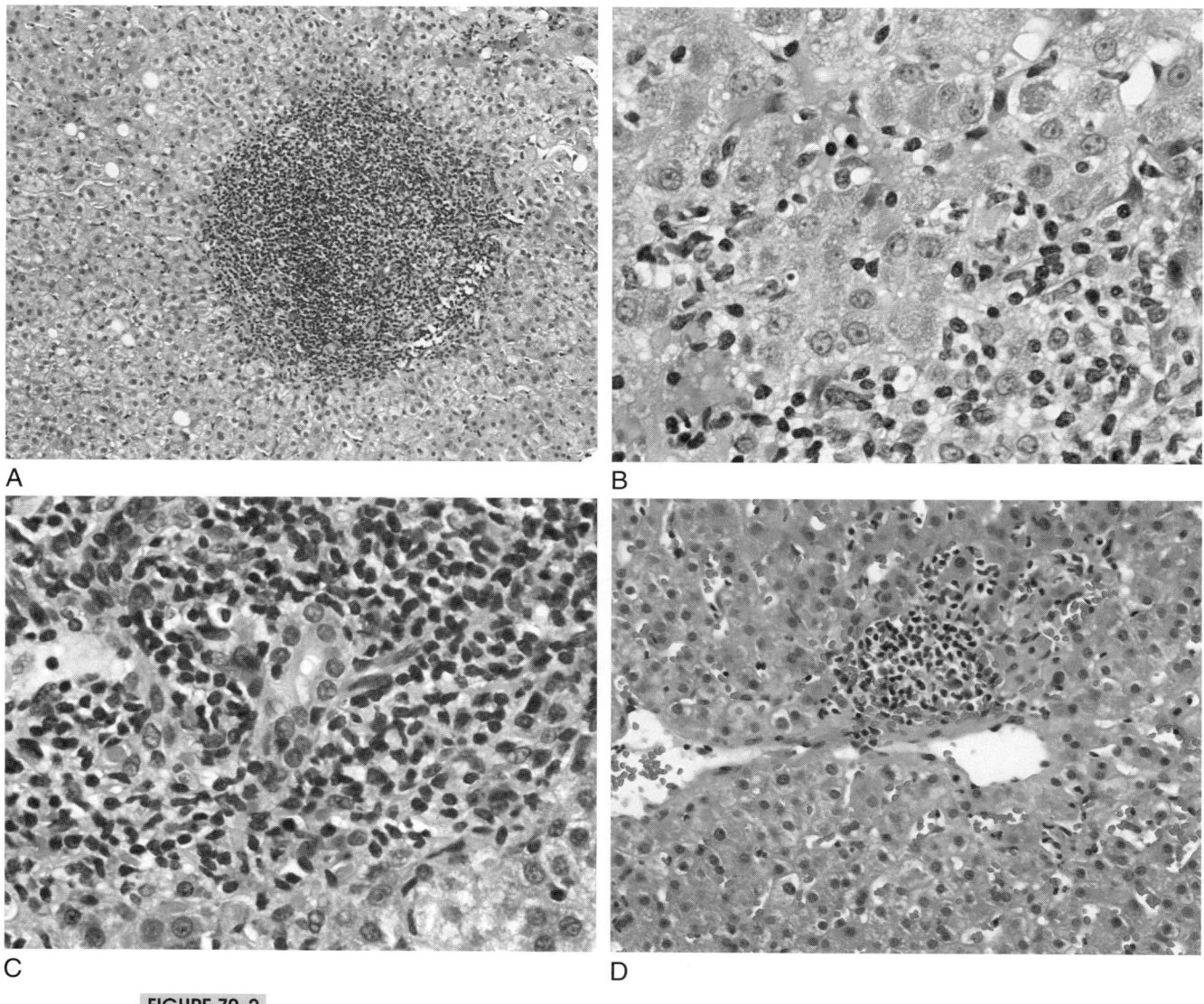

A

B

C

D

FIGURE 70–2

Chronic hepatitis C. **A,** Nodular portal infiltrate with interface activity typical of chronic hepatitis C,
native liver (H&E ×100). **B,** Interface activity with disruption of the limiting plate, allograft liver (H&E ×400).
C, Lymphocytic infiltration of the bile duct, native liver (H&E ×400). **D,** Perivenular activity in hepatitis C,
native liver (H&E ×200).

results in a similar finding (confluent necrosis). Again, identification of convincing endothelial injury along with subendothelial lymphocytes is very helpful in establishing a diagnosis of AR (see Fig. 70–3D).

Arterial Endotheliitis. Subendothelial lymphocytic inflammation in the arterioles of small and medium-sized portal areas is rarely seen in AR. In our experience, it occurs only in the setting of severe AR with extensive and obvious venous endotheliitis.

Interface and Lobular Activity. As described earlier, interface and lobular activity is generally interpreted as histological evidence of recurrent hepatitis C. However, interface and lobular activity may be seen in cases of

severe AR. They are in fact criteria that are used to distinguish moderate from severe AR.[31]

In many cases the distinction between hepatitis C and AR is straightforward, particularly in the first few months after transplantation, when the histological findings of hepatitis C are predominantly lobular with less portal infiltrates. However, as the portal infiltrates of hepatitis C become more prominent, the distinction can become more difficult. Often, interpretation becomes an exercise in weighing the various findings. If there is clear-cut hepatocellular apoptosis and interface activity but only a few eosinophils, mild bile duct infiltration, and questionable endotheliitis, a diagnosis of AR is not warranted. However, if there is an extensive eosinophilic infiltrate,

Table 70–1. HISTOLOGICAL CHARACTERISTICS OF ACUTE REJECTION VERSUS THOSE OF RECURRENT DISEASE

	Acute Rejection	Hepatitis C	Primary Biliary Cirrhosis	Primary Sclerosing Cholangitis
Portal infiltrate	Mixed, with lymphocytes, neutrophils, and eosinophils. Diffuse, not nodular	Predominantly lymphocytic, often nodular	Lymphoplasmacytic, dense, may be nodular, may be centered on bile duct. Edema and neutrophils in some cases	Predominantly lymphocytic or lymphoplasmacytic. Edema and neutrophils in some cases
Bile ducts	Variable infiltration by lymphocytes from mild to marked, with epithelial injury from mild to severe	Mild infiltration by lymphocytes with mild epithelial injury	Variable infiltration and injury from mild to florid duct lesion	Variable from normal to lymphocytic infiltrate to periductal edema and fibrosis
Portal veins	Swollen or pyknotic endothelium, detached from basement membrane by subendothelial inflammatory cells	Lymphocytes may encroach endothelium from the stroma or adhere to the luminal aspect of the cell	Lymphocytes may encroach endothelium from the stroma or adhere to the luminal aspect of the cell	Lymphocytes may encroach endothelium from the stroma or adhere to the luminal aspect of the cell
Interface	Only in severe acute rejection	Minimal in early recurrence, variable from mild to marked with chronicity	Ductal metaplasia and or interface activity is often present	Ductal metaplasia and or interface activity is often present
Lobules	Inflammation and cellular injury only in severe acute rejection	Predominant in early recurrence, variable later	± Activity, variable	± Activity, variable
Central vein	Endothelitis as above ± perivenular inflammation and necrosis	± Small perivenular aggregates of lymphocytes and plasma cells ± hepatocellular necrosis. Rarely extensive	Generally uninvolved; however, perivenular activity is seen in cases with a prominent component of hepatitis (autoimmune hepatitis)	Generally uninvolved; however, perivenular activity is seen in cases with a prominent component of hepatitis (autoimmune hepatitis)

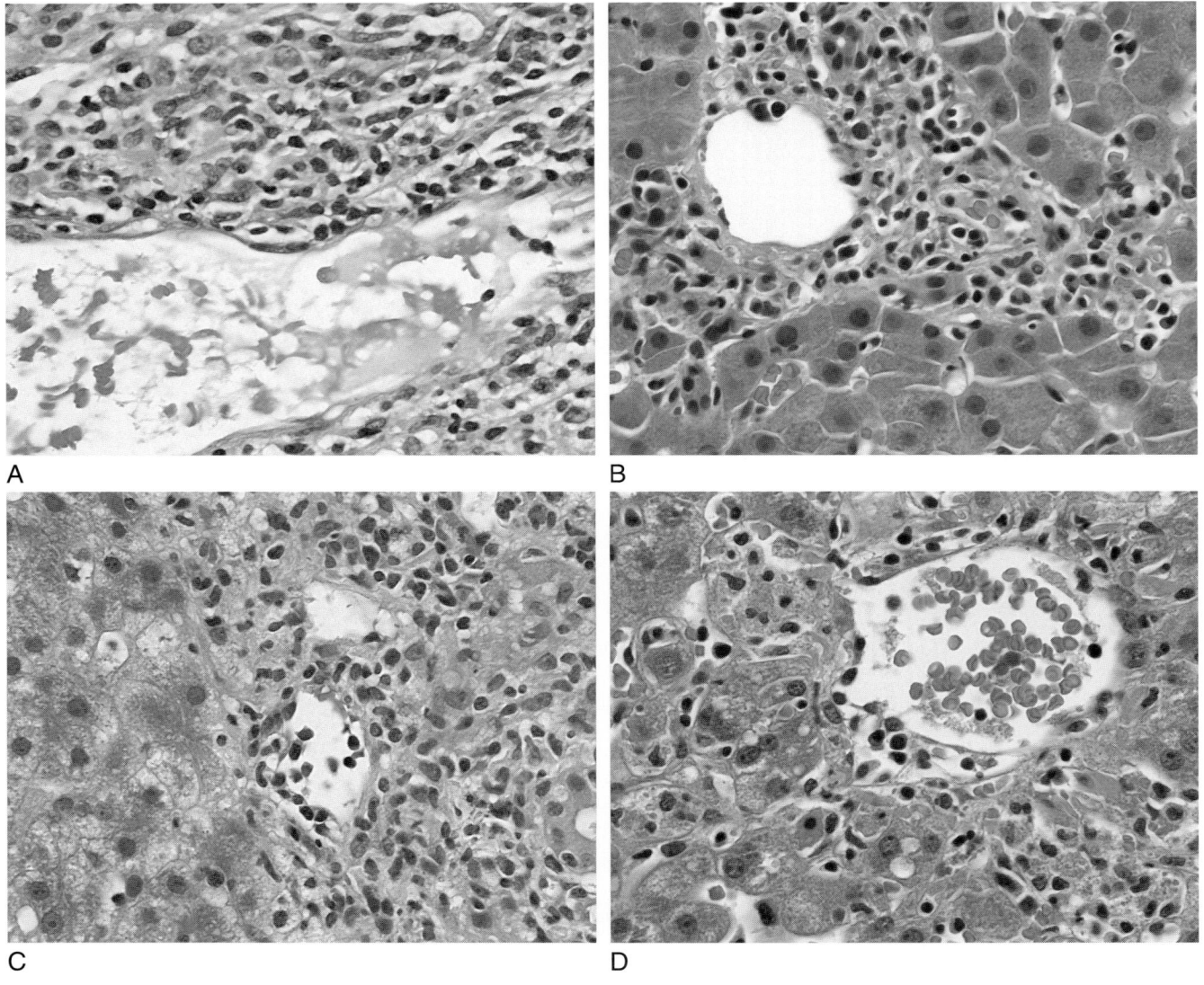

A

B

C

D

FIGURE 70–3

Endotheliitis. **A,** Subendothelial lymphocytic inflammation in hepatitis C in native liver (H&E ×400).
B, Minimal portal vein endotheliitis with a single lymphocyte beneath the endothelium (H&E ×400).
C, More obvious portal vein endotheliitis (H&E ×400). **D,** Central vein endotheliitis (H&E ×400).

bile duct infiltrates, or convincing endotheliitis (or any combination of these findings), a diagnosis of AR should be considered even if rounded lymphoid aggregates and extensive interface activity are present.

Because increased immunosuppression is detrimental to transplant patients with hepatitis C,[18] it is our practice to "raise the bar" for a diagnosis of AR when features of hepatitis C are present. We are willing to err on the side of undercalling AR rather than overdiagnosing AR in these patients.

It is our practice to report the findings as follows:

AR, no support for recurrent hepatitis C—the typical features of AR are present, without interface or lobular activity.

Recurrent hepatitis consistent with hepatitis C with activity, no AR—typical features of hepatitis C are present with or without mild bile duct infiltration by lymphocytes, no or few eosinophils, and no convincing portal or central endotheliitis.

Recurrent hepatitis consistent with hepatitis C with activity, cannot rule out mild AR (indeterminate for AR)—typical features of hepatitis C are present along with more marked lymphocytic infiltration of bile ducts or moderate eosinophilic infiltrates (or both), perivenular lymphocytes, but no convincing portal or central endotheliitis.

Recurrent hepatitis C and AR—lymphoid nodules or interface and lobular activity (or both) are present,

bile ducts are not apparent on routine histochemical stains, immunohistochemistry with pankeratin or cytokeratin 7 is often helpful in evaluating for bile duct atrophy or loss.

When advanced fibrosis from hepatitis C has occurred, the scarring process may obliterate the portal areas and result in loss of the interlobular bile ducts. Neovascularization is often present, as well as extensive ductular reaction in many cases. Biopsy material may simply be inadequate to evaluate for duct atrophy or loss. In these cases it is our practice to include a diagnostic line stating that CR cannot be excluded.

Fibrosing Cholestatic Hepatitis

FCH is a rare, aggressive form of recurrent hepatitis B and hepatitis C characterized by cholestasis and rapid graft loss.[8,46] Despite reports of successful treatment,[47-52] such graft loss is a serious concern. FCH is thought to be an unusual complication of immunosuppression[51,53-55]; it was first described in kidney,[56-58] heart, and bone marrow transplant patients and subsequently reported in the liver transplant setting. It is thought to result from unchecked viral replication with extensive hepatocellular injury. Indeed, unlike the usual viral hepatitis, in which the cytopathic injury is mediated by an immune response, FCH may result from direct cytolysis of hepatocytes by virus. Clinically, it resembles rapidly progressive BDO. Serological studies for hepatitis B virus (HBV) antigens or HCV RNA may be helpful in distinguishing FCH from BDO.

Biopsy specimens in patients with FCH demonstrate extensive hepatocellular injury in the form of ballooning change and apoptosis. There is extensive cholestasis with bile present in hepatocytes, Kupffer cell aggregates, and canaliculi (Fig. 70-4). In patients with hepatitis B, immunohistochemical studies for hepatitis B surface antigen (HBsAg) demonstrate cytoplasmic staining of nearly all hepatocytes. Although extensive Kupffer cell hypertrophy is prominent, there is generally mild lymphocytic infiltration of the lobules. Portal tracts are expanded, extensive ductular reaction is present at the interface, and in many cases, there is surprisingly little lymphocytic infiltrate. Lymphoid nodules may be entirely absent. Portal-to-portal bridging fibrosis occurs rapidly, and because regeneration is minimal, the pattern resembles that of rapidly progressing BDO. The primary differential diagnosis is thus BDO, which is not usually accompanied by such extensive hepatocellular injury. Nonetheless, FCH is a diagnosis of exclusion, and, particularly in hepatitis C, in which reliable histological markers of viral proteins or RNA are not readily available, imaging studies to rule out BDO should be performed.

Epstein-Barr Virus Infection versus Recurrent Hepatitis C

Liver transplantation is rarely complicated by Epstein-Barr virus (EBV) infection and posttransplant lymphoproliferative disorder. Graft involvement by EBV may be manifested as a mass lesion, as atypical lymphocytic infiltrates in the portal tracts, or as extensive sinusoidal infiltration by lymphocytes, thereby simulating hepatitis C.[59,60] Marked cytological atypia, the presence of numerous plasma cells, and clinical features such as fever, lymphadenopathy, and diarrhea should raise the possibility of EBV infection. Immunohistochemistry can be used to confirm the diagnosis (see Chapters 69 and 71).

Hepatitis C–Positive Donors

Organs from HCV-positive donors have been used in HCV-positive recipients.[22,61-64] A number of studies have now demonstrated that there is no effect on long-term outcome when compared with HCV-negative recipients.[22,65-67] Knowledge of donor status is helpful when interpreting biopsy specimens taken soon after transplantation. Portal tracts may contain dense lymphoid clusters characteristic of chronic hepatitis C. These clusters should not be taken as evidence of recurrent disease because they represent a histological abnormality of donor origin.

Hepatitis C in Living Donor Transplantation

Adult-to-adult living donor liver transplantation has gained popularity because of the shortage of deceased donor organs. There was initial concern that recurrent hepatitis C would be more aggressive in living donor liver transplantation and result in the rapid development of cirrhosis.[68] Recent studies, with up to 1-year follow-up, have not demonstrated any difference in outcome, histological activity, or stage of fibrosis.[69,70] Long-term studies are under way.

Treatment of Hepatitis C in the Transplant Liver

More and more data are demonstrating that as in native livers infected with HCV, antiviral treatment in the transplant setting is effective in treating hepatitis C. Not only have sustained viral responses[71] been achieved in many patients, there has also been improvement in histological grade[20,27,72] and stage (regression of fibrosis). It should be noted, however, that even in patients

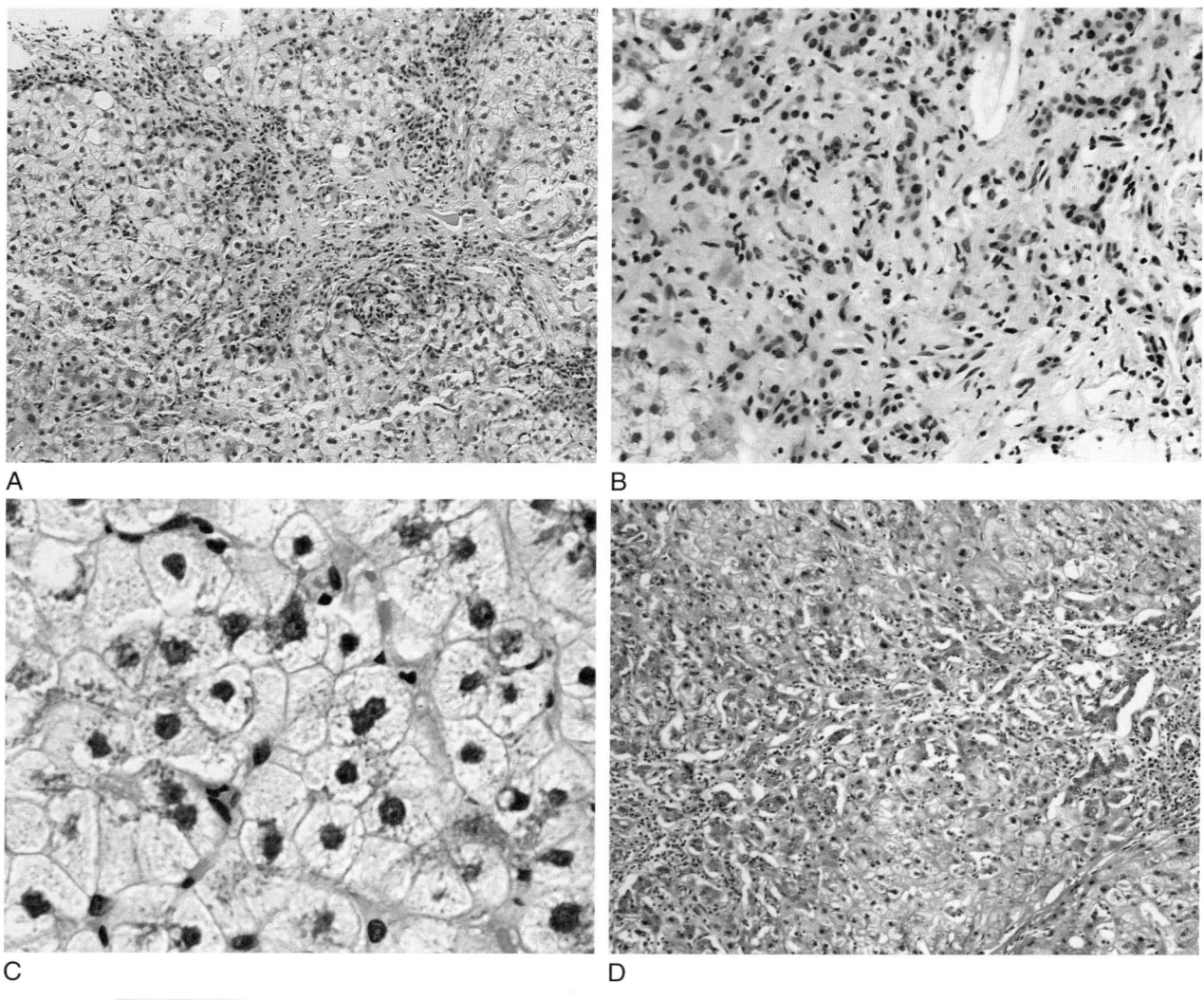

FIGURE 70–4

Fibrosing cholestatic hepatitis (FCH). **A,** Irregular portal expansion and diffuse parenchymal ballooning change in a biopsy specimen from a cardiac transplant patient with hepatitis C (H&E ×100). **B,** Portal area in the same biopsy specimen; note the cholangioles and relative paucity of inflammatory cells (H&E ×200). **C,** Diffuse hepatocellular ballooning change in the same specimen (H&E ×400). **D,** Failed liver transplant in a patient with FCH and hepatitis C. Bridging fibrosis is accompanied by an extensive ductular reaction reminiscent of biliary obstruction (H&E ×100).

with a sustained viral response, portal inflammation, interface activity, and lobular activity can persist even when viral RNA levels in serum by PCR are negative.

There are reports of severe rejection occurring in patients during treatment with interferon,[73-76] but rigorous studies to determine the frequency of this event have not yet been published.

Recurrent Hepatitis B

With the combined use of nucleoside analogues and hepatitis B immune globulin, the recurrence rate of hepatitis B in allografts is presently less than 10%.[77-80]

Recurrence is now seen primarily in the setting of noncompliance or with "breakthrough" strains of virus.[81-84] Viral recurrence can be diagnosed by serological studies for HBsAg or by quantitative PCR for viral DNA. When biopsies are performed, they demonstrate varying degrees of interface and lobular hepatitis from mild to severe to FCH (see earlier). Immunohistochemical studies can be used to confirm recurrent hepatitis B but are not generally necessary because the diagnosis has been established by serological studies. Rare cases of recurrent hepatitis B that are serologically negative but positive for surface or core antigen (or both) by immunohistochemistry have been seen (personal communication, S. Geller). Furthermore, immunohistochemistry is very helpful in cases in which serological studies are incomplete or unavailable to the pathologist at the time of biopsy. Immunohisto-chemistry is therefore warranted in any patient with unexplained hepatitis in an allograft, particularly in a patient transplanted for hepatitis B. The histological findings are similar to those of hepatitis C, and the differential diagnosis is similar. The presence of characteristic "ground-glass" hepatocytes is helpful in distinguishing hepatitis B from other forms of dysfunction; however, immunohistochemistry is more sensitive and specific.

Recurrent Autoimmune Hepatitis

Autoimmune hepatitis (AIH) recurs in up to 50% of patients.[85-91] Patients who undergo liver transplantation for AIH are at greater risk for AR and CR, thus necessitating higher levels of immunosuppression. Nonetheless, the long-term prognosis is comparable to that of transplantation for other causes.[92,93] AIH can recur at any time after transplantation, and the severity of such recurrent disease is variable.

The diagnosis of recurrent AIH is based on serological, biochemical, and histological studies, although recurrent AIH has been demonstrated in protocol biopsy material from patients with normal biochemical studies.[89,94] The differential diagnosis of recurrent AIH is similar to that for viral hepatitis, but it is not fraught with the same anxiety of misdiagnosis because treatment of AR in patients with AIH has not been demonstrated to have the same negative impact on graft survival as does treatment in patients with viral hepatitis. Nonetheless, because treatment of recurrent AIH is not identical to treatment of AR, caution must still be exercised.

The histology of recurrent AIH (Fig. 70–5) is similar to that of AIH in the native liver; however, serological and biochemical studies remain very helpful.[90,95,96] Early recurrence may be manifested as lobular hepatitis with scattered apoptosis, clusters of lymphocytes and Kupffer cells, and sinusoidal lymphocytes.[97] Most biopsy specimens demonstrate portal lymphocytic infiltrates, some with an extensive plasma cell component, and interface activity (see Fig. 70–5). The presence of plasma cell clusters at the interface with surrounding parenchyma is a helpful finding but is not always seen.[85,91,94,98] Infiltration of bile ducts may be prominent in recurrent AIH and is therefore of limited use in differentiating AIH from AR. The presence of eosinophils and portal vein endotheliitis strongly favors AR. Perivenular necroinflammatory activity accompanied by hemorrhage is more common in AIH than in other forms of chronic hepatitis.[99,100] This lesion may be difficult to distinguish from central vein endotheliitis. If convincing endotheliitis—as characterized by the separation of swollen endothelial cells from the underlying stroma with subendothelial lymphocytes—is not identified, the cause of the perivenular injury can be difficult to determine. In these cases, examination of other structures may provide a clue to the nature of the process. Interface activity, plasma cells, and other forms of lobular activity all favor AIH, whereas significant eosinophilia and portal vein endotheliitis favor AR (see Table 70–1).

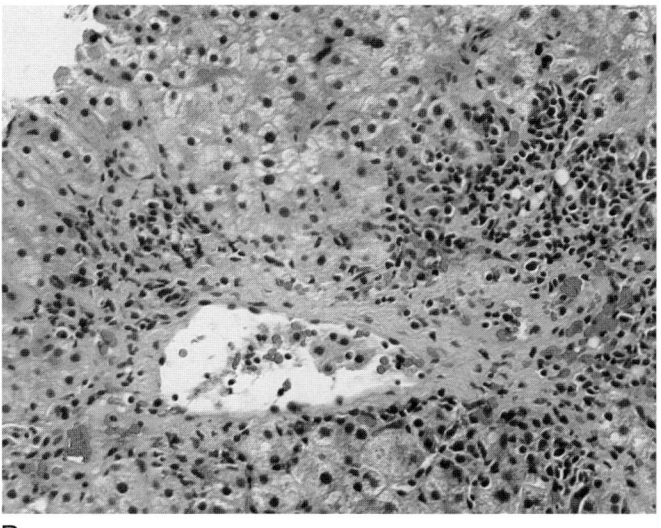

A   B

FIGURE 70–5

Recurrent autoimmune hepatitis. **A**, Extensive interface activity with a plasma cell component (H&E ×400). **B**, Extensive perivenular necroinflammatory activity, but not endotheliitis (H&E ×200).

Autoimmune Hepatitis versus Chronic Rejection

Distinction of AIH from CR is often straightforward (see Table 70–2). As described earlier for hepatitis C, CR is a paucicellular process characterized by atrophy and loss of interlobular bile ducts.[45] The presence of significant infiltrates, interface activity, and lobular activity favors AIH over CR. However, if the findings associated with AIH are accompanied by significant atrophy or loss of bile ducts, the diagnosis becomes more problematic. Is the bile duct loss in these cases secondary to a component of CR that accompanied the AIH, or is the bile duct loss secondary to a component of "autoimmune cholangitis"?

The pattern of fibrosis associated with recurrent AIH is similar to that in native livers, and any standard staging system can be used to report the degree of fibrosis.[32-35] Again, as in hepatitis C, portal-to-portal bridging is not generally seen in uncomplicated CR and favors chronic AIH; perivenular fibrosis favors CR.

Recurrent Primary Biliary Cirrhosis

Recurrence of PBC in liver allografts has been a controversial subject but is now well accepted.[101] Reports of recurrence with the typical histological features of PBC had appeared in the early literature,[102,103] but a large retrospective study failed to differentiate between recurrent PBC and CR in explanted livers.[104] More recent large studies have convincingly demonstrated recurrent disease.[105-109] The difficulty in establishing a diagnosis of recurrent disease arises in part from the extensive overlap between the features of PBC and those of AR and CR.[110] The recurrence rate (8% to 30%[105-109]) is difficult to determine without protocol biopsies because histological alterations may precede biochemical evidence of recurrence.[111] Furthermore, because the inflammatory lesions of PBC exist along a spectrum, the recurrence rate is influenced by the histological criteria used for diagnosis.[101]

Recurrent PBC (Fig. 70–6) can be reliably diagnosed in the presence of florid duct lesions and granulomas.

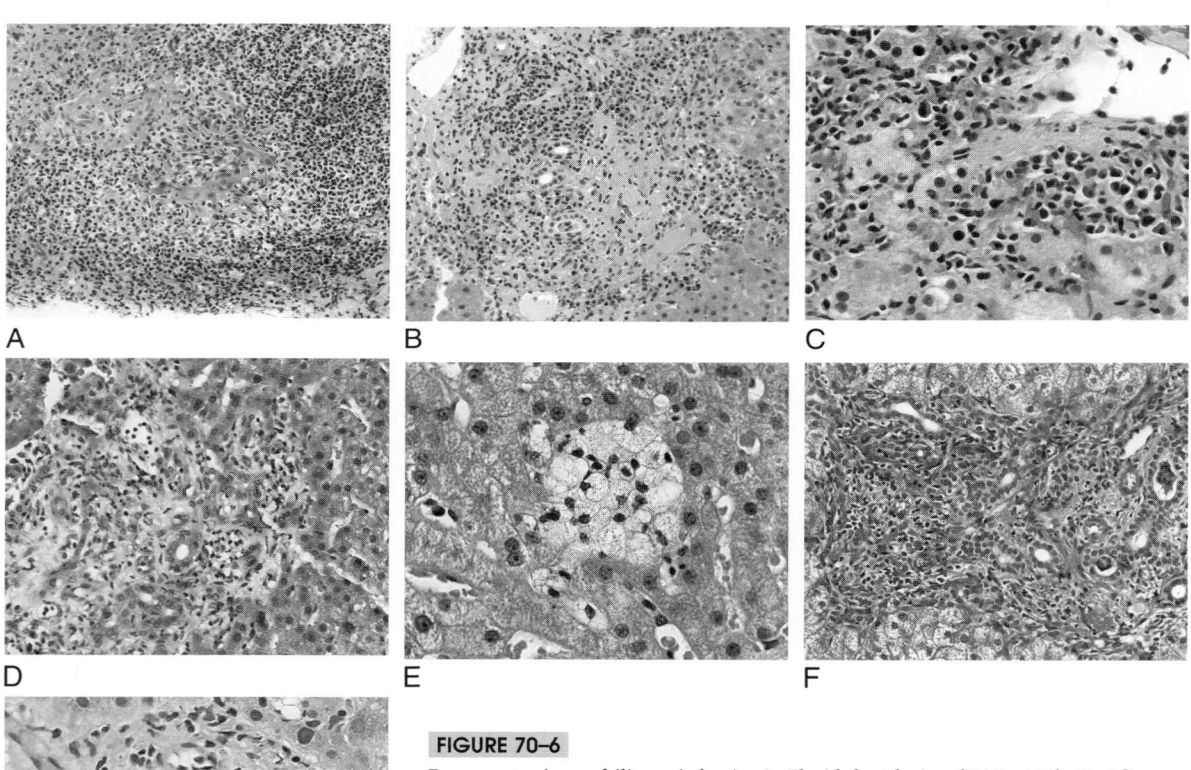

FIGURE 70–6

Recurrent primary biliary cirrhosis. **A,** Florid duct lesion (H&E ×200). **B,** Adjacent portal area in the same biopsy specimen. Note the relatively mild lymphocytic infiltration of bile ducts and the predominance of interface activity with plasma cells as in autoimmune hepatitis (H&E ×200). **C,** Same biopsy specimen with acinar zone III activity and a plasma cell component, as in autoimmune hepatitis (H&E ×400). **D,** Irregular edematous expansion of the portal tract (H&E ×200). **E,** Cluster of foamy macrophages (H&E ×400). **F,** Irregular portal fibrosis with ductular reaction (Masson trichrome ×200). **G,** Bile duct atrophy with minimal inflammation in a patient with primary biliary cirrhosis. This portal area resembles chronic rejection (H&E ×400).

Florid duct lesions are characterized by dense lymphoid infiltrates centered on the bile ducts with marked infiltration by lymphocytes and epithelial cell injury in the form of vacuolization or necrosis. Granulomas (which are seen in some cases) may be portal or lobular; when portal, they may be a component of the destructive lesion. Less specific, but common, features of PBC include portal lymphoplasmacytic infiltrates with mild biliary injury, interface activity, and occasionally lobular activity. The presence of significant numbers of plasma cells in portal infiltrates may be indicative of recurrent PBC.[112] Ductular reaction is often present and may raise the possibility of BDO. Mild infiltrates and bile duct injury may be difficult to distinguish from AR. Eosinophils and endotheliitis favor AR, whereas granulomas, interface and lobular activity, and plasma cell infiltrates favor PBC (see Table 70–1).

The inflammatory duct lesions of PBC are quite variable, not only between patients but also between individual portal areas in a single biopsy specimen. A specimen may contain normal portal areas; portal areas with mild mononuclear infiltrates, with or without bile duct infiltration and injury; portal areas with or without interface activity; portal areas with edema, ductular reaction, and neutrophils; and portal areas with florid duct lesions and granulomas. Adequate sampling is therefore imperative.

Finally, because PBC may recur months to years after transplantation and AR is relatively uncommon after 1 year, significant infiltrates in the portal areas more than 1 year after transplantation are more likely to represent recurrent PBC than AR unless the patient has a history of noncompliance.

Primary Biliary Cirrhosis versus Chronic Rejection

Because both CR and PBC result in atrophy and loss of interlobular ducts (see Fig. 70–6), distinction on needle core biopsy specimens can be extremely challenging (see Table 70–2).[104,113] PBC cannot be ruled out if one sees the typical features of CR, namely, ductopenia, minimal infiltrates, perivenular fibrosis, and lobular aggregates of foamy or bile-laden Kupffer cells. However, most cases of advanced PBC are not so diffusely uniform in appearance, and portal areas often demonstrate various stages of disease, some with ductopenia, others with significant infiltrates, and yet others with florid duct lesions or ductular reaction. This heterogeneity of inflammatory lesions favors PBC over CR. As described for other recurrent diseases, the presence of portal-to-portal bridging fibrosis favors recurrent disease over uncomplicated CR. Finally, in explant or autopsy specimens, the presence of foam cell arteritis indicates that there is at least a component of CR.

Recurrent Primary Sclerosing Cholangitis

Recurrence of PSC has been particularly difficult to establish and somewhat controversial given the fact that the transplant liver is not infrequently complicated by BDO. Complications that result in BDO include both strictures at the anastomotic site and intrahepatic strictures secondary to hepatic artery thrombosis or stenosis. Nonanastomotic biliary strictures developing in patients with normal hepatic artery studies might be assumed to be secondary to recurrent PSC.[114] More convincingly, it has been documented that biliary strictures identified by cholangiography occur at a greater frequency in patients transplanted for PSC than for other causes.[115,116] The recurrence rate of PSC is estimated at 9% to 30%.[117-120] Overall survival in patients transplanted for PSC, excluding those with cholangiocarcinoma at the time of transplantation, is comparable to that in patients transplanted for non-PSC causes.[121]

The histology of recurrent PSC in the transplant liver is similar to that in the native liver.[118,122,123] Findings of BDO are most helpful; however, occasional biopsy samples will instead demonstrate features suggestive of chronic hepatitis. Further complicating biopsy evaluation, the histological findings are not uniformly distributed such that adjacent portal areas can have quite different appearances. It is important to remember that PSC is primarily a disease of larger bile ducts and that the findings in the small portal tracts sampled in biopsy material are secondary to (usually) unsampled large-duct disease. Edematous expansion of portal areas, in particular, concentric, periductal edema, is one of the earliest and more specific manifestations of BDO (Fig. 70–7). The inflammatory infiltrate is variable and in the early stages may be predominantly neutrophils. Neutrophils within duct lumens or surrounding bile ducts are characteristic of BDO and are a very helpful finding. Portal areas may contain elongated, serpentine ductules, or there may be a ductular reaction at the interface.

With progression of PSC, portal areas demonstrate fibrous expansion and ductular reaction at the interface with the surrounding parenchyma. Interlobular and septal bile ducts are variable in appearance. They may be normal, may be infiltrated by lymphocytes, may be atrophic, may demonstrate a thickened basement membrane, and occasionally may be associated with concentric "onion skin" fibrosis characteristic of PSC. With progression, the interlobular and septal ducts may disappear and be replaced by a dense collagenous scar. The development of bridging fibrosis and cirrhosis may make diagnosis more difficult as portal structures become more difficult to identify. Cholestasis is generally a late finding in PSC, so the absence of identifiable bile does not preclude a diagnosis of PSC.

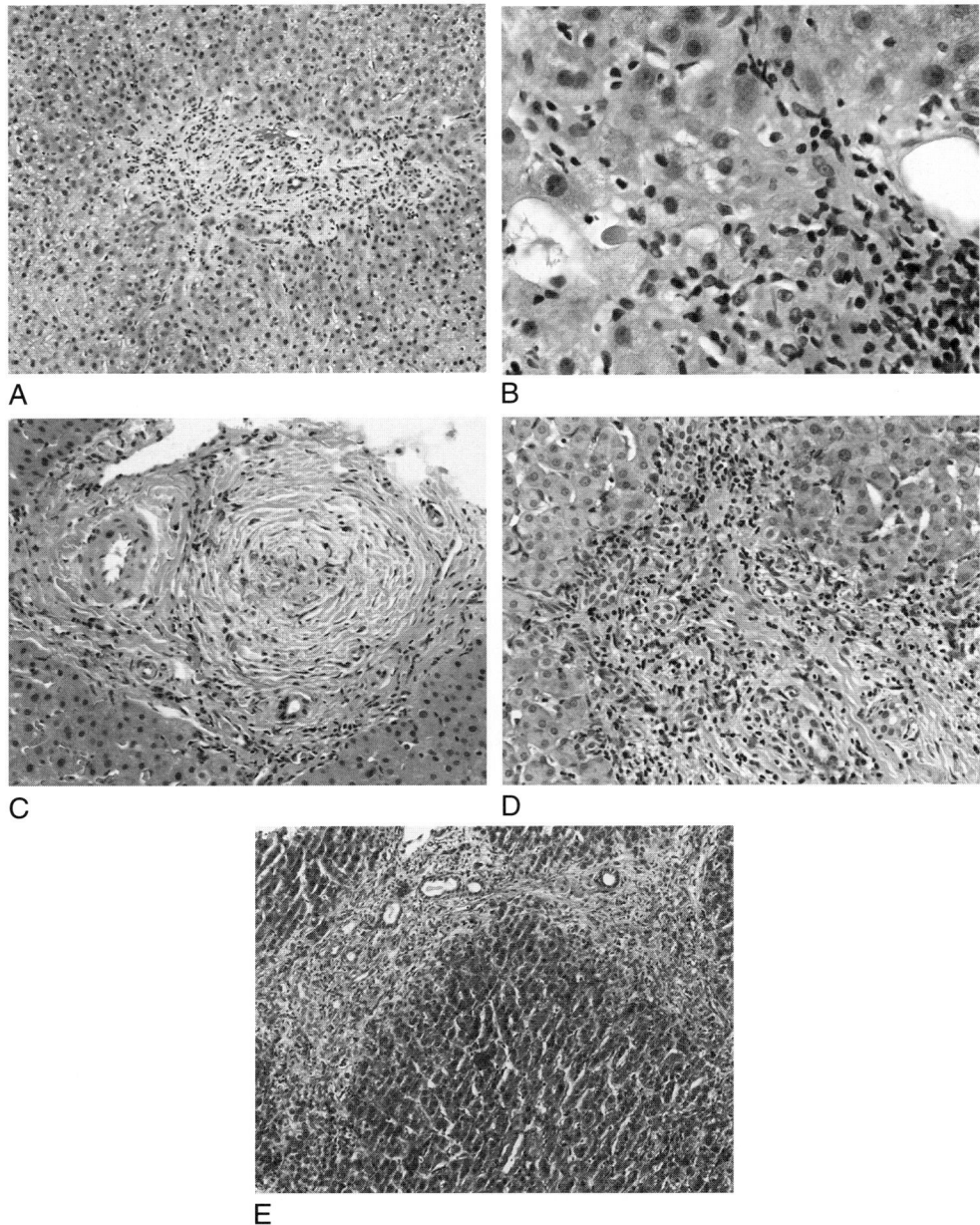

FIGURE 70-7

Recurrent primary sclerosing cholangitis (PSC). **A,** Edematous expansion of a portal area in PSC (H&E ×100). **B,** Interface activity resembling chronic hepatitis in recurrent PSC (H&E ×400). **C,** Concentric edema/fibrosis with bile duct loss/scarring (H&E ×200). **D,** Irregular portal fibrosis with ductular reaction typical of bile duct obstruction (H&E ×200). **E,** Bridging biliary fibrosis in PSC (Masson trichrome ×100).

As mentioned previously, some portal areas in PSC may demonstrate features suggestive of chronic hepatitis with predominantly lymphocytic or lymphoplasmacytic infiltrates, interface activity, and normal-appearing bile ducts. These findings should prompt an effort to rule out viral and medication/herbal-related hepatitis and, most importantly, AIH. AIH/PSC overlap syndrome has been well described in native livers[124]

and more recently in transplant livers.[123] A histological picture suggestive of chronic hepatitis in a PSC patient should trigger a serological workup for AIH and, of course, de novo viral hepatitis.

It is important to remember that recurrent PSC is a diagnosis of exclusion; other causes of BDO must be ruled out. Because bile duct strictures may be secondary to hepatic artery compromise, a diagnosis of recurrent

PSC should be considered very carefully in the setting of hepatic artery thrombosis or in those with radiographic evidence of hepatic artery compromise.

Recurrent Primary Sclerosing Cholangitis versus Acute Rejection

Distinction of recurrent PSC from AR is generally straightforward. Whereas PSC can recur at any point after transplantation, AR is unusual after 1 year. A mixed portal infiltrate with eosinophils favors AR, as does endotheliitis. However, infiltration of bile ducts by lymphocytes is common to both processes and is thus not helpful in making the distinction between AR and recurrent PSC. As described earlier, features of BDO or chronic hepatitis favor recurrent PSC (see Table 70–1).

Recurrent Primary Sclerosing Cholangitis versus Chronic Rejection

Distinction of recurrent PSC from CR is also generally uncomplicated (see Table 70–2). As described earlier, CR is a paucicellular process that results in atrophy and loss of interlobular bile ducts with minimal portal fibrosis. PSC may also result in atrophy and loss of interlobular bile ducts.[125] When this is the case, however, other features of PSC that are not present in CR should be apparent. Such features include portal inflammation, ductular reaction, portal fibrosis (ranging from mild to cirrhosis), periductal fibrosis, and collagenous scars in place of the bile duct.

Recurrent Alcoholic Liver Disease and Nonalcoholic Steatohepatitis

Recurrence of alcoholic steatohepatitis and nonalcoholic[126-132] steatohepatitis (NASH) is well documented. The histological differential diagnosis is relatively straightforward because there is little overlap between the features of AR and CR with steatohepatitis. Difficulty may, however, arise after a histological diagnosis of steatohepatitis is made because of the inability to accurately distinguish between alcoholic and nonalcoholic hepatitis in most cases.[133] Our practice is to report the diagnosis of steatohepatitis and allow the clinician to determine which of the numerous clinical associations are relevant for this form of liver dysfunction.

The clinicopathological diagnosis of recurrent NASH in the transplant liver is further complicated by the fact that many patients who received transplants for presumed cryptogenic cirrhosis may have had NASH,[134,135] the histological features of which were not present in the explanted organ (so-called burned-out NASH). It is therefore difficult to determine with certainty whether a diagnosis of steatohepatitis in a patient transplanted for cryptogenic cirrhosis represents recurrent NASH, de novo NASH, de novo alcoholic liver disease, or even recurrent alcoholic liver disease.

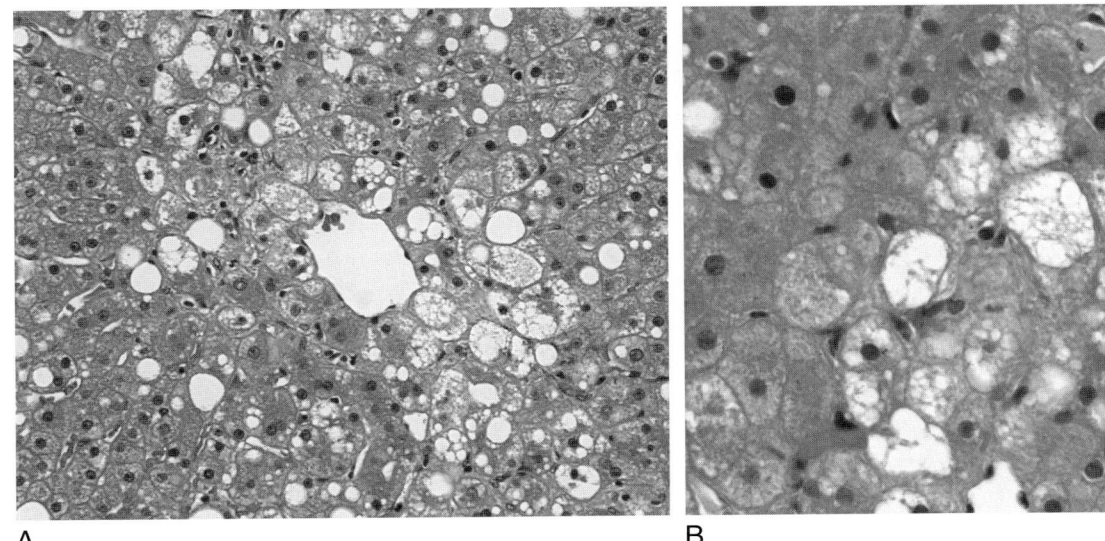

A   B

FIGURE 70–8

Recurrent alcoholic steatohepatitis. **A**, Steatosis and ballooning change in a patient transplanted for ethanol-related liver disease who admits to drinking (H&E ×200). **B**, Ballooning change in the same patient (H&E ×400).

Continued

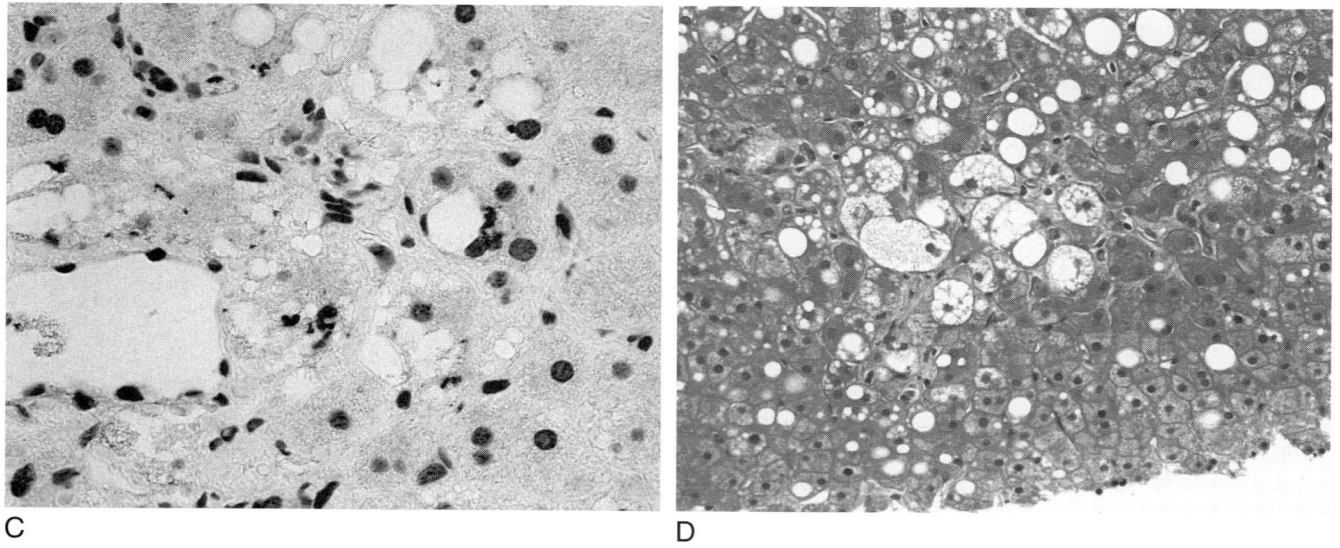

C

D

FIGURE 70–8, cont'd

Recurrent alcoholic steatohepatitis. **C,** Ubiquitin stain highlighting Mallory bodies, which were not appreciated on routine histochemical stains (immunoperoxidase for ubiquitin ×400). **D,** Early lobular, pericellular fibrosis characteristic of steatohepatitis (Masson trichrome ×200).

Steatohepatitis is characterized by varying degrees of steatosis, ballooning change, lobular inflammation, Mallory bodies, and a characteristic pattern of sinusoidal fibrosis that begins in acinar zone III.[133,136,137] Steatosis is primarily macrovesicular with varying degrees of microvesicular steatosis. Mallory bodies are "ropey," eosinophilic cytoplasmic inclusions that are generally present in cells with ballooning change. They can be prominent and easily identified or wispy and difficult to identify with routine histochemistry. Immunohistochemistry for ubiquitin can be used to highlight Mallory bodies in questionable cases (Figs. 70–8 and 70–9).[138] Mallory bodies tend to be more prominent in alcoholic liver disease than in NASH; however, the distinction is

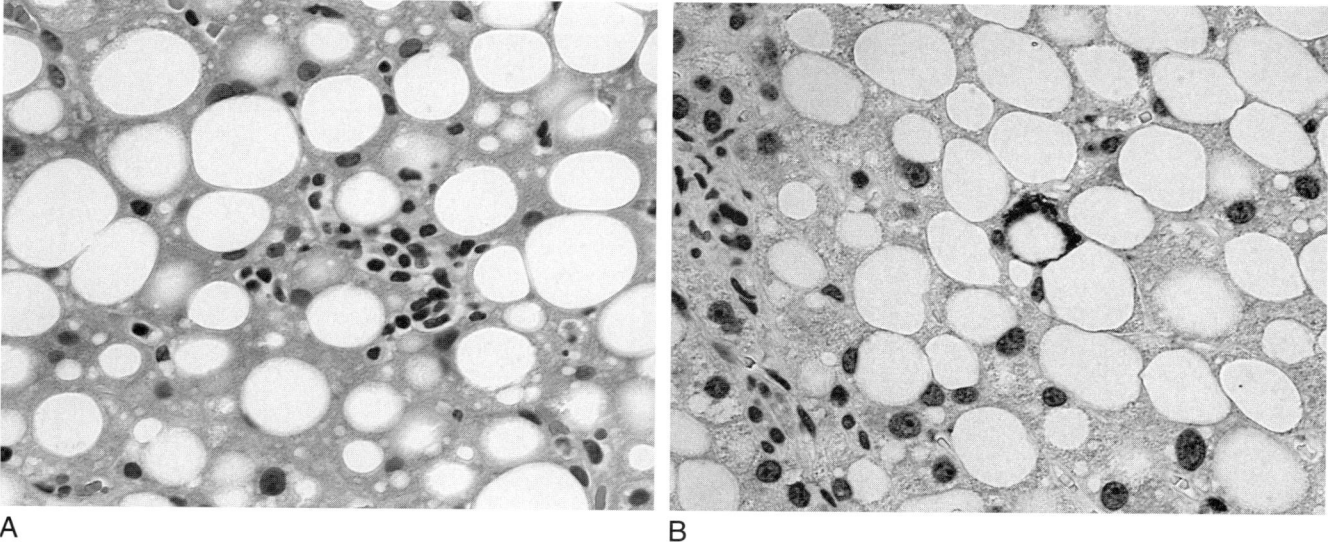

A

B

FIGURE 70–9

Recurrent nonalcoholic steatohepatitis in a diabetic patient transplanted for presumed α_1-antitrypsin disease. The native liver had extensive steatosis in addition to features of α_1-antitrypsin disease. **A,** Extensive steatosis and rare lobular clusters of mononuclear cells in a biopsy performed for elevated aspartate and alanine transaminase 1 year after transplantation (H&E ×400). **B,** Ubiquitin stain highlighting Mallory bodies, which were not appreciated on routine histochemical stains (immunoperoxidase for ubiquitin ×400).

not always reliable. Inflammation in steatohepatitis is primarily lobular and mononuclear, and neutrophils may be present, particularly surrounding cells with Mallory bodies. Neutrophils tend be more prominent in alcoholic liver disease than in NASH. The fibrosis of steatohepatitis begins in the lobule, usually in acinar zone III. It is irregular in distribution, sinusoidal, and pericellular. When well developed, it is often referred to as "spidery fibrosis."

The exact diagnostic criteria for steatohepatitis have not been widely agreed on; however, the presence of steatosis and some indicator of progressive disease is usually required.[139] The diagnosis is most easily established when there is steatosis and Mallory bodies or when there is steatosis and sinusoidal fibrosis in zone III. If a biopsy specimen demonstrates steatosis and mild patchy lobular mononuclear inflammation without ballooning change, Mallory bodies, or perivenular fibrosis, a diagnosis of steatohepatitis may not be warranted, especially in transplant patients. Follow-up biopsies may be necessary to establish a diagnosis of steatohepatitis, particularly in patients with hepatitis C, who often have steatosis in liver biopsy samples. A diagnosis of steatohepatitis should be made in a patient with hepatitis C only if there is a predominance of lobular activity and either convincing evidence of Mallory bodies or fibrosis of the pattern characteristic of steatohepatitis. Even then, it is difficult to be certain how much injury is secondary to hepatitis C as opposed to the fatty process.

Grading and Staging of Steatohepatitis

The inflammatory activity and hepatocellular injury in steatohepatitis can be graded and the degree of fibrosis quantified (staged) according to the system of Brunt and coworkers devised for native liver biopsy specimens.[140]

Pearls and Pitfalls

- Because the recurrence rate of HCV is nearly 100%, the differential diagnosis on biopsy once HCV has recurred is not recurrent HCV versus rejection. It is recurrent HCV versus recurrent HCV *and* rejection
- The grading of acute rejection is based on the amount of inflammation and the degree of hepatocellular injury in non–HCV-infected grafts. The presence of hepatitis is not accounted for in the grading scheme for rejection. Therefore, when there are infiltrates and injury due to HCV, the grading of rejection is difficult if not impossible.

Pearls and Pitfalls—cont'd

- The histological feature most useful in determining whether acute rejection is present in the setting of recurrent HCV is endotheliitis.
- PCR of peripheral blood for HCV does not correlate well with histologic activity.
- Fibrosing cholestatic hepatitis is a diagnosis of exclusion and requires negative cholangiographic studies.
- A diagnosis of recurrent AIH is made based on interface and lobular activity. A diagnosis of rejection is based primarily on endotheliitis. Both recurrent AIH and rejection are often accompanied by extensive bile duct infiltration by lymphocytes.
- Ductopenia without significant inflammation is compatible with both recurrent PBC and chronic rejection.
- Ductopenia with significant portal inflammation favors recurrent PBC over chronic rejection.
- Recurrent PSC cannot be reliably distinguished form other forms of biliary obstruction on needle biopsy specimens.

References

1. Knoop M, Lusebrink R, Langrehr JM, et al: Incidence and clinical relevance of recurrent hepatitis C infection after orthotopic liver transplantation. Transpl Int 7(Suppl 1):S221-S223, 1994.
2. Martin P, Munoz SJ, Di Biscegli AM, et al: Recurrence of hepatitis C virus infection after orthotopic liver transplantation. Hepatology 13:719-721, 1991.
3. Feray C, Samuel D, Thiers V, et al: Reinfection of liver graft by hepatitis C virus after liver transplantation. J Clin Invest 89:1361-1365, 1992.
4. Wright TL, Donegan E, Hsu HH, et al: Recurrent and acquired hepatitis C viral infection in liver transplant recipients. Gastroenterology 103:317-322, 1992.
5. Ascher NL, Lake JR, Emond J, Roberts J: Liver transplantation for hepatitis C virus–related cirrhosis. Hepatology 20(1 Pt 2):24S-27S, 1994.
6. Sallie R, Cohen AT, Tibbs CJ, et al: Recurrence of hepatitis C following orthotopic liver transplantation: A polymerase chain reaction and histological study. J Hepatol 21:536-542, 1994.
7. Konig V, Bauditz J, Lobeck H, et al: Hepatitis C virus reinfection in allografts after orthotopic liver transplantation. Hepatology 16:1137-1143, 1992.
8. Ferrell LD, Wright TL, Roberts J, et al: Hepatitis C viral infection in liver transplant recipients. Hepatology 16:865-876, 1992.
9. Boker KH, Dalley G, Bahr MJ, et al: Long-term outcome of hepatitis C virus infection after liver transplantation. Hepatology 25:203-210, 1997.
10. Shiffman ML, Contos MJ, Luketic VA, et al: Biochemical and histologic evaluation of recurrent hepatitis C following orthotopic liver transplantation. Transplantation 57:526-532, 1994.
11. Mateo R, Demetris A, Sico E, et al: Early detection of de novo hepatitis C infection in patients after liver transplantation by reverse transcriptase polymerase chain reaction. Surgery 114:442-448, 1993.

12. Gugenheim J, Baldini E, Mazza D, et al: Recurrence of hepatitis C virus after liver transplantation. Transpl Int 7(Suppl 1):S224-S226, 1994.

13. Lumbreras C, Delgado R, Fuertes A, et al: Clinical significance of hepatitis C virus (HCV) infection in liver transplant recipients. Role of serology and HCV RNA detection. Dig Dis Sci 39:965-969, 1994.

14. Vargas V, Comas P, Castells L, et al: Incidence and outcome of hepatitis C virus infection after liver transplantation. Transpl Int 7(Suppl 1):S216-S220, 1994.

15. Fukumoto T, Berg T, Ku Y, et al: Viral dynamics of hepatitis C early after orthotopic liver transplantation: Evidence for rapid turnover of serum virions. Hepatology 24:1351-1354, 1996.

16. Greenson JK, Svoboda-Newman SM, Merion RM, Frank TS: Histologic progression of recurrent hepatitis C in liver transplant allografts. Am J Surg Pathol 20:731-738, 1996.

17. Guido M, Fagiuoli S, Tessari G, et al: Histology predicts cirrhotic evolution of post transplant hepatitis C. Gut 50:697-700, 2002.

18. Sheiner PA, Schwartz ME, Mor E, et al: Severe or multiple rejection episodes are associated with early recurrence of hepatitis C after orthotopic liver transplantation. Hepatology 21:30-34, 1995.

19. Sugo H, Balderson GA, Crawford DH, et al: The influence of viral genotypes and rejection episodes on the recurrence of hepatitis C after liver transplantation. Surg Today 33:421-425, 2003.

20. Abdelmalek MF, Firpi RJ, Soldevila-Pico C, et al: Sustained viral response to interferon and ribavirin in liver transplant recipients with recurrent hepatitis C. Liver Transpl 10:199-207, 2004.

21. Ahmad J, Dodson SF, Demetris AJ, et al: Recurrent hepatitis C after liver transplantation: A nonrandomized trial of interferon alfa alone versus interferon alfa and ribavirin. Liver Transpl 7:863-869, 2001.

22. Ahmed A, Keeffe EB: Hepatitis C virus and liver transplantation. Clin Liver Dis 5:1073-1090, 2001.

23. Alberti AB, Belli LS, Airoldi A, et al: Combined therapy with interferon and low-dose ribavirin in posttransplantation recurrent hepatitis C: A pragmatic study. Liver Transpl 7:870-876, 2001.

24. Andreone P, Gramenzi A, Cursaro C, et al: Interferon-alpha plus ribavirin and amantadine in patients with post-transplant hepatitis C: Results of a pilot study. Dig Liver Dis 33:693-697, 2001.

25. Berenguer M, Wright TL: Treatment strategies for recurrent hepatitis C after liver transplantation. Clin Liver Dis 3:883-899, 1999.

26. Bizollon T, Ducerf C, Trepo C: New approaches to the treatment of hepatitis C virus infection after liver transplantation using ribavirin. J Hepatol 23(Suppl 2):22-25, 1995.

27. Bizollon T, Ahmed SN, Radenne S, et al: Long term histological improvement and clearance of intrahepatic hepatitis C virus RNA following sustained response to interferon-ribavirin combination therapy in liver transplanted patients with hepatitis C virus recurrence. Gut 52:283-287, 2003.

28. Dickson RC, Caldwell SH, Ishitani MB, et al: Clinical and histologic patterns of early graft failure due to recurrent hepatitis C in four patients after liver transplantation. Transplantation 61:701-705, 1996.

29. Baiocchi L, Tisone G, Palmieri G, et al: Hepatic steatosis: A specific sign of hepatitis C reinfection after liver transplantation. Liver Transpl Surg 4:441-447, 1998.

30. Feray C, Gigou M, Samuel D, et al: The course of hepatitis C virus infection after liver transplantation. Hepatology 20:1137-1143, 1994.

31. Banff schema for grading liver allograft rejection: An international consensus document. Hepatology 25:658-663, 1997.

32. Ishak K, Baptista A, Bianchi L, et al: Histological grading and staging of chronic hepatitis. J Hepatol 22:696-699, 1995.

33. Batts KP, Ludwig J: Chronic hepatitis. An update on terminology and reporting. Am J Surg Pathol 19:1409-1417, 1995.

34. Desmet VJ, Gerber M, Hoofnagel JH, et al: Classification of chronic hepatitis: Diagnosis, grading and staging. Hepatology 19:1513-1520, 1994.

35. Knodell RG, Ishak KG, Black WC, et al: Formulation and application of a numerical scoring system for assessing histological activity in asymptomatic chronic active hepatitis. Hepatology 1:431-435, 1981.

36. Tillery W, Demetris J, Watkins D, et al: Pathologic recognition of preservation injury in hepatic allografts with six months follow-up. Transplant Proc 21:1330-1331, 1989.

37. Aardema KL, Nakhleh RE, Terry LK, et al: Tissue quantification of hepatitis C virus RNA with morphologic correlation in the diagnosis of recurrent hepatitis C virus in human liver transplants. Mod Pathol 12:1043-1049, 1999.

38. Park YN, Boros P, Zhang DY, et al: Serum hepatitis C virus RNA levels and histologic findings in liver allografts with early recurrent hepatitis C. Arch Pathol Lab Med 124:1623-1627, 2000.

39. Sreekumar R, Gonzalez-Koch A, Maor-Kendler Y, et al: Early identification of recipients with progressive histologic recurrence of hepatitis C after liver transplantation. Hepatology 32:1125-1130, 2000.

40. Nuovo GJ, Holly A, Wakely P Jr, Frankel W: Correlation of histology, viral load, and in situ viral detection in hepatic biopsies from patients with liver transplants secondary to hepatitis C infection. Hum Pathol 33:277-284, 2002.

41. Demetris AJ, Eghtesad B, Marcos A, et al: Recurrent hepatitis C in liver allografts: Prospective assessment of diagnostic accuracy, identification of pitfalls, and observations about pathogenesis. Am J Surg Pathol 28:658-669, 2004.

42. Shuhart MC, Bronner MP, Gretch DR, et al: Histological and clinical outcome after liver transplantation for hepatitis C. Hepatology 26:1646-1652, 1997.

43. Chopra KB, Demetris AJ, Blakolmer K, et al: Progression of liver fibrosis in patients with chronic hepatitis C after orthotopic liver transplantation. Transplantation 76:1487-1491, 2003.

44. Testa G, Crippin JS, Netto GJ, et al: Liver transplantation for hepatitis C: Recurrence and disease progression in 300 patients. Liver Transpl 6:553-561, 2000.

45. Demetris A, Adams D, Bellamy C, et al: Update of the International Banff Schema for Liver Allograft Rejection: Working recommendations for the histopathologic staging and reporting of chronic rejection. An international panel. Hepatology 31:792-799, 2000.

46. Walker N, Apel R, Kerlin P, et al: Hepatitis B virus infection in liver allografts. Am J Surg Pathol 17:666-677, 1993.

47. Lo CM, Cheung ST, Ng IO, et al: Fibrosing cholestatic hepatitis secondary to precore/core promoter hepatitis B variant with lamivudine resistance: Successful retransplantation with combination adefovir dipivoxil and hepatitis B immunoglobulin. Liver Transpl 10:557-563, 2004.

48. Beckebaum S, Malago M, Dirsch O, et al: Efficacy of combined lamivudine and adefovir dipivoxil treatment for severe HBV graft reinfection after living donor liver transplantation. Clin Transplant 17:554-559, 2003.

49. Jung S, Lee HC, Han JM, et al: Four cases of hepatitis B virus–related fibrosing cholestatic hepatitis treated with lamivudine. J Gastroenterol Hepatol 17:345-350, 2002.

50. Walsh KM, Woodall T, Lamy P, et al: Successful treatment with adefovir dipivoxil in a patient with fibrosing cholestatic hepatitis and lamivudine resistant hepatitis B virus. Gut 49:436-440, 2001.

51. Munoz De Bustillo E, Ibarrola C, Colina F, et al: Fibrosing cholestatic hepatitis in hepatitis C virus–infected renal transplant recipients. J Am Soc Nephrol 9:1109-1113, 1998.

52. Toth CM, Pascual M, Chung RT, et al: Hepatitis C virus–associated fibrosing cholestatic hepatitis after renal transplantation: Response to interferon-alpha therapy. Transplantation 66:1254-1258, 1998.

53. Benner KG, Lee RG, Keefe EB, et al: Fibrosing cytolytic liver failure secondary to recurrent hepatitis B after liver transplantation. Gastroenterology 103:1307-1312, 1992.

54. Boletis JN, Delladetsima JK, Makris F, et al: Cholestatic syndromes in renal transplant recipients with HCV infection. Transpl Int 13(Suppl 1):S375-S379, 2000.

55. Bonino F, Brunetto MR: Possible immunopathogenesis for fibrosing cholestatic hepatitis. Gastroenterology 106:822-823, 1994.

56. Chen CH, Chen PJ, Chu JS, et al: Fibrosing cholestatic hepatitis in a hepatitis B surface antigen carrier after renal transplantation. Gastroenterology 107:1514-1518, 1994.

57. Lam PW, Wachs ME, Somberg KA, et al: Fibrosing cholestatic hepatitis in renal transplant recipients. Transplantation 61:378-381, 1996.

58. Zylberberg H, Carnot F, Mamzer MF, et al: Hepatitis C virus–related fibrosing cholestatic hepatitis after renal transplantation. Transplantation 63:158-160, 1997.

59. Alshak NS, Jiminez AM, Gedebou M, et al: Epstein-Barr virus infection in liver transplantation patients: Correlation of histopathology and semiquantitative Epstein-Barr virus–DNA recovery using polymerase chain reaction. Hum Pathol 24:1306-1312, 1993.

60. Langnas AN, Markin RS, Inagaki M, et al: Epstein-Barr virus hepatitis after liver transplantation. Am J Gastroenterol 89:1066-1070, 1994.

61. Sheiner PA, Mor E, Schwartz ME, Miller CM: Use of hepatitis C–positive donors in liver transplantation. Transplant Proc 25:3071, 1993.

62. Wright TL: Liver transplantation for chronic hepatitis C viral infection. Gastroenterol Clin North Am 22:231-242, 1993.

63. Fishman JA, Rubin RH, Koziel MJ, Periera BJ: Hepatitis C virus and organ transplantation. Transplantation 62:147-154, 1996.

64. Bouthot BA, Murthy BV, Schmid CH, et al: Long-term follow-up of hepatitis C virus infection among organ transplant recipients: Implications for policies on organ procurement. Transplantation 63:849-853, 1997.

65. Salizzoni M, Lupo F, Zamboni F, et al: Outcome of patients transplanted with liver from hepatitis C–positive donors. Transplant Proc 33:1507-1508, 2001.

66. Testa G, Goldstein RM, Netto G, et al: Long-term outcome of patients transplanted with livers from hepatitis C–positive donors. Transplantation 65:925-929, 1998.

67. Ghobrial RM, Steadman R, Gornbein J, et al: A 10-year experience of liver transplantation for hepatitis C: Analysis of factors determining outcome in over 500 patients. Ann Surg 234:384-393, discussion 393-394, 2001.

68. Rodriguez-Luna H, Vargas HG, Sharma P, et al: Hepatitis C virus recurrence in living donor liver transplant recipients. Dig Dis Sci 49:38-41, 2004.

69. Van Vlierberghe H, Troisi R, Colle I, et al: Hepatitis C infection–related liver disease: Patterns of recurrence and outcome in cadaveric and living-donor liver transplantation in adults. Transplantation 77:210-214, 2004.

70. Gaglio PJ, Malireddy S, Levitt BS, et al: Increased risk of cholestatic hepatitis C in recipients of grafts from living versus cadaveric liver donors. Liver Transpl 9:1028-1035, 2003.

71. Mukherjee S, Rogge J, Weaver LK, Schafer DF: Pilot study of pegylated interferon alfa-2b and ribavirin for recurrent hepatitis C after liver transplantation. Transplant Proc 35:3042-3044, 2003.

72. Nair S, Khan S, Loss G, et al: Treatment of recurrent hepatitis C in liver transplant recipients: Is there any histologic benefit? Liver Transpl 9:354-359, 2003.

73. Feray C, Samuel D, Gigou M, et al: An open trial of interferon alfa recombinant for hepatitis C after liver transplantation: Antiviral effects and risk of rejection. Hepatology 22:1084-1089, 1995.

74. Min AD, Bodenheimer HC Jr: Does interferon precipitate rejection of liver allografts? Hepatology 22:1333-1335, 1995.

75. Jain A, Demetris AJ, Manez R, et al: Incidence and severity of acute allograft rejection in liver transplant recipients treated with alfa interferon. Liver Transpl Surg 4:197-203, 1998.

76. Saab S, Kalmaz D, Gajjar NA, et al: Outcomes of acute rejection after interferon therapy in liver transplant recipients. Liver Transpl 10:859-867, 2004.

77. Terrault NA, Vyas G: Hepatitis B immune globulin preparations and use in liver transplantation. Clin Liver Dis 7:537-550, 2003.

78. Anselmo DM, Ghobrial RM, Jung LC, et al: New era of liver transplantation for hepatitis B: A 17-year single-center experience. Ann Surg 235:611-619, discussion 619-620, 2002.

79. Ben-Ari Z, Mor E, Tur-Kaspa R: Experience with lamivudine therapy for hepatitis B virus infection before and after liver transplantation, and review of the literature. J Intern Med 253:544-552, 2003.

80. Chu CJ, Fontana RJ, Moore C, et al: Outcome of liver transplantation for hepatitis B: Report of a single center's experience. Liver Transpl 7:724-731, 2001.

81. Seehofer D, Rayes N, Bechstein WO, et al: [Treatment of recurrent hepatitis B infection after liver transplantation. A retrospective analysis of 200 liver transplantations based on hepatitis B–associated liver diseases.] Z Gastroenterol 38:773-783, 2000.

82. Terrault NA, Zhou S, McCory RW, et al: Incidence and clinical consequences of surface and polymerase gene mutations in liver transplant recipients on hepatitis B immunoglobulin. Hepatology 28:555-561, 1998.

83. Tillmann HL, Trautwein C, Bock T, et al: Mutational pattern of hepatitis B virus on sequential therapy with famciclovir and lamivudine in patients with hepatitis B virus reinfection occurring under HBIg immunoglobulin after liver transplantation. Hepatology 30:244-256, 1999.

84. Pruett TL, McCory R: Hepatitis B immune globulin: The US experience. Clin Transplant 14(Suppl 2):7-13, 2000.

85. Devlin J, Donaldson P, Portmann B, et al: Recurrence of autoimmune hepatitis following liver transplantation. Liver Transpl Surg 1:162-165, 1995.

86. Neuberger J: Recurrence of primary biliary cirrhosis, primary sclerosing cholangitis, and autoimmune hepatitis. Liver Transpl Surg 1(5 Suppl 1):109-115, 1995.

87. Prados E, Cuervas-Mons V, de la Mata M, et al: Outcome of autoimmune hepatitis after liver transplantation. Transplantation 66:1645-1650, 1998.

88. Gotz G, Neuhaus R, Bechstein WO, et al: Recurrence of autoimmune hepatitis after liver transplantation. Transplant Proc 31:430-431, 1999.

89. Milkiewicz P, Hubscher SG, Skiba G, et al: Recurrence of autoimmune hepatitis after liver transplantation. Transplantation 68:253-256, 1999.

90. Ratziu V, Samuel D, Sebagh M, et al: Long-term follow-up after liver transplantation for autoimmune hepatitis: Evidence of recurrence of primary disease. J Hepatol 30:131-141, 1999.

91. Ayata G, Gordon FD, Lewis WD, et al: Liver transplantation for autoimmune hepatitis: A long-term pathologic study. Hepatology 32:185-192, 2000.

92. Vogel A, Heinrich E, Bahr MJ, et al: Long-term outcome of liver transplantation for autoimmune hepatitis. Clin Transplant 18:62-69, 2004.

93. Neuberger J: Transplantation for autoimmune hepatitis. Semin Liver Dis 22:379-386, 2002.

94. Hubscher SG: Recurrent autoimmune hepatitis after liver transplantation: Diagnostic criteria, risk factors, and outcome. Liver Transpl 7:285-291, 2001.

95. Hayashi M, Keefe EB, Krams SM, et al: Allograft rejection after liver transplantation for autoimmune liver diseases. Liver Transpl Surg 4:208-214, 1998.

96. Narumi S, Hakamada K, Sasaki M, et al: Liver transplantation for autoimmune hepatitis: Rejection and recurrence. Transplant Proc 31:1955-1956, 1999.

97. Sempoux C, Horsmans Y, Lerut J, et al: Acute lobular hepatitis as the first manifestation of recurrent autoimmune hepatitis after orthotopic liver transplantation. Liver 17:311-315, 1997.

98. Neuberger J, Portmann B, Calne R, Williams R: Recurrence of autoimmune chronic active hepatitis following orthotopic liver grafting. Transplantation 37:363-365, 1984.

99. Te HS, Koukoulis G, Ganger DR: Autoimmune hepatitis: A histological variant associated with prominent centrilobular necrosis. Gut 41:269-271, 1997.

100. Bach N, Thung SN, Schaffner F: The histological features of chronic hepatitis C and autoimmune chronic hepatitis: A comparative analysis. Hepatology 15:572-577, 1992.

101. Sylvestre PB, Batts KP, Burgart LJ, et al: Recurrence of primary biliary cirrhosis after liver transplantation: Histologic estimate of incidence and natural history. Liver Transpl 9:1086-1093, 2003.

102. Neuberger J, Portmann B, Macdougall BR, et al: Recurrence of primary biliary cirrhosis after liver transplantation. N Engl J Med 306:1-4, 1982.

103. Weaver GA, Franck WA, Streck WF: Recurrence of primary biliary cirrhosis after liver transplantation. N Engl J Med 306:1235-1236, 1982.

104. Demetris AJ, Markus BH, Esquivel C, et al: Pathologic analysis of liver transplantation for primary biliary cirrhosis. Hepatology 8:939-947, 1988.

105. Polson RJ, Portmann B, Neuberger J, et al: Evidence for disease recurrence after liver transplantation for primary biliary cirrhosis. Clinical and histologic follow-up studies. Gastroenterology 97: 715-725, 1989.

106. Balan V, Batts KB, Porayko MK, et al: Histological evidence for recurrence of primary biliary cirrhosis after liver transplantation. Hepatology 18:1392-1398, 1993.

107. Hubscher SG, Elias E, Buckels JA, et al: Primary biliary cirrhosis. Histological evidence of disease recurrence after liver transplantation. J Hepatol 18:173-184, 1993.

108. Liermann Garcia RF, Evangelista Garcia C, McMaster P, Neuberger J: Transplantation for primary biliary cirrhosis: Retrospective analysis of 400 patients in a single center. Hepatology 33:22-27, 2001.

109. Khettry U, Anand N, Faul PN, et al: Liver transplantation for primary biliary cirrhosis: A long-term pathologic study. Liver Transpl 9:87-96, 2003.

110. Portmann BC: Recurrence of primary biliary cirrhosis after transplantation. The pathologist's view. Eur J Gastroenterol Hepatol 11:633-637, 1999.

111. Van de Water J, Gerson LB, Ferrell LD, et al: Immunohistochemical evidence of disease recurrence after liver transplantation for primary biliary cirrhosis. Hepatology 24:1079-1084, 1996.

112. Sebagh M, Farges O, Dubel L, et al: Histological features predictive of recurrence of primary biliary cirrhosis after liver transplantation. Transplantation 65:1328-1333, 1998.

113. Lerut JP, Zimmermann A, Gertsch P: Late graft dysfunction after liver transplantation for primary biliary cirrhosis: Disease recurrence versus chronic graft rejection. Am J Gastroenterol 89:1896-1898, 1994.

114. Kubota T, Thomson A, Clouston AD, et al: Clinicopathologic findings of recurrent primary sclerosing cholangitis after orthotopic liver transplantation. J Hepatobiliary Pancreat Surg 6: 377-381, 1999.

115. Sheng R, Campbell WL, Zajko AB, Baron RL: Cholangiographic features of biliary strictures after liver transplantation for primary sclerosing cholangitis: Evidence of recurrent disease. AJR Am J Roentgenol 166:1109-1113, 1996.

116. Harrison RF, Davies MH, Neuberger JA, Hubscher SG: Fibrous and obliterative cholangitis in liver allografts: Evidence of recurrent primary sclerosing cholangitis? Hepatology 20:356-361, 1994.

117. Liden H, Norrby J, Firman S, Olausson M: Liver transplantation for primary sclerosing cholangitis—a single-center experience. Transpl Int 13(Suppl 1):S162-S164, 2000.

118. Graziadei IW, Wiesner RH, Batts KP, et al: Recurrence of primary sclerosing cholangitis following liver transplantation. Hepatology 29:1050-1056, 1999.

119. Rai RM, Boitnott J, Klein AS, Thuluvath PJ: Features of recurrent primary sclerosing cholangitis in two consecutive liver allografts after liver transplantation. J Clin Gastroenterol 32:151-154, 2001.

120. Wiesner RH: Liver transplantation for primary sclerosing cholangitis: Timing, outcome, impact of inflammatory bowel disease and recurrence of disease. Best Pract Res Clin Gastroenterol 15:667-680, 2001.

121. Goss JA, Shackleton CR, Farmer DG, et al: Orthotopic liver transplantation for primary sclerosing cholangitis. A 12-year single-center experience. Ann Surg 225:472-481, discussion 481-483, 1997.

122. Vera A, Moledina S, Gunson B, et al: Risk factors for recurrence of primary sclerosing cholangitis of liver allograft. Lancet 360:1943-1944, 2002.

123. Khettry U, Keaveny A, Goldar-Najafi A, et al: Liver transplantation for primary sclerosing cholangitis: A long-term clinicopathologic study. Hum Pathol 34:1127-1136, 2003.

124. van Buuren HR, van Hoogstraten HJE, Terkivatan T, et al: High prevalence of autoimmune hepatitis among patients with primary sclerosing cholangitis. J Hepatol 33:543-548, 2000.

125. Jeyarajah DR, Netto GJ, Lee SP, et al: Recurrent primary sclerosing cholangitis after orthotopic liver transplantation: Is chronic rejection part of the disease process? Transplantation 66:1300-1306, 1998.

126. Kim WR, Poterucha JJ, Porayko MK, et al: Recurrence of nonalcoholic steatohepatitis following liver transplantation. Transplantation 62:1802-1805, 1996.

127. Carson K, Washington MK, Treem WR, et al: Recurrence of nonalcoholic steatohepatitis in a liver transplant recipient. Liver Transpl Surg 3:174-176, 1997.

128. McCaughan GW: Recurrence of nonalcoholic steatohepatitis (NASH) post–liver transplantation. Liver Transpl Surg 3:683, 1997.

129. Molloy RM, Komorowski R, Varma RR: Recurrent nonalcoholic steatohepatitis and cirrhosis after liver transplantation. Liver Transpl Surg 3:177-178, 1997.

130. Charlton M, Kasparova P, Weston S, et al: Frequency of nonalcoholic steatohepatitis as a cause of advanced liver disease. Liver Transpl 7:608-614, 2001.

131. Contos MJ, Cales W, Sterling RK, et al: Development of nonalcoholic fatty liver disease after orthotopic liver transplantation for cryptogenic cirrhosis. Liver Transpl 7:363-373, 2001.

132. Sanjeevi A, Lyden E, Sunderman B, et al: Outcomes of liver transplantation for cryptogenic cirrhosis: A single-center study of 71 patients. Transplant Proc 35:2977-2980, 2003.

133. Brunt EM: Alcoholic and nonalcoholic steatohepatitis. Clin Liver Dis 6:399-420, vii, 2002.

134. Ayata G, Gordon FD, Lewis WD, et al: Cryptogenic cirrhosis: Clinicopathologic findings at and after liver transplantation. Hum Pathol 33:1098-1104, 2002.

135. Poonawala A, Nair SP, Thuluvath PJ: Prevalence of obesity and diabetes in patients with cryptogenic cirrhosis: A case-control study. Hepatology 32:689-692, 2000.

136. Ludwig J, McGill DB, Lindor KD: Review: Nonalcoholic steatohepatitis. J Gastroenterol Hepatol 12:398-403, 1997.

137. Ludwig J, Viggiano TR, McGill DB, Oh BF: Nonalcoholic steatohepatitis: Mayo Clinic experiences with a hitherto unnamed disease. Mayo Clin Proc 55:434-438, 1980.

138. Banner BF, Savas L, Zivny J, et al: Ubiquitin as a marker of cell injury in nonalcoholic steatohepatitis. Am J Clin Pathol 114: 860-866, 2000.

139. Brunt EM: Nonalcoholic steatohepatitis: Definition and pathology. Semin Liver Dis 21:3-16, 2001.

140. Brunt EM, Janney CJ, Di Bisceglie AM, et al: Nonalcoholic steatohepatitis: A proposal for grading and staging the histological lesions. Am J Gastroenterol 94:2467-2474, 1999.

Transplant-Related Malignancies

JOSEPH F. BUELL
THOMAS M. BEEBE
MICHAEL J. HANAWAY
MARK J. THOMAS
STEVEN M. RUDICH
E. STEVE WOODLE

Classification of transplant-related
  malignancies   1150

Donor-transmitted malignancy   1150
  Tumor transmission from donors with central
    nervous system lesions   1150
  Non–central nervous system donor tumor
    transmission   1151

Potential cause of de novo cancers   1151

Incidence of de novo malignancies after
  transplantation   1152
  Incidence of de novo malignancies in liver
    transplant recipients   1152
  Overview of malignancies reported to the
    Israel Penn International Transplant Tumor
    Registry   1153

De novo nonlymphoid malignancies   1153
  Cancer of the skin and lips   1154
  Kaposi's sarcoma   1154
  Carcinoma of the vulva and perineum   1155

Posttransplant lymphoproliferative disorder   1155

Liver transplantation for malignancy   1157
  Hepatocellular cancer   1157
  Cholangiocarcinoma   1159
  Metastatic neuroendocrine tumors   1160

Rare primary liver tumors   1160
Liver metastases   1160

Recurrence of preexisting malignancy   1161
  Tumors with low recurrence   1161
  Tumors with intermediate recurrence rates   1161
  Tumors with high recurrence rates   1162

Posttransplant cancer screening   1162

The increased risk of cancer associated with chronic immunosuppression in organ transplant recipients is well recognized.[1-3] The largest experience with posttransplant malignancies has involved renal allograft recipients, many of whom have follow-up periods approaching 30 years. In contrast to the patterns of neoplasms observed in kidney recipients, a rather different pattern of activity has been observed in the comparatively smaller experience involving liver allograft recipients. In this chapter the authors review the overall experience in liver transplant recipients and examine the differences between tumor occurrence in kidney and liver recipients.

Most conditions in which a state of profound immunosuppression exists are associated with an increased risk of malignancy.[4] Individuals with known congenital defects in antibody production or immune response mechanisms have been noted to experience a higher incidence of non-Hodgkin's lymphoma (NHL), leukemia, and certain other malignancies.[4,5] In states of acquired immunodeficiency, such as acquired immunodeficiency syndrome (AIDS), a higher incidence of skin and lymphatogenous malignancies such as Kaposi's sarcoma (KS) and NHL is found.[5] Within the immunosuppressed transplant recipient population, the risk of cancer is increased threefold to fourfold, with some individual cancers associated with up to a 100-fold increased risk in comparison to the general population.[3,6] Furthermore, the effect of immunosuppression is thought to be cumulative over time such that the incidence of malignancy reaches 20% to 70% in all solid-organ recipients by 20 years after transplantation (Fig. 71–1).[7] With the exception of skin cancer, malignancies encountered in the general population have not been associated with an increased frequency in the immunosuppressed transplant population. However, malignancies with known viral origin are more frequently encountered in the presence of immunosuppression: posttransplant lymphoproliferative disease (Epstein-Barr virus), KS (human herpesvirus-8 [HHV-8]), and cervical and vulvar cancer (human papillomavirus).

The most commonly observed malignancy in transplant recipients is skin cancer. Several distinct differences have been noted between skin malignancies appearing in immunosuppressed patients and those found in the general population. Skin malignancies in transplant recipients tend to appear at an earlier age, occur in multiple sites, and often have multiple recurrences.[8,9] In contrast to the general population, transplant recipients have a higher incidence of squamous cell cancer (SCC) than basal cell cancer (BCC).[10] The Israel Penn International Transplant Tumor Registry (IPITTR), founded by Israel Penn, M.D., and formerly referred to as the Cincinnati Transplant Tumor Registry (CTTR), has accrued data on transplant-related malignancies for more than 3 decades. After Dr. Penn's

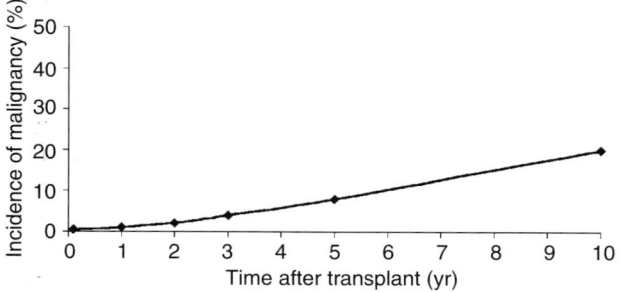

FIGURE 71–1

Incidence of malignancy in transplant recipients related to years of immunosuppression reported by the Scientific Registry of Transplant Recipients.

passing, the registry, renamed in his honor, was computerized and preserves his vision of providing a consultation service to caregivers and transplant centers worldwide.

Classification of Transplant-Related Malignancies

Penn classified transplant-related malignancies into one of three broad categories:

1. Donor-transmitted malignancy: a malignancy with a genetically confirmed donor source that is transferred to an organ recipient through the donor allograft and results in local or metastatic disease.

2. Recurrence of preexisting recipient malignancy: a previous or active malignancy that was treated in the recipient before transplantation and subsequently recurs after transplantation. Recurrence in these patients is due largely to the effects of immunosuppression, which may increase the incidence of recurrence or diminish the interval to tumor recurrence.

3. De novo malignancy: malignancies that occur after transplantation in patients with no previous history of the specific malignancy.

Donor-Transmitted Malignancy

Tumor Transmission from Donors with Central Nervous System Lesions

In the early years of transplantation, before the inception of laws establishing brain death criteria, organs were frequently procured from donors with active malignancies, which resulted in all-to-frequent transmission of the donor cancer to the recipient.[10,11] Today, because of the lessons learned from early misadventures, high-risk donors are readily identified and their use avoided, thus making donor-transmitted malignancies a rare occurrence. Over a period of 3 decades, Israel Penn catalogued more than 250 cases involving organs from donors with a history of malignancy. Penn examined tumor histology, donor risk factors, tumor manifestations, and recipient outcome in each case in which transmission of a donor malignancy occurred. Although most recipients remained disease free, some were less fortunate, with cancers developing that were highly suggestive of donor origin.

The most common tumors encountered in potential donors with malignancies are central nervous system (CNS) tumors.[12-14] A recent study from the IPITTR

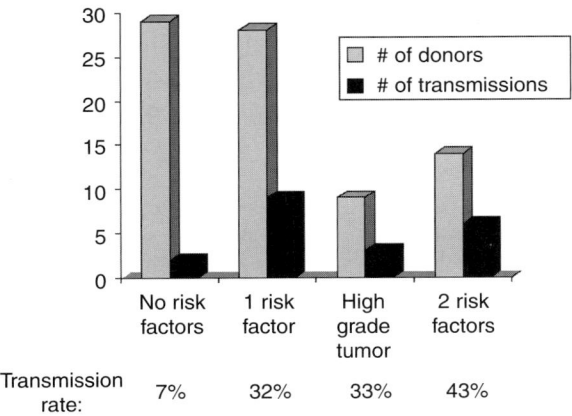

FIGURE 71–2

Impact of donor risk factors on transmission rates of central nervous system malignancy in organ recipients.

evaluated risk factors present in cases involving donor transmission. The study identified an overall tumor transmission rate of 23% but found that the presence of one or more risk factors, including high tumor grade, use of ventriculoperitoneal or ventriculoatrial shunting, or extensive craniotomy, increased the incidence of transmission to 53% whereas the absence of identifiable risk factors reduced the incidence of donor transmission to 7% (Fig. 71–2).[15]

Non–Central Nervous System Donor Tumor Transmission

Some donor tumor histological characteristics have been identified as having a propensity for high rates of transmission from donor to recipient.[11,12,16] Choriocarcinoma, a gynecological malignancy, has been associated with a 93% tumor transmission rate and a 64% mortality rate. Malignant melanoma has been noted to have similarly high rates of tumor transmission (74%) and mortality (58%).[16] Moreover, recurrent malignant melanoma from a superficial lesion has been witnessed as late as 15 years after surgical excision in both the general and transplant populations.

Renal cell carcinoma (RCC) has a demonstrated track record of transmission from donor to recipient.[17] In a study examining 70 donors with previous or undetected RCC, a 61% incidence of donor transmission was identified, with the majority being confined to the allograft.[18,19] Early identification and detection of interval growth, which occurred from 3 to 36 months after transplantation, permitted successful intervention and resection. The accompanying 15% patient mortality rate is suggestive of a tumor biology that is less aggressive than that of melanoma and choriocarcinoma. Tumors with the most favorable prognoses, which consequently pose the least risk for tumor transmission,

were those that had low-grade histology and were void of extracapsular or vascular invasion. This has been demonstrated in a series of transplant recipients who received kidneys with RCC that was identified at the time of harvest, excised ex vivo, and subsequently implanted into the respective recipients.[11,16-18] In none of the 14 patients in the series, whose mean tumor size was 2.1 cm with tumor grades of either Fuhrman grade I/IV or II/IV, did tumor transmission occur.

In the United States, lung cancer remains one of the most common causes of cancer-related death in the general population. The use of donors with previous lung malignancies was associated with a 43% tumor transmission rate and a 32% percent mortality rate, and therefore their use as donors should be avoided.[20,21] At the 2003 American Society of Transplant Surgeons consensus conference, the incidence of nodal or metastatic disease from colon cancer with a primary tumor classification of T1 was reported to be less than 1%. With primary tumors classified as T2 or T3, the incidence increases and overall survival decreases until 7 years has elapsed after resection. Thus, the convening body concluded that the risks associated with the use of donors with a primary tumor classification of T1 are acceptable whereas donors with T2 or T3 lesions should have a minimum 7-year disease-free interval and, even then, should be used with caution.[22] Limited data exist on the use of donor organs from patients with previous or active breast malignancies.[20] A recent review from the IPITTR identified a donor tumor transmission rate of 29% from donors with invasive breast cancer.[23] Cases involving in situ breast carcinoma, such as ductal (DCIS) and lobular carcinoma (LCIS), displayed no evidence of donor transmission. As with melanoma, breast cancer has a notorious reputation for late and aggressive recurrence. For this reason, the use of donors with a history of breast cancer should be limited to those with noninvasive forms such as DCIS and LCIS. Based on data from a series of transplant recipients with histories of preexisting breast malignancy, it may also be permissible to use donors with low-stage invasive lesions and an extended disease-free interval.

Potential Cause of De Novo Cancers

Transplant-related malignancies arise from a complex interplay of factors. Chronic immunosuppression may severely depress components of a solid-organ recipient's native immune system, such as natural killer cells.[24,25] The function of these cells is surveillance and destruction of neoplastic cells that arise from either viral or carcinogenic stimulation. Chronic antigen stimulation by antibodies from transplanted organs, repeat infections, or transfusions of blood or related products may overly stimulate a partially depressed immune system and result in the development of a transplant-related lymphoma.[24,25] Alternatively, impaired feedback mechanisms may fail to control the degree of immune response, which may also lead to unrestrained lymphoid proliferation with resultant lymphoma.[26] Moreover, once this loss of regulation occurs, the defensive capabilities of the immune system are weakened, and other nonlymphoid neoplasms may then appear.

The short induction time of certain malignancies suggests that viruses may play a catalytic role in these immunosuppressed patients. There is strong evidence linking Epstein-Barr virus with NHL, not only in transplant patients but also in patients with primary immunodeficiency disease or AIDS.[26,27] Thus far, little evidence has linked other viruses (human T-cell lymphotropic virus type I, HHV-6) to these cancers. Another group of viruses strongly suspected as being causative agents of carcinoma of the uterine cervix, vulva, perineum, anus, and possibly the skin are the human papillomaviruses.[28-30] Some viruses, most notably HHV-8, have been linked to KS.[31-33] Hepatitis B virus and possibly hepatitis C virus may contribute to the high incidence of hepatocellular cancer (HCC) in kidney transplant recipients. Mounting evidence that viruses may cause cancer in humans reinforces the need for development of vaccines, such as hepatitis B vaccine, to protect susceptible populations from cancer.

Immunosuppressive agents that may directly damage recipient DNA, such as azathioprine, cyclophosphamide, and cyclosporine, are thought to contribute to the development of certain malignancies.[24,25,34,35] Immunosuppressive agents may potentiate the effects of other carcinogens, such as sunlight, in causing carcinoma. Genetic factors may influence susceptibility to malignancy by affecting carcinogen metabolism, interferon secretion, response to viral infections, or regulation of the immune response by the major histocompatibility complex. Although some studies have linked certain HLA groups to either increased susceptibility or resistance to the development of KS, others contradict this notion. In a study of organ recipients with de novo KS that included 135 patients with HLA-A and HLA-B typing and 67 with HLA-DR typing, no significant difference was found among the groups when ethnicity was considered.[32] Fifty-six percent of the patients were Italian, Greek, Jewish, or Arabic.

Incidence of De Novo Malignancies after Transplantation

Tumors such as invasive uterine cervical carcinoma and carcinoma of the lung, breast, and prostate appear with similar frequency in both the general and transplant populations.[1,2,36] Only two types of cancer common to the general population are encountered with greater frequency in the transplantation population, those being SCC and lymphoma. Whereas the overall percentage of nonmelanoma skin cancer (32%) was very similar to that observed in the general population (30%), the incidence of SCC was markedly increased.[13,24,34] Certain cancers appear with greater frequency in the transplant population than in the general population: lymphoma, 23% versus 5%; lip cancer, 7% versus 0.3%; KS, 6% versus a negligible incidence; carcinoma of the kidney, 5% versus 2%; carcinoma of the vulva and perineum, 4% versus 0.5%; hepatobiliary tumors, 2.6% versus 1.4%; and sarcomas (excluding KS), 1.6% versus 0.5%.[34,35,37,38]

Incidence of De Novo Malignancies in Liver Transplant Recipients

In a review of the CTTR data collected during the previous 2 decades, Penn made several observations concerning de novo tumors in liver transplant recipients.[39] In his review, Penn compared several different posttransplant malignancies found in liver recipients with those seen after kidney transplantation.[39] As opposed to kidney transplant recipients, in whom skin cancer accounted for the highest percentage of de novo tumors among these recipients in the registry, posttransplant lymphoproliferative disorder (PTLD) was reported to occur more frequently than skin cancer after liver transplantation. Penn postulated that heightened immunosuppression after liver transplantation resulted in a greater risk for early PTLD than would otherwise be expected in kidney transplant recipients. It should also be noted that 23% of the liver transplant recipients in Penn's data series were from the pediatric population, in whom the development of nonlymphoid malignancies after transplantation is less likely to occur.

In a recent study of 888 liver transplant recipients, skin cancer was identified as the most common nonlymphoid tumor, with an estimated incidence of 1.6%. Nonmelanoma lesions were predominant, with SCC demonstrating a fourfold prevalence over BCC (the converse of which is seen in the general population).[40] After skin cancer, sarcoma and prostate and colon cancer were the most common malignancies, with an estimated incidence of 0.6%, 0.5%, and 0.3%, respectively. A follow-up report concluded that the estimated overall incidence of de novo malignancy was higher in liver transplant recipients than in the general population.[41]

In another large series, the Berlin group found that lymphoid and nonlymphoid cancer, including PTLD, skin cancer, and cervical or uterine neoplasia (or both), occurred at similar frequency after liver transplantation (incidence of 1.5%).[42] No clear correlation was found to exist between agents used for induction or maintenance immunosuppression and cancer risk. A subsequent study that examined 1007 recipients with 39 malignancies (17 skin, 13 PTLD, 9 uterine/cervical) estimated the risk of cancer to be 4% 5 years after transplantation.[43]

The largest and most comprehensive single-center study of de novo malignancy after liver transplantation was conducted by the University of Pittsburgh, which examined two patient cohorts to characterize the risk for and behavior of cancer. In the first study, 1000 consecutive adult and pediatric liver recipients were monitored prospectively over a mean of 93 months. The study confirmed skin cancer as the most common nonlymphoid malignancy, followed by gastrointestinal, genitourinary, pulmonary, oropharyngeal, and breast malignancy.[44,45] Statistical analysis estimated a 7.6-fold increase in oropharyngeal cancer and a 1.7-fold increase in pulmonary malignancy over the predicted incidence found in the general population.[46] A later study from the University of Pittsburgh examined 3192 adult liver recipients who underwent transplantation between 1981 and 1998 in an effort to characterize PTLD after liver transplantation.[47] The incidence of PTLD in the adult group was 2.9%, which was significantly lower than the incidence in children (9.7%). The median time from liver transplantation to the diagnosis of PTLD was shorter in children than in adults (8.1 months versus 15 months). Lymph nodes were the most common site of disease in PTLD at the time of diagnosis in adults (50%), followed by the gastrointestinal tract (42%), liver and spleen (20.6%), lungs (20.6%), and CNS (6.5%). Analysis of variables indicated that grade I PTLD (versus grades II to IV) and PTLD with a single-site location of disease were associated with more favorable survival. Most of the patients in whom PTLD was diagnosed died of PTLD itself (44%), infection (23%), multisystem organ failure (5%), or graft failure (5%). This study remains the

reference point for a single-center experience in the study of PTLD after liver transplantation. The experience of the IPITTR with de novo malignancy after liver transplantation is outlined in the next section.

Overview of Malignancies Reported to the Israel Penn International Transplant Tumor Registry

The incidence of individual malignancies varies among transplant types (Table 71-1). Contrary to Penn's initial reports, which included both adults and children, current IPITTR data on adult recipients after liver transplantation indicate that skin cancer was reported more frequently than PTLD. This observation is congruent with the findings of the Berlin single-center study presented earlier.[42] Penn observed that the patterns of malignancy differ among different types of transplant recipients. However, current data indicate that the frequency of nonlymphoid tumors after liver transplantation is very similar to that reported for other organ transplant recipients. The dramatic differences in the reported frequency of PTLD among kidney, liver, and pancreas recipients may reflect the voluntary nature of reporting inherent in registries such as the IPITTR. The remainder of the discussion focuses on lymphoid and nonlymphoid malignancies.

De Novo Nonlymphoid Malignancies

A total of 269 males and 166 females with de novo nonlymphoid cancer after liver transplantation were reported to the IPITTR. Cancer of the skin was the predominant de novo malignancy (37%) reported in liver recipients, followed by PTLD (26%), colon cancer (5.7%), cervical cancer (2.3%), and vulvar/perineal cancer (1.6%). The median age at diagnosis of de novo nonlymphoid malignancies ranged from 44.2 to 62.6 years of age,

Table 71-1. IPITTR REPORTING FREQUENCY OF DE NOVO TUMORS IN RENAL, LIVER, AND PANCREAS TRANSPLANT RECIPIENTS

	Renal (n = 7200)	Hepatic (n = 434)	Pancreas (n = 113)
Skin cancer	2819 (39%)	160 (37%)	42 (38%)
PTLD	828 (12%)	114 (26%)	52 (46%)
Kaposi's sarcoma	314 (4%)	6 (1.4%)	2 (1.8%)
Cervical cancer	278 (4%)	10 (2.3%)	2 (1.8%)
Renal cell cancer	276 (4%)	3 (0.7%)	2 (1.8%)
Vulvar/perineal cancer	207 (3%)	7 (1.6%)	6 (5.3%)
Colon cancer	265 (4%)	25 (5.7%)	0

IPITTR, Israel Penn International Transplant Tumor Registry; PTLD, posttransplant lymphoproliferative disorder.

Table 71–2. AGE AT DIAGNOSIS AND MEDIAN TIME FROM TRANSPLANTATION TO DIAGNOSIS FOR NONLYMPHOID CANCER AFTER LIVER TRANSPLANTATION

Type of Tumor	Number	Median Age at Diagnosis (yr)	Median Time from Transplantation to Diagnosis (mo)
Skin	160	57.1	26.3
SCC	64	58.2	33.2
BCC	59	54.7	24.5
SCC/BCC	17	58.9	22
Melanoma	4	62.6	72.6
Solid (nonskin)	191	57.3	22.8
Colon Ca	33	57.2	27.8
Lung Ca	29	59.3	24.5
Breast Ca	11	55	21.7
Cervical Ca	10	44.2	17.7

BCC, basal cell carcinoma; Ca, cancer; SCC, squamous cell carcinoma.

with the majority of tumors occurring in the fifth decade of life (Table 71–2). The median time from transplantation to diagnosis of cancer ranged from 17.7 to 72.6 months, with most malignancies developing within 36 months after transplantation. The reported frequency of BCC was similar to that for SCC, which was similar to Penn's initial observation in kidney transplant recipients. In contrast, BCC is more common than SCC in the general population by a factor of 5 to 1.[24,37,38] Of note, although perhaps not surprising, survival was significantly longer in patients with skin versus all other de novo solid-tumor malignancies or PTLD (Fig. 71–3). Overall, an updated analysis of IPITTR data indicates that skin cancer was reported more frequently than PTLD, with improved survival over all other de novo solid tumors and PTLD.

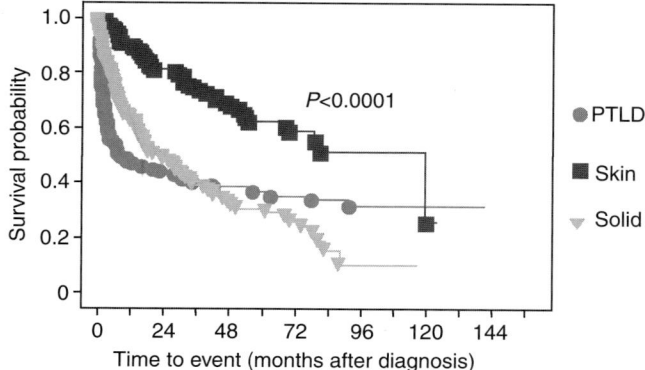

FIGURE 71–3

Kaplan-Meier survival curves for liver transplant recipients in whom skin cancer, solid tumor, and posttransplant lymphoproliferative disorder (PTLD) were diagnosed after transplantation.

Cancer of the Skin and Lips

Cancer of the skin is the most common malignancy (37%) reported in the transplant population, with the incidence varying in proportion to the degree of sun exposure.[8,9,24,25] In regions with limited exposure, a 4- to 7-fold increase was observed, which increased to 21-fold in those residing in more sun-exposed locations. The majority of these malignancies were SCC. Exposure to sunlight, although significant, is not the sole determining factor. The surprisingly high incidence of SCC reported from areas with low levels of sunlight such as Canada, Sweden, and Scotland may be related to malignant changes in papillomavirus-induced cutaneous warts or the influence of immunosuppression, as well as sun exposure and other possible factors.[24,25] The incidence of skin cancer increased with the length of follow-up after transplantation, thus suggesting a dose response to chronic immunosuppression.[36]

In transplant patients, skin cancers demonstrated some unusual features not seen in their general population counterparts. BCC outnumbered SCC in the general population by 5 to 1, but the reverse was true in transplant recipients, in whom SCC outnumbered BCC by 1.8 to 1.[8,9] In the general population, SCC commonly occurs in people in their sixth and seventh decade of life, but the mean age range of occurrence in transplant patients was 30 to 40 years. Transplant recipients also suffered from a remarkably high incidence of multiple skin cancers (present in at least 42%), with some recipients experiencing more than 100 occurrences. Such a phenomenon in the general population is limited to those receiving excessive exposure to sunlight.

SCC was noted to be more aggressive in transplant recipients than in the general population. Metastasis to the lymph nodes occurred in 161 (6%) of the 2739 patients, with 75% of the metastases occurring from SCC and only 16% from melanoma.[24,25] Eight percent originated from Merkel cell tumors, and less than 1% were from BCC.[32] Remarkably, 137 (5%) of the 2739 affected individuals died of their skin malignancies; 61% of the deaths resulted from SCC, whereas 32% resulted from melanoma, 5% from Merkel cell tumor, and 1% from BCC.[9,24,38] In contrast to these findings, most lymph node metastases and deaths from metastatic skin cancer in the general population result from melanoma.

Kaposi's Sarcoma

Before the now-epidemic level of AIDS seen in the United States, the 6% incidence of KS in organ transplant recipients was much higher than that found in the general population, in whom it accounted for a mere 0.02% to 0.07% of all cancers. An epidemiological study showed a 400- to 500-fold increase in the incidence of KS in kidney transplant recipients when compared with controls of the same ethnic origin.[31,32] The high incidence of KS in this worldwide series of patients is similar to that observed in tropical Africa, where the disease occurs endemically and accounts for between 3% and 9% of all malignancies. KS affected males more frequently than females (2.9:1), but not to the extent as the 9:1 to 15:1 ratio found in the general population. KS occurred most often in transplant patients of Arabic, Jewish, African, or Mediterranean (mostly eastern or southern) ancestry.[31,32,38] Sixty-one percent were affected by nonvisceral KS confined to the skin or oropharyngeal or laryngeal mucosa. The remaining 39% demonstrated a broad spectrum of visceral involvement that primarily affected the gastrointestinal tract and lungs. Of the 182 patients with nonvisceral disease, 178 (98%) had lesions confined to the skin, with 4 (2%) involving the mouth or oropharynx. Of the 117 patients with visceral disease, 26 (22%) had no concomitant skin involvement, but 4 (3%) had involvement of the oral mucosa, which provided a readily available site for biopsy and diagnosis of the disease.[31,32,38]

Complete posttreatment remissions were seen in 84 of 182 patients with nonvisceral disease (46%). Remarkably, 27 (32%) of these remissions occurred as a result of a reduction or cessation of immunosuppressive therapy alone. Episodic recurrences of KS were identified in patients in whom immunosuppressive therapy was reduced/discontinued initially, but later resumed. Only 22 of 117 (19%) patients with visceral involvement experienced complete remission, 12 (55%) instances of which occurred in response to reduction/cessation of immunosuppressive therapy only.[31,32] Reduction of immunosuppression in these patients with KS was not without a price, however; more than half the patients thus treated lost the function of their kidney allografts. Seventy-four patients (63%) with visceral KS died, with 54 (73%) of the deaths considered cancer related.

Carcinoma of the Vulva and Perineum

The increased incidence of anogenital malignancies reported to the IPITTR is in keeping with an epidemiological study in which it was shown that the incidence of such malignancies in kidney transplant recipients is increased 100-fold in comparison to controls.[2,5] Of the 194 patients, females outnumbered males by 2.5:1, in contrast to most other posttransplant cancers, in which males outnumbered females by more than 2:1.

Two thirds of the patients had invasive lesions that occurred at a much earlier age (average age, 42 years) than in their counterparts from the general population (average age, between 50 and 70 years). Some transplant recipients acknowledged a history of condyloma acuminatum, or genital warts caused by human papillomavirus, before development of the neoplasm, and thus condyloma should be regarded as a premalignant disease in these patients. Some women had multicentric lesions involving not only the vulva and perineum but also the vagina, uterus, and cervix. Although many patients with carcinoma of the vulva and perineum responded well to local or extensive excision of their disease, some died of metastases despite undergoing abdominoperitoneal resection or radical vulvectomy.[28,29]

Posttransplant Lymphoproliferative Disorder

One hundred fourteen adult liver recipients who were reported to the IPITTR with a diagnosis of PTLD were evaluated retrospectively. This series was composed of 63 males and 51 females reported from transplant centers around the United States who underwent liver transplantation in the last decade. The median age at diagnosis was 50.7 years (range, 18.1 to 70.2 years), and the median time from liver transplantation to diagnosis of PTLD was 5.4 months (range, 1 to 140 months). The most frequent causes of liver failure in patients with PTLD were alcoholic liver disease (18%), infectious hepatitis (17%) and primary biliary cirrhosis (14%). A single site of PTLD involvement was only slightly more prevalent than multiple-site involvement (55% versus 45%). PTLD involvement at the time of diagnosis was most commonly identified in the liver allograft and lymph nodes, followed by the gastrointestinal tract, CNS, and spleen (Fig. 71–4). Interestingly, among liver recipients in whom PTLD developed, 64% succumbed to progressive malignancy as compared with 5.4% who

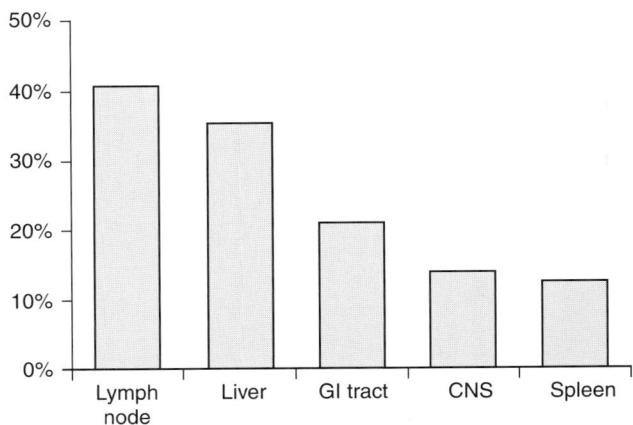

FIGURE 71–4

Sites of involvement of posttransplant lymphoproliferative disorder after liver transplantation.

Table 71-3. CAUSES OF DEATH IN LIVER TRANSPLANT RECIPIENTS WITH PTLD

Cause of Death	Number	Median Survival Time (mo)
PTLD	47 (64%)	1.3 (0–12.1)
Infection	10 (13.5%)	1.8 (0.1–41.7)
Unknown	7	2.8 (0–91.6)
Liver failure/rejection	4 (5.4%)	8.5 (0–27.6)
Cardiac	2	70.3 (62.7–77.9)
Multisystem organ failure	2	31.0 (29.5–34.3)
Intracranial hemorrhage	1	9.6
Hepatitis	1	0.2

PTLD, posttransplant lymphoproliferative disorder.

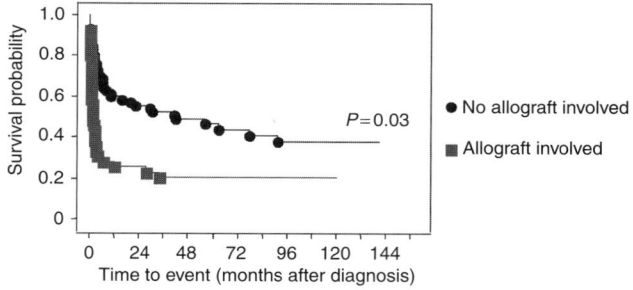

FIGURE 71–6

Kaplan-Meier analysis of survival in patients with liver allograft posttransplant lymphoproliferative disorder (PTLD) and PTLD not involving the liver at the time of diagnosis.

died of liver failure/rejection (Table 71–3). This finding suggests that liver recipients in whom PTLD develops may not have undergone adequate reduction or cessation of immunosuppression, possibly because of a fear of potential allograft rejection on the part of clinicians managing patient care.

In a recent multivariate analysis that examined survival after the development of PTLD in liver transplant recipients, patients with multiple-site involvement of PTLD at the time of diagnosis experienced poorer overall survival than did those with single-site involvement (Fig. 71–5).[47a] Allograft involvement with PTLD was also independently associated with decreased survival (Fig. 71–6). This finding is in contrast to other reports suggesting that allograft involvement was not a predictor of death.[47-51] A diagnosis of PTLD involving the CNS correlated with the worst prognosis in liver transplant recipients, with no survivors being identified (Fig. 71–7). This association between CNS PTLD and mortality has been observed in all other allograft recipients.[47] Neither previous use of antilymphocyte preparations such as OKT3 or antilymphocyte globulin for induction or rejection therapy nor the choice of individual calcineurin inhibitor (tacrolimus versus cyclosporine) had

an impact on survival. Therapeutic approaches for the treatment of PTLD, including chemotherapy, radiation therapy, or both, did not significantly alter survival. However, reduction or discontinuation of immunosuppression as monotherapy or as a component of multimodality therapy approached, but did not reach statistical significance in prolonging survival (Fig. 71–8).

The results of this analysis of PTLD after liver transplantation were similar to those of studies from other centers. Results from a University of Pittsburgh study also indicated that a single site of PTLD at the time of diagnosis confers superior long-term survival.[47] Both studies confirmed that lymph nodes were the most common site of occurrence and that most patients who died did so after succumbing to PTLD. Although the IPITTR experience with PTLD in pancreas and kidney transplants also found CNS involvement at the time of diagnosis to be a predictor of poor outcome, there was no apparent correlation between allograft involvement and poor survival in this recipient group.[47] Similar to findings in the liver recipient series, this analysis found no clear link between specific immunosuppressive medications and outcome.

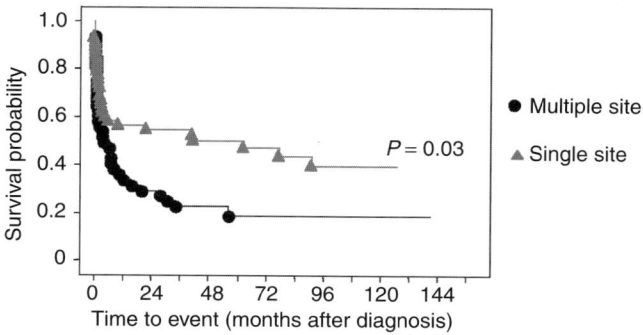

FIGURE 71–5

Kaplan-Meier analysis of survival in patients with single and multiple sites of involvement of posttransplant lymphoproliferative disorder.

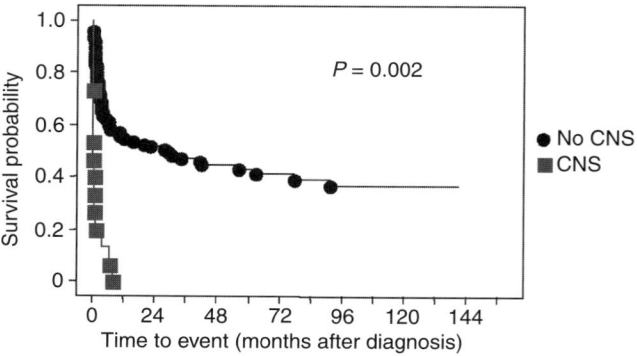

FIGURE 71–7

Kaplan-Meier analysis of survival in liver transplant patients with and without central nervous system posttransplant lymphoproliferative disorder at the time of diagnosis.

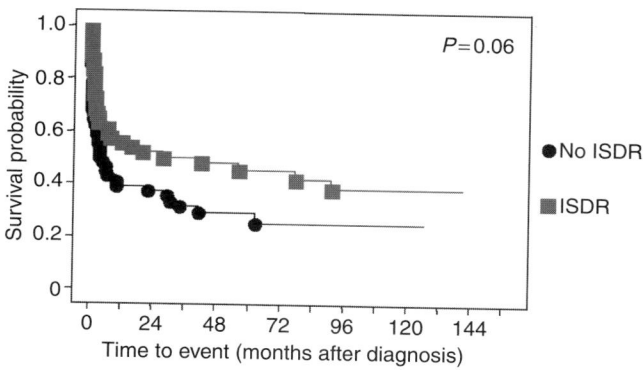

FIGURE 71-8

Kaplan-Meier analysis of survival in liver transplant patients who were or were not treated with reduction/discontinuation of immunosuppression (ISDR).

A review of cases reported to the IPITTR determined that cancer of the skin is the most commonly reported de novo malignancy found in liver recipients, followed by PTLD and cancer of the colon, cervix, and vulvar/perineal region. SCC and BCC were more prevalent than KS or melanoma, with survival after the diagnosis of cutaneous cancer found to be superior to that after PTLD and de novo solid tumors. Single-site involvement of PTLD was found to be predictive of better overall survival, which correlated closely with results from large, single-center studies of PTLD, and as seen in studies of PTLD in other organ types, CNS involvement is a predictor of poor survival.

Liver Transplantation for Malignancy

Tumors of the liver are an inhomogeneous group that arise from the liver parenchyma or bile duct or through deposition of metastatic disease. Worldwide, HCC accounts for the vast majority of primary hepatic tumors (80% to 90%). HCC, which affects males more so than females, is most commonly (60% to 80%) seen in patients who have preexisting liver disease, with those having hepatitis B or C or hemachromatosis being at greatest risk. Other end-stage liver diseases that can lead to HCC include alcoholic cirrhosis, schistosomal infestation, and homozygous α_1-antitrypsin deficiency. The pathogenesis of HCC, which is thought to result from proto-oncogene activation and suppressor gene inactivation during hepatocyte replication, may be related to chronic liver injury, adenomatous hyperplasia, or dysplastic nodules, which also result from such genetic alterations. Eventually, over a period varying between several months and years, dedifferentiation occurs, beginning with well-differentiated HCC and subsequently progressing to poorly differentiated HCC.[52] Traditionally, treatment of HCC has involved surgical

intervention for both early and advanced stages of the disease. Several methods ranging from local destruction (cryotherapy, thermal ablation, and ethanol injection) to major resection (hepatectomy) have been used with varying degrees of success. Because of the significant perioperative mortality associated with the performance of hepatectomy, the utility of such procedures in Child's B or C patients is limited. Despite surgical intervention, whose curative potential for many types of malignancy is well known, postinterventional malignancies often develop in patients with HCC. These malignancies may occur either as recurrent malignancy that develops in the previously resected tumor bed or, even more commonly, as a secondary primary in the diseased liver. From a therapeutic perspective, total hepatectomy with complete excision, regional lymphadenectomy, and liver replacement is the most viable option for reducing postinterventional malignancy formation. In 1991, reporting on a series of 365 patients with unresectable HCC, Penn identified an 18% 5-year survival rate for the series, with the main cause of mortality being recurrent HCC. Since that time, several studies have resulted in the refinement of recipient criteria to better improve outcomes. More current studies, looking at the use of surgical resection in HCC, report 5-year survival rates between 28% and 44% with resection,[53,54] whereas survival rates after transplantation have been reported to be as high as 69%.[55]

The sharp rise in the frequency of diagnosis of HCC in North America over the past decade, whether before or incidental to transplantation, has largely been due to the rising incidence of hepatitis C. HCC, which has risen 75% since 1993, is now ranked the fifth leading cause of cancer worldwide.[56]

Hepatocellular Cancer

In the late 1960s and 1970s, liver transplantation was frequently performed in patients with advanced HCC because of the lack of alternative therapies. Lack of refined recipient selection criteria led to liver transplantation in many HCC patients with large tumor burdens or advanced stages of disease involvement (T3 and T4). Because of dismal long-term survival and organ shortages, recipient selection was switched to include only those with nonmalignant causes. During this era, efforts to improve survival led to closer examination of tumor characteristics and patient selection criteria, which resulted in the exclusion of patients with lesions greater than 5 cm in size or those with large bilobar cancers. The Milan group further specified the selection criteria to exclude (1) tumors greater than 5 cm in diameter, (2) more than three lesions present in the entire liver, (3) disease progression outside the liver, or (4) invasion of tumor into the "large" blood vessels, as signified by new onset of portal vein thrombosis. Implementation of the Milan group selection criteria has led to reduced recurrence rates and improved recipient survival.

Since implementation of the Model for End-Stage Liver Disease/(Model for) Pediatric End-Stage Liver Disease (MELD/PELD) scoring schema, the prevalence of HCC patients has risen. This increase may in part be due to the fact that screening for tumors in liver transplant candidates has become a critical part of transplant evaluation, since increased priority is given to patients with higher MELD/PELD scores, which increase between 8 and 14 points in the presence of HCC. Abdominal imaging with ultrasonography, computed tomography, or magnetic resonance imaging should be performed every 4 to 6 months while awaiting transplantation. Serum α-fetoprotein (AFP) measurements should be a routine part of the pretransplant workup. Although there are many causes of elevated AFP, AFP levels that remain elevated warrant further evaluation to rule out HCC. AFP measurements every 3 to 6 months while on the waitlist should be considered a routine part of pretransplant care.

Resection before Transplantation

Patients with early HCC and well-preserved liver function who undergo partial liver resection and remain eligible for "salvage transplantation" have 5-year survival rates that rival those of liver transplant recipients.[57] Of 611 HCC patients evaluated between 1989 and 2001, 36 who underwent partial hepatic resection also met the criteria for orthotopic liver transplantation (OLT). Most of these patients were Child's class A, with 78% having histological cirrhosis. There was one death, a hepatic morbidity rate of 10%, and a 5-year survival rate in resected patients of 69%. At a median follow-up of 35 months, recurrent HCC had developed in 20 of the 36 resected patients, with only 1 then considered ineligible for transplantation. Although the data did not present the specific survival outcomes in patients with hepatitis C or the risk for progressive liver failure after resection, in patients with minimal evidence of end-stage liver disease, the study argues that resection followed by salvage liver transplantation in those with recurrent HCC is a sound approach.

How does the survival rate of patients with HCC and cirrhosis who undergo liver transplantation compare with that in transplant recipients with cirrhosis alone? Figueras and colleagues reported results from a prospective study of 174 patients, 38 with pretransplant HCC and 136 with no evidence of malignancy.[58] Median follow-up in both groups was longer than 24 months. Five-year actuarial survival rates were virtually identical in both groups, 63% in those with HCC and 68% in those without malignancy ($P = .84$).

Min reviewed 55 patients who underwent transplantation for hepatitis C with accompanying HCC.[59] A comparison of the results in an equal number of matched control subjects found allograft and patient survival to be equivalent between the groups. These results, along with those from other published works, indicate that concomitant HCC and cirrhosis or end-stage liver disease does not reduce survival after transplantation when compared with those undergoing liver replacement for cirrhosis alone.

Is liver transplantation as effective as other treatment modalities for HCC? As early as 1991, Iwatsuki and associates did not find any difference in survival between transplantation and resection groups when HCC was not associated with cirrhosis.[60] The study, which reported on 533 patients with HCC, 46 of whom did not have cirrhosis, concluded that liver transplantation should be the treatment of choice for HCC confined to the liver when HCC is unresectable or when hepatic function is compromised (or both).[61] A significant survival benefit was found for transplantation over resection, transarterial chemoembolization (TACE), and percutaneous ethanol injection. This study was one of the first to stratify survival according to known factors affecting outcome.

Factors Affecting Tumor Recurrence

Observations of pretransplant recurrence of HCC at sites of both previous biopsy and radiofrequency ablation suggest that tumor seeding may occur along tract sites. This possibility has placed biopsy confirmation of HCC, for the purpose of enabling candidates to receive favorable MELD points, at the center of contention. Tumor recurrence after transplantation, although most commonly involving the liver, may also be manifested as pulmonary metastasis. Although the risk of recurrence is particularly high within the first 3 years after transplantation, recurrence beyond 5 years has also been observed. Prognostic factors for tumor recurrence include vascular or lymphatic invasion, tumor size greater than 5 cm, bilobar disease, and the absence of cirrhosis. In a multivariate analysis of tumor characteristics predictive of recurrence, stage IV (TNM) disease classification was the only factor to independently predict recurrence or mortality.[62] The investigators compared OLT outcomes between two groups, cirrhotics with HCC and those without HCC, and found identical results after transplantation; median follow-up for the series was 6 years.[62] In the initial Mazzaferro series, 48 cirrhotic patients with either stage I or stage II HCC underwent transplantation and achieved a 75% 4-year survival rate.[63]

The authors concluded that careful patient selection, excluding those with large tumors and extrahepatic involvement, is the key to acceptable long-term outcomes. A review from an international tumor registry examined the impact of tumor characteristics on outcome in 422 liver transplant recipients.[64] Tumor size (<5 cm), absence of vascular or lymphatic invasion, and low histological grade all had a significant impact on improvement in long-term outcome. The diagnosis of tumors in explants, where 29% of the tumors in 52 patients were identified incidentally, was also examined.[65] Actuarial 5-year survival rates, calculated for OLT recipients with stage I to III disease and for those without disease, were 79% and 84%, respectively. Researchers from Taiwan recently reported that the p53 gene mutation may help identify patients with HCC who are at greater risk for recurrence.[66]

One of the challenges stemming from the heterogeneous nature of the patient population and discrepancies in transplant outcomes has been difficulty in finding prognostic indicators of poor outcome. A report in 2000 of the Pittsburgh experience with transplantation for HCC suggested a new scoring system to predict the success of liver replacement in patients with HCC.[67] They analyzed clinical and pathological risk factors in 344 HCC patients who underwent OLT at their institution between 1981 and 1998. Through multivariate analysis, three factors were independently identified as being significant predictors of a poor prognosis: tumor size (largest: >5 cm), presence of vascular invasion, and bilobar distribution. They reported mean survival rates of 73%, 58.8%, 49.4%, and 32.7% at 1, 3, 5, and 10 years, respectively, for 69 patients who underwent OLT for HCC; minimum follow-up for the series was 36 months.[68] Tumors were found to recur in 39 (56.6%) patients during the follow-up period. Factors associated with increased tumor recurrence included tumor size greater than 5 cm, more than five nodules, vascular invasion, stage IV (TNM) disease, and the absence of cirrhosis.

Adjuvant Therapy

Adjuvant therapy after liver transplantation has often been considered ineffective, and the prognosis after recurrent disease is dismal. Chemotherapeutic regimens are based on doxorubicin (Adriamycin) chemotherapy, and the use of local therapy such as radiotherapy for local recurrence is still largely anecdotal. Most centers markedly decrease the level of immunosuppression to improve host tumor responsiveness while hoping to not precipitate an acute rejection episode. In a small pilot study by Mazzaferro and coworkers[63] involving 20 patients, doxorubicin alone and in combination with cisplatin was used to treat recurrent disease after transplantation, with encouraging results.[69-71]

In 1997 a group reported an investigation involving the use of preoperative TACE in 111 patients undergoing liver transplantation for HCC.[70] A key observation in the study was a 50% downsizing of tumors larger than 3 cm in diameter, which occurred in 54% of the patients receiving TACE and resulted in a 71% 5-year disease-free survival rate after transplantation. In almost 30% of patients with nearly total tumor necrosis, a disease-free 5-year survival rate approaching 90% was obtained. These results, among the most encouraging noted to date, suggest a significant advantage for patients who respond to this type of adjuvant therapy. Further randomized clinical trials to investigate the use of TACE before transplantation are warranted.

A study from Virginia University monitored 32 patients with pretransplant HCC who underwent a protocol consisting of either radiofrequency ablation or TACE, followed by infusion of doxorubicin and cisplatin to the liver before OLT. After nearly 3 years of patient follow-up, a 100% patient survival rate with only one recurrence has been reported.

Impact of Incidental Hepatocellular Cancer

Currently, up to 40% of HCC found in transplant patients is discovered incidentally, which means that the lesions were detected during routine pathological examination of the explanted organ after transplantation.[64] Data from the Scientific Registry of Transplant Recipients (SRTR) on 21,823 liver transplants performed between July 1994 and December 1999 indicate very little survival difference between patients with known malignancies and those whose malignancies are discovered incidentally. One-, 3-, and 5-year survival rates were 81.0%, 66.2%, and 57.0%, respectively, for those with known malignancy and 81.6%, 68.8%, and 59.3%, respectively, for those with malignancies that were discovered incidentally. Among patients who received transplants for nonmalignant diseases, 1-, 3-, and 5-year survival rates were 84%, 77.8%, and 72.6%, respectively. It should be noted that the SRTR data do not include staging information. Lack of staging stratification of the patients in the study, coupled with the heterogeneous mix of tumor histology in addition to HCC, may account for the significant differences in long-term survival between registry data and data from many single-center studies.

In an analysis of the effect of tumor characteristics on outcome by Klintmalm, the incidental discovery of tumors did not result in a survival benefit.[64] The explanation postulated that undetected lesion growth during the prolonged waiting period before transplantation made the incidental HCCs more prone to recurrence than those that were identified and treated before OLT.

Cholangiocarcinoma

Liver transplant candidates with primary sclerosing cholangitis are at greater risk for the development of both colon cancer and cholangiocarcinoma. Cholangiocarcinoma is manifested in at least two variations. The central extrahepatic variety, also commonly referred to as a Klatskin tumor, is localized mainly to the major bile duct bifurcation at the hepatic hilum. The peripheral intrahepatic variety, which arises from small biliary radicles within the liver parenchyma, is sometimes referred to as cholangiocellular carcinoma. Detection with imaging techniques or serological markers (CA 19-9) has proved unreliable, and although the development of biliary ductal dilatation in at-risk patients may herald the onset of cholangiocarcinoma, pretransplant diagnosis of this malignancy has remained notoriously difficult. Consequently, because of its tendency to disseminate along lymphatic channels and nerves, cholangiocarcinoma remains a clear contraindication to liver transplantation.

The majority of clinical studies have reported poor survival after liver replacement for cholangiocarcinoma, with 1-, 2-, and 5-year survival rates ranging between 53% and 72%, 32% and 48%, and 17% and 25%, respectively. Tumor recurrence, with its corresponding mortality, is the usual explanation for such dismal survival rates. As with HCC, most recurrences appear early, usually within 2 to 3 years after transplantation, with the liver and lungs being the predominant sites of recurrent disease. The largest series of patients (n = 25) to undergo liver transplantation for bile duct carcinoma experienced an overall 5-year survival rate of just 17%. Longer survival was identified in patients with negative lymph nodes and early tumor stages. Several centers have reported attempts to increase the oncological efficacy of the operation by combining total hepatectomy and lymphadenectomy with pancreaticoduodenectomy and liver transplantation (multivisceral resection and cluster transplantation), but the results remain unconvincing.[72]

The incidence of biliary tract carcinoma in primary sclerosing cholangitis is estimated at between 10% and 36%. Lesions discovered incidentally in the explant rather than before liver replacement pose an even greater problem.[73] Because tumors that have remained undetected until transplantation are often at an advanced stage, outcomes in such cases are generally poor. For this reason, the "best" solution presently available is to advocate early transplantation in the course of this illness.

A recent report from the Mayo Clinic has provided some optimism in the treatment of cholangiocarcinoma with liver transplantation.[73a] Their approach, which achieved a 5-year survival rate of 87% in a very select patient population, centers on the pretransplant treatment of isolated bifurcation tumors with external beam radiation and bolus fluorouracil.

Metastatic Neuroendocrine Tumors

In contrast to other malignancies of the liver, neuroendocrine tumors, whether primary or metastatic to the liver, behave less aggressively and replicate more slowly.

Many transplant centers believe that select patients with localized hepatic disease can benefit from liver transplantation, although this approach remains controversial.[74] Before transplantation, the majority of these patients received surgical, chemotherapeutic, or radiotherapeutic intervention, either alone or in varying combinations, for primary lesions of the small bowel or pancreas. Despite good intermediate survival, tumor recurrence in the liver was common. Although recurrence-free survival rates at 5 years were less than 25%, overall recipient survival rates approached 50%, comparable to that for patients with severe hepatitis C reinfection. In a single-center series of 12 patients who underwent OLT for neuroendocrine malignancies, the 5-year survival rate was 81%.[75] Given these outcomes and the capability of transplantation to offer symptomatic relief, with good patient selection, neuroendocrine cancer isolated to the liver need not be an absolute contraindication to transplantation.

Rare Primary Liver Tumors

Included in the category of rare primary tumors of the liver, which on occasion may warrant transplantation, are neoplasms of epithelial origin, such as epithelioid hemangioendothelioma and hepatoblastoma, and mesenchymal lesions, such as sarcoma and hemangiosarcoma. Because of their infrequent appearance and difficulties associated with definitive diagnosis, the data available on these malignancies appear either as limited series or as part of a larger series in which more common tumors are addressed.

Epithelioid hemangioendothelioma is a tumor with distinctive pathological characteristics. In a 1988 report on the largest series to date, Marino and colleagues reported a 5-year disease-free survival rate of 76%, although it was noted that recurrent disease eventually developed in nearly all recipients.[76] Liver transplantation should not be ruled out a priori for patients with epithelioid hemangioendothelioma. Hepatoblastoma is the most commonly encountered childhood malignancy of the liver. Systemic chemotherapy with doxorubicin and cisplatin is administered as first-line therapy to reduce tumor size. In patients with residual disease deemed amenable to hepatic resection, surgical intervention may be used.[77] The largest experience with liver transplantation for hepatoblastoma, which included 12 pediatric cases, was published in 1991. The authors reported a 2-year survival rate of 58% and cited early tumor stage and absence of extrahepatic disease as factors contributing to prolonged disease-free survival.[78]

Liver Metastases

In the Western world, secondary hepatic malignancies are more prevalent than primary liver malignancies.

Less than 40% of those afflicted will be eligible for surgery, which is unfortunate because hepatic resection is the only treatment that offers a significant survival benefit (approximately 30% at 5 years). In the largest series of patients to undergo liver transplantation for secondary malignancy it was reported that 25 of 30 patients had unresectable metastases from colorectal cancer. Seventeen of these recipients lived beyond 3 months; median survival improved markedly to 32 months in the absence of lymphatic spread. The 5-year actuarial survival rate for the series was 16%.[79]

With short- and intermediate-term results being so poor, most transplant physicians agree that liver transplantation for metastatic disease cannot be justified. In a select group of patients with neuroendocrine tumors, namely, those without extrahepatic involvement, liver replacement for palliative purposes may be worthy of consideration.

Recurrence of Preexisting Malignancy

As the age of patients being considered for transplantation increases, the number of candidates with either previous or active malignancies will also increase. Data addressing the impact of immunosuppression on preexisting malignancies must be evaluated to more accurately determine the point at which, after curative intervention has been undertaken, immunosuppressive agents can be safely introduced with minimal risk of inducing recurrence. Penn approached this particular problem in a creative and functional manner by segregating these malignancies into categories based on low, medium, and high rates of recurrence.

Dr. Penn's recommendations were based on findings in 1137 transplant recipients with previous or active malignancies at the time of transplantation.[18,20,21,48,80] Two hundred thirty-nine patients experienced recurrent disease (21%). The effect of interval waiting times was readily apparent, with 54% (128 cases) of tumor recurrences occurring in patients with intervals between treatment and transplantation shorter than 2 years. In patients with a 2- to 5-year wait interval, the percentage decreased to 33% (80 cases). Beyond 5 years, the recurrence rate declined to 13%.

Tumors with Low Recurrence

Incidentally discovered RCC was found to have the lowest incidence (<7%) of tumor recurrence.[21,23] An initial series of small, asymptomatic RCCs discovered incidentally at the time of bilateral nephrectomy demonstrated a 0% recurrence rate. In contrast, RCCs that were either symptomatic or demonstrated evidence

of extracapsular or neurovascular involvement had a recurrence rate approaching 25%.

Patients with histories of uterine or cervical cancer experienced few tumor recurrences when they underwent transplantation before a 5-year waiting period. However, several recurrences were found in individuals who received a transplant after a 5-year wait. Closer inspection of these cases suggests that the reported occurrences may actually have been secondary primary lesions that occurred under the effect of immunosuppression. In the male population, few cases of recurrent testicular cancer were noted to occur. This finding was especially true in patients with early-stage disease, in whom no recurrences were observed. Unfortunately, the majority of patients reported to the registry were transplanted after a median wait interval of 150 months. Finally, thyroid cancer also displayed few tumor recurrences, with Hürthle cell and low-grade papillary carcinoma being among the histological types that were most favorable to nonrecurrence (Table 71–4).

Tumors with Intermediate Recurrence Rates

Tumors found to have an intermediate (8% to 22%) incidence of recurrence include lymphoma, Wilms'

Table 71-4. RISK OF RECURRENCE OF CANCER AFTER LIVER TRANSPLANTATION

	Number of Patients	Recurrence Rate (%)	Treated >5 yr before Transplantation
Low Risk			
Incidental RCC	72	1	0
Uterine	26	4	50
Testicular	43	5	58
Cervical	93	6	54
Thyroid	54	7	38
Intermediate Risk			
Lymphoma	37	11	76
Wilms'	78	13	33
Prostate	33	18	34
Colon	53	21	42
High Risk			
Breast	90	23	51
Symptomatic RCC	222	27	22
Bladder	55	29	22
Sarcoma	17	29	24
Skin	25	53	11

RCC, renal cell carcinoma.

tumor, prostate and colon cancer, and melanoma.[21,23] The majority of patients with these cancers had waiting times longer than 5 years. Recurrence of colon and prostate cancer most directly related to tumor stage (see Table 71–4).

Tumors with High Recurrence Rates

Several aggressive malignancies were found to have high rates of recurrence (>23%). Included in this category are soft tissue sarcomas, breast cancer, and symptomatic RCC.[21,23,48,80,81] Recurrence in patients with soft tissue sarcomas was based on tumor grade. Transplant recipients who suffered tumor recurrence all had high-grade sarcomas; the overall incidence of recurrence among high-grade lesions was 43%. In breast cancer survivors, tumor recurrence has been reported many years after the patient's primary disease had been treated. Individuals with stage I and stage II breast cancer saw limited recurrence, with rates of 6% and 8%, respectively. In stage III patients, tumor recurrence was a staggering 64%, with a corresponding 5-year survival rate of 14%. In the case of RCC, patients with the highest recurrence rates were those with symptomatic lesions (80%) or bilateral cancer (25%).

Several malignancies have a demonstrated a propensity for multifocal recurrence, whether as local recurrence or as secondary primaries. Transitional cell carcinoma of the bladder and nonmelanoma skin cancer often occur as metachronous, multifocal lesions rather than as extensions of a localized primary lesion. Although the majority of skin and bladder cancers are considered nuisance malignancies, a small number were found to be manifested as advanced local disease or as nodal metastasis (see Table 71–4).

Posttransplant Cancer Screening

Individuals at risk for the development of female malignancies such as breast cancer should undergo routine screening based on their age and risk factors. The most important risk factors for the development of breast cancer are a history of previous breast cancer or a first-degree relative in whom breast cancer has developed. If a risk factor or factors exist, mammography should be initiated before 50 years of age. Annual or biennial mammography is otherwise recommended after the age of 50 and should be performed in addition to routine self-examination. Annual Papanicolaou smears should also be obtained as part of routine monitoring for cervical cancer.[82]

Males older than 40 years should undergo routine screening for prostate cancer. Serum prostate-specific

Table 71–5. POSTTRANSPLANT CANCER SCREENING

Breast

Women > 50 yr: mammogram every 1–2 yr

Women < 50 yr at high risk (family history or previous cancer): mammogram every 1–2 yr

Cervical

Women > 18 yr: Papanicolaou smear every year

Prostate

Men > 40 yr: rectal examination and prostate-specific antigen every year

Colorectal

Recipients > 50 yr: fecal blood test yearly and flexible sigmoidoscopy every 5 yr

Skin

Annual self-examination and biopsy of all suspicious lesions

antigen, which has a sensitivity approaching 70%, should be incorporated as part of routine screening. Colorectal screening should begin at 50 years of age in all transplant recipients unless there is a history of familial colon cancer, polyps, or inflammatory bowel disease. Testing for fecal occult blood should be performed annually, with flexible sigmoidoscopy or full colonoscopic examination being performed every 5 years. In addition to regular self-examination, screening for skin cancer should include an annual routine examination by the patient's primary care physician or dermatologist, with early biopsy being performed on all suspicious lesions (Table 71–5).[81]

Pearls and Pitfalls

Pearls

- Evaluate potential recipients for all previous malignancies and identify their stage and therapy.

- High-risk donors should be selected carefully by diligent survey of the patient's history and intraoperative evaluation of the donor.

- Posttransplant lymphoproliferative disorder should be managed as though it were a spectrum of diseases, with treatment ranging from antiviral therapy, reduction of immunosuppression, and use of biological agents, to systemic chemotherapy.

- De novo skin and solid-organ malignancies should be aggressively treated surgically, and maintenance immunosuppression should be modified.

Pearls and Pitfalls—cont'd

Pitfalls

- Donors with high-grade brain tumors, surgical shunts, or extensive craniotomies should be avoided.
- Donors with a history of melanoma should be avoided.
- Recipients with Kaposi's sarcoma or advanced stage (III/IV) carcinoma should be avoided.
- Not all patients with posttransplant lymphoproliferative disorder should receive systemic chemotherapy.

References

1. Penn I: Cancers in renal transplant recipients. Adv Ren Replace Ther 7:147-156, 2000.
2. Penn I: Post-transplant malignancy: The role of immunosuppression. Drug Saf 23:101-113, 2000.
3. Penn I: Occurrence of cancers in immunosuppressed organ transplant recipients. Clin Tranpl 147-148, 1998.
4. Diehl V, Hauch PM, Harris NL: Hodgkin's disease. In DeVita VT, Hellman S, Rosenberg SA (eds): Cancer Principles and Practice of Oncology. Philadelphia, Lippincott Williams & Wilkins, 2001, pp 2339-2387.
5. Yarchoan R, Little RF: Immunosuppression-related malignancies. In DeVita VT, Hellman S, Rosenberg SA (eds): Cancer Principles and Practice of Oncology. Philadelphia, Lippincott Williams & Wilkins, 2001, pp 2575-2996.
6. Hojo M, Morimoto T, Maluccio M, et al: Cyclosporine induces cancer progression by a cell-autonomous mechanism. Nature 397:530-534, 1999.
7. 2001 Annual Report of the US Organ Procurement and Transplantation Network and the Scientific Registry for Transplant Recipients: Transplant Data 1991-2002. Department of Health and Human Services, Health Resources and Services Administration, Office of Special Programs. Division of Transplantation, Rockville, MD; United Network for Organ Sharing, Richmond, VA; University Renal Research and Education Association, Ann Arbor, MI.
8. Dreno B, Mansat E, Legoux B, Litoux P: Skin cancers in transplant patients. Nephrol Dial Transplant 13:1374-1379, 1998.
9. Gupta AK, Cardella CJ, Habeman HF: Cutaneous malignant neoplasms in patients with renal transplants. Arch Dermatol 122:1288-1293, 1986.
10. Penn I: Donor transmitted disease: Cancer. Transplant Proc 23:2629-2631, 1991.
11. Penn I: Malignancy transmitted from the organ donor. Graft 1(Suppl I):19-20, 1998.
12. Kauffman HM, McBride MA, Delmonico FL: First report of the United Network for Organ Sharing Transplant Tumor Registry: Donors with a history of cancer. Transplantation 70:1747-1751, 2000.
13. Kauffman HM, McBride MA, Cherikh WS, et al: Transplant tumor registry: Donor related malignancies. Transplantation 74:358-362, 2002.
14. Chui AKK, Herbertt K, Wang LS, et al: Risk of tumor transmission in transplantation from donors with primary brain tumors: An Australian and New Zealand Registry report. Transplant Proc 31:1266-1267, 1999.
15. Buell JF, Trofe J, Sethuraman G, et al: Donors with central nervous system malignancies: Are they truly safe? Transplantation 76:340-343, 2003.
16. Penn I: Transmission of cancer from organ donors. Ann Transplant 2(4):7-12, 1997.
17. Buell JF, Beebe TM, Gross TG, et al: Can donor kidneys with small renal cell cancers be safely transplanted? Am J Transplant 3:176, 2003.
18. Penn I: Kidney transplantation following treatment of tumors. Transplant Proc 18(Suppl 3):16-20, 1986.
19. Penn I: Primary kidney tumors before and after renal transplantation. Transplantation 59:480-485, 1995.
20. Penn I: Evaluation of transplant candidates with pre-existing malignancies. Ann Transplant 2(4):14-17, 1997.
21. Penn I: Evaluation of the candidate with a previous malignancy. Liver Transpl Surg 2(Suppl 1):109-113, 1996.
22. Adams R: The impact of breast or colon cancer. Paper presented at the Third Annual ASTS Winter Symposium, January 24-26, 2003, Miami Beach, FL.
23. Buell JF: Israel Penn International Transplant Tumor Registry. Paper presented at the Third Annual ASTS Winter Symposium, January 24-26, 2003, Miami Beach, FL.
24. Penn I: Immunosuppression and skin cancer. Clin Plast Surg 7:361-368, 1980.
25. Penn I: Cancer and kidney transplantation. In Toledo-Pereyra LH (ed): Kidney Transplantation. Philadelphia, FA Davis, 1988, pp 205-214.
26. Rosenberg SA: Principles of cancer management: Biologic therapy. In DeVita VT, Hellman S, Rosenberg SA (eds): Cancer Principles and Practice of Oncology. Philadelphia, Lippincott Williams & Wilkins, 2001, pp 307-344.
27. Paya CV, Fung JJ, Nalesnik MA, et al: Epstein-Barr virus–induced posttransplant lymphoproliferative disorders. Transplantation 68:1517-1525, 1999.
28. Crum CP, Abbott DW, Quade BJ: Cervical cancer screening: From the Papanicolaou smear to the vaccine era. J Clin Oncol 21(10 Suppl):224-230, 2003.
29. Yoo SS, Whitmore SE: A human papillomavirus type 16 vaccine. N Engl J Med 348:1402-1405, 2003.
30. Brown MR, Noffsinger A, First MR, et al: HPV subtype analysis in lower genital tract neoplasms of female renal transplant recipients. Gynecol Oncol 70:220-224, 2000.
31. Frances C: Kaposi's sarcoma after renal transplantation. Nephrol Transplant 13:2768-2773, 1998.
32. Penn I: Kaposi's sarcoma in transplants recipients. Transplantation 64:669-673, 1997.
33. Penn I: The changing pattern of post-transplant malignancies. Transplant Proc 23:1101-1103, 1991.
34. Buell JF, Gross TG, Beebe TM, et al: Cancer after renal transplantation. In Cohen E (ed): Cancer and the Kidney. (in press)
35. Hartevelt MM, Vavinck JN, Kootte AM, et al: Incidence of skin cancer after renal transplantation in The Netherlands. Transplantation 49:506-509, 1990.
36. Sayegh MH, Brennan DC: Development of malignancy following solid organ transplantation. Up to Date Online [serial online]. June 25, 2001, version 10:1.
37. Penn I: Skin disorders in organ transplant recipients: External anogenital lesions [editorial]. Arch Dermatol 133:221-223, 1997.
38. Penn I: Post-transplant kidney cancers and skin cancers (including Kaposi's sarcoma). In Schmähl D, Penn I (eds): Cancer in Organ Transplant Recipients. Berlin, Springer-Verlag, 1991, pp 46-53.
39. Penn I: Post transplantation de novo tumors in liver allograft recipients. Liver Transpl Surg 1:52-59, 1996.

40. Kelly DM, Emere S, Guy SR, et al: Liver transplant recipients are not at increased risk for nonlymphoid solid organ tumors. Cancer 6:1237-1243, 1998.
41. Sheiner PA, Magliocca JF, Bodain CA, et al: Long-term medical complications in patients surviving greater or equal to five years after liver transplant. Transplantation 69:781-789, 2000.
42. Jonas S, Rayes N, Neumann U, et al: De novo malignancies after liver transplantation using tacrolimus-based protocols or cyclosporine-based quadruple immunosuppression with an interleukin-2 receptor antibody or antithymocyte globulin. Cancer 80:1141-1150, 1997.
43. Scheiner P: Paper presented at the Seventh Congress of the International Liver Transplantation Society, Berlin, July 12, 2001.
44. Jain AB, Yee LD, Nalesnik MA, et al: Comparative incidence of de novo nonlymphoid malignancies after liver transplantation under tacrolimus using surveillance epidemiologic end result data. Transplantation 66:1193-2000, 1998.
45. Jain A, DiMartini A, Kashyap R, et al: Long-term follow-up after liver transplantation for alcoholic liver disease under tacrolimus. Transplantation 70:1335-1335, 2000.
46. Ries LA: SEER Cancer Statistical Review, 1973-1993: Tables and Graphs. Bethesda, MD, National Cancer Institute, 1996.
47. Jain A, Nalesnik M, Reyes J, et al: Posttransplant lymphoproliferative disorders in liver transplantation: A 20-year experience. Ann Surg 4:429-437, 2002.
47a. Hanaway MJ, Buell JF, Rudich S, et al: Am J Transplant 3:211, 2003.
48. Penn I: Recurrence of malignant disease post transplantation [letter]. Transpl Immunol 12(3):10-11, 1996.
49. Buell JF, Hanaway MJ, Trofe J, et al: Post-transplant lymphoproliferative disorder in liver transplant recipients: Comparison between children and adults. Am J Transplant 2:438, 2002.
50. Trofe J, Buell JF, First MR, et al: The role of immunosuppression in lymphoma. Recent Results Cancer Res 159:55-66, 2002.
51. Hanaway MJ, Buell JF, Trofe J, et al: De novo liver malignancy after liver transplantation. Liver Transpl 7(6):C-39, 2001.
52. Hemming AW, Langer B, Sheiner P, et al: Aggressive surgical management of fibrolamellar hepatocellular carcinoma. J Gastrointest Surg 1:342-346, 1997.
53. Poon RT, Fan ST, Lo CM, et al: Improving survival results after resection of hepatocellular carcinoma: A prospective study of 377 patients over 10 years. Ann Surg 234:63-70, 2001.
54. Fan ST, Lai EC, Lo CM, et al: Hospital mortality of major hepatectomy for hepatocellular carcinoma associated with cirrhosis. Arch Surg 130:198-203, 1995.
55. Llovet JM, Fuster J, Bruix J: Intention-to-treat analysis of surgical treatment for early hepatocellular carcinoma: Resection versus transplantation. Hepatology 30:1434-1440, 1999.
56. Watson RW: The rising incidence of hepatocellular carcinoma. N Engl J Med 340:734-750, 1999.
57. Cha C, Dematteo RP, Blumgart LH: Surgical therapy for hepatocellular carcinoma. Adv Surg 38:363-376, 2004.
58. Figueras J, Jaurrieta E, Valls C, et al: Survival after liver transplantation in cirrhotic patients with and without hepatocellular carcinoma: A comparative study. Hepatology 25:1485-1489, 1997.
59. Min AD, Saxena R, Thung SN, et al: Outcome of hepatitis C patients with and without hepatocellular carcinoma undergoing liver transplant. Am J Gastroenterol 93:2148-2153, 1998.
60. Iwatsuki S, Starzl TE, Sheahan DG, et al: Hepatic resection versus transplantation for hepatocellular carcinoma. Ann Surg 214:221-229, 1991.
61. Colella G, Bottelli R, De Carlis L, et al: Hepatocellular carcinoma: Comparison between liver transplantation, resective surgery, ethanol injection, and chemoembolization. Transpl Int 11(Suppl 1):S193-S196, 1998.
62. Herrero JI, Sangro B, Quiroga J, et al: Influence of tumor characteristics on the outcome of liver transplantation among patients with liver cirrhosis and hepatocellular carcinoma. Liver Transpl 7:631-636, 2001.
63. Mazzaferro V, Regalia E, Doci R, et al: Liver transplantation for the treatment of small hepatocellular carcinomas in patients with cirrhosis. N Engl J Med 334:693-699, 1996.
64. Klintmalm GB: Liver transplantation for hepatocellular carcinoma: A registry report of the impact of tumor characteristics on outcome. Ann Surg 228:479-490, 1998.
65. Bechstein WO, Guckelberger O, Kling N, et al: Recurrence-free survival after liver transplantation for small hepatocellular carcinoma. Transpl Int 11(Suppl 1):S189-S192, 1998.
66. Jeng KS, Sheen IS, Chen BF, Wu JY: Is the p53 gene mutation of prognostic value in hepatocellular carcinoma after resection? Arch Surg 135:1329-1333, 2000.
67. Iwatsuki S, Dvorchik I, Marsh JW, et al: Liver transplantation for hepatocellular carcinoma: A proposal of a prognostic scoring system. J Am Coll Surg 191:389-394, 2000.
68. Schlitt HJ, Neipp M, Weimann A, et al: Recurrence patterns of hepatocellular and fibrolamellar carcinoma after liver transplantation. J Clin Oncol 17:324-331, 1999.
69. Olthoff KM, Rosove MH, Shackleton CR, et al: Adjuvant chemotherapy improves survival after liver transplantation for hepatocellular carcinoma. Ann Surg 221:734-743, 1995.
70. Majno PE, Adam R, Bismuth H, et al: Influence of preoperative transarterial Lipiodol chemoembolization on resection and transplantation for hepatocellular carcinoma in patients with cirrhosis. Ann Surg 226:688-703, 1997.
71. Stone MJ, Klintmalm GB, Polter D, et al: Neoadjuvant chemotherapy and liver transplantation for hepatocellular carcinoma: A pilot study in 20 patients. Gastroenterology 104:196-202, 1993.
72. Tzakis AG, Todo S, Madariaga J, et al: Upper-abdominal exenteration in transplantation for extensive malignancies of the upper abdomen—an update. Transplantation 51:727-728, 1991.
73. Nashan B, Schlitt HJ, Tusch G, et al: Biliary malignancies in primary sclerosing cholangitis: Timing for liver transplantation. Hepatology 23:1105-1111, 1996.
73a. Heimbach JK, Haddock MG, Alberts SR, et al: Transplantation for hilar cholangiocarcinoma. Liver Transpl 10(10 Suppl 2):S65-S68, 2004.
74. Lehnert T: Liver transplantation for metastatic neuroendocrine carcinoma: An analysis of 103 patients. Transplantation 66:1307-1312, 1998.
75. Lang H, Oldhafer KJ, Weimann A, et al: Liver transplantation for metastatic neuroendocrine tumors. Ann Surg 225:347-354, 1997.
76. Marino IR, Todo S, Tzakis AG, et al: Treatment of hepatic epithelioid hemangioendothelioma with liver transplantation. Cancer 62:2079-2084, 1988.
77. Tagge EP, Tagge DU, Reyes J, et al: Resection, including trasplantation, for hepatoblastoma and hepatocellular carcinoma: Impact on survival. J Pediatr Surg 27:292-297, 1992.
78. Koneru B, Flye MW, Busuttil RW, et al: Liver transplantation for hepatoblastoma. The American experience. Ann Surg 213:118-121, 1991.
79. Muhlbacher F, Huk I, Steininger R, et al: Is orthotopic liver transplantation a feasible treatment for secondary cancer of the liver? Transplant Proc 23(1 Pt 2):1567-1568, 1991.
80. Penn I: The effect of renal transplantation in patients with a history of curative cancer therapy. In Stewart THM, Wheelock EF (eds): Cellular Immune Mechanisms and Tumor Dormancy. CRC Press, Boca Raton, FL, 1992, pp 239-260.
81. Kasiske BL, Cangro CB, Hariharan S, et al: The evaluation of renal transplantation candidates: Clinical practice guidelines. Am J Transplant 1(Suppl 2):1-95, 2002.
82. Amare D, Buell JF: Management of malignancy after renal transplantation. The Transplant Nephrology Community Outreach Program at the University of Alabama School of Medicine, April 2003.

X

Immunology of Liver Transplantation

Rejection After Transplantation

GERALD S. LIPSHUTZ

NANCY L. ASCHER

JOHN P. ROBERTS

Models used to define rejection   1168

Cellular basis for liver allograft rejection   1169

CD4+ cells and rejection   1171

HLA antigens and rejection   1172

Antibody-mediated liver rejection   1173

Nitric oxide production in acute rejection   1174

Role of cytokines in liver allograft
    rejection   1174

Hepatitis C and hepatic allograft rejection   1175

Methods of diagnosis of acute liver
    transplant rejection   1176

Grading of rejection on biopsy   1177

Liver transplantation is recognized as optimal therapy for acute and chronic end-stage liver disease and metabolic disease. Results today are excellent, with 1- and 5-year patient survival rates of up to 90% and 75%,[1] depending on the status of the patient and center-related factors. However, the frequency of acute rejection after transplantation ranges from 30% to 70%[2-6] within the first year of transplantation, with the highest incidence in the first 7 to 10 days[6] and the vast majority of episodes occurring in the first 1 to 2 months after transplantation.[7] Long-term, single episodes of acute rejection do not impair hepatic function[8,9]; however, recurrent episodes may result in permanent damage to the liver allograft.[10]

Hepatic allograft rejection is classified into acute and chronic rejection based on timing, reversibility, and the histological features of the inflammatory infiltrate.[11] The features of both types of rejection can occur at any time and in combination, and thus the terms *acute* and *chronic* seem inappropriate at times.[11] The term *acute cellular rejection* better defines the histological features of a portal-based hepatitis, nonsuppurative destructive cholangitis, and endotheliitis (Snover's triad). Conversely, the main histological feature of "chronic rejection" is progressive bile duct destruction that leads to a decrease in the number of interlobular and septal bile ducts (ductopenia), frequently seen without significant inflammation.[11] In addition, progressive intimal and subintimal inflammation of second and third order hepatic arterial branches occurs, resulting in obliterative endarteritis[12] and ischemia of zone 3 hepatocytes and interlobular bile ducts.[13] Approximately 10% of liver allograft recipients who develop acute cellular rejection do go on to develop severe ductopenic (chronic) rejection.[14] These patients may ultimately require retransplantation because of chronic rejection.

Acute cellular rejection (ACR) is a T-cell–mediated response. The targets of this response are major and minor histocompatibility antigens on cells.[15] Factors known to affect cell-mediated immunity may influence the incidence of rejection.[16] Rejection is more likely to occur in younger patients, black patients,[17] those who undergo transplantation for autoimmune disease,[18] those with fulminant hepatic failure, transplants with fewer HLA-DR matches, cold ischemia times of 15 hours or longer, donor age of 30 years or older,[19] recipients with hepatitis C infection,[20] and in those with less severe liver disease. The original disease also affects the incidence of rejection. For example, rates of acute cellular rejection in patients with alcoholic liver disease are lower than in patients with primary biliary cirrhosis.[21] This difference may be a result of the nutritional state of the recipient,[16] as alcoholic cirrhotic patients are often severely malnourished.[22] Conversely, the prior targets of the immune system in the patient with primary biliary cirrhosis, the bile ducts, may predispose to rejection.

Rat models[23] of liver allograft tolerance show that graft acceptance is characterized by the presence of nondestructive cellular infiltrates. These infiltrates are histologically indistinguishable from the characteristic periportal infiltrates that characterize acute cellular rejection.[24] The cellular infiltrate seen with rejection may not always be a bad thing. It has been proposed that mild acute rejection in the human liver allograft without biochemical hepatic dysfunction represents an analogous situation to the rat.[25] This lymphocyte trafficking may be contributing to the development of immunological tolerance.

This chapter presents current ideas regarding the mechanisms of liver allograft rejection.

Models Used to Define Rejection

The definition of rejection is a composite one, derived from human and animal data. In vitro study of cells, direct histological examination of the allograft, and animal models of acute rejection are the main methods used to understand the mechanisms underlying acute liver transplant rejection. In some animal models of transplantation, immunosuppressive agents are used to prevent or modify rejection. When immunosuppressive agents with known mechanisms of actions are used in these settings, the relative importance of a specific mechanism may be assigned based on the known effects of that agent.

Because the understanding of rejection is based on various models, it is important to be aware of the limitations of a given model relative to our total concept of the transplantation process. In vitro coculture systems such as cell-mediated cytotoxicity define potential cellular interactions and have proved invaluable in the definition and characterization of helper T cells, cytotoxic T cells, and antigen-presenting cells (APC). The in vitro system is limited, however, because the coculture environment allows for optimization of culture conditions and the relevant cytokines. As such, it may not reflect the in vivo response in which cytokines may be absent or at low levels and the precursor cells may be compartmentalized rather than in direct proximity with each other or with host antigen. The technique of limiting dilution analysis, for example, maximizes the number of stimulator cells and culture nutrients to facilitate determination of a limited number of responder cells. Although a small number of specific cells can be expanded under such conditions, they may not be readily identified in an in vivo system.

As an alternative to isolated in vitro models, one can remove cells from the graft and examine their functional capacity in vitro. In this way the cells can be activated to undergo the immunological events occurring in the graft and then be examined in vitro. The cells of interest could be recovered from peripheral blood or biopsy specimens or by using more novel techniques such as allogeneic-coated sponge matrix allografts.[26,27] For example, the ability of the cells found in the peripheral blood after transplantation to damage target cells sharing major histocompatibility antigens with the donor can be studied. The cells may be used directly in a cytotoxicity assay if enough cells can be removed. Using this approach, one is dependent on the adequacy of the in vitro assay to infer the in vivo function of the cell. If only a few cells can be removed directly, they may be cultured in vitro to expand the population. This approach has been criticized because the in vitro culturing and expansion are done in the presence of donor antigen and therefore may select for recipient cells with reactivity against donor antigen.

Examination of the histological features of acute cellular rejection allows for a recording of the rejection response; the presence of a cell type is used to infer that the cell plays an important role in the rejection process. Examination of the histological picture does not help us understand the cell-cell interaction or the specific mechanisms of the immune response. As methods for determining the state of activation of a cell improve, the inferences regarding the role of a given cell type may become more accurate. The use of immunohistochemistry is expanding rapidly with the ability to examine tissue for a wide number of proteins. This field may make important contributions to our understanding of the rejection process.

Animal models[28] may be limited because of different responses to alloantigen in different species, different sensitivity to immunosuppression, variation in the toxicity profile of agents in different species, tolerance to portal revascularization, and the ease with which tolerance is induced in some models. Perhaps the models that have the greatest potential to define specific cellular mechanisms are those in which the host animal is depleted of responding cells and is subsequently repopulated with one or more specific cell types or clones (i.e., adoptive transfer experiments). Although this approach does not address the issue of the compartmentalization of cells or cytokines within the host, it is useful for screening cell types that can injure allografts.

The mouse is frequently used in models to define allograft response. Although the ability to perform liver transplantation in the mouse is limited, some investigators have achieved success in this area[29] and found that success after liver transplantation did not follow major histocompatibility complex (MHC) disparity between donor and recipient as would be predicted by in vitro coculture studies. Because of the technical difficulties involved in the liver transplantation procedure, the rat is the model most frequently used to study liver allograft response. The rat, which has been a common model for the testing of factors related to liver preservation and transplantation, does not require rearterialization for successful liver transplantation. Rat donor-recipient combinations vary widely in the kinetics of the rejection response and the ability to induce tolerance[24,30]; the explanation for this variability is unclear but must be borne in mind by investigators planning to study a specific treatment modality.

A short course of immunosuppressive therapy in the rat can lead to long-term graft acceptance without the need for further therapy.[31] The mechanism by which this state of unresponsiveness develops is unknown and must be critically examined in the light of the emerging information regarding the development of human chimeras following solid-organ transplantation.[32] Rejection has been described extensively in rat liver allografts; the histological differences in the high responder versus the low responder are mainly in the kinetics of the rejection response[24] and in different patterns of infiltrating cells. Rejection has also been described in larger animal models[33]; these findings offer the advantage of being more clinically relevant because, unlike most rat liver allografts, allograft tolerance with a short course of immunosuppression is not to be expected with canine and porcine grafts.

Another factor that separates animal studies from the experience in humans is the historical exposure to infectious agents. Exposure to infectious agents in specific pathogen-free laboratory rodents can be controlled, unlike in large nonhuman primates and human patients. This acquired immune history may result in a heterologous immune response—specifically, virally induced alloreactive memory—that is a potent barrier to tolerance induction.[34,35] Thus, an understanding of the human liver allograft response depends on a composite of animal models and observations and of the histological patterns and response to treatment seen in liver transplant patients.

Cellular Basis for Liver Allograft Rejection

The histological characteristics of acute rejection[2-5,36,37] are based on the presence of a largely portal-based inflammatory cell infiltrate with injury to liver components. The early targets of acute cellular liver transplant rejection are the bile duct epithelium and the venous endothelium. If allowed to progress, hepatocytes may demonstrate signs of injury, either from direct immune attack or as an effect of vascular injury and subsequent ischemia.

The lymphocyte is the predominant cell type involved in acute cellular rejection. Liver allograft rejection is mediated by a primary response of T lymphocytes, followed by a mixed inflammatory infiltrate. The lymphocyte population contains both CD4+ and CD8+ cells,[38,39] and once activated, these cells proliferate, differentiate, and secrete cytokines. The appearance of CD4+ lymphocytes within the portal tracts predicts rejection even before biochemical evidence is present.[40] At the time of the rejection response (as defined by injury to the small bile ducts and elevated serum alkaline phosphatase levels), the predominant lymphocyte within the portal tracts displays the CD8+ phenotype. Acute rejection and chronic rejection correlate with the presence of CD8+ rather than CD4+ cells within portal tracts.[39] Investigators at the Mayo Clinic found an association between the patterns of the inflammatory response and the response to treatment of rejection.[41] These investigations indicate that CD4+ cells are important in initiating and amplifying the immune response and that CD8+ cells have an important effector role in the rejection process.

The other cells present within the portal tracts are considered to be part of a nonspecific inflammatory response. Their appearance likely reflects the influence of local cytokines in the inflammatory response. Polymorphonuclear neutrophils appear in the setting of rejection but also appear with acute cholangitis and cytomegalovirus (CMV) infection. Neutrophils may be the predominant cell type in late or partially treated rejection, which can make the differential diagnosis of rejection versus biliary disease particularly difficult.

Eosinophils are a frequent feature of liver allograft rejection, although the relative number of these cells is generally less than 5%. Peripheral eosinophilia has also been identified in kidney and liver allograft recipients with acute rejection.[42,43] CD4[+] T helper 2 (T$_H$2) cells secrete interleukin (IL)-5, which attracts eosinophils to the portal triads, causing further inflammation and injury. The identification of message for IL-5 in rejecting liver allografts supports the role of eosinophils in liver graft rejection.[44,45] The predictive value of the *blood* eosinophil count in the diagnosis of acute cellular rejection and the value as a marker of response to treatment has been examined.[46] An elevated eosinophil count has a positive predictive value for acute cellular rejection of the liver, whereas a normal count generally excludes moderate or severe rejection. There is interest in using peripheral eosinophilia as a marker to differentiate between rejection and recurrent hepatitis C.[46]

Macrophages and plasma cells make up the remainder of the cells present at the graft site. The macrophages are presumed to be part of a nonspecific inflammatory response. Plasma cells have not been tested in terms of antibody specificity. There is some interest in using the pattern of peripheral blood lymphocytes to predict liver allograft rejection. In general, the study of peripheral blood lymphocytes as a marker of acute rejection is of limited value in recipients of liver, kidney, and heart allografts.[47-50]

Class I MHC molecules (human leukocyte antigen [HLA] A, B, and C) are expressed on all nucleated cells. They consist of a 44-kD heavy chain noncovalently linked to β_2-microglobulin. Class II MHC molecules (HLA DR, DP, DQ) contain a 34-kD alpha chain and a 29-kD beta chain. These molecules are normally expressed on APCs (macrophages and dendritic cells), activated T and B cells, and Kupffer cells. According to classic models, CD4[+] cells recognize antigens (i.e., exogenous peptides) in the context of MHC class II antigen, and CD8[+] cells recognize antigens (i.e., endogenous or viral antigens) in the context of class I antigens. Essential to the initiation of acute cellular rejection is recipient T-cell recognition of allo-MHC-peptide complexes on donor APCs. Transplanted livers contain large numbers of donor APCs and these serve as the primary stimulation of the recipient's alloreactive T-cell receptors.[13]

Ibrahim and colleagues[51] and Dollinger and colleagues[52] analyzed rejecting versus nonrejecting specimens according to cell phenotype and location using markers of cell activation. Proliferation of mononuclear leukocytes inside the liver allograft was a prominent feature of acute rejection; they were located predominantly in the portal tracts at the site of the inflammatory infiltrate and found to decrease in response to treatment with corticosteroids. Increased numbers of portal CD3[+] T cells were found in rejecting compared with nonrejecting liver grafts.[51] The increased number of CD3[+] cells could be accounted for mainly by an increased number of CD8[+] cells. Examination of the CD45 marker revealed an increase in memory cells

(CD45 RO[+]) but not in "naïve cells" (CD45 RA)[51]; these were located periportally.[52] CD8[+] T lymphocytes, CD57[+] natural killer cells, and CD68[+] macrophages, however, were located intraparenchymally throughout the lobules, whereas CD20[+] B lymphocytes were present only in some of the portal tracts.[52] It is believed that the CD8[+] cells that are present cause graft injury via cytolytic activity directed against donor alloantigen. This scheme is consistent with classic models of cytotoxic effector cells that are dependent on helper T cells for differentiation and maturation.[53]

Other investigations have found that early acute rejection is also characterized by a higher expression of CD4[+] CD7[+] and CD8[+] CD38[+] T lymphocytes in the liver than in peripheral blood. Moreover, a preferential proinflammatory (T helper 1 [T$_H$1] cell [see the next section, "CD4[+] Cells and Rejection"]) cytokine profile was related to liver-resident T lymphocytes in comparison with corresponding plasma. However, in the patients without acute rejection, CD4[+] CD7[+] T lymphocytes were higher in blood than in liver and the T$_H$2-like cytokine profile characterized these subjects. These studies suggest that a preferential T$_H$1 immune mechanism operates in a local fashion and may be involved in acute rejection.[54]

Investigations by Ibrahim[51] at Duke University Medical Center support an effector role of memory CD8[+] cells. These cells may be independent of the requirement of CD4[+] cell-based help and capable of maturation and cytolytic function in the presence of inflammatory mediators and cytokines. The central role of the lymphocyte in acute liver allograft rejection is also supported by the Pittsburgh group led by Zeevi and Duquesnoy.[55,56] These investigators were able to culture clones of antidonor reactive cells from small liver biopsy specimens in the setting of acute rejection, but they were unsuccessful when rejection was not present. Although lymphocytes infiltrated the biopsy specimens of patients with hepatitis, the lymphocytes were much more resistant to in vitro propagation compared with cells in the biopsy specimens of patients with rejection. This work was confirmed by Kolbeck and colleagues[57] in liver transplant recipients.

Other investigators have shown similar antidonor activity of cells cultured from rejecting kidney allografts.[58-60] The reactive clones identified in this work demonstrated antidonor cytolytic activity and were directed against either class II or class I HLA cells of the donor. That lymphocytes from biopsy specimens showing no rejection could also be propagated with alloreactivity demonstrates the particular conditions used: donor alloantigen in the form of the liver tissue and exogenous IL-2 favor alloreactive lymphocyte proliferation. The work from the Pittsburgh group in liver and cardiac allograft recipients indicates that the presence of antidonor reactive cells within biopsy specimens may precede evidence of injury to specific liver or heart targets. Additional examination of this point is important, because there is considerable debate regarding the appropriate treatment of a patient whose liver biopsy specimen demonstrates inflammation in the absence of bile duct injury.

The induction of tolerance in liver transplantation is associated with an increased rate of apoptosis of T lymphocytes in the portal inflammatory infiltrate and the presence of an intragraft T_H2-like T-cell population.[61] Kupffer cells reside in the hepatic sinusoids and are believed to be able to directly interact with circulating T lymphocytes. As such, Kupffer cells may play a unique role in immunomodulation. Recent investigation demonstrates that the Kupffer cells can suppress T-cell proliferation in vitro in mixed leukocyte reactions.[61] In addition, Kupffer cells express functional Fas ligand and can induce apoptosis of Fas-positive cells. This process can be blocked by the addition of neutralizing anti-Fas ligand antibody. Using an allogeneic liver transplant model, Sun and colleagues[61] demonstrated that Kupffer cells recovered from chronically accepted hepatic allografts have increased Fas ligand messenger ribonucleic acid (mRNA) and protein expression. In addition, they have a greater ability to induce apoptosis of alloreactive T cells as compared with Kupffer cells obtained from animals with acute rejection. Furthermore, they demonstrated that Kupffer cells not only induce apoptosis of T cells but also regulate cytokine production and the T_H2/ T helper 3 (T_H3)-like cytokine mRNA expression in allogeneic mixed lymphocyte reaction. Finally, they were able to demonstrate that administration of Kupffer cells derived from allogeneic transplants with spontaneous tolerance in rats actually prolong the survival of hepatic allografts in animals with acute rejection.[61]

CD4+ Cells and Rejection

Clinical observation supports the concept that CD4+ cells have a central role in liver allograft rejection by acting through CD8+ effector cells; agents that act through suppression of IL-2 production and release, such as cyclosporine and tacrolimus, play a major role in inhibition of the rejection response.[62] T helper (T_H) cells have been categorized as T_H1 or T_H2 based on a function and cytokine profile. These cytokines result in the activation, proliferation, and differentiation of other lymphocytes.[63] These cells have been implicated in tolerance induction to organ allografts and in acute cellular rejection.[64-66] When CD4+ T_H0 cells are activated, IL-2, IL-4, and interferon (IFN)-γ are secreted. This activation results in two phenotypes:

1. T_H1 cells—producing IL-2, IFN-α, tumor necrosis factor-alpha/beta (TNF-α/β), and supporting cellular responses, including acute allograft rejection (generating cytotoxic T lymphocytes and activating macrophages)

2. T_H2 cells—producing IL-4, IL-5, IL-6, IL-10, and IL-13, and supporting humoral (antibody-mediated [immunoglobulin (Ig)G1 and IgE]) responses

In addition, these cytokines may counteract ACR by suppressing delayed-type hypersensitivity and inhibiting activation of macrophages induced by T_H1 cells. In this way, these subsets of cells regulate one another, which may relate to the observation that either cellular or antibody-mediated responses predominate in a given immune response.[67]

In infection models, the susceptibility of a host to infection can be decreased by conversion of a phenotype from T_H2 to T_H1.[68] The converse might also be expected. In long-surviving hepatic allografts in animals, a T_H2 cytokine profile appears to predominate and T_H1 cytokines are absent; in rejecting grafts, the T_H1 cytokine profile predominates.[69] IL-10 may be instrumental in this shift in phenotype necessary to achieve a state of tolerance. It acts to downregulate the expression of the costimulatory molecule B7, diminishing T-cell activation,[70] and may also induce T-cell anergy.[71] Other laboratory investigations demonstrate that 1,25-$(OH)_2$ vitamin D_3 may also be important in this shift to the T_H2 type cytokine profile.[72]

In vitro models of immune response using human or murine cells also support a central role for CD4+ cells and strong supporting roles for macrophages (or antigen-presenting cells) and cytotoxic lymphocytes. Lafferty's two-signal hypothesis is well accepted:[73] donor antigen provides one signal and antigen-presenting cells provide a second signal to stimulate responder CD4+ cells effectively. These cells elaborate cytokines, the most important of which is IL-2, which, in turn, stimulates the proliferation of additional CD4+ cells and the proliferation and maturation of CD8+ cells via newly expressed IL-2 receptors.[74] Both CD4+ T cells and CD8+ T cells can act as cytotoxic T lymphocytes. However, analysis indicates that the CD8+ cells are the primary effector cells that infiltrate the bile ducts and cause apoptosis (CD8-to-CD4 ratio of 5:1).[13,75,76] Mature cytolytic CD8+ cells can damage donor tissue through contact and the release of active enzymes.[77]

The in vitro models of immunoactivity have generally used lymphoid cells such as splenocytes for all three components of the immune response: responder cells, stimulator cells, and target cells. These studies have been invaluable in defining a central role for CD4+ cells, an essential role for antigen-presenting cells, and an effector role for cytolytic cells. These models have also been important in defining the role of the MHC antigens in stimulating the development of proliferative and cytolytic responses and in defining the specificity of the effector function. Nonetheless, the applicability of in vitro studies to organ transplantation may be served better by substituting parenchymal cells for the stimulator cells and target cells. Lymphoid cells from the graft may serve as the sensitizing antigen at the graft site, or they may migrate out of the graft and elicit host sensitization at another site.[78] Graft parenchymal cells may provide sensitization of the host by having their antigens indirectly presented through host antigen-presenting cells. Because the graft is damaged as a result of the rejection response, one would assume that the donor parenchymal cells represent an appropriate target for the antidonor response seen in rejection. Using the mixed lymphocyte hepatocyte coculture system, purified murine hepatocytes or nonparenchymal cells (Kupffer cells, epithelial cells, and endothelial cells) can stimulate the development of specific antidonor cytotoxic cells.[79,80] Because hepatocytes express only class I antigens on their surfaces, using purified hepatocytes as simulators requires the presence of antigen-presenting cells within the responder cell population; removal of these antigen-presenting cells abrogates the cytolytic response. Work by Bumgardner and colleagues[81,82] demonstrated that the immune response to murine parenchymal and nonparenchymal cells involves both direct and indirect antigen presentation. The cytotoxic response of lymphocytes that develop in mixed lymphocyte-hepatocyte coculture is generally tested with blast targets sharing MHC antigens with the stimulating hepatocytes in a chromium[51] release assay. Hepatocytes may also be used as targets, but instead of using chromium labeling, transaminase release from injured hepatocytes has been monitored.

HLA Antigens and Rejection

The distribution of HLA antigens in the liver allograft parallels the histological pattern of rejection observed. Most of the inflammatory response seen in rejection is localized to the portal tracts, where a mixed inflammatory cell infiltrate is seen with damage to the bile duct epithelium and venous endothelium. This damage results in an elevated alkaline phosphatase level detected in the serum.[83] The apparent target cells within the portal tracts—bile duct epithelium and vascular endothelium—are rich in class I and class II antigens.[84] Central vein endothelium is another characteristic target of the rejection response, and these cells also express both class I and class II antigens.

These data raise the question of why there is only scant inflammation in the parenchyma relative to the portal tracts in liver graft rejection. An explanation is related to the distribution of liver blood flow. The portal tract region receives the richest blood supply, so

cells in this region may be more exposed to host cells that can respond to graft antigens and cause graft damage. This mechanical explanation does not account for the endotheliitis seen in the central vein endothelium. Another possible explanation for the distribution of inflammatory cells seen in acute hepatic allograft rejection is that the parenchymal cells are immunogenic but release substances on injury that inhibit the immune response. The question has been raised as to whether arginase released from hepatocytes prevents immune activation and proliferation.[85] It is noteworthy that Kupffer cells within parenchymal sinusoids are rich in class I and class II antigen expression but are not generally a target for the immune response.

The importance of class I expression in the stimulation of an immune response is demonstrated by the β_2-microglobulin–deficient mouse. This animal lacks β_2-microglobulin and as such is unable to assemble and express class I antigen. When hepatocytes from these animals are used to stimulate a mixed lymphocyte-hepatocyte coculture, no cytotoxicity is generated. Similarly, islet grafts from β_2-microglobulin–deficient donor mice are prolonged in streptozocin-treated, H2-disparate mice.[86] These results indicate the importance of class I antigen expression in allograft rejection. These data do not negate the importance of class II–positive cells; class II–positive cells of donor origin may present antigen directly. Alternatively, class I–positive donor cells may work through host class II–positive cells to effect sensitization. These data raise the question of why there is only scant inflammation in the parenchyma relative to the portal tracts in liver graft rejection, given the presence of class I antigen on hepatocytes. One explanation may be that bile duct epithelium and venous endothelium, which express both class I and class II antigens, display a greater density of class I antigen than do the hepatocytes. Another possibility is that the combination of class I and II, which are both expressed on bile duct epithelium and endothelium, is more immunogenic. Alternatively, the endothelium may be more immunogenic as a result of adhesion molecules that are elaborated.

Conversely, hepatocytes are rarely the target cell of the acute rejection response, except in late rejection; they express only scant amounts of class I antigen on their surface and do not generally express class II antigen.[87,88] Sole expression of class I is also apparent in hepatocytes that have been purified from whole livers; this is true for human[89] as well as murine[90] hepatocytes. During acute rejection, human livers demonstrate increased class I expression.[91] Class II expression cannot be induced in hepatocytes cocultured with sensitized lymphocytes or with IFN-γ, which is known to enhance class II expression on the surface of other cells.[90] There are numerous examples in a variety of animal models associating MHC antigen expression and rejection.[92-94] The relative importance of class I versus class II expression as it relates to the triggering of the immune response remains in debate.[95,96]

One would anticipate that the expression of HLA antigens in some way triggers the rejection response and that HLA disparity between donor and recipient correlates with rejection. The dependence of rejection on HLA disparity is well established in kidney transplantation with improved results with better HLA matching and recipients matched for six HLA antigens.[97] The relationship between HLA matching and liver transplantation results is controversial. At present, no attempt has been made to match donors and recipients according to their shared MHC antigens. Although there are some conflicting reports, a few new series associate HLA class I matching with a decrease in the frequency of acute rejection after liver transplantation. The Wisconsin group found that matching at MHC class I but not class II predicted graft survival in humans.[98] Pittsburgh researchers observed that class I or class II compatibility was associated with decreased graft survival, although fewer grafts were lost secondary to rejection.[99] These findings have been interpreted as consistent with an increased susceptibility to viral infections (increased CMV risk when HLA DR is well-matched[100]) and graft-versus-host disease when the donor and recipient are well-matched. In addition, the same study showed a positive correlation between class I matching and graft success.[1,101]

It has been observed experimentally that class I MHC antigen may be shed by allograft organs and in particular by the allograft liver. Donor-type MHC class I antigen has been identified in the serum of liver transplant recipients; however, it decreases with removal of the liver.[102] A method was developed to identify serum HLA class I antigen rapidly using a solid-phase, enzyme-linked immunoassay.[103] Liver and heart transplant recipients demonstrated a higher than pretransplantation level of circulating soluble class I antigen after transplantation, with transient increases at times of rejection and infection. It may be that the soluble class I antigens are effective in neutralizing preformed antidonor cytotoxic antibodies. In the laboratory, allochimeric class I molecules bearing donor-type class I sequences induce donor-specific tolerance to cardiac allografts.[104]

Antibody-Mediated Liver Rejection

Antibodies have had an uncertain role in liver allograft rejection. Initial reports of successful transplantations in the setting of a positive cross-match indicated that successful transplantation could be done in the presence of anti–donor-HLA antibody.[105,106] More recently, it was determined that transplantation outcome in the setting

of a positive cross-match is inferior to transplantation outcome in the setting of a negative cross-match,[107,108] particularly in female patients.[109] It was found in the largest series of liver allograft recipients with a positive cross-match that the liver allograft failure rate was higher in the first 4 weeks after transplantion when there was a positive T-cell cross-match. This difference disappeared in the second year after transplantation. In addition, T-cell–positive cross-match patients were more likely to suffer from sepsis in the early period after transplant. These investigators concluded that the cross-match should not be used to decide against transplantation but to identify a high-risk group of patients that require closer follow-up.[109]

The relative resistance of the liver to antibody-mediated injury and its protective ability on other grafts (e.g., kidney) is unexplained. This might be partly explained by the architecture of the liver: an organ with a double blood supply and a less vasoreactive venous system.[110] This might also explain why there are only a few reports of hyperacute rejection of the liver in humans.[111] Experimental models and patient experiences demonstrate that the transplanted liver is capable not only of resisting hyperacute rejection but also of absorbing antibodies from the circulation.[112,113]

The clinical pattern seen with ABO-incompatible grafts may represent an important form of antibody-mediated liver allograft rejection.[114] Although short-term results from these grafts are satisfactory, the long-term results are poor, particularly in adult recipients. We have observed a consistent pattern in adult recipients: initial biopsies reveal a periportal infiltrate consistent with mild pericholangitis. Periductular inflammation progresses, and the inflammation extends into the parenchyma. This process progresses to eventual hepatocyte necrosis. At retransplantation, these patients have demonstrated an inflammatory process within the arterial wall of the main hepatic artery and its major branches. Hepatic artery compromise and even thrombosis may be present in small vessels, and necrosis is present within the liver parenchyma; the main hepatic artery has been patent in these cases. The pericholangitis presumably reflects relative ischemia of the bile duct system. This is borne out by the frequency of intrahepatic bile duct strictures in these patients. Still investigational, a protocol of intraportal infusion therapy after transplantation with methylprednisolone, prostaglandin E_1, and gabexate mesylate may decrease the incidence of these vascular or biliary complications.[115] ABO-incompatible liver allografts have been more successful in pediatric patients, particularly in those who are younger than 3 years of age. In younger children, this success may be explained by the lack of antibody against ABO antigens.

The use of living related liver transplantation may further enable investigators to delineate the importance of

MHC antigens in the immune response to human liver. One study aimed to assess the influence of HLA compatibility in a large series of pediatric living related liver transplants.[116] A total of 321 pediatric patients who underwent ABO-identical or ABO-compatible primary transplants from a parental donor were examined for graft survival and rejection episodes. Kasahara and colleagues found that the overall 1- and 5-year graft survivals were 85.7% and 84.1%, respectively. The 5-year graft survivals in HLA 0, HLA 1, HLA 2, and HLA 3 mismatch groups (A, B, and DR) were not statistically different. The overall incidence of rejection during the follow-up period (median 66 months) was 46.1%, and no significant difference was found in the incidence of rejection among the groups.[116] Thus there does not appear to be supportive evidence at present for any beneficial effect of HLA matching in pediatric living related liver transplantation.

Nitric Oxide Production in Acute Rejection

Nitric oxide (NO) is a gaseous molecule produced by NO synthases, a group of P450-like enzymes.[117] These enzymes convert L-arginine and oxygen into L-citrulline and NO. NO, an immunomodulatory molecule, has been proposed as a mediator of acute cellular rejection in the liver allograft in animal models.[118] Plasma levels of NO metabolites and allograft-inducible NO synthase mRNA and protein levels are all increased in animal models of acute rejection, events that are not present with immunosuppression.[119-121] Certain immunosuppressive agents (i.e., calcineurin inhibitors) decrease NO synthesis.[117,122] Increases in liver nitrotyrosine staining, a marker of the reactive oxidant species peroxynitrite, is prominent in animal models of cellular rejection, but not with pharmacological immunosuppression. This has led some to conclude that the role of NO in cellular rejection, while unclear, is likely to be of an injurious nature.[118]

In humans, similar conclusions associating NO with acute cellular rejection have been made.[123,124] NO production during hepatic allograft rejection has been observed.[124] Hepatocytes are the main cellular source for NO production. Plasma levels of NO metabolites are increased during acute cellular rejection when compared with chronic rejection or stable graft function.[125] By immunohistochemistry, inducible nitric oxide synthase (iNOS) expression in patients with acute cellular rejection is significantly stronger than in patients without rejection.[124] After treatment with corticosteroids, iNOS expression decreases as treatment results in downregulation of intrahepatic iNOS expression. NO levels appear to correspond to rejection severity. They do not appear to be increased after liver resection surgery alone.[123,125]

Role of Cytokines in Liver Allograft Rejection

It is increasingly clear that the molecules elaborated by activated inflammatory cells are important in cell-cell interactions. These cytokines have important positive and negative effects on other cells as well. Many cytokines have been identified with myriad regulatory roles; the same cytokine may have different effects on other cells, depending on the specific conditions and the presence of other cytokines.[126-128] In vitro models demonstrate important roles for IL-1, IL-2, IL-2 receptors, IL-4, IL-6, IL-10, IFN-γ, and TNF in expansion and development of the proliferative and cytotoxic response. The role of cytokines in allograft rejection has been approached by the examination of systemic levels of cytokines or of cytokine levels at the graft site. Identification of systemic cytokines provides a straightforward method for identifying pathological changes and would be a convenient noninvasive way to diagnose rejection.

An important issue to be considered is whether the findings are specific to the rejection response. The group at the University of California at Los Angeles has noted increased levels of systemic TNF in individuals with acute liver allograft rejection.[129] However, levels were also elevated in patients with viral and bacterial infections. The raised TNF levels preceded biochemical evidence of rejection by 1 to 2 days. Imagawa and colleagues[130] used anti-TNF antibody treatment in rats to effect allograft prolongation; they also found a beneficial effect of antibody to lymphotoxin and the greatest graft prolongation when these two antibody treatments were combined. IL-6 enhances the differentiation of B cells and cytotoxic T cells and induces IL-2–receptor expression.[131,132] Ohzato and colleagues[133] measured serum IL-6 levels in monkeys undergoing liver transplantation. They found that the monitoring of serum IL-6 suggested acute hepatic rejection and preceded biochemical indications. This study did not include animals with viral infections to delineate the specificity of these findings. The authors hypothesized that the origin of the serum IL-6 was monocytes, although histological confirmation with immunoperoxidase staining was not available. Hamilton and colleagues[134] examined the prognostic significance of endotoxin, TNF-α, and IL-6 in humans undergoing liver transplantation. Endotoxin levels did not correlate with complications, but high TNF-α immediately on reperfusion was associated with rejection. The authors suggested that TNF-α might promote the binding of host lymphocytes to graft endothelium or induce the expression of MHC antigens within the graft, or both. A high intraoperative IL-6 level was predictive of viral or bacterial infections in this series.

As with TNF, elevations of the IL-2 receptor are not specific, for elevations were also seen with infections. In kidney transplant recipients, infection and rejection may be differentiated by the use of a combination of IL-2 receptor observations and serum creatinine assays.[135] Elevated levels of the IL-2 receptor during acute rejection speaks for its central role in allograft rejection. The central role of IL-2 and the IL-2 receptor was the basis for human trials using antibody to the IL-2 receptor.[136] Because eosinophils are frequently a prominent cell type in human liver allograft rejection and IL-5 is a known growth factor for cytotoxic lymphocytes, we hypothesized that eosinophils at the graft site produce IL-5, which, in turn, enhances the development of cytotoxic T cells. It is unlikely that IL-5 plays a central role in rejection. Its presence in the context of therapy that inhibits IL-2 production and release (i.e., cyclosporine or tacrolimus) speaks for a central IL-2 role and an accessory role for other cytokines.

IL-15, like IL-2, is produced in macrophages. Plasma levels and in situ expression of IL-15 are elevated during liver rejection, in particular with steroid-resistant acute cellular and chronic rejection. Studies in vitro demonstrate that IL-15 production is not inhibited by corticosteroids or calcineurin inhibitors.[137]

Hepatitis C and Hepatic Allograft Rejection

Recurrent hepatitis C is a major problem, and effective therapy is needed to prevent both progression of hepatitis C and recurrence in the graft to avoid retransplantation.[138] Recurrent infection of the allograft with hepatitis C virus (HCV) is universal and is an important cause of fibrosis and cirrhosis after liver transplantation. Histological recurrence develops in at least 50% of patients within the first year after transplantation.[139] The use of recombinant IFN in combination with ribavirin holds promise in overcoming recurrent hepatitis C.[138]

Acute rejection and recurrent HCV infection can occur in the same patient, and both can be detected in a single liver biopsy.[140-142] There is substantial histological overlap between recurrent HCV infection and cellular rejection. Histological examination of both acute rejection and recurrent HCV infection can demonstrate portal inflammation, ductal damage, and apoptosis of hepatocytes, as both conditions are associated with bile duct injury and portal lymphocytic infiltration. Endotheliitis, a sign of rejection, is sometimes present in biopsy specimens with recurrent HCV.[141,143] These findings often make the diagnosis of recurrent hepatitis C or acute rejection (or both) difficult. Unfortunately, these two conditions require opposite therapeutic management.

Many groups have attempted to develop methods (histological, biochemical, or serum based) to distinguish these two entities. In general, features such as steatosis, lobular inflammation, and spotty necrosis favor recurrent hepatitis C.[144,145] One group compared the histology of acute rejection and recurrent HCV infection by evaluating 44 histological changes in lobules and portal tracts. Although they found that several portal tract changes were significantly associated with acute rejection, there were no specific histological correlates to recurrent hepatitis C infection.[144] Others have favored recurrent HCV infection when sinusoidal dilatation, steatosis, chronic portal inflammation, Kupffer cell activation, spotty necrosis, or acidophil bodies[144,145] were detected on biopsy.

The criteria for the diagnosis of acute rejection described in the Banff International Consensus Document[146] consist of cholangiolitis, mixed portal inflammation, and endotheliitis. Hepatocyte necrosis is classified only as a finding in severe acute rejection. We closely examine liver biopsy specimens for acidophil bodies (i.e., necrotic or apoptotic hepatocytes) along with examining the serum to determine the quantitative viral RNA load to then favor the diagnosis of recurrent HCV or acute rejection.

Data from other institutions suggests that this may be the best way to differentiate the two conditions. One group demonstrated that there are twice as many acidophil bodies in the initial stage of recurrent HCV infection versus acute rejection (average of 55 per centimeter in recurrent HCV versus 21 per centimeter for rejection).[147] Others have found a significant CD8+ and CD57+ (natural killer) cellular infiltrate with cell-to-cell contact between HCV-infected hepatocytes and immune cells. This finding was then followed by a subsequent peak in hepatocyte apoptosis and proliferation at the time of acute hepatitis.

Several groups of researchers have proposed quantitative detection of HCV RNA as a tool for distinguishing recurrent hepatitis C from acute rejection.[148,149] Overlap in values does exist but HCV RNA levels are a useful adjunct to histological examination to distinguish between recurrent HCV and acute rejection. There is a peak in serum viral load at the time of detection of the initial biochemical hepatitis.[150] In liver transplant recipients with HCV and elevated transaminase levels, HCV RNA levels are statistically higher in patients with recurrent HCV than in patients with acute rejection.[151] Patients with low HCV RNA levels are unlikely to have recurrent HCV, whereas patients with recurrent HCV tend to have high HCV RNA levels.

Examination of the intrahepatic gene response by gene microarray technology to distinguish recurrent HCV from cellular rejection has been performed.[152] This group found less than a 1% difference at the mRNA level between the two conditions: acute rejection showed a relatively increased expression of immune activation genes (TNF, granzyme B, and complement components) and MHC complex classes I and II.[152] Other investigators have found that IL-3, matrix metalloprotease (MMP)-9, tissue inhibitors of metalloprotease (TIMP)-1, TNF, IL-10, clusterin, and transforming growth factor (TGF)-1 to -3 were differentially expressed in allograft rejection specimens when compared with those with viral hepatitis or stable graft function.[153]

Zekry and colleagues[154] examined the T_H1- and T_H2-like gene expression and found that acute rejection in the setting of HCV infection was more like acute rejection in non–HCV-infected patients and was associated with increases in IL-10 and IL-4 gene expression, rather than the IL-2/INF/TNF response seen more in chronic HCV infection alone. Studying immunoglobulin levels, one group found that serum IgM anti-HCV levels increased (or changed from negative to positive) in cases with recurrent hepatitis C at the time of aminotransferase elevation yet remained unchanged in cases of acute rejection.[155] Although not used routinely, these tests may ultimately assist in this distinction (Table 72–1).

The presence of hepatitis C in liver allograft recipients should cause reevaluation of which maintenance immunosuppression is selected. Both the incidence and severity of recurrent hepatitis C may be related to corticosteroids when used either as maintenance immunosuppression or in the context of treating rejection. The King's College group was among the first to raise the issue of prednisone in maintenance immunosuppression in patients with hepatitis C.[156] Reasons for this concern included the known stimulation of viral replication by corticosteroids in nontransplantation patients, the increase in viremia seen with pulse steroid therapy, and the suggestion that treatment of rejection was associated with acceleration of recurrent hepatitis C.[157]

As a result, the King's College group discontinued the use of steroid therapy 6 months after liver transplantation.

Methods of Diagnosis of Acute Liver Transplant Rejection

A variety of clinical signs and symptoms may be observed with liver allograft rejection. These include fever, malaise, abdominal pain, and hepatosplenomegaly. Unfortunately, however, none of these are specific for rejection, nor are they common manifestations. Liver allograft function may remain stable in many patients found to have focal or mild histological features of rejection on liver biopsy even without treatment. Acute cellular rejection may be suspected with elevation of serum transaminase, alkaline phosphatase, or bilirubin levels, or any combination.[158] Unfortunately, none of these serum markers is sensitive or specific for distinguishing rejection from other causes of allograft dysfunction.[7] In addition, there is no correlation between the serum values and histological abnormalities.[159]

Liver transplant rejection is best diagnosed through the use of a percutaneous allograft biopsy rather than through reliance on biochemical parameters; generally, alternative methods are perceived to be nonspecific.[160] The use of percutaneous biopsy as the gold standard[7] has been reaffirmed in a study from the University of Michigan.[161] These investigators confirmed earlier observations that the biochemical pattern could not differentiate histopathological characteristics and that two or more pathological processes could frequently coexist.

There have been efforts to develop noninvasive methods for diagnosing rejection to avoid the complications of biopsy (e.g., bleeding). One technique, fine-needle aspiration biopsy (FNAB) of the liver allograft or collecting cells from bile, is based on an understanding of the cells involved in rejection. FNAB of the graft is increasingly recognized as a useful method in the diagnosis of rejection by the identification of activated mononuclear cells. It has been also used successfully to examine the response of rejection to immunosuppressive therapy.[162,163] In addition to determing the cell type that is present, examination of mediators of rejection can be performed. For example, cytotoxic T lymphocytes release granzyme B, a serine protease that participates in the perforin-dependent pathway of T-cell–based cytotoxicity; granzyme can be detected in acute hepatic allograft rejection. Granzyme-expressing cells in FNAB specimens are significantly increased during clinically acute rejection episodes. However, granzyme B also tends to be increased during subclinical rejection episodes and cytomegalovirus infections and thus its use is limited. FNAB is also limited by the lack of

Table 72–1. DIFFERENTIATION OF HEPATITIS C VIRUS INFECTION ALONE VERSUS HEPATITIS C VIRUS INFECTION AND ACUTE CELLULAR REJECTION

Feature	HCV Alone	HCV and Acute Rejection
Intrahepatic T_H1 cytokines	++	+
Intrahepatic T_H2 cytokines	±	++
Endotheliitis	±	+++
Bile duct damage	±	++
Lymphocyte portal tract infiltration	++	++
Eosinophils in portal tract infiltrate	-	++
Steatosis	++	±
Acidophil Bodies	+++	+++
Serum HCV RNA	+++	+++

Modified from McCaughan GW, Zekry A. Pathogenesis of hepatitis C virus recurrence in the liver allograft. Liver Transpl 8(Suppl 1):S7, 2002.
HCV, hepatitis C virus.

cytoarchitecture present from biopsy specimens. Consequently, this technique cannot be used to predict features of chronic rejection such as fibrosis and decreases in numbers of bile duct cells.

Exfoliative urinary cytological examination has been used to diagnose acute rejection of kidney and pancreas allografts.[164] Similarly, bile cytological examination has been used to diagnose acute liver transplant rejection.[165-167] The presence of a high cell density within the bile sediment and polymorphonuclear leukocytes appears to characterize acute rejection. Roberti and colleagues[168] examined the use of sequential bile specimens in patients who demonstrated a number of different pathological processes after liver transplantation. Although the first few days after transplantation were associated with a mild degree of ischemic injury and a high number of inflammatory cells in bile samples, after that time an increase in inflammatory cells was highly specific for acute rejection (95%). Unlike previous investigations, this study found that lymphoblastoid cells, rather than polymorphonuclear neutrophils, were associated with rejection. In most centers, however, biliary cytological examination is not used routinely.

Grading of Rejection on Biopsy

To overcome weaknesses of different systems of grading acute cellular rejection, an international consensus panel met in Banff, Canada in 1995 and developed the Banff schema[146] (Table 72–2). The schema has two components. First, there is a "rejection activity index" (RAI) that grades the severity of portal inflammation, bile duct

Table 72–2. BANFF CLASSIFICATION

Rejection Activity Index

Category	Criteria	Score
Portal inflammation	Mostly lymphocytic inflammation involving, but not noticeably expanding, a minority of triads	1
	Expansion of all or most of the triads by a mixed infiltrate containing lymphocytes with occasional blasts, neutrophils, and eosinophils	2
	Marked expansion of most or all of the triads by a mixed infiltrate containing numerous blasts and eosinophils with inflammatory spillover into the periportal parenchyma	3
Bile duct inflammation/damage	A minority of the ducts are cuffed and infiltrated by inflammatory cells and show only mild reactive changes such as an increased nuclear-to-cytoplasmic ratio of the epithelial cells	1
	Most or all of the ducts are infiltrated by inflammatory cells; more than an occasional duct shows degenerative changes such as nuclear pleomorphism, disordered polarity, and cytoplasmic vacuolization of the epithelium	2
	Same as for a score of 2, with most or all of the ducts showing degenerative changes or focal luminal disruption	3
Venous endothelial inflammation	Subendothelial lymphocytic infiltration involving some, but not a majority, of the portal and/or hepatic venules	1
	Subendothelial infiltration involving most or all of the portal and/or hepatic venules	2
	Same as for a score of 2, with moderate or severe perivenular inflammation that extends into the perivenular parenchyma and is associated with perivenular hepatocyte necrosis	3

Total score = sum of the components to provide a final rejection score, which is then converted to a histological grade: 0-2, no rejection; 3, borderline; 4-5, mild rejection; 6-7, moderate rejection; 8-9, severe rejection

Global Assessment

Category	Criteria
Indeterminate	Portal inflammatory infiltrate that fails to meet the criteria for the diagnosis of acute rejection
Mild	Rejection infiltrate in a minority of triads that is generally mild and confined within the portal spaces
Moderate	Rejection infiltrate involving most or all of the triads
Severe	As above for moderate, with spillover into periportal areas and moderate to severe perivenular inflammation that extends into the hepatic parenchyma and is associated with perivenular hepatocyte necrosis

From Demetris A, Batts K, Dhillon A, et al: Banff schema for grading liver allograft rejection: An international consensus document. Hepatology 25:658, 1997.

damage, and venous endothelial damage. Each category is given a score of 0 to 3, providing a total score of 0 to 9. Second, there is a "global assessment" that provides a verbal grade based on the overall appearance of the biopsy specimen with particular weight provided by the severity of portal tract inflammation.[169]

Pearls and Pitfalls

- The early targets of acute cellular liver transplant rejection are the bile duct epithelium and the venous endothelium.

- Three major histological features are associated with cellular rejection:
  - Endotheliitis
  - Portal triads with mixed infiltrates (predominantly mononuclear but may also contain neutrophils and eosinophils)
  - Destructive or nondestructive nonsuppurative cholangitis involving interlobular biliary epithelium

- CD4 + T cells are prominent mediators of acute cellular rejection.

- An elevated eosinophil count has a positive predictive value for acute cellular rejection of the liver, whereas a normal count generally excludes moderate or severe rejection.

- There is no consistent biochemical pattern that predicts acute cellular rejection; a noninvasive scheme of ultrasonography (to rule out vascular and bile duct pathology) may need to be followed by biopsy.

- Although variable, acute cellular rejection is characterized by a rise in alkaline phosphatase and bilirubin levels, with less increase in aminotransferase levels.

- The beneficial effect of acute cellular rejection is controversial, but has been suggested by those who think a balance between host-versus-graft and graft-versus-host reactions is eventually achieved.

References

1. Chung SW, Greig PD, Cattral MS, et al: Evaluation of liver transplantation for high-risk indications. Br J Surg 84:189, 1997.
2. Snover DC, Sibley RK, Freese DK, et al: Orthotopic liver transplantation: A pathological study of 63 serial liver biopsies from 17 patients with special reference to the diagnostic features and natural history of rejection. Hepatology 4:1212, 1984.
3. Ray RA, Lewin KJ, Colonna J, et al: The role of liver biopsy in evaluating acute allograft dysfunction following liver transplantation: A clinical histologic correlation of 34 liver transplants. Hum Pathol 19:835, 1988.
4. Ascher NL, Stock PG, Bumgardner GL, et al: Infection and rejection of primary hepatic transplant in 93 consecutive patients treated with triple immunosuppressive therapy. Surg Gynecol Obstet 167:474, 1988.
5. Demetris AJ, Lasky S, Van Thiel DH, et al: Pathology of hepatic transplantation: A review of 62 adult allograft recipients immunosuppressed with a cyclosporine/steroid regimen. Am J Pathol 118:151, 1985.
6. Fisher LR, Henley KS, Lucey MR: Acute cellular rejection after liver transplantation: Variability, morbidity, and mortality. Liver Transpl Surg 1:10, 1995.
7. Batts KP: Acute and chronic hepatic allograft rejection: Pathology and classification. Liver Transpl Surg 5(Suppl 1):S21, 1999.
8. Demetris AJ, Ruppert K, Dvorchik I, et al: Real-time monitoring of acute liver-allograft rejection using the Banff schema. Transplantation 74:1290, 2002.
9. Seiler CA, Renner EL, Czerniak A, et al: Early acute cellular rejection: No effect on late hepatic allograft function in man. Transpl Int 12:195, 1999.
10. Dousset B, Conti F, Cherruau B, et al: Is acute rejection deleterious to long-term liver allograft function? J Hepatol 29:660, 1998.
11. Wiesner RH, Ludwig J, van Hoek B, Krom RA: Current concepts in cell-mediated hepatic allograft rejection leading to ductopenia and liver failure. Hepatology 14:721, 1991.
12. Demetris AJ, Murase N, Ye Q, et al: Analysis of chronic rejection and obliterative arteriopathy. Possible contributions of donor antigen-presenting cells and lymphatic disruption. Am J Pathol 150:563, 1997.
13. Vierling JM: Immunology of acute and chronic hepatic allograft rejection. Liver Transpl Surg 5(Suppl 1):S1, 1999.
14. Soin AS, Rasmussen A, Jamieson NV, et al: Cyclosporine levels in the early posttransplant period: Predictive of chronic rejection in liver transplantation? Transplant Proc 27:1129, 1995.
15. Germain RN: MHC-dependent antigen processing and peptide presentation: Providing ligands for T lymphocyte activation. Cell 76:287, 1994.
16. Bathgate AJ, Hynd P, Sommerville D, Hayes PC: The prediction of acute cellular rejection in orthotopic liver transplantation. Liver Transpl Surg 5:475, 1999.
17. Maggard M, Goss J, Ramdev S, et al: Incidence of acute rejection in African-American liver transplant recipients. Transplant Proc 30:1492, 1998.
18. Neuberger J, Adams D: What is the significance of acute liver allograft rejection? J Hepatol 29:143, 1998.
19. Wiesner RH, Demetris AJ, Belle SH, et al: Acute hepatic allograft rejection: Incidence, risk factors, and impact on outcome. Hepatology 28:638, 1998.
20. Neuberger J: Incidence, timing, and risk factors for acute and chronic rejection. Liver Transpl Surg 5(Suppl 1):S30, 1999.
21. Farges O, Saliba F, Farhamant H, et al: Incidence of rejection and infection after liver transplantation as a function of the primary disease: Possible influence of alcohol and polyclonal immunoglobulins. Hepatology 23:240, 1996.
22. Caregaro L, Alberino F, Amodio P, et al: Malnutrition in alcoholic and virus-related cirrhosis. Am J Clin Nutr 63:602, 1996.
23. Kobayashi E, Kamada N, Goto S, Miyata M: Protocol for the technique of orthotopic liver transplantation in the rat. Microsurgery 14:541, 1993.
24. Knechtle SJ, Wolfe JA, Burchette J, et al: Infiltrating cell phenotypes and patterns associated with hepatic allograft rejection or acceptance. Transplantation 43:169, 1987.
25. Calne R: WOFIE hypothesis: Some thoughts on an approach toward allograft tolerance. Transplant Proc 28:1152, 1996.

26. Ascher NL, Ferguson RM, Hoffman R, Simmons RL: Partial characterization of cytotoxic cells infiltrating sponge matrix allografts. Transplantation 27:254, 1979.

27. Ascher NL, Chen S, Hoffman RA, Simmons RL: Maturation of cytotoxic T cells within sponge matrix allografts. J Immunol 131:617, 1983.

28. Rosengard BR, Ojikutu CA, Guzzetta PC, et al: Induction of specific tolerance to class I-disparate renal allografts in miniature swine with cyclosporine. Transplantation 54:490, 1992.

29. Tian Y, Rudiger HA, Jochum W, Clavien PA: Comparison of arterialized and nonarterialized orthotopic liver transplantation in mice: Prowess or relevant model? Transplantation 74:1242, 2002.

30. Yamaguchi Y, Harland RC, Wyble C, Bollinger RR: The role of class I major histocompatibility complex antigens in prolonging the survival of hepatic allografts in the rat. Transplantation 47:171, 1989.

31. Ochiai T, Nakajima K, Nagata M, et al: Studies of the induction and maintenance of long-term graft acceptance by treatment with FK506 in heterotopic cardiac allotransplantation in rats. Transplantation 44:734, 1987.

32. Starzl TE, Demetris AJ, Trucco M, et al: Systemic chimerism in human female recipients of male livers. Lancet 340:876, 1992.

33. Williams JW, Peters TG, Haggitt R, et al: Cyclosporin A in orthotopic canine hepatic transplants. J Surg Res 32:576, 1982.

34. Adams AB, Williams MA, Jones TR, et al: Heterologous immunity provides a potent barrier to transplantation tolerance. J Clin Invest 111:1887, 2003.

35. Adams AB, Pearson TC, Larsen CP: Heterologous immunity: An overlooked barrier to tolerance. Immunol Rev 196:147, 2003.

36. Hubscher SG: Histological findings in liver allograft rejection—new insights into the pathogenesis of hepatocellular damage in liver allografts. Histopathology 18:377, 1991.

37. Demetris AJ, Qian SG, Sun H, Fung JJ: Liver allograft rejection: An overview of morphologic findings. Am J Surg Pathol (Suppl 1):49, 1990.

38. McCaughan GW, Davies S, Waugh J, et al: Cell surface phenotype of mononuclear cells infiltrating bile ducts during acute and chronic liver allograft rejection. Transplant Proc 21:2201, 1989.

39. Perkins JD, Wiesner RH, Banks PM, et al: Immunohistologic labeling of infiltrating T lymphocytes in hepatic allografts: A rejection indicator. Transplant Proc 19:2474, 1987.

40. Perkins JD, Rakela J, Sterioff S, et al: Immunohistologic pattern of the portal T-lymphocyte infiltration in hepatic allograft rejection. Mayo Clin Proc 64:565, 1989.

41. Perkins JD, Rakela J, Sterioff S, et al: Results of treatment in hepatic allograft rejection depend on the immunohistologic pattern of the portal T lymphocyte infiltrate. Transplant Proc 20:223, 1988.

42. Foster PF, Sankary HN, Hart M, et al: Blood and graft eosinophilia as predictors of rejection in human liver transplantation. Transplantation 47:72, 1989.

43. Kormendi F, Amend WJ Jr: The importance of eosinophil cells in kidney allograft rejection. Transplantation 45:537, 1988.

44. Martinez OM, Burke EC, Alan TJ, Ascher NL: Allogeneic hepatocytes stimulate the production of immunoregulatory molecules in mixed lymphocyte hepatocyte cultures. Transplant Proc 23:805, 1991.

45. Martinez OM, Krams SM, Sterneck M, et al: Intragraft cytokine profile during human liver allograft rejection. Transplantation 53:449, 1992.

46. Barnes EJ, Abdel-Rehim MM, Goulis Y, et al: Applications and limitations of blood eosinophilia for the diagnosis of acute cellular rejection in liver transplantation. Am J Transplant 3:432, 2003.

47. Vaessen LM, Baan CC, Ouwehand AJ, et al: Acute rejection in heart transplant patients is associated with the presence of committed donor-specific cytotoxic lymphocytes in the graft but not in the blood. Clin Exp Immunol 88:213, 1992.

48. Morris PJ, Carter NP, Cullen PR, et al: Role of T-cell-subset monitoring in renal-allograft recipients. N Engl J Med 306:1110, 1982.

49. Herrod HG, Williams J, Dean PJ: Alterations in immunologic measurements in patients experiencing early hepatic allograft rejection. Transplantation 45:923, 1988.

50. Cosimi AB, Colvin RB, Burton RC, et al: Use of monoclonal antibodies to T-cell subsets for immunologic monitoring and treatment in recipients of renal allografts. N Engl J Med 305:308, 1981.

51. Ibrahim S, Dawson DV, Killenberg PG, Sanfilippo F: The pattern and phenotype of T-cell infiltration associated with human liver allograft rejection. Hum Pathol 24:1365, 1993.

52. Dollinger MM, Howie SE, Plevris JN, et al: Intrahepatic proliferation of "naive" and "memory" T cells during liver allograft rejection: Primary immune response within the allograft. FASEB J 12:939, 1998.

53. Weiss A, Imboden JB: Cell surface molecules and early events involved in human T lymphocyte activation. Adv Immunol 41:1, 1987.

54. Cuomo O, Perrella O: Immune response in liver transplantation: Is there a preferential pattern in acute rejection? Int J Immunopathol Pharmacol 12:63, 1999.

55. Fung JJ, Zeevi A, Starzl TE, et al: Functional characterization of infiltrating T lymphocytes in human hepatic allografts. Hum Immunol 16:182, 1986.

56. Saidman SL, Demetris AJ, Zeevi A, Duquesnoy RJ: Propagation of lymphocytes infiltrating human liver allografts. Correlation with histologic diagnosis of rejection. Transplantation 49:107, 1990.

57. Kolbeck PC, Wood RP, Markin RS: The immunopathology and clinical relevance of lymphocyte cultures in liver transplantation. Mod Pathol 6:307, 1993.

58. Mayer TG, Fuller AA, Fuller TC, et al: Characterization of in vivo-activated allospecific T lymphocytes propagated from human renal allograft biopsies undergoing rejection. J Immunol 134:258, 1985.

59. Nocera A, Barocci S, Valente U, et al: In vitro characterization of a donor-specific cytolytic T cell line established from human lymphocytes homing in a rejected kidney allograft. Transplantation 41:135, 1986.

60. Moreau JF, Bonneville M, Peyrat MA, et al: T lymphocyte cloning from rejected human kidney allografts. Growth frequency and functional/phenotypic analysis. J Clin Invest 78:874, 1986.

61. Sun Z, Wada T, Maemura K, et al: Hepatic allograft-derived Kupffer cells regulate T cell response in rats. Liver Transpl 9:489, 2003.

62. Bunjes D, Hardt C, Rollinghoff M, Wagner H: Cyclosporin A mediates immunosuppression of primary cytotoxic T cell responses by impairing the release of interleukin 1 and interleukin 2. Eur J Immunol 11:657, 1981.

63. O'Garra A: Cytokines induce the development of functionally heterogeneous T helper cell subsets. Immunity 8:275, 1998.

64. Mosmann TR, Cherwinski H, Bond MW, et al: Two types of murine helper T cell clone. I. Definition according to profiles of lymphokine activities and secreted proteins. J Immunol 136:2348, 1986.

65. Mosmann TR, Coffman RL: TH1 and TH2 cells: Different patterns of lymphokine secretion lead to different functional properties. Annu Rev Immunol 7:145, 1989.

66. Strom TB, Roy-Chaudhury P, Manfro R, et al: The Th1/Th2 paradigm and the allograft response. Curr Opin Immunol 8:688, 1996.

67. Mosmann TR, Moore KW: The role of IL-10 in crossregulation of TH1 and TH2 responses. Immunol Today 12:A49, 1991.

68. Sadick MD, Heinzel FP, Holaday BJ, et al: Cure of murine leishmaniasis with anti-interleukin 4 monoclonal antibody. Evidence for a T cell-dependent, interferon gamma-independent mechanism. J Exp Med 171:115, 1990.

69. Wren SM, Wang SC, Thai NL, et al: Evidence for early Th 2 T cell predominance in xenoreactivity. Transplantation 56:905, 1993.

70. Li J, Yang Y, Inoue H, et al: The expression of costimulatory molecules CD80 and CD86 in human carcinoma cell lines: Its regulation by interferon gamma and interleukin-10. Cancer Immunol Immunother 43:213, 1996.

71. Groux H, Bigler M, de Vries JE, Roncarolo MG: Interleukin-10 induces a long-term antigen-specific anergic state in human CD4$^+$ T cells. J Exp Med 184:19, 1996.

72. Zhang AB, Zheng SS, Jia CK, Wang Y: Effect of 1,25-dihydroxyvitamin D3 on preventing allograft from acute rejection following rat orthotopic liver transplantation. World J Gastroenterol 9:1067, 2003.

73. Lafferty KJ, Prowse SJ, Simeonovic CJ, Warren HS: Immunobiology of tissue transplantation: A return to the passenger leukocyte concept. Annu Rev Immunol 1:143, 1983.

74. Cantrell DA, Smith KA: Transient expression of interleukin 2 receptors. Consequences for T cell growth. J Exp Med 158:1895, 1983.

75. Krams SM, Martinez OM: Apoptosis as a mechanism of tissue injury in liver allograft rejection. Semin Liver Dis 18:153, 1998.

76. Patel T, Gores GJ: Apoptosis in liver transplantation: A mechanism contributing to immune modulation, preservation injury, neoplasia, and viral disease. Liver Transpl Surg 4:42, 1998.

77. Landegren U, Ramstedt U, Axberg I, et al: Selective inhibition of human T cell cytotoxicity at levels of target recognition or initiation of lysis by monoclonal OKT3 and Leu-2a antibodies. J Exp Med 155:1579, 1982.

78. Larsen CP, Morris PJ, Austyn JM: Migration of dendritic leukocytes from cardiac allografts into host spleens. A novel pathway for initiation of rejection. J Exp Med 171:307, 1990.

79. Bumgardner GL, Chen S, Hoffman R, Ascher NL: Responder T-cell subsets and antigenic stimulus in mixed lymphocyte-hepatocyte culture. Curr Surg 46:20, 1989.

80. So SK, Wilkes LM, Platt JL, et al: Purified hepatocytes can stimulate allospecific cytolytic T lymphocytes in a mixed lymphocyte-hepatocyte culture. Transplant Proc 19:251, 1987.

81. Bumgardner GL, Chen S, Almond PS, et al: Cell subsets responding to purified hepatocytes and evidence of indirect recognition of hepatocyte major histocompatibility complex class I antigen. I. The role of L3T4$^+$ T cells in the development of allospecific cytotoxicity in hepatocyte-sponge matrix allografts. Transplantation 53:857, 1992.

82. Bumgardner GL, Chen S, Almond PS, et al: Cell subsets responding to purified hepatocytes and evidence of indirect recognition of hepatocyte major histocompatibility complex class I antigen. II. In vitro-generated "memory" cells to class I$^+$ class II-hepatocytes. Transplantation 53:863, 1992.

83. Hockerstedt K, Lautenschlager I, Ahonen J, et al: Diagnosis of acute rejection in liver transplantation. J Hepatol 6:217, 1988.

84. Takacs L, Szende B, Monostori E, et al: Expression of HLA-DR antigens on bile duct cells of rejected liver transplant. Lancet 2:1500, 1983.

85. Bumgardner GL, Ascher N, Chen S: Immunosuppressive factors in hepatocyte and liver cytosol. Surg Forum 30:391, 1989.

86. Osorio RW, Ascher NL, Jaenisch R, et al: Isolation of functional MHC class I-deficient islet cells. Transplant Proc 25:968, 1993.

87. Daar AS, Fuggle SV, Fabre JW, et al: The detailed distribution of HLA-A, B, C antigens in normal human organs. Transplantation 38:287, 1984.

88. Steinhoff G, Wonigeit K, Pichlmayr R: Analysis of sequential changes in major histocompatibility complex expression in human liver grafts after transplantation. Transplantation 45:394, 1988.

89. Burke EC, Martinez OM, Freise CE, et al: MHC expression on human hepatocytes before and after isolation. Transplant Proc 23:1428, 1991.

90. Clemmings SM, Alan TJ, Bumgardner GL, Ascher NL: Lack of class II antigen expression on hepatocytes profoundly affects CTL development in vitro and in vivo. Transplant Proc 23:817, 1991.

91. So SK, Platt JL, Ascher NL, Snover DC: Increased expression of class I major histocompatibility complex antigens on hepatocytes in rejecting human liver allografts. Transplantation 43:79, 1987.

92. Hayry P: Intragraft events in allograft destruction. Transplantation 38:1, 1984.

93. Tilney NL, Notis-McConarty J, Strom TB: Specificity of cellular migration into cardiac allografts in rats. Transplantation 26:181, 1978.

94. Warren HS, Simeonovic CJ, Dixon JE, et al: Sensitized Lyt-2$^+$ T cells trigger rejection of grafts expressing class I major histocompatibility complex alloantigens. Transplant Proc 18:310, 1986.

95. Faustman D, Hauptfeld V, Lacy P, Davie J: Prolongation of murine islet allograft survival by pretreatment of islets with antibody directed to Ia determinants. Proc Natl Acad Sci U S A 78:5156, 1981.

96. Stock PG, Meloche M, Ascher NL, et al: Generation of allospecific cytolytic T-lymphocytes stimulated by pure pancreatic beta-cells in absence of Ia$^+$ dendritic cells. Diabetes 38(Suppl 1):161, 1989.

97. Cecka JM, Cho YW, Terasaki PI: Analyses of the UNOS Scientific Renal Transplant Registry at three years—early events affecting transplant success. Transplantation 53:59, 1992.

98. Knechtle SJ, Kalayolu M, D'Alessandro AM, et al: Histocompatibility and liver transplantation. Surgery 114:667, 1993.

99. Markus BH, Fung JJ, Gordon RD, et al: HLA histocompatibility and liver transplant survival. Transplant Proc 19(Suppl 3):63, 1987.

100. Seehofer D, Rayes N, Tullius SG, et al: CMV hepatitis after liver transplantation: Incidence, clinical course, and long-term follow-up. Liver Transpl 8:1138, 2002.

101. Yagihashi A, Kobayashi M, Noguchi K, et al: HLA matching effect in liver transplantation. Transplant Proc 24:2432, 1992.

102. Davies HS, Pollard SG, Calne RY: Soluble HLA antigens in the circulation of liver graft recipients. Transplantation 47:524, 1989.

103. Rhynes VK, McDonald JC, Gelder FB, et al: Soluble HLA class I in the serum of transplant recipients. Ann Surg 217:485, 1993.

104. Singer JS, Mhoyan A, Fishbein MC, et al: Allochimeric class I MHC molecules prevent chronic rejection and attenuate alloantibody responses. Transplantation 72:1408, 2001.

105. Iwatsuki S, Iwaki Y, Kano T, et al: Successful liver transplantation from crossmatch-positive donors. Transplant Proc 13:286, 1981.

106. Gordon RD, Fung JJ, Markus B, et al: The antibody crossmatch in liver transplantation. Surgery 100:705, 1986.

107. Takaya S, Bronsther O, Iwaki Y, et al: The adverse impact on liver transplantation of using positive cytotoxic crossmatch donors. Transplantation 53:400, 1992.

108. Batts KP, Moore SB, Perkins JD, et al: Influence of positive lymphocyte crossmatch and HLA mismatching on vanishing bile duct syndrome in human liver allografts. Transplantation 45:376, 1988.

109. Charco R, Vargas V, Balsells J, et al: Influence of anti-HLA antibodies and positive T-lymphocytotoxic crossmatch on survival and graft rejection in human liver transplantation. J Hepatol 24:452, 1996.

110. Flye MW, Duffy BF, Phelan DL, et al: Protective effects of liver transplantation on a simultaneously transplanted kidney in a highly sensitized patient. Transplantation 50:1051, 1990.

111. Bird G, Friend P, Donaldson P, et al: Hyperacute rejection in liver transplantation: A case report. Transplant Proc 21:3742, 1989.

112. Fung J, Makowka L, Tzakis A, et al: Combined liver-kidney transplantation: Analysis of patients with preformed lymphocytotoxic antibodies. Transplant Proc 20(Suppl 1):88, 1988.

113. Margreiter R, Kornberger R, Koller J, et al: Preliminary results with combined hepatorenal transplantation. Transplant Proc 19:3552, 1987.

114. Gordon RD, Iwatsuki S, Esquivel CO, et al: Experience with primary liver transplantation across ABO blood groups. Transplant Proc 19:4575, 1987.

115. Tanabe M, Shimazu M, Wakabayashi G, et al: Intraportal infusion therapy as a novel approach to adult ABO-incompatible liver transplantation. Transplantation 73:1959, 2002.
116. Kasahara M, Kiuchi T, Uryuhara K, et al: Role of HLA compatibility in pediatric living-related liver transplantation. Transplantation 74:1175, 2002.
117. Shah V, Kamath PS: Nitric oxide in liver transplantation: Pathobiology and clinical implications. Liver Transpl 9:1, 2003.
118. Yamaguchi Y, Okabe K, Matsumura F, et al: Peroxynitrite formation during rat hepatic allograft rejection. Hepatology 29:777, 1999.
119. Langrehr JM, Murase N, Markus PM, et al: Nitric oxide production in host-versus-graft and graft-versus-host reactions in the rat. J Clin Invest 90:679, 1992.
120. Kuo PC, Alfrey EJ, Abe KY, et al: Cellular localization and effect of nitric oxide synthesis in a rat model of orthotopic liver transplantation. Transplantation 61:305, 1996.
121. Goto M, Yamaguchi Y, Ichiguchi O, et al: Phenotype and localization of macrophages expressing inducible nitric oxide synthase in rat hepatic allograft rejection. Transplantation 64:303, 1997.
122. Schaffer MR, Fuchs N, Proksch B, et al: Tacrolimus impairs wound healing: A possible role of decreased nitric oxide synthesis. Transplantation 65:813, 1998.
123. Ioannidis I, Hellinger A, Dehmlow C, et al: Evidence for increased nitric oxide production after liver transplantation in humans. Transplantation 59:1293, 1995.
124. Romero M, Garcia-Monzon C, Clemente G, et al: Intrahepatic expression of inducible nitric oxide synthase in acute liver allograft rejection: Evidence of modulation by corticosteroids. Liver Transpl 7:16, 2001.
125. Devlin J, Palmer RM, Gonde CE, et al: Nitric oxide generation. A predictive parameter of acute allograft rejection. Transplantation 58:592, 1994.
126. Ranges GE, Figari IS, Espevik T, Palladino MA Jr: Inhibition of cytotoxic T cell development by transforming growth factor beta and reversal by recombinant tumor necrosis factor alpha. J Exp Med 166:991, 1987.
127. Thornhill MH, Wellicome SM, Mahiouz DL, et al: Tumor necrosis factor combines with IL-4 or IFN-gamma to selectively enhance endothelial cell adhesiveness for T cells. The contribution of vascular cell adhesion molecule-1-dependent and -independent binding mechanisms. J Immunol 146:592, 1991.
128. Halloran PF, Cockfield SM, Madrenas J: The mediators of inflammation (interleukin 1, interferon-tau, and tumor necrosis factor) and their relevance to rejection. Transplant Proc 21:26, 1989.
129. Imagawa DK, Millis JM, Olthoff KM, et al: The role of tumor necrosis factor in allograft rejection. I. Evidence that elevated levels of tumor necrosis factor-alpha predict rejection following orthotopic liver transplantation. Transplantation 50:219, 1990.
130. Imagawa DK, Millis JM, Olthoff KM, et al: The role of tumor necrosis factor in allograft rejection. II. Evidence that antibody therapy against tumor necrosis factor-alpha and lymphotoxin enhances cardiac allograft survival in rats. Transplantation 50:189, 1990.
131. Kishimoto T, Hirano T: Molecular regulation of B lymphocyte response. Annu Rev Immunol 6:485, 1988.
132. Wong GG, Clark SC: Multiple actions of interleukin 6 within a cytokine network. Immunol Today 9:137, 1988.
133. Ohzato H, Monden M, Yoshizaki K, et al: Serum interleukin-6 levels as an indicator of acute rejection after liver transplantation in cynomolgus monkeys. Surg Today 23:521, 1993.
134. Hamilton G, Prettenhofer M, Zommer A, et al: Intraoperative course and prognostic significance of endotoxin, tumor necrosis factor-alpha and interleukin-6 in liver transplant recipients. Immunobiology 182:425, 1991.
135. Colvin RB, Preffer FI, Fuller T, et al: A critical analysis of serum and urine interleukin 2 receptor assays in renal allograft recipients. Transplant Proc 21:1863, 1989.
136. Cantarovich D, Le Mauff B, Hourmant M, et al: Prophylactic use of a monoclonal antibody (33B3.1) directed against interleukin 2 receptor following human renal transplantation. Am J Kidney Dis 11:101, 1988.
137. Conti F, Frappier J, Dharancy S, et al: Interleukin-15 production during liver allograft rejection in humans. Transplantation 76:210, 2003.
138. Wiesner RH, Rakela J, Ishitani MB, et al: Recent advances in liver transplantation. Mayo Clin Proc 78:197, 2003.
139. Firpi RJ, Abdelmalek MF, Soldevila-Pico C, et al: Combination of interferon alfa-2b and ribavirin in liver transplant recipients with histological recurrent hepatitis C. Liver Transpl 8:1000, 2002.
140. Prieto M, Berenguer M, Rayon JM, et al: High incidence of allograft cirrhosis in hepatitis C virus genotype 1b infection following transplantation: Relationship with rejection episodes. Hepatology 29:250, 1999.
141. Ferrell LD, Wright TL, Roberts J, et al: Hepatitis C viral infection in liver transplant recipients. Hepatology 16:865, 1992.
142. Mueller AR, Platz KP, Berg T, et al: Association between hepatitis and rejection: Upregulation of cytokines and extracellular matrix parameters. Transplant Proc 29:2843, 1997.
143. Dhillon AP, Dusheiko GM: Pathology of hepatitis C virus infection. Histopathology 26:297, 1995.
144. Petrovic LM, Villamil FG, Vierling JM, et al: Comparison of histopathology in acute allograft rejection and recurrent hepatitis C infection after liver transplantation. Liver Transpl Surg 3:398, 1997.
145. Khettry U, Robiou C, Jenkins R, et al: Recurrent hepatitis C in liver allografts: Early histologic indicators. Intern J Surg Pathol 6:197, 1998.
146. Demetris A, Batts K, Dhillon A, et al: Banff schema for grading liver allograft rejection: An international consensus document. Hepatology 25:658, 1997.
147. Saxena R, Crawford JM, Navarro VJ, et al: Utilization of acidophil bodies in the diagnosis of recurrent hepatitis C infection after orthotopic liver transplantation. Mod Pathol 15:897, 2002.
148. Duvoux C, Pawlotsky JM, Cherqui D, et al: Serial quantitative determination of hepatitis C virus RNA levels after liver transplantation. A useful test for diagnosis of hepatitis C virus reinfection. Transplantation 60:457, 1995.
149. Aardema KL, Nakhleh RE, Terry LK, et al: Tissue quantification of hepatitis C virus RNA with morphologic correlation in the diagnosis of recurrent hepatitis C virus in human liver transplants. Mod Pathol 12:1043, 1999.
150. Gane EJ, Naoumov NV, Qian KP, et al: A longitudinal analysis of hepatitis C virus replication following liver transplantation. Gastroenterology 110:167, 1996.
151. Gottschlich MJ, Aardema KL, Burd EM, et al: The use of hepatitis C viral RNA levels in liver tissue to distinguish rejection from recurrent hepatitis C. Liver Transpl 7:436, 2001.
152. Sreekumar W, Gores G, Rosen C, et al: Differential gene expression patterns in HCV infected allografts during acute cellular rejection [abstract]. Hepatology 32:260A, 2000.
153. Tannapfel A, Geissler F, Witzigmann H, et al: Analysis of liver allograft rejection related genes using cDNA-microarrays in liver allograft specimen. Transplant Proc 33:3283, 2001.
154. Zekry A, Bishop GA, Bowen DG, et al: Intrahepatic cytokine profiles associated with posttransplantation hepatitis C virus-related liver injury. Liver Transpl 8:292, 2002.
155. Ciccorossi P, Filipponi F, Oliveri F, et al: Increasing serum levels of IgM anti-HCV are diagnostic of recurrent hepatitis C in liver transplant patients with ALT flares. J Viral Hepat 10:168, 2003.
156. Gane EJ, Portmann BC, Naoumov NV, et al: Long-term outcome of hepatitis C infection after liver transplantation. N Engl J Med 334:815, 1996.

157. Sheiner PA, Schwartz ME, Mor E, et al: Severe or multiple rejection episodes are associated with early recurrence of hepatitis C after orthotopic liver transplantation. Hepatology 21:30, 1995.

158. McCaughan GW, Zekry A: Pathogenesis of hepatitis C virus recurrence in the liver allograft. Liver Transpl 8(Suppl 1):S7, 2002.

159. Abraham SC, Furth EE: Receiver operating characteristic analysis of serum chemical parameters as tests of liver transplant rejection and correlation with histology. Transplantation 59:740, 1995.

160. Williams JW, Peters TG, Vera SR, et al: Biopsy-directed immunosuppression following hepatic transplantation in man. Transplantation 39:589, 1985.

161. Henley KS, Lucey MR, Appelman HD, et al: Biochemical and histopathological correlation in liver transplant: The first 180 days. Hepatology 16:688, 1992.

162. Lautenschlager I, Hockerstedt K, Hayry P: Fine-needle aspiration biopsy in the monitoring of liver allografts. Transpl Int 4:54, 1991.

163. Lautenschlager I, Hockerstedt K, Taskinen E, et al: Fine-needle aspiration biopsy in the monitoring of liver allografts. I. Correlation between aspiration biopsy and core biopsy in experimental pig liver allografts. Transplantation 46:41, 1988.

164. Kubota K, Reinholt FP, Tyden G, Groth CG: Recent experience with pancreatic juice cytology in monitoring pancreatic graft rejection. Transplant Proc 21:3643, 1989.

165. Topalidis T, Bechstein WO, Bohmann C, et al: New preparation method for bile cytology in liver transplantation: Diagnosis of rejection. Transplant Proc 25:1979, 1993.

166. Oldhafer KJ, Gubernatis G, Ringe B, Pichlmayr R: Experience with bile cytology after liver transplantation. Transplant Proc 22:1524, 1990.

167. Kubota K, Ericzon BG, Reinholt FP: Diagnosis of liver transplant rejection by bile cytology. Transplant Proc 22:1521, 1990.

168. Roberti I, Lieberman KV, Manzarbeitia C, et al: Evidence that the systematic analysis of bile cytology permits monitoring of hepatic allograft rejection. Transplantation 54:471, 1992.

169. Ormonde DG, de Boer WB, Kierath A, et al: Banff schema for grading liver allograft rejection: Utility in clinical practice. Liver Transpl Surg 5:261, 1999.

Cell Migration, Chimerism, and Graft Acceptance, with Particular Reference to the Liver*

THOMAS E. STARZL
NORIKO MURASE
ANTHONY J. DEMETRIS
MASSIMO TRUCCO
BIJAN EGHTESAD
PAULO FONTES
KAREEM ABU-ELMAGD
AMADEO MARCOS
JOHN J. FUNG

"Accidental" immunosuppression-aided
   tolerance   1184
   After kidney transplantation   1184
   After liver transplantation   1186

The question of donor leukocyte
   chimerism   1186
   Chimeric allografts   1186
   Systemic chimerism   1186

A unified view of transplantation   1189

A paradigm shift   1192

The development of tolerogenic
   immunosuppression   1193

The clinical transplantation of tissues and organs was viewed as a biologically unsound objective until Billingham, Brent, and Medawar showed in 1953 that transplant tolerance could be acquired.[1] The crucial observation was that immunologically immature neonatal mice whose bone marrow–derived hematolymphopoietic cells had been replaced by those of an adult donor (donor leukocyte chimerism) could accept skin grafts from the original cell donor strain but from no other. The demonstration in 1955 by Main and Prehn of similar tolerance in radiation chimeras (i.e., cytoablated bone marrow mouse recipients) established the experimental model that led directly to clinical bone marrow transplantation (Fig. 73–1, right).[2] The donor-specific tolerance in the mouse models, humans, and all other

*This work was supported by National Institutes of Health grants DK 29961 and DK 64207.

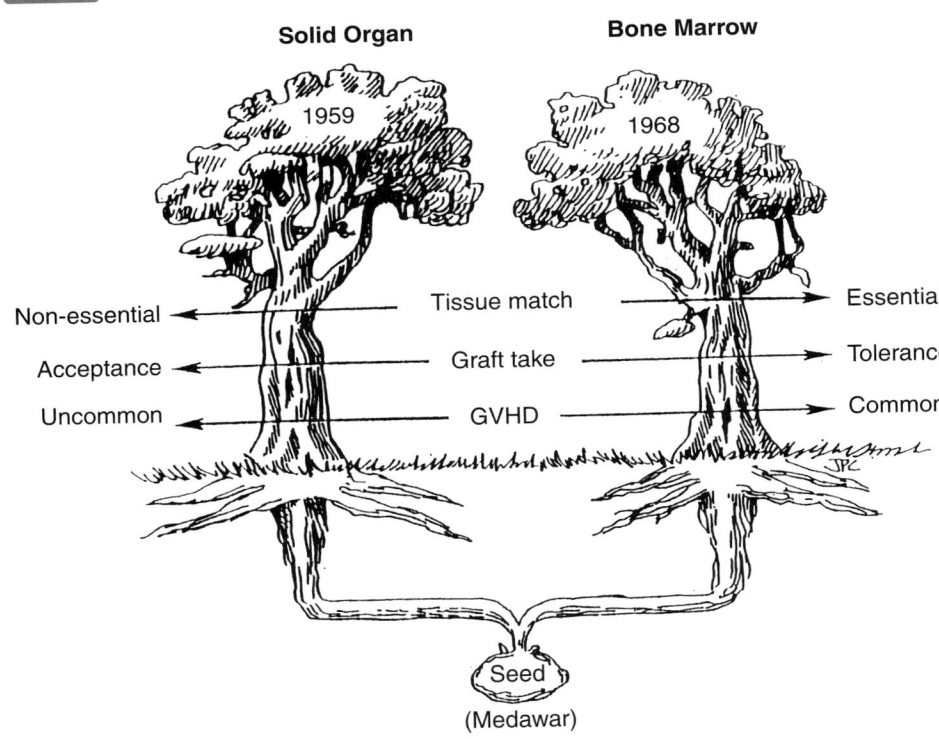

Solid Organ   **Bone Marrow**

FIGURE 73–1

The developmental tree of bone marrow (**right**) and whole-organ transplantation (**left**) after it was demonstrated by Gibson and Medawar during World War II that rejection is an immunological response. GVHD, graft-versus-host disease. (From Starzl TE, Demetris AJ, Trucco M, et al: Cell migration and chimerism after whole-organ transplantation: The basis of graft acceptance. Hepatology 17:1127-1152, 1993.)

tested species obviously involved donor leukocyte chimerism–associated mechanisms.

In contrast to this bench-to-bedside development, organ transplantation was accomplished first in irradiated humans and subsequently refined in stepwise empirical advances that were made possible by a small number of progressively more potent immunosuppressive agents, used singly or in various combinations. Because neither bone marrow nor any other kind of donor hematolymphopoietic cells were given, the enigmatic mechanisms of organ engraftment were assumed to be independent of leukocyte chimerism (see Fig. 73–1, left). When it was discovered in 1992 that long-surviving human organ recipients had low levels of donor leukocyte chimerism,[3,4] it could be suggested that bone marrow and organ transplantation were variations on the same theme. Before this, however, there had been clues that organ engraftment was a state of variable tolerance that in some cases became dependent on immunosuppression.

"Accidental" Immunosuppression-Aided Tolerance

After Kidney Transplantation

With Sublethal Total-Body Irradiation. The first two successful transplantations of kidney allografts in the world (in any species) were carried out in Boston[5] and Paris[6] in January and June 1959 (see Table 1–2 in Chapter 1). Both recipients of fraternal twin kidneys were conditioned with 450 R of total-body irradiation before transplantation. Although the patients were not treated afterward with maintenance immunosuppression, they had continuous renal function until they died of cancer 20 and 26 years later. These results were never duplicated. By 1963, pretransplant cytoablation was abandoned for organ transplantation, with further advances left up to drug development.

Using Pharmacological Immunosuppression. The effective use of drug therapy depended on exploitation of two qualities of the adaptive immune response that were first recognized at the University of Colorado in 1962-1963 in kidney transplant recipients who were treated before transplantation as well as afterward with azathioprine monotherapy, with high doses of prednisone added only for the treatment of rejection (Fig. 73–2A).[7] The first key observation was that kidney rejection was a highly reversible event, as had been predicted from the results of canine experiments (see Chapter 1). Second, rejection was frequently succeeded by what appeared to be variable partial tolerance.

Tolerance was inferred from a rapidly declining need for maintenance immunosuppression after successful treatment of rejection (see Fig. 73–2A). Nine (20%) of the 46 patients who received kidney allografts from living related donors over a period of approximately 14 months beginning in the autumn of 1962 retained

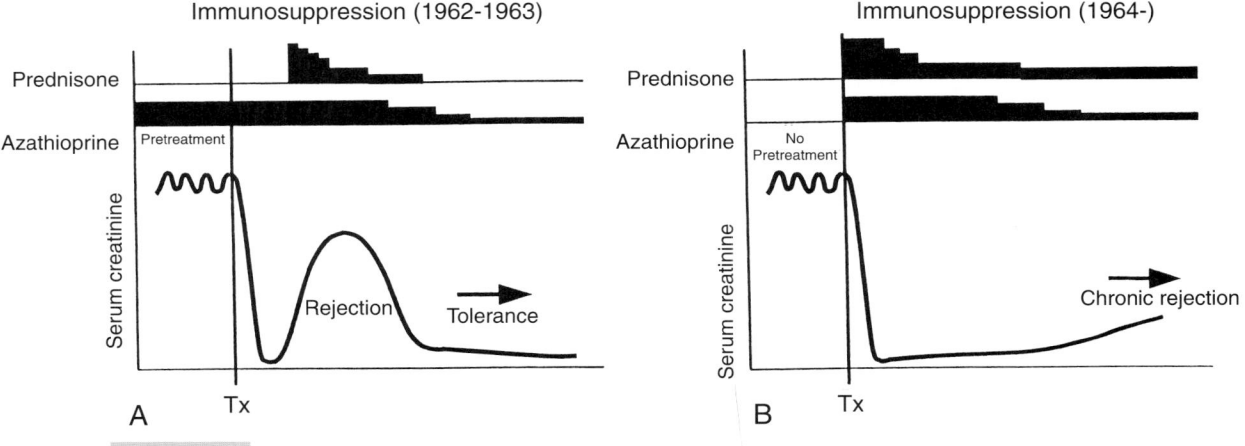

FIGURE 73–2

A, Empirically developed immunosuppression used for kidney transplant recipients in 1962 and 1963. Azathioprine was given before as well as after transplantation. Note the reversal of rejection with the addition of prednisone to azathioprine. More than a third of a century later, it was realized that the immuno-suppression had been in compliance with the two tolerogenic principles of immunosuppression depicted in Figure 73–15A: recipient pretreatment and minimum posttransplant immunosuppression. **B,** Treatment revisions made by 1964 that unwittingly violated both principles. Pretreatment was de-emphasized or eliminated, and high-dose multiagent immunosuppression was given prophylactically instead of as needed. Acute rejection was more efficiently prevented, but the type of drug-free tolerance shown in **A** was no longer observed.

their grafts for the next 4 decades, all but 1 with normal function throughout. Eight of the nine recipients are still alive and bear the longest surviving kidney allografts in the world today. Importantly, seven of the nine eventually stopped taking all immunosuppression for periods ranging from 2½ to 39 years without undergoing rejection (Fig. 73–3).[8]

Two changes were then made in management (see Fig. 73–2B). In December 1963, pretreatment with azathioprine was de-emphasized because of immuno-suppression-associated infectious complications that had delayed or prevented transplantation. In addition, high doses of prednisone were routinely instituted at the time of surgery rather than as needed (see Fig. 73–2B).[9] The second "reform" was prompted by a 15% incidence of loss of kidney allografts to acute rejection that could not be reversed. When the early loss of kidneys was dramatically reduced, the changes in management

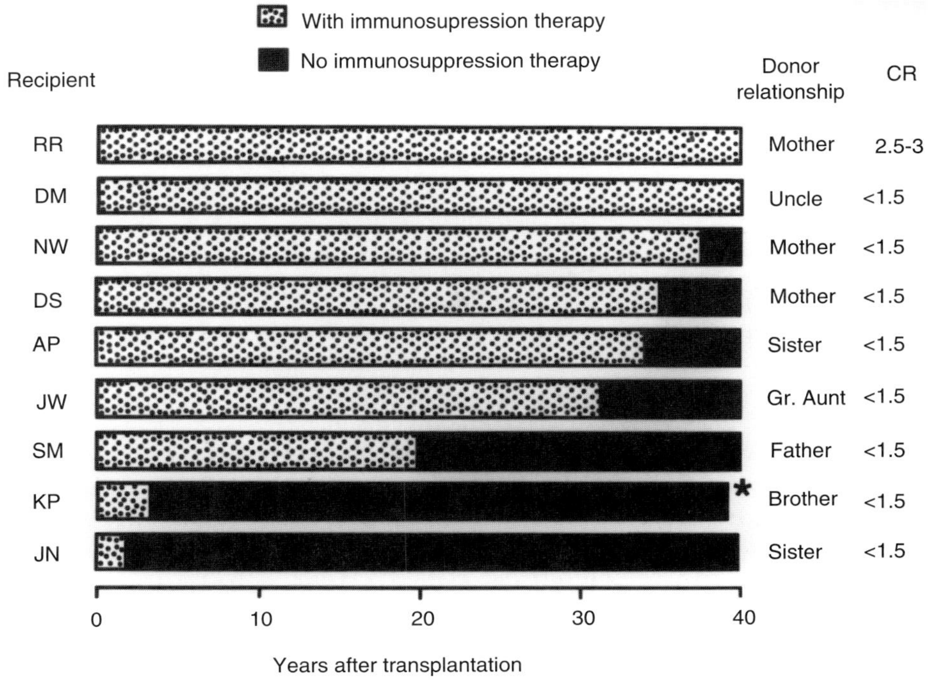

FIGURE 73–3

Nine (20%) of the 46 living donor kidney recipients treated at the University of Colorado over a 14-month period beginning in autumn 1962 whose grafts functioned for 4 decades. The solid portion of the *horizontal bars* depicts the time without immuno-suppression. Note that the current serum creatinine concentration is nor-mal in all but one patient. *Asterisk,* murdered: kidney allograft normal at autopsy. (From Starzl TE: The saga of liver replacement, with particular refer-ence to the reciprocal influence of liver and kidney transplantation [1955-1967]. J Am Coll Surg 195:587-610, 2002.)

With immunosuppression therapy

No immunosuppression therapy

Recipient		Donor relationship	CR
RR		Mother	2.5-3
DM		Uncle	<1.5
NW		Mother	<1.5
DS		Mother	<1.5
AP		Sister	<1.5
JW		Gr. Aunt	<1.5
SM		Father	<1.5
KP		* Brother	<1.5
JN		Sister	<1.5

Years after transplantation

appeared to be justified. The policy of heavy prophylactic immunosuppression with multiple agents (often called "induction") quickly became the accepted worldwide standard of treatment. Inexplicably, no comparable cluster of drug-free renal recipients was ever produced again, in Colorado or anywhere else.

After Liver Transplantation

In contrast, groups of drug-free liver recipients continued to be observed, but only during four periods. The first was in the 1970s as described in Chapter 1 and more completely elsewhere.[8] During this time, baseline immunosuppression with azathioprine (or cyclophosphamide) was combined with a short course of preoperative and postoperative antilymphocyte globulin (ALG) and the sparing use of prednisone. Tolerant liver recipients were also produced after the advent of calcineurin inhibitor drugs, but almost exclusively in 1979-1980 and 1989-1990 in Denver and Pittsburgh, just after cyclosporine[10] and tacrolimus,[11,12] respectively, were introduced clinically as monotherapy, with prednisone added only for breakthrough rejection. When multidrug prophylactic immunosuppression was used in subsequent cases, drug-free tolerance was no longer seen. The fourth group of tolerant liver patients was produced recently in Kyoto, Japan, where many pediatric recipients of partial livers from parental donors were successfully weaned from a steroid-sparing tacrolimus-based regimen,[13] similar to that originally used in 1989-1990.[12]

The Question of Donor Leukocyte Chimerism

The drug-free state of these human organ recipients, as well as animal organ recipients treated with a short course of immunosuppression, was called "operational tolerance" or designated by other terms. The reason was the conclusion "by consensus" as early as 1963 that the mechanisms of organ engraftment were different from the donor leukocyte chimerism–associated mechanisms of the mouse tolerance models.[1,2] Because of the dramatic clinical differences between the two types of procedures (see Fig. 73–1), this conclusion seemed inescapable. In retrospect, however, there was always reason to question whether this distinction was justified.

Chimeric Allografts

In 1950, Woodruff and Woodruff postulated that the reduced antigenicity of experimental endocrine grafts (adaptation) during their residence in the anterior chamber of the eye was due to replacement of certain elements of the graft, including "stromal" cells.[14] The concept that transplants become donor-recipient composites was subsequently validated with skin grafts in the first stage of classic parking experiments in mice.[15,16] Unequivocal evidence that whole-organ grafts underwent such a transformation was obtained in 1968 in livers from male deceased donors that had been transplanted to female recipients at the University of Colorado.[17,18] It was shown with karyotyping that the hepatocytes and the endothelium of the major blood vessels of the transplants retained their donor sex whereas the bone marrow–derived passenger leukocytes, including Kupffer cells, were largely replaced with recipient female cells. The changes were complete within 100 postoperative days (Fig. 73–4B).

Similar leukocyte replacement was later seen in transplanted rat organs after stage I parking experiments,[19-21] but this phenomenon was model specific, that is, demonstrable only with immunologically "weak" strain combinations. Thus, the leukocyte replacement in the human liver allograft was considered to be a unique feature of hepatic transplantation. This illusion was dispelled in 1991 by studies of rat[22] and human[23] intestinal allografts. The intestinal epithelium and vascular endothelium remained donor specific, but the lymphoid, dendritic, and other leukocytes in the lamina propria, Peyer's patches, and mesenteric nodes were mostly replaced by recipient cells of the same lineage. The suspicion that comparable events must be occurring during engraftment of other kinds of organs was confirmed in the 1990s by studies of human kidney[24,25] and thoracic organ allografts[26,27] and even in models of concordant organ xenotransplantation.[28] Thus, the image shown in Figure 73–4B was applicable to all engrafted organs.

Systemic Chimerism

Circumstantial Evidence. Until the 1990s it was widely assumed that the donor leukocytes that were missing from transplanted organs had undergone immune destruction with selective preservation of the specialized parenchymal cells (Fig. 73–5). Contrary to this view, earlier indirect evidence suggested that at least some of the passenger leukocytes had merely relocated in the recipient. This information was largely ignored, forgotten, or misinterpreted. In the earliest example, skin tests for tuberculin, histoplasmin, blastomycin, and coccidioidin, as well as tests for mumps, candidiasis, and trichophytosis immunity, were performed in the first wave of Colorado kidney recipients in 1962-1963 and in their donors.[29] Recipients whose skin reactions were negative preoperatively became positive at a 77% rate after receiving transplants from skin test–positive donors (Fig. 73–6). Failure of transfer

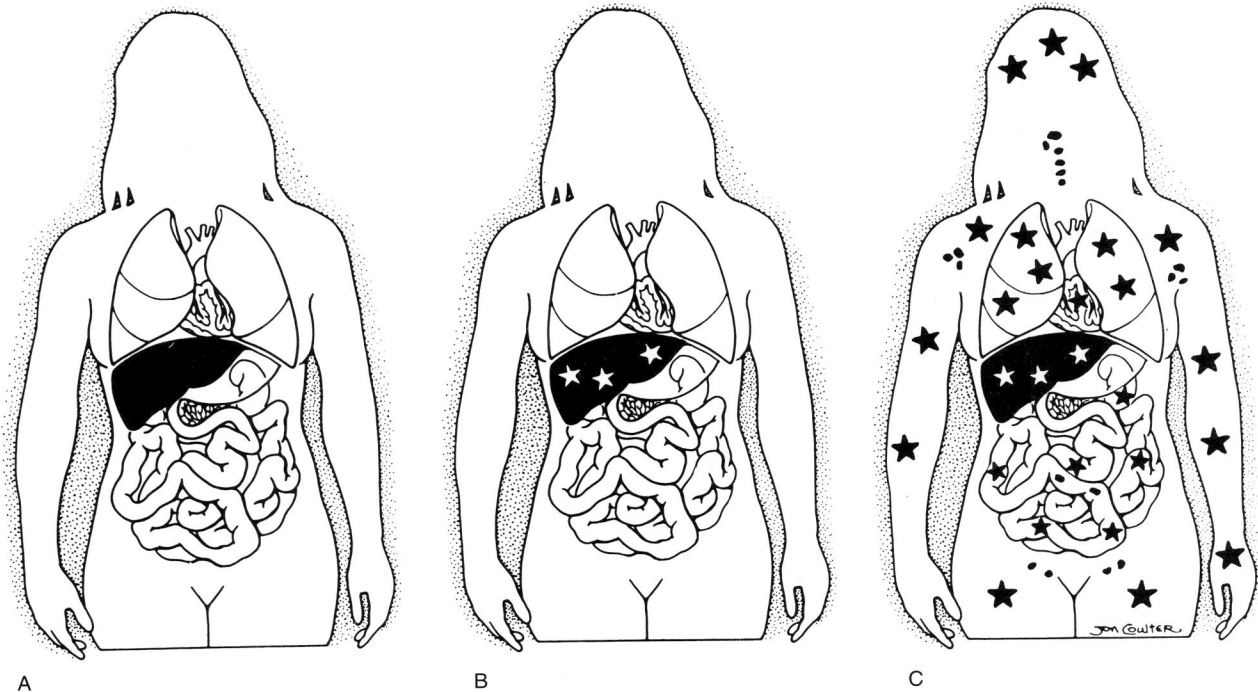

FIGURE 73–4

Steps in the understanding of liver transplantation. **A**, Historical view of the organ as a defenseless island in a hostile recipient sea. **B**, Recognition in 1969 that the liver graft became a genetic composite (organ chimera). **C**, Discovery in 1992 that organ recipients have systemic chimerism. (From Starzl TE, Demetris AJ, Trucco M, et al: Cell migration and chimerism after whole-organ transplantation: The basis of graft acceptance. Hepatology 17:1127-1152, 1993.)

Organ engraftment

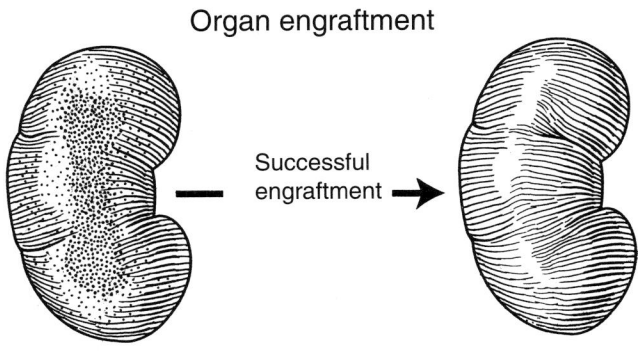

Successful engraftment →

▦ Passenger leukocytes   ▤ Specialized kidney cells

FIGURE 73–5

Left, The passenger leukocytes of bone marrow origin present in all organs are symbolized by a bone silhouette within a kidney. **Right**, Disappearance of these cells from a successfully engrafted organ and their replacement by similar recipient white cells. It was widely assumed until the 1990s that successful engraftment meant that the donor leukocytes had been selectively destroyed by the host-versus-graft response with selective preservation of parenchymal cells. (From Starzl TE: Organ transplantation: A practical triumph and epistemologic collapse. Proc Am Philos Soc 147: 226-245, 2003.)

of skin test positivity usually meant that the kidney had been promptly rejected.

It was suggested in 1964 that the acquisition of positive skin test findings could have been ". . . caused by the *adoptive transfer* of donor cellular immunity by leukocytes in the renal graft vasculature and hilar lymphoid tissue."[29] This explanation was considered implausible, however, in part because the kidney was thought to contain very few leukocytes. In addition, large-scale cell migration after organ transplantation was not part of the conceptual framework at the time. Further evidence of adoptive immunity was obtained in 1969 in human liver recipients whose blood analysis revealed new donor immunoglobulin types.[18,30] More support came in 1984 with the observation that anti–red cell antibodies (isoagglutinins) of apparently donor origin were responsible for the hemolysis seen in recipients of ABO-compatible but not ABO-identical livers.[31]*

---

*In an anecdotal modern example of adoptive transfer, Henri Bismuth successfully transplanted the liver from a brain-dead donor who had suffered a fatal allergic reaction from peanuts. Some months later, the otherwise well recipient reported potentially life-threatening symptoms after peanut consumption. The problem was resolved with peanut abstinence.[32]

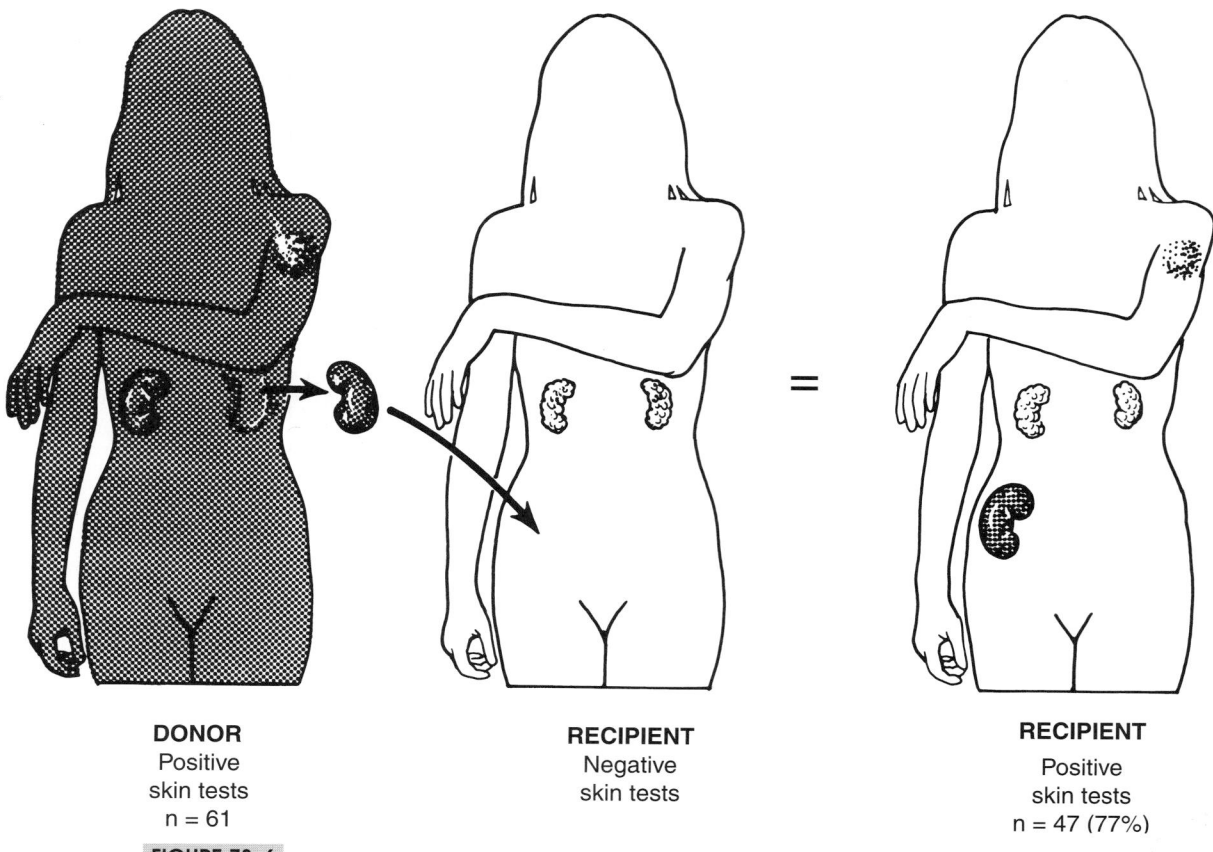

DONER
Positive
skin tests
n = 61

RECIPIENT
Negative
skin tests

=

RECIPIENT
Positive
skin tests
n = 47 (77%)

FIGURE 73–6

Adoptive transfer of positive skin test results from kidney donors to recipients in patients at the University of Colorado, 1962 to 1964.[29] (From Starzl TE, Demetris AJ, Trucco M, et al: Cell migration and chimerism after whole-organ transplantation: The basis of graft acceptance. Hepatology 17:1127-1152, 1993.)

In the meanwhile, there was mounting appreciation that cell migration is a striking phenomenon after the transplantation of all whole organs. Cell migration was first reported in 1981 by Nemlander and Hayry in their studies on the kinetics of rejecting experimental kidney grafts.[33] The donor cells that departed the organ were the donor hematolymphopoietic (passenger) leukocytes of bone marrow origin (including dendritic cells[34,35]) that had been postulated by Snell[36] to be the principal cause of allograft immunogenicity. Finally, in 1991, Murase and colleagues[37,38] showed with flow cytometry that the leukocytes leaving small bowel and multivisceral allografts in rat recipients treated with a short course of tacrolimus rapidly migrate in large numbers through vascular routes to widely distributed host lymphoid tissues.

The migration created a state of unstable mixed blood chimerism for 30 to 45 days during which up to 20% of the recipient circulating mononuclear cells were of donor origin. The findings were not associated with lethal or even detectable graft-versus-host disease (GVHD), except in a few GVHD-prone strain combinations.[37-39] The rodent data were supplemented

by studies of human bowel recipients in whom the flood of cells into the recipient blood was directly correlated with the rapid disappearance of passenger leukocytes from the transplant (Fig. 73–7).[23,40] Because the circulating donor cells rapidly diminished within a few weeks and became undetectable by flow cytometry after 30 to 60 days in both rodent and human recipients, the conviction of most observers was that the donor cells had now been eliminated.

Direct Evidence. The next and, as it turned out, decisive step, between April and July 1992, was to look for donor hematolymphopoietic cells in the blood and tissues of 30 human recipients of kidneys and livers whose successful transplantation had been performed 3 to 29 years earlier (Fig. 73–8).[3,4,24,41] The study was made feasible by the distinctive qualities of two chromosomes. The presence of the X or Y chromosome in the tissues or blood of recipients of grafts from donors of the opposite sex was considered strong evidence of systemic chimerism. Alternatively, probes were used that detected HLA alleles of chromosome 6.

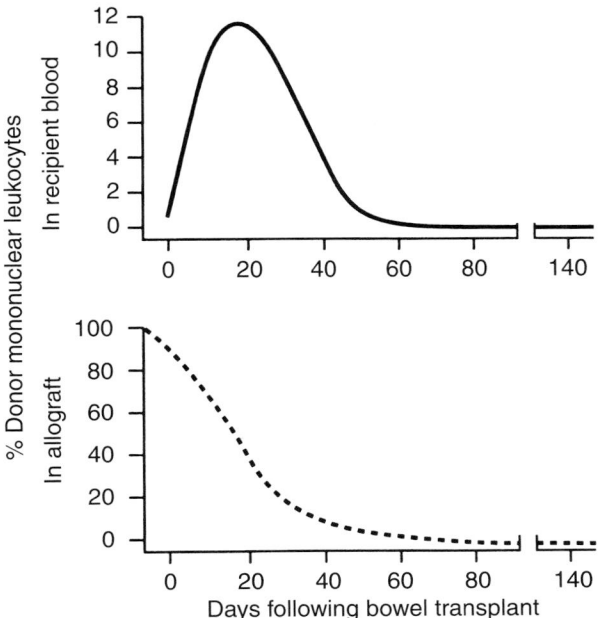

FIGURE 73–7

Dynamic events during intestinal engraftment. **Upper panel**, Surge of migratory donor mononuclear leukocytes in the recipient blood during the first 2 or 3 weeks after transplantation. **Lower panel**, Contemporaneous disappearance of passenger leukocytes from the allograft; they are replaced by recipient cells of the same lineage. (Adapted from Starzl TE, Murase N, Thomson AW, et al: Immunity and tolerance are related, and governed by antigen migration and localization. Transplant Proc 31:1406-1411, 1999.)

Cytostaining allowed detection of the location and morphological characterization of the phenotypically distinct donor and recipient cells. Polymerase chain reaction could distinguish donor from recipient DNA at a sensitivity limit of 1 donor cell per 10^5 recipient cells.[3,4,41]

Low-level multilineage donor leukocyte chimerism (microchimerism) was found in all 30 patients in one or more locations, including the skin, lymph nodes, heart, lungs, spleen, intestine, kidneys, bone marrow, and thymus. At any given site, donor leukocytes were present in larger numbers in liver recipients than in kidney recipients studied at comparable posttransplant times. With the persistence of donor cells for as long as 30 years, it was inferred that hematolymphopoietic precursor and stem cells were part of the passenger leukocyte population of organ grafts. The results in the human studies were congruent with a soon to be large body of experimental evidence[22,37-39,42-52] that changed the generic portrait of a successfully treated organ recipient to that depicted in Figure 73–4C.

A Unified View of Transplantation

As early as 1992, however, a grand design could already be pieced together whose very simplicity had cloaked its existence and delayed its discovery. It was deduced that alloengraftment of both bone marrow cells and organs began immediately after implantation and consisted of ". . . responses of co-existing donor and recipient [white] cells, each to the other, causing reciprocal clonal exhaustion, followed by peripheral clonal deletion" (Fig. 73–9).[3,4] After transplantation, the two responses begin as passenger leukocytes start their selective migration to host lymphoid organs,[33-35] where they induce a donor-specific response.

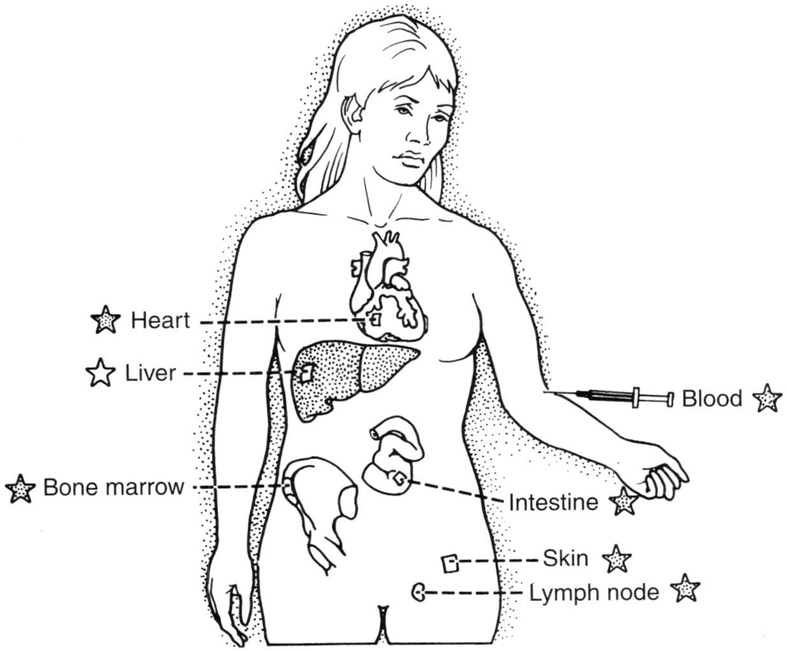

FIGURE 73–8

Host sites sampled in 1992 in studies of the longest-surviving kidney and liver recipients in the world. Donor leukocyte chimerism was looked for in host blood, skin, and lymph nodes, as well as in the allograft (here a liver) of all patients. In selected recipients, biopsy samples were also taken from the heart, intestine, other organs, or bone marrow. (From Starzl TE: The birth of clinical organ transplantation. J Am Coll Surg 192:431-446, 2001.)

☆ Heart
☆ Liver
Blood ☆
☆ Bone marrow
Intestine ☆
Skin ☆
Lymph node ☆

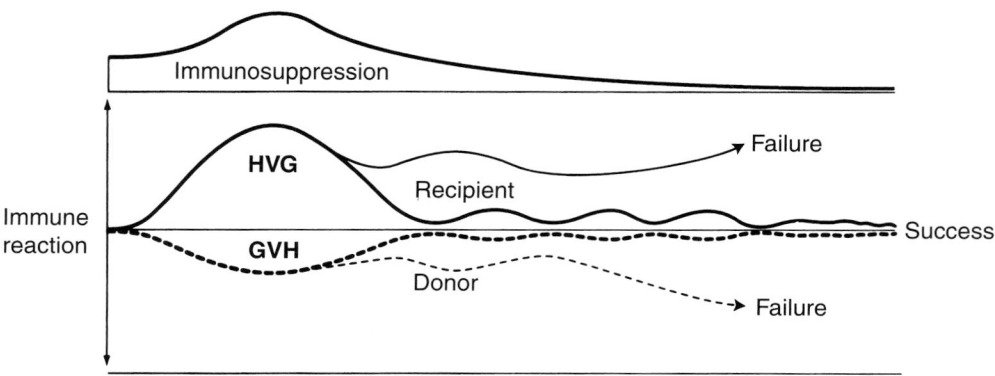

FIGURE 73–9

Contemporaneous host-versus-graft (HVG) (*upright curves*) and graft-versus-host (GVH) (*inverted curves*) responses after organ transplantation. If some degree of reciprocal clonal exhaustion is not induced and maintained (usually requiring protective immunosuppression), one cell population will destroy the other. In contrast to the generally dominant HVG reaction of organ transplantation (shown here), the GVH reaction is usually dominant in a cytoablated bone marrow recipient. Therapeutic failure with either type of transplantation implies an inability to control one, the other, or both of the responses. (Reprinted, by permission, from Starzl TE, Zinkernagel RM: Antigen localization and migration in immunity and tolerance. N Engl J Med 339:1905-1913, 1998.)

The donor cells found years later in the nonlymphoid as well as lymphoid sites shown in Figure 73–8 were obviously derived from pluripotential passenger leukocytes that were later proved to be a component of the passenger leukocyte population.[48,53,54]

Exhaustion and deletion of the dominant response of organ transplantation (the upright curve in Fig. 73–9) corresponded to the characteristic acute immunological crisis and resolution first observed 30 years earlier in our Colorado kidney recipients.[7] In clinical practice and in most experimental models, a protective umbrella of immunosuppression is required to prevent one cell

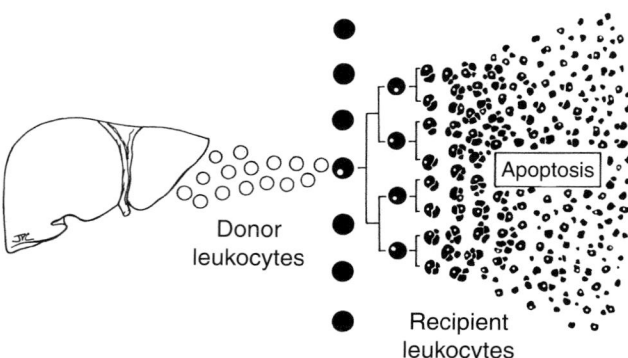

FIGURE 73–10

Clonal exhaustion-deletion, the seminal mechanism of organ engraftment and acquired tolerance. Persistence of some donor cells is a prerequisite for maintenance of the variable deletional tolerance induced by the initial surge of donor cells. (From Starzl TE: The saga of liver replacement, with particular reference to the reciprocal influence of liver and kidney transplantation [1955-1967]. J Am Coll Surg 195:587-610, 2002.)

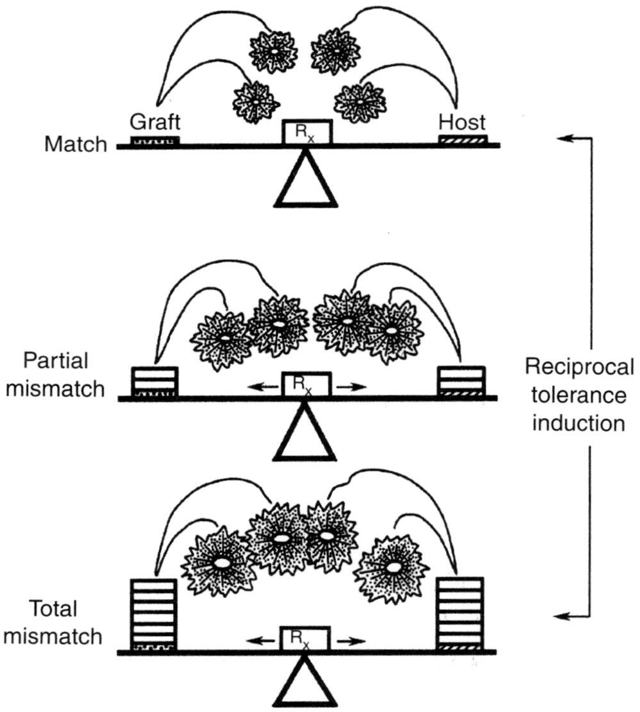

FIGURE 73–11

Reciprocal clonal exhaustion-deletion of the host-versus-graft and graft-versus-host responses is a buffer against rejection on the one hand and graft-versus-host disease on the other. R$_x$, iatrogenic immunosuppression. (Modified from Starzl TE, Demetris AJ, Murase N, et al: Donor cell chimerism permitted by immunosuppressive drugs: A new view of organ transplantation. Immunol Today 14:326-332, 1993.)

population from destroying the other before deletion can occur. However, deletion occurs without treatment in some pig,[55-58] rat,[59,60] and mouse[45] models of spontaneous organ tolerance. The allograft in most (but not all) of these experimental models is the liver with its large quantity of passenger leukocytes (Fig. 73–10).

Pretransplant cytoablation of the bone marrow recipient simply reversed the proportions of donor and recipient cells. The resulting transfer of immune dominance to the graft (the inverted response curve in Fig. 73–9) explained all the differences between bone marrow and organ transplantation (see Fig. 73–1). As long as the balance of the two response arms was not excessively disrupted and if both cell populations were equally immunosuppressed (as was the empirically developed policy of organ transplantation), the "nullification" effect of the reciprocal tolerance induction (Fig. 73–11) accounted for the poor prognostic value of HLA matching for organ transplantation[61] and the rarity of GVHD after the engraftment of immunologically active organs such as the intestine and liver.[4,39,44]

The foregoing interpretation of our findings generated a controversy that is only now reaching resolution. Historically, the events set in motion by transplantation had been defined in the context of a single immune response. In the organ recipient (Fig. 73–12A), this was the host-versus-graft reaction. The subsidence of the response that occurred with engraftment had been attributed to theoretical mechanisms that did not require the presence of donor leukocyte chimerism.

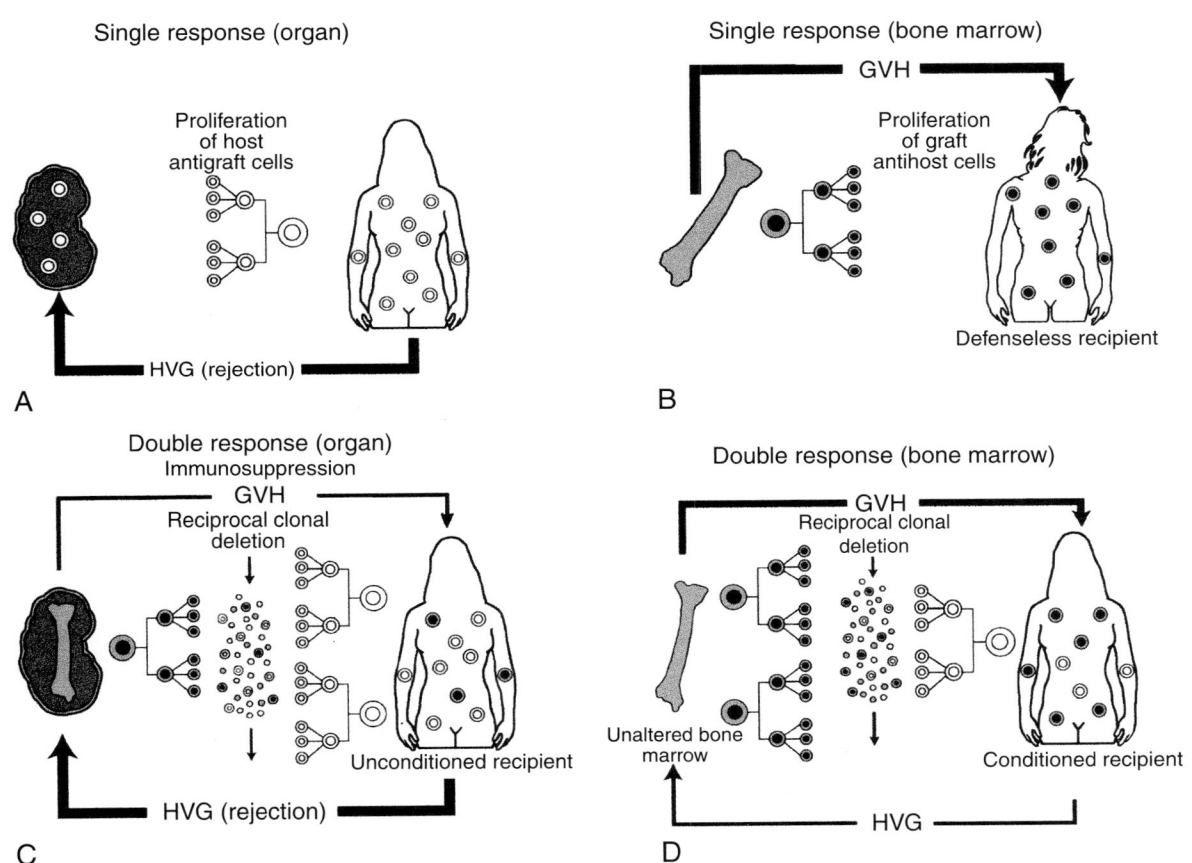

FIGURE 73–12

Old (**A** and **B**) and new views (**C** and **D**) of transplantation recipients. **A**, Early conceptualization of immune mechanisms in organ transplantation in terms of a unidirectional host-versus-graft (HVG) response. Although this conceptualization readily explained organ rejection, it limited possible explanations of organ engraftment. **B**, Mirror image of **A** depicting the early understanding of successful bone marrow transplantation as complete replacement of the recipient's immune system by that of the donor, with the potential complication of an unopposed lethal unidirectional graft-versus-host (GVH) response, that is, rejection of the recipient by the graft. **C**, Our current view of bidirectional and reciprocally modulating immune responses of coexisting immune-competent cell populations leading to organ engraftment despite a usually dominant HVG reaction. The transplanted organ, which initially loses most of its passenger leukocytes, apparently remains an important site for donor precursor and stem cells. **D**, Our currently conceived mirror image of **C** with reversal of the size proportions of the reciprocally modulating donor and recipient populations of immune cells after successful bone marrow transplantation.

Bone marrow transplantation had also been viewed from the perspective of an all-or-none response. Here, either the host rejected the infused cells, or the graft rejected the recipient (GVHD) (see Fig. 73–12B). This unidirectional response doctrine had already been brought into question in 1989, however, by the demonstration that essentially all bone marrow recipients who had ostensibly complete donor leukocyte chimerism actually had a small residual population of their own hematolymphopoietic cells (see Fig. 73–12D).[62,63]

With the discovery in 1992 of microchimerism in organ recipients, it was self-evident that successfully treated organ and bone marrow recipients were mirror images in every way (compare panels C and D in Fig. 73–12). Moreover, it could be persuasively argued that both kinds of engraftment were dependent on the same donor leukocyte chimerism–associated mechanisms.

A Paradigm Shift

The revised view of transplantation depicted in Figures 73–9 through 73–12 explained previously enigmatic observations in experimental models of transplantation and essentially all events seen in clinical practice (see Fig. 73–1). What was not apparent, however, was how the microchimeric donor cells managed to survive in the organ recipient and why, as we had postulated, their persistence was essential for long-term survival of the transplanted organ. Answers to these questions awaited a collaboration with Rolf Zinkernagel, the Swiss pathologist and 1996 Nobel Laureate (Fig. 73–13), that began in the summer of 1997.

A quarter of a century earlier, Zinkernagel and Doherty had demonstrated that noncytopathic (i.e., intracellular) microorganisms are controlled primarily by cytolytic or interleukin-releasing T lymphocytes that recognize as "non-self" host cells displaying complexes composed of self–major histocompatibility complex (MHC) molecules plus peptides derived from the infecting microorganism.[64] Allograft rejection was the apparent transplantation equivalent of this host-versus-pathogen adaptive immune response. However, the specific mechanisms leading to the asymptomatic "carrier state" after such infections and to the presumably analogous "acceptance" of allografts had remained enigmatic.

In 1996 and 1997, Zinkernagel had proposed in several publications that the adaptive immune response to viruses and other noncytopathic organisms was determined by the migration patterns of the pathogen.[65-68] This theory matched our conclusion that leukocyte migration plus relocation was the key event in organ engraftment.[3,4] Except for the different antigens of interest, we had independently described the same thing. Joining forces, we now explained how the small numbers of residual donor leukocytes could survive in the organ recipient and how this microchimerism could maintain the clonal exhaustion-deletion induced at the outset. We also emphasized that these donor cells could have the undesired effect of sustaining alloimmunity.[69]

Our larger objective, however, was to formulate a general principle of immune regulation that would more firmly place transplantation and infection on common ground and would apply in all other circumstances of immune reactivity or nonreactivity (e.g., tumor immunity and self-nonself discrimination). In essence, our hypothesis was that *immune responsiveness or nonresponsiveness to a given antigen is governed by migration and localization of the specific antigen.*[69] In this paradigm, previously postulated mechanisms of immune regulation (e.g., suppressor, veto, or T regulatory cells; self perpetuating cytokine mixtures; and idiotypic antibodies) were not essential, singly or in combination.

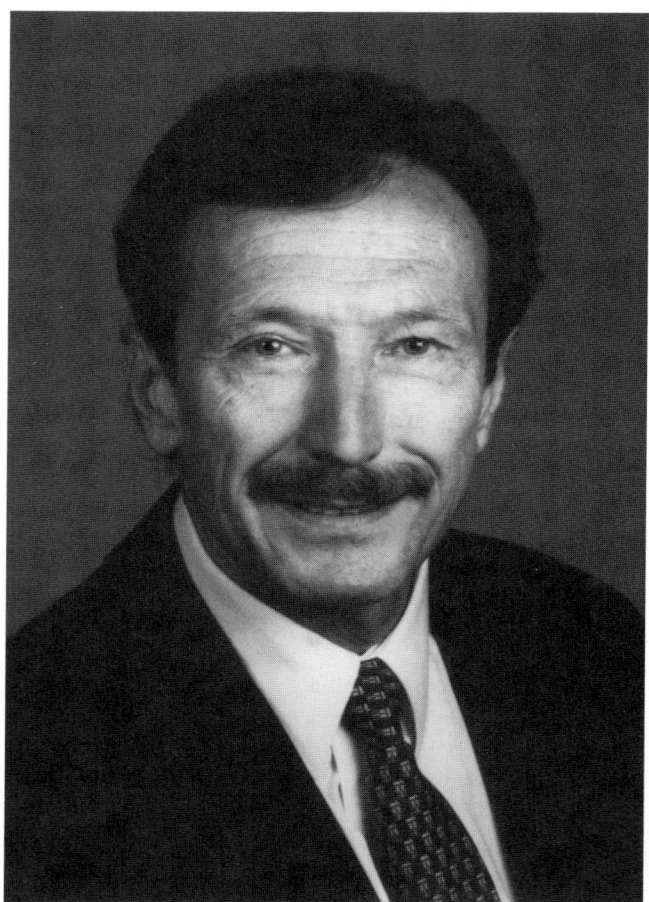

FIGURE 73–13

Rolf Zinkernagel (1944-). Swiss scientist whose discovery (with Peter Doherty) of the mechanisms of the adaptive immune response to noncytopathic microorganisms earned the Nobel Prize in 1996. (From Starzl TE: Organ transplantation: A practical triumph and epistemologic collapse. Proc Am Philos Soc 147: 226-245, 2003.)

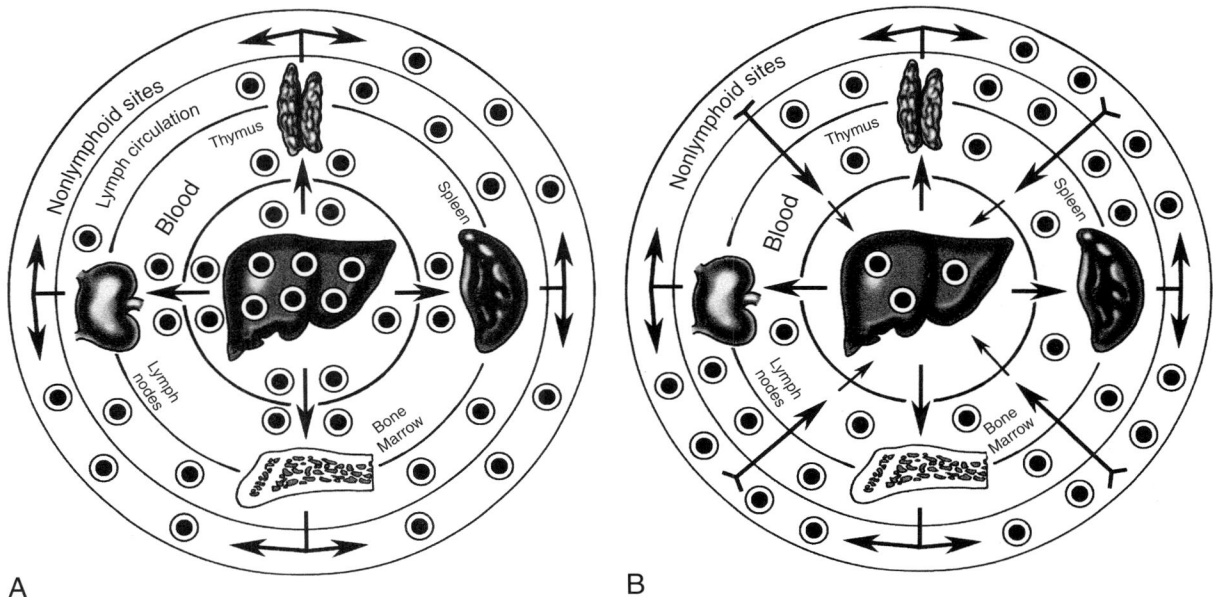

FIGURE 73–14

The migration routes of passenger leukocytes of transplanted organs are similar to those of infused bone marrow cells. **A,** Selective migration at first to host lymphoid organs. After 15 to 30 days, surviving leukocytes begin to secondarily move to nonlymphoid sites. **B,** Establishment of reverse traffic by which the exhaustion-deletion induced at the outset can be maintained.[69,70] See text.

Instead, alloengraftment could be accounted for by two straightforward mechanisms, both of which were regulated by antigen migration and localization. The first was immune ignorance, in which antigen that fails to reach host lymphoid organs or find refuge in privileged nonlymphoid sites is not recognized. The second mechanism was clonal exhaustion and deletion of the response induced by antigen that reaches organized lymphoid destinations (i.e., lymph nodes, spleen, bone marrow, and in lower mammalian species, the thymus). All outcomes after organ transplantation could be readily explained by the collaboration of these mechanisms.[69,70]

Beginning within a few minutes of transplantation, passenger leukocytes (i.e., hematolymphopoietic cells of bone marrow origin) begin to leave the organ graft and migrate selectively to host lymphoid organs. After 15 to 30 days, cells that have escaped destruction or have avoided lymphatic pathways and lymphoid sites begin to move to nonlymphoid niches (including the organ allograft[50,51]) that are relatively inaccessible to effector cells and neutralizing antibodies (Fig. 73–14A). By 60 days, the primary and secondary migration is relatively complete. The survival advantage of leukocytes in "protected" locations is similar to that of residual microorganisms after a spreading infection. From these sites where they may be forgotten or "ignored," or both, donor cells can migrate back to the host lymphoid organs and sustain the clonal exhaustion-deletion

induced at the outset (see Fig. 73–14B). If the initial tolerance is high grade, passage of cells from lymphoid to lymphoid compartment may be completely unrestricted.[69,70]

The Development of Tolerogenic Immunosuppression

If the hypothesis was correct, immunosuppression "permitted" the practical use of clinical transplantation because it reduced the alloimmune response into a deletable range, not because it was able to eliminate this response. We now proposed that the variable immunosuppression-aided tolerance exemplified by organ engraftment could be made more complete by adhering to two simple therapeutic principles.[70] The first principle was recipient pretreatment to decrease overall responsiveness before arrival of the alloantigen and thereby bring the anticipated antidonor response into a more deletable range (Fig. 73–15A).

The second principle was the minimal use of posttransplant immunosuppression. Here, the objective was to make the antidonor response still more deletable while preventing irreversible immune damage to the transplanted organ (see Fig. 73–15A). Too much treatment after transplantation in an effort to

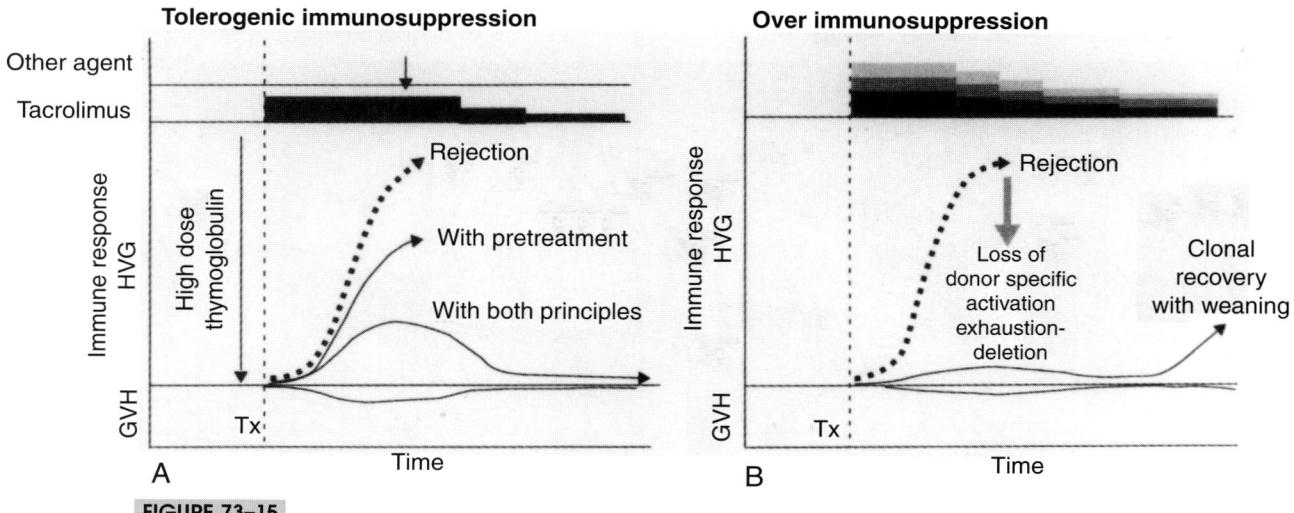

FIGURE 73–15

A, Conversion of rejection (*thick dashed arrow*) to an immune response that can be exhausted and deleted. Such conversion is done by combining pretreatment with minimal posttransplant immunosuppression. **B**, If the clonal response is eliminated by excessive posttransplant immunosuppression, the exhaustion-deletion shown in **A** may be precluded, thus making subsequent graft survival dependent on permanent high-dose immunosuppression. GVH, graft versus host; HVG, host versus graft; Tx, transplantation.

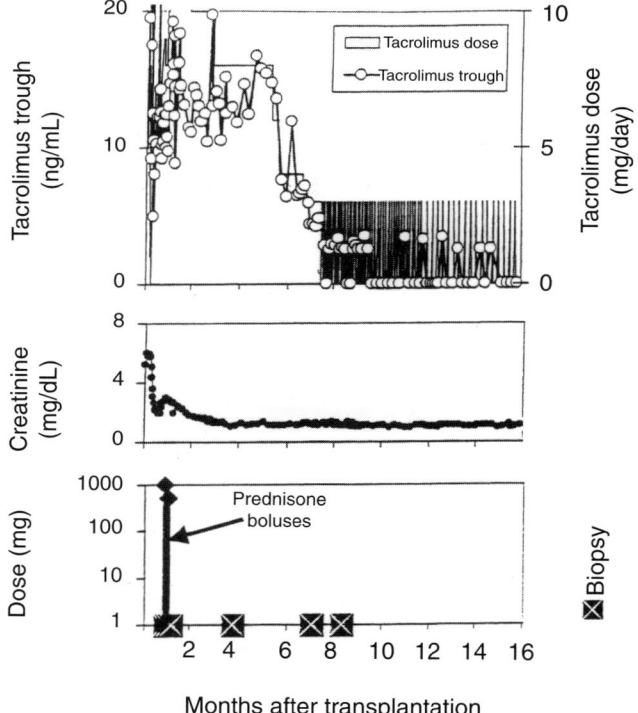

FIGURE 73–16

Course of treatment of a deceased donor kidney recipient. Biopsy-proven rejection (Banff 1A) in the third week was treated with boluses of 1.0 g and 0.5 g prednisolone. Similar findings in later biopsy specimens were not associated with renal function changes and were not treated. Instead, weaning was begun at 7 months. Now beyond 2 years, treatment remains one dose of tacrolimus per week.

reduce the incidence of rejection to zero would predictably shut down the donor-specific clonal activation on which the desired exhaustion-deletion depends (see Fig. 73–15B). In an initially overtreated recipient, therefore, subsequent attempts to reduce immunosuppression and allow restoration of global immune reactivity would permit parallel recovery of the undeleted clone and thereby commit the patient to lifetime dependence on unacceptably heavy maintenance immunosuppression (see Fig. 73–15B).

Given that immunosuppression is a two-edged sword, the worldwide practice of starting heavy multidrug immunosuppression on the day of transplantation was a systematic error that had been passed on from generation to generation of transplant physicians and surgeons for the last 40 years. The error was introduced *after* compilation of the cluster of highly tolerant Colorado kidney recipients depicted in Figure 73–3. These pioneer patients had been managed in accordance with both therapeutic principles (see Fig. 73–2A). Because of pretransplant infections, pretreatment with azathioprine (Imuran) was de-emphasized. In addition, to avoid graft loss from acute rejection, heavy multidrug immunosuppression was instituted on the day of surgery (see Fig. 73–2B). This antitolerogenic policy of prophylactic immunosuppression became the state of the art for organ transplantation by 1964 and has remained so ever since.

Reform required a counterintuitive return to 1962-1963, but armed this time with better drugs.

Beginning in July 2001, pretreatment was provided with a superior ALG (thymoglobulin) or with a broadly reacting monoclonal antibody (alemtuzumab [Campath]). Posttransplant monotherapy was given with tacrolimus. As expected, cyclosporine or rapamycin could be substituted for tacrolimus in the event of tacrolimus toxicity. Other agents (including prednisone) were added only in the event of breakthrough rejection and for as brief a period as possible. After approximately 4 months, weaning was begun in patients who were on stable baseline monotherapy. After several weeks or months, tacrolimus doses were progressively spaced: every other day, then three times per week, twice per week, and in many cases, once per week by 1 year (Fig. 73–16).

This strategy has been used for the treatment of more than 1000 kidney, liver, intestine, pancreas, and lung recipients, the first 200 of whom have been reported.[71,72] Except for the organ-specific functions, the pattern of treatment and convalescence has been the same for all organs (Fig. 73–17). The quality of life of these patients, including freedom from complications of immunosuppression, has exceeded anything ever systematically achieved before except in the very first kidney recipients of 40 years ago.

This experience has had the effect of validating the paradigm of transplantation immunology proposed in 1998.[69] Recognition that immune regulation is by antigen migration and localization has many implications

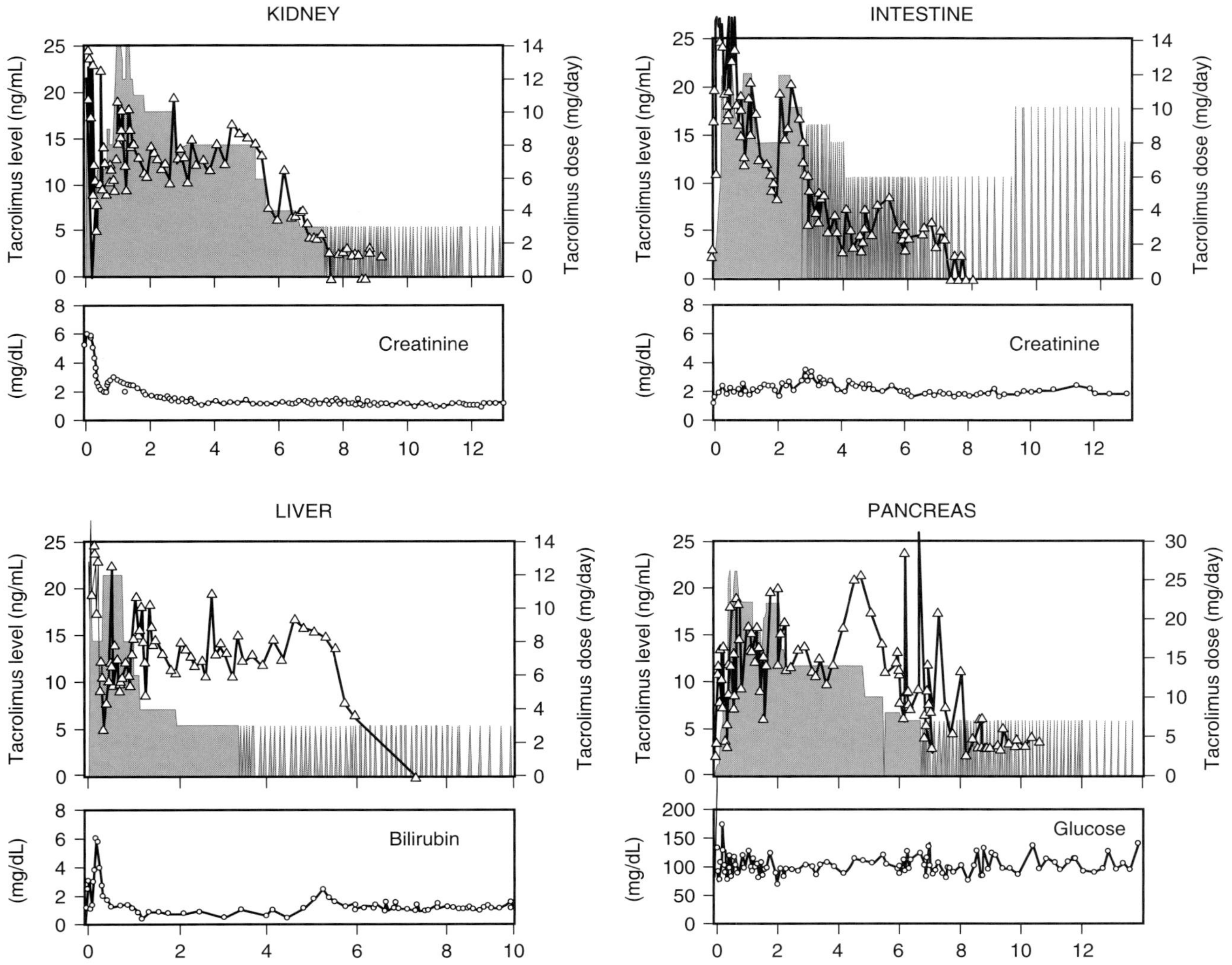

FIGURE 73–17

First-year posttransplant courses of kidney, liver, intestine, and pancreas recipients under the current immunosuppressive protocol. All four patient groups were taking one dose of tacrolimus per week by 1 year and were still maintained on this treatment at or beyond 2 years.

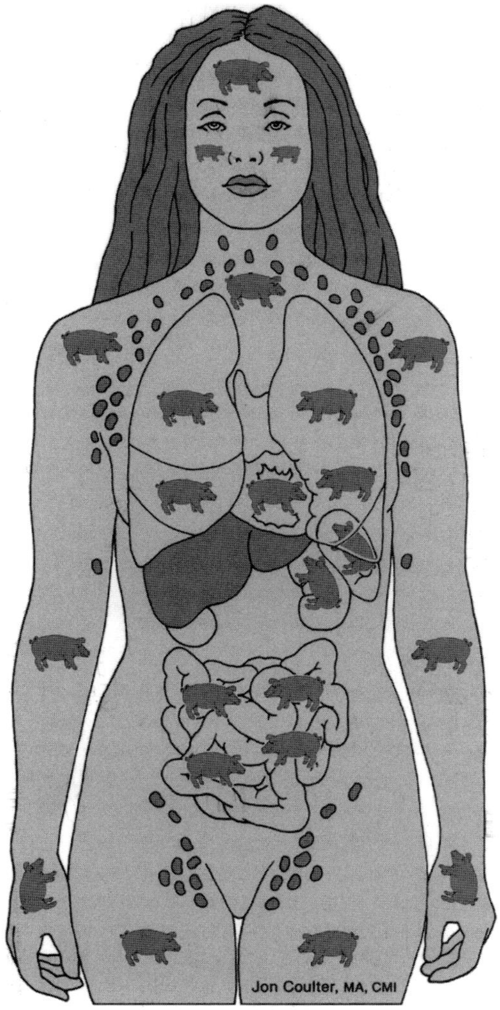

FIGURE 73–18

Successful xenotransplantation will be based on the same mechanisms and rules of human-to-human allotransplantation. The pig profiles represent disseminated porcine passenger leukocytes. (From Starzl TE: Organ transplantation: A practical triumph and epistemologic collapse. Proc Am Philos Soc 147:226-245, 2003.)

for improved immunotherapy in other fields: infectious disease, vaccinology, oncology, and autoimmunity. As for transplantation in the future, pigs are currently being produced with knockout of their αGal gene.[73] More genetic modifications will undoubtedly be needed. However, the engraftment mechanisms and therapeutic principles almost certainly will be the same when xenotransplantation comes to the clinic. The crucial migratory antigen will be the transgenic pig leukocytes (Fig. 73–18).

References

1. Billingham RE, Brent L, Medawar PB: "Actively acquired tolerance" of foreign cells. Nature 172:603-606, 1953.
2. Main JM, Prehn RT: Successful skin homografts after the administration of high dosage X radiation and homologous bone marrow. J Natl Cancer Inst 15:1023-1029, 1955.
3. Starzl TE, Demetris AJ, Murase N, et al: Cell migration, chimerism, and graft acceptance. Lancet 339:1579-1582, 1992.
4. Starzl TE, Demetris AJ, Trucco M, et al: Cell migration and chimerism after whole-organ transplantation: The basis of graft acceptance. Hepatology 17:1127-1152, 1993.
5. Murray JE, Merrill JP, Dammin GJ, et al: Study of transplantation immunity after total body irradiation: Clinical and experimental investigation. Surgery 48:272-284, 1960.
6. Hamburger J, Vaysse J, Crosnier J, et al: Transplantation of a kidney between nonmonozygotic twins after irradiation of the receiver. Good function at the fourth month. Presse Med 67:1771-1775, 1959.
7. Starzl TE, Marchioro TL, Waddell WR: The reversal of rejection in human renal homografts with subsequent development of homograft tolerance. Surg Gynecol Obstet 117:385-395, 1963.
8. Starzl TE: The saga of liver replacement, with particular reference to the reciprocal influence of liver and kidney transplantation (1955-1967). J Am Coll Surg 195:587-610, 2002.
9. Starzl TE: Pretreatment with prednisone. In Starzl TE (ed): Experience in Renal Transplantation. Philadelphia, WB Saunders, 1964, pp 171-178.
10. Starzl TE, Klintmalm GBG, Porter KA, et al: Liver transplantation with use of cyclosporin A and prednisone. N Engl J Med 305:266-269, 1981.
11. Starzl TE, Todo S, Fung J, et al: FK 506 for human liver, kidney and pancreas transplantation. Lancet 2:1000-1004, 1989.
12. Todo S, Fung JJ, Starzl TE, et al: Liver, kidney, and thoracic organ transplantation under FK 506. Ann Surg 212:295-305, 1990.
13. Takatsuki M, Uemoto S, Inomata Y, et al: Weaning of immunosuppression in living donor liver transplant recipients. Transplantation 72:449-454, 2001.
14. Woodruff MFA, Woodruff HG: The transplantation of normal tissues: With special reference to auto- and homotransplants of thyroid and spleen in the anterior chamber of the eye, and subcutaneously, in guinea pigs. Phil Trans B 234:559-581, 1950.
15. Steinmuller D: Immunization with skin isografts taken from tolerant mice. Science 158:127-129, 1967.
16. Elkins WL, Guttmann RD: Pathogenesis of a local graft versus host reaction: Immunogenicity of circulating host leukocytes. Science 159:1250-1251, 1968.
17. Porter KA: Pathology of the orthotopic homograft and heterograft. In Starzl TE (ed): Experience in Hepatic Transplantation. Philadelphia, WB Saunders, 1969, pp 427-437.
18. Kashiwagi N, Porter KA, Penn I, et al: Studies of homograft sex and of gamma globulin phenotypes after orthotopic homotransplantation of the human liver. Surg Forum 20:374-376, 1969.
19. Hart DNJ, Winearls CG, Fabre JW: Graft adaptation: Studies on possible mechanisms in long-term surviving rat renal allografts. Transplantation 30:73-80, 1980.
20. Lechler RI, Batchelor JR: Restoration of immunogenicity to passenger cell–depleted kidney allografts by the addition of donor-strain dendritic cells. J Exp Med 155:31, 1982.
21. Armstrong HE, Bolton EM, McMillan I, et al: Prolonged survival of actively enhanced rat renal allografts despite accelerated cellular infiltration and rapid induction of both class I and class II MHC antigens. J Exp Med 165:891-907, 1987.
22. Murase N, Demetris AJ, Matsuzaki T, et al: Long survival in rats after multivisceral versus isolated small bowel allotransplantation under FK 506. Surgery 110:87-98, 1991.
23. Iwaki Y, Starzl TE, Yagihashi A, et al: Replacement of donor lymphoid tissue in human small bowel transplants under FK 506 immunosuppression. Lancet 337:818-819, 1991.
24. Starzl TE, Demetris AJ, Trucco M, et al: Chimerism and donor specific nonreactivity 27 to 29 years after kidney allotransplantation. Transplantation 55:1272-1277, 1993.
25. Randhawa PS, Starzl TE, Ramos H, et al: Allografts surviving for 26-29 years following living related kidney transplantation:

Analysis by light microscopy, in situ hybridization for the Y chromosome, and anti-HLA antibodies. Am J Kidney Dis 24:72-77, 1994.

26. Fung JJ, Zeevi A, Kaufman C, et al: Interactions between bronchoalveolar lymphocytes and macrophages in heart-lung transplant recipients. Hum Immunol 14:287-294, 1985.

27. Demetris AJ, Murase N, Starzl TE: Donor dendritic cells in grafts and host lymphoid and non-lymphoid tissues after liver and heart allotransplantation under short term immunosuppression. Lancet 339:1610, 1992.

28. Valdivia LA, Demetris AJ, Langer AM, et al: Dendritic cell replacement in long-surviving liver and cardiac xenografts. Transplantation 56:482-484, 1993.

29. Wilson WEC, Kirkpatrick CH: Immunologic aspects of renal homotransplantation. In Starzl TE (ed): Experience in Renal Transplantation. Philadelphia, WB Saunders, 1964, pp 239-261.

30. Kashiwagi N: Special immunochemical studies. In Starzl TE (ed): Experience in Hepatic Transplantation. Philadelphia, WB Saunders, 1969, pp 394-407.

31. Ramsey G, Nusbacher J, Starzl TE, Lindsay GD: Isohemagglutinins of graft origin after ABO-unmatched liver transplantation. N Engl J Med 311:1167-1170, 1984.

32. Legendre C, Caillat-Zucman S, Samuel D, et al: Transfer of symptomatic peanut allergy to the recipient of a combined liver-and-kidney transplant. N Engl J Med 337:822-824, 1997.

33. Nemlander A, Soots A, von Willebrand E, et al: Redistribution of renal allograft–responding leukocytes during rejection. II. Kinetics and specificity. J Exp Med 156:1087-1100, 1982.

34. Larsen CP, Morris PJ, Austyn JM: Migration of dendritic leukocytes from cardiac allografts into host spleens. A novel route for initiation of rejection. J Exp Med 171:307-314, 1990.

35. Demetris AJ, Qian S, Sun H, et al: Early events in liver allograft rejection. Am J Pathol 138:609-618, 1991.

36. Snell GD: The homograft reaction. Annu Rev Microbiol 11:439-458, 1957.

37. Murase N, Demetris AJ, Woo J, et al: Lymphocyte traffic and graft-versus-host disease after fully allogeneic small bowel transplantation. Transplant Proc 23:3246-3247, 1991.

38. Murase N, Demetris A, Woo J, et al: Graft versus host disease (GVHD) after BN to LEW compared to LEW to BN rat intestinal transplantation under FK 506. Transplantation 55:1-7, 1993.

39. Tanabe M, Murase N, Demetris AJ, et al: The influence of donor and recipient strains in isolated small bowel transplantation in rats. Transplant Proc 26:4325-4332, 1994.

40. Starzl TE, Murase N, Thomson AW, et al: Immunity and tolerance are related, and governed by antigen migration and localization. Transplant Proc 31:1406-1411, 1999.

41. Starzl TE, Demetris AJ, Trucco M, et al: Chimerism after liver transplantation for type IV glycogen storage disease and type I Gaucher's disease. N Engl J Med 328:745-749, 1993.

42. Murase N, Kim DG, Todo S, et al: FK 506 suppression of heart and liver allograft rejection II: The induction of graft acceptance in rat. Transplantation 50:739-744, 1990.

43. Murase N, Demetris AJ, Kim DG, et al: Rejection of the multivisceral allografts in rats: A sequential analysis with comparison to isolated orthotopic small bowel and liver grafts. Surgery 108:880-889, 1990.

44. Demetris AJ, Murase N, Fujisaki S, et al: Hematolymphoid cell trafficking, microchimerism, and GVHD reactions after liver, bone marrow, and heart transplantation. Transplant Proc 25:3337-3344, 1993.

45. Qian S, Demetris AJ, Murase N, et al: Murine liver allograft transplantation: Tolerance and donor cell chimerism. Hepatology 19:916-924, 1994.

46. Murase N, Starzl TE, Tanabe M, et al: Variable chimerism, graft versus host disease, and tolerance after different kinds of cell and whole organ transplantation from Lewis to Brown-Norway rats. Transplantation 60:158-171, 1995.

47. Lu L, Rudert WA, Qian S, et al: Growth of donor-derived dendritic cells from the bone marrow of murine liver allograft recipients in response to granulocyte/macrophage colony-stimulating factor. J Exp Med 182:379-387, 1995.

48. Murase N, Starzl TE, Ye Q, et al: Multilineage hematopoietic reconstitution of supralethally irradiated rats by syngeneic whole organ transplantation: With particular reference to the liver. Transplantation 61:1-4, 1996.

49. Qian S, Lu L, Fu F, et al: Apoptosis within spontaneously accepted mouse liver allografts: Evidence for deletion of cytotoxic T cells and implications for tolerance induction. J Immunol 158:4654-4661, 1997.

50. Terakura M, Murase N, Demetris AJ, et al: Lymphoid/non-lymphoid compartmentalization of donor leukocyte chimerism in rat recipients of heart allografts, with or without adjunct bone marrow. Transplantation 66:350-357, 1998.

51. Sakamoto T, Ye Q, Lu L, et al: Donor hematopoietic progenitor cells in non myeloablated rat recipients of allogeneic bone marrow and liver grafts. Transplantation 67:833-840, 1999.

52. Ichikawa N, Demetris AJ, Starzl TE, et al: Donor and recipient leukocytes in organ allografts of recipients with variable donor-specific tolerance: With particular reference to chronic rejection. Liver Transpl 6:686-702, 2000.

53. Taniguchi H, Toyoshima T, Fukao K, Nakauchi H: Presence of hematopoietic stem cells in the adult liver. Nat Med 2:198-203, 1996.

54. Starzl TE, Murase N, Thomson A, Demetris AJ: Liver transplants contribute to their own success. Nat Med 2:163-165, 1996.

55. Cordier G, Garnier H, Clot JP, et al: La greffe de foie orthotopique chez le porc. Mem Acad Chir (Paris) 92:799-807, 1966.

56. Peacock JH, Terblanche J: Orthotopic homotransplantation of the liver in the pig. In Read AE (ed): The Liver. London, Butterworth, 1967, p 333.

57. Calne RY, White HJO, Yoffa DE, et al: Observations of orthotopic liver transplantation in the pig. BMJ 2:478-480, 1967.

58. Calne RY, Sells RA, Pena JR, et al: Induction of immunological tolerance by porcine liver allografts. Nature 223:472-474, 1969.

59. Zimmerman FA, Davies HS, Knoll PP, et al: Orthotopic liver allografts in the rat. Transplantation 37:406-410, 1984.

60. Kamada N, Brons G, Davies HS: Fully allogeneic liver grafting in rats induces a state of systemic nonreactivity to donor transplantation antigens. Transplantation 29:429-431, 1980.

61. Starzl TE, Rao AS, Trucco M, et al: Explanation for loss of the HLA matching effect. Transplant Proc 27:57-60, 1995.

62. Przepiorka D, Thomas ED, Durham DM, Fisher L: Use of a probe to repeat sequence of the Y chromosome for detection of host cells in peripheral blood of bone marrow transplant recipients. Am J Clin Pathol 95:201-206, 1991.

63. Wessman M, Popp S, Ruutu T, et al: Detection of residual host cells after bone marrow transplantation using non-isotopic in situ hybridization and karyotype analysis. Bone Marrow Transplant 11:279-284, 1993.

64. Zinkernagel RM, Doherty PC: The discovery of MHC restriction. Immunol Today 18:14, 1997.

65. Zinkernagel RM: Immunology taught by viruses. Science 271:173-178, 1996.

66. Zinkernagel RM, Ehl S, Aichele P, et al: Antigen localization regulates immune responses in a dose- and time-dependent fashion: A geographical view of immune reactivity. Immunol Rev 156:199-209, 1997.

67. Zinkernagel RM, Hengartner H: Antiviral immunity. Immunol Today 18:258-260, 1997.

68. Zinkernagel RM, Bachmann MF, Kundig TM, et al: On immunologic memory. Annu Rev Immunol 14:333-367, 1996.

69. Starzl TE, Zinkernagel R: Antigen localization and migration in immunity and tolerance. N Engl J Med 339:1905-1913, 1998.

70. Starzl TE, Zinkernagel RM: Transplantation tolerance from a historical perspective. Nat Rev Immunol 1:233-239, 2001.

71. Starzl TE, Murase N, Abu-Elmagd K, et al: Tolerogenic immunosuppression for organ transplantation. Lancet 361:1502-1510, 2003.

72. Shapiro R, Jordan M, Basu A, et al: Kidney transplantation under a tolerogenic regimen of recipient pre-treatment and low-dose postoperative immunosuppression, with subsequent weaning. Ann Surg 238:520-525, discussion 525-527, 2003.

73. Phelps CJ, Koike C, Vaught TD, et al: Production of α1,3-galactosyltransferase–deficient pigs. Science 299:411-414, 2003.

ABO, Tissue Typing, and Cross-match Incompatibility in Liver Transplantation

J. MICHAEL CECKA
ELAINE F. REED

ABO blood groups and natural antibodies   1200
  Liver transplantation in ABO-nonidentical
    recipients   1200
  Deliberate ABO-incompatible liver
    transplantations from living donors   1202
  Hemolytic disease after ABO-compatible
    transplantation   1202

Human leukocyte antigens (HLA) and anti-HLA
  antibodies   1203
  Cross-match compatibility in liver
    transplantation   1203
  HLA compatibility effects on liver
    transplantation   1204
  Graft-versus-host disease   1205

Conclusions   1206

The ABO blood group antigens and the human leukocyte antigens (HLA) encoded by the major histocompatibility gene complex represent substantial barriers to transplantation of tissues and organs between individuals. The antigens of these two systems are expressed on most cells in the body and antibodies directed against either ABO or HLA antigens of the donor can cause severe damage to the graft. The allogeneic donor HLA antigens themselves are major targets of rejection reactions. The important roles of ABO, tissue typing, and cross-match incompatibilities in transplantation were recognized early in the experience with kidney transplants. Most ABO-incompatible kidney transplants reported between 1955 and 1964 were rapidly and irreversibly rejected[1-3] because of anti-blood-group antibodies in the recipient's circulation. As a result of those early experiences, all organs are now transplanted to ABO-identical or -compatible recipients with few exceptions. By the mid-1960s, it was also clear that patients who had circulating antidonor HLA antibodies at the time of transplantation experienced irreversible hyperacute rejection of their kidney graft.[4,5] Screening tests to identify sensitized patients awaiting a transplant who are most at risk and cross-match tests, which are now routinely performed at the time of kidney transplantation to determine whether circulating anti-HLA antibodies directed against donor HLA antigens are present, have nearly eliminated hyperacute rejection of transplanted kidneys. Thus, circulating antibodies to graft ABO or HLA antigens caused rapid kidney graft loss, characterized by renal artery thrombosis, neutrophil infiltrates, intimal fibrin deposition, and cortical necrosis.[6,7] Similar observations of hyperacute rejections were subsequently reported in recipients of hearts, lungs, and livers.

The importance of prospectively selecting HLA-compatible donor kidneys for transplantation is considerably more controversial. Transplanting HLA-matched kidneys consistently results in superior long-term graft survival when compared with HLA-mismatched organs, whether the kidney is from a living or a deceased donor,[8,9] because reducing the allogeneic targets of rejection reactions reduces the likelihood of rejection after the transplant. HLA compatibility has been favored in the allocation of deceased donor kidneys in the United States and Europe for many years,[9,10] but few attempts have been made to find HLA-compatible donor hearts, lungs, or livers for patients awaiting these life-saving organs.

Despite the general acceptance of the roles of ABO and HLA antigens and antibodies in organ and tissue transplantation based on these early observations, a preponderance of data now suggests that liver transplants are exceptional with regard to the rules of ABO and HLA. The liver is a massive organ compared with a kidney or a heart, and with its dual blood supply and capacity for regeneration, it appears to be less susceptible to irreparable immune damage than other organs. After more than 30 years of experience and more than 112,000 liver transplantations worldwide, controversy remains regarding the importance of the ABO and HLA antigen systems in transplantation of the liver. Clearly, the effects of ABO, HLA, and cross-match incompatibilities are more complex as they apply to liver transplantation than to other organ transplants. This chapter summarizes the current status of histocompatibility for ABO and HLA in liver transplantation.

ABO Blood Groups and Natural Antibodies

A detailed description of blood groups and their genetics is beyond the scope of this chapter (for a review, see reference 11). Structurally, the ABO blood group antigens are carbohydrates that specific transferases add to core saccharides attached to glycolipids or glycoproteins. Blood group A individuals have the terminal trisaccharide [GalNAcα_{1-3} (Fucα_{1-2}) Galβ]–, blood group B individuals have [Galα_{1-3} (Fucα_{1-2}) Galβ]–, and blood group O individuals lack the terminal sugar and have only the disaccharide [Fucα_{1-2} Galβ]–. These structures are added to four core polysaccharide chains.

Approximately 20% of blood type A individuals with European ancestry have a transferase that adds the GalNAcα_{1-3} (Fucα_{1-2}) Galβ– trisaccharide to only two of the core chains, resulting in a lower density of blood group A determinants in the tissues. These individuals have blood group A2, a subgroup of blood group A.

Individuals develop natural antibodies against the A and B structures that differ from their own. Thus, blood group A and O individuals have circulating antibodies against blood group B, and blood group O and B individuals have antibodies against blood group A. Blood group O individuals can make antibodies to both A and B antigens because they display neither, and blood group AB individuals do not make antibodies to the A or B antigens because they display both. Individuals with blood group A2 do not produce anti-A antibodies even though expression of the antigen is limited. Although the stimulus for blood group antibodies is not well established, many factors may affect the titer of antibody, which can vary widely among individuals of the same type.[12]

Liver Transplantation in ABO-Nonidentical Recipients

Matching donor livers with recipients for ABO blood groups to avoid damage from natural blood group antibodies is not difficult. The blood groups are evenly distributed among liver donors and liver transplant candidates (Table 74–1). The less common blood groups B and AB constitute only approximately 10% and 3% of donors and candidates, respectively. Thus, the donor pool is considerably more limited for patients with these less common types. ABO-incompatible transplants have been performed in emergency situations when a compatible donor is not available, and unlike the outcome of other ABO-incompatible organ transplants, hyperacute rejection of the ABO-incompatible liver rarely occurs.[13]

Table 74-1. ABO BLOOD GROUP DISTRIBUTIONS AMONG CANDIDATES AWAITING A LIVER TRANSPLANTATION ON JUNE 13, 2003 AND AMONG LIVER DONORS JANUARY TO JUNE 2003

Group	Donors		Candidates	
A	501	35.7%	6,138	35.6%
B	144	10.3%	1,973	11.4%
O	722	51.4%	8,645	50.2%
AB	37	2.6%	481	2.8%
Total	1,404		17,237	

Based on UNOS/OPTN data as of June 13, 2003. Retrieved from www.unos.org.

Even in cases when there was a hyperacute rejection, the process proceeded at a slower pace than for kidneys.

Although hyperacute rejection is rare, the literature shows that ABO-identical liver transplants have had the best prospects for survival. Initially, a large retrospective study of 671 liver transplants performed in Pittsburgh,[14] of which 91 were ABO compatible and 31 were incompatible, revealed a substantially higher graft failure rate among the ABO-nonidentical grafts. The authors recommended that the use of ABO-nonidentical grafts should be limited to small children for whom few suitable donors were available or to patients in urgent need of transplantation. This policy has been largely followed with respect to ABO. Rydberg[15] reviewed the results of 400 ABO-incompatible liver transplantations performed between 1986 and 2000 and reported in 24 different studies and concluded that ABO-incompatible liver transplantations were substantially less successful than ABO-compatible liver transplants. Rydberg noted that children younger than 3 years whose immature immune system may be more forgiving than that of adults might be an exception to this trend.

Recent data from the United Network for Organ Sharing (UNOS) Organ Procurement and Transplantation Network (OPTN) (Fig. 74–1) also show that recipients of ABO-compatible or ABO-incompatible livers between 1995 and 2000 had poorer outcomes than recipients of ABO-identical organs. The graft survival rates at 6 months ranged from 83% for ABO-identical to 76% for ABO-compatible and 66% for ABO-incompatible livers. Five years after transplantation the differences in graft survival rates remained essentially the same, suggesting that the deleterious effect of ABO differences manifests early within the first year after transplantation and that there is no additional long-term disadvantage associated with ABO-nonidentical transplants. Thus, liver graft survival rates for recent ABO-incompatible transplants performed at centers throughout the United States was approximately 15% lower at 5 years than from ABO-compatible donors overall. It is noteworthy that among these 25,507 deceased donor liver transplants performed in the United States between 1995 and 2000, ABO nonidentical transplants were not common. Only 9% of liver transplants were performed from ABO-nonidentical but compatible donors, and fewer than 2% were from ABO-incompatible donors.

The often urgent nature of ABO-compatible and -incompatible transplants could explain the poorer outcomes in these combinations. However, two early studies compared ABO-identical, -compatible, and -incompatible transplants done in urgent situations and found that the 35% to 45% lower 2-year survival rate of ABO-incompatible grafts was not a result of the emergency conditions under which the transplantation was performed.[16,17] In fact, the incompatible grafts in each case were lost early and immunoglobulin and complement components were readily identified on sinusoidal cells and arterial endothelium, indicating a clear humoral component to the graft failures. This conclusion was supported by a subsequent analysis comparing 31 ABO-incompatible transplants with 199 ABO-compatible emergency transplants at the University of California at Los Angeles (UCLA),[18] which revealed a significantly increased incidence of rejection, thrombosis, and biliary stricture among incompatible graft recipients, resulting in a 20% lower 1-year graft survival rate. Most recently, a study of 229 highly urgent liver transplantations in Scandinavia[19] noted that patients who received an ABO-identical graft had significantly higher patient survival rates than did those who received ABO-compatible (n = 76) or -incompatible livers (n = 10). In this study, which included transplants performed in five countries during 1990 to 2001, the authors noted that the outcomes for highly urgent transplants had improved during the course of the study, but that ABO compatibility produced superior results throughout.

Liver allocation algorithms often provide for mandatory sharing of livers for highly urgent patients, allowing ABO-compatible and even ABO-incompatible offers. However, such prioritizations may disadvantage other less urgent patients, particularly blood group O patients. Eurotransplant reported a simulation study that suggests that a restricted ABO matching policy provides the optimal balance for both urgent and elective patients from the allocation perspective. Under this system, blood group O livers are offered to blood group O or B patients and blood group A livers are offered to blood group A or AB patients.[20] The UNOS in the United States uses a similar policy. Blood group O livers are allocated first to blood group O patients,

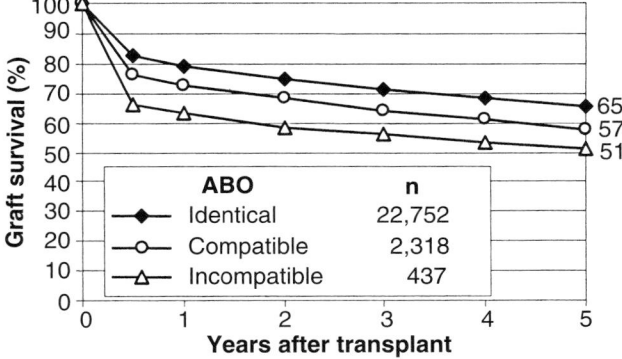

FIGURE 74–1

Five-year graft survival rates for first graft recipients of deceased donor livers according to ABO blood group compatibility. (Based on data from the UNOS/OPTN Registry for US transplants performed between 1995 and 2000. Retrieved on July 11, 2003 from www.unos.org.)

then livers are allocated to blood group B patients who are ranked according to their medical condition. A point system is used to promote ABO-identical combinations over ABO-compatible and ABO-incompatible transplantations.

Despite the poorer survival rates for ABO-incompatible transplantations, many survive and function well. This observation contrasts sharply with the results for inadvertent ABO-incompatible kidney transplants, nearly all of which have failed very early after the transplant.[21] When ABO-incompatible transplants are performed inadvertently or in urgent situations, there is no time to assess the suitability of the recipient to receive an incompatible organ. However, the results of ABO-incompatible transplantations might be improved when the incompatibility is anticipated and the recipient can be conditioned in advance.

Deliberate ABO-Incompatible Liver Transplantations from Living Donors

During the 1980s, a small number of deliberate ABO-incompatible kidney transplantations were undertaken when a willing, medically suitable living donor was available, but ABO incompatibility presented a barrier. Alexandre[22] and others demonstrated that when the titer of ABO antibody could be reduced through plasmapheresis or adsorption, transplantations across the ABO barrier could be performed successfully. As interest in living donor organ transplants has grown, exploring the limits of transplanting across the ABO barrier has again become an issue. The most experience with deliberate ABO-incompatible liver transplants may be in Asia, specifically in Japan, where the lack of deceased donor livers limits the availability of liver transplantation to those with a living donor. Living donor transplantations in ABO-compatible and -incompatible combinations are frequently performed after conditioning the patient to reduce the likelihood of early antibody-mediated damage. Conditioning's goal is to reduce the titer of anti-A or anti-B antibody in the patient prior to transplantation and to prevent its rapid rebound in the early posttransplant period. This has been accomplished by plasmapheresis,[23-27] often accompanied by splenectomy,[25,27] immunosuppressant drugs,[24,25] and other approaches,[28,29] with monitoring of antibody titers. Most studies agree that an antibody titer of less than 1:8 is sufficiently low to avoid most problems.

Despite these preparations, however, there remains a high risk of failure as several of these studies have reported a 40% to 60% early graft loss rate among recipients of ABO-incompatible living donor liver transplants.

The most encouraging results were obtained by Hanto,[27] who reported no immunological graft losses in 14 patients after a combination of pre- and posttransplant total plasma exchange and splenectomy with quadruple immunosuppression.

Interestingly, anti-ABO blood group antibodies may return to high levels after the transplant without causing apparent damage to the graft. Alexandre[22] first described this phenomenon, called *accommodation*, in recipients of deliberate ABO-incompatible kidneys. The mechanism underlying graft accommodation remains unclear. Platt[30] proposed three possible mechanisms for this phenomenon, postulating that either the antibody or the antigen was somehow modulated on the graft or, alternatively, that the graft itself becomes resistant to the damaging effects of antibody. There is some evidence to support the latter possibility that cells exposed to low levels of antibody may express antiapoptotic genes early after exposure[31,32] and that accommodated grafts acquire a distinct phenotype characterized by expression of tumor necrosis factor-alpha (TNF-α), transforming growth factor-beta$_1$ (TGF-β_1), SMAD5, protein kinase GFRA1, and MUC1, 3 months or more after successful transplantation.[33]

Transplants of A2 livers to O recipients appear to be safe without augmented immunosuppression or restrictions with regard to anti-A antibody titers, according to a study of six such transplants at Mt. Sinai Medical Center in New York City.[34] Similar results have been reported for kidney transplantations,[35] although some early rejections and failures have prompted caution regarding transplants of A2 kidneys to O patients with high anti-A antibody titers.

Hemolytic Disease After ABO-Compatible Transplantation

The recipient's natural anti–blood group antibodies are an important consideration in preparing for an ABO-incompatible liver transplant. However, anti–blood group antibodies may also complicate ABO-compatible (O to A, O to B, and O to AB) and -incompatible (A to B and B to A) liver transplantations. Hemolytic reactions develop in some patients as a result of antibodies produced by passenger lymphocytes in the graft against the recipient's blood group antigens. The hemolytic reactions vary in their severity from mild to serious.[36-38] These "graft-versus-host" blood group reactions are often self-limiting because the antibody-producing plasma cells transplanted with the graft have a limited life span and are not replaced. The occurrence of hemolytic reactions is rare and is not limited to cases involving transplanted livers[39] nor to the major ABO blood groups.[40,41] Donors with very high antibody titers against ABO or other blood group antigens may pose a special threat.[42]

HLA Antigens and Anti-HLA Antibodies

The HLA antigens comprise a series of cell surface glycoproteins that play an integral role in the normal immune response. The class I HLA-A, -B, and -C antigens are present on all nucleated cells in the body and the class II HLA-DR and -DQ antigens have a restricted tissue distribution limited to B lymphocytes, macrophages, monocytes, and dendritic cells. The class II antigens can be induced on activated T lymphocytes and on endothelial cells. The HLA molecules normally function in antigen presentation to T lymphocytes in initiating an immune response. HLA molecules incorporate peptides from degraded intracellular (in the case of class I) or extracellular (class II) proteins. When the peptides are derived from pathogens or toxins, an immune response can be initiated when T lymphocytes recognize the foreign peptides in the context of the HLA molecules' surface. Not surprisingly, allogeneic HLA antigens on the graft with peptides of donor origin display a large array of potential targets for immune elimination. In fact, these donor HLA molecules are the major targets of immune rejection reactions.

As with the ABO blood group antigens, circulating antidonor HLA antibodies represent a risk to the graft. Unlike the natural ABO blood group antibodies, anti-HLA antibodies are produced as a result of direct immunization with allogeneic HLA molecules. This occurs most commonly through pregnancies during which the mother is exposed to paternal HLA alloantigens from the fetus. Not all pregnancies cause antibody production, but the incidence increases directly with the number of pregnancies.[43] Other immunizing events, such as blood transfusions or previous transplants, may provide additional allogeneic stimulation for multiparous women as well as for females who have not been pregnant and for males. Severe infections, particularly when associated with surgical procedures, may also stimulate anti-HLA antibody production.[44]

Although avoiding HLA antigen differences between the donor and recipient would prevent potential anti-HLA antibody damage to the transplanted liver, finding an HLA-matched liver for a sensitized patient is not an option because of the remarkable polymorphism of the HLA antigens. The most common HLA phenotype occurs at a rate of approximately 1 per 250 individuals and most phenotypes are far less common. It is not difficult to identify those candidates who are sensitized against HLA antigens and in many cases to identify the specific HLA antigens to which they have circulating antibody.

Cross-match–incompatible donors can be avoided for elective transplantations, or treatments can be altered to mitigate antibody-mediated damage when a cross-match–incompatible donor must be used.

Cross-match Compatibility in Liver Transplantation

The role of anti-HLA antibodies in liver transplantation is not well understood. Early data suggested that the liver—with its large size relative to the recipient and its regenerative capacity—was resistant to damage by antidonor HLA antibodies. Hyperacute rejection was clearly demonstrated in two liver-kidney transplant recipients[45] and a presensitized liver recipient,[46] but the progress of the rejection in the liver was slower than that observed for the kidney. Interestingly, at least one of these earliest documented hyperacute rejections occurred in a patient who had no detectable antidonor antibodies using the technologies that were available at the time. The cross-match test was devised to detect preformed antidonor HLA antibodies, which cause hyperacute rejection of kidney grafts in a very high percentage of patients transplanted with a cross-match–incompatible kidney. The original test based on lymphocytotoxicity has been modified and improved to be more sensitive and more specific over the years, but the results of liver transplantation in the face of a positive cross-match have not been uniformly poorer than the results of transplants with a negative cross-match.[47] Conflicting results for liver transplants in the face of a positive cross-match continue to appear.[48,49] Many of the earliest studies may have been complicated by offsetting losses as a consequence of other causes such as surgical complications and primary nonfunction. Nevertheless, some studies noted higher initial nonfunction rates among recipients with preformed antidonor antibodies.[50,51] Other studies found increased and earlier bile duct complications associated with anti-HLA antibodies.[52] Many studies have reported an increased incidence of rejection episodes in cross-match–positive combinations.

Because the cross-match tests used at different centers at different times have different sensitivities, it could be argued that the conflicting results surrounding cross-matches for liver transplants were a result of differences in the methods used to detect antibody. A recent study of 465 consecutive liver transplantations[53] designed to measure the concentration of antibody (using the very sensitive flow cytometry method) on liver outcomes reported that 91 patients with a positive cross-match had fewer early graft losses than did those with a negative cross-match and did not have an increased incidence of rejection. No differences in graft or patient survival rates were noted when comparing the cross-match–positive and –negative patients. However, patients with higher antibody concentrations more often had steroid-resistant rejections (31%) than those with low (4%) or no antibody (8%). These results suggest that the liver is more resistant to antidonor HLA antibody-mediated damage than other organs, but that the graft and patient survival may differ depending on how well different centers manage rejection.

The literature indicates that between 7% and 33% of liver candidates are overtly sensitized to allogeneic HLA antigens.[47] Often these are female patients with children or patients who have had previous surgeries with accompanying blood transfusions or other exposures to allogeneic HLA antigens. Patients at risk of being sensitized might benefit from a screening test to determine whether or not they have preformed antibody and its titer and specificity. Even when cross-matches are performed retrospectively, the information may provide advance notice of an increased likelihood of rejection.

In the case of living donor or reduced-size livers, the impact of preformed antibody might be greater. This result has been convincingly demonstrated in rats.[54] In the clinical experience, one study from Kyoto[55] noted that four of five flow cross-match–positive recipients of living donor livers experienced early acute rejections that required higher steroid doses than did those among recipients of a cross-match–negative graft. More to the point, a study of 43 adult-to-adult small-for-size grafts in Korea[56] identified 4 patients with a positive cross-match against their donors, all of whom were women and all of whom died of multiorgan failure after early acute rejection episodes. Three of these patients had received "extra small" grafts with a graft recipient weight ratio of less than 0.8%. In some cases, plasmapheresis has been used in recipients of living donor livers with a positive cross-match[24] and although anti-HLA antibody titers were reduced, it was difficult to determine whether plasmapheresis affected the outcome. At least one study[57] suggests that anti-HLA antibodies that persist after transplantation may be harmful. This observation raises the question of whether the strength or persistence of the response, rather than the specificity or titer of the antibody, might be the important factor determining the effect of antibody on liver transplantations.

Overcoming a positive cross-match in broadly sensitized patients awaiting a kidney transplant recently received considerable attention based on two approaches using intravenous immunoglobulin (IVIg) preparations.[58-60] The mechanism by which high-dose IVIg or low-dose IVIg in combination with plasmapheresis modulates the antibody response is unclear, and multiple mechanisms may operate in both types of treatment. However, when antibodies are reduced following either treatment, kidney transplants may be performed across a positive cross-match without hyperacute rejection.

HLA Compatibility Effects on Liver Transplantation

There has been no widespread effort to allocate livers to HLA-compatible recipients. Although the quality of HLA compatibility was incorporated into the allocation algorithm for distributing kidneys at both the national and local levels, there were no data to support the use of HLA for livers when the OPTN first established national organ allocation systems in the United States during the late 1980s. Had there been supporting data, logistic considerations would have limited interest in sharing livers for more histocompatible recipients. At that time, the low tolerance for prolonged ischemia was considered a major barrier to sharing livers over a wide geographical area. Local waiting lists were small, which would make finding good matches unlikely, and the fact that organ size and the severity of the patient's illness would clearly trump histocompatibility concerns effectively placed HLA low on the list of priorities. Nevertheless, interest in the immunology of transplantation has prompted a number of studies on the effects of HLA compatibility in liver transplantation. The results of these studies, while offering little support for efforts to prospectively select more histocompatible liver transplant donors, have revealed a number of interesting relationships between HLA and graft outcome. There are a variety of situations when knowing the HLA antigens of the donor and recipient could be useful in evaluating a potential liver donor.

Even the largest of the studies of HLA-matching effects is hampered by the fact that few HLA-compatible transplantations have been performed by chance.[61-63] As Fig. 74–2 indicates, only 29 and 91 of the 15,603 liver transplants performed in the United States between 1995 and 2000 with HLA types reported to the OPTN/UNOS Registry had no or only one HLA-A, -B, or -DR mismatch, respectively. The results for these liver transplants show no clear pattern that would suggest a survival advantage for more HLA-compatible liver transplantations. In fact, those few recipients of livers with zero to one HLA mismatches had generally (although not significantly) poorer survival.

Most studies of HLA and liver transplantation agree that having fewer HLA mismatches, particularly DR mismatches, is associated with fewer rejection episodes. Thus, the expectation that the alloimmune response against the transplanted liver would be weaker with fewer HLA differences between the donor and recipient appears to be correct. However, other effects of HLA in liver transplant recipients may complicate the story.

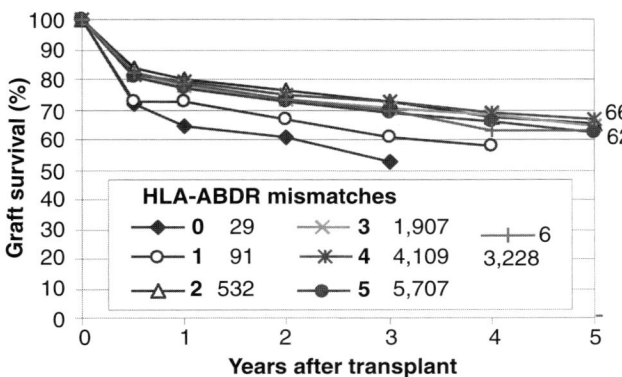

FIGURE 74–2

Five-year graft survival rates for first graft recipients of deceased donor livers according to the number of HLA-A, -B, and -DR mismatches. (Based on data from the UNOS/OPTN Registry for U.S. transplants performed between 1995 and 2000. Retrieved on July 11, 2003 from www.unos.org.)

Early analyses of HLA matching in liver recipients failed to demonstrate any survival advantage among recipients of better HLA-matched grafts; in fact, an initial analysis of more than 500 liver recipients[61] revealed consistently poorer survival among those who received a liver with no mismatches at any of the individual HLA-A, -B, or -DR loci. The authors reported that although the more poorly HLA-matched grafts were more likely to fail because of rejection, the better matched grafts suffered a higher rate of graft loss because of primary nonfunction or other causes. The results prompted the authors to speculate a dualistic effect of HLA matching in liver transplantations. On the one hand, HLA incompatibilities produced more rejection episodes and failures to rejection. On the other hand, disease-associated autoimmune mechanisms might cause recurrent damage to the transplanted liver when the new liver was more compatible. Because the targets of these autoimmune responses were likely to be viral or other peptides associated with the patient's own HLA antigens, the HLA-compatible transplanted liver would readily display these same targets, resulting in rapid autoimmune damage. Although little was known of the targets of autoimmune liver disease, patients with primary biliary cirrhosis, sclerosis, cholangitis, and autoimmune active hepatitis had primary immune causes. Subsequently, this group analyzed 355 liver transplant recipients and noted an increased incidence of *Cytomegalovirus* hepatitis among patients matched for one or two HLA-DR antigens with their donor.[64]

A more recent analysis of 446 liver transplants from the Australian National Liver Transplantation Unit[63] corroborated the prediction, showing that patients with autoimmune liver diseases had better graft survival when fewer donor HLA antigens were matched with the recipient, whereas those whose liver disease did not have an autoimmune component had better outcomes when fewer HLA antigens were mismatched. A study of 227 patients who underwent transplantation because of hepatitis C at UCLA that was reported at the American Society for Transplantation Congress in 2003[65] noted a significantly higher and more rapid recurrence rate for hepatitis C viral disease among patients who received a more HLA-compatible liver transplantation.

A large study of 924 liver transplant recipients from the Charite in Berlin[66] found significantly poorer survival of better HLA-DR–matched grafts among patients transplanted for primary sclerosing cholangitis as well as for recipients with autoimmune hepatitis, although the latter results did not reach statistical significance. In contrast, the same group's earlier retrospective analysis of 84 transplantations for hepatitis B virus (HBV) cirrhosis found better graft survival and fewer cases of HBV reinfection among recipients with one or two HLA-B locus compatibilities as compared with those who were completely mismatched.[67] The authors proposed that antiviral medications effectively controlled reinfection, eliminating the "dualistic effect" of HLA matching.

Even though most studies identify a trend toward fewer rejections with more HLA antigens matched between the donor and recipient, it is difficult to provide a clinical guideline. In most cases, "better" HLA-matched livers had up to four HLA-A, -B, and -DR antigens mismatched, and those that were poorly matched had five or six antigens mismatched. The association between HLA-DR mismatches and early rejection episodes has been most consistently reported. Thus, when there is no autoimmune disease or autoimmune damage to the liver, a better HLA-DR–matched graft should reduce the incidence and severity of early acute rejection. When recurrent autoimmune disease is a concern, an HLA-DR–mismatched liver might reduce the likelihood or speed of recurrence. Such considerations are possible for less urgent patients awaiting a deceased donor liver and when evaluating potential living related donors.

Graft-versus-Host Disease

Graft-versus-host disease (GVHD) following liver transplantation is a rare but often fatal complication that results from engraftment of alloreactive donor T lymphocytes carried in the graft. Since the first description of a case of liver GVHD in 1988,[68] fewer than 50 cases have been reported,[69-76] usually as case reports, although a series of 13 cases was recently reported from a single center.[76] The incidence from that particular study was approximately 1%, although the authors cautioned that the problem may be underdiagnosed because the characteristic fever, skin rash, diarrhea, and pancytopenia are difficult to distinguish from cytomegalovirus (CMV) disease or from drug reactions. Most cases have been confirmed by demonstrating a high proportion of donor lymphocytes in the circulation, usually by performing HLA typing of lymphocytes from peripheral blood or skin lesions and identifying and quantifying donor HLA antigens.

The clinical features of the liver GVHD closely resemble those of transfusion-associated GVHD, except that the transplanted liver is unaffected. HLA antigen differences between the recipient and the liver donor are the targets of GVH reactions, as they are targets of graft rejection by the host. Indeed, HLA compatibility (i.e., fewer mismatches) has been identified as a significant factor in both liver-associated and transfusion-associated GVHD. The potential for this complication may be exacerbated when there is a one-way mismatch between the donor and recipient, setting up a situation in which the donor lymphocytes respond to allogeneic differences in the recipient but the graft is matched with the recipient, providing no allogeneic targets for a reciprocal response.[77] Consider the case of transfusion-associated GVHD that occurred in a man who received a fresh blood transfusion from his grandson.[78] HLA typing showed the grandfather to be A2,26 B38,44, DR4,–, DQ3,– and the grandson donor to be A26,–, B38,–, DR4,–, DQ3,–. The donor and recipient shared one HLA haplotype (A26, B38, DR4, DQ3) and the donor was homozygous for these antigens. Thus, the grandson's cells could respond to the A2 and B44 antigens of the grandfather, but there were no strong allogeneic donor HLA antigens that might have elicited a response from the grandfather. Such clear cases are extremely rare when the donors are genetically unrelated individuals; however, within a family, the incidence of one-way mismatches could be rather high. Living liver donors should be HLA typed prospectively to identify homozygosity and to avoid such one-way mismatches (or even unbalanced mismatches when more recipient than donor antigens differ).

Most reported cases of liver GVHD do not involve one-way mismatches, however, and other factors clearly play important roles as well. The difference between the donor's and recipient's ages is also a risk factor,[76] particularly when the donor is substantially younger than the recipient; this may be related to the older senescent recipient immune system being more easily suppressed than the younger, more vigorous immune system of the donor.

UNOS has collected data on GVHD as a cause of death since 1994. Table 74–2 shows the numbers and percentages of deaths reported as caused by GVHD as reported to UNOS through December 2002. Deaths attributed to GVHD were rare, occurring in far less than

Table 74–2. INCIDENCE OF DEATHS CAUSED BY GRAFT-VERSUS-HOST DISEASE (GVHD) AMONG ADULT RECIPIENTS OF LIVER TRANSPLANTATION REPORTED TO UNOS BETWEEN 1995 AND 2002

Event	Type of Donor		
	Deceased	Living	Total
Transplants	31,332	1,149	32,481
Deaths	7,090	161	7,251
GVHD	38	3	41
Percentage of transplants	0.1%	0.3%	0.1%
Percentage of deaths*	0.5%	1.9%	0.6%

*P = .06
Based on data reported to the UNOS/OPTN Registry for U.S. transplants as of October 1, 2003. Retrieved from www.unos.org.

1% of liver transplant recipients and accounting for less than 1% of deaths among liver transplant recipients. Although the number of GVHD deaths was small, a higher percentage occurred among recipients of living donor grafts (1.9%). This preliminary trend supports the idea that one-way or partially mismatched grafts would occur more frequently among recipients of grafts from a related donor than from a genetically unrelated donor and that the risk of GVHD would be higher.

It will be more important to evaluate the degree and nature of HLA incompatibilities between the recipient and donor when evaluating a potential living related donor to avoid the most blatant one-way mismatches and to be aware of the potential for GVH complications after the transplant.

Conclusions

The transplanted liver is less susceptible to acute immune injury than are other organs for reasons that may relate to its size and capacity to regenerate, the fact that large quantities of soluble HLA antigens are shed by the liver that may neutralize or block cells and antibodies, or to other mechanisms that are more subtle. The early findings that the liver was resistant to hyperacute rejection by preformed anti-ABO and HLA antibodies may have been affected by the large volumes of blood that were exchanged during the surgery. Still, it is clear that antibodies against donor ABO or HLA can damage the liver and should be avoided whenever possible to reduce early dysfunction, stubborn rejection, and probably chronic problems that have not been explored in any systematic way. There are indications that with smaller grafts from splitting or from living donors, the actions of antibodies may play a larger role in the outcome.

Although prospective HLA matching for recipients undergoing liver transplantation is not likely to benefit many patients, there are indications that patients whose liver disease has an autoimmune cause might benefit from avoiding donors with the same HLA antigens to reduce the likelihood and speed with which their disease could recur. Similarly, liver damage caused by immunity against viral infections may recur more rapidly when the liver graft is HLA matched with the recipient, introducing the same targets for the antiviral response.

Acknowledgments

We thank Sara Taranto and Alan Ting for providing the UNOS/OPTN information on the effects of HLA and ABO on liver transplantation outcomes, and for analyzing the reported incidence of GVHD as a cause of death among recipients undergoing liver transplantation in the United States.

Pearls and Pitfalls

- Pretransplantation assessment of liver candidates is complicated by the often urgent nature of liver transplantation.

- Many consider testing for HLA and sensitization to be an unnecessary expense to obtain information that will be of little importance in selecting a donor. Although HLA incompatibilities and antibodies have little effect on the overall outcome of liver transplantations and would warrant little consideration in urgent transplantations, there are certainly instances when knowing that a patient has antidonor HLA antibodies or knowing the HLA types of the donor and recipient is helpful.

- A small fraction of candidates for liver transplantation are sensitized against HLA antigens; they are readily identified by a simple and inexpensive test. It is likely that a single test will suffice unless events occur while the patient is waiting that might provoke an immune response, such as transfusions, surgery, or infections requiring antibiotics.

- HLA typing may be helpful in avoiding one-way HLA mismatches that can predispose to GVHD complications. These tests should be performed on all patients for whom a living related donor is evaluated.

References

1. Hume DM, Merrill JP, Miller BF, Thorn GW: Experience with transplantation in the human: Report of nine cases. J Clin Invest 34:327-382, 1955.
2. Murray JE, Merrill JP, Dammin GJ, et al: Study on transplantation immunity after total body irradiation: Clinical and experimental investigation. Surgery 48:272-284, 1960.
3. Starzl TE, Marchioro TL, Holmes JH, et al: Renal homografts in patients with major donor recipient blood group incompatibilities. Surgery 55:195-200, 1964.
4. Patel R, Terasaki PI: Significance of the positive crossmatch test in kidney transplantation. N Engl J Med 280:735-739, 1969.
5. Kissmeier-Nielsen F, Olsen S, Peterson VP, Fjeldborg O: Hyperacute rejection of kidney allografts associated with preexisting humoral antibodies against donor cells. Lancet 2:662-665, 1966.
6. Wilbrandt R, Tung KSK, Deodhar SD, et al: ABO blood group incompatibility in human renal transplantation. Am J Clin Pathol 51:15-23, 1969.
7. Porter KA: The effects of antibodies on human renal allografts. Transplant Proc 8:189-197, 1976.
8. Gjertson DW, Cecka JM: Living unrelated donor kidney transplantation. Kidney Int 58:491-499, 2000.
9. Takemoto SK, Terasaki PI, Gjertson DW, Cecka JM: Twelve years experience with shipping HLA-matched cadaver kidneys for transplantation. N Engl J Med 343:1078-1084, 2000.
10. Persijn GG, De Meester JM: Demand, supply and allocation in Eurotransplant. Ann Transplant 2:26-33, 1997.
11. Watkins WM: The ABO blood group system: Historical background. Transfus Med 11:243-265, 2001.
12. Cecka JM, Breidenthal SE, Terasaki PI: Low anti-A and anti-B titers in some type O patients may permit renal transplantation across the ABO barrier. Transplant Proc 19:4507-4510, 1987.
13. Starzl TE, Koep LJ, Halgrimson CG, et al: Fifteen years of clinical liver transplantation. Gastroenterology 77:375-388, 1979.
14. Gordon RD, Iwatsuki S, Esquivel CO, et al: Liver transplantation across ABO blood groups. Surgery 100:342-348, 1986.
15. Rydberg L: ABO incompatibility in solid organ transplantation. Transfus Med 11:325-342, 2001.
16. Demetris AJ, Jaffe R, Tzakis A, et al: Antibody-mediated rejection of human orthotopic liver allografts. Am J Pathol 132:489-502, 1988.
17. Gugenheim J, Didier S, Reynes M, Bismuth H: Liver transplantation across ABO blood group barriers. Lancet 336:519-523, 1990.
18. Lo CM, Shaked A, Busuttil RW: Risk factors for transplantation across the ABO barrier. Transplantation 58:543-547, 1994.
19. Bjoro K, Ericzon BG, Kirkegaard P, et al: Highly urgent liver transplantation: Possible impact of donor-recipient ABO matching on the outcome after transplantation. Transplantation 75:347-353, 2003.
20. de Meester J, Bogers M, de Winter H, et al: Which ABO-matching rule should be the decisive factor in the choice between a highly urgent and an elective patient? Transpl Int 15:431-435, 2002.
21. Cook DJ, Graver B, Terasaki PI: ABO incompatibility in cadaver kidney allografts. Transplant Proc 19:4549-4552, 1987.
22. Alexandre GPJ, Squifflet JP, DeBruyere M, et al: Present experiences in a series of 26 ABO-incompatible living donor renal allografts. Transplant Proc 19:4538-4542, 1987.
23. Takayama J, Ohkohchi N, Oikawa T, et al: Living related liver transplantation in patients with ABO incompatibility. Transplant Proc 30:3504-3506, 1998.
24. Hashimoto T, Kondo S, Suzuki T, et al: Strategy for ABO-incompatible living-related liver transplantation. Transplant Proc 32:2104-2106, 2000.
25. Kawagishi N, Ohkohchi N, Fujimori K, et al: Antibody elimination by apheresis in living donor liver transplant recipients. Ther Apher 5:449-454, 2001.

26. Kozaki K, Kasahara M, Oike F, et al: Apheresis therapy for living-donor liver transplantation: Experience for apheresis use for living-donor liver transplantation at Kyoto University. Ther Apher 6:478-483, 2002.

27. Hanto DW, Fecteau AH, Alonso MH, et al: ABO-incompatible liver transplantation with no immunological graft losses using total plasma exchange, splenectomy and quadruple immunosuppression: Evidence for accommodation. Liver Transpl 9:22-30, 2003.

28. Fang WC, Saltzman J, Rososhansky S, et al: Acceptance of an ABO-incompatible mismatched (AB(+) to O(+)) liver allograft with the use of daclizumab and mycophenolate mofetil. Liver Transpl 6:497-500, 2000.

29. Tanabe M, Shimazu M, Wakabayashi G, et al: Intraportal infusion therapy as a novel approach to adult ABO-incompatible liver transplantation. Transplantation 73:1959-1961, 2002.

30. Platt JL, Vercellotti GM, Dalmasso AP, et al: Transplantation of discordant xenografts: A review of progress. Immunol Today 11:450-456, 1990.

31. Salama AD, Delikouras A, Pusey CD, et al: Transplant accommodation in highly sensitized patients: A potential role for Bcl-xL and alloantibody. Am J Transplant 1:260-269, 2001.

32. Soares MP, Lin Y, Sato K, et al: Accommodation. Immunol Today 20:434-437, 1999.

33. Park WD, Grande JP, Ninova D, et al: Accommodation in ABO-incompatible kidney allografts, a novel mechanism of self-protection against antibody-mediated injury. Am J Transplant 3:952-960, 2003.

34. Fishbein TM, Emre S, Guy SR, et al: Safe transplantation of blood type A2 livers to blood type O recipients. Transplantation 67:1071-1073, 1999.

35. Nelson PW, Landreneau MD, Luger AM, et al: Ten-year experience in transplantation of A2 kidneys into B and O recipients. Transplantation 65:256-260, 1998.

36. Ramsey G. Nusbacher J, Starzl T, et al: Isohemagglutinins of graft origin after ABO-unmatched liver transplantation. N Engl J Med 311:1167-1170, 1984.

37. Kunimasa JI, Yurugi K, Ito K, et al: Hemolytic reaction due to graft-versus-host (GVH) antibody production after liver transplantation from living donors: A report of two cases. Jpn J Surg 28:857-861, 1998.

38. Au WY, Lo CM, Fan ST, et al: Life-threatening ABO-mediated hemolysis after cadaveric orthotopic liver transplantation. Transplantation 74:285-286, 2002.

39. Ramsey G: Red cell antibodies arising from solid organ transplants. Transfusion 31:76-86, 1991.

40. Hareuveni M, Merchav H, Austerlitz N, et al: Donor anti-Jk(a) causing hemolysis in a liver transplant recipient. Transfusion 42:363-367, 2002.

41. Au WY, Lo CM, Hawkins BR, et al: Evan's syndrome complicating graft-versus-host disease after cadaveric liver transplantation. Transplantation 72:527-528, 2001.

42. Bracey AW: Anti-A of donor origin in three recipients of organs from the same donor. Vox Sang 53:181-183, 1987.

43. Opelz G, Graver B, Mickey MR, Terasaki PI: Lymphocytotoxic antibody responses to transfusions in potential kidney transplant recipients. Transplantation 32:177-183, 1981.

44. John R, Leitz K, Schuster M, et al: Immunologic sensitization in recipients of left ventricular assist devices. J Thorac Cardiovasc Surg 125:587-591, 2003.

45. Starzl TE, Demetris AJ, Todo S, et al: Evidence for hyperacute rejection of human liver grafts: The case of the canary kidneys. Clin Transpl 3:37-45, 1989.

46. Hanto DW, Snover DC, Noreen HJ, et al: Hyperacute rejection of a human orthotopic liver allograft in a presensitized patient. Clin Transpl 1:304-310, 1987.

47. Donaldson PT, Williams R: Crossmatching in liver transplantation. Transplantation 62:789-794, 1997.

48. Bishara A, Brautbar C, Eid A, et al: Is presensitization relevant to liver transplant outcome? Hum Immunol 63:742-750, 2002.

49. Neumann UP, Lang M, Moldenhauer A, et al: Significance of a T-lymphocytotoxic crossmatch in liver and combined liver-kidney transplantation. Transplantation 71:1163-1168, 2001.

50. Ogura K, Terasaki PI, Koyama H, et al: High one-month graft failure rates in flow cytometry crossmatch-positive recipients. Clin Transpl 8:111-115, 1994.

51. Katz SM, Kimball PM, Ozaki C, et al: Positive pre-transplant crossmatches predict early graft loss in liver allograft recipients. Transplantation 57:616-620, 1994.

52. Takaya S, Jain A, Uagihashi A, et al: Increased bile duct complication and/or chronic rejection in crossmatch positive human liver allografts. Transplant Proc 31:2028-2031, 1999.

53. Scornik JC, Soldevilla-Pico C, Van der Werf WJ, et al: Susceptibility of liver allografts to high or low concentrations of preformed antibodies as measured by flow cytometry. Am J Transplant 1:152-156, 2001.

54. Astarcioglu I, Cursio R, Reynes M, Gugenheim J: Increased risk of antibody-mediated rejection of reduced-size liver allografts. J Surg Res 87:258-262, 1999.

55. Takakura K, Kiuchi T, Kasahara M, et al: Clinical implications of flow cytometry crossmatch with T or B cells in living donor liver transplantation. Clin Transpl 15:309-316, 2001.

56. Suh KS, Kim SB, Chang SH, et al: Significance of a positive cytotoxic crossmatch in adult-to-adult living donor transplantation using small graft volume. Liver Transpl 12:1109-1112, 2002.

57. Manez R, Kelly RH, Kobayashi M, et al: Immunoglobulin G antibodies in clinical liver transplantation: Studies toward further defining their significance. Hepatology 21:1345-1349, 1995.

58. Jordan S, Tyan D, Czer L, Toyoda M: Immunomodulatory actions of intravenous immunoglobulin (IVIG): Potential applications in solid organ transplant recipients. Pediatr Transplant 2:92-105, 1998.

59. Montgomery RA, Zachary AA, Racussen LC, et al: Plasmapheresis and intravenous immunoglobulin provides effective rescue therapy for refractory humoral rejection and allows kidneys to be successfully transplanted into crossmatch-positive recipients. Transplantation 70:887-895, 2000.

60. Gloor JM, DeGoey SR, Pineda AA, et al: Overcoming a positive crossmatch in living-donor kidney transplantation. Am J Transplantation 3:1017-1023, 2003.

61. Markus BH, Duquesnoy RJ, Gordon RD, et al: Histocompatibility and liver transplant outcome: Does HLA exert a dualistic effect? Transplantation 46:372-377, 1988.

62. Nikaein A, Backman L, Jennings L, et al: HLA compatibility and liver transplant outcome: Improved patient survival by HLA and crossmatching. Transplantation 58:786-792, 1994.

63. Doran TJ, Geczy AF, Painter D, et al: A large, single center investigation of the immunogenetic factors affecting liver transplantation. Transplantation 69:1491-1498, 2000.

64. Manez R, White LT, Linden P, et al: The influence of HLA matching on cytomegalovirus hepatitis and chronic rejection after liver transplantation. Transplantation 55:1067-1071, 1993.

65. Carmody IC, Ghobrial RM, Gjertson DW, et al: Impact of HLA matching on hepatitis C recurrence following orthotopic liver transplantation [abstract]. Am J Transplant 3(Suppl 5): 518, 2003.

66. Neumann UP, Guckelberger O, Langrehr JM, et al: Impact of human leukocyte matching in liver transplantation. Transplantation 75:132-137, 2003.

67. Neumann UP, Langrehr JM, Naumann U, et al: Impact of HLA-compatibilities in patients undergoing liver transplantations for HBV-cirrhosis. Clin Transpl 16:122-129, 2002.

68. Burdick JF, Vogelsang GB, Smith WJ, et al: Severe graft-versus-host disease in a liver transplant patient. N Engl J Med 318:689-691, 1988.
69. Rosen CB, Ng CS, Moore SB, et al: Clinical and pathological features of graft-versus-host disease after liver transplantation: A case report and review of the literature. Clin Transpl 7:52-58, 1993.
70. Whitington PF, Rubin CM, Alonzo EM, et al: Complete lymphoid chimerism and chronic graft-vs-host-disease in an infant recipient of a hepatic allograft from an HLA-homozygous parental living donor. Transplantation 62:1516-1519, 1996.
71. Au WY, Ma SK, Kwong YL, et al: Graft-versus-host disease after liver transplantation: Documentation by fluorescent in situ hybridization and human leukocyte antigen typing. Clin Transpl 14:174-177, 2000.
72. Lehner F, Becker T, Sybrecht L, et al: Successful outcome of acute graft-versus-host disease in a liver allograft recipient by withdrawal of immunosuppression. Transplantation 73:307-310, 2002.
73. Arrieta A, Maruri N, Rinon M, et al: Confirmation of graft-versus-host disease by HLA typing after liver transplantation. Transplant Proc 34:278-279, 2002.
74. Knox KS, Behnia M, Smith LR, et al: Acute graft-versus-host disease of the lung after liver transplantation. Liver Transpl 8:968-971, 2002.
75. Nemoto T, Kubota K, Kita J, et al: Unusual onset of chronic graft-versus-host disease after living-related liver transplantation from a homozygous donor. Transplantation 75:733-736, 2003.
76. Smith DM, Agura E, Netto G, et al: Liver transplant-associated graft-versus-host disease. Transplantation 75:118-126, 2003.
77. Kasahara M, Kiuchi T, Uryuhara K, et al: Role of HLA compatibility in pediatric living-related liver transplantation. Transplantation 74:1175-1180, 2002.
78. Petz LD, Calhoun L, Yam P, et al: Transfusion-associated graft-versus-host disease in immunocompetent patients: Report of a fatal case associated with transfusion of blood from a second-degree relative, and a survey of predisposing factors. Transfusion 33:742-750, 1993.

XI

Immunosuppression

75

Induction and Maintenance of Immunosuppression

SRINATH CHINNAKOTLA
GORAN B. KLINTMALM

Immunobiology of acute rejection   1214

Individual immunosuppressants   1215
    Corticosteroids   1215
    Cyclophosphamide   1217
    Azathioprine   1218
    Mycophenolate mofetil   1218
    Leflunomide   1219
    Cyclosporine   1220
    Tacrolimus (FK506)   1221
    Sirolimus   1222
    Antibody therapies   1222
    Monoclonal antibodies   1223

Developing therapeutic strategies to maximize
    outcomes in special populations or
    conditions   1226
    Recipient groups   1226

Conclusions   1230

Liver transplant outcomes have improved progressively over the last decade, with current 1- and 5-year survival rates reported by the United Network for Organ Sharing (UNOS) to be approximately 80% and 70%, respectively.[1] Advances in surgical technique have contributed to better early outcomes, and advances in immunosuppression have contributed significantly to improved long-term survival.

The first success in controlling rejection was reported by Starzl and coauthors in the early 1960s when a combination of azathioprine and prednisone was used in living related kidney transplants.[2] The next advance was made in the late 1960s and early 1970s with the introduction of antilymphocyte globulin (ALG). The early liver transplants performed in Colorado were maintained with azathioprine and steroids, and subsequently ALG was also used.[3] A striking improvement in the results of liver transplantation was made in 1978 when cyclosporine was used in combination with steroids, with or without azathioprine, in primary immunosuppressive protocols by Calne and colleagues.[4,5] In 1989, tacrolimus (FK506) was first used in clinical studies for both rejection prophylaxis and rescue therapy for persistent rejection.[6] Subsequently, the results of multicenter trials evaluating the use of tacrolimus for primary immunosuppression in liver transplants were reported in 1994.[7] However, both cyclosporine and tacrolimus were associated with significant nephrotoxicity and neurotoxicity.

By the end of the previous millennium, the introduction of several new agents such as mycophenolate mofetil (MMF), sirolimus, leflunomide, and monoclonal antibodies offered medications that avoid nephrotoxicity and neurotoxicity. These new medications (Fig. 75–1) provide several agents from which to choose; however, they carry other side effects, largely gastrointestinal and hematological in nature. Since individual patients or groups of patients differ in their immune responsiveness and comorbidity, management of immunosuppression protocols should be individualized to account for these differences. The infusion of new medications to the immunosuppression armamentarium has allowed clinicians to tailor the medication regimen to achieve improved outcomes, both for prevention and treatment of rejection as well as for reduced side effects and optimized effects or control of comorbid conditions. Thus, this chapter outlines the various immunosuppressive agents currently used and their common adverse effects. Additionally, examples are presented of protocols developed for specific groups of liver transplant recipients to provide effective immunosuppression with minimal toxic side effects.

Immunobiology of Acute Rejection

The exact mechanism of the immunological barrier to acceptance of allogeneic tissues and organs is not completely known. However, immune responses can be compartmentalized into alloantigen recognition, lymphocyte activation, clonal expansion, and graft inflammation (Table 75–1).

The immune response categories provide the framework for understanding the mechanism of the proposed sites of action of the immunosuppressive drugs and the clinical approach to immunosuppressive therapy.[8] The immune response begins with antigen recognition (see Fig. 75–1). Progression from alloantigen recognition to cellular activation depends on the presence of several stimulatory signals presented to the T cell. Once T cells are activated, a cascade of intracellular responses are initiated, mediated partially through intracellular calcium and numerous promoters directed at enhanced transcription of the interleukin-2 (IL-2) gene. Although several cytokines are involved, IL-2 is the key juncture in the transplant immune response, and a number of drugs designed to inhibit IL-2 transcription have been developed, including immunophilin-binding agents. Once selected by the process of antigen presentation and IL-2/growth factor expression, the individual T cells that have responded undergo a burst of proliferative activity. Drugs such as MMF, azathioprine, and sirolimus inhibit the proliferation of T cells. When their population is expanded, these T cells perform their regulatory and cytotoxic functions as would be predicted by the immune response to infection. The effector arm

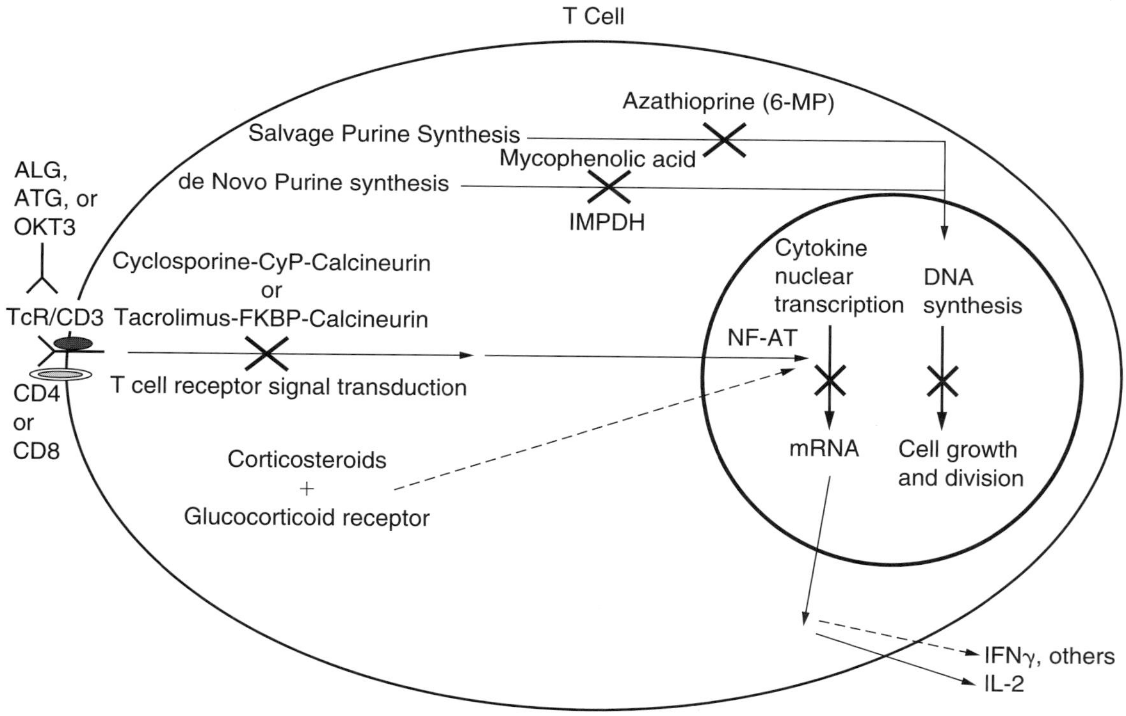

FIGURE 75–1

Mechanism of immunosuppressive agents.

Table 75-1. IMMUNOLOGICAL RESPONSE TO IMMUNOSUPPRESSIVE MEDICATIONS USED IN TRANSPLANTATION

Phase of Immune Response	Immune System Requisites	Current Clinical Interventions	Cellular Mediator
Alloantigen recognition	Presentation in context of MHC molecules	Antilymphocyte antibodies	APC
		Blood or marrow cell infusion	
Lymphocyte activation	Two inciting stimuli to transcribe IL-2, IL-12, and IFN-γ	Immunophilin-binding agents: cyclosporine and tacrolimus	T lymphocytes
		Monoclonal antibodies*	
Clonal expansion	IL-2 and IL-2R expression	Mycophenolate mofetil, azathioprine, sirolimus, cyclophosphamide	T lymphocyte
Graft inflammation	Adhesion molecule and chemokine expression	Steroids, antilymphocyte antibodies	T lymphocytes, non-specific cytotoxic cells

*Certain monoclonal antibodies recognizing CD4, CD28, the IL-2 receptor, and the like may have efficacy in downregulating or altering the lymphocyte response to alloantigen.
APC, antigen-presenting cell; IFN, interferon; IL-2R, interleukin-2 receptor.
From Valente JI, Wesley JA: Immunobiology of renal transplantation. Surg Clin North Am 78:1-26.

of the de novo immune response to allograft antigens is principally cellular and requires the adherence and transvascular migration of immune cells into the graft to become manifested. Cytokines are released at the site of rejection and recruit these nonspecific inflammatory cells, whose presence in tissues causes graft inflammation and damage. The damage occurs through a number of routes, including the release of perforins, destructive enzymes, and vasoactive and toxic mediators and direct cell-mediated cytotoxicity. This injury is clinically acute cellular rejection, which is manifested histologically as venulitis and bile duct damage.

Individual Immunosuppressants

Corticosteroids

Corticosteroids remain a cornerstone of many immunosuppressive regimens. Low doses of prednisone have for many years been a critical component of maintenance posttransplant immunotherapy, whereas larger doses of both prednisone and methylprednisolone are often used as first-line treatment of acute allograft rejection (Table 75-2). The immunosuppressive properties of steroids are related to their ability to suppress antibody and complement binding and to reduce the synthesis of key immunomodulating cytokines such as IL-2 and interferon-γ.[9] Additionally, steroids inhibit macrophage secretion of IL-1, a key element in antigen presentation and initiation of acute allograft rejection.

Four major corticosteroid compounds are used in liver transplantation: hydrocortisone, prednisone, prednisolone, and methylprednisolone. Prednisone is rapidly absorbed from the gastrointestinal tract; however, liver metabolism of prednisolone is required for biological activity. Thus, the bioavailability of prednisone is approximately 80% and is diminished in patients with liver insufficiency. In the case of methylprednisolone (the intravenous form), a succinate moiety is present and must be hydrolyzed by the liver for steroid activity.[10] In addition, this compound has multiple active metabolites, which prolongs its biological half-life.

Table 75-2. TYPICAL STEROID DOSING REGIMENS FOR USE IN LIVER TRANSPLANTATION: THE CLASSIC TAPER USED IN COMBINATION WITH CYCLOSPORINE AND AZATHIOPRINE

Time Period	Drug	Double-Drug Regimen*	Triple-Drug Regimen†
Intraoperative	Hydrocortisone	1 g IV	1 g IV
Postoperative	Prednisolone		
Day 1	Prednisolone	50 mg q6h	60 mg q12h
Day 2	Prednisolone	40 mg q6h	50 mg q12h
Day 3	Prednisolone	30 mg q6h	40 mg q12h
Day 4	Prednisolone	20 mg q6h	30 mg q12h
Day 5	Prednisolone	20 mg q12h	20 mg q12h
Day 7	Prednisolone	15 mg q12h	20 mg q24h
Day 30	Prednisolone		15 mg q24h
Day 60	Prednisolone	15 mg q24h	10 mg q24h
Day 180	Prednisolone	12.5 mg q24h	5 mg q24h
Day 360	Prednisolone	10 mg q24h	5 mg q24h

*Generally used in combination with cyclosporine or tacrolimus.
†Generally used in combination with azathioprine and cyclosporine or tacrolimus.

Table 75-3. MAJOR SIDE EFFECTS OF IMMUNOSUPPRESSIVE AGENTS (AS SEEN AT BAYLOR UNIVERSITY MEDICAL CENTER)

Agent	Bone Marrow Suppression	Hyperlipidemia	Hypertension	Neurotoxicity	Osteoporosis	Posttransplant Diabetes	Nephrotoxicity	Gastrointestinal
						Side Effects		
Azathioprine	+++							++
Mycophenolate mofetil	++							+++
Leflunomide	++							+
Sirolimus	++	+++						+
Corticosteroids		+	++		++	+		+
Cyclosporine		+	+	++	+	+	++	
Tacrolimus		+	++	+++	+	++	+++	+

Table 75–4. STEROID DOSING FOR TREATMENT OF ACUTE CELLULAR REJECTION (BAYLOR UNIVERSITY MEDICAL CENTER)

Condition	Postoperative Day	Steroid Dosing
Hepatitis B and C	1	1 g methylprednisolone IV
	2	1 g methylprednisolone IV
	3 to 10	Taper IV: 100 → 80 → 60 → 40 → 20 → 15 → 12.5 → 10 mg/day
All other patients	1	1 g methylprednisolone IV
	2	1 g methylprednisolone IV
	3 to 8	Taper IV: 200 → 160 → 120 → 80 → 40 → 20 mg/day

Oral and intravenous doses of prednisolone are equivalent because no liver metabolism is required for steroid activity. Steroid activity is primarily inactivated by liver metabolism through reduction and conjugation, together with urinary excretion.[11] Thus, changes in liver function may markedly influence the activation, metabolism, and elimination of corticosteroids. Studies in liver transplant recipients have shown that metabolism of prednisolone is slower in liver transplant recipients than in nontransplant patients. This finding may be related to the lower cytochrome P450 activity and may help explain the immunological effectiveness of low-dose prednisone regimens in this group of patients.[11]

Numerous side effects are associated with steroid therapy (Table 75–3). Long-term use can lead to glucose intolerance or diabetes mellitus, fluid retention and hypertension, hyperlipidemia, osteopenia, cataracts, cushingoid appearance, cosmetic changes (acne, hirsutism, skin fragility with ecchymoses), weight gain, susceptibility to infection, impaired wound healing, amenorrhea in women, and growth inhibition in pediatric patients. Even in the short term, high doses of steroids are associated with aseptic bone necrosis and myopathy, as well as de novo diabetes mellitus, cushingoid appearance, weight gain, impaired wound healing, and infections. Quality of life in transplant recipients can also be impaired by steroid-related side effects such as emotional instability, personality changes, manic/depressive psychoses, and insomnia. Steroid use also increases the risk for cardiovascular disease by promoting diabetes mellitus or glucose intolerance, hypertension, and hyperlipidemia. The use of steroids in the immediate postoperative period reduces the requirement for pain medication.

As originally designed, the majority of immunosuppression protocols in transplantation typically begin with a high burst of steroid therapy followed by a stepwise dose reduction. More recently, several modified steroid-dosing protocols have been designed to avoid some of the adverse effects of steroids. For example, lower doses of steroids may be indicated in transplant recipients with hepatitis C because recurrence after liver transplantation is directly related to steroid exposure (Table 75–4). A rapid taper in steroid dosage is recommended for this group of patients, with steroids being discontinued in most patients by 60 days after transplantation. Conversely, higher steroid doses are used in patients with autoimmune hepatitis without discontinuation because rapid taper and withdrawal may result in acute cellular rejection and recurrent autoimmune hepatitis, respectively (see Table 75–6).

Pearls and Pitfalls

- Recurrence of hepatitis C after liver transplantation may be related to steroid exposure.
- Steroid metabolism is slower in liver transplant recipients; thus, even low-dose steroids are immunologically effective.

Cyclophosphamide

Cyclophosphamide (Cytoxan) is a nitrogen mustard derivative that is broadly classified as an alkylating agent. Its mechanism of action is disruption of cellular growth and mitosis by interfering with DNA replication and transcription of RNA, which ultimately results in disruption of nucleic acid function. Cyclophosphamide is activated by liver microsomal (P450 mixed-function oxidase) enzymes. Similar to azathioprine, antimitotic activity is greatest in rapidly proliferating cells.

Cyclophosphamide is rapidly absorbed after oral administration, with the maximum plasma concentration occurring at about 1 hour.[12] Minute quantities of cyclophosphamide and its metabolites appear to be distributed throughout the body, including cerebrospinal fluid, breast milk, and synovial fluid. In vivo protein binding generally ranges from 0% to 10%, but protein binding of alkylating metabolites is greater than 50%.

The serum half-life of cyclophosphamide after intravenous administration is 4 to 6.5 hours. Approximately 15% of the drug is excreted unchanged in urine.

Myelosuppression, primarily leukopenia, is the usual dose-limiting toxicity of cyclophosphamide and occurs to a greater extent than with azathioprine therapy. Alopecia is to be expected to some degree in all patients. Gastrointestinal toxicity (nausea, vomiting, diarrhea) is also expected. Other long-term side effects include malignancy, teratogenesis, and decreased reproductive capability. Cyclophosphamide was used earlier as an immunosuppressive agent but is now used mainly in chemotherapy regimens for cancer treatment.

Pearls and Pitfalls

- Used in earlier immunosuppression protocols but now used mainly in chemotherapy regimens.

Azathioprine

Azathioprine (Imuran) is an imidazole derivative of mercaptopurine that is rapidly metabolized to 6-mercaptopurine, as well as several other active and inactive metabolites. Azathioprine is an antimetabolite and acts as a purine analogue that is incorporated into cellular DNA and inhibits purine nucleotide synthesis and metabolism.[12] Rapidly dividing cells such as T and B lymphocytes are most susceptible. Thus, azathioprine acts early during the proliferative phase of the cell cycle and inhibits primary cell-mediated humoral responses.[12]

In use for more than 30 years, azathioprine has been a key component of triple immunosuppressive regimens. Myelosuppression remains the most common side effect of azathioprine, with more than 50% of transplant recipients experiencing varying degrees of hematological toxicity.[13] The antimitotic effect of azathioprine on gastrointestinal epithelium can cause nausea, oral mucosal ulcerations, and esophagitis. There is also a reported increased incidence of skin cancer in patients receiving azathioprine long-term.[14] Azathioprine is not neurotoxic, nor is it nephrotoxic (see Table 75–3).

Azathioprine is available in both intravenous and oral dosage forms. Because the drug is readily absorbed after oral administration, intravenous dosing is the same as oral dosing. Initial daily doses of 2 to 3 mg/kg are used when azathioprine is the primary immunosuppressive agent. Maintenance doses larger than 1 to 2 mg/kg/day

are rarely tolerated in combination therapy. Azathioprine should be given as a single dose, not to exceed 200 mg/day. Since myelosuppression is dose dependent, the azathioprine dosage should be adjusted in accordance with the patient's total white cell count. The dose is reduced when there are rapid decreases in white cells or the white cell count is less than 5000 cells/mL. The dose should be withheld or reduced to 25 mg/day with white cell counts of less than 3000 cells/mL. Allopurinol inhibits the principal metabolic pathway of azathioprine (oxidative metabolism of mercaptopurine by xanthine oxidase). Thus, concomitant administration of allopurinol increases both the magnitude of immunosuppression and the hematological toxicity associated with azathioprine therapy. It is strongly recommended that concomitant therapy be avoided. One of the most attractive aspects of azathioprine is its lack of nephrotoxicity. Azathioprine is very useful in patients who are being treated with a triple-drug immunosuppression regimen and do not tolerate MMF because of severe gastrointestinal side effects.

Pearls and Pitfalls

- Myelosuppression is the major side effect.
- Does not cause nephrotoxicity or neurotoxicity.
- Useful substitute in patients who do not tolerate MMF because of gastrointestinal side effects.
- Avoid concomitant use of allopurinol.

Mycophenolate Mofetil

MMF (CellCept) is the 2-morpholinoethyl ester of mycophenolic acid (MPA), which is produced by several species of *Penicillium*.[15,16] MMF is converted to MPA in the liver by ester hydrolysis and is most commonly used in transplantation to inhibit cellular proliferation.[17]

The major advantage of MPA over azathioprine is its relatively selective effect on lymphocyte activation. This effect is due to two aspects of the drug's mechanism: inhibition of purine synthesis and selective inhibition of inosine monophosphate dehydrogenase II. In purine synthesis, guanosine and adenosine (the two purine nucleotides synthesized via the de novo pathway) are inhibited by MPA. With these vital DNA substrates depleted, lymphocytes are unable to proliferate. In contrast, cells other than lymphocytes can use the salvage pathway to produce adequate quantities of guanosine monophosphate and adenosine monophosphate by recycling the guanine and adenine already present in the cell. The second mechanism is that MPA more selectively inhibits inosine monophosphate dehydrogenase II, which is predominantly used by proliferating lymphocytes. MMF has also been shown to have antiviral activity against hepatitis C virus (HCV), similar to ribivarin.[18,19] The common side effects of MMF are gastrointestinal and hematological (see Table 75–3). Gastrointestinal side effects include mild ileus, gastritis, nausea, and vomiting. The most frequently seen hematological side effects are leukopenia, thrombocytopenia, and occasional pancytopenia. As with other immunosuppressive agents, opportunistic infections are common, especially cytomegalovirus (CMV).[20,21] Doses of 2000 mg/day or higher, as were used in these reports, were shown to be most efficacious. No significant nephrotoxicity, neurotoxicity, or hepatotoxicity was observed.

Available in oral dosage forms, the bioavailability of MMF is about 20%. Doses of 1000 mg twice daily are used in combination therapy. The gastrointestinal side effects are dose dependent (as established in renal transplantation trials). When gastrointestinal side effects are significant and other causes are ruled out, the first step in dose adjustment would be to give the same amount of drug three or four times a day (e.g., 750 mg three times daily or 500 mg four times daily). This step alone frequently reduces the gastrointestinal side effects. If the change in dosing frequency does not result in improvement in side effects, reducing the dosage by 50% (500 mg twice daily) is advised. Most patients will tolerate a dose reduction; discontinuation of the drug is rarely necessary for control of side effects. Recently, an enteric-coated preparation, mycophenolate sodium (Myfortic), has been developed with the aim of reducing gastrointestinal side effects. Mycophenolate sodium allows delayed release of the active agent into the small intestine, unlike MMF, which immediately releases MPA into the stomach. The dose is 360 mg of mycophenolate sodium, which is equivalent to 500 mg of MMF.[22,23]

The use of MMF in liver transplantation has been studied by several investigators.[24-29] When MMF in combination with tacrolimus and steroids was compared with tacrolimus and steroids alone, patient and graft survival was similar. However, a trend toward fewer episodes of rejection, lower need for steroids, and better perioperative renal function occurred in patients treated with the triple-therapy combination.[29]

MMF displays considerable versatility in transplant recipients. Clinicians have successfully used MMF as rescue therapy to treat liver rejection and also to allow early steroid withdrawal.[24-28] Additionally, MMF has been used as a renal-sparing agent by allowing dose reduction of calcineurin inhibitors when they are administered together.[30] Recent data also indicate that a higher dose of MMF (1500 mg twice daily) is beneficial in preventing disease recurrence in patients transplanted for hepatitis C.

Pearls and Pitfalls

- Versatile agent used in triple-drug immunosuppression protocols and renal-sparing protocols.
- Does not cause nephrotoxicity or neurotoxicity.
- Gastrointestinal adverse side effects are common, but usually respond to dose adjustment.
- High-dose MMF (1500 mg twice daily) may have antiviral activity against HCV.

Leflunomide

Leflunomide (Arava) is a member of the family of drugs called malonitrilamides. These compounds have a variety of biological activities, many of which have been linked to their ability to reversibly block dihydroorotate dehydrogenase, an enzyme required for de novo pyrimidine synthesis in lymphocytes and other cells, and their inhibition of selected tyrosine kinases.[31] A large volume of experimental data have been published on the ability of leflunomide to control and reverse acute rejection.[32-36] The more recently observed inhibitory effects of leflunomide on herpesvirus replication, specifically CMV, add a new dimension to its evaluation in transplant patients.[37,38] Leflunomide itself is a prodrug and is essentially undetectable in blood after oral dosing. The active metabolite (A77 1726) forms as a result of hydrolytic opening of the isoxazole side ring. In human blood, the active metabolite is almost exclusively confined to plasma or serum, with less than 5% found in the formed elements of blood. The active metabolite has a half-life of approximately 5 to 15 days in kidney transplant recipients.[39]

A recent study evaluating the use of leflunomide in 53 stable liver and kidney transplant recipients showed that it possesses substantial immunosuppressive potency. When dosed to serum levels higher than 100 µg/mL, side effects appeared in approximately 25% to 35% of patients. The principal side effects were anemia and elevation of liver enzymes in liver recipients.[39] Other reported side effects include rash, gastrointestinal symptoms, and pancreatitis. Observations from these 53 patients demonstrated no other evidence of leflunomide-related organ damage, such as neurological or renal toxicity, lipid changes, glucose changes, or significant hematological changes other than anemia.[39] Although further studies are needed to substantiate these findings, leflunomide has the potential to be an immunosuppressive agent without nephrotoxicity or neurotoxicity. Its use may be similar to that of MMF and azathioprine.

Cyclosporine

Cyclosporine is a cyclic endecapeptide with potent immunosuppressive activity that is isolated from the soil fungi *Cylindrocarpon lucidum*.[4] The potent properties of cyclosporine were reported shortly after it was isolated. It has been found to bind several cytosolic proteins, with cyclophilin, a ubiquitous cytosolic protein, suggested as the primary receptor.[40] Cyclosporine primarily affects the T-cell immune response by blocking production of IL-2. Inhibition of IL-2 activity is associated with a decreased response to class I and II antigens, which are critical for the rejection cascade. Cyclosporine inhibits gene transcription for IL-2, interferon-γ, IL-3, IL-4, c-myc, c-fos, and other genes required for differentiation and proliferation of T and B lymphocytes.[4] Cyclosporine is not cytotoxic and does not significantly inhibit the myeloid or erythroid cell lines. The selective immunosuppressive activity of cyclosporine has resulted in significantly reduced rejection rates and improved patient and graft survival after liver transplantation.[41] In earlier formulations, the bioavailability of the orally administered conventional formulation of cyclosporine (Sandimmune) was variable, but with the recent introduction of the microemulsion, nonaqueous form (Neoral), bioavailability is excellent. After oral administration, cyclosporine is variably absorbed via the lymphatic system in the proximal jejunum and achieves peak serum or whole blood levels within 2 to 4 hours.[12] Once absorbed, cyclosporine is widely distributed, with adipose, pancreatic, adrenal, kidney, and liver tissues having the highest concentrations.[12] The metabolism of cyclosporine is primarily hepatic and occurs via the monooxygenase P450 system. It is predominantly excreted via biliary secretion.[4] In liver failure, in which the liver is unable to metabolize cyclosporine or excrete its metabolites, the potential for dangerous toxicity should be recognized. Cyclosporine has an average half-life of 27 hours (range, 10 to 40 hours). Drugs that stimulate the P450 system, such as rifampin, isoniazid, phenytoin, phenobarbital, carbamazepine, and quinolones, will increase cyclosporine metabolism and decrease blood levels.[42,43] In contrast, drugs that inhibit or are metabolized by the hepatic enzyme system

(such as erythromycin, ketoconazole, diltiazem, verapamil, high doses of corticosteroids, nonsteroidal anti-inflammatory agents, and oral contraceptives) may increase blood levels and result in increased toxicity.[43] A dose-dependent interaction between cyclosporine and fluconazole has been reported.[44]

Nephrotoxicity and hypertension remain the most important side effects of cyclosporine (see Table 75-3). Its nephrotoxicity can be classified into four distinct patterns: (1) acute reversible decrease in kidney function as a result of vasoconstriction, (2) acute tubular dysfunction caused by high blood concentrations, (3) an idiosyncratic acute vasculopathy, and (4) the development of chronic irreversible functional impairment with associated morphological and histological changes.[42-46] Neurological side effects include paresthesias, tremors, headaches, hallucinations, and confusion.[47] Seizures and convulsions have been reported in patients receiving intravenous cyclosporine. Hypertrichosis and gingival hyperplasia resulting in significant cosmetic discomfort can be troublesome in pediatric and younger patients.[48] Less commonly reported side effects include hepatotoxicity, nausea, vomiting, neutropenia, thrombocytopenia, anemia, allergic reactions, tinnitus, myalgia, and arthralgia.

Oral cyclosporine is initiated at a dose of 5 mg/kg twice daily. Daily trough levels are monitored to avoid too little or too much immunosuppression, as well as kidney, liver, and neurological toxicity. For liver transplant patients receiving double immunosuppression regimens, levels are maintained between 250 and 400 ng/mL for the first 1 to 3 months postoperatively. Thereafter, levels of 200 to 300 ng/mL are maintained. Many institutions use lower target levels, such as 200 to 250 ng/mL for induction followed by 100 to 200 ng/dL for maintenance. In patients receiving a triple-dose regimen, levels of 200 ng/mL in the first 3 months and 150 ng/mL thereafter are adequate. Cyclosporine therapy is withheld for 48 to 72 hours in liver transplant recipients with oliguric renal failure. Reliance is placed on MMF and steroids to establish an adequate degree of immunosuppression. Cyclosporine is introduced gradually after kidney function is restored.

Special Considerations in the Use of Generic Cyclosporine

In the United States, the patent for cyclosporine expired in September 1995. This opened the door for the development of several generic cyclosporine formulations. To date, the following generic cyclosporine products have been approved by the Food and Drug Administration (FDA): Eon cyclosporine (cyclosporine capsules, Eon Labs), Gengraf Capsules (cyclosporine capsules, Abbott Laboratories), and Pliva cyclosporine (cyclosporine capsules, Pliva, Inc.).

Several factors influence cyclosporine pharmacokinetics in transplant patients, including age, disease, race or ethnicity, gender, diet, and intraindividual and interindividual variation in metabolism and enteric transport processes. The possible impact of pharmacokinetic differences on transplant outcome has been studied in renal transplant patients receiving different cyclosporine formulations. Low drug exposure, more than high drug exposure, predisposed patients to acute rejection episodes.[49,50] Even greater pharmacokinetic differences were observed in four independent blinded crossover studies in which maintenance renal transplant immunosuppression was alternated between the Neoral microemulsion and the corn oil–based (conventional) Sandimmune formulations.[51-54] The trials showed that absorption was lower, area-under-the-curve values were lower, and the incidence of nephrotoxicity was higher with the conventional Sandimmune formulations.[51-54]

The potential adverse impact of substituting generic drugs is now well recognized. Currently, the FDA requires the demonstration of bioequivalence of generic drugs to proprietary drugs in healthy subjects. The consensus report of the American Society of Transplantation's Conference on Immunosuppressive Drugs and the Use of Generic Immunosuppressants, though supporting the availability of efficacious, less expensive generic cyclosporine, stated that caution should be exercised with its use in potentially at-risk populations, especially African Americans and pediatric patients.[55] Transplant physicians should institute appropriate monitoring whenever therapy is switched between generic formulations and proprietary drugs. The National Kidney Foundation White Paper also recommends that patients be well informed about generic substitutes so that they can participate in treatment choices.[56] Based on our own experience with these generic drugs, they were not equivalent. We advise against their use in our institution.

Pearls and Pitfalls

- A striking improvement in the results of liver transplantation was made in 1978 when cyclosporine was introduced into immunosuppressive protocols.

- Nephrotoxicity remains the most important adverse side effect.

- Generic substitution of the drug should be undertaken with caution, especially in high-risk patients such as children and African Americans.

Tacrolimus (FK506)

Tacrolimus (Prograf) is a macrolide compound with potent immunosuppressive properties that was isolated from *Streptomyces tsukubaensis*.[57] In the laboratory, tacrolimus inhibits the mixed-lymphocyte reaction, the formation of IL-2 by T lymphocytes, and the formation of other soluble mediators, including IL-3 and interferon-γ. As an immunosuppressive agent, tacrolimus is approximately 100 times more potent than cyclopsorine.[6,58-61] Oral availability of tacrolimus ranges from 5% to 67%, with a mean value of 27%.[62] An oral dose of 0.15 mg/kg results in peak plasma concentrations of 0.4 to 3.7 ng/mL. Like cyclosporine, tacrolimus is primarily metabolized in the liver through the cytochrome P450 system. It has a high volume of distribution and is not dialyzable.

Starzl and colleagues in 1989 first reported the successful use of tacrolimus in rescue therapy for liver allografts failing conventional therapy.[6] Subsequently, several investigators evaluated tacrolimus in liver transplant recipients. The U.S. multicenter trial, which randomized 478 patients to receive either tacrolimus- or cyclosporine-based immunosuppression, showed that tacrolimus was associated with significantly fewer episodes of acute, corticosteroid-resistant, or refractory rejection.[7] The European multicenter trial also showed similar findings, in addition to a lower incidence of chronic rejection and infection.[63] However, in both trials, tacrolimus was associated with a higher incidence of adverse effects. Long-term follow-up of patients receiving tacrolimus-based immunosuppression showed that tacrolimus was safe and effective for long-term maintenance immunosuppression with a low incidence of late acute rejection, chronic rejection, and de novo malignancies.[64,65] Tacrolimus was also well tolerated by pediatric patients.[65]

The adverse effects of tacrolimus are similar to those of cyclosporine, the most significant being nephrotoxicity and neurotoxicity (see Table 75–3). The neurotoxicity observed in patients treated with tacrolimus ranges from mild symptoms such as headaches, insomnia or somnolence, and tremors to severe symptoms, including incapacitating headaches, dysarthria, obtundation, seizures, and coma. In such patients, it is very important to stop tacrolimus therapy and switch to cyclosporine. Tacrolimus is also known to cause hypertension, but to a lesser extent than cyclosporine does. In addition, the incidence of diabetes mellitus is higher with tacrolimus than with cyclosporine. Other side effects include hyperlipidemia, nausea, diarrhea, abdominal pain, and pruritus. The half-life of cyclosporine (6 to 15 hours) is prolonged to 26 to 74 hours in patients receiving tacrolimus, thus contraindicating simultaneous use of the two drugs in the same patient.[66]

The recommended initial oral dosage of tacrolimus is 0.05 mg/kg every 12 hours. Initial blood levels in liver transplant recipients are maintained between 10 and 15 ng/mL, and later levels of 8 to 10 ng/mL are adequate. In patients receiving a triple-drug regimen, tacrolimus levels of 5 ng/mL are appropriate. Aggressive dosage reduction in the setting of poor liver function or in patients with poor renal function is recommended. Elderly patients and those with preexisting neurological conditions appear to be more susceptible to tacrolimus-associated toxicity.

Pearls and Pitfalls

- Very potent agent, almost 100 times more potent than cyclosporine.
- The most frequently and the principal agent used for maintenance immunosuppression in liver transplantation.
- Nephrotoxicity and neurotoxicity are the main adverse side effects.
- Neurotoxicity can be very subtle and consists of somnolence, headaches, and dysarthria or severe symptoms such as seizures. In such patients, it is very important to stop tacrolimus therapy and switch to cyclosporine.

Sirolimus

Sirolimus (Rapamune) is a macrocyclic triene antibiotic produced by *Streptomyces* species isolated from soil samples collected on Easter Island in 1975.[67,68] Sirolimus was originally developed as an anticandidal and antitumor agent.[69,70] The mechanism of action of sirolimus involves binding to FK-binding protein 25. It inhibits a variety of cytokine-mediated, protein kinase C–triggered, and lymphokine-mediated signal transduction pathways, particularly those triggered by IL-2 or IL-6.[71] The overall effect of these actions is interference with progression of T cells from the G_1 to the S phase of the cell cycle. The primary side effects of sirolimus are reversible: dose-related decrease in platelet counts, less pronounced leukopenia, hyperlipidemia, arthralgia, interstitial pneumonitis, and diarrhea.[72-75] Delayed wound healing has been reported in some patients.[76] There are no reports of nephrotoxicity or neurotoxicity from sirolimus.[72-75] Thus, the main advantage of sirolimus is that it is a potent immunosuppressant without nephrotoxicity or neurotoxicity and, moreover, it is not associated with side effects such as hypertension or induction of diabetes mellitus. Additionally, novel uses for the drug have been identified, especially its use as an antitumor agent in

hepatocellular carcinoma (HCC), and recently, sirolimus-coated coronary stents have shown considerable promise for prevention of neointimal proliferation, restenosis, and associated clinical events in coronary revascularization.[77] It is likely that sirolimus-coated stents or oral sirolimus may be useful in hepatic artery stenosis in liver transplantation. The most important benefit with the use of rapamycin is its renal-sparing ability, thus making this drug an attractive long-term alternative to calcineurin inhibitors as maintenance immunosuppression. Several studies in renal transplant recipients have shown that the use of sirolimus permits early cyclosporine withdrawal and can result in improved kidney function.[74] In a recent report, stable liver transplant recipients with renal dysfunction were converted to a sirolimus-based regimen.[78] Even late conversion appeared to be effective, and improved kidney function was demonstrated as measured by improvement in the glomerular filtration rate.[78] We start with a loading dose of 5 mg orally and continue with a maintenance dose of 2 to 3 mg/day. In the immediate posttransplant period, we try to achieve levels of 10 to 20 ng/dL and, after 3 months, maintain levels of 5 to 10 ng/dL.

Pearls and Pitfalls

- Attractive long-term alternative to calcineurin inhibitors (tacrolimus and cyclosporine) in patients with renal dysfunction as a result of calcineurin toxicity.
- Delays wound healing and should be avoided in patients with nonhealing wound infections.
- The ability of sirolimus to inhibit metastatic tumor growth and angiogenesis in an in vivo mouse model suggests that it may potentially benefit liver transplant recipients with hepatocellular carcinoma.

Antibody Therapies

Polyclonal Antibodies

Antithymocyte globulin (ATG) (Thymoglobulin) and ALG are polyclonal antibody preparations with different degrees of immunoglobulin purity that are produced by immunizing animals with lymphocytes from different sources (Table 75–5).

After immunization of the selected animals, sera are harvested and processed to obtain purified globulin. Processing generally involves extensive adsorption with nonlymphoid cells to remove contaminating

Table 75-5. CHARACTERISTICS OF POLYCLONAL ANTIBODY THERAPIES USED IN TRANSPLANTATION IMMUNOSUPPRESSION

	Thymoglobulin (SangStat)	Atgam
Immunogen	Thymus	Thymus
Species	Rabbit	Equine
Dosage (mg/kg/day)	1.0-1.5	10-30
CD2	+	++
CD3	+	++
CD4	±	+++
CD8	++	++
CD11a	±	++
CD18	+	++
CD28	±	+

Data from references 79-81.

antibodies (e.g., hemolysins), as well as fractionation to obtain the IgG portion of serum that contains the immunosuppressive component. Nevertheless, more than 95% of the final product consists of irrelevant equine or rabbit globulin, and it is estimated that only about 2% of the administered antibodies are specifically reactive with human T lymphocytes.[79]

The two commonly used polyclonal antibodies are shown in Table 75–5. Polyclonal antibody preparations are best administered via a central venous line. A painful chemical phlebitis can be associated with peripheral administration through low-flow veins.

There appear to be at least three mechanisms of action by which polyclonal antibodies exert their immunosuppressive effect. In vivo administration of polyclonal antibodies results in profound lymphopenia. One mechanism is classic complement-mediated cell lysis. The targeted cells include CD2, CD3, CD4, CD8, CD11a, CD25, CD40, and CD54.[79-81] Another likely mechanism of action includes the uptake of opsonized T cells by the reticuloendothelial system. A third mechanism by which polyclonal antibodies could exert immunosuppressive properties is through masking or modulation of essential surface receptors on lymphocytes that remain in the circulation but whose function is blocked. After cessation of lymphocyte therapy, repopulation of peripheral lymphocytes occurs within 3 to 10 days.

The reported incidence and severity of clinical reactions after the administration of polyclonal antibodies have varied with the preparation used. Fever, often in association with significant chills and sometimes diarrhea, develops during the initial infusion in the majority of patients. Intensive evaluation of these first-dose reactions has shown that they correlate with the release of cytokines, including tumor necrosis factor, IL-1, IL-6, and interferon-γ.[82] Thrombocytopenia or anemia of

varying severity, or both, have been reported in up to 30% of patients. These side effects are generally dose related and usually respond to modest dose reduction or stopping the concomitant administration of MMF or azathioprine. Thrombocytopenia mainly occurs from low levels of contaminating antiplatelet antibodies.[83] Less common side effects include nausea, diarrhea, serum sickness, arthralgia, hypotension, dyspnea, seizures, and anaphylaxis. An increased incidence of CMV infection and posttransplant lymphoproliferative disorder has been reported.

ATG has been used for induction and treatment of steroid-resistant acute cellular rejection in liver transplantation. Tchervenkov and associates retrospectively studied 57 liver transplant recipients who received induction with ATG and found a reduced incidence of acute rejection. In addition, in selected patients with renal failure, induction with ATG allowed a delay in the introduction of cyclosporine, thus allowing renal recovery.[84] Eason and colleagues performed a randomized prospective trial comparing induction with ATG and maintenance with tacrolimus and MMF without using steroids and showed that a similar incidence of acute cellular rejection was achieved while avoiding steroids.[85] ATG is administered over a 4-hour period as an intravenous infusion through a central line because infusion through a peripheral line can cause severe phlebitis. The dose is 1.5 mg/kg/day for 10 to 14 days. Before the first two doses, premedication with 1 g hydrocortisone, 25 mg diphenhydramine, and 650 mg acetaminophen should be administered to prevent cytokine release syndrome. Dose reduction by 50% is recommended when the white cell count drops to between 2000 and 3000 cells/mL or the platelet count drops to 50,000 to 75,000 cells/mL. Withholding the dose is recommended if the platelet count is less than 50,000 cells/mL or the white cell count is less than 2000 cells/mL. All patients receiving ATG should also receive CMV prophylaxis.

Pearls and Pitfalls

- Very potent polyclonal antibody, useful for steroid-resistant rejection.
- Thrombocytopenia and leukopenia are common dose-related side effects.

Monoclonal Antibodies

The production of monoclonal antibodies is based on two well-established observations. First, each B lymphocyte and its expanded clone produce a single specific antibody in an immunized animal. However, they have a very short life span when cultured ex vivo. Second, malignant myeloma cells can be grown permanently in culture but produce antibodies with no predefined specificity. The key breakthrough in monoclonal antibody technology occurred in 1975 when Kohler and Milstein succeeded in fusing these two cell types, thus combining the essential properties of specific antibody secretion and permanent cell growth.[86]

Muromonab-CD3 (Orthoclone OKT3) is the most frequently used monoclonal antibody in liver transplantation. More recent refinements have led to the development of humanized monoclonal antibodies,[87] and basiliximab and daclizumab are the commonly used humanized monoclonal antibodies in liver transplantation. Humanized antibodies have been developed in an attempt to overcome the human antimouse response observed in most patients receiving monoclonal antibodies of murine origin. These human antimouse antibodies cause rapid clearance of the murine antibody from the recipient's circulation, thereby reducing therapeutic efficacy and possibly precluding sequential courses of murine antibody. Furthermore, humanized monoclonal antibodies are less likely to induce the cytokine release syndrome, and the effective half-life of the administered agent is greatly prolonged in the circulation of recipients.[87-90]

Orthoclone OKT3

Muromonab-CD3 was the first monoclonal antibody approved for use in solid-organ transplantation. It is most frequently used for the treatment of steroid-resistant rejection, rejection prophylaxis in special situations, and induction therapy in the posttransplant period.[91] OKT3 is directed against the CD3-antigen complex found on all mature human T cells.[92] It is a highly effective, yet potentially toxic, drug. OKT3 binds to one of the 20-kD subunits of the CD3 complex, an intrinsic part of the T-cell receptor. Subsequent deactivation of the CD3 complex causes the T-cell receptor to undergo endocytosis and be lost from the cell surface. The T cells become ineffectual, and within an hour, they become opsonized and are removed from the circulation into the reticuloendothelial system. OKT3 also blocks the function of killer T cells in the allograft, which have an important role in generating the rejection response.[92]

The standard dose of OKT3 is 5 mg given as an intravenous bolus. The standard course consists of a daily dose of 5 mg for 10 to 14 days. Administration of OKT3 is nearly always accompanied by a cytokine release syndrome characterized by symptoms such as fever, dyspnea, nausea, vomiting, chest pain, diarrhea, tremor, wheezing, headache, tachycardia, chills, and

hypertension.[93] This flu-like syndrome, termed the cytokine release syndrome, occurs most notably during the initial two to three doses of OKT3. In general, the onset of cytokine release syndrome occurs within 1 hour of drug administration, and it usually resolves in 4 to 6 hours; cessation of muromonab-CD3 is not generally required. The incidence and severity of the symptom complex may be variably affected by changes in the infusion rate or dose, by pretreatment with antipyretics or steroids, or by histamine receptor blockade. However, no strategy has been successful in totally preventing the syndrome. One of the most serious side effects, pulmonary edema, may be prevented by patient diuresis before drug administration and the demonstration of no preexisting pulmonary edema or pleural effusions on chest radiographs taken within 24 hours before injection. It is recommended that the patient be premedicated with 1 g hydrocortisone, 25 mg diphenhydramine, and 650 mg acetaminophen. After the first dose, only diphenhydramine (25 mg) and acetaminophen (650 mg) are used for premedication. Other reported complications include headache, aseptic meningitis, increased incidence of infections such as Epstein-Barr virus and CMV infection, and posttransplant lymphoproliferative disorder. If aseptic meningitis or diarrhea develops, premedication with 100 mg of hydrocortisone before each OKT3 infusion is highly effective.

Recently, the use of OKT3 has been associated with an increased risk for recurrent hepatitis C in patients transplanted for hepatitis C–related cirrhosis. The effectiveness of OKT3 may need to be monitored during the course of therapy because of the potential for the development of antibodies, which may abrogate its action and allow for the reappearance of potent CD3-positive T cells. Antibodies may be directed against the antibody itself (anti-idiopathic), against the IgG protein subclass (anti-isotypic), and against the mouse protein of origin (antimurine). During the effective course of OKT3, the percentage of CD3-positive T cells falls precipitously within 24 to 48 hours from approximately 60% to less than 5%. Failure of the CD3-positive percentage to fall or a fall followed by a rapid rise indicates the appearance of blocking antibodies. Monitoring the absolute lymphocyte count is recommended in all patients undergoing OKT3 treatment. In patients who have a rise in the absolute lymphocyte count of more than 500 cells/mL, monitoring to ensure that the CD3 count remains under 300 cells/mL is recommended. If the absolute lymphocyte count increases to more than 500 cells/mL, we double the OKT3 dose to 10 mg/day, which seems to effectively overwhelm the developing neutralizing antibodies and maintain the immunosuppressive effect. We usually also see a fall in lymphocyte counts.

Interleukin-2 Inhibitors

Basiliximab (Simulect) and daclizumab (Zenapax) are chimeric monoclonal antibodies, a new class of recently introduced medications that inhibit IL-2 receptors (IL-2Rs) and thereby affect T-cell activation. The chimeric structure of the antibodies has both prolonged the half-life and reduced the immunogenicity of these compounds.[87,88]

Basiliximab is produced from a genetic construct of variable regions of a murine anti-CD25 monoclonal antibody (RTF5) and constant regions of human IgG1 heavy and κ light chains.[94] Basiliximab binds to the alpha chain of IL-2R with an affinity approximating that of IL-2 itself and, therefore, is a potent inhibitor of IL-2–mediated T-cell proliferation. Resting T cells, which do not express IL-2Rα, are not affected. Early clinical studies have shown that basiliximab is well tolerated, with no evidence of significant toxicity. The optimal dose of basiliximab is 20 mg intravenously the day of transplantation, followed by a second dose on day 4 after transplantation.[94-97] Administered in accordance with this schedule, basiliximab achieves consistent suppression of CD25 for a period of 30 to 45 days.[95] A multicenter study evaluating the safety and efficacy of basiliximab in 101 liver transplant recipients showed that the use of basiliximab was safe, without injection site reactions, anaphylaxis, or cytokine release syndrome. When compared with historical controls, this study also showed that adding basiliximab to triple-immunosuppressive therapy reduces the incidence of acute rejection episodes with no clinically significant increase in adverse effects.[97]

Daclizumab is very similar to basiliximab. The clinical difference between the two IL-2 inhibitors is that basiliximab has higher affinity for the receptor than daclizumab does. Analysis of the safety and pharmacodynamics of daclizumab in 28 liver transplant recipients showed that a two-dose regimen of 1 mg/kg within 6 hours of transplantation, followed by a second dose of 0.5 mg/kg on day 4, provided effective blockade of IL-2Rα for at least 14 days after transplantation. No major clinical side effects such as cytokine release syndrome, neurotoxicity, or nephrotoxicity were reported in the study.[98] However, Roche Pharmaceuticals (in a personal communication) recently reported that severe acute anaphylaxis has been observed on both initial exposure and re-exposure to daclizumab.[99] Based on unpublished pharmacokinetic data, dramatic shortening of the half-life and Cmax occurs in liver transplant patients (Roche Pharmaceuticals); we have therefore used higher dosing of daclizumab (2 mg/kg on day 1, 2 mg/kg on day 3, and 1 mg/kg on day 8 after transplantation). We believe that this change in pharmacokinetics is due to loss of the drug in blood and fluid, which occurs routinely in post–liver transplant patients. Preliminary data with such dosing have been excellent.

The main advantage of basiliximab and daclizumab is their ability to provide effective immunosuppression without clinical side effects such as cytokine release syndrome, neurotoxicity, or nephrotoxicity. Daclizumab may be a very useful agent in a liver recipient who has renal dysfunction, is taking pressors, and will not tolerate OKT3 induction and cytokine release syndrome. Daclizumab, MMF, and steroids can be successfully used as initial immunosuppression in liver transplant recipients with impaired renal function.[100] However, after 7 to 8 days, as renal function improves, calcineurin inhibitors should be introduced; otherwise, there may be a risk of incurring acute rejection and steroid-resistant acute rejection.[101]

Developing Therapeutic Strategies to Maximize Outcomes in Special Populations or Conditions

The cardinal challenge for clinicians is to define optimal therapeutic strategies for using the recently broadened range of immunotherapeutic agents. The ideal protocol should effectively prevent rejection and minimize side effects. Although it is difficult to predict how an individual will react to a particular drug, we can reasonably predict how a group of patients would react to a specific group of drugs. Patients who have a higher immunological response need more intensive immunosuppression to optimize outcome. Other patients are at higher risk for recurrent disease. Patients with specific comorbid conditions (such as acute renal failure, hepatorenal syndrome, acute tubular necrosis, hepatic encephalopathy, and others) are more susceptible to toxic drug effects and may be permanently debilitated if subjected to particular drugs immediately after transplantation (Table 75–6). The side effect profile of the individual drugs must also be considered.

Experienced clinical transplant teams, by combining data from clinical trials and their own experience, have developed protocols for incorporating the newer medications with the established ones for tailoring treatments to individual requirements. Examples of protocols provided in this text have been developed by clinicians at Baylor University Medical Center (Dallas) in 1992. The protocols were developed to achieve the following goals: (1) prevention of acute cellular rejection, (2) avoidance of drug toxicity, (3) prevention of exacerbation of existing morbidity, and (4) minimization of medication side effects. These protocols have been implemented and are familiar to and easily followed by transplant fellows, coordinators, and hospital personnel. The protocols should be considered guidelines; individual patients may have idiosyncratic reactions to specific agents and may need individual changes in any particular protocol.

Recipient Groups

Acute Oliguric/Prerenal Failure

Renal dysfunction after liver transplantation decreases patient and graft survival.[102] Patients who have preoperative renal dysfunction or hepatorenal syndrome are more likely to experience renal dysfunction.[102] A study of 834 patients indicated that 1-mg/dL increases in serum creatinine above baseline at 4 weeks, 3 months, and 1 year were independent risk factors for the development of chronic renal failure and end-stage renal disease.[102] Thus, effort should be undertaken to normalize renal function as quickly as possible after liver transplantation. Furthermore, patients with hepatorenal syndrome have abnormal renal vasoconstriction, which could be aggravated by the early addition of calcineurin inhibitors, drugs that cause vasoconstriction.[103,104] Thus, it is not hard to speculate that renal failure would develop in patients who have reduced kidney function at the time of transplantation and are then treated with calcineurin inhibitors. Various strategies have been used to minimize renal dysfunction in this group of patients. One approach is to use MMF and corticosteroids only and avoid tacrolimus for up to 72 to 96 hours after transplantation in patients with acute oliguric and pretransplant renal failure (see Table 75–6). In the protocol, if renal function improves, low-dose tacrolimus (levels at 5 ng/dL) is begun along with the maximum tolerated MMF dose to minimize nephrotoxicity.[105] MMF monotherapy is associated with serious acute rejection.[106] If renal function does not improve, we begin OKT3 for 2 weeks. In patients who were receiving renal replacement therapy before transplantation, immunosuppression is initiated with OKT3 and MMF; as kidney function improves, we introduce tacrolimus.

We have increasingly used sirolimus in this group of patients after OKT3 therapy is discontinued but have yet to incorporate this drug into our standard protocols.

Pearls and Pitfalls

- Tacrolimus and cyclosporine can be safely withheld for 48 to 72 hours after liver transplantation in a patient with acute renal failure to help in recovery of renal function. MMF and corticosteroids are adequate immunosuppression for this period.

- Sirolimus does not cause nephrotoxicity and is increasingly being used in renal-sparing protocols as a replacement for calcineurin inhibitors.

Fulminant Hepatic Failure

Patients transplanted for fulminant hepatic failure (FHF) can have varied causes of liver failure, such as a drug (acetaminophen overdose) or viral cause; in addition, they are younger, have severe encephalopathy (to meet the requirements for transplantation), and have poor preoperative renal function.[107-111] In the early posttransplant period, this group of patients has poor tolerance of agents with neurotoxic or nephrotoxic side effects. Both tacrolimus and cyclosporine are

Table 75-6. BAYLOR UNIVERSITY MEDICAL CENTER LIVER TRANSPLANTATION IMMUNOSUPPRESSION PROTOCOLS

	Standard	Autoimmune Hepatitis	Viral Hepatitis (B and C)	Acute Oliguric Renal Failure	Fulminant Hepatic Failure	Hepatoma
Tacrolimus or cyclosporine	Tacrolimus, 0.05 mg/kg PO bid Level: Week 1–2: 15 ng/dL (Elderly > 60 yr: 5–10 ng/dL) Week 3 to mo 3: 8–12 ng/dL > 3 mo: 5–10 ng/dL	Tacrolimus, 0.05 mg/kg PO bid Level: Week 1–2: 10–20 ng/dL (Elderly > 60 yr: 5–10 ng/dL) Week 3 to mo 3: 10–15 ng/dL > 3 mo: 5–10 ng/dL	Tacrolimus, 0.05 mg/kg PO bid Level: Week 1–2: 10–15 ng/dL Week 3 to mo 3: 8–12 ng/dL > 3 mo: 3–5 ng/dL	No tacrolimus for up to 72–96 hr until UOP > 50–100 mL/hr. If still oliguric, begin OKT3, 5 mg IV qd for 5–10 days. Begin tacrolimus when UOP > 100 mL/hr using routine doses/level	OKT3, 5 mg IV qd for 5–10 days; when awake begin tacrolimus at routine doses/level	Neoral, 5 mg/kg PO bid Level: 150–200
3rd Agent MMF or sirolimus	None	Sirolimus, 5 mg PO qd and levels 5–10	MMF, 1500 mg PO bid	MMF, 1000 mg PO bid for 7 days	MMF, 1000 mg PO bid for 7 days	Sirolimus, 5 mg PO qd and levels 5–10
Steroids	Preop: 40 mg IV	Preop: 40 mg IV	Preop: 40 mg IV	Preop: 40 mg IV	Preop: 40 mg IV	Preop: 40 mg IV
	Intraop: 1 g methylprednisolone (SM)	Intraop: 1 g methylprednisolone (SM)	Intraop: 1 g methylprednisolone (SM)	Intraop: 1 g methylprednisolone (SM)	Intraop: 1 g methylprednisolone (SM)	Intraop: 1 g methylprednisolone (SM)
	Postop:	Postop:	Postop:	Postop:	Postop:	Postop:
	100 mg day1	100 mg day1	100 mg day1	100 mg day1	100 mg day1	100 mg day1
	80 mg day 2	80 mg day 2	80 mg day 2	80 mg day 2	80 mg day 2	80 mg day 2
	60 mg day 3	60 mg day 3	60 mg day 3	60 mg day 3	60 mg day 3	60 mg day 3
	40 mg day 4	40 mg day 4	40 mg day 4	40 mg day 4	40 mg day 4	40 mg day 4
	Prednisolone PO	Prednisolone PO	Prednisolone PO	Prednisolone PO	Prednisolone PO	Prednisolone PO
	20 mg day 5	20 mg day 5	20 mg day 5	20 mg day 5	20 mg day 5	20 mg day 5
	15 mg day 14	15 mg day 90	15 mg day 6	15 mg day 14	15 mg day 14	15 mg day 14
	12.5 mg day 21	10 mg day 180	10 mg day 7	12.5 mg day 21	12.5 mg day 21	12.5 mg day 21
	10 mg day 28	7.5 mg day 270	5 mg day 14	10 mg day 28	10 mg day 28	10 mg day 28
	7.5 mg day 60	5 mg day 360	2.5 mg day 30	7.5 mg day 60	7.5 mg day 60	7.5 mg day 60
	5 mg day 90	Do not d/c steroids	d/c day 60	5 mg day 90	5 mg day 90	5 mg day 90
	2.5 mg day 360			2.5 mg day 360	2.5 mg day 360	2.5 mg day 360
	2.5 mg qod day 390			2.5 mg qod day 390	2.5 mg qod day 390	2.5 mg qod day 390
	d/c day 420			d/c day 420	d/c day 420	d/c day 420

d/c, discontinue; MMF, mycophenolate mofetil; SM, methylprednisolone (Solumedrol); UOP, urinary output.

neurotoxic and best avoided until the encephalopathy has cleared. It is impossible to assess drug neurotoxicity in comatose patients. In addition, this group of patients may have some renal impairment at the time of transplantation, and thus avoidance of nephrotoxicity from calcineurin inhibitors may be desirable. For these reasons, use of antibody therapy (such as OKT3) for induction may be beneficial (see Table 75–6). Calcineurin inhibitors are introduced at a low dose only after the patient is awake and can answer questions. Usually at that time, renal function is also improved.

Patients with FHF have a significantly higher incidence of acute rejection (84% versus 56%).[111,112] The incidence of steroid-resistant rejection is also higher (8.7% versus 4.5%) than in patients transplanted electively.[112] Among FHF patients, the European multicenter trial demonstrated that tacrolimus reduces the incidence of acute rejection when compared with cyclosporine treatment. Patients treated with tacrolimus also tended to have a lower incidence of infection.[112] After the immediate postoperative period, no significant differences in adverse events attributable to the immunosuppressive drugs were found in FHF patients when compared with those who were transplanted electively.[112] Thus, we use three drugs (tacrolimus, MMF, and steroids) for maintenance immunosuppression to provide a higher level of immunosuppression (see Table 75–6).

Pearls and Pitfalls

- Both tacrolimus and cyclosporine are best avoided until encephalopathy is cleared. Antibody induction may be beneficial in this group of patients.
- Patients with FHF experience a significantly higher incidence of acute rejection and will require higher doses of maintenance immunosuppression.

Viral Hepatitis

Liver disease from hepatitis C is emerging as the most common indication for liver transplantation.[113] The rate of histological recurrence of hepatitis C after transplantation varies from 40% to 60%, and viremia is almost universal (75% to 95%).[114-120] Several studies have been performed to identify risk factors for recurrence. There is a strong correlation between the number of rejection episodes, exposure to corticosteroids, and histological recurrence of hepatitis C.[121] Data from the National Institute of Diabetes and Digestive and Kidney Diseases have also shown that greater average daily

steroid dosages were independently associated with increased mortality and graft loss in these patients.[122] Thus, it appears that decreasing steroid exposure in this group of patients may reduce the incidence of recurrence. Protocols such as the one provided in this text, including an early taper of steroids, may be beneficial in patients with hepatitis C (see Table 75–6). Additionally, a lower dose of steroids is recommended for treating acute cellular rejection.

Data summarizing the effect of different types of immunosuppression on the outcome of posttransplant infection have been conflicting.[120-124] However, tacrolimus-based double therapy was found to be associated with a lower incidence of acute rejection and steroid-resistant rejection and better survival than cyclosporine-based triple therapy was.[125-128]

The antiviral properties of MMF remain controversial. Data from some centers have not shown a significant benefit of MMF in decreasing recurrence of hepatitis C.[129,130] However, recent data have shown that use of continuous high-dose MMF (>1.5 g/day) is associated with a lower incidence of recurrence and progression of recurrent disease. HCV RNA levels and the incidence of fibrosis were significantly lower in the MMF group, thus suggesting that MMF may have clinically relevant antiviral activity.[30,31] Thus, incorporation of MMF into the immunosuppression regimen for patients with hepatitis C seems prudent and may be beneficial in an effort to avoid the use of steroids in this group (see Table 75–6). Several studies are now under way to provide a more definitive answer to the question of optimal immunosuppression for liver recipients with hepatitis C.

Pearls and Pitfalls

- There is a strong correlation between the number of rejection episodes, exposure to corticosteroids, and histological recurrence of hepatitis C.
- Early taper of steroids and lower doses of steroids may be beneficial in patients with hepatitis C.
- Higher-dose MMF (1500 mg orally twice daily) may have antiviral activity against hepatitis C.

Malignancies

According to the International Registry of Hepatic Tumors in Liver Transplantation, half the posttransplant morbidity is caused by recurrent HCC.[131] One reason for the high recurrence rate in posttransplant patients is immunosuppression.[132] Furthermore, this group of patients does not have an increased incidence of rejection or comorbid conditions such as nephrotoxicity or neurotoxicity.

Experimental data suggest that sirolimus may reduce the risk of cancer development while simultaneously providing effective immunosuppression. Sirolimus has been shown to inhibit the growth of human hepatoma cell lines by up to 74% at a low concentration of 5 ng/dL when compared with controls. This low concentration is a clinically attainable serum level in view of the daily dose of 2 to 5 mg.[133] Tumor inhibition is achieved either by cell cycle arrest or by induction of apoptosis, whereas tacrolimus was shown to stimulate the growth of cancer cells.[134-138] Sirolimus has also been found to inhibit tumor angiogenesis in a mouse model.[139]

Cyclosporine may likewise have protective benefits in patients with a history of HCC. Studies using HCC cell lines to characterize the in vitro chemomodulatory properties of cyclosporine have shown that cyclosporine, at levels found in the plasma of post-transplant patients, enhances doxorubicin cytotoxicity in MDR1+ human hepatoma cells.[140,141] These findings support the use of cyclosporine in recipients with HCC. Thus, a combination of sirolimus and cyclosporine in patients transplanted for HCC may be beneficial (see Table 75–6).

Pearls and Pitfalls

- Immunosuppression is an important cause of the high recurrence rate of tumors after transplantation.
- Sirolimus has been shown to inhibit the growth of hepatoma cells in in vitro studies and inhibit tumor angiogenesis in in vivo animal models and thus has potential benefit in liver transplant recipients with HCC.

Autoimmune Liver Disease

Patients who undergo transplantation for autoimmune liver disease have an increased incidence of rejection.[142] A report by Klintmalm and colleagues of 45 patients monitored for a median of 2.4 years (range, 1 to 11 years) showed that patients with autoimmune hepatitis experienced more rejection (80% versus 60%) than controls did with no increase in the incidence of steroid-resistant rejection requiring antibody therapy.[143] Several other studies have also demonstrated that patients transplanted for autoimmune hepatitis

have a higher incidence of rejection, as high as 83%.[144-146] The incidence of moderate or severe rejection episodes requiring antibody therapy is likewise high.[147,148] Tacrolimus therapy is associated with a lower incidence of rejection in this group and has also been reported to be a potential treatment of autoimmune chronic hepatitis.[147,148] As a group, these patients have not demonstrated a higher incidence of nephrotoxicity, neurotoxicity, or sepsis. Thus, it appears that the use of tacrolimus at higher levels, steroids, and a third agent (MMF or sirolimus) in this group of patients would be beneficial (see Table 75–6).

It may be prudent to maintain patients with autoimmune liver disease on higher doses of steroids in the first year, primarily because the incidence of acute cellular rejection is higher during this period.[143] Recurrence of autoimmune liver disease is also common in the first year after transplantation.[142,143,149,150] Although some transplantation protocols have called for reducing steroid dosages during the first posttransplant year, there are reports of recurrent disease in many patients.[142,143,151,152] However, some programs in which patients have been maintained on steroids have indicated a low rate of recurrent disease.[143] Therefore, maintaining patients on a 5-mg/day steroid regimen indefinitely may have beneficial effects (see Table 75–6). Because patients with primary biliary cirrhosis and primary sclerosing cholangitis also have a possible autoimmune cause with a recognized recurrence rate of 15%, it may be prudent to treat them similar to patients with autoimmune hepatitis.[153,154]

Pearls and Pitfalls

- Recipients with autoimmune liver disease have an increased incidence of acute rejection.
- Use of tacrolimus at higher levels, steroids, and a third agent (MMF or sirolimus) in this group would be beneficial.
- Recurrence of autoimmune disease in the allograft may be reduced by maintaining this group of patients on steroids (5 mg) indefinitely.

Elderly Patients

Previous studies have shown that elderly recipients (>60 years of age), especially those hospitalized before transplantation, have poor graft and patient survival when compared with younger recipients.[155-157] The causes of mortality in elderly patients after liver transplantation are unrelated to transplantation. They typically do not lose their liver allografts to rejection.[156] Elderly recipients also have a higher incidence of posttransplant renal failure and neurological complications and infections.[157] However, the incidence of acute rejection in this group is lower that in younger transplant recipients (<60 years).[157] In patients older than 60 years, it may be beneficial to use two drugs for immunosuppression and maintain lower levels of tacrolimus with the aim of minimizing nephrotoxicity and neurotoxicity without increasing the risk for acute rejection (see Table 75–6). Avoidance of MMF, which is known to increase the incidence of infectious complications after transplantation, may also be desirable.[29]

Pearls and Pitfalls

- Elderly patients have a lower incidence of rejection and a higher incidence of neurological complications and infection. Maintain lower levels of immunosuppression (tacrolimus levels of 5 to 8 ng/dL).

Conclusions

The quest for the perfect immunosuppression for liver transplant recipients continues. Although several potent agents are available, the existing drugs continue to have serious toxicities, the most important of which are nephrotoxicity, neurotoxicity, bone marrow suppression, and gastrointestinal side effects. The growth of liver transplantation over the last 20 years has allowed clinicians to identify groups of patients with particular immune responsiveness and comorbid conditions related to specific disease states and conditions. Such identification, together with the expanded cache of therapeutic agents, has resulted in the development of regimens specific to a patient's condition, as well as reduced rates of rejection, increased graft and patient survival, and fewer comorbid conditions than ever before. However, the quest for further improvement in long-term graft and patient survival and continued improvement in rates of comorbidity will, it is hoped, stimulate researchers and pharmaceutical companies to continue developing products for these patients.

References

1. URREA, UNOS: 2002 Annual Report of the U.S. Organ Procurement and Transplantation Network and the Scientific Registry of Transplant Recipients: Transplant Data 1992-2001 [Internet]. Rockville, MD, HHS/HRSA/OSP/DOT, 2003 [modified 2003 Feb 18; cited 2003 Nov 4]. Available from http://www.optn.org/data/annualReport.asp.

2. Starzl TE, Maarchioro TL, Waddell WR: The reversal of rejection in human renal homografts with subsequent development of homograft tolerance. Surg Gynecol Obstet 117:385, 1963.

3. Starzl TE, Groth CG, Brettschneider L, et al: Orthotopic homotransplantation of the human liver. Ann Surg 168:392-415, 1968.

4. Borel JF, Feurer C, Gulber HU, Stahelin H: Biological effects of cyclosporine A: A new lymphocyte agent. Agents Actions 6:486, 1976.

5. Calne RY, White DJG, Thiru S, et al: Cyclosporine A in patients receiving renal allografts from cadaver donors. Lancet 2:1323-1327, 1978.

6. Starzl TE, Todo S, Fung J, et al: FK 506 for liver, kidney, and pancreas transplantation. Lancet 2:1000-1004, 1989.

7. A comparison of tacrolimus (FK 506) and cyclosporine for immunosuppression in liver transplantation: The U.S. Multicenter FK506 Liver Study Group. N Engl J Med 331:1110-1115, 1994.

8. Valente JI, Wesley JA: Immunobiology of renal transplantation. Surg Clin North Am 78:1-26, 1998.

9. Hayes JM: The immunobiology and clinical use of current immunosuppressive therapy for renal transplantation. J Urol 149:437-448, 1993.

10. Hayes RC Jr: Adrenocorticotropic hormone, adrenocortical steroids and their synthetic analogs inhibitors of the synthesis and actions of adrenocortical hormones. In Gilman AG, Rall TW, Nies AS, Taylor P (eds): Goodman and Gilman's The Pharmacological Basis of Therapeutics, 8th ed. New York, Pergamon Press, 1990, p 1431.

11. Jeng S, Chanchairujira T, Jusko W, Steiner R: Prednisone metabolism in recipients of kidney or liver transplants and in lung recipients receiving ketoconazole. Transplantation 75:792-795, 2003.

12. American Society of Hospital Pharmacists: AHFS Drug Information 93. Bethesda, MD, American Society of Hospital Pharmacists, 1993.

13. Rossi SJ, Schroeder TJ, Hariharan S, First MR: Prevention and management of the adverse effects associated with immunosuppressive therapy. Drug Saf 9:104-131, 1993.

14. Blohme I, Brynger H: Malignant disease in renal transplant patients. Transplantation 39:23-25, 1985.

15. Platz KP, Sollinger HW, Hullett DA, et al: RS-61443, a new potent immunosuppressive agent. Transplantation 51:27-31, 1991.

16. Sollinger HW, Eugi EM, Allison AC: RS-61443: Mechanism of action, experimental and early clinical results. Clin Transplant 5(Suppl):523-526, 1991.

17. Allison AC, Eugui EM, Sollinger HW: Mycophenolate mofetil (RS61443): Mechanism of action and effects in transplantation. Transplant Rev 7:129-139, 1993.

18. Neyts J, Meerbach A, McKenna P, De Clercq E: Use of yellow fever virus vaccine strain 17D for the study of strategies for the treatment of yellow fever virus infections. Antiviral Res 30:125-132, 1996.

19. Neyts J, Andrei G, De Clercq E: The antiherpes virus activity of H2G[(R)-9-[4-hydroxy-2-(hydroxymethyl) butyl] guanine] is markedly enhanced by the novel immunosuppressive agent mycophenolate mofetil. Antimicrob Agents Chemother 42:3285-3289, 1998.

20. Sollinger HW, Deierhoi MH, Belzer FO, et al: RS-61433: Phase I clinical trial and pilot rescue study. Transplantation 53:428-432, 1992.

21. Deierhoi MH, Sollinger HW, Diethelm AG, et al: One-year follow-up results of phase I trial of mycophenolate mofetil (RS-61443) in cadaveric renal transplantation. Transplant Proc 25:693-694, 1993.

22. Gabradi S, Tran JL, Clarkson MR: Enteric-coated mycophenolate sodium. Ann Pharmacother 37:1685-1693, 2003.

23. Granger DK: Enteric coated mycophenolate sodium: Results of two pivotal global multicenter trials. Transplant Proc 33:341-344, 2001.

24. Klintmalm GB, Ascher NL, Busuttil RW, et al: RS 61443 for treatment-resistant human liver rejection. Transplant Proc 25:697, 1993.

25. Freise CE, Herbert M, Osorio RW, et al: Maintenance immunosuppression with predinsone and RS-61443 alone following liver transplantation. Transplant Proc 25:1758-1759, 1993.
26. Eckoff DE, McGuire BM, Frenette LR, et al: Tacrolimus (FK 506) and mycophenolate mofetil combination therapy versus tacrolimus in adult liver transplantation. Transplantation 65:180-187, 1998.
27. Paterson DL, Singh N, Panebiano A, et al: Infectious complications occurring in liver transplant recipients receiving mycophenolate mofetil. Transplantation 65:180-187, 1998.
28. Stegall MD, Wachs ME, Everson G, et al: Prednisone withdrawal 14 days after liver transplantation with mycophenolate. Transplantation 64:1755-1760, 1997.
29. Jain A, Kashyap R, Dodson F, et al: A prospective randomized trial of tacrolimus and prednisone versus tacrolimus, prednisone and mycophenolate mofetil in primary adult liver transplantation: A single center report. Transplantation 72:1091-1097, 2001.
30. Fasola CG, Netto GJ, Jennings LW, et al: Recurrence of hepatitis C in liver transplant recipients treated with mycophenolate mofetil. Transplant Proc 34:1563-1564, 2002.
31. Fasola CG, Netto GJ, Christensen LL, et al: Delay of hepatitis C recurrence in liver transplant recipients: Impact of mycophenolate mofetil on transplant recipients with severe acute rejection or with renal dysfunction. Transplant Proc 34:1561-1562, 2002.
32. Chong ASF, Lui W, Shen J, et al: In vitro activity of leflunomide: Pharmacokinetics, analyses and mechanism of immunosuppression. Transplantation 52:527, 1999.
33. Williams JW, Xiao F, Foster P, et al: Leflunomide in experimental transplantation: Control of rejection and alloantibody production, reversal of acute rejection and interaction with cyclosporine. Transplantation 57:1223, 1994.
34. Foster PF, Xiao F, Kociss K, et al: Leflunomide immunosuppression in rat small intestinal transplantation. Transplant Proc 26:1599, 1994.
35. Morris RE, Huang X, Cao W, et al: Leflunomide (HWA 486) and its analog suppress T and B cell proliferation in vitro, acute rejection, ongoing rejection and antidonor antibody synthesis in mouse, rat, and cynomolgus monkey transplant recipients as well as arterial intimal thickening after balloon catheter injury. Transplant Proc 27:445, 1995.
36. Ostraat O, Qi ZQ, Tufveson G, et al: The effects of leflunomide and cyclosporin A on rejection of cardiac allografts in the rat. Scand J Immunol 47:828, 1998.
37. Waldman WJ, Knight DA, Lurain NS, et al: Novel mechanism of inhibition of human cytomegalovirus by the experimental immunosuppressive agent, leflunomide. Transplantation 68:814, 1999.
38. Waldman WJ, Knight DA, Blinder L, et al: Inhibition of cytomegalovirus in vitro and in vivo by the experimental immunosuppressive agent leflunomide. Intervirology 42:412, 1999.
39. Williams JW, Mital D, Chong A, et al: Experiences with leflunomide in solid organ transplantation. Transplantation 73:358-366, 2002.
40. Jarrell BE, Moritz MJ, Radomski J: Cyclosporine. In Maddrey WC (ed): Transplantation of the Liver. New York, Elsevier, 1988, p 249.
41. Starzl TE, Klintmalm GB, Porter KA, et al: Liver transplantation with use of cyclosporine A and prednisone. N Engl J Med 305:266-269, 1981.
42. Rossi SJ, Schroeder TJ, Hariharan S, First MR: Prevention and management of the adverse effects associated with immunosuppressive therapy. Drug Saf 9:104, 1993.
43. Lake KD: Cyclosporine drug interactions: A review. Cardiac Surg 2:617, 1988.
44. Lopez-Gil JA: Fluconazole-cyclosporine interaction: A dose-dependent effect? Ann Pharmacother 27:427, 1993.
45. Barry JM: Immunosuppressive drugs in renal transplantation. A review of the regimens. Drugs 44:554-566, 1992.
46. Kahan BD: Cyclosporine nephrotoxicity: Pathogenesis, prophylaxis, therapy, and prognosis. Am J Kidney Dis 8:323-331, 1986.
47. McManus R, Ohair D, Schwriger J, et al: Cyclosporine-associated central neurotoxicity after heart transplantation. Ann Thorac Surg 53:326-327, 1992.
48. Pan WL, Chan CP, Huang CC, Lai MK: Cyclosporine-induced gingival overgrowth. Transplant Proc 24:1393-1394, 1992.
49. Kovarik J, Bredenbach T, Gerbeau C, et al: Disposition and immunodynamics of basiliximab in liver allograft recipients. Clin Pharmacol Ther 54:203, 1993.
50. Lindholm A, Welsch M, Rutzky L, Kahan BD: The adverse impact of high cyclosporine clearance rates on the incidences of acute rejection and graft loss. Transplantation 55:985-993, 1993.
51. Kovarik JM, Mueller EA, Van Bree JB, et al: Cyclosporine pharmacokinetic and variability from a microemulsion formulation—a multicenter investigation in kidney transplant patients. Transplantation 58:658-663, 1994.
52. Kahan BD, Dunn J, Fitts C, et al: Reduced inter- and intrasubject variability in cyclosporine pharmacokinetics in renal transplant recipients treated with a microemulsion formulation in conjunction with fasting, low-fat meals or high-fat meals. Transplantation 59:505-511, 1995.
53. Wahlberg J, Wilcezk HE, Fauchald P, et al: Consistent absorption of cyclosporine from a microemulsion formulation assessed in stable renal transplant recipients over a one-year study period. Transplantation 60:648, 1995.
54. Keowen PA: Therapeutic strategies for optimal use of novel immunosuppressants. Transplant Proc 28:2147, 1999.
55. Alloway RR, Issacs R, Lake K, et al: Report of the American Society of Transplantation conference on immunosuppressive drugs and the use of generic immunosuppressants. Am J Transplant 3:1211-1215, 2003.
56. Drug substitution in transplantation: A National Kidney Foundation White Paper. Am J Kidney Dis 33:389-397, 1999.
57. Kino T, Hatanaka H, Miyata S, et al: FK-506, a novel immunosuppressant isolated from a Streptomyces. II. Immunosuppressive effect of FK-506 in vitro. J Antibiot (Tokyo) 40:1256-1265, 1987.
58. Sigal NH, Lin CS, Siekierka JJ: Inhibition of human T cell activation by FK 506, rapamycin, and cyclosporine A. Transplant Proc 23(2 Suppl 2):1-5, 1991.
59. Jiang H, Suguo H, Takahara S, et al: Combined immunosuppressive effect of FK 506 and other immunosuppressive agents on PHA- and CD3-stimulated human lymphocyte proliferation in vitro. Transplant Proc 23:2933-2936, 1991.
60. Chen-Woan M, Zerbe TR, Zeevi A, et al: Diminished lymphocyte growth from endomyocardial biopsies from cardiac transplant patients on FK 506 immunosuppression. Transplant Proc 23:2941-2942, 1991.
61. Kawauchi M, Van Arsdell G, Alonso de Begona J, et al: Flow cytometric analysis of lymphocyte populations in FK 506–treated newborn goats. Transplant Proc 23:2970-2971, 1991.
62. Venkataramanan R, Jain A, Warty VS, et al: Pharmacokinetics of FK 506 in transplant patients. Transplant Proc 23:2736-2740, 1991.
63. Randomised trial comparing tacrolimus (FK506) and cylcosporin in prevention of liver allograft rejection. European FK506 Multicenter Liver Study Group. Lancet 344:423-428, 1994.
64. Wiesner RH: A long term comparison of tacrolimus (FK506) versus cyclosporine in liver transplantation: A report of the United States FK506 Study Group. Transplantation 66:493-499, 1998.
65. Jain A, Reyes J, Kashyap R, et al: What have we learned about primary liver transplantation under tacrolimus immunosuppression? Long-term follow-up of the first 1000 patients. Ann Surg 230:441-448, 1999.
66. Venkataramanan R, Jain A, Cadoff E, et al: Pharmacokinetics of FK 506: Preclinical and clinical studies Transplant Proc 22:52-56, 1990.

67. Vezina C, Kudelski A, Seghal SN: Rapamycin (AY-22,989), a new antifungal antibiotic. I. Taxonomy of the producing streptomycete and isolation of the active principle. J Antibiot (Tokyo) 28:721-726, 1975.

68. Sehgal SN, Baker H, Vezina C: Rapamycin (AY-22,989), a new antifungal antibiotic. II. Fermentation, isolation and characterization. J Antibiot (Tokyo) 28:727-732, 1975.

69. Douros J, Suffness M: New antitumor substances of natural origin. Cancer Treat Rev 8:63-87, 1981.

70. Eng CP, Sehgal SN, Vezina C: Activity of rapamycin (AY-22,989) against transplanted tumors. J Antibiot (Tokyo) 37:1231-1237, 1984.

71. Khan BD: Immunosuppressive agents acting upon lymphokine synthesis and signal transduction. Clin Transplant 7:113-125, 1993.

72. Morelon E, Stern M, Israel-Biet D, et al: Characteristics of sirolimus-associated interstitial pneumonitis in renal transplant patients. Transplantation 72:787, 2001.

73. Trotter J, Wachs M, Trouillot T, et al: Dyslipidemia during sirolimus therapy in liver transplant recipients occurs with concomitant cyclosporine but not with tacrolimus. Liver Transpl 7:401-408, 2001.

74. Johnson R, Kreis H, Oberbauer R, et al: Sirolimus allows early cyclosporine withdrawal in renal transplantation resulting in improved renal function and lower blood pressure. Transplantation 72:777, 2001.

75. Watson C, Friend P, Jamieson N, et al: Sirolimus a potent new immunosuppressant for liver transplantation. Transplantation 67:505-509, 1999.

76. Guilbeau J: Delayed wound healing with sirolimus after liver transplant. Ann Pharmacother 36:1391-1395, 2002.

77. Morice MC, Serruys PW, Sousa JE, et al: Randomized study with the sirolimus-coated bx velocity balloon-expandable stent in the treatment of patients with de novo native coronary artery lesions. N Engl J Med 346:1770-1771, 2002.

78. Sanchez E, Onaca N, Thomas M, et al: Rapamune conversion in long-term liver transplant patients: Continued improvement in measured glomerular filtration rate two years after transplant. Submitted for publication.

79. Bonnefoy-Berard N, Vincent C, Revillard JP: Antibodies against functional leukocyte surface molecules in polyclonal anti-lymphocyte and antithymocyte globulins. Transplantation 51:669-673, 1991.

80. Rebellato LM, Gross U, Verbanac KM, Thomas KM: A comprehensive definition of the major antibody specificities in polyclonal rabbit antithymocyte globulin. Transplantation 57:685-694, 1994.

81. Bourdage JS, Hamlin DM: Comparative polyclonal antithymocyte globulin and antilymphocyte/antilymphoblast globulin anti-CD antigen analysis by flow cytometry. Transplantation 59:1194-1200, 1995.

82. Debets JMH, Leunissen KML, van Hooff HJ, et al: Evidence of involvement of tumor necrosis factor in adverse reactions during treatment of kidney allograft rejection with antithymocyte globulin. Transplantation 47:487-492, 1989.

83. Henricsson A, Husburg B, Bergentz SE: The mechanism behind the effect of ALG on platelets in vivo. Clin Exp Immunol 29:515-522, 1977.

84. Tchervenkov J, Flemming C, Guttmann RD, des Gachons G: Use of thymoglobulin induction therapy in prevention of acute graft rejection episodes following liver transplantation. Transplant Proc 29(7A):13S-15S, 1997.

85. Eason JD, Loss GE, Blazek J, et al: Steroid-free liver transplantation using rabbit antithymocyte globulin induction: Results of a prospective randomized trial. Liver Transpl 7:693-697, 2001.

86. Kohler G, Milstein C: Continuous cultures of fused cells secreting antibody of predefined specificity. Nature 256:495-497, 1975.

87. Winter G, Milstein C: Man-made antibodies. Nature 349:293-299, 1991.

88. Alegre ML, Peterson LJ, Xu D, et al: A non-activating "humanized" anti-CD3 monoclonal antibody retains immunosuppressive properties in vivo. Transplantation 57:1537-1543, 1994.

89. Alegre ML, Lennschow DJ, Bluestone JA: Immunomodulation of transplant rejection using monoclonal antibodies and soluble receptors. Dig Dis Sci 40:58-64, 1995.

90. Vincenti F, Lantz M, Birnbaum J, et al: A phase I trial of humanized anti–interleukin 2 receptor antibody in renal transplantation. Transplantation 63:33-38, 1997.

91. Solomon H, Gonwa TA, Mor E, et al: OKT3 rescue for steroid-resistant rejection in adult liver transplantation. Transplantation 55:87-91, 1993.

92. Cosimi AB: Clinical development of Orthoclone OKT3. Transplant Proc 19(2 Suppl 1):7-16, 1987.

93. Jeyarajah DR, Thistlethwaite JR Jr: General aspects of cytokine-release syndrome: Timing and incidence of symptoms. Transplant Proc 25(2 Suppl 1):16-20, 1993.

94. Amlot PL, Rawings E, Fernando ON, et al: Prolonged action of a chimeric interleukin-2 receptor (CD25) monoclonal antibody used in cadaveric renal transplantation. Transplantation 60:748-756, 1995.

95. Kovarik J, Wolf P, Cisterne JM, et al: Disposition of basiliximab, an interleukin-2 receptor monoclonal antibody, in recipients of mismatched cadaver renal allografts. Transplantation 64:1701-1705, 1997.

96. Kovarik JM, Rawlings E, Sweny P, et al: Prolonged immunosuppressive effect and minimal immunogenicity from chimeric (CD25) monoclonal antibody SDZ CHI 621 in renal transplantation. Transplant Proc 28:913-914, 1996.

97. Calmus Y, Scheele JR, Gonzalez-Pinto I, et al: Immunoprophylaxis with basiliximab, a chimeric anti–interleukin-2 receptor monoclonal antibody, in combination with azathioprine-containing triple therapy in liver transplant recipients. Liver Transpl 8:123-131, 2002.

98. Koch M, Niemeyer G, Patel I, et al: Pharmacokinetics, pharmacodynamics and immunodynamics of daclizumab in two-dose regimen in liver transplantation. Transplantation 73:1640-1646, 2002.

99. Personal communication from Roche.

100. Emre S, Gondolesi G, Polat K, et al: Use of daclizumab as initial immunosuppression in liver transplant recipients with impaired renal function. Liver Transpl 7:220-225, 2001.

101. Hirose R, Roberts JP, Quan D, et al: Experience with daclizumab in liver transplantation: Renal transplant dosing without calcineurin inhibitors is insufficient to prevent acute rejection in liver transplantation. Transplantation 69:307-311, 2000.

102. Gonwa TA, Mai ML, Melton LB, et al: End-stage renal disease (ESRD) after orthotopic liver transplantation (OLTX) using calcineurin-based immunotherapy: Risk of development and treatment. Transplantation 72:1934-1939, 2001.

103. de Mattos AM, Olyaei AJ, Bennett WM: Nephrotoxicity of immunosuppressive drugs: Long-term consequences and challenges for the future. Am J Kidney Dis 35:333-346, 2000.

104. Gines P, Arroyo V: Hepatorenal syndrome. J Am Soc Nephrol 10:1833-1839, 1999.

105. Gonwa TA, Klintmalm GB, Levy M, et al: Impact of pretransplant renal function on survival after liver transplantation. Transplantation 59:361-365, 1995.

106. Stewart SF, Hudson M, Talbot D, et al: Mycophenolate mofetil monotherapy in liver transplantation. Lancet 357:609-610, 2001.

107. Ohmori S, Shiraki K, Inoue H, et al: Clinical characteristics and prognostic indicators of drug-induced fulminant hepatic failure. Hepatogastroenterology 50:1531-1534, 2003.

It remains unclear whether induction with antilymphocyte preparations can achieve long-term reduction in immunosuppression in children. The largest pediatric experience is from the Hanover group, which reported an 11.5% incidence of rejection with the use of basiliximab induction combined with low-dose cyclosporine, MMF, and early weaning of steroids.[8] A decreased incidence of acute rejection was also reported in children after a single dose of daclizumab combined with MMF and prednisone for induction, with a delay in initiation of tacrolimus until day 7 after transplantation.[54] Because neither of these studies were randomized with a control group, it is difficult to foresee what the long-term benefits might be. One benefit of antibody induction therapy is seen in children with renal impairment. In these children a delay in starting CNI therapy has been demonstrated to potentiate the recovery of renal function.[55]

The Pittsburgh group is using a polyclonal antibody, antithymocyte globulin, in innovative protocols designed to allow minimization or complete withdrawal of immunosuppression. Preliminary results in children after liver transplantation have shown that with a two-dose regimen consisting of a pretransplant and early posttransplant dose of antithymocyte globulin, tacrolimus, and no steroids, the incidence of rejection was acceptable and the frequency of tacrolimus dosing could be reduced to once per day in some patients within the first year after transplantation.[56]

Rejection

An analysis of rejection in 1902 first pediatric liver transplant recipients from the SPLIT registry showed that rejection occurred most often in the first 3 months.[26] The cumulative rejection rates were 0.45 at 3 months, and they increased only modestly to 0.59 at 24 months (Fig. 76–3). The median time to first rejection was 16 days, the average number of rejection episodes per patient per year was 0.51, more that one rejection episode occurred in 18.5% of children, and steroid-resistant rejection was relatively unusual and occurred in 11.2% of children. High-dose steroids were the most common treatment of rejection. Antilymphocyte preparations such as antithymocyte globulin or OKT3 were used as initial treatment in 8.3% of first rejection episodes and 3.8% of second rejection episodes but increased to 11.4% if patients experienced more than three rejection episodes. When Kaplan-Meier probabilities of rejection over time were examined for various factors, there was a trend toward less rejection in children younger than 6 months and in recipients of living donor grafts, findings also reported by other investigators.[21,57,58] In a multivariate analysis, initiation

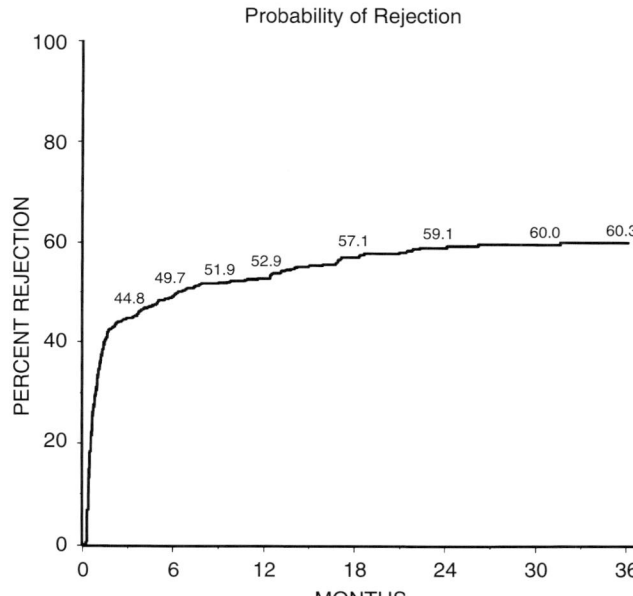

Probability of Rejection

FIGURE 76–3

Kaplan-Meier probability of rejection over the first 24 months after a first liver transplant. (From McDiarmid S, Anand R, Lindblad AS, SPLIT Research Group: Studies of pediatric liver transplantation: 2002 update. An overview of demographics, indications, timing, and immunosuppressive practices in pediatric liver transplantation in the United States and Canada. Pediatr Transplant 8:284-294, 2004.)

of immunosuppression with tacrolimus as opposed to cyclosporine was the only factor that showed a significantly lower probability of rejection at 6 months, 51% versus 64% ($P = .01$).[31] At the time of last follow-up, however, no difference in patient or graft survival was noted in those who underwent tacrolimus or cyclosporine induction.

Somewhat surprisingly, the incidence of rejection in pediatric recipients of living related grafts has not been shown to be significantly less than in recipients of deceased donor grafts despite better HLA compatability.[59-61] In one study the incidence of rejection was similar, but the severity of rejection was less in recipients of living donor grafts than in those who received deceased donor grafts.[57] Therefore, in general, pediatric transplant programs do not alter their immunosuppressive protocols for living donor as compared with deceased donor grafts.

Late acute rejection carries a different prognosis than early rejection does.[62,63] It is frequently associated with low levels of immunosuppression, which are often related to noncompliance. The diagnosis may be delayed and the liver biopsy specimen more difficult to interpret because of features of hepatitis and centrilobular venulitis and necrosis.[64,65] In addition, the response to steroids can be suboptimal, and some authors have reported an increased risk of progression to chronic rejection.[66]

Chronic rejection appears to be increasingly rare, and some investigators attribute this decline in chronic rejection to the increasing use of tacrolimus in pediatric liver transplantation. In reviewing the extensive use of tacrolimus in Pittsburgh, Jain and coauthors[67] reported that chronic rejection, defined histologically as vanishing bile duct syndrome, occurred in 3.1% of 1048 tacrolimus-treated patients and was virtually absent in pediatric recipients.[68] A study of risk factors for chronic rejection in 385 pediatric liver recipients at the University of Chicago found that recipients of deceased donor organs, African Americans, patients with two or more episodes of rejection, patients with posttransplant lymphoproliferative disease (PTLD) and cytomegalovirus (CMV) disease, and those with autoimmune hepatitis as the indication for transplantation had a significantly higher risk for chronic rejection.[69]

Understanding the consequences of rejection may be a more important subject for study than the incidence of rejection. In contrast to kidney and heart allografts, a liver allograft is often described as an immunologically privileged organ.[70] Evidence continues to accumulate that rejection, particularly if steroid sensitive and occurring early after transplantation, appears to have no long-term adverse effects on either graft function or survival.[71-73] As noted earlier, no prospective randomized trial that investigated a new immunosuppressive drug for use after liver transplantation has shown a significant improvement in patient or graft survival despite significant improvements in rejection and even steroid-resistant rejection. In fact, a few adult studies and one pediatric study purport that rejection itself may have a beneficial effect on patient survival. Wiesner and colleagues[72] showed that one episode of rejection resulted in a small, but statistically significant improvement in patient survival 36 months after liver transplantation. An investigation of long-term graft function in adult liver recipients by Dousset and coworkers[71] showed that one episode of rejection had no influence on graft function 1 year after transplantation. In children registered in the SPLIT database, rejection, listed as either present or absent, within 6 months after transplantation was associated with a significantly lower risk for death or graft loss. However, when analyzed as a time-varying parameter, rejection, either one or more than one episode versus no episodes, lost its effect on patient and graft survival.[74] In a multivariate analysis of many factors affecting posttransplant survival, the predicted effect of one versus no episodes of rejection approached significance for patient survival, $P = .06$.[73] The intriguing finding that some rejection may in fact be protective of graft function and survival raises the question that a controlled amount of immune activation may actually be necessary to delete clones of recipient-derived lymphocytes injurious to the graft.[75]

Treatment of Rejection

Treatment of rejection varies little between children and adults after liver transplantation. Any effective alternative that avoids prolonged or repeated courses of high-dose steroids is advantageous to children. Steroid-sparing strategies that are used in children include converting cyclosporine therapy to tacrolimus at the onset of the first rejection episode[76] or simply increasing tacrolimus levels in children primarily treated with tacrolimus.

Steroid-resistant rejection appears to be less common than previously, but it is still problematic to treat. The efficacy of OKT3, a murine monoclonal antibody directed against the CD3 complex receptor common to all T cells, is undisputed. A success rate of 75% to 80% has been reported in series combining adult and pediatric patients,[6,77,78] and OKT3 was associated with a lower retransplantation rate for rejection. OKT3 is administered only intravenously and for short courses of 10 to 14 days.[79,80] However, two studies comparing OKT3 treatment in children and adults[13,81] reported a lower success rate in pediatric patients. One study attributed the lower success of OKT3 in reversing rejection in children to a high incidence of antimurine antibody formation (67% of patients) and the need for dose increases in the majority to maintain low CD3$^+$ cell counts.[13]

The newer IL-2R monoclonal antibodies have been used almost exclusively for induction. However, a recent study using basiliximab for steroid-resistant rejection reported success in all five children in whom it was used.[82]

The addition of MMF[49] or sirolimus[83] in children with resistant rejection has had variable success. Conversion from cyclosporine to tacrolimus is more successful for acute rejection than for chronic rejection.[84,85] Once serum bilirubin is higher than 10 mg/dL, successful control of resistant rejection is unlikely.

Changing Ideas and Future Directions in Immunosuppression Therapy

Our better understanding of the consequences of rejection and increasing awareness of the detriments of overimmunosuppression have instigated a change in thinking about both new induction immunosuppression strategies in children and long-term maintenance therapy. New induction therapies should no longer strive to keep decreasing the incidence of rejection, but rather provide enough immunosuppression to control damaging rejection and thereby protect graft function and survival without the added risks of unnecessary immunosuppression, including infection, de novo malignancy, and the long-term toxicities of CNIs, particularly nephrotoxicity. The ultimate, but difficult-to-achieve, goal of induction therapy will be to use methods that facilitate the development of donor-specific tolerance and thereby allow patients eventual freedom from all immunosuppression and its attendant toxicities.

Minimizing long-term maintenance immunosuppression has recently become the focal point of new studies. Investigators who care for children are increasingly concerned about the consequences of decades of exposure to immunosuppression. What are the risks of de novo malignancy, renal failure, and long-term central nervous system toxicity for a 40-year-old who received a transplant at the age of 1 year? Although this question is still unanswerable, a sense of the impact of long-term immunosuppression can be appreciated by examining the causes of late graft loss in children. Now that a substantial number of children have lived more than 10 years after transplantation, some even more than 20 years, causes of graft failure in very long-term survivors are only just becoming apparent. Unlike their adult liver recipient counterparts, in whom recurrent disease and extrahepatic degenerative diseases have a powerful impact on late patient and graft loss,[86] in children virtually all late losses are related to immunosuppression, either too little or, more often, too much. Graft or patient loss from underimmunosuppression is often a result of noncompliance, whereas sepsis, PTLD, lymphomas, and other de novo malignancies are the result of too much immunosuppression. Several large pediatric liver transplant centers have reported strikingly similar results. Sudan and associates[4] showed that sepsis, noncompliance, and graft failure were the most common causes of death 1 year after transplantation in pediatric liver recipients. Ryckman and colleagues[87] also showed that after 3 months sepsis was the most common cause of subsequent death. In Fridell and coworkers' study[88] of 279 children, sepsis was the most common cause of death in children who died after 1 year, followed by PTLD. In the experience of the pediatric liver transplant program at the University of California at Los Angeles (UCLA),[89] of 285 children surviving more than 1 year, 2.4% (7 children) died at a mean of 5.2 years after liver transplantation. Five of the seven deaths were directly attributable to immunosuppression: lymphoma in two, sepsis in two, and chronic rejection in one. Recently, the Brussels group[3] has also analyzed late graft loss in more than 400 children. They likewise found the complications and implications of long-term immunosuppressive therapy to be the most important factors influencing graft loss: infection in 21.2%, PTLD in 21%, and chronic rejection in 17%. The consistent theme that the effects of long-term immunosuppression are implicated in most of the causes of late patient and graft loss is having

a disquieting effect on the transplant physicians who hold the stewardship of decades of life after transplantation for their young patients. This realization is forcing a reevaluation of immunosuppression practices both from the time of transplantation to decades after the procedure.

As discussed earlier, steroid withdrawal was the first step toward achieving the goal of less long-term immunosuppression. Complete steroid avoidance is the extension of this concept. Steroid avoidance protocols rely on the use of either polyclonal or monoclonal antibody therapy because of high rejection rates in patients given monotherapy with either cyclosporine or tacrolimus.[90] In the only randomized controlled trial of steroid avoidance in liver transplant recipients (all adults) reported to date, induction with thymoglobulin (a polyclonal, depleting antilymphocyte preparation), MMF, and tacrolimus was compared with an induction regimen consisting of tacrolimus, MMF, and steroids. The incidence of biopsy-proven rejection in the steroid-free thymoglobulin group was 20.5% versus 32% in controls. Although success has not yet been reported in pediatric liver transplantation, several centers are beginning the practice of complete steroid avoidance. Optimism that this approach may be successful has been fueled by studies in pediatric kidney recipients. Induction with a prolonged course of daclizumab[91] or with an antilymphocyte preparation[92] combined with MMF and a CNI resulted in a low incidence of rejection, thus challenging the long-held belief that long-term steroid therapy is essential for kidney graft survival. Preliminary results from a steroid-free protocol using basiliximab induction combined with tacrolimus and MMF in pediatric liver recipients are promising.[93]

Steroid withdrawal or even avoidance of steroids does not appear to be dependent on a fundamental change in our current reliance on CNIs for maintenance immunosuppression. As yet, no replacements for CNIs appear promising as primary therapy. Sirolimus (rapamycin) has a mechanism of action distinct from that of the CNIs, and although it may cause hyperlipidemia and thrombocytopenia, it is not nephrotoxic or neurotoxic,[94] thus making it particularly attractive for use in children.[95] The first randomized trial of sirolimus after liver transplantation was conducted in adults. The group receiving sirolimus, cyclosporine, and prednisone had a lower incidence of rejection than did the control group treated with tacrolimus and steroids.[96] However, safety issues related to an observed increased incidence of vascular thrombosis, particularly hepatic artery thrombosis, has precluded further multicenter, randomized trials, especially any including pediatric liver recipients, who are already at increased risk for hepatic artery thrombosis. Single-center reports have been much more encouraging about the role of sirolimus in induction therapy after liver transplantation. In 56 adult liver transplant recipients, the incidence of rejection in patients receiving sirolimus combined with low-dose tacrolimus was 14%, with only one episode of hepatic artery thrombosis.[97] Trotter and colleagues[98] successfully used sirolimus as induction therapy combined with tacrolimus and only 3 days of steroids, with a reported 30% incidence of rejection. To date, no sirolimus study has yet reported successful early withdrawal of a CNI. The reported use of sirolimus in pediatric liver transplant patients has been limited to mostly rescue therapy. Sirolimus has been used to replace CNIs in small numbers of children with unacceptable toxicity from the CNIs[99] or as primary therapy in a few selected patients.[83]

Further progress in substantially decreasing immunosuppression and its attendant long-term toxicities will require finding ways to minimize or even stop the use of CNIs and, ultimately, all immunosuppression. Two transplant programs have now reported their results of withdrawing all immunosuppression in children after liver transplantation, despite an inability to predict the children in whom this strategy might be successful. Interestingly, the 25% and 26% incidence of rejection during and after weaning was remarkably similar in both authors' experience, although one program used deceased donor grafts[9] and the other used living related (usually parental) donors.[10] Neither study reported graft loss as a result of weaning. However, acute rejection could occur as long as 4 years after all immunosuppression is stopped, thus implying that long-term, close surveillance of these patients is essential and that the "tolerant" state may be reversible. As attractive as the concept of freedom from all immunosuppression is, the major factor contributing to the reluctance of many transplant physicians to initiate complete withdrawal of immunosuppression systematically in their patients is the inability to evaluate whether the host is truly nonresponsive to the allograft. Although studies are in progress to develop a so-called tolerance assay, no such assays have yet proved reliable in the clinical setting.

In addition to attempts to withdraw "conventional" immunosuppression, there is increasing impetus to design innovative induction protocols that may promote tolerance to the allograft. As our knowledge of the complexities of both the initial and ongoing recipient response to the allograft evolves,[100] as well as the role of donor-derived hematopoietic cells, it is becoming apparent that some of our current immunosuppressive strategies may be antitolerogenic. It is increasingly being appreciated that some immune activation is necessary for induction of tolerance and that it may be mediated by IL-2 and tumor necrosis factor.[101] What role, therefore, do cyclosporine and tacrolimus, both of which decrease IL-2 production, or IL-2R blocking monoclonal antibodies have in abrogating tolerizing mechanisms?[102]

Clonal depletion and clonal exhaustion of alloreactive T cells appear to be central to the induction and maintenance of tolerance.[103] The role of the large number of donor-derived passenger lymphocytes in the liver graft that quickly migrate to peripheral lymphoid tissue may be important in initiating a "graft-versus-host" response, thus aiding in containment of the host's response to the graft.[104] Likewise, methods to achieve early depletion of host T cells could be very important, hence the recent upsurge in interest in using depleting antibodies or other conditioning treatments in induction regimens.[105] Clearly, the amount as well as timing of depleting strategies is crucial. If balance between the host-versus-graft reaction and the graft-versus-host reaction is lost, either rejection or clinical graft-versus-host disease will be the consequence.[75]

Early clinical trials are also under way to investigate another immune pathway important to induction of tolerance. Blockade of the costimulatory pathway of T-cell activation has been shown in animal models to be an effective inducer of tolerance. One promising biological agent now entering clinical trials is CTLA4-Ig, which blocks the costimulatory interaction between CD28 and B7.[106,107]

Pharmacokinetics of Immunosuppressive Drugs in Pediatric Patients

The use of new immunosuppressive drugs in pediatric transplant recipients has often been limited by lack of pharmacokinetic data—especially in the very young children who constitute the largest segment of the pediatric liver transplant population.

The pharmacokinetics of immunosuppressive drugs is substantially different in children and adults. The assumption cannot be made that the pharmacokinetic information obtained from adult trials during drug development is applicable to children. For example, as was learned with the early use of both cyclosporine and tacrolimus, extrapolation of drug doses to children based on average adult doses resulted in subtherapeutic blood levels in children. In fact, it may be that the dose of some drugs should be adjusted to surface area, a more accurate reflection of body mass in small children, rather than by weight.

Apart from the generalization that children tend to metabolize drugs more rapidly than adults do because of increased hepatic enzyme activity,[108] other mechanisms have been invoked to explain pharmacokinetic differences in pediatric liver recipients. Changes in hepatic blood flow, which generally decreases with age,[109] may affect drug extraction and therefore clearance. Another possibility is that because some drugs such as cyclosporine are strongly bound to lipoproteins and lipoprotein concentrations increase with age, there is a resultant decrease in the free fraction of cyclosporine, which theoretically reduces the hepatic clearance of cyclosporine. Shortened bowel length, which decreases the area available for drug absorption, was shown to play a role in cyclosporine absorption in children with a Roux-en-Y choledochojejunostomy after liver transplantation.[110] Because this procedure is the most usual method of biliary reconstruction in small children, including all those with biliary atresia, this factor may be more important than previously thought.

Pediatric patients also have a higher propensity for diarrheal illness than adults do. Diarrhea quickly reduces circulating serum cyclosporine levels,[111] which in turn may induce rejection. Cyclosporine levels must be restored either by increasing the oral dose or (rarely) by giving intravenous cyclosporine. In contrast, tacrolimus levels frequently increase, even into the toxic range, with viral enteritis. This finding has been best described in association with rotavirus infection.[112,113] The loss of P-glycoprotein in damaged or sloughed enterocytes is one proposed explanation. P-glycoprotein is expressed on intestinal epithelial cells and regulates drug absorption by actively transporting drug out of the enterocyte back into the lumen of the intestine. Another explanation is that intestinal expression of cytochrome P4503A4 is decreased in damaged enterocytes and, as a result, the metabolism of tacrolimus is decreased.[114]

It is essential that parents be counseled that they must notify the transplant center if diarrhea persists beyond 24 hours. In addition, pediatricians should be aware that management of diarrhea in a posttransplant child taking either cyclosporine or tacrolimus requires a different approach than in a normal child. Hospitalization may be needed to quickly normalize hydration and electrolytes and manage dosing of cyclosporine or tacrolimus.

When compared with adult liver transplant patients, children are more likely to be treated with other drugs that may dramatically alter levels of cyclosporine and tacrolimus. Cyclosporine and tacrolimus share virtually the same profile of interactions with drugs that either decrease or increase their levels. Of particular importance in children after liver transplantation is use of the commonly prescribed macrolide antibiotics erythromycin and clarithromycin. Both decrease cyclosporine and tacrolimus clearance by competing with cytochrome P450, and the resultant rise in cyclosporine and tacrolimus levels is sometimes high enough to precipitate acute nephrotoxicity.[115,116] Because erythromycin is commonly prescribed for children with impetigo, otitis media (e.g., Pediazole, which contains erythromycin plus sulfamethoxazole), and *Mycoplasma* pneumonia, this potentially serious interaction is quite commonly seen.

A safer alternative is azithromycin, which does not appear to affect CNI drug levels. Although less often used in children, ketoconazole administered for severe fungal infection has a similar effect.[117,118] If the use of these drugs cannot be avoided, it is wise to decrease the CNI dose by about 50% concurrently, with close follow-up of CNI levels.

The converse problem, subtherapeutic cyclosporine and tacrolimus levels, which may precipitate rejection, occurs most often when anticonvulsants are initiated without an increase in cyclosporine or tacrolimus doses. The most commonly used anticonvulsants in children, phenobarbital, phenytoin, carbamazepine, and valproic acid, all induce cytochrome P450 and therefore increase cyclosporine and tacrolimus clearance.[118] The same mechanism applies to rifampin, and with the recent resurgence of tuberculosis, this drug may be used more frequently in the postoperative care of transplant patients.[119,120]

It must also be remembered that when patients are weaned off such medications, CNI levels may abruptly rise into the toxic range.

Cyclosporine

The original formulation of cyclosporine (Sandimmune) is a highly lipid-soluble compound with unpredictable and relatively poor bioavailability; it is metabolized in the liver by cytochrome P4503A. In the early use of Sandimmune for pediatric liver recipients, it became clear that children required much higher doses per kilogram to achieve the same therapeutic blood levels as their adult counterparts.[121,122] Even in adult patients, cyclosporine has an erratic pharmacokinetic profile characterized by inconsistent oral absorption with a mean bioavailability of only 27%.[123,124] In contrast, oral absorption in pediatric liver transplantation patients ranged from less than 5% to 18%.[109,121] Other studies confirmed that as age increased, both cyclosporine clearance and the volume of distribution decreased.[111]

Development of the microemulsion form of cyclosporine, Neoral, was a major advance in overcoming some of the variability in the pharmacokinetics of Sandimmune. A 1:1 conversion from Sandimmune to Neoral in stable pediatric liver recipients resulted in significant increases in total drug exposure, measured as area under the concentration curve (AUC) and as the mean maximum blood concentration of Neoral, by 66% and 109%, respectively.[125] Significantly improved bioavailability was also demonstrated in pediatric liver recipients immediately after transplantation.[126] The increased bioavailability of Neoral correlated with a significantly lower incidence of rejection, without increased toxicity, in a randomized, controlled trial of pediatric liver recipients receiving either Sandimmune

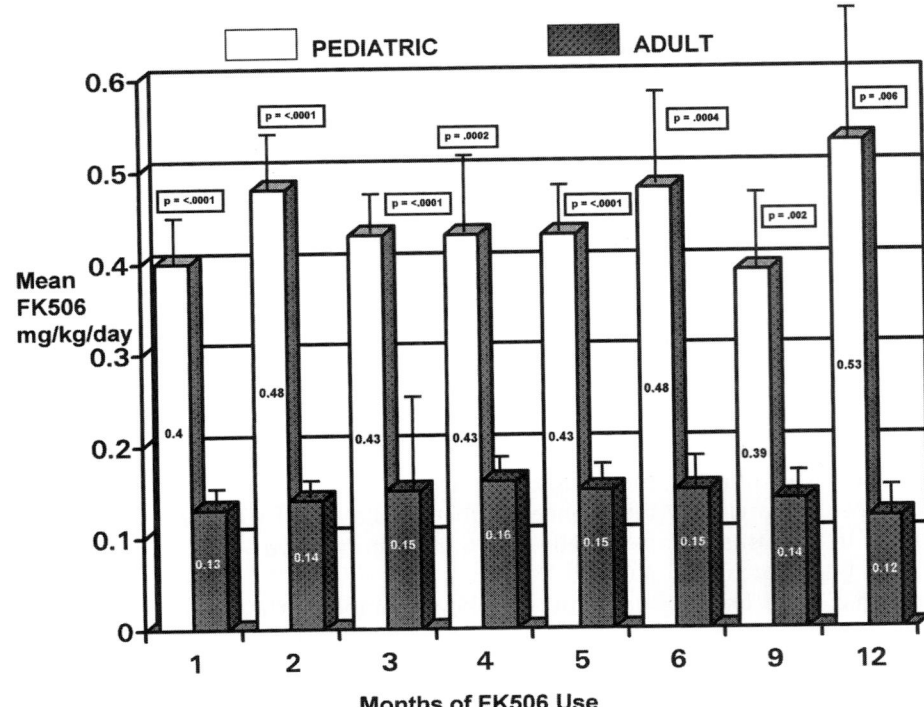

PEDIATRIC   **ADULT**

Mean FK506 mg/kg/day

p = <.0001   0.4
p = <.0001   0.48
p = .0002   0.43
p = <.0001   0.43
p = <.0001   0.43
p = .0004   0.48
p = .002   0.39
p = .006   0.53

0.13   0.14   0.15   0.16   0.15   0.15   0.14   0.12

1   2   3   4   5   6   9   12

Months of FK506 Use

FIGURE 76–4

Comparison of pediatric and adult tacrolimus doses (mg/kg/day) over the first 12 months after transplantation. Pediatric patients required significantly more tacrolimus at each time point in comparison to adults. The mean trough levels were not significantly different (data not shown). (From McDiarmid SV, Colonna JO 2nd, Shaked A, et al: Differences in oral FK506 dose requirements between adult and pediatric liver transplant patients. Transplantation 55:1328-1332, 1993.)

or Neoral in the early posttransplant period.[127] Moreover, the weak correlation with trough levels (Cmin) and AUC for Sandimmune was significantly improved with Neoral.[128,129] Children with fat malabsorption, such as cystic fibrosis patients,[130] could more easily achieve therapeutic levels. African American children, a population known to have poor cyclosporine bioavailability, had an increase in AUC with conversion to Neoral. This improvement was most evident in children 1 to 5 years of age, whose AUC increased by an average of 164%.[131] An additional advantage was that the presence of a draining bile tube did not appear to decrease levels to the extent seen with Sandimmune.[132] The improved bioavailability of Neoral should be considered when converting children without known malabsorption from Sandimmune to Neoral. A 1:1 conversion led to evidence of toxicity[133] even if the trough levels were kept constant, thus leading some authors to recommend a 1:0.75 conversion ratio between Sandimmune and Neoral in stable patients.[134,135]

Tacrolimus

The pharmacokinetics of tacrolimus in children shares several similarities with that of cyclosporine. Tacrolimus, like cyclosporine, is primarily metabolized in the liver and uses the cytochrome P4503A system.[136] In addition, it has the same drug reactions seen with cyclosporine.[137]

As with cyclosporine, soon after the introduction of tacrolimus, three centers reported that the oral dose per kilogram of tacrolimus required to maintain a therapeutic level is up to five times higher in children than in adults, especially those younger than 5 years.[138-140] In one report a mean pediatric dose of 0.46 mg/kg/day versus a mean adult dose of 0.13 mg/kg/day was needed to achieve the same blood levels (Fig. 76–4).[139] The discrepancy between adults and children regarding intravenous tacrolimus was not quite as pronounced, although intravenous doses up to two times higher than those for adults have been required in children.[140] These data suggest that the impaired gastrointestinal absorption in children as opposed to adults may play an important role in the difference in dose requirement.

Some of the first pharmacokinetic studies of tacrolimus were performed by the Pittsburgh group.[141] After an intravenous infusion, the half-life is variable and ranges from 3.5 to 40.5 hours with a mean of 8.7 hours. The volume of distribution is large, thus indicating an extensive extravascular compartment.[142] In contrast to cyclosporine, tacrolimus is a relatively high-clearance drug and is associated in plasma with the lipoprotein-deficient fraction.[142] In adults, the average bioavailability of tacrolimus was 27% but ranged from 5% to 67%.[142,143] In comparison, the Pittsburgh group noted that in children the half-life of tacrolimus was 2 times shorter, its clearance 2 to 4 times more rapid, and the volume of distribution 1.8 times higher than in adult patients in the early postoperative period.[141] In some patients the drug appeared to be absorbed continuously over a long period, whereas in others, the peak level was achieved rapidly. Tacrolimus absorption, unlike that of cyclosporine, appears to be independent of bile in the intestinal lumen, so a draining biliary T tube does not affect tacrolimus levels.[144] Differences in gastric emptying, or the inability of tacrolimus to dissolve in the aqueous fluid environment of the stomach, are possible explanations for this variation.

Used intravenously, tacrolimus has a high incidence of both nephrotoxicity and neurotoxicity. Despite considerable interpatient variability in oral absorption, oral tacrolimus, even in the immediate posttransplant period, can quite quickly achieve therapeutic levels. Intravenous tacrolimus is not recommended for induction treatment because of its associated toxicities.[145,146]

An interesting observation recently made and especially relevant to pediatric recipients of partial grafts is that the pharmacokinetic patterns of tacrolimus retain the characteristics of the age of the donor, not the recipient. It is well established that tacrolimus doses may need to be two to five times higher in children than in adults to achieve the same blood trough levels.[139,140,147] Therefore, lower doses of tacrolimus can be expected to be needed by a pediatric recipient of a partial graft from an adult as opposed to a pediatric graft.[148]

Mycophenolate Mofetil

Although used quite commonly in children after liver transplantation, very few studies have examined the pharmacokinetics of the active compound mycophenolic acid (MPA) in children after liver transplantation. Wide interpatient variability in MPA pharmacokinetics has been reported. In a study of stable pediatric liver transplant recipients, trough concentrations of MPA reliably predicted the AUC. Comedication with cyclosporine required higher MMF doses to achieve equivalent trough levels when compared with tacrolimus.[149] In 100 pediatric renal recipients aged 3 months to 18 years, MPA pharmacokinetics did not seem to vary with age.[150]

Useful pharmacokinetic studies in pediatric liver recipients have recently been published for basilixumab,[151] tacrolimus oral suspension,[147] and sirolimus.[152]

Therapeutic Drug Monitoring in Children

The general principles of therapeutic drug monitoring are similar in adults and children. Monitoring of cyclosporine and tacrolimus levels helps in both avoiding toxicity and ensuring a therapeutic range.[153,154] Acute nephrotoxicity correlates with high levels (measuring

either the parent drug plus metabolites or the parent drug alone), especially in the early posttransplant period.[155] In a long-term analysis of renal function in children, a glomerular filtration rate (GFR) less than 90 mL/min/1.73 m^2 resulted in significantly higher cyclosporine levels (by high-performance liquid chromatography).[156] Although the method and matrix (whole blood versus plasma) for monitoring varies between centers, most agree that in the early posttransplant period, a cyclosporine whole blood level of 150 to 300 ng/mL and a tacrolimus whole blood level of 8 to 15 ng/mL represent the therapeutic range. By 1 year after transplantation, target levels are 100 to 150 ng/mL for cyclosporine and 3 to 5 ng/mL for tacrolimus.

Although it is now well accepted that the best measure of drug exposure is the AUC, such studies are often difficult to perform in young children because of the requirement for multiple, timed blood samples. Abbreviated AUC estimates, using two or three time points, have been shown to have acceptable accuracy and are more suited to pediatric studies. For tacrolimus, the correlation with AUC and trough levels is good, so other surrogate measures for AUC are not needed in clinical practice. In comparison, trough concentrations of cyclosporine (Neoral) do not provide an accurate estimate of total drug exposure. Studies in adult liver[157] and kidney[158] recipients have shown that peak cyclosporine concentrations measured 2 hours after a dose (C_2 monitoring) are an accurate reflection of the AUC between 0 and 4 hours (AUC_{0-4}) after a dose. This 4-hour time interval is when interpatient variability is greatest. Adjusting Neoral doses to the C_2 rather than the trough level increased the efficacy and decreased the toxicity of Neoral. There is now preliminary evidence from studies in pediatric renal recipients[159] and one study in pediatric liver recipients[160] that C_2 levels are also an accurate surrogate for AUC_{0-4}. In children, it remains to be determined what the therapeutic target level for C_2 should be and how it may differ by age, organ type, and time after transplantation.

The liver plays a central role in the metabolism of MMF and its metabolites.[159] Changes in liver function after liver transplantation would be expected to alter the pharmacokinetics of MMF. However, monitoring of MPA levels in liver recipients is not commonly practiced, and the therapeutic range is not well established for MPA in either children or adults. In children, monitoring of MPA levels has been performed only in renal transplant recipients.[150]

Therapeutic monitoring of monoclonal antibody preparations raises some difficult questions. As was seen in the early experience with OKT3, the recommended dose was quite arbitrary and based on two weight ranges: less than 25 and more than 25 kg.[161] When serum OKT3 levels were measured, the recommended dose was subsequently shown to be inadequate in some patients.[13,162] Use of the newer monoclonal antibodies directed against IL-2R is no more scientific. Different doses per kilogram (daclizumab), doses based on less than 40 kg or more than 40 kg (basiliximab), different time intervals between doses, and different durations of therapy make it difficult to compare results between studies. In the past, monitoring of monoclonal antibodies has relied on measuring expression of the targeted receptor on peripheral blood lymphocytes. For example, if the absolute number of CD3$^+$ cells was less that 25/mm^3, it was thought to correlate with OKT3 efficacy. However, this approach assumes that expression of the target molecule correlates with function. For monitoring of IL-2R monoclonal antibodies, saturation of IL-2R can be assessed by measuring CD25 expression. However, CD25 is directed against only the alpha chain of the receptor, and thus it is implied that not all function of the receptor is blocked. Measuring monoclonal antibody serum levels is more cumbersome but, as was shown for OKT3, may be more helpful in guiding dosing.

Long-Term Risks of Immunosuppression in Children after Liver Transplantation

Long-term immunosuppression, regardless of the protocol used, always carries a risk of increased susceptibility to infection and the appearance of de novo malignancy. Most immunosuppressive regimens for children after liver transplantation now seek to discontinue steroid treatment early and avoid the long-term use of either MMF or azathioprine unless specifically indicated. Therefore, the most important drug-specific risks of long-term immunosuppression relate to the use of CNIs. Cyclosporine and tacrolimus are equally nephrotoxic and neurotoxic, and both also increase the risk of cardiovascular disease by contributing to hypertension, hyperlipidemia, and the de novo onset of diabetes. Also to be considered in children are the effects of immunosuppression on growth and cognitive function.

Nephrotoxicity

Renal impairment remains the most serious complication of our continued reliance on long-term CNI use.[163] In the 1990s, reports appeared that renal impairment after pediatric liver transplantation was quite common, more serious than expected, and not significantly different between cyclosporine- and tacrolimus-treated patients.[164-167] Furthermore, it was increasingly realized that relying only on serum creatinine as a serial measure of renal function underestimated the severity of the problem[168,169] and that the GFR was the most valid measurement.[170] Even calculated GFR, most often using the Schwartz formula, was shown to overestimate the true GFR.[124,171,172] The use of timed isotope plasma clearance methods for the measurement of GFR made GFR studies much more practical in children because the difficulties of performing timed, prolonged urine collections were eliminated.[173] However, relatively few studies of true GFR in children after liver transplantation have been performed, and most have not been conducted serially over years of CNI exposure. We reported that 73% of cyclosporine-treated children after liver transplantation had a true GFR of less than 70 mL/min/1.73 m^2. In children treated for 12 to 24 months, the mean GFR was 79 mL/min/1.73 m^2; it fell significantly to 52 mL/min/1.73 m^2 in children treated for longer than 24 months.[156] A progressive fall in GFR was also reported by Berg and coauthors,[172] who found that after liver transplantation children had lower GFRs than normal children did. Children requiring antihypertensive drugs and children who underwent transplantation for metabolic disease had the lowest GFRs. Taking the available evidence together, in the first year after transplantation the fall in GFR appears to be somewhat variable and also dependant on pre-transplant renal function. There seems to be a general consensus that early renal impairment induced by CNI use is often reversible and that dose reduction can be beneficial.[174,175] Although less well documented, at some point renal impairment appears to become irreversible. What is unknown is when that transition occurs, if it is predictable, and whether it is avoidable. Recent data from more than 10 years of exposure to CNIs in adult liver transplant recipients are concerning. Gonwa and colleagues[176] showed that 13 years after transplantation, 9.5% of 834 adult liver recipients were maintained on dialysis or had required a kidney transplant. Although pediatric recipients may start off with better renal function and have a greater functioning nephron mass than their adult counterparts do, even if by 20 years after transplantation children show similar degrees of renal impairment as the adults in Gonwa and colleagues' study, the chances become worrisome that renal failure will develop in early adulthood in a substantial number of children who receive a liver transplant before their fifth birthday.

Several observations lend credence to the idea that long-term renal impairment is not being overstated. In children who undergo retransplantation after several years of CNI exposure, unexpected degrees of renal failure often develop when exposed to higher CNI levels after retransplantation. Children in whom even mild dehydration develops as part of an acute intercurrent illness years after transplantation may have unusually high creatinine levels. There is also a considerable number of children who become hypertensive after liver transplantation. Studies in pediatric liver recipients have reported a 17% to 33% incidence of hypertension requiring therapy.[167,172,177] Hypertension in the early posttransplant period is relatively common and may be compounded by steroid use, but earlier steroid withdrawal may well improve this early-onset hypertension. In the SPLIT database,[178] although about a third of children were receiving antihypertensive medication 1 year after transplantation, this number fell to 16% at 24 months after transplantation. Hypertension requiring medication beyond a year after transplantation or occurring as a new-onset problem several years after transplantation may carry an entirely different prognosis than early hypertension does. The extent of this problem in children a decade or more after liver transplantation is not known. There is a notable lack of studies investigating renal function in children more than 10 years after transplantation. Such investigation will probably require a collaborative effort between several centers whose pediatric liver transplant programs began in the 1980s. As discussed in detail earlier, some currently available alternatives to CNIs have been used in pediatric liver transplantation to ameliorate long-term CNI-induced nephrotoxicity. The strategy most often used is to markedly reduce doses of CNIs or eliminate them altogether and add either MMF or sirolimus. Although improvement in renal function has been shown after such changes,[83,179] it is unclear whether such strategies can improve long-established renal impairment secondary to many years of CNI exposure. Until we are able to safely minimize CNI exposure or develop strategies to avoid CNI use altogether—if not initially after transplantation, then after the first year or two—renal impairment with the long-term threat of renal failure will continue to cast a shadow over the long-term prognosis of pediatric liver transplantation.

Neurotoxicity

The early neurotoxic effects of CNIs are well known.[180,181] The risk of neurotoxicity developing may be related to polymorphisms in the multidrug-resistant gene.[182] What is not yet understood is the effect of decades of exposure to such neurotoxins. How might development, cognitive function, and personality be affected? Studies of quality of life, development, and cognitive function after pediatric liver transplantation have produced troubling results. In an early study, children after liver transplantation had significantly lower nonverbal intelligence, lower academic achievement, and poorer scores for learning and memory than did children with cystic fibrosis.[183] Other investigators found learning problems in 26% of children,[184] and 50% were functioning at least one grade level lower than expected.[185] In a study of children with biliary atresia

who received transplants before 2 years of age, 35% demonstrated developmental delays.[184] Conversely, neurodevelopmental outcome after more than 4 years of follow-up appeared to be within normal limits in 25 children who received transplants before 1 year of age.[186]

Cardiovascular Risk

Cardiovascular risk is of increasing concern in adult recipients.[187] The triad of hypertension, hyperlipidemia, and de novo diabetes, all associated with the use of immunosuppression, substantially increases the risks for cardiovascular complications. There is some evidence that at least with cyclosporine therapy, lipid profiles in children may be abnormal. In one study, 50% of children had serum cholesterol levels greater than the 75th percentile.[188] The implications of childhood hypercholesteremia for later risk of cardiovascular events in adulthood are concerning.

To date, very few studies have investigated cardiovascular risk specifically in pediatric liver transplant recipients. For tacrolimus-treated children after liver transplantation, there appears to be a tendency to lower lipid levels,[7] but an increased risk for de novo diabetes as compared with cyclosporine-treated children has been reported for pediatric heart and kidney recipients.[189,190] However, this finding has not been well established in properly controlled studies in pediatric liver recipients.

De Novo Malignancies

PTLDs, including true lymphomas such as Burkitt's, Hodgkin's and non-Hodgkin's lymphoma, are still the most important neoplasms occurring after pediatric liver transplantation and are associated with substantial mortality. As the potency of our immunosuppressive strategies has increased, so has the incidence of PTLD, which has ranged from 2% to 27%.[191-194] This observation was made with the introduction of cyclosporine,[193] OKT3,[195-197] and tacrolimus.[192,194,198] In addition, the time to its appearance has shortened.[197] PTLD in children is almost always an Epstein-Barr virus (EBV)-driven B-cell proliferation that causes a spectrum of disease ranging from relatively benign lymphohyperplasia to true lymphoma. The initial symptoms and signs are protean, and PTLD can involve virtually any organ, including the graft itself.[199] Apart from immunosuppression, risk factors for PTLD are primary EBV infection after transplantation, young age, an EBV-negative recipient receiving an EBV-positive organ, and CMV infection.[200-202] Many clinicians draw a distinct difference between true lymphomas such as Burkitt's, Hodgkin's and non-Hodgkin's and PTLD. PTLD is almost always a B-cell–driven proliferation seen more often within the first 2 years after transplantation, is highly associated with primary EBV infection, and is usually successfully treated by withdrawal of immunosuppression.[203] In contrast, the true lymphomas generally occur years after transplantation, often in patients maintained on low-dose immunosuppression, and although the tumor cells show EBV expression, viremia, as measured by polymerase chain reaction (PCR) in peripheral blood, is often not demonstrable. Even though lymphomas tend to occur late, rapid evolution of a polymorphous proliferation to a typical monoclonal Burkitt lymphoma has been described.[204] The true lymphomas carry a much worse prognosis than early PTLD does.[201] They do not respond to antiviral drugs or withholding of immunosuppression and require chemotherapy for treatment.[204] Moreover, no good surveillance strategies appear effective, other than routine physical examination and rapid evaluation of suspicious lesions or changes in overall clinical status.

Both the incidence and mortality of PTLD occurring in the early posttransplant period has decreased over the past several years,[205,206] with a decline from between 40% and 70%[200,207,208] to between 10% and 20%.[209,210] This decrease appears to be directly attributable to the increasing use of surveillance for EBV viremia by serial EBV PCR determinations in peripheral blood, particularly when it became clear that monitoring EBV serological status was not useful.[211] Several investigators have reported that a rising EBV PCR copy number is an indictor of increasing viral load and is an important monitoring tool for the detection of primary EBV infection or reactivation,[212-214] which can then be treated preemptively. There is also general agreement that although a rising EBV PCR is not specific for PTLD, it is quite sensitive.[212-214] Allen and associates[215] demonstrated that the virus load had 69% sensitivity and 76% specificity for PTLD, whereas we showed 100% sensitivity and 27% specificity.[205]

A variety of prophylaxis regimens against EBV infection, such as ganciclovir, acyclovir, or CMV hyperimmune globulin (also shown to have high levels of EBV antibodies), alone or in combination, are commonly used, particularly in high-risk recipients, specifically, EBV-naïve recipients of EBV-positive grafts. If prophylaxis fails, preemptive treatment of a rising EBV PCR copy number before clinical disease has occurred appears to be very important to prevent progression to PTLD. Lowering immunosuppression, with or without the use of antiviral drugs or CMV hyperimmune globulin, is the key to preemptive management.[216] In the UCLA experience, a combination of prevention and preemptive therapy using ganciclovir for both prophylaxis and preemptive treatment, along with lowering of immunosuppression, has reduced the incidence of PTLD from 10% to 5% and, more recently, to less than 1%.[205] The role of antiviral therapy in the management of a rising viral load, or once PTLD has been diagnosed, is disputed. It is generally thought that the lytic phase of the virus, against which antiviral drugs are effective, occurs early and is short lived. However, increasing evidence suggests that lytic replication can occur sporadically in up to 45% of patients with PTLD.[217]

Further advances in the management of PTLD have focused on when it is appropriate to reintroduce immunosuppression and thus avoid rejection. The basic tenant behind stopping immunosuppression is to allow the host's natural EBV-specific T-cell response to reappear and limit the disease. At the same time, antidonor T-cell responses are also likely to be reactivated. By using an enzyme-linked immunospot (Elispot) methodology, which allows a determination of T-cell function by the production of interferon from cytotoxic T cells,[218,219] investigators have timed when T-cell specificity reappears and becomes of sufficient strength to potentially cause rejection.[220] At this point immunosuppression can be restarted.

New therapies for PTLD unresponsive to reduction of immunosuppression or for EBV-related lymphomas include anti-CD20 (a receptor found on most B cells) monoclonal antibodies and the injection of in vitro–expanded autologous EBV-specific cytotoxic T cells.[221] Although the most commonly used anti-CD20 monoclonal antibody in use, rituximab, has proved successful in treating lymphomas,[222] its role in PTLD is less clear.[223] Profound and prolonged B-cell depletion occurs after rituximab use, thus exposing the patient to additional risks of other infections.[224] The drawback of autologous injection of EBV-specific cytotoxic T cells is that they are most efficiently grown from patients who already have EBV infection, but even then, up to 30 days may be necessary before enough cells can be cultured. Ways to expand EBV-specific T cells in EBV-naïve recipients are being explored.[225]

PTLD and lymphomas are not the only EBV-driven tumors seen after pediatric liver transplantation. EBV-associated spindle cell smooth muscle tumors[226] and leiomyosarcomas[227] have also been described.

As yet, other de novo malignancies in children after liver transplantation have not been extensively reported. Kaposi's sarcoma[228] and fibrosarcomas have been described.[229] However, there is concern that with more years of immunosuppressive exposure, skin cancer and other solid-organ tumors, which are already reported to be increased in adult liver recipients[230,231] in comparison to the normal population, will also develop in young adults who received transplants as children.

Growth

Poor nutrition as a consequence of chronic liver disease depresses linear growth.[232] However, successful liver transplantation does not necessarily guarantee accelerated growth.[35,36,233] In the early results of pediatric liver transplantation, it was noted that less than 50% of children showed catch-up growth even with normal liver function.[35] Although the causes of poor linear growth after liver transplantation are multifactorial,[234] the ongoing use of steroids, even at low doses, can be expected to have a deleterious effect on growth after transplantation.[235] It is still not known at what critical steroid dose per kilogram that the growth-retarding effects of steroids are manifested. Nocturnal growth hormone secretion may be affected by steroids,[236] and a steroid-mediated increase in hypothalamic somatostatin secretion has been described.[237] Clearly, children requiring frequent high doses of steroids to control rejection are at particular risk for growth retardation. Although only one small prospective controlled trial of complete steroid withdrawal in children[39] has been reported, several single-center experiences have noted a positive effect on posttransplant growth with steroid reduction to alternate days[41] or complete steroid withdrawal.[40,42,238,239]

As a result, steroid withdrawal, first practiced in Europe,[40] is now commonplace, and steroid-avoidance protocols are being advocated for children after liver transplantation. Successful steroid withdrawal does not appears to be dependent on whether Neoral or tacrolimus is the primary immunosuppressant.

Immunosuppression and Infection: Special Considerations for Pediatric Liver Recipients

Depressed T- and B-cell function as a consequence of long-term immunosuppression makes pediatric liver transplant recipients especially vulnerable to infection. Of particular importance are the common viral illnesses of childhood. These usually benign, self-limited conditions can become disseminated in an immunocompromised host and cause severe illness and even death. This potential for severe morbidity and mortality particularly applies to the herpesviruses, measles, and several of the common respiratory viruses.

Cytomegalovirus and Epstein-Barr Virus Infection

Because the majority of pediatric liver recipients are younger than 5 years, primary herpes viral infections after liver transplantation are a particular problem. Primary CMV and EBV infections generally have their greatest impact in the first months after transplantation, when immunosuppression is at its peak.[240] However, the risk of CMV and EBV infection causing disease has been substantially reduced by the use of prophylactic strategies. For both viruses, variable courses of

ganciclovir, given either orally or intravenously, acyclovir, and CMV hyperimmune globulin have been reported to be efficacious.[241-246] Although in adults oral ganciclovir is more effective than oral acyclovir[245] for CMV prophylaxis, in children oral ganciclovir has poor and highly variable absorption.[247] The more favorable pharmacokinetics of oral valganciclovir offers promise for use in children as a substitute for intravenous ganciclovir.[248]

Successful treatment of CMV disease depends on early recognition, and serial measurements of CMV viral load can be useful in guiding treatment.[244] CMV disease in an immunosuppressed transplant recipient carries significant morbidity and mortality and is discussed in more detail in Chapter 64, "Infections after Liver Transplantation."[249,250] As CMV disseminates, the liver is often infected and may show evidence of clinical disease.[251] Several issues are relevant to pediatric patients. Because the incidence of seropositivity increases with age, pediatric recipients are more likely to be seronegative at the time of transplantation.[252] Risk factors for the development of CMV disease include a seronegative recipient and a seropositive donor (primary infection), the use of monoclonal or polyclonal antibodies (e.g., OKT3, antilymphocyte globulin), and retransplanation.[249,253-255] The incidence of CMV disease in pediatric transplant patients has been reported to range from 27.7% to 35%.[254,256] Primary infection occurred in 19% and reactivation in 47% in the study of Salt and colleagues.[257] With the increased use of reduced-sized grafts from older donors and even living related grafts, there is more risk that a seronegative child will receive an organ from a seropositive older donor. Therefore, primary infection is more likely to develop in children after transplantation. Increased awareness of this problem will allow appropriate prophylactic regimens to be implemented. Effective prophylaxis has been achieved with acyclovir or ganciclovir with or without immune globulin.[241,252,258,259] Early treatment with ganciclovir (10 mg/kg/day intravenously) was effective in 87% of patients with CMV disease.[249]

Like CMV infection, EBV infection is common in childhood and is characterized by latency, liver involvement, and the potential for reactivation.[260] About 50% of children are seropositive before transplantation.[195] In Lamy and colleagues' study, 63% of seronegative children had converted within 2 to 3 months of transplantation, with a further 22.5% showing evidence of reactivation.[196] The usual clinical features of EBV disease in a normal host—adenopathy, pharyngitis, tonsillitis, hepatitis, splenomegaly, and purpura—may be more severe in an immunocompromised patient, with an increased risk for atypical lymphocyte transformation and proliferation. However, of greatest concern, as discussed earlier, is the potential for EBV-driven lymphoproliferative disease in immunosuppressed patients. The spectrum of findings ranges from generalized lymphadenopathy with a usually polyclonal B-cell expansion, which can be easily controlled by lowering immunosuppression, to a highly malignant monoclonal lymphoma, which can be rapidly fatal.[201]

Varicella

After liver transplantation, a child without a history of chickenpox and with negative varicella antibodies is susceptible to posttransplant chickenpox. From studies of other immunosuppressed children, varicella can be a life-threatening and even fatal illness, with mortality ranging from 7% to 50%.[261,262] Systemic dissemination affecting the lungs, central nervous system, liver, musculature, and heart has been well described.[263-265] Therefore, when an unprotected pediatric liver transplant patient is exposed to chickenpox, varicella-zoster immune globulin should be given intramuscularly in a dose of one vial per 10 kg within 96 hours of contact with the infected case.[266] If chickenpox does develop, the child should be hospitalized and receive intravenous acyclovir (500 mg/m^2 per dose every 8 hours) until the last lesion is crusted over.[267] Impaired kidney function mandates lowering of the dose. Oral acyclovir alone is not indicated because of its poor bioavailability and the risk of dissemination in immunocompromised children.[268]

Varicella vaccine is a live attenuated herpesvirus.[269] In normal children it is both safe and efficacious and prevents chickenpox in 87% of household-exposed children.[270] It is not recommended in immunosuppressed children, although in studies of immunocompromised leukemic patients,[271-273] there was no evidence of ongoing viral replication and no increased incidence of herpes zoster. This vaccine has not been studied, either for efficacy or safety, in patients with solid-organ transplants. In the absence of an approved vaccine for varicella after transplantation, varicella vaccine should be given before transplantation whenever possible. Improved efficacy with the use of a two-dose varicella vaccine regimen has been reported in children with chronic renal failure.[274]

Recently, there has been increasing awareness of clinical illness caused by herpesvirus 6 and 7, either as primary or as reactivated infection. Infection with herpesvirus 6, the virus responsible for roseola, is the best characterized in transplant recipients and may cause fever, rash, hepatitis, and encephalopathy.[275] These findings are particularly important for very young children undergoing transplantation, who are likely to have had no previous exposure to these viruses. Interestingly, coinfection with CMV and herpesvirus 6 and 7 has been demonstrated.[276-278]

Common respiratory viruses may still prove devastating if they become disseminated and invasive in newly transplanted children. Adenovirus, parainfluenza virus, and influenza virus are the biggest threats because they may induce a lethal necrotizing pneumonitis.[279,280] To date, antiviral therapies against these viruses have had only limited efficacy.

Of the seasonal infections, two are important because of the availability of specific preventive measures. Each fall the general population is exposed to a new influenza epidemic of varying severity. Because influenza virus can be associated with severe disease in immunocompromised hosts, routine, yearly influenza vaccination is recommended for transplanted children and each family member.[281]

Although the humoral immune response to influenza vaccine has been reported to be lower in transplanted patients than in healthy controls, protection rates of 92% to 95% were observed in a study of liver transplant patients.[282]

Respiratory syncytial virus (RSV) infections may cause severe disease in immunosuppressed children. No randomized studies in transplanted children have specifically addressed the efficacy of prophylaxis with either the pooled human RSV immune globulin preparation or palivizumab, a monoclonal antibody directed against the F protein of the virus.[283,284] Some centers routinely give prophylaxis with palivizumab against RSV infection over the winter months to children younger than 2 years.

Adenovirus infection, usually associated with mild upper respiratory tract infection in immunocompetent children, may cause fulminant hepatitis or necrotizing pneumonitis in the early posttransplant period, when immunosuppression is at its peak.[279,285,286] Serotypes 1, 2, and 5 are most often implicated, with type 5 being highly associated with hepatitis. In a retrospective study of 484 pediatric transplant patients,[285] there was a 10% incidence of adenovirus infection occurring at a mean of 25 days after transplantation. Invasive infection developed in 41% of these children with a subsequent mortality of 45%. In this study an increased incidence of invasive adenovirus was associated with the recent use of OKT3. Management of severe adenovirus infection is largely supportive, but aggressive reduction in immunosuppression is essential, even to the point of stopping cyclosporine and azathioprine entirely.[286] No specific antiviral therapy is available, although there have been occasional reports of some adenoviruses sensitive to ganciclovir. More recently, promising reports of the efficacy of ribavirin suggest that this drug may be the best option.[287] The source of the adenovirus may be primary infection from the environment, reactivation within the host, or possibly transmission from the donor.

The incidence of measles has surged in the last several years as immunization practices have become less rigorous.[288] The measles-mumps-rubella (MMR) vaccine is composed of three live attenuated viruses. The standard teaching that live vaccines should be avoided in immunosuppressed patients has recently been challenged by recommendations that measles vaccine can be safely administered to children suffering from human immunodeficiency virus.[289] Two small studies reported that immunization with MMR after liver transplantation was safe.[290,291] However, in one study less than half the children achieved protective antibodies.[290] The usual practice is to avoid MMR after transplantation and give pooled human immune globulin (0.5 mL/kg up to 15 mL) within 6 days of exposure.[292] The recommended age for administration of MMR is usually 15 months, but in a pretransplant child, the vaccine can be administered even at 9 months of age. A measles antibody titer can be checked to see whether protection was induced.

Poliomyelitis has also increased in incidence in the past years. Although not as protective as the oral vaccine, the killed Salk vaccine can be safely given either just before or after liver transplantation. The attenuated poliovirus in the oral formulation is no longer recommended in the United States for prevention of polio because of reported cases of wild-type polio, presumably contracted from vaccination. However, in countries still using the live poliovirus vaccination, it should be remembered that the virus can be excreted in the stool for up to 1 month in immunocompetent children and is a source of possible infection. Therefore, siblings of transplanted children should also receive the killed polio vaccine, and young children in whom transplantation is imminent should not be given oral polio vaccine.[289]

Vaccination Recommendations in Immunosuppressed Children

Vaccination is an essential component of preventive medicine and of crucial importance for children both before and after liver transplantation.[293] However, before transplantation many children with end-stage liver disease are malnourished and chronically ill and are therefore in a state of relative immune hyporesponsiveness, which may preclude a protective antibody response to vaccines.[294] With the exception of the live polio vaccine, usual childhood vaccinations should be aggressively pursued up until the time of transplantation. Transplantation should be deferred if a live virus vaccine has been given 4 to 6 weeks before the proposed transplant procedure.

Hepatitis B vaccination should be a priority.[295] However, the protective hepatitis B surface antibody may not develop in chronically ill patients. It is important that all children immunized for hepatitis B in infancy have a confirmed positive antibody response before transplantation. If not, reimmunization is recommended and may require a double-dose accelerated regimen.[296]

Hepatitis A vaccination is not yet routinely recommended for all children. However, in children older than 2 years in whom transplantation is likely, hepatitis A vaccination should be given. There is no contraindication to

vaccination after liver transplantation, although in one adult study the seroconversion rate was significantly lower than in controls,[297] so documenting the presence of protective antibody is necessary to assess efficacy.

After transplantation, vaccination can be recommenced once the child is an outpatient and preferably when steroid doses are being weaned. With the exception of the live vaccines (MMR, varicella, oral polio, bacille Calmette-Guérin vaccine), there is no contraindication to the standard recommendations for immunization of children.[289,298] In addition, the polysaccharide pneumococcal vaccine should be given after the age of 2 years and repeated at 5-year intervals, although in a study of adults, rapidly waning levels were reported after transplantation.[299] Children with asplenia or functional hyposplenia are at particular risk for overwhelming pneumococcal infection. All should receive both the conjugated and the polysaccharide pneumococcal vaccine, as well as a daily dose of penicillin or amoxicillin. The conjugated vaccine may be more immunogenic than the polysaccharide vaccine.[300] Hepatitis A[297] and B[301] vaccination can be given after transplantation (although preferably before transplantation), but development of the protective antibody must be determined. Meningococcal vaccine should be routinely given to children who are asplenic, as well as to teenagers entering college. The influenza vaccine should be given yearly in the fall.

Passive immunization is usually less effective but may ameliorate clinical illness. The use of zoster immune globulin was described earlier. Pooled human immune globulin is indicated for exposure to measles, mumps, and hepatitis A.

Particular care should be taken to adequately protect an immunocompromised child traveling to foreign countries.[302] The yellow fever and oral typhoid vaccines are both live vaccines and should not be given.

The current fear of a bioterrorist attack has led to recommendations for vaccinations in both healthy and immunosuppressed populations. Of the two most likely agents that might be used, smallpox and anthrax, only for smallpox is there a readily available supply of vaccine. However, the smallpox vaccine is a live vaccine and should be given to immunocompromised patients only if they are directly exposed.[303] For anthrax there is a killed vaccine available (and others in development) that would be safe in immunosuppressed patients, but currently only limited stocks are available.[304]

Special Considerations for Teenage Recipients

The hormonal storms of adolescence and the increased societal pressures of modern living unfortunately do not spare the liver transplant patient. The teenager's fight for identity combined with a heightened awareness of body image makes continued compliance with the routine daily medication regimens imposed by adults a natural target for rebellion. Knowing that the medications themselves may adversely alter physical appearance only adds fuel to the fire. Coupled with adolescents' common perception of their own invincibility, a healthy teenage liver transplant patient may wrongly conclude that the rules of daily immunosuppressive therapy can be safely broken. The resulting rejection is frequently diagnosed late because the teenager typically seeks no help until a parent or teacher notices jaundice. Such advanced rejection is often difficult to control, and frequently retransplantation becomes inevitable.

Preteens also appear to be at risk. De Bolt and coauthors[305] reported that children between 6 and 11 years of age had lower scores for social, scholastic, and physical function than healthy children did. In a large study of psychosocial adjustment in 146 patients monitored at a single center, Tornqvist and associates[306] found that older children, particularly boys, had more psychosocial adjustment problems than healthy children did. Girls perceived themselves to be less scholastically competent than their peers, whereas boys had significantly lower perceptions of their self-worth and athletic competency. The same center also reported that earlier age at transplantation was associated with higher scores for aggressive behavior and lower scores for activities and competence. The longer after transplantation, the more problems mothers reported with somatic complaints, anxiety, depression, and issues involving competence and social activities.[307] These findings shed light on the increasingly recognized problem of noncompliance in teenagers, which in this author's experience has now become a heart-breaking cause of patient death.

Such compliance issues are the single most serious and time-consuming problem that a physician managing an adolescent faces. From the physician's perspective, understanding this phenomenon is difficult and hampered by few studies providing guidance. The most published information relates to teenagers after kidney transplantation. Ettenger and colleagues described an incidence of 50% noncompliance in pediatric renal transplant patients with an associated rejection rate of 71% and graft loss rate of 13%.[308] Noncompliance was most common in teenagers, and the authors emphasize that early detection of a noncompliant teenager, before graft dysfunction occurs, is very difficult.

Several clues can tip off an astute physician that noncompliance is becoming a problem before the graft is affected. Unexpectedly low cyclosporine or tacrolimus levels are an obvious sign. However, sudden fluctuations in previously stable cyclosporine levels, particularly unusually high levels, may indicate that the patient has doubled up the previous day's dose knowing that a level will be checked at the following clinic visit. The same patient may show alternating high and low levels seemingly not responding to drug adjustments made by physicians.

A good history, sometimes obtained from the patient but often from a parent, is worth the time spent. Taking medications at increasingly erratic times ("I was too busy," "I was out with my friends," "Is it O.K. to take my cyclosporine at 3:00 AM?") is a danger sign. Noting when patients should be due for refills can help determine whether doses are being missed. Refusal to take medication under supervision and parents who choose to turn over all responsibility to their teenagers are also indicators. Missed clinic appointments, arriving late to avoid seeing their physician, changes in school performance or behavior at home, and new, perhaps less supportive friends are also clues.

Apart from the normal, if difficult-to-handle behavior patterns of adolescents, clinical depression may develop in some patients and may be manifested as noncompliance.[309] All too frequently this diagnosis is made only when the teenager is admitted deeply jaundiced and with irreversible rejection. Retransplantation with intensive psychiatric support is one option. However, most centers have had the tragic experience of the rare teenager, usually with a fractured social support system, who leaves the medical system and chooses to die instead. Intervention before such outcomes is clearly desirable but very difficult to provide.

In monitoring a teenage liver transplant patient several practical issues can be addressed. Sensitivity to questions regarding body image is needed. Steroid-induced exacerbations of acne should be aggressively treated. Periodontic care for gum hypertrophy secondary to the use of cyclosporine is appropriate, and consideration of conversion to tacrolimus, which does not have this side effect, may be suitable. Hirsutism, also secondary to cyclosporine, is especially troublesome in a teenage girl, and if depilatories are not sufficient, tacrolimus is another alternative, although temporary hair thinning may be induced. Adolescents may frequently rediscover, with dismay, their abdominal scar. In some, plastic surgical repair may even be sought.

The clinic visit is a time to reinforce the concepts of safe sexual practices and lifestyle choices. Teenagers must be educated that their risk for contracting sexually transmitted disease is likely to be higher than for their peers. Although abstinence from alcohol may be the most desirable goal, counseling teenagers that alcohol intake must be strictly limited is appropriate. Apart from the obvious dangers in any illicit drug use, transplanted teenagers should know that contaminating substances, such as microorganisms in street drugs, may be of particular harm to them.

For teenage girls, counseling to prevent or perhaps plan pregnancy is essential. After successful liver transplantation, menstrual cycles will begin by 3 months in

57% of previously amenorrheic young women and by 5 months in 80%.[310] In general, oral contraceptives should be avoided in sexually active young women because of the associated risk of hepatic adenoma.[311] However, if compliance with any other regimen is not likely, oral contraceptive use is a better alternative than an unwanted pregnancy.

Practical Problems in Pediatric Immunosuppression

The practicalities of administering essential medications to a young child on a daily basis try the ingenuity of doctors and parents alike. Not only are the number and frequency of such drugs formidable, but the ability of a young child to take solid-phase drugs is severely limited. Many of the drugs needed in pediatric transplantation are formulated to serve the needs of adults. The cooperation of a pediatric pharmacist in creating suspensions of drugs not commercially available and in appropriate concentrations to allow very small doses is essential. Commonly used medications that require suspension are azathioprine (50-mg tablets suspended in a concentration of 10 mg/1 mL) and acyclovir (200-mg tablets suspended to a concentration of 200 mg/5 mL). Another problem encountered is that pharmacies outside the transplant center are often unwilling to formulate suspensions, and consultation with the transplant pharmacist is needed.

Parents must receive education and practical advice before discharge regarding not only administration of the essential immunosuppressive agents but also their common side effects. In addition, parents are frequently asked to give a wide array of other drugs, particularly in the early posttransplant period. Being able to discern the essential from the nonessential is helpful to parents in planning dosage schedules. Because an unwilling child will frequently spit out medications or may vomit after taking several drugs, guidelines for repeat administration of the immunosuppressive drugs are needed. We advise that if vomiting or spitting up occurs within 1 hour of the dose, the whole dose should be repeated.

The medication schedule of school-age children should be arranged, if at all possible, to avoid medications at school. Frequent trips to the school nurse reinforce to children, their peers, and their teachers that they are vulnerable. However, the school nurse should be adequately informed by the transplant center of a child's immunosuppressive drugs, doses, and common side effects in case of an emergency. In addition, the nurse should be advised that the child's parents should be notified immediately if any illness occurs in the child, particularly of a febrile nature. The school nurse also plays an essential role in informing parents of outbreaks of any communicable diseases in the immediate contact group of the transplanted child, such as chickenpox, measles, and hepatitis A.

Finally, it is important to include small pediatric liver recipients in trials of potentially important new immunosuppressive agents. Careful pharmacokinetic studies and the development of suitable oral formulations are essential. Studies that are designed to meet these sometimes rigorous conditions will allow pediatric transplant recipients safe and timely access to improvements in immunosuppressive therapy.

Acknowledgement

The author wishes to thank Dinora Duarte for her invaluable expertise in preparation of this work.

References

1. Ettenger RB, Blifeld C, Prince H, et al: The pediatric nephrologist's dilemma: Growth after renal transplantation and its interaction with age as a possible immunologic variable. J Pediatr 6:1022-1025, 1987.
2. Kimball PM, Kerman RH, Portman R, et al: Pediatric patients have poorer renal allograft survival and stronger immune responses than adults. Paper presented at a meeting of the American Society of Transplant Physicians, Chicago, Illinois, 1991, p 138.
3. Wallot MA, Mathot M, Janssen M, et al: Long-term survival and late graft loss in pediatric liver transplant recipients—a 15-year single-center experience. Liver Transpl 8:615-622, 2002.
4. Sudan DL, Shaw BWJ, Langnas AN: Causes of late mortality in pediatric liver transplant recipients. Ann Surg 227:289-295, 1998.
5. Starzl TE, Klintmalm GBG, Porter KA, et al: Liver transplantation with use of cyclosporine and prednisone. N Engl J Med 305:266-269, 1981.
6. Colonna JO, Goldstein LI, Brems JJ, et al: A prospective study on the use of monoclonal anti-T3-cell antibody (OKT3) to treat steroid-resistant liver rejection. Arch Surg 122:1120-1123, 1987.
7. McDiarmid SV, Busuttil RW, Ascher NL, et al: FK506 (tacrolimus) compared with cyclosporine for primary immunosuppression after pediatric liver transplantation. Transplantation 59:530-536, 1995.
8. Ganschow R, Broering DC, Stuerenburg I, et al: First experience with basiliximab in pediatric liver graft recipients. Pediatr Transplant 5:353-358, 2001.
9. Broelsch CE, Emond JC, Whitington PF, et al: Application of reduced-size liver transplants as split grafts, auxiliary orthotopic grafts, and living related segmental transplants. Ann Surg 212:368-377, 1990.
10. Takatsuki M, Uemoto S, Inomata Y, et al: Weaning of immunosuppression in living donor liver transplant recipients. Transplantation 72:449-454, 2001.
11. McDiarmid SV, Millis MJ, Terasaki P, et al: Induction of immunosuppression in pediatric orthotopic liver transplantation. Clin Transpl 5:174-180, 1991.
12. Ettenger RB: Age and the immune response in pediatric renal transplantation. Eur J Pediatr 151:S7-S8, 1992.
13. McDiarmid SV, Busuttil RW, Terasaki P, et al: OKT3 treatment of steroid-resistant rejection in pediatric liver transplant recipients. J Pediatr Gastroenterol Nutr 14:86-91, 1992.
14. Yanase Y, Tango T, Okumura K, et al: Lymphocyte subsets identified by monoclonal antibodies in healthy children. Pediatr Res 20:1147-1151, 1986.

15. Scornik JC, Pfaff WW, Howard RJ, et al: Increased antibody responsiveness to blood transfusions in pediatric patients. Transplantation 58:1361-1365, 1994.

16. Sokal E, Veyckemans F, de Ville de Goyet J, et al: Liver transplantation in children less than 1 year of age. J Pediatr 117:205-210, 1990.

17. Goldstein G, Fuccello AJ, Norman DJ, et al: OKT3 monoclonal antibody plasma levels during therapy and the subsequent development of host antibodies to OKT3. Transplantation 42:507-511, 1986.

18. Schroeder TJ, First MR, Mansour ME, et al: Antimurine antibody formation following OKT3 therapy. Transplantation 49:48-51, 1990.

19. Payne H, Herrod G, Williams J: Evaluation of immune status in pediatric recipients of hepatic orthografts. J Pediatr Surg 23:825-828, 1988.

20. Woodle ES, Millis JM, So SKS, et al: Liver transplantation in the first three months of life. Transplantation 66:606-609, 1998.

21. Murphy MS, Harrison R, Davies P, et al: Risk factors for liver rejection: Evidence to suggest enhanced allograft tolerance in infancy. Arch Dis Child 75:502-506, 1996.

22. Martin S, Anand R, Lindblad A, et al: Studies of pediatric liver transplantation 2002: Patient and graft survival and rejection in pediatric recipients of a first liver transplant in the United States and Canada. Pediatr Transplant 8:273-283, 2004.

23. Tejani A, Stablein D, Alexander S, et al: Analysis of rejection outcomes and implications—a report of the North American Pediatric Renal Transplant Cooperative Study. Transplantation 59:500-504, 1995.

24. Bauer J, Thul J, Kramer U, et al: Heart transplantation in children and infants: Short-term outcome and long-term follow-up. Pediatr Transplant 5:457-462, 2001.

25. Balzer DT, Moorhead S, Saffitz JE, et al: Utility of surveillance biopsies in infant heart transplant recipients. J Heart Lung Transplant 14:1095-1101, 1995.

26. McDiarmid S, Anand R, Lindblad AS, SPLIT Research Group: Studies of pediatric liver transplantation: 2002 update. An overview of demographics, indications, timing, and immunosuppressive practices in pediatric liver transplantation in the United States and Canada. Pediatr Transplant 8:284-294, 2004.

27. Kelly D, Jara P, Rodeck B, et al: Tacrolimus dual therapy versus cyclosporine-microemulsion triple therapy in paediatric liver transplantation: Results from a multicentre randomized trial. Am J Transplant 2(Suppl 3):351, 2002.

28. Jain A, Mazariegos G, Kashyap R, et al: Pediatric liver transplantation. A single center experience spanning 20 years. Transplantation 73:941-947, 2002.

29. Jain A, Mazariegos G, Kashyap R, et al: Comparative long-term evaluation of tacrolimus and cyclosporine in pediatric liver transplantation. Transplantation 70:617-625, 2000.

30. Cao S, Cox KL, Berquist W, et al: Long-term outcomes in pediatric liver recipients: Comparisons between cyclosporin A and tacrolimus. Pediatr Transplant 3:22-26, 1999.

31. McDiarmid SV, Anand R: Outcome of cyclosporine- and tacrolimus-treated pediatric patients enrolled in the SPLIT registry. Transplantation 69:388, 2000.

32. Reding R: Tacrolimus in pediatric liver transplantation. Pediatr Transplant 6:447, 2002.

33. McDiarmid SV: The use of tacrolimus in pediatric liver transplantation. J Pediatr Gastroenterol Nutr 26:90-102, 1998.

34. Reding R: Steroid withdrawal in liver transplantation. Transplantation 70:405-410, 2000.

35. Moukarzel AA, Najm I, Vargas JV, et al: Prediction of long-term linear growth following liver transplantation. Transplant Proc 22:1558-1559, 1990.

36. Chin SE, Shepherd RW, Cleghorn GJ, et al: Survival, growth and quality of life in children after orthotopic liver transplantation: A 5 year experience. J Paediatr Child Health 27:380-385, 1991.

37. Sarna S, Laine J, Sipila I, et al: Differences in linear growth and cortisol production between liver and renal transplant recipients on similar immunosuppression. Transplantation 60:656-661, 1995.

38. Sarna S, Sipila I, Vihervuori E, et al: Growth delay after liver transplantation in childhood: Studies of underlying mechanisms. Pediatr Res 38:366-372, 1995.

39. McDiarmid SV, Farmer DA, Goldstein LI, et al: A randomized prospective trial of steroid withdrawal after liver transplantation. Transplantation 60:1443-1450, 1995.

40. Margarit C, Martinez-Ibanez V, Tormo R, et al: Maintenance immunosuppression without steroids in pediatric liver transplantation. Transplant Proc 21:2230-2231, 1989.

41. Superina R, Acal L, Bilik R, Zaki A: Growth in children after liver transplantation on cyclosporine alone or in combination with low-dose azathioprine. Transplant Proc 25:2580, 1993.

42. Dunn SP, Falkenstein K, Lawrence JP, et al: Monotherapy with cyclosporine for chronic immunosuppression in pediatric liver transplant recipients. Transplantation 57:544-547, 1994.

43. Dmitrewski J, Ayres S, Gunson BK, et al: Steroid withdrawal 3 months after liver transplantation—does FK506 confer any advantages over cyclosporine? Transpl Int 7:S85-S87, 1994.

44. Washburn K, Speeg KV, Esterl R, et al: Steroid elimination 24 hours after liver transplantation using daclizumab, tacrolimus, and mycophenolate mofetil. Transplantation 72:1675-1679, 2001.

45. Stegall MD, Wachs ME, Everson G, et al: Prednisone withdrawal 14 days after liver transplantation with mycophenolate: A prospective trial of cyclosporine and tacrolimus. Transplantation 64:1755-1760, 1997.

46. Eason JD, Loss GE, Blazek J, et al: Steroid-free liver transplantation using rabbit antithymocyte globulin induction: Results of a prospective randomized trial. Liver Transpl 7:693-697, 2001.

47. Birnbaum AH, Benkov KJ, Pittman NS, et al: Recurrence of autoimmune hepatitis in children after liver transplantation. J Pediatr Gastroenterol Nutr 25:20-25, 1997.

48. Renz JF, Rosenthal P, Frankel W, et al: Mycophenolate mofetil, microemulsion cyclosporine, and prednisone as primary immunosuppression for pediatric liver transplant recipients. Pediatr Transplant 2:91, 1998.

49. Chardot C, Nicoluzzi JE, Janssen M, et al: Use of mycophenolate mofetil as rescue therapy after pediatric liver transplantation. Transplantation 71:224-229, 2001.

50. Freise CE, Hebert M, Osorio RW, et al: Maintenance immunosuppression with prednisone and RS-61443 alone following liver transplantation. Transplant Proc 25:1758-1759, 1993.

51. McDiarmid SV, Busuttil RW, Levy P, et al: The long-term outcome of OKT3 compared with cyclosporine prophylaxis after liver transplantation. Transplantation 52:91-97, 1991.

52. Kelly DA: The use of anti–interleukin-2 receptor antibodies in pediatric liver transplantation. Pediatr Transplant 5:386-389, 2001.

53. Hirose R, Roberts JP, Quan D, et al: Experience with daclizumab in liver transplantation: Renal transplant dosing without calcineurin inhibitors is insufficient to prevent acute rejection in liver transplantation. Transplantation 27:307-311, 2000.

54. Heffron TG, Pillen T, Smallwood GA, et al: Single-dose induction with daclizumab immediately after liver transplantation in pediatric patients. Transplant Proc 33:1449, 2001.

55. Arora N, McKiernan PJ, Beath SV, et al: Concomitant basiliximab with low-dose calcineurin inhibitors in children post-liver transplantation. Pediatr Transplant 6:214-218, 2002.

56. Mazariegos G, Rakesh S, Smith A, et al: Rabbit anti-thymocyte globulin (rATG) induction therapy for pediatric steroid-free liver transplantation. Am J Transplant 3:453, 2003.

57. Alonso EM, Piper JB, Echols G, et al: Allograft rejection in pediatric recipients of living related liver transplants. Hepatology 23:40-43, 1996.

58. Broering DC, Mueller L, Ganschow R, et al: Is there still a need for living-related liver transplantation in children? Ann Surg 234:713-722, 2001.

59. Kasahara M, Kiuchi T, Uryuhara K, et al: Role of HLA compatibility in pediatric living-related liver transplantation. Transplantation 74:1175-1180, 2002.

60. Reding R, de Ville de Goyet J, Delbeke I, et al: Pediatric liver transplantation with cadaveric or living related donors: Comparative results in 90 elective recipients of primary grafts. J Pediatr 134:280-286, 1999.

61. Toyoki Y, Renz JF, Mudge C, et al: Allograft rejection in pediatric liver transplantation: Comparison between cadaveric and living related donors. Pediatr Transplant 6:301, 2002.

62. D'Antiga L, Dhawan A, Portman B, et al: Late cellular rejection in pediatric liver transplantation: Aetiology and outcome. Transplantation 73:80-84, 2002.

63. Anand AC, Hubscher SG, Gunson BK, et al: Timing, significance, and prognosis of late acute liver allograft rejection. Transplantation 60:1098-1103, 1995.

64. Allen KJ, Rand EB, Hart J, Whitington PF: Prognostic implications of centrilobular necrosis in pediatric liver transplant recipients. Transplantation 65:692-698, 1998.

65. Krasinskas AM, Ruchelli ED, Rand EB, et al: Central venulitis in pediatric liver allografts. Hepatology 33:1141-1147, 2001.

66. Sellers M, Singer A, Maller E, et al: Incidence of late acute rejection and progression to chronic rejection in pediatric liver recipients. Transplant Proc 29:428-429, 1997.

67. Jain A, Demetris AJ, Kashyap R, et al: Does tacrolimus offer virtual freedom from chronic rejection after primary liver transplantation? Risk and prognostic factors in 1,048 liver transplantations with a mean follow-up of 6 years. Liver Transpl 7:623-630, 2001.

68. Jain A, Mazariegos G, Pokharna R, et al: Almost total absence of chronic rejection in primary pediatric liver transplantation under tacrolimus. Transplant Proc 34:1968-1969, 2002.

69. Gupta P, Hart J, Cronin D, et al: Risk factors for chronic rejection after pediatric liver transplantation. Transplantation 72:1098-1102, 2001.

70. Gao Z, McAllister VC, Williams GM: The "privileged" liver and hepatic tolerogenicity. Repopulation of liver endothelium by bone-marrow–derived cells. Liver Transpl 7:918-920, 2001.

71. Dousset B, Conti F, Cherruau B, et al: Is acute rejection deleterious to long-term liver allograft function? J Hepatol 29:660-668, 1998.

72. Wiesner RH, Demetris AJ, Belle SH, et al: Acute hepatic allograft rejection: Incidence, risk factors, and impact on outcome. Hepatology 28:638-645, 1998.

73. McDiarmid S, Anand R, SPLIT Research Group: A multivariate analysis of factors affecting patient and graft survival after pediatric transplantation. Am J Transplant 3(Suppl 5):307, 2003.

74. McDiarmid S, Anand R, SPLIT Research Group: Immunosuppression, rejection and the effect on outcome in children after liver transplantation. Liver Transpl 9:C-47, 2003.

75. Starzl TE, Zinkernagel RM: Antigen localization and migration in immunity and tolerance. N Engl J Med 339:1905-1913, 1998.

76. Millis JM, Cronin DC, Newell KA, et al: Successful use of tacrolimus for initial rejection episodes after liver transplantation. Transplant Proc 30:1407-1408, 1998.

77. Cosimi AB, Cho SI, Delmonico FL, et al: A randomized clinical trial comparing OKT3 and steroids for treatment of hepatic allograft rejection. Transplantation 43:91-95, 1987.

78. Fung JJ, Markus BH, Gordon R, et al: Impact of Orthoclone OKT3 on liver transplantation. Transplant Proc 19:37-44, 1987.

79. Goldstein G: Overview of the development of Orthoclone OKT3: Monoclonal antibody for therapeutic use in transplantation. Transplant Proc 19:1-6, 1987.

80. Tsoukas CD, Valentine M, Lotz M, et al: The role of the T3 molecular complex in antigen recognition and subsequent activation events. Immunol Today 5:311, 1984.

81. Woodle ES, Thistlethwaite JR, Emond JC, et al: OKT3 therapy for hepatic allograft rejection. Transplantation 51:1207-1212, 1991.

82. Aw MM, Taylor RM, Verna A, et al: Basiliximab (Simulect) for the treatment of steroid-resistant rejection in pediatric liver transplant recipients: A preliminary experience. Transplantation 75:796-799, 2003.

83. Sindhi R, Webber S, Venkataramanan R, et al: Sirolimus for rescue and primary immunosuppression in transplanted children receiving tacrolimus. Transplantation 72:851-855, 2001.

84. Reyes J, Jain A, Mazariegos G, et al: Long-term results after conversion from cyclosporine to tacrolimus in pediatric liver transplantation for acute and chronic rejection. Transplantation 69:2573-2580, 2000.

85. McDiarmid SV, Klintmalm GB, Busuttil RW: FK506 conversion for intractable rejection of the liver allograft. Transpl Int 6: 305-312, 1993.

86. Abbasoglu O, Levy MF, Brkic BB, et al: Ten years of liver transplantation: An evolving understanding of late graft loss. Transplantation 64:1801-1807, 1997.

87. Ryckman FC, Alonso MH, Bucuvalas JC, Balistreri WF: Long-term survival after liver transplantation. J Pediatr Surg 34: 845-849, 1999.

88. Fridell JA, Jain A, Reyes J, et al: Causes of mortality beyond 1 year after primary pediatric liver transplant under tacrolimus. Transplantation 74:1721-1724, 2002.

89. McDiarmid S, Busuttil RW, Goss J, et al: Causes of late graft dysfunction, re-transplantation (RE-TX) and death after pediatric (OLT) orthotopic liver transplantation. Liver Transpl Surg 3:C-47, 1997.

90. Rolles K, Davidson BR, Burroughs AK: A pilot study of immunosuppressive monotherapy in liver transplantation: Tacrolimus versus microemulsified cyclosporin. Transplantation 68: 1195-1209, 1999.

91. Sarwal MN, Yorgin PD, Alexander S, et al: Promising early outcomes with a novel, complete steroid avoidance immunosuppression protocol in pediatric renal transplantation. Transplantation 72:13-21, 2001.

92. Birkeland SA, Larsen K-G, Rohr N: Pediatric renal transplantation without steroids. Pediatr Nephrol 12:87-92, 1998.

93. Reding R, Gras J, Sokal E, et al: Steroid-free liver transplantation in children: A pilot study in 20 pediatric recipients. Am J Transplant 3:452, 2003.

94. Neuhaus P, Klupp J, Langrehr JM: mTOR inhibitors: An overview. Liver Transpl 7:473-484, 2001.

95. Kahan BD: The potential role of rapamycin in pediatric transplantation as observed from adult studies. Pediatr Transplant 3:175-180, 1999.

96. Wiesner R, Klintmalm G, McDiarmid S, Rapamune Liver Transplant Study Group: Sirolimus immunotherapy results in reduced rates of acute rejection in de novo orthotopic liver transplant recipients. Am J Transplant 2:464, 2002.

97. McAlister VC, Peltekian KM, Malatjalian DA, et al: Orthotopic liver transplantation using low-dose tacrolimus and sirolimus. Liver Transpl 7:701-708, 2001.

98. Trotter JF, Wachs M, Bak T, et al: Liver transplantation using sirolimus and minimal corticosteroids (3-day taper). Liver Transpl 7:343-351, 2001.

99. Sindhi R, Ganjoo J, McGhee W, et al: Preliminary immunosuppression withdrawal strategies with sirolimus in children with liver transplants. Transplant Proc 34:1972-1973, 2002.

100. Li XC, Strom TB: Mechanisms of tolerance. In Norman DJ, Turka LA (eds): Primer on Transplantation. Mt Laurel, New Jersey, American Society of Transplantation, 2001, pp 34-42.

101. Bishop GA, McCaughan GW: Immune activation is required for the induction of liver allograft tolerance: Implications for immunosuppressive therapy. Liver Transpl 7:161-172, 2001.

102. Smiley ST, Csizmadia V, Gao W, et al: Differential effects of cyclosporine A, methylprednisolone, mycophenolate, and rapamycin on CD154 induction and requirement for NFκB. Indications for tolerance induction. Transplantation 70:415-419, 2000.

103. Sharland A, Yan Y, Wang C, et al: Evidence that apoptosis of activated T cells occurs in spontaneous tolerance of liver allografts and is blocked by manipulations which break tolerance. Transplantation 68:1736-1745, 1999.

104. Starzl TE, Demetris AJ, Trucco M, et al: Cell migration and chimerism after whole-organ transplantation: The basis of graft acceptance. Hepatology 17:1127-1152, 1993.

105. Kimikawa M, Sachs DH, Colvin RB, et al: Modifications of the conditioning regimen for achieving mixed chimerism and donor-specific tolerance in cynomolgus monkeys. Transplantation 64:709-716, 1997.

106. Cheung ST, Tsui TY, Wang WL, et al: Liver as an ideal target for gene therapy: Expression of CTLA4Ig by retroviral gene transfer. J Gastroenterol Hepatol 17:1008-1014, 2002.

107. Sho M, Sandner SE, Najafian N, et al: New insights into the interactions between T-cell costimulatory blockade and conventional immunosuppressive drugs. Ann Surg 236:667-675, 2002.

108. Rane A, Wilson JT: Clinical pharmacokinetics in infants and children. Clin Pharmacokinet 1:2-24, 1976.

109. Burckart GJ, Ptachcinski RJ, Venkataramanan R, et al: Cyclosporine trough concentration monitoring in liver transplant patients. Transplant Proc 18:188-193, 1986.

110. Whitington PF, Emond JC, Whitington SH, et al: Small-bowel length and the dose of cyclosporine in children after liver transplantation. N Engl J Med 322:733-738, 1990.

111. Yee GC, Lennon TP, Gmur DJ, et al: Age-dependent cyclosporine: Pharmacokinetics in marrow transplant recipients. Clin Pharmacol Ther 40:438-443, 1986.

112. Fruhwirth M, Fischer H, Simma B, et al: Rotavirus infection as cause of tacrolimus elevation in solid-organ–transplanted children. Pediatr Transplant 5:88-92, 2001.

113. Berengue JI, Lopez-Espinoza JA, Ortega-Lopez J, et al: Two- to three-fold increase in blood tacrolimus (FK506) levels during diarrhea in liver-transplanted children. Clin Transplant 17:249-253, 2003.

114. Mittal N, Thompson JF, Kato T, Tzakis AG: Tacrolimus and diarrhea: Pathogenesis of altered metabolism. Pediatr Transplant 5:75, 2001.

115. Jensen CWB, Flechner SM, Van Buren CT, et al: Exacerbation of cyclosporine toxicity by concomitant administration of erythromycin. Transplantation 43:263-270, 1987.

116. Gonwa TA, Nghiem DD, Schulak JA, Corry RJ: Erythromycin and cyclosporine. Transplantation 41:797-799, 1986.

117. Cockburn I: Cyclosporine A: A clinical evaluation of drug interactions. Transplant Proc 18:50-55, 1986.

118. Scott JP, Higenbottam TW: Adverse reactions and interactions of cyclosporine. Med Toxicol Adverse Drug Exp 3:107-127, 1988.

119. Al-Sulaiman MH, Dhar JM, Al-Khader AA: Successful use of rifampicin in the treatment of tuberculosis in renal transplant patients immunosuppressed with cyclosporine. Transplantation 50:597-598, 1990.

120. Van Buren CT, Wideman CA, Reid M: The antagonistic effect of rifampicin upon cyclosporine bioavailability. Transplant Proc 16:1642-1645, 1984.

121. Burckart GJ, Starzl TE, Williams L, et al: Cyclosporine monitoring and pharmacokinetics in pediatric liver transplant patients. Transplant Proc 17:1172-1175, 1985.

122. Margarit C, Martinez-Ibanez V, Potau N, et al: Cyclosporine in pediatric liver transplantation: Is there a therapeutic blood level that abrogates rejection? Transplant Proc 20:369-374, 1988.

123. Venkataramanan R, Burckart GJ, Ptachcinski RJ: Pharmacokinetics and monitoring of cyclosporine following orthotopic liver transplantation. Semin Liver Dis 5:357-368, 1985.

124. Evans GO, Griffiths PD: Limitations concerning the use in children of the relationship between plasma creatinine and body height to derive glomerular filtration rate. Ann Clin Biochem 18:295-298, 1981.

125. Dunn S, Cooney G, Sommerauer J, et al: Pharmacokinetics of an oral solution of the microemulsion formulation of cyclosporine in maintenance pediatric liver transplant recipients. Transplantation 63:1762-1767, 1997.

126. Dunn SP, Cooney GF, Kulinsky A, et al: Absorption characteristics of a microemulsion formulation of cyclosporine in de novo pediatric liver transplant recipients. Transplantation 60:1438-1442, 1995.

127. Alvarez F, Atkison PR, Grant DR, et al: NOF-11: A one-year pediatric randomized double-blind comparison of Neoral versus Sandimmune in orthotopic liver transplantation. Transplantation 69:87-92, 2000.

128. Melter M, Rodeck B, Kardorff R, et al: Pharmacokinetics of cyclosporine in pediatric long-term liver transplant recipients converted from Sandimmune to Neoral. Transpl Int 10:419-425, 1997.

129. Renz JF, Mudge CL, Heyman MB, et al: Donor selection limits use of living-related liver transplantation. Hepatology 22:1122-1126, 1995.

130. Pescovitz MD, Puente JG, Jindal RM, et al: Improved absorption of cyclosporine for microemulsion in a pediatric liver transplant recipient with cystic fibrosis. Transplantation 61:331-333, 1996.

131. Cooney GF, Dunn SP, Sommerauer J, et al: Improved cyclosporine bioavailability in black pediatric liver transplant recipients after administration of the microemulsion formulation. Liver Transpl Surg 5:112-118, 1999.

132. Superina RA, Strong DK, Acal LA, DeLuca E: Relative bioavailability of Sandimmune and Sandimmune Neoral in pediatric liver recipients. Transplant Proc 26:2979-2980, 1994.

133. Laine J, Hoppu K, Jalanko H, et al: Kidney function after 1:1 conversion to the cyclosporine microemulsion formulation in children with liver allografts. Transplantation 63:1768-1772, 1997.

134. van Mourik ID, Thomson M, Kelly DA: Comparison of pharmacokinetics of Neoral and Sandimmune in stable pediatric liver transplant recipients. Liver Transpl Surg 5:107-111, 1999.

135. D'Agostino D, Gimenez M, Yamaguchi B, et al: Conversion and pharmacokinetic studies of a microemulsion formulation of cyclosporine in pediatric liver transplant patients. Transplantation 62:1068-1071, 1996.

136. Moochhala SM, Lee EJD, Earnest L, et al: Inhibition of drug metabolism in rat and human liver microsomes by FK506 and cyclosporine. Transplant Proc 23:2786-2788, 1991.

137. Shah IA, Whitling PH, Omar G, et al: FK506 metabolism and drug interactions. Effects of FK506 on human hepatic microsomal cytochrome P-450–dependent drug metabolism in vitro. Transplant Proc 23:2783, 1991.

138. Uemoto S, Tanaka K, Honda K, et al: Experience with FK506 in living-related liver transplantation. Transplantation 55:288-292, 1993.

139. McDiarmid SV, Colonna JO, Shaked A, et al: Differences in oral FK506 dose requirements between adult and pediatric liver transplant patients. Transplantation 55:1328-1332, 1993.

140. Jain A, Fung JJ, Venkataramanan R, et al: Comparative study of cyclosporine and FK506 dosage requirement in adult and pediatric orthotopic liver transplantation. Transplant Proc 23:2763-2766, 1991.

141. Venkataramanan R, Jain A, Cadoff E, et al: Pharmacokinetics of FK506: Preclinical and clinical studies. Transplant Proc 22:52-56, 1991.

142. Venkataramanan R, Jain A, Warty VS, et al: Pharmacokinetics of FK506 in transplant patients. Transplant Proc 23:2736-2740, 1991.

143. Ericzon BG, Ekqvist B, Groth CG, Sawe J: Pharmacokinetics of FK506 during maintenance therapy in liver transplant patients. Transplant Proc 23:2775-2776, 1991.

144. Jain A, Venkataramanan R, Cadoff E, et al: Effect of hepatic dysfunction and T tube clamping on FK506 pharmacokinetics and trough concentrations. Transplant Proc 22:57-59, 1990.

145. Esquivel CO, So SK, McDiarmid SV, et al: Suggested guidelines for the use of tacrolimus in pediatric liver transplant patients [letter]. Transplantation 61:847-848, 1996.

146. Cacciarelli TV, Esquivel CO, Cox KL, et al: Oral tacrolimus (FK506) induction therapy in pediatric orthotopic liver transplantation. Transplantation 61:1188-1192, 1996.

147. MacFarlane GD, Venkataramanan R, McDiarmid SV, et al: Therapeutic drug monitoring of tacrolimus in pediatric liver transplant patients. Pediatr Transplant 5:119-124, 2001.

148. Staatz CE, Taylor PJ, Lynch SV, et al: Population pharmacokinetics of tacrolimus in children who receive cut-down or full liver transplants. Transplantation 72:1056-1061, 2001.

149. Brown NW, Aw MM, Mieli-Vergani G, et al: Mycophenolic acid and mycophenolic acid glucuronide pharmacokinetics in pediatric liver transplant recipients: Effect of cyclosporine and tacrolimus comedication. Ther Drug Monit 24:598-606, 2002.

150. Bunchman T, Navarro M, Broyer M, et al: The use of mycophenolate mofetil suspension in pediatric renal allograft recipients. Pediatr Nephrol 16:978-984, 2001.

151. Kovarik JM, Gridelli BG, Martin S, et al: Basiliximab in pediatric liver transplantation: A pharmacokinetic-derived dosing algorithm. Pediatr Transplant 6:224-230, 2002.

152. Sindhi R, Webber S, Goyal J, et al: Pharmacodynamics of sirolimus in transplanted children receiving tacrolimus. Transplant Proc 34:1960, 2002.

153. Hamilton G, Muhlbacher F, Steininger R, et al: Cyclosporine A nephrotoxicity in liver graft recipients: Determination of nephrotoxic cyclosporine blood concentrations in liver graft recipients as defined by the HPLC and RIA tests. Transplant Proc 19:4045-4048, 1987.

154. Kohlhaw K, Wonigeit K, Schafer O, et al: Association of very high blood levels of cyclosporine metabolites with clinical complications after liver transplantation. Transplant Proc 21:2232-2233, 1989.

155. Tredger JM, Steward CM, Williams R: Cyclosporine blood levels—an evaluation of radioimmunoassay with selective monoclonal or polyclonal antibodies and high-performance liquid chromatography in liver transplant recipients. Transplantation 46:681-686, 1988.

156. McDiarmid SV, Ettenger RB, Hawkins RA, et al: The impairment of true glomerular filtration rate in long-term cyclosporine-treated pediatric allograft recipients. Transplantation 49:81-85, 1990.

157. Grant D, Kneteman N, Tchervenkov J, et al: Peak cyclosporine levels (Cmax) correlate with freedom from liver graft rejection: Results of a prospective, randomized comparison of Neoral and Sandimmune for liver transplantation (NOF-8). Transplantation 67:1133-1137, 1999.

158. Canadian Neoral Renal Transplantation Study Group: Absorption profiling of cyclosporine microemulsion (Neoral) during the first 2 weeks after renal transplantation. Transplantation 72:1024-1032, 2001.

159. Dello Strologo L, Campagnano P, Federici G, Rizzoni G: Cyclosporine A monitoring in children: Abbreviated area under curve formulas and C2 level. Pediatr Nephrol 13:95-97, 1999.

160. Dunn S, Falkenstein K, Cooney G: Neoral C2 monitoring in pediatric liver transplant recipients. Transplant Proc 33:3094-3095, 2001.

161. Goldstein G, Kremer AB, Barnes L, Hirsch RL: OKT3 monoclonal antibody reversal of renal and hepatic rejection in pediatric patients. J Pediatr 111:1046-1050, 1987.

162. McDiarmid SV, Millis M, Terashita G, et al: Low serum OKT3 levels correlate with failure to prevent rejection in orthotopic liver transplant patients. Transplant Proc 22:1774-1776, 1990.

163. Shapiro R, Weismann I, Mandel H, et al: Primary hyperoxaluria type 1: Improved outcome with timely liver transplantation: A single-center report of 36 children. Transplantation 72:428-432, 2001.

164. McDiarmid SV, Colonna JO, Shaked A, et al: A comparison of renal function in cyclosporine- and FK506-treated patients after primary orthotopic liver transplantation. Transplantation 56:847-853, 1993.

165. Fung JJ, Abu-Elmagd K, Jain A, et al: A randomized trial of primary liver transplantation under immunosuppression with FK506 vs cyclosporine. Transplant Proc 23:2977-2983, 1991.

166. Laine J, Krogerus L, Fyhrquist F, et al: Renal function and histopathologic changes in children after liver transplantation. J Pediatr 125:863-869, 1994.

167. Bartosh SM, Alonso EM, Whitington PF: Renal outcomes in pediatric liver transplantation. Clin Transplant 11:354-360, 1997.

168. Tomlanovich S, Golbetz H, Perlroth M, et al: Limitations of creatinine in quantifying the severity of cyclosporine-induced chronic nephropathy. Am J Kidney Dis 8:332-337, 1986.

169. Walser M, Drew HH, LaFrance ND: Creatinine measurements often yield false estimates of progression in chronic renal failure. Kidney Int 34:412-418, 1988.

170. Davies JG, Taylor CM, White RHR, Marshall T: Clinical limitations of the estimation of glomerular filtration rate from height/plasma creatinine ratio: A comparison with simultaneous ^{51}Cr edetic acid slope clearance. Arch Dis Child 57:607-610, 1982.

171. McDiarmid SV, Ettenger RB, Fine RN, et al: Serial decrease in glomerular filtration rate in long-term pediatric liver transplantation survivors treated with cyclosporine. Transplantation 47:314-318, 1989.

172. Berg UB, Ericzon BG, Nemeth A: Renal function before and long after liver transplantation in children. Transplantation 72:631-637, 2001.

173. Waller DG, Keast CM, Fleming JS, Ackery DM: Measurement of glomerular filtration rate with technetium-99m DTPA: Comparison of plasma clearance techniques. J Nucl Med 28:372-377, 1987.

174. Chapman JR, Griffiths D, Harding NGL, Morris PJ: Reversibility of cyclosporine nephrotoxicity after three months treatment. Lancet 1:125-130, 1985.

175. Wheatley HC, Datzman M, Williams JW, et al: Long-term effects of cyclosporine on renal function in liver transplant recipients. Transplantation 43:641-647, 1987.

176. Gonwa TA, Mai ML, Melton LB, et al: End-stage renal disease (ESRD) after orthotopic liver transplantation (OLTX) using calcineurin-based immunotherapy. Risk of development and treatment. Transplantation 72:1934-1939, 2001.

177. Marsden CD: Wilson's disease. Q J Med 65:959-966, 1987.

178. SPLIT Research Group: Studies of Pediatric Liver Transplantation (SPLIT): Year 2000 outcomes. Transplantation 72:463-476, 2001.

179. Aw MM, Samaroo B, Baker AJ, et al: Calcineurin-inhibitor related nephrotoxicity—reversibility in paediatric liver transplant recipients. Transplantation 72:746-749, 2001.

180. Lopez OL, Martinez AJ, Torre-Cisneros J: Neuropathologic findings in liver transplantation: A comparative study. Transplant Proc 23:3181-3182, 1991.

181. Mueller AR, Platz KP, Bechstein WO, et al: Neurotoxicity after orthotopic liver transplantation. A comparison between cyclosporine and FK506. Transplantation 58:155-170, 1994.

182. Yamauchi A, Ieiri I, Kataoka Y, et al: Neurotoxicity induced by tacrolimus after liver transplantation: Relation to genetic

polymorphisms of the ABCB1 (MDR1) gene. Transplantation 74:571-572, 2002.

183. Stewart S, Hiltebeitel C, Nici J, et al: Neuropsychological outcome of pediatric liver transplantation. Pediatrics 87:367-376, 1991.

184. Wayman KI, Cox KL, Esquivel CO: Neurodevelopmental outcome of young children with extrahepatic biliary atresia 1 year after liver transplantation. J Pediatr 131:894-898, 1997.

185. Zitelli BJ, Miller JW, Gartner C Jr, et al: Changes in life-style after liver transplantation. Pediatrics 82:173-180, 1988.

186. van Mourik ID, Beath SV, Brook GA, et al: Long-term nutritional and neurodevelopmental outcome of liver transplantation in infants aged less than 12 months. J Pediatr Gastroenterol Nutr 30:269-275, 2000.

187. Johnston SD, Morris JK, Cramb R, et al: Cardiovascular morbidity and mortality after orthotopic liver transplantation. Transplantation 73:901-906, 2002.

188. McDiarmid SV, Gornbein JA, Fortunat M, et al: Serum lipid abnormalities in pediatric liver transplant patients. Transplantation 53:109-115, 1992.

189. Hathout EH, Chinnock RE, Johnston JK, et al: Pediatric posttransplant diabetes: Data from a large cohort of pediatric heart-transplant recipients. Am J Transplant 3:994-998, 2003.

190. Al-Uzri A, Stablein DM, A Cohn R: Posttransplant diabetes mellitus in pediatric renal transplant recipients: A report of the North American Pediatric Renal Transplant Cooperative Study (NAPRTCS). Transplantation 72:1020-1024, 2001.

191. Ganschow R, Schulz T, Meyer T, et al: Low incidence of posttransplant lymphoproliferative disease in children with low-dose immunosuppression after liver transplantation. Transplant Proc 34:1961-1962, 2002.

192. Younes BS, McDiarmid SV, Martin MG, et al: The effect of immunosuppression on posttransplant lymphoproliferative disease in pediatric liver transplant patients. Transplantation 70:94-99, 2000.

193. Penn I: The changing pattern of posttransplant malignancies. Transplant Proc 23:1101-1103, 1991.

194. Cox KL, Lawrence-Miyasaki LS, Garcia-Kennedy R, et al: An increased incidence of Epstein-Barr virus infection and lymphoproliferative disorder in young children on FK506 after liver transplantation. Transplantation 59:524-529, 1995.

195. Renard TH, Andrews W, Foster ME: Relationship between OKT3 administration, EBV seroconversion, and the lymphoproliferative syndrome in pediatric liver transplant recipient. Transplant Proc 23:1473-1476, 1991.

196. Lamy M, Favart AM, Cornu C, et al: Epstein-Barr virus infection in 59 orthotopic liver transplant patients. Med Microbiol Immunol 179:137-144, 1990.

197. Alfrey EJ, Friedman AL, Grossman RA, et al: A recent decrease in the time to development of monomorphous and polymorphous posttransplant lymphoproliferative disorder. Transplantation 54:250-253, 1992.

198. McDiarmid SV, Klintmalm GBG, Busuttil RW: FK506 conversion for intractable rejection of the liver allograft. Transpl Int 6:305-312, 1993.

199. Rustgi VK: Epstein-Barr viral infection and posttransplantation lymphoproliferative disorders. Liver Transpl Surg 1:100-108, 1995.

200. Sokal EM, Caragiozoglou T, Lamy M, et al: Epstein-Barr virus serology and Epstein-Barr virus–associated lymphoproliferative disorders in pediatric liver transplant recipients. Transplantation 56:1394-1398, 1993.

201. Ho M, Jaffe R, Miller G, et al: The frequency of Epstein-Barr virus infection and associated lymphoproliferative syndrome after transplantation and its manifestations in children. Transplantation 45:719-727, 1988.

202. Walker RC, Paya CV, Marshall WF, et al: Pretransplantation seronegative Epstein-Barr virus status is the primary risk factor for posttransplantation lymphoproliferative disorder in adult heart, lung, and other solid organ transplantations. J Heart Lung Transplant 14:214-221, 1995.

203. Cacciarelli TV, Green M, Jaffe R, et al: Management of posttransplant lymphoproliferative disease in pediatric liver transplant recipients receiving primary tacrolimus (FK506) therapy. Transplantation 66:1047-1052, 1998.

204. Smets F, Vajro P, Cornu C, et al: Indications and results of chemotherapy in children with posttransplant lymphoproliferative disease after liver transplantation. Transplantation 69:982-984, 2000.

205. McDiarmid SV, Jordan S, Lee GS, et al: Prevention and preemptive therapy of posttransplant lymphoproliferative disease in pediatric liver recipients. Transplantation 66:1604-1611, 1998.

206. Jain A, Nalesnik M, Reyes J, et al: Posttransplant lymphoproliferative disorders in liver transplantation: A 20-year experience. Ann Surg 236:429-437, 2002.

207. Newell KA, Alonso EM, Whitington PF, et al: Posttransplant lymphoproliferative disease in pediatric liver transplantation. Transplantation 62:370-375, 1996.

208. Malatack JJ, Gartner JC, Urbach AH, Zitelli BJ: Orthotopic liver transplantation, Epstein-Barr virus, cyclosporine, and lymphoproliferative disease: A growing concern. J Pediatr 118:667-675, 1991.

209. Cacciarelli TV, Green M, Jaffe R, et al: Management of posttransplant lymphoproliferative disorder (PTLD) in pediatric liver transplant recipients receiving primary tacrolimus (FK 506) therapy. Liver Transpl Surg 3:C-47, 1997.

210. McDiarmid S, Goss J, Seu P, et al: One hundred children treated with tacrolimus after primary orthotopic liver transplantation. Transplant Proc 30:1397-1398, 1998.

211. Wagner H-J, Fischer L, Jabs WJ, et al: Longitudinal analysis of Epstein-Barr viral load in plasma and peripheral blood mononuclear cells of transplanted patients by real-time polymerase chain reaction. Transplantation 74:656-664, 2002.

212. Riddler SA, Breinig MC, McKnight JL: Increased levels of circulating Epstein-Barr virus (EBV)-infected lymphocytes and decreased EBV nuclear antigen antibody responses are associated with the development of posttransplant lymphoproliferative disease in solid-organ transplant recipients. Blood 84:972-984, 1994.

213. Savoie A, Perpete C, Carpentier L, et al: Direct correlation between the load of Epstein-Barr virus–infected lymphocytes in the peripheral blood of pediatric transplant patients and risk of lymphoproliferative disease. Blood 83:2715-2722, 1994.

214. Kenagy DN, Schlesinger Y, Weck K, et al: Epstein-Barr virus DNA in peripheral blood leukocytes of patients with posttransplant lymphoproliferative disease. Transplantation 60:547-554, 1995.

215. Allen U, Hebert D, Petric M, et al: Utility of semiquantitative polymerase chain reaction for Epstein-Barr virus to measure virus load in pediatric organ transplant recipients with and without posttransplant lymphoproliferative disease. Clin Infect Dis 33:145-150, 2001.

216. Holmes RD, Orban-Eller K, Karrer FR, et al: Response of elevated Epstein-Barr virus DNA levels to therapeutic changes in pediatric liver transplant patients: 56-month follow-up and outcome. Transplantation 74:367-372, 2002.

217. Hopwood PA, Brooks L, Parratt R, et al: Persistent Epstein-Barr virus infection: Unrestricted latent and lytic viral gene expression in healthy immunosuppressed transplant recipients. Transplantation 74:194-202, 2002.

218. Savoldo B, Goss J, Liu Z, et al: Generation of autologous Epstein-Barr virus–specific cytotoxic T cells for adoptive immunotherapy in solid organ transplant recipients. Transplantation 72:1078-1086, 2001.

219. Savoldo B, Huls MH, Liu Z, et al: Autologous Epstein-Barr virus (EBV)-specific cytotoxic T cells for the treatment of persistent active EBV infection. Blood 100:4059-4066, 2002.

220. Smets F, Latinne D, Bazin H, et al: Ratio between Epstein-Barr viral load and anti–Epstein-Barr virus specific T-cell response as a predictive marker of posttransplant lymphoproliferative disease. Transplantation 73:1603-1610, 2002.

221. Heslop HE, Rooney CM: Adoptive cellular immunotherapy for EBV lymphoproliferative disease. Immunol Rev 157:218-222, 1997.

222. Dotti G, Rambaldi A, Fiocchi R, et al: Anti-CD20 antibody (rituximab) administration in patients with late occurring lymphomas after solid organ transplant. Haematologica 86:618-623, 2001.

223. Zompi S, Tulliez M, Conti F, et al: Rituximab (anti-CD20 monoclonal antibody) for the treatment of patients with clonal lymphoproliferative disorders after orthotopic liver transplantation: A report of three cases. J Hepatol 32:521-527, 2000.

224. Suzan F, Ammor M, Ribrag V: Fatal reactivation of cytomegalovirus infection after use of rituximab for a post-transplantation lymphoproliferative disorder. N Engl J Med 345:1000, 2001.

225. Savoldo B, Cubbage ML, Durett AG, et al: Generation of EBV-specific CD4 + cytotoxic T cells from virus-naive individuals. J Immunol 168:909-918, 2002.

226. Lee ES, Locker J, Nalesnik M, et al: The association of Epstein-Barr virus with smooth-muscle tumors. N Engl J Med 332:19-25, 1995.

227. Timmons CF, Dawson DB, Richards CS, et al: Epstein-Barr virus–associated leiomyosarcomas in liver transplantation recipients. Origin from either donor or recipient tissue. Cancer 76:1481-1489, 1999.

228. Yokois NU, Perlman EJ, Colombani P, et al: Kaposi's sarcoma presenting as a protracted multisystem illness in an adolescent liver transplant recipient. Liver Transpl Surg 3:541-544, 1997.

229. Danhaive O, Ninane J, Sokal E, et al: Hepatic localization of a fibrosarcoma in a child with a liver transplant. J Pediatr 120:434-437, 1992.

230. Fung JJ, Jain A, Kwak EJ, et al: De novo malignancies after liver transplantation: A major cause of late death. Liver Transpl 7:S109-S118, 2001.

231. Jain AB, Yee LD, Nalesnik MA, et al: Comparative incidence of de novo nonlymphoid malignancies after liver transplantation under tacrolimus using surveillance epidemiologic end result data. Transplantation 66:1193-1200, 1998.

232. Moukarzel AA, Najm I, Vargas JV, et al: Effect of nutritional status on outcome of orthotopic liver transplantation in pediatric patients. Transplant Proc 22:1560-1563, 1990.

233. Laine J, Homlberg C, Sipila I, et al: Growth and renal function after liver transplantation in children. Transplant Proc 24:398-400, 1992.

234. McDiarmid SV, Gornbein JA, DeSilva P, et al: Factors affecting growth after pediatric liver transplantation. Transplantation 67:404-411, 1999.

235. Blodgett FM, Burgin L, Iezzoni D, et al: Effects of prolonged cortisone therapy on the statural growth, skeletal maturation and metabolic status of children. N Engl J Med 254:636-641, 1956.

236. Pennisi AJ, Costin G, Phillips LS, et al: Somatomedin and growth hormone studies in pediatric renal allograft recipients who receive daily prednisone. Am J Dis Child 133:950-954, 1979.

237. Giustina A, Girelli A, Alberti D, et al: Effects of pyridostigmine on spontaneous and growth hormone–releasing hormone stimulated growth hormone secretion in children on daily glucocorticoid therapy after liver transplantation. Clin Endocrinol 35:491-498, 1991.

238. Sarna S, Hoppu K, Neuvonen PJ, et al:. Methylprednisolone exposure, rather than dose, predicts adrenal suppression and growth inhibition in children with liver and renal transplants. J Clin Endocrinol Metab 82:75-77, 1997.

239. Diem HV, Sokal EM, Janssen M, et al: Steroid withdrawal after pediatric liver transplantation: A long-term follow-up study in 109 recipients. Transplantation 75:1664-1670, 2003.

240. Green M: Viral infections and pediatric liver transplantation. Pediatr Transplant 6:20-24, 2002.

241. Stratta RJ, Shaefer MS, Cushing KA, et al: Successful prophylaxis of cytomegalovirus disease after primary CMV exposure in liver transplant recipients. Transplantation 51:90-97, 1991.

242. Mellon A, Shepherd RW, Faoagali JL, et al: Cytomegalovirus infection after liver transplantation in children. J Gastroenterol Hepatol 8:540-544, 1993.

243. King SM, Superina R, Andrews W, et al: Randomized comparison of ganciclovir plus intravenous immune globulin (IVIG) with IVIG alone for prevention of primary cytomegalovirus disease in children receiving liver transplants. Clin Infect Dis 25:1173-1179, 1997.

244. Norris S, Kosar Y, Donaldson N, et al: Cytomegalovirus infection after liver transplantation: Viral load as a guide to treating clinical infection. Transplantation 74:527-531, 2002.

245. Rubin RH, Kemmerly SA, Conti D, et al: Prevention of primary cytomegalovirus disease in organ transplant recipients with oral ganciclovir or oral acyclovir prophylaxis. Transpl Infect Dis 2:112-117, 2000.

246. Winston DJ, Imagawa DK, Holt CD, et al: Long-term ganciclovir prophylaxis eliminates serious cytomegalovirus disease in liver transplant recipients receiving OKT3 therapy for rejection. Transplantation 60:1357-1360, 1995.

247. Pescovitz MD, Brook B, Jindal RM, et al: Oral ganciclovir in pediatric transplant recipients: A pharmacokinetic study. Clin Transplant 11:613-617, 1997.

248. Pescovitz M: Oral ganciclovir and pharmacokinetics of valganciclovir in liver transplant patients. Transpl Infect Dis 1:31-34, 1999.

249. Stratta RJ, Shaeffer MS, Markin RS, et al: Cytomegalovirus infection and disease after liver transplantation. An overview. Dig Dis Sci 37:673-688, 1992.

250. Dummer JS: Cytomegalovirus infection after liver transplantation: Clinical manifestations and strategies for prevention. Rev Infect Dis 12:S767-S775, 1990.

251. Griffiths PD: Cytomegalovirus and the liver. Semin Liver Dis 4:307-313, 1984.

252. Dussaix E, Wood C: Cytomegalovirus infection in pediatric liver recipients. A virological survey and prophylaxis with CMV immune globulin and early DHPG treatment. Transplantation 48:272-274, 1989.

253. King SM, Petric M, Superina RA, et al: Cytomegalovirus infections in pediatric liver transplantation. Am J Dis Child 144:1307-1310, 1990.

254. Gorensek MJ, Carey WD, Vogt D, Goormastic M: A multivariate analysis of risk factors for cytomegalovirus infection in liver-transplant recipients. Gastroenterology 98:1326-1332, 1990.

255. Hooks MA, Perlino CA, Henderson JM, et al: Prevalence of invasive cytomegalovirus disease with administration of muromonab CD-3 in patients undergoing orthotopic liver transplantation. Ann Pharmacother 26:617-620, 1992.

256. Stratta RJ, Shaefer MS, Markin R, et al: Clinical patterns of cytomegalovirus disease after liver transplantation. Arch Surg 124:1443-1450, 1989.

257. Salt A, Sutehall G, Sargaison M, et al: Viral and *Toxoplasma gondii* infections in children after liver transplantation. J Clin Pathol 43:63-67, 1990.

258. Boudreaux JP, Hayes DH, Mizrahi S, et al: Decreasing incidence of serious cytomegalovirus infection using ganciclovir prophylaxis in pediatric liver transplant patients. Transplant Proc 25:1872, 1993.

259. Freise CE, Pons V, Lake J, et al: Comparison of three regimens for cytomegalovirus prophylaxis in 147 liver transplant recipients. Transplant Proc 23:1498-1500, 1991.

260. White NJ, Juel-Jensen BE: Infectious mononucleosis hepatitis. Semin Liver Dis 4:301-306, 1984.

261. Feldman S, Hughes WT, Daniel CB: Varicella in children with cancer: Seventy-seven cases. Pediatrics 56:388-397, 1975.

262. Finkel KC: Mortality from varicella in children receiving adrenocorticosteroids and adrenocorticotropin. Pediatrics 28:436-441, 1961.

263. Morgan ER, Smalley LA: Varicella in immunocompromised children. Am J Dis Child 137:883-885, 1983.

264. Alonso EM, Fox AS, Franklin WA, Whitington PF: Postnecrotic cirrhosis following varicella hepatitis in a liver transplant patient. Transplantation 49:650-653, 1990.

265. Patti ME, Selvaggi KJ, Kroboth FJ: Varicella hepatitis in the immunocompromised adult: A case report and review of the literature. Am J Med 88:77-80, 1990.

266. Varicella-zoster infections. In Peter G (ed): Report of the Committee of Infectious Diseases. Elk Grove Village, IL, American Academy of Pediatrics, 1991, pp 517-521.

267. Antiviral drugs. In Peter G (ed): Report of the Committee of Infectious Diseases. Elk Grove Village, IL, American Academy of Pediatrics, 1991, p 579.

268. Deen JL, Blumberg DA: Infectious disease considerations in pediatric organ transplantation. Semin Pediatr Surg 2:218-234, 1993.

269. Takahashi M: Clinical overview of varicella vaccine: Development and early studies. Pediatrics 78:736-741, 1986.

270. White CJ, Kuter BJ, Hildebrand CS, et al: Varicella vaccine (VARIVAX) in healthy children and adolescents: Results from clinical trials, 1987 to 1989. Pediatrics 87:604-610, 1991.

271. Lawrence R, Gershon AA, Holzman R, Steinberg SP: The risk of zoster after varicella vaccination in children with leukemia. N Engl J Med 3:543-548, 1988.

272. Plotkin SA: Hell's fire and varicella-vaccine safety. N Engl J Med 318:573-575, 1988.

273. Gershon AA, Steinberg SP, Gelb L: Live attenuated varicella vaccine use in immunocompromised children and adults. Pediatrics 78:757-762, 1986.

274. Furth SL, Fivush BA:. Varicella vaccination in pediatric kidney transplant candidates. Pediatr Transplant 6:97-100, 2002.

275. Humar A, Kumar D, Caliendo AM, et al: Clinical impact of human herpesvirus 6 infection after liver transplantation. Transplantation 73:599-604, 2002.

276. Razonable RR, Paya CV: The impact of human herpesvirus-6 and -7 infection on the outcome of liver transplantation. Liver Transpl 8:651-658, 2002.

277. DesJardin JA, Cho E, Supran S, et al: Association of human herpesvirus 6 reactivation with severe cytomegalovirus-associated disease in orthotopic liver transplant recipients. Clin Infect Dis 33:1358-1362, 2001.

278. Lautenschlager I, Lappalainen M, Linnavuori K, et al: CMV infection is usually associated with concurrent HHV-6 and HHV-7 antigenemia in liver transplant patients. J Clin Virol 25:S57-S61, 2002.

279. Koneru B, Jaffe R, Esquivel CO, et al: Adenoviral infections in pediatric liver transplant recipients. JAMA 258:489-492, 1987.

280. Breinig MK, Zitelli B, Starzl TE, Ho M: Epstein-Barr virus, cytomegalovirus, and other viral infections in children after liver transplantation. J Infect Dis 156:273-279, 1987.

281. Gross PA, Lee H, Wolff JA, et al: Influenza immunization in immunosuppressed children. J Pediatr 72:29-32, 1979.

282. Burbach G, Bienzle U, Stark K, et al: Influenza vaccination in liver transplant recipients. Transplantation 67:753-755, 1999.

283. Pollack P, Groothuis JR: Development and use of palivizumab (Synagis): A passive immunoprophylactic agent for RSV. J Infect Chemother 8:201-206, 2002.

284. Weisman LE: Current respiratory syncytial virus prevention strategies in high-risk infants. Pediatr Int 44:475-480, 2002.

285. Michaels MG, Green M, Wald ER, Starzl TE: Adenovirus infection in pediatric liver transplant recipients. J Infect Dis 165:170-174, 1992.

286. Cames B, Rahier J, Burtomboy G, et al: Acute adenovirus hepatitis in liver transplant recipients. J Pediatr 120:33-37, 1992.

287. Gavin PJ, Katz BZ: Intravenous ribavirin treatment for severe adenovirus disease in immunocompromised children. Pediatrics 110:e9, 2002.

288. Gindler JS, Atkinson WL, Markowitz LE, Hutchins SS: Epidemiology of measles in the United States in 1989 and 1990. Pediatr Infect Dis J 11:841-846, 1992.

289. Recommendations of the Advisory Committee on Immunization Practices (ACIP): Use of vaccines and immune globulins for persons with altered immunocompetence. MMWR Morb Mortal Wkly Rep 42(RR-4):1-18, 1993.

290. Rand EB, McCarthy CA, Whitington PF: Measles vaccination after orthotopic liver transplantation. J Pediatr 123:87-89, 1993.

291. Kano H, Mizuta K, Sakakihara Y, et al: Efficacy and safety of immunization for pre– and post–liver transplant children. Transplantation 74:543-550, 2002.

292. Measles. In Peter G (ed): Report of the Committee of Infectious Diseases. Elk Grove Village, IL, American Academy of Pediatrics, 1991, pp 308-323.

293. Burroughs M, Moscona A: Immunization of pediatric solid organ transplant candidates and recipients. Clin Infect Dis 30:857-869, 2000.

294. Pesanti EL: Immunologic defects and vaccination in patients with chronic renal failure. Infect Dis Clin North Am 15:813-832, 2001.

295. Van Thiel DH, el-Ashmawy L, Love K, et al: Response to hepatitis B vaccination by liver transplant candidates. Dig Dis Sci 37:1245-1249, 1992.

296. Arslan M, Wiesner RH, Sievers C, et al: Double-dose accelerated hepatitis B vaccine in patients with end-stage liver disease. Liver Transpl 7:314-320, 2001.

297. Arslan M, Wiesner RH, Poterucha JJ, Zein NN: Safety and efficacy of hepatitis A vaccination in liver transplantation recipients. Transplantation 72:272-276, 2001.

298. Marshall GS, Barbour SD: Meaningful immunization for the immune-deficient child. Contemp Pediatr 109-124, 1989.

299. McCashland TM, Preheim LC, Gentry MJ: Pneumococcal vaccine response in cirrhosis and liver transplantation. J Infect Dis 181:757-760, 2000.

300. Kumar D, Rotstein C, Miyata G, et al: Randomized, double-blind, controlled trial of pneumococcal vaccination in renal transplant recipients. J Infect Dis 187:1639-1645, 2003.

301. Duca P, Del Pont JM, D'Agostino D: Successful immune response to a recombinant hepatitis B vaccine in children after liver transplantation. J Pediatr Gastroenterol Nutr 32:168-170, 2001.

302. Ericsson CD: Travellers with pre-existing medical conditions. Int J Antimicrob Agents 21:181-188, 2003.

303. Dropulic LK, Rubin RH, Bartlett JG: Smallpox vaccination and the patient with an organ transplant. Clin Infect Dis 36:786-788, 2003.

304. Spencer RC: *Bacillus anthracis*. J Clin Pathol 56:182-187, 2003.

305. DeBolt AJ, Stewart SM, Kennard BD, et al: A survey of psychosocial adaptation in long-term survivors of pediatric liver transplants. Child Health Care 24:79-96, 1995.

306. Tornqvist J, Van Broeck N, Finkenauer C, et al: Long-term psychosocial adjustment following pediatric liver transplantation. Pediatr Transplant 3:115-125, 1999.

307. Schwering KL, Febo-Mandl F, Finkenauer C, et al: Psychological and social adjustment after pediatric liver transplantation as a function of age at surgery and of time elapsed since transplantation. Pediatr Transplant 1:99-100, 1997.

308. Ettenger RB, Rosenthal T, Marik J, et al: Cadaver renal transplantation in children: Long-term impact of new immunosuppressive strategies. Clin Transplant 5:197-203, 1991.

309. Kiley DJ, Lam CS, Pollak R: A study of treatment compliance following kidney transplantation. Transplantation 55:51-56, 1993.

310. Cundyl TF, O'Grady JG, Williams R: Recovery of menstruation and pregnancy after liver transplantation. Gut 31:337-338, 1990.

311. Greer T: Hepatic adenoma and oral contraceptive use. J Fam Pract 28:322-326, 1989.

312. McDiarmid SV, Colonna JO 2nd, Shaked A, et al: Differences in oral FK506 dose requirements between adult and pediatric liver transplant patients. Transplantation 55:1328-1332, 1993.

77

Treatment of Acute and Chronic Rejection

IAN C. CARMODY
PAULINE W. CHEN

Acute rejection   1264
  Immune mechanisms and pathology   1264
  Clinical findings and diagnosis   1264
  Treatment   1266
  Pediatric population   1270
  Outcomes   1270

Late acute rejection   1270

Chronic rejection   1270
  Immune mechanisms and pathology   1270
  Clinical findings and diagnosis   1271
  Treatment   1271

Hyperacute rejection   1271
  Immune mechanisms and pathology   1272
  Clinical findings and diagnosis   1272
  Treatment   1272

Future   1272

Conclusions   1272

Advances in the treatment of rejection have mirrored the evolution of liver transplantation. In the earliest days of transplantation, clinical outcomes were marred by fatal complications related to ischemia, preservation injury, surgical technique, and infection. Grafts that would survive long enough to succumb to rejection were rare. Moreover, tackling rejection was not yet part of the transplant paradigm, and organs that did survive were eventually ruined by rejection. Despite the first successful transplantation of kidneys between identical twins, theoretical immunologists and other naysayers predicted devastating consequences of transplantation between individuals who were not genetically identical.[1-4]

During the late 1960s and early 1970s, however, considerable progress was made in the surgical technique and selection and postoperative care of transplant patients. Early work in immunosuppression began changing the landscape of clinical transplantation. Surgeons started to transplant successfully and consistently between unrelated individuals. With these improvements, the notion of halting or even reversing the rejection process came to the fore. Notable advances were achieved in the area of pharmacological modulation of the immune system. Immunosuppression, at first akin to an unwieldy hammer, became more precise and directed at specific steps in the immunological process. The advent of less toxic medications, such as cyclosporine and later tacrolimus, revolutionized transplantation of all organs. Concurrently, the side effects of these medications, often apparent only after long-term use, were tempered, and new, less toxic immunosuppressive protocols were devised. With these discoveries, liver transplantation, once an experimental modality, became the accepted standard of care for most patients suffering from end-stage liver disease.[5,6]

Currently, long-term graft survival is a reality. As a consequence, there continues to be new research and developments in the treatment of rejection. Like many of the early once-fatal complications, the diagnosis of rejection has become less devastating and significantly less ominous. In the quotidian life of the long-term liver transplant patient, morbidity from the chronic use of immunosuppressive agents is beginning to surpass rejection as the major concern. Even chronic rejection is now responsible for only a small proportion of graft loss and mortality, whereas immunosuppression-related sequelae such as sepsis, atherosclerosis, renal failure, and post-transplant malignancy form the overwhelming concerns.[7]

In this chapter we review the treatment of several forms of rejection after liver transplantation. Because preceding chapters have reviewed the pathology of rejection and the pharmacology of immunosuppressive agents in detail, we concentrate here on the treatment of rejection.

Rejection can be classified as acute, late acute, chronic, and hyperacute. Each of these processes requires a thoughtful therapeutic approach. Acute rejection is the most common form of rejection and usually responds well to steroid therapy. Chronic rejection was once believed to be irreversible, but over the past decade there have been improvements in its treatment. Late acute rejection represents the continuum between acute and chronic rejection. Hyperacute rejection is rare, but extremely rapid, and can lead to graft loss.

Acute Rejection

The definition of acute rejection (AR) has evolved over the past 40 years. Broadly defined as graft inflammation, AR represents immunological injury elicited as a consequence of the genetic disparity between donor and recipient. AR can develop anytime from several days to more than a week after transplantation, with the peak incidence occurring between 8 and 10 days after transplantation. The vast majority of AR episodes take place within the first 3 months after transplantation.[8] AR is the most common form of rejection and, fortunately, the most responsive to treatment. Some authors have documented the incidence of AR in orthotopic liver transplantation to be as high as 70%. Moreover, after a first diagnosis of AR, 20% of patients subsequently experience a second attack, and 4% eventually have a third episode.[9-11]

When compared with other solid-organ transplant patients, AR develops in liver transplant patients with equal or greater frequency. Fortunately for this group of patients, the sequelae of AR in liver grafts are generally less significant than in other solid organs. This difference may be due to the protective mechanisms and regenerative capabilities of the liver. In fact, the liver itself may be an immune modulator. The liver's capacity to affect the immune system is most dramatically illustrated by its impact on other organs in combined transplants. Patients who receive combined grafts consisting of a liver with any other organ tend to have lower rates of all forms of rejection. Although it remains unclear why the liver lessens the impact of the immune system on transplanted organs in general, and the concept is controversial, proposed mechanisms include the development of chimerism by soluble HLA secreted by the liver graft.[12]

Additionally, the liver differs from other solid organs in the experimental observation of tolerance. Experimental hepatic tolerance was first recognized in 1965 when liver grafts transplanted between outbred pigs survived without immunosuppression.[13] In later animal studies, Calne and colleagues demonstrated the immunomodulatory effect of liver transplantation when isogenic skin grafts had prolonged subsequent survival.[14,15] In humans, there have been anecdotal reports of tolerance developing in transplanted patients who were weaned from, or noncompliant with, immunosuppressive therapy.[16]

Several risk factors for the development of AR have been established. The most common risk factor is inadequate immunosuppression, with AR being more likely to develop in patients who are not receiving or absorbing adequate immunosuppression. Other important risk factors include having an underlying autoimmune disease, being the female recipient of a male donor organ, and having fewer HLA matches at the DR locus.[17,18] The type of immunosuppression used may also have an impact on the development of AR; patients who receive tacrolimus have lower rates of rejection than those who receive cyclosporine.[18]

Immune Mechanisms and Pathology

AR is mediated predominantly by effector (killer) T cells that develop in response to donor antigens from the transplanted organ. This inflammation initially affects the biliary epithelium and subsequently the hepatocytes. Histological examination of liver tissue reveals a mixed cellular infiltrate composed predominantly of lymphocytes localized to the portal tracts and the central vein areas. Early histological changes, however, are often nonspecific and may be confused with recurrent hepatitis C infection. With time or severity, damage to bile ducts and to the central vein endothelium occurs.

Clinical Findings and Diagnosis

Most cases of AR are manifested as asymptomatic biochemical changes. These biochemical changes almost always occur before clinical signs and symptoms and

Table 77–1. SIGNS AND SYMPTOMS OF ACUTE REJECTION

Fever

Malaise

Abdominal pain

Ascites

Hepatomegaly

Anorexia

are a manifestation of the cholestatic inflammation first affecting the biliary epithelium and subsequently the hepatocytes. Accordingly, subtle increases can first be seen in bilirubin, alkaline phosphatase, and γ-glutamyltransferase. Shortly thereafter, a rise in serum transaminase levels is seen. Although no absolute biochemical parameters can currently be used to define an episode of rejection, clinicians base their suspicions on a relative rise in numbers, the amount of time elapsed since transplantation, and the underlying disease.

Clinical findings tend to appear later in the course of rejection and reflect more significant injury to the graft. These signs and symptoms can include fatigue, fever, malaise, abdominal pain, decreased bile output, increasing ascites, and hepatomegaly (Table 77–1). If bile is available for inspection through a T tube, it may be lighter in color and less viscous.

The "gold standard" for the diagnosis of AR is percutaneous liver biopsy.[19] Although invasive, this diagnostic procedure affords the greatest sensitivity and specificity in the diagnosis of AR. However, percutaneous liver biopsy is not without risk. Although bleeding is the most common complication, serious hemorrhagic complications can occur in 0.06% to 0.35% of cases. Other complications include pneumothorax, hemobilia, peritonitis, perforated viscus, and the development of an arteriovenous fistula. The risk of sustaining any of these complications is about 2%, and the risk of death hovers between 0.009% and 0.1%.[20-22] Because the most common complication is bleeding, clinicians should attempt to correct any coagulopathy before performing this procedure.

On occasion, despite percutaneous biopsy, the diagnosis of rejection can remain in doubt, particularly since other causes of acute inflammation in the liver can be confused with AR. Most frequently, cytomegalovirus (CMV) infection and recurrence or persistence of hepatitis C make the diagnosis of AR quite difficult. Treating presumptive AR with increased immunosuppression can be devastating if, in fact, the actual diagnosis is hepatitis C. In these situations, repeat biopsy before treatment may be of help.

Protocol biopsies in the postoperative period are advocated in some centers as a way to treat rejection more effectively. By increasing sensitivity and specificity,

protocol biopsies allow one to diagnose AR while it is still at the subclinical level. The underlying assumption in performing protocol biopsies is that early diagnosis and treatment of AR may be of benefit. Although no multicenter randomized controlled trial has ever been conducted, some centers treat based on histological criteria without biochemical evidence of graft dysfunction. These preemptive efforts have not been conclusively shown to be beneficial in liver transplant patients. Recent data suggest that this approach may be overly cautious and may lead to overtreatment. From 15 studies of patients undergoing protocol biopsies, 302 patients were identified who had histological, but no biochemical evidence of rejection. Of these patients, only 36 subsequently experienced clinical rejection, 7 of which were steroid resistant and 9 of which were chronic rejection.[11]

Despite the sensitivity and specificity of percutaneous liver biopsy, the procedure remains an invasive one with all the attendant risk of morbidity and mortality. Numerous investigators have searched for safer and less invasive diagnostic methods, as well as ones that would potentially diagnose AR at an earlier time point. Some centers have tried fine-needle aspiration.[23-26] However, no large randomized controlled studies have examined this issue in liver transplant patients. Although the smaller bore of the fine needle may result in less trauma, this risk may be amplified by the need to perform multiple passes because insufficient quantity of tissue may be obtained with a single pass.[27] In addition, the subtle changes of early AR may be missed because of sampling error, with a subsequent delay in diagnosis and treatment. "Overcalling" AR can also occur and result in a needless increase in immunosuppression with its attendant morbidity. Moreover, in cases in which chronic rejection is also being considered, fine-needle aspiration has no diagnostic role because a core needle biopsy is required to more accurately assess hepatic histology.[28]

Biliary aspirates from indwelling T tubes, cytokine profiling, histological analysis of cellular aspirates, cellular Fas ligand analysis, and isotope scanning, along with other noninvasive technologies, have also been investigated in the laboratory and the clinic. All these methods, however, have been hampered by suboptimal sensitivity or specificity because of similarities between AR and other forms of acute inflammation.[29-39] Recently, quantification of granzyme expression in fine-needle aspirates has been investigated with moderate success.[40] Although this technique has been used with a high level of accuracy for the diagnosis of AR in renal allografts,[41] the presence of CMV infection appears to decrease the accuracy of this method in liver transplants.

Thus, despite numerous attempts to use noninvasive techniques over the past 20 years, none of these diagnostic methods have been validated or meet the sensitivity and specificity of percutaneous liver biopsy.

Table 77–2. DIFFERENTIAL DIAGNOSIS OF ACUTE REJECTION
First Month after Transplantation
Vascular complications
Hepatic artery thrombosis
Portal vein thrombosis
Vena cava/hepatic vein obstruction
Biliary leak
Preservation injury
Intra-abdominal sepsis
First Year after Transplantation
Infection
Hepatitis C persistence/recurrence
Intrahepatic abscess
Opportunistic infections: cytomegalovirus, Epstein-Barr virus, herpes simplex virus
Biliary complications
Stricture
Cholangitis
Drug toxicity
Longer than 1 Year after Transplantation
Chronic rejection
Recurrent disease
Autoimmune hepatitis
Primary sclerosing cholangitis
Posttransplant lymphoproliferative disease
Steatohepatitis

Table 77–3. POTENTIAL CAUSES OF REJECTION
Malabsorption
Vomiting
Diarrhea
T-tube losses
Fistula output
Immunosuppression
Underdosing
Steroid-weaning protocols
Noncompliance
Adverse effects
Psychosocial issues
Concomitant disease
Infection
Recurrent disease
Drug interactions

Core needle liver biopsy remains the procedure of choice for the diagnosis of AR.

Before initiating treatment of AR, other diagnoses should be considered (Table 77–2). Potentially confounding differential diagnoses are often time dependent. Within the first month after transplantation, other possible diagnoses include preservation injury, early hepatic artery thrombosis, portal vein thrombosis, biliary leak, CMV infection, and intra-abdominal sepsis. After the early postoperative period until approximately a year after transplantation, recurrence or persistence of hepatitis C, drug toxicity, biliary strictures, and opportunistic infections may be confused with AR. After the first year, late mimics of AR can include late hepatic artery thrombosis, recurrent autoimmune hepatitis, recurrent primary sclerosing cholangitis, chronic rejection, and posttransplant lymphoproliferative disorder (PTLD). Once treatment has started, every effort should be made to also eliminate or decrease potentially aggravating factors (Table 77–3). Conditions such as diarrhea and drug interactions can lead to suboptimal levels of immunosuppression and hamper effective therapy and resolution of AR. As many as 50% of patients suffering from AR may have one or more of these aggravating factors.[42]

Treatment

After the diagnosis of AR is established, therapy first consists of optimization of maintenance immunosuppression (Fig. 77–1). The dosage of the patient's mainstay calcineurin inhibitor can be increased, and other immunosuppressive agents such as mycophenolate mofetil, azathioprine, and rapamycin, if not currently being taken, can also be added. If the AR does not appear to respond to these initial measures, intravenous and high-dose steroid therapy can be implemented. Antilymphocytic antibodies and newer agents such as interleukin-2 receptor antagonists (IL-2RAs) are reserved for rarer cases of steroid-resistant AR or for the occasional severe case of untreated AR.

Such treatment is associated with a constellation of potential toxicities, including a risk of excessive immunosuppression and infection. Of concern as well is the risk for PTLD. These risks and benefits must be considered in each individual case. Although treatment of the AR episode will ameliorate or reduce symptoms, liver grafts generally do not suffer from long-term sequelae as a result of early episodes of AR. Unlike renal allografts, there is no direct correlation between the number of AR episodes and long-term graft or patient survival. (There is some controversy about these statements.) Generally, however, once AR is diagnosed from histological and clinical or biochemical evidence, the benefits of treatment outweigh the risks.

After AR is adequately treated, maintenance immunosuppression may be changed or increased for

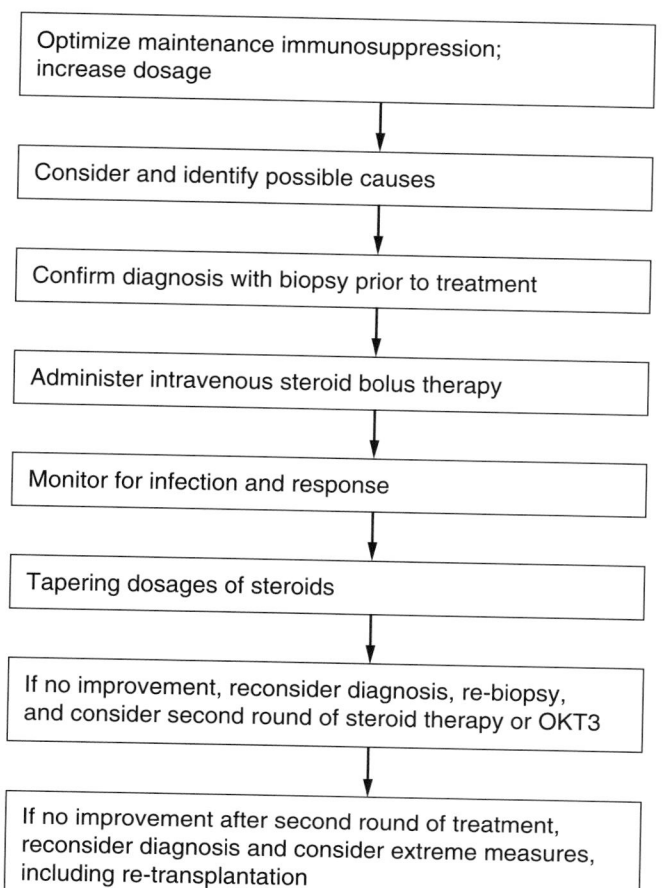

FIGURE 77–1

Treatment of acute rejection.

Table 77–4. POTENCY AND HALF-LIVES OF COMMONLY USED GLUCOCORTICOIDS		
Agent	Potency	Half-Life
Hydrocortisone (Solu-Cortef)	1	90 min
Prednisone	4–5	60 min
Prednisolone	4–5	200 min
Methylprednisolone (Solu-Medrol)	6–7	240 min

to use them sparingly. In AR, however, corticosteroids remain first-line therapy.

Mechanism of Action. Corticosteroids are 21-carbon steroid hormones derived from the metabolism of cholesterol, and their efficacy is dependent on the presence of a hydroxyl group on carbon 11. Corticosteroids have nonspecific anti-inflammatory effects. After binding to high-affinity receptors in cytoplasm, the steroid-receptor complex enters the nucleus and binds to DNA. Transcription is triggered, with the eventual synthesis of proteins. The upregulated proteins that result from steroid binding are responsible for many of the anti-inflammatory effects. Among the many immunosuppressive effects of corticosteroids: phagocytosis by neutrophils and monocytes is inhibited and disruption of T-cell activation occurs.

Current Use. No consensus has been reached on the optimal form, dosage, or length of treatment with corticosteroids. Trials have been conducted to compare different protocols of steroid therapy, and unfortunately, it is difficult to extrapolate general conclusions from these small and heterogeneous reports.[43,44] Moreover, not all steroids are equivalent in strength, and their relative potencies should be known to the administering clinician (Table 77–4).

One possible protocol for steroid treatment is given in Table 77–5. Regardless of which steroid protocol is used, several caveats should be observed. Given the debilitated state of the liver in AR, the steroid chosen should not be dependent on hepatic metabolism for its

several months to reduce the probability of relapse. For patients being treated with cyclosporine-based immunosuppressive regimens, changing maintenance therapy to tacrolimus may also help treat and decrease the incidence of acute and chronic rejection.[18] Other immunosuppressive agents may be added, and patients previously receiving dual therapy may temporarily be maintained on triple or even quadruple therapy.

Pediatric patients in whom AR is diagnosed have very specific concerns in their treatment, and these issues are reviewed later.

Corticosteroids

History. Corticosteroids were first used clinically for transplantation of renal allografts during the early 1960s. For many years, corticosteroids remained a mainstay of immunosuppressive therapy and ceded their major role only when calcineurin inhibitors were accepted into regular clinical practice in the mid-1980s. Over the past 4 decades, the panoply of complications related to long-term use has led most transplant centers

Table 77–5. STEROID TREATMENT PROTOCOL FOR ACUTE REJECTION	
Day 1	Solu-Medrol, 1000 mg IVPB × 1 over 1-hr period
Day 2	Solu-Medrol, 1000 mg IVPB × 1 over 1-hr period
Day 3	Solu-Medrol, 50 mg IVP q6h × 4 doses
Day 4	Solu-Medrol, 40 mg IVP q6h × 4 doses
Day 5	Solu-Medrol, 30 mg IVP q6h × 4 doses
Day 6	Solu-Medrol, 20 mg IVP q6h × 4 doses
Day 7	Solu-Medrol, 20 mg IVP q12h × 2 doses
Day 8	Resume prednisone, 20 mg PO qd

IVP, intravenous push; IVPB, intravenous piggyback.

active form. The half-life should be long enough to afford reversal of the rejection process but not so long that long-term steroid side effects are introduced. Finally, the steroid should have as little mineralocorticoid effect as possible to avoid sodium retention, weight gain, and hypertension.

The most common initial step in the treatment of AR is a series of intravenous steroid boluses administered over a 3-day period, followed by a scheduled tapering dosage of an oral steroid. Intravenous steroid administration is used initially because this route of administration results in the fastest and most consistent serum levels. Usually well tolerated, this treatment protocol can be administered to outpatients, but it may be associated with increased rates of sepsis and an accelerated progression to cirrhosis in patients with hepatitis C.[45] While undergoing treatment, patients should be regularly assessed for both clinical and biochemical responses. Approximately 90% of patients with AR respond to steroid treatment.

In patients without clinical or biochemical improvement, ongoing rejection should be suspected. A second percutaneous liver biopsy should be performed and liver histology re-examined. Patients whose biopsy findings continue to be consistent with rejection may have steroid-resistant AR, and other treatment options must be entertained. Occasionally, these patients are first treated with another course of intravenous steroid therapy, particularly if they have responded in the distant past or if there is evidence of even slight improvement. However, for the most part, patients with steroid-resistant AR are treated with other therapeutic modalities, and their overall outcomes tend to be worse than those of patients who respond to steroid treatment.

Antilymphocyte Antibodies

History. Early immunosuppression tended to have more generalized effects on the immune system. The development of antilymphocyte antibodies, however, allowed clinicians to target the immune system more selectively. The first antilymphocyte antibodies were obtained by using the serum of animals (e.g., horses or rabbits) challenged with recipient lymphocytes. These early antibody preparations, called antilymphocyte antibodies or antilymphocytic globulins (ALGs), were polyclonal with a broad and relatively unselective spectrum of activity against the immune system.

Initial attempts to use ALG were complicated by occasional severe anaphylactic-like reactions because of the presence of foreign animal haptens. As laboratory techniques improved, a "second generation" of more selective antilymphocyte antibodies was created, which resulted clinically in a reduction in anaphylactic-like reactions and more selective lysis.

Mechanism of Action. Antilymphocyte antibodies have been shown to work indirectly through complement-dependent lysis of lymphoid cells. In homogeneous monoclonal antibody preparations, such activity is directed against a single surface structure on the lymphoid cells. Monoclonal anti-CD3 antibodies are the most commonly used antilymphocyte antibody. Directed against the CD3 component of the T-cell receptor, these monoclonal antibodies have been shown to be quite potent and able to lyse a significant fraction of CD3-positive lymphocytes within minutes of administration. Patients who receive multiple administrations of this antibody have a significantly increased risk of infection and malignancy. Consequently, these agents tend to be reserved for either induction immunosuppression in high-risk patients or, more commonly, salvage therapy in patients with steroid-resistant AR or chronic rejection.[46]

OKT3. OKT3 (Orthoclone) is the most frequently used antilymphocyte antibody in the treatment of AR. The effectiveness of OKT3 in cases of steroid-resistant AR has been well documented.[47] Most commonly, OKT3 is administered intravenously at a dose of 5 mg/day for 7 to 14 days, and patients require hospitalization during this period. In addition to assessment of response, these patients require surveillance for potential complications, as well as premedication with steroids, acetaminophen, and antihistamines to reduce common reactions to the drug. Response to OKT3 therapy is evaluated by clinical assessment, measurement of transaminase levels, and in some centers, quantification of serum CD3 cell levels. The vast majority of patients with AR respond to either steroids or OKT3.

Antilymphocyte/Antithymocyte Globulin. ALG (Thymoglobulin) and antithymocyte globulin (ATG) are less commonly used antilymphocyte antibody preparations. Generally considered a second choice, ALG/ATG is used when treatment with monoclonal antibodies is not suitable because of the presence of recipient antibodies. ALG/ATG preparations contain a diverse repertoire of antibodies; thus, variations in effectiveness between batches frequently occurs. These products are often administered as daily 4-hour infusions, and the treatment duration varies from 1 to 2 weeks depending on the preparation and response. Dosing and specifications vary with the different commercial preparations. After a treatment course, antibodies may develop against the foreign proteins in these preparations.

Complications. Therapy with antilymphocyte antibodies, particularly OKT3, may be accompanied by significant complications. During the first two doses, the patient's course can be complicated by cytokine release syndrome. Though relatively rare, symptoms of this syndrome mimic anaphylactic reactions and range from fever to pulmonary edema and frank hypotension. Anaphylactic reactions have been documented with polyclonal ALG preparations, but the cytokine release syndrome is presumed to be secondary to lysis of lymphoid cell populations and tends to occur with the more selective OKT3.

Significant neutropenia or thrombocytopenia may develop from the use of antilymphocyte antibodies, particularly with less specific preparations. Antibodies against neutrophil or platelet antigens can result in white cell counts of less than 3000 and platelet counts of less than 50,000. When such significant drops occur, many centers decrease the dose of the antilymphocyte antibody preparation to half until the counts rise to a less critical level.

Anti-OKT3 antibodies may develop in patients who have previously received OKT3 therapy. These antibodies are directed against the species-specific antigen on the Fc portion of the OKT3 antibody. Patients who receive the newer "humanized" monoclonal antibodies, in which the Fc portion of the antibody is human, are less prone to the development of anti-OKT3 antibodies. Patients who received the older preparations in the past and have such antibodies are less likely to respond to OKT3 therapy.

Finally, repeated use of OKT3 or ALG/ATG has been shown to be a risk factor for the development of PTLD.[46] This increased incidence of PTLD is believed to be secondary to excessive immunosuppression, and in some centers retransplantation is preferable to multiple OKT3 treatment courses in liver transplant patients.

Interleukin-2 Receptor Antagonists

IL-2RAs are a relatively new class of immunosuppressive medications. IL-2 has been known to be a key mediator in T-cell proliferation. T cells, sensitized by the presence of donor antigen, require IL-2 to proliferate. IL-2RA preparations block IL-2 receptors, thus preventing T-cell proliferation and effecting a specific form of immunosuppression. Moreover, like the "third-generation" antilymphocyte antibodies, IL-2RAs with humanized Fc portions have been developed, thus decreasing the incidence of species-specific antibodies. The binding region, however, remains of murine origin.

IL-2RAs have been evaluated primarily as induction agents for immunosuppression rather than as therapy for AR. In preliminary studies with basiliximab as an induction agent, there appears to be a decrease in the rate of AR, including steroid-resistant AR, but also an increase in the rate of chronic rejection.[48,49] Although cytokine release syndrome has not been seen with IL-2RAs, a reduction in efficacy has been noted with repeated use. Despite the humanized Fc portions of these antibodies, their destruction is apparently antibody mediated.

Optimizing Immunosuppression

AR usually occurs because of suboptimal serum levels of immunosuppression. After successful treatment of an episode of AR, the issue of adequate baseline immunosuppression needs to be addressed long term. As a result of individual patient variation and disease-specific factors, some patients need to maintain higher dosage levels.[50] When increasing the dosage, clinicians should also be aware of the resultant higher risk of adverse reactions from these medications.

Other options include changing the mainstay medication of immunosuppression from one calcineurin inhibitor to another. The most commonly performed substitution is conversion of cyclosporine to tacrolimus therapy; less frequently, patients are switched from tacrolimus to cyclosporine therapy. Another strategy is to add a third agent to double-drug therapy. Potential third agents include mycophenolate mofetil, azathioprine, and rapamycin. By adding a third agent, it is anticipated that not only will the risk of any future AR episodes be lessened but the freedom to potentially decrease the dosages of the other two immunosuppressive medications will also be gained.

Desperate Situations

On occasion, a patient with severe AR will not respond steroids, antilymphocyte antibodies, or IL-2RA. In such desperate situations, extreme measures may be taken, including graft irradiation, the use of powerful lymphotoxic drugs, the use of exchange resins, or retransplantation. Patients who eventually require retransplantation because of severe AR subsequently tend to have worse graft survival. Fortunately, AR requiring such extreme measures is rare.

Complications Arising from Therapy

Patients undergoing antirejection therapy are at increased risk for complications secondary to increased immunosuppression (Table 77–6). Concomitant opportunistic infections may develop and are often difficult to diagnose given the immunosuppressed status of the patient. Treatment with corticosteroids may also lead to subsequent adrenal insufficiency; this diagnosis should be considered in any hypotensive posttransplant patient.

Table 77–6. COMPLICATIONS AFTER ACUTE REJECTION THERAPY

Opportunistic infection

Posttransplant lymphoproliferative disease

Steroid withdrawal

Malaise, depression

Higher doses of immunosuppression, especially anti-lymphocyte preparations, increase the risk for subsequent PTLD.[51,52] A patient's mental health status may also be affected during and after a bout of AR. Depression or posttraumatic stress disorder may develop in some patients, and management should include psychiatric evaluation and treatment.[53]

Pediatric Population

Pediatric liver transplant patients have multiple considerations that require particular notice. Whereas some of these issues stem from differences in pediatric and adult pathophysiology, others are psychosocial in origin.

AR in children can be preceded, accompanied, or followed by diseases and symptoms that may adversely affect the rejection process. Pediatric patients, for example, are more likely than adult patients to harbor viral infections or to suffer from diarrhea or vomiting. Such perturbations in the gastrointestinal tract can lead to malabsorption of orally absorbed immunosuppressive agents.

Because of deleterious effects on growth, children with liver transplants are more likely to be weaned off corticosteroids. The balance of growth considerations versus adequate immunosuppression is a delicate one, and pediatric patients being weaned off steroids may run an increased risk of AR. At the same time, long-term high-dose immunosuppression, with or without steroids, can predispose children to PTLD.

As these children become adolescents, noncompliance may become a particularly important issue. Noncompliance should be considered in teenagers with AR. This form of AR usually develops later than other types of AR, and unfortunately, it is often refractory to steroid therapy. Changing the immunosuppressive regimen occasionally eliminates noncompliance in such patients.[54]

Children who suffer AR while receiving cyclosporine-based immunosuppression are now more commonly treated by converting to a tacrolimus-based regimen. Success rates of up to 80% have been seen with such conversion.[55] In children with AR that does not respond to steroid therapy, monoclonal antibody therapy with OKT3 can be used. However, such treatment has been associated with a high risk for viral complications.

Outcomes

Effective treatment of AR decreases patient symptoms and is often associated with improved quality of life. In kidney transplant patients, episodes of AR predispose the allograft to chronic rejection and graft loss.

Although rare cases of refractory AR can progress to chronic rejection in liver transplant patients, recent data suggest that the occurrence of early AR in liver allografts does not affect patient or graft survival.[9] Interestingly enough, mild AR has even been reported to be associated with increased patient and graft survival.[10]

Late Acute Rejection

Late acute rejection (LAR) occurs more than 30 days after liver transplantation and may develop in 15% to 20% of patients. When compared with AR, LAR appears to be a more virulent form of rejection. Factors predisposing patients to LAR include underlying liver disease, decreased immunosuppression, and poor compliance. Histological features, such as centrilobular necrosis, tend to be more atypical, and initial misdiagnosis occasionally occurs. Consequently, LAR is frequently associated with a delay in diagnosis, and such delay often results in decreased response to initial steroid treatment. One study showed as few as 50% of treated patients responding to steroids.[56]

Treatment of LAR generally follows the same algorithm as treatment of AR.

Chronic Rejection

Chronic rejection (CR) differs from AR in many aspects. Although CR has been documented in liver grafts as early as a month after transplantation, it does not generally occur until at least several months afterward. Episodes of AR are not necessarily portents of CR, but CR is often preceded by one or more episodes of AR, usually the steroid-resistant type.[57] A more insidious process, CR carries a worse prognosis than AR does and more frequently results in graft failure with eventual loss.

Although the overall incidence of CR has been decreasing, CR resulting in graft failure still occurs in about 3% to 4% of liver transplant patients.[58] The causes are multifactorial.[59] Patients at risk for CR include those with autoimmune liver disease and those with a history of previous CR resulting in graft loss necessitating retransplantation. Additionally, there appears to be an association between CR and CMV infection or African American heritage.[60]

Immune Mechanisms and Pathology

Though not as well understood as AR, CR is believed to be a result primarily of the cellular arm of the immune response. Although the humoral arm does have a small role, cellular-mediated injury is directed at antigens that have increased expression on the vascular endothelium and biliary ducts. The bile ducts in a transplanted liver graft are already uniquely sensitive to hypoxia. Immune-mediated vascular injury leads to a more ischemic state of the bile ducts. Thus, the bile ducts are attacked not only directly by the immunological process of CR but also indirectly. These processes result in progressive ductopenia, or loss of small bile ducts, on serial histological examination. This finding is an ominous one and earned CR the moniker of "vanishing bile duct syndrome."

Histological diagnosis of CR is more difficult than AR. CR is characterized most consistently by ductopenia. Other findings include fibrosis in the portal area, arteriopathy, minimal lymphoid infiltrates, centrilobular degeneration, and venulitis. Early CR may exhibit only minimal changes, and depending on the amount of fibrosis and bile ducts visualized, CR may be diagnosed only when biopsies are examined serially. In contrast, AR usually has a much more obvious preponderance of infiltrating lymphocytes.

Clinical Findings and Diagnosis

The clinical features of CR are usually more insidious than those of AR. Other than the more common occurrence of jaundice in CR, the signs and symptoms may be the same as those of AR. Additionally, CR patients usually have had a longer period of graft function preceding rejection, and this history can make the diagnosis of CR a surprising one.

Like AR, the diagnosis is confirmed by percutaneous liver biopsy. Histological examination also allows the clinician to rule out other more treatable or concomitant conditions.

Treatment

CR was once believed to lead to inevitable end-stage liver disease. Not surprisingly, given its success with AR, intravenous high-dose corticosteroid therapy was the focus of early treatment efforts. Such therapy no longer has a role in CR and is, in fact, discouraged. Steroids have little or no impact on CR, and their use, with all the attendant side effects, only renders the patient a worse candidate for retransplantation. Fortunately, newer medications such as tacrolimus have not only decreased the incidence of CR but have also aided in modulating the progression of CR (Fig. 77–2).

Because of its effectiveness, tacrolimus has become the mainstay of immunosuppressive therapy in most liver transplant programs. With most centers now using tacrolimus, the general incidence of CR is decreasing.

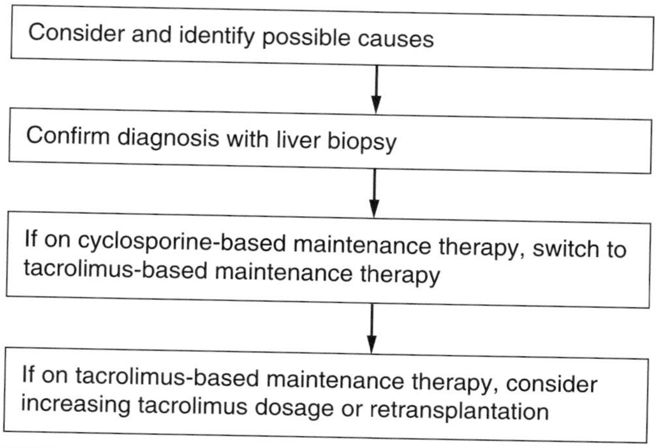

FIGURE 77–2

Treatment of chronic rejection.

However, there are still patients with CR who respond to tacrolimus as salvage therapy. These patients tend to have mild to moderate cholestasis, their CR is diagnosed at least 3 months after transplantation, and they are not taking tacrolimus at the time of diagnosis.[61] Some CR patients already taking tacrolimus may respond to increased dosages and serum levels.

Tacrolimus is not without a significant side effect profile. It may lead to the development of de novo diabetes or exacerbate a preexisting diabetic condition. Renal toxicity is a prominent side effect as well and has resulted in temporary or even permanent renal failure. Moreover, there can be significant neurotoxicity associated with the use of tacrolimus. Tremors and seizures can occur, as well as frank psychosis and aphasia necessitating a change to a cyclosporine-based immunosuppression regimen.

Finally, adding another immunosuppressive agent to a patient's standing maintenance therapy can also be of some use. These third agents can be added to the patient's baseline tacrolimus or cyclosporine and steroids, and they include medications such as mycophenolate mofetil, azathioprine, and rapamycin.

Hyperacute Rejection

Hyperacute rejection (HAR) is rare after liver transplantation. Although the exact reason is unclear, the relative paucity of HAR in liver versus other solid-organ transplants may be related to the liver's immunomodulatory capabilities. In fact, the transplanted liver may serve as a protective organ. In combined-organ transplants, it has been shown that a liver graft can protect a simultaneously transplanted kidney from HAR.[62]

HAR is a condition marked by an extremely rapid onset. Occurring within minutes to hours of reperfusion,

HAR leads to rapid graft loss and is associated with high mortality. Because HAR is so rare in liver transplantation, it is difficult to identify high-risk groups preoperatively.

Immune Mechanisms and Pathology

HAR is caused by preformed cytotoxic anti-HLA class I (IgG) or anti-ABO blood group antibodies.[63] They may occur as a result of previous exposure to antigens from blood transfusion or pregnancy. These complement-binding cytotoxic antibodies are directed against graft cellular antigens. Histological examination reveals antibodies bound to the endothelial cell surfaces of arterioles.[64]

Clinical Findings and Diagnosis

Signs and symptoms of HAR reflect immediate postoperative graft failure (Table 77–7). Elevated liver function test values, coagulopathy, lack of bile production, postoperative coma, and acidosis may be manifestations of HAR. Other causes of acute graft failure such as hepatic artery thrombosis, primary graft nonfunction, and portal vein thrombosis should be ruled out first before making the diagnosis of HAR. The diagnosis is occasionally delayed until a graft hepatectomy is performed and histological examination of the explant confirms the deposition of preformed antibodies.

Treatment

No effective treatment is available for HAR. Preventive measures include ABO matching.

Future

Treatment strategies for rejection after liver transplantation have evolved considerably. Although current immunosuppression is highly effective, there is still a need to improve treatment options. Liver transplant patients tend to be maintained on immunosuppressive

therapy chronically, and the long-term effects of such maintenance therapy can be significant. It is hoped that in the future, new immunosuppressive medications will eliminate not only rejection but also the current side effect profile of such drugs. Although immunosuppressive regimens now tend to be grossly fitted to specific patients, future approaches to clinical management may include regimens that are tailored to underlying diagnoses or genetic makeup. In addition, efforts are being made to develop highly selective drugs that will affect only those elements of the immune system that respond unfavorably to donor antigens.

Other areas of work include improved diagnostic and monitoring methods. Presumably, the ideal diagnostic test would be noninvasive, economical, and highly accurate, thus leading to earlier diagnosis and potentially improved outcomes and patient care. Improved methods of titrating immunosuppression and monitoring bioavailability could result in a more consistently suppressed immune state and consequently a lower incidence of rejection.

There has been a surge of new basic science discoveries in transplant immunology, but work still needs to be done in translating that knowledge into clinically relevant therapy. For example, genetic polymorphism for the production of various cytokines is known to exist.[66] Some of these polymorphisms appear to be associated with a higher risk for rejection.[66] How this information translates into the clinical realm—which patients should be monitored or treated differently—remains unclear.

Conclusions

Although the holy grail of transplantation, immune tolerance, still remains a theoretical ideal, tremendous strides have been made in the treatment of rejection. AR is the most common form of rejection in liver transplant patients. For the most part, it is readily reversible with steroid treatment. Occasionally, AR is resistant to steroid therapy, and other forms of treatment, specifically, monoclonal antibody therapy or IL-2RA therapy, may need to be used. In the rare case of steroid-resistant rejection, monoclonal antibody therapy is often effective. LAR is treated in a similar manner but tends to have a poorer response rate to steroids, presumably because of delay in diagnosis.

The incidence of CR has decreased since the introduction of tacrolimus. Treatment in patients undergoing cyclosporine-based maintenance therapy may involve switching to tacrolimus or adding another immunosuppressive agent.

HAR is rare in liver transplantation. Although no effective treatment is available, preventive measures such as ABO matching should be used.

Table 77–7. HYPERACUTE REJECTION CRITERIA
Immediate graft failure, excluding all other causes
Manifested similar to primary nonfunction
Immune deposits, IgG and IgM, on the hepatic veins and sinusoids
Donor-specific antibodies in the graft, though often difficult to visualize

Pearls and Pitfalls

- Rejection is diagnosed by graft dysfunction and biopsy.
- Ninety-five percent of acute rejection episodes respond to steroids.
- Not every patient and disease require the same level of immunosuppression.
- "Rejection" not responding to treatment may indicate a missed diagnosis.
- Rejection and infection may coexist.
- Consider noncompliance as a cause of rejection in teenagers.
- Steroids can exacerbate the overall condition of a patient with chronic rejection.

References

1. Starzl TE: Experience in Renal Transplantation. Philadelphia, WB Saunders, 1964.
2. Starzl TE, Marcioro TL, Waddell WR: The reversal of rejection in human renal homografts with subsequent development of homograft tolerance. Surg Gynecol Obstet 117:385-394, 1963.
3. Goodwin WE, Kauffman JJ, Mimms MM, et al: Human renal transplantation: Clinical experience with 6 cases of renal homotransplantation. J Urol 89:13-21, 1965.
4. Murray JE, Merril JP, Harrison JH, et al: Prolonged survival of human-kidney homografts by immunosuppressive drug therapy. N Engl J Med 268:1315-1323, 1963.
5. Borel JF, Fuerer C, Magnee C, et al: Effects of the new antilymphocytic peptide cyclosporine A in animals. Immunology 32:1017-1025, 1977.
6. Calne RY, White DJH, Thiru S, et al: Cyclosporine A in patients receiving renal allografts from cadaver donors. Lancet 2:1323-1327, 1978.
7. Abbasoglu O, Levy MF, Brkic BB, et al: Ten years of liver transplantation: An evolving understanding of late graft loss. Transplantation 64:1801-1807, 1997.
8. Klintmalm GB, Nery JR, Husberg BS, et al: Rejection in liver transplantation. Hepatology 10:978-985, 1989.
9. Fisher L, Henry K, Lucey M: Acute cellular rejection after liver transplantation: Variability, morbidity, and mortality. Liver Transpl Surg 1:101-115, 1995.
10. Wiesner RH, Demetris AJ, Belle SH, et al: Acute hepatic allograft rejection: Incidence, risk factors and impact on outcome. Hepatology 28:638-645, 1998.
11. Bartlett A, Ramadas R, Furness S, et al: The natural history of acute histologic rejection without biochemical graft dysfunction in orthotopic liver transplantation: A systematic review. Liver Transpl 8:1147-1153, 2002.
12. Smith NA, Naziruddin B, Pointdexter NJ, et al: Liver transplant recipient sera derived soluble HLA mediates allele specific CTL apoptosis. Transplantation 69:157-162, 2000.
13. Garnier H, Clot J, Bertrand M: Liver transplantation in the pig: Surgical approach. C R Acad Sci Paris 260:5621-5623, 1965.
14. Calne RY, Sells RA, Pena JR, et al: Induction of immunological tolerance by porcine liver allografts. Nature 233:472-474, 1969.
15. Calne R: WOFIE hypothesis: Some thoughts on an approach to allograft tolerance. Transplant Proc 28:1152, 1996.
16. Mazariegos GV, Reyes J, Marino IR, et al: Weaning immunosuppression in liver transplant recipients. Transplantation 63:243-249, 1997.
17. Berlakovich GA, Imhof M, Karner-Hanusch J, et al: The importance of the effect of underlying disease on rejection outcomes following liver transplantation. Transplantation 61:554-560, 1996.
18. Busuttil RW, McDiarmid S, Klintmalm GB, et al: A comparison of tacrolimus and cyclosporine for immunosuppression in liver transplantation. N Engl J Med 331:1110-1115, 1994.
19. Williams J, Peters T, Vera S, et al: Biopsy-directed immunosuppression following hepatic transplantation in man. Transplantation 39:589-596, 1985.
20. Piccinino T, Sagnelli E, Pasquale G, et al: Complications following percutaneous liver biopsy: A multicenter retrospective study on 68,276 biopsies. J Hepatol 2:165-173, 1986.
21. Froehlich F, Lamy O, Fried M, et al: Practice and complications of liver biopsy: Results of a nationwide survey in Switzerland. Dig Dis Sci 38:1480-1484, 1993.
22. McGill DB, Rakela J, Zinsmeister AR, et al: A 21-year experience with major hemorrhage after percutaneous liver biopsy. Gastroenterology 99:1396-1400, 1990.
23. Kwekkeboom J, Zondervan PE, Kuijpers MA, et al: Fine-needle aspiration cytology in the diagnosis of acute liver rejection after liver transplantation. Br J Surg 90:246-247, 2003.
24. Lautenschlager I, Hockstertedt K, Hayry P: Fine-needle aspiration biopsy in the monitoring of liver allografts. Transpl Int 4:54-61, 1991.
25. Von Willebrand E, Hayry P: Reproducibility of the fine-needle aspiration biopsy: Analysis of 93 double biopsies. Transplantation 38:314-316, 1984.
26. Carbonnel F, Samuel D, Reynes M, et al: Fine-needle aspiration biopsy of human liver allografts; correlation with liver histology for the diagnosis of acute rejection. Transplantation 50:704-706, 1990.
27. Ali G, Lubcke R, Schlup M, et al: Evaluation of a new fine needle technique in routine percutaneous liver biopsy. N Z Med J 103:184-186, 1990.
28. Hayry P, Lautenschlager I: Fine-needle aspiration biopsy in transplantation pathology. Semin Diagn Pathol 9:232-237, 1992.
29. Warle MC, Metsellar HJ, Hop WCJ, et al: Early differentiation between rejection and infection in liver transplant patients by serum and biliary cytokine parameters. Transplantation 75:146-151, 2003.
30. Adams DH, Wang L, Hubscher SG, et al: Soluble interleukin-2 receptors in serum and bile of liver transplant recipients. Lancet 1:469-471, 1989.
31. Platz KP, Mueller AR, Rossaint R, et al: Cytokine pattern during rejection and infection after liver transplantation—improvements in postoperative monitoring? Transplantation 62:1441-1450, 1996.
32. Imagawa DK, Millis JM, Olthoff KM, et al: The role of tumor necrosis factor in allograft rejection. Transplantation 50:219-225, 1990.
33. Lautenschlager I, Hockerstedt K, Hayry P, et al: Fine needle aspiration in the monitoring of liver allografts. Transpl Int 4:54-61, 1991.
34. Schlitt HJ, Nashan B, Ringe B, et al: Differentiation of liver graft dysfunction by transplant aspiration cytology. Transplantation 51:786-793, 1991.
35. Wiesner RH: Advances in diagnosis, prevention and management of hepatic allograft rejection. Clin Chem 40:2174-2185, 1994.
36. Baan CC, Metselaar HJ, Mol WM, et al: Intragraft IL-4 mRNA expression is associated with down-regulation of liver graft rejection. Clin Transplant 10:542-549, 1996.
37. Moench C, Uhrig A, Thies J, et al: Chemokines: Reliable markers for diagnosis of rejection and inflammation following orthotopic liver transplantation. Transplant Proc 33:3293-3294, 2001.

38. Janssen H, Lange R, Erhard J, et al: Serum bile acids in liver transplantation—early indicator for acute rejection and monitor for antirejection therapy. Transpl Int 4:429-437, 2001.

39. Tannapel A, Geissler F, Witzigmann H, et al: Analysis of liver allograft rejection related genes using cDNA microarray in liver allograft specimen. Transplant Proc 33:3283-3284, 2001.

40. Kuiff MM, Kwekkeboom J, Kuijpers MA, et al: Granzyme expression in fine needle aspirates from liver allografts is increased during acute rejection. Liver Transpl 8:952-956, 2002.

41. Pascoe MD, Marshall SE, Welsh KI, et al: Increased accuracy of renal allograft rejection diagnosis using combined perforin, granzyme B, and Fas ligand fine-needle aspiration immunocytology. Transplantation 69:2547-2553, 2000.

42. Anand AC, Hubscher SG, Gunson BK, et al: Timing, significance and prognosis of late acute liver allograft rejection. Transplantation 60:1098-1103, 1995.

43. Wiesner RH, Ludwig J, Krom RAF, et al: Treatment of early cellular rejection following liver transplantation with intravenous methylprednisolone—the effect of dose on response. Transplantation 58:1053-1056, 1994.

44. Evans RW, Manninen DL, Dong FB, et al: Immunosuppressive therapy as a determinant of transplantation outcome. Transplantation 55:1297-1305, 1993.

45. Charlton M, Seaberg E: Impact of immunosuppression and acute rejection on recurrence of hepatitis C: Results of the National Institute of Diabetes and Digestive and Kidney Diseases Liver Transplantation Database. Liver Transpl Surg 5(Suppl):S107-S114, 1999.

46. Swinnen L, Costanzo-Nordin M, Fisher S, et al: Increased incidence of lymphoproliferative disorder after immunosuppression with the monoclonal antibody OKT3 in cardiac transplant patients. N Engl J Med 323:1723-1728, 1990.

47. Wall WJ, Ghent CN, Roy A, et al: Use of monoclonal antibody as induction therapy for control of rejection in liver transplantation. Dig Dis Sci 40:52-57, 1995.

48. Glaneman M, Langrehr JM, Raakow R, et al: Anti–IL-2 receptor BT563 versus placebo: A randomised trial for induction therapy after liver transplantation. Transplant Proc 30:2159-2160, 1998.

49. Langrehr JM, Lohmann R, Raakow R, et al: Chronic rejection after orthotopic liver transplantation is increased under induction therapy with interleukin-2 receptor antibody BT563. Transplant Proc 33:2290-2291, 2001.

50. Boillot O, Viale JP, Gratadour P, et al: Reversal of early acute rejection with increased doses of tacrolimus in liver transplantation. Transplantation 66:1182-1185, 1998.

51. Trofe J, Buell JR, First MR, et al: The role of immunosuppression in lymphoma. Recent Results Cancer Res 159:55-66, 2002.

52. Cockfield SM: Identifying the patient at risk for post-transplant lymphoproliferative disorder. Transpl Infect Dis 3:70-78, 2001.

53. Rothenhausler HB, Ehrentraut S, Kapfhammer HP, et al: Psychiatric and psychosocial outcome of orthotopic liver transplantation. Psychother Psychosom 71:285-297, 2002.

54. McDiarmid SV: Management of the pediatric liver transplant patient. Liver Transpl 7(11 Suppl 1):S77-S86, 2001.

55. Sokal EM, Gleghorn G, Goulet O, et al: Liver and intestinal transplantation in children: Working group report of the First World Congress of Pediatric Gastroenterology, Hepatology, and Nutrition. J Pediatr Gastroenterol Nutr 35(Suppl 2):S159-S172, 2002.

56. Mor E, Gonwa TA, Husberg BS, et al: Late-onset acute rejection in orthotopic liver transplantation—associated risk factors and outcome. Transplantation 54:821-824, 1992.

57. Hayry P: Chronic rejection: An update on the mechanisms. Transplant Proc 30:3993-3995, 1998.

58. Neuberger J: Incidence, timing and risk factors for acute and chronic rejection. Liver Transpl Surg (Suppl) S30-S36, 1999.

59. Wiesner RH, Batts KP, Krom RAF: Evolving concepts in the diagnosis, pathogenesis, and treatment of chronic rejection. Liver Transpl Surg 5:388-400, 1999.

60. van Hoek B, Wiesner RH, Krom RA, et al: Severe ductopenic rejection following liver transplantation: Incidence, time of onset, risk factors, treatment, and outcome. Semin Liver Dis 12:41-50, 1992.

61. Sher LS, Cosenza CA, Michel J, et al: Efficacy of tacrolimus as rescue therapy for chronic rejection in orthotopic liver transplantation. Transplantation 64:258-263, 1997.

62. Fung JJ, Mackowka L, Griffin M, et al: Successful sequential liver-kidney transplantation in patients with preformed lymphocytic antibodies. Clin Transpl 1:187-194, 1987.

63. Imagawa DK, Noguchi K, Iwaki Y, et al: Hyperacute rejection following ABO-compatible orthotopic liver transplantation—a case report. Transplantation 54:1114-1117, 1992.

64. Kissmeyer-Nielsen F, Olsen S, Petersen VP, Fjeldborg O: Hyperacute rejection of kidney allografts associated with pre-existing humoral antibodies against donor cells. Lancet 2:662-665, 1966.

65. Hutchinson I, Pravicia V, Sinnott P: Genetic regulation of cytokine synthesis: Consequences for acute and chronic rejection. Graft 1:186-192, 1998.

66. Suthanthiran M: Altered cytokine synthesis and the fate of the transplanted organ: Is DNA destiny? Graft 1:173-174, 1998.

Novel Immunosuppressive Agents

RYUTARO HIROSE
FLAVIO VINCENTI

Overall strategy   1275

The old and the new   1276

Biological agents—antibodies and fusion
   proteins   1276
   Antibodies/biological agents   1277
   Antiproliferatives   1280
   FTY720   1281

Summary   1281

The advent of a large array of immunosuppressants has greatly expanded the armamentarium used by transplant physicians and surgeons to prevent and treat liver allograft rejection. The availability of these drugs has been an important factor in the excellent short- and long-term outcomes achieved in liver transplantation. However, these drugs continue to lack specificity, many require frequent therapeutic drug monitoring, and all are associated with acute and chronic toxicity. Although the liver is considered a relatively "tolerogenic" organ, we have yet to attain the "Holy Grail" of transplantation (i.e., transplantation tolerance) in any meaningful or consistent manner. As such, liver transplant recipients are still currently being sentenced to a lifelong course of chronic immunosuppression. Small molecules, biological agents such as antibodies and fusion proteins, and corticosteroids continue to play a central role in the immunosuppressive regimens used in liver transplantation. In addition, a number of novel immunosuppressive agents have been used in preclinical and clinical trials and show promise for use in the near future. Our objective in this chapter is to present novel immunosuppressive agents and attempt to gaze into the crystal ball and predict future developments in the immunosuppressive front.

Overall Strategy

As in all solid-organ transplants, the general strategy of using a combination of synergistic medications to maximize efficacy and minimize toxicity remains the hallmark of most immunosuppressive regimens. Most commonly, this approach has included the use of corticosteroids, an antiproliferative agent, and a calcineurin inhibitor such as cyclosporine or tacrolimus. Using this combinatorial approach, transplant physicians have sought effective prophylaxis against acute allograft rejection while at the same time minimizing specific toxicities such as calcineurin inhibitor–induced nephrotoxicity and neurotoxicity or bone marrow suppression by antiproliferative agents, as well as steroid-induced bone disease, hyperlipidemia, and posttransplant diabetes. Despite this laudable theoretical goal, toxicity from immunosuppressive agents is common and at times threatens the quality and quantity of life of liver transplant recipients.

The goals of immunosuppression in liver transplantation differ slightly from those of other solid-organ transplants. In general, liver transplant recipients receive less overall immunosuppression than do recipients of other organs. Although acute rejection episodes are generally to be avoided, they do not portend as ominous an outcome as in other transplants. Unlike the scenario in renal transplantation, where every episode of acute cellular rejection has a significant negative impact on long-term allograft survival, acute rejection can have a minimal impact on long-term liver function and liver allograft survival.[1] Higher rejection rates are thus tolerated. In addition, the very conditions that are considered contraindications for transplantation of other organs, such as malignancy (e.g., hepatocellular carcinoma) and chronic active infection (e.g., hepatitis C), are in fact the most common indications for liver transplantation. The impact of immunosuppression on the potential recurrence of these diseases cannot be overemphasized. Finally, the side effects from standard chronic immunosuppressive regimens affect liver transplant recipients as much as, if not more than, other solid-organ transplant recipients. For example, a recent study demonstrated that the cumulative incidence of renal insufficiency in liver transplant patients 5 years after transplantation is 18.1%.[2]

Recently, much emphasis has been placed on avoiding corticosteroids and using calcineurin inhibitor–sparing protocols to minimize and further reduce long-term side effects. Many of the newer immunosuppressive agents on the market today are being used in just this manner.

The Old and the New

The use of cyclosporine and subsequently tacrolimus has revolutionized solid-organ transplantation and specifically transplantation of the liver. With the use of calcineurin inhibitors, graft and patient survival rates approaching 90% were made possible. Without question, both cyclosporine and tacrolimus are effective antirejection agents. There are conflicting data, however, regarding the optimal calcineurin inhibitor to use for liver transplantation. Overall, the side effect profiles of the two drugs, although overlapping, are not identical, and clinical judgment based on the individual patient is probably warranted. The use of corticosteroids and their short- and long-term toxicities are well documented. Finally, the antiproliferative drugs azathioprine and mycophenolate mofetil (MMF) are also in widespread use, and their mechanism of action and clinical use have been covered elsewhere (see Chapter 75, "Induction and Maintenance of Immunosuppression"). Biological agents such as antilymphocyte antibodies have been in clinical use for more than 3 decades as well. Polyclonal antibody preparations continue to be in use, as well as monoclonal antibodies (mAbs) with a variety of targets. The rabbit polyclonal antibody thymoglobulin has been used in steroid-free regimens in liver transplantation with some success.[3,4] The newer mAbs and biological agents have greater specificity than the prototypical example OKT3 does, and they have shown some promise in the arena of calcineurin inhibitor and steroid elimination, as well as tolerance induction protocols.

Biological Agents—Antibodies and Fusion Proteins

The specificity and selectivity of new biological agents render them less toxic than the oral maintenance drugs, and thus they could possibly replace maintenance immunosuppressants associated with long-term toxicity, such as corticosteroids and the calcineurin inhibitors. Figure 78–1 demonstrates some of the targets of the newer biological agents. The recently introduced anti–interleukin-2 receptor (IL-2R) mAbs are the prototype of future biological agents; they are selective and safe and induce prolonged biological effects. IL-2R mAbs have been used with a variety of maintenance immunosuppression regimens. Another major thrust of the new biological agents in clinical development is costimulatory blockade. The first results from attempts to block CD40-CD154 with anti-CD154 mAbs were disappointing. Anti-CD154 therapy in renal transplant trials was associated with thromboembolic events and acute rejection. Attempts at blocking the CD28-B7s (CD80-CD86) pathway are currently under way with the receptor fusion protein LEA29Y, a second-generation CTLA4-Ig, and humanized mAbs to CD80 and CD86. The lymphocyte function antigen LFA-1, an adhesion molecule that also participates in costimulation, has likewise been targeted with a mAb that binds to the CD11a chain of LFA-1. Efalizumab, a humanized anti-CD11a mAb, was shown in a phase I trial to be potentially effective in renal transplantation. A humanized anti-CD45 RB mAb is currently in preclinical studies and will probably be

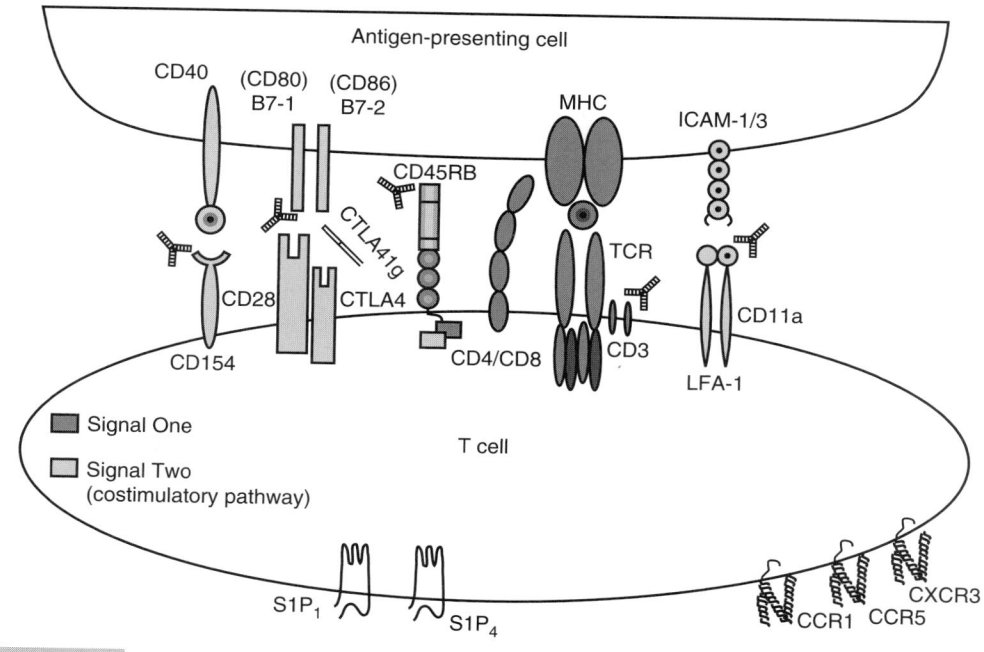

FIGURE 78-1

Cell surface targets for novel immunosuppressive agents. (From Vincenti F: What's in the pipeline? New immunosuppressive drugs in transplantation. AM J Transplant 2:898-903, 2002.)

tested in a phase I trial of renal transplantation within 1 year. Although excellent results with anti-CD45 RB mAbs have been achieved in experimental transplantation, the mechanism of action of anti-CD45 RB mAbs remains to be determined. Several antibodies that are approved for nontransplant indications are currently being used in single-center clinical trials in renal transplantation, including alemtuzumab (Campath 1H), a humanized anti-CD52 mAb; rituximab, an anti-CD20 chimeric mAb; and infliximab, an anti–tumor necrosis factor-α chimeric mAb. Specifically, several groups have published their preliminary experience with Campath 1H in kidney and more recently in liver transplantation.[5,6] This promising and interesting new agent elicits long-term T-lymphocyte depletion in humans. In addition, several humanized mutagenized anti-CD3 mAbs—huOKT3, aglycosyl CD3, and HuM291—have been used in limited trials in renal transplantation but have yet to undergo formal clinical development. Humanized mAbs and receptor fusion proteins offer the potential of providing renal transplant recipients with a novel algorithm for immunosuppression that relies on chronic intermittent intravenous administration of safe, nontoxic agents instead of maintenance oral drug therapy.

Antibodies/Biological Agents

Anti–Interleukin-2 Receptor

Recent technological advances in molecular biology have made possible the ability to create fusion proteins

and chimeric or humanized mAbs. Targeting the alpha chain of the high-affinity IL-2R with genetically modified mAbs has met with success in solid-organ transplantation. The high-affinity IL-2R is a heterotrimer made up of alpha, beta, and gamma chains. The beta and gamma chain are constitutively expressed by T cells, whereas the alpha chain (CD25) is found on activated T cells. Because the alpha chain is expressed on activated human T cells and not on resting or naïve T cells, by blocking CD25 one would ostensibly be targeting only activated T cells responding to an immunological stimulus, such as an allograft. This selective action would potentially result in less global, less nonspecific immunosuppression. Murine mAbs were developed against CD25 and used in clinical trials, including one trial in liver transplantation. To circumvent the development of antimurine, anti-idiotype immunity, chimeric and humanized versions have been developed. The two antibodies that are currently used in clinical transplantation are basiliximab and daclizumab. Clinical trials of chimeric and humanized anti-CD25 mAbs in kidney transplantation have been conducted, and a significant reduction in acute rejection rates was observed with the use of these antibodies. No increase in the rate of infectious complications or malignancies has been reported to date with either agent. These antibodies are remarkable for their distinct lack of toxicity and side effects, which of course, is in stark contrast to antilymphocyte agents such as OKT3 and thymoglobulin. Other studies in renal transplantation have included steroid-sparing regimens.

Two large series of liver transplant patients receiving basiliximab have recently been reported. Both studies demonstrated acceptable rates of rejection, but with less benefit in patients with hepatitis C. Calmus and coauthors reported the results of a single-arm open-label multicenter trial of basiliximab in which 101 patients received basiliximab in conjunction with cyclosporine, azathioprine, and corticosteroids.[7] They found an overall rejection rate of 22.8% at 6 months, with more rejection episodes in patients with hepatitis C (9/31 = 29.0%). These rejection rates are well within the acceptable range, and the authors state that this rate is better than the historical control rate from another trial of cyclosporine, azathioprine, and prednisone. The authors also reported excellent 1-year patient and graft survival rates of 90.1% and 88.1%, respectively, and no anaphylactic reactions or other major side effects related to the infusion of basiliximab. Neuhaus and associates presented the results of a large multicenter randomized, double-blind, placebo-controlled phase III trial in which 381 recipients received either two doses of 20 mg basiliximab or placebo in addition to cyclosporine and corticosteroids.[8] The randomization was stratified according to hepatitis C virus (HCV) status. The primary endpoint to be measured in the study was the acute rejection rate at 6 months. This is the largest randomized controlled study with the use of an IL-2R mAb in liver transplantation published to date. The biopsy-proven rejection rate at 6 months was 35.1% in the basiliximab-treated group and 43.5% in the placebo group (P = not significant). With further subgroup analysis, the difference in rejection rates was more notable in patients who were HCV negative. In fact, 6-month rejection rates in HCV-positive patients were slightly higher in the basiliximab arm than in the placebo arm (39.1% versus 36.2%, P = .911).

The effect on the incidence of recurrent hepatitis C is of major concern with any additional immunosuppressive agent that is used. These findings are further confounded by the well-documented fact that recurrent hepatitis C and rejection are often extremely difficult to distinguish from each other on a histological basis. This difficulty could clearly influence the reported rates of rejection or recurrent hepatitis C (or both). Although immunosuppression is associated with increased susceptibility to viral infection, some authors have suggested that the hepatocyte and cellular damage in viral hepatitis is immune mediated and have even gone as far as treating recurrent hepatitis C with daclizumab. In any event, with the data available, it is unclear whether these agents should be used in the setting of hepatitis C.

There are theoretical concerns about targeting CD25. Many immunologists have shown renewed interest in the phenomenon of regulatory or suppressor T cells. Several groups have reported on the immunomodulatory characteristics of CD4+, CD25+ regulatory T cells in inhibiting both in vitro T-cell responses and in vivo phenomenon such as autoimmunity in rodent models. By inhibiting the activity of these regulatory T cells, one can envision augmenting rather than inhibiting an immune response such as transplant rejection. In general, these concerns have not been borne out by clinical experience. It is, however, of note that in the absence of any calcineurin inhibitor for longer than 1 week after transplantation, the use of daclizumab in liver transplantation was met with little success and a high incidence of steroid-resistant rejection.[9]

The fact that acute rejection can occur despite adequate saturation of the alpha chain of IL-2R may have implications regarding the mechanisms and molecules involved in immune activation during allograft rejection. The beta-gamma dimeric intermediate-affinity IL-2Rs may still be able to bind IL-2 and induce signaling to activate T cells. Alternatively, other cytokines such as IL-15 may have redundant roles and activate T cells independent of IL-2.

Are there certain subgroups of patients who may benefit from the use of anti–IL-2R antibodies? Several groups have reported on the safety and efficacy of the use of daclizumab in liver transplantation, specifically in the setting of renal insufficiency when it is desirable to avoid the nephrotoxic calcineurin inhibitors. Eckoff and coworkers reported a nonrandomized pilot study of 39 patients who received daclizumab after liver transplantation; 7 of 39 patients (18%) experienced acute rejection at 6 months.[10] Emre and coauthors published a report of 25 patients with impaired renal function who had acceptable outcomes as well.[11] The anti–IL-2R antibodies used in clinical practice have been associated with a significant decrease in the incidence of acute rejection in renal transplantation. The data in liver transplantation are less clear. The most notable characteristic of these agents is their remarkable lack of major side effects.

Overall, the use of anti–IL-2R antibodies appears to be safe and effective. A potentially useful role seems to be in the not uncommon scenario of renal insufficiency or neurological compromise in liver transplant recipients, which may preclude the use of full-dose calcineurin inhibitors. However, it seems that caution must be exercised if calcineurin inhibitors are completely avoided. In a multicenter trial of calcineurin inhibitor avoidance in kidney transplantation in which the regimen consisted of daclizumab, MMF, and steroids, the rejection rate was 48% at 6 months.[12] Similarly, in a pilot study of daclizumab with MMF and steroids in liver transplantation, rejection rates were extremely high unless calcineurin inhibitors were started at least at a low dose within a week of transplantation.[9] Further studies of calcineurin inhibitor avoidance with the use of other agents, such as sirolimus, in combination are warranted. Another potential arena in which these antibodies may prove useful in liver transplantation is in steroid avoidance. Basiliximab has been used successfully in this context in renal transplantation, and a recent presentation demonstrated potential promise in liver transplantation with the use of daclizumab in one arm of a clinical trial (HCV 3 trial) in which daclizumab, tacrolimus, MMF, but no steroids were administered. Interestingly, the 3-month rejection rate in this arm is reported to be less than 9% (unpublished data).

Costimulatory Blockade

The underlying concept behind costimulatory blockade is the notion that to fully stimulate and activate a T cell, at least two signals from an antigen-presenting cell are required: (1) stimulation of the T-cell receptor by a major histocompatibility complex molecule–antigenic peptide complex and (2) stimulation of costimulatory molecules such as CD28 by ligands (e.g., B7). In fact, if a T cell receives a signal through the T-cell receptor without signal 2, functional inactivation or deletion of that T cell results. This finding was the impetus behind the development of agents such as anti-CD154 (anti-CD40L) and CTLA4-Ig. This strategy resulted in nothing less than spectacular outcomes in preclinical models.[13,14] Unfortunately, in human trials, use of these agents has met with mixed results. The most dramatic failure in the recent past is Biogen's anti-CD154 (hu5C8). Despite impressive experimental evidence, a phase I trial with humanized hu5C8 was halted after the occurrence of thromboembolic events, as well as failure of immunosuppression efficacy (five of seven

patients had rejection episodes). IDEC Pharmaceutical had started clinical trials with another humanized anti-CD154, IDEC131 (targeting a different epitope than hu5C8 does), in patients with autoimmune diseases, but these studies are unlikely to be extended to organ transplantation. A more promising approach may be to target CD40 directly.

LEA29Y (CTLA4-Ig)

CTLA4-Ig is a fusion protein that consists of the extracellular domain of CTLA4 fused with the Fc portion of human immunoglobulin. LEA29Y is a second-generation CTLA4-Ig (extracellular domain of CTLA4 and the Fc domain of IgG1) with increased binding avidity to CD80 (2-fold) and CD86 (4-fold) and approximately 10-fold more effectiveness in vitro than CTLA4-Ig on a per-dose basis in inhibiting T-cell effector function. A phase I/II trial is currently under way in primary renal transplantation with an immunosuppression regimen based on preclinical studies performed by Drs. Chris Larsen and Tom Pearson at Emory University (unpublished results). The phase I study randomized 217 primary renal transplant patients to three treatment groups; groups 1 and 2 are being treated with LEA29Y, basiliximab (20 mg on days 0 and 4), MMF (2 g), and conventional steroid therapy (Fig. 78–2). Patients randomized to group 3 serve as controls and are being treated with a standard regimen consisting of basiliximab (20 mg on days 0 and 4), cyclosporine, MMF, and steroids. Patient enrollment in this trial has been completed. The acute rejection rate at 6 months was comparable

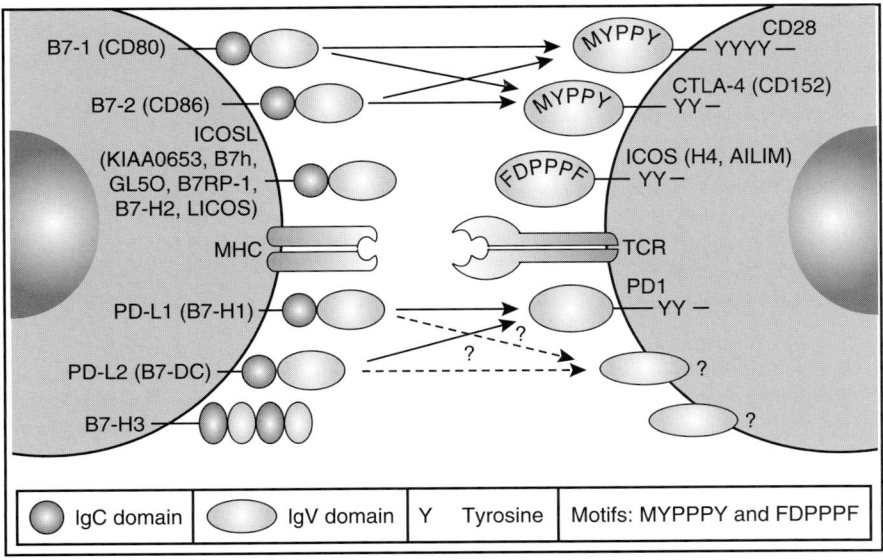

FIGURE 78–2

Schematic of costimulatory molecules. (From Sharp A, Freeman G: The B7-CD28 superfamily. Nat Rev Immunol 2:116-126, 2002.)

between patients treated with LEA29Y and cyclosporine. This study may provide an important clue to the clinical efficacy achieved by blocking a single track of the costimulatory pathway. It is possible, however, that effective clinical blockade of the costimulatory signal may require disruption of several targets within the pathway (see Fig. 78–2).

Antiproliferatives

The current antiproliferative agents in standard practice in liver transplantation include azathioprine and MMF, which are covered in Chapter 75. The most recently introduced antiproliferative agents include mTOR inhibitors (Fig. 78–3).

mTOR Inhibitors—Sirolimus and Everolimus

Sirolimus (rapamycin; Rapamune) is a macrocyclic lactone produced by *Streptomyces hygroscopicus*.[15] Both sirolimus (rapamycin) and everolimus, a related derivative, act as antiproliferative agents and are recent additions to the immunosuppressive regimens of solid-organ transplant recipients. These agents act by binding the intracellular receptor FKBP-12, but unlike tacrolimus (which shares the same intracellular receptor), they do *not* inhibit calcineurin. Rather, the rapamycin–FKBP-12 complex binds and inhibits the activity of a large molecule with kinase activity termed the mammalian target of rapamycin (mTOR). mTOR is a kinase that is intricately involved in the signal transduction pathways downstream to many growth factor receptors, including IL-2R. Specifically, mTOR is a kinase that is downstream to the phosphatidyl inositol 3 (PI3) kinase/AKT/protein

kinase B pathway and is known to phosphorylate substrates such as p70S6 kinase, which in turn phosphorylates the 40S ribosomal protein S6. In addition, phosphorylation of other substrates such as initiation factor 4E–binding protein 1 (4E-BP1) is also mediated by mTOR. The activity of cyclin-dependent kinases is also inhibited by rapamycin. The overall effect of inhibition of mTOR is cell cycle arrest as a result of a block in the transition from G_1 to S phase. This activity has been demonstrated in lymphocytes, as well as many tumor cells.

The efficacy of sirolimus and everolimus as immunosuppressives has been demonstrated in randomized clinical trials in kidney transplantation.[16-18] The experience with sirolimus is more extensive in this regard. Overall, a reduction in acute rejection rates was demonstrated in these trials with the use of sirolimus versus placebo or azathioprine.

The use of sirolimus in transplant patients is associated with a dose-dependent increase in serum cholesterol and triglycerides that may require treatment.[19-22] Although immunotherapy with sirolimus per se is not nephrotoxic, patients treated with cyclosporine plus sirolimus, as well as those treated with tacrolimus and sirolimus, have impaired renal function when compared with patients treated with cyclosporine and either azathioprine or placebo. Renal function must therefore be monitored closely in such patients. Partly responsible may be an overall increase in total exposure to calcineurin inhibitors as a result of the combination of drugs. Thus, one should consider dose reduction of calcineurin inhibitors when the concomitant administration of sirolimus is introduced to prevent nephropathy.

The use of sirolimus in liver transplantation remains somewhat controversial. Concern has been raised

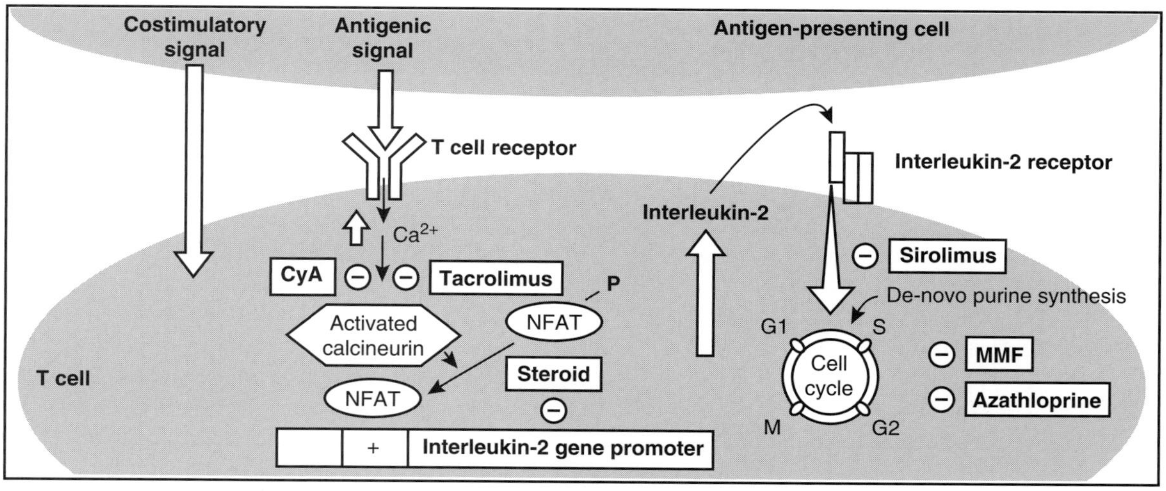

FIGURE 78-3

Stages of T-cell activation and targets for immunosuppressive agents. CyA, cyclosporine A; MMF, mycophenolate mofetil; NFAT, nuclear factor of activated T cells. (From Denton MD, Magee CC, Sayegh MH: Immunosuppressive strategies in transplantation. Lancet 353:1083-1091, 1999.)

about the development of hepatic artery thrombosis during clinical trials involving the de novo use of sirolimus in liver transplantation. This led to a "black box warning" against the use of sirolimus in the de novo management of fresh post–liver transplant patients. In addition, wound healing issues have been raised with the use of sirolimus in the perioperative period. An increased rate of lymphoceles in renal transplant recipients was noted. Despite these concerns, several publications have favorably reported the use of sirolimus in liver transplant recipients, and subsequent published experience has not noted an increase in hepatic artery thrombosis.

An interesting effect of rapamycin is its well-documented antitumor activity, presumably by a mechanism very similar to its effect on immunocytes. However, additional evidence has shown that angiogenesis is inhibited as well, possibly because of inhibition of the activity of such transcriptional factors as HIF-1a and a resultant decrease in the elaboration of angiogenic molecules such as vascular endothelial growth factor. In the future, it may be feasible to predict which tumors may be sensitive to inhibition by mTOR inhibitors, for example, by examining the status of the PI3 kinase/AKT pathway in these tumors.

Other Antiproliferatives

Several antiproliferative agents are being developed in renal transplantation, including JAK3 inhibitors, FK778, and VX497. FK778, a new oral immunosuppressive agent under development by Fujisawa Healthcare, is an analogue of the active metabolites of leflunomide. FK778 has a unique mechanism of action, specifically, binding to dihydro-orotate dehydrogenase and inhibiting de novo pyrimidine biosynthesis, thereby blocking T- and B-cell proliferation and strongly suppressing IgM and IgG antibody production. In addition, FK778 appears to have antiviral effects in vitro against a number of viruses, including cytomegalovirus and polyomavirus. FK778 is currently in a phase II trial in Europe. A new, rationally designed inhibitor of inosine monophosphate dehydrogenase, VX-497, with a mechanism of action similar to that of MMF has been developed by Vertex and used in clinical studies in patients with psoriasis and hepatitis C. Despite encouraging preclinical studies in renal transplantation in dogs however, its clinical development in transplantation remains in doubt.

FTY720

FTY720 is a novel immunomodulatory drug with a unique mechanism of action. It is a synthetic structural analogue of myriocin, a metabolite of an ascomycete. FTY720 shares structural and functional homology with sphingosine-1-phosphate (S1P), a natural ligand to several G-protein–coupled receptors. FTY720 displays a novel mechanism of action characterized by sequestration of lymphocytes into secondary lymphoid organs without affecting their function.[23] FTY720-monophosphate (FTY720-P), the active form of the drug, acts as an agonist and signals via the S1P receptor family, $S1P_1$ and $S1P_4$ on lymphocytes, the effect of which is to block egress of lymphocytes from lymph nodes and Peyer's patches. This sequestration reduces migration of effector cells to inflammatory tissues and graft sites. In a recently published study, 20 stable renal transplant recipients receiving a cyclosporine-based regimen were treated with single oral doses of FTY720 ranging from 0.25 to 3.5 mg.[24] FTY720 was well tolerated with no serious adverse events except for transient asymptomatic bradycardia after 10 of 24 doses. The elimination half-life ranged from 89 to 157 hours, independent of the dose. FTY720 pharmacodynamics was characterized by reversible transient lymphopenia within 6 hours, the nadir being 42% of the baseline value. The lymphocyte count returned to baseline within 72 hours in all dosing cohorts except the highest. The interim results of two FTY720 trials were reported but not yet published. The first study assessed the efficacy of four different maintenance doses of FTY720 (0.25, 0.5, 1, 2.5 mg) in 155 patients concomitantly treated with cyclosporine and prednisone. The incidence of acute rejection ranged from 38% to 11%. The second trial was performed in patients at risk for delayed graft function, and the immunosuppression regimen consisted of FTY720, 2 mg, everolimus, 2 mg, and prednisone. The results from these studies were promising, and FTY720 is currently in phase III trials.

To date, there has yet to be a published large clinical trial in liver transplantation, but such studies are, by report, being designed.

Summary

New immunosuppressive agents that are in development have taken advantage of the recently expanded understanding of the interaction of immune cells with endothelium, the elucidation of novel signaling mechanisms, and the molecules responsible for normal trafficking of immune cells. This understanding has led to the use of agents that interfere with or alter immune cells by exploiting these various pathways. In some cases, these agents may result in more specific immunosuppression, whereas others may result in diversion of the immune response from the allograft while preserving systemic immunity. In addition, some of these agents may provide the added benefit of ameliorating ischemia-reperfusion injury, in which (like rejection) leukocyte–endothelial cell interactions are thought to play a key role.

A decade of spectacular innovation in maintenance immunosuppression drugs has resulted in dramatic reductions in acute rejection and improvement in short- and long-term outcomes in solid-organ transplantation. Although true tolerance (i.e., maintenance of allograft function with no immunosuppression) has still not been achieved, reduction or elimination of the use of certain classic immunosuppressants with their long-term toxicities is well within our grasp.

References

1. Wiesner RH, Demetris AJ, Belle SH, et al: Acute hepatic allograft rejection: Incidence, risk factors, and impact on outcome. Hepatology 28:638, 1998.
2. Ojo AO, Held PJ, Port FK, et al: Chronic renal failure after transplantation of a nonrenal organ. N Engl J Med 349:931, 2003.
3. Eason JD, Blazek J, Mason A, et al: Steroid-free immunosuppression through thymoglobulin induction in liver transplantation. Transplant Proc 33:1470, 2001.
4. Eason JD, Nair S, Cohen AJ, et al: Steroid-free liver transplantation using rabbit antithymocyte globulin and early tacrolimus monotherapy. Transplantation 75:1396, 2003.
5. Ciancio G, Burke GW, Gaynor JJ, et al: The use of Campath-1H as induction therapy in renal transplantation: Preliminary results. Transplantation 78:426, 2004.
6. Tzakis AG, Tryphonopoulos P, Kato T, et al: Preliminary experience with alemtuzumab (Campath-1H) and low-dose tacrolimus immunosuppression in adult liver transplantation. Transplantation 77:1209, 2004.
7. Calmus Y, Scheele JR, Gonzalez-Pinto I, et al: Immunoprophylaxis with basiliximab, a chimeric anti–interleukin-2 receptor monoclonal antibody, in combination with azathioprine-containing triple therapy in liver transplant recipients. Liver Transpl 8:123, 2002.
8. Neuhaus P, Clavien PA, Kittur D, et al: Improved treatment response with basiliximab immunoprophylaxis after liver transplantation: Results from a double-blind randomized placebo-controlled trial. Liver Transpl 8:132, 2002.
9. Hirose R, Roberts JP, Quan D, et al: Experience with daclizumab in liver transplantation: Renal transplant dosing without calcineurin inhibitors is insufficient to prevent acute rejection in liver transplantation. Transplantation 69:307, 2000.
10. Eckhoff DE, McGuire B, Sellers M, et al: The safety and efficacy of a two-dose daclizumab (Zenapax) induction therapy in liver transplant recipients. Transplantation 69:1867, 2000.
11. Emre S, Gondolesi G, Polat K, et al: Use of daclizumab as initial immunosuppression in liver transplant recipients with impaired renal function. Liver Transpl 7:220, 2001.
12. Vincenti F, Ramos E, Brattstrom C, et al: Multicenter trial exploring calcineurin inhibitors avoidance in renal transplantation. Transplantation 71:1282, 2001.
13. Kenyon NS, Chatzipetrou M, Masetti M, et al: Long-term survival and function of intrahepatic islet allografts in rhesus monkeys treated with humanized anti-CD154. Proc Natl Acad Sci U S A 96:8132, 1999.
14. Kirk AD, Burkly LC, Batty DS, et al: Treatment with humanized monoclonal antibody against CD154 prevents acute renal allograft rejection in nonhuman primates. Nat Med 5:686, 1999.
15. Vezina C, Kudelski A, Sehgal SN: Rapamycin (AY-22,989), a new antifungal antibiotic. I. Taxonomy of the producing streptomycete and isolation of the active principle. J Antibiot (Tokyo) 28:721, 1975.
16. Ciancio G, Burke GW, Gaynor JJ, et al: A randomized long-term trial of tacrolimus/sirolimus versus tacrolimus/mycophenolate mofetil versus cyclosporine (NEORAL)/sirolimus in renal transplantation. II. Survival, function, and protocol compliance at 1 year. Transplantation 77:252, 2004.
17. Ciancio G, Burke GW, Gaynor JJ, et al: A randomized long-term trial of tacrolimus and sirolimus versus tacrolimus and mycophenolate mofetil versus cyclosporine (NEORAL) and sirolimus in renal transplantation. I. Drug interactions and rejection at one year. Transplantation 77:244, 2004.
18. MacDonald AS: A worldwide, phase III, randomized, controlled, safety and efficacy study of a sirolimus/cyclosporine regimen for prevention of acute rejection in recipients of primary mismatched renal allografts. Transplantation 71:271, 2001.
19. Murgia MG, Jordan S, Kahan BD: The side effect profile of sirolimus: A phase I study in quiescent cyclosporine-prednisone–treated renal transplant patients. Kidney Int 49:209, 1996.
20. Trotter JF, Wachs ME, Trouillot TE, et al: Dyslipidemia during sirolimus therapy in liver transplant recipients occurs with concomitant cyclosporine but not tacrolimus. Liver Transpl 7:401, 2001.
21. Legendre C, Campistol JM, Squifflet JP, et al: Cardiovascular risk factors of sirolimus compared with cyclosporine: Early experience from two randomized trials in renal transplantation. Transplant Proc 35:151S, 2003.
22. Chueh SC, Kahan BD: Dyslipidemia in renal transplant recipients treated with a sirolimus and cyclosporine–based immunosuppressive regimen: Incidence, risk factors, progression, and prognosis. Transplantation 76:375, 2003.
23. Brinkmann V, Pinschewer DD, Feng L, et al: FTY720: Altered lymphocyte traffic results in allograft protection. Transplantation 72:764, 2001.
24. Budde K, Schmouder RL, Brunkhorst R, et al: First human trial of FTY720, a novel immunomodulator, in stable renal transplant patients. J Am Soc Nephrol 13:1073, 2002.

XII

Survival and Results

Outcome Predictors in Liver Transplantation

R. MARK GHOBRIAL
GORAN B. KLINTMALM

Principles of organ allocation   1286

Model for End-Stage Liver Disease   1286
   MELD and pretransplant mortality   1287
   MELD and posttransplant survival   1287
   MELD dilemma   1287

Outcome parameters after primary orthotopic
   liver transplantation   1288
   Donor characteristics   1288
   Recipient factors   1289
   Operative variables   1290
   Postoperative indicators   1290

Outcome parameters after
   retransplantation   1291
   Survival predictors after repeat orthotopic
     liver transplantation   1291
   Early versus late retransplantation   1292
   Retransplantation outcomes in recipients
     with hepatitis C versus those without
     hepatitis C   1292
   Retransplantation and MELD   1293
   Approaches to improve retransplantation
     outcomes   1294

Posttransplant survival models   1294
   Retransplantation models   1294
   Model for posttransplant survival   1295

Prospectus   1296

Since 1987, the rate of new registration to the United Network for Organ Sharing (UNOS) waiting list has far exceeded the growth of deceased donor (DD) liver organs. Less than 5000 DD livers are available annually, yet close to 19,000 patients currently await liver transplantation.[1] Despite adopting minimal listing criteria[2] and expanding the definitions of acceptable liver organ grafts, the current disparity between supply and demand has both exponentially increased median waiting times and linearly increased waiting list deaths, which reached 1600 in 2000 (Fig. 79–1). The growing scarcity of donor organs in conjunction with the increasing pool of potential recipients awaiting liver transplantation has also added to the number of patients undergoing transplantation as urgent-status recipients.[3]

The disparity between DD organs and orthotopic liver transplantation (OLT) candidates has highlighted the debate in organ allocation. On first glance, transplantation of recipients who exhibit the greatest need may provide a logical approach. However, survival benefits in critically ill recipients are poor when compared with nonurgent patients (Fig. 79–2),[4-7] thereby reducing the benefits of a very scarce organ resource. Such debate must therefore be guided by understanding the factors that predict survival outcome before transplantation. Application of such factors may allow the development of a nonbiased objective approach to patient and organ selection that can tailor organ distribution to appropriate transplant candidates to ensure

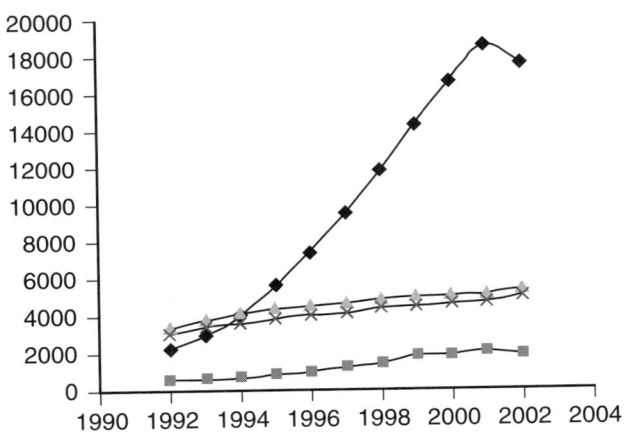

FIGURE 79–1

Shortage of deceased donor organs in the United States. The number of new registrations for liver transplantation (*diamonds*) has increased exponentially, whereas the number of available deceased donor livers (*x*) and the overall number of liver transplantations (*triangles*) have exhibited modest increases. The number of patient deaths (*squares*) on the waiting list has increased linearly during the past decade.

successful outcomes. The following text highlights the guiding principles of organ distribution and the factors that influence outcome after liver transplantation.

Principles of Organ Allocation

Two seemingly opposing principles for liver allocation have been advocated: efficiency of organ use and urgency of need.[8] The first implies transplantation into low-risk recipients where the best results are achieved, whereas the second favors organ diversion to high-risk patient cohorts. If sufficient liver organ allografts were available for transplantation, application of the

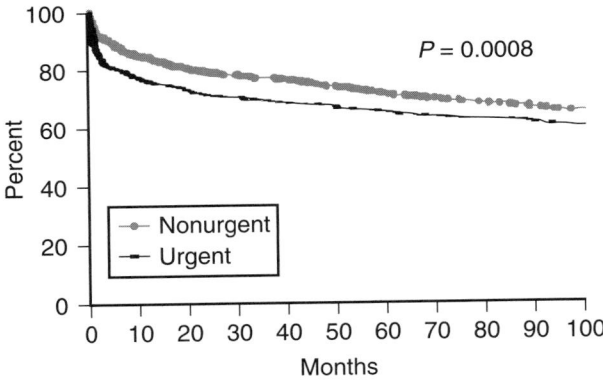

FIGURE 79–2

Recipient survival after transplantation based on urgent versus nonurgent UNOS status.

urgency-of-need principle alone would be well suited for organ allocation. However, the aforementioned scarcity of DD organs in conjunction with mounting deaths on waiting lists and failure of one in five adult primary liver grafts within the first year after transplantation[9] argues that organ distribution based on posttransplant survival outcome may provide the best benefit to our patients.

Over the last 2 decades, the organ allocation system has become strongly biased toward the severity of illness.[2-3] Additionally, recent adoption of the Model for End-Stage Liver Disease (MELD),[10,11] which is a strong predictor of death in patients on waiting lists, as the basis for national organ allocation may increase the percentage of urgent patients receiving DD transplants and further minimize the survival outcomes of a limited organ resource.

In 1998, the Department of Health and Human Services (DHHS) issued the final rule[12] in which the principles that govern operation of the Organ Procurement and Transplant Network (OPTN) were defined. Included were the following guidelines: (1) organs should be allocated to transplant candidates based on medical urgency, (2) the role of waiting times should be minimized, and (3) attempts should be made to avoid futile transplants and promote the efficient use of our scarce organ resource. Thus, the policy for organ distribution calls for a balance between disease severity and expected outcomes. To date, this balance remains an elusive goal for the transplant community. Furthermore, the definition of "futile transplantation" has lacked objective criteria.

Successful development of preoperative models that accurately predict patient survival after liver transplantation has therefore become a crucial concern of the liver transplant community. Such models will allow (1) balancing outcomes with severity of disease so that "futile" transplantation is not performed and (2) implementation of objective criteria for "delisting" of transplant candidates when expected OLT outcomes fall below an established survival threshold, as proposed by an amendment to the final rule of the DHSS.[12]

Model for End-Stage Liver Disease

MELD is a continuous disease severity scale that was originally designed to assess short-term prognosis in patients with hepatic cirrhosis who underwent a transjugular intrahepatic portosystemic shunt (TIPS) procedure. Since then, it has been shown to predict short-term survival in patients awaiting liver transplantation.[10] Application of a liver allocation policy by New England transplant centers that used a continuous severity scale, like the MELD system, and de-emphasized waiting time for status 2B candidates resulted in a significant reduction in overall deaths on the waitlist.[13] Liver allocation policy in the United States has therefore changed to a MELD-based continuous disease severity scale with minimal weight given to waiting time in an effort to better prioritize DD liver transplant candidates. A question therefore arises regarding the accuracy of the MELD as a pretransplant and posttransplant outcome predictor.

MELD and Pretransplant Mortality

The validity of the model was determined by the c-statistic (concordance-equivalent to the area under the receiving operating curve [ROC]), which indicates the probability of the risk of death in randomly selected patients in a defined time frame. A c-statistic of 1 indicates perfect correlation, whereas 0.5 is the result of chance alone.[10] A c-statistic of 0.8 to 0.9 indicates excellent correlation, and one greater than 0.7 is useful. The MELD model was validated in a variety of settings, including hospitalized and outpatient patients with cirrhosis, in whom the c-statistic ranged from 0.78 to 0.87. The ROC of MELD in predicting pretransplant mortality at 3 months far exceeded the previously used Child-Turcotte-Pugh classification (Fig. 79–3).[14] Currently, the MELD score is based on objective laboratory values, including serum creatinine, bilirubin, and the international normalized ratio. Inclusion of additional complications of portal hypertension such as ascites, bleeding, encephalopathy, or spontaneous bacterial peritonitis to the laboratory values in MELD did not increase its accuracy. Similarly, addition of the cause of liver disease did not affect the MELD c-statistic. Thus, the MELD score provides the best available 3-month mortality estimate from liver disease.

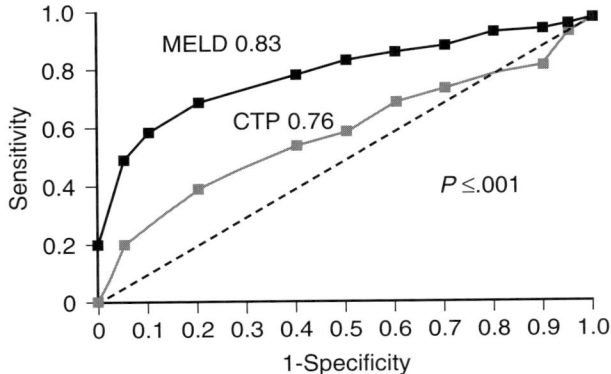

FIGURE 79–3

The area under the receiving operating curve (ROC) for the MELD score compared with the Child-Turcotte-Pugh score for 3-month mortality.

Table 79–1. CORRELATION OF PRETRANSPLANT MELD SCORE WITH POSTTRANSPLANT SURVIVAL

MELD	Number	Survival (%)		
		3 mo	12 mo	24 mo
< 15	340	94.7	89.4	85.8
15–24	226	90.27	85.4	82.3
≥ 25	103	84.47	75.7	74.7
P value		.003	.002	.031

MELD, Model for End-Stage Liver Disease.

MELD and Posttransplant Survival

Although the MELD system is efficient at predicting 3-month mortality from liver disease, it is unclear whether it can predict posttransplant survival. This issue has been addressed by several studies.[11,15-17] In the first study, the Baylor group showed progressively lower patient survival benefits with rising MELD scores, as demonstrated in Table 79–1. One year after transplantation, recipients with MELD scores higher than 25 exhibited survival rates of 75% as opposed to 89.4% in patients with MELD scores lower than 15 (P = .003).[17] Similar results were shown by another large study from the University of California at Los Angeles (UCLA), where survival of patients with a MELD score higher than 25 was significantly lower than in those with MELD scores lower than 25 at the time of OLT (P < .001, Fig. 79–4A).[15] Evaluation of the results of the first year of implementation of the MELD allocation system by Freeman and colleagues[16] clearly demonstrated a nationwide adjusted increased risk for mortality with increasing MELD scores (see Fig. 79–4B). However, MELD prediction of mortality within 3 months after OLT has a c-statistic of only 0.62 (95% confidence interval, 0.55 to 0.69).[10] Therefore, although these results suggest a relationship between the MELD score and postoperative patient survival, they also suggest that the MELD score alone is not able to accurately predict posttransplant deaths.

MELD Dilemma

The inability of the MELD score to accurately predict posttransplant outcomes has led to a dilemma, since its application may not satisfy the "final rule" parameter of avoiding futile transplantation. Specifically, two issues arise. First, if desperately ill candidates with MELD scores higher than 40 are continuously prioritized for transplantation, more futile transplantations will be performed, since it has been already shown that such candidates have an unacceptably high risk for death at OLT (see Fig. 79–4B). To resolve this issue, a consensus was reached to cap the MELD score at a maximum of 40 points so that

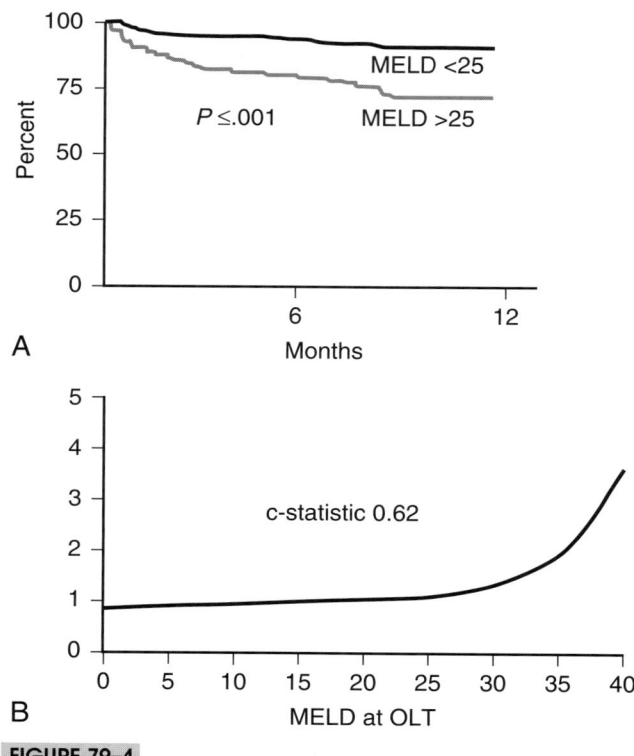

FIGURE 79-4

Model for End-Stage Liver Disease (MELD) score as a predictor of posttransplant survival. **A**, Recipient survival after transplantation based on pretransplant MELD score. **B**, Increased relative risk of mortality 3 months after transplantation with rising MELD scores.[16] Such correlation achieves a c-statistic of 0.62.[10]

without providing an additional advantage of organ allocation.

The second issue is the multitude of other variables that may affect OLT outcomes in addition to the MELD score. For instance, transplantation in patients with a high MELD score may not be futile if a young organ is used, whereas transplantation in another recipient with an extended criteria donor may not be successful despite a low MELD score. This issue can be addressed only if other recipient and graft variables are taken into account, as discussed in the ensuing sections.

Outcome Parameters after Primary Orthotopic Liver Transplantation

Many studies have critically examined[4-7,18-37] the variables associated with transplantation outcomes in different patient populations after primary OLT or retransplantation. In general, such variables can be artificially divided into donor, recipient, operative, and postoperative factors (Table 79–2). However, many of these factors have been shown to exhibit dynamic interactions that ultimately determine the outcome of OLT.[38] The following discussion aims to dissect the relative importance of each of these variables.

Donor Characteristics

Several single-center studies have attempted to define donor variables associated with poor function and,

candidates with MELD scores higher than 40 get no additional priority. This modification allows centers to attempt transplantation of desperately ill candidates

Table 79-2. FACTORS IMPLICATED AS A CAUSE OF POOR OUTCOME AFTER ORTHOTOPIC LIVER TRANSPLANTATION

Donor	Preoperative	Operative	Postoperative
Age	Urgent UNOS status	Blood loss	Elevated ALT
Weight/BMI	MELD score	Blood product use	Elevated AST
Gender compatibility	Age	Bile production	Serum bilirubin
ABO status	Renal dysfunction	Urine output	Serum creatinine
Length of hospitalization	Mechanical ventilation	Warm ischemia	Prothrombin time
Use of pressors	Serum bilirubin		
Downtime	Prothrombin time		
Liver function	Mechanical ventilation		
Sodium level	Ascites		
Reduced/split grafts	AST/ALT		
NHB status	Malnutrition		
Steatosis	Coma score		
Cold ischemia			

ALT, alanine transaminase; AST, aspartate transaminase; BMI, body mass index; NHB, non–heart-beating; MELD, Model for End-Stage Liver Disease; UNOS, United Network for Organ Sharing.

ultimately, graft failure and patient death after OLT.[16,17,24,31] However, these studies exhibited wide variability and seemingly opposing results in the factors reported to influence graft function after OLT. One study that examined 365 DD grafts between 1985 and 1990 identified donor weight above 100 kg as the only variable associated with increased 3-month graft loss (P <.01).[31] Prolonged donor hospital stay (>3 days), donor age older than 50 years, or cold ischemia time longer than 12 hours did not affect the outcome. In marked contrast, another study reported donor age (>30 years) and donor hospitalization (>3 days) to be associated with significantly higher rates of graft failure.[39] Similarly, a multivariate analysis of split-liver grafts identified donor hospital stay longer than 5 days as the most significant predictor of graft failure and recipient death.[6] Another large study that analyzed 340 OLTs demonstrated that donor plasma sodium concentrations higher than 155 mmol/L and ABO incompatibility were independent predictors of patient and graft survival.[40] Such variability in these studies was probably caused by the type of analysis performed (univariate versus multivariate), definitions of graft nonfunction, the donor parameters examined, and the donor populations used by the center.[24] Furthermore, operative factors such as warm ischemia time and the condition of the recipient may further influence the outcome,[38] since transplantation of an extended criteria DD liver graft into a stable recipient may prove to be successful whereas use of a similar graft in an urgent patient may be associated with graft failure and death.

A collective review of the literature revealed at least 15 donor variables that may be associated with poor graft survival and increased risk of recipient death. Such variables included donor age, sex, race, weight, gender, ABO status, cause of brain death, length of hospital stay, pulmonary insufficiency, use of pressors, cardiac arrest, blood chemistry, cold preservation time, fat in the liver, and sodium level.[24] A critical analysis of all such donor variables by Strasberg and associates[24] divided donor factors into absolute and relative risks (Table 79–3). Severe macrosteatosis (>60%) and cold preservation longer than 30 hours were the main absolute donor risk factors. Relative risk factors were moderate steatosis (30% to 60%), cold preservation longer than 12 hours, and donor age older than 50 years.

Table 79-3. DONOR ABSOLUTE AND RELATIVE RISK FACTORS ASSOCIATED WITH LIVER GRAFT FAILURE

Factor	Relative Risk	Absolute Risk
Cold preservation time	> 12 hr	≥ 30 hr
Fat in liver	30%–60%	> 60%
Age	> 50 yr	None

Recipient Factors

The influence of patient selection on survival after transplantation has been recognized and extensively investigated since the early days of liver transplantation.[32,41] Perhaps the first to mathematically correlate such a relationship was Shaw and coworkers in an analysis in 1985.[41] In this study, recipients were assigned a score based on the degree of coma, malnutrition, ascites, and previous surgery. Additional points were assigned if recipients had a history of sepsis, bleeding, or spontaneous bacterial peritonitis. With the use of a regression analysis model, 6-month mortality highly correlated with increased operative blood loss, coma score, malnutrition score, serum bilirubin, prothrombin time, and date of transplantation. Significant blood loss was encountered in patients with high coma and ascites scores. Prospective validation of this scoring system in 180 adult and pediatric OLTs revealed that the patients scoring highest were likely to die of causes related to preoperative morbidity.[32,42]

The deleterious effects of advanced recipient illness on posttransplant survival have been well documented by surrogate markers such as UNOS status and MELD score, as well as by multiple objective parameters such as recipient age, renal impairment, coagulation parameters, mechanical ventilation, and liver function (see Table 79–2).[4-6,9,19-21,23,27,32,34-36] A study from UCLA that included more than 3000 transplants performed over the past decade clearly demonstrated the association of poor survival with urgent-status patients (see Fig. 79–2), whereas another study from the same group indicated that pretransplant MELD scores higher than 25 are predictive of significantly lower survival after transplantation (see Fig. 79–4A).[15] Nevertheless, as previously discussed, neither UNOS status nor MELD score alone can predict posttransplant survival with a high degree of accuracy that allows delisting of patients to avoid futile transplantation.

Perhaps the most objective parameter indicating advanced liver disease is the degree of pretransplant renal impairment. The predictive value of preoperative renal function on postoperative OLT survival has been extensively investigated by the Baylor University Medical Center group.[34-36] Data from 569 consecutive OLTs demonstrated that patients with hepatorenal syndrome (HRS) have significantly decreased actuarial survival 5 years after liver transplantation when compared with patients without HRS (P <.03). Furthermore, end-stage renal disease developed in 10% of patients with HRS after OLT versus 0.8% of patients without HRS (P <.005). Another early study, in 1986, that was based on 93 consecutive OLTs demonstrated that of seven variables that predicted survival, elevated serum creatinine was associated with the greatest risk for mortality after OLT.[20] A preoperative serum creatinine concentration of either less than or greater than 1.72 mg/dL accurately predicted survival or death, respectively, in 79% of cases.

The aforementioned observations have been validated by multiple studies in large patient cohorts.[4-6,9,19,21,34-36,38] Cuervas-Mons and coworkers[20] found that preoperative serum creatinine alone was the strongest predictor of death after transplantation. Similarly, pretransplant creatinine was shown to be related to early postoperative sepsis and hospital death.[43] The analysis by Seaberg and colleagues[9] on the UNOS registry confirms the independent effect of renal function on survival after OLT. In a study from UCLA that included 1148 consecutive OLTs,[19] five variables were found to be independent predictors of outcome after primary transplantation. Identified recipient factors included recipient age, serum creatinine, and requirement for mechanical ventilation. However, donor age and sodium levels were also found to affect post-OLT outcome. Another study from UCLA that evaluated survival indicators based on more than 25,000 recipients from UNOS data sets demonstrated advanced recipient age, creatinine, bilirubin, and prothrombin time to be strong predictors of patient death after OLT.[38] Nevertheless, the development by the latter study of a model that predicted post-OLT survival with significant accuracy required the use of donor and operative factors that were also shown to exhibit independent effects on OLT survival outcome.[38] Thus, the best outcomes may be achieved by "tailoring-matching" organs based on their quality to recipients according to their severity of illness.

One unifying theme that emerges from the many studies that have examined variables associated with posttransplant survival is the lack of correlation between the cause of the liver disease and short-term posttransplant survival.[4,5,7] Interestingly, the prognostic indicators outlined by Ricci and collaborators[30] for patients with cholestatic liver disease were similar to those detected in the UCLA survival model for recipients with hepatitis C.[5] Such indicators included recipient age, serum creatinine, UNOS status, and Child's class. These findings underscore that the condition of the patient at the time of transplantation may be the primary determinant of survival after OLT.

Taken together, all these data indicate that surrogate markers for critically ill recipients such as urgent UNOS status and MELD score or other objectively defined recipient variables are important predictors of survival outcome after transplantation. However, despite the clear identification of such poor prognostic indicators, objective parameters for patient delisting, which are based only on the severity of liver disease, have not yet been established. To date, there are only a few absolute recipient contraindications for OLT[19,24]: extrahepatic malignancy, uncontrolled sepsis, and irreversible multiple organ system failure.

Operative Variables

Perhaps operative parameters were the first variables to be investigated for their correlation with poor outcomes. Early studies demonstrated the negative impact of an increased requirement for blood transfusions in OLT recipients.[41] A more recent study associated the lack of immediate bile production, platelet transfusions of 20 U or more, and urine output less than 2.0 mL/kg/hr with an increased incidence of graft failure.[44] The deleterious effect of prolonged warm ischemia time on the outcome of transplantation has been well established.[24,45] Analysis of survival after split-liver transplantation indicated decreased survival with warm ischemia time longer than 35 minutes,[6] and examination of the UNOS database over the past decade demonstrated an association of increased warm ischemia time with reduced patient survival.[38]

Despite the demonstrated effect of operative parameters on recipient survival, they were seldom incorporated in survival models. Such reluctance is based on the perceived absence of their pretransplant predictive value. However, of all intraoperative parameters, warm ischemia time is one factor that may be incorporated into pretransplant models, since its value is well identified in all transplant centers. Based on UNOS data, warm ischemia time for U.S. centers over the past decade has remained stable at an average of 51 minutes.[38]

Postoperative Indicators

A difficult quagmire that is faced after transplantation is determination of the need for urgent retransplantation in the face of allograft dysfunction. Immediate postoperative variables have therefore been investigated in an effort to predict the development of early graft failure and the need for retransplantation. A prospective study from the University of Pittsburgh attempted to reconstruct several models by using logistic regression analysis of data available on postoperative day 2 or 3.[21] Several models were constructed and evaluated for their overall accuracy, goodness of fit, and area under the curve. The best overall model for prediction of graft failure was the one generated from postoperative day 3 data. This model had a predictive accuracy of 92.7% and included serum bilirubin, prothrombin time, and creatinine. The authors concluded that despite a high predictive value, the models generated did not exhibit the high discriminative power that is needed for routine clinical use. To date, our ability to predict early graft dysfunction and requirement for allograft retransplantation immediately after OLT is based more on clinical acumen than solid objective criteria.

Outcome Parameters After Retransplantation

The association of re-OLT with poor survival outcome has been well defined by many investigators.[4,7,21,23,26-28,38,46-51] Since the early days of liver transplantation, re-OLT has been associated with high death rates as reported by Shaw and coauthors.[51] Because of ethical concerns, the debate has shifted from retransplantation for early graft loss to the validity of re-OLT for recurrent disease in general and recurrent hepatitis C in particular. On the one hand, concerns are based on poor survival outcomes after retransplantation, the scarcity of DD organ resources, continued deaths of primary OLT candidates on the waiting list, and the predicted increased requirements for re-OLT in transplant recipients with recurrent hepatitis C. On the other hand, the arguments for re-OLT in recipients with hepatitis C are the limited efficacy of antiviral therapy and the fact that re-OLT becomes the only viable option for patients with allograft failure. Furthermore, in selected patients, retransplantation may be accompanied by good short-term survival outcomes when performed in the early stages of recurrence.[46]

Survival Predictors After Repeat Orthotopic Liver Transplantation

To date, most of the relevant data have been single-center experiences (Table 79–4). In an analysis of 418 hepatic retransplantations performed at the University of Pittsburgh from 1987 to 1993, seven independent variables were found to be associated with graft failure within the first year after retransplantation.[26] These factors included female donor gender, recipient age, mechanical ventilation, serum creatinine, and bilirubin. Evaluation of 299 patients at 1, 5, and 10 years who underwent retransplantation at UCLA for a variety of indications revealed survival rates of 62%, 47%, and 45% from the date of the first OLT (Fig. 79–5) and rates of 55%, 47%, and 44% from the date of the second transplant, respectively.[7] During the same time interval, primary OLT achieved 83%, 74%, and 68% patient survival rates at 1, 5, and 10 years (see Fig. 79–5). By bivariate and multivariate analysis, variables that significantly influenced survival outcome in all 299 patients who underwent retransplantation included recipient age ($P < .03$), interval to retransplantation ($P < .005$), total number of grafts ($P < .007$), and recipient UNOS status ($P < .015$). Recipient primary diagnosis and indication for retransplantation were not found to influence survival.[7] Examination of the UNOS database, which included 1356 retransplantations, by Rosen and Martin,[28] as well as other single-center studies from the United Kingdom,[27] France,[53] and the United States,[47] provided very similar data (see Table 79–4). Among the different predictive factors, recipient age, urgent status, and recipient serum creatinine and serum bilirubin appear to exhibit the most significant predictive power. Other important indicators have also been identified, including cold ischemia time, use of blood products, ventilator status, and interval to re-OLT. However, since most investigators attempted to construct re-OLT models based on preoperative data elements, the effects of the liver allograft itself on

Table 79–4. PREDICTORS OF SURVIVAL AFTER LIVER RETRANSPLANTATION

Reference	Number	Prognostic Factors	Comments
Powelson,[50] 1993	71	Interval to re-OLT	Single-center experience
Doyle,[26] 1996	418	Donor gender, recipient age, mechanical ventilation, creatinine, bilirubin	Single-center experience
Wong,[27] 1997	70	Age, UNOS status, inpatient status, creatinine, bilirubin	Single-center experience
Markman,[18] 1999	299	Age, interval to transplantation, total number of grafts, UNOS status	Single-center experience
Kim,[52] 1999	447	Interval to re-OLT	Single center, PBC, PSC
Rosen,[28] 1999	1356	Age, bilirubin, creatinine, UNOS status, cause of graft failure (PNF versus non-PNF)	UNOS database
Facciuto,[47] 2000	48	Age, serum creatinine, intraoperative blood products	Single-center experience
Azoulay,[53] 2002	139	Age, serum creatinine, urgency of transplantation	Single-center experience

OLT, orthotopic liver transplantation; PBC, primary biliary cirrhosis; PNF, primary nonfunction; PSC, primary sclerosing cholangitis; UNOS, United Network for Organ Sharing.

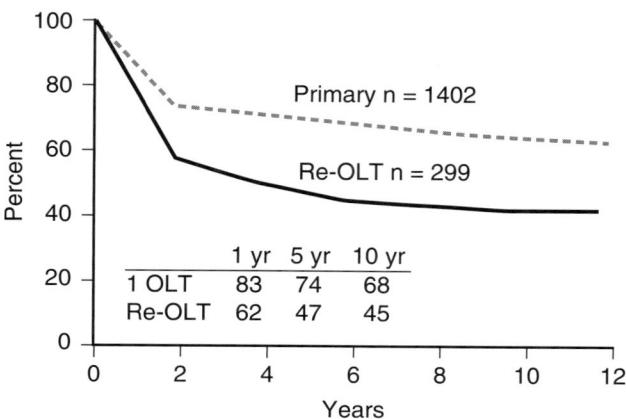

FIGURE 79–5

Recipient survival after retransplantation versus primary transplantation.

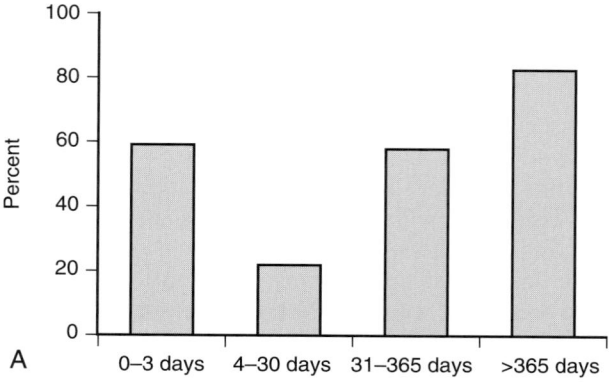

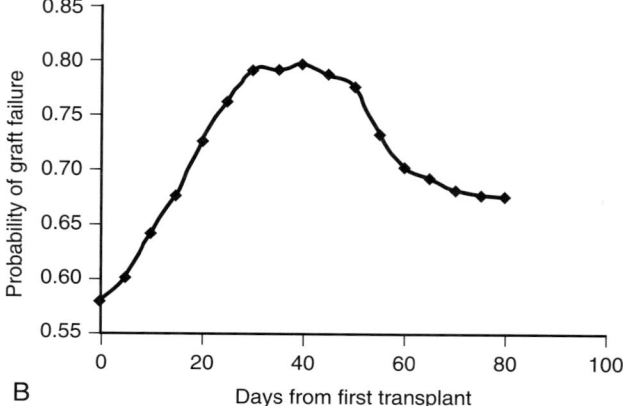

FIGURE 79–6

Effect of the time interval until retransplantation on survival outcome. **A**, One-year survival estimates of retransplant recipients based on the time interval from the first transplant. **B**, Probability of graft failure after retransplantation as a function of the time elapsed from primary transplantation.

retransplantation outcomes have not been fully studied. Ironically, even the most experienced surgeons may not attempt long-term redo transplantations unless a high-quality graft is available.

Early versus Late Retransplantation

A difficulty often faced in evaluating retransplantation outcomes is the distinction between re-OLT performed for early graft failure versus delayed re-OLT undertaken for recurrent disease, chronic rejection, or other late complications of transplantation. The persisting question is whether the risk of death after early re-OLT is different from that after delayed retransplantation. The series from the Mayo Clinic,[52] which was limited to patients with cholestatic liver disease, suggested better survival outcomes when retransplantation was performed within 30 days after primary OLT. More detailed analyses were performed by at least three other large studies. The first, from the New England group (Fig. 79–6A),[50] demonstrated a 1-year survival rate of 57% for re-OLTs performed within 3 days of the primary transplant. Recipient survival dropped to 24% and afterward increased to 54% when the time intervals were 4 to 30 and 31 to 365 days, respectively. The best 1-year survival rates of 83% were obtained when re-OLTs were performed after 1 year. In agreement was the report by UCLA,[7] which demonstrated worst survival in patients retransplanted between 8 and 30 days. The study from the University of Pittsburgh (see Fig. 79–6B)[26] similarly showed that the probability of graft failure after retransplantation steadily increased from 0.58 at day 0 to reach a maximum of 0.8 at day 38, followed by a slow decline thereafter. Taken together, these data demonstrate that survival within the first week after re-OLT may be equivalent to that after delayed retransplantation. The highest survival risk is

predicted for patients within these two aforementioned groups.

Retransplantation Outcomes in Recipients with Hepatitis C versus Those Without Hepatitis C

Initial reports on poor outcomes associated with retransplantation for recurrent hepatitis C and the suggestion that viral reinfection may negatively influence the prognosis of re-OLT questioned the wisdom of the procedure.[46,54] However, retransplantation carries a worse prognosis than primary OLT does for all indications. Evaluation of 299 patients who underwent retransplantation at UCLA[7] for a variety of indications revealed that the recipient's primary diagnosis at re-OLT and the reason for retransplantation were not found to influence survival. In another study by the same group, retransplantation for recurrent hepatitis C achieved 1- and 2-year survival rates of 60%, equivalent to survival rates after retransplantation for other indications.[4,7] These studies therefore suggest that the results of retransplantation for recurrent hepatitis C are not different from the results of retransplantation for other causes in recipients without hepatitis C.

At least two studies have suggested that the prognosis after re-OLT for recurrent hepatitis C is inferior to that after retransplantation performed for other indications in patients without hepatitis C.[47,54] The first report,[47,55] which analyzed predictors of mortality after late retransplantation (>6 months after initial OLT), demonstrated that patients retransplanted for recurrent hepatitis C had poorer survival rates (57% and 43%) than did patients retransplanted for other indications (81% and 74%) at 6 months and 1 year, respectively. Although this difference was not statistically significant ($P < .09$), it may be clinically relevant, since most of the deaths occurred within the first 90 days after re-OLT. Only one patient died because of recurrent hepatitis C, the death occurring 161 days after retransplantation. The independent predictors of 90-day mortality identified by the study included preoperative creatinine higher than 2 mg/dL, recipient age older than 50 years, and the intraoperative use of blood products. Thus, the initial high mortality observed with re-OLT for recurrent hepatitis C may reflect the poor preoperative condition of the patient and failure to identify the predictors of poor prognosis in patients undergoing retransplantation.[55]

The second study[54] analyzed UNOS data on 1539 patients, including 357 hepatitis C–positive adult recipients undergoing liver retransplantation. Kaplan-Meier analysis demonstrated significantly diminished survival rates in the hepatitis C–positive group at 1, 3 and 5 years, 57%, 55%, and 54%, as compared with 65%, 63%, and 61%, respectively, in the hepatitis C–negative group ($P < .0038$; relative risk, 1.36). Multivariate logistic regression analysis of the subgroup of hepatitis C–positive patients undergoing retransplantation for graft failure not caused by primary nonfunction identified preoperative serum bilirubin and serum creatinine as significant independent predictors of death after re-OLT. Additionally, only 7 of 207 (3.4%) patients undergoing retransplantation died of recurrent hepatitis C in their second allografts. Despite the inherent limitations of this study caused by incomplete data sets from the UNOS registry, it underscores the fact that the preoperative condition of the patient, not recurrent hepatitis C, is the primary determinant of survival after re-OLT. Additionally, the conclusions from this study were in direct contrast to those of another more recent report by Watt and colleagues,[48] which was also based on the UNOS registry. Whereas the former study made comparisons between hepatitis C and all non–hepatitis C patients regardless of the primary diagnosis, the group from the University of Nebraska stratified non–hepatitis C recipients into subgroups based on the

cause of the liver disease. Only recipients with hepatitis B and patients with autoimmune disease exhibited better survival rates than patients with hepatitis C after re-OLT. There were no significant survival differences after retransplantation between hepatitis C–positive, cryptogenic, cholestatic, or alcoholic liver disease patients when adjusted for age and MELD scores. These results are in support of other single-center experiences in which the recipient primary diagnosis was not found to influence survival after re-OLT.

Thus, in the final assessment, most authors would agree that regardless of the underlying cause of the liver disease, the primary indicator for re-OLT survival is the recipient's severity of illness.[4,7,38,46,55,56] The initial lack of recognition that recurrence of hepatitis C could lead to frank graft failure and the delay in retransplantation until patients were severely ill and debilitated from recurrent disease may account for the poor early results of retransplantation for recurrent hepatitis C. Nevertheless, the impact of recurrent disease on long-term survival is yet to be determined.

Retransplantation and MELD

In contrast to the UNOS classification, adoption of the MELD scores for organ allocation has provided a unique opportunity for objective stratification of retransplant candidates based on the severity of illness.[10] Analysis of MELD scores for 2129 patients undergoing re-OLT from 1996 to 2002 by the University of Nebraska group[48] in which causes of early retransplantation were excluded revealed very important findings. First, survival after re-OLT decreased with increasing preoperative MELD scores (Table 79–5). Patients who underwent retransplantation at a MELD score less than 20 exhibited 1-year survival rates between 73% and 81%. The best survival outcomes of 81% to 83% were achieved when

Table 79–5. RECIPIENT SURVIVAL AFTER RETRANSPLANTATION BASED ON MELD SCORES

MELD Score	Cause	1-Year Survival (%)
< 10	HCV	83
	Non-HCV	81
11–20	HCV	65
	Non-HCV	73
21–25	HCV	62
	Non-HCV	81
26–30	HCV	57
	Non-HCV	64
> 30	HCV	42
	Non-HCV	55

HCV, hepatitis C virus.

retransplantation was performed at a MELD score less than 10. One-year survival rates after re-OLT were decreased to approximately 60% in both non–hepatitis C patients with MELD scores higher than 25 and hepatitis C–positive recipients with MELD scores higher than 20. Most concerning was the extremely poor survival rate of approximately 50% in re-OLT patients with a MELD higher than 30. Second, the mean MELD scores for re-OLT in patients with and without hepatitis C were 21.7 and 21.5, respectively. Taken together, these data indicate that a large proportion of patients currently undergo re-OLT at MELD scores that are associated with high mortality. Therefore, at a given MELD score, re-OLT may be associated with a significantly higher death rate than is the case with primary transplantation. To improve re-OLT–associated outcomes, retransplantation must be undertaken at lower MELD scores than those used for primary OLT recipients.

Approaches to Improve Retransplantation Outcomes

The demonstrated impact of higher MELD scores on poor survival after retransplantation leaves the transplant community with tough decisions to improve re-OLT survival outcomes. One seemingly straightforward approach is to define a MELD score with an acceptable survival rate after retransplantation below which re-OLT should be discouraged, such as 60% at 1 year. However, survival outcomes have been shown to be dependent on additional variables other than those defined by MELD. Use of MELD as the sole indicator for re-OLT survival may therefore be insufficient. A logical alternative approach is to adopt a transplant model that predicts posttransplant survival and apply such a model to re-OLT candidates. However, it may not be plausible that re-OLT patients would receive their organs based on predicted survival outcomes after transplantation whereas primary transplant patients would receive organs based on the principle of prevention of death as predicted by the MELD criteria. One could therefore argue a third approach in which both primary OLT and re-OLT candidates receive organs based on expected survival rather than the current allocation based on MELD-predicted pretransplant mortality. A fourth approach is to award re-OLT candidates additional MELD points to allow retransplantation to occur at a lower biological MELD score that is consistent with acceptable survival rates. The study by Watt and coworkers[48] correlated a biological MELD score of less than 20 with acceptable survival outcomes for re-OLT candidates. With any of the aforementioned approaches, efficient use of organs argues in favor of establishing criteria for appropriate patient selection so that re-OLT is not performed under desperate circumstances.

Posttransplant Survival Models

Over the last few years, alternative scoring systems have been developed by using proportional hazard or logistic regression analysis of the plethora of previously discussed variables. Ideally, these models could be used to identify a subset of candidates with poor survival outcomes so that "futile" transplantation can be avoided. Unlike the discrete variables previously used in the Child-Turcotte-Pugh scoring systems, the newer mathematical models use continuous variables. Although more complicated, continuous variables eliminate subjective bias and address the "ceiling" effect, which limits the numerical score of a given risk factor despite its continuous progression.[28] Application of the MELD score as an indicator of pretransplant mortality, in conjunction with posttransplant outcome-predicting models, would maximize recipients' benefits from transplantation. However, two issues remain before such models could be applied to clinical practice. First, the accuracy of outcome prediction must be sufficiently high to allow application to the individual patient. Second, a consensus must be developed by the transplant community to determine the lower range of acceptable survival, such as 60% to 65% at 1 year, below which transplantation or re-OLT, or both, should not be undertaken. The following discussion focuses on a few models that have undergone some degree of validation.

Retransplantation Models

The first model by Rosen and Martin[28] addressed poor outcomes after re-OLT by assigning a mortality risk score based on pretransplant variables. These factors included recipient age, creatinine, bilirubin, cause of graft failure (primary nonfunction versus non–primary nonfunction), and a UNOS status coefficient (status 1, −0.261; status 2, −0.463; status 3, −1.07). Risk scores of the selected population exhibited a normalized distribution. Calculated risk scores for individual patients assigned re-OLT recipients into low-, medium- and high-risk groups (P <.0001). Although the model-predicted survival was not statistically different from observed survival after re-OLT, this model has not yet undergone stringent validation. Additionally, the UNOS status used by the model is a rather subjective assessment that may reduce its strength. Furthermore, the model has not incorporated allograft elements that have been shown to independently have an impact on re-OLT outcome.[38] Another retransplantation model similarly used a 5-point scoring system that excluded UNOS status and the cause of graft loss and incorporated recipient age, creatinine, bilirubin, cold ischemia time, and ventilation status.[18] Although originally developed in an

Table 79-6. MODELS OF POSTTRANSPLANT SURVIVAL

Reference	Model	Comments
Rosen,[28] 1999	Risk score = 0.024 (recipient age) + 0.112 $\sqrt{\text{bilirubin}}$ + 0.230 (log$_e$ creatinine) + 0.947 (cause of graft failure) + UNOS coefficient	Retransplantation model based on UNOS database, 900 re-OLT recipients
Markmann,[18] 1999	Risk score = 0.726 cold ischemia + 0.561 ventilator status + 0.0292 serum bilirubin + 0.202 serum creatinine + 0.526 age group	Retransplantation model based on UCLA database, 150 re-OLT recipients
Ghobrial,[38] 2002	Risk score = 0.0084 donor age + 0.019 recipient age + 0.816 log creatinine + 0.0044 warm ischemia + 0.659 (if second transplant) + 0.10 log bilirubin + 0.0087 PT + 0.01 cold ischemia	Universal model based on UNOS data set, 25,000 primary OLT and re-OLT recipients

OLT, orthotopic liver transplantation; PT, prothrombin time; UCLA, University of California at Los Angeles; UNOS, United Network for Organ Sharing.

analysis of 150 re-OLT recipients at UCLA, it has been validated in UNOS data sets and Baylor University Medical Center patient populations. However, in the UNOS cohort, actual survival was higher according to the Cox model, which may question its applicability to broader populations. Although these differences may have been attributed to missing elements in the UNOS database, stringent validation is required.

Model for Posttransplant Survival

Taking into account multiple recipient, allograft, and surgical variables that are available readily preoperatively, the UCLA group has defined a universal model for liver transplant survival (MLTS) that attempts to define survival after both primary transplantation and retransplantation.[38] This model incorporates recipient age, donor age, recipient creatinine, recipient total bilirubin, prothrombin time, retransplantation, and warm and cold ischemia times (Table 79–6). The mean warm ischemia time is a well-documented value for the surgical team, and the expected cold ischemia time could be easily calculated before transplantation.

Two methods were used for MLTS validation. Mortality risk scores were calculated for individual patients and used to stratify transplant recipients into five risk groups. The risk score cutoff values dividing the patients were chosen so that each quintile would contain a roughly equal number of patients. As shown in Table 79–7, the mean mortality score exhibited a sequential increase from the first patient quintile with a mean risk score of 1.33 to 2.59 in the fifth quintile. The model's ability to stratify patients by risk scores was validated by the observed relative risk of death, which increased sequentially from 1.0 in the first quintile to 3.89 in the fifth quintile. Additionally, the model-predicted relative risk of death was identical to the observed relative risk of death throughout all quintiles. Furthermore, the model-predicted survival was identical to the actual Kaplan-Meier survival estimates for the entire UNOS population and subpopulations, including UNOS non–hepatitis C recipients, UNOS hepatitis C recipients, and UCLA hepatitis C recipients.[38] The second validation methodology included the c-statistic, which was estimated at 0.69 and 0.67 at 3 and 12 months, respectively. The MELD score is generally believed to exhibit a high c-statistic of 0.8 to 0.87 and 0.78 to 0.87 at 3 months and 1 year, respectively.[10] However, these high c-statistic estimates were achieved with only small sample sizes of 282 to 491 patients. When the MELD score was applied to a larger sample size of 1179, the c-statistic dropped to 0.78 and 0.73 at 3 months and 1 year, respectively. In a much larger patient population, the MELD c-statistic may even decline further. Thus, the c-statistic of 0.69 achieved by

Table 79-7. PREDICTED AND OBSERVED RISK FOR DEATH IN THE UCLA MODEL OF POST-OLT SURVIVAL

Quintile	Number of Patients	Mean Model Mortality Score	Model Relative Risk	Observed Relative Risk
1	5153	1.33	1.0	1.0
2	5154	1.64	1.37	1.38
3	5155	1.85	1.69	1.66
4	5155	2.08	2.14	2.23
5	5155	2.59	3.52	3.89

OLT, orthotopic liver transplantation; UCLA, University of California at Los Angeles.

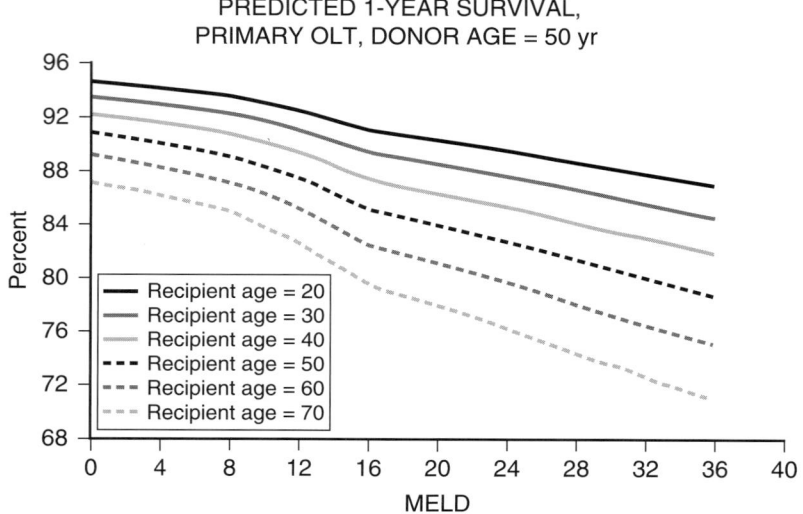

PREDICTED 1-YEAR SURVIVAL,
PRIMARY OLT, DONOR AGE = 50 yr

FIGURE 79–7

Predicted 1-year recipient survival estimates for primary orthotopic liver transplant recipients of different ages and with different MELD scores based on the UCLA model for posttransplant survival. The examples provided assume mean cold and warm ischemia times of 12 hours and 51 minutes, respectively.

this universal model in the heterogeneous UNOS population of more than 25,000 patients provides an extremely useful model.

Two modifications to this model were adopted. To facilitate its use, the MELD score was substituted for preoperative serum creatinine, serum bilirubin, and prothrombin time. Second, to increase its sensitivity, the risk of death imposed by re-OLT was reassessed, since retransplantation was shown to exhibit a different risk based on the time interval from the first transplant.[7,26,50] Accordingly, re-OLT within the first 7 days after the first transplant markedly increased the risk of death (hazard ratio [HR] of 1.53), whereas re-OLT within 7 to 30 or past 30 days doubled the risk of death (HR of 2.153 and 2.131). Therefore, by holding warm and cold ischemia times at median levels, post–re-OLT survival can be accurately computed for an individual patient at 3 and 12 months after transplantation based on the MELD score and recipient and donor ages. As shown in Figure 79–7, a 50-year-old primary OLT candidate with a MELD score of 28 should achieve an expected survival rate of 82% at 1 year. In contrast, a 20-year-old receiving a similar graft would exhibit a 90% survival rate. When delayed retransplantation is considered, a different picture emerges. A 50-year-old re-OLT candidate with a MELD score of 28 exhibits a 1-year survival rate of 75% if a 30-year-old donor organ is used, which drops to 64% if a 50-year-old donor organ is used (Table 79–8). Furthermore, the same 50-year-old patient, if retransplanted at a MELD score of 36, would exhibit a 59% survival estimate at 1 year. As demonstrated in Table 79–8, to achieve a survival benefit of greater than 65%, the 50-year-old donor is best used in 30- to 40-year-old re-OLT recipients at any MELD score or in 50-year-old candidates with a MELD score of 24 or less. Re-OLT

should be avoided in older recipients or 50-year-old patients with MELD scores higher than 28. Thus, this model has the ability to tailor organ needs to recipients based on the severity of disease and expected outcomes. Nevertheless, prospective validation is still required.

Prospectus

Continued outcomes research and application of sophisticated mathematical models to liver transplantation have allowed the identification of multiple factors that influence the survival of patients with liver disease before or after transplantation. The current

Table 79–8. PREDICTED PATIENT SURVIVAL BASED ON MELD SCORES AND RECIPIENT AGE AFTER RE-OLT WITH A 50-YEAR-OLD DECEASED DONOR GRAFT*†

MELD	Recipient Age (yr)				
	30	40	50	60	70
20	77	73	68	**64**	**58**
24	75	71	66	**61**	**55**
28	73	69	**64**	**58**	**53**
32	71	67	**62**	**56**	**50**
36	69	65	**59**	**54**	**48**
40	67	**63**	**57**	**52**	**45**

*Calculations are based on median cold and warm ischemia times of 12 hours and 51 minutes, respectively.
†Expected survival rate estimates less than 65% are in boldface.
MELD, Model for End-Stage Liver Disease; OLT, orthotopic liver transplantation.

MELD allocation system, which predicts pretransplant mortality, was the wellspring of this effort. At present, much attention is directed to developing models that accurately predict posttransplant survival. The use of outcome-predicting models, in conjunction with MELD, would maximize recipients' benefits from a limited donor organ pool. An inherent difficulty in creating pretransplant models that predict posttransplant survival based on recipient pretransplant variables alone stems from the effect of the allograft and the surgical procedure on posttransplant outcomes. An accurate posttransplant survival model must therefore account for surgical and allograft interactions in addition to recipient characteristics. What seemed like an impossible task a few years ago appears to be within grasp in the immediate future. Nevertheless, to apply such models, a consensus must be reached among transplant physicians that defines "futile" transplantation in general and accepted survival outcomes in particular below which transplantation is to be avoided. As recipients with hepatitis C enter their second decade after OLT, it is likely that graft failure and retransplantation issues will become more challenging. Such issues can be resolved only by collecting multicenter data to accurately define factors that influence retransplantation, determine long-term outcomes of the procedure, establish early patient selection criteria, improve re-OLT outcomes, and perhaps establish parameters for delisting of OLT/re-OLT candidates.

Pearls and Pitfalls

- Survival after transplantation is based on recipient characteristics and donor and operative variables. MELD alone cannot accurately predict survival after OLT.

- Critically ill and advanced-age recipients require good-quality grafts to maximize their chance for survival.

- Re-OLT for early graft failure should be performed as soon as possible within a 7-day period to reduce the chance of mortality after transplantation.

- Delayed retransplantation may produce survival outcomes similar to those of re-OLT performed for early graft failure. Late re-OLT produces good survival outcomes when performed in patients with MELD scores lower than 20.

- Further definition of "futile" transplantation and application of posttransplant outcome predictors to organ allocation are warranted to maximize the benefits of a scarce organ resource.

References

1. United Network for Organ Sharing website (http://wwwew3.att.net/ UNOS), accessed April 2002.
2. Lucey MR, Brown KA, Everson GT, et al: Minimal criteria for placement of adults on the liver transplant waiting list: A report of a national conference organized by the American Society of Transplant Physicians and the American Association for the Study of Liver Diseases. Liver Transpl 3:628, 1997.
3. Federal Register (FR Doc 98-8191) 42 CFR Part 121, April 2, 1998, p 16296.
4. Ghobrial RM, Farmer DG, Baquerizo A, et al: Orthotopic liver transplantation for hepatitis C: Outcome, effect of immunosuppression and causes of retransplantation during an eight-year single center experience. Ann Surg 229:824-833, 1999.
5. Ghobrial RM, Steadman R, Gornbein J, et al: A ten-year experience of liver transplantation for hepatitis C: Analysis of factors determining outcome in over 500 patients. Ann Surg 234:384-394, 2001.
6. Ghobrial RM, Yersiz H, Farmer D, et al: Predictors of survival after in vivo split liver transplantation: Analysis of 110 consecutive cases. Ann Surg 232:312-323, 2000.
7. Markmann JF, Markowitz JS, Yersiz H, et al: Long-term survival after retransplantation of the liver. Ann Surg 226:408-418, discussion 418-420, 1997.
8. Bronsther O, Fung JF, Tzakis A, et al: Prioritization and organ distribution for liver transplantation. JAMA 271:140-143, 1994.
9. Seaberg EC, Belle SH, Beringer KC, et al: Liver transplantation in the United States from 1987-1998: Updated results from the Pitt-UNOS liver transplant. In Cecka M, Terasaki P (eds): Clinical Transplants. Los Angeles, UCLA Tissue Typing Laboratory, 1998.
10. Wiesner RH, McDiarmid SV, Kamath PS, et al: MELD and PELD: Application of survival models in liver allocation. Liver Transpl 7:567-580, 2001.
11. Kamath PS, Wiesner RH, Malinchoc M, et al: A model to predict survival in patients with end-stage liver disease. Hepatology 33:464-470, 2001.
12. Organ procurement and transplantation network—HRSA. Final rule with comment period. Fed Reg 63:16296-16338, 1998.
13. Freeman RB, Roher RJ, Katz E, et al: Preliminary results of a liver allocation plan using a continuous medical severity score that de-emphasizes waiting time. Liver Transpl 7:173-178, 2001.
14. Wiesner R, Edwards E, Freeman R, et al: UNOS liver disease severity score committee. Model for end-stage liver disease (MELD) and allocation of donor livers. Gastroenterology 124:91-96, 2003.
15. Saab S, Wang V, Ibrahim AB, et al: MELD score predicts 1-year patient survival post-transplantation. Liver Transpl 9:473-476, 2003.
16. Freeman R, Weisner RH, Edwards E, et al: UNOS/OPTN liver and intestine transplantation committee. Results of the first year of the new liver allocation plan. Liver Transpl 10:7-15, 2004.
17. Onaca NN, Levy MF, Sanchez EQ, et al: A correlation between pretransplantation MELD score and mortality in the first two years after liver transplantation. Liver Transpl 9:117-123, 2003.
18. Markmann JF, Gornbein J, Markowitz J, et al: A simple model to predict survival after retransplantation of the liver. Transplantation 67:422-430, 1999.
19. Markmann JF, Markmann JW, Markmann DA, et al: Preoperative factors associated with outcome and their impact on resource use in 1148 consecutive primary liver transplants. Transplantation 72:1113-1122, 2001.
20. Cuervas-Mons V, Millan I, Gavaler JS, et al: Prognostic value of preoperatively obtained clinical and laboratory data in predicting survival after liver transplantation. Hepatology 6:922-927, 1986.
21. Doyle HR, Marino IR, Jabbour N, et al: Early death or retransplantation in adults after orthotopic liver transplantation. Can outcome be predicted? Transplantation 57:1028-1036, 1994.

22. Gonzalez FX, Rimola A, Grande L, et al: Predictive factors of early postoperative graft function in human liver transplantation. Hepatology 20:565-573, 1994.

23. Doyle HR, Dvorchik I, Mitchell S, et al: Predicting outcomes after liver transplantation. Ann Surg 219:408-415, 1994.

24. Strasberg SM, Howard TK, Molmenti EP, Hertl M: Selecting donor livers: Risk factors for poor function after orthotopic liver transplantation. Hepatology 20:829-838, 1994.

25. Doyle HR, Marino IR, Morelli F, et al: Assessing risk in liver transplantation. Ann Surg 224:168-177, 1996.

26. Doyle HR, Morelli F, McMichael J, et al: Hepatic retransplantation—an analysis of risk factors associated with outcome. Transplantation 61:1499-1505, 1996.

27. Wong T, Devlin J, Rolando N, et al: Clinical characteristics affecting the outcome of liver transplantation. Transplantation 64:878-882, 1997.

28. Rosen HR, Martin P: A model to predict survival following liver retransplantation. Hepatology 29:365-370, 1999.

29. Showstack J, Katz PP, Lake JR, et al: Resource utilization in liver transplantation. JAMA 281:1381-1386, 1999.

30. Ricci P, Therneau TM, Malinchoc M, et al: A prognostic model for the outcome of liver transplantation in patients with cholestatic liver disease. Hepatology 25:672-677, 1997.

31. Mor E, Klintmalm GB, Gonwa TA, et al: The use of marginal donors for liver transplantation. A retrospective study of 365 liver donors. Transplantation 53:383-386, 1992.

32. Shaw BW Jr: The candidate in the intensive care unit: Assessing risk. Liver Transpl Surg 2(5 Suppl 1):21-24, 1996.

33. Testa G, Crippin JS, Netto GJ, et al: Liver transplantation for hepatitis C: Recurrence and disease progression in 300 patients. Liver Transpl 6:553-561, 2000.

34. Gonwa TA, Klintmalm GB, Levy M, et al: Impact of pretransplant renal function on survival after liver transplantation. Transplantation 59:361-365, 1995.

35. Levy MF, Goldstein RM, Husberg BS, et al: Baylor update: Outcome analysis in liver transplantation. Clin Transpl 161-173, 1993.

36. Gonwa TA, Morris CA, Goldstein RM, et al: Long-term survival and renal function following liver transplantation in patients with and without hepatorenal syndrome—experience in 300 patients. Transplantation 51:428-430, 1991.

37. Ploeg RJ, D'Alessandro AM, Knechtle SJ, et al: Risk factors for primary dysfunction after liver transplantation: A multivariate analysis. Transplantation 55:807-813, 1993.

38. Ghobrial RM, Gornbein J, Steadman R, et al: Pretransplant model to predict posttransplant survival in liver transplant patients. Ann Surg 236:315-323, 2002.

39. Greig PD, Froster J, Superina RA, et al: Donor-specific factors predict graft function following liver transplantation. Transplant Proc 22:2072-2073, 1990.

40. Figuras J, Busquets J, Grande L, et al: The deleterious effect of donor high plasma sodium and extended preservation in liver transplantation. A multivariate analysis. Transplantation 61:410-413, 1996.

41. Shaw BW Jr, Wood RP, Gordon RD, et al: Influence of selected patient variables and operative blood loss on six-month survival following liver transplantation. Semin Liver Dis 5:385-393, 1985.

42. Shaw BW, Wood P, Stratta RJ, et al: Stratifying the cause of death in liver transplant recipients. An approach to improving survival. Arch Surg 124:895-900, 1989.

43. Baliga P, Merion RM, Turcotte JG, et al: Preoperative risk factor assessment in liver transplantation. Surgery 112:704-710, 1992.

44. Markmann JF, Markmann JW, Desai NM, et al: Operative parameters that predict the outcomes of hepatic transplantation. J Am Coll Surg 196:556-572, 2003.

45. Mimeault R, Grant D, Ghent C, et al: Analysis of donor and recipient variables and early graft function after orthotopic liver transplantation. Transplant Proc 21:3355, 1989.

46. Ghobrial RM: Retransplantation for recurrent hepatitis C. Liver Transpl 8(10 Suppl 1):S38-S43, 2002.

47. Facciuto M, Heidt D, Guarrera J, et al: Retransplantation for late liver graft failure: Predictors of mortality. Liver Transpl 6:174-179, 2000.

48. Watt KDS, Lyden ER, McCashland TM: Poor survival after liver retransplantation. Is hepatitis C to blame? Liver Transpl 9:1019-1024, 2003.

49. Biggins SW, Beldecos A, Rabkin JM, Rosen HR: Retransplantation for hepatic allograft failure: Prognostic models and ethical considerations. Liver Transpl 8:313-322, 2002.

50. Powelson JA, Cosimi AB, Lewis WD, et al: Hepatic retransplantation in New England—a regional experience and survival model. Transplantation 55:802-806, 1993.

51. Shaw BW, Gordon RD, Starzl TE: Hepatic retransplantation. Transplant Proc 28:264-271, 1985.

52. Kim WR, Wiesner RH, Poterucha JJ, et al: Hepatic retransplantation in cholestatic liver disease: Impact of the interval to retransplantation on survival and resource utilization. Hepatology 30:395-400, 1999.

53. Azoulay D, Linhares MM, Huget E, et al: Decision for retransplantation: An experience- and cost-analysis. Ann Surg 236:713-721, discussion 721, 2002.

54. Rosen H, Martin P: Hepatitis C infection in patients undergoing liver retransplantation. Transplantation 66:1612, 1998.

55. Sheiner PA: Hepatitis C after liver transplantation. Semin Liver Dis 20:201-209, 2000.

56. Ghobrial RM: Retransplantation for recurrent hepatitis C in the model for end-stage liver disease era: How should we or shouldn't we? Liver Transpl 9:1025-1027, 2003.

U.S. Trends in Liver Transplantation, 1988 to 2001

IDRIS V.R. EVANS
STEVEN H. BELLE

Methods   1300

Results   1300
  Recipient characteristics   1300
  Waiting time   1309
  Demographics   1309
  Primary liver disease   1309
  Patient's location while awaiting
    transplantation   1311
  Cold ischemia time   1312
  Laboratory values   1312

Donor characteristics   1312
  Demographics   1312
  Recipient-donor matching
    characteristics   1313

Outcome analysis—crude survival
  percentages   1313

Outcome analysis—multivariable
  modeling   1314

Discussion   1319

The first human liver transplantation was attempted at the University of Colorado by Dr. Thomas Starzl in 1963.[1] The recipient was a 3-year-old boy with biliary atresia, although the operation was not completed owing to fatal hemorrhaging. None of the first seven recipients whose transplantations were performed in Denver, Boston, and Paris over the next 3 years survived more than 23 days following transplantation. In 1967 and 1968, with the use of better immunosuppressive agents and organ preservation techniques, more transplantations were attempted. Although several of these transplantations resulted in initial success, within 2.5 years all of the patients had died. By 1980, with cyclosporine being used as an immunosuppressive agent, patient survival dramatically increased, leading to an increase in liver transplantation so that by 1983 more than 500 procedures had been performed in the United States and Western Europe.[2] The growing use of liver transplantation led to a National Institutes of Health (NIH)–sponsored Consensus Development Conference, which recommended that a "registry or clearinghouse be established for collection and evaluation of all available data on liver transplantation."[2] As a result, the National Institute of Diabetes and Digestive and Kidney Diseases (NIDDK)–sponsored Liver Transplantation Database was established in 1985 for the purpose of developing a database to collect information on candidates for liver transplantation, and information about recipients and their donors, the operation, and sequelae.[3,4]

In addition, the National Organ Transplant Act of 1984[5] mandated a national registry of all solid-organ transplantations performed in the United States. In 1987, the United Network for Organ Sharing (UNOS), in collaboration with four existing solid-organ transplantation registries (kidney, liver, heart, and pancreas) began operating the Scientific Transplant Registries. The UNOS Scientific Liver Transplant Registry (SLTR) was operated from the Department of Epidemiology at the University of Pittsburgh Graduate School of Public Health from its inception until 1998, at which time it was transferred to UNOS in Richmond, Virginia. Throughout its history, the SLTR has obtained information from centers that perform liver transplantation in the United States to document information about the recipients of all liver transplantations performed in the United States. This information is collected when candidates are listed with UNOS to await a donor, at transplantation, 6 months after transplantation, and at annual transplantation anniversaries until retransplantation, at which time the follow-up schedule converts to the time following the most recent transplantation.

Since the SLTR began operation, there have been numerous changes affecting liver transplantation recipients, for example, new immunosuppressive regimens and preservation solutions have been developed and used, schema for allocating donor livers to eligible recipients have undergone modifications owing, in part, to increased waiting times for candidates, and living donors are more common as a result of the relative shortage of donor livers compared with people waiting for liver transplantation. This chapter documents changes in recipient and donor characteristics over the 14-year period from 1988 to 2001. It also examines patient and retransplantation-free survival over the same period.

Methods

The initial data set provided by UNOS (OPTN data created October 31, 2002) included information about all liver transplantations performed in the United States between 1987 and 2002. Because data collection began in October 1987 and the data set was requested in 2002, ascertainment was incomplete in those 2 years. Therefore analyses were restricted to transplantations occurring between 1988 and 2001. Pediatric (younger than age 16 years) and adult recipients were examined separately.

To determine changes over time, descriptive statistics were calculated: proportions for categorical variables and means or medians for continuous variables. In calculating proportions, the number of known responses was used as the denominator. To determine if there were trends in the distributions of discrete variables over time, the Cochran-Armitage trend test was applied. To enable this test to be applied to discrete variables with multiple levels (such as race), indicator variables were created for each level. Categorical variables examined in this manner included type of transplantation, race, primary liver disease, location awaiting transplantation, and recipient-donor gender match and blood type match. Moving average plots were constructed for continuous variables to visualize the relationship with year of transplantation. For example, the moving average of adult recipient's age at transplantation by year of transplantation demonstrated a quadratic relationship, whereas albumin levels for both adult and pediatric patients were related linearly to year of transplantation. The determination of trends for continuous variables involved constructing a simple linear regression model of the variable of interest, possibly transformed to linearize the relationship, regressed over year of transplantation so that the resultant slope could be analyzed for significance and direction. For all analyses, a P value of less than .05 indicated statistical significance.

To address the hypothesis that survival improved over time, we designated the main variable of interest in the analyses as year of transplantation. Initially, crude survival rates for each year of transplantation were calculated by using the product limit method,[6] and the Wilcoxon test[7] was used to determine whether there were statistically significant differences in survival rates by year of transplantation. Multivariable proportional hazards regression models[8] were used to estimate the strength of association, as measured by the hazard ratio (or relative risk) for failure, of each independent variable with the outcomes of patient death or the combined end point of patient death or retransplantation (graft failure), respectively. All variables were included in the final models except for recipient ethnicity, donor ethnicity, cold ischemia time, waiting time, and the laboratory measurements (creatinine, bilirubin, albumin, and prothrombin time). These variables were excluded because of the large number of missing observations for each, thereby maximizing the number of recipients included in the model. To determine whether a continuous variable should be included as originally measured, or whether categories or transformations should be used, separate models containing each form of the variable were compared and the model that had the lowest Akaike information criterion (AIC) value was reported. The AIC statistic examines the likelihood and number of parameters in the model and attempts to balance parsimony, that is, a model with fewer parameters and a more complex model with a larger likelihood.

Results

Recipient Characteristics

Between 1988 and 2001, 51,292 liver transplantations for 45,880 recipients were reported to UNOS. Twelve transplantations were performed for eleven individuals

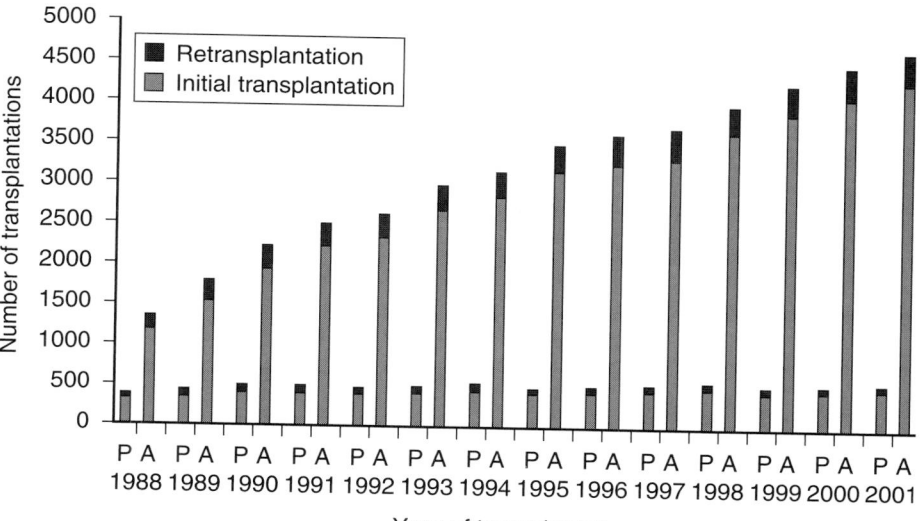

FIGURE 80-1

Numbers of liver transplantations by year for pediatric (P) and adult (A) recipients.

whose ages were unknown at transplantation, so they could not be classified as adult or pediatric recipients. Excluding these cases, there were 44,442 transplantations (87%) performed for 40,055 adult recipients (87%) and 6838 transplantations for 5814 pediatric recipients (younger than age 16 years).

Among adults, there was a consistent increase in the annual number of transplantations from 1338 in 1988 to 4638 in 2001, an increase of 247% (Fig. 80–1). The number of transplantations for pediatric recipients did not increase consistently and peaked at 548 in 1998, a 46% increase from the nadir year of 1988.

The number of retransplantations also increased among adults (from 157 in 1988 to 384 in 2001), but not to the extent that the number of initial transplantations did (145% vs. 247%, respectively). Therefore, the percentage of retransplantations among adults declined over time (Table 80–1). Across all years, 9.9% of transplantations in adults were retransplantations, ranging from a high of 14.1% in 1989 to a low of 8.3% in 2001. The number of retransplantations among children ranged from 46 in 1988 to 94 in 1994, with no apparent trend, although the percentage of retransplantations, as with adults, generally decreased over time. The percentages of retransplantation were higher among pediatric recipients than among adult recipients, with 15.0% of children receiving a retransplantation across all years (range, 20.0% in 1989 to 11.6% in 2001).

The percentage of transplantations among adults involving organs in addition to the liver ranged from 1.8% in 1993 to 3.5% in 1997, with no apparent trend over time (see Table 80–1). Across all years, 2.6% of liver transplantations performed on adults were multiorgan transplantations. The organ most commonly transplanted along with the liver among adults each year was the kidney, and the proportion of such recipients increased noticeably after 1990, reaching the peak

of 95.1% of all multiorgan transplantations in 1994. The percentage of multiorgan transplantations including a heart or intestine in addition to the liver increased from 0.0% in 1988 to 16.5% in 2001, whereas the proportion of liver-pancreas transplantations dropped markedly from 35.5% in 1988 to 0.7% in 2001. Only nine liver transplantations among adults also involved lung transplantation over the 14-year period.

There was an overall increase in the percentage of procedures performed each year in pediatric patients involving organs in addition to the liver, from a nadir of 0.5% in 1989 to 9.4% in 2001. Overall, 5.2% of the transplantations performed on children involved the transplantation of organs in addition to the liver. The most common multiorgan transplantation among pediatric recipients between 1988 and 1990 was liver-kidney, after which the intestine was the most common additional organ transplanted. Hearts and lungs were rarely transplanted along with the livers in pediatric recipients, whereas the percentage of multiorgan transplantations involving the pancreas ranged between 0.0% and 27.9% each year.

The first partial liver transplantation performed for an adult recipient was reported to UNOS in 1993. Less than 1.0% of transplantations for adult recipients used a partial liver until 1999, when the percentage nearly tripled in 1 year from 0.7% in 1998 to 2.0%. The percentage of transplantations among adult recipients that used a partial liver more than doubled over the next 2 years such that in 2001 more than 5.0% of transplantations among adults involved a partial liver. At least 1.0% of transplantations for adult recipients used a split liver each year from 1997 to 2001, during which time the percentage doubled from 1.4% to 2.9%. Until 1998, more split-liver than partial-liver procedures were performed for adults; however, between 1999 and 2001 the relative frequency reversed.

Text continued on p. 11

Table 80-1. SURGICAL, RECIPIENT, AND DONOR CHARACTERISTICS

No. Transplantations Performed

Adult														
Adult	1338	1770	2206	2474	2601	2953	3127	3461	3584	3667	3958	4217	4448	4638	44442
% retransplantations	11.7	14.1	12.8	11.1	11.1	10.1	10.0	9.5	10.0	10.3	8.6	8.4	8.6	8.3	9.9
Pediatric	375	431	484	479	462	487	524	471	489	514	548	506	525	543	6838
% retransplantations	12.3	20.0	19.2	18.4	15.2	16.0	17.9	13.0	13.5	14.2	13.0	14.0	12.2	11.6	15.0

Year

Variable	1988	1989	1990	1991	1992	1993	1994	1995	1996	1997	1998	1999	2000	2001	TOTAL
MULTIORGAN RECIPIENTS (%)															
Adult recipients	2.3	2.7	2.2	1.9	2.3	1.8	2.6	2.4	3.2	3.5	2.6	2.2	2.9	3.0	2.6
Pediatric recipients	1.1	0.5	2.1	2.1	3.0	4.3	4.2	4.9	7.6	8.4	7.8	7.9	7.2	9.4	5.2
TYPE (%)															
Adult Recipients															
Partial liver	0.0	0.0	0.0	0.0	0.0	0.2	0.3	0.1	0.3	0.2	0.7	2.0	3.7	5.2	1.2
Split technique	0.2	0.3	0.2	0.3	<0.1	0.2	0.4	0.2	0.9	1.4	1.3	1.8	2.4	2.9	1.1
Reduced technique	0.0	0.0	0.0	<0.1	<0.1	0.0	0.0	0.0	0.0	0.1	0.0	0.0	0.0	<0.1	<0.1
Whole liver	99.8	99.7	99.8	99.7	99.9	99.6	99.3	99.7	98.8	98.2	98.0	96.2	93.9	91.8	97.6
Unknown (#)	0	0	0	0	0	0	0	0	3	3	8	67	105	117	303
Pediatric Recipients															
Partial liver	0.0	0.2	0.0	0.6	7.8	13.3	33.7	29.3	28.7	26.9	18.8	19.4	20.5	18.3	16.1
Split technique	3.5	4.9	2.7	1.1	1.1	1.9	3.6	2.8	7.2	10.4	14.4	15.9	16.7	15.9	7.4
Reduced technique	0.0	0.5	2.9	4.2	5.2	5.2	1.5	0.0	0.2	0.0	0.2	0.0	0.0	0.2	1.4
Whole liver	96.5	94.4	94.4	94.1	85.9	79.6	61.2	67.9	63.8	62.7	66.6	64.7	62.8	65.6	75.0
Unknown (#)	0	0	2	5	1	7	1	0	5	15	15	41	46	40	178
WAITING TIME: MEDIAN (DAYS)															
Adult recipients	17.0	22.0	21.0	32.0	48.0	62.5	71.0	79.0	106.0	125.0	159.0	164.0	180.5	176.0	87.0
Unknown (#)	415	405	410	198	155	129	51	44	70	52	33	36	50	36	2084
Pediatric recipients	38.0	45.0	37.0	38.5	52.0	82.0	45.0	63.0	57.0	50.0	56.0	60.0	66.0	65.5	54.0
Unknown (#)	136	154	174	67	63	48	29	19	27	29	28	28	29	21	852
Demographics															
SEX (%)															
Females—adult recipients	48.8	45.8	44.7	45.3	43.0	44.0	41.4	42.1	41.2	40.9	37.3	38.0	37.7	35.2	40.7
Females—pediatric recipients	51.7	51.0	50.8	52.0	48.1	53.0	53.1	50.5	47.6	49.4	53.5	51.4	52.0	56.7	51.6

RACE (%)

Adult Recipients

White	89.0	88.3	89.0	89.0	88.0	88.1	88.3	88.3	87.4	86.7	86.9	86.5	86.5	87.5
Black	7.8	6.6	5.9	5.8	6.0	7.0	6.8	6.6	7.3	7.6	7.5	7.8	7.8	7.1
Asian	2.0	2.8	2.8	2.8	3.9	2.6	2.3	2.8	3.0	3.5	3.4	2.8	3.2	3.0
Other	1.2	2.2	2.3	2.3	2.6	2.7	2.9	2.3	2.2	2.2	2.2	2.9	3.2	2.4
Unknown (#)	5	9	17	12	5	12	10	1	1	3	1	4	14	94

Pediatric Recipients

White	78.2	77.1	74.8	80.4	74.4	76.3	76.1	74.3	71.4	73.3	74.3	77.4	73.0	75.5
Black	16.2	15.4	19.1	16.1	18.2	19.5	19.1	16.3	21.9	20.0	18.6	17.0	19.7	18.1
Asian	2.7	4.4	2.3	0.8	2.2	1.9	2.5	5.1	2.9	2.0	3.4	2.5	3.9	2.8
Other	3.0	3.0	3.7	2.7	5.2	2.3	2.3	4.2	3.9	4.8	3.8	3.1	3.2	3.6
Unknown (#)	4	3	3	0	1	1	0	0	0	2	1	2	5	22

ETHNICITY (%)

Adult Recipients

Hispanic/Latino	10.0	9.6	14.0	15.1	13.7	11.9	11.0	12.2	10.1	11.0	10.9	12.1	12.1	11.5
Unknown (#)	647	834	1070	1193	806	602	355	77	30	51	49	23	16	5790

Pediatric Recipients

Hispanic/Latino	22.5	25.5	21.5	24.9	24.8	20.4	20.1	19.0	16.8	15.2	14.7	22.6	23.1	19.9
Unknown (#)	162	200	223	222	151	134	67	12	6	8	9	4	3	1209

MEAN AGE (YR)

Adult recipients	43.1	44.9	45.9	47.4	47.1	48.2	48.6	48.4	49.4	48.4	49.7	50.0	50.3	48.4
Adult recipients—>60 years (%)	8.0	8.8	11.0	14.9	14.4	15.2	16.0	14.2	16.8	14.8	15.9	16.2	16.2	15.0
Pediatric recipients	4.0	3.5	4.1	3.9	4.0	4.1	3.7	4.4	4.1	3.8	4.0	4.0	4.4	4.0

Primary Liver Disease

Adult Recipients (%)

Chronic hepatitis C	14.9	13.7	16.2	19.2	20.5	24.2	24.1	23.8	23.6	24.9	27.9	31.5	31.7	24.9
Alcoholic liver disease	11.1	17.2	20.8	19.7	19.5	17.3	16.6	15.2	14.0	13.1	13.0	11.9	11.8	14.9
Chronic cryptogenic cirrhosis	10.2	11.4	10.9	10.7	10.8	9.9	10.4	11.0	11.0	10.0	9.7	9.7	8.3	10.0
PSC	11.0	11.5	8.8	10.0	9.4	9.4	8.4	8.2	8.3	7.8	6.0	6.0	6.1	8.0
PBC	15.8	10.2	10.4	10.5	9.0	10.1	9.3	8.1	7.6	6.9	5.2	5.0	4.6	7.6
AHN	9.2	8.5	7.9	5.9	6.2	5.5	6.1	6.1	6.0	8.0	8.9	9.4	8.5	7.5
Unknown	1.7	1.7	2.2	2.5	2.7	2.0	2.2	2.0	2.5	2.8	2.8	2.9	2.0	2.3

Continued

Table 80-1. SURGICAL, RECIPIENT, AND DONOR CHARACTERISTICS—cont'd

Variable	1988	1989	1990	1991	1992	1993	1994	1995	1996	1997	1998	1999	2000	2001	Total
-Hepatitis C	3.6	2.5	2.6	0.9	0.7	0.7	1.6	1.6	1.3	1.9	2.6	2.9	3.2	3.2	2.1
-Hepatitis B	1.8	2.4	1.6	1.1	1.2	1.0	0.8	1.0	0.7	1.4	1.3	1.1	1.4	1.0	1.2
-Drug induced	1.3	1.1	0.9	0.6	1.0	1.3	0.9	1.0	0.9	0.8	0.8	0.8	0.8	0.8	0.9
-Other	0.3	0.3	0.1	0.3	0.3	0.2	0.3	0.3	0.4	0.7	1.0	1.2	1.0	1.4	0.7
-Hepatitis A	0.5	0.5	0.5	0.5	0.3	0.3	0.3	0.2	0.2	0.4	0.3	0.1	0.1	0.1	0.3
Alcoholic liver disease + hepatitis C	0.0	0.1	0.2	0.8	2.2	3.0	5.1	7.7	8.6	7.9	8.2	7.6	6.4	6.5	5.5
Miscellaneous	6.4	5.8	4.4	4.3	4.2	2.5	3.4	3.1	4.2	5.0	5.5	6.0	6.4	7.3	5.0
Chronic hepatitis B	6.7	7.1	6.8	6.1	5.0	4.4	3.2	4.2	4.2	4.1	4.0	4.5	3.2	4.0	4.5
Chronic autoimmune cirrhosis	3.8	3.2	3.9	4.6	5.4	5.8	5.7	5.1	4.8	4.5	4.5	3.5	3.5	3.4	4.4
Metabolic disease	4.2	4.3	4.1	3.4	4.1	3.6	4.0	3.8	3.9	3.8	3.0	2.9	3.0	3.0	3.5
α_1-Antitrypsin deficiency	1.4	2.0	1.4	0.9	1.4	1.7	1.2	1.7	1.7	1.4	1.3	1.2	1.2	1.4	1.4
-Hemochromatosis	0.9	1.0	0.9	0.8	1.0	0.9	1.0	0.9	1.4	0.9	0.7	0.7	0.7	0.6	0.9
-Wilson's disease	1.3	1.1	1.3	1.1	1.0	0.7	1.1	0.7	0.4	0.8	0.6	0.3	0.6	0.5	0.7
-Other	0.6	0.2	0.5	0.6	0.7	0.3	0.7	0.5	0.4	0.7	0.4	0.7	0.5	0.5	0.5
Primary liver malignancy	6.3	6.3	5.0	4.2	3.0	3.2	2.6	3.1	3.1	2.9	2.5	3.1	3.1	3.5	3.4
Other chronic diseases	0.5	0.9	0.7	0.6	0.8	0.8	0.9	0.9	0.7	1.0	1.1	0.9	1.1	1.3	0.9
Unknown (#)	0	0	0	0	0	0	0	0	0	0	1	0	0	5	6
Primary Liver Disease															
Pediatric Recipients (%)															
Biliary atresia	58.1	60.6	55.2	54.3	51.1	52.4	52.1	49.9	49.9	42.6	41.8	41.9	37.5	36.6	48.3
AHN	9.1	7.4	13.2	12.1	13.2	10.9	11.1	10.6	12.3	12.6	13.0	16.7	11.9	10.0	11.8
-Unknown	2.3	2.8	5.0	8.8	7.8	7.7	7.4	7.7	9.3	8.0	8.2	12.5	8.8	7.0	7.6
-Other	0.3	0.0	0.4	0.4	2.6	1.0	1.5	1.1	1.2	1.6	2.6	2.0	1.7	1.8	1.3
-Hepatitis C	2.7	2.3	3.9	1.5	0.9	0.6	0.4	0.6	0.4	0.8	0.9	0.8	0.2	0.2	1.1
-Drug induced	1.9	0.9	2.1	0.4	1.3	1.0	1.0	0.8	0.2	1.6	0.4	1.0	1.0	0.6	1.0
-Hepatitis A	1.9	0.9	1.0	0.8	0.4	0.6	0.6	0.2	0.4	0.6	0.7	0.4	0.2	0.4	0.6
-Hepatitis B	0.0	0.5	0.8	0.2	0.2	0.0	0.2	0.2	0.8	0.0	0.2	0.0	0.0	0.0	0.2
Metabolic Diseases	13.0	12.5	9.0	12.0	10.6	11.3	11.5	15.3	12.2	13.7	8.7	9.8	10.3	10.1	11.3
α_1-Antitrypsin deficiency	8.5	7.9	6.2	6.3	3.9	6.8	6.3	7.2	4.9	5.4	3.3	3.0	2.1	2.8	5.2
-Other	1.3	2.6	1.4	3.3	1.9	2.7	1.7	3.4	3.1	4.3	3.1	3.4	4.2	3.7	2.9
-Wilson's disease	1.6	0.9	0.4	0.6	1.3	0.2	1.1	1.5	0.8	0.6	0.4	0.8	1.3	1.5	0.9

–Tyrosinemia	1.6	0.9	0.4	0.6	1.3	0.2	1.1	1.5	0.8	0.6	0.8	1.3	1.5	0.9
–Primary oxalosis	0.0	0.0	0.4	0.8	1.1	1.4	1.1	1.3	1.4	1.4	1.0	0.8	0.2	0.9
–Hemochromatosis	0.0	0.2	0.2	0.4	1.1	0.0	0.2	0.4	1.2	1.4	0.8	0.6	0.4	0.5
Miscellaneous	2.4	2.1	2.1	3.8	4.5	4.1	5.9	3.6	4.9	5.8	9.9	17.4	18.1	7.1
Genetic disorders	6.1	8.8	9.1	5.4	7.8	7.0	5.9	8.1	6.5	6.6	5.0	5.7	6.5	6.8
–Cystic fibrosis	2.1	0.2	1.7	1.7	1.7	0.8	0.8	2.1	2.2	1.2	1.6	1.5	2.0	1.6
–Other	2.9	7.4	5.8	3.3	4.5	5.7	4.2	3.2	3.9	4.1	2.4	3.6	3.3	4.1
–Congenital hepatic fibrosis	1.1	1.2	1.7	0.4	1.5	0.4	1.0	2.8	0.4	1.4	1.0	0.6	1.1	1.1
TPN-HILD	0.8	0.0	0.8	1.5	1.5	2.1	3.8	4.7	5.3	7.2	5.4	6.7	7.4	4.0
Chronic cryptogenic cirrhosis	4.3	4.2	3.7	4.4	3.0	2.3	3.1	4.5	3.1	4.1	3.0	2.7	2.8	3.4
Primary liver malignancy	1.9	0.9	2.1	1.9	1.7	3.7	1.9	1.9	2.0	3.5	4.4	3.6	4.3	2.7
Chronic autoimmune cirrhosis	1.1	0.9	0.8	0.6	2.4	2.7	2.1	1.5	1.2	1.8	1.6	2.7	2.8	1.8
Other chronic diseases	0.8	0.2	1.9	0.8	1.1	1.2	1.3	0.4	0.8	1.6	1.6	0.6	1.1	1.1
Chronic hepatitis C	1.9	0.9	0.8	0.8	0.6	1.2	1.1	0.8	1.4	0.4	0.2	1.1	1.3	0.9
Unknown (#)	0	3	0	0	0	0	0	0	0	0	3	2	2	7

Location Awaiting Transplantation (%)

Adult Recipients

Not hospitalized	40.7	39.5	48.3	55.9	55.6	59.8	58.0	53.5	51.4	47.3	63.5	64.4	61.8	56.3
Hospitalized, non ICU	28.1	24.1	22.6	19.2	21.5	19.8	22.0	26.2	28.9	30.5	13.4	11.1	13.7	20.2
ICU, no life support	10.5	12.1	10.9	8.9	7.4	7.5	8.4	8.1	8.1	11.6	13.0	14.6	15.0	11.0
On life support	20.7	24.4	18.2	16.0	15.5	12.9	11.6	12.1	11.6	10.6	10.1	9.9	9.5	12.5
Unknown (#)	0	3	0	1	0	1	6	9	21	21	58	61	121	335

Pediatric Recipients

Not hospitalized	40.8	37.1	39.9	45.9	43.9	48.7	42.7	47.6	45.7	45.8	51.9	53.1	51.8	46.6
Hospitalized, non-ICU	22.1	18.3	20.0	21.7	20.1	22.2	22.3	25.7	22.1	24.4	15.7	13.4	15.4	19.6
ICU, no life support	9.9	14.4	15.7	10.6	11.0	11.5	13.7	11.9	12.2	13.8	15.9	16.1	18.0	13.7
On life support	27.2	30.2	24.4	21.7	24.9	17.7	21.2	14.9	20.0	16.1	16.5	17.4	14.8	20.1
Unknown (#)	0	0	0	0	0	0	0	0	5	5	9	3	10	34

MEAN COLD ISCHEMIA TIME (DAYS)

Adult recipients	10.3	11.7	11.7	11.5	11.3	10.9	10.3	9.5	8.9	9.1	8.6	8.0	7.6	9.6
Less than 12 hours (%)	71.0	62.2	61.9	64.0	71.4	74.3	80.5	85.9	87.8	88.0	89.5	91.7	93.7	82.0
Unknown (#)	88	91	113	113	126	139	121	154	145	253	771	953	997	4399

Continued

Table 80-1. SURGICAL, RECIPIENT, AND DONOR CHARACTERISTICS—cont'd

Variable	1988	1989	1990	1991	1992	1993	1994	1995	1996	1997	1998	1999	2000	2001	TOTAL
Pediatric recipients	10.4	11.6	12.1	12.0	11.4	11.9	10.7	9.8	9.0	8.9	8.1	7.5	7.1	7.3	9.8
Less than 12 hours (%)	70.6	61.2	61.8	63.6	69.8	71.0	76.0	85.7	85.0	88.1	87.7	90.2	93.9	94.8	79.2
Unknown (#)	32	65	78	56	68	73	41	30	61	59	52	97	85	77	874
CREATININE LEVEL ≥ 2 mg/dL (%)															
Adult recipients	17.7	18.5	19.8	15.6	18.3	16.2	16.0	15.4	15.0	15.9	14.8	15.7	14.7	14.0	15.9
Unknown (#)	22	38	4	6	9	11	22	27	58	69	89	145	156	241	897
Pediatric recipients	3.3	3.8	3.7	5.4	3.9	3.5	4.8	3.9	4.6	3.2	3.9	2.7	4.6	3.3	3.9
Unknown (#)	9	15	2	2	5	1	7	5	13	19	14	31	29	52	204
MEAN ALBUMIN LEVEL (g/dL)															
Adult recipients	2.9	3.0	3.0	3.0	3.0	3.0	3.0	2.9	2.9	2.9	2.8	2.8	2.8	2.8	2.9
Unknown (#)	233	283	129	62	127	200	202	231	256	282	275	334	338	396	3348
Pediatric recipients	3.2	3.2	3.2	3.2	3.2	3.2	3.1	3.2	3.2	3.1	3.2	3.0	3.0	3.1	3.2
Unknown (#)	42	32	15	9	27	30	18	24	42	50	32	46	44	50	461
BILIRUBIN LEVEL															
Adult recipients >10 mg/dL (%)	40.5	35.8	33.6	28.5	27.2	25.6	24.6	23.3	21.6	21.5	19.9	19.1	18.5	17.6	23.5
Adult recipients, mean	11.8	10.4	10.5	9.2	9.2	8.6	8.7	8.3	7.7	7.8	7.5	7.0	6.9	6.7	8.2
Unknown (#)	28	40	10	6	10	20	48	41	86	106	115	147	145	223	1025
Pediatric recipients >10 mg/dL (%)	58.1	56.8	56.3	54.6	55.5	49.4	51.8	50.0	49.7	45.5	44.2	46.5	45.7	46.1	50.5
Pediatric recipients, mean	14.4	14.1	14.0	14.0	13.5	12.7	13.5	13.0	12.9	12.0	11.1	11.3	11.3	11.4	12.7
Unknown (#)	5	7	1	1	6	3	7	7	18	22	14	37	24	40	192
PROTHROMBIN TIME, MEAN (SECONDS)															
Adult recipients	16.4	15.6	16.3	16.1	16.4	16.3	16.2	16.5	16.5	16.5	17.3	17.4	17.0	17.5	16.6
Unknown (#)	134	116	39	59	93	141	115	182	289	402	537	1163	1954	2791	8015
Pediatric recipients	17.1	16.9	16.7	16.8	17.6	16.7	17.0	17.0	18.0	18.4	18.2	18.3	17.7	18.2	17.4
Unknown (#)	38	33	15	16	37	38	21	40	64	95	117	150	168	230	1062
Donor Characteristics															
Sex (%)															
Females—donors for adults	35.8	32.8	35.1	34.9	36.6	36.5	36.9	39.7	39.3	39.6	41.2	40.9	42.4	40.1	38.7
Unknown (#)	8	3	0	0	0	0	0	0	0	0	0	0	1	0	12
Females—donors for pediatrics	41.3	39.0	42.1	42.6	42.9	39.4	44.5	43.5	46.6	45.3	43.4	45.8	40.2	47.3	43.2

Unknown (#)	2	0	0	0	0	0	0	0	0	0	0	0	0	0	2
RACE (%)															
White—donors for adults	90.8	90.1	89.7	89.1	87.8	87.2	86.9	85.9	85.7	85.2	86.9	86.5	86.0	85.1	86.8
Black—donors for adults	7.4	7.7	9.0	9.3	10.1	10.9	10.8	11.8	11.9	12.1	11.0	10.7	11.2	11.7	10.8
Asian—donors for adults	0.4	1.1	0.8	1.0	1.2	1.2	1.7	1.3	1.4	1.7	1.3	1.6	1.6	1.7	1.4
Other—donors for adults	1.4	1.1	0.5	0.6	0.9	0.7	0.6	1.0	0.9	1.0	0.8	1.2	1.2	1.4	1.0
Unknown (#)	0	0	0	0	0	0	3	1	0	3	0	12	10	0	29
White—donors for pediatrics	85.9	82.8	80.8	85.4	81.0	79.7	82.2	82.3	83.6	82.7	81.2	83.0	79.5	81.2	82.1
Black—donors for pediatrics	12.0	12.8	17.1	12.5	17.3	18.5	15.1	14.7	13.9	14.4	16.8	12.8	16.9	15.7	15.1
Asian—donors for pediatrics	0.8	1.9	0.6	0.6	0.9	1.2	1.9	0.6	1.6	2.5	0.7	1.8	1.7	1.3	1.3
Other—donors for pediatrics	1.3	2.6	1.4	1.5	0.9	0.6	0.8	2.3	0.8	0.4	1.3	2.4	1.9	1.8	1.4
Unknown (#)	0	0	0	0	0	0	1	1	0	1	5	5	3	0	16
ETHNICITY (%)															
Hispanic/Latino—donors for adults	9.1	12.7	11.7	14.5	11.3	10.4	8.1	8.6	8.4	9.4	9.8	10.3	10.6	11.4	10.1
Unknown (#)	583	769	1048	1178	752	460	103	17	33	22	34	24	10	0	5033
Hispanic/Latino—donors for pediatrics	12.1	12.3	15.2	18.1	13.2	13.3	9.6	11.8	12.2	14.9	11.1	15.2	13.2	17.1	13.4
Unknown (#)	193	203	214	209	143	96	22	4	7	5	7	6	3	0	1112
MEAN AGE (YR)															
Donors for adults	25.3	28.2	30.2	30.9	33.0	33.4	33.9	34.8	36.2	36.3	37.5	38.2	38.3	38.5	35.1
Donors for adults—>60 years (%)	0.0	0.5	1.5	2.9	5.6	7.6	8.3	9.3	10.5	11.1	12.4	12.9	12.5	12.2	9.0
Unknown (#)	13	6	0	1	5	0	2	0	0	0	1	8	13	28	77
Donors for pediatrics	5.8	7.3	10.4	10.5	13.2	12.4	14.7	12.5	14.5	14.3	14.1	16.8	15.9	15.3	12.9
Donors for pediatrics—≥30 years (%)	3.2	5.8	9.3	12.5	15.4	12.3	18.5	14.4	19.4	16.8	16.0	24.8	23.4	20.5	15.6
Unknown (#)	3	2	0	0	0	0	0	0	0	1	9	10	7	6	38

Continued

Table 80-1. SURGICAL, RECIPIENT, AND DONOR CHARACTERISTICS—cont'd

Variable	1988	1989	1990	1991	1992	1993	1994	1995	1996	1997	1998	1999	2000	2001	TOTAL
Matching Characteristics															
GENDER (RECIPIENT-DONOR) (%)															
Adult Recipients															
Male-male	36.5	39.5	41.4	39.6	39.0	38.3	40.5	37.6	38.6	37.7	39.9	39.1	39.0	41.6	39.3
Male-female	14.7	14.8	14.0	15.1	18.0	17.7	18.1	20.2	20.2	21.4	22.8	22.9	23.3	23.3	20.0
Female-female	21.1	18.1	21.1	19.8	18.6	18.7	18.8	19.4	19.2	18.2	18.4	18.0	19.1	16.8	18.7
Female-male	27.7	27.7	23.5	25.5	24.4	25.3	22.6	22.7	22.0	22.7	18.9	20.1	18.6	18.3	22.0
Unknown (#)	8	3	0	0	0	0	0	0	0	0	0	0	1	0	12
Pediatric Recipients															
Male-male	27.3	30.4	30.0	27.6	30.3	27.7	26.1	27.0	28.2	29.8	25.7	26.3	27.8	22.5	27.5
Male-female	20.6	18.6	19.2	20.5	21.6	19.3	20.8	22.5	24.1	20.8	20.8	22.3	20.2	20.8	20.9
Female-female	20.6	20.4	22.9	22.1	21.2	20.1	23.7	21.0	22.5	24.5	22.6	23.5	20.0	26.5	22.4
Female-male	31.4	30.6	27.9	29.9	26.8	32.9	29.4	29.5	25.2	24.9	30.8	27.9	32.0	30.2	29.2
Unknown (#)	2	0	0	0	0	0	0	0	0	0	0	0	0	0	0
ABO MATCHING (%)															
Adult Recipients															
Identical	87.6	87.1	88.1	89.1	89.3	91.2	92.3	90.1	90.5	88.7	89.9	89.7	90.8	88.8	89.7
Compatible	9.5	10.7	9.0	9.0	8.4	7.4	6.7	8.5	8.0	9.6	8.4	8.7	8.6	10.4	8.7
Incompatible	2.9	2.2	2.9	1.9	2.3	1.4	1.0	1.4	1.6	1.7	1.7	1.5	0.6	0.8	1.5
Unknown (#)	15	9	3	2	5	5	1	0	0	0	1	0	3	0	44
Pediatric Recipients															
Identical	76.6	76.5	80.6	78.0	78.6	79.1	83.4	83.0	85.3	80.0	82.8	84.4	79.2	82.5	80.9
Compatible	15.6	15.4	12.2	14.9	15.4	16.0	11.8	14.0	10.4	16.3	12.8	11.3	17.5	15.8	14.2
Incompatible	7.8	8.2	7.2	7.1	6.1	4.9	4.8	3.0	4.3	3.7	4.4	4.3	3.2	1.7	4.9
Unknown (#)	3	2	0	1	0	0	0	0	0	0	0	0	0	0	6

AHN, acute hepatic necrosis; ICU, intensive care unit; PBC, primary biliary cirrhosis; PSC, primary sclerosing cholangitis; TPN-HILD, total parenteral nutrition–hyperalimentation-induced liver disease.

Reduced livers were reported in only six transplantations for adults during this 14-year period.

Each year, there were more partial-liver and split-liver procedures performed for pediatric recipients than for adult recipients. The first transplantation involving a partial liver for a pediatric recipient was reported in 1989, and the number of transplantations involving partial livers increased dramatically until 1994, when more than one third of pediatric liver transplantations used a partial liver. Over the next several years, there was a decrease in the percentage of transplantations using partial livers among pediatric recipients as the percentage of procedures involving a split liver increased. The percentage of pediatric liver transplantations using split livers was never greater than 5.0% until 1996 when 7.2% of the transplantations involved a split liver, after which time the percentage increased steadily, reaching 16.7% in 2000. The surge in 1996 of split-liver transplantations among children is timed to the publication of a study carried out on the data collected by the European Split Liver Registry program[9] that concluded that a split-liver technique could be more successful than originally believed. Reduced livers accounted for between 1.5% and 5.2% of transplantations in children between 1990 and 1993, but have been used rarely since then.

Waiting Time

In 1988, the median waiting time was 17 days for adult recipients and 38 days for pediatric recipients, but waiting time data were not available for 31% of adults and 36% of children. The medians of waiting times for pediatric recipients were longer than for adults until 1993, but more than 4% of adult recipients and 9% of pediatric recipients had unknown waiting times each year. Since 1994, these data were more complete and median waiting times were consistently longer for adult recipients than for pediatric recipients. By 2001, one half of adult recipients waited approximately 6 months or more for transplantation, whereas one half of pediatric recipients waited at least 2 months for transplantation.

Demographics

Overall, fewer than one half of the transplantations among adult recipients were performed on women, whereas more than one half of pediatric liver transplantations were performed on female children. The fraction of liver transplantations among adult recipients that were performed on women decreased steadily from less than one half in 1988 to about one third in 2001 (see Table 80–1). The percentage of transplantations in female children did not show a significant

trend over the period, ranging from 48.1% in 1992 to 56.7% in 2001.

The percentage of transplantations for white recipients decreased over time for both adults and children while, correspondingly, there was an increase over time in the percentages of procedures performed for both black and Asian recipients among both adults and children. The percentage of transplantations performed for Asian recipients was similar for adult and pediatric recipients each year, but the percentage of transplantations for white recipients was greater among adults than among children every year, and the percentage of transplantations for black recipients was greater among children than among adults every year.

Before April 1994, data on race and ethnicity were collected together as one variable, after which they were recorded separately. Since April 1994, the percentage of transplantations for adult recipients who were Hispanic has been between 10.1% and 12.2%, whereas 14.7% to 23.1% of pediatric liver transplantations were for Hispanics.

The mean age for adult recipients increased steadily from 43.1 years in 1988 to 50.3 years in 2001. The percentage of transplantations for adults older than 60 years more than doubled from 8.0% in 1988 to the highest percentage of 16.8% in 1996, and then remained at about the same level. Pediatric recipients' ages averaged between 3.5 and 4.4 years. The percentage of transplantations for children in the extreme age groups increased over time, with the percentage of procedures for children younger than 1 year increasing from 23.2% in 1988 to 30.2% in 2001, and the percentage of transplantations for children ages 9 to 16 years increased from 13.9% in 1988 to 21.5% in 2001.

Therefore, adult liver transplantations were increasingly performed for male, nonwhite, older recipients, whereas pediatric liver transplantations became more common among nonwhite recipients and those children in the youngest and oldest age groups.

Primary Liver Disease

The most common indication for a liver transplantation among adults was hepatitis C, including acute and chronic, and with and without alcoholic liver disease (ALD). Non-A, non-B hepatitis was included as hepatitis C in all years. Overall, hepatitis C accounted for 32.5% of all liver transplantations among adults, with three fourths of these being for patients with chronic hepatitis C. The percentage of transplantations for adults caused by chronic hepatitis C more than doubled from 14.9% in 1988 to 31.7% in 2001, by far the largest increase in primary liver disease over the period examined. This substantial increase in chronic hepatitis C, coupled with the 3.5-fold increase in the number of transplantations performed for adults over time, meant that there were more than seven times as many transplantations resulting from chronic hepatitis C in 2001 (n = 1471) than in 1988 (n = 200).

Alcoholic liver disease with or without hepatitis C was the next most common indication for transplantation among adult recipients (20.4%). Of these, approximately one fourth of the adult recipients had concomitant hepatitis C–induced liver damage. The percentage of transplantations for adults with alcoholic liver disease and hepatitis C peaked at 8.6% in 1996, decreasing to 6.5% in 2001. The percentage of transplantations for adults whose primary liver disease was ALD without hepatitis C peaked at 20.8% in 1990, decreasing to 11.8% by 2001.

The third most common reason for a liver transplantation in adults, cryptogenic cirrhosis, accounted for 10.0% of liver transplantations, but unlike hepatitis C and ALD, the percentage of transplantations resulting from cryptogenic cirrhosis did not have a consistent trend over time.

The cholestatic diseases of primary sclerosing cholangitis (PSC) and primary biliary cirrhosis (PBC) were the fourth and fifth most common indications for liver transplantation among adults (8.0% and 7.6%, respectively). The percentages of transplantations for both of these diseases decreased over time.

Overall, acute hepatic necrosis (AHN) accounted for 7.5% of transplantations among adult recipients with no consistent trend in percentages over time. The most common cause of AHN from 1988 to 1990 was hepatitis C, after which "unknown etiology" was ascribed most often, until 1998 when hepatitis C again became the most common form of AHN and remained so for the next 3 years. Overall, AHN of unknown etiology accounted for slightly more transplantations (2.3%) than did acute hepatitis C (2.1%).

Miscellaneous diagnoses, including secondary biliary cirrhosis (SBC), genetic disorders, biliary atresia, Budd-Chiari syndrome, bile duct cancers, and tumors, accounted for 5.0% of transplantations performed among adult recipients.

The percentages of adult liver transplantations caused by chronic hepatitis B or chronic autoimmune cirrhosis were similar (4.5% and 4.4%, respectively), with neither showing a consistent trend in percentages over time. The percentage of transplantations for each disease peaked before 1994.

Metabolic diseases (α_1-antitrypsin deficiency, hemochromatosis, Wilson's disease, and others) were the primary liver disease for adult recipients in 3.5% of transplantations, with 40% of these transplantations caused by α_1-antitrypsin deficiency. There was no consistent trend in the percentages of transplantations resulting from the individual metabolic disease diagnoses over time, although as a whole, the percentage of

transplantations for adult recipients with metabolic disease decreased slightly after 1994. Except for 1991, when Wilson's disease was the most common metabolic liver disease, α_1-antitrypsin deficiency was the most common metabolic disease each year.

Primary liver malignancies (PLMs) were the primary indication for 3.4% of transplantations among adult recipients, with the highest percentages occurring in 1988 and 1989.

Almost half of all pediatric liver transplantations resulted from biliary atresia, although the percentage decreased from 58.1% in 1988 to 36.6% in 2001. Acute hepatic necrosis was the second most common primary liver disease leading to pediatric liver transplantations (11.8%) with unknown etiology accounting for nearly 65% of those transplantations. There was no consistent trend over time in the percentages of either the individual AHN diagnoses (unknown etiology, hepatitis C, drug-induced, hepatitis A, hepatitis B, and "other") or AHN as a whole. The third most common indication for pediatric liver transplantation was metabolic disease (11.3%), with 46% of those transplantations involving children who had α_1-antitrypsin deficiency. Up until 1999, α_1-antitrypsin deficiency was the most common metabolic disease each year; however, rarer forms of metabolic disease (i.e., other than Wilson's disease, tyrosinemia, primary oxalosis, and hemochromatosis) were the metabolic diseases most often ascribed in the last 3 years of the time period. The percentage of transplantations among children caused by metabolic diseases fluctuated between 9.0% and 15.3% each year.

Miscellaneous diagnoses (PBC, PSC, SBC, Budd-Chiari syndrome, bile duct cancers, and benign tumors) were each rare indications for pediatric liver transplantation. However, together they were the fourth most frequent indication overall for liver transplantation among children (7.1%). The percentage of transplantation for these diagnoses nearly doubled in 1998 (from 5.8% to 10.6%) and again in 2000 (from 9.9% to 17.4%). This was mostly the result of the increase in the number of pediatric transplantations performed because of the "other" diagnosis category provided by UNOS, which does not indicate the specific liver disease.

Genetic disorders as an indication for pediatric liver transplantation were only slightly less common than the miscellaneous diagnoses (6.8%). Cystic fibrosis or congenital hepatic fibrosis was the genetic disorder in 40% of such transplantations, although neither disease was ever the most common genetic disorder in any year of the study period. There was no significant trend over time in the percentage of pediatric transplantations performed for a genetic disorder.

The sixth most common indication for liver transplantation in children was total parenteral nutrition–hyperalimentation–induced liver disease (TPN-HILD, 4.0%). The percentage of procedures performed in children as a result of this indication increased from less than 1.0% before 1991 to 7.4% in 2001. This increase parallels the increase of multiorgan transplantations seen among pediatric recipients. In fact, 55% of all children who underwent multiorgan transplantation did so because of TPN-HILD. This is not surprising given that TPN is important in medical care; however, it is associated with gastrointestinal complications,[10] which if severe enough can necessitate transplantation of the small bowel,[11] explaining why the intestine increased as the organ most often transplanted in addition to the liver among pediatric recipients.

The only form of chronic liver disease in children that accounted for more than 2.0% of the procedures was cryptogenic cirrhosis (3.4%). The percentage of transplantations performed because of this indication varied over time, as did the percentage of pediatric liver transplantations performed for chronic autoimmune cirrhosis, "other" chronic diseases, chronic hepatitis C, and, subsequently, chronic liver disease as a whole. Chronic hepatitis C, which was the most common indication for adult liver transplantation, was the indication for less than 1.0% of pediatric liver transplantations. Primary liver malignancies were the indication for 2.7% of all pediatric liver transplantations.

In summary, only for the indication of hepatitis C did the percentage of adult liver transplantations increase, so much so that by 2001, nearly one in every three transplantations was caused by this indication. Among pediatric recipients, almost one of every two transplantations was performed on a child with biliary atresia, but the percentage of transplantations for this indication decreased over time so that by 2001, only 37% of transplantations for children were caused by biliary atresia. The greatest percentage increase of pediatric liver transplantations was for the miscellaneous diagnoses, followed by TPN-HILD.

Patient's Location While Awaiting Transplantation

The variable of where the patient resides while awaiting transplantation is influenced, in large part, by how ill the candidate was while awaiting transplantation and by admission policies that differ across centers and have changed within most centers between 1988 and 2001. The percentage of adult liver transplantations for recipients who awaited transplantation outside of a hospital increased (40.7% in 1988 to 64.4% in 2000), as did the percentage of transplantations for adult recipients who were in an intensive care unit (ICU) but not on life support (10.5% in 1988 to 15.0% in 2001). Similar trends occurred among pediatric recipients, with the percentage of transplantations for recipients awaiting transplantation outside of a hospital increasing from 40.8% in 1988 to 53.1% in 2000. Approximately 10.0% of pediatric liver transplantations in 1988 were for recipients who awaited transplantation while in an ICU but not on life support. This percentage increased to 18.0% by 2001.

The length of time that a recipient waited for transplantation differed according to their location while awaiting transplantation, reflecting allocation policies that gave preference to sicker recipients and waiting list mortality for the sickest patients who did not receive transplantation. Across all years, the median waiting time for adult recipients who were not hospitalized was 140 days as compared with adult recipients on life support, half of whom waited only 4 days or less (Fig. 80–2). Similarly, the median waiting time for non-hospitalized pediatric recipients was 106.5 days, whereas half of the pediatric recipients on life support waited 5 days or less. If those recipients with an acute form of liver disease are excluded, the respective

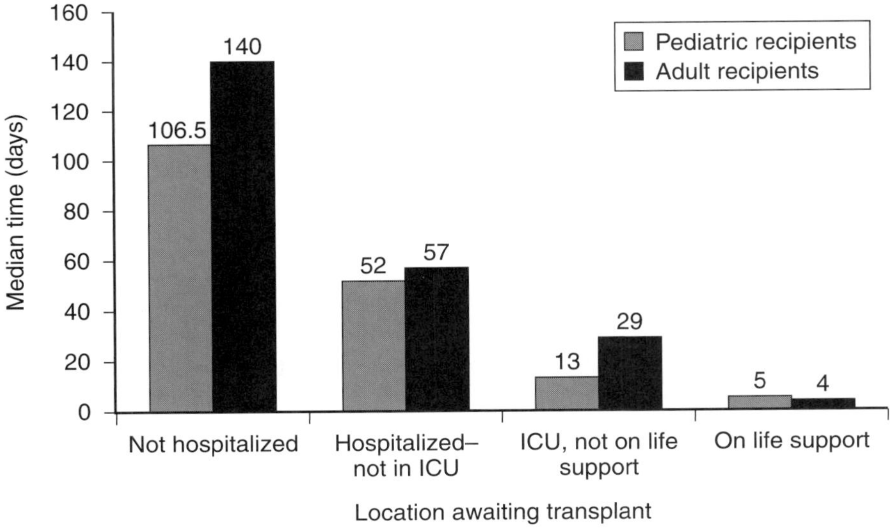

FIGURE 80–2

Median waiting time for recipients by location while awaiting transplantation.

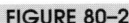

median waiting times for each location prior to transplantation are slightly longer; however, the association still exists between waiting time and location prior to transplantation.

Cold Ischemia Time

Cold ischemia time is the time interval that begins when the organ is cooled with a cold perfusion solution during the organ procurement surgery and ends when the organ is reperfused in the recipient. The number of adult liver transplantations performed in which the cold ischemia time was missing increased markedly from 145 (4.0%) in 1996 to 997 (21.5%) in 2001. The number of pediatric liver transplantations reported that had missing cold ischemia times fluctuated slightly over the period (between 30 in 1995 and 97 in 1999). For liver transplantations among both adult and pediatric patients, the average cold ischemia time increased slightly from 1988 to 1990 and then decreased steadily. For procedures among adult recipients, the highest average cold ischemia time of 11.7 hours occurred in 1989 and 1990, decreasing to 7.6 hours by 2001. For transplantations among pediatric patients, the highest average cold ischemia time of 12.1 hours occurred in 1990, decreasing to 7.3 hours by 2001. The percentage of transplantations for adult recipients that used a liver with a cold ischemia time of less than 12 hours decreased from 71% in 1988 to 62% in 1990 and then increased steadily afterward so that in 2001, 94% of livers used in adult liver transplantation had a cold ischemia time of less than 12 hours. Similarly, the percentage of transplantations for pediatric recipients that involved a liver with a cold ischemia time of less than 12 hours decreased from 71% in 1988 to 61% in 1989 and then increased steadily to 95% by 2001.

Laboratory Values

Creatinine is a protein produced by muscle, which is released into the blood and filtered by the kidney. Thus, high serum creatinine levels indicate poor kidney function, which may be caused by liver disease. The percentage of transplantations for adult recipients whose serum creatinine level was 2 mg/dL or greater decreased from 19.3% in 1990 to 14.0% in 2001. There was not a consistent trend over time in the percentage of procedures performed for pediatric recipients with a serum creatinine level of 2 mg/dL or greater. However, the proportion of transplantations for children with a creatinine level of at least 2 mg/dL (3.9%) was much smaller than for transplantations for adult recipients (15.9%), which is expected given that children generally have lower creatinine levels than adults do.

Albumin is a protein manufactured by the liver, and low levels can be indicative of poor liver function. There was no consistent trend in the mean albumin levels of adult or pediatric recipients over time, but pediatric recipients had consistently higher average levels of albumin than did adult recipients.

Bilirubin is a waste product of the degradation of hemoglobin, a process performed by the liver. Bilirubin is presented as both a dichotomous and a continuous variable because the moving average plots for adult recipients indicated a noticeable increase in risks around a bilirubin level of 10 mg/dL, whereas the continuous form was most appropriate based on the moving average plot for pediatric recipients. As evident by either form of the variable, bilirubin levels for both adult and pediatric recipients decreased over time, with children consistently having a higher bilirubin level than did adults.

Prothrombin time is a measure of how well the blood clots. The liver is responsible for the manufacture of the proteins involved in clot formation, so increased prothrombin time is reflective of poor liver function. There were no consistent trends over time in the mean prothrombin times for either adult or pediatric recipients, although pediatric recipients consistently had higher mean prothrombin times than did adults. The number of missing prothrombin time values increased over time for both adult and pediatric recipients.

Donor Characteristics

Demographics

For both adult and pediatric recipients, male donors were more common than female donors. Furthermore, the proportion of transplantations among adults using livers from male donors increased slightly over time. In every year but 2000, the percentage of transplantations for pediatric recipients using a liver from a female donor was greater than the percentage of procedures for adult recipients using a liver from a female donor (see Table 80–1).

The percentage of procedures among adult recipients that involved livers from white donors decreased gradually over time. Livers from white donors were more common for transplantations among adult recipients than for transplantations among pediatric recipients each year, whereas livers from black donors were more common for transplantations among pediatric recipients than for transplantations among adult recipients. The percentage of procedures that used livers from Asian donors was similar for both adult and pediatric recipients each year.

Beginning in 1989 and continuing to 2001, there were more livers from black donors being used in transplantations for adult recipients than there were transplantations being performed for black adult recipients each year. The number of transplantations for white adult recipients and the number of adult liver transplantations using livers from white donors were similar each year, whereas the number of procedures performed for Asian adult recipients always outnumbered the number of procedures among adult recipients that used livers from Asian donors. In every year, there were more liver transplantations among pediatric recipients that used livers from white donors than there were liver transplantations for white pediatric recipients, and more pediatric liver transplantations for black recipients than there were pediatric liver transplantations that involved livers from black donors. As with adult liver transplantations, there were more transplantations for Asian pediatric recipients than there were procedures performed that used livers from Asian donors.

Every year from 1990 onward, there were more liver transplantations performed for Hispanic adult recipients than there were livers from Hispanic donors being used in adult liver transplantations. Hispanics undergoing pediatric liver transplantation always outnumbered pediatric liver transplantations involving livers from Hispanic donors. In every year but 1989 there was a higher percentage of livers from Hispanic donors being used in pediatric liver transplantations than in adult liver transplantations.

The livers used for the procedures among adult recipients came from progressively older donors over time, with the average donor age increasing from 25.3 years in 1988 to 38.5 years in 2001. This was primarily a result of a steady increase in the proportion of livers from donors older than 60 years, from 0% in 1988 to 12.2% in 2001. Among pediatric recipients, the mean donor age fluctuated with the percentage of donors who were older than 30 years. Overall, there was a substantial increase in mean donor age from 5.8 years in 1988 to 15.3 years in 2001, with the highest mean age of 16.8 years occurring in 1999. This increase in donor age is attributable to the increased use of split-liver transplantations and living donor transplantations, because the mean age of the split-liver donors was 22.8 years and the mean age of the living donors was 24.8 year, as compared with a mean deceased donor age of 8.7 years.

Recipient-Donor Matching Characteristics

As would be expected by the increase in the percentage of adult liver transplantations among male recipients and the increase in the percentage of transplantations among adult recipients who used livers obtained from female donors, there was an increase in the percentage of transplantations in which an adult male recipient received a liver from a female donor over time (14.7% in

1988 to 23.3% in 2001) and a decrease in the percentage of transplantations in which an adult female recipient received a liver from a male donor (27.7% in 1988 to 18.3% in 2001). Among pediatric liver transplantations, there was no consistent trend in the percentage of recipient-donor gender matches over time.

As would be expected, blood type matching was related to the recipient's location before transplantation. Although 94.5% of transplantations for adult recipients who were not hospitalized while awaiting transplantation used a liver from a donor with an identical blood type, only 73.8% of transplantations for adult recipients waiting in an ICU and on life support used a donor organ with an identical blood type match (Fig. 80-3). Transplantations for children who were not hospitalized before transplantation had a recipient-donor identical blood match 88.4% of the time, whereas only 67.9% of transplantations for children in an ICU and on life support used a liver from a donor with the same blood type as the recipient.

The percentage of adult recipients with the same blood type as their donor ranged from 87% to 92% over time, whereas the percentage of adult recipients whose blood type was incompatible with their donor decreased from 2.9% in 1988 to 0.8% in 2001. Similar relationships were found for pediatric recipients, although the percentage of recipients with the same blood type as their donor was lower among transplantations for pediatric recipients than among transplantations for adult recipients.

Outcome Analysis—Crude Survival Percentages

As mentioned previously, the focus of the analysis is to determine whether survival improved over time. Table 80-2 displays the survival (patient and graft) percentages by year of transplantation for adult and pediatric recipients separately at 1 day, 1 week, 1 month, 3 months, 6 months, 1 year, 2 years, 5 years, and 10 years after transplantation. The crude patient and graft survival percentages were higher for adults and children who became recipients in the latter part of the period examined when compared with those recipients who underwent transplantation earlier. The results of the Wilcoxon test indicated that survival, both patient and graft, improved over time for both adult and pediatric recipients.

The greatest drop in survival percentages for both adult and pediatric recipients occurs within the first 3 months after transplantation as a function of perioperative mortality and early retransplantations. The average drop in adult patient survival in each year during the first 3 months was 11.4%, which is greater than the average drop in patient survival of 10.3% in the following 21 months. The difference is even greater for

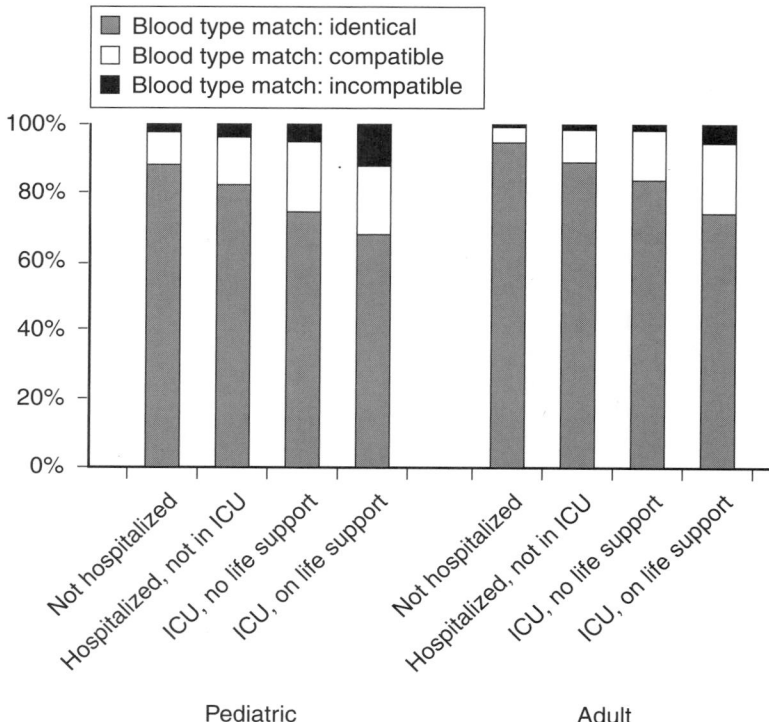

FIGURE 80-3

Blood type match according to location awaiting transplantation.

adult graft survival, with the percentage dropping 15.1% on average within the first 3 months as compared with 10.6% from 3 months to 2 years after transplantation. However, the disparity is even more drastic in pediatric recipients. Patient survival decreased an average of 13.4% in the first 3 months, which is nearly two times greater than the average decrease of 7.0% that occurred from 3 months to 2 years after transplantation. Graft survival dropped more than two times as much in the first 3 months after transplantation (18.8%) than it did from 3 months to 2 years after transplantation (8.1%).

Outcome Analysis— Multivariable Modeling

As evidenced by hazard ratios for death of greater than 1, factors independently associated with reduced survival among adult recipients were receiving organs in addition to a liver, a split liver, undergoing retransplantation, being black (as compared with being white), awaiting transplantation in a hospital or ICU (as compared with not being hospitalized), receiving a liver from an older donor, being a male recipient of a liver from a female donor, and receiving a liver from a donor of a different blood type (Table 80-3). Furthermore, recipients whose indication for transplantation was primary liver malignancy had significantly worse survival than the comparison group of recipients whose indication for

liver transplantation was chronic hepatitis C. Conversely, recipients whose indication for liver transplantation was cryptogenic cirrhosis, PSC, PBC, AHN, chronic hepatitis B, autoimmune cirrhosis, α_1-antitrypsin deficiency, or Wilson's disease all had better survival than patients whose transplantation resulted from chronic hepatitis C. There was no significant difference in survival between those whose indication was chronic hepatitis C and those whose indication was ALD. Adults who were older at the time of transplantation had greater risks of mortality, whereas the lowest risks of death were observed in those recipients who were in their late 20s or early 30s (Fig. 80-4). When adjusting for all of these factors, many of which changed over time, there was a 4% reduction in risk of death each year as year of transplantation increased.

Although some effect sizes changed (e.g., for split livers, the hazard ratio for death or retransplantation was 1.65 compared with 1.23 for death, and for incompatible blood type the hazard ratio for death or retransplantation was 1.30 compared with 1.06 for death), in general, the results for graft failure were similar to those for death among adult recipients.

As with patient death, the results of the multivariable modeling indicate that the risk of graft failure among adult recipients became significantly lower over time.

For pediatric recipients, multiorgan transplantation, retransplantation, being black, awaiting transplantation in the hospital or ICU, receiving a liver from an older

Table 80-2. ADULT AND PEDIATRIC RECIPIENT CRUDE SURVIVAL PERCENTAGES BY YEAR OF TRANSPLANTATION

Adult Recipients—Patient Survival

Follow-up Time	1988	1989	1990	1991	1992	1993	1994	1995	1996	1997	1998	1999	2000	2001
1 day	96	98	97	97	98	98	98	98	98	99	98	98	98	98
1 wk	94	96	96	96	96	97	97	97	98	97	98	97	97	98
1 mo	89	90	91	91	92	93	94	93	94	94	95	94	94	95
3 mo	83	83	86	86	88	89	90	90	90	91	91	90	91	92
6 mo	79	80	82	83	85	86	88	87	87	89	89	88	89	90
1 yr	76	76	79	80	82	83	85	83	84	86	86	85	86	86
2 yr	72	72	74	76	78	79	81	79	80	81	81	81	82	NA
5 yr	64	65	67	67	68	71	73	71	71	NA	NA	NA	NA	NA
10 yr	53	51	53	53	53	NA	NA	NA	NA	NA	NA	NA	NA	NA

Adult Recipients—Graft Survival

Follow-up Time	1988	1989	1990	1991	1992	1993	1994	1995	1996	1997	1998	1999	2000	2001
1 day	96	97	97	97	97	98	98	98	98	98	98	97	98	98
1 wk	92	93	93	93	94	95	96	94	96	95	95	95	95	96
1 mo	85	86	87	87	88	90	90	89	90	90	91	91	91	92
3 mo	79	80	82	81	84	86	87	86	86	87	87	87	88	89
6 mo	76	77	78	78	81	84	84	83	82	84	85	84	85	86
1 yr	73	73	75	74	78	80	80	79	78	81	82	81	82	82
2 yr	69	69	71	70	74	76	76	75	74	76	77	77	78	NA
5 yr	61	62	63	62	65	66	67	66	66	NA	NA	NA	NA	NA
10 yr	49	48	49	49	50	NA	NA	NA	NA	NA	NA	NA	NA	NA

Pediatric Recipients—Patient Survival

Follow-up Time	1988	1989	1990	1991	1992	1993	1994	1995	1996	1997	1998	1999	2000	2001
1 day	98	98	99	98	99	98	99	99	99	98	99	98	99	98
1 wk	95	93	97	95	95	95	97	98	95	96	96	94	96	96
1 mo	88	87	92	89	91	91	93	95	91	92	91	91	93	93
3 mo	82	81	88	84	85	87	87	90	87	87	87	88	89	90
6 mo	79	79	85	81	83	84	83	88	85	83	85	85	87	89
1 yr	78	77	83	80	81	80	81	86	82	81	83	83	85	87
2 yr	75	76	82	77	79	77	79	85	79	78	80	80	84	NA
5 yr	71	74	79	73	77	74	77	80	75	NA	NA	NA	NA	NA
10 yr	69	72	76	70	72	NA	NA	NA	NA	NA	NA	NA	NA	NA

Pediatric Recipients—Graft Survival

Follow-up Time	1988	1989	1990	1991	1992	1993	1994	1995	1996	1997	1998	1999	2000	2001
1 day	98	98	98	97	98	98	99	99	98	97	98	97	99	97
1 wk	93	89	94	90	91	94	94	97	91	92	92	91	94	94
1 mo	83	80	84	83	86	88	85	91	85	87	86	86	89	88
3 mo	77	74	80	77	81	83	80	86	82	82	81	82	86	86
6 mo	74	71	77	74	79	81	76	84	80	77	79	80	82	84
1 yr	73	70	76	72	77	77	73	81	77	74	77	78	80	81
2 yr	70	69	74	69	74	72	71	78	73	71	73	74	78	NA
5 yr	66	65	72	66	69	68	68	75	67	NA	NA	NA	NA	NA
10 yr	62	63	67	61	61	NA	NA	NA	NA	NA	NA	NA	NA	NA

NA, not available.

Table 80-3. HAZARD RATIOS (HR) AND 95% CONFIDENCE INTERVALS (CI) FOR DEATH AND GRAFT FAILURE OF ADULT RECIPIENTS USING MULTIVARIABLE PROPORTIONAL HAZARDS MODELS (N = 38,482)

Variable	Death		Graft Failure	
	HR	95% CI	HR	95% CI
Year of transplantation	0.96	(0.95, 0.97)	0.962	(0.957, 0.967)
Multiorgan transplantation recipient	1.35	(1.21, 1.50)	1.22	(1.10, 1.35)
TYPE OF TRANSPLANTATION (BASELINE: WHOLE)				
Split	1.23	(1.02, 1.49)	1.65	(1.40, 1.94)
Reduced	1.29	(0.32, 5.15)	1.50	(0.37, 6.00)
Partial	1.07	(0.87, 1.32)	1.40	(1.18, 1.66)
Received more than 1 liver transplantation	1.82	(1.72, 1.92)	NOT APPLICABLE	
Demographics				
RACE (BASELINE: WHITE)				
Black	1.37	(1.28, 1.47)	1.28	(1.20, 1.37)
Asian	1.01	(0.91, 1.13)	0.99	(0.90, 1.10)
Other	0.88	(0.77, 1.01)	0.91	(0.81, 1.03)
RECIPIENT AGE (YEARS)*				
Continuous	0.99	(0.98, 1.00)	0.98	(0.97, 0.99)
Quadratic	1.0003	(1.0002, 1.0004)	1.0003	(1.0002, 1.0004)
PRIMARY LIVER DISEASE (BASELINE: CHRONIC HEPATITIS C)				
Alcoholic liver disease	0.95	(0.90, 1.01)	0.89	(0.84, 0.94)
Chronic cryptogenic cirrhosis	0.85	(0.80, 0.91)	0.84	(0.79, 0.90)
Primary sclerosing cholangitis	0.64	(0.59, 0.70)	0.72	(0.67, 0.77)
Primary biliary sclerosis	0.55	(0.51, 0.60)	0.60	(0.55, 0.65)
Acute hepatic necrosis—hepatitis C	0.87	(0.76, 0.99)	0.88	(0.77, 0.99)
Acute hepatic necrosis—hepatitis B	0.82	(0.68, 0.97)	0.84	(0.71, 0.99)
Acute hepatic necrosis—drug-induced	0.79	(0.65, 0.96)	0.77	(0.64, 0.92)
Acute hepatic necrosis—other	1.07	(0.83, 1.38)	0.99	(0.78, 1.25)
Acute hepatic necrosis—hepatitis A	0.73	(0.53, 1.02)	0.71	(0.52, 0.98)
Acute hepatic necrosis—unknown etiology	0.84	(0.73, 0.96)	0.83	(0.73, 0.94)
Alcoholic liver disease + hepatitis C	1.03	(0.94, 1.12)	0.99	(0.91, 1.07)
Chronic hepatitis B	0.88	(0.80, 0.96)	0.90	(0.82, 0.98)
Chronic autoimmune cirrhosis	0.73	(0.66, 0.81)	0.74	(0.67, 0.81)
Metabolic disease—α_1-antitrypsin deficiency	0.63	(0.52, 0.75)	0.66	(0.56, 0.77)
Metabolic disease—hemochromatosis	1.03	(0.86, 1.23)	1.07	(0.90, 1.26)
Metabolic disease—Wilson's disease	0.43	(0.32, 0.59)	0.56	(0.44, 0.72)
Metabolic diseases—other	0.86	(0.66, 1.12)	0.77	(0.60, 0.99)
Primary liver malignancy	1.65	(1.52, 1.80)	1.45	(1.34, 1.58)
Other chronic diseases	1.09	(0.91, 1.30)	0.99	(0.83, 1.18)
Miscellaneous	1.08	(0.98, 1.19)	0.98	(0.90, 1.08)
LOCATION AWAITING TRANSPLANTATION (BASELINE: NOT HOSPITALIZED)				
Hospitalized—not in ICU	1.23	(1.18, 1.29)	1.19	(1.14, 1.24)
ICU, not on life support	1.33	(1.25, 1.42)	1.28	(1.21, 1.36)
On life support	1.83	(1.72, 1.94)	1.77	(1.67, 1.88)
Donor Characteristics				
Donor age (years)	1.007	(1.006, 1.009)	1.011	(1.010, 1.012)

Table 80–3. HAZARD RATIOS (HR) AND 95% CONFIDENCE INTERVALS (CI) FOR DEATH AND GRAFT FAILURE OF ADULT RECIPIENTS USING MULTIVARIABLE PROPORTIONAL HAZARDS MODELS (N = 38,482)—cont'd

Variable	Death		Graft Failure	
	HR	95% CI	HR	95% CI
DONOR RACE (BASELINE: WHITE)				
Black	1.05	(0.99, 1.11)	1.18	(1.12, 1.25)
Asian	1.01	(0.86, 1.18)	1.14	(0.99, 1.32)
Other	1.21	(1.00, 1.46)	1.16	(0.97, 1.38)
Matching Characteristics				
GENDER MATCHING (BASELINE: MALE RECIPIENT—MALE DONOR)				
Male recipient—female donor	1.06	(1.01, 1.12)	1.14	(1.09, 1.19)
Female recipient—female donor	1.02	(0.96, 1.07)	1.02	(0.97, 1.07)
Female recipient—male donor	1.01	(0.96, 1.06)	1.02	(0.97, 1.07)
BLOOD TYPE (BASELINE: IDENTICAL)				
Compatible	1.14	(1.07, 1.22)	1.08	(1.02, 1.15)
Incompatible	1.06	(0.91, 1.23)	1.30	(1.14, 1.48)

*See Figure 80-4.

donor, a black donor, and a male recipient receiving a liver from a female donor are independently associated with higher mortality (Table 80–4). Younger and older children had higher risks of death than those children in the middle, with the youngest children having the highest risk of mortality (Fig. 80–5). Neither type of transplantation nor blood type match was significantly associated with pediatric recipient mortality.

Relative to biliary atresia, the only indication for transplantation among children with a lower risk of mortality was α_1-antitrypsin, whereas there were several indications that were significantly associated with higher risks of mortality (see Table 80–4). The highest hazard ratio for death was for TPN-HILD, followed by chronic hepatitis C, and cystic fibrosis.

As with pediatric mortality, the indication of TPN-HILD, relative to biliary atresia, was associated with the highest hazard ratio for graft failure among pediatric recipients of any of the indications for transplantation. Primary liver malignancies, miscellaneous diagnoses, and AHN of unknown etiology were also associated with elevated risks of graft failure compared with biliary atresia. As with mortality, the only indication with a smaller risk of graft failure than biliary atresia was α_1-antitrypsin.

The need for life support before transplantation, being black or receiving a liver from a black donor, multiorgan transplantation, split-liver transplantations, male recipients receiving a liver from a female donor, and incompatible blood type matches were all independently associated with increased risk of pediatric graft failure.

FIGURE 80–4

Hazard ratios for death and graft failure relative to an adult recipient age 48* years.

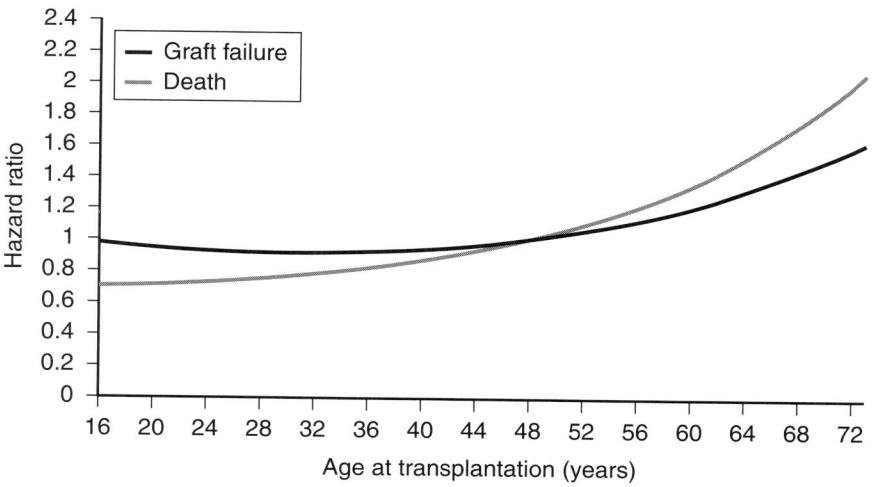

*Mean age of adult recipients

Table 80-4. HAZARD RATIOS (HR) AND 95% CONFIDENCE INTERVALS (CI) FOR DEATH AND GRAFT FAILURE OF PEDIATRIC RECIPIENTS USING MULTIVARIABLE PROPORTIONAL HAZARDS MODELS (N = 5447)

Variable	Death HR	Death 95% CI	Graft failure HR	Graft failure 95% CI
Year of transplantation	0.95	(0.93, 0.97)	0.96	(0.95, 0.97)
Multiorgan transplantation recipient	1.84	(1.40, 2.41)	1.34	(1.04, 1.72)
TYPE OF TRANSPLANTATION (BASELINE: WHOLE)				
Split	0.96	(0.76, 1.22)	1.38	(1.14, 1.66)
Reduced	0.73	(0.44, 1.19)	0.93	(0.63, 1.38)
Partial	1.12	(0.94, 1.33)	1.12	(0.97, 1.29)
Received more than 1 liver transplantation	2.29	(2.01, 2.61)	NOT APPLICABLE	
Demographics				
RACE (BASELINE: WHITE)				
Black	1.30	(1.13, 1.50)	1.23	(1.09, 1.39)
Asian	0.98	(0.69, 1.39)	0.87	(0.63, 1.19)
Other	1.22	(0.91, 1.63)	1.10	(0.85, 1.42)
RECIPIENT AGE (YEARS)*				
Continuous	0.85	(0.81, 0.89)	0.90	(0.86, 0.93)
Quadratic	1.009	(1.006, 1.012)	1.006	(1.004, 1.009)
PRIMARY LIVER DISEASE (BASELINE: BILIARY ATRESIA)				
Acute hepatic necrosis—hepatitis C	0.98	(0.55, 1.72)	1.26	(0.82, 1.92)
Acute hepatic necrosis—drug-induced	2.09	(1.32, 3.30)	1.41	(0.92, 2.16)
Acute hepatic necrosis—hepatitis A	1.17	(0.62, 2.22)	1.37	(0.80, 2.36)
Acute hepatic necrosis—hepatitis B	0.71	(0.26, 1.93)	0.69	(0.28, 1.69)
Acute hepatic necrosis—unknown	1.64	(1.32, 2.05)	1.27	(1.04, 1.55)
Acute hepatic necrosis—other	1.53	(1.00, 2.34)	1.20	(0.81, 1.77)
Metabolic disease—α_1-antitrypsin deficiency	0.57	(0.38, 0.85)	0.63	(0.46, 0.85)
Metabolic disease—Wilson's disease	0.94	(0.46, 1.94)	0.64	(0.35, 1.19)
Metabolic disease—tyrosinemia	0.58	(0.32, 1.03)	0.68	(0.43, 1.08)
Metabolic disease—primary oxalosis	1.63	(0.95, 2.79)	1.56	(0.95, 2.56)
Metabolic disease—hemochromatosis	1.49	(0.81, 2.75)	1.11	(0.62, 1.98)
Metabolic diseases—other	1.11	(0.77, 1.59)	1.01	(0.75, 1.37)
Genetic disorders—other	1.23	(0.93, 1.62)	1.02	(0.79, 1.30)
Genetic disorder—cystic fibrosis	2.43	(1.61, 3.67)	1.40	(0.96, 2.06)
Genetic disorder—congenital hepatic fibrosis	0.94	(0.51, 1.73)	1.06	(0.65, 1.71)
TPN-HILD	3.02	(2.29, 3.98)	2.47	(1.91, 3.20)
Chronic cryptogenic cirrhosis	1.06	(0.73, 1.53)	1.16	(0.87, 1.54)
Primary liver malignancy	2.10	(1.56, 2.81)	1.64	(1.26, 2.13)
Chronic autoimmune cirrhosis	1.54	(1.00, 2.37)	1.21	(0.83, 1.75)
Chronic hepatitis C	2.56	(1.52, 4.31)	1.57	(0.97, 2.54)
Other chronic diseases	1.09	(0.61, 1.94)	1.40	(0.88, 2.22)
Miscellaneous	1.54	(1.20, 1.99)	1.43	(1.15, 1.77)
LOCATION AWAITING TRANSPLANTATION (BASELINE: NOT HOSPITALIZED)				
Hospitalized—not in ICU	1.16	(1.00, 1.34)	1.14	(1.01, 1.30)
ICU, not on life support	1.14	(0.95, 1.37)	1.14	(0.97, 1.33)
On life support	2.14	(1.82, 2.52)	1.88	(1.62, 2.17)

Table 80-4. HAZARD RATIOS (HR) AND 95% CONFIDENCE INTERVALS (CI) FOR DEATH AND GRAFT FAILURE OF PEDIATRIC RECIPIENTS USING MULTIVARIABLE PROPORTIONAL HAZARDS MODELS (N = 5447)—cont'd

Variable	Death		Graft failure	
	HR	95% CI	HR	95% CI
Donor Characteristics				
DONOR AGE (YEARS)				
Continuous	1.009	(1.004, 1.014)		
Quadratic†			1.0002	(1.0001, 1.0003)
DONOR RACE (BASELINE: WHITE)				
Black	1.31	(1.13, 1.51)	1.38	(1.22, 1.57)
Asian	0.90	(0.55, 1.47)	1.07	(0.72, 1.59)
Other	0.73	(0.41, 1.29)	0.80	(0.49, 1.30)
Matching Characteristics				
GENDER MATCHING (BASELINE: MALE RECIPIENT—MALE DONOR)				
Male recipient—female donor	1.18	(1.01, 1.38)	1.17	(1.02, 1.33)
Female recipient—female donor	1.01	(0.86, 1.19)	1.00	(0.87, 1.15)
Female recipient—male donor	1.02	(0.88, 1.18)	1.05	(0.92, 1.20)
BLOOD TYPE (BASELINE: IDENTICAL)				
Compatible	1.09	(0.93, 1.28)	1.11	(0.97, 1.27)
Incompatible	1.23	(0.97, 1.54)	1.33	(1.09, 1.63)

*See Figure 80-5.
†See Figure 80-6.

Older and younger children experienced greater risks of graft failure than those children in the middle age group (see Fig. 80-5). Older donor age was associated with increased risk of pediatric graft failure, although the relationship is quadratic (Fig. 80-6) as opposed to the linear relationship seen with pediatric mortality, indicating that the risk of graft failure increases more rapidly with donor age than does patient death.

Children who became recipients more recently had better patient and graft survival than did children who became recipients earlier in the study period.

Discussion

Among the greatest challenges in liver transplantation today is the limited deceased donor pool. Efforts to

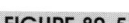

FIGURE 80-5

Hazard ratios for death and graft failure relative to a pediatric recipient age 4* years.

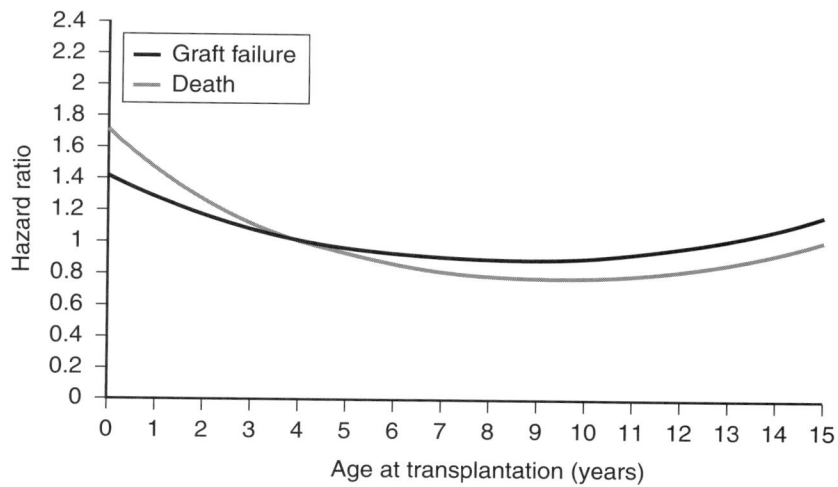

* Mean age of pediatric recipients

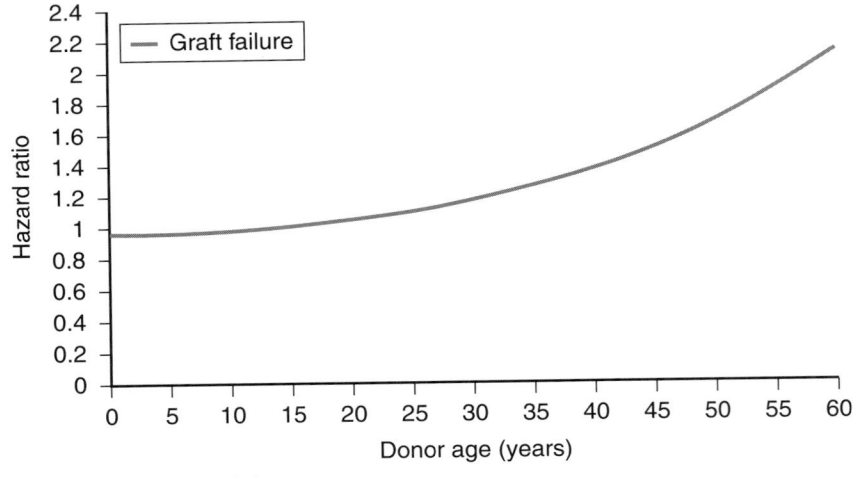

FIGURE 80–6

Hazard ratio for graft failure relative to a pediatric recipient whose donor was age 13* years.

* Mean age of donors

expand the donor pool have manifested in the increased use of livers from older donors and increasing use of alternative procedures including split livers and living donors, especially for pediatric recipients. Older donors were associated with poorer survival in both adult and pediatric recipients, a relationship that has been reported previously.[12,14] However, Hoofnagle and associates[13] found that the reduction in survival occurred mainly among recipients of livers from older donors (>50 years old) that the surgeon assessed to be of fair or poor quality. Because of the organ shortage, then, it is difficult to justify excluding donors solely on the basis of age, especially when recent studies[15,16] demonstrate that successful liver transplantation is possible with livers from donors older than 80 years of age.

Adult recipients of split livers had a higher risk of mortality and graft failure than did adult recipients of whole livers, whereas pediatric recipients of split livers experienced a higher risk of graft failure than did pediatric recipients of whole livers. Split livers among adult recipients are still a relatively new procedure. The relative inexperience with the technique among adults may partially explain, along with unique complications, why split-liver procedures are associated with an increased risk in mortality in adults, but not among children. Because there is a learning curve for liver transplantation,[17] it is not surprising that results from the newer surgical techniques are somewhat poorer than those from whole-liver transplantations. Partial-liver transplantations were associated with poorer graft survival in adults, but were not significantly associated with mortality in adults, or with either mortality or graft failure in children. As with split-liver transplantations, the success of partial-liver transplantations among adult recipients is still being explored and a learning curve exists.[18] Although alternative surgical techniques appear to be more successful for children

than for adult recipients, with further time and research one may expect the adult recipient population to benefit as much as pediatric recipients from alternative techniques, the use of which should also alleviate some of the donor shortage now being experienced.

Care needs to be taken when interpreting the effects of partial-liver transplantations and split-liver transplantation because there may have been some confusion on the part of those completing the data collection forms. In addition to a variable indicating type of surgery, the UNOS dataset also contained a variable that indicated whether the donor was living or deceased. A cross-tabulation of these two variables revealed that 173 (of 986) split transplantations involved living donors, and 678 (of 1627) partial liver transplantations involved deceased donors. Parenthetically, 31 (of 48,094) whole liver transplantations were indicated as being from a living donor. These inconsistencies highlight the potential difficulties of working with a large, public database if analysts do not examine data critically and thoroughly.

Another evolution in liver transplantation is the drastic increase in the percentage of adult recipients who undergo transplantation for chronic hepatitis C with or without concomitant ALD. Liver transplantation was less successful only when indicated for patients with primary liver malignancies rather than with chronic hepatitis C and was more successful for several other indications (see Table 80–3). The recurrence of hepatitis C is nearly universal, thus necessitating retransplantation (which is also associated with increased risks of mortality). The impact of recurrent hepatitis C on the success of retransplantation is controversial; some studies indicate that outcomes are worse,[19] whereas a report has been published that the effect of hepatitis C on mortality is no greater than most other indications for retransplantation.[20] The increasing use of liver transplantation for the indication of TPN-HILD among pediatric recipients may become problematic, as it is associated with higher risks of death and graft failure, as is multiorgan transplantation, a consequence of the progression of TPN-HILD. The most common indication for pediatric liver transplantation, biliary atresia, not only is decreasing in prevalence but also is quite successfully treated by liver transplantation.

Recipient age at transplantation has changed over time. Adult recipients have become older even as older age among adult recipients is found to be detrimental to survival, as reported by others.[21,22] Pediatric recipients have become both increasingly younger (younger than 2 years old) and older (9 to 16 years old) at transplantation, with these age groups experiencing the poorest survival.

Despite the changes in recipient and donor characteristics, several of which negatively influence recipient's outcomes, both patient and graft survival improved over time for both adult and pediatric recipients. This improvement is consistent with the experiences of liver transplant recipients in Europe.[23] The exact reasons for the improvement in survival is not revealed through these analyses, although refinements in surgical techniques, changes in recipient and donor selection, and improvements in immunosuppressive therapy and postoperative care are likely to have contributed.

Overall, liver transplantation has become the accepted treatment for end-stage liver disease, and significant advances in both procedure and postoperative care have been achieved. The ever-increasing shortage of donor livers is the most daunting problem; however, success has already been achieved in alternative procedures among pediatric recipients, transplantations involving older recipients, and transplantations involving older donors. Critical topics for current and future research include expanding the donor pool for adult recipients, maintaining the health of living donors, changing immunosuppressive regimens, and managing the recurrence of hepatitis C.

Pearls and Pitfalls

- Hepatitis C as an indication for transplantation for adults has substantially increased, such that one of three transplantations in 2001 were for this indication.

- Biliary atresia, although the most common indication for liver transplantation among children, decreased from more than one half of the recipients in 1988 to slightly more than one third in 2001.

- Despite poorer outcomes with increasing age, adult recipients in 2001 were significantly older than adult recipients in 1988.

Pearls and Pitfalls—cont'd

- There has been a substantial increase in the use of split-liver and partial-liver transplantations for adult recipients.

- Despite changes in both recipient and donor characteristics, some of which are associated with poorer outcomes, patient and graft survival improved over time for both adult and pediatric recipients.

- Analyzing data and reporting results without carefully examining the data being used.

References

1. Starzl TE: History of liver and other splanchnic organ transplantation. In Busuttil RW, Klintmalm GB (eds): Transplantation of the Liver. Philadelphia: Saunders, 1996, pp 3-22.
2. National Institutes of Health Consensus Development Conference on Liver Transplantation: National Institutes of Health Consensus Development Conference Statement: Liver transplantation, June 20-23, 1983. Hepatology 4:107S-110S, 1984.
3. Detre KM, Belle SH, Carr MA, et al: A report from The NIDDK Liver Transplantation Database. In Terasaki PI (ed): Clinical transplants 1989. Los Angeles: UCLA Tissue Typing Laboratory, 1989, pp 129-141.
4. Wei YL, Detre KM, Everhart, JE: The NIDDK Liver Transplantation Database. Liver Transpl Surg 3:10-22, 1997.
5. The National Organ Transplant Act (1984 Public Law 98-507), approved October 19, 1984.
6. Kaplan EL, Meier P: Nonparametric estimation from incomplete observations. J Am Stat Assoc 53:457-481, 1958.
7. Kalbfleisch JD, Prentice RL: The statistical analysis of failure time data. New York: John Wiley and Sons, 1980.
8. Cox DR: Regression models and life tables (with discussion). J Royal Stat Soc B 34:187-220, 1972.
9. de Ville de Goyet J: Split liver transplantation in Europe—1988 to 1993. Transplantation 59:1371-1376, 1995.
10. Jordinson M, Goodlad RA, Brynes A, et al: Gastrointestinal responses to a panel of lectins in rats maintained on total parenteral nutrition. Am J Physiol Gastrointest Liver Physiol 276:G1235-G1242, 1999.
11. Fryer J, Pellar S, Ormond D, et al: Mortality in candidates waiting for combined liver-intestine transplant exceeds that for other candidates waiting for liver transplants. Liver Transpl 9: 1067-1084, 2003.
12. Marino IR, Doyle HR, Aldrighetti L, et al: Effect of donor age and sex on the outcome of liver transplantation. Hepatology 22: 1754-1762, 1995.
13. Hoofnagle JH, Lombardero M, Zetterman RK, et al: Donor age and outcome of liver transplantation. Hepatology 24:89-96, 1996.
14. Rull R, Vidal O, Momblan D, et al: Evaluation of potential liver donors: limits imposed by donor variables in liver transplantation. Liver Transpl 9:389-393, 2003.
15. Cescon M, Grazi GL, Ercolani G, et al: Long-term survival of recipients of liver grafts from donors older than 80 years: Is it achievable? Liver Transpl 9:1174-1180, 2003.

16. Filipponi F, Romagnoli J, Urbani L, et al: Transplantation of a ninety-three-year-old donor liver. Case report. Hepato-gastroenterology 50:510-511, 2003.

17. Belle SH, Detre KM, Beringer KC: The relationship between outcome of liver transplantation and experience in new centers. Liver Transpl Surg 1:347-353, 1995.

18. Bak T, Wachs M, Trotter J, et al: Adult-to-adult living donor transplantation using right-lobe grafts: Results and lessons learned from a single-center experience. Liver Transpl 7:680-686, 2001.

19. Yoo HY, Maheshwari A, Thuluvath PJ: Retransplantation of liver: Primary graft nonfunction and hepatitis C virus are associated with worse outcome. Liver Transpl 9:897-904, 2003.

20. Watt KDS, Lyden ER, McCashland TM: Poor survival after liver retransplantation: Is hepatitis C to blame? Liver Transpl 9: 1019-1024, 2003.

21. Bjoro K, Hockerstedt K, Ericzon BG, et al: Liver transplantation in patients over 60 years of age. Transpl Int 13:S165-S170, 2000.

22. Herrero JI, Lucena JF, Quiroga J, et al: Liver transplant recipients older than 60 years have lower survival and higher incidence of malignancy. Am J Transplant 3:1407-1412, 2003.

23. Adam R, McMaster P, O'Grady JG, et al: Evolution of liver transplantation in Europe: Report of the European Liver Transplant Registry. Liver Transpl 9:1231-1243, 2003.

Long-Term Functional Recovery and Quality of Life: Childhood, Adulthood, Employment, Pregnancy, and Family Planning

MARLON F. LEVY
TERIANNE COWLING
GORAN B. KLINTMALM

Assessing function and health-related
  quality of life   1324

Preoperative status   1324

Inpatient postoperative recovery   1326

Outpatient postoperative recovery   1326

Employment after liver transplantation   1327

Pediatric recipients   1327

Pregnancy after liver transplantation   1329

With the now commonplace application and clinical access of orthotopic liver transplantation, focus on the procedure has, in many places, broadened to include questions of monetary costs, resource utilization, and social impact. Issues such as health-related quality of life, long-term functional recovery (i.e., employment and societal reintegration), and psychosocial adjustment of patients and their families are being critically examined with regularity in the literature. Such concerns are not trivial. In some countries, particularly in the United States, increasing medical costs and tight health care budgets have forced scrutiny of the allocation of limited resources. For example, the legislature of the late 1980s in the state of Oregon diverted some public funding away from organ transplantation in favor of prenatal care for Medicaid participants.[1] Although Oregon has since reinstated funding for organ transplantation among its Medicaid recipients, that state has gone on to take the lead in rationing health care services for its financially indigent population.[2] In truth, some patients have fallen victim to their newly found well-being. Many individuals, despite being healthy, have been unable to find work or health insurance coverage because of prejudice against assumed higher medical costs.[3,4] The primary hindrance many transplant recipients face regarding a return to work is the potential loss of health insurance or disability income.[5] Although the Health Insurance Portability and Accountability Act of 1996 was developed with this obstacle in mind,[6] documentation of these patients' successes is needed to help increase transplant recipients' work opportunities as well as their insurability after transplantation. Demonstrating the success of resource-intensive procedures through outcomes such as increased life expectancy, improved health-related quality of life, and cost-effectiveness of treatment has become the responsibility of physicians and medical institutions alike.

Assessing Function and Health-Related Quality of Life

Quality of life eludes strict definition. Campbell and colleagues have most succinctly termed it "the satisfaction of needs."[7] Although a complete review of functional assessment methods and tools is beyond the scope of this discussion, a summary of the development of quality of life assessment among the transplant population is in order. With the recognition in the early 1980s that liver transplantation had moved out of the experimental phase came the impetus to catalogue and quantify the changes in functional status and quality of life brought on by that intervention. Before that time, the National Center for Health Statistics quantified patient disability by assessing life years, institutional days, activity limitation days, presence of acute or chronic illnesses, bed disability days, and days lost from work because of illness.[8] Despite this broad approach, experts in the field of functional assessment and disease impact found the system wanting.[9]

In the early 1980s, the National Institutes of Health funded through one of its agencies the development of a quality of life survey tool with the goal of being able to evaluate changes in a patient's functional assessment and quality of life after liver transplantation.[10] With this came the National Institute of Diabetes and Digestive and Kidney Diseases Liver Transplantation Database Quality of Life (NIDDK LTD QOL) questionnaire, which was designed to be a survey instrument administered to patients before transplantation and again at desired time points following transplantation (months and years).[11] It incorporated patient demographics, global measures of satisfaction, and several functional assessment indices, drawing heavily on the work of established researchers in the field.[7,12-14] In fact, central to the concept of quantification of

performance is the work of Karnofsky and Burchenal,[15] which originally addressed that of cancer patients several decades ago. The Karnofsky Performance Status Scale remains a key method of measuring patient physical functioning (Table 81–1).[16]

Aside from Karnofsky's seminal work, many other health assessment measures were incorporated into the creation of the NIDDK LTD QOL questionnaire. The Activities of Daily Living Scale developed by Katz and colleagues[17] was an early and is now a well-established method for quantifying performance. The Sickness Impact Profile (SIP), a diagnosis- and prognosis-neutral measure of health-related dysfunction, has also spawned many of the Quality of Life Form questions.[18,19] The concepts of symptom burden and symptom distress can claim the SIP as a direct ancestor. The NIDDK LTD QOL questionnaire has, since its inception, undergone multiple revisions and modifications both as a whole and at the individual transplantation centers where it was disseminated. Its application as a data gathering tool may perhaps be restricted to single-center use in which longitudinal tracking of patients is the most practical.

Beyond the research tools that help define and quantify health-related quality of life come, of course, the clinician's impressions of the patient at the bedside. A less scientific but no less important marker of end-stage liver disease and the attendant need for transplantation is the loss of the individual's ability to function. Although this loss may come from the extremes of mental loss (encephalopathy) and physical loss (muscle mass and strength loss), the end result is the same. The full-time worker must reduce the workload to part time or must stop work altogether; the homemaker can no longer manage the home, raise the children, or pursue commonplace tasks; and most individuals must sleep at midday, every day, to avoid succumbing to exhaustion. Many liver transplantation candidates have volunteered in the course of their evaluation that they could no longer "go on living like this."

Preoperative Status

Although some candidates for liver transplantation remain quite functional up to the time of surgery, most experience the ravages of end-stage liver disease. Encephalopathy, weakness, lethargy, intractable ascites and peripheral edema, anorexia, bouts of peritonitis, and pneumonia all affect health-related quality of life in a profoundly negative way. Often a severely depleted nutritional state, as measured by muscle wasting, grip strength, or body mass index is evident (see Chapter 33, *"Nutritional Aspects of Adult Liver Transplantation"*). Up to one half of liver transplantation candidates can

Table 81-1. KARNOFSKY PERFORMANCE STATUS SCALE

General Category	Index	Specific Criteria
Able to carry on normal activities, no special care needed	100	Normal, no complaints, no evidence of disease
	90	Able to carry on normal activity; minor signs or symptoms of disease
	80	Normal activity with effort; some signs or symptoms of disease
Unable to work, able to live at home and care for or to do work most personal needs; varying amounts of assistance needed	70	Cares for self, unable to carry on normal activity or to do work
	60	Requires occasional assistance from others, but able to care for most needs
	50	Requires considerable assistance from others and frequent medical care
Unable to care for self, requires institutional or hospital care or equivalent; disease may be rapidly progressing	40	Disabled, requires special care and assistance
	30	Severely disabled, hospitalization indicated; death not imminent
	20	Very ill and hospitalization necessary; active supportive treatment necessary
	10	Moribund
	0	Dead

From Mor V, Laliberle L, Morris JN, Wiemann M. The Karnofsky Performance Status Scale: An examination of its reliability and validity in a research setting. Cancer 53:2002-2007, 1984. Used with permission.

be expected to be bedridden for more than 1 week during the final few weeks before transplantation. Nearly one third will be disabled or unable to work because of their illness.[20]

Before evaluating the changes brought by liver transplantation on health-related quality of life, quantification of a patient's pretransplantation state is a must. This task is not always easy, given the myriad diagnoses leading to end-stage liver failure. Further, liver failure can and does manifest itself in a variety of ways, each of which may have a different impact on health-related quality of life. In the first large scale study specifically assessing the impact of chronic liver disease on quality of life, Tarter and colleagues[21] evaluated a cohort of 306 prospective liver transplantation candidates using the SIP. Included in this study were only those patients whose chronic liver disease had exceeded 3 years in duration. However, we are not informed as to how many of these patients actually became candidates for transplantation or how long before transplantation the SIP was completed. Self-perception of lifestyle, on which the SIP is based, can certainly change over time amid a chronic illness; nonetheless, some observations are worth noting. The scores on the SIP did not correlate with the subjects' clinical rating of severity using

medical criteria such as the Child-Turcotte classification.[21] A pattern of quality of life impairment could also not be linked to a particular diagnostic group. The authors surprisingly noted scores not as low as would normally be expected for patients with a fatal illness. Perhaps patient selection and exclusion criteria influenced these results.

Other instruments that assess health-related quality of life have been applied to pretransplantation patients, including the Karnofsky Performance Status Scale, the Activities of Daily Living Scale, the Nottingham Health Profile, and the Index of Well-Being.[22-24] These studies have highlighted the low level of experienced well-being, decreased physical functioning, numerous physical disturbances, and increased psychological distress characterizing the pretransplantation state. Although physical functioning status was noted to be substantially impaired before transplantation, as indicated by a low Karnofsky Performance Status Scale rating, the ability to perform activities of daily living appeared to be only modestly impaired.[22] Other investigators have documented severely impaired daily functioning in this patient population.[20-23] The sometimes disparate results obtained in these pretransplantation quality-of-life studies serve to highlight the inhomogeneity of the liver transplantation candidate population.

Inpatient Postoperative Recovery

The return to normalcy of life among liver transplant recipients begins long before the patient is discharged from the hospital. The recipient is usually weak and nutritionally depleted, with minimal muscle mass. Aggressive physical therapy is often required, initially on an inpatient basis but subsequently on an outpatient basis. Patients may on occasion spend days or weeks in an inpatient rehabilitation hospital before being able to carry on independent activities of daily living. Common specific physical ailments of the immediate posttransplantation period include incisional pain, low back pain, muscle weakness—especially of the proximal limb girdles—and ulnar nerve neurapraxias on the side of the axillary bypass access. Commonly, proper nutrition either as oral supplements or as enteral tube feedings provides the necessary shift from a catabolic to an anabolic state.

Psychosocial distress and, on occasion, frank psychotic breaks are not unusual in patients or their families. Orientation to reality, patient education, and supportive nursing care are all critical to early normalization of emotional well-being. On occasion, pharmacological intervention with antidepressants, anxiolytics, or sedatives, as well as psychiatric therapy is necessary.

Outpatient Postoperative Recovery

Over the past 20 to 25 years, health-related quality-of-life research has taken on more importance in the field of transplantation. Kidney and heart recipients have been the subject of some benchmark work in this field. Evans and associates were the first to address quality of life issues both in kidney transplant patients and in those with end-stage kidney failure. They used the SIP, the Index of Psychological Affect, the Index of Overall Life Satisfaction, the Index of Well-Being, and the Karnofsky Performance Status Scale to outline the gains achieved with transplantation.[13,25] Simmons and associates, again addressing kidney transplantation, conceptualized assessment of quality of life along three major dimensions: physical, emotional, and social well-being.[14] In doing so, they built on a variety of scores, indices, and scales developed by Evans, Rosenberg, Bradburn, and Campbell.[7,13,26-28] Lough and coworkers,[29] concerned with quality of life in heart transplant recipients, made use of symptom frequency and distress scales to conclude that adaptation to symptoms led to lower distress over time.

A growing body of work specifically addresses health-related quality-of-life changes after liver transplantation, although some of these studies are limited in that they examined patients only postoperatively. By using the Nottingham Health Profile, Lowe and colleagues[30] found a high level of quality of life among liver transplant recipients—indeed broadly similar to levels expected in the general population. Subjects in this study, similar to the general population in age and sex, were found to have a higher incidence of difficulties relating to physical mobility but fewer emotional burdens. Foley and colleagues,[31] citing results with symptom frequency and symptom distress scales, found no correlation between these and quality of life. They placed more importance on perceived negative changes in life, including a change for the worse in patient's financial status. Tarter and others[32] reported that liver transplantation surgery results in a sharp improvement in quality of life relative to one's pretransplant status, although improvement does not reach that of a recipient's premorbid status.

In a large prospective study examining health-related quality of life before and after liver transplantation, Levy and associates[33] noted significant improvements in health-related quality of life by the first year after transplantation, which were sustained to at least 5 years after transplantation. Bravata and coworkers[34] conducted a meta-analysis of numerous studies that assessed health-related quality of life following liver transplantation. Forty-nine studies involving 3576 adult patients who had undergone liver transplantation between 1963 and 1996, assessing either pretransplant and posttransplant data or data from a comparison group, were included in the analysis. Findings revealed impairment in health-related quality of life before liver transplantation and improvement in health-related quality of life following liver transplantation. At a mean of 27.9 months after transplantation, the most significant improvements were observed in physical health, sexual functioning, performance of daily activities, and overall quality of life. Smaller improvements were noted in psychological and social functioning. Others have noted a lower quality of life among older liver transplant recipients and among those who had recently undergone transplantation (less than 1 year)[35]; however, findings from a large multicenter study have refuted both of these observations.[36]

Measures intent on quantifying the neuropsychiatric impact of liver disease and the attendant recovery expected have also been reported. The question of reversibility of pretransplantation encephalopathy prompted an evaluation of liver transplant recipients 3 years after the procedure.[37] Chronic liver disease among subjects had predated transplantation by 45 months. In comparison with an age-matched and sex-matched control group of patients with Crohn's disease, liver transplant recipients were found to be similar to controls in measures of intelligence, attention and concentration, logical and figural memory, social organization, and language capacities. The group of transplant recipients was noted to be superior in motor skills, highlighting the integrity of the cerebellum. On the whole, patients with Crohn's disease were judged to exhibit more hypochondriacal tendencies. Liver transplant recipients and Crohn's disease patients did not differ on measures of intelligence, language, attention, concentration, spatial organization, memory, or learning. Performance on these various aspects of cognitive functioning by both groups separately measured in the "normal" ranges when compared with normative or standardized test values. Psychiatric status and social functioning, although similar in both groups, differed from historically compared healthy individuals in showing more anxiety, somatic distress, frustration, depression, worry, and social withdrawal.

Other studies substantiate posttransplantation improvements in cognitive functioning resulting in nearly normative values by 1 year after transplantation.[32] Nonetheless, subtle neurobehavioral deficits in daily life may persist. Standard psychometric tests have been used to measure neurocognitive functioning and mental state as early as 3 months after transplantation.[38] Overt psychiatric morbidity appears to be no more frequent among liver transplant recipients than among the general population.[22,39] Recovery of cerebral function is the norm after liver transplantation.

Employment after Liver Transplantation

A fundamental goal of liver transplantation is the return of patients to the mainstream of society. For many patients, a hallmark of this recovery is their resumption of pretransplantation activities such as working for pay. Transplant recipients who are employed have been noted to have a higher quality of life than those who are not employed.[40-42] Among individuals with traumatic brain injury, a strong positive correlation has been found between employment and perceived quality of life, social integration within the community, and participation in home and leisure activities.[43-46] Barriers to posttransplantation employment have been examined in the literature. These include a patient's self-perception of functional status, fear of the loss of health insurance and Social Security disability benefits, fear of denied health insurance coverage at a new job, hiring discrimination against individuals with adverse medical histories, limited education and/or work skills, and the perceived inability to maintain a rigid or full-time work schedule following transplantation.[3,4,47-49] Quantifying the employment status of transplant recipients is a difficult task. Although some recipients may not be working for pay, they may be quite busy with other activities such

as caring for a home and family, attending school, or participating in volunteer work. The wide variation in activity levels, together with the various types of employment, precludes easy comparisons.

A review of the world literature reveals a limited number of reports that address work status after transplantation (Table 81-2). These reports are disparate in patient population, sample size, length of follow-up, and definitional use of the term "employed." Only a few mention pretransplantation work status. Because the term employed has been defined differently by different investigators, comparisons between studies to determine an appropriate "average" or "common" rate of posttransplantation employment has not been possible.[33,48-50]

In addition to working for pay, liver transplant recipients are actively involved in homemaking, academic study, support of loved ones through financial and/or caregiving efforts, and participation in structured social or community groups and activities, including volunteer work.[51] In a study examining societal reintegration after transplantation, investigators found that both alcohol-related and non–alcohol-related liver transplant recipients had reentered society to become active and productive members. No significant differences were noted between the two groups in their level of participation in the aforementioned activities except for social activities, wherein a greater percentage of non–alcohol-related transplant recipients reported participation in structured social activities compared with alcohol-related transplant recipients.

Pediatric Recipients

Quality-of-life assessment gains another dimension when the pediatric liver transplant recipient is considered. Unlike most of their adult counterparts, pediatric patients face the added posttransplantation burdens of physical, emotional, and metabolic (endocrine) growth. Future school and work performance is also a concern. All too often, the pretransplantation period is marked by months or years of chronic illness, debility, and delayed academic development.

Early reports of patients receiving cyclosporine immunosuppressive therapy held out the promise of low-dose steroid regimens. Before the use of cyclosporine, severely inhibited growth and development patterns were linked to the use of high-dose steroids.[52] Optimism regarding low-dose steroid use among pediatric patients proved to be warranted, as most children have exhibited linear growth following transplantation.[53-55] Sixty percent of pediatric liver transplant recipients exhibit catch-up growth, both in height and weight, following transplantation.[55] Catch-up growth has been noted to occur between 6 and 24 months after transplantation, with no differences noted

Table 81–2. REPORTED EMPLOYMENT AMONG LIVER TRANSPLANT RECIPIENTS

Transplantation Center	Pretransplantation Employment	Posttransplantation Employment	Posttransplantation Follow-up
Denver 1979 (Starzl et al.[79])	N/A	10 of 12 adults returned to work (8) or school (2)	>1 yr
Pittsburgh 1985 (Iwatsuki et al.[80])	N/A	12 of 14 adults working full time or homemakers	>5 yr
Memphis 1987 (Williams et al.[81])	N/A	13 of 28 full-time, 7 of 28 full-time homemakers	>1 yr
UCLA 1988 (Colonna et al.[82])	32% full-time or part-time	75% full-time or part-time	16 mo
Pittsburgh 1988 (Tarter et al.[32])	N/A	35% full-time, 9% part-time, 29% homemakers	>1 yr
Mayo Clinic 1989 (Eid et al.[83])	N/A	26 of 46 full-time, 16 of 46 full-time homemakers, 4 of 16 "did not work"	21 mo
UCLA 1989 (Wolcott et al.[35])	N/A	48% part-time, 25% full-time	>4 mo
Pittsburgh 1990 (Robinson et al.[84])	45% full-time or part-time	48% full-time or part-time, 26% homemakers	3 yr
Birmingham 1992 (Commander et al.[39])	19%	19% full-time	6 mo
Toronto 1993 (Adams et al.[85])	N/A	40% full-time, 17% part-time	3 yr
Dallas 1993 (Levy et al.[86])	65%	61% full-time or part-time	2 yr
Dallas 1995 (Levy et al.[33])	62% full time or part time	58% working full-time or part-time (current/recent)	2 yr
		70% working full-time or part-time (current/recent)	5 yr
North Carolina 1998 (Hunt et al.[87])	83%	31% returned to full employment	approx. 18-24 mo
Dallas 2004 (Cowling et al.[51])	N/A	33% (working full-time or part-time) alcohol-related transplant recipients	≥2 yr (median = 52 mos)
Dallas 2004 (Cowling et al.[51])	N/A	38% (working full-time or part-time) non–alcohol-related transplant recipients	≥2 yr (median = 52 mo)

N/A, not applicable.

between female and male patients.[56] Codoner-Franch and colleagues[56] have reported that both girls and boys experienced a normal pubertal growth spurt and normal development of secondary sexual characteristics after transplantation. All adolescent girls experienced regular menstrual cycles; one delivered a normal infant 6 years following liver transplantation. Linear growth has been seen in nearly all children after transplantation and does not appear to be influenced by cause of liver disease, with the exception of fulminant hepatic failure. Low-dose use of corticosteroids, administered on an alternate-day basis, have been found to contribute to growth improvement among pediatric liver transplant recipients.[56] After following multivariate analyses of factors potentially influencing pediatric growth following transplantation, some investigators have suggested that although pediatric liver transplant recipients do show some potential for catch-up growth, normal heights are not achieved by the majority of children following liver transplantation when compared with age- and sex-matched peers.[57] These authors concluded that the most important factors detrimental to linear growth are older age at the time of transplantation, Z scores (standardized height scores) greater than −2.0 at transplant, fulminant hepatic failure, tumor, and posttransplantation complications causing graft dysfunction.

Findings regarding academic progress among pediatric transplant patients are also available. At 2 to 5 years after transplantation, 77% of all pediatric patients are reportedly in age-appropriate grade levels or only 1 year behind (51% age-appropriate level; 26%

1 year behind).[58] Another 12% are reportedly 2 years behind their appropriate class level. Zitelli and colleagues[58] in Pittsburgh studied 65 long-term survivors of pediatric liver transplantation with standardized measures of intelligence. In a subgroup of patients and their parents, researchers also investigated child development, motor skills, behavior, and parent-child interactions. Further, certain pretransplantation and posttransplantation markers of morbidity were compared. On the whole, surviving liver transplant recipients experienced fewer admissions and fewer number of days in the hospital and were taking fewer medications each day than in the examined pretransplantation period. All of these differences reached statistical significance. Before transplantation, children were found to have poorer overall behavior than that expected for age-matched children who had not had transplant surgery. Parents described these children as overly dependent, complaining, and demanding prior to transplantation. Likewise, relationships with siblings before transplantation were often described as problematic. After transplantation, overall behavior of the recipients was considered improved, including behavior related to sibling relationships. Transplantation also led to improvements in the child's social maturity, school separation behavior, locomotion, and self-help areas. Notably, before transplantation children were found to be behind their peers in motor skills, which were predominantly brought up to age-appropriate levels after transplantation. Cognitive skills were not found to be altered by transplantation; the average intelligence quotient (IQ) was 92 before transplantation and 93 after transplantation (at least 1 year later). Zitelli and colleagues did report a lack of complete normalcy in the lives of children who undergo transplantation. The patients remained overprotected by their families, parental anxieties continued to be heightened, and some parents reported defiant behavior and aggression in their children. Enuresis, especially nocturnal, was six times more prevalent than in age-matched healthy children. Parental divorce rates (one couple in six) were quite comparable with those reported for other families with chronically ill children.[59]

What emerges from this research is a picture of the severe functional and social impairment of children with liver disease, an impairment very successfully (although not completely) corrected by a successful transplantation. It is of note that not all investigators agree with the work of Zitelli and colleagues, citing study limitations and contradictory findings.[60] However, this research takes an important step in defining health-related quality of life as improved by liver transplantation. Accepted standardized measures of IQ, behavior, and social interactions are applied and analyzed to give concrete measures of success, bringing

better definition to a field sometimes viewed as nebulous.

Pregnancy After Liver Transplantation

An important component of the restoration of quality of life and of normalcy (however defined) after liver transplantation is parenthood. Many women who undergo transplantation are still of childbearing age. Often with patients in end-stage liver failure, pregnancy or its prevention is not a concern. However, just as women are very often amenorrheic before transplantation, a successful transplant almost uniformly leads to a prompt return of normal menstrual cycles.[61] Conception in one female transplant recipient has been documented as occurring as early as 3 weeks after liver transplantation.[62]

Medical experience has shown that despite the administration of medications and changes in maternal physiology among female transplant recipients, successful pregnancy can be sustained.[63] Children born to female transplant recipients are more likely to be premature and/or small for their gestational age when compared with children of male transplant recipients.[64] Offspring of male transplant recipients appear to be comparable to those of the general population.[63]

Data specifically addressing the teratogenicity of standard immunosuppressants among humans are limited. The incidence of structural malformation in offspring born to female transplant recipients treated with cyclosporine falls within the range expected for the general population.[65] Two cases of structural malformations have been noted in the offspring of female transplant recipients having been exposed to mycophenolate mofetil during pregnancy; however, data are limited and not sufficient to determine the incidence of a specific malformation.[65] No problem patterns have been detected among offspring of male transplant recipients treated with mycophenolate mofetil.[65] No difference has been noted in the type or incidence of pregnancy complications before or after the widespread use of cyclosporine, and no specific pattern of malformation among newborns has been reported in association with cyclosporine use.[63,64] Although cyclosporine is known to cross the placental barrier and to be excreted into breast milk, indications are that the neonate's level of exposure is minimal and some physicians permit breast-feeding among female transplant recipients under their care.[66,67] Breast-feeding is not recommended during the use of azathioprine, as small amounts have been detected in breast milk.[68]

Few data exist regarding the use of tacrolimus (FK-506; Prograf) among pregnant women, although some reports have suggested that complications associated with pregnancy are less common among women treated with tacrolimus-based immunosuppressive therapy than with cyclosporine-based immunosuppressive therapy.[69,70] In a study examining 27 pregnancies among 21 female liver transplant recipients who were administered tacrolimus, a lower incidence of hypertension and preeclampsia occurred compared with earlier reports of transplant recipients who received cyclosporine-based therapy.[71] Transient kidney damage and hyperkalemia were noted in 36% of the newborns, presumably due to tacrolimus crossing the placental barrier.[67] A lower rate of both hypertension and preeclampsia has been noted in transplant recipients administered tacrolimus-based therapy when compared with the use of Neoral (or cyclosporine).[72] In addition, slightly greater mean birth weights and a smaller percentage of low birth weight have been observed in the offspring of tacrolimus-treated mothers as compared with the offspring of mothers treated with Neoral (or cyclosporine). There have been no reports of increased birth defects or growth retardation among newborns of mothers receiving tacrolimus, but too few data have been gathered to conclusively declare use of this drug harmless during pregnancy.

Although data continue to accrue on pregnancy in liver transplant recipients, some lessons may be learned from the larger amount of data available on kidney transplant recipients. Davison[73] reported on more than 2300 pregnancies in nearly 1600 female renal transplant recipients. Of these conceptions, 40% did not continue beyond the first trimester, although the majority of the abortions were therapeutic (27%), not spontaneous (13%). Ninety-two percent of pregnancies that had reached the second trimester ended successfully. Permanent renal impairment occurred in 15% of the pregnancies. A 30% chance of developing hypertension or preeclampsia, or both, was noted among subjects. Although about one half of infants born to renal transplant recipients are expected to be of normal size and gestational age, 45% to 60% can be expected to be delivered preterm, with 20% to 30% of pregnancies resulting in offspring being small for their gestational age.[73,74]

Pregnancy in renal transplant recipients appears to have no lasting impact on the health of the mother. In a case-controlled evaluation of 18 previously pregnant females a mean of 12 years after delivery, no differences in graft function, blood pressure, or graft or patient survival were noted when compared with nonpregnant kidney transplant recipients.[75] In a comparison of 57 newborns born to renal transplant recipients who were receiving azathioprine and 94 newborns born to mothers taking cyclosporine, those babies born to mothers on azathioprine had a significantly higher birth weight than those on cyclosporine, with no incidence of congenital malformation in either group.[76]

The first large study focusing on pregnancy among female liver transplant recipients was reported from Pittsburgh.[77] Twenty pregnancies among 17 liver transplant recipients were examined. Twelve of the women were noted to have normal biochemical parameters of liver function, whereas the others had some enzyme elevation before delivery. One case of biopsy proven rejection resolved spontaneously without treatment. Thirteen of the 20 infants were delivered by cesarean section, 11 of those prematurely. Toxemia of pregnancy and early rupture of membranes were the primary indications for cesarean section. Seven births were delivered vaginally, all being full term. All mothers delivered without complications and remained well, with the exception of one who died of lymphoma 2.5 years after delivery (nearly 4 years after transplantation). All of the children were reported as alive and well, having reached normal developmental milestones, except for one child who exhibited immature speech development.

Although successful pregnancies have become the rule among transplant recipients, it should be noted that pregnancy in the female liver transplant recipient is considered high risk, requiring close surveillance by a coordinated team of health care personnel.[72] Patient monitoring should include frequent blood chemistry and drug level tests, ultrasonography, liver biopsies when needed, and screenings for infection. Both mother and fetus should be monitored for cytomegalovirus infection. With stable liver and kidney function, pregnancy is typically well tolerated in the female liver transplant recipient. A small group of liver recipients may experience worsening graft function during pregnancy, especially those with viral hepatitis or cytomegalovirus infection, leading to increased risk to both mother and newborn.[72]

Many female patients seek advice on the safest times to pursue pregnancy or, more often, on the safest means of contraception. In our center, as in most others, couples wanting to conceive a child are asked to wait 2 years after transplantation to allow for complete recovery from surgery, stabilization of immunosuppression, reduction in steroid use, and optimal patient longevity. Liver transplant recipients who are well 2 years after transplantation have an excellent chance of longevity.[78] For patients wishing contraception, barrier methods are the preferred choice. Oral contraceptives are relatively contraindicated because of the risks of thromboembolism, cholestasis, exacerbated hypertension, and interference in cyclosporine metabolism. Intrauterine devices also are discouraged because of their increased risk of infection and documented 13% incidence of bacteremia on insertion.[73] Contraceptive methods that are safe and efficacious should be practiced by all those wishing to avoid pregnancy because a return to fertility is the rule following liver transplantation.

Pearls and Pitfalls

- Health-related quality-of-life assessment typically focuses on physical, psychological, and cognitive functioning, symptom distress and frequency, and social and emotional well-being. Employment is sometimes assessed in addition to health-related quality of life.

- Liver transplantation results in a sharp improvement in quality of life relative to the pretransplant status, although improvement does not appear to reach that of the premorbid status.

- Following transplantation, liver recipients return to society to become active and productive members, participating in employment, homemaking, supporting others through financial or caregiving efforts, academic study, social and community involvement, and volunteer work.

- Although cognitive functioning has been noted to approach normative values by 1 year after transplantation, subtle neurobehavioral deficits may persist.

- The majority of pediatric transplant recipients exhibit linear growth following transplantation.

- Among pediatric liver transplant recipients, use of low-dose corticosteroids administered on an alternate-day basis contributes to growth improvement.

- Some investigators have suggested that although pediatric liver transplant recipients show some potential for catch-up growth, normal heights are not achieved by most children following liver transplantation when compared with age-matched and sex-matched peers.

- Pediatric liver transplantation has led to improvements in recipients' overall behavior, social maturity, school separation behavior, locomotion, and self-help areas.

- A successful transplant almost uniformly leads to a prompt return of normal menstrual cycles.

- Children born to female transplant recipients are more likely to be premature and/or small for their gestational age when compared with children of male transplant recipients. Offspring of male transplant recipients appear to be comparable to those of the general population.

Pearls and Pitfalls—cont'd

- Although successful pregnancies have become the rule among transplant recipients, pregnancy in the female liver transplant recipient is considered high risk and requires close surveillance by a coordinated team of health care personnel.

- Patient monitoring should include frequent blood chemistry and drug level tests, ultrasonography, liver biopsies when needed, and screening for infection. Both mother and fetus should be monitored for cytomegalovirus infection.

- With stable liver and kidney function, pregnancy is typically well-tolerated in the liver transplant recipient.

References

1. Welch HG, Larson EB: Dealing with limited resources. The Oregon decision to curtail funding for organ transplantation. N Engl J Med 319:171-173, 1988.
2. Oregon Health Plan Administrative Rules. Salem, Oregon Office of Medical Assistance Programs, 1995.
3. Pennington JC: Quality of life following liver transplantation. Transplant Proc 21:3514-3516, 1989.
4. Gutkind L: Life after transplantation. Transplant Proc 20 (suppl 1):1092-1099, 1988.
5. Carter JM, Winsett RP, Rager D, et al: A center-based approach to a transplant employment program. Prog Transplant 10:204-208, 2000.
6. Paris W, Harrison J, Diercks M, et al: The new health insurance law and its potential impact on transplant programs and recipients. J Transpl Coord 7:157-158, 1997.
7. Campbell A, Converse PE, Rodgers NL: The quality of American life: Perceptions, evaluations, and satisfactions. New York, Russell Sage Foundation, 1976.
8. Kovar MG, La Croix AZ: Aging in the eighties, ability to perform work-related activities (data from the Supplement on Aging to the National Health Interview Survey, United States, 1984: Advance Data from Vital and Health Statistics No. 136, DHHS Pub. No. [PHS] 87-1250). Hyattsville, Md, National Center for Health Statistics, 1987.
9. Itoh M, Lee MHM: The epidemiology of disability as related to rehabilitation medicine and rehabilitation. In Kottke FJ, Lehmann JF (eds.) Krusen's handbook of physical medicine and rehabilitation, 4th ed. Philadelphia, WB Saunders, 1990, pp 215-233.
10. Wei YL, Detre KM, Everhart JE: The NIDDK liver transplantation database. Liver Transpl Surg 3:10-22, 1997.
11. Belle SH, Porayko MK, Hoofnagle JH, et al: Changes in quality of life after liver transplantation among adults. National Institute of Diabetes and Digestive and Kidney Diseases (NIDDK) Liver Transplantation Database (LTD). Liver Transpl Surg 3:93-104, 1997.
12. Bradburn NM: The structure of psychological well-being. Chicago: Aidine Press, 1969.
13. Evans RW, Manninen DL, Garrison LP, et al: The quality of life of patients with end-stage renal disease. N Engl J Med 312:553-559, 1985.

14. Simmons RG, Abress L, Anderson CR: Quality of life after kidney transplantation. A prospective, randomized comparison of cyclosporine and conventional immunosuppressive therapy. Transplantation 45:415-421, 1988.
15. Karnofsky DA, Burchenal JH: The clinical evaluation of chemotherapeutic agents in cancer. In McLeod CM (ed.) Evaluation of chemotherapeutic agents. New York, Columbia University Press, 1949, pp 191-205.
16. Hirsch D, Grabois M, Dectra N: Rehabilitation of the cancer patient. In De Lisa JA (ed.) Rehabilitation Medicine—Principles and Practice. Philadelphia, JB Lippincott, 1988, pp 660-670.
17. Katz S, Ford AB, Moskowitz RW, et al: The index of ADL: A standardized measure of biological and psychosocial function. JAMA 185:914-918, 1963.
18. Gilson BS, Gilson JS, Bergner M, et al: The Sickness Impact Profile: Development of an outcome measure of health care. Am J Public Health 65:1304-1310, 1975.
19. Bergner M, Bobbitt RA, Pollard WE, et al: The Sickness Impact Profile: Validation of a health status measure. Med Care 14: 57-67, 1976.
20. Levy MF, Husberg B, Gonwa T, et al: Social impact of liver transplantation: Pretransplant quality of life [abstract]. Presented at the annual meeting of the American Society of Transplant Physicians, Chicago, May 1992.
21. Tarter RE, Switala J, Arria A, et al: Impact of liver disease on daily living in transplantation candidates. J Clin Epidemiol 44:1079-1083, 1991.
22. Bonsel GJ, Essink-Bot ML, Klompmakier IJ, et al: Assessment of the quality of life before and following liver transplantation. Transplantation 53:796-800, 1992.
23. Geevarghese SK, Bradley AE, Wright JK, et al: Outcomes analysis in 100 liver transplantation patients. Am J Surg 175:348-353, 1998.
24. Price CE, Lowe D, Cohen AT: Prospective study of the quality of life in patients assessed for liver transplantation: Outcome in transplanted and not transplanted groups. J R Soc Med 88: 130-135, 1995.
25. Evans RW: Quality of life assessment and the treatment of end-stage renal disease. Seattle, Batelle Human Affairs Research Centers, 1990.
26. Rosenberg M, Simmons RG: Black and white self-esteem: The urban school child. Washington, DC, American Sociological Association, 1972.
27. Rosenberg M: Society and the adolescent self-image. Princeton, NJ, Princeton University Press, 1965.
28. Bradburn NM: The structure of psychological well-being. Chicago, Aldine, 1969.
29. Lough ME, Lindsey AM, Shinn JA, et al: Impact of symptom frequency and symptom distress on self-reported quality of life in heart transplant recipients. Heart Lung 16:193-200, 1987.
30. Lowe D, O'Grady JG, McEwen J, et al: Quality of life following liver transplantation: A preliminary report. J R Coll Physicians Lond 24:43-46, 1990.
31. Foley TC, Davis CP, Conway PA: Liver transplant recipients: Self report of symptom frequency, symptom distress, quality of life. Transplant Proc 21:2417, 1989.
32. Tarter RE, Erb S, Biller PA, et al: The quality of life following liver transplantation: A preliminary report. Gastroenterol Clin North Am 17:207-217, 1988.
33. Levy MF, Jennings L, Abouljoud MS, et al: Quality of life improvements at one, two, and five years after liver transplantation. Transplantation 59:515-518, 1995.
34. Bravata DM, Olkin U, Barnato A, et al: Health-related quality of life after liver transplantation: A meta-analysis. Liver Transpl Surg 5:318-331, 1999.
35. Wolcott D, Norquist G, Busuttil R: Cognitive function and quality of life in adult liver transplant recipients. Transpl Proc 21: 3563, 1989.
36. Williams L, Wood GP: Perceived quality of life in adult liver transplant recipients [abstract]. Presented at Dilemmas in Organ Transplantation, Omaha, Neb, October 1991.
37. Tarter RE, Van Thiel DH, Hepedus AM, et al: Neuropsychiatric status after liver transplantation. J Lab Clin Med 103:776-782, 1984.
38. Riether AM, Smith SL, Lewison BJ, et al: Quality-of-life changes and psychiatric and neurocognitive outcome after heart and liver transplantation. Transplantation 54:444-450, 1992.
39. Commander M, Neuberger J, Dean C: Psychiatric and social consequences of liver transplantation. Transplantation 53:1038-1040, 1992.
40. Tart JS: Quality of life in liver transplant recipients [abstract]. Presented at Dilemmas in Organ Transplantation, Omaha, Neb, October 1991.
41. Winsett RP: Posttransplant quality of life: A decade of descriptive studies leading to practice interventions. Posttransplant QOL Intervention Study Group. J Transpl Coord 8:236-240, 1998.
42. Hathaway DK, Winsett RP, Johnson C, et al: Post kidney transplant quality of life prediction models. Clin Transplant 12:168-174, 1998.
43. O'Neill J, Hibbard MR, Brown M, et al: The effect of employment on quality of life and community integration after traumatic brain injury. J Head Trauma Rehabil 13:68-79, 1998.
44. Heineman AW. Whiteneck GG: Relationships among impairment, disability, handicap, and life satisfaction in persons with traumatic brain injury. J Head Trauma Rehabil 10:54-63, 1995.
45. Webb DR, Wrigley M, Yoels W, et al: Explaining quality of life for persons with traumatic brain injuries two years after injury. Arch Phys Med Rehabil 76:1113-1119, 1995.
46. Melamed S, Groswasser Z, Stern MJ: Acceptance of disability, work involvement and subjective rehabilitation status of traumatic brain-injured (TBI) patients. Brain Inj 6:233-243, 1992.
47. Thomas DJ: Returning to work after liver transplant: Experiencing roadblocks. J Transpl Coord 6:134-138, 1996.
48. Paris W, Woodbury A, Thompson S, et al: Social rehabilitation and return to work after cardiac transplantation—a multicenter survey. Transplantation 53:433-438, 1992.
49. Hunt CM, Tart JS, Dowdy E, et al: Effect of orthotopic liver transplantation on employment and health status. Liver Transpl Surg 2:148-153, 1996.
50. Cowling T, Jung G, Molmenti EP, et al: Social reintegration after liver transplantation for alcohol-related liver disease. Transplantation 67:S246, 1999.
51. Cowling T, Jennings LW, Goldstein RM, et al: Societal reintegration after liver transplantation: Findings in alcohol-related and non–alcohol-related transplant recipients. Ann Surg 239:93-98, 2004.
52. Starzl TE, Iwatsuki S, Malatack JJ, et al: Liver and kidney transplantation in children receiving cyclosporine A and steroids. J Pediatr 100:681-686, 1992.
53. Gartner JC, Zitelli BJ, Malatack JJ, et al: Orthotopic liver transplantation in children: Two-year experience with 47 patients. Pediatrics 74:140-145, 1984.
54. Urbach AH, Gartner JC, Malatack JJ, et al: Linear growth following pediatric liver transplantation. Am J Dis Child 141:544-549, 1987.
55. Andrews WS, Wanek E, Fyock B, et al: Pediatric liver transplantation: A 3-year experience. J Pediatr Surg 24:77-82, 1989.
56. Codoner-Franch P, Bernard O, Alvarez F: Long-term follow-up of growth in height after successful liver transplantation. J Pediatr 124:368-373, 1994.
57. McDiarmid SV, Gornbein JA, DeSilva PJ, et al: Factors affecting growth after pediatric liver transplantation. Transplantation 67:404-411, 1999.

58. Zitelli BJ, Miller JW, Gartner JC Jr, et al: Changes in lifestyle after liver transplantation. Pediatrics 82:173-180, 1988.
59. Sabbeth BF, Leventhal JM: Marital adjustment to chronic childhood illness: A critique of the literature. Pediatrics 73:762-768, 1984.
60. Bradford R: Children's psychological health status—the impact of liver transplantation: A review. J R Soc Med 84:550-553, 1991.
61. Cundy TF, O'Grady JG, Williams R: Recovery of menstruation and pregnancy after liver transplantation. Gut 31:337-338, 1990.
62. Laifer SA, Darby MJ, Scantlebury VP, et al: Pregnancy and liver transplantation. Obstet Gynecol 76:1083-1088, 1990.
63. Armenti VT, Moritz MJ, Radomski JS, et al: Pregnancy and transplantation. Graft 3:59-63, 2000.
64. Armenti VT, Ahlswede KM, Ahlswede BA, et al: Data from the National Transplantation Pregnancy Registry. Philadelphia, Thomas Jefferson University, 1993.
65. Armenti VT, Radomski JS, Moritz MJ, et al: Reports from the National Transplantation Pregnancy Registry (NTPR): Outcomes of pregnancy after transplantation. Clin Transpl 97-105, 2001.
66. Ziegenhagen DJ, Crombach G, Dieckmann M, et al: Pregnancy during cyclosporine medication following a kidney transplant. Dtsch Med Wochenschr 113:260-262, 1988.
67. Nyberg G, Haljamae U, Frisenette-Fich C, et al: Breast-feeding during treatment with cyclosporine. Transplantation 65:253-255, 1998.
68. Product Information Imuran (R), 2003.
69. Jain A, Venkataramanan R, Lever J, et al: FK506 and pregnancy in liver transplantation patients. Transplantation 56:1588-1589, 1993.
70. Casele HL, Laifer SA: Association of pregnancy complications and choice of immunosuppressant in liver transplant patients. Transplantation 65:581-583, 1998.
71. Jain A, Venkataramanan R, Fung JJ, et al: Pregnancy after liver transplantation under tacrolimus. Transplantation 64:559-565, 1997.
72. Armenti VT, Herrine SK, Radomski JS, et al: Pregnancy after liver transplantation. Liver Transpl 6:671-685, 2000.
73. Davison JM: Dialysis, transplantation, and pregnancy. Am J Kidney Dis 17:127-132, 1991.
74. Davison JM: Pregnancy in renal allograft recipients: Prognosis and management. Bailliere's Clin Obstet Gynaecol 1:1027-1045, 1987.
75. Sturgiss SN, Davison JM: Effect of pregnancy on long-term function of renal allografts. Am J Kidney Dis 19:167-172, 1992.
76. Toma H, Kazunari T, Tokumoto T: Pregnancy on long-term function of renal allografts. Am J Kidney Dis 19:167-172, 1992.
77. Scantlebury V, Gordon R, Tzakis A, et al: Childbearing after liver transplantation. Transplantation 49:317-321, 1990.
78. Backman L, Gibbs J, Levy MF, et al: Causes of late graft loss after liver transplantation. Transplantation 55:1078-1082, 1993.
79. Starzl TE, Koep U, Schröter GPJ, et al: The quality of life after liver transplantation. Transplant Proc 11:252-256, 1979.
80. Iwatsuki S, Shaw BW, Starzl TE: Five-year survival after liver transplantation. Transplant Proc 17:259-263, 1985.
81. Williams JW, Vera S, Evans LS: Socioeconomic aspects of hepatic transplantation. Am J Gastroenterol 82:1115-1119, 1987.
82. Colonna JO, Brems JJ, Hiatt JR, et al: The quality of survival after liver transplantation. Transplant Proc 20(suppl 1):594-597, 1988.
83. Eid A, Steffen R, Porayko MK, et al: Beyond a year after liver transplantation. Mayo Clin Proc 64:446-450, 1989.
84. Robinson LR, Switala J, Tarter RE, et al: Functional outcome after liver transplantation: A preliminary report. Arch Phys Med Rehabil 71:426-427, 1990.
85. Adams PC, Ghent CN, Grant DR, et al: The effect of age on quality of life following liver transplantation [abstract]. Presented at the Second Congress of the International Liver Transplant Society, Toronto, October 1993.
86. Levy MF, Jennings L, Goldstein RM, et al: Quality of life changes two years after liver transplantation [abstract]. Presented at the annual meeting of the American Association for the Study of Liver Disease, Chicago, November 1993.
87. Hunt CM, Camargo CA Jr, Dominitz JA, et al: Effect of postoperative complications on health and employment following liver transplantation. Clin Transplant 12:99-103, 1998.

Results: Survival and Quality of Life After Orthotopic Liver Transplantation in Children

CARLOS O. ESQUIVEL

Preoperative risk factors   1336

Patient age   1337

Diagnosis   1337
   Cholestatic liver disease   1337
   Metabolic disorders   1340
   Mass-occupying lesions   1340
   Injury to the liver   1341

Immunosuppression   1341

Allograft size   1342
   Reduced-size liver transplantation   1342
   Split-liver transplantation   1343
   Living-related transplantation   1343

Retransplantation   1344

Combination liver transplantation   1346

Hepatic dysfunction   1347
   Vascular complications   1348
   Biliary tract complications   1348

Quality of life after transplantation   1348

Comment   1350

Human liver transplantation was first attempted in 1963 in a child with extrahepatic biliary atresia.[1] At the time the best candidates for liver transplantation were children with biliary atresia or patients with advanced liver malignancy because of the absence of therapeutic options for such patients with terminal diseases. The indications for liver transplantation in children expanded as the outcomes of this treatment improved following the introduction of cyclosporine in 1980.[2-5] The new problem became the shortage of organs from deceased donors because such donors were mostly of school age, but the children in need of liver transplantation were mostly preschoolers. The pressing need for pediatric donors paved the way to impressive advances in the surgical techniques of liver transplantation. The lack of donors led to the use of reduced-size (cut down) livers. This, in turn, resulted in the development of techniques currently applied for splitting livers from deceased donors as well as the procurement of segments or lobes from living donors.

During the last few years, other important advances in pediatric liver transplantation have involved the creation of effective and safer immunosuppressive protocols, including the elimination of steroids that are well known to have devastating side effects, particularly in children. It is clear that liver transplantation in children is not only a life-saving procedure but also a therapeutic modality that improves the child's quality of life. This chapter reviews the outcomes, including quality of life, of liver transplantation in children.

Preoperative Risk Factors

The child's medical condition at the time of liver transplantation may have a direct bearing on the outcome of the procedure. Poor prognostic factors are the presence of ascites, hypocholesterolemia (< 100 mg/dL), low albumin level, renal dysfunction, prolonged international normalized ratio (INR), and severe malnutrition.[6,7] A retrospective analysis of patients with three or more organ system failures showed that only 25% recovered after liver transplantation.[8] Certain intraoperative factors may also be associated with a poor outcome, including large volumes of blood transfusions, portal vein thrombosis or agenesis, hepatic artery anomalies, previous operations in the right upper quadrant, and, possibly, the level of expertise of the surgical team.[9-12]

The use of organs from ABO-incompatible donors has prognostic significance depending on the age of the child at the time of transplantation. The recipients of such grafts are high-risk patients who receive these livers under desperate, nonelective circumstances, so it is difficult to distinguish the effect of tissue incompatibility from that of the patient's medical condition at the time of transplantation. Decreased patient and graft survival has been observed in one group of children who received ABO-incompatible grafts, and similar results have been noted in two studies of adult and pediatric patients at the University of Pittsburgh.[13-15] A 46% rate of graft failure at 1 month as compared with the 11% rate for ABO-compatible organs has been reported.[15] In contrast, the Minnesota group achieved patient and graft survival rates of 76% and 60%, respectively.[16] The Stanford team was the first to suggest that the age of the patient at the time of transplantation may correlate with outcomes of ABO-incompatible combinations.[17] In a series of 2 adolescents and 12 children younger than the age of 3 years, both of the former died compared with just 1 of the latter. Only 1 of the surviving 11 patients required retransplantation for chronic rejection. Patient and graft survival in this cohort was similar to that among recipients of ABO-compatible grafts. There were no cases of hyperacute rejection noted in this study.[17] The use of incompatible grafts has also been seen in living donor liver transplantation.[18] A report from the University of Kyoto demonstrated that patients younger than 1 year of age did well with ABO-incompatible grafts. In contrast, older children receiving ABO-incompatible liver allografts experienced a high incidence of hepatic necrosis, biliary strictures, and graft loss. The 5-year patient survival was 80%, 76%, and 59% for ABO identical, ABO mismatched but compatible, and ABO mismatched incompatible, respectively. According to the age of the patients at the time of transplantation, the 5-year patient survival was 76% for children younger than 1 year of age, 68% for children between the ages of 1 and 8 years, 53% for children between the ages of 8 and 16 years, and only 22% for patients older than 16 years of age.[18] One plausible explanation for these results relates to the very young age of the patients and the possibility that their immature immune systems were more tolerant of the grafts. Furthermore, the Kyoto group demonstrated that young children have very low levels of anti-ABO titers before transplantation.[18] These data indicate that ABO-incompatible donors may be safely used in young children. In contrast, the prognosis is poor in older children, and measures to lower the anti-ABO titers must be implemented to minimize the risk of complications. Such measures may include plasmapheresis and intensive immunosuppression after transplantation. In terms of HLA compatibility, a positive T-cell cross-match has been observed to be associated with a high incidence of acute rejection, increased use of steroids, and graft loss.[19-21] In contrast, a positive B cell cross-match had no clinical significance.[21]

In response to the scarcity of liver allografts in the United States, the Department of Health and Human Services issued a rule that allocation be performed according to medical urgency. The model for end-stage liver disease (MELD) was thus created to prioritize the allocation of livers to adult recipients.[22] A similar method was created for the pediatric patient population (PELD).[23] To calculate the PELD score, the following parameters are entered into a mathematical formula: age (<1 year), growth retardation, and serum albumin, creatinine, and INR concentrations. This model was found to predict mortality (0.92 for death and 0.82 for "death-moved to ICU."[7] A retrospective analysis of the PELD score on patients with biliary atresia was conducted by a group from Yokohama, Japan.[24] PELD, particularly in combination with the Child-Pugh score was found to be a good predictor of patient mortality. However, they also observed that in children with biliary atresia who died before transplantation, PELD was not a predictor of patient mortality. There were other risk factors not included in the mathematical formula, such as acute cholangitis or gastrointestinal variceal bleeding. Further, an analysis of outcomes after liver transplantation in children was also performed by using the Pediatric Risk of Mortality (PRISM) as well as PELD scores.[25] PELD score was associated with the length of stay after transplantation but not with mortality or ICU length of stay. In contrast, PRISM was associated with patient mortality at 1 year, length of ICU stay, and days of ventilatory support in the ICU. PRISM is a score based on the patient's physiological condition, and it is an excellent predictor of the patient's hospital course and mortality.

Table 82-1 shows many factors other than the ones mentioned earlier that may influence the outcome of

Table 82-1. RISK FACTORS SPECIFIC TO THE UNDERLYING DISEASE AMONG INDICATIONS FOR PEDIATRIC LIVER TRANSPLANTATION

Disease	Risk Factors
Cholestatic Liver Disease	
Biliary atresia	Hypoplastic or absent portal vein
	Preduodenal portal vein
	Situs inversus
	Multiple operations in the upper abdomen
	Liver abscess and/or bilomas
Alagille syndrome	Pulmonary hypertension
Metabolic Disorders	
Tyrosinemia	Hepatocellular carcinoma
Cystic fibrosis	*Aspergillus* colonization
	Chronic sinusitis
Neonatal hemochromatosis	Cardiac failure
Wilson's disease	Fulminant liver failure
	Hemolysis
Methylmalonic acidemia	Renal failure
	CNS injury
Crigler-Najjar syndrome, type 1	CNS injury
OTC deficiency	CNS injury
Citrullinemia	CNS injury
Glycogen storage disease	Hepatocellular carcinoma
	Adenomatosis
	CNS injury
Liver Injury	
Acute fulminant hepatitis	Coma stage III/IV
	Abnormal MRI of brain
	Multiple organ system failure
Chronic hepatitis C or B	Hepatocellular carcinoma
Mass-Occupying Lesions	
Hepatoblastoma	Gross vascular invasion
	Metastatic disease
	Previous hepatectomy
Hepatocellular carcinoma	Gross vascular invasion
	Metastatic disease
Giant hemangioendothelioma	Congestive heart failure
	Respiratory distress

CNS, central nervous system; MRI, magnetic resonance imaging; OTC, ornithine transcarbamylase.

surgery yet are not considered in the calculation of risk. Co-existing hepatocellular carcinoma, hypoxia due to hepatopulmonary syndrome, pulmonary hypertension in Alagille syndrome, intrinsic renal disease, and the cytomegalovirus (CMV) status of both the donor and recipient are some examples of such factors. The final recommendation for transplantation candidacy must be based on a careful individual assessment, weighing all the benefits of surgery against all the risks.

Patient Age

In the early days of transplantation, infants had a lower survival rate than that of older children, but advances in the field have narrowed the gap between these two groups.[26-28] In several published series, young age at the time of transplantation was associated with a poor outcome. At Stanford, neither age at the time of transplantation nor weight appears to have any bearing on patient survival.[29] As Figure 82–1A illustrates, the difference between children younger than 6 months of age and older children did not reach statistical significance. Conversely, as Figure 82–1B illustrates, graft survival was compromised in children younger than 6 months of age and the difference compared with older children was statistically significant. Furthermore, in a retrospective analysis, the experience of three large pediatric transplant programs (University of California, Los Angeles [UCLA], University of Chicago, and Stanford) demonstrated that the 1- and 2-year actuarial patient survival in children younger than the age of 3 months at the time of transplantation was 60% for both, and the 1- and 2-year actuarial graft survival for this cohort of patients was 60% and 42%, respectively.[30] Several factors may be responsible for this improvement, but perhaps the most important may be the reduced incidence of hepatic artery thrombosis. Thrombosis used to occur at a rate as high as 40%, making it the most common cause of graft failure and a significant contributing factor in patient death.[11,31] However, today its rate has dropped to less than 10% as a result of improvements in the surgical technique including the use of microsurgery techniques, postoperative thrombosis prophylaxis with antiplatelet agents or other anticoagulants, better methods of organ procurement and transplantation, better immunosuppression, and the more frequent use of segmental transplantation from live or deceased donors.[4,5,11,32]

Diagnosis

Cholestatic Liver Disease

Secondary biliary cirrhosis resulting from extrahepatic biliary atresia is the most common indication for liver

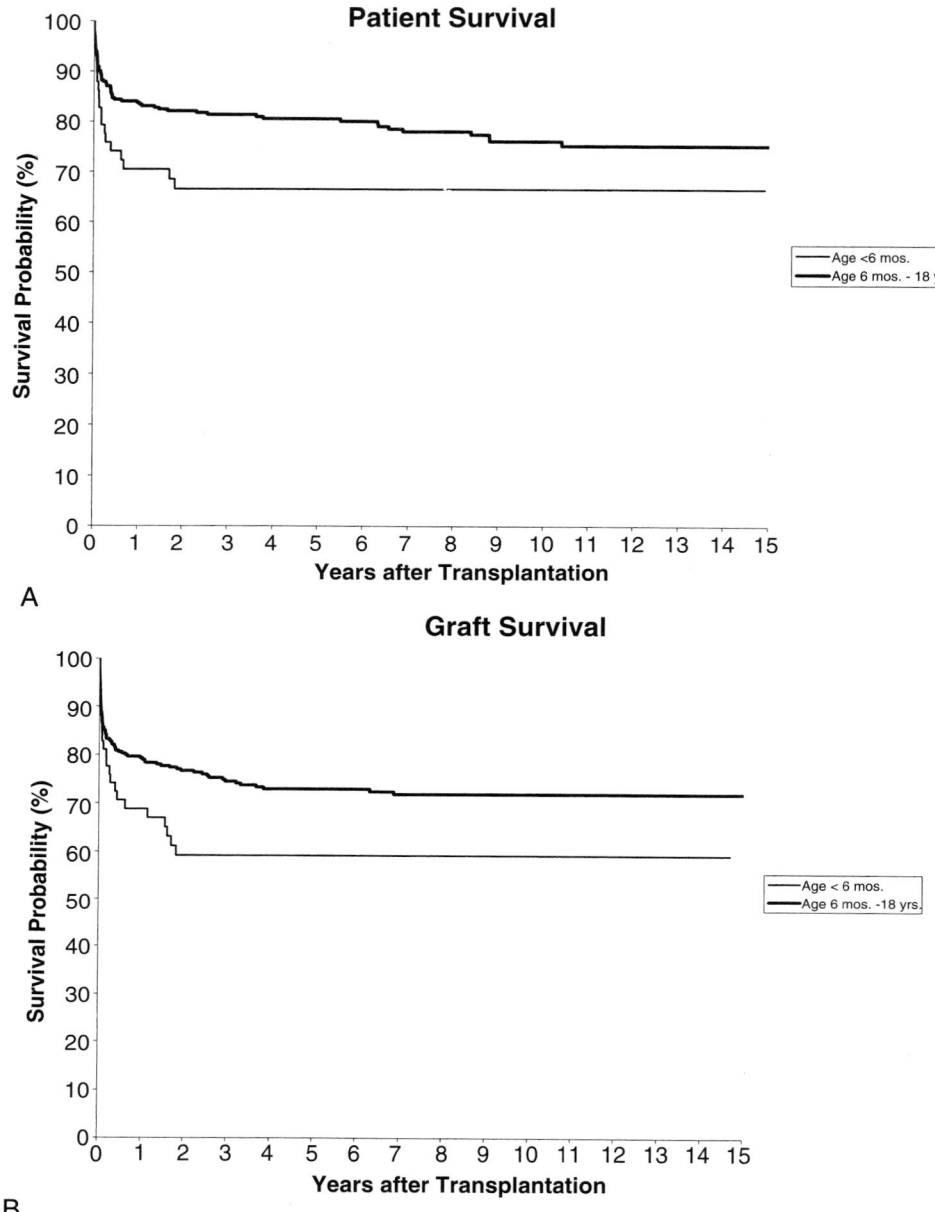

Patient Survival

Graft Survival

A

B

FIGURE 82-1

A, Actuarial patient survival in pediatric liver transplant recipients at Lucile Salter Packard Children's Hospital at Stanford. The difference in patient survival did not reach statistical significance ($P = .0656$). **B,** The actuarial graft survival; the difference between the two age groups did reach statistical significance ($P = .0477$).

transplantation in children, with metabolic disease being a distant second.[33] However, underlying liver disease has little if any effect on patient and graft survival. Children with biliary atresia once had the poorest results but now enjoy survival rates that do not differ statistically from children with metabolic disorders.[34-37] Figure 82–2 illustrates the results of a comparison of the patient and graft survival for biliary atresia with metabolic disorders at my institution. Morbidity in children with biliary atresia is significant, but it is similar to that of children who have undergone transplantation for other indications. This morbidity is caused by the young age of these patients, many of whom have been subjected to several operations before transplantation.[9,10,33-37]

Previous operation in the upper right quadrant is associated with significant morbidity after liver transplantation. The hepatectomy may be a formidable task in some of the children—especially those who have had multiple revisions of the portoenterostomy. Portoenterostomy is indicated in patients with biliary atresia because it may provide some of these children with temporary relief from the effects of the disease, allowing them to grow and become better surgical candidates for liver transplantation if they need it later on.[35,36] However, if the portoenterostomy fails, revision should not be attempted, as it is usually unsuccessful and may jeopardize a future transplant. Instead, the patient should be referred to a transplant center for evaluation.

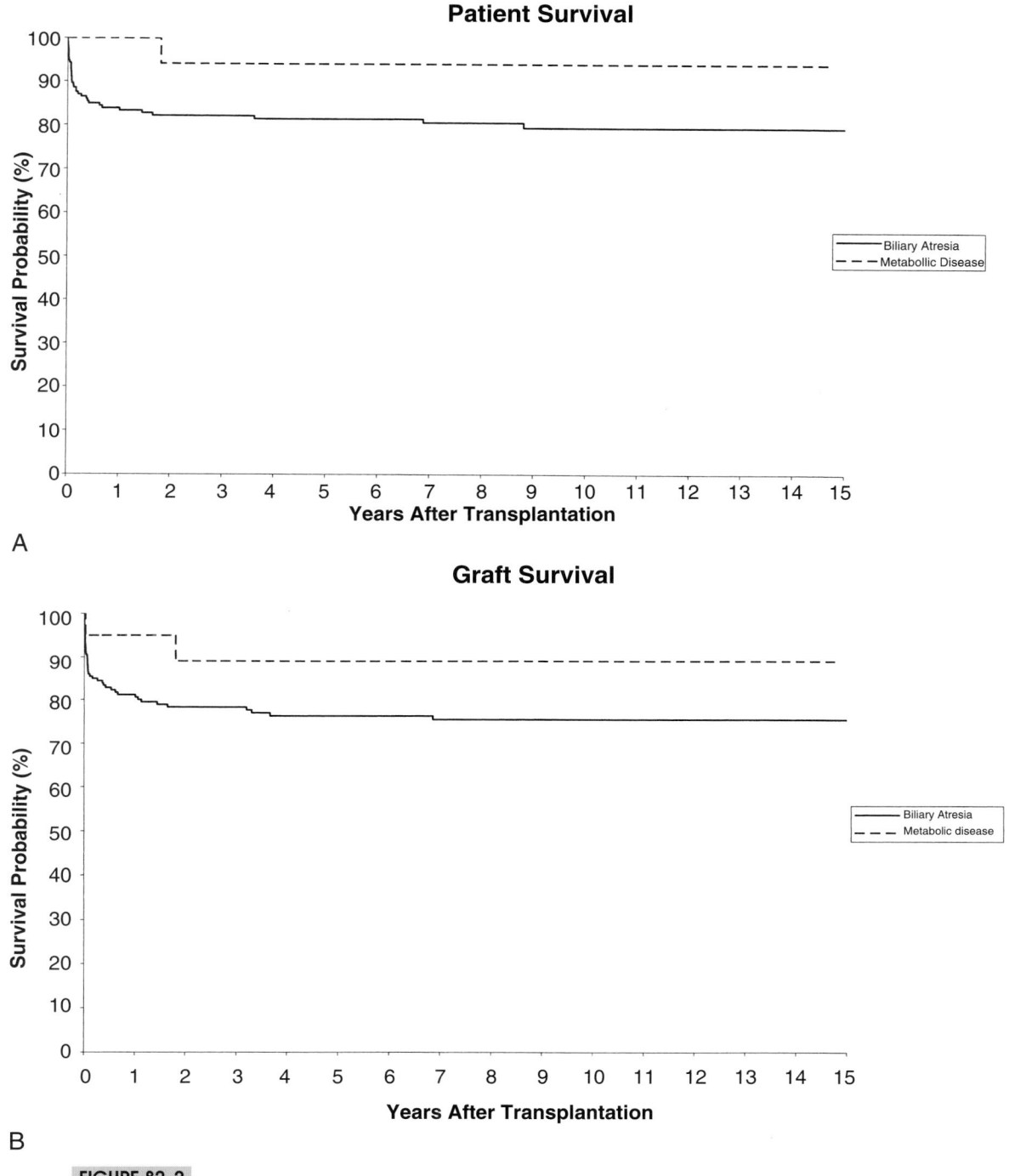

FIGURE 82–2

A, Comparison of actuarial patient survival of liver transplantation for biliary atresia and metabolic disorders. The difference was not significant ($P = .1301$). **B,** The actuarial graft survival; the difference between the two indications was not statistically significant ($P = .1980$).

Another approach still under scrutiny is to perform a percutaneous or laparoscopic liver biopsy in a child suspected of having biliary atresia. If the biopsy shows severe fibrosis with bridging and a nodular architecture, the portoenterostomy procedure is aborted and the patient is referred for liver transplantation because the outcome with portoenterostomy is expected to be dismal. In a retrospective study of 30 children with biliary atresia and severe hepatic fibrosis at the time of the portoenterostomy, the overall survival was 18% at 2 years and 0% at 10 years. This approach would avoid unnecessary surgery in some patients with biliary atresia.[38]

The polysplenia syndrome is a variant of biliary atresia associated with multiple spleens, preduodenal portal vein, intestinal malrotation, and absence of the vena cava. There are also variations within this syndrome. Affected children appear to have a high complication rate after liver transplantation. The hepatectomy is usually easier, since the vena cava is absent, but the reconstruction of the preduodenal vein may pose a technical challenge. Some of these patients also have situs inversus. In our experience and that of others, segmental transplants from deceased or living donors is an excellent solution to the spatial problems associated with situs inversus.[39,40]

Patients with Alagille syndrome are also reported to have a poorer rate of survival because of their propensity for severe peripheral pulmonic stenosis and associated pulmonary hypertension.[41] However, awareness of this complication and proper perioperative management can ensure a successful outcome. Five children have undergone transplantation for this problem at my institution, and all are alive and doing well.

Metabolic Disorders

Hepatic replacement is a good therapeutic option for children with certain metabolic disorders based in the liver. These metabolic disorders fall into two categories: first, those associated with liver injury resulting in acute or chronic liver failure and second, those diseases not associated with intrinsic liver disease but a metabolic defect that results in injury of other organs. A significant phenomenon is the recipient's conversion to the donor phenotype after undergoing transplantation for an inborn error of metabolism based in the liver (e.g., tyrosinemia, α_1-antitrypsin deficiency, and type 1 hyperoxaluria, among others); this represents an actual correction of the metabolic defect.[42-44] The timing of transplantation is critical to ensure good outcomes. Living donor liver transplantation has been used effectively for the treatment of several metabolic disorders based in the liver.[45-51]

Mass-Occupying Lesions

Liver replacement for primary hepatic malignancy is an infrequent indication for liver transplantation in children. Nevertheless, hepatoblastomas account for 75% of the malignant tumors of the liver. In the series reported by Koneru and colleagues,[52] the 2-year patient survival was 58%; those individuals who had undergone previous hepatic resection or laparotomy appeared to have a poorer prognosis, suggesting either that tumor seeding may influence the outcome or perhaps that these tumors had "more malignant behavior." Furthermore, the International Society of Pediatric Oncology (SIOP)

conducted a prospective study in which liver transplantation was a therapeutic option for patients with unresectable tumors (primary liver transplantation) or for those who experienced recurrence after resection.[53] The protocol consisted of four to six courses of chemotherapy followed by resection or transplantation. A total of 12 children (7 primary and 5 rescue liver transplantations) underwent transplantation. The overall patient survival of these 12 children was 75% and 66% at 5 and 10 years, respectively. More importantly, the patient survival was 85.7% among children who underwent primary liver transplantation and 40% among children who underwent rescue transplantation. The same authors performed an analysis of the world experience and observed that the overall survival at 6 years after primary liver transplantation was 82%, and 30% for rescue liver transplantation. The authors also noted that children who present with pulmonary metastases may become suitable candidates for liver transplantation if the metastatic lesions clear with chemotherapy. An important observation in the SIOP and world experience was that for patients whose liver tumors cannot be adequately resected (i.e., close to the tumor margins), liver transplantation may be the treatment of choice.[53]

A small hepatocellular carcinoma is occasionally found in the explanted liver of a child who has undergone liver transplantation for other indications, but recurrence of malignancy rarely occurs in such cases, and a successful outcome can usually be expected.[54] It should be emphasized that several hepatic disorders that may result in ongoing cellular damage may lead to hepatocellular carcinoma (Table 82–2). Epithelioid hemangioendothelioma is an infrequent indication for

Table 82–2. HEPATIC DISORDERS ASSOCIATED WITH HEPATOCELLULAR CARCINOMA IN CHILDREN

Metabolic Disease
Hereditary tyrosinemia
α_1-Antitrypsin deficiency
Glycogen storage disease, types I, III, and IV
Chronic Active Hepatitis; Cirrhosis
Hepatitis B infection
Hepatitis C infection
Cholestatic Liver Disease
Alagille syndrome
Familial cholestatic cirrhosis (Byler's disease)
Biliary atresia
Parenteral nutrition
Other
Congenital hepatic fibrosis
Neonatal iron storage disease
Fanconi anemia (androgen-treated)

hepatic transplantation in children. These patients may present with respiratory failure from pulmonary restriction secondary to the large liver tumors impinging on the diaphragm. In more advanced cases, these children develop congestive heart failure. Transplantation is a life-saving treatment and the prognosis is excellent.[55]

Injury to the Liver

Hepatitis B is a rare indication for liver transplantation in children.[33] As in adults, the patient's prognosis depends on their infectivity at the time of transplantation. Recurrence of hepatitis B may be prevented by the long-term administration of hepatitis B immunoglobulin accompanied by antiviral drugs. Hepatitis C is also an infrequent indication for liver transplantation in children.[56-58] The course of the disease, including recurrence and subsequent liver failure, follows the same characteristics as in adult patients infected with hepatitis C virus. The experience with the use of interferon and ribavirin in children is almost nonexistent. The UCLA team treated with interferon-2α 12 children with de novo hepatitis C after transplantation. A disappointing 15% response rate was observed.[58]

Aside from hepatitis B, malignancy, and hepatitis C, very few of the liver diseases treated by hepatic transplantation have the potential to recur in the allograft. There have been several reports of recurrence of autoimmune hepatitis, and there has been one case of recurrence of blue sea histiocytosis.[59,60] Several children with cystic fibrosis have undergone successful hepatic transplantation, and recurrence of the liver disease has been observed in none.[61] Among frequent indications for liver transplantation in children, several potential risk factors linked to the underlying liver disease may influence the outcomes after hepatic replacement as shown in Table 82–3.

Immunosuppression

Significant progress has been made in the immunosuppressive management of pediatric patients following

Table 82–3. INDICATIONS FOR RETRANSPLANTATION AT LUCILE SALTER PACKARD CHILDREN'S HOSPITAL

Indication	No. Patients	%
Rejection	12	23
Vascular complications	17	33
Primary graft nonfunction	10	19
Recurrent disease	7	13
Miscellaneous	6	12
Total	52	100

hepatic transplantation, as shown in Figure 82–3. The main goal of new immunosuppressive regimens has been the elimination of steroids because of their devastating side effects, particularly in children, or the complete withdrawal of immunosuppression.[62-65] The ultimate goal is to achieve tolerance, and efforts are being made to reach this goal.[66] Cyclosporine was responsible for bringing transplantation from the dark ages into the limelight. Many programs continue to use cyclosporine as the main drug for maintenance of immunosuppression, but tacrolimus is a newer agent that has been demonstrated to be a good alternative for maintenance of immunosuppression in pediatric liver transplantation. In terms of patient and graft survival, U.S. and European trials comparing tacrolimus and cyclosporine did not show any significant difference between the two.[67,68] However, the profile of side effects was somewhat different. Tacrolimus is associated with a much lower incidence of hypertension (33%) compared with cyclosporine (66%). Other side effects observed with cyclosporine but not with tacrolimus were hirsutism and gingival hyperplasia.[67] These advantages over cyclosporine are particularly important in the management of pediatric transplant patients, particularly when children reach school age or when they become more interested in their own body image.[69] In individual center studies comparing cyclosporine with tacrolimus in pediatric liver transplantation, tacrolimus immunosuppression was associated with improved patient and graft survival and lower rates of acute rejection, steroid resistant rejection, and retransplantation. However, in many of these studies, cyclosporine was given in the conventional formula preparation. In more recent studies using microemulsion (better absorption), no difference was demonstrated in the incidence of acute or chronic rejection between the two drugs. Neurotoxicity, nephrotoxicity, and resistance to insulin are side effects observed with both drugs.[70-75] Tacrolimus is also associated with food allergies, including angioedema.[76,77] The incidence of this complication is about 10%, and conversion to cyclosporine is often needed in affected patients. Another problem unique to pediatric patients—especially small children—is the difficulty in achieving therapeutic levels of cyclosporine or tacrolimus. This difficulty results from either rapid metabolism of the drug or poor absorption, or both.[78,79] On the basis of surface area, children often need higher doses of tacrolimus than adult patients do, and this may be the result of rapid metabolism of the drug and not absorption problems. Measures to increase blood levels of these drugs such as the concomitant administration of fluconazole, diltiazem, and vitamin E have met with some success.[80-82]

Several steroid-sparing protocols are under investigation. Some of these protocols include the use of monoclonal antibodies (e.g., anti-interleukin-2) or polyclonal

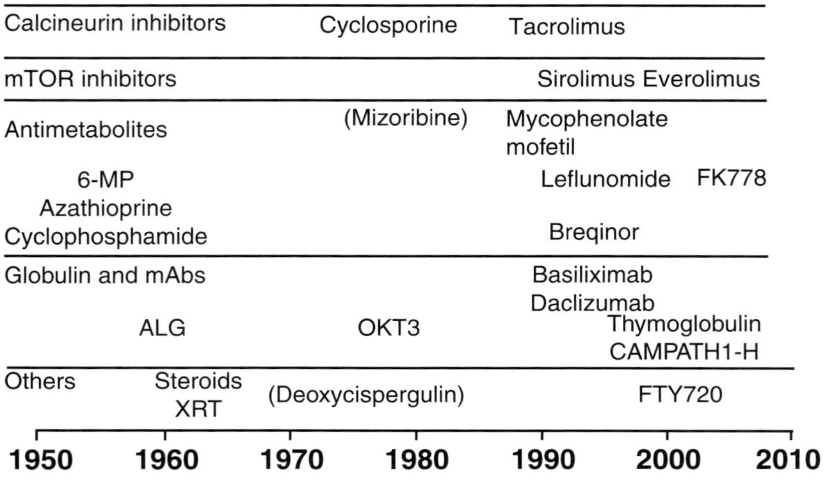

Calcineurin inhibitors	Cyclosporine	Tacrolimus	
mTOR inhibitors			Sirolimus Everolimus
Antimetabolites		(Mizoribine)	Mycophenolate mofetil
6-MP Azathioprine Cyclophosphamide			Leflunomide FK778 Breqinor
Globulin and mAbs			Basiliximab Daclizumab
	ALG	OKT3	Thymoglobulin CAMPATH1-H
Others	Steroids XRT	(Deoxycispergulin)	FTY720

1950   1960   1970   1980   1990   2000   2010

FIGURE 82–3

The last 2 decades have been a period of many advances in the understanding of the mechanisms of rejection in solid organ transplantation resulting in the discovery of new immunosuppressive agents (From Furukawa H, Todo S: Evolution of immunosuppression in liver transplantation: Contribution of cyclosporine. Transplant Proc 36:S274-S284, 2004.)

antibodies (antithymocyte globulin).[83-86] In addition, these protocols may include a second drug for maintenance such as mycophenolate mofetil (MMF) or sirolimus.[87,88]

A prospective study to wean patients from immunosuppression after liver transplantation demonstrated that in one of five patients, immunosuppression was successfully discontinued, but 20% of the patients experienced rejection following discontinuation of the medications and the remaining patients were still in the middle of the weaning program.[65] A similar study was also carried out in living donor liver transplantation. Twenty-four (38.1%) of 65 patients were successfully weaned from immunosuppression with a median drug-free period of 23.5 months. Sixteen patients (25.4%) required the reinitiation of immunosuppression because of onset of acute rejection. The remaining patients were still in the weaning process at the time of preparation of this chapter.[63]

The preferred immunosuppressive protocol at Stanford consists of tacrolimus monotherapy. Eighty percent of our pediatric patients are successfully weaned from steroids by the end of the first year after transplantation. Proponents of double or triple drug therapy claim that the addition of MMF or sirolimus provides more intense immunosuppression without increasing the rate of infection.[87] These drugs may be used to spare the use of steroids and to reduce the dosage of calcineurin inhibitors with the goal of protecting renal function. Patients who experience frequent episodes of rejection may also benefit from the more intense immunosuppression resulting from the addition of MMF or sirolimus, but most of this experience comes from trials in adult patients. Azathioprine, a nonselective immunosuppressant, is quickly falling out of favor because of its toxicity on the bone marrow, pancreas, and liver. The administration of the monoclonal interleukin-2 inhibitors, antithymocyte globulin (ATG),

or the polyclonal OKT3 as induction therapy has been reported to be of benefit in pediatric liver transplantation.[83-86] The goal of this type of induction therapy is to provide effective immunosuppression without calcineurin inhibitors during the initial postoperative period.[83] Patients with postoperative acute tubular necrosis or resolving hepatorenal syndrome benefit most from this measure, as it allows the recovery of kidney function.

Allograft Size

Reduced-Size Liver Transplantation

The shortage of small donors in pediatric liver transplantation is a significant problem that surgeons have attempted to alleviate by using segments or lobes from living or deceased donors.[89-92] Reduced-size liver transplantation, first reported by Bismuth and Houssin in 1984, was initially used only in emergency transplantation.[89] In this setting, it achieved surprisingly high patient survival rates of 44% to 50%, encouraging its use in more elective cases.[93] As a result of its more liberal application, the patient survival rate rose to more than 80%, matching that for full-size liver transplantation.[93-99] In my experience, infants benefit most from this procedure. Survival of reduced-size grafts was significantly better than that of full-size grafts in this pediatric subpopulation.[28] Early in its development, graft ischemia and vascular occlusion were among the most frequent complications. Equally problematic if not more so was size disparity, but this could be remedied by performing a more extensive resection to ensure a donor-to-recipient weight ratio of no more than 5:1.[99] Bleeding, bilomas, and portal vein thrombosis were complications related to the procedure itself, which was associated with an increased number of reoperations. Conversely, this technique expanded the size of the donor pool for small pediatric recipients, thereby decreasing the mortality rate on waiting lists and the rate of hepatic artery thrombosis.[28,89] To date, the incidence of infection and rejection for this procedure is similar to those for full-size liver transplantation.[28] Further, hepatic monosegments have been reported to be successful in transplantation in newborns, with a reported patient survival of 80% at 1 year.[100] The problem with monosegmental transplantation is a 20% incidence of hepatic artery thrombosis.[100]

Reduced-size liver transplantation addressed the shortage of donor organs for children by drawing from the pool of donors for the older patient population. Thus, it failed to relieve the donor shortage overall, but it laid the groundwork for other innovative modalities such as split-liver transplantation and living-related transplantation (see Chapters 41 and 42).

Split-Liver Transplantation

In split-liver transplantation, the liver is divided into two portions for transplantation into two recipients.[101] The technique for division of the liver parenchyma may be carried out ex situ or in situ.[102,103] Initially, the procedure was performed ex situ (back-table split), but the outcome of the transplant was often compromised by biliary leaks, vascular thrombosis, and graft ischemia, the complications being caused by anatomic variation in most instances.[104] The rates of patient and graft survival were discouragingly poor, the retransplantation rate was high, and some began to question the virtue of the procedure at all.[105] Houssin and others reported having achieved satisfactory results with this procedure by radiographically visualizing the biliary tree and hepatic artery of the liver allograft before dividing the parenchyma.[106] According to these authors, visualization allows anomalies to be diagnosed so that appropriate steps may be taken to avoid compromising the segments to be transplanted when dividing the liver. They reported immediate patient and graft survival rates of 75% and 67%, respectively, but with significant morbidity and a 25% incidence of hepatic artery thrombosis.[106] In response to the increased morbidity observed with the ex situ technique, Broelsch and collaborators introduced the concept of in situ splitting of the liver.[104] Proponents of this technique claim to obtain better grafts by proper identification of vascular and biliary tract anomalies in the hepatic hilum, improved hemostasis after reperfusion by meticulous ligation of vessels and bile ducts on the raw surface during the partitioning of the liver, and shorter preservation time. Conversely, the in situ technique has the drawback of lengthening the donor operation, which may render the donor unstable and may create logistical problems in small community hospitals.

The outcomes of split-liver transplantation differ greatly depending on factors such as the quality of the donor (and possibly age as well), the medical urgency of the recipient, and the expertise of the surgical team. By using a modified ex situ technique, the group from Birmingham, United Kingdom reported a 1-year graft survival of 78% and vascular complications of 3.3% compared with their historical controls of 59% graft survival at 1 year and 20% vascular complication rate.[102] The results of pediatric recipients of ex situ split liver transplantation reported by Deshpande and coauthors from London, showed an actuarial patient survival of 93.5% and 88.1% at 1 and 3 years, respectively. The actuarial graft survival at 1 and 3 years was 89.7% and 86.1%, respectively.[107] The vascular complication rate was 7.5% and the biliary complication rate was 8.7%.[107] UCLA recently reported its experience with 100 split livers that yielded 165 grafts used at its own institution and 25 other grafts allocated to other centers in the United States.[108] Of recipients of the 165 grafts used at UCLA, 105 were recipients of the left lateral segment (LLS). Of these, 33 grafts failed (20%)—15 within 1 week of transplantation. Although compared with their own experience with living donor liver transplantation and whole-liver transplantation, the graft survival was not statistically significant, and it is of concern that the actuarial graft survival at 1 and 3 years for the split LLS was 68% and 64%, respectively. For the split-extended right lobe the 1 year graft survival was 69%.[108] These outcomes were discouraging considering that the average donor age was 20.9 ± 8.2 years and that the donor was free from other risk factors. The European experience with split-liver transplantation revealed a 20% retransplantation rate with split livers compared with 10% with other types of transplants.[103] Support for the concept of split-liver transplantation does exist, but outcomes must improve before transplant teams will fully embrace this type of procedure. In a survey of the U.S. experience with split-liver transplantation, only 45% of 83 teams that responded to the survey had experience with split-liver transplantation and of these, two thirds had performed fewer than five procedures.[109] Further, the share of split grafts among centers in this analysis was only 4%.[109]

Even if it is associated with greater morbidity, split-liver transplantation may be the most effective means of expanding the donor pool provided that it can achieve the same rate of patient survival as that for full-size liver transplantation. The most recent reports by individual centers are encouraging, as they indicate progress toward that goal.

Living-Related Transplantation

The concept of living-related liver transplantation was derived from the experience with reduced-size organ transplantation. As in the latter technique, a portion of a liver is used for grafting; however, it is taken from a living rather than a deceased donor.[90,91] Initially, hepatic artery thrombosis was the most common technical complication, but this problem could almost always be resolved by using meticulous microsurgical techniques or by placing an interposition vascular graft from the supraceliac aorta.[32,110-112] Minimal morbidity has been observed among the living donors of left lateral segments, but this does not mean that the procedure is without the risk of serious complications, such as injury to the common bile duct, bleeding requiring the transfusion of nonautologous blood, infections, reoperations, and death.[93,113,114]

The outcomes in pediatric recipients of living donor liver transplants are excellent. The actuarial patient survival at 1 year at my institution is 90% with very little attrition thereafter. Similar results have been reported by other centers throughout the world[115-119] The outcomes in children are superior to those noted among adult recipients of living donor liver transplants.[120] Morbidity in living donor liver transplantation (LDLT) such as vascular and biliary tract complications occur significantly less often in pediatric than in adult recipients.[121-123] The most common indication in living donor pediatric recipients is biliary atresia. However, LDLT has been used successfully for the treatment of several metabolic disorders such as Wilson's disease, tyrosinemia, familial cholesterolemia, ornithine transcarbamylase (OTC) deficiency, propionic acidemia and α_1-antitrypsin deficiency, Crigler-Najjar syndrome type 1, and citrullinemia.[45-49] In many of these cases, the donor was a heterozygous parent and a good outcome was the norm. Other unusual diagnostic indications for LDLT in children are Alagille syndrome, fulminant hepatic failure, and retransplantation.[124-128] Retransplantation with living donor liver has taken place mostly in Asia, where the only opportunity for an urgent transplant is a living donor, since transplantation with organs from deceased donors is not fully accepted by the public.[129] Fulminant hepatic failure and ICU-bound patients in multiorgan system failure were not considered suitable candidates for LDLT in the past. Today, these conditions are moving into the mainstream because of the outstanding results with LDLT in such difficult circumstances.[125,126]

Split-liver and living-related transplantation as well as using organs across the ABO barrier have almost solved the organ shortage problem in pediatric liver transplantation. The mortality rate of small pediatric patients on waiting lists is less than 1%. Living donor liver transplantation has benefited infants most, achieving excellent rates of patient and graft survival (Fig. 82–4). In contrast, graft survival in split-liver transplantation is significantly lower than that of LDLT and full-size liver transplantation, particularly in small children.

To maximize its potential, this procedure should be performed only by teams with experience in liver resection and transplantation in small children (see Chapter 41). An unexpected problem that has been encountered at my institution is the difficulty of finding suitable living donors. Many are unwilling to participate because of concern for their own safety, and almost two thirds of those who do volunteer have been excluded because of anatomic anomalies, intrinsic hepatic disease, or psychosocial contraindications.

Retransplantation

The retransplantation rate in whole-liver transplantation averages 10%, and the most common indications at my institution are listed in Table 82–3. Rejection used to account for one half of all pediatric retransplantations, but it has become a less frequent and serious problem since the introduction of new and potent immunosuppressive drugs.[3,72,73,127,128] Retransplantation for rejection is usually an elective procedure. It has a 2-year patient survival rate of 60% to 70%—a fairly good prognosis that can be attributed to the patient's relatively stable medical condition at the time of operation. The 2-year patient survival rate following retransplantation for hepatic artery thrombosis—the most common technical complication for which retransplantation is performed—is approximately 50%.[31,129] The cause of death in such cases is usually sepsis. Primary graft nonfunction is associated with the poorest prognosis of all, with a 1-year patient survival rate of approximately 20%.[130] The incidence of primary graft nonfunction is rising because of more liberal use of split livers as well as the use of organs from donors based on extended donor criteria. Affected patients deteriorate so quickly that they are often moribund at the time of retransplantation. Recurrence of the underlying liver disease is seldom an indication for retransplantation in children.

Although retransplantation improves the rate of patient survival among transplant recipients overall, an individual patient's chances of survival decline with the number of retransplantations; the likelihood of survival declines by about 20% after the first retransplantation (Fig. 82–5), and the gap widens with each successive attempt. Currently, the incidence of retransplantation in children varies between 0% and 20%, depending on the medical urgency, the diagnostic indication for retransplantation, the size of the allograft, and donor availability.[30,37,108,109] In Japan, for example, retransplantation is almost impossible because of the shortage of deceased donors. In such circumstances, LDLT may be the only option. In a recent report from the University of Kyoto, the retransplantation rate was 4%.[129] The indications for transplantation were chronic rejection (35.7%), chronic cholangitis (21.4%), and

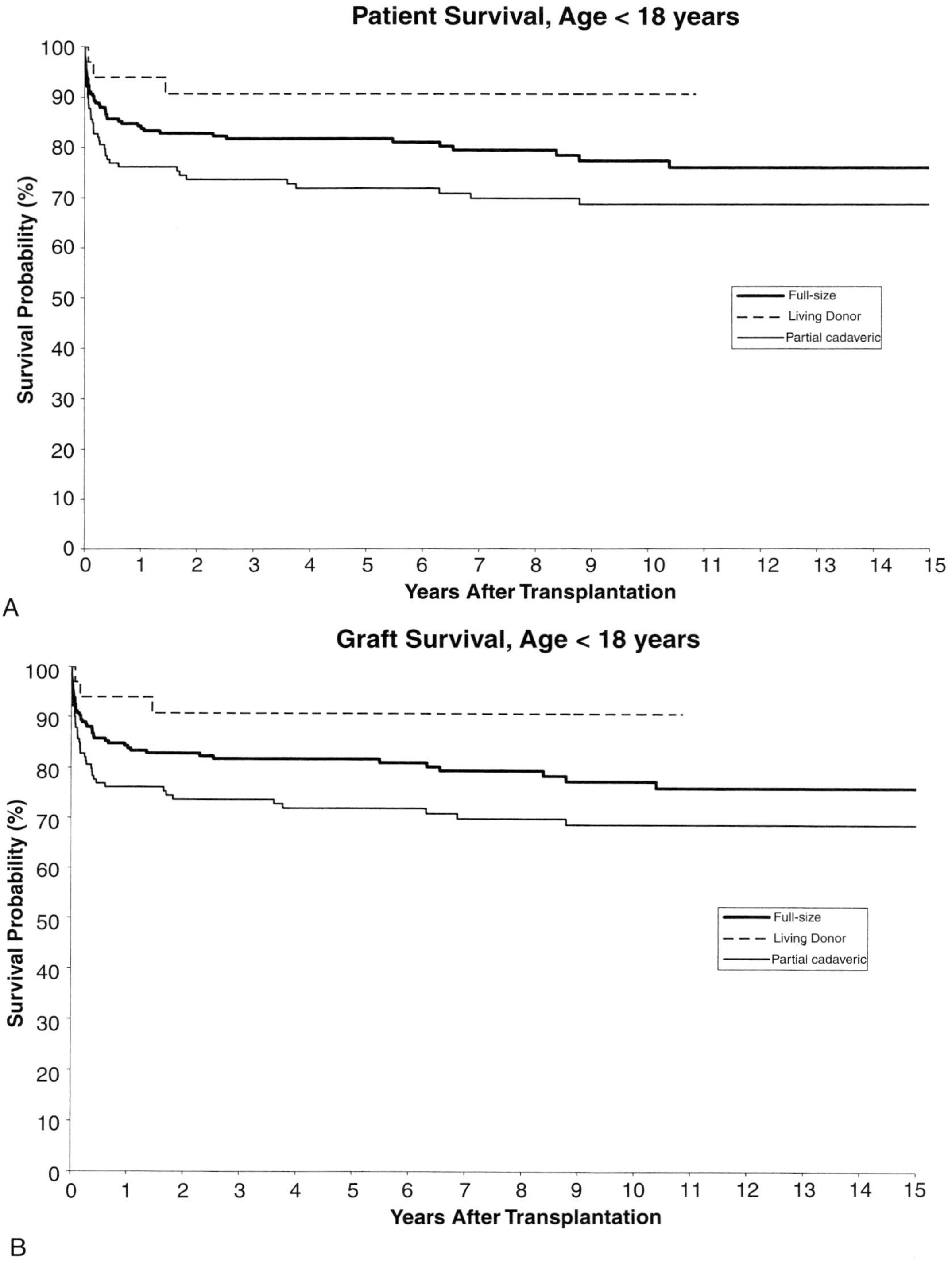

FIGURE 82–4

This figure shows a comparison of actuarial patient (**A**) and graft (**B**) survival of full-size liver transplantation compared with segmental liver transplantation from live and deceased donors at Lucile Salter Packard Children's Hospital at Stanford. The only statistically significant difference was between segmental living donor transplantation and segmental deceased donor transplantation ($P = .0268$).

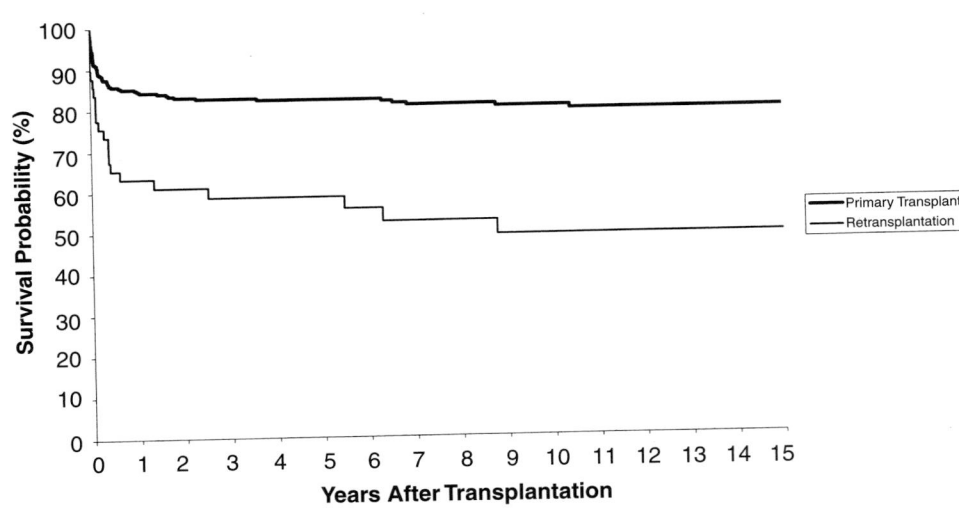

Patient Survival, Primary Transplant vs. Retransplantation

A

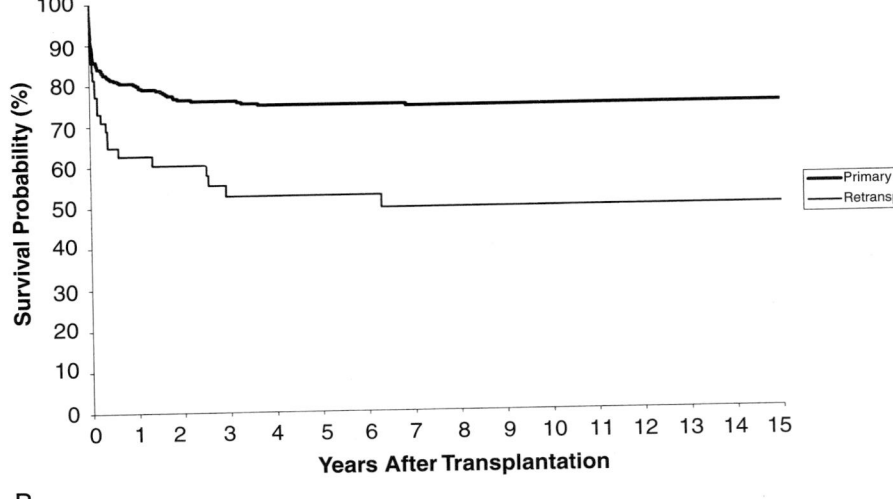

Graft Survival, Primary Transplant vs. Retransplantation

B

FIGURE 82-5
A, Actuarial patient survival associated with primary liver transplantation and retransplantation in children at Lucile Salter Packard Children's Hospital. The difference was highly significant ($P < .0001$). **B,** Depicts the actuarial graft survival and the difference was also significant ($P = .0007$).

vascular complications (25%). Of all these indications, vascular complications were associated with the worst prognosis after living donor liver retransplantation.[129] The patient survival were primary LDLT was 82.7%, 82.1%, and 80.6%, at 1, 3, and 5 years, respectively. In contrast, the patient survival after living donor liver retransplantation was 47.6% at 1 year and remained unchanged at 5 years.[129]

Combination Liver Transplantation

Certain medical conditions may require the need for combination transplants (Table 82–4). A simultaneous

liver and kidney transplantation is the most common multiorgan transplant procedure performed in children. Primary hyperoxaluria is a metabolic disorder based in the liver. Children with this disease have normal liver function; however, they develop complications from the deposition of oxalate crystals in the kidneys, bones, and other organs. Often these children develop renal failure early in life. The treatment of choice is the transplantation of the liver to correct the metabolic defect accompanied by kidney transplantation. At Stanford, a proper timing for transplantation as well as aggressive fluid management during the postoperative period resulted in 100% patient and graft survival.[131] Other indications for combined liver-kidney transplantation are cirrhosis with associated renal disease (e.g., tyrosinemia),

Table 82-4. TRANSPLANTATION OF LIVER WITH OTHER ORGANS IN CHILDREN

	Diagnostic Indications	Outcomes and Comments
Liver-kidney	Primary oxalosis	Excellent prognosis;. fluid challenge very important for elimination of oxalate crystals after transplantation
	Liver failure and intrinsic renal disease	Often in the setting of retransplantation accompanied by calcineurin inhibitor–induced toxicity
Liver-intestine	Short gut syndrome and TPN- induced liver failure	Challenging posttransplantation management; patient and graft survival of 75% in experienced hands
Multivisceral	Extensive thrombosis of splanchnic venous system	Infection, rejection, and PTLD occur often and may be life-threatening complications; patient and graft survival of 50% at 1 year
	Familial polyposis and TPN induced liver failure	
Liver-heart-lung	Cystic fibrosis	1-yr actuarial survival of 70%
Liver-lung	Hepatopulmonary syndrome	Bleeding and infection are common complications
Liver-heart	Hypercholesterolemia	Successful outcomes in a few anecdotal reports

PTLD, posttransplantation liver disease; TPN, total parenteral nutrition.

hepatic allograft failure with drug-induced nephrotoxicity, hepatorenal syndrome, and methylmalonic acidemia.[132]

A serious complication of total parenteral nutrition (TPN) in patients with short gut syndrome is the development of liver failure. Once these patients develop liver failure the prognosis is grim, with a life expectancy of less than 1 year. A combined liver-intestine transplant is a life-saving procedure for this type of patient. The 1-year patient and graft survival reported by the International Intestinal Transplant Registry was 50% and 40%, respectively.[133] The outcomes with multivisceral transplantation (stomach, duodenum, small intestine, liver, and pancreas) are definitely worse, with a 1-year patient and graft survival of 40% and 30%, respectively. Further, the concomitant existence of liver failure in intestinal transplantation is a predictor of good outcome. Patients with short gut syndrome should undergo isolated intestinal transplantation at the onset of liver dysfunction. Currently, the expected 1-year patient survival for isolated intestinal transplantation is 80%.[134-136]

Other combination transplants including the liver are rarely performed; they are liver-heart-lung transplantation, liver–double-lung transplantation, and liver-heart transplantation.[137-140] Table 82–4 lists the indications for these types of operations and the outcomes.

Hepatic Dysfunction

Following transplantation, a series of events may take place that can result in hepatic dysfunction (Table 82–5), and these events must be assessed rapidly and managed properly if good results are to be obtained.[141]

Thus, children with hepatic dysfunction undergo a thorough evaluation, which includes radiological studies, liver biopsies, and exploratory laparotomies, when necessary. The most common problems observed in pediatric hepatic transplantation are discussed herein. It is important to remember that these complications may involve any organ system and have the potential to be life-threatening.

Liver biopsies are used to establish rejection, which, if present, should be treated aggressively. An effective immunosuppressive regimen decreases the likelihood of rejection, but it also renders the patient more susceptible to infection.[34-36,142] Such infections are a frequent cause of posttransplantation hepatic dysfunction, and those caused by bacteria account for almost one half of all episodes.[34-36,142,143] Pediatric patients usually

Table 82-5. COMMON CAUSES OF LIVER DYSFUNCTION AFTER HEPATIC TRANSPLANTATION

Medical Causes

Acute or chronic rejection

Recurrence of liver disease

TPN-induced cholestasis

Drug-induced toxicity

Systemic sepsis

Hemolysis

Surgical Causes

Vascular complications

Biliary tract complications

Preservation-reperfusion injury

Small-for-size graft

lack suitable peripheral veins for daily blood withdrawal and drug administration and, therefore, need the kind of prolonged central venous access provided by an indwelling catheter. Understandably, then, catheter sepsis is the most common bacterial infection in this population. Treatment consists of catheter removal and appropriate antibiotic therapy.

Once common, the incidence of viral and fungal infections has decreased considerably because of improved prophylaxis and the judicious use of immunosuppressive therapy. CMV infection must always be ruled out in a child with hepatic dysfunction who has recently been treated with high-dose steroids and monoclonal and polyclonal antibodies.[144,145] The reported incidence of CMV disease varies from 9% to 18%.[144-146] The chances of infection are reduced with the prophylactic administration of ganciclovir, the use of CMV-negative blood products in CMV-negative recipients, and the use of hyperimmune globulin.[144-146]

Epstein-Barr virus hepatitis is uncommon among pediatric liver transplant recipients, having a reported incidence of approximately 1% to 2%, but it should be part of the differential diagnosis of posttransplantation hepatic dysfunction.[147] The clinical findings are variable. Some patients present with fever and shaking chills and quickly develop acute liver failure. In other patients, the infection can be asymptomatic, being discovered only when a liver biopsy specimen is obtained as part of the workup for mild transaminase elevation.[147-149] Treatment consists of withdrawing immunosuppression and administering ganciclovir and CD-20 antibody (rituximab), should the cells be positive for CD-20 on immunohistological evaluation.[150]

Adenoviral hepatitis (type 5) has been observed in pediatric liver transplant recipients but, interestingly, not in adult patients.[151] The histological features of this infection are pathognomonic and consist of "punch out" lesions surrounded by giant cells. Other viruses associated with hepatic dysfunction after liver transplantation include influenza virus types A and B, respiratory syncytial virus, and herpesvirus.

Vascular Complications

As mentioned earlier, hepatic artery thrombosis is a significant cause of morbidity and mortality in pediatric liver transplant recipients.[11,152,153] Three distinct categories of presentation have been observed in these children.[152] In the first, extensive areas of necrosis develop in the liver 7 to 10 days after surgery. These infarctions may liquefy, forming bilomas that become infected as a result of continuity with the jejunal limb of the choledochojejunostomy, and gas-forming gangrene has occasionally been observed. Patients with this problem deteriorate rapidly and die quickly unless

retransplantation is carried out. Patients in the second category develop ischemia of the bile ducts and, eventually, segmental stenosis. In such cases, the hepatic artery thrombosis may have been missed initially, and the patient may present months later with acute cholangitis.[154] Patients in the third category develop necrosis of the extrahepatic biliary system, which leads to a bile leak and peritonitis.[152]

Portal vein thrombosis is seldom observed in liver transplantation with whole organs, but it does occur with deceased or living donor segmental transplantation. When it does occur, the clinical presentation can vary from no overt symptoms to progressive liver failure. If diagnosed early, thrombectomy and portal vein reconstruction may salvage the graft. Stenosis of the portal vein anastomosis, which results in portal hypertension and hypersplenism, has also been remedied by revision of the anastomosis or percutaneous transhepatic balloon dilation of the stenosis. In some patients stenting the stenosis may be necessary.[155,156]

Biliary Tract Complications

Bile duct complications should be part of the differential diagnosis if the patient develops graft dysfunction.[121,157,158] The presence of a bile leak or intrahepatic strictures of the biliary system strongly suggest hepatic artery thrombosis, and proper steps should be taken to rule out bile duct complications. An anastomotic stricture may be treated with balloon dilation or surgical revision. A much greater problem is posed by intrahepatic strictures. A recent report suggests that surgery to remove the extrahepatic biliary system and create a portoenterostomy may provide adequate biliary drainage.[154] Ursodeoxycholic acid has been used in some patients, but its efficacy has yet to be demonstrated. Retransplantation is the definitive treatment for these patients.

Hepatic dysfunction as a result of primary graft nonfunction occurs immediately after transplantation but varies in presentation with the extent of preservation injury. Likewise, it has been suggested that there is a high incidence of rejection among patients who have received grafts with significant harvesting injury.[159] When rejection and technical complications have been ruled out, other causes of liver dysfunction, such as hemolysis and drug-induced hepatitis, should be suspected.[141]

Quality of Life After Transplantation

Now that more than 80% of these children can expect to survive, more attention is being paid to the patient's quality of life. Stewart and coworkers[160] compared intellectual and motor function, social competence, and growth in 29 children before and 1 year after liver transplantation. Motor and mental functioning for the series as a whole was no different 1 year after operation, but approximately 40% to 50% of the children whose motor and mental functioning was delayed before transplantation moved into the normal range after surgery. These changes were not statistically significant, however. Those children whose mental or motor functioning was delayed were more likely to have developed liver disease early on (during the first year of life) compared with children who had late-onset disease. Early onset of liver disease thus appeared to have a pernicious effect on intellectual function. All of the children experienced a significant improvement in social competence after liver replacement. Body weight, head circumference, and anthropometrics improved as well, but not the linear growth rate. This study clearly illustrates the detrimental effect of corticosteroids.[160] In a different study of 27 children who had undergone liver transplantation for biliary atresia—vitamin E deficiency, serum albumin, serum bilirubin, and patient height and weight were factors implicated in the poor developmental outcome observed in some.[161]

A study of mental and motor development of 25 young recipients of liver transplants was carried out at my institution.[162] These children, who were scheduled to undergo liver replacement before the age of 3 years, were evaluated before transplantation and at 3 and 12 months after transplantation. The average age at the time of transplantation was 12.5 months (range, 1 to 36 months), and the indication for surgery in each case was end-stage liver disease secondary to extrahepatic biliary atresia. Psychomotor development was measured on the Spence-Wayman Quality of Movement Scales, and mental development was evaluated on the Bayley Scales of Infant Development. At 3 months after transplantation, 7 of the children were considered normally developed, with the scores on both scales being above 85; 13 of the children were in the "suspect" range, with one score below 85 and the other score above 85; and 5 children were rated as being abnormally developed, with both scores being below 85. At 12 months, the children had regained their pretransplantation level of mental development, attaining near-average scores on the Bayley Scales. Their psychomotor developmental level was similar to what it was before transplantation, but it was still 1 standard deviation below the norm. Serum albumin and length of hospital stay appeared to be most closely associated with developmental outcome at 12 months.[162]

An interesting study was a comparison of the quality of life of liver transplant recipients with children with cystic fibrosis, a chronic disease.[163] Twenty-eight pediatric liver transplant recipients (age range, 4 to 18 years) were evaluated 1 year after operation and compared with 18 patients with cystic fibrosis to study the effect of chronic illness. The liver transplant recipients had lower academic achievement; lower scores on nonverbal intelligence tests; lower scores on tests evaluating abstract concept formation, learning, and memory; and poorer visual, spatial, and motor skills. The two groups scored no differently on tests that assess alertness and motor function, perceptual motor function, and sensory-perceptual function. However, on tests that measure intellectual and academic function, the liver transplant recipients scored lower on nearly every variable, including performance IQ, reading, spelling, and arithmetic; verbal IQ was the only measure on which the groups performed at the same level. Their social skills were comparable to those of the children with cystic fibrosis, as they performed equally well in group situations. Six of the 24 school-age children in the liver transplant group and 1 of the 14 children with cystic fibrosis were in special education programs. The difference in school placement was not statistically significant. However, the numbers are misleading, as 12 additional transplant recipients would have been candidates for special education had discrepancy between IQ and academic standard been used as the criterion for placement. The implication of these numbers is that liver transplant recipients are expected to perform at a lower level. This study suggests that children with end-stage liver disease are alert and able to concentrate but have problems related to abstract thinking and logical analysis. Thus, they may have unrecognized neuropsychological deficits and, for that reason, should always be evaluated for their need to participate in educational programs that will maximize their potential.[163]

Other studies have also demonstrated a good quality of life among the majority of pediatric liver transplant recipients.[164-167] Nonetheless, a fraction of patients may experience academic and psychosocial disabilities. Further, similar findings have been observed in pediatric liver recipients of living donors.[168] As children grow, they become more concerned about their own health and body image and they experience less pleasure than ordinary teenagers and this may result in a poor relationship with peers.[69,169] The support of the family and the transplant team play an important role in the patient's quality of life.[170,171]

The use of steroids has a detrimental effect on the growth of children after transplantation.[172-177] The weight catch-up growth is often better than the height catch-up growth. Other factors that may impair growth in children following liver transplantation are retransplantation, diagnosis of tumor, posttransplantation liver disease (PTLD), and low baseline Z scores.[172-175]

A troublesome problem is noncompliance of liver recipients, particularly adolescents. An analysis of noncompliance carried out at Stanford demonstrated that 37% of 98 teenagers admitted noncompliance.

Interestingly, 43% of the noncompliant group received the liver transplant as an adolescent compared with only 26% in the compliant group. Further, six patients in the noncompliant group required retransplantation because of chronic rejection compared with none in the compliant group. This analysis showed that the adolescent more at risk for noncompliance was a female who had the liver transplant as a teenager.

The incidence of hearing loss in children after hepatic replacement is significant, being reported at 15%. This is presumably because children with chronic liver disease who undergo transplantation are often exposed to ototoxic drugs.[178] Hearing impairment is known to interfere with the patients' well-being. These children with hearing loss may experience problems with speech and language development, learning, and social adaptation.

In general, the results in terms of quality of life and growth are encouraging, but they suggest that pediatric liver transplant recipients may require speech and physical therapy, special educational programs, and careful follow-up. Further research in this area must examine other factors that may influence development, including drugs, family dynamics, and the specific kind and severity of the liver disease.

Comment

Improvements in surgical technique for both the donor and recipient, more effective organ preservation, and the advent of potent immunosuppressive agents have markedly improved patient and graft survival. The consequences of chronic end-stage liver disease in children are devastating. Patients have problems associated with portal hypertension and the effects of malabsorption, particularly in chronic cholestatic liver disease. The growth failure and rickets that develop in children with biliary atresia are typical examples of such problems. Children with hopelessly advanced liver disease must therefore be promptly referred to a transplant center before the onset of irreversible sequelae. Fortunately, liver transplantation is now routinely performed in many transplant centers worldwide, and long-term survival can be expected in at least 80% to 85% of cases. The use of segmental grafts from living or deceased donors, as well as using organs across the ABO groups, has almost eliminated mortality on pediatric waiting lists.

The future of pediatric liver transplantation will most certainly involve the pursuit of immunotolerance and the implementation of minimally invasive surgery among living liver donors for pediatric recipients.[179] Although new immunosuppressive agents are highly selective in their action, their side effects are significant. Sequelae from chronic or acute liver failure, the potential complications following hepatic replacement, and the side effects of medications may result in learning disabilities, which in turn may predispose to noncompliance when children reach adolescence and begin to assume a more active role in their own medical management. Follow-up with great attention to the child's needs will ensure a good outcome as they transition into adulthood.

Pearls and Pitfalls

- The age of the child has no bearing on patient survival except for infants younger than 6 months.

- ABO-incompatible grafts may be performed under special circumstances in children younger than 2 years of age.

- In terms of graft survival, living donor grafts are associated with better outcomes than full-size deceased donor grafts and these, in turn, have better results than split-liver deceased donor grafts.

- Side-effects of cyclosporine are similar to those of tacrolimus with the exception of hirsutism and gingival hyperplasia observed with cyclosporine use. These two side effects are troublesome, particularly among teenagers who are more concerned about self-image.

- The majority of pediatric liver transplant recipients may be weaned from steroids.

- The quality of life in pediatric liver transplant recipients is excellent in the majority of patients. However, a few children may have neuropsychological deficits that require special education programs.

- Noncompliance may become a problem when children reach adolescence. The adolescent more at risk for noncompliance is a female who underwent liver transplantation as a teenager.

References

1. Starzl TE, Marchioro TL, Von Kaulla K, et al: Homotransplantation of the liver in humans. Surg Gynecol Obstet 117:659-676, 1963.
2. Calne RY, Rolles K, White DJG, et al: Cyclosporin A initially as the only immunosuppressant in 34 recipients of cadaveric organs: 32 kidneys, 2 pancreases, and 2 livers. Lancet 2:1033-1036, 1979.
3. Starzl TE, Iwatsuki S, Van Thiel DH, et al: Evolution of liver transplantation. Hepatology 2:614-636, 1982.
4. Starzl TE, Iwatsuki S, Esquivel CO, et al: Refinements in the surgical technique of liver transplantation. Semin Liver Dis 5:349-356, 1985.
5. Kalayoglu M, Sollinger HW, Stratta RJ, et al: Extended preservation of the liver for clinical transplantation. Lancet 1:617-619, 1988.
6. Malatack JJ, Schald DJ, Urbach AH, et al: Choosing a pediatric recipient of orthotopic liver transplantation. J Pediatr 111:479-489, 1987.

7. McDiarmid SV, Anand R, Lindblad AS, et al: Development of a pediatric end-stage liver disease score to predict poor outcome in children awaiting liver transplantation. Transplantation 74:173-181, 2002.

8. Esquivel CO, Koneru B, Todo S, et al: Is multiple organ failure a contraindication for liver transplantation in children? Transplant Proc 19:47-48, 1987.

9. Cuervas-Mons V, Rimola A, Van Thiel DH, et al: Does previous abdominal surgery alter the outcome of pediatric patients subjected to orthotopic liver transplantation? Gastroenterology 90: 853-857, 1986.

10. Meister RK, Esquivel CO, Cox KL, et al: The influence of porto enterostomy with stoma on morbidity in pediatric patients with biliary atresia undergoing orthotopic liver transplantation. J Pediatr Surg 28:387-390, 1993.

11. Mazzaferro V, Esquivel CO, Makowka L, et al: Factors responsible for hepatic artery thrombosis after pediatric liver transplantation. Transplant Proc 21:2466-2467, 1989.

12. Stock PG, Estrin JA, Fryd DS, et al: Factors influencing early survival after liver transplantation. Am J Surg 157:215-219, 1989.

13. Renard TH, Andrews WS: An approach to ABO-incompatible liver transplantation in children. Transplantation 53:116, 1992.

14. Gordon RD, Iwatsuki S, Esquivel CO, et al: Liver transplantation across ABO blood groups. Surgery 100:342-349, 1986.

15. Demetris AJ, Jaffe R, Tzakis A, et al: Antibody-mediated rejection of human liver allografts: Transplantation across ABO blood groups. Transplant Proc 21:2217-2220, 1989.

16. Fischel RJ, Ascher NL, Payne WD, et al: Pediatric liver transplantation across ABO blood group barriers. Transplant Proc 21:2221-2222, 1989.

17. Cacciarelli TV, So SK, Lim J, et al: A reassessment of ABO incompatibility in pediatric liver transplantation. Transplantation 60:757-760, 1995.

18. Egawa H, Oike F, Buhler L, et al: Impact of recipient age on outcome of ABO-incompatible living-donor liver transplantation. Transplantation 77:403-411, 2004.

19. Demetris AJ, Nakamura K, Yagihashi A, et al: A clinicopathological study of human liver allograft recipients harboring preformed IgG lymphocytotoxic antibodies. Hepatology 16:671-681, 1992.

20. Charco R, Vargas V, Balsells J, et al: Influence of anti-HLA antibodies and positive T-lymphocytotoxic crossmatch on survival and graft rejection in human liver transplantation. J Hepatol 24:452-459, 1996.

21. Takakura K, Kiuchi T, Kasahara M, et al: Clinical implications of flow cytometry crossmatch with T or B cells in living donor liver transplantation. Clin Transplant 15:309-316, 2001.

22. Kamath PS, Wiesner RH, Malinchoc M, et al: A model to predict survival in patients with end-stage liver disease. Hepatology 33:464-470, 2001.

23. Freeman RB Jr, Wiesner RH, Harper A, et al: The new liver allocation system: Moving toward evidence-based transplantation policy. Liver Transpl 8:851-858, 2002.

24. Shinkai M, Ohhama Y, Take H, et al: Evaluation of the PELD risks core as a severity index of biliary atresia. J Pediatr Surg 38: 1001-1004, 2003.

25. Carroll CL, Goodman DM, Superina RA, et al: Timed pediatric risk of mortality scores predict outcomes in pediatric liver transplant recipients. Pediatr Transplant 7:289-295, 2003.

26. Esquivel CO, Koneru B, Karrer F, et al: Liver transplantation before 1 year of age. J Pediatr 110:545-548, 1987.

27. Sokal EN, Veyckernans F, de Ville de Goyet J, et al: Liver transplantation in children less than 1 year of age. J Pediatr 17:205, 1990.

28. Esquivel CO, Nakazato P, Concepcion W, et al: The impact of liver reduction in pediatric liver transplantation. Arch Surg 126:1278, 1991.

29. Cox K, Nakazato P, Berquist W, et al: Liver transplantation in infants weighing less than 10 kilograms. Transplant Proc 23:1579-1580, 1991.

30. Woodle ES, Millis JM, So SKS, et al: Liver transplantation in the first three months of life. Transplantation 66:606-609, 1998.

31. Stevens LH, Emond JC, Piper JB, et al: Hepatic artery thrombosis in infants. A comparison of whole livers, reduced-size grafts, and grafts from living-related donors. Transplantation 53:396-399, 1992.

32. Inomoto T, Nishizawa F, Sasaki H, et al: Experiences of 120 microsurgical reconstructions of hepatic artery in living related liver transplantation. Surgery 119:20-26, 1996.

33. Esquivel CO, Iwatsuki S, Gordon RD, et al: Indications for pediatric liver transplantation. J Pediatr 111:1039-1045, 1987.

34. Busuttil RW, Seu P, Millis JM, et al: Liver transplantation in children. Ann Surg 213:48-57, 1991.

35. Ryckman F, Fisher R, Pedersen S, et al: Improved survival in biliary atresia patients in the present era of liver transplantation. J Pediatr Surg 28:382-386, 1993.

36. Kalayoglu M, D'Alessandro AM, Knetchtle SJ, et al: Long-term results of liver transplantation for biliary atresia. Surgery 114: 711-718, 1993.

37. Diem HV, Evrard V, Vinh HT, et al: Pediatric liver transplantation for biliary atresia: Results of primary grafts in 328 recipients. Transplantation 75:1692-1697, 2003.

38. Weerasooriya VS, White FV, Shepherd RW: Hepatic fibrosis and survival in biliary atresia. J Pediatr 144:123-125, 2004.

39. Kawamoto S, Strong RW, Lynch SV: Liver transplantation in the presence of situs inversus totalis: Application of reduced-size graft. Liver Transplant Surg 1:23-25, 1995.

40. Sugawara Y, Makuuchi M, Takayama T, et al: Liver transplantation from situs inversus to situs inversus. Liver Transpl 7:829-830, 2001.

41. Png K, Veyckemans F, De Kock M, et al: Hemodynamic changes in patients with Alagille's syndrome during orthotopic liver transplantation. Anesth Analg 89:1137-1142, 1999.

42. Starzl TE, Zitelli BJ, Shaw BW Jr, et al: Changing concepts: Liver replacement for hereditary tyrosinemia and hepatoma. J Pediatr 106:604-606, 1985.

43. Hood JM, Koep LH, Peters RL, et al: Liver transplantation for advanced liver disease with alpha-1-antitrypsin deficiency. N Engl J Med 302:272-275, 1980.

44. Esquivel CO, Marino R, Fioravanti V, et al: Liver transplantation for metabolic disease of the liver. Gastroenterol Clin North Am 17:167-175, 1988.

45. Shirahata Y, Ohkohchi N, Kawagishi N, et al: Living-donor liver transplantation for homozygous familial hypercholesterolemia from a donor with heterozygous hypercholesterolemia. Transpl Int 16:276-279, 2003.

46. Yorifuji T, Muroi J, Uematsu A, et al: Living-related liver transplantation for neonatal-onset propionic acidemia. J Pediatr 137:572-574, 2000.

47. Astarcioglu I, Karademir S, Gulay H, et al: Primary hyperoxaluria: Simultaneous combined liver and kidney transplantation from a living related donor. Liver Transpl 9:433-436, 2003.

48. Sato S, Fuchinoue S, Kimikawa M, et al: Sequential liver-kidney transplantation from a living-related donor in primary hyperoxaluria type 1 (oxalosis). Transplant Proc 35:373-374, 2003.

49. Liu PP, de Villa VH, Chen YS, et al: Outcome of living donor liver transplantation for glycogen storage disease. Transplant Proc 35:366-368, 2003.

50. Al Shurafa H, Wali S, Chehab MS, et al: Living related liver transplantation for Crigler-Najjar syndrome in Saudi Arabia. Clin Transplant 16:222-226, 2002.

51. Ban K, Sugiyama N, Sugiyama K, et al: A pediatric patient with classical citrullinemia who underwent living-related partial liver transplantation. Transplantation 71:1495-1497, 2001.

52. Koneru B, Flye MW, Busuttil RW, et al: Liver transplantation for hepatoblastoma. The American experience. Ann Surg 213:118, 1991.

53. Otte JB, Pritchard J, Aronson DC, et al: Liver transplantation for hepatoblastoma: Results from the International Society of Pediatric Oncology (SIOP) Study SIOPEL-1 and review of the world experience. Pediatr Blood Cancer 42:74-83, 2004.

54. Iwatsuki S, Gordon RD, Shaw BW Jr, et al: The role of liver transplantation in cancer therapy. Ann Surg 202:401-407, 1985.

55. Egawa H, Berquist W, Garcia-Kennedy R, et al: Respiratory distress from benign liver tumors: A report of two unusual cases treated with hepatic transplantation. J Pediatr Gastroenterol Nutr 19:114-117, 1994.

56. Dussaix E, de Paillette L, Laurent-Puig P, et al: Hepatitis C virus infection in pediatric liver transplantation. Transplantation 55:795-798, 1993.

57. Nowicki MJ, Ahmad N, Heubi JE, et al: The prevalence of hepatitis C virus (HCV) in infants and children after liver transplantation. Dig Dis Sci 39:2250-2254, 1994.

58. McDiarmid SV, Conrad A, Ament ME, et al: De novo hepatitis C in children after liver transplantation. 66:311-318, 1998.

59. Neuberger J, Portmann B, Calne R, et al: Recurrence of autoimmune chronic active hepatitis following orthotopic liver grafting. Transplantation 37:363-365, 1984.

60. Gartner JC Jr, Bergman I, Malatack JJ, et al: Progression of neurovisceral storage disease with supranuclear ophthalmoplegia following orthotopic liver transplantation. Pediatrics 77:104-106, 1986.

61. Kayler LK, Merion RM, Lee S, et al: Long-term survival after liver transplantation in children with metabolic disorders. Pediatr Transplant 6:295-300, 2002.

62. McDiarmid SV, Farmer DA, Goldstein LI, et al: A randomized prospective trial of steroid withdrawal after liver transplantation. Transplantation 60:1443-1450, 1995.

63. Takatsuki M, Uemoto S, Inomata Y, et al: Weaning of immunosuppression in living donor liver transplant recipients. Transplantation 72:449-454, 2001.

64. Diem HV, Sokal EM, Janssen M, et al: Steroid withdrawal after pediatric liver transplantation: A long-term follow-up study in 109 recipients. Transplantation 75:1664-1670, 2003.

65. Mazariegos GV, Reyes J, Marino IR, et al: Weaning of immunosuppression in liver transplant recipients. Transplantation 63:243-249, 1997.

66. Thomson AW, Mazariegos GV, Reyes J, et al: Monitoring the patient off immunosuppression. Conceptual framework for a proposed tolerance assay study in liver transplant recipients. Transplantation 72:S13-S22, 2001.

67. McDiarmid SV, Busuttil RW, Ascher NL, et al: FK506 (tacrolimus) compared with cyclosporine for primary immunosuppression after pediatric liver transplantation. Result from the U.S. Multicenter Trial. Transplantation 59:530-536, 1995.

68. Furukawa H, Todo S: Evolution of immunosuppression in liver transplantation: Contribution of cyclosporine. Transplant Proc 36:2745-2845, 2004.

69. Kelly DA: Strategies for optimizing immunosuppression in adolescent transplant recipients: A focus on liver transplantation. Paediatr Drugs 5:177-183, 2003.

70. Cao S, Cox KL, Berquist W, et al: Long-term outcomes in pediatric liver recipients: Comparison between cyclosporine A and tacrolimus. Pediatr Transplant 3:22-26, 1999.

71. Jain A, Mazariegos G, Kashyap R, et al: Comparative long-term evaluation of tacrolimus and cyclosporine in pediatric liver transplantation. Transplantation 70:617-625, 2000.

72. Jain A, Mazariegos G, Pokharna R, et al: The absence of chronic rejection in pediatric primary liver transplant patients who are maintained on tacrolimus-based immunosuppression: A long-term analysis. Transplantation 75:1020-1025, 2003.

73. Gupta P, Hart J, Cronin D, et al: Risk factors for chronic rejection after pediatric liver transplantation. Transplantation 72:1098-1102, 2001.

74. Dunn SP, Falkenstein K, Lawrence JP, et al: Monotherapy with cyclosporine for chronic immunosuppression in pediatric liver transplant recipients. Transplantation 57:544-547, 1994.

75. Jain A, Mazariegos G, Kashyap R, et al: Reasons why some children receiving tacrolimus therapy require steroids more than 5 years post liver transplantation. Pediatr Transplant 5:93-98, 2001.

76. Lykavieris P, Frauger E, Habes D, et al: Angioedema in pediatric liver transplant recipients under tacrolimus immunosuppression. Transplantation 75:152-155, 2003.

77. Romero R, Abramowsky CR, Pillen T, et al: Peripheral eosinophilia and eosinophilic gastroenteritis after pediatric liver transplantation. Pediatr Transplant 7:484-488, 2003.

78. Burckhart GJ, Starzl TE, Williams L, et al: Cyclosporine monitoring and pharmacokinetics in pediatric liver transplant patients. Transplant Proc 17:1172, 1985.

79. Wallemacq PE, Verbeeck RK: Comparative clinical pharmacokinetics of tacrolimus in paediatric and adult patients. Clin Pharmacokinet 40:283-295, 2001.

80. Sokol RJ, Johnson KE, Karren FM, et al: Improvement of cyclosporin absorption in children after liver transplantation by means of water-soluble vitamin E. Lancet 338:212, 1991.

81. Baciewicz AM, Baciewicz FA Jr: Cyclosporine pharmacokinetic drug interactions. Am J Surg 157:264-271, 1989.

82. Christians U, Jacobsen W, Benet LZ, et al: Mechanisms of clinically relevant drug interactions associated with tacrolimus. Clin Pharmacokinet 41:813-851, 2002.

83. Kelly DA: The use of anti-interleukin-2 receptor antibodies in pediatric liver transplantation. Pediatr Transplant 5:386-389, 2001.

84. Busuttil RW: Use of orthoclone OKT$_3$ for prophylaxis in liver transplantations and its re-use in liver allograft rejection. Transplant Proc 21(suppl 12):19-23, 1989.

85. Heffron TG, Pillen T, Smallwood GA, et al: Pediatric liver transplantation with daclizumab induction. Transplantation 75:2040-2043, 2003.

86. Aw MM, Taylor RM, Verma A, et al: Basiliximab (Simulect) for the treatment of steroid-resistant rejection in pediatric liver transplant recipients: A preliminary experience. Transplantation 75:796-799, 2003.

87. Renz JF, Lightdale J, Mudge C, et al: Mycophenolate mofetil, microemulsion cyclosporine, and prednisone as primary immunosuppression for pediatric liver transplant recipients. Liver Transpl Surg 5:136-143, 1999.

88. Markiewicz M, Kalicinski P, Teisseyre J, et al: Rapamycin in children after liver transplantation. Transplant Proc 35:2284-2286, 2003.

89. Bismuth H, Houssin D: Reduced-size orthotopic liver graft in hepatic transplantation in children. Surgery 95:367-370, 1984.

90. Raia S, Nery JR, Mies S: Liver transplantation from live donors. Lancet 2:497, 1989.

91. Strong RW, Lynch SV, Ong TH, et al: Successful liver transplantation from a living donor to her son. N Engl J Med 322:1505, 1990.

92. Broelsch CE, Emond JC, Thistlethwaite JR, et al: Liver transplantation including the concept of reduced-size liver transplants in children. Ann Surg 208:410-420, 1988.

93. Broelsch CE, Emond JC, Thistlethwaite JR, et al: Liver transplantation with reduced-size donor organs. Transplantation 45:519-523, 1988.

94. Ong TH, Lynch SV, Pillay SP, et al: Reduced-size orthotopic liver transplantation in children: An experience with seven cases. Transplant Proc 21:2443, 1989.

95. Otte JB, de Ville de Goyet J, Sokal E, et al: Size reduction of the donor liver is a safe way to alleviate the shortage of size-matched organs in pediatric liver transplantation. Ann Surg 211:146-157, 1990.

96. Kalayoglu M, D'Alessandro AM, Sollinger HW, et al: Experience with reduced-size liver transplantation. Surg Gynecol Obstet 171:139-147, 1990.

97. Broelsch CE, Whitington PF, Emond JC: Evolution and future perspectives for reduced-size hepatic transplantation. Surg Gynecol Obstet 171:353-359, 1990.

98. Houssin D, Soubrane O, Boillot O, et al: Orthotopic liver transplantation with a reduced-size graft: An ideal compromise in pediatrics? Surgery 111:532-541, 1992.

99. Soubrane O, Dousset B, Ozier Y, et al: The choice of the reduction technique for orthotopic liver transplantation (OLT) in children using a reduced-size graft. Transplant Proc 22:1487-1488, 1990.

100. Kasahara M, Kaihara S, Oike F, et al: Living-donor liver transplantation with monosegments. Transplantation 76:694-696, 2003.

101. Pichlmayr R, Ringe B, Gubernatis G, et al: Transplantation of one donor liver to two recipients (splitting transplantation): A new method for further development of segmental liver transplantation. Langenbecks Arch Surg 373:127-130, 1988.

102. Noujaim HM, Gunson B, Mayer DA, et al: Worth continuing doing ex situ liver graft splitting? A single-center analysis. Am J Transplant 3:318-323, 2003.

103. Malagó M, Hertl M, Testa G, et al: Split-liver transplantation: Future use of scarce donor organs. World J Surg 26:275-282, 2002.

104. Broelsch CE, Emond JC, Whitington PF, et al: Application of reduced-size liver transplants as split grafts, auxiliary orthotopic grafts, and living-related segmental transplants. Ann Surg 212:368-377, 1990.

105. Merion RM, Campbell DA: Split-liver transplantation: One plus one doesn't always equal two. Hepatology 14:572-574, 1991.

106. Houssin D, Boillot O, Soubrane O, et al: Controlled liver splitting for transplantation in two recipients: Technique, results, and perspectives. Br J Surg 80:75-80, 1993.

107. Deshpande RR, Bowles MJ, Vilca-Melendez H, et al: Results of split liver transplantation in children. Ann Surg 236:248-253, 2002.

108. Yersiz H, Renz JF, Farmer DG, et al: One hundred in situ split-liver transplantations—A single center experience. Ann Surg 238:496-507, 2003.

109. Renz JF, Emond JC, Yersiz H, et al: Split-liver transplantation in the United States: Outcomes of a national survey. Ann Surg 239:172-181, 2004.

110. Emond JC, Heffron TG, Kortz EO, et al: Improved results of living-related liver transplantation with routine application in a pediatric program. Transplantation 55:835-840, 1993.

111. Inomata Y, Tanaka K, Okajima H, et al: Living related liver transplantation for children younger than one year old. Eur J Pediatr Surg 6:148-151, 1996.

112. Hatano E, Terajima H, Yabe S, et al: Hepatic artery thrombosis in living related liver transplantation. Transplantation 64:1443-1446, 1997.

113. Shimahara Y, Awane M, Yamaoka Y, et al: Analyses of the risk and operative stress for donors in living-related partial liver transplantation. Transplantation 54:983-988, 1992.

114. Lo CM: Complications and long-term outcome of living liver donors: A survey of 1,508 cases in five Asian centers. Transplantation 75(suppl 3):S12-S15, 2003.

115. Ozawa K, Uemoto S, Tanaka K, et al: An appraisal of pediatric liver transplantation from living relatives. Ann Surg 216:547-553, 1992.

116. Broering DC, Mueller L, Ganschow R, et al: Is there still a need for living-related liver transplantation in children? Ann Surg 234:713-721, 2001.

117. McDiarmid SV, Davies DB, Edwards EB: Improved graft survival of pediatric liver recipients transplanted with pediatric-aged liver donors. Transplantation 70:1283-1292, 2000.

118. Fujita S, Tanaka K, Tolunaga Y, et al: Living-related liver transplantation for biliary atresia. Clin Transplant 7:571-577, 1993.

119. Roberts JP, Hulbert-Shearon TE, Merion RM, et al: Influence of graft type on outcomes after pediatric liver transplantation. Am J Transplant 4:373-377, 2004.

120. Goldstein MJ, Salame E, Kapur S, et al: Analysis of failure in living donor liver transplantation: Differential outcomes in children and adults. World J Surg 27:356-364, 2003.

121. Egawa H, Inomata Y, Uemoto S, et al: Biliary anastomotic complications in 400 living related liver transplantations. World J Surg 25:1300-1307, 2001.

122. Adam R, McMaster P, O'Grady JG, et al: Evolution of liver transplantation in Europe: Report of the European Liver Transplant Registry. Liver Transpl 9:1231-1243, 2003.

123. Nakamura T, Tanaka K, Kiuchi T, et al: Anatomical variations and surgical strategies in right lobe living donor liver transplantation: Lessons from 120 cases. Transplantation 73:1896-1903, 2002.

124. Kasahara M, Kiuchi T, Inomata Y, et al: Living-related liver transplantation for Alagille syndrome. Transplantation 75:2147-2150, 2003.

125. Tanaka K, Uemoto S, Inomata Y, et al: Living-related liver transplantation for fulminant hepatic failure in children. Transpl Int 7(suppl 1):S108-S110, 1994.

126. Liu CL, Fan ST, Lo CM, et al: Live donor liver transplantation for fulminant hepatic failure in children. Liver Transpl 9:1185-1190, 2003.

127. Mack CL, Ferrario M, Abecassis M, et al: Living donor liver transplantation for children with liver failure and concurrent multiple organ system failure. Liver Transpl 7:890-895, 2001.

128. Liu CL, Fan ST, Lo CM, et al: Living-donor liver transplantation for high-urgency situations. Transplantation 75(suppl 3):S33-S36, 2003.

129. Ogura Y, Kaihara S, Haga H, et al: Outcomes for pediatric liver retransplantation from living donors. Transplantation 76:943-948, 2003.

130. Achilleos OA, Mirza DF, Talbot D, et al: Outcome of liver retransplantation in children. Liver Transplant Surg 5:401-406, 1999.

131. Millan MT, Berquist WE, So SK, et al: One hundred percent patient and kidney allograft survival with simultaneous liver and kidney transplantation in infants with primary hyperoxaluria: Single center experience. Transplantation 76:1458-1463, 2003.

132. van't Hoff WG, Dixon M, Taylor J, et al: Combined liver-kidney transplantation in methylmalonic acidemia. J Pediatr 132:1043-1044, 1998.

133. http://www.intestinaltransplantregistry.org.

134. Grant D, Abu-Elmagd K, Reyes J, et al: 2003 Report of the Intestine Transplant Registry: A new era has dawned. (Submitted for publication.)

135. Horslen SP, Sudan DL, Iyer KR, et al: Isolated liver transplantation in infants with end-stage liver disease associated with short bowel syndrome. Ann Surg 235:435-439, 2002.

136. Kato T, Mittal N, Nishida S, et al: The role of intestinal transplantation in the management of babies with extensive gut resections. J Pediatr Surg 38:145-149, 2003.

137. Starzl TE, Bilheimer DW, Bahnson HT, et al: Heart-liver transplantation in a patient with familial hypercholesterolaemia. Lancet 1:1382-1383, 1984.

138. Couetil JPA, Soubrane O, Houssin DP, et al: Combined heart-lung-liver, double lung-liver, and isolated liver transplantation for cystic fibrosis in children. Transpl Int 10:33-39, 1997.

139. Dennis CM, McNeil KD, Dunning J, et al: Heart-lung-liver transplantation. J Heart Lung Transplant 15:536-538, 1996.

140. Couetil JPA, Houssin DP, Soubrane O, et al: Combined lung and liver transplantation in patients with cystic fibrosis—A 4½ year experience. J Thorac Cardiovasc Surg 110:1415-1423, 1995.

141. Esquivel CO, Jaffe R, Gordon RD, et al: Liver rejection and its differentiation from other causes of graft dysfunction. Semin Liver Dis 5:369-374, 1985.

142. Ascher NL, Stock PG, Bumgardner GL, et al: Infection and rejection of primary hepatic transplant in 93 consecutive patients treated with triple immunosuppression therapy. Surg Gynecol Obstet 167:474-484, 1988.

143. George DL, Arnow PM, Fox A, et al: Patterns of infection after pediatric liver transplantation. AJDC 146:924-929, 1992.

144. Bronsther O, Makowka L, Jaffe R, et al: Occurrence of cytomegalovirus hepatitis in liver transplant patients. J Med Virol 24:423-434, 1988.

145. Stratta RJ, Shaefer MS, Markin RS, et al: Clinical patterns of cytomegalovirus disease after liver transplantation. Arch Surg 124:1443-1450, 1989.

146. Winston DJ, Busuttil RW: Randomized controlled trial of sequential intravenous and oral ganciclovir versus prolonged intravenous ganciclovir for long-term prophylaxis of cytomegalovirus disease in high-risk cytomegalovirus-seronegative liver transplant recipients with cytomegalovirus-seropositive donors. Transplantation 77:305-308, 2004.

147. Randhawa PS, Markin RS, Starzl TE, et al: Epstein-Barr virus-associated syndromes in immunosuppressed liver transplant recipients: Clinical profile and recognition on routine allograft biopsy. Am J Surg Pathol 14:538-547, 1990.

148. Telenti A, Smith TF, Ludwig J, et al: Epstein-Barr virus and persistent graft and dysfunction after liver transplantation. Hepatology 14:282, 1991.

149. Garcia-Kennedy R, Lennette E, Concepcion W, et al: Epstein-Barr infections in liver transplant recipients. Hepatology 14:76, 1991.

150. Serinet MO, Jacquemin E, Habes D: Anti-CD20 monoclonal antibody (rituximab) treatment for Epstein-Barr virus-associated, B-cell lymphoproliferative disease in pediatric liver transplant recipients. J Pediatr Gastroenterol 34:389-393, 2002.

151. Koneru B, Jaffe R, Esquivel CO, et al: Adenoviral infections in pediatric liver transplant recipients. JAMA 258:489-492, 1987.

152. Tzakis AG, Gordon RD, Shaw BW Jr, et al: Clinical presentation of hepatic artery thrombosis after liver transplantation in the cyclosporine era. Transplantation 40:667-671, 1985.

153. Shaked A, McDiarmid SV, Harrison RE, et al: Hepatic artery thrombosis resulting in gas gangrene of the transplanted liver. Surgery 111:462-465, 1992.

154. Langnas AN, Stratta RJ, Wood RP, et al: The role of intrahepatic cholangiojejunostomy in liver transplant recipients after extensive destruction of the extrahepatic biliary system. Surgery 112:712-718, 1992.

155. Koneru B, Esquivel CO, Bowen AD, et al: Early detection and management of portal vein thrombosis after hepatic transplantation: Report of a case. Clin Transplant 2:214-215, 1988.

156. Scantlebury VP, Zajko AB, Esquivel CO, et al: Successful reconstruction of late portal vein stenosis after hepatic transplantation. Arch Surg 124:503-505, 1989.

157. Heffron TG, Pillen T, Welch D, et al: Biliary complications after pediatric liver transplantation revisited. Transplant Proc 35:1461-1462, 2003.

158. Gondolesi GE, Varotti G, Florman SS, et al: Biliary complications in 96 consecutive right lobe living donor transplant recipients. Transplantation 77:1842-1848, 2004.

159. Howard TK, Klintmalm GB, et al: The influence of preservation injury on rejection in the hepatic transplant recipient. Transplantation 49:103, 1990.

160. Stewart SM, Vauy R, Waller DA, et al: Mental and motor development, social competence, and growth one year after successful pediatric liver transplantation. J Pediatr 114:574-581, 1989.

161. Stewart SM, Vauy R, Waller DA, et al: Mental and motor correlates in patients with end-stage biliary atresia awaiting liver transplantation. Pediatrics 79:882-888, 1987.

162. Wayman KI, Cox KL, Esquivel CO: Neurodevelopmental outcome of young children with extrahepatic biliary atresia 1 year after liver transplantation. J Pediatr 131:894-898, 1997.

163. Stewart SM, Hiltebertel C, Nici J, et al: Neuropsychological outcome of pediatric liver transplantation. Pediatrics 87:367-376, 1991.

164. Alonso EM, Neighbors K, Mattson C, et al: Functional outcomes of pediatric liver transplantation. J Pediatr Gastroenterol Nutr 37:155-160, 2003.

165. Zamberlan KE: Quality of life in school-age children following liver transplantation. Matern Child Nurs J 20:167-229, 1992.

166. Burdelski M, Nolkemper D, Ganschow R, et al: Liver transplantation in children: Long-term outcome and quality of life. Eur J Pediatr 158(suppl 2):S34-S42, 1999.

167. Midgley DE, Bradlee TA, Donohoe C, et al: Health-related quality of life in long-term survivors of pediatric liver transplantation. Liver Transpl 6:333-339, 2000.

168. Ohkohchi N, Orii T, Kawagishi N, et al: Quality of life of pediatric patients receiving living donor liver transplantation in long-term follow-up period. Transplant Proc 33:3610-3613, 2001.

169. Manificat S, Dazord A, Cochat P, et al: Quality of life of children and adolescents after kidney or liver transplantation: Child, parents' and caregiver's point of view. Pediatr Transplant 7:228-235, 2003.

170. Qvist E, Jalanko H, Holmberg C: Psychosocial adaptation after solid organ transplantation in children. Pediatr Clin North Am 50:1505-1519, 2003.

171. Stone RD, Beasley PJ, Treacy SJ, et al: Children and families can achieve normal psychological adjustment and a good quality of life following pediatric liver transplantation: A long-term study. Transplant Proc 29:1571-1572, 1997.

172. Urbach AH, Gartner JC Jr, Malatack JJ, et al: Linear growth following pediatric liver transplantation. Am J Dis Child 141:547-549, 1987.

173. Asonuma K, Inomata Y, Uemoto S, et al: Growth and quality of life after living-related liver transplantation in children. Pediatr Transplant 2:3-5, 1998.

174. McDiarmid SV, Gornbein JA, DeSilva PJ, et al: Factors affecting growth after pediatric liver transplantation. Transplantation 67:404-411, 1999.

175. Bartosh SM, Thomas SE, Sutton MM, et al: Linear growth after pediatric liver transplantation. J Pediatr 135:624-631, 1999.

176. Chin SE, Shepherd RW, Cleghorn GJ, et al: Survival, growth and quality of life in children after orthotopic liver transplantation: A 5 year experience. J Paediatr Child Health 27:380-385, 1991.

177. D'Antiga L, Moniz C, Buxton-Thomas M, et al: Bone mineral density and height gain in children with chronic cholestatic liver disease undergoing transplantation. Transplantation 73:1788-1793, 2002.

178. Bucuvalas JC, O'Connor A, Buschle K, et al: Risk of hearing impairment in pediatric liver transplant recipients: A single center study. Pediatr Transplant 7:265-269, 2003.

179. Cherqui D, Soubrane O, Husson E, et al: Laparoscopic living donor hepatectomy for liver transplantation in children. Lancet 359:392-396, 2002.

Future Developments in Liver Transplantation

Genetic Modulation in Transplantation

HEIDI YEH

ABRAHAM SHAKED

Gene transfer technologies   1358
  Viral vectors   1358

Graft modification   1359
  Immunosuppressive cytokines   1359
  Secreted fusion proteins   1360
  Reduction of ischemic injury and
    apoptosis   1360

Recipient modification   1361

Summary   1362

Gene therapy encompasses a broad range of techniques aimed at controlling cellular phenotypes by modifying genetic material. The many different delivery systems represent tradeoffs among efficiency of transduction, stability of expression, and tissue selectivity. Approaches to gene therapy can be broadly divided into germline and somatic cell modification. Germline manipulation occurs at the level of the reproductive system or during the early stages of embryonic development, resulting in permanent changes to the genetic material of all cells of an organism in a heritable pattern. Somatic modification results in alterations only to specific cells in an organism, which do not get passed on.

The most obvious application of such technology is the introduction of exogenous DNA to replace absent or defective sequences. This would presumably convert the dysfunctional cell and its associated disease state to a functional cell and, hopefully, a return to relative health for the patient. Examples of such introduction include the low density lipoprotein (LDL) receptor in familial hypercholesterolemia or the cystic fibrosis transmembrane conductance regulator (CFTR) gene in cystic fibrosis. Sometimes cells with normal genetic material still fail to prevent disease. For example, the immune system can fail to eradicate cancer cells that express aberrant proteins. In such cases, the goal of genetic modulation is to augment normal cell function. Many human anticancer gene therapy strategies seek to enhance immune-mediated antitumor responses with a variety of genes, including those encoding cytokines.

On occasion, normal cellular function is not only inadequate but also detrimental. This is true in autoimmune diseases and, of course, in the field of transplantation. Liver allograft survival is limited by immune-mediated rejection and ischemic-reperfusion injury, both of which involve physiological pathways that normally help maintain homeostasis. The use of gene therapy to improve outcomes after solid-organ transplantation is, therefore, driven by our understanding of immunity, tolerance, and organ injury.

Recognition of nonself antigens expressed on transplanted tissue initiates a cascade of humoral and cellular immune responses, ending finally in graft rejection. Currently, this response is blunted by pharmaceutical agents that nonspecifically suppress the immune system. The disadvantages of systemic immunosuppression are easy to predict and have been borne out by experience; the most dreaded complications of the antirejection regimen are the development of uncontrolled infections and increased rates of malignancy. The myriad side effects of immunosuppressive drugs, including hirsutism, hypertension, diabetes, and renal failure, also make them unappealing.

Gene therapy is being explored as an approach to rejection prevention based on targeted immunosuppression. In fact, the transplant setting offers a unique advantage to gene therapy; the graft can be efficiently transduced before transplantation by donor pretreatment or by ex vivo gene delivery during cold preservation, thereby sidestepping the problem of directed gene delivery. One can easily imagine the creation of a local immunosuppressive zone by transducing only the graft with sequences encoding immunosuppressive cytokines or soluble forms of receptor ligands. These soluble ligands could bind alloreactive immune cells entering the graft and either block activating receptors or bind inhibitory receptors. Such an environment could even give rise to true immunological tolerance, making the continued expression of immunosuppressive proteins unnecessary.

There is also interest in inducing tolerance by genetically modifying the immune cells of the recipient. For the most part, this has been explored by expressing donor antigens in bone marrow cells, thymus, or other antigen-presenting cells (APCs). These strategies require pretreatment of the recipient and extensive genetic workup of the donor, so the time involved in such processing has precluded these options from being clinically useful. However, these strategies may represent opportunities to avoid long-term immunosuppression, with pharmacological immunosuppression being used only initially while preparations are being made to induce tolerance.

Another early event leading to liver graft dysfunction is ischemia-reperfusion injury, which is antigen independent. Ischemia-reperfusion injury is especially important in the setting of organ shortage and interest in suboptimal organs: small for size, steatotic, and non–heart-beating donor livers. Although the use of University of Wisconsin (UW) cold storage solution has largely limited the damage sustained during cold ischemia, significant insult can occur during organ reperfusion. These effects have been attributed to free radical production in the presence of oxygen and cytokine release in response to cellular injury. It is of note that increased cellular injury may also make grafts more immunogenic, so the use of gene products to block oxygen free radical production and cytokine release could improve graft function both immediately and in the long term.

There are several basic prerequisites for gene therapy to be clinically applicable to liver transplantation. First, genes that improve graft survival without causing significant side effects must be identified. Second, systems of efficient gene delivery to the whole liver or specific liver cell populations must be available. Third, functional protein must be synthesized, although long-term expression may be less of an issue in the prevention of reperfusion injury and the induction of tolerance. Finally, it would be preferable to complete transduction and modification in the short period available between the time of donor identification and the time of transplantation. This article discusses some of the specific gene transfer techniques that may become useful in liver transplantation, as well as gene products and strategies that may contribute to prolonged graft survival.

Gene Transfer Technologies

Gene delivery systems can be categorized into three types: naked DNA, DNA associated with a carrier particle, and DNA packaged in a virus. Naked DNA can be transfected by precipitation onto gold particles and using a gene gun, liposomes to carry the DNA through the cell and nuclear membranes, Ca_2PO_4 precipitation, or electrical impulses to make the cell membrane porous (electroporation).[1] Carrier particles are most often specific ligands, such as asialoglycoproteins, which can be coupled to the DNA to enhance uptake in hepatocytes that express the asialoglycoprotein receptor.[2,3] Although cultured cells grown in monolayers or single-cell suspensions can be easily transfected by any method, organ-directed gene transfer requires biological vectors that can be injected into the vasculature and thereby gain access to all the cells of the organ.

Viral Vectors

This section briefly describes some of the common viral vectors used in gene therapy.

Retrovirus

Retrovirus particles contain a double-stranded RNA (ribonucleic acid) genome and reverse transcriptase packaged in a capsule. [4] They enter target cells via receptor-mediated endocytosis, but the proteins involved in this interaction are not well characterized. Once internalized, viral RNA is converted to DNA (proviral DNA) via the reverse transcriptase, and the proviral DNA then enters the nucleus and randomly integrates into the genome. The ability of proviral DNA to enter the nucleus and integrate is dependent on cellular mitosis, presumably because the nuclear membrane breaks down during cell division, allowing the proviral DNA to enter.

The wild-type retrovirus then uses the cellular machinery for production of RNA and envelope proteins, which are then assembled into new virions. Successful virion assembly requires a specific packaging sequence on the RNA strand. Retroviruses used for gene therapy protocols are replication defective, that is, they are able to infect cells without being able to make additional copies of themselves. These genomes are constructed by using DNA cloning techniques that replace endogenous viral sequences required for capsid production with the target gene of interest. The virus particles are then produced in a packaging cell line, which already contains an integrated viral genome that encodes all the capsid proteins, but lacks the packaging sequence. The viral genome of interest is, therefore, packaged into a capsid produced from sequences from a separate viral genome that is itself unable to be packaged. When these virions infect the target cells, which presumably have not been previously infected with a retrovirus supplying the missing capsid proteins, they can integrate into the host genome but cannot produce new virus.

Retroviruses are useful because their genomes are easy to manipulate and they integrate stably into the genome, presumably resulting in long-term expression. This property is also associated with the theoretical risk of insertional mutagenesis at the site of integration. Other disadvantages include the inability of retroviruses to infect all target cell populations efficiently, a problem that is particularly difficult to address because the receptors involved in endocytosis have not been identified. In addition, these viruses cannot infect cells that are not actively dividing. Although adult human liver cells do retain the capacity to divide, as in regeneration following injury or resection and in culture, the requirement for active division has limited the use of retroviral gene transfer in the liver transplantation setting. There has been recent interest in lentiviruses, which are also retroviruses but do not have the absolute requirement for cell proliferation necessary to infect cells.

Adenovirus

The majority of gene therapy work has centered on adenovirus vectors, in particular types 2 and 5.[5] The human adenovirus contains 35 to 40 kb of double-stranded DNA. It is internalized by receptor-mediated endocytosis and then transported to the nucleus, where it is not incorporated into the host genome but remains as an extrachromosomal DNA-histone complex. Because of this, the human adenovirus is subject to degradation by cellular nucleases and therefore has a limited life span. In addition, expression of viral proteins results in a brisk inflammatory response by the host, further contributing to transient gene expression.

Adenoviral vectors are popular because they are easy to grow and purify and generally result in high levels of gene expression. Unlike retroviral vectors, adenoviral vectors can infect resting cells. Strains currently in use are rendered replication incompetent by deletion of the E1a and E1b genes, which are required for replication of viral DNA and expression of structural proteins. Deletion of other sequences may make adenoviral vectors less immunogenic as well.

One problem with viral-mediated gene transfer as used in experiments is that control groups are usually injected with adenovirus carrying an inert marker gene, such as β-galactosidase. As a result, it is unclear whether the improvement in graft function and survival reflects a decrease in damage caused by physiological factors or in damage caused by the pathogenicity and antigenicity of the viral vector. If differences in treatment groups are actually a result of the former, the advantages seen in the laboratory would not translate into improved patient outcomes, since no virus at all is used at baseline in a therapeutic human transplantation.

Graft Modification

Immunosuppressive Cytokines

Interleukin (IL)-10 was first discovered as the product of T_H2 cells, which could inhibit the production of the proinflammatory cytokines IL-2 and interferon (IFN)-γ. Local expression of IL-10 in a transplanted liver might result in decreased rejection, which is known to depend on IL-2 production. Transduction of donor ACI liver grafts with adenovirus containing the IL-10 gene resulted in in vivo levels of expression sufficient to suppress bidirectional mixed lymphocyte reaction (MLR) in vitro.[6] Subsequent experiments showed that transduction of liver allografts 24 to 48 hours before transplantation resulted in prolonged graft survival, with peak IL-10 levels in the first week following transplantation.[7] Interestingly, the timing of viral infection in relation to transplantation was crucial to the success of the gene transfer, which will be important to keep in mind when translating this technology to the clinical setting.

A multifunctional protein, transforming growth factor-beta (TGF-β) inhibits the proliferation and activation of T lymphocytes and is presumably another candidate for the prevention of allograft rejection. Although transduction of cardiac allografts with TGF-β prolongs cardiac allograft survival,[8] results in liver transplantation have been limited to demonstrating that adenoviral constructs containing the TGF-β gene can efficiently infect liver allografts during cold preservation time and result in high levels of expression up to 1 week after transplantation.[9] There has not been convincing evidence of prolonged vascularized liver allograft survival.

IL-4 is a T_H2 immunosuppressive cytokine, the role of which in allograft rejection has been investigated. Although some studies show that IL-4 production is associated with decreased rejection,[10] other studies show that intragraft IL-4 levels are not correlated with graft survival at all.[11] More in keeping with the latter result are experiments showing that IL-4 gene transfer to the liver is associated with hepatitis and dose-dependent mortality.[12] However, this was a T-cell–independent event and was related rather to apoptosis of the hepatocytes, suggesting that IL-4 may have a direct toxicity to the liver that precludes its use as an immunosuppressant.

Secreted Fusion Proteins

An approach to suppressing antiallograft lymphocytes would be to interfere with the ligand-receptor interactions required for the activation of T cells. Many immune signals are transmitted via cell surface proteins that require cell-cell contact rather than secreted cytokines that are soluble in serum. These contacts occur between APCs and the effector T cells. To disrupt T-cell receptors from binding their ligands, one strategy has been to engineer a soluble form of the receptor, which then binds to all the available ligands, thereby preventing the ligand from binding to functional signaling receptors on the surface of lymphocytes. This has been applied to the CD40/CD154 pairing. CD40 is a costimulatory molecule, the engagement of which is required at the time of antigen recognition to prevent a state of anergy. The extracellular domain of CD40 can be attached to the Fc portion of an immunoglobulin (Ig) G molecule, which converts it from a membrane protein to a soluble secreted protein. Adenoviral constructs expressing the fusion proteins have been given to rat liver allografts, both before and after transplantation, resulting in long-term, strain-specific tolerance.[13,14]

An alternative strategy was used in the case of the CD28/CD80/86 pathway. CD28 normally binds and activates CD80/86, another costimulatory signal required

to prevent T-cell anergy. CTLA-4, another membrane protein, which exists in much lower concentrations but binds CD80/86 with higher affinity, not only prevents the activation signal from being transmitted but also sends an inhibitory signal. Adenoviral constructs containing CTLA-4-Ig sequences were used to transduce cold-preserved rat liver allografts. Expression of CTLA-4-Ig was associated with indefinite graft survival and donor-specific tolerance.[15] Another group succeeded in getting gene expression with a retroviral construct by performing partial transplants to induce liver regeneration and cell division.[16]

Reduction of Ischemic Injury and Apoptosis

The supply of suitable donor livers has not kept up with increasing demand. Extending the donor pool by splitting organs between recipients, using non–heart-beating donors, or transplanting steatotic livers would begin to address this problem. However, such suboptimal grafts are particularly susceptible to ischemia-reperfusion injury, leading to a high risk of graft loss. Although current harvest and preservation protocols protect normal donor livers reasonably well, gene therapy is being pursued as an adjunct for expanded criteria grafts so that their use will be clinically feasible.

One approach to reducing liver injury is to prevent the formation of oxygen-derived free radicals. Oxygen free radicals can be generated by free Fe^{2+}. Ferritin binds Fe^{2+}, thus indirectly functioning as an antioxidant molecule. Investigators have found that overexpression of the ferritin heavy chain gene results in decreased hepatocellular damage after transplantation into syngeneic recipients.[17] Apoptosis in vivo was inhibited not only in the hepatocytes but also in the endothelial cells.

Once free radicals are produced, there are many enzymes that function to neutralize them so that they cannot cause further damage. The most commonly studied endogenous free radical scavenger in liver transplant models is the Cu/Zn-superoxide dismutase (SOD). The Cu/Zn-SOD degrades oxygen free radicals but has a short half-life if given exogenously. Adenoviral vectors encoding the Cu/Zn-SOD gene were used to infect rat donors that had received the regular diet, a high-fat diet, or an ethanol-containing high-fat diet. Free radical adducts were increased in the ethanol-fed rats following transplantation, but pretreatment with the vector resulted in a blunting of this increase as well as an increase in graft survival.[18]

Heme-oxygenase-1 (HO-1) is another molecule that confers protection against oxidative stress. Fatty livers from obese Zucker rats were transplanted into lean Zucker rats after being treated in vivo with adenoviral constructs containing the HO-1 gene. Graft survival and function were both improved when compared with controls[19] and seemed to be related to prevention of CD95/FasL-mediated apoptosis.[20] The same group also found that overexpression of the HO-1 gene was associated with decreased lymphocytic infiltrates, high levels of IL-4 and IL-10, and lower levels of IL-2 and IFN-γ,[21] suggesting that decreasing cellular damage is also associated with less of an inflammatory response.

Obviously, the acute inflammatory response to ischemia-reperfusion injury would be associated with even greater injury to the liver. Macrophages play an important role early in this response, producing a number of inflammatory mediators. IL-13 is a potent suppressor of macrophage function, so investigators have used adenovirus to transfer the IL-13 gene into rat livers and then stressed them with both warm and cold ischemia.[22] In the warm ischemia model, which involved in situ ischemia followed by reperfusion, Ad-IL-13 resulted in decreased hepatocyte damage, as measured by serum transaminase levels. In the cold ischemia model, involving ex vivo cold ischemia followed by transplantation, IL-13 gene transfer was associated with prolonged graft survival.

To block the CD40/CD154 pairing, which is part of the costimulation pathway in CD4+ T cells, Ke and colleagues transfected rat livers with Ad-CD40Ig and then subjected the livers to 24 hours of cold ischemia time before transplantation.[23] They found that Ad-CD40Ig treatment doubled graft survival at 2 weeks. This was correlated with increased mRNA expression of the inhibitory cytokines IL-4/IL-13 and decreased levels of the activating cytokines IL-2/IFN-γ as well as with lower serum transaminase levels and sinusoidal congestion and necrosis. In an interesting feedback loop, HO-1 expression was enhanced in Ad-CD40Ig–treated transplants. As expected, hepatocyte apoptosis as measured by several parameters was decreased in the treated group.

The end result of both ischemia-reperfusion injury and the inflammatory response is necrosis and apoptosis; thus the interest in bcl-2, an antiapoptotic molecule that regulates mitochondrial membrane permeability. Attempts to improve organ preservation by modifying liver grafts to overexpress bcl-2 have been made, showing decreased apoptosis and liver injury.[24,25] However, graft survival was not examined in these studies. Of course, bcl-2 is overexpressed in B-cell lymphomas[26] and overexpression in liver cells, especially in a setting of immunosuppression, could lead to increased rates of malignancy.

Recipient Modification

Dendritic cells play an important role in stimulating the immune system. However, dendritic cells express only the appropriate surface molecules necessary to provide a costimulatory signal to T cells if they, in turn, have been activated by "danger signals" such as proinflammatory cytokines, microbial products, or stress hormones.[27] Failure to send the "second signal" results in T-cell anergy/apoptosis[28] or even in differentiation into regulatory cells[29] that can actively suppress conventional T cells. Genetic modification of dendritic cells to prevent their maturation into professional APCs is a potential way to induce tolerance.

Dendritic cells (DC), by virtue of their proximity to the effector T cells, are also useful as carriers of immunosuppressive cytokines or "killer" molecules. Fas-ligand, which induces apoptosis in Fas-positive T cells, has been liposomally transfected into donor DCs.[30] These DCs were then injected into allogeneic mice prior to heart transplantation, resulting in prolonged graft survival. However, this required more than 2 weeks of pretreatment before transplantation, making it less useful in deceased donor liver transplants and in bone marrow–derived DCs, and making it prohibitive in living related transplants. Others have transduced a donor DC line with Ad-CTLA4Ig and injected them into recipients together with islets and shown marginally prolonged survival.[31] Peripheral blood–modified DCs from humans infected with Ad-IL-10 have been used in a skin graft model onto humanized NOD-SCID (severe combined immunodeficient) mice, resulting in decreased rejection according to histological evaluation at days 7 and 14.[32] Similar experiments in mice renal allografts performed with Ad-IL-10 and Ad-TGF-β show similar potential.[33]

It is known that donor-specific tolerance can be induced by mixed cellular chimerism achieved by an allogeneic bone marrow transplant.[34] This may not be a practical way of inducing tolerance routinely because of the morbidity of pretransplantation ablation procedures, as well as the potential for inducing graft-versus-host disease. However, investigators have used a retroviral construct to transduce bone marrow–derived cells with an allogeneic major histocompatibility complex (MHC) class I in mice, resulting in tolerance to skin grafts from mice of that MHC class I type.[35] Another group performed similar experiments with an adenovirus construct and cardiac allografts.[36] Although these experiments were performed with the standard harvest and ablation protocols, the use of a gene rather than whole cells does remove the risk of graft-versus-host disease. In addition, there is a suggestion that the use of peripheral lymphoid cells (T cells) rather than bone marrow cells may be sufficient, making it a more attractive option clinically. This option would be particularly useful if xenogeneic transplants ever become a viable source of organs because the transplant antigens would be well defined and identical for all transplants, rather than each donor having to be individually characterized and a new genetic construct having to be made for each donor.

B cells can also function as tolerogenic APCs. This has been studied, especially in autoimmune diseases such as experimental allergic encephalomyelitis, the animal model of multiple sclerosis; and NOD (nonobese diabetic) mice, the animal model of type I diabetes. One group used a retroviral construct expressing myelin basic protein or insulin fused to IgG as a tolerogenic carrier, which was then used to transduce B cells.[37] Unlike bone marrow protocols, no ablation was required. They were able to ameliorate both the encephalitis as well as the hyperglycemia. We can imagine carrying this idea over to the transplant setting and using allogeneic MHC molecules fused to the IgG to induce tolerance to allografts. This approach may work even in patients who have already undergone transplantation; an established response in these autoimmune models was actually subdued, as opposed to merely preventing an immune response from starting.

Rather than relying on existing mechanisms for inducing tolerance, there are also techniques to actively kill donor-specific T cells. Chimeric receptors can be constructed that fuse the extracellular domain of an MHC I molecule to a T-cell receptor (TCR) signaling domain.[38] When a T cell modified to express this receptor is pulsed with a specific antigen to present in the MHC molecule, it can then lyse precursor cytotoxic T-lymphocyte (CTL) specific for that antigen. In a transplant setting, we could pulse such a modified T cell with liver cell lysates, generate a repertoire of T cells that alloantigen-specific CTL would bind via their TCR, resulting in lysis of the CTL. In addition to the obvious logistical limitations of this approach, memory CTLs were resistant to lysis.

Summary

Options for improving graft survival after liver transplantation are increasing as we expand our understanding of ischemia-reperfusion injury and immune-mediated rejection. Concurrently, new vectors and transfection techniques offer many approaches for deploying our understanding. Although we have much greater experience in graft modification, investigations are also being undertaken in recipient modification with gene therapy, with the ultimate goal of expanding the donor pool and limiting the use of nonspecific immunosuppression.

References

1. Larregina AT, Morelli AE, Tkacheva O, et al: Highly efficient expression of transgenic proteins by naked DNA-transfected dendritic cells through terminal differentiation. Blood 103:811-819, 2004.

2. Cristano RJ, Smith LC, Woo SL: Hepatic gene therapy: Adenovirus enhancement of receptor-mediated delivery and expression in primary hepatocytes. Proc Natl Acad Sci U S A 88:2122-2126, 1991.

3. Wu GY, Wilson JM, Shalaby F, et al: Receptor-mediated gene delivery in vivo. Partial correction of genetic analbuminemia in Nagase rats. J Biol Chem 266:14338-14342, 1991.

4. Raper S: Human gene therapy. In Greenfield LJ (ed): Surgery, Scientific Principles and Practice. Philadelphia, Lippincott-Raven, pp 507-510.

5. Raper S: Human gene therapy. In Greenfield LJ (ed): Surgery, Scientific Principles and Practice. Philadelphia, Lippincott-Raven, pp 513-514.

6. Drazan KE, Wu L, Olthoff KM, et al: Transduction of hepatic allografts achieves local levels of viral IL-10 which suppress alloreactivity in vitro. J Surg Res 59:219-223, 1995.

7. Tashiro H, Shinozaki K, Yahata H, et al: Prolongation of liver allograft survival after interleukin-10 gene transduction 24-48 hours before donation. Transplantation 70:336-339, 2000.

8. Chavin KD, Lihui Q, Tahara H, et al: Gene transfer of TGF-beta and viral IL-10 prolong cardiac allograft survival. Surg Forum XLIII:407-409, 1992.

9. Drazan KE, Olthoff KM, Wu L, et al: Adenovirus-mediated gene transfer in the transplant setting: Early events after orthotopic transplantation of liver allografts expressing TGF-beta1. Transplantation 62:1080-1084, 1996.

10. Baan CC, Metselaar HJ, Mol WM, et al: Intragraft IL-4 mRNA expression is associated with down-regulation of liver graft rejection. Clin Transplant 10:542-549, 1996.

11. Lang T, Krams SM, Martinez OM: Production of IL-4 and IL-10 does not lead to immune quiescence in vascularized human organ grafts. Transplantation 62:776-780, 1996.

12. Guillot C, Coathalem H, Chetritt J, et al: Lethal hepatitis after gene transfer of IL-4 in the liver is independent of immune responses and dependent on apoptosis of hepatocytes: A rodent model of IL-4–induced hepatitis. J Immunol 166:5225-5235, 2001.

13. Nomura M, Yamashita K, Murakami M, et al: Induction of donor-specific tolerance by adenovirus-mediated CD40Ig gene therapy in rat liver transplantation. Transplantation 73:1403-1410, 2002.

14. Chang GJ, Liu T, Feng S, et al: Targeted gene therapy with CD40Ig to induce long-term acceptance of liver allografts. Surgery 132:149-156, 2002.

15. Olthoff KM, Judge TA, Gelman AE, et al: Adenovirus-mediated gene transfer into cold-preserved liver allografts: Survival pattern and unresponsiveness following transduction with CTLA4Ig. Nat Med 4:194-200, 1998.

16. Cheung ST, Tsui TY, Wang W, et al: Liver as an ideal target for gene therapy: Expression of CTLA4Ig by retroviral gene transfer. J Gastroenterol Hepatol 17:1008-1014, 2002.

17. Berberat PO, Katori M, Kaczmarek E, et al: Heavy chain ferritin acts as an antiapoptotic gene that protects livers from ischemia reperfusion injury. FASEB J 17:1724-1726, 2003.

18. Lehmann TG, Wheeler MD, Schwabe RF, et al: Gene delivery of Cu-/Zn-superoxide dismutase improves graft function after transplantation of fatty livers in the rat. Hepatology 32:1255-1264, 2000.

19. Coito A, Buelow R, Shen XD, et al: Heme oxygenase-1 gene transfer inhibits inducible nitric oxide synthase expression and protects genetically fat Zucker rat livers from ischemia-reperfusion injury. Transplantation 74:96-102, 2002.

20. Ke B, Buelow R, Shen XD, et al: Heme oxygenase-1 gene transfer prevents CD95/Fas ligand-mediated apoptosis and improves liver allograft survival via carbon monoxide signaling pathway. Hum Gene Ther 13:1189-1199, 2002.

21. Ke B, Shen XD, Melinek J, et al: Heme oxygenase-1 gene therapy: A novel immunomodulatory approach in liver allograft recipients? Transplant Proc 33:581-582, 2001.

22. Ke B, Shen XD, Lassman CR, et al: Interleukin-13 gene transfer protects rat livers from antigen-independent injury induced by ischemia and reperfusion. Transplantation 75:1118-1123, 2003.

23. Ke B, Shen XD, Gao F, et al: Gene therapy for liver transplantation using adenoviral vectors: CD40-CD154 blockade by gene transfer

of CD40Ig protects rat livers from cold ischemia and reperfusion injury. Mol Ther 9:38-45, 2004.

24. Bilbao G, Contreras JL, Gomez-Navarro J, et al: Genetic modification of liver grafts with an adenoviral vector encoding the Bcl-2 gene improves organ preservation. Transplantation 67: 775-783, 1999.

25. Yamabe K, Shimizu S, Kamiike W, et al: Prevention of hypoxic liver cell necrosis by in vivo human bcl-2 gene transfection. Biochem Biophys Res Commun 243:217-223, 1998.

26. Ngan BY, Chen-Levy Z, Weiss LM, et al: Expression in non-Hodgkin's lymphoma of the bcl-2 protein associated with the t(14;18) chromosomal translocation. N Engl J Med 318:1638-1644, 1988.

27. Matzinger P: The danger model: A renewed sense of self. Science 296:301-305, 2002.

28. Jenkins MK, Chen CA, Jung G, et al: Inhibition of antigen-specific proliferation of type 1 murine T-cell clones after stimulation with immobilized anti-CD3 monoclonal antibody. J Immunol 144: 16-22, 1990.

29. Jonuleit H, Schmitt E, Schuler G, et al: Induction of interleukin 10-producing, non-proliferating CD4+ T cells with regulatory properties by repetitive stimulation with allogeneic immature human dendritic cells. J Exp Med 192:1213-1222, 2000.

30. Min WP, Gorczynski T, Huang XY, et al: Dendritic cells genetically engineered to express Fas ligand induce donor-specific hyporesponsiveness and prolong allograft survival. J Immunol 164:161-167, 2000.

31. O'Rourke RW, Kang SM, Lower JA, et al: A dendritic cell line genetically modified to express CTLA4-Ig as a means to prolong islet allograft survival. Transplantation 69:1440-1446, 2000.

32. Coates PT, Krishnan R, Kireta S, et al: Human myeloid dendritic cells transduced with an adenoviral interleukin-10 gene construct inhibit human skin graft rejection in humanized NOD-scid chimeric mice. Gene Ther 8:1224-1233, 2001.

33. Gorczynski RM, Bransom J, Cattral M, et al: Synergy in induction of increased renal allograft survival after portal vein infusion of dendritic cells transduced to express TGF-beta and IL-10, along with administration of CHO cells expressing the regulatory molecule OX-2. Clin Immunol 95:182-189, 2000.

34. Ildstad ST, Sachs DH: Reconstitution with syngeneic plus allogeneic or xenogeneic bone marrow leads to specific acceptance of allografts or xenografts. Nature 307:168-170, 1984.

35. Tian C, Bagley J, Iacomini J: Expression of antigen on mature lymphocytes is required to induce T cell tolerance by gene therapy. J Immunol 179:3771-3776, 2002.

36. Fry JW, Morris PJ, Wood KJ: Adenoviral transfer of a single donor-specific MHC class I gene to recipient bone marrow cells can induce specific immunological unresponsiveness in vivo. Gene Ther 9:220-226, 2002.

37. Melo ME, Qian J, El-Amine M, et al: Gene transfer of Ig-fusion proteins into B cells prevents and treats autoimmune diseases. J Immunol 168:4788-4795, 2002.

38. Nguyen P, Geiger TL: Antigen-specific targeting of CD8+ T cells with receptor-modified T lymphocytes. Gene Ther 10:594-604, 2003.

Xenotransplantation and the Liver*

JEFFREY L. PLATT

IRA J. FOX

Rationale for xenotransplantation   1366

Source of organs   1366

Applications of xenotransplantation
of the liver   1367
　Orthotopic liver transplantation   1367
　Auxiliary (or heterotopic) liver
　　transplantation   1367
　Hepatocyte transplantation   1368
　Ex vivo perfusion and hepatic assist
　　devices   1368

Hurdles to xenotransplantation of the liver   1369

Immunological hurdles to
xenotransplantation   1369
　Hyperacute rejection   1369
　Acute vascular rejection   1371
　Antibody depletion and
　　accommodation   1371
　Cellular rejection   1372
　Formation of immune complexes   1372
　Sensitization   1372

Physiological hurdles to
xenotransplantation   1372
　Infection   1373

Benefits and barriers to liver perfusion and liver
assist devices   1373

Concluding remarks on the prospects for
xenotransplantation of the liver   1374

A severe shortage of human livers for allotransplantation has sparked interest in the potential use of animals in lieu of humans as a source of livers—that is, xenotransplantation. Xenotransplantation might also provide a means by which recurrence of hepatitis might be averted. Among the types of xenografts that might be undertaken are extracorporeal "xenoperfusion" or perfusion of devices containing xenogeneic hepatocytes, auxiliary liver transplants, bridge liver transplants, and hepatocyte transplants. The hurdles to xenotransplantation of the liver include the immune response of the recipient against the graft, incompatibility of the graft with complex physiological and biochemical systems of the recipient, and the possibility of transferring infectious agents from the graft to the recipient. Recent progress in characterizing and overcoming these hurdles has encouraged some optimism regarding the ultimate application of xenotransplantation for the treatment of human disease.

Organ transplantation is the preferred therapy for patients with irreversible failure of the liver, kidneys, pancreas, heart, and lungs. Although some patients with hepatic failure may recover, many die while waiting for an organ transplant, making the shortage of human organs and tissues the most pressing problem in transplantation today. In 2002, 6076 waiting-list individuals

*Work in the authors' laboratories is supported by grants from the National Institutes of Health (HL52297 and AI49472).

died—approximately 10% of patients waiting for organ transplants in the United States. Of 16,929 individuals waiting for liver transplants, 1756 died. Put another way: 5325 liver transplants were performed in the United States in 2002; one third as many patients died as underwent transplantation.[1] In addition, the problem is not getting better; the percentage of those waiting for transplants who die is increasing.[2] Those at particular risk of death are young children and adults with acute liver failure who require immediate transplantation. Although the need for liver transplantation will decrease with improvements in the care of patients with liver disease, particularly hepatitis C, a more comprehensive solution to the problem will require the development of artificial organs or the development of another source of organs for transplantation. The use of animals as a source of organs and tissues for transplantation, called *xenotransplantation,* is thus a way that transplantation can realize its full potential as an approach to treating human disease. This chapter reviews the various ways that xenotransplantation can be used to treat hepatic disease and the obstacles barring such use.

Rationale for Xenotransplantation

The primary rationale for xenotransplantation is to address the shortage of human livers for transplantation. Beyond this reason, however, xenotransplantation offers several other advantages. First, xenotransplantation offers a potential way to avoid recurrence of the disease that caused failure of the autogenous organ. Thus, xenotransplantation might be used to address liver failure caused by hepatitis B or hepatitis C, as these viruses would inevitably infect and might destroy a human liver transplant but evidently do not infect animal livers.[3,4] To avert such reinfection and because donors are limited, Starzl and colleagues[5,6] transplanted the livers of baboons into patients with hepatitis.

As a second potential advantage, animals might be used as a source of hepatocytes for treatment of a metabolic defect. Some metabolic defects, such as Crigler-Najjar syndrome type 1 and severe familial hypercholesterolemia, have been treated by transplantation of the whole liver,[7] even though the structure and most functions of the native liver are intact. These defects might instead be treated by hepatocyte transplantation, leaving the native liver in place to provide all other functions. Such an approach using human hepatocytes has been reported.[8,9] Because human livers are in short supply, some authors advocate the use of xenogeneic hepatocytes for this purpose.[10]

The third potential advantage of xenotransplantation is that it might offer a means of gene delivery that could overcome some of the current hurdles to gene therapy.[11,12] In animals such as pigs, but not in humans, genetic material can be introduced into the nucleus of the fertilized egg and become incorporated into the genome of the egg. The transgenic animal derived from that egg and suitably bred progeny may express the transgene, potentially in all cells, and thus the gene product can be delivered by transplanting xenogeneic cells (or organs). As an extension of this method of gene delivery, targeted changes can be made in the genomic DNA of cultured cells (such changes might include knocking genes out or substituting genes) and the nucleus of cultured cells can be transferred by various means to an enucleated egg. Such a transfer, called *cloning,* can be used to produce a line of animals with known changes in genetic material,[13-15] including expression of transgenes. Those cells or organs might then be transplanted as a means of gaining expression of the gene. These technologies are discussed subsequently.

Source of Organs

The most suitable species to use as a source of xenografts is believed to be a nonhuman primate such as the chimpanzee or baboon. In the early 1960s, Reemtsma[16] transplanted a series of chimpanzee kidneys into patients with renal failure, and in the early 1990s, Starzl[5] transplanted baboon livers into two patients with liver failure. The renal and liver xenografts maintained the survival of patients for up to 9 months. However, enthusiasm for using nonhuman primates as a source of organs for xenotransplantation has waned in recent years for several reasons. First, the number of nonhuman primates, especially of a size suitable to provide organs for adult humans, is limited. Although a chimpanzee or baboon might provide a liver of a size suitable for infants or children, the size of the baboon (a baboon generally weighs less than 20 kg) is too small for its liver to be optimal for many adults. Second, nonhuman primates may harbor viruses, such as the herpes viruses, which could be lethal if transmitted to humans. Nonhuman primates might also harbor retroviruses, some of which are incompletely characterized.[17] Third, current technology for genetic manipulation would be difficult to undertake in primates, and the use of nonhuman primates as a source of livers for xenotransplantation might provoke social opposition.

Because of the problems listed previously, most investigators today focus on using lower mammals, particularly pigs, as a source of organs and tissues for xenotransplantation. One such reason for focusing on the pig is that these animals are available in large numbers and the organs are of suitable size for use in large adult patients. Another reason for focusing on pigs is that these animals present a relatively limited risk of zoonosis, and the liver of a pig may resist infection by agents that cause viral hepatitis. A third reason for favoring the use of pigs as a source of organs for xenotransplantation is that pigs can be genetically engineered.[18,19]

Applications of Xenotransplantation of the Liver

Xenogeneic livers might be used in various ways to treat diseases of the liver. The potential applications of xenogeneic livers are discussed briefly in the following sections.

Orthotopic Liver Transplantation

Orthotopic allotransplantation of the liver is the most effective treatment for hepatic failure. The indications for orthotopic liver transplantation include acute and chronic liver failure, metabolic liver diseases, and unresectable malignant tumors.[20,21] Liver allotransplantation is occasionally performed for a variety of metabolic disorders, including Crigler-Najjar syndrome, ornithine transcarbamylase deficiency, and familial homozygous hypercholesterolemia.[21] The indications for orthotopic liver xenotransplantation may be similar to those for allotransplantation. However, additional indications might include temporary transplantation as a bridge for certain patients awaiting a human liver allograft and as a transplant that would avert reinfection by hepatitis viruses.[22]

There have been 12 cases of clinical orthotopic liver xenotransplantation since 1966,[23-25] including 4 cases of chimpanzee-to-human, 7 cases of baboon-to-human, and 1 case of pig-to-human xenografts (Table 84–1). The chimpanzee-to-human xenografts functioned for only 1 to 9 days, perhaps limited more by the surgical, medical, and immunosuppressive therapies available in that era than by the biology of the graft. The more recent cases were two patients with hepatic failure caused by hepatitis B who received liver xenografts from baboons that functioned for 26 days and 70 days without evidence of reinfection by hepatitis virus.[5,36,37]

Although nonhuman primate livers have been used with some success, use of lower mammals such as the pig as a source of livers for xenotransplantation also provokes controversy. Most concern has been voiced about the possibility that such organs could convey zoonotic agents to the recipients, although, as discussed further on, there is no evidence that infectious agents have been passed from pigs to humans in the course of ex vivo liver perfusion.[38] Also of concern is the possibility that the products secreted by a

Table 84-1. ATTEMPTS AT CLINICAL LIVER XENOTRANSPLANTATION

Year	Donor	Type	Survival days	Reference
1966	Chimpanzee	Heterotopic	<1	26
1969	Chimpanzee	Orthotopic	9	27
	Chimpanzee	Orthotopic	<2	25
1969	Baboon	Heterotopic	<1	28
1970	Baboon	Heterotopic	3	29
1970	Baboon	Heterotopic	<1	30, 31
1971	Baboon	Heterotopic	<1	32
1971	Baboon	Heterotopic	3	33
1974	Chimpanzee	Orthotopic	14	24
1992	Baboon	Orthotopic	70	5, 22, 34
1993	Baboon	Orthotopic	26	22, 34
1993	Pig	Heterotopic	<2	30, 35

Adapted from Taniguchi S, Cooper DKC: Clinical xenotransplantation: A brief review of the world experience. In Cooper DKC, Kemp E, Platt JL, White DJG (eds): Xenotransplantation: The Transplantation of Organs Between Species. Berlin: Springer, 1997, p 779, with permission.

xenogeneic liver would inadequately replace human products and that components of complex cascades of enzymes, such as coagulation and complement systems secreted by xenogeneic livers, might actually cause systemic pathophysiology.[3,12,39] Although such incompatibilities may be unavoidable, the limited clinical and experimental evidence suggests that the incompatibilities may not pose an absolute barrier to success. Makowka and colleagues[40] transplanted a porcine liver as a heterotopic auxiliary graft into a patient with fulminant decompensation of autoimmune hepatitis. Although metabolic function of the porcine graft was reported, the patient died of neurological complications 34 hours later. Calne and coworkers[41,42] and Martinez and colleagues[43] reported that orthotopic porcine liver xenografts can provide life-supporting hepatic function for a period of days.

Auxiliary (or Heterotopic) Liver Transplantation

Auxiliary, or heterotopic, liver transplantations are accomplished by inserting the graft beside, or in continuity with, the recipient's own liver.[20] This operation is usually performed for patients with fulminant or subfulminant hepatic failure, but is not routinely performed for metabolic liver diseases,[44,45] as auxiliary liver transplantation in this setting requires banding of the portal vein to prevent shunting of portal blood away from the graft. The purpose of these transplants is to retain the native liver in case of graft failure or spontaneous recovery or for future gene therapy. Auxiliary liver transplantation,[23] including the most recent pig-to-human transplant,[40] is clearly feasible but is technically difficult. What may limit application as much as the technical hurdles is that the number of human livers available for this purpose is limited. Auxiliary transplantation by using an expendable liver, such as a xenograft, might enable the treatment of metabolic diseases, leaving the native liver to carry out most physiological functions.[45] With the clinical outcome of xenotransplantation of the liver still uncertain, for reasons discussed in subsequent paragraphs, auxiliary transplantation of the xenogeneic liver might also be an early step in evaluating the feasibility of clinical xenotransplantation.

Hepatocyte Transplantation

Another approach to liver xenotransplantation involves transplantation of isolated hepatocytes into the recipient's liver or spleen. One especially compelling indication for hepatocyte transplants might be in the treatment of metabolic diseases of the liver. In this case, the structure and most functions of the native hepatic parenchyma are normal; the hepatocytes are needed for only limited purposes. For example, in 1998, Fox and colleagues[8] and Lake[46] reported the treatment of the Crigler-Najjar syndrome type I by hepatocyte allotransplantation.

The main barrier to hepatocyte transplantation is finding a source of the large number of hepatocytes needed for the procedure. Allogeneic hepatocytes might be obtained from donors who are unsuitable for providing whole-liver transplants. Ideally, isolated human hepatocytes might be stored and used as needed.[47] However, human hepatocytes obtained for this purpose may survive and function poorly. At best, function in the new environment may not be optimal until days have elapsed. Another potential limitation is that the anatomic positioning of the cells may not permit optimal secretion of bile. However, recent reports on intrasplenic use of rat and porcine hepatocytes to reverse chronic liver failure in rats would suggest that this type of transplant could be used for short periods to enhance survival.[48-50]

Xenotransplantation of hepatocytes would overcome the problem of limited availability and questionable quality of human cells and might obviate the need for preservation. Presumably, xenogeneic hepatocytes could be available when needed. Another important advantage of hepatocyte xenotransplantation is that animal sources could be genetically engineered to express needed enzymes or receptors at high levels. Another advantage is that the immune hurdles to hepatocyte xenotransplantation are less than those to whole-liver transplantation, and a further decrease in such hurdles might be achieved by encapsulation of the cells. Still another advantage may be the opportunity to use fetal cells, if such cells are needed.

Possible applications of hepatocyte xenotransplantation have been explored in experimental models. Gunsalus and colleagues[10] showed that porcine hepatocytes introduced into the liver of Watanabe rabbits, which have a genetic defect in low-density lipoprotein (LDL) receptors causing severe hypercholesterolemia, brings about a substantial lowering of blood cholesterol. Other potential applications were recently reviewed.[51,52] The major barrier to hepatocyte xenotransplantation may be the incompatibility of secreted donor proteins with proteins of the recipient.[53]

Ex Vivo Perfusion and Hepatic Assist Devices

The perfusion of blood through intact livers and through hepatic assist devices has gained attention in recent years as potential approaches to treatment of fulminant hepatic failure and exacerbation of chronic liver disease. Although the use of such procedures is not transplantation, the indications, limitations, and risks of such treatments have a bearing on transplantation, warranting brief consideration here.

Perfusion of intact livers has been carried out for decades with only limited success[54]; however, recent advances in perfusion technologies, including the ability to oxygenate the perfused blood, has allowed the procedure to be applied with lower risk and, perhaps, greater efficacy.[55,56] We have successfully supported patients with fulminant hepatic failure for up to 8 days by using ex vivo perfusion of porcine livers.[55,57] The livers continuously secreted bile; however, even the best results using extracorporeal liver perfusion are not equal to that of liver transplantation for several possible reasons. Components of the circuitry, including membranes, filters, tubings and so on, may activate leukocytes, leading to cytokine release. Function of the perfused organs may be limited by inflammatory and immune reactions.[58,59] Finally, perfusion of the extracorporeal organ with systemic, rather than portal, blood may prevent optimal hepatic function.

An appealing alternative to the use of intact livers is the perfusion of a device containing hepatocytes encased in a permeable membrane. A number of such devices have been described, among them being a porcine hepatocyte–based "bioartificial liver."[60] The advantage of liver perfusion or the use of bioartificial liver systems is that either can, in principle, be applied immediately and require little surgical manipulation of the patient. Another advantage is that neither commits the patient to transplantation and immunosuppression, should there be the possibility of recovery of the patient's native liver.[61] Whether bioartificial devices can function as well as the perfused, intact liver and whether devices can replace hepatic function for prolonged periods is still unclear. Controlled trials using bioartificial livers containing porcine hepatocytes have not revealed definitive improvement in survival of treated patients over conventional intensive care. However, improvements in the design of these devices may yield better results.[62]

Hurdles to Xenotransplantation of the Liver

Although xenotransplantation of the liver or hepatocytes would address significant needs, it is prevented by significant hurdles. These hurdles include the immunological response of the recipient to the liver or liver cells, leading to the destruction of foreign cells; the inherent limitation of the xenogeneic liver or the device to restore the physiological status in the treated patient; and the possibility of transferring infectious agents from the perfused liver or device to the treated patient and, potentially, beyond. Subsequent text describes the potential applications of xenotransplantation for the treatment of liver disease and the factors that stand as a barrier to this and other related types of therapy.

To a large extent, the nature and severity of these hurdles depends on the type of transplant used.[63] The biological properties of xenografts are determined, in part, by the way in which the graft is connected with the circulation of the recipient and by the origin of the microenvironment surrounding donor cells. Because whole-organ transplants are carried out by primary anastomosis of donor and recipient blood vessels, the vascular system consists entirely of donor blood vessels. The interaction of the host immune system with donor blood vessels gives rise to a series of rejection responses, which are depicted in Figure 84–1A. These responses constitute a severe barrier to xenotransplantation and will be discussed in detail subsequently. Conversely, whole-organ xenografts have the advantage of providing their own microenvironment. The hepatocytes are situated in proper orientation and in apposition to appropriate extracellular matrix. Thus, an intact organ can function nearly immediately on transplantation and is not constrained by incompatibilities between parenchymal cells and the microenvironment. Grafts of isolated cells, such as hepatocytes, derive their vascular supply and microenvironment from the recipient. The recipient blood vessels, particularly the endothelial lining of blood vessels, pose a barrier between the immune system of the recipient and the transplanted cells. Because of this barrier, the types of rejection observed resemble more closely the types of

rejection seen in allotransplants, and the severity is much less than the severity of whole-organ xenografts (see Fig. 84–1B). Conversely, the dependence of hepatocyte transplants on the microenvironment of the recipient poses a severe hurdle to normal functioning of the cells. Hepatocytes may survive and function poorly in a foreign microenvironment because cells are not provided with the growth factors and extracellular matrix components needed.

The risk of infectious disease may also vary with the type of transplant used. Patients treated by using xenoperfusion or with hepatic assist devices are not generally subjected to immunosuppression and are treated only transiently. Therefore, the risk of infection is generally perceived to be lower than that in the organ transplant recipient.

Immunological Hurdles to Xenotransplantation

All foreign transplants, particularly xenografts, would appear to provoke an immune response.[64] This response includes humoral- and cell-mediated immunity. What happens as a consequence of this response depends very much on the nature of the graft, that is, whether the graft consists of isolated cells such as hepatocytes or tissues on the one hand or intact organs such as the whole liver on the other. Unfortunately, few studies have been conducted on hepatocyte and whole-liver xenotransplantation; therefore, much of what follows must be inferred from experiences with experimental xenotransplantation of the heart and kidney. Figure 84–1 shows a model for the immunological hurdles to xenotransplantation of vascularized organs.

Hyperacute Rejection

Porcine hearts and kidneys transplanted into primates and, perhaps, into humans are subject to hyperacute rejection.[65] The histopathological features of hyperacute rejection include interstitial hemorrhage and thrombosis, the thrombi consisting largely of platelets. Hyperacute rejection of renal and cardiac xenografts is initiated by the binding of xenoreactive natural antibodies, mainly immunoglobulin (Ig)M, to the endothelial cells of blood vessels in the transplanted organ.[66] These xenoreactive natural antibodies can be found in the blood of all immunocompetent individuals without a known history of sensitization. In humans, Old World monkeys, and apes, xenoreactive natural antibodies predominantly recognize Galα1-3Gal, a sugar expressed on the cells of lower mammals.[67] Antibodies binding to Galα1-3Gal activate the complement system, and it is complement that mediates hyperacute rejection.

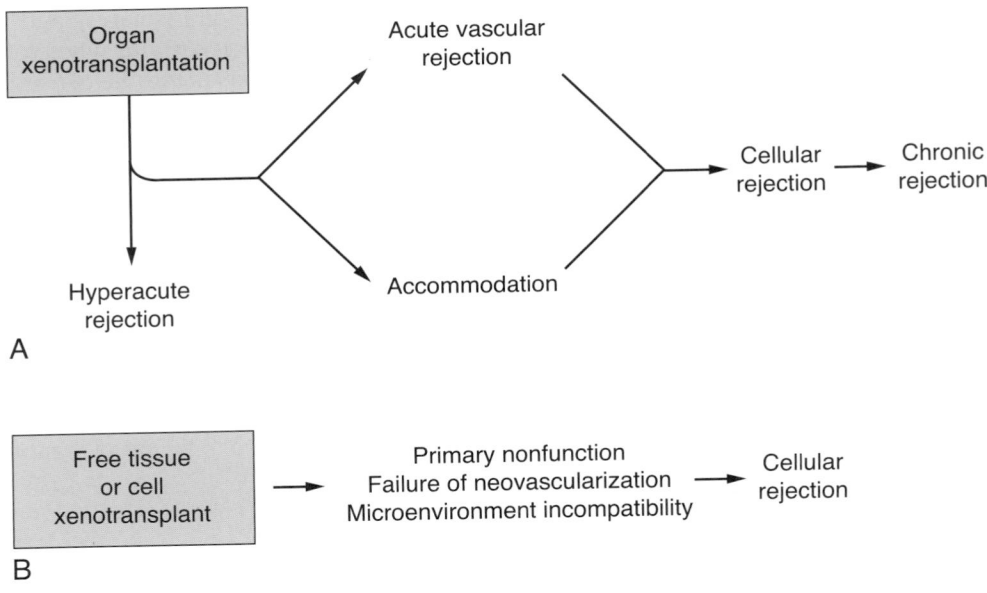

FIGURE 84–1

Biological hurdles for xenotransplantation. **A,** Organ transplantation between unmodified disparate species leads to hyperacute rejection. If hyperacute rejection is averted by depletion of xenoreactive natural antibodies or inhibition of the complement system, the xenograft may be subject to acute vascular rejection or "accommodation" may occur. If acute vascular rejection is prevented, the graft will be subject to cellular rejection or chronic rejection. **B,** Tissue or cell xenotransplants are subject to failure caused by primary nonfunction that may reflect failure of engraftment or a very rapid immune response. If primary nonfunction is bypassed and the tissue or cells engraft, they are then subject to cellular rejection. Humoral rejection is not usually considered a hurdle to cell transplantation because the blood vessels of recipient origin hinder humoral elements from reaching the graft. However, small amounts of antidonor antibodies and complement might, in principle, impair graft function. (Adapted from Nagayasu T, Platt JL: Progress in xenotransplantation. Graft 1:19-24, 1998.)

Liver xenografts may be less susceptible than kidney or heart xenografts to hyperacute rejection. The basis for such lower susceptibility to hyperacute rejection is uncertain. Some have suggested that livers may be intrinsically resistant to complement-mediated injury.[55] Consistent with this concept was the finding of Calne and colleagues[41,42] that hyperacute rejection did not occur in a series of pig livers transplanted into baboons; rather, the orthotopic liver xenografts functioned for a day or more. In the clinical setting, an important factor in decreasing susceptibility to hyperacute rejection may be the lower levels of complement found in patients with hepatic failure.[58] In a series of porcine livers perfused by the blood of human subjects with fulminant hepatic failure, we observed that the treated patients had very low or undetectable levels of complement in the blood, and small amounts of complement deposition was observed in the perfused porcine livers.[58] The livers did undergo hemorrhagic changes that bear resemblance to hyperacute rejection; however, in the absence of complement, these changes must reflect some process other than hyperacute rejection. Further, although livers may resist hyperacute rejection, hyperacute rejection can be induced in experimental models.[68,69]

A special example of hyperacute rejection may be the immune and inflammatory reactions that occur in livers perfused by human blood for treatment of acute hepatic failure, as discussed previously. In naïve experimental animals, xenogeneic perfusion has been associated with thrombosis and severe fibrin deposition on the endothelium of the perfused organ.[70] This thrombotic reaction may be initiated by components of the device but also may result from incompatibility between human coagulation proteins and the xenogeneic cells.[71] For example, we have found that human thrombin and protein C are incompatible with porcine thrombomodulin.[72]

If hyperacute rejection were to pose a serious hurdle to xenotransplantation of the liver, there are methods that can effectively avert this process. These methods include depletion of xenoreactive natural antibodies[73] and inhibition of complement activation.[74] Inhibition of complement activation can be achieved by administration of complement inhibitors, such as cobra venom factor,[74] soluble complement receptor type I,[75] and gamma globulin[76]; all of these approaches prevent hyperacute rejection of cardiac or renal xenografts and allow graft function for days. The safest and most effective way to prevent hyperacute rejection, however, is to express human complement regulatory proteins, such as decay accelerating factor (DAF), which inhibits complement at the levels of C3 and CD59, which then inhibits complement at the levels of C8 and C9 in the transplant.[77] Expression of human complement regulatory proteins can be achieved by developing transgenic pigs through microinjection of DNA constructs into fertilized eggs.[78] Expression of even very low levels of DAF and CD59 are sufficient to prevent hyperacute rejection[79-81] and allow graft function for days to weeks. The reason transgenic organs have proved so successful is that they overcome incompatibility of complement regulation between species.[77,82] These results not only underscore the importance of complement dysregulation as a pathogenetic factor in xenotransplantation but also point to a useful strategy for protecting the graft against complement-mediated injury.

Although porcine hearts and kidneys expressing human complement regulatory proteins may resist the most devastating manifestations of vascular rejection, this approach may have certain limitations in the transplantation of porcine livers. One limitation may turn out to be porcine complement secreted by porcine hepatocytes. These "heterologous" complement components might cause damage to recipient tissues owing to the lack of species-specific control of complement activation. Another limitation is that a pig liver, transgenic for human complement regulatory proteins, might interfere with the ability of porcine complement regulatory proteins to inhibit pig complement deposited in the xenograft.

Some investigators have focused on inhibiting or reducing the expression of the galα1-3 gal antigen as an approach to preventing hyperacute rejection.[83] By using homologous recombination in embryonic stem cells, the gene for α1,3-galactosyl transferase, which catalyzes synthesis of Galα1-3Gal, has been knocked out.[84] Recently, the same gene in pigs has also been knocked out. Thus, homologous recombination was carried out in cultured cells and the nuclei of the cells were transferred to enucleated eggs, a procedure that leads to cloning.[13-15] However, it is not yet known whether eradication of antigen expression will prevent hyperacute rejection.[85]

Acute Vascular Rejection

When hyperacute rejection of cardiac and renal xenografts is averted, the xenograft becomes susceptible to acute vascular rejection,[86] so named because of its resemblance to acute vascular rejection of allografts.[87] Acute vascular rejection may be the first type of rejection seen in orthotopic liver xenotransplants across humoral barriers, such as those posed by blood group antigens.[88] The typical histological features of acute vascular rejection, sometimes called *delayed xenograft rejection*, include endothelial swelling, ischemia, and diffuse intravascular thrombosis (the thrombi consisting primarily of fibrin). These histological features are similar to those of acute vascular rejection of allografts.

Acute vascular rejection of xenografts and allografts is usually triggered by the binding of antidonor antibodies to the graft.[89,90] In addition, antidonor antibodies and other factors, such as complement activation, natural killer cells, and inflammatory cells, have been thought to play a pathogenetic role in acute vascular rejection.[91,92] What is critical to understanding acute vascular rejection and to developing therapeutic strategies is the finding that depletion of antidonor antibodies can delay or prevent acute vascular rejection.[90] Thus, what appears most critical is the antibody-antigen reaction that initiates the rejection process.

Overcoming acute vascular rejection is currently a major objective in the field of xenotransplantation. Three approaches would seem to hold some promise: (1) transient depletion of antidonor antibodies, allowing development of accommodation; (2) induction of immunological tolerance; and (3) genetic engineering to decrease expression of donor antigen.

Antibody Depletion and Accommodation

When acute vascular rejection is temporarily averted, a state of accommodation may occur in which a graft seems to be protected from humoral reactions with the antidonor antibodies present in the circulation.[77] This condition was first observed in ABO-incompatible kidney allografts[93,94] when anti–blood group antibodies were depleted from the blood of transplant recipients and prolonged survival of allografts was observed, despite the return of antidonor antibodies to the circulation and the presence of an intact complement system. Accommodation and graft function for years are now routinely achieved in ABO-incompatible renal allografts.[95]

The means by which accommodation prevents humoral injury to organ transplants is unclear. Accommodation arises as a result of a change in the properties of antidonor antibodies, a change in the antigen, or an acquired resistance of blood vessels to humoral injury. Many now believe that accommodation results from expression of genes, such as heme oxygenase-1 or CD59, which seem to protect grafts from humoral injury, either by preventing apoptosis[96] or complement-mediated injury.[97,98]

Accommodation has been observed in experimental xenografts. Depletion of recipient Ig during the days following xenotransplantation of porcine hearts expressing human DAF and CD59 allowed accommodation and, thus, weeks to greater than a month of graft survival with little tissue injury to be achieved.[90,99] Efforts are under way in various laboratories to facilitate accommodation by inducing genes, such as heme oxygenase-1, that help tissues resist injury.[96,100]

Cellular Rejection

When hyperacute and acute vascular rejection are averted, xenografts become subject to cell-mediated rejection. In allotransplantation, cell-mediated rejection is controlled by immunosuppressive therapy. It is still unknown whether cell-mediated responses in xenografts might be more severe and less responsive to immunosuppressive therapy. The intensity of this immune response may reflect several factors, including the wide variety of foreign antigens expressed in the graft, the amplifying effects of a humoral response, and especially antibodies that might be elicited against foreign proteins. The cellular immune response and its impact on liver xenografts have not been studied in detail. Work in allografts suggests that although hepatocytes can elicit immune responses[101,102] the cellular response selectively targets the bile ducts and vessels. This concept is consistent with our own experience in the transplantation of xenogeneic hepatocytes, that is, the hepatocytes elicit a response but are relatively resistant to cell-mediated injury.[50]

Given the potential strength of the T-cell response to xenotransplantation and the potential importance of elicited antibodies, some have suggested that the success of xenotransplantation may depend on the generation of immunological tolerance.[103] One approach to this end may involve transplanting bone marrow of donor origin.[103,104] The transplanted bone marrow may cause apoptosis of donor-reactive T-cell precursors in the thymus or mature T cells in the periphery, or it may inhibit responses by mature donor-reactive T cells. Another strategy may involve the transplantation of donor thymus tissue, which helps fashion a T-cell repertoire that does not react with cells of donor origin.[105] How effective these or other strategies would be in bridging the immunological barrier to transplanting porcine organs into humans is not known, as enduring transplantation of porcine hematopoietic cells in non-human primates has not been achieved.

Another aspect of the cellular immune response in xenotransplantation involves the potential importance of natural killer cells, which are "naturally" activated lymphocytes that can destroy foreign cells and tumor cells. Natural killer cells accumulate in xenografts and, for various reasons, may exhibit a high level of cytotoxicity for xenogeneic cells.[106] The relative importance of natural killer cell–mediated injury is yet to be determined; however, these cells are curiously absent from many vascularized xenografts.

Conversely, the liver would seem to exhibit immunosuppression properties not manifested by other organs.[107] To the extent that these properties are manifested across species, the need for extraordinary measures to control T-cell responses may be correspondingly reduced.

Formation of Immune Complexes

Another immunological hurdle to xenotransplantation may be the formation of immune complexes, owing to humoral reaction with proteins or carbohydrates secreted from the graft. Immune complexes may form when antibodies in the blood of the treated patient bind material secreted by the transplanted organ or cells or by the perfused organ or device. These responses may generate inflammatory mediators that can injure the transplant. In addition to this effect, the immune complexes may incite systemic injury to the treated patient. We have recently reported that immune complexes can form following organ xenotransplantation,[108] and it is highly likely that such complexes will form from the products secreted by foreign hepatocytes. In the case of lung xenotransplants, the major immune reaction involves recognition of Galα1-3Gal by foreign antibodies. Combination of natural antibodies with Galα1-3Gal is also likely to be the dominant reaction when liver perfusion is first applied in a given patient. Because the individuals treated by hepatic assist or liver perfusion may not be immunosuppressed, it is likely that sensitization to foreign proteins will also occur, allowing the formation of other types of immune complexes with repeated treatments. Other protein-protein interactions, such as the reaction of porcine von Willebrand factor with human platelet Ib receptors, could lead to medical complications, such as thrombocytopenia, and need to be considered as potential hazards.

Sensitization

Another category of immune response to the transplant that could pose a hurdle to the application of xenotransplantation is sensitization of the patient to potential allogeneic donors. Thus, the immune response to antigens carried by the xenograft, such as swine histocompatibility antigens, might cross-react with human alloantigens such as human leukocyte antigen (HLA). Should cross-reactive responses occur, xenotransplantation or hepatic assist devices or liver perfusion could erect a hurdle to subsequent allotransplantation.

Physiological Hurdles to Xenotransplantation

Progress in addressing some of the immune obstacles to xenotransplantation has now brought into focus questions as to what extent xenografts can function in different species. Preliminary studies indicate that the kidney of a pig can provide a physiological replacement for a human kidney and that the porcine heart and lungs may be capable of providing hemodynamic and pulmonary support, respectively, in primates.[109,110] However, there may be defects in physiology across species, especially defects in the function of the liver, which will preclude normal physiology. One potential problem is that some protein-protein reactions between species do not function well.[92] We previously found that human thrombin and protein C are incompatible with porcine thrombomodulin, leading to a defect in the generation of activated protein C and, thus, potentially to a thrombotic diathesis.[72] In a reversed situation, it is reasonable to believe that porcine thrombin and protein C might be incompatible with human thrombomodulin. Porcine complement proteins, expressed by the liver, might also prove incompatible with the complement inhibitory proteins expressed on recipient human cells, thereby making those cells susceptible to complement-mediated injury.[111] Beyond these concerns is the possibility that more subtle defects will pose a relative hurdle. For example, Donato and colleagues[112] observed vitamin B_{12} deficiency in long-term (1-year) hepatic xenografts between monkeys and baboons. Conversely, porcine livers have proved capable of addressing the most severe manifestations of liver failure.[55,113] Therefore, many of the physiological differences between humans and pigs may be relative rather than absolute hurdles. Further, xenograft function might be improved through genetic engineering to correct specific molecular defects.

Infection

Successful allotransplantation requires a balance between immunosuppression, which is necessary to maintain graft function, and the risks associated with opportunistic infectious diseases and tumors. In xenotransplantation, similar or perhaps more rigorous immunosuppression might be required than in allotransplantation and, therefore, the risk of opportunistic infection will be the same or higher. In addition, the porcine graft may carry unusual infectious organisms to which the recipient might not otherwise be exposed at such high levels. As a result, another hurdle to the success of xenotransplantation becomes the potential transmission of infectious agents from the graft to the recipient. Despite these problems, the risks associated with infection may, in principle, be lower in xenotransplantation than in allotransplantation because it is possible in xenotransplantation to screen the donor for infectious agents and eliminate those agents from the sources of transplants.

There still remains concern about the possible transmission of certain microbial agents into the recipient. Patience and colleagues[114] showed that a C-type retrovirus, endogenous to the pig, could be activated in pig cells, which leads to the release of particles that can infect human cell lines. Nyberg and coworkers[115] found that, depending on porcine size, devices containing porcine hepatocytes might also release porcine endogenous retrovirus (PERV). Endogenous retroviruses, being part of the genome, cannot be eliminated by means other than genetic engineering. Concern about PERV has decreased recently, however, because studies in various clinical settings, including the study of patients whose blood was perfused through porcine livers, has failed to reveal any evidence that the virus can be transmitted to human cells in vivo.[38,116] Despite these results, rigorous follow-up is still necessary to determine whether other yet to be identified agents might pose some risk.

The risk of zoonosis, as such, is thought to be heightened for xenotransplants because the recipient of a xenotransplant has animal cells in continuity with the cells of the recipient for protracted periods and, in part, because the recipient is treated with immunosuppressive agents. These risks, however, are effaced in the case of liver perfusion and the use of hepatic assist devices because these procedures do not involve protracted contact between the cells of the animal and the cells of the recipient and because the patient would not be immunosuppressed. Thus, the condition of exposure to animal tissues in the course of xenoperfusion or the use of xeno assist devices is not substantively different from the contact that occurs between the blood of human and animal cells in the course of animal husbandry, slaughtering, and other similar conditions. Clearly, there is a finite risk of zoonosis. However, if the source of tissues and organs is suitably screened, this risk may be less than the risk attendant to exposure to pigs under occupational circumstances.

Benefits and Barriers to Liver Perfusion and Liver Assist Devices

The potential benefits and barriers to application of liver perfusion and xeno assist devices are distinct from liver xenotransplantation. These issues have been presented in detail.[117] To a large extent, the immunological features of xenotransplantation focus on the fate of the transplanted organ—the fate of the patient being, in general, inextricably linked with the fate of the organ. In contrast to this perspective, however, the issues of greatest import for the use of xenogeneic devices are not so much related to the fate of the devices as they are to the function of the device and complications experienced by the patient. The immune response of the patient to the cells in a hepatic assist device might lead, in principle, to three categories of complications. These categories shall be referred to as (1) rejection,

(2) immune complexes, and (3) sensitization. These terms do not fully describe the range of issues to be considered, but are intended, rather, to represent various problems that can be explained from the perspective of the immune system.

The permeable membrane associated with hepatic assist devices isolates the hepatocytes, to a certain extent, from the immune system of the recipient. Accordingly, the major immune reactions visited on a perfused or transplanted foreign organ would not occur in the protected barrier of the hepatic assist device. Still, some types of injury to the cells may occur, and for the purposes of this review, injury will be equated with "rejection." Although most elements of humoral immunity and, clearly, the elements of cellular immunity would be prevented from contacting the foreign cells, anaphylatoxins, the molecular weight of which is less than 10,000 kDa, generated in the vicinity of the device might well pass any membrane and alter hepatocyte function. Depending on the size of the membrane used, it is possible that some immunoglobulins could also permeate it. Some immune reactions may occur outside the device, owing to the binding of antibodies to proteins secreted from xenogeneic hepatocytes, thereby leading to engagement of the complement system. These reactions, although potentially not severe or even fatal, might add to ischemic injury caused by the limited accessibility of the foreign cells to the treated blood of the patient.

Concluding Remarks on the Prospects for Xenotransplantation of the Liver

There has been significant progress in defining the immunological hurdles to xenotransplantation, although less is known about the immunological hurdles to xenotransplantation of the liver. Of equal or greater significance than the immunological hurdles to xenotransplantation of the liver may be the physiological hurdles. Incompatibility between porcine and human proteins would seem to pose a significant barrier. The dimensions of the immunological or physiological barrier may be addressed, in part, by a careful analysis of the responses to therapy by xenoperfusion and liver assist devices. Of particular interest will be trials in which the intact porcine liver is connected to the circulation of human patients. Whether liver injury persists despite genetic manipulations already undertaken, and whether that injury is caused by the perfusion procedure itself or by mechanisms that would apply to a whole-organ transplant, are salient questions. Unlikely to be answered by this analysis, however, is the question of the elicited immune response to xenotransplantation because the patients treated with devices or liver perfusion generally do not receive immunosuppressive therapy, whereas xenotransplant recipients would receive such therapy. How well the intact porcine organ or a liver assist device is able to maintain the physiological functioning of the patient, and the extent to which proteins emitted from porcine cells interfere with the complement and coagulation cascades, will give important clues to disturbances that might arise following liver xenotransplantation.

The next logical step toward the clinical application of liver xenotransplantation might be the use of a xenogeneic auxiliary liver as a temporary means of maintaining hepatic function in patients with the prospect for recovery of liver function. Such a procedure might avoid orthotopic liver transplantation and, at the same time, offer important clues regarding the extent to which genetic manipulations and immunosuppressive therapy could control the detrimental effects of the immune system of the host on the porcine liver. Use of an auxiliary liver would also provide important information regarding infectious risks and subtle physiological defects. Despite the multiple avenues of progress during the present decade, however, it is difficult to escape the conclusion that full replacement of the human liver with an animal liver may be a more difficult undertaking than replacement of other organs. Clearly, the studies described herein will provide important insights about whether this concern or a more optimistic view is appropriate.

References

1. U.S. Department of Health and Human Services: 2001 Annual Report of the U.S. Organ Procurement and Transplantation Network and the Scientific Registry for Transplant Recipients: Transplant Data 1991-2000. Rockville, MD; United Network for Organ Sharing, Richmond, VA; University Renal Research and Education Association, Ann Arbor, MI. Accessed December 9, 2002 at: http://www.optn.org//data/annualReport.asp.
2. U.S. Department of Health and Human Services: 1999 Annual Report of the U.S. Scientific Registry of Transplant Recipients and the Organ Procurement and Transplantation Network: Transplant Data 1989-1998. (2000, February 21). Rockville, MD and Richmond, VA: HHS/HRSA/OSP/DOT and UNOS. Accesed November 10, 2001 at: http://www.unos.org/Data/anrpt_main.htm.
3. Kanazawa A, Platt JL: Prospects for xenotransplantation of the liver. Semin Liver Dis 20:511, 2000.
4. Kanai N, Platt JL: Xenotransplantation of the liver. Clin Liver Dis 4:731, 2000.
5. Starzl TE, Fung J, Tzakis A, et al: Baboon-to-human liver transplantation. Lancet 341:65, 1993.
6. Starzl TE, Valdivia LA, Murase N, et al: The biological basis of and strategies for clinical xenotransplantation. Immunol Rev 141:213, 1994.
7. Van Thiel DH, Wright HI, Fagiuoli S, Gavaler JS: Unusual indications for liver transplantation. In Busuttil RW, Klintmalm GB (eds): Transplantation of the Liver. Philadelphia, Saunders, 1996, p 151.

8. Fox IJ, Chowdhury JR, Kaufman SS, et al: Treatment of the Crigler-Najjar syndrome type I with hepatocyte transplantation. N Engl J Med 338:1422, 1998.

9. Muraca M, Gerunda G, Neri G, et al: Hepatocyte transplantation as a treatment for glycogen storage disease type 1a. Lancet 359: 317, 2002.

10. Gunsalus JR, Brady DA, Coulter SM, et al: Reduction of serum cholesterol in Watanabe rabbits by xenogeneic hepatocellular transplantation. Nat Med 3:48, 1997.

11. Blau HM, Springer, ML: Muscle-mediated gene therapy. N Engl J Med 333:1554, 1995.

12. Platt JL: New directions for organ transplantation. Nature 392(Suppl):11, 1998.

13. Dai Y, Vaught TD, Boone J, et al: Targeted disruption of the alpha1,3-galactosyltransferase gene in cloned pigs. Nat Biotechnol 20:251, 2002.

14. Lai L, Kolber-Simonds D, Park KW, et al: Production of α-1, 3-galactosyltransferase knockout pigs by nuclear transfer cloning. Science 295:1089, 2002.

15. Phelps CJ, Koike C, Vaught TD, et al: Production of alpha 1, 3-galactosyltransferase-deficient pigs. Science 299:411, 2003.

16. Reemtsma K, McCracken BH, Schlegel JU, et al: Renal heterotransplantation in man. Ann Surg 160:384, 1964.

17. Allan JS: Xenotransplantation at a crossroads: Prevention versus progress. Nat Med 2:18, 1996.

18. White D, Wallwork J: Xenografting: Probability, possibility, or pipe dream? Lancet 342:879, 1993.

19. Platt JL, Logan JS: Use of transgenic animals in xenotransplantation. Transplant Rev 10:69, 1996.

20. Kelly DA, Mayer D: Liver transplantation. In Kelly DA (ed) Diseases of the Liver and Biliary System in Children. Oxford, Blackwell Science, 1999, p 293.

21. Rosen HR, Shackeleton CR, Martin P: Indications for and timing of liver transplantation. In Martin P, Friedman LS (eds): The Medical Clinics of North America: Management of Chronic Liver Disease, vol. 80. Philadelphia, WB Saunders, 1996, p 1069.

22. Starzl TE, Tzakis A, Fung JJ, et al: Prospects of clinical xenotransplantation. Transplant Proc 26:1082, 1994.

23. Taniguchi S, Cooper DKC: Clinical xenotransplantation—a brief review of the world experience. In Cooper DKC, Kemp E, Platt JL, White DJG (eds): Xenotransplantation, 2nd ed. Berlin, Springer-Verlag, 1997, 776.

24. Starzl TE, Putnam CW, Porter KA, et al: Progress in and deterrents to orthotopic liver transplantation, with special reference to survival, resistance to hyperacute rejection, and biliary duct reconstruction. Transplant Proc 6:129, 1974.

25. Giles GR, Boehmig HJ, Amemiya H, et al: Clinical heterotransplantation of the liver. Transplant Proc 2:506, 1970.

26. Starzl TE, Marchioro TL, Faris TD, et al: Avenues of future research in homotransplantation of the liver with particular reference to hepatic supportive procedures, antilymphocyte serum, and tissue typing. Am J Surg 112:391, 1966.

27. Starzl TE: Orthotopic heterotransplantation. In Experience in Hepatic Transplantation. Philadelphia, WB Saunders, 1969, p 408.

28. Bertoye A, Essais de traitement de certaines infuggisances hepatiques graves par greffe hepatique heterlogue. Lyon Medical 222:345, 1969.

29. Leger L, Chapuis Y, Lenriot JP: Heterotopic graft of baboon liver in a patient with fulminating hepatitis. Chirurgie 96:249, 1970.

30. Marion P: Les transplantations cardiaques et les transplantations hepatiques. Lyon Medical 222:585, 1969.

31. Marion P, Bertoye A, Mikaeloff P, et al: Treatment of hepatic coma by auxiliary heterologous transplantation. Chirurgie 96:152, 1970.

32. Pouyet M, Berard P: 2 cases of true heterotopic transplantation of the baboon liver in malignant acute hepatitis. Lyon Chirurgical 67:288, 1971.

33. Motin J: Quoted in: Dubernard JM, Bonneau M, Latour M: Heterographs in primates. Villeurbanne, Fondation Merieux. 42, 1974.

34. Starzl TE, Murase N, Tzakis AG, et al: Clinical xenotransplantation. Xenotransplantation 1:3, 1994.

35. Makowka L, Wu GD, Hoffman A, et al: Immunohistopathologic lesions associated with the rejection of a pig-to-human liver xenograft. Transplant Proc 26:1074, 1994.

36. Starzl TE: Liver transplantation. Gastroenterology 112:288, 1997.

37. Fung J, Rao A, Phil D, Starzl TE: Clinical trials and projected future of liver xenotransplantation. World J Surg 21:956, 1997.

38. Paradis K, Langford G, Long Z, et al: Search for cross-species transmission of porcine endogenous retrovirus in patients treated with living pig tissue. Science 285:1236, 1999.

39. Hammer C: Physiological obstacles after xenotransplantation. Ann N Y Acad Sci 862:19, 1998.

40. Makowka L, Cramer DV, Hoffman A, et al: The use of a pig liver xenograft for temporary support of a patient with fulminant hepatic failure. Transplantation 59:1654, 1995.

41. Calne RY, White HJO, Herbertson BM, et al: Pig-to-baboon liver xenografts. Lancet 1:1176, 1968.

42. Calne RY, Davis DR, Pena JR, et al: Hepatic allografts and xenografts in primates. Lancet 1:103, 1970.

43. Martinez OM, Krams SM, Sterneck M, et al: Intragraft cytokine profile during human liver allograft rejection. Transplantation 53:449, 1992.

44. Kayler LK, Merion RM, Lee S, et al: Long-term survival after liver transplantation in children with metabolic disorders. Pediatr Transplant 6:295, 2002.

45. Rela M, Muiesan P, Vilca-Melendez H, et al: Auxiliary partial orthotopic liver transplantation for Crigler-Najjar syndrome type I. Ann Surg 229:565, 1999.

46. Lake JR: Hepatocyte transplantation. N Engl J Med 338:1463, 1998.

47. Wang X, Andersson R: Hepatocyte transplantation: a potential treatment for acute liver failure. Scand J Gastroenterol 30:193, 1995.

48. Kobayashi N, Fujiwara T, Westerman KA, et al: Prevention of acute liver failure in rats with reversibly immortalized human hepatocytes. Science 287:1258, 2000.

49. Kobayashi N, Ito M, Nakamura J, et al: Hepatocyte transplantation in rats with decompensated cirrhosis. Hepatology 31:851, 2000.

50. Nagata H, Ito M, Cai J, et al: Treatment of cirrhosis and liver failure in rats by hepatocyte xenotransplantation. Gastroenterology 124:422, 2003.

51. Hoopes CW, Platt JL: Hepatocyte transplantation: History, immunology, and potential for clinical application. Biotech Lab Int 3:11, 1998.

52. Edge ASB, Gosse ME, Dinsmore J: Xenogeneic cell therapy: Current progress and future developments in porcine cell transplantation. Cell Transplant 7:525, 1998.

53. Wakizaka Y, Miki T, Rao AS, et al: Correction of congenital hyperbilirubinemia in homozygous Gunn rats by xenotransplantation of hamster livers. Xenotransplantation 4:262, 1997.

54. Abouna GM, Kirkley JR, Hull CJ, et al: Treatment of hepatic coma by extracorporeal pig-liver perfusion. Lancet 1:64, 1969.

55. Chari RS, Collins BH, Magee JC, et al: Treatment of hepatic failure with ex vivo pig-liver perfusion followed by liver transplantation. N Engl J Med 331:234, 1994.

56. Abouna GM: Extracorporeal xenogeneic liver perfusion for the treatment of hepatic failure. In Cooper DKC, Kemp E, Platt JL, White DJG (eds): Xenotransplantation: The Transplantation of Organs and Tissues Between Species, 2nd ed. Berlin, Springer-Verlag, 1997.

57. Horslen SP, Hammel JM, Fristoe LW, et al: Extracorporeal liver perfusion using human and pig livers for acute liver failure. Transplantation 70:1472, 2000.

58. Collins BH, Chari RS, Magee JC, et al: Mechanisms of injury in porcine livers perfused with blood of humans with fulminant hepatic failure. Transplantation 58:1162, 1994.

59. Yu PB, Parker W, Everett M, et al: Immunochemical properties of anti-Galα1-3Gal after sensitization with xenogeneic tissues. J Clin Immunol 19:116, 1999.

60. Watanabe FD, Mullon CJ, Hewitt WR, et al: Clinical experience with a bioartificial liver in the treatment of severe liver failure. A phase I clinical trial. Ann Surg 225:484, 1997.

61. Bismuth H, Figueiro J, Samuel D: What should we expect from a bioartificial liver in fulminant hepatic failure? Artif Organs 22:26, 1998.

62. Busse B, Gerlach JC: Bioreactors for hybrid liver support: historical aspects and novel designs. Ann N Y Acad Sci 875:326, 1999.

63. Cascalho M, Platt JL: Xenotransplantation and other means of organ replacement. Nat Rev Immunol 1:154, 2001.

64. Cascalho M, Platt JL: The immunological barrier to xenotransplantation. Immunity 14:437, 2001.

65. Platt JL: Hyperacute xenograft rejection. Medical Intelligence Unit. RG Landes, Austin, TX, 1995.

66. Platt JL, Fischel RJ, Matas AJ, et al: Immunopathology of hyperacute xenograft rejection in a swine-to-primate model. Transplantation 52:214, 1991.

67. Galili U, Clark MR, Shohet SB, et al: Evolutionary relationship between the natural anti-Gal antibody and the Galα1-3Gal epitope in primates. Proc Nat Acad Sci U.S.A. 84:1369, 1987.

68. Knechtle SJ, Kolbeck PC, Tsuchimoto S, et al: Hepatic transplantation into sensitized recipients: Demonstration of hyperacute rejection. Transplantation 43:8, 1987.

69. Merion RM, Colletti LM: Hyperacute rejection in porcine liver transplantation: I. Clinical characteristics, histopathology, and disappearance of donor-specific lymphocytotoxic antibody from serum. Transplantation 49:861, 1990.

70. Shiraisha M, Oshiro T, Taira K, et al: Improved hepatic microcirculation by human soluble urinary thrombomodulin in the xeno-perfused porcine liver. Transplantation 71:1046, 2001.

71. Robson SC, Cooper DKC, d'Apice AJF: Disordered regulation of coagulation and platelet activation in xenotransplantation. Xenotransplantation 7:166, 2000.

72. Lawson JH, Daniels L, Platt JL: The evaluation of thrombomodulin activity in porcine to human xenotransplantation. Transplant Proc 29:884, 1997.

73. Lin SS, Kooyman DL, Daniels LJ, et al: The role of natural anti-Galα1-3Gal antibodies in hyperacute rejection of pig-to-baboon cardiac xenotransplants. Transplant Immunol 5:212, 1997.

74. Leventhal JR, Dalmasso AP, Cromwell JW, et al: Prolongation of cardiac xenograft survival by depletion of complement. Transplantation 55:857, 1993.

75. Pruitt SK, Kirk AD, Bollinger RR, et al: The effect of soluble complement receptor type 1 on hyperacute rejection of porcine xenografts. Transplantation 57:363, 1994.

76. Magee JC, Collins BH, Harland RC, et al: Immunoglobulin prevents complement mediated hyperacute rejection inswine-to-primate xenotransplantation. J Clin Invest 96:2404, 1995.

77. Platt JL, Vercellotti GM, Dalmasso AP, et al: Transplantation of discordant xenografts: A review of progress. Immunol Today 11:450, 1990.

78. Logan JS, Martin MJ: Transgenic swine as a recombinant production system for human hemoglobin. Methods Enzymol 231:435, 1994.

79. McCurry KR, Kooyman DL, Alvarado CG, et al: Human complement regulatory proteins protect swine-to-primate cardiac xenografts from humoral injury. Nat Med 1:423, 1995.

80. Byrne GW, McCurry KR, Martin MJ, et al: Transgenic pigs expressing human CD59 and decay-accelerating factor produce an intrinsic barrier to complement-mediated damage. Transplantation 63:149, 1997.

81. Cozzi E, Yannoutsos N, Langford GA, et al: Effect of transgenic expression of human decay-accelerating factor on the inhibition of hyperacute rejection of pig organs. In Cooper DKC, Kemp E, Platt JL, White DJG (eds): Xenotransplantation: The Transplantation of Organs and Tissues Between Species, 2nd ed. Berlin, Springer-Verlag, 1997, p 665.

82. Dalmasso AP, Vercellotti GM, Platt JL, Bach FH: Inhibition of complement-mediated endothelial cell cytotoxicity by decay accelerating factor: Potential for prevention of xenograft hyperacute rejection. Transplantation 52:530, 1991.

83. Sandrin MS, Fodor WL, Mouhtouris E, et al: Enzymatic remodelling of the carbohydrate surface of a xenogeneic cell substantially reduces human antibody binding and complement-mediated cytolysis. Nat Med 1:1261, 1995.

84. Thall AD, Malý P, Lowe JB: Oocyte Galα1,3Gal epitopes implicated in sperm adhesion to the zona pellucida glycoprotein ZP3 are not required for fertilization in the mouse. J Biol Chem 270:21437, 1995.

85. Platt JL: Knocking out xenograft rejection. Nat Biotechnol 20:231, 2002.

86. Leventhal JR, Matas AJ, Sun LH, et al: The immunopathology of cardiac xenograft rejection in the guinea pig-to-rat model. Transplantation 56:1, 1993.

87. Porter KA: Renal transplantation. In Heptinstall RH (ed): Pathology of the Kidney, vol. 3, 4th ed. Boston, Little Brown, 1992, p 1799.

88. Gugenheim J, Samuel D, Reynes M, Bismuth H: Liver transplantation across ABO blood group barriers. Lancet 336:519, 1990.

89. Platt JL, Lin SS, McGregor CGA: Acute vascular rejection. Xenotransplantation 5:169, 1998.

90. Lin SS, Weidner BC, Byrne GW, et al: The role of antibodies in acute vascular rejection of pig-to-baboon cardiac transplants. J Clin Invest 101:1745, 1998.

91. Bach FH, Winkler H, Ferran C, et al: Delayed xenograft rejection. Immunol Today 17:379, 1996.

92. Lawson JH, Platt JL: Molecular barriers to xenotransplantation. Transplantation 62:303, 1996.

93. Chopek MW, Simmons RL, Platt JL: ABO-incompatible renal transplantation: Initial immunopathologic evaluation. Transplant Proc 19:4553, 1987.

94. Bannett AD, McAlack RF, Morris M, et al: ABO incompatible renal transplantation: A qualitative analysis of native endothelial tissue ABO antigens after transplant. Transplant Proc 21: 783, 1989.

95. Gloor JM, Lager DJ, Moore SB, et al: ABO-incompatible kidney transplantation using both A2 and non-A2 living donors. Transplantation 75:971, 2003.

96. Bach FH, Hancock WW, Ferran C: Protective genes expressed in endothelial cells: A regulatory response to injury. Immunol Today 18:483, 1997.

97. Dalmasso AP, He T, Benson BA: Human IgM xenoreactive antibodies can induce resistance of porcine endothelial cells to complement-mediated injury. Xenotransplantation 3:54, 1996.

98. Dorling A, Stocker C, Tsao T, et al: In vitro accommodation of immortalized porcine endothelial cells: Resistance to complement-mediated lysis and down-regulation of VCAM expression induced by low concentrations of polyclonal human IgG antipig antibodies. Transplantation 62:1127, 1996.

99. Lin SS, Hanaway MJ, Gonzalez-Stawinski GV, et al: The role of anti-Galα1-3Gal antibodies in acute vascular rejection and accommodation of xenografts. Transplantation (Rapid Communication) 70:1667, 2000.

100. Parker W, Saadi S, Lin SS, et al: Transplantation of discordant xenografts: A challenge revisited. Immunol Today 17:373, 1996.

101. Bumgardner GL, Chen S, Hoffman R, et al: Afferent and efferent pathways in T cell responses to MHC class I+, II− hepatocytes. Transplantation 47:163, 1989.

102. Bumgardner GL, Orosz CG: Unusual patterns of alloimmunity evoked by allogeneic liver parenchymal cells. Immunol Rev 174:260, 2000.

103. Sachs DH, Sablinski T: Tolerance across discordant xenogeneic barriers. Xenotransplantation 2:234, 1995.

104. Ildstad ST, Vacchio MS, Markus PM, et al: Cross-species transplantation tolerance: Rat bone marrow–derived cells can contribute to the ligand for negative selection of mouse T cell receptor Vb in chimeras tolerant to xenogeneic antigens (mouse + rat → mouse). J Exp Med 175:147, 1992.

105. Zhao Y, Swenson K, Sergio JJ, et al: Skin graft tolerance across a discordant xenogeneic barrier. Nat Med 2:1211, 1996.

106. Inverardi L, Samaja M, Motterlini R, et al: Early recognition of a discordant xenogeneic organ by human circulating lymphocytes. J Immunol 149:1416, 1992.

107. Starzl TE, Demetris AJ, Murase N, et al: Cell migration, chimerism, and graft acceptance. Lancet 339:1579, 1992.

108. Holzknecht ZE, Coombes S, Blocher BA, et al: Evidence of immunocomplex formation in pulmonary xenografts. Transplant Proc 32:1141, 2000.

109. Lawson JH, Platt JL: Xenotransplantation: Prospects for clinical application. In Owen W, Pereira B, Sayegh M (eds): Dialysis and Transplantation: A Companion to Brenner and Rector's The Kidney. Philadelphia, WB Saunders, 2000, p 653.

110. Daggett CW, Yeatman M, Lodge AJ, et al: Total respiratory support from swine lungs in primate recipients. J Thor Cardiovasc Surg 115:19, 1998.

111. Edwards J: Complement activation by xenogeneic red blood cells. Transplantation 31:226, 1981.

112. Donato MF, Arosio E, Berti E, et al: Immunopathology of liver allografts and xenografts in nonhuman primates. Transplant Proc 25:850, 1993.

113. Desille M, Corcos L, L'Helgoualc'h A, et al: Detoxifying activity in pig livers and hepatocytes intended for xenotherapy. Transplantation 68:1437, 1999.

114. Patience C, Takeuchi Y, Weiss RA: Infection of human cells by an endogenous retrovirus of pigs. Nat Med 3:282, 1997.

115. Nyberg SL, Hibbs JR, Hardin JA: Transfer of porcine endogenous retrovirus across hollow fiber membranes: Significance to a bioartificial liver. Transplantation 67:1251, 1999.

116. Patience C, Patton GS, Takeuchi Y, et al: No evidence of pig DNA or retroviral infection in patients with short-term extracorporeal connection to pig kidneys. Lancet 352:699, 1998.

117. Platt JL: Xenoassistance devices for the treatment of hepatic failure: Challenges and controversies. Transplant Proc 32:2693, 2000.

Hepatocyte Transplantation in Liver Disease

VIVEK DIXIT

Hepatocyte transplantation: transplantation
sites   1380

Hepatocyte transplantation: experimental
studies   1380

Intraperitoneal transplantation
of hepatocytes   1381

Microcarrier-attached hepatocytes   1381

Microencapsulated hepatocytes   1381

Clinical experience with hepatocyte
transplantation   1383

Transplantation of isolated healthy hepatocytes to supplement failing or deficient liver function is an innovative technique that offers a variety of important applications. Treatment of liver disease by transplantation of healthy hepatocytes can also have significant implications for organ replacement therapy. When compared with whole-organ transplantation, it is a technically simple procedure that offers numerous advantages. It may be possible in the future for relatives of patients to donate small samples of liver cells for transplantation, or one whole liver could be used to treat many patients. Unlike whole organs, hepatocytes can also be cryopreserved for future use. During the past 2 decades, various experimental approaches for transplantation of healthy isolated hepatocytes, with previously limited success, were investigated with very promising results. Recent clinical studies on transplanted hepatocytes suggest considerable promise in hepatocyte transplantation being able to provide a full range of liver functions in the short term. Sustained long-term replacement of hepatic function remains a problem, however.

A normal functioning liver is essential to maintain metabolic balance and survival. Severe injury or substantial impairment of liver function will rapidly result in serious consequences that often lead to death. The current "gold standard" for treating such patients is whole-organ liver transplantation. Since its pioneering days in the early 1960s, advances in surgical techniques and immunosuppression therapeutics have made liver transplantation the only reliable therapeutic option for patients with severe, life-threatening liver disease.[1] This progress has resulted in liver transplantation being offered to a wide assortment of patients with liver disease who previously may not have been considered candidates for this procedure. Thus, the tremendous success of liver transplantation has progressively outpaced the supply of donor livers such that in 2002, of the nearly 17,500 patients listed for liver transplantation, only about 5000 received transplants.[2] Despite attempts to abate the demand for donor livers by using split-liver grafts and the more controversial living related donor grafts, the endemic shortage of donor livers for transplantation has remained unchanged.[3]

Treatment of disease by implanting functional cells and tissue into the body has long been a dream in medicine. The use of bone marrow and pancreatic islet cells in cancer and diabetes, respectively, attests to this fact. Hence, among the various technologies that are currently being developed to overcome the persistent shortage of donor livers for transplantation, hepatocyte transplantation holds considerable promise as a viable therapeutic modality. Since the first experimental report on hepatocyte transplantation for correcting hyperbilirubinemia in rodents in 1976,[4] this technology has overcome major obstacles related to hepatocyte isolation, handling, culture, and transplantation techniques. The main stumbling block in procuring a high yield of metabolically active, isolated hepatocyte cells was overcome when enzymatic digestion of the liver became possible.[5] This seminal development ushered in an era of hepatocyte transplantation for treating a spectrum of liver diseases ranging from acute liver failure to chronic metabolic liver disease.[6] Subsequent development of suitable animal models, cell culture, and transplantation techniques has made the procedure feasible, and recently, several preliminary clinical studies of this technology have been performed.[7] Hepatocyte transplantation holds many advantages over whole-organ transplantation in that it is a nonsurgical procedure with relatively low risk and minimal morbidity.[7] Furthermore, a high yield of pure isolated hepatocytes can now be readily obtained from donor organs and cryopreserved for later use. In this regard, donor organs deemed unsuitable for orthotopic liver transplantation for a variety of reasons can likewise be salvaged and used to obtain isolated hepatocytes. Finally, recent experience suggests that it may also be possible to treat several patients with hepatocytes isolated from a single donor.[8]

Hepatocyte Transplantation: Transplantation Sites

Several hepatocyte transplantation sites have been reported in the literature. Among the first sites studied was the liver itself, via the intraportal route. This site was intuitively considered ideal because it represented an optimal environment for the hepatocytes to implant and become incorporated into liver tissue. However, initial experience with this technique led to accumulation of hepatocyte aggregates in distal portal branches, sinusoids, and central veins, thereby resulting in extensive hepatic necrosis, severe portal hypertension, and pulmonary hypertension.[9] The procedure has since been further modified, and hepatocytes were delivered to the portal vein by first injecting them into the spleen.[8] Subsequently, embolization of the transplanted hepatocytes from the spleen and entry into the portal circulation resulted in minimal portal blockage and congestion. Other hepatocyte transplantation sites have included subcutaneous tissue, intracapsular dorsal fat pads, muscle, peritoneum, renal capsule, and lungs.[10,11] Among the aforementioned transplantation sites, only the spleen and peritoneal cavity have shown any real measure of success. Both routes of hepatocyte transplantation have their proponents, but it appears that in the preclinical experimental setting, the intraperitoneal route may be by far the most advantageous for short-term liver replacement therapy. Intraperitoneal transplantation is a simple technique that causes negligible trauma to the recipient animal. The intraperitoneal route also allows several orders of magnitude greater quantities of hepatocytes to be transplanted than with the intrasplenic route.[12] Recently, technological refinements have facilitated slow controlled infusion of hepatocytes directly into the portal circulation, and this technique has now become the preferred method to deliver hepatocytes to the liver.

Hepatocyte Transplantation: Experimental Studies

Pioneering studies on hepatocyte transplantation were first carried out by Ebata and coworkers.[13] This group developed the intrasplenic transplantation technique whereby a small suspension of isolated hepatocytes were injected directly into the splenic pulp. The hepatocytes then attached to the splenic red pulp to form hepatic cords and sinusoids. Splenic white pulp did not support the proliferation of implanted hepatocytes. Frequently, some embolization of transplanted hepatocytes into the liver was observed, but this was not carefully investigated at the time and was considered a detriment to the procedure. It was only later realized that slow embolization of hepatocytes into the liver might provide a convenient method to deliver hepatocytes to the liver. The pioneering studies of Ebata and colleagues demonstrated the formation of a "hepatized" spleen 1 year after the transplantation of syngeneic hepatocytes. The transplanted hepatocytes were able to correct the inherited glucuronyl transferase deficiency in Gunn rats,[14] but the procedure was deemed impractical because only about 3% of the spleen was incorporated with liver tissue and it took nearly a year to hepatize the spleen. Studies in those days were also primarily aimed at providing liver support during acute liver failure, and the small amount of liver tissue in the spleen was insufficient to provide adequate liver support.

Intraperitoneal Transplantation of Hepatocytes

Subsequent to the development of intrasplenic hepatocyte transplantation, intraperitoneal transplantation techniques were developed that also demonstrated encouraging but temporary results.[2,15] It was not widely recognized then that the peritoneal milieu did not offer a suitable attachment environment for the anchorage-dependent hepatocytes, thus limiting their life span and functionality. Intraperitoneal transplantation of hepatocytes did not advance further until the development of microcarrier and microencapsulation technology for transplantation. These techniques provided suitable substrates for hepatocytes to attach to and function more effectively. With advances in microcarrier and microencapsulation techniques, intraperitoneally transplanted isolated hepatocytes have shown tremendous promise in being able to assume the full range of liver functions in several animal models of severe liver disease.[10,16-19]

Microcarrier-Attached Hepatocytes

Microcarriers have been used in tissue culture and biotechnology for more than a decade. However, their application in cell transplantation studies is recent.[10,19,20] Microcarriers provide an essential attachment substratum for hepatocytes. Their enormous surface area–to-volume relationship facilitates the transplantation of huge quantities of hepatocytes in very small volumes of microcarrier suspension. The first cell transplantation studies with microcarrier-attached hepatocytes were reported by Demetriou and coauthors, who demonstrated the feasibility of restoration of deficient liver function in two animal models of congenital metabolic liver defects: hyperbilirubinemia and analbuminemia.[10] In these studies, intraperitoneal transplantation of microcarrier-attached hepatocytes into hyperbilirubinemic Gunn rats and analbuminemic Nagase rats resulted in a significant fall in bilirubin levels and an increase in albumin levels in the respective animal models. Furthermore, the decrease in bilirubin in Gunn rats was accompanied by a concurrent increase in the level of bilirubin conjugates in the bile of the recipient animals, thus indicating

function of the transplanted hepatocytes. In cross-species experiments with isolated human hepatocytes, this group demonstrated similar results in these animal models.[21] They also showed that intraperitoneally transplanted microcarrier-attached hepatocytes could significantly improve the survival of rats undergoing 90% partial hepatectomy,[18] thereby demonstrating that the transplanted hepatocytes provided significant metabolic support to maintain life.

Subsequently, several investigators successfully demonstrated a reduction in cholesterol levels of up to 50% in hyperlipidemic rabbits and a reduction in serum low-density lipoprotein (LDL) levels in congenitally hyperlipidemic Watanabe rabbits after the intraperitoneal transplantation of microcarrier-attached hepatocytes.[19] It was also shown that hepatocyte transplantation could prevent the formation of atherosclerotic plaque in the aorta.[22] In addition, intraperitoneal transplantation of microcarrier-attached hepatocytes has been shown to significantly improve the long-term survival of rats with galactosamine-induced fulminant hepatic failure.[23] In ongoing studies to improve the effectiveness of hepatocyte attachment and function, investigators developed highly efficient hepatocyte immobilization techniques with the use of biologically modified polyhydroxyethylmethacrylate (PHEMA) microcarriers to allow greater than 75% coverage of the microcarriers, in contrast to the approximately 25% coverage with collagen-coated dextran microcarriers used in previous studies.[24] Thus, data from several centers strongly suggest that intraperitoneally transplanted, microcarrier-attached hepatocytes can provide significant metabolic support in animal models of both acute and chronic (congenital) metabolic liver disease. However, without adequate immunosuppression, hepatocyte rejection remains a significant problem.[10,20]

Microencapsulated Hepatocytes

Microencapsulation techniques for hepatocyte transplantation evolved after the successful experiments with microcarrier-attached hepatocytes just described. This technique circumvents the need for immunosuppression through the microencapsulation of hepatocytes within a semipermeable membrane that allows substrate and product to exchange freely but prevents the encapsulated hepatocytes from escaping the microcapsule. Microencapsulation technology was derived from Chang's pioneering work[25] and the more recent application of this technique by Sun and coworkers[26] for encapsulating islets of Langerhans. Briefly, microcapsules are synthetic, spherical polymeric structures that are composed of ultrathin semipermeable membranes of cellular dimensions. The microcapsule membrane can be prepared from various polymers; its contents can consist of tissue or cells, enzymes, or other biologically active material.[27] The membrane prevents the contents of the microcapsule from leaking out and causing immunological reactions, but it still allows those contents to interact freely in biological reactions. Additionally, the membrane keeps unwanted substances, such as cells and antibodies, from entering the microcapsule.

In contrast to the microcarrier studies described in the preceding section, in which hepatocytes are cultured on the exterior surface of collagen-coated microcarriers, hepatocytes are microencapsulated within a three-dimensional collagen matrix separated from the external environment by a semipermeable membrane. This three-dimensional orientation has been suggested to play an important role in the maintenance of hepatocyte function through improved cell-cell interaction.[28] Thus, microencapsulation provides a unique and innovative technique for the transplantation of foreign tissue and cells that eliminates the need for immunosuppression. Indeed, microencapsulation techniques have now been successfully used to transplant a variety of cells, such as islets of Langerhans[29] for the treatment of diabetes in rats, parathyroid cells for a bioartificial parathyroid,[30] and adrenal cortex cells for neurological disorders.[31]

The feasibility of microencapsulated hepatocyte transplantation for the replacement of liver function has been demonstrated by several groups in various animal models of fulminant hepatic failure and congenital metabolic liver disease.[16,17,32-34] In controlled experiments involving the well-characterized galactosamine-induced fulminant hepatic failure rat model,[35] transplantation of microencapsulated hepatocytes significantly increased survival time by twofold when transplanted during the late stages of liver failure.[36] Furthermore, in the same animal model, transplanted microencapsulated hepatocytes significantly increased the overall survival rate of rats when compared with untreated control animals or control animals treated with empty microcapsules. It is noteworthy that the animals in the aforementioned studies received no immunosuppression. Since fulminant hepatic failure essentially requires support only during the critical phase of liver injury, these studies demonstrated the effectiveness of microencapsulated hepatocyte transplantation for short-term liver support.

To demonstrate the long-term effectiveness of microencapsulated hepatocytes, studies similar to those performed with microcarrier-attached hepatocytes were conducted in the Gunn rat model. This animal model is congenitally deficient in the liver enzyme bilirubin uridine diphosphate (UDP)-glucuronyl transferase and is unable to conjugate bilirubin; as a result, Gunn rats have lifelong, nonhemolytic unconjugated hyperbilirubinemia.[37] A number of studies have now

conclusively demonstrated that transplanted microencapsulated hepatocytes can significantly lower the level of hyperbilirubinemia in Gunn rats after just a single transplantation.[16,17] Additionally, as was the case with microcarrier-attached hepatocytes, the decrease in serum bilirubin levels was paralleled by an increase in conjugated bilirubin in bile.[17,28] These studies effectively demonstrated that transplanted microencapsulated hepatocytes were as competent as transplanted unencapsulated, microcarrier-attached hepatocytes in providing liver function in Gunn rats.[10,16,17] However, unlike the latter, microencapsulated hepatocytes offered the advantage of circumventing the need for immunosuppression.[10,17]

One of the main drawbacks observed in hepatocyte transplantation studies (with both microcarrier-attached hepatocytes and microencapsulated hepatocytes) is that transplanted hepatocytes have limited (4 to 6 weeks) functional viability in the peritoneal cavity of Gunn rats.[10,38] It has been suggested that the decline in functional viability of microencapsulated hepatocytes may be related to the specific attachment requirements of hepatocytes.[28] Hence, by using attachment substrates such as Matrigel, a mouse sarcoma-derived complex of proteins that closely resembles liver basement membrane proteins, a significant increase in the functional viability of transplanted microencapsulated hepatocytes was reported.[28] Other methods to improve long-term functional viability may be achieved through coculture techniques.[39]

If microencapsulated hepatocyte transplantation is to be considered a therapeutic option for acute and chronic liver disease, the long-term fate of the hepatocytes after transplantation must be considered. Investigators have now examined the fate of microencapsulated hepatocytes for 6 months after intraperitoneal transplantation.[38] It was observed that microencapsulated hepatocytes are stable and function adequately for up to 6 to 8 weeks after transplantation. Thereafter, the membrane surrounding the microcapsule deteriorates, and the microcapsule physically breaks down.[38] It has been speculated that degeneration of microencapsulated hepatocytes (autolysis) leads to ionic and pH changes within the microcapsule microenvironment.[38] These pH changes may weaken the alginate-polylysine copolymer membrane of the microcapsule by altering charges on the molecules that form the membrane. Thus, the observation of degenerative changes in the microcapsules beginning 2 months after transplantation suggests that repeated transplantation may be necessary for the long-term effectiveness of microencapsulated hepatocytes.[40] In a subsequent 6-month-long study, repeated monthly transplantation of microencapsulated hepatocytes into Gunn rats, performed before the previous month's microencapsulated hepatocyte transplant began to deteriorate, produced a prolonged and sustained decrease in serum bilirubin levels.[40] In contrast, the control rats that received empty microcapsules experienced no reduction in hyperbilirubinemia.

For microencapsulated hepatocyte transplantation to provide a viable form of artificial liver support (e.g., a bridge to transplantation), it must be simple and convenient to use. Large quantities of healthy microencapsulated hepatocytes must be readily available for transplantation when required. In concept, a facility akin to a blood bank in which microencapsulated hepatocytes could be stored and used as needed would be ideal. Cryopreservation is a standard procedure for preserving various cell types and can be used effectively to store microencapsulated hepatocytes. It has been demonstrated that cryopreserved, microencapsulated hepatocytes function as well as freshly prepared, nonfrozen microencapsulated hepatocytes both in vitro and in vivo.[17] Thus, transplantation of cryopreserved microencapsulated hepatocytes can provide a convenient therapeutic option for the management of fulminant hepatic failure, as well as inborn errors of metabolism, without the need for immunosuppression.

Despite encouraging studies with microencapsulated and microcarrier-attached hepatocytes, it now appears that such techniques may be useful only for providing temporary liver support. Because of the limited life span of primary hepatocyte culture, multiple transplantations of microcarrier or microencapsulated hepatocytes are required, which may not be ideally suited for the clinical setting. The accumulation of microcarriers and breakdown products of microcapsules may present a safety concern not suitable for patients with severe liver disease. Thus, attention has again focused on transplanting hepatocytes directly into the liver via the intraportal route. Recent clinical studies have also demonstrated that the previous fears of portal vein obstruction by transplanted hepatocytes are not justified, provided that slow controlled infusion of hepatocytes can be accomplished.

Clinical Experience with Hepatocyte Transplantation

A tremendous number of controlled animal experiments over the past 3 decades have enabled implementation of the first of several hepatocyte transplantation trials in humans. The early hepatocyte transplantation trials in humans were uncontrolled and resulted in variable outcomes. The patient population also varied, which did not facilitate good comparison among the various clinical studies that were being conducted worldwide. Furthermore, the spectrum of liver disease in the patients studied ranged from end-stage liver cirrhosis to fulminant hepatic failure and congenital metabolic liver disease. The number of hepatocytes transplanted also differed significantly, as did the source of

hepatocytes and the site of transplantation. Nevertheless, the results were encouraging and have prompted other more carefully designed trials that have on the whole validated the promises of the earlier experimental observations in animals.

The first clinical trials of hepatocyte transplantation were reported by Mito and Kusano, who injected isolated human hepatocytes into the spleen of 10 Japanese patients with liver cirrhosis or chronic hepatitis.[14] Although some transient improvement was noted initially, no obvious clinical improvement was observed in the patients studied. However, a year later in 1994, investigators in India conducted a study in which seven patients with fulminant hepatic failure of different causes were intraperitoneally transplanted with approximately 60 million hepatocytes isolated from aborted fetuses.[41] In this trial, fetal hepatocytes were pooled from fetuses ranging in gestational age from 26 to 34 weeks. Unmatched control patients did not receive hepatocyte transplantation and consisted of those who did not consent to the procedure. Investigators found a significant difference in the survival of patients treated with hepatocyte transplantation (48%) and matched controls (33%). In patients who survived, a decrease in blood ammonia and bilirubin levels was observed. No beneficial effects were seen with regard to the prothrombin time. Investigators observed 100% survival in patients treated during the early stages (grade III) of hepatic encephalopathy, in contrast to those treated in the late stages (grade IV), who all died. The investigators of this study concluded that fetal hepatocyte transplantation produced a beneficial effect on patient outcome when hepatocyte transplantation was performed earlier in the clinical course of the disease.

In the United States, approximately 19 acute liver failure patients have been treated with hepatocyte transplantation, primarily as a bridge to transplantation.[42,43] Patients were infused with approximately 10 million to 10 trillion allogeneic hepatocytes obtained from deceased donor livers. Hepatocytes were infused into either the splenic artery or the portal vein. In some cases, hepatocytes were infused into the portal vein via transjugular catheterization. As was expected from the nature of these experimental clinical trials and the small patient population, the results were largely inconclusive. Although functionally viable hepatocytes were identified in the spleen and liver, it was unclear whether there was any engraftment of the hepatocytes in the liver. No improvement in synthetic liver function was observed in the first few days after hepatocyte transplantation. However, some clinical benefit was observed in anecdotal reports, such as improvement in the level of encephalopathy, intracranial pressure, serum ammonia levels, prothrombin time, cerebral perfusion pressure, and cardiovascular stability. The wide range in the number of hepatocytes transplanted further clouds the issue of possible benefit derived from the hepatocytes. Infusing very large numbers of hepatocytes directly into the splenic artery causes impairment of blood flow in the liver and may have resulted in the detrimental outcome in some patients who died of sepsis.[44] Overall, of the 19 patients who underwent hepatocyte transplantation for acute liver failure, 7 were successfully bridged to liver transplantation, 2 recovered completely, and 10 died because of complications resulting from hepatocyte transplantation. In patients who survived long enough to receive whole-organ transplants, the average survival time was approximately 4 ± 3 days (mean $\pm$ SD). In patients who died while waiting for a transplant, the mean survival time was approximately 4.5 ± 2.5 days.

Approximately 18 patients with decompensated chronic liver failure have been treated with hepatocyte transplantation therapy worldwide.[8,14,43] As was the modus operandi in patients with acute liver failure, hepatocytes were transplanted into the liver either via direct portal vein infusion or via the splenic artery, the latter being the more frequent route of administration. Hepatocyte transplantation via the splenic artery was preferable from a safety standpoint because it resulted in reduced obstruction of liver blood flow. The hepatocyte infusions from deceased donors were well tolerated and ranged from 10 to 100 million hepatocytes per patient. Although engraftment of hepatocytes was visualized in the spleen, the therapy did not affect the clinical outcome. Some anecdotal observations from a small group of patients who underwent transjugular intrahepatic portosystemic shunting showed resolution of their encephalopathy and anuria. Overall, the procedure was safely performed with no morbidity or mortality.

A small group of patients with a diversity of inherited liver-based metabolic diseases have also been treated with hepatocyte transplantation therapy. The first attempt at treating an inherited metabolic liver disease with hepatocyte transplantation was made in the context of ex vivo gene therapy for familial hypercholesterolemia. This trial was based on preclinical experimental studies with LDL receptor–deficient Watanabe heritable hyperlipidemic (WHHL) rabbits.[45] Here, primary WHHL hepatocytes harvested from these animals were transduced with a recombinant retrovirus expressing the human LDL receptor gene and then transplanted back into the donor rabbit; the technique resulted in a long-term reduction in serum LDL levels.[46-48] In human trials, primary hepatocytes isolated from surgically resected liver segments from the patient were similarly transduced with an LDL receptor expressing a retroviral vector and then retransplanted back into the patient via the portal vein. A small trial involving four patients demonstrated a modest reduction in plasma cholesterol levels and persistence of the transplanted cells and transgene function. It was observed that the low level of transduction of primary hepatocytes by the retroviral vectors and the small number of cells transplanted may have contributed to the low response to therapy. Although the procedure did not result in a useful reduction in LDL levels, the trial established the feasibility of hepatocyte transplantation and the longevity of the transplanted cells.[49]

Subsequently, other investigators have transplanted allogeneic hepatocytes to correct liver-based metabolic disorders, including urea cycle disorder (ornithine transcarbamylase [OTC] deficiency), α_1-antitrypsin deficiency, glycogen storage disease type 1a, infantile Refsum's disease, and Crigler-Najjar syndrome type 1.[50-54] Isolated hepatocyte transplantation appeared to result in temporary relief of the hyperammonemia and protein intolerance attributable to OTC deficiency. Transient metabolic stability was achieved, but was lost after 11 days, presumably as a result of rejection of the transplanted cells because of insufficient immunosuppression.[50] Hepatocyte transplantation was performed in an adult patient who had glycogen storage disease type 1a and severe fasting hypoglycemia. Nine months after the infusion of 2 billion viable hepatocytes via an indwelling portal vein catheter, the patient achieved long-term improvement in blood glucose control, eats a normal diet, and can fast for 7 hours without experiencing hypoglycemia.

Refsum's disease affects growth of the myelin sheath on nerve fibers in the brain.[53] The disease affects both males and females, and symptoms of the disorder may include vision impairment, peripheral neuropathy, ataxia, impaired hearing, and bone and skin changes. Combinations of approximately 2 billion fresh and cryopreserved hepatocytes were successfully transplanted into a 4-year-old girl with infantile Refsum's disease. Total bile acids and abnormal dihydroxycoprostanoic acid markedly decreased in the patient's serum, indicative of resolution of cholestasis and repopulation of liver cells. Pipecolic acid decreased by 40% and the c26:c22 fatty acid ratio by 36% after 18 months. Detection of donor chromosome sequences on biopsy specimens after transplantation indicated engraftment.

Crigler-Najjar syndrome is another metabolic liver disorder that has been successfully treated with hepatocyte transplantation.[54] In this inherited disorder, bilirubin in the liver cannot be converted to bilirubin glucuronide because of a deficiency of bilirubin UDP-glucuronyl transferase. In the clinical trial, a 10-year-old patient was transplanted with approximately 7.5 billion hepatocytes ($\approx$5% of the hepatic mass) by three infusions through a percutaneously placed portal vein catheter. The patient's serum bilirubin levels, which averaged 27 mg/dL, were dramatically reduced by 50% to 60% after hepatocyte transplantation. Analysis by high-performance liquid chromatography revealed that before hepatocyte transplantation therapy, the patient's bile contained predominantly unconjugated bilirubin with only a trace of bilirubin monoglucuronide. After hepatocyte transplantation therapy, significant amounts of bilirubin monoglucuronide and diglucuronide could be detected in the bile of this patient. Furthermore, when compared with pretransplant biopsy specimens, hepatic bilirubin UDP-glucuronyl transferase activity had increased nearly 14-fold to 110 pmol/hr/g protein ($\approx$5.5% of the normal level). Unequivocal evidence of function of the transplanted human hepatocytes was demonstrated when long-term engraftment showed persistent bilirubin UDP-glucuronyl transferase activity, as measured by analysis of duodenal bile aspirates even 30 months after a single session of hepatocyte transplantation.[55] This patient has since undergone successful auxiliary liver transplantation.

These experimental and clinical studies have clearly demonstrated that hepatocyte transplantation is a convenient alternative to liver transplantation, especially for the treatment of rare inborn errors of metabolism. The efficacy of hepatocyte transplantation in treating acute liver failure and chronic liver disease is still unclear. To achieve meaningful conclusions in this regard, more research and controlled clinical studies are need. In addition, several technical matters, such as optimal transplantation sites, also need to be resolved. The liver presently appears to be an ideal location, and optimal ways to deliver substantial amounts of hepatocytes to this location without causing hepatic obstruction are needed. The question of using adult versus fetal hepatocytes is controversial and needs to be resolved in a scientific setting. Furthermore, the increasing scientific interest in hepatic stem cell technology may provide yet another source for hepatocyte transplantation. This potential source should be able to provide a stable and uniform population of cells for liver replacement therapy. Finally, alternative technology such as liver tissue engineering is appearing on the horizon and could transform liver transplantation as it currently stands. Recent studies have demonstrated that such engineering is a viable option that needs further investigation.[56,57] Certainly, whole-organ liver transplantation will remain the gold standard for the foreseeable future. However, the growing shortage of liver organs available for transplantation, the escalating cost of the transplantation procedure, and the increasing number of patients who are listed each year for liver transplantation will eventually spur the development of new and exciting therapies.

References

1. Carithers RL Jr: Liver transplantation. Liver Transpl 6:122-135, 2000.
2. United Network for Organ Sharing (http://www.unos.org).
3. Cronin DC, Millis M, Siegler M: Transplantation of liver grafts from living donors into adults—too much, too soon. N Engl J Med 344:1633-1637, 2001.
4. Matas AJ, Sutherland DER, Steffes MW, et al: Hepatocellular transplantation for metabolic deficiencies: Decrease of plasma bilirubin in Gunn rats. Science 192:892-894, 1976.
5. Berry MN, Friend DS: High-yield preparation of isolated rat liver parenchymal cells. J Cell Biol 43:506-520, 1969.
6. Dixit V: Development of a bioartificial liver using isolated hepatocytes. Artif Organs 18:371-384, 1994.
7. Fox IJ, Chowdhury JR: Hepatocyte transplantation. J Hepatol 40:878-886, 2004.
8. Strom SC, Chowdhury JR, Fox IJ: Hepatocyte transplantation for the treatment of human disease. Semin Liver Dis 19:39-48, 1999.
9. Rivas P, Fabrega AJ, Schwartz D, et al: Preservation and transplantation of purified canine hepatocytes. Transplant Proc 24:2833-2836, 1992.
10. Demetriou AA, Whiting JF, Feldman D, et al: Replacement of liver function in rats by transplantation of microcarrier-attached hepatocytes. Science 233:1190-1192, 1986.
11. Fuller BJ: Transplantation of isolated hepatocytes. A review of current ideas. J Hepatol 7:368-376, 1988.
12. Selden C, Darby H, Hodgson HJF: Further observations on the survival, proliferation and function of ectopically implanted syngeneic and allogeneic liver cells in rat spleen. Eur J Gastroentrol Hepatol 3:607-611, 1991.
13. Ebata H, Kusano M, Onishi T, et al: Liver regeneration utilizing isolated hepatocytes transplanted into the rat spleen. Surg Forum 29:338-340, 1978.
14. Mito M, Kusano M: Hepatocyte transplantation in man. Cell Transplant 2:65-74, 1993.
15. Makowka L, Falk RE, Rotstein LE, et al: Cellular transplantation in the treatment of experimental hepatic failure. Science 210:901-903, 1980.
16. Dixit V, Darvasi R, Arthur M, et al: Restoration of liver function in Gunn rats without immunosuppression using transplanted microencapsulated hepatocytes. Hepatology 12:1342-1349, 1990.
17. Dixit V, Darvasi R, Arthur M, et al: Cryopreserved microencapsulated hepatocytes: Transplantation studies in Gunn rats. Transplantation 55:616-622, 1993.
18. Demetriou AA, Reisner A, Sanchez J, et al: Transplantation of microcarrier-attached hepatocytes into 90% partial hepatectomized rats. Hepatology 8:1006-1009, 1988.
19. Weiderkehr JC, Kondos GT, Pollak R: Hepatocyte transplantation for the low-density lipoprotein receptor–deficient state. Transplantation 50:466-476, 1990.
20. Demetriou AA, Levenson SM, Novikoff PM, et al: Survival, organization, and function of microcarrier-attached hepatocytes transplanted in rats. Proc Natl Acad Sci U S A 83:7475-7479, 1986.
21. Moscioni AD, Chowdhury JR, Barbour R, et al: Human liver cell transplantation: Prolonged function in athymic-Gunn and athymic-analbuminemic hybrid rats. Gastroenterology 96:1546-1551, 1989.
22. Rozga J, Demetriou AA: Intraportal hepatocyte transplantation. In Mito M, Sawa M (eds): Hepatocyte Transplantation. Basel, Karger Landes Systems, 1997, pp 47-66.
23. Nagaki M, Kano T, Muto Y, et al: Effects of intraperitoneal transplantation of microcarrier-attached hepatocytes in D-galactosamine-induced acute liver failure rats. Gastroenterol Jpn 25:78-87, 1990.
24. Dixit V, Piskin E, Arthur M, et al: Hepatocyte immobilization on PHEMA microcarriers and its biologically modified forms. Cell Transplant 1:391-399, 1992.
25. Chang TMS: Semipermeable microcapsules. Science 146:524-525, 1964.
26. Sun AM, Cai ZH, Shi ZQ, et al: Microencapsulated hepatocytes as a bioartificial liver. Trans Am Soc Artif Intern Organs 32:39-41, 1986.
27. Chang TMS: Artificial cells in medicine and biotechnology. Appl Biochem Biotechnol 10:5-24, 1984.

28. Dixit V, Darvasi R, Arthur M, et al: Improved function of micro-encapsulated hepatocytes in a hybrid bioartificial liver support system. Artif Organs 16:336-341, 1992.

29. Lacy PE, Hegre OD, Gerasidimi-Vazeou A, et al: Maintenance of normoglycemia in diabetic mice by subcutaneous xenografts of encapsulated islets. Science 254:1782-1784, 1991.

30. Fu XW, Sun AM: Microencapsulated parathyroid cells as a bio-artificial parathyroid. Transplantation 47:432, 1989.

31. Aebischer P, Tresco PA, Winn SR, et al: Long-term cross-species brain transplantation of a polymer-encapsulated dopamine-secreting cell line. Exp Neurol 111:267, 1991.

32. Cai ZH, Shi ZQ, Sherman M, Sun AM: Development and evaluation of a system of microencapsulation of primary rat hepatocytes. Hepatology 10:855-860, 1989.

33. Bruni S, Chang TMS: Hepatocytes immobilized by microencapsulation in artificial cells: Effects on hyperbilirubinemia in Gunn rats. Biomat Artif Cells Artif Organs 17:403-411, 1989.

34. Miura Y, Akimoto T, Kanazawa H, Yagi K: Synthesis and secretion of protein by hepatocytes entrapped within calcium alginate. Artif Organs 10:460-465, 1986.

35. Dixit V, Chang TMS: Brain edema and the blood brain barrier in galactosamine-induced fulminant hepatic failure rats: An animal model for evaluation of liver support systems. ASAIO Trans 36:21-27, 1990.

36. Wong H, Chang TMS: Bioartificial liver: Implanted artificial cells microencapsulated living hepatocytes increases survival of liver failure rats. Int J Artif Organs 9:335-336, 1986.

37. Yeary RA, Grothaus RH: The Gunn rat as an animal model in comparative medicine. Lab Animal Sci 21:362-366, 1971.

38. Dixit V, Arthur M, Gitnick G: A morphological and functional evaluation of transplanted isolated encapsulated hepatocytes following long-term transplantation in Gunn rats. Biomater Artif Cells Immobilization Biotechnol 21:119-133, 1993.

39. Guguen-Guillouzo C, Clement B, Baffet G, et al: Maintenance and reversibility of active albumin secretion by adult rat hepatocytes co-cultured with another liver epithelial cell type. Exp Cell Res 143:47-54, 1983.

40. Dixit V, Arthur M, Gitnick G: Repeated transplantation of microencapsulated hepatocytes for sustained correction of hyperbilirubinemia in Gunn rats. Cell Transplant 1:275-279, 1992.

41. Habibullah CM, Syed IH, Qamar A, Taher-Uz Z: Human fetal hepatocyte transplantation in patients with fulminant hepatic failure. Transplantation 58:951-977, 1994.

42. Strom SC, Fisher RA, Thompson MT, et al: Hepatocyte transplantation as a bridge to orthotopic liver transplantation in terminal liver failure. Transplantation 63:559-569, 1997.

43. Bilir BM, Guinette D, Karrer F, et al: Hepatocyte transplantation in acute liver failure. Liver Transpl 6:32-40, 2000.

44. Fisher RA, Strom SC: Human hepatocyte transplantation: Biology and therapy. In Berry M, Edwards A (eds): The Hepatocyte Review. London, Kluwer, 2000.

45. Grossman M, Rader DJ, Muller DW, et al: A pilot study of ex vivo gene therapy for homozygous familial hypercholesterolemia. Nat Med 1:1148-1154, 1995.

46. Chowdhury JR, Grossman M, Gupta S, et al: Long term improvement of hypercholesterolemia after ex vivo gene therapy in LDL-receptor deficient rabbits. Science 254:1802-1805, 1991.

47. Grossman M, Raper SE, Kozarsky K, et al: Successful ex vivo gene therapy directed to the liver in a patient with familial hypercholesterolemia. Nat Genet 6:335-341, 1994.

48. Raper SE: Hepatocyte transplantation and gene therapy. Clin Transplant 9:249-254, 1995.

49. Raper SE, Grossman M, Rader DJ, et al: Safety and feasibility of liver-directed ex vivo gene therapy for homozygous familial hypercholesterolemia. Ann Surg 223:116-126, 1995.

50. Horslen SP, McCowan TC, Goertzen TC, et al: Isolated hepatocyte transplantation in an infant with a severe urea cycle disorder. Pediatrics 111:1262-1267, 2003.

51. Strom SC, Fisher RA, Rubinstein WS, et al: Transplantation of human hepatocytes. Transplant Proc 29:2103-2106, 1997.

52. Muraca M, Gerunda G, Neri D, et al: Hepatocyte transplantation as a treatment for glycogen storage disease type 1a. Lancet 359:317-318, 2002.

53. Sokal EM, Smets F, Bourgois A, et al: Hepatocyte transplantation in a 4-year-old girl with peroxisomal biogenesis disease: Technique, safety, and metabolic follow-up. Transplantation 76:735-738, 2003.

54. Fox IJ, Chowdhury JR, Kaufman SS, et al: Treatment of the Crigler-Najjar syndrome type I with hepatocyte transplantation. N Engl J Med 338:1422-1426, 1998.

55. Lee SW, Wang X, Chowdhury NR, Roy-Chowdhury J: Hepatocyte transplantation: State of the art and strategies for overcoming existing hurdles. Ann Hepatol 3:48-53, 2004.

56. Takimoto Y, Dixit V, Arthur M, Gitnick G: De novo liver tissue formation in rats using a novel collagen-polypropylene scaffold. Cell Transplant 12:413-421, 2003.

57. Dixit V, Elcin YM: Liver tissue engineering: Successes & limitations. Adv Exp Med Biol 534:57-67, 2003.

New Approaches in Immunosuppression

MARTIN HERTL
A. BENEDICT COSIMI

New biological agents   1388
  Campath-1H   1389
  Humanized OKT3 preparations—HuOKT3γ
    (Ala-Ala), HuM291   1390
  CD3 Immunotoxin   1391
  MEDI-507   1391

Anti-CD154/CD40   1391

CTLA4-Ig and LEA29Y   1392

Intravenous immunoglobulin   1393

Rituximab   1393

New pharmacological regimens and
  agents   1393
  Steroid withdrawal and avoidance   1394
  Drug minimization—"prope" tolerance   1394
  FK778   1395
  FTY720   1396

Everolimus   1396

Calcineurin-free protocols   1397

Immunological approaches   1397
  Mixed chimerism   1397
  Total lymphoid irradiation and donor bone
    marrow   1399

Conclusion   1399

The ultimate goal of immunosuppressive therapy is to produce in the recipient a state of tolerance of only those histoincompatible antigens presented by the donor, while retaining normal responsiveness to all other specificities. That this immunological state could be realized was observed more than 50 years ago in dizygotic cattle[1] and neonatal mice.[2] Since then, numerous strategies for inducing transplant tolerance have been developed (Fig. 86–1). Until recently, successful application of these approaches was limited to rodent models. As a result, the initial development of clinical transplantation relied upon identification of pharmacological or biological agents that globally suppressed immune responses (Table 86–1), even though, because of their nonspecificity, administration of such agents could be predicted to result in considerable morbidity. Subsequently, remarkable improvement in allograft survival rates and lower morbidity rates have been achieved as a result of the continued identification of new products that have progressively provided more selective suppression of host responses (Table 86–2).

Over the past 3 decades, most programs tended to rely upon induction therapy with as many as four or five agents, followed by maintenance therapy with two or three drugs. A more recent trend is toward induction therapy (with antilymphocyte preparations or interleukin (IL)-2 receptor antagonists) followed by "drug minimization" maintenance, the objective being to limit the use of steroids and calcineurin inhibitors. Nevertheless, the mainstay of current treatment is

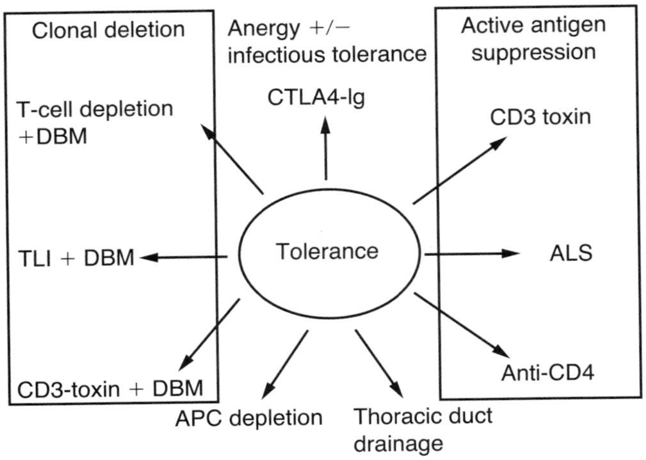

FIGURE 86–1
Possible strategies to induce tolerance. ALS, antilymphocyte serum;
APC, antigen-presenting cell; DBM, donor bone marrow;
TLI, T-lymphocyte infusion.

still steroids, calcineurin inhibitors, azathioprine, or
mycophenolate mofetil and OKT3 (Ortho Biotech) or
antithymocyte globulin (rabbit) (Thymoglobulin).[3]

Despite the improved immunosuppressive options
now available, approximately 20% to 30% of patients
undergoing orthotopic liver transplantation (OLT) are
treated for acute rejection within the first year. This
incidence has decreased from earlier reports (45% to
50% in the early 1990s), but adverse effects (e.g., bone
marrow suppression, rapid recurrence of hepatitis
C virus [HCV], posttransplantation liver disease [PTLD],
and diabetes, among others) continue to limit the rehabilitation of these recipients. No immunosuppressive

regimen has consistently produced long-term allograft
survival *free* of acute or chronic rejection. Therefore,
the ultimate goal, as for recipients of any allograft, continues to be the achievement of tolerance induction.
Only preliminary trials of tolerance induction are currently underway. Thus, this chapter mainly summarizes
those approaches that use regimens that attempt to
replace current agents without anticipating complete
drug withdrawal. Most human studies cited are of recipients of kidney transplantation. Some of the newer agents
and monoclonal antibodies (mAbs), however, are still at
the preclinical level and, therefore, primate studies are
reported as well. Rodent studies have the disadvantage of
being too far removed from clinical application, and for
that reason such studies are rarely included in this summary. This review summarizes the current status of only
those (a) new biological agents, (b) new pharmacologic
agents or regimens, and (c) tolerance-induction strategies
that have been or seem likely to be soon incorporated
into clinical practice.

New Biological Agents

The use of biological agents in clinical immunosuppressive protocols has progressed from polyclonal,
antilymphoid antibody preparations in the 1960s to
mAbs in the 1980s and 1990s, and now to more specifically designed protein molecules. This approach to
controlling immune responses is particularly attractive
because these agents exhibit unique therapeutic properties that, in contrast to conventional chemical immunosuppressants, selectively target immunocompetent cells.

Table 86–1. IMMUNOSUPPRESSIVE MILESTONES AND SUBSEQUENT MODIFICATIONS*

Clinical Introduction	Initial Product	Modification
1958	Irradiation	
1960	Steroids	
1961	Azathioprine	
1966	ALS	ATG, RATG
1978	Cyclosporine (Sandimmune)	Neoral, Gengraf, etc.
1980	OKT3	**HuM291, HuOKT3γ (Ala-Ala)**
1989	Tacrolimus	Sustained-release Prograf
1993	Mycophenolate (Myfortic)	Enteric-coated MMF
1998	**Tolerance**	**"Prope" Tolerance**
1999	Rapamycin	**Everolimus**
2000	Anti-IL2R	
2004	**FK778, FTY720, LEA29Y, alemtuzumab (Campath-1H), rituximab**	
Under Evaluation	**Anti-CD154, IVIg, MEDI-507**	

*__Bold__ formatted items are discussed in the chapter.
ALS, antilymphocyte serum; ATG, antithymocyte globulin; RATG, rabbit ATG.

Table 86-2. SPECIFICITY OF IMMUNOSUPPRESSIVE APPROACHES

Clinical Application	Degree of Unresponsiveness	Protocols Possible
1950s	Nonspecific	Aza, steroids, X-ray
1960s	Mononuclear cells	ALS
1970s	T cells	ATG, OKT3, CYA
1980s	T-cell subsets	mAbs (CD4, 8, 25, etc.)
1990s	T cells	MMF, FK506, rapamycin, Campath
2000s	Cellular responses, donor-specific "tolerance"	Anti-CD154, LEA29Y, mixed chimerism, TLI + DBM

ALS, antilymphocyte serum; ATG, antithymocyte globulin; Aza, azathioprine; CYA, cyclosporine A; mAbs, monoclonal antibodies; MMF, mycophenolate mofetil, TLI + DBM, total lymphoid irradiation + donor bone marrow.

These agents can, under some circumstances, even promote immune tolerance, which can be defined as an acquired state of antigen-specific unresponsiveness that is durable in the absence of chronic immunosuppression. This was first observed by Monaco and colleagues,[4] who showed that tolerance could be produced with thymectomy and antilymphocyte serum in adult mice, and continues to be pursued today in strategies designed to induce tolerance in humans.[5] The following approaches are currently in solid-organ transplantation clinical trials but have not yet been incorporated into routine practice.

Campath-1H

Campath-1H (alemtuzumab, anti-CD52) is a humanized mAb (IgG1) against CD52, which is located on thymocytes, lymphocytes, monocytes, macrophages, and the epithelial cells lining the male reproductive tract. The physiological function of CD52 is not known. Because CD52 is located on all lymphocytes, the effects of Campath-1H encompass both T and B cells.

Campath-1H has been evaluated for nearly a decade in a range of clinical trials including treatment or prevention of transplant rejection.[6] Renewed interest in this antibody was stimulated by the report of a study by Calne,[7] which indicated that a state of stable graft acceptance was observed in the majority of patients treated with Campath-1H and only minimal-dose conventional immunosuppression (sometimes referred to as "prope" tolerance, see subsequent text). In that trial, 31 patients received kidneys from deceased donors.[8] Immunosuppression was started after the transplantation procedure with an intravenous injection of 20 mg Campath-1H, followed by a second dose 24 hours later. On postoperative day 3, cyclosporine A (CYA) alone was added to the immunosuppressive regimen at a dose providing trough levels of approximately 75 to125 ng/mL. At follow-up of 15 to 28 months, 29 patients had sustained allograft function and no serious infections or malignancies were observed. Six patients had experienced acute rejections, which were successfully reversed. One patient died of congestive heart failure; 27 patients remained on low-dose CYA monotherapy.

In a similar drug minimization study by Knechtle and coworkers,[9] 40 mg of Campath-1H was given before kidney transplantation in 29 patients, followed by sirolimus monotherapy. The rate of early humoral rejection (5 of 29) was remarkable, with one patient losing the graft. This single anti-CD52 mAb dose, therefore, proved to be ineffective in blocking B-cell responses. In another pilot study performed at the National Institutes of Health (NIH),[10] Campath-1H was administered at a dosage of 0.3 mg/kg/day for 3 to 5 days to seven renal allograft recipients. Methylprednisolone was given with the first three doses; no other immunosuppressive agents were used. Peripheral lymphocyte counts decreased within 1 hour after initiating Campath-1H and returned gradually beginning 1 month after transplantation. Monocyte counts declined more gradually and recovered faster than the lymphocyte counts. Rejection requiring institution of conventional therapy was diagnosed in all patients between weeks 3 and 4, despite persisting, profound T-cell depletion. On evaluation of biopsy specimen, macrophage infiltration was the predominant histological picture.

Nishida and colleagues reported the use of Campath-1H in intestinal transplant recipients where very encouraging results were achieved. Only mild, easily controlled rejection was observed in 13 consecutive recipients, 11 of who were surviving at 1 year. This approach has been extended by the same group to multivisceral and liver transplant recipients. Campath-1H was typically administered in four doses of 0.3 mg/kg. Several patients in the multivisceral group had rejections that required steroid or OKT3 treatment, but none of the liver transplant recipients experienced rejection episodes after a follow-up period of 47 to 189 days. Infectious complications were not more common than in their previous experience. The authors concluded that steroid administration can, therefore, be limited to only the treatment of rejection episodes in patients who have received Campath-1H, except for intestinal transplant alone recipients who apparently require low-dose steroid treatment to maintain normal graft function.[6]

There has also been limited experience with Campath-1H therapy in a lung transplant recipient in whom repeated rejection episodes were unresponsive to steroids, tacrolimus, and intravenous immunoglobulins. Campath-1H was then administered at an initial dose of 3 mg/kg (significantly higher than doses in previous studies), followed by doses of 10, 30, and 30 mg on days 2, 3, and 4, respectively. The patient subsequently remained free of clinical and histopathological evidence of rejection after 8 months of follow-up. However, T-cell levels remained severely depressed, indicating that profound and long-lasting lymphocyte depletion can be observed following treatment with this agent.[11]

In summary, Campath-1H is a well-tolerated humanized mAb that has been shown to profoundly deplete B and T lymphocytes, but apparently it does not lead to an increased incidence of viral infections. Because of the long-lasting lymphopenia produced by this agent, maintenance immunosuppression has been successfully accomplished in many patients with single-drug conventional therapy. To date, however, successful withdrawal of all immunosuppressive therapy (tolerance induction) has not been accomplished. It appears to be a promising agent for induction, especially since it lacks the typical side effects of calcineurin inhibitors (nephrotoxicity and neurotoxicity). The long-term consequences of persisting T- and B-cell depletion remain to be established.

Humanized OKT3 Preparations— HuOKT3γ (Ala-Ala), HuM291

CD3, an immunoglobulin complex of five membrane-bound polypeptide chains, is closely associated with the T-cell receptor (TCR). The cytoplasmic tail of CD3 contains the "immunoreceptor tyrosine-based activation motif" (ITAM), which is crucial for signal transduction. When a major histocompatibility complex (MHC)–peptide complex binds to the TCR, a signal cascade is initiated leading to activation of "nuclear factor of activated T cells" (NF-AT), which in turn upregulates transcription and expression of the many genes necessary for T-cell proliferation.

Because T cells devoid of CD3 are unable to respond to alloantigen stimulation, biological agents that target this cell-surface immunoglobulin would be expected to effectively limit immune responses. OKT3, the first mAb developed for clinical use, confirmed this hypothesis.[12] This agent was first shown more than 20 years ago to reverse even steroid-resistant rejection. Limitations to its use include the development of antibodies to the murine molecule and adverse reactions of fever, chills, and nausea in response to the massive cytokine release

associated with initial administration of OKT3. This has fostered extensive studies that seek approaches that could remodel the antibody molecule to reduce the likelihood of these adverse effects while maintaining its remarkable immunosuppressive efficacy. Alegre and colleagues[13] genetically engineered the OKT3 molecule to produce a humanized mAb with specific mutations that result in reduced Fc-receptor binding activity— HuOKT3γ (Ala-Ala). These modifications provide not only a less immunogenic molecule but also a reduced likelihood of T-cell activation—which is largely responsible for the cytokine-release adverse effects. In a phase 1 study, this agent reversed rejection in five of seven renal or renal-pancreas recipients with minimal first-dose reactions and no evidence of anti-OKT3 antibody production.[14] The authors concluded that these encouraging observations support the conduct of additional trials with HuOKT3γ (Ala-Ala) which, in fact, are currently under way.[15]

Cole and coworkers[16] have designed another mouse mAb specific for the human CD3 complex. M291, the mouse anti-CD3 antibody, was humanized, producing HuM291, the binding capability of which is limited to the CD3 complex of humans and chimpanzees. HuM291 (visilizumab) induces apoptosis in activated T cells. Its human Ig2 isotype confers the longest half-life among human immunoglobulins and also reduces M291's ability to bind to complement. Like HuOKT3γ (Ala-Ala), HuM291 does not bind to the Fc receptor and, thus, is less likely to be associated with cytokine-release adverse reactions.

Initial clinical evaluation included treatment of graft-versus-host disease (GVHD) after bone marrow transplantation (BMT). In a series of 17 patients, there were 7 complete remissions and 3 partial remissions observed.[17] In another study, Norman and associates[18] evaluated the T-cell-depleting effects and toxicity of HuM291 in patients awaiting living donor kidney transplantation. Despite the theoretical advantages of this designer molecule, 30% to 70% of patients still experienced mild-to-moderate headache, chills, nausea, fever, and vomiting. Doses of 0.0015 to 0.015 mg/kg provided significant T-cell depletion, beginning 2 to 6 hours after the first dose, and lasting 4 to 8 days in the lower dose group and 8 to 13 days in the highest dose group. They concluded that this humanized mAb is better tolerated than OKT3, while retaining its potent pharmacological function with respect to depleting circulating CD2$^+$ and CD3$^+$ T cells.

In summary, genetic engineering technology has already produced at least two new anti-CD3 mAb preparations that may provide comparable therapeutic effects, but fewer of the complications associated with OKT3 administration. The ultimate role for these agents in future immunosuppressive protocols will depend upon the results of ongoing clinical trials.

CD3 Immunotoxin

Another possible approach to improving the efficacy of OKT3 is to prepare a conjugate, coupling a toxin to the mAb. Because of the antibody's high affinity for the CD3 receptor, the toxin would be delivered primarily to T cells. Anti-CD3 immunotoxin was developed in the mid-1990s by conjugating an antimonkey CD3 mAb to the mutant diphtheria toxin protein, CRM9. This diphtheria toxin has a 300-fold lower toxicity than the wild type. The immunotoxin depletes CD2$^+$ and CD3$^+$ lymphocytes from peripheral blood and lymph nodes to less than 1% of pretreatment levels, while the relative percentage of CD20$^+$ peripheral blood cells increases.[19] In nonhuman primate renal or islet transplant recipients this immunotoxin has, to date, shown inconsistent potential to facilitate tolerance induction.[20,21] When administering the drug at the time of transplantation, stimulation of alloantibody-producing B cells was observed with the consequent production of antidonor immunoglobulin. This was controlled by adding mycophenolate mofetil (MMF) and prednisone therapy.[22,23] A caveat for the clinical application of this approach is the report of occasional neurotoxicity in swine treated with a comparable immunotoxin. The observed neurotoxicity resembled diphtheria toxin–induced polyneuropathy.[24] Widespread clinical application of this approach, therefore, seems unlikely unless a reliable tolerance-inducing protocol can be defined.

MEDI-507

MEDI-507 (AlloMune component II) is a humanized anti-CD2 mAb of IgG1 subclass derived from the rat antibody parent BTI-322. CD2, also known as lymphocyte function associated antigen-2 (LFA-2), is an adhesion and signal transduction molecule expressed on T cells and most natural killer (NK) cells. Inhibition of CD2 signaling has been shown to result in T-cell apoptosis or anergy.[25] Because of limited cross-reactivity with other species, preclinical evaluation of MEDI-507 was possible only in chimpanzees, in which prolonged depletion of T cells was observed.

Initial clinical studies were undertaken in living donor kidney transplant recipients for whom MEDI-507 was used as induction therapy. Peripheral T-cell depletion, similar to that observed in chimpanzees, was noted and early rejection episodes were uncommon (unpublished observations). The most commonly reported side effects were lymphopenia, fever, and malaise. Because the profound and durable T-cell depletion produced by MEDI-507 suggested that it might be a useful agent for tolerance induction, most subsequent studies have been in this area.

Spitzer and colleagues[26] added MEDI-507 to a regimen consisting of thymic irradiation, cyclophosphamide, CYA, BMT, and posttransplantation donor lymphocyte infusion (DLI) in patients with chemorefractory hematological malignancies. MEDI-507 was well tolerated, leading to profound T-cell depletion that lasted for more than 2 months. No GVHD was encountered; however, because of graft loss in the first cohort of patients, the MEDI-507 was administered earlier prior to BMT in a subsequent group. This approach reduced the incidence of bone marrow rejection but significant GVHD was encountered. A third cohort, therefore, received MEDI-507 at the same time-points, but the bone marrow was modified to yield a CD34$^+$ T-cell enriched preparation. With this approach, excellent engraftment was observed and GVHD was avoided in all patients. On the basis of these studies we have now initiated a study of tolerance induction in haplo-identical kidney transplant recipients (see subsequent section, "Mixed Chimerism").

Anti-CD154/CD40

The first signal in a T-cell–mediated immune response is provided by antigen binding to the specific TCR; the second or costimulatory signal is received by T cells after interacting with the antigen-presenting cells (APCs). For full activation of T cells, both TCR-mediated and simultaneously delivered costimulatory signals are necessary. Without the costimulatory signals, allo-activated T-cells cannot effectively produce essential cytokines and abortive activation results. Attempts to block these costimulatory pathways, therefore, have been studied extensively as potential approaches to not only immunosuppression, but also tolerance induction. Among its costimulatory signals that have been identified, the CD40/CD40 ligand (CD154) and the CD28 or CTLA4/CD8086 pathways have been determined to be of central importance. CD154 is upregulated on activated T cells and serves as the ligand for the CD40 complex expressed on APCs. The interactions between CD154 and CD40 on endothelial cells are crucial in E-selectin and intercellular adhesion molecule (ICAM) upregulation and allograft rejection.

Kirk and colleagues[27] evaluated the humanized mAb against CD154, hu5C8, in a rhesus monkey renal transplant model. Monotherapy with this agent provided rejection-free survival for more than 100 days with no clinically evident side effects. When the antibody was combined with CTLA4-Ig, even longer-term survival was achieved, although most recipients still rejected their allografts. The investigators then evaluated chronic administration of hu5C8 in rhesus monkeys treated for several months.[28] This regimen led to renal allograft survival of more than 1 year, initially thought to represent tolerance induction. However, most recipients did eventually develop alloantibody and chronic rejection. No delays in wound healing, infections, or malignancies were observed, despite the fact that all animals were cytomegalovirus (CMV) positive before transplantation. These observations led the investigators to conclude that costimulatory blockade could revolutionize clinical approaches to rejection control.

More recently, the same group[29] combined another humanized mAb, IDEC-131, with rapamycin and donor-specific transfusions (DST) given to rhesus monkey skin transplant recipients. Their rationale was that DST-activated T cells would be eliminated in the presence of rapamycin. The investigators observed skin graft survival of 7 months in these recipients, including up to 4 months following cessation of immunosuppression. Knechtle[30] converted rhesus monkey renal allograft recipients to hu5C8, 60 days after transplantation and initial treatment with conventional immunosuppression consisting of steroids, MMF, and CYA. As in the previous studies, these authors noted prolonged, but not indefinite, allograft survival.

On the basis of these encouraging findings, clinical trials of anti-CD154 mAb therapy were undertaken in patients with both renal transplantation and autoimmune diseases such as psoriasis, idiopathic thrombocytopenic purpura, and systemic lupus erythematosus. These initial trials were halted when an unusually high incidence of thromboembolic complications was noted to be associated with the administration of anti-CD154.[31] Although Koyama and coworkers had observed similar thrombophilia in cynomolgus monkeys after kidney transplantation, the remarkable immunomodulatory properties of the costimulatory blocking agents encouraged these investigators to continue evaluation of anti-CD154 mAbs. They have now developed a protocol of administration, which appears to prevent the thromboembolic complications.[32]

In summary, blocking the CD40/CD154 pathway by anti-CD154 mAbs markedly prolongs allograft survival even long beyond the point of discontinuation of therapy. Unfortunately, the clinical promise of this therapeutic approach has been delayed by the observation of thromboembolic complications in the initially treated patients. Ongoing preclinical studies have now demonstrated that inhibition of platelet aggregation is an effective approach to controlling this thrombophilia, so that resumption of clinical trials may be possible in the near future.

CTLA4-Ig and LEA29Y

Manipulation of the CD28/CD80, 86 pathway has been mainly evaluated with the use of cytotoxic T-lymphocyte-associated protein 4 (CTLA4)-Ig fusion molecules.

Although such agents would be expected to inhibit both the costimulatory CD28/CD80, 86 and the regulatory CTLA4/CD80, 86 signals, the overall effect of CTLA4-Ig administration has been suppression of immune responses. CTLA4-Ig consists of the extracellular domain of CTLA4 and a fragment of the Fc domain of IgG1. LEA29Y is a second-generation molecule based on CTLA4-Ig, changed in two amino acid residues. Its affinity for CD80 and CD86 is not only greater than that of CD28 but also about twofold higher than CTLA4-Ig. Because CD28 must interact with CD80 and CD86 on APCs for full T-cell activation, LEA29Y administration interrupts the immune response by competitive inhibition. LEA29Y is active only in primates. Intravenous injections of LEA29Y at single doses up to 90 mg/kg or repeated doses of up to 50 mg/kg in cynomolgus monkeys were not associated with any significant signs of drug-related toxicity. In the repeat-dose studies, minimal reversible decreases in serum IgG levels and minimal to moderate reversible lymphoid depletion of splenic and/or lymph node germinal centers occurred. These were considered to be pharmacological effects of the drug and not clinically significant. Functional recovery of the immune system after 26 weeks of dosing followed by an 8-week drug-free period was demonstrated.

Adams and coworkers[33] investigated islet cell rejection in rhesus monkeys receiving either rapamycin and IL-2 receptor antibody alone or in conjunction with LEA29Y. Animals receiving the basic immunosuppression rejected the islets within 1 week, whereas addition of LEA29Y prolonged islet allograft survival to a mean of 204 days. Significant side effects were not encountered. In a preclinical renal transplant model, the same investigators observed prolongation of kidney survival to more than 6 months when LEA29Y was combined with CellCept (mycophenolate mofetil) and steroid therapy (personal communication).

LEA29Y has been evaluated in healthy volunteers in a phase I protocol; in a phase II protocol, in subjects with active rheumatoid arthritis; and in an ongoing phase II trial of renal allograft recipients randomized to receive either CYA or LEA29Y in conjunction with mycophenolate and steroids. In the phase I trial, 30 healthy volunteers received single intravenous infusions of LEA29Y at doses up to 20 mg/kg. The drug was well tolerated. All reported adverse events were of mild or moderate intensity. Subjects with active rheumatoid arthritis were randomized to LEA29Y, CTLA4-Ig, or placebo treatment.[34] Again, the drug was well tolerated. Initial efficacy evaluation revealed that less than 7% of LEA29Y-treated subjects discontinued therapy because of progressive disease, in contrast to more than 30% in the placebo group. Ongoing assessment of the renal allograft trial has been so encouraging that a multi-institution phase III study has been developed and will begin enrollment soon. This agent, therefore, could soon become available for clinical protocols designed to minimize or even exclude the use of calcineurin inhibitors.

Intravenous Immunoglobulin

Although conventional therapeutic protocols are effective for suppressing cellular responses to alloantigen stimulation, control of humoral immunity remains a challenge. In contrast to kidney allografts, the liver has proved to be relatively resistant to antibody-mediated injury. In fact, there have been reports of combined renal and liver transplants in highly sensitized recipients, in which the liver protected the kidney from hyperacute rejection despite a pretransplantation-positive cross-match.[35] Nevertheless, accelerated, presumably antibody-mediated, liver rejection has been reported[36] and earlier experience had suggested inferior liver allograft survival in highly sensitized recipients compared to that in their nonsensitized counterparts.[37] Current practice, however, has established that aggressive therapeutic measures will usually control humoral rejection in liver allografts and the pretransplantation presence of cytotoxic antibodies, therefore, should not be deleterious to survival.[38] Therapy for such rejection may include plasmapheresis and intravenous immunoglobulin (IVIg) in conjunction with intensive T-cell suppression, which was initially shown to provide effective rescue from refractory humoral rejection in renal allografts.[39] IVIg is a pooled human plasma product compiled of greater than 90% intact IgG. Several mechanisms of action have been suggested to explain the immunomodulatory effects of IVIg,[40] including negative signaling via Fc receptors that downregulates B-cell antibody production and neutralization via anti-idiotypes of circulating antibodies. Doses as high as 2 g/kg have been administered, with humoral rejection being successfully reversed in greater than 80% of renal allograft recipients.[41] More recently, IVIg has been used in preemptive protocols administered to highly sensitized renal allograft candidates.[42,43] Transplantation of such patients was previously hampered by the need to find a compatible organ lacking any of the human leukocyte antigen (HLA) specificities recognized by the recipient's antibodies. As a result, the waiting time for these patients was, at best, much prolonged; and many could never receive a transplant. IVIg therapy has now been shown to eliminate positive cross-matches. Jordan and colleagues at the UCLA School of Medicine[42] originally studied such protocols. In patients with potential living donors, 2 g/kg was administered and the cross-match was repeated immediately after the IVIg infusion. If the result was negative, the patient underwent transplantation within 1 to 3 days. For deceased donor candidates, an IVIg test dose was administered to confirm that

in vitro inhibition occurred. IVIg was then administered for 4 months before transplantation, with another dose given 1 month after transplantation. Thirty-one percent of the successfully transplanted recipients developed rejection episodes; however, only three grafts were lost to rejection. Patient and graft survival rates at 2 years were 97.6% and 89.1%, respectively. Thus this approach now allows successful renal transplantation of highly sensitized patients for whom it was previously contraindicated. As noted previously, this has not proved to be necessary for sensitized liver allograft recipients who can typically be managed by transplantation, even in the presence of a positive cross-match. Such recipients are monitored more closely in the postoperative period, and treatment for humoral rejection is added only if necessary.

Rituximab

Rituximab, a chimeric mouse/human mAb directed against the CD20 specificity, provides greater than 90% peripheral blood B-cell depletion following the first administered dose. Rituximab was initially evaluated in patients with rheumatoid arthritis in whom accumulative dosages as high as 2 g have been administered. This resulted in profound B-cell depletion, which was sustained for several months. These observations suggested that this mAb might be uniquely efficacious for treatment of B-cell–initiated humoral rejection. Several recent reports have now confirmed this hypothesis.[9,44] As with IVIg summarized previously, rituximab is also being evaluated in preemptive therapeutic protocols designed to interrupt alloantibody production in highly sensitized renal transplant candidates. Again, this particular issue is of lesser consequence for liver allograft recipients; however, the obvious efficacy of rituximab in such trials indicates that it will probably play an increasingly important role in many future immunosuppressive protocols.

New Pharmacological Regimens and Agents

In contrast to biological preparations, pharmacological agents are rather nonselective in their effects on immune responses. However, since immunomodulation often requires simultaneous interruption of many pathways at the same time, most of which were undefined until recently, the relative nonspecificity of these agents was essential for the development of early immunosuppressive protocols. These agents, in fact, have proven to be remarkably effective, admittedly at a cost of well-recognized side-effects (e.g., neurotoxicity, nephrotoxicity, diabetes, hirsutism, and posttransplantation lymphoproliferative disorder [PTLD]) that limit rehabilitation or contribute to mortality following otherwise successful organ transplantation. To address these limitations, a number of trials attempting to avoid or wean drugs from earlier regimens have been undertaken.

Steroid Withdrawal and Avoidance

The adverse effects of steroids are many and are largely dose related. These effects can greatly limit the recipient's quality of life, especially in the pediatric population, where permanent growth retardation does not occur infrequently. Numerous attempts have been made to reduce doses or even to withdraw steroid therapy early after liver transplantation. The results of these efforts remained mixed over the past 2 decades, when most patients had been maintained on triple-drug regimens typically including CYA, azathioprine (Imuran), and prednisone. Prednisone withdrawal from such protocols was regularly shown to provide a number of benefits but was found, not infrequently, to increase the risk of rejection and even graft loss. This observation was sufficiently evident in some renal allograft trials that patient enrollment was stopped early when excess rejection (30% in the withdrawal group versus 10% in control) was noted.[45]

In contrast, several uncontrolled trials with tacrolimus-based immunosuppression initially suggested that successful liver transplantation could be accomplished without the use of steroids.[46] The first report of a controlled randomized trial of steroid-free immunosuppressive therapy in liver transplantation came from Eason and colleagues.[47] In 119 liver transplant recipients they compared rabbit antithymocyte globulin (RATG), beginning intraoperatively, to methylprednisolone (1 g during the anhepatic phase, then weaned to 20 mg daily by postoperative day 6 and discontinued after 3 months). Patients in both groups received tacrolimus and MMF. MMF was discontinued in both groups after 3 months, with long-term suppression being tacrolimus monotherapy. The incidence of acute rejection was 25% in RATG-treated patients and 31% in the steroid group, in all cases occurring within the first 30 days after transplantation. Interestingly, CMV infection (5% versus 23%) and new-onset diabetes mellitus (2% versus 14%) were significantly lower in the RATG-treated group. Patient survival in HCV-negative and HCV-positive patients was similar, although there was a trend toward more fibrosis and cirrhosis within 2 years after the transplant in the steroid-treated group (21% versus 11%, respectively). These observations have encouraged more widespread adoption of steroid-sparing, tacrolimus-based immunosuppressive protocols. The approach is especially attractive for recipients whose underlying disease is HCV, reactivation of which is greatly enhanced by high-dose steroids. An additional consideration is the ample animal data indicating that peritransplant steroid administration impairs the induction of tolerance. The underlying mechanism remains undefined, but one hypothesis is that steroids interfere with regulatory dendritic cell activity in the thymus. We have been evaluating a therapeutic protocol in which HCV-positive liver transplant recipients receive RATG induction and no steroids. Initial observations indicate that this approach leads to a low incidence of rejection, lower levels of viral replication, and a significant delay in the posttransplantation HCV recurrence rate compared to conventional triple-drug immunosuppression (unpublished data). An excellent summary of approaches to steroid-free immunosuppression is provided in a recent review by Hricik.[48]

Drug Minimization—"Prope" Tolerance

Although graft loss from early acute rejection is now uncommon, chronic rejection, particularly following heart or kidney transplantation, leads to graft loss in more than 50% of recipients after 5 to 10 years. In liver transplantation there is less likelihood of chronic rejection, but the recipient faces the complications of life-threatening infection, disease recurrence (e.g., viral hepatitis), and the myriad of adverse effects of chronic immunosuppression. Nearly 5% of patients more than 5 years out after liver transplantation develop chronic renal failure; and, increasingly, cardiac events develop as a result of the steroid and calcineurin inhibitor–induced hypertension and hyperlipidemia. Therefore, the current goal in liver transplantation, as in heart and kidney transplantation, is to develop protocols that provide minimal long-term exposure to immunosuppressive drugs (Table 86–3).

As initially observed by Starzl, long-term surviving liver allograft recipients have sometimes discontinued all immunosuppressive therapy without rejection of the allograft.[49] Subsequent trials of deliberate weaning of immunosuppressive agents has confirmed that some 15% to 30% of patients can successfully come off of all immunosuppression 5 or more years after the transplant procedure (see reference 50 for overview). For example, Mazariegos and colleagues reported the outcome in 95 patients who were 8.4 ± 4.4 years out after liver or liver-kidney transplantation.[51] Eighteen patients (19%) had been drug-free for 10 months to 4.8 years, another 18 patients had biopsy-proven acute rejection, necessitating reinstitution of immunosuppression. The remaining patients were still in the weaning process. There was no rejection-related death; two patients died during the study from immunosuppression-related morbidity. In that study the weaning process was azathioprine first, steroids next, and last, calcineurin inhibitors. Later the protocol was changed to weaning calcineurin inhibitors first, followed by azathioprine and prednisone. Oike and others[52] reported the outcome of 67 patients who

Table 86-3. DRUG MINIMIZATION TRIALS ("PROPE" TOLERANCE)

Induction (ref)	Planned Monotherapy	Success	Reject	Off IS
Campath-1H[8]	CYA	27/31	6/31	0
Campath-1H[9]	Rapa	20/24	8/24 (CD4+)	0
Campath-1H + infliximab[53]	Delayed rapa	13/15	15/15	0
Thymoglobulin[54]	FK506	30/50	> 50%	0
Thymoglobulin[56]	Rapa	10/11	3/11	0
HuM291 (huOKT3γ (Ala-Ala)) (unpublished)	Rapa	In progress		

IS, immunosuppression.

had been stable without evidence of rejection more than 2 years after liver transplantation. Sixteen of these patients (24%) achieved a drug-free state; eight had experienced rejection episodes; the remainder of patients were still being weaned.

Unfortunately, no assay is currently available to distinguish this subset of operationally tolerant long-term survivors from the much larger majority in whom rejection ensues, even at this late date. As a result, essentially all liver allograft recipients have been advised that they must continue immunosuppression indefinitely. Now the development of increasingly powerful immunosuppressive agents has encouraged a new approach intended to induce profound peritransplant T-cell depletion, which, it is hoped, might more reliably induce the type of operational tolerance that has been observed in the sporadic liver allograft recipients following long-term treatment with conventional therapy. Initial preclinical and clinical studies emphasized that monotherapy with antibodies, such as those listed in Table 86–2, resulted in an unacceptably high incidence of rejection.[10,53] Thus, the clinical approach has been to add to the antibody induction regimen, chronic administration of minimal and it is hoped nontoxic, doses of maintenance pharmacological therapy. This was initially devised by Calne, who termed the resulting immunological state "prope" or "almost" tolerance.[7] As detailed earlier, that trial combined alemtuzumab (Campath-1H) with low dosage CYA in deceased donor renal allograft recipients with very encouraging results. The following summary reviews some of the observations that have emerged from the various protocols currently exploring this strategy.

Again, as noted earlier, Knechtle and others have evaluated, in 29 renal allograft recipients, a drug minimization protocol similar to that used by Calne, except that Campath-1H induction was combined with rapamycin rather than CYA monotherapy.[9] After a follow-up of 3 to 29 months, only one allograft had been lost. However, the authors reported biopsy-proven rejection within the first month in eight of the recipients. Of greatest concern was the observation of pathological features consistent with antibody-mediated allograft injury in five of the patients. This unacceptably high incidence of early humoral rejection prompted a halt to this trial and modification of the regimen by the addition of tacrolimus. Complete drug withdrawal had not been attempted in any recipient.

Starzl and coworkers have subsequently used a similar approach in recipients of various deceased donor organs,[54] in which monotherapy with tacrolimus was continued after initial induction with high-dose RATG and prednisone. When available, donor bone marrow (DBM) was also infused. Preliminary reports of this regimen in kidney, pancreas, bowel, and liver recipients noted a rather high incidence of what was interpreted as acute rejection on protocol biopsies (more than 50% in renal recipients) but excellent overall graft and patient survival.[55] Sirolimus, prednisone, and OKT3 were added for episodes of rejection. Graft survival was 89% and patient survival 95% at 1 year. Forty-three of 72 recipients with functioning primary grafts were receiving spaced-dose tacrolimus with every-other-day, twice-weekly, or even once-weekly dosing. There was no apparent benefit derived from DBM infusion. No patients had had complete withdrawal of immunosuppression.

A similar approach using RATG induction with maintenance sirolimus monotherapy is being evaluated by Kirk and associates.[56] The investigators also noted a high incidence of early but reversible rejection ultimately leading to good long-term function without the need for chronic steroid or calcineurin inhibitor treatment in most patients. Maintenance immunosuppression, however, could not be withdrawn from any patient.

These and other similar approaches using the humanized OKT3 mAbs (discussed previously) for T-cell depletion have emphasized that many patients are chronically overimmunosuppressed by currently used protocols. Unfortunately, however, no combination of T-cell depletion and conventional pharmacological therapy studied to date has been found to reliably induce tolerance.

FK778

FK778 (malononitrilamide 715) is a promising member of a new class of low-molecular-weight immunosuppressive agents that are derivatives of leflunomide.

FK778 acts as an antimetabolite that blocks T- and B-cell function by inhibiting the dihydroorotate dehydrogenase, a key enzyme in de novo pyrimidine synthesis. Qi and colleagues57 administered FK778 to Velvet monkey renal allograft recipients either with or without tacrolimus. The best results were achieved with tacrolimus starting at the time of transplantation and FK778 given on postoperative day 7. Interestingly, giving both drugs together at the time of transplantation did not yield similarly prolonged allograft survival, despite the long half-life of FK778 of 15 to 18 days. It was speculated that tacrolimus was probably most effective in blocking T-cell–related acute rejection, which occurs 3 to 4 days after transplantation and that FK778 acted synergistically by inhibiting B-cell proliferation that peaks at 7 days after transplantation. This anti–B-cell activity makes this class of immunosuppressive agents extremely attractive; however, no clinical trials have yet been reported.

FTY720

FTY720 is a synthetic low-molecular-weight compound with potent immunosuppressive properties. Its mechanism of action, which is distinct from that of the calcineurin inhibitors (CNIs), provides synergistic effects with tacrolimus and CYA but without increased toxicity. In vitro data suggest that FTY720, an agonist of the sphingosine-1-phosphate receptor, increases chemokine-dependent lymphocyte trafficking from the peripheral blood into secondary lymphoid tissue, thereby reducing the recruitment of activated lymphocytes into the allograft. In conjunction with CNIs, FTY720 has provided adequate suppression even for islet xenotransplantation.[58] In a rat heart transplant model with donor-specific blood transfusion, Koshiba and associates[59] found that FTY720 and CYA given for more than 90 days completely prevented chronic rejection. Neither drug given alone abrogated chronic injury. Kimura and coworkers used FTY720 in a small-bowel transplant model. All rats in the control group died 7 to 10 days after small-bowel transplantation, whereas the mean survival in FTY720-treated recipients was greater than 60 days.[60] Comparably encouraging observations in canine and nonhuman primate renal allograft recipients have now led to clinical trials incorporating FTY720 into conventional therapeutic protocols. In a randomized, placebo-controlled phase I study, patients at least 1 year after renal transplantation received once-daily doses of 0.125 to 5 mg FTY720 or placebo for 28 days. FTY720 led to a 30% to 80% reduction in peripheral blood lymphocyte counts within 4 hours of initial administration with return to near-normal levels within 24 to 96 hours in a dose-dependent fashion. The major potential advantage offered by FTY720 is its lack of nephrotoxicity,

neurotoxicity, and marrow suppressive function, none of which was observed in this trial.[61] Of concern has been the potential for cardiac side effects, particularly bradycardia, which has been sporadically observed but was not confirmed in this clinical trial.

The ultimate clinical utility of FTY720 remains difficult to predict but will be clarified by phase III randomized trials currently under way. Of particular potential interest for liver transplantation is the recently reported observation that FTY720 may ameliorate biochemical and histological manifestations of hepatic ischemia and reperfusion injury.[62] Presumably the mechanism is related to removal from the circulation of T lymphocytes as mediators of the ischemia-reperfusion process.

Everolimus

Everolimus (Certican) is a recently discovered proliferation signal inhibitor derived from sirolimus (rapamycin). Sirolimus binds to cytoplasmic immunophilins (FKBP-12), resulting in arrest of cell cycle progression at the $G_1 \rightarrow S$ transition. Everolimus also binds to FKBP-12, but its affinity is about threefold weaker than that of rapamycin.[63] Nevertheless, in rat models of glomerulonephritis, the efficacy was similar between the two drugs. In rat kidney allograft experiments, everolimus-treated recipients did not show rejection during an observation period of 80 days, whereas all animals in the rapamycin group showed severe cellular rejection. In a rat heterotopic heart transplant model, a combined CYA and everolimus therapeutic regimen led to long-term graft survival.[63] Everolimus has also been shown to be effective in preventing chronic graft nephropathy, probably related to its apoptosis-enhancing properties.[64]

Everolimus/full-dose CYA was compared with MMF/CYA in a multicenter study[65] of adult patients undergoing kidney transplantation. The major side effects of everolimus/CYA were hyperlipidemia and hypercholesterolemia, which were observed in almost 50% of patients. Everolimus showed equal efficacy to MMF in terms of incidence of rejection and patient and graft survival but was associated with a higher median serum creatinine level. This has prompted an ongoing subsequent study using everolimus in combination with reduced-dose CYA.

Kahan and coworkers[66] compared different doses of everolimus in conjunction with CYA and corticosteroids in renal transplant recipients. A dosage of 1, 2, or 4 mg/day led to biopsy-proven acute rejection episodes within the first 6 months in 32.4%, 14.7%, and 25.7% of recipients, respectively. The incidence of viral and fungal infections was found to be higher in the group treated with 4 mg/day everolimus.

In a cardiac transplant study, 634 patients were randomly assigned to receive either everolimus (1.5 mg or

3 mg/day) or azathioprine (1 to 3 mg/kg/day) in conjunction with CYA and corticosteroids. The endpoints were death, graft loss or retransplantation, grade 3A biopsy-proven acute rejection, or rejection with hemodynamic compromise. In the group receiving 3 mg/day of everolimus, only 27% reached the endpoints at 6 months compared with 36% of patients receiving 1.5 mg everolimus and 40.6% of patients in the azathioprine group. Of major interest was the finding on intravascular ultrasonography of reduced intimal thickness 12 months after transplantation in the everolimus-treated groups. CMV infections were also significantly reduced in the everolimus groups compared with the azathioprine group (7.7% and 7.6% versus 21.5%, respectively). Rates of bacterial infections were higher in the 3-mg everolimus group compared with the azathioprine group.[67]

In conclusion, everolimus may offer a new treatment option, with its particular attraction being its potential to limit the likelihood of chronic rejection. This is illustrated by its already observed capacity to delay vasculopathy in heart transplant recipients. However, the agent seems to have an adverse effect profile similar to that of the original drug sirolimus, including hyperlipidemia and bone marrow depression. Ongoing studies are under way to delineate further the possible benefits of this new immunosuppressive agent.

Calcineurin-Free Protocols

Currently, essentially every treatment regimen includes a CNI as part of the therapeutic protocol. Unfortunately, nephrotoxicity associated with CNI administration results in impaired renal function in 5% to 9% of extrarenal transplant recipients receiving CYA or tacrolimus. The goal, therefore, has been to define effective maintenance immunosuppressive protocols that minimize long-term administration of these agents. At this point it remains unclear whether the safest approach is to use CNI-free suppression immediately after transplantation or to convert liver allograft recipients later in the follow-up period, or to maintain recipients on CNI indefinitely. Stewart and associates[68] attempted to convert liver transplant recipients, who developed renal failure while receiving CYA therapy, to MMF monotherapy. Although the renal failure improved in all patients, the trial was stopped when three of five patients receiving monotherapy developed rejection necessitating retransplantation.

Schlitt and coworkers[69] reported a similar experience. In their study, 5 of 14 patients developed liver function abnormalities 2 to 3 months after conversion to MMF, 3 of whom had biopsy-proven rejection. All patients with rejection were restarted on CNI with successful reversal of rejection.

Similar observations have been reported in kidney transplant recipients for whom almost all studies noted better renal function in the non-CNI arm, but the benefit was often offset by an increased rate of acute rejection.

As detailed previously (see "New Biological Agents"), LEA29Y is one of the most promising new agents that could allow development of effective CNI-free immunosuppression. Its major limitation, however, is the requirement for chronic parenteral administration. For the future, the challenge remains to identify patients who will do well after minimization of immunosuppressants. Clearly, a reliable assay for monitoring each patient's immune status would limit the likelihood of immunosuppressant-related complications. Unfortunately, at this point, such assays remain in the developmental stage.

Immunological Approaches

Mixed Chimerism

More than a decade ago, it was reported that induction of complete hematopoietic chimerism with myeloablative therapy and bone marrow transplantation in humans provides tolerance to subsequently implanted renal allografts. Thus, patients who developed renal failure after a previous allogeneic BMT for treatment of hematological malignancies were able to receive a kidney transplant from the same donor with no requirement for immunosuppression.[70] However, the infectious and GVHD-derived morbidity associated with the myeloablative conditioning required to accomplish these successful bone marrow transplantations precludes the routine application of this approach to induction of tolerance for patients undergoing solid-organ transplantation. Clearly, a state of mixed chimerism would be preferable, in which the presence of donor-derived elements induces tolerance while host-type APCs maintain normal immunocompetence.

Confirmation of the validity of such a strategy began with the finding by Ildstad and Sachs[71] in 1984 that mice reconstituted with a mixture of donor- and recipient-strain bone marrow following myeloablative conditioning became specifically tolerant of skin allografts from the bone marrow donor. The lethal total-body irradiation (TBI) used in these initial "proof of concept" studies was subsequently replaced with nonmyeloablative therapeutic protocols, including T-cell–depleting mAbs and local thymic irradiation.[72] Such conditioning regimens have been observed to provide transient T-cell depletion, to allow engraftment of the DBM, and to result in multilineage chimerism and donor-specific tolerance indistinguishable from that observed in mixed chimeras prepared by lethal irradiation.

We have extended this approach to the induction of renal allograft tolerance through mixed chimerism in

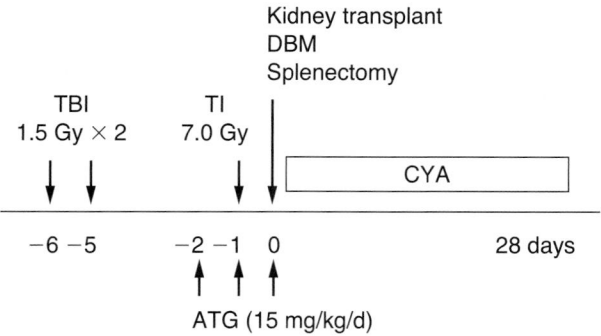

FIGURE 86-2

Conditioning protocol for inducing mixed chimerism and renal allograft tolerance in cynomolgus monkeys. ATG, horse antithymocyte globulin (ATGAM); CYA, cyclosporin A; DBM, donor bone marrow; TI, thymic irradiation; TBI, total-body irradiation.

nonhuman primates.[73] Some of the monkeys studied initially[74] have maintained normal allograft function with no evidence of chronic rejection for as long as 10 years after discontinuation of immunosuppressive therapy.

Elements of the initial preparative regimen included TBI (1.5 Gy × 2), local thymic irradiation (7 Gy), antithymocyte globulin (ATGAM), splenectomy, DBM, and a 1-month course of CYA therapy following transplantation (Fig. 86-2). Recipients conditioned with this regimen typically developed multilineage chimerism detectable by flow cytometry over the first several weeks; approximately 70% survived long term. The recipients showed donor-specific hyporesponsiveness in vitro and accepted skin grafts from the original kidney donor while rapidly rejecting allografts from third-party animals. Most importantly, there has been no evidence of chronic renal allograft rejection in sequential renal allograft biopsies, a highly unusual observation among currently reported nonhuman primate tolerance trials. In addition, no GVHD was observed in any recipient, most likely because of the continued presence of residual T-cell–depleting ATGAM in the serum of the recipient at the time of DBM infusion, and possibly also reflecting the inherently decreased susceptibility of mixed chimeras to GVHD.[75]

The remarkable efficacy of the tolerant state produced in these animal models and the lack of serious toxicity observed in long-term survivors suggested that mixed chimerism might provide a reliable strategy for achieving solid-organ acceptance without chronic immunosuppression in humans. Initial application of this concept was undertaken by Sykes and colleagues[76] and Spitzer and coworkers[77] in patients receiving HLA-matched and mismatched BMT for the treatment of refractory hematological malignancies. In these studies, the therapeutic regimen outlined in Figure 86-2 was modified by replacing TBI with cyclophosphamide (200 mg/kg) in order to provide more cytoreductive capability for the malignancy. Donor chimerism and

striking antitumor responses were achieved in more than 80% of the treated patients. Severe GVHD did not prove to be a major limitation for HLA-matched donor-recipient pairs. Acute GVHD or graft loss, however, did develop after HLA-mismatched DBM transplantation, indicating that the initial protocol did not provide sufficient donor or recipient T-cell depletion. The regimen was, therefore, further modified to include MEDI-507 (see earlier), in place of ATGAM, for haplo-identical bone marrow transplantation.[26] All of these observations proved to be crucial for the development of the first clinical trials of deliberate induction of mixed lymphohematopoietic chimerism to provide allotolerance of a solid-organ transplant.

The first patients chosen for induction of renal allograft tolerance were individuals with an available HLA-matched donor and end-stage renal disease (ESRD) secondary to multiple myeloma.[78] The dual indication attempt to induce tolerance and need for neoplasia treatment presented by these patients made them especially appropriate candidates for such innovative therapy. The first of the six individuals treated to date was entered into the protocol in October 1998. The conditioning regimen for these patients is shown in Figure 86-3. The treatment was modified from that used for treatment of malignancy alone (see Fig. 86-2), in view of their impaired renal function. Therefore, patients with ESRD received only 120 mg/kg of cyclophosphamide. CYA was begun on day 1 and continued postoperatively with the plan to discontinue it at 2 to 3 months postoperatively. This was accomplished in five of the six patients between days 40 and 77. One patient was continued on CYA until day 380 because of facial and truncal erythematous rash consistent with mild GVHD.

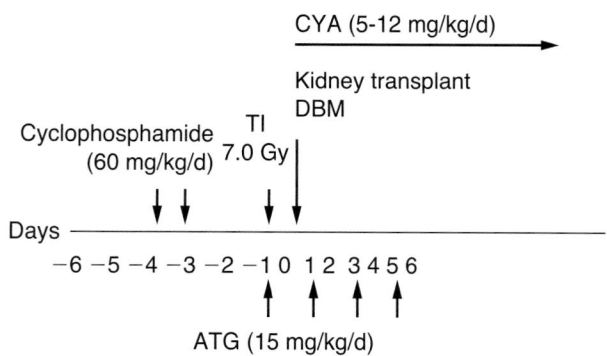

FIGURE 86-3

Conditioning regimen used in patients with multiple myeloma and end-stage renal disease. The therapeutic regimen of the animal experiments was modified by replacing TBI with cyclophosphamide (120 mg/kg) in order to provide more cytoreductive capability for the malignancy. ATG, antithymocyte globulin; CYA, cyclosporine A; DBM, donor bone marrow; TBI, total-body irradiation; TI, thymic irradiation.

In all patients, renal function was normalized within 48 hours. Despite discontinuation of all immunosuppressive therapy, there has been no evidence of rejection in any patient. Long-term kidney allograft function has remained normal except in one patient in whom persistent multiple myeloma has resulted in recurrent cast nephropathy.

In summary, of the six patients followed to date over periods of 8 months to more than 5 years, all have developed apparent renal allograft tolerance, five have stable or complete remission of the myeloma, and mild GVHD was observed in only two patients who were converted with DLI to full donor chimerism in an effort to control their myeloma. As in the nonhuman primate recipients, there has been no evidence of chronic rejection observed in sequential allograft biopsies, despite withdrawal of all immunosuppressive therapy for up to 5 years.

Encouraged by the consistently successful induction of allograft tolerance in the first trial, we more recently extended this approach to patients with ESRD without malignancy and without an available HLA-matched donor. We designed a treatment protocol for this study on the basis of observations made in our earlier nonhuman primate studies and in the clinical therapeutic trials for hematological malignancies.[26,76,77] These studies had shown that treatment with MEDI-507 instead of ATGAM could minimize the risk of GVHD,[26] but still achieve the same kind of transient mixed chimerism that was effective in inducing tolerance in monkeys.[73] Except for this substitution and the absence of DLI, the conditioning for these recipients was identical to that for recipients with multiple myeloma.

To date, three patients have entered this study. Although it is still too early to evaluate the long-term results, the data in at least two of these patients are encouraging with regard to the likely establishment of tolerance.

Total-Lymphoid Irradiation and Donor Bone Marrow

Nonmyeloablative total-lymphoid irradiation (TLI) followed by transplantation of granulocyte colony stimulating factor (G-CSF)-stimulated DBM progenitor cells has been successfully used to control hematological or lymphoid malignancies. The group at Stanford University[79] has extended this approach to solid-organ transplantation. They transfused CD34$^+$ (stem cell)-enriched donor peripheral blood mononuclear cells into four patients receiving an HLA-mismatched kidney. Induction immunosuppression included RATG (1.5 mg/kg) followed by TLI beginning on day 1 for a total of 10 doses (800 cGy). Prednisone was started at day 0 and CYA was started 3 days before infusion of the donor cells.

The CD34$^+$ cells were administered after the last TLI treatment on postoperative day 11. Mixed chimerism developed in three of four patients; in two of these patients, all immunosuppression was weaned. Both patients subsequently required reinstitution of therapy when acute rejection was diagnosed. None of the patients developed GVHD or any significant infectious complications from this intense treatment except for one patient with herpes zoster at 6 months.

This study, as well as others aforementioned, show that the century-long quest, namely, the successful transplantation of organs or tissues without the need for chronic immunosuppression, might enter its final stage. The holy grail of transplantation immunology, the reliable establishment of long-term stable tolerance, now appears to be imminent.

None of these approaches has yet been studied in liver allograft recipients. However, in view of the observation that a state of operational tolerance is most often observed after a period of chronic immunosuppression in liver transplant recipients, one might anticipate that deliberate induction of tolerance might be most successful with this organ.

Conclusion

With the large number of immunosuppressive agents already available or now under evaluation, the clinician is challenged to define the optimal protocol for induction and maintenance therapy for each recipient. This chapter has reviewed newer approaches that seem promising for clinical application in the near future. This review emphasizes that current strategies, in contrast to earlier four- and five-drug regimens, are increasingly directed toward selective immunomodulation, drug minimization, and even complete drug withdrawal. For the first time in the 50-year history of clinical transplantation, recipients are being conditioned with the intention of providing long-term allograft acceptance without the requirement for ongoing immune therapy. In fact, a handful of patients has now provided proof of concept for this approach, suggesting that the long sought dream of tolerance may soon become reality for increasing numbers of human allograft recipients.

References

1. Owen RD: Immunogenetic consequences of vascular anastomoses between bovine twins. Science 102:400-401, 1945.
2. Billingham RE, Brent L, Medawar PB: Actively acquired tolerance of foreign cells. Nature 172:603-606, 1953.
3. Helderman JH, Bennett WM, Cibrik DM, et al: Immunosuppression: Practice and trends. Am J Transplant 3(Suppl 4):41-52, 2003.
4. Monaco AP, Wood ML, Russell PS: Studies on heterologous antilymphocyte serum in mice. III. Immunological tolerance and chimerism produced across the H2-locus with adult thymectomy and antilymphocyte serum. Ann N Y Acad Sci 129:190-209, 1996.

5. Spitzer TR, Delmonico F, Tolkoff-Rubin N, et al: Combined histocompatibility leukocyte antigen–matched donor bone marrow and renal transplantation for multiple myeloma with end-stage renal disease: The induction of allograft tolerance through mixed lymphohematopoietic chimerism. Transplantation 68:480-484, 1999.

6. Tzakis A, Kato S, Nishida S, et al: Preliminary experience with Campath 1H (C1H) in intestinal and liver transplantation. Transplantation 75:1227-1231, 2003.

7. Calne R: Prope tolerance: A step in the search for tolerance in the clinic. World J Surg 24:793-796, 2000.

8. Calne R, Moffatt SD, Friend PJ, et al: Campath 1H allows low-dose cyclosporine monotherapy in 31 cadaveric renal allograft recipients. Transplantation 681:613-1616, 1999.

9. Knechtle SJ, Pirsch JD, Fechner JH, et al: Campath-1H induction plus rapamycin monotherapy for renal transplantation: Results of a pilot study. Am J Transplant 3:722-730, 2003.

10. Kirk AD: Less is more: Maintenance minimization as a step toward tolerance. Am J Transplant 3:643-645, 2003.

11. Reams BD, Davis RD, Curl J, et al: Treatment of refractory acute rejection in a lung transplant recipient with Campath 1H. Transplantation 74:903-904, 2002.

12. Cosimi AB, Burton RC, Colvin RB, et al: Treatment of acute renal allograft rejection with OKT3 monoclonal antibody. Transplantation 32:535-539, 1981.

13. Alegre ML, Peterson LJ, Xu D, et al: A non-activating "humanized" anti-CD3 monoclonal antibody retains immunosuppressive properties in vivo. Transplantation 57:1537-1543, 1994.

14. Woodle ES, Xu D, Zivin RA, et al: Phase I trial of a humanized, Fc receptor nonbinding OKT3 antibody, huOKT3γ1 (Ala-Ala) in the treatment of acute renal allograft rejection. Transplant Proc 68:608-616, 1999.

15. Hering BJ, Kandaswamy R, Harmon JV, et al: Transplantation of cultured islets from two-layer preserved pancreases in type 1 diabetes with anti-CD3 antibody. Am J Transplant 4:390-401, 2004.

16. Cole MS, Stellrecht KE, Shi JD, et al: HuM291, a humanized anti-CD3 antibody, is immunosuppressive to T cells while exhibiting reduced mitogenicity in vitro. Transplantation 68:563-571, 1999.

17. Carpenter JR, Appelbaum FR, Corey L, et al: A humanized non-FcR-binding anti-CD3 antibody, visilizumab, for treatment of steroid-refractory acute graft-versus-host disease. Blood 99:2712-2719, 2002.

18. Norman DJ, Vincenti F, De Mattos AM, et al: Phase I trial of HuM291, a humanized anti-CD3 antibody, in patients receiving renal allografts from living donors. Transplantation 70:1707-1712, 2000.

19. Hamawy MM, Tsuchida M, Cho CS, et al: Immunotoxin FN18-CRM9 induces stronger T cell signaling than unconjugated monoclonal antibody FN18. Transplantation 72:496-503, 2001.

20. Fechner JH, Vargo DJ, Geissler EK, et al: Split tolerance induced by immunotoxin in a rhesus kidney allograft model. Transplantation 63:1339-1345, 1997.

21. Contreras JL, Wang PX, Eckhoff DE, et al: Peritransplant tolerance induction with anti-CD3-immunotoxin: A matter of proinflammatory cytokine control. Transplantation 65:1159-1169, 1998.

22. Armstrong N, Buckley P, Oberley T, et al: Analysis of primate renal allografts after T-cell depletion with anti-CD3-CRM9. Transplantation 66:5-13, 1998.

23. Fechner JH, Dong Y, Hong X, et al: Graft survival in a rhesus renal transplant model after immunotoxin-mediated T-cell depletion is enhanced by mycophenolate and steroids. Transplantation 72:581-587, 2001.

24. Gargollo P, Yamada K, Esnaola N, et al: Neuropathy in miniature swine after administration of the mutant diphtheria toxin–based immunotoxin, pCD3-CRM9. Transplantation 72:818-822, 2001.

25. Branco L, Barren P, Mao S-Y, et al: Selective deletion of antigen-specific, activated T cells by a humanized MAB to CD2 (MEDI-507) is mediated by NK cells. Transplantation 68:1588-1596, 1999.

26. Spitzer TR, McAfee SL, Dey BR, et al: Nonmyeloablative haploidentical stem-cell transplantation using anti-CD2 monoclonal antibody (MEDI-507)-based conditioning for refractory hematologic malignancies. Transplantation 75:1748-1751, 2003.

27. Kirk AD, Harlan DM, Armstrong NN, et al: CTLA4-Ig and anti-CD40 ligand prevent renal allograft rejection in primates. Proc Natl Acad Sci U S A 94:8789-8794, 1997.

28. Kirk AD, Burkly LC, Batty DS, et al: Treatment with humanized monoclonal antibody against CD154 prevents acute renal allograft rejection in nonhuman primates. Nat Med 5:686-693, 1999.

29. Xu H, Montgomery SP, Preston EH, et al: Studies investigating pretransplant donor-specific blood transfusion, rapamycin, and the CD154-specific antibody IDEC-131 in a nonhuman primate model of skin allotransplantation. J Immunol 170:2776-2782, 2003.

30. Cho CS, Burkly LC, Fechner JH, et al: Successful conversion from conventional immunosuppression to anti-CD154 monoclonal antibody costimulatory molecule blockade in rhesus renal allograft recipient. Transplantation 72:587-597, 2001.

31. Kirk AD, Knechtle SJ, Sollinger HW, et al: Preliminary results of the use of humanized anti-CD154 in human renal allotransplantation. Am J Transplant 1(Suppl):190, 2001.

32. Koyama I, Kawai T, Andrews D, et al: Thrombophilia associated with anti-CD154 monoclonal antibody treatment and its prophylaxis in nonhuman primates. Transplantation 77:460-462, 2004.

33. Adams AB, Shirasugi N, Durham M, et al: Calcineurin inhibitor–free CD28 blockade–based protocol protects allogeneic islets in nonhuman primates. Diabetes 51:265-270, 2002.

34. Moreland LW, Alten R, Van den Bosch F, et al: Costimulatory blockade in patients with rheumatoid arthritis. Arthritis Rheum 46:1470-1479, 2002.

35. Flye MW, Duffy BF, Phelan DL, et al: Protective effects of liver transplantation on a simultaneously transplanted kidney in a highly sensitized patient. Transplantation 50:1051-1054, 1990.

36. Hanto DW, Snover DC, Sibley RK, et al: Hyperacute rejection of a human orthotopic liver allograft in a presensitized recipient. Clin Transplant 1:304-310, 1987.

37. Takaya S, Bronsther O, Iwaki Y, et al: The adverse impact on liver transplantation of using positive cytotoxic crossmatch donors. Transplantation 53:400-406, 1992.

38. Goggins WC, Fisher RA, Kimball PM, et al: The impact of a positive crossmatch upon outcome after liver transplantation. Transplantation 62:1794-1798, 1996.

39. Pascual M, Saidman S, Tolkoff-Rubin N, et al: Plasma exchange and tacrolimus-mycophenolate rescue for acute humoral rejection in kidney transplantation. Transplantation 66:1460-1464, 1998.

40. Kazatchkine MD, Kaveri SV: Advances in immunology: Immunomodulation of autoimmune and inflammatory diseases with intravenous immune globulin. N Engl J Med 345:747-755, 2001.

41. Rocha PN, Butterly DW, Greenberg A, et al: Beneficial effect of plasmapheresis and intravenous immunoglobulin on renal allograft survival of patients with acute humoral rejection. Transplantation 75:1490-1495, 2003.

42. Jordan SC, Vo A, Bunnapradist S, et al: Intravenous immune globulin treatment inhibits crossmatch positivity and allows for successful transplantation of incompatible organs in living-donor and cadaver recipients. Transplantation 76:631-636, 2003.

43. Montgomery RA, Zachary AA, Racusen LC, et al: Plasmapheresis and intravenous immune globulin provides effective rescue therapy for refractory humoral rejection and allows kidneys to be successfully transplanted into cross-match–positive recipients. Transplantation 70:887-895, 2000.

44. Aranda JM, Scornik JC, Normann SJ, et al: Anti-CD20 monoclonal antibody (rituximab) therapy for acute cardiac humoral rejection: A case report. Transplantation 73:907-910, 2002.

45. Group SWS: Steroid withdrawal in kidney transplant recipients on cyclosporine and mycophenolate mofetil—a prospective randomized study. Transplantation 68:1865-1874, 1999.

46. Pirenne J, Aerts R, Koshiba T, et al: Steroid-free immunosuppression during and after liver transplantation—a 3-yr follow-up report. Clin Transplant 17:177-182, 2003.

47. Eason JD, Nair S, Cohen AJ, et al: Steroid-free liver transplantation using rabbit antithymocyte globulin and early tacrolimus monotherapy. Transplantation 75:1396-1399, 2003.

48. Hricik DE: Steroid-free immunosuppression in kidney transplantation: An editorial review. Am J Transplant 2:19-24, 2002.

49. Starzl TE, Murase N, Demetris AJ, et al: Lessons of organ-induced tolerance learned from historical clinical experience. Transplantation 77:926-929, 2004.

50. Riordan SM, Williams R: Tolerance after liver transplantation: Does it exist and can immunosuppression be withdrawn? J Hepatol 31:1106-1119, 1999.

51. Mazariegos GV, Reyes J, Marino IR, et al: Weaning of immunosuppression in liver transplant recipients. Transplantation 63:243-249, 1997.

52. Oike F, Yokoi A, Nishimura E, et al: Complete withdrawal of immunosuppression in living donor liver transplantation. Transplant Proc 34:1521, 2002.

53. Kirk AD, Hale G, Mannon RB, et al: Results from a human renal allograft tolerance trial evaluating the humanized CD52-specific monoclonal antibody alemtuzumab (Campath-1H). Transplantation 76:120-129, 2003.

54. Starzl TE, Murase N, Albu-Elmaghd K, et al: Tolerogenic immunosuppression for organ transplantation. Lancet 361:1502-1510, 2003.

55. Matas AJ: What's new and what's hot in transplantation: Clin Sci ATC 2003. Am J Transplant 3:1465-1473, 2003.

56. Swanson SJ, Hale DA, Mannon RB, et al: Kidney transplantation with rabbit antithymocyte globulin induction and sirolimus monotherapy. Lancet 360:1662-1664, 2002.

57. Qi S, Zhu S, Xu D, et al: Significant prolongation of renal allograft survival by delayed combination therapy of FK778 with tacrolimus in nonhuman primates. Transplantation 75:1124-1128, 2003.

58. Maeda A, Goto M, Zhang J, et al: Immunosuppression with FTY720 and cyclosporine A inhibits rejection of adult porcine islet xenografts in rats. Transplantation 75:1409-1414, 2003.

59. Koshiba T, Van Damme B, Rutgeerts O, et al: FTY720, an immunosuppressant that alters lymphocyte trafficking, abrogates chronic rejection in combination with cyclosporine A. Transplantation 75:945-952, 2003.

60. Kimura T, Hasegawa T, Nakai H, et al: FTY720 reduces T-cell recruitment into murine intestinal allograft and prevents activation of graft-infiltrating cells. Transplantation 75:1469-1474, 2003.

61. Kahan BD, Karlix JL, Ferguson RM, et al: Pharmacodynamics, pharmacokinetics, and safety of multiple doses of FTY720 in stable renal transplant patients: A multicenter, randomized, placebo-controlled, phase I study. Transplantation 76:1079-1084, 2003.

62. Anselmo DM, Amersi FF, Shen XD, et al: FTY720 pretreatment reduces warm hepatic ischemia reperfusion injury through inhibition of T-lymphocyte infiltration. Am J Transplant 2:843-849, 2002.

63. Schuler W, Sedrani R, Cottens S, et al: SDZ RAD, a new rapamycin derivative: Pharmacological properties in vitro and in vivo. Transplantation 64:36-42, 1997.

64. Lutz J, Zou H, Liu S, et al: Apoptosis treatment of chronic allograft nephropathy with everolimus. Transplantation 76:508-515, 2003.

65. Kovarik JM, Kaplan B, Silva HT, et al: Pharmacokinetics of an everolimus-cyclosporine immunosuppressive regimen over the first 6 months after kidney transplantation. Am J Transplant 3:606-613, 2003.

66. Kahan BD, Kaplan B, Lorber MI, et al: RAD in de novo renal transplantation: Comparison of three doses on the incidence and severity of acute rejection. Transplantation 71:1400-1406, 2001.

67. Eisen H, Tuzcu EM, Dorent R, et al: Everolimus for the prevention of allograft rejection and vasculopathy in cardiac transplant recipients. N Engl J Med 349:847-858, 2003.

68. Stewart SF, Hudson M, Talbot D, et al: Mycophenolate mofetil monotherapy in liver transplantation. Lancet 357:609-610, 2001.

69. Schlitt HJ, Barkann A, Boeker KHW, et al: Replacement of calcineurin inhibitors with mycophenolate mofetil in liver transplant patients with renal dysfunction: A randomised controlled study. Lancet 357:587-591, 2001.

70. Dey B, Sykes M, Spitzer TR: Outcomes of recipients of both bone marrow and solid organ transplants: A review. Medicine (Baltimore) 77:355-369, 1998.

71. Ildstad ST, Sachs DH: Reconstitution with syngeneic plus allogeneic or xenogeneic bone marrow leads to specific acceptance of allografts or xenografts. Nature 307:168-170, 1984.

72. Sharabi Y, Sachs DH: Mixed chimerism and permanent specific transplantation tolerance induced by a nonlethal preparative regimen. J Exp Med 169:493-502, 1989.

73. Kawai T, Cosimi AB, Colvin RB, et al: Mixed allogeneic chimerism and renal allograft tolerance in cynomolgus monkeys. Transplantation 59:256-262, 1995.

74. Huang CA, Fuchimoto Y, Scheier-Dolberg R, et al: Stable mixed chimerism and tolerance using a nonmyeloablative preparative regimen in a large-animal model. J Clin Invest 105:173-181, 2000.

75. Wekerle T, Sykes M: Mixed chimerism as an approach for the induction of transplantation tolerance. Transplantation 68:459-467, 1999.

76. Sykes M, Preffer F, Saidman SL, et al: Mixed lymphohematopoietic chimerism is achievable following non-myeloablative therapy and HLA-mismatched donor marrow transplantation. Lancet 353:1755-1759, 1998.

77. Spitzer TR, McAfee S, Sackstein R, et al: The intentional induction of mixed chimerism and achievement of anti-tumor responses following non-myeloablative conditioning therapy and HLA-matched donor bone marrow transplantation for refractory hematologic malignancies. Biol Blood Bone Marrow 6:309-320, 2000.

78. Buhler LH, Spitzer TR, Sykes M, et al: Induction of kidney allograft tolerance after transient lymphohematopoietic chimerism in patients with multiple myeloma and end-stage renal disease. Transplantation 74:1405-1409, 2002.

79. Millan M, Shizuru JA, Hoffmann P, et al: Mixed chimerism and immunosuppressive drug withdrawal after HLA-mismatched kidney and hematopoietic progenitor transplantation. Transplantation 73:1386-1391, 2002.

Ischemia-Reperfusion Injury of the Liver

CONSTANTINO FONDEVILA
RONALD W. BUSUTTIL
JERZY W. KUPIEC-WEGLINSKI

Molecular mechanisms of hepatic ischemia-reperfusion injury   1404
Nitric oxide and endothelin   1404
Cytokines and chemokines   1405
Complement   1406
Lipid mediators   1406
Oxygen free radicals   1406

Cellular mechanisms of hepatic ischemia-reperfusion injury   1406
Cell cascades   1406
Mechanisms of cell death during
   reoxygenation   1406
Sinusoidal endothelial cell injury during
   hepatic preservation   1407
Neutrophil response during reperfusion:
   cellular adhesion molecules   1407
Role of Kupffer cells   1408
Role of T cells   1408

Adenosine and ischemic preconditioning   1409

Heme oxygenase system   1409
Role of carbon monoxide in the regulation of
   hepatic blood flow after ischemia-
   reperfusion injury   1411
Heme oxygenase induction—a novel strategy
   to prevent hepatic ischemia-reperfusion
   injury   1411

Future research   1412

The damage to the liver caused by ischemia-reperfusion (I-R) represents a continuum of processes that culminates in hepatocellular injury. These processes are triggered when the liver is transiently deprived of oxygen and reoxygenated and can occur in a number of clinical settings, such as those associated with low-flow states, diverse surgical procedures, or during the organ procurement for transplantation. In fact, I-R injury to the liver, an antigen-independent component of "harvesting" insult, represents an important problem affecting transplantation. It causes up to 10% of early organ failure, and can lead to a higher incidence of both acute and chronic liver graft rejection.[1] Factors concerning the donor, operative technique, and the recipient all contribute to I-R injury. Donor livers may be subjected to various types of stress such as ischemia caused by hypotension or drug-induced liver dysfunction, rendering them more susceptible to I-R injury.

I-R injury contributes to the acute shortage of livers available for transplantation because of the higher susceptibility of expanded criteria livers to ischemic insult. Indeed, steatotic liver grafts, implicated directly in primary graft nonfunction or dysfunction, are more susceptible to I-R insult, as compared with normal livers.[2] Operative factors that may contribute to reperfusion injury relate primarily to the technical issues, such as reduced portal venous or hepatic arterial inflow, and to the length of the cold and warm ischemic times. Cold ischemic storage and reperfusion of liver result in ultrastructural changes, which become more prominent with increasing storage time. These changes include widening of endothelial fenestrations, sinusoidal endothelial cell vacuolization, retraction of cellular processes, and sinusoidal denudation. Biopsy specimens obtained from human liver grafts at different stages after transplantation reveal signs of sinusoidal endothelial as well as Kupffer cell activation. These signs are visible at the end of the preservation period and become more prominent after revascularization.[3] Apoptosis is also frequently evident in postreperfusion biopsy specimens from liver allografts.[4]

Although reperfusion alone after short periods of cold ischemia is usually well tolerated, it becomes critical for the manifestation of injury that originates during deep and prolonged hypothermia, which can cause alterations in cytoskeleton and organelle structures of cells and disrupts the membrane electrical potential gradient, thereby resulting in ion redistribution. I-R injury to the endothelium affects the delicate balance that maintains homeostasis in the microcirculation with attraction, activation, adhesion, and migration of polymorphonuclear neutrophils (PMNs), causing local tissue destruction by release of proteases and oxygen free radicals (OFRs). The severity of hepatic I-R injury is also related to the duration of the procedure, episodes of intraoperative hypotension, and the degree of splanchnic ischemia. Some of these factors can be controlled; however, the dramatically increasing shortage of donor organs motivates the use of suboptimal livers (such as livers from non–heart-beating donors (NHBDs) or from high-risk donors), which are much more susceptible to I-R injury.[5]

The majority of organs available for transplantation come from brain-dead donors. Brain death induces a number of physiological and metabolic changes in the tissues and is associated with hemodynamic instability and upregulation of inflammatory mediators. It is a potentially detrimental process that predisposes deceased donor organs to increased I-R injury and alloreactivity after transplantation. It has been demonstrated in experimental models that brain death induces progressive liver dysfunction.[6] It seems that superior results might be achieved by using living donors because in this situation one can avoid the effect of the events that occur otherwise during and subsequent to brain death. Interest in NHBDs has been renewed owing to organ shortage and better techniques for procurement and preservation. However, I-R injury causes severe graft injury in NHBD grafts[7] with late structural and functional deterioration.[8] Strategies to decrease I-R injury in NHBD organs are essential to expanding the donor pool.

Because many of the donor risk factors for a poor outcome after transplantation are not remediable,

developing therapies for I-R injury is of critical importance. Minimizing the adverse effects of I-R injury could significantly increase the number of patients that may successfully undergo liver transplantation. Prevention of preservation injury is important, not only to reduce the incidence of primary nonfunction but also to diminish the likelihood of late sequelae and suboptimal graft function related to preservation injury. However, at present there is no treatment available to prevent hepatic I-R injury. As intervention on more than one level is most likely needed to allow the recovery of cellular and organ function, extensive research efforts to better understand the mechanisms of hepatic I-R injury are warranted. There is now a renewed interest in studies that should potentially lead to better appreciation of the complex molecular basis of hepatic I-R injury.

Molecular Mechanisms of Hepatic Ischemia-Reperfusion Injury

Nitric Oxide and Endothelin

Impaired blood flow within individual sinusoids secondary to stellate cell contraction is seen during the early reperfusion period. Endothelin-1 (ET-1) elicits stellate cell contraction in a dose-dependent manner. It has been suggested that I-R injury is a result of an imbalance between ET-1 and nitric oxide (NO) levels during the reperfusion period. Indeed, increased concentration of ET-1 in both plasma and hepatic parenchyma in the early stages of hepatic reperfusion has been correlated with a decrease in liver blood flow.[9] In experimental models, liver pretreatment with ET-1 receptor antagonists (bosentan, tezosentan) has been shown to exert protective effects against I-R–induced endothelial damage, thereby improving sinusoidal hemodynamics-oxygenation and decreasing inflammatory response.[10,11]

NO was identified as endothelium-derived relaxing factor in 1987, which diffuses freely across cell membranes and acts intracellularly by activation of guanylate cyclase. However, a number of other physiological actions in addition to vasodilator effects have been attributed to NO, including inflammatory and platelet activity reduction, decrease in the expression of cytokines and adhesion molecules, protection of the mitochondria, and induction of heat shock proteins (HSPs).[12] NO has also been shown to react with superoxide to form the potent oxidant peroxynitrite.[13] NO is generated in the liver by constitutively expressed endothelial nitric oxide synthase (eNOS) as well as by inducible nitric oxide synthase (iNOS). Although eNOS is expressed selectively in sinusoidal endothelial cells (ECs), iNOS can be transcriptionally upregulated in EC, hepatocytes, and other liver cells.

NO concentration is low during the first few hours of reperfusion. This is a result of low intracellular levels of nicotinamide-adenine dinucleotide phosphate (NADPH) and oxygen (cofactors required for NO synthesis) after the ischemic period, and the release of a large amount of arginase, which breaks down L-arginine (the precursor required for NO synthesis). In experimental models, blockade of the L-arginine/NO pathway significantly increased necrotic and apoptotic cell death in the transplanted graft, whereas L-arginine supplementation and NO synthesis decreased necrotic and apoptotic cell death and ameliorated liver transplant preservation injury.[14,15]

Immediately after hepatic reperfusion in human orthotopic liver transplantation (OLT), high amounts of arginase are released from the graft, and this has been shown to result in depletion of L-arginine at 30 minutes after the onset of reperfusion. Significant production of NO is unlikely to occur until 6 hours from the onset of reperfusion, as this requires induction of NOS, which takes 4 to 6 hours. eNOS-derived NO is responsible for maintaining liver blood flow, inducing vasodilation at the level of sinusoid and presinusoidal sites. However, excessive NO formation by iNOS may lead to peroxynitrite-induced injury as well as systemic effects, such as hypotension and shock.[16]

Cytokines and Chemokines

An excessive inflammatory response is clearly recognized as a key mechanism of injury during reperfusion. Proinflammatory cytokines and chemokines are responsible for PMN recruitment and the subsequent PMN-induced oxidant stress during the later reperfusion phase. Moreover, stimulation of primed Kupffer cells by complement factors causes the continuous activation of these macrophages. Kupffer cell- and neutrophil-induced oxidant stress stimulated by cytokines is an important factor in vascular and parenchymal cell injury during reperfusion.[17] Activated PMNs release proteases, their cytotoxic mediators, which can act locally without the interference of plasma antiproteases owing to inactivation of antiproteases by reactive oxygen species (ROS). The postischemic oxidant stress can enhance the expression of genes such as tumor necrosis factor-α (TNF-α), iNOS, heme oxygenase-1 (HO-1), CXC chemokines, and adhesion molecules. Furthermore, ROS can promote reperfusion injury at least in part through stimulation of the transcription nuclear factor-κ B (NF-κB) and activating protein-1 (AP-1).[18]

TNF-α and interleukin (IL)-1 are the two cytokines most commonly implicated in hepatic I-R injury.

Both cytokines induce IL-8 synthesis and upregulate the expression of adhesion molecules (such as selectins and β integrins) favoring leukocyte–sinusoidal EC interactions,[19] which result in additional cytokine production. TNF-α induces the local generation of a chemokine—epithelial neutrophil activating protein-78—which plays an important part in PMN chemotaxis and activation and induces Kupffer cells to generate superoxide radicals.[20] IL-1 induces Kupffer cells to produce TNF-α and also upregulates free radical production by PMNs. The role of both cytokines in hepatic I-R injury is further confirmed by experiments in which their neutralization following treatment with antiserum, monoclonal antibodies, or receptor antagonists decreased the severity of reperfusion injury, as evidenced by decreased PMN infiltration and parenchymal damage.[21] IL-12 also supports the inflammatory response and postischemic injury. Studies with neutralizing antibodies or with IL-12–deficient mice showed that IL-12 formation is important for prolonged TNF-α and interferon (IFN)-γ formation, both of which promote PMN-dependent injury during reperfusion.[22]

Chemokine formation is induced by cytokines in Kupffer cells and hepatocytes. Chemokines are important in hepatic I-R injury because of their ability to recruit PMNs into the postischemic liver. The most relevant chemokines involved in I-R injury are neutrophil chemoattractant CXC chemokines MIP-2 and KC; CXCR3 chemokine IL-10; and cytokine-induced neutrophil chemoattractant-1 (CINC-1), a member of the IL-8 family.[23] Selective overexpression of CINC-1 in hepatocytes induced a chemotactic gradient, which caused not only PMN sequestration in sinusoids but also transmigration and injury.[24] IL-8, which also promotes accumulation of PMN in liver sinusoids, has the capacity to upregulate Mac-1, a surface adhesion molecule that allows PMN migration into the liver tissue.[25]

Some cytokines, however, such as IL-6, IL-10, and IL-13 may exert an inhibitory effect on I-R injury. Indeed, IL-6 can downregulate TNF-α mRNA during reperfusion, and it promotes hepatocyte regeneration.[26] IL-10 controls the inflammatory response by exerting an inhibitory effect on transcriptional NF-κB. It has been shown that recombinant murine IL-10 suppresses mRNA expression of TNF-α, chemokines, and intercellular adhesion molecules, thereby attenuating hepatic reperfusion injury in mice.[27] Cytoprotection rendered by virally induced IL-13 in a clinically relevant rat hepatic cold I-R injury model was accomplished via decreased apoptosis/induction of antiapoptotic/antioxidant molecules.[28] Furthermore, the anti-inflammatory effect of IL-13 is also exerted through the activation of signal transducer and activator of transcription-6 (STAT-6) pathway.[29] Secretory leukocyte protease inhibitor (SLPI) is another protein that may protect against I-R injury by reducing TNF formation and inhibiting proteases released by PMNs.[30]

Complement

The activation of complement represents a critical event during hepatic I-R injury. Indeed, the complement cascade can be rapidly activated by the extensive release of cellular proteins during the early reperfusion period. Complement factors, such as C5a, upregulate the Mac-1 receptor on circulating PMNs and cause their recruitment into sinusoids. C5a also primes and activates PMNs and Kupffer cells for reactive oxygen formation.[31] In addition to the proinflammatory effect, the assembled membrane attack complex can directly cause cell injury. Therefore, blocking complement activation effectively reduces the inflammatory response, microcirculatory disturbances, and cell injury.[32]

Lipid Mediators

Platelet-activating factor (PAF) levels increase significantly after 12 hours of reperfusion and reach a peak after 24 hours of reperfusion, at the time of maximal hepatic injury. PAF is formed mainly by EC and can prime PMNs for generation of superoxide. In addition, PAF is a potent activator of the β_2-integrin Mac-1 and of adherence-dependent reactive oxygen formation. PAF receptor antagonists exert beneficial effects against reperfusion injury through reduced PMN activation and reduced microvascular damage.[33] Leukotriene B$_4$ (LTB$_4$) is a potent chemotactic factor that may contribute to the amplification of PMN response during reperfusion.[34] Lipid peroxidation products are also important chemotactic factors for neutrophils. This mechanism may be responsible for the propagation of the inflammatory injury during reperfusion, especially at times when many peptide mediators are no longer generated. Lipid-soluble antioxidants and iron chelators can reduce the inflammatory response and reperfusion injury by reducing the signal (lipid peroxidation products) for continued PMN recruitment.[35]

Oxygen Free Radicals

Oxygen free radicals (OFRs) are probably one of the earliest and most important components of tissue injury after reperfusion of ischemic organs. The major OFRs include the superoxide radical, hydroxyl, and hydrogen peroxide. The prime sources of OFR production in ischemic livers include cytosolic xanthine oxidase (XOD), Kupffer cells, and adherent PMNs. OFR-induced injury targets proteins, enzymes, nucleic acids, cytoskeleton, cell membranes, and lipid peroxides, resulting in decreased mitochondrial function and lipid peroxidation. In addition to the inactivation of antiproteases and the direct cytotoxic effects, OFRs can promote reperfusion injury through stimulation of NF-κB and AP-1.[36]

The EC damage caused by OFRs leads to the loss of microvascular integrity and decreased blood flow. Endogenous antioxidant compounds, such as superoxide dismutase, catalase, glutathione, α-tocopherol, and beta-carotene, may all limit the effects of OFRs, but these systems can quickly become overwhelmed by large OFR quantities. Antioxidants can also attenuate proinflammatory gene expression through inhibition of NF-κB and AP-1 activation.[37] Potential strategies to attenuate OFR-mediated injury may involve gene vectors. Indeed, recombinant adenoviral delivery of superoxides significantly reduced acute I-R hepatic damage in mice.[38] Another strategy may be the incorporation of superoxides or antioxidants such as allopurinol, desferroxiamine, or glutathione into organ preservation solution to provide EC protection.

Cellular Mechanisms of Hepatic Ischemia-Reperfusion Injury

Cell Cascades

The process of I-R injury to the liver combines interrelated factors that produce a cascade of events that lead ultimately to hepatic failure (Fig. 87–1). Ample evidence suggests that activation of Kupffer cells, PMNs, ECs, and ROSs are all critical in the pathogenesis of I-R injury.[39] The final consequence of these interrelated processes is structural tissue alterations causing hepatocellular dysfunction. The histopathological changes that occur in ischemic liver after reperfusion include cellular swelling, vacuolization, EC disruption, and PMN infiltration. Significant microcirculatory changes reducing organ perfusion occur, reaching maximum levels within 48 hours of reperfusion. In viable organs that recover from the I-R insult, these changes decline and normalization of hepatic architecture is seen within 2 weeks of reperfusion.[40] It seems that nonparenchymal cells (Kupffer, EC, and Ito cells) are more susceptible to "cold" I-R injury than hepatocytes are. Apoptotic cell death of sinusoidal ECs, as well as coagulative necrosis, increases after cold storage followed by reperfusion of liver grafts.[41]

Mechanisms of Cell Death During Reoxygenation

Apoptosis and necrosis occur after I-R injury, and both appear linked to an excess of intracellular OFR production. Apoptosis depends on the availability of cellular adenosine triphosphate (ATP), so reoxygenation could potentiate apoptosis by restoring cellular energy.

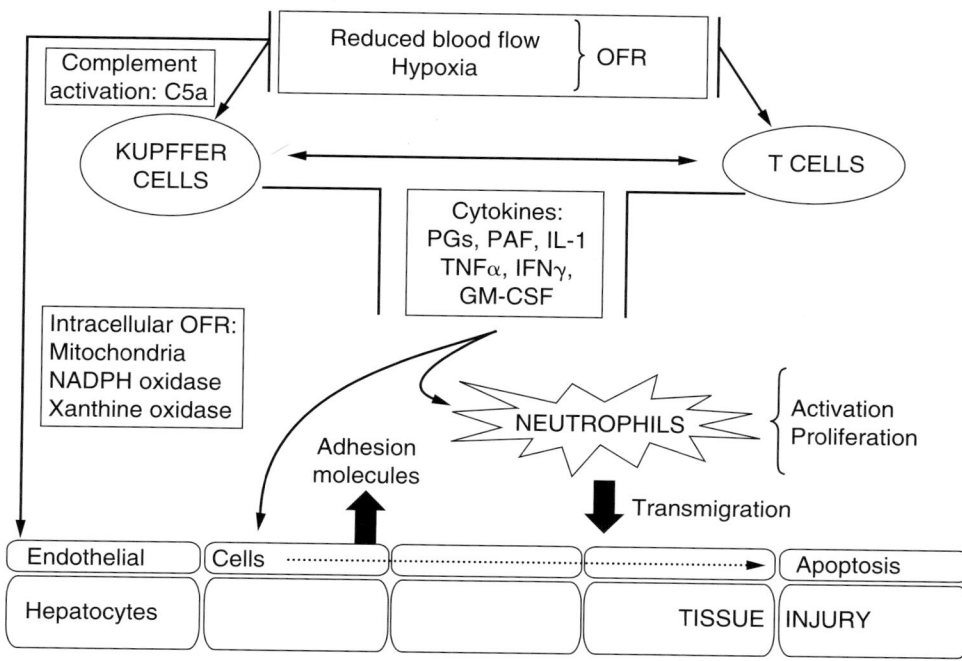

FIGURE 87-1

The cascade of cellular events in liver I-R injury. Free radicals generated during the acute phase of I-R injury initiate the inflammatory cascade that gives rise to the subacute-phase response, characterized by infiltration and activation of polymorphonuclear neutrophils (PMNs) in the liver shortly after reperfusion. Activation of Kupffer cells and T lymphocytes promotes PMN recruitment, assisted by increased endothelial expression of adhesion molecules such as intercellular adhesion molecule-1 (ICAM-1). Activated Kupffer and T cells secrete an array of cytokines that stimulate each other to amplify organ destruction.

Bcl-2 inhibits hydrogen peroxide production and its overexpression allows cells to adapt to ROS overproduction.[42] NF-κB augments apoptosis by suppressing the antiapoptotic Bcl-2 expression in hypoxia.[43] Bax and p53 are induced in some cell types that undergo apoptosis after hypoxia. Bax protein translocates to mitochondria during reoxygenation and triggers cell death. Mitochondria are involved in posthypoxic apoptosis through increased OFR production and cytochrome *c* release. Apoptosis after reoxygenation is also associated with activation of caspase-3 and -9, and both caspase inhibition and Bcl-2 overexpression inhibit apoptosis.[44] Inhibition of apoptosis, because of the lack of energy owing to hypoxia-induced ATP depletion, may predispose to necrosis, and both mechanisms of cell death typically overlap. Cells are capable of undergoing necrosis directly after reoxygenation, since necrosis is also related to increased OFR.[44]

Sinusoidal Endothelial Cell Injury During Hepatic Preservation

The first consequence of I-R injury is tissue anoxia that disturbs the intracellular energy metabolism and the enzyme function, thereby resulting in depletion of ATP, accumulation of intracellular sodium, and cellular edema. The energy state at reperfusion is an indicator of cell recovery. Reperfusion can rescue the cell, but it also induces further injury that starts as microcirculatory flow disturbances, manifested by red blood cells (RBCs), PMNs, and platelet adhesion to EC and sinusoidal congestion. The response of the hepatic endothelium to

I-R is a significant causative factor, with EC the least tolerant to I-R of the nonparenchymal liver cells.

Hypothermia during cold preservation causes morphological changes in some sinusoidal cells such that they become rounded, detached, and slough into the sinusoidal lumen. Some proteases, such as matrix metalloproteinases (gelatinases), seem to play an important role in mediating the endothelial changes during hypothermia. In fact, the injury to the sinusoidal EC during cold ischemia is an active process, possibly involving angiogenic factors and proteases and resulting in digestion of the connective tissue matrix. An important target might be fibronectin, a key molecule linking collagen to the sinusoidal lining cell membrane integrin.[45,46]

During the early phases of reperfusion, apoptosis of sinusoidal ECs may also represent the principal mechanism of injury. Molecules linking EC to each other or to perisinusoidal matrix may play a critical role in cell viability. However, other molecules could induce apoptosis of the sinusoidal EC after reperfusion, such as OFR, TNF-α, increased cytoplasmic calcium concentration, calpain proteases, caspases, sphingosine derivates, mitogen-activated protein kinases (MAPK), and products from adherent leukocytes and platelets.[47]

Neutrophil Response During Reperfusion: Cellular Adhesion Molecules

EC become activated during I-R to express an array of surface adhesion molecules and major histocompatibility complex (MHC) antigens, priming the endothelium for further PMN interactions. In fact, initial tethering of PMNs in sinusoidal venules requires expression of selectins on ECs and interaction with their counter-receptors on PMNs. In venular endothelial cells P- and E-selectin as well as ICAM-1 and VCAM-1 can be upregulated transcriptionally.[48] Subsequent activation of β_1 and β_2 integrins on PMNs by chemotactic factors leads to the firm PMN adhesion on the EC surface. The severe vascular injury during reperfusion also induces aggregation of platelets, which can adhere through a selectin-dependent mechanism.[49] Indeed, PMNs may adhere to platelets as well as to ECs. The accumulation and activation of PMNs exacerbate microcirculatory disturbances and finally are followed by extravasation and migration to the inflammatory site. Once extravasation and transmigration have occurred, there is little doubt about the destructive capabilities of the PMNs that elaborate toxic enzymes such as elastase, serine protease, and metalloproteinases, but they can also produce OFRs. The PMN-induced injury to the hepatocyte results from adhesion between the two cells, mediated by β_2 integrins and ICAM-1 expressed on hepatocytes.[50] Increased expression of ICAM-1 can be induced by various proinflammatory cytokines, such as TNF-α and IL-1, so it is not surprising that I-R injury leads to increased expression of ICAM-1 within the liver.[51] Anti-ICAM-1 antibodies have been used effectively to attenuate liver injury after transplantation in experimental models.[52] Indeed, recombinant P-selectin glycoprotein ligand (PSGL)-Ig mediated early blockade of P-selectin–PMN interactions and significantly decreased I-R–induced hepatocyte injury.[53] Thus, treatment of rats with rPSGL-Ig improved liver function; diminished PMN infiltration, as evidenced by decreased myeloperoxidase (MPO) activity; ameliorated cardinal histological features of hepatocyte injury; and diminished intragraft mononuclear cell infiltration, as well as expression of macrophage/T_H1-type proinflammatory cytokines.

Role of Kupffer Cells

Another nonparenchymal cell involved in hepatic I-R injury is the Kupffer cell, the resident macrophage found in the sinusoidal space of the liver, which appears to be relatively resistant to ischemia yet becomes activated during reperfusion. When activated, it produces an array of factors, including proinflammatory cytokines—prostaglandins (PGs), PAF, IL-1, TNF-α, IL-6, and interferon (IFN)-γ—and OFRs that act as direct cytotoxins to EC and hepatocytes; induce changes in cell membrane receptors on hepatocytes, ECs and PMNs; activate other Kupffer cells and PMNs; and may induce chemotactic gradients for PMNs.[54] Furthermore, Kupffer cells appear to be very active in

clearing apoptotic bodies shed by the adjacent apoptotic sinusoidal ECs.[41]

Role of T Cells

It has been postulated that prolonged ischemia results in allografts that are more "immunogenic" and, therefore, more susceptible to T-cell immune responses. In fact, evidence is mounting about the importance of T cells in mediating both short- and long-term damage during I-R injury, which in turn could explain why I-R contributes to poor late allograft function.[55] The contributory role of lymphocytes in hepatic I-R is likely multifactorial. The attenuation of hepatocellular injury following I-R systemic immunosuppression (cyclosporine A [CYA], FK506) suggests the involvement of T lymphocytes in the pathophysiology of the injury.[56] The data are supported by findings in T-cell–deficient (nude) mice,[57,58] as well as in rats in which treatment with FTY720 prevented hepatic I-R insult in parallel with massive redistribution of recirculating T cells from host peripheral blood into the lymph node compartment.[59] The adherence of lymphocytes in hepatic sinusoids occurs early during reperfusion and impairs liver function following prolonged cold ischemic times[60] but circulating CD4+ T lymphocytes may act as a cellular mediator in the subacute PMN recruitment following hepatic I-R injury.[61] In addition, the protective effects of anti-inflammatory IL-10 in models of I-R injury relate not only to the inhibition of Kupffer cell cytokine release but also to the inhibition of resident T cells.[62]

All of these results are consistent with an emerging paradigm on the pivotal role of T cells in the mechanism of I-R injury. However, the question remains as to how T cells become activated during I-R insult, which by definition is an antigen (Ag)-independent event. Indeed, liver sinusoidal ECs constitutively express molecules necessary for Ag presentation (CD80/CD86, CD40) and can function as antigen-presenting cells (APCs) for CD4+ and CD8+ T cells.[63] These ECs do not need to undergo maturation for acquisition of APC function but can undergo endocytosis and can present antigen to T cells outside the lymphatic environment.[64] Moreover, liver-infiltrating T cells express cytokines, chemokines, and adhesion molecules that may result in increased T-cell adhesion to ECs. As liver is involved in the clearance of foreign antigens and toxic products from the gastrointestinal tract, it is plausible that liver sinusoidal ECs present "foreign" antigens and activate T lymphocytes during hepatic I-R injury. It is of interest to note that both CD28-B7 and CD154-CD40 T-cell costimulation pathways are important in the mechanism of hepatic I-R injury.[57] Moreover, disruption of the signal transducer and activator of transcription-4

(STAT-4) pathway results in cytoprotection,[58] consistent with the benefits of inducing type-2 IL-13 in rat liver model of cold ischemia followed by OLT.[28]

Adenosine and Ischemic Preconditioning

Adenosine is an endogenous compound produced by the action of various enzymes on ATP, adenosine diphosphate (ADP), and adenosine monophosphate (AMP). Increased levels of extracellular adenosine are thought to confer cytoprotection on ischemic tissue. In fact, augmentation of endogenous adenosine improves survival, hepatic tissue blood flow, liver function, and liver histological status in animal models of hepatic I-R.[65] The doubling in cold liver preservation time from 9 to 20 hours with the introduction of University of Wisconsin (UW) solution has been attributed partly to its adenosine content.

Ischemic preconditioning refers to a phenomenon in which tissues are rendered resistant to the deleterious effects of I-R by previous exposure to brief periods of vascular occlusion. The protective effects were first described in the myocardium and have also been demonstrated in the liver. The protective effect of ischemic preconditioning is believed to result, at least in part, from the release of adenosine to the ischemic tissue (Fig. 87–2).[66] In ischemic preconditioning, an elevated extracellular adenosine concentration induces the activation of adenosine A2 receptors. This, in turn, by induction of NO synthesis confers cytoprotection on ischemic tissue. The administration of adenosine deaminase or adenosine A2-receptor antagonist abolishes the protective effect of ischemic preconditioning in the liver.[67] Liver ischemic preconditioning also reduced xanthine accumulation and conversion of xanthine dehydrogenase (XDH) to xanthine oxidase (XOD), thereby preventing postischemic OFR generation and hepatic injury.[68]

Heme Oxygenase System

Heme oxygenases (HOs) are ubiquitous enzymes that catalyze the initial and rate-limiting steps in the oxidative degradation of heme into biliverdin, carbon monoxide (CO), and free iron (Fig. 87–3). This oxidation reaction involves a sequence of transformations that consumes three molecules of oxygen and seven electrons, provided by NADPH-cytochrome P450 reductase. Biliverdin is reduced to bilirubin by bilirubin reductase, and the free iron is used in intracellular metabolism or sequestered in ferritin. It is believed that the byproducts derived from the catalysis of heme by HO, namely biliverdin, bilirubin, ferritin accumulated from released

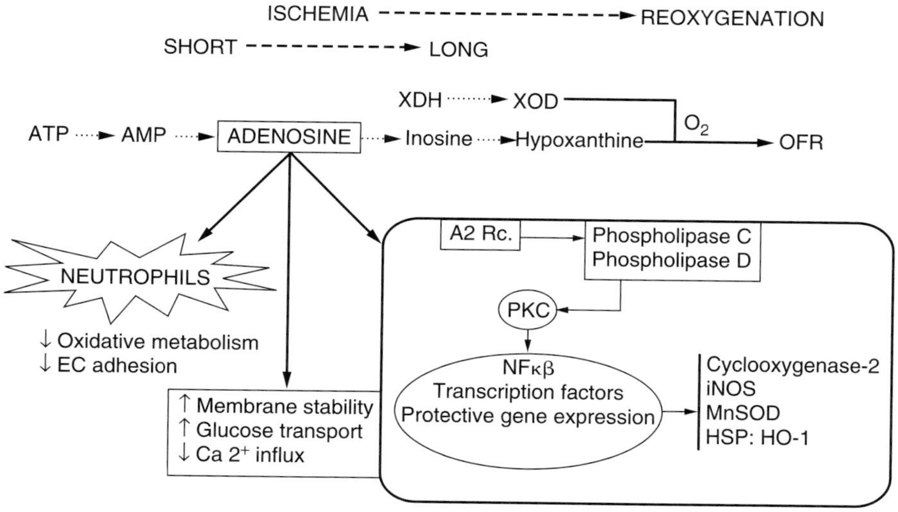

FIGURE 87–2

Protective mechanisms of ischemic preconditioning. Adenosine, released during ischemic preconditioning, inhibits PMN oxidative metabolism and adhesion to endothelial cells (ECs), increases membrane stability and energy production by promoting glucose transport, and reduces Ca^{2+} influx through the activation of ATP-dependent K^+ channels. Furthermore, adenosine binds to its receptor and activates membrane-bound phospholipase C and D. These phospholipases can activate specific isoforms of protein kinase (PK)C. PKC migrates to the nucleus, inducing nuclear transcription factors like nuclear factor-κ B (NF-κB) and the expression of protective genes. Several proteins have been proposed as possible effectors, including cyclooxygenase-2, inducible nitric oxide syntase (iNOS), antioxidant enzymes (Mn-SOD), and heat shock proteins (HSPs).

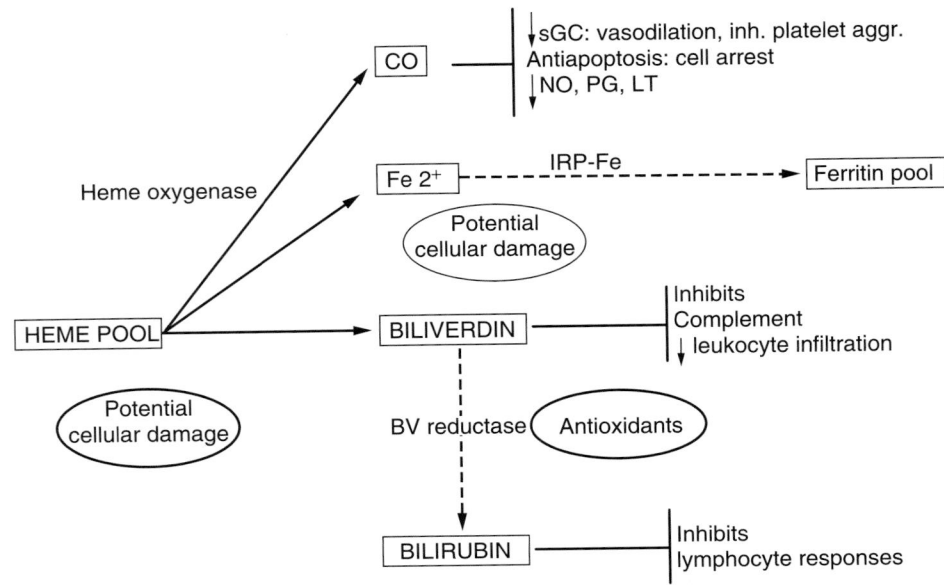

FIGURE 87–3

Mechanism of cytoprotection rendered by heme degradation. Microsomal heme oxygenase (HO) catalyzes the rate-limiting step in heme metabolism that produces carbon monoxide (CO), free iron (Fe^{2+}), and biliverdin. CO stimulates soluble guanylyl cyclase (sGC) of smooth muscle cells and platelets, leading to vasodilation or prevention of platelet aggregation; it also induces cell arrest and interferes with cyclooxygenase, lipoxygenase, and NO synthase, resulting in the reduction of NO and prostaglandins (PGs, LT). The released iron is transiently available for both pro-oxidant and regulatory processes. Fe^{2+} binds to the iron regulatory protein (IRP), releasing the Fe-IRP complex from ferritin mRNA, thereby increasing its translation. Biliverdin, which inhibits the complement in vitro and leukocyte recruitment, is reduced to bilirubin by soluble enzyme reductase. Both act as scavengers of oxygen free radicals (OFRs) to protect cells against oxidative stress. Bilirubin may also decrease systemic lymphocyte activation and proliferation.

iron, and finally CO, can all mediate the physiological effects of HO-1.[69] Three HO isoforms have been identified: the inducible HO-1, also known as HSP 32, the constitutive HO-2, and the not fully defined HO-3. HO-1 activity can be induced by various stimuli that have the capacity to provoke oxidative stress, such as hyperthermia, hypoxia, and radiation, and is considered to be one of the most sensitive indicators of cellular oxidative injury.

The transcriptional regulation of the HO-1 gene by oxidants led to the hypothesis that HO-1 provides a cellular defense mechanism during oxidative stress.[70] Moreover, in the context of diminishing concentrations of intracellular antioxidants such as glutathione, the potential of oxidants to induce the HO-1 gene is increased.[71] This upregulation of HO-1 is thought to be a protective response to cellular stress following ischemia, inflammation, and radiation, thereby preventing the deleterious effects of heme, which promotes lipid peroxidation and free radical formation. Activation of the HO system could then afford a cytoprotective function during the cascade of events triggered by I-R. In addition, recent findings have led to a redefinition of the HO pathway as not just anti-oxidative, but as a more complex and coordinated cytoprotective and immunomodulatory system.[72]

Hemoglobin constitutes the main source of extracellular heme protein. RBCs are one of the cell types most susceptible to damage by OFR. In I-R injury, damaged RBCs increase their deformity and aggregate, thereby increasing blood viscosity and flow resistance. When lysis occurs, released free heme exacerbates the oxidative process generating OFRs and a harmful iron chelate, which may promote deleterious cellular processes such as oxidative membrane damage. The hepatic microvascular disturbance in I-R injury is characterized by a reduction in sinusoidal RBC velocity after reperfusion, which progresses to extravasation of RBCs and petechial bleeds, indicating marked injury of liver sinusoidal ECs. Further progression of the endothelial damage may result in focal hemorrhage, hepatocellular dysfunction, and ultimate organ failure.[73] Different approaches may be envisioned to ameliorate this process as well as the resultant I-R injury: reduction of intravascular hemoglobin levels, administration of hemopexin (heme-binding protein) that may work as a scavenger of heme in reperfused tissue, and promotion of heme degradation by means of the HO system.[74] The beneficial function of HO as a heme removal mechanism is twofold: first, in the avoidance of heme's deleterious effect in membrane lipid peroxidation, and second, in the consumption of oxygen molecules to decrease OFR generation.

The bile pigment biliverdin is produced as a consequence of the heme degradation by HO, and then reduced to bilirubin. Bilirubin formed in tissues is normally processed for elimination by hepatic conjugation and biliary excretion. By scavenging various OFRs, both biliverdin and bilirubin are considered endogenous antioxidants that protect cells from oxidative injury as effectively as α-tocopherol does. In addition, biliverdin can modulate leukocyte infiltration by altering the expression of adhesion molecules in liver endothelial cells in an endotoxin model and it also inhibits human complement in vitro.[75,76]

Reduced iron released during HO-mediated heme degradation becomes available for regulatory processes, especially ferritin synthesis. Although both free heme and free iron are pro-oxidant species, the released iron is less likely to accumulate in membranes and may have more pathways available for redistribution and neutralization. Therefore, the potential catalysis of oxidative reactions by iron is limited through its sequestration by ferritin.[69]

Role of Carbon Monoxide in the Regulation of Hepatic Blood Flow After Ischemia-Reperfusion Injury

CO, released directly from heme, may act as a regulatory molecule in different cellular and biological processes, similarly to the function of nitric oxide (NO). Both can activate soluble guanylate cyclase (sGC), thereby leading to smooth muscle relaxation, which contributes to endothelium vasodilatation, and may explain the CO-mediated cytoprotection mechanism against I-R injury. CO allows maintenance of microcirculatory blood flow by inhibiting the vasoconstriction seen otherwise during reperfusion.[9] The activation of the cyclic guanosine monophosphate (cGMP) pathway also provides CO with the ability to inhibit platelet aggregation, and thus diminishes the microvascular thrombosis associated with I-R injury. Another CO cytoprotective mechanism against hepatic I-R injury may include suppression of iNOS,[77] downregulation of some proinflammatory cytokines via the mitogen-activated protein kinases pathway (MAPK),[78] and inhibition of EC apoptosis.[79]

The effects and down-stream mechanisms of CO on cold I-R injury have been studied recently in a clinically relevant isolated perfusion rat liver model.[80] After 24 hours of cold storage, rat livers perfused ex vivo for 2 hours with blood supplemented with CO showed significantly decreased portal venous resistance and increased bile production, as compared with control livers perfused with blood devoid of CO. These beneficial effects correlated with improved liver function

(serum glutamic-oxaloacetic transferase [SGOT] levels) and diminished histological features of hepatocyte injury (Banff's score). The CO-mediated cytoprotective effects were iNOS and cGMP independent, but p38 MAPK dependent. Moreover, adjunctive use of zinc protoporphyrin, a competitive HO inhibitor, has revealed that exogenous CO could fully substitute for endogenous HO-1 in preventing hepatic I-R insult. Hence, HO-1–mediated cytoprotection against hepatic I-R injury depends on the generation of, and can be substituted by, exogenous CO. Indeed, regimens that use exogenous CO should be revisited, as they may have potential applications in preventing and mitigating I-R injury, and thereby expanding the liver donor pool for clinical transplantation.

Heme Oxygenase Induction—A Novel Strategy to Prevent Ischemia-Reperfusion Injury

Given the multifactorial cytoprotective properties of the HO system, its use as a novel strategy to prevent I-R injury has been studied extensively.[72] Exogenous HO-1 overexpression exerts potent cytoprotective functions in a number of hepatic I-R injury transplant models. HO-1 induction by pharmacological means (e.g., cobalt protoporphyrin, hemin, pyrrolidine dithiocarbamate) or genetic engineering maintains tissue architecture, preserves organ function, and leads to prolonged graft survival (Table 87–1).[81-83] Moreover, OLTs in animals overexpressing HO-1, primarily by infiltrating macrophages,[82] exhibit less macrophage infiltration in the portal areas and depressed iNOS expression.[77] It is of interest to note that local expression of antiapoptotic Bcl-2 and Bag-1 increases in well-functioning OLTs, whereas caspase-3 protein expression is markedly diminished. Clearly, HO-1 induction exerts striking hepatic cytoprotection against I-R insult in association with the modulation of pro- and antiapoptotic pathways.

In the clinical setting, however, there may be several barriers to using the HO system because there are no known reagents that specifically induce HO activity, and the unintended effects of treatment with nonspecific HO-1 inducers would likely represent a disadvantage.[72] Although adenoviral-based HO-1 gene transfer has been attempted in vivo, the efficiency of viral transfection is organ dependent. CO may represent a candidate for treatment of transplant patients against I-R injury, but its therapeutic window must be carefully considered because inhalation of high levels can be toxic or even lethal. An alternative to gaseous CO is the use of methylene chloride. This compound metabolizes exclusively into CO and CO_2 and has been shown to exert immunosuppressive effects in the rat liver allotransplant model.[84] Biliverdin and reduced bilirubin

Table 87–1. HO-1 CYTOPROTECTION IN EXPERIMENTAL MODELS OF HEPATIC ISCHEMIA–REPERFUSION INJURY

Model	Inducing/Inhibiting agent	Outcome	Reference No.
Rat	CoPP, Ad-HO-1/ZnPP	Improved function, prolonged survival	81
Rat	Fasting	Prolonged survival	85
Rat	CoPP	Improved function, prolonged survival	82
Rat	CO/ZnPP	Improved function	80
Rat	Ad-HO-1	Prolonged survival	77
Mouse	T-cell deficiency, CD154-blockade/SnPP	Improved function	57
Mouse	STAT-4 disruption/SnPP	Improved function	58
Rat	PDTC	Improved function, prolonged survival	83
Rat	Ad-IL-13/ZnPP	Improved function, prolonged survival	28

Ad-HO-1, adenoviral HO-1; Ad-IL, adenoviral IL; CO, carbon monoxide; CoPP, cobalt protoporphyrin; HO, heme oxygenase; PDTC, pyrrolidine dithiocarbamate; STAT-4, signal transducer and activator of transcription-4; SnPP, tin protoporphyrin; ZnPP, zinc protoporphyrin.

may also represent possible candidates for clinical application. Preliminary data at our laboratory show that biliverdin exerted protective effects in stringent rat liver models of I-R injury, as evidenced by improved portal blood flow and bile production and reduction of hepatocellular damage. In addition, there is improved survival in a syngeneic rat OLT model after prolonged cold ischemia. However, the excess bilirubin can cause neurotoxicity and can act as a lytic agent binding to erythrocyte membranes.[69] Hence, the therapeutic window of biliverdin should be considered before its clinical use.

Future Research

The primary nonspecific injury (such as I-R injury) to the donor organ induces events of the two distinct immunological defense systems: (1) a more broadly directed innate immune host defense (evolutionary directed normally against infections), resulting in (2) a definite adaptive immune host defense that ultimately leads to a specific graft injury (i.e., rejection). Indeed, I-R may create a milieu of inflammation that operates as a "danger" signal in OLTs, and in analogy to the infectious agent–induced inflammation, it may initiate a state of innate immunity by activating the host toll-like receptor (TLR) system. The environmental challenges may lead to degradation of potential agonists, such as soluble heparan sulfate proteoglycan, which may then deliver activation signals via TLR on dendritic cells. The question arises as to whether there are any endogenous ligands on autologous damaged cells that activate the TLR system in response to oxidative injury during hepatic I-R injury. As discussed earlier, cold ischemia, the most prominent component of the hepatic I-R insult, affects primarily liver sinusoidal ECs. Indeed, hyaluronic acid (HA), metabolized almost exclusively by EC, is considered a dependable marker of liver endothelial function. Hence, it is plausible that HA provides a triggering signal to activate TLR complex (primarily TLR4) on Kupffer cells during I-R injury. Conversely, HO-1 expression may inhibit HA, with resultant hepatocytoprotection. Future dissection of HA-TLR cross-talk should provide important insights into the mechanisms of hepatic I-R injury, and the rationale for the development of novel and much needed therapeutic modalities based on the concept that hepatic I-R injury represents a case of host innate immunity.

References

1. Henderson JM: Liver transplantation and rejection: An overview. Hepatogastroenterology 46(Suppl 2):1482-1484, 1999.
2. Koneru B, Dikdan G: Hepatic steatosis and liver transplantation current clinical and experimental perspectives. Transplantation 73:325-330, 2002.
3. Carles J, Fawaz R, Hamoudi NE, et al: Preservation of human liver grafts in UW solution. Ultrastructural evidence for endothelial and Kupffer cell activation during cold ischemia and after ischemia-reperfusion. Liver 14:50-56, 1994.
4. Borghi-Scoazec G, Scoazec JY, Durand F, et al: Apoptosis after ischemia-reperfusion in human liver allografts. Liver Transpl Surg 3:407-415, 1997.
5. Rull R, Vidal O, Momblan D, et al: Evaluation of potential liver donors: Limits imposed by donor variables in liver transplantation. Liver Transpl 9:389-393, 2003.
6. Van der Hoeven JA, Lindell S, van Schilfgaarde R, et al: Donor brain death reduces survival after transplantation in rat livers preserved for 20 hr. Transplantation 72:1632-1636, 2001.
7. Garcia-Valdecasas JC, Tabet J, Valero R, et al: Evaluation of ischemic injury during liver procurement from non–heart-beating donors. Eur Surg Res 31:447-456, 1999.
8. Laskowski IA, Pratschke J, Wilhelm MM, et al: Early and late injury to renal transplants from non–heart-beating donors. Transplantation 73:1468-1473, 2002.
9. Pannen BH: New insights into the regulation of hepatic blood flow after ischemia and reperfusion. Anesth Analg 94:1448-1457, 2002.
10. Scommotau S, Uhlmann D, Loffler BM, Involvement of endothelin/nitric oxide balance in hepatic ischemia/reperfusion injury. Langenbecks Arch Surg 384:65-70, 1999.

11. Uhlmann D, Armann B, Gaebel G, et al: Endothelin A receptor blockade reduces hepatic ischemia/reperfusion injury after warm ischemia in a pig model. J Gastrointest Surg 7:331-339, 2003.
12. Wang Y, Vodovotz Y, Kim PK, et al: Mechanisms of hepatoprotection by nitric oxide. Ann N Y Acad Sci 962:415-422, 2002.
13. Squadrito GL, Pryor WA: Oxidative chemistry of nitric oxide: The roles of superoxide, peroxynitrite, and carbon dioxide. Free Radic Biol Med 25:392-403, 1998.
14. Valero R, Garcia-Valdecasas JC, Net M, et al: L-Arginine reduces liver and biliary tract damage after liver transplantation from non–heart-beating donor pigs. Transplantation 70:730-737, 2000.
15. Yagnik GP, Takahashi Y, Tsoulfas G, et al: Blockade of the L-arginine/NO synthase pathway worsens hepatic apoptosis and liver transplant preservation injury. Hepatology 36:573-581, 2002.
16. Serracino-Inglott F, Virlos IT, Habib NA, et al: Differential nitric oxide synthase expression during hepatic ischemia-reperfusion. Am J Surg 185:589-595, 2003.
17. Jaeschke H: Molecular mechanisms of hepatic ischemia-reperfusion injury and preconditioning. Am J Physiol Gastrointest Liver Physiol 284:G15-G26, 2003.
18. Fan C, Zwacka RM, Engelhardt JF: Therapeutic approaches for ischemia/reperfusion injury in the liver. J Mol Med 77:577-592, 1999.
19. Pober JS: Activation and injury of endothelial cells by cytokines. Pathol Biol 46:159-163, 1998.
20. Shibuya H, Ohkohchi N, Tsukamoto S, Satomi S: Tumor necrosis factor–induced, superoxide-mediated neutrophil accumulation in cold ischemic/reperfused rat liver. Hepatology 26:113-120, 1997.
21. Shito M, Wakabayashi G, Ueda M, et al: Interleukin 1 receptor blockade reduces tumor necrosis factor production, tissue injury, and mortality after hepatic ischemia-reperfusion in the rat. Transplantation 63:143-148, 1997.
22. Lentsch AB, Yoshidome H, Kato A, et al: Requirement for interleukin-12 in the pathogenesis of warm hepatic ischemia/reperfusion injury in mice. Hepatology 30:1448-1453, 1999.
23. Colletti LM, Kunkel SL, Walz A, et al: The role of cytokine networks in the local liver injury following hepatic ischemia/reperfusion in the rat. Hepatology 23:506-514, 1996.
24. Maher JJ, Scott MK, Saito JM, Burton MC: Adenovirus-mediated expression of cytokine-induced neutrophil chemoattractant in rat liver induces a neutrophilic hepatitis. Hepatology 25:624-630, 1997.
25. Detmers PA, Lo SK, Olsen-Egbert E, et al: Neutrophil-activating protein 1/interleukin 8 stimulates the binding activity of the leukocyte adhesion receptor CD11b/CD18 on human neutrophils. J Exp Med 171:1155-1162, 1990.
26. Camargo CA Jr, Madden JF, Gao W, et al: Interleukin-6 protects liver against warm ischemia/reperfusion injury and promotes hepatocyte proliferation in the rodent. Hepatology 26:1513-1520, 1997.
27. Yoshidome H, Kato A, Edwards MJ, Lentsch AB: Interleukin-10 suppresses hepatic ischemia/reperfusion injury in mice: Implications of a central role for nuclear factor kappaB. Hepatology 30:203-208, 1999.
28. Ke B, Shen XD, Lassman CR, et al: Interleukin-13 gene transfer protects rat livers from antigen-independent injury induced by ischemia and reperfusion. Transplantation 75:1118-1123, 2003.
29. Yoshidome H, Kato A, Miyazaki M, et al: IL-13 activates STAT6 and inhibits liver injury induced by ischemia/reperfusion. Am J Pathol 155:1059-1064, 1999.
30. Lentsch AB, Yoshidome H, Warner RL, et al: Secretory leukocyte protease inhibitor in mice regulates local and remote organ inflammatory injury induced by hepatic ischemia/reperfusion. Gastroenterology 117:953-961, 1999.
31. Jaeschke H, Farhood A, Bautista AP, et al: Complement activates Kupffer cells and neutrophils during reperfusion after hepatic ischemia. Am J Physiol 264:G801-G809, 1993.
32. Chavez-Cartaya RE, DeSola GP, Wright L, et al: Regulation of the complement cascade by soluble complement receptor type 1. Protective effect in experimental liver ischemia and reperfusion. Transplantation 59:1047-1052, 1995.
33. Walcher F, Marzi I, Fischer R, et al: Platelet-activating factor is involved in the regulation of pathological leukocyte adhesion after liver transplantation. J Surg Res 61:244-249, 1996.
34. Hughes H, Farhood A, Jaeschke H: Role of leukotriene B4 in the pathogenesis of hepatic ischemia-reperfusion injury in the rat. Prostaglandins Leukot Essent Fatty Acids 45:113-119, 1992.
35. Liu P, Vonderfecht SL, McGuire GM, et al: The 21-aminosteroid tirilazad mesylate protects against endotoxin shock and acute liver failure in rats. J Pharmacol Exp Ther 271:438-445, 1994.
36. Jaeschke H: Reactive oxygen and mechanisms of inflammatory liver injury. J Gastroenterol Hepatol 15:718-724, 2000.
37. Zwacka RM, Zhou W, Zhang Y, et al: Redox gene therapy for ischemia/reperfusion injury of the liver reduces AP1 and NF-kappaB activation. Nat Med 4:698-704, 1998.
38. Zhou W, Zhang Y, Hosch MS, et al: Subcellular site of superoxide dismutase expression differentially controls AP-1 activity and injury in mouse liver following ischemia/reperfusion. Hepatology 33:902-914, 2001.
39. Farmer DG, Amersi F, Kupiec-Weglinski JW, Busuttil RW: Current status of ischemia and reperfusion injury in the liver. Transplant Rev 14:106-126, 2000.
40. Ikeda T, Yanaga K, Kishikawa K, et al: Ischemic injury in liver transplantation: Difference in injury sites between warm and cold ischemia in rats. Hepatology 16:454-461, 1992.
41. Gao W, Bentley RC, Madden JF, Clavien PA: Apoptosis of sinusoidal endothelial cells is a critical mechanism of preservation injury in rat liver transplantation. Hepatology 27:1652-1660, 1998.
42. Esposti MD, Hatzinisiriou I, McLennan H, Ralph S: Bcl-2 and mitochondrial oxygen radicals. New approaches with reactive oxygen species–sensitive probes. J Biol Chem 274:29831-29837, 1999.
43. Matsushita H, Morishita R, Nata T, et al: Hypoxia-induced endothelial apoptosis through nuclear factor-κB (NF-κB)-mediated bcl-2 suppression: In vivo evidence of the importance of NF-κB in endothelial cell regulation. Circ Res 86:974-981, 2000.
44. Li C, Jackson RM: Reactive species mechanisms of cellular hypoxia-reoxygenation injury. Am J Physiol Cell Physiol 282:C227-C241, 2002.
45. Upadhya AG, Harvey RP, Howard TK, et al: Evidence of a role for matrix metalloproteinases in cold preservation injury of the liver in humans and in the rat. Hepatology 26:922-928, 1997.
46. Amersi F, Shen XD, Moore C, et al: Fibronectin-α4β1 integrin-mediated blockade protects genetically fat Zucker rat livers from ischemia/reperfusion injury. Am J Pathol 162:1229-1239, 2003.
47. Clavien PA: Sinusoidal endothelial cell injury during hepatic preservation and reperfusion. Hepatology 28:281-285, 1998.
48. Jaeschke H: Cellular adhesion molecules: Regulation and functional significance in the pathogenesis of liver diseases. Am J Physiol 273:G602-G611, 1997.
49. Yadav SS, Howell DN, Steeber DA, et al: P-Selectin mediates reperfusion injury through neutrophil and platelet sequestration in the warm ischemic mouse liver. Hepatology 29:1494-1502, 1999.
50. Nagendra AR, Mickelson JK, Smith CW: CD18 integrin and CD54-dependent neutrophil adhesion to cytokine-stimulated human hepatocytes. Am J Physiol 272:G408-G416, 1997.
51. Farhood A, McGuire GM, Manning AM, et al: Intercellular adhesion molecule 1 (ICAM-1) expression and its role in neutrophil-induced ischemia-reperfusion injury in rat liver. J Leukoc Biol 57:368-374, 1995.

52. Nakano H, Nagasaki H, Barama A, et al: The effects of N-acetylcysteine and anti-intercellular adhesion molecule-1 monoclonal antibody against ischemia-reperfusion injury of the rat steatotic liver produced by a choline-methionine-deficient diet. Hepatology 26:670-678, 1997.

53. Amersi F, Farmer DG, Shaw GD, et al: P-selectin glycoprotein ligand-1 (rPSGL-Ig)-mediated blockade of CD62 selectin molecules protects rat steatotic liver grafts from ischemia/reperfusion injury. Am J Transplant 2:600-608, 2002.

54. Shiratori Y, Kiriyama H, Fukushi Y, et al: Modulation of ischemia-reperfusion–induced hepatic injury by Kupffer cells. Dig Dis Sci 39:1265-1272, 1994.

55. Takada M, Chandraker A, Nadeau KC, et al: The role of the B7 costimulatory pathway in experimental cold ischemia/reperfusion injury. J Clin Invest 100: 1199-1203, 1997.

56. Matsuda T, Yamaguchi Y, Matsumura F, et al: Immuno-suppressants decrease neutrophil chemoattractant and attenuate ischemia/reperfusion injury of the liver in rats. J Trauma 44: 475-484, 1998.

57. Shen XD, Ke B, Zhai Y, et al: CD154-CD40 T-cell costimulation pathway is required in the mechanism of hepatic ischemia/reperfusion injury, and its blockade facilitates and depends on heme oxygenase-1–mediated cytoprotection. Transplantation 74: 315-319, 2002.

58. Shen XD, Ke B, Zhai Y, et al: Stat4 and Stat6 signaling in hepatic ischemia/reperfusion injury in mice: HO-1 dependence of Stat4 disruption–mediated cytoprotection. Hepatology 37:296-303, 2003.

59. Anselmo DM, Amersi FF, Shen XD, et al: FTY720 pretreatment reduces warm hepatic ischemia reperfusion injury through inhibition of T-lymphocyte infiltration. Am J Transplant 2:843-849, 2002.

60. Clavien PA, Harvey PR, Sanabria JR, et al: Lymphocyte adherence in the reperfused rat liver: Mechanisms and effects. Hepatology 17:131-142, 1993.

61. Zwacka RM, Zhang Y, Halldorson J, et al: CD4(+) T-lymphocytes mediate ischemia/reperfusion-induced inflammatory responses in mouse liver. J Clin Invest 100:279-289, 1997.

62. Le Moine O, Louis H, Demols A, et al: Cold liver ischemia-reperfusion injury critically depends on liver T cells and is improved by donor pretreatment with interleukin 10 in mice. Hepatology 31:1266-1274, 2000.

63. Knolle PA, Uhrig A, Hegenbarth S, et al: IL-10 down-regulates T cell activation by antigen-presenting liver sinusoidal endothelial cells through decreased antigen uptake via the mannose receptor and lowered surface expression of accessory molecules. Clin Exp Immunol 114:427-433, 1998.

64. Knolle PA, Gerken G, Loser E, et al: Role of sinusoidal endothelial cells of the liver in concanavalin A–induced hepatic injury in mice. Hepatology 24:824-829, 1996.

65. Zhang S, Jin MB, Zhu Y, et al: Effect of endogenous adenosine augmentation on ischemia and reperfusion injury to the liver. Transplant Proc 29:1336-1337, 1997.

66. Cutrin JC, Perrelli MG, Cavalieri B, et al: Microvascular dysfunction induced by reperfusion injury and protective effect of ischemic w-preconditioning. Free Radic Biol Med 33:1200-1208, 2002.

67. Peralta C, Hotter G, Closa D, et al: The protective role of adenosine in inducing nitric oxide synthesis in rat liver ischemia preconditioning is mediated by activation of adenosine A2 receptors. Hepatology 29:126-132, 1999.

68. Fernandez L, Heredia N, Grande L, et al: Preconditioning protects liver and lung damage in rat liver transplantation: Role of xanthine/xanthine oxidase. Hepatology 36:562-572, 2002.

69. Ryter SW, Tyrrell RM: The heme synthesis and degradation pathways: Role in oxidant sensitivity. Heme oxygenase has both pro- and antioxidant properties. Free Radic Biol Med 28:289-309, 2000.

70. Applegate LA, Luscher P, Tyrrell RM: Induction of heme oxygenase: A general response to oxidant stress in cultured mammalian cells. Cancer Res 51:974-978, 1991.

71. Lautier D, Luscher P, Tyrrell RM: Endogenous glutathione levels modulate both constitutive and UVA radiation/hydrogen peroxide inducible expression of the human heme oxygenase gene. Carcinogenesis 13:227-232, 1992.

72. Katori M, Busuttil RW, Kupiec-Weglinski JW: Heme oxygenase-1 system in organ transplantation. Transplantation 74:905-912, 2002.

73. Menger M, Vollmar B, Glasz J, et al: Microcirculatory manifestations of hepatic ischemia/reperfusion injury. In Messmer K, Menger M (eds): Liver Microcirculation and Hepatobiliary Function, Progress in Applied Microcirculation. Basel, Karger, 1993, 106-124.

74. Katori M, Anselmo DM, Busuttil RW, Kupiec-Weglinski JW: A novel strategy against ischemia and reperfusion injury: Cytoprotection with heme oxygenase system. Transpl Immunol 9: 227-233, 2002.

75. Vachharajani TJ, Work J, Issekutz AC, Granger DN: Heme oxygenase modulates selectin expression in different regional vascular beds. Am J Physiol Heart Circ Physiol 278:H1613-H1617, 2000.

76. Nakagami T, Toyomura K, Kinoshita T, Morisawa S: A beneficial role of bile pigments as an endogenous tissue protector: Anti-complement effects of biliverdin and conjugated bilirubin. Biochim Biophys Acta 1158:189-193, 1993.

77. Coito AJ, Buelow R, Shen XD, et al: Heme oxygenase-1 gene transfer inhibits inducible nitric oxide synthase expression and protects genetically fat Zucker rat livers from ischemia-reperfusion injury. Transplantation 74:96-102, 2002.

78. Otterbein LE, Bach FH, Alam J, et al: Carbon monoxide has anti-inflammatory effects involving the mitogen-activated protein kinase pathway. Nat Med 6:422-428, 2000.

79. Brouard S, Otterbein LE, Anrather J, et al: Carbon monoxide generated by heme oxygenase 1 suppresses endothelial cell apoptosis. J Exp Med 192:1015-1026, 2000.

80. Amersi F, Shen XD, Anselmo D, et al: Ex vivo exposure to carbon monoxide prevents hepatic ischemia/reperfusion injury through p38 MAP kinase pathway. Hepatology 35:815-823, 2002.

81. Amersi F, Buelow R, Kato H, et al: Upregulation of heme oxygenase-1 protects genetically fat Zucker rat livers from ischemia/reperfusion injury. J Clin Invest 104:1631-1639, 1999.

82. Kato H, Amersi F, Buelow R et al: Heme oxygenase-1 overexpression protects rat livers from ischemia/reperfusion injury with extended cold preservation. Am J Transplant 1:121-128, 2001.

83. Tsuchihashi S, Tamaki T, Tanaka M, et al: Pyrrolidine dithio-carbamate provides protection against hypothermic preservation and transplantation injury in the rat liver: The role of heme oxygenase-1. Surgery 133:556-567, 2003.

84. Ke B, Buelow R, Shen XD, et al: Heme oxygenase 1 gene transfer prevents CD95/Fas ligand-mediated apoptosis and improves liver allograft survival via carbon monoxide signaling pathway. Hum Gene Ther 13:1189-1199, 2002.

85. Uchida Y, Tamaki T, Tanaka M, et al: De novo protein synthesis induced by donor nutritional depletion ameliorates cold ischemia and reperfusion injury in the rat liver. Transplant Proc 32:1657-1659, 2000.

Extracorporeal Xenogeneic Liver Support

RAVI S. CHARI
WILLIAM C. MEYERS
MARLON F. LEVY

Historical review of xenogeneic liver
   perfusion   1416

Technical considerations   1417

Ex vivo liver function   1418

Immunological considerations   1419

Clinical results   1419

Recent experience   1420

Summary   1421

Since publication of the first edition of this textbook, the field of extracorporeal hepatic support has seen both progress and setbacks. At the bedside, much more focus is being placed on bioartificial livers wherein "cartridges" loaded with hepatocytes (porcine or human) provide the necessary hepatocyte mass to detoxify the blood of patients in liver failure (see Chapter 89). In preclinical or clinical studies, focus has been on advances in creating transgenic animals (pigs) capable, it is hoped, of being physiologically and immunologically compatible enough with humans to serve as organ donors. This chapter outlines some of the challenges in achieving clinically reliable means of extracorporeal hepatic support with whole-organ perfusion.

With total absence of the liver, life can be sustained for up to 24 or 36 hours by maintenance of the blood glucose concentration, albumin, and clotting factors, as well as by antibiotic prophylaxis and nutritional supplementation (total parenteral nutrition). Other functions of the liver that are less well understood and poorly characterized, such as its role in encephalopathy, can be managed to a limited degree by empirical therapeutic regimens. Nonetheless, most patients with fulminant liver failure die unless further measures are instituted. The exact cause of death in these circumstances is not known definitely, but the role of the liver in toxin metabolism (e.g., ammonia, mercaptans, fatty acids, and free phenols) is critical. Absent recovery of the failed liver or transplantation, patients with fulminant liver failure die of cerebral edema and decreased cerebral perfusion leading to brain death.[1] Currently, the preferred treatment of refractory fulminant liver failure is liver transplantation (see also Chapter 11, "Transplantation for Fulminant Hepatic Failure").[2] However, many patients in fulminant failure are not suitable for liver transplantation because of concomitant infection, neoplasm, ongoing alcoholism, or other organ failure.[3,4] In this setting, mortality rates would be improved if a system of adequate liver support were available until such time that the patient's own (native) liver could recover from the insult sustained.

An "artificial liver" that provides the same level of support for patients with liver failure as hemodialysis does for patients with kidney failure does not exist. Indeed, many techniques of artificial liver support have been tried over the past 40 years, including hemodialysis,[5] hepatodialysis,[6] activated charcoal hemoperfusion,[7,8] exchange transfusion,[9] and plasmapheresis with plasma exchange.[10] These systems, however, do not address the principal clinical problem: loss of functioning hepatocytes. Myriad functions are performed by the liver and individual hepatocytes, including synthesis of protein, elimination of toxins, metabolism of many substances, and maintenance of nutritional status and immunocompetence. To address the need for hepatocyte function, some systems have included extracorporeal heterologous or homologous liver perfusion[11,12] or cross-circulation.[13,14]

Systems combining biological material with synthetic material have been developed as well (see also Chapter 89, "Development of Bioartificial Liver").[15] Of these systems for liver support, it has been believed that extracorporeal liver perfusion is the most rapid and effective method of replacing normal liver function.[16] Initially, complex systems, short perfusions, and a paucity of immunological agents limited the effectiveness of the procedure. Today, improved preservation techniques, improved circuitry, and better understanding of xenogeneic immunology may make extracorporeal liver perfusion an important adjuvant to the treatment of liver disease and the study of xenogeneic reactions. Furthermore, bridge-to-transplantation models using transgenic porcine livers may allow testing of the transgenic liver's safety and efficacy outside the context of (and short of) actual transplantation.

Historical Review of Xenogeneic Liver Perfusion

The use of an extracorporeal liver as a method of temporary liver support in liver failure is based on experimental work first reported by Otto and coauthors in 1958.[17] In the decade after this report was published, a number of studies involving various animal donor species were performed in the clinical arena. Eiseman and colleagues[11] were the first to report the use of this technique. Eight patients underwent 11 porcine liver perfusions with an arteriovenous circuit. Neurological improvement was appreciated after all but one perfusion. The longest survival was 13 days; this patient underwent three separate perfusions. Perfusion times ranged from 70 minutes to 6 hours and 10 minutes.

After this report, data from a number of centers confirmed these findings (Table 88–1). One interesting report described the use of 16 livers (10 pigs, 3 baboons, and 1 each from a calf, monkey, and human) to support a single patient hepatorenally for 76 days.[26] Coma was reversed eight times with these multiple ex vivo perfusions. Pig proteins synthesized by the donor liver were present in the patient's serum and persisted for approximately 23 days. One episode of anaphylaxis was described. To avoid this complication, livers from other species were used for a 6-week period while the levels of pig antibody decreased. Subsequent perfusions combining corticosteroid pretreatment were performed successfully.

Isolated heterologous bovine perfusion was first reported in 1970 by Condon and associates.[19] Only two of the seven patients in this series showed neurological improvement despite improvement in biochemical profile in all. There were no survivors in this series. In 1973, Abouna and colleagues reported the accumulated experience with 33 clinical liver hemoperfusions for the treatment of 21 episodes of deep liver coma in 10 patients by using an ex vivo perfusion technique; four different animal species were used in this series.[20]

Table 88–1. HISTORY OF EX VIVO XENOPERFUSION

Year	Investigator	Description
1958	Otto et al.[17]	Canine model of ex vivo liver perfusion
1966	Sen et al.[18]	Ex vivo liver alloperfusion
1965	Eiseman et al.[11]	Ex vivo porcine liver perfusion
1970	Condon et al.[19]	Ex vivo calf liver perfusion
1973	Abouna et al.[20]	Ex vivo baboon liver perfusion
1980	Lie[21] and Tung et al.[22]	German experience of ex vivo liver perfusion
1994	Chari et al.[23]	Ex vivo liver perfusion followed by allotransplantation
2000	Levy et al.[24]	Transgenic (hCD55/59) ex vivo perfusion followed by allotransplantation
2001	Tector et al.[25]	Ex vivo liver perfusion

This extensive work highlighted the importance of the duration of perfusion and described the immunological aspects of xenoperfusion.[20] Lie performed detailed studies of xenogeneic liver perfusion in Germany from 1973 to 1981. He reported a 50% survival rate in his series of 34 hemoperfusions involving 32 baboon livers and 2 human livers for acute liver failure.[21] Tung and coworkers[22] reported a survival rate of 17%. In the latter, 21 perfusions using livers from 14 pigs, 8 baboons, and 1 calf were carried out in 12 patients for 17 cases of coma.

In the early 1980s, as orthotopic liver transplantation (OLT) became widely available, this procedure established itself as the treatment of choice for appropriate patients with fulminant liver failure. Thereafter, enthusiasm for ex vivo liver perfusion dropped off. More recently, it has become apparent that OLT is not the appropriate treatment for all patients in liver failure. Furthermore, critical organ donor shortages preclude the timely use of OLT in some patients. With the development of a small-volume extracorporeal venovenous bypass circuit incorporating a membrane oxygenator, successful allotransplantation after porcine liver perfusion has led to recovery of a patient.[23,24] In this new era, improved understanding of the immunological interactions may allow strategies for prolonging ex vivo xenogeneic livers, thereby increasing the probability of survival and possibly decreasing the demand for OLT.

Technical Considerations

One of the most critical elements of ex vivo perfusion, as with OLT, is the technical success of the liver retrieval operation.[27] Historically, the donor liver was removed and perfused with cold lactated Ringer's solution on a back table.[11,28] It was known that the perfusion techniques were inadequate and in part responsible for the relatively short perfusion times.[29] Today, retrieval of porcine livers is almost exactly like that of a human liver for OLT. Catheters are placed in the abdominal aorta and directly into the portal vein; in the pig, perfusion of both the portal and arterial routes is superior to perfusion of the portal vein alone.[30] The superior mesenteric artery is ligated. Preservation with 4° C University of Wisconsin solution is performed. The volume of perfusate is based on the approximate liver mass: 2 L for 20- to 40-kg pigs.[31] Care must be taken to ensure hemostasis at the time of explantation because the liver will be perfused during anticoagulation of the patient. The cystic duct is ligated, but the gallbladder is not removed.

Patient preparation begins as soon as the decision is made that ex vivo liver perfusion is appropriate. Informed consent from family members on the basis of an institutional review board–approved protocol should be obtained before the perfusion. Arterial and pulmonary artery (Swan-Ganz) pressure catheters are inserted. At the clinician's discretion and capability, an intracranial pressure catheter may be placed before perfusion. Baseline neurological examination is well documented before commencement of perfusion; an electroencephalogram is optional. Circuits described before 1990 were mostly arteriovenous types; priming volumes were large (from 3 U of blood[32] to 2.5 L[33]), and hypotension often accompanied initiation of the circuit.[11,28] More recently, the development of a venovenous circuit with a small circuit volume has addressed many of the technical problems with earlier systems.[23] The latter system requires the placement of venous catheters in the iliac or jugular veins for inflow and outflow to the circuit. Moreover, this system has less hemodynamic effect on the patient on initiation of the circuit.[34]

Much of the emphasis of previous research has been in the area of perfusion parameters (Table 88-2). These data are now widely accepted and applied regardless of the system used to perfuse the ex vivo liver. Tait and colleagues showed that total liver blood flow less than 0.2 mL/g of liver mass per minute is associated with cessation of bile flow.[35] Optimal conditions for nonpulsatile perfusion of the isolated liver are (1) flow greater than 0.5 mL/g of liver per minute if the portal vein alone is perfused and (2) flow of 0.2 to 0.5 mL/g of liver per minute for both the hepatic artery and portal vein perfusion.[35] Simultaneous perfusion of the hepatic artery and portal vein is preferred.[24]

These data were based on oxygen utilization, ammonia, and sulfobromophthalein (Bromsulphalein) clearance and bile production. Cuello-Mainard and coworkers used the arteriovenous difference to establish an optimal portal flow of 0.75 to 1.0 mL/g of liver per minute of oxygenated blood.[36] Hardison[37] and Winkler[38] and their associates maintained the need for perfusion flow of 1.0 mL/g of liver per minute in isolated portal vein perfusion. Winkler and colleagues[38]

Table 88-2. TECHNICAL CONSIDERATIONS IN EX VIVO LIVER PERFUSION

Parameter	Consideration
Blood flow	Isolated portal flow: 0.5–1.0 mL/g of liver per min
	Arterial and portal routes: 0.2–0.5 mL/g of liver per min
Temperature	Inflow: 37° C–38° C
Portal pressure	10–15 mm Hg
Hepatic venous pressure	<5 mm Hg
Blood conditions	pH 7.40
	$P_{O_2} > 95$ mm Hg; oxygen saturation > 95%
	$P_{CO_2} \approx 40$ mm Hg
Anticoagulation	Activated clotting time ≈ 200 sec

also showed that the differences in bile flow and indo-cyanine green elimination are relatively small, and Eiseman's data confirmed that flow rates greater than 0.9 mL/g of liver per minute perfusion via the portal vein alone fulfill the metabolic demands of the liver. Drapana and coworkers demonstrated that perfusion through the portal vein alone results in diminished oxygen consumption and an inability to metabolize lactic and pyruvic acid.[39] They also noted that single-vessel (portal) perfusion is probably adequate in the clinical setting because some liver function is maintained even by a dying liver. Other investigators advocate perfusion of both the porcine portal vein and the hepatic artery.[24] Inflow temperatures are maintained at 37°C to 38°C,[11,35,40,41] and portal inflow pressure should be maintained less than 49 cm H_2O[38] or 10 to 15 mm Hg.[42] If parallel arterial and venous perfusion is undertaken, arterial flow should be pulsatile and as low as 0.15 mL/g of liver per minute.[40] The blood perfusing the liver should have an oxygen saturation greater than 95% and normal partial pressure of carbon dioxide and oxygen.[43] The extracorporeal liver appears to be extremely sensitive to decreased pH.[34] Previous work has supported the need to dilute the blood perfusate to increase perfusion flow.[44] However, more recent work has not shown such dilution to be necessary.[23] Heparin is administered before perfusion to achieve an activated clotting time of approximately 200 seconds. Heparin-bonded tubing may also be used.

On the outflow end, return is most easily accomplished by one catheter (8 to 10 French) in the suprahepatic vena cava. The pressure on this side of the liver should be less than 5 mm Hg. Transhepatic vascular pressure gradients across the liver between the portal vein and the suprahepatic vena cava should be maintained in the range of 12 to 14 mm Hg.[32] Return of blood is facilitated by raising the liver 30 to 40 cm above the level of the patient. In some recent circuit designs, posthepatic pumps have been used to return the blood to the patient and maintain low posthepatic circuit pressure (I. Fox, personal communication, May 1993) (Fig. 88-1), although some successful perfusions have not incorporated this feature.[24] Ex vivo livers produce 4 to 8 mL of ascites per minute,[11,28] and the degree of ascites appears to be directly proportional to outflow tract occlusion.[43]

A variety of positions and containers have been used in the past: warmed water baths, warmed baths with paddles to simulate respiratory movements,[38] warmed containers with the liver on a moving diaphragm,[20] warmed saline baths with the liver suspended from the vena cava to simulate the position in the pig,[41] or simply a sterile box or basin.[19,34] Although some advocate positioning as being important,[41] none have shown a particular position to be significantly better. Table 88-2 summarizes the main technical considerations of ex vivo liver perfusion.

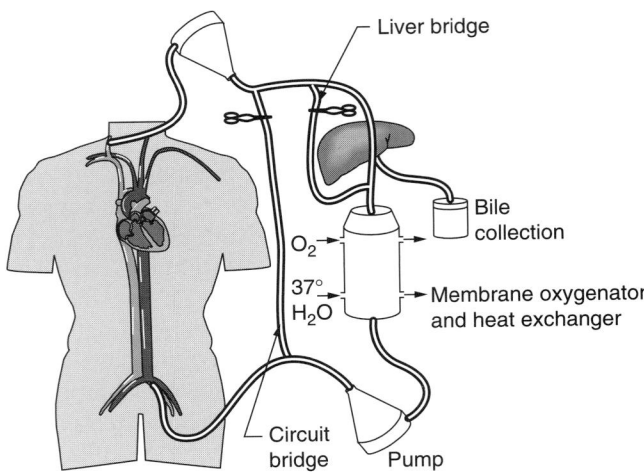

FIGURE 88-1

Ex vivo circuit design using venovenous bypass, an extracorporeal membrane oxygenator, and a post–ex vivo liver pump.

Ex Vivo Liver Function

Table 88-3 outlines some of the tests and parameters used in experimental or clinical liver perfusion to assess liver viability and function. Various other parameters on performance of the ex vivo liver can also be examined during the perfusion period, including tests of liver damage (increases in transaminases and potassium, weight gain of the liver, poor appearance) and liver function (oxygen uptake, bile flow, excretion and metabolism of various compounds). Functional parameters are more important because function determines the usefulness of the perfused liver, and function and damage assessments are not necessarily complementary.[45]

Tygstrup and colleagues compared the function of ex vivo perfused livers with that of in vivo livers.[33] They concluded that an ex vivo liver cannot be considered to be functionally identical to an in vivo liver and

Table 88-3. INDICES OF LIVER FUNCTION
Bile production
Oxygen consumption
Clearance of lactate
Lactate-pyruvate ratio
Bilirubin excretion
Galactose clearance
Indocyanine green clearance
Iodine 131 rose bengal elimination
Sulfobromophthalein clearance
Plasma ammonia and bilirubin
Liver appearance

that the metabolic capacity of the perfused liver should be considered to be at most only about two thirds that of the intact liver. Blood ammonia and urea nitrogen concentrations after ammonium citrate loads were studied in the isolated perfusion model[46]; the efficacy of clearance was remarkable even in the most cyanotic and degenerate-looking livers. This result suggested that the mechanism of ammonia conversion of the liver was durable. By itself, however, ammonia clearance did not reflect the integrity of function of the ex vivo perfused liver.[47] Liem's studies supported Eiseman's observations, as well as reported data concerning the efficiency of iodine 131 rose bengal elimination, sulfobromophthalein retention, serum galactose disappearance, and oxygen utilization.[48] Interestingly, bile flow persisted when all these functions remained intact.

Oxygen consumption rates at the initiation of perfusion were reported to start at 181 μL/100 mg/hr.[44] This value decreases as perfusion continues and liver viability and function decline.[44,48] Ramsoe and others suggested galactose elimination as an indicator of functional liver mass.[45] Sulfobromophthalein has been said to be a poor test of function of the isolated liver,[42] although confirmation of this finding is lacking. Indocyanine green as an indicator of liver function has also been studied. In Eiseman's experience with pig liver preservation, the most sensitive liver function test under ex vivo conditions was indocyanine green excretion followed by bile flow, oxygen uptake, and ammonia uptake. Others found bile flow and indocyanine green to be no more sensitive than bile flow alone in estimating liver function.[49] Bile flow is a very direct measure and varies from 1 to 27 mL/hr.[11] Bile salt clearance is highly correlated with bile flow.[45] Flow of bile increases significantly with arterial versus portal perfusion.[11] The sensitivity of bile as a marker of function may be increased if the concentration of bilirubin in bile is known.[50] Through their own experiments, Abouna and colleagues[47] concluded that bile output and oxygen consumption were good indicators of overall liver function. Clearance of lactate, the lactate-pyruvate ratio, and the rate of elimination of galactose were also sensitive liver function indices. In contrast, surface redox potential was not useful as an index of viability of an extracorporeal liver during hemoperfusion.[51] Liver appearance alone has not correlated with function inasmuch as livers that appeared cyanotic after 3 hours maintained function.[11]

Immunological Considerations

Results of pathological examination of porcine livers after ex vivo perfusion vary. Some authors reported a normal anatomic appearance, vascular pattern, and hepatocyte structure after perfusion lasting 5 to 9 hours,[20,52] whereas others reported centrilobular congestion and hemorrhage, as well as areas of necrosis.[39,53] In porcine livers, extensive intraparenchymal neutrophil accumulation has also been noted[23,54]; less has been appreciated in baboon livers.[26,55] Immunofluorescence studies on porcine livers have shown variable deposits of immunoglobulin (IgM or natural antibody), complement or complement activation products, and fibrinogen.[20,56] Complement has been implicated in hyperacute rejection of xenografts in other models,[57-59] but its role in rejection of xenoperfused livers is less clear.[56,60] Baboon livers perfused for 12 to 24 hours show less evidence of damage, but immunoglobulin and complement were still detected to a variable degree.[20]

The immunological reaction of the patient to the liver has also been studied. Bibler and associates have shown the presence of protein of bovine origin in the plasma of dogs after temporary ex vivo bovine liver perfusion,[61] and similar results were shown in calves perfused with porcine livers.[54] Norman and colleagues demonstrated that the circulating porcine antigens absent before perfusion and present in increasing amounts after serial perfusion were porcine albumin and α- and $α_2$-globulin.[28] In addition to these antigens, clotting factors are produced by the ex vivo liver.[20] The amount of these proteins in the patient's serum was directly related to the length of the perfusion time.[62] No patient showed a demonstrable antibody response to these circulating antigens. Abouna and coauthors reported a clinical anaphylactic reaction in one patient when repeated porcine perfusion was attempted 12 days after the first series of four consecutive liver perfusions.[26] Studies in which skin grafts were taken from the liver donor pigs and applied to the calves demonstrated that a degree of immunological tolerance was produced as a result of exposure to large amounts of antigen.[54] Circulating antibody has been studied and found to decrease after perfusion.[21] Many other questions remain unanswered, such as those concerning the nature of rejection of the ex vivo liver and the long-term effects on patients undergoing porcine liver perfusion. Data from more recent studies investigating pig liver perfusion may help uncover the answers to these and other questions, and strategies aimed at prolonging the duration of perfusion and function may be developed from such studies.[23]

Clinical Results

Clinically, two parameters have been used to judge the success of perfusion: (1) recovery of consciousness and (2) survival. It was also apparent that the maximum metabolic benefit of porcine perfusion occurs within the first 4 hours[34] and rarely beyond 6 hours. With baboon livers, perfusion times were longer.[20,21] It has been postulated that volume of flow and length of perfusion time are the most important determinants of clinical outcome in ex vivo xenoperfusion[20]; thus, perfusion with livers capable of lasting longer (i.e., baboon livers) may yield better results.

From the onset, it was evident that the ex vivo liver had a remarkable capacity to clear ammonia.[11,24] Bilirubin also decreased during the course of almost all liver perfusions. However, it became clear that rectification of the biochemical profile did not always correlate with recovery of consciousness.[11,20,28,62,63] Table 88–4 outlines the results of larger series reported in the literature. The difficulty in interpreting the results of recovery from coma is in part due to the subjective assessment of coma grade and inconsistencies in scales and individual grading. The data, however, do point out that with respect to neurological improvement, there is a success rate of approximately 45% for an individual perfusion. Neurological recovery is not coincidental with perfusion and may lag by 3 to 6 hours.[63] Electroencephalographic changes were observed by Ranek and coworkers,[64] but no specific alteration was associated with change in coma after xenoperfusion. It is apparent that although the data from Table 88–4 predate the advent of clinical transplantation, transplantation might have helped many patients who otherwise recovered neurologically but had insufficient remaining liver mass to effect regeneration.

Other biochemical parameters have been studied to determine the functional results of xenoperfusion in the clinical setting. However, very few data have been gathered to find indices correlating ex vivo liver function and clinical outcome. Within the bile of porcine or baboon perfused ex vivo liver, human bile salts[50,65] and human proteins have been found.[28] Immunopheresis of the biliary proteins has demonstrated α-, β-, and γ-globulin, all of human origin. Bilirubin and bile acids are both excreted in bile[28,65]; neither, however, appears to influence coma status or patient outcome.[50] Branched-chain amino acids have been shown to be unaltered by xenoperfusion, whereas aromatic amino acids decreased by 10%.[55] Of the ammonia-genic amino acids, threonine, serine, and lysine have been shown to have only minor fluctuations, whereas glutamine and histidine decreased significantly.[55] Others have demonstrated a statistically significant increase in the ratio of branched-chain amino acids to aromatic amino acids; free fatty acids in plasma are significantly reduced by extracorporeal livers, but they have no correlation with coma grade, nor are changes in their concentrations predictive of outcome.[66]

Serious complications have been uncommon. Hypotension on initiation of the arteriovenous circuits has been alluded to earlier in the chapter. Moreover, anaphylaxis has been described only once in the literature.[20] Thrombocytopenia resulting from sequestration within the parenchyma of the liver has been described by several authors.[3,54,64] Air embolism in a non–closed-circuit system has also been described.[20] After perfusion, hypocoagulable states, stress ulceration, and gastrointestinal hemorrhage are the major complications; these problems, however, are infrequent.[18] Blood transfusion and clotting factor replacement therapy are routine with almost every perfusion.

Recent Experience

Clinical extracorporeal whole-organ perfusion was performed less often in the early part of this century, although some reports continue to appear in the literature.[24,25] The most comprehensive of these reports comes from the Baylor group in Dallas, where transgenic (hD55/hCD59) porcine livers were used as a bridge to

Table 88–4. RESULTS OF LIVER PERFUSION IN 10 STUDIES

Author	Year	No. of Patients	No. of Perfusions	Species	Survivors	Change in Coma
Eiseman et al.[11]	1965	8	11	Pig	0	10
Norman et al.[28]	1966	5	15	Pig	0	Coma not documented
Watts et al.[63]	1967	3	6	Pig	1	3
Bertrand et al.[62]	1968	10	15	Pig	2	9
Condon et al.[19]	1970	7	14	Cow	0	2
Ranek et al.[64]	1971	5	5	Pig	0	0
Abouna et al.[20]	1973	10	32	Pig, baboon, cow	2	13
Lie[21]	1980	14	29	Baboon	6	14
Tung et al.[22]	1980	12	21	Pig, baboon	1	12
Fischer et al.[55]	1980	8	41	Baboon	1	8
Total		82	189		13	71*

*The total excludes the results of Norman and colleagues.[28]

transplantation for two young patients in deep coma from fulminant hepatic failure. These patients, after 7 and 10 hours of perfusion, respectively, were successfully transplanted with human livers and have sustained a normal posttransplant course. Of note is that in neither of these patients, despite massive parenteral exposure to transgenic porcine tissue, have any porcine endogenous retrovirus antibodies developed.[24] The transgenic nature of these livers may have afforded both immunological and morphological protection to the livers not seen in nontransgenic organs exposed to human blood. Interest in xenotransplantation in general and whole-organ work in particular has fallen under considerable regulatory scrutiny in the United States and is not a reality in any other country.[67]

Extensive preclinical work has been conducted in the last few years by the Cambridge group and others to assess the performance of the porcine liver in an isolated perfusion circuit, usually in a normothermic environment with sanguine perfusion.[68-74] This body of work strongly suggests that viable hepatic support can be sustained for at least 72 hours in a carefully controlled physiological environment (temperature, oxygenation, supplemental bile salts, prostaglandins) with maintenance of acid-base balance, continued hepatic protein synthesis (complement and factor V), and histologically demonstrated good preservation of the liver with no overall architectural change.

The nontransgenic porcine liver, when perfused with human blood under these conditions, does indeed suffer significant immunological damage. The Cambridge group showed that over the course of 72 hours of extracorporeal perfusion of porcine livers with human blood, the hematocrit fell progressively to as low as 2.5% of starting values, a phenomenon not seen with perfusion using porcine blood. Both porcine complement and immunoglobulin were found in human blood after xenoperfusion, along with porcine antibodies with specificity for human leukocyte antigens. With increasing duration of perfusion, 40% of the xenoperfusions showed increasing titers of porcine antibodies with specificity for HLA, thus suggesting a response primed by porcine lymphocytes and the ability of porcine livers to generate both a humoral and a cellular graft-versus-host response to human cells.[70] A significant hurdle to the widespread use of porcine livers for extracorporeal whole-organ liver support, however, probably remains activation of the complement cascade by either the classical or the alternative pathway when human blood is exposed to antigens of the porcine vascular endothelium. Although liver failure patients may be a bit less susceptible to this phenomenon,[25] complement activation remains a major concern.[75,76]

Experimentally, there is evidence that porcine livers transgenic for complement regulatory proteins (principally hCD55) may possess some protection from immunological destruction inherent in cross-species sanguineous perfusion. The group from London, Ontario, showed that hDAF livers perfused with human blood had a lower alanine transaminase level, less protein and albumin loss, lower bilirubin levels in the perfusate, less weight gain, and greater bile acid production than did wild-type livers perfused with human blood. This transgene seemed to confer superior function and histology, thus suggesting some protection from hyperacute rejection and a better donor source than wild-type pigs for extracorporeal liver support.[71] The Cambridge group reports similar results.[73]

An interesting development of this research is the application that may come from the effort of sustaining healthy liver function in these perfusion circuits. The interest in the non–heart-beating donor in the United States (DCD donor, or donor after cardiac death) is merging with these perfusion experiments.[77] Indeed, the point has been made that normothermic sanguineous perfusion can "rescue" a liver after a period (1 hour) of warm ischemia in a way not possible with simple cold storage in University of Wisconsin solution. As with kidneys, perfusion of the liver yet may find its place in the clinical environment.[74,78]

Summary

Ex vivo extracorporeal xenogeneic liver perfusion represents a rapid and effective method of replacing liver function in patients with liver failure. Livers of many species have been used, and experimental and clinical data on perfusion parameters, patient reactions, and immunological outcomes have accumulated over the last 30 years. Bile flow, oxygen consumption, and the appearance of the liver are indices of liver viability and function. Initially, complex systems, short perfusions, and a paucity of immunological agents limited the effectiveness of the procedure. Today, improved preservation techniques, improved circuitry, and better understanding of xenogeneic immunology may make extracorporeal xenogeneic liver perfusion an important adjuvant to the treatment of liver disease and the study of xenogeneic reactions. The techniques developed and our understanding of the performance of the perfused liver may contribute to future work in xenotransplantation or to current work in organ preservation before transplantation.

References

1. Lee W: Acute liver failure. N Engl J Med 329:1862-1872, 1993.
2. Tarter R, Switala J, Arria A, et al: Quality of life before and after orthotopic hepatic transplantation. Arch Intern Med 151:1521-1529, 1991.
3. Busuttil RW, Colonna JO II, Hiatt JR, et al: The first 100 liver transplants at UCLA. Ann Surg 206:387-402, 1987.

4. Leventhal R, Berman D, Lasky S, et al: Liver transplantation: Initial experience in the Veterans Administration. Dig Dis Sci 35:673-680, 1990.

5. Opolon P, Rapin JR, Huget C, et al: Hepatic failure coma treated by polyacrylamide membrane hemodialysis. Trans Am Soc Artif Intern Organs 22:701-710, 1976.

6. Kimoto S: The artificial liver experiments and clinical applications. ASAIO Trans 5:102-110, 1959.

7. Gazzard BG, Weston JM, Murray-Lyon IM, et al: Charcoal hemoperfusion in the treatment of fulminant hepatic failure. Lancet 1:1301-1307, 1974.

8. O'Grady JG, Gimson AE, O'Brien CJ, et al: Controlled trials of charcoal hemoperfusion and prognostic factors in fulminant hepatic failure. Gastroenterology 94:1186-1192, 1988.

9. Lee C, Tink A: Exchange transfusion in hepatic coma: Report of a case. Med J Aust 1:40-42, 1958.

10. Sabin S, Merrit JA: Treatment of hepatic coma in cirrhosis by plasmapheresis and plasma infusion (plasma exchange). Ann Intern Med 68:1-7, 1968.

11. Eiseman B, Liem DS, Raffucci F: Heterologous liver perfusion in treatment of hepatic failure. Ann Surg 162:329-345, 1965.

12. Abouna GM, Cook JS, Fisher LM, et al: Treatment of acute hepatic coma by ex vivo baboon and human liver perfusions. Surgery 71:537-546, 1972.

13. Burnell JM, Dawborn JK, Epstein MD, et al: Acute hepatic coma treated by cross-circulation or exchange transfusions. N Engl J Med 276:935-943, 1967.

14. Swift JE, Ghent WR, Beck IT: Direct hepatic cross circulation in hepatic coma in man. Can Med Assoc J 97:1435-1445, 1967.

15. Nyberg SI, Shatford RA, Hu W-S, et al: Hepatocyte culture systems for artificial liver support: Implications for critical care medicine (bioartificial liver support). Crit Care Med 20:1157-1168, 1992.

16. Matsushita M, Nose Y: Artificial liver. Artif Organs 10:378-384, 1986.

17. Otto JJ, Pender JC, Geary JH, et al: The use of a donor liver in experimental animals with elevated blood ammonia. Surgery 43:301-309, 1958.

18. Sen PK, Bhalerao RA, Parulkar GP, et al: Use of isolated perfused cadaveric liver in the management of hepatic failure. Surgery 59:774-781, 1966.

19. Condon RE, Bombek CT, Steigmann F: Heterologous bovine liver perfusion therapy of acute hepatic failure. Am J Surg 119:147-154, 1970.

20. Abouna GM, Fisher LM, Kendrick AP, et al: Experience in the treatment of hepatic failure by intermittent liver hemoperfusions. Surg Obstet Gynecol 137:741-752, 1973.

21. Lie TS: Treatment of acute hepatic failure by extracorporeal hemoperfusion over human and baboon liver. In Brunner G, Schmidt FW (eds): Artificial Liver Support. Berlin, Springer-Verlag, 1980, pp 268-273.

22. Tung LC, Haring R, Weber D, et al: Experience in the treatment of hepatic coma by extracorporeal liver perfusion. In Brunner G, Schmidt FW (eds): Artificial Liver Support. Berlin, Springer-Verlag, 1980, pp 274-279.

23. Chari RS, Collins BH, Magee JC, et al: Xenogeneic ex-vivo liver perfusion: Prolonged hepatic support followed by successful liver transplantation. N Engl J Med 331:234-237, 1994.

24. Levy MF, Crippin J, Sutton S, et al: Liver allotransplantation after extracorporeal hepatic support with transgenic (hCD55/hCD59) porcine livers: Clinical results and lack of pig-to-human transmission of the porcine endogenous retrovirus. Transplantation 69:272-280, 2000.

25. Tector AJ, Berho M, Fridell JA, et al: Rejection of pig liver xenografts in patients with liver failure: Implications for xeno-transplantation. Liver Transpl 7(2):82-89, 2001.

26. Abouna GM, Serrou B, Boehmig HG, et al: Long-term hepatic support by intermittent multi-species liver perfusions. Lancet 1:391-396, 1970.

27. Norman JC, Franco FO, Brown M, et al: Techniques of obtaining and preparing the porcine liver in experimental and clinical temporary ex-vivo perfusion. J Surg Res 6:117-120, 1966.

28. Norman JC, Saravis CA, Brown ME, et al: Immunological observations in clinical heterologous (xenogeneic) liver perfusions. Surgery 60:179-190, 1966.

29. Abouna GM: Pig liver perfusion with human blood. Br J Surg 55:761-768, 1968.

30. Marino IR, De Luca G, Celli S, et al: Comparison of combined portal-arterial versus portal perfusion during liver procurement. Transplant Proc 20:578-587, 1988.

31. Isai H, Sheil AGR, Bell R, et al: A comparison of UW solution with and without hydroxyethyl starch for liver perfusion using isolated porcine liver perfusion model. Transplant Proc 22:2152-2153, 1990.

32. Norman JC, Brown M, Saravis CA, et al: Perfusion techniques in temporary human-isolated ex-vivo porcine cross circulation. J Surg Res 6:121-125, 1966.

33. Tygstrup N, Funding J, Juul-Nielsen J, et al: The function of the isolated perfused and in-vivo pig liver. Scand J Gastroenterol 9(Suppl):131-138, 1971.

34. Eiseman B, van Wyk J, Griffen WO: Methods of extracorporeal hepatic assist. Surg Obstet Gynecol 123:522-530, 1966.

35. Tait IB, van Wyk J, Eiseman B: Optimal hepatic perfusion at low flow perfusion. Surg Forum 16:294-296, 1965.

36. Cuello-Mainard L, Vasquez-Quintana E, Raffucci-Arce FL: Determination of optimal flow during ex-vivo liver perfusion. Surg Forum 16:290-293, 1965.

37. Hardison WG, Greene EA, Norma JC: The viability and effect of flow upon function of the in vivo perfused pig liver. J Lab Clin Med 69:246-255, 1967.

38. Winkler K, Juul-Nielsen J, Hansen IR, et al: The relation between function and perfusion of the isolated pig liver. Scand J Gastroenterol 9(Suppl):139-147, 1971.

39. Drapana T, Zemel R, Vang JO: Hemodynamics of the isolated perfused pig liver: Metabolism according to routes of perfusion and rate of flow. Ann Surg 164:522-528, 1966.

40. Tait IB, Eiseman B: Perfusion dynamics for extracorporeal hepatic assist. Arch Surg 93:131-141, 1966.

41. Tauber J, Bircher J, Halperin A, et al: Substitution of the liver: A physiologic approach to the technique of isolated pig liver perfusion. Rev Eur Etude Clin Biol 16:917-924, 1971.

42. Ham JM, Pirola RC, Davidson GM, et al: Pig liver perfusion for the treatment of acute hepatic coma. Surg Obstet Gynecol 127:543-549, 1968.

43. Norman JC, Brown M, Ackroyd FW, et al: Effect of increasing outflow occlusion on the rate and composition of ascites formation by the isolated perfused porcine liver. Surg Forum 16:276-277, 1965.

44. Norman JC, Covelli VH, Hardisson WG, et al: Experimental studies related to clinical xenogeneic liver perfusions. Transplantation 5:809-819, 1967.

45. Ramsoe K, Juul-Nielsen J, Hansen RI, et al: The functional pattern of the isolated perfused pig liver. Scand J Gastroenterol 9(Suppl):149-154, 1971.

46. Eiseman B, Knipe P, McColl HA, et al: Isolated liver perfusion for reducing blood ammonia. Arch Surg 83:45-51, 1961.

47. Abouna GM, Ashcroft T, Dale G, et al: The assessment of function of the isolated liver perfused with homologous blood [abstract]. Br J Surg 55:388, 1968.

48. Liem DS, Watluch TI, Eiseman B: Function of the ex-vivo pig liver perfused with human blood. Surg Forum 15:90-91, 1964.

49. Strebel HH, Stirnemann H, Tauber J, et al: Die Leitstungsfahigkeit der Schweineleber in situ und bei heterologer Perfusion. Langenbecks Arch Klin Chir 325:1118-1122, 1969.

50. Sommoggy SV, Schleicher P, Rakette S, et al: Clearance of bilirubin and bile acids from the serum of patients treated with

extracorporeal baboon liver perfusion. In Brunner G, Schmidt FW (eds): Artificial Liver Support. Berlin, Springer-Verlag, 1980, pp 286-292.

51. Kim BR, Gunderman K-J, Kimura K, et al: Surface redox potential and vitality of an extracorporeal liver during hemoperfusion. In Brunner G, Schmidt FW (eds): Artificial Liver Support. Berlin, Springer-Verlag, 1980, pp 310-317.

52. Eiseman B: Treatment of hepatic coma by extracorporeal liver perfusion. Ann R Coll Surg Engl 38:329-348, 1965.

53. Collins BH, Chari RS, Magee JC, et al: Mechanisms of injury in porcine livers perfused with blood of patients with fulminant hepatic failure. Transplantation 58:1161-1171, 1994.

54. Abouna GM, Aschroft T, Muckle TJ, et al: Heterologous extracorporeal hepatic support: Haemodynamic, biochemical and immunological observations. Br J Surg 57:213-220, 1970.

55. Fischer M, Botterman P, Sommoggy SV, et al: Functional capacity of extracorporeal baboon liver perfusion. In Brunner G, Schmidt FW (eds): Artificial Liver Support. Berlin, Springer-Verlag, 1980, pp 280-285.

56. Collins BH, Chari RS, Magee JC, et al: Immunopathology of porcine livers perfused with blood of humans with fulminant hepatic failure. Transplant Proc 27:280-281, 1995.

57. Platt JL, Fischel RJ, Matas AJ, et al: Immunopathology of hyperacute xenograft rejection in a swine-to-primate model. Transplantation 52:214-220, 1991.

58. Platt JL, Vercellotti GM, Dalmasso AP, et al: Transplantation of discordant xenografts: A review of progress. Immunol Today 11:449-456, 1991.

59. Platt JL, Bach FH: The barrier to xenotransplantation. Transplantation 52:937-947, 1991.

60. Lim SML, Heng KK, Poh LH, et al: A study of the xenogeneic response in an isolated liver perfusion circuit: Preliminary observations. Transplant Proc 24:581-582, 1992.

61. Bibler DD Jr, Condon RE, Nyhus LM: Effect of heterologous liver perfusion on dogs in experimental hepatic insufficiency. Surg Forum 16:286-288, 1965.

62. Bertrand L, Romieu C, Pujol H, et al: Assistance hepatique a l'homme par perfusion du foie de porc. Presse Med 68:2459-2462, 1968.

63. Watts JM, Douglas MC, Dudley HAF, et al: Heterologous liver perfusion in acute hepatic failure. BMJ 2:341-345, 1967.

64. Ranek L, Hansen RI, Jilden M, et al: Pig liver perfusion in the treatment of acute hepatic failure. Scand J Gastroenterol 9(Suppl):161-169, 1971.

65. Hardison WG, Norman JC: Ex vivo pig liver perfusion for acute hepatic failure: Bile salt composition of pig bile during perfusion. Medicine (Baltimore) 46:97-102, 1967.

66. Gunderman K-J, Olek K, Uhlhaas S, Lie TS: The influence of baboon liver hemoperfusion on serum levels of amino acids and free fatty acids in patients with acute liver failure. In Brunner G, Schmidt FW (eds): Artificial Liver Support. Berlin, Springer-Verlag, 1980, pp 293-300.

67. Salomon DR: The U.S. Public Health Service guideline for xenotransplantation: Advances and limitations. Xenotransplantation 20:88-89, 2003.

68. Peter SD, Imber CJ, Kay J, et al: Hepatic control of perfusate homeostasis during normothermic extracorporeal preservation. Transplant Proc 35:1587-1590, 2003.

69. Imber CJ, St Peter SD, De Cenarruzabeitia IL, et al: Optimisation of bile production during normothermic preservation of porcine livers. Am J Transplant 2:593-599, 2002.

70. Rees MA, Butler AJ, Davies HF, et al: Porcine livers perfused with human blood mount a graft-versus-"host" reaction. Transplantation 73:1460-1467, 2002.

71. Luo Y, Levy G, Ding J, et al: HDAF transgenic pig livers are protected from hyperacute rejection during ex vivo perfusion with human blood. Xenotransplantation 9:36-44, 2002.

72. Butler AJ, Rees MA, Wight DG, et al: Successful extracorporeal porcine liver perfusion in 72 hr. Transplantation 73:1212-1218, 2002.

73. Rees MA, Butler AJ, Chavez-Cartaya G, et al: Prolonged function of extracorporeal hDAF transgenic pig livers perfused with human blood. Transplantation 73:1194-1202, 2002.

74. St Peter SD, Imber CJ, Lopez I, et al: Extended preservation of non–heart-beating donor livers with normothermic machine perfusion. Br J Surg 89:609-616, 2002.

75. Tector AJ, Fridell JA, Ruiz P, et al: Experimental discordant hepatic xenotransplantation in the recipient with liver failure: Implications for clinical bridging trials. J Am Coll Surg 191:54-64, 2000.

76. Tector AJ, Chen X, Soderland C, et al: Complement activation in discordant hepatic xenotransplantation. Xenotransplantation 5:257-261, 1998.

77. D'alessandro AM, Hoffmann RM, Knechtle SJ, et al: Liver transplantation from controlled non–heart-beating donors. Surgery 128:579-588, 2000.

78. Schon MR, Kollmar O, Wolf S, et al: Liver transplantation after organ preservation with normothermic extracorporeal perfusion. Ann Surg 233:114-123, 2001.

Development of Bioartificial Liver

WING S. CHEUNG
JOSEPH P. VACANTI

The motivation for developing a
 bioartificial liver   1425

Addressing the issue of organ shortage   1426
 Current surgical approaches   1426
 Xenotransplantation   1426
 Hepatocyte transplantation   1426

Bioartificial liver   1427
 Non–cell-based approach   1427
 Cell-based bioartificial liver   1428
 Clinical trials   1430
 Bioreactor design   1432
 Cell source   1432
 Animal models and preclinical
  evaluation   1433

Cell replacement approach   1433

Biodegradable polymer and tissue
 engineering   1433

The road ahead   1434

The Motivation for Developing a Bioartificial Liver

Acute liver failure (ALF) remains a highly morbid and increasingly costly disease. Twenty-five million Americans, or 1 in 10, are afflicted with liver disease, and about 20,300 individuals die of the disease each year.[1] The medical cost of treating liver failure is estimated at $8 billion per year. Regardless of the initiating event, hepatocyte injury and eventual necrosis leads to loss in synthetic, metabolic, regulatory, and elimination functions essential to sustain the patient's life. Complications include rapid and progressive encephalopathy, cerebral edema, cardiovascular and pulmonary failure, renal failure, infection, and life-threatening sepsis. Currently, many of these processes and complications are treated with medical therapies in the intensive care setting. However, unlike other organ failure such as renal failure, the only established permanent medical treatment is orthotopic liver transplantation (OLT).

Advances in liver transplantation have significantly improved the survival of ALF patients. However, despite the advances in surgical techniques, anesthesia, and immunosuppression therapies, transplantation is still an imperfect treatment. Long-term immunosuppression has complications and occasional failures, in some instances requiring retransplantation. Immunosuppressed patients are more prone to opportunistic infections and certain cancers, including posttransplantation lymphoproliferative disorder (PTLD) and others such as skin cancer, cervical cancer, and colon cancer.[2] Nevertheless, new discoveries and improvements in immunosuppression and methods to develop tolerance may eventually overcome these complications and side effects. However, the greatest shortfall of whole-organ transplantation is the scarcity of donor organs. Currently there are 17,000 patients on the waiting list for a liver. Although 5261 underwent liver transplantation in 2001, another 1861 died while waiting for a matching organ donor.[3] The incidence of liver disease such as hepatitis C is increasing, and thus the number of patients awaiting a liver is outgrowing the available organs.

Clinicians and scientists have devised diverse support treatments for ALF. Among these various efforts is the bioartificial liver (BAL), which would support a patient in ALF until a transplantable organ becomes available. This has proved to be an engineering feat that unfortunately lags behind the success of other artificial organ systems, such as renal dialysis, extracorporeal membrane oxygenators (ECMOs), and left ventricular assist devices (LVADs). As discussed in this chapter, the engineering of an artificial liver poses many challenges, including biomechanical, cell source, infectious, immunological, and biomaterial. Despite these challenges, great progress has been made in this area, with a handful of BALs having already undergone clinical trials.

Addressing the Issue of Organ Shortage

Current Surgical Approaches

The first surviving orthotopic liver transplant in a human was performed in 1967 by Dr. Starzl in Denver, Colorado.[4] During the following decade, more transplantations were performed in the United States and in Europe. However, these procedures met with limited success, mostly owing to the inadequacy of immunosuppression. Then, with the discovery of cyclosporine in the late 1970s, the field of transplantation advanced rapidly. Surgical techniques became more standardized and new potent immunosuppressive agents were introduced. With these advancements, surgical liver transplantation has become the mainstream treatment for end-stage liver disease.

Despite ongoing scientific advances in transplantation, an almost insurmountable challenge has been to expand the list of available donor livers. Several surgical approaches have been developed to address the issue of organ scarcity or to use some kind of bridge until an organ becomes available. These developments include new surgical approaches such as living donor liver transplantation (LDLT) in which a living donor gives part of his or her liver to a smaller recipient,

usually a pediatric patient. Another development is partial-liver transplantation, which allows a single adult deceased donor liver to be transplanted into one adult patient and one pediatric patient. A similar approach is auxiliary partial orthotopic liver transplantation (APOLT) in which a portion of a patient's diseased liver is removed and replaced with a portion of normal liver. This surgical technique has been proposed as a bridge until a full-sized liver becomes available for permanent transplantation.[5] Still, these surgical developments have made only a small impact on increasing the number of available transplantable organs, prompting scientists to look beyond the human pool as a source of livers.

Xenotransplantation

Xenogeneic sources for organs are enticing, since there would appear to be a limitless supply of organs, or at least not a shortage given the current demand. However, xenotransplantation has its own obstacles, mainly that of immunogenicity and the current incompatibility of porcine proteins with human recipients. Another concern is that of zoonosis, the transmission of animal diseases to humans. This has been a growing concern with the recent attention on human immunodeficiency virus (HIV, which supposedly started in monkeys), mad cow disease, Creutzfeldt-Jakob disease, and others. Still, much research is being conducted in this area in the hope that animals can become an endless source of healthy livers for human transplantation. New cases of animal-to-human liver transplantations have, in fact, been performed with moderate success.[6,7] Despite these efforts, there are no large human clinical trials planned owing to significant government policy and ethical issues.[8,9]

Hepatocyte Transplantation

In the 1970s, preclinical studies in animals involved hepatocyte transplantation into liver, spleen, and other ectopic sites. These early studies showed that these transplanted hepatocytes organized into normal liver architecture and maintained hepatocyte function such as albumin synthesis, glycogen storage, bilirubin conjugation, and cytochrome P450 function. One study showed an immortalized hepatocyte cell line that was transplanted into rat livers integrated into hepatic cords or spleen, which was able to protect the recipient from hyperammonemia-induced hepatic encephalopathy.[10] These initial results were promising and were seen also as a potential means of gene therapy. If directly transplanted hepatocytes can survive in vivo, these cells could undergo in vitro gene transduction prior to transplantation. Individuals with genetic disorders such as hereditary tyrosinemia, Wilson's disease, or α_1-antitrypsin deficiency who may not be in liver failure can benefit from direct hepatocyte cell transplantation.[11-13] One clinical trial in humans demonstrated that when hepatocytes were injected into the spleen, they could still be detected up to 11 months after implantation. In another study at the College of Virginia, 11 patients received injections of hepatocytes into the spleen. This study demonstrated overall survival of 3.8 ± 3.3 days in patients who underwent OLT, and 4.6 ± 2.5 days in patients who died awaiting OLT. Although these results did not differ significantly from those of control patients who did not receive hepatocyte transplants and had survival rates of 2.8 ± 2.5 days, other parameters such as blood ammonia levels, cerebral blood flow, and encephalopathy improved.[14] The concept that cell suspensions or partial organs could be means of liver replacement was significant for the development of BALs.

Bioartificial Liver

Along with the instrumental progress in making existing organs and hepatocytes more available and transplantable, similar developments have been made to create a BAL. Significant scientific progress has been made in this area and significant efforts are still being made to develop a fully functional and reliable BAL. Already there have been a small number of case reports and clinical trials. However, given the intricacies and complexity of the liver with its myriad functions, a commercially available BAL is still a work in progress.

The goal of a BAL is a system that can support and replace normal liver function during the period of ALF while a patient is awaiting an organ to become available or until the native liver recovers from an acute reversible injury. Although these devices may not increase the number of transplantable livers, they could increase the survival of patients in ALF as they await a liver. BALs could also keep patients alive while allowing the native liver to regenerate from a reversible injury, perhaps obviating the need for transplantation. Along the same reasoning, these devices could lay the foundation for developing a long-term hepatic dialysis device similar to that of renal dialysis devices. This may thereby decrease the number of patients who require liver transplantation as a definitive therapy.

To temporarily or permanently replace and support the damaged native liver, a BAL must fulfill a number of crucial functions: (1) synthesize proteins such as clotting factors; (2) produce and secrete bile, regulate and store carbohydrate, fat, and maintain protein metabolism; and (3) detoxify the blood of various waste and xenobiotics. Approaches to fulfill these functional criteria can be categorized into either non–cell-based procedures such as dialysis, charcoal hemoperfusion, and immobilized enzymes or procedures that are cell based by incorporating living hepatocytes.

Non–Cell-Based Approach

Initial non–cell-based approaches have focused on the function of blood or plasma detoxification. Motivations behind these approaches stem from the many biochemical indicators for ALF. The theory is that if the biochemical abnormalities can be corrected by an extracorporeal dialysis system, a majority of the liver's function can be replaced.

Borrowing from the success of renal hemodialysis, early studies sought to eliminate toxins accumulated in fulminant hepatic failure by simple hemodialysis. Macromolecules are eliminated from the blood through a porous membranes that is permeable to molecules of a specified size. However, conventional low-flux dialysis membranes used in renal dialysis did not prove to be successful in ameliorating liver failure. Trials with higher-flux membranes and the use of poly(acrylonitrile) proved more promising. Nonetheless, clinical trials with hemodialysis alone did not improve overall survival when compared with medical treatment alone.[15-17]

Continuous hemofiltration is another noncellular approach. Unlike hemodialysis, it is a lower pressure system that uses venovenous systems. One clinical trial using this system had moderate success in acting as a bridge for a small number of patients until transplantation or until spontaneous recovery.[18] Another clinical trial with 68 patients combined hemofiltration with plasma exchange and resulted in a 56% survival rate without liver transplantation.[19] However, other clinical trials using similar methods showed benefits in improving hepatic encephalopathy but did not improve survival.[20]

Hemoperfusion involves removing toxins from blood by passing blood through an ion exchange column or charcoal particles. Clinical trials using charcoal hemoperfusion for patients with grade III encephalopathy showed a 65% survival rate. However, patients with grade IV encephalopathy did not show these benefits, with survival rates at only 20%.[21] Standard medical and intensive care therapy produces a survival rate of 15%. A combination of plasma filtration and hemoperfusion first separates plasma from blood and then passes it through an adsorbent device rather than exposing blood directly to an adsorbent column. This process reduces the destruction of platelets and reduces bleeding complications associated with hemoperfusion. Another non–cell-based adsorption method is albumin dialysis. Albumin normally binds many proteins and toxins. A small number of studies showed some potential for this therapy as a bridge to transplantation with medical therapy.

High-volume plasma or whole-blood exchange transfusions also have been investigated.[22] However, these studies showed that large volumes of blood or plasma had to be exchanged each day. Given the limitation of these resources and their associated complications, these methods could not be permanent options.

The commonality with all these non–cell-based techniques was the promising initial results, but all of them ultimately provided only limited survival benefits.[23] The liver not only functions as a filter for toxins but is also responsible for the synthesis of many important proteins such as all the clotting factors, albumin, transferrin, ferritin, α_1-antitrypsin; regulation of carbohydrates, fats, and proteins; detoxification of the ammonia product of nitrogen metabolism; and breakdown of drugs and alcohol. Nevertheless, in the late 1990s there was a U.S. Food and Drug Administration (FDA)-approved Liver Dialysis Unit (LDU) marketed by HemoTherapies.[24] Along these lines, other researchers have sought to create bioartificial livers, which include cellular components so that these important functions can be included as part of the device.[25]

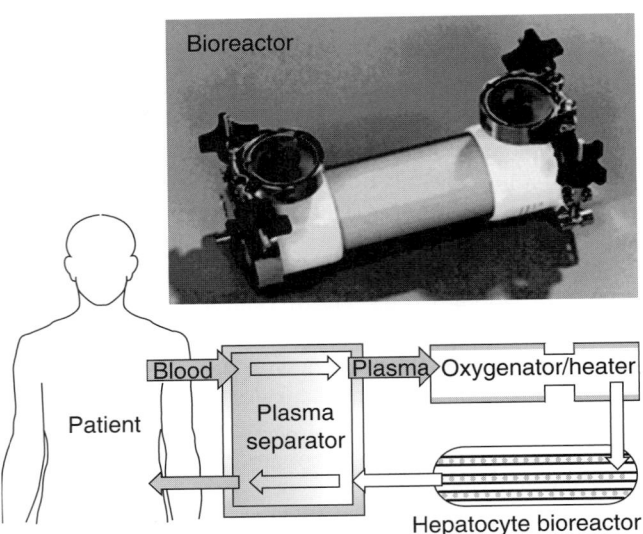

FIGURE 89–1

General scheme of a bioartificial liver assist system connected to the patient's circulation. In contrast to the shown AMC-bioreactor at the top, other types of bioreactors need an extra oxygenator in the plasma circuit. (From Strain AJ, Neuberger JM: A bioartificial liver—state of the art. Science 295:1005-1009, 2002.

Cell-Based Bioartificial Liver

The first attempts to include cellular components into BALs date back to the 1960s when in one study patients with stage IV encephalopathy had their blood perfused through porcine livers.[26,27] Other such ex vivo perfusion studies included livers from other sources such as baboons, humans, calves, and monkeys. These studies demonstrated improvements in encephalopathy but not in survival. The next approach was to use only slices or chunks of liver tissue so that there was increased surface area for tissue and blood contact without the complication of clotting small vessels. The patient's blood was percolated through a device housing these liver slices. These studies showed chemical improvements such as lower blood toxins and increased synthetic factors. Unfortunately, these liver chunks and slices suffered ischemic injury given that this method could not adequately provide oxygen and nutrients to the tissue, since it did not have direct blood perfusion through its capillary bed. Despite these early limited successes and the inability to prove definitive significant effects on improving survival, the idea of incorporating the important contributions of cellular components have paved the way to the next generation of BALs.

Given the complexity of the liver and its numerous functions, the idea that a filtration device could temporarily replace all liver functions was too simplistic. Since the 1960s, researchers have investigated the idea of adding cellular components to these devices (Fig. 89-1). The use of metabolically active hepatocytes in these systems allows for functional replacement without actually having to identify and mimic the exact biochemical process from the myriad possible functions of the liver. In fact, the first report of a BAL tested on a patient used rabbit liver cells. Since then hepatocytes have been used in suspension, encapsulated in microcapsules or hollow fibers, and grown on microcarriers or polymer networks.[28] Sources of hepatocytes have included pig, monkey, and rabbit. Primary human hepatocytes from nonimplantable livers have also been tested. However, given the limited availability of human livers, most studies were done using nonhuman cell types, most notably primary porcine hepatocytes. Recently, an immortalized human hepatocyte cell line, HepG2, a cell line initially derived from a human hepatoblastoma, has become available, and this cell source has also been used. Unfortunately, despite the incredible regenerative ability of the liver in vivo, hepatocytes from primary harvests do not propagate well outside the body. In addition, it has been widely reported that primary hepatocytes lose their differentiation and key hepatic functions once in culture. For this reason, researchers have been forced to use cell sources from other animals and cell lines such as HepG2.

To date, four BAL systems have been studied in either stage 1 or stage 2 clinical trials. They can be categorized by the cell types or by the support system. HepatAssist by Circe Biomedical (Lexington, MA) is a hollow-fiber system (Fig. 89–2). Porcine hepatocytes are seeded onto dextran beads, which are placed in the extrafiber space of a hollow-fiber cartridge. Rather than directly perfusing the blood into these hollow fibers, the blood is first centrifuged to separate the plasma from its cellular components. The plasma is then

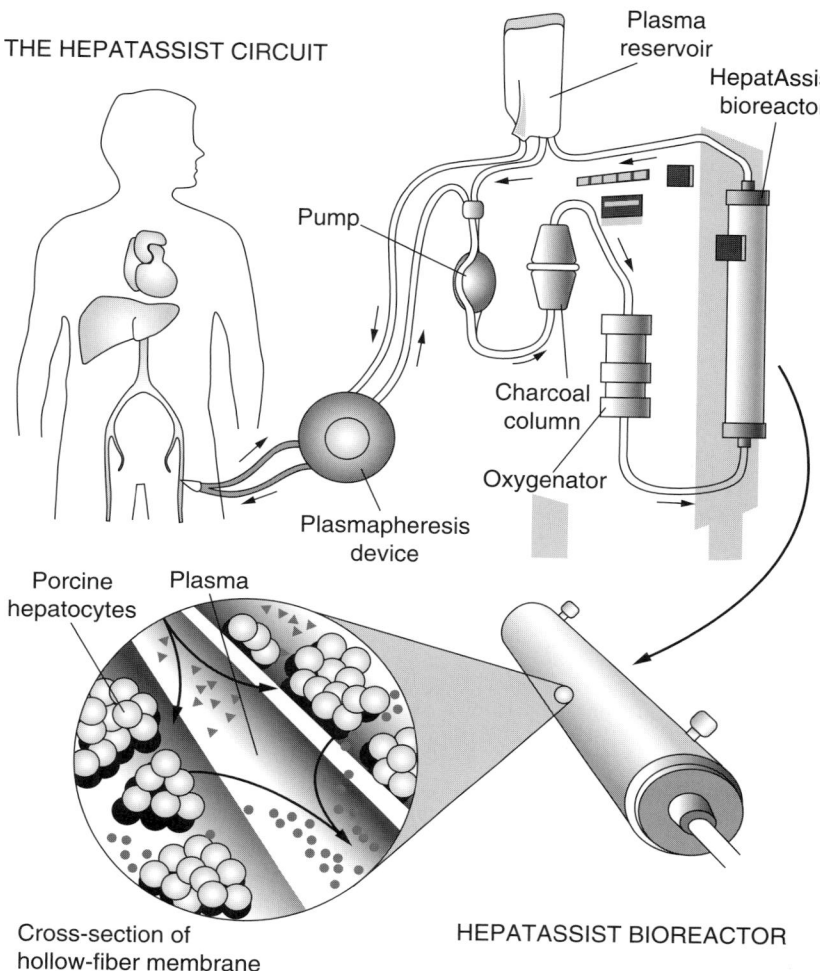

THE HEPATASSIST CIRCUIT

Plasma reservoir

HepatAssist bioreactor

Pump

Charcoal column

Oxygenator

Plasmapheresis device

Porcine hepatocytes

Plasma

Cross-section of hollow-fiber membrane through which plasma flows

HEPATASSIST BIOREACTOR

FIGURE 89–2

Schematic of the HepatAssist Device using hollow-fiber networks. (From http://bms. brown.edu/curriculum/b108/liver/Circepg.htm.)

passed through an activated cellulose charcoal column, an oxygenator, and a heater, before finally entering the hollow fiber system to interface with the hepatocytes. After this interface, the detoxified plasma with its renewed proteins is recombined with the blood. Patients are placed on the HepatAssist for 6 hours each day while they are in ALF. The duration of treatment— continuous versus periodic—is dependent on the measurable biochemical activity during the treatment period and the safety of long-term plasmapheresis or anticoagulation specific to the experiences of each device.

ELAD (Extracorporeal Liver Assist Device) is another BAL system marketed by VitaGen, Inc. (La Jolla, CA). This system uses the human HepG2/C3a immortalized cell line. Like the HepatAssist, it also uses hollow fiber–based cartridges to house hepatocytes (Fig. 89–3). Likewise, it perfuses the plasma component rather than whole blood through the hollow fibers. However, unlike the HepatAssist, patients

are placed on ELAD continuously while they are in acute liver failure.

BLSS (Bioartificial Liver Support System) made by Excorp Medical, Inc (Oakdale, MI) was developed by Sussman and colleagues at Baylor College of Medicine. BLSS uses porcine hepatocytes seeded in the extrafiber space of hollow-fiber cartridges. Unlike the other systems, however, BLSS perfuses the cartridges with whole blood. The blood is warmed and oxygenated. Heparin is administered only if necessary, since most ALF patients are commonly coagulopathic. In addition to the nutrients from the blood, the hepatocytes also receive a nutrient stream from another source. Patients are maintained on this system 12 hours each day.

Developments of BAL are not restricted to the United States. The Charite Institute for Transplantation and Organ Regeneration (Berlin, Germany) developed a modular BAL called MELS (Modular Extracorporeal Liver Support) (Fig. 89–4). MELS has three components: the hepatocyte-housing component; the detox module,

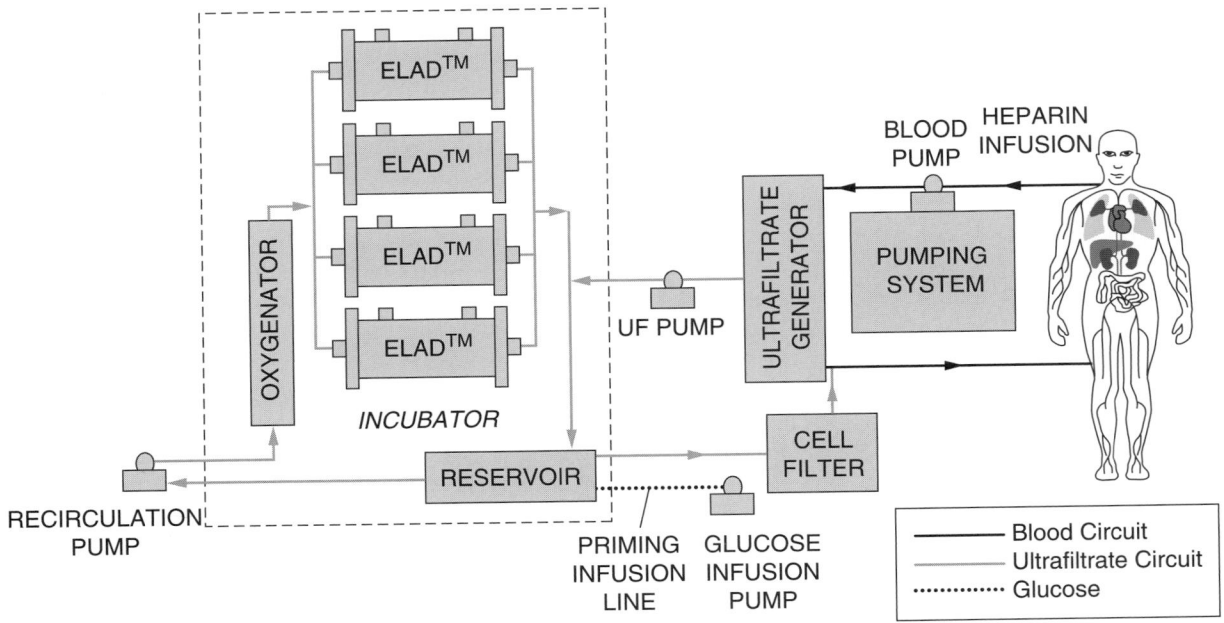

FIGURE 89–3

ELAD device from VitaGen depicting multiple hepatocyte housing units.
(From http://bms.brown.edu/Courses/BI108/BI108_2002_Groups/liver/webpage/vitagenpg.htm)

which is an albumin dialysis system that removes albumin and any albumin-bound toxins; and the optional renal dialysis system for renal failure that often accompanies severe liver failure known as hepatorenal syndrome. Hepatocytes used in MELS are human hepatocytes harvested from donors that are unsuitable for whole-organ orthotopic transplantation, often secondary to steatosis, cirrhosis, or trauma. After collagenase perfusion separation, hepatocytes are seeded onto a fiber system.[29]

Clinical Trials

There have been several clinical trials of the aforementioned BALs for treating ALF since the late 1980s. Most of these studies demonstrate the safety of BAL (Table 89–1). The primary side effect noted in most of these studies is bleeding secondary to anticoagulation or hemoperfusion-associated coagulopathy. However, clinical efficacy in prolonging survival of ALF patients has been more difficult to demonstrate.

The HepatAssist device underwent phase I and II/III clinical trials. The results of phase I clinical trials that included 20 patients with severe ALF were reported in 1996.[30] Patients in this study were categorized into two groups: group 1 (n = 12) were patients with fulminant hepatic failure but no history of chronic liver failure and were all candidates for OLT, group 2 (n = 8) were patients with chronic underlying liver disease who

developed acute exacerbation and were not candidates for OLT, owing to sepsis, multiorgan failure, or alcoholism. All group 1 patients were successfully "bridged" to OLT. These patients seemed to tolerate the treatments well with minimal adverse effects. The most common observation was an improvement in neurologic dysfunction such as reversal of decerebrate state and an increase in level of responsiveness. There were also improvements in several metabolic and biochemical parameters: ammonia, transaminase, and bilirubin levels. All patients in group 1 survived. Group 2 patients behaved differently. Only two patients survived from the acute exacerbation to later qualify for OLT. In general, there was only a transient beneficial effect from treatment with the HepatAssist device. These trials suggest that BAL is not yet a permanent solution for anhepatic states if the native liver has no ability to recover. In addition to these findings, the authors also reported no adverse reactions to the porcine hepatocytes.[31] Given these encouraging results, a phase II/III clinical trial with 171 patients in the United States and Europe ensued. Unfortunately, the study was halted prior to completion because of an inability to prove clinical efficacy. Nonetheless, smaller clinical studies in the United States and abroad using HepatAssist are still being reported.[32,33]

The ELAD system also underwent a phase I/II clinical trial.[34] Patients with fulminant liver failure of their native liver or their transplanted liver were divided into experimental and control groups in a randomized fashion.

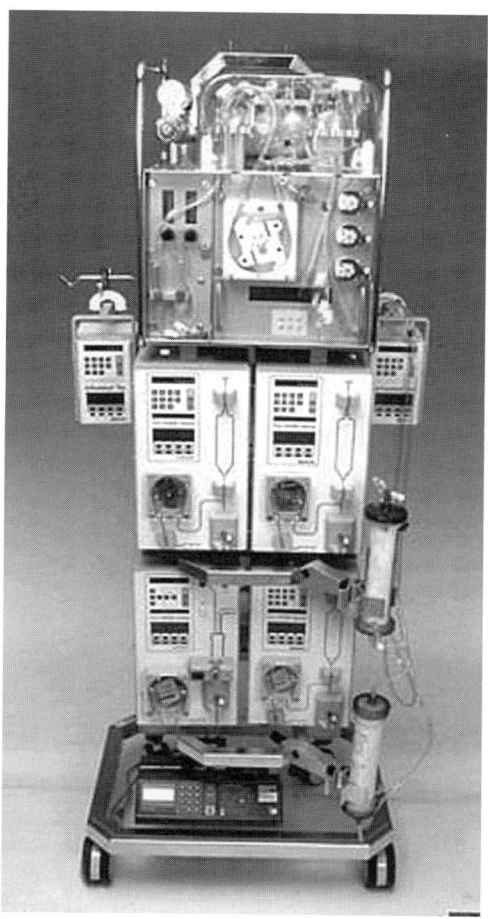

FIGURE 89–4

Picture of MELS/BELS devices. (From http://www.hybrid-organ.com.)

tachycardia, tachypnea, and pyrexia. These results demonstrated the potential for the ELAD to be an efficacious liver support device. However, the clinical trial was halted owing to lack of funding because VitaGen, Inc., the company marketing ELAD, had financial problems. Given the promising initial results, however, interest and efforts in ELAD continues as Vital Therapies, Inc. recently acquired Vitagen in hopes of furthering these studies.[35]

The BLSS system has been undergoing clinical trials as well. Researchers and Excorp have reported preclinical trials in canine models with promising results.[36] They reported the use of the BLSS on a 41-year-old woman with fulminant hepatic failure. Markers for liver failure—ammonia, lactate, and total bilirubin—decreased.[37] In an earlier report of four patients, these investigators demonstrated safety of the BLSS in patients with ALF of any cause. Side effects or complications included hypoglycemia and transient hypotension, both of which are medically treatable.[38] In addition, they also reported improvements in the patients' neurological status.

The MELS system has completed preclinical trials with hepatectomized pigs and is poised to enter clinical trials. BELS (Berlin Extracorporeal Liver Support) system, an earlier model of MELS, had already undergone a small phase I trial of eight patients with ALF. All eight patients underwent transplantation after treatment with BELS for 7 to 46 hours.[39] The MELS system is currently in human clinical trials. By November 2000, three patients with acute liver disease were treated successfully with the MELS system and underwent transplantation.[40]

By the late 1990s, many of the companies that had spearheaded the advancement of BAL had financial difficulties. Although all had reported phase I and II clinical trials, the fact that there were no readily marketable products made it difficult for them to overcome their financial situation. Consequently, many of the BAL companies filed for bankruptcy. Progression to large phase III clinical trials was delayed mainly because of this situation. However, with some corporate restructuring, interest in BAL technology is re-emerging. In fact, there are plans for a large phase III human clinical trial for the ELAD system.

Of the 15 patients in the experimental group, a bridge to transplantation or recovery was successful in 12 patients. Five of 9 patients in the control group received a transplant or recovered. Safety aspects of the ELAD system were also studied and established. Of the 24 patients, there were only two major complications. One patient developed coagulopathy secondary to disseminated intravascular coagulation (DIC), and another had a possible immune reaction marked by

Table 89–1. SUMMARY OF THE FOUR BIOARTIFICIAL LIVERS THAT UNDERWENT CLINICAL TRIALS					
Device	Company	Cell Type	Research Group	Clinical Trial Phase	Perfusion
HepatAssist	Circe Biomedical	Cryopreserved porcine hepatocytes	Demetriou[66]	II/III	Plasma perfusion
ELAD	Vital Therapies	Hep G2/C3a (human hepatoma)	Sussman[67]	I/II	Plasma perfusion
MELS	Charite Virchow Clinic	Primary porcine hepatocytes	Gerlach[29]	I	Plasma perfusion
BLSS	Excorp Medical	Primary porcine hepatocytes	Patzer[36]	I/II	Whole-blood perfusion

Most of these devices are designed so that there is a barrier between the patient's plasma and the hepatocytes through semipermeable membranes. This limits the immune reactions against these various cell types. The major concern in using nonhuman cell types is the possibility of zoonosis. However, early animal studies and human clinical trials have not shown this to occur. For instance, porcine endogenous retrovirus (PERV) has not been shown to pass from BAL to human subjects in these studies. This was shown for the BLSS system where the effluent from the system was tested for PERV. Although the proviral and mitochondrial DNA could occasionally be detected, no viral particles were detected. Moreover, the HEK-293 cells were exposed to the effluent, and no HEK cells were effectively infected. In addition, five patients who underwent BLSS treatment were studied for PERV infection by using reverse transcriptase polymerase chain reaction (RT-PCR) and were found not to carry the virus.[41] One design feature of the BLSS that could be significant in preventing viral particle transmission into the effluent plasma is the use of a 0.4-μm porous membrane. Nevertheless, larger and longer studies will need to be carried out to further confirm these initial promising results.

Bioreactor Design

The process of isolating and culturing many cells is not trivial, especially given the large oxygen and metabolic requirements of active hepatocytes. Moreover, it is necessary to immobilize these hepatocytes to preserve their functionality. The challenge is to create a substrate on which hepatocytes can cluster allow for efficient mass transfer of nutrients and sufficient oxygen delivery. Most researchers and engineers working on BAL devices have used flat-sheet or hollow-fiber membrane for these purposes (Figs. 89–5 and 89–6). In attempts to preserve hepatocyte phenotype and functionality, researchers have investigated the effect of improving the microenvironment. Most BALs use hollow-fiber systems that allow for cell attachment but may not be optimal for oxygen or nutrient delivery. The flat-plate design allows for better oxygen delivery but may not allow for three-dimensional architecture or easy scalability. Improvements in mass transport to and from hepatocytes in these systems may improve sustained hepatocyte viability and function.[42]

Cell Source

In order to replace the function of a failed native liver, researchers have estimated that a BAL will need about one third to one half of the liver mass of an adult human.

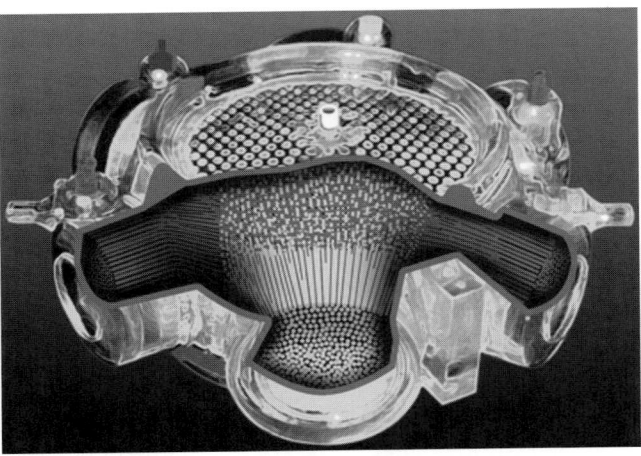

FIGURE 89–5

Schematic of numerous hollow-fiber networks to supply nutrients and oxygen to hepatocytes. (From Sauer IM, Obermeyer N, Kardassis D, et al: Development of a hybrid liver support system. Ann N Y Acad Sci 944:308-319, 2001.)

This translates to a minimum of 10^{10} hepatocytes. Currently, these large quantities of cells have been derived from animal and human livers that are of inadequate quality for whole-organ transplantation and cell lines.

The use of the HepG2 cell line is an intriguing concept in that is a human cell line, but it has its own immunological and safety concerns, since it is an immortalized cell line from a hepatoma. The likelihood of an acute rejection is diminished given that it is akin to a homotransplant. However, given that it is derived from a tumor cell line may cause concern for tumorigenicity and transformation. There is also a concern as

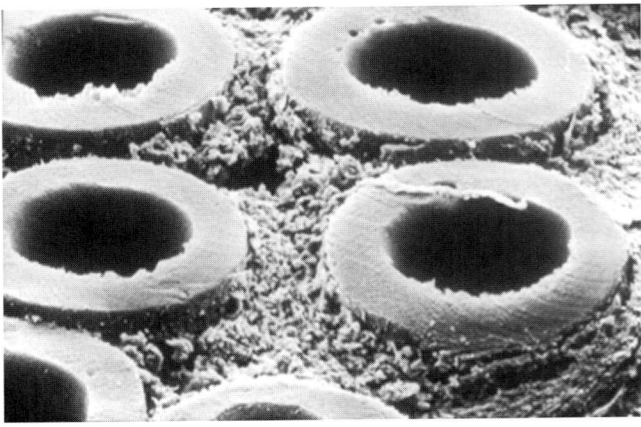

FIGURE 89–6

Scanning electron micrograph of the hollow-fiber networks supplying a dense growth of hepatocytes. (From Sauer IM, Obermeyer N, Kardassis D, et al: Development of a hybrid liver support system. Ann N Y Acad Sci 944:308-319, 2001.)

to whether these immortalized cell lines retain sufficient function for complete liver replacement. A possible solution would be to combine various cell lines to complement their functions. Nonetheless, BALs with HepG2 cells have already been used in small clinical trials that have been approved by the FDA.

Thus far, the safety of BAL has been shown in numerous studies. However, the more grave and pressing issue of efficacy is still questionable. Because of the small number of clinical trials, not a single BAL has been shown to increase survival with any statistical rigor. The only compelling beneficial effect to date has been an improvement in encephalopathy. Perhaps this single clinical improvement may be reason enough to implement BAL, given that hepatic encephalopathy is a serious concern in end-stage liver failure. Moreover, with larger clinical trials and further improvements in the development of BALs, these systems may prove to have more significant clinical effects that the current small trials were not able to show.

Animal Models and Preclinical Evaluation

Along with the efforts made in human clinical trials, various researchers are also verifying and improving on the concept of BALs in animal models with ALF. Viral, toxic, ischemic, and bacterial models can give varying results among different animal models of ALF. Hepatectomy does not provide for regeneration or liver recovery studies. Nonetheless, numerous animal models and trials have been carried out, mostly using hepatectomy or ischemia. Most studies demonstrate efficacy of BALs in reducing encephalopathy. ELADs with HepG2 cells were used on dogs with acetaminophen-induced fulminant hepatic failure; results showed not only marked mental status improvement but also improvement in clotting time and albumin synthesis.[43] However, survival times among treatment, and even control, groups varied significantly among research groups. Given the heterogenous nature of the animal model and results, interpreting these initial results and extrapolating them to human trials has proved difficult. Nonetheless, continued efforts in creating a consistent animal model for the testing of BALs may prove to be a useful preclinical tool given the even more heterogeneous nature of human clinical trials and the various BALs available.

Cell Replacement Approach

During the time that BALs were being developed, other groups studied the possibilities of hepatocyte transplantation. The liver has an incredible regenerative ability.[44] This ability was even told in the Greek story of Prometheus, who was sentenced to eternal punishment for having stolen fire from heaven and given it to mankind by having small portions of his liver eaten daily by an eagle only to have the liver regenerate.[45] Counting on this ability to grow, direct cell transplantation may allow for transplanted cells to proliferate and replace the injured hepatocytes. There has been limited success in injecting hepatocytes into the portal vein, spleen, peritoneum, and lung.[46,47] Cell transplantation could also pave the way for directed gene therapy for specific inherited diseases.[48,49] However, hepatocyte proliferation did not occur to such an extent that liver function could be completely replaced. There are many regulators and factors that affect liver growth and regeneration, much of which are still not completely understood.[50,51]

Biodegradable Polymer and Tissue Engineering

A potential alternative to using BAL to act as a bridge for a patient with liver failure until OLT is to perform transplantation immediately with a tissue-engineered liver. Tissue engineering applies the principles of engineering and life sciences toward the development of biological substitutes for replacing damaged tissue or organs. Researchers have made significant advances in the engineering of various tissues, including skin, cartilage, and teeth.[52] The focus in liver tissue engineering has been the use of biodegradable scaffolds as a template for hepatocytes to grow on.[53] Progress has been made in animal models in which polymers seeded with hepatocytes were successfully implanted into animals by using the omentum as a source for blood supply.[54] These cells have demonstrated viability and functionality.[55] Experiments have been carried out in rats, dogs, and pigs.[56-60] However, the potential to transplant a tissue-engineered liver is still years away from any clinical trials.

The most current advancement in tissue engineering is the use of MicroElectoMechanial Systems (MEMS) technology to design and fabricate a vascular network of channels. Prevascularized liver devices are designed by using a computational model that simulates the microfluidics and fractal topology of native microvasculature. The fluidic network is then etched onto a silicon wafer by using MEMS technology. The pattern is then transferred to polydimethylsiloxane polymer using replica molding. This vascular network communicates with a parenchymal compartment via a nanoporous membrane, which allows for mass transport of nutrients and oxygen. This is an improvement on the polymer-based system, since each vascular network and parenchymal compartment can be overlaid to create a three-dimensional construct with an intrinsic vascular network at each layer. This modular design also allows the construct to be of any size and not be inhibited by nutrient diffusion (Fig. 89–7). Hepatocytes have been shown to survive and maintain synthetic and drug metabolism function.[61] Specifically, hepatocytes in these devices are able to synthesize albumin and ferritin and elaborate cytochrome P450 function. Investigators are currently working on further characterizing these tissue-engineered liver devices and to begin animal studies to test whether these implantable liver devices can sustain an anhepatic small animal.[62]

Concurrently, these devices are being generated in biodegradable polymers so that they can be implanted long term. Because the backbone of these devices naturally degrades within the recipient, the hepatocytes and supporting cells such as vascular endothelial cells and biliary duct cells can then take form and continue to grow along with the recipient. This principle of an immediately viable and proliferative liver device will be especially important in the pediatric patient population, for which liver donors are severely lacking owing to not only human leukocyte antigen (HLA)–matching criteria but also size criteria. In the adult patient population, a biodegradable liver device will also be advantageous in that the host will ultimately have a fully cellular and biological liver with no foreign material.

A better understanding of and improvement of hepatocyte survival and function will lead to better nonimplantable BALs and tissue-engineered devices.[63] The scientific concepts learned from BALs naturally leads to a miniaturized implantable BAL. The current trend in tissue engineering is to use a prevascularized platform to grow large sheets of hepatocytes, which can then be stacked into three-dimensional arrays.[64] Advancement in both BAL and tissue engineering promises to resolve the problem of our current severe donor liver organ shortage.

The Road Ahead

The initial design of a BAL dates back to 1963 when Yukihiko Nose used canine liver slices to treat a patient with fulminant hepatic failure.[65] Since then, there have been significant advances in whole-organ transplantation and in the development of hybrid BALs. Despite the milestones that have already been reached, to date no single BAL has gained significance in the clinical setting. Four BAL systems have undergone clinical trials with promising initial results. However, as noted earlier, most of the companies sponsoring and manufacturing these BALs experienced some financial setbacks in the late 1990s, mainly because of lack of funding and the high cost of clinical trials. Safety and efficacy will remain the major questions as progress in these technologies is made. Further studies and larger clinical trials are still being planned, and alternative

TISSUE ENGINEERED LIVER

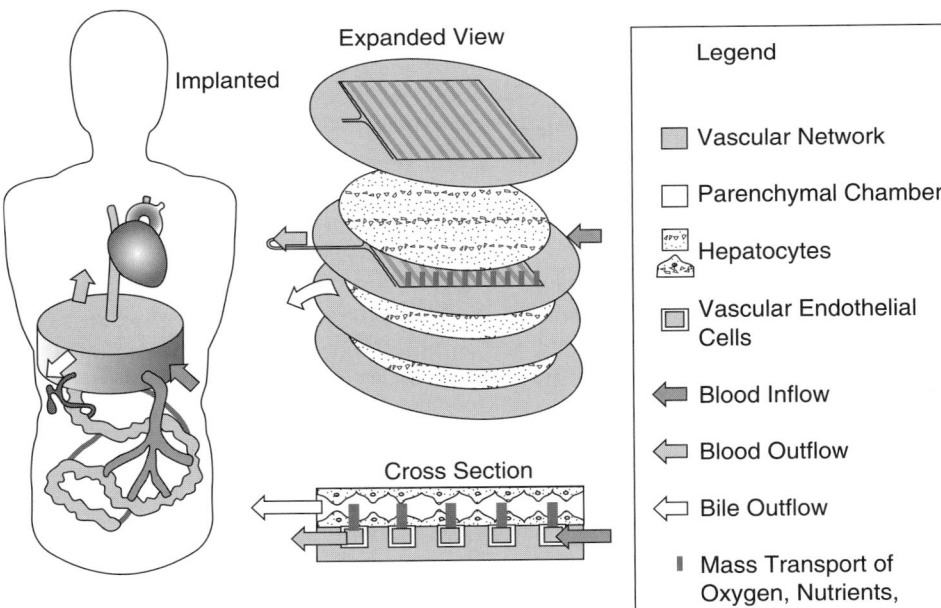

FIGURE 89–7

Conceptualization of tissue-engineered liver device with a built-in microvascular network and parenchymal cells. (From Sevy A, Kulig K, Vacanti P: Tissue engineering of the liver. In Wnek GE, Bowlin GL (eds): Encyclopedia of Biomaterials and Biomedical Engineering. New York, Marcel Dekker, 2004, pp 1570–1579.)

approaches are also emerging from the pipeline. In addition, the increasing incidence of liver disease and the still unsolved organ shortage problems are forcing clinicians and scientists to look more closely at the salient issues that preclude BALs from wider adoption in the clinical setting. These issues can be focused in the areas of bioreactor design, cell source, cell culturing and nurturing, and standardized protocols for implementation in patients. For now, OLT remains the main mode of therapy for ALF. However, cell-based therapies in the form of BAL, cell transplantation, or tissue engineering promise not only an alternative to OLT but also a possible solution to the organ shortage problem.

Pearls and Pitfalls

- Bioartificial livers (BALs) act as a bridge for patients with acute liver failure (ALF) until a transplantable liver becomes available.

- BALs use a cell-based approach to replace vital liver function that is not automatically achieved in a plasma filtration device alone.

- Cell sources from humans, animals, or human cell lines allow for a more flexible supply of cells than a transplantable organ does.

- BALs have been demonstrated to be safe in multiple clinical trials for ALF.

- BALs have demonstrated efficacy in ameliorating ALF hepatic encephalopathy.

- Four BALs have undergone stage I and II clinical trials and are still under continued investigation for possible stage III trials.

- BAL is not a long-term solution to end-stage liver disease or OLT.

- Maintaining prolonged hepatocyte viability and function within an artificial environment in a cost-effective manner is a challenge.

- Development of an effective BAL requires a good understanding of cell culture and cell biology.

- Choice of a better cell source is still being investigated.

- Safety of BALs has been shown, but true efficacy in prolonging patient survival has not yet been demonstrated.

- There is a significant cost in further clinical trials or full implementation of BALs in transplantation centers.

References

1. American Liver Foundation. www.liverfoundation.org/db/articles/1008. Accessed January 2005.
2. Maddrey WC, Schiff ER, Sorrell MF (eds): Transplantation of the Liver. Philadelphia, Lippincott, Williams & Wilkins, 2000.
3. UNOS. www.unos.org. Last accessed September 2003.
4. Starzl TE, Groth CG, Brettschneider L, et al: Orthotopic homotransplantations of the human liver. Ann Surg 168:392–415, 1968.
5. Boudjema K, Bachellier P, Wolf P, et al: Auxiliary liver transplantation and bioartificial bridging procedures in treatment of acute liver failure. World J Surg 26:267-274, 2002.
6. Starzl TE, Fun J, Tzakis A, et al: Baboon to human liver transplant. Lancet 341:65–71, 1993.
7. Michaels MG, Jenkins FJ, George KS, et al: Detection of infectious baboon cytomegalovirus after baboon-to-human liver xenotransplantation. J Virol 75(6):2825–2828, 2001.
8. Archer K, McLellan F: Controversy surrounding proposed xenotransplant trial. Lancet 359:949, 2002.
9. Butler D: Europe is urged to hold back on xenotransplant clinical trials. Nature 397:281-282, 1999.
10. Schumacher IK, Okamoto R, Kim B-H, et al: Transplantation of conditionally immortalized hepatocytes to treat hepatic encephalopathy. Hepatology 24(2):337–343, 1996.
11. Gilbert JC, Takada T, Stein J, et al: Cell transplantation of genetically altered cells on biodegradable polymer scaffolds in syngeneic rats. Transplantation 56:423-427, 1993.
12. Fontaine M, Hensen LK, Thompson S, et al: Transplantation of genetically altered hepatocytes using cell-polymer constructs. Transplant Proc 25:1002-1004, 1993.
13. Raper SE, Wilson JM: Cell transplantation in liver-directed gene therapy. Cell Transplant 12:381-400, 1993.
14. Strom S, Chowdhury J, Fox I: Hepatocyte transplantation for the treatment of human disease. Semin Liver Dis 19:39-48, 1999.
15. McLaughlin B, Tosone C, Custer L, Mullon C: Overview of extracorporeal liver support system and clinical results. Ann N Y Acad Sci 875:310-325, 1999.
16. Opolon P: Large pore hemodialysis in fulminant hepatic failure. In Brunner G, Schmidt FW (eds): Artificial Liver Support. New York, Springer-Verlag, 1981, pp 126-131.
17. Opolon P, Rapin J, Huguet C, et al: Hepatic failure coma (HFC) treated by polyacrylonitrile membrane (PAN) hemodialysis (HD). Trans Am Soc Artif Intern Organs 22:701-710, 1976.
18. Rakela J, Kurtz S, McCarthy J, et al: Postdilution hemofiltration in the management of acute hepatic failure. Blood Purif 11:163-169, 1988.
19. Yoshiba M, Inoue K, Sekyama K, Koh I: Favorable effect of new artificial liver support on survival of patients with fulminant hepatic failure. ASAIO J 42:233-235, 1996.
20. Inaba S, Kishikawa T, Zaitsu A, et al: Continuous haemoperfusion for fulminant hepatic failure [letter]. Lancet 338:1342-1343, 1991.
21. Gimson A, Braude S, Mellon P, et al: Earlier charcoal haemoperfusion in fulminant hepatic failure. Lancet 2:681-683, 1982.
22. Kondrup J, Almdal T, Vilstrup H, Tygstrup N: High volume plasma exchange in fulminant hepatic failure. Int J Artif Organs 15:669-676, 1992.
23. Stange J, Mitzner S: A carrier-mediated transport of toxins in a hybrid membrane. Safety barrier between a patient's blood and bioartificial liver. Int J Artif Organs 19:677-691, 1996.
24. Ash SR: Powdered sorbent liver dialysis and pheresis in treatment of hepatic failure. Ther Apher 5:404-416, 2001.
25. O'Grady JG, Gimson AES, O'Brien CJ, et al: Controlled trials of charcoal hemoperfusion and prognostic factors in fulminant hepatic failure. Gastroenterology 94:1186-1192, 1988.
26. Norman J, Saravis C, Brown M, McDermott W: Immunochemical observation in clinical heterologous (xenogeneic) liver perfusion. Surgery 60:179-190, 1966.

27. Lewis JD, Hussey CV, Varma RR, Darin JC: Exchange transfusion in hepatic coma: Factors affecting results, with long-term follow-up data. Am J Surg 129:125-129, 1975.

28. Langer R, Vacanti JP: Tissue engineering. Science 260:920-925, 1993.

29. Sauer IM, Gerlach J: Thoughts and progress: Modular extracorporeal liver support. Artif Organs 26:703-733, 2002.

30. Chen SC, Hewitt WR, Watanabe FD, et al: Clinical experience with a porcine hepatocyte-based liver support system. Int J Artif Organs 19:664-669, 1996.

31. Watanabe FD, Mullon CJ, Hewitt WR, et al: Clinical experience with a bioartificial liver in the treatment of severe liver failure—A phase I clinical trial. Ann Surg 225:484-491, 1997.

32. Watanabe FD, Arnout WS, Ting P, et al: Artificial Liver. Transplant Proc 31:371-373, 1999.

33. Samuel D, Philippe I, Feray C, et al: Neurological improvements during bioartificial liver sessions in patients with acute liver failure awaiting transplantation. Transplantation 73:257-264, 2002.

34. Millis JM, Cronin DC, Johnson R, et al: Initial experience with the modified extracorporeal liver-assist device for patients with fulminant hepatic failure: System modifications and clinical impact. Transplantation 74:1735-1746, 2002.

35. Vital Therapies acquires the assets of Vitagen. Available at www.pharmalicensing.com. Last accessed October 2, 2003.

36. Patzer JF, Mazariegos GV, Lopez R: Preclinical evaluation of the Excorp Medical, Inc. Bioartificial Liver Support System. J Am Coll Surg 195:299-310, 2002.

37. Mazariegos GV, et al: First clinical use of a novel bioartificial liver support system (BLSS). Am J Transplant 2:260-266, 2002.

38. Mazariegos GV, Kramer DJ, Lopez RC, et al: Safety observations in phase I clinical evaluation of the Excorp Medical Bioartificial Liver Support System after the first four patients. ASAIO J 47(5):471–475, 2001.

39. Busse B, Smith MD, Gerlarch JC: Treatment of acute liver failure: Hybrid liver support. A critical overview. Langenbecks Arch Surg 384:588-599, 1999.

40. Sauer IM, Obermeyer N, Kardassis D: Development of a hybrid liver support system. Ann N Y Acad Sci 944:308-319, 2001.

41. Pitkin Z, Mullon C: Evidence of absence of porcine endogenous retrovirus (PERV) infection in patients treated with a bioartificial liver support system. Artif Organs 23:829-833.

42. Allen JW, Bhatia SN: Improving the next generation of bioartificial liver devices. Semin Cell Dev Biol 13:447-454, 2002.

43. Kelly JH, Sussman NL: The hepatix extracorporeal liver assist device in the treatment of fulminant hepatic failure. ASAIO J 40:83-85, 1994.

44. Zieve L, Anderson WR, Lindblad S: Course of hepatic regeneration after 80% to 80% resection of normal rat liver. J Lab Clin Med 105:331-336, 1985.

45. Schwab G: Gods and Heroes: Myths and Epics of Ancient Greece. New York, Pantheon Books, 1946.

46. Woods RJ, Parbhoo S: An explanation for the reduction in bilirubin levels in congenitally jaundiced Gunn rats after transplantation of isolated hepatocytes. Eur Surg Res 13:278, 1981.

47. Sandbicher P, Then P, Vogel W, et al: Hepatocellular transplantation into the lung for temporary support of acute liver failure in the rat. Gastroenterology 102:605-609, 1992.

48. Strom SC, Chowdhury JR, Fox IJ: Hepatocyte transplantation for the treatment of human disease. Semin Liver Dis19:39-48, 1999.

49. Raper SE, Wilson JM: Cell transplantation in liver-directed gene therapy. Cell Transplant 2:381-400, 1993.

50. Fausto N, Mead JE: Regulation of liver growth: Protooncogenes and transforming growth factors. Lab Invest 60:4-13, 1989.

51. Kaufmann PM, Sano K, Uyuma S, et al: Heterotopic hepatocyte transplantation: Assessing the impact of hepatotrophic stimulation. Transplant Proc 26:2240-2241, 1994.

52. Langer R, Vacanti J: Tissue engineering. Science 260:920-926, 1993.

53. Davis MW, Vacanti JP: Toward development of an implantable tissue engineered liver. Biomaterials 17:365-370, 1996.

54. Kim SS, Utsunomiya H, Koski JA, et al: Survival and function of hepatocytes on a novel three dimensional synthetic biodegradable polymer scaffold with an intrinsic network of channels. Ann Surg 228:8-13, 1998.

55. Johnson LB, Aiken J, Mooney D, et al: The mesentery as a laminated vascular bed hepatocyte transplantation. Cell Transplant 3:273-281, 1994.

56. Yang MB, Vacanti JP, Inger DE: Hollow fibers for hepatocyte encapsulation and transplantation: Studies of survival and function in rats. Cell Transplant 3:373-385, 1994.

57. Takeda T, Murphy S, Uyama S, et al: Hepatocyte transplantation in swine using prevascularized polyvinyl alcohol sponges. Tissue Eng 1:253-262, 1995.

58. Mooney D, Vacanti JP: Tissue engineering using cells and synthetic polymers. Transplant Rev 7:153-162, 1993.

59. Cusick RA, Sano K, Lee H, et al: Heterotopic fetal rat hepatocyte transplantation on biodegradable polymers. Surg Forum 156:658-661, 1995.

60. Kaihara S, Vacanti JP: Tissue engineering: Toward new solutions for transplantation and reconstructive surgery. Arch Surg 134:1184-1188, 1999.

61. Cheung WS, Borenstein J, Kaazempur-Mofrad M, et al: Hepatocyte and endothelial cell survival in a tissue engineered human liver device with its own vascular network. J Am Coll Surg (Suppl 3):S1, 2003.

62. Cheung WS, Borenstein J, Kaazempur-Mofrad M, et al: Development of an implantable tissue-engineered liver device with a vascular network of channels co-cultured with human hepatocytes and human microvascular endothelial cells. Am J Transplant 3(Suppl 5):160, 2003.

63. Bhatia SN, Balis UJ, Yarmush ML, Toner M: Probing heterotypic cell interactions: Hepatocyte function in microfabricated co-cultures. J Biomater Sci Polym Ed 9:1137-1160, 1998.

64. Kaihara S, Borenstein J, Koka R, et al: Silicon micromachining to tissue engineer branched vascular channels for liver fabrication. Tissue Eng 6:105-117, 2000.

65. Nose Y, Schamaun M, Kantrowitz A: An experimental artificial liver utilizing extracorporeal metabolism with sliced or granulated canine liver. Trans Am Soc Artif Intern Organs 9:358–362, 1963.

66. Demitriou AA, Brown RS, Busuttil R: Prospective, randomized, multicenter controlled trial of bioartificial liver in treating acute liver failure. Ann Surg 239(5):660–667, 2004.

67. Sussman NL, Gislason GT, Conlin CA, et al: The Hepatix expracorporeal liver assist device: Initial clinical experience. Artif Organs 18(5):390–396, 1994.

Index

Note: Page numbers followed by f indicate figures; those followed by t indicate tables.

A

Aagenaes syndrome, 314
  bile duct paucity in, 306t
Abdominal aorta cannulation, in donor
    operation, 549-550, 550f, 554
Abdominal aortic aneurysm,
    unanticipated, technical
    implications of, 554
Abdominal pain, 1041
  chronic, 1048t
  in Budd-Chiari syndrome, 251
  incision, 1041
  postoperative, 604, 836, 1041
    in living donors, 715
    pediatric, 884t, 885
Abdominal wall, anterior, 25
Abdominal wall transplantation,
    798-800, 799f, 799t
Abdominothoracic fistula, 937
ABO blood group antigens,
    1200-1203
  distribution of, 1200, 1200t
  graft compatibility with, 1078, 1173,
      1199. See also Cross-matching.
  hemolytic disease and, 1202-1203
  in living donor transplants, 643,
      1202
  transplant outcome and, 1173-1174,
      1200, 1201-1202, 1201f
    in children, 1336
  in organ allocation algorithms,
      1201-1202
  natural antibodies to, 1200
  structure of, 1200
Abscess
  biliary, 463f, 464, 937, 938f. See also
      Biliary complications.
    treatment of, 944
  brain, 1032, 1032f
Abstinence, alcohol, before transplan-
    tation, 99-100
Academic achievement. See Cognitive
    function.
Acamprosate, for alcoholism, 270
Accommodation, in ABO-incompatible
    transplantation, 1202
ACE inhibitors
  diarrhea from, 875
  in hepatorenal syndrome, 897
Acetaminophen
  hepatotoxicity of
    acute hepatic failure from, 45

fulminant hepatic failure from,
    161, 162, 163
  with antithymocyte globulin, 1223
  with OKT3, 1223
Acetic acid, for hepatic malignancy, 103
N-Acetylcysteine, for graft failure, 924
Acid-base imbalances, 902-903, 902t.
    See also Acidosis; Alkalosis.
  in brain-dead donors, 518, 519t
  in renal disease, 417, 596
Acidosis
  in renal disease, 417, 596
  metabolic, 902, 902t
  respiratory, 902, 902t
Acne, posttransplant, 1051t, 1252
Acquired immunodeficiency syndrome
    (AIDS). See Human immunodefi-
    ciency virus (HIV) infection.
Acremonium infection, posttransplant,
    975
Activities of daily living, patient
    education for, 1046, 1048t-1049t
Activities of Daily Living Scale, 1324,
    1325
Activity and exercise, posttransplant,
    1051t
Acute hepatic failure. See Hepatic
    failure, acute.
Acute hepatic necrosis. See Hepatic
    necrosis.
Acute respiratory distress syndrome,
    592, 847
Acute tubular necrosis, 420
  after liver-kidney transplant, 810
Acute vascular reaction,
    in xenotransplantation, 1371
Acyclovir
  for cytomegalovirus prophylaxis,
      979, 980t
  for varicella zoster virus infection,
      981, 1250
  immunosuppressant interactions
      with, 972t
  seizures and, 1023
Ad-CD40Ig, 1361
Adefovir
  for hepatitis B
    after transplantation, 123
    in recurrent infection, 1008
    with lamivudine resistance, 118, 119
  immunosuppressant interactions
      with, 972t
  resistance to, 1008, 1009

Adenocarcinoma. See also Cancer.
  mucin-secreting, 222
Adenoma, hepatic
  in glycogen storage diseases, 350-351
  transplantation for, 282
Adenosine, in preservation injury,
    562-563, 1409, 1409f
Adenosine triphosphate (ATP), in
    preservation injury, 562-563
Adenosine-citrate-dextrose, for
    salvaged blood, 600
Adenoviral vectors, 1359
Adenovirus infection, 982
  after small bowel/liver
      transplantation, 796
  donor-transmitted, 1094-1095, 1094f
  in allograft, 1094-1095, 1094f
  in children, 1250, 1348
Adhesiolysis, in living related liver
    transplant, 631-632, 632f, 642
Adhesion molecules, hepatic
    expression of, 1069t
Adhesions, after Kasai portoenterostomy,
    631-632, 632f, 642
Adolescents. See also Children.
  graft rejection in, 1252
  immunosuppression for, 1251-1253
    noncompliance with, 1252, 1270,
        1349-1350
  jaundice in, 304t
  liver disease in, 304t-305t
  psychosocial issues in, 862, 1251-1252
  quality of life in, 1251-1253,
      1349-1350. See also Quality of
      life.
  sexual development in, 1328
Adrenal insufficiency, in fulminant
    hepatic failure, prognostic value
    of, 169
Adult living donor transplantation. See
    Living donor liver transplantation.
Adult respiratory distress syndrome,
    592, 847
African Americans. See Race/ethnicity.
Age
  donor, 521-522
    graft failure and, 918
    hepatitis C progression and,
        150-151
    hepatitis C recurrence and, 1002
    in living related donor transplant,
        632
    trends in, 1307t, 1309

Age (*Continued*)
recipient
as transplant contraindication, 107
in patient selection, 107, 387-388
pediatric transplant outcome and, 1337, 1338f
transplant outcome and, 402
trends in, 1303t, 1313
Akinetic mutism, 1024-1025
Ala Ala (HuOKT3γ), 1390
Alagille syndrome, 308-310
bile duct paucity in, 306, 306t, 308
clinical features of, 308, 308t, 309t
congenital heart disease with, 291
inheritance of, 309
living related donor transplant and, 634
molecular biology of, 308-309
preoperative risk factors in, 1337t
prognosis of, 309-310
transplantation for, 289, 294, 310
outcome in, 1340
treatment of, 310
Alanine glyoxylate aminotransferase deficiency, 276
Alanine transaminase
allograft function and, 838
in biliary atresia, 326
in preservation injury, 1072
postoperative, 866
Albumin
serum
postoperative, 866
trends in, 1306t, 1312
with paracentesis, for ascites, 479
Alcohol
abstinence from, before transplantation, 99-100, 271
in autoimmune hepatitis, 198t
in cirrhosis progression, 132
in patient selection, 99
Alcoholic liver disease, 265-272, 895t, 1110
alcoholism in, 265, 267-268. *See also* Alcoholism.
cirrhosis in, 50
posttransplant mental status and, 1030
preservation injury and, 562
recurrent, 1101t, 1110, 1143-1145, 1144f, 1443f
retransplantation for, 770, 770f
risk factors for, 99, 267, 267t
transplantation for, 98-100, 99f, 266-270
abstinence before, 99-100, 271
alcoholic relapse after, 268-269, 401, 1067t, 1110
ethical aspects of, 266, 388
historical perspective on, 266
patient support in, 271-272
quality of life in, 268
referral biases in, 268
results of, 266
timing of, 266
trends in, 1303t, 1310
Alcoholism, 265, 267-268, 400-401
acetaminophen in, fulminant hepatic failure from, 163
as transplant contraindication, 107, 266, 388, 400-401
cirrhosis from, 50

diagnosis of, 401
hepatic encephalopathy in, 1020
hepatitis C in, 151, 265
in alcoholic liver disease, 265, 267-268
neuropsychiatric outcomes and, 1020
patient selection and, 266, 388, 400-401
posttransplant mental status and, 1030
posttransplant relapse in, 268-269, 401, 1067t, 1110
psychiatric evaluation in, 401
transplant outcome and, 400-401
treatment of, 270, 401
in transplant patients, 269-271
pharmacological, 270
preventive, 270
psychosocial, 270
Alemtuzumab, 1277, 1389-1390
in small bowel/liver transplantation, 794
Alkaline phosphatase
in autoimmune hepatitis, 198t
in biliary atresia, 326
postoperative, 866
Alkalosis, 902-903, 902t
in renal disease, 417, 596
metabolic, 902-903, 902t
postoperative, pediatric, 856
respiratory, 902, 902t
Alloengraftment
antigen migration/localization in, 1192, 1193
clonal exhaustion-deletion responses in, 1189-1192, 1190f, 1191f
donor-recipient responses in, 1189-1192, 1190f, 1191f
Allograft(s). *See also* Donor/donation; Organ(s).
ABO-incompatible, antibody-mediated rejection in, 1079, 1173-1174
acceptance of, 1183-1196, 1192
accommodation in, 1202
adaptive immune response of, 10, 1192
adenoviral infection in, 1094-1095, 1094f
anatomic types of, 714-715, 714f
back-table preparation of, 554-556, 555f, 556f
bacterial infection of, 1089-1090
biopsy of
for biliary complications, 934
for rejection, 1176-1177, 1265
small bowel, 794
chimeric, 1186, 1186f. *See also* Chimerism.
Couinaud segment II/III, 28-29, 28f-32f, 31, 40
cytomegalovirus hepatitis in, 1090-1091, 1091f, 1092
dysfunction of. *See also* Allograft(s), primary nonfunction of.
diagnosis of, 869-870
Epstein-Barr virus hepatitis in, 1092-1094, 1093f
extended-criteria, retransplantation and, 769
failure of. *See* Allograft failure.
function of
assessment of, 838-840
immunosuppression and, 871

impaired. *See* Allograft failure; Allograft(s), primary nonfunction of; Allograft rejection.
in children, 885
infections and, 871-872
initial poor, 916-926. *See also* Allograft failure.
monitoring of, 866-873
biopsy in, 870-871, 870f
laboratory studies in, 866-869, 867t
wall chart in, 868f-869f, 869
nutrition and, 872-873
positive signs of, 603
fungal infection of, 1067t, 1089-1090
genetically modified, 1359-1361
good-functioning, signs of, 603
hemiliver, 40
surgical anatomy for, 31-35, 33f-39f, 38, 40
hepatic steatosis in, 681, 918-919
hepatic vein complications in, 1075-1076, 1076f
hepatitis in. *See also under* Hepatitis.
hepatitis A in, 1095
hepatitis B in, 1090, 1095-1096. *See also* Hepatitis B.
hepatitis C coinfection with, 1100
treatment of, 122-123, 123t
hepatitis C in, 143, 1090, 1096-1100, 1098f, 1099f
antiviral therapy for, 153-155, 154t
treatment of, 1137-1138
hepatitis D in, 1095, 1096
hepatitis G in, 1100
herpes simplex hepatitis in, 1091-1092, 1092f
infection of, 871-872, 965-966, 1067t, 1068
large-for-size
compartment syndrome and, 782
in living donor living transplant, 604, 704-705, 705f
volumetric lobar analysis for, 704-705, 705f
in living related liver transplant, 635, 641, 641f
living donor. *See* Living donor liver transplantation, allograft in.
living related donor, 298, 635-636, 635f, 641, 641f
multivisceral, 7-8, 9f. *See also* Multivisceral transplantation.
partial. *See* Auxiliary liver transplantation, partial orthotopic.
peripheral sensitization in, 1066
preservation of. *See* Organ preservation.
primary nonfunction of, 603, 779, 916-926. *See also* Allograft failure.
definition of, 916
diagnosis of, 779, 839, 917
etiology of, 917-922
in children, 859, 1348
incidence of, 916
postoperative management of, 838-839
predictors of, 922-923
presentation of, 779
prevention of, 923-924
retransplantation for, 768-769, 769f, 772
treatment of, 779, 924-925

Allograft(s) *(Continued)*
  recurrent disease in, 1058, 1059t, 1067t,
    1100, 1101t-1104t, 1104-1111
  reduced-size, 16, 23. *See also* Split-liver
    transplantation.
    anatomy of, 27, 27f
      hilar dissection for, 27-28, 27f, 28f
      pitfalls in, 40
  rejection of. *See* Allograft rejection.
  renal failure impact on, 906-907
  reuse of, 524
  rewarming of, hepatitis C recurrence
    and, 151
  septicemia affecting, 1111-1112
  size of. *See also* Allograft, reduced-size;
    Small-for-size syndrome.
    compartment syndrome and, 782
    in living donor transplant, 657-658,
      661, 663, 664-665, 676, 681-682
      volumetric lobar analysis for,
        704-705, 705f
    in pediatric transplantation, 297-298,
      635-636, 1342-1343
  skin, survival of, 9
  split, 524. *See also* Split-liver
    transplantation.
  systemic disease affecting, 1111-1112
  tolerance of. *See* Tolerance.
  varicella-zoster virus hepatitis in, 1092
  vascular complications in, 1073-1076.
    See also Thrombosis.
  viral infection of, 1090-1100
Allograft failure, 915-926
  N-acetylcysteine for, 924
  blocking of ischemia-reperfusion injury
    for, 925
  causes of, 917-923, 1071-1100
    immunological, 1066, 1067t
    in children, 1241
  cholestasis and, 1005
  continuum of, 916, 916t
  definition of, 915-916
  diagnosis of, 917
  donor-related factors in, 918
  early, predictors of, 1290
  expanded criteria and, 1061,
    1062t-1063t, 1064
  graft hepatectomy for, 924
  hemodynamic stability and, 921
  hepatitis B and, 1005
  hepatitis C and, 1005
  hepatitis C reinfection and, 1001
  in children, 1241
  liver-assist devices for, 925. *See also*
    Extracorporeal liver support.
  long-term changes and, 1111
  noncompliance and, in adolescents, 1252
  outcome analysis for, 1314-1319,
    1315t-1319t
  pathology of, 1060
  plasmapheresis for, 924-925
  predictors of, 922-923, 1290. *See also*
    Outcome prediction.
  preservation injury and, 922. *See also*
    Preservation injury.
  prevention of, 923-924
  primary nonfunction and, 603, 916. *See
    also* Allograft, primary nonfunction of.

procurement-related factors in, 922
prostaglandins for, 924
recipient-related factors in, 922
rejection and, 922, 1088, 1240. *See also*
  Allograft rejection.
reperfusion injury and, 922, 925
retransplantation after, 767-775, 924.
  See also Retransplantation.
risk factors for, 918t
small-for-size syndrome and, 916,
  919-921, 925
terminology for, 916, 916t
treatment of, 923-925
vs. autoimmune hepatitis, 206-207, 206t
Allograft rejection, 999-1000, 1043t,
    1058-1112, 1167-1178
  ABO incompatibility and, 1079,
    1173-1174, 1200
  acute, 1066, 1067t, 1068, 1080-1084,
      1264-1270
    antibody-mediated injury in, 1079
    causes of, 999t
    cellular, 1067t, 1081, 1081f, 1082f,
        1167-1168
      antithymocyte globulin for, 1223
    centrilobular-based, 1076
    clinical features of, 1080, 1176
    definition of, 1167
    diagnosis of, 1265-1266
    differential diagnosis of, 1083-1084,
        1266, 1266t
    early, 1082
    grading of, 1082-1083, 1083t, 1084t
    graft survival and, 1264
    histopathology of, 1081-1083, 1081f,
        1082f
    immune mechanisms in, 1264
    immunological effector phase of, 1068,
        1068f, 1080
    in children, 1236-1237, 1239, 1270
    in preservation injury, 1073
    inflammation in, 1080
    late-onset, 999-1000, 999t, 1270
      in children, 1239
      treatment of, 1270
    necrotizing arteritis in, 1082, 1082f
    noncompliance and, 1252, 1270
    outcomes in, 1270
    pathophysiology of, 1080, 1264
    perivenular inflammation in, 1082, 1082f
    prevention of, 1080, 1269. *See also*
      Immunosuppression.
    risk factors for, 1080, 1264
    severe, 1269
    signs and symptoms of, 1264-1265,
        1265t
    treatment of, 1266-1270
      agents in, 1266-1269
      complications of, 1269-1270, 1269t
      in desperate situations, 1269
    vascular, in xenotransplantation, 1371
    vs. biliary tract obstruction/cholangitis,
        1077
    vs. hepatitis B, 1083, 1096
    vs. primary sclerosing cholangitis, 1143
  adaptive immune response in, 1192
  antibody-mediated, 1067t, 1078-1080,
      1173-1174, 1199, 1200-1203, 1201f

ABO-incompatible grafts and,
    1173-1174, 1200-1203
  clinical features of, 1078-1079
  differential diagnosis of, 1079-1080
  histopathology of, 1079
  pathophysiology of, 1078
antidonor cytolytic activity in, 1170-1171
antigenic targets of, 1067t, 1068-1069,
    1069t
Banff classification for, 1177-1178, 1177t
bile duct injury in, 1130-1131
biopsy in, 1176-1177
causes of, 999t, 1071-1100, 1266, 1266t
CD4+ cells and, 1169, 1170, 1171-1172
chronic, 1067t, 1084-1089, 1270-1271
  bile ducts in, 1085, 1087-1088, 1087f
  clinical features of, 1086, 1086t, 1271
  cytokine excess theory of, 1085
  cytomegalovirus hepatitis and,
      1090, 1091
  definition of, 1084, 1167
  diagnosis of, 1088, 1271, 1272
  differential diagnosis of, 1088-1089
  early, 1082, 1082f, 1086-1087,
      1086t, 1088
  fibrosis in, 1085-1086, 1088
  from acute rejection, 1070
  hepatic artery in, 1087, 1088
  hepatitis C in, 1100
  histology of, 1271
  histopathology of, 1086-1088, 1087f
  immune mechanisms in, 1270-1271
  immunolymphatic theory of, 1085
  in children, 1240
  in primary sclerosing cholangitis, 190
  incidence of, 1270
  late, 1084, 1086-1088, 1086t, 1087f
  loss of supporting architecture theory
      of, 1085
  monitoring of, 1272
  pathology of, 1270-1271
  pathophysiology of, 1085-1086
  premature senescence theory of,
      1085-1086
  prevention of, 1271
  retransplantation for, 1088
  risk factors for, 1048t, 1084-1085
  staging of, 1086t, 1089
  tacrolimus for, 1271
  treatment of, 1270-1271, 1271f
  vs. autoimmune hepatitis, 1140
  vs. primary sclerosing cholangitis, 1143
  vs. recurrent hepatitis C, 1136-1137,
      1136t
  vs. recurrent primary biliary
      cirrhosis, 1141
classification of, 1078, 1135
clinical features of, 1080, 1086, 1086t, 1176
cross-matching and, 1173-1174. *See also*
    Cross-matching.
cytokines in, 1174-1175, 1359-1360
diagnosis of, 1176-1177
direct allorecognition in, 1069-1070
ductopenic. *See* Allograft rejection.
endothelial cells in, 1069
endotheliitis in, 1131-1132, 1134f
grading of, 1177-1178, 1177t
graft survival and, 922, 1240

Allograft rejection (Continued)
granzyme in, 1176, 1265
hepatitis C and, 1002, 1005, 1083, 1100,
1130-1137, 1133t, 1134f, 1136t,
1175-1176, 1176t, 1228
histology of, 1169-1171, 1169-1172
histopathological grading of, 1070
HLA antigens and, 1172-1173
hyperacute, 1173, 1271-1272, 1272t
in xenotransplantation, 1369-1371,
1370f
postoperative management of, 840
immune response in, 1065, 1068f, 1080,
1085, 1168-1173, 1214-1215, 1214f,
1264, 1393
in autoimmune hepatitis, 1229
in autoimmune liver disease, 204, 205,
206, 1108, 1229
in cancer, 1228-1229
in children, 1236-1237, 1239-1240, 1270,
1347-1348
graft survival and, 1240
treatment of, 1240
in dogs, 7, 8f
in elderly, 1229-1230
in fulminant hepatic failure, 1226-1228
in liver-kidney transplant, 811
in xenotransplantation, 1369-1371
acute vascular rejection in, 1371
cellular rejection in, 1372
hyperacute rejection in, 1369-1371, 1370f
indirect allorecognition in, 1070-1071
inexorable course of, 7
inflammatory response in, 1172
interface/lobular activity in, 1132,
1134-1135
interferon and, 1005
late acute, 999-1000, 999t, 1270
in children, 1239
treatment of, 1270
lymphocytes in, 1169-1172
mechanisms of, 1168-1175
MHC molecules in, 1067t, 1068-1069, 1069t
models of, 1168-1169
nitric oxide production in, 1174
noncompliance and, 1252, 1270
outcome of, 1240
overview of, 1167-1168
pathology of, 7, 8f
portal inflammatory infiltrates in, 1130
prevention of. See Immunosuppression.
rejection activity index for, 1083, 1084t
renal disease and, 1226
risk for, 1000-1001, 1077-1078, 1168
severe, 1269
treatment of, 1263-1273, 1271, 1271f
agents in, 1266-1269
complications of, 1269-1270, 1269t
for acute rejection, 1266-1270
for chronic rejection, 1270-1271
for late acute rejection, 1270
future trends in, 1272
in desperate situations, 1269
vs. autoimmune hepatitis, 205
vs. hepatitis C, 1099-1100
vs. recurrent hepatitis C, 1130-1132,
1133t, 1134-1135, 1134f

Alloimmunity, in posttransplant
hepatitis C, 146
Allopurinol
azathioprine and, 1218
for gout, 996
Alopecia, 1051t
Alternative and complementary therapies,
safety of, 399
Alveolar-arterial oxygen gradient,
calculation of, 412-413
Alzheimer type II astrogliosis, 1034
Amikacin, immunosuppressant interactions
with, 972t
Amino acid disorders, 344-349
tyrosinemia, 344-346, 347f, 372-373
urea cycle defects, 346-348
Amino acids, in protein metabolism, 491,
495-496
Aminoglycosides
acute tubular necrosis from, 894
immunosuppressant interactions
with, 972t
Δ-Aminolevulinic acid, in erythropoietic
protoporphyria, 243-244, 244f
Aminotransferase, serum, in autoimmune
hepatitis, 196, 200, 202
Ammonia. See also Hyperammonemia.
postoperative levels of, 866
Amphotericin B
for fungal prophylaxis, 976t, 977
for posttransplant aspergillosis,
977-978
for posttransplant candidiasis, 977
immunosuppressant interactions
with, 972t
prophylaxis with, 872
Ampicillin-sulbactam, for antibacterial
prophylaxis, 985t
Ampullary dysfunction, 940-941, 941f.
See also Biliary complications.
treatment of, 947
Amyloidosis, 399
hereditary, transplantation for, 239-240,
240f
results of, 245, 246t
Amylopectin deposition, in type IV
glycogen storage disease, 349
Analgesics, 598, 604, 855
for children, 855, 884t, 885
pharmacokinetics/pharmacodynamics
of, 598
Anastomosis. See also specific types.
complications of, 1073-1074,
1076-1077
leakage from, after pediatric
transplant, 332
Anemia
antiviral therapy and, 135
aplastic, in pediatric transplantation, 294
polyclonal antibodies and, 1223
Anencephalic organ donation, ethical
aspects of, 384-385
Anesthesia, 589-604
cardiovascular system and, 591
coagulopathy and, 595-596
fluid management and, 603
hepatic encephalopathy and, 590

hepatopulmonary syndrome and, 594
in anhepatic phase, 601-602
in children, 604
in donor management, 598
in living donor transplant, 683
in neohepatic phase, 602-603
in preanhepatic phase, 601
in venovenous bypass, 602
increased intracranial pressure and,
590-591
induction of, 601
metabolic disorders and, 596-597
monitoring during, 599, 600f
overview of, 589-600
pharmacokinetics/pharmacodynamics
in, 598-599
postoperative care and, 603-604
preoperative assessment for, 590-597
pulmonary hypertension and, 592-594
rapid infusion devices and, 599-600
renal function and, 594-595
technique for, 601
thermal homeostasis and, 600-601
venous access for, 599
ventilation in, 601
Aneurysms
false
arterial anastomotic, after small
bowel/liver transplant, 796
hepatic artery, 458, 958-959
hemobilia from, 468
hepatic artery, 458-459
extrahepatic, 459
false, 459, 468
intrahepatic, 459
splenic artery, rupture of, 341
unanticipated abdominal aortic, technical
implications of, 554
Angiography. See also Cholangiography;
Cholangiopancreatography.
computed tomography, 704
for hepatic artery thrombosis,
956, 956f
in living donor transplant, 707-710,
708f, 709f
in portal vein thrombosis, 744
digital subtraction, in posttransplant
evaluation, 459, 460f, 461f
hepatic artery
in posttransplant evaluation, 452-459,
453f-459f
in pretransplant evaluation, 447-448
for living donor transplant,
707-709
in thrombosis, 841f
in antibody-mediated rejection, 1079
in brain death determination, 517
in posttransplant evaluation
of hepatic artery, 456-457
of portal vein, 459, 460f
magnetic resonance, 704
for biliary complications, 935
in biliary atresia, 326
in cholangiocarcinoma, 189
in portal vein thrombosis, 744
in posttransplant evaluation, 465
of portal vein, 459, 459f

Angiography (Continued)
  in pretransplant evaluation, 451-452, 452f
    in living donor transplant, 704, 711
  superior mesenteric, in posttransplant evaluation, 459, 460f, 461f
Angiomas, pleural spider, 407, 408
Angioplasty
  balloon, for portal vein stenosis, 461
    after living related liver transplant, 643
  percutaneous transluminal, for hepatic artery stenosis, 457
Angiosarcoma, in children, 375-376
Angiotensin-converting enzyme (ACE) inhibitors
  diarrhea from, 875
  in hepatorenal syndrome, 897
Animal donors. See Xenotransplantation.
Anthrax, immunization for, in children, 1251
Anti-ABO blood group antibodies, 1200
  accommodation to, 1202
Antibiotics
  for bacterial cholangitis, 188
  for spontaneous bacterial peritonitis, 133
  immunosuppressant interactions with, 972t, 1243
  posttransplant
    for children, 884, 884t
    for infection, 871-872
    for specific bacterial infections, 971-972, 972t
    for suspected bacterial sepsis, 971
  prophylactic, 877, 971
Antibody(ies)
  antidonor, 1078, 1199-1200, 1203
  anti-HLA, in liver transplantation, 1203-1204
  anti–interleukin-2 receptor, 1276-1279
  antilymphocyte, 12, 871, 1213, 1222-1223, 1268-1269. See also Antibody therapy.
    for rejection, 1268-1269
      in children, 1240
    in induction, 871, 1222-1223
      in children, 1238-1239
  anti-MHC lymphocytotoxic, 1078
  antimitochondrial
    in autoimmune hepatitis, 198t
    in primary biliary cirrhosis, 178, 179, 183
    in recurrent primary biliary cirrhosis, 1106
  antinuclear, in autoimmune hepatitis, 196, 198t, 200
  anti–tumor necrosis factor, 1277
  in accommodation, 1202, 1371
  in graft rejection, 1173-1174, 1240, 1268-1269
  monoclonal. See Monoclonal antibodies.
  polyclonal, 871, 1222-1223, 1223t, 1268
    for children, 1238-1239
  preformed, in living donors, 1204
  to ABO blood group antigens, 1200
    accommodation to, 1202
  to hepatitis C, 130
Antibody depletion, in xenotransplantation, 1371

Antibody therapy, 871, 1222-1225, 1223t, 1268-1269, 1276-1280
  complications of, 1268-1269
  development of, 1268
  for children, 1341-1342
    for rejection, 1240
    in induction, 1238-1239
    therapeutic monitoring of, 1245-1246
  for hepatitis C progression, 149
  for rejection, 1268-1269
    in children, 1240
  in induction, 1222-1225
    in children, 1238-1239
  mechanism of action in, 1268
  monoclonal antibodies in, 871, 1223-1225, 1268-1269, 1390-1393. See also Monoclonal antibodies.
  novel agents in, 1276-1280
  polyclonal antibodies in, 871, 1222-1223, 1238-1239, 1268
Antibody-mediated rejection, 1067t, 1078-1080, 1173-1174, 1199, 1200-1203, 1201f
  ABO-incompatible grafts and, 1173-1174, 1200-1203
  clinical features of, 1078-1079
  differential diagnosis of, 1079-1080
  histopathology of, 1079
  pathophysiology of, 1078
Anti-CD 154/CD40, 1391-1392
Anti-CD monoclonal antibodies, 1276-1279, 1360, 1389-1390
  for small bowel/liver transplant, 794
Anticoagulation
  for hepatic artery thrombosis, 957
  for salvaged blood, 600
  in Budd-Chiari syndrome, 257, 258
  intraoperative, in donor operation, 549
    in children, 556-557
    in living related liver transplant, 637
    in two-adult split-liver transplant, 651
  prophylactic, for portal vein thrombosis, 748
Anticonvulsants, calcineurin inhibitors and, 1243
Antidepressants
  safety of, 398-399, 1024
  with interferon alfa, 400
Antiepileptics, calcineurin inhibitors and, 1243
Antifungal agents
  immunosuppressant interactions with, 972t
  prophylactic, 436, 975-977, 976t
Antigen(s)
  in rejection, 206, 1068-1069, 1069t, 1067t
    direct presentation of, 1069-1070
    indirect presentation of, 1070-1071
  microbial, in primary biliary cirrhosis, 178
Antigen-presenting cells, in graft rejection, 206, 1168, 1170
Anti-hepatitis B core immunoglobulin M, in fulminant hepatic failure, 164
Antihistamines, for pruritus, 188

Anti-HLA antibodies, in liver transplantation, 1203-1204
Antihyperlipidemics
  adverse effects of, 501t, 997
  indications for, 997
Antihypertensives, 998
Anti–interleukin-2 receptor antibodies, 1276-1279. See also Basiliximab; Daclizumab.
Anti–liver-cytosol type 1 autoantibodies, in autoimmune hepatitis, 200-201
Anti–liver-kidney microsome 1, in autoimmune hepatitis, 197, 198t, 199, 200
Antilymphocyte antibodies, 871, 1213, 1222-1223, 1223t, 1268-1269. See also Antibody therapy.
  for rejection, 1268-1269
    in children, 1240
  in induction, 871, 1222-1223
    in children, 1238-1239
Antilymphocyte globulin, 1213, 1222-1223, 1268. See also Antibody therapy.
  development of, 12
  for rejection, 1268-1269
  infection risk from, 968
Anti-MHC lymphocytotoxic antibodies, in rejection, 1078
Antimitochondrial antibody
  in autoimmune hepatitis, 198t
  in primary biliary cirrhosis, 178, 179, 183
  in recurrent primary biliary cirrhosis, 1106
Antinuclear antibodies, in autoimmune hepatitis, 196, 198t, 200
Antioxidant properties
  of biliverdin, 1409, 1411-1412
  of ferritin, 1360
  of heme-oxygenase-1, 1360
Antioxidants, 1360-1361
  adverse effects of, 501t
  for neonatal iron storage disease, 357
Antiproliferatives, 1280-1281
Antipsychotics
  adverse effects of, 1022
  for delirium, 1022
Antiresorptive agents, for osteoporosis, 483, 997
  in primary biliary cirrhosis, 183-184
Antiretroviral therapy
  fulminant hepatic failure from, 164
  transplantation indications and, 108
Antiseizure agents, calcineurin inhibitors and, 1243
Anti–soluble liver antigen/anti–liver-pancreas antigen, in autoimmune hepatitis, 196
Antithrombotic therapy, in Budd-Chiari syndrome, 257-259, 259f
Antithymocyte globulin, 1222-1223, 1223t, 1268. See also Antibody therapy.
α_1-Antitrypsin deficiency, 339-341, 1102t
  bile duct paucity in, 306t
  extrahepatic, neonatal, 305t
  pulmonary dysfunction and, 410-411
  transplantation for, 103, 293, 338t, 341
α_1-Antitrypsinogen deficiency, 895t
Anti–tumor necrosis factor antibody, 1277

Antiviral therapy, 872
  for Epstein-Barr virus, in children, 1248
  for hepatitis B, 122-123
    after transplantation, 118-119, 119t,
      120t, 121f, 123t
    before transplantation, 118
    in recurrent infection, 1008, 1009
  for hepatitis C, 134-136, 136t
    after transplantation, 153
    before transplantation, 152-153
    in recurrent infection, 153-155, 154t
  for herpes simplex virus infection,
    980-981
  immunosuppressant interactions
    with, 972t
Anxiety, 398-399, 1023-1024
Anxiolytics, safety of, 399
Aortic aneurysm, unanticipated, technical
  implications of, 554
Apes, as donors, 19, 1366. *See also*
  Xenotransplantation.
Aplastic anemia, in pediatric
  transplantation, 294
Apoptosis, of liver cells, 47-48, 49f
  in ischemia-reperfusion injury, 1360,
    1406-1407
Apoptotic bodies, vs. preservation
  injury, 1073
Aprotinin
  for fibrinolysis, 596
  thrombosis from, 834, 841
Arcuate ligament syndrome, 842,
  953-954, 954f
ARDS, 592, 847
Arginine vasopressin, in hormonal
  resuscitation, for brain-dead donors,
  518, 519t
Arginosuccinate synthetase deficiency, 348
Arrhythmias, 415
  in brain-dead donors, 517t
  postoperative, 846
Arterial blood gas values
  in intensive care, 834, 834t
  in pretransplant evaluation, 412-413
Arterial complications, 953-960
  arcuate ligament syndrome, 953-954
  hepatic artery thrombosis, 954-958. *See
    also* Hepatic artery, thrombosis of.
  steal syndrome, 954
Arterial portography, in posttransplant
  evaluation, 459
Arterialization, hepatic, 820
Arteriography. *See* Angiography.
Arteriolar endotheliitis, in rejection vs.
  recurrent hepatitis C, 1132
Arteriosclerosis. *See* Atherosclerosis.
Arteriovenous malformations, in children,
  transplantation for, 374
Arteritis, necrotizing, in acute rejection,
  1082, 1082f
Arthritis
  free rheumatoid, 1360
  in primary biliary cirrhosis, 179
Artificial liver. *See* Bioartificial liver.
Ascites, 397-398
  hepatic hydrothorax and, 406-407
  in biliary atresia, 328

  in decompensated cirrhosis, 132-133
  nutritional aspects of, 491
  postoperative, pediatric, 886-887
  pretransplant management of, 478-479
  refractory, 479
  treatment of, 418-419, 478-479
Asialoglycoprotein receptor, in autoimmune
  hepatitis, 200
Asian Americans. *See* Race/ethnicity.
Aspartate transaminase
  allograft function and, 838
  in biliary atresia, 326
  in preservation injury, 1072
  postoperative, 866
Aspergillosis, 436
  central nervous system, 1032, 1034
  posttransplant, 973-974, 973t
    prophylaxis for, 976, 977, 1045
    risk factors for, 967
    timing of, 966, 966f
    treatment of, 977-978
  pretransplant evaluation/management of,
    965, 967
Aspiration biopsy. *See also* Biopsy.
  for allograft rejection, 1176-1177, 1265
Aspirin
  for portal vein thrombosis
    prophylaxis, 748
  in Budd-Chiari syndrome, 257-258, 259f
  postoperative, pediatric, 884, 884t
Asplenia, with situs inversus, 756, 756f
Astrogliosis, Alzheimer type II, 1034
Atgam, 1222-1223, 1223t
Atherosclerosis. *See also* Cardiovascular
  disease; Coronary artery disease.
  posttransplant, 501
  pretransplant evaluation of, 414-417
  unanticipated, technical implications
    of, 554
Atovaquone, for *Pneumocystis carinii*
  prophylaxis, 985
ATP, in preservation injury, 562-563
ATP8B1, in progressive familial intrahepatic
  cholestasis, 311
Atracurium, metabolism of, 599
Atypical antipsychotics, for delirium, 1022
Autoantibodies
  in de novo autoimmune hepatitis, 207
  in recurrent autoimmune hepatitis, 1107
  in recurrent primary biliary cirrhosis, 1106
Autoimmune disease
  acute hepatic failure from, 44t
  in cell death, 47
  liver disease in, 200. *See also* Hepatitis,
    autoimmune.
  primary biliary cirrhosis as, 179, 1106
Autoimmune polyendocrinopathy,
  candidiasis, ectodermal dystrophy
  (APECED), in autoimmune
  hepatitis, 199
Autotransplantation, intestinal, 800
Auxiliary liver transplantation, 13, 170,
  778, 815-828
  allografts for, 27, 27f
  animal models of, 5-6, 5f
  disease recurrence after, 824
  for chronic liver failure, 827

  for fulminant hepatic failure, 170,
    816-826
  for metabolic disease, 816, 826
  for small-for-size syndrome, 816, 826
  graft function after, 822-824
  graft removal after, 823-824
  heterotopic, 817-818, 817f
    advantages and disadvantages of,
      817-818
    technique of, 817, 817f
    with portal vein arterialization, 818-
      821, 819f
  history of, 815-817
  immunosuppression withdrawal after,
    823-824
  indications for, 816
  liver regeneration after, 816, 821, 823
  outcomes in, 824-826, 825t
  overview of, 815-816
  partial orthotopic, 13, 778, 818, 818f
    allografts for, 27, 27f
    animal models of, 5-6, 5f
    left, 822
    right, 822
  patient selection for, 821-822, 821t
  postoperative care in, 822-823
  postoperative course in, 822-823
  problems and complications of, 820-823,
    820t
  technique for, 816-821
    selection of, 822, 827f
  vs. orthotopic transplantation, 815-816,
    821, 827f
  with intestinal transplant, 827
  xenotransplantation in, 1367-1368,
    1374
Azathioprine, 1218
  dosage of, 1218
  for autoimmune hepatitis, 201, 202, 202t,
    203
    after transplantation, 204
  immunosuppression with, 15f, 1185,
    1185f, 1218. *See also*
    Immunosuppression.
    allopurinol and, 1218
    animal models of, 10
    infections from, 968
  in hepatitis C progression, 149
  in pregnancy, 877
  mechanism of action of, 1218
  neurotoxicity of, 1033
  side effects of, 1033, 1216t, 1218

B

B cells. *See also* Lymphocyte(s).
  donor, 1066
  Epstein-Barr virus in, 1092
  in gene therapy, 1362
  in tolerance induction, 1362
Baboons, xenotransplantation with, 19,
  1366. *See also* Xenotransplantation.
Bacillus cereus, fulminant hepatic failure
  from, 165
Back-table allograft preparation, 554-556,
  555f, 556f
Back-table biopsy, 1065

Bacteremia
  donor transmission of, 435
  postoperative, 848
  posttransplant, 969, 971
    timing of, 966f
Bacterial infections. *See also specific types.*
  as transplant contraindication, 434-435
  in allograft, 1089-1090
  in children
    cholestasis in, 314, 315
    posttransplant, 861, 861t, 887, 887t
  in cholangitis, 188
  in donor, 435, 523
  posttransplant, 431t, 968-972, 1045,
    1089-1090
    from multidrug-resistant bacteria,
      969-970
    in children, 861, 861t, 887, 887t
    in immediate postoperative period, 848
    incidence of, 968-969
    pathogens in, 969-970, 969t
    prophylaxis for, 971, 984, 985t
    treatment of, 971-972, 972t
  pretransplant evaluation for, 434-435
  prophylaxis for, 431t, 971, 984, 985t,
    1045
  transplantation for, 279
Bacterial peritonitis. *See* Peritonitis.
Balloon angioplasty, for portal vein
  stenosis, 461
  after living related liver transplant, 643
Balloon dilatation, for biliary strictures,
  466-467, 467f, 944, 946
  after living related liver transplant, 643
Balloon tamponade, for variceal bleeding,
  478, 508
Band ligation, for variceal bleeding, 478, 508
Banff grading system, of acute rejection,
  1082-1083, 1083t
Basal energy expenditure,
  posttransplant, 496
Basiliximab, 1225, 1277-1279. *See also*
  Immunosuppression.
  for children
    for rejection, 1240
    in induction, 1238, 1241
    therapeutic monitoring of, 1246
  for small bowel/liver transplant, 794
  infection risk from, 968
Bathing, with T tube, 1042t
Beauveria infection, posttransplant, 975
Behavioral interventions, for alcoholism,
  270, 271
Behçet's syndrome, Budd-Chiari syndrome
  from, 281
BELS system, 778, 1431, 1431f, 1431t.
  See also Bioartificial liver.
Benzoate, for hyperammonemia, 480
Benzodiazepine receptor antagonists, for
  hepatic encephalopathy, 480-481
Benzodiazepines
  hepatic encephalopathy and, 1022
  postoperative, pediatric, 855
β-blockers, for variceal bleeding
  prophylaxis, 476-477
Bicaval anastomosis, alternatives to,
  750-7511

Bile acid
  excretion of, in progressive familial
    intrahepatic cholestasis type 2, 312
  metabolism of, 24
    inborn errors of, 313, 1102t
      bile duct paucity in, 306t
Bile acid–binding resins, 997
  adverse effects of, 501t
Bile collections, 937, 938f. *See also* Biliary
  complications.
  treatment of, 944
Bile duct(s). *See also* Biliary tract.
  anatomy of
    standard, 57-58, 677f, 681
    variations in, 616, 665, 680-681, 681f
  common, 27f, 33
    stenosis of, 842, 842f
  complications affecting. *See* Biliary
    complications.
  dilation of, 464-465, 464f, 465f
    in acute rejection, 1081
    in chronic rejection, 1085, 1087-1088,
      1087f
    in cytomegalovirus infection, 306t, 1091
    in recurrent primary biliary cirrhosis,
      1107
    in split-liver transplant, 616
  inflammation of. *See* Cholangitis.
  injury to
    in rejection vs. recurrent hepatitis C,
      1130-1131
    ischemic posttransplant, 190
  paucity of, 306, 306t, 308
  reconstruction of, 585-587, 586f, 603,
    930. *See also* Biliary reconstruction.
    in living related liver transplant, 641
    in recipient hepatectomy and grafting,
      585-587, 586f, 603
  segmental variation of, 29, 30f-31f, 31
  stenosis of, 842, 842f
    transplantation for, 282
Bile duct cells, in preservation injury,
  1071-1072
Bile ductopenia, transplantation for, 282
Bile leaks, 463-464, 936-937. *See also*
  Biliary complications.
  diagnosis of, 934-935
  early, 936-937, 936f
  in children, 332, 886, 1348
  in living donor transplant, 695
    in donors, 716, 751
    in recipients, 695
  in living related liver transplant,
    463-464, 642
  in two-adult split-liver transplant, 651
  late, 937
  pathophysiology of, 932-934
  postoperative, 844
  treatment of, 943-944
  T-tubes and, 1042, 1042t
Bile peritonitis, T-tube and, 1042
Bilhemia, 942. *See also* Biliary complications.
Biliary abscess, 463f, 464, 937, 938f.
  See also Biliary complications.
  treatment of, 944
Biliary anastomosis, 61, 585-587, 586f, 603.
  See also Biliary reconstruction.

in living related liver transplant, 641
leakage from. *See* Bile leaks.
Biliary atresia, 305, 305t, 323-333
  as primary pediatric transplant indication,
    1304t, 1310
  associated abnormalities in, 324-325,
    330, 331f
  biopsy for, 1339
  classification of, 325
  clinical forms of, 324-325
  complications of, 327-328
  diagnosis of, 325-327, 1339
  differential diagnosis of, 325-327
  etiology of, 324
  fetal, 324-325
  histologic features of, 325
  historical perspective on, 323-324
  incidence of, 324
  Kasai portoenterostomy for, 292-293,
    323-324, 325, 328-329. *See also*
    Kasai portoenterostomy.
  living related liver transplant for, 629-645
  medical management of, 327-328
  nutritional effects of, 296, 296f
  polysplenia syndrome and, 324-325, 1340
  postnatal form of, 324-325
  preoperative risk factors in, 1337t
  signs and symptoms of, 325
  situs inversus and, 756
  transplantation for, 104, 289, 291, 292,
    329-333. *See also specific procedures.*
    as primary therapy, 329
    complications of, 330-331
    indications for, 329
    outcomes in, 1337-1340, 1339f
    results of, 332-333, 332t
    technical aspects of, 329-330, 331f
  vena cava anomalies in, 750
Biliary casts, 941-942. *See also* Biliary
  complications.
  treatment of, 947
Biliary cirrhosis. *See* Cirrhosis, primary
  biliary.
Biliary complications, 462-468, 929-948,
  1076-1077
  ampullary dysfunction, 940-941, 941f, 947
  bile collection/biliary abscess, 463f, 464,
    937, 938f, 944
  bile leaks, 62, 463-464, 651, 695, 716, 751,
    936-937, 943. *See also* Bile leaks.
  bilomas, 463f, 464, 937, 938f, 944
  cholangiography for, 934-935
  clinical features of, 934, 1076-1077
  diagnosis of, 868, 934-936
  differential diagnosis of, 1077
  epidemiology of, 930-932, 931t
  fistulas, 937
  graft biopsy for, 934
  graft rejection and, 999t
  hemobilia, 468, 942, 947
  hepatobiliary scintigraphy for, 935
  histopathology of, 1077
  in children, 332, 468, 1348
  in deceased-donor transplant, 931t
  in living donor transplant
    in donors, 715, 716
    in recipients, 695, 932, 933t

Biliary complications *(Continued)*
  in living related liver transplant, 642, 931
  in split-liver transplant, 931, 931t
  ischemic-type, 939, 946, 948
  mucocele, 942, 947
  overview of, 929-930
  pathophysiology of, 932-934, 1076
  reconstructive techniques and, 930-932, 931t
  serum markers of, 934
  strictures, 939-940, 939f, 944-947, 945f, 946f
  treatment of, 942-947
  T-tube and, 930-931
  types of, 930t
  ultrasonography for, 934
  with bilioenteric anastomosis, 942
Biliary distention, posttransplant, 464-465, 464f, 465f
Biliary drainage catheter, persistent hemobilia through, 468
Biliary fistulas, 937
Biliary mucocele, 942
  treatment of, 947
Biliary papillomatosis, transplantation for, 283
Biliary reconstruction, 61, 585-587, 586f, 603, 930. *See also* Biliary anastomosis.
  in living related liver transplant, 641
  in recipient hepatectomy and grafting, 585-587, 586f, 603
Biliary sludge, 466, 466f, 941-942. *See also* Biliary complications.
  treatment of, 467-468, 947
Biliary stenosis. *See also* Biliary tract, obstruction of.
  after living related liver transplant, 643
Biliary stents, 468
  complications from, 466, 930
  for ampullary dysfunction, 947
  for leaks, 943, 943f
  for strictures, 944, 946, 946f
Biliary stones, 941-942, 941f. *See also* Biliary complications.
  treatment of, 947
Biliary strictures, 190-192, 465-468, 937-938. *See also* Biliary complications; Biliary tract, obstruction of.
  anastomotic, 939, 939f
    treatment of, 944, 945f
  balloon angioplasty for, 466-467, 467f
  biliary sludge and, 942
  biliary stones and, 942
  extrahepatic, 1043t
  hepatic artery thrombosis and, 939
  hilar, treatment of, 946
  in children, 1348
  in living donor transplant, 695
  in living related liver transplant, 643
  intrahepatic, 1043t
  nonanastomotic, 939-940, 939f
    treatment of, 944-947, 946f
  pathophysiology of, 939-940
  postoperative, 844-845, 844f
  treatment of, 944-947, 946f, 1043t
  T-tubes and, 930-931, 939, 939f

Biliary tract, 34. *See also* Bile duct(s).
  anatomy of, 57-58, 677f, 680
    variations in, 665, 680-681, 681f, 710-711, 710f, 711f
    vascular, 58
  cancer of. *See* Cholangiocarcinoma.
  complications of. *See* Biliary complications.
  disorders of, acute hepatic failure due to, 44t
  fungal infection of, transplantation for, 280
  granuloma of, 1081
  imaging studies of, 462-468
  in antibody-mediated rejection, 1078-1079
  in chronic rejection, 1087-1088, 1087f
  in partial allograft, 27
  infections of, posttransplant, 848
    timing of, 966f
  ischemia of, 1076
  obstruction of, 1067t, 1076-1077. *See also* Biliary strictures.
    cholangitis with, 1077
    differential diagnosis of, 1077
    hepatic artery thrombosis with, 1075
    posttransplant, 190-192, 191f, 192f, 464-468, 464f-467f, 651
      in children, 332, 860
    radiographic diagnosis of, 464-468, 464f-467f
    treatment of, 466-468, 467f
    vs. acute rejection, 1083-1084
    vs. allograft hepatitis C, 1099
    vs. chronic rejection, 1088-1089
    vs. preservation injury, 1073
    vs. recurrent hepatitis C, 1135
  partial external diversion procedures on, in progressive familial intrahepatic cholestasis, 311-312
  physiology of, 57-58
Biliary tumors. *See also* Cholangiocarcinoma.
  imaging of, 212
Biliary vascular communications, management of, 468
Bilioenteric anastomosis
  complications of, 942
  indications for, 942
Bilirubin
  antioxidant properties of, 1410, 1411
  serum
    in antibody-mediated rejection, 1079
    in autoimmune hepatitis, 200
    in biliary complications, 934
    in preservation injury, 1072
    in rejection, 7, 8f
    in transplantation, 11f
    trends in, 1306t, 1312
  synthesis of, 1409, 1410
Bilirubin metabolism, disorders of, 353-354
Biliverdin
  antioxidant properties of, 1409, 1411-1412
  in ischemia-reperfusion injury, 1409, 1411-1412
  therapeutic applications of, 1411-1412

Bilomas, 463f, 464, 937, 938f. *See also* Biliary complications.
  treatment of, 944
Bioartificial liver, 778-779, 1425-1435
  alternatives to, 1426-1427, 1433-1434
  animal models for, 1433
  bioreactor design for, 1432, 1432f
  BLS system, 778, 1429-1432, 1431f, 1431t
  cell replacement approach for, 1433
  cell sources for, 1432-1433
  clinical trials of, 1430-1432, 1431t
  efficacy of, 1433
  ELAD system, 778, 1429-1431, 1430f, 1431t
  future directions for, 1434-1435
  hemodialysis and, 1427
  hemoperfusion in, 1427
  HepatAssist device, 778, 925, 1428-1429, 1429f, 1430, 1431t
  implantable, 1433-1434, 1434f
  MELS/BELS system, 1430-1431, 1431f, 1431t
  non cell–based approach for, 1427-1433
  organ shortage and, 1426
  porcine hepatocytes in, 1368-1369
  preclinical evaluation of, 1433
  rationale for, 1425-1426
  safety of, 1433
  tissue engineering and, 1433-1434, 1434f
  types of, 778-779, 925, 1428-1430, 1429f-1431f, 1431t
  vs. hepatocyte transplantation, 1427, 1433
  vs. xenotransplantation, 1426
Bioartificial Liver Support System (BLS), 1429-1432, 1431f, 1431t. *See also* Bioartificial liver; Extracorporeal liver support.
Biodegradable polymers, in tissue engineering, 1433-1434, 1434f
Biopsy
  allograft, 934
    for biliary complications, 934
    for rejection, 1176-1177, 1265
    in small bowel/liver transplant, 794
  aspiration, 1176-1177, 1265
  gastrointestinal, in posttransplant lymphoproliferative disease, 797
  hepatic. *See* Liver, biopsy of.
  renal, indications for, 421, 422
Bisphosphonates, for osteoporosis, 483, 997
  in primary biliary cirrhosis, 183-184
BK virus infection, posttransplant, 982
Blacks. *See* Race/ethnicity.
Bladder cancer, recurrent, 1161t, 1162
Blastomycosis, 436
  posttransplant, 973, 975
Bleeding. *See also* Hemorrhage.
  gastrointestinal, in biliary atresia, 328
  postoperative, 604
Bleeding disorders, 595-596
Blood cells, intrahepatic production of, 24
Blood clotting. *See under* Coagulation.
Blood count, in intensive care, 834, 834t
Blood groups. *See* ABO blood group antigens; Cross-matching.
Blood salvage systems, 600

Blood studies, in routine surveillance, 1040, 1040t
Blood transfusions. *See* Transfusions.
BLS system, 778, 1429-1432, 1431f, 1431t. *See also* Bioartificial liver; Extracorporeal liver support.
Body image, in adolescents, 1252, 1349
Body mass index. *See also* Graft-recipient body weight ratio.
  in living donor transplant, 661
Body temperature
  in brain-dead donors, 518-519
  intraoperative, 600-601
Body weight. *See* Body mass index; Weight.
Bone disease. *See also* Osteopenia/osteoporosis.
  in autoimmune hepatitis, 203
  in primary biliary cirrhosis, 179, 183-184
  in primary sclerosing cholangitis, 188
  management of, 997
  metabolic, in primary biliary cirrhosis, 179
  posttransplant, 502, 996-997
  pretransplant management of, 483
Bone marrow
  cells from, in liver regeneration, 46
  in Budd-Chiari syndrome, 254, 255t
  in myeloproliferative disorders, 259
Bone marrow suppression, azathioprine-related, 1218
Bone marrow transplantation
  donor leukocyte chimerism in, 1191-1192, 1191f
  experimental model for, 1183, 1184f
  for erythropoietic protoporphyria, 245, 256t
  for mucopolysaccharidoses, 359
  for tolerance induction, 1361, 1395
  in drug-minimization immunosuppression, 1395
  in xenotransplantation, 1372
  living donor transplantation after, 669
  with total-lymphoid irradiation, 1399
Botanicals, safety of, 399
Brachial plexus neuropathy, 601
Brain abscess, 1032, 1032f
Brain damage, in children, after transplantation, 294
Brain death
  confirmatory tests for, 516-517
  determination of, 382-383, 516-517
  donation and, 63, 64, 517-520
  donor management in, 518-520
  graft failure and, 921
  medical complications of, 517-518, 517t
  physiological effects of, 517-518, 517t
  preservation injury and, 562
Brain tumors, donor-transmitted, 1150-1151
Breast cancer
  donor-transmitted, 1151
  recurrent, 1161t, 1162
  screening for, 1162, 1162t
Breast-feeding
  immunosuppression and, 1329
  postoperative, 878
Bretschneider's (HTK) solution, 568, 569
  preservation injury and, 566

Budd-Chiari syndrome, 249-261, 895t
  as living donor transplant contraindication, 665
  biopsy in, 251, 256
  bone marrow findings in, 254, 255t
  clinical presentation of, 251
  diagnosis of, 251, 253t
  etiology of, 250, 250t
  factor V Leiden mutation in, 260
  fulminant hepatic failure in, pretransplant management for, 172, 173
  histology of, 251, 251f
  imaging of, 251-253, 252f, 253f
  immunosuppression in, 257
  myeloproliferative disorders and, 250, 254, 259-260, 259f, 280
    antithrombotic therapy for, 257-259, 259f
  pathology of, 250-251
  pathophysiology of, 250-251
  polycythemia vera and, 254, 258, 260
  portosystemic shunting for, 254-256
  protein C deficiency and, 243f
  prothrombin gene mutation in, 260-261
  recurrent, postoperative management of, 843
  sarcoidosis and, 261
  segmental anatomy in, 26
  thrombosis in, 250, 257
  transplantation for, 103, 254-257, 280-281
    antithrombotic therapy after, 257-259, 259f
    contraindications to, 254-256
    indications for, 254-256
    patient characteristics in, 254, 255t
    results of, 254-255, 257
    surgical procedure in, 256-257
  venal caval webs in, 250, 280
  veno-occlusive disease in, 250-251
Burkitt's lymphoma. *See* Lymphoma; Posttransplant lymphoproliferative disorder.
Byler's disease, 310-312, 311t
  bile duct paucity in, 306t
Bypass
  coronary artery, with liver transplantation, 591
  ileal, for familial homozygous hypercholesterolemia, 276
  venovenous. *See* Venovenous bypass.
Bypass seroma, 1043t

C

C4d deposits, in antibody-mediated rejection, 1079
CA 19-9, in cholangiocarcinoma, 475
Calcineurin headache, 874, 1023
Calcineurin inhibitors. *See also* Cyclosporine; Immunosuppression; Tacrolimus.
  adverse effects of, 996, 997, 1019-1025
  avoidance of, 1397
  depression and, 1024
  drug interactions with, 906
    in children, 1243
  for autoimmune hepatitis, after transplantation, 204

  for children, 884, 1237, 1238, 1243-1245, 1244f, 1341-1342, 1342f
  for liver-kidney transplantation, 806
  headaches from, 874
  hyperglycemia and, 501-502, 996
  hypertension and, 500-501, 998
  in de novo autoimmune hepatitis, 207
  nephrotoxicity of, 905
  neurotoxicity of, 845, 846, 874, 1019-1025
  seizures from, 845-846
  therapeutic monitoring of, in children, 1245
Calcitonin, for osteoporosis, in primary biliary cirrhosis, 183-184
Calcium
  abnormalities of, 901
    postoperative, 837-838
  supplemental
    for autoimmune hepatitis, 203
    for osteopenia/osteoporosis, 483
    for primary biliary cirrhosis, 183
    for primary sclerosing cholangitis, 188
Calcium channel blockers, for posttransplant hypertension, 998
Calculi, biliary, 941-942, 941f. *See also* Biliary complications.
  treatment of, 947
Calpain, in preservation injury, 563-564, 564f, 567
Campath-1H, 1277, 1389-1390
  for small bowel/liver transplant, 794
Cancer, 1149-1163
  as donation contraindication, 521, 1150-1151
  biliary. *See* Cholangiocarcinoma.
  bladder, recurrent, 1161t, 1162
  brain, donor-transmitted, 1150-1151
  breast
    donor-transmitted, 1151
    recurrent, 1161t, 1162
    screening for, 1162, 1162t
  central nervous system, donor-transmitted, 1150-1151
  cervical
    recurrent, 1161, 1161t
    screening for, 1162, 1162t
  chemotherapy for. *See* Chemotherapy.
  colorectal. *See* Colorectal cancer.
  donor-transmitted, 1150-1151
  etiology of, 1151-1152
  graft rejection in, 1228-1229
  hepatocellular. *See* Hepatocellular carcinoma.
  immunosuppression and, 1152, 1227t, 1228-1229, 1247-1248
  in children, 290-291
    transplant outcome in, 1340-1341
  Kaposi's sarcoma, 1154-1155
  liver, 211-227. *See also* Hepatic malignancy.
  liver transplant for, 1157-1161
  lung, donor-transmitted, 1151
  lymphatic, 999. *See also* Posttransplant lymphoproliferative disorder.
    in children, 1247-1248
    recurrent, 1161-1162, 1161t

Cancer (Continued)
  metastatic, 233-236. See also Liver,
    metastases to.
  transplant for, 1160-1161
  pathogenesis of, 1151-1152
  posttransplant, 999, 1046
    graft rejection and, 999t
    prevention of, 1229
    screening for, 1162, 1162t
    transplant type and, 1153
  prevention of, patient education for, 1051t
  primary hepatic, 211-227. See also
    Cholangiocarcinoma; Epithelioid
    hemangioendotheliomas; Hepatic
    malignancy; Hepatocellular
    carcinoma.
    in children, 367-376
  prostate, recurrent, 1161-1162, 1161t
  recurrent preexisting, 1161-1162, 1161t
  renal cell, donor-transmitted, 1151
  skin, 999, 1150-1154. See also Skin cancer.
    donor-transmitted, 1151
  testicular, recurrent, 1161, 1161t
  thyroid, recurrent, 1161, 1161t
  transplant-related
    classification of, 1150
    de novo, 1151-1155
      incidence of, 1152-1153, 1153t
      nonlymphoid, 1153-1155
    donor-transmitted, 1150-1151
    incidence of, 1150f
    overview of, 1149-1150
    posttransplant lymphoproliferative
      disorder and. See Posttransplant
      lymphoproliferative disorder.
  unanticipated, in donor operation,
    553-554
  uterine, recurrent, 1161, 1161t
  viruses and, 1152
  vulvar/perineal, 1155
Cancer antigen 19-9,
  in cholangiocarcinoma, 189
Candidiasis, 436
  posttransplant, 972-973, 973t
    prophylaxis for, 976, 977
    timing of, 966, 966f
    treatment of, 977
  pretransplant evaluation/management
    of, 965
Cannulation. See Catheterization.
Cantilie's line, 25
Capsofungin
  for fungal prophylaxis, 976-977
  for posttransplant aspergillosis, 978
  immunosuppressant interactions
    with, 972t
Caput medusae, 25
Carbamoyl-phosphate synthetase
  deficiency, 347-348
Carbohydrate metabolism, 492, 492t
Carbon monoxide, in ischemia-reperfusion
  injury, 1411
Carcinoembryonic antigen, in
  cholangiocarcinoma, 189
Carcinoids, metastatic, transplantation
  for, 224
Carcinoma. See Cancer.

Cardiac arrest, donor, biopsy in, 1064
Cardiac arrhythmias, 415
  in brain-dead donors, 517t
  postoperative, 846
Cardiac disease
  anesthesia and, 591
  as transplant contraindication,
    107-108, 417
  congenital, with Alagille syndrome, 291
  in fulminant hepatic failure, 171t
  posttransplant, 501
  pretransplant evaluation of, 414-417
  transplantation in, 414-417
Cardiac function. See also Heart.
  pretransplant evaluation of, 414, 415-417
Cardiac stress testing, pretransplant,
  416-417
Cardiac transplantation, with liver
  transplant, in children, 1347, 1347t
Cardiomegaly, in children, transplantation
  in, 291
Cardiomyopathy, 415
  anesthesia and, 591
Cardiovascular disease
  anesthesia and, 591
  as transplant contraindication,
    107-108, 417
  immunosuppression and, 1247
  in fulminant hepatic failure, 171t
  posttransplant, 501, 997-998
  pretransplant evaluation of, 414-417
  transplantation in, 414-417
  unanticipated, operative implications
    of, 554
Cardiovascular function, in brain-dead
  donors, 517t, 518, 519t
Cardiovascular system
  postoperative management of,
    in children, 857
  preoperative monitoring of, 591
Caspase(s)
  in apoptosis, 47
  in preservation injury, 567
Caspase-8, RNA interference of, 48
Casts, biliary, 941-942. See also Biliary
  complications.
  treatment of, 947
Catheter
  biliary drainage, persistent hemobilia
    through, 468
  intravenous, posttransplant infection from
    in children, 1347-1348
    timing of, 966f
Catheter care, in nutritional support, 1042
Catheterization
  abdominal aorta, in donor operation,
    549-550, 550f, 554
  femoral vein, in recipient hepatectomy, 578
  portal vein, in recipient hepatectomy,
    578-579
  pulmonary artery
    intraoperative, 599
    preoperative, 591
Cavocaval anastomosis, 750-751
Cavocavostomy, infrahepatic vena, 751
Cavoportal hemitransposition, 747, 747f
CD3 immunotoxin, 1391

CD4+ cells
  in children, 1236
  in graft rejection, 1169, 1170, 1171-1172
  in hepatitis C, 130
CD8+ cells
  in graft rejection, 1169, 1170
  in hepatitis C, 130
Cefotaxime, for spontaneous bacterial
  peritonitis, 479
Ceftizoxime, for antibacterial prophylaxis,
  985t
Cell(s)
  death of, 47-48
  migration of, in transplantation,
    1183-1196, 1189f
Cell adhesion molecules, in ischemia-
  reperfusion injury, 1407-1408
Cell cycle, in liver regeneration, 46
Cell lines, for liver-support devices,
  1432-1434
Cell savers, 600
Cell surface death receptors, 47
Cellular immunity. See also Immune
  response; Immunity.
  adoptive transfer of, 1186-1187, 1188f
  in autoimmune hepatitis, 199
  in hepatitis C, 130
Celsior solution, 568
Center for Medicare and Medicaid Service,
  64, 65f
Central nervous system. See also Brain.
  Aspergillus infection of,
    posttransplant, 974
  diseases of, in children, transplantation
    in, 291
  infections of, 970-971, 1032, 1032f
    immunosuppression and, 972t
Central pontine myelinosis, 845, 1024-1025,
  1031-1032, 1031f, 1032f, 1034, 1048t
Central vein endotheliitis, in rejection vs.
  recurrent hepatitis C, 1131-1132
Cephalosporins, 972t
  for spontaneous bacterial peritonitis, 479
Cerebral edema
  in fulminant hepatic failure, 597-598, 1025
    irreversible, 597-598
  postoperative, 1025, 1035
    in children, 854
  preoperative, 590-591, 597-598
Cerebral function monitoring,
  intraoperative, 599
Cerebral hemorrhage, 1031, 1034
Cerebral infarction, 1031, 1034
Cerebral perfusion pressure, postoperative,
  in children, 855
Cerebrovascular accidents,
  postoperative, 846
Cervical cancer
  recurrent, 1161, 1161t
  screening for, 1162, 1162t
Chelating agents
  for neonatal iron storage disease, 357
  for Wilson's disease, 343
Chemical pleurodesis, for hepatic
  hydrothorax, 407
Chemoembolization, transarterial, 212
  for hepatocellular carcinoma, 103, 1159

Chemokines
    in acute rejection, 1068, 1068f, 1070
    in ischemia-reperfusion injury, 1405
Chemotherapy
    diarrhea from, 875
    for cholangiocarcinoma, 223
    for hepatic malignancy, 211-212, 224-225
    for hepatoblastoma, 1160
        in children, 368-369
    for hepatocellular carcinoma, 221, 1159
Chest radiography, in pretransplant
        evaluation, 406, 411
Chickenpox. *See* Varicella-zoster virus
        infection.
Child-Pugh score, 1294
    in alcoholic liver disease, 99
    in lamivudine therapy, 118
    in listing, 97, 98
    in living donor transplantation, 111
    vs. MELD score, 1287, 1287f
Children. *See also* Adolescents; Infants *and*
        specific disorders and procedures.
    adenovirus infection in, 1250, 1348
    biliary atresia in. *See* Biliary atresia.
    biliary complications in, 332, 468, 1348
    catheter sepsis in, 1347-1348
    cholangitis in
        portoenterostomy for, 292-293
        transplantation for, 104, 290
    cholestasis in. *See* Cholestasis,
        in children.
    cirrhosis in
        as transplant indication, 1305t, 1311
        in cholestasis syndromes, 294-295
    cytomegalovirus infection in, 296, 314,
        1249-1250, 1348
    developmental delays in,
        immunosuppression and, 1247,
        1327-1339, 1349
    Epstein-Barr virus infection in, 296,
        1247-1248, 1348
    fever in
        posttransplant, 887, 887t
        pretransplant evaluation of, 436-437
    graft failure in, 1241
    graft rejection in, 1236-1237, 1239-1240,
        1270, 1347-1348
    growth retardation in, corticosteroids
        and, 1248-1249, 1327-1328
    hemangioendotheliomas in, 374-375,
        473-475, 1337t, 1340-1341
    hepatic artery thrombosis in, 331, 332,
        859-860, 860t, 957-958, 1337, 1348
    hepatitis B in, 1341
    hepatitis C in, 1341
    hepatoblastoma in, 105, 367-371, 1337t,
        1340-1341
        transplantation for, 105, 367-371, 1160
        outcome in, 1340
    hepatocellular carcinoma in, 367,
        371-372, 1337t
        associated disorders in, 1340, 1340t
    immunosuppression in, 1235-1253,
        1341-1342. *See also*
        Immunosuppression, for children.
    intracranial pressure in, 854-855
    jaundice in, 304t, 316

liver disease in
    causes of, 304t-305t
    complications of, 296
    malignant, 367-376
    metabolic, 291, 337-359. *See also*
        Metabolic diseases.
    nonprogressive, 289
    parenchymal, 296, 296f
    treatment of, before transplantation, 291
mechanical ventilation in, weaning from,
        856-857, 856t, 885
nutrition support in, 315-316. *See also*
        Nutrition support.
organ procurement from, 556-558
pharmacokinetics in, 1242-1246
portal vein thrombosis in, 748, 1348
postoperative intensive care for, 853-862.
        See also Intensive care, pediatric.
postoperative pain in, 854t, 855,
        884t, 885
posttransplant lymphoproliferative
        disorder in, 1247-1248
primary graft nonfunction in, 859, 1348
psychosocial issues in, 862, 1251-1252
quality of life in, 1327-1329, 1348-1350
small bowel/liver transplantation in.
        See also Small bowel/liver
        transplantation.
    history of, 787-788
    indications for, 789, 789t, 1305t, 1311
total parenteral nutrition in. *See* Total
        parenteral nutrition.
transplantation in, 18-19, 287-299, 374,
        629-645, 715, 717. *See also*
        specific indications.
    ABO-incompatible, 1201
    allograft function after, 885
    anesthesia in, 604
    aplastic anemia after, 294
    ascites after, 886-887
    auxiliary, 778
    biliary complications in, 1348
    combination, outcome in, 1346-1347,
        1347t
    complications of, 331-332, 886
    considerations in, 287-288
    contraindications to, 291-292
    Couinaud segment II/III allograft for,
        28-29, 28f-32f, 31
    cross-matching in, 1336. *See also*
        Cross-matching.
    disease recurrence after, 1341
    donors for, 297-298
    ethical issues in, 629-630
    evaluation before, 295-297, 295t
    fever after, 887, 887t
    for nonprogressive liver disease, 289
    for secondary liver disease, 290
    for vascular disorders, 291-292, 374-376
    graft size and, 297-298, 635-636,
        1342-1343. *See also* Small-for-size
        syndrome.
    growth and, 296
    hearing loss after, 1350
    hemiliver allograft for, 31
    hemodynamic status after, 885-886
    hepatic artery thrombosis after, 331

hepatic dysfunction after, 1347-1348,
        1347t
HIV infection and, 292
immunosuppression after. *See*
        Immunosuppression, for children
        and specific agents.
improvements in, 287
in infection, 292
indications for, 104-105, 288-291, 288t
    trends in, 1304t-1305t, 1310-1311
infection after, 296
laboratory abnormalities after, 886, 886t
large-for-size allograft in, 604, 635,
        641, 641f
living donor, 18-19, 298, 629-644,
        1343-1344. *See also* Living related
        liver transplantation.
malnutrition in, 296, 296f
multivisceral, 790, 1347, 1347t
non–heart-beating donor, 538-539
nutrition after, 887
operative technique in, 604
organ allocation for, 72-75, 73t, 74f, 75f
outcomes in, 1335-1348
    allograft size and, 1342-1343
    hepatic dysfunction and, 1346-1347,
        1347t
    in combination transplants,
        1346-1347, 1347t
    in living related transplant,
        1343-1344, 1345f
    in retransplantation, 1344-1346, 1346f
    in split-liver transplant, 1343
    neurological, 291
    patient age and, 1337, 1338f
    preoperative risk factors and,
        1336-1337, 1337t. *See also*
        Pediatric End-Stage Liver
        Disease (PELD) score.
    primary liver disease and, 1337-1341
oversized liver in, 604
partial allograft for, 16, 23. *See also*
        Auxiliary liver transplantation,
        partial orthotopic.
PELD score in, 71-75, 97-98, 296,
        1336. *See also* Pediatric End-Stage
        Liver Disease (PELD) score.
poor prognostic factors in, 1336
postoperative care for, 881-888
    course of, 887-888
    in intensive care unit, 853-862, 883.
        See also Intensive care, pediatric.
    operative factors affecting, 883
    preoperative factors affecting,
        881-882
    standardized orders in, 883-885, 884t
postoperative pain in, 854t, 855,
        884t, 885
preoperative care for, 881
preoperative risk factors for,
        1336-1337, 1337t. *See also*
        Pediatric End-Stage Liver Disease
        (PELD) score.
PRISM score in, 1336-1337
reduced-size graft in, 16, 23, 298,
        1342-1343. *See also* Split-liver
        transplantation.

Children (Continued)
   anatomy of, 27, 27f
      hilar dissection for, 27-28, 27f, 28f
      pitfalls in, 40
   referral for, 295
   results of, 288
   retransplantation after, 105, 768,
      1344-1346. See also
      Retransplantation.
      indications for, 1341t
   split-liver, 19, 609-625, 1343. See also
      Split-liver transplantation.
   surgical innovations for, 296-297
   trends in. See Liver transplantation,
      trends in.
   vascular complications in, 331-332, 1348
   varicella-zoster immune globulin for, for
      postexposure prophylaxis, 432
   vascular lesions in, 373-376
Child-Turcotte-Pugh score, 68, 68t, 71,
   1294. See also Child-Pugh score.
Chimerism
   in allograft, 1186, 1186f
   in transplantation, 1183-1196, 1361,
      1397-1399, 1398f
   leukocyte, 1186-1189
      donor, 1184, 1191-1192, 1191f
      systemic, 1186-1189, 1187f-1189f
   mixed, induction of, 1397-1399, 1398f
Chimpanzees, xenotransplantation with,
   19, 1366. See also Xenotransplantation.
Cholangiocarcinoma, 222-223
   bile duct, recurrent, 1101t
   chemotherapy for, 223
   extrahepatic, 222, 1159-1160
   imaging of, 212-213, 213f, 214f, 223
   in primary sclerosing cholangitis, 101,
      189, 1160
      survival rates and, 189-190
   intrahepatic, 214, 1160
   peripheral, 222
   posttransplant stricture in, 466
   pretransplant evaluation/management of,
      451, 965
   psychological aspects of, 399
   recurrent, 1101t, 1160
   screening for, in primary sclerosing
      cholangitis, 475
   survival in, 1160
   transplantation for, 101, 223,
      1159-1160
   vs. hepatocellular carcinoma, 215
Cholangiocytes, 45t
Cholangiography
   computed tomographic, 704
   endoscopic retrograde
      for biliary complications, 934-935,
         942-943, 946
      postoperative, 868
   for biliary complications, 934-935
   for biliary leaks, 463-464, 934-935
   in posttransplant evaluation, 462-465, 935
   in pretransplant evaluation, 451
   intraoperative, in living donor transplant,
      683, 689
   magnetic resonance, 704
      for biliary complications, 935

   in biliary atresia, 326
   in posttransplant evaluation, 465
   percutaneous transhepatic, 931, 934-935
      for bile leaks, 943-944
      hemobilia and, 942
      in biliary obstruction, 467-468
      in recurrent primary sclerosing
         cholangitis, 191, 191f
      postoperative, 868
   T-tube, in posttransplant evaluation, 462,
      462f, 464f, 465, 465f
Cholangiolitis, in preservation injury, 1073
Cholangiopancreatography
   endoscopic retrograde, 133, 710-711
      postoperative, 868
   magnetic resonance, 704
      for biliary complications, 935
      for cholangiocarcinoma, 189
      pretransplant, for living donor
         transplant, 711
Cholangiopathy, obstructive, vs. hepatitis,
   1077, 1100
Cholangitis, 1043t
   after portoenterostomy, 327-328, 329
   ascending, in children
      portoenterostomy for, 292-293
      transplantation in, 292
   bacterial, 188
      pretransplant evaluation/management
         of, 434
   biliary tract obstruction with, 1077
   nonsuppurative destructive, in primary
      biliary cirrhosis, 179
   primary sclerosing, 187-192
      characteristics of, 187-188
      cholangiocarcinoma in, 101,
         189-190, 1160
      cholangiocarcinoma screening in, 475
      chronic rejection in, 190
      in children, transplantation for, 104, 290
      inflammatory bowel disease in, 187,
         188-189, 190, 476, 1109
      osteodystrophy in, 188
      pretransplant management of, 431t,
         475-476
      pruritus in, 188
      recurrent, 190-192, 191f, 192f,
         1009-1010, 1076, 1101t, 1109-1110,
         1141-1143, 1142f
         cholangiography of, 191, 191f
         histology of, 191, 192f, 1133t,
            1136, 1136t
         retransplantation for, 770
         vs. rejection, 1143
      survival models for, 189
      transplantation for, 101
         biliary strictures after, 190-192,
            191f, 192f
         chronic/ductopenic rejection in, 190
         complications of, 190-192
         inflammatory bowel disease after, 190
         survival after, 189-190
      trends in, 1303t, 1310
   T-tubes and, 930-931
   vs. preservation injury, 1073
Choledochocholedochostomy, 16, 930-931
   advantages of, 930

   complications of, 929-948. See also
      Biliary complications.
   indications for, 930
   postoperative assessment of, 868
   Roux-en-Y, 61
   stents in, 930
   T-tube in, 930. See also T-tube(s).
Choledochojejunal anastomosis, 1076-1077
Choledochojejunostomy, 16, 930-931
   complications of, 929-948. See also
      Biliary complications.
   for situs inversus transplant patients,
      760f, 763
   in recipient hepatectomy and grafting, 586
   indications for, 931
   postoperative assessment of, 868
   Roux-en-Y
      bacterial infection after, 970
      for primary sclerosing cholangitis, 189
   stents in, biliary obstruction from, 466
Cholestasis. See also Jaundice.
   allograft failure and, 1005
   fatal familial, in Greenland Eskimos, 313
   hepatocanalicular, in preservation injury,
      1073, 1074f
   hereditary, with lymphedema, 314
   in children, 303, 305-316, 325-327, 326t,
      327f, 332
      benign recurrent intrahepatic, 313-314
      bile duct paucity in, 305-306, 306t
      classification of, 310, 311t
      differential diagnosis of, 303-305,
         304t-305t, 325-327, 326t, 327f
      diseases associated with, 304, 304t-305t
      in Alagille syndrome, 308-310, 308t
      in biliary atresia, 316, 1337-1338
      in infectious hepatitis, 314-315
      in neonatal hepatitis, 306-307, 307t,
         308t, 326-327
      in North American Indians, 313
      preoperative risk factors in, 1337t
      total parenteral nutrition–associated,
         315-316
      transplantation for, 17, 82, 101,
         104-105, 294-295, 316-317
         outcomes in, 1337-1340, 1339f
      treatment of, 316
   neonatal, 304, 305, 305t
      differential diagnosis of, 325-327,
         326t, 327f
   postoperative, after Kasai
      portoenterostomy, 328
   primary, 895t
   progressive familial intrahepatic, 310
      cirrhosis in, 294-295
      type 1, 310-312, 311t
      type 2, 311t, 312
      type 3, 311t, 312-313
   pruritus in, 328
   recurrent, 1009
   transplantation for, 17, 101, 104-105,
      294-295, 316-317
      in children, 882
      outcomes in, 1337-1340, 1339f
Cholestasis familiaris groenlandica, 313
Cholesterol, elevated serum. See Familial
   hypercholesterolemia; Hyperlipidemia.

Cholesterol ester storage disease, 353
Cholestyramine, for pruritus, 188, 482
Choriocarcinoma, donor-transmitted, 1151
Chromosomal disorders, bile duct paucity in, 306t
Chronic fatigue, 1048t
Chrysosporium infection, posttransplant, 975
Cigarette smoking, 401-402
    posttransplant, 1052t
Cirrhosis
    alcohol use in, 132
    alcoholic, 50. *See also* Alcoholic liver disease.
    ascites in, 132-133
    clinical manifestations of, 44t, 48-50, 132-133
    cryptogenic, 895t
        as transplant indication, 1303t, 1310
            in children, 1305t, 1311
        nonalcoholic steatohepatitis, 1110
        trends in, 1303t, 1305t, 1310, 1311
    definition of, 44
    development of, 55
        biopsy histology and, 151
    etiology of, 44t, 50
    fibrosis in. *See* Hepatic fibrosis.
    focal biliary, in cystic fibrosis, 279
    glomerulonephritis in, 894
    hemophilia and, transplantation for, 241-243, 242f
    hepatic failure from, 132
    hepatitis B and, 50, 1095
    hepatitis C and, 50, 131-132, 132t, 143, 144, 983, 1096-1097
        decompensation in, 132-134, 132t, 136
        hepatocellular carcinoma in, 134
        survival in, 132, 132f
        treatment of, 135-136, 136t, 144
    hepatocytes in, 44
    hepatorenal syndrome and, 419-420, 481-482
    in autoimmune hepatitis, 196, 201
    in children
        as transplant indication, 1305t, 1311
        in cholestasis syndromes, 294-295
    in cystic fibrosis, 355
    in hepatocellular carcinoma, 132, 214, 215
    living donor transplantation for, 111
    malnutrition in, 483-484
    nonalcoholic fatty liver and, 50
    North American Indian, 313
    pathogenesis of, 50-55, 50f, 51f, 52t
    portal hypertension in. *See* Portal hypertension.
    portal vein thrombosis with, 1075
    primary biliary, 177-184, 895t
        antimitochondrial antibody in, 178, 179, 183, 1106
        antinuclear antibody–negative, 179
        asymptomatic, 178
        autoimmunity and, 179, 200, 1106, 1107
        causes of, 178
        clinical features of, 178-179
        complications of, 179
        diagnosis of, 179
        epidemiology of, 177-178

hepatocellular carcinoma in, 179
        histology of, 179
        humoral immunity in, 178
        in children, transplantation for, 288-289
        in cystic fibrosis, 355
        in primary sclerosing cholangitis, 187
        microbial antigens in, 178
        natural history of, 179-180
        pretransplant management of, 475
        prognosis of, 179-180
        pruritus in, 482-483
        pulmonary dysfunction in, 410
        recurrent, 183, 1009-1010, 1101t, 1105-1107, 1140-1141, 1140f
            autoantibodies in, 1106
            clinical features of, 1106
            differential diagnosis of, 1107
            histology of, 1133t, 1136, 1136t
            histopathology of, 1106-1107, 1106f
            pathophysiology of, 1105-1106
            retransplantation for, 770
            vs. chronic rejection, 1141
            vs. hepatitis C, 1100
        symptomatic, 178-179, 178t
        transplantation for, 101, 180-184
            bone disease after, 183-184
            de novo autoimmune hepatitis after, 207
            MELD score in, 182-183
            outcome of, 180-182, 181f, 182f
            quality of life after, 182, 182f
            treatment of, 180
            trends in, 1303t, 1310
            ursodeoxycholic acid for, 177, 180
    renal disease in, 419-420, 481-482
    renal function in, 892
    spontaneous bacterial peritonitis in, 132, 133
    transplantation for, 99f, 132
    variceal bleeding in. *See* Variceal bleeding.
Cirrhotic cardiomyopathy, anesthesia and, 591
Clarithromycin
    calcineurin inhibitors and, 1243
    immunosuppressant interactions with, 972t, 1243
Clichy criteria, for fulminant hepatic failure, 167-168
Clindamycin, immunosuppressant interactions with, 972t
Clinical nurse coordinator, 439-446
    as transplant committee member, 443-445
    goals of, 439-440
    in end-stage liver disease, 439-446
    in pretransplant evaluation, 440-443
    in referral process, 440, 441f
Clonal exhaustion-deletion, 1193
    after transplantation, 1189-1190, 1190f
    reciprocal, 1190f, 1191
Clonidine, for hypertension, 873
Coagulation disorders, 595-596. *See also specific disorders.*
    antilymphocyte antibodies and, 1269
    in brain-dead donors, 517t
    in fulminant hepatic failure, 597-598
    intraoperative management of, 596, 599, 600f, 603

monitoring for, 596, 599, 600f
    monoclonal antibodies and, 1223
    neurologic complications and, 1031
    postoperative, 604
    thrombotic. *See* Thrombosis.
    transplantation for, 241-243, 242f, 243f
Coagulation factors, hepatic synthesis of, 595, 595t
Coagulation, monitoring of, 596, 599, 600f
Coagulative necrosis, vs. preservation injury, 1073
Coagulopathy. *See* Coagulation disorders.
Coccidioidomycosis
    posttransplant, 973, 973t, 975
    prophylaxis for, 431t, 436, 965
    pretransplant evaluation/management of, 965
Cognitive function, 1020, 1030, 1326-1327. *See also* Hepatic encephalopathy; Neuropsychiatric outcomes.
    assessment of, 398, 1327
    in children, immunosuppression and, 1247, 1328-1329, 1349
Coil embolotherapy, for hepatopulmonary syndrome, 482
Cold ischemia, 1071, 1072. *See also* Ischemia.
    duration of
        as outcome predictor, 922, 1289, 1289t
        trends in, 1305t-1306t, 1312
    injury from. *See* Ischemia-reperfusion injury; Preservation injury.
Cold perfusion, in organ preservation. *See* Organ preservation, cold perfusion in.
Cold preservation injury, 562-565. *See also* Preservation injury.
Cold storage solutions. *See* Preservation solutions.
Cold symptoms, over-the-counter medications for, 1047t
Colonoscopy, in primary sclerosing cholangitis, 188-189
Colorectal cancer
    donor-transmitted, 1151
    hepatic metastases from
        transplantation for, 235, 235f, 1161
        treatment alternatives for, 235-236
    in ulcerative colitis with primary sclerosing cholangitis, 476
    recurrent, 1161-1162, 1161t
    screening for, 1162, 1162t
Common bile duct, 27f, 33. *See also* Bile duct(s).
    stenosis of, 842, 842f
Compartment syndrome, hepatic infarction and, 782
Complement
    in ischemia-reperfusion injury, 1406
    in xenotransplantation, 1370-1371, 1373
Complementary therapies, safety of, 399
Complete blood count, in intensive care, 834, 834t
Compliance. *See* Noncompliance.
Complications, postoperative. *See* Postoperative complications.
Computed tomographic cholangiography, 704

Computed tomographic segmental volume
    analysis, 704-705
Computed tomography
    in hepatic volumetric analysis,
        704-705, 705f
    in posttransplant evaluation, of biliary
        tract, 464-465, 465f
    in pretransplant evaluation, 448-450, 449f
        for living donor transplant, 704-711
    liver attenuation index and, 705-707
    multidetector, 704
    of biliary complications, 935
    of Budd-Chiari syndrome, 252, 252f
    of hepatic malignancy, 212, 212f-214f
    of hepatic tumors, 212, 448
Computed tomography angiography, 704
    for hepatic artery thrombosis, 956, 956f
    in living donor transplant, 707-710,
        708f, 709f
    in portal vein thrombosis, 744
Congenital heart disease, with Alagille
    syndrome, 291
Congenital malformations,
    immunosuppression and, 1329
Congenital TORCH infections, vs. biliary
    atresia, 325-326
Consciousness, alterations in, posttransplant,
    1021-1022, 1030
Consent, 520
    for living donor transplant, 734
    for living related liver transplant, 629-630
    presumed, 386
Constipation, over-the-counter medications
    for, 1047t
Continuous renal replacement therapy, for
    hepatorenal syndrome, 898-899
Continuous venovenous hemodialysis,
    intraoperative, 595
Contraception, 1052t, 1252-1253, 1330
Contraindications. See Liver transplantation,
    contraindications to.
Copper metabolism, in Wilson's disease,
    341-342. See also Wilson's disease.
Coronary artery bypass grafting, with liver
    transplantation, 591
Coronary artery disease. See also
    Cardiovascular disease.
    anesthesia and, 591
    posttransplant, 501, 997-998
    pretransplant evaluation of, 414-417
Coronary ligament
    left, 25
    right, 25
Corticosteroids, 1215-1217. See also
    Immunosuppression.
    bone loss and, 502, 997, 997f, 1217.
        See also Osteopenia/osteoporosis.
    depression and, 1024, 1217
    dosage of, 1215-1217, 1215t, 1217t, 1227t
    for autoimmune hepatitis, 201, 202,
        202t, 203
        after transplantation, 204
    for biliary atresia, 327-328
    for brain-dead donors, 518
    for children
        growth retardation and, 1248-1249,
            1327-1328, 1349

    taper for, 1238
    withdrawal/avoidance of, 1241-1242,
        1248-1249
    for graft rejection, 1267-1268, 1267t
    for small bowel/liver transplantation,
        794, 794t
    glucose metabolism and, 501-502
    hepatitis C progression and, 149
    hepatitis C recurrence and, 1001, 1217
    hyperlipidemia and, 500, 500t, 1217
    hypertension and, 998, 1216t, 1217
    infections from, 968
    mechanism of action of, 1267
    metabolism of, 1215-1217
    neurotoxicity of, 1022, 1033, 1217
    obesity and, 500, 999, 1217
    protocols for, 1215t, 1227t
    recurrent primary biliary cirrhosis and, 183
    side effects of, 203, 502, 997, 997f,
        1216t, 1217t
    taper for, 1215t, 1217, 1217t
        in children, 1238
    withdrawal/avoidance of, 1394
        in pediatric immunosuppression,
            1241-1242, 1248-1249
Costimulatory blockade, in
    immunosuppression, 1276, 1279,
    1391-1932
Cough, over-the-counter medications
    for, 1047t
COX-2 inhibitors, in hepatorenal
    syndrome, 897
Cramps, muscle, 1049t
    quinine sulfate for, 478
Creatinine, serum
    as outcome predictor, 1289-1290
    in end-stage liver disease, 892
    in MELD score, 73
    trends in, 1306t, 1312
CREST (calcinosis, Raynaud's
    phenomenon, esophageal dysmotility,
    sclerodactyly, telangiectasia)
    syndrome, in primary biliary
    cirrhosis, 179
Crigler-Najjar syndrome, 353-354, 354f,
    1103t
    hepatocyte transplant for, 338-339, 1384
    liver transplant for, 105, 290, 338t
Critical Pathway for the Organ Donor,
    519-520, 519t
Cross-matching, 12, 1199, 1203-1205, 1205f.
    See also ABO blood group antigens;
    Human leukocyte antigen(s) (HLA).
    graft rejection and, 1173-1174
    in kidney transplantation, 1200
    in liver transplantation, 1204-1205, 1205f
    in liver-kidney transplantation, 804-805
    in living related donor transplantation,
        634-635
    in pediatric transplantation, 1173-1174
    intravenous immunoglobulin and, 1393
    transplant outcome and, 1173-1174,
        1200-1202, 1201f
        in children, 1336
    trends in, 1308t, 1313, 1314f
Crude survival percentages, 1313-1314, 1315t
Cryosurgery, for hepatic malignancy, 212

Cryptococcosis
    posttransplant, 973, 973t, 974
        prophylaxis for, 965, 976
        timing of, 966, 966f
    pretransplant evaluation/management
        of, 965
Cryptogenic cirrhosis, 895t
    as transplant indication, 1303t, 1310
        in children, 1305t, 1311
    nonalcoholic steatohepatitis, 1110
    trends in, 1303t, 1305t, 1310, 1311
Cryptosporidiosis, prophylaxis for, 1045
C-statistic, 1287
CTLA4-Ig (LEA29Y), 1276, 1279-1280,
    1392-1393
CTP score, for hepatitis C, 137-138
Cu/Zn superoxide dismutase, 1360
Cyclophosphamide, 9, 1217-1218. See also
    Immunosuppression.
    for small bowel/liver transplantation,
        794, 794t
    mechanism of action of, 1217
    metabolism of, 1217-1218
    side effects of, 1218
Cyclosporine, 14-15, 15f, 1220-1221.
    See also Calcineurin inhibitors;
    Immunosuppression.
    adverse effects of, 996, 997, 1019-1025
    antibiotic interactions with, 972t
    avoidance of, 1397
    depression and, 1024
    diabetes and, 874
    dosage of, 1220
    drug interactions with, 906, 1220
        in children, 1243
    emulsion form of, 1243-1244
        for hepatoma, 1227t
        therapeutic monitoring of, 1245-1246
    for autoimmune hepatitis, 203
        after transplantation, 204
    for children, 884, 1237-1238, 1243-1244,
        1341, 1342
    for hepatocellular carcinoma, 1229
    for liver-kidney transplantation, 806
    generic formulations of, 1220-1221
    gout and, 996
    headaches from, 874, 1023
    hepatitis C recurrence and, 1001
    hirsutism and, 1051t, 1252
    hyperglycemia and, 501-502, 996
    hyperlipidemia and, 500, 500t
    hypertension and, 500-501, 873, 998, 1220
    in Budd-Chiari syndrome, 257
    in de novo autoimmune hepatitis, 207
    in pregnancy, 877, 1329-1330
    infections from, 968
    leukoencephalopathy and, 1033, 1033f
    mechanism of action of, 1220
    metabolism of, 1220
        in children, 1243-1244
    nephrotoxicity of, 904-906, 1220
    neurotoxicity of, 845, 874, 1019-1025,
        1023t, 1033
    obesity and, 499-500
    pharmacokinetics of, 1221
        in children, 1243-1244
    postoperative regimen with, 871

Cyclosporine (*Continued*)
  protocols for, 1227t
  renal function and, 874
  seizures from, 845-846, 1023
  side effects of, 1216t, 1220
  therapeutic monitoring of,
    in children, 1245
  with sirolimus, 906, 1222
Cyst(s), hepatic
  imaging of, 213
  in polycystic kidney disease, liver/kidney
    transplant for, 908
Cystic artery, 33
Cystic fibrosis, 354-355, 1104t
  bile duct paucity in, 306t
  focal biliary cirrhosis in, 279
  pretransplant evaluation in, 411
  quality of life in, 1349
  transplantation for, 105, 279, 338t, 355
Cystinosis, 1104t
Cytoablation, immunosuppression by, 8-9, 9t
Cytochrome P450, in drug metabolism, 598
Cytokine release syndrome, 1224
  prevention of, 1223
Cytokines
  immunosuppressive, 1359-1360
  in acute hepatic failure, 48
  in alcoholic liver disease, 267
  in autoimmune hepatitis, 199
  in graft rejection, 1068, 1068f, 1070, 1071,
    1085, 1174-1175, 1214, 1214f, 1215t,
    1359-1360
  in hepatic fibrosis, 51, 52t
  in hepatitis B, 1095
  in hepatocyte growth, 58
  in ischemia-reperfusion injury, 566,
    567, 1405
Cytomegalovirus hyperimmune globulin, 872
Cytomegalovirus infection
  bile duct effects of, 306t, 1091
  congenital, vs. biliary atresia, 325
  gastrointestinal, 979
  hepatic artery thrombosis from, 1090
  hepatic failure from, 279
  hepatitis C recurrence and, 1002-1003
  hepatitis from
    in allograft, 1090-1092, 1091f
    neonatal, 305t
    posttransplant, 978
  herpesvirus 6/7 and, 432
  in children, 296, 1249-1250, 1348
    cholestasis in, 314
  in donor, 431, 978
  pneumonia from, 978-979
  posttransplant, 978-979
    diagnosis of, 979
    in children, 861-862
    incidence of, 978
    management of, 979
  pretransplant evaluation/management of,
    431, 431t, 965
  reactivation of, 431, 431t
  timing of, 966, 966f, 978
  prophylaxis for, 431, 431t, 872, 965,
    979-980, 980t, 985, 985t, 1044,
    1044t, 1045, 1045t
    in children, 884, 884t, 1249

Cytomegaly, vs. adenoviral hepatitis, 1094
Cytopenia, antiviral therapy and, 135
Cytotoxic T-lymphocytes, 1362, 1392-1393

D

Daclizumab, 1225, 1277-1279. *See also*
    Immunosuppression.
  for children, 1238
  for recurrent hepatitis C, 1278
  in small bowel/liver transplant, 794, 794t
  infection risk from, 968
  therapeutic monitoring of, in children,
    1246
Dapsone, for *Pneumocystis carinii*
    prophylaxis, 985, 985t
Deafness, after pediatric transplant, 1350
Death. *See also* Brain death.
  determination of, 382-383
Deferoxamine, in preservation solutions, 568
Degenerative nodules, magnetic resonance
    imaging of, 451
Delirium, postoperative, 845, 1021-1022, 1022t
Dendritic cells
  donor, 1065-1066
  in gene therapy, 1361
  in immune response, 1361
  in recipient, 1361
Dental care, 1052t
Dental procedures, prophylaxis for, 877
Depression, 398-399, 483, 1023-1024,
    1048t
  in adolescents, 1252
  symptoms of, 1048t
Derivative diisopropyl iminodiacetic acid
    (DISIDA) scans, in posttransplant
    evaluation, 455
Des-γ-carboxy prothrombin, in hepatocellu-
    lar carcinoma, 215
Developmental delays, immunosuppression
    and, 1247, 1327-1339, 1349
Dexamethasone, in super-rapid non–
    heart-beating transplant, 537
Dextran, for portal vein thrombosis
    prophylaxis, 748
Diabetes mellitus
  posttransplant, 501-502, 995-996
  transplant outcome in, 501
Dialysis
  bioartificial liver in, 1427
  for hepatorenal syndrome, 420, 898-899
  in MELD score, 73, 75
  intraoperative continuous venovenous,
    595, 603
  postoperative, 847
  pediatric, 858
Diaphragm, surgical anatomy of, 25
Diarrhea, 1048t
  in children, immunosuppression and, 1243
  over-the-counter medications for, 1047t
  postoperative, 875
Diatheses, hemorrhagic
  transplantation for, 243
  transplant-related transmission of, 245
Diet. *See also* Nutrition.
  in hepatic encephalopathy, 480
  liquid, 496

posttransplant
  long-term guidelines for, 502-503, 502t
  short-term guidelines for, 495-496
posttransplant guidelines for, 495-496,
    502-503, 502t
pretransplant, 494-495, 495t
sodium-restricted
  for ascites, 479
  in posttransplant period, 501
weight loss
  for nonalcoholic steatohepatitis, 1011
  pretransplant, 402
Digital subtraction arteriography, in post-
    transplant evaluation, 459, 460f, 461f
Diltiazem, for hypertension, 873
Diphenhydramine
  with antithymocyte globulin, 1223
  with OKT3, 1223
Disability issues, 1051t
Discharge
  assessment criteria for, 1039t
  contraindications to, 1040t
  patient education for, 1039, 1039t.
    See also Patient education.
DISIDA scans, in posttransplant
    evaluation, 455
Disseminated intravascular coagulation,
    595-596
Distal splenorenal shunts, 509, 749
  for variceal bleeding, 509
  preexisting, intraoperative management
    of, 749
Diuretics, for ascites, 418, 478-479
DNA
  in gene delivery systems, 1358
  naked, 1358
Dobutamine stress echocardiography,
    preoperative, 417, 591
Dog
  antilymphocyte globulin trials in, 12
  drug-induced immunosuppression in, 10
  kidney transplantation in, 10
  liver transplantation in
    auxiliary, 5-6, 5f
    orthotopic, 6, 6f
    prerequisites for, 7, 8f
    tolerogenicity in, 12, 13f
  multivisceral transplantation in, 8, 9f
  rejection in, 7, 8f
Domino (sequential) transplantation, 524
Donor bone marrow progenitor cells,
    transplantation of. *See also* Bone
    marrow transplantation.
  with total-lymphoid irradiation, 1399
Donor operation, 545-558. *See also*
    Hepatectomy.
  anesthesia in, 598
  arterial reconstruction in, 556, 557f, 558f
  arterial variations in, 556
  back-table preparation in, 554-556,
    555f, 556f
  cold dissection in, 551-553, 551f-553f
  cold perfusion in
    preparation for, 547-550, 548f-550f
    technique for, 550-551
  hemodynamic instability in, 554
  in children, 556-558

Donor operation (Continued)
  in non–heart-beating donor transplant, 536-538, 537f, 554
  preoperative preparation in, 546-547
  special circumstances in, 553-554
  unanticipated abdominal aortic aneurysm in, 554
  unanticipated atherosclerotic disease in, 554
  unanticipated peritonitis in, 553
  with prior median sternotomy, 554
Donor/donation. See also Allograft(s); Organ(s).
  absolute vs. relative risk factors for, 523-524
  age of. See Age, donor.
  allocation sequence for, 72, 73t
  anencephalic, ethical aspects of, 384-385
  animal. See Xenotransplantation.
  anti-HBc-positive, biopsy of, 1064-1065
  anti-hepatitis C status of, 151
  cancer transmission by, 1150-1151
  consent for, 520
  contraindications to
    absolute, 521, 524, 1061
    relative, 521-523, 524, 1061
  coordination of, 520
  critical pathway for, 519-520, 519t
  cytomegalovirus from, 978
  deceased
    biopsy for, 1061, 1062t-1063t, 1064
      back-table, 1065
    ethical aspects of, 381-383, 1060-1061, 1061t, 1064-1065, 1064f
    expanded criteria for, 1061, 1062t-1063t, 1064
    frozen section biopsy of, 1060-1061, 1061t, 1064-1065, 1064f
  dendritic cells of, 1065-1066
  determination of death for, 382-383
  direct stimulation in, 1066, 1066f
  ethical aspects of, 382-386, 539-540
  evaluation at time of procurement for, 523-524
  extended criteria for, 521-523
  family objections to, 386
  gender and, 1306t, 1312-1313
  Good Samaritan, 668-669
  hepatitis C–positive, 145, 1137
  HIV-infected, 982-983
  HLA-compatible, 1200
  identification of, 520
  immune response of, 1065-1066, 1066f
  in hepatic malignancy, 224, 225
  in hepatocellular carcinoma, 217-218
  in non–heart-beating donor liver transplant, 525-526, 536, 539-542. See also Non–heart-beating donor liver transplantation.
  in pediatric transplantation, 297-298. See also Children, transplantation in.
  in split-liver transplant, 524, 610-611. See also Split-liver transplantation.
  infection transmission from, 429-437, 523, 965-966
  leukocyte chimerism in, 1184

  living, 18-19, 524-525, 630-636. See also Living donor liver transplantation; Living related liver transplantation.
    ABO-incompatible, 1202
    antibody-mediated rejection in, 1078
    biopsy of, 1065
    ethical aspects of, 383-384, 729-738
    preformed antibody in, 1204
  macrovesicular steatosis in, 1064, 1064f
  marginal, 17-18, 217
  nondirected, 668-669
  obese, allograft from, 839
  operative procedures for. See Organ procurement.
  organ shortage and, 17-19, 382, 521, 522f. See also Organ(s), shortage of.
  paid, 384
  parent-to-child. See Living related liver transplantation.
  passenger leukocytes of, 1065-1066, 1070
  pathological evaluation of, 1060-1065
  pediatric, 556-558
  presumed consent of, 386
  pretransplant evaluation of, 546. See also Pretransplant evaluation.
  race/ethnicity and, 1307t, 1312-1313
  rate of, 520, 520f
  recipient and, clonal exhaustion-deletion responses between, 1189-1192, 1190f, 1191f
  required request laws for, 386
  selection of, 521
  withdrawal of support for, 536, 536t, 537f, 540-541
  xenograft, ethical aspects of, 384-385
Dopamine
  for hepatorenal syndrome, 897-898, 898t
  for postoperative pediatric fluid management, 858
Doppler probe, implantable, 331, 331f
Doppler ultrasonography. See also Ultrasonography.
  in brain death determination, 516-517
  in posttransplant evaluation, 452-455, 453f-455f
    of hepatic artery, 457, 458f, 955-956, 958
    of portal vein, 459, 459f
  in pretransplant evaluation, 447-448
Dorsal splenorenal shunt, 509
Drainage catheter, persistent hemobilia through, 468
Drainage, T-tube. See T-tube(s).
Drug(s). See also specific drugs and drug families.
  acute hepatic failure from, 44t
  adverse reactions to
    allograft effects of, 1112
    vs. graft-versus-host disease, 1089
  for alcoholism, 270
  for outpatients, 1045-1046, 1047t-1049t
  hepatotoxic, in autoimmune hepatitis, 198t, 199
  immunosuppression with. See Immunosuppression.
  nephrotoxic, 419

  over-the-counter, patient instructions for, 1047t
Drug abuse, fulminant hepatic failure from, 164
Drug interactions
  patient education for, 1043-1044
  renal failure from, 905-906
  with lipid-lowering agents, 501t
Drug metabolism
  in elderly, 1227t, 1229-1230
  in liver disease, 598-599
Drug-resistant bacteria, posttransplant infection from, 969-970
Ductopenia, vs. chronic rejection, 1089
Ductus venosus, 24
Duodenum, 25
  transplantation of. See Small bowel/liver transplantation.
Dysfibrinogenemia, 595-596
Dyskinesias, posttransplant, 1024-1025
Dyslipidemia, 351-353
  in primary biliary cirrhosis, 179
Dyspepsia
  in living donors, 715
  over-the-counter medications for, 1047t
Dysplastic nodules, computed tomography of, 450
Dysrhythmias, 415
  in brain-dead donors, 517t
  postoperative, 846

E
Echinocandins, for fungal prophylaxis, 976-977
Echinococcus granulosus infection, transplantation for, 280
Echocardiography
  dobutamine stress, preoperative, 417, 591
  in brain-dead donors, 519t
  in pretransplant evaluation
    of cardiac function, 416, 417, 591
    of pulmonary function, 406, 407, 408, 409, 413
  transesophageal, preoperative, 591
Echovirus, in children, cholestasis in, 315
Eck's fistula
  pathophysiology of, 13
  reverse, 7f
Ecstasy, fulminant hepatic failure from, 164
Edema
  cerebral. See Cerebral edema.
  posttransplant, 1048t
  pulmonary, postoperative, 846-847
    in children, 856
Efalizumab, 1276
Effector molecules, in reperfusion injury, 566
ELAD system, 778, 1429, 1430-1431, 1430f, 1431t. See also Bioartificial liver; Extracorporeal liver support.
Elastic band ligation, for variceal bleeding, 478, 508
Elderly
  age of as contraindication, 107
  graft rejection in, 1229-1230

Elderly *(Continued)*
  immunosuppression in, 1227t, 1229-1230
  transplant outcome in, 402
Electrocardiography, pretransplant, 415-416
Electrocautery, in recipient hepatectomy, 576, 577
Electroencephalography
  in brain death determination, 516
  in hepatic encephalopathy, 590
Electrolyte imbalances, 900-902
  in brain-dead donors, 517t, 518, 519t
  in preservation injury, 563
  in renal disease, 417-418
  postoperative, 496, 837-838
    mental status alterations and, 1030
    pediatric, 858, 858t
Embolization
  hepatocyte, 1380-1381
  of thrombi. *See* Thromboembolism.
  therapeutic
    for biliary vascular communications, 468
    for hepatopulmonary syndrome, 482
Embryology, 24
Emergency department care, postdischarge, indications for, 1041, 1041t
Emergency hepatectomy, 783-784
  for necrotic liver, 778
  indications for, 783
  technique for, 783-784, 784f
Employment, posttransplant, 1327, 1328t
Encephalitis, posttransplant, 1032
Encephalopathy. *See* Hepatic encephalopathy.
Endocrine disorders
  bile duct paucity in, 306t
  neonatal, 305t
Endoscopic band ligation, for variceal bleeding, 478, 508
Endoscopic retrograde cholangiography (ERC). *See also* Cholangiography.
  for biliary complications, 934-935, 942-943, 946
  postoperative, 868
Endoscopic retrograde cholangiopancre-atography (ERCP), 133, 710-711
  of common bile duct stenosis, 842, 842f
  postoperative, 868
Endoscopic sclerotherapy, for variceal bleeding
  for prophylaxis, 476
  for treatment, 477, 508
Endoscopic sphincterotomy
  for ampullary dysfunction, 947
  for bile stones, 947
Endoscopy, for hepatitis C, 133
Endothelial cells, 45t
  in rejection, 1069
Endotheliitis, 1081
  in rejection vs. recurrent hepatitis C, 1131-1132, 1134f
Endothelin-1
  in hepatic fibrosis, 54
  in ischemia-reperfusion injury, 567, 1404
Endotracheal intubation, 601
  extubation in, 835-836, 836t
    pediatric, 856-857, 856t, 885

End-stage liver disease. *See* Hepatic failure; Liver disease, end-stage.
End-stage renal disease. *See* Renal failure.
Energy metabolism, 491-492, 492t
Engraftment, intestinal, leukocyte migration in, 1188, 1189f
Enteral feeding. *See also* Nutrition support.
  after small bowel/liver transplant, 795
  liver disease in, 778
  necrotizing enterocolitis and, 795
  posttransplant, 496-498, 587, 873
  pretransplant, 493-495
  tube placement for, 587
Enteritis, after small bowel/liver transplantation, 796
Enterobacteriaceae, posttransplant infection from, 969, 969t, 970, 971-972
Enterococcal infections, posttransplant, 969, 969t
Enterocolitis, after small bowel/liver transplantation, 796
Enzymes, liver, elevated, with biliary complications, 934
Eosinophils, in graft rejection, 1169-1170
Epithelioid hemangioendotheliomas, 223-224, 375, 375t
  imaging of, 214f
  in children, 473-475, 1337t, 1340-1341
  transplant for, 1160
Epoprostenol, for pulmonary/portopulmonary hypertension, 409, 592, 593
Epstein-Barr virus infection
  clinical features of, 1092-1093
  differential diagnosis of, 1093-1094
  disorders related to, 1094
  hepatitis from, 1090
    clinical features of, 1092-1093
    differential diagnosis of, 1093-1094
    histopathology of, 1093, 1093f
    in allograft, 1092-1094
    pathophysiology of, 1092
    vs. cytomegalovirus infection, 1091
  histopathology of, 1093, 1093f
  in allograft, 1092-1094
  in children, 1348
    posttransplant, 296, 1247-1250
  pathophysiology of, 1092
  posttransplant, 981
    in children, 296, 1247-1250
    timing of, 966, 966f
  posttransplant lymphoproliferative disorder and, 431, 965, 981, 1093, 1093f, 1247-1248
    in children, 1247-1248
  pretransplant evaluation/management of, 432-433, 965
  prophylaxis for, 431t, 432, 1044, 1045
    in children, 1248
  vs. recurrent hepatitis C, 1137
Epstein-Barr virus RNA, in situ hybridization for, 1093, 1093f, 1094
Erythrocyte savers, 600
Erythrocytes, in ischemic-reperfusion injury, 1410

Erythromycin
  calcineurin inhibitors and, 1243
  for antibacterial prophylaxis, 985t
  immunosuppressant interactions with, 972t, 1243
Erythropoietic protoporphyria, 243-245, 244f, 1104t
  transplantation for, 245, 246t, 277
Escherichia coli infection, in children, cholestasis in, 315
Eskimos, fatal familial cholestasis syndrome in, 313
Esophageal varices
  bleeding from. *See* Variceal bleeding.
  in decompensated cirrhosis, 133
Esophagogastroduodenoscopy, for esophageal varices, 508
Esophagogastrostomy, in multivisceral transplant, 793-794
Estrogen, for osteopenia/osteoporosis, 183, 483
Ethanol. *See also* Alcohol.
  for hepatic malignancy, 103, 212
Ethical issues, 381-392
  in living donor liver transplantation, 382-386, 669, 729-738. *See also* Living donor liver transplantation, ethical issues in.
  in living related liver transplantation, 629-630
  in non–heart-beating liver transplantation, 539-540
  in organ donation and procurement, 381-386
  in patient selection, 266, 387-390, 730-732
  in resource allocation, 390-392, 768
  in retransplantation, 768, 772
  in transplant team expertise, 734-735
  in withdrawal of support, 539-540
Etidronate, for osteoporosis, in primary biliary cirrhosis, 183
Eurocollins solution, 567-568, 569
Europe, organ allocation in, 79-81, 80f, 80t
Eurotransplant Liver Allocation System, 81, 87-90, 88f, 89t
Everolimus, 1280-1281, 1396-1397
  postoperative regimen with, 871
Evoked cerebral potentials, in brain death determination, 516
Ex vivo perfusion systems. *See* Extracorporeal liver support.
Exercise and activity, posttransplant, 1051t
Exfoliative urinary cytology, in graft rejection, 1177
Extracellular matrix
  in cirrhosis, 50
  in hepatic fibrosis, 51, 52t
  in hepatic injury, 51
  transforming growth factor-β effects on, 54
Extracorporeal Liver Assist Device (ELAD), 778, 1429, 1430-1431, 1430f, 1431t
Extracorporeal liver support, 10, 11f, 570, 778-779, 816, 1368-1369, 1373-1374
  bioartificial liver in, 778-779, 1368-1369, 1425-1435. *See also* Bioartificial liver.

Extracorporeal liver support (Continued)
  cell sources for, 779, 1368-1369,
    1373-1374, 1432-1433, 1432f
  for graft failure, 925
  for hepatic necrosis, 778
  hepatocyte transplantation with,
    in fulminant hepatic failure, 173
  history of, 1416-1417, 1416t
  immunological considerations in, 1419
  limitations of, 816
  liver function indices in, 1418-1419, 1418t
  perfusion parameters in, 1417-1418, 1417t
  porcine liver in, 779, 1368-1369,
    1373-1374, 1417, 1419, 1421
  recent experience with, 1420-1421,
    1420t
  results of, 1419-1421, 1420t
  technical considerations in, 1417-1418,
    1417t
Extradural pressure monitoring,
    in fulminant hepatic failure, 171
Extubation, 835-836, 836t
  pediatric, 856-857, 856t, 885

F

Factor V Leiden mutation
  in Budd-Chiari syndrome, 260
  transmission of, transplantation in, 245
  transplantation for, 243, 243f
Falciform ligament, 25, 25f
False aneurysms
  arterial anastomotic, after small
    bowel/liver transplant, 796
  hepatic artery, 458, 958-959
    hemobilia from, 468
Famciclovir
  for hepatitis B
    after transplantation, 122-123
    before transplantation, 118
    in recurrent infection, 1009
  resistance to, 123, 280
Familial amyloidosis, 399
  transplantation for, 239-240, 240f
    results of, 245, 246t
Familial hypercholesterolemia, 351-352,
    351f, 1103t. See also Hyperlipidemia.
  transplantation for, 276
    hepatocyte, 1384
Family objections, to organ donation, 386
Famotidine, for pediatric gastrointestinal
    ulcers, 858-859
Fanconi syndrome, in tyrosinemia, 344
Fas
  expression of, knocking down of, 48, 49f
  in acute hepatic failure, 47-48, 49f
  in hepatocyte apoptosis, 47-48
Fas ligand, 47
Fasciculations, 1024
Fat malabsorption, 492, 492t
Fatal familial cholestasis syndrome, in
    Greenland Eskimos, 313
Fatigue
  chronic, 1048t
  in autoimmune hepatitis, 200
  in primary biliary cirrhosis, 178
  posttransplant, 1025

Fatty acid metabolism, impaired,
    transplantation for, 278
Fatty liver. See also Alcoholic liver disease;
    Cirrhosis.
  alcoholic, recurrent, 1110, 1143, 1143f-1144f
    grading of, 1145
  nonalcoholic. See Nonalcoholic fatty
    liver/nonalcoholic steatohepatitis.
  postoperative, 839
Federal funding, for transplantation, 390-392
Feeding. See Diet; Nutrition support.
Femoral vein cannulation, in recipient
    hepatectomy, 578
Fentanyl
  for postoperative pain, 855, 884t, 885
  in anesthesia, 601
Ferritin, antioxidant properties of, 1360
Ferrochelatase, in erythropoietic
    protoporphyria, 244, 244f, 277
α-Fetoprotein
  in hepatocellular carcinoma, 101-102,
    134, 215
  in pediatric hepatic malignancy, 291
Fever
  posttransplant, 1045, 1046t
    in children, 887, 887t
  pretransplant evaluation of, 436-437
Fibric acid derivatives, 997
  adverse effects of, 501t
Fibrinolysis, intraoperative management of,
    596, 599, 600f, 603
Fibrosing cholestatic hepatitis, 122, 1006,
    1137, 1183f. See also Cholestasis.
  adefovir dipivoxil for, 123
  differential diagnosis of, 1099
  in allograft hepatitis B, 1096
  in allograft hepatitis C, 1097-1098, 1099f
  vs. preservation injury, 1073
Fibrosis. See Hepatic fibrosis.
FIC1 gene, in progressive familial
    intrahepatic cholestasis, 311
Final Rule, 66, 66t
Fine-needle aspiration biopsy. See also
    Biopsy.
  for allograft rejection, 1176-1177, 1265
Fissures, hepatic, 26, 26f
Fistulas
  abdominothoracic, 937
  biliary, 937
  Eck's
    pathophysiology of, 13
    reverse, 7f
FK506. See Tacrolimus.
FK778, 1281, 1395-1396
Flaviviridae, 129
Fluconazole
  for fungal prophylaxis, 975-976, 976t,
    985, 985t
  immunosuppressant interactions
    with, 972t
Fluid management
  in brain-dead donors, 518
  in renal disease, 418-419
  in variceal bleeding, 477, 508
  intraoperative, 601, 603
  postoperative, 846-847
    pediatric, 858, 883-884, 884t

Flumazenil, for hepatic encephalopathy,
    480-481
Fluoroquinolones
  for decompensated cirrhosis, 133
  for spontaneous bacterial peritonitis, 479
5-Fluorouracil, for cholangiocarcinoma, 223
Focal nodular hyperplasia, 282
  imaging of, 213
  transplantation for, 282
Focal pontine leukoencephalopathy,
    posttransplant, 1031, 1031f-1033f,
    1034
Foreign nationals, as transplant
    recipients, 390
Fractures, pathologic, 996-997. See also
    Osteopenia/osteoporosis.
Fratricide, 48
Free radical scavengers, 603
Free radicals, 1360-1361
  in ischemia-reperfusion injury, 1406
  in preservation injury, 563, 603
Free rheumatoid arthritis, 1360
Fructosemia, 349
FTY720, 1281, 1396
Fulminant hepatic failure. See Hepatic
    failure, fulminant.
Fulminant hepatitis, 124, 130, 163-164
Fumarylacetoacetate hydrolase (FAH)
    deficiency, in tyrosinemia, 344
Functional status. See Quality of life.
Fungal infections, 435-436. See also specific
    types, e.g., Candidiasis.
  biliary tract, transplantation for, 280
  in allograft, 1067t, 1089-1090
  posttransplant, 848, 972-978, 1067t,
    1089-1090
    clinical features of, 973-975
    diagnosis of, 974, 975
    in children, 861
    management of, 975
    pathogens in, 972-973, 973t
    prophylaxis for, 436, 872,
      975-977, 976t, 984-985, 985t,
      1044, 1044t
    treatment of, 977-978
  pretransplant evaluation/management of,
    435-436, 436t
Furosemide, for ascites, 418, 478-479
Fusarium infection, posttransplant, 975
Fusion proteins, 1276-1277, 1360

G

G6PD deficiency, 349-350
GABA, in hepatic encephalopathy, 590
α-Gal epitope, in xenotransplantation, 19
Galactomannan assay, in aspergillosis
    diagnosis, 974
Galactosemia, 349
  neonatal, 305t
β-Galactosidofructose, for hepatic
    encephalopathy, 133
Gallbladder fossa, 25, 25f
Gamma globulin, in autoimmune
    hepatitis, 198t
Gamma-aminobutyric acid (GABA),
    in hepatic encephalopathy, 590

Ganciclovir
 for cytomegalovirus prophylaxis, 979-980, 980t, 985, 985t
 for Epstein-Barr virus, in children, 1248
 for hepatitis B, after transplantation, 122
 for postoperative cytomegalovirus infection, 872
 immunosuppressant interactions with, 972t
 seizures and, 1023
Gastric artery, left, 28
Gastric motility
 decreased, 1048t
 in living donors, 715
Gastric varices
 bleeding from. See Variceal bleeding.
 in decompensated cirrhosis, 133
Gastric wall adhesions, in living related liver transplant, 631-632, 632f, 642
Gastroesophageal reflux disease, 1048t
Gastrogastrostomy, in multivisceral transplant, 793-794
Gastrohepatic ligament, 24, 25
Gastrointestinal bleeding, in biliary atresia, 328
Gastrointestinal tract
 cytomegalovirus infection of, posttransplant, 979
 decontamination of, for infection prophylaxis, 984
 pretransplant management of, in fulminant hepatic failure, 172t
Gaucher's disease, 352
Gemfibrozil, 997
 for hyperlipidemia, 997
Gender
 donor status and, 1306t, 1309
 recipient status and, 387-388, 1302t, 1312-1313
Gene(s)
 in autoimmune hepatitis, 199
 in liver regeneration, 46, 58
Gene therapy, 1357-1362
 applications of, 1357-1358
 for accommodation, 1371
 for metabolic disorders, 339
 for tolerance induction, 1357-1358, 1361-1362, 1371. See also Tolerance induction.
 gene transfer techniques in, 1358-1359
 graft modification in, 1359-1361
 indications for, 1357-1358
 overview of, 1357-1358
 recipient modification in, 1361-1362
 transgenic animals in, 1415
 viral vectors in, 1358-1359
 xenotransplantation in, 1361, 1366. See also Xenotransplantation.
Genetic disorders, acute hepatic failure from, 44t
Gentamicin
 for antibacterial prophylaxis, 985t
 immunosuppressant interactions with, 972t
Geotrichum infection, posttransplant, 975
Geriatric patients. See Elderly.
Gingival hyperplasia, 1052t, 1252

Glomerular filtration rate
 in end-stage liver disease, 892
 postoperative, 836, 873
 in children, immunosuppression and, 1246
 pretransplant measurement of, 418
Glomerulonephritis
 acute renal failure from, 894
 hepatitis C–related, 807
Glucose, blood, in liver rejection, 7, 8f
Glucose intolerance, postoperative, 874
Glucose metabolism, 492, 596
 in fulminant hepatic failure, 597
 in preservation injury, 562
 posttransplant, 492, 501-502, 596, 995-996
Glucose-6-phosphate dehydrogenase deficiency, 349-350
γ-Glutamyl transpeptidase (GGTP)
 in biliary atresia, 326
 in preservation injury, 1072
 postoperative, 866
γ-Glutamyltransferase, elevated
 as donation contraindication, 524
 in biliary complications, 934
Glutathione-S-transferase, antibodies to, in de novo autoimmune hepatitis, 207
Glycogen storage diseases, 338t, 349-351, 373, 895t, 1102t. See also Metabolic diseases.
 hepatocyte transplant for, 351, 1384
Glycolysis, in fulminant hepatic failure, 162
Good Samaritan donation, 668-669
Gout, posttransplant, 996, 1049t
G-protein–coupled receptor ligands, in hepatic fibrosis, 52t
Graft(s)
 arterial, 16
 for hepatic artery thrombosis, 956
 hepatic. See Allograft(s).
 vascular interposition, complications of, 1074
 venous, 16
 for portal vein thrombosis, 745-747, 747f
Graft-recipient body weight ratio, 658, 664, 682, 704
 segmental volume analysis and, 704-705, 705f
Graft-versus-host disease (GVHD), 1043t, 1089, 1205-1206, 1206t
 after multivisceral transplantation, 8
 after small bowel/liver transplantation, 797
 bile duct paucity in, 306t
 deaths from, 1206, 1206t
 diarrhea from, 875
 HLA mismatches in, 1206
 humanized OKT3 for, 1390
 postoperative, 866
Graft-versus-host reaction, 1189, 1190f
Granuloma
 peribiliary, 1081
 vs. adenoviral hepatitis, 1094
Granzyme, in graft rejection, 1176, 1265
Greenland Eskimos, fatal familial cholestasis syndrome in, 313

Growth factors
 for hepatitis C, 135
 in hepatic fibrosis, 51, 52t
 in hepatocyte, 58
 in liver regeneration, 46
Growth retardation, corticosteroids and, 1248-1249, 1327-1328, 1349
Gustation, impaired, 1025

H
Hair loss, 1051t
Hallucinations, visual, 1023
Haloperidol, postoperative, 875-876
Hamartomas, mesenchymal, transplantation for, 282
Hazard ratios, in outcome analysis, 1314, 1316t-1319t
Headache
 calcineurin, 874, 1023
 chronic, 1048t
 posttransplant, 874-875, 1023
Health care spending, future of, 391-392
Hearing loss, after pediatric transplant, 1350
Heart. See also under Cardiac.
 iron deposition in, 241
 monitoring of, in intensive care, 834, 834t, 835
 transplantation of, 14, 14t
Heartburn, over-the-counter medications for, 1047t
Heart-liver transplantation, in children, 1347, 1347t
Heat preconditioning, 569
Hemangioendotheliomas, 223-224, 375, 375t
 imaging of, 214f
 in children, 1337t, 1340-1341
 infantile, 374-375
 transplantation for, 1160
Hemangiomas
 cavernous, imaging of, 213
 giant, transplantation for, 281
 hepatic, transplantation for, 282
 in children, transplantation for, 374
Hematin, for erythropoietic protoporphyria, 245
Hematological disorders. See also specific disorders, e.g., Amyloidosis, hereditary.
 transplantation for, 239-246
 results of, 245, 246t
Hematological system, pretransplant management of, in fulminant hepatic failure, 172t
Hematolymphoid cells, 1065
Hematolymphopoietic cells, donor, in transplant recipient, 1188-1189, 1189f
Hematoma, intra-abdominal, postoperative, 868
Hematopoiesis, intrahepatic, 24
Heme oxygenase(s)
 cytoprotective effects of, 1410-1411, 1410f, 1412t
 in ischemia-reperfusion injury, 1409-1412
 in ischemic preconditioning, 569

Heme oxygenase-1
  in accommodation, 1371
  in ischemic preconditioning, 569
Heme, synthesis of, in erythropoietic
    protoporphyria, 243, 244f
Hemiliver, 40
  definition of, 26
  left, 27
  right, 27
  surgical anatomy for, 31-35, 33f-39f,
    38, 40
Hemobilia, 942. See also Biliary
    complications.
  persistent, 468
  treatment of, 947
Hemochromatosis, 1050t, 1104t
  hereditary, 240-241, 242f
    transplantation for, 103, 241
      results of, 245, 246t
  pretransplant management of, 475
  secondary, 241, 242f
Hemodialysis. See Dialysis.
Hemodynamic monitoring,
    intraoperative, 599
Hemoglobinuria, paroxysmal nocturnal,
    Budd-Chiari syndrome from, 254
Hemolytic disease, after ABO-compatible
    transplantation, 1202-1203
Hemoperfusion, bioartificial liver in, 1427
Hemophilia, 1103t
  cirrhosis in, transplantation for,
    241-243, 242f
  hepatitis C in, 242
  HIV infection in, 242
  transplantation for, results of, 245, 246t
Hemorrhage. See also Bleeding.
  cerebral, 1031, 1034
  postoperative, 604, 840-841
    in children, 860
  variceal. See Variceal bleeding.
Hemorrhoids, 1048t
Heparin
  in Budd-Chiari syndrome, 257, 258
  intraoperative infusion of
    in donor operation, 549
      in children, 556-557
      in living related liver transplant, 637
      in two-adult split-liver transplant, 651
Heparin effect, intraoperative management
    of, 603
HepatAssist device, 778, 925, 1428-1429,
    1429f, 1430, 1431t. See also
    Bioartificial liver; Extracorporeal liver
    support.
Hepatectomy
  donor, 545-558. See also Donor operation.
  emergency, 783-784
    for necrotic liver, 778
    indications for, 783
    technique for, 783-784, 784f
  left, 26
  liver regeneration after, 46
  native specimens from, pathology of,
    1059-1060, 1060f
  recipient, 575-587. See also Recipient
    hepatectomy and grafting.
  right, 26

total
  for hepatic malignancy, 211
  in fulminant hepatic failure, 597
  with temporary end-to-side portocaval
    shunt, 60f
  vascular anatomy and, 58, 59f
Hepatic adenomas
  in glycogen storage diseases, 350-351
  transplantation for, 282
Hepatic arterial revascularization, 956
Hepatic artery
  anatomy of
    segmental, 29f
    standard, 677f, 678, 708, 708f
    variations in, 58, 59f, 614f, 678, 679f
      in living donor transplant, 665,
        678-679, 679f, 707-709, 709f
      in living related liver transplant,
        635-636, 636f
      in split-liver transplant and, 613-614,
        614f, 615
      operative implications of, 556, 557f
  aneurysms of
    extrahepatic, 459
    false, 459, 958-959
      hemobilia from, 468
    intrahepatic, 459
  anomalies of, with situs inversus, 756, 756f
  biliary system supply by, after
    transplantation, 190
  erosion bleeding of, 937
  imaging of
    in posttransplant evaluation, 452-459,
      453f-459f
    in pretransplant evaluation, 447-448
      for living donor transplant, 707-709
    in chronic rejection, 1087, 1088, 1089
    in split-liver transplant, 613-614, 614f, 615
  infarction of
    imaging of, 455-456, 456f
    postoperative, 839-840, 839t, 840f
  left, 29
    in hemiliver allograft, 32
    segmental branches of, 28, 28f, 29f
  middle, 679, 679f
  posttransplant complications in, 452-459,
    453f-459f
  proper, 27, 27f, 28f
  reconstruction of, 584-585, 584f, 585f, 603
    in living related liver transplant,
      640-641, 640f
  replaced, 28, 28f
  resistive index for, 779
  right, 27, 27f, 28f
    accessory, 32, 34f
    in hemiliver allograft, 32, 33f
  rupture of, 959
  stenosis of, 958
    percutaneous transluminal angioplasty
      for, 457, 457f
    posttransplant, 455-457, 456f, 842
      in children, 859
  thrombosis of, 841, 954-958, 1058, 1067t
    after living related liver transplant,
      641-642
    angiography of, 841f
    biliary strictures and, 939, 1075

clinical features of, 458, 780, 955,
    955t, 1074
  cytomegalovirus infection and, 1090
  diagnosis of, 457-458, 485f, 955-956,
    955f
  differential diagnosis of, 1075
  evaluation of, 867
  histopathology of, 1074, 1074f, 1075f
  imaging of, 457-458, 485f, 955-956,
    955f, 956f, 959f
  incidence of, 954-955
  infarction and, 455-459, 778, 780.
    See also Hepatic infarction.
  microscopic findings in, 780
  pathophysiology of, 1074
  recurrent, 957
  retransplantation for, 768, 769, 769f,
    772, 780, 955, 956
  risk factors for, 780, 958t
  treatment of, 458, 459f, 642, 780, 955f,
    956, 959f, 1043t
  vs. allograft hepatitis C, 1099
  with biliary tract obstruction, 939, 1075
Hepatic artery anastomosis, 584-585, 584f,
    585f, 603
  in living related liver transplant, 640-641,
    640f
Hepatic chords, 24
Hepatic duct
  common, 27, 27f, 28f, 33
    bifurcation of, 34, 34f
  left, 29, 34
    posterior right hepatic duct from, 34, 35f
  right, 34
    posterior branch of, 34, 35f
Hepatic encephalopathy, 397-398
  immunosuppression in, 1226-1228, 1227t
  posttransplant, 835, 1019-1025, 1029-1035.
    See also Neuropsychiatric outcomes.
  anesthesia and, 590
  benzodiazepines and, 1022
  clinical features of, 479-480
  diagnosis of, 480
  in acute hepatic failure, 44
  in alcoholic patients, 1020
  in autoimmune hepatitis, 199
  in decompensated hepatitis C, 133-134
  in fulminant hepatic failure, 162, 167,
    597-598
  mental status alterations and, 1029-1030
  pathogenesis of, 480
  pathophysiology of, 1019-1020
  precipitating factors in, 480
  pretransplant management of, 479-481,
    597-598
  risk factors for, 1030
  subclinical, 1020
Hepatic failure. See also specific disorders.
  acute, 43, 44-48
    clinical manifestations of, 44-45, 44t
    definition of, 44
    development of, 55
    etiology of, 44t, 45
    Fas in, 47-48, 49f
    in children, transplantation for, 294
    King's College criteria for, 86t
    liver regeneration after, 46-47

Hepatic failure *(Continued)*
  living donor transplant in, 668
  pathogenesis of, 45-48, 45t
  transplantation for, 279-280
  treatment of, 55
  cellular basis of, 43-55
  chronic, 43
    auxiliary liver transplant for, 827
  enteral nutrition–related, 788-789
  from cirrhosis, 132
  fulminant, 597-598, 895t
    acetaminophen toxicity and, 161, 162, 163
    auxiliary liver transplant for, 170, 816-817, 821-826
    Bacillus cereus emetic toxin and, 165
    causes of, 161, 162-165, 821-822
      transplantation rates and, 169
    classification of, 821
    definition of, 161, 162, 821
    encephalopathy in, 162, 167
    extracorporeal therapy for, 173, 778-779, 816, 1368-1369, 1373-1374, 1415-1421. *See also* Extracorporeal liver support.
    graft rejection and, 1226-1228
    hepatitis B and, 124, 162, 163-164, 169
    hepatitis C and, 130, 164
    hepatitis D and, 164, 169
    hepatitis E and, 169
    hepatitis viruses and, 163-164
    immunosuppression in, 1226-1228, 1227t
    jaundice in, 162
    lymphomatous infiltration in, 173
    multiorgan dysfunction in, 162
    neurological sequelae of, 1035
    orthotopic liver transplant for, 821
    pathophysiology of, 597
    perioperative management of, 597-598
    prognostic criteria for, 165-169
    recurrent, 169-170
    signs and symptoms of, 597-598
    spontaneous survival in, 161, 162
    transplantation for, 104, 161-173
      auxiliary partial, 170
      cause/waiting time in, 169
      Clichy criteria in, 167-168
      cost-effectiveness of, 170
      hepatocyte, 173, 1384
      in children, 882
      King's College criteria in, 165-167, 165t, 166t
      living donor, 720
      living related, 170-171
      medical management before, 171-173, 171t-172t
      outcome in, 169-171
      selection criteria for, 165-169
      survival after, 161-162
    viral infection and, 163, 279
      recurrent, 169
  in children, transplantation for, 288-289, 288t, 289t, 294, 882
  molecular basis of, 43-55
  quality of life and, 1324-1325

    renal dysfunction in, 420, 421t
    subfulminant, 44
Hepatic fibrosis
  alcohol in, 132
  congenital, transplantation for, 295
  endothelin-1 in, 54
  hepatitis C and, 144
    treatment of, 135, 136, 136t
  in children, transplantation for, 295
  in chronic rejection, 1085-1086, 1088
  in living donor allograft, 111
  in recurrent hepatitis C, 1136
  injury and, 50-53, 51f, 52t
  location of, 55
  mediators of, 51-53, 52t
  perivenular, vs. chronic rejection, 1089
  platelet-derived growth factor in, 53
  prevention of, 55
  signaling pathways in, 53-54
  transforming growth factor-β in, 54
Hepatic hydrothorax, pretransplant management of, 406-407, 412, 482
Hepatic infarction
  clinical manifestations of, 778
  compartment syndrome and, 782
  hepatic artery thrombosis and, 455-459, 778, 780
  hepatic vein thrombosis and, 781-782
  hilar vessel compression and, 782-783
  honeymoon period in, 778
  imaging of, 455-456, 456f, 778
  inferior vena cava thrombosis and, 781
  necrosis and, 777-778. *See also* Hepatic necrosis.
  portal vein thrombosis and, 781
  postoperative, 839-840, 839t, 840f
  prognosis in, 778
  thromboembolism and, 783
  treatment of, 778
Hepatic iron index, in hereditary hemochromatosis, 241
Hepatic lymphangiomatosis, transplantation for, 282-283
Hepatic malignancy. *See also specific types,* e.g., Hepatocellular carcinoma.
  acetic acid for, 103
  adjuvant therapy for, 212
  ethanol for, 103, 212
  imaging of, 212-214, 212f-214f, 448-452, 449f, 452f
  immunosuppression for, 225, 235
  in children, 105, 290-291, 367-376
  metastatic. *See* Liver, metastases to.
  psychological aspects of, 399
  rare types of, transplantation for, 1160
  recurrent
    after transplantation, 211, 224
    prophylaxis for, 225
  stage of, transplantation and, 1105
  transplantation for, 17, 101-103, 211
    adjuvant therapy with, 224, 225
    bridge treatment before, 225
    donors for, 225
    for rare tumors, 1160
    in children, 105, 290-291, 367-376
    results of, 224-225, 226

    treatment of
      chemotherapy in, 211-212, 224-225
      decision making in, 226f, 227
      historical perspective on, 211-212
      locoregional, 218, 218t, 225
      radiofrequency ablation in, 103, 212
      unanticipated, in donor operation, 553-554
    vascular, in children, 375-376, 375t
Hepatic necrosis, 777-784
  as transplant indication, 1303t, 1310
  auxiliary liver transplant for, 778
  compartment syndrome and, 782
  emergency hepatectomy for, 778
  hepatic vein thrombosis and, 781-782
  hilar vessel compression and, 782-783
  in herpes simplex hepatitis, 1092, 1092f
  inferior vena cava thrombosis and, 781
  liver-assist devices for, 778-779
  of liver cells, 47-48
  portal vein thrombosis and, 781
  primary graft nonfunction and, 779
  regeneration after, 816
  trends in, 1303t, 1310
  vs. adenoviral hepatitis, 1094
Hepatic nodules
  degenerative, magnetic resonance imaging of, 451
  dysplastic, computed tomography of, 450
  regenerative
    computed tomography of, 450
    magnetic resonance imaging of, 451
Hepatic portoenterostomy. *See* Kasai portoenterostomy.
Hepatic resection. *See also* Hepatectomy.
  for hepatoblastoma, in children, 368-370
Hepatic segmental volume analysis, 704-705
Hepatic steatosis, 839
  after transplantation, 151
  as donation contraindication, 522
  in donor allograft, 918-919
  in living donor transplant, 681
  macrovesicular
    in donor, 1064, 1064f
    preservation injury in, 1071, 1072
    quantification of, 705-707
  prepreservation injury and, 562
Hepatic tumors. *See* Hepatic malignancy *and specific types.*
Hepatic vein
  anastomosis of, in living related liver transplant, 638-639, 639f
  anatomy of
    standard, 677f, 679
    variations in, 679-680, 680f
      in living donor transplant, 665, 710-711, 710f
  complications of, in allograft, 1075-1076, 1076f
  embryonic common, 24
  imaging of
    in posttransplant evaluation, 454, 454f, 461-462
    in pretransplant evaluation, 447-448
  in split-liver transplant, 615
  injury to, 59
    immune-mediated, 1076

Hepatic vein (Continued)
  left, 24, 28, 38, 39f
    variation of, 31, 32f
  middle, 24, 34-35, 36f
    broad, anterior, 38, 39f
    in living donor allograft, 680
  outflow obstruction of, 1075-1076, 1076f
  reconstruction of, in living related liver
      transplant, 638-639, 639f
  right, 24, 35, 37f-39f, 38
    accessory, 38, 39f
    short, posterior, 38, 39f
  segmental course of, 26
  stenosis of, 1075-1076, 1076f
    after living related liver transplant, 642
  thrombosis of, 781-782. See also Budd-
      Chiari syndrome.
    antithrombotic therapy for, 257-259,
        259f
    as contraindication to living donor
        transplant, 665
    in hepatocellular carcinoma, 451
    postoperative, 843
Hepatic venography, in Budd-Chiari
    syndrome, 253, 253f
Hepatic volumetric analysis, 704-705
Hepatic-assist devices. See Extracorporeal
    liver support.
Hepatitis, 895t
  adenoviral, in allograft, 1094-1095, 1094f
  alcoholic. See Alcoholic liver disease.
  as transplant contraindication, 431t, 475
  autoimmune, 195-207, 895t, 1050t
    alcohol in, 198t
    aminotransferase in, 196, 200, 202
    antibodies in, 196, 198t, 200-201
    cirrhosis in, 196, 201
    clinical manifestations of, 199-201
    de novo, 206-207, 206t, 1010
    diagnosis of, 196-197, 197t, 198t
    diclofenac associated, 199
    encephalopathy in, 199
    epidemiology of, 196
    extrahepatic, autoimmune-mediated
        syndromes in, 200
    graft rejection in, 204, 205, 206,
        1108, 1229
    hepatocellular carcinoma in, 196
    histology of, 201
    historical perspective on, 195-196
    idiopathic chronic, 196
    immunoserological subclassifications
        of, 197, 198t, 199
    immunosuppression for, 196, 203-204,
        1227t, 1229
    in acute rejection, 1108
    in recurrent primary biliary
        cirrhosis, 1107
    laboratory findings in, 200-201
    pathophysiology of, 199
    pretransplant management of, 476
    primary biliary cirrhosis in, 200
    recurrent, 204-206, 205t, 1009-1010,
        1067t, 1101t, 1139, 1139f
      clinical features of, 1108
      diagnosis of, 1107-1108
      differential diagnosis of, 1108

  histology of, 1108, 1108f
  pathophysiology of, 1107-1108
  retransplantation for, 770
  risk factors for, 1108
  vs. rejection, 205
  relapse of, 202-203
  survival in, 196
  transplantation for, 204
  treatment of, 201-204, 201f, 202t
    adjunctive, 203
    failure of, 203
  viral infection in, 198t, 199
  vs. chronic rejection, 1140
  vs. hepatitis C, 1100
cytomegalovirus. See also
    Cytomegalovirus infection.
  in allograft, 1090-1092, 1091f
  neonatal, 305t
  posttransplant, 978
Epstein-Barr virus. See Epstein-Barr virus
    infection.
fibrosing cholestatic, 122, 1006, 1137,
    1183f. See also Cholestasis.
  adefovir dipivoxil for, 123
  differential diagnosis of, 1099
  in allograft hepatitis B, 1096
  in allograft hepatitis C, 1097-1098, 1099f
  vs. preservation injury, 1073
fulminant, 124, 130, 163-164, 280. See
    also Hepatic failure, fulminant.
herpes simplex, 432. See also Herpes
    simplex virus infection.
  in allograft, 1091-1092, 1092f
idiopathic posttransplant, 196, 1110-1111
immunization for, 1008-1009
in allograft, hepatitis delta coinfection
    with, 1095, 1096
in children, transplantation for, 105
interface, 201, 203
lobular, in allograft, 1098
lupoid, 196
neonatal, 305, 305t
  cholestasis in, 314-315
  familial, 306, 307
  idiopathic, 306-307
  sporadic, 307
  transplantation for, 307, 307t, 308t
  vs. biliary atresia, 325-326
non-A, non-B, 129. See also Hepatitis C.
  non-C, fulminant, transplantation
      for, 280
non-A-E, aplastic anemia in, 294
opportunistic viruses and, 1090
piecemeal (periportal), 201
postinfantile giant cell, recurrent, 1105
preservation injury and, 562
pretransplant evaluation/management of,
    432-433, 965
prophylaxis for, 431t
recurrent, 1067t
  treatment of, 1009
varicella-zoster virus, 431t, 432, 1090.
    See also Varicella-zoster virus
    infection.
  in allograft, 1092
  vs. chronic obstructive
      cholangiopathy, 1077

Hepatitis A
  acute hepatic failure from, 45
  fulminant, 125, 162, 163. See also
      Hepatitis, fulminant.
    transplantation for, 280
  immunization for
    posttransplant, 1008-1009
    pretransplant, 436, 474
  in allograft, 1095
  pretransplant evaluation/management
      of, 433
  recurrent, 1101t
    fulminant hepatic failure from, 169
  transplantation for, 124-125, 280, 433
  trends in, 1304t, 1310
Hepatitis B, 895t
  acute hepatic failure from, 45
    Fas in, 48
  antiviral therapy for, 122-123
    posttransplant, 118, 965
    pretransplant, 118-119, 119t,
        120t, 121f
  as transplant contraindication, 431t, 475
  chronic, 1005
    fulminant, 124
    prevalence of, 1005
    race/ethnicity and, 1005
  cirrhosis from, 50, 1095
  drug-resistant, 118, 119, 122-123, 125,
      279-280, 1008, 1009
  famciclovir-resistant, 123, 280
  fibrosing cholestatic, 122, 1006
  fulminant, 124, 162, 163-164. See also
      Hepatitis, fulminant.
    transplantation for, 123-124
  graft infection with, treatment of,
      122-123
  hepatitis C with, disease severity/
      progression in, 151
  hepatitis D with, 124
    in fulminant hepatic failure, 164
  hepatocellular carcinoma in, 215
  immunization for
    in children, 1251
    in living donors, 668
    posttransplant, 1008-1009, 1045
    pretransplant, 436, 474
  immunosuppression and, 1227t
  in allograft, 1095-1096
    hepatitis C coinfection with, 1100
    posttransplant infection and, 1006
    treatment of, 122-123, 123t
  in children, 1341
    transplantation in, 292
  in donor, 433, 523, 965
  in living donors, 668
  lamivudine-resistant, 118, 119, 122-123,
      125, 279-280
  mutant forms of, hepatic failure from,
      279-280
  posttransplant, 983
    de novo, 1006
    recurrent. See Hepatitis B, recurrent.
  pretransplant evaluation of, 432-433, 965
  pretransplant management of, 431t,
      432-433, 475, 965
  prophylaxis for, 1045

Hepatitis B (*Continued*)
  recurrent, 100, 115, 116, 983, 1005-1009,
    1090, 1095, 1101t, 1138-1139
    antiviral therapy for, 118-119, 119t,
      120t, 121f, 122-123
    clinical features of, 1095
    differential diagnosis of, 1096
    fibrosing cholestatic, 122, 1006
    frequency of, 1006
    fulminant hepatic failure from, 169
    hepatitis D with, 124
    histopathology of, 1095-1096
    immune globulin prophylaxis for,
      116-118, 117t
    outcome of, 122
    pathogenesis of, 1006
    pathophysiology of, 1095
    prophylaxis for, 116-122, 1006-1009,
      1007f, 1007t, 1095
    rates of, 116-117, 117t
    retransplantation for, 123, 769-770
    risk factors for, 115, 1006
    timing of, 1006
    treatment of, 122, 125, 1009, 1104
    vs. acute rejection, 1083, 1096
    vs. posttransplant de novo infection,
      1006
  transplantation for, 100, 116-124,
    432-433
    allograft failure and, 1005
    drug-resistance and, 118
    indications for, 116
    outcome in, 123-124, 432-433,
      1005-1006
    patient classification in, 119
    treatment of, allograft reinfection
      after, 1095
  trends in, 1304t, 1310
  vs. cytomegalovirus infection, 1091
Hepatitis B core antigen
  in allograft, 1095, 1096
  in fulminant hepatic failure, 164
  in recurrence, 122
Hepatitis B e antigen, in recurrence, 116, 122
Hepatitis B immune globulin
  discontinuation of, reinfection and, 119,
    121-122
  for recurrent infection, 1006-1008, 1007t
  immunization with, 1045
  long-term safety of, 117-118
  postoperative, 877
  prophylaxis with, 100, 115, 116-118, 117t,
    119, 121f, 965, 1045
    for hepatitis C reinfection, 152
  resistance to, 1007-1008
  with lamivudine, 115, 119, 120t, 125,
    1008
Hepatitis B surface antigen
  immunization with, 1008
  in allograft, 1095, 1096
  in fulminant hepatic failure, 164
  in hepatitis D, 124
  in recurrence, 122
  lamivudine effects on, 116
  mutations in, hepatitis B immune
    globulin resistance and, 1007
  prophylaxis and, 121f

Hepatitis C, 129-138, 895t
  acute, 130t, 131
  antiviral therapy for, 134-136, 136t,
    153-155, 154t, 1002-1003
    after transplantation, 153
    before transplantation, 152-153
    in recurrent infection, 153-155, 154t
    posttransplant, 1003-1004
    pretransplant, 1003
  as primary transplant indication, 1304t,
    1309-1310
  cellular immunity in, 130
  characteristics of, 130, 130t
  cholestatic, 1097
  chronic, 130-131, 130t
    antiviral therapy for, 134-136, 135t
    cirrhosis from, 50, 131-132, 132t,
      143, 144
      decompensation in, 132-134, 132t
      hepatocellular carcinoma in, 134
      survival in, 132, 132f
      treatment of, 135-136, 136t, 144
    hepatocellular carcinoma from, 134, 144
    transplantation for, 144-145
    transplantation for, 136-137, 137f,
      137t, 144
  cirrhosis from, 50, 131-132, 132t, 143,
    144, 983, 1096-1097
    decompensation in, 132-134, 132t, 136
    hepatocellular carcinoma in, 134
    survival in, 132, 132f
    treatment of, 135-136, 136t, 144
  discovery of, 129
  encephalopathy in, 133-134
  fulminant hepatic failure from, 130, 164
  genotypes of, 130
    disease severity and, 150
  glomerulonephritis in, 807
  graft failure in, 1005
  graft rejection in
    immunosuppression for, 149
    vs. recurrence, 146
  growth factors for, 135
  hepatitis B with, disease severity/
    progression in, 151
  hepatocellular carcinoma in, 215
  heterogeneity of, disease progression
    and, 150
  immunosuppression and, 1227t, 1228
  in alcoholism, 151, 265
  in allograft, 143, 1090, 1096-1100, 1098f,
    1099f. See also Hepatitis C, recurrent.
    hepatitis B coinfection with, 1100
    treatment of, 1137-1138
  in children, 1341
    transplantation in, 292
  in chronic rejection, 1100
  in donor, 145, 433, 523, 965, 1137
  in hemophilia, 242
  in immunocompromise, 147
  in living donor transplant, 1137
  incidence/prevalence of, 131, 144, 1096
    increasing, posttransplant care
      coordination and, 1046-1050
  mycophenolate mofetil for, 1228
  natural history of, 131, 131f, 143, 144
  pathogenesis of, 130

posttransplant, 143, 145-152, 983-984,
  1090. See also Hepatitis C, recurrent.
  alloimmunity in, 146
  antiviral therapy for, 153
  disease severity/progression in,
    147-148, 148t
    donor-related variables in, 150-151
    external factors in, 151-152
    histology-related variables in, 151
    host-related variables in, 148-150
    surgery-related variables in, 151
    virus-related variables in, 149, 150
  histology of, 146-147
  infection sources in, 145
  natural history of, 146-147, 147f
  prophylaxis for, 152
  survival in, 147, 148f
  treatment of, 984
posttransplant diabetes and, 996
pretransplant evaluation/management of,
  433, 965
pretransplant management of, 431t, 475
prophylaxis for, 152
psychological aspects of, 399-400
recurrent, 100, 965, 983-984, 1000-1005,
  1101t, 1104, 1129-1138. See also
  Hepatitis C, posttransplant.
  after living donor transplant, 667-668
  allograft failure and, 1001
  antiviral therapy for, 153-155, 154t,
    1002-1003
    posttransplant, 1003-1004
    pretransplant, 1003
  bile duct injury in, 1130-1131
  chronic, 1098, 1098f
  clinical factors in, 1002-1003
  clinical features of, 1097-1098
  corticosteroids and, 1217
  daclizumab for, 1278
  diagnosis of, 145
  differential diagnosis of, 1099-1100
  donor factors in, 1002
  endotheliitis in, 1131-1132, 1134f
  fibrosing cholestatic hepatitis in, 1097,
    1098, 1099f
  fibrosis in, 1136
  genotype in, 1097, 1098
  grading of, 1135
  graft rejection and, 1002-1003, 1005,
    1083, 1130-1137, 1133t, 1134f,
    1136t, 1175-1176, 1176t, 1228
  histology of, 145-146, 146t, 1130,
    1131f, 1132f
  histopathology of, 1098-1099,
    1098f, 1099f
  immunosuppression and, 1001, 1176,
    1227t, 1228-1229
  in living donor allograft, 111
  interface/lobular activity in, 1132,
    1134-1135
  OKT3 and, 1224
  pathophysiology of, 1097
  polymerase chain reaction for,
    1135-1136
  portal inflammatory infiltrates in, 1130
  prophylaxis for, 1003, 1005
  recipient factors in, 1002

Hepatitis C (Continued)
  retransplantation for, 144, 155, 770
    outcome predictors for, 1292-1293
  risk factors for, 1001, 1002t, 1097
  severity of, 1001-1002, 1002t
  timing of, 1000-1001, 1001f
  treatment of, 144. See also Hepatitis C,
    antiviral therapy for.
  trends in, 1304t, 1309-1310
  viral factors in, 1001-1002
  viral load and, 1000-1001
  vs. bile duct obstruction, 1135
  vs. Epstein-Barr virus, 1137
  vs. graft rejection, 146, 1083, 1099-1100,
    1130-1132, 1133t, 1134-1137, 1134f,
    1136t, 1175-1176, 1176t
  vs. preservation injury, 1135
risk factors for, 1050t
RNA levels in, allograft disease and, 150
routine surveillance for, 1050t
screening for, frozen section histology in,
  1064
severity of
  alcoholism and, 151
  transplantation need and, 137-138
transfusion-associated, 131
transplantation for, 100, 144-145, 433
trends in, 1304t, 1309-1310
vs. autoimmune hepatitis, 1100
vs. cytomegalovirus infection, 1091
vs. Epstein-Barr virus hepatitis,
  1093-1094
vs. recurrent primary biliary cirrhosis, 1100
vs. rejection, 1099-1100
Hepatitis C immune globulin, 1005
  for hepatitis C reinfection, 152
Hepatitis D
  hepatitis B with, fulminant hepatic
    failure from, 164
  in allograft, 1095, 1096
  recurrent, 124, 1101t
    fulminant hepatic failure from, 164, 169
  transplantation for, 124
Hepatitis E
  fulminant, transplantation for, 280
  recurrent, fulminant hepatic failure
    from, 169
Hepatitis G, in allograft, 1100
Hepatobiliary scintigraphy,
  posttransplant, 935
Hepatobiliary system
  diseases of, neonatal, 305
  origination of, 24
Hepatoblastoma, 367-371. See also Hepatic
  malignancy.
  preoperative risk factors in, 1337t
  transplantation for, 105, 367-371, 1160
    outcome in, 1340
Hepatocellular carcinoma, 214-222. See also
  Hepatic malignancy.
  α-fetoprotein levels in, 101-102, 134, 215
  as incidental finding, 1157, 1159
  biopsy of, 102, 215
  chemotherapy for, 221, 1159
  cirrhosis in, 132, 214, 215
  clinical presentation of, 215-216
  diagnosis of, 102, 215-216, 1157

epidemiology of, 214-215, 1157
hepatitis and, 215
hepatitis B and, 215
hepatitis C and, 134, 144, 215
  transplantation for, 144-145
imaging of, 212, 448
  computed tomography in, 212,
    448-450, 449f
  magnetic resonance imaging in, 450-451
immunosuppression for, 225, 1228-1229
in autoimmune hepatitis, 196
in children, 290-291, 367, 371-372, 1337t
  associated disorders in, 1340, 1340t
  transplant outcome in, 1340
in primary biliary cirrhosis, 179
in tyrosinemia, 291, 372-373
incidence of, 214, 214t, 1157
living donor transplant for, 666
natural history of, 131f
organ allocation in, 75, 1157-1158
pathogenesis of, 1157
postinterventional malignancy in, 1157
prognosis of, 217-218
psychological aspects of, 399
recurrent, 219, 224, 1101t, 1157, 1158-1159
resection of, 218
staging of, 102, 216, 216t, 217, 217t
transarterial chemoembolization for, 103
transplantation for, 101-103, 218-222,
  1157-1159
  adjuvant therapy with, 218-219, 1159
  chemotherapy with, 221
  contraindications to, 211
  donor pool in, 217-218
  frequency of, 1158
  historical perspective on, 221, 221t
  in children, 367, 371-372
  living-donor, 102, 666
  MELD score in, 102
  outcomes in, 1158, 1159
  patient selection for, 75, 1157-1158
  prognostic factors in, 221-222, 221t, 1159
  radiofrequency ablation with, 221
  recurrence after, 219, 224, 1101t, 1157,
    1158-1159
  results of, 218-219, 219t, 220f, 221,
    221f, 224-225
  therapy before, 102-103
  tumor resection before, 1158
treatment of, 103, 218, 218t, 221, 1157
tumor markers for, 215
tyrosinemia and, 345-346
vs. cholangiocarcinoma, 215
Hepatocholangiocarcinoma. See also
  Hepatic malignancy.
  mixed, incidence of, 214
Hepatocyte(s)
  apoptosis of, 47
    Fas-mediated, 47-48, 49f
  bile formation in, 24
  biodegradable scaffolds for, 1433
  for liver-assist devices, 779, 1368-1369,
    1373-1374, 1432-1433, 1432f. See
    also Extracorporeal liver support.
  growth of, 58
    methods of, 1432-1434, 1432f
  in cirrhosis, 44

in gene therapy, 339
in liver regeneration, 46
in preservation injury, 1073, 1074f
in tissue-engineered liver, 1433-1434
injury response of, 51
necrosis of, 47-48. See also Hepatic
    necrosis.
    in adenoviral hepatitis, 1094, 1094f
  porcine. See Porcine hepatocytes/liver.
  replication of, 46
  role of, 45t
Hepatocyte growth factor
  in acute hepatic failure, 46
  in liver regeneration, 46
Hepatocyte transplantation, 1379-1385,
    1426-1427, 1433
  as bridge to transplantation, 1383-1384
  cell sources for, 1380, 1385
  clinical experience with, 1383-1385
  experimental studies of, 1380-1381
  for fulminant hepatic failure, 173, 1384
  for glycogen storage diseases, 351, 1384
  for hyperlipidemia, 1381, 1384
  for metabolic diseases, 338-339, 351,
    1384-1385
  for urea cycle defects, 347, 1384
  for Wilson's disease, 344
  hepatocyte embolization in, 1380-1381
  history of, 1380-1381
  in xenotransplantation, 1368
  indications for, 1383-1385
  intraperitoneal, 1380, 1381
  intraportal, 1380
  intrasplenic technique in, 1380-1381
  sites of, 1380
  with microcarrier-attached hepatocytes,
    1381
  with microencapsulated hepatocytes,
    1381-1383
Hepatoduodenal ligament, 25
Hepatoiminodiacetic acid scans. See HIDA
  scans.
Hepatolenticular degeneration.
  See Wilson's disease.
Hepatoma
  Budd-Chiari syndrome and, 256
  magnetic resonance imaging of, 212f, 213f
  treatment of, 1227t
Hepatomegaly, in idiopathic neonatal
  hepatitis, 306
Hepatopulmonary syndrome, 407-409, 594
  as transplant contraindication,
    107-108, 409
  as transplant indication, 594
  classification of, 594
  diagnosis of, 407-408, 594
  natural history of, 594
  pathogenesis of, 408-409
  perioperative management of, 594
  perioperative mortality in, 594
  portopulmonary hypertension and,
    409, 594
  postoperative, 848
  pretransplant management of, 482, 594
  reversibility of, 409
  signs and symptoms of, 594
  transplant outcome and, 409

Hepatorenal ligament, 25
Hepatorenal syndrome, 419-420, 595,
    895-900
  classification of, 896, 896t
  diagnosis of, 895-896, 896t
  pathogenesis of, 896-897
  perioperative management of, 595
  postoperative assessment for, 836-837
  predictive variables in, 896, 896t
  pretransplant management of,
    481-482, 595
  renal failure in, 806
  transplantation for
    outcome of, 1289
    results of, 909-910
  treatment of, 897-899, 898t, 899t, 900f
Hepatotoxicity
  acetaminophen
    acute hepatic failure from, 45
    fulminant hepatic failure from,
      161, 162, 163
  isoniazid, 964
Herbal remedies, safety of, 399
Hereditary fructosemia, 349
Hereditary hemochromatosis, 240-241,
    242f. See also Hemochromatosis.
  pretransplant management of, 475
  transplantation for, 103, 241
    results of, 245, 246t
Hereditary hemorrhagic telangiectasia,
    transplantation for, 281
Heredofamilial amyloidosis, 399
Hernias
  in living donors, 715
  incisional, 1043t
Herniation, cerebral. See also Cerebral
    edema.
  postoperative pediatric, 854
Herpes simplex virus infection
  bile duct paucity in, 306t
  congenital, vs. biliary atresia, 325-326
  fulminant, hepatic failure from, 279
  hepatitis from, 1090
    in allograft, 1091-1092, 1092f
    in children, cholestasis in, 314
    neonatal, 305t
  pretransplant evaluation/management
    of, 432
  prophylaxis for, 431t, 432, 1044, 1045
  reactivation of, 432, 980-981
    timing of, 966, 966f
  vs. cytomegalovirus infection, 1091
Herpes zoster infection, posttransplant, 981
Herpesvirus infections
  in children, 1250
  posttransplant, 981-982
    prophylaxis for, 430-432, 431t
  pretransplant evaluation/management of,
    430-432
Heterotaxia, 756. See also Situs inversus.
  liver transplantation in
    results of, 757-759, 759t
    technical aspects of, 759-763, 760f-762f
Heterotopic auxiliary liver transplantation.
    See Auxiliary liver transplantation.
HFE gene, 240-241
H-grafts, for variceal bleeding, 509

HIDA scans
  for bile leaks, 463, 464f
  in biliary atresia, 326
  in posttransplant evaluation, 455
    of biliary tract, 463, 464, 464f
    of hepatic artery, 455-456, 456f
High stomal output, after small bowel/liver
    transplantation, 795
Highly sensitized patients, intravenous
    immunoglobulin for, 1393
Hilar anatomy, 27-28, 28f, 40, 677f
  replaced, 28, 28f
Hilar dissection, 27f
Hilar fissure, transverse, 25, 25f
Hilar vessels, compression of, hepatic
    infarction and, 782-783
Hirsutism, 1051t, 1252
Hispanics. See also Race/ethnicity.
  living donor liver transplant in, 664
Histamine blockers, postoperative,
    for children, 884, 884t
Histidine-tryptophanketoglutarate (HTK)
    solution, 568, 569
    preservation injury and, 566
Histoplasmosis
  posttransplant, 973, 973t, 975
  pretransplant evaluation/management
    of, 965
  prophylaxis for, 431t, 436, 965
HIV. See Human immunodeficiency virus
    (HIV) infection.
HLA. See Human leukocyte antigen(s) (HLA).
HMG-CoA reductase inhibitors, 501t, 997
  adverse effects of, 501t
Hodgkin's disease. See Lymphoma;
    Posttransplant lymphoproliferative
    disorder.
Home care, 1040-1042
  nutrition support in, 1041-1042
  wound care in, 1041-1042
Homograft, tolerance of, 10
Hormonal resuscitation, in brain-dead
    donors, 518, 519t
Hormone replacement therapy, for
    osteoporosis, 483
  in primary biliary cirrhosis, 183
Host-versus-graft reaction, 1189, 1190f, 1191
HTK solution, 566, 568, 569
  preservation injury and, 566
HuM291, 1390
Human immunodeficiency virus (HIV)
    infection
  antiretroviral therapy for
    fulminant hepatic failure from, 164
    transplantation indications and, 108
  as transplant contraindication, 108,
    431t, 433
  in donor, 433-434, 982-983
  in hemophilia, 242
  in hepatitis C progression, 149
  posttransplant, 982-983
  pretransplant evaluation/management of,
    433, 964-965
  transplantation in, 433-434
    in children, 292
Human leukocyte antigen(s) (HLA),
    1199-1200, 1203-1206

  allogeneic, 1203
    sensitization to, 1204
  class I, 1203
  class II, 1203
  in graft rejection, 1170, 1174
  in graft-versus-host disease, 1206
  matching of. See also Cross-matching.
    in kidney transplantation, 1200
    in liver transplantation, 1204-1205, 1205f
    in living related donor transplant,
      634-635
    trends in, 1313
Human leukocyte antigen (HLA) B, in match-
    ing, hepatitis C recurrence and, 150
Human leukocyte antigen (HLA) B14, in
    hepatitis C progression, 149
Human leukocyte antigen (HLA) BDRB1*04,
    in hepatitis C progression, 149
Human leukocyte antigen (HLA) DR,
    mismatches with, outcome and, 1205
    in children, 1336
Human leukocyte antigen (HLA) DR3,
    in autoimmune hepatitis, 197, 199
    rejection in, 205-206
Human leukocyte antigen (HLA) DR4,
    in autoimmune hepatitis, 197, 199
    rejection in, 205-206
Human T-lymphotropic viruses (HTLV), 434
Humanized OKT3, 1390
Humoral immunity. See also Immune
    response; Immunity.
    in autoimmune hepatitis, 199
    in primary biliary cirrhosis, 178
HuOKT3γ, 1390
Hyaluronic acid, in ischemia-reperfusion
    injury, 1412
Hydatid cyst disease, transplantation for, 280
Hydrocortisone, 1215-1217, 1215t. See also
    Corticosteroids.
  with antithymocyte globulin, 1223
  with OKT3, 1223
Hydrothorax, hepatic, pretransplant
    management of, 406-407, 412, 482
3-Hydroxyacyl-coenzyme A dehydrogenase
    deficiency, long-chain, transplantation
    for, 278
3β-Hydroxy-steroid dehydrogenase
    deficiency, 313
Hydroxyurea, in Budd-Chiari syndrome,
    257-258, 259f
Hyperacute rejection, 1173, 1271-1272,
    1272t. See also Allograft rejection.
  in xenotransplantation, 1369-1371, 1370f
  postoperative management of, 840
Hyperalimentation. See Nutrition support.
Hyperammonemia
  in hepatic encephalopathy, 480
    management of, 480
  in urea cycle defects, 346-348
  postoperative, 866
Hypercalcemia, 901
Hypercholesterolemia. See also
    Hyperlipidemia.
  familial, 351-352, 351f, 1103t
    transplantation for, 276
    hepatocyte, 1384
  in primary biliary cirrhosis, 179

Hypercoagulable states, 595-596
  prophylaxis for, 596
Hyperglycemia
  in brain-dead donors, 517t
  patient teaching for, 1049t
  posttransplant, 1049t
Hyperhomocysteinemia, posttransplant, 501
Hyperkalemia, 900-901. *See also* Potassium
    imbalance.
  perioperative management of, 596-597
  postoperative, 837
Hyperlipidemia, 351-352, 351f
  drug therapy for, adverse effects of, 501t
  hepatocyte transplant for, 1381, 1384
  immunosuppression and, 500, 500t, 997
  in familial hypercholesterolemia, 276,
    351-352, 351f, 1103t, 1384
  in primary biliary cirrhosis, 179
  lifestyle modification for, 1049t
  posttransplant, 500, 500t, 997-998
Hypermagnesemia. *See* Magnesium
    imbalance.
Hypernatremia. *See also* Sodium imbalance.
  donor, prophylaxis for, 547-549
Hyperoxaluria, 806-807, 895t, 1103t
  liver transplant for, 276, 290, 338t, 807
  liver-kidney transplant for, 355-357,
    806-807, 809-810, 908-909, 1346
  type I, 276, 355-357, 357f, 806-807
  type II, 807
Hyperphosphatemia, prognostic value of,
    in acetaminophen-related hepatic
    injury, 168
Hypersplenism, in biliary atresia, 328
Hypertension, 1049t
  cyclosporine-related, 873, 998, 1220
  headaches from, 874
  in children, 857
    immunosuppression and, 857, 1246-1247
  in pregnancy, 1330
  intracranial
    in fulminant hepatic failure, 597-598,
      1035
    monitoring/management of, 590-591,
      597-598, 1035
    in children, 854-855
  portal. *See* Portal hypertension.
  portopulmonary, 409-410, 592-594. *See
    also* Portopulmonary hypertension.
  posttransplant, 500-501, 604, 846, 873, 998
    in children, 857
  pulmonary. *See* Pulmonary hypertension.
  treatment of, 998
Hyperuricemia, posttransplant, 996, 1049t
Hyperventilation, for increased intracranial
    pressure, 590-591
Hypocalcemia, 901
  postoperative, 837
  in children, 858
Hypocoagulable states, 595-596
Hypoglycemic agents, for posttransplant
    diabetes mellitus, 996
Hypokalemia, 900. *See also* Potassium
    imbalance.
  in renal disease, 418
  postoperative, 837
    in children, 858

Hypomagnesemia, 901, 1049t. *See also*
    Magnesium imbalance.
  postoperative, 837
    in children, 858
Hyponatremia. *See also* Sodium imbalance.
  ascites and, pretransplant management
    of, 478-479
  donor, graft failure and, 921
  in brain-dead donors, 517t, 518
  in renal disease, 417-418
  perioperative management of, 596
  postoperative, 837
    pediatric, 858
  pretransplant, 900
Hypophosphatemia, 901
  postoperative, pediatric, 858
Hypotension, in brain-dead donors, 517t
Hypothermia
  in brain-dead donors, 518-519
  prevention of, 600-601
Hypovolemia, vascular isolation in, 59, 60f
Hypoxanthine, in preservation injury, 563
Hypoxemia
  as transplant contraindication, 414
  pretransplant evaluation of, 411-413
Hypoxia
  causes of, 594
  in cell death, 47
  in heptopulmonary syndrome, 594

I

IDA scans
  for bile leaks, 463, 464f
  in posttransplant evaluation
    of biliary tract, 463, 464, 464f
    of hepatic artery, 455-456, 456f
IDEC-131, 1392
Idiopathic neonatal hepatitis. *See* Hepatitis,
    neonatal.
IgG, in autoimmune hepatitis, 198t
Ileal bypass, for familial homozygous
    hypercholesterolemia, 276
Imaging studies. *See* Radiological
    evaluation *and specific techniques.*
Iminodiacetic acid scans. *See* IDA scans.
Imipenem-cilistatin, immunosuppressant
    interactions with, 972t
Immune cells, 45t
Immune complexes, in xenotransplantation,
    1372
Immune deposits, in antibody-mediated
    rejection, 1079
Immune globulin
  hepatitis B. *See* Hepatitis B immune
    globulin.
  hepatitis C, 1005
    for reinfection, 152
  intravenous, 1393
  varicella-zoster, for postexposure
    prophylaxis, 432, 1044, 1045
Immune ignorance, 1193
Immune response. *See also* Immunity.
  adaptive, in allograft, 10, 1192
  antigen migration/localization in, 1192
  biopsy and, 1065-1071
  cytomegalovirus effects on, 979

  in allograft rejection, 1065, 1068f, 1080,
    1085, 1168-1173, 1214-1215, 1214f,
    1264, 1393
  in children, 1236-1237
  in ischemia-reperfusion injury, 1361, 1412
  in rejection, 1065, 1168-1173
  in xenotransplantation, 1369-1372
  sensitization in, 1066
  to immunosuppression, 1214-1215, 1215t
Immune system
  diseases of
    bile duct paucity in, 306t
    recurrent, 1104-1105
  in chronic rejection, 1085
  recipient, 1066, 1066f
Immunity. *See also* Immune response.
  cellular
    adoptive transfer of, 1186-1187, 1188f
    in autoimmune hepatitis, 199
    in hepatitis C, 130
  humoral
    in autoimmune hepatitis, 199
    in primary biliary cirrhosis, 178
    in hepatitis C progression, 149-150
  transfer of, to graft, 1191
Immunization
  for anthrax, in children, 1251
  for children, 296, 432, 436, 1250-1251
  for hepatitis A
    in children, 1251
    pretransplant, 474
  for hepatitis B, 1008-1009
    in children, 1251
    in living donors, 668
    posttransplant, 1045
    pretransplant, 436, 474
  for influenza, 1045
    in children, 1250, 1251
    posttransplant, 877
  for measles, 436, 1250-1251
  for smallpox, 1045, 1045t
    in children, 1251
  for varicella, 432, 1044, 1045, 1250
  pneumococcal, 1251
  postoperative, 877
  pretransplant, 436, 474
    for children, 296, 432, 436
  viral shedding from, infection risk from,
    877, 1044-1045, 1250-1251
  with live attenuated vaccines,
    contraindications to, 877, 1250-1251
Immunocompromise, hepatitis C in, 147
Immunodeficiency, in hepatitis C
    progression, 148, 148t
Immunoglobulin. *See also* Immune globulin.
  intravenous, 1393
Immunoglobulin G, in autoimmune
    hepatitis, 198t
Immunosuppression, 871, 1184-1186, 1185f,
    1193-1195, 1193-1196, 1194f, 1195f,
    1213-1230. *See also specific drugs.*
  adverse effects of, 1046, 1046t-1049t
    in children, 1241, 1246-1249, 1327-1329,
      1341, 1349
  antiproliferatives in, 1280-1281
  bone loss and, 502
  breast-feeding and, 1329